Fishman's
Pulmonary Diseases and Disorders

Volume 2

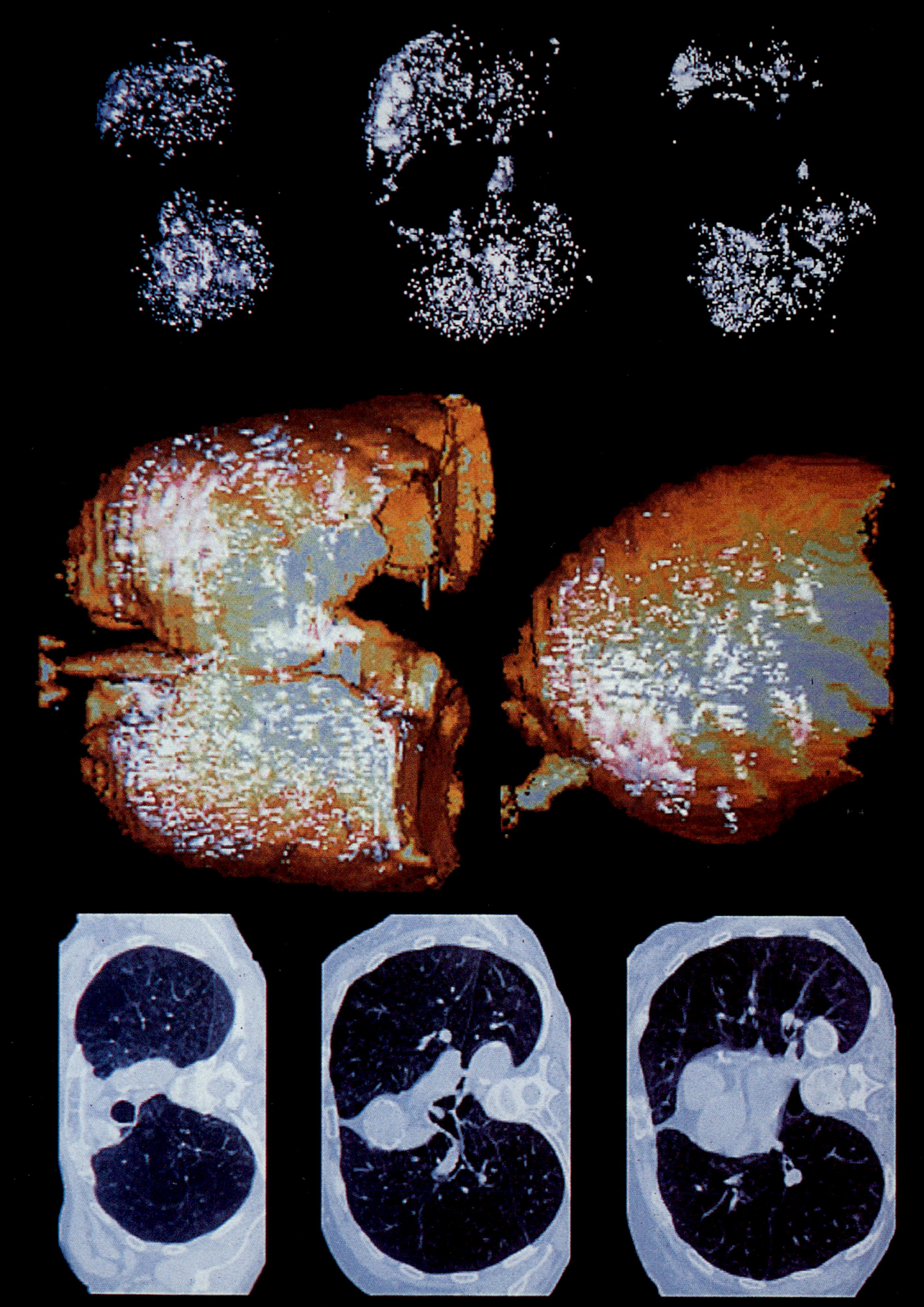

Frontispiece: Legend appears on page v.

Fishman's
Pulmonary Diseases and Disorders
Third Edition

Volume 2

EDITOR-IN-CHIEF

Alfred P. Fishman, M.D.

William Maul Measey Professor of Medicine
University of Pennsylvania Medical Center
Philadelphia, Pennsylvania

SECTION EDITORS

Jack A. Elias, M.D.

Chief, Pulmonary and Critical Care Medicine
Yale University School of Medicine
New Haven, Connecticut

Jay A. Fishman, M.D.

Infectious Diseases Unit
Massachusetts General Hospital-East
Charlestown, Massachusetts

Michael A. Grippi, M.D.

Vice Chairman, Clinical Affairs
University of Pennsylvania Medical Center
Philadelphia, Pennsylvania

Larry R. Kaiser, M.D.

Director, Lung Transplant
Division of Cardiothoracic Surgery
University of Pennsylvania Medical Center
Philadelphia, Pennsylvania

Robert M. Senior, M.D.

Professor, Jewish Hospital
Washington University Medical Center
St. Louis, Missouri

McGraw-Hill
Health Professions Division

New York   St. Louis   San Francisco   Auckland   Bogotá   Caracas   Lisbon   London   Madrid
Mexico City   Milan   Montreal   New Delhi   San Juan   Singapore   Sydney   Tokyo   Toronto

McGraw-Hill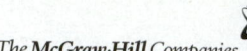
A Division of The **McGraw·Hill** *Companies*

Fishman's
Pulmonary Diseases and Disorders

1234567890 DOWDOW 9987

ISBN 0-07-911167-X (set)
ISBN 0-07-021179-5 (volume 1)
ISBN 0-07-021180-9 (volume 2)

This book was set in Times Roman by York Graphic Services, Inc.
The editors were J. Dereck Jeffers and Lester A. Sheinis;
the production supervisors were Robert R. Laffler and Helene G. Landers;
the text designer was Marsha Cohen / Parallelogram;
the cover designer was Edward R. Schultheis;
the indexer was Irving Condé Tullar.
R. R. Donnelley & Sons Company was printer and binder.
This book is printed on acid-free paper.

Library of Congress Cataloging-in-Publication Data

Fishman's pulmonary diseases and disorders / editor-in-chief, Alfred P. Fishman; section
editors, Jack A. Elias . . . [et al.].—3rd ed.
     p. cm.
   Rev. ed. of: Pulmonary diseases and disorders. 2nd ed. c1988.
   Includes bibliographical references and index.
   ISBN 0-07-911167-X (set).—ISBN 0-07-021179-5 (v. 1).—ISBN 0-07-021180-9 (v. 2)
   1. Lungs—Diseases. I. Fishman, Alfred P. II. Elias, Jack A. III. Pulmonary diseases and
disorders. IV. Title: Pulmonary diseases and disorders.
   [DNLM: 1. Lung Diseases. WF 600 F537 1997]
RC756.P826 1997
616.2′4—DC20
DNLM/DLC
for Library of Congress   96-26303

Front cover: Lateral view of resin cast of left human lung, with airways (yellow), pulmonary
arteries (red), and pulmonary veins (blue) filled out to fine lobular branches. *(Courtesy of
Dr. H. C. Walter Weber, Department of Anatomy, University of Bern, Switzerland.)*

Alfred P. Fishman, M.D.

To Linda, Hannah; Mark, Martha, Eric; Sarah; Jay, Gayle, Aaron, and Brian

Jack A. Elias, M.D.

To Sandy, Lauren, Alma, and Gabby

Jay A. Fishman, M.D.

To Aaron, Brian, and Gayle

Michael A. Grippi, M.D.

To Barbara, Kristen, and Amy

Larry R. Kaiser, M.D.

To Ruthy, Jeffrey, and Jonathan

Robert Senior, M.D.

To Jerry Flance, Jack Pierce, and Martha

FRONTISPIECE: Quantification of regional emphysema by three-dimensional maps of the lungs using newer CT techniques. *Left column:* High-resolution CT (HRCT) scans through upper, middle, and lower lobes. Areas of emphysema characterized by hypoattenuation and diminished pulmonary vasculature. *Center column:* Single breath-holding spiral CT scan. Three-dimensional shaded-surface displays. Areas of emphysema appear in white. *Top.* Both lungs, frontal projection. *Bottom.* Left lung, lateral projection. Distribution of emphysema is heterogeneous affecting predominantly the upper and middle zones. *Right column:* High-resolution CT (HRCT). Regional, three-dimensional axial projections of the upper, middle, and lower thirds of the lungs. The brightest areas correspond to the regions with highest concentrations of emphysema. *Right lung.* Emphysema occupies 23% of the total lung volume. *From top-to-bottom:* Emphysema occupies 43% of top third, 20% of middle third, and 17% of lower third. *Left lung.* Emphysema occupies 15% of the total lung volume. *From top-to-bottom:* 25%, 17%, and 7%, respectively. *(Courtesy of Krishanu B. Gupta, M.D., Ph.D., and Warren B. Gefter, M.D., Department of Radiology, University of Pennsylvania Medical Center.)*

Contents

Section 3
The Lungs in Different Physiological States

Section 4
Lung Immunology

Section 5
Lung Injury and Repair

Part Three

SYMPTOMS AND SIGNS OF RESPIRATORY DISEASE / 359

Section 6
Clinical Approach to the Patient

Section 7
Diagnostic Procedures

Part Four
OBSTRUCTIVE LUNG DISEASES / 643

Section 8
Chronic Obstructive Pulmonary Disease

Section 9
Asthma

Section 10
Other Obstructive Disorders

Part Seven

INTERSTITIAL AND INFLAMMATORY LUNG DISEASES / 1035

Section 13
Immunologic and Interstitial Diseases

Section 14
Depositional and Infiltrative Disorders

Part Eight

ALVEOLAR DISEASES / 1191

Part Nine

DISORDERS OF THE PULMONARY CIRCULATION / 1231

Part Ten

DISORDERS OF THE PLEURAL SPACE / 1387

APPENDIXES

Part Fifteen
NEOPLASMS OF THE LUNGS / 1693

Section 15
Cancer of the Lungs

Section 16
Lymphoproliferative Disorders

Section 19
Special Hosts and Opportunistic Infections

Section 20
Specific Microorganisms

Section 21
Mycobacterial Infections

Part Seventeen
ACUTE RESPIRATORY FAILURE / 2523

Section 22
Lung Failure

Section 23
Respiratory Pump Failure

Section 24
Management and Therapeutic Interventions

APPENDIXES

Contributors

MASAZUMI ADACHI, M.D., SC.D.
Director of Laboratories,
Isaac Albert Research Institute,
Kingsbrook Jewish Medical Center,
Brooklyn, New York
(Chapter 78)

ABASS ALAVI, M.D.
Professor of Radiology,
Chief, Nuclear Medicine,
Department of Radiology,
University of Pennsylvania,
Philadelphia, Pennsylvania
(Chapter 35)

STEVEN ALBELDA, M.D.
Associate Professor of Medicine,
Pulmonary and Critical Care Division,
University of Pennsylvania Medical Center,
Philadelphia, Pennsylvania
(Chapter 92)

MURRAY D. ALTOSE, M.D.
Professor of Medicine,
Chief of Staff,
Case Western Reserve University,
VA Medical Center,
Cleveland, Ohio
(Chapter 10)

MICHEL AOUN, M.D.
Attending Physician,
Department of Medicine,
Institut Jules Bordet,
Brussels, Belgium
(Chapter 123)

CARLOS A. ARES, M.D.
Pulmonary and Critical Care Medicine,
Winthrop Pulmonary Associates, PC,
Mineola, New York
(Chapter 110)

DONALD ARMSTRONG, M.D.
Chief, Infectious Disease Service,
Memorial Sloan-Kettering Cancer Center,
New York, New York
(Chapter 146)

JOHN R. BACH, M.D.
Professor and Chair,
Department of Pulmonary Medicine and Rehabilitation,
UMD-New Jersey Medical School,
University Hospital,
Newark, New Jersey
(Chapter 99)

ANN SULLIVAN BAKER, M.D.[†]
Associate Professor of Medicine, HMS,
Infectious Disease Unit,
Massachusetts General Hospital,
Boston, Massachusetts
(Chapter 126)

JOHN G. BARTLETT, M.D.
Professor of Medicine and Chief,
Division of Infectious Disease,
Johns Hopkins University School of Medicine,
Baltimore, Maryland
(Chapter 129)

† Deceased.

MICHAEL F. BEERS, M.D.
Assistant Professor of Medicine,
Institute for Environmental Medicine,
University of Pennsylvania School of Medicine,
Philadelphia, Pennsylvania
(Chapter 172)

JEFFREY S. BERMAN, M.D.
Associate Professor of Medicine
Chief, Pulmonary and Critical Care Medicine,
Pulmonary Center,
Boston University School of Medicine,
Boston, Massachusetts
(Chapter 21)

ALAN L. BISNO, M.D.
Chief, Medical Service,
Miami VA Medical Center,
Miami, Florida
(Chapter 142)

PETER D. BITTERMAN, M.D.
Professor of Medicine,
Division of Pulmonary and Critical Care Medicine,
University of Minnesota,
Minneapolis, Minnesota
(Chapter 27)

CHARLES D. BLANKE, M.D.
Assistant Professor of Medicine,
Division of Medical Oncology,
Vanderbilt University School of Medicine,
The Vanderbilt Clinic,
Nashville, Tennessee
(Chapter 114)

CHRISTINE A. BLASKI, M.D.
Division of Pulmonary, Critical Care, and Occupational Medicine,
University of Iowa Hospitals and Clinics,
Iowa City, Iowa
(Chapter 61)

ALAN B. BLOCH, M.D., M.P.H.
Medical Epidemiologist,
Division of Tuberculosis Elimination,
National Center for HIV, STD, TB Prevention,
Centers for Disease Control and Prevention,
Atlanta, Georgia
(Chapter 161)

SIDNEY S. BRAMAN, M.D.
Professor of Medicine,
Brown University School of Medicine,
Rhode Island Hospital,
Providence, Rhode Island
(Chapter 52)

PETER H. BURRI, M.D.
Professor and Chairman
Institute of Anatomy
University of Bern
Bern, Switzerland
(Chapter 5)

MICHAEL E. BURT, M.D., PH.D.
Attending Surgeon,
Thoracic Surgery Department,
Memorial Sloan-Kettering Cancer Center,
New York, New York
(Chapter 117)

WILLIAM W. BUSSE, M.D.
Professor, Department of Medicine,
Head, Allergy and Clinical Immunology,
Clinical Science Center,
University of Wisconsin Hospital and Clinics,
Madison, Wisconsin
(Chapter 47)

JAY C. BUTLER, M.D.
Assistant Chief, Respiratory Diseases,
Division of Bacterial and Mycotic Diseases,
National Center for Infectious Disease, Centers for
Disease Control and Prevention,
Atlanta, Georgia
(Chapter 153)

EDWARD J. CAMPBELL, M.D.
Associate Professor of Medicine,
Division of Respiratory, Critical Care, and Occupational Pulmonary Medicine,
University of Utah,
Salt Lake City, Utah
(Chapter 19)

DAVID M. CENTER, M.D.
Professor of Medicine
Chief, Pulmonary and Critical Care Medicine,
Boston University School of Medicine,
The Pulmonary Center,
Boston, Massachusetts
(Chapter 21)

RICHARD E. CHAISSON, M.D.
Director, AIDS Service,
Division of Infectious Diseases,
Johns Hopkins University,
Baltimore, Maryland
(Chapter 163)

NEIL S. CHERNIACK, M.D.
Director, Clinical Affairs,
Dean's Office,
Case Western Reserve University,
Cleveland, Ohio
(Chapter 11)

JOHN W. CHRISTMAN, M.D.
Assistant Professor of Medicine,
Division of Pulmonary Medicine,
Vanderbilt University School of Medicine,
Nashville, Tennessee
(Chapter 166)

JOHN P. CHUTE, M.D.
National Cancer Institute–Navy Medical Oncology Branch,
National Naval Medical Center,
Bethesda, Maryland
(Chapter 116)

JAMES M. CLARK, M.D., PH.D.
Clinical Associate Professor of Environmental Medicine in Pharmacology,
Institute for Environmental Medicine,
University of Pennsylvania,
Philadelphia, Pennsylvania
(Chapter 64)

J. ALLEN D. COOPER, JR., M.D.
Associate Professor of Medicine,
Chief, Pulmonary Section,
University of Alabama at Birmingham,
Birmingham, Alabama
(Chapter 60)

ANTHONY CORBET, M.B.B.S.
Clinical Professor of Pediatrics,
University of Texas Health Science Center,
San Antonio, Texas
(Chapter 169)

ROBERT O. CRAPO, M.D.
Medical Director, Pulmonary Laboratory,
LDS Hospital,
Salt Lake City, Utah
(Chapter 19)

ROBERT S. CRAUSMAN, M.D.
Director, Internal Medicine Residency Program,
Memorial Hospital of Rhode Island,
Pawtucket, Rhode Island
(Chapters 76, 77)

STEPHEN W. CRAWFORD, M.D.
Associate Professor of Medicine,
Critical Care Director,
University of Washington,
Fred Hutchinson Cancer Research Center,
Seattle, Washington
(Chapter 137)

GERARD JOSEPH CRINER, M.D.
Associate Professor of Medicine,
Director, Pulmonary and Critical Care Medicine,
Temple University Hospital,
Philadelphia, Pennsylvania
(Chapters 98, 171)

ARTHUR M. DANNENBERG, JR., M.D., PH.D.
Professor, Environmental Health Sciences, Molecular Microbiology and
Immunology, and Epidemiology
Johns Hopkins School of Hygiene and Public Health,
Baltimore, Maryland
(Chapter 160)

DAVID M. DAUGHTON, M.S.
Behavioral Researcher,
Pulmonary and Critical Care Division,
University of Nebraska Medical Center,
Omaha, Nebraska
(Chapter 45)

PAUL T. DAVIDSON, M.D.
Director, Tuberculosis Control,
Public Health Programs and Services,
Los Angeles County Department of Health Services,
Los Angeles, California
(Chapter 164)

RICHARD O. DAVIES, D.V.M., PH.D.
Professor of Physiology,
Animal Biology,
University of Pennsylvania,
Philadelphia, Pennsylvania
(Chapter 101)

MALCOLM M. DECAMP, JR., M.D.
Assistant Professor of Surgery,
Division of Thoracic Surgery,
Brigham and Women's Hospital,
Boston, Massachusetts
(Chapter 95)

MARC DECRAMER, M.D., PH.D.
Professor of Medicine,
Respiratory Division,
University Hospitals,
Leuven, Belgium
(Chapter 3)

HORACE M. DELISSER, M.D.
Assistant Professor of Medicine,
Pulmonary and Critical Care Division,
University of Pennsylvania Medical Center,
Philadelphia, Pennsylvania
(Chapter 40)

RICHARD A. DEREMEE, M.D.
Professor of Medicine,
Mayo Medical School, Mayo Clinic,
Rochester, Minnesota
(Chapter 86)

CLIFFORD S. DEUTSCHMAN, M.D.
Associate Professor of Anesthesia,
University of Pennsylvania Medical Center,
Philadelphia, Pennsylvania
(Chapter 168)

LISA L. DEVER, M.D.
Assistant Professor,
Department of Medicine, VAMC,
Division of Infectious Diseases,
UMD-New Jersey Medical School,
East Orange, New Jersey
(Chapter 119)

GORDON M. DICKINSON, M.D.
Professor of Medicine,
Division of Infectious Diseases,
University of Miami School of Medicine,
Miami, Florida
(Chapter 142)

FRANCIS W. DIPIERRO, M.D.
Instructor, Department of Surgery,
University of Pennsylvania School of Medicine,
Philadelphia, Pennsylvania
(Chapter 105)

ROBERT J. DOWNEY, M.D.
Attending Thoracic Surgeon,
Director, Surgical Critical Care,
Memorial Sloan-Kettering Cancer Center,
New York, New York
(Chapter 104)

MARLENE DURAND, M.D.
Assistant in Medicine,
Infectious Disease Unit,
Massachusetts General Hospital,
Boston, Massachusetts
(Chapter 126)

JEFFREY D. EDELMAN, M.D.
Pulmonary and Critical Care Division,
University of Pennsylvania Medical Center,
Philadelphia, Pennsylvania
(Chapter 58)

JACK A. ELIAS, M.D.
Professor and Chief,
Pulmonary and Critical Care Medicine,
Department of Internal Medicine,
Yale University School of Medicine,
New Haven, Connecticut
(Chapter 20)

PAUL E. EPSTEIN, M.D.
Chief, Pulmonary Division,
Graduate Hospital,
Philadelphia, Pennsylvania
(Chapter 41)

ALAN M. FEIN, M.D.
Director, Pulmonary and Critical Care Medicine,
Winthrop Pulmonary Associates, PC,
Mineola, New York
(Chapter 110)

STEVEN H. FEINSILVER, M.D.
Director, Pulmonary and Critical Care Medicine, Training Program,
Winthrop Pulmonary Associates, PC,
Mineola, New York
(Chapter 110)

GREGORY A. FILICE, M.D.
Chief, Infectious Disease Section,
VA Medical Center,
Associate Professor of Medicine,
University of Minnesota Medical School,
Minneapolis, Minnesota
(Chapter 146)

SYDNEY M. FINEGOLD, M.D.
Staff Physician, Medical Services,
Department of Veterans Affairs Medical Center,
Los Angeles, California
(Chapter 130)

JAMES E. FISH, M.D.
Director, Pulmonary and Critical Care Medicine,
Jefferson Medical College,
Philadelphia, Pennsylvania
(Chapter 50)

ALFRED P. FISHMAN, M.D.
William Maul Measey Professor of Medicine,
Department of Rehabilitation Medicine,
University of Pennsylvania Medical Center,
Philadelphia, Pennsylvania
(Chapters 1, 16, 28, 30, 36, 42, 55, 75, 82, 83, 84, 109)

JAY ALAN FISHMAN, M.D., F.A.C.P.
Associate Physician,
Infectious Diseases Unit,
Massachusetts General Hospital-East,
Charlestown, Massachusetts
(Chapters 130, 133, 134, 135, 136, 138, 150)

HENNING A. GAISSERT, M.D.
Assistant Professor of Surgery,
Brown University School of Medicine,
Rhode Island Hospital,
Providence, Rhode Island
(Chapter 52)

GREGORY P. GEBA, M.D.
Assistant Professor of Medicine,
Pulmonary and Critical Care Medicine,
Yale University School of Medicine,
New Haven, Connecticut
(Chapter 49)

CHARLES F. P. GEORGE, M.D.
Associate Professor of Medicine,
University of Western Ontario,
Director of Sleep Laboratory,
London Health Sciences Centre–Victoria Campus,
London, Ontario, Canada
(Chapter 103)

RONALD B. GEORGE, M.D.
Professor and Chairman, Department of Medicine,
Louisiana State University,
Shreveport, Louisiana
(Chapter 44)

ANDREW N. GOLDBERG, M.D.
Assistant Professor,
Department of Otorhinolaryngology,
Hospital of the University of Pennsylvania,
Philadelphia, Pennsylvania
(Chapter 102)

STANLEY GOLDFARB, M.D.
Vice Chairman, Network Development,
Department of Medicine,
University of Pennsylvania Medical Center,
Philadelphia, Pennsylvania
(Chapter 15)

MITCHELL GOLDMAN, M.D.
Assistant Professor of Medicine,
Department of Medicine,
Wishard Memorial Hospital,
Indianapolis, Indiana
(Chapter 149)

DANIEL M. GOODENBERGER, M.D.
Associate Professor of Medicine,
Washington University School of Medicine,
St. Louis, Missouri
(Chapter 87)

JONATHAN GOTTLIEB, M.D.
Pulmonary and Critical Care Medicine
Thomas Jefferson University Hospital
Philadelphia, Pennsylvania
(Chapter 175)

STEPHEN B. GREENBERG, M.D.
Professor and Vice Chairman,
Department of Medicine,
Baylor College of Medicine,
Houston, Texas
(Chapter 151)

JEFFREY K. GRIFFITHS, M.D., M.P.H., T.M.
Assistant Professor of Medicine,
Tufts University School of Medicine,
Director, Microbiology,
St. Elizabeth's Medical Center,
Brighton, Massachusetts
(Chapter 155)

MICHAEL A. GRIPPI, M.D.
Associate Professor of Medicine,
Vice Chairman, Clinical Affairs,
University of Pennsylvania Medical Center,
Philadelphia, Pennsylvania
(Chapters 36, 40, 165)

PRABODH K. GUPTA, M.D.
Director, Cytopathology and Cytometry,
Pathology and Laboratory Medicine,
University of Pennsylvania Medical Center
Philadelphia, Pennsylvania
(Chapter 33)

IMAD Y. HADDAD, M.D.
Assistant Professor of Pediatrics,
University of Alabama at Birmingham,
Birmingham, Alabama
(Chapter 26)

JOHN HANSEN-FLASCHEN, M.D.
Associate Professor and Chief,
Pulmonary and Critical Care Division,
University of Pennsylvania Medical Center,
Philadelphia, Pennsylvania
(Chapter 179)

C. WILLIAM HANSON III, M.D.
Assistant Professor of Anesthesia, Surgery, and Internal Medicine,
University of Pennsylvania Medical Center,
Philadelphia, Pennsylvania
(Chapter 174)

WILLIAM D. HARDIN, JR., M.D.
Associate Professor of Surgery and Pediatrics,
The Children's Hospital of Alabama,
Birmingham, Alabama
(Chapter 140)

HOWARD M. HELLER, M.D.
Instructor in Medicine,
Harvard Medical School,
Massachusetts Institute of Technology,
Medical Department,
Cambridge, Massachusetts
(Chapter 157)

HARRY R. HILL, M.D.
Professor, Departments of Pathology and Pediatrics,
Head, Division of Clinical Immunology and Allergy,
University of Utah School of Medicine,
Salt Lake City, Utah
(Chapter 139)

MICHAEL P. HLASTALA, PH.D.
Professor, Physiology and Biophysics,
Pulmonary and Critical Care Medicine,
University of Washington,
Seattle, Washington
(Chapter 14)

ANN D. HOROWITZ, PH.D.
Instructor of Pediatrics,
Children's Hospital Medical Center,
Division of Pulmonary Biology,
Cincinnati, Ohio
(Chapter 7)

LEONARD D. HUDSON, M.D.
Head, Pulmonary and Critical Care Medicine,
University of Washington,
Harborview Medical Center,
Seattle, Washington
(Chapter 167)

SUZANNE S. HURD, PH.D.
Director, Division of Lung Diseases,
National Heart, Lung, and Blood Institute, National Institutes of Health,
Bethesda, Maryland
(Chapter 182)

BRIAN V. JEGASOTHY, M.D.
Professor and Chairman,
Department of Dermatology,
University of Pittsburgh,
Pittsburgh, Pennsylvania
(Chapter 29)

WALDEMAR G. JOHANSON, JR., M.D.
Professor and Chairman,
Department of Medicine,
UMD-New Jersey Medical School,
Newark, New Jersey
(Chapter 119)

BRUCE E. JOHNSON, M.D.
National Cancer Institute,
Navy Medical Oncology Branch,
National Naval Medical Center,
Bethesda, Maryland
(Chapter 116)

DAVID H. JOHNSON, M.D.
Director,
Vanderbilt University School of Medicine,
Division of Medical Oncology,
The Vanderbilt Clinic,
Nashville, Tennessee
(Chapter 114)

LARRY R. KAISER, M.D.
Associate Professor of Surgery,
Department of Surgery,
University of Pennsylvania Medical Center,
Philadelphia, Pennsylvania
[Chapters 39, 96, 105, 113 (Part I)]

KUSHAGRA KATARIYA, M.D.
Chief Resident,
Department of Surgery,
Beth Israel Medical Center,
New York, New York
(Chapter 115)

STEVEN M. KELLER, M.D.
Chief, Division of Thoracic Surgery,
Director, David B. Kriser Lung Cancer Center,
Department of Surgery,
Beth Israel Medical Center,
New York, New York
(Chapter 115)

MARK A. KELLEY, M.D.
Professor of Medicine,
Vice Dean for Clinical Affairs,
University of Pennsylvania Medical Center,
Philadelphia, Pennsylvania
(Chapters 84, 180)

STEVEN G. KELSEN, M.D.
Professor of Medicine and Physiology,
Temple University Hospital,
Philadelphia, Pennsylvania
(Chapters 98, 171)

DAVID KENT, M.D.
Chief Medical Resident,
The Cambridge Hospital,
Cambridge, Massachusetts
(Chapter 141)

JEFFREY A. KERN, M.D.
Associate Professor of Medicine,
Department of Internal Medicine,
University of Iowa Hospitals and Clinics,
Iowa City, Iowa
(Chapter 107)

GARY T. KINASEWITZ, M.D.
Professor of Medicine, Physiology, and Biophysics,
University of Oklahoma,
Oklahoma City, Oklahoma
(Chapter 88)

TALMADGE E. KING, JR., M.D.
Senior Faculty Member,
Vice Chairman for Clinical Affairs,
Department of Medicine,
National Jewish Center for Immunology and Respiratory Medicine,
Denver, Colorado
(Chapters 54, 76, 77)

JEAN A. KLASTERSKY, M.D.
Professor and Chief of Medicine,
Department of Medicine,
Institut Jules Bordet,
Brussels, Belgium
(Chapter 123)

ROBERT A. KLOCKE, M.D.
Professor and Chairman,
Department of Medicine,
State University of New York at Buffalo,
Buffalo, New York
(Chapter 13)

MICHAEL I. KOTLIKOFF, PH.D., D.V.M.
Professor and Chairman, Animal Biology,
School of Veterinary Medicine,
University of Pennsylvania,
Philadelphia, Pennsylvania
(Chapter 6)

ROBERT M. KOTLOFF, M.D.
Assistant Professor of Medicine,
Pulmonary and Critical Care Medicine,
University of Pennsylvania Medical Center,
Philadelphia, Pennsylvania
(Chapter 170)

MEIR H. KRYGER, M.D.
Professor of Medicine,
Director, Sleep Research,
St. Boniface Hospital Research Center,
Winnipeg, Manitoba, Canada
(Chapter 103)

LESZEK KUBIN, PH.D.
Research Associate Professor,
Department of Animal Biology,
School of Veterinary Medicine,
Philadelphia, Pennsylvania
(Chapter 101)

STEVEN L. KUNKEL, PH.D.
Professor, Department of Pathology,
University of Michigan Medical School,
Ann Arbor, Michigan
(Chapter 24)

SUKHAMAY LAHIRI, PH.D.
Professor, Department of Physiology,
University of Pennsylvania School of Medicine,
Philadelphia, Pennsylvania
(Chapter 63)

KENNETH S. LANDRETH, PH.D.
Professor, Department of Microbiology and Immunology,
West Virginia University,
Mary Barb Randolph Cancer Center,
Morgantown, West Virginia
(Chapter 23)

PAUL N. LANKEN, M.D.
Associate Professor of Medicine,
Medical Intensive Care Unit,
University of Pennsylvania Medical Center,
Philadelphia, Pennsylvania
(Chapter 181)

JAMES W. LEATHERMAN, M.D.
Associate Professor of Medicine,
Pulmonary and Critical Care Medicine,
University of Minnesota,
Hennepin County Medical Center,
Minneapolis, Minnesota
(Chapter 79)

CLAUDE LENFANT, M.D.
Director, National Heart, Lung, and Blood Institute,
National Institutes of Health,
Bethesda, Maryland
(Chapter 182)

LESLIE A. LITZKY, M.D.
Assistant Professor of Medicine,
Department of Pathology and Laboratory Medicine,
University of Pennsylvania,
Philadelphia, Pennsylvania
(Chapters 92, 111)

JACOB S. LOKE, M.D.
Clinical Professor of Medicine,
Pulmonary Medicine,
Yale University School of Medicine,
New Haven, Connecticut
(Chapter 65)

WALKER A. LONG, M.D.
Associate Professor of Pediatrics,
Pediatric Cardiology Division,
University of North Carolina,
Chapel Hill, North Carolina
(Chapter 169)

JOSEPH P. LYNCH III, M.D.
Professor of Internal Medicine,
The University of Michigan Medical Center,
Ann Arbor, Michigan
(Chapters 70, 79)

MITCHELL MACHTAY, M.D.
Assistant Professor,
Department of Radiation Oncology,
University of Pennsylvania Medical Center,
Philadelphia, Pennsylvania
[Chapter 113 (Part III)]

ADEL A. F. MAHMOUD, M.D., PH.D.
The John H. Hord Professor and Chairman,
Department of Medicine,
University Hospitals of Cleveland,
Cleveland, Ohio
(Chapter 156)

SAVVAS C. MAKRIDES, PH.D.
Director of Molecular Biology,
T Cell Sciences, Inc.,
Needham, Massachusetts
(Chapter 9)

SCOTT MANAKER, M.D., PH.D.
Assistant Professor of Medicine and Pharmacology,
Pulmonary and Critical Care Division,
University of Pennsylvania,
Philadelphia, Pennsylvania
(Chapter 173)

MITCHELL L. MARGOLIS, M.D.
Chief, Pulmonary Division,
Philadelphia VA Medical Center,
Philadelphia, Pennsylvania
(Chapter 112)

JOHN J. MARINI, M.D.
Professor of Medicine,
University of Minnesota,
St. Paul Ramsey Medical Center,
St. Paul, Minnesota
(Chapter 177)

THOMAS J. MARRIE, M.D.
Professor of Medicine,
Victoria General Hospital,
Department of Medicine, Infectious Diseases,
Halifax, Nova Scotia, Canada
(Chapter 127)

SADIS MATALON, PH.D.
Professor, Department of Anesthesiology,
University of Alabama at Birmingham,
Birmingham, Alabama
(Chapter 26)

C. GLEN MAYHALL, M.D.
Department of Internal Medicine,
University of Texas Medical Branch at Galveston,
Galveston, Texas
(Chapter 143)

F. DENNIS McCOOL, M.D.
Associate Professor of Medicine,
Pulmonary Division,
Memorial Hospital of Rhode Island,
Pawtucket, Rhode Island
(Chapter 97)

PAUL B. McCRAY, JR., M.D.
Associate Professor,
Department of Pediatrics,
University of Iowa College of Medicine,
Iowa City, Iowa
(Chapter 8)

VINCENT G. McDERMOTT, M.B., M.R.C.P.I., F.R.C.R.
Assistant Professor of Radiology,
Department of Diagnostic Radiology,
Duke University Medical Center,
Durham, North Carolina
(Chapter 34)

DAVID S. McKINSEY, M.D.
Clinical Associate Professor of Medicine,
University of Kansas School of Medicine,
Research Medical Center,
Kansas City, Missouri
(Chapter 142)

GEOFFREY McLENNAN, M.B.B.S., F.R.A.C.P.
Associate Professor of Medicine,
Pulmonary and Critical Care Medicine,
University of Iowa Hospitals and Clinics,
Iowa City, Iowa
(Chapter 107)

JOSEPH L. MELNICK, M.D., PH.D.
Distinguished Service Professor of Virology,
Division of Molecular Virology,
Baylor College of Medicine,
Houston, Texas
(Chapter 154)

SAUMIL N. MERCHANT, M.D.
Assistant Professor, Otology and Laryngology,
Assistant Surgeon in Otolaryngology,
Massachusetts Eye and Ear Infirmary,
Boston, Massachusetts
(Chapter 126)

LOUIS F. METZGER, R.P.F.T.
Administrative Director,
Center for Sleep and Respiratory Neurobiology,
University of Pennsylvania Medical Center,
Philadelphia, Pennsylvania
(Chapter 36)

JAMES L. MICHEL, M.D., PH.D.
Assistant Professor of Medicine,
Microbiology and Molecular Genetics,
Channing Laboratory,
Harvard Medical School,
Boston, Massachusetts
(Chapter 125)

JAMES S. MILLEDGE, M.D.
Emeritus,
Clinical Research Centre,
Northwick Park Hospital,
Harrow, Middlesex, England
(Chapter 63)

WALLACE T. MILLER, M.D.
Professor of Radiology,
University of Pennsylvania,
Philadelphia, Pennsylvania
(Chapter 32)

DAVID R. MOLLER, M.D.
Assistant Professor of Medicine,
Director, Sarcoid Clinic,
Johns Hopkins School of Medicine,
Baltimore, Maryland
(Chapter 69)

ADRIAN R. MORRISON, D.V.M., PH.D.
Professor of Behavioral Neuroscience,
School of Veterinary Medicine,
University of Pennsylvania,
Philadelphia, Pennsylvania
(Chapter 100)

MAURICE A. MUFSON, M.D.
Professor and Chairman,
Department of Medicine,
Marshall University School of Medicine,
Huntington, West Virginia
(Chapter 145)

DAVID M. MURPHY, M.D.
Clinical Associate Professor of Medicine
Chief, Pulmonary Medicine Department,
Deborah Heart and Lung Center,
Browns Mills, New Jersey
(Chapter 55)

EDWARD A. NARDELL, M.D.
Chief, Pulmonary Medicine,
Assistant Professor of Medicine, HMS,
The Cambridge Hospital,
Cambridge, Massachusetts
(Chapter 141)

RONALD LEE NICHOLS, M.D.
William Henderson Professor of Surgery,
Department of Surgery,
Tulane University Medical Center,
New Orleans, Louisiana
(Chapter 140)

JERRY A. NICK, M.D.
Instructor, Division of Pulmonary Sciences and Critical Care Medicine,
Worthen Lab,
National Jewish Center,
Denver, Colorado
(Chapter 25)

MICHAEL S. NIEDERMAN, M.D.
Associate Professor of Medicine,
Director, Critical Care Subsection,
Pulmonary and Critical Care Unit,
Winthrop-University Hospital,
Mineola, New York
(Chapter 122)

RICHARD H. OCHS, M.D.
Adjunct Clinical Professor and Director,
Department of Pathology and Laboratory Medicine,
Bryn Mawr Hospital,
Bryn Mawr, Pennsylvania
(Chapter 75)

ELIZABETH A. OLEK, D.O.
Instructor in Medicine,
Infectious Diseases Section,
Boston University Medical Center Hospital,
Boston, Massachusetts
(Chapter 147)

A. FUSON ONER-EYUBOGLU, M.D.
Instructor in Medicine,
Pulmonary and Critical Care Medicine,
University of Pennsylvania Medical Center,
Philadelphia, Pennsylvania
(Chapter 162)

IDA M. ONORATO, M.D.
Chief, Surveillance and Epidemiologic Investigations Branch,
Division of TB Elimination, Centers for Disease Control and Prevention,
Atlanta, Georgia
(Chapter 158)

ALLAN I. PACK, M.D., PH.D.
Professor of Medicine,
Center for Sleep and Respiratory Neurobiology,
University of Pennsylvania Medical Center,
Philadelphia, Pennsylvania
(Chapters 11, 101, 102)

HAROLD I. PALEVSKY, M.D.
Associate Professor of Medicine,
Pulmonary and Critical Care Division,
University of Pennsylvania Medical Center,
Philadelphia, Pennsylvania
(Chapter 84)

REYNOLD A. PANETTIERI, JR., M.D.
Assistant Professor of Medicine,
Pulmonary and Critical Care Division,
University of Pennsylvania Medical Center,
Philadelphia, Pennsylvania
(Chapter 6)

JOHN E. PARKER, M.D.
Division of Respiratory Disease Studies,
National Institute for Occupational Safety and Health,
Morgantown, West Virginia
(Chapter 59)

DAVID E. PARRY, M.D.
Instructor, Allergy and Clinical Immunology,
University of Wisconsin Hospital and Clinics,
Madison, Wisconsin
(Chapter 47)

MARK S. PASTERNACK, M.D.
Chief, Pediatric Infectious Disease Unit,
Massachusetts General Hospital,
Charlestown, Massachusetts
(Chapter 128)

ROY PATTERSON, M.D.
Chief of Allergy and Immunology,
Northwestern University Medical School,
Chicago, Illinois
(Chapter 51)

CYNTHIA S. PAYNE, M.D.
Assistant Professor of Radiology,
Department of Diagnostic Radiology,
Duke University Medical Center,
Durham, North Carolina
(Chapter 34)

ANDERS PERSSON, M.D., PH.D.
Assistant Professor of Medicine,
Respiratory and Critical Care Division,
Barnes-Jewish Hospital (North Campus),
St. Louis, Missouri
(Chapter 81)

JAY I. PETERS, M.D.
Associate Professor of Medicine,
Department of Medicine,
University of Texas Health Sciences Center,
Audie Murphy VA,
San Antonio, Texas
(Chapter 91)

STEPHEN P. PETERS, M.D., PH.D.
Professor of Medicine,
Jefferson Medical College,
Philadelphia, Pennsylvania
(Chapter 50)

EDWARD L. PETSONK, M.D.
Chief of Clinical Section,
Division of Respiratory Disease Studies,
National Institute for Occupational Safety and Health,
Morgantown, West Virginia
(Chapter 59)

KATHLEEN D. PFEFFER, M.D.
Assistant Professor of Medicine,
Division of Pulmonary Medicine,
Department of Pediatrics,
University of Utah School of Medicine,
Salt Lake City, Utah
(Chapter 139)

GERALD B. PIER, PH.D.
Associate Professor of Medicine,
Microbiology and Molecular Genetics,
Harvard Medical School,
Channing Laboratory,
Boston, Massachusetts
(Chapter 125)

GIUSEPPE G. PIETRA, M.D.
Professor, Pathology and Laboratory Medicine,
Division of Anatomic Pathology,
University of Pennsylvania Medical Center,
Philadelphia, Pennsylvania
(Chapter 118)

SUSAN K. PINGLETON, M.D.
Professor of Medicine,
Pulmonary and Critical Care Medicine,
University of Kansas Medical Center,
Kansas City, Kansas
(Chapter 178)

BRUCE R. PITT, PH.D.
Professor of Pharmacology,
University of Pittsburgh School of Medicine,
Pittsburgh, Pennsylvania
(Chapter 26)

JOHN POPOVICH, JR., M.D.
Division Head,
Division of Pulmonary and Critical Care Medicine,
Henry Ford Hospital,
Detroit, Michigan
(Chapter 18)

PIETER E. POSTMUS, M.D.
Department of Pulmonology,
Free University Hospital,
Amsterdam, The Netherlands
(Chapter 108)

JOE B. PUTNAM, JR., M.D.
Associate Professor of Surgery,
Thoracic and Cardiovascular Surgery,
The University of Texas,
M.D. Anderson Cancer Center
Houston, Texas
(Chapter 93)

GANESH RAGHU, M.D.
Associate Professor of Medicine,
Pulmonary and Critical Care Medicine,
University of Washington Medical Center,
Seattle, Washington
(Chapter 68)

DONALD G. RAIBLE, M.D.
Associate Professor of Medicine,
Medical College of Pennsylvania and Hahnemann University,
Philadelphia, Pennsylvania
(Chapter 22)

CARRIE A. REDLICH, M.D.
Associate Professor of Medicine,
Pulmonary and Critical Care Medicine,
Yale University School of Medicine,
New Haven, Connecticut
(Chapter 56)

STEPHEN I. RENNARD, M.D.
Chief, Pulmonary and Critical Care Medicine,
University of Nebraska Medical Center,
Omaha, Nebraska
(Chapter 45)

HERBERT Y. REYNOLDS, M.D.
J. Lloyd Huck Professor of Medicine,
Department of Medicine,
Milton S. Hershey Medical Center,
The Pennsylvania State University,
Hershey, Pennsylvania
(Chapter 20)

ELIZABETH A. RICH, M.D.
Associate Professor of Medicine,
Division of Pulmonary and Critical Care Medicine,
Case Western Reserve University,
Cleveland, Ohio
(Chapter 152)

RENÉE RIDZON, M.D.
Medical Epidemiologist,
Division of TB Elimination,
Centers for Disease Control,
Atlanta, Georgia
(Chapter 158)

ANDREW L. RIES, M.D.
Professor of Medicine,
Associate Director, Pulmonary Rehabilitation,
University of California Medical Center,
San Diego, California
(Chapter 46)

JEAN E. RINALDO, M.D.
Professor of Medicine,
Division of Pulmonary Medicine,
Vanderbilt University School of Medicine,
Nashville, Tennessee
(Chapter 166)

JOHN R. ROBERTS, M.D.
Assistant Professor of Surgery,
University of Pennsylvania Medical Center,
Philadelphia, Pennsylvania
(Chapter 96)

KENNETH B. ROBERTS, M.D.
Assistant Professor,
Department of Therapeutic Radiology,
Yale University School of Medicine,
New Haven, Connecticut
(Chapter 72)

CYNTHIA ROBINSON, M.D.
Assistant Professor, Pulmonary and Critical Care,
University of Pennsylvania,
Philadelphia, Pennsylvania
(Chapter 53)

KEITH M. ROBINSON, M.D.
Vice Chairman for Clinical Services,
Department of Rehabilitation Medicine,
University of Pennsylvania Medical Center,
Philadelphia, Pennsylvania
(Chapter 80)

CAROLYN L. ROCHESTER, M.D.
Assistant Professor of Medicine,
Section of Pulmonary and Critical Care,
Yale University School of Medicine,
New Haven, Connecticut
(Chapter 74)

DUDLEY F. ROCHESTER, M.D.
Professor Emeritus,
Department of Medicine,
University of Virginia,
Charlottesville, Virginia
(Chapter 97)

SARA ROCKWELL, PH.D.
Professor, Department of Therapeutic Radiology and Cancer Center,
Yale University School of Medicine,
New Haven, Connecticut
(Chapter 72)

WILLIAM N. ROM, M.D.
Professor of Medicine and Environmental Medicine,
Pulmonary and Critical Care Medicine,
Bellevue,
New York University Medical Center,
New York, New York
(Chapter 57)

JESSE ROMAN, M.D.
Chief, Pulmonary and Critical Care Section,
Department of Medicine,
Atlanta VA Medical Center,
Decatur, Georgia
(Chapter 4)

MILTON D. ROSSMAN, M.D.
Professor, Pulmonary and Critical Care,
University of Pennsylvania Medical Center,
Philadelphia, Pennsylvania
(Chapters 58, 162)

ROBERT H. RUBIN, M.D., F.A.C.P., F.C.C.P.
Chief, Transplantation Infectious Disease,
Massachusetts General Hospital,
Boston, Massachusetts
(Chapter 138)

MARK E. RUPP, M.D.
Assistant Professor of Medicine,
Department of Internal Medicine,
University of Nebraska Medical Center,
Omaha, Nebraska
(Chapter 131)

WILLIAM A. RUTALA, PH.D., M.P.H.
Professor of Medicine,
University of North Carolina,
Chapel Hill, North Carolina
(Chapter 143)

UNA S. RYAN, PH.D.
Vice President of Research,
T Cell Services, Inc.,
Needham, Massachusetts
(Chapter 9)

ANN V. SACKS, B.S., R.P.F.T.
Associate Director,
Pulmonary and Critical Care Medicine,
University of Pennsylvania Medical Center,
Philadelphia, Pennsylvania
(Chapter 36)

STEVEN A. SAHN, M.D.
Professor, Pulmonary and Critical Care Medicine,
Medical University of South Carolina,
Charleston, South Carolina
(Chapter 90)

EDWARD Y. SAKO, M.D., PH.D.
Assistant Professor,
Department of Surgery,
Division of Cardiothoracic Surgery,
The University of Texas Health Sciences Center at San Antonio,
San Antonio, Texas
(Chapter 91)

KEVIN E. SALHANY, M.D.
Assistant Professor,
Division of Anatomic Pathology,
University of Pennsylvania Medical Center,
Philadelphia, Pennsylvania
(Chapter 118)

JONATHAN M. SAMET, M.D.
Professor and Chairman,
Department of Epidemiology,
Johns Hopkins School of Hygiene and Public Health,
Baltimore, Maryland
(Chapter 62)

GERARDO S. SAN PEDRO, M.D.
Associate Professor of Clinical Medicine,
Pulmonary and Critical Care Medicine,
Louisiana State University Medical Center,
Shreveport, Louisiana
(Chapter 44)

WILLIAM T. SAUSE, M.D., F.A.C.R.
Associate Professor of Radiology,
University of Utah,
LDS Hospital,
Salt Lake City, Utah
[Chapter 113 (Part III)]

THOMAS F. SCANLIN, M.D.
Professor, Pediatrics,
Abramson Pediatric Center,
Children's Hospital of Philadelphia,
Philadelphia, Pennsylvania
(Chapter 53)

EDWARD S. SCHULMAN, M.D.
Professor of Medicine,
Allegheny University Hospital, Hahnemann Division,
Pulmonary and Critical Care Medicine,
Philadelphia, Pennsylvania
(Chapter 22)

DANIEL P. SCHUSTER, M.D.
Associate Professor of Medicine and Radiology,
Department of Internal Medicine,
Washington University School of Medicine,
St. Louis, Missouri
(Chapter 85)

MARK R. SCHUYLER, M.D.
Professor of Medicine,
Chief, Medical Service,
VA Medical Center,
Albuquerque, New Mexico
(Chapter 71)

RICHARD J. SCHWAB, M.D.
Assistant Professor of Medicine,
Medical Director, Penn Center for Sleep Disorders,
Hospital of the University of Pennsylvania,
Philadelphia, Pennsylvania
(Chapter 102)

DAVID A. SCHWARTZ, M.D.
Associate Professor,
Director, Occupational Medicine,
University of Iowa College of Medicine,
Iowa City, Iowa
(Chapter 61)

MARVIN I. SCHWARZ, M.D.
Professor of Medicine,
Head, Division of Pulmonary Sciences and Critical Care Medicine,
University of Colorado Health Services Center,
Denver, Colorado
(Chapter 73)

ROBERT M. SENIOR, M.D.
Dorothy R. and Hubert C. Moog Professor of Pulmonary Diseases in Medicine,
Washington University Medical Center,
Barnes-Jewish Hospital (North Campus),
St. Louis, Missouri
(Chapter 43)

STEVEN D. SHAPIRO, M.D.
Associate Professor of Medicine,
Barnes-Jewish Hospital (North Campus),
St. Louis, Missouri
(Chapter 43)

KUMAR SHARMA, PH.D.
Assistant Professor of Medicine,
Thomas Jefferson University,
Philadelphia, Pennsylvania
(Chapter 15)

MICHAEL S. SIMBERKOFF, M.D.
Chief, Infectious Diseases Section,
Veteran Affairs Medical Center,
New York, New York
(Chapter 124)

TONY P. SMITH, M.D.
Professor of Radiology,
Department of Diagnostic Radiology,
Duke University Medical Center,
Durham, North Carolina
(Chapter 34)

KENNETH P. STEINBERG, M.D.
Assistant Professor of Medicine,
University of Washington,
Harborview Medical Center,
Seattle, Washington
(Chapter 167)

DANIEL H. STERMAN, M.D.
Instructor of Medicine,
University of Pennsylvania Medical Center,
Philadelphia, Pennsylvania
(Chapters 38, 92)

ROBERT M. STRIETER, M.D.
Professor of Internal Medicine,
Division of Pulmonary and Critical Care Medicine,
University of Michigan,
Ann Arbor, Michigan
(Chapter 24)

ALAN M. SUGAR, M.D.
Associate Professor of Medicine,
Boston University Medical Center Hospital,
Boston, Massachusetts
(Chapter 147)

MORTON N. SWARTZ, M.D.
Professor of Medicine,
Infectious Diseases Unit,
Massachusetts General Hospital,
Boston, Massachusetts
(Chapters 121, 132)

ERIK R. SWENSON, M.D.
Associate Professor of Medicine,
Pulmonary Section,
University of Washington,
VA Medical Center,
Seattle, Washington
(Chapter 14)

LYNN T. TANOUE, M.D.
Assistant Professor of Medicine,
Yale School of Medicine,
Pulmonary and Critical Care Medicine,
New Haven, Connecticut
(Chapter 66)

C. RICHARD TAYLOR, PH.D.†
Charles P. Lyman Professor of Biology,
Museum of Comparative Zoology,
Harvard University,
Cambridge, Massachusetts
(Chapter 2)
†Deceased.

RICHARD TEPLICK, M.D.
Associate Professor of Anesthesia,
Department of Anesthesia,
Massachusetts General Hospital,
Boston, Massachusetts
(Chapter 133)

KAREN J. TIETZE, PHARM.D.
Associate Professor of Clinical Pharmacy,
Philadelphia College of Pharmacy and Science,
Philadelphia, Pennsylvania
(Chapter 173)

MARTIN J. TOBIN, M.D.
Professor and Chief,
Pulmonary and Critical Care Division,
Loyola University of Chicago,
Maywood, Illinois
(Chapter 176)

GALEN B. TOEWS, M.D.
Professor of Internal Medicine,
Chief, Pulmonary Medicine,
The University of Michigan Medical Center,
Ann Arbor, Michigan
(Chapters 70, 120)

JOSEPH F. TOMASHEFSKI, JR., M.D.
Associate Professor of Pathology,
Case Western Reserve University,
Metro Health Medical Center,
Cleveland, Ohio
(Chapter 160)

JOSEPH TREAT, M.D.
Division of Hematology-Oncology,
Department of Medicine,
University of Pennsylvania,
Philadelphia, Pennsylvania
[Chapter 113 (Part II)]

PETER G. TUTEUR, M.D.
Associate Professor of Medicine,
Pulmonary and Critical Care Division,
Washington University School of Medicine,
St. Louis, Missouri
(Chapter 31)

MICHAEL UNGER, M.D.
Clinical Professor of Medicine,
Thomas Jefferson University,
Philadelphia, Pennsylvania
(Chapter 38)

MARK J. UTELL, M.D.
Professor, Medicine and Environmental Medicine,
Director, Pulmonary and Occupational Medical Units,
Strong Memorial Hospital,
University of Rochester School of Medicine,
Rochester, New York
(Chapter 62)

FRITS VAN DER KUYP, M.D., M.P.H.
Controller,
Tuberculosis for Cuyahoa County,
Metrohealth Medical Center,
Cleveland, Ohio
(Chapter 159)

EMANUEL N. VERGIS, M.D.
Instructor in Medicine,
University of Pittsburgh,
Infectious Disease Section,
VA Medical Center,
Pittsburgh, Pennsylvania
(Chapter 144)

PETER D. WAGNER, M.D.
Professor of Medicine,
Department of Medicine,
University of California / San Diego,
La Jolla, California
(Chapter 12)

JOHN C. WAIN, M.D.
Associate Visiting Surgeon,
Thoracic Surgery Unit,
Massachusetts General Hospital,
Boston, Massachusetts
(Chapter 106)

DAVID J. WEBER, M.D., M.P.H.
Associate Professor of Medicine,
Infectious Disease Division,
University of North Carolina,
Chapel Hill, North Carolina
(Chapter 143)

KARL T. WEBER, M.D.
Professor and Chairman, Internal Medicine,
Division of Cardiology,
University of Missouri at Columbia,
Columbia, Missouri
(Chapter 37)

EWALD R. WEIBEL, M.D.
Professor Emeritus of Anatomy,
University of Berne,
Fondation Maurice E. Müller,
Berne, Switzerland
(Chapter 2)

ARNOLD N. WEINBERG, M.D.
Professor of Medicine, H.M.S.,
Medical Director
Massachusetts Institute of Technology,
Health Services,
Cambridge, Massachusetts
(Chapter 157)

SCOTT T. WEISS, M.D.
Professor of Medicine,
Director, Respiratory and Environmental Epidemiology,
Channing Laboratory, Brigham and Women's Hospital,
Harvard Medical School,
Boston, Massachusetts
(Chapter 48)

DAVID N. WEISSMAN, M.D.
Associate Professor of Medicine,
Pulmonary and Critical Care Medicine,
West Virginia Health Sciences Center,
Robert C. Byrd Center,
Morgantown, West Virginia
(Chapter 23)

MICHAEL J. WELSH, M.D.
Professor of Medicine and Physiology and Biophysics
Howard Hughes Medical Institute
Department of Internal Medicine
University of Iowa College of Medicine,
Iowa City, Iowa
(Chapter 8)

CHRISTINE H. WENDT, M.D.
Assistant Professor of Medicine,
University of Minnesota,
Minneapolis, Minnesota
(Chapter 27)

L. JOSEPH WHEAT, M.D.
Professor of Medicine,
Division of Infectious Diseases,
Wishard Memorial Hospital,
Indianapolis, Indiana
(Chapters 148, 149)

BRIAN J. WHIPP, PH.D., D.SC.
Professor of Physiology,
University of London,
St. George's Hospital Medical School,
London, England
(Chapter 17)

JEFFREY A. WHITSETT, M.D.
Professor of Pediatrics,
Division of Pulmonary Biology,
Children's Hospital Medical Center,
Cincinnati, Ohio
(Chapter 7)

NEVIN W. WILSON, M.D.
Associate Professor of Pediatrics,
Department of Pediatrics,
West Virginia University,
Health Science Center,
Morgantown, West Virginia
(Chapter 23)

RICHARD H. WINTERBAUER, M.D.
Head, Pulmonary and Critical Care Medicine,
Virginia Mason Medical Center,
Seattle, Washington
(Chapter 89)

ERIC T. WITTBRODT, PHARM.D.
Assistant Professor of Clinical Pharmacy,
Philadelphia College of Pharmacy and Science,
Philadelphia, Pennsylvania
(Chapter 173)

DANIEL WORSLEY, M.D.
Assistant Professor of Radiology,
Division of Nuclear Medicine,
Department of Radiology,
Vancouver General Hospital,
Vancouver, Canada
(Chapter 35)

G. SCOTT WORTHEN, M.D.
Department of Medicine,
National Jewish Center for Immunology and Respiratory Medicine,
Denver, Colorado
(Chapter 25)

CAMERON D. WRIGHT, M.D.
Assistant Professor of Surgery,
Howard Medical School,
Massachusetts General Hospital,
Boston, Massachusetts
(Chapter 94)

DAVID J. WYLER, M.D.
Professor of Medicine,
Tufts University School of Medicine,
Division of Geographic and Infectious Diseases,
New England Medical Center,
Boston, Massachusetts
(Chapter 155)

VICTOR L. YU, M.D.
Professor of Medicine,
University of Pittsburgh,
Chief, Infectious Disease Section,
Veterans Affairs Medical Center,
Pittsburgh, Pennsylvania
(Chapter 144)

SHERIF R. ZAKI, M.D., PH.D.
Chief, Molecular Pathology and Ultrastructure Activity,
Division of Viral and Rickettsial Diseases,
Centers for Diseases Control and Prevention,
Atlanta, Georgia
(Chapter 153)

RALPH J. ZITNIK, M.D.
Assistant Professor of Medicine,
Pulmonary and Critical Care Medicine,
Department of Internal Medicine,
Yale University School of Medicine,
New Haven, Connecticut
(Chapter 67)

RICHARD D. ZOROWITZ, M.D.
Director, Stroke Rehabilitation,
Department of Rehabilitation Medicine,
University of Pennsylvania Medical Center,
Philadelphia, Pennsylvania
(Chapter 80)

Preface

This edition deserves a special word of explanation since it marks a radical departure from the two previous editions, not so much in format as in editorial lineup and, as an inevitable result, in content. Instead of a single editor, there is now an editor-in-chief abetted by five associate editors, each one of whom is expert in at least one domain of chest medicine.

Looking back, we may find it rewarding for the sake of perspective to recapitulate the changing scene in pulmonary medicine that the two previous editions had addressed. In 1980, when the first edition appeared after several years of preparation, pulmonary medicine was reveling in its solid substrates of anatomy and pathology buttressed by physiology. Quantification was in the air and science was providing fresh insights into the mechanisms of disease. Previous preoccupation with infectious disease had given way to a pervasive interest in pulmonary function testing and derangements in pulmonary mechanics; new therapeutic modalities were evolving based on the improved understanding of the mechanisms of disease. Chronic obstructive pulmonary disease (COPD) and diffuse interstitial diseases were recognized by epidemiologic and clinical studies to be widespread and formidable problems that needed to be addressed. Prevention focused on smoking as a prime cause of both COPD and of lung cancer. The scientific meetings and journals took on new life, and all concerned in the science or clinical aspects of pulmonary medicine were proud of the distinguished leaders: Wallace Fenn, Hermann Rahn, Cournand and Richards, Julius Comroe. The first edition reflected the solid base in structure-function and the promising vistas opened by respiratory physiology.

The second edition eight years later moved into higher gear. By then, structure-function was solidly in place as a foundation for new advances in related fields. Immunology had found its feet in pulmonary medicine aided by hypersensitivity diseases, chemotherapy, and the spread of AIDS. Biochemistry had paved the way for studies of vital substances, such as pulmonary surfactant. Genetic diseases, such as cystic fibrosis and alpha-1-antitrypsin deficiency, were attracting attention in molecular terms. Clinical medicine received an enormous boost from the newer technologies: bronchoscopy, imaging, mechanical ventilation. Sleep disorders were incorporated into the purview of pulmonary medicine. Critical care medicine became a burgeoning subset of pulmonary medicine that took advantage of virtually all advances in both the understanding of pulmonary diseases and its management.

This glimpse from the rearview mirror brings us back to a look at this edition, which, in dealing with the present state of pulmonary medicine, also looks ahead toward leading edges, where advances in understanding, knowledge, and their applications are to be anticipated. This goal is in keeping with the recent report by the American Thoracic Society which sets forth "the major problems in lung disease and possible pathways to their solution." The report, entitled "Future Directions for Research on Diseases of the Lung," is reassuring to the editors of the third edition in that each target listed in this report is dealt with substantively and expertly in this book. As expected, the third edition envisages even larger and brighter horizons in the years ahead because of the clear and discerning visions of the individual contributors who write in their chapters about their special fields of interest.

The experience and knowledge of each of the editors have been directed at ensuring that the specialized, as well as the general, aspects of pulmonary medicine have been expertly covered and well presented. Although the book is now a collective arbeit, discussion and debate among the editors and authors have led to a work integrated by a meeting of the minds. By the process of peer review, the book aspires to provide a readable and balanced coverage of what is latest and most meaningful in pulmonary diseases and disorders.

I have already indicated how much this book owes to the experts who comprise the editorial board. Clearly, they would have little to work with were it not for the splendid chapters contributed by the individual authors. Nor would the book be as well orchestrated were it not for the leadership (and prodding) of J. Dereck Jeffers, editor-in-chief at McGraw-Hill, who has been the shepherd for all three editions, latterly promoting camaraderie and productivity among the editors while ensuring that deadlines were met.

I owe a great deal to those close to home. Alice K. Glover handled the preparation of the book with great skill and speed, moving its pages along from manuscript to page proof. Betsy Ann Bozzarello freed time for me to devote to the book while catalyzing the efforts of others. Roger Webb continued to infiltrate the text with his telltale drawings, and Daniel Barrett was once again on continuing standby alert, ready and available to pitch in as needed.

My family provided the encouragement and peace of mind that such an effort inevitably calls for. My wife, Linda, was unwavering in her tolerance and support. My daughter, Hannah, who is trying her own hand at writing, was both impressed by the enormity of the undertaking and indulgent about anyone who would embark on such a venture. My sons, Mark and Jay, shared my conviction that this book is in keeping with our shared academic convictions. Their spouses, Gayle and Martha, helped to create the setting and frame of mind in which this book was put together.

Alfred P. Fishman, M.D.

Fishman's
*Pulmonary Diseases
and Disorders*
Volume 2

PART ELEVEN

DISEASES OF THE MEDIASTINUM

CHAPTER 93

THE MEDIASTINUM: OVERVIEW, ANATOMY, AND DIAGNOSTIC APPROACH

Joe B. Putnam, Jr.

The mediastinum lies centrally within the chest and spans the region vertically from the thoracic inlet to the diaphragmatic hiatus, transversely between the parietal pleura, and coronally between the sternum and vertebral column. Diseases of the mediastinum may affect any or all structures within the chest, with diverse effects both clinically and anatomically. Many patients, however, are asymptomatic, with the mediastinal mass found on routine screening chest radiograph. The location and mass effect on the heart or great vessels, the tracheobronchial tree, the esophagus, and nerves and other structures may produce specific clinical symptoms and may narrow the differential diagnosis. With the advent of the routine plain chest radiograph, computed tomography of the chest, magnetic resonance imaging, and various other diagnostic studies, the diagnosis of mediastinal lesions can be made more frequently and accurately.[34] Histologic diagnosis by fine-needle aspiration or open biopsy and complemented by immunohistochemistry and electron microscopy enhances accurate diagnosis and improves subsequent treatment decisions.

The clinician must be aware of the many problems that may arise from diseases affecting the mediastinal structures and the relationship of these diseases to mediastinal anatomy.[18] Primary and metastatic neoplasms will occur in the mediastinum, and further evaluation of the patient may be needed. Benign masses (bronchogenic cysts, pericardial cysts), diaphragmatic hernias, and local extensions of other problems (lung cancer, goiter, infections, etc.) may occur. The clinical presentation of the patient with mediastinal diseases may range from asymptomatic, with the mass simply identified on screening chest radiograph, to hypoxia and acute respiratory distress, superior vena cava syndrome, or hemodynamic instability. Symptoms may be specifically related to invasion of defined mediastinal structures. Treatment for these symptoms requires evaluation of the extent of disease, diagnosis and staging, and an assessment of the benefits to be achieved with various treatment options. A multidisciplinary approach to the problem will require the skills of surgeons, physicians, pediatricians, radiologists, nuclear medicine radiologists, pathologists, and radiation oncologists.

Radiographic examination of the mediastinum has been used widely for investigating the location and the extent of mediastinal masses within the thorax. Classically, a plain chest radiograph taken in two planes (posteroanterior and lateral) provided basic information on the location of a mediastinal mass. Based on the embryologic development of cervicothoracic organs and anatomy, a broad differential diagnosis can be obtained when the radiographic findings are correlated with the anatomy of structures within the mediastinum. Computed tomography or magnetic resonance imaging (or both) will routinely complement the chest radiograph. Other imaging techniques may incorporate specific biologic features of the mass.

Clinical staging of the patient (defined as all studies obtained before initiation of definitive therapy) is required for all mediastinal masses. The clinical presentation of the patient, the radiographic findings, and the location of the tumor all assist the clinician, who must consider the potential for neoplasia and infections, as well as anatomic, congenital, or traumatic causes. Diagnosis of mediastinal masses may require histologic or other laboratory evaluation. Cytology (from fine-needle aspiration), core biopsy, or open (surgical) biopsy may be required for complete staging if neoplasia is suspected, as the treatment of mediastinal masses may be determined from histology and clinical staging.

ANATOMY

The mediastinum contains all soft-tissue thoracic organs with the exception of the two lungs (Fig. 93-1). The mediastinal structures are separated from the thoracic cavity by the parietal pleura. The mediastinum is not fixed to the rigid thoracic structures and therefore can shift from its normal midline position by pressure (blood, air) or by compression from tumors. Acute displacement may impair venous return to the heart and may be fatal. Tumors that penetrate this pleura, by definition, invade the mediastinum. The paravertebral sulcus is a part of the hemithorax and not a true part of the mediastinum; however, the close juxtaposition of the mediastinal structures to the paravertebral sulcus and the radiographic appearances of tumors and abnormalities in this area typically allow these lesions to be grouped together with discussions of the mediastinum.

The thoracic inlet provides the superior limit of the mediastinum (Fig. 93-2A). The first ribs and clavicles provide excellent protection to the great vessels (arteries and veins), trachea, and esophagus as they traverse the thoracic inlet. The great veins lie in a retrosternal position, behind the manubrium and anterior to the great arteries. The thoracic duct enters into the posterior aspect of the junction of the left internal jugular and subclavian veins (Fig. 93-2B). Other important anatomic structures are the phrenic and recurrent laryngeal nerves bilaterally. Tumors in this area are further confined by the limited space within the thoracic inlet and may affect breathing by compression of the trachea.

The diaphragm (Fig. 93-3) provides the inferior border to the mediastinum and separates the thorax from the abdomen. Phrenic nerve injury or paralysis may manifest itself in elevation of the hemidiaphragm.

The structures within the mediastinum may be grouped together in various "compartments." Structures within each compartment may be defined by gross anatomy. The radiographic appearance of a mediastinal mass may be clinically correlated on the basis of its location within the mediastinum.

MEDIASTINAL COMPARTMENTS

The mediastinum can be empirically divided into various areas or compartments, which contain certain structures and may serve to focus the clinician or surgeon's differential diagnosis and diagnostic evaluation (Fig. 93-4A). No single concept covers all nuances of diseases within the mediastinum, as the boundaries of the mediastinal compartments are empiric. Mediastinal diseases may affect one or more compartments. Shields has divided

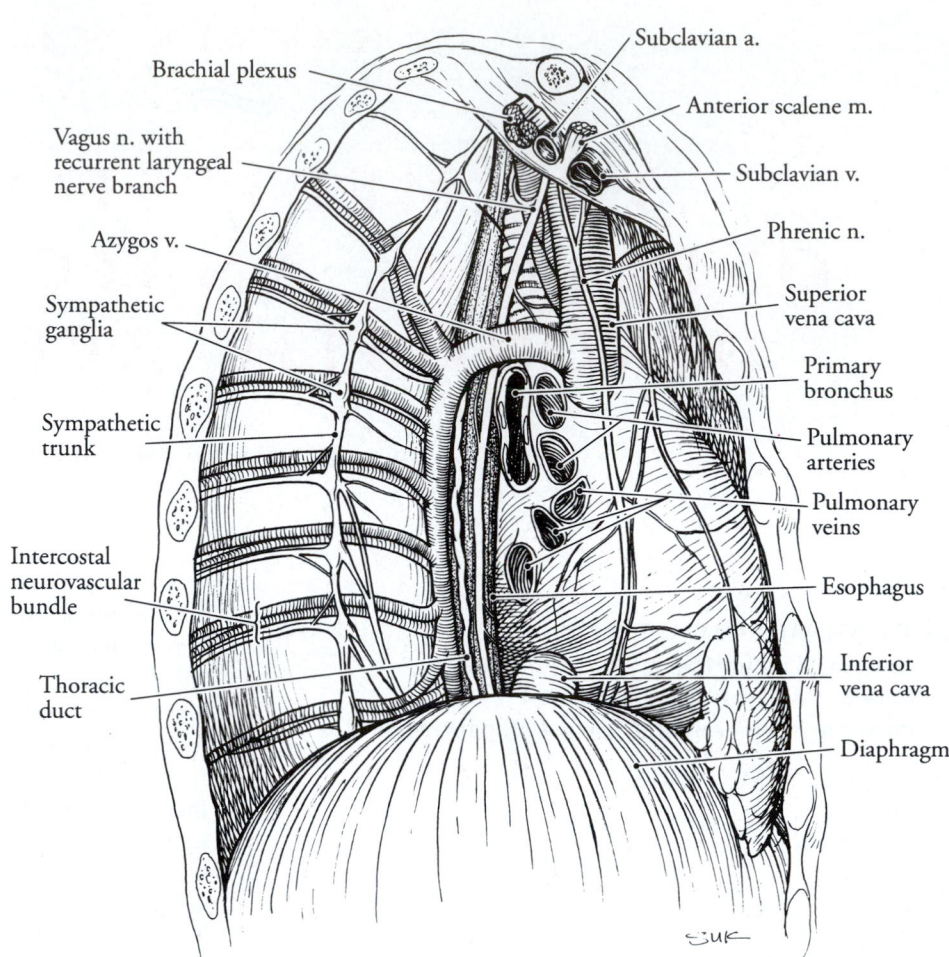

FIGURE 93-1 The mediastinum as seen from the right thorax. The right lung has been removed.

the mediastinum into three compartments that extend vertically from the diaphragm to the thoracic inlet and has provided a simple and understandable model to define the origin of the mediastinal mass (Fig. 93-4B).[42] Specific structures or embryologic remnants lie within each compartment and may give rise to different mediastinal masses (Tables 93-1 and 93-2).

Anterior Compartment

The anterior compartment is defined by the posterior surface of the sternum, the pericardium posteriorly, and the visceral pleurae laterally (at the apposition of the pleura and pericardium). Tumors of the anterior mediastinum include thymomas (Fig. 93-5), lymphomas (Fig. 93-6),[46] germ cell neoplasms, goiters, and primary carcinomas. Tissue is frequently required for diagnosis of lymphoma; fine-needle aspirate is usually inadequate. Thyroid goiter or thyroid tumors may be located in the superior retrosternal space (Fig. 93-7). Substernal goiter may be generally resected from a cervical incision. Thyroid carcinoma may invade tissues of the thoracic inlet. Claviculectomy or median sternotomy may be needed to remove the tumor and associated lymph node tissue.

For the surgeon, thymomas usually are the most common neoplasm of the anterior mediastinum, and lymphomas are second; for the radiologist, however, lymphoma and Hodgkin's disease are the most common mediastinal masses. The peak incidence

TABLE 93-1

Potential Mediastinal Diseases within the Mediastinal Compartments

Anterior Compartment	Visceral Compartment	Posterior Compartment
Thymomas	Congenital cysts	Neurogenic tumors
Thymolipomas	Bronchogenic cyst	Arising from peripheral nerves
Carcinoid tumors	Enteric duplication cyst	Neurilemmoma (schwannoma)
Thymic cyst	Pericardial cyst	Malignant schwannoma
Thyroid (aberrant)	Miscellaneous (thoracic duct,	Neurofibroma
Germ cell tumors	neuroenteric cyst)	Neurosarcoma
Teratomas	Primary cardiac/vascular tumors	Arising from sympathetic ganglia
Seminomas	Myxomas	Ganglioneuroma
Choriocarcinomas	Sarcomas	Ganglioneuroblastoma
Embryonal cell carcinoma	Miscellaneous cardiac sarcomas	Neuroblastoma
Malignant lymphomas	Lymphoma	Arising from paraganglia/receptors
Giant lymph node hyperplasia	Neural crest tumors	Pheochromocytomas
Teratomas	Pheochromocytoma	Paraganglioma (chemodectoma)
Parathyroid adenoma	Paraganglioma	Lymphoma
Parathyroid carcinoma		Mesenchymal tumors/soft-tissue
Mesenchymal tumors and soft-		sarcomas
tissue sarcomas		
Lipomas		
Liposarcomas		
Fibromas		
Fibrosarcomas		
Mesothelioma		
Lymphovascular tumors		
Lymphangiomas or		
cystic hygromas		
Hemangioma		
Angiosarcoma		
Primary carcinoma		

of thymomas occurs between the ages of 40 and 60. Germ cell neoplasms include benign and malignant teratomas, choriocarcinoma, seminoma, and embryonal cell neoplasm.[37] These are primary tumors (not metastases) that derive from primitive germ cells that have migrated to the mediastinum during ontogenesis.[7] Teratomas frequently occur in young adults. The gonads are the most common primary site, followed by the mediastinum. Most are benign, but 20 percent are malignant.[7] Malignant teratomas may produce high serum levels of α-fetoprotein and carcinoembryonic antigen. Lymphomas frequently occur in the anterior mediastinum. Endocrine disease of the thyroid and parathyroid may occur in the anterior mediastinum as a result of their

TABLE 93-2

Relative Frequency of Various Mediastinal Tumors and Cysts in Adults and Children

Adults	Percentage	In Children	Percentage
Histology	24	Histology	39.7
Neurogenic tumor	21.8	Neurogenic tumor	14.1
Thymoma	13.1	Lymphoma	13.5
Lymphoma	12.3	Germ cell tumors	10
Germ cell tumors	12.2	Mesenchymal tumor	6.1
Enterogenous cysts	7.98	Preliminary malignancies	12.2
Pericardial cysts	8.5	Cysts, other	1.1
Miscellaneous	100	Pericardial cysts	3.3

In adults, roughly 75% of mediastinal masses are benign and 25% malignant. In children, approximately 50% are benign and 50% malignant.
Incidence of mediastinal tumors often results from large surgical series compiled over one or more decades. Series have been published from the early 1950s to the present. Diagnostic imaging, histologic diagnostic techniques, and surgical procedures have evolved considerably during the past 40 years, influencing the ability of the surgeon to improve selection of appropriate patients for treatment and to pathologically confirm the disease present within the mediastinum. Above is an approximation of incidence of mediastinal masses from various surgical series.

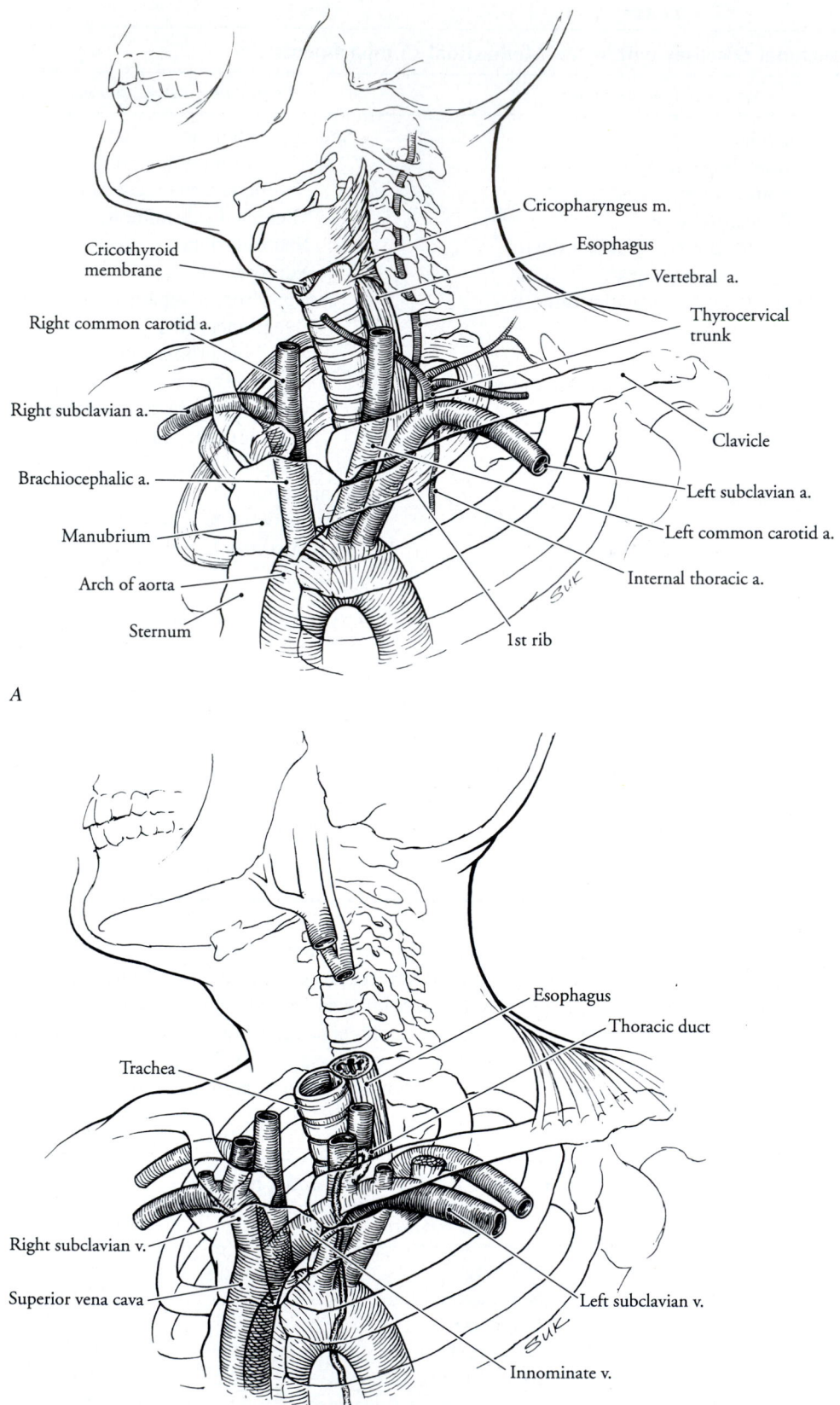

FIGURE 93-2 The thoracic inlet. *A.* The superior border of the mediastinum is the thoracic inlet—a bony ring to protect the vessels, airway, and esophagus. *B.* The larynx is cut away to demonstrate the close apposition between the posterior membranous trachea and the esophagus. The great veins are shown overlying the aorta and great arteries. The thoracic duct enters the vasculature posteriorly at the level of the innominate and left subclavian veins.

anatomic position in the adult (substernal goiter) or embryologic development. Rarely, carcinoid tumors may be found within the thymus.[40] Primary carcinomas of the mediastinum are rare but occasionally present as an invasive mass initially thought to be a thymoma. The distinction between thymic carcinoma and thymoma is made by the pathologist. Giant lymph node hyperplasia ("Castleman's disease") is an uncommon and a benign process. Soft-tissue sarcomas or mesenchymal tumors may also occur in this compartment.

Middle (Visceral) Compartment

The visceral compartment (Fig. 93-8) includes the thoracic inlet superiorly and extends from the pericardium anteriorly to the anterior surface of the vertebrae posteriorly. Tumors of the heart and great vessels are found in the visceral compartment, as are, more commonly, tumors of the trachea and main-stem bronchi and esophagus.[22] Benign lesions such as pericardial cysts (Fig. 93-9) and bronchogenic cysts (Fig. 93-10) may also occur within this compartment.[8] These cysts are not connected to the tracheobronchial tree or with the esophagus. Infection may occur in these cysts. Resection is indicated to exclude malignancy. Other benign diseases, such as aortic aneurysms and left ventricular aneurysms, may be identified.

Posterior (Paravertebral Sulci) Compartment

This compartment is bounded by the visceral compartment anteriorly and the costophrenic angles laterally. It includes the posterolateral space lateral to the spine, the sympathetic chain, the thoracic spinal nerve roots, and some posterior lymph nodes (Fig. 93-11).

In most series, neurogenic tumors are the most common primary tumor of the mediastinum (20 percent incidence); approximately 25 percent are malignant in adults, 50 percent in children. These series are historical, however, and often fail to account for the influences of improvements in diagnostic imaging so critical for treatment

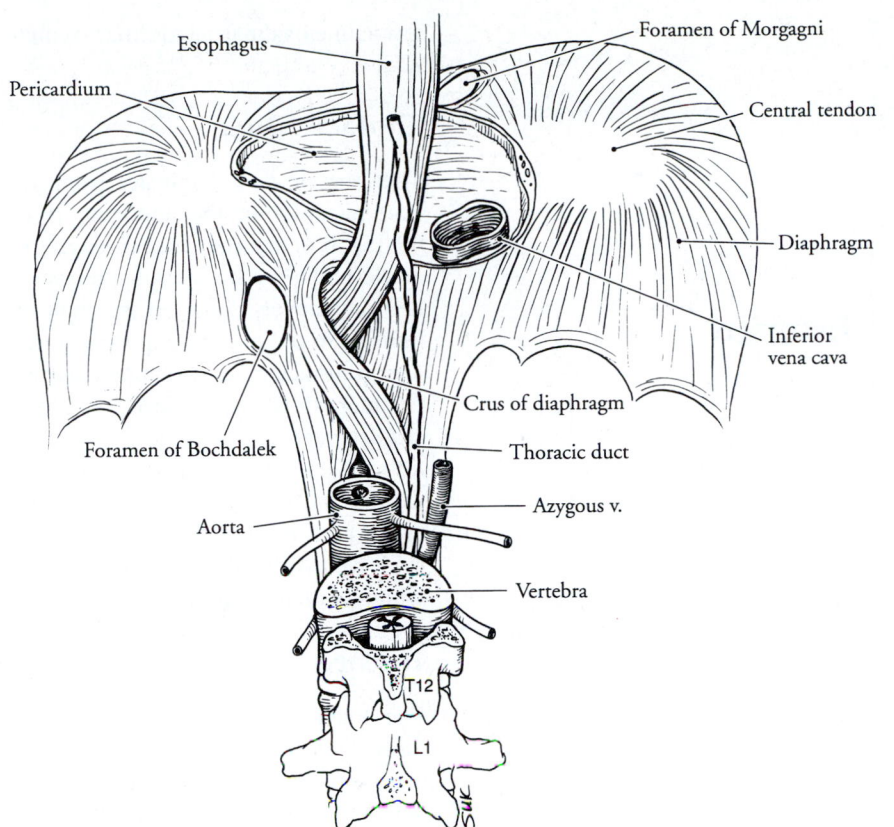

FIGURE 93-3   Posterior view of the diaphragm. The anterior aspect of the vertebral bodies is identified. The hemiazygous and thoracic ducts are identified. The thoracic duct is formed by the cisterna chyli as it enters the chest through the anterior aspect of the aortic hiatus. Posteriorly the location of a Bochdalek hernia and anteriorly the location of a Morgagni hernia are shown. Note the relationship of the aortic hiatus and esophageal hiatus, and the entrance of the inferior vena cava.

ANATOMIC STRUCTURES

Mediastinal structures may be conveniently placed into a particular mediastinal compartment that correlates to a varying degree with the radiographic appearance of the mass.

Thyroid

Diseases of the thyroid are more commonly considered with lesions of the head and neck. However, an enlarged thyroid gland may extend to the level of the thoracic inlet or potentially through the thoracic inlet to lie in a retrosternal position within the anterior compartment. The blood supply arises from the superior and inferior thyroid arteries in the neck and course downward. Frequently the surgeon may remove a retrosternal thyroid from a cervical approach, as the substernal goiter does not invade other mediastinal structures. Occasionally, these large glands are associated with tracheal compression; at times, pressure on the recurrent laryngeal nerve may result in left vocal chord paresis or even paralysis (Fig. 93-6) or produce tracheomalacia. Patients may come to medical attention because of stridor or dyspnea on exertion. If a thyroid carcinoma invades mediastinal structures, it may be necessary to resect a portion of the clavicle or perform a median sternotomy to facilitate optimal resection of the neoplasm as well as to enhance cervical and mediastinal lymphadenectomy.

Parathyroids

The superior parathyroids arise from the fourth pharyngeal pouch. These generally are behind the upper pole of the thyroid gland. The inferior parathyroids, arising from the third pharyngeal pouch, generally move in an inferior direction, at times with the thymus (also a derivative of the third pharyngeal pouch)—which explains the occasional position of parathyroid tissue within the thymus gland. The inferior parathyroids may be found within the mediastinum, in the thymus gland, and in unusual positions behind the esophagus or in the tracheoesophageal groove. Parathyroid adenomas or parathyroid carcinomas may arise within the neck or anterior mediastinum, depending on the location of the gland.

Thymus

The thymus lies within the anterior compartment of the mediastinum and is responsible for most primary epithelial tumors of the anterior mediastinum. The gland develops from the third pharyngeal pouch

decisions. Neurogenic tumors account for about 28 percent of mediastinal tumors in children. These tumors are located within the paravertebral sulcus and may erode into the adjacent vertebra or rib, causing pain (Fig. 93-12). Paravertebral sulcus tumors may produce symptoms as a result of compression or functional hormonal activity. Schwannomas or neurilemmomas are the most common neurogenic tumor. Neurofibromas arise from the nerve sheath and fibers and occur in middle-aged patients. In children, ganglioneuroma is the most common neurogenic tumor. Neurogenic tumors (20 percent of all tumors, 28 percent of tumors in children) include benign and malignant neoplasms of the sympathetic ganglia, cells of the peripheral nerve sheaths, and paraganglioma and chemoreceptor cell tumors. Ganglioneuromas and neuroblastomas may produce diarrhea, flushing, and diaphoresis. Neurilemmomas and neurosarcomas may produce insulin, resulting in hypoglycemia. Surgical resection of these neurogenic tumors is usually the procedure of choice.

The embryologic development of the neural crest cells forms an embryologic and anatomic basis of neuroendocrine tumors in the mediastinum. One percent of pheochromocytomas occur within the mediastinum. Symptoms may result from catecholamine production, which may be alleviated by surgical resection. Chemodectomas or paragangliomas may arise from chemoreceptor tissues around the aorta and great vessels, including the carotid, and are quite vascular.

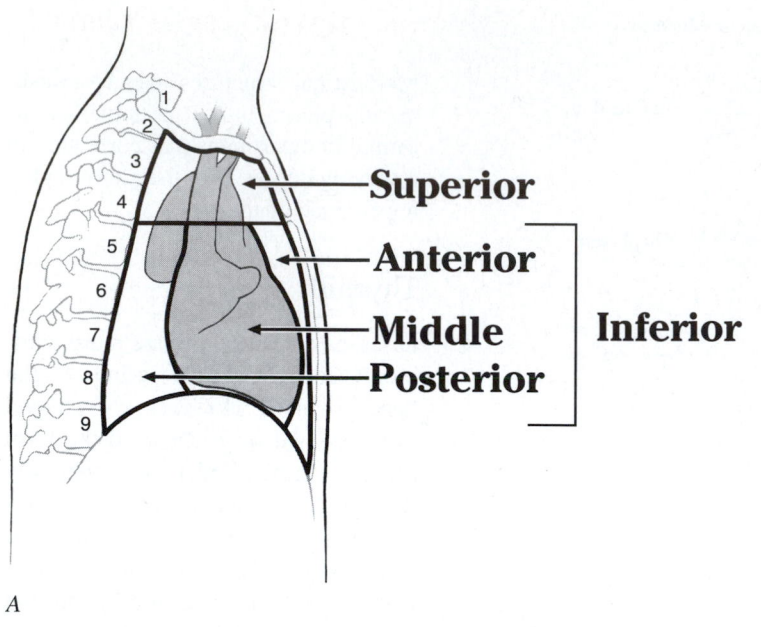

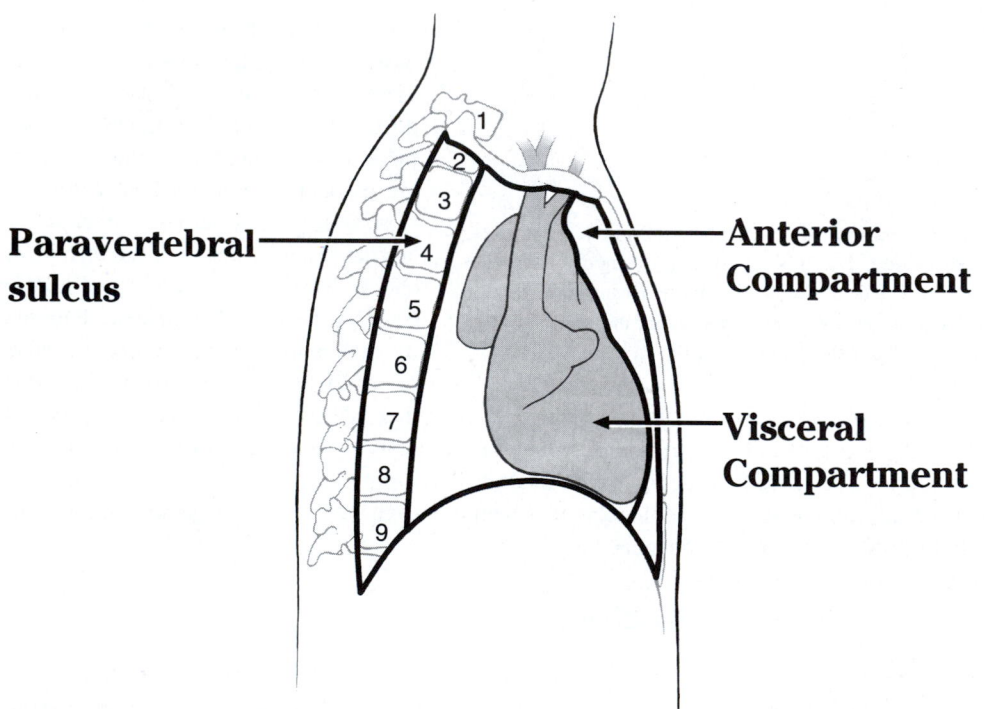

FIGURE 93-4 Compartments of the mediastinum. Various proposals for correlating radiographic mediastinal densities to an anatomic compartment. *A.* A four-compartment model for the mediastinum. *B.* A three-compartment model for the mediastinum for proposed general use.

and extends inferiorly to reside in the upper portion of the anterior mediastinum, anterior to the great vessels. The thymus gland is composed of a right and left lobe. The thymus varies in size and may extend farther into the right or left chest and also may extend inferiorly for a variable extent. The right and left lobes of the thymus extend well into the neck—an important point to consider when one is performing thymectomy for myasthenia gravis in which a total thymectomy is key.

The blood supply of the thymus derives from the internal mammary arteries, and the venous drainage goes to the innominate vein and internal thoracic veins. Lymph drainage is via lower cervical lymph nodes as well as the internal mammary, an-terior mediastinal, and hilar lymph nodes.

Thoracic Duct

The thoracic duct originates from the cisterna chyli in the abdomen (Fig. 93-13). It enters the chest through the aortic hiatus in an anterolateral position and travels above to the right of midline in the chest along the antero-lateral surface of the vertebral column. At approximately the level of T5, it crosses over to the left to empty posteriorly into the junction of the left jugular and subclavian veins. Because of its proximity to the esophagus, it may be disrupted during dissection, with a resultant chylothorax.

Trachea

The trachea enters the mediastinum through the thoracic inlet in front of the esophagus and behind the great vessels (Figs. 93-2A and 93-9). It extends approximately 12 to 13 cm before it bifurcates into the right and left main-stem bronchi. The right main-stem bronchus extends more vertically before giving off the right upper-lobe bronchus. The left main-stem bronchus obliquely bifurcates under the aortic arch. The subcarinal space contains lymph nodes, which are a common site for metastatic disease in lung cancer. The tracheal blood supply is segmental and originates from the inferior thyroid and the bronchial arteries. Branches from the vagal nerves provide innervation.

Heart and Great Vessels

The heart and great vessels also lie within the middle (visceral) mediastinum (Fig. 93-9). The innominate artery is the first branch of the aortic arch and subsequently branches into the right subclavian and right carotid arteries. The left carotid artery and the left subclavian artery most commonly arise as separate trunks. The great veins, the innominate vein, and the superior vena cava lie anterior to these structures. The azygous vein joins the superior vena cava on the right at the level of approximately T3-T4 laterally. The ligamentum arteriosum, the remnant of the ductus arteriosum, courses between the aorta and the central portion of the pulmonary artery. The ligamentum is attached to the proximal left main pulmonary artery. The left recurrent laryngeal nerve courses around the ligamentum and then "recurs" in the tracheoesophageal nerve. The inferior vena cava enters the thorax through the medial portion of the diaphragm.

Esophagus

The esophagus extends from the cricopharyngeus muscle to the gastro-esophageal junction (Fig. 93-8). It traverses the neck, thorax, and abdomen. The esophagus enters the mediastinum approximately 4 to 5 cm below the cricopharyngeus muscle and extends approximately 15 to 20 cm within the mediastinum. The esophagus and the posterior membranous trachea are adjacent to one another, although a potential plane does exist between these two structures. The esophagus crosses behind the origin of the left main-stem bronchus. After it passes this level, the esophagus deviates somewhat to the right of midline to pass along the right anterior lateral aspect of the vertebral column. The esophagus enters the abdomen through the esophageal hiatus. The vagus nerves descend along the esophagus in an anterior (left vagus) and a posterior (right vagus) location. Small branches extend from the vagus nerve to innervate the distal esophagus and stomach. The blood supply is segmental in the neck, chest, and abdomen. A dense plexus of vessels in the esophageal submucosa provides excellent vascularization of the organ along its entire length.

Lymph Nodes

Lymph nodes lie throughout the mediastinum. The critical lymph nodes within the mediastinum drain the head and neck, the lungs, and the esophagus. Infections or malignant cells may drain to these middle mediastinal lymph nodes, which may enlarge and be easily visible on a computed tomographic scan. Regional metastases from lung cancer to the mediastinal lymph nodes signify a more biologically aggressive tumor with a significant likelihood for disseminated disease and should prompt a multimodality approach to treatment.[21,24,36,38,39] Enlarged mediastinal lymph nodes should be sampled with one of a variety of approaches to document the presence, or absence, of metastatic disease.[13]

In the United States, the American Thoracic Society lymph node map is used to identify lymph nodes within the mediastinum (Fig. 93-14). As can be inferred from the figure, particular nodal stations drain particular areas of the lung.[26]

A mediastinoscopy is typically performed through a cervical

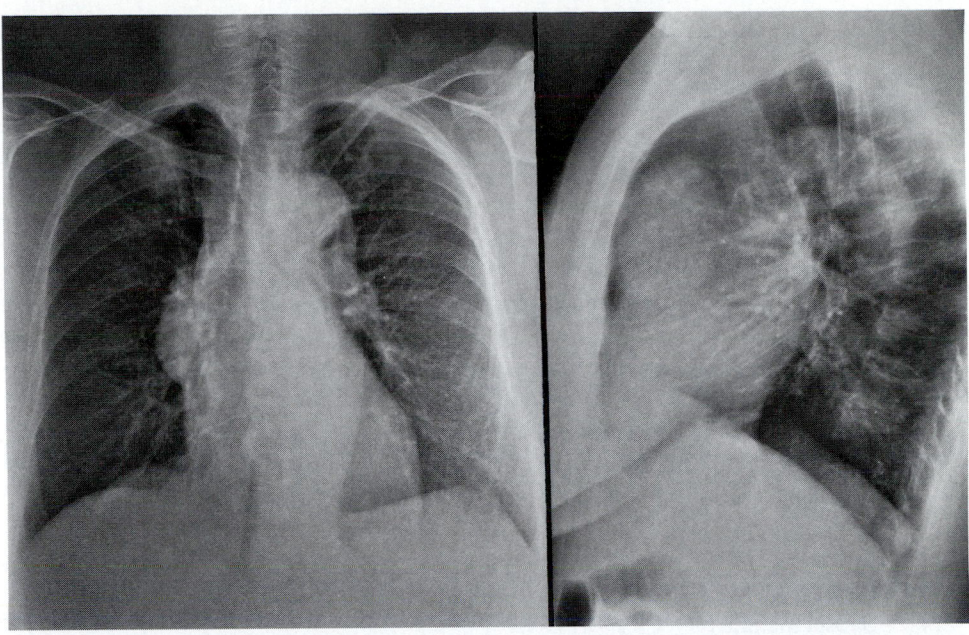

A

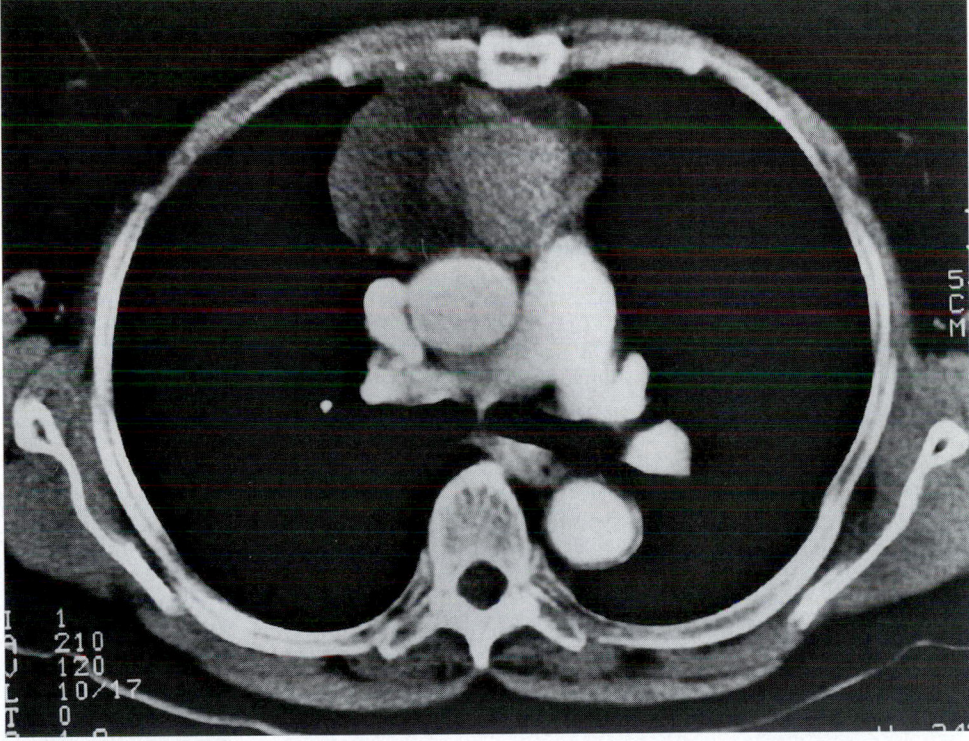

B

FIGURE 93-5 Thymoma. *A* and *B*. Thymoma typically affects the anterior mediastinum and may be predisposed to either the right or left side.

incision made just above the sternal notch to document the histologic status of the superior mediastinal lymph nodes (Table 93-3). Other procedures, such as the Chamberlain procedure (anterior mediastinotomy) or an extended mediastinoscopy or VATS (video-assisted thoracic surgery, a minimally invasive procedure), may be used as adjuncts to standard cervical mediastinoscopy.[19] Bilateral mediastinal lymph nodes at levels 2 and 4 as well as levels 7 and 10 are all accessible through the mediastinoscopy, and finding metastatic tumor in these nodes often changes treatment recommendations.[38,39]

TABLE 93-3

Mediastinal Lymph Node Designations

N2 Lymph nodes
2R	Right upper paratracheal, above the bottom level of innominate vein
2L	Left upper paratracheal above aortic arch
4R	Right lower paratracheal
4L	Left lower paratracheal
5	Aortopulmonary
6	Anterior aortic (anterior mediastinal, ventral to ligamentum arteriosum)
7	Subcarinal
8R	Right paraesophageal
8L	Left paraesophageal
9R	Right pulmonary ligament
9L	Left pulmonary ligament

N1 Lymph nodes
11	Interlobar
12	Lobar
13	Segmental
14	Subsegmental

Neurogenic Structures

The phrenic nerve enters the thorax through the thoracic inlet, coursing along the anterior aspect of the anterior scalene muscle. The phrenic nerves on both sides are composed of branches of cervical nerves 2, 3, 4, and 5. On the right side, the phrenic nerve runs along the right anterolateral aspect of the superior vena cava. The nerve enters the diaphragm, and the fibers course radially to innervate the diaphragm. On the left side, the left phrenic nerve runs along the pericardium anterior to the hilar vessels before it enters the diaphragm.

The vagus nerves enters the thoracic inlet through the carotid sheath. It lies in front of the subclavian artery and behind the innominate artery on the right. The right recurrent laryngeal nerve loops around the innominate artery and then back up to the larynx to innervate the right vocal chord. The vagus nerve continues posteriorly in the tracheoesophageal groove to innervate the trachea and the esophagus. On the left side, the vagus nerve enters the thorax through the thoracic inlet and, as it exits the carotid sheath, courses along the anterior aspect of the aortic arch. The recurrent laryngeal nerve arises from the vagus nerve and courses around the ligamentum arteriosum and continues back up the tracheoesophageal groove to innervate the left vocal cord. The left vagus nerve continues within the mediastinum along the esophagus.

The spinal nerve roots leave the neural foramina and bifurcate to send a branch as intercostal nerve, which innervates the skin and intercostal musculature and a branch to the sympathetic ganglion (Fig. 93-11). The thoracic sympathetic trunk is composed of several ganglia that lie along the ribs. The most superior ganglion is the stellate ganglion and lies at the level of T1 within the posterosuperior portion of the thorax.

CLINICAL MANIFESTATIONS AND DIAGNOSIS

Benign lesions predominate as asymptomatic lesions (more than 90 percent) and commonly are found on screening chest radiographs (Table 93-4). Surgical resection of all mediastinal masses without diagnosis may be considered; however, the added

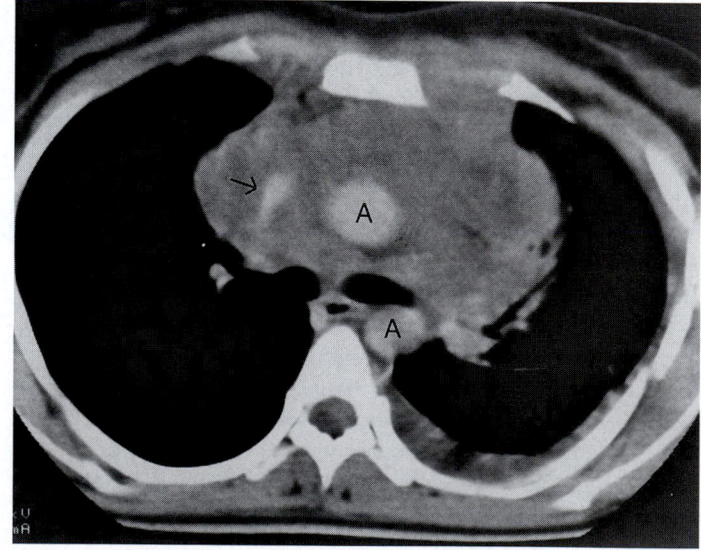

A   *B*

FIGURE 93-6   Mediastinal lymphoma. *A.* PA and lateral chest radiograph demonstrates a large multilobulated anterior mediastinal mass in a previously healthy 26-year-old woman. The patient presented with shortness of breath and cough, which did not resolve with antibiotics. A chest radiograph was performed. *B.* CT scan of the chest demonstrated extensive spread of the mass in the anterior mediastinum, completely surrounding the aorta and superior vena cava, with compression of the tracheobronchial tree. Vascular structures with contrast can be easily identified.

TABLE 93-4

Clinical Problems and Symptoms of Mediastinal Tumors

Superior vena cava syndrome	Obstruction of superior vena cava
Hoarseness	Recurrent laryngeal nerve paralysis
Horner's syndrome	Compression of the stellate ganglion
Diaphragmatic paralysis	Phrenic nerve paralysis
Chylothorax	Obstruction of thoracic duct
Dysphagia	Compression of the esophagus
Dyspnea, cough	Compression of the trachea or tracheobronchial tree by mediastinal shift from tumor
Dyspnea	Phrenic nerve paralysis
Pericardial tamponade	Compression of the heart from lymphoma, pericardial effusion
Arrhythmias	Cardiac compression or involvement of myocardium with tumor
Back pain	Paravertebral sulcus tumor eroding into rib or vertebrae
Stroke, hypertension	Pheochromocytoma
Gynecomastia	beta-HCG production from germ cell tumor
Mental confusion	Hypercalcemia from mediastinal parathyroid adenoma or carcinoma
Weakness/myasthenia gravis	Thymoma

value of surgery may be low and may subject the patient to a small but finite risk of an operation that can be avoided. Today, the accurate diagnosis of a mediastinal mass may be obtained in many ways and may not require general anesthesia.

Diagnostic Imaging

Plain film radiography continues to provide valuable discriminatory information to the clinician. The plain chest radiograph, taken in two planes (posteroanterior and left lateral), provides basic information about location of the mass within the mediastinum, with the lateral view providing most of the information.

Fluoroscopy assists in evaluating the effects of the mediastinal mass on diaphragm movement. To evaluate phrenic nerve paralysis, the "sniff test" may be performed. Under fluoroscopy, the patient forcibly "sniffs" with the mouth closed while the radiologist determines whether paradoxical elevation of the diaphragm occurs.

Arteriography or venography may be used to evaluate the mediastinal vessels—specifically, whether luminal invasion is present—and the relationship of the mediastinal mass to the vessel(s) in question. This study may be required if surgical resection is anticipated but usually adds little to information provided by computed tomography or magnetic resonance imaging.

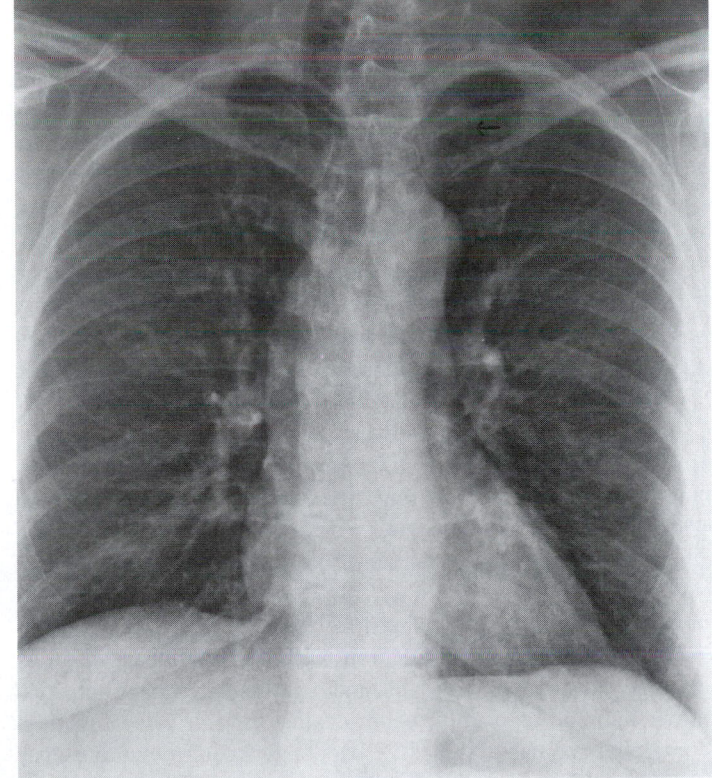

A

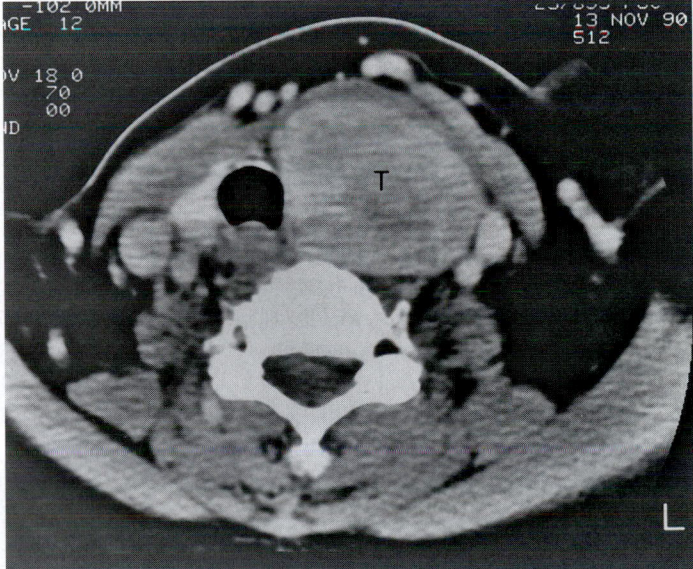

B

FIGURE 93-7   Retrosternal thyroid. A patient with shortness of breath was identified as having a left cervical mass that displaced the trachea laterally and extended into the thoracic inlet. PA chest radiograph (*A*) shows the tracheal shift, and a CT scan (*B*) confirms the evidence of an enlarged left thyroid. A thyroid scan showed the thyroid extending into the chest. The patient underwent thyroidectomy requiring a median sternotomy for resection.

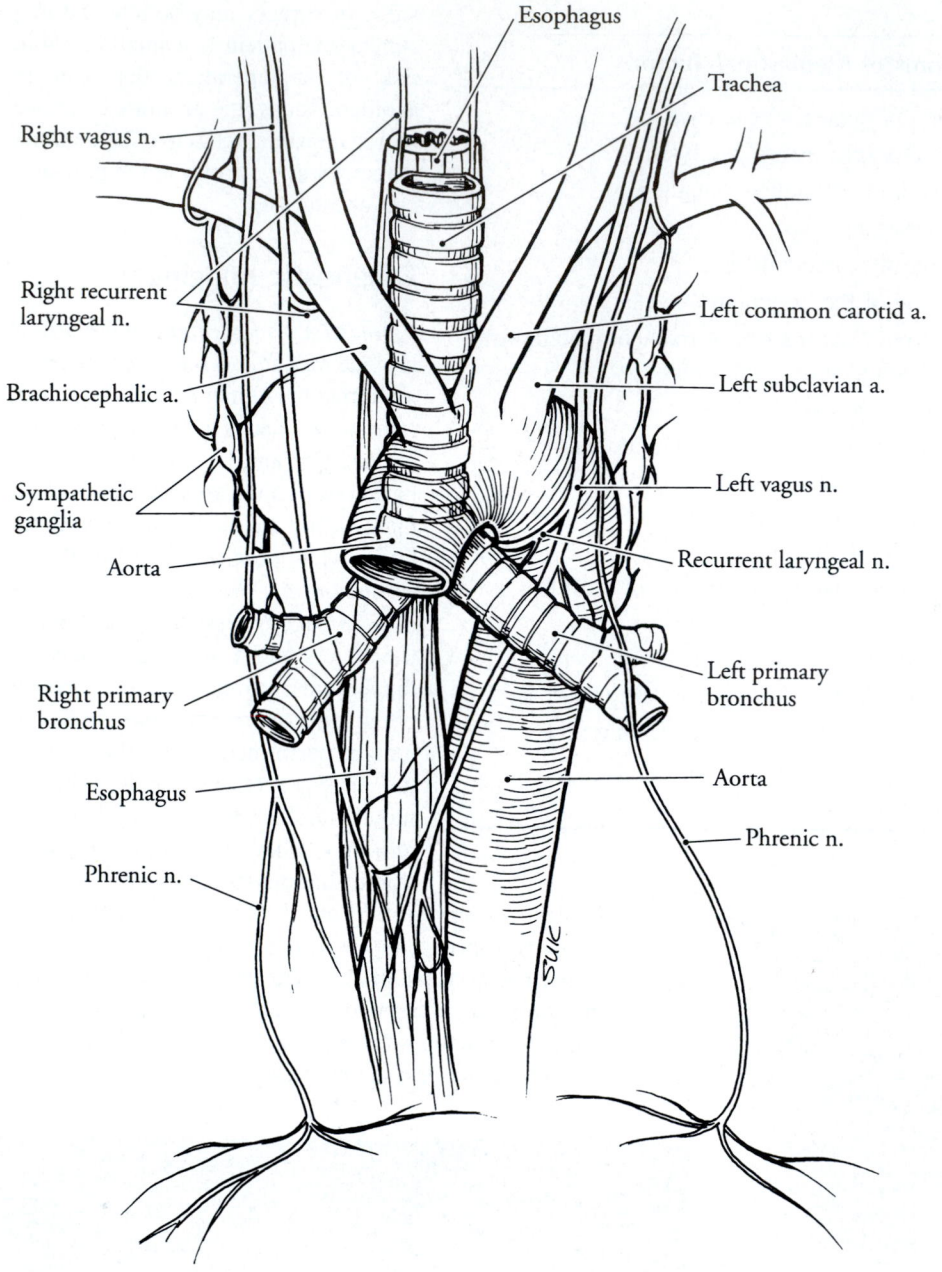

FIGURE 93-8 Visceral (middle) mediastinum. A cutaway view of the visceral (middle) mediastinum with the heart removed to reveal the relationships of the esophagus, trachea, and aorta. The middle mediastinum consists of the heart, great vessels, tracheobronchial tree, esophagus, and neural structures. The vagus nerves and the recurrent laryngeal nerves are shown, the right looping around the distal innominate artery and the left looping around the aorta at the level of the ligamental arteriosum. The phrenic nerves are shown, as are the stellate ganglia. Mediastinal tumors compressing these structures may produce symptoms by obstructing or compressing these structures.

Computed tomography of the chest (chest CT) adds considerably to the information provided by plain chest radiographs.[32] Excellent resolution of mediastinal structures is achieved routinely with modern computed tomographic equipment. The sensitivity of chest CT is 3 to 5 mm, although its specificity may be limited at that level.[45] Anterior and posterior mediastinal soft-tissue masses are readily apparent as the contrasting tissue densities are more discernible. Location of the mass and tissue density characteristics (solid, cystic, mixed, calcified) are easily delineated. Determining invasion remains difficult, and the CT scan is poor at differentiating between abutment and invasion. Intravascular contrast

to opacify vessels defines the relationship of the great vessels to a mediastinal mass. For paravertebral sulcus tumors, chest CT is standard and usually complemented by magnetic resonance imaging to evaluate the neural foramina and the spinal canal.

Magnetic resonance imaging (MRI) provides additional information over and above the chest CT, especially for posterior lesions.[6,10,44,47,48] As blood flow is visualized as a void, given its continuous motion, masses that may abut or surround vessels can be specifically noted. With an anterior mediastinal mass such as a thymoma, MRI helps evaluate invasion of the pulmonary artery, innominate vein, or superior vena cava. However, final assessment of resectability can be made only at operation.

MRI and chest CT are complementary studies. Both studies have diagnostic imaging advantages and disadvantages. Various studies have compared CT and MRI for mediastinal masses or enlarged lymph nodes.[2,3,12,28,30] In a patient with a superior sulcus tumor invading the mediastinum at the thoracic inlet, the chest CT nicely demonstrates chest wall invasion and mediastinal lymph node enlargement. The MRI may better evaluate the extent of brachial plexus involvement, assess the likelihood of vascular involvement, assess involvement of a vertebral body and the neural foramina, and show extradural extension of disease. The MRI costs significantly more than chest CT but provides the additional ability to view sagittal and coronal reconstructions, which are extremely useful in certain situations.

Ultrasound used via transthoracic (transcutaneous) or transesophageal routes can identify masses overlying the heart[28] and generally tell whether a mass is solid or cystic. Most transcutaneous echocardiography is used for evaluation of cardiac chamber filling, overall heart function (ejection fraction), and presence or absence of fluid around the heart. Transesophageal ultrasound can be used to better evaluate mitral valve function, contiguous mediastinal masses, esophageal carcinoma, presence of enlarged lymph nodes,[15,35,43,52] and aortic dissection. Ultrasound is inexpensive and readily available. Its ability to provide detailed anatomic information is frequently lacking unless there is involvement of the heart or esophagus, in which case additional studies are required. Chest CT and MRI scans are anatomically more accurate for most mediastinal masses.

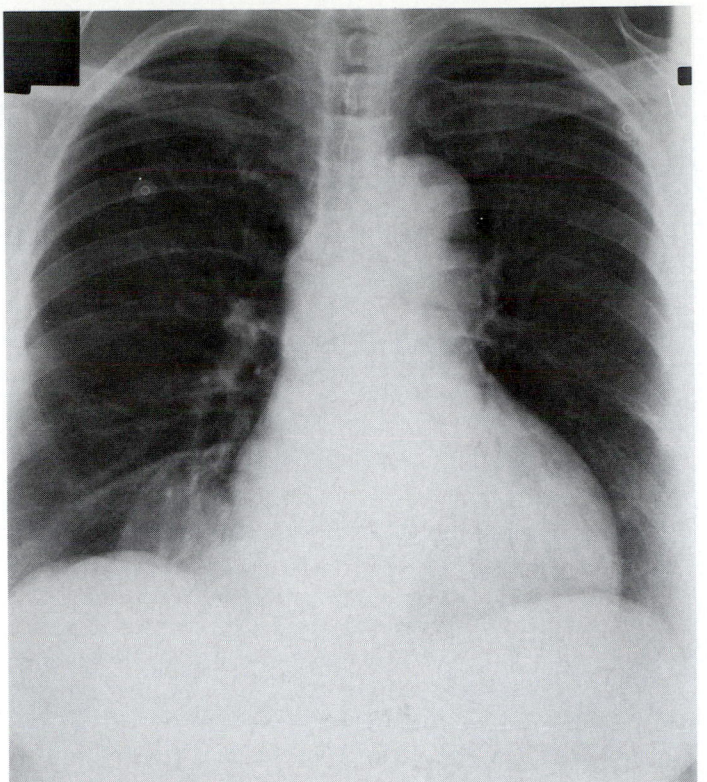

A

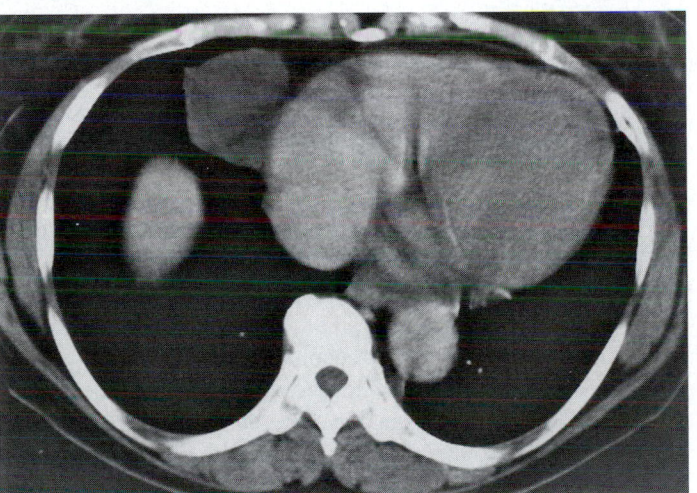

B

FIGURE 93-9 Pericardial cyst. *A.* Pericardial cyst may be identified by its characteristic location in the anterior mediastinum in the costophrenic angle. Typically the superior is a well-demarcated density with the PA and lateral chest radiograph. *B.* A CT scan confirms the radiographic appearance of the mass. Diagnosis with needle aspiration will facilitate both diagnosis and treatment. Should the mass recur, a definitive resection would be warranted.

Nuclear medicine studies rely on the ability of a mass to take up specific radionuclides. Radioactive iodine (^{131}I) may be taken up by a functional thyroid tumor or substernal goiter,[29] which confirms the diagnosis. Gallium 67 scans may aid in the diagnosis of lymphoma. Indium 111–labeled leukocytes can identify localized infections within the mediastinum. Single-photon emission computed tomography (SPECT) uses the nuclear medicine energy source within the patient in a manner similar to the radiation energy used in CT. Better localization of a functional mass within the mediastinum may result. A functional mediastinal

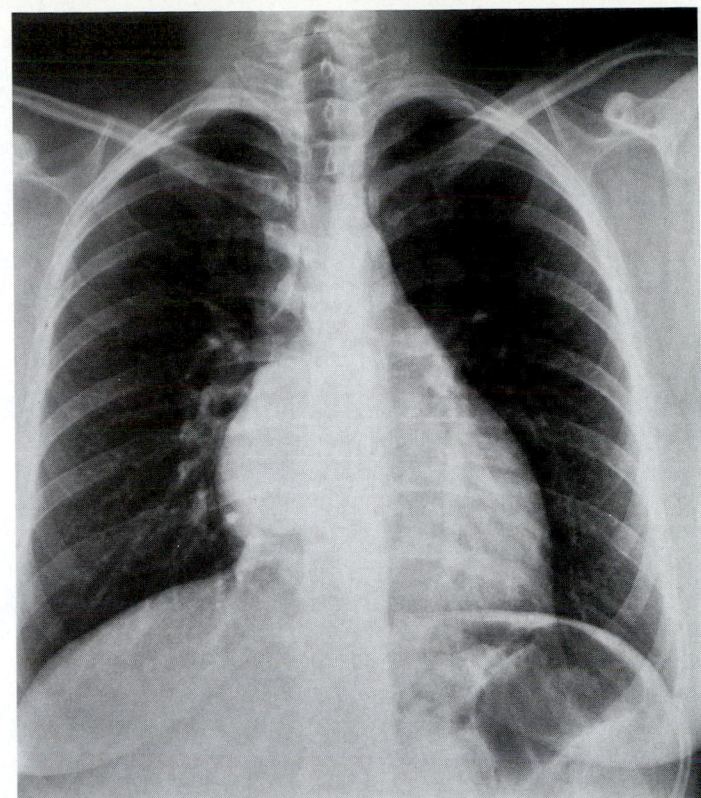

A

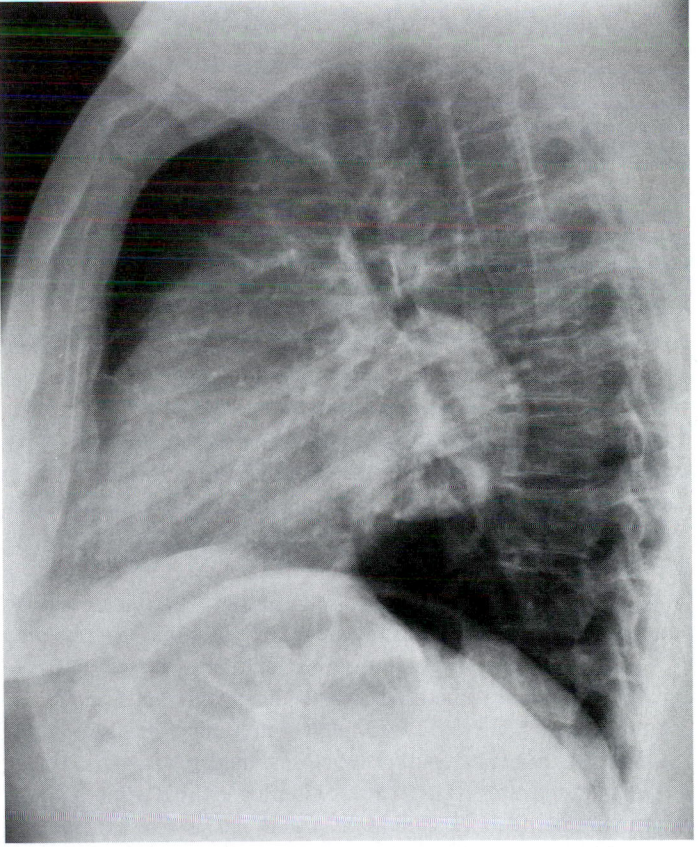

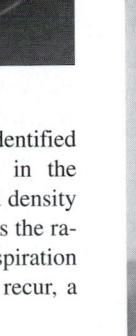

B

FIGURE 93-10 Bronchogenic cyst. Bronchogenic cysts may be identified as a middle mediastinal mass, which can be visualized on both the PA and lateral chest radiograph. CT scan (*A*) or MRI scan (*B*) may be considered for further delineation of the density of the mass and its location within the mediastinum and potential involvement with other mediastinal structures. The mass is generally well circumscribed, and it is not connected to the bronchus. It should be removed to prevent further infectious complications.

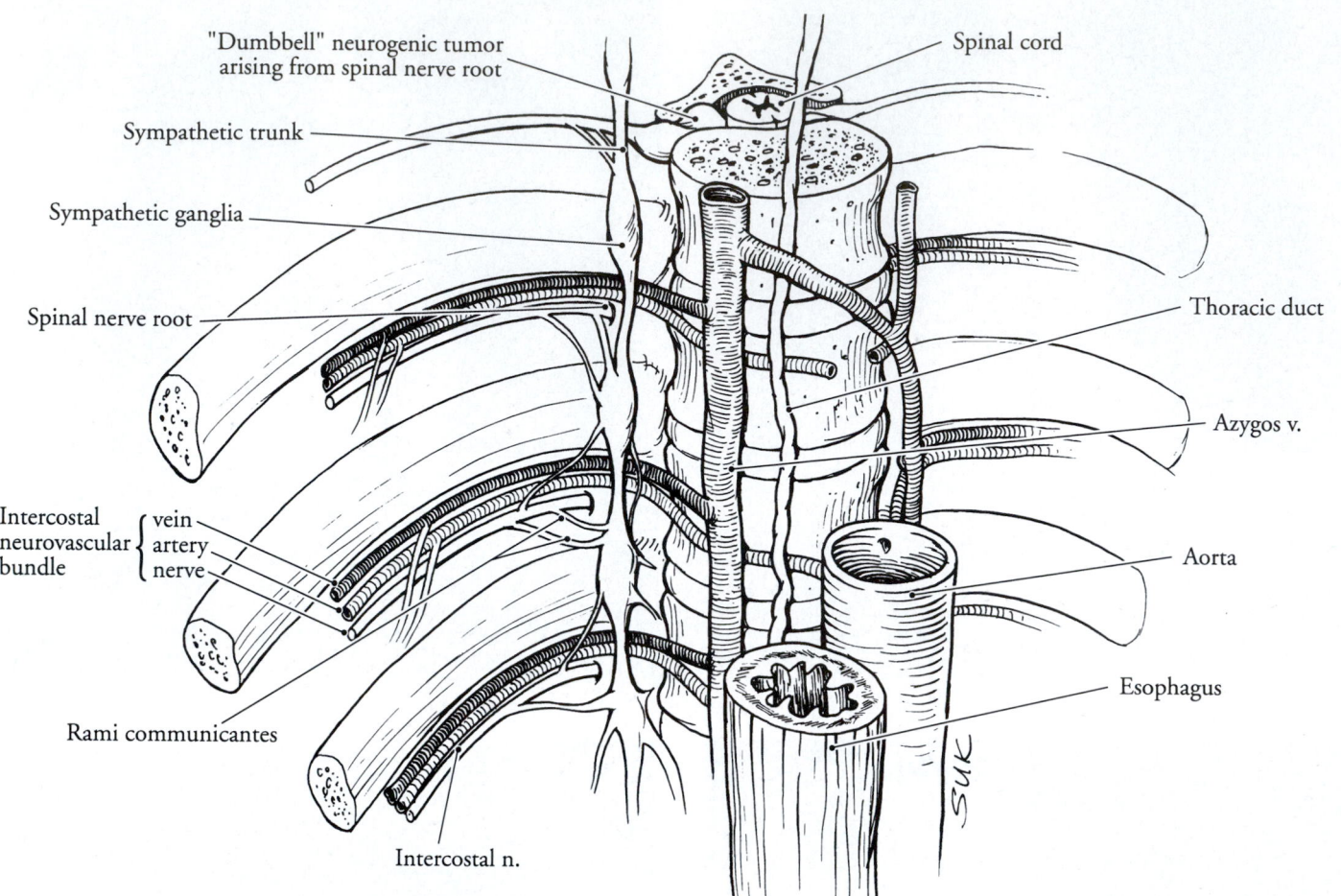

FIGURE 93-11   Paravertebral sulcus. A cutaway view of the paravertebral sulcus is shown. The nerve root exits through the neural (intervertebral) foramen. The sympathetic ganglia and the intercostal nerves are shown. The sympathatic ganglia are related by the sympathetic trunk. A "dumbbell" tumor may arise from the spinal root, producing symptoms and impinging on the neural (intervertebral) foramen.

pheochromocytoma may be imaged in this manner. Positron emission tomography (PET) scan takes advantage of the propensity of tumor cells to take up more glucose than normal tissues. Specially labeled radioactive glucose can be injected into a patient with a known neoplasm. Metastases, smaller than routinely detected on other imaging techniques (such as chest CT or MRI), may be identified from their differential and increased utilization of glucose. The routine use of PET scans is limited by a lack of availability of equipment and definitive clinical trials to validate the diagnostic accuracy. Selenomethionine 75 scans may be helpful in identifying parathyroid adenomas or thymic cysts, and ^{99m}Tc-pertechnetate scans may be used to detect ectopic gastric mucosa. ^{131}I-metaiodobenzylguanidine may be used for localizing functional pheochromocytomas and paragangliomas.[41]

Other diagnostic techniques combining radiographic and nuclear medicine techniques can be performed to assist in localizing mediastinal masses and to improve clinical staging. Some mediastinal masses may secrete specific hormones or biologic markers. Parathyroid adenomas or functioning parathyroid carcinomas may cause hypercalcemia and secrete parathormone, which can be detected with great accuracy by radioimmunoassay. Venous sampling can also localize the dysfunctional parathyroid.[25] Mediastinal pheochromocytomas are rare (less than 1 percent of all pheochromocytomas) and may produce hypertension

from production of various catecholemines that may be detected in serum and urine.[41] Germ cell neoplasms may produce alpha-fetoprotein (αFP) (embryonal cell carcinoma) or beta–human chorionic gonadotropin (βHCG) (choriocarcinoma). For that reason, all young men with anterior mediastinal masses should have the levels of these markers determined. Thymic carcinoids may be part of a multiple endocrine neoplasia (MEN) syndrome. Commonly, Cushing's syndrome results from ectopic production of adrenocorticotropic hormone (ACTH) by these thymic carcinoids.

Posterior neurogenic tumors such as ganglioneuromas and neuroblastomas may have associated symptoms of diarrhea and abdominal bloating or hypertension and flushing. Hypoglycemia has been associated with neurilemmomas and neurosarcomas secondary to increased insulin levels. Children with a paravertebral sulcus tumor should undergo evaluation for increased epinephrine and norepinephrine. As symptoms frequently occur, surgical extirpation has been recommended for both benign and malignant neurogenic tumors. Immediate resection may provide both diagnosis and treatment if the mass is smaller and easily resectable.

Histologic Diagnosis

Various techniques may be used to obtain sufficient tissue for definitive diagnosis.[11] Bronchoscopy or esophagoscopy (both

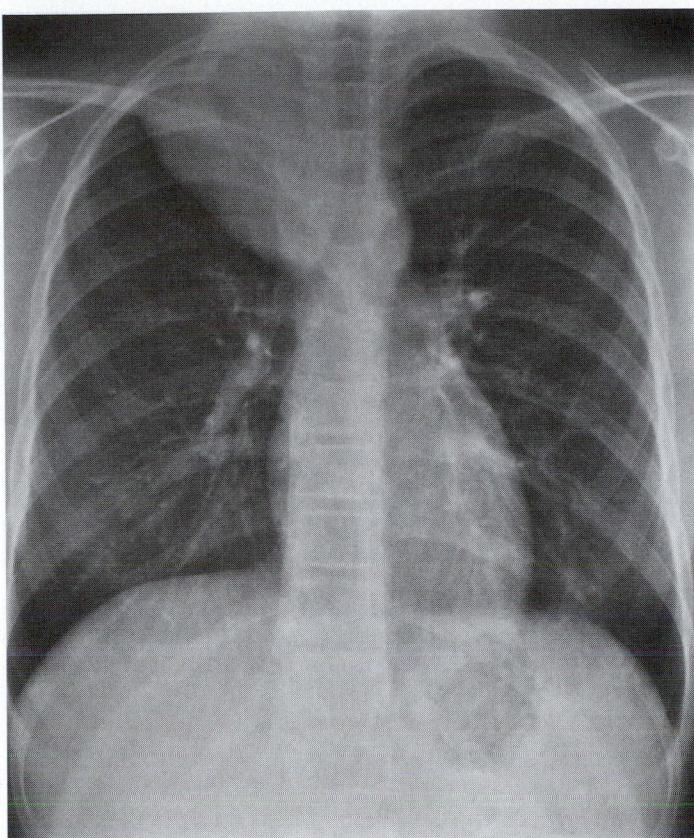

A

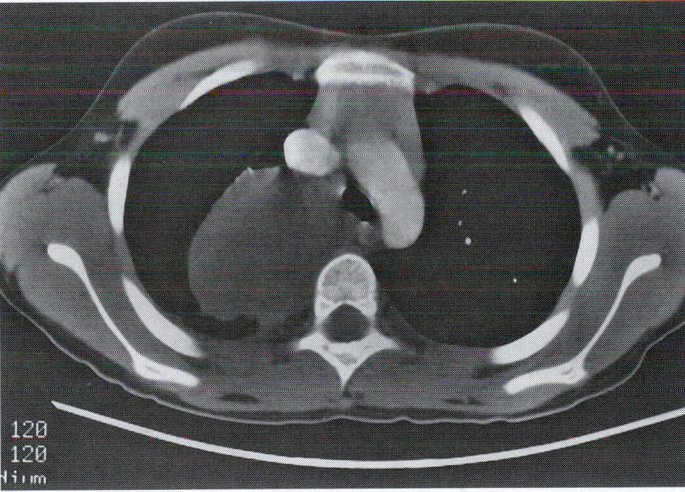

B

FIGURE 93-12 Neurogenic tumor. The chest radiograph (*A*) and the CT scan (*B*) demonstrate a paravertebral sulcus mass, a neurogenic tumor of the posterior mediastinum, with compression medially and ventrally of the mediastinal contents. A ganglioneuroblastoma was identified within the tissue. The mass was resected.

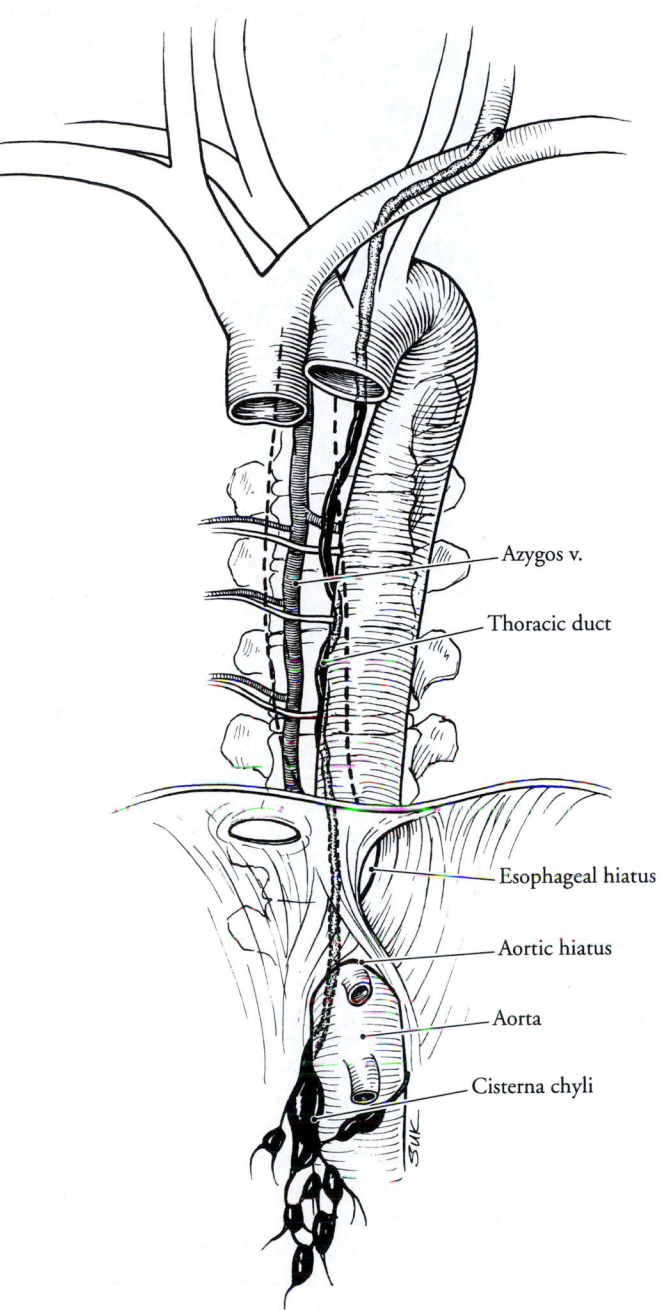

FIGURE 93-13 Posterior mediastinum. Posterior visceral mediastinum with the esophagus, trachea, and great vessels removed; the anterior aspect of the vertebral bodies is identified. The hemiazygous and thoracic ducts are identified. The thoracic duct is formed by the cisterna chyli as it enters into the chest through the anterior aspect of the aortic hiatus. It begins to the right of midline and traverses to the left of midline at approximately the T5 level. Tumors may block this thoracic duct or may compromise chyle flow and, in so doing, create chylothorax. Compression of the azygous system does not tend to produce symptoms.

rigid and flexible) may be helpful in evaluating dyspnea or dysphagia, respectively.

Fine-needle aspiration or needle biopsy of a mediastinal mass may provide sufficient tissue for diagnosis of thymic carcinoma or other epithelial neoplasms (Fig. 93-15).[1,27,33,49] In a recent study of 141 patients with mediastinal masses evaluated over a 15-year period, a diagnosis was obtained with needle biopsy in 92 percent.[51] Ninety-four of 95 patients with malignancy were correctly classified. To make a definitive diagnosis of lymphoma, larger amounts of tissue than are obtained with needle biopsy usually are required, so that phenotypic marker studies can be performed and the lymphoma accurately typed.

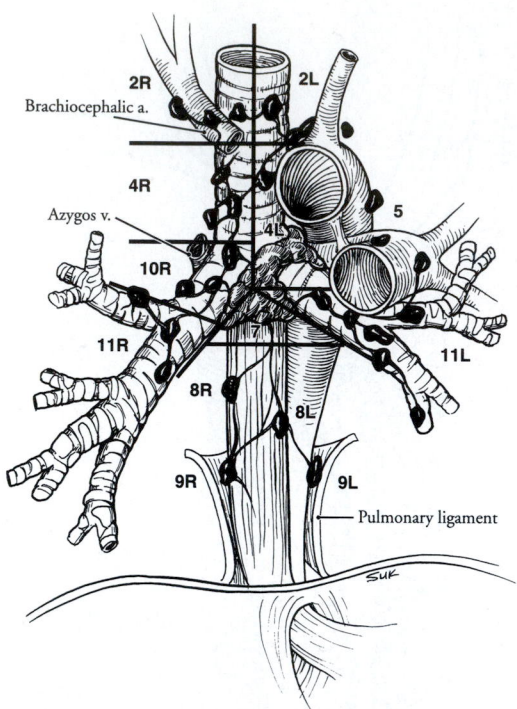

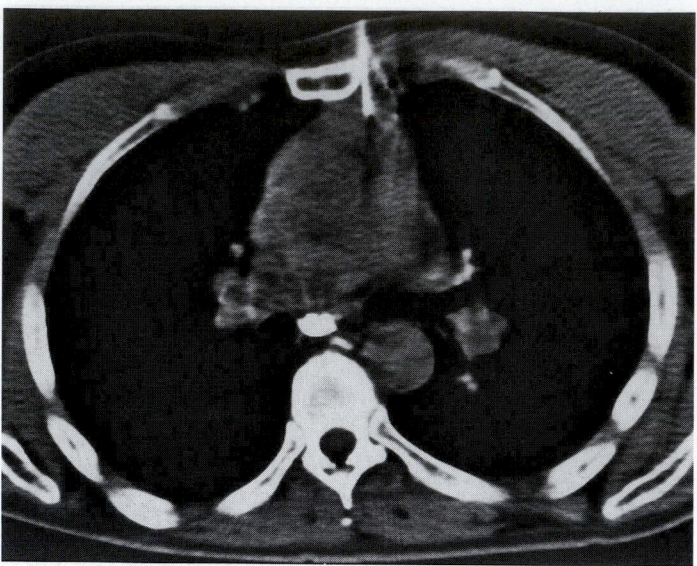

FIGURE 93-15 Needle biopsy. Needle biopsy of an anterior mediastinal mass is shown, with the needle tract identified just adjacent to the sternum. Histologic and cytologic evaluation of these masses may yield critical diagnostic information.

FIGURE 93-14 Mediastinal lymph node map (American Thoracic Society). This mediastinal lymph node map is in common use in the United States to define lymph nodes in relationship to their location within the mediastinum. N2 (mediastinal) lymph nodes in the high peritracheal area above the innominate artery, level 2; paratracheal, level 4; hilar nodes medial to the pleural reflection, level 10; and intralobar lymph nodes, 11. Subcarinal lymph nodes (level 7) may be sampled by mediastinoscopy or surgically removed from either the right or the left side; on the left side, level 2 nodes are paratracheal nodes above the level of the aortic arch, level 4 lymph nodes are paratracheal nodes to the left of the lower trachea between the trachea and the aorta; level 5 lymph nodes are aortopulmonary window/subaortic lymph nodes; and level 6 nodes (not shown) are the anterior aortic or intramediastinal lymph nodes. Lymph nodes along the esophagus are level 8 and, within the pulmonary ligament, level 9. Tumors from the left lower lobe may metastasize to regional lymph nodes and progress in a systematic way to the left hilar nodes and the subcarinal nodes, and from there to the right paratracheal lymph nodes. With a left lower lung cancer, and histologically confirmed right-sided lymph nodes, the patient would be considered to have N3 lymph nodes and have a stage designation of IIIB.

Cervical or supraclavicular lymph node biopsy, anterior mediastinotomy, or core needle biopsy may be required. Invasive intrathoracic biopsy (via thoracoscopy[14] or open thoracotomy) may be required. Needle tract seeding with implants from malignant thymoma are rare.[23]

Mediastinoscopy has been safely used to evaluate specific areas within the superior mediastinum and has been used most extensively for diagnosis of enlarged mediastinal lymph nodes.[4,5,17,31,50]

The anterior mediastinotomy, or "Chamberlain procedure," was introduced in 1966 to complement cervical mediastinoscopy.[19] Anterior mediastinotomy was developed to assess lymph nodes in the aortopulmonary window and left para-aortic

area. The procedure can be used on either side to obtain tissue from an anterior mediastinal mass or a centrally located mass within the hilum. Access to the mediastinum is gained by excising the second costal cartilage in a subperichondrial plane. The internal mammary vessels are either protected or ligated and the pleura is reflected laterally so that the surgeon stays in an extrapleural plane. Anterior mediastinotomy often is the procedure of choice for a diffuse anterior mediastinal mass.[9]

Extended cervical mediastinoscopy may be used for sampling lymph nodes in the aortopulmonary window but is not widely practiced.[12]

Thoracoscopy (or VATS) complements mediastinoscopy as a staging procedure for lung cancer but also may be used to obtain tissue for diagnosis or staging.[16,20] Therapeutic use of VATS for excision of certain mediastinal lesions may be considered, but the cost, "learning curve," and complications generally limit the use of this procedure for treatment of diseases to certain major centers (although expertise with the techniques seems to be increasing). For mediastinal masses, a tissue diagnosis may be obtained in up to 86 percent of patients without a standard open procedure.[14]

Median sternotomy or thoracotomy provides a direct visual approach to the mediastinum and may be used for biopsy, staging, or resection of a wide range of mediastinal lesions. Median sternotomy or thoracotomy remains the "gold standard" for definitive surgical treatment of a mediastinal mass but should be reserved for lesions that are resectable. One would like to avoid performing a median sternotomy only to find that the lesion is a lymphoma. For many lesions, it is best to obtain diagnostic material with an incisional biopsy before proceeding with thoracotomy or median sternotomy. For all but well-encapsulated lesions, a diagnosis should be established before attempts at definitive resection.

REFERENCES

1. Adler OB, Rosenberger A, Peleg H: Fine-needle aspiration biopsy of mediastinal masses: Evaluation of 136 experiences. *AJR Am J Roentgenol* 140:893–896, 1983.
2. Batra P, Herrmann C Jr, Mulder D: Mediastinal imaging in myasthenia gravis: Correlation of chest radiography, CT, MR, and surgical findings. *AJR Am J Roentgenol* 148:515–519, 1987.
3. Buy JN, Ghossain MA, Poirson F, et al: Computed tomography of mediastinal lymph nodes in nonsmall cell lung cancer: A new approach based on the lymphatic pathway of tumor spread. *J Comput Assist Tomogr* 12:545–552, 1988.
4. Carlens E: Mediastinoscopy: A method for inspection and tissue biopsy in the superior mediastinum. *Dis Chest* 36:343–352, 1959.
5. Carlens E: *Mediastinoscopy*. Odense, Denmark, Odense University Press, 1971.
6. Cohen AM, Creviston S, LiPuma JP, et al: Nuclear magnetic resonance imaging of the mediastinum and hili: early impressions of its efficacy. *AJR Am J Roentgenol* 141:1163–1169, 1983.
7. Cox JD: Primary malignant germinal tumors of the mediastinum: A study of 24 cases. *Cancer* 36:1162–1168, 1975.
8. Dais RD, Oldham HN, Sabiston DC: Primary cysts and neoplasms of the mediastinum: Recent changes in clinical presentation, methods of diagnosis, management, and results. *Ann Thorac Surg* 44:229–237, 1987.
9. Elia S, Cecere C, Giampaglia F, Ferrante G: Mediastinoscopy vs. anterior mediastinotomy in the diagnosis of mediastinal lymphoma: A randomized trial. *Eur J Cardiothorac Surg* 6:361–365, 1992.
10. Gamsu G, Sostman D: Magnetic resonance imaging of the thorax. *Am Rev Respir Dis* 139:254–274, 1989.
11. Ginsberg RJ: Evaluation of the mediastinum by invasive techniques. *Surg Clin North Am* 67:1025–1035, 1987.
12. Ginsberg RJ, Rice TW, Goldberg M, et al: Extended cervical mediastinoscopy: A single staging procedure for bronchogenic carcinoma of the left upper lobe. *J Thorac Cardiovasc Surg* 94:673–678, 1987.
13. Johnston MR: Invasive staging of the mediastinum. *World J Surg* 17:700–704, 1993.
14. Kern JA, Daniel TM, Tribble CG, et al: Thoracoscopic diagnosis and treatment of mediastinal masses. *Ann Thorac Surg* 56:92–96, 1993.
15. Kobayashi H, Danbara T, Sugama Y, et al: Observation of lymph nodes and great vessels in the mediastinum by endoscopic ultrasonography. *Jpn J Med* 26:353–359, 1987.
16. Landreneau RJ, Hazelrigg SR, Mack MJ, et al: Thoracoscopic mediastinal lymph node sampling: Useful for mediastinal lymph node stations inaccessible by cervical mediastinoscopy. *J Thorac Cardiovasc Surg* 106:554–558, 1993.
17. Luke WP, Pearson FG, Todd TRJ, et al: Prospective evaluation of mediastinoscopy for assessment of carcinoma of the lung. *J Thorac Cardiovasc Surg* 91:53–56, 1986.
18. Marchevsky AM: *Surgical Pathology of the Mediastinum*, 2d ed. New York, Raven, 1992.
19. McNeill TM, Chamberlain JM: Diagnostic anterior mediastinotomy. *Ann Thorac Surg* 2:532–539, 1966.
20. Morrissey B, Adams H, Gibbs AR, Crane MD: Percutaneous needle biopsy of the mediastinum: Review of 94 procedures. *Thorax* 48:632–637, 1993.
21. Mountain CF: A new international staging system for lung cancer. *Chest* 89(Suppl):225S–233S, 1986.
22. Murphy MC, Sweeney MS, Putnam JB Jr, et al: Surgical treatment of cardiac tumors: A 25-year experience. *Ann Thorac Surg* 49:612–617, 1990.
23. Nagasaka T, Nakashima N, Nunome H: Needle tract implantation of thymoma after transthoracic needle biopsy. *J Clin Pathol* 46:278–279, 1993.
24. Naruke T, Tomoyuki G, Tsuchiya R, Suemasu K: Prognosis and survival in resected lung carcinoma based on the new international staging system. *J Thorac Cardiovasc Surg* 96:440–447, 1988.
25. Nilsson BE, Tisell LE, Jansson S, et al: Parathyroid localization by catheterization of large cervical and mediastinal veins to determine serum concentrations of intact parathyroid hormone. *World J Surg* 18:605–611, 1994.
26. Nohl-Osler HC: An investigation of the anatomy of the lymphatic drainage of the lungs as shown by the lymphatic spread of bronchial carcinoma. *Ann R Coll Surg Engl* 51:157–176, 1972.
27. Noppen MM, De Mey J, Meysman M, et al: Percutaneous needle biopsy of localized pulmonary, mediastinal, and pleural diseased tissue with an automatic disposable guillotine soft-tissue needle: Preliminary results. *Chest* 107:1615–1620, 1995.
28. Nyman R, Rehn S, Glimelius B, et al: Magnetic resonance imaging, chest radiography, computed tomography and ultrasonography in malignant lymphoma. *Acta Radiol* 28:253–262, 1987.
29. Park HM, Tarver RD, Siddiqui AR, et al: Efficacy of thyroid scintigraphy in the diagnosis of intrathoracic goiter. *Am J Radiol* 148:527–529, 1987.
30. Patterson GA, Ginsberg RJ, Poon PY, et al: A prospective evaluation of magnetic resonance imaging, computed tomography, and mediastinoscopy in the preoperative assessment of mediastinal node status in bronchogenic carcinoma. *J Thorac Cardiovasc Surg* 94:679–684, 1987.
31. Pearson FG, Nelems JM, Henderson RD, et al: The role of mediastinoscopy in the selection of treatment for bronchial carcinoma with involvement of superior mediastinal lymph nodes. *J Thorac Cardiovasc Surg* 54:382–390, 1972.
32. Picus D, Balfe DM, Koehler RE, et al: Computed tomography in the staging of esophageal carcinoma. *Radiology* 146:433–438, 1983.
33. Powers CN, Silverman JF, Geisinger KR, Frable WJ: Fine-needle aspiration biopsy of the mediastinum: A multi-institutional analysis. *Am J Clin Pathol* 105:168–173, 1996.
34. Pugatch RD: Radiologic evaluation in chest malignancies: A review of imaging modalities. *Chest* 107(Suppl):294S–297S, 1995.
35. Rice TW, Boyce GA, Sivak MV, et al: Esophageal carcinoma: Esophageal ultrasound assessment of preoperative chemotherapy. *Ann Thorac Surg* 53:972–977, 1992.
36. Riquet M: Anatomic basis of lymphatic spread from carcinoma of the lung to the mediastinum: Surgical and prognostic implications. *Surg Radiol Anat* 15:271–277, 1993.
37. Rosai J, Levine GD: *Tumors of the Thymus*, 2d ser, fasc 13 ed. Washington, DC, Armed Forces Institute of Pathology, 1975.
38. Rosell R, Gómez-Codina J, Camps C, et al: A randomized trial comparing preoperative chemotherapy plus surgery with surgery alone in patients with non–small cell lung cancer. *New Engl J Med* 330:153–158, 1994.
39. Roth JA, Fossella F, Komaki R, et al: A randomized trial comparing perioperative chemotherapy and surgery with surgery alone in resectable stage III non–small cell lung cancer. *J Natl Cancer Inst* 86:673–680, 1994.
40. Salyer WR, Salyer DC, Eggleston JC: Carcinoid tumors of the thymus. *Cancer* 37:958–973, 1976.
41. Shapiro B, Sisson J, Kalff V, et al: The location of middle mediastinal pheochromocytomas. *J Thorac Cardiovasc Surg* 87:814–820, 1984.
42. Shields TW: *Mediastinal Surgery*. Philadelphia, Lea and Febiger, 1991.

43. Shorvon PJ: Endoscopic ultrasound in oesophageal cancer: The way forward. *Clin Radiol* 42:149–151, 1990.

44. Siegel MJ: Chest applications of magnetic resonance imaging in children. *Top Magn Reson Imaging* 3:1–23, 1990.

45. Steinfeld AD, Glicksman AS: Postoperative adjuvant mediastinal radiation in lung cancer. *J Surg Oncol* 26:154–157, 1984.

46. Vaeth JM, Moskowitz SA, Green JP: Mediastinal Hodgkin's disease. *AJR Am J Roentgenol* 126:123–126, 1976.

47. Webb WR: Magnetic resonance imaging of the hila and mediastinum. *Cardiovasc Intervent Radiol* 8:306–313, 1986.

48. Weinreb JC, Naidich DP: Thoracic magnetic resonance imaging. *Clin Chest Med* 12:33–54, 1991.

49. Westcott JL: Needle aspiration biopsy of pulmonary, hilar, and mediastinal masses. *Clin Chest Med* 5:365–377, 1984.

50. Westcott JL, Henschke CI, Berkmen Y: MR imaging of the hilum and mediastinum: Effects of cardiac gating. *J Comput Assist Tomogr* 9:1073–1078, 1985.

51. Zafar N, Moinuddin S: Mediastinal needle biopsy: A 15-year experience with 139 cases. *Cancer* 76:1065–1068, 1995.

52. Ziegler K, Sanft C, Zeitz M, et al: Evaluation of endosonography in TN staging of oesophageal cancer. *Gut* 32:16–20, 1991.

CHAPTER 94

NONNEOPLASTIC DISORDERS OF THE MEDIASTINUM

Cameron D. Wright

ANATOMY

Boundaries

The mediastinum is defined as the potential space between the two pleural cavities bounded by the sternum anteriorly, the vertebral column posteriorly, the thoracic inlet superiorly, and the diaphragm inferiorly (Fig. 94-1). The major mediastinal structures are the heart and great vessels, the trachea and main bronchi, and the esophagus, all closely related to one another and connected by loose connective tissue. Hence, air or infection can disseminate widely throughout the mediastinal space, contained laterally only by the mediastinal pleural reflections. The mediastinum communicates with both the neck and the retroperitoneum, and these portals can also serve as routes of egress from the mediastinum. Fascial planes connect the neck, mediastinum, and retroperitoneum and thus facilitate movement of air or infection from one location to another.

Compartments

Several subdivisions of the mediastinum have been emphasized in the surgical and radiologic literature with no uniform agreement. Most commonly, three compartments are proposed: anterior, middle (visceral), and posterior (paravertebral sulcus) (Fig. 94-2). The boundaries of these divisions are not agreed upon, further emphasizing their nonanatomic origins. Shields proposed a simple three-compartment subdivision in 1972, which makes both anatomic and surgical sense.[27] The anterior compartment is bounded by the sternum and the anterior surface of the pericardium and great vessels. The middle (visceral) compartment extends from the posterior limit of the anterior compartment to the anterior surface of the vertebral columns and then to the thoracic inlet. The posterior compartment (paravertebral sulcus) extends from the anterior surface of the vertebral column to the anterior surface of the paravertebral ribs. The structures in these compartments are listed in Table 94-1. The pericardial sac is the only true compartment of the mediastinum and it provides a strong barrier to infection. Subdividing the mediastinum into compartments proves most helpful when one is interpreting a plain radiograph where a mediastinal mass is present. Knowledge of the contents of the involved compartment facilitates arriving at a proper diagnosis.

Lymphatics

The mediastinal lymphatic system proves to be quite complex and variable. Mediastinal lymph nodes are interconnected; thus, involvement of one group of lymph nodes in a pathological process frequently leads to involvement of other groups. Like subdividing the mediastinum into compartments, naming individual nodal stations is somewhat arbitrary and leads to the mistaken notion that these nodal stations are discrete. To the contrary, the mediastinum is covered in a dense network of lymphatic vessels and lymph nodes with no predictable boundaries. Nonetheless, there are commonly accepted nodal stations that have clinical importance, especially in the staging of lung can-

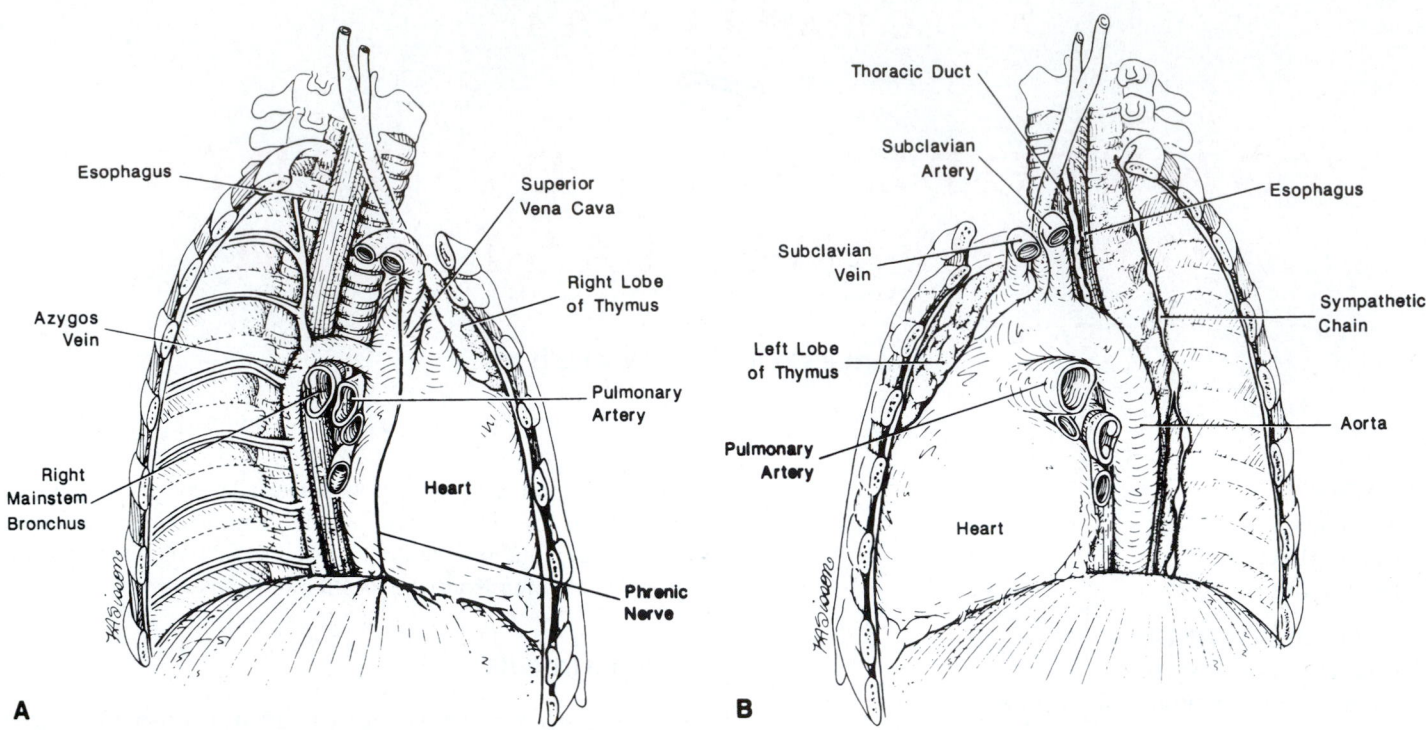

FIGURE 94-1 *A.* Lateral view of the mediastinum as seen through a right thoracotomy. *B.* Lateral view of the mediastinum as seen through a left thoracotomy. *(From LoCicero,[15] with permission.)*

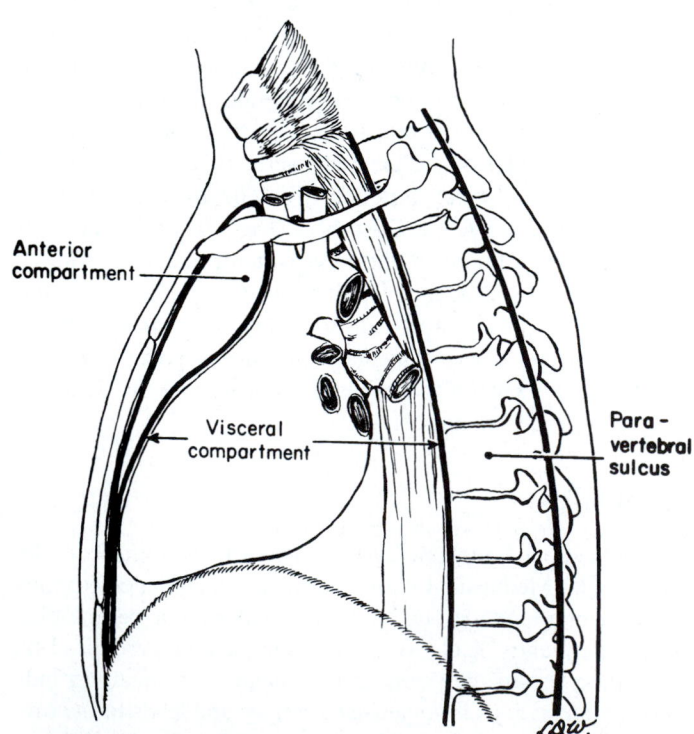

FIGURE 94-2 Compartments of the mediastinum. Note continuity of visceral (middle) compartment with the neck and retroperitoneum. *(From Shields,[1] with permission.)*

cer. The lymph node map proposed by Naruke in 1978 has been widely accepted and serves as a standard for communication of lymph node involvement (Fig. 94-3).[22]

PNEUMOMEDIASTINUM

Pneumomediastinum (mediastinal emphysema) is an uncommon condition but now is being seen with increasing frequency due to the common use of mechanical ventilation—specifically, certain modes of mechanical ventilation. Air (or gas) outside the normal confines of the respiratory and gastrointestinal tracts is always abnormal and always requires an explanation. Treatment is directed at the underlying abnormality if one can be identified.

Anatomic Considerations

Pneumomediastinum, when present, is frequently associated with other forms of extraalveolar air, including pulmonary interstitial emphysema, pneumopericardium, pneumothorax, subcutaneous emphysema, pneumoretroperitoneum, and pneumoperitoneum. The key to understanding the distribution of extraalveolar air lies in the recognition of the common fascial planes that unite these areas. In the neck, the deep layer of the deep cervical fascia ensheathes the trachea and esophagus as they descend into the mediastinum. The trachea and esophagus are thus enclosed in this visceral space; therefore air or infection can readily travel from the mediastinum to the neck or retroperitoneum (Fig. 94-4). This fascial plane extends into the hilum of the lung and merges with the bronchovascular sheaths that surround the terminal bronchioles, arteries, and veins. The bronchovascular sheath also

TABLE 94-1

Contents of Mediastinal Compartments

Anterior	Middle	Posterior
Thymus gland	Pericardium	Azygous and hemiazygous veins
Pericardial fat	Heart	Thoracic duct
Lymph nodes	Trachea and main bronchus	Symphathetic trunk
	Esophagus	
	Aorta	
	Phrenic and vagus nerves	Intercostal nerves
	Lymph nodes	

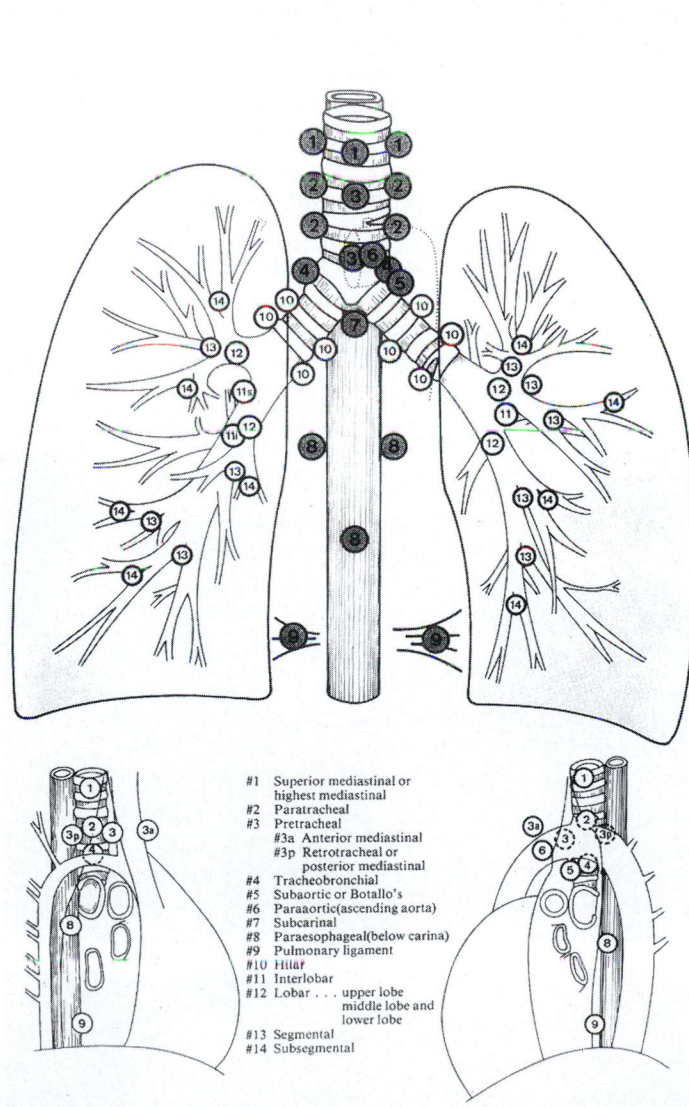

#1 Superior mediastinal or highest mediastinal
#2 Paratracheal
#3 Pretracheal
    #3a Anterior mediastinal
    #3p Retrotracheal or posterior mediastinal
#4 Tracheobronchial
#5 Subaortic or Botallo's
#6 Paraaortic(ascending aorta)
#7 Subcarinal
#8 Paraesophageal(below carina)
#9 Pulmonary ligament
#10 Hilar
#11 Interlobar
#12 Lobar . . . upper lobe
                middle lobe and
                lower lobe
#13 Segmental
#14 Subsegmental

FIGURE 94-3 Lymph node groups of the lungs and mediastinum. *(From Naruke,[2] with permission.)*

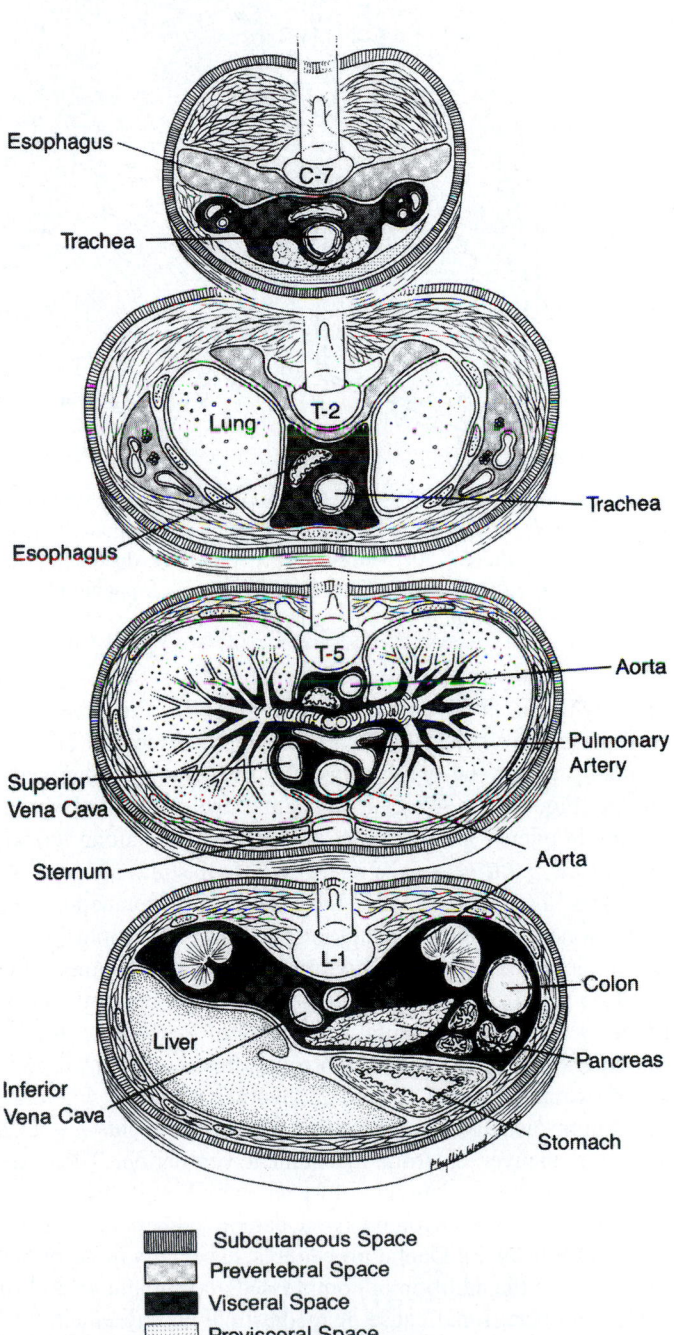

- Subcutaneous Space
- Prevertebral Space
- Visceral Space
- Previsceral Space

FIGURE 94-4 Soft tissue compartments of the neck, thorax, and abdomen demonstrating continuity of visceral space between regions. *(From Maunder et al,[19] with permission.)*

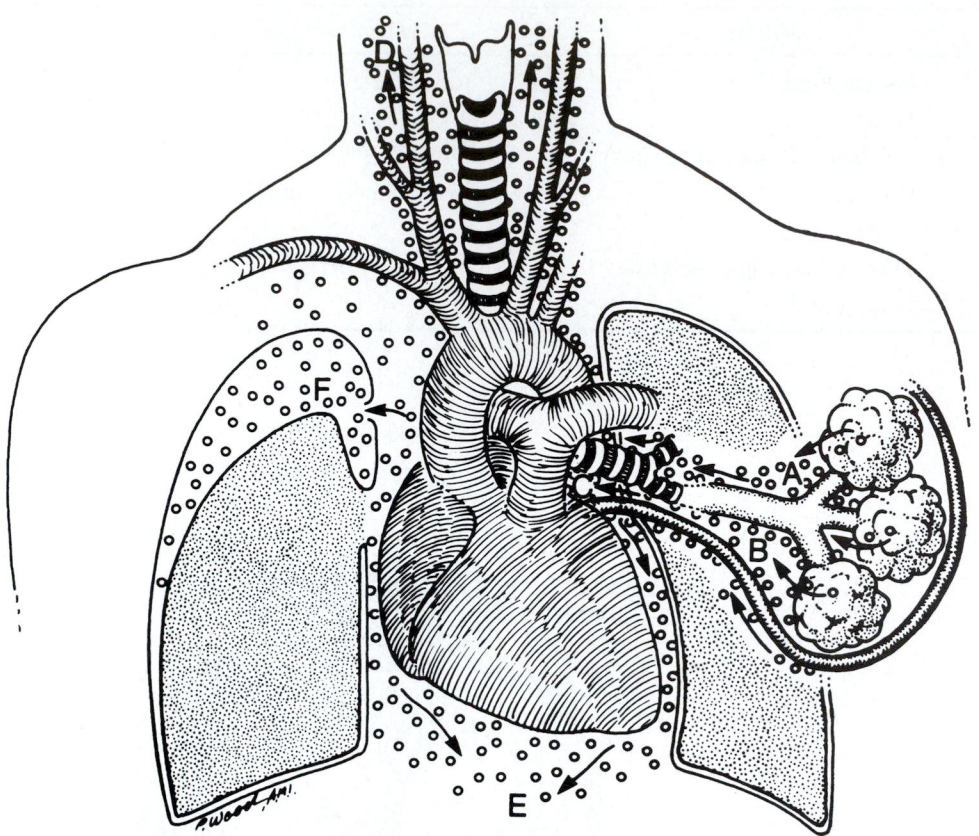

Hamman, in 1939, described crepitation synchronous with the heartbeat in these patients.[12] The majority of patients with spontaneous pneumomediastinum have predisposing factors that cause elevated airway pressure, which leads to alveolar rupture. Most commonly, this results from straining against a closed glottis, as during vomiting, coughing, or exercising. Other mechanisms include sudden and/or severe increases in lung volume, as occur during marijuana smoking, inhaling of cocaine, and/or during a seizure. Localized airway obstruction from tumor, foreign bodies, asthma, or parenchymal lung disease can also cause alveolar rupture. An accurate history is most important in order to define the mechanism in a particular patient.

Spontaneous pneumomediastinum almost always presents with substernal pain, often pleuritic, which may radiate to the neck or back. Patients may experience either separately or in combination dyspnea, dysphagia, odynophagia, and dysphonia.[25] Air in the subcutaneous tissues of the neck produces a characteristic change in voice quality, a higher-pitched nasal tone, that the

FIGURE 94-5   Possible routes of air following alveolar disruption. Air from the alveolus (*A*) enters perivascular interstitium (*B*), dissecting proximally within bronchovascular sheath toward mediastinum (*C*). As mediastinal pressure rises, decompression occurs in cervical (*D*), subcutaneous, and retroperitoneal (*E*) soft tissue spaces. A pneumothorax is possible if the pleura (*F*) is ruptured. (*From Maunder et al,[19] with permission.*)

merges with and is continuous with the pericardium. After alveolar rupture, air enters the perivascular interstitium and dissects proximally within the bronchovascular sheath toward the mediastinum (Fig. 94-5). Air can then enter the pericardial space, resulting in pneumopericardium, or it may dissect along the adventia of the great vessels (Fig. 94-6). Mediastinal air can also decompress by extension into the cervical, subcutaneous, and retroperitoneal spaces. A pneumomediastinum that ruptures into the free pleural space results in a pneumothorax. Pneumothorax may also result from air dissecting out toward the visceral pleural surface of the lung and rupturing. Macklin, in 1944, in an elegant experimental cat model, confirmed this theory of progression of extraalveolar air following alveolar rupture.[17] Pneumomediastinum usually results from a ruptured alveolus due to a Valsalva maneuver or from mechanical ventilation. There are many other possible sources, however, which must be considered when one is confronted by a patient with pneumomediastinum (Table 94-2). Dental procedures, especially those on the mandible with the addition of compressed air to maintain a clear field, are an occasional cause of mediastinal emphysema.[4]

Spontaneous Pneumomediastinum

Idiopathic spontaneous pneumomediastinum is a rare self-limited condition that most commonly affects young adult men.[1]

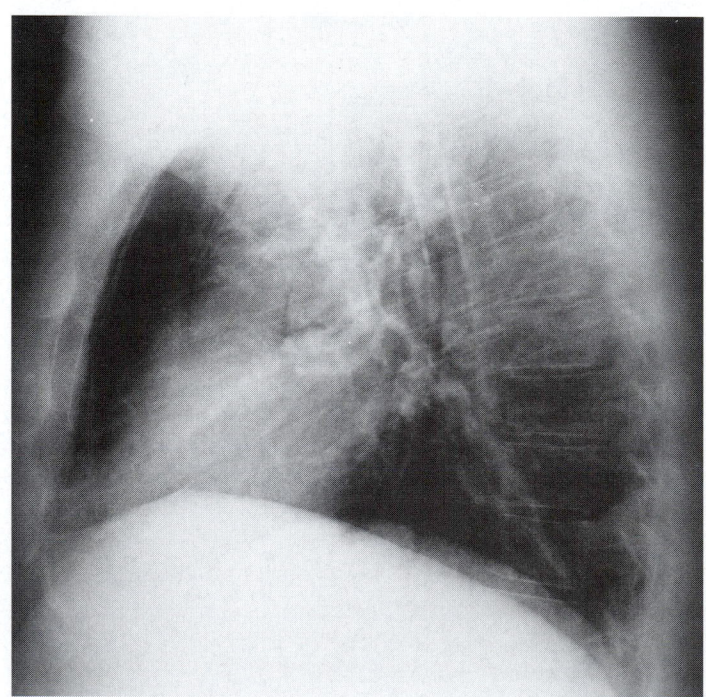

FIGURE 94-6   Lateral radiograph of a middle-aged patient with an acute asthma attack requiring hospital admission. Mediastinal air is seen outlining the aorta and esophagus. This resolved spontaneously.

experienced clinician easily recognizes. Examination often reveals palpable subcutaneous emphysema in the neck. Auscultation of the chest may reveal a crunching or clicking sound heard over the pericardium, synchronous with the heartbeat (Hamman's sign). Low-grade fever is present in about one-third of cases and mild leukocytosis in about one-half.[25] Nonspecific electrocardiographic changes, such as ST-T wave changes and ST elevation, may also be present. A chest radiograph usually demonstrates a thin radiolucent strip along a mediastinal fascial plane, most commonly along the left heart border. The aortic knob may be highlighted as well (Fig. 94-6). Computed tomography (CT) is more sensitive in detecting air then plain radiographs (Fig. 94-7). Air may be evident deep in the neck as well as in the subcutaneous tissue.

The differential diagnosis is broad and includes musculoskeletal, pleural, pulmonary, cardiac, and esophageal causes. While most patients who present are not acutely ill, the occasional patient may suffer an acute, catastrophic onset with hypotension and hemodynamic compromise. Esophageal perforation is the condition most likely to be confused with spontaneous mediastinal emphysema. Worrisome features suggesting esophageal perforation include recent esophageal instrumentation, a history of esophageal problems, severe retching, the presence of a pleural effusion, or shock. A contrast esophagogram should be obtained immediately if there is any question of an esophageal perforation, since a delay in making this diagnosis often proves fatal. A high index of suspicion regarding esophageal perforation should always be present whenever a patient presents with mediastinal emphysema.

Treatment of spontaneous mediastinal emphysema is supportive and is primarily directed at pain relief and reassurance. Appropriate management of contributing causes such as foreign bodies, asthma, and parenchymal lung disorders should be instituted. The patient should be followed both clinically and radiographically to exclude another cause for mediastinal emphysema and to detect a possible pneumothorax. Prompt resolution is the rule. Supplemental oxygen to hasten reabsorption (similar to that proposed for pneumothorax) has been reported but is probably not necessary. Needle aspiration or skin incision to relieve subcutaneous emphysema is almost never necessary. Prophylactic tube thoracostomy is unnecessary. For patients who present with minimal findings and a clear inciting factor (such as coughing),

only a short period of observation in the emergency department is required.

Pneumomediastinum Associated with Mechanical Ventilation

Mechanical ventilation is commonly associated with pneumomediastinum and may often lead to life-threatening tension pneumothorax. Alveolar rupture results from high peak inspiratory pressures with subsequent elevated alveolar pressure associated with abnormal airways or parenchyma (decreased compliance). Classic predisposing factors include high tidal volumes, high levels of positive end-expiratory pressure, and "fighting" the ventilator. Air trapping with occult positive end-expiratory pressure (auto-PEEP) is probably an underrecognized cause of barotrauma.[8] It is not clear if one mode of ventilation (pressure-controlled versus volume-limited) is associated with a decreased incidence of barotrauma.

TABLE 94-2

Etiology of Pneumomediastinum

Upper respiratory tract
  Head and neck infection
  Fracture of facial bones
  Trauma to hypopharynx and larynx (especially intubation)
  Dental procedures (especially mandibular)
Lower respiratory tract
  Trauma
  Bronchoscopy, especially therapeutic bronchoscopy (i.e., YAG laser and rigid core-out and transbronchial biopsy)
Lung
  Trauma
  Surgery
  Spontaneous alveolar rupture
    Straining and Valsalva maneuver
    Local airway obstruction
    Scuba diving
    Mechanical ventilation
Gastrointestinal tract
  Esophageal perforation
  Perforated viscus
Infection
  Acute mediastinitis
  Descending necrotizing mediastinitis
Air from outside the body
  Trauma
  Surgery (especially mediastinoscopy, tracheostomy, and sternotomy)
  Pneumoperitoneum (especially with laparoscopic hiatus hernia repair)

SOURCE: Adapted from Pierson,[23] with permission.

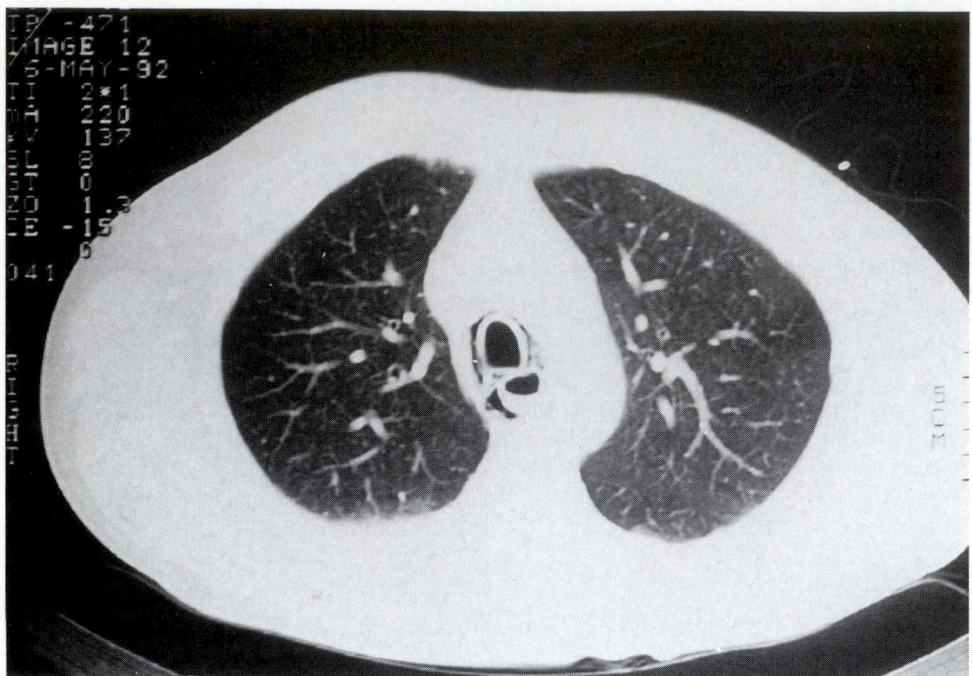

FIGURE 94-7 Computed tomography of man with 8-h-old postemetic esophageal rupture. Posteroanterior radiograph was normal. Mediastinal air is seen outlining trachea and esophagus.

Unlike spontaneous mediastinal emphysema, pneumomediastinum occurring in a patient on mechanical ventilation is potentially catastrophic because of its frequent association with tension pneumothorax. The chest radiograph should be closely examined to detect even a small pneumothorax and, if such is present, tube thoracostomy promptly performed. Obviously, a sudden deterioration marked by hypotension and increased pulmonary pressures should prompt immediate attention with insertion of unilateral or bilateral chest tubes, depending on the clinical examination. The issue of prophylactic tube insertion is controversial and unresolved. At the least, a thoracostomy tray should be kept at the patient's bedside and the nursing staff reminded of the signs of a pneumothorax in a mechanically ventilated patient. If a physician is not readily available around the clock, it may be advisable to perform bilateral prophylactic tube thoracostomy in certain patients. Removing the patient from mechanical ventilation as soon as possible is appropriate. As this is seldom possible, efforts should be directed at minimizing alveolar distension as much as possible. These efforts include relief of bronchospasm, minimizing "fighting" the ventilator, reducing tidal volume and positive end-expiratory pressure, and manipulation of inspiratory flow and timing to reduce auto-PEEP.

Pneumopericardium

Pneumopericardium as a form of barotrauma is much more frequent in neonates, presumably due to immature fascial planes. Hemodynamically significant tamponade is also much more likely to occur in infants rather than adults and has resulted in collapse and death.[6] Pericardial drainage with a subxyphoid tube should be performed promptly in the neonate. In the adult, drainage should be performed only if there is hemodynamic embarrassment.

ACUTE MEDIASTINITIS

Acute mediastinitis is a life-threatening disorder that causes severe morbidity in the afflicted patient. All three mediastinal compartments can be affected; the anterior compartment most commonly after sternotomy for cardiac surgery, the middle compartment usually from esophageal perforation, and the posterior compartment from direct extension from the lung or spine. Instrumental perforation of the esophagus is the most common cause of acute mediastinitis in the United States. A summary of the causes of acute mediastinitis is presented in Table 94-3.

Mediastinitis from Esophageal Perforation

Instrumental perforation of the esophagus now accounts for almost one-half of all esophageal perforation.[14] Perforation is more common after rigid esophagoscopy, dilation of a stricture, and pneumatic dilation for achalasia, but it also occurs after variceal sclerosis, esophageal tube placement (nasogastric, Sengstaken-Blakemore, and salivary bypass tubes), and simple flexible esophagoscopy. Boerhaave's syndrome (postemetic rupture) was described in 1724 but still represents a diagnostic challenge and remains a major consideration in patients with otherwise unexplained mediastinitis (Fig. 94-8). Patients usually present with the abrupt onset of severe substernal chest pain, which is pleuritic after forceful vomiting or retching. Dyspnea is common even in the absence of pneumothorax. Shock develops quickly and the patient usually appears gravely ill. Examination reveals tachypnea, tachycardia, fever, hypotension, splinting of the chest and abdomen, and cervical emphysema. Radiographic findings may show cer-

TABLE 94-3

Etiology of Acute Mediastinitis

Esophageal perforation
    Instrumental
    Postemetic (Boerhaave's syndrome)
    Trauma
    Foreign body
    Operative injury
    Caustic ingestion
    Cancer
    Direct extension
Tracheobronchial perforation
Descending necrotizing mediastinitis
Direct extension (pulmonary and pancreatitis)
Poststernotomy mediastinitis
Anthrax mediastinitis

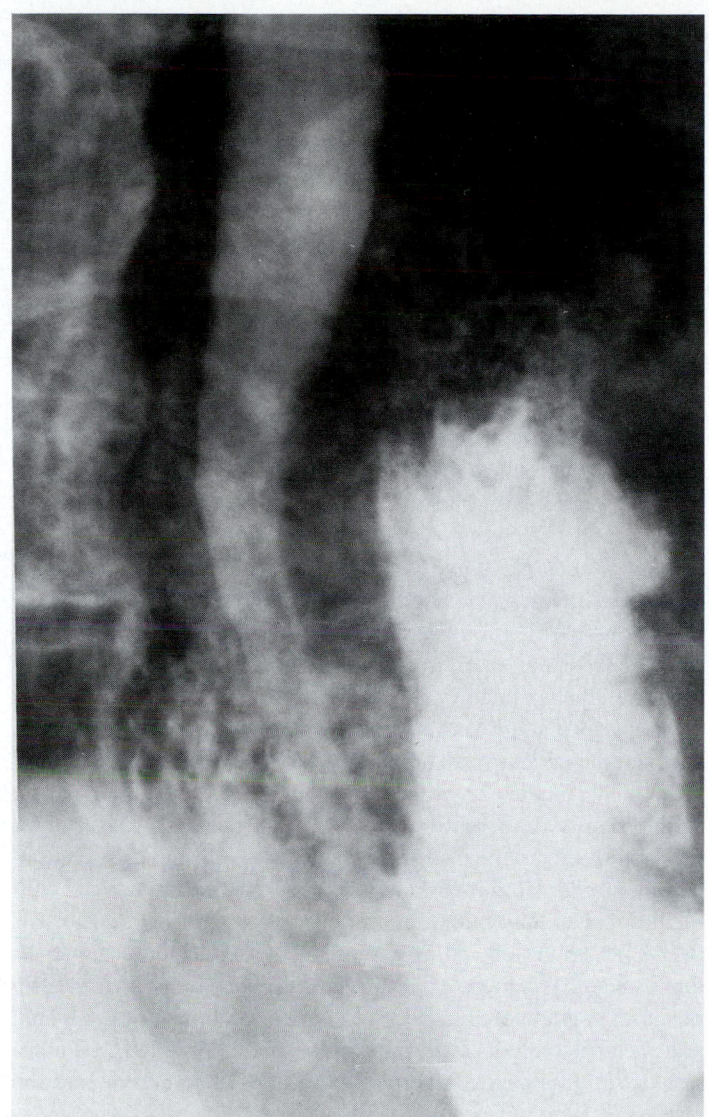

FIGURE 94-8   Water-contrast esophagogram of a patient with Boerhaave's syndrome. Note extensive extravasation of contrast and mediastinal emphysema.

vical or mediastinal emphysema, pneumothorax, and (commonly) pleural effusion. Noncontrast radiographic studies are normal in 10 to 30 percent of cases of esophageal perforation. A contrast esophagogram (usually with water-soluble contrast) should be performed immediately when the diagnosis is suspected, but one should be aware that this study has a false-negative rate of 10 percent. Flexible esophagoscopy is the definitive study in a patient in whom esophageal perforation is suspected but who has a negative esophagogram. Prompt diagnosis and, therefore, a high index of suspicion are essential, as the incidence of complications and the mortality rate are directly dependent on the time elapsed between perforation and treatment.[14] The differential diagnosis is broad and includes perforated ulcer, acute pancreatitis, myocardial infarction, pneumonia, aortic dissection, pulmonary embolism.

Treatment should be instituted urgently and involves surgical debridement of necrotic tissue, secure closure of the perforation, correction of any distal obstruction, and wide drainage, usually per-

formed through a left thoracotomy.[31] Appropriate broad-spectrum antibiotics with anaerobic coverage and the maintenance of proper nutrition are also integral components of the management plan. Esophagectomy is occasionally required in the presence of a perforated, nondilatable stricture, a destroyed esophagus where direct repair is not possible, or cancer. Nonoperative treatment is *rarely* appropriate but may be instituted in highly selected cases (i.e., contained, asymptomatic instrumental perforations) where a significant interval has passed and the patient is clinically stable. Mortality is less than 10 percent if the perforation is recognized and repaired within 24 h, whereas mortality rises to 30 to 40 percent if more than 24 h has elapsed between perforation and repair.[14,31] The mortality rises even higher with advanced age of the patient.

Tracheobronchial Perforation

Tracheobronchial perforation is rare and is most commonly seen following trauma or instrumentation. Severe mediastinitis is rare after tracheobronchial disruption, presumably due to the less noxious nature of its contents and better containment. Intubation is now the most frequent cause of tracheobronchial injury, but it should be avoidable with gentle and proper technique. Blood in the airway, airway obstruction (infrequent), subcutaneous and mediastinal emphysema, and pneumothorax are the common presenting signs. Prompt recognition and operative repair are necessary and yield excellent results, although small tears in the cervical trachea may often be managed with antibiotics alone, without operation.

Descending Necrotizing Mediastinitis

Mediastinitis occasionally develops after severe deep cervical infections that originate from the oropharynx.[30] Most patients present with a mixed aerobic and anaerobic infection. Previously these infections had a fulminant, often lethal course with mortality as high as 40 percent. Extension of the cervical infection down the prevertebral or visceral space into the mediastinum leads to this syndrome of descending necrotizing mediastinitis. Computed tomography should be performed on all severe neck infections to identify signs of mediastinitis that may not be clinically apparent. Aggressive surgical drainage (cervical, substernal, and transthoracic) and antibiotics have reduced mortality, though prompt management is essential.

Mediastinitis from Direct Extension

Necrotizing pneumonias may cause mediastinitis by direct extension and is more common in immunocompromised patients. Aspergillosis of the posterior mediastinum has been reported with increasing frequency and is highly lethal.[29] Treatment involves reversal of immunosuppression (if possible), appropriate antibiotic therapy, and surgical drainage and debridement.

Pancreatitis can extend from the retroperitoneum into the mediastinum and present as a mediastinal process with evidence of mediastinitis. Pancreatic pseudocysts can also erode into the mediastinum and cause pleural effusions with elevated amylase levels.[13] Treatment is directed at providing adequate drainage of the pseudocyst, usually internal drainage into the stomach. The pleural effusion(s) may require tube thoracostomy drainage.

Poststernotomy Mediastinitis

Sternal wound infection with resulting mediastinitis is a relatively new entity, which emerged in the era of modern cardiac surgery. The incidence remains low at 0.5 to 1 percent of all sternotomies, but such infection is a source of major morbidity, prolonged hospital stay, and significant mortality (0 to 30 percent; average, 15 percent).[11,24] Multivariate analysis has demonstrated that prolonged preoperative stay, reoperation, blood transfusions, and reexploration for bleeding are significant risk factors.[16] The presence of diabetes mellitus and use of internal thoracic artery grafts (which may devascularize the sternum) also are significant risk factors.[11] Organisms commonly isolated include *Staphylococcus epidermidis* and *aureus,* various gram-negative organisms, as well as *Candida* species and atypical mycobacteria. The etiology appears to be a combination of intraoperative contamination and hematogenous seeding of mediastinal clot in the early postoperative period. Breaks in technique during the operation or inadequate sterilization of instruments before it probably cause the majority of these infections.

Most patients have an insidious presentation with low-grade fever and leukocytosis, wound problems (erythema, drainage, sternal instability), and eventually bacteremia. Infections caused by gram-negative organisms tend to present earlier than those caused by gram-positive organisms. Most infections occur within the first or second week following the operative procedure. A high index of suspicion must be maintained so that an early diagnosis can be made and appropriate treatment instituted. Wound aspiration, local wound exploration, and a CT scan aid in making the diagnosis. Exploration in the operating room remains the definitive diagnostic maneuver and material should be obtained for culture at that time if it has not been obtained before or has been unrevealing.

If the infection is relatively early and the bony sternum appears viable, debridement, drainage, and saline (or antibiotic) irrigation with reclosure are indicated. Although it may seemingly violate time-honored surgical principles (leaving contaminated wounds open, to close by secondary intention), primary closure of the early infected sternum yields excellent results in many patients if adequate debridement is carried out. Proper and prolonged antibiotic therapy is, of course, necessary. Reported mortality rates approach zero for these early infections if managed appropriately.[21] Late sternal wound infections with mediastinitis present a more formidable challenge, in part due to the extensive sternal osteomyelitis and necrotic soft tissue which, when debrided, result in significant dead space, which creates a favorable environment for continued bacterial proliferation and persistent infection. Most surgeons favor extensive sternal debridement, usually with total sternal excision and rotation of pectoralis muscle flaps (bilateral) or transposition of gastrocolic omentum to fill the dead space with viable tissue. The presence of prosthetic material, such as sutures, Teflon pledgets, or prosthetic grafts further complicates the problem and may lead to catastrophic hemorrhage with a fatal outcome. Mediastinitis in the presence of a prosthetic aortic graft is a particularly disastrous complication.

Anthrax Mediastinitis

Anthrax, caused by *Bacillus anthracis,* is found almost exclusively in the Middle East, with farm animals as the primary reservoir. The inhalation of anthrax spores allows entry into the lungs with subsequent transport to the mediastinal lymph nodes by alveolar macrophages. A hemorrhagic mediastinitis may ensue and quickly cause death.[3] Gram-positive bacilli are present in tissue specimens, and penicillin is the drug of choice for this extremely rare disease.

CHRONIC MEDIASTINITIS

Granulomatous mediastinitis is a disease of the mediastinal lymph nodes usually resulting from infection by *Histoplasma capsulatum* and occasionally from tuberculosis or other fungi.[20] In certain areas of the country (Mississippi river valley) where *Histoplasma* is endemic, this disease is fairly common. Coalescence of caseous mediastinal lymph nodes can result in a single large mass that incites a considerable fibrotic response, which can result in encapsulation and produce a mediastinal granuloma. The right paratracheal area is the most common site for development of an encapsulated mass as described. When calcification is absent and the patient presents with what appears to be mediastinal adenopathy, a tissue diagnosis is required to exclude malignancy. With progressive increase in the size of this "benign" mass, compression of the trachea, superior vena cava, or esophagus can occur. In a report from the Mayo Clinic, 34 percent of patients with mediastinal granuloma went on to develop mediastinal fibrosis over a 2-year period.[24] Based on reports such as these, most authors suggest that there exists a spectrum of disease ranging from mediastinal granuloma to fibrosing mediastinitis. Caseating lymph nodes can also erode into and rupture in the esophagus, be associated with esophageal diverticula (Fig. 94-9), and erode into the airway, causing obstruction or bleeding.

Mediastinal granulomas should be excised if symptomatic. Although complete excision is possible, the intense surrounding fibrosis places important structures at risk for operative injury. Evacuation of the granulomatous mass is usually a safer option. Specimens for culture and special stains should be obtained at the time of operation, but organisms can rarely be identified or grown in culture.[20,26]

Mediastinal lymph nodes involved by the granulomatous process may become calcified as individual masses and—because of the proximity of lymph nodes to the tracheobronchial tree—ultimately erode into the airway. This erosion into the airway, if it occurs, does so over a prolonged period of time and may remain asymptomatic, only to be noted if a bronchoscopy is performed for some other indication. The presence of calcified lymph node masses within the bronchi is referred to as *broncholithiasis* and may also present with symptoms of obstruction or bleeding. Symptomatic broncholithiasis should prompt bronchoscopy for documentation of findings only. Rarely, if ever, should broncholiths be removed bronchoscopically, the exception being the occasional "stone" that is completely free within the bronchus. An effort to remove a broncholith that is not completely detached from the wall of the bronchus may be accompanied by catastrophic hemorrhage due to the close proximity of pulmonary artery branches to the bronchus. Most symptomatic broncholiths should be removed at thoracotomy, where the pulmonary artery may be managed. These can be extremely difficult and hazardous operations and should be carried out by thoracic surgeons experienced in the management of granulomatous disease. Usually lobectomy or segmentectomy is required, since removal of the calcified mass will almost certainly take a portion of the bronchial wall.

Fistulas occurring between the trachea and esophagus or esophagus and mediastinum should be closed and reinforced with viable tissue. There is no consensus regarding management of large asymptomatic mediastinal granulomas but some have recommended excision to forestall the development of fibrosing mediastinitis. This, however, remains controversial.

Fibrosing Mediastinitis

Fibrosing mediastinitis may cause a variety of clinical syndromes due to the compression and/or erosion of vital mediastinal structures by the dense fibrous tissue reaction that is present. While the syndrome itself is rare, the commonly presumed causative agents—*Histoplasma* and (rarely) *Mycoplasma tuberculosis*—are relatively ubiquitous. Other very rare causes include other fungi, silicosis, the drug methysergide, autoimmune disorders, and familial multifocal fibrosclerosis.[5,16] Goodwin proposed the currently accepted (by most) hypothesis that fibrosing mediastinitis results from a delayed hypersensitivity reaction to fungal, mycobacterial, or other antigens.[9] Pathological features include the presence of dense fibrotic tissue surrounding the trachea and hila of the lungs, often extending into contiguous structures. Compression of the airway, pulmonary arteries, or veins may occur because of this process. Histologic features include dense hyalinized collagenous tissue, aggregates of plasma cells and lymphocytes, and occasionally granulomas. Cultures are almost always negative, as are special stains for organisms.

Symptoms are primarily caused by compression of vital mediastinal structures. Fibrosis around the right peritracheal area commonly causes superior vena cava syndrome. Subcarinal fibrosis can extend posteriorly to encase the esophagus or extend laterally to involve the pulmonary veins. Hilar fibrosis can obstruct either the tracheobronchial tree or pulmonary arteries (Fig. 94-10). Rarely, constrictive pericarditis or obstruction of the trachea or proximal main bronchi can also occur. The signs and symptoms may progress over a period of time.

Superior Vena Caval Syndrome

The most common mediastinal compression syndrome seen in fibrosing mediastinitis is the superior vena cava (SVC) syndrome, occurring in 20 to 50 percent of the patients.[9,26] While, in the vast majority of cases, SVC syndrome is due to malignant disease, fibrosing mediastinitis is the most common benign cause. Patients present with cervical venous distension; edema and plethora of the face, neck, and arms; and central nervous system complaints such as headache and visual disturbances. Men often note as a first sign that their collar size increases and symptoms are worse upon bending over. Because this syndrome

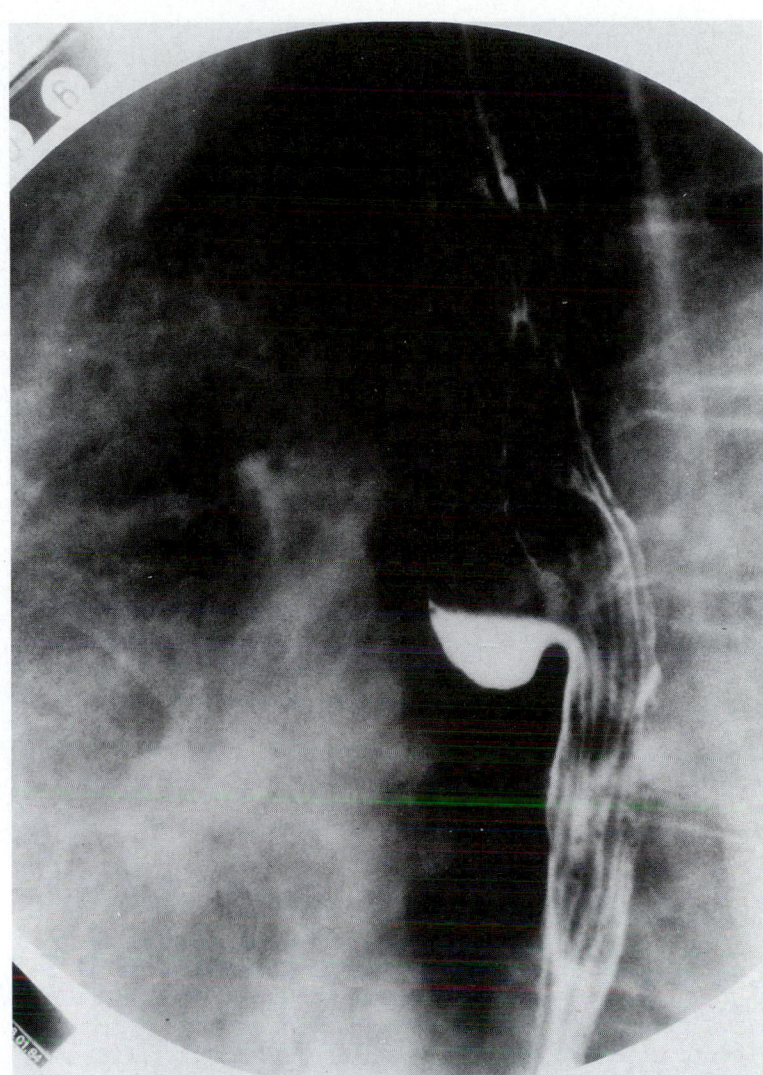

FIGURE 94-9   Barium swallow of elderly woman with a history of treated tuberculosis with symptomatic diverticulum of midesophagus adjacent to the subcarinal lymph nodes.

is usually of gradual onset, venous collaterals develop over the anterior chest wall and provide adequate decompression in many patients (Fig. 94-11). Confirmation of the diagnosis of SVC syndrome is easily made with contrast CT or venography, demonstrating blockage of contrast at the thoracic inlet and the presence of collateral vessels. Bilateral upper extremity venograms demonstrate the precise anatomy of the involved veins and are helpful if surgical decompression is contemplated. Surgical bypass is reserved for patients with intractable symptoms and is performed by connecting an unobstructed large brachiocephalic vein to the right atrial appendage with either saphenous vein or an externally supported polytetrafluoroethylene graft. Favorable long-term results have been reported.[28] Percutaneous angioplasty and stenting of a stenotic superior vena cava has been reported, but long-term follow-up is limited.[28]

Other Compression Syndromes

Tracheobronchial compression is also common and leads to dyspnea, obstructive pneumonias, wheezing, hemoptysis, cough, and

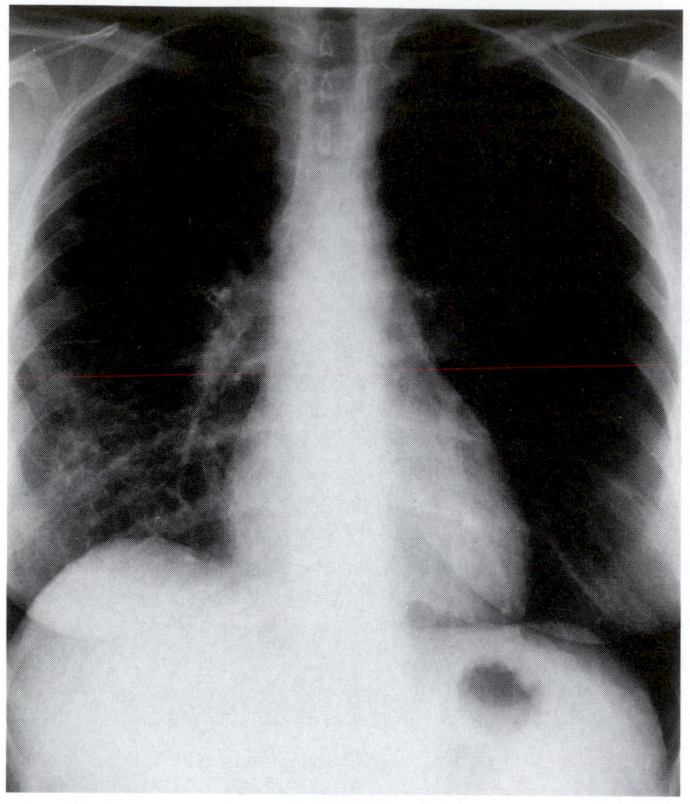

A

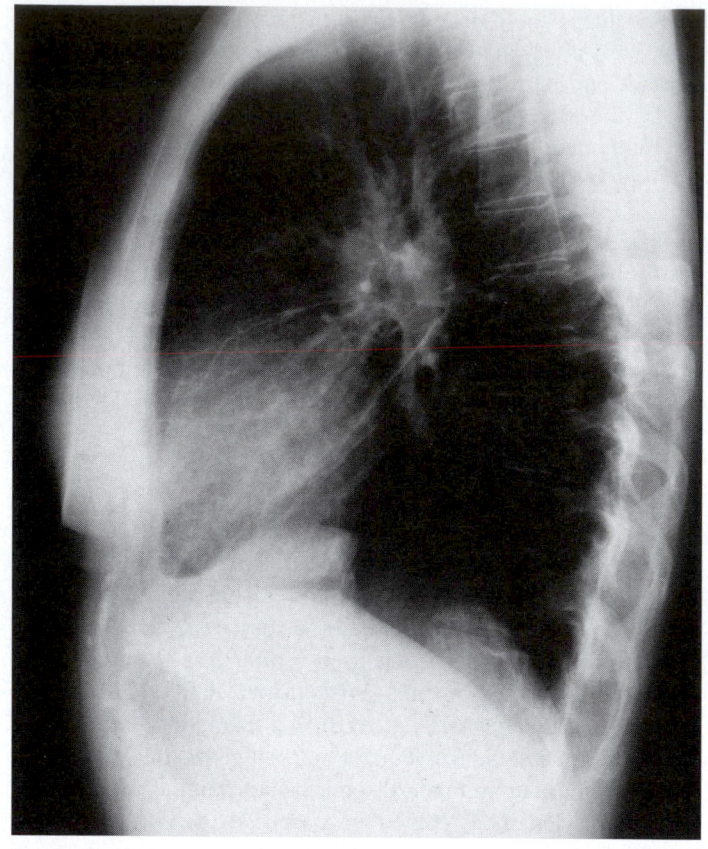

B

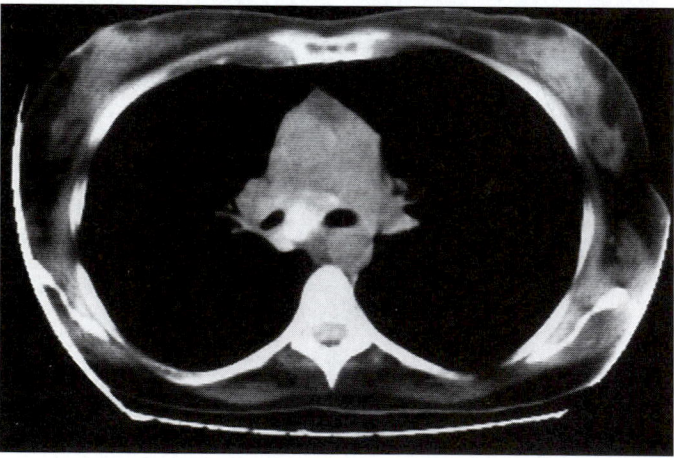

C

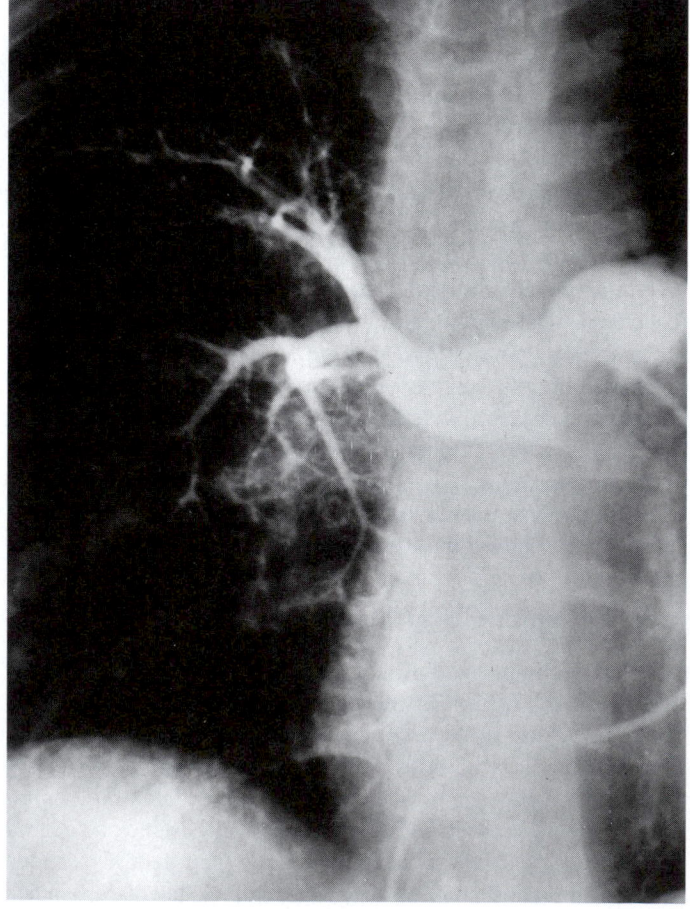

D

FIGURE 94-10 Mediastinal fibrosis due to histoplasmosis in a middle-aged nurse with narrowing of the trachea and main bronchi as well as occlusion of the right pulmonary artery. *A.* Posteroanterior radiograph demonstrating focal infiltrate in right lower zone with right hilar fullness. *B.* Lateral radiograph demonstrating a mass centered around the carina with mild narrowing of the distal trachea. *C.* Computed tomography shows calcified mass around bronchus intermedius with mild compression of bronchus. *D.* Pulmonary angiogram demonstrates complete occlusion of right pulmonary artery beyond the anterior trunk due to mediastinal fibrosis. The left pulmonary artery was moderately narrowed. *E.* Oblique tomogram demonstrating narrowing of distal trachea and left main bronchus. *F.* Oblique tomogram demonstrating narrowing of right bronchus intermedius with large mass of lymph nodes anterior and posterior to the airway.

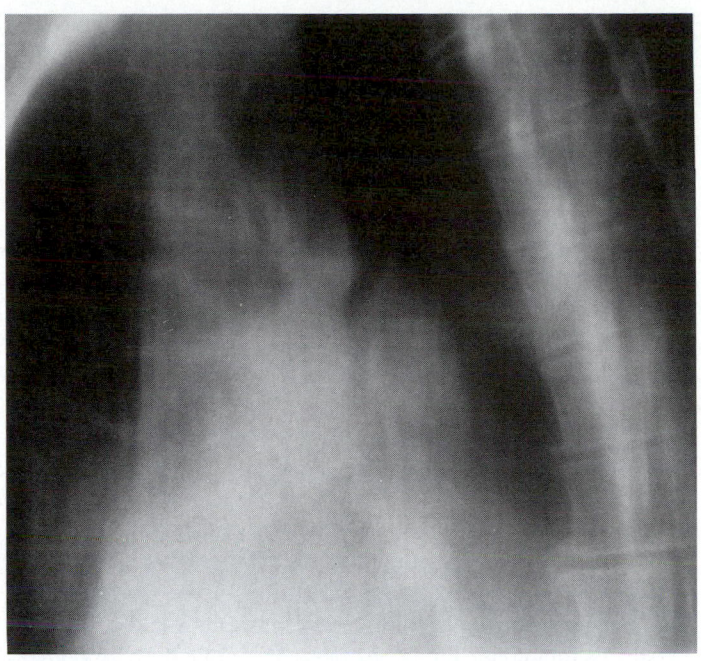

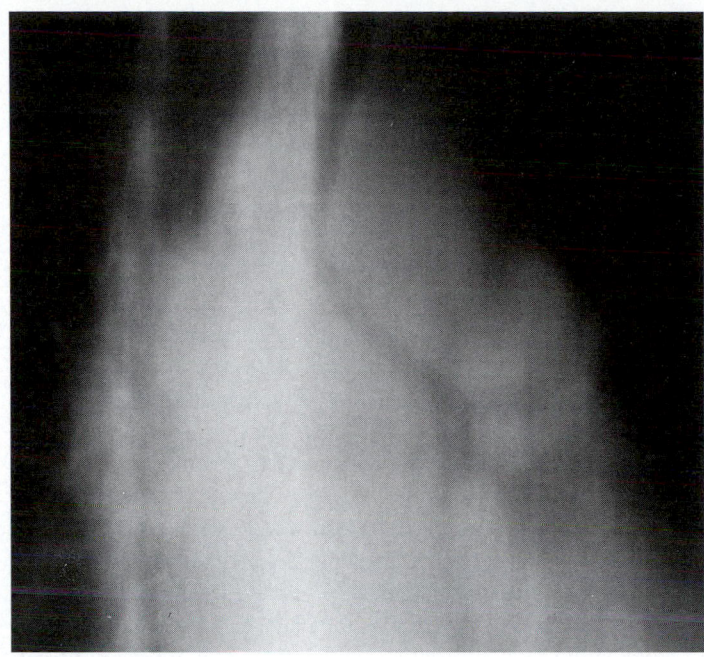

E

F

FIGURE 94-10 *(Cont.)*

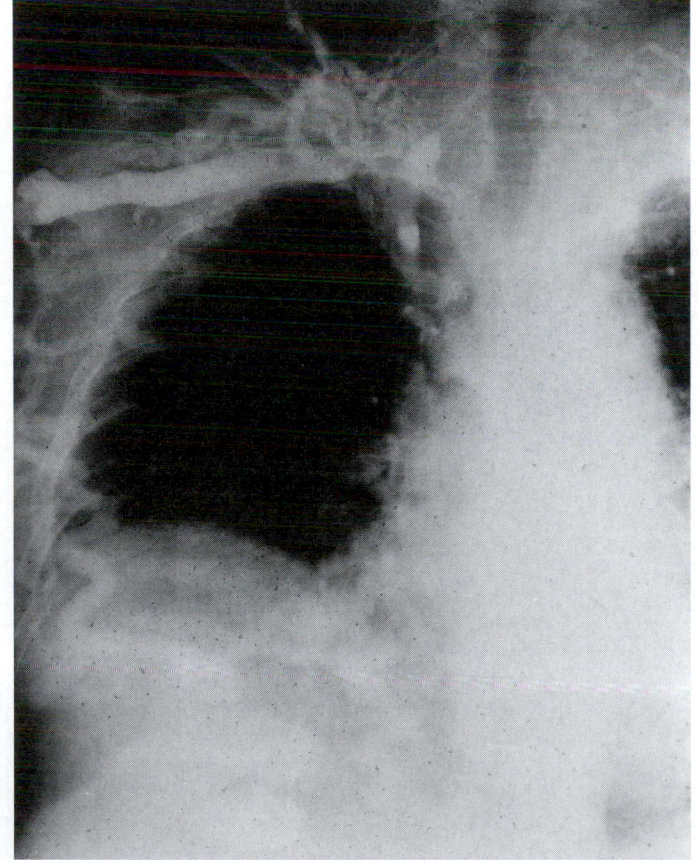

FIGURE 94-11 Patient with SVC syndrome secondary to mediastinal fibrosis due to histoplasmosis. Numerous dilated and tortuous collateral veins present on the chest wall are characteristic of chronic SVC obstruction.

the middle lobe syndrome (Fig. 94-10). A localized stenotic area can sometimes be dilated but often pulmonary resection is required, usually of the right middle and, occasionally, lower lobes.[18] Resection is the procedure of choice if chronic infection has been present. Bronchoplastic procedures are sometimes appropriate if lung parenchyma remains normal.[18] The placement of stents into the trachea and/or mainstem bronchi may allow for adequate management of a compressed airway. A Y-bifurcation stent and individual stents (Schneider Wallstent) placed in the trachea or bronchi are available. Airway management must be individualized based on findings at bronchoscopy.

Complete or partial unilateral or bilateral pulmonary artery obstruction can result from fibrosing mediastinitis (Fig. 94-10). Dyspnea and signs of right heart failure can be present. The differential diagnosis should include chronic pulmonary thromboembolism. The fibrosis may also extend to involve the pulmonary veins, producing pulmonary venooclusive disease. Patients can present with complaints similar to those of patients presenting with mitral stenosis: dyspnea, cough, and hemoptysis. Surgical correction of these disorders is rarely possible due to the extreme fibrosis present around the vessels. If the situation is unilateral, a pneumonectomy may be an alternative.

Esophageal obstruction is not uncommon in fibrosing mediastinitis, and the middle third of the esophagus is most frequently involved because of its relationship to the subcarinal space. Dilation, enucleation of scar, and resection are therapeutic options. Fistulas may also occur between the subcarinal lymph nodes and the esophagus or into the tracheobronchial tree.[8,18] Operative treatment for fistula formation is directed at closing the fistula and separating structures with viable tissue such as muscle. An esophageal diverticulum may form from inflammatory adherence to the subcarinal lymph nodes but is usually asymptomatic (Fig. 94-9).

Corticosteroids have not proven of benefit in fibrosing mediastinitis despite its obvious inflammatory nature. The majority of reports of treatment with chemotherapeutic agents directed against the suspected causative organism have been negative. Urschel reported success in six patients who were treated with prolonged ketoconazole therapy.[28] Patients were selected based on an elevated sedimentation rate and histoplasmosis complement fixation titer and were given ketoconazole following appropriate surgical decompression. These patients likely are not typical or representative of most with fibrosing mediastinitis but rather closer in the spectrum to those with granulomatous mediastinitis.

MISCELLANEOUS MEDIASTINAL PATHOLOGY

Foramen of Morgagni Hernias

Hernias occurring through the foramen of Morgagni are rare causes of cardiophrenic angle masses (Fig. 94-12). This hernia results from failure of the normal fusion of the diaphragmatic components during embryologic development. Small hernias are usually asymptomatic but large ones can contain the entire omentum, transverse colon, and even stomach and thus cause symptoms. Symptoms include substernal discomfort and dyspnea; rarely, they may point to intestinal obstruction. The diagnosis is now easily confirmed by CT and operative repair is always indicated.

Mediastinal Repositioning in Postpneumonectomy Syndrome

Following pneumonectomy, airway compression may be caused by extreme mediastinal shift and rotation, manifest by herniation and overdistension of the remaining lung.[10] The problem occurs rarely but is more common after right pneumonectomy. It may also occur after left pneumonectomy, especially in the presence of a right aortic arch. The problem has been particularly noted in children but also occurs in younger adults. When extreme shift of the mediastinum occurs after pneumonectomy, compression of the main bronchus occurs against the aorta and/or vertebral column (Fig. 94-13). Patients may develop disabling dyspnea, stridor, and recurrent pulmonary infections.

Computed tomography confirms the diagnosis, and pulmonary function studies generally show severe obstruction, flattened flow-volume loops, and an elevated ratio of residual volume to total lung capacity. Bronchoscopy delineates the extent of airway compression and is helpful in assessing any malacia that may be present. Operative repair is indicated and consists of mediastinal repositioning through the original thoracotomy incision by placing expandable saline breast prostheses (Fig. 94-13). In the absence of severe malacia, airway compression is relieved and clinical results are excellent. Management of residual airway malacia is troublesome and is probably best handled by internal stenting.

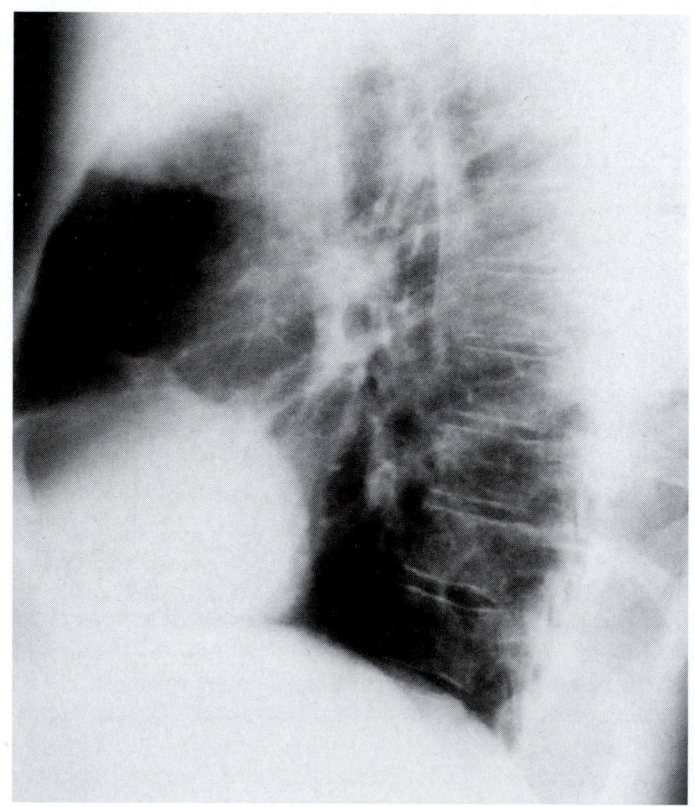

A   *B*

FIGURE 94-12   Foramen of Morgagni hernia. This man presented with substernal discomfort and heaviness. Incarcerated omentum was present in the hernia sac. *A*. Posteroanterior radiograph demonstrating large, smooth mass obscuring the right cardiophrenic angle. *B*. Lateral radiograph showing large, smooth substernal mass.

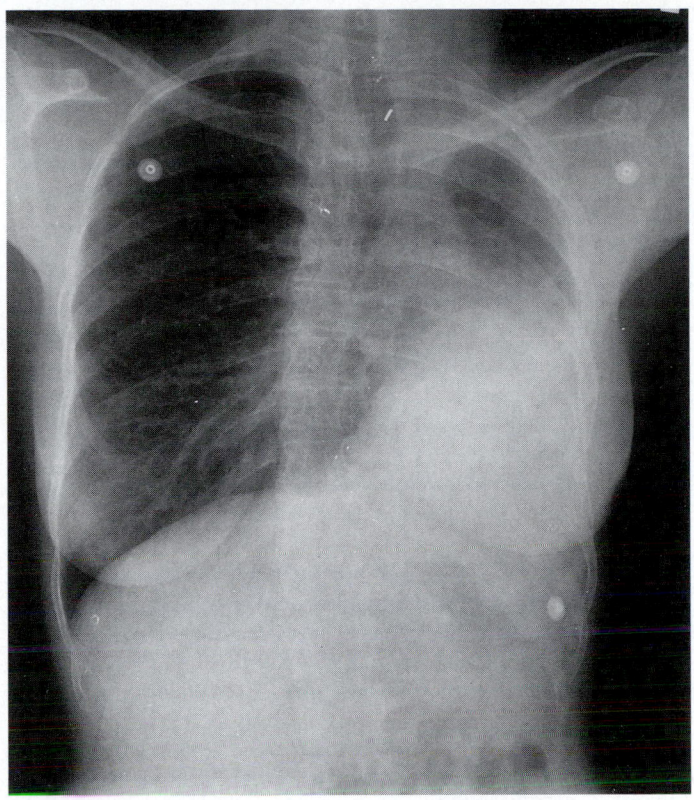

A

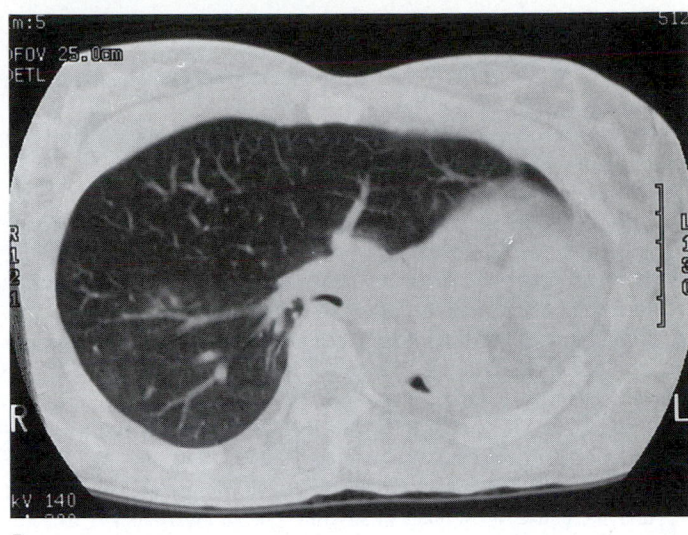

B

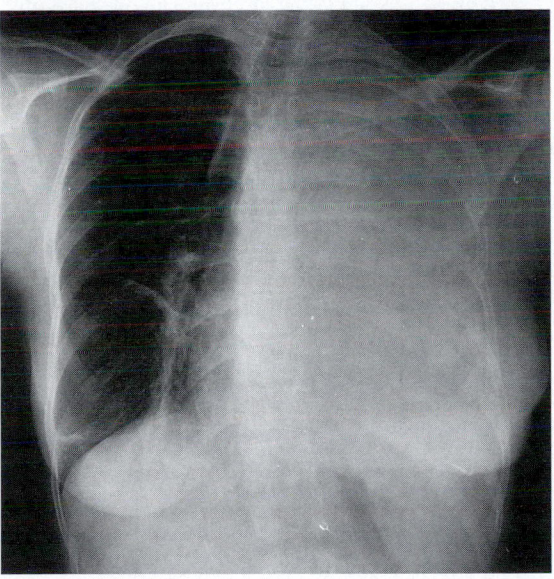

C

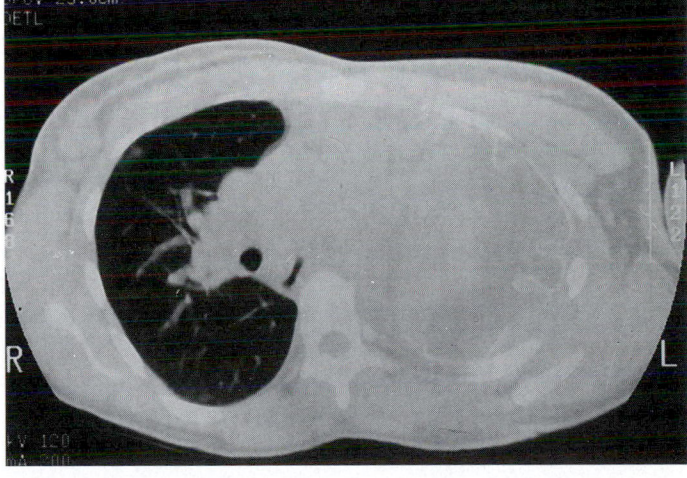

D

FIGURE 94-13 Thirty-year-old woman with previous left carinal pneumonectomy for granular cell tumor with postpneumonectomy syndrome. She presented with worsening dyspnea, which worsened with recumbency. She became asymptomatic after mediastinal repositioning. *A.* Posteroanterior radiograph demonstrating marked overexpansion of right lung with mediastinal shift. Right tracheobronchial tree appears narrowed. *B.* Computed tomography scan confirming severe compression of right bronchus intermedius against the spine. *C.* Posteroanterior radiograph early after mediastinal repositioning with 1000 mL of saline implants. *D.* Computed tomography scan at level of bronchus intermedius after mediastinal repositioning demonstrating relief of bronchial compression.

Spontaneous Mediastinal Hemorrhage

Spontaneous mediastinal hemorrhage is quite rare.[28] Mediastinal hemorrhage due to aortic dissection, contained rupture of a thoracic aortic aneurysm, or iatrogenic injury is much more common. Symptoms are usually of sudden onset and consist of sub-sternal pain, dyspnea, and rarely hemodynamic compromise. The hemorrhage is usually brief and self-limited. Treatment is supportive and secondary causes of mediastinal hemorrhage must be excluded. Mediastinal fibrosis has rarely been reported following mediastinal hemorrhage.

REFERENCES

1. Abolnik I, Losser IS, Brewer R: Spontaneous pneumomediastinum: A report of 25 cases. *Chest* 100:93–95, 1991.
2. Benson MS, Pierson DJ: Auto-PEEP during mechanical ventilation of adults. *Respir Care* 33:557–565, 1988.
3. Brochman PS: Inhalation anthrax. *Ann NY Acad Sci* 353:83–93, 1980.
4. Cole FH, Cole FH, Duckworth HK: Mediastinal emphysema secondary to dental restoration. *Ann Thorac Surg* 52:139–140, 1991.
5. Comings DE, Skubi KB, Eyer JV, Motulsky AG: Familial multifocal fibrosclerosis. *Ann Intern Med* 66:884–892, 1967.
6. Cummings RG, Wesley RLR, Adams DH, Lowe JE: Pneumopericardium resulting in cardiac tamponade. *Ann Thorac Surg* 37:511–517, 1984.
7. Epstein AM, Klassen KP: Spontaneous superior mediastinal hemorrhage. *J Thorac Cardiovasc Surg* 39:740, 1960.
8. Goenka MK, Gupta NM, Kochhar R, et al: Mediastinal fibrosis: An unusual cause of esophageal stricture. *J Clin Gastroentrol* 20:331–333, 1995.
9. Goodwin RA, Mickell JA, Des Prez RM: Mediastinal fibrosis complicating healed primary histoplasmosis and tuberculosis. *Medicine* 51:227–246, 1972.
10. Grillo HC, Shepard JO, Mathisen DJ, Kanarek DJ: Postpneumonectomy syndrome: Diagnosis, management and results. *Ann Thorac Surg* 54:638–651, 1992.
11. Grossi EA, Esposito R, Harris LJ, et al: Sternal wound infections and use of internal mammary artery grafts. *J Thorac Cardiovasc Surg* 102:342–347, 1991.
12. Hamman L: Spontaneous mediastinal emphysema. *Bull Johns Hopkins Hosp* 64:1–21, 1939.
13. Johnston RH, Owensby LC, Vargus GM, Garcia-Rinaldi R: Pancreatic pseudocyst of the mediastinum. *Ann Thorac Surg* 41:210, 1986.
14. Jones WG, Ginsberg RJ: Esophageal perforation: A continuing challenge. *Ann Thorac Surg* 53:534–543, 1992.
15. LoCicero J: Median sternotomy and thoracotomy, in Shields TW (ed): *Mediastinal Surgery.* Philadelphia, Lea & Febiger, 1991, p 95.
16. Logerstrom CF, Mitchell HG, Graham BS, Hammon JW: Chronic fibrosing mediastinitis and superior vena caval obstruction from blastomycosis. *Ann Thorac Surg* 54:764–765, 1992.
17. Macklin MT, Macklin CC: Malignant interstitial emphysema of the lungs and mediastinum as an important occult complication in many respiratory diseases and other conditions: An interpretation of the clinical literature in the light of laboratory experiment. *Medicine* 23:281–358, 1944.
18. Mathisen DJ, Grillo HC: Clinical manifestation of mediastinal fibrosis and histoplasmosis. *Ann Thorac Surg* 54:1053–1058, 1992.
19. Maunder RJ, Pierson DJ, Hudson LD: Subcutaneous and mediastinal emphysema. *Arch Intern Med* 144:1447–1453, 1984.
20. Mole TM, Glover J, Shepard MN: Scherosing mediastinitis: A report on 18 cases. *Thorax* 50:280–283, 1995.
21. Molina JE: Primary closure for infected dehiscence of the sternum. *Ann Thorac Surg* 55:459–463, 1993.
22. Naruke T, Suemasu K, Ishikawa S: Lymph node mapping and curability at various levels of metastasis in resected lung cancer. *J Thorac Cardiovasc Surg* 76:832–839, 1978.
23. Pierson DJ: Pneumomediastinum, in Murray JF, Nadal JA (eds): *Textbook of Respiratory Medicine.* Philadelphia, Saunders, 1994, p 2251.
24. Diner DE, Payne WS, Bernatz PE, Pairolero PC: Mediastinal granuloma and fibrosing mediastinitis. *Chest* 75:320–324, 1979.
25. Ralph-Edwards C, Pearson FG: Atypical presentation of spontaneous pneumomediastinum. *Ann Thorac Surg* 58:1758–1760, 1994.
26. Schowengerdt CG, Suyemoto R, Main FB: Granulomatous and fibrous mediastinitis: A review and analysis of 180 cases. *J Thorac Cardiovasc Surg* 57:365–379, 1969.
27. Shields TW: The mediastinum and its compartments, in Shields TW (ed): *Mediastinal Surgery.* Philadelphia, Lea & Febiger, 1991, p 4.
28. Urschel HC, Razzuk MA, Netto GJ, et al: Sclerosing mediastinitis: Improved management with histoplasmosis titer and ketoconazole. *Ann Thorac Surg* 50:215–221, 1990.
29. Wells WJ, Fox AH, Theodore PR, et al: Aspergillosis of the posterior mediastinum. *Ann Thorac Surg* 57:1240–1243, 1994.
30. Wheatley MJ, Stirling MC, Kirsh MM, et al: Descending necrotizing mediastinitis: Transcervical drainage is not enough. *Ann Thorac Surg* 49:780–784, 1990.
31. Wright CD, Mathisen DJ, Wain JL, et al: Reinforced primary repair of thoracic esophageal perforation. *Ann Thorac Surg* 60:245–249, 1995.

CHAPTER 95

CONGENITAL CYSTS OF THE MEDIASTINUM: BRONCHOPULMONARY FOREGUT ANOMALIES

Malcolm M. DeCamp, Jr.

Mediastinal masses represent a diverse collection of tumors arising from, and associated with, each of the organs found in the thorax. Cystic lesions account for up to 25 percent of reported mediastinal masses.[13] These cysts may be congenital or acquired or may represent cystic degeneration of a previously solid tumor. In this chapter, we focus on congenital cystic lesions within the mediastinum, specifically addressing bronchopulmonary anomalies arising from the foregut. We briefly consider simple cysts arising from or associated with the thymus and pericardium. Many other solid mediastinal neoplasms (dermoids, teratomas, thymomas, parathyroid adenomas, and thyroid goiters) may present with cystic components. These lesions are discussed in other chapters.

ANATOMY

Cysts arise in each of the three distinct anatomic regions of the mediastinum (see Chapter 96).

The *anterosuperior compartment* extends from the manubrium and the first rib inferiorly to the diaphragm. The anterior border of this region is the posterior sternal table, and the posterior margin includes the pericardium and the innominate vein. Endocrine lesions, such as thyroid goiters and cystic adenomas of the parathyroid gland, as well as thymic cysts, are found in this compartment.

The *middle mediastinum* is the site of origin of most bronchopulmonary foregut cysts. The boundaries of the middle mediastinum include the pericardial reflections superiorly and anteriorly and the diaphragm inferiorly. The posterior margin of the middle mediastinum is the anterior border of the spine. Pericardial cysts, as well as bronchogenic cysts, are found in this region.

The *posterior mediastinum* extends from the superior aspect of the first thoracic vertebral body inferiorly to the diaphragm. Its anterior border is the ventral aspect of the vertebral bodies, and it extends posteriorly to the articulation of the vertebral transverse process with each rib. The posterior mediastinum includes both costovertebral sulci and segmental nerve roots as well as the sympathetic chain. The structures found within the posterior compartment include the esophagus, both vagus nerves, the thoracic duct and azygous vein, as well as the descending aorta. Neuroenteric cysts as well as some esophageal duplication cysts are found in this area. Lesions that arise primarily within the mediastinum may extend above the chest into the neck[16] or below the diaphragm into the retroperitoneum,[19] where they present as extrathoracic mass lesions.

EPIDEMIOLOGY

In reported series of mediastinal masses, the prevalence of primary cysts ranges from 10 to 25 percent and has remained steady for the past 5 decades (Table 95-1).[3,5,13,25,44] Some minor heterogeneity over this time span is accounted for by variations in the ages of patients reported in each series. For example, the relatively low 9 percent incidence of cysts in one series from the 1970s reflects a predominance of adults in this series.[5]

TABLE 95-1

Prevalence of Primary Cysts in Reported Series of Mediastinal Tumors over the Past 50 Years

Year	n	Mediastinal Cysts (%)	Reference
1952	101	20	Sabiston & Scott[44]
1963	92	24	Heimberger et al[25]
1972	209	9	Benjamin et al[5]
1987	400	25	Davis et al[13]
1993	257	18	Azarow et al[3]

The etiology and distribution of cystic mediastinal masses are different in children and adults. Cysts of foregut origin account for only half of the lesions found in adults, whereas they constitute nearly 90 percent of cystic lesions reported in pediatric series (Table 95-2).[20,23,26,38,55] Conversely, pericardial cysts account for up to one-third of all cystic lesions in adults.[34,36] True pericardial cysts are exceedingly rare in children.[10,23] Among congenital lesions of the foregut and tracheobronchial tree seen in children—including pulmonary sequestrations, congenital lobar emphysema, cystic adenomatoid malformations, arteriovenous malformations, and bronchial atresias—simple foregut cysts (bronchogenic, enterogenous, and neurenteric) compose between 13 and 29 percent of reported cases.[4,8,12]

Although the relative frequencies of cystic and solid mediastinal masses have remained fairly constant, the advent of cross-sectional imaging techniques, such as computed tomography (CT) and magnetic resonance imaging (MRI), has increased the detection of all mediastinal lesions.

BRONCHOGENIC CYSTS

Embryology and Terminology

The primitive foregut gives rise to a variety of aerodigestive organs and tissues, beginning with the pharynx and subsequently giving rise to the larynx, upper and lower respiratory tracts, esophagus, stomach, proximal duodenum, liver, pancreas, and associated ducts (see Chapter 5). Cystic malformations of foregut origin may have a variety of epithelial linings that reflect the embryologic tissues from which they are derived. The lung bud develops caudally from the laryngotracheal tube, beginning in the fourth week of gestation. By the fifth week, the single bud has divided into right and left main bronchi, which grow into the surrounding splanchnic mesenchyme and are destined to become bronchial cartilage and smooth muscle as well as visceral pleura. Dichotomous branching of the primitive bronchi continues until

TABLE 95-2

Origin of Mediastinal Cysts

Cyst Type	All Ages (n = 289)	Pediatric Only (n = 52)
Bronchogenic	32%	54%
Enteric	15%	35%
Pericardial	35%	2%
Other	18%	9%

SOURCE: Based on Fontenelle et al,[20] Haller et al,[23] Heimburger and Battersby,[26] Pokorny and Sherman,[38] and Whittaker and Lynn.[55]

about the 24th week, when the terminal bronchioles begin to give rise to primitive alveoli.[27,31]

Throughout this period of embryogenesis, abnormal bronchi and bronchioles may form larger saccular structures, which are clinically recognized as bronchogenic cysts. Such saccular malformations may be invested by their own splanchnic mesenchyme (neopleura). Usually abutting on the trachea, carina, or hilum, they are termed *mediastinal bronchogenic cysts* (Figs. 95-1 and 95-2). Less frequently, these lesions are contained within the pulmonary parenchyma. Rarely do they maintain communication with the respiratory tract. Malformations within the lung are termed *intrapulmonary bronchogenic cysts* (Fig. 95-3).[27,29] Some investigators believe that mediastinal bronchogenic cysts arise early in the cycle of bronchial branching, whereas intrapulmonary bronchogenic cysts represent derangements later in fetal development.[15] Because they uniformly arise before alveoli form (at 28 weeks), bronchogenic cysts have no gas exchange potential even if their bronchial communications persist.

Presentation and Diagnosis

Most patients with bronchogenic cysts have symptoms at the time of diagnosis.[5,25,43] Eraklis and colleagues[17] noted life-threatening respiratory compromise in 70 percent of infants with foregut cysts. Mass effects from the cysts, which caused compression, "ball valving," or differential ventilation, were the predominant causes of distress. These neonates were often cyanotic, with wheezing or stridor, and their radiographs demonstrated inhomogeneous aeration, lobar collapse, and/or mediastinal shift. In series of nonneonatal children, up to 95 percent had symptoms. Especially in the older children, signs and symptoms of infection led the list of problems.[39]

In adults, symptomatic bronchogenic cysts are less common. In the 1950s, a report of a large series indicated that symptoms were present in about one-third of patients.[44] Most of the complaints were due to pain, cough, and dyspnea.[37,44] In more recent series, 75 to 95 percent of patients were without symptoms when the lesions were detected.[4,46] Many patients who are followed without treatment develop subtle, local symptoms and/or signs of secondary infection.

The presence of a bronchogenic cyst is suggested by plain chest radiographs in up to two-thirds of cases in any age group.[22] The usual appearance is that of a 2- to 10-cm ovoid, smooth, homogeneous mass that abuts on the mediastinum or hilum or splays the carina. An air-fluid level connotes either persistent bronchial communication or secondary infection of the cyst (Fig. 95-3). As mentioned above, some cysts (especially in infants) may exert a mass effect, causing airway compression, parenchymal atelectasis, or cardiovascular compression (Fig. 95-2B).[21] In 60 to 65 percent of patients, posteroanterior and lateral plain chest radiographs make it possible to diagnose these lesions and to document their precise location.[39]

Ultrasonography has been helpful in confirming the cystic nature of mediastinal lesions in infants and children. Prenatal

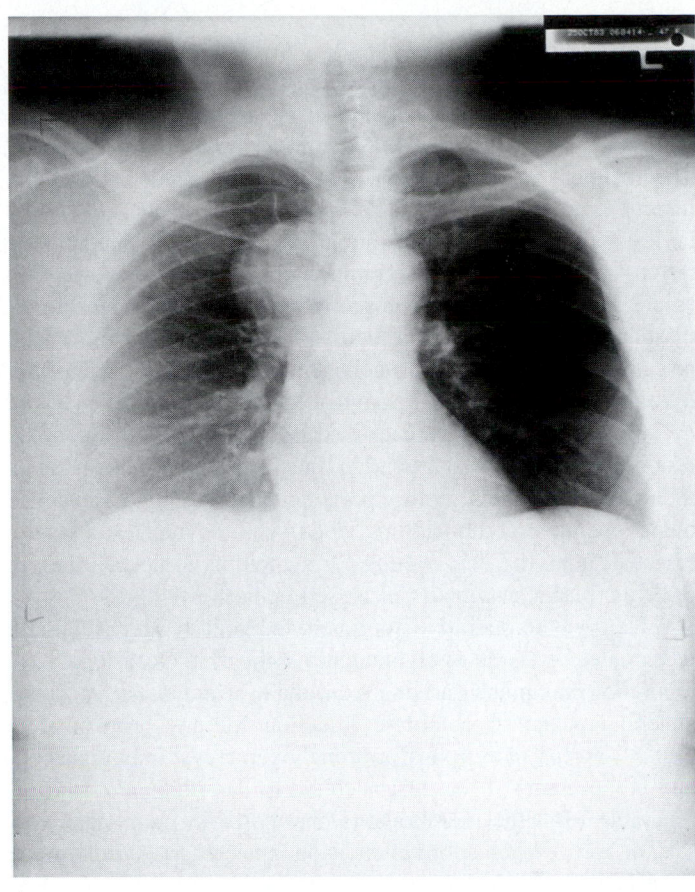

A

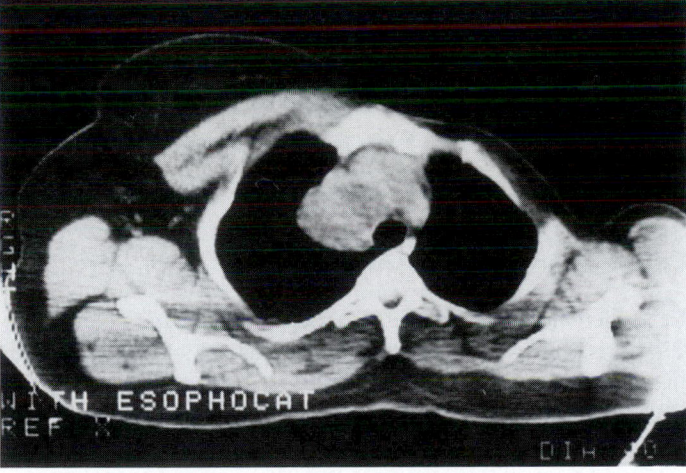

B

FIGURE 95-1   *A*. Posteroanterior radiograph of a smooth-walled paratracheal bronchogenic cyst. *B*. Computed tomogram of the same paratracheal bronchogenic cyst. Note that the cyst contents are somewhat heterogeneous but generally of lower density than the surrounding mediastinal structures.

diagnosis is also feasible.[57] Such forewarning allows for the expeditious management of these infants at the time of delivery, when most quickly develop symptoms after the lungs are inflated. In the adult, because air within the large lungs is a poor conductor of sound, surface ultrasonography has little to offer in the acoustic visualization of suspected bronchogenic cysts.

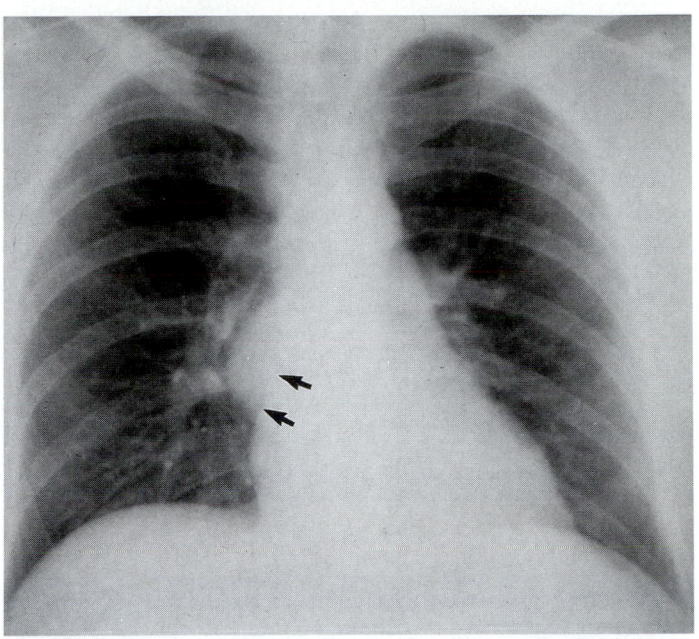

A

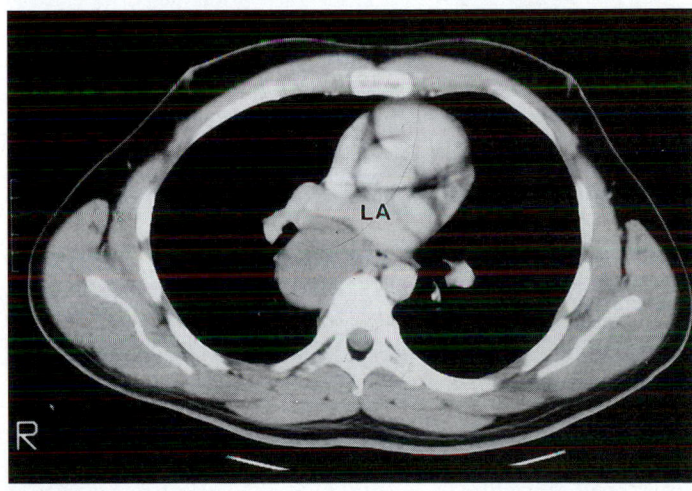

B

FIGURE 95-2   *A*. Posteroanterior radiograph of a smooth-walled subcarinal bronchogenic cyst. Note that the cyst is distinct from the right heart border (arrows). *B*. Contrast-enhanced axial CT image of the homogenous, subcarinal bronchogenic cyst. This patient presented with atrial dysrhythmia attributed to left atrial (LA) compression by the cyst. [*From DeCamp MM Jr, Swanson SJ, Sugarbaker DJ: The mediastinum, in Baue AE, Geha AS, Hammond GL, et al (eds), Glenn's Thoracic and Cardiovascular Surgery, 6th ed. Stamford, CT, Appleton & Lange, 1996, pp 643–663.*]

Cross-sectional imaging techniques, using either CT or MRI, have become the diagnostic procedures of choice for investigating mediastinal masses. These methods provide helpful details of cyst structure, including the density and type of cyst fluid, amount of calcium in the cyst wall, vascularity of the cyst, and the relationships of the cyst to adjacent mediastinal structures. MRI and CT are probably equally useful in the diagnosis of mediastinal-based cysts. CT is superior for the examination of intrapulmonary cysts because of its ability to delineate more sharply the cystic lesion from the surrounding air-filled parenchyma (Figs. 95-1, 95-2, and 95-3).[33,40]

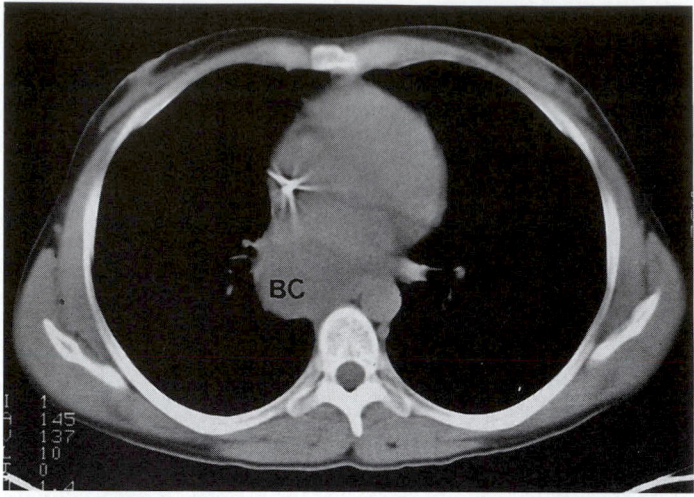

A

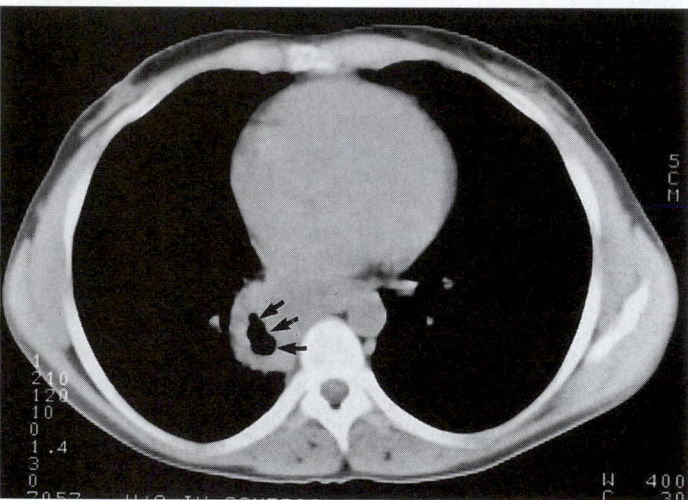

B

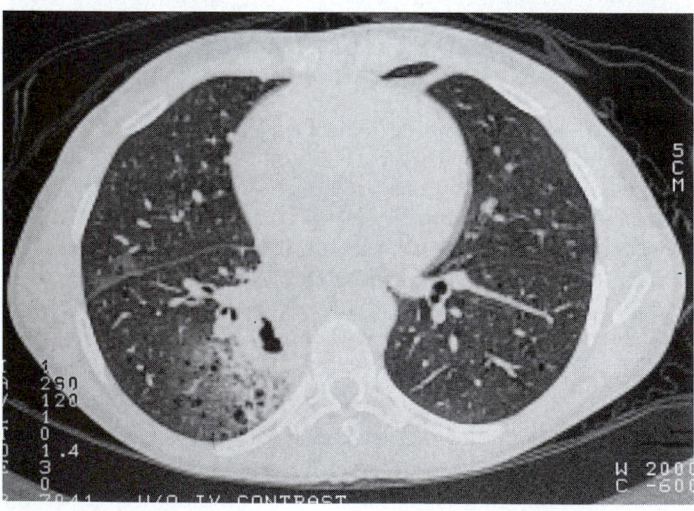

C

FIGURE 95-3 *A.* Nonenhanced CT image of an asymptomatic bronchogenic cyst (BC). *B.* Nonenhanced CT image of the same cyst after 6 months of expectant management. The cyst has "cavitated" (arrows) indicative of secondary infection. *C.* Axial CT image with "lung windows" of the infected, intraparenchymal bronchogenic cyst. Note the associated right lower lobe pneumonitis surrounding the cyst, not appreciated by the "mediastinal" window in image *B.*

Therapy

Bronchogenic cysts are the most commonly treated mediastinal foregut anomaly. They accounted for 60 percent of all mediastinal lesions reported by the Mayo Clinic over a 40-year period.[56] The treatment options for bronchogenic cysts include observation, resection, and aspiration. One option for asymptomatic simple cystic lesions is continued observation (see below). All symptomatic lesions should be removed.[9] Traditionally, a thoracotomy was necessary. Recently, videothoracoscopy has been used to resect mediastinal cysts.[24] Urschel and Horan[50] have described piecemeal resection of a mediastinal bronchogenic cyst using a Carlens mediastinoscope introduced through a small suprasternal incision.

Two large clinics advocate resection for even asymptomatic lesions.[47,37] They report a trend in time for asymptomatic patients to develop symptoms. Both reports document a higher incidence of perioperative complications when symptomatic lesions were resected, implying that waiting for symptoms to develop before resection places patients at increased operative risk.

Whatever the operative approach, the goal of surgery should be complete excision of all elements of the cyst. Occasional case reports of malignancy arising from the cyst mucosa support the general concept of complete resection for any bronchogenic cyst.[7,35] Partial resection of a bronchogenic cyst may occasionally be necessary if the cyst is found to be adherent to and inseparable from the membranous airway, main pulmonary vessels, or aorta. When subtotal excision is necessary, symptomatic recurrences requiring reexcision have been reported.[42]

Aspiration of a cyst to confirm a benign diagnosis and to instill a sclerosing agent (ethanol or bleomycin) has been used to manage some cysts. Reports of long-term follow-up for this approach to both the diagnosis and therapy of bronchogenic cysts are scant. However, it may represent a useful form of therapy for inoperable patients.[28,30]

ENTEROGENOUS CYSTS

Embryology and Terminology

Enterogenous cysts are also termed *esophageal duplications.* They arise from the elongating esophagus, which separates from the respiratory tract in about the fifth week of gestation (see Chapter 5). As with most intestinal duplications, enterogenous cysts represent failure of normal recanalization during embryogenesis. Most esophageal duplications are of the closed and cystic type. Rarely are they tubular, and communication is preserved with the alimentary tract.[31]

Presentation and Diagnosis

Nearly 75 percent of esophageal duplication cysts are recognized in childhood. For unclear reasons, there is a two-to-one predilection for cysts to be on the right side.[54] Symptoms commonly include cough and dyspnea and occasionally stridor. These are clearly related to a mass effect by the cyst on the nearby respiratory tract. Dysphagia is surprisingly infrequent. In asymptomatic patients, the most common clue leading to this diagnosis is the coexistence of other gastrointestinal duplication(s). Unlike bronchogenic cysts, which are always lined with respiratory mucosa, enterogenous cysts may have a variety of epithelial linings, including the squamous epithelium native to the esophagus. However, most esophageal duplications have a glandular epithelium with a subset that contains gastric mucosa containing parietal cells capable of acid secretion. The finding of an acid-secreting mucosa in 60 percent of patients with enterogenous cysts lends credence to other case reports of cyst hemorrhage and rupture.[32]

Esophageal duplications usually present radiographically as smooth-walled, posterior mediastinal lesions at the base of the right hemithorax (Fig. 95-4A). A barium swallow demonstrates deviation of the lumen around the cyst, but rarely shows communication with it (Fig. 95-4B). Proximal esophageal dilatation is not common because the cysts usually are not obstructive. In patients with suspected duplication, a technetium pertechnetate nuclear scan may suggest the presence of ectopic gastric mucosa within the chest.[45] Cross-sectional imaging (CT or MRI) is almost routinely employed to characterize the contents of a cyst and to define the relationship of the cyst to contiguous structures (Fig. 95-4C). Endoesophageal ultrasound has provided a useful, minimally invasive tool to investigate these lesions and to allow sampling of cyst contents to confirm that the lesion, in an otherwise asymptomatic patient, is benign.[51]

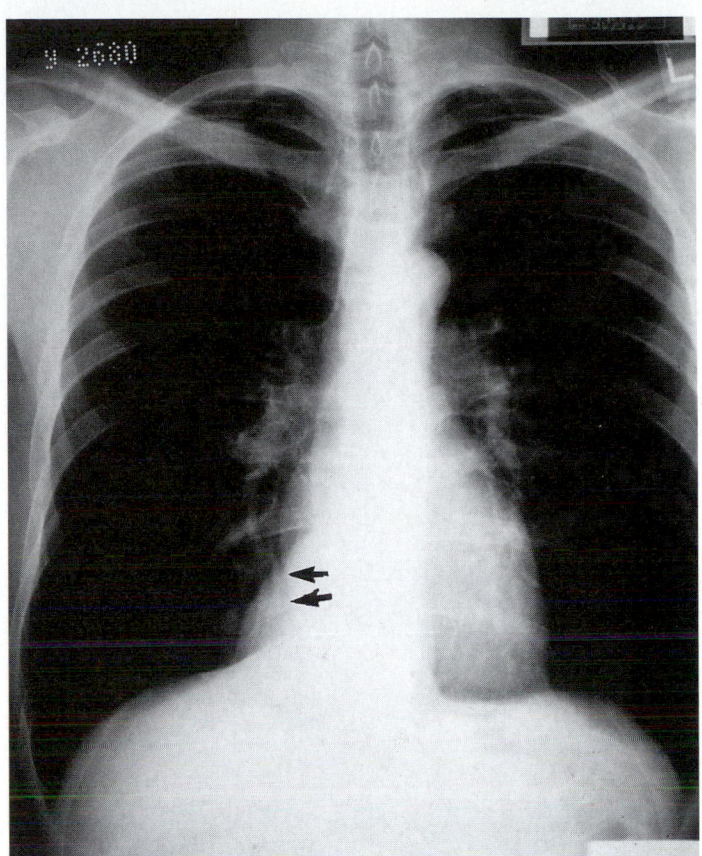

A

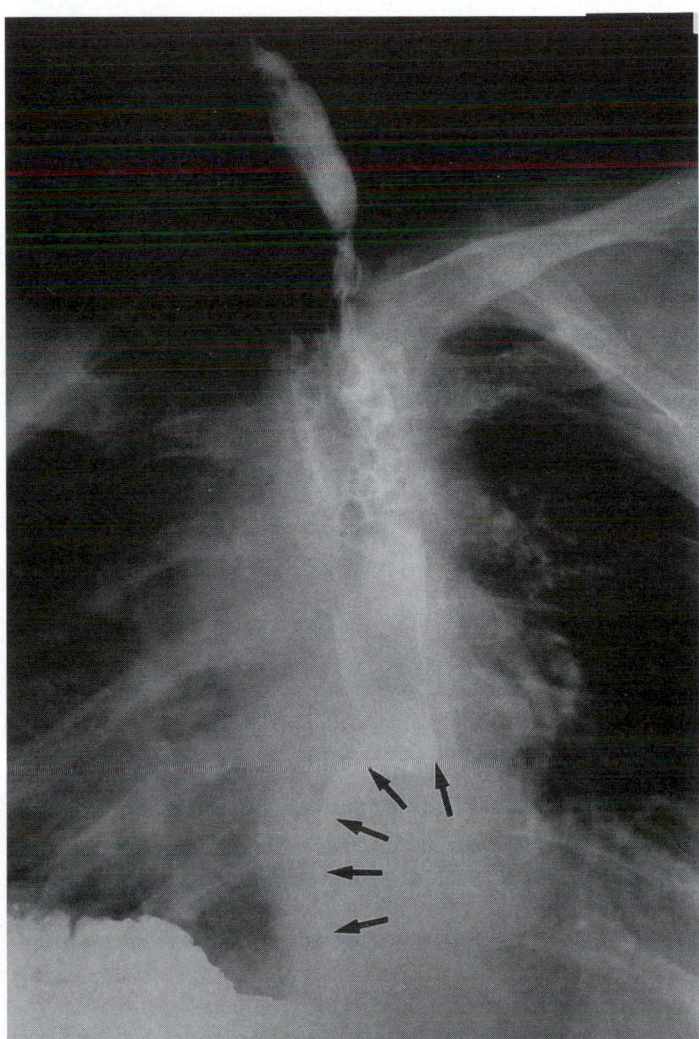

B

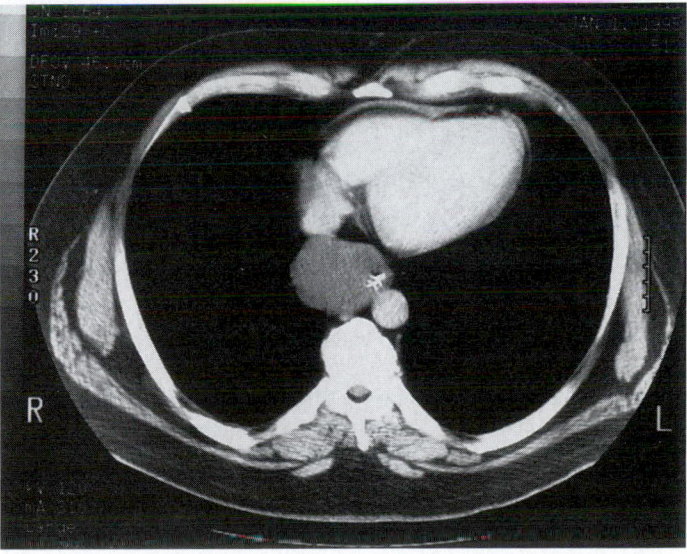

C

FIGURE 95-4 *A.* Frontal radiograph demonstrating smooth-walled posterior mediastinal mass consistent with an enterogenous cyst. The lesion is easily separable from the right heart border (arrows). *B.* Barium esophogram of the same patient demonstrating deviation of the true esophageal lumen around the smooth extramucosal lesion, found at resection to be an enterogenous cyst (esophageal duplication). *C.* Oral and intravenous contrast-enhanced CT image of the enterogenous cyst. The lesion is radiographically inseparable from the esophagus but free of all cardiac structures.

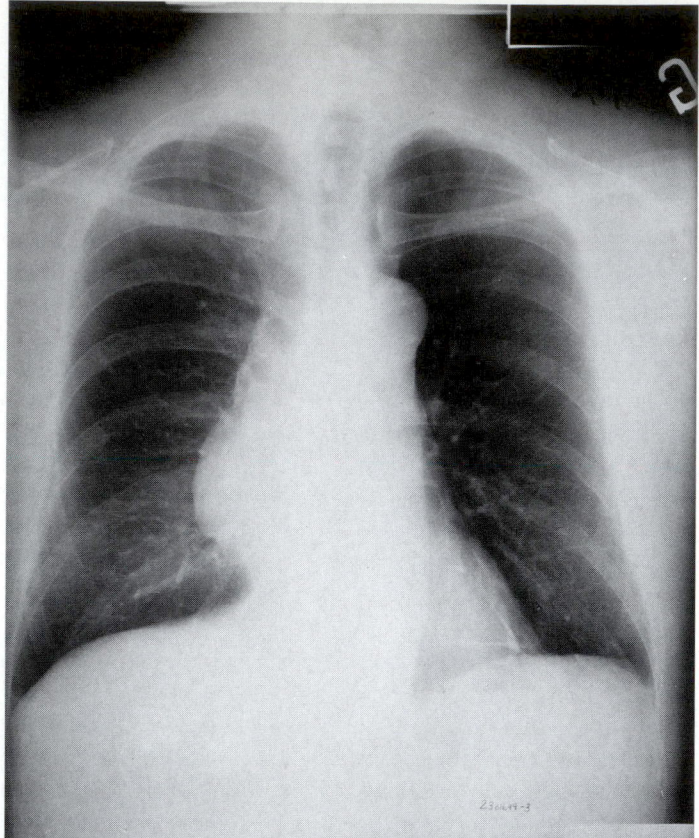

A

B

FIGURE 95-5 *A.* Frontal radiograph of an anterior mediastinal mass inseparable from the right heart border. *B.* Axial CT image of this mass demonstrates its thick, focally calcified (arrows) wall containing homogenous nonenhancing fluid. At resection what was feared to be a teratoma was found to be a thymic cyst. [*From DeCamp MM Jr, Swanson SJ, Sugarbaker DJ: The mediastinum,* in Baue AE, Geha AS, Hammond GL, et al (eds), *Glenn's Thoracic and Cardiovascular Surgery, 6th ed. Stamford, CT, Appleton & Lange, 1966, pp 643–663.*]

Therapy

As in the case of bronchogenic cysts, esophageal duplications are likely to become infected in time. The common occurrence of gastric mucosa within the enterogenous cyst predisposes to spontaneous hemorrhage and/or ulceration. Because of existing symptoms or the natural history of the cyst to become symptomatic, resection is recommended for all enterogenous cysts.

Such lesions can be approached through a standard thoracotomy or, at experienced centers, with the videothoracoscope.[14] Despite the lack of communication with the esophageal lumen, cyst resection may leave defects in the esophageal wall that must be meticulously repaired. The esophagus should be closed primarily in layers, and the repair should be reinforced with a locally procured flap of vascularized tissue. Options for buttressing, such as esophageal repair, include the pericardial fat pad, pleura, intercostal muscle, the pericardium itself, or omentum. A case report documenting the occurrence of an adenocarcinoma in an esophageal duplication, which was carefully followed for a long time, underscores the need for resection of these lesions at the time of diagnosis.[35]

NEURENTERIC CYSTS

Embryology and Terminology

During the third week of normal embryogenesis, the notochord should separate from the primitive foregut (see Chapter 5). If this separation is incomplete, the mesodermal masses, which normally encircle the neural tube, cannot enclose it and vertebral anomalies arise. The attached foregut often spawns an associated mediastinal enteric cyst.[2,48] The bony abnormalities may include butterfly vertebrae, hemivertebrae, and anterior spina bifida.[22] When enterogenous cysts are found associated or contiguous with vertebral anomalies, the cyst is considered neurenteric.

Presentation and Diagnosis

Neurenteric cysts are exceedingly rare. Virtually all present in childhood. More than half of afflicted children have CNS complaints or findings. These include back pain, motor deficits of a lower extremity, and gait disturbance.[22,48] The diagnosis is usually made after detection of vertebral anomalies on the chest radiograph. CT can define the specifics of bony abnormalities and demonstrate extension of the cystic lesion into the spinal canal. This study must often be combined with the injection of intrathecal contrast in order to obtain a CT myelogram. MRI has recently supplanted CT myelography. Because of its ability to image in the axial, coronal, and sagittal planes and the availability of gadolinium as an enhancing agent, MRI provides a complete, noninvasive assessment of the bony abnormality, the intraspinal extent of the cyst, and the degree of spinal cord or nerve root compression associated with a neurenteric cyst.[22,53] Any suspected neurenteric cyst warrants an MRI evaluation of both the thoracic spine and posterior mediastinum.

Therapy

This form of congenital cyst accounts for only 5 to 10 percent of all foregut lesions.[26] These cysts are consistently associated with some bony anomaly of the spine. The spectrum of vertebral anomalies extends from fused vertebrae to include butterfly or hemivertebrae. The vertebral abnormality is usually cephalad to the cystic lesion, since the esophagus descends (or the pharynx ascends) during fetal development.[27] Careful imaging of suspected neuroenteric cysts is paramount for successful extirpation. MRI is useful to exclude extension of the cystic component into a neural foramen or the spinal canal proper and to exclude an associated meningocele.[22] Such findings would require a staged resection employing a posterior neurosurgical approach

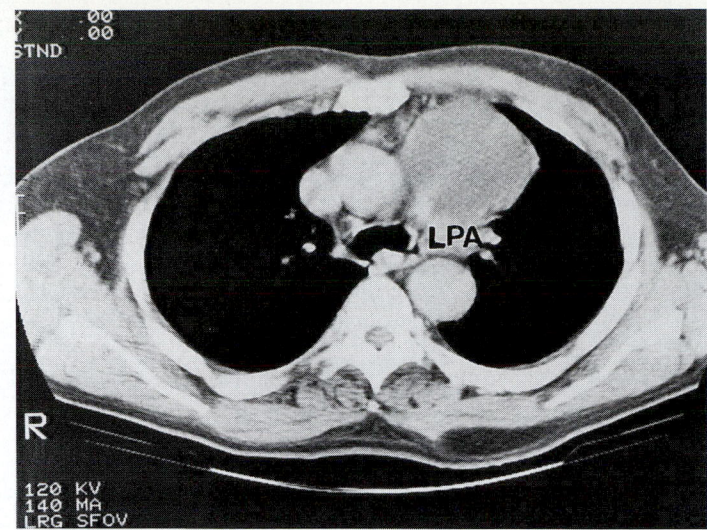

A

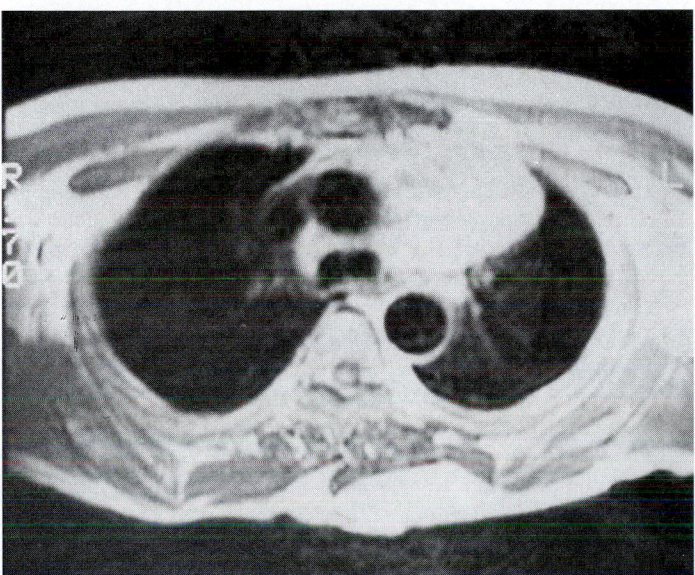

B

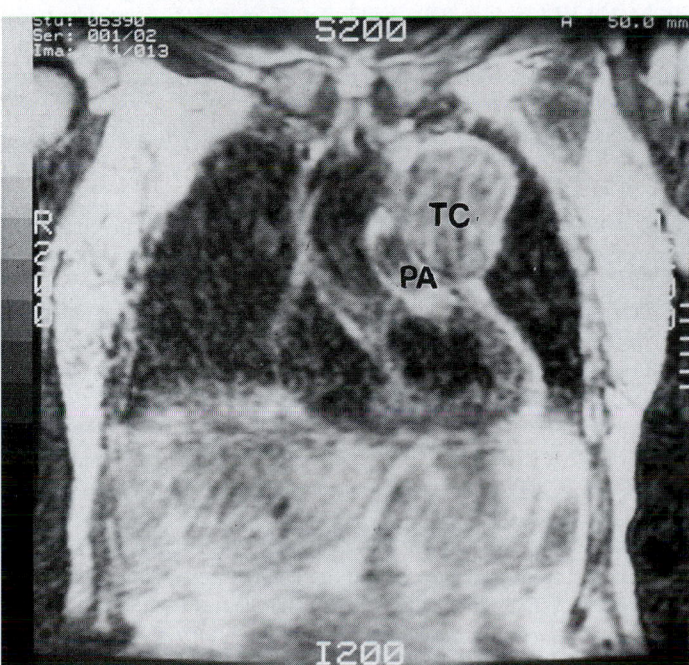

C

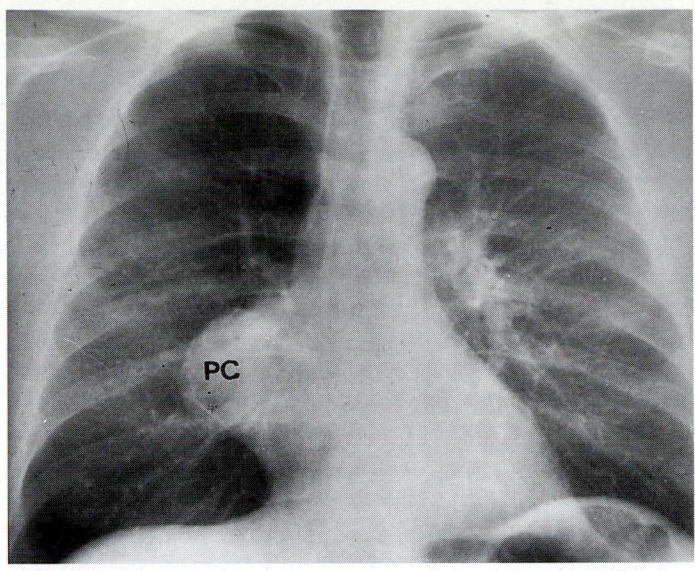

FIGURE 95-7 Frontal radiograph of a mediastinal mass, isodense with and inseparable from the right heart border. Thoracoscopy showed this to be a broadly based pericardial cyst (PC).

first, to decompress the cord or its nerve roots, followed by resection of the mediastinal component by standard thoracotomy or video-assisted technique.[1]

THYMIC CYSTS

The thymus is derived from the third pharyngeal pouch (see Chapter 5). Its development is incomplete at birth, and the gland continues to grow throughout childhood into adolescence. Cysts within the gland are thought to occur during adulthood, when gland architecture involutes and central cells degenerate and are replaced by fat.[41]

Thymic cysts are rare congenital or acquired lesions embryologically derived from the pharyngeal pouches. Although thymic cysts are benign, they must be distinguished from thymomas, germ cell tumors, and lymphomas—all of which may have areas of cystic degeneration.[6,49] These cysts arise in the anterior mediastinum (Fig. 95-5) and may extend to the middle mediastinal compartment, especially in the aortopulmonary window (Fig. 95-6). Both CT and MRI demonstrate clear tissue plains separating the cyst from other vital structures (Figs. 95-5 and 95-6). In older people, benign cysts may degenerate and present as a complex, thickened cystic mass with calcified walls that contain heterogeneous fluid (Fig. 95-5). Such lesions are easily confused with a mediastinal teratoma. Excision using an open or video-assisted technique excludes other, more worrisome histologies and is curative.[41]

PERICARDIAL CYSTS

Pericardial cysts are exceedingly rare in children, suggesting that they may be acquired. However, their common position at or near the cardiophrenic angles suggests a possible embryologic defect,

FIGURE 95-6 Equivalent axial-enhanced CT (*A*) and axial MRI (*B*) images of an aortopulmonary window mass that appears to compress if not invade the left pulmonary artery (LPA). Coronal MR image (C) of the same lesion demonstrating an intact tissue plane separating the benign thymic cyst (TC) from the pulmonary artery (PA).

whereby fusion of the pleuropericardial membranes and the septum transversum of the developing diaphragm is incomplete.[31]

Pericardial cysts are simple, smooth-walled cystic lesions (Fig. 95-7) that are commonly located at the lateral basal edge of the pericardium, where it fuses with the diaphragm. They can be mistaken for foramen of Morgagni hernias or prominent pericardial fat pads. They can be differentiated from more solid mediastinal tumors by CT scanning with a computer analysis of the radiographic density of cyst fluid.[18] Pericardial cysts characteristically contain clear, low-density serous fluid; hence their synonym, "spring water cysts." They have no malignant potential and, after aspiration has confirmed the diagnosis, can be followed clinically. Resection should be reserved for cysts that cause symptoms (hemodynamic compromise, arrhythmia, atelectasis) or for change in radiographic appearance over time.[11,52] Because a cyst often overlies a phrenic nerve, an unroofing procedure or subtotal resection is acceptable therapy if total excision would jeopardize diaphragmatic function. Rarely do pericardial cysts erode into vital structures. Such cases suggest secondary infection of the cyst and may require circulatory support for safe extirpation.[11]

REFERENCES

1. Allen MS, Payne WS: Cystic foregut malformation in the mediastinum. *Chest Surg Clin North Am* 2:89–106, 1992.
2. Alrabeeah A, Gillis DA, Giacomantonio M, Lau H: Neurenteric cysts—a spectrum. *J Pediatr Surg* 23:752–754, 1988.
3. Azarow KS, Pearl RH, Zurcher R, et al: Primary mediastinal masses: A comparison of adult and pediatric populations. *J Thorac Cardiovasc Surg* 106:67–72, 1993.
4. Bailey PV, Tracy T Jr, Connors RH, et al: Congenital bronchopulmonary malformations: Diagnostic and therapeutic considerations. *J Thorac Cardiovasc Surg* 99:597–602, 1990.
5. Benjamin SP, McCormack LJ, Effer DB, Grover LK: Primary tumors of the mediastinum. *Chest* 62:297–303, 1972.
6. Benjamin SP, McCormack LJ, Effler DB, et al: Primary lymphatic tumors of the mediastinum. *Cancer* 30:708–712, 1972.
7. Bernheim J, Griffel B, Versano S, Bruderman I: Mediastinal leiomyosarcoma in the wall of a bronchial cyst (letter). *Arch Pathol Lab Med* 104:221, 1980.
8. Bogers AJ, Hazebroek FW, Molenaar J, Bos E: Surgical treatment of congenital bronchopulmonary disease in children. *Eur J Cardiothorac Surg* 7:117–120, 1993.
9. Bolton JW, Shahian DM: Asymptomatic bronchogenic cysts: What is the best management? *Ann Thorac Surg* 53:1134–1137, 1992.
10. Bower RJ, Kiesewetter WB: Mediastinal masses in infants and children. *Arch Surg* 112:1003–1009, 1977.
11. Chopra PS, Duke DJ, Pellett JR, Rahko PS: Pericardial cyst with partial erosion of the right ventricular wall. *Ann Thorac Surg* 51:840–841, 1991.
12. Coran AG, Drongowski R: Congenital cystic disease of the tracheobronchial tree in infants and children: Experience with 44 consecutive cases. *Arch Surg* 129:521–527, 1994.
13. Davis RD Jr, Oldham HN Jr, Sabiston DC Jr: Primary cysts and neoplasms of the mediastinum: Recent changes in clinical presentation, methods of diagnosis, management and results. *Ann Thorac Surg* 44:229–237, 1987.
14. DeCamp MM, Jaklitsch MT, Mentzer SJ, et al: The safety and versatility of video-thoracoscopy: A prospective analysis of 895 consecutive cases. *J Am Coll Surg* 81:113–120, 1995.
15. DeFossez SM, DeLuca SA: Bronchogenic cysts. *Am Fam Physician* 39:129–132, 1989.
16. Downey RJ, Cerfolio RJ, Deschamp C, et al: Mediastinal parathyroid cysts. *Mayo Clin Proc* 70:946–950, 1995.
17. Eraklis AJ, Griscom NT, McGovern JB: Bronchogenic cysts of the mediastinum in infancy. *Nev Engl J Med* 281:1150–1155, 1969.
18. Feigin DS, Fenoglio JJ, McAllister HA, Madewell JE: Pericardial cysts: A radiologic-pathologic correlation and review. *Radiology* 125:15–20, 1977.
19. Foerster HM, Sengupta EE, Montag AG, Kaplan EL: Retroperitoneal bronchogenic cyst presenting as an adrenal mass. *Arch Pathol Lab Med* 115:1057–1059, 1991.
20. Fontenelle LJ, Armstrong RG, Stanford W, et al: The asymptomatic mediastinal mass. *Arch Surg* 102:98–102, 1971.
21. Fratellone PM, Coplan N, Friedman M, Stelzner P: Hemodynamics compromise secondary to a mediastinal bronchogenic cyst. *Chest* 106:610–612, 1994.
22. Haddon MJ, Bowen A: Bronchopulmonary and neurenteric forms of foregut anomalies: Imaging for diagnosis and management. *Radiol Clin North Am* 29:241–254, 1991.
23. Haller JA Jr, Mazur DO, Morgan WW Jr: Diagnosis and management of mediastinal masses in children. *J Thorac Cardiovasc Surg* 58:385–393, 1969.
24. Hazelrigg SR, Landreneau RJ, Mack MJ, Acuff TE: Thoracoscopic resection of mediastinal cysts. *Ann Thorac Surg* 56:659–660, 1993.
25. Heimberger I, Battersby JS, Vellios F: Primary neoplasms of the mediastinum: A fifteen-year experience. *Arch Surg* 86:978–984, 1963.
26. Heimburger IL, Battersby JS: Primary mediastinal tumors of childhood. *J Thorac Cardiovasc Surg* 50:92–103, 1965.
27. Heithoff KB, Sane SM, Williams HJ, et al: Bronchopulmonary foregut malformations: A unifying etiological concept. *Am J Roentgenol* 126:46–55, 1976.
28. Johnston SR, Adam A, Allison DJ, et al: Recurrent respiratory obstruction from a mediastinal bronchogenic cyst. *Thorax* 47:660–662, 1992.
29. Kirwan WO, Walbaum PR, McCormack RJ: Cystic endothoracic derivatives of the foregut and their complications. *Thorax* 28:424–428, 1973.
30. Malde HM, Kedar RP, Chadda DJ: Ethanol sclerosis of a mediastinal cyst. *Can Assoc Radiol J* 44:310–312, 1993.
31. Moore KL: *The Developing Human: Clinically Oriented Embryology.* Philadelphia, Saunders, 1977.
32. Nakahara F, Fujii Y, Miyoshi S, et al: Acute symptoms due to a huge duplication cyst ruptured into the esophagus. *Ann Thorac Surg* 50:309–311, 1990.
33. Nakata H, Nakayama C, Kimoto T, et al: Computed tomography of mediastinal bronchogenic cysts. *J Comput Assist Tomogr* 6:733–738, 1982.
34. Oldham HN Jr, Sabiston DC Jr: Primary tumors and cysts of the mediastinum. *Monogr Surg Sci* 4:243–279, 1967.
35. Olsen JB, Clemmensen O, Andersen K: Adenocarcinoma arising in a foregut cyst of the mediastinum. *Ann Thorac Surg* 51:497–499, 1991.
36. Parish JM, Rosenow EC III, Muhm JR, Rosenow EC: Mediastinal masses: Clues to interpretation of radiological studies. *Postgrad Med* 76:173–186, 1984.
37. Patel SR, Meeker DP, Biscotti CV, et al: Presentation and management of bronchogenic cysts in the adult. *Chest* 106:79–85, 1994.
38. Pokorny WJ, Sherman JO: Mediastinal masses in infants and children. *J Thorac Cardiovasc Surg* 68:869–875, 1974.
39. Ramenofsky ML, Leape LL, McCauley RG: Bronchogenic cyst. *J Pediatr Surg* 14:219–224, 1979.

40. Rappaport DC, Herman SJ, Weisbrod GL: Congenital bronchopulmonary diseases in adults: CT findings. *AJR Am J Roentgenol* 162: 1295–1299, 1994.

41. Rastegar H, Arger P, Harken AH: Evaluation and therapy of mediastinal thymic cyst. *Am Surg* 46:236–238, 1980.

42. Read CA, Moront M, Carangelo R, et al: Recurrent bronchogenic cyst: An assessment for complete surgical excision. *Arch Surg* 126: 1306–1308, 1991.

43. Ribet ME, Copin MC, Gosselin B: Bronchogenic cysts of the mediastinum. *J Thorac Cardiovasc Surg* 109:1003–1010, 1995.

44. Sabiston DC Jr, Scott HW Jr: Primary neoplasms and cysts of the mediastinum. *Ann Surg* 136:777–797, 1952.

45. Sfakianakis GN, Conway JJ: Detection of ectopic gastric mucosa in Meckel's diverticulum and in other aberrations by scintigraphy: 1. Pathophysiology and 10-year clinical experience. *J Nucl Med* 22:647–654, 1981.

46. St.-Georges R, Deslauriers J, Duranceau A: Clinical spectrum of bronchogenic cysts of the mediastinum and lung in the adult. *Ann Thorac Surg* 52:6–13, 1991.

47. Suen HC, Mathisen DJ, Grillo HC, et al: Surgical management and radiological characteristics of bronchogenic cysts. *Ann Thorac Surg* 55:476–481, 1993.

48. Superina RA, Ein SH, Humphreys RP: Cystic duplications of the esophagus and neurenteric cysts. *J Pediatr Surg* 19:527–530, 1984.

49. Suster S, Rosai J: Cystic thymomas: A clinicopathologic study of ten cases. *Cancer* 69:92–97, 1992.

50. Urschel JD, Horan TA: Mediastinoscopic treatment of mediastinal cysts. *Ann Thorac Surg* 58:1698–1700, 1994.

51. Van Dam J, Rice TW, Sivak MV Jr: Endoscopic ultrasonography and endoscopically guided needle aspiration for the diagnosis of upper gastrointestinal tract foregut cysts. *Am J Gastroenterol* 87: 762–765, 1992.

52. Vlay SC, Hartman AR: Mechanical treatment of atrial fibrillation: Removal of a pericardial cyst by thoracoscopy. *Am Heart J* 129: 616–618, 1995.

53. von Schulthess GK, McMurdo K, et al: Mediastinal masses: MR imaging. *Radiology* 158:289–296, 1986.

54. Whitaker JA, Deffenbaugh LD, Cooke AR: Esophageal duplication cyst. *Am J Gastroenterol* 73:329–332, 1980.

55. Whittaker LD, Lynn HB: Mediastinal tumors and cysts in the pediatric patient. *Surg Clin North Am* 58:893–904, 1973.

56. Wychulis AR, Payne WS, Clagett OT, Woolner LB: Surgical treatment of mediastinal tumors: A 40 year experience. *J Thorac Cardiovasc Surg* 62:379–392, 1971.

57. Young G, L'Heureux PR, Krueckeberg ST, Swanson DA: Mediastinal bronchogenic cyst: Prenatal sonographic diagnosis. *AJR Am J Roentgenol* 152:125–127, 1989.

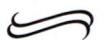

ACQUIRED LESIONS OF THE MEDIASTINUM: BENIGN AND MALIGNANT

John R. Roberts / Larry R. Kaiser

HISTORY

MEDIASTINAL COMPARTMENTS
Anterosuperior Compartment
Middle Compartment
Posterior Compartment

EPIDEMIOLOGY AND INCIDENCE

SIGNS AND SYMPTOMS

INVESTIGATION OF MEDIASTINAL MASSES
Noninvasive Diagnostic Procedures
Invasive Biopsy Procedures

MEDIASTINAL INFECTIONS
Transsternal Esophageal Procedures
Esophageal Perforations
Acute Descending Necrotizing Mediastinitis

LESIONS MASQUERADING AS MEDIASTINAL TUMORS
Substernal Goiter
Cystic Hygromas
Lesions Originating from the Thoracic Skeleton
Extramedullary Hematopoiesis
Vascular Lesions
Esophageal Lesions
Pulmonary Lesions
Subdiaphragmatic Lesions

ANTERIOR MEDIASTINAL NEOPLASMS
Lesions of the Thymus
Tumors of Lymph Nodes
Germ Cell Tumors

MIDDLE MEDIASTINAL MASSES
Bronchogenic Cysts
Esophageal Cysts
Neuroenteric Cysts
Mesothelial Cysts

POSTERIOR MEDIASTINAL MASSES
Neurogenic Tumors
Tumors of Nerve Sheath Origin

ENDOCRINE TUMORS
Mediastinal Pheochromocytoma
Parathyroid Adenomas

OTHER MEDIASTINAL TUMORS
Mesenchymal Tumors
Fatty Tumors

SUPERIOR VENA CAVA SYNDROME

Lesions that originate in the mediastinum are rare compared to the diverse lesions that can involve the mediastinum secondarily. Although neoplasms of the mediastinum are diverse, they have in common a single clinical manifestation: widening of the mediastinum on the chest radiograph taken in the upright position. This shared feature has not lent itself readily to differential diagnosis. In recent years, however, the advent of computed tomography (CT) and magnetic resonance imaging (MRI) has greatly enhanced the evaluation and subsequent treatment of these lesions.

The mediastinum extends from the thoracic inlet to the diaphragm superoinferiorly and from pleural space to pleural space (Fig. 96-1). Contained within it are heart, aorta, brachiocephalic vein, esophagus, tracheobronchial tree, and elements of the autonomic nervous system and the lymphatic system. Further, various endocrine organs may project into it, distant malignancies may metastasize to it, and infectious processes can manifest themselves within it.

This chapter focuses on lesions that either originate in the mediastinum or represent disease processes of the mediastinum.

HISTORY

The history of the diseases of the mediastinum derives mostly from the impact of study of three specific entities—substernal goiters, ectopic parathyroid glands, and myasthenia gravis. Substernal extension of goiters into the mediastinum was first described in the middle of the eighteenth century. Billroth described resection of goiters in 1869.[6] Kocher subsequently reported 1000 thyroidec-

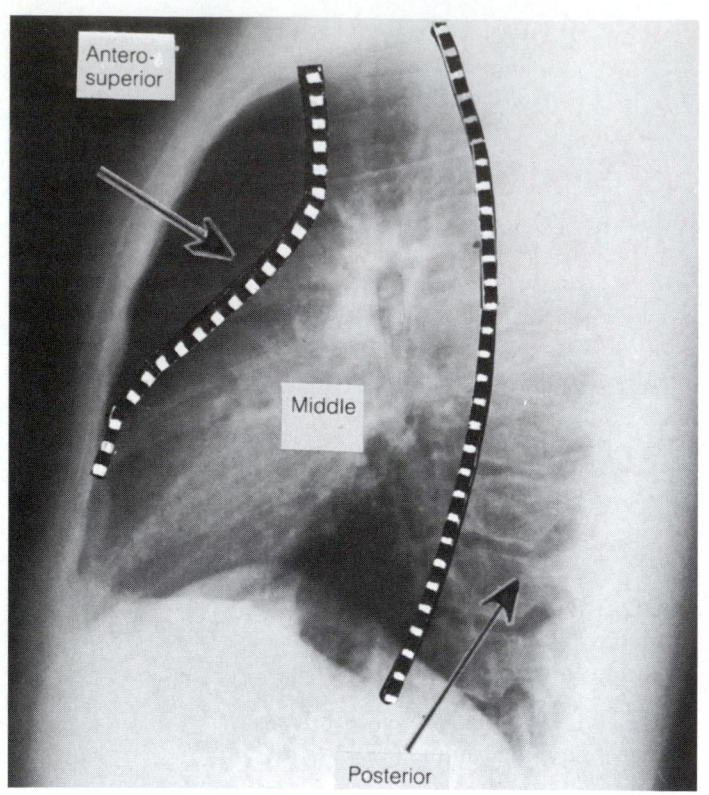

A

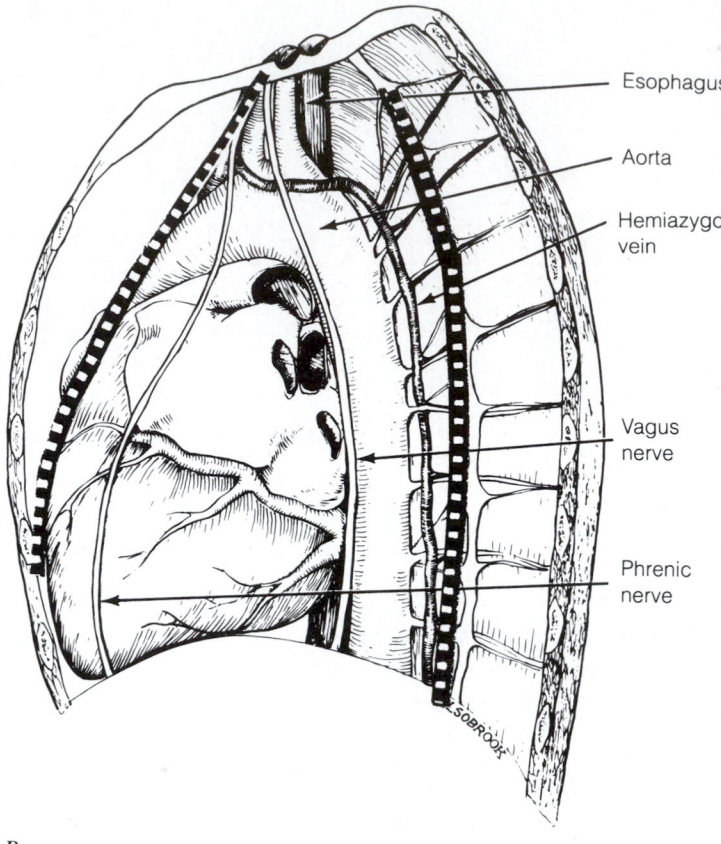

Esophagus

Aorta

Hemiazygos vein

Vagus nerve

Phrenic nerve

B

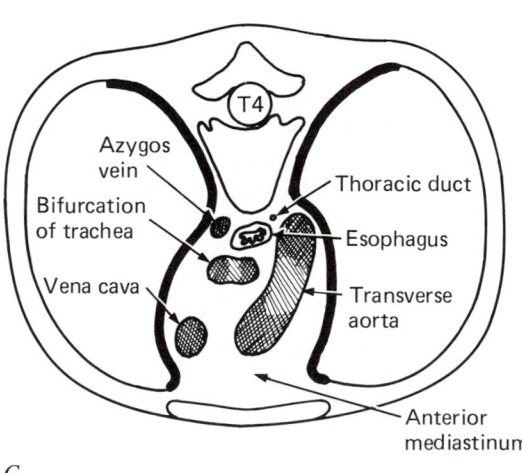

C

FIGURE 96-1 Compartments of the mediastinum. *A.* Lateral radiograph of chest. *B.* Schematic representation of the contents of the three mediastinal compartments. *C.* Cross sections of the thorax at T4 (left) and T8 (right) to show relative positions of mediastinal structures.

[*Based on the data of Lyerly and Sabiston, Primary neoplasms and cysts of the mediastinum, Fishman (ed) Pulmonary Diseases and Disorders, 2d ed. New York, McGraw-Hill, 1988, with permission.*]

tomies and he described techniques for removing substernal goiters.[35] Churchill first described recognition of ectopic mediastinal parathyroid glands, and Creswell and Wells subsequently reported a series of more than 6000 patients who underwent parathyroidectomy. Two percent of those patients required sternotomy for resection of a parathyroid gland in the mediastinum.[13]

Early knowledge of myasthenia gravis also developed largely from the work of German clinicians, who described the symptom triad of ptosis, dysarthria, and weakness in the late 1800s. Jolly unified these findings and coined the term *myasthenia gravis pseudoparalytica* in 1885.[29]. Laquer and Weigert connected the manifestations of myasthenia gravis to thymic disease in 1901.[36] Not until 1974, however, were the autoimmune aspects of the disease clarified when Almon and colleagues described serum antibodies to the acetylcholine receptor.[3]

Blalock's performed the first thymic resection via median sternotomy at Johns Hopkins Hospital in 1936.[7] In 1944, Blalock reported a series of 20 patients who had undergone thymic resection and advocated thymectomy for patients with myasthenia gravis.[7] This approach has an appreciable mortality, however, so a transcervical approach for patients with nonthymomatous myasthenia gravis is now preferred in some clinics.

MEDIASTINAL COMPARTMENTS

The mediastinum has been variably described by different authors. As shown in Fig. 96-1, the simplest system divides the mediastinum into three compartments: anterosuperior, visceral (or middle), and paravertebral (or posterior).

Anterosuperior Compartment

This compartment extends from the manubrium and the first ribs to the diaphragm. Its posterior border is defined by the anterior aspect of the pericardium inferiorly and curves posteriorly to include the arch of the aorta and great vessels. Structures contained within it include the ascending aorta, the superior vena cava, the azygous vein, the thymus gland, lymph nodes, fat, connective tissue, transverse aorta, and great vessels (Table 96-1). Common major lesions contained within the anterosuperior mediastinal compartment are thymomas, lymphomas, and germ cell tumors (Table 96-1; Fig. 96-2). Less common lesions are tumors of mesenchymal origin, vascular lesions, and displaced thyroid or parathyroid glands.

Middle Compartment

The middle compartment is also called the visceral compartment (Fig. 96-1). The superior pericardial reflection defines the superior border, while the diaphragm defines the inferior border. The posterior border extends to the spine. Contained within this compartment are the heart and pericardium, trachea and major bronchi, pulmonary vessels, lymph nodes, fat, and connective tissue (Table 96-1). Lesions contained within the visceral compartment include cysts of the foregut, primary and secondary tumors of the lymph nodes, and, less commonly, pleural, pericardial, neuroenteric and gastroenteric cysts (Table 96-1, Fig. 96-2).

Posterior Compartment

The posterior compartment is also called the paravertebral compartment. It extends from the superior aspect of the first thoracic vertebral body to the diaphragm anteriorly and then posteriorly to the posterior-most curvature of the ribs (Fig. 96-1). Contained within it are the sympathetic chain, vagus nerves, esophagus, thoracic duct, various lymph nodes, and the descending aorta. Lesions contained within it are primarily tumors of neurogenic ori-

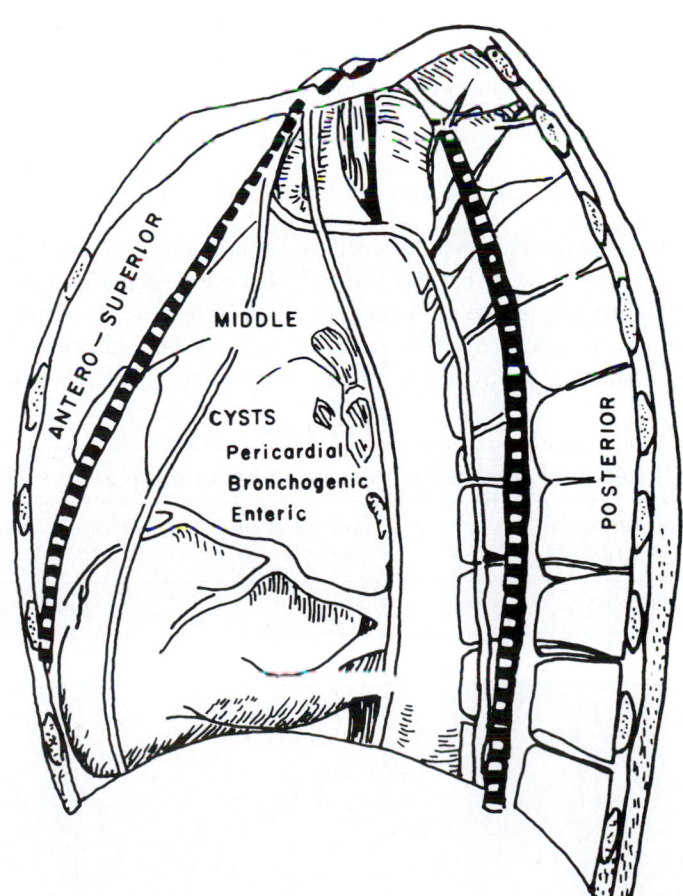

TUMORS
  THYMOMAS
    Benign
    Malignant
  LYMPHOMAS
    Hodgkin's disease
    Lymphocytic lymphoma
    Lymphocytic /
      histiocytic lymphoma
    Histiocytic lymphoma
    Undifferentiated lymphoma
  TERATODERMOIDS
    Benign
    Malignant
  GERM CELL TUMORS
    Seminoma
    Embryonal carcinoma
    Choriocarcinoma
  PARATHYROID ADENOMA

NEUROGENIC TUMORS
  Neurofibroma
  Neurilemoma
  Neurosarcoma
  Ganglioneuroma
  Ganglioneuroblastoma
  Neuroblastoma
  Chemodectoma
  Pheochromocytoma

ANTERO-SUPERIOR MIDDLE CYSTS Pericardial Bronchogenic Enteric POSTERIOR

FIGURE 96-2 Most common location of specific neoplasms and cysts within the subdivisions of the mediastinum.

TABLE 96-1

Structures and Lesions in the Three Compartments of the Mediastinum

Structures	Common Lesions	Rare Lesions
Anterosuperior compartment		
Ascending aorta	Thymomas	Vascular lesions
Superior vena cava	Lymphomas	Mesenchymal tumors
Azygous vein	Germ cell tumors	Endocrine tumors
Thymus gland		
Lymph nodes		
Transverse and great vessels		
Connective tissue		
Middle compartment		
Heart and pericardium	Foregut cysts	Pleural and pericardial cysts
Trachea and bronchi	Lymphatic tumors	Neuroenteric and gastro-
Pulmonary vessels		enteric cysts
Connective tissue		
Posterior Compartment		
Sympathetic chain	Tumors of neurogenic	Vascular tumors
Vagus nerves	origin	Mesenchymal tumors
Esophagus		Lymphatic lesions
Thoracic duct		
Lymph nodes		
Descending aorta		

101 primary cysts and neoplasms of the mediastinum presenting at Johns Hopkins Hospital from July 1933 to July 1951.[53] Heimberger and coworkers described 92 mediastinal lesions over a 15-year period.[26] Benjamin and colleagues described a series of 209 patients in 1972,[5] Davis and coworkers a series of 400 patients in 1986,[16] Cohen and associates a series of 230 patients in 1991,[12] and Azanow's team a series of 257 patients in 1993.[4] Results of the six series presented in Table 96-2 show a relative increase in the proportion of lymphomas and relative stability in the proportion of neurogenic tumors, cysts, and thymomas. The reason for the increased incidence of lymphomas is unclear.

Great differences exist between children and adults with respect to the location of mediastinal lesions. In adults, 65 percent of the lesions arise in the anterosuperior, 10 percent in the middle, and 25 percent in the posterior compartments; this distribution is reversed in children, in whom 28 percent of lesions arise in the anterosuperior, 10 percent in the middle, and 62 percent in the

gin. Less common is a potpourri of lesions including vascular tumors, mesenchymal tumors, and lymphatic lesions (Table 96-1; Fig. 96-2).

posterior compartments.[4] In general, the incidence of posterior lesions is higher in children, whereas anterior lesions predominate in adults.

EPIDEMIOLOGY AND INCIDENCE

The mix of mediastinal lesions in adults has changed considerably during the past 5 decades: As may be seen in Table 96-2, significant changes have occurred in the proportions of thymoma and lymphoma, while the proportions of other lesions have remained relatively stable.[3,5,6,8,15,30] Sabiston and Scott examined

SIGNS AND SYMPTOMS

Approximately half of all mediastinal lesions are asymptomatic and are detected on chest radiographs taken for unrelated reasons. The absence of symptoms suggests that a lesion is benign, whereas the presence of symptoms suggests malignancy. The percentage of patients with symptoms from mediastinal masses

TABLE 96-2

Histology of Mediastinal Masses as Reported over Five Decades

Histology	Sabiston and Scott (1952)[53]	Heimberger et al (1963)[26]	Benjamin et al (1972)[5]	Davis et al (1987)[16]	Cohen et al (1991)[12]
n	101	92	209	400	230
			Frequency, % of total		
Cysts	17	24	9	25	20
Neurogenic	20	21	23	14	17
Thymic	17	10	16	17	24
Lymphoma	11	9	15	15	16
Germ cell	9	10	13	10	10
Mesenchymal	1	4	11	6	7
Endocrine	2	8	11	3	2
Other	23	14	2	10	4

closely parallels, or equals, the percentage of malignant lesions (Table 96-2). In adults, 48 to 62 percent of lesions are symptomatic, whereas the percentage of symptomatic lesions is higher in children—58 to 78 percent. Since the incidence of symptoms parallels the incidence of malignancy, a child with a mediastinal mass is considerably more likely to have a malignancy than is an adult with a mediastinal mass.

The most common symptoms are cardiorespiratory—in particular, chest pain and cough. Other manifestations are heaviness in the chest, dysphagia, dyspnea, hemoptysis, signs of superior vena caval obstruction with facial swelling, and cyanosis (Table 96-3). Recurrent respiratory infections are a common complaint. As is discussed below in greater detail, several mediastinal lesions are associated with other clinical syndromes—thymoma with myasthenia gravis, red-cell aplasia, hypogammaglobulinemia, and nonthymic cancers; Hodgkin's disease with recurrent fevers; and von Recklinghausen's disease with neurofibromas.

INVESTIGATION OF MEDIASTINAL MASSES

Mediastinal masses commonly present on routine chest radiographs obtained for other purposes. History and physical examination are occasionally useful in diagnosis, especially in patients with one of the rarer symptoms (e.g., hoarseness and Horner's syndrome). The age of the patient can also narrow diagnostic possibilities. However, the chest radiograph remains the most important lead to diagnosis, followed by CT of the chest; the latter has revolutionized the diagnosis and evaluation of mediastinal masses and should be part of the routine workup of a mediastinal mass. In contrast to CT, standard tomography offers little beyond that afforded by chest radiographs and is rarely indicated.

Noninvasive Diagnostic Procedures

COMPUTED TOMOGRAPHY

As noted above, chest CT should be routine for all suspected or confirmed mediastinal masses. Although CT is poor with respect to distinguishing between cystic and solid structures, it provides excellent examination of the mediastinum. Indeed, the diagnosis of certain lesions—such as aortic aneurysms, mediastinal lipomatosis, and pericardial fat pads—is so straightforward with CT that further search or biopsy is not necessary (Fig. 96-3).[50] CT scanning is the most common technique used to obtain fine-needle aspiration (FNA) biopsies and to provide information about invasion. Additionally, if biopsy or resection is indicated, CT can assist in the selection of the surgical approach (left chest, right chest, mediastinoscopy, or median sternotomy). Finally, chest CT may aid in the use of anesthesia.[38]

MAGNETIC RESONANCE IMAGING

MRI is superior to CT imaging in three specific circumstances: when preoperative determination of a tumor's invasion of vascular or neural structures is crucial, when coronal or radial body sections are necessary, and when contrast material cannot be given intravenously because of renal disease or known allergy to contrast (Fig. 96-4).[63] Gadolinium can be used to provide additional vascular contrast with MRI but is generally unnecessary because the high inherent contrast between mediastinal masses and cardiovascular structures generally suffices to define those masses. For lesions below the aortic arch, electrocardiographic gating can improve image quality. The ability to perform T_1- and T_2-weighted images allows discrimination of mediastinal masses from mediastinal fat on T_1-weighted images and from the heart and chest wall on T_2-weighted images. The use of the combination of these sequences can usually clearly delineate mediastinal masses from surrounding soft tissues. Finally, all neoplasms have higher T_1 and T_2 values than inflammatory lesions, with bronchogenic carcinoma generating the greatest T_1 and T_2 values. The difference between T_1 and T_2 values for bronchogenic carcinoma and chronic inflammatory processes has been shown to be highly significant ($p < 0.001$).[63]

For lesions close to the thoracic inlet, MRI is probably better than CT at identifying invasion of the brachial plexus and vertebral foramina. Similarly, MRI can clarify lesions at the inferior aspect of the mediastinum that invade the diaphragm (Fig. 96-4). It is the method of choice for evaluation of neurogenic lesions, vascular anomalies, and anomalies of the aortic arch. However, MRI also has some disadvantages: longer times for acquisition of data, greater expense, and unavailability at some institutions. Also, patients are less likely to comply with MRI because of claustrophobia and difficulties inherent in lying still for longer periods.

ULTRASONOGRAPHY

Ultrasonography is used in some clinics to determine the nature of the mediastinal mass, particularly whether it is cystic or solid; in other clinics, it is used to direct fine-needle biopsies.[25] Although the value of ultrasound in differentiating cystic and solid masses is recognized, the use of ultrasound has probably been supplanted in most institutions by CT, MRI, and radionuclide scintigraphy. It is particularly use-

TABLE 96-3

Common Symptoms and Their Mechanisms in Patients with Mediastinal Lesions

Symptom	Mechanism
Cough	Airway narrowing, compression
Chest pain	Chest wall invasion, neural invasion
Dyspnea	Airway compromise, pericardial tamponade, pleural effusions, pulmonary stenosis, congestive heart failure
Hemoptysis	Bronchogenic carcinoma, airway invasion, pulmonary stenosis, congestive heart failure
Dysphagia	Esophageal narrowing/obstruction, esophageal motor dysfunction
Hoarseness	Vocal cord paralysis
Facial swelling	Superior vena cava syndrome

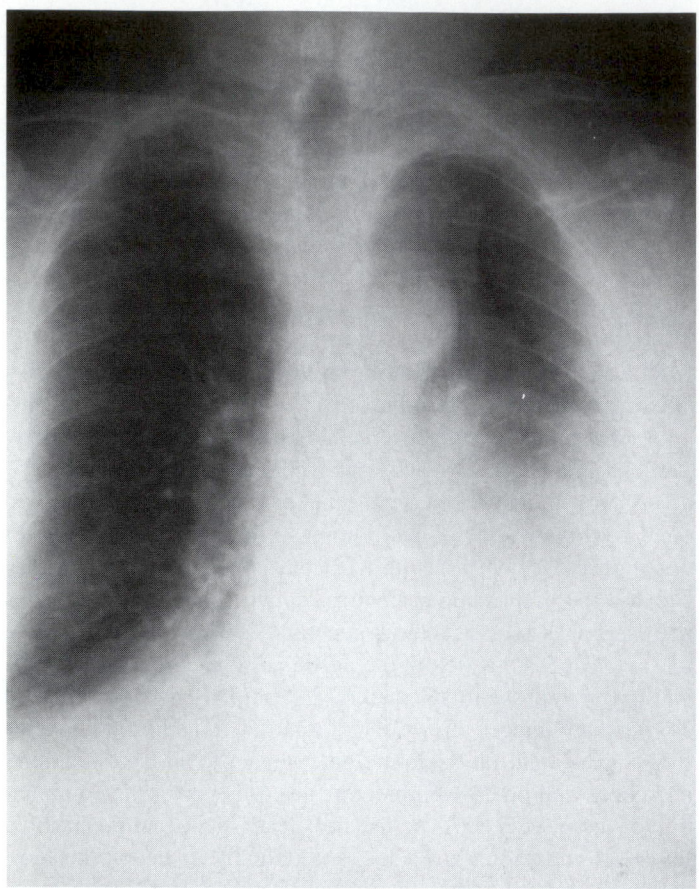

A

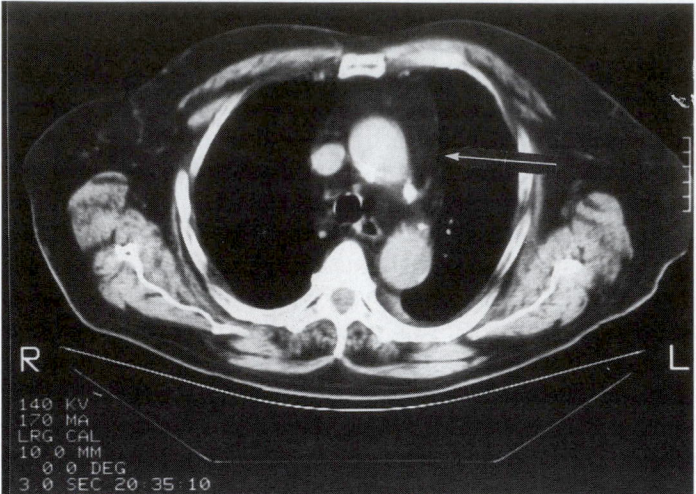

B

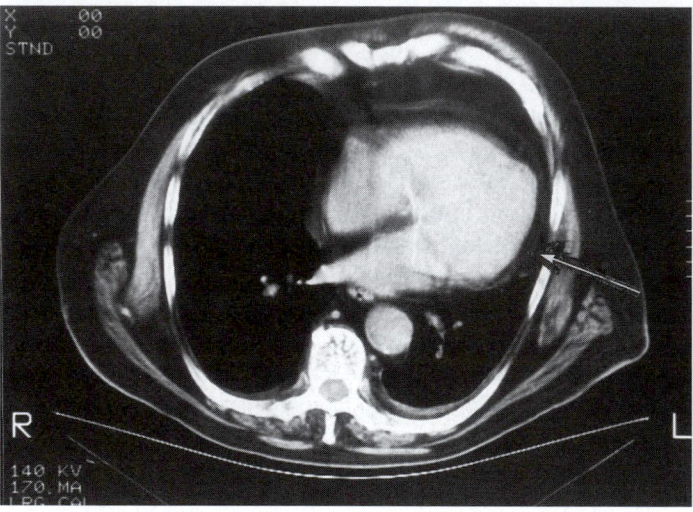

C

FIGURE 96-3 Mediastinal lipomatosis. *A.* PA radiograph of an 82-year-old woman with urinary incontinence and bladder infection. Chest radiograph shows a widened mediastinum with apparent pleural collection. *B.* Chest CT at level of aortic arch showing normal mediastinum except for diffuse fatty infiltration (arrow). *C.* Chest CT at the level of the heart demonstrating cardiomegaly and mediastinal fatty infiltration (arrow).

ful in evaluating masses in children because lying still is not as critical. Additionally, endoscopic ultrasound is increasingly useful in evaluating lesions of the esophagus and various periesophageal structures.

RADIONUCLIDES

Several radionuclide agents are useful in evaluating mediastinal masses (Table 96-4). Thyroid scintigraphy with ^{131}I or ^{123}I may be helpful in patients with obscure substernal anterosuperior compartment lesions. While reports in the surgical literature generally find thyroid scans to be nondiagnostic for substernal thyroids,[31,54] Park and colleagues found a sensitivity of 93 percent, specificity of 100 percent, and overall accuracy of 94 percent for thyroid scintigraphy when performed using current techniques.[48] Technetium use in the mediastinum is complicated because the salivary glands secrete technetium, which is swallowed, so the entire esophagus is invariably positive. However, technetium can help to identify rests of gastric mucosa in the esophagus if scanning is performed immediately after several glasses of liquid are swallowed to clear the esophagus.

[131]I-metaiodobenzylguanine can help to identify pheochromocytomas or functioning paragangliomas anywhere in the body, including the mediastinum. Subsequent CT or MRI scanning is necessary to delineate the anatomy of "hot spots" identified in this way. Selenomethionine scans can localize parathyroid adenomas and thymic cysts. Finally, gallium 67 scanning has been used to distinguish benign from malignant anterior mediastinal masses, especially to differentiate lymphomas from benign le-

T A B L E   9 6 - 4

Radionuclides in the Evaluation of Mediastinal Masses

Radionuclide	*Mediastinal Mass*
[131]I or [123]I	Substernal goiter
[131]I-metaiodobenzylguanine	Pheochromocytoma
Gallium 67	Lymphoma
Selenomethionin	Parathyroids
Technetium	Ectopic gastric mucosa

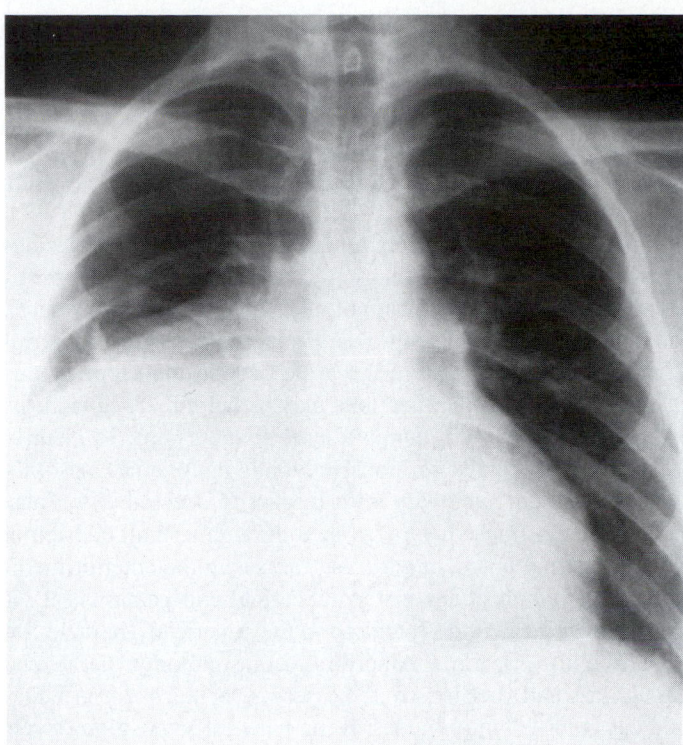

A

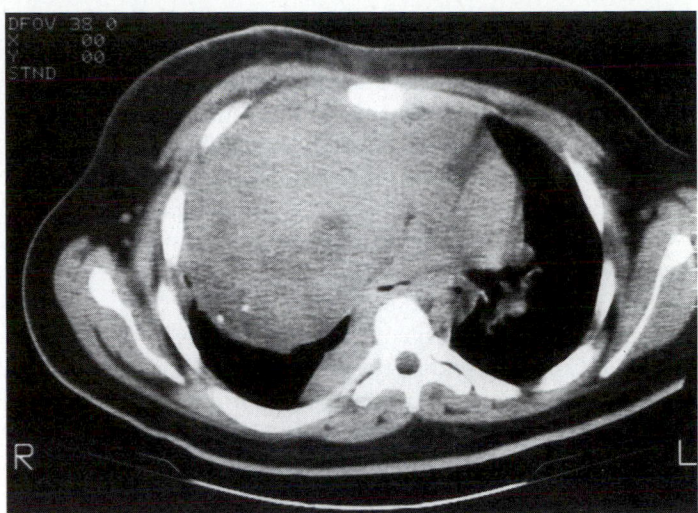

B

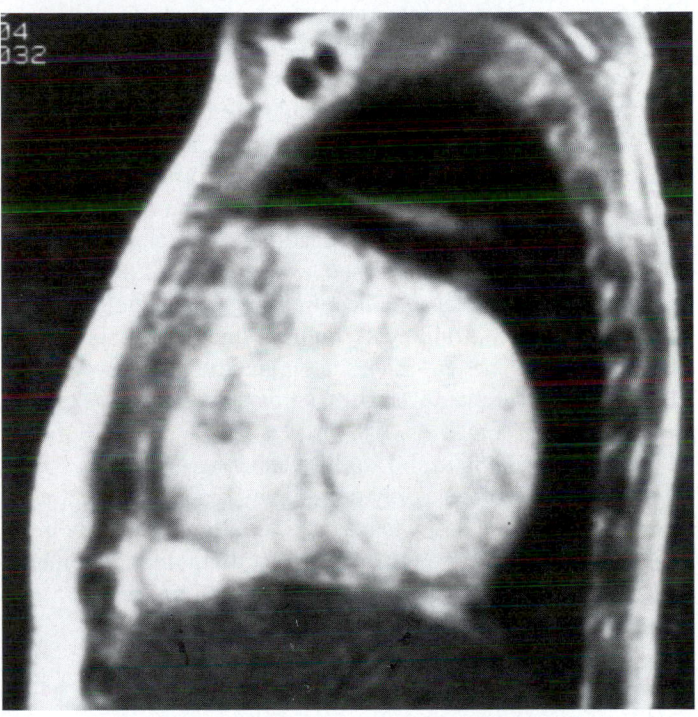

C

FIGURE 96-4   Comparison of CT and MRI in evaluation of mediastinal masses. Nineteen-year-old man with a 1-month history of fever, heaviness in the chest, and cough. Examination revealed a tall, very thin man with dystrophic testes (habitus consistent with Klinefelter's syndrome). Serum AFP was 32,000 and βHCG was 25,000. *A.* PA radiograph of the chest reveals large mediastinal mass projecting into right hemithorax. *B.* CT at the level of the diaphragm demonstrates an inhomogeneous mass. Diaphragmatic invasion could not be assessed. *C.* Sagittal MRI view demonstrates the mass apparently contained by the diaphragm (arrows). Biopsy demonstrated embryonal cell carcinoma. This patient received high-dose cisplatin, vinblastine, and bleomycin, with resultant regression of tumor and normalization of serum markers. Subsequent resection revealed a mature teratoma.

sions.[21] Institutional expertise in the use of these markers and interpretation of the data they yield are at least as important as the choice of diagnostic technique.

BIOCHEMICAL MARKERS

All patients with anterior mediastinal masses, particularly young men, should have determinations of levels of alphafetoprotein (AFP), beta human chorionic gonadotropin (βHCG), and carcinoembryonic antigen (CEA). Serum levels of AFP, βHCG, or both increase in the presence of nonseminomatous malignant germ cell tumors or of some teratomas and carcinomas.

Pheochromocytomas are accompanied by increases in serum catecholamines and in several urinary products—e.g., catecholamines, vanillylmandelic acid, and homovanillic acid. These markers are more valuable in following patients after treatment—i.e., to detect recurrence—than in screening. The levels of these substances should be determined in patients who present with flushing, tachycardia, or headache for which there are no other explanations. Some paravertebral masses—such as paragangliomas, ganglioneromas, and some neuroblastomas—can also elaborate norepinephrine and epinephrine.

Invasive Biopsy Procedures

The decision to biopsy mediastinal masses is not straightforward. Biopsy before resection is not necessary in some cases and potentially harmful in others. The likelihood of a positive biopsy depends on several factors: (1) the presence, or absence, of local symptoms; (2) the location and extent of the lesion; (3) the presence, or absence, of various tumor markers; and (4) gallium uptake by the lesion. (Methods of biopsy are discussed below.)

Locally asymptomatic lesions should not undergo biopsy before removal if they do not extend beyond the anterior compartment, show no increase in levels of tumor markers, and do not take up gallium. In particular, biopsy of a clinically suspected well-encapsulated thymoma should be avoided because it may cause spillage of tumor cells and prevent resection of an early-stage neoplasm from being curative. For patients with symptoms of locally invasive disease—such as severe chest pain, dyspnea, cough, dysphagia, pleural effusion, and superior vena caval obstruction—incisional or fine-needle aspiration biopsy (FNAB) before surgery is mandatory. These lesions are usually malignant and require chemotherapy or radiotherapy as primary or definitive therapy, rather than resection.

Bulky adenopathy should always undergo biopsy, since surgical intervention is seldom the primary means for treating these lesions. Most lesions in the anterosuperior mediastinum can be easily accessed by mediastinoscopy or FNA while lesions in the posterior mediastinum are amenable to FNA or thoracoscopic techniques. Lesions in the middle mediastinum (visceral), just deep to the sternum, can be sampled by way of subxyphoid mediastinoscopy, whereas other middle-mediastinal lesions require FNA or thoracoscopic techniques.

It is critical to perform biopsy on patients with mediastinal masses in whom levels of AFP, βHCG, or CEA are increased. The treatment of choice for patients with these clinical features—i.e., with the features of metastatic non–small cell bronchogenic carcinoma or nonseminomatous germ cell tumors—is chemotherapy followed by surgical resection. Occasionally, chemotherapeutic treatment for oncologic emergencies may be initiated on the basis of increased levels, per se, of tumor markers. In contrast, increased concentrations of catecholamines in serum or urine contraindicate biopsy, since disturbance of a pheochromocytoma or pharmacologically active paraganglioma before preparation with alpha and beta blockade is dangerous.

Gallium uptake is useful in differentiating lymphomas from thymoma.[21] Gallium is avidly taken up by lymphomas and other inflammatory processes, whereas it is usually taken up by bronchogenic carcinomas, rarely taken up by thymomas, and unpredictably taken up by carcinoids and germ cell tumors.

METHOD OF BIOPSY

FNAB may fail to obtain diagnostic tissue, especially in patients with lymphoma. FNAB is diagnostic in approximately 75 percent of mediastinal masses, though it lacks the precision to stage mediastinal and pulmonary malignancies. Heilo obtained a diagnosis in 84 percent of 62 patients undergoing ultrasound-guided core needle biopsy.[25] It is important to emphasize that the primary benefit of FNAB in this group of patients is to prevent needless surgical intervention. Accordingly, in a candidate for surgery, a diagnosis other than lymphoma, small cell carcinoma, or stage IIIB non–small cell bronchogenic carcinoma will not obviate surgery, since all other diagnoses of solid tumor require surgical staging or resection. In a group of 35 patients in whom diagnostic tissue was obtained, ultrasound-guided needle biopsy prevented subsequent surgery in only 17 patients.[25]

Patients with potential early thymomas should not undergo FNAB, as the procedure may spread tumor cells along needle tracks, thereby preventing subsequent curative surgery. Although

a core biopsy may suffice for the diagnosis of a specific lymphoma, most often more invasive and definitive approaches—such as cervical mediastinoscopy, anterior or parasternal mediastinoscopy, and videothoracoscopy—are necessary. In summary, FNAB is inconsistently useful for diagnosis of diseases of the mediastinum, and its use must be carefully assessed. However, complications of FNAB are rare.

Surgical approaches to obtain tissue from mediastinal lesions include cervical mediastinoscopy, extended cervical mediastinoscopy, anterior mediastinotomy (Chamberlain procedure), subxyphoid mediastinoscopy, and videothoracoscopy. Descriptions of these specific techniques are beyond the scope of this chapter, but some generalizations may be helpful. The diagnosis of lymphoma usually requires a large tissue sample to identify the subtype, especially for non-Hodgkin's lymphomas. Also, lesions at different sites vary with respect to accessibility. Thus, cervical mediastinoscopy, performed through a small incision in the suprasternal notch, can sample masses in the anterior mediastinum or lymph nodes in the subcarinal and paratracheal location (levels 1, 2, 3, 4, 7, and 10 in the American Thoracic Society staging system). Anterior mediastinotomy performed through a small incision over the second or third rib on either side can sample lymph nodes in the para-aortic position (levels 5 and 6) or anteriormediastinal masses. These procedures can be performed in the outpatient setting, have a very low complication rate, and do not delay chemotherapy or radiotherapy. A portion of the specimen should be kept fresh for formal evaluation of T- and B-cell subpopulations and a sample of any enlarged node sent for culture.

The use of mediastinoscopy to sample large masses that compromise the airway or elicit clinical signs of superior vena caval obstruction may be problematic. However, mediastinoscopy can still be useful with cautious anesthetic management (awake intubation and extubation).[38,56] Mediastinoscopy poses no greater risk of bleeding for patients with superior vena caval syndrome than for normal persons undergoing mediastinoscopy.

Subxyphoid mediastinoscopy, performed through an incision below the xyphoid process, is an unusual procedure. It is used to obtain biopsies of tissues located inferiorly in the mediastinum. Videothoracoscopic approaches to either the left or right side of the mediastinum are straightforward and obtain adequate tissue samples with minimal morbidity. However, thoracoscopic biopsies are not currently being done as outpatient procedures.

MEDIASTINAL INFECTIONS

Mediastinal infections can present as mediastinal masses. The various infections that can present in this way fall into four groups: (1) mediastinitis, secondary to transsternal cardiac procedures; (2) acute perforation of the esophagus secondary to vomiting, tumor, or attempts at esophageal dilation; (3) acute descending necrotizing mediastinitis resulting from descent of oral infectious processes into the mediastinum; and (4) upward extension of a subdiaphragmatic infectious process into the mediastinum by way of the various tissue planes that connect the mediastinum with the retroperitoneum and the peritoneum. Of these categories, the first two are the most common. Diagnosis of mediastinitis after surgery on the mediastinum is uncomplicated.

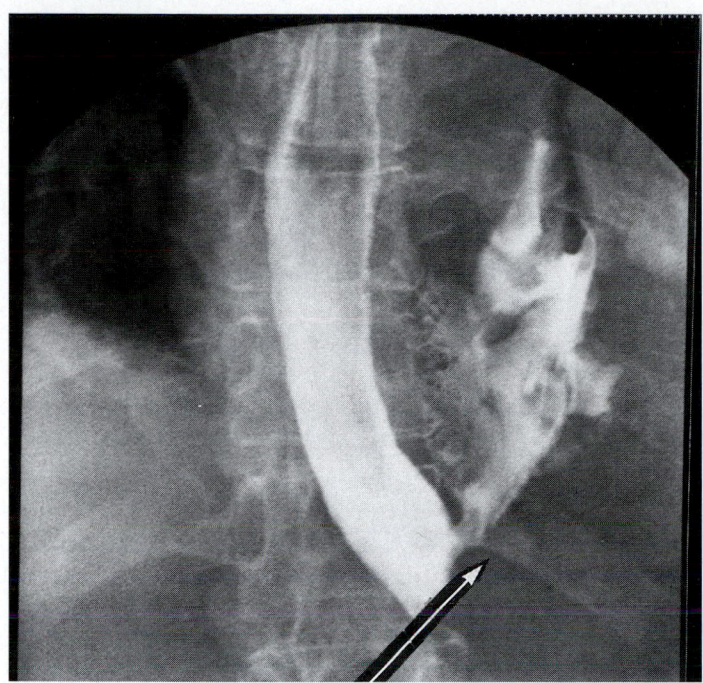

A

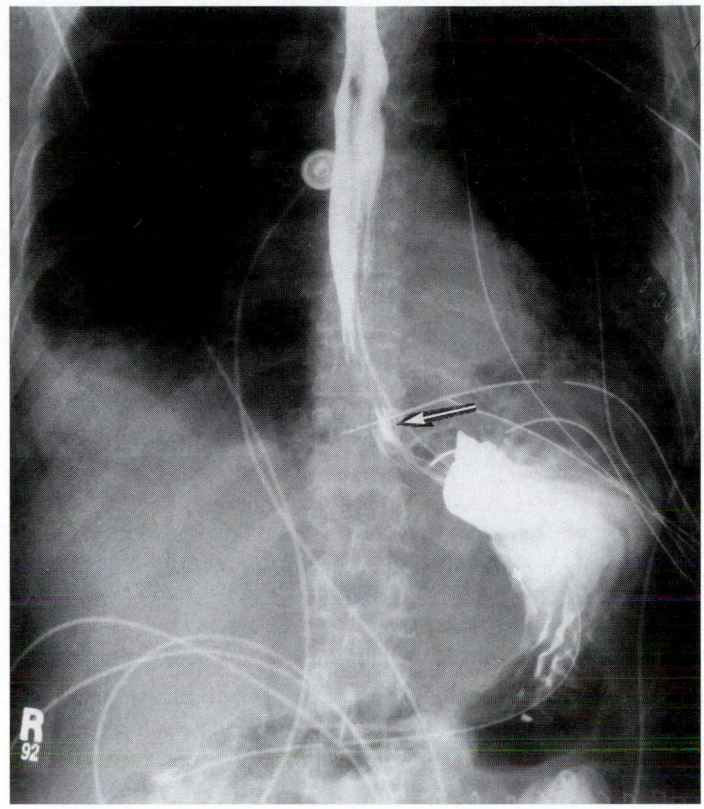

B

FIGURE 96-5   Esophageal tear with communication to pleura. Sixty-three-year-old woman with multiple myeloma receiving chemotherapy in inpatient setting. After an episode of vomiting, she developed a left pleural effusion and leukopenia (WBC of 500). *A.* Contrast study reveals leak into left chest (arrow). *B.* Postoperative film after primary repair reveals normal flow of contrast.

Transsternal Cardiac Procedures

The diagnosis of mediastinitis after surgery on the mediastinum is evident. The therapeutic approach is described in surgical texts.

Esophageal Perforations

Acute infections of the mediastinum caused by esophageal disease are usually due to esophageal perforation from retching or vomiting, malignancy, ingestion of a foreign body, or diagnostic or therapeutic instrumentation (Fig. 96-5). Along with clinical suspicion, two radiologic criteria are helpful in establishing the diagnosis: pneumomediastinum and pleural effusion. In distal esophageal perforations, the pleural effusion typically presents on the left side, whereas midesophageal and proximal esophageal lesions typically present with right-sided pleural effusions. Although pneumomediastinum is invariably present after an esophageal perforation, it does not localize well to the site of perforation because of dissection along tissue planes. A swallow of water-soluble contrast can confirm the diagnosis of esophageal perforation. If the swallow fails to reveal the perforation, it is repeated with a small amount of dilute barium. Although water-soluble contrast is safer from the standpoints of infection and surgery, barium affords a more detailed examination and can disclose a small perforation that is not identified by a water-soluble agent.

In general, the treatment of an esophageal perforation is surgical drainage and repair of the perforation. However, appropriate timing for repair has been debated: the older surgical litera-ture holds that a perforation more than 24 h old should be repaired only after diversion of the cervical esophagus. The more recent literature indicates that many of the late-presenting perforations can be repaired without diversion. Finally, small perforations that drain back into the gastrointestinal tract without significant soilage of the mediastinum or larger injuries that can be well drained by tube thoracostomy can be treated with antibiotics as long as the patient shows no signs of sepsis. Such fistulas that are managed without surgery may either heal spontaneously or require surgical repair at a later date.

Acute Descending Necrotizing Mediastinitis

Acute descending necrotizing mediastinitis is a complication of cervical, pharyngeal, or oropharyngeal abscesses. Odontogenic diseases (molar abscesses, peritonsillar abscesses, retropharyngeal abscesses, Ludwig's angina, and adult epiglottitis) and iatrogenic injury are the most common causes (Fig. 96-6). The infections are mixed, and culture may grow aerobic beta-hemolytic streptococcus, *Bacteroides,* peptostreptococcus, or anaerobic streptococci. Initial treatment usually entails the use of antibiotics and cervical drainage. Should these measures fail, mediastinitis can develop within 48 h.

There are no pathognomonic radiographic manifestations. Mediastinal involvement is suggested by widening of the retrocervical space with an air-fluid level, anterior displacement of the tracheal air column on lateral neck or chest radiographs, mediastinal emphysema, or the loss of the normal lordosis of the cervical spine. A CT scan of the chest and neck can verify the presence of a descending mediastinitis.

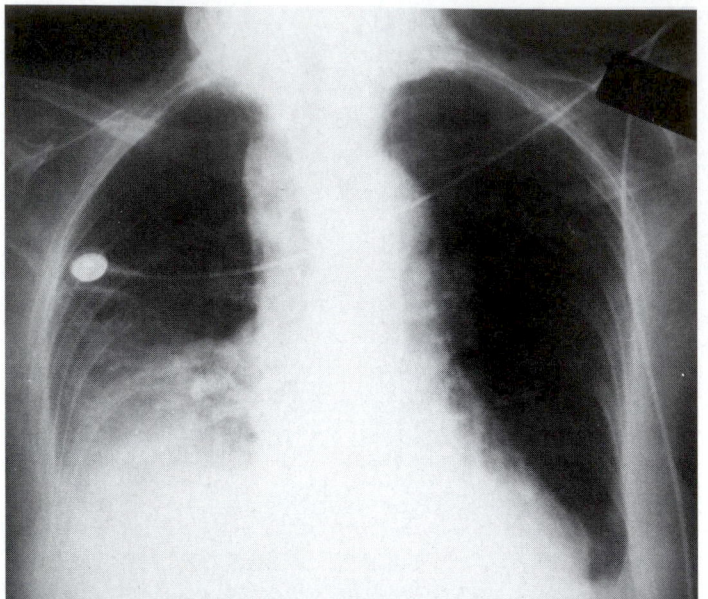

A

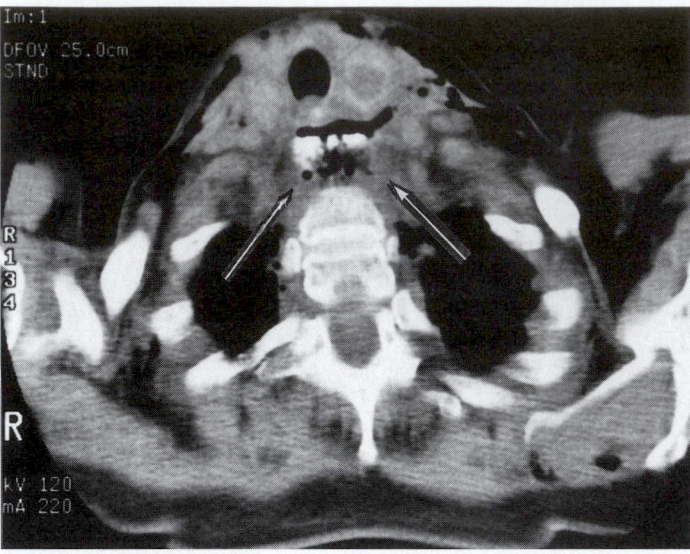

C

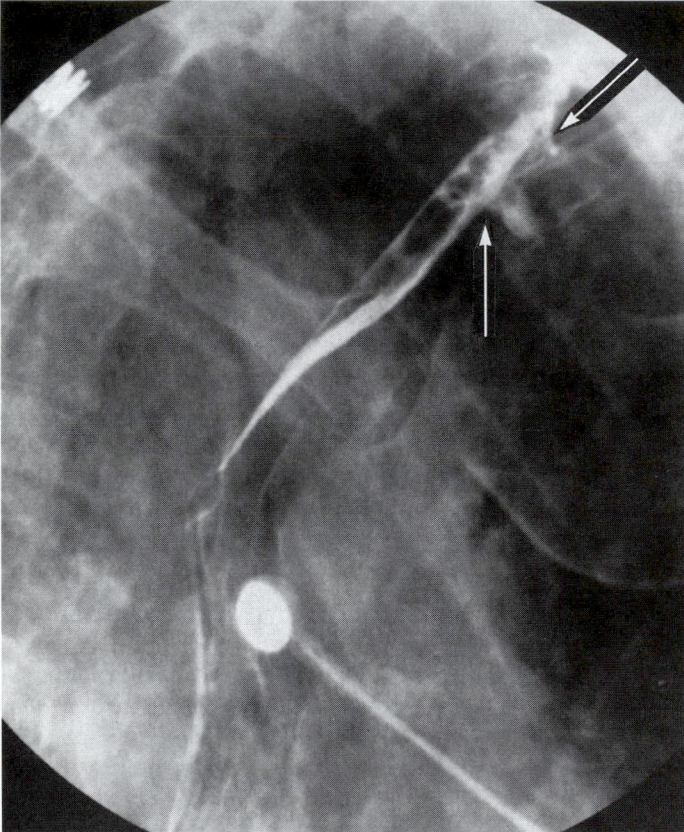

B

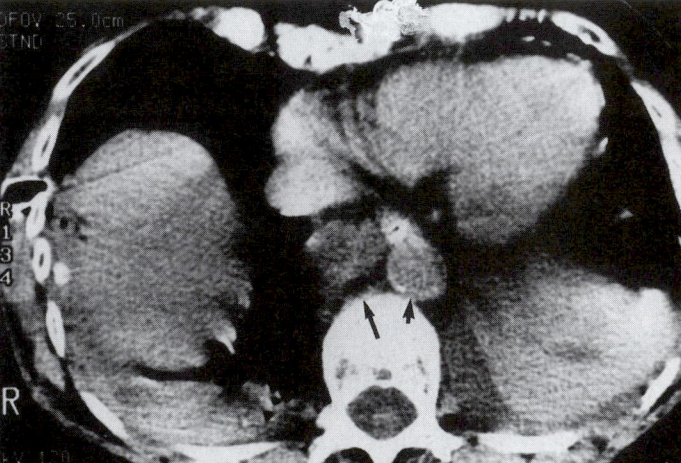

D

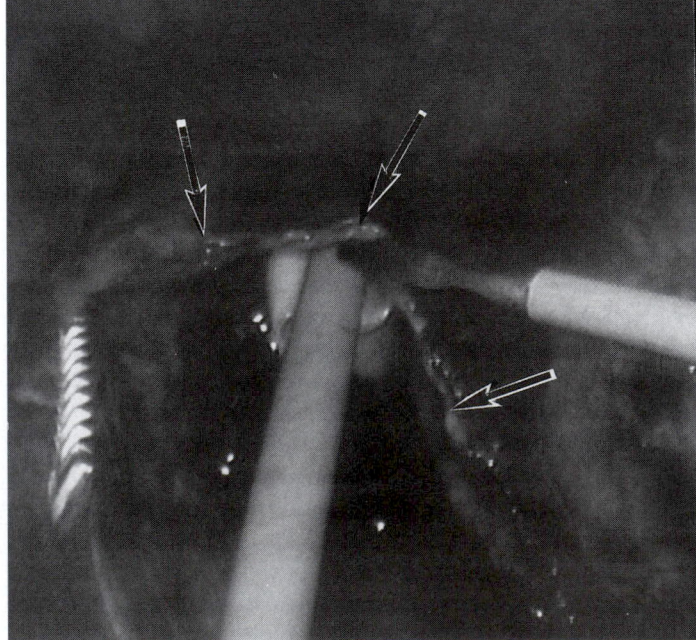

E

FIGURE 96-6 Acute descending necrotizing mediastinitis. Sixty-nine-year-old woman developed cervical neck mass and subcutaneous emphysema 96 h after attempted esophagoscopy. *A.* PA radiograph reveals a widened mediastinum with pneumomediastinum and pleural effusion. *B.* Contrast study demonstrates leak in the proximal esophagus (arrows). *C.* CT scan at the thoracic inlet reveals 5-cm irregular abscess (arrows). *D.* CT scan of chest close to the diaphragm reveals that the abscess extends the length of the chest (arrows). *E.* Combined thoracoscopic and cervical drainage resulted in clearing of the abscess (arrows).

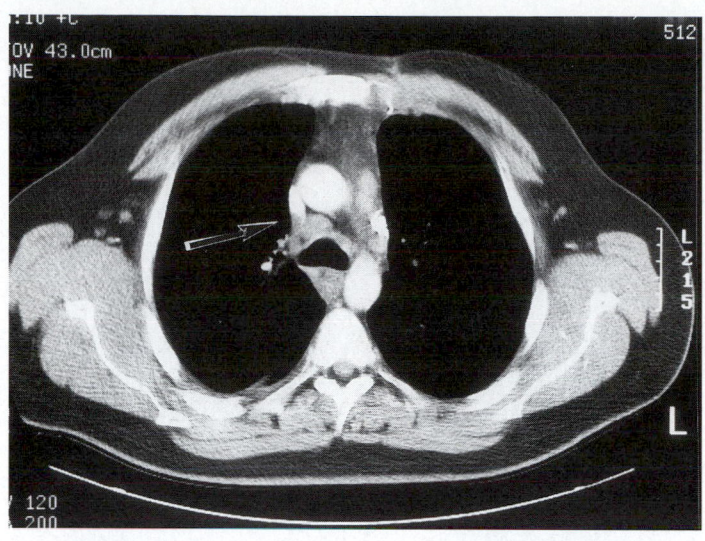

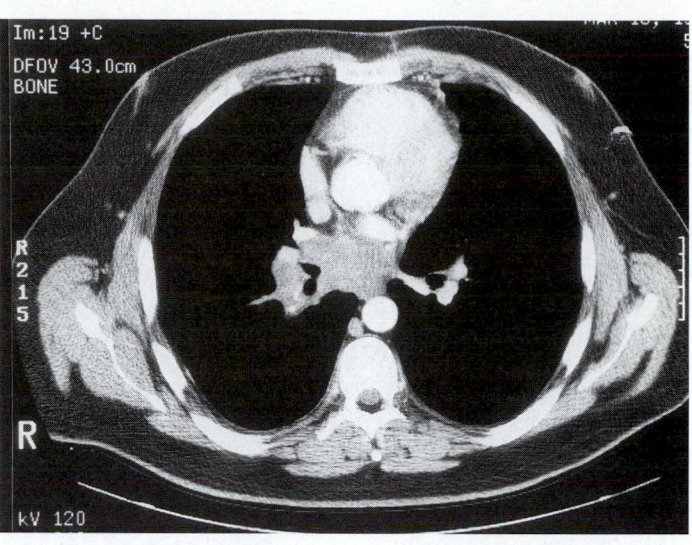

A

B

FIGURE 96-7   Chronic fibrosing mediastinitis. Thirty-year-old man with malaise and one episode of hemoptysis. Chest radiograph is normal. *A.* Chest CT at the level of the carina reveals paratracheal mass (arrow) surrounding the airway. *B.* The same process extends along the airways into inferior mediastinum. Mediastinoscopy was done to perform biopsy. Patient was treated successfully with steroids.

The mainstays of treatment are broad-spectrum antibiotics, surgical drainage, and tracheostomy. Antibiotics should be chosen to cover gram-negative, gram-positive, and anaerobic organisms. Cervical drainage is often the definitive treatment: careful review of the chest CT scan can indicate whether more invasive approaches are necessary. Bilateral anterior mediastinotomies may be sufficient if the infection has not progressed below the fourth thoracic vertebra. Soft, pliable drains prevent erosion into major neck vessels. Subxyphoid drainage may be necessary if the anterior space is affected. Extensive infections can be treated successfully by wide drainage of the mediastinum.[65]

The role of tracheostomy in treatment is debatable. A tracheostomy can protect the airway, especially in patients with significant cervical inflammation and edema. Despite aggressive treatment, reported mortality ranges up to 40 percent. Death can result from pulmonary sepsis, blood vessel erosion and exsanguination, and intracranial infection. A high level of suspicion that mediastinitis may be present and early surgical management are critical for successful outcome.

SUBACUTE MEDIASTINITIS

The incidence of subacute mediastinitis is increasing in the growing population of immunocompromised patients. This diagnosis applies only to patients with mild and evanescent symptoms (e.g., substernal pain, fever, and night sweats) and with an identifiable anterior or visceral mediastinal mass. In immunocompetent patients, the most common causes are histoplasmosis and tuberculosis. Mycotic infections are rare. In immunocompromised patients, the most common causes are *Mycobacterium avium-intracellulare* and *Mycobacterium tuberculosis.* Gallium scintigraphy or indium-labeled leukocyte scintigraphy may be useful in identifying subacute infections early in their course but is less effective in more chronic infections.

CHRONIC MEDIASTINITIS

Patients with chronic mediastinal infections often have cough, hemoptysis, fever, and dysphagia. Causes of chronic mediastinal infections are granulomatous lymphadenopathies, such as tuberculosis; fungal infections, such as histoplasmosis and coccidiomycosis; sarcoidosis; and Wegener's granulomatosis. Whereas tuberculosis was the most frequent cause in the early twentieth century, now fungal infections cause most chronic mediastinal infections. The diagnosis requires biopsy and culture.

Complications of chronic mediastinal infections are uncommon. Airway compromise may require surgical relief. Seventy-five percent of all benign obstructions of the superior vena cava result from mediastinal granulomatous disease. Calcified lymph nodes may erode into airway (bronchiolithiasis) and require removal. Most symptoms resulting from *benign* lesions that cause obstruction of the superior vena cava resolve with time. Medical treatment consists of diuretics, anticoagulation, and observation. In contrast, malignant obstruction of the superior vena cava requires urgent nonsurgical treatment.

CHRONIC FIBROSING MEDIASTINITIS

This entity is also referred to as chronic sclerosing mediastinitis, chronic granulomatous mediastinitis, or chronic idiopathic mediastinitis. It differs from chronic mediastinitis in its compression and obliteration of vessels, bronchi, or esophagus (Fig. 96-7). In keeping with the supposition that chronic fibrosing mediastinitis (CFM) is the result of infection, cultures of mediastinal tissue sometimes grow *Histoplasma capsulatum* or *M. tuberculosis.* Most instances of CFM involve the vicinity of the thoracic duct and its main tributaries. Most patients have strongly positive gallium scans and serum reactions to *Histoplasma* antigens.

Patients with CFM present with a chronic smoldering inflammatory process that deposits woody, fibrous tissue throughout the visceral compartment of the mediastinum. This

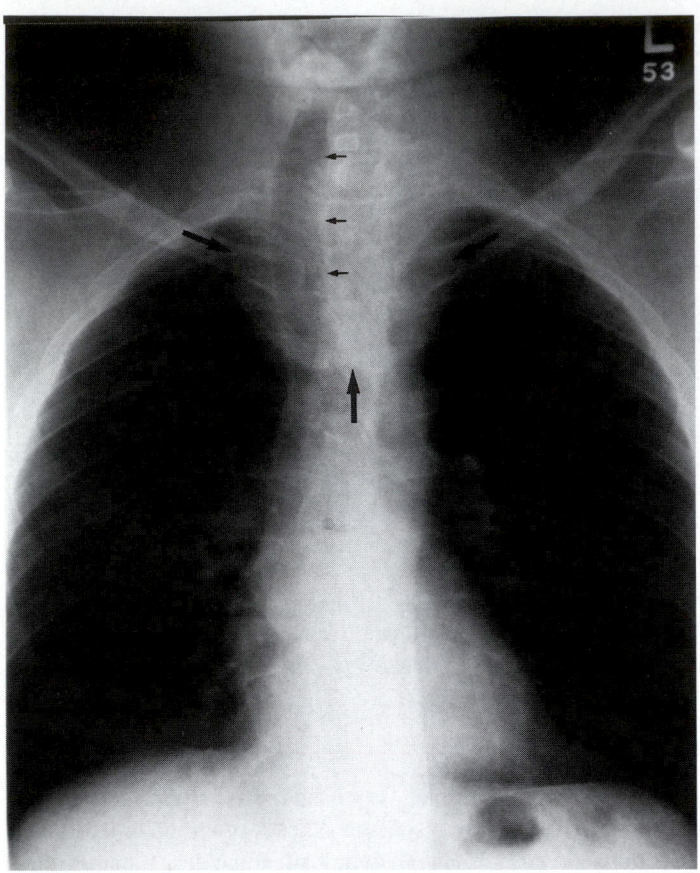

A

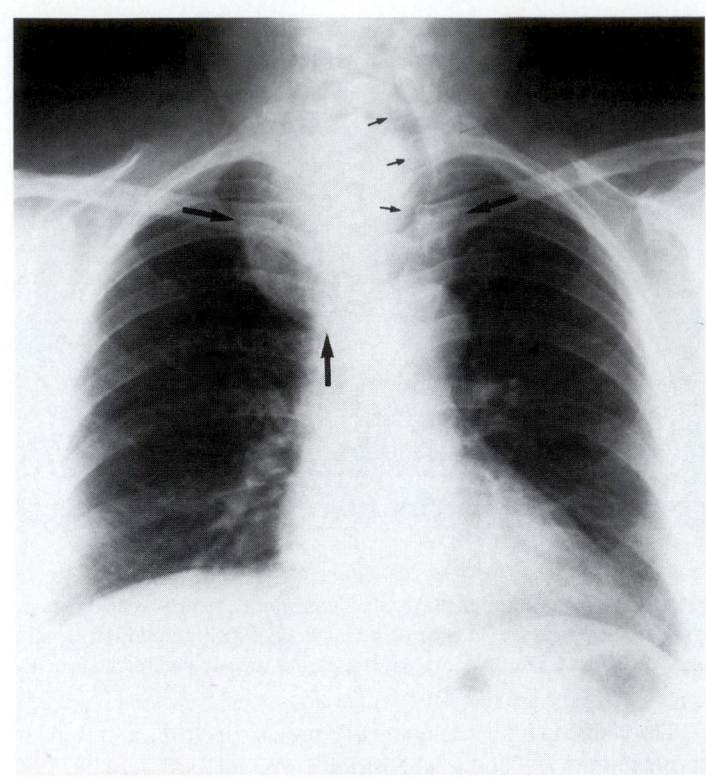

B

FIGURE 96-8 Substernal goiter. *A.* Substernal thyroid in 33-year-old man (arrow). He underwent subsequent uncomplicated thyroidectomy by way of collar incision. *B.* Substernal thyroid in 67-year-old woman with diabetes and congestive heart failure (arrows). Thyroid suppression was followed by a decrease in the size of the goiter.

fibrous tissue extends beyond lymph node boundaries. A diagnosis of CFM is appropriate only if the process includes obstruction of one of the major airways, pulmonary arteries, pulmonary veins, or esophagus. Occasionally, patients have similar fibrotic processes elsewhere—e.g., in the retroperitoneal space, the orbit (orbital pseudotumor), or the thyroid (Riedel's struma). The diffuse fibrosis, which also occurs in patients with systemic lupus erythematosus or rheumatoid disease or those who have received methysergide, suggests an immune mechanism.

Clinical features are puzzling, and the disorder may be self-limiting. The highest incidence of CFM is in young adults, primarily in white women 19 to 25 years of age, who develop the disease three times more often than do men of the same age. Sixty percent of patients have symptoms that depend on the structures affected. The radiologic findings are variable. The superior mediastinal shadow may be abnormally wide because of an asymmetric mass that projects into either hemithorax. In some instances in which the chest radiograph is normal, a CT scan may demonstrate compression of the trachea, arterial compression, or other abnormalities. Contrast venograms, anteriograms, or MRI can document vascular obstruction even when CT scans are unrevealing. Bronchoscopy and mediastinoscopy are usually sufficient to obtain tissue for diagnosis, although thoracotomy may be necessary. Esophagoscopy can be diagnostic in patients

with dysphagia. Any tissue obtained should be cultured for mycobacteria and fungus. Serum sent for complement fixation studies for histoplasmosis and coccidiomycosis can contribute to the diagnosis. Culture and histologic evaluation of material for fungal and acid-fast organisms are essential but often unrewarding; they may be negative even in patients who later respond to antibacterial treatment.

TREATMENT

In a series of 22 patients with CFM, 13 had superior vena caval obstruction, 3 had dysphagia, 3 had stridor and dyspnea, 2 had pericardial involvement, and 1 had pulmonary artery obstruction.[26] Ketoconazole improved outcomes in patients with high titers for histoplasmosis (greater than 1:32). It is recommended before resection because its use may obviate surgery in some patients and improve outcome in patients who require surgery. Amphotericin is of value only for acute infections. Medical treatment, using steroids, has not been effective in reversing the fibrotic process.

Because major surgical resections entail a high morbidity and mortality, they are worthwhile only when other measures have failed. Superior vena caval replacement by spiral vein graft may be useful for patients with localized superior vena caval obstruction and unremitting symptoms.[19] In a series of 18 patients who underwent major surgical resections for CFM, there were four deaths, most of them in patients who required carinal pneumonectomy.[44]

LESIONS MASQUERADING AS MEDIASTINAL TUMORS

Substernal Goiter

Substernal goiters usually present as anterosuperior mediastinal masses (Fig. 96-8) even though ectopic thyroid tissue can also be found in retrotracheal and retroesophageal locations. Essentially all substernal thyroids descend into the mediastinum from the neck; primary mediastinal thyroids are vanishingly rare. Two-thirds of patients with a substernal goiter complain of a neck mass. Most are otherwise asymptomatic. Twenty-five percent complain of dyspnea or dysphagia. The occurrence of symptoms does not herald malignancy.[54] CT and MRI scans are the most useful studies in the diagnosis and evaluation of these lesions. Modern radioactive ^{131}I scans can delineate the substernal goiter, although there is some debate about the incidence of false-negative scans.[48,54] A combined analysis of available studies indicates that modern techniques of thyroid scintigraphy are diagnostic of most substernal goiters.

Three recent studies, with 50 to 80 patients included in each, dealt with the evaluation and resection of substernal goiters.[2,31,54] These reports indicate that even the most bulky lesions can be resected through cervical incisions: The lesion usually does not extend beyond the uppermost portion of the anterosuperior compartment, and ligation of the vascular supply in the neck allows delivery of the mediastinal goiter to the neck. In these series, six patients (3.3 percent) required median sternotomy or thoracotomy along with cervical incision to achieve resection. There were no deaths due to surgery in any of the series. Three patients in one series had significant intraoperative bleeding. The overall major complication rate was 1.6 percent; the rate of minor complications was 15.4 percent.

The reported incidence of malignancy has ranged from 2.5 to 21 percent. These data are particularly pertinent to the decision to recommend surgery for asymptomatic substernal goiters. Everyone would support resection if 21 percent of all substernal goiters were malignant. Unfortunately, FNAB was seldom successful in identifying the lesions that ultimately proved to be malignant. Weighing in the balance the frequency of malignancy (about 2 to 20 percent), the potential danger of acute airway obstruction, and the relative safety of the surgical procedure, surgical excision seems reasonable even in asymptomatic patients.[31] This balance in favor of surgery can obviously be tilted against it by the presence of medical complications.

Cystic Hygromas

Mediastinal lymphangiomas typically extend from cervical cystic hygromas along the phrenic nerve into the chest. Cystic hygromas may be evident at birth or may not be discovered until later in life. Symptoms are caused by infection, hemorrhage, or continued growth. Resection is accomplished by combined cer-

vicomediastinal approaches. Some of these lesions gradually regress spontaneously without surgical intervention. Sclerosis (e.g., injection of tetracycline) is possible but is generally not effective.

Lesions Originating from the Thoracic Skeleton

Most skeletal lesions in the mediastinum are bony tumors that project from the thoracic spine. Chordomas of the spine are ectopic embryonic remnants of primitive notochords that may be manifest in the paravertebral sulcus. CT scanning usually shows destruction of vertebral bodies in association with soft tissue mass. These tumors are malignant and require extensive excision and reconstruction of the spinal cord. As a rule, 5-year survival is poor.

Other lesions associated with the thoracic skeleton are paravertebral abscesses caused by staphylococcal hematogenous infections of paraspinal muscles, similar to retroperitoneal abscesses. The treatment of these is the same as for all infectious lesions—i.e., drainage and appropriate antibiotic treatment.

An anterior meningocele may occur in the paravertebral sulcus. These are generally asymptomatic masses discovered incidentally on CT scan. They may be confused with primary neurogenic tumors. Patients with anterior meningoceles often have peripheral neurofibromatosis, skeletal abnormalities, or both. Myelography or MRI is crucial in the diagnosis of these lesions. If the diagnosis is made preoperatively, no treatment is needed unless symptoms become manifest.

Extramedullary Hematopoiesis

Hematopoietic tissue can present in the mediastinum, typically in the posterior mediastinum. This process of extramedullary hematopoiesis develops as a compensatory mechanism in patients with abnormal bone marrow function. It may be manifest in several organs, such as the adrenals, liver, lymph nodes, and lungs. Large masses of extramedullary hematopoiesis are designated as erythroblastoma and myelolipoma. Consideration of this diagnosis is appropriate in patients with blood dyscrasias, especially thalassemia, who present with mediastinal masses. The tissue is pathologically characteristic, so FNAB is often diagnostic. Resection is not indicated if the diagnosis is made preoperatively.[11]

Vascular Lesions

Vascular lesions in the mediastinum may be either arterial or venous lesions and either pulmonary or systemic.[30] Validation of lesions suspected of being vascular requires either angiography or MRI scanning to avoid dangerous biopsy. Appropriate therapy depends on the diagnosis.

Esophageal Lesions

Several benign esophageal lesions—such as diverticula, duplications, large leiomyomas, hiatal hernias, and achalasia—may present as mediastinal masses. Esophageal carcinoma with extramural spread, bulky adenopathy, or contained perforation can manifest as bulky visceral or posterior mediastinal masses. Chest CT scan with oral contrast can differentiate most of these lesions. Formal contrast studies and esophagoscopy are reserved for puzzling circumstances.

Pulmonary Lesions

Pulmonary lesions may manifest primarily as mediastinal masses, particularly as mediastinal adenopathy. Small cell lung cancer often presents as bulky adenopathy with either a small or an involuted primary lesion. Extralobar sequestration may also present on the chest radiograph as a paramediastinal mass in a patient with recurrent pneumonia.

Subdiaphragmatic Lesions

Subdiaphragmatic lesions may present as mediastinal masses. The gastrointestinal tract (typically the stomach) may herniate through the esophageal hiatus posteriorly (to form a hiatal hernia) or through the foramen of Morgagni anteriorly. Pancreatic pseudocysts rarely present as mediastinal masses; they occur in patients with characteristic histories of previous pancreatitis or known abdominal pancreatic pseudocysts. These lesions should be drained by laparotomy rather than thoracotomy.

ANTERIOR MEDIASTINAL NEOPLASMS

Lesions of the Thymus

THYMOMA

Thymomas appear benign histologically even when they are invasive. They derive from either cortical or medullary epithelial cells. They are the most common of the thymic malignancies (Table 96-5). Five histologic grades have been described, based on lymphocytic infiltration: lymphocytic, lymphoepithelial (mixed), epithelial, spindle cell, and unclassified.[52] Thus, a *lymphocytic thymoma* consists of 67 to 80 percent lymphocytes. *Mixed thymomas* are tumors with 50 percent lymphocytes and 50 percent epithelial cells. In *epithelial thymomas,* 67 to 80 percent of the cells are epithelial cells. *Spindle cell tumors* have a

TABLE 96-5

Thymic Malignancies

Thymoma
Thymic carcinoma
   Low grade: squamous cell carcinoma, mucoepidermoid, basaloid
   High grade: small cell, undifferentiated, sarcomatoid, clear cell
Thymic carcinoid
Oat cell carcinoma of thymus
Thymic hyperplasia

TABLE 96-6

Staging of Thymic Malignancies

Stage	Description	10-yr Survival (%)
I	Encapsulated tumors without gross or microscopic invasion	85–100
II	Capsular or pleural invasion	60–84
III	Macroscopic invasion of surrounding tissues (lung, pericardium, vena cava, or aorta)	21–77
IVA	Disseminated disease within the chest	26–47
IVB	Distant metastases	Unknown

SOURCE: Adapted from: Masoaka et al.[43]

characteristic appearance, and *unclassified tumors* are typically too undifferentiated to classify. The number of mitotic figures in these tumors is very low, so cytologic preparations always appear benign.

A second classification depends on the relative predominance of thymic medullary or thymic cortical cells.[32,42] Medullary tumors are less aggressive, with rare recurrences, while cortical thymomas (and the most aggressive subtype, thymic carcinoma) tend to recur and metastasize. Differentiation between lymphomas and thymomas can be difficult without substantial tissue and often cannot be made with needle biopsy.

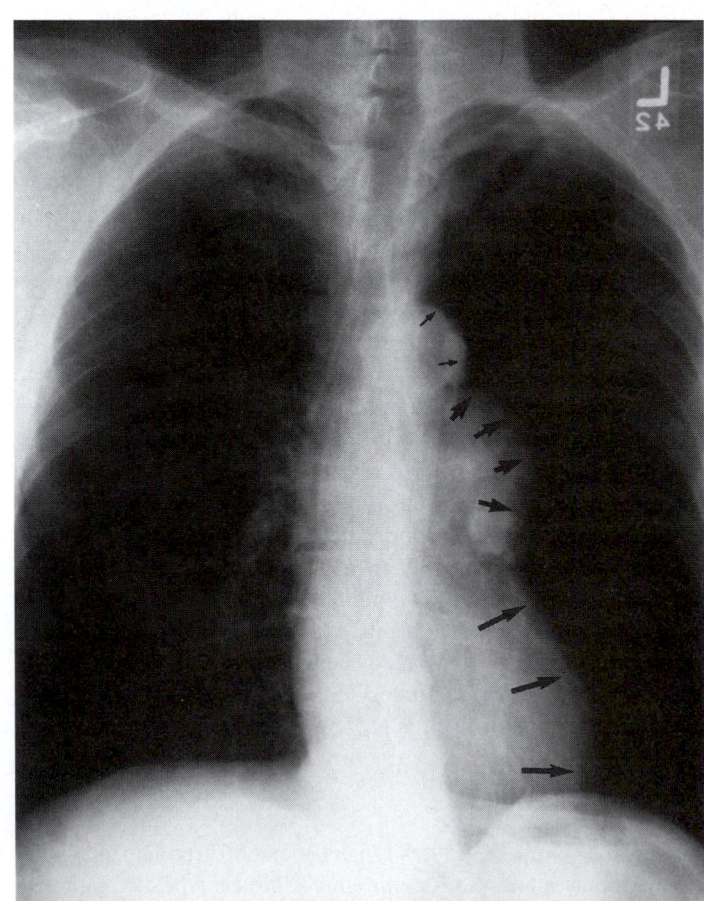

A

FIGURE 96-9

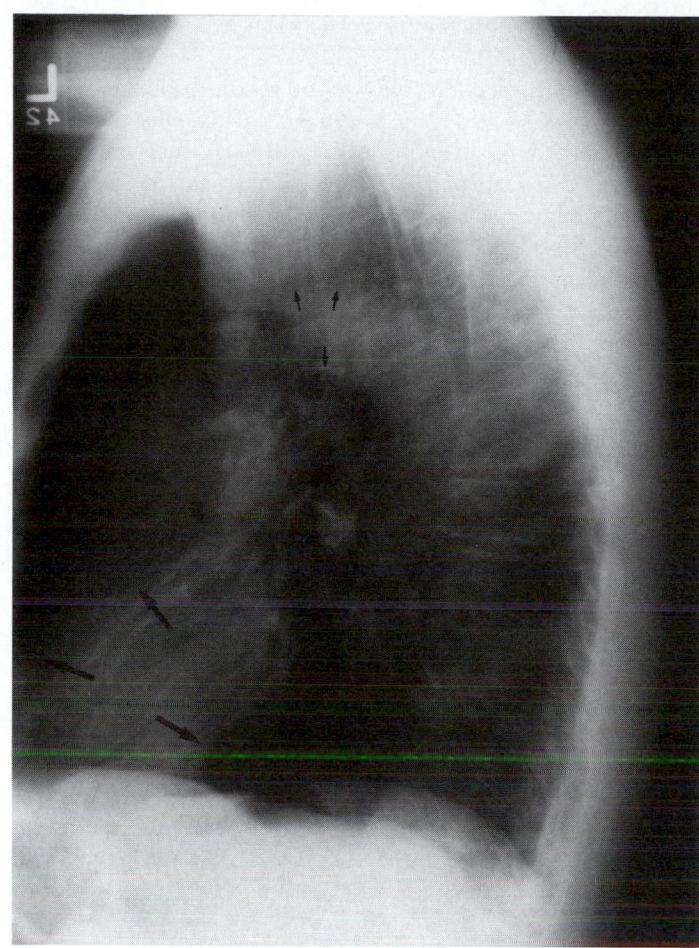

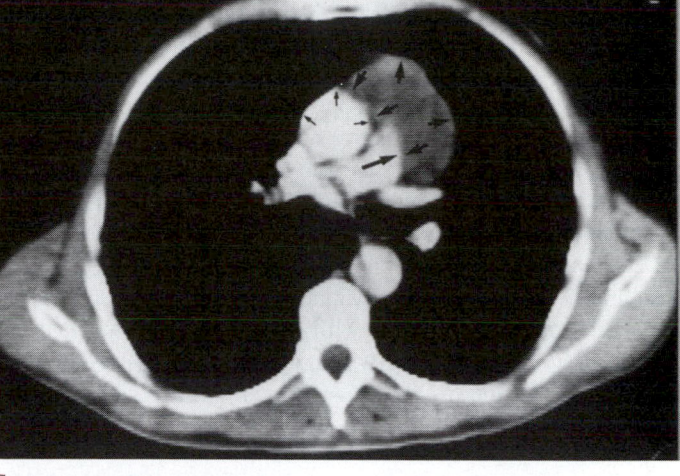

C

B

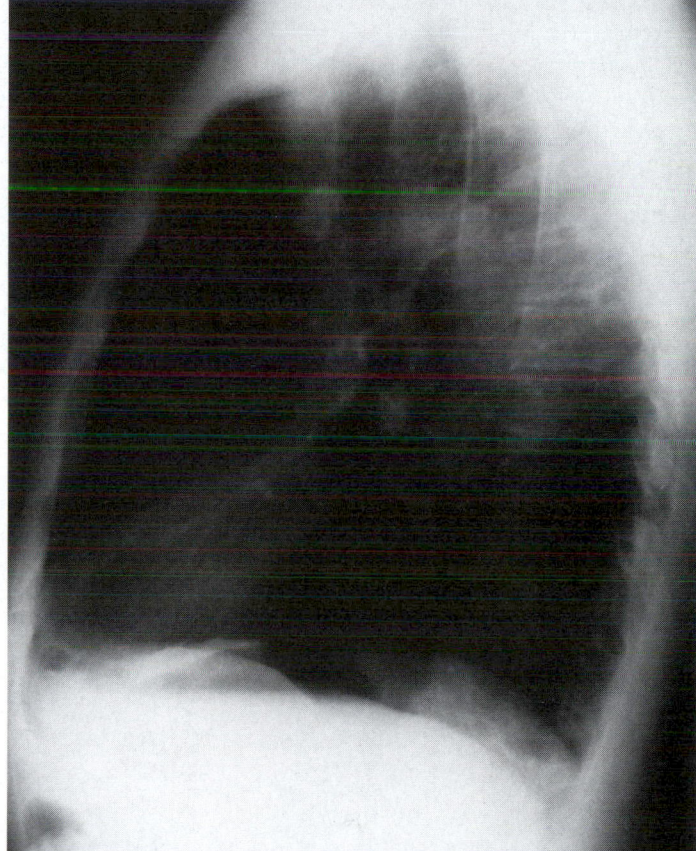

E

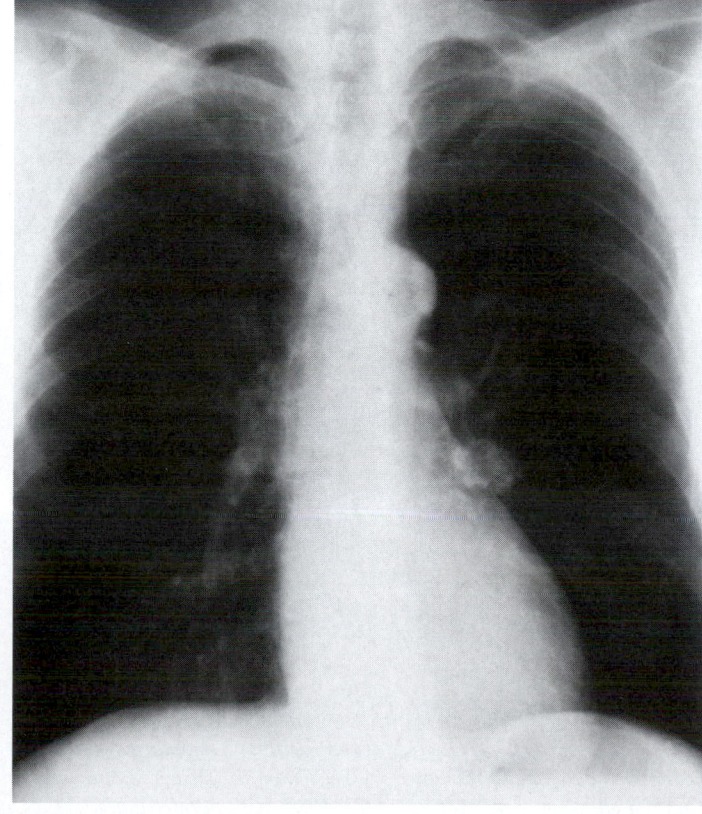

D

FIGURE 96-9 *(Cont.)*   Thymoma. Sixty-two-year-old man after successful treatment of gastric cancer and aortic aneurysm. *A* and *B*. PA and lateral radiographs demonstrate an anterior mediastinal mass projecting into left hemithorax (arrows). *C*. CT scan demonstrates 4-cm mass abutting thoracic aorta (arrows). No obvious invasion. *D* and *E*. Postoperative films showing remaining calcified lymph nodes but no thymoma.

Tumor stage at the time of treatment indicates prognosis better than tumor grade. Table 96-6 lists the most common staging mechanism applied to thymic malignancies. Stage I lesions are generally considered benign. Tumor-node-metastasis (TNM) staging has not been widely adopted. A peculiar characteristic of the benign histologic appearance of many of these lesions is that invasion of adjacent structures, and thus the stage of the tumor, can usually be more easily determined by the surgeon at the time of operation than by the pathologist at the time of microscopy.

Thymoma is the most common primary neoplasm of the mediastinum, comprising approximately 15 percent of all thymic lesions. These tumors occur with equal frequency in men and women 40 to 60 years of age. Seventy-five percent present in the anterior mediastinum; more than 90 percent are visible on the chest radiograph.

The mainstay of therapy, even for extensive lesions, is surgical resection (Figs. 96-9 and 96-10). In a series of 141 patients who underwent resection followed by routine radiotherapy (30 Gy in 3 weeks to 50 Gy in 6 weeks),[46] those who underwent complete resections, even up to stage III, had survival rates of 100 percent at 5 years and 94.7 percent at 10 and 15 years. There was no difference between stages as long as the resection was complete. Most surgeons, even those experienced in thoracoscopy, recommend median sternotomy for the procedure. Another study reported 5- and 10-year survivals of 74 percent and 57 percent, respectively, following a treatment regimen that included surgery and postoperative radiotherapy for all patients and postoperative chemotherapy for some patients with high-grade lesions. For patients who had total resection, the reported 5-year survival was 89 percent.[1,43]

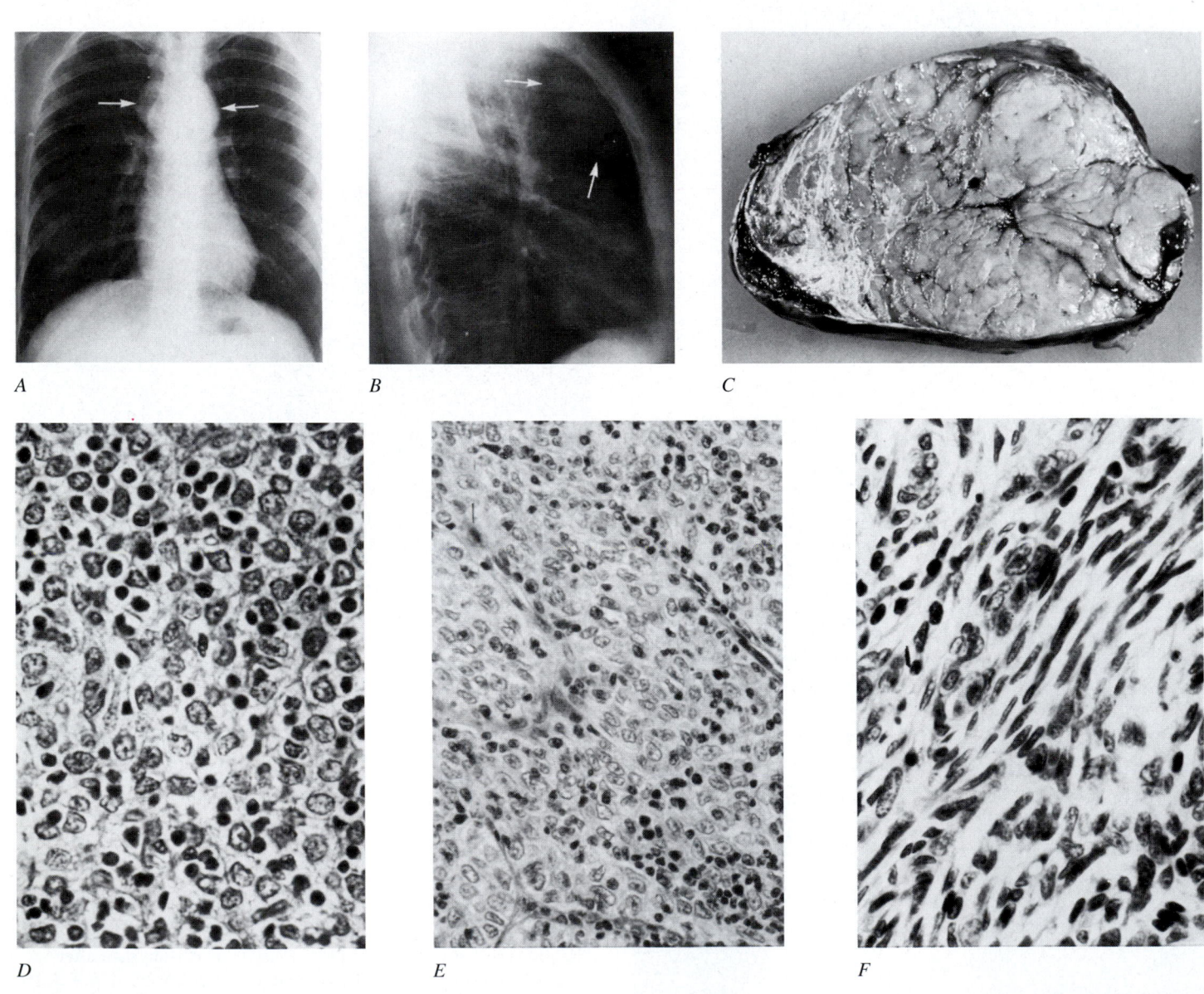

A   *B*   *C*

D   *E*   *F*

FIGURE 96-10   Benign thymoma of anterior mediastinum. *A* and *B*. Radiographic appearance of thymoma. *C*. Gross appearance of a benign thymoma. The tumor has a thick fibrous capsule. *D* to *F*. Varied histologic appearances of thymomas. In *D*, the cells are mixed epithelial (large cells with clear nuclei) and lymphocytic, ×250. In *E*, epithelial cells predominate, ×224. In *F*, the predominant cells are spindles, ×248. [*Based on data of Lyerly and Sabiston, Primary neoplasms and cysts of the mediastinum, in Fishman (ed), Pulmonary Diseases and Disorders, 2d ed. New York, McGraw-Hill, 1988, with permission.*]

TABLE 96-7

Paraneoplastic Syndromes Associated with Thymoma

Well established (proven)
  Myasthenia gravis
  Pure red-cell aplasia
  Acquired hypogammaglobulinemia
  Nonthymic cancers
Less well established (associated)
  Pancytopenia
  Lambert-Eaton
  Peripheral neuropathies
  CNS changes
  Multiple endocrine defects
  Multiple rheumatologic disorders
  Nephrotic syndrome

Most recurrences are local, either in the pleural space or in the mediastinum. Distant recurrences, when they do develop, are most often in bone. Recurrences are potentially curable, requiring several therapeutic methods, including repeated surgical exploration. Reexploration and successful resection were reported for 23 patients who had recurrence of thymoma after previous complete resections.[33]

All patients in whom an invasive thymoma has been resected should receive postoperative radiotherapy, which is strongly recommended for all but stage I patients. Surgery alone yields a recurrence rate of 28 percent, whereas radiation and surgery together yield a recurrence rate of 3 percent.[14] Whether noninvasive and encapsulated thymomas respond to irradiation is unsettled. Dosage is usually 3500 to 5000 rads over 3 to 6 weeks. A dosage of more than 5000 rads does not increase the response rate but does increase the frequency of complications.

Patients with thymomas, even when the disease is unresectable, recurrent, or metastatic, often respond to treatment with cisplatin, doxorubicin, and cyclophosphamide. In an intergroup study of 22 patients with locally unresectable or metastatic disease, there were 3 complete and 11 partial responses, for a total response rate of 70 percent. The median survival of all patients was 59 months; three patients remained disease-free after 3 years of follow-up.[40]

Paraneoplastic Syndromes Myasthenia gravis is the most common thymoma-associated systemic syndrome.[34] Many other syndromes may also be related to thymoma. Table 96-7 lists the four well-established syndromes and some others that are less characteristically associated.

The most commonly used clinical staging classification is shown in Table 96-8. Patients with myasthenia gravis present with muscle weakness that intensifies with repetitive activity. The pathophysiology of myasthenia gravis entails the autoimmune-mediated binding of antibodies to the acetylcholine receptor, followed by their lysis by complement-mediated factors. Striking clinical improvement may occur after thymectomy without any change in measurable immune parameters, including the absence of change in the serum levels of autoantibodies. Unfortunately, the likelihood of improvement after thymectomy is significantly less for patients with thymomas.

No randomized studies have demonstrated a benefit of thymectomy for any group or subgroup of patients with myasthenia gravis, with or without thymomas. In a series of 149 patients with juvenile myasthenia gravis who were followed for a median of 17 years, half of the patients who underwent thymectomy sustained complete remission, whereas only one-third of the medically treated patients had the same response.[51] The patients who underwent thymectomy also had slightly improved long-term survival. Because of such information, thymectomy has become standard for patients with myasthenia gravis, except for those who have only ocular symptoms.

Myasthenia gravis is present in approximately one-third of patients with thymomas. This disorder may either precede or follow the development of thymoma by many years. Any type of thymic tumor may occur in patients with myasthenia gravis. Patients with thymoma and myasthenia gravis derive less neurologic benefit from resection than do those with myasthenia gravis without a thymoma.[55]

Among patients with myasthenia gravis without thymomas, remission can be expected in one-quarter to one-half: in about 20 percent, remissions are completely drug-free; in up to 30 percent, remission is maintained by drugs—i.e., a combined remission rate of 50 percent.[34] Improvement can be expected in one-third to one-half of patients; no change is evident in 10 percent, and a rare patient gets worse after surgery.[17] Patients with myasthenia gravis and thymoma fare more poorly after resection than do those without a thymoma: their symptomatic improvement after surgery is poorer, with combined remission rates of only 30 percent, and there is considerable risk of recurrence of the thymoma. Combined cervical and mediastinal incisions have been recommended to accomplish a maximal thymectomy.[28]

TABLE 96-8

Osserman Clinical Staging Classification for Myasthenia Gravis

Group 1 Ocular myasthenia gravis
  A   Ocular symptoms, stable for 4 years
  B   Ocular symptoms only, with history of generalized
        symptoms
Group 2 Generalized myasthenia gravis
  A   Mild generalized
        Ocular weakness gradually spreading to skeletal involvement
        Respiratory and bulbar muscles not affected
  B   Moderate generalized
        Progression to generalized involvement of skeletal and
          bulbar muscles
        Dysarthria, dysphagia, difficult mastication
  C   Severe generalized
        Skeletal and bulbar muscle weakness
        Respiratory muscle involvement

SOURCE: Adapted from Blossmon et al.[10]

Postoperative radiotherapy decreases the recurrence rate after resection. Radiation therapy without resection can worsen myasthenia gravis. The dose of radiotherapy should be 3500 to 5000 rads.

Red-cell aplasia occurs in 5 percent of patients with thymomas. It is a rare disorder that results in a severe normochromic normocytic anemia. Erythroid precursors in the bone marrow are decreased or absent, so reticulocytosis is markedly decreased. Thirty-three to 50 percent of patients with red-cell aplasia have thymomas. Thymectomy produces remissions in approximately 40 percent of patients. It is more likely to be effective in patients with thymoma or thymic enlargement (remissions in up to 50 percent of patients) than in patients without thymomas.

Hypogammaglobulinemia occurs in 5 to 10 percent of patients with thymomas. It is more common in patients with both thymoma and rheumatoid arthritis, ulcerative colitis, many cytopenias, and some extrathymic cancers. Thymectomy has not proved beneficial.

Extrathymic cancers develop in up to 20 percent of patients who survive thymoma, most commonly as lymphomas, bronchogenic carcinomas, and thyroid cancers. The management of these patients should be determined by the extrathymic malignancy and not by the previous thymoma.

THYMIC CARCINOMA

These are epithelial neoplasms of thymic origin with considerably more cytologic and architectural features of malignancy than manifested by thymomas. Several subtypes exist, with significant differences in outcomes after surgical resection. In 60 patients who underwent surgery with or without adjuvant chemoradiotherapy, the 5-year survival rate was 33 percent.[60] As may be seen in Table 96-5, patients with low-grade lesions (squamous cell carcinoma, mucoepidermal carcinoma, and basaloid carcinoma) sustained a 95 percent cure rate. However, treatment of high-grade lesions (lymphoepithelioid lesions, small cell or neuroendocrine lesions, clear cell and sarcomatoid carcinomas, and anaplastic tumors) yielded only a 15 percent long-term survival.[60] All high-grade lesions should be considered for resection, followed by postoperative chemotherapy, since the more malignant group of tumors may respond to cisplatin-based regimens.[64] These malignancies often are positive for Epstein-Barr virus (EBV) or demonstrate EBV-associated nuclear antigens in carcinoma cells. However, not all thymic carcinomas demonstrate a linkage to EBV.

THYMIC CARCINOID

These are distinctly uncommon neuroendocrine cell neoplasms that may present with a paraneoplastic syndrome. Patients in whom the tumors have a small cell appearance on histology need postoperative chemotherapy; those in whom the histology is carcinoid require resection alone.

THYMOLIPOMAS

These are tumors of fatty tissue within the thymus gland. They are benign tumors that masquerade as cardiomegaly. If the di-

agnosis is made preoperatively, they are best followed with CT scans and do not require resection. However, concern about possible malignancy usually necessitates resection.

THYMIC HYPERPLASIA

True hyperplasia is a large bulky benign tumor that most commonly presents in young boys with massive thymic enlargement. This true hyperplasia occurs in children after treatment of other malignancies and recovery from other systemic disease states. It is a common form of presentation in patients who develop bulky thymus glands after treatment for Hodgkin's lymphoma.

Tumors of Lymph Nodes

Together, lymphomas and metastatic cancer constitute the most common mediastinal masses. The anterior mediastinum not only is the most common site of primary mediastinal lymphomas but also can be invaded by cervical or visceral disease.

LYMPHOMA

Lymphomas constitute 10 to 14 percent of mediastinal masses in adults. They make up 20 percent of anterosuperior mediastinal masses and 20 percent of middle mediastinal masses, ranking second in frequency in both compartments. Lymphomas are rare in the posterior mediastinum. The numerous classifications proposed for lymphoma are generally no better for determining prognosis or managing patients than is simple classification into either Hodgkin's or non-Hodgkin's lymphoma.

Fully 20 to 30 percent of patients with lymphoma are asymptomatic, even with bulky malignant disease. Of the symptomatic patients, 60 to 70 percent have symptoms of local invasion and 30 to 35 percent have systemic symptoms, including fever, weight loss, and pruritus (so-called B type symptoms). Local symptoms include chest heaviness, discomfort, and cough. Tracheal or bronchial compression can cause associated wheezing or stridor. Dysphagia is an unusual complaint. Superior vena cava syndrome is a rare presentation.

Diagnosis requires significant tissue samples. FNA biopsies are not adequate in most circumstances, although the yield improves with radiologic (ultrasound or CT) techniques that target specific areas of the mediastinal mass. The yield is relatively low, but so is the complication rate. Therefore, an attempt is reasonable, especially in patients for whom general anesthesia is problematic. Biopsies under local anesthesia of more accessible cervical nodes or of mediastinal nodes by mediastinoscopy or anterior mediastinotomy (under general anesthesia) have the greatest yield.

MEDIASTINAL HODGKIN'S DISEASE

The age distribution of patients with mediastinal Hodgkin's disease is bimodal—20 to 30 years of age or greater than 50 years of age. Among young adults, men and women are affected equally, although mediastinal lymphoma is more common in older men than in older women. The nodular sclerosing subtype of Hodgkin's disease accounts for almost 90 percent of patients

TABLE 96-9

Ann Arbor Staging System for Hodgkin's Disease

Stage	Characteristics
I	One lymph node region on either side of the diaphragm
II	Two or more lymph node regions on the same side of the diaphragm
III	Two or more lymph node regions on both sides of the diaphragm
IV	Diffuse or disseminated organ involvement

who present with mediastinal invasion. Of these, half have only mediastinal disease and the other half have mediastinal disease with associated neck disease. Systemic symptoms of night sweats, fever, malaise, and weight loss are common. Mild local symptoms such as pain and cough are not uncommon. Severe local symptoms, such as superior vena cava syndrome, are very uncommon.

Chest radiographs reveal superior mediastinal masses that typically arise in the anterior or visceral compartment. In 108 patients with newly diagnosed Hodgkin's disease, CT of the chest disclosed a predictable pattern of contiguous spread: the disease typically began in the anterior mediastinal/paratracheal area and spread to the other mediastinal lymph node groups and subsequently to the hila and into the lungs.[18] So predictable was this pattern of spread that the demonstration of noncontiguous or skip disease should prompt consideration of diagnoses other than Hodgkin's disease. Furthermore, impairment of lungs or pericardium consistently occurred only when the diameter of the mediastinal mass was greater than 30 percent of the thoracic diameter.

This consistent progression of Hodgkin's disease of the mediastinum correlates with the staging of the disease. Table 96-9 depicts the Ann Arbor staging system for Hodgkin's disease. In stages IA and IIA, mediastinal irradiation alone is used. In the more advanced stages, chemotherapy is combined with radiotherapy (Fig. 96-11). Different clinics use somewhat different therapeutic approaches.[27] Most patients (70 to 85 percent, depending on the stage of disease at presentation) respond to treatment with long-term disease-free survivals. Chemotherapy is so effective against Hodgkin's disease that relapses can be treated effectively.

NON-HODGKIN'S LYMPHOMA

Whereas about 75 percent of patients with Hodgkin's disease present with mediastinal disease, only 5 percent of patients with non-Hodgkin's lymphoma present with mediastinal involvement.[18] Abdominal lymph nodes, cervical lymph nodes, and lymphoid tissue of Waldeyer's ring are more commonly affected than are mediastinal nodes. Large irregular anterior and superior mediastinal masses are common and are often associated with large pleural effusions, large pericardial effusions, and large pulmonary parenchymal changes. Because lymph nodes other than mediastinal nodes and body fluids are more accessible, mediastinoscopic biopsy is not usually necessary.

Radiation alone is poor treatment for non-Hodgkin's lymphoma because the disease spreads in a less predictable manner than does Hodgkin's disease (Fig. 96-12). These malignancies may consist of T cells, B cells, diffuse large cell lymphomas, or lymphoblastic lymphomas. Because of the aggressive nature of these lymphomas, a modified staging system (Table 96-10) has been proposed for non-Hodgkin's lymphomas (*lymphocytic lymphomas*).[41]

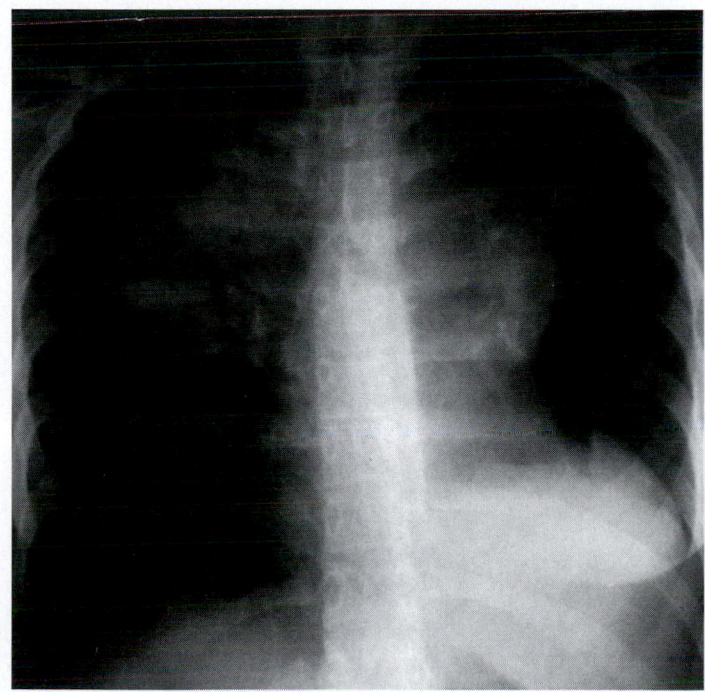

A

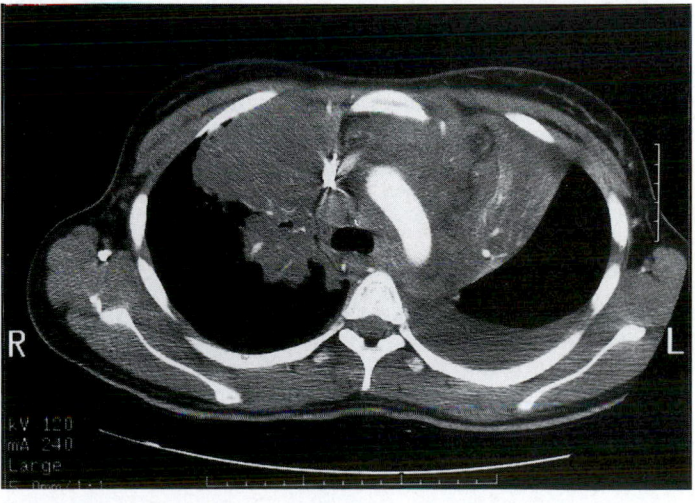

B

FIGURE 96-11 Hodgkin's disease. *A.* Bulky mediastinal mass demonstrated to be Hodgkin's disease by mediastinoscopy. *B.* Chest CT demonstrates bulky mediastinal mass and pleural effusion. The mass disappeared in response to combination chemotherapy and radiotherapy. The patient is well at 18 months.

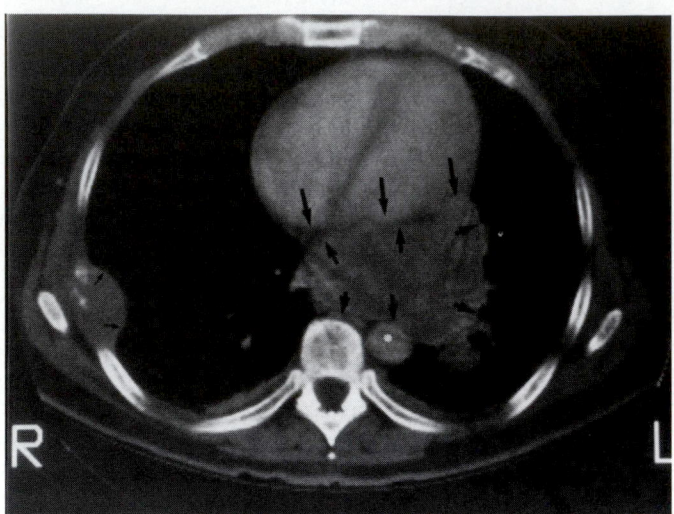

FIGURE 96-12   Non-Hodgkin's lymphoma. Chest CT shows large middle and posterior mediastinal mass with distant metastasis to a rib in the contralateral chest. This skip involvement is typical of non-Hodgkin's lymphoma.

Radiation therapy is effective in treatment for patients with early-stage low-grade lymphoma. In some patients it may be curative (10 years disease-free survival rates of 50 to 60 percent). Chemotherapy may improve results in this group of patients. Patients with advanced low-grade lymphoma may not benefit from treatment. Indeed, no treatment has demonstrated consistent ability to induce a long-term disease-free survival or to alter the natural history of the disease in these patients. Most oncologists would treat patients with Ann Arbor stage III disease with combinations of chemotherapy and radiotherapy, anticipating a 10-year survival of 40 percent.

The treatment of a localized lymphoma that appears histologically to be aggressive consists of combination chemotherapy, either with or without radiation therapy of the affected field. Stages I and II patients can expect 5-year disease-free survival rates of 80 to 100 percent. The benefit of radiotherapy is unclear, as comparisons between patients who receive radiotherapy and those who do not demonstrate no differences in survival. Patients with advanced aggressive disease clearly benefit from combination chemotherapy and can expect survival rates of 35 percent at 10 years.

CASTLEMAN'S DISEASE

Castleman's disease (giant lymph node hyperplasia) is characterized by mass lesions that occur most often in the anterosuperior mediastinum (52 percent) and less often (26 percent) in the neck, abdomen, and axilla. The mass is a vascular tumor often surrounded by lymphadenopathy. This arrangement makes CT useful diagnostically, since CT may reveal lymphadenopathy surrounding an encapsulated mass that enhances brightly and is distinct from the aorta.

The term is applied to three lesions that are histologically distinct: hyaline vascular, plasma cell, and generalized. The first two represent localized disease, whereas the third refers to multicentric (generalized) disease (Fig. 96-13).

Hyaline vascular Castleman's disease comprises 90 percent of cases. It is a localized lesion found incidentally in asymptomatic patients. Surgical excision is the treatment of choice; radiotherapy has not been effective. The plasma cell variant, also localized, is much less common. Patients are much more likely to have symptoms and present with fever, fatigue, weight loss, and hemolytic anemia. The sedimentation rate is often high and associated with hypergammaglobulinemia, which results from the production of interleukin 6 by the hyperplastic lymph nodes. Resection is the treatment of choice in order to prevent malignant degeneration.

Generalized, or multicentric, Castleman's disease has the histologic features of both localized forms. The disease occurs in older patients, who typically present with severe systemic symptoms, generalized lymphadenopathy, and hepatosplenomegaly. The mortality from this disease is 50 percent, and the median survival is 27 months. Progression to lymphoma is common. The diagnosis of lymphoma is made from biopsy, and treatment is directed at managing the lymphoma.

SARCOIDOSIS

Sarcoidosis often presents with mediastinal or hilar adenopathy that is characterized histologically by noncaseating granulomas. The typical patient is in the third or fourth decade of life, is asymptomatic, and has been found to have a mediastinal mass consistent with adenopathy. Some patients present with fatigue and malaise or with complaints referable to particular organ systems. Cough and dyspnea are common; the most common sites of extrapulmonary involvement are the eyes (uveitis, conjunctivitis, and retinitis) and the skin (nodules, plaques, and erythema nodosum). The clinical and laboratory features of sarcoidosis are described elsewhere in this book (see Chapter 69). Chest radiograph typically (in 80 percent of patients with this disease) shows bilateral hilar and mediastinal adenopathy, often accompanied by parenchymal involvement of the lungs.

The diagnosis is one of exclusion but

TABLE 96-10

NCI Modified Staging for Intermediate and High-Grade Lymphomas

Stage	Characteristics
I	Localized nodal or extranodal disease (Ann Arbor stage I or IB)
II	Two or more sites of disease or a localized extranodal site plus draining nodes with *none* of the following:
	Performance status <70
	B symptoms
	Any mass >10 cm in diameter
	Serum LDH >500
	Three or more extranodal sites of disease
III	Stage II plus any poor prognostic factors

SOURCE: From DeVita VT Jr et al: Lymphatic lymphomas, in: DeVita VT Jr, Hellman S, Rosenberg SA (eds), *Cancer: Principles of Oncology,* 3d ed., Philadelphia, Lippincott, 1989.

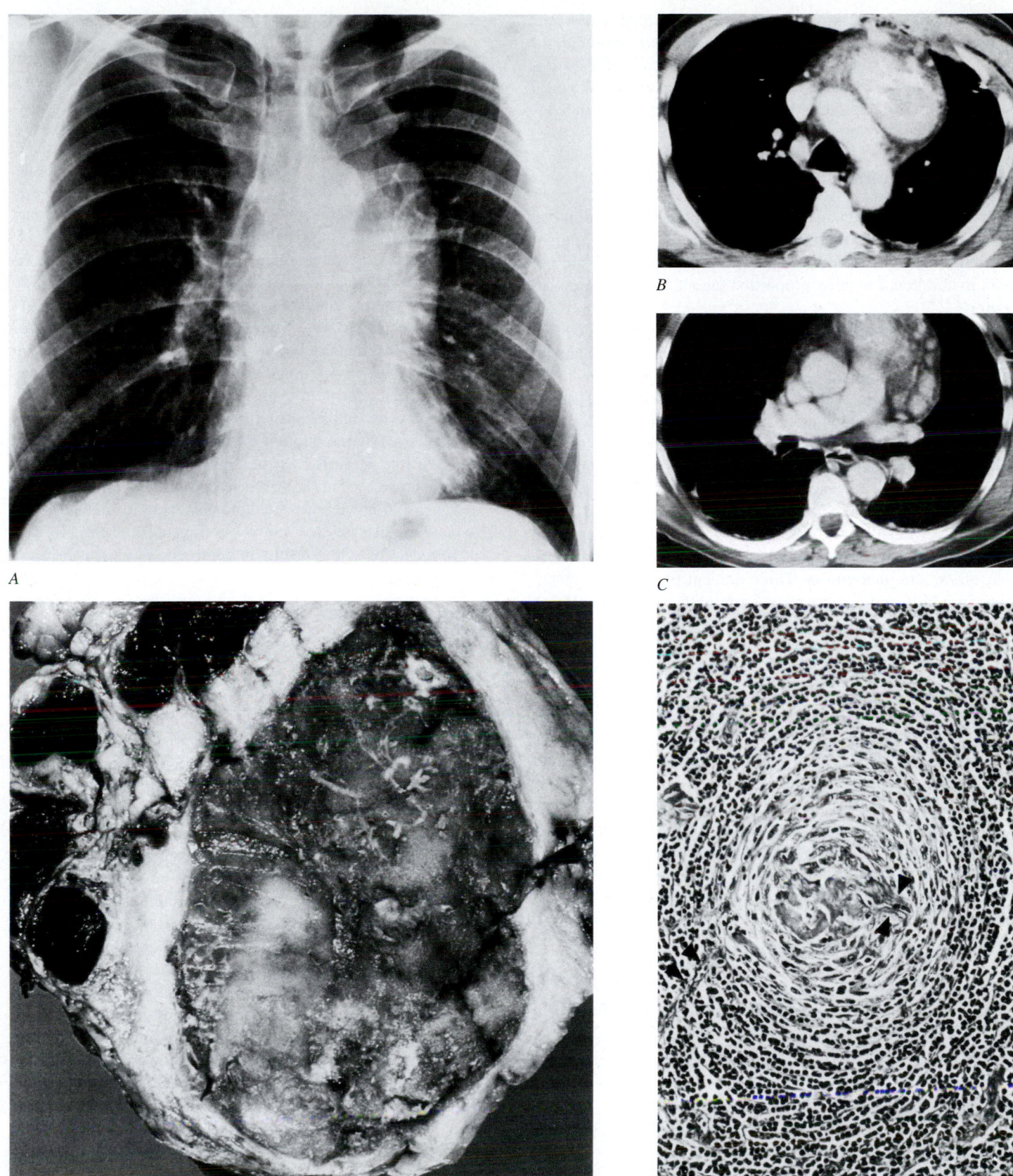

FIGURE 96-13   Giant lymph node hyperplasia (Castleman's disease). *A.* Posteroanterior radiograph. Lobulated superoanterior mediastinal mass extending into the left hemithorax and containing areas of dense calcification (that were quite striking on the lateral chest radiograph). *B* and *C.* CT scans reveal enhancing mass that extends throughout the anterior mediastinum as far as the orgin of the pulmonary artery. The mass contains calcifications and is surrounded inferiorly by multiple lymph nodes. *D.* Excised specimen. Maximum diameter of 13.5 cm. Thick, fibrous capsule that also envelopes adjacent, anthracotic lymph nodes. *E.* Histologic appearance. Many lymphoid follicles with prominent germinal centers. The germinal centers are permeated by radially oriented capillaries and surrounded by concentrically arranged lymphocytes.

may require biopsy of skin lesions or the mediastinal nodes. Part of the tissue obtained by biopsy is smeared and cultured for acid-fast or other likely organisms. The condition of most patients improves, or remains stable, without treatment. About 20 percent suffer progressive pulmonary impairment, with an overall mortality at 5 years of 4 percent.

Germ Cell Tumors

Both benign and malignant teratomas are classified as germ cell tumors. They are the fourth most common lesion in the adult mediastinum. Most lesions in the adult (60 to 80 percent) are benign; in children, a smaller proportion (about 57 percent) are benign.

Mediastinal germ cell tumors are of several types. *Benign teratomas* constitute 70 percent of the lesions in children and 60 percent of the lesions in adults. The predominant malignant lesions are *seminomas,* which constitute 50 percent of all malignant lesions. Nonseminomatous malignant lesions include a mix of tumors: malignant teratomas, malignant teratocarcinomas, yolk sac tumors, endodermal sinus tumors, choriocarcinomas, and embryonal cell carcinomas (Table 96-11).

All types of germ cell tumors that have been found in the testes have been reported to occur in the mediastinum. Nonetheless, compared to testicular tumors, extragonadal germ cell tumors are uncommon. Three percent of all germ cell tumors in adults and 7 percent of germ cell tumors in children are extragonadal. An even smaller percentage (1 to 2 percent) of germ cell tumors originate in the mediastinum. Blood levels of alpha-fetoprotein (AFP) and human chorionic gonadotropin (HCG) should be determined for all patients in whom malignant germ cell tumors are suspected. Mediastinal metastasis is common in testicular neoplasms. In weighing the possibility of a germ cell tumor, a primary testicular tumor should always enter into the differential diagnosis because cells responsible for mediastinal germ cell tumors may derive from germ cell rests that migrated to the mediastinum from the urogenital ridge. Metastases from the testes, however, are unlikely. Germ cell tumors usually develop along the body midline in the cranium, mediastinum, retroperitoneum, and presacral areas.

BENIGN GERM CELL TUMORS (TERATOMAS)

These tumors are of multiple tissues that are foreign to the part of the body in which they develop. They consist of a disorganized mixture of derivatives of the three germinal layers—ectoderm, mesoderm, and endoderm. Consequently, they may contain elements of skin and its appendages, bone, cartilage, intestinal and respiratory epithelium, and neurovascular tissue. About 80 percent of these lesions are benign. A dermoid cyst (benign cystic teratoma) is a variant that contains sebaceous material within a lining of squamous epithelium.

The lesions occur most often in adolescents or adults; the incidence is about equal in males and females. In one series of 86 patients in whom benign mediastinal teratomas had been resected, the mean age was 28 years.[37] About one-third of the patients are asymptomatic, but symptoms are likely to develop if the cysts become infected and erode into the pericardial space, the pleural space, or a bronchus. Occasionally, episodes of hypoglycemia occur in patients with benign mediastinal teratomas and are relieved by resection of the tumor. Approximately a third of these lesions are calcified. In the series of 86 patients, all of the surgical deaths (5 of 86) occurred before 1945. If the benign lesions were completely resected, no postoperative radiation was given and the disease-free interval averaged 10 years.[37] In general, complete resection results in cure.

MALIGNANT GERM CELL TUMORS

The origin of malignant germ cell tumors is unclear. The several different types behave differently and require different therapies.

Malignant Mediastinal Teratomas   Malignant teratomas typically include elements of mature (benign) teratoma, immature teratoma, choriocarcinoma, yolk sac carcinoma, embryonal carcinoma, and seminoma in various proportions. These tumors produce either AFP or HCG, the presence of either of which is diagnostic for malignant as opposed to benign tumor. In a series of eight patients, neoadjuvant chemotherapy resulted in a decrease in hormone levels. Two regimens—one with vincristine, methotrexate, bleomycin, and cisplatin and the other with etoposide, dactinomycin, and cyclophosphamide—were given. Six of the eight patients subsequently underwent resection; one patient, who had residual tumor, also received postoperative chemotherapy. One surgical patient died eight months after surgery; the others were alive and well 13 to 136 months after the start of treatment. The two patients who were treated medically died 1 and 15 months, respectively, after the operation.[49]

Mediastinal Seminomas   The embryologic origins of mediastinal seminomas are unclear. One theory holds that they derive from somatic cells of the bronchial cleft. The other holds that they derive from extragonadal or em-

TABLE 96-11

Mediastinal Germ Cell Tumors

Histology	Primary Treatment Method	Overall 5-year Survival (%)
Benign teratomas	Surgical resection	>90
Malignant teratomas	Chemotherapy + surgical resection	~50
Seminomas		
Metastatic	Cisplatin-based chemotherapy	60–85
Resectable	Surgery + radiation + cisplatin chemotherapy	>90
Nonseminomatous lesions	Cisplatin-based chemotherapy	30–50

SOURCE: Table compiled from Parker et al;[49] Dulmet et al;[20] Logothetis CJ, Samuels ML, Selig DE, et al: *J Clin Oncol* 3:316–325, 1985; Goss PE, Schwertfeger L, Blackstein ME, et al: *Cancer* 73:1971–1979, 1994.

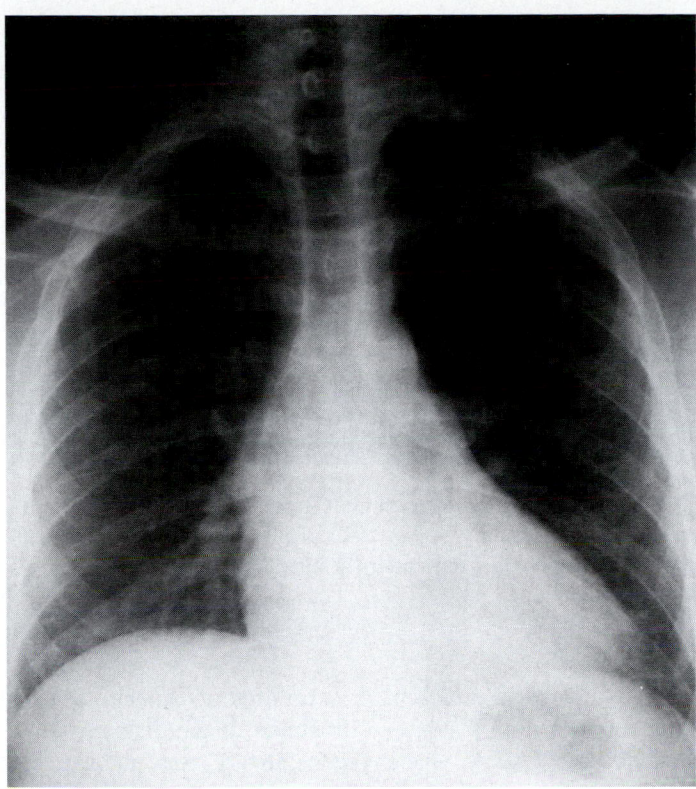

A

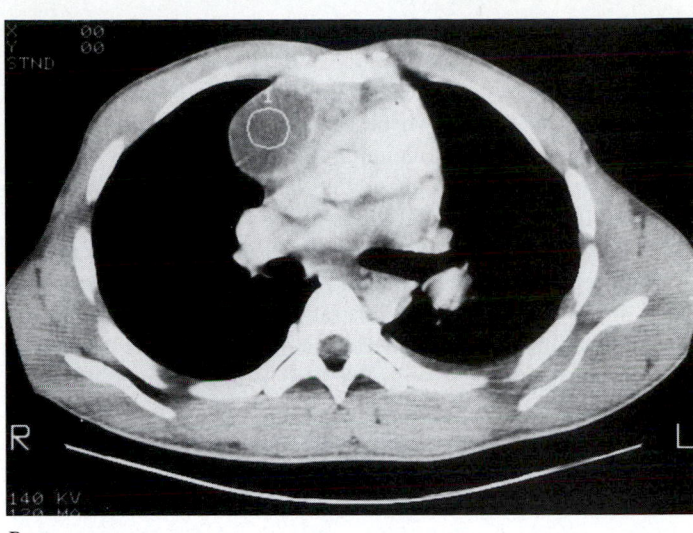

B

FIGURE 96-14 Mediastinal seminoma. Twenty-nine-year-old man, HIV positive, with generalized malaise and 5- to 10-pound weight loss. *A.* Chest radiograph reveals inferior mediastinal enlargement. *B.* Chest CT shows homogeneous mass within thymic fat.

bryonic yolk sac germ cells arrested near the developing thymus in the course of their migration along the urogenital ridge to the gonad.

Pure seminomas constitute 50 percent of all germ cell tumors of the mediastinum. They occur principally in men 20 to 40 years of age (Fig. 96-14); fewer than 5 percent occur in women. Mediastinal seminomas are the most common of the malignant germ cell tumors of the mediastinum. They often present with intrathoracic metastases that preclude excision. A CT scan of the testicles is necessary to rule out a primary lesion that originates in the testicles. Serum levels of AFP and HCG rarely increase in patients with mediastinal seminomas; if their levels are increased, another diagnosis is likely.

Seminomas are very radiosensitive. Radiotherapy is appropriate primary therapy for early-stage lesions, as is surgical resection. Criteria for resectability are that the patient is asymptomatic, that the mass is confined to the anterior mediastinum, and that neither intrathoracic nor distant metastases are present. Only complete resections contribute to cure or palliation. Even after complete resection, radiation (4500 to 5000 rads) improves outcome.

Chemotherapy benefits patients whose lesions appear histologically to be particularly malignant and therefore suggest a high risk of failure. The regimens most commonly used are vinblastine, bleomycin, and cisplatin. Chemotherapy given to patients with disseminated disease can yield 5-year disease-free survivals of 60 to 90 percent.[22,39] Extensive disease and prior radiotherapy presage poorer prognosis.

In a series of 41 patients with advanced abdominal seminoma who were reevaluated after treatment with cisplatin-based chemotherapy, 23 were found to have a residual mass; in 14 of these patients, the mass was greater than 3 cm in diameter. Nineteen of the patients with residual lesions underwent subsequent excision or biopsy. In 6 of the 14 patients in whom the residual mass was greater than 3 cm, viable seminoma was found. These observations suggested that patients in whom the residual mass is greater than 3 cm in diameter should receive follow-up treatment with either radiotherapy or additional chemotherapy, depending on the clinical situation.[45]

Nonseminomatous Tumors   These tumors are less common than seminomatous malignant germ cell tumors. They form in the anterior mediastinal compartment. Nonseminomatous tumors present with symptoms of compression or invasion of local thoracic structures. Patients also have systemic symptoms of weight loss, fatigue, and fever. In 85 to 95 percent, there is one site of distant metastasis. Serum HCG or AFP greater than 500 mg/ml is diagnostic of nonseminomatous malignant germ cell tumors (Fig. 96-4). Nonseminomatous malignant germ cell tumors include pure and mixed embryonal carcinomas, teratocarcinomas, choriocarcinomas, and endodermal sinus (or yolk sac) tumors.

The typical patient is a young male (median age of 35 years). In all patients with these tumors, βHCG or AFP levels in serum are increased. Nonseminomatous tumors usually have a heterogeneous density on CT scan, whereas seminomas tend to have a homogeneous density. They can present with pleural effusions. These tumors are relatively more frequent in patients with Kleinfelter's syndrome.

Embryonal carcinomas occur in both adults and children and are clinically similar to seminomas.

Choriocarcinomas typically present in young adult men, half of whom have gynecomastia. This results from production of βHCG by the tumor. Therefore, βHCG is a tumor marker in these patients and helps in following the course and recurrence of the disease.

Endodermal sinus (yolk sac) tumors form in both adults and children. They occur infrequently in the mediastinum and more commonly in sacrococcygeal teratomas and in the gonads. They produce AFP no matter where they are located; the blood level of this protein helps in following therapy.

Teratocarcinomas are mixed-cell lesions. They are similar to embryonal and endodermal sinus tumors in that they occur in adults and children and may present with distant metastases.

Management of these tumors does not require surgery initially, since the lesions are generally unresectable at presentation. Treatment with chemotherapy and radiotherapy is the mainstay. More aggressive regimens, particularly the addition of cisplatin, improve the results of treatment of extragonadal nonseminomatous tumors. In such responders who are left with a residual mass, resection is appropriate. Testicular tumors are more chemosensitive than all extragonadal tumors, and retroperitoneal tumors are more sensitive than mediastinal tumors. The chemotherapy regimens include bleomycin, cisplatin, vinblastine, and etoposide. These regimens can yield complete response rates of 40 to 60 percent and 30 to 50 percent long-term survivors (Table 96-11).[20]

Patients with nonseminomatous germ cell tumors, especially those with yolk sac or embryonal cell carcinoma in combination with teratoma, are prone to develop hematologic neoplasms. The median time to development of the hematologic malignancy (usually megakaryoblastic leukemia or malignant histiocytosis) is 6 months. Thirteen of 16 reported patients developed the second hematologic malignancy within 1 year after the diagnosis of the mediastinal germ cell tumor. The course of the hematologic malignancy is particularly virulent. Although all these patients had received cisplatin, it could not be implicated as the etiologic agent because reviews of large numbers of patients who received cisplatin for other malignancies have revealed no similar hematologic malignancies. A marking isochromosome (12p) in the mediastinal germ cell tumor and in the associated leukemic blasts in one patient has suggested that these tumors may arise from a common progenitor cell.[47]

Any mass that remains after chemotherapy should be resected if two conditions are met: The patient has had a good response to the chemotherapy, and levels of tumor markers in serum fall to normal. Any tumor left behind is usually a benign teratoma or necrotic tumor mass that can degenerate and redevelop malignancy. If the tumor markers do not fall but the tumor shrinks, surgery is of no benefit.

A few mediastinal germ cell tumors are composed of a single cell type. Testicular biopsy or testicular CT is necessary in patients with such mediastinal germ cell tumors to rule out a primary testicular neoplasm. Testicular biopsy is indicated if a mass is palpated, if high-resolution ultrasound is abnormal, and if CT demonstrates involvement of pelvic or retroperitoneal lymph nodes.

MIDDLE MEDIASTINAL MASSES

Bronchogenic Cysts

Mediastinal cysts constitute 20 percent of all mediastinal masses, and bronchogenic cysts make up 60 percent of all mediastinal

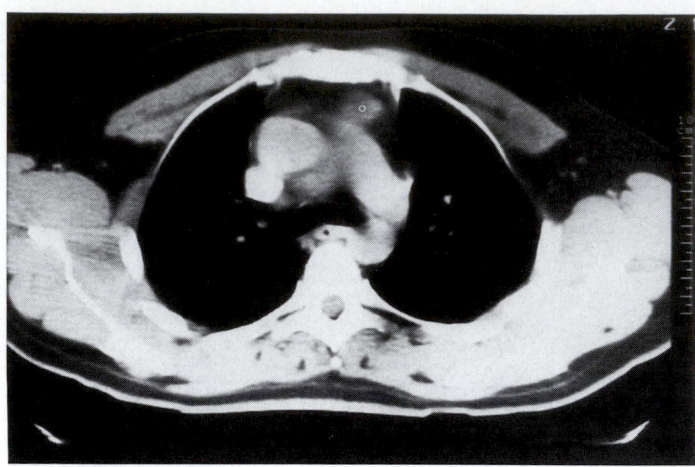

FIGURE 96-15   Bronchogenic cyst. CT scan obtained to evaluate dull chest ache. The lesion was thoracoscopically excised, and the patient was discharged home 2 days after the operation.

cysts. Symptoms are present in two-thirds of patients, usually from compression of adjacent structures. If the diagnosis of a bronchogenic cyst is made preoperatively and patients are asymptomatic, observation is an appropriate course. If there is any question of malignancy—based on radiographic appearance, positive cytology, or evidence of enlargement or recurrence—the lesion should be resected. The presence of symptoms—especially pain, cough, or hemoptysis—suggests the advisability of resection. The presence of an air-fluid level indicates connection with the bronchopulmonary tree and the likelihood of recurrent infection and indicates that resection is in order. Symptoms tend to develop with time, and resection at an asymptomatic stage may be best in healthy subjects. Also, malignancy or infection can develop in these cysts if the decision is made to observe instead of operating. Video-assisted techniques offer the opportunity to resect less threatening lesions with low morbidity (Fig. 96-15).

In 86 patients followed for 20 years at the same institution, 20 of whom had bronchogenic cysts of the lung and 66 of the mediastinum, 33 percent were asymptomatic at the time of operation. At operation in these 86 patients, fistulization, ulceration, hemorrhage, or infection was found in 33 percent of the resected lesions. Overall, the experience indicated that 82 percent of these patients had a bronchogenic cyst that was symptomatic, complicated, or both. There were no surgical deaths, and one major complication ensued (reintubation and ultimate tracheostomy for respiratory failure). In view of these results, the authors recommended resection of all bronchogenic cysts, asymptomatic or not.[58]

Esophageal Cysts

Esophageal cysts are periesophageal lesions that are smooth and possess some form of gastroesophageal epithelial lining. Diagnosis is possible with esophageal ultrasound, chest CT scan, or contrast studies of the upper gastrointestinal tract. Resection is the therapy of choice, whether by thoracoscopic or open tech-

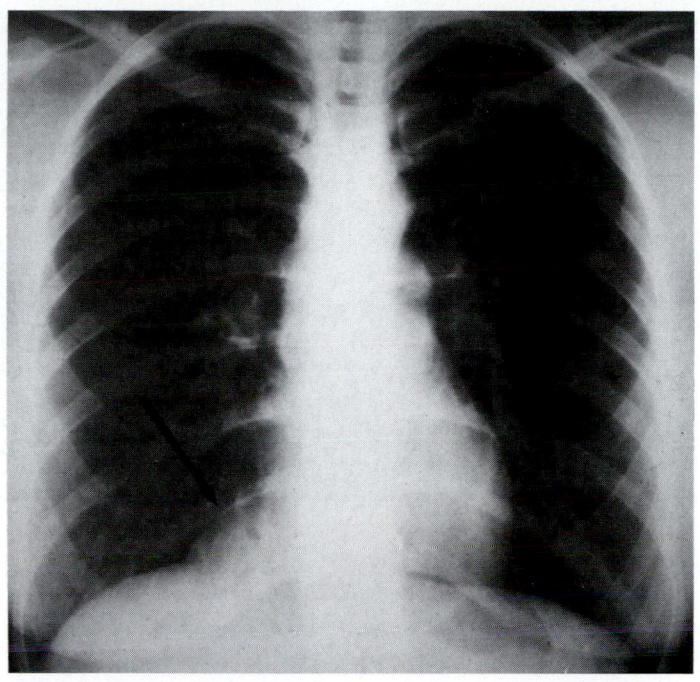

A

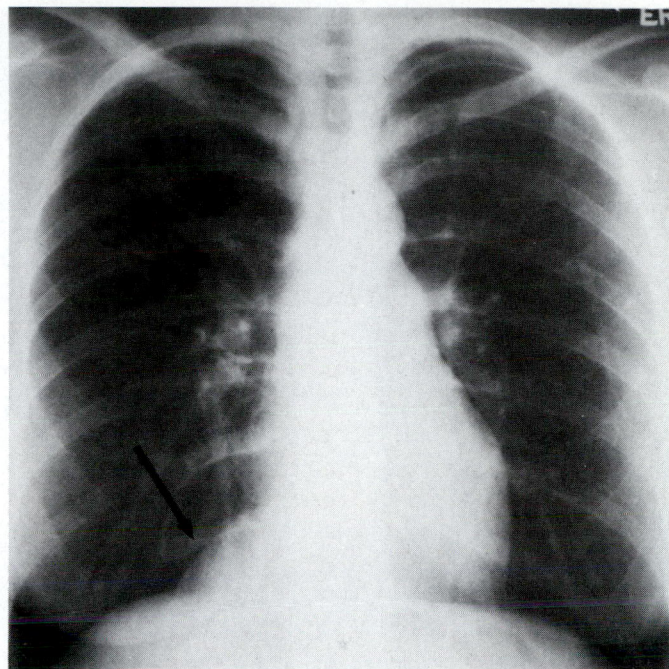

B

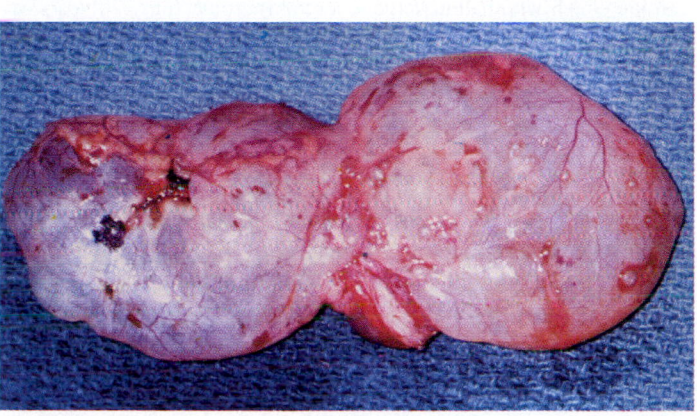

C

FIGURE 96-16   Pericardial cyst. *A.* Posteroanterior radiograph when patient was first seen. Arrows outline cyst. *B.* Three years later. *C.* Specimen removed at surgery.

nique. The site of the resection should be buttressed with vascularized tissue.

Neuroenteric Cysts

Neuroenteric cysts make up 5 to 10 percent of foregut lesions and are associated with vertebral anomalies. They possess not only endodermal but also ectodermal or neurogenic elements. They are usually connected by a stalk to the meninges and spinal cord. They present in infants before 1 year of age and are uncommon in adults. A CT scan showing a cystic mediastinal lesion with an associated vertebral abnormality—such as congenital scoliosis, hemivertebrae, and spina bifida—should prompt consideration of neuroenteric cysts.

Mesothelial Cysts

Mesothelial cysts have been described as pericardial, pleuropericardial, spring water, cardiophrenic, and simple cysts.

PERICARDIAL OR PLEUROPERICARDIAL CYSTS

Pericardial cysts are commonly located in the cardiophrenic angles. They have fibrous walls and contain clear, watery fluid. Mesothelial cysts are benign, and if the diagnosis is secure, resection is not necessary. If symptoms develop or if the lesions cannot be differentiated from hernias, bronchogenic cysts, or sequestra, resection is necessary (Fig. 96-16).

THORACIC DUCT CYSTS

These cysts are rare. They may arise at any level of the thoracic duct but do not retain a communication with the thoracic duct. The lesion may distort the trachea or esophagus. Observation is appropriate if the diagnosis can be made preoperatively, since there is no malignant potential. Ligation of the thoracic duct may be necessary to resect a thoracic duct cyst.

POSTERIOR MEDIASTINAL MASSES

Neurogenic Tumors

The most common masses in both children and adults used to be neurogenic tumors. In recent decades, although these tumors continue to be the most common malignancy in children, in adults they have become less common than either thymomas or lymphomas. They now represent approximately 15 percent of all mediastinal masses in adults. Furthermore, in adults, the malignancy rate of neurogenic tumors is less than 10 percent (and

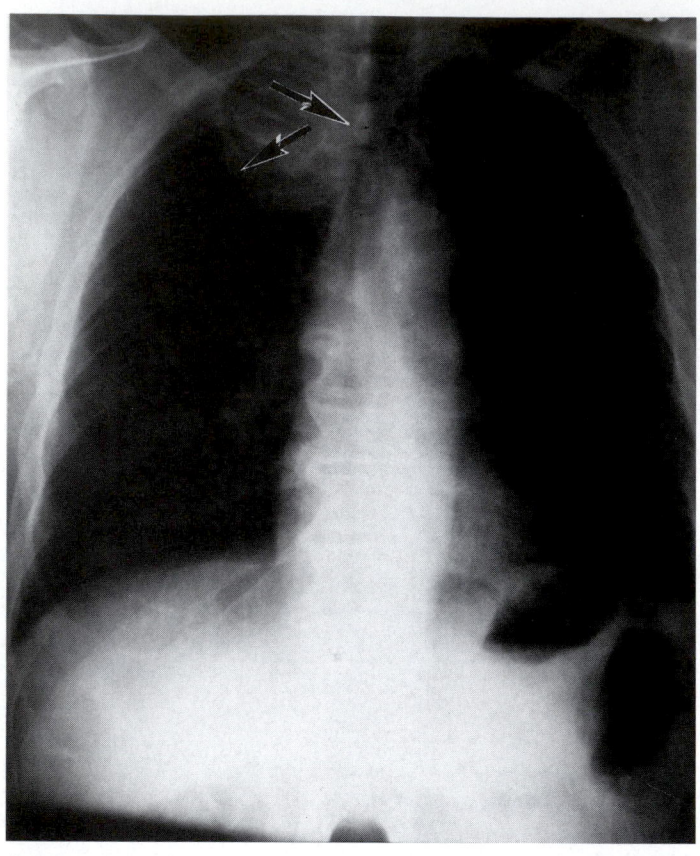

A

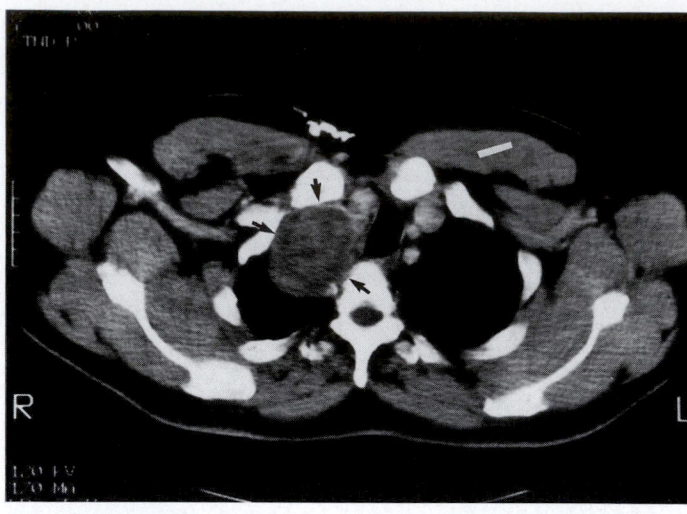

B

FIGURE 96-17   Schwannoma. PA radiograph of 67-year-old man with chronic cough who had undergone a total thyroidectomy 20 years earlier. *A.* Chest radiograph demonstrates superior mediastinal mass projecting into the right hemithorax. *B.* Lesion high in thoracic inlet abutting anterior and posterior chest walls.

probably only 1 to 2 percent). In children, fully 50 percent of these lesions are malignant.

Neurogenic tumors develop from the embryonic neural crest cells around the spinal ganglia and from either sympathetic or parasympathetic components. Almost all these lesions form in the paravertebral sulci in association with intercostal nerves. Lesions can also develop from vagus and phrenic nerves. Most of the lesions are asymptomatic, although some patients manifest symptoms of spinal cord compression or have cough, dyspnea, chest wall pain, and hoarseness. Horner's syndrome is an unusual presentation.

Most patients with neurogenic tumors are asymptomatic, so the initial diagnosis is usually made on chest radiographs obtained for other reasons. A rare patient may present with a pheochromocytoma or a chemically active neuroblastoma or neuroganglia. In all symptomatic patients, serum catecholamine levels and 24-h urine levels of homovanillic acid and vanillylmandelic acid should be determined.

CT scanning is necessary to rule out intraspinal extension along the vertebral nerve roots (so-called dumbbell tumors). These patients often present with symptoms of spinal cord compression. About 10 percent of patients with mediastinal neurogenic tumors have extension through a vertebral foramen.[1] Although the vast majority of these lesions are benign, approximately 1 to 2 percent are malignant. The CT scan typically shows a smoothly rounded homogeneous density abutting the vertebral column. For patients with dumbbell extensions through the intravertebral foramina or lesions abutting on the thoracic vessels, MRI may be useful in demonstrating involvement

of the vertebral column and extension into the spinal cord. Nerve sheath tumors account for 65 percent of all mediastinal neurogenic tumors. Widening of the intervertebral foramen calls for myelography to determine whether there is involvement of the spinal cord. Combined laminectomy and thoracic resection at the same site has been popularized by Grillo's team.[24]

Tumors of Nerve Sheath Origin

Benign lesions are classified as either neurilemoma (schwannoma) or neurofibromas (Fig. 96-17). Neurilemomas are more common than neurofibromas. Twenty-five to 40 percent of patients with nerve sheath tumors have multiple neurofibromatosis (von Recklinghausen's disease).

Malignant tumors (neurogenic sarcomas or malignant schwannomas) are unusual. The incidence of malignancy is greater in tumors that are part of von Recklinghausen's disease (10 to 20 percent).

Neurilemomas are well encapsulated, firm, and grayish tan. Melanotic schwannomas are grossly pigmented, and most of them extend into the spinal cord.

In general, the prognosis with any malignant tumor of nerve sheath origin is poor. Neurogenic sarcomas occur at the extremes of age—in the first and second decades of life and in the sixth and seventh decades. They represent less than 10 percent of all thoracic neurogenic tumors. The primary method of treatment is resection, by either thoracotomy or video-assisted thoracic resection. CT scanning is necessary to identify any intraspinal extension. If intraspinal extension is present, it should be resected at the same time with neurosurgical assistance. Postoperative radiation is always given.

So-called dumbbell tumors are neurogenic tumors that extend through the intravertebral foramen into the spinal column. Akwari and associates found that 9.8 percent of patients with mediastinal neurogenic tumors had extension through an intervertebral foramen.[1] These patients present with symptoms of spinal cord compression. MRI is useful to delineate vertebral column impairment and intraspinal extension.

TUMORS OF AUTONOMIC NERVOUS SYSTEM

Neuroblastomas and ganglioneuroblastomas typically occur in children and are rare in adults. They are malignant and should be resected if identified.

ENDOCRINE TUMORS

Mediastinal Pheochromocytoma

These tumors usually cause no symptoms. Occasionally, however, they do present with varying degrees of hypertension, diabetes, and hypermetabolism. The tumors produce epinephrine, norepinephrine, or both. Vanillylmandelic acid and homovanillic acid are the chief urinary excretion products, but epinephrine and norepinephrine may also be secreted in the urine. Normal levels of vanillylmandelic acid in the urine are 2 to 9 mg/24 h. Normal levels of epinephrine in the urine should be less than 50 μg/24 h; normal norepinephrine levels in urine should be less than 150 μg/24 h.

Large masses may be visible on the chest radiograph, but in most patients CT scans are necessary to visualize the tumors. On MRI, a nonhomogeneous mass with a flow void will be visualized. ^{131}I-metaiodobenzylguanidine scintigraphy is particularly useful for mediastinal lesions: it can be used to localize lesions not seen on other scans.[57]

The tumors may produce functioning peptides that can cause Cushing's syndrome, secretory diarrheas, and polycythemia vera. In the thorax, they probably derive from neuroendocrine cells and typically develop in the paravertebral sulci. Treatment requires surgical excision. However, the patient should first undergo alpha blockade with phenoxybenzamine for 1 week and then beta blockade with metoprolol or propranolol. Typically, the fluid volume of these patients is contracted and will normalize during the period of alpha blockade. For emergency surgery, simultaneous alpha and beta blockade and fluid restoration are necessary.

Parathyroid Adenomas

Normal parathyroid glands occur in abnormal positions in 20 percent of the population—in the lower part of the neck, in the thymic capsule, or in the anterior mediastinum. Approximately 20 percent of parathyroid adenomas localize to the mediastinum: 80 percent in the anterior mediastinum and 20 percent in the visceral compartment. It is unusual to be able to identify these lesions either by chest radiography or by CT scan. Usually, a search in the mediastinum begins only after a negative neck exploration

for hyperparathyroidism. After a negative exploration of the neck, further search using MRI, technetium scanning, thallium scanning, single photon emission computed tomography (SPECT) scanning, and venous sampling for parathyroid hormone can help to localize the lesion.

OTHER MEDIASTINAL TUMORS

Mesenchymal Tumors

These tumors constitute approximately 2 percent of all tumors that occur in the mediastinum. More than half of these mesenchymal lesions are malignant, however, and they run the entire gamut of soft tissue tumors. Their management resembles that of soft tissue tumors in the rest of the body; resection is indicated if possible.

Fatty Tumors

Some fatty tumors, if they can be reliably identified before surgery, do not require resection. Lipomatosis is overgrowth of mature fat seen as a widening of the mediastinum (Fig. 96-3). It results from exogenous obesity, steroids, or Cushing's disease and should not be resected. Lipomas can form in the mediastinum and do not require resection unless they appear to be growing rapidly. Large lipomas can cause respiratory embarrassment and may require resection for symptomatic reasons.

Lipomoblastomatosis is an unusual benign lesion seen principally in children. It is associated with fatty overgrowth in the mediastinum and compression of structures. It should be resected. *Liposarcomas* of the mediastinum are rare. On CT scanning, the density of these masses is midway between that of fat and water. The lesions are large and ill defined. They cause local symptoms, including superior vena caval obstruction and tracheobronchial compression. They should be resected.

SUPERIOR VENA CAVA SYNDROME

In the first part of the twentieth century, the most common causes of the superior vena cava (SVC) syndrome were benign mediastinal diseases, specifically syphilitic aneurysms. Currently, malignant tumors, such as lymphoma, bronchopulmonary cancers, thymic malignancies, and germ cell tumors of the mediastinum, account for more than 90 percent of all SVC obstructions. Lung cancer is most common, especially small cell cancer, although lymphoma is also common. Other malignancies are rare. Five to 10 percent of cases of SVC obstruction are due to benign causes. Most result from invasive monitoring techniques, such as the placement of central venous lines, Swan-Ganz catheters, and interventional techniques, such as the placement of pacemakers and central venous catheters for chemotherapy.

Congestion of venous outflow from the head, neck, and upper extremities results in swelling of the face, neck, arms, and upper chest. Patients may have headaches, dizziness, tinnitus, and a bursting sensation. In addition, the face may appear cyanotic even though capillary refill is normal. Venous hypertension in SVC syndrome may lead to serious consequences (e.g., jugular venous and cerebrovascular thrombosis). Therefore, this syndrome requires urgent treatment.

Chest radiography may show mediastinal widening but is non-specific. CT scanning, using intravenous contrast, can document the SVC syndrome but must show opacification of the SVC above the mass and nonopacification below to establish the diagnosis. Thrombosis, compression, and invasion of the SVC are common causes. If the CT scan is nondiagnostic, bilateral phlebography using arm veins may demonstrate caval obstruction, especially for the SVC syndrome that is secondary to chronic fibrosing mediastinitis or indwelling intravenous catheters or pacemaker leads. Radioactive iodine scans may be useful for SVC obstruction secondary to goiter.

In order to obtain tissue for diagnosis, FNAB may be diagnostic. Experienced surgeons and anesthesiologists can perform mediastinoscopy safely in this group of patients.[38] Intraoperative complications, including bleeding, are rare, but the airway management is complicated. Patients with the SVC syndrome, or any large anterior mediastinal mass, often must be intubated and extubated while awake so that airway obstruction can be prevented during the surgical procedure.

If the underlying disease is malignant, it is important to obtain tissue from the mediastinal neoplasm causing the SVC syndrome in order to direct therapy. Because the SVC syndrome may cause cerebral venous thrombosis, it is an oncologic emergency. In patients with respiratory or neurologic symptoms, treatment without tissue diagnosis may be necessary. The treatment of choice is very high-dose radiation therapy: 3000 to 4000 rads for 4 days.

Additional medical measures include salt restriction, diuretic treatment, steroid administration, and anticoagulation. Although radiotherapy is the mainstay of treatment, patients with small cell carcinoma, lymphoma, and undifferentiated carcinoma may benefit from the addition of chemotherapy. Intravascular stenting with expandable venous stents (Gianturco or Palmaz) has been successful in many patients and is appropriate therapy for poor-risk patients who do not respond to radiotherapy. Surgical resection is aggressive therapy but is appropriate in good-risk patients. In a series of 22 patients who underwent resection of lung cancers (n = 6) and malignant mediastinal tumors (n = 16), combined with resection of the SVC and subsequent reconstruction, the mortality was modest (4.5 percent) and the survival rates surprisingly good: the overall actuarial survival rate was 48 percent at 5 years. The survival rate of patients with mediastinal tumors was 60 percent at 5 years.[15]

For benign causes of SVC syndrome, treatment must be tailored to the specific origin. Substernal goiters should be resected. Aneurysmal disease causing SVC syndrome requires cardiopulmonary bypass and repair. Anticoagulation and antibiotic administration are the best initial treatments of idiopathic thrombophlebitis or septic thrombophlebitis and iatrogenic thrombosis of the SVC. Failure of these approaches calls for the use of fibrinolytic agents such as urokinase and streptokinase.

The treatment of SVC syndrome in patients with chronic fibrosing mediastinitis is controversial. Replacement of the SVC with vein[19] or ringed polytetrafluoroethylene (PTFE) grafts is possible, but the technique is reserved for severe symptoms recalcitrant to medical treatment. The best approach in this case is median sternotomy. Unless the benign process continues to progress, however, most symptoms will resolve without surgery as collaterals develop.

REFERENCES

1. Akwari OE, Payne WS, Onofrio BM, et al: Dumbbell neurogenic tumors of the mediastinum. *Mayo Clin Proc* 53:353–358, 1978.
2. Allo MD, Thompson NW: Rationale for the operative management of substernal goiters. *Surgery* 94:969–977, 1983.
3. Almon RR, Andrew CG, Appel SH: Serum globulin in myasthenia gravis: Inhibition of α-bungarotoxin binding to acetylcholine receptors. *Science* 186:55–57, 1974.
4. Azanow KS, Pearl RH, Zurcher R, et al: Primary mediastinal masses: A comparison of adult and pediatric populations. *J Thorac Cardiovasc Surg* 106:67–72, 1993.
5. Benjamin SP, McCormack LJ, Effler DB: Primary lymphatic tumors of the mediastinum. *Cancer* 30:708–712, 1972.
6. Billroth T: Geschwulster der Schiddr use. *Chir Klin Zurich* 67–89, 1869.
7. Blalock A: Thymectomy in the treatment of myasthenia gravis: Report of 20 cases. *J Thorac Surg* 13:316–339, 1944.
8. Blalock A, Mason MF, Morgan HJ, Riven SS: Myasthenia gravis and tumors of the thymic region. *Ann Surg* 110:544–561, 1939.
9. Blalock A, Mason MF, Morgan HJ, et al: Myasthenia gravis and tumors of the thymic regions: Report of a case in which the tumor was removed. *Ann Surg* 110:544–561 1939.
10. Blossmon GB, Ernstoff RM, Howells GA, et al: Thymectomy for myasthenia gravis. *Arch Surg* 128:855–862, 1993.
11. Cantinella FP, Boyd AD, Spencer FRC: Intrathoracic extramedullary hematopoiesis simulating anterior mediastinal tumor. *J Thorac Cardiovasc Surg* 89:580–584, 1985.
12. Cohen AJ, Thompson L, Edwards FH, Bellamy RF: Primary cysts and tumors of the mediastinum. *Ann Thorac Surg* 51:378–386, 1991.
13. Creswell LL, Wells SA: Mediastinal masses originating in the neck. *Chest Surg Clin North Am* 2:23–78, 1992.
14. Crucitti F, Doglietto GB, Bellantone R, et al: Effects of surgical treatment in thymoma with myasthenia gravis: Our experience in 103 patients. *J Surg Oncol* 50:43–46, 1992.
15. Dartevelle PG, Chapelier AR, Pastorino U, et al: Long-term follow-up after prosthetic replacement of the superior vena cava combined with resection of mediastinal-pulmonary malignant tumors. *J Thorac Cardiovasc Surg* 102:259–265, 1991.
16. Davis RD, Oldham HN, Sabiston DC: Primary cysts and neoplasms of the mediastinum: Recent changes in clinical presentation, methods of diagnosis, management and results. *Ann Thorac Surg* 44: 229–237, 1987.
17. DeFilippi VJ, Richman DP, Ferguson MK: Transcervical thymectomy for myasthenia gravis. *Ann Thorac Surg* 57:194–197, 1994.
18. Diehl LF, Hopper KD, Giguere J, et al: The pattern of intrathoracic Hodgkin's disease assessed by computed tomography. *J Clin Oncol* 9:438–443, 1991.
19. Doty DB, Doty JR, Jones KW: Bypass of superior vena cava: Fifteen years' experience with spiral vein graft for obstruction of superior vena cava caused by benign disease. *J Thorac Cardiovasc Surg* 99:889–896, 1990.
20. Dulmet EM, Macchiarini P, Suc B, Verlely JM: Germ cell tumors of the mediastinum: A 30-year experience. *Cancer* 72:1894–1901, 1993.
21. Ferguson MK, Lee E, Skinner DB, Little AG: Selective operative approach for diagnosis and treatment of anterior mediastinal masses. *Ann Thorac Surg* 44:583–586, 1987.
22. Fossa SD, Borge L, Aass N, et al: The treatment of advanced metastatic seminoma: Experience in 55 cases. *J Clin Oncol* 5:1071–1077, 1987.
23. Frist WH, Thirumalai S, Doehring CB, et al: Thymectomy for the myasthenia gravis patient: Factors influencing outcome. *Ann Thorac Surg* 57:334–338, 1994.

24. Grillo HC, Ojemann RG, Scannell JG, Zervas NT: Combined approach to "dumbbell" intrathoracic and intraspinal neurogenic tumors. *Ann Thorac Surg* 36:402–407, 1983.

25. Heilo A: Tumors in the mediastinum: US-guided histologic core-needle biopsy. *Radiology* 189:143–146, 1993.

26. Heimberger IL, Battersby JS, Vellios F: Primary neoplasms of the mediastinum: A 15-year experience. *Arch Surg* 86:978–985, 1963.

27. Hoppe RT, Coleman CN, Cox RS, et al: The management of stage I–II Hodgkin's disease with irradiation alone or combined modality therapy: The standard experience. *Blood* 59:455–465, 1982.

28. Jaretzki IIIA, Wolff M, Jaretzki A: "Maximal" thymectomy for myasthenia gravis. Surgical anatomy and operative technique. *J Thorac Cardiovasc Surg* 96:711–716, 1988.

29. Jolly F: Über myasthenia gravis pseudoparalytica. *Berl Klin Wochenschr* 32:1–7, 1885.

30. Kelley MJ, Mannes EJ, Rawin CE: Mediastinal masses of vascular origin. A review. *J Thorac Cardiovasc Surg* 76:559–572, 1978.

31. Katlic MR, Grillo HC, Wang C: Substernal goiter: Analysis of 80 patients from Massachusetts General Hospital. *Am J Surg* 149:283–287, 1985.

32. Kirchner T, Muller-Hermelink HK: New approaches to the diagnosis of thymic epithelial tumors. *Prog Surg Pathol* 70:167–189, 1989.

33. Kirschner PA: Reoperation for thymoma: Report of 23 cases. *Ann Thorac Surg* 49:550–555, 1990.

34. Kirschner PA: Myasthenia gravis, in: Shields TW (ed), *Mediastinal Surgery*. Philadelphia, Lea & Febiger, 1991, pp 339–369.

35. Kocher T: Bericht über ein zweites tousend Kropfexcisionen. *Arch Klin Chir* 64:454–471, 1901.

36. Laquer L, Weigert C: Beitrage zur Lehyre von de Erbschen Krankheit. I: Uber de Erbschen Krankheit (myasthenia gravis) (Laquer). II: Pathologisch-anatomischer Beitrag zur Erbschen Krankheit (myasthenia gravis) (Weigert). *Zentralbl Neurochir* 20:594–612, 1901.

37. Lewis BD, Hurt RD, Payne WS, et al: Benign teratomas of the mediastinum. *J Thorac Cardiovasc Surg* 86:727–731, 1983.

38. Lewis RJ, Sisler GE, MacKenzie JW: Mediastinoscopy in advanced superior vena cava obstruction. *Ann Thorac Surg* 32:458–462, 1981.

39. Loehrer PJ, Birch R, Williams SD, et al: Chemotherapy of metastatic seminoma: The Southeastern Cancer Study Group experience. *J Clin Oncol* 5:1212–1220, 1987.

40. Loehrer PJ, Perez CA, Roth LM, et al: Chemotherapy for advanced thymoma: Preliminary results of an intergroup study. *Ann Intern Med* 113:520–524, 1990.

41. Longo DL, Mauch P, Devita VT, et al: *"Lymphocytic Lymphomas"* in Cancer: Principles and Practice of Oncology, 4th ed., Philadelphia, JB Lippincott, 1993, pp 1859–1927.

42. Marino M, Müller-Hermelink HK: Thymoma and thymic carcinoma: Relation of thymoma epithelial cells to the cortical and medullary differentiation of the thymus. *Virchows Arch [A]* 407:119–149, 1985.

43. Masaoka A, Monden Y, Nakahara K, Tanioka T: Follow-up study of thymomas with special reference into their clinical stages. *Cancer* 48:2485–2492, 1981.

44. Mathisen DJ, Grillo HC: Clinical manifestation of mediastinal fibrosis and histoplasmosis. *Ann Thorac Surg* 54:1053–1058, 1992.

45. Motzer R, Bosl G, Heelan R, et al: Residual mass: An indication or further in patients with advanced seminoma following systemic chemotherapy. *J Clin Oncol* 5:1064–1070, 1987.

46. Nakahare K, Ohno K, Hashimoto J, et al: Thymoma: Results with complete resection and adjuvant postoperative irradiation in 141 consecutive patients. *J Thorac Cardiovasc Surg* 95:1041–1047, 1988.

47. Nichols CR, Roth BJ, Heerema N, et al: Hematologic neoplasia associated with primary mediastinal germ-cell tumors. *New Engl J Med* 322:1425–1429, 1990.

48. Park H-M, Tarver RD, Siddiqui AR, et al: Efficacy of thyroid scintigraphy in the diagnosis of intrathoracic goiter. *Am J Roentgenol* 148:527–529, 1987.

49. Parker D, Holford CP, Begent RHJ, et al: Effective treatment for malignant mediastinal teratoma. *Thorax* 38:897–902, 1983.

50. Pugatch RD, Faling LJ, Robbins AH, Spira R: CT diagnosis of benign mediastinal abnormalities. *Am J Roentgenol* 134:685–694, 1980.

51. Rodriguez M, Gomez MR, Howard FM Jr, Taylor WF: Myasthenia gravis in children: Long-term follow-up. *Ann Neurol* 13:504–510, 1983.

52. Rosai J, Levine GD: Tumors of the thymus, in *Atlas of Tumor Pathology,* 2nd series, fascicle 13. Washington, DC, Armed Forces Institute of Pathology, 1976, pp 55–99.

53. Sabiston DC, Scott HW: Primary neoplasms and cysts of the mediastinum. *Ann Surg* 136:777–797, 1951.

54. Sanders LE, Rossi RL, Shahian DM, Williamson WA: Mediastinal goiters: The need for an aggressive approach. *Arch Surg* 127:609–613, 1992.

55. Saunders DB, Scoppetta C: The treatment of patients with myasthenia gravis. *Neurol Clin North Am* 12:343–369, 1994.

56. Shamberger RC, Holzma RS, Griscow NT, et al: CT quantitation of tracheal cross-sectional areas as a guide to the surgical and anesthetic management of children with anterior mediastinal masses. *J Pediatr Surg* 26:138–143, 1991.

57. Shapiro B, Sisson J, Kalff V, et al: The location of middle mediastinal pheochromocytomas. *J Thorac Cardiovasc Surg* 87:814–820, 1994.

58. St. Georges R, Deslauriers J, Duranceau A, et al: Clinical spectrum of bronchogenic cysts of the mediastinum and lung in the adult. *Ann Thorac Surg* 52:6–13, 1991.

59. Sugarbaker DJ: Thoracoscopy in the management of anterior mediastinal masses. *Ann Thorac Surg* 56:653–656, 1993.

60. Suster S, Rosai J: Thymic carcinoma: A clinicopathologic study of 60 cases. *Cancer* 67:1025–1032, 1991.

61. Urschel HC, Razzuk MA, Netto GJ, et al: Sclerosing mediastinitis: Improved management and histoplasmosis titer and ketoconazole. *Ann Thorac Surg* 50:215–221, 1990.

62. Van Dam J, Rice TW, Sivak MV: Endoscopic ultrasonography and endoscopically guided needle aspiration for the diagnosis of upper gastrointestinal tract foregut cysts. *Am J Gastroenterol* 87:762–765, 1991.

63. Von Schulthess GK, McMurdo K, Tscholakoff D, et al: Mediastinal masses: MR imaging. *Radiology* 158:289–296, 1986.

64. Weide LG, Ulbright TM, Loehrer PJ, Williams SD: Thymic carcinoma: A distinct clinical entity responsive to chemotherapy. *Cancer* 71:1219–1223, 1993.

65. Wheatley MJ, Stirling MC, Kirsh MM, et al: Descending necrotizing mediastinitis: transcervical drainage is not enough. Ann Thorac Surg 49:780–784, 1990.

PART TWELVE

DISORDERS OF THE CHEST WALL, DIAPHRAGM, AND SPINE

CHAPTER 97

NONMUSCULAR DISEASES OF THE CHEST WALL

F. Dennis McCool / Dudley F. Rochester

The chest wall consists of the abdomen, the bony structure of the rib cage, the respiratory muscles, and the spine and its articulations. It is one of the components of the inspiratory pump, and its normal function is needed for effective ventilation. Consequently, diseases in any of the structures that make up the chest wall may, by themselves or in combination with other disease processes, interfere with ventilation and lead to respiratory failure. The diseases of the chest wall that most profoundly embarrass ventilatory function are kyphoscoliosis and restrictive disease due to previous thoracoplasty. Flail chest may result in respiratory failure especially when there is associated lung contusion. Other diseases that involve the bones of the rib cage or the spinal column, such as pectus excavatum or carinatum and ankylosing spondylitis, have much less of an impact on ventilatory capacity. Diseases directly involving the respiratory muscles also impair ventilatory function and are discussed in Chapter 98. Obesity is included in this section because of its profound effects on the mechanical properties of the chest wall.

KYPHOSCOLIOSIS

Diagnosis and Etiology

Kyphoscoliosis is a disease of the spine and its articulations. It is a common disorder, with the incidence of mild spinal deformities being as great as 1 in 1000 and of more severe spinal deformity as much as 1 in 10,000 in the United States. Since severe spinal deformities are clinically apparent, kyphoscoliosis is an easily recognizable cause of respiratory failure. Despite decades of investigation, some aspects of cardiorespiratory failure in kyphoscoliosis are unresolved. For example, areas that need further clarification include determining the impact of sleep-related events on the clinical course of kyphoscoliosis, evaluating the impact of correctional surgery on lung function, and determining which interventions are best in treating respiratory failure.

The deformation of the spine in this disorder characteristically consists of a lateral displacement or curvature (scoliosis) or an anteroposterior angulation (kyphosis) or both (Fig. 97-1).

Kyphosis may at times exist as an isolated deformity—for example, in elderly patients with osteoporosis. However, scoliosis is almost always associated with kyphosis and the rotation of the spine around its long axis. The lateral and rotatory movement of the spine may create severe distortion of the ribs, which consist of wide separation of the interspaces posteriorly and crowding of the interspaces anteriorly. The deformations of the spinal column and ribs can be readily appreciated on chest radiographs and their severity determined by measurement the acute angle formed by the two limbs of the convex primary curvature (Fig. 97-2). This angle, referred to as the *Cobb angle*, is used to assess severity of the disease. A Cobb angle greater than 100° is considered a severe deformity. This angle also has been used to determine prognosis and to predict the effects of disease on lung function and the risk of developing respiratory failure.

As many as 80 percent of the cases of kyphoscoliosis are idiopathic, often beginning in childhood. Idiopathic kyphoscoliosis may be caused by defects in the vertebrae themselves or in the vertebral connective tissue. Hereditary factors also may play a role in the development of idiopathic kyphoscoliosis, although their exact role is undefined. Kyphoscoliosis may be a sequela of other disease processes. Secondary kyphoscoliosis is often due to a number of diseases that affect the vertebrae, the vertebral connective tissue, or the neuromuscular system supporting the spinal column (Table 97-1). The most common cause of secondary kyphoscoliosis is neuromuscular disease such as polio or muscular dystrophy, whereas other forms of secondary kyphoscoliosis—such as Marfan's syndrome, osteomalacia, and post-thoracoplasty—are much less common.

By its very nature, severe kyphoscoliosis is easily recognizable on physical examination. In children and adolescents, however, the changes in spinal curvature may be subtle, and the spine should be carefully inspected for signs of mild scoliosis. Because of the rotation of the vertebrae in scoliosis, the curvature of the vertebral column is much greater than that of the palpable spinous processes, and only radiographs can reveal the true severity. The dorsal hump seen on examination is due to the angu-

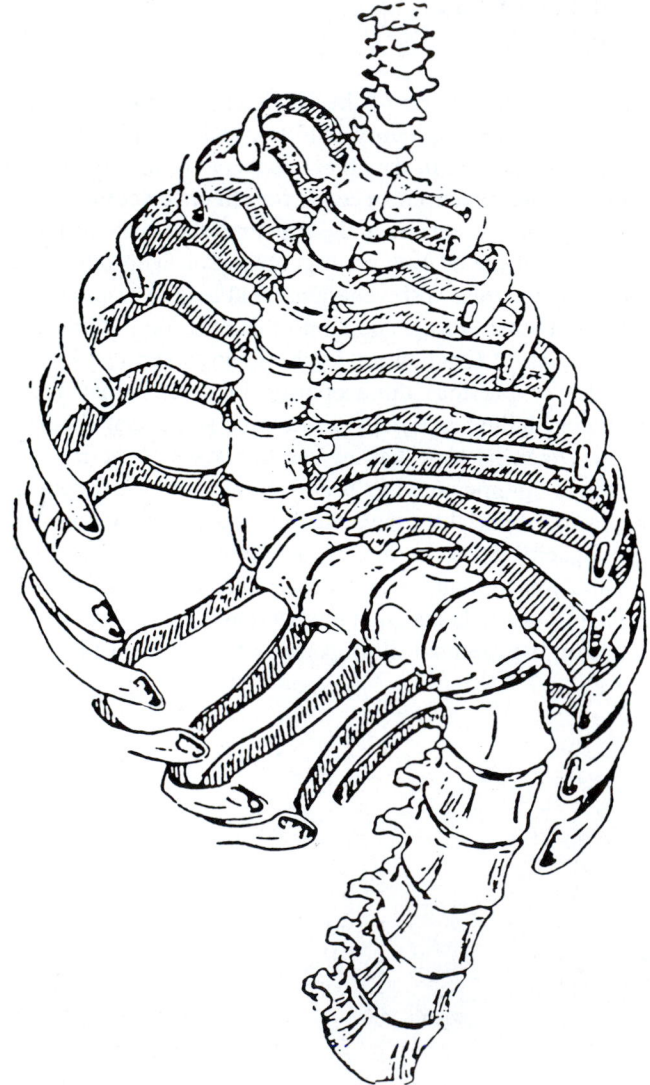

FIGURE 97-1   Schematic representation of the rotation of the spine and rib cage seen with scoliosis. (*Based on data of Bergofsky et al,[4] with permission.*)

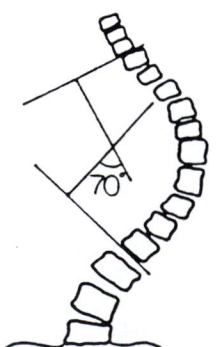 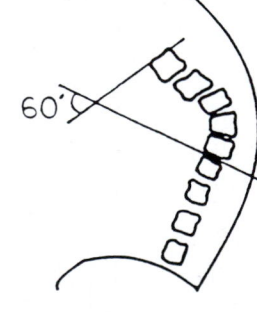

Posteroanterior   Lateral

FIGURE 97-2   Schematic of the posteroanterior radiograph depicting the lines constructed to measure the Cobb angle of scoliosis and lines drawn on the lateral radiograph to measure the Cobb angle of kyphosis. (*Based on data of Rochester and Findley in:* Textbook of Respiratory Medicine. *Murray and Nadel, (eds), Philadelphia, WB Saunders, 1988, p 1942.*)

TABLE 97-1

Causes of Kyphoscoliosis

Idiopathic
Neuromuscular disease
   Muscular dystrophy
   Poliomyelitis
   Cerebral palsy
   Friedreich's ataxia
Vertebral disease
   Osteoporosis
   Osteomalacia
   Vitamin D–resistant rickets
   Tuberculous spondylitis
   Neurofibromatosis
Disorders of connective tissue
   Marfan's syndrome
   Ehlers-Danlos syndrome
   Morequio's syndrome
Thoracic cage abnormality
   Thoracoplasty
   Empyema

lated ribs rather than to the spine. With severe degrees of kyphoscoliosis, right-sided heart failure may be present, and patients will have cyanosis, distended neck veins, peripheral edema, or hepatomegaly. Chest radiographs are useful in evaluating the degree of spinal deformity; however, their utility is limited in evaluating the mediastinum, cardiac size, and pulmonary infiltrates because of the spinal rotation.

Pathophysiology

Severe kyphoscoliosis has a profound impact on pulmonary function.[3] Among the chest wall diseases, it produces the most severe restrictive pattern. Total lung capacity (TLC) can be markedly reduced, with relative preservation of residual volume (RV) (Fig. 97-3). Accordingly, vital capacity (VC) is reduced and the RV/TLC ratio is elevated. The combination of a reduced VC and increased RV/TLC ratio may at times be mistakenly attributed to superimposed obstructive disease.

   Since TLC is set by the ability of the inspiratory muscles to overcome the recoil of the respiratory system, either a reduction of chest wall compliance or inspiratory muscle weakness will decrease TLC. Both factors may be operant in kyphoscoliosis. In adults with kyphoscoliosis, chest wall compliance (C_{CW}) may be reduced to only 20 to 30 percent of predicted. The reduction in

C_{CW} can be related to the degree of spinal deformity[3] as follows:

$$C_{CW} (L/cmH_2O) = 0.211 - 0.0015 \times \text{Cobb angle} \qquad (1)$$

Accordingly, angles of greater than 100° would profoundly reduce C_{CW}. In contrast to that in adults, chest wall compliance is normal in children, even in those with severe spinal deformity.[11] A stiff chest wall would also diminish the resting position of the chest wall, which would in turn reduce functional residual capacity (FRC).

   The reductions in lung compliance (C_L) that are reported in these patients are not as profound as the reductions in C_{CW}, but they also contribute to the restrictive process. Changes in C_L are a consequence of the relatively immobile chest wall and not disease of the lung parenchyma itself. Stiffening of the chest wall leads to a reduction in lung compliance by reducing FRC, thereby shifting tidal breathing to a flatter portion of the volume-pressure curve of the lung, and promoting microatelectasis because of the inability to fully expand the lung.

   Inspiratory muscle weakness also may contribute to the restrictive process. However, the prevalence of inspiratory muscle weakness is unknown. In young patients with mean scoliosis angles of approximately 50°, both maximal voluntary static inspiratory and expiratory pressures (PI_{max} and PE_{max}) are decreased to 70 and 80 percent of control, respectively,[54] with the impairment in strength independent of the degree of spinal curvature. In older patients with somewhat more scoliosis, PI_{max} is about 50 percent of predicted in eucapnic patients and 25 percent of predicted in hypercapnic patients (Fig. 97-4).[39] The reductions in maximal inspiratory and expiratory strength may be due not to intrinsic muscle disease but to changes in geometry of the chest wall affecting the mechanical advantage of the inspiratory muscles. In contrast to the above-mentioned studies, no alteration of maximal inspiratory pressures was found in children,[11] and the reduction of respiratory muscle function may not be a

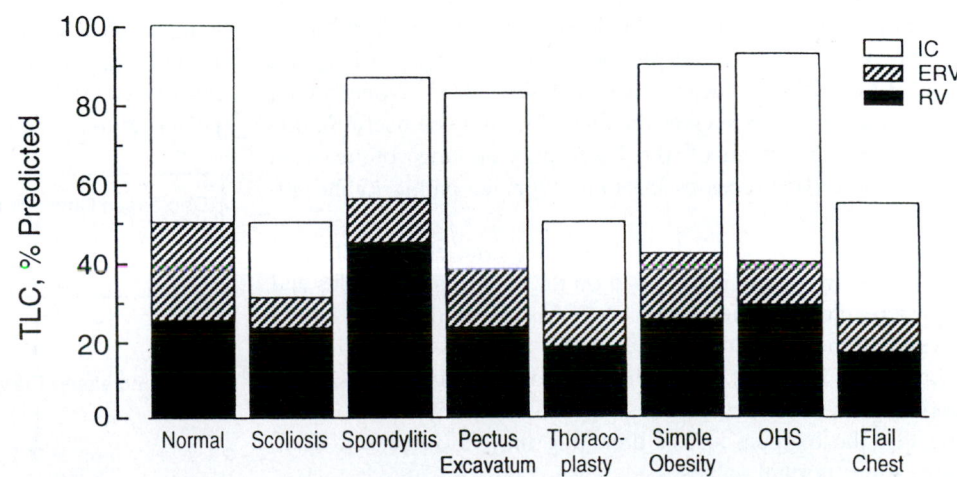

FIGURE 97-3 Representative values of TLC and its subdivisions for varied disorders of the chest wall, including ankylosing spondylitis (AS), kyphoscoliosis (KS), pectus excavatum (PE), thoracoplasty (TP), flail chest (FC), simple obesity (SO), and obesity hypoventilation syndrome (OHS).

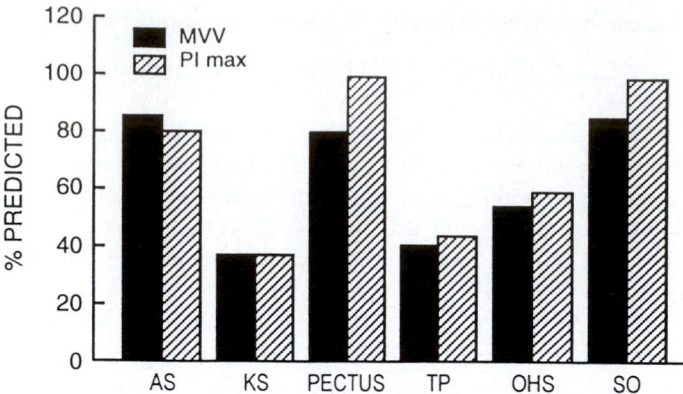

FIGURE 97-4 Representative values of inspiratory muscle performance in varied chest wall disorders. Abbreviations as in Fig. 97-3.

regular feature of scoliosis in adults.[57] The preservation of strength in some people may be related to increases in maximal diaphragm tension due to the strength-training effect of the large elastic loads imposed by the deformed chest wall.

In adults with idiopathic kyphoscoliosis, the severity of the restrictive process is proportional to the severity of spinal deformity. The relationship between these two factors has been described as follows:

$$VC\ (\%\ predicted) = 87.6 - 0.338 \times (Cobb\ angle) \quad (2)$$

Accordingly, someone with a Cobb angle of 100° would have a reduction in vital capacity to only 54 percent of predicted.[3] Other investigators have similarly demonstrated that patients with angles greater than 90° have their VC reduced to less than 50 percent of predicted and those with angles between 60 and 90° have milder reductions of VC (to 64 percent of predicted). In contrast to the adults with idiopathic scoliosis, patients with secondary kyphoscoliosis do not exhibit as strong a correlation between VC and the degree of spinal deformity. In these patients, confounding factors such as neuromuscular weakness may have a more profound effect on vital capacity than mild to moderate degrees of spinal deformity. Similarly, in a group of adolescents with idiopathic scoliosis and mild reductions in VC, VC correlated more closely with indices of respiratory muscle strength (PI_{max} and PE_{max}) than with the degree of spinal curvature.[54] Nonetheless, predictive equations such as the one above may be useful in differentiating the effects of spinal deformity on lung volume from other restrictive processes in adults with idiopathic kyphoscoliosis.

With kyphoscoliosis, the reduced lung and chest wall compliances increase the elastic load on the respiratory muscles and therefore increase the inspiratory pressure needed to inhale a given volume (Pbreath). Consequently, the work of breathing is increased (Fig. 97-5). Since the work of breathing is positively correlated with the oxygen cost of breathing,[41] it is not surprising that the oxygen cost of breathing may be increased up to three times normal values.

The increased elastic load that is imposed with every breath may place these patients at risk of developing inspiratory muscle fatigue. As noted above, Pbreath is increased because of the

reduction in respiratory system compliance, and PI_{max} may be reduced because of inspiratory muscle weakness. In healthy persons, inspiratory muscle fatigue occurs during inspiratory resistive loaded breathing when the ratio of Pbreath to PI_{max} exceeds 0.5. Patients with kyphoscoliosis may approach this ratio when intercurrent illnesses either increase Pbreath or decrease PI_{max}. Another risk factor for developing fatigue is the heightened oxygen cost of breathing. The oxygen cost of breathing in kyphoscoliosis is approximately five times normal.[3] Healthy subjects are at risk of developing fatigue when the oxygen cost of breathing is increased in this range.[41]

To compensate for the increased load on the inspiratory muscles, central drive to the muscles may be increased, and/or these patients may adopt a rapid shallow breathing pattern. In young scoliotics without ventilatory failure, the tidal volume is inversely proportional to ventilatory drive as measured by mouth occlusion pressure ($P_{0.1}$). The advantages of low tidal volumes are that the work per breath may be minimized, thereby reducing the ratio of Pbreath to PI_{max} and lowering the risk of developing inspiratory muscle fatigue, and that the sense of respiratory effort is reduced by lowering the ratio of Pbreath to PI_{max}. Disadvantages of adopting this breathing pattern include the potential to develop microatelectasis, an increase in dead-space ventilation, and an increase in the oxygen cost of breathing.

The reduction in expiratory flow rates that are seen in kyphoscoliosis are usually not related to intrinsic airway disease but reflect the overall restrictive process. Indeed, specific airway conductance is usually normal or even increased despite the reduction in lung volumes.[3] The increase in airway conductance may be explained, in part, by increased radial tension on the airways due to the increased elastic recoil of the lung. Airway obstruction may in some cases occur as a consequence of the change in geometry of the airways or as a result of a mediastinal structure, such as the aorta impinging on the tracheal wall.

Hypoxemia in patients with severe kyphoscoliosis is due to ventilation-perfusion mismatch or to underlying atelectasis and shunt. Ventilation-perfusion mismatch appears to be dependent on the degree of spinal curvature occurring more frequently in patients with scoliosis angles greater than 65°, but the maldistribution of ventilation appears to be independent of whether the hemithorax is concave or convex. Hypoventilation worsens hypoxemia and may be associated with further widening of the alveolar-arterial oxygen difference. With severe kyphoscoliosis, persistent hypoxemia leads to pulmonary vasoconstriction, right

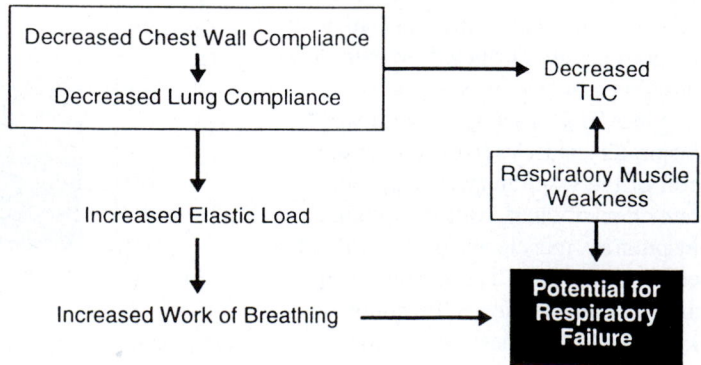

FIGURE 97-5 Changes in respiratory mechanics with kyphoscoliosis.

ventricular hypertrophy, and cor pulmonale. Proliferation of pulmonary artery smooth muscle or compression of the pulmonary vascular bed by deflated lung may further increase pulmonary artery pressure at rest or during exercise.

Exercise capacity in patients with mild to moderate kyphoscoliosis may be limited. In general, the lower the FVC, FEV_1, and MVV, the lower the maximal oxygen consumption (V_{O_2max}).[32] Depending on the severity of the scoliosis, maximal oxygen consumption may be reduced to approximately 60 to 80 percent of predicted. With mild to moderate kyphoscoliosis (Cobb angle between 25° and 70°), the breathing pattern response to exercise is similar to that seen in normal subjects, with the ratio of maximal tidal volume to vital capacity (VT/VC) reaching 0.5 and the ratio of maximal ventilation to maximal voluntary ventilation (VE_{max}/MVV) reaching 70 percent.[32] In a group of adolescent scoliotics whose exercise and ventilatory capacities as well as respiratory muscle strength were on average 80 to 85 percent of normal, exercise capacity was related to muscle mass and strength as well as to the degree of ventilatory impairment.[31] Since ventilatory control is often normal and the anaerobic threshold near 50 percent of the maximal oxygen consumption, the impairment of exercise performance found in adolescents and adults with moderate scoliosis can be attributed to deconditioning and lack of regular aerobic exercise rather than to ventilatory limitation or impaired chemoreceptor sensitivity.

Clinical Course

Patients with idiopathic kyphoscoliosis usually live into the sixth decade. Those who are younger than 35 years tend to be asymptomatic even though they may have severe degrees of kyphoscoliosis. In contrast, middle-aged patients with severe idiopathic kyphoscoliosis tend to develop dyspnea, decreased exercise tolerance, and acute respiratory infections and are at risk for developing respiratory failure. The onset of respiratory failure is insidious, and its incidence is variable, accounting for less than 1 percent of chronic ventilatory failure in adults. When respiratory failure occurs, it is often attributed to the spinal deformity. However, the cause of respiratory failure is often multifactorial and should not be attributed solely to the skeletal deformity when the Cobb angle is less than 100°. Coincident factors such as inspiratory muscle weakness, advanced age, disordered ventilatory control, sleep-disordered breathing, intrinsic airway disease and underlying cardiac disease, also may predispose these patients to respiratory failure.

The degree of spinal deformity is the factor that has traditionally been considered as heralding the onset of respiratory failure and has been most extensively studied. Early studies found that kyphosis and scoliosis angles of at least 100° were associated with a significant risk of developing respiratory failure and that the effects of kyphosis and scoliosis were additive.[3] Alternatively, severe scoliosis (Cobb angle over 100°) in the absence of significant kyphosis (Cobb angle less than 20°) usually did not bring about ventilatory failure. However, the notion that the degree of spinal deformity is a key factor in the development of respiratory failure has been challenged. First, patients may survive into the seventh decade with minimal or mild cardiorespiratory impairment despite Cobb angles greater than 105°. Second, there may be no correlation between the severity of hypercapnia and the degree of thoracic deformity.[39] Despite these findings, the important role of reduced chest wall compliance in the pathophysiology of respiratory dysfunction and the correlation between the chest wall deformity and chest wall compliance implies that the degree of spinal deformity is a key factor in the development of respiratory failure.

Other factors that may predict the eventual development of respiratory failure are the age of onset, the origin of kyphoscoliosis, and the presence of inspiratory muscle weakness (Fig. 97-6). When the spinal deformity develops before the age of 7, it is more likely to lead to respiratory failure than when the disease develops in adolescence. Whether the cause of kyphoscoliosis is a harbinger of respiratory failure remains controversial. In some series, the cause of kyphoscoliosis was found to augur respiratory failure, with paralytic kyphoscoliosis and the associated inspiratory muscle weakness contributing to a more progressive course.[3] Other studies found no such association.[39] Just as respiratory muscle weakness may contribute to hypercapnic ventilatory failure, the converse may also be true—namely, hypercapnia may weaken the inspiratory muscles and worsen respiratory failure.

Impaired ventilatory control has also been considered a factor contributing to respiratory failure. However, patients with kyphoscoliosis usually have normal or slightly low ventilatory responses to CO_2,[32] and if the response is reduced, the magnitude of reduction is proportional to the degree of mechanical limitation imposed by the chest wall. Thus, the decrement in ventilatory response to CO_2 resembles that of external resistive loading and can be attributed to the restricted respiratory system rather than to any inherent problem with respiratory control. Moreover, ventilatory drive as assessed by $P_{0.1}$ is increased in

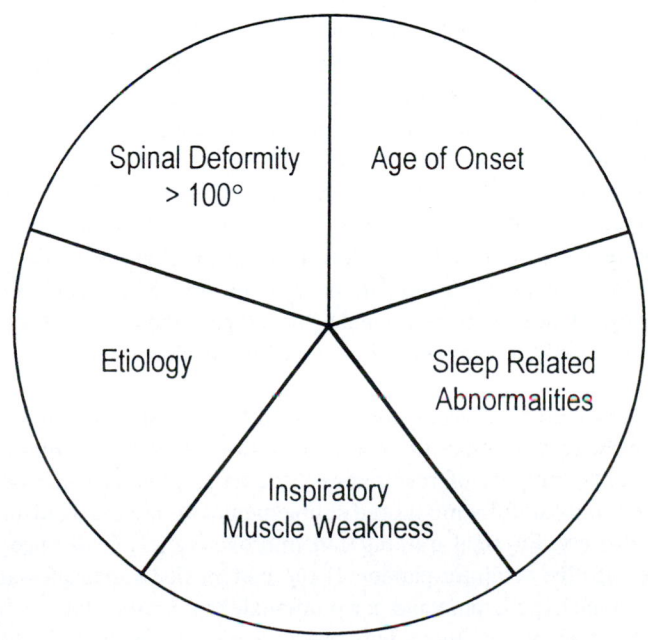

FIGURE 97-6   Factors predisposing patients with kyphoscoliosis to respiratory failure.

young scoliotics. However, the effects of aging and its influence on central ventilatory control need further clarification in this population.

Sleep-disordered breathing may also contribute to the development of respiratory failure. Several studies have documented significant nocturnal hypoventilation and oxyhemoglobin desaturation in kyphoscoliotic patients, usually occurring during REM sleep. Hypoventilation may be due to a combination of decreased neural drive to the intercostal and accessory muscles during REM sleep and decreased chest wall compliance. While awake, patients with kyphoscoliosis may rely more on the intercostal and accessory muscles to assist the diaphragm in displacing the stiff chest wall than normally. With REM sleep, the intercostal and accessory muscles become hypotonic, and hypoventilation may ensue. The degree of oxyhemoglobin desaturation during sleep in these patients appears to be more severe than that seen during sleep in patients with chronic obstructive pulmonary disease (COPD) or interstitial lung disease. A second cause of nocturnal hypoventilation is recurrent episodes of obstructive sleep apnea.[19] Distortion of the upper-airway anatomy in kyphoscoliosis may predispose these patients to intermittent airway obstruction during REM-induced hypotonia of the pharyngeal muscles; however, the incidence of this disorder in patients with kyphoscoliosis is not increased over that in the general population. Regardless of mechanism, recurrent hypercarbia and hypoxemia during sleep may potentiate the daytime development of hypercarbia, cor pulmonale, and respiratory muscle dysfunction. Since sleep-related disorders represent a potentially treatable or reversible cause of respiratory failure, they should be evaluated in patients with kyphoscoliosis developing CO_2 retention.

Treatment

GENERAL MEASURES

In general, patients with mild to moderate degrees of kyphoscoliosis have an excellent prognosis, with little impairment of breathing or overall lifestyle. These patients do not require special treatment to prevent ventilatory failure and are not significantly different from a control population with regard to symptoms or the loss of lung volume with aging. Pregnancy usually poses no added risk of respiratory complications. With severe degrees of kyphoscoliosis accompanied by reductions in vital capacity to less than 1 L, however, the risk of respiratory complications may be high, and patients may be advised to avoid pregnancy. Once cor pulmonale develops, the prognosis is considerably worse, and without treatment, death generally occurs within a year (Fig. 97-7).

The medical therapy for adults with kyphoscoliosis is both preventive and supportive. Immunization, adequate hydration, prompt treatment of respiratory infections, avoidance of sedatives, and carefully monitored supplemental O_2 are the mainstays of therapy. Physical training can improve exercise tolerance in the inactive scoliotic patient. If the patient decompensates and develops hypercapnia and cor pulmonale, respiratory failure can be treated conservatively with chest physiotherapy, bronchodilators, oxygen therapy, and diuretics if needed. When using oxygen, adult patients with moderately severe kyphoscoliosis and

chronic ventilatory failure experience less exercise desaturation and dyspnea.[43]

IPPB

Intermittent positive pressure breathing (IPPB) should be part of the conservative approach, as its benefits in this patient population include improvement in lung mechanics, resting arterial P_{CO_2}, and oxygenation, which lasts up to 4 h following treatment.[53] IPPB probably acts by decreasing microatelectasis, thereby increasing lung compliance and decreasing the work of breathing. With prolonged IPPB therapy, the improvement in vital capacity may persist for up to 9 months. The acute effects of IPPB, however, have not been shown to be as efficacious in other diseases associated with diminished respiratory system compliance and have little effect on improving chest wall compliance.[40] In cases of acute respiratory failure refractory to the measures described above, positive-pressure ventilation with a volume cycle ventilator is needed to treat hypoventilation and hypoxemia.

NONINVASIVE VENTILATION

Nocturnal negative-pressure ventilation with devices such as cuirass and body wrap ventilators can be used to treat chronic respiratory failure. These devices have proved beneficial by relieving dyspnea, pulmonary hypertension, and right ventricular failure and improving blood gas composition (Fig. 97-

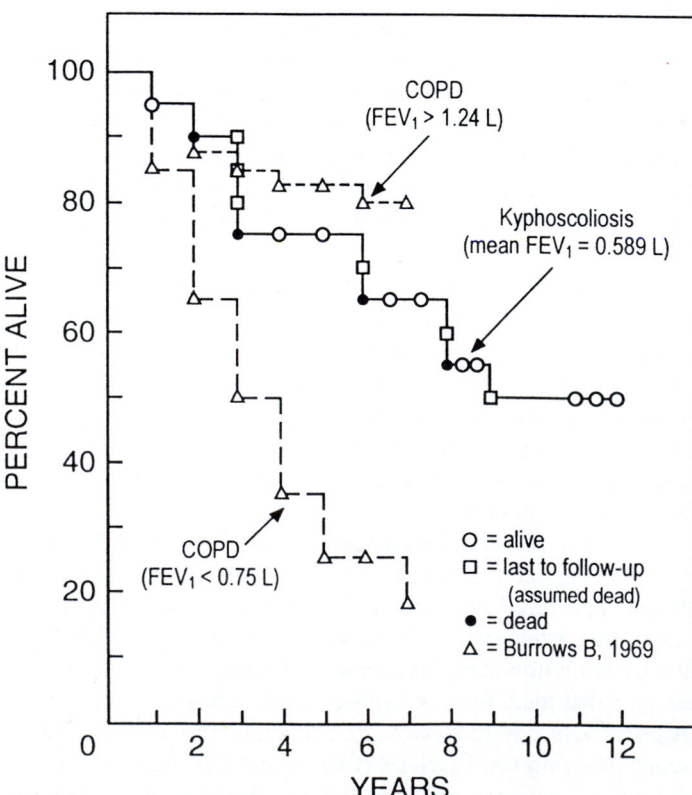

FIGURE 97-7 Patients with kyphoscoliosis who had a previous episode of cor pulmonale have a prognosis that is similiar to that of patients with mild COPD but better than that of patients with severe COPD. (*Based on data of Libby et al.[38]*)

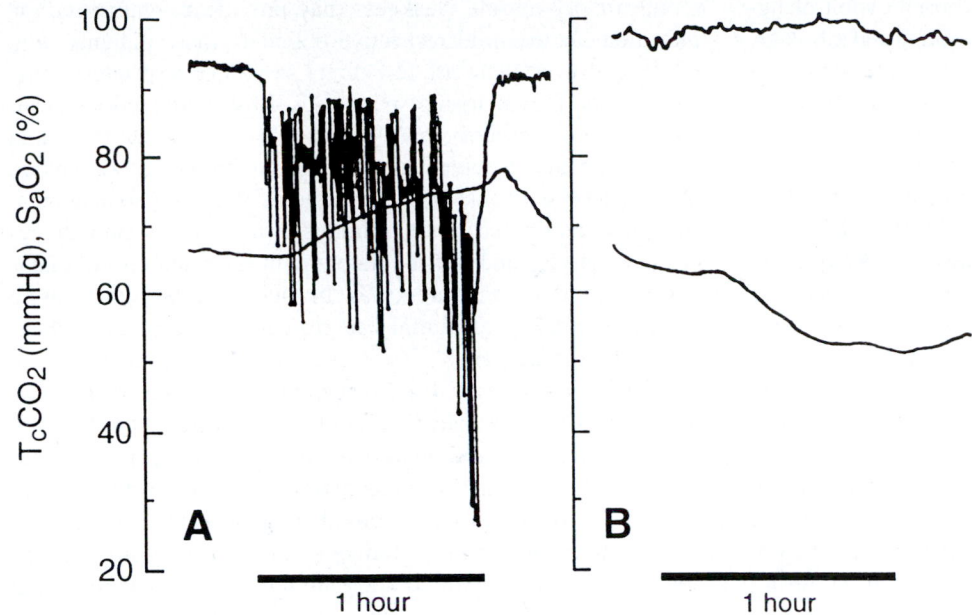

FIGURE 97-8   Recordings of arterial oxyhemoglobin saturation (Sa_{O_2}) and transcutaneous carbon dioxide tension (Tc_{CO_2}) in a patient with kyphoscoliosis during REM sleep. *A.* With no ventilator support, there is oxyhemoglobin desaturation and CO_2 retention. *B.* With nasal positive pressure ventilation these changes are prevented. *(Based on data of Ellis et al.[18])*

8).[19] Another benefit of long-term nocturnal ventilation with negative-pressure devices is a marked reduction in the need for hospitalization. Disadvantages of using negative-pressure devices include the induction of upper-airway obstruction during sleep and the need to custom fit a cuirass to the deformed chest wall.

Nocturnal positive-pressure ventilation has yielded benefits similar to those noted for negative-pressure ventilation—namely, increased tidal volume, improved alveolar ventilation, reduced work of breathing, improved respiratory muscle strength, normalized sleep patterns, and improved quality of life.[3,18,19] Initially, positive-pressure assistance was delivered through a tracheostomy with portable ventilators. With proper care, patients could be maintained with a tracheostomy on a portable ventilator for decades. However, to avoid the complications of tracheostomy, positive pressure is now more commonly delivered via nasal or face mask. The mechanism of improvement in pulmonary function with positive-pressure ventilation may be related to reversing atelectasis, improving compliance, or resting the observed decrease in diaphragmatic EMG activity, reduction in negative esophageal pressure swings, and improved synchronization between rib cage and abdomen motion noted during non-invasive ventilation. In addition, nocturnal ventilation ay benefit these patients by reducing both obstructive and nonobstructive sleep-related events.[18] Long-term nocturnal ventilation has resulted in improved gas exchange, ventilation, cardiac function, and activities of daily living.[18] In addition, long-term nocturnal non-invasive positive-pressure ventilation in 105 patients with kyphoscoliosis decreased hospitalizations for respiratory illnesses, improved quality of life, and improved sleep quality.[36]

SPINAL SURGERY

Since the degree of spinal deformity is associated with the development of respiratory failure in idiopathic kyphoscoliosis, surgical therapy has been used as an early intervention in hope of stabilizing the spine. Immediately after surgery, pulmonary function deteriorates, with reductions of chest wall and respiratory system compliance of 20 to 129 percent. This deterioration in respiratory mechanics is thought to be due to rib cage trauma and changes in chest wall caliper.

Despite several years of observation, the long-term benefits of spinal surgery on pulmonary function remain controversial. In adults, it is generally accepted that surgical procedures are not useful in improving pulmonary function. In children and adolescents, however, there may be a role for corrective surgery. Following Harrington rod instrumentation and spinal fusion, lung function improved in children and adolescents 18 months after surgery.[14] In women with an average curvature of 58°, there was a 12 percent improvement in vital capacity 3 years after surgery.[24] Other studies, however, demonstrate no improvement in lung function. In a group of 222 patients over the age of 20, spinal fusion and Harrington rod placement did not significantly improve the FVC, FEV_1, or resting arterial PO_2, and there were associated complications.[56]

To summarize, patients with severe kyphoscoliosis have impaired lung function and are at risk of developing respiratory failure. Although the degree of spinal distortion certainly plays a significant role in the pathogenesis of respiratory failure, there is no clear consensus on which other factors portend progression to respiratory failure. The decreased respiratory system compliance imposes an elastic load on the respiratory muscles and increases the work of breathing. Since inspiratory muscle weakness may accompany kyphoscoliosis, the combination of the increased elastic load and muscle weakness may result in inspiratory fatigue and further aggravate respiratory failure. In addition, sleep-related dysfunction may also contribute to daytime hypercapnia, cor pulmonale, and pulmonary hypertension. Even after the development of cardiorespiratory failure, conservative measures coupled with the use of IPPB and positive-pressure ventilation delivered via a tracheostomy or noninvasively, relieve symptoms, reduce hospitalization, and improve prognosis.

ANKYLOSING SPONDYLITIS

Diagnosis and Etiology

Ankylosing spondylitis is a rheumatic disease of unknown origin that invades the axial skeleton and commonly afflicts males.

Chronic inflammation results in fibrosis and ossification of ligamentous structures of the spine, sacroiliac joint, and rib cage. These inflammatory changes result in rigidity of the spine and limitation of rib cage mobility due to bony ankylosis of the costovertebral and sternoclavicular joints. There is a genetic predisposition, as 95 percent of Caucasians with primary ankylosing spondylitis have the HLA-B27 antigen. Conversely, approximately 20 percent of Caucasians with HLA-B27 will manifest some features of ankylosing spondylitis. Ankylosing spondylitis is common in that 1 percent of Caucasians may have both HLA-B27 antigen and meet some of the clinical criteria for ankylosing spondylitis. Systemic manifestations occur in as many as 10 to 20 percent of patients with long-term ankylosing spondylitis and include iritis, aortic insufficiency, heart block, diastolic dysfunction, and peripheral arthritis.

Clinically, ankylosing spondylitis is characterized by chronic low back pain with limitation of spinal motion and of rib cage expansion. The rib cage often moves less than 2.5 cm as measured at the level of the fourth intercostal space during a vital-capacity maneuver. Respiratory complaints such as dyspnea and chest wall pain are uncommon and may be related to chest wall restriction, kyphosis, or to upper-lobe fibrobullous disease. Occasionally, some patients experience mild exercise intolerance. Respiratory failure is uncommon unless the patient has underlying lung disease, diaphragm dysfunction, or cardiac disease.

Pathophysiology

Altered respiratory mechanics are a consequence of the severe restriction of rib cage mobility. As with kyphoscoliosis, chest wall and total respiratory system compliance is reduced in ankylosing spondylitis, and chest wall resistance is increased. In contrast to that in kyphoscoliosis, lung compliance is generally normal. Although the reduction in respiratory system compliance is similar to that seen in kyphoscoliosis, there is only a mild restriction in TLC and VC (Fig. 97-3).[22,60] TLC is reduced on average to 80 percent of predicted, and its reduction is proportional to the radiographic severity of the spinal ankylosis. VC is generally reduced to 70 percent of predicted, and the reduction in VC has been positively correlated with the lack of rib cage expansion, with disease activity and duration,[22] and with spinal mobility.[60] Since the rib cage is often fixed in an inspiratory position, both FRC and RV may be increased above the predicted levels. An increase in the RV/TLC ratio may be mistakenly interpreted as coincident obstructive disease in these patients.

With the development of osteoporosis, kyphosis may also occur; at times, it can produce modest spinal deformity and may contribute to the mild restrictive process. Elderly patients with osteoporosis and a moderate degree of kyphosis (spinal angles of 46 to 80°) have diminished vertical and lateral excursions of the rib cage and a mild reduction in vital capacity.[15] However, there is no correlation between the kyphosis angle and vital capacity in ankylosing spondylitis because posterior fusion of the ribs may play a greater role in limiting rib expansion and vital capacity than the degree of kyphosis.

Inspiratory muscle weakness may provide an alternative explanation for the mild restrictive deficit in these patients (Fig. 97-4). However, there are few direct studies of respiratory muscle function in ankylosing spondylitis. Modest reductions in inspiratory and expiratory muscle strength (reductions of PI_{max} and PE_{max} to 56 and 76 percent, respectively, of predicted) were noted in 30 patients with ankylosing spondylitis.[60] Since maximal pressures may be limited by the muscles of the rib cage and the accessory muscles and not the diaphragm, the reduction in maximum inspiratory pressures may be due to intercostal muscle atrophy secondary to diminished rib cage mobility and not diaphragm dysfunction.

Diaphragm function has been indirectly evaluated in ankylosing spondylitis by partitioning of inhaled volume changes between the rib cage and abdomen. As rib cage expansion is severely limited with ankylosing spondylitis, most of the volume change is through the diaphragm-abdomen pathway. Since these patients have only a mild reduction in vital capacity, the diaphragm apparently can compensate quite well for the reduced rib cage excursion. Indeed, these patients may have greater displacement of the diaphragm caudally and greater outward motion of the abdominal wall during tidal breathing than controls. Consequently, diaphragm shortening must be greater for a given tidal volume in anklyosing spondylitis. The combination of increased diaphragm shortening and decreased chest wall compliance would increase the work done by the diaphragm and potentially provide a training stimulus for the diaphragm.

Exercise capacity may be mildly reduced in patients with ankylosing spondylitis and may in part be limited by inspiratory muscle performance. Changes in intercostal and diaphragm EMG signals suggestive of fatigue have been seen during exercise. However, the lack of correlation between the limitation of chest wall expansion and $\dot{V}_{O_2max}$ or exercise tolerance suggests that exercise tolerance was not limited by the cardiac or respiratory systems but by deconditioning.[3]

Gas exchange is usually unimpaired in these patients, and the Pa_{O_2} either normal or slightly decreased. If there is a reduction in diffusion capacity, it can usually be accounted for by the reduction in lung volume.[60] With the exception of apical fibrobullous disease, regional ventilation is normal despite restriction of the rib cage.

Approximately 1 percent of patients with ankylosing spondylitis will develop fibrobullous upper-lobe disease, which is characterized by nonspecific chronic inflammation and fibrosis of the alveolar walls. This complication occurs predominantly in males with long-standing disease and may unpredictably progress from minimal upper-lobe interstitial infiltrates to marked fibrosis, honeycombing, and cavity formation. Fibrobullous disease may mimic tuberculosis and should be recognized so that unnecessary antituberculosis therapy can be obviated. These patients are usually asymptomatic, although they are at risk for developing spontaneous pneumothorax and becoming infected with *Aspergillus* or atypical mycobacterial disease. Fibrobullous disease often poses a management problem. Although there may be relief of symptoms, corticosteroids do not prevent the progression of the disease. Because thoracic surgery for fibrobullous disease is complicated by bronchopleural fistula in 50 to 60 percent of patients, it is recommended only for the treatment of major hemoptysis.

Treatment

The medical therapy for adult patients with ankylosing spondylitis is both preventive and supportive. Tobacco use should be avoided and baseline chest radiographs and spirometry obtained. Referral to a pulmonologist is advised for evaluation of abnormal chest radiographs, deteriorating pulmonary function, hypoxemia, or hypercapnia. Cardiorespiratory fitness and spinal mobility should be enhanced by institution of exercise and physiotherapy programs. The results of pulmonary rehabilitation have been equivocal, demonstrating either improvement in pulmonary function following breathing exercise or no change in pulmonary function despite improved chest wall and spinal mobility. Since these patients already have compensated for the reduced chest wall mobility by increasing the contribution of the diaphragm-abdomen pathway to tidal volume, improvements in spinal mobility may not improve absolute lung volumes but instead may alter the partitioning of volume between the rib cage and abdomen. Such a redistribution of volume would decrease diaphragm shortening for a given tidal volume and thus reduce diaphragm work.

Upper-airway obstruction is an infrequent complication of ankylosing spondylitis and is due to involvement of the cricoarytenoid cartilage. When it occurs, patients may present with hoarseness or stridor. If intubation is required, it should be done with caution, as such patients are at an increased risk for spinal cord injury.

To summarize, ankylosing spondylitis is a chronic inflammatory disease that may limit spinal flexion and rib cage expansion. However, the diaphragm adequately compensates for the reduced rib cage mobility, as only mild reductions of VC and TLC are reported. The reduction of maximum inspiratory pressures may be attributed to atrophy of the intercostal muscles rather than to diaphragm dysfunction. The mild degree of ventilatory restriction may contribute to exercise intolerance.

THORACOPLASTY

Diagnosis and Etiology

Surgically induced collapse of the lung was a mainstay of antituberculous therapy before the advent of effective chemotherapy. Of the surgical procedures employed, thoracoplasty was one of the most common and was frequently used for treating cavitary pulmonary tuberculosis and empyema. Thoracoplasty entailed removal of a number of ribs and intercostal muscles. However, the first rib was often retained in hopes of retarding the subsequent development of spinal deformity. In recent years, thoracoplasty has been used to a limited extent to treat postpneumonic and postresectional empyema.

When the procedure was performed in the 1940s and 1950s, postoperative mortality was high, but survivors were thought to have a good life expectancy. Indeed, many patients who underwent this procedure are still alive. However, the survivors often develop restrictive disease due to distortion of the chest wall, pleural thickening, and secondary scoliosis. Although these patients may remain asymptomatic for more than a decade after the surgery, they eventually present with dyspnea on exertion,

and respiratory failure may occur in as many as half of the long-term survivors of thoracoplasty. It may occur acutely over days or weeks or chronically over years. Risk factors associated with the development of respiratory failure included preoperative cavitary disease, advanced age at the time of operation, a previous surgically induced pneumothorax on the opposite side, and the male sex.[54] The risk is greater in patients who underwent thoracoplasty than in those who underwent pneumonectomy alone. Long-term follow-up of patients with previous thoracoplasty reveals that they have a higher mortality than controls (Fig. 97-9).[28,47] Of 171 patients who were operated on between 1951 and 1953, more than one-third had died by 1987.[46] Of the 65 deaths, 19 were due to respiratory failure; 8 survivors had developed respiratory failure.

Pathophysiology

Of the disorders affecting the chest wall, thoracoplasty is second only to kyphoscoliosis in producing a severe restrictive pattern (Fig. 97-3). However, the degree of restriction does not correlate with the extent of thoracoplasty (number of ribs removed or the number of surgical stages).[6] The restrictive pattern is due primarily to a reduction in respiratory system compliance, but other factors—such as progressive lung fibrosis related to underlying granulomatous disease, fibrothorax, phrenic nerve damage, scoliosis, and previous lung resection—may also contribute to the reduced lung volumes. The restrictive process may worsen with

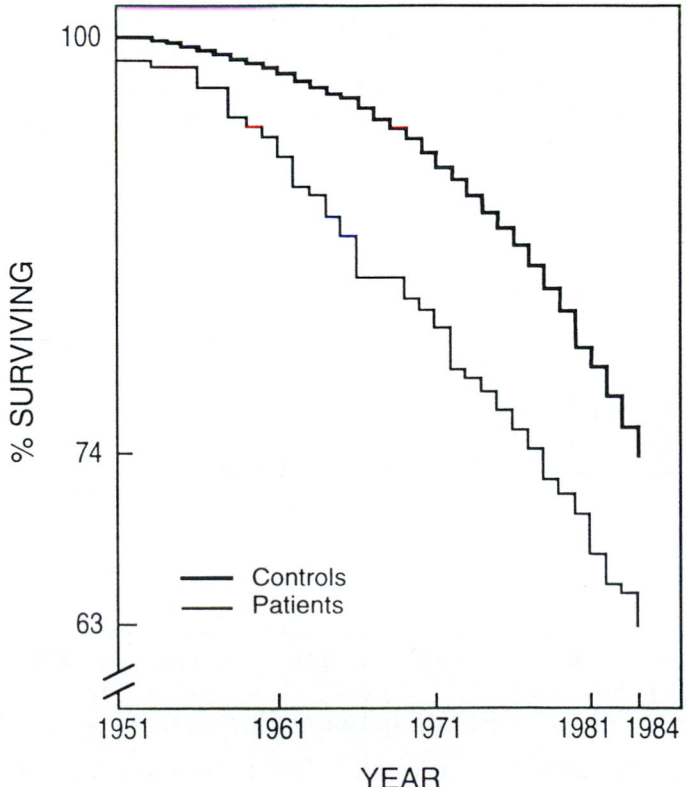

FIGURE 97-9   Survival rates for patients with thoracoplasty (thin line) and controls (thick line). *(Based on data of Phillips et al.[47])*

time because of progressive scoliosis or the progressive reductions of respiratory system compliance that normally occur with aging. The restrictive pattern seen in patients several years after surgery is characterized by a reduction in VC and TLC to 40 to 70 percent of predicted. RV and FRC are reduced to 70 and 90 percent of predicted, respectively.

As with other restrictive processes, the FEV_1 is reduced. Unlike the situation in other restrictive diseases of the chest wall, however, coincident airflow obstruction is common, with a prevalence ranging from 34 to 51 percent.[6] When airflow obstruction is present, FEV_1/FVC ratio is reduced, the RV/TLC ratio is increased, and the obstructive process usually is not reversible. Airway obstruction may be due to chronic bronchitis from cigarette smoking; however, other factors, such as chronic bronchitis from old tuberculous lung disease, may be operant. The obstructive component becomes more common with aging and is more severe in patients with CO_2 retention, hypoxemia, or complaints of dyspnea. Determining the presence and severity of airflow obstruction may help identify those at greater risk for developing respiratory failure (Fig. 97-10).

The elastic and resistive loads imposed by the respiratory system and airways increase the work of breathing. The observations that the oxygen cost of breathing is three to four times higher in these patients than in controls and is of the same magnitude as that seen in kyphoscoliosis[55] are consistent with the notion that the work of breathing is increased. The increased oxygen cost of breathing may also be attributed to inspiratory muscle inefficiency. Chronic airflow obstruction, which occurs in half of these patients, leads to hyperinflation, which in turn reduces inspiratory muscle efficiency.

Gas exchange may be impaired in these patients, leading to severe hypoxemia and hypercarbia. Diffusing capacity is moderately reduced but when corrected for lung volume, it is within the normal range.[6] With exercise, however, the diffusing capacity fails to increase appropriately, indicating an irreversibly restricted pulmonary vascular bed. Cor pulmonale can develop in this disease and may be due to hypoxemia or medial hypertrophy of the pulmonary arteries.

Patients with thoracoplasty frequently complain of reduced exercise tolerance and, when tested, have a diminished $\dot{V}_{O_2max}$.[46] The reduced $\dot{V}_{O_2max}$ correlates with reductions in maximal ventilation during exercise and with the baseline FEV1. These findings and the observation that these patients stopped exercise before reaching 85 percent of their predicted maximal heart rate suggest that exercise is limited by diminished ventilatory capacity.

Treatment

As with other restrictive processes of the chest wall, treatment is supportive, with the use of domiciliary oxygen and treatment of intercurrent infections. In addition, any obstructive component should be vigorously treated. Positive-pressure ventilation has been used acutely to treat respiratory failure and relieve hypoxemia and hypercapnia. Noninvasive positive- or negative-pressure ventilation also has been employed in the management of chronic respiratory failure. Its benefits include reducing the work of breathing, alleviating respiratory muscle fatigue, relieving dyspnea, and improving sleep-induced desaturation.[28] With long-term ventilation, improvements in VC, MIP, MEP, and arterial blood gases occurred soon after initiation of therapy, but they did not improve further or deteriorate thereafter (Fig. 97-11). In addition, long-term nocturnal noninvasive domiciliary ventilation improves prognosis.[28] Even with nocturnal ventilatory assistance, however, mortality is greater than in a control population, with a survival of 55 percent 7 years after initiation of treatment (Fig. 97-12).

FLAIL CHEST

Diagnosis and Etiology

The term "flail chest" denotes a condition in which a segment of the rib cage is disconnected from the rest of the chest and deforms markedly with quiet breathing. It is produced by double fractures of three or more contiguous ribs or combined sternal and rib fractures, has been reported to occur in 12 to 20 percent of patients with blunt chest wall trauma, and may lead to respiratory failure. The most common cause of flail chest is blunt chest trauma following falls or automobile accidents. Flail chest may also occur following pathologic fractures such as those due to multiple myeloma, following chest compression during cardiopulmonary resuscitation, or following total sternectomy.

Mortality from chest trauma is generally high, ranging from 7 to 14 percent. However, when flail chest is seen in the chest trauma patient, mortality is increased further.[25] In a series of 1026 multiple-trauma patients, the mortality for those with flail chest was 68.6 percent, compared to a 27.1 percent mortality for the entire group. This high mortality could be attributed in part to associated injuries such as fractures of long bones or vertebrae, head trauma, rupture of the aortic arch or other arteries, and laceration of the liver or spleen. Other pulmonary complications, which occur in approximately 60 percent of patients with

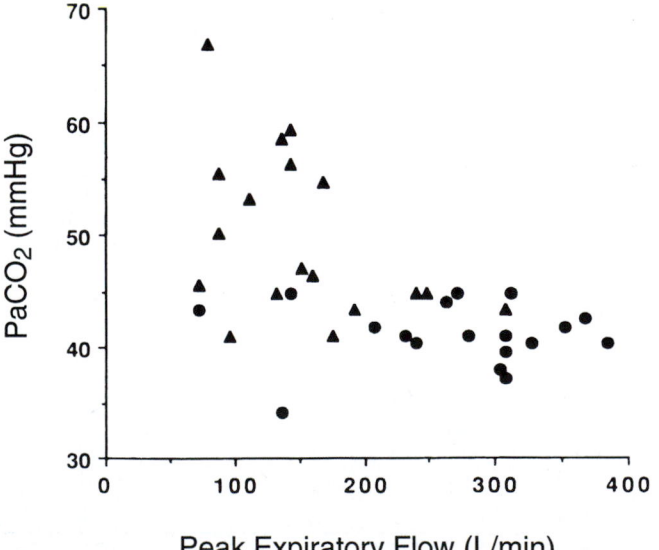

FIGURE 97-10 The development of airways obstruction, as assessed by a reduction of peak expiratory flow, is associated with an increased risk of CO_2 retention in patients after thoracoplasty. *(Based on data of Phillips et al.[47])*

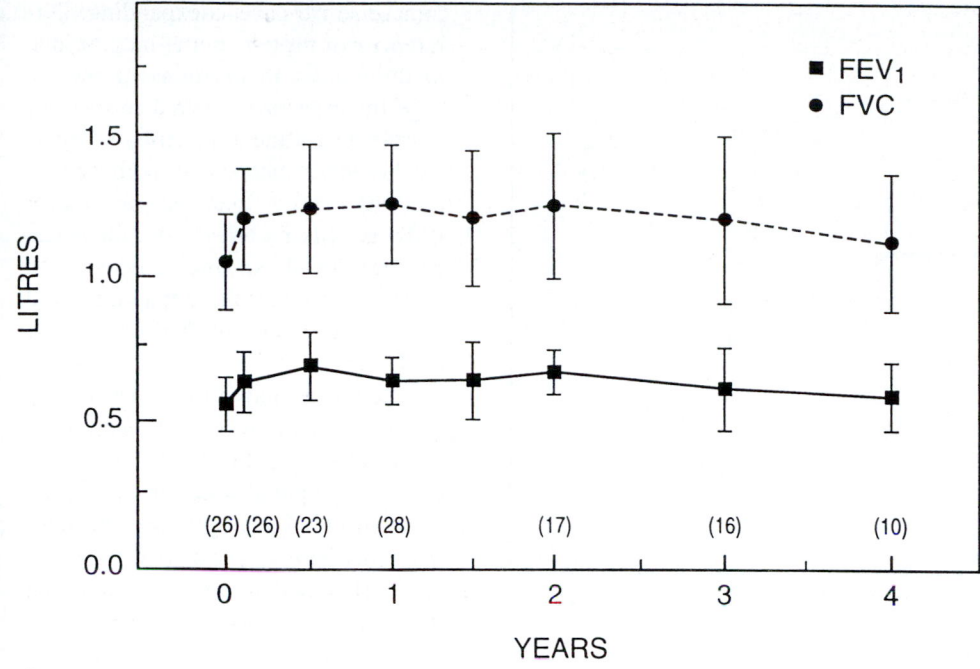

A

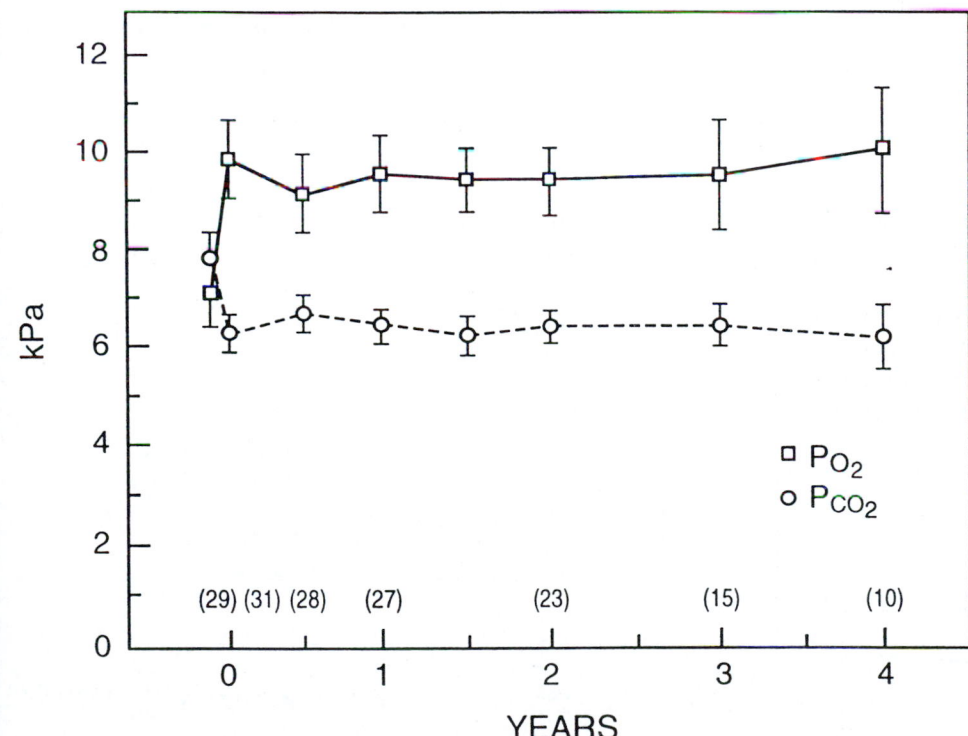

B

FIGURE 97-11 Nocturnal cuirass or nasal positive pressure ventilation produces immediate improvements in FVC and FEV (*A*) and arterial blood gases (*B*), which are sustained for up to 4 years. (*Based on data of Jackson et al.*[28])

of pulmonary contusion has also been shown to result in respiratory failure.[1] Although the chest radiograph is better at detecting bone injuries, the chest CT scan detects more pulmonary contusions than the chest radiograph. However, the contusions seen on chest radiograph may be more clinically significant.

Long-term disability is relatively common following chest trauma. In one series, symptoms consisting of chest tightness, chest pain, or dyspnea occurred in more than half of 32 patients following traumatic flail chest injury, and only 12 had returned to full-time work.[35] Despite the occurrence of symptoms, there are only a few studies of long-term follow-up of respiratory function in patients with flail chest. Initially, FRC and VC are reduced following flail chest injury and either recover to baseline values within 6 months[33] or remain mildly reduced.[35] In contrast, patients with pulmonary contusion may have reductions in FRC for up to 4 years (Fig. 97-13). The persistent reduction in FRC in patients with lung contusion may be due to fibrous changes in the previously contused area, as demonstrated by CT scan. Thus, flail chest without pulmonary contusion may cause short-term but not long-term respiratory dysfunction.

Pathophysiology

In contrast to other processes affecting the chest wall, there are only a limited number of studies evaluating the effects of flail chest on respiratory system mechanics. Normally, the passive recoil of the rib cage, the insertional actions of the intercostal muscles and diaphragm, and abdominal pressures permit the ribs to expand in a uniform fashion during inspiration. On the other hand, lowering pleural pressure during inspiration is deflationary to the rib cage. With flail chest, the multiple rib fractures uncouple part of the chest wall from the inspiratory actions of the intercostal and accessory muscles. Consequently, during inspiration the negative intrathoracic pressure is unopposed and may displace the uncoupled part of the rib cage inward. Any reduction in lung compliance due to pulmonary contusion or microatelectasis or an increase in airway resistance will increase the degree of negative pleural pressure during inspira-

flail chest, are pulmonary contusion, hemothorax, and pneumothorax. Lung contusion itself has just as high a mortality (56 percent) as flail chest in multiple-trauma patients.

The harmful effects of blunt chest injuries on gas exchange are related primarily to pulmonary contusion and pain rather than to the flail segment per se. However, flail chest in the absence

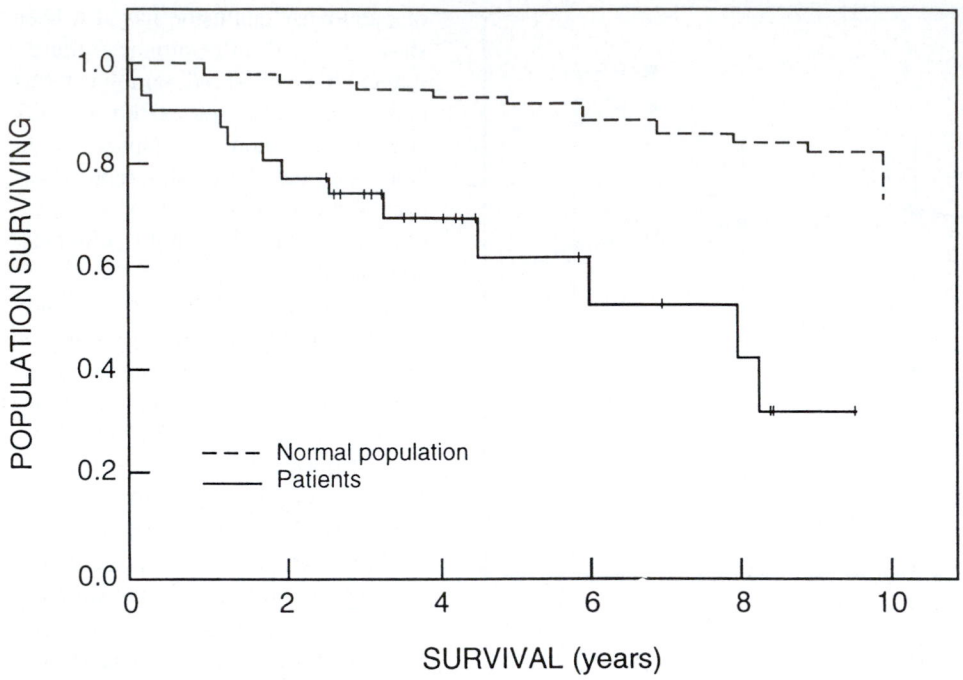

FIGURE 97-12 Survival of 32 postthoracoplasty patients treated with cuirass or positive-pressure nasal ventilation compared to a control population. Half of the patients survived for 6 to 8 years. *(Based on data of Jackson et al.[28])*

transverse rib cage is expanding. Differences in these patterns may be due to differences in locations of the rib cage fractures or to altered respiratory muscle recruitment patterns. Support for the latter mechanism comes from the observation that the inspiratory EMG activity recorded from the external intercostals of the affected area were increased by more than threefold in a canine model of flail chest (Fig. 97-15).[10]

Paradoxical motion of the chest wall will increase the work of breathing by two mechanisms (Fig. 97-16). First, because of the paradoxical motion of the chest wall, the inspiratory muscles must shorten more for a given tidal volume. This added muscle shortening represents extra work but is not reflected as an increase in tidal volume and therefore is not measured as work by standard techniques. Second, regional reductions in lung compliance

tion and worsen paradoxical chest wall motion. During expiration, pleural pressure becomes more positive, and the flail segment can be seen to move outward.

Different patterns of chest wall distortion may be seen in patients with flail chest (Fig. 97-14).[59] Paradoxical motion may occur between the rib cage and abdomen or within the rib cage itself. Patterns that have been described include inward displacement of the lower rib cage as the transverse rib cage and abdomen are expanding, inward displacement of the transverse rib cage as the lower rib cage and abdomen are expanding, and inward displacement of the lower rib cage and abdomen as the

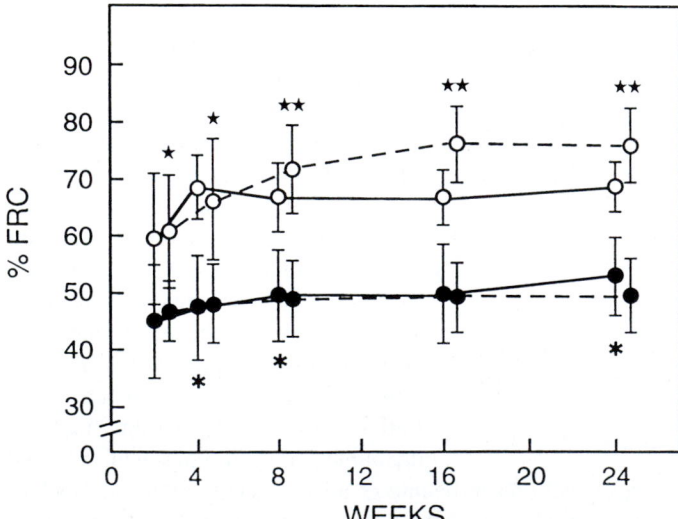

FIGURE 97-13 Following blunt chest wall trauma, FRC is reduced. During the ensuing 6 months, FRC approaches normal values in patients with flail chest alone (FC). When pulmonary contusion complicates flail chest (FC + PC), FRC remains well below predicted values. *(Based on data of Kishikawa et al.[33])*

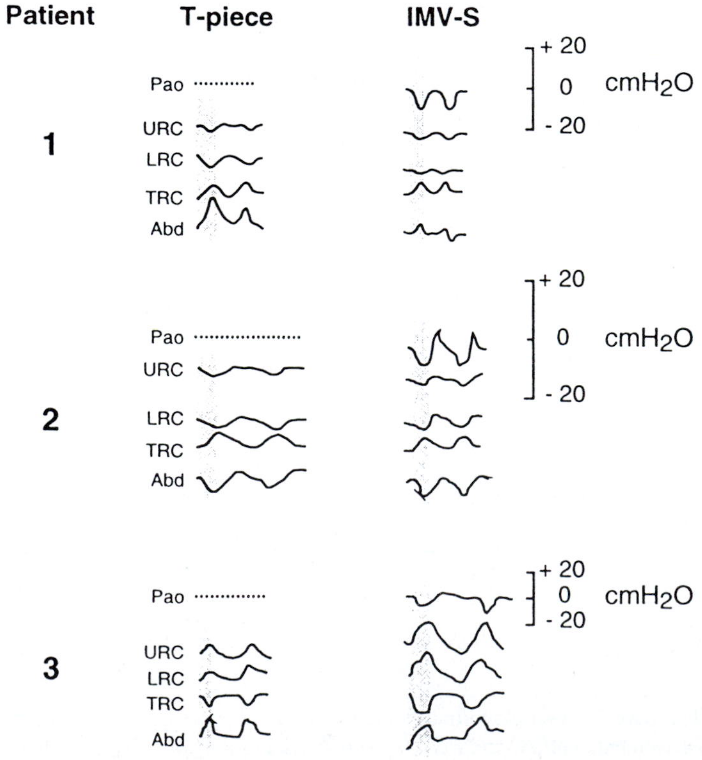

FIGURE 97-14 Representative tracings of chest wall dimensions. URC and LRC = upper and lower rib cage anteroposterior diameters; TRC = transverse diameter of the lower rib cage; Abd = abdomen A-P, and Pao = pressure at the airway opening. The shaded area represents inspiration. Each of the three patients with flail chest shows a distinct pattern of chest wall distortion: paradoxical inward motion of the URC and LRC (patient 1), paradoxical inward motion of the URC, LRC and Abd (patient 2), and paradoxical inward motion of the TRC (patient 3). During spontaneous breaths on an IMV circuit (IMV-S), there is distortion of the chest wall in all patients. *(Based on data of Tzelepis et al.[59])*

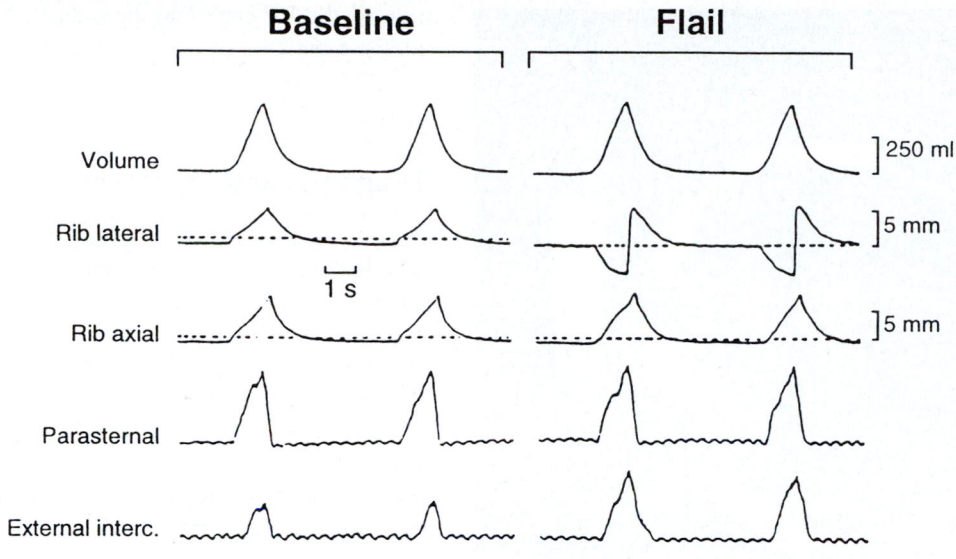

FIGURE 97-15   Following flail injury in an animal model (right panel), the EMG activity of the external intercostal of the flail segment is increased and axial displacement of the ribs preserved. The increased EMG activity may be reflexly mediated. *(Based on data of Cappelo et al.[10])*

due to coincident pulmonary contusion increase the pleural pressure needed to inhale. In this instance, the added work could be measured.

The oxygen cost of breathing also may be increased in these patients because of the increased work of breathing and possibly because of inefficiency of the inspiratory muscles. The efficiency of breathing is reduced when the inspiratory muscles operate over shorter lengths. Diaphragm inefficiency due to the added diaphragm shortening would then be expected in flail chest. The combination of increased work of breathing and decreased efficiency of breathing increases the energy demand of the inspiratory muscles and will predispose them to fatigue. Hypoxemia due to atelectasis or contusion would further predispose the muscles to inspiratory muscle fatigue by reducing energy supplies.

Treatment

Therapy for flail chest includes measures to control pain, assistance with mechanical ventilation if necessary, and possibly sta-

bilizing the flail segment. Adequate pain relief is imperative not only for patient comfort but also because it reduces splinting and improves tidal volume, vital capacity, and the clearance of respiratory secretions by cough. It can be accomplished by direct intercostal nerve blocks or by use of epidural anesthesia.

The need for stabilizing the flail segment is controversial. Initially, tape, strappings, and external devices were applied to the chest wall to stabilize the flail segment. Alternatively, positive-pressure ventilation was used to stabilize the flail segment. Such "pneumatic splinting" consisted of tracheostomy with a 3 to 5-week period of mechanical ventilation. This approach had been the mainstay of therapy directed at stabilizing the flail segment since its introduction in 1956, but mortality remained high. In a series of 543 patients treated with tracheostomy and continuous mechanical ventilation, mortality was 31 percent.[51] Mortality and morbidity were also affected by the mode of mechanical ventilation. In one large series, the mortality averaged 18 percent for continuous mechanical ventilation and 6 percent for intermittent mandatory ventilation (IMV).[58] In contrast, patients who were not mechanically ventilated had no mortality. The morbidity also was significantly lower when there was either no mechanical ventilation or ventilation with IMV instead of continuous ventilation. Consequently, ventilator management was not recommended to be used primarily as a means of providing a pneumatic splint to stabilize the chest wall but for treating respiratory failure when it accompanies flail chest.

The use of devices to fixate the flail segment externally to avoid prolonged periods of mechanical ventilation has been reevaluated. Devices such as a chest cuirass used to deliver constant negative extrathoracic pressure[27] or an acrylic frame[1] have been used postoperatively in a limited number of patients to fix the flail segment. These devices reduced symptoms of pain, improved ventilatory function, and facilitated weaning from mechanical ventilation when paradoxical motion of the anterior chest wall occurred following total sternectomy. Thus, in selective patients with major chest wall resection, temporary external chest wall stabilization may enable patients to be sustained without mechanical ventilatory assistance; however, this assertion needs to be tested in larger numbers of patients.

When respiratory failure develops, the mode of mechanical ventilation should be chosen so as to impose the least resistive or elastic load. Such loads in patients with flail chest will make pleural pressure swings more negative, worsen chest wall distortion, and increase the oxygen cost of breathing during spontaneous breaths. Although IMV has been frequently used as a

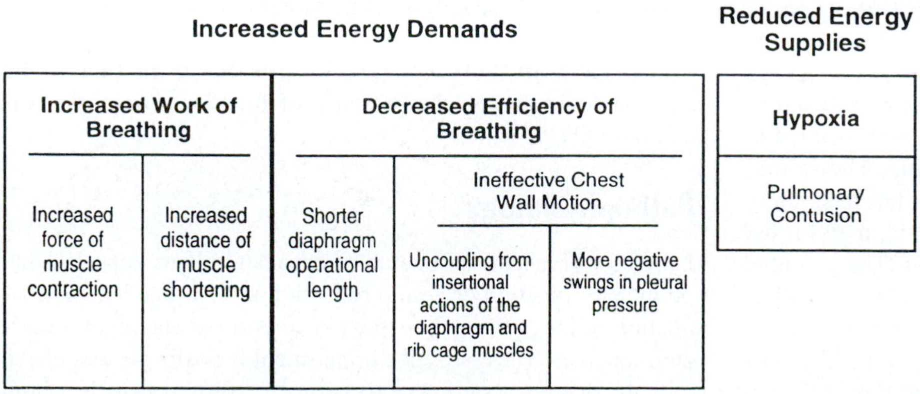

Increased Energy Demands					Reduced Energy Supplies
Increased Work of Breathing		**Decreased Efficiency of Breathing**			
			Ineffective Chest Wall Motion		**Hypoxia**
Increased force of muscle contraction	Increased distance of muscle shortening	Shorter diaphragm operational length	Uncoupling from insertional actions of the diaphragm and rib cage muscles	More negative swings in pleural pressure	Pulmonary Contusion

FIGURE 97-16   Pathophysiology of flail chest.

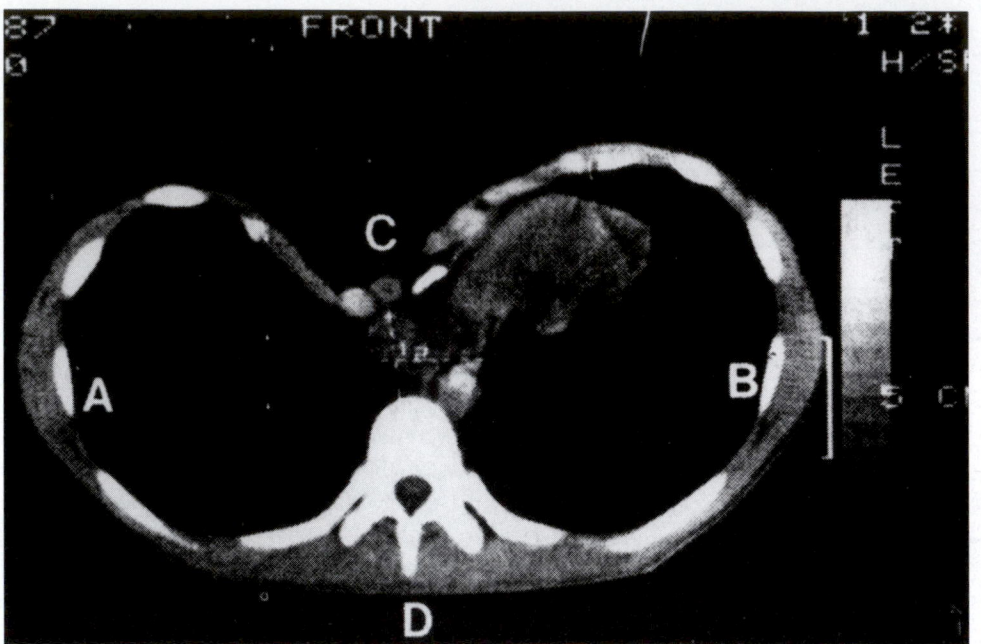

FIGURE 97-17 Chest CT of a patient with pectus excavatum. The anteroposterior diameter is markedly decreased in the midline (C-D). The ratio of the transverse (A-B) to anteroposterior diameter of the rib cage is 7.6, much greater than the ratio of 3.25 that is commonly used to select patients for surgery. *(Based on data of Haller et al, Ann Surg 209:578-582, 1989.)*

mode of ventilating patients with flail chest once respiratory failure ensues, spontaneous breaths through the added resistance of the IMV circuit may aggravate chest wall distortion. The use of a low-impedance system such as high-flow continuous positive airway pressure (CPAP) has been shown to produce less chest wall distortion than an IMV circuit.[59] Such modes may reduce the likelihood of developing inspiratory muscle fatigue and thus may be preferred to IMV for weaning. A randomized, controlled trial of CPAP versus mechanical ventilation in patients who had similar degrees of blunt thoracic trauma showed that patients treated with CPAP had significantly fewer days of treatment, intensive care, and total hospitalization.[5] Pressure support ventilation may be an alternative means of reducing the load imposed by the endotracheal tube during spontaneous breaths, but the effects of this mode on chest wall distortion have not been evaluated.

To summarize, flail chest in combination with pulmonary contusion carries a high risk of acute respiratory failure and is associated with a high mortality. It adversely affects chest wall mechanics in the following manner: (1) vital capacity is reduced owing to inward displacement of the rib cage; (2) the work of breathing is increased; (3) the energy demands of the inspiratory muscles are heightened; and (4) gas exchange is worsened by underlying pulmonary contusion. Flail chest may result in respiratory failure because of increases in the work of breathing and a reduction in the efficiency of breathing. The serious complications that accompany trauma, such as adult respiratory distress syndrome, tracheal injury, and pneumonia, may further increase the mortality in this patient population. The essential components of treatment include pain control and mechanical ventilation for respiratory failure. In attempts to wean these patients, modes of ventilation should be used that reduce the elastic and resistive loads on the respiratory system. External fixa-

tion of the rib cage may be indicated in some patients.

PECTUS EXCAVATUM

Diagnosis and Treatment

Pectus excavatum is a disorder in which the sternum is abnormally depressed. It is the most common chest wall deformity seen by pediatricians and primary care providers. The incidence is approximately 8 per 1000, and it occurs three times more often in boys than girls. Pectus excavatum may be due to a defect in the connective tissue surrounding the sternum and is occasionally associated with connective-tissue disorders such as Marfan's syndrome. In one large series, a family history of pectus deformity was present in 41 percent of these persons.[23] Pectus carinatum, a disorder in which the sternum is protuberant, is less common than pectus excavatum. It is of unknown origin and may be associated with congenital heart disease, severe childhood asthma, and rickets.

As with kyphoscoliosis and ankylosing spondylitis, the degree of chest wall deformity with pectus excavatum has been assessed with radiographic techniques. With lateral chest radiographs, the ratio of the transthoracic diameter to the sternovertebral distances and the absolute distance between the posterior aspect of the lower sternum and the anterior face of the vertebral column have been used as indices of chest wall deformity. With CT scans, the ratio of the transverse to AP diameter of the inner chest wall at the level of the deepest sternal depression has been used to assess the degree of chest wall deformity (Fig. 97-17). These indices have been used to select patients for surgical correction and also have been correlated with pulmonary function.

The most frequent complaint in patients with pectus deformity is an unattractive chest wall. However, as many as 30 to 70 percent of these patients may have additional respiratory complaints—most commonly dyspnea on exertion, particularly during athletic activities. Other symptoms are chest pain and frequent respiratory infections.[23] Scoliosis can be associated with pectus excavatum and was noted in 15 percent of 252 patients. Congenital heart disease was seen 4 percent of the time in the same series, although the presence of functional murmurs was common (31 percent).[23]

Pathophysiology

Patients with pectus carinatum or excavatum have either normal pulmonary function or a mild reduction in TLC and VC. The reduction in lung volumes is more severe in patients with associated scoliosis. The restrictive impairment is positively associated with the degree of sternal depression.[30,44] FRC is usually within the normal range, and RV may be slightly elevated or normal. Although the rib cage is deformed, its mobility is not impaired during quiet breathing or exercise.[42] Unlike kyphoscoliosis, in which lung compliance is reduced as a result of limited chest wall mobility, lung compliance would be expected to be within normal limits unless these patients develop intrinsic lung disease. Indeed, the limited measures of lung compliances that are available are within normal limits.[12,17] Although complaints of exercise intolerance are very common, exercise performance may be normal or only mildly diminished.[64] A small fraction of patients have a reduction in exercise tolerance and an increase in the oxygen consumption for a given work rate.[12]

Treatment

A transverse to AP diameter ratio of greater than 3.25, as assessed by CT scanning, is often used as one of the criteria to select patients for surgical correction. There is no question that surgical repair can provide cosmetic benefits. Subjective improvement in exercise tolerance and relief of dyspnea have also been noted following surgery. However, despite the marked improvements in the radiologic appearance of the pectus deformity and the subjective improvements in exercise tolerance, the physiological benefits of corrective surgery are questionable. Some studies have shown that pulmonary function can be improved following surgery,[9] whereas others have shown no improvement or even a reduction in pulmonary function either within the first year[30,64] or several years after surgical repair.[16,44] The impaired lung function following surgery has been attributed to abnormal chest wall mechanics due to articular changes in the sternal and parasternal areas. The postoperative reduction in lung function may be greatest in those with the mildest restrictive deficit. Discrepancies among studies regarding the benefits of surgery may be related to differences in the severity of the deformity, surgical techniques, length of time following the operation, and the effects of growth on pulmonary function.

The effects of surgery on exercise tolerance are also controversial. Some investigators report an improvement in $\dot{V}_{O_2max}$ and exercise tolerance following surgical correction.[9] One controlled study, however, found no differences in $\dot{V}_{O_2max}$, minute ventilation at maximal exercise, and cardiac output following surgery.[64]

To summarize, pectus deformities are often accompanied by complaints of exercise intolerance but are associated with only mild reductions in TLC and VC. Surgical repair for cosmetic reasons may be justified, with radiographic techniques used to assist in patient selection. Following surgery, there is often symptomatic improvement but no change in aerobic capacity and often a reduction in TLC and VC several years after surgery. The above-described studies evaluated changes in function in either young adolescents or adults. Whether younger patients may benefit from surgical correction because of the continued growth of the thorax in adolescence is unknown.

OBESITY

Diagnosis and Etiology

Obesity refers to an excess of body fat. It is a serious medical problem that affects as many as one-fourth of the adults living in the United States. Body fat usually constitutes 15 to 20 percent of the body mass in healthy men and 25 to 30 percent in healthy women. Body fat composition can be assessed by direct techniques such as densitometry, measurement of total body potassium, and the inhalation of fat-soluble inert gases or by indirect techniques such as skinfold measurements and weight-to-height ratios. Obesity also can be defined in terms of risk to life by utilizing tables of desirable weight for height and age (Metropolitan Life Insurance Co.). This section focuses on the effects of obesity on respiratory mechanics, respiratory muscle function, and control of breathing. The obesity hypoventilation syndrome and its relation to obstructive sleep apnea are covered in detail in Chapter 102.

The severity of obesity can be assessed by calculating weight as a percentage of ideal body weight, the ratio of weight to height (WT/Ht), or body mass index (BMI), which is the ratio of WT/Ht^2. Exceptions to use of this rule would be marked localized edema such as ascites or anasarca. Obesity is considered mild when body weight lies between 120 and 150 percent of ideal body weight, or the BW/Ht ratio is between 0.4 and 0.6, or the BMI lies between 28 and 40 kg/m^2. Obesity is severe when body weight is greater than 150 percent of ideal, the BW/Ht ratio is greater than 0.6, or the BMI is greater than 40 kg/m^2. Values for WT/Ht of 0.8 and 1.0 kg/cm correspond to body weights of approximately 200 and 250 percent of ideal, respectively. The advantage of the WT/Ht ratio and BMI over calculating the percentage of ideal body weight is that no tables of height and weight are needed. The weight-to-height ratios, however, fail to differentiate between increases in body weight due to muscularity and those due to obesity. Most respiratory studies of obesity have employed subjects with weights greater than 150 percent of ideal body mass.

Obese persons have increased fat-free mass, body cell mass, and total body water as well as increased fat mass and body weight (Table 97-2). The increase in resting energy expenditure in obesity is proportional to the increase in fat-free mass and body cell mass, and the ratio of energy expenditure to fat-free

TABLE 97-2

Body Composition in Obesity

Variable	Normals	Mild Obesity	Severe Obesity
Body mass index (kg/m^2)	23	34	50
Body fat (%)	22	35	45
Body weight (kg)	65	96	132
Fat-free mass (kg)	51	63	72
Body cell mass (kg)	27	32	36
Total body water (L)	38	44	49
Resting energy expenditure (watts)	68	86	96

Note increases in fat-free mass, body cell mass, and total body water. Resting energy expenditure is proportional to fat-free mass.
SOURCE: Modified from Verga et al.[61]

mass is the same in mild and severe obesity as it is in normal-weight subjects.[37,61]

In regard to its effects on the respiratory system, patients are classified as exhibiting either simple obesity or the obesity hypoventilation syndrome (OHS). OHS is characterized by CO_2 retention and is frequently accompanied by obstructive sleep apnea. Patients with simple obesity are eucapnic, and men with simple obesity often have obstructive sleep apnea. Both groups often complain of exercise intolerance and dyspnea on exertion. In addition, they are at increased risk for developing postoperative complications such as pneumonia and atelectasis.

Pathophysiology

The effects of obesity on lung volumes have been extensively studied.[49] Patients with simple obesity may have either a mild restrictive ventilatory pattern or normal lung volumes. Generally, with simple obesity there is no restrictive ventilatory defect unless the body mass index is greater than 60 kg/m^2. In this circumstance, VC may be reduced by 25 percent but TLC and FRC can still be within the range of normal. When TLC is reduced in patients with a BMI less than 60 kg/m^2, other explanations of the restrictive process should be sought. In mildly obese men, expiratory reserve volume (ERV) is inversely proportional to BMI even though all other lung volumes are normal. In addition, mildly obese men whose obesity is more centrally distributed have lower values of FVC, FEV$_1$, and TLC than those with more peripheral obesity.[13] In OHS, TLC is 20 percent smaller and VC and MVV are 40 percent smaller than in simple obesity. ERV is reduced to 60 percent of that predicted in simple obesity and to 35 percent of that predicted in OHS. ERV is most severely impaired when the BMI exceeds 60 kg/m^2. The above-mentioned studies indicate that the adverse effects of obesity on pulmonary function cannot be entirely explained by the absolute load of adipose on the chest wall, as similar degrees of obesity in simple obesity and OHS result in very different patterns of lung volume changes.

Obesity generally lowers chest wall and total respiratory system compliance, and, as with TLC, compliance is more severely affected in OHS.[49] In simple obesity, chest wall and total respiratory system compliances are generally 80 and 90 percent of values obtained in normal subjects—even when the body weight/height ratio and the body mass index are as high as 1.2 kg/cm and 80 kg/m^2, respectively. In contrast, with OHS, the chest wall and total respiratory system compliance are generally only 37 and 44 percent of normal. The changes in compliance are thought to be due to weight pressing on the thorax and abdomen, thereby imposing an elastic load. The excess weight also may impose a threshold-type load on the chest wall; pleural pressure must be lowered to a sufficient degree before inspiratory flow can ensue. The threshold load then appears as though it were a resistance to flow rather than a change in compliance. The reduced respiratory system compliance is due not only to the reduced chest wall compliance but also to a reduction in lung compliance.[45] Factors that would decrease lung compliance in obese patients include an increased pulmonary blood volume and closure of dependent airways. It is generally decreased by approximately 25 percent in simple obesity and 40 percent in OHS.

Airway and respiratory system resistances are increased in patients with obesity, in part because of the reduction in lung volume. After correcting for the reduced lung volume, specific airway conductance may be near normal or reduced to 50 to 70 percent of normal.[49] Although specific airway conductance is diminished, the FEV$_1$/FVC ratio is normal in simple obesity and in OHS. Thus, the source of the increased airways resistance appears to lie in lung tissue and small airways rather than in the large airways. Chest wall and total respiratory system resistances are also increased in simple obesity and OHS, with those resistances being higher in OHS. Total respiratory system resistance, determined by the forced oscillation technique, is higher than normal in simple obesity. Moreover, respiratory resistance increases when obese subjects shift from upright to supine, but the mechanism of the postural change in resistance and reactance is not clear.[65]

The increased elastic and resistive loads imposed by the lung and chest wall, along with the threshold load imposed by the fatty deposits around the abdomen, require a greater reduction of pleural pressure to achieve a given tidal volume. Accordingly, the work of breathing is increased in both simple obesity and OHS. However, since respiratory system compliance and resistance are impaired to a greater degree in OHS, the work of breathing is greater in OHS than in simple obesity. Compared to normals, the work of breathing is 60 percent higher in simple obesity and may be as much as 250 percent higher in OHS. The increased work is accompanied by an increase in the oxygen cost of breathing. Accordingly, the oxygen cost of breathing is four times normal in simple obesity and nearly 10 times normal with OHS.[49]

Gas exchange is often impaired in obese persons. Severely obese patients commonly have a widened alveolar-arterial oxygen tension gradient. However, hypoxemia may be mild or absent in simple obesity. In contrast, the P_{O_2} is lower than normal in OHS. In both simple obesity and OHS, hypoxemia becomes more pronounced when the person assumes the supine position. Mechanisms leading to hypoxemia include ventilation-perfusion mismatching and shunting. In OHS, hypoventilation further aggravates hypoxemia. In general, with obesity the lung bases are well perfused but poorly ventilated, owing to airway closure and alveolar collapse. This has practical consequences. In anesthetized, normal-weight patients who received 100 percent oxygen, it took 6 min of apnea for the Sa_{O_2} to fall to 90 percent, as compared to less than 2 min of apnea in obese subjects.[29] The single-breath–diffusing capacity is usually normal in simple obesity and slightly reduced in OHS. The physiological dead space (VD) and the ratio of dead space to tidal volume (VD/VT) are normal.[49]

Metabolism is increased in obesity, thereby increasing carbon dioxide production and oxygen consumption. At rest, obese subjects consume approximately 25 percent more oxygen than nonobese subjects.[50] Consequently, during breath-holding, the alveolar P_{O_2} falls much faster in obese subjects than in normals, with the magnitude of fall in P_{O_2} correlating with the severity of obesity. However, the increase in oxygen consumption per kilogram of body weight in obese subjects is lower than the increase per kilogram in subjects with a normal distribution of body fat.

Since the work of breathing is increased in both simple obesity and in OHS, one would expect an increase in ventilatory drive to compensate for the increased load on the respiratory muscles. Indeed, respiratory drive may be increased in simple obesity but is clearly abnormal in OHS.[49] The observation that P_{CO_2} can be lowered to a normal level by voluntary hyperventilating in OHS can be taken as evidence of abnormal ventilatory control. This notion is supported by more direct studies of respiratory drive. The ventilatory response to carbon dioxide ($\Delta \dot{V}_E / \Delta P_{CO_2}$) is generally reduced by approximately 40 percent in simple obesity and 65 percent in OHS. In contrast, the ventilatory response to hypoxia, the resting $P_{0.1}$, and V_T/T_I may be normal or higher than normal in simple obesity. In addition, $P_{0.1}$ increases normally with C_{O_2} inhalation in simple obesity. Values for $P_{0.1}$ in overt OHS are unavailable. However, respiratory muscle electrical (EMG) responses to inhaled gas mixtures should parallel the mouth occlusion pressure response. As with $P_{0.1}$, the diaphragm EMG response to inhalation of CO_2 is elevated in simple obesity. In contrast, the EMG response to CO_2 in OHS, which should also be elevated, is low, lying in the normal range. The finding that $P_{0.1}$ in former OHS patients is the same as in simple obesity indicates that these changes are in part reversible.

Obese patients may alter their breathing pattern to compensate for the increased load placed on the respiratory system. During quiet breathing, the respiratory rate of simple obesity subjects is approximately 40 percent higher than in normal subjects. The increased rate is accomplished by shortening both T_I and T_E, so that the duration of T_I as a fraction of the total breath time (T_{TOT}) is normal. In contrast to the increase in breathing frequency, tidal volume is normal in simple obesity at rest and during maximal exercise. Patients with OHS also exhibit higher breathing frequencies while maintaining TI/T_{TOT} in the normal range. In the person with OHS, breathing frequency is 25 percent higher than in the person with simple obesity. In contrast, tidal volume is 25 percent lower than in simple obesity.[49] The rapid shallow breathing pattern in OHS worsens gas exchange in these subjects.

Inspiratory and expiratory muscle strength is generally normal in simple obesity.[49] In severely obese subjects, however, there may be a mild degree of inspiratory muscle weakness, perhaps related to overstretching the diaphragm.[52] Nonetheless, in the person with simple obesity, the inspiratory muscles are strong enough to overcome the mild reduction in lung and chest wall compliance so that total lung capacity is not reduced. In OHS, inspiratory muscle strength may be reduced by 40 percent.[49] The cause of inspiratory muscle weakness with OHS is unknown. One possibility is that inspiratory muscle training may occur in simple obesity and not in OHS. With OHS, the level of daily ventilation may be lower owing to tolerance of higher levels of CO_2 and to relative inactivity. Consequently, the added resistive and elastic loads provide less of a training stimulus in OHS. Second, in the person with OHS, diaphragm contractility may be impaired. A single case report describes fatty infiltration of the diaphragm in a patient with OHS who died in cardiorespiratory failure.[20]

Animal studies also indicate that diaphragm contractility may be impaired. In one group of obese rats, there was a 20 to 30 percent reduction in muscle mass, an 8 to 20 percent reduction in fiber diameters, and a reduction of twitch tension by 21 percent even after normalizing for the reduced muscle cross-sectional area.[8] In morbidly obese Zucker rats, the diaphragms contained 30 percent more type I and 28 percent fewer type IIa fibers, and the cross-sectional areas of the type I and type IIa fibers were increased by 60 percent.[21] As a result of the remodeling, diaphragms of obese rats were 29 percent thicker, 9 percent shorter and generated 13 percent lower tetanic force.

Exercise capacity is near normal in simple obesity with values for $\dot{V}_{O_2 max}$ and $\dot{V}_{E max}$ approaching 90 percent of predicted.[50] When oxygen consumption at maximal exercise is related to body weight, however, $\dot{V}_{O_2 max}$ (in milliliters per kilogram) is only 60 percent normal and is inversely correlated with the percentage of body fat. Obese subjects have a higher minute ventilation, respiratory rate, heart rate, and oxygen consumption during treadmill exercise than normals, but they have a lower $\dot{V}O_2$ at anaerobic threshold. There may be hypoventilation and oxyhemoglobin desaturation at the onset of exercise. Exercise efficiency may be reduced in simple obesity, since at a given work rate, the oxygen consumption tends to be higher. The cardiac response is within the normal range with simple obesity. The increment in heart rate over time parallels that seen in healthy young persons. With weight loss, the metabolic demands are reduced. Consequently, CO_2 production and alveolar ventilation during exercise fall by 12 to 22 percent.

Obesity is strongly associated with obstructive sleep apnea. Analysis of data from four studies shows that obstructive sleep apnea occurs in approximately 19 percent of obese subjects with body mass indices ranging from 41 to 50 kg/m²; the prevalence is 49 percent in males versus 8 percent in females (Table 97-3).[7,34,48,62] The $P_{0.1}$ at rest and both the $P_{0.1}$ and ventilatory responses to hypercapnic stimuli were above normal in obese women and normal in obese men.[34] The ventilatory response to inhaled CO_2 is higher, and the awake Pa_{CO_2} and TLC are lower, in eucapnic obese patients (body mass index of 34 kg/m²) with sleep apnea than in equally obese patients without sleep apnea.[26] The severity of obstructive sleep apnea in both men and women correlates with upper-body obesity as reflected by triceps and subscapular skinfold thicknesses, but not with body mass index. In addition, men had a greater degree of

TABLE 97-3

Prevalence of Obstructive Sleep Apnea (OSA) in Simple Obesity

Source	BMI	Female OSA/Total	Male OSA/Total	Combined OSA/Total
Kunimoto et al. (1988)[34]	41	2/14	4/8	6/22
Rajala et al. (1991)[48]	50	1/14	11/13	12/27
Broussole et al. (1994)[7]	>30	13/37	22/46	35/83
Vgontzas et al. (1994)[62]	47	6/200	20/50	26/250
Pooled series	~45	22/265	57/117	73/382
OSA prevalence	(%)	8.3	48.7	20.7

Note that OSA occurs six times more often in obese men than in obese women.
BMI = body mass index.

TABLE 97-4

Respiratory Pathophysiology of Simple Obesity and Obesity Hypoventilation Syndrome

Variable	Units	Nl	SO	OHS
BW	(% ideal)	105	195	201
BW/Ht	(Kg/cm)	0.42	0.75	0.78
BMI	(Kg/m^2)	24	45	46
TLC	% predicted	100	95	83
C_{RS}	L/cm H$_2$O^{-1}	0.11	0.05	0.06
R_{RS}	cm H$_2$O L^{-1} sec^{-1}	1.2	4.0	7.8
Work	J/L	0.43	0.74	1.64
MVV	L/min	159	129	89
PI$_{max}$	cm H$_2$O	100	95	60

NOTE: Nl = normal; SO = simple obesity; OHS = obesity hypoventilation syndrome; BW = body weight; Ht = height; BMI = body mass index; TLC = total lung capacity; C_{RS} = respiratory system compliance; R_{RS} = respiratory system resistance; MVV = maximal voluntary ventilation; PImax = maximal inspiratory pressure.

upper-body obesity than women, and for a given degree of upper-body obesity, men had more severe obstructive sleep apnea.

Treatment

The optimal treatment for obesity would seem to be weight loss, but it is difficult for patients to lose weight and even harder for them to remain at the lower weight. Insight into the problem was provided by a study showing that losing weight decreases total energy expenditure in both normal and obese subjects, whereas the opposite is true with weight gain.[37] In other words, the body has a tendency to resist changes in weight in either direction. Patients who have undergone various types of gastric stapling, banding, or bypass procedures all lose weight in the first year, but after 10 years more than half have regained part or all of the lost weight.[63]

The effects of weight loss—either by dietary means, small-bowel bypass, or gastric surgery—on pulmonary function have been well described.[49] With weight loss in the range of 40 kg, there is either no change or a small increase in VC, TLC, or compliance. However, there is a 75 percent increase in ERV, which is a consequence of both changes in FRC and RV. As a result of the increase in FRC and RV, there is better ventilation to the lung bases and improved gas exchange. P$_{O_2}$ may be increased by 4 to 8 mmHg in the person with simple obesity. The improvement in gas exchange is more pronounced in those whose body weight is reduced to less than 130 percent of ideal. In OHS, the effects of weight loss on ERV and FRC are even more pronounced. VC increases as well and is correlated with the degree of weight loss. Gas exchange is also improved following weight loss in OHS. The Pa$_{O_2}$ increases, and the decrease in Pa$_{CO_2}$ is positively correlated with weight loss. Ketosis induced by fasting increases the $\Delta\dot{V}E/\Delta P_{CO_2}$ in OHS.

Weight loss in the range of 20 to 30 percent was associated with a 12 percent loss of lean body mass, a 9 percent reduction in PE$_{max}$, a 26 percent reduction in oxygen consumption during exercise, and a 10 percent increase in MVV.[49] Respiratory control remains essentially unaltered following weight loss. A further benefit of weight loss is the abatement of obstructive sleep apnea. The episodes of apnea are diminished, and there is an improvement in daytime Pa$_{CO_2}$ and Pa$_{O_2}$.[48]

With persistent hypercapnia, nocturnal noninvasive mechanical ventilation has been employed in an attempt to improve daytime function. Negative-pressure ventilation can improve nocturnal oxygenation, but it often aggravates upper-airway obstruction during sleep. Alternatively, positive-pressure ventilation has been attempted in patients with simple obesity and OHS. This can be delivered as either CPAP or intermittent positive-pressure ventilation by nose mask. The advantage of positive-pressure ventilation is the improvement in sleep quality. Complications from delivering positive-pressure ventilation by mask include skin erosion and nasal stuffiness or sinusitis. These complications by be averted by using a lip seal device to deliver long-term positive-pressure ventilation.

To summarize, an equal degree of obesity may have profoundly different effects on the respiratory system (Table 97-4). In simple obesity, VC and TLC may be slightly decreased. In the obese hypoventilation syndrome, these lung volumes may be markedly reduced. Similarly, in simple obesity, respiratory system compliance may be somewhat low and accompanied by a modest increase in respiratory system resistance, whereas in OHS the changes are more severe. In simple obesity, the inspiratory muscle strength is well preserved, whereas in OHS the inspiratory muscles are somewhat weak and the ventilatory drive does not increase in keeping with the increased work of breathing. As a consequence of the increased work of breathing, the oxygen cost of breathing is increased in both simple obesity and OHS. Both simple obesity and OHS are associated with obstructive sleep apnea, which is much more prevalent in men than in women. Treatment consists of weight loss, which causes dramatic improvement in pulmonary function in both groups but more so in OHS. In addition, noninvasive positive-pressure ventilation can maintain oxygenation and relieve upper-airway obstruction.

REFERENCES

1. Ali J, Harding B, deNiord R: Effect of temporary external stabilization on ventilator weaning after sternal resection. *Chest* 95:472–473, 1989.
2. Baydur A, Gilgoff I, Prentice W, et al: Decline in respiratory function and experience with long-term assisted ventilation in advanced Duchenne's muscular dystrophy. *Chest* 97:884–889, 1990.
3. Bergofsky EH: Thoracic deformities, in Roussos C (ed), *The Thorax.* New York, Dekker 1995, pp 1915–1950.
4. Bergofsky EH, Turino GM, Fishman AP: Cardiorespiratory failure in kyphoscoliosis. *Medicine (Baltimore)* 38:263–317, 1959.
5. Bolliger CT, van Eeden SF: Treatment of multiple rib fractures: Randomized control trial comparing ventilatory and nonventilatory management. *Chest* 97:943–948, 1990.

6. Bredin CP: Pulmonary function in long-term survivors of thoracoplasty. *Chest* 95:18–20, 1989.

7. Broussolle C, Piperno D, Gormand F, et al: [Sleep apnea syndrome in obese patients: Are there any predictive factors?] [French]. *Rev Med Interne* 15:161–165, 1994.

8. Burbach JA, Schlenker EH, Goldman M: Characterization of muscles from aspartic acid obese rats. *Am J Physiol* 249:R106–R110, 1985.

9. Cahill JL, Lees GM, Roberston HT: A summary of preoperative and postoperative cardiorespiratory performance in patients undergoing pectus excavatum and carinatum repair. *J Pediatr Surg* 19:430–433, 1984.

10. Cappello M, Yuehua C, DeTroyer A: Rib cage distortion in a canine model of flail chest. *Am J Respir Crit Care Med* 151:1481–1485, 1995.

11. Caro CG, DuBois AB: Pulmonary function in kyphoscoliosis. *Thorax* 16:282–290, 1961.

12. Castile R, Staats B, Westbrook P: Symptomatic pectus deformities of the chest. *Am Rev Respir Dis* 126:564–568, 1982.

13. Collins LC, Hoberty PD, Walker JF, et al: The effect of body fat distribution on pulmonary function tests. *Chest* 107:1298–1302, 1995.

14. Cooper DM, Rojas J, Mellins RB, et al: Respiratory mechanics in adolescents with idiopathic scoliosis. *Am Rev Respir Dis* 130:16–22, 1984.

15. Culham EG, Jimenez HA, King CE. Thoracic kyphosis, rib mobility, and lung volumes in normal women and women with osteoporosis. *Spine* 19:1250–1255, 1994.

16. Derveaux L, Clarysse I, Ivanoff I, Demedts M: Preoperative and postoperative abnormalities in chest x-ray indices and in lung function in pectus deformities. *Chest* 95:850–856, 1989.

17. Donnelly PM, Daxini BV, Bye PT. The upper limit of alveolar capillary recruitment in a young man with lung growth impairment. *Eur Respir J* 7:1371–1375, 1994.

18. Ellis ER, Grunstein RR, Chan S, et al: Noninvasive ventilatory support during sleep improves respiratory failure in kyphoscoliosis. *Chest* 94:811–815, 1988.

19. Eveloff SE, McCool FD. Disorders of the chest wall: Implications for respiratory failure, in Marini JJ, Roussos C (eds), *Ventilatory Failure*. Berlin, Springer, 1991, pp 219–239.

20. Fadell EJ, Richman AD, Ward WW, Hendon JR. Fatty infiltration of respiratory muscles in the Pickwickian syndrome. *New Engl J Med* 266:861–863, 1962.

21. Farkas GA, Gosselin LE, Zhan W-Z, et al: Histochemical and mechanical properties of diaphragm muscle in morbidly obese Zucker rats. *J Appl Physiol* 77:2250–2259, 1994.

22. Feltelius N, Hedenstrom H, Hillerdal G, Hallgren R: Pulmonary involvement in ankylosing spondylitis. *Ann Rheum Dis* 45:736–740, 1986.

23. Fonkalsrud EW, Salman T, Guo W, Gregg JP: Repair of pectus deformities with sternal support. *J Thorac Cardiovasc Surg* 107:37–42, 1994.

24. Gagnon S, Jodoin A, Martin R: Pulmonary function test study and after spinal fusion in young idiopathic scoliosis. *Spine* 14:486–490, 1989.

25. Gaillard M, Herve C, Mandin L, Raynaud P. Mortality prognostic factors in chest injury. *J Trauma* 30:93–96, 1990.

26. Gold AR, Schwartz AR, Wise RA, Smith PL: Pulmonary function and respiratory chemosensitivity in moderately obese patients with sleep apnea. *Chest* 103:1325–1329, 1993.

27. Hartke RH Jr, Block AJ: External stabilization of flail chest using continuous negative extrathoracic pressure. *Chest* 102:1283–1285, 1992.

28. Jackson M, Smith I, King M, Shneerson J: Long term non-invasive domiciliary assisted ventilation for respiratory failure following thoracoplasty. *Thorax* 49:915–919, 1994.

29. Jense HG, Dubin SA, Silverstein PI, O'Leary-Escolas U: Effect of obesity on safe duration of apnea in anesthetized patients. *Anesth Analg* 72:89–93, 1991.

30. Kaguraoka H, Ohnuki T, Itaoka T, et al: Degree of severity of pectus excavatum and pulmonary function in preoperative and postoperative periods. *J Thorac Cardiovasc Surg* 104:1483–1488, 1992.

31. Kearon C, Viviani GR, Killian KJ: Factors influencing work capacity in adolescent idiopathic thoracic scoliosis. *Am Rev Respir Dis* 148:295–303, 1993.

32. Kesten S, Garfinkel SK, Wright T, Rebuck AS: Impaired exercise capacity in adults with moderate scoliosis. *Chest* 99:663–666, 1991.

33. Kishikawa M, Yoshioka T, Shimazu T, et al: Pulmonary contusion causes long-term respiratory dysfunction with decreased functional residual capacity. *J Trauma* 31:1203–1210, 1991.

34. Kunimoto F, Kimura H, Tatsumi K, et al: Sex differences in awake ventilatory drive and abnormal breathing during sleep in eucapnic obesity. *Chest* 93:968–976, 1988.

35. Landercasper J, Cogbill TH, Lindesmith LA: Long-term disability after flail chest injury. *Trauma* 24:410–414, 1984.

36. Leger P, Bedicam JM, Cornette A, et al: Nasal intermittent positive pressure ventilation: Long-term follow-up in patients with severe chronic respiratory insufficiency. *Chest* 105:100–105, 1994.

37. Leibel RL, Rosenbaum M, Hirsch J: Changes in energy expenditure resulting from altered body weight. *New Engl J Med* 332:621–628, 1995.

38. Libby DM, Briscoe WA, Boyce B, Smith JP: Acute respiratory failure in scoliosis or kyphosis. *Am J Med* 73:532–538, 1982.

39. Lisboa C, Moreno R, Fava M, Ferretti R: Inspiratory muscle function in patients with severe kyphoscoliosis. *Am Rev Respir Dis* 132:48–52, 1985.

40. McCool FD, Mayewski RJ, Shayne DS, et al: Intermittent positive pressure breathing in patients with respiratory muscle weakness: Alterations in total respiratory system compliance. *Chest* 90:546–552, 1986.

41. McCool FD, Tzelepis GE, Leith DE, Hoppin FG, Jr: Oxygen cost of breathing during fatiguing inspiratory resistive loads. *J Appl Physiol* 66:2045–2055, 1989.

42. Mead J, Sly P, Lesouef P, et al: Rib cage mobility in pectus excavatum. *Am Rev Respir Dis* 130:1223–1228, 1985.

43. Meecham-Jones DJ, Paul EA, Bell JH, Wedzicha JA: Ambulatory oxygen therapy in stable kyphoscoliosis. *Eur Respir J* 8:819–823, 1995.

44. Morshuis W, Folgering H, Barentsz J, et al: Pulmonary function before surgery for pectus excavatum and at long-term follow-up. *Chest* 105:1646–1652, 1994.

45. Pelosi P, Croci M, Ravagnan I, et al. Total respiratory system, lung, and chest wall mechanics in sedated-paralyzed postoperative morbidly obese patients. *Chest* 109:144–151, 1996.

46. Phillips MS, Kinnear WJM, Shaw D, Shneerson JM: Exercise responses in patients treated for pulmonary tuberculosis by thoracoplasty. *Thorax* 44:268–274, 1989.

47. Phillips MS, Kinnear WJM, Shneerson JM: Late sequelae of pulmonary tuberculosis treated by thoracoplasty. *Thorax* 42:445–451, 1987.

48. Rajala R, Partinen M, Sane T, et al: Obstructive sleep apnoea syndrome in morbidly obese patients. *J Intern Med* 230:125–129, 1991.

49. Rochester DF: Obesity and abdominal distention, in Roussos C (ed), *The Thorax*. New York, Dekker 1995, pp 1915–1950.

50. Salvadori A, Fanari P, Mazza P, et al: Work capacity and cardiopulmonary adaptation of the obese subject during exercise testing. *Chest* 101:674–679, 1992.

51. Shackford SR, Smith DE, Zarins CD, et al: The management of flail chest: A comparison of ventilatory and nonventilatory treatment. *Am J Surg* 132:759–762, 1976.

52. Sharp JT, Druz WS, Kondragunta VR. Diaphragmatic responses to body position changes in obese patients with obstructive sleep apnea. *Am Rev Respir Dis* 133:32–37, 1986.

53. Sinha R, Bergofsky EH: Prolonged alteration of lung mechanisms in kyphoscoliosis by positive-pressure hyperinflation. *Am Rev Respir Dis* 106:47–57, 1972.

54. Smyth RJ, Chapman KR, Wright TA, et al: Pulmonary function in adolescents with mild idiopathic scoliosis. *Thorax* 39:901–904, 1984.

55. Sridhar MK, Carter R, Lean ME, Banham SW. Resting energy expenditure and nutritional state of patients with increased oxygen cost of breathing due to emphysema, scoliosis and thoracoplasty. *Thorax* 49:781–785, 1994.

56. Swank S, Lonstein J, Moe J, et al: Surgical treatment of adult scoliosis. *J Bone Joint Surg [Am]* 63:268–287, 1981.

57. Szeinberg A, Canny GJ, Rashed N, et al: Forced vital capacity and maximal respiratory pressures in patients with mild and moderate scolioses. *Pediatr Pulmonol* 4:8–12, 1988.

58. Trinkle JK, Richardson JD, Franz JL, et al: Management of flail chest without mechanical ventilation. *Ann Thorac Surg* 19:355–363, 1975.

59. Tzelepis GE, McCool FD, Hoppin FG Jr: Chest wall distortion in patients with flail chest. *Am Rev Respir Dis* 140:31–37, 1989.

60. Vanderschueren D, Decramer M, van den Dael P, et al: Pulmonary function and maximal transrespiratory pressure in ankylosing spondylitis. *Ann Rheum Dis* 48:632–635, 1989.

61. Verga S, Buscemi C, Caimi C: Resting energy expenditure and body composition in morbidly obese, obese and control subjects. *Acta Diabetol* 31:47–51, 1994.

62. Vgontzas AN, Tan TL, Bixler EO, et al: Sleep apnea and sleep disruption in obese patients. *Arch Intern Med* 154:1705–1711, 1994.

63. Wolfel R, Gunther K, Rumenapf G, et al: Weight reduction after gastric bypass and horizontal gastroplasty for morbid obesity. Results after 10 years. *Eur J Surg* 160:219–225, 1994

64. Wynn S, Driscol D, Ostrom N, et al: Exercise cardiorespiratory function in adolescents with pectus excavatum. *J Thorac Cardiovasc Surg* 99:41–47, 1990.

65. Yap JCH, Watson RA, Gilbey S, Pride NB: Effects of posture on respiratory mechanics in obesity. *J Appl Physiol* 79:1199–1205, 1995.

CHAPTER 98

EFFECTS OF NEUROMUSCULAR DISEASES ON VENTILATION

Gerard Joseph Criner / Steven G. Kelsen

Neuromuscular diseases comprise a diverse group of disorders that vary markedly in etiology, rate of progression, pattern of respiratory involvement, prognosis, and therapy. Neuromuscular disorders impair the respiratory system as a vital pump; however, depending on the particular disease, the respiratory pump may be impaired at the level of the central nervous system (e.g., cerebral cortex or brain stem), spinal cord, peripheral nerve, neuromuscular junction, or respiratory muscle (Table 98-1).

The pattern of ventilatory impairment among these disorders is highly dependent on the specific neuromuscular disease. For example, some disorders may impair ventilation at only one level (e.g., isolated diaphragm paralysis) or simultaneously affect it at different levels (e.g., multiple sclerosis). Additionally, the severity of impairment may be minimal and totally resolve with time and proper treatment (e.g., Guillain-Barré syndrome) or is characterized by relentless progression to eventual respiratory death (e.g., amyotrophic lateral sclerosis). Moreover, some neuromuscular diseases concomitantly affect several structures (e.g., swallowing dysfunction in poliomyelitis, interstitial lung disease in polymyositis), increasing ventilatory workload in patients who already have diminished ventilatory reserve.

This chapter describes the etiology, pathophysiology, and treatment of ventilatory dysfunction in neuromuscular diseases.

RESPIRATORY PATHOPHYSIOLOGY

Substantial information exists concerning the ventilatory function of patients with neuromuscular disease at rest and during sleep, as well as the effects on maximum static inspiratory and expiratory efforts, and responses associated with these disorders to hypoxic and hypercapnic challenges. In general, the response of the respiratory system to moderate or severe neuromuscular disease is relatively stereotyped. The typical features are a reduced forced vital capacity, reduced respiratory muscle strength, and, in some cases, malfunction of the neurons that control breathing.

Control of Breathing

The breathing pattern is often abnormal in patients with neuromuscular disease. In comparison with healthy subjects, patients with respiratory muscle weakness have a low tidal volume and a high respiratory rate[4] that persists in response even to hypoxic or hypercapnic challenge.[5] Moreover, this rapid, shallow breathing pattern is not due to abnormalities in gas exchange (i.e., hypoxemia or hypercapnia) but is more likely to be due to severe muscle weakness and/or disordered afferent and efferent output in motoneurons impaired by the underlying neuromuscular disease.[5]

Changes in ventilation can be used to evaluate ventilatory drive in subjects with normal lung and respiratory muscle mechanics. However, ventilation is not a good index of respiratory

TABLE 98-1

Levels of Respiratory System Dysfunction Induced by Neuromuscular Diseases and Conditions

Level	Disease or Condition
Upper motoneuron	
Cerebral	Vascular accidents
	Cerebellar atrophy
	Trauma
Spinal cord	Trauma
	Tumor
	Syringomyelia
	Mulitple sclerosis
Lower motoneuron	
Anterior horn cells	Poliomyelitis
	Spinal muscle atrophy
	Amyotrophic lateral sclerosis
Motor nerves	Cardiac surgery
	Charcot-Marie-Tooth disease
	Diabetes
	Polyneuropathy
	Toxins
	Guillain-Barré syndrome
	Neuralgia amyotrophy
	Critical illness polyneuropathy
Neuromuscular junction	Myasthenia gravis
	Eaton-Lambert syndrome
	Botulism
	Organophosphate poisoning
	Drugs
Muscle	Dystrophy
	Acid maltase deficiency
	Malnutrition
	Corticosteroids
	Polymyositis

motor activity in subjects with significant respiratory muscle weakness because the thoracic bellows cannot perform increased work of breathing. Decreased ventilatory response to hypoxic or hypercapnic challenge in these patients could indicate abnormalities in afferent information from diseased respiratory muscles, abnormal lung or chest wall mechanics, or upper motoneuron dysfunction, rather than an abnormality in the central control of breathing. In some neuromuscular diseases, degenerative changes in the muscle spindle, impaired afferent stimulation from abnormal stretch reflexes in the muscle spindles, or decreased mechanoreceptor output from tendons may explain the altered breathing pattern.[4]

Measurement of mouth occlusion pressure ($P_{0.1}$), the pressure generated during the first 100 ms of inspiration, is relatively independent of inspiratory effort and therefore is a more reliable estimate of central ventilatory drive independent of respiratory muscle mechanics. $P_{0.1}$ is maintained or increased in patients with neuromuscular disease despite substantial muscle weakness.[5,57] The relationship between respiratory mechanics, respiratory muscle strength, and control of ventilation has been ex-

amined in patients with neuromuscular diseases in comparison with healthy control subjects.[4] Although patients had 37 percent and 52 percent reductions in maximum inspiratory and expiratory mouth pressures, respectively, their $P_{0.1}$ was 66 percent greater than that of controls.

Similar findings were encountered when normal subjects had acute muscle weakness induced by curarization.[37] After severe muscle weakness was induced, significant increases in $P_{0.1}$ were observed during hypercapnic challenge. Partial curarization of spontaneously breathing cats also produced a marked increase in phrenic nerve discharge despite a substantial decrease in minute ventilation. These studies indicate that under conditions of substantial respiratory muscle weakness, ventilation is not a reliable measure of central respiratory drive, and that central respiratory drive, at least when measured by $P_{0.1}$, is usually well preserved.

Respiratory Muscle Function

Patients with neuromuscular disease who develop significant respiratory muscle weakness may demonstrate fatigue, dyspnea, impaired control of secretions, recurrent lower respiratory tract infections, acute or chronic presentations of respiratory failure, pulmonary hypertension, and cor pulmonale.

The pattern, prognosis, and degree of respiratory muscle weakness attributable to a neuromuscular disorder are varied. They depend on the level of neuromuscular system impairment, the prognosis of the underlying disorder, and whether therapy is available. Patients with neuropathy, such as Guillain-Barré syndrome, tend to have less severe respiratory muscle weakness than patients with lower motoneuron lesions or neuromuscular junction disorders, such as myasthenia gravis. Even when respiratory muscle dysfunction is observed, all respiratory muscles are not equally impaired, and the course of the underlying neuromuscular disease and degree of respiratory and nonrespiratory muscle impairment can be very different between patients with the same disease. In some neuromuscular disorders, respiratory muscle weakness is the only presentation of an underlying disease (i.e., neuralgia amyotrophy of the diaphragm); in the case of muscular dystrophy, significant respiratory muscle weakness may occur only late in the disease course. Severe, relentless, progressive dysfunction of the respiratory muscles may occur, as in amyotrophic lateral sclerosis, or be characterized by exacerbations and relapses (e.g., multiple sclerosis). Finally, respiratory muscle weakness may completely reverse with time (phrenic nerve injury after open heart surgery) or with therapy (plasmapheresis in myasthenia gravis).

A significant number of patients with severe respiratory muscle weakness due to chronic neuromuscular disease do not complain of dyspnea or have any respiratory complaints despite profound weakness.[16,63] Examination of pulmonary function in 29 patients with moderate neuromuscular disease who had no respiratory complaints found that eight patients had severe reductions in inspiratory and expiratory mouth pressures (46 percent and 29 percent of predicted, respectively).[16]

Severe inspiratory and expiratory muscle weakness was also found in 50 percent of 30 asymptomatic patients with stable chronic neuromuscular disease.[63] Reductions in inspiratory and expiratory mouth pressures did not correlate with general muscle strength assessment; however, the type of neuromuscular disease and distribution of general muscle weakness both correlated with respiratory muscle impairment. Patients with myopathy, rather than polyneuropathy, whose involvement produced proximal rather than distal limb muscle weakness, were more likely to have significant respiratory muscle weakness. Pulmonary symptoms correlated poorly with evidence of respiratory muscle weakness.

Explanations for the lack of pulmonary complaints in these two studies despite significant muscle weakness are not clear. Patients with chronic and severe neuromuscular disease are usually sedentary and incapable of exertion and, therefore, seldom stress the respiratory system—which may explain their lack of symptoms.

The rapid, shallow breathing pattern found in patients with respiratory muscle weakness may be due to decreased respiratory muscle force generation, but it may also be due to changes in lung and chest wall elastic recoil. A decrease in inspiratory muscle tone may lead to unopposed lung elastic recoil, which reduces lung volume and produces chronic changes in chest wall tone and distensibility. Once inspiratory muscle strength decreases to approximately 30 percent of normal, abnormalities in gas exchange (manifested primarily by hypercapnia) commonly occur.[10]

Expiratory muscle weakness is also commonly observed in patients with neuromuscular disease. It causes ineffectual cough and impaired secretion clearance, which in some patients leads to recurrent lower respiratory tract infections. In normal persons, dynamic compression of the central intrathoracic airways by large changes in pleural pressure generated by forceful contraction of the expiratory muscles acts to propel secretions proximally, where they can be expectorated. As expiratory muscle weakness progresses, pleural pressures generated during coughing efforts are reduced and airway clearance is impaired.[18]

Lung and Chest Wall Mechanics

A characteristic hallmark of chronic neuromuscular disease is a decreased vital capacity (VC). The VC is reduced as a consequence of respiratory muscle weakness, and the decrease in VC parallels the progression of the underlying disease, but the magnitude of the reduction in VC is greater than expected solely on the basis of the reduction in respiratory muscle force. The sigmoidal shape of the pressure-volume curve would suggest that large reductions in pressure initially produce only small reductions in lung volume. In 25 patients with a variety of neuromuscular diseases, De Troyer found that reductions in VC were much greater than expected, solely based on the reductions in inspiratory muscle strength (Fig. 98-1).[17]

Similar results were observed in studies on the effect of curare on maximum static pressure-volume relationships in normal volunteers.[57] It appears that in addition to muscle weakness, alterations in the mechanical properties of the lung and chest wall contribute to the reduced VC. Using the mean deflationary pressure-volume curve of the lung in 25 patients with moderate to severe neuromuscular disease, De Troyer and colleagues found, on average, a 40 percent decrease in lung compliance (Fig. 98-2).[17] Because of the hysteresis of the pressure-volume curve obtained by static expiratory maneuvers, a reduction in static compliance achieved on full inspiration alters the position of

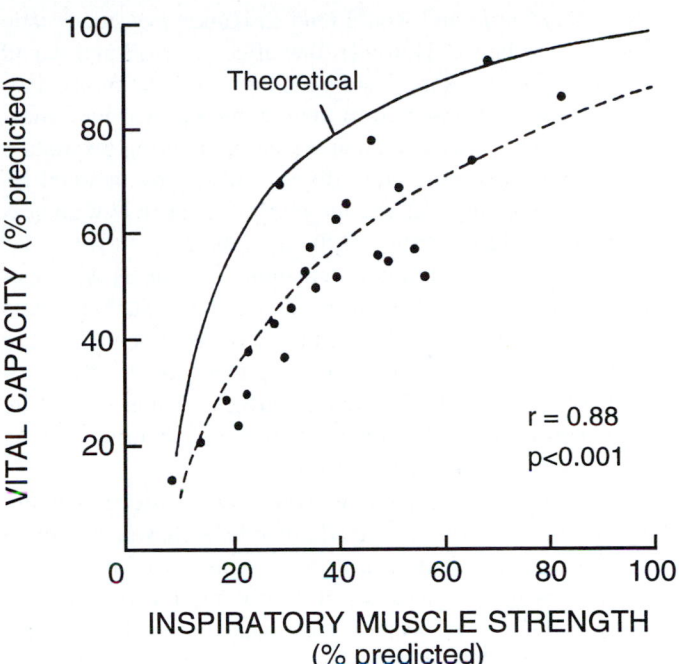

FIGURE 98-1 The solid curve represents the theoretic effect of respiratory muscle weakness on vital capacity (VC) on the assumption that the relaxation pressure-volume characteristic of the lung and chest wall are normal and that the inspiratory and expiratory muscles are uniformly involved. Dashed curve is the logarithmic regression calculated in 25 patients with neuromuscular disease (closed circles). Data suggest that loss of lung volume is out of proportion to the degree of inspiratory muscle weakness. *(Based on data of De Troyer,[17] with permission.)*

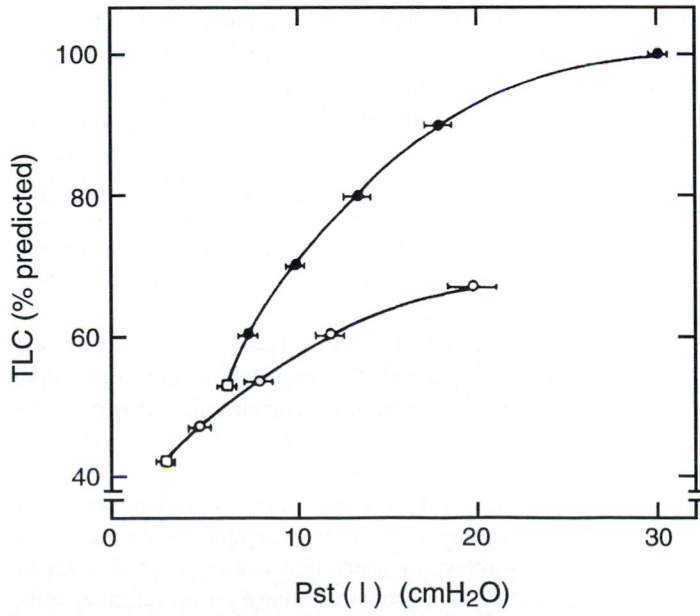

FIGURE 98-2 Static expiratory pressure-volume curve in patients with neuromuscular disease and respiratory muscle weakness. Open circles represent average data in 25 patients. Volume is displayed on the Y axis as a percentage of predicted total lung capacity (TLC). Closed circles represent mean predicted values. In patients, absolute lung volume was decreased for any given transpulmonary pressure. *(Based on data of De Troyer,[17] with permission.)*

the expiratory curve and would tend to reduce measured static expiratory compliance. However, this effect is small and would not account for the significant reductions in expiratory pulmonary compliance observed in their study. Furthermore, measurements of static lung compliance measured during inspiration in patients with neuromuscular diseases also show marked reductions,[32] suggesting that chronic respiratory muscle weakness changes the elastic properties of the lung itself.

The cause of reduced lung distensibility in patients with neuromuscular disease is unknown. Several causes—such as failed maturation of normal lung tissue in the presence of childhood or congenital neuromuscular diseases, the presence of micro- or macroatelectasis, increased alveolar surface tension caused by breathing chronically at low tidal volumes, and alteration in lung tissue elasticity—have been proposed.

Impaired lung maturation is unlikely, since patients who develop neuromuscular disease in adulthood also have a reduction in VC that is disproportionate to the magnitude of respiratory muscle weakness. The presence of micro- and macroatelectasis also appears untenable, because most patients who have significant reductions in VC do not have alveolar collapse on chest radiograph or chest computed tomography. In the minority of patients who have atelectasis on radiographic examination, the areas of atelectasis are usually insufficient to account for the reductions in lung compliance. Studies in rats and in dogs demonstrate that breathing at small tidal volumes is associated with reductions in lung compliance and may promote increased alveolar surface tension. In experimental models of increased alveolar surface tension, a few deep inspirations rapidly restored lung distensibility. Although rapid and shallow breathing patterns are encountered in patients with chronic severe neuromuscular disease, mechanical hyperinflation of the lung does not restore lung distensibility. Therefore, increased alveolar surface tension is not considered the principal cause of reduced lung compliance in patients with chronic neuromuscular disease.

Theoretically, a reduction in lung tissue elasticity may also contribute to a reduction in lung compliance in patients with neuromuscular disease, but there is no evidence that lung collagen, elastin, and other matrix proteins change in these diseases. Currently, the reason for the reduction in lung compliance in patients with chronic neuromuscular disease is unknown and awaits further study.

Many studies indicate that chest wall compliance is decreased by approximately 30 percent in patients with chronic neuromuscular disorder.[26,28] In 16 patients with chronic neuromuscular diseases (e.g., spinal cord injury, Duchenne muscular dystrophy, and myasthenia gravis), the weighted spirometer technique was used to examine chest wall compliance in comparison with that of 20 healthy control subjects.[28] The weighted spirometer technique delivers an airway pressure that causes an increment in thoracic volumes so as to construct the pressure-volume relationship. In 12 of these patients, chest wall compliance was reduced (Fig. 98-3). Based on the contour of the pressure-volume curve of the normal relaxed chest wall at lower lung volumes, a reduction in functional residual capacity (FRC), as seen in patients with chronic neuromuscular diseases, may in itself reduce static chest wall compliance. However, in other disorders in which FRC is decreased owing to parenchymal lung disease (i.e.,

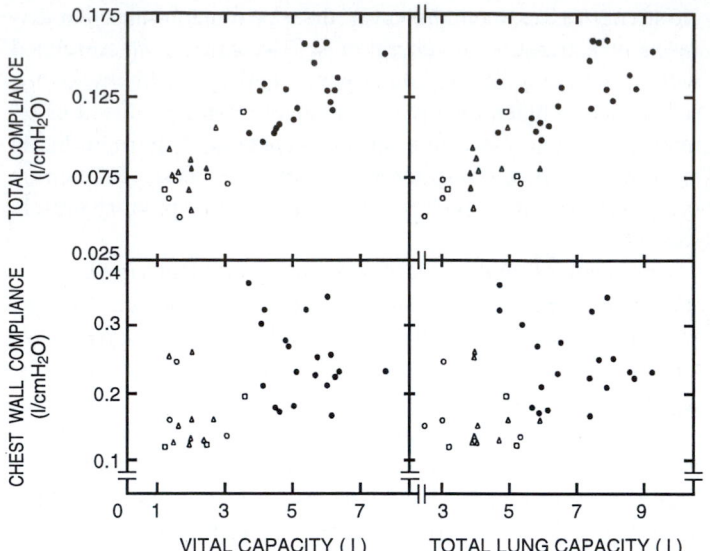

FIGURE 98-3   Relationships between total respiratory system compliance and VC and TLC (upper panels) and between chest wall compliance and VC and TLC (lower panels) in 16 patients with chronic neuromuscular diseases (open symbols) compared to 20 healthy controls (closed circles). Triangles symbolize patients who are quadriplegic, squares symbolize patients who are paraplegic, and 4 patients had generalized neuromuscular diseases (circles). In patients, total respiratory system and chest wall compliance were significantly reduced. *(Based on data of Estenne et al,[28] with permission.)*

pulmonary fibrosis), a reduction in chest wall compliance has not been demonstrated. The mechanism for the reduction in chest wall compliance in patients with chronic neuromuscular disease has not been definitely established, but limitations in respiratory excursions have been proposed to lead to increased rib cage stiffness by decreasing the viscoelasticity of chest wall structures (i.e., tendons, ligaments, and costovertebral and costosternal articulations). Regardless of the mechanism, it appears that a reduction in chest wall compliance, along with a decrease in lung compliance, contributes to the marked decrease in VC observed in patients with neuromuscular disease.

Although reductions in VC appear to be clearly established in patients with chronic neuromuscular disease, data examining the effect of chronic neuromuscular disease on FRC and residual volume (RV) are contradictory. FRC has been reported to be unchanged, decreased,[17] or mildly increased. Similarly variable results have been reported for RV.[20,32] Discrepancies between these studies could be explained by differences in the types, severity, and stages of neuromuscular diseases studied or body positions in which testing was performed. However, in two separate studies, patients with a wide variety of chronic neuromuscular diseases, all studied in a similar seated position, were found to have approximately 20 percent reductions in FRC but normally predicted values of RV.[17,32] Furthermore, confirmation of these findings was demonstrated in eight patients with myasthenia gravis given pyridostigmine, which acutely decreased FRC by approximately 15 percent without any significant change in RV.[19] Further corroboration of the maintenance of RV and reduction in FRC in states of respiratory muscle weakness was again demonstrated when normal subjects partially curarized were found to have a reduction in FRC and no change in RV.[21]

On the basis of the above data, it appears that patients with chronic neuromuscular disease have moderate reductions in VC and total lung capacity (TLC) that are associated with a moderate decrease in FRC and a normal RV (Table 98-2). The decrease in VC not only is due to respiratory muscle weakness but also appears to result from decreased lung and chest wall compliance.

Sleep-Related Breathing Disturbances

Breathing during sleep is often abnormal in patients with neuromuscular disease. Impaired sleep quality and hypopnea and hypercapnia related to rapid eye movement (REM) sleep are frequent.[11,58,59] Patients with chronic neuromuscular disease of various causes have significant and numerous episodes of nocturnal desaturation, which are most prevalent during REM sleep and are characterized by hypoventilation rather than upper-airway obstruction (Fig. 98-4).[11] Of six patients, 16 to 22 years of age, with advanced Duchenne muscular dystrophy, randomized to breathing either air or oxygen on two consecutive nights, five demonstrated significant oxygen desaturation during REM sleep and approximately 35 percent reductions in minute ventilation compared to their baseline awake values.[59] Furthermore, severity of diaphragmatic dysfunction was related to degree of oxygen desaturation.

Several hypotheses have been proposed to explain nocturnal desaturation.[18] Patients with chronic neuromuscular diseases develop an even more rapid and shallow breathing pattern during REM sleep. A rapid and shallow breathing pattern leads to increased dead-space ventilation, which promotes hypercapnia and worsened oxygenation. Reductions in ventilatory drive may be accentuated during sleep in patients with underlying neuromuscular disease—especially in those who have preexisting abnormalities of ventilatory control, which may further contribute to worsened nocturnal hypoventilation.

It has been hypothesized that patients with neuromuscular disease, especially with diaphragmatic dysfunction, may be more prone to nocturnal desaturation during REM sleep. Intercostal muscle and accessory respiratory muscle activity during REM sleep are depressed, with a greater contribution of the diaphragm required for maintenance of eucapnia and oxygenation. Support for this hypothesis comes from studies that have found diaphragm dysfunction to be highly correlated with the presence

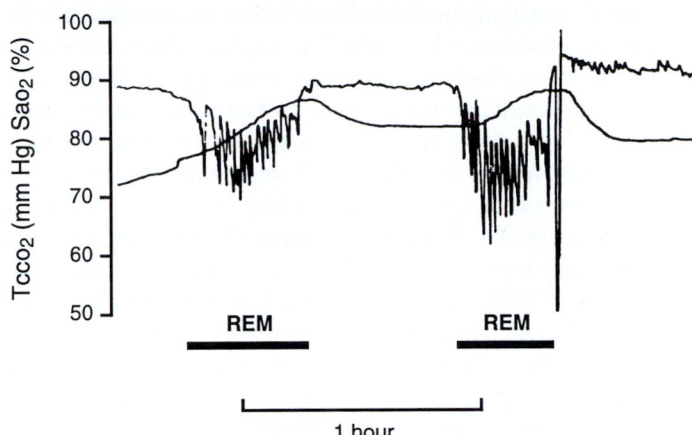

FIGURE 98-4 Oxygen desaturation and hypercapnia in REM sleep shown from a recording of an all-night sleep study. Transcutaneous carbon dioxide ($TcCO_2$) is shown in the smooth solid line; arterial hemoglobin oxygen saturation (SaO_2) is shown in the line with sharp deflections. *(From data of Bye et al,[11] with permission.)*

and magnitude of REM-related oxygen desaturation.[11] A direct relation has been found between the lowest SaO_2 value measured during REM sleep and the percentage fall in VC measured between the erect and supine positions, using the latter measurements as an index of diaphragm weakness.[11] Similarly, among patients who have paradoxical abdominal movement, signifying a decrease in diaphragmatic contribution to ventilation, a greater oxygen desaturation in both REM and non-REM sleep is observed. In contrast, patients with isolated diaphragmatic dysfunction with intact accessory muscle function are not predisposed to severe nocturnal hypoventilation.[40] Accordingly, severe hypoventilation may become evident only when diaphragmatic weakness is found in the background of global accessory and intercostal muscle weakness, or when ventilatory reserve is severely reduced for other reasons, such as asthma or chronic obstructive pulmonary disease (COPD).

Abnormalities in nocturnal gas exchange are harbingers of problems in daytime gas exchange. Hypoventilation during sleep precedes the appearance of daytime hypercapnia,[11] and patients with the most impaired gas exchange during REM sleep have the greatest degree of daytime hypercapnia. Moreover, patients with normal nocturnal gas exchange are unlikely to have abnormal daytime values. Noninvasive (e.g., nasal positive-pressure ventilation, external negative-pressure ventilation) or invasive (e.g., positive-pressure ventilation by tracheostomy) mechanical ventilation improves nocturnal gas exchange and sleep quality, with simultaneous improvement in daytime gas exchange.[31]

Two theories have been proposed to explain the sustained improvements in gas exchange during daytime spontaneous breathing in patients with chronic neuromuscular disease who receive nocturnal ventilatory support.

TABLE 98-2

Characteristic Changes in Respiratory Mechanics in Patients with Neuromuscular Disease

Central drive:	Rapid shallow breathing pattern
	Decreased ventilatory response to hypoxic or hypercapnic challenge
	Normal or increased $P_{0.1}$ to hypoxic or hypercapnic challenge
Lung volumes:	Decreased vital capacity (VC)
	Decreased inspiratory capacity (IC)
	Decreased functional residual capacity (FRC)
	Decreased expiratory reserve volume (ERV)
	Maintained residual volume (RV)

One theory states that nocturnal ventilation rests chronically fatigued respiratory muscles, thereby permitting improved spontaneous ventilation and gas exchange. Although several studies have demonstrated that noninvasive ventilation provides inspiratory muscle rest, data are lacking to demonstrate chronic inspiratory muscle fatigue in patients with neuromuscular disease, or that mechanical ventilation consistently increases respiratory muscle strength. An alternative hypothesis suggests that nocturnal ventilatory support lowers the central respiratory center CO_2 set point and, thereby, sets the central controller to maintain a lower spontaneous daytime CO_2 level. This hypothesis is supported by studies showing that after several weeks of chronic nocturnal ventilation, hypoventilation was less severe in nocturnal studies without ventilation than it had been on baseline nights before chronic intermittent ventilation.[33a] Moreover, interruption of successful nocturnal noninvasive ventilation in patients with neuromuscular disease and chronic respiratory failure results in a return of nocturnal hypoventilation and symptoms of impaired gas exchange without evidence of respiratory muscle dysfunction.[36] To date, neither of the above theories has been established conclusively, and further investigation is warranted, as one or the other, or both, may be valid in different patients.

ASSESSMENT OF RESPIRATORY FUNCTION

Patients with significant respiratory muscle impairment may range from being totally asymptomatic to having moderate dyspnea at rest or, in some cases, overt respiratory failure. Some patients with neuromuscular disease may have significant weakness of the respiratory muscles and be asymptomatic, whereas others may present with ventilatory failure without an established history of a neuromuscular disease.[18,25,63] In the latter patients, the diagnosis of neuromuscular disease may initially be entertained only after difficulty is encountered in weaning the patient from mechanical ventilation. A detailed history and physical examination, coupled with appropriate diagnostic tests, enable the physician to diagnose the presence and type of neuromuscular disease and its effect on the respiratory system. The following section reviews features of the history and physical exam and the diagnostic studies considered useful in the assessment of respiratory function in patients with neuromuscular disease.

Clinical History

The signs and symptoms of respiratory muscle weakness due to a neuromuscular disease are usually nonspecific and of limited value. Moreover, the clinical manifestations of respiratory muscle dysfunction depend on the specific muscle or muscles affected and the extent of their impairment. In conditions of mild weakness, or in the early stages of neuromuscular disease, the patient may be totally asymptomatic. As respiratory muscle weakness progresses, however, dyspnea on exertion, followed by dyspnea at rest, occurs. Disturbed sleep and daytime hypersomnolence resulting from nocturnal hypoventilation may occur, and if the expiratory muscles are affected, patients may have impaired cough and repeated lower respiratory tract infections. As respiratory muscle weakness becomes more severe, hypercarbia or hypoxemia becomes evident and respiratory failure may ensue, requiring ventilatory support.

The clinical history is invaluable in that it may be the first clue that a neuromuscular disease is the cause of the patient's pulmonary dysfunction. A history is also useful in characterizing the type of neuromuscular disease that is present. Dyspnea, alveolar hypoventilation, and impaired cough with or without recurrent lower respiratory tract infections may be the first clinical clues that a neuromuscular disease is present. Impaired swallowing due to bulbar symptoms and the presence of peripheral limb muscle weakness are indications that one is dealing with a disseminated neuromuscular disease, prompting the appropriate diagnostic workup.

To provide an organized approach to direct the clinical history taking and physical examination of patients with neuromuscular disease, Table 98-1 characterizes the types of neuromuscular disease that present at different levels of the neuromuscular system. Table 98-3 describes the innervation of different groups of respiratory muscles.

Physical Examination

Although the physical exam may yield normal results in patients with early or mild impairment of the respiratory system, patients with more established disease often demonstrate tachypnea at rest. Further clinical information on the nature of the underlying disease and the extent of underlying muscle impairment can be gleaned from the pattern of respiratory muscle contraction in both seated and supine positions. Respiratory rate should be recorded, along with any evidence of nasal flaring, intercostal muscle retraction, or palpable evidence of contraction of the sternocleido-

TABLE 98-3

Innervation of the Respiratory Muscles

Muscle Group	Innervation Level	Nerve
Upper airway		
Palate, Pharynx	IX, X, XI	Glossopharyngeal, vagus, spinal accessory
Genioglossus	XII	Hypoglossal
Inspiratory		
Diaphragm	C3-5	Phrenic
Scalenes	C4-8	
Parasternal intercostals	T1-7	Intercostal
Sternocleidomastoid	XI, C1, C2	Spinal accessory
Lateral external intercostals	T1-12	Intercostal
Expiratory		
Abdominal	T7-L1	Lumbar
Internal intercostals	T1-12	Intercostal

SOURCE: Modified from Rochester and Esau.[56]

mastoid and scalene muscles. Furthermore, inward paradoxical motion of the rib cage or abdomen should be sought, as its presence may indicate a respiratory workload that is greater than the patient's respiratory muscle strength, or evidence of severe weakness of the diaphragm as a result of the underlying neuromuscular disease. Besides gross paradoxical movement of the rib cage or abdominal compartments, asynchronous compartmental movements (e.g., one compartment moving faster than the other) may be early evidence of impaired respiratory pump performance.

The hallmark finding of severe diaphragm weakness or paralysis is paradoxical inward movement of the abdomen with inspiration. In the presence of severe diaphragm weakness, the upper abdomen moves inward when the upper rib cage moves outward—in stark contrast to the normal pattern of synchronized outward movements of the rib cage and abdominal compartments. Besides paradoxical movement of the upper abdomen, a marked increase in respiratory rate, accompanied by progressive accessory muscle use, and increased dyspnea occur when patients assume the recumbent position due to hypoxemia, hypercapnia, and placing the accessory inspiratory muscles at mechanical disadvantage. Upon reassuming the upright posture, patients may have palpable phasic contractions of the abdominal expiratory muscles. Physiologically, this inward movement of the abdomen on expiration enables passive outward movement of the upper abdomen and diaphragm descent during expiratory muscle relaxation in early inspiration.

Besides a detailed examination of the respiratory musculature and breathing pattern, the physical exam should include a complete neuromuscular examination to exclude systemic involvement. Inspection for atrophy or fasciculations of respiratory and nonrespiratory muscles may point to a lower motoneuron disease. The presence of scoliosis may contribute to the development of a restrictive ventilatory pattern.

Radiographic Assessment

In patients with severe inspiratory muscle weakness or bilateral diaphragm paralysis, maximum inspiration is limited and lung volume appears reduced on chest radiograph. Unilateral hemidiaphragm paralysis produces an elevated hemidiaphragm on the affected side.

Fluoroscopy is often used in the assessment of diaphragm paralysis, with the patient making a forceful sniff in the supine position. In unilateral diaphragm paralysis, a positive "sniff" test may demonstrate paradoxical upward movement of the affected hemidiaphragm.[45] However, "sniff" tests have a false-positive rate as high as 6 percent in normal persons.[1] The use of the "sniff" test to diagnose bilateral diaphragm paralysis is limited by compensatory abdominal muscle contraction. With abrupt cessation of abdominal muscle contraction during early inspiration, the abdominal contents descend caudally. The abdominal wall moves outward, and the diaphragm will then appear to descend caudally, at least radiographically. Besides the fact that passive diaphragm descent due to active abdominal muscle contraction is a limitation during fluoroscopy, the fluoroscopic observational field used to examine the diaphragm is limited because of the small visual band that encompasses only the diaphragmatic dome

and adjacent ribs. If rib cage rostral movement exceeds diaphragm ascent, the diaphragm will appear to descend lower than the thorax; that may falsely suggest the presence of diaphragm shortening.[45]

Arterial Blood Gas Analysis

Arterial blood gas abnormalities usually occur only in patients with severe respiratory muscle weakness. Hypoxemia is usually mild and may occur as a result of microatelectasis and subsequent intrapulmonary shunting or ventilation-perfusion mismatch. In addition, patients with impaired muscle strength have impaired cough and may retain secretions that further contribute to the development of hypoxemia. Measurement of arterial oxyhemoglobin saturation by pulse oximetry, which has become an extremely common laboratory test for oxygenation, is an insensitive indicator of hypoventilation. In patients with mild to moderate respiratory muscle weakness, the value of solely measuring the level of oxygenation is limited and may be misleading.

Hypercarbia is an insensitive measure of respiratory muscle strength. The Pa_{CO_2} does not increase until respiratory muscle strength (measured by maximum inspiratory and expiratory mouth pressures) is less than 50 percent of predicted. In patients with severe respiratory muscle weakness, however, an elevation in Pa_{CO_2} may be evident. Examination of the bicarbonate and pH values may help determine whether an acute or chronic respiratory acidosis is present. Because daytime hypercarbia is usually followed by nocturnal hypoventilation, the presence of daytime hypercarbia should prompt investigation of the breathing pattern and gas exchange during sleep, so that appropriate therapy (e.g., nocturnal supplemental oxygen or noninvasive ventilation) can be implemented.

Respiratory Muscle Strength

MAXIMUM MOUTH PRESSURES

Maximum static inspiratory and expiratory mouth pressures, measured at the airway opening during a voluntary contraction against an occluded airway, are the simplest and most commonly performed tests of respiratory muscle strength. Although several methods exist, the technique of Black and Hyatt[7] is still the most widely used. In this technique, mouth pressures are measured by a handheld manometer with the patient seated upright with a nose clip on. During these maneuvers, the patient purses the lips inside a circular wide-bore rubber mouthpiece, which prevents perioral air leakage. This small orifice (2 mm in diameter, 15 mm in length) is placed in the circuit to minimize the contribution of the facial muscles to airway pressure and to keep the glottis open. Maximum inspiratory pressures ($P_{I_{max}}$) are measured near residual volume after maximal expiration, while maximal expiratory pressures ($P_{E_{max}}$) are measured at or near total lung capacity. In each case, efforts are maintained for at least 1 s. Maximum inspiratory and expiratory mouth pressures in normal males and females are listed in Table 98-4. Reported values in normal subjects vary widely and may be due to differences in techniques between different studies or a learning effect in subjects who perform these maneuvers.[7,13,44,45,54,55,65]

TABLE 98-4

Reported Values for Maximum Static Airway Pressures in Normal Adults

Study	Sex	# of Subjects	Age Range (Years)	PI_{max} (cmH$_2$O)	PE_{max} (cmH$_2$O)
Black & Hyatt, 1969[7]	Males	60	20–54	124±22	233±42
	Females	60	20–54	87±16	152±27
Rinqvist, 1966[54]	Males	100	18–83	130±32	237±46
	Females	100	18–83	98±25	165±30
Leech et al, 1983[44]	Males	325	17–35	114±36	154±82
	Females	480	15–35	71±27	94±33
Rochester & Arora, 1983[55]	Males	80	19–49	127±28	216±41
	Females	121	19–49	91±25	138±39
Vincken et al, 1987[62]	Males	46	16–79	105±25	140±38
	Females	60	16–79	71±23	89±24
Cook et al, 1964[13]	Males	17	18–47	133±39	237±45
	Females	9	18–32	100±19	146±34
Wilson et al, 1984[65]	Males	48	19–65	106±31	148±34
	Females	87	18–65	73±22	93±17

Values are mean ± standard deviation.

A major factor affecting PI_{max} is lung volume. PI_{max} is greatest at residual volume, whereby the inspiratory muscles are at greatest mechanical advantage and the outward elastic recoil of the respiratory system is maximum. On the other hand, measurement of PE_{max} is greatest at total lung capacity because expiratory muscles are at greatest mechanical advantage and inward elastic recoil of the respiratory system is greatest (Fig. 98-5). Only at functional residual capacity, where the respiratory system recoil pressures measured at the airway opening are zero, are maximum inspiratory and expiratory mouth pressures solely a function of the pressure generated by actively contracting respiratory muscles (Pmus).

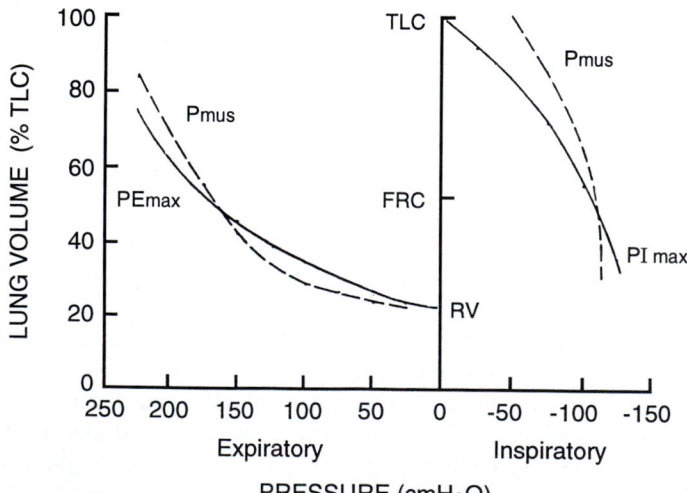

FIGURE 98-5 The effect of lung volume on maximum respiratory pressures (PI_{max} and PE_{max}) measured at the airway opening displayed by solid lines. Both PI_{max} and PE_{max} are made up of two components: the pressure generated by the respiratory muscles (Pmus, dashed lines) and the recoil pressure of the respiratory system. At FRC, both PE_{max} and PI_{max} are equal to Pmus.

Changes in lung volume due to chest wall or lung pathology may have important effects on the generation of maximum respiratory pressures in patients. For example, patients with COPD and significant hyperinflation have a larger FRC and residual volume than normal subjects; therefore, PI_{max} performed at FRC or RV usually results in lower values than in age- and sex-matched normal subjects. Likewise, a reduction in total lung capacity due to restrictive ventilatory diseases may result in a reduction in measured values for PE_{max}. Therefore, it is important to realize that in patients with pathologically altered lung volumes, all or part of the reduction in mouth pressures may be due to inspiratory muscle mechanical disadvantage.

Maximum inspiratory and expiratory mouth pressures in patients with neuromuscular diseases range from normal to severely reduced.[8,16,25,63] Patients may have significant respiratory muscle weakness without any pulmonary complaints, and no correlation exists between respiratory muscle strength and the presence of generalized nonrespiratory muscle weakness.[63] When PI_{max} falls below 30 cmH$_2$O, ventilatory failure commonly ensues.

TRANSDIAPHRAGMATIC PRESSURE MEASUREMENT

While maximum static airway pressures are useful measures of global respiratory muscle strength, they fail to assess individual respiratory muscle function. Since the diaphragm is the primary muscle of inspiration, and may be susceptible to isolated disease (e.g., phrenic nerve paralysis after open heart surgery or idiopathic diaphragm paralysis), specific testing of diaphragm strength is desirable in some patients. Assessment of diaphragm strength is made by measuring gastric (Pga) and endoesophageal (Pes) pressures with balloon-tipped catheters placed in the stomach and midesophagus, respectively. Transdiaphragmatic pressure (Pdi) is then calculated as the algebraic subtraction of Pes from Pga (Pdi=Pga–[Pes]).

Maneuvers to elicit maximum transdiaphragmatic pressures (Pdi$_{max}$) have been the subject of intensive study. Earlier studies measured Pdi during maximum static inspiratory efforts against a closed airway (e.g., Müller's maneuver) at FRC or RV. However, this maneuver results in submaximal diaphragm activation, with the degree of activation varying widely from subject to subject. Several studies have demonstrated significant intraindividual variability, with a coefficient of variation as high as 40 percent in measurement of Pdi_{max} during Müller's maneuver. When five maneuvers to measure Pdi_{max} in 35 subjects (10 normal, 13 with restrictive lung disease, and 12 with COPD) were compared,[39] a combined maneuver of active expulsion with superimposed Müller's maneuver yielded the most reproducible and maximal transdiaphragmatic pressure. The mechanism for the highest and most reproducible pressures found during combined expulsive-Müller's maneuver were not conclusively shown, but changes in diaphragm shape during the expulsive phase of the maneuver favorably affect force generation.

PHRENIC NERVE STIMULATION

A crucial factor in the measurement of diaphragm strength is the ability to consistently obtain maximal activation of the diaphragm during volitional efforts. Electrophrenic stimulation is a method that has been recently utilized to consistently activate the diaphragm. Although phrenic nerve stimulation as a means of providing artificial respiration in patients has been known since the 1950s, its application in assessing diaphragm contractile function was not studied until the past decade. Besides assessing diaphragm strength, this technique has the added advantage of assessing phrenic nerve conduction and excluding the possibility of phrenic nerve injury in patients with diaphragm weakness of unknown origin.

The phrenic nerve is stimulated in the neck near the posterior border of the sternocleidomastoid muscle, at the level of the cricoid cartilage, where the phrenic nerves are most superficial. Stimulation may be performed either transcutaneously with surface electrodes or percutaneously with needle or wire electrodes. Stimulation of the phrenic nerves must be supramaximal with regard to voltage and current. Supramaximal conditions are ensured by increasing the stimulus intensity until maximum diaphragm muscle action potential (DMAP) or Pdi is achieved. The DMAP is then checked periodically throughout the study to ensure that consistent stimulation is maintained.

The most commonly used technique of electrophrenic stimulation now employs a frequency of one pulse per s to measure Pdi during a single unfused twitch contraction (e.g., Pdi_{TWITCH}). Pdi_{TWITCH} has also been used to assess maximal static Pdi indirectly by the twitch occlusion technique. In this method, single twitches are superimposed on progressively stronger voluntary Pdi contractions. As voluntary effort and Pdi increase, the increment in Pdi produced during the twitch (the twitch deflection superimposed on the Pdi) decreases (Fig. 98-6A). When there is no discernible Pdi_{TWITCH} deflection, it is assumed that the diaphragm is maximally activated and voluntary Pdi represents Pdi_{max}. Several investigators have proposed a method for estimating Pdi_{max} during submaximal voluntary efforts from the inverse linear relationship between the amplitude of the superimposed twitch and Pdi measured during volitional effort.[6] The extrapolation of the line of this relation-

ship to the X axis has been interpreted as representing maximum static Pdi (Fig. 98-6B).

Few studies have directly assessed Pdi_{TWITCH} in patients with suspected diaphragm weakness. Bilateral Pdi_{TWITCH} was measured in the supine position in 20 normal subjects and 10 patients with diaphragm weakness due to a variety of causes.[50] In addition, maximum Pdi during a forceful sniff (Pdi_{SNIFF}) was measured in the seated position. Pdi_{SNIFF} was used as an index of Pdi_{max} because of its relative ease of performance and reproducibility, even though higher values for transdiaphragmatic pressure are usually obtained with other maneuvers.[39] Pdi_{TWITCH} ranged from 9 to 33 cmH_2O in the controls and from 3 to 27 cmH_2O in the 10 patients. Six of the patients

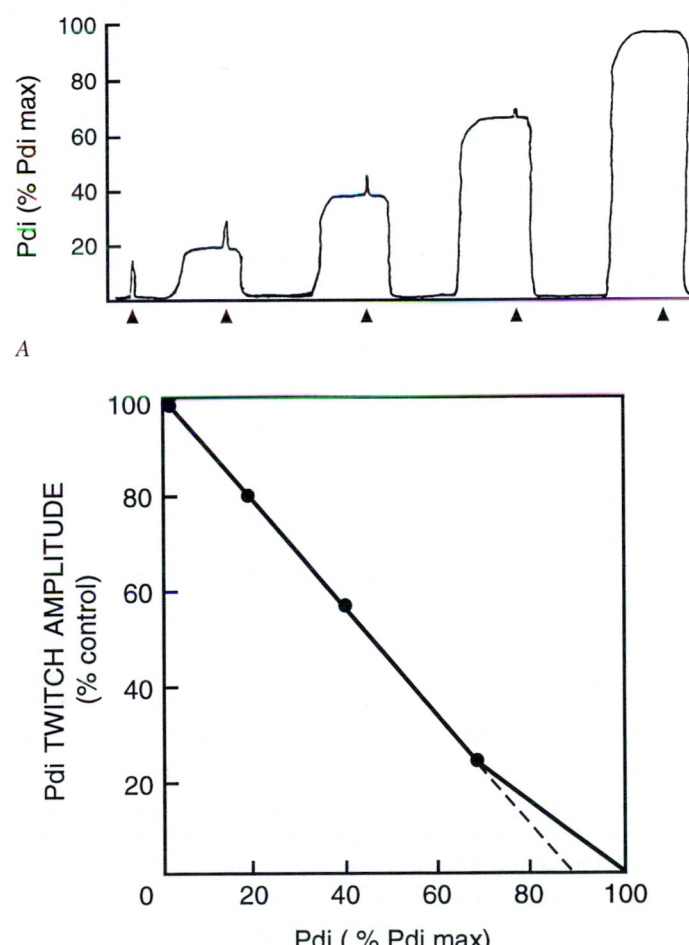

FIGURE 98-6   *A.* Illustration of a typical Pdi tracing during twitch occlusion study. As Pdi increases during volitional efforts, the superimposed Pdi deflection during a phrenic nerve 1-Hz stimulation (twitch) decreases. At 100 percent of Pdi_{max}, the diaphragm is maximally activated and no superimposed twitch is seen. Arrows on the horizontal axis mark indicate the phrenic nerve twitches. *B.* Data from *A* plotted as Pdi_{TWITCH} amplitude versus voluntary Pdi. Using linear regression, Pdi_{max} can be extrapolated from results obtained during submaximal efforts. It has been suggested that extrapolation performed from Pdi values below 70 percent of maximum may underestimate Pdi_{max} by approximately 10 percent (dashed line).

had Pdi$_{TWITCH}$ values within the range of those of the control group. All control subjects had a normal maximum Pdi$_{SNIFF}$ value, whereas all neuromuscular patients demonstrated a reduced Pdi$_{SNIFF}$. Although the patients tended to demonstrate a lower Pdi$_{TWITCH}$ than the controls (14 versus 21 cmH$_2$O), there was no significant difference in Pdi$_{TWITCH}$ between the two groups. The authors concluded that the Pdi$_{TWITCH}$ is a relatively insensitive test for diagnosing diaphragm weakness given the wide overlap in Pdi$_{TWITCH}$ values between the patient and control groups. Moreover, the Pdi$_{TWITCH}$ values were found to be clearly out of the normal range only when weakness was very severe.

Because of the relative invasiveness of electrophrenic stimulation of the diaphragm, and the large coefficient of variation in some studies when Pdi was measured during maximal volitional efforts, some investigators prefer measuring maximum inspiratory pressures during a sniff maneuver.[43] In this technique, the subject performs a vigorous sniff against an unoccluded airway. During such an effort, the nose acts as a Starling resistor, thereby generating intrathoracic pressures against an occluded airway. Some investigators argue that this maneuver approaches a more natural respiratory effort than other types of maneuvers used to measure maximum inspiratory pressures and thus should be easily mastered by patients and more reproducibly performed by technicians.

Measurement of positive pleural pressures during a forceful cough (Pes$_{COUGH}$) has also been proposed as a measure of expiratory muscle strength. Pes$_{COUGH}$ has been shown to decrease in parallel with PE$_{max}$ when expiratory muscle weakness is induced by progressive curarization. This technique has also been used in the evaluation of cough strength after thoracotomy.

ANALYSIS OF RIB CAGE AND ABDOMINAL MOTION

During normal tidal breathing, the chest and abdominal compartments move synchronously in an outward direction, owing to diaphragm contraction decreasing pleural pressure and increasing abdominal pressure. In situations where the diaphragm is severely paretic or paralyzed, however, the flaccid diaphragm cannot counterbalance the negative changes in pleural pressure generated by contraction of the inspiratory muscles of the neck and rib cage. Instead of moving normally in a caudad direction, the flaccid diaphragm moves paradoxically cephalad into the thorax. This change in diaphragm motion gives rise to a paradoxical inward motion of the upper abdomen indicative of severe diaphragm weakness or paralysis.

Changes in rib cage and abdominal pressure, or volume displacement during respiration, can provide important information about diaphragm strength. Partitioning of respiration can be examined from changes in abdominal and pleural pressures, as proposed by Macklem and colleagues.[47] Changes in abdominal and pleural pressures during inspiration, expressed as the ratio of delta Pab:delta P$_{PL}$, are normally negative as pleural pressure becomes more negative and abdominal pressure becomes more positive. This ratio has a maximum value of +1 when the diaphragm does not contribute to inspiration and is valid only if the expiratory muscles do not contribute significantly to the pressures being generated. Alternatively, the partitioning of ventilation can be noninvasively measured by compartmental changes in rib cage and abdominal volume by respiratory inductance plethysmography or magnetometry.

Spirometry

Respiratory muscle weakness induced by neuromuscular disease produces a restrictive pattern on spirometric testing with a reduction in VC. As previously mentioned, the reduced VC is commonly out of proportion to the reduction in maximal respiratory muscle force. Reductions in lung and chest wall compliance also probably contribute. Moreover, because of the contour of the pressure-volume curve, large reductions in respiratory muscle forces have to occur before VC is significantly reduced. A decrease in VC greater than 25 percent on moving from the upright to supine postures has been used as a sign of diaphragmatic weakness and a greater likelihood of sleep-related hypoventilation.[2,15]

Forced expiratory volume in 1 s (FEV$_1$) and measurements of midexpiratory flow rates (FEF$_{25-75}$ or FEF$_{50}$) are often greater than normal predicted values in patients with neuromuscular disease.[56] The supranormal increases in midexpiratory flow rates appear to be due to the fact that maximum expiratory flow can be achieved over most of the vital capacity with low driving pressures. Further increases in expiratory flow may occur in patients with neuromuscular diseases due to increased lung recoil. Two independent studies.[19,21] have shown that partial curarization in normal subjects produces a decrease in peak expiratory flow with an increase in midexpiratory flow rates compared to baseline. Moreover, in patients with myasthenia gravis in their baseline state of weakness before the administration of pyridostigmine, midexpiratory flow rates are increased over the range of vital capacity when referenced to absolute lung volume (Fig. 98-7).

Flow-Volume Loops

Changes in the configuration of the flow-volume loop occur in various neuromuscular diseases. These changes reflect respiratory muscle weakness or malfunction of upper-airway muscles.

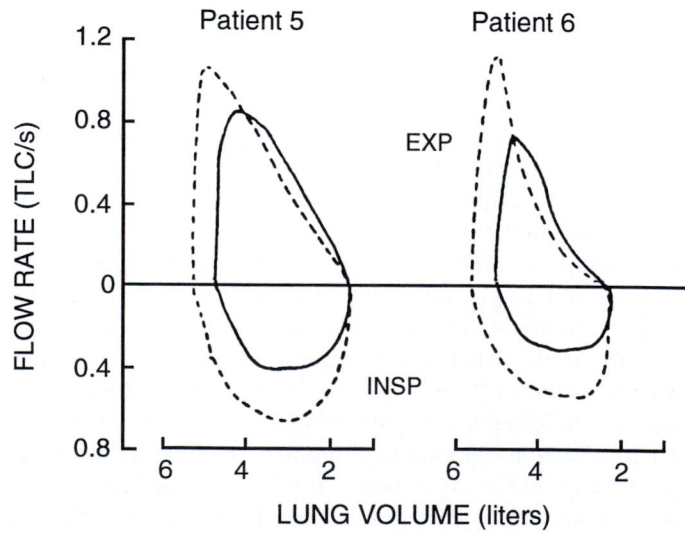

FIGURE 98-7 Two representative patients with myasthenia gravis and respiratory muscle weakness illustrating the effect of anticholinesterase therapy on maximum expiratory and inspiratory flow-volume curves. Solid curves represent pretreatment data; dashed curves were obtained following the injection of pyridostigmine. (*From DeTroyer and Borenstein,[19] with permission.*)

"Sawtoothing" of the flow contour is seen in extrapyramidal disorders affecting upper-airway muscles. Similarly, plateauing of the inspiratory flow wave form indicative of extrathoracic airway obstruction has been described in vocal cord paralysis caused by extrapyramidal neuromuscular disorders. An abnormal flow-volume curve is significantly more common in patients with clinically apparent bulbar muscle involvement (90 percent versus 15 percent, respectively), and the presence of an abnormal flow-volume loop predicted bulbar and upper muscle involvement by a neuromuscular disease with a high sensitivity and specificity.[64] A characteristic flow-volume contour showing involvement of the upper-airway muscles by motor neuron disease is shown in Fig. 98-8.

Among patients with stable, chronic neuromuscular disease, the flow-volume loop is significantly more disturbed in those with respiratory muscle weakness, and these abnormalities correlate with reduced mouth pressures.[64] Several features of flow-volume loop configuration correlate with reduced maximum static inspiratory and expiratory mouth pressures: a reduced peak expiratory flow, decreased slope of the ascending limb of the maximum expiratory curve, a dropoff of forced expiratory flow near residual volume, and a reduction in forced inspiratory flow at 50 percent of vital capacity (Fig. 98-9). A flow-volume loop score composed of the above parameters has a high degree of specificity and 90 percent sensitivity in predicting respiratory muscle weakness.[64]

Lung Volumes

A restrictive ventilatory pattern is demonstrated in patients with neuromuscular disease. A reduced TLC[25,56] and a normal or re-

duced FRC are common.[17] The RV is usually elevated and is a sign of expiratory muscle weakness.

Maximum Voluntary Ventilation

Maximum voluntary ventilation (MVV) is an index of respiratory muscle endurance in the presence of normal expiratory flow rates. This appears to be appropriate in patients with neuromuscular disease, since airway resistance and FRC are usually within the normal range. Values for MVV correlate with respiratory muscle strength and may be even more sensitive than VC in detecting respiratory muscle weakness.

SELECTED NEUROMUSCULAR DISEASES

A helpful approach toward understanding how specific neuromuscular diseases affect the respiratory system is to localize the

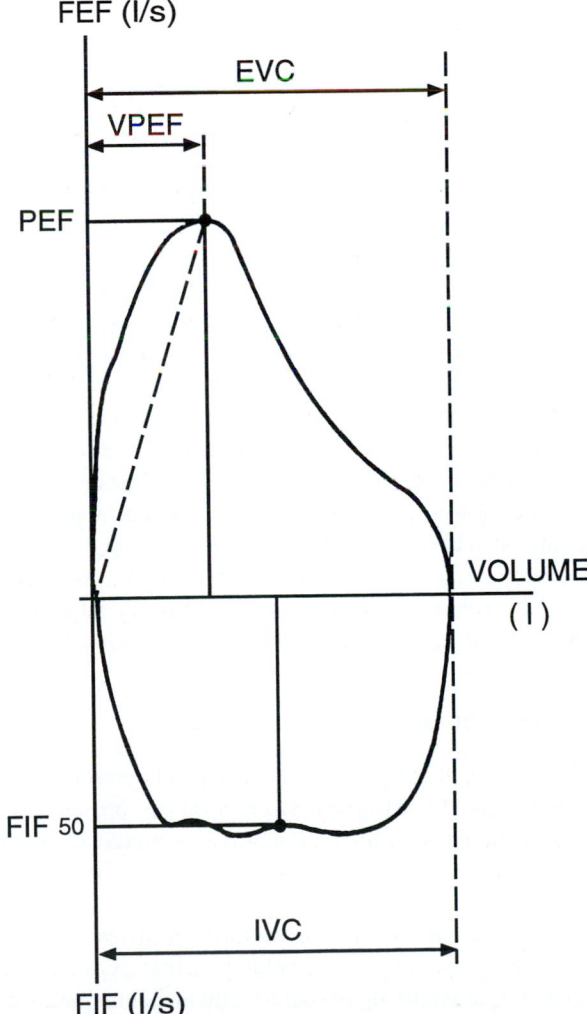

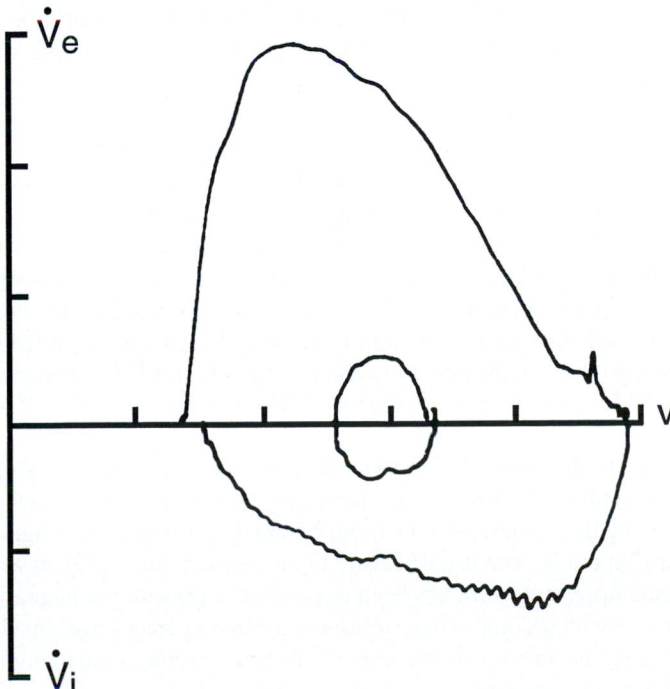

FIGURE 98-8 Flow-volume loop in a patient with motor neuron disease, showing inspiratory flow oscillation and inspiratory flow limitation. Subdivisions on volume and flow axis represents 1 L, flow axis 1 L per s. *(Based on data of Vincken et al,[62] with permission.)*

FIGURE 98-9 Representative flow-volume loop of a patient with chronic neuromuscular disease, showing different-volume loop parameters indicative of respiratory muscle weakness. These parameters quantify the effects of respiratory muscle strength on the effort-dependent portions of the flow-volume loop. These four parameters are peak expiratory flow (PEF); ratio of PEF to the exhaled volume at which PEF was achieved, rapid vertical drop of forced expiratory flow at residual volume, and forced midinspiratory flow. *(Based on data of Vincken et al,[64] with permission.)*

anatomic involvement of the respiratory system. A detailed description of the neuroanatomy of respiration is outside the scope of this chapter (see Chapter 11). In general, however, neuromuscular disorders can be broken down into disorders that involve the upper motoneuron, the lower motoneuron, or the muscle itself.

Lesions that arise in the cerebral cortex, brain stem, or spinal cord are classified as upper motoneuron lesions and are characterized by an increase in muscle tone or spasticity, the presence of an extensor plantar response, and increased reflex activity. Lesions in the lower motoneuron system demonstrate flaccidity, depressed reflexes, muscular fasciculations, and atrophy. The location and character of the patient's weakness may enable one to identify the exact site of the lesion in the lower motoneuron system (i.e., the anterior horn cell, the peripheral nerve, the neuromuscular junction, or the muscle itself).

The following describes the effect of specific neuromuscular diseases on the respiratory system and makes recommendations for treatment.

Upper Motoneuron Lesions

STROKE

Hemispheric ischemic strokes reduce chest wall and diaphragm movement on the side contralateral to the cerebral insult. Decreased diaphragm excursion with stroke correlates with diaphragmatic cortical representation identified by transcranial magnetic stimulation. Bilateral hemispheric strokes are also associated with Cheyne-Stokes respiration, which is progressive hyperventilation alternating with hypoventilation and ending in apnea (see Chapter 11). This breathing pattern may result from increased responsiveness to carbon dioxide as a result of interruption of normal cortical inhibition. The significance of Cheyne-Stokes respiration to stroke remains unclear but appears to be more common with bilateral than unilateral insults. Besides its effects on an alteration of breathing pattern, up to 50 percent of patients with strokes may have signs of pulmonary aspiration due to dysfunction of upper-airway muscles that protect the airway.

SPINAL CORD INJURY

The degree of respiratory impairment depends on the level and extent of the spinal cord injury. High cervical cord lesions (C1 to C3) cause paralysis of the diaphragmatic, intercostal, scalene, and abdominal muscles. Because all respiratory muscle activity is lost except for accessory and bulbar muscle function, high cervical cord injuries almost always require ventilatory assistance. In some patients, spontaneous breathing can be accomplished by glossopharyngeal breathing or diaphragmatic pacing because the phrenic nerve motoneurons (C3 to C5) remain intact.

Middle cervical cord (C3 to C5) lesions destroy the phrenic motoneurons and prohibit the use of phrenic nerve pacing. Patients with more caudal lesions (i.e., C4 to C5 level) have an improved chance to wean from ventilator support compared to those with more cranial lesions. (Forty percent of patients with C3 lesions remain ventilator dependent.) Patients with lower cervical (C6 to C8) and upper thoracic (T1 to T6) cord lesions have in-

tact diaphragm and neck accessory muscle action, but have denervated intercostal and abdominal muscles. These patients usually require ventilatory support only during the period immediately after the injury and rarely require long-term ventilation.

In a study of C5 or lower spinal cord–injured patients, inspiratory muscle strength was reduced to approximately 60 percent of predicted but was dependent on the level of cord injury.[3] In this study, PI_{max} values in low cervical, midthoracic, and lower thoracic–upper lumbar lesions were 61 percent, 69 percent, and 75 percent of predicted, respectively, whereas PE_{max} values were 30 percent, 32 percent, and 54 percent of predicted, respectively. The lower PE_{max} values were explained by a paralysis of abdominal and intercostal muscles, resulting in reduced cough and decreased clearance of bronchial secretions. Abdominal muscle paralysis probably accounts for an abnormally compliant abdomen in patients with lower spinal cord injury, which is in stark contrast to the 30 percent reduction in chest wall compliance believed due to abnormal rib cage stiffness.[26]

Patients with spinal cord injuries also have alterations in thoracoabdominal motion during tidal breathing that is further accentuated by changing from the erect to supine position. In quadriplegic patients with relatively intact diaphragm function, the distribution of respiratory muscle weakness results in paradoxical inward motion of the upper rib cage during inspiration, owing to weakness of the parasternal and scalene muscles. This pattern of abnormal thoracoabdominal movement is more marked in the supine than in the upright position. Patients with high quadriplegia (above C3 to C5) may be able to sustain short periods of spontaneous respiration because of inspiratory activity of the sternocleidomastoid and trapezius muscles. Phasic inspiratory electromyographic (EMG) activity has been observed in the platysma, mylohyoid, and sternohyoid muscles. Analysis of rib cage motion in these patients shows increased upper rib cage diameter, due to the inspiratory action of the neck accessory muscles pulling the sternum cranially and expanding the upper rib cage.

The distribution of muscle paralysis in low cervical cord spinal patients also has a profound effect on the performance of forced expiratory maneuvers. In contrast to healthy normal subjects, in whom VC is moderately decreased on assuming the supine position, in quadriplegic patients there is a paradoxical increase in FVC in the supine compared to seated position without a significant increase in TLC. In 14 quadriplegic patients (C4 to C7), there was a 16 percent increase in VC on changing from the upright to supine position and a reduction in RV (29 percent) and TLC (on average, 6 percent).[27] The mechanism believed to be responsible for the increase in VC in supine quadriplegic patients is the hydrostatic effect of abdominal contents, causing cephalad displacement and diaphragm lengthening and thereby placing the diaphragm on a more favorable portion of its length-tension curve. The use of elastic binders when quadriplegics assume upright posture has been advocated to prevent the increase in abdominal compliance. Abdominal binding may have physiological benefit by maintaining diaphragm precontraction length in a more optimum position on its length-tension curve.[49]

It was previously believed that all expiratory muscles were paralyzed in lower cervical cord injuries. However, studies[22] of C5 to C8 quadriplegics indicate that phasic EMG activity of the clavicular portion of the pectoralis major is associated with a marked decrease in the anteroposterior diameter of the upper rib cage. This portion of the pectoralis muscle receives innervation from fibers originating from the C5 to C6 cord level. With the arms placed at the subject's side, contraction of the caudate head of the pectoralis major causes caudal displacement of the manubrium sterni and upper rib cage. This expiratory action has been shown to decrease expiratory reserve volume (ERV) by 60 percent when the shoulders are held in abduction. After 6 weeks of pectoralis muscle isometric training, patients with low quadriplegia can have a marked increase in maximum pectoralis muscle isometric strength and a significant reduction in ERV.[28] Conceivably, therefore, training of this muscle could improve the effectiveness of cough in patients with low spinal cord injury.

In the months following spinal cord injury, pulmonary function typically improves. In patients with spinal injuries below the C5 level, VC is approximately 30 percent of predicted in the first week after injury, but increases to 45 percent of predicted by the fifth week and by the fifth month to approximately 60 percent of predicted.[43] Improvements in VC have been attributed to spasticity developing in previously flaccid intercostal and abdominal muscles, thereby increasing the rigidity of the thorax and abdomen and improving diaphragm force generation.

PARKINSON'S DISEASE

Parkinson's disease is due to degeneration of neurons in the substantia nigra. It has a prevalence in the United States of approximately 200 cases per 100,000 people. Parkinson's disease can be either primary (e.g., idiopathic) or secondary, as in postencephalitic parkinsonism associated with the influenza pandemic, or part of more generalized disorder, such as multiple system atrophy or drug abuse with MPTP (1-methyl-4-phenyl-1,2,3,6-tetrahydropyridine).

Respiratory abnormalities are common in Parkinson's disease, with pneumonia being the most common cause of death.[10a] A substantial problem with Parkinson's disease is glottic muscle dysfunction. An abnormal flow-volume loop contour showing regular or irregular flow oscillations commonly occurs. On direct fiberoptic visualization of the upper airway, these oscillations correspond to rhythmic involuntary movements of glottic and subglottic structures. Physiological evidence of upper-airway obstruction may be present. Impairment of the upper-airway muscles is occasionally severe enough to cause upper-airway obstruction. In addition to the presence of oscillations in flow, a rounding-off of the peak of the midexpiratory flow-volume curve, a lowered peak expiratory flow rate, and a delayed appearance of peak expiratory flow have been observed in Parkinson's patients.[9] These results have been interpreted as evidence for less coordinated or less "explosive" respiratory muscle contractions.

Patients with mild to moderate Parkinson's disease are able to perform simple single respiratory efforts (e.g., measurements of lung volume and maximum static inspiratory pressures) but have difficulty performing more complex, repetitive ventilatory efforts (e.g., sustaining inspiratory resistive loads to exhaustion and performing maximum unloaded breathing efforts).[61] Performance of repetitive respiratory tasks is associated with an in-

creased work of breathing when compared to that of an age-matched control group. These findings are similar to derangements in task performance exhibited by peripheral skeletal muscle groups in Parkinson's patients.

Treatment (e.g., with apomorphine) significantly improves neurologic scores, maximum expiratory pressures, and peak inspiratory flow. In summary, Parkinson's disease results in problems in coordination and activation of upper-airway and chest wall muscles that may result in functional glottic obstruction and/or failed coordination of repetitive respiratory tasks. These abnormalities are favorably treated with antiparkinsonian medications.

MULTIPLE SCLEROSIS

Multiple sclerosis (MS) is a demyelinating disorder of the central nervous system, characterized clinically by remissions and relapses of clinical symptoms due to disseminating CNS lesions. MS is the most common neurologic disease afflicting young adults, with an estimated prevalence of 250,000 to 300,000 cases in the United States in 1990. The cause of the disease is unknown, although epidemiologic evidence points to genetic and environmental factors. Classic clinical symptoms include paresthesias, motor weakness, diplopia, blurred vision, dysarthria, bladder incontinence, and ataxia.

Symptoms are typically aggravated by an increase in temperature, which precipitates conduction block in partly demyelinated fibers. The disease course may be remitting and relapsing, or chronic and progressive. Pathologically, the lesions of MS have a predilection to invade the periventricular white matter of the cerebral hemispheres, optic nerves, brain stem, and cervical spinal cord.

Because MS can cause focal lesions anywhere in the central nervous system, different patterns of respiratory impairment can occur. Impairment of the respiratory centers and the medulla can cause failure of automatic breathing (Ondine's curse), apneustic breathing, paroxysmal hyperventilation, obstructive sleep apnea, or neurogenic pulmonary edema.[11a] The three most common respiratory manifestations of MS are respiratory muscle weakness, bulbar dysfunction, and abnormalities in respiratory control.

Acute respiratory failure rarely occurs in this disease, but it can occur because of severe demyelination of the cervical cord. Diaphragmatic paralysis resulting in respiratory insufficiency has also been reported. Even with severe disability and impaired respiratory muscle strength, patients with MS seldom complain of dyspnea. This paucity of respiratory complaints may be due to restricted motor activities and greater expiratory than inspiratory muscle dysfunction. Clinical signs that may be helpful in predicting respiratory muscle impairment are weak cough and inability to clear secretions, limited ability to count on a single exhalation, and upper extremity involvement. Advanced MS is frequently complicated by aspiration, atelectasis, and pneumonia.

Pulmonary dysfunction correlates with the severity of the disease and the functional capacity of the patient. Ambulatory patients have normal FVC, MVV, and maximum expiratory pressures, but these values are severely reduced in bedridden patients. In patients who are wheelchair bound with upper-extremity impairment, moderate reductions in FVC, MVV, and maximum expiratory pressure are found. Patients who are quadriplegic with prominent bulbar involvement are at high risk for the development of acute respiratory failure.

Treatment of MS includes ACTH, high-dose corticosteroids, immunosuppressive agents, such as cyclophosphamide and azathioprine, intravenous immunoglobulin therapy, and plasmapheresis. ACTH and prednisone have been shown to hasten the resolution of clinical symptoms in controlled trials. Methylprednisone, 1 mg daily for 5 days with or without prednisone taper, may be helpful in MS patients with severe respiratory complications. Plasmapheresis resolves clinical symptoms in patients with severe acute exacerbation and relapsing/remitting types of MS in acute exacerbation. Beneficial effects of intravenous immunoglobulin have been reported in a patient with quadriplegia and respiratory failure following an attack of MS. Additional studies are required before this mode of therapy can be advocated.

Lower Motoneuron Lesions

POLIOMYELITIS

In the early part of the 20th century, poliomyelitis was the most common cause of lower motor neuron disease in the United States. Paralytic poliomyelitis is the most devastating respiratory presentation of poliomyelitis infection and is preceded by a period of fever and mild illness. After several days of mild fever and myalgia, symptoms disappear; then, 5 to 10 days later, fever reoccurs with signs of meningeal irritation and asymmetric flaccid paralysis. Respiratory motor nuclei may be directly involved, resulting in diaphragmatic or other respiratory muscle dysfunction. In 6 to 25 percent of paralytic cases, bulbar symptoms may arise, increasing the risk of upper-airway obstruction, pooling of pharyngeal secretions, and pulmonary aspiration. Moreover, the central respiratory centers can be directly affected, resulting in irregular respirations.

In contrast to Guillain-Barré syndrome, sensation is intact. Tendon reflexes are significantly diminished or absent. Cerebrospinal fluid analysis shows a pleocytosis associated with mild protein elevation, and electroneuromyography shows widespread patchy denervation.

Fifteen to 30 percent of adults with paralyzing infection die, and treatment overall is supportive. Many patients require aggressive ventilatory and hemodynamic support during the acute phases of their illness. As temporarily damaged nerve cells regain function, recovery begins and may continue for as long as 6 months. Paralysis persisting beyond that point is permanent, however, and may be associated with complaints of severe pain, which sometimes recurs years after the illness.

Some patients develop progressive muscle weakness 20 to 30 years after the initial infection; this has been termed "postpolio syndrome." Symptoms vary from mild to moderate deterioration of function, with fatigue, joint pain, or weakness that may progress to muscle atrophy. The weakness tends to progress slowly, with an average decline in muscle strength of approximately 1 percent a year. The pathogenesis appears to be due to dysfunction of surviving motor neurons, with slow disintegration of axonal terminals eventually leading to muscle denervation.

AMYOTROPHIC LATERAL SCLEROSIS

Amyotrophic lateral sclerosis (ALS) is a chronic, degenerative neurologic disorder characterized by death of motoneurons in the cerebral cortex and spinal cord. The result is a combination of upper and lower motoneuron dysfunction, manifested by spasticity and hyperreflexia, muscle wasting, weakness, and fasiculations. It has an incidence of approximately 1 to 2 cases per 100,000 people. Males are more commonly affected than females—by a 2:1 ratio. Most cases are sporadic, but approximately 5 to 10 percent of cases demonstrate an autosomal dominant inheritance pattern. Recent reports incriminate abnormal glutamate metabolism as a potential cause in the development of sporadic ALS. Glutamate has been shown to exert specific neurotoxic effects and induces neuronal degeneration, both in vivo and in vitro. A familial form of ALS has been localized to chromosome 20, and a defect in gene coding for superoxide dismutase has been identified in some families.

The usual clinical presentation is progressive weakness of the distal extremities, although earlier involvement of the bulbar and respiratory muscles may occur. Respiratory muscle impairment is usually evident in the more advanced stages of the disease. Abnormalities in pulmonary function are apparent, even in patients with mild extremity weakness.[37a] Progression of respiratory impairment is much faster in ALS than in other chronic neuromuscular disorders. Serial lung function studies in ALS patients show progressive reduction in FVC and MVV. In contrast to patients with other neurologic disorders, however, patients with ALS usually have a normal or slightly elevated FRC, transpulmonary pressures at FRC are generally normal rather than decreased, and RV is usually increased and continues to rise as the disease progresses with maintenance of a normal TLC. These changes are thought to be due to earlier involvement of the abdominal musculature, with preservation of intercostal and diaphragm function. Support for these physiological findings comes from pathologic studies that show a more pronounced loss of motoneurons in the lumbosacral and lower thoracic spinal segments than in the upper and midthoracic regions.

The shape of the flow-volume curve may also pinpoint the subgroup of ALS patients with greater weakness of the expiratory muscles. In patients with severe expiratory muscle weakness, the flow-volume curve near RV shows a sharp drop in flow, such that the maximum expiratory curve has a concave appearance. This group of ALS patients usually have lower maximum expiratory pressures, smaller VC, reduced expiratory reserve volume, and a higher RV than do ALS patients with more-normal-appearing flow-volume curves.

Severe respiratory muscle weakness, particularly intercostal muscle and diaphragm weakness, has resulted in some ALS presenting with respiratory insufficiency as the initial symptom.

Treatment of the respiratory complications of ALS includes a high index of suspicion for impaired swallowing due to bulbar involvement. Difficulty in swallowing food or even saliva predisposes ALS patients to a markedly high risk for pulmonary aspiration. Special swallowing precautions, earlier placement of enteral feeding tubes, or antisialogues may be required.

In one study, the administration of theophylline to eight ALS patients for 3 days increased respiratory muscle strength after periods of resistive breathing, with a 28 percent increase in negative inspiratory pressure, a 10 percent increase in VC, and a 12 percent increase in peak inspiratory flow rate.[57a]

Overall, however, ALS is a progressive and fatal neuromuscular disease, and all patients will eventually develop respiratory failure; ventilatory assistance will therefore need to be considered. In some cases, noninvasive forms of ventilatory support may be feasible, but in most cases, airway intubation is required because of bulbar dysfunction impairing cough and the inability to clear secretions. Long-term ventilatory support is infrequently applied in ALS patients, but decisions must be made on an individual basis.

A recent prospective, randomized, controlled trial showed that the antiglutamate agent riluzole induced a significant improvement in survival and decreased the rate of deterioration in muscle strength in comparison to a placebo.[6a] Further investigation is indicated to determine whether antiglutamate therapy has a potential role in this heretofore incurable disease.

Disorders of Peripheral Nerves

Phrenic nerve dysfunction can be a significant cause of respiratory weakness in patients with neuromuscular diseases due to a variety of causes.

DIAPHRAGM PARALYSIS

Unilateral or bilateral diaphragm paralysis following phrenic nerve injury can result from cardiac surgery, trauma, mediastinal tumors, infections of the pleural space, or forceful manipulation of the neck. Phrenic nerve injury during open heart surgery is one of the most common causes of unilateral and bilateral diaphragm paralysis and is due either to cold exposure during cardioplegia or to mechanical stretching of the phrenic nerve during surgery. Diaphragm paralysis may also be seen with a variety of motoneuron diseases, myelopathies, neuropathies, and myopathies.

Bilateral diaphragm paralysis is characterized by a severe restrictive ventilatory impairment, with VC being frequently less than 50 percent of predicted in the upright position and a further reduction of 25 percent or more in VC in the supine position.[45] TLC is also markedly decreased, as well as FRC and static pulmonary compliance.[15,58] In most patients with nontraumatic bilateral diaphragm paralysis, the most important clinical feature is orthopnea out of proportion to the severity of the underlying cardiopulmonary disease.

In patients with nontraumatic bilateral diaphragm paralysis, the diagnosis usually goes unrecognized until they present with cor pulmonale or cardiorespiratory failure.[12] A chest radiograph showing elevation of both hemidiaphragms with volume loss and/or atelectasis at the lung bases is common. The diagnosis of bilateral diaphragm paralysis should be considered when any of the following four abnormalities is present: (1) a 40 percent or greater reduction in VC in the supine compared to upright position; (2) fluoroscopically observed paradoxical movements of both hemidiaphragms during a "sniff" test; (3) absence of phrenic latency on phrenic nerve conduction velocity tests or lack of EMG evidence of spontaneous diaphragm activity; and (4) trans-

diaphragmatic pressure two standard deviations below the expected mean for normal subjects with paradoxical inward abdominal motion during maximum inspiratory efforts.[12]

Because in most patients bilateral diaphragm paralysis occurs in the context of global respiratory muscle impairment, measurements of PI_{max} and PE_{max} may be sufficient to arouse suspicion of diaphragm paralysis as a cause of the patient's complaints. With diaphragm paralysis, a marked reduction in PI_{max} with preservation of PE_{max} should be found, and in general, there is a correlation between maximum inspiratory pressures and Pdi_{SNIFF}. Reductions in Pdi_{SNIFF} to less than 30 cmH$_2$O are accompanied by orthopnea, a supine decrease in VC, and the presence of abdominal paradox. In most cases, the presence of severe bilateral diaphragm weakness can be diagnosed from physical exam, measurements of VC in the upright and supine positions, and PI_{max} and PE_{max}. In cases where the diagnosis is uncertain, or when definite documentation is desired, measurement of transdiaphragmatic pressures, phrenic nerve conduction times, EMG activity, or transdiaphragmatic pressures during phrenic nerve stimulation may be desired. An elevation in $PaCO_2$, particularly in the supine position in patients with diaphragm paralysis has been reported,[15,58] but is not consistent.[40]

Hemidiaphragm paralysis is more common than bilateral paralysis and is usually diagnosed from unilateral elevation of the hemidiaphragm on chest radiograph. Most disorders reported as causing bilateral diaphragm paralysis have also been reported as causes of unilateral paralysis (e.g., cervical spondylosis, spine cord injury, poliomyelitis, and muscular dystrophy). Other, more specific causes of unilateral diaphragm paralysis are pneumonia, trauma from central vein cannulation, and viral infections of the cervical nerve roots.

Patient complaints and physical exam abnormalities in unilateral diaphragm paralysis are usually the same as with bilateral diaphragm paralysis but are less striking. Orthopnea is a frequent complaint, but it is less dramatic than in patients with bilateral paralysis. Moreover, physical exam findings are nonspecific, but occasionally may show paradoxical inward motion of the paralyzed hemidiaphragm with a reduction in breath sounds at the affected lung base and an increase in percussible dullness. The alveolar arterial oxygen gradient may be increased with mild hypoxemia due to the reduction in ventilation and perfusion of the lower lobe on the affected side.

Tests of diaphragm function are intermediate between those in patients with bilateral diaphragm paralysis and normal predicted values. VC in the upright posture may be reduced to 74 to 81 percent of predicted, with a fall in VC also present in the supine compared to erect position, but of lesser magnitude than in patients with bilateral diaphragm paralysis. In patients with right hemidiaphragm paralysis, the fall in VC may be almost twice as great (19 percent versus 10 percent) in comparison with left-sided paralysis, owing to the weight of the liver further encroaching on lung volume. Maximum inspiratory mouth pressures are frequently reduced to approximately 50 to 62 percent of normal. Similar reductions are also found in maximum Pdi measured during maximum static voluntary efforts and during maximum sniff.[41]

Treatment of patients with bilateral diaphragm paralysis is similar to that of other patients with chronic neuromuscular diseases. Eliminating nocturnal hypoventilation, especially during REM sleep, is warranted, and the implementation of noninvasive ventilation, especially positive-pressure ventilation, may be indicated. In some cases of symptomatic unilateral hemidiaphragm elevation, surgical plication of the affected hemidiaphragm may relieve symptoms and improve FVC and transdiaphragmatic pressure.

GUILLAIN-BARRÉ SYNDROME

Guillain-Barré syndrome (GBS) precipitates respiratory failure more often than any other peripheral neuropathy. It is an acute idiopathic polyneuritis with an annual incidence of 0.6 to 1.9 cases per 100,000 people. It usually presents as paresthesia and ascending paralysis of the lower extremities with absent deep tendon reflexes in a symmetrical distribution. Objective findings of sensory loss are variable, and the degree of motor weakness can range from mild paresis to complete paralysis. Maximum weakness of the lower extremities occurs within 2 weeks in 50 percent of cases, and 90 percent of cases reach their nadir in weakness by 4 weeks. After the nadir is reached, patients remain at that level for an additional 1 to 4 weeks before recovery begins. Facial, ocular, and oropharyngeal muscles may be impaired as well as the respiratory muscles. Respiratory muscle weakness and, specifically, severe diaphragm weakness may be found in patients with GBS.[60a]

The distribution of muscle weakness between respiratory and nonrespiratory muscles is not uniform in GBS, and peripheral muscle strength does not correlate with the presence or absence of respiratory muscle weakness; however, ventilatory failure correlates with diaphragmatic weakness.

The impairment on respiratory tests in GBS is similar to that for other generalized neuromuscular diseases. A decline in FVC and maximum inspiratory and expiratory mouth pressures, impairment in nocturnal gas exchange during REM sleep, and the onset of hypercapnia detected by arterial blood gas analysis have all been reported in symptomatic GSB patients. An FVC of 12 to 15 cc/kg is a sign of imminent respiratory failure in GBS. Hypercapnia is a late sign of respiratory failure, with the average Pa_{CO_2} at the time of intubation 43 mmHg when FVC is less than 12 cc/kg.

Respiratory treatment of GBS patients is mainly supportive. Since bulbar involvement, leading to swallowing dysfunction, increases the propensity for pulmonary aspiration, special precautions for feeding and control of upper-airway secretions may be required. Moreover, earlier intubation and assisted ventilation may be indicated to avoid complications that arise from progressive respiratory failure, overwhelming pulmonary infections, or both. Aggressive pulmonary toilet, including repeated bronchoscopy, may be needed to decrease atelectasis and the incidence of nosocomial pneumonia.[34b]

In two multicenter trials, plasmapheresis (250 cc/kg every 2 days, for a total of five treatments), using either albumin or fresh frozen plasma as replacement fluids, produced short-term benefits in earlier motor recovery, ambulation, reduction in number of patients who required assisted ventilation, and shortened the duration of mechanical ventilation.[30a] Plasmapheresis should be started within 2 weeks of the onset of symptoms or earlier, if possible. In patients with rapidly deteriorating clinical symptoms, however, plasmapheresis may still offer some benefit, even if the duration of the disease is greater than 3 weeks. Intravenous immunogammoglobulin (IVIG), given within 2 weeks after the onset of GBS, may also be effective therapy.[61a] However, further study is required before IVIG is established as an accepted treatment in GBS.

CRITICAL ILLNESS POLYNEUROPATHY

A recently recognized clinical entity characterized by polyneuropathy presenting as prolonged weakness of the distal extremities in critically ill patients has been reported.[66] Patients with this syndrome have no history of neuropathy, but are characterized by having a prolonged stay in an intensive care unit, documented sepsis, and clinical and laboratory findings consistent with multiple organ failure. About 30 percent of patients have difficulty being weaned from mechanical ventilation, and 70 percent have evidence of peripheral neuropathy. EMG studies in these patients show a reduction in the amplitude of the compound muscle action potential without significant prolongation of stimulus latency, suggesting primarily axonal nerve damage rather than a demyelinating process.

The clinical course for most of these patients is usually benign; however, clinical recovery of nerve function is usually prolonged, and it may be 6 months to 1 year before complete recovery occurs.

The exact mechanism for axonal damage in this syndrome is unknown. Possible causes include nerve toxins released during episodes of multiple system organ failure, antibiotics impairing neuromuscular transmission, protracted use of neuromuscular blocking agents, and hyperglycemia causing nerve ischemia by endovascular shunting.

Disorders of the Neuromuscular Junction

MYASTHENIA GRAVIS

Myasthenia gravis is an autoimmune disorder characterized by impaired transmission of neural impulses across the neuromuscular junction due to the production of antibodies directed against the acetylcholine receptor. The prevalence of myasthenia gravis is estimated to be approximately 1 in 10,000 people, with a 2-to-1 female-to-male predominance. It occurs more often in younger than older adults. The typical myasthenic patient presents with fluctuating muscular weakness, with improvement after rest and the administration of anticholinesterase agents (e.g., edrophonium chloride). Ocular, facial, and neck muscles are commonly affected, but patients who have the most severe respiratory involvement have either acute fulminating or late severe classifications of myasthenia gravis.[67]

In patients with moderate, generalized myasthenia gravis, pulmonary function studies before the administration of edrophonium chloride reveal a mild reduction in FVC and moderate reductions in both maximum inspiratory (approximately 46 percent of predicted) and expiratory (reduced to approximately 48 percent of predicted) mouth pressures. Because of increased lung recoil pressure, normal or supranormal values of maximal expiratory flow are seen in relation to lung recoil pressure or absolute lung volume.

Acute respiratory failure usually occurs in the setting of a myasthenic crisis or cholinergic crisis or as the initial presentation of the disease. A myasthenic crisis refers to worsening of the basic underlying disease, usually precipitated by decreased anticholinesterase medication, surgery, administration of neuromuscular blocking medication, and emotional upset. The most common complications of myasthenic crisis are respiratory failure and recurrent pneumonias due to aspiration from bulbar involvement and impaired cough. The mean duration of mechanical ventilation in myasthenia gravis in a series of 22 patients (12 postoperative myasthenic or cholinergic crises, four myasthenic crises, two cholinergic crises, and four other medical disorders) was 8 days, with six patients (32 percent) requiring tracheostomy for prolonged mechanical ventilation.[34] Of the 22 patients, 21 survived and were totally weaned from ventilatory support over 1 to 32 days. Clinical parameters useful in predicting the development of postoperative respiratory failure include the severity of the disease (e.g., acute fulminating or late severe categories of myasthenia gravis), a low preoperative VC, and bulbar symptoms.

The treatment of myasthenia gravis includes the use of anticholinesterase agents, high-dose corticosteroids, thymectomy, and plasmapheresis in patients refractory to steroid or immunosuppressive therapy. Anticholinesterase agents are the first line of treatment. Most patients improve significantly with anticholinesterase agents, but only a few regain normal function. Remissions can be induced in up to 80 percent of patients with the use of corticosteroids. However, corticosteroids may cause temporary worsening of muscle weakness, usually on the sixth to 10th day of therapy, and close observation for signs of respiratory insufficiency is advisable. Other immunosuppressive agents (e.g., cyclosporine and azathioprine) may be useful with or without concomitant corticosteroids.

In retrospective studies, thymectomy improves survival and relieves clinical symptoms, even in the absence of thymoma. In patients with thymoma, thymectomy is also indicated because the risk for malignant transformation is high in patients less than 55 years of age. In up to 80 percent of myasthenia gravis patients without thymoma, clinical improvement after thymectomy occurs during prolonged follow-up.

Plasmapheresis produces a temporary reduction in acetylcholine receptor antibody level and may be helpful in patients with respiratory failure not responding to anticholinesterase and immunosuppressive agents. Four patients with respiratory failure refractory to conventional therapy were successfully weaned from mechanical ventilation following plasmapheresis.[34a]

EATON-LAMBERT SYNDROME

Eaton-Lambert syndrome is a rare myasthenialike disorder resulting from a reduction in neurotransmitter release from presynaptic terminals that develops in association with tumor (especially small cell lung carcinoma). Although patients may respond weakly to administration of edrophonium chloride, the disease is differentiated from myasthenia gravis by the predominant involvement of limb and girdle muscles compared to the ocular and bulbar muscle involvement in myasthenia gravis. Respiratory muscle weakness is often detected on pulmonary function tests, but respiratory failure is infrequent.

BOTULISM

Botulism is a rare disorder caused by the *Clostridium botulinum* toxin. It occurs as a result of eating improperly cooked food, wound contamination by the organism, or, especially in infants, the absorption of toxin from the GI tract. There are eight types of toxins, although human diseases are usually caused by type A, B, or E.

Botulinum toxin binds to the calcium channel in presynaptic terminals, impairing neuromuscular transmission of acetylcholine. GI symptoms predominate early in the disease, followed by neurologic impairment, including descending paralysis of the neck, trunk, and limb muscles. Weakness of the respiratory muscles requiring mechanical ventilation is frequent, especially with botulinum type A toxins. Spirometry usually reveals a restrictive ventilatory defect, and recovery from respiratory muscle weakness may take months, often requiring prolonged mechanical ventilation. The average duration of ventilatory support for type A poisoning is 58 days, in contrast to 26 days for type B botulism. Exertional dyspnea and poor exercise tolerance may persist, even with normal lung function.

Muscular Dystrophies and Acquired Myopathies

Respiratory function may be significantly affected by a variety of inherited muscle disorders and acquired myopathies (Table 98-5).[46] The inherited muscular dystrophies refer to a heterogeneous group of progressive, degenerative, hereditary skeletal muscle diseases that cause severe muscle weakness, eventually

TABLE 98-5

Myopathies Likely to Produce Respiratory Abnormalities

Inherited Myopathies	Acquired Myopathies
Muscular Dystrophies	Inflammatory (dermatomyositis, polymyositis)
Duchenne	Systemic lupus erythematosus
Myotonic	Endocrine myopathies
Fascioscapulohumeral	Thyroid dysfunction
Limb-girdle	Hyperadrenocorticism
Oculopharyngeal	Acute steroid myopathy
Congenital myopathies	Electrolyte disorders
Nemaline myopathy	Rhabdomyolysis
Centronuclear myopathy	
Metabolic myopathies	
Acid maltase deficiency	
Mitochondrial myopathies	

SOURCE: Modified from Lynn et al.[46]

resulting in repeated pneumonias, respiratory failure, and, in some cases, death. Respiratory failure, often accompanied by pneumonia, contributes to death in more than 75 percent of patients with Duchenne's muscular dystrophy.[60]

Inherited Myopathies

DUCHENNE'S MUSCULAR DYSTROPHY

Duchenne's muscular dystrophy (DMD) is the best characterized of these heredofamilial muscle diseases. This disease is transmitted by an X-linked recessive gene, although approximately one-third of cases arise from spontaneous mutation. The disease is due to the mutation of the gene for skeletal protein dystrophin, a subsarcolemmal protein believed to play a major role in providing structural integrity in the muscle cell surface membrane. Approximately 30 to 40 percent of the normal amount of dystrophin must be expressed in order to prevent major myopathic symptoms. The diagnosis is confirmed by demonstrating mutation of the dystrophin gene in DNA from peripheral leukocytes, or an absence or abnormality in dystrophin in muscle biopsy samples.

Symptoms usually present in early childhood. Gait disturbances and delayed motor development are common manifestations, with proximal weakness resulting in an exaggerated lumbar lordosis. Most patients are wheelchair bound by the age of 12 to 15 years, with death occurring around the age of 20 years as a result of progressive respiratory failure and pneumonia. Kyphoscoliosis commonly develops as a result of severe muscle weakness and further contributes to a restrictive ventilatory deficit. Pulmonary symptoms are often minimal early on, despite significant weakness of the respiratory muscles. Maximum inspiratory pressure is reduced at all lung volumes in patients with DMD and declines with time. FVC increases with growth during the first decade and may mask early respiratory muscle dysfunction before it plateaus and progressively decreases about 5 to 6 percent per year after 12 years of age (Fig. 98-10). Reductions in maximum inspiratory pressure, therefore, occur early in the clinical course of DMD and may precede the reduction observed in VC. Inspiratory muscle weakness does not necessarily parallel the development of expiratory muscle weakness. Maximum expiratory mouth pressures are substantially lower than maximum inspiratory mouth pressures, possibly leading to a marked decrease in the effectiveness of cough.

Despite severe and progressive muscle weakness, hypercapnia is uncommon in patients with DMD in the absence of pulmonary infections. The absence of hypercapnia despite severe muscle weakness is believed to be due to relative preservation of diaphragm function until very late in the illness. Once hypercapnia occurs, however, the course is rapidly progressive, and mean survival is approximately 10 months.

Since ventilation is heavily dependent on diaphragmatic function in DMD patients, severe nocturnal hypoventilation may occur during REM sleep, when activity of chest wall and neck muscles is markedly attenuated. Indeed, REM hypoventilation has been documented in DMD patients—even in those who have normal daytime gas exchange. Sleep-related hypoxemia may contribute to respiratory insufficiency and the development of cor pulmonale.

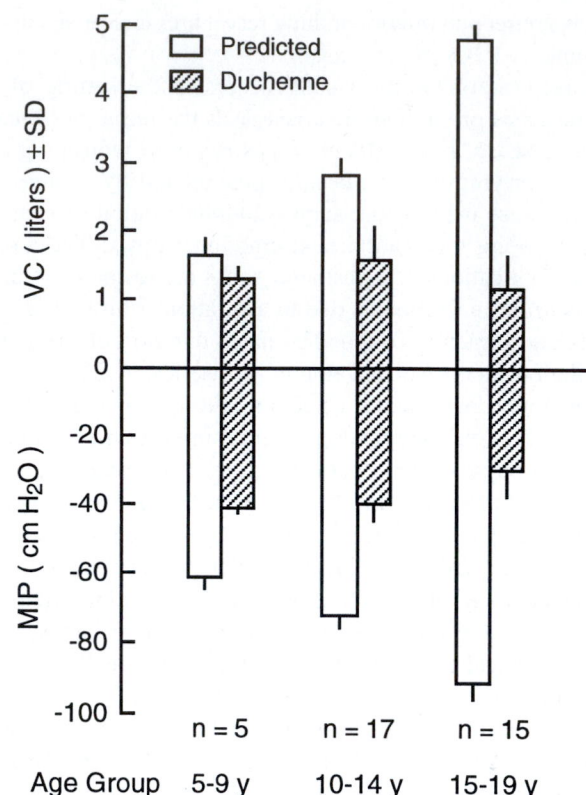

FIGURE 98-10   Mean vital capacity (VC) and maximum static inspiratory pressures (MIP) in 37 DMD patients in three age groups (shaded bars) in comparison to normal predicted values (unshaded bars). MIP decreases gradually as DMD progresses, despite body growth, whereas VC increases until patients reach their early teens. *(Based on data of Smith et al,[60] with permission.)*

Management of patients with DMD is mainly supportive. Ambulation should be maintained and encouraged as long as possible to retard the development of scoliosis. Surgical correction may attenuate the scoliotic contribution to the fall in VC and improve patient morale and quality of life overall. However, the downward trend in VC continues despite spine surgical stabilization. General physiotherapy may be helpful in preventing contractures. Maintenance of proper nutrition, with an emphasis on weight control, is important. Patients with DMD have a propensity to become overweight through a combination of inactivity, reduced energy requirements, and a misguided desire to improve muscle bulk by overeating.[60] Some authors have emphasized a high-protein (more than 80 g protein daily), low-calorie diet, aiming to achieve a body weight somewhat lower than the ideal weight in patients of a similar height and normal muscle mass.

Since chest infections are a serious complication in DMD patients, patients with poor cough and severe respiratory muscle weakness must be treated with physiotherapy, postural drainage, appropriate antibiotics, and vaccination for pneumococcal pneumonia and influenza.

In some patients, assisted ventilation is required once respiratory insufficiency or symptoms of sleep-related breathing disorders are present. Intermittent facial positive-pressure ventilation prolongs survival and may attenuate the decline in FVC and

MVV. Longer-term follow-up of DMD patients treated with noninvasive ventilation demonstrates that pulmonary function continues to deteriorate 3 to 4 years after the initiation of noninvasive ventilation, with patients requiring longer periods of ventilation and/or transition to tracheostomy with positive-pressure ventilation.[51]

Two recent studies suggest that prednisone treatment is beneficial. In a randomized, double-blind, controlled 6-month trial of prednisone in 103 boys, age 5 to 15 years, with DMD, patients were assigned to one of three regimens: prednisone 0.5 mg/kg per day, prednisone 1.5 mg/kg per day, or placebo.[52] Both prednisone groups showed significant improvements in muscle strength and functional scores. After 6 months of therapy, patients randomized to high-dose prednisone had an improvement in time needed to stand, climb stairs, or lift weights, and a significantly larger FVC (1.7 versus 1.5 L), compared to the placebo group. In the other study, of 93 DMD boys given 0.75 mg of prednisone daily over a 2-year period, there were improvements in strength (e.g., FVC and MVV maneuvers) throughout the 2 years.[30] Although these results are preliminary, they are encouraging and suggest that corticosteroid therapy may have a potential future role in DMD.

Gene therapy may be applicable to DMD in the future. Preliminary animal studies examining adenovirus-mediated in vivo gene transfer to dystrophic mouse diaphragm suggest that the adenovirus vector delivery of functional dystrophin gene to impaired muscle may be feasible therapy.[53]

MYOTONIC DYSTROPHY

Myotonic dystrophy is the most common form of hereditary muscular dystrophy in adults, with an estimated incidence of 1 in 8000 people. The gene responsible for the disease is located on the long arm of chromosome 19 and demonstrates an autosomal dominant inheritance pattern. Symptoms usually present during adolescence and in early adulthood, although the syndrome may be recognized as early as infancy.

Respiratory muscle weakness is common and can be severe, despite mild limb muscle weakness.[46] Myotonia of the respiratory muscles contributes to an increased work of breathing by increasing inspiratory impedance. Studies have suggested that the presence of a chaotic breathing pattern may explain the higher prevalence of chronic hypercapnia in patients with myotonic dystrophy than in patients with other forms of muscular dystrophy. Support for these findings came from studies that showed abnormal ventilatory responses to hypercapnic challenges in patients with myotonic dystrophy. However, more recent studies that have used mouth occlusion pressures ($P_{0.1}$) have revealed normal or supranormal responses in $P_{0.1}$ in patients with myotonic dystrophy compared to controls. These data seem to suggest that prior studies showing hypercapnia in patients with myotonic dystrophy underestimated the severity of respiratory muscle weakness by itself as a limitation in the ability to mount a normal ventilatory response. The chaotic breathing pattern observed in some patients with myotonic dystrophy has been suggested to be related to disordered afferent information from diseased muscle spindles.

Patients with myotonic dystrophy are particularly susceptible

to development of respiratory failure with general anesthesia and sedatives. Postoperative respiratory monitoring is essential if surgery or the use of these agents is required. Pharyngeal and laryngeal dysfunction increase the risk of aspiration. Sleep-related breathing disturbances are common and may include both central and obstructive forms of sleep apnea. Nocturnal positive-pressure ventilation should be tried when hypercapnia and hypoxemia are present.

FACIOSCAPULOHUMERAL DYSTROPHY

Other inherited adult muscular dystrophies are facioscapulohumeral dystrophy (FSH) and limb-girdle dystrophy. FSH is an autosomal dominant dystrophy that primarily affects muscles of the face and the proximal portion of the upper extremities. FVC is significantly reduced in patients with FSH, although facial weakness complicates spirometric assessment. In 20 percent of patients with FSH, the disease affects pelvic girdle and trunk muscles, sometimes impairing respiratory function.

LIMB-GIRDLE DYSTROPHY

Limb-girdle dystrophy is a heterogeneous group of autosomal dominant recessive disorders. The disease usually becomes evident in the second or third decade of life. Several case reports have documented the development of chronic hypercapnia in patients with limb-girdle dystrophy who have severe diaphragm weakness or bilateral diaphragm paralysis as the basis for hypercapnia.[58] However, not all patients with limb-girdle dystrophy develop hypercapnia. Most patients have moderate respiratory muscle weakness with normal gas exchange.

ACID MALTASE DEFICIENCY

Two metabolic myopathies, acid maltase deficiency and mitochondrial myopathy, have received attention as potential causes of respiratory failure. Acid maltase deficiency is a type I glycogen storage disease due to the deficiency of the lysosomal enzyme responsible for hydrolysis of both the α_{1-4} and α_{1-6} linkages of glycogen. The disease presents in three clinical forms: infantile, childhood, and adult. In adult-onset disease, onset usually occurs after 20 years of age and presents with progressive proximal muscle weakness. The diagnosis may be difficult to establish in some patients, as respiratory failure or sleep-related complaints, secondary to respiratory deterioration during REM sleep, may be the initial presentation.

Diagnostic studies include elevated serum muscle enzymes, myopathic changes on electromyography, and vacuoles filled with lysosomal breakdown products on muscle biopsy. A report that a weight-reducing, high-protein diet improved respiratory function in a patient with an acid maltase deficiency has not been confirmed, and treatment remains supportive.

MITOCHONDRIAL MYOPATHY

Mitochondrial myopathy represents a new, heterogeneous group of disorders that affect mitochondrial function and may present as complex multisystem disorders. Three mitochondrial disorders have been described, with brain and striated muscle being the predominant organs affected: (1) Kearns-Sayre syndrome; (2) myoclonic epilepsy, "ragged red fibers," and mitochondrial myopathy; and (3) encephalopathy, lactic acidosis, and strokelike episodes.[46] The clinical manifestations may be broad and include myalgia and exercise intolerance, proximal muscle weakness, and external ophthalmoplegia with unexplained respiratory failure. All three disorders are characterized by hypoventilation and depressed responses to hypoxia and hypercapnia and, in some cases, unexplained respiratory failure. Skeletal muscle biopsy establishes the diagnosis of mitochondrial myopathy by showing "ragged red fibers," which are accumulations of mitochondria identified with modified trichrome staining. Treatment is in general supportive. Once identified, patients should be cautioned regarding the use of sedatives, and special attention is required when sedation or surgery is planned.

Acquired Myopathies

Acquired myopathies include inflammatory polymyopathies (polymyositis and dermatomyositis), systemic lupus erythematosus, endocrine myopathies (hyper- or hypothyroidism), hyperadrenocorticism, electrolyte disturbances, rhabdomyolysis, and the use of high-dose exogenous corticosteroids, with or without concomitant use of neuromuscular blocking agents.

INFLAMMATORY MYOPATHIES

Pulmonary complications are the major cause of morbidity and mortality in dermatomyositis and polymyositis. These include interstitial pneumonitis, pulmonary vasculitis, recurrent aspiration from oropharyngeal dysfunction, and, rarely, hypoventilatory failure from respiratory muscle weakness. Respiratory failure is uncommon in the inflammatory myopathies and is usually due to clinically significant interstitial lung disease. Ten to 30 percent of patients with inflammatory myopathies have interstitial lung disease, manifested by dyspnea, nonproductive cough, and hypoxemia, with radiographic evidence of diffuse interstitial lung disease and impaired gas exchange.[23]

Corticosteroids may be successful in the treatment of interstitial pneumonitis and myositis. Successful treatment appears to be enhanced by early initiation of therapy, as patients in later stages of the disease become more refractory to corticosteroids and cytotoxic agents.

SYSTEMIC LUPUS ERYTHEMATOSUS

Diaphragm dysfunction and respiratory muscle weakness with small lung volumes occur without apparent involvement of the peripheral skeletal muscles in patients with systemic lupus erythematosus (SLE).[32] This syndrome has been called "the shrinking lung syndrome." Decreased lung volumes appear not to be due to parenchymal lung disease or phrenic neuropathy but, rather, to a myopathic process affecting diaphragm strength. It is estimated that approximately 25 percent of SLE patients have diaphragm weakness, even in the absence of a generalized myopathy.[46]

STEROID MYOPATHY

Although a syndrome of acute myopathy secondary to high-dose steroid use was first described almost 20 years ago, the development of severe respiratory muscle weakness and prolonged respiratory failure following the use of high-dose steroids has received renewed interest.[38] Most patients have received neuromuscular blocking agents, along with high-dose steroids, before weakness becomes evident. Some patients require months of mechanical ventilation before eventual recovery. The serum CPKs are often normal, and EMG data show nonspecific changes. Overall, it is difficult to incriminate specific neuromuscular blocking agents or steroids as the only factors responsible for myopathic changes because an underlying severe illness, undernutrition, multiple medications, and disuse atrophy are usually concurrent. Additional investigation is required to identify the mechanism(s) and determine the exact incidence and pathogenesis of this disorder.

TREATMENT

Principles of Management

Principles in management of respiratory dysfunction in patients with neuromuscular disease include (1) preventive therapies designed to minimize the impact of impaired secretion clearance and alveolar hypoventilation on gas exchange and lower respiratory tract infections and (2) stabilization of patients who develop acute or chronic presentations of respiratory failure (see Chapter 99).

Because patients with neuromuscular disease usually have nonpulmonary symptoms and signs before the onset of respiratory problems, preventive actions can be taken to preserve their respiratory status. In neuromuscular disorders causing bulbar dysfunction, swallowing precautions and airway control measures are required. With advanced bulbar symptoms, upper-airway control with a cuffed tracheostomy tube may be needed to protect the airway and facilitate suction of lower respiratory tract secretions, averting atelectasis and pneumonia. In patients with impaired cough, assisted coughing (e.g., ancillary hand thrust in the substernal location to increase intrathoracic pressure and expel secretions mouthward) may be helpful, along with postural drainage and the use of incentive spirometry.

Preventive Therapies

INTERMITTENT POSITIVE-PRESSURE BREATHING

There is no evidence for a beneficial effect of intermittent positive-pressure breathing on respiratory system compliance or lung volumes and static pulmonary compliance in patients with chronic neuromuscular disorders.

RESPIRATORY MUSCLE TRAINING

Inspiratory and expiratory muscle training may be helpful in some neuromuscular diseases. One could hypothesize that respiratory muscle weakness is key to the development of respiratory tract infections and ventilatory failure in patients with chronic neuromuscular disease. Besides weakened muscles, a reduction in lung and chest wall compliance and, in some cases, the presence of hypoxemia and hypercapnia all act to increase ventilatory workload in patients who already have markedly diminished ventilatory pump capacity. Strengthening weakened respiratory muscles relieves cough, improves secretion clearance, and increases ventilatory capacity.

Respiratory muscle training improves strength and ventilatory endurance in normal subjects and in patients with pulmonary diseases. Several uncontrolled studies, performed in patients with muscular dystrophy, showed that inspiratory muscle training may improve respiratory muscle endurance and strength.[24,49]

Some authors have questioned the wisdom of training respiratory muscles of patients with significant neuromuscular dysfunction. Breathing through resistive loads may be harmful and perhaps further damage or tire already weakened respiratory muscles.[18] Also, the training techniques do not apply to upper-airway and pharyngeal musculature.

The effects of inspiratory muscle training have also been examined in quadriplegic patients, who may be a more appropriate group for respiratory muscle training because, although weakened, their respiratory muscles are normal. In small numbers of quadriplegic patients, 6 to 16 weeks of inspiratory resistive training improved inspiratory muscle strength and endurance,[35] and 6 weeks of pectoralis muscle isometric training significantly increased expiratory reserve volume in C6 to C8 quadriplegic patients.[28] Such increases in expiratory reserve volume suggest that these patients may have a more effective cough. Although these changes may be physiologically beneficial, no study has correlated such improvements with better clinical outcome. Accordingly, the therapeutic value of inspiratory muscle training remains speculative.

Mechanical Ventilation

In patients with severe respiratory impairment, mechanical ventilation may be indicated to augment or supplant spontaneous breathing. Overall, indications for mechanical ventilation are shown in Table 98-6. Comparisons of the situations in which invasive or noninvasive mechanical ventilation is applicable are summarized in Table 98-7. The types of ventilation available and their advantages and disadvantages are provided in Table 98-8. Patients who present with the onset of severe dyspnea, CO_2 retention, and moderate to severe hypoxemia require intubation and mechanical ventilation. In patients with acute respiratory failure who are awake, alert, and able to control their airway and do not have copious secretions, noninvasive ventilation (e.g., positive-pressure ventilation with a face mask rather than an endotracheal or tracheostomy tube) may obviate intubation (see Chapter 10).

In some patients, the onset of respiratory failure is insidious, manifested by the gradual onset of dyspnea, daytime hypersomnolence, morning headaches, nightmares, enuresis, and easy fatigability. In patients with these symptoms, arterial blood gas analysis is warranted, especially if vital capacity falls below 1.5 to 1 L. Daytime measurements may be misleading, however, because impaired gas exchange may occur only during REM sleep. Nocturnal oximetry or a full polysomnogram should be considered to exclude the presence of nocturnal hypoventilation. In patients who have chronic hypoventilation, uncompensated respiratory acidosis, hypoxemia refractory to supplemental oxygen, or worsening symptoms such as easy fatigability and morning headaches, the implementation of nocturnal mechanical ventilation should be anticipated (Table 98-6).

In most cases, noninvasive forms of ventilatory support should be considered first. Since the polio epidemic in the 1940s and '50s, correction of nocturnal and daytime hypoventilation with a range of noninvasive ventilators—including Drinker respirators, cuirasses, and poncho-wrap ventilators—has supported patients' nocturnal and daytime gas exchange for months to years. Although these types of ventilators are relatively inexpensive, durable, and successful, there are limitations to their use (Table 98-8).

Negative-pressure ventilators function by intermittently applying subatmospheric pressure to the thorax and abdomen that increases transpulmonary pressure and inflates the lung. The ef-

---

TABLE 98-6

Indications for Mechanical Ventilation in Patients with Neuromuscular Diseases

Acute respiratory failure
 Severe dyspnea
 Marked accessory muscle use
 Copious secretions
 Unstable hemodynamic state
 Hypoxemia refractory to supplemental O_2
 Acute severe gas exchange disturbances (increased Pa_{CO_2} with pH ≤ 7.25)
Chronic respiratory failure
 Symptoms of nocturnal hypoventilation (e.g., morning headaches, decreased energy, nightmares, enuresis)
 Dyspnea at rest or increased work of breathing impairing sleep
 Cor pulmonale due to hypoventilation, $Pa_{CO_2} > 45$, pH < 7.32 after treating reversible conditions
Nocturnal desaturation ($Sa_{O_2} < 88\%$) despite supplemental O_2 therapy

---

TABLE 98-7

Invasive Versus Noninvasive Mechanical Ventilation in Patients with Neuromuscular Disease

Invasive Ventilation (endotracheal or tracheostomy tube and positive-pressure ventilation)	*Noninvasive Ventilation (no airway cannulation)*
Copious secretions	Awake, cooperative patient
Inability to control upper airway	Good airway control
Inability to tolerate or failure of noninvasive ventilation	Minimal secretions
Impaired cognition	Hemodynamic stability
Unstable hemodynamics	Reversible cause of respiratory failure

TABLE 98-8

Types of Noninvasive and Alternative Forms of Ventilation Used in Patients with Neuromuscular Disease

Tank	Advantages	Disadvantages
Negative-pressure ventilators	Familiar and dependable	Cumbersome
Tank	No airway cannulation	Induces obstructive apnea
Pulmowrap	Can significantly augment ventilation	Constrains body posture
Cuirass	Rare hemodynamic concerns	Bulky (tank)
	Simple devices	Limits nursing care
		Controlled ventilation
Positive-pressure by mask or mouthpiece	Averts upper-airway obstruction, pressure preset, leak compensates	Attachment bothersome
	Patient initiated machine breaths	Leaks
		Aerophagia
		Skin breakdown
Glossopharyngeal breathing	Decreases ventilator dependency	Learning curve
		Limited ventilation
Diaphragmatic pacing	Decreases ventilator dependency	Expensive
		Upper-airway obstruction
		Requires surgery
		Diaphragm fatigue

ficacy of negative-pressure ventilation is determined by thoracic and abdominal compliance, as well as the surface area over which negative pressure is applied. Tank ventilators are the most efficient form of negative-pressure ventilators and cuirass ventilators, less so, since tank ventilators surround a greater thoracic and abdominal surface area. Although tank ventilators are very reliable, they are large, cumbersome, and claustrophobia inducing for patients and markedly interfere with nursing care. Chest cuirasses and poncho-wrap ventilators are more portable than tank ventilators, but both require that the patient remain recumbent, induce a rocking motion in the lower posterior thoracic spine, and may induce discomfort and pressure sores at areas of skin contact. Moreover, all forms of negative-pressure ventilation tend to induce obstructive sleep apnea due to upper-airway collapse during a mechanically delivered breath. This problem is overcome by noninvasive positive-pressure ventilation, whereby positive pressure applied to the upper airway acts as a pneumatic stent that maintains a patent upper airway during a machine-delivered breath.

Rocking beds and pneumobelts—abdominal displacement ventilators—have been used as ventilatory assist devices in patients with mild to moderate ventilatory failure. Both devices augment diaphragmatic motion by displacing the abdominal viscera against gravity. The rocking bed consists of a mattress on a motorized platform that rocks in an arc of 40 degrees with the patient lying recumbent. As the bed rocks with the head dependent, gravity induces the abdominal contents and diaphragm to move cranially, thereby assisting exhalation. In the next cycle, as the bed tilts upward, gravity acts to move the diaphragm and abdominal contents in a caudad direction, thereby assisting inspiration. The bed rocks between 12 and 24 times per minute and may be adjusted to optimize patient comfort and achieve minute ventilation targets.

The pneumobelt is an inflatable bladder that is worn over the anterior abdomen and connected to a positive-pressure ventilator that intermittently inflates it. With a patient seated upright, bladder inflation increases intra-abdominal pressure, forcing the diaphragm cephalad and thereby inducing active exhalation. When the bladder deflates, gravity moves the abdominal contents and diaphragm caudally, thereby facilitating passive inspiration. Tidal volume can be augmented by increasing bladder inflation pressures to target goals.

Both devices should be considered methods to assist ventilation in impaired patients rather than mechanical ventilators to replace ventilation in iller subjects. Both devices are limited by their constraints on patient posture. The rocking bed is bulky, stationary, and limited by the degree of ventilatory assistance that it provides. Similarly, the pneumobelt requires that the patient use it in the upright position, the amount of ventilatory assistance provided is limited, and some patients complain of pain and discomfort when high bladder inflation pressures are required to sufficiently augment ventilation.

Recently, several studies have examined the application of noninvasive positive-pressure ventilation given only at night, or intermittently throughout the 24-hour period using nasal, oronasal, or mouthpiece attachment. Several authors have shown significant improvements in daytime gas exchange after 3 months of nocturnal ventilation, with the mean increase in Pa_{O_2} approximately 15 mmHg and the decrease in Pa_{CO_2} approximately 14 mmHg. Beneficial effects of chronic intermittent noninvasive ventilation, besides better gas exchange, include abatement in patients' symptoms and improvement in functional status. There is an inconsistent effect on increasing maximum inspiratory and expiratory mouth pressures and lung volumes.

The exact mechanisms for the improvement with chronic intermittent noninvasive ventilation in daytime gas exchange in patients with neuromuscular diseases are unknown, but several hypotheses have been proposed: (1) respiratory muscle resting treats patients who suffer from chronic intermittent fatigue; (2) preventing nocturnal hypoventilation resets the central respiratory center Pa_{CO2} threshold; (3) there is improved ventilation-perfusion matching; and (4) improved lung and chest wall compliance decreases the work of breathing.

Although none of the above mechanisms has been established as a conclusive mechanism for the improvement in gas exchange observed in these patients following noninvasive ventilation, resetting of the central controller Pa_{CO2} level appears to be the most tenable. The presence of chronic inspiratory muscle fatigue has never been proved in any patient group, and other studies have shown that intermittent positive-pressure breathing does not decrease the incidence of atelectasis or improve lung volume. Whatever the mechanism(s), however, all studies reported to date show that noninvasive positive-pressure ventilation improves gas exchange and alleviates symptoms of nocturnal hypoventilation in patients with chronic neuromuscular diseases.

Other Forms of Ventilatory Assistance

In certain patients with neuromuscular diseases, glossopharyngeal breathing and diaphragmatic pacing may be important aids to augment ventilation.

GLOSSOPHARYNGEAL BREATHING

Intermittent glossopharyngeal breathing—using oral, pharyngeal, and laryngeal muscles—may augment ventilation (see Chapter 10).[14] Short periods of spontaneous ventilation are possible once patients have mastered this technique. With glossopharyngeal breathing, the patient gulps in air by lowering and raising the tongue against the palate in a pistonlike fashion, thereby injecting air into the trachea. After practice, patients may be able to gulp approximately 50 to 150 cc of air every half second. Patients may then repeat gulps in series without preventing air from escaping into the trachea so that, with repeated gulping, a tidal volume of approximately 500 to 600 cc may be achieved. With repeating series of gulps, a normal minute ventilation can be achieved for short periods. Although this technique is difficult for some patients, patients with high spinal cord injuries, postpolio syndrome, and other neuromuscular diseases successfully utilize this technique.

DIAPHRAGMATIC PACING

To increase independence from mechanical ventilation, diaphragmatic pacing may be a treatment option in selected patients. Although phrenic nerve pacing by external stimulation has been well documented since the late 1940s, long-term phrenic nerve stimulation did not become a reality until a small implantable electrode and receiver were developed in the late 1960s. Diaphragmatic pacing consists of a radiofrequency transmitter and an antenna that discharges stimulatory signals to a receiver that, when activated by radiofrequency waves, transmits electrical impulses to an electrode placed over the phrenic nerve. Surgery is required to implant the electrodes and receiver. Elec-

trode implantation around the phrenic nerves can be achieved by a cervical or thoracic approach; however, the thoracic approach is preferred, to ensure stimulation of all phrenic nerve roots while avoiding the brachial plexus. The subcutaneous receiver is usually placed in the lower anterolateral rib cage to allow it to be superficial, but in an area where soft-tissue movement is limited.

Diaphragmatic pacing has a number of potential limitations, including its high cost (approximately $20,000), the potential to fail abruptly, the development of upper-airway obstruction, and the induction of diaphragm fatigue. On the other hand, successful implantation allows patients to be independent from ventilatory support for prolonged periods, and to speak more freely.

The main group of patients who appear to benefit from diaphragmatic pacing are ventilator-dependent patients following high cervical cord injury.[33] Approximately one-third of patients with high cervical spinal cord injuries may be suitable for this type of treatment. Although short-term improvements are noted in terms of ventilator independence and improvement in functional status, no long-term studies demonstrating efficacy have been published to date.[52a]

REFERENCES

1. Alexander C: Diaphragm movements and the diagnosis of diaphragmatic paralysis. *Clin Radiol* 17:79–83, 1966.
2. Allen SM, Hunt B, Green M: Fall in vital capacity with posture. *Br J Dis Chest* 79:267–271, 1985.
3. Arora NS, Suratt PM, Rochester DF: Respiratory muscle and ventilatory function in spinal cord injury. *Clin Res* 26:443–444, 1978.
4. Baydur A: Respiratory muscle strength and control of ventilation in patients with neuromuscular disease. *Chest* 99:330–338, 1991.
5. Begin R, Bureau MA, Lupien L, Lemieux B: Control and modulation of respiration in Steinert's myotonic dystrophy. *Am Rev Respir Dis* 121:281–289, 1980.
6. Bellemare F, Bigland-Ritchie B: Assessment of human diaphragm strength and activation using phrenic nerve stimulation. *Respir Physiol* 58:263–277, 1984.
6a. Bensimon G, Lacomblez L, Meininger V: A controlled trial of riluzole in amyotrophic lateral sclerosis. *New Engl J Med* 330:585–591, 1994.
7. Black LF, Hyatt RE: Maximal respiratory pressures normal values and relationship to age and sex. *Am Rev Respir Dis* 99:696–702, 1969.
8. Black LF, Hyatt RE: Maximal static respiratory pressures in generalized neuromuscular disease. *Am Rev Respir Dis* 103:641–649, 1971.
9. Bogaard JM, Hovestadt A, Meerwaldt J, et al: Maximal expiratory and inspiratory flow-volume curves in Parkinson's disease. *Am Rev Respir Dis* 139:610–614, 1989.
10. Braun NMT, Rochester DF: Muscular weakness and respiratory failure. *Am Rev Respir Dis* 119:123–125, 1979.
10a. Brown LK: Respiratory dysfunction in Parkinson's disease. *Clin Chest Med* 15:715–727, 1994.
11. Bye PTP, Ellis ER, Issa FG, et al: Respiratory failure and sleep in neuromuscular disease. *Thorax* 45:241–247, 1990.
11a. Carter JL, Noseworthy JH: Ventilatory dysfunction in multiple sclerosis. *Clin Chest Med* 15:693–703, 1994.
12. Chan CK, Loke J, Virgulto JA, et al: Bilateral diaphragmatic paralysis: Clinical spectrum, prognosis, and diagnostic approach. *Arch Phys Med Rehabil* 69:976–979, 1988.
13. Cook CD, Mead J, Orzalesi NM: Static volume-pressure characteristics of the respiratory system during maximal efforts. *J Appl Physiol* 19:1016–1022, 1964.

14. Dail CW, Affeldt JE, Collier CR: Clinical aspects of glossopharyngeal breathing. *JAMA* 158:445–449, 1953.

15. Davis J, Goldman M, Loh L, Casson M: Diaphragm function and alveolar hypoventilation. *Q J Med* 177:87–100, 1976.

16. Demedts M, Beckers J, Rochette F, Bulcke J: Pulmonary function in moderate neuromuscular disease without respiratory complaints. *Eur J Respir Dis* 63:62–67, 1982.

17. De Troyer A: Lung volume restriction in patients with respiratory muscle weakness. *Thorax* 35:603–610, 1980.

18. De Troyer A, Estenne M: The respiratory system in neuromuscular disorders, in Roussos C (ed), *The Thorax*. New York, Marcel Dekker, 1995, pp 2177–2212.

19. De Troyer A, Borenstein S: Acute changes in respiratory mechanics after pyridostigmine injection in patients with myasthenia gravis. *Am Rev Respir Dis* 121:629–638, 1980.

20. De Troyer A, Borenstein S, Cordier R: Analysis of lung volume restriction in patients with respiratory muscle weakness. *Thorax* 35:603–610, 1980.

21. De Troyer A, Basternier-Geens J: Effects of neuromuscular blockade on respiratory mechanics in conscious man. *J Appl Physiol* 1162–1168, 1979.

22. De Troyer A, Estenne M, Heilporn A: Mechanism of active expiration in tetraplegic subjects. *New Engl J Med* 314:740–744, 1986.

23. Dickey BF, Myers AR: Pulmonary disease in polymyositis/dermatomyositis. *Semin Arthritis Rheum* 14:60–76, 1984.

24. DiMarco AF, Kelling JS, DiMarco MS, et al: The effects of inspiratory muscle training on respiratory muscle function in patients with muscular dystrophy. *Muscle Nerve* 8:284–290, 1985.

25. Dolmage TE, Avendano MA, Goldstein RS: Respiratory function during wakefulness and sleep among survivors of respiratory and nonrespiratory poliomyelitis. *Eur Respir J* 5:864–870, 1992.

26. Estenne M, De Troyer A: The effects of tetraplegia on chest wall statics. *Am Rev Respir Dis* 134:121–124, 1986.

27. Estenne M, De Troyer A: Mechanism of the postural dependence of vital capacity in tetraplegic subjects. *Am Rev Respir Dis* 135:367–371, 1987.

28. Estenne M, Heilporn A, Delhez L, et al: Chest wall stiffness in patients with chronic respiratory muscle weakness. *Am Rev Respir Dis* 128:1002–1007, 1983.

29. Estenne M, Knoop C, Vanvaerenbergh J, et al: The effect of pectoralis muscle training in tetraplegic subjects. *Am Rev Respir Dis* 139:1218–1222, 1989.

30. Fenichel GM, Florence JM, Pestronk A, et al: Long-term benefit from prednisone therapy in Duchenne muscular dystrophy. *Neurology* 41:1874–1877, 1991.

30a. French Cooperative Group on Plasma Exchange in Guillain-Barré Syndrome: Efficiency of plasma exchange in Guillain-Barré syndrome: Role of replacement fluids. *Ann Neur* 22:753–761, 1987.

31. Garay SM, Turino GM, Goldring RA: Sustained reversal of chronic hypercapnia in patients with alveolar hypoventilation syndrome. *Am J Med* 70:269–274, 1981.

32. Gibson GJ, Pride NB, Newsom D, Loh LC: Pulmonary mechanics in patients with respiratory muscle weakness. *Am Rev Respir Dis* 115:389–395, 1977.

33. Glenn WW, Hogan JF, Phelps ML: Ventilatory support of the quadriplegic patient with respiratory paralysis by diaphragm pacing. *Surg Clin North Am* 60:1055–1078, 1980.

33a. Goldstein RS, Molotiu N, Skrastins R, et al: Reversal of sleep-induced hypoventilation and chronic respiratory failure by nocturnal negative pressure ventilation in patients with restrictive ventilatory impairment. *Am Rev Resp Dis* 135:1049–1055, 1987.

34. Gracey DR, Divertie MB, Howard FM: Mechanical ventilation for repiratory failure in myasthenia gravis. *Mayo Clin Proc* 58: 597–602, 1983.

34a. Gracey DR, Howard FM, Divertie MB: Plasmapheresis in the treatment of ventilator-dependent myasthenia gravis patients: report of four cases. *Chest* 86:739–743, 1984.

34b. Gracey DR, McMihan JC, Divertie MB, Howard FM: Respiratory failure in Guillain-Barré syndrome. *Mayo Clin Proc* 57:742–746, 1982.

35. Gross D, Ladd HW, Riley EJ, et al: The effect of training on strength and endurance of the diaphragm in quadriplegia. *Am J Med* 68:27–35, 1980.

36. Hill NS, Eveloff SE, Carlisle CC, Goff, SG: Efficacy of nocturnal nasal ventilation in patients with restrictive thoracic disease. *Am J Med* 63:223–232, 1977.

37. Holle RHO, Shoene RB, Pavlin EJ: Effect of respiratory muscle weakness on P0.1 induced by partial curarization. *J Appl Physiol* 57:1150–1157, 1984.

37a. Kaplan LM, Hollander D: Respiratory dysfunction in amyotrophic lateral sclerosis. *Clin Chest Med* 15:675–681, 1994.

38. Kupfer Y, Okrent DG, Twersky RA, et al: Disuse atrophy in a ventilated patient with status asthmaticus receiving neuromuscular blockage. *Crit Care Med* 15:795–797, 1987.

39. Laporta D, Grassino A: Assessment of transdiaphragmatic pressure in humans. *J Appl Physiol* 58:1469–1476, 1996.

40. Laroche C, Carroll N, Moxham J, Green M: Clinical significance of severe isolated diaphragm weakness. *Am Rev Respir Dis* 138:862–866, 1988.

41. Laroche CM, Mier AK, Moxham J, Green M: Diaphragm strength in patients with recent hemidiaphragm paralysis. *Thorax* 43:170–174, 1988.

42. Laroche C, Mier AK, Moxham J, Green M: The value of sniff esophageal pressures in the assessment of global inspiratory muscle strength. *Am Rev Respir Dis* 138:598–603, 1988.

43. Ledsome JR, Sharp JM: Pulmonary function in acute cervical cord injury. *Am Rev Respir Dis* 124:41–44, 1981.

44. Leech JA, Ghezzo H, Stevens D, Becklake MR: Respiratory pressures and function in young adults. *Am Rev Respir Dis* 128:17–23, 1983.

45. Loh L, Goldman M, Davis JN: The assessment of diaphragm function. *Medicine* 56:165–169, 1977.

46. Lynn DJ, Woda RP, Mendell JR: Respiratory dysfunction in muscular dystrophy and other myopathies. *Clin Chest Med* 15:661–674 1994.

47. Macklem PT, Gross D, Grassino A, Roussos C: Partitioning of inspiratory pressure swings between diaphragm and intercostal/accessory muscles. *J Appl Physiol* 44:200–208, 1978.

48. Martin AJ, Stern L, Yeates J, et al: Respiratory muscle training in Duchenne dystrophy. *Med Child Neurol* 28:314–318, 1986.

49. McCool FD, Pichurko BM, Slustky A, et al: Changes in lung volume and rib cage configuration with abdominal binding in quadriplegia. *J Appl Physiol* 60:1198–1202, 1986.

50. Mier A, Brophy C, Moxham J, Green M: Twitch pressures in the assessment of diaphragm weakness. *Thorax* 44:990–996, 1989.

51. Mohr CH, Hill NS. Long-term follow-up of nocturnal ventilatory assistance in patients with respiratory failure due to Duchenne-type muscular dystrophy. *Chest* 97:91–96, 1990.

52. Mendell JR, Moxley RT, Griggs RC, et al: Randomized, double-blind six-month trial of prednisone in Duchenne's muscular dystrophy. *New Engl J Med* 320:1592–1597, 1989.

52a. Moxham J, Shneerson JM: Diaphragmatic pacing. *Am Rev Resp Dis* 148:S33–S36, 1993.

53. Petrof BJ, Acsadi G, Jani A, et al: Efficiency and functional consequences of adenovirus-mediated in vivo gene transfer to normal

and dystrophic (mdx) mouse diaphragm. *Am J Respir Cell Mol Biol* 13:508–517, 1995.

54. Rinqvist T: The ventilatory capacity in healthy adults: An analysis of causal factors with special reference to the respiratory forces. *Scand J Clin Lab Invest* 18(Suppl 88):1–111, 1966.

55. Rochester DF, Arora NS: Respiratory muscle failure. *Med Clin North Am* 67:573–598, 1983.

56. Rochester DF, Esau SA: Assessment of ventilatory function in patients with neuromuscular disease. *Clin Chest Med* 15:751–763, 1994.

57. Saunders NA, Rigg JR, Campbell EJ: Effect of curare on maximum static PV relationships of the respiratory system. *J Appl Physiol* 44:589–595, 1978.

57a. Schiffman PL, Belsh JM: Effect of inspiratory resistance and theophylline on respiratory muscle strength in patients with amyotrophic lateral sclerosis. *Am Rev Resp Dis* 139:1418–1423, 1989.

58. Skatrud J, Iber C, McHugh W, et al: Determinants of hypoventilation during wakefulness and sleep in diaphragmatic paralysis. *Am Rev Respir Dis* 121:587–593, 1980.

59. Smith PEM, Calverley PMA, Edwards RHT: Hypoxemia during sleep in Duchenne's muscular dystrophy. *Am Rev Respir Dis* 137:884–888, 1988.

60. Smith PEM, Edwards RHT, Evans GA, Campbell EJM. Practical problems in the respiratory care of patients with muscular dystrophy. *New Engl J Med* 316:1197–1205, 1987.

60a. Teitelbaum JS, Borel CO: Respiratory dysfunction in Guillain-Barré syndrome. *Clin Chest Med* 15:705–714, 1994.

61. Tzelepis GE, McCool FD, Friedman JH, Hoppin FG: Respiratory muscle dysfunction in Parkinson's disease. *Am Rev Respir Dis* 138:266–271, 1988.

61a. Van der Meche FGA, Schmitz PIM, The Dutch Guillain-Barré Study Group: A randomized trial comparing intravenous immune globulin and plasma exchange in Guillain-Barré syndrome: *New Engl J Med* 326:1123–1129, 1992.

62. Vincken W, Elleker G, Cosio G: Detection of upper airway muscle involvement in neuromuscular disorders using the flow-volume loop. *Chest* 90:52–57, 1986.

63. Vincken W, Elleker MG, Cosio MG: Determinants of respiratory muscle weakness in stable chronic neuromuscular disorders. *Am J Med* 82:53–58, 1987.

64. Vincken WG, Elleker MG, Cosio MG: Flow-volume loop changes reflecting respiratory muscle weakness in chronic neuromuscular disorders. *Am J Med* 83:673–680, 1987.

65. Wilson, Cooke NT, Edwards RHT, Spiro SG: Predicted normal values for maximal respiratory pressures in Caucasian adults and children. *Thorax* 39:535–538, 1984.

66. Young GB: Neurologic complications of systemic illness. *Neur Clin* 13:645–658, 1995.

67. Zulueta JJ, Fanburg BL: Respiratory dysfunction in myasthenia gravis. *Clin Chest Med* 15:683–691, 1994.

CHAPTER 99

PULMONARY REHABILITATION IN NEUROMUSCULAR DISEASES

John R. Bach

PATHOPHYSIOLOGY

PHYSICAL MEDICINE AIDS
  The Inspiratory Muscle Aids
  The Expiratory Muscle Aids
  Glossopharyngeal Breathing (GPB)

RESPIRATORY MUSCLE ASSISTANCE PROTOCOLS
  Prevention of Pulmonary Morbidity
  Decannulation and Conversion to Noninvasive
    Respiratory Aids

Most patients with ventilatory dysfunction caused by a combination of respiratory muscle weakness, paralysis, or mechanical dysfunction of the chest wall are not treated until they develop respiratory distress. At this stage, they are generally managed as though they had obstructive disease of the airways or intrinsic lung disease. Accordingly, they are given supplemental oxygen, bronchodilators, and chest physical therapy and, occasionally, prophylactic tracheostomy. Nocturnal, bilevel positive airway pressure (BPAP) may be used, but typically at pressures inadequate to support alveolar ventilation, to rest the inspiratory muscles, or to provide deep enough breaths to assist in coughing.[5] This scenario almost inevitably leads to respiratory failure, hospitalization, and to endotracheal intubation for ventilatory support. Eventually, weaning from the ventilator using some combination of synchronized intermittent mandatory ventilation (SIMV), assist-control along with pressure support ventilation, or positive end-expiratory pressure (PEEP), and supplemental oxygen usually fails, and a tracheostomy is performed.

It is essential to recognize that therapeutic modalities designed for other respiratory diseases are inappropriate for patients with ventilatory impairments due to neuromuscular disorders. For example, bronchodilators are rarely useful and can augment anxiety and increase the tachycardia that is common in myopathic patients. Theophylline, often given to relieve diaphragmatic fatigue, may actually increase or delay recovery from diaphragmatic fatigue in the presence of hypercapnia and hypoxia[33] and lead to other adverse side effects.[20]

Oxygen therapy also poses problems of a higher risk of pulmonary morbidity, rate of hospitalizations, and mortality than that which occurs with the use of ventilatory assistance or with no treatment at all.[4,15] Oxygen therapy may obscure recognition of mucous plugging because it tends to compensate for the hypoxemia associated with its use. Oxygen therapy may prolong hypopneas and apneas during rapid eye movement (REM) sleep and in individuals with Duchenne muscular dystrophy (DMD) who still have good ventilatory function.[38] Oxygen therapy also appears to supress the reflex muscular activity, mediated by the central nervous system, needed for effective, nocturnal, noninvasive intermittent positive pressure ventilation (IPPV).[8]

Translaryngeal intubation, tracheostomy, and tracheal suction are commonly used for patients with Duchenne muscular dystrophy and other neuromuscular conditions even though such patients rarely require such interventions as long as they have sufficient oropharyngeal muscle function to speak and swallow.

Since patients are seldom introduced to the idea of noninvasive ventilatory assistance, most are uninformed about this option when they are asked to consider endotracheal intubation or tracheostomy. Those who refuse prophylactic tracheostomy predictably develop acute respiratory failure, usually as the result of their inability to clear airway secretions during intercurrent upper respiratory tract infections. Typically, many patients who say they will refuse, ultimately agree to intubation and tracheostomy under duress of a respiratory crisis. Since only the use of noninvasive inspiratory and expiratory aids can prevent respiratory failure, it is not surprising that few patients with alveolar hypoventilation due to progressive neuromuscular disease avoid respiratory failure.

Until the late 1950s, negative pressure body ventilators (NPBVs) were the predominant methods of ventilatory support. However, because they were only practical and effective while the user was recumbent and because placement of an indwelling tracheostomy tube facilitated the management of airway secretions during episodes of acute respiratory failure, tracheostomy and translaryngeal suctioning of airway secretions have been widely used since then. Nevertheless, in most instances of alveolar hypoventilation, tracheostomy is both unnecessary and undesirable[1,3,4] because of the difficulties, complications, and expense associated with maintaining an indwelling tracheostomy tube. Noninvasive options for ventilatory support and recent advances in the noninvasive handling of airway secretions have provided more expedient and effective approaches to these patients.

PATHOPHYSIOLOGY

The reader is referred to Chapters 97 and 98 for detailed discussions of the physiological disturbances associated with nonmuscular chest wall and neuromuscular disorders that affect ventilation.

Any combination of respiratory muscle weakness and paralysis can lead to alveolar hypoventilation. Mechanical dysfunction of the chest wall and lungs associated with thoracic deformities, extreme obesity, and abdominal distension, and the use of improperly fitting thoracolumbar orthoses, can also produce respiratory failure. In addition, hypopharyngeal collapse or other upper airway narrowing during sleep can exacerbate alveolar hypoventilation. In individuals with these types of disorders, respiratory failure may be precipitated by an acute respiratory infection, fatigue,[31] bronchial mucous plugging, pulmonary infiltrations, atelectasis, pleural disease, and pneumothorax.

Patients with advanced respiratory muscle insufficiency who are breathing spontaneously, adapt a breathing pattern of rapid, shallow inspirations coupled with the inability to take occasional deep breaths. This pattern can lead to microatelectasis in as little as 1 h.[32] If unrelieved, chronic microatelectasis, and decreased chest wall elasticity, ensues.[18,21] Decreased pulmonary compliance initially results from microatelectasis but ultimately from increased stiffness of the chest wall and lung tissues themselves.[21] Suboptimal treatment of acute respiratory tract infections leads to pulmonary scarring that can cause further loss of compliance as can kyphosis and scoliosis.

Respiratory muscle dysfunction, combined with increased work of breathing, can lead to alveolar hypoventilation. In the context of neuromuscular disorders, hypercapnia is a consequence of rapid shallow breathing[10] and usually occurs when the vital capacity decreases to less than about 55 percent of predicted.[13,14] Hypercapnia itself can contribute to decreasing respiratory muscle strength.[27,38] The risk of pulmonary morbidity and mortality from acute respiratory failure correlates with increasing hypercapnia.[12,24]

If alveolar hypoventilation is not corrected by appropriate use of inspiratory muscle aids, respiratory control centers reset to accommodate increasing carbon dioxide tensions,[8] and there is a compensatory retention of bicarbonate by the kidneys. The resulting increase in bicarbonate levels in the central nervous system contributes to depression of the ventilatory response to hypoxia and hypercapnia. Besides permitting worsening of the global alveolar hypoventilation, decreased ventilatory responsiveness seems to decrease the effectiveness of treatment of the hypercapnia by the nocturnal use of noninvasive IPPV.[8]

Patients with respiratory muscle dysfunction often have concomitant weakness of expiratory and oropharyngeal muscles which decrease peak flows during a cough.[13,23] If peak cough flows do not exceed 3 L/s, cough will be inadequate to eliminate airway secretions.[3] Peak cough flows are significantly re-

duced in patients who cannot take or cannot receive and hold a breath greater than 1.5 L.[28] Peak cough flow is also decreased in patients in whom airflow is decreased because of dysfunction of the expiratory muscles or irreversible airway obstruction caused by tracheal stenosis, laryngeal incompetence, postintubation vocal cord adhesions or paralysis, or chronic obstructive pulmonary disease. For patients with airway obstruction, the airway secretions that develop during upper respiratory tract infections and after surgical anesthesia often result in mucous plugging followed by acute respiratory failure and pneumonia. Smoking, the presence of an endotracheal cannula, or bronchorrhea for any reason, all increase the tendency to develop mucous plugging. Mucous plugging often results in intubation and repeated bronchoscopy and can lead to tracheostomy. The latter further reduces peak flows during coughing. During routine suctioning of the airways, the catheter often fails to enter the left main stem bronchus, thereby leading to continued plugging and increased morbidity.

For patients with respiratory muscle dysfunction, arterial hypoxemia and hypercapnia occur initially during REM sleep.[35] In time, the blood-gas abnormalities gradually extend throughout most of sleep and eventually throughout daytime hours.[37] Nocturnal arterial hypoxemia, with an oxyhemoglobin saturation of less than 85 percent, often occurs in patients in whom arterial Pa_{CO_2} is greater than 50 mmHg while awake.[34] The cough reflex is also suppressed during sleep, which is when mucous plugs are most likely to cause sudden hypoxia and respiratory dysfunction. Normocapnic arterial hypoxemia is also common,[24] most likely reflecting ventilation-perfusion imbalance associated with microatelectasis and pulmonary fibrosis.

Medications such as calcium channel blockers, aminoglycosides, steroids, and benzodiazepines can reduce the ventilatory response to hypercapnia and hypoxemia and exacerbate alveolar hypoventilation. Beta blockers may increase airway resistance. Malnutrition, acidosis, electrolyte disturbances, cachexia, infection, fatigue, and muscle disuse or overuse can all exacerbate ventilatory insufficiency.

Most patients with progressive neuromuscular weakness develop alveolar hypoventilation insidiously.[13] The decreases in myoneural function that occur with normal aging can contribute to the problem. Most often, alveolar hypoventilation is first recognized largely because of bronchial mucous plugging, when an intercurrent respiratory infection triggers acute respiratory failure. However, on occasion, chronically hypercapnia patients complain of symptoms of hypoventilation or experience respiratory arrest without any obvious precipitating cause. Ventilatory failure can also develop suddenly or over a period of hours or days in patients with acute cervical myelopathies, Guillain-Barré syndrome, myasthenia gravis, acute poliomyelitis, or multiple sclerosis.

PHYSICAL MEDICINE AIDS

Alveolar hypoventilation and inability to clear airway secretions lead to respiratory complications, hospitalizations, and even death. Many patients are hospitalized, intubated, bronchoscoped, and mechanically ventilated and weaned on numerous occasions before institution of physical medicine inspiratory and expiratory muscle aids eliminates further episodes.

Inspiratory and expiratory muscle aids are methods and devices that involve the manual or mechanical application of forces to the body or intermittent pressure changes to the airways to assist respiratory muscle function. Devices that act on the body include body ventilators that create atmospheric pressure changes around the thorax and abdomen or that apply force directly to the body to mechanically displace respiratory muscles. Devices that apply intermittent pressure changes directly to the airway include bilevel positive airway pressure machines and positive and negative pressure ventilators. Blowers, including continuous positive airway pressure (CPAP) machines, do not directly assist inspiratory muscle function unless they are used to insufflate the lungs intermittently and the patient exhales to atmospheric pressure. Table 99-1 summarizes the criteria necessary for successful implementation of long-term use of noninvasive inspiratory and expiratory muscle aid alternatives to tracheostomy. The conditions for which these criteria are most often met are listed in Table 99-2.

The Inspiratory Muscle Aids

NEGATIVE PRESSURE BODY VENTILATORS (NPBVS)

Negative pressure body ventilators intermittently generate a subatmospheric pressure around the thorax and abdomen to assist, or support, the inspiratory effort. Tank ventilators consist of a cylinder or chamber (e.g., the iron lung) that envelopes the body up to the neck. Negative pressure is created in the chamber by motorized bellows. This results in passive lung insufflation. Iron lungs continue to be manufactured and used in the United States, England, Germany, and Italy, and in some centers they continue to be the mainstay of intensive care ventilatory support.[16] Today, for portable iron lungs and most other NPBVs, the negative pressure is created not by a motorized bellows, but by pumps or negative pressure ventilators that can cycle negative and, at times, positive pressure as well.

Chest-shell and wrap-style ventilators envelop the thorax and abdomen. Negative pressure ventilators cycle subatmospheric pressure under the shell or grid to assist the inspiratory effort. For wrap-style ventilators, the grid and the body under it are covered by a wind-proof jacket that is sealed around the neck and extremities. Although more time-consuming to don than the chest-shell, they can be more effective because of more complete covering of the thorax and abdomen. Although chest-shell ventilators

---

TABLE 99-1

Criteria for Successful Use of Noninvasive Ventilatory Support for Neuromusculoskeletal Disorders

1. Patient cooperative and no use of heavy sedation or narcotics
2. No substance abuse or convulsions
3. Peak cough flows greater than 3 L/s, unassisted or assisted
4. Adequate swallowing without aspiration of airway secretions
5. Arterial blood gases return to adequate levels ($Pa_{O_2} \geq 60$ mmHg, Pa_{CO_2} normal) with use of noninvasive ventilatory support alone
6. No mechanical obstacles to using IPPV interfaces (e.g., facial fractures or interfering devices)

TABLE 99-2

Neuromusculoskeletal Disorders for Which Noninvasive IPPV Has Proved Effective for Total Ventilatory Support

Myopathies

Muscular dystrophies
   Dystrophinopathies (Duchenne and Becker dystrophies)
   Other muscular dystrophies (limb-girdle, Emery-Dreifuss, facioscapulohumeral, congenital, childhood autosomal recessive, and myotonic dystrophy)
Other myopathies
   Congenital and metabolic myopathies (e.g. acid maltase deficiency)
   Inflammatory myopathies (e.g. polymyositis)

Neurological Disorders

Motor neuron diseases and spinal muscular atrophy
Poliomyelitis
Neuropathies
   Hereditary sensory motor neuropathies
   Phrenic neuropathies associated with cardiac hypothermia, surgical or trauma
   Guillain-Barré syndrome
Multiple sclerosis
Myelopathies
Myasthenia gravis
Tetraplegia associated with pancuronium bromide

Sleep-Disordered Breathing

Central and congenital hypoventilation syndromes
Obesity hypoventilation

Skeletal Pathology

Kyphoscoliosis
Osteogenesis imperfecta

can be used while the patient is sitting, their use has been largely supplanted by the more practical intermittent abdominal pressure ventilator (IAPV), noninvasive IPPV methods, and, at times, by glossopharyngeal breathing (GPB).

Negative pressure body ventilators are particularly suitable for overnight ventilatory support and have been used for decades to sustain alveolar ventilation in patients with little or no vital capacity. However, in the 1970s, when pulse oximetry became available, it was found that bouts of arterial hypoxemia occurred while they were in use, apparently due to episodes of airway collapse. As the patient ages and pulmonary compliance decreases, NPBVs can become ineffective and are associated with the development of systemic hypertension. The patients then need to be switched to more effective inspiratory muscle aids.[7] Furthermore, except for the iron lung and PortaLung, NPBVs are usually ineffective in patients with severe scoliosis or extreme obesity. Moreover, back pain is common, particularly in patients using a chest-shell or wrap-style ventilator in whom greater than 60 cm H_2O of negative pressure is often needed.

An alternative to NPBVs is the rocking bed ventilator which applies force directly to the body in order to create, or increase, diaphragm excursions. It assists alveolar ventilation by rocking the patient through an arc of 15 to 30 degrees, allowing gravity to displace cyclically the abdominal contents, and therefore, the diaphragm. Although it is still being used for ventilatory support and can provide as much as 1000-ml tidal volumes for some patients without a measurable vital capacity, it is generally not as effective as NPBVs.[22]

Today, NPBVs are best used to support alveolar ventilation for patients with little, or unmeasurable, vital capacity during tracheal extubation or removal of a tracheostomy tube while transitioning to the 24-h use of other noninvasive aids;[4] NPBVs are also occasionally useful for patients during episodes of nasal congestion who would otherwise be using nocturnal, nasal IPPV (Fig. 99-1).[4] Since noninvasive IPPV methods are more versatile, convenient, and effective and are not associated with and can alleviate upper airway instability, they are the preferred methods of ventilatory support for patients in whom ventilation is primarily impaired and who satisfy the criteria indicated in Table 99-1. Comprehensive discussions on body ventilators are available elsewhere.[4]

NONINVASIVE IPPV

Noninvasive IPPV is the preferred method for 24-h ventilatory support, especially for patients for whom intermittent abdominal pressure ventilation is ineffective for daytime use.[1] IPPV can be delivered noninvasively via oral,[7] nasal,[19,27,30] or oral-nasal interfaces.[30]

MOUTHPIECE IPPV

Until the mid-1950s, when iron lungs had to be opened to permit nursing care, patients who had no breathing capability received IPPV via a dome that enclosed their heads. This is ironic, since these patients, unless unresponsive or severely impaired cognitively, could have received ventilatory support via simple mouthpieces. Although it was originally used in 1956 to provide

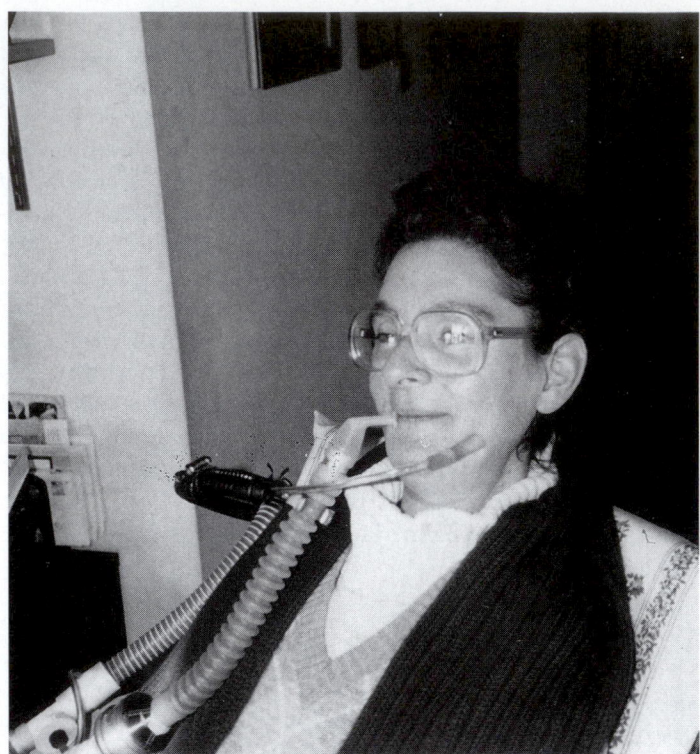

FIGURE 99-1 Postpoliomyelitis patient with no measurable vital capacity since 1954 using intermittent positive pressure ventilation delivered via a mouthpiece fixed adjacent to the sip and puff controls of her motorized wheelchair since 1957.

daytime ventilatory support in patients who left their iron lungs, mouthpiece IPPV was first described in 1969.[4]

IPPV is delivered via a mouthpiece held between the lips and teeth. The mouthpiece is usually maintained close to the mouth by either a telephone holder or by a metal clamp attached to the wheelchair or fixed onto motorized wheelchair controls (sip and puff, chin, or tongue control) (Fig. 99-1).

Mouthpiece IPPV is used as needed to maintain alveolar ventilation. Since high tidal volumes are delivered, even patients with little vital capacity need to take only a few deep insufflations per minute. They can vary their tidal volumes and, in addition, they can air-stack subsequent insufflations and deeply expand the lungs to increase voice volume, to increase peak cough flows, and to help maintain pulmonary compliance. The ultimate goal of air stacking is to approach the predicted inspiratory capacity and in doing so to increase the maximum insufflation capacity (MIC).

In learning to use mouthpiece IPPV, the patient has to learn palatal movements in order to prevent leakage out of the nose during insufflation and to open the glottis during each assisted breath. This can be difficult for patients who are being transferred from IPPV via a tracheostomy (tracheostomy IPPV) to noninvasive IPPV, because reflex glottic opening and dilation of the hypopharynx are lost during tracheostomy IPPV. Often patients are thought to have tracheal stenosis or other reasons for upper airway obstruction before they learn to reopen the glottis in order to enable IPPV. This is not usually a problem after translaryngeal tracheal intubation. Adequate neck rotation and oromotor function are also necessary for the patient to grab the mouthpiece and receive IPPV without leakage out of the mouth or nose during insufflation. To prevent the latter, the soft palate must elevate to seal off the nasopharynx.

Once it was appreciated that patients could retain their mouthpieces while asleep in their wheelchairs, some patients began to use simple mouthpiece IPPV for overnight aid as well. This approach proved effective in sustaining alveolar ventilation and optimizing quality of life even for patients with no use of their extremities or measurable vital capacity. Over a period of 40 years, simple mouthpiece IPPV has proved to be the most convenient, reliable, and effective method of daytime assisted ventilation. Mouthpiece IPPV can be used alone or in combination with other noninvasive ventilatory assist methods for up to 24 h of ventilatory support.[7]

LIPSEAL IPPV

Although many patients with little autonomous ventilatory capacity maintained alveolar ventilation during sleep using simple mouthpiece IPPV, a problem remained in that these patients experienced frequent, and at times severe, arterial hypoxemia during periods of leakage during insufflation. In 1972, the *lipseal* became available (Fig. 99-2). The lipseal holds the mouthpiece firmly in the mouth and minimizes air insufflation leakage around the mouthpiece and out of the mouth. Lipseal IPPV has been used for nocturnal ventilatory support by more than 150 patients, many for more than 20 years.[7] Orthodontic bite plates and custom-fabricated acrylic lipseals can increase comfort and efficacy and eliminate risk of severe orthodontic deformity.

Generally, nasal leakage during nocturnal lipseal IPPV does not lead to hypoventilation because high ventilatory insufflation volumes (1200 to more than 2000 ml at times) are used to compensate for nasal leakage, and the conditioned reflexes that occur during sleep assure adequate ventilatory support. However, about 3 percent of lipseal IPPV users have periods of excessive leakage that result in arousals with shortness of breath. This problem can be corrected by sealing the nose with a clip or cotton pledgets.[7]

Besides orthodontic deformities, other potential difficulties include aerophagia and allergy to the plastic lipseal. Abdominal distention often occurs sporadically. The air passes as flatus once the patient is mobilized in the morning. When severe, a rectal tube can usually decompress the colon.

NASAL IPPV

The idea of delivering IPPV noninvasively through the nostrils as an alternative to mouthpiece IPPV for resting the inspiratory muscles of patients with muscular dystrophy was first suggested in 1982. Nocturnal nasal IPPV has since become a conventional approach to temporarily relieving nocturnal hypoventilation. Originally, IPPV was delivered using urinary drainage catheters, with the cuffs inflated in both nostrils. Subsequently, nasal CPAP masks were used as the nasal interfaces. Since 1984, a variety of CPAP masks have become commercially available. Each design applies pressure differently to the paranasal area. Since it is impossible to predict which model will be most effective and comfortable for any particular patient, various models are tried for every user. Many patients use different styles on alternate nights to vary skin contact pressure. Custom-molded nasal interfaces,[27,30] which can be obtained both commercially (Fig. 99-3) or in specialized centers (Fig. 99-4), are important alternatives to CPAP masks.[30]

Because patients generally prefer to use mouthpiece IPPV or the IAPV for daytime aid,[7] nasal IPPV is most practical only for nocturnal use. Daytime nasal IPPV can be used by those who cannot grab or retain a mouthpiece because of oral muscle weakness, inadequate jaw opening, or insufficient neck movement. Therefore, 24-h nasal IPPV is a viable alternative to tracheostomy even for some patients with severe lip and oropharyngeal muscle weakness.[4]

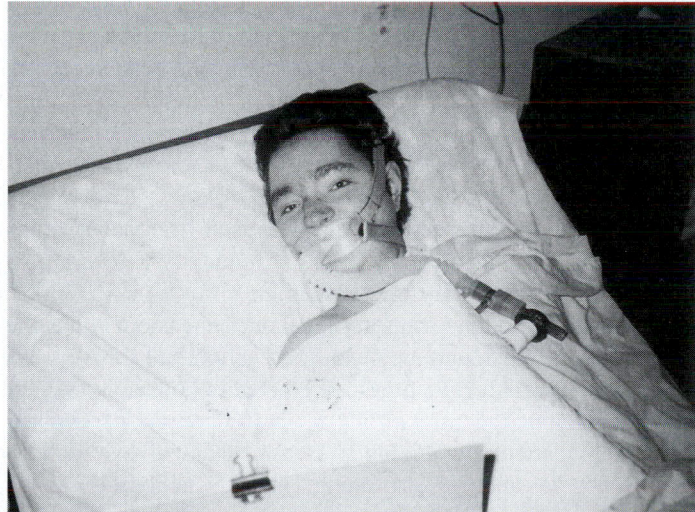

FIGURE 99-2   Duchenne muscular dystrophy patient who has required 24-h ventilatory support for 14 years and currently has less than 2 min of ventilator-free breathing ability. For nocturnal ventilatory support he uses mouthpiece intermittent positive pressure ventilation (IPPV) with lipseal retention.

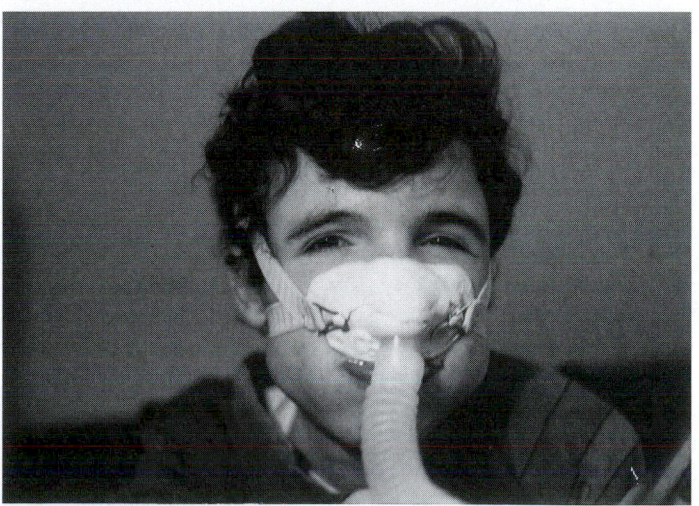

FIGURE 99-3   Duchenne muscular dystrophy patient with no ventilator-free breathing ability and inadequate lip strength to use mouthpiece IPPV who used 24-h nasal IPPV, alternating use of various nasal interfaces, for 7 years before succumbing to a pneumothorax.

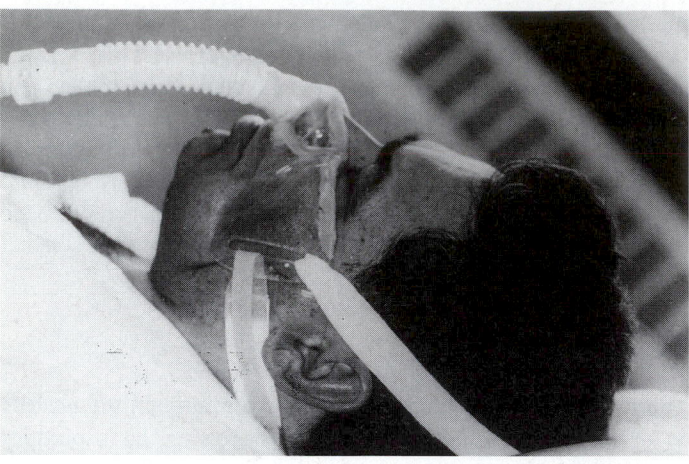

FIGURE 99-4 Patient with severe chronic alveolar hypoventilation due to kyphoscoliosis who has used a low-profile custom acrylic nasal interface for nocturnal nasal intermittent positive pressure ventilation for the last 8 years.[30]

ORAL-NASAL INTERFACES

Oral-nasal interfaces were described for long-term supported ventilation in 1989.[21] Since nasal and lipseal interfaces are effective for long-term nocturnal IPPV, strap-retained oral-nasal interfaces are generally unnecessary for this purpose. However, strapless oral-nasal interfaces (SONIs) with bite-plate retention have been used in Europe since 1985. Not only do these interfaces provide an essentially airtight seal for the delivery of IPPV, but simple tongue thrust is all that is necessary to expel them.[4] The bite-plate retention is also useful for patients living alone who are unable to independently don straps (Fig. 99-5). Unfortunately, these interfaces are difficult and time-consuming to construct, and adequate and stable dentition is necessary to use them.

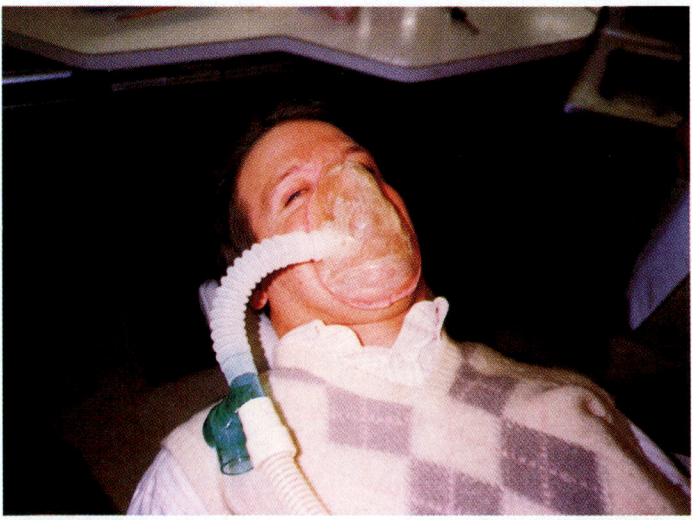

FIGURE 99-5 Patient with cervical spine injury in 1957 who developed late-onset ventilatory failure and has been a ventilator user since 1982. Here he is seen using a strapless oral-nasal interface.

INTERMITTENT ABDOMINAL PRESSURE VENTILATOR (IAPV)

The IAPV involves the intermittent inflation of an elastic air sac that is contained in a corset or belt worn beneath the patient's outer clothing (Fig. 99-6). The sac is inflated by a positive pressure ventilator. Bladder action moves the diaphragm upward, causing a forced exsufflation. During bladder deflation, the abdominal contents and diaphragm return to the resting position, and inspiration occurs passively. A trunk angle of 70 to 80 degrees from the horizontal is ideal for the effectiveness of the IAPV. The patient who has any inspiratory capacity or is capable of glossopharyngeal breathing can add autonomous tidal volumes to the mechanically assisted inspirations. The IAPV generally augments tidal volumes by about 300 ml, but volumes as high as 1200 ml have been reported.[6] Patients with less than 1 h of ventilatory-free breathing ability often prefer to use the IAPV rather than noninvasive IPPV during daytime hours.[6] The IAPV is usually inadequate in the presence of scoliosis or obesity.

The Expiratory Muscle Aids

As in the case of inspiratory muscle aids, expiratory muscle assistance can be applied to the body as manual thrusts, or pressure changes can be applied directly to the airway to create forced exsufflations to increase peak cough flows. There are at least 12 methods of manually assisted coughing.[29] For patients with less than 1.5 L of vital capacity, peak cough flows can be considerably increased by maximal insufflations before manually assisted coughing.[2] A manual resuscitator, positive pressure blower, intermittent positive pressure breathing (IPPB) machine, or portable ventilator can be used to deliver the deep insufflations.

Peak cough flows can also be considerably increased by the use of mechanical insufflation-exsufflation (MI-E). This entails the delivery of a maximal positive pressure insufflation followed by a sudden decrease in pressure, usually from about +40 cm H_2O to −40 cm H_2O, via a translaryngeal tube, a tracheostomy tube, or an oral-nasal interface. Insufflation pressures should be increased gradually for patients who have not been receiving maximal insufflations on a routine basis. One treatment consists of about five cycles of MI-E followed by a period of normal breathing or ventilator use for 20 to 30 s to avoid hyperventilation. The treatments continue until no further secretions are expulsed and any arterial hypoxemia caused by mucous plugs is reversed. MI-E may be required as frequently as every 5 to 15 min during respiratory tract infections.

When used through a translaryngeal or tracheostomy tube, the tube cuff is inflated, and a concomitant abdominal thrust is unnecessary. Since effective flows are created in both right and left airways without the discomfort or airway trauma of tracheal suctioning, patients invariably prefer mechanical insufflation-exsufflation to tracheal suctioning; indeed suctioning can be discontinued entirely for most patients.[5]

When mechanical insufflation-exsufflation is used via an oral-nasal interface, an abdominal thrust applied during the exsufflation cycle further increases peak cough flows and airway secretion expulsion.[2] Care must be taken not to apply abdominal thrusts to a full stomach. Although no medications are usually

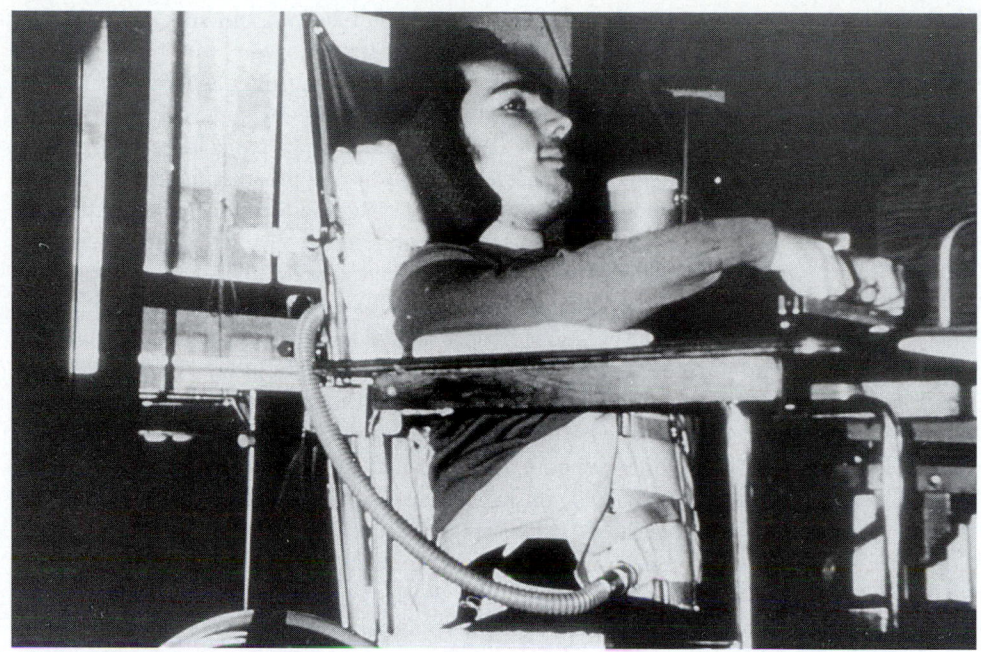

FIGURE 99-6 High-level spinal-cord-injured patient who used tracheostomy intermittent positive pressure ventilation 24 h a day for 2 years before switching to 24-h noninvasive aids. He used an intermittent abdominal pressure ventilator during daytime hours (seen here) and lipseal IPPV overnight.

required for effective MI-E, in neuromuscular ventilator users with respiratory tract infections, liquefaction of sputum using heated aerosol treatments can facilitate exsufflation when secretions are inspissated.

The efficacy of MI-E has been demonstrated both clinically and in animal models. Vital capacity, airflow rates, and arterial oxygenation, when abnormal, improve immediately with clearing of mucous plugs by MI-E.[2,11] Except for painful stretching of the rib cage musculature of patients receiving deep insufflations for the first time, and the appearance of bradycardias in acutely injured high-level spinal cord patients in spinal shock, no untoward effects have been reported in thousands of applications of MI-E.[2] It is not helpful when patients cannot cooperate sufficiently to keep the airway open, when there is a fixed upper airway obstruction, or when upper airway dilator muscles cannot maintain sufficient patency to allow for adequate expiratory flows.[25] These limitations are seen most often in advanced bulbar amyotrophic lateral sclerosis and severe spinal muscular atrophy patients.

Glossopharyngeal Breathing (GPB)

Both inspiratory and, indirectly, expiratory muscle function can be assisted by glossopharyngeal breathing. This technique, first recognized and described in the early 1950s as an aid for coughing,[7] involves the use of the tongue and pharyngeal muscles to add to an inspiratory effort by projecting (gulping) boluses of air past the glottis. The glottis closes with each gulp. One breath usually consists of 6 to 9 gulps of 60 to 200 ml each. It is important to monitor the efficacy of GPB during the training period by spirometry, measuring the milliliters of air per gulp, gulps per

breath, and breaths per minute. An excellent training video is available.[17]

Glossopharyngeal breathing is taught to patients with less than 1 L of vital capacity. Effectively used, it enables patients to attain maximum insufflations without the need for a blower or ventilator for air stacking. GPB can provide individuals without respiratory muscle function with normal alveolar ventilation for hours and perfect safety when not using a ventilator or in the event of sudden ventilator failure day or night.

Although severe oropharyngeal muscle weakness can limit the usefulness of GPB, some ventilator users with Duchenne muscular dystrophy have been able to use GPB successfully.[9] Approximately 60 percent of ventilator users who have no breathing ability while off the ventilator but who have good oropharyngeal muscle function can use GPB for ventilator-free breathing time.[4] Unfortunately, few health care professionals are familiar with the technique, and GPB is rarely useful in the presence of an indwelling tracheostomy tube. The safety and versatility afforded by effective GPB are key reasons to eliminate tracheostomy in favor of noninvasive aids.

RESPIRATORY MUSCLE ASSISTANCE PROTOCOLS

Patient evaluation includes assessment for symptoms of global alveolar hypoventilation, measurements of vital capacity (in sitting and recumbent positions), maximum insufflation capacity, peak cough flows unassisted and assisted, oxyhemaglobin saturation (Sa_{O_2}), and, at times, end-tidal CO_2 in the sitting and in recumbent positions. Symptoms can include daytime drowsiness, morning headaches, fatigue, impaired concentration, frequent sleep arousals, anxiety, and nightmares. Oxygen saturation is monitored overnight when any symptoms, daytime hypercapnia, or arterial hypoxemia are noted, or whenever the vital capacity is substantially less when supine or the patient is more short of breath when supine than when sitting. Arterial blood gases need not be evaluated in the stable patient. Nocturnal oximetry is done using an oximeter that collates the data hourly and prints it out in a form that is easy for quantitative comparisons. When arterial oxyhemoglobin desaturation is present in a patient who is suspected of hypoventilation and who is not troubled by airway secretions, the ability of the patient to normalize arterial oxygen saturations by voluntarily increasing ventilation is assessed. When airway secretions are present and assisted peak cough flows are marginal (3 to 4 L/s), airway secretion clearance is assisted with the use of MI-E. Vital capacity and arterial oxygenation should be observed to increase as bronchial mucous is eliminated by MI-E.

Prevention of Pulmonary Morbidity

Patients with less than 50 percent of predicted normal vital capacity, when measured sitting or supine, or with assisted peak cough flows that are less than 5 L/s, risk developing acute respiratory failure during intercurrent respiratory tract infections or any events that might tax respiratory musculature. Often such patients fail to wean from ventilators after surgical anesthesia.

Patients at risk for ventilatory failure are taught how to receive IPPV via mouthpieces and nasal interfaces. They are provided with a manual resuscitator and placed on a regimen of air-stacking exercises several times per day. They and their care providers are taught manually assisted coughing and mechanical insufflation-exsufflation. Patients also receive an oximeter and are instructed to monitor their SaO_2 during respiratory tract infections and any events which cause undue fatigue or shortness of breath. Whenever SaO_2 decreases below 95 percent, the patient is taught to consider the possibilities of artifact, the presence of alveolar hypoventilation, and bronchial mucous plugging. If hypoventilation and especially airway secretions are not managed in a timely manner with the use of respiratory muscle aids, a decrease in baseline SaO_2 below 92 percent often signals pneumonia or other acute pulmonary complications that necessitate hospitalization, oxygen therapy, and possibly intubation. Although it is common for the baseline SaO_2 of properly managed patients to decrease to 92 percent temporarily, particularly when febrile, pneumonia and gross atelectasis are rare, and hospitalization is only infrequently indicated irrespective of the extent of need for ventilatory support. Family members and personal care attendants invariably pay greater attention at home to the management of airway secretions and assisted coughing than do personnel in intensive care units.

Patients often require 24-h noninvasive IPPV during intercurrent respiratory tract infections and wean to nocturnal-only IPPV. Patients with few or minimal symptoms of alveolar hypoventilation often wish to discontinue nocturnal IPPV until the next acute event. Return of unaided nocturnal mean SaO_2 to 94 percent or greater generally indicates that IPPV can be safely discontinued. However, a mean nocturnal SaO_2 that is 2 to 3 percent higher when using IPPV than when sleeping unaided attests to the benefits of continuing nocturnal IPPV. The clinician should recognize that when discontinuing nocturnal IPPV, mean nocturnal SaO_2 can progressively decrease over a period of days to weeks, signaling the approach of respiratory failure.

Decannulation and Conversion to Noninvasive Respiratory Aids

When converting patients from tracheostomy to noninvasive IPPV, the vital capacity and ability to breathe are not crucial. However, assisted peak cough flows must exceed 3 L/s. A cuffed, fenestrated tracheostomy tube is placed (the cuff is needed for MI-E), and the patient practices receiving IPPV via a mouthpiece or nasal interface. Once adept at mouthpiece IPPV, a tracheostomy button can be placed and assisted peak cough flows assessed with the patient using mouthpiece IPPV. If assisted peak cough flows cannot exceed 3 L/s with the site buttoned, the tracheostomy tube should not be removed.[3]

The most difficult task of transition from tracheostomy to noninvasive IPPV is facilitating tracheostomy site closure while providing effective IPPV. Soft silicon ovals are commercially available that, when used with figure-of-eight dressings, cover the site while minimizing the need for taping the skin.[4] Although negative pressure body ventilators can be used as a bridge to ventilate the patient's lungs until the tracheostomy site closes, patients are now decannulated and converted directly to noninvasive IPPV. The tracheostomy site usually closes in 24 to 78 h. If not closed after 7 days, the site is sutured closed. Although noninvasive IPPV is the predominant method of ventilatory support, patients with little vital capacity may decide to use an IAPV for daytime support. Once the tracheostomy site is closed, peak cough flows can be measured more accurately, and the patient is taught glossopharyngeal breathing.

Because patients who transfer from invasive to noninvasive IPPV invariably prefer the latter for safety, convenience, comfort, improved speech, swallowing, sleep, appearance, and overall,[1] it might be argued that every ventilator user with neuromuscular disease and greater than 3 L/s of peak cough flow should be transferred to noninvasive aids. In practice, however, only patients who are good candidates for learning glossopharyngeal breathing should be transferred to noninvasive IPPV. Patients with very weak oropharyngeal musculature should only be transferred when they have had serious difficulties with their tracheostomy tubes. Thus, the majority of ventilator users with spinal cord injury, postpoliomyelitis, and non-Duchenne myopathies should be switched to noninvasive inspiratory aids as part of routine rehabilitation procedure.

REFERENCES

1. Bach JR: A comparison of long-term ventilatory support alternatives from the perspective of the patient and care giver. *Chest* 104:1702–1706, 1993.
2. Bach JR: Update and perspectives on noninvasive respiratory muscle aids: Part 2—the expiratory muscle aids. *Chest* 105:1538–1544, 1994.
3. Bach JR: Amyotrophic lateral sclerosis: predictors for prolongation of life by noninvasive respiratory aids. *Arch Phys Med Rehabil* 76:828–832, 1995.
4. Bach JR: Prevention of morbidity and mortality with the use of physical medicine aids, in Bach JR (ed), *Pulmonary Rehabilitation: The Obstructive and Paralytic Conditions.* Philadelphia, Hanley & Belfus, 1996, pp 303–329.
5. Bach JR: Illustrative case studies of respiratory management, in Bach JR (ed), *Pulmonary Rehabilitation: The Obstructive and Paralytic Conditions.* Philadelphia, Hanley & Belfus, 1996, pp 331–346.
6. Bach JR, Alba AS: Total ventilatory support by the intermittent abdominal pressure ventilator. *Chest* 99:630–636, 1991.
7. Bach JR, Alba AS, Saporito LR: Intermittent positive pressure ventilation via the mouth as an alternative to tracheostomy for 257 ventilator users. *Chest* 103:174–182, 1993.
8. Bach JR, Robert D, Leger P, Langevin B: Sleep fragmentation in kyphoscoliotic individuals with alveolar hypoventilation treated by nasal IPPV. *Chest* 107:1552–1558, 1995.

9. Baydur A, Gilgoff I, Prentice W, et al: Decline in respiratory function and experience with long-term assisted ventilation in advanced Duchenne's muscular dystrophy. *Chest* 97:884–889, 1990.

10. Begin P, Grassino A: Inspiratory muscle dysfunction and chronic hypercapnia in chronic obstructive pulmonary disease. *Am Rev Respir Dis* 143:905–912, 1983.

11. Bickerman HA: Exsufflation with negative pressure: elimination of radiopaque material and foreign bodies from bronchi of anesthetized dogs. *Arch Int Med* 93:698–704, 1954.

12. Boushy SF, Thompson HK Jr, North LB, et al: Prognosis in chronic obstructive pulmonary disease. *Am Rev Respir Dis* 108:1373–1383, 1973.

13. Braun NMT, Arora MS, Rochester DF: Respiratory muscle and pulmonary function in polymyositis and other proximal myopathies. *Thorax* 38:616–623, 1983.

14. Canny GJ, Szeinberg A, Koreska J, Levison H: Hypercapnia in relation to pulmonary function in Duchenne muscular dystrophy. *Pediatr Pulmonol* 6:169–171, 1989.

15. Chailleux E, Fauroux B, Binet F, et al: Predictors of survival in patients receiving domiciliary oxygen therapy or mechanical ventilation: A 10-year analysis of ANTADIR Observatory. *Chest* 109:741–749, 1996.

16. Corrado A, Gorini M, De Paola E: Alternative techniques for managing acute neuromuscular respiratory failure. *Semin Neurol* 15:84–89, 1995.

17. Dail CW, Affeldt JE: Glossopharyngeal breathing [video]. Los Angeles, Department of Visual Education, College of Medical Evangelists, 1954.

18. De Troyer A, Deisser P: The effects of intermittent positive pressure breathing on patients with respiratory muscle weakness. *Am Rev Respir Dis* 124:132–137, 1981.

19. Ellis ER, Bye PTP, Bruderer JW, Sullivan CE: Treatment of respiratory failure during sleep in patients with neuromuscular disease, positive-pressure ventilation through a nose mask. *Am Rev Respir Dis* 135:148–152, 1987.

20. Esau SA: The effect of theophylline on hypoxic, hypercapnic hamster diaphragm muscle in vitro. *Am Rev Respir Dis* 143:954–959, 1991.

21. Estenne M, De Troyer A: The effects of tetraplegia on chest wall statics. *Am Rev Respir Dis* 134:121–124, 1986.

22. Goldstein RS, Molotiu N, Skrastins R, et al: Assisting ventilation in respiratory failure by negative pressure ventilation and by rocking bed. *Chest* 92:470–474, 1987.

23. Griggs RG, Donohoe KM, Utell MJ, et al: Evaluation of pulmonary function in neuromuscular disease. *Arch Neurol* 38:9–12, 1981.

24. Inkley SR, Oldenburg FC, Vignos PJ Jr: Pulmonary function in Duchenne muscular dystrophy related to stage of disease. *Am J Med* 56:297–306, 1974.

25. Juan G, Calverley P, Talamo C: Effect of carbon dioxide on diaphragmatic function in human beings. *New Engl J Med* 310:874–879, 1984.

26. Kobavashi I, Perry A, Rhymer J, et al: Relationships between the electrical activity of genioglossus muscle and the upper airway patency: A study in laryngectomised subjects. *Respir Crit Care Med* 149:A148, 1994.

27. Leger P, Jennequin J, Gerard M, Robert D: Home positive pressure ventilation via nasal mask for patients with neuromuscular weakness or restrictive lung or chest-wall disease. *Respir Care* 34:73–79, 1989.

28. Leith DE: Lung biology in health and disease: Respiratory defense mechanisms, part 2, in Brian JD, Proctor D, Reid L (eds), *Cough.* New York, Dekker, 1977, pp 545–592.

29. Massery M: Manual breathing and coughing aids. *Phys Med Rehabil Clin N Am* 7:407–422, 1996.

30. McDermott I, Bach JR, Parker C, Sortor S: Custom-fabricated interfaces for intermittent positive pressure ventilation. *Int J Prosthodont* 2:224–233, 1989.

31. Mier-Jedrzejowicz A, Brophy C, Green M: Respiratory muscle weakness during upper respiratory tract infections. *Am Rev Respir Dis* 138:5–7, 1988.

32. Miller WF: Rehabilitation of patients with chronic obstructive lung disease. *Med Clin N Am* 51:349–361, 1967.

33. Moxham J: Aminophylline and the respiratory muscles: An alternative view. *Clin Chest Med* 9:325–336, 1988.

34. Ohtake S: Nocturnal blood gas disturbances and treatment of patients with Duchenne muscular dystrophy. *Kokyu To Junkan* 38:463–469, 1990.

35. Redding GJ, Okamoto GA, Guthrie RD, et al: Sleep patterns in nonambulatory boys with Duchenne muscular dystrophy. *Arch Phys Med Rehabil* 66:818–821, 1985.

36. Rochester DF, Braun NMT: Determinants of maximal inspiratory pressure in chronic obstructive pulmonary disease. *Am Rev Respir Dis* 132:42–47, 1985.

37. Smith PEM, Edwards RHT, Calverley PMA: Ventilation and breathing pattern during sleep in Duchenne muscular dystrophy. *Chest* 96:1346–1351, 1989.

38. Smith PEM, Edwards RHT, Calverley PMA: Oxygen treatment of sleep hypoxemia in Duchenne muscular dystrophy. *Thorax* 44:997–1001, 1989.

PART THIRTEEN

SLEEP AND SLEEP DISORDERS

CHAPTER 100

THE STAGES OF SLEEP

Adrian R. Morrison

WHAT IS SLEEP?

WHY SLEEP?

AUTONOMIC REGULATION DURING SLEEP

ANATOMIC SUBSTRATE AND PHYSIOLOGICAL
 MECHANISMS OF SLEEP

THE NATURE OF REM

Approximately 45 years ago, two reports published within a few years of each other revolutionized our thinking about sleep and wakefulness. In 1949, Moruzzi and Magoun[30] reasoned, on the basis of results with electrical stimulation of the brainstem, that its central core, the reticular formation, contained the elements essential for arousal and, consequently, wakefulness (Fig. 100-1). Previously the view had been that various stimuli operated on the cerebrum via the "classic" long sensory pathways to arouse the individual. Moruzzi and Magoun recognized that the multisynaptic complexity of the reticular formation lay at the heart of consciousness.

Nonetheless, the idea persisted, until 4 years later, that only wakefulness required active participation of the nervous system. At that time, Aserinsky and Kleitman[2] reported periods during sleep in which the EEG resembled that of wakefulness. They also observed the rapid eye movements that give this stage of sleep its name, rapid-eye-movement (REM) sleep, and reported that vivid dreams occurred then. Clearly, more than a simple withdrawal of sensory influences had to be involved in the changes from wakefulness to sleep. As a result of this insight, the dominant view of sleep shifted from regarding it as a *passive* process to the belief in *active* processes that still prevails. Kleitman had previously been a proponent of the earlier view, arguing that it was the mechanism of wakefulness, not sleep, that required explanation.

Sleep disorders medicine began to emerge as a clinical specialty just a generation ago. Thanks to the earlier recognition of the "curious" state of REM and then a considerable amount of basic research aimed at unraveling its mechanisms and those of sleep in general, various medical specialities began to recognize that serious disease can accompany this seemingly peaceful portion of daily life. Previously, sleep was almost exclusively an interest of psychiatrists. Of course, pulmonary physicians now play a major role in sleep disorders medicine.

This chapter focuses on the mechanisms underlying the daily alternation of sleep and wakefulness. Emphasis is placed on emerging ideas about the organization of a largely hidden portion of our lives, particularly ideas that push us beyond conventional thought. Physician readers of this chapter should keep in mind the tremendous debt that sleep disorders medicine owes to animal-based research and that such research has been a particular target of animal rights activism.[27a]

WHAT IS SLEEP?

Sleep is a period of bodily rest characterized by reduced awareness of the environment, a species-specific posture, and for most species, a particular sleep place. During each period of sleep, mammals cycle between two phases, non–rapid-eye-movement (NREM) sleep and REM, with NREM always preceding a bout of REM. In humans, the cycle length averages 90 min, although NREM and REM are not evenly distributed through the night[8] (Fig. 100-2). Cycle length varies directly with brain weight; hence, the family dog or cat cycles between NREM and REM more frequently, about every 25 min, as well as having multiple sleep periods.[50]

The physiological characteristics of the two phases of sleep are dramatically different. Figure 100-3 illustrates the appearance of the human electroencephalogram (EEG) during the four stages of NREM in which there are lower-frequency EEG waves than in wakefulness. In other mammals, NREM is not as well individuated into different stages, but the largest-amplitude, lowest-frequency waves occur as the animal approaches REM (Fig. 100-4C). A most striking feature is the similarity in appearance of the waking and the REM EEG patterns in humans and animals: low-amplitude, high-frequency waves (Fig. 100-4A and D).

Another event that characterizes REM can be detected in animals with deeply implanted electrodes. Just before and during REM, large-amplitude waves appear in recordings from the lateral geniculate body (Fig. 100-4C and D). They are termed ponto-geniculo-occipital (PGO) waves, after the sites in which they were first recorded. Rather than being part of a REM-generating mechanism, as first thought, they appear to be another sign of the "peculiar" brain alertness that is an essential feature of REM.[26] These waves are discussed further below, under "The Nature of REM."

Behaviorally, REM is recognized by body twitches, rapid eye movements, and irregularity in rate and depth of respiration. Electromyographic (EMG) recordings of postural muscles reveal a striking generalized atonia, the result of the postsynaptic inhibition of spinal motor neurons.[9] Excitatory barrages briefly overcome this inhibition, leading to the muscle twitches. In contrast, NREM is characterized by behavioral quiescence with residual

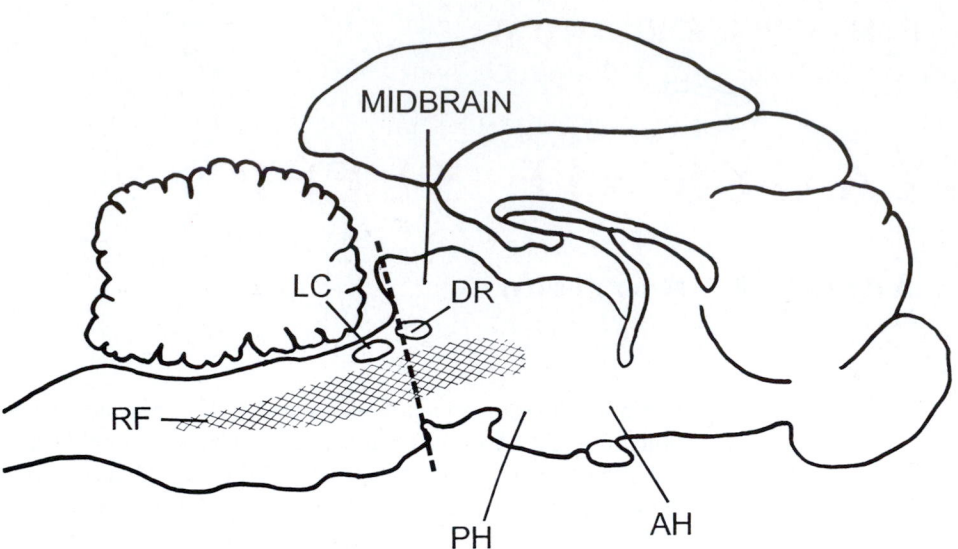

FIGURE 100-1 Diagrammatic representation of structures that may be key to sleep regulation. The interrupted line marks the level of decerebration that still permits expression of all the peripheral aspects of REM. The locus ceruleus (LC) actually lies laterally in the pons, while the dorsal raphe nuclei (DR) are midline structures. AH = anterior hypothalamus; PH = posterior hypothalamus; RF = reticular formation. *(From Morrison,[27] with permission.)*

muscle tone and very regular, deep breathing. A further distinction is a marked suppression of hypothalamic regulation of homeostasis in REM[35] (see "Autonomic Regulation during Sleep," below).

Many aspects of sleep have been experimentally manipulated in animals (cats and rats in particular), with the result that we have a much greater understanding of the mechanisms that might be altered in human sleep pathology now than we did even 20 years ago. Currently, there are two naturally occurring animal models under study: obstructive sleep apnea in the English bulldog[13] and narcolepsy in Doberman pinschers.[31] Also, an experimental animal preparation (see "The Nature of REM," below) led to the discovery of REM behavior disorder, which is characterized by REM episodes in which patients express their dreams physically.[42]

Birds also exhibit brief periods of REM as well as NREM. Evidence for REM in other classes of vertebrates is not as clear. A feature linking birds and mammals is their homeothermy. Because hypothalamic control of thermoregulation is suspended in REM, converting mammals briefly into "poikilotherms," it may be that poikilotherms (i.e., fish, amphibians, and reptiles), do not have the means or the "need" to express this or other features of REM.

The echidna, which is a nonplacental, nonmarsupial mammal (a monotreme), has always complicated the picture, because in it no evidence for REM could be found. Recently, Siegel et al.[43] found that the echidna's brainstem neural activity presented a composite picture of the two phases during sleep: that is, the decreased discharge rate of NREM and the increased variability of firing rate of REM were accompanied by EEG synchronization. Thus, NREM and REM may have differentiated later from this primordial state in mammals.

Just as sleep is not uniform among different groups of animals, its characteristics also vary with age. Human infants, for example, sleep in a polyphasic pattern for much of the time. During the first year of life, their sleep consolidates into one major period with shorter naps. In parallel fashion, REM, which occupies a large portion of sleep at birth—as much as 90 percent in some species—decreases to about 25 percent of total sleep time as wakefulness increases with maturity. This percentage remains relatively constant into old age, although the total amount of sleep decreases.[8] However, because neural activity in infant animal sleep resembles that of the undifferentiated sleep state of the primitive echidna,[43] we may question whether it is appropriate to speak of a very high REM percentage in newborns.

WHY SLEEP?

Unlike other behaviors, the actual function of sleep remains a subject for debate. Thinking in broad terms, some have suggested that energy is saved when an animal has nothing better to do or that there is a survival value for certain prey species to nestle out of harm's way. Other aspects of life to which sleep contributes, according to some, are consolidation of memory and improved learning. Of course, one feels better or restored after a night's sleep. But what has been "restored," and how?

A possible way out of the dilemma would be to focus on sleep not as a *be-*

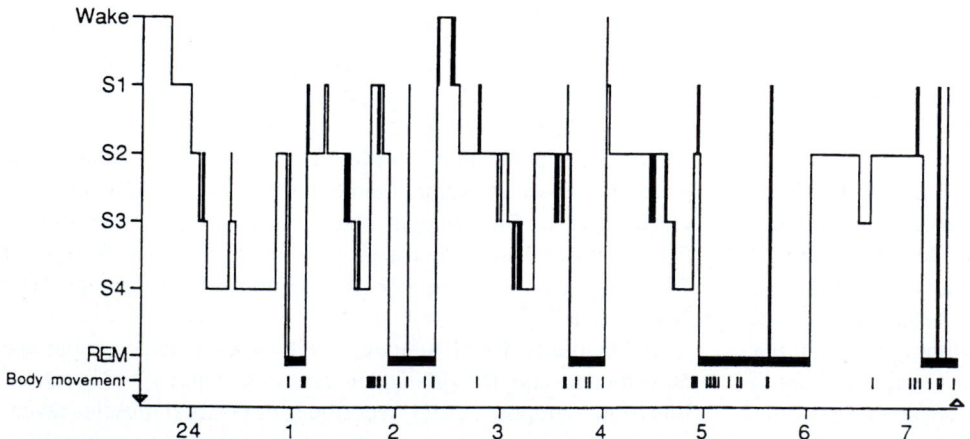

FIGURE 100-2 The progression of sleep stages across a single night's sleep of a normal young adult. The histogram was drawn on the basis of continuous recordings scored in 30-s epochs. *(From Carskadon and Dement,[8] with permission.)*

havior (like feeding, which happens only during wakefulness), but as a *state* that can subserve multiple functions (just as the waking state does). Indeed, the dramatic physiological differences between NREM and REM suggest this, and the many theories of the function of sleep tacitly acknowledge the idea: they generally present a hypothesis accounting for only one phase. For example, a recent well-supported, well-reasoned theory posits that NREM is essential for replenishment of cerebral glycogen stores, although some less efficient restoration may occur in REM.[7] Likewise, another tightly constructed theory, in this case for REM, notes that noradrenergic neurons become progressively inactive in sleep and are totally silent during REM. Because noradrenaline serves the important role of improving the efficacy of transmission at synapses where it coexists with other transmitters, REM would function to allow restoration of depleted noradrenergic receptors.[44]

Returning to a larger theme, the survival value of a stage of sleep,

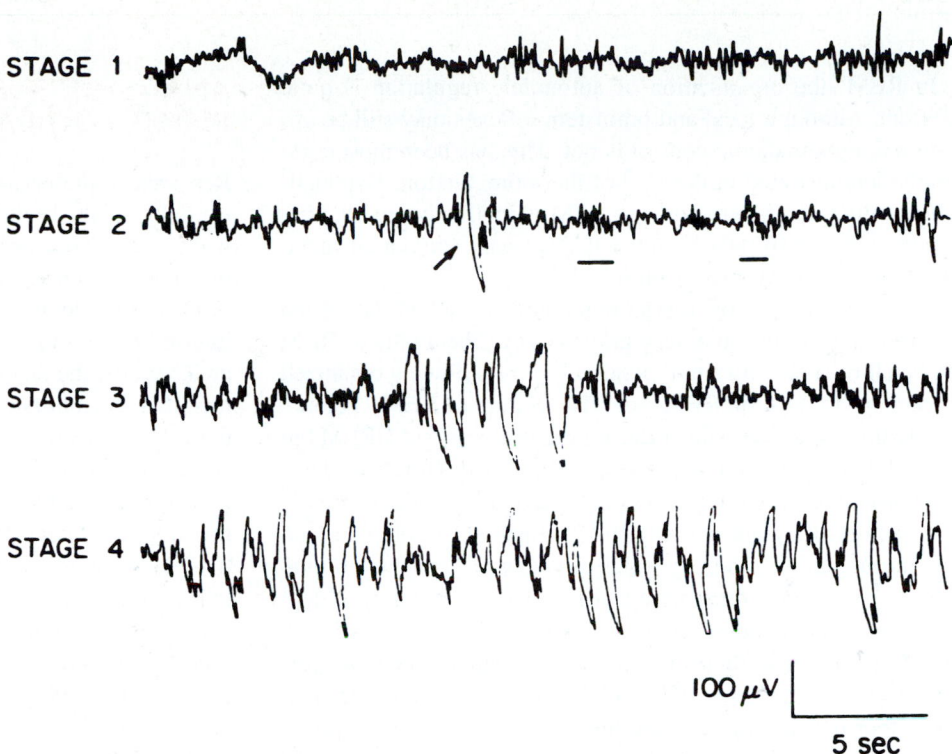

FIGURE 100-3 Electroencephalographic tracings recorded from a normal young adult demonstrating the four stages of NREM sleep. In the stage 2 recording, the arrow points to a characteristic K complex and the underlining to sleep spindles. *(From Carskadon and Dement,[8] with permission.)*

REM, in which an animal is depressed sensorially, paralyzed, and poorly regulated homeostatically remains to be explained. Although humans on antidepressant medication can go without REM for extended periods without severe physiological changes, rats die after several weeks of near-total REM deprivation and within 3 weeks of near-total sleep deprivation. They are hypothermic and eat more yet lose weight.[39] The reduced homeostatic regulation of normal REM may rest vital, undetermined processes in small animals.

AUTONOMIC REGULATION DURING SLEEP

Pulmonologists will be particularly interested that two major changes in autonomic regulation occur during sleep. One of them is predictable or at least not surprising: an increase in parasympathetic activity over that in the sympathetic system. The second is truly remarkable, though: suppression if not abolition of homeostatic regulation by the hypothalamus in REM.[35]

When an animal passes from wakefulness to NREM, the metabolic and behavioral demands on the body are obviously reduced. The heartbeat becomes slower and more regular. This is one sign that parasympathetic tone has increased; cutting the sympathetic nerves to the

heart has little effect, indicating that central parasympathetic neurons increase their activity in sleep.[5] Respiration slows and becomes more regular in NREM, but the normal compensatory mechanisms remain unchanged other than a moderate reduction in sensitivity to CO_2 and O_2. Normal thermoregulatory mechanism—such as panting, shivering and appropriate vascular changes—occur as well.[35]

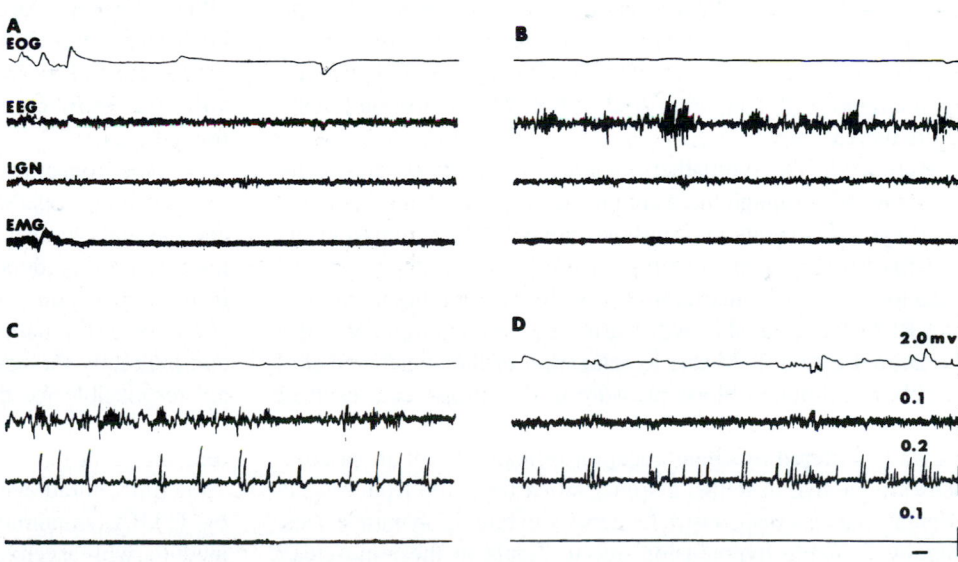

FIGURE 100-4 Characteristics of the states of sleep in the cat: *A.* Quiet wakefulness. *B.* NREM. *C.* Transition to REM. *D.* REM. EOG = eye movements; EEG = electroencephalogram; LGN = recordings of spontaneous PGO waves in the lateral geniculate body in *(C)* and *(D)*; EMG = electromyographic recordings in the dorsal cervical muscles. Note the decreasing muscle tone at the end of the transition period and throughout REM. Time = 1 s. *(From Morrison,[26] with permission.)*

In REM, the organization of autonomic regulation is quite different. Although local and brainstem reflexes may still be operational, hypothalamic control is not. This has been most completely demonstrated in the case of thermoregulation. Hypothalamic cooling and heating during REM is ineffective in eliciting responses normally associated with heat gain (increased metabolic rate) and heat loss (panting).[10,34]

The suppression of thermoregulation in REM has been demonstrated further in a very graphic way. The atonia of REM can be eliminated with small pontine lesions, allowing organized movements to occur in REM (see "The Nature of REM," below). Cats with such lesions shiver during wakefulness and NREM but cease shivering as soon as they enter REM without atonia. They also leave their protective curled posture and lose piloerection.[12] Furthermore, they are actually more sensitive to cold and heat than normal animals during wakefulness, which further emphasizes the disruption of thermoregulation that occurs during REM.[1]

These indirect measures have been supplemented by direct recordings of single thermosensitive hypothalamic neurons during different behavioral states. Cold- and warm-sensitive neurons either increase or decrease their rate of firing as a response to hypothalamic cooling or warming during wakefulness and NREM, but the majority lose their sensitivity in REM.[32] Thus, the preoptic hypothalamic drive of thermoregulatory effectors is lost in REM.

Alterations in respiratory control occur during REM, and there is evidence that the hypothalamus no longer modulates lower reflexes. Electrical stimulation in the hypothalamus that elicits inflation- and deflationlike effects during wakefulness and NREM will no longer do so in REM; in contrast, vagal stimulation remains effective, indicating that the brainstem circuits are not altered in REM.[33] Tone in upper airway muscles is diminished during NREM and virtually absent during REM; the atonia during REM of the upper airway and intercostal muscles imposes a considerable burden on respiration. The respiratory rhythm is disrupted by irregularities in rate and depth of respiration due to the excitatory barrages responsible for muscle twitches in postural muscles. Ventilatory responses to hypercapnia are depressed, and, compared to NREM, the arousal threshold is increased.[35]

Activity in the sympathetic nerves of cats drops drastically during REM, although there are phasic increases that accompany rapid eye movements and muscle twitches.[6] As a consequence, paradoxical responses in skin temperature occur, due to passive reductions in vasoconstrictor or vasodilator tone upon entrance into REM (e.g., the skin will warm in a cool environment after the animal enters REM due to relaxation of the constricted skin vessels).[36] Although blood pressure in cats drops as a result of bradycardia and vasodilation in the gastrointestinal beds, the decrease is buffered by chemoreceptor reflexes.[11] Not all vascular beds are passive in REM: a spinal reflex triggered from muscle afferents induces vasoconstrictor activity in hind-limb muscle beds, thereby reducing hypotension due to atonia in these muscles.[3]

Blood pressure increases during REM in rats and humans. In the former, this increase is a consequence of an increase in the sensitivity of the baroreceptor reflex; a similar mechanism has been invoked to account for the pressor response in humans as well. Heart rate sometimes increases in humans.[21]

ANATOMIC SUBSTRATE AND PHYSIOLOGICAL MECHANISMS OF SLEEP

Research in the earlier part of this century pointed to the diencephalon as the region critical for the organization of the sleep-wake cycle. This view was supported by (1) the association of insomnia or somnolence with pathological changes in the anterior or posterior hypothalamus after encephalitis in humans, (2) elicitation of sleep in cats by electrical stimulation of the preoptic area, and (3) the results of experimental hypothalamic lesions in rats that corroborated the human disease observations.[48] Yet until the discovery of REM, the prevailing opinion pictured sensory inflow as the governing factor.

In 1962, emphasis shifted to the hindbrain because of an important experiment designed to determine the area of the brain that plays the predominant role in REM regulation. Jouvet found that even after removal of the brain rostral to the pons (i.e., decerebration), major elements of REM continued to appear periodically; indeed, rapid eye movements and atonia even overcame decerebrate rigidity. Transection caudal to the pons eliminated all signs of REM.

An additional discovery, the identification of neurons using serotonin (the dorsal raphe nucleus) or noradrenaline (the locus ceruleus) as transmitters with widespread connections extending to the cerebral cortex, further focused attention on the pons as the key region for regulating all of sleep. A series of experiments involving destruction of these neurons and/or pharmacological manipulations led to the hypothesis that serotonin regulates NREM and noradrenaline, REM.[18] Although the monoamine hypothesis of sleep regulation stimulated a number of important experiments, it eventually had to be abandoned because recordings of serotonergic and noradrenergic neurons revealed that these neurons begin to reduce their firing rates when cats pass from wakefulness to NREM, becoming almost totally inactive during REM.[24] Thus, their roles can only be permissive (i.e., allowing REM to occur as a result of their inactivity). There is, however, the possibility (probability in my view) that the changes are an effect of more complex processes leading to sleep that involve the rostral brain, and we shall shortly consider the reasons for thinking so.

Another transmitter, acetylcholine, clearly plays an active role in REM processes. Many studies have demonstrated that acetylcholine and agonists (e.g., carbachol), will induce REM when injected into the dorsal pons.[23] A cluster of cholinergic neurons in the dorsal pons and midbrain are the natural source of the cholinergic stimulation. Two effects are clear: they excite directly and indirectly the neurons in the medullary inhibitory area that are responsible for the postsynaptic inhibition of spinal motor neurons in REM,[9] and they induce the changes in thalamic neurons that contribute to the waking pattern of the EEG.[46] At the same time, noradrenergic and serotonergic neurons are inhibited by GABA-containing neurons.[23] Cholinergic neurons in the medulla with ascending projections also appear to play a facilitatory role in the generation of REM.[15]

Cholinergic stimulation of thalamocortical neurons by mesopontine cholinergic cells changes them from the burst-firing mode that underlies the EEG spindles and slow waves characterizing NREM to a tonic-firing mode with an increased transfer function. Cholinergic neurons in the basal forebrain play a parallel role in the cortex. Evidence is also mounting that glutamatergic systems play a parallel role in EEG activation.[46] Because noradrenergic neurons in the pontine locus ceruleus also change the firing mode of thalamocortical neurons in parallel with the nearby mesopontine cholinergic neurons and glutamatergic neurons,[46] their silence in REM is possibly an important feature distinguishing mental activity of wakefulness from REM. In terms of maintaining wakefulness and counteracting sleep-promoting activity of the anterior hypothalamus, histaminergic projections from the posterior hypothalamus may play a significant role.[20]

Although EEG patterns allow us to detect the various sleep stages, they do not as accurately reflect the type of mental activity occurring during sleep as some still present it. Initially, REM was equated with "dream sleep," and many still accept this convenient distinction. The similarity of the REM EEG pattern to that of wakefulness and the vividness of REM dreams (bizarre, perhaps, but still wakinglike) make this a tidy classification. Unfortunately (for the sake of simplicity), mental activity is frequently reported from NREM awakenings, and it can resemble REM dreams, although REM and NREM mental activity can be discriminated on the basis of perceptual vividness and thematic coherence. (The earliest experiments finding few or no dreams in reports from NREM awakenings were designed in ways that were biased against collection of NREM dreams.) Furthermore, stage 1 NREM and REM have similar EEG patterns, yet reports of mental activity are quite different.[38]

The elements within the various patterns of neural activity underlying the dramatically different EEG patterns of NREM and REM that determine dreaming in humans remain uncertain.[37] A recent candidate is the fast, spontaneous EEG rhythm between 20 and 40 Hz observed during attentive waking behavior and REM and also during the depolarizing phases of slow brainwave oscillations occurring in NREM.[47] Because the mesopontine cholinergic neurons that induce fast rhythms are spontaneously active in REM and are responsible for PGO waves (a sign of alerting, remember), they may provide the conditions that make the REM dream invariably vivid. However, the dangers of relating specific electrophysiological events to complex mental activities should be obvious.

How the caudal brainstem cholinergic neurons normally "affect" the expression of REM is not known. At first blush, they do not seem to require the rostral brain: decerebrate cats spontaneously exhibit REM atonia and the pontine component of PGO waves,[17] and carbachol injection is also effective in decerebrate cats.[9] Absence of noradrenaline must be a factor, because noradrenergic blockers will also induce the REM state in the same way that cholinergic agonists do.[49] A reduction of serotonergic influence is likely a factor as well.

The forebrain is, of course, involved in sleep regulation, as the early work indicated. Many lesion, stimulation and unit recording studies in the basal forebrain have demonstrated its importance for the onset of sleep (i.e., NREM).[24,48] The suprachiasmatic nucleus has a role in the timing of sleep occurrence.[25] But is there a greater role for the forebrain in REM initiation than current wisdom, based on early decerebration experiments, dictates? Two observations led us to propose that the initiation

of REM in *intact* animals might well require interactions among fore- and hindbrain mechanisms:[28] (1) Decerebrate cats can be induced to enter a REM-like state by a number of stimuli not normally sleep-promoting, such as passing a stomach tube, inserting a rectal probe, opening the mouth, and hypothermia.[17,19] Consequently, the brainstem, lacking modulation by rostral structures, appears to be in an unstable, supersensitive state. (2) In the normal cat, homeostatic mechanisms usually regulated by the hypothalamus are suppressed during REM,[35] and the same could be argued for the decerebrate cat. Clearly, a central reorganization in the hypothalamus and/or other rostral structures must take place at or before the transition from non-REM to REM. Given the decerebrate cat's abnormal propensity to enter REM, midbrain transection might well serve as a substitute for the suppression of forebrain control that we argue precedes natural REM.

These ideas do not deny the important role played in REM by the caudal brainstem but imply that full understanding of the mechanisms initiating and maintaining REM requires a more global outlook. Indeed, recent investigations have revealed interesting effects of forebrain manipulations of REM. Simultaneous infusion of carbachol into cholinoceptive regions of the basal forebrain and the pons significantly reduced the ability of the latter to generate a REM-like state.[4] Further, the posterior hypothalamus influences the generation of REM via descending neural pathways; ibotenic acid lesions induced a 300 percent increase in REM during the first postinjection day and released the same reflex-induced episodes seen after decerebration.[40] A selective enhancement of REM for several days (more episodes rather than lengthened episodes) follows bilateral ibotenic acid lesions of the thalamic nucleus centralis lateralis.[22] And infusion of serotonin into the amygdala will cause a change of state or arousal in significantly more trials in REM compared to NREM.[41]

In concluding this section, it should be noted that rarely, if ever, have workers considered the possibility that sleep changes after various manipulations might be secondary to changes in thermosensitivity, other sensory thresholds, blood gases, etc.

THE NATURE OF REM

Earlier, we observed that a variety of answers have been proposed for the question "What does REM do for the individual?" But no one asks "Why does REM occur in the form that it does?" In other words, can one make physiological sense out of the characteristics observed or is there no coherent organization? As a seemingly disparate assemblage, one finds the REM EEG resembling the waking EEG: the almost total paralysis, the ineffectual muscle twitches, the rapid eye movements, and, of course, the depression of homeostasis. A mechanistic explanation brings order out of this assortment and also leads to a broader view of the pontine tegmentum, a region that has assumed so much importance in sleep research.

The premise is that the brain in REM resembles to a surprising degree the brain of an individual during alert wakefulness when he or she orients to a novel or unexpected stimulus.[26] From this point of view one can begin to make sense of the apparently unrelated features of REM—in particular, the reticular activation, the atonia, and the depressed homeostasis.

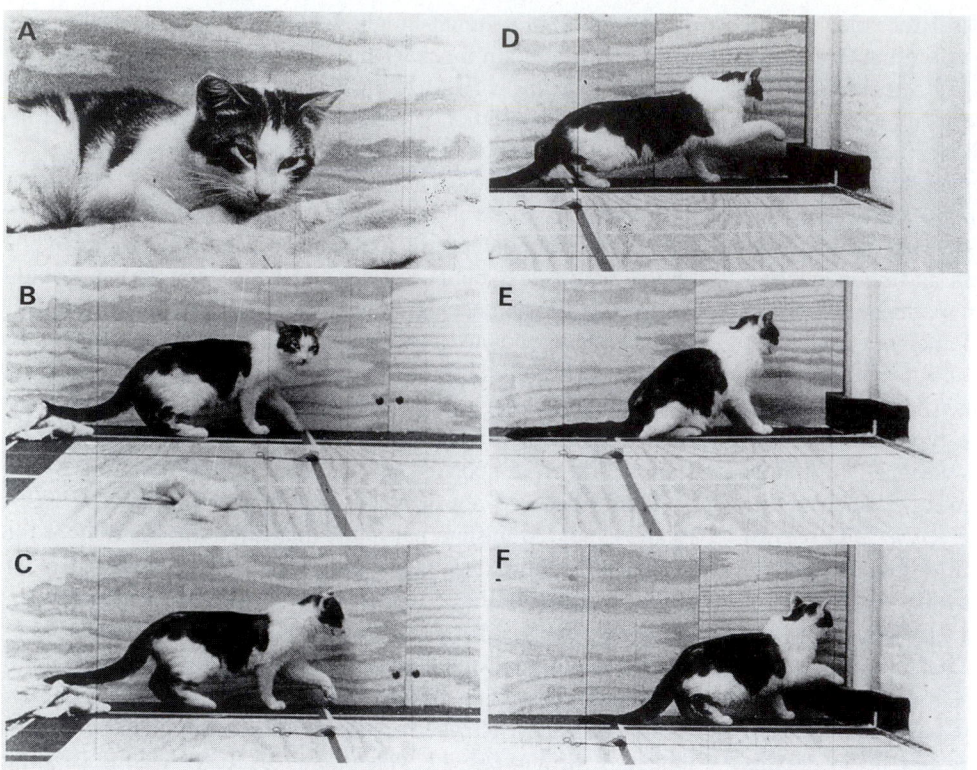

FIGURE 100-5   Film sequence of behavior during one episode of REM without atonia. Note the relaxed nictitating membranes in the eyes in the enlargement in (*A*). Hindlimb and axial support was not as good as when the cat was awake. (*From Hendricks et al.,*[14] *with permission.*)

duced by auditory stimuli or electrical stimulation of the reticular formation.[16] Their occurrence is associated with an increase in information transfer through the lateral geniculate body.

Taken together, these observations support the concept of an "alert" brain in REM. This counterintuitive idea becomes less so if one is open to the suggestion that in REM, the brain is focused upon itself and the world of dreams. Interestingly, though, cats show the same degree of orientation to an external sound source in REM without atonia as they do when awake.[29]

In addition, we have proposed a linkage between the "alert" brain and atonia in REM on the basis of a behavioral observation and a concept:[28] the observation is that when an awake animal orients to an unexpected stimulus its ongoing behavior ceases for an instant; the concept is that nature is a parsimonious organizer, very often using the same structures and mechanisms in slightly different ways for various tasks. The respiratory system is a good example of the latter, for the airway and lungs are used for respiration, phonation, and temperature regulation.

Therefore, the extreme motor inhibition in REM can be explained in a mechanical way as an inevitable link between an exaggerated, continuing state of "orienting" and the suppression of motor activity. Moreover, the brain seems to employ the same structures and mechanisms in both wakefulness and REM, but not identically, of course (Fig. 100-6). Rather than global activation during alert wakefulness, one should see in the dorsal pontine tegmentum selective activation of neurons associated with specific movements, not driving them but modulating the set of muscle contractions and relaxations for movement from any posture in response to a sudden stimulus. There are, in fact, such neurons.[45] Thus, the dorsal pons, the focus of so much attention from sleep researchers, is probably more generally involved in any behaviors dependent upon abrupt input into the reticular formation.

To begin with, certain features are common to REM and alert wakefulness: the EEG pattern; synchronous waves recorded from the hippocampus, called theta rhythm; an increase in brain temperature during orienting and REM; and suppression of panting and shivering in both states. Two additional observations made in the laboratory reinforce this line of reasoning.

1. As briefly noted above, the atonia of REM can be eliminated in cats by small lesions in the pontine tegmentum that destroy a complex of cells and fibers that normally excite the medullary inhibitory area of cats.[14,18] In such animals, behavior during REM consists largely of orienting, searching, or startle unassociated with any obvious external stimuli. Depending on lesion site,[14] some cats can even walk during "REM without atonia," although their axial and hindlimb support does not equal that of waking (Fig. 100-5). REM without atonia completely replaces normal REM—permanently in some cases; while in others there is gradual recovery to a more normal-appearing REM. Other than the lack of skeletal muscle paralysis, REM without atonia is identical to normal REM.

2. The PGO waves that normally appear spontaneously just prior to and throughout REM in recordings from the lateral geniculate body of cats can be elicited by loud sounds in NREM and REM.[26] These waves will occur in wakefulness after stimulation with sound, and others have recently reported that intracellular recordings from geniculate neurons are the same during the spontaneous waves and those in-

WAKEFULNESS

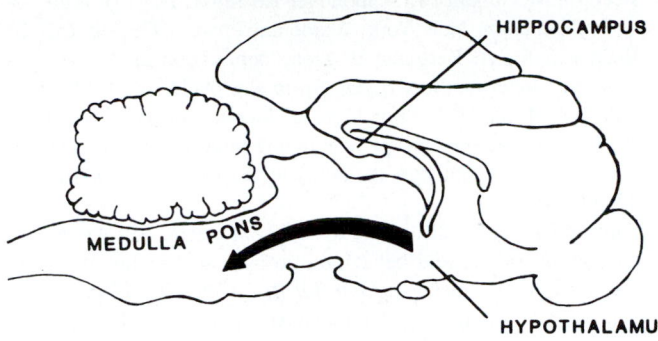

NREM SLEEP

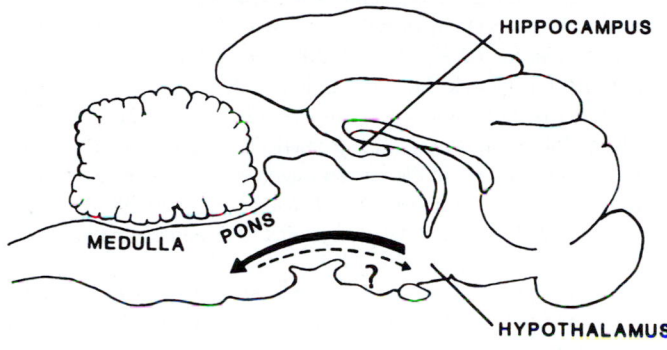

REM SLEEP AND ORIENTING

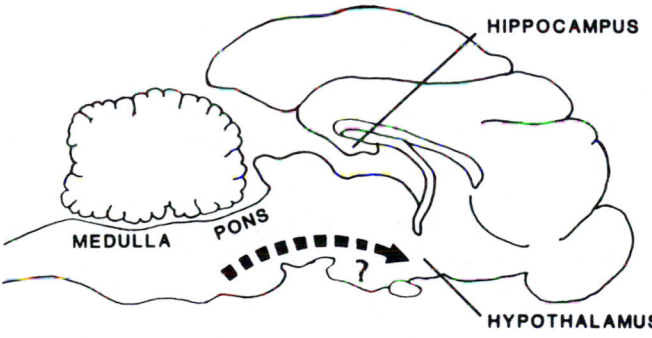

FIGURE 100-6   Diagrammatic representation of the changing control from the forebrain as an individual passes from NREM to REM when hypothalamic control is suppressed. The same shift in control may occur briefly during orienting in wakefulness. (*From Morrison,*[27] *with permission.*)

REFERENCES

1. Amini-Sereshki L, Morrison AR: Effects of pontine tegmental lesions that induce paradoxical sleep without atonia on thermoregulation in cats during wakefulness. *Brain Res* 384:23–28, 1986.
2. Aserinsky E, Kleitman N: Regularly occurring periods of eye motility, and concomitant phenomena during sleep. *Science* 118:273–274, 1953.
3. Baccelli G, Guazzi M, Mancia G, Zanchetti A: Central and reflex regulation of sympathetic vasoconstrictor activity of limb muscles during desynchronized sleep in the cat. *Circ Res* 35:625–635, 1974.
4. Baghdoyan HA, Spotts JL, Snyder SG: Simultaneous pontine and basal forebrain microinjections of carbachol suppress REM sleep. *J Neurosci* 13:229–242, 1993.
5. Baust W, Bohnert B: The regulation of heart rate during sleep. *Exp Brain Res* 7:169–180, 1969.
6. Baust W, Weidinger H, Kirchner F: Sympathetic activity during natural sleep and arousal. *Arch Ital Biol* 106:379–390, 1968.
7. Bennington JH, Heller HC: Restoration of brain energy metabolism as the function of sleep. *Prog Neurobiol* 45:347–360, 1995.
8. Carskadon MA, Dement WC: Normal human sleep: An overview, in Kryger MH, Roth T, Dement WC (ed): *Principles and Practice of Sleep Medicine.* Philadelphia, Saunders, 1994, pp 16–25.
9. Chase MH, Morales FR: The control of motoneurons during sleep, in Kryger MH, Roth T, Dement WC (ed): *Principles and Practice of Sleep Medicine.* Philadelphia, Saunders, 1994, pp 163–175.
10. Glotzbach SF, Heller HC: Central nervous regulation of body temperature during sleep. *Science* 194:537–539, 1976.
11. Guazzi M, Zanchetti A: Blood pressure and heart rate during natural sleep of the cat and their regulation by carotid sinus and aortic reflexes. *Arch Ital Biol* 103:789–817, 1965.
12. Hendricks JC: Absence of shivering in the cat during paradoxical sleep without atonia. *Exp Neurol* 75:700–710, 1982.
13. Hendricks JC, Kline LR, Kowalski RJ, et al: The English bulldog: A natural model of sleep-disordered breathing. *J Appl Physiol* 63:1344–1350, 1987.
14. Hendricks JC, Morrison AR, Mann GL: Different behaviors during paradoxical sleep without atonia depend on pontine lesion site. *Brain Res* 239:81–105, 1982.
15. Holmes CJ, Jones BE: Importance of cholinergic, gabaergic, serotonergic and other neurons in the medial medullary reticular formation for sleep-wake states studied by cytotoxic lesions in the cat. *Neuroscience* 62:1179–1200, 1994.
16. Hu B, Steriade M, Deschenes M: The cellular mechanisms of thalamic ponto-geniculo-occipital waves. *Neuroscience* 31:25–35, 1989.
17. Jouvet M: Recherches sur les structures nerveuses et les mécanismes responsables des différentes phases du sommeil physiologique. *Arch Ital Biol* 100:125–206, 1962.
18. Jouvet M: The role of monoamines and acetylcholine-containing neurons in the regulation of the sleep-waking cycle. *Ergeb Physiol* 64:166–307, 1972.
19. Jouvet M, Buda C, Sastre JP: Hypothermia induces a quasi-permanent paradoxical sleep state in pontine cats, in Malan A, Canguilhem B (eds): *Living in the Cold.* London, John Libbey, 1989, pp 487–498.
20. Lin JS, Sakai K, Jouvet M: Hypothalamo-preoptic histaminergic projections in sleep-wake control in the cat. *Euro J Neurosci* 6:618–625, 1994.
21. Mancia G, Zanchetti A: Cardiovascular regulation during sleep, in Orem J, Barnes CD (eds): *Physiology in Sleep.* New York, Academic Press, 1980, pp 1–55.
22. Marini G, Gritti I, Mancia M: The role of some thalamic nuclei in sleep mechanisms: Evidence from chemical lesions in the cat, in Mancia M, Marini G (eds): *The Diencephalon and Sleep.* New York, Raven Press, 1990, pp 279–292.
23. McCarley RW, Greene RW, Rainnie D, Portas CM: Brainstem neuromodulation and REM sleep. *Semin Neurosci* 7:341–354, 1995.
24. McGinty DJ, Szymusiak R: Neuronal unit activity patterns in behaving animals: Brainstem and limbic system. *Annu Rev Psychol* 39:135–168, 1988.
25. Moore-Ede MC, Sulzman FM, Fuller CA: *The Clocks That Time Us.* Cambridge, MA, Harvard University Press 1982.
26. Morrison AR: Brainstem regulation of behavior during sleep and wakefulness, in Sprague JM, Epstein AN (eds): *Progress in Psychobiology and Physiological Psychology.* New York, Academic Press, 1979, vol 8, pp 91–131.

27. Morrison AR: Update in Fishman AP (ed): *Pulmonary Diseases and Disorders.* New York, McGraw-Hill, 1992, pp 237–247.

27a. Morrison AR: Understanding (and misunderstanding) the animal rights movement in the United States, in DeDeyn PP (ed): *The Ethics of Animal and Human Experimentation.* London, John Libbey, 1994, pp 93–106.

28. Morrison AR, Reiner PB: A dissection of paradoxical sleep, in McGinty DJ, Drucker-Colin R, Morrison A, Parmeggiani PL (eds): *Brain Mechanisms of Sleep.* New York, Raven Press, 1985, pp 97–110.

29. Morrison AR, Sanford LD, Ball WA, et al: Stimulus-elicited behavior in rapid eye movement sleep without atonia. *Behav Neurosci* 109:972–979, 1995.

30. Moruzzi G, Magoun HW: Brainstem reticular formation and activation of the EEG. *Electroencephalogr Clin Neurophysiol* 1:455–473, 1949.

31. Nishino S, Reid M, Dement WC, Mignot E: Neuropharmacology and neurochemistry of canine narcolepsy. *Sleep* 17:584–592, 1994.

32. Parmeggiani PL, Azzaroni A, Cevolani D, Ferrari G: Responses of anterior hypothalamic neurons to direct thermal stimulation during wakefulness and sleep. *Brain Res* 269:382–385, 1983.

33. Parmeggiani PL, Calasso M, Cianci T: Respiratory effects of preoptic anterior hypothalamic electrical stimulation during sleep in cats. *Sleep* 4:7–82, 1981.

34. Parmeggiani PL, Franzini C, Lenzi PL, Zamboni G: Threshold of respiratory responses to preoptic heating during sleep in freely moving cats. *Brain Res* 52:189–201, 1973.

35. Parmeggiani PL, Morrison AR: Alterations in autonomic functions during sleep, in Loewy AD, Spyer KM (eds): *Central Regulation of Autonomic Functions.* Oxford, England, Oxford University Press, 1990, pp 367–386.

36. Parmeggiani PL, Zamboni G, Cianci T, Calasso M: Absence of thermoregulatory vasomotor responses during fast wave sleep in cats. *Electroencephalogr Clin Neurophysiol* 42:372–380, 1977.

37. Pivik RT: Tonic states and phasic events in relation to sleep mentation, in Arkin AM, Antrobus JS, Ellman SJ (eds): *The Mind in Sleep: Psychology and Psychophysiology.* Hillsdale, NJ, Erlbaum, 1978, pp 245–271.

38. Rechtschaffen A: The psychophysiology of mental activity during sleep, in McGuigan FJ, Schoonover RS (eds): *The Psychophysiology of Thinking.* New York, Academic Press, 1973, pp 153–205.

39. Rechtschaffen A, Bergman B: Sleep deprivation in the rat by the disk-over-water method. *Behav Brain Res* 69:55–63, 1995.

40. Sallanon M, Sakai K, Buda C, et al: Increase of paradoxical sleep induced by microinjections of ibotenic acid into the ventrolateral part of the posterior hypothalamus in the cat. *Arch Ital Biol* 126:87–97, 1988.

41. Sanford LD, Tejani-Butt SM, Ross RJ, Morrison AR: Amygdaloid control of alerting and behavioral arousal in rats: Involvement of serotonergic mechanisms. *Arch Ital Biol* 13:81–99, 1995.

42. Schenck CH, Bundlie SR, Patterson AL, Mahowald MW: Rapid eye movement sleep behavior disorder: A treatable parasomnia affecting older adults. *JAMA* 257:1786–1789, 1987.

43. Siegel JM, Manger PR, Nienhuis R, et al: Echidna contains REM and NREM aspects in a single sleep state: Implications for the evolution of sleep. *J Neurosci.* 16:3500–3506, 1996.

44. Siegel JM, Rogawski MA: A function for REM sleep: Regulation of noradrenergic receptor sensitivity. *Brain Res Rev* 13:213–233, 1988.

45. Siegel JM, Tomaszewski KS: Behavioral organization of reticular formation—studies in the unrestrained cat: I. Cells related to axial, limb, eye, and other movements. *J Neurophysiol* 50:696–716, 1983.

46. Steriade M: Neuromodulatory systems of thalamus and neocortex. *Semin Neurosci* 7:361–370, 1995.

47. Steriade M, Gloor P, Llinás R, et al: Basic mechanisms of cerebral rhythmic activities. *Electroencephalogr Clin Neurophysiol* 76:481–508, 1990.

48. Sterman MB, Shouse MN: Sleep "centers" in the brain: The preoptic basal forebrain area revisited, in McGinty DJ, Drucker-Colin R, Morrison A, Parmeggiani PL (eds): *Brain Mechanisms of Sleep.* New York, Raven Press, 1985, pp 277–299.

49. Tononi G, Pompeiano M, Gianni S, Pompeiano O: Enhancement of desynchronized sleep signs after microinjection of the beta-adrenergic antagonist propranolol in the dorsal pontine tegmentum. *Arch Ital Biol* 126:119–123, 1988.

50. Zepelin H: Mammalian sleep, in Kryger MH, Roth T, Dement WC (eds): *Principles and Practice of Sleep Medicine.* Philadelphia, Saunders, 1994, pp 69–80.

CHAPTER 101

CHANGES IN THE CARDIORESPIRATORY SYSTEM DURING SLEEP

Allan I. Pack / Leszek Kubin / Richard O. Davies

CHANGES IN VENTILATION AND VENTILATORY CONTROL DURING NREM SLEEP

PERIODICITIES OF VENTILATION IN LIGHT NREM SLEEP

CHANGES IN CARDIOVASCULAR VARIABLES DURING NREM SLEEP

CHANGES IN VENTILATION DURING REM SLEEP

CHANGES IN THE CARDIOVASCULAR SYSTEM IN REM SLEEP

LESSONS FROM THE CARBACHOL MODEL

CONCLUSION

Sleep is associated with profound changes in cardiorespiratory control. These changes are not only of intrinsic interest but also highly relevant to sleep-related breathing disorders and to certain disorders of the cardiovascular system. There is increasing realization that unique cardiopulmonary events during sleep can have a major impact on daytime functioning. Thus, we are moving into an era in which variables such as arterial and pulmonary pressures will be considered not as values at a single point in time; rather, the whole 24-h rhythm of these variables will be of clinical interest. This chapter reviews what we know about the changes in cardiorespiratory control with sleep and, where relevant, points out the clinical implications with particular emphasis on the obstructive sleep apnea syndrome. As described elsewhere in this volume, normal sleep consists of several cycles of four successively occurring stages of non–rapid eye movement (NREM) sleep, followed by a period of rapid eye movement (REM) sleep (see Chapter 100). The changes in cardiorespiratory control vary among the different stages.

CHANGES IN VENTILATION AND VENTILATORY CONTROL DURING NREM SLEEP

During NREM sleep, ventilation declines; it becomes regular in stages 3 and 4 sleep. In stages 1 and 2 of NREM sleep, however, ventilation is more likely to be variable and, in certain persons, periodic breathing with cycles of waxing and waning in ventilation occur (see below).

One of the important principles of the effect of sleep on respiratory control is that sleep differentially affects the activity of the muscles of the respiratory pump and the dilator muscles of the upper airway, with changes in the latter being more profound.[10,37] There are exceptions to this rule: in particular, the activity of some laryngeal muscles is profoundly suppressed during sleep, whereas that of others is not.[24,25] Overall, however, one major reason for the reduction in ventilation in NREM sleep is an increase in resistance secondary to a decrease in activity of the dilator muscles of the upper airway, especially in the pharyngeal region. However, no change occurs in the transdiaphragmatic pressure difference during inspiration, a measure of diaphragmatic function (Fig. 101-1). As a consequence of this decrease in ventilation in NREM sleep, Pa_{CO_2} rises, typically from its normal value of 40 mmHg to 45 to 46 mmHg. The magnitude of this increase in Pa_{CO_2} is a function of the responsiveness of the system to CO_2 during wakefulness[8]: subjects with low ventilatory responses to CO_2 have larger increases in Pa_{CO_2} than do subjects with high responses (Fig. 101-2). Parallel to this increase in Pa_{CO_2}, the Pa_{O_2} falls. In normal persons, who are operating on the flat part of the oxygen saturation curve, the Pa_{O_2} does not fall to a level where significant desaturations occur. However, in persons with low Pa_{O_2} during wakefulness, who operate closer to the "knee" of the oxygen saturation curve, this fall in Pa_{O_2} during sleep may lead to a significant hypoxemia. For example, patients with chronic obstructive pulmonary disease may require supplemental oxygen during sleep but not during wakefulness.

Another major change that occurs during NREM sleep is an increase in the CO_2 apnea threshold.[42] This apnea threshold is the Pa_{CO_2} at which there is insufficient chemical drive and ventilation ceases. During wakefulness, Pa_{CO_2} can be reduced by assisted ventilation to values as low as 20 mmHg and rhythmic ventilation will be maintained;[6,40] thus, the CO_2 apnea threshold during wakefulness is extremely low. In contrast, during NREM sleep, the Pa_{CO_2} need be reduced only to values close to the normal awake Pa_{CO_2} (38 to 40 mmHg) and

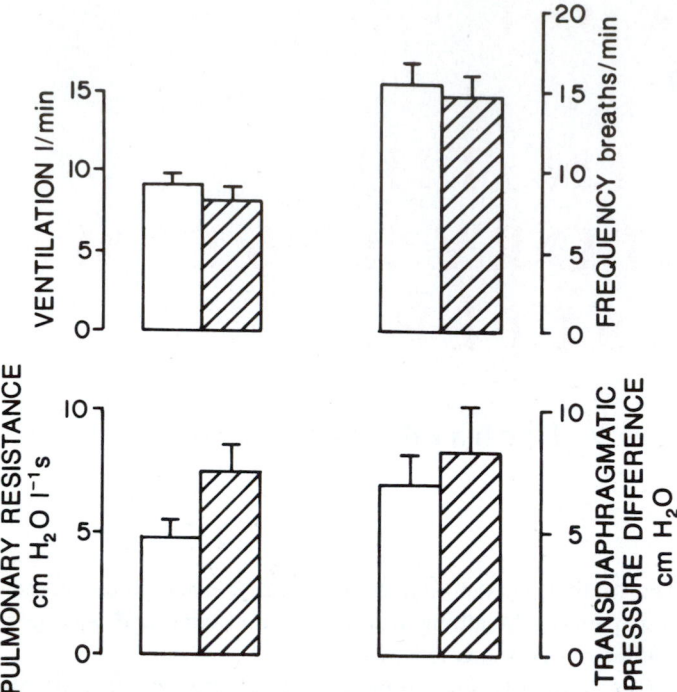

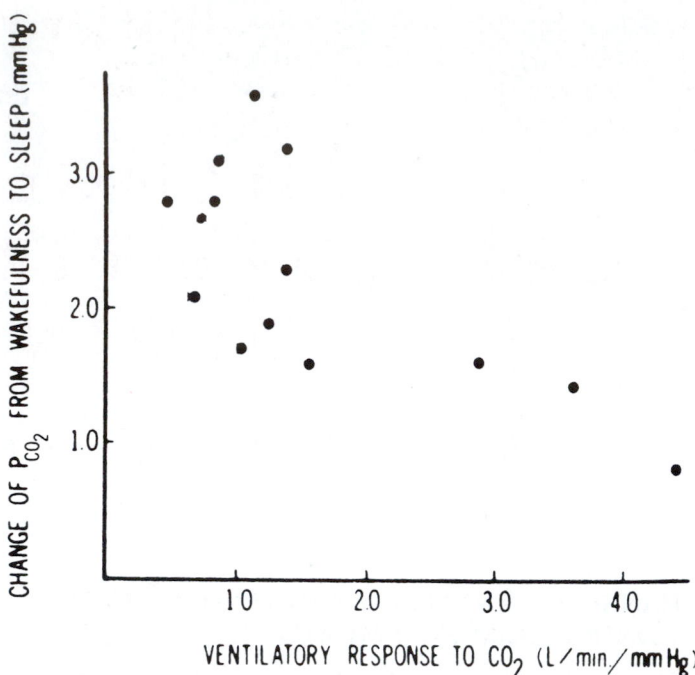

FIGURE 101-1   Changes in ventilation, respiratory frequency, total pulmonary resistance, and transdiaphragmatic pressure between wakefulness and stages 3 and 4 NREM sleep in normal subjects. (*Based on data of Skatrud and Dempsey,[43] with permission.*)

FIGURE 101-2   Relationship between the increase in P_{CO_2} that occurs in normal subjects in going from wakefulness to stages 1 and 2 NREM sleep and the CO_2 ventilatory response in wakefulness. Persons with the lowest ventilatory responses show the largest change in P_{CO_2} in going to sleep. (*From Gothe et al,[8] with permission.*)

ventilation will cease. Thus, the normal increase in Pa_{CO_2} that occurs during NREM sleep is often necessary to maintain rhythmic ventilation.

This NREM sleep–related increase in apnea threshold has profound implications. In situations where ventilation is stimulated—for example, by hypoxia—Pa_{CO_2} may be reduced below the apnea threshold typical for normoxic conditions, creating a state of increased vulnerability to central apneas. It is likely that unexplained central apnea during sleep occurs in association with hypocapnia.[50] If this is the mechanism for these apneas, increase in the Pa_{CO_2} should abolish them. Instances have been reported of persons with central apnea in whom apnea was relieved when they breathed air enriched with low concentrations of CO_2.

The specific cellular and neurochemical mechanisms for this NREM sleep–related change in the apnea threshold are currently unknown. Conceptually, however, it may be considered within the same category as the so-called wakefulness stimulus for breathing.[6,40] Brain-stem neuronal groups, such as the locus coeruleus and raphe nuclei, in which the major transmitters are norepinephrine and serotonin, respectively, decrease their activity with sleep. Since both these transmitters have important excitatory effects at various levels of the central respiratory control system, these neuronal groups may represent one component of the wakefulness stimulus. This possibility still needs to be elucidated. An alternative postulate is that ventilation is controlled by different neural circuits during sleep than during wakefulness.

In addition to the change in the apnea threshold to Pa_{CO_2}, the slope of the response to P_{CO_2} decreases during sleep.[1] Such a decrease may result either from a decrease in central CO_2 sensitivity (e.g., due to state-dependent changes in the activity or membrane properties of CO_2-sensitive neurons in the brain stem) or from the reduced activity at the respiratory motor output (e.g.,

due to the sleep-related withdrawal of the excitatory effect of the wakefulness stimulus on respiratory motoneurons or their premotor cells). Although a reduction in excitability at motoneuronal levels does occur, the evidence for state-dependent changes in central CO_2 sensitivity is much less compelling. Overall, however, the progressive declines in the ventilatory response to CO_2 are smaller in stages 1 and 2 than in stages 3 and 4 NREM sleep.[1] They must contribute to the hypoventilation that occurs during sleep by making the system less able to compensate for the increase in upper-airway resistance.

A compromised upper airway and the chronic occurrence of obstructive apneic episodes during sleep are associated with a host of important changes in the control of upper-airway patency, and in the control of breathing in general, that are only beginning to be described and understood. Thus, it appears that the amount of activity present in upper-airway muscles during wakefulness is higher in patients with sleep apnea (and in English bulldogs) than in normal subjects (and control dogs).[14,27] (The English bulldog is a natural animal model of obstructive sleep apnea.[12]) This increase in activity is an expected compensatory mechanism that helps maintain the airway patent in the face of anatomic narrowing. Of interest is that this compensatory mechanism is much weaker or unable to function during sleep; consequently, the sleep-related decrements in airway muscle tone appear to be larger in sleep apneics than in normals.[28] Another peripheral, rather than central, phenomenon highly relevant for the efficacy with which upper-airway muscles can maintain the airway patent is the occurrence of injury to the upper-airway muscles in the sleep apnea syndrome.[36] The underlying cause is probably the large forces that these muscles have to generate in order to resolve repeated nocturnal airway obstructions. The presence of upper-airway muscle injury suggests that a vicious cycle may take place in the natural progression of the disease, whereby an initial injury imposes an even higher demand on the remaining unaltered muscle fibers and leads to further, accelerated muscle injury.

PERIODICITIES OF VENTILATION IN LIGHT NREM SLEEP

Periodic (oscillatory) ventilation is more likely to occur during light NREM sleep (stages 1 and 2) than in slow-wave sleep (stages 3 and 4). This is highly relevant to the problem of obstructive sleep apnea; most apneas occur in stages 1 and 2 sleep. If a subject with sleep apnea is able to enter stages 3 and 4 NREM sleep, regular ventilation resumes and apneas are less likely to occur. Oscillatory ventilation is also typically observed during hypoxia, as in lung disease or at high altitude, and in certain cardiovascular diseases.

Ventilation may be periodic because of particular dynamic properties of the chemical feedback system that controls respiration.[17] As in any feedback system, the critical determinants of this unstable (oscillatory) behavior are the overall response (gain) of the control system and the time delay (phase lag) between the plant and the controller. For the respiratory system, the plant is the gas exchange apparatus in the lung; the controllers are the chemoreceptors, peripheral and central; and the controlled variables are the arterial blood-gas tensions, Pa_{CO_2} and Pa_{O_2}. Thus, in the case of the respiratory control system, this time delay is that between the lung and the sensors, the peripheral and central chemoreceptors.

The importance of this delay is illustrated in Fig. 101-3 for a situation in which a disturbance to the ventilatory control system leads to a change in Pa_{CO_2}. If there is no delay, the control system responds immediately to this perturbation by adjusting ventilation to correct the change in Pa_{CO_2} (Fig. 101-3A). In contrast, if there is a delay in the feedback loop, the controller may act to sustain the cyclical disturbance (Fig. 101-3B); this is because during the time it takes the altered Pa_{CO_2} level to reach the sensor, the controller may make an inappropriate correction. For example, when the Pa_{CO_2} in the blood leaving the lung is low, the controller should respond by reducing ventilation, returning the Pa_{CO_2} to the regulated value. If, however, the delay is such that by the time the low Pa_{CO_2} signal reaches the sensor, the Pa_{CO_2} of the blood leaving the lung is already higher (e.g., due to the presence of an external perturbation or already existing oscillations, as in Fig. 101-3B), the controller will act incorrectly to reduce ventilation and further increase the Pa_{CO_2}. Such a situation promotes a self-sustaining periodic ventilation. Thus, the time delay determines not only whether periodic ventilation will or will not occur but also the period of this oscillation.

Periodic ventilation would not occur if the control system failed to respond, or responded weakly, to these perturbations. Thus, the gain of the response of the system is as important as the magnitude of the delay in determining whether unstable operation of the ventilatory control system will occur. This gain is usually defined as the product of the response of the controller (the change in ventilation per unit change in Pa_{CO_2}—i.e., CO_2 *sensitivity*) and the gain of the plant (the change in Pa_{CO_2} per unit change in ventilation—i.e., the *overall loop gain*).

Periodic breathing occurs in clinical situations, particularly in hypoxic subjects (e.g., patients with lung disease) and normal sojourners at high altitude: hypoxia increases the gain of the response of the controller, making the system more unstable. The period of the oscillations in ventilation induced by hypoxia is on the order of 20 s—i.e., much shorter than those typically seen in patients with obstructive sleep apnea. Abnormally increased circulatory time, which prolongs the delay between the lung and chemoreceptors, can also produce an unstable system and ventilatory periodicities. This mechanism is likely to be responsible, at least in part, for the ventilatory oscillations that occur during sleep in patients with severe congestive heart failure (Cheyne-Stokes respiration).

In addition to these mechanisms that are related to instability of the chemical control system for ventilation, *state instability* can produce sleep-related oscillations in ventilation;[17] state instability is defined as periodic changes in the stages of sleep that cause discrete and periodic changes in the level of the wakefulness stimulus to ventilation. At the onset of sleep, there are, as discussed in the preceding section, decreases in ventilation and increases in upper-airway resistance that cause an increase in Pa_{CO_2}; the increase in Pa_{CO_2} may, in turn, directly or indirectly interfere with the normal progression of the sleep cycle. For example, an abrupt change in sleep state may occur as a re-

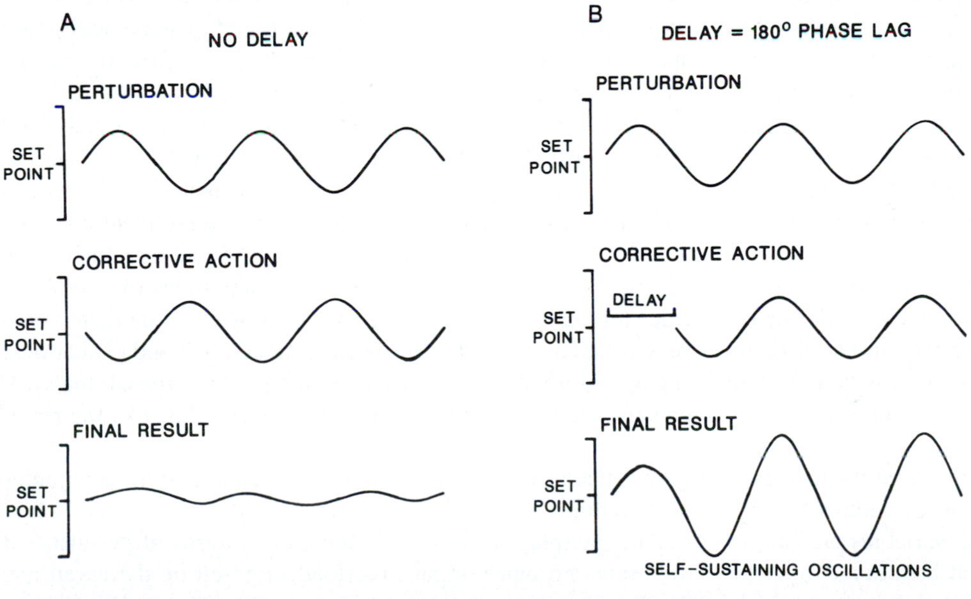

FIGURE 101-3 Implications for a control system with a delay between the plant and the control system. The left panel *(A)* shows how a control system will respond to a sinusoidal perturbation when there is no delay. The perturbation is essentially neutralized. The right panel *(B)* shows how a control system acts if it has a delay that results in the corrective action being 180° out of phase with the perturbation. In this case, the controller's action acts to sustain, and not to neutralize, the original sinusoidal perturbation.

sult of airflow limitation and increased respiratory effort, leading to an awakening to a lighter stage of sleep—i.e., to an arousal.[4] Upon arousal, ventilation increases, upper-airway resistance decreases, and Pa_{CO_2} drops. The subject returns to sleep, and the whole cycle may repeat itself. This state instability is more likely to arise if the ventilatory response to CO_2 is low, since the Pa_{CO_2} increases more at sleep onset and is more apt to drive the level of respiratory effort to a point at which an arousal from sleep occurs.[17] The period of ventilatory oscillation caused by this mechanism is longer than that seen with chemical instability—i.e., around 60 to 90 s. This mechanism, we believe, predominates in producing the sleep apnea syndrome and periodic breathing in patients with low ventilatory responses to CO_2 (e.g., patients with hypothyroidism, in whom central and obstructive apneas are common).

CHANGES IN CARDIOVASCULAR VARIABLES DURING NREM SLEEP

The cardiovascular system also undergoes stereotypical changes in performance during NREM sleep. Heart rate and blood pressure decrease successively during the progressively deeper stages of NREM sleep.[2] Respiratory sinus arrhythmia, consisting of heart rate accelerations during inspiration and decelerations during expiration, is enhanced during NREM sleep. This enhancement is most pronounced in persons in whom vagal control of the heart rate is more marked. In these persons, both slowing and deepening of the respiratory pumping movements (pulmonary and airway mechanoreflex mechanisms) and changes in the relative contribution of the central vagal and sympathetic control of the heart rate favor central control.

In slow-wave sleep, mean blood pressure may be around 15 to 20 mmHg lower than in wakefulness. Thus, during sleep there is considerable "unloading" of the cardiovascular system (Fig. 101-4). This decrease in blood pressure is largely the result of a fall in cardiac output, since overall peripheral resistance changes little. The fall in cardiac output is, in turn, explained by the reduced heart rate, since stroke volume shows no consistent change with sleep. Heart rate falls from a typical value of 70 beats per minute in quiet wakefulness to 48 to 50 beats per minute in slow-wave sleep. This change in heart rate is related to both increased vagal efferent activity and reduced sympathetic outflow to the heart.[15,45]

The effects of sleep do not, however, affect the blood flow to all peripheral vascular beds identically. For some vascular beds (e.g., mesenteric and renal), there is little change in blood flow in NREM sleep. Maintenance of blood flow in these beds is the result of vasodilatation to compensate for the reduced arterial pressure. In contrast, blood flow to the muscle vascular bed declines during sleep while that to the brain increases; the increase in brain blood flow is not uniform in all brain structures.

These normal changes in cardiovascular variables are interfered with in patients with sleep-disordered breathing. In such patients, as a result of their apneic episodes, mean arterial blood pressure does not decrease with sleep.[44] Since this increased blood pressure is present over many hours, it represents an increased load to the left ventricle in terms of its total 24-h performance. During an obstructive episode, blood pressure in-

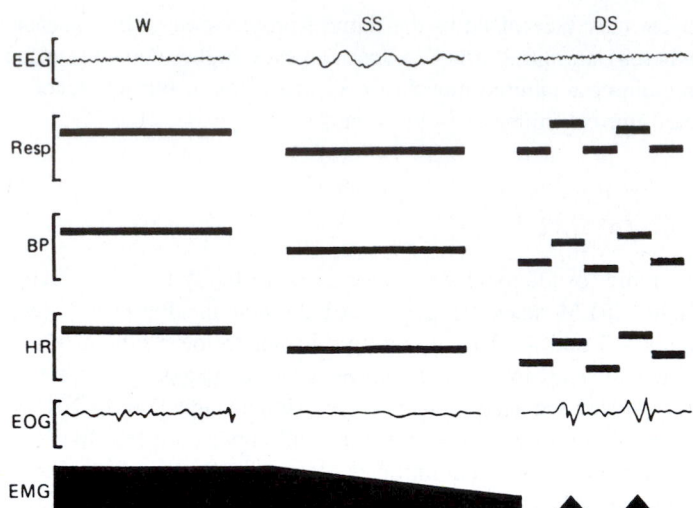

FIGURE 101-4 Schematic representation of cardiovascular changes during NREM sleep and REM sleep. The traces show a schematic of the electroencephalogram (EEG), mean ventilation (Resp), mean blood pressure (BP), mean heart rate (HR), electrooculogram (EOG), and electromyographic activity of neck muscles (EMG). Data are illustrated from wakefulness and from slow-wave and REM sleep. The decline in ventilation, blood pressure, and heart rate in slow-wave sleep are illustrated, as is the marked variability of these measures in REM sleep. *(Modified from Coote,[2] with permission.)*

creases, apparently because of the progressive hypoxia.[32] During the apneic episode, sympathetic outflow, recorded from the peroneal nerve in sleep apnea patients, increases progressively.[44] A further, often dramatic, increase in blood pressure occurs at the termination of apnea, apparently related predominantly to the arousal from sleep.[38] The tonically elevated arterial blood pressure during sleep and its dramatic transient swings probably contribute to the development of arterial hypertension, which is very common in sleep apnea patients.[35] Although patients with sleep apnea seem to have increased sympathetic outflow during the day, the mechanism leading to this increase is not known.[44]

When breathing is periodic, as discussed above, arterial blood pressure also shows large fluctuations within the same period. They are caused through three distinct mechanisms: (1) periodically changing venous return and cardiac output resulting from the cyclical alterations in the magnitude of pressure changes in the thorax; (2) periodically changing magnitudes of cardiovascular reflexes originating in the heart, lungs, and thoracic blood vessels and arterial and central chemoreceptors; and (3) periodic changes in the level of arousal. With regard to arousal, the sympathetic output to the heart and skeletal muscles, like the respiratory motor output, is under an excitatory influence of the brainstem reticular formation analogous to the wakefulness stimulus for breathing.[15,30]

The interplay of these mechanisms, in terms of perfusion of the brain and other organs, the load imposed on the heart, and combination of excitatory and suppressant effects on both respiratory and sympathetic output, is very complex. Although animal studies, in which selected components of these complex events can be studied in isolation from other factors, are helpful in gaining a better insight into the relative importance of these distinct mechanisms, most of those experiments are performed under anesthesia, which adds another confounding factor. Thus, comprehensive models of the operation of the cardiovascular and respiratory systems during periodic breathing are still difficult to design. It is important to note, however, that the large transient increases in arterial blood pressure—for example, at the end of an apneic episode but before its resolution—cause a reflex inhibition of central respiratory activity mediated by arterial baroreceptors.[39] The presence of this inhibitory influence highlights the dramatic nature of opposing effects on breathing that take place just around the time the apneic episode is resolved.

CHANGES IN VENTILATION DURING REM SLEEP

The changes in ventilation that occur during REM sleep are more complex than those in NREM sleep. REM sleep is a singular stage of the sleep–wake cycle. During REM sleep, the cortical EEG shows the same highly active, desynchronized pattern as in wakefulness, and there are flurries of activation

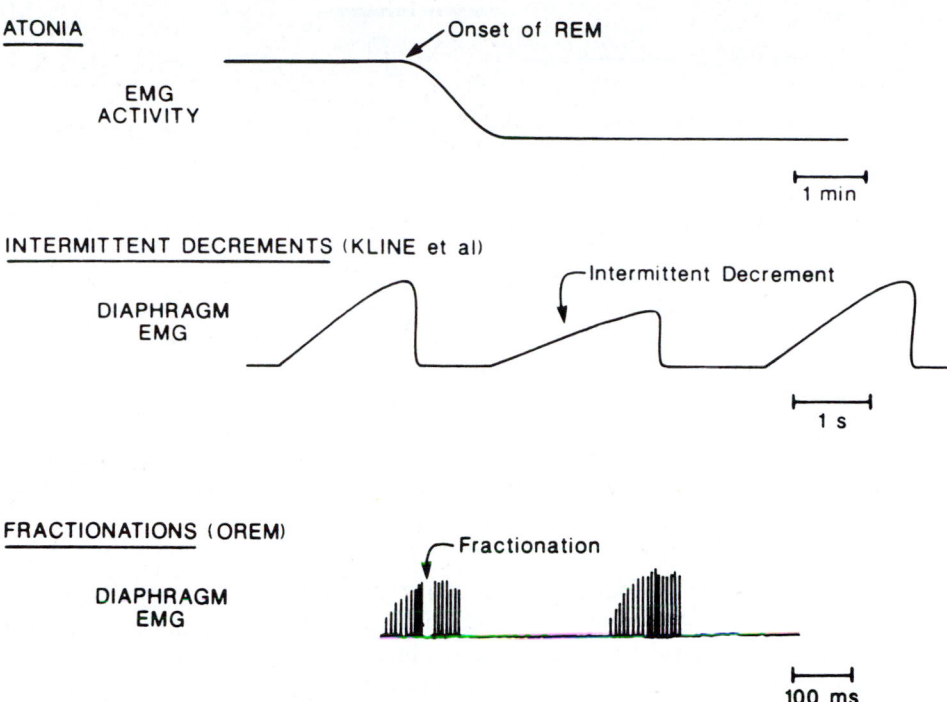

FIGURE 101-5 Schematic representation of the changes in the activity of the diaphragm during REM sleep. Top panel: The atonia that occurs in REM sleep. (While this is most pronounced for postural and limb muscles, even in the diaphragm some motor units cease firing throughout REM sleep.) Middle panel: Intermittent decrements in motor activity, first described by Kline et al,[20] that occur in association with the phasic events of REM sleep. These decrements occur over a period of seconds to minutes. Bottom panel: Fractionations in diaphragm activity that also occur in association with the phasic events of REM sleep. Fractionations, first described by Orem,[33] are brief pauses in activity that last for about 10 to 40 msec.

(phasic events) such as pontogeniculo-occipital (PGO) waves (large-voltage waves having a characteristic configuration that can be recorded in the pons, lateral geniculate nucleus, and occipital cortex), bursts of eye movements, and twitches of skeletal muscles (see Chapter 100). Most skeletal muscles are, however, actively paralyzed in this stage, so normal persons do not live out their dreams. Both the phasic changes and the tonic suppression of motor activity affect cardiorespiratory control.

Associated with the flurries in activity, such as eye movements, are phasic changes in ventilation: increases in ventilation occur from increases in respiratory rate, and reductions in ventilation accompany slowing of the respiratory rate.[20,31] Despite this profound breath-to-breath variability in normal persons during REM sleep, the average ventilation changes very little compared to wakefulness. The phasic changes in ventilatory output affect the rib cage more than the abdomen; hence, when compartmental ventilation is measured, rib cage ventilation decreases more.[31]

Studies of the electromyographic activity of respiratory muscles—i.e., both the pump muscles such as the diaphragm and the upper-airway dilator muscles—provide insights into the nature of these changes.[20,48] They show that the normal pattern of muscle activation can be profoundly disturbed during REM sleep. A number of processes occur with different time courses (Fig. 101-5). *First*, individual motor units, including those in the diaphragm, may cease firing throughout the whole REM sleep episode. This represents a "tonic" change in REM sleep. *Second*,

episodes of either decreases or increases in motor output to respiratory muscles may occur over several respiratory cycles; these have been called *intermittent decrements* or *intermittent increments*.[20,31] An example of an intermittent decrement of diaphragmatic activity is illustrated in Fig. 101-5. In normal human subjects, intermittent decrements during eye movements can also markedly decrease the motor output to the genioglossus muscle (Fig. 101-6).[48] *Third*, on an even shorter time scale are the so-called fractionations—i.e., brief pauses in diaphragmatic activity in association with the phasic events of REM sleep (Fig. 101-5).[13,33] These pauses in activity are around 10 to 40 msec in duration, tend to occur in clusters, and are associated with PGO waves.

The changes in respiratory motor output associated with these phasic events during REM sleep do not uniformly affect all motor units in a muscle. For example, simultaneous recordings from two different sites in the diaphragm show that activity in one site may be markedly suppressed, while the activity of the other is not.[11] Such asynchronous activation of respiratory muscles is a unique feature of REM sleep. Given such changes, it is not surprising that in subjects prone to sleep apnea, profound apneas can occur in relationship to these phasic events. This relationship has been found to occur in the English bulldog, an animal that exhibits naturally occurring obstructive sleep apnea as a result of its craniofacial anatomy (Fig. 101-7).[13]

In addition to transient inhibitory events, intermittent accelerations of the respiratory rate and periods of excitation also oc-

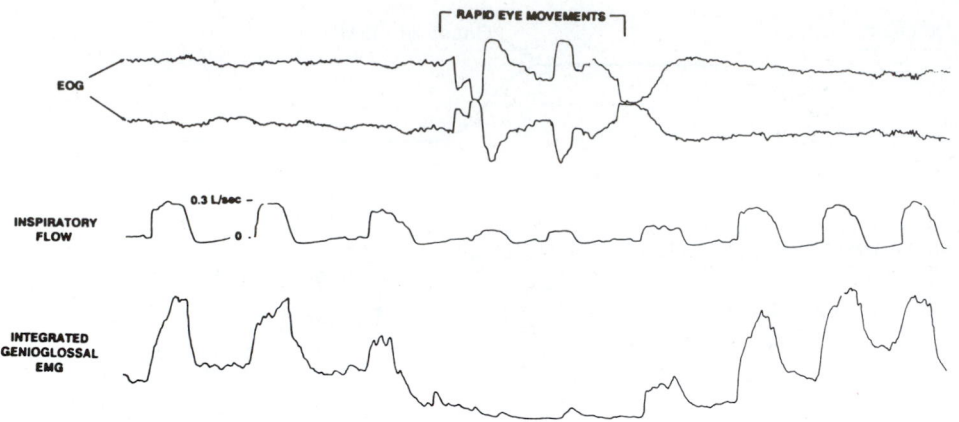

FIGURE 101-6   Intermittent decrement in the activity of the genioglossus muscle in a normal human during the phasic eye movements of REM sleep. *(Based on data of Wiegand et al,[48] with permission.)*

cur during REM sleep in both pump and upper-airway muscles.[2,20,31] Some central respiratory neurons in the brain stem show a strong enhancement of activity, even when respiratory motoneurons are relatively suppressed.[33,34] Such excitatory phenomena may, to some degree, reduce the likelihood of airway obstructions during REM sleep in sleep apnea patients. In addition, however, apneas in stages 1 and 2 sleep resulting in arousals can limit the natural progression of the sleep cycle from NREM to REM sleep, and apneas in REM can also prematurely terminate this state. The deprivation of REM sleep that results from these disturbances is responsible for the large increase in the amounts of REM sleep seen in some patients when they are first treated with continuous positive airway pressure.[16] This failure to obtain an adequate amount of REM sleep may account for the frequently held view that airway obstructions are primarily a problem of NREM sleep. On the other hand, apneic episodes and the resulting oxygen desaturations that occur during REM sleep are longer lasting and more severe than those during NREM sleep.[5] Similarly, the observation that in mild cases of sleep apnea, apneic episodes occur predominantly in REM sleep shows that this stage of sleep represents the period with the highest vulnerability to airway obstructions.

CHANGES IN THE CARDIOVASCULAR SYSTEM IN REM SLEEP

Just as variability of respiration occurs in association with the phasic events of REM sleep, so do variabilities occur in the cardiovascular system.[2] Periods of tachycardia and bradycardia are found (Fig. 101-4). The bradycardia can, at

times, be intense even in normal subjects, and episodes of sinus arrest have been described (Fig. 101-8).[9] Likewise, bidirectional fluctuations in blood pressure occur. Blood pressure can rise to levels above that found in wakefulness, although it can also decline to levels below that found in slow-wave sleep. As in NREM sleep, changes in heart rate play the major role in the changes in blood pressure, with alterations in stroke volume playing little, if any, role.

Marked fluctuations in sympathetic outflow occur in REM sleep; these are reflected in peroneal nerve activity in humans.[45] As noted above, the changes in sympathetic nerve activity do not affect the output to all vascular beds in the same way.[2,7] The activity in some sympathetic outflows (e.g., renal) may decrease, while that in vasoconstrictor fibers to skeletal muscle increases.[2] Thus, there are differential effects of REM sleep on blood flow to different organs. In particular, there are increases in blood flow to the brain in REM sleep. These increases are different for different brain structures and in different species.[7] Different changes also occur during REM sleep in different vascular beds in association with phasic events. For example, coronary blood flow in dogs shows surges in association with the phasic events of REM sleep. These surges are largely abolished following removal of

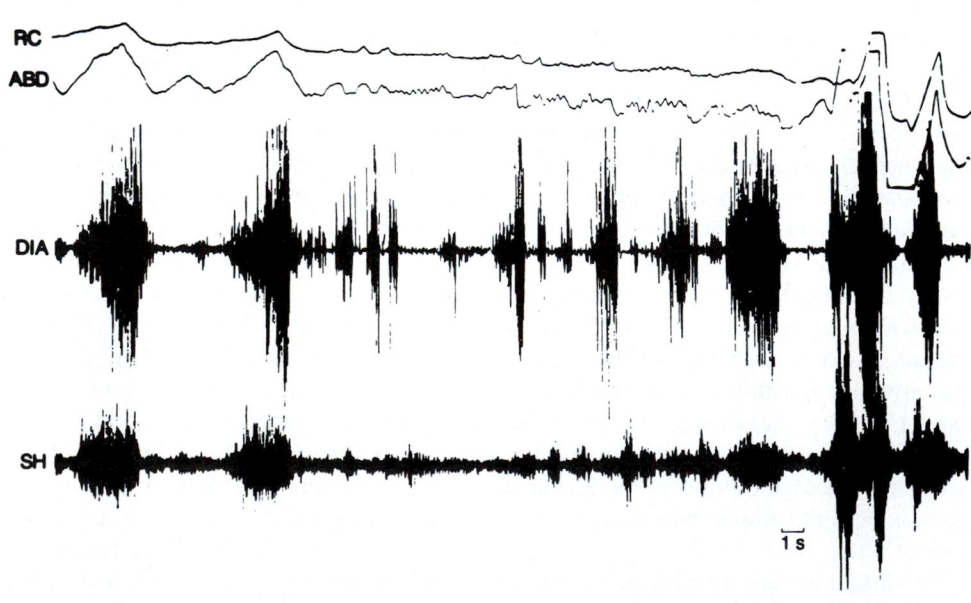

FIGURE 101-7   Apnea in an English bulldog during the phasic events of REM sleep. From top to bottom: rib cage motion (RC), abdominal motion (ABD), diaphragm electromyogram (DIA), and sternohyoid electromyogram (SH). During the apnea, considerable suppression and disorganization of the motor activity occur in both the diaphragm and a representative upper airway muscle—i.e., the sternohyoid. The apnea is terminated by an arousal from REM sleep. While these changes in motor activity occur in normal individuals, they have important consequences in individuals who are predisposed to the development of apnea because of orofacial anatomic factors. *(From Hendricks et al,[13] with permission.)*

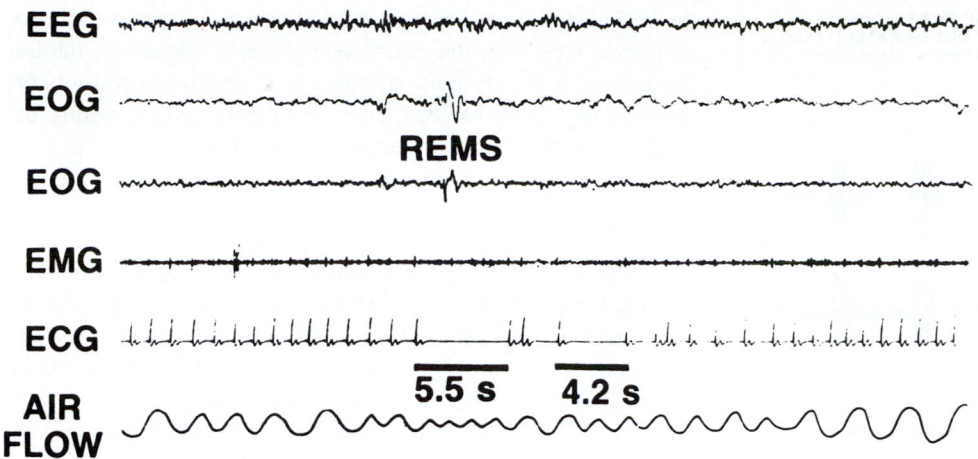

FIGURE 101-8   Sinus arrest in a normal person during REM sleep. Profound changes in the cardiovascular system can occur in association with the phasic events of REM sleep. Although this example is not particularly common, it does show how intense the "normal" cardiovascular changes can be in REM sleep. (*From Guilleminault et al,[9] with permission.*)

the sympathetic outflow to the heart. Of interest is that in dogs with an induced coronary stenosis, phasic increases in blood flow are converted to phasic decrements.[19] Thus, these normal physiological changes in REM sleep may play an important role in precipitating adverse cardiovascular events. A number of disturbing phenomena occur during sleep in patients with cardiovascular disease. These include arrhythmias, nocturnal angina, and episodes of paroxymal nocturnal dyspnea in patients with left ventricular dysfunction. The role that "normal" physiological changes in sleep play in precipitating these events in persons with compromised cardiovascular function remains to be determined. Moreover, we do not know why acute events such as myocardial infarction, stroke, and sudden death are more common in the hours immediately after the normal sleep period.

LESSONS FROM THE CARBACHOL MODEL

It is apparent from the preceding two sections that cardiorespiratory control during REM sleep is extremely complex, owing to the presence of a number of state-specific excitatory and inhibitory influences. Further complications arise when airway obstructions occur and acutely activate reflex mechanisms, while also producing long-term adaptive (and maladaptive—e.g., airway muscle injury and hypertension) changes in the cardiorespiratory system. Simplified models have been used in an attempt to understand these processes better.

With regard to the neural processes occurring during REM sleep, one animal model makes it possible to activate selected components of REM sleep in a controlled laboratory environment. The model is based on the finding that REM sleep phenomena originate, and are orchestrated, in the brain stem, with a major role played by the neurotransmitter acetylcholine (see Chapter 100).[41] In particular, microinjections of a cholinergic agonist—carbachol—into a specific region of the dorsal pons produce in intact, chronically instrumented animals a state very similar to REM sleep; in contrast, lesions of this region result in a major reduction in the amount of REM sleep and in long-term abolition of the tonic postural atonia characteristic of this state.[47]

Moreover, major signs of REM sleep, such as postural atonia, eye movements, and PGO-like waves, occur periodically in the brain stem and spinal cord of a "reduced" preparation in which the rostral parts of the central nervous system have been acutely or chronically removed (decerebration).[41] As in intact animals, carbachol is extremely effective in producing the signs of REM sleep in this preparation.

Taking advantage of the fact that REM sleep phenomena can be produced pharmacologically, extensive studies of the neural mechanisms relevant for cardiorespiratory control during REM sleep have been performed in recent years using pontine carbachol injections in both intact, chronically instrumented and decerebrate animals.[18,26] In the course of those studies, it became apparent that carbachol injections activate only selected phenomena of REM sleep. In particular, postural atonia and the simultaneous tonic suppression of respiratory motor output are consistently present, whereas muscle twitches and short timescale variabilities in the respiratory rate and respiratory motor output are absent. Thus, the carbachol-induced, REM sleep–like state represents a particularly useful model of the suppressant influences of REM sleep on breathing. Significantly, the ability to investigate those influences in animals in which only the fictive respiratory motor output is measured by recording from respiratory nerves, while the animal is paralyzed and pulmonary gas exchange is maintained constant by artificial ventilation, allows one to assess the central effects of activation of the pontine cholinergic mechanisms relevant for REM sleep in isolation from respiratory reflexes.

Three important findings have emerged from the studies using the reduced (artificially ventilated, paralyzed, decerebrate cats) carbachol model of REM sleep atonia. First, recordings from multiple upper-airway and pump muscle nerves have shown that, following pontine carbachol injections, there is a highly stereotyped pattern of suppression across different respiratory motor outputs: phrenic nerve activity is suppressed the least, whereas activities of the hypoglossal nerve (innervating the genioglossus and other tongue muscles) and expiratory intercostal nerve are suppressed the most. Figure 101-9 shows typical records from these three nerves before and after pontine carbachol injection.[18] The fact that this pattern of suppression is consistent with that seen during natural REM sleep suggests that state-specific central mechanisms, rather than reflexes, play a major role in shaping the behavior of respiratory motor output during REM sleep.

Second, studies of the neurochemical mechanisms of the carbachol-induced suppression of hypoglossal motoneurons have shown that a state-specific inhibition mediated by inhibitory amino acid neurotransmitters such as glycine or GABA is not a major mechanism of suppression of activity in hypoglossal motoneurons.[21] This is in contrast to postural motoneurons of the

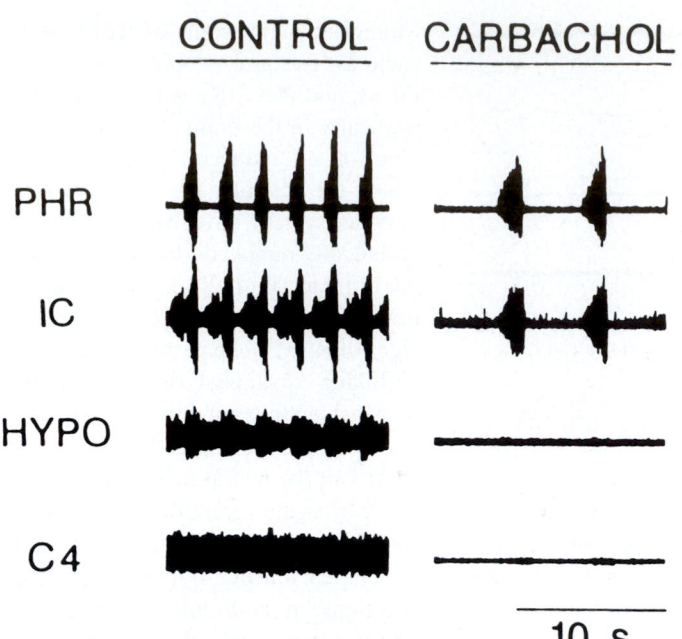

CONTROL   CARBACHOL

PHR

IC

HYPO

C4

10 s

FIGURE 101-9 Carbachol microinjection into the pons to activate maximally one component of the brain-stem circuitry involved in the generation of the phenomena of REM sleep. Arterial blood gases were maintained constant by artificial ventilation. The figure illustrates the hierarchic effect of carbachol microinjection on the different motor outputs. Phrenic nerve activity (top panel) is least affected, intercostal activity (middle panel) is more affected, and hypoglossal nerve activity (second panel from bottom) is massively suppressed. The suppression of hypoglossal nerve activity is similar to that for a branch of C4 (bottom panel) to a postural neck muscle. *(Based on data of Kimura et al,[18] with permission.)*

hindlimbs, where glycinergic inhibition has been shown to be the most important mechanism mediating the postural atonia during both natural REM sleep and the carbachol-induced atonia in a reduced preparation.[29] Thus, even though tonic suppression of postural and upper airway motor tones occurs simultaneously during REM sleep, the respective neurochemical mechanisms are different.

Finally, one neurochemical component of the suppression of hypoglossal nerve activity has been identified. It consists of a withdrawal of a serotoninergic excitation that these motoneurons apparently need in order to maintain a normal, wakefulnesslike level of activity. One line of evidence for this mechanism is that local microinjections into the hypoglossal motor nucleus,[23] as well as systemic administrations in English bulldogs,[46] of serotoninergic antagonists such as methysergide and ritanserin reduce the spontaneous activity of hypoglossal motoneurons. Another line of evidence comes from the finding that the extracellular level of serotonin (5-HT) in the hypoglossal nucleus region is reduced during the carbachol-induced atonia.[22] Consistent with this evidence, cells have been identified in the midline of the medulla (raphe nuclei), whose activity decreases during the carbachol-induced atonia; the location and properties of these cells are consistent with what is known about the properties of brain-stem cells containing and releasing 5-HT.[49] Such evidence points to the serotoninergic system as a potential target for pharmacologic treatments of obstructive sleep apnea. With

the recent explosion of new data about the diversity of serotoninergic receptors, the emergence of new evidence for the importance of 5-HT in many diseases, and new research tools offered by molecular biology, such treatments may be within the reach of the modern pharmaceutical industry.

CONCLUSION

The changes in the cardiorespiratory system during sleep have profound implications for cardiorespiratory control in sleep apnea syndromes and other diseases. Sleep-related respiratory disorders affect a large percentage of our society (see Chapter 102). Moreover, the normal processes that occur during sleep can augment the effects of other diseases that affect the respiratory system. This is true both for intrinsic disorders affecting the lung and for neuromuscular disease. At present, the respiratory consequences of sleep in health and disease are better described and understood than those of the cardiovascular system.

REFERENCES

1. Bulow K: Respiration and wakefulness in man. *Acta Physiol Scand* 59(Suppl 209):1–110, 1963.
2. Coote JH: Respiratory and circulatory control during sleep. *J Exp Biol* 100:223–244, 1982.
3. Deegan PC, McNicholas WT: Pathophysiology of obstructive sleep apnoea. *Eur Respir J* 8:1161–1178, 1995.
4. Dempsey JA, Smith CA, Harms CA, et al: Sleep-induced breathing instability. *Sleep* 19:236–247, 1996.
5. Findley LJ, Wilhoit SC, Suratt PM: Apnea duration and hypoxemia during REM sleep in patients with obstructive sleep apnea. *Chest* 87:432–436, 1985.
6. Fink BR, Hanks EC, Ngai SH, Papper EM: Central regulation of respiration during anesthesia and wakefulness. *Ann NY Acad Sci* 109:892–900, 1963.
7. Franzini C, Zoccoli G, Cianci T, Lenzi P: Sleep-dependent changes in regional circulation. *News Physiol Sci* 11:274–280, 1996.
8. Gothe B, Altose MD, Goldman MD, Cherniack NS: Effect of quiet sleep on resting and CO_2-stimulated breathing in humans. *J Appl Physiol* 50:724–730, 1981.
9. Guilleminault C, Pool P, Motta J, Gillis AM: Sinus arrest during REM sleep in young adults. *New Engl J Med* 311:1006–1010, 1984.
10. Haxhiu MA, van Lunteren E, Mitra J, Cherniack NS: Comparison of the response of diaphragm and upper airway dilating muscle activity in sleeping cats. *Respir Physiol* 70:183–193, 1987.
11. Hendricks JC, Kline LR: Differential activation within costal diaphragm during rapid-eye-movement sleep in cats. *J Appl Physiol* 70:1194–1200, 1991.
12. Hendricks JC, Kline LR, Kovalski RJ, et al: The English bulldog: A natural model of sleep-disordered breathing. *J Appl Physiol* 63:1344–1350, 1987.
13. Hendricks JC, Kovalski RJ, Kline LR: Phasic respiratory muscle patterns and sleep-disordered breathing during rapid eye movement sleep in the English bulldog. *Am Rev Respir Dis* 144:1112–1120, 1991.
14. Hendricks JC, Petrof BJ, Panckeri K, Pack AI: Upper airway dilating muscle hyperactivity during non–rapid eye movement sleep in English bulldogs. *Am Rev Respir Dis* 148:185–194, 1993.
15. Horner RL, Brooks D, Kozar LF, et al: Immediate effects of arousal from sleep on cardiac autonomic outflow in the absence of breathing in dogs. *J Appl Physiol* 79:151–162, 1995.

16. Issa FG, Sullivan CE: The immediate effects of nasal continuous positive airway pressure treatment on sleep pattern in patients with obstructive sleep apnea syndrome. *Electroencephalogr Clin Neurophysiol* 63:10–17, 1986.

17. Khoo MCK, Gottschalk A, Pack AI: Sleep-induced periodic breathing and apnea: A theoretical study. *J Appl Physiol* 70:2014–2024, 1991.

18. Kimura H, Kubin L, Davies RO, Pack AI: Cholinergic stimulation of the pons depresses respiration in decerebrate cats. *J Appl Physiol* 69:2280–2289, 1990.

19. Kirby DA, Vernier RL: Differential effects of sleep stage on coronary hemodynamic function during stenosis. *Physiol Behav* 45:1017–1020, 1989.

20. Kline LR, Hendricks JC, Davies RO, Pack AI: Control of activity of the diaphragm in rapid-eye-movement sleep. *J Appl Physiol* 61:1293–1300, 1986.

21. Kubin L, Kimura H, Tojima H, et al: Suppression of hypoglossal motoneurons during the carbachol-induced atonia of REM sleep is not caused by fast synaptic inhibition. *Brain Res* 611:300–312, 1993.

22. Kubin L, Reignier C, Tojima H, et al: Changes in serotonin level in the hypoglossal nucleus region during carbachol-induced atonia. *Brain Res* 645:291–302, 1994.

23. Kubin L, Tojima H, Davies RO, Pack AI: Serotonergic excitatory drive to hypoglossal motoneurons in the decerebrate cat. *Neurosci Lett* 139:243–248, 1992.

24. Kuna ST, Insalaco G, Villeponteaux RD: Arytenoideus muscle activity in normal adult humans during wakefulness and sleep. *J Appl Physiol* 70:1655–1664, 1991.

25. Kuna ST, Smickley JS, Vanoye CR, McMillan TH: Cricothyroid muscle activity during sleep in normal adult humans. *J Appl Physiol* 76:2326–2332, 1994.

26. Lydic R, Baghdoyan HA: Cholinergic pontine mechanisms causing state-dependent respiratory depression. *News Physiol Sci* 7:220–224, 1992.

27. Mezzanotte WS, Tangel DJ, White DP: Waking genioglossal electromyogram in sleep apnea patients versus normal controls (a neuromuscular compensatory mechanism). *J Clin Invest* 89:1571–1579, 1992.

28. Mezzanotte WS, Tangel DJ, White DP: Influence of sleep onset on upper-airway muscle activity in apnea patients versus normal controls. *Am J Respir Crit Care Med* 153:1880–1887, 1996.

29. Morales FR, Engelhardt JK, Soja PJ, et al: Motoneuron properties during motor inhibition produced by microinjection of carbachol into the pontine reticular formation of the decerebrate cat. *J Neurophysiol* 57:1118–1129, 1987.

30. Morgan BJ, Crabtree DC, Puleo DS, et al: Neurocirculatory consequences of abrupt change in sleep state in humans. *J Appl Physiol* 80:1627–1636, 1996.

31. Neilly JB, Gaipa EA, Maislin G, Pack AI: Ventilation during early and late rapid-eye-movement sleep in normal humans. *J Appl Physiol* 71:1201–1215, 1991.

32. O'Donnell CP, Ayuse T, King ED, et al: Airway obstruction during sleep increases blood pressure without arousal. *J Appl Physiol* 80:773–781, 1996.

33. Orem J: Neuronal mechanisms of respiration in REM sleep. *Sleep* 3:251–267, 1980.

34. Orem J: Central respiratory activity in rapid eye movement sleep: Augmenting and late inspiratory cells. *Sleep* 17:665–673, 1994.

35. Pack AI: Obstructive sleep apnea. *Adv Intern Med* 39:517–567, 1994.

36. Petrof BJ, Hendricks JC, Pack AI: Does upper airway muscle injury trigger a vicious cycle in obstructive sleep apnea? A hypothesis. *Sleep* 19:465–471, 1996.

37. Remmers JE, de Groot WJ, Sauerland EK, Anch AM: Pathogenesis of upper airway occlusion during sleep. *J Appl Physiol* 44:931–938, 1978.

38. Ringler J, Garpestad E, Basner RC, Weiss JW: Systemic blood pressure elevation after airway occlusion during NREM sleep. *Am J Respir Crit Care Med* 150:1062–1066, 1994.

39. Saupe KW, Smith CA, Henderson KS, Dempsey JA: Respiratory and cardiovascular responses to increased and decreased carotid sinus pressure in sleeping dogs. *J Appl Physiol* 78:1688–1698, 1995.

40. Shea SA: Behavioural and arousal-related influences on breathing in humans. *Exp Physiol* 81:1–26, 1996.

41. Siegel JM: Brainstem mechanisms generating REM sleep, in Kryger MH, Roth T, Dement WC (eds), *Principles and Practice of Sleep Medicine*. Philadelphia, Saunders, 1994, pp 125–144.

42. Skatrud JB, Dempsey JA: Interaction of sleep state and chemical stimuli in sustaining rhythmic ventilation. *J Appl Physiol* 55:813–822, 1983.

43. Skatrud JB, Dempsey JA: Airway resistance and respiratory muscle function in snorers during NREM sleep. *J Appl Physiol* 59:328–335, 1985.

44. Somers VK, Dyken ME, Clary MP, Abboud FM: Sympathetic neural mechanisms in obstructive sleep apnea. *J Clin Invest* 96:1897–1904, 1995.

45. Somers VK, Dyken ME, Mark AL, Abboud FM: Sympathetic-nerve activity during sleep in normal subjects. *New Engl J Med* 328:303–307, 1993.

46. Veasey SC, Panckeri KA, Hoffman EA, et al: The effects of serotonin antagonists in an animal model of sleep-disordered breathing. *Am J Respir Crit Care Med* 153:776–786, 1996.

47. Webster HH, Jones BE: Neurotoxin lesions of the dorsolateral pontomesencephalic tegmentum-cholinergic cell area in the cat: II. Effects upon sleep-waking states. *Brain Res* 458:285–302, 1988.

48. Wiegand L, Zwillich CW, Wiegand D, White DP: Changes in upper airway muscle activation and ventilation during phasic REM sleep in normal men. *J Appl Physiol* 71:488–497, 1991.

49. Woch G, Davies RO, Pack AI, Kubin L: Behaviour of raphe cells projecting to the dorsomedial medulla during carbachol-induced atonia in the cat. *J Physiol (Lond)* 490:745–758, 1996.

50. Xie A, Rutherford R, Rankin F, et al: Hypocapnia and increased ventilatory responsiveness in patients with idiopathic central sleep apnea. *Am J Respir Crit Care Med* 152:1950–1955, 1995.

CHAPTER 102

SLEEP APNEA SYNDROMES

Richard J. Schwab / Andrew N. Goldberg / Allan I. Pack

Sleep-disordered breathing is an extremely common medical disorder that is associated with considerable morbidity. Sleep apnea has been recognized as an important clinical condition only for the past 30 years.[27] However, sleep apnea syndromes have probably existed for centuries. Features of these disorders were described in ancient Greek literature and by William Shakespeare. In 1836, Charles Dickens wrote *Posthumous Papers of the Pickwick Club,* in which he described the classic findings of the Pickwickian syndrome in the character Joe, the "fat boy." In Dickens' novel, the reader is introduced to Joe as follows: "And on the box sat a fat and red-faced boy, in a state of somnolency." Sir William Osler is credited with being first to discern, in 1918, the relationship between obesity and Pickwickian syndrome. However, it was not until 1956 that Burwell and colleagues[4] described the relationship between alveolar hypoventilation and the Pickwickian syndrome. In 1966, Gastaut and associates[12] demonstrated the occurrence of recurrent apneas during sleep and suggested that these apneas resulted in sleep disruption and daytime sleepiness. Over the past 30 years, sleep apnea has proved to be an extremely common disorder. In addition, the pathogenesis of sleep apnea has begun to be understood, and effective diagnostic and treatment options have been developed for this common disorder.

DEFINITIONS

Sleep-disordered respiration is present when there are recurrent episodes of cessation of respiration (apnea) or decrements in airflow (hypopneas) during sleep.

Apnea is cessation of airflow for at least 10 s. An apnea can be obstructive (no airflow but continued respiratory effort), central (airflow and respiratory effort are both absent), or mixed. A mixed apnea is one that starts as a central event but then becomes obstructive during the same episode. Most patients with obstructive sleep apnea have both obstructive and mixed apneas.

Hypopnea is a decrement in airflow of 50 percent or more associated with a 4 percent fall in oxygen saturation or an electroencephalographic arousal. Hypopnea can produce clinical consequences identical with those of apnea, although apnea may be associated with greater oxyhemoglobin desaturations.[14] The term *sleep hypopnea syndrome* was introduced to take the hypopneas into account.[14]

The respiratory disturbance index (RDI)—the number of apneas plus hypopneas per hour of sleep, also called the apnea/hypopnea index—has become the standard by which to define and quantify the severity of obstructive sleep apnea. An RDI of more than 15 events per hour is indicative of obstructive sleep apnea. In general, as the RDI increases, so does the severity of symptoms.

The obstructive sleep apnea syndrome is said to be present when the RDI is greater than 15 events per hour and the patient has both daytime and nighttime symptoms.[14] Obstructive sleep apnea can either coexist with three other syndromes (obesity-hypoventilation syndrome, central sleep apnea, the upper-airway resistance syndrome) or occur independently. Persons with obstructive sleep apnea usually do not have hypercapnia (arterial P_{CO_2} greater than 45 mmHg) during wakefulness.

The obesity-hypoventilation syndrome (also known as the Pickwickian syndrome) usually coexists with obstructive sleep apnea. The syndrome consists of obesity, usually morbid, and, in contrast with the obstructive sleep apnea syndrome, chronic hypoventilation with daytime hypercapnia (Pa_{CO_2} over 45). Characteristic findings in patients with obesity-hypoventilation syndrome include arterial hypoxemia during wakefulness, hypersomnolence, pulmonary hypertension with chronic right heart failure, and nocturnal hypoventilation. The diagnosis of obesity-hypoventilation syndrome can be confirmed by demonstration of an increase in Pa_{CO_2} of greater than 10 mmHg during sleep. Although sleep apnea is usually present in such patients, the degree of apnea may not be severe. Obesity is a risk factor for both the obesity-hypoventilation syndrome and sleep apnea. Therefore, it is not surprising that the two often coexist.

Central sleep apnea is much less common than obstructive sleep apnea and is often associated with an underlying neurologic condition. It is characterized by repeated episodes of apnea during sleep that occur in the absence of respiratory muscle effort. Persons with central sleep apnea complain, as do those with obstructive sleep apnea, of daytime sleepiness secondary to sleep fragmentation from the apneic events. The pathogenesis of central sleep apnea is related to transient abnormalities of central drive to the respiratory muscles. The diagnosis of central sleep apnea is made by polysomnography, which demonstrates recurrent episodes of apnea in the absence of motion of the chest wall and abdomen.[54]

Upper-airway resistance syndrome can cause symptoms similar to those of obstructive sleep apnea.[15] This syndrome is characterized by repeated arousals secondary to increased upper-airway resistance (or crescendo snoring).[15] At the end of the episode of crescendo snoring, arousal occurs with an abrupt decrease in upper-airway resistance, so that snoring disappears, albeit temporarily. In the upper-airway resistance syndrome, there are no apneas or significant decreases in oxyhemoglobin saturation. It is proposed that the arousals in the upper-airway resistance syndrome, analogous to arousals from apneas or hypopneas, result in sleep fragmentation and daytime sleepiness. The incidence and prevalence of the upper-airway resistance syndrome are unknown.[36,52]

SPECTRUM OF SLEEP-DISORDERED BREATHING

Obstructive sleep apnea should be regarded as a continuum—a spectrum of diseases from snoring to the obesity-hypoventilation syndrome (Pickwickian syndrome) (Fig. 102-1). Snoring should not be considered normal; it is often the first manifestation of sleep-disordered breathing. This concept of a continuum of abnormality is important, since it is likely, although not proven, that the natural history of sleep-disordered breathing follows this continuum. Weight gain or loss may be a factor that moves a person along this continuum of sleep-disordered breathing. Weight gain

is an important risk factor for sleep apnea and the Pickwickian syndrome.[51] Persons may also shift position on the continuum rather abruptly. For example, alcohol can worsen the degree of sleep-disordered breathing, since it preferentially suppresses the activity of upper airway dilator muscles. Alcohol, sedatives, or hypnotics can cause a normal person to snore during sleep and turn a patient who snores into a patient with obstructive apneas during sleep. Treatment of sleep-disordered breathing—e.g., with nasal continuous positive airway pressure (CPAP)—is expected to move patients along the continuum. It is possible, however, that although apneas are abolished with CPAP, the patients may not move sufficiently along the continuum to remove all abnormalities: they are left with the residual upper airway-resistance syndrome or snoring. Such patients may remain symptomatic and excessively sleepy despite treatment with nasal CPAP.

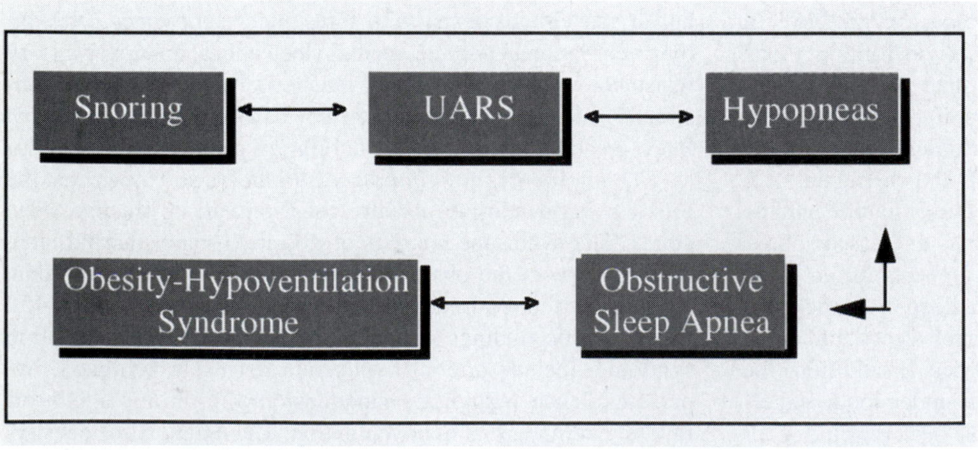

OBSTRUCTIVE SLEEP APNEA

Pathogenesis

The pathogenesis of obstructive sleep apnea includes both an anatomic and a neurologic component. The upper airway may be narrowed anatomically, even during wakefulness, by enlarged soft tissue structures (increased size of the tongue, soft palate, or lateral pharyngeal walls) or by bony abnormalities (retrognathia, micrognathia). Such narrowing predisposes the airway to collapse during sleep.

The upper airway is an extremely complicated structure that performs several different physiological functions, including vocalization, respiration, and deglutition. The biomechanical relationships of the various muscles (more than 24 have been described) that enable the upper airway to perform these functions are not well understood. However, the upper airway can be subdivided into three regions: (1) *nasopharynx* (region between the nasal turbinates and hard palate); (2) *oropharynx,* which can be subdivided into the retropalatal (also called the velopharynx) and retroglossal regions; and (3) *hypopharynx* (region from the base of the tongue to the larynx). These regions are demonstrated in Fig. 102-2, which displays a midsagittal magnetic resonance image (MRI) of a normal subject in which the retropalatal and retroglossal regions of the oropharynx are outlined. In addition, this midsagittal image highlights the tongue and soft palate, which are important anteroposterior soft tissue structures of the upper airway.

The important lateral upper-airway soft tissue structures—the lateral pharyngeal walls and lateral parapharyngeal fat pads just outside the walls of the pharynx—are demonstrated in the axial MRI of the retropalatal region of a normal subject shown in Fig. 102-3. In persons with sleep apnea, collapse of the airway can occur in the retropalatal or retroglossal region or at both sites. Although the location of collapse varies between subjects, in a given subject it tends to be reproducible from episode to episode.

FIGURE 102-1   Spectrum of sleep-disordered breathing. UARS = upper airway resistance syndrome.

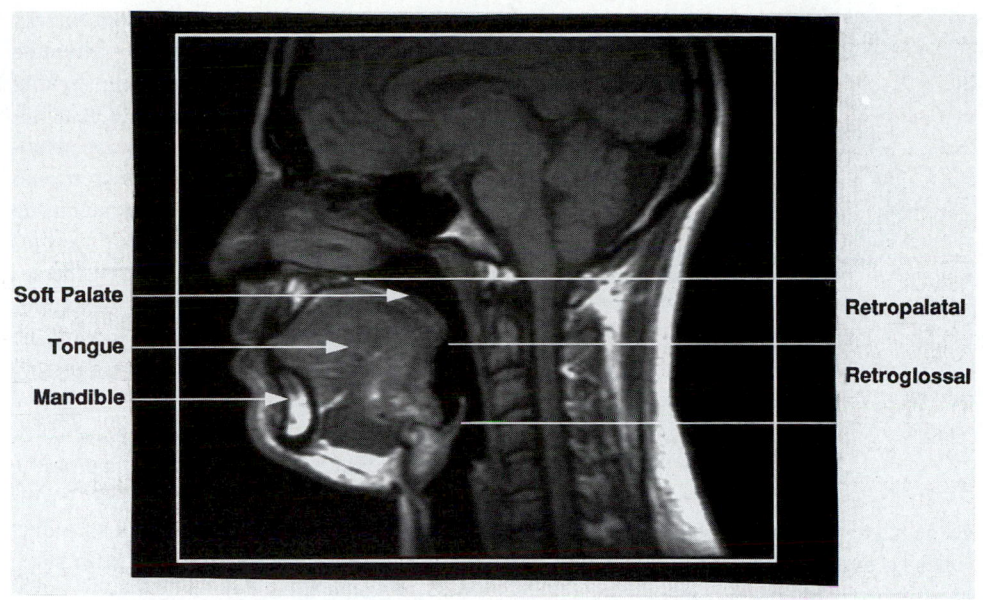

FIGURE 102-2 Midsagittal magnetic resonance (MR) image in a normal subject demonstrating the anatomic regions of the upper airway and relevant soft tissue structures. The retropalatal region is defined from the level of the hard palate and the distal margin of the soft palate; the retroglossal region is defined from the distal margin of the soft palate and the base of the epiglottis. In obstructive sleep apnea, obstruction can occur in the retropalatal or retroglossal levels or at both locations.

Imaging studies, using computed tomography or magnetic resonance techniques, have provided insight into the pathogenesis of obstructive sleep apnea.[36,43] During wakefulness, upper-airway caliber is, in general, smaller in patients with sleep apnea than in normal subjects, and the shape of the upper airway in apneic subjects differs from that of normal subjects (Fig. 102-4). In the normal airway, the major axis is oriented in the lateral,

horizontal dimension. In apneic subjects, the lateral diameter of the airway is considerably reduced, while the anteroposterior diameter is relatively preserved. Thus, the airway of the apneic patient is oriented more in the anteroposterior dimension. It is believed that the apneic airway configuration (Fig. 102-4) adversely affects the activity of the upper-airway muscles, predisposing to airway closure during sleep.[28]

This lateral narrowing of the airway indicates that soft tissue structures lateral to the airway may be important in modulating airway caliber. The two primary structures lateral to the upper airway are the lateral pharyngeal walls and lateral parapharyngeal fat pads (Fig. 102-3). Obesity or, more specifically, increased neck size is a risk factor for sleep apnea.[7,51,56] Weight loss causes the upper airway to become less collapsible and to improve sleep-disordered respiration.[51] For this reason, it has been hypothesized that increased adipose tissue deposited in the lateral parapharyngeal fat pads may lead to airway narrowing by compressing the airway. However, a recent study demonstrated that the lateral narrowing of the upper airway in apneic persons is explained by increased thickness of the lateral pharyngeal walls, not by compression of the walls by the parapharyngeal fat pads.[46] Fig. 102-5 compares axial images at the minimum airway area (retropalatal region) in a normal subject with those of a patient with sleep apnea. The airway area and width are smaller in the apneic patient; moreover, the lateral pharyngeal walls are thicker. The basis for the increased thickness of the lateral pharyngeal walls in apneic subjects is unknown. Other imaging studies have demonstrated that the total volume of fat surrounding the upper airway is greater in apneic than in normal persons, suggesting that fat deposition in the neck plays a role in the pathogenesis of obstructive sleep apnea. However, it does not appear that obesity predisposes to the development of apnea by compressing the lateral pharyngeal airway walls. Although the lateral pharyngeal walls are larger in patients with sleep apnea, several imaging studies have indicated that tongue size and soft-palate area and length are also larger in these patients. The pathogenesis of the increase in size of these soft tissue structures of the upper airway is unknown, but possible etiologic mecha-

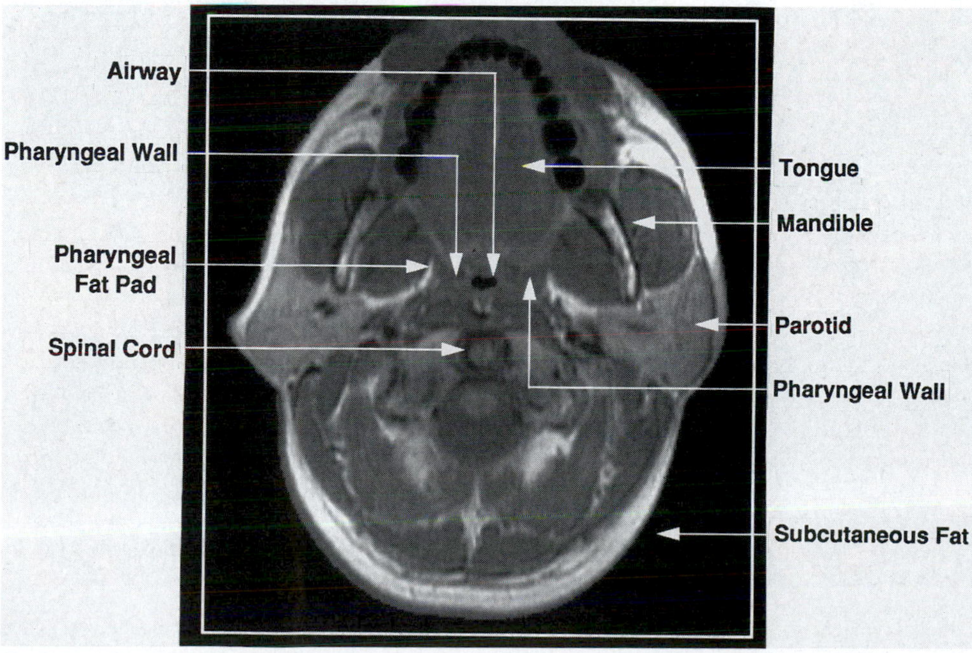

FIGURE 102-3 Axial MR image at the retropalatal level in a normal subject. The relevant soft tissue and bony structures surrounding the upper airway are highlighted. The tissues immediately lateral to the airway are the lateral pharyngeal walls and the parapharyngeal fat pads.

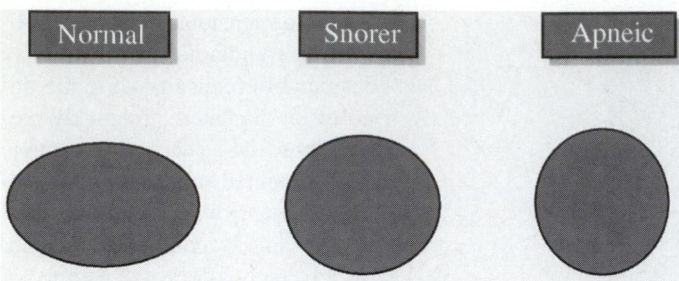

FIGURE 102-4 Schematic diagram of upper-airway configuration in a normal subject, a snorer, and an apneic subject. The normal airway has a horizontal orientation, with the largest diameter being the lateral diameter. The apneic airway is narrowed laterally, with its longest axis being in the anteroposterior. The airway of the snorer is intermediate between these two.

nisms include edema as a result of the large negative pressure generated in the upper airway during sleep, obesity, and genetic factors. Not only is the size of these soft tissue structures important but the biomechanical interrelationships between the tongue, soft palate, and lateral pharyngeal walls also have to be taken into account in the pathogenesis of obstructive sleep apnea.

The upper airway should not be considered to be a structure with static dimensions. The size of the upper airway depends on the phase of the respiratory cycle.[44] During wakefulness, changes in the dimensions of the upper airway during respiration can be considered to occur in four distinct phases (Fig. 102-6). In phase 1, at the onset of inspiration, the area of the upper airway in-

creases, presumably reflecting the activation of upper-airway dilator muscles at the onset of inspiration. In phase 2, the area of the upper airway is maintained relatively constant throughout the remainder of inspiration. Therefore, there appears to be a balance between the action of negative intraluminal pressure, tending to collapse the airway, and the activity of airway dilator muscles, tending to enlarge the airway. Phase 3 marks the beginning of expiration. At this time, the activity of airway dilator muscles decreases and the airway widens, presumably because of the action of positive intraluminal pressure at the beginning of expiration. In Phase 4, airway dimensions decrease rapidly toward the end of expiration: the airway appears headed toward its resting position, where it is no longer kept open either by the positive intraluminal pressure (at the onset of expiration, or phase 3) or by the phasic action of airway dilator muscles (during inspiration, or phases 1 and 2). Thus, the airway may be particularly vulnerable to collapse at the end of expiration. Airway closure during expiration has been reported to occur in patients with sleep apnea.[44]

During wakefulness, activation of airway dilator muscles protects the airway from collapse. In patients with sleep apnea, activation of these muscles increases during wakefulness to compensate for the anatomic compromise of the airway. This compensation is lost during sleep. In non-REM (NREM) sleep, both the tonic and phasic activation of airway dilator muscles decrease during inspiration. This decrease is probably secondary to reduced activation of the relevant motoneurons as a consequence of a decrease in excitation by central brain-stem path-

Normal   **Apneic**

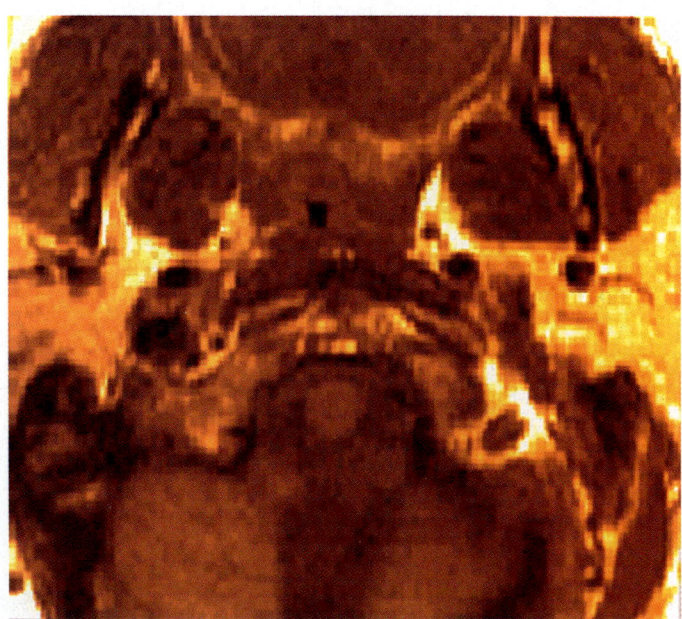

FIGURE 102-5 Comparison of a cross-sectional image in the retropalatal region in a normal subject (left panel) and in an apneic subject (right panel). The left side of the picture shows a volumetric rendering of the head with a segmented airway as obtained by our image analysis software. Oblique sections (perpendicular to the airway) are displayed in a normal subject and an apneic subject at the retroplatal level. The apneic airway is smaller, with the major difference being in the lateral dimension. This lateral narrowing is explained by the increased thickness of the lateral walls, which is evident in these figures.

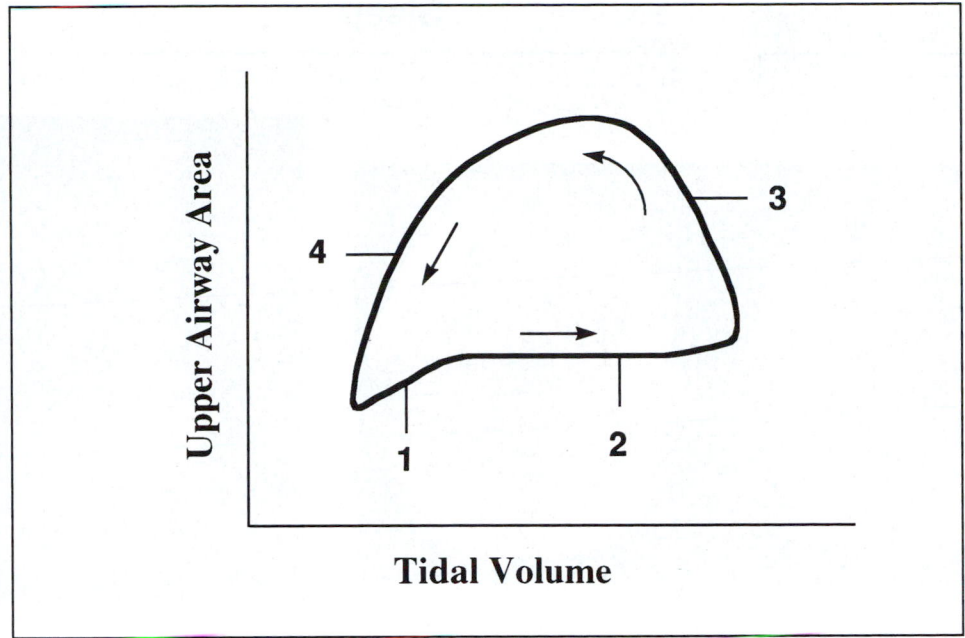

FIGURE 102-6   Schematic diagram of upper-airway area as a function of tidal volume during inspiration and expiration in patients with sleep apnea. Four distinct phases in the respiratory cycle are recognized: phase 1 = early inspiration; phase 2 = remainder of inspiration; phase 3 = early expiration; and phase 4 = late expiration. For further details, see text.

in the genesis of airway closure during apnea. The dynamic changes in airway size with respiration may differ during sleep from those during wakefulness. In particular, the neuromechanical mechanism that maintains airway size relatively constant during inspiration may be lost during sleep, so that the airway narrows during the inspiratory phase of the respiratory cycle. Therefore, during sleep, narrowing of the airway may occur during the inspiratory phase of the cycle as well as during the later part of expiration.

Epidemiology and Risk Factors

Sleep apnea is an extremely common disorder. This has been demonstrated in studies in the United States, Europe, Israel, and Australia. The largest, most comprehensive study was conducted in Wisconsin—the Wisconsin Sleep Cohort Study.[56] This study, conducted on

ways during sleep. This excitatory input is mediated by serotonin from raphe cells. The decrease in firing from these cells during sleep may be important in decreasing activation of upper-airway dilator muscles. Alteration in peripheral reflexes also contributes to the failure to compensate for anatomic compromise of the airway. During wakefulness, negative pressure inside the airway activates upper-airway dilator muscles by a reflex mechanoreceptor feedback loop. This reflex is markedly decreased, and indeed can be lost, during NREM sleep, contributing to the decrease in airway dilator muscle activity that occurs in patients with sleep apnea. In REM sleep, these changes in airway dilator muscle activity can be even more pronounced. In particular, in association with the phasic REM events, activity of the airway dilator muscles can be completely suppressed. It is not surprising, therefore, that in patients with sleep apnea, these disturbances can be most profound during REM sleep.

In summary, the decrease in activation of airway dilator muscles during sleep leads to a decrease in airway size both in normal subjects and in patients with sleep apnea (Figs. 102-7 and 102-8). This reduction in airway size is due to a decrease in both the anteroposterior and the lateral dimensions, the decrease in the latter being the larger. Sleep is associated with increased thickening of the lateral walls surrounding the airway. This suggests that the lateral pharyngeal walls play a role

state employees in Wisconsin, found that in 9 percent of middle-aged men and 4 percent of middle-aged women, the RDI exceeded 15 events per hour. If nighttime and daytime symptoms (excessive sleepiness) were included in the definition of sleep apnea, 4 percent of middle-aged men and 2 percent of middle-aged women manifested sleep apnea. Thus, obstructive sleep apnea is a common clinical disorder; as such, it has major public health implications.[37]

The epidemiologic studies show a male predominance: the disorder is twice as common in males as in females. However, early reports from clinical studies indicated an 8- to 9-fold in-

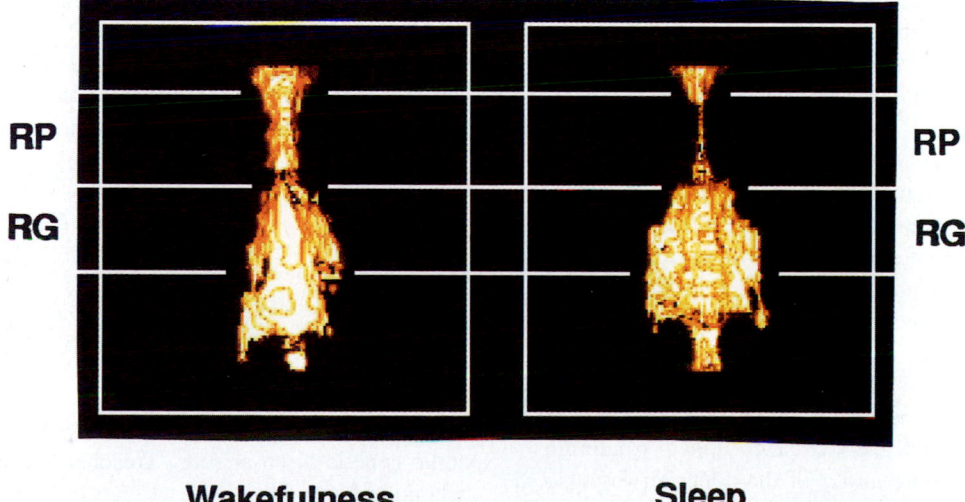

FIGURE 102-7   Three-dimensional surface renderings of the upper airway demonstrating state-dependent changes in upper-airway volume in a normal subject. Airway caliber narrows significantly during sleep in the retropalatal region. RP = retropalatal region; RG = retroglossal region.

Wakefulness   ## Sleep

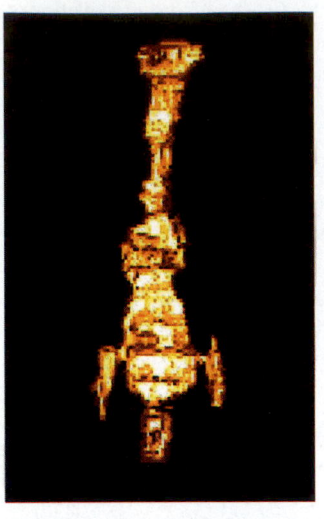
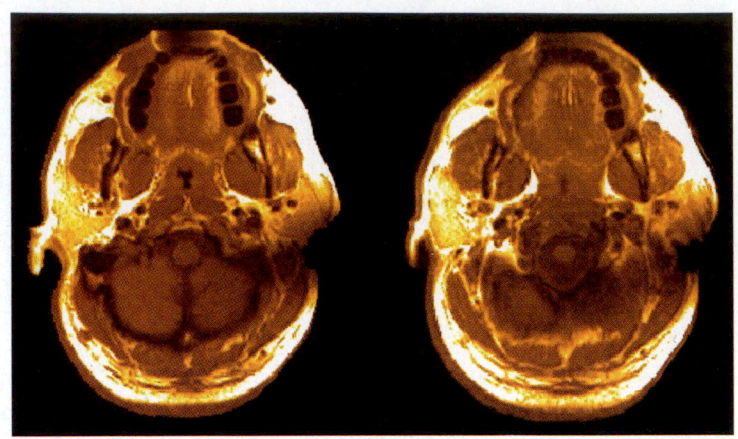
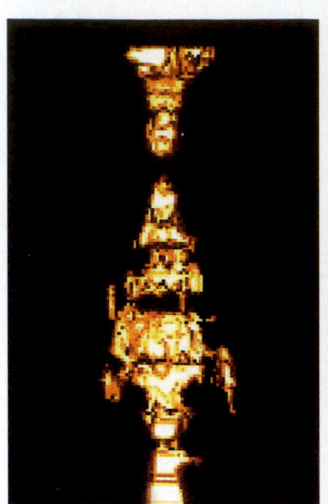

3D Airway   **Retropalatal Axial Sections**   **3D Airway**

FIGURE 102-8 Axial MR images (middle pictures) at the retropalatal level and volumetric surface rendered images of the entire upper airway in an apneic subject during wakefulness and sleep. In this person, the retroglossal region increases in size during sleep.

crease in case rates of obstructive sleep apnea in males. This marked difference in male/female ratios between epidemiologic studies and clinical reports is probably due to two factors: (1) once a disorder is labeled as predominantly a male condition, physicians may be less likely to think about it in women and, hence, less likely to refer women to sleep disorders centers; and (2) symptoms appear to differ between males and females: women are less likely to complain of sleepiness but more likely to complain of nonspecific fatigue.[16]

Epidemiologic studies also reveal the major risk factors for the disorder (Table 102-1). The major risk factor, at least in adults, is obesity. In the Wisconsin Sleep Cohort Study,[56] the prevalence of sleep apnea tripled in association with an increase in body mass index by one standard deviation. Not surprisingly, fat in the neck plays the largest role. In population studies, neck (or collar size) is the best indicator of the presence of sleep apnea.[7] Approximately 30 percent of snoring males with a collar size larger than 17 inches will have obstructive sleep apnea. Because of this relationship to neck size, measurement of neck size should be part of the routine physical examination. Neck size in women is less well investigated, but when it is over 15 inches, it increases the risk for sleep apnea.[16]

Obesity is not the only risk factor for obstructive sleep apnea. Anatomic abnormalities of the upper airway also play a role. These include soft tissue abnormalities such as tonsillar and adenoidal hypertrophy. In children, this appears to be the major risk factor for ap-

nea, although formal epidemiologic prevalence studies have not been conducted in this age group. Nasal abnormalities, such as nasal septal deviation, also increase the risk of apnea. Structural bony abnormalities, such as micrognathia and retrognathia, are also known risk factors. Genetic factors are also included among the risk factors for obstructive sleep apnea. Specific genetic disorders are associated with sleep apnea. These include genetic craniofacial disorders (e.g., Treacher Collins syndrome, Down syndrome, Apert's syndrome, achondrophasia) in which the upper airway is anatomically compromised. In these disorders, obstructive sleep apnea syndrome is both common and severe.

Even without a specific gene defect, genetic factors play a role. For example, relatives of a person with sleep apnea have approximately twice the normal risk of having sleep apnea.[31,38] This increased risk is not simply explained by obesity. Indeed, relatives of nonobese patients with sleep apnea have increased risk of sleep apnea.[31] However, in these relatives there are un-

TABLE 102-1

Risk Factors for Obstructive Sleep Apnea

Gender (male/female, 2:1)
Obesity (>120% ideal body weight)
Neck size (collar size >17 in. in males, >15 in. in females)
Tonsillar hypertrophy
Nasal septal deviation
Retrognathia, micrognathia
Specific genetic diseases (e.g., Treacher Collins, Down syndrome, Apert's syndrome, achondrophasia, etc.)
Genetic predisposition (as yet unexplained)
Endocrine disorders (e.g., hypothyroidism, acromegaly)
Alcohol, sedatives, or hypnotics

derlying structural differences: the relatives have longer, larger soft palates and more retroposed maxillas and mandibles. It seems likely that, as in other disorders, a number of specific genes, individually or in combination, may increase the risk of sleep apnea.

Endocrine disorders can also be accompanied by apnea. Hypothyroidism is associated with an increased prevalence of both obstructive and central apnea; the macroglossia of hypothyroidism contributes to this high frequency. Also, in persons who have previously undergone thyroid surgery, the prevalence of sleep apnea is increased, presumably because of damage to the muscular apparatus that controls the upper airway. Sleep apnea syndrome is also common and often severe in acromegalic patients, presumably because of the large tongue coupled with other structural changes in the upper airway.

Alcohol, which reduces upper-airway muscle tone, and sedatives or hypnotics, which reduce the arousal mechanism, exacerbate obstructive sleep apnea.

Each of these risk factors needs to be considered in the examination of a patient with obstructive sleep apnea. It is important to uncover why a particular patient has developed sleep apnea. Although routine in-depth evaluation of the upper airway by fiberoptic techniques and screening for hypothyroidism with thyroid function tests are not required in every patient, the physician should be ready to perform such studies, particularly in patients in whom the origin of the sleep apnea is not entirely clear.

Clinical Presentation

The diagnosis of obstructive sleep apnea is not difficult to make: the symptoms are typical and the major risk factor is relatively obvious. Patients with sleep apnea have both nighttime and daytime symptoms (Table 102-2), which can be uncovered by a careful sleep history. As a rule, persons with sleep apnea usually do not report difficulty in falling asleep, although some complain of insomnia. They report frequent nocturnal awakenings and sleep fragmentation. Occasionally they report waking up snorting or gasping, but more often they wake up to urinate; nocturnal naturesis is part of the pathophysiology of obstructive sleep apnea. The nocturia is probably related to the large negative swings in pleural pressure that occur during the obstructive apneic episodes. These episodes stretch the right atrial wall and

TABLE 102-2

Obstructive Sleep Apnea

Loud, habitual snoring
Witnessed apneas
Nocturnal awakening
Gasping or choking episodes during sleep
Nocturia
Unrefreshing sleep, morning headaches
Excessive daytime sleepiness
Automobile or work-related accidents
Irritability, memory loss, personality change
Decreased libido

thereby increase the production of atrial naturetic factor. Indeed, patients with sleep apnea may seek urologic help, with nocturia as their presenting complaint.

Bed partners provide more information about the events occurring during sleep, and a careful history from a bed partner is an important part of the evaluation of all patients with sleep apnea. Bed partners will report snoring. Typically, the snoring has persisted for many years. The snoring of obstructive sleep apnea is both loud (it can be heard in an adjacent room) and habitual (it occurs nightly). The loudness may be such that bed partners have been driven to sleeping in another room. The bed partners may also have witnessed apneas and the loud snorts or gasps that occur at the end of the apneic episodes. Occasionally, during the arousal that terminates the apneic event, the bed partner may witness arm flailing or other gross movements.

As a result of these repetitive apneic events, persons with sleep apnea have extremely fragmented sleep that results in less slow-wave sleep (stages 3 and 4 sleep or delta sleep) and REM sleep than in age-matched controls. Thus, persons with sleep apnea do not feel refreshed when they awaken in the morning. Morning headaches are relatively uncommon; instead, morning headache suggests hypercapnia and a manifestation of the obesity-hypoventilation syndrome.

Persons with sleep apnea commonly report difficulty in getting going in the morning. During the day, patients with sleep apnea are excessively sleepy. Persons with mild disease generally feel tired and drowsy during the day but do not fall asleep; however, they do fall asleep in the evening as soon as they sit down to watch TV or read the newspaper. Patients with severe disease fall asleep inappropriately in many circumstances (e.g., in face-to-face conversation, on the telephone, while eating). Thus, their sleepiness is relatively uncontrollable. Driving is particularly problematic in patients with sleep apnea, and it is important to question patients carefully about falling asleep while driving or at traffic lights. Sleep apnea patients often report feeling drowsy while driving and having to pull over to nap. They may report having actually fallen asleep while driving and left the road or had a crash. A common history is that people with sleep apnea fall asleep in the car while waiting at red lights. In general, sleepiness in these people is directly related to the severity of sleep apnea. A standard instrument (the Epworth Sleepiness Scale) is a useful tool in clinical practice to assess the degree of self-rated sleepiness (Table 102-3).[24] A value above 10 is considered abnormal. The Epworth Sleepiness Scale score is usually high in patients with sleep apnea and lowers with treatment of sleep apnea. The Epworth Sleepiness Scale score has been reported to correlate with the degree of physiological sleepiness as measured by the multiple sleep latency test.[24]

Persons with sleep apnea have other impairments. They report difficulties in paying attention, in memory, and with concentration and ambition. These difficulties often interfere with their ability to function at work. They also report limiting social contact because of their fear of sleepiness and falling asleep. Patients with sleep apnea may be irritable, and their spouses may report personality changes. Sexual dysfunction is common (e.g., diminished libido even though men with apnea can obtain an erection). Persons with sleep apnea may note nocturnal palpitations or skipped heartbeats.

TABLE 102-3

Epworth Sleepiness Scale

In contrast to just feeling tired, how likely are you to doze off or fall asleep in the following situations? (This refers to your usual life in recent times. Even if you have not done some of these things recently, try to work out how they would have affected you.) Use the following scale to choose the most appropriate number for each situation:

0 = Would never doze
1 = Slight chance of dozing
2 = Moderate chance of dozing
3 = High chance of dozing

Situation	*Chance of Dozing*
Sitting and reading	_____
Watching TV	_____
Sitting inactive a public place (e.g., in a theater or at a meeting)	_____
As a passenger in a car for an hour without a break	_____
Lying down to rest in the afternoon when circumstances permit	_____
Sitting and talking to someone	_____
Sitting quietly after lunch without alcohol	_____
In a car, while stopping for a few minutes in traffic	_____

The predominant clinical manifestations of obstructive sleep apnea reflect the risk factors: obesity (particularly of the upper body); increased neck size (greater than 17 inches in men and greater than 15 inches in women, measured at the cricothyroid membrane); crowded oropharynx (tonsillar hypertrophy and enlargement of soft palate, uvula, and tongue, as well as lateral peritonsillar narrowing); retrognathia; and micrognathia. The consequences of the disorder may also be manifest in hypertension and, in severe cases, cardiac arrhythmias, pulmonary hypertension, edema, and polycythemia. Pulmonary hypertension and right heart failure develop in a subgroup of patients with severe sleep apnea; most of these patients have the obesity-hypoventilation syndrome. In mild obstructive sleep apnea, persistent pulmonary hypertension does not occur.

Diagnosis

The diagnosis of obstructive sleep apnea is made by polysomnography—i.e., a sleep study. Variables are recorded while the subject is asleep: electroencephalogram (EEG); electrooculogram (EOG), for monitoring eye movements; electromyogram (EMG), for muscle tone (all three of these variables allow the stage of sleep to be determined); respiratory airflow; respiratory effort (e.g., by bands placed around the chest and abdomen); arterial oxygen saturation; snoring intensity; electrocardiogram; and EMG of the anterior tibialis muscles, to monitor for presence of periodic leg movements during sleep (Fig. 102-9). From such records, apneas, hypopneas, and snoring-related arousals are scored. The RDI is calculated from the number of apneas plus hypopneas per hour.

A typical diagnostic polysomnography study entails a whole night of recording during sleep. Patients found to have sleep apnea return on a subsequent night for a second sleep study, during which the level of CPAP necessary to abolish sleep-related breathing events is determined (see below). Effort has been made to compress both of these components, diagnostic and therapeutic, into one night of study, "a split-night study."[21] The scientific rationale for split-night polysomnography is that the RDI in the first half of the night is highly indicative of that for the whole night of study; in addition, split-night studies are more cost-effective than two-night studies. Split-night polysomnography is effective in approximately 78 percent of patients;[21] in some patients, difficulties in optimizing the CPAP make it necessary to add another night to complete the study. Although concerns remain about whether CPAP titrations performed over half the night are suboptimal and whether subsequent CPAP compliance is worse with this abbreviated approach, there are no data to support these reservations.

SLEEP APNEA

Screening

Techniques to screen for the disorder would have to be inexpensive. Both standardized questionnaires (e.g., the Multivariable Apnea Prediction [MAP])[21] and simple tests, such as oximetry during the night,[36] have been evaluated. Three questions about nighttime events seem to offer the best predictive power for the presence of sleep apnea.[30] The three questions have the same form: during the past month, have you had, or have you been told about, the following symptom: snorting or gasping; loud snoring; or breathing stops, choking or struggling for breath? The frequency of occurrence is indicated as follows: never (0); rarely, less than once per week (1); once or twice per week (2); three or four times per week (3); five to seven times per week (4); or don't know. The total symptom score is computed; when it is combined with a measure of the major risk factor for sleep apnea (i.e., obesity), as evaluated by the body mass index (BMI), a pretest likelihood of apnea can be calculated (Fig. 102-10).[30] At high values of BMI, the presence of symptoms does not add predictive power, since the risk factor for the disorder (obesity) is so dominant. However, at lower or intermediate values of BMI, the symptom score affects the calculated likelihood of apnea.

Although questionnaires may be useful, they cannot yet be recommended for routine screening for obstructive sleep apnea. Once suspicion is aroused, however, individuals should be ques-

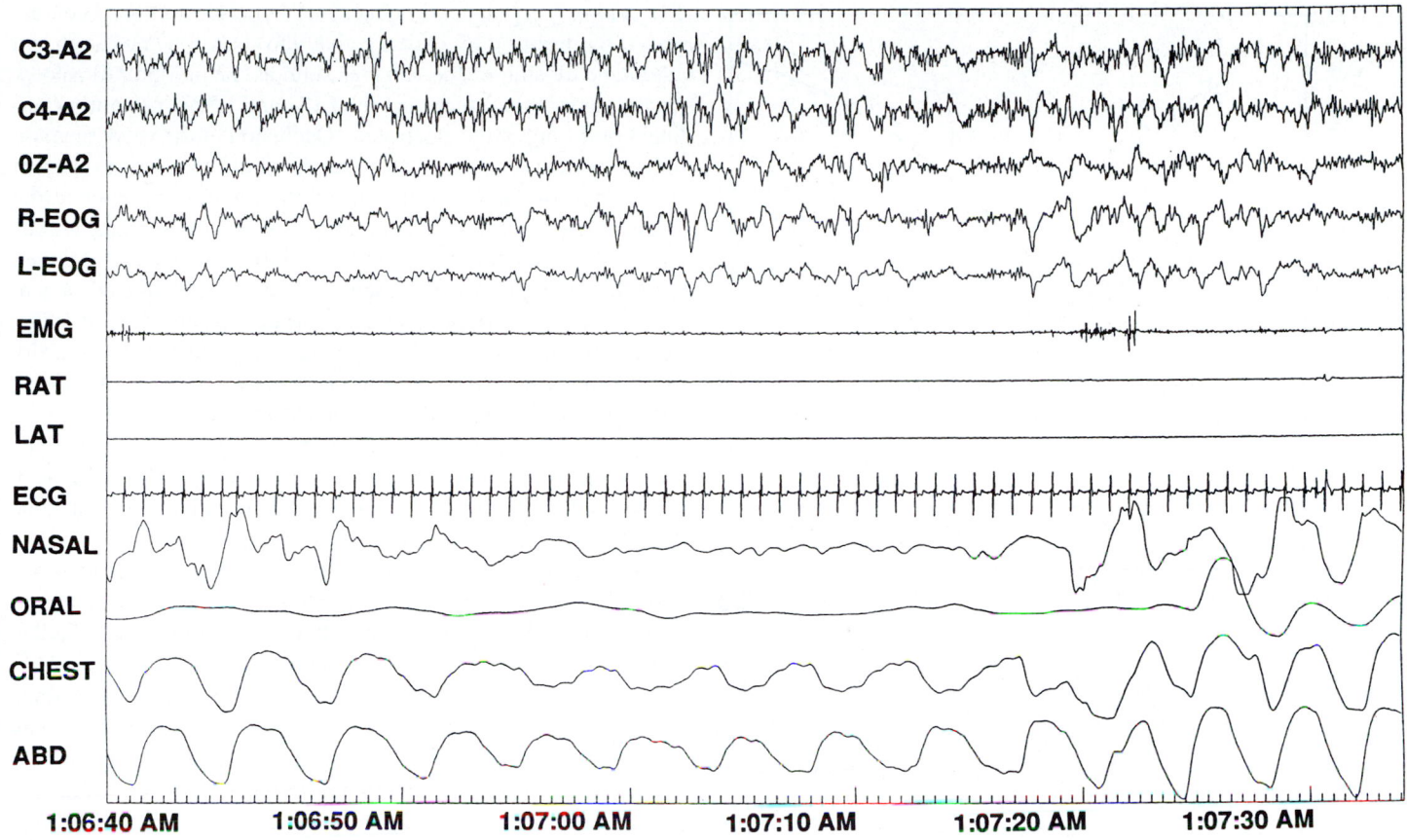

FIGURE 102-9 Example of an obstructive apneic episode in a patient with sleep apnea syndrome. The polysomnography traces from the top down are as follows: three EEG channels (C3-A2, C4-A2, OZ-A2); two EOG channels (R and L); submental EMG (EMG); right and left anterior tibialis EMG (RAT, LAT); electrocardiogram (ECG); nasal and oral airflow; chest and abdominal motion (CHEST and ABD). During the apneic episodes, there is abnormal airflow (both oral and nasal), with paradoxical motion of the rib cage and abdomen. At the end of the apneic episode, there is a burst of EMG activity at the arousal. Following arousal, respiration resumes with synchronous movements of the rib cage and abdomen.

tioned for symptoms of sleep apnea, and a measurement of neck size should be made. Standard questionnaires such as the Multivariable Apnea Prediction and the Epworth Sleepiness Scale are available for investigating the possibility of obstructive sleep apnea. The indications for evaluating the possibility of sleep apnea are outlined in Table 102-4. Questions about sleep disorders should be part of the review of systems in *all* patients.

Consequences

The consequences of obstructive sleep apnea syndrome can be broadly divided into those related to excessive sleepiness and those related to the cardiovascular system. Excessive daytime sleepiness produces a number of problems for patients with sleep apnea, among which the most serious is vehicular crashes.[10] Studies in driving simulators and in simple tests such as Steer-Clear, which is a modified reaction-time test, indicate that sleep apnea impairs driving ability. Recently it was demonstrated that patients with sleep apnea can be as impaired in driving skills as are those with blood alcohol concentrations in excess of legal limits.[13]

Persons who carry the diagnosis of sleep apnea have three to seven times the crash rates of control groups.[10] This increased crash risk has been confirmed in the Wisconsin Sleep Cohort Study.[56] In this prevalence study, however, fewer than 10 percent of the large number of people who had been found to have the sleep apnea syndrome were being treated for the disorder.

This increased risk of vehicular crashes places an important responsibility on both the patient and the physician. The physician needs to determine whether the patient is medically competent to continue to drive. While sleep apnea is dealt with by broad, relatively vague rules about driving in most states, it is specifically listed in two states (Texas and California) and in all Canadian provinces as a disorder that requires physicians to report patients with this disorder to state motor vehicle authorities. Concern has been expressed about whether such a regulation will have the desired effect of reducing vehicular crashes or whether it will discourage persons with sleep apnea from seeking treatment for fear of losing their drivers' licenses.

This topic has been addressed by the American Thoracic Society (ATS), which has recommended against categorical reporting of all patients.[1] The ATS recommends, instead, that physicians report sleep apnea patients to departments of motor vehicles only if they have had a crash caused by falling asleep at the wheel or if they have refused treatment for their disorder. The ATS statement highlights the importance of documenting

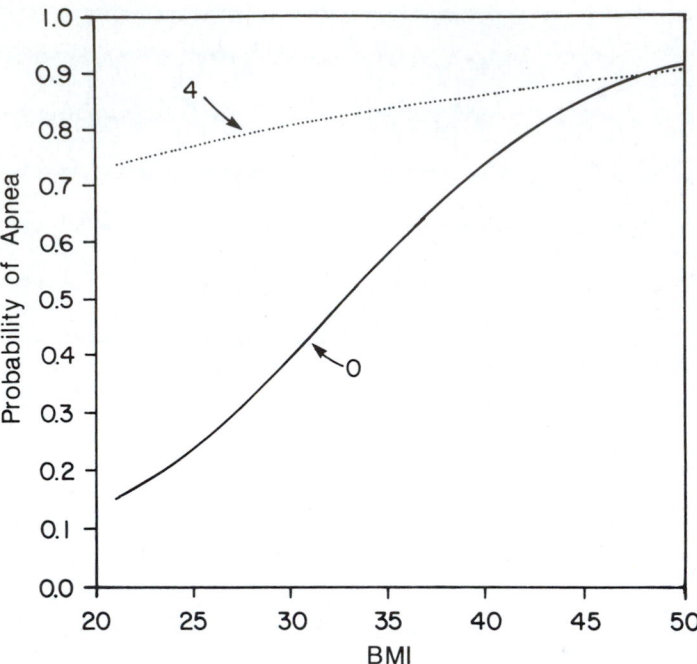

FIGURE 102-10 Relationship between likelihood of apnea and body mass index (BMI). The curves shown are for a person with no symptoms of apnea (curve labeled zero) and for a person with frequent loud snoring, snorting, and gasping, and witnessed apneas (curve labeled four). At high levels of BMI, there is a high probability of sleep apnea with or without symptoms. At lower levels of weight, the frequently occurring symptoms make a significant difference in the likelihood of apnea. *(Based on data of Maislin et al,[30] with permission.)*

that the individual patient with sleep apnea was counseled about the dangers of driving. The patient must be made aware of his or her responsibility in this regard: in one legal case, a patient with sleep apnea who had failed to use his CPAP was in a crash that caused a fatality; the person was charged and convicted of vehicular homicide.

In addition to automobile crashes as a consequence of apnea, there are a number of cardiovascular consequences. The first of these is hypertension. Sleep apnea syndrome is common among patients with essential hypertension, and hypertension is common among patients with the sleep apnea syndrome.[3,55] But since obesity is a risk factor for both conditions, the precise role of sleep apnea has been difficult to identify in human studies.[6,18]

TABLE 102-4

When to Consider Whether Sleep Apnea Is Likely to Be Present

Routine history and physical
Evaluation of new patient, particularly in the following circumstances:
    Hypertension
    Obesity
    Myocardial infarction
    Cerebrovascular accident
    Driver involved in an automobile crash
    Evaluation for preoperative anesthesia

The role of sleep apnea in genesis of hypertension has been assessed by insertion of a silent valve into the trachea of dogs and automatic closing of the valve as soon as the animal fell asleep. A computer system recorded the EEG and EMG, permitting on-line monitoring of the sleep state. Occlusion of the valve resulted in an obstructive apnea that, in time, produced an arousal from sleep. The computer system sensed the arousal and opened the valve, thereby terminating the apnea. With this system, repetitive obstructive apneas were induced during sleep and continued for a few months. During each experimentally induced apnea, blood pressure increased; arousal was accompanied by an additional large increase in blood pressure. Particularly noteworthy was an increase in *daytime* blood pressure during wakefulness. After several weeks, mean daytime blood pressure had increased by about 15.0 mmHg; this increment disappeared after the animals no longer experienced the experimentally induced apneas. These studies provide strong evidence that obstructive apneas during sleep increase daytime blood pressure.[3]

The mechanisms mediating these blood pressure changes are currently being studied by recording peripheral sympathetic nerve activity from the peroneal nerve in humans. Such studies suggest that the increase in blood pressure during the apnea is mediated by an increase in sympathetic nerve activity secondary to hypoxemia.[36,50] What's more interesting is that these studies reveal that patients with sleep apnea have increased sympathetic activity during the day—an increase that is reversed when the patients are treated with nasal CPAP. The basis for this "hangover" effect in sympathetic activity from these nighttime events to the daytime is unknown, but recurrent hypoxemia may play a role.[34]

The period at the termination of apnea is a particularly vulnerable time for the cardiovascular system. At this time, there is a high sympathetic outflow and blood pressure is high. Nonetheless, oxygen delivery to the heart is compromised, owing to the large fall in oxygen content that occurs during the apneic event. Thus, the oxygen-starved heart is pumping into a highly constricted circulation with a large increase in afterload.

Sleep apnea is associated with increased risk of myocardial infarction.[20] Also, tachy- and bradyarrhythmias and episodes of complete heart block occur in patients with sleep apnea, suggesting that sleep apnea can increase mortality from cardiovascular events.[17,37] However, this relationship has not yet been proved.

Sleep apnea may also be a risk factor for stroke. Loud, habitual snoring, a common symptom of sleep apnea, is associated with about twice the normal risk of stroke.[36] Sleep apnea is also common in persons who have recently had a stroke. However, it is difficult in such studies to ascertain whether the sleep apnea led to the stroke or vice versa.

Treatment

Currently, the first line of treatment for sleep apnea syndrome is medical management. The medical treatments for obstructive sleep apnea are listed in Table 102-5.

TABLE 102-5

Medical Treatment of Obstructive Sleep Apnea

General measures
  Avoidance of alcohol, sedatives, and hypnotics
  Weight loss
  Other (less effective) measures
    Pharmacologic agents
    Oxygen therapy
    Nasal dilators
Specific measures
  Position therapy
  Positive airway pressure
    CPAP
    Bilevel systems
    Auto-CPAP
  Oral appliances

GENERAL MEASURES

Patients with sleep apnea should avoid alcohol, sedatives, and hypnotics. Alcohol reduces upper-airway dilator muscle tone and increases the severity of snoring and apneas. As indicated above, it moves people along the continuum of abnormality in the direction of increasing severity. Thus, alcohol in the evening should be avoided by all patients with sleep apnea. Hypnotics and sedatives depress arousal mechanisms, thereby prolonging the apneas and causing greater oxygen desaturation.

Weight loss decreases the severity of obstructive sleep apnea and lessens the collapsibility of the upper airway. Indeed, very moderate reductions in weight improve upper-airway function.[51] Unfortunately, weight loss is difficult to achieve and maintain for these patients. Nonetheless, weight management programs should be recommended for all obese patients with obstructive sleep apnea. Bariatric surgery was proposed for patients with severe sleep apnea, but long-term results have been disappointing. Thus, in general, bariatric surgery is not recommended for patients with sleep apnea. Neuropharmacologic approaches to treating obesity are currently under investigation.

MEASURES WITH LIMITED EFFICACY

Pharmacologic approaches to treat sleep apnea have been disappointing.[19] Acetazolamide and medroxyprogesterone, both of which increase ventilatory drive, have been tried in the treatment of sleep apnea syndrome. Acetazolamide is useful for treating central sleep apnea but not for obstructive sleep apnea. Although medroxyprogesterone can reduce arterial P_{CO_2} in hypoventilation syndromes, it has no role in the management of obstructive sleep apnea.[36]

Protriptyline has also been used for the treatment of sleep apnea. Originally thought to work by increasing upper-airway tone, it has since been shown to exert its primary effect by decreasing the amount of REM sleep, when apneas are often more frequent. The anticholinergic side effects of protriptyline, including dry mouth, constipation, and urinary retention, have caused this agent to be reserved for the occasional patient for whom the apnea is primarily REM related.

Oxygen therapy also has a limited role in the treatment of sleep apnea syndrome. Although oxygen can reduce the degree of desaturation during the apneic event by increasing the "store" of oxygen in the lung, it does not, in general, abolish the apneas. Indeed, oxygen therapy, by improving blood oxygenation, delays the arousal threshold, thereby prolonging the apneas so that sleep fragmentation persists and the patient continues to experience excessive daytime sleepiness. Thus, supplemental oxygen has a limited role in managing sleep apnea syndrome. For the occasional patient who fails other forms of therapy, however, improvement in arterial oxygenation may be helpful in avoiding cardiovascular complications.

Nasal dilators such as Breathe Right have been proposed as a treatment for snoring and sleep apnea. However, since snoring and airway obstruction during apneas occur in the retropalatal or retroglossal region, nasal dilators are not effective in treating patients with sleep apnea syndrome.

SPECIFIC MEDICAL THERAPIES

Positional Therapy

In some patients, apneas may be totally position dependent—i.e., apneas occur in the supine but not in the lateral decubitus position. Position-dependent sleep apnea can be easily diagnosed by polysomnography, which demonstrates a high RDI in the supine position but not in the lateral decubitus position. For patients with position-dependent sleep apnea, symptoms may be alleviated by sleeping in the lateral decubitus position. Position therapy can be accomplished by sewing pockets for one or two tennis balls in the back of patients' nightshirts in the attempt to prevent them from assuming the supine position. Devices to train people to sleep in the lateral position have been described.[36] The long-term efficacy of position therapy is unknown. In general, patients who have significant symptoms or severe sleep apnea should not be treated with this approach.

CPAP and Its Modifications

At present, the *treatment of choice* for patients with obstructive sleep apnea is nasal CPAP (Fig. 102-11). CPAP has the advantage of being noninvasive and has been shown to reduce the number of apneic and hypoxic episodes during sleep and to reduce daytime sleepiness and improve neuropsychiatric function in patients with obstructive sleep apnea.[33]

CPAP operates by providing a pneumatic splint for the airway, thereby preventing collapse during sleep, when upper-airway dilator muscle activity is low. The effect of CPAP on upper-airway caliber and the surrounding soft tissue structures is shown in Fig. 102-12. CPAP increases airway caliber in the retropalatal and retroglossal regions; in particular, it increases the lateral dimensions of the airway and thins the lateral pharyngeal walls.[47]

The optimal CPAP pressure is determined by technologists during polysomnography. Typically, 5 to 20 cmH$_2$O is the pressure needed to abolish apneas, snoring, and oxyhemoglobin desaturations in all positions and during REM sleep.

CPAP is usually applied through a nasal mask or nasal pillows, which insert into the nostrils (Fig. 102-11). It is important

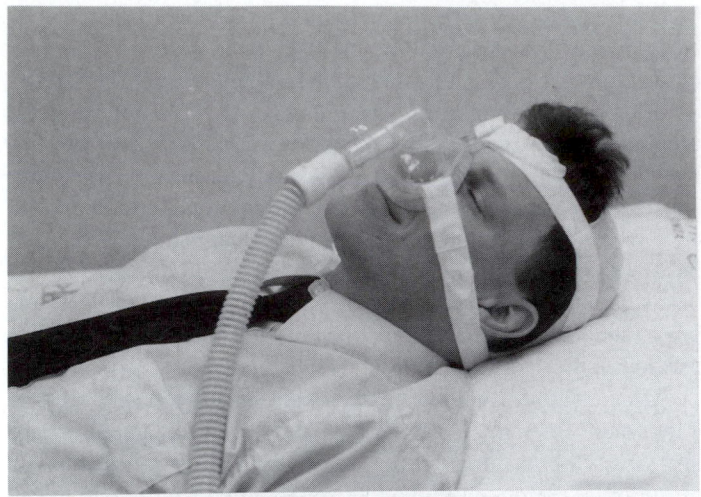

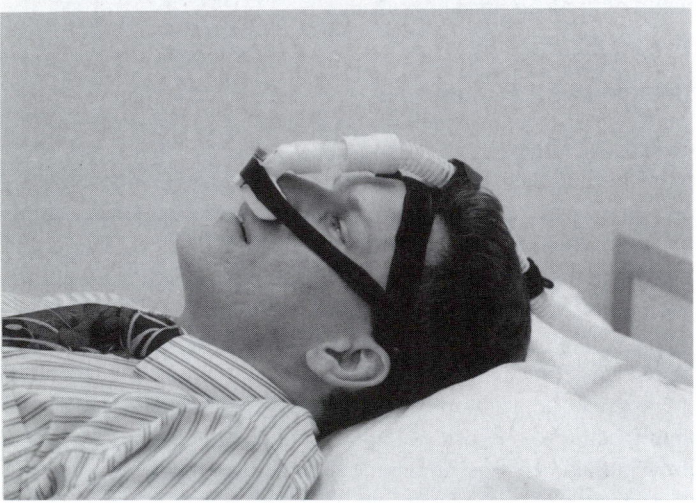

FIGURE 102-11 Example of a subject connected to a CPAP machine. The top panel shows the patient wearing a CPAP mask that covers the nose. The bottom panel demonstrates the patient using nasal pillows that insert directly into the nostrils. With both types of device, it is essential to ensure a good seal with no leaks.

to ensure that the patient has a well-fitting connection to the CPAP machine, with no air leaks. Mouth leaks render CPAP ineffective, since the high flow through the nose generated by the CPAP machine escapes through the mouth. Such leaks often cause the patient to complain of an extremely dry mouth while using the CPAP unit. Mouth leaks can be managed by prescription of a chin strap to keep the mouth closed during sleep.

Full face masks that cover the nose and mouth are also available. If a patient wearing such a mask should regurgitate, however, aspiration may occur. Therefore, full face masks are used relatively infrequently, most often in patients who have persistent mouth leaks while on CPAP. A number of different nasal masks are available for the application of CPAP. Compliance with the use of different masks can vary considerably. The next generation of CPAP masks are "gel" masks, which hold promise of being better tolerated by patients with sleep apnea than the currently available mask.

Although CPAP use is associated with few serious complications, it does elicit a number of complaints (Table 102-6). Most

of these can be alleviated. Nasal irritation and rhinitis can be treated by initial humidifying of the CPAP system; if these difficulties persist, nasal steroids may be helpful. Claustrophobia may be relieved by a switch from nasal mask to nasal pillows. Aerophagia can be treated with changes in body position or mask type. Occasional instances have been reported of more serious side effects, such as severe epistaxis, meningitis, and pneumocephalus.

The major problem with CPAP is not serious side effects but, rather, in achieving adherence to the therapy. On average, usage of CPAP has been for about 4.5 to 5.0 h per night.[26,39] However, this average conceals the fact that there are distinct subgroups of users: one group, comprising about 60 percent of the total, consists of patients who use CPAP almost every night for more than 6 h a night; these are the "regular users." The remainder, the "irregular users," frequently "skip" their CPAP: on some nights, they make no attempt to use the device. Even on nights when they do use CPAP, they do so for only a few hours. The irregular users, who constitute about 40 percent of all those for whom CPAP is prescribed, are essentially "CPAP failures."

The bases for CPAP failures are not well understood. Failure to adhere to a CPAP regimen is apparently unrelated to the severity of disease as measured by the RDI. Patients who only snore, with minimal apnea, also tend to be poorly compliant. Nor does usage of CPAP relate to the prescribed pressure or to the frequency of most of the "nuisance" side effects noted in Table 102-6, other than claustrophobia.

Instead, whether patients adhere to CPAP appears to be related to degree of sleepiness when first evaluated and to the symptomatic benefit that patients experience in response to therapy.

CPAP manufacturers are making changes in the CPAP units in an attempt to improve patient compliance. For example, CPAP machines with a "ramp feature" enable the patient to fall asleep with the CPAP mask in place while little or no airway pressure is applied; airway pressure is then gradually increased over a 15- to 45-min period. Although this concept is attractive in principle, no data exist to show improved adherence or reduced CPAP failures with this approach.

A newer technique for delivering positive airway pressure allows independent regulation of the inspiratory positive airway pressure (IPAP) and expiratory positive airway pressure (EPAP). However, bilevel systems are more expensive than conventional CPAP systems, and the algorithms to adjust the inspiratory and expiratory pressures are essentially empiric. There are no stud-

TABLE 102-6

Side Effects of CPAP

Nocturnal arousals
Rhinitis, nasal irritation, and dryness
Aerophagia
Mask and mouth leaks
Facial skin discomfort
Difficulty in exhaling
Claustrophobia
Chest and back pain

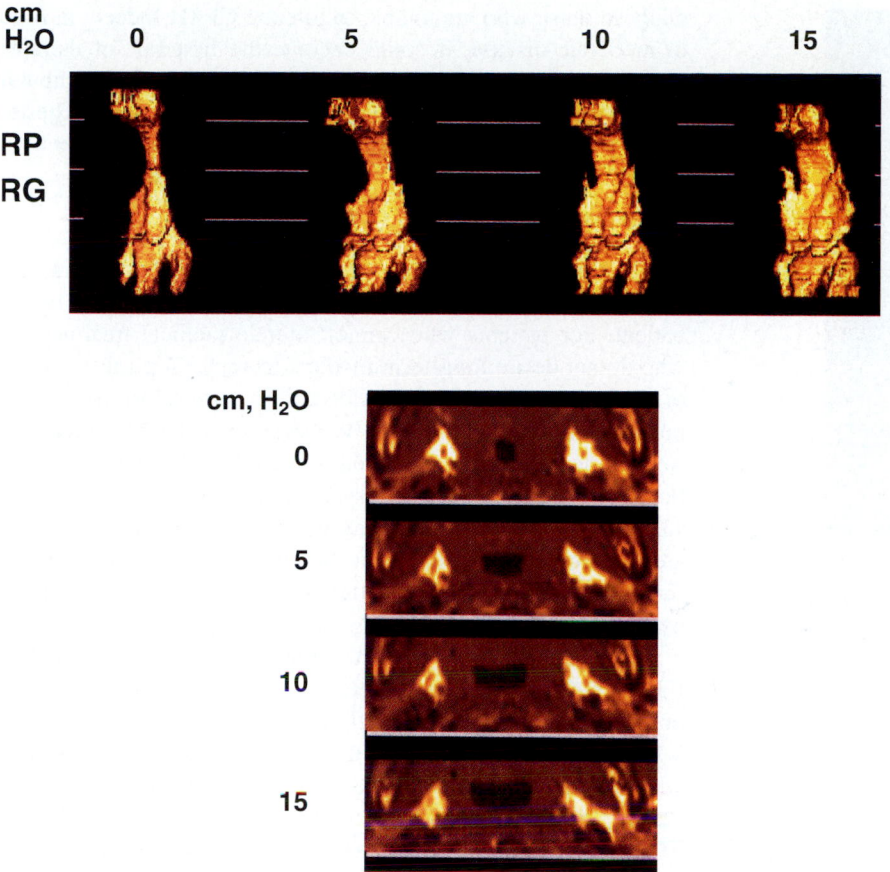

FIGURE 102-12   *Top:* Three-dimensional surface renderings of the upper airway demonstrating the effect of progressive increase in CPAP pressure (0–15 cmH₂O) on upper-airway volume. CPAP significantly increases airway volume in the retropalatal (RP) and retroglossal (RG) regions. *Bottom:* Soft tissue images in the same patient in the retropalatal region at analogous levels of CPAP. With increasing CPAP there is a progressive increase in the size of the upper airway, particularly in the lateral dimension. There is little movement of the parapharyngeal fat pads (white structures lateral to the airway) but progressive thinning of the lateral pharyngeal walls.

fects; and auto-CPAP eliminates the prospect of inadequate prescription of CPAP levels, which may change with weight gain or loss.

These devices are more expensive than conventional CPAP units. Moreover, although attractive in principle, auto-CPAP has not yet been sufficiently tested with respect to failure rates.[32]

Intraoral Devices

Oral appliances are an effective noninvasive alternative to CPAP in patients with mild to moderate sleep apnea.[42] There are a large number of devices, some of which reposition the mandible, while others maintain the tongue in a forward position (tongue-retaining devices). The most common and best-studied appliances are the mandibular advancing devices (Fig. 102-14). These devices may be particularly effective in patients with retrognathia and micrognathia. For these devices to treat sleep apnea effectively, the mandible should be advanced to 50 to 75 percent of the maximal forward protrusion of the jaw. Cephalometrics have shown that the mandibular advancing devices advance and rotate the mandible and increase the size of the posterior airway space.

In most patients, dental appliances lessen but do not abolish obstructive sleep apnea and snoring. In many pa-

ies evaluating the relative efficacy of different levels of IPAP or EPAP in abolishing apneic events. A comparison of adherence to a bilevel system (BiPAP) and CPAP failed to disclose any difference between the two after the introductory phase was passed.[39] Consequently, bilevel systems are now reserved for patients who cannot tolerate CPAP, especially for those who experience difficulties with exhalation or chest pain as a result of the hyperinflation produced by the applied positive pressure.

The newest modification in CPAP systems is auto-CPAP.[32] These CPAP machines adjust the CPAP pressure throughout the night rather than delivering one fixed pressure. They are based on the detection of apneas, snoring, or inspiratory flow limitation; the last is a sensitive indicator that the airway is narrowing and occurs before the presence of apnea (Fig. 102-13).

The idea of automatic adjustment of CPAP pressures throughout the night to abolish apneas and hypopneas is attractive on several counts: changes in position and in the stages of sleep affect the occurrence and severity of apnea; alcohol, sedatives, and infections of the upper airway affect the level of CPAP that is required to abolish apneas and hypopneas; the use of lower mean pressure in the auto-CPAP may reduce pressure-related side ef-

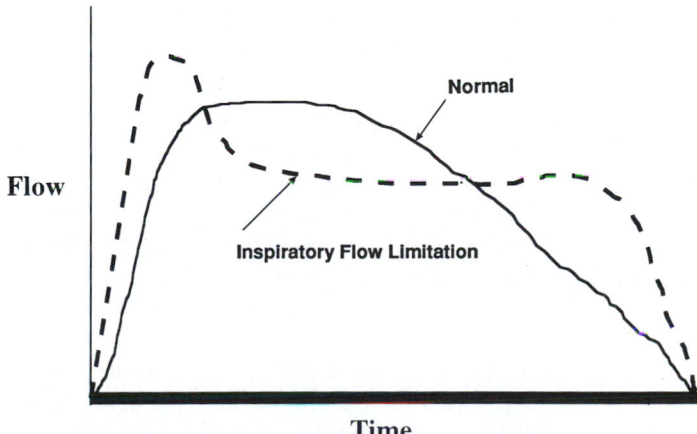

FIGURE 102-13   Schematic showing the normal pattern of airflow during inspiration and what occurs when there is inspiratory flow limitation. In the latter, the flow quickly reaches a level that is maintained relatively constant throughout inspiration. The pattern of airflow can be detected by computers built into CPAP machines.

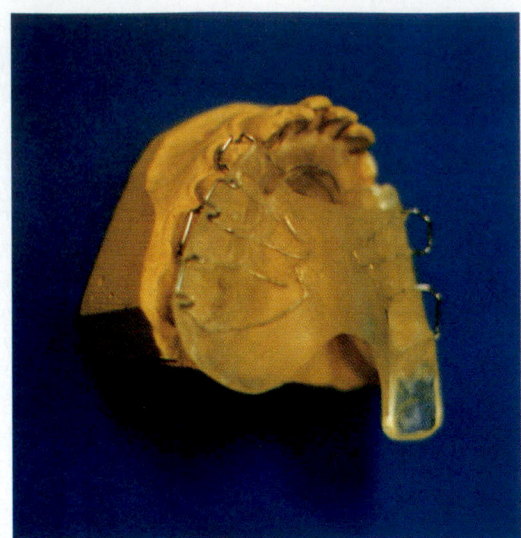

FIGURE 102-14   Example of a mandibular repositioning device. This device fits on the upper and lower teeth; it is worn during sleep and results in anterior motion of the mandible, with consequent enlargement of the airway.

tients treated with an oral appliance, the RDI still remains high, with more than 20 events per hour after treatment.[42]

Currently, oral appliances are used predominantly in persons with mild to moderate disease—i.e., an RDI of 15 to 40 events per hour. Adjusting the degree of mandibular advancement can be cumbersome. Currently, the degree of anterior repositioning begins with clinical assessment by the practitioner. A sleep study is then used to determine whether this degree of advancement is effective. Newer devices are enabling adjustments to be made more simply, and algorithms are evolving in which adjustments are based on the patient's own report or on that of his or her bed partner about snoring and on use of simple tests, such as overnight oximetry, at home. Nonetheless, adjustment can still be long and arduous.

The side effects of oral appliances include excessive salivation, dental misalignment, and pain in, or damage to, the temporomandibular joint. Data about long-term outcomes from the use of oral appliances are sparse. No data exist about adherence to this form of therapy. However, new monitoring devices for adherence are under development.

Despite these uncertainties, there are encouraging reports about the use of intraoral devices in patients with mild to moderate sleep apnea. In two recent studies, a crossover design was used to compare the use of CPAP and the intraoral device in patients with mild sleep apnea.[5,9] Although CPAP produced larger improvements in the respiratory disturbance indices during sleep, more patients expressed satisfaction with the intraoral device; when given the choice, more chose this form of therapy than chose CPAP. Thus, the intraoral device seems destined to play a major role in patients with mild to moderate sleep apnea, espe-

cially in those who are unable to tolerate CPAP. Indeed, in mild to moderate disease, it could become the first line of therapy. Improvements in the ability to adjust the degree of mandibular repositioning will be helpful, as will new, simpler approaches to determining the optimal degree of mandibular advancement.

SURGICAL TREATMENT

Since obstructive sleep apnea is a chronic and often progressive disease, it requires long-term therapy that is well tolerated by the patient. For patients who cannot tolerate medical treatment or who do not desire long-term medical therapy, surgical treatment of sleep apnea should be considered. The full set of options for nonsurgical treatment should be discussed with the patient before surgical treatment is started. Physical examination, fiberoptic laryngoscopy, and upper-airway imaging assist in locating the areas of obstruction so that surgical procedures can target these areas. After each procedure in the surgical treatment of apnea, polysomnography is used to determine whether significant apnea remains.

Adults choose upper-airway surgery for a variety of reasons. For example, even though weight loss can relieve apnea in the obese patient, weight loss is difficult to maintain. Although CPAP is effective in combating obstructive sleep apnea, it is associated with side effects and many patients are unable to tolerate the device. For psychological or sociologic reasons, patients may not be able to adapt to CPAP or an oral appliance as long-term treatment options. In certain adult patients, adjunctive surgical treatment, such as septoplasty or other nasal surgery, may be necessary to improve the tolerance to CPAP. In children, in whom the risk factors differ from those of adults, surgical treatment, such as tonsillectomy or adenoidectomy, is very effective.[2]

Critical evaluation of the airway is critical for surgical success. Evaluation includes a clinical, fiberoptic, and often radiographic examination (cephalometrics or MRI) to determine as accurately as possible the principal site of obstruction. Currently, these evaluations are performed during wakefulness, raising questions about their value in pinpointing sites of obstruction during sleep.

Classification of Obstructive Sites

Evaluation of the airway for sites of obstruction extends from the nose through the glottis. Nasal abnormalities can affect the soft tissues of the nose, septum, turbinates, and nasal cavity and can be a source of obstruction that exacerbates apnea or acts as an obstacle to the use of CPAP. Rhinitis, sinusitis, and nasal polyps can also contribute to nasal obstruction and poor CPAP compliance. In the oral cavity and oropharynx, retrognathia, micrognathia, size of the tongue, palate and uvular length, tonsillar hypertrophy, and prominent pharyngeal walls need to be evaluated. Examination of the neck—including notation of the position of the larynx, distance from the larynx to the mandible, palpation of the thyroid, and neck thickness (collar size)—also offers valuable information. Fiberoptic laryngoscopy is performed to visualize the nasopharynx, oropharynx, hypopharynx, and larynx. The degree of collapse on negative inspiration (the Mueller maneuver), although not a direct indicator of the site of obstruction during sleep, suggests likely sites of obstruction.

This examination is used to classify the level of obstruction: oropharyngeal (type I), oropharyngeal and hypopharyngeal (type II), or only hypopharyngeal (type III). Different surgical procedures have been proposed for patients with different levels of obstruction (Table 102-7).[40,49]

The abnormal anatomy and physiology pose challanges to both the anesthesiologist and the surgeon. Maintenance of the airway during induction and emergency can be difficult. Untoward reactions to narcotics and anesthetics can exacerbate the obstruction and make airway management on induction and emergence difficult. Postoperatively, some patients manifest an exacerbation of obstructive sleep apnea. Compromise of the airway in the perioperative period is a serious threat. CPAP is used in the postoperative period until surgical success is confirmed.

Surgical Approaches

Based on the physical examination and ancillary studies, a systematic approach to the process of surgical selection has been developed.[40] "Phase I" refers to the use of uvulopalatopharyngoplasty (UPPP) or genioglossus advancement with hyoid myotomy (GAHM), depending on the site of obstruction. Patients with an oropharyngeal obstruction (type I) are candidates for UPPP; patients with a hypopharyngeal obstruction (type III) undergo GAHM. Patients with obstruction in both sites (type II) undergo simultaneous UPPP and GAHM.

"Phase II" refers to maxillomandibular advancement osteotomy for forward advancement of the jaws. Patients who fail phase I go on to phase II surgery. The success rate of this form of surgery is higher than that for all types of surgery for apnea except tracheostomy. However, many patients refuse to undergo this type of surgery. Other procedures (described below) can be used in selected patients in whom specific anatomic abnormalities are identified. Polysomnography after any of the surgical procedures is critical to determine whether sleep apnea persists.

Uvulopalatopharyngoplasty (UPPP) is the most common surgical procedure for adult obstructive sleep apnea. It was introduced into the United States in 1981 by Fujita and colleagues.[11] UPPP entails removal of excessive mucosa and tissue from the palate and palatopharyngeal arch. The underlying musculature of the palate is left intact, and the uvula is shortened or amputated. The tonsils, if present, are removed at the time of this procedure, and the remaining mucosa is trimmed and sutured together. Successful treatment is reported to vary from 19 to 86 percent for patients with obstructive sleep apnea.[41] UPPP is 90

percent effective in decreasing snoring. The success rate in patients undergoing UPPP appears to be partly related to the site of obstruction: patients with retropalatal obstruction experience better results than those with retroglossal obstruction. The preoperative presence of tonsils has been associated with improved success of UPPP.

It is critical to avoid overresection or underresection during UPPP. Overresection carries the threat of velopalatal insufficiency. Transient uvulopalatal insufficiency is common in the postoperative period, but it rarely persists. Pain on swallowing and pain with speech are regular occurrences for 1 to 2 weeks after UPPP. Medications to relieve pain must be administered with caution because of the possibility of exacerbating sleep apnea. Hemorrhage after UPPP occurs in 2 to 4 percent of patients, an incidence similar to that of hemorrhage in tonsillectomy. Late complications of UPPP include pharyngeal discomfort, tightness or dryness, the sensation of food catching in the throat, and difficulty in initiating swallowing. Disturbances in taste, numbness of the tongue, and nasopharyngeal stenosis occur occasionally. Despite the wide range of potential complications and side effects, in practice UPPP is generally well tolerated and uneventful. However, patients who fail UPPP tolerate CPAP less well than before surgery because surgical reduction of the soft palate leads to mouth leaks at relatively low levels of pressure.

Laser-assisted uvulopalatoplasty (LAUP) is a new procedure that has been developed to treat snoring in the outpatient setting. The procedure entails reshaping the palate and tonsillar pillars in one to seven serial sessions (typically two or three) under local anesthesia. Each session lasts approximately 15 min and is generally well tolerated; the incidence of complications is low.[25] Pain following the procedure is significant but of less magnitude than that after UPPP. The procedure is successful in reducing snoring in 90 percent of patients.[25] However, the success rate in patients with obstructive sleep apnea or the upper-airway resistance syndrome is not yet clear. Although there seems to be a group of patients with obstructive sleep apnea whose condition improves after the procedure, as manifested by a decrease in RDI and relief of symptoms of apnea, a process for sorting out these patients preoperatively has not been developed. One concern that remains to be discounted is that LAUP may result in a "silent," nonsnoring apneic.

Other Surgical Procedures Advancement of the genioglossus muscle with hyoid myotomy, sliding mortise genioplasty, mandibular osteotomy, and maxillomandibular advancement osteotomy are among the procedures that can be utilized in patients with abnormalities of the bony framework of the jaws or retroglossal obstruction. Each of these procedures advances the bony framework of the mandible or maxilla, which, in turn, advances the tongue and soft tissues of the pharynx anteriorly, thereby improving the airway. In some patients, tracheostomy may be necessary to ensure a safe airway in the perioperative period. If tracheostomy is not deemed necessary, CPAP is used in the postoperative period.

Other procedures (Table 102-7) are available to improve the airway or to improve CPAP compliance. Nasal surgery, while helpful as an adjunct to other procedures, or to improve CPAP compliance, is rarely effective, per se, for obstructive apnea. The role of linguaplasty is yet to be defined. Patients with macro-

---

TABLE 102-7

Surgery for Obstructive Sleep Apnea

Nasal surgery (septoplasty, sinus surgery, and others)
Tonsillectomy ± adenoidectomy
Uvulopalatopharyngoplasty (UPPP)
Laser-assisted uvulopalatoplasty (LAUP)
Linguaplasty
Genioglossus advancement with hyoid myotomy (GAHM)
Sliding genioplasty
Maxillomandibular advancement osteotomy
Tracheostomy

glossia may be candidates for a tongue reduction, usually in conjunction with another surgical procedure.

Tracheostomy, because it bypasses the upper airway, is virtually 100 percent effective in eliminating apnea. Until recent years, it was the only reliable surgical procedure for obstructive sleep apnea. Unfortunately, it requires changes in lifestyle and impairs the patient's quality of life. It is generally reserved for patients with very severe obstructive sleep apnea who have failed medical or surgical therapy and manifest malignant arrhythmias or cardiac failure.

Tracheostomy can be performed in the traditional fashion, with the creation of a stoma that will close with decannulation; or a more permanent stoma can be made by directly sewing skin to the mucosa of the trachea. The permanent stoma provides an epithelium-lined tract from the skin to the trachea that will not close. Although most patients adjust to the presence of a tracheostomy, in some, depression is a problem.

MANAGEMENT OF OTHER DISORDERS

Obesity-Hypoventilation Syndrome

Obesity-hypoventilation syndrome (Pickwickian syndrome) is characterized by the combination of obesity, hypoventilation, and daytime hypercapnia (Pa_{CO_2} over 45). Patients with the obesity-hypoventilation syndrome present with resting hypoxemia and hypercapnia, hypersomnolence, pulmonary hypertension, and chronic right heart failure. The Pickwickian syndrome usually coexists with obstructive sleep apnea. Patients with obesity-hypoventilation syndrome have a characteristic pattern on nocturnal oximetry that differs from that of obstructive sleep apnea (Fig. 102-15).

The diagnosis of obesity-hypoventilation syndrome can be confirmed by demonstrating a nocturnal increase in arterial P_{CO_2} greater than 10 mmHg (Table 102-8). The obesity-hypoventila-

TABLE 102-8

Diagnostic Features of Obesity-Hypoventilation Syndrome

Clinical presentation
    Daytime manifestations of hypercapnia (e.g., chronic fatigue and morning headache)
    Cor pulmonale and right heart failure
Laboratory findings
    Hypercapnia during wakefulness (Pa_{CO_2} >45 mmHg)
    Hypoxemia during wakefulness and sleep (Sa_{O_2} <90%)
    Increase in Pa_{CO_2} during sleep (>10 mmHg)
    Respiratory acidosis during sleep (pH <7.3)
    Nocturnal oximetry demonstrating persistent oxyhemoglobin desaturation
    Polysomnography demonstrating concomitant obstructive sleep apnea or evidence of hypoventilation

tion syndrome probably has many causes and may involve impaired central respiratory drive, ventilatory muscle dysfunction, adverse effects of obesity on pulmonary function, ventilation–perfusion mismatch, and compromised respiratory neuromuscular capacity. The ob/ob mouse, in which obesity is genetically determined by a lack of functioning leptin, exhibits hypercapnia without evidence of sleep apnea. Patients with obstructive sleep apnea, unlike those with the Pickwickian syndrome, do not develop hypercapnia during wakefulness, indicating that their level of ventilation over 24 h is appropriate for their metabolic needs.

The management of obesity-hypoventilation syndrome requires adequate ventilatory support and treatment of coexisting medical conditions. The administration of supplemental oxygen, per se, lengthens apneas and exacerbates the respiratory acidosis. Diuretics and cardiotonic agents relieve right-sided congestive heart failure.[23] However, the treatment of choice for the obesity-hypoventilation syndrome is nocturnal noninvasive ventilation administered through a nasal or oral face mask.[32,53] A protocol that can be used is outlined in Table 102-9.

Nocturnal noninvasive ventilation in patients with the obesity-hypoventilation syndrome corrects daytime and nighttime hypoxemia and hypercapnia, alleviates sleep fragmentation, rests the respiratory muscles, reduces pulmonary artery pressures, and improves right ventricular function. Symptoms also resolve: daytime hypersomnolence decreases, energy levels increase, morn-

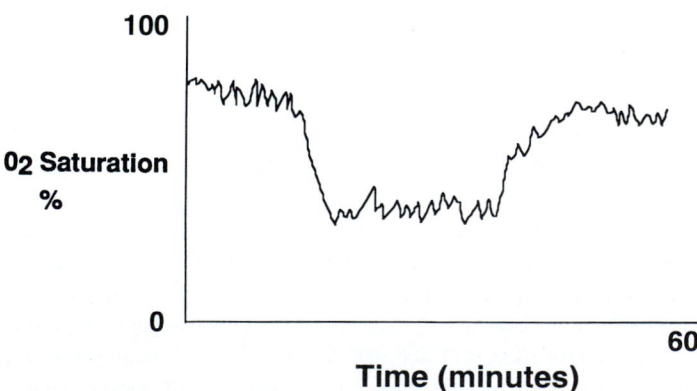

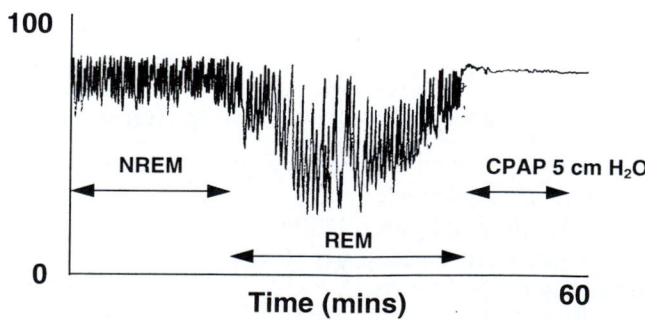

FIGURE 102-15   Example of typical tracings of oxygen saturation in a patient with obesity-hypoventilation syndrome (left panel) and a different patient with obstructive sleep apnea (right panel). The former shows an episode of sustained desaturation. In obstructive sleep apnea there are frequent episodic desaturations (saw tooth pattern) that are more profound in REM sleep and abolished by CPAP.

TABLE 102-9

Protocol for Nocturnal Noninvasive Ventilation in Patients with Obesity-Hypoventilation Syndrome

Setup
Semielective admission to ICU/stepdown unit
    Mean length of stay 4–5 days to adjust nocturnal ventilation
    Obtain appropriate fitting CPAP mask, nasal pillows, or oronasal mask
    Chin strap may be necessary to keep the mouth closed
Parameters for volume-cycled ventilator
Mode
    Assist control mode
    Intermittent mandatory ventilation (IMV); pressure can be added
Tidal volume
    For most patients, 10 ml/kg
    Obese patients (>100 kg), 5–7 ml/kg
Respiratory rate
    Start with 12 breaths per minute
    Adjust rate and/or tidal volume to obtain appropriate Pa_{CO_2} (40–50 mmHg during wakefulness)
F_{IO_2}
    In patients with a normal A–a (ΔP_{O_2}), room air ($F_{IO_2} = 21$) usually is sufficient
    Aim to maintain arterial O_2 saturation >92%
Monitoring nasal ventilation
Exhaled volume
    Although exhaled volume should theoretically equal tidal volume (V_T), because of leaks in the system, exhaled volume is often $<V_T$
    Increase V_T until exhaled volume equals desired V_T
Sa_{O_2}
    Oximeters are required to adjust F_{IO_2}; keep $Sa_{O_2} \geq 92\%$
Pa_{CO_2}
    An indwelling arterial line should be used
    Arterial blood gases should be checked frequently during sleep (every 2 h) to determine Pa_{CO_2} and make appropriate ventilator adjustments

---

ing headaches are relieved, and pulmonary hypertension and right heart failure abate. Conventional volume- or pressure-cycled ventilators may be used for noninvasive ventilation. However, volume-cycled nasal ventilation is the method of choice because pressure-cycled ventilators may not provide a large enough inspiratory pressure in obese persons to ensure an adequate tidal volume. Pressure-cycled ventilation may require inspiratory pressures of 30 to 40 cmH$_2$O to decrease the Pa_{CO_2}. Nonetheless, regardless of the mode of ventilation, the minute ventilation should be adjusted to maintain a normal arterial P_{CO_2}. For patients with severe hypercapnia, the minute ventilation should be increased gradually over several nights to avoid a precipitous drop in the arterial P_{CO_2} and concomitant metabolic alkalosis. Mouth leaks during nasal ventilation should be treated by adding a chin strap or switching to a full face mask.

Central Sleep Apnea

Central sleep apnea is a much less common disorder than obstructive sleep apnea. It is usually associated with an underlying neurologic disorder.[54] In central sleep apnea, repeated episodes of apnea occur during sleep in the absence of respiratory muscle effort (Fig. 102-16). Central sleep apnea may be idiopathic or associated with a number of neurologic conditions, including Shy-Drager syndrome, myasthenia gravis, autonomic dysfunction, neuromuscular disease, bulbar poliomyelitis, brain-stem infarction, and encephalitis. In addition, central sleep apnea can occur in a variety of disorders with chronic alveolar hypoventilation and in persons who are newly exposed to high altitude. Finally, the elderly may manifest central sleep apnea without obvious neurologic dysfunction. Patients with central sleep apnea have clinical features that range from daytime sleepiness to end-stage pulmonary hypertension and right heart failure. These patients complain of daytime sleepiness secondary to sleep fragmentation due to the central apneas.

The diagnosis of central sleep apnea is made by overnight polysomnography demonstrating repeated episodes of apnea without motion of the chest wall and abdomen. These apneic episodes may result in hypoxia, hypercapnia, and acidemia. CPAP may not be effective for the treatment of central sleep apnea, since the airway remains patent even though it may narrow somewhat because of the loss of motor output to respiratory muscles. The treatment of choice for central sleep apnea is nocturnal nasal noninvasive ventilation, which imposes an "on call" respiratory rate that abolishes the central apneas. Pressure-cycled ventilation with a bilevel system and backup respiratory rate is usually effective in abolishing the central apneas. Ventilatory stimulants, such as acetazolamide, have not proved useful for conventional central sleep apnea even though they are effective in treating central apneas associated with high altitude.

Upper-Airway Resistance Syndrome

The upper-airway resistance syndrome is characterized by recurrent arousals secondary to increased upper-airway resistance (crescendo snoring).[15] However, questions have been raised about whether episodes of crescendo snoring are simply hypopneas—i.e., whether the upper-airway resistance syndrome is simply another name for the sleep hypopnea syndrome. In the upper-airway resistance syndrome, repeated arousals occur because of snoring or increased upper-airway resistance. These arousals may fragment sleep and cause daytime sleepiness. Sleep fragmentation in nonapneic snorers is a risk factor for systemic hypertension.[27]

In order to make the diagnosis of the upper-airway resistance syndrome, a polysomnogram using an esophageal balloon is nec-

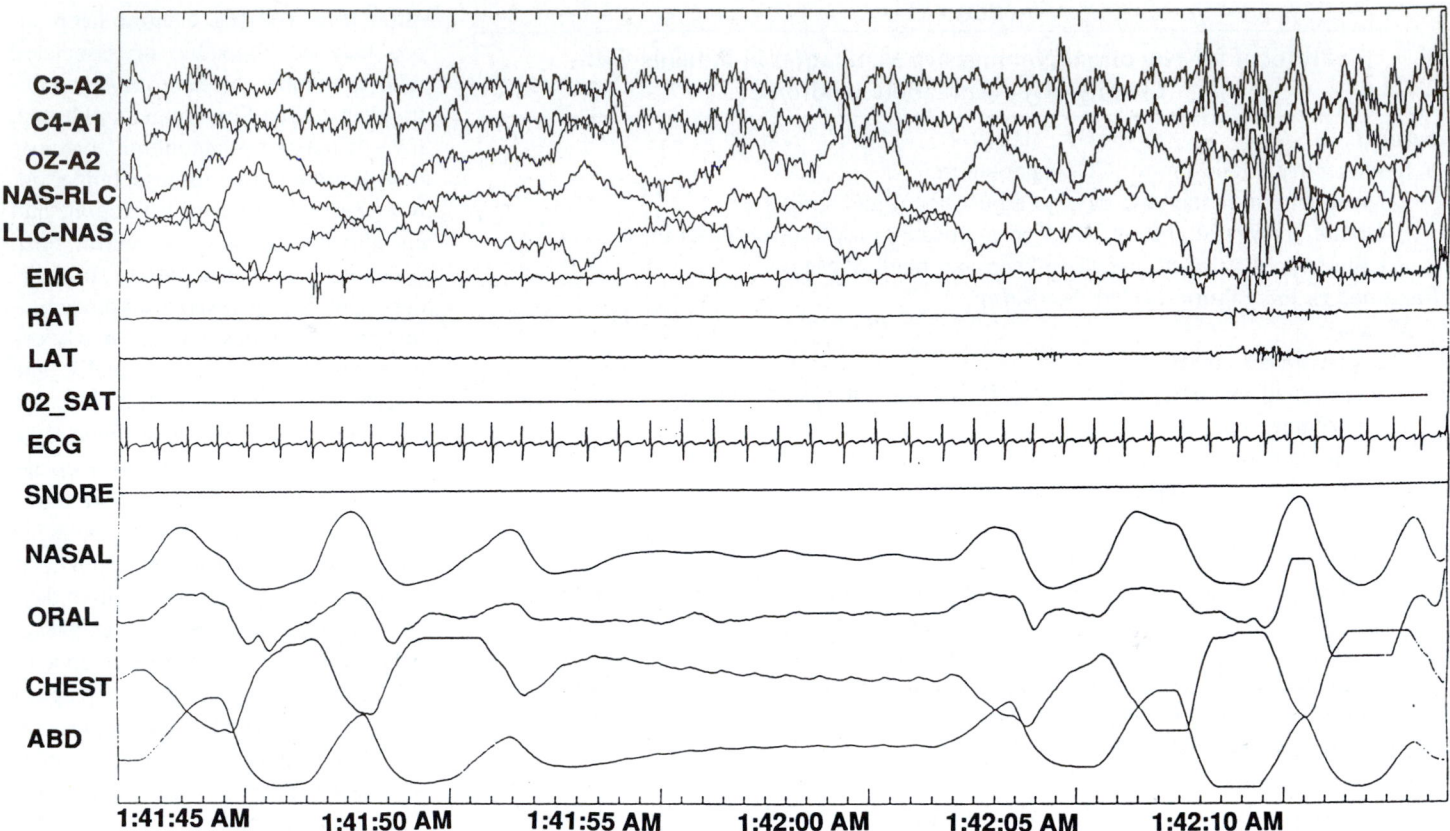

FIGURE 102-16 Example of a central apnea. The polysomnography traces from the top down are as follows: three EEG channels (C3-A2, C4-A2, OZ-A2); two EOG channels (NAS-RLC and LLC-NAS); submental EMG (EMG); right and left anterior tibialis EMG (RAT, LAT); oxyhemoglobin saturation (O_2 SAT); electrocardiogram (ECG); snoring channel (SNORE), nasal and oral airflow; chest and abdominal motion (CHEST and ABD). During the apneic episodes, there is abnormal airflow (both oral and nasal) without rib cage and abdomen motion. At the end of the apneic episode, there is a burst of EMG activity at the arousal.

essary. Since most sleep laboratories do not use esophageal balloons, arousals associated with episodes of snoring have been substituted for the invasive technique (Fig. 102-17). It seems likely, however, that the use of snoring-related arousals to diagnose the upper-airway resistance syndrome underestimates the prevalence of this disorder. If the snoring-related arousal index is greater than 15 per hour, the diagnosis of upper-airway resistance syndrome should be entertained. The current treatment of choice for the upper-airway resistance syndrome is nasal CPAP. Dental appliances, and possibly upper-airway surgery, including laser-assisted palatoplasty, may be effective therapeutic interventions.

CARDIOPULMONARY DISORDERS THAT ARE EXACERBATED DURING SLEEP

Sleep can exacerbate such disorders as asthma, chronic obstructive pulmonary disease (COPD), coronary artery disease, and congestive heart failure. Two-thirds of all asthmatics develop nocturnal bronchoconstriction; the cause of the bronchoconstriction is unknown. These asthmatic patients have been labeled "morning dippers" and manifest falls in FEV_1 and a peak flow of 50 percent during sleep. Nocturnal bronchoconstriction is most common in unstable asthmatics or in those recovering from recent asthmatic attacks. These nocturnal asthmatic attacks are not related to a specific sleep stage.[8] Asthmatic patients admitted to the hospital should be expected to experience decrements in expiratory flow rates during sleep. Therefore, weaning of an asthmatic from the ventilator should be performed cautiously at night. Long-acting bronchodilators given before sleep help to prevent nocturnal bronchoconstriction.[45]

The condition of patients with COPD often deteriorates at night. Arterial oxyhemoglobin saturations during sleep in patients with COPD may approach 10 to 35 percent; hypoxemic episodes are especially severe during REM sleep. Hypercapnia can also be exacerbated during sleep in patients with COPD; the hypercapnic episodes are also more severe during REM sleep than during NREM sleep. Cardiac arrhythmias (i.e., atrial and ventricular atopy) and cardiac ischemia (i.e., ST depressions on the electrocardiogram) can also be significant problems in COPD patients. Oxygen administration reverses most of these cardiac abnormalities. Patients with a wide variety of lung diseases—including interstitial lung disease, cystic fibrosis, restrictive lung disease, and chest wall disease (e.g., kyphoscoliosis)—develop hypoxemia during sleep.

Relatively little is known about the effect of sleep on cardiovascular disease. Ischemic episodes and arrhythmias frequently occur during sleep. Nocturnal angina is common and occurs at about the same frequency in REM sleep as in NREM sleep. Patients with nocturnal angina should be suspected of

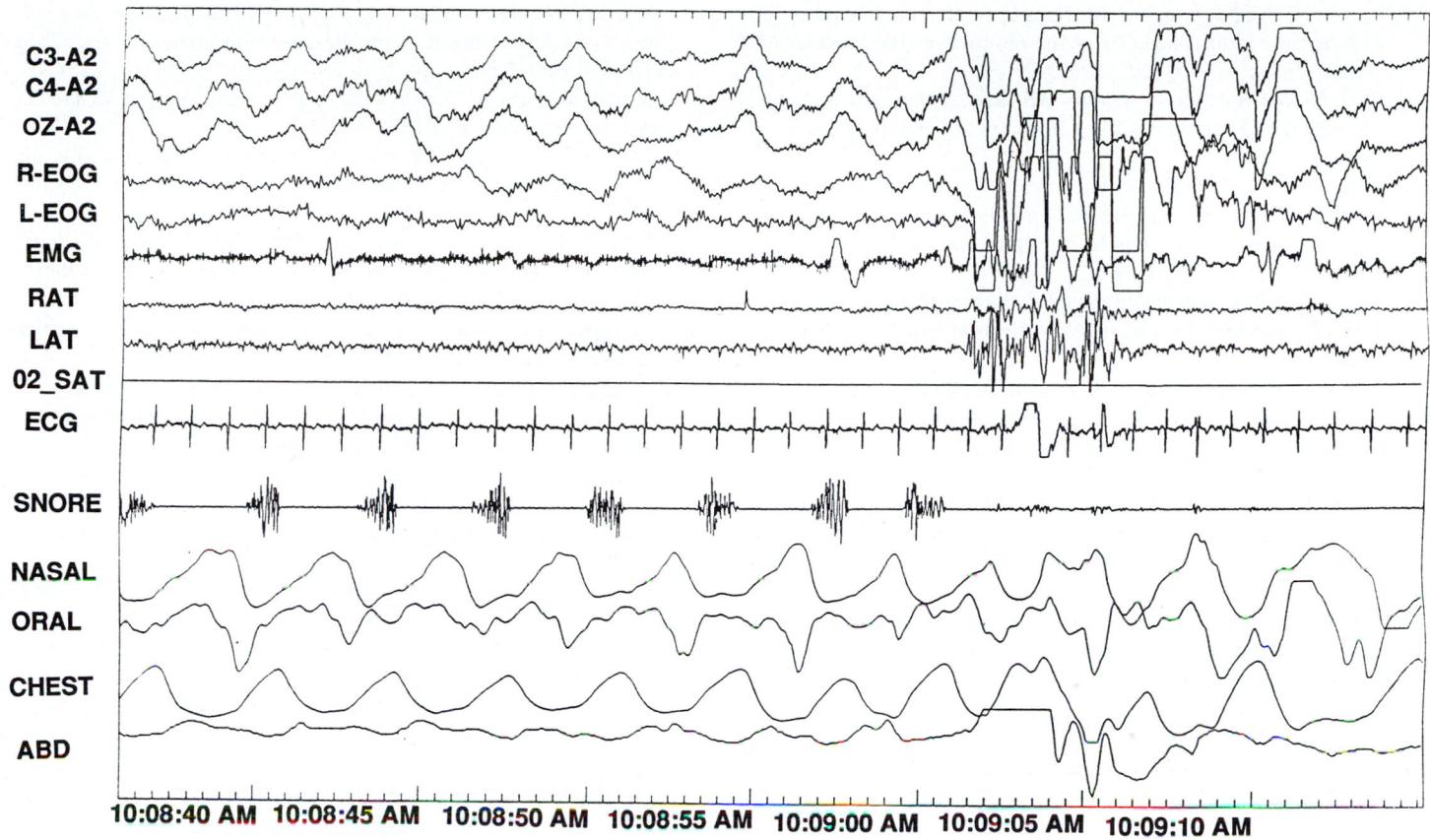

FIGURE 102-17   Example of an episode of increased upper-airway resistance in a patient with upper-airway resistance syndrome. The traces are similar to those in previous figures. Particular attention should be paid to snoring channel (SNORE). At the beginning of the trace, there is snoring present on each inspiration. Toward the end of the trace, there is an obvious arousal, with movement artifact on the EEG/EOG traces and activity recorded on both right (RAT) and left (LAT) anterior tibialis EMG. With the arousal there is some increase in airflow, but the most obvious change is the abolition of snoring as a consequence of the reduction in upper-airway resistance.

having obstructive sleep apnea. Although myocardial infarction seems to have a circadian propensity to occur between 6:00 A.M. and 12:00 noon, the mechanism underlying this relationship is unclear.[36,48] Ventricular arrhythmias may increase, decrease, or remain unchanged during sleep; no relationship has been shown between the stage of sleep and the behavior of ventricular arrhythmias.[48]

Patients with congestive heart failure have a high incidence of sleep-disordered breathing. The primary risk factor for sleep-disordered breathing is the severity of left ventricular dysfunction. In a recent study, 45 percent of patients with stable, treated congestive heart failure demonstrated moderate to severe sleep-disordered breathing.[22] The mean RDI was 44 events per hour. These apneas were primarily central events that were associated with ventricular arrhythmias. They were accompanied by an increased number of arousals and significant oxyhemoglobin desaturations. In a follow-up study, theophylline improved sleep-disordered breathing in patients with congestive heart failure by decreasing the number of apneas and the duration of the episodes of oxyhemoglobin desaturation.[53]

Cheyne-Stokes respiration is common in patients with congestive heart failure (New York Heart Association class 3 or 4). In these patients, it is found primarily in stages 1 and 2 NREM sleep and not during the deeper stages of delta sleep or REM sleep. The respiratory irregularity causes fragmentation in the pattern of sleep, manifested by a decrease in total sleeping time, a decrease in the duration of delta sleep, and frequent arousals. CPAP may be an effective therapy for patients with Cheyne-Stokes respiration and congestive heart failure.[35] A randomized trial of the use of CPAP in treatment of congestive heart failure is currently under way.

REFERENCES

1. American Thoracic Society: Sleep apnea, sleepiness and driving risk. *Am J Respir Crit Care Med* 150:1463–1473, 1994.
2. Brooks LJ: Treatment of otherwise normal children with obstructive sleep apnea. *Ear Nose Throat J* 72:77–79, 1993.
3. Brooks D, Horner RL, Kozar LF, et al: Obstructive sleep apnea as a cause of systemic hypertension: Evidence from a canine model. *J Clin Invest* 99:106–109, 1997.
4. Burwell CS, Robin ED, Whaley RD, Bickelmann AG: Extreme obesity associated with alveolar hypoventilation—A Pickwickian syndrome. *Am J Med* 21:811–818, 1956.
5. Clark GT, Blumenfeld I, Yoffe N, et al: A crossover study comparing the efficacy of continuous positive airway pressure with anterior mandibular positioning devices on patients with obstructive sleep apnea. *Chest* 109:1477–1483, 1996.
6. Coy TV, Dimsdale JE, Ancoli-Israel S, Clausen JL: The role of sleep-disordered breathing in essential hypertension. *Chest* 109:890–895, 1996.

7. Davies RJ, Ali NJ, Stradling JR: Neck circumference and other clinical features in the diagnosis of the obstructive sleep apnoea syndrome. *Thorax* 47:101–105, 1992.

8. Douglas NJ: Asthma, in Kryger MH, Roth T, Dement WC (eds), *Principles and Practice of Sleep Medicine.* Philadelphia, Saunders, 1994, pp 748–757.

9. Ferguson KA, Ono T, Lowe AA, et al: A randomized crossover study of an oral appliance vs nasal-continuous positive airway pressure in the treatment of mild–moderate obstructive sleep apnea. *Chest* 109:1269–1275, 1996.

10. Findley LJ, Levinson MP, Bonnie RJ: Driving performance and automobile accidents in patients with sleep apnea. *Clin Chest Med* 13:427–435, 1992.

11. Fujita S, Conway W, Zorick F, Roth T: Surgical correction of anatomic abnormalities in obstructive sleep apnea syndrome: Uvulopalatopharyngoplasty. *Otolaryngol Head Neck Surg* 89:923–934, 1981.

12. Gastaut H, Tassinari CA, Duron B: Polysomnographic study of the episodic diurnal and nocturnal (hypnic and respiratory) manifestations of the Pickwick syndrome. *Brain Res* 2:167–186, 1966.

13. George CF, Boudreau AC, Smiley A: Simulated driving performance in patients with obstructive sleep apnea. *Am J Respir Crit Care Med* 154:175–181, 1996.

14. Gould GA, Whyte KF, Rhind GB, et al: The sleep hypopnea syndrome. *Am Rev Respir Dis* 137:895–898, 1988.

15. Guilleminault C, Stoohs R, Clerk A, et al: A cause of excessive daytime sleepiness: The upper airway resistance syndrome. *Chest* 104:781–787, 1993.

16. Guilleminault C, Stoohs R, Kim Y-D, et al: Upper airway sleep-disordered breathing in women. *Ann Intern Med* 122:493–501, 1995.

17. He J, Kryger MH, Zorick FJ, et al: Mortality and apnea index in obstructive sleep apnea: Experience in 385 male patients. *Chest* 94:9–14, 1988.

18. Hla KM, Young TB, Bidwell T, et al: Sleep apnea and hypertension: A population-based study. *Ann Intern Med* 120:382–388, 1994.

19. Hudgel DW: Pharmacologic treatment of obstructive sleep apnea. *J Lab Clin Med* 126:13–18, 1995.

20. Hung J, Whitford EG, Parsons RW, Hillman DR: Association of sleep apnoea with myocardial infarction in men. *Lancet* 336:261–264, 1990.

21. Iber C, O'Brien C, Schluter J, et al: Single night studies in obstructive sleep apnea. *Sleep* 14:383–385, 1991.

22. Javaheri S, Parker TJ, Wexler L, et al: Occult sleep-disordered breathing in stable congestive heart failure. *Ann Intern Med* 122:487–492, 1995.

23. Javaheri S, Parker TJ, Wexler L, et al: Effect of theophylline on sleep-disordered breathing in heart failure. *New Engl J Med* 335:562–567, 1996.

24. Johns MW: A new method for measuring daytime sleepiness: The Epworth sleepiness scale. *Sleep* 14:540–545, 1991.

25. Krespi YP, Pearlman SJ, Keidar A: Laser-assisted uvula-palatoplasty for snoring. *J Otolaryngol* 23:328–334, 1994.

26. Kribbs NB, Pack AI, Kline LR, et al: Objective measurement of patterns of nasal CPAP use by patients with obstructive sleep apnea. *Am Rev Respir Dis* 147:887–895, 1993.

27. Lavie P, Herer P, Peled R, et al: Mortality in sleep apnea patients: A multivariate analysis of risk factors. *Sleep* 18:149–157, 1995.

28. Leiter JC: Upper airway shape: Is it important in the pathogenesis of obstructive sleep apnea? *Am J Respir Crit Care Med* 153:894–898, 1996.

29. Lofaso F, Coste A, Gilain L, et al: Sleep fragmentation as a risk factor for hypertension in middle-aged nonapneic snorers. *Chest* 109:896–900, 1996.

30. Maislin G, Pack AI, Kribbs NB, et al: A survey screen for prediction of apnea. *Sleep* 18:158–166, 1995.

31. Mathur R, Douglas NJ: Family studies in patients with the sleep apnea-hypopnea syndrome. *Ann Intern Med* 122:174–178, 1995.

32. Meurice JC, Marc I, Series F: Efficacy of auto-CPAP in the treatment of obstructive sleep apnea/hypopnea syndrome. *Am J Respir Crit Care Med* 153:794–798, 1996.

33. Meyer TJ, Hill NS: Noninvasive positive pressure ventilation to treat respiratory failure. *Ann Intern Med* 120:760–770, 1994.

34. Morgan BJ, Crabtree DC, Palta M, Skatrud JB: Combined hypoxia and hypercapnia evokes long-lasting sympathetic activation in humans. *J Appl Physiol* 79:205–213, 1995.

35. Naughton MT, Liu PP, Bernard DC, et al: Treatment of congestive heart failure and Cheyne-Stokes respiration during sleep by continuous positive airway pressure. *Am J Respir Crit Care Med* 151:92–97, 1995.

36. Pack AI: Obstructive sleep apnea. *Ann Intern Med* 39:517–567, 1994.

37. Phillipson EA: Sleep apnea—A major public health problem. *New Engl J Med* 328:1271–1273, 1993.

38. Redline S, Tishler PV, Tosteson TD, et al: The familial aggregation of obstructive sleep apnea. *Am J Respir Crit Care Med* 151:682–687, 1995.

39. Reeves-Hoché MK, Hudgel DW, Meck R, et al: Continuous versus bilevel positive airway pressure for obstructive sleep apnea. *Am J Respir Crit Care Med* 151:443–449, 1995.

40. Riley RW, Powell NB, Guilleminault C: Obstructive sleep apnea syndrome: A review of 306 consecutively treated surgical patients. *Otolaryngol Head Neck Surg* 108:117–125, 1993.

41. Schechtman KB, Sher AE, Piccirillo JF: Methodological and statistical problems in sleep apnea research: The literature of uvulopalatopharyngoplasty. *Sleep* 18:659–666, 1995.

42. Schmidt-Nowara W, Lowe A, Wiegand L, et al: Oral appliances for the treatment of snoring and obstructive sleep apnea: A review. *Sleep* 18:501–510, 1995.

43. Schwab RJ: Radiographic imaging in the diagnostic evaluation of sleep apnea, in Weinberger SE (ed), UpToDate (4.3) in *Pulmonary and Critical Care Medicine,* electronic media, 1996.

44. Schwab RJ, Gefter WB, Hoffman EA, et al: Dynamic upper airway imaging during awake respiration in normal subjects and patients with sleep disordered breathing. *Am Rev Respir Dis* 148:1385–1400, 1993.

45. Schwab RJ, Getsy JE, Pack AI: Central nervous system failure including sleep disorders, in Carlson RW, Geheb MA (eds), *The Principles and Practice of Medical Intensive Care.* Philadelphia, Saunders, 1993, pp 773–786.

46. Schwab RJ, Gupta KB, Gefter WB, et al: Upper airway and soft tissue anatomy in normal subjects and patients with sleep-disordered breathing: Significance of the lateral pharyngeal walls. *Am J Respir Crit Care Med* 152:1673–1689, 1995.

47. Schwab RJ, Pack AI, Gupta KB, et al: Upper airway and soft tissue structural changes induced by CPAP in normal subjects. *Am J Respir Crit Care Med* 154:1106–1116, 1996.

48. Shepard JW Jr: Hypertension, cardiac arrhythmias, myocardial infarction, and stroke in relation to obstructive sleep apnea. *Clin Chest Med* 13:437–458, 1992.

49. Sher AE, Schechtman KB, Picirillo J: The efficacy of surgical modifications of the upper airway in adults with obstructive sleep apnea syndrome. *Sleep* 19:156–177, 1996.

50. Somers VK, Dyken ME, Claray MP, Abbound FM: Sympathetic neural mechanisms in obstructive sleep apnea. *J Clin Invest* 96:1897–1904, 1995

51. Strobel RJ, Rosen RC: Obesity and weight loss in obstructive sleep apnea: A critical review. *Sleep* 19:104–115, 1996.

52. Strollo PJ Jr, Rogers RM: Obstructive sleep apnea. *New Engl J Med* 334:99–104, 1996.

53. Trudo F, Schwab RJ: Obesity-hypoventilation syndrome, in Lanken PN, Manaker S, Hanson WC (eds), *The Intensive Care Unit Manual.* Philadelphia, Saunders. In press.

54. White DP: Central sleep apnea, in Kryger MH, Roth T, Dement WC (eds), *Principles and Practice of Sleep Medicine.* Philadelphia, Saunders, 1994, pp 630–642.

55. Working Group on OSA and Hypertension: Obstructive sleep apnea and blood pressure elevation: What is the relationship? *Blood Press* 2:166–182, 1993.

56. Young T, Palta M, Dempsey J, et al: The occurrence of sleep-disordered breathing among middle-aged adults. *New Engl J Med* 328:1230–1235, 1993.

CHAPTER 103

DIFFERENTIAL DIAGNOSIS AND EVALUATION OF SLEEPINESS

Meir H. Kryger / Charles F. P. George

THE PHENOMENON OF SLEEPINESS

QUANTIFYING SLEEPINESS

FACTORS AFFECTING SLEEPINESS
    Quantity of Sleep
    Sleep Quality
    Circadian Rhythms
    Medications

PREVALENCE OF EXCESSIVE DAYTIME SLEEPINESS

EVALUATING THE SLEEPY PATIENT
    Approach and Differential Diagnosis

Excessive daytime sleepiness is a common problem affecting large segments of the population. Epidemiologic surveys have shown that 4 to 5 percent of the population complain of excessive sleepiness,[1,2] and there is increasing evidence that sleepiness plays a part in both industrial and road traffic accidents.[3] Over the past 10 to 12 years, research has provided increased understanding of, among other sleep disorders, obstructive sleep apnea (OSA). With the recognition that sleep apnea alone affects about 2 to 4 percent of the population,[4] and with increasing awareness of sleep disorders by the general public, respiratory physicians, by necessity, are dealing more and more with sleep apnea and other sleep disorders. In recognition of the need for training pulmonary physicians in sleep disorders, in 1994 the American Thoracic Society published recommendations for training in sleep medicine (available through the ATS office). It is therefore clear that pulmonary physicians need to better understand and treat excessive daytime sleepiness whatever its cause.

THE PHENOMENON OF SLEEPINESS

Sleepiness is both a subjective and an objective phenomenon, a constellation of sensations and a physiological state with stereotypical behaviors. As such, it is sometimes difficult to define, and its measurement (see below) depends on the circumstances. Sleepiness can be reflected by any or all of the following: heaviness of the eyelids, mild burning or itching of the eyes, difficulty keeping the eyes open, heaviness in the arms or legs, reluctance to move, loss of initiative, loss of interest in surroundings, and difficulty with concentration. These sensations are accompanied by behavioral changes such as rubbing the eyes, yawning and stretching, and nodding the head, and by generally reduced motor functions such as speech, facial expression, and body movement. Indeed, the average sleepy person often exhibits a face with a glazed, blank, or even "dopey" expression.

Sleepiness also can be considered a physiological state like hunger or thirst. Just as hunger and thirst are physiological states that occur with fasting and are satisfied by eating and drinking, sleepiness is produced by sleep restriction or deprivation and is reversed or satisfied by sleep. The factors that produce and influence sleepiness will be detailed below; they include such obvious factors as time since last asleep, previous amount of sleep, continuity of sleep, and normal 24-hour circadian influences. These factors determine the physiological state of sleepiness (or the physiological sleep tendency). Environmental stimuli influence this state and can determine, up to a point, whether or not this sleepy tendency will be manifested. For example, heavy meals, warm rooms, boring lectures, or monotonous tasks are usually considered soporific activities or situations. In these situations, a person might feel sleepy and, perhaps, might fall asleep. Yet the environmental factors themselves do not cause the sleepiness; they only allow it to be expressed. Equally, the same degree of physiological sleep tendency might go unnoticed when environmental stimulation occurs in the form of a life-threatening situation. In other words, the degree to which sleepiness is experienced or evident in behavior is determined by the underlying physiological sleep tendency (or the need for sleep) and environmental factors, which interact to make manifest the sleep tendency or sleep propensity.

While it is accepted that sleepiness is a physiological state, the physiological substrates of this state have not been identified. Neurotransmitters such as serotonin, acetylcholine, and the catecholamines have been implicated in the sleep/wake mechanism along with a variety of other sleep-inducing substances.[5] While much research is ongoing, the understanding of the neurochemicals responsible for sleep, sleepiness, and loss of alertness are still far from clear.

QUANTIFYING SLEEPINESS

The sensation of sleepiness is often difficult to quantify, as are other subjective symptoms, such as pain or shortness of breath.

All of these subjective sensations mean different things to different people, and are modified by factors including motivation, external stimulation, and competing needs. What constitutes extreme sleepiness for one person may be only mild sleepiness for another and depend on the situation in which it occurs.

The degree of sleepiness can be judged or measured in many ways. Measurements of performance after sleep loss intuitively should reflect daytime sleepiness, since most people report decreased performance after a sleepless night. Previously it was felt that only performance tests that were prolonged and monotonous were sensitive to sleep loss.[6] However, the work of Dinges[7]—using his Psychomotor Vigilance Task (PVT)—demonstrates that if the signal rate is high and the response measure sufficiently sensitive, repetitive tasks of only 10-min duration will expose the limits of performance in sleepy persons. Performance decrements resulting from sleep deprivation (or sleep disorders such as sleep apnea) can be observed in such a task if results are analyzed over time. This time-on-task or vigilance decrement may be observed as evidence of fatigue even in well-motivated subjects with adequate prior sleep, and it manifests itself as a shallow decline in performance as time-on-task increases. When the subject is sleep deprived, it is impossible to sustain attention long enough to maintain peak performance throughout the entire task. Sleep loss increases the rate of decline in performance.

While the effects of sleepiness on performance may occur in a dose-dependent fashion in normals (i.e., the more sleep deprived, the more sleepy and the worse the performance), performance decrements in patients who are sleepy because of an underlying sleep disorder may be accounted for by factors other than sleepiness. We have been studying driving performance in sleep apnea patients using a divided attention task that integrates the two essential features of driving: tracking and visual search.[8] While it is clear that many sleep apneics have poor performance (equal to or worse than normals impaired by alcohol), sleepiness, as measured by the Multiple Sleep Latency Test (see below), accounts for less than 25 percent of the variance in tracking performance.

Subjective reports may be used to quantify sleepiness, but statements such as "I feel sleepy" and "I feel very sleepy" often do not distinguish between feelings caused by a high physiological sleep tendency and those resulting from muscular fatigue, depressed mood, or a general lack of energy. Thus, several subjective sleepiness scales have been developed. The first to receive widespread use was the Stanford Sleepiness Scale (SSS),[9] a seven-point self-rating scale ranging from 1 (alert, wide awake) to 7 (almost in reverie, sleep onset soon). It has been shown to correlate with the performance of mental tasks and to demonstrate changes in sleepiness with sleep loss. However, unlike normal persons who are experimentally sleep deprived, patients with more chronic sleep deprivation (such as sleep apnea) cannot be accurately tested with the SSS. Some patients who have an obvious overwhelming physiological sleep tendency may claim to be only mildly sleepy, yet fall asleep before your eyes. This was first observed in the early 1970s by Dement and colleagues,[10] and was a stimulus for that group to develop more objective measures of sleepiness (see below). It is clear that over a period of months or years, many sleep apnea patients lose their frame of reference with regard to normal alertness and cannot distinguish major changes in sleepiness. Thus, the subjective report of sleepi-ness (using the SSS) by people who are chronically and severely sleep deprived is not reliable. Recently other scales have been introduced, including the Karolinska Sleepiness Scale (KSS)[11] and the more widely used Epworth Sleepiness Scale (ESS).[12]

The KSS is a nine-point scale ranging from 1 (very alert) to 9 (very sleepy, fighting sleep, making an effort to keep awake), with verbal descriptions of every second point. Like the SSS, the KSS requires the subject to integrate and translate a number of sensations to a continuum that is fairly abstract despite the verbal description. Ratings obtained with these scales may be affected by the situation where the scale is presented (at rest or during performing a task) and how the subject relates his or her perception to that particular time or place. Nonetheless, both the SSS and the KSS show high correlations with performance. The KSS was also found to be strongly related to EEG and electro-oculographic signs of sleepiness.[13]

The newest and most widely used subjective measure of sleepiness is the ESS (see Table 103-1). The ESS was designed to measure sleep propensity in a single, standardized way and is based on questions relating to eight situations, some known to be very soporific. The questions are self-administered, and subjects are asked to rate on a 0–3 scale how likely they are to doze off in the situation based on their usual habits. The ESS tries to overcome the fact that people have different daily routines, some facilitating and others preventing daytime sleep. ESS scores have shown significant correlations with mean sleep latency in the MSLT (see below)[12] and have distinguished groups of patients with disorders of excessive sleepiness such as narcolepsy, OSA, and idiopathic hypersomnolence. It has also correlated significantly with the apnea/hypopnea index (AHI).[14] The ESS has a high test-retest reliability and a high level of internal reliability[15] in normals and patients with sleep apnea.[16] Johns has further examined the utility of measuring sleepiness in different situations using the ESS.[17] His results suggest that individual measurements of sleep propensity (i.e., sleepiness) entail three components of variation: a general characteristic of the subject (the average sleep propensity), a general characteristic of the situation in which the sleepiness or sleep propensity is measured (its soporific nature), and a third component that is specific for both subjects and situation.

In an effort to have an objective, reliable, and reproducible measure of physiological sleep tendency, the Multiple Sleep Latency Test (MSLT) has been developed and standardized.[18] Performed at intervals throughout the day, the MSLT measures the time to sleep onset, as determined by the EEG. This test is based on the assumption that, given the proper surroundings, physiological sleep tendency will be expressed; it has an intuitive appeal in that if one patient is more sleepy than the other, the sleepier patient should fall asleep more quickly. Patients are instrumented to record the EEG, electro-oculogram (EOG), and electromyogram (EMG); they are put in a quiet, darkened, temperature-controlled room, and are asked to lie quietly, close the eyes, and try to fall asleep. Naps are scheduled at 2-hour intervals, with 20 min allowed for sleep to occur; the average sleep latency of the naps represents the result of the MSLT. Since sleepiness follows a circadian rhythm (see below), one nap is insufficient to document and quantify daytime sleepiness. Accordingly, a minimum of four and a maximum of six naps are

TABLE 103-1

The Epworth Sleepiness Scale

NAME: _____

Today's Date: _____   Your age (years) _____

Your sex (male = M; female = F) _____

How likely are you to doze off or fall asleep in the following situations, in contrast to feeling just tired? This refers to your usual way of life in recent times. Even if you have not done some of these things recently, try to work out how they would have affected you. Use the following scale to chose the *most appropriate number* for each situation.

    0 = would *never* doze
    1 = *slight* chance of dozing
    2 = *moderate* chance of dozing
    3 = *high* chance of dozing

Situation	Chance of dozing
Sitting and reading	_____
Watching TV	_____
Sitting inactive in a public place (e.g., in a theater or at a meeting)	_____
As a passenger in a car for an hour without a break	_____
Lying down to rest in the afternoon when circumstances permit	_____
Sitting and talking to someone	_____
Sitting quietly after a lunch without alcohol	_____
In a car, while stopped for a few minutes in the traffic	_____

recommended. The MSLT is a reliable, reproducible test that has been validated in a number of sleep deprivation experiments in normal subjects and in a variety of clinical conditions with patients who have disorders such as narcolepsy and sleep apnea.[19–21] An important advantage of the MSLT is that patient motivation cannot counteract the effects of previous sleep loss on sleep latency. That is, while most people can be motivated to compensate for reduced performance after sleep deprivation, motivation cannot overcome an increased pressure for sleep, particularly when the patient is in bed in a darkened room.[22]

An alternative to the MSLT is the Maintenance of Wakefulness Test (MWT).[23] This is a variation on a theme in which subjects sit in a chair in a darkened room and are requested to remain awake for 20 (or 40) min. This test was developed on the assumption that the ability to fall asleep and the ability to stay awake are two separate phenomena. The MWT has undergone further tests of validity,[24,25] and Sangal and colleagues compared the results of MSLT and MWT done on the same day in 258 patients with a variety of sleep disorders. Of interest, they found some patients with low MSLT scores were able to stay awake on the MWT; conversely, some patients failed to stay awake when asked to do so (MWT) but were unable to fall asleep quickly on the MSLT. The authors suggested that the discordant results call into question the exclusive use of the MSLT in making clinical decisions about disability relating to sleep tendency. The results of factor analysis suggest that MSLT measures sleep tendency while the MWT measures ability to stay awake. However, as Johns points out,[17] Sangal's results and his own demonstrate the problem of extrapolating the results from one test situation to another. No one situational sleep tendency or propensity can accurately represent a subject's average sleep propensity in daily life. While the total ESS gives an estimate of this average sleep propensity on the basis of eight life situations, there is currently no gold standard with which to compare that estimate. The ESS is an inexpensive way to assess sleepiness in large numbers of patients with chronic sleep disorders, but like all other methods for measuring sleepiness, it has its limitations, particularly when one is trying to make individual decisions based on group data.

There are ongoing efforts to use EEG measures to improve the ease of objectively measuring sleepiness. The Alpha Attenuation Test (AAT), recently developed by Stampi,[26,27] is based on the observation that when a person drifts into sleepiness, the power spectrum in the alpha frequency band of the EEG (8 to 12 Hz) increases with the eyes open but tends to decrease with the eyes closed. The alertness level (or alpha attenuation coefficient, AAC) is defined as the ratio of the mean alpha power with eyes closed to the mean alpha power with eyes open. The higher the ACC, the greater the alertness level. The AAT has been validated in sleep-restricted normals and in patients with narcolepsy and correlates strongly with the MSLT. Compared to the MSLT, the AAT has the advantage of being fast (it requires only 6 min of recording), minimally intrusive, easily administered, and a purely objective measure of sleepiness. While these features make the AAT a valuable tool in lab and field research, its utility in clinical settings has yet to be determined.

FACTORS AFFECTING SLEEPINESS

Sleepiness is determined by the quantity of sleep and the quality and type of sleep, interacting with circadian rhythms or drugs that patients may be taking.

Quantity of Sleep

The amount of nocturnal sleep has a strong relationship to the degree of daytime sleepiness. Partial or total sleep deprivation is followed by increased daytime sleepiness in normal persons.[19,21] Furthermore, sleep restriction will become cumulative over time and lead to increasing daytime sleepiness.

The work of Carskadon and Dement demonstrates the effect of sleep restriction on sleep latency (Fig. 103-1). When the sleep of young adults was reduced by 2 hours a night on consecutive nights, sleepiness (as measured by the MSLT) progressively increased over 7 days.[21] Even as little as 1 h per night of sleep loss will accumulate over time and lead to daytime sleepiness—a fact

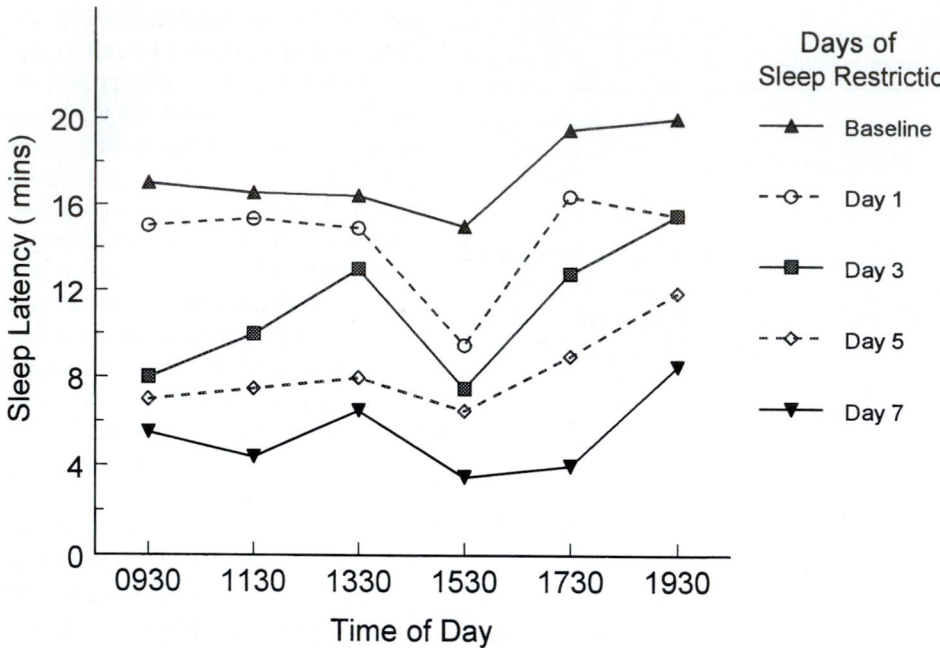

FIGURE 103-1 Average daily sleep latency test scores for young adults when nighttime sleep was reduced by 2 h a night for 7 consecutive nights. (Adapted from Dement WC, Carskadon MA: An essay on sleepiness, in Boldy-Moulinier M (ed): *Actualitiés en Médécine Expérimentale, en Hommage au Prof D Passouant.* Montpellier, Euromed, 1981, pp 47–71.)

subjects. Within the group of 120 young subjects, 12 healthy, nonsmoking men aged 21 to 35 years had a mean sleep latency of less than 6 min on MSLT testing, while another 12 had an MSLT of greater than 16 min. These subjects had baseline testing and then extended their sleep period time from 8 to 10 h over 6 days. Repeat testing on days 1, 3, and 6 showed stepwise increases in MSLT and performance testing for both subgroups. These data support the notion that chronic voluntary sleep restriction produces objective sleepiness that may or may not be perceived by the subject.

Sleep Quality

Sleep quality is perceived to be abnormal when sleep is decreased or discontinuous. Disrupting sleep continuity—i.e., causing arousal from sleep, either experimentally or by sleep disorders—affects the quality of sleep and results in increased physiological sleep tendency.[32,33] An arousal can be defined as a brief (3 to 15 s) speeding up of the EEG, or as a burst of alpha activity occasionally accompanied by transient increases in skeletal muscle tone. These typically do not result in awakening as defined by standard sleep staging criteria or behavioral indicators.[34] Sleep studies can identify various causes of arousal, such as recurrent obstructive apnea, leg movements, or pain, in some but not all cases. A common exception is the patient with chronic obstructive pulmonary disease (COPD) who has frequent arousals from sleep in the absence of obstructive apnea or leg movements. Patients with COPD often experience oxygen desaturation during sleep, and this is a potential stimulus for arousal. However, arousal frequency is unchanged when supplemental oxygen is given and desaturation is prevented, so the stimulus is still undefined.[35] Nonetheless, compared with age-matched controls, COPD patients have discontinuous sleep and poor sleep efficiency (defined as percentage of time actually asleep in bed). This might be expected to lead to daytime sleepiness, but the sleep latency of COPD patients has not yet been measured systematically.

generally not appreciated. Each person has a certain biologic sleep need, and the specific amount varies from one subject to the next. Regardless of cultural or environmental factors, most adults sleep between 7 and 8 h per day,[28] but the old adage that we must sleep 8 h each night is not true for everyone. Some people require more than 8 h, and others less; even Siamese twins show an independence of sleep needs.[29] In the absence of pathology, normal human sleep length varies between 6 and 9 h, although some people require less. It would be ideal to require a minimum amount of sleep to allow maximum productivity in work and adequate time for social pursuits. Indeed, some investigators believe that Western society predisposes to sleep deprivation. With economic and social constraints, the sleep period is the time most encroached on, potentially leading to daytime sleepiness.

That voluntary sleep restriction or insufficient sleep causes daytime sleepiness has been demonstrated by Roehrs and colleagues.[30] Among all prominent features differentiating this group of patients with insufficient sleep from those with narcolepsy was the report, obtained from the sleep history, of a disparity between the amount of sleep on weekdays and that on weekends. People with insufficient sleep typically have a much longer sleep period on weekends (by 2 h or more).

Most patients consider their weekly sleep loss trivial and assume that it is recovered on weekends. However, while recovery from a single experimental sleep restriction occurs in a couple of nights, it is not likely that repeated episodes of sleep deprivation can be compensated for in just one night. Further work by Roehrs and colleagues has elaborated on this point.[31] They studied a large group of normal subjects without complaints of daytime sleepiness and observed that young subjects (particularly college students) had shorter sleep latencies than did older

Auditory stimuli presented externally to normal subjects during sleep can produce arousal; repetitive presentation of such stimuli can produce daytime sleepiness. Several studies have shown decreased performance and increased sleepiness the day after repetitive arousal,[36,37] with the degree of daytime sleepiness related to the frequency of nocturnal sleep disruption. Bonnet awakened young adults from sleep every 1, 10, or 150 min and measured daytime sleep latency and performance. Not surprisingly, the shortest sleep latency occurred after the most fragmented nocturnal sleep.[37] This increased sleepiness will result even if the stimulus is only sufficient to produce EEG signs of arousal, without full wakefulness.[32]

Circadian Rhythms

If sleep latency is measured every 2 h over a complete 24-h day, a biphasic pattern of sleep tendency becomes obvious. Figure 103-2 displays the work of Richardson and colleagues, who used active, elderly subjects from a local senior citizens' recreation center and young adults from a university community, none of whom had sleep complaints.[38] On three consecutive days and nights in the sleep lab, sleep latency was recorded at 2-h intervals. During the normal nocturnal sleep period, patients were awakened for 15 min and then allowed to go back to sleep. This and other work clearly demonstrates that there are two peaks and troughs of sleepiness over a 24-h period. Not surprisingly, the times of increased sleepiness are during the nocturnal hours and during the daytime hours (in the midafternoon between 2 and 4 p.m.). This circadian rhythm of sleepiness is present in all age groups, although the time of the peak rhythm may vary. The circadian rhythm of sleepiness is similar to other circadian rhythms in that it possesses an endogenous periodicity that can be affected by environmental influences that fine-tune or entrain the rhythm. Even in the absence of these environmental cues (such as awakening time, alarm clock, degree of light or darkness, food and stimulants, social contact), rhythms show a persistent periodicity. The circadian rhythm of temperature is extremely stable. Temperatures fall in the late afternoon, are lowest during the middle of the sleep period, and rise before morning awakening. The temperature rhythm synchronizes most closely with sleepiness. Although the amplitude of body temperature and sleep latency rhythms differ considerably, no other biologic rhythms correlate so well in time.[39]

Two other examples of the influence of circadian rhythms on sleepiness are obvious. The first is that associated with shift work,[40] and the second is due to transcontinental travel (jet lag).[41] Workers with a normal nocturnal sleep period and a previously stable circadian sleepiness rhythm suddenly will have a trough of sleepiness during the middle of their night work period. They will attempt to stay awake, while the circadian influences will promote sleep. Not surprisingly, performance may suffer.

Medications

Drug effects on sleep can be significant and can either promote sleep and sleepiness or increase wakefulness and alertness. Not surprisingly, sedative drugs increase sleepiness. Benzodiazepine hypnotics are widely used to help people get to sleep at night. Many objective studies confirm the ability of hypnotics to shorten sleep latency at bedtime. When given during the day, they will promote sleep. However, the daytime carryover effect of nocturnal sedation is not always recognized.[42] This effect occurs most commonly with long-acting benzodiazepines, but it may occur with other medications as well. Alcohol consistently shortens sleep onset and produces sedation, whether given at night or during the day. Drugs that produce sleepiness include antihistamines, which are used in allergy and pulmonary practice. Many of the early H_1 antihistamines, such as diphenhydramine and chlorpheniramine, have been shown to reduce the MSLT.[43] Some newer antihistamines, such as terfenadine and astemizole, do not produce objective sleepiness. The more lipid-soluble drugs (e.g., diphenhydramine and chlorpheniramine) penetrate the central nervous system more easily and therefore are more likely than less lipid-soluble drugs to produce sedation. Other medications with high lipid solubility have been reported to produce daytime sedation; the most common of these are the beta-blocker drugs. There are no controlled, objective studies of sleep latency with this type of drug, and sleepiness from these medications is based on reports of side effects.

The effect of a particular drug in producing sleepiness also depends on the background level of sleepiness or alertness. This has been demonstrated by Lumley and colleagues,[44] who gave either ethanol or caffeine to 18 normal sleeping young men in the morning and then measured their daytime alertness or sleepiness with the MSLT. One might expect ethanol to produce daytime sleepiness and caffeine to increase sleep latency during the day. To alter the background level of sleepiness, subjects received the drugs after having spent 5, 8, or 11 h in bed the previous night. Subjects were consistently sleepier after ethanol than after caffeine ingestion, but it was noted that fully rested subjects (those having spent 11 h in bed) did not show sleepiness after taking ethanol. In other words, the sedative effects of drugs such as alcohol can be enhanced by increased back-

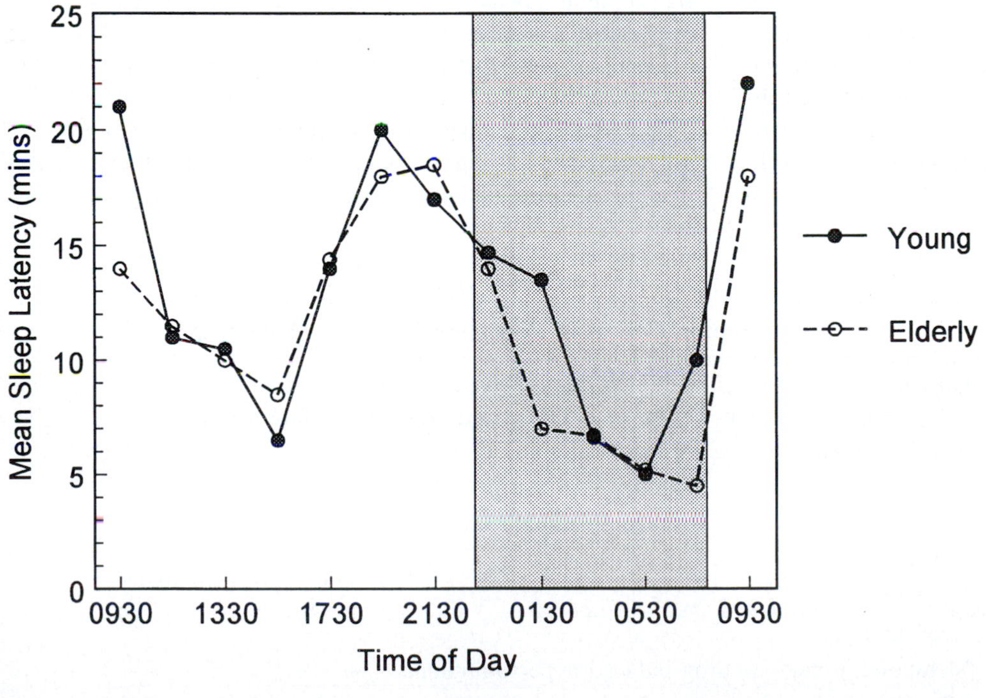

FIGURE 103-2   Sleep latency (mean) as a function of time of day for young subjects (filled circles) and elderly subjects (open circles). *Stippled area* denotes nighttime sleep period. (Adapted from Richardson GS, Carskadon MA, Orav EJ, et al: *Sleep* 5:882–92, 1982.)

ground sleepiness. Thus, a driver who is sleepy to start with may be as vulnerable after just one or two drinks as a previously alert driver who has become legally intoxicated.

Stimulants such as amphetamine, methylphenidate, and pemoline increase alertness. These are most often used in the treatment of narcolepsy but are also used, quite inappropriately, by truck drivers trying to keep awake when driving over long distances. It is our anecdotal experience that many sleepy truck drivers actually have sleep apnea and are not particularly helped by stimulant medications. Caffeine, probably the most widely used stimulant, can reduce daytime sleepiness and transiently increase alertness. Excessive caffeine intake also paradoxically may cause a degree of daytime sleepiness. This occurs when caffeine levels persist into nocturnal hours and promote difficulties with sleep onset and increased awakenings during sleep.

PREVALENCE OF EXCESSIVE DAYTIME SLEEPINESS

Few studies have adequately addressed the complaint of daytime sleepiness. Prevalence rates revealed by questionnaire surveys or reports from sleep laboratories vary between 0.3 and 4 to 4.5 percent. These figures suggest that daytime sleepiness is less common than insomnia, which has an estimated prevalence of 14 to 35 percent. However, in a sample of 8000 patients at a large sleep/wake disorders center, Coleman found that hypersomnia was a more common problem than insomnia.[45] Symptoms of excessive daytime somnolence vary according to sample, the number of people investigated, the type of questions used, and the center. McGhie and Russell reported that 0.5 percent of 2466 Scottish subjects reported "too much sleep."[46] The prevalence of "hypersomnia" among 1006 households in Los Angeles was 4.2 percent.[1] Of 1502 industrial workers in Israel, 4.9 percent had "excessive daytime somnolence" and 7.8 percent reported falling asleep regularly during at least two of six passive activities.[2] Of 2552 Finnish army recruits, 9.5 percent answered affirmatively when asked, "Do you consider yourself more sleepy during the daytime than your friends or workmates?"[47] In addition, "daytime sleepiness" was reported by 16.2 percent of 1138 male subjects aged 18 to 23 years in a questionnaire distributed in Milan.[48] More recently, the prevalence of excessive daytime somnolence was investigated in 58,162 draftees in the French army; 14.1 percent reported occasional daytime sleep episodes, 3.8 percent reported one or two daily episodes, and 1.1 percent reported more than two daily episodes.[49] Of the total sample, 5 percent considered the sleep periods to be affecting their lives. A multivariate analysis showed five independent factors related to excessive daytime sleepiness: use of hypnotics, sleep difficulties, irregular sleep/wake schedule, snoring, and hours of sleep.

The Wisconsin study by Young and colleagues was the first to formally determine the prevalence of sleepiness as a function of sleep apnea. This landmark study demonstrated that at least 2 percent of middle-aged women and 4 percent of middle-aged men had OSA and symptoms of excessive daytime sleepiness.[4] While there may have been other causes for the daytime sleepiness besides OSA, it is clear that sleep apnea is responsible for a great deal of the daytime sleepiness in North America.

EVALUATING THE SLEEPY PATIENT

Approach and Differential Diagnosis

Keeping in mind the factors that determine daytime sleepiness, the sleep history can be individualized and can be very helpful in narrowing the differential diagnosis (Table 103-2). One should always question the patient about his or her nocturnal sleep, looking specifically at sleep onset time, sleep period time, number of awakenings, and time of rising in the morning. Sleep onset phenomena such as sleep paralysis and hypnagogic hallucinations often suggest a diagnosis of narcolepsy, although these sometimes occur in apneics who are severely sleep deprived. A history of loud snoring or stopped breathing during sleep is suggestive of sleep apnea, particularly if the snoring is cyclical rather than continuous, with periods of loud snoring or snorting alternating with quiet intervals. Since insufficient sleep may be the cause of sleepiness, it is important to ask if there is any difference in the amount of sleep required during the week compared with that on weekends. Equally important is whether the patient has any changes in subjective sleepiness on weekends or holidays compared with weekdays.

In some instances, more information will be obtained from the spouse (or bed partner) or from a sleep/wake diary, since not all people are aware of the severity of their sleepiness. Moreover, patients may not understand the importance of good sleep hygiene; the diary can serve as a reminder for patients to be diligent about it.

In estimating the degree of daytime sleepiness, it is useful to ask when and during what activities the patient experiences sleepiness. Is the patient sleepy on awakening in the morning,

---

TABLE 103-2

Common Causes of Persistent Daytime Sleepiness

Obstructive sleep apnea and other sleep-disordered breathing conditions
  (e.g., neuromuscular weakness with nocturnal respiratory failure)

Narcolepsy/cataplexy syndrome

Sleep-related movement disorders
  (e.g., periodic limb movement disorder, bruxism, etc.)

Depression

Postviral fatigue

Head injury

Metabolic, toxic, and drug-induced hypersomnolence

Idiopathic hypersomnolence

Insufficient sleep

Circadian rhythm sleep disorders

or is it only by midday? Does the patient fall asleep while doing things or only when inactive? Driving to and from work are important times when sleepiness may become obvious, particularly while the person is waiting at a railroad crossing or stoplight. Episodes of automatic behavior, related to "microsleeps," often occur while one is driving. Do patients nap during the day, and if so, is the nap refreshing? Many patients with sleep apnea are still sleepy or foggy after a nap, whereas patients with narcolepsy most often feel refreshed immediately upon awakening.

Since drugs can have a profound effect on sleep and sleepiness, a careful drug history is mandatory in the assessment of sleepiness. The clinician must remember to include queries not only about drugs that specifically affect sleep (hypnotics, sedatives, or other psychoactive medications) but also about substances that may not be considered to have any effect on sleep or waking. In particular, alcohol is a known precipitant or exaggerating factor for sleep apnea; patients will often report that they feel much worse the day after ingesting alcohol despite having had a nonintoxicating dose.

Apart from a general physical exam, one should pay particular attention to the size of the jaw, face, and upper airway, looking for obvious skeletal abnormalities—particularly retrognathia or micrognathia. One then carefully examines the upper airway, looking for nasal obstructions such as a deviated nasal septum or inflammatory allergic polyps; then, one examines the oropharynx, looking at the size of the tongue, the position of the soft palate, and the size of the uvula; finally one examines the larynx to rule out upper-airway tumors or other obstructing lesions. While the typical sleep apnea patient will be the obese plethoric man with a thick neck, it is important to remember that examination of the awake, upright airway may bear no relationship to what happens when the patient is supine and asleep. Thus, the diagnosis of sleep apnea usually is confirmed by nocturnal polysomnography.

The patient who has a history of snoring and daytime sleepiness but has no sleep apnea during his or her nocturnal study must undergo an objective measure of daytime sleepiness, because some patients who claim to have substantial daytime somnolence are simply looking for compensation. Also, some OSA patients will remain sleepy despite adequate treatment of their apnea, and an additional sleep disorder may coexist. Again, daytime quantification of sleepiness will be necessary. The only disadvantage of the MSLT is that it is an inefficient test. Compared with objective measurements of airflow (i.e., and FEV_1), which take seconds to perform and interpret, the MSLT takes almost a whole day and provides only one piece of information. Until better tests are developed and validated, however, the MSLT will continue as a standard, albeit time-inefficient, objective measure of daytime sleepiness.

REFERENCES

1. Bixler ED, Kales A, Soldatos CR, et al: Prevalence of sleep disorders in the Los Angeles metropolitan area. *Am J Psychiatry* 136: 1257–1262, 1979.
2. Lavie P: Sleep habits and sleep disturbances in industrial workers in Israel. *Sleep* 4:147–158, 1982.
3. Mitler MM, Carskadon MA, Czeisler CA, et al: Catastrophes, sleep, and public policy: Consensus report. *Sleep* 11:100–109, 1988.
4. Young T, Palta M, Dempsey J, et al: The occurrence of sleep disordered breathing among middle-aged adults. *New Engl J Med* 338: 1230–1235, 1993.
5. Inoue S: Sleep substances: Their roles and evolution, in Inoue S, Borbely AA (eds), *Endogenous Sleep Substances and Sleep Regulation.* Tokyo, Japan Scientific Societies Press, 1985, pp 3–12.
6. Wilkinson RT: Sleep deprivation: Performance tests for partial and selective sleep deprivation, in Abt LE, Reiss BF (eds), *Progress in Clinical Psychology,* vol 8. New York, Grune & Stratton, 1968, pp 28–43.
7. Dinges DF: Probing the limits of functional capability: The effects of sleep loss on short duration tasks. In Broughton RG, Ogilvie RD (eds), *Sleep, Arousal and Performance.* Boston, Birkhauser, 1992, pp 177–188.
8. George CFP, Boudreau AC, Smiley S: Simulated driving performance in patients with obstructive sleep apnea. *Am J Respir Crit Care Med* (in press).
9. Hoddes E, Zarcone V, Smythe H, et al: Quantification of sleepiness: A new approach. *Psychophysiology* 10:431–436, 1978.
10. Dement WC, Carskadon MA, Richardson GW: Excessive daytime sleepiness in the sleep apnea syndrome, in Guilleminault C, Dement WC (eds): *Sleep Apnea Syndrome.* New York, Alan R Liss, 1978, pp 23–46.
11. Akerstedt T, Gillberg M: Subjective and objective sleepiness in the active individual. *Int J Neurosci* 52:29–37, 1990.
12. Johns MW: A new method for measuring daytime sleepiness: The Epworth Sleepiness scale. *Sleep* 14:540–545, 1991.
13. Gillberg M, Kecklund G, Akerstedt T: Relations between performance and subjective rating of sleepiness during a night awake. *Sleep* 17:236–241, 1994.
14. Johns MW: Daytime sleepiness, snoring, and obstructive sleep apnea: The Epworth Sleepiness Scale. *Chest* 103:30–36, 1993.
15. Johns MW: Reliability and factor analysis of the Epworth Sleepiness Scale. *Sleep* 15:376–381, 1992.
16. Ferguson KA, Flaherty BA, George CFP: The Epworth Sleepiness Scale and obstructive sleep apnea: Reproducibility over time. *Sleep Res* 24: 232, 1995.
17. Johns MW: Sleepiness in different situations measured by the Epworth Sleepiness Scale. *Sleep* 17:703–710, 1994.
18. Carskadon MA, Dement WC, Mitler MM, et al: Guidelines for the multiple sleep latency test (MSLT): A standard measure of sleepiness. *Sleep* 9:519–524, 1986.
19. Carskadon MA, Dement WC: Nocturnal determinants of daytime sleepiness. *Sleep* 5:573–581, 1982.
20. Richardson GS, Carskadon MA, Flagg W, et al: Excessive daytime sleepiness in man: Multiple sleep latency measurement in narcoleptic and control subjects. *Electroencephalogr Clin Neurophysiol* 45:621–627, 1978.
21. Carskadon MA, Dement WC: Cumulative effects of sleep restriction on daytime sleepiness. *Psychophysiology* 18:107–113, 1981.
22. Hartse KM, Roth T, Zorick FJ: Daytime sleepiness and daytime wakefulness: The effect of instruction. *Sleep* 5:S107–118, 1982.
23. Mitler MM, Gujavarty KS, Browman CP: Maintenance of wakefulness test: A polysomnographic technique for evaluating treatment efficacy in patients with excessive somnolence. *Electroencephalogr Clin Neurophysiol* 53:658–661, 1982.
24. Poceta JS, Timms RM, Jeong D-U, et al: Maintenance of wakefulness test in obstructive sleep apnea. *Chest* 101:893–897, 1992.
25. Sangal RB, Thomal L, Mitler MM: Maintenance of wakefulness test and multiple sleep latency test: Measurement of different ability in patients with sleep disorders. *Chest* 101:898–902, 1992.
26. Stampi C, Stone P, Michimori A: The alpha attenuation test: A new quantitative method for assessing sleepiness and its relationship to the MSLT. *Sleep Res* 22:115, 1993.

27. Stampi C, Michimori A, Aguirre A: Optimization of the alpha attenuation test for the objective assessment of sleepiness. *Sleep Res* 23:469, 1994.

28. Browman CP, Gordon GC, Tepas DI, et al: Reported sleep and drug use of workers: A preliminary report. *Sleep Res* 6:111, 1977.

29. Webb WB: The sleep of conjoined twins. *Sleep* 1:205–211, 1978.

30. Roehrs T, Zorick F, Sicklesteel J, et al: Excessive daytime sleepiness associated with insufficient sleep. *Sleep* 6:319–325, 1982.

31. Timms V, Roehrs T, Zwyghuizen-Doorenbos A, et al: Sleep extension in sleepy and alert individuals. *Sleep Res* 12:449–457, 1982.

32. Stepanski E, Lamphere J, Badia P, et al: Sleep fragmentation and daytime sleepiness. *Sleep* 7:18–26, 1984.

33. Levine B, Roehrs T, Stepanski E, et al: Fragmenting sleep diminishes its recuperative value. *Sleep* 10:590–599, 1987.

34. Rechtschaffen A, Kales A (eds): *A Manual of Standardized Terminology, Techniques and Scoring for Sleep Stages of Human Subjects.* Los Angeles, UCLA Brain Research Institute/Brain Information Service, 1968.

35. Fleetham J, West P, Mezon B, et al: Sleep, arousals and oxygen desaturation in chronic obstructive pulmonary disease. *Am Rev Respir Dis* 126:429–433, 1982.

36. Bonnet MH: Effect of sleep disruption on sleep performance and mood. *Sleep* 8:11–19, 1985.

37. Bonnet MH: Performance and sleepiness as a function of frequency and placement of sleep disruption. *Psychophysiology* 23:263–271, 1986.

38. Richardson GS, Carskadon MA, Orav EJ, et al: Circadian variation of sleep tendency in elderly and young adult subjects. *Sleep* 5:S82–92, 1982.

39. Czeisler CA, Zimmerman JC, Ronda JH, et al: Timing of REM sleep is coupled to the circadian rhythm of body temperature in man. *Sleep* 2:328–346, 1980.

40. Akerstedt T: Sleepiness as a consequence of shift work. *Sleep* 11:17–34, 1988.

41. Nicholson AN, Pascoe PA, Spencer MB, et al: Nocturnal sleep and daytime alertness of aircrew after transamerican flights. *Aviat Space Environ Med* 57(suppl 12):B43–52, 1986.

42. Roth T, Roehrs T: Determinants of residual effects of hypnotics. *Accid Anal Prev* 17:291–296, 1985.

43. Nicholson AN, Stone BM: Antihistamines: Impaired performance and the tendency to sleep. *Euro J Clin Pharmacol* 30:27–32, 1986.

44. Lumley M, Roehrs T, Asker D, et al: Ethanol and caffeine effects on daytime sleepiness/alertness. *Sleep* 10:306–312, 1987.

45. Coleman RM: Diagnosis, treatment and follow-up of about 8000 sleep/wake disorder patients, in Guilleminault C, Lugaresi E (eds): *Sleep/Wake Disorders: Natural History, Epidemiology and Long-Term Evolution.* New York, Raven, 1983, pp 87–97.

46. McGhie A, Russell SM: The subjective assessment of normal sleep patterns. *J Ment Sci* 8:642–654, 1962.

47. Partinen M: Sleeping habits and sleep disorders of Finnish men before, during and after military service. *Ann Med Milit Fenn* 57(suppl 1):96, 1982.

48. Lugaresi E, Cirignotta F, Zucconi M, et al: Good and poor sleepers: An epidemiological survey of the San Marino population, in Guilleminault C, Lugaresi E (eds), *Sleep/Wake Disorders: Natural History, Epidemiology and Long-Term Evolution.* New York, Raven, 1983, pp 1–12.

49. Billiard M, Alperovitch A, Perot C, et al: Excessive daytime somnolence in young men: Prevalence and contributing factors. *Sleep* 10:297–305, 1987.

PART FOURTEEN

SURGICAL ASPECTS OF PULMONARY MEDICINE

CHAPTER 104

PERIOPERATIVE CARE OF THE PATIENT UNDERGOING LUNG RESECTION

Robert J. Downey

Patients undergoing lung resection usually present with reduced pulmonary capacity, which is worsened by the surgical procedure. During the perioperative period, many factors, almost all of them iatrogenic, conspire to create pulmonary complications. Estimates of the overall surgical mortality for pulmonary resection range in large series from 2 to 4 percent.[11,17] The estimated mortality increases with the size of the resection—from less than 1 percent for a wedge resection, to 2 to 3 percent for a lobectomy, and to 6 to 8 percent for a pneumonectomy.

As may be expected from the estimated surgical mortality for lung resection, the morbidity associated with these operations is also high: complications are estimated to occur in 36 to 75 percent of patients undergoing pneumonectomy and 41 to 50 percent after lobectomy. The major causes of complications and death after pulmonary procedures include respiratory failure and pneumonia, myocardial infarction and arrhythmias, bronchopleural fistula and empyema, and pulmonary embolus.

This review deals with the following: (1) the assessment of preoperative and predicted postoperative lung function, (2) the factors that combine to reduce cardiopulmonary capacity during the perioperative period, (3) the routine postoperative management of the patient undergoing lung resection, and (4) the potential complications, some common and some rare, that may be encountered.

PREOPERATIVE ASSESSMENT AND OPTIMIZATION

Lung Function

Assessment of the ability of a patient to undergo a planned resection of the lung begins at the first encounter with the patient. Probably the most important, but least tangible, factor is a patient's willingness to undergo the sheer hard work of recuperation from a thoracic surgical procedure. A study performed by the Lung Cancer Study Group[42] suggested that the patient's attitude toward his or her malignancy was the best indicator of long-term survival. A patient who appears to be unwilling to participate in his recovery should be allowed ample opportunity to explore reasonable alternative therapies, such as radiation.

An extraordinary range of preoperative pulmonary function tests have been investigated in an attempt to delineate the risk to any one patient.[3,13,31] Unfortunately, preoperative tests presage only a small percentage of postoperative complications, and most complications appear to be random events visited on the patient and surgeon. In a study of 476 patients operated on over 12 years, only three of seven preoperative risk factors for morbidity and mortality were found to have a significant association with mortality; these were age over 60 years, pneumonectomy, and the presence of ventricular premature contractions on the preoperative electrocardiogram.[23] All risk factors analyzed together accounted for only 12 percent of the risk of mortality. The surgeon's impression of surgical risk, a skill honed over time, remains the most useful tool for selecting patients for resectional surgery.

At the time of initial visit, an attempt to establish the amount and character of sputum production, the presence or absence of an effective cough, and a patient's ability to climb a flight of stairs of fixed height[5,34] often provide a clear picture of the ability of a patient to undergo surgery. Patients with preoperative arterial hypercapnia are apt to have pulmonary hypertension and are poor candidates for pneumonectomy, but they may be able to tolerate a lobectomy. Pulmonary function tests, in particular the FEV_1, in combination with lobar perfusion scans, allow prediction of postresectional FEV_1 to within approximately 100 ml (Fig. 104-1). A postresectional FEV_1 less than 40 percent of predicted or less than 800 ml is cause for concern. A study of the DL_{CO} in 165 patients who underwent lung resection identified it as the most important indicator of postoperative pulmonary complications or death.[13] Another study focused on the maximal oxygen consumption (MVO_2): an MVO_2 of 20 ml/kg/min was associated with fewest complications, whereas an MVO_2 under 15 ml/kg/min was associated with 75 percent of the postoperative morbidity.

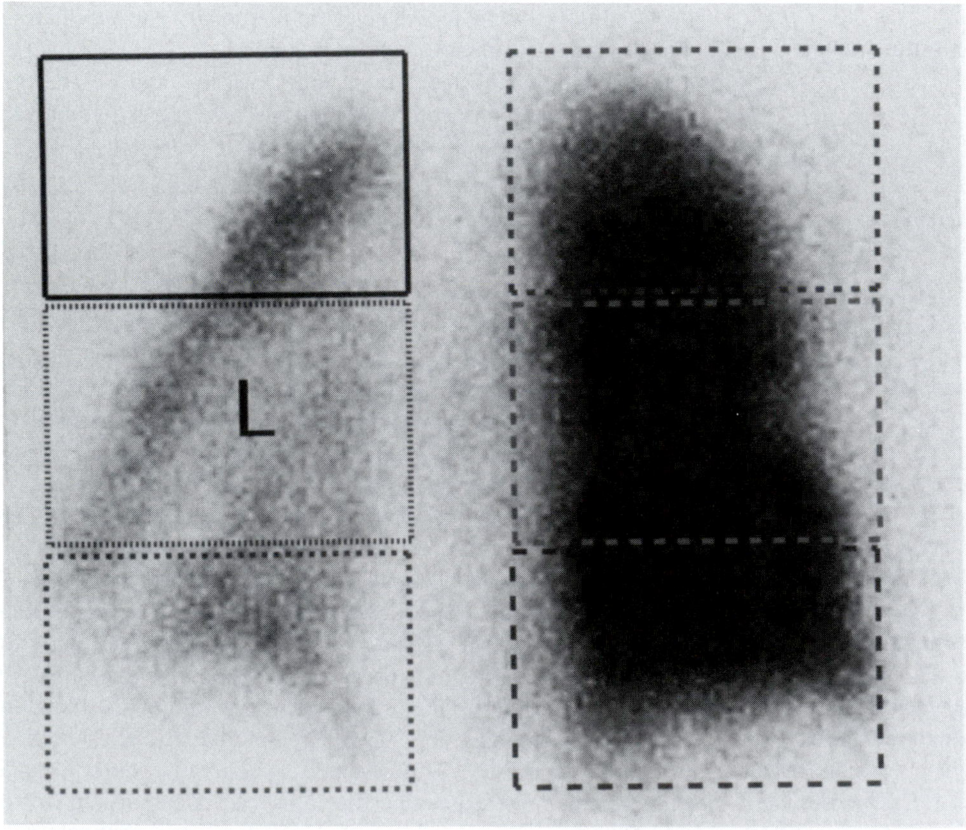

Optimization of Preoperative Pulmonary Function

Essentially all patients presenting for resection of lung malignancies have some degree of chronic airflow obstruction. A variety of medical therapies are designed to improve pulmonary function.[31,45] Optimization of pulmonary function begins with smoking cessation.[8,16] Even a short period of abstinence from cigarettes can improve the effectiveness of mucociliary transport.[15] Heavy smokers also maintain levels of carboxyhemoglobin that interfere with oxygen transport and delivery to peripheral tissues.[21] However, the optimal time after smoking cessation for repair of the airway to be undertaken is unclear. Studies of patients undergoing abdominal surgery and coronary artery bypass surgery suggest that 8 weeks of abstinence is necessary to achieve a significant decrease in pulmonary complications.[19,53]

In patients with evidence of reversible airway obstruction on pulmonary function tests, or with episodes of symptoms suggestive of airflow obstruction, nebulized albuterol appears to be of benefit. Mucostasis, if present, may warrant the addition of mucolytics such as *N*-acetylcysteine, with due regard to the possible side effect of bronchoconstriction. Methylxanthines are added only for refractory cases. Similarly, although the condition of patients with reversible airflow obstruction generally improves with steroids, prednisone or other corticosteroids should be added reluctantly, because of their effects on wound healing and rate of infection. If steroids are deemed necessary, the dosage in the postoperative period should be as low as possible. Patients who produce purulent sputum should be treated with oral antibiotics directed at the organism identified.

PERIOPERATIVE FACTORS REDUCING LUNG FUNCTION

Despite the varieties of pathology that are encountered and the procedures performed on a thoracic surgical service, the course of postoperative recovery often follows a fairly predictable trajectory. After the thoracic surgical procedure, there is a period of recovery marked by reduced activity and recumbency. Recognition of the unfavorable effects of prolonged inactivity has prompted a shift to rapid remobilization, particularly in the early postoperative period. However, almost all hospitalized patients undergo a period of reduced activity. Therefore, the physiological consequences of decreased activity and lack of changes in posture form a background for the pathophysiological processes caused by the underlying illness and the surgical procedure.

FIGURE 104-1 Quantitative perfusion lung scan showing the majority of the pulmonary blood flow going to the right lung.

Bed Rest and Respiratory Function

In normal adults, mismatches between alveolar ventilation and blood flow are small. In bed-ridden postoperative patients, however, ventilation and perfusion are badly matched.

The zones of the upright lung are considered in Chapter 12.[27,55] Placing a normal patient in a recumbent position leads to changes in all lung volumes except the tidal volume. In a normal person, a change from upright to supine position decreases the vital capacity by 2 percent, total lung capacity by 7 percent, closing volume by 10 percent, residual volume by 19 percent, expiratory reserve volume by 46 percent, and functional residual capacity (FRC) by 30 percent.[10] The decrements in volume that accompany changes to other than the supine position are small. In normal subjects, the FRC decreases by only 17 percent after a move from the upright to the lateral decubitus position.[30] The closing volume has been shown to be relatively independent of posture. However, the FRC decreases by about 20 percent in the supine position—an amount that may be sufficient to cause the closing volume to exceed the end-tidal volume, thereby resulting in closure of basilar alveoli. These alveoli remain closed for the initial portions of the next inhalation, while the ventilation is shunted to the open apical alveoli.

It is interesting that these changes might be *less* in patients with chronic pulmonary disease. Thus, in patients with chronic airflow obstruction, a decrease in FRC of only 3.5 percent accompanied a move from upright to supine position and a decrease of only 1.9 percent accompanied the move from the supine to the lateral decubitus position.[30] Finally, although arterial oxygen saturation decreased significantly in supine normal subjects, it did not do so in patients with significant airflow obstruction.

The degree to which changes described above affect gas exchange has been only partly studied. In normal young males after 10 days of bed rest, Pa_{O_2} decreased by 9 mmHg and the alveolar-arterial difference in P_{O_2} by 10 mmHg, without change in Pa_{CO_2}.[7] Such changes, which would probably not be important in normal young people, might take on greater significance in a patient with chronic obstructive pulmonary disease (COPD).

Bed Rest and Cardiac Function

Upon standing, approximately 500 ml of blood shifts from the upper to the lower body. Upon assumption of the supine position, central venous return increases, resulting in a decrease in heart rate, peripheral vasodilatation, increased renal blood flow, and diuresis. Within an average of 24 h, the diuresis causes a 5 percent decrease in plasma volume, which continues to fall by 10 percent in 6 days and 20 percent in 14 days.[20]

A wide variety of experimental subjects and protocols have been used to examine the cardiovascular effects of prolonged immobilization.[12] Orthostatic intolerance is common after prolonged bed rest. This is attributable, at least in part, to the depletion in intravascular volume noted above, possibly compounded by an increase in venous pooling in the lower extremities because of an increase in venous compliance after bed rest. Prolonged recumbency also blunts cardiac responsiveness to rapid changes in posture. Bed rest increases the resting heart rate by 4 to 15 beats a minute; after bed rest, the increase in heart rate during exercise is more pronounced. For example, normal volunteers experienced an increase in heart rate to approximately 129 beats a minute during submaximal exercise; after bed rest, the same exercise drove the heart rate to approximately 165 beats a minute.[49]

Alterations in Lung Function Secondary to Surgery

Superimposed on the physiological substrate of inactivity and recumbency described above, the thoracic surgery patient experiences major alterations in chest wall compliance and discomfort, which lead to an increased work of breathing that is independent of the amount of resected lung.[43] Manipulation of the lung leads to "bruising"; reexpansion of a lung that has been collapsed for surgery is imperfect, so microscopic or even macroscopic areas of atelectasis persist. Fluid or blood clots in the pleural cavity may compress the lung parenchyma. Inhalational anesthesia depresses mucociliary transport.[15] Mechanical changes alter the work of breathing. Thoracotomy alone was found to decrease chest wall compliance to 47 percent of preoperative levels and to increase work of breathing to 143 percent of preoperative levels.[36] As a result, vital capacity and oxygen saturation fall significantly in the first few postoperative days.[4,46] Pain, among other factors, leads to diminished cough. Cough pressures were found to decrease to 29 percent of preoperative levels after surgery and to increase only to 50 percent of preoperative levels by the seventh postoperative day.[6]

ROUTINE POSTOPERATIVE CARE OF THE PATIENT UNDERGOING LUNG RESECTION

Extubation and Postoperative Supplemental Oxygen

Almost every patient undergoing lung resection at the Memorial Sloan-Kettering Cancer Center is able to be extubated in the operating room and is brought to the postanesthesia care unit breathing spontaneously. Reintubation in the immediate postoperative period is rare. If prolonged intubation is anticipated, however, the double-lumen endotracheal tube is replaced by a single-lumen endotracheal tube of sufficient size to permit introduction of an adult bronchoscope. For extubation, standard criteria are followed: vital capacity more than 10 ml/kg, respiratory rate less than 30 breaths per minute, and normal arterial blood gases.

Supplemental oxygen is supplied in the postoperative period if the patient's arterial oxygen saturation, measured by pulse oximetry, is less than 92 percent, either at rest or during exercise. The routine administration of increased concentrations of oxygen may be counterproductive, since each appliance attached to the patient hinders incrementally the patient's mobility.

Pain Control

The patient with reduced pulmonary reserve can ill afford the additional burden of a painful chest wall, which limits ambulation and cough. Following thoracotomy, all patients should receive either epidural administration of a local anesthetic or a narcotic or patient-controlled intravenous analgesia, using either morphine or Demerol. The complications associated with epidural opiates are numerous and include pruritus, ileus, urinary retention, and respiratory depression. Epidural analgesia does improve pulmonary function in the postthoracotomy patient and, despite concerns about complications, should not be withheld from the patient in whom pulmonary function is markedly impaired. Most of patients appear to tolerate postthoracotomy pain well with the use of a patient-controlled anesthesia alone, particularly if a short course of oral ketorolac is used as an adjunct. In the late postoperative period, oral medications, such as Percocet, are usually sufficient.

Antibiotics

Wound infection following thoracotomy is rare. However, infectious complications, such as empyema and pneumonia, are not uncommon following lung resection, and prophylactic antibiotics are often given in an attempt to reduce the incidence of these complications.[48] Currently, it is recommended that a broad-spectrum antibiotic, such as cefazolin, be administered within 1 h of the skin incision, and continued for 24 to 48 h. Subsequent antibiotic administration should be based on clinical factors such as fever, radiographic infiltrates, leukocytosis, and sputum Gram's stain and culture results. There is no need to provide antibiotic coverage simply because a chest tube is in place.

A study that examined the relationship between pulmonary flora and postoperative infections found that *Hemophilus influenzae* was the most common organism identified from sputum at the time of surgery and that the risk of pneumonia in culture-positive patients was 10-fold that of patients with culture-negative secretions.[52] However, the cultured organisms were sensitive to the antibiotic that was administered, suggesting that the administration of antibiotics may be less important than careful pulmonary toilet in preventing postoperative pneumonia.

Fluids, Electrolytes, and Oral Intake

A routine lung resection is not associated with large fluid losses intraoperatively or sequestration of volume in the third space postoperatively. Most patients should leave the operating room relatively euvolemic. Administration of intravenous fluids consisting of 5% dextrose and 0.45% normal saline at 50 to 75 ml/h until the patient begins to take oral fluids is usually adequate to maintain intravascular fluid volume. Oral intake should be resumed as soon as the patient is able to take fluids by mouth. Urine output should be maintained at 0.5 to 1 ml/kg of body weight an hour in order to preserve renal function. Some surgeons practice aggressive diuresis with the goal of reducing secretions. However, it is not clear that a lower volume of thick, tenacious secretions is preferable to a higher volume of thin secretions that are more readily cleared. Ideally, diuresis would be guided by measurements of intravascular volume. Measurements of central venous pressure correlate poorly with intravascular volume, though, and many surgeons are reluctant to insert

Swan-Ganz catheters into patients after lung resection, particularly after pneumonectomy, because of the possibility of disruption of a pulmonary artery closure. Even if a Swan-Ganz balloon-tipped catheter has been safely introduced into a patient postoperatively, the data should be interpreted with caution, because the inflated balloon may have occluded a significant portion of the remaining pulmonary vascular bed, thereby artificially increasing right ventricular afterload and decreasing cardiac output.

Blood transfusion is not necessary unless the hematocrit is less than 24 percent or if bleeding should continue. Transfusion of 250 ml of packed red blood cells increases the intravascular volume by 750 to 1000 ml, because of the movement of extravascular volume into the intravascular space due to plasma oncotic forces. The increase in intravascular volume may be more dangerous than a low hematocrit. Furthermore, the intraoperative administration of blood is probably immunosuppressive and may be associated with a decrease in frequency of 5-year disease-free intervals.[18]

Chest Tube Management

Chest tube placement is routine after thoracotomy to enable drainage of blood, serum, and air from the pleural space. After a wedge excision, usually only one apical chest tube is required. However, two apical tubes are preferable for an upper lobectomy and one apical and one basilar tube for a lower lobectomy. Chest tubes are connected to suction for the first night after surgery and then to water seal. Daily chest radiographs are performed to ensure that effective removal of air and fluid is being achieved. If increased air in the pleural space is seen after a tube has been connected to water seal, suction drainage should be reestablished, usually for 36 h, before another attempt at water seal drainage is attempted. Daily management should include "stripping" the tubes in the attempt to remove clots, examination of all connections to ensure their integrity, and maintaining appropriate water levels in all drainage bottles.

Postpneumonectomy space drainage is managed differently from postlobectomy drainage. After pneumonectomy, the position of the mediastinum is a major concern. Shift of the mediastinal structures either into the pneumonectomy cavity or toward the residual lung can lead to either hemodynamic or respiratory compromise. To allow "balancing" of the mediastinum after a pneumonectomy, most surgeons leave a single chest tube in the pleural cavity (Fig. 104-2). This tube can be removed in the operating room after the patient has been returned to the supine position and is hemodynamically stable. Alternatively, the tube can be removed in the recovery room or on the nursing unit once it is clear that the patient is not bleeding. If the mediastinum is shifted significantly after the chest tube is removed, air can be aspirated from, or introduced into, the pneumonectomy cavity by a needle inserted through an intercostal space. This is only rarely necessary, but occasionally it can relieve respiratory distress or an unexplained tachycardia. Potential complications include bleeding and contamination of the pneumonectomy space.

For resections other than pneumonectomy, chest tubes are removed when there is no air leak and fluid output has decreased

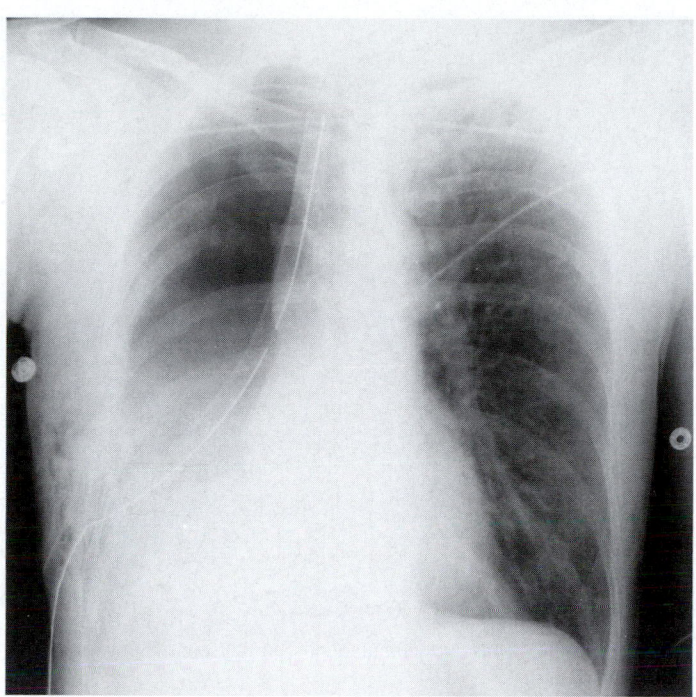

FIGURE 104-2   Chest radiograph taken in the early postoperative period following right pneumonectomy with a chest tube draining the pneumonectomy space. Note the midline position of the mediastinum.

to less than 200 ml a day. Removal is performed while the patient performs a Valsalva maneuver; an occlusive dressing is maintained over the site for 36 h. Patients should be advised that it is not uncommon to have additional drainage after lysis of intrathoracic blood clots has occurred; this drainage is thin, pink, and self-limited and occurs on approximately the seventh to tenth postoperative day.

Excessive chest tube output in the first 24 h after surgery is worrisome as a sign of persistent intrathoracic bleeding. In patients without a bleeding disorder, losses in excess of 200 ml per hour that continue for more than 4 to 6 h require surgical reexploration. Confirmation that the drainage is blood can be obtained by hematocrit quantification on a small sample drawn directly from the chest tube.

Excessive drainage that persists for several days after surgery suggests the possibility of injury to the thoracic duct or other major lymph channel. When such an injury has occurred, the drainage is clear and the volume may decrease initially. As the patient resumes a normal diet, however, the volume increases and the character of the liquid changes from serosanguineous to creamy. Often, the diagnosis is apparent from only an examination of the pleural drainage containers. That the fluid is lymph is confirmed by performing a cell count on the liquid and demonstrating a markedly elevated lymphocyte count without a commensurate number of red blood cells.

Following chemical confirmation that the liquid is chyle, the initial management of a thoracic duct injury is to deny the patient food by mouth and to provide total parenteral nutrition. If drainage decreases in response to this management, the patient should receive a high-fat meal before the chest tube is removed in order to confirm that the leak has closed. If drainage remains

greater than 500 ml a day for 5 to 7 days, surgical reexploration is indicated to ligate the thoracic duct.

COMPLICATIONS AFTER LUNG RESECTION

Atelectasis and Pneumonia

Atelectasis, with or without superimposed pneumonia, is the most common postoperative complication following thoracic surgery (Fig. 104-3). As previously mentioned, risk factors for the development of atelectasis include advanced age, obesity, and the continued use of tobacco.

Routine measures directed toward the minimization of postoperative atelectasis should be initiated early in the preoperative period and include education, smoking cessation, and the use of incentive spirometry. Postoperatively, the most important measures are deep-breathing techniques, incentive spirometry, early ambulation, and bronchoscopy as needed to relieve retention of secretions.

The mainstays in the prevention of atelectasis are deep inspiratory respiratory maneuvers performed either with or without an incentive spirometer. Carefully supervised programs of these maneuvers have been shown to reduce the incidence of atelectasis after laparotomy.

Chest physical therapy, although widely practiced, is of unclear benefit, is often poorly administered, and imposes a considerable physiological load on the already compromised patient. Its use should be reserved for the patient with obstructive atelectasis secondary to mucous impaction in a major airway. Chest physical therapy increases oxygen consumption and carbon diox-

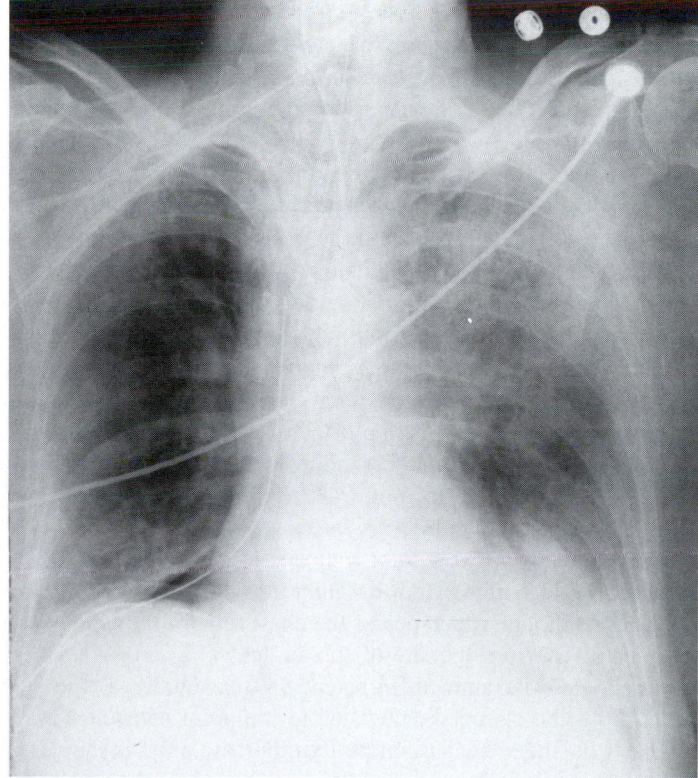

FIGURE 104-3   Left upper-lobe infiltrate following a right-sided pulmonary resection.

ide production to approximately 40 percent above resting values.[54] Of interesting is that the decrease in arterial oxygen levels was less in patients with preoperative arterial hypoxemia, so that with careful monitoring, chest physical therapy, if indicated, should not be withheld from marginal patients.[38] For many patients with major obstruction of the airway, bronchoscopy is a preferred alternative. With current noninvasive blood pressure monitoring and pulse oximetry, bronchoscopy can be performed routinely at the bedside with excellent results. Tracheal suctioning can cause appreciable arterial hypoxemia, is uncomfortable, and is performed blindly without the ability to direct the catheter to specific regions of the airway. For these reasons, tracheal suctioning has largely been supplanted by bronchoscopy.

Air Leaks and Subcutaneous Emphysema

Division of the lung parenchyma always leads to macroscopic or microscopic "bleeding" of air from the cut lung surface. Usually, these leaks seal within a few days after surgery, either as the result of adherence of the lung to the parietal pleura or by deposition of proteinaceous fluid on the lung surface. Occasionally, air leaks persist. Different clinics define a "prolonged leak" differently but usually in terms of 7 to 10 days. It is important that the chest tube drainage system be examined daily to ensure that it is an actual air leak and not a loose connection that allows air to enter the system. The simplest way to establish that a leak is from within the thorax is to temporarily clamp the chest tube at the skin surface: if the leak persists while the clamp occludes the tube, the leak is "from the system" and all connections should be secured.

Surgical reexploration for small leaks is rarely indicated, since manipulation of the lung in a search for leaks may create as many leaks as are closed. Instead, the patient should be advised that most small leaks will eventually close without surgical intervention, even if he or she has to be sent home with a chest tube in place with a one-way Heimlich valve attached. Unfortunately, the continued passage of air from the lung through the pleural space probably increases the incidence of empyema. However, most of these infections respond to drainage and antibiotics.

Large air leaks in the immediate postoperative period are most worrisome as a possible sign of inadequate closure or disruption of a bronchus. Bronchoscopy should be done urgently to clarify whether the bronchial stump is indeed intact. If disruption is found, surgical reexploration with closure of the stump, reinforcement with a pedicled flap of pericardium, intercostal muscle, omentum, or other material, and wide drainage of the pleural cavity should be performed in order to minimize the chances of ongoing pleural infection.

Occasionally, massive subcutaneous emphysema may occur if either the loss of air from the lung into the pleural cavity exceeds the drainage capacities of the chest tube or the tube is positioned away from the site of the air leak (Fig. 104-4). Chest tubes should be examined for patency. Occasionally, a tube will be found to be clamped or twisted to the point of occlusion. If a tube is occluded because of an intrathoracic plug, it should be stripped; if this fails to reestablish patency, the tube should be opened and suctioned, using sterile technique, with a nasotracheal suction catheter. Some surgeons irrigate an occluded tube

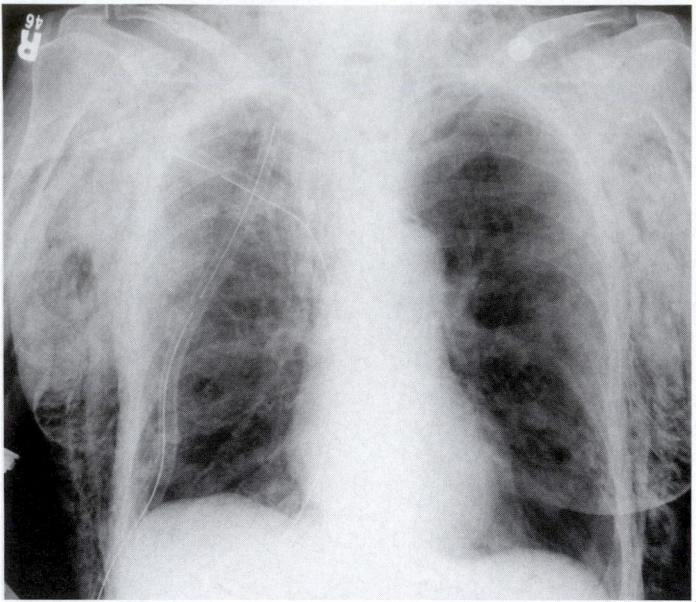

FIGURE 104-4　Massive subcutaneous emphysema following a pulmonary resection.

with sterile saline, but because of the possibility of infectious contamination, it is unclear whether this technique is advisable. If all methods fail to reestablish patency of a chest tube, the tube should be removed and a new one inserted.

Although uncomfortable and disfiguring, massive subcutaneous emphysema is rarely life-threatening. However, two dangerous situations can arise. First, in patients with tracheostomies, the tube can be displaced into the subcutaneous tissues if the skin is elevated up and away from the tracheal opening. Second, circumferential massive lifting of the skin around the thorax can lead to restriction of normal outward excursions of the rib cage excursion, limiting tidal volume—as in the case of limitation imposed by circumferential eschar in a burn patient. Such emergency situations may require the placement of small skin incisions, usually in an infraclavicular location.

Supraventricular Tachycardias

For many years, it has been appreciated that thoracotomy is commonly associated with the postoperative development of supraventricular arrhythmias.[29] Recent studies suggest that supraventricular tachycardias occur in 17 to 20 percent of all patients undergoing lobectomy or pneumonectomy.[50] The development of supraventricular arrhythmias after pneumonectomy is a marker for perioperative morbidity and mortality. Indeed, in one study, of 236 pneumonectomy patients, 25 percent of patients developing atrial fibrillation died within 30 days.[25] The cause of the dysrhythmias is almost certainly multifactorial; suggested factors include intrapericardial resection, hypoxemia, hyperadrenergic tone, and atrial distention.

Digitalis has been proposed as a prophylactic measure against the development of dysrhythmias. However, the potential toxicities of this drug are well known, and it is not clear that the risks outweigh the benefits. Conflicting results have been reported with the prophylactic use of verapamil after thoracotomy.[29] Preliminary data from a recent trial compared the routine postoperative administration of digoxin with diltiazem after pneumonectomy for the prevention of supraventricular arrhythmias. The incidence of supraventricular arrhythmias was 29 percent in the digitalized group, 21 percent in the untreated historical controls, and 0 percent in the diltiazem-treated group.[1] Despite these trials, it is not clear that reduction in the occurrence of arrhythmias will translate into overall improved outcomes, since the arrhythmia may simply be a marker of greater underlying physiological disarray rather than a cause of morbidity in itself. If supraventricular arrhythmias arise in the postoperative period, the preferred method of treatment is the use of adenosine, verapamil, or digoxin to control the rate and to relieve symptoms in accord with standard cardiologic practice.

Right Ventricular Failure

In the patient with normal pulmonary vasculature, pneumonectomy is remarkably well tolerated. Despite removal of one-half of the pulmonary vascular bed, the remaining pulmonary vasculature is sufficiently compliant to accommodate the entire cardiac output without the development of either pulmonary edema or right ventricular overload. In the patient with COPD, pulmonary hypertension often develops, but it is usually mild, with mean pulmonary artery pressures of around 20 to 35 mmHg and a normal cardiac output. Although the end-diastolic filling pressure of the right ventricle is generally normal at rest in the patient with COPD, he or she is apt to manifest inability to increase cardiac output during exercise.[33]

It is possible that some patients with postoperative complications after lung resection experience an acute exacerbation of pulmonary arterial hypertension that leads to right ventricular failure and a decrease in cardiac output. Several reports bear on this possibility. One study, based on the use of thermodilution catheters, found that the right ventricular end-diastolic volume increased from 153 to 177 ml, and that the right ventricular ejection fraction decreased from 45 to 36 percent in the first few postoperative days.[39] Another, using echocardiography, found that patients who developed supraventricular arrhythmias after lung resection had a significant increase in the velocity of the tricuspid regurgitant jet, whereas those who underwent lung resection without arrhythmias did not.[2] A third study of patients undergoing pneumonectomy was unable to find any hemodynamic variable or pulmonary function test that augured early morbidity.[38] It did, however, indicate that a right ventricular ejection fraction of less than 35 percent, pulmonary vascular resistance greater than 200 dyne · s/cm^5, and a pulmonary vascular resistance/right ventricular ejection fraction ratio equal to or greater than 5.0 indicated long-term cardiopulmonary disability. No studies have been reported of patients suffering severe complications, such as pneumonia, in the remaining lung after pneumonectomy to determine whether right ventricular failure is a component of the cardiopulmonary dysfunction.

A better understanding of the alterations in right ventricular function might lead to modification in patient management.[28] For example, the anesthetic technique might be altered. In a recent study concerning ventilation of one lung, the administration of propofol was associated with sustained decrease in right ventricular ejection fraction and mean cardiac output as compared with the administration of isoflurane.[22] The use of proper anesthetic agents might minimize the additive effects of hypoxic pulmonary vasoconstriction and surgical resection of the pulmonary vascular bed. In principle, numerous therapies are available to lessen the burden on the right ventricle in the postoperative period. Among the agents proposed are nitric oxide,[41] adenosine,[14] calcium channel blockers,[32] dopamine,[9] and mechanical devices.[47] However, none of these has yet been put to the test.

Postpneumonectomy Pulmonary Edema

Postpneumonectomy pulmonary edema is a rare but lethal complication of pneumonectomy.[57] For several reasons, the patient who has undergone pneumonectomy is thought to be at increased risk of pulmonary edema. First, although the removal of one lung is well tolerated if the pulmonary vasculature is normal, if preexisting pulmonary vascular disease is present, the reduced pulmonary vascular bed may be unable to accommodate the cardiac output without an inordinate increase in pulmonary arterial pressure. Second, disruption of lymphatics associated with mediastinal lymph node dissection may interfere significantly with the clearance of fluid from the lung. In the presence of these two predisposing factors, overzealous administration of fluid may lead to the formation of lethal pulmonary edema.

The clinical presentation of postpneumonectomy pulmonary edema is that of a relatively uneventful initial 24- to 48-h postoperative period, followed by a relentlessly increasing need for respiratory support, usually culminating in death within 24 to 48 h. The pulmonary edema progresses despite aggressive efforts to effect a diuresis and other supportive measures (Fig. 104-5). Current therapy is directed at limiting the administration of fluids perioperatively and providing supportive measures if the complication should arise.

Empyema/Bronchopleural Fistulas

Empyema is a rare complication after pulmonary resection and can usually be managed with continued pleural drainage. If empyema occurs later in the postoperative period (3 to more than 6 weeks), surgical intervention may be required to decorticate the lung in order to allow it to fill the pleural space or to drain a fixed space. Disruption of a bronchial closure after lung resection occurs in less than 5 percent of patients.[51] Although dehiscence of a lobar bronchus occurs occasionally after lobectomy, it rarely presents a challenge in management. Usually, chest tube drainage and antibiotics are all that is necessary; rarely is further surgical intervention required. Seldom, if ever, is there need to reclose a bronchus unless a technical problem becomes evident in the early postoperative period. Dehiscence of the bronchial stump following a bilobectomy may require complete pneumonectomy.

Infection in a postpneumonectomy space presents far greater challenges in management.[44] Infections may occur with or without a bronchopleural fistula, but in either case, early management is the same. The typical patient with an infected pneumonectomy space usually returns for the first postoperative visit complaining of poor appetite, fatigue, low-grade fevers, and continued weight loss. If there is no communication with the

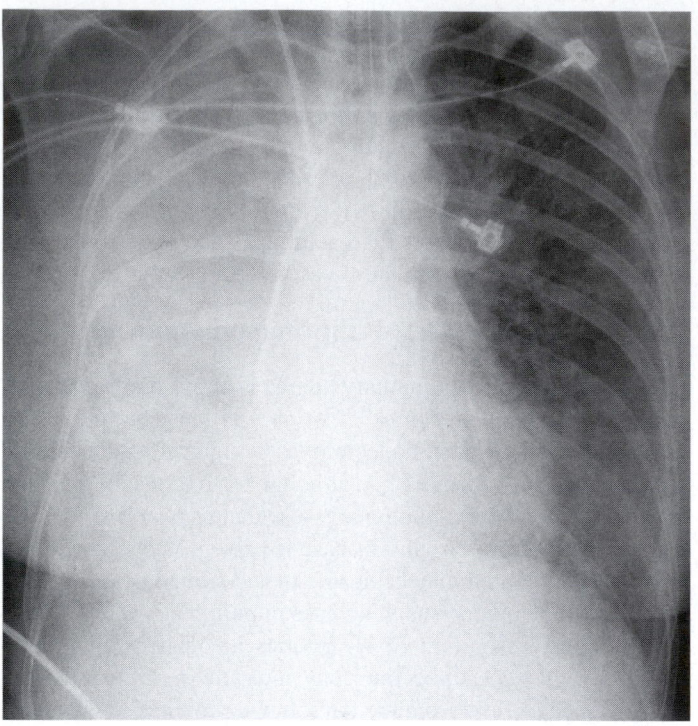

FIGURE 104-5 Postpneumonectomy pulmonary edema with onset 48 h after extrapleural pneumonectomy. There is a diffuse interstitial infiltrate present that was heralded by the insidious development of hypoxemia in this otherwise healthy 60-year-old woman.

bronchus, no significant amount of sputum will be produced and the space may be filled as expected. The fluid in the space should be sampled under sterile conditions and sent for Gram's stain and culture. The patient with a bronchial stump dehiscence may complain of production of watery brown sputum, and the chest radiograph demonstrates a decrease in the fluid level as compared with the level seen on the radiograph at the time of discharge from the hospital. Both situations require drainage of the pneumonectomy space by means of a chest tube initially, followed by an open-window thoracostomy that entails resection of segments of rib in the most dependent area of the space and sewing the skin edges to the thickened pleural edges (Fig. 104-6). The window needs to be large and correctly positioned in the most dependent portion of the space in order to effect unobstructed drainage.

Rarely is it necessary or advisable to attempt to close a disrupted bronchial stump unless a complication, indicating a technical problem, occurs in the early postoperative period (within the first 7 days). With an early stump breakdown, operation is indicated to resuture the bronchus and to buttress the closure with a muscle flap. Most bronchial stump disruptions occur late, as described above, and the leak itself is a secondary problem best dealt with by an open drainage procedure. Most of the bronchial leaks are small and can be assessed by bronchoscopy performed at the time of the open-window thoracostomy. These leaks usually close gradually after the establishment of effective drainage of the infected space. Occasionally, complete bronchial stump dehiscence may occur, resulting in the loss of a considerable amount of expired air, so that speech is difficult.

Once the open-window thoracostomy is created, most patients begin to gain weight and regain strength. Over time, the open window begins to close as the space contracts. There is no hurry to close an open-window thoracostomy, and many patients adjust well to its presence. Minimal care is required; a dry dressing, changed once or twice daily, is worn over the opening. The wound is not packed. After several months, depending on the patient's overall status, the window may be closed, usually by the transposition of a muscle flap to obliterate the remaining space.[35] A small residual air leak is not a contraindication to closing the window with a transposed muscle flap. Either the latissimus dorsi or serratus anterior muscle may be used, depending on which was divided at the initial thoracotomy. The pectoralis major muscle may also be used. These procedures often are done in collaboration with a plastic surgeon.

Subarachnoid–Pleural Fistulas

Subarachnoid–pleural fistulas are unusual. They occur most often after trauma but may also complicate thoracic surgical procedures if dissection in the costovertebral angle or excessive trac-

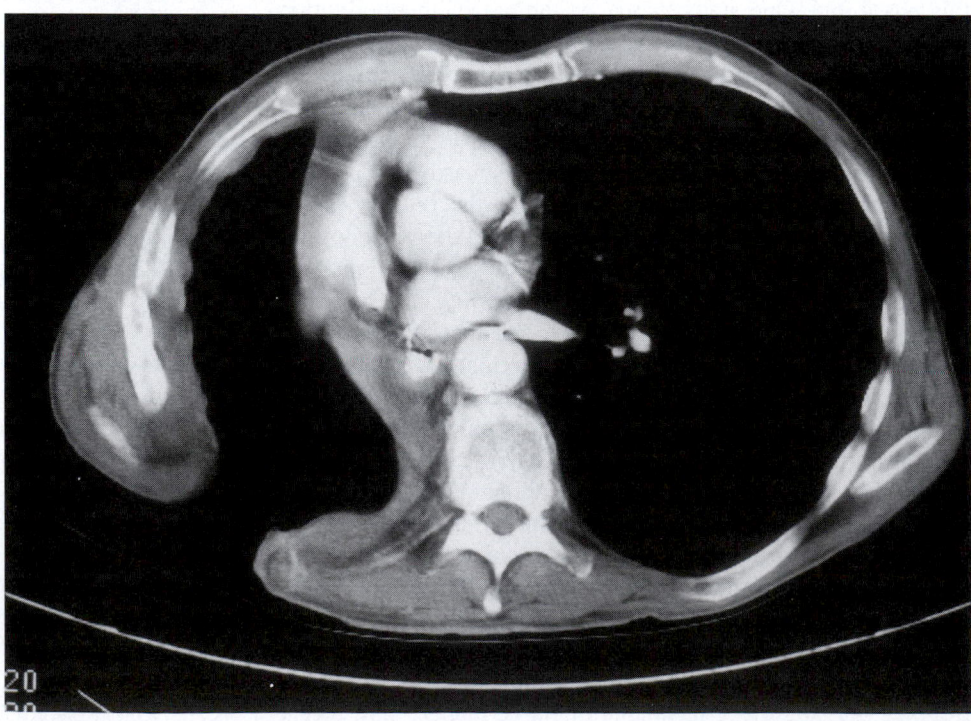

FIGURE 104-6 An open-window thoracostomy seen on CT scan. The window needs to be large and in the most dependent location.

tion avulses a thoracic nerve root from its dural sleeve.[37] The most common setting for this to occur is during resection of malignancies invading either the posterior chest wall or the vertebral column; however, retraction of the ribs for exposure during a standard posterolateral thoracotomy may generate sufficient traction to avulse a nerve root. The presence of a communication between the subarachnoid and pleural spaces allows for the bidirectional movement of cerebrospinal fluid and pleural fluid: during inspiration, low intrathoracic pressure sucks cerebrospinal fluid into the thorax; during expiration, elevated thoracic pressure forces air and potentially contaminated material into the subarachnoid space. A chest tube placed next to the fistulous tract may increase loss of cerebrospinal fluid. As a result, patients may develop headaches, meningismus, paresis, seizures, hemorrhagic infarcts, and obtundation leading to death. Cerebrospinal fluid analysis may be bizarre, owing to the entry of serosanguineous fluid into the subarachnoid space.

The diagnosis of a communication between the subarachnoid and pleural spaces is suggested by visualization of a pneumocephalus on skull radiographs. More specifically, the fistulous communication may be delineated by contrast CT myelography. The time between thoracotomy and the clinical diagnosis of the fistula ranges from 5 to 8 weeks. The unpredictable nature of the neurologic sequelae mandates that surgical closure of the dura be carried out as soon as the diagnosis is confirmed.

Postpneumonectomy Syndrome

Postpneumonectomy syndrome is a rare complication manifested by cough and dyspnea on exertion that usually follows right pneumonectomy. It is due to progressive mediastinal shift with compression of the left main-stem bronchus by the vertebral column. The underlying cause of this complication of pneumonectomy is herniation of the contralateral lung into the vacant pleural space, causing compression of the main-stem bronchus between the aorta, the pulmonary artery, or the vertebral column (Fig. 104-7). Repair is directed toward repositioning and stabilizing the mediastinum in the midline by a combined procedure of cardiopexy and placement of pliable, variable-volume tissue expanders into the empty pleural space.[40] Cardiopexy alone probably provides insufficient protection against recurrence. Before surgical repositioning, it can be difficult to assess whether significant tracheomalacia is present in the compressed segment. Persistent airway narrowing and symptoms of obstruction following correction of mediastinal shift may require placement of an airway stent or reoperation for resection of the affected bronchial segment.

Pulmonary Torsion

During a pulmonary resection, an extensive dissection is usually performed around the hilum for division of the pulmonary vessels. In addition, after an upper lobectomy, the inferior pulmonary ligament is divided to allow the lower lobe to rise within the pleural space to obliterate the residual apical space. Unfortunately, the increased mobility of these structures can, on rare occasions, lead to torsion of all or part of the residual lung, causing venous outflow obstruction and, possibly, pulmonary gan-

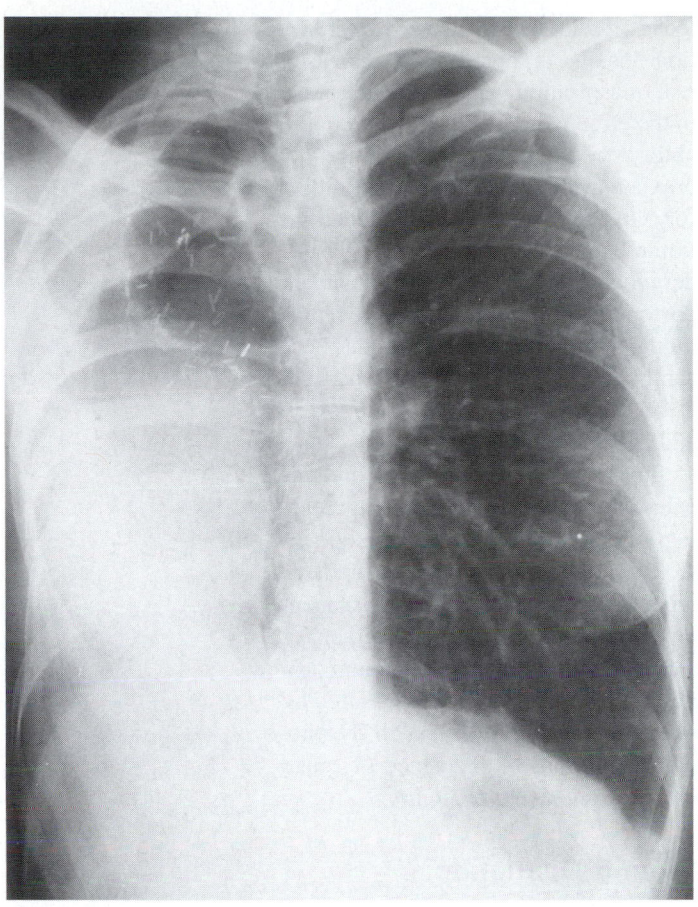

FIGURE 104-7 Marked shift of the mediastinum with hyperinflation of the left lung and tethering of the left main-stem bronchus over the vertebral column, characteristic of postpneumonectomy syndrome.

grene.[56] The middle lobe with complete fissures is at highest risk, although any portion of residual lung can be affected (Fig. 104-8).[26] In order to reduce the risk of middle-lobe torsion, sutures or staples are used to secure the middle lobe to the remaining lobe following right upper or lower lobectomy.

Pulmonary torsion may be suggested by the radiographic finding of consolidated lung, in association with fever, leukocytosis, and purulent, occasionally bloody sputum. Bronchoscopy may be helpful if a twisted bronchus can be demonstrated. The treatment is immediate surgical exploration with rerotation of the affected lung, followed by fixation to surrounding structures. If the lung is not viable, lobectomy or completion pneumonectomy may be required.

Recurrent Laryngeal Nerve Injury

In a patient with lung cancer, the recurrent laryngeal nerves are vulnerable to injury because of either direct invasion by malignancy or injury during surgical manipulation. The left vagus nerve is at greater risk than the right because of its course from the neck down into the left aspect of the mediastinum and across the aortic arch before giving off the left recurrent laryngeal nerve at the level of the inferior border of the aortic arch (Fig. 104-9). The nerve passes around the ligamentum arteriosum and "recurs" along the left tracheoesophageal groove. If either nerve is affected, unilateral vocal cord dysfunction results in hoarseness, increased risk of aspiration, and marked decrease in the effectiveness of cough and in the ability to clear secretions. A neuropraxia may resolve within weeks or last for 6 to 9 months. For the patient with limited pulmonary reserve who has undergone surgery, with its attendant postoperative transient decrease in pulmonary function, vocal cord paralysis can be a devastating problem and may mean the difference between recovery and respiratory failure.

Surgical correction of unilateral vocal cord paralysis is becoming increasingly popular.[24] Techniques include injection of Gelfoam for temporary medialization, Teflon for permanent medialization, or surgical placement of a hand-crafted silicone elastomer implant. The success rate, as measured by symptomatic improvement in dysphonia, aspiration, or incidence of pneumonia, exceeds 90 percent.

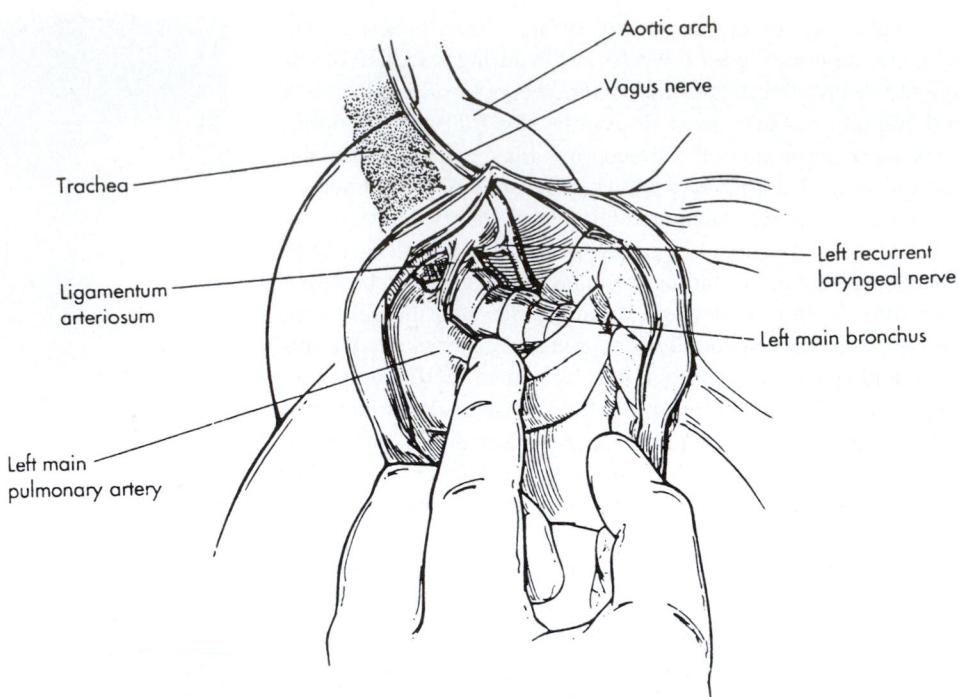

FIGURE 104-9   Location of the left recurrent laryngeal nerve as it takes its origin from the vagus nerve at the level of the aortic arch. Note its position relative to the ligamentum arteriosum.

Wound Disruption

Disruption of a posterolateral thoracotomy wound is a distinctly uncommon event. Limited areas of separation of the skin and, less commonly, of the underlying musculature are usually attributable to malnourishment that leads to poor wound healing and to bony prominences that place an excessive amount of pressure on one portion of the incision. Limited skin dehiscence responds to local wound care alone.

Disruption of the rib closure with intact overlying skin is a more serious problem, since it can lead to respiratory insufficiency—particularly in the early postoperative period, when the mediastinum is still mobile. Cough becomes ineffective, as expired air is forced out not through the vocal cords but into the extrapleural space. Effective ventilation may also be impaired to the point of hypoxia and hypercarbia. Chest wall dehiscence in the early postoperative period requires reexploration, debridement, and reclosure of the wound.

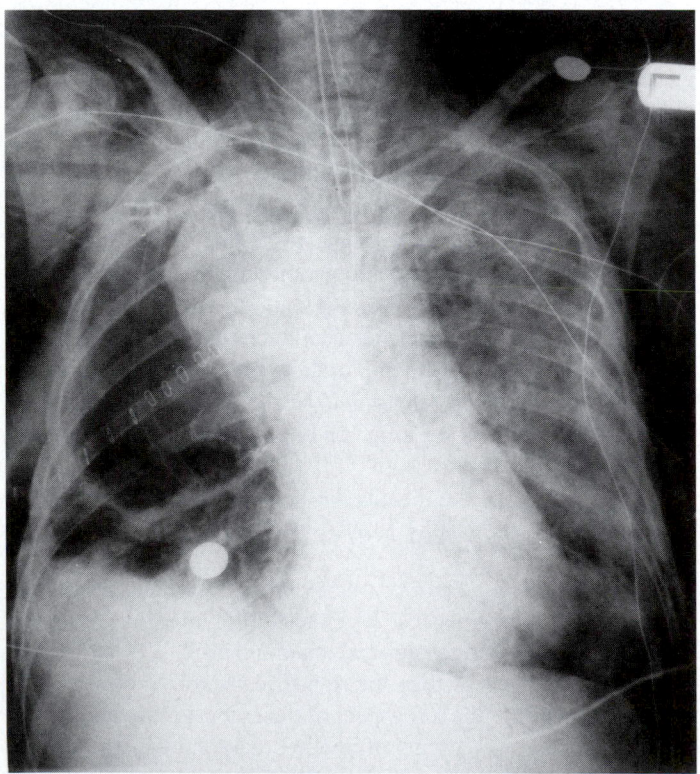

FIGURE 104-8   Consolidation of the right middle lobe caused by torsion following right upper lobectomy.

REFERENCES

1. Amar D: Personal communication.
2. Amar D, Burt ME, Roistacher N, et al: Value of perioperative Doppler echocardiography in patients undergoing major lung resection. *Ann Thorac Surg* 61:516–520, 1996.
3. Bechard D, Wetstein L: Assessment of exercise oxygen consumption as preoperative criterion for lung resection. *Ann Thorac Surg* 44:344–349, 1987.
4. Bolton JW, Weiman DS: Physiology of lung resection. *Clin Chest Med* 14:293–303, 1993.
5. Bolton JW, Weiman DS, Haynes JL, et al: Stair climbing as an indicator of pulmonary function. *Chest* 92:783–788, 1987.
6. Byrd RB, Burns JR: Cough dynamics in the post-thoracotomy state. *Chest* 67:654–657, 1975.
7. Cardus D: O$_2$ alveolar-arterial tension difference after ten days recumbency in man. *J Appl Physiol* 23:934–937, 1967.

8. Chalon J, Tayyab M, Ramanathan S: Cytology of respiratory epithelium as a predictor of respiratory complications after operations. *Chest* 67:32–35, 1975.

9. Chan TY: Low-dose dopamine in severe right heart failure and chronic obstructive pulmonary disease. *Ann Pharmacother* 29:493–496, 1995.

10. Craig DB, Wahba WM, Don HF: Airway closure and lung volumes in surgical positions. *Can Anaesth Soc J* 18:92–99, 1971.

11. Deslauriers J, Ginsberg RJ, Dubois P, et al: Current operative mortality associated with elective surgical resection for lung cancer. *Can J Surg* 32:335–339, 1989.

12. Dietrick JE, Whedon GD, Shorr E: Effects of immobilizations upon various metabolic and physiologic functions of normal men. *Am J Med* 4:3–36, 1948.

13. Ferguson MK, Little L, Rizzo L, et al: Diffusing capacity predicts morbidity and mortality after pulmonary resection. *J Thorac Cardiovasc Surg* 96:894–900, 1988.

14. Fullerton DA, Jones SD, Grover FL, McIntyre RC: Adenosine effectively controls pulmonary hypertension after cardiac operations. *Ann Thorac Surg* 61:1118–1124, 1996.

15. Gamsu G, Singer MM, Vincent HH, et al: Postoperative impairment of mucous transport in the lung. *Am Rev Respir Dis* 114:673–679, 1976.

16. Gerrard JW, Cockcroft DW, Mink JT, et al: Increased nonspecific bronchial reactivity in cigarette smokers with normal lung function. *Am Rev Respir Dis* 122:577–581, 1980.

17. Ginsberg RJ, Hill LD, Eagan RT, et al: Modern 30-day operative mortality for surgical resections in lung cancer. *J Thorac Cardiovasc Surg* 86:654–658, 1983.

18. Hyman N, Foster RS Jr, DeMeules JE, Costanza MC: Blood transfusion and survival after lung cancer. *Am J Surg* 149:502–507, 1985.

19. Jackson CV: Preoperative pulmonary evaluation. *Arch Intern Med* 148:2120–2127, 1988.

20. Johnson PC, Driscoll TB, Carpenter WR: Vascular and extravascular fluid changes during six days of bed rest. *Aerospace Med* 42:875–878, 1971.

21. Kambam JR, Chen LH, Hyman SA: Effect of short-term smoking halt on carboxyhemoglobin levels and P50 values. *Anesth Analg* 65:1186–1188, 1986.

22. Kellow NH, Scott AD, White SA, Feneck RO: Comparison of the effects of propofol and isoflurane anaesthesia on right ventricular function and shunt fraction during thoracic surgery. *Br J Anaesth* 75:578–582, 1995.

23. Kohman LJ, Meyer JA, Ikings PM, Oates RP: Random versus predictable risks of mortality after thoracotomy for lung cancer. *J Thorac Cardiovasc Surg* 91:551–554, 1986.

24. Kraus DH, Ali MK, Ginsberg RJ, et al: Vocal cord medialization for unilateral paralysis associated with intrathoracic malignancies. *J Thorac Cardiovasc Surg* 111:334–341, 1996.

25. Krowka MJ, Pairolero PC, Trastek VF, et al: Cardiac dysrhythmia following pneumonectomy: Clinical correlates and prognostic significance. *Chest* 91:490–495, 1987.

26. Kucich VA, Villareal JR, Schwartz DB: Left upper lobe torsion producing pulmonary torsion following lower lobe resection. *Chest* 95:1146–1147, 1989.

27. Laver MB, Hallowell P, Goldblatt A: Pulmonary dysfunction secondary to heart disease: Aspects relevant to anesthesia and surgery. *Anesthesiology* 33:161–192, 1970.

28. Lewis JW Jr, Bastanfar M, Gabriel F, Mascha E: Right heart function and prediction of respiratory morbidity in patients undergoing pneumonectomy. *J Thorac Cardiovasc Surg* 108:169–175, 1994.

29. Lindgren L, Lepantalo M, von Knorring J, et al: Effect of verapamil on right ventricular pressure and atrial tachyrhythmia after thoracotomy. *Br J Anaesth* 66:205–211, 1991.

30. Marini JJ, Tyler ML, Hudson LD, et al: Influence of head-dependent positions on lung volume and oxygen saturation in chronic airflow obstruction. *Am Rev Respir Dis* 129:101–105, 1984.

31. Martinez FJ, Paine R III: Medical evaluation of the patient with potentially resectable lung cancer, in Pass HI, Mitchell JB, Johnson DH, Turrisi AT (eds), *Lung Cancer: Principles and Practice.* Philadelphia, Lippincott-Raven, 1996, pp 511–534.

32. Mols P, Huynh CH, Deschamps P, et al: Acute effect of nifedipine on systolic and diastolic ventricular function in patients with chronic obstructive pulmonary disease. *Chest* 103:1381–1384, 1993.

33. Oliver RM, Fleming JS, Waller DG: Right ventricular function at rest and during exercise in chronic obstructive pulmonary disease. *Chest* 103:74–80, 1993.

34. Olsen GN, Bolton JW, Weiman DS, Hornung CA: Stair climbing as an exercise to predict the postoperative complications of lung resection: Two years' experience. *Chest* 99:587–590, 1991.

35. Pairolero PC, Arnold PG, Trastek VF, et al: Postpneumonectomy empyema: The role of intrathoracic muscle transposition. *J Thorac Cardiovasc Surg* 99:958–968, 1990.

36. Peters RM, Wellons HA Jr, Htwe TM: Total compliance and work of breathing after thorocotomy. *J Thorac Cardiovasc Surg* 57:348–355, 1969.

37. Pollack IF, Pang D, Hall WA: Subarachnoid-pleural and subarachnoid-mediastinal fistulae. *Neurosurgery* 26:519–525, 1990.

38. Pryor JA, Webber BA, Hodson ME: Effect of chest physiotherapy on oxygen saturation in patients with cystic fibrosis. *Thorax* 45:77, 1990.

39. Reed CE, Spinale FG, Crawford FA Jr: Effect of pulmonary resection on right ventricular function. *Ann Thorac Surg* 53:578–582, 1992.

40. Riveron FA, Adams C, Lewis JW, et al: Silastic prosthesis plombage for right pneumonectomy syndrome. *Ann Thorac Surg* 50:465–466, 1990.

41. Rossaint R, Falke KJ, Lopez F, et al: Inhaled nitric oxide for the adult respiratory distress syndrome. *New Engl J Med* 328:399–405, 1993.

42. Ruckdeschel J, Piantadosi S: Quality of life in lung cancer surgical adjuvant trials. *Chest* 1066(Suppl):324S–328S, 1994.

43. Sabanathan S, Eng J, Mearns AJ: Alterations in respiratory mechanics following thoracotomy. *J R Coll Surg Edinb* 35:144–145, 1990.

44. Sabanathan S, Richardson J: Management of postpneumonectomy bronchopleural fistulae: A review. *J Cardiovasc Surg (Torino)* 35:449–457, 1994.

45. Schulz V: Preoperative treatment of chronic obstructive lung disease, in: Peters RM, Toledo J (eds), *Current Topics in General Thoracic Surgery: An International Series,* vol 2: *Perioperative Care.* Amsterdam, Elsevier, 1992.

46. Siebecker K, Sadler P, Mendenhall J: Postoperative ear oximeter studies on patients who have undergone pulmonary resection. *J Thorac Surg* 36:88–94, 1958.

47. Slater JP, Goldstein DJ, Ashton RC Jr, Levin HR, et al: Right-to-left veno-arterial shunting for right circulatory failure. *Ann Thorac Surg* 60:978–985, 1995.

48. Tarkka M, Polela R, Lepojarvi M, et al: Infection prophylaxis in pulmonary surgery: A randomized prospective study. *Ann Thorac Surg* 44:508–513, 1987.

49. Taylor HL, Henschel A, Brozek J, et al: Effects of bed rest on cardiovascular function and work performance. *J Appl Physiol* 2:223–235, 1949.

50. van Migehem W, Tits G, Demuynck K, et al: Verapamil as prophylactic treatment for atrial fibrillation after lung operations. *Ann Thorac Surg* 61:1083–1086, 1996.

51. Vester SR, Faber LP, Kittle CF, et al: Bronchopleural fistula after stapled closure of bronchus. *Ann Thorac Surg* 52:1253–1257, 1991.

52. Wansbrough-Jones MH, Nelson A, New L, et al: Bronchoalveolar lavage in the prediction of post-thoracotomy chest infection. *Eur J Cardiovasc Surg* 5:433–434, 1991.

53. Warner MA, Offord KP, Warner ME, et al: Role of preoperative cessation of smoking and other factors in postoperative pulmonary complications: A blinded prospective study of coronary artery bypass patients. *Mayo Clin Proc* 64:609–616, 1989.

54. Weissman C, Kemper M, Damask MC, et al: Effect of routine intensive care interactions on metabolic rate. *Chest* 86:815–818, 1984.

55. West JB: *Ventilation-Blood Flow and Gas Exchange,* 3d ed. Philadelphia, Lippincott, 1977.

56. Wong PS, Goldstraw P: Pulmonary torsion: A questionnaire survey and a survey of the literature. *Ann Thorac Surg* 54:286–288, 1992.

57. Zeldin RA, Normandin D, Landtwing D, Peters RM: Postpneumonectomy pulmonary edema. *J Thorac Cardiovasc Surg* 87:359–365, 1984.

THORACIC TRAUMA

L a r r y   R .   K a i s e r   /   F r a n c i s   W .   D i P i e r r o

Chest trauma can be classified as either blunt or penetrating. *Blunt injury* most commonly results from motor vehicle accidents but may also result from falls or beatings. *Penetrating injuries* are the result of stab or gunshot wounds and occasionally of impalement.

The approach to diagnosis and treatment of injuries to the chest depends greatly on the mechanism of injury which influences the incidence and type of associated injuries. Most, if not all, gunshot wounds of the chest require thoracotomy for management, whereas blunt injury usually is managed nonoperatively. The possibility of associated injuries, especially to the abdomen, must also be kept in mind and thoroughly investigated prior to initiating a treatment plan. This is especially important for penetrating injuries which occur in the so-called intermediate zone, where the chest, abdomen, or both may be involved. An injury of the anterior chest in the fifth intercostal space may not involve intrathoracic structures, but the damage may be confined solely to the abdomen.

The type of weapon as well as the site of injury is particularly important. The physician managing a penetrating chest injury needs to know what type of knife was used because it is crucial to know the length of the blade in order to assess the possibility of visceral injury in either the chest or abdomen. Likewise for gunshot wounds, it is important to know the type of gun used to better address the potential extent and severity of the resultant injury. Often a determination of the type of gun may be made based on the appearance of the bullet seen on radiographic studies.

Physicians managing patients with chest injuries must be prepared to make quick but accurate judgments and decisions and to act on them. With the development of trauma systems in most cities, more critically injured patients are surviving long enough to make it to the hospital, and the time spent prior to taking the patient to the operating room may make the difference between survival and mortality. The thoracic surgeon should be involved as soon as the patient arrives in the emergency room, although many chest injuries will not require operation.

INITIAL MANAGEMENT

Ensuring Airway Patency and Breathing

The initial goal in resuscitation of any patient sustaining a traumatic injury is to establish adequate oxygenation and ventilation. Of primary importance is the establishment of a patent airway. Objects commonly found obstructing the airway following chest trauma include the patient's tongue, teeth, blood, secretions, or vomitus. Foreign objects as well as intrinsic laryngeal tissue, as in laryngeal fracture, can also obstruct the airway. As initial management, an oropharyngeal or nasopharyngeal airway can be inserted to maintain patency of the airway. Endotracheal intubation may be performed for apnea, to protect the airway from blood or secretions, or for hyperventilation in cases of severe head trauma. In cases of severe maxillofacial injury, a tracheostomy may need to be performed.

Once patency of the airway has been established, it must be verified that breathing is adequate. The patient's chest is fully exposed and inspected for evidence of rise and fall with respiration. In the intubated patient, a carbon dioxide monitor can be connected to the endotracheal tube in order to establish that gas exchange is adequate and that the tube is properly situated. Mechanical ventilation may be instituted as necessary.

Emergency Department Interventions

Once adequate oxygenation and ventilation have been established, the primary resuscitation effort must rule out other life-threatening chest injuries. Simple, open, and tension pneumothoraces, hemothoraces, and pericardial tamponade are injuries that require immediate attention.

SIMPLE PNEUMOTHORAX

Simple pneumothorax is created when a tear in the pleura allows entry of air into the pleural space with resultant loss of negativity in intrathoracic pressure. If an injury to the lung parenchyma produces an airleak, the air accumulates in the pleural space with each breath markedly increasing intrathoracic pressure, thereby shifting the mediastinum toward the opposite hemithorax (Fig. 105-1). This so-called tension pneumothorax is immediately life-threatening because of the limitation of vena caval blood flow which results in hypotension, tachycardia, and cardiac arrest.

Treatment of simple pneumothorax requires insertion of a chest tube into the pleural space under sterile conditions, usually through the fifth or sixth intercostal space in the anterior axillary line, and connection of the tube to suction. In cases of tension pneumothorax, the pressure is initially relieved by placement of a standard 16 gauge needle in the anterior second intercostal space in the midclavicular line. This maneuver is followed by placement of a chest tube for definitive management.

TENSION PNEUMOTHORAX

The diagnosis of tension pneumothorax should always be considered in a patient who has sustained penetrating chest trauma. It is less likely to occur after blunt trauma. In this circumstance, the likelihood of its occurrence increases with the severity of the injury to the chest wall (e.g., when rib fractures puncture the lung parenchyma). A high index of suspicion for tension pneumothorax should be maintained while remembering that insertion of a large bore needle into the second intercostal space may result in injury to the lung if the diagnosis is incorrect.

Clinical findings that support the diagnosis of tension pneumothorax include hypotension, absent breath sounds on the in-

volved side with tympany on percussion, tracheal deviation toward the opposite side, and difficulty in mechanically ventilating the patient because of high airway pressures. Once the diagnosis of tension pneumothorax is suspected, treatment should be initiated immediately without waiting for chest radiograph confirmation. A rush of air exiting via the needle confirms the diagnosis as treatment is initiated. It should always be kept in mind that not every pneumothorax that results from trauma is a tension pneumothorax.

PNEUMOTHORAX AND OPEN CHEST WOUND

When a pneumothorax is associated with an open chest wound after penetrating trauma, initial management is designed to restore a seal to the thoracic cavity. This is accomplished by applying a sterile occlusive dressing to the wound immediately followed by placement of a chest tube. The dressing allows some air to escape from the pleural space but does not allow air from the outside to enter.

HEMOTHORAX

Both blunt and penetrating injuries of the chest may be associated with hemothorax, but this finding is far more common following penetrating trauma. Absence of breath sounds over the injured hemithorax and dullness to percussion are the characteristic physical findings. When the quantity of blood in the chest is small, the chest radiograph, which is usually taken as an anteroposterior film while the patient is supine, may only show haziness on the involved side (Fig. 105-2). On rare occasion, he-

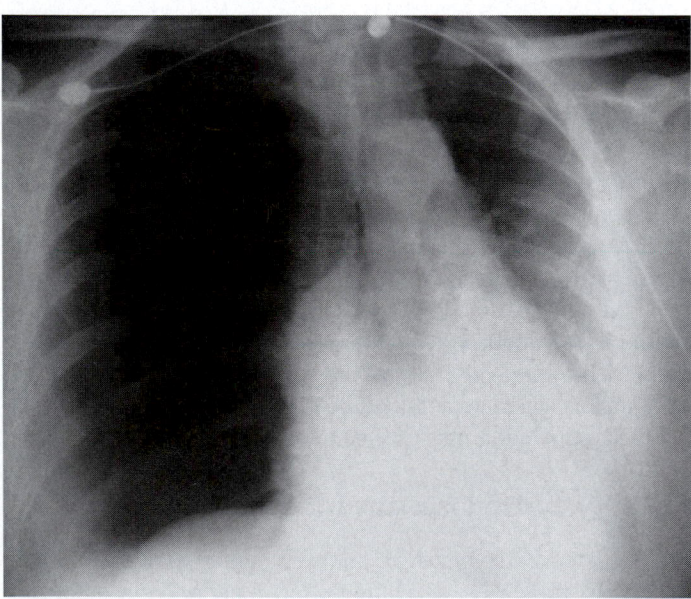

FIGURE 105-1 Right tension pneumothorax. Note the marked shift of the mediastinum to the left and the total absence of lung markings on the right.

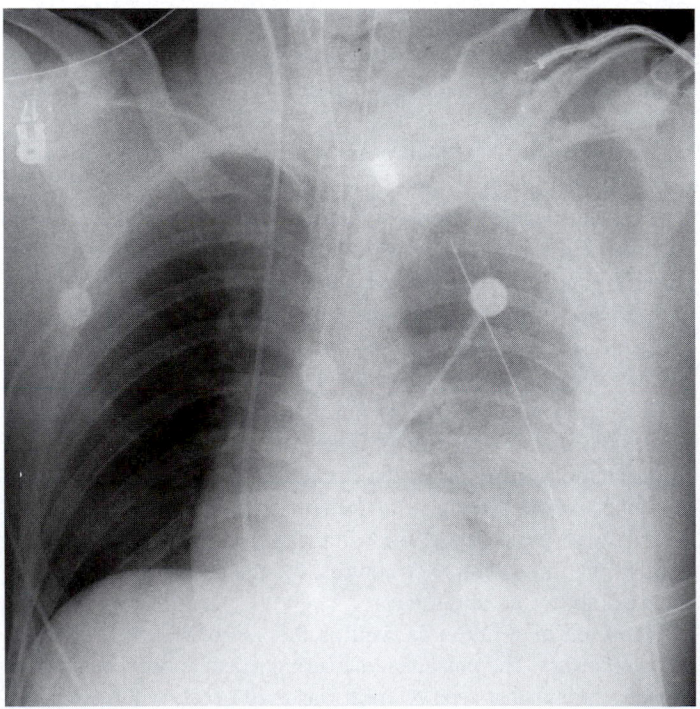

FIGURE 105-2 Hemothorax following a penetrating wound to the left chest showing the characteristic haziness seen on a supine film. The blood has been incompletely drained despite placement of a large-bore chest tube.

mothorax, which is usually the result of injury to the lung parenchyma, can reproduce the physiological disturbances of a tension pneumothorax by increasing intrapleural pressure. Injury to the pulmonary artery or veins or the aorta is usually fatal before the patient reaches the hospital, but occasionally these patients do reach the emergency room. This type of massive exsanguination is usually obvious because of the clinical findings, and immediate transfer to the operating room is mandatory for any chance to save the patient's life.

For the more common type of hemothorax, which is due to lung parenchymal injury, a large-bore (36 Fr or greater) chest tube should be inserted, and blood volume replacement should be initiated simultaneously. Additional therapeutic maneuvers are based on the documentation of continued blood loss. Depending upon the extent of parenchymal injury, bleeding may have ceased by the time the chest tube is inserted. Thus, after the accumulated blood has drained, little, if any, further drainage will occur. If blood continues to drain, and the patient is hypotensive and tachycardic in spite of volume replacement, exploration of the chest is indicated. An intraabdominal injury should be ruled out; if suspected, the appropriate procedures initiated. Even in the hemodynamically stable patient, if blood continues to drain from the chest tube at a rate of greater than 200 ml/h for 2 or 3 h, the patient should be surgically explored. Following chest tube insertion, if the decision is made to observe the patient, a chest radiograph should be repeated within several hours of the insertion to ensure that blood is not accumulating in the chest.

CARDIAC INJURY

Penetrating injury to the chest may involve not only the pulmonary parenchyma but also, not infrequently, the heart. Many patients with these injuries live long enough to make it to the hospital despite evidence of cardiac tamponade which can be managed temporarily by massive replacement of the blood volume. Cardiac tamponade results when the intrapericardial pressure becomes high enough to impede the low-pressure venous return to the heart resulting in circulatory collapse. Aspiration of as little as 10 to 20 ml of blood from the pericardial space often relieves intrapericardial pressure sufficiently to restore adequate circulation until the patient can be transported to the operating room for definitive repair of the inciting injury to the myocardium, usually the right atrium or ventricle. On rare occasion, blunt chest injury may cause cardiac tamponade. However, although myocardial rupture secondary to blunt trauma is usually fatal, an occasional patient with rupture of the atrium will survive to reach the emergency room.

EMERGENCY ROOM THORACOTOMY

Occasionally, a patient with a penetrating injury to the chest who arrives at the emergency department loses vital signs soon after arrival. A thoracotomy performed in the emergency room allows immediate control of an exsanguinating thoracic injury and enables open cardiac massage while the patient is being transported to the operating room. The decision to perform an emergency room thoracotomy is a difficult one and requires consideration of the time required to transport the patient to the operating room

in the particular hospital. Indications for emergency room thoracotomy vary from institution to institution. In general, emergency center thoracotomy is indicated in patients with exsanguinating chest injury who become pulseless after arrival but in whom some myocardial electrical activity persists. The procedure is rarely indicated in the patient who arrives without vital signs, since the success rate in resuscitating these individuals is dismal. Application of a clamp across the thoracic aorta, open cardiac massage, and simultaneous volume replacement are all performed once the chest is opened in order to restore blood flow to the brain and heart. If the hemorrhage originates in part from the pulmonary hilum, a vascular clamp or the surgeon's hand can be placed across the hilum. In addition, for penetrating cardiac wounds, the pericardium is opened and the injury repaired.

The survival rates for patients undergoing emergency center thoracotomy is less than 10 percent. Feliciano and coworkers[4] reported an 8.1 percent survival rate with 335 emergency center thoracotomies performed over a 7-year period. In most series, the procedure has been successful most often in patients with stab wounds as opposed to gunshot wounds and in patients in whom the injury is confined to the chest.

BLUNT THORACIC TRAUMA

Tracheobronchial Injuries

Isolated injury to the tracheobronchial tree is unusual because of the proximity of other major structures, specifically, the great vessels. However, it does occur occasionally. Tracheal disruption may follow blunt injury to the neck and is usually identified by the presence of subcutaneous emphysema. Intuitively, it is not obvious how an individual can survive after complete disruption of the cervical trachea. However, survival is due to the pretracheal fascia, which ensheathes the trachea and is stout enough to preserve sufficient integrity of the airway to allow air to pass into the distal trachea, albeit with some difficulty.

The more common injury to the tracheobronchial tree that results from blunt trauma is disruption of a mainstem bronchus, usually resulting from sudden deceleration either as a result of a motor vehicle accident or fall. Since the left mainstem bronchus and carina are tethered by the aortic arch, sudden deceleration of this fixed structure may result in a tear or total disruption of either the right or left main bronchus. Blunt injuries causing tracheobronchial disruption are often associated with simultaneous injuries to adjacent structures including the great vessels (especially the descending thoracic aorta), the esophagus, the manubrium, the mandible, and the cervical spine. Usually such coincident injuries are fatal. Those patients with a tracheobronchial injury who do survive long enough to reach the hospital usually have only the isolated injury, implying individuals with other injuries have already died in the field. The isolated tracheobronchial injury occurs most often in young people in whom the blood vessels, including the aorta, are somewhat more compliant than the tracheobronchial tree, so that these vessels remain intact despite trauma to the chest which disrupts the tracheobronchial tree.

How tracheobronchial injuries present clinically depends on the type of injury. Rupture of the airways resulting from blunt trauma commonly presents with subcutaneous emphysema, although this manifestation may be too subtle to appreciate by clinical examination. Other associated findings include hemoptysis, respiratory distress, change in voice, pneumothorax, or hemothorax. Pneumothorax is only present if the airway rupture communicates with the pleural space, a circumstance which does not always occur because of the dense, fibroconnective tissue around the carina and mainstem bronchi. In fact, more commonly, the only finding, even in the presence of complete bronchial disruption, is the presence of deep cervical or mediastinal air that is only appreciated on the chest radiograph (Fig. 105-3). The diagnosis of airway rupture has to be suspected if the small amount of mediastinal or cervical emphysema displayed by the chest radiograph is to be detected by physical examination. Detection of mediastinal or cervical emphysema is rendered more difficult by the rarity of tracheobronchial injuries (i.e., no more than 2 to 3 per year) seen in major trauma centers.

As noted above, pneumothorax may follow bronchial disruption, but the evidence of an airway injury is usually not apparent until after a chest tube is placed. When suction is applied to the chest tube, the patient may become significantly more dyspneic, a situation which is only relieved by discontinuing the suction. Also, as a consequence of the large air leak, the lung expands incompletely despite increasing suction. Although the combination of these findings almost ensures the diagnosis, bronchoscopy should always be done even if suspicion is low that the airway is injured. Bronchoscopy clearly delineates the injury and confirms the location, information that is crucial for planning the operative approach.

Management of the patient with tracheobronchial injury begins with making sure that the patient has a reliable airway. In patients with suspected injury to the cervical or mediastinal trachea, intubation of the trachea beyond the injury is performed under direct vision under bronchoscopic guidance. If airway injury is not suspected, blind endotracheal intubation may suffice but may result in further problems. Tracheostomy should be avoided if at all possible. In patients with unilateral bronchial injury, intubation of the opposite main bronchus is desirable.

Airway Ruptures

Airway ruptures occur in transverse, longitudinal, or in combined directions. The most common tracheal injury occurs between tracheal rings. Longitudinal injuries occur along the membranous portion of the airways. Most tracheobronchial ruptures occur within 2.5 cm of the carina, and the trachea or bronchi may be completely disrupted.

The principles of managing airway rupture include debridement of devitalized tissue and primary repair for tracheobronchial injuries. Lesions of the distal trachea, carina, and the right mainstem bronchus are approached via a right thoracotomy. This approach also provides excellent exposure of the proximal left main bronchus, but the way in which an injury on the left should be managed is greatly influenced by the bronchoscopic findings. A partial disruption of the proximal left mainstem bronchus is usually approached by way of a right thoracotomy with mobilization of the carina. Complete disruption on the left usually should be managed by way of a left thoracotomy. Exposure of the proximal left main bronchus from the left side is difficult because of the aortic arch. Often the arch must be encircled and retracted superiorly in order to gain adequate exposure. Division of the ligamentum arteriosum also facilitates exposure of the left main bronchus at its origin.

The bronchus is either repaired or reanastomosed with sutures so as to be airtight. Rarely is pulmonary resection required, although lobectomy may have to be carried out if a lobar bronchus is involved. Pneumonectomy should never be required unless the lung parenchyma has been virtually destroyed. In cases involving complex injuries to the distal trachea, carina, or mainstem bronchi, providing adequate oxygenation and ventilation during the operation without the use of cardiopulmonary bypass may be difficult, but this is distinctly unusual.[12] Usually the airway is managed just as it is in elective carinal or main bronchial sleeve resections, scrupulously avoiding the use of extracorporeal oxygenation and systemic heparinization.

Pulmonary Contusion

Pulmonary contusion occurs during blunt thoracic trauma as the force of impact is transferred through the chest wall to the lung parenchyma. The anatomic manifestation of contusion is disruption of alveolar-capillary interfaces and resultant collection of blood and protein in the interstitium and alveoli. Both the physiologic derangements and the presentation of patients with this type of injury are variable and range from asymptomatic to severe hypoxia and the need for mechanical ventilation. This variability in presentation reflects the fact that contusion often occurs with associated injuries that require resuscitative measures which can add to the anatomic insult. Also, the extent of the contusion may be quite variable.

In a classic series of experiments,[10,14] Trinkle and colleagues studied the effects of crystalloid versus colloid resuscitation on

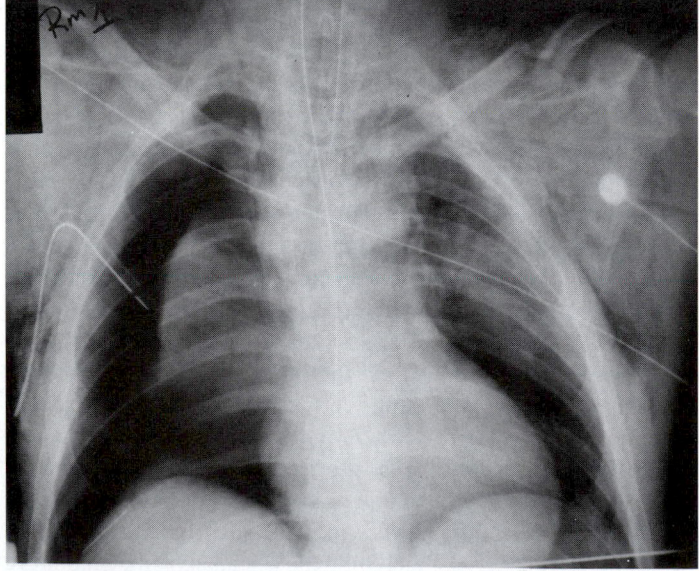

FIGURE 105-3 Traumatic rupture of the right main bronchus following a motor vehicle accident. This radiograph demonstrates the classic findings of a pneumothorax which fails to resolve despite chest tube placement and subcutaneous and mediastinal air. Often the findings are more subtle.

the severity of pulmonary contusions in dogs. To mimic the clinical situation where pulmonary injury is often associated with significant blood loss from associated injuries, the dogs also underwent blood loss that called for restoration of blood volume. Crystalloid intravenous fluid resulted in more severe pulmonary damage than did the use of colloidal solutions. In addition, mechanical ventilation and furosemide therapy decreased the severity of the pulmonary lesion. Hence, in patients suspected of having extensive pulmonary contusion, restoration of blood volume using crystalloid should be accomplished carefully in order to avoid increasing the injury.

In addition to associated injuries, preexisting medical conditions greatly influence the course of patients with pulmonary contusions. Patients with chronic obstructive pulmonary disease, heart failure, or renal failure are predisposed to shunting in the involved segment of lung parenchyma and should be mechanically ventilated at the first suggestion of systemic hypoxemia. Similarly, the degree of pulmonary vascular reactivity influences the severity of injury from pulmonary contusion and the subsequent clinical course.[17] Pulmonary vasoconstriction occurs after pulmonary contusion, apparently serving to reduce that intrapulmonary shunt created by perfusing injured, poorly ventilated parenchyma. Patients unable to vasoconstrict adequately experienced larger shunt fractions than do those with more reactive pulmonary vasoconstriction. Although the value of classifying patients as "good vasoconstrictors" or "bad vasoconstrictors" is not clear, the distinction may help to determine treatment strategies, including the decision to abandon conservative management and to proceed with limited pulmonary resection.

Pulmonary laceration often complicates pulmonary contusion. In the transfer of energy to the chest wall during blunt trauma, shear forces are often generated that are capable of tearing the lung. Although most lacerations resolve spontaneously, elastic recoil of the lung can extend the laceration and form a cavity or a pulmonary pseudocyst. Potential complications of these cysts include infection, abscess formation, hemoptysis, air leak, adult respiratory distress syndrome (ARDS), and death. Although secondary infection of these pseudocysts is rare, it does occur and is treated in the same way as uncomplicated lung abscesses with sputum culture, directed antibiotic therapy, and pulmonary toilet. Failure of an infected pseudocyst to respond requires either surgical drainage and debridement or drainage via a percutaneous catheter introduced with the guidance of computed tomograph (CT).[5]

The findings on chest radiograph in pulmonary contusion range from small nodular patchy infiltrates to frank consolidation involving a significant portion of the pulmonary parenchyma (Fig. 105-4). These findings become evident within a few hours of injury in the classic presentation of pulmonary contusion. The usefulness of the chest radiograph in the management of contused lung is limited by the time lag between the appearance of abnormalities in gas exchange and the appearance of the injury on chest radiograph. Nonetheless, the chest radiograph is valuable in following resolution. Chest CT scans define the extent of injury more accurately than do chest radiographs and can allow rapid classification and quantification of pulmonary parenchymal damage.[16]

The management of pulmonary contusion consists mainly of adequate analgesia and pulmonary toilet along with supplemen-

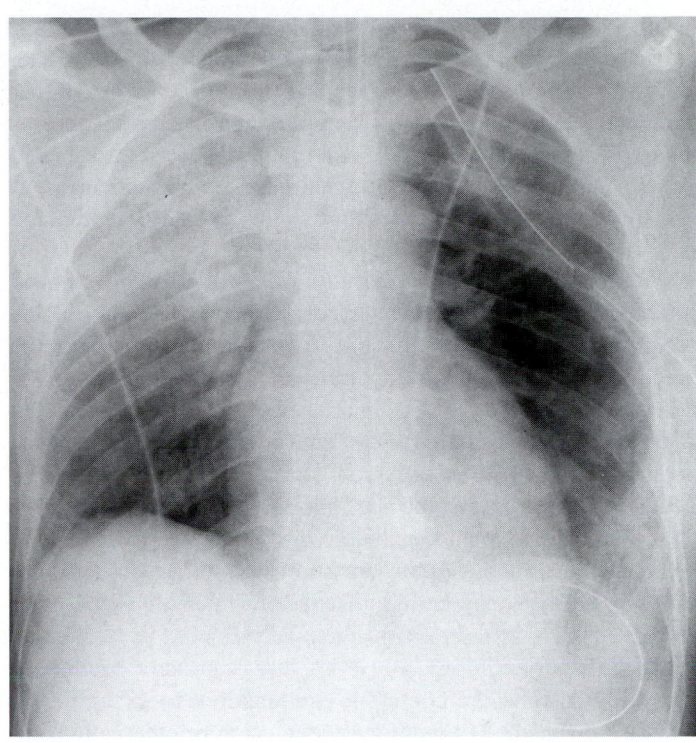

FIGURE 105-4 Right pulmonary contusion following blunt chest trauma associated with left-sided rib fractures.

tal oxygen as needed. Endotracheal intubation and mechanical ventilation may be required depending on the extent of the contusion and the presence of associated injuries. Avoidance of overhydration is particularly important. Serial chest radiographs can be used to follow the course of a pulmonary contusion until it resolves, although clinical evidence of improved gas exchange is really the bottom line as far as the patient is concerned.

Rib Fracture and Flail Chest

Blunt trauma to the chest may fracture ribs or produce flail chest.

RIB FRACTURE

The designation "simple rib fracture" usually refers to a nondisplaced fracture of a rib without injury to the lung or pleura. The most common mechanism for simple rib fractures is direct impact such as occurs in a fall or in a motor vehicle accident. Clinically, simple rib fractures may present with manifestations ranging from pain isolated to the involved rib to pneumonia secondary to splinting and hypoventilation caused by the pain. This latter circumstance is more likely in the elderly patient with osteoporosis, obstructive pulmonary disease, or malnutrition. Point tenderness is present over the fracture site, and a step-off may be palpated at the point where the fractured ends overlap. However, the physical findings are often more subtle.

Physical examination in the awake patient is usually sufficient to make the diagnosis of rib fracture. Chest radiographs obtained during the initial evaluation of a trauma patient in the emergency room usually are anteroposterior views taken with the patient supine, and rib fractures are often missed. Since the management of isolated simple rib fractures consists of analgesia and pulmonary toilet, attempting to ensure a radiographic diagnosis with oblique views or special rib views may not be necessary. In patients with underlying lung disease, the anteroposterior chest radiograph is most useful in establishing the absence of associated injuries, such as pulmonary contusion and pneumothorax.

The management of rib fractures may, at times, be dictated in part by which ribs and how many are injured. Fracture of the first or second ribs requires significant force and can be associated with major vascular or nerve injury as a result of the proximity of these ribs to the subclavian vessels and the brachial plexus. Although fractures of these two ribs are not necessarily an indication for an arteriogram,[7] certain associated injuries do require angiographic study. Abnormalities in pulse or in the neurologic examination of the upper extremities or a hematoma at the base of the neck should prompt an arteriogram. Other indications include palpable displacement of the first rib and a widened mediastinum on the chest radiograph. Fracture of the lower ribs may be associated with injury to the liver or spleen.

Regardless of etiology, all rib fractures caused by trauma require repeated chest radiographic examinations to screen for radiographic evidence of pulmonary contusion or other complication such as hemothorax. Pulmonary complications of rib fractures can result from pain and splinting and include retained secretions, atelectasis, ventilatory failure in patients with limited pulmonary reserve, and empyema.

The cornerstone of the management of rib fractures is the management of secretions. This can only be accomplished by adequate analgesia. Options for analgesia with rib fractures include narcotics and intercostal nerve blocks.

Rib fractures often accompany other injuries. In a series of 711 patients with rib fractures evaluated over a 5-year period, 94 percent had associated injuries, 32 percent had a pneumothorax or a hemothorax, 26 percent had a pulmonary contusion, and 12 percent died.[18] Thus, information underscores the importance of knowing the mechanism of injury and the high likelihood of additional injuries either in the chest or elsewhere.

FLAIL CHEST

Flail chest is an even better indicator of extensive injury. It occurs when a section of the chest wall becomes unstable because of multiple rib fractures (Fig. 105-5). This segment moves paradoxically with respiration causing respiratory embarrassment. There has been a continuing debate regarding whether the segmental, paradoxical chest wall motion or the underlying lung contusion is responsible for the ventilatory abnormalities seen in these patients. The force of the injury required to cause a flail segment causes a significant contusion, and it is likely that the contused lung contributes most significantly to the derangement in gas exchange.

Because of the evolving views concerning the pathophysiological mechanism, the treatment of flail chest has changed dramatically over the years. The early approach reflected the belief that the chest wall deformity was responsible for the ventilatory compromise and consisted of external stabilization of the chest wall with sandbags. Operations were also performed for internal

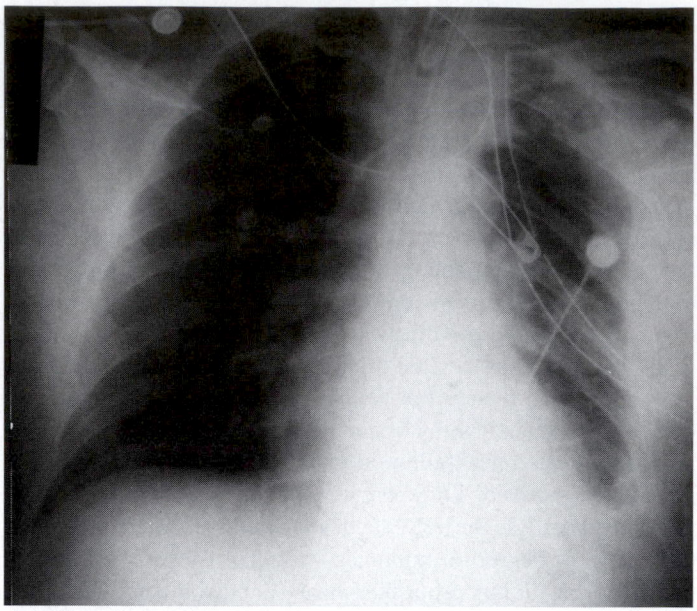

FIGURE 105-5   Left flail chest following blunt trauma.

fixation of the flail segment. Subsequently, internal pneumatic stabilization with positive pressure ventilation was used in a further effort to prevent the paradoxical chest wall motion produced by spontaneous respiration. Patients were intubated and ventilated even when gas exchange was reasonable.

In time, more attention was directed toward the underlying pulmonary contusion as the significant pathophysiological mechanism. Trinkle tested this concept by treating one group of chest trauma patients with flail chest using positive-pressure ventilation while treating a second group with a standard pulmonary contusion which included restriction of fluids and relief of pain.[15] Length of hospitalization was shorter and incidence of complications significantly less in the group treated without mechanical ventilation.

Current treatment for flail chest avoids mechanical ventilation until mandated by standard criteria. There is no physiological reason to institute positive-pressure ventilation solely to prevent paradoxical chest wall motion. Management is directed toward the pulmonary contusion and control of pain. Continuous epidural analgesia has proven to be an excellent adjunct in the overall management of these patients, since the relief of pain lessens splinting, improves chest wall mechanics, and decreases the risk of atelectasis and pneumonia. Aggressive pulmonary toilet and secretion management are also important in the overall management of these patients.

If a segment of the chest wall is completely disrupted, operative fixation may provide a necessary adjunct. In this injury, the bellows mechanism of the chest is severely disordered by the major skeletal deformity which consists of complete separation of the ribs from each other with maintenance only of the integrity of the overlying skin. In this injury, the flail is severe, and operative repair with wire stabilization of the flail segment and reconstruction of the chest wall is often necessary for restoration of the bellows.

Sternal Fracture

Sternal fracture most commonly occurs during motor vehicle accidents in which there is direct impact of the anterior chest on the steering wheel. Paramedics often report damage to the steering wheel in accidents that produce these injuries. Sternal fractures also are occasionally associated with single or multiple costochondral dislocations. The association of these two injuries can lead to flail chest with paradoxical motion of the sternum during spontaneous respiration. Other injuries associated with sternal fracture include flexion injuries of the vertebral column, tracheobronchial rupture, aortic disruption, and myocardial contusion or rupture. Isolated sternal injury is a relatively rare injury, since the force required to fracture the sternum usually results in other injury, which is often fatal.

When first seen, the awake, conversant patient with a sternal fracture often complains of pain. Inspection of the chest wall often reveals ecchymosis or abrasion of the skin overlying the sternum; a chest wall deformity may be visible. Palpation of the sternum and the costochondral junctions may reveal point tenderness and a crepitance or step-off over the fracture. Sternal fractures are difficult to detect on anterior or oblique films.[2] Patients suspected of having a sternal fracture should have lateral views with a specific request for sternal views. In the patient with multiple injuries who is unable to tolerate many diagnostic studies, the diagnosis can be made based safely on physical examination. Sternal fractures most commonly extend either through the body of the sternum or occur at the junction of the manubrium and body.

Simple undisplaced sternal fractures require no treatment. Displaced fractures with overlapping fragments may require operative reduction, debridement, and direct wire fixation. Claviculosternal dislocations may compress the structures traversing the thoracic inlet including the trachea, major vessels, and the brachial plexus. Treatment of the sternal fracture may need to be delayed depending on the presence of other associated injuries.

Diaphragmatic Injury

Injury to the diaphragm should be considered in any penetrating or blunt injury to the chest, abdomen, or lower back.[13] The injury is easily detectable at the time of laparotomy but is often overlooked in the heat of the moment when dealing with intraabdominal hemorrhage (Fig. 105-6). When a diaphragmatic injury is noted, primary suture repair of the rent usually suffices, but occasionally repair with prosthetic mesh is required. Regardless of etiology, all diaphragmatic injuries should be repaired

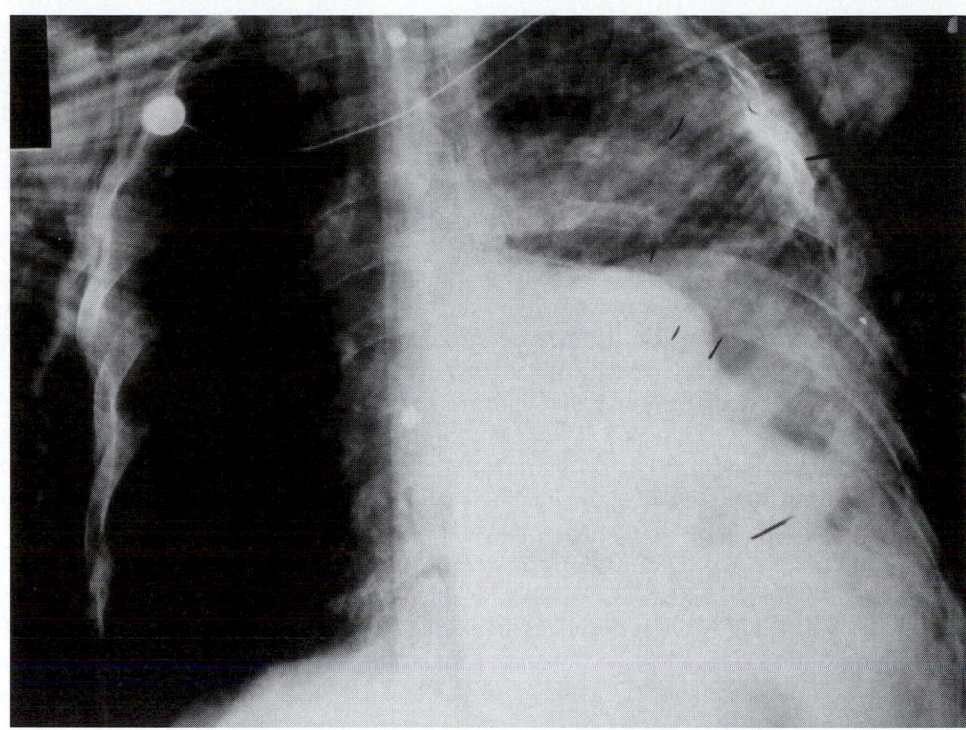

FIGURE 105-6   Ruptured left hemidiaphragm following a motor vehicle accident. Note the subcutaneous emphysema and the loss of diaphragm contour on the left. The contents of the left side of the abdomen are in the left chest.

because there is a significant risk of incarceration and possible strangulation of abdominal viscera through the hernia as well as pulmonary compromise secondary to compression.

In those patients who do not undergo emergency laparotomy, the diagnosis can be delayed for several months or even years. Diaphragmatic injuries can occur with penetrating injuries as well as from blunt trauma, although the injuries incurred from a blunt mechanism tend to produce larger rents in the diaphragm. Patients with missed diaphragm injuries often complain of midepigastric pain or symptoms of bowel obstruction as abdominal viscera herniate into the chest. Examination may reveal a scaphoid abdomen without significant tenderness to palpation. Auscultation of the chest may reveal bowel sounds. The chest radiograph shows what appears to be an elevated hemidiaphragm, hydrothorax, hydropneumothorax, an air-fluid level, and evidence of abdominal viscera. These findings are most often seen on the left side because, after right-sided diaphragmatic injuries, the liver protects the abdominal viscera from herniating into the right chest. Occasionally, the liver itself may herniate after right-sided injuries. An easy diagnostic test is the introduction of a nasogastric tube. If the tube coils into the left chest, the diagnosis of gastric herniation through the diaphragmatic injury is made, and operation is indicated for repair of the diaphragm and restoration of the abdominal contents into the abdomen. Similarly, an upper gastrointestinal series or barium enema can be performed to evaluate the viscera with respect to herniation into the chest. If the diagnosis is made relatively quickly after herniation, the abdominal approach can be used for repair. If the diagnosis is made before incarceration but well after the initial herniation, the repair is performed through the left chest, since there are often adhesions to the lung as a result of chronic inflammation. As mentioned above, almost all these injuries occur on the left side with only the occasional diaphragmatic injury seen on the right.

PENETRATING INJURY OF THE LUNG

Penetrating injuries of the lung occur from stab or gunshot wounds. An occasional impalement injury may also be seen. The degree of injury sustained by the lung ranges from small lacerations caused by knife injuries to massive destruction with shotgun blasts (Fig. 105-7). In addition, the type of firearm used will define the amount of injury. Specifically, high-velocity missiles such as those used during wartime and, more recently in urban areas, are more likely to produce severe damage than the typical low velocity missiles used by civilians. High-velocity bullets create a blast effect, producing a large temporary cavity within the tissues hit by the bullet.[3] Although it may not be evident initially, the ultimate extent of injury caused by such forces is often extensive because of the associated pulmonary contusion from the blast effect. Low-velocity bullets are more likely to produce wounds that have a cross-sectional area about the size of the bullet and the blast effect is relatively less than that produced by high-velocity bullets.

In a series of 1168 patients with penetrating injuries to the thoracic cavity, only 6 percent of these required operative repair of pulmonary parenchymal or hilar injuries.[11] Of 384 patients with gunshot wounds, 283 (74 percent) were managed with chest tubes alone. Similarly, of 784 patients with stab wounds to the thorax, 602 (77 percent) required only a chest tube. Mortality for those requiring only a chest tube was 0.7 percent. In contrast, mortality for those with hilar injuries was

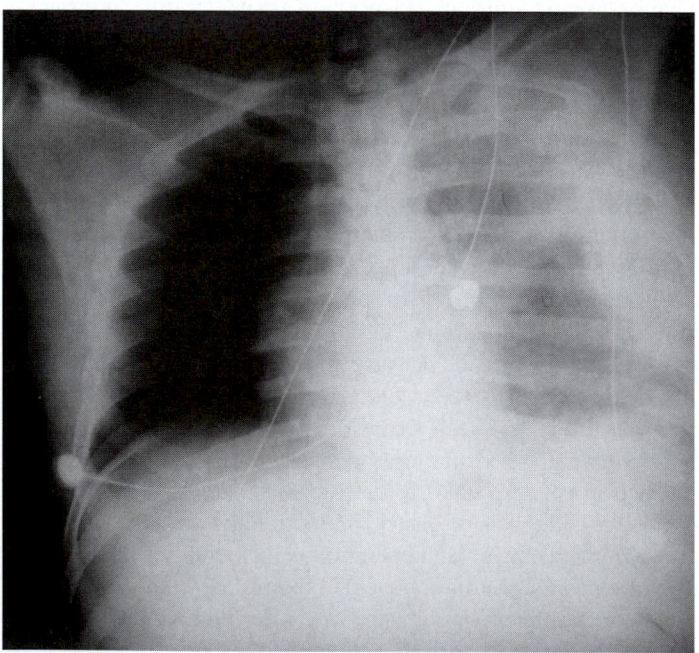

FIGURE 105-7 Gunshot wound to the left chest demonstrating a large hemothorax present on admission to the emergency room prior to chest tube placement. The amount of blood in the chest and the continued drainage of blood determine whether exploration of the chest is indicated.

30 percent, and, for those with injuries requiring lung resection, mortality was 28 percent. Thus, most civilian penetrating thoracic injuries can be managed with tube thoracostomy alone because of relatively minimal injury to lung parenchyma. Hilar injury or significant parenchymal injury requiring resection carries a high mortality.

The management of penetrating thoracic injury begins with placement of a chest tube. One indication for operation in such patients is an initial drainage of 2 L or more of blood. Clinical signs are particularly important. The patient who remains hypotensive following volume replacement should be explored. In those with less initial drainage, continuing drainage of 150 to 200 ml of blood every hour for 3 to 4 h is another indication for operation. Additional indications include hemoptysis, shock, and cardiac tamponade. Options for treatment include direct suture repair of the lung, wedge resection, or formal anatomic resection, such as lobectomy. Great effort is made to preserve pulmonary parenchyma, and resection is reserved for those cases where there is significant destruction of lung tissue or injury to a pulmonary artery. Everything possible is done to avoid pneumonectomy which, in this situation, is associated with mortality greater than 60 percent.

ARDS AFTER CHEST TRAUMA

The adult respiratory distress syndrome often complicates chest trauma, and its clinical manifestations are similar to those that occur in patients with ARDS after insults that do not involve trauma. Several injuries and their sequelae have been implicated in the etiology of ARDS. Among these are the following clinical factors often found in the chest trauma patient: sepsis syndrome, pulmonary contusion, aspiration of gastric contents, multiple emergency transfusions, and multiple major fractures.[8] In addition, the risk of ARDS has been found to be most closely related to the number of risk factors present (18 percent with one factor, 85 percent with three or more factors).[9] Hence, any chest trauma patient admitted with clinical risk factors of ARDS should be followed closely so that appropriate treatment can be administered promptly. In addition, although these risk factors are only associated with ARDS rather than causative, they should receive prompt treatment with the goal of minimizing any potential causative role they could have.

Mechanically Assisted Ventilation

As with other etiologies, the mainstay of treatment of ARDS in the patient with chest trauma revolves around the use of assisted ventilation (see Chapters 176, 177), i.e., volume ventilation and positive end-expiratory pressure (PEEP). By increasing the number of ventilated alveoli, thereby increasing the functional residual capacity (FRC), the shunt fraction ($\dot{Q}s/\dot{Q}t$) is decreased, and arterial oxygenation improves. The target usually established for the $\dot{Q}s/\dot{Q}t$ ratio is < 0.2. The goals of this scheme for ventilatory management are to adjust the fraction of inspired oxygen (FIO_2) and the level of PEEP to the lowest values capable of supporting adequate oxygenation. In the rare patient with severe chronic lung disease, bronchopleural fistula, or such severe ARDS that oxygenation using this approach is not successful, high-frequency jet ventilation, extracorporeal membrane oxygenation (ECMO), and simultaneous independent lung ventilation remain as options.

High-Frequency Jet Ventilation

In high-frequency jet ventilation, a small cannula is inserted into the airway and brief high-pressure jets of air are used to ventilate the lungs. As the jet of air enters the bronchus it pulls air along by the Venturi effect, thereby determining the inspiratory volume. Typical ventilator settings include tidal volumes of 1 ml to 3 ml per kg and rates of 100 to 200 breaths per minute. The advantage of this mode of ventilation is the avoidance of the high-peak airway pressures produced by PEEP. Results obtained with this technique have not been consistent from clinic to clinic. Hurst and colleagues[6] used both high-frequency jet ventilation (HFJV) and the related high-frequency percussive ventilation (HFPV) in trauma patients with injury to multiple organ systems. This combination combines the mechanism of HFJV with the ability to change airway pressure phasically. They found that HFJV improved CO_2 elimination more effectively than did the intermittent mandatory ventilation/continuous positive airway pressure (IMV/CPAP) mode of ventilation. In addition, HFPV improved PaO_2 and reduced $PaCO_2$ at lower peak, mean, and end-expiratory pressures. In contrast, Albelda and coworkers[1] studied the use of HFJV in patients with bronchopleural fistulae and found no clear benefit with the technique in these patients. The utility of HFJV in chest trauma patients remains to be completely elucidated, but it is available as an option in patients with severe barotrauma from PEEP.

Extracorporeal Membrane Oxygenator (ECMO)

Yet another option in the chest trauma patient with recalcitrant ARDS is extracorporeal membrane oxygenator. This technique is not yet used routinely in adult patients with severe ARDS. One reason that ECMO has produced variable results in this population is that these patients often have major multiorgan system dysfunction in addition to their pulmonary dysfunction. If these other conditions are not corrected, the likelihood of survival is low despite the ability to oxygenate and ventilate using ECMO. The role of ECMO in the adult population with ARDS remains to be defined.

Ventilation of Each Lung Separately

Simultaneous ventilation of each lung separately involves the use of one separate ventilator for each lung using a double lumen endobronchial tube. The ventilators can function in either synchronous and asynchronous modes. The technique is used in conditions of unilateral severe lung disease, such as postunilateral lung transplantation or unilateral severe pulmonary contusion.

CONCLUSION

For purposes of classification, a distinction must be made between blunt and penetrating trauma to the chest, yet the management of many of these injuries, no matter what the cause, is similar. An injury confined to the chest most often results in a favorable outcome; the difficulty lies in the fact that most chest trauma is associated with other injuries. Many multiple-injury patients with chest trauma never make it to the hospital. Those who do must be managed by a team of individuals consisting of trauma and thoracic surgeons as well as physicians trained in critical care. The initial management of patients with thoracic trauma often requires quick and accurate decisionmaking such as in the case of the patient who presents with a tension pneumothorax. It behooves all physicians who deal with critically ill patients to be familiar with the care of patients with chest trauma.

REFERENCES

1. Albelda SM, Hansen-Flaschen JH, Taylor E, et al: Evaluation of high-frequency jet ventilation in patients with bronchopleural fistulas by quantification of the airleak. *Anaesthesia* 63:551–55, 1985.
2. Dee PM: The radiology of chest trauma. *Radiol Clin North Am* 30:291–306, 1992.
3. DeMuth WE Jr: High velocity bullet wounds of the thorax. *Am J Surg* 115:606–625, 1968.
4. Feliciano DV, Bitondo CG, Cruse PA, et al: Liberal use of emergency center thoracotomy. *Am J Surg* 152:654–659, 1986.
5. Gincherman Y, Luketich JD, Kaiser LR: Successful nonoperative management of secondarily infected pulmonary pseudocyst: case report. *J Trauma* 38(6):960–963, 1995.
6. Hurst JM, Branson RD, DeHaven CB: The role of high-frequency ventilation in posttraumatic respiratory insufficiency. *J Trauma* 27:236–242, 1987.
7. Lazrove S, Harley DP, Grinnell VS, et al: Should all patients with first rib fracture undergo arteriography? *J Thorac Cardiovasc Surg* 83:532–537, 1985.
8. Maunder RJ: Clinical prediction of the adult respiratory distress syndrome. *Clin Chest Med* 6:413–426, 1985.
9. Pepe PE, Potkin RT, Reus DH, et al: Clinical predictors of the adult respiratory distress syndrome. *Am J Surg* 144:124–130, 1982.
10. Richardson JD, Franz JL, Grover FL, Trinkle JK: Pulmonary contusion and hemorrhage—crystalloid versus colloid replacement. *J Surg Res* 16:330–336, 1974.
11. Robison PD, Harman PK, Trinkle JK, Grover FL: Management of penetrating lung injuries in civilian practice. *J Thorac Cardiovasc Surg* 95:184–190, 1988.
12. Symbas PN, Justicz AG, Ricketts RR: Rupture of the airways from blunt trauma: treatment of complex injuries. *Ann Thorac Surg* 54:177–183, 1992.
13. Symbas PN, Vlasis SE, Hatcher CR Jr: Blunt and penetrating diaphragmatic injuries with or without herniation of organs into the chest. *Ann Thorac Surg* 42:153–162, 1986.
14. Trinkle JK, Furman RW, Hinshaw MA, et al: Pulmonary contusion—pathogenesis and effect of various resuscitative measures. *Ann Thorac Surg* 54:177–183, 1992.
15. Trinkle JK, Richardson JD, Franz JL, et al: Management of flail chest without mechanical ventilation. *Ann Thorac Surg* 19:355–363, 1975.
16. Wagner RB, Jamieson PM: Pulmonary contusion—evaluation and classification by computed tomography. *Surg Clin North Am* 69(1):31, 1989.
17. Wagner RB, Slivko B, Jamieson PM, et al: Effect of lung contusion on pulmonary hemodynamics. *Ann Thorac Surg* 52:51–58, 1991.
18. Ziegler DW, Agarwal NN: The morbidity and mortality of rib fractures. *J Trauma* 37(6):975–979, 1994.

CHAPTER 106

LUNG TRANSPLANTATION

John C. Wain

Lung transplantation has been used as a successful therapeutic intervention for a variety of end-stage pulmonary parenchymal and vascular diseases over the past 15 years. Advances in recipient and donor selection, surgical technique, and postoperative management have improved early survival. The criteria for the use of either isolated lung transplantation or heart–lung transplantation continue to be defined, with the role for heart–lung transplantation lessening over the past decade. A relative shortage of donor organs has been the major constraint on wider application of this treatment. In addition, chronic rejection in the pulmonary allograft, manifested as obliterative bronchiolitis, remains a major obstacle to long-term patient survival.

HISTORY

Pioneering efforts in experimental lung transplantation were undertaken in the 1940s and 1950s. Demikhov performed a variety of experiments involving transplantation of pulmonary lobes and heterotopic heart–lung transplantation in dogs.[12] These experiments demonstrated the technical feasibility of such procedures. In addition, the heart and the lung in heart–lung grafts pursued different functional courses, foreshadowing the differing rates of rejection of the heart and the lungs that were seen in combined heart–lung transplants performed clinically more than 3 decades later.[12] Metras reported the results of left-lung transplantation in the dog and presciently emphasized technical factors that are now used clinically for isolated lung transplantation.[29] Subsequent experimental studies showed that the transplanted lung could provide ventilation for the recipient.[18]

Clinical lung transplantation was undertaken first by Hardy in 1963.[19] The procedure consisted of a left single-lung transplant performed for a carcinoma of the left lung that involved the hilum. The patient survived for 18 days, dying of renal failure and malnutrition. This effort demonstrated that a transplanted lung could function for the short term in a patient and stimulated further clinical and experimental efforts. Between 1963 and 1978, however, at least 38 attempts were made at isolated lung transplantation, and only one patient survived to hospital discharge.[13] The particular patient had undergone a right single-lung transplant for silicosis; he developed a bronchial anastomotic stricture and succumbed to sepsis and chronic rejection 8 months after transplantation. The remaining patients in this 15-year experience all died postoperatively. The major cause of mortality beyond the first postoperative week in these patients was bronchial dehiscence. In addition, most of the patients were greatly debilitated at the time of the procedure, frequently ventilator dependent or in a state of multisystem and multiorgan failure, hindering their ability to survive. It was appreciated that in many of these patients, the available immunosuppressive regimens, which relied on high-dose corticosteroids (2 mg/kg of prednisone per day), significantly compromised postoperative healing of the bronchus and further potentiated the adverse effects of preexisting conditions.

The problem of bronchial healing was related to the relative ischemia of the donor bronchus, which followed revascularization of the lung graft without reestablishment of bronchial circulation. One technical approach to this problem was the development of a procedure for combined heart–lung transplantation, allowing for maintenance of collateral bronchial circulation from the coronary circulation and mediastinal tissues. Although the operation was performed primarily for patients with end-stage cardiac failure due to pulmonary hypertension, the initial report of successful heart–lung transplantation demonstrated the feasibility of this approach in obtaining healing of the airway and confirmed the ability of the transplanted lung to provide long-term respiratory function.[37] Subsequently, heart–lung transplantation has been performed for numerous pulmonary parenchymal diseases, including emphysema and bilateral septic lung disease, such as cystic fibrosis.

An alternative technique for improving bronchial healing was to optimize the bronchial–pulmonary collateral circulation by limiting the length of the donor bronchus and to revascularize the bronchial circulation extrinsically by wrapping the anastomosis with omentum. In addition to these technical measures, the avoidance of high-dose steroid immunosuppressive regimens, made possible by the use of cyclosporine, was shown to improve bronchial anastomotic healing.[16] These advances, combined with the selection of well-conditioned recipients with pulmonary fibrosis, whose pathophysiology favored perfusion and ventilation of the allograft, culminated in the clinical success of isolated single-lung transplantation.[45] Further efforts were made to perfect a technique for isolated double-lung transplantation to expand this approach to patients with bilateral septic lung disease. The initial clinical success of an en bloc double-lung transplant procedure was tempered by a significant incidence of bronchial anastomotic complications.[34] However, further modification of the technique, by either direct bronchial revascularization or bilateral sequential single-lung transplantation, has provided satisfactory results.[9,32]

It has since been shown that despite initial concerns about the physiology of allograft ventilation, isolated single-lung transplantation is also appropriate for patients with end-stage chronic obstructive pulmonary disease (COPD).[27] Isolated single- and double-lung transplantation has also been successfully applied to patients with primary pulmonary hypertension or Eisenmenger's syndrome (with correction of the congenital shunt), for whom combined heart–lung transplantation was initially devised.[33,15] As the utility of isolated lung transplantation for these pulmonary diseases has been demonstrated, the need for heart–lung transplantation has diminished.

RECIPIENT SELECTION

General Considerations

The evaluation of a potential candidate for lung transplantation should include a complete assessment of cardiopulmonary function and of the patient's general health, in addition to a thorough evaluation of psychosocial status. A battery of screening tests are required, as well as evaluation by members of the transplant team, including pulmonologists, cardiologists, thoracic surgeons, psychiatrists, and social workers (Table 106-1). Contingent on the patient's status, this evaluation can be completed in many instances on an outpatient basis. A coordinated review of the results of these studies by the multidisciplinary transplant team serves to assure that the best candidates are accepted as potential transplant recipients.

Lung transplantation is a treatment of last resort. Potential recipients should be patients with an end-stage pulmonary parenchymal or vascular disease who have a limited life expectancy and for whom no effective alternative therapy is available. The life expectancy of potential recipients is related to both the underlying disease process and the degree of reduction in activities of daily living resulting from the disease, with significant secondary alterations in the patient's psychosocial status. The variable rates of progression of the diseases for which lung transplantation is performed and the variety of supportive therapies available dictate that many specific criteria are related to a specific disease state. However, since the average waiting time in the United States for donor lungs is more than 550 days, a *life expectancy of 2 years or less* is considered a critical criterion for patients who deserve further evaluation as potential transplant recipients. Sufficient debility to result in a *New York Heart Association class III or class IV* status is also a general indicator of a potential transplant candidate. As physical rehabilitation is an important component of posttransplant therapy, it is important that all potential recipients be able to participate in such a *rehabilitation program*. Although most patients with parenchymal diseases also engage in a preoperative rehabilitation program, patients with pulmonary vascular disease cannot do so because of the considerable risks of such preoperative therapy. For these patients, participation in rehabilitation programs is generally deferred until after the transplant procedure. However, an appropriate psychological and emotional context can be promoted by regular preoperative participation in a patient support group (Table 106-2).

Absolute contraindications to lung transplantation include *bone marrow failure* and *hepatic cirrhosis,* the latter to be distinguished from reversible hepatic dysfunction due to right heart failure, which resolves following lung transplantation. In exceptional circumstances, combined liver and lung transplantation may be contemplated, although the risks of such a procedure are likely to be prohibitive. An *active malignancy precluding long-term survival,* which in the case of most solid tumors implies a disease-free survival beyond 5 years, is also an absolute contraindication. Because of the current limited supply of donor lungs, other significant life-limiting disorders also stand as a proscription against lung transplantation (Table 106-3).

A host of additional factors may be considered relative contraindications to lung transplantation. The age of the recipient may be a significant factor in view of the limited number of donor organs and the presumed subclinical organ dysfunction associated with the aging process that increases the potential for postoperative complications. As the latter factor is variable, a "physiological age" rather than a strict chronologic criterion is appropriate. The type of transplant procedure also influences the significance of age as a contraindication. (Isolated single-lung transplantation is more suitable for older patients because of its lower risk.) Other contraindications are evidence of psychosocial instability that would preclude compliance with the necessary posttransplant regimens and active use of tobacco products

TABLE 106-1

Recipient Evaluation for Lung Transplantation

Hematology
  Complete blood count with differential, platelet count, PT, PTT, ESR
Chemistry
  Na, K, Cl, CO_2, BUN, Cr, glucose, osmolality, uric acid, Ca, P, Mg, total protein, albumin, globulin, amylase, bilirubin (direct, indirect), alkaline phosphatase, SGOT, LDH, CPK, triglycerides, cholesterol, HDL/LDL
Renal function
  Urinalysis, 24 h for calcium and creatinine
Endocrine
  TSH, LH, FSH, vitamin D, testosterone (males), estradiol (females)
Infectious disease
  Sputum (Gram's stain, C+S, fungal smear and culture, AFB smear and culture), CMV, hepatitis B (antigen/antibody), hepatitis C, herpes, varicella, EBV, HIV, rapidplasma reagin, toxoplasma PPD, mumps, *Candida* skin tests
Immunology
  ABO blood type and cross match, MHC typing, HLA sensitization (PRA screen)
Radiology
  Chest radiograph (AP, lateral), high-resolution chest CT scan, quantitative V/Q scan, quantitative bone density, abdominal ultrasonography, sinus CT*
Cardiology
  ECG, echocardiogram with pulse Doppler imaging, right heart catheterization, left heart catheterization[†]
Pulmonary
  Pulmonary function tests (spirometry, lung volumes, DLCO), Baird level II exercise test[‡]

*Septic lung disease.
[†]If >50 years of age, coronary artery disease or LVEF <45%.
[‡]Excluding patients with pulmonary hypertension.

during the wait for transplantation. Obesity or cachexia can increase the risk for perioperative morbidity. The same is true of the continued need for high doses of steroid therapy (e.g., more than 20 mg of prednisone per day).

Respiratory failure requiring mechanical ventilation before transplantation also increases the likelihood of complications. Most centers will not consider a new patient for evaluation who is completely ventilator dependent or has acutely deteriorated and become ventilator dependent. However, patients who have a chronic need for partial ventilatory assistance or those who have been accepted as transplant candidates and require assisted ventilation because of progression of their native disease may still be considered potential recipients for a limited time. Prolonged mechanical ventilation results in colonization of the lower respiratory tract with significant microbiologic pathogens and a degree of deconditioning and protein wasting that significantly increases the perioperative risk of transplantation.

Chronic renal disease may affect eligibility for lung transplantation. All immunosuppressive regimens have some element of renal insufficiency as a complication of therapy, as do many of the antimicrobial regimens required for the management of these patients. As with irreversible hepatic dysfunction, combined renal and lung transplantation may be considered, but the potential risks of the procedure, particularly in the context of the shortage of donor lungs, require careful consideration. In most patients, severe preexisting renal insufficiency is a contraindication for lung transplantation.

Severe peripheral vascular disease may be a limiting factor in selecting candidates because of the occasional need for cardiopulmonary support in the perioperative period by either partial cardiopulmonary bypass (CPB) or extracorporeal membrane oxygenation (ECMO) via the femoral or subclavian routes. Peripheral vascular disease is also frequently associated with significant coronary or aortic disease, which may greatly increase the morbidity and mortality of the lung transplant procedure. Finally, transplantation in patients with gangrenous changes in the extremities due to peripheral vascular disease is contraindicated because of the potential for systemic spread of the infectious process during immunosuppression.

Postoperatively, patients require an aggressive rehabilitation program to complete their immediate recovery and to achieve maximum functional capacity. Severe preexisting osteoporosis or severe chest wall deformity may complicate these efforts, owing to difficulties with bone fractures, pain management, and ambulatory status. Careful consideration is required before patients with such preexisting disease are accepted for transplantation. In addition, chronic steroid immunosuppressive therapy causes bone loss in all patients and will exacerbate the complications

TABLE 106-2

General Indications for Lung Transplantation

End-stage pulmonary parenchymal and/or vascular disease
  Projected life expectancy <2 years
  NYHA class III or IV functional level
  Rehabilitation potential
  Disease-specific mortality exceeding transplant-specific mortality over 1–2 years

TABLE 106-3

Contraindications to Lung Transplantation

Absolute Contraindications
  Bone marrow failure
  Hepatic cirrhosis
  Active malignancy precluding long-term survival
  Other life-limiting condition

Relative Contraindications
  Physiological age
    >65 for single-lung transplantation
    >60 for bilateral-lung transplantation
    >55 for heart–lung transplantation
  Psychosocial instability
  Tobacco use within 6 months
  Weight outside acceptable range (obesity or cachexia)
  Prednisone use >20 mg/day or 40 mg q.o.d.
  Mechanical ventilation
  Intrinsic renal disease
  Significant peripheral vascular disease
  Symptomatic osteoporosis
  Severe chest wall deformity
  Sputum with panresistant bacteria or *Aspergillus*
  Active hepatitis B or C infection

of prior osteoporosis. Close attention to bone density and calcium homeostasis is required postoperatively in all lung transplant patients on chronic steroid therapy. Most of them benefit from calcium supplementation and/or alendronate to offset the steroid effect.

Infectious diseases have a profound effect on the morbidity and mortality of lung transplantation.[3] Colonization of the respiratory tract with potential pathogens in patients with end-stage pulmonary disease requires careful assessment of anatomic changes in the airways and determination of antimicrobial susceptibility. Significant anatomic abnormalities that preclude mechanical drainage of secretions in either the upper or lower respiratory tract should be dealt with preoperatively (e.g., drainage of chronic sinusitis in patients with cystic fibrosis) or at the time of the transplantation (e.g., removal of the lung containing a focal area of bronchiectasis). Most bacterial flora in transplant candidates have a pattern of antibiotic sensitivity that can be identified preoperatively in order to define a perioperative antibiotic regimen. However, *Pseudomonas cepaciae*, a pathogen found in approximately 15 percent of patients with cystic fibrosis, is often highly resistant to antimicrobials and is a relative contraindication to transplantation unless a suitable pattern of antibiotic sensitivity can be identified before transplantation. *Aspergillus fumigatus* and other *Aspergillus* species are also common pathogens in the sputum of patients with septic lung disease or COPD. A history of *Aspergillus* in the sputum of a potential transplant recipient requires prophylactic perioperative therapy with amphotericin B to eliminate the potential for an invasive infection postoperatively.

Viral diseases in a potential lung transplant recipient can also have a significant impact on the outcome of transplantation. Active hepatitis B or C in the lung transplant candidate increases

both early and late mortality because of the effect of hepatic dysfunction on perioperative complications and the accelerated progression of these diseases in patients requiring chronic immunosuppression. Cytomegalovirus (CMV), a DNA-type virus that is incorporated into the host genome, can cause both a systemic illness and a pneumonitis in immunosuppressed patients. The serologic CMV status of the recipient is therefore an important determination to make before transplantation. While some centers prefer to match donor and recipient CMV status as a strategy for minimizing perioperative complications, the use of preemptive prophylactic ganciclovir therapy has been shown to eliminate CMV disease in transplant patients.[1] However, some strains of CMV are resistant to ganciclovir, and because the occurrence of CMV disease is a significant risk factor for morbidity and mortality, ongoing surveillance for CMV based on antigenemia assays and transbronchial lung biopsy is required.[3,14]

Immunologic study of potential transplant candidates includes assessment of ABO status and cross matching for transfusion. All patients are currently matched to donors by ABO status, most commonly with ABO-identical donors; virtually all patients require some transfusion in the perioperative period. MHC status is also assessed preoperatively, primarily for use in studies of postoperative outcome, such as the effect of HLA–DR mismatching or donor–recipient microchimerism on chronic rejection.[4,24] Screening for sensitization to HLA antigens is also done at some centers. Pregnancy, blood transfusion, or prior transplantation can lead to HLA sensitization. Before transplantation, potential recipients who show a response of more than 15 percent to the panel of antigens will require a direct lymphocytotoxic cross match with any potential donor before transplantation.

Specific Disease States

The rate of progression of the specific diseases is an important factor in the timing of the evaluation and selection of potential transplant recipients. The most common indication for lung transplantation is *obstructive lung disease,* with COPD accounting for 30 percent of all lung transplants and emphysema due to α_1-antitrypsin deficiency accounting for 15 percent of all lung transplants. Patients with these diseases, who demonstrate chronic airway obstruction on pulmonary function tests, tend to remain relatively stable for long periods. Although lung transplantation provides marked symptomatic and functional palliation for these patients, it remains to be proved that lung transplantation improves survival. The FEV_1 after administration of a bronchodilator is an excellent predictor of the severity of the disease and is useful, along with assessment of resting Pa_{O_2} and Pa_{CO_2}, in estimating survival before transplantation. A postbronchodilator FEV_1 of less than 25 percent of the predicted value, particularly if associated with significant hypoxemia or hypercarbia, heralds a shortened survival, thereby identifying patients who may be transplant candidates (Table 106-4). Death during the wait for transplantation is rare in these patients, occurring in less than 5 percent of cases. This may be due in part to two factors: their participation in a graduated rehabilitation program while they await transplantation, which may maintain or even increase the patients' functional capacity, and the institution of oxygen therapy, which improves survival in patients with obstruc-

TABLE 106-4

Disease-Specific Indications for Lung Transplantation

Obstructive Lung Disease—FEV_1 <25% predicted, postbronchodilator
  Chronic obstructive pulmonary disease
  α_1-Antitrypsin deficiency
Restrictive Lung Disease
  Idiopathic pulmonary fibrosis—FVC <50% predicted, Pa_{O_2} <50 mmHg, Pa_{CO_2} >45 mmHg
    Pulmonary artery hypertension
    No response to steroid therapy
  Interstitial lung disease
    Sarcoidosis
    Desquamative interstitial pneumonitis
    Lymphangioleiomyomatosis
    Chemotherapy- or radiation therapy–related fibrosis
    Collagen vascular disorders with primarily pulmonary involvement
    Eosinophilic granuloma or histiocytosis X
    Alveolar microlithiasis
Septic Lung Disease
  Cystic fibrosis—FEV_1 <30% predicted, FVC ≤40% predicted, Pa_{O_2} <60 mmHg, room air
  Bilateral bronchiectasis
    Hypogammaglobulinemia
    Postinfectious (childhood measles, pertussis, postpneumonia, or tuberculosis)
    Immotile cilia syndrome—Kartagener's syndrome
    Allergic bronchopulmonary aspergillosis
Pulmonary Vascular Disease
  Primary pulmonary hypertension—symptomatic disease
  Eisenmenger's syndrome

tive lung disease. Supplemental oxygen should be started early and continued throughout the pretransplantation period, along with serial assessments of oxygen consumption based on estimates obtained from the 6-min walk test.[5]

Restrictive lung diseases are the indication for lung transplantation in 20 percent of patients who undergo lung transplantation. The most common cause is idiopathic pulmonary fibrosis (IPF), which accounts for 15 percent of lung transplant patients, whereas a variety of interstitial lung diseases with mixed physiological characteristics account for the remainder (Table 106-4).

The end-stage fibrotic lung is characterized by severe destruction of gas exchange units, distortion and dilatation of the airways with development of cystic lesions, and replacement of the lung with nondistensible fibrous tissues. The work of breathing in these patients may be increased five times above normal because of the increased elastic load. The vital capacity in patients with pulmonary fibrosis is severely reduced, as is the functional residual capacity (FRC), which is a better indicator of disease severity than total lung capacity. Dead-space ventilation is increased, and may actually increase further during exercise. A marked reduction in diffusing capacity is always present, commonly with some degree of alveolar hyperventilation; as the disease becomes increasingly severe, hypercapnia occurs during exercise and later at rest. Extensive intrapulmonary shunting of blood flow is seen, resulting in hypoxemia and, in later stages, pulmonary hypertension. Progression of the disease may be variable, but patients often deteriorate precipitously and severely, developing progressive hypoxemia and pulmonary hypertension.

As a result, the mortality of these patients while they await transplantation is more than 20 percent. Criteria for considering IPF patients for of transplantation include severe dyspnea, forced vital capacity (FVC) less than 50 percent of predicted, resting arterial hypoxemia or hypercarbia, and pulmonary hypertension. However, a downhill clinical course despite adequate medical therapy is the best individual indication for transplantation.

Because airway obstruction is frequently a component of the lung disease in some patients with interstitial lung disease, an FEV_1 of less than 30 percent of predicted may be an additional useful criterion. Two other factors in patients with interstitial lung disease are also important: many of these diseases are systemic, and the effects of the disease on extrapulmonary organs may result in a sufficient number of relative contraindications to exclude the patient from consideration for transplantation; and a number of these diseases, including sarcoidosis and lymphangiomyomatosis, have been shown to recur in the lung graft, underscoring the need for particularly cautious screening of such patients as potential candidates for transplantation.

Septic lung disease, including cystic fibrosis and other types of bronchiectasis, accounts for 15 to 20 percent of patients undergoing lung transplantation. Candidates with focal or unilateral disease can often be managed with medical treatment or surgical resection of the affected area. In most patients, however, the disease is bilateral or systemic, and the natural history is one of recurrent infection and progressive pulmonary failure. It is important to attempt to establish a cause of the bronchiectasis before transplant evaluation, because of the impact of systemic diseases on management before and after transplantation (Table 106-4). Cystic fibrosis can be diagnosed with a sweat test or from genotyping. Serum immunoglobulin levels should be measured and a careful assessment for evidence for a systemic illness—such as rheumatoid arthritis, ulcerative colitis, or immotile cilia syndrome—should be undertaken. Primary infectious causes, such as tuberculosis and allergic bronchopulmonary aspergillosis, should be identified and treated appropriately before transplantation. Finally, any suggestion of aspiration as a primary or secondary factor demands further investigation, including a barium swallow.

Many of these patients demonstrate significant short-term improvements in response to aggressive medical therapy, which includes postural drainage, intravenous and inhaled antibiotics, and nutritional supplementation. Once medical therapy has been optimized, however, a pattern of more frequent hospitalizations for "clean-outs," continued weight loss, and progressive functional impairment is indicative of a patient who has a limited life span and should be given priority for transplantation. Cystic fibrosis patients with an FEV_1 under 30 percent of the predicted value, a Pa_{O_2} under 55 mmHg, or a Pa_{CO_2} greater than 50 mmHg have a 2-year mortality of 50 percent; the FEV_1 appears to be the most sensitive predictive factor.[25,38] Any patient with septic lung disease who manifests these criteria should be further evaluated as a potential transplant recipient. While the patient is awaiting transplantation, close medical follow-up is required, and all of the patient's therapeutic regimen (e.g., postural drainage, DNAse therapy) should be continued. Serial study of sputum microbiology is important for assessing changes in flora. Aerosolized broad-spectrum antibiotic therapy (e.g., colistin 150 mg via nebulizer twice a day) reduces the bacterial load while minimizing the potential for renal toxicity; in some cases, it may transiently improve functional capacity. In the event of progressive hemoptysis, bronchial artery embolization can provide adequate short-term control of the bleeding without significantly compromising technical aspects of the transplant procedure. Finally, institution of nasal ventilation in the patient who is approaching respiratory failure has been shown to prolong viability without adversely affecting the outcome of transplantation. Application of these measures generally ensures that fewer than 20 percent of cystic fibrosis patients will die while awaiting lung transplantation. However, because of the shortage of donor organs and the variability in the progression of the disease, donation of a lung from a dying related donor may warrant consideration for some patients. Initial results of this approach, using bilateral isolated lobar transplants from two donors, have been encouraging for patients with cystic fibrosis, without entailing donor mortality or significant morbidity.[41]

Pulmonary vascular disease, either primary pulmonary hypertension (PPH) or secondary pulmonary hypertension due to Eisenmenger's syndrome, accounts for 10 to 15 percent of patients requiring isolated lung transplantation and for 45 to 50 percent of patients requiring heart–lung transplantation. The criteria for identifying patients who may require transplantation relate to the risks of death due to the underlying disease. On the basis of data from the National Heart, Lung, and Blood Institute registry, patients with PPH have an estimated life span of 2.8 years from the time of cardiac catheterization. In this study popula-

tion, sudden death occurred in 26 percent; in 46 percent, death was due to progressive right ventricular failure. At 5 years, only 34 percent of patients were alive.[10] From this registry, it is apparent that a NYHA class III or IV functional status, an elevated central venous pressure, a decreased cardiac index, and an elevated *mean* pulmonary artery pressure correlate with a poor prognosis. Episodes of near-syncope, syncope, or near-death, which tend to occur later in the course of the disease, are also associated with mortality. It should be noted, however, that alleviation of symptoms or physiological abnormalities by medical therapy using high-dose calcium channel blockers or prostacyclin infusions in PPH patients may significantly modify the natural history of the disease. Therefore, symptomatic patients with PPH who do not respond to medical therapy are the ones best considered for transplantation. Although identical data concerning the natural history of patients with Eisenmenger's syndrome are not available, similar clinical criteria and evidence of a declining functional status associated with progressive right heart failure are indications for transplantation in these patients.

The decision about whether a patient should undergo isolated lung transplantation or heart–lung transplantation may be difficult. However, with the relative shortage of suitable heart–lung donor blocs, and a mortality of 20 to 25 percent among patients with significant pulmonary hypertension who are awaiting lung transplantation, an increasing number of patients with pulmonary vascular disease have undergone isolated lung transplantation. The results with isolated lung transplantation are similar to those with heart–lung transplantation for pulmonary vascular disease provided that there is no significant left ventricular dysfunction [i.e., absence of cardiomyopathy, left ventricular ejection fraction (LVEF) at least 45 percent], that right ventricular *diastolic* function is maintained (i.e., right ventricular end-diastolic (RVEDP) of 15 mmHg or under), and that there are no incorrectable structural abnormalities. Of interest, the presence of severe right ventricular systolic dysfunction [i.e., right ventricular ejection fraction pressure (RVEF) of 20 percent or less] does not appear to affect the results of isolated lung transplantation, and the severe tricuspid regurgitation and pulmonary valvular regurgitation that are present in virtually all patients preoperatively resolve almost immediately after isolated lung transplantation. Patients with Eisenmenger's syndrome who have a shunt defect that can be corrected at the time of transplantation are also candidates for isolated lung transplantation.[15] Heart–lung transplantation is primarily limited to patients with either significant biventricular dysfunction (e.g., severe valvular cardiomyopathy) or incorrectable congenital heart defects.

TRANSPLANT PROCEDURE SELECTION

Except for patients with bilateral septic lung disease or severe pulmonary arterial hypertension, single-lung transplantation (SLT) is optimal for the majority of end-stage pulmonary diseases that require transplantation.[8,27,45] SLT is associated with a shorter wait for donor lungs before transplantation and a lower morbidity and mortality rate after transplantation than other lung transplant procedures performed for the same recipient diagnoses. The surgical mortality for SLT ranges from 3 to 10 percent, relating to the specific transplant indication, the presence or absence of pulmonary hypertension, and the intraoperative need for cardiopulmonary bypass.

Double-lung transplantation (DLT) is the procedure of choice for patients with bilateral septic lung disease, such as cystic fibrosis, or for patients with pulmonary arterial pressures that are at near-systemic levels from either primary or secondary causes. Some centers also favor the use of DLT for patients with emphysema who are less than 50 years of age.[8] Typically, however, surgical mortality is higher for DLT than for SLT, ranging from 10 to 15 percent. Surgical mortality is probably higher because of the number of patients with septic lung disease treated by DLT—patients who are at greater risk for complications. Notably, at most large centers, perioperative morbidity from other than infectious complications, including acute graft failure and bronchial dehiscence, is similar for SLT and DLT. For patients with pulmonary vascular disease, DLT is favored over SLT for patients with the higher levels of pulmonary artery (PA) pressures (e.g., systolic PA at least 90 mmHg or mean PA at least 65 mmHg) and more advanced right ventricular dysfunction (e.g., RVEF 20 percent or less).

Combined heart–lung transplantation (HLT) has been used successfully for virtually all end-stage pulmonary diseases that require transplantation. However, with the perfection of the techniques of SLT and DLT and in light of the significant limitations in supply of donor organs, the use of HLT has focused on patients with significant refractory right ventricular *diastolic* dysfunction (e.g., RVEDP more than 15 mmHg), significant intrinsic left ventricular dysfunction, or Eisenmenger's syndrome and irreparable shunt defects.[9] The surgical mortality for HLT at large centers is about 15 percent; typically, it is higher than the surgical mortality for SLT or DLT for similar disease states (Table 106-5).

DONOR SELECTION

The most significant factor limiting wider application of lung transplantation is the supply of donor organs. Unlike other solid organs used for transplantation, the lung is exposed, before brain death, to environmental contamination, including both microbiologic pathogens and toxic substances, which may significantly impair its functional capabilities. The microbiologic aspects of this exposure are accentuated by the endotracheal intubation that is a necessary aspect of donor management. In addition, aspiration of oropharyngeal or gastric contents is a common occurrence during the events preceding brain death.

Nearly half of all comatose patients will develop pneumonia within 1 week of intubation, probably owing to a combination of these factors. Brain death itself may also lead to neurogenic pulmonary edema. In cases of trauma that lead to brain death, significant injury to the thorax may occur, or the volume replacement required for the resuscitation of these patients may limit the suitability of the lungs for subsequent transplantation. As a result, only about 25 percent of cadaveric organ donors are potential lung donors.

Criteria for lung donation are meant to identify donors with evidence of good gas exchange in the absence of infection of the airways or parenchyma (Table 106-6). A donor age of less than 60 years and a history of smoking for less than 20 to 30 pack-years are important. Both increasing age and prolonged tobacco use are known to correlate directly with anatomic alterations in the pulmonary parenchyma—which, despite preservation of gas exchange function in the donor, may result in impaired graft function in the recipient. Chest radiograph should reveal a normal lung on the side of the proposed lung donation. Unilateral pneumonia or parenchymal trauma does not preclude use of the contralateral lung for transplantation in most circumstances. No major thoracic surgery should have been performed on the side of proposed donation, not only because of potential technical limitations but also because such a history usually suggests either a major anatomic abnormality (e.g., prior lobectomy) or pathology (e.g., malignant neoplasm), which would preclude donation.

Finally, the size of the donor lungs, based on direct measurement or correlated to body surface area as estimated by donor height, is a useful parameter for one to use when selecting lungs for a particular recipient. Generally, the donor lungs should be within 25 to 30 percent of the *predicted* size of the recipient's lungs. Since most recipients have significant abnormalities in lung volume, the predicted size of an ideal recipient lung, estimated from the recipient's body surface area, should be used for comparison. A donor lung larger than these measurements can be volume reduced at the time of transplantation, whereas a donor lung smaller than these measurements should usually be avoided.

Adequate gas exchange has been defined as a Pa_{O_2} greater than 300 mmHg on mechanical ventilation, with an F_{IO_2} of 1.0 and positive end-expiratory pressure (PEEP) at least 5 cm H_2O. Minute ventilation should be adjusted to achieve normocarbia, with a tidal volume of 10 to 15 ml/kg and an appropriate respiratory rate. If a unilateral

---

TABLE 106-5

Indications for Specific Lung Transplant Procedures

Single-lung transplantation (SLT)
  Obstructive lung disease
  Restrictive lung disease
  Unilateral septic lung disease
  Primary pulmonary hypertension
  Eisenmenger's syndrome with a correctable shunt defect
Double-lung transplantation (DLT)
  Obstructive lung disease (patient <50 years old)
  Bilateral septic lung disease
  Primary pulmonary hypertension
  Eisenmenger's syndrome with a correctable shunt defect
Combined heart–lung transplantation (HLT)
  Refractory right ventricular end-diastolic dysfunction (RVEDP >15 mmHg)
  Significant intrinsic left ventricular dysfunction (LVEF <45%)
  Significant coronary artery disease, not amenable to nonsurgical interventions
  Eisenmenger's syndrome with an irreparable shunt defect

TABLE 106-6

Characteristics of a Suitable Lung Donor

Age <60 years
Cigarette smoking <30 pack-years
No significant prior thoracic surgery on the side of the donor lung
Normal chest radiograph of the donor lung
Adequate gas exchange of the donor lung
    Pa_{O_2} >300 mmHg on $F_{I_{O_2}}$ 1.0, PEEP ≥5 cm
    Pv_{O_2} >450 mmHg on $F_{I_{O_2}}$ 1.0, PEEP ≥5 cm
Bronchoscopic evaluation demonstrating absence of mucosal inflammation
No significant pulmonary trauma or anatomic abnormalities

pulmonary process is present, however, a lower Pa_{O_2} may be acceptable because of the possibility of mixing of venous blood from the two lungs at the level of the left atrium. In this circumstance, intraoperative evaluation of unilateral gas exchange by sampling from the ipsilateral pulmonary vein for determination of P_{O_2} can be used to determine that the prospective donor lung is satisfactory.[35]

All lung donors will have some evidence of colonization of the lower respiratory tract by potential pathogens owing to the requisite endotracheal intubation, which bypasses the defense mechanisms of the upper airway. A distal tracheitis is uniformly present after 72 h of intubation. Therefore, a sputum Gram's stain revealing polymorphonuclear leukocytes or multiple bacterial forms does not necessarily imply invasive infection. For this reason, bronchoscopy is a critical step in the evaluation of any potential lung donor. Bronchoscopy allows inspection of the large airways for the presence of aspirated debris as well as assessment of the character of the secretions and the status of the bronchial mucosa. A finding of diffuse bronchial mucosal inflammation is significant, even if only a limited amount of aspirated debris or secretions are present. However, purulent secretions without significant mucosal inflammation in the presence of a clear chest radiograph and preserved gas exchange generally indicate a suitable lung for donation. A potassium hydroxide smear for fungal organisms is also a part of the routine evaluation of the lung donor, although as with the Gram's stain, the mere presence of fungal organisms does not preclude lung donation. In most cases, the presence of potential pathogens in the donor sputum by either Gram's stain or fungal smear requires preemptive modification of the recipient's antimicrobial regimen if such lungs are used for transplantation. At some centers, this treatment is begun by the administration of intravenous or aerosolized antimicrobial therapy to the donor before extraction of the lungs.[26]

The donor evaluation is completed by intraoperative inspection of the pleural space and lung.[44] Occasionally, unsuspected parenchymal trauma is evident in the form of a bloody pleural effusion or a pulmonary contusion. The donor lung should also be studied for evidence of unsuspected bullous disease or mass lesions. Excisional biopsy and intraoperative pathologic evaluation of any parenchymal mass lesion should be carried out. Finally, the anesthesiologist should be directed to maintain adequate tidal volumes and PEEP during intraoperative ventilation to preserve optimal function of the donor lung before its removal.

The appropriateness of a potential lung donor should always be interpreted in the context of the recipient's disease and clinical status. Older patients, patients with diseases such as COPD (in whom lung transplantation may be largely palliative), and patients with a sudden clinical deterioration, such as those who have recently been placed on mechanical ventilation, may all benefit from transplantation with a lung that does not fulfill all the criteria of an optimal donor lung. Most frequently, the criteria relating to cigarette smoking and Pa_{O_2} are breeched in these circumstances. The results have generally been satisfactory in such recipients, suggesting that the use of these "compromised" lung donors may partly address the problem of donor organ shortage.[42] It has also been shown that the effect of the functional status of the donor lung is most significant in the first 24 h after transplantation, and that subsequent graft function depends primarily on factors related to the recipient.[39] However, the potential effects of using compromised lung on long-term issues, such as the incidence of rejection, is not known. In addition, these studies have underscored that patients with pulmonary hypertension, who are the most difficult to manage postoperatively, are best served by transplantation with noncompromised lungs from optimal donors.

LUNG PRESERVATION

The ideal method of pulmonary preservation has not yet been identified. With current techniques, however, satisfactory graft function can be obtained after ischemic intervals as long as 6 to 8 h. As with other vascularized solid organs used for transplantation, the lung consists of a heterogeneous population of cells, of which the vascular endothelial cell appears to be the most sensitive to ischemia. Ischemic injury to the pulmonary vascular endothelium increases its permeability and results in pulmonary edema, the common end point for assessment of injury in models of pulmonary preservation techniques. Hypothermia is the major method used clinically to limit ischemic injury to these cells. The lung also has some unique biologic and physical characteristics that distinguish it from other solid organ transplants: although it has an absolute requirement for aerobic metabolism, the lung is capable of using ambient oxygen for the metabolism of glucose, even during the ischemic state.[11] In addition, the effective size of the pulmonary vascular bed and the thermal conductivity of the lung can be manipulated by the state of lung inflation. Current clinical methods of lung preservation make use of these characteristics to optimize graft function following an ischemic interval.

Two techniques are currently being used for lung preservation, core cooling and hypothermic flush perfusion. *Extracorporeal core cooling* (ECC) is a technique that has been used primarily for procurement of heart–lung donor blocs, commonly in conjunction with multiorgan procurement at abdominal sites. ECC consists of systemic heparinization of the donor and institution of full CPB by means of a transpericardial approach. The donor is cooled to 15°C (rectal temperature). Ventricular fibrillation typically develops during this maneuver, and the heart is decompressed through the left ventricle. CPB is then discontinued, and the heart–lung bloc is harvested and transported in a cold ischemic state with the lungs inflated. No flush solutions are used, although the lungs are essentially being flushed by cooled autologous blood during the time of CPB. Safe ischemic times of 6 h or more have been reported with adequate pulmonary function. It is of interest that while oxygenation in lungs preserved by ECC appears to be somewhat less optimal than in those preserved by hypothermic flush techniques, the pulmonary vascular resistance upon reperfusion of the lungs following ECC is generally lower than that seen upon reperfusion of lungs obtained by flush techniques.

Hypothermic flush perfusion is the method most commonly used for pulmonary preservation in clinical practice. This technique consists of flushing the pulmonary vasculature with a cold solution after systemic heparinization of the donor, followed by extraction and transport of the lungs inflated with 100 percent oxygen. A cold intracellular solution with an osmolarity slightly higher than that of serum is used. Euro-Collins' solution, modified by the addition of magnesium sulfate (4 meq/L) and 65 ml of 50 percent dextrose to each liter, is the most commonly used solution. University of Wisconsin solution has also been used and at some centers appears to provide superior preservation. A volume of 50 to 60 ml/kg of donor body weight, delivered via large-bore pulmonary artery cannula over 4 to 5 min, is the preferred technique of administration.

The state of inflation of the lungs is important in obtaining optimal perfusion of the pulmonary vasculature by the flush solution, for the effects both of rapid cooling and of direct cellular preservation by the solution itself. Intraoperatively, maintaining a tidal volume similar to that used during the initial donor assessment is important. The addition of PEEP during the procurement procedure maintains FRC and the desired state of inflation of the donor lungs. PEEP also increases the intra-alveolar release of surfactant, minimizing pulmonary compliance abnormalities after implantation of the donor lungs. Ventilation is continued throughout the period of lung perfusion to maintain the effective size of the pulmonary vascular bed. Maintenance of an F_{IO_2} of 1.0 during the procurement is also useful, particularly at the time of lung extraction, to provide an oxygen-rich ambient environment for metabolic activity of the lung during the ischemic interval. The lungs are extracted and transported in a state of inflation that approximates end-tidal inspiration. Some consideration should be given to the fact that the donor lungs may be transported by aircraft, in which a fall in atmospheric pressure may result in further inflation of the lungs. Overinflation of the donor lungs is to be avoided, as this leads to increased capillary permeability and postimplantation pulmonary edema.

The administration of prostanoids, either prostaglandin E_1 (PgE_1) or prostacyclin, into the pulmonary circulation before flush perfusion has been shown to improve lung preservation. The mechanism of action of prostanoids includes dilation of the pulmonary vasculature, allowing for better distribution of the flush solution, and decreased leukocyte adhesiveness, which can abrogate the initial events of reperfusion injury. Most commonly in North America, PgE_1 is used as a bolus (500 μg) into the pulmonary circula-

tion, with or without the addition of similar amounts of PgE_1 directly to the flush solution. The use of prostanoids in combination with intracellular flush solutions has been shown to provide pulmonary preservation equivalent, if not superior, to that with the use of extracellular-type flush solutions alone.

Most flush solutions are administered at a temperature of 4°C, while topical cooling is carried out by filling of the pleural cavity with iced crystalloid solution. After extraction, the lungs are immersed in crystalloid and packed in ice, resulting in a transport temperature of 1 to 4°C. Some studies have shown that lung preservation is superior when a more moderate hypothermia with a temperature of 10°C is used. However, because of the concerns regarding the deleterious effects of flush and storage temperatures greater than 10°C, and the difficulties in maintaining this temperature during the procurement procedure, clinical flush perfusion continues to be performed at the lower temperature ranges.

Experimental work has identified numerous adjuncts to the techniques currently used for pulmonary preservation that have the potential for prolonging ischemic intervals. A significant part of the lung injury seen after ischemia has been shown to be due to the phenomenon of reperfusion, which is initiated by leukocyte adhesion to endothelial cells and the production of oxygen-derived free radicals and peroxides. Measures that diminish this response, in addition to the use of prostanoids, include donor leukocyte depletion, the administration of antibodies to block adhesion molecules, the use of inhaled nitric oxide, and the inclusion of oxygen radical scavengers, such as superoxide dismutase or catalase, to the flush solution. In addition, methods of increasing the resistance of cells to ischemic injury, such as the induction of heat shock proteins, have been shown to be beneficial in other organs and may be of some use in lung preservation. Evidence of the effect of these manipulations on tolerable ischemic intervals in clinical lung transplantation awaits additional study.[6,30]

TECHNIQUES OF LUNG TRANSPLANTATION

Anesthetic Management

Proper perioperative management of the recipient is crucial to obtain the best outcome following lung transplantation. Close cooperation and understanding between the anesthesiology and surgical teams are essential. An appreciation of the unique aspects of the physiology of the various types of lung transplant recipient is also important. Patients with COPD have reduced expiratory flow rates, air trapping, and increased lung volumes. In advanced states, chronic pulmonary artery hypertension develops and leads to cor pulmonale in 10 to 40 percent of patients. These patients are usually oxygen dependent, dyspneic, orthopneic, and quite anxious. Following endotracheal intubation, extreme care should be taken to allow adequate expiratory time for emptying of the lungs, avoiding the cardiovascular instability caused by "pulmonary tamponade" due to progressive air trapping in the lungs and reduction of ventricular filling. Tension pneumothorax due to rupture of bullae can also occur but is relatively uncommon. Patients with *restrictive lung disease* have progressive fibrosis of the lung tissue, with secondary hypoxemia and progressive pulmonary hypertension. Patients with these diseases have an increased work of breathing and are oxygen dependent and extremely dyspneic before transplantation. Many of these patients will have evidence of cor pulmonale at the time of transplantation and will not tolerate occlusion of the pulmonary artery during implantation of the donor lung without the support of cardiopulmonary bypass. Careful and repeated assessment of filling pressures and cardiac output is required to allow prompt interventions in such patients.

Patients with *septic lung disease* demonstrate primarily the abnormalities in pulmonary function seen in patients with obstructive airway disease. However, these recipients have excessive copious purulent secretions, which can exacerbate air trapping and also contribute to marked V/Q abnormalities—particularly during single-lung ventilation. Careful management of double-lumen endotracheal tubes to avoid contamination of the contralateral lung graft and attention to bronchopulmonary hygiene to avoid obstruction of the lumens of these tubes are needed in these patients. Finally, recipients with *pulmonary vascular disease* who present for transplantation have marginally compensated cor pulmonale and are extremely dyspneic and anxious. Patients with PPH become oxygen dependent late in the course of their disease, although oxygen is commonly administered to these patients to lessen the hypoxic contribution to their pulmonary hypertension. For this reason, oxygen therapy should be continued throughout the time of preoperative preparation and line placement to avoid abrupt right heart dysfunction. Because these patients have normal pulmonary mechanics, they generally tolerate mechanical ventilation well. Patients with Eisenmenger's syndrome are well adapted to chronic hypoxemia. In these patients, supplemental oxygen does not reverse the hypoxemia and may even worsen arterial hypoxemia by eliciting systemic vasodilatation and increasing right-to-left shunting.

All lung transplant procedures should be performed with CPB available on standby. However, CPB is best avoided in cases of septic lung disease or when there are known extensive intrapleural adhesions, to avoid excessive bleeding complications. If CPB is required, the routine use of aprotonin infusions has been shown to reduce the likelihood of postoperative hemorrhage due to excessive fibrinolysis and the requirement for transfusion.[47] No specific preoperative factors can be used to predict the need for CPB—with the exception of either PPH or Eisenmenger's syndrome, for which CPB is requisite for the procedure. For other lung transplant recipients, assessment of the need for CPB is best made intraoperatively by trial clamping of the pulmonary artery, followed by assessment of hemodynamic parameters, oximetry, and, if available, ventricular function testing by transesophageal echocardiography. Progressive deterioration in these parameters requires unclamping of the pulmonary artery and an attempt to optimize factors such as preload, inotropic support, PaO_2, $PaCO_2$, and pulmonary vascular resistance. If repeat trial clamping of the pulmonary artery is still not tolerated, plans for CPB are made. Typically, cannulation after systemic heparinization is via the femoral vessels for SLT and via a transpericardial approach for patients undergoing DLT or HLT.

Single-Lung Transplantation

The approach to SLT requires an initial decision regarding the side of implantation. Most commonly, the native lung with the

least pulmonary function based on preoperative V/Q scans is excised. In some patients, however, specific technical factors, such as a prior pleurodesis, may override this factor. When the function of the two lungs is equal or when the need for CPB is anticipated, the right side is preferred because of the greater ease of surgical exposure and the institution of CPB via the ascending aorta and right atrium. A right-sided approach also facilitates exposure for closure of intracardiac defects in patients with Eisenmenger's syndrome. Despite the potential differences in size of the right and left hemithorax, there does not appear to be any long-term difference in outcome following right or left SLT.

Most often, exposure for SLT is via a generous posterolateral thoracotomy through the fifth intercostal space or the bed of the excised fifth rib. When elective CPB via the right hemithorax is planned, the use of a fourth interspace may facilitate placement of the cannulae. The ipsilateral groin is included in the surgical field in the event that cannulation of the femoral vessels is required for partial CPB. Although the use of femoral sites for cannulation requires repair of the vessels after removal of the cannulae, it does provide a site for additional venous drainage with use of intrathoracic cannulation sites. Femoral cannulation sites also provide access for conversion to ECMO support if acute graft failure occurs immediately after implantation. Occasionally, when the repair of an associated intracardiac defect requires an anterior approach, a median sternotomy may be used for right SLT in patients with Eisenmenger's syndrome.

The donor lung is prepared for implantation and then wrapped in sponges soaked with cold crystalloid solution and placed into the hemithorax. The bronchial anastomosis is performed first. Although a variety of techniques have been described, the essential points are to minimize the length of both the donor and recipient bronchi to preserve collateral blood supply and to achieve some degree of anastomotic overlap. The smaller bronchus, most commonly the donor bronchus, is telescoped into the larger bronchus with either a technique of interrupted sutures or a combination of running sutures on the membranous wall and interrupted sutures on the anterior wall in a figure-eight or horizontal mattress fashion. Polyfilament absorbable suture (e.g., 4-0 polyglactin) or monofilament suture, either absorbable (e.g., polydioxanone) or nonabsorbable (e.g., polypropylene), may be used. The anastomosis is then covered by either local peribronchial tissue or local pedicled flaps of thymic tissue or pericardial fat (Fig. 106-1).

The order of the vascular anatomoses can vary even though the pulmonary artery anastomosis is frequently the more technically difficult to perform. A continuous 5-0 polypropylene suture is used for each anastomosis, leaving the ends untied for de-airing upon reperfusion of the lung. For the pulmonary artery anastomosis, the length of the donor and recipient vessels requires careful assessment to avoid kinking. For the left atrial anastomosis, the confluence of the recipient pulmonary veins is incised to create a left atrial cuff. Occasionally, dissection in the interatrial groove is required to allow more proximal placement of the vascular clamp on the recipient left atrium (Fig. 106-2). After completion of these anastomoses, the lung is gently reinflated. Perfusion of the lung graft is then reestablished, initially in an antegrade fashion, evacuating air via the left atrial suture line. The atrial clamp is removed, with the atrial suture line under a fluid

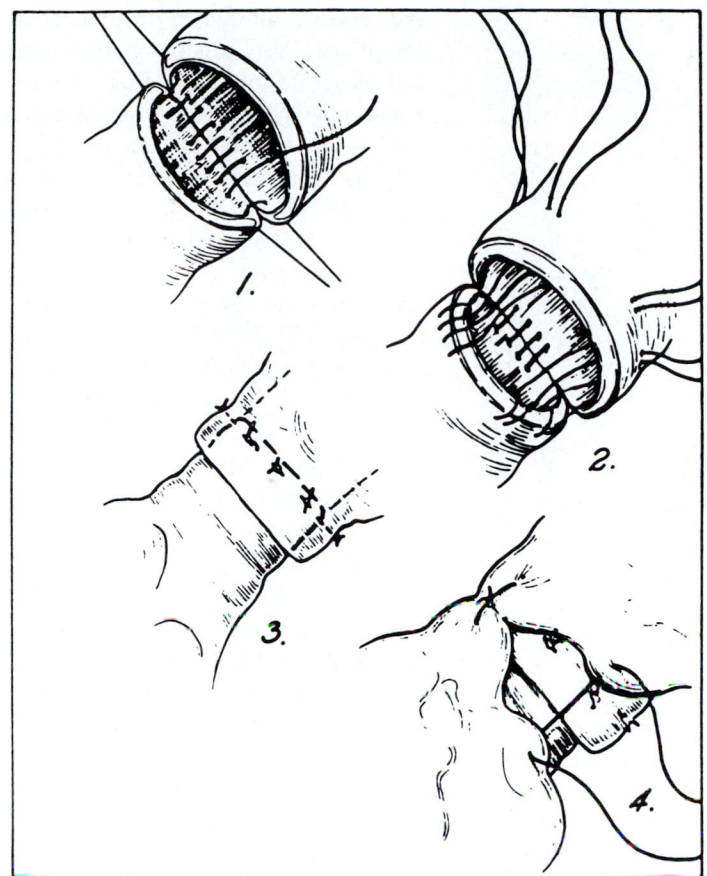

FIGURE 106-1 Bronchial anastomosis for lung transplantation. A technique of approximation using stay sutures at the junction of the cartilaginous and membranous walls is shown. A running suture is used for the membranous wall (1), followed by an interrupted suture technique of horizontal mattress sutures on the cartilaginous wall to achieve telescoping of the donor into the recipient bronchus (2). Significant anastomotic overlap is achieved with this technique (3), with additional anastomotic coverage obtained by approximation of peribronchial and mediastinal tissues about the site (4). *(From Pearson: Thoracic Surgery. New York, Churchill Livingstone, 1995, with permission.)*

level to prevent entrainment of air into the left heart. Ventilation of the donor lung is resumed, and after a few minutes to allow the vascular suture lines to adapt to the distention caused by increased flow, these suture lines are secured. Hemostasis is then obtained, two chest tubes are placed, and the chest is closed in a standard fashion. Following reintubation with a single-lumen tube, flexible bronchoscopy is completed to inspect the bronchial anastomosis and clear the airway of blood or residual secretions.

Double-Lung Transplantation

The most frequently performed DLT procedure is that of bilateral sequential SLT. This procedure has a significantly lower incidence of bronchial complications than the *en bloc* DLT procedure, and is technically less difficult to perform than *en bloc* DLT with simultaneous bronchial artery revascularization. The exposure for bilateral sequential lung transplantation is via bilateral anterolateral thoracotomies through the fourth or fifth intercostal space, connected by a transverse sternotomy—the so-called clam

shell incision (Fig. 106-3). The incision provides adequate exposure for mobilization of intrapleural adhesions, even after previous pulmonary resections or pleurodesis, and also provides excellent access for institution of CPB and correction of intracardiac defects. In most patients, the entire incision is made at the beginning of the procedure, and both lungs are completely mobilized. For patients with emphysema who undergo DLT, however, the contralateral hemithorax may be left closed until after the first lung graft is implanted; this sequence minimizes the tendency to overinflation of the native lung that may occur during the initial implantation procedure. The mobilization and pneumonectomy of the native lung and the implantation of the lung graft are conducted in the same manner as described for SLT. Thymic and anterior mediastinal tissue on a superiorly based vascular pedicle may be mobilized for coverage of the bronchial anastomoses.[32,36]

Living related lung transplantation is most commonly performed as a bilateral sequential transplant procedure using the clam shell incision. Cardiopulmonary bypass is instituted electively after the recipient native lungs are mobilized. Each of the donor lobes is implanted at the recipient hilum. Typically, there is little discrepancy in size between the *lobar* bronchus and pulmonary vein of the donor (usually an adult) and the *main* bronchus and left atrium of the typical pediatric recipient. The order of the anastomoses (bronchus first) and the technique are the same as for cadaveric SLT and DLT. Overinflation of the lobar graft is more likely than with a cadaveric allograft and may contribute to postoperative pulmonary edema. A marked size discrepancy between the lobar allograft and the recipient hemithorax is uncommon; if present, the descrepancy should be treated conservatively (e.g., by avoiding chest tube suction rather than by aggressive surgical measures such as thoracoplasty). In all cases, sufficient remodeling of the thorax or hyperinflation of the lobar grafts will occur to obliterate any residual pleural space.[41]

Heart–Lung Transplantation

Either a standard median sternotomy or a clam shell incision may be used for HLT. The latter provides better access for mobilization of intrapleural incisions and is particularly useful for recipients with septic lung disease or prior pulmonary procedures. Following institution of CPB, the lungs are removed by an extrapericardial approach using successive stapling of the bronchovascular structures at the pulmonary hila.

The donor right atrium is incised from the inferior vena cava to the right atrial appendage. Inspection is made for the presence of an atrial septal defect and for adequate closure of the superior vena cava. The donor bloc is positioned by passing the lungs into the pleural spaces via the retrophrenic pedicles. If a tracheal anastomosis is utlized, the posterior pericardium is incised between the ascending aorta and superior vena cava to expose the distal trachea and, after the donor and recipient tracheas have been trimmed, a distal tracheal anastomosis is performed. Some centers prefer bilateral bronchial anastomoses at the mediastinal pleural reflection, using a telescoping technique as described for SLT. This approach obviates dissection in the posterior mediastinum and may be associated with fewer anastomotic complications. The right atrial anastomosis is completed, followed by

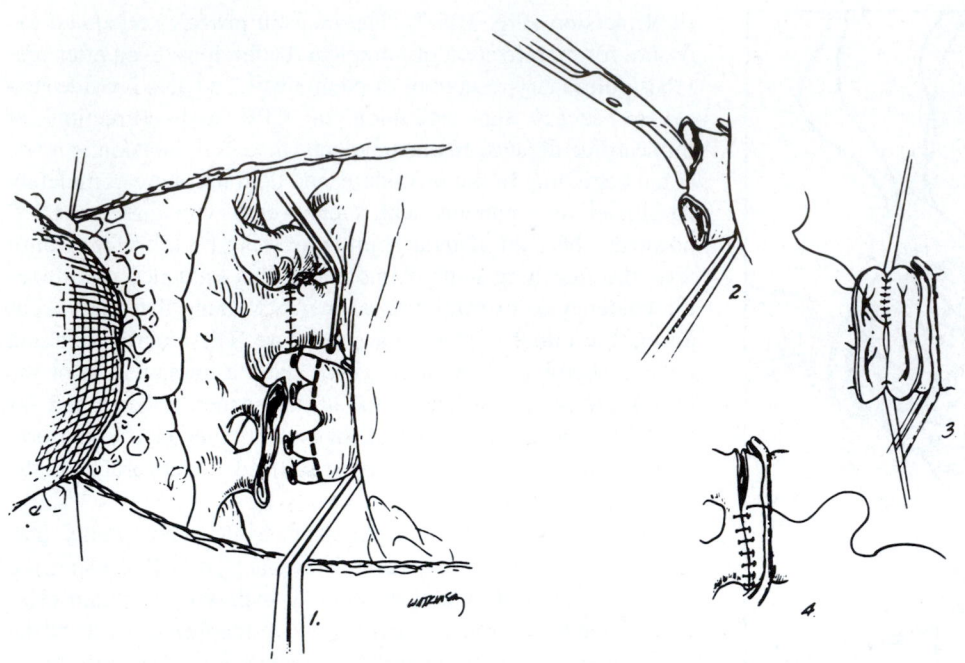

FIGURE 106-2   Implantation of the donor lung at the right hilum. 1. The bronchial anastomosis is performed first, followed by the vascular anastomoses. A clamp is placed on the proximal pulmonary artery, and the anastomosis is performed distal to the first upper-lobe arterial branch in the recipient, which has been ligated. A clamp is placed on the left atrium intrapericardially. 2. After excision of the pulmonary vein stumps, the confluence of the pulmonary veins is incised to create a cuff of left atrium for anastomosis. 3. Atrial anastomosis is performed with a running monofilament suture following approximation with stay sutures superiorly and inferiorly. 4. On completion of the anastomosis, the sutures are left untied until lung reinflation and antegrade reperfusion is completed to evacuate air from the donor vasculature. *(From Shields: General Thoracic Surgery. Philadelphia, Lea & Febiger, 1994, with permission.)*

the aortic anastomosis. The aortic cross clamp is removed, and after reinflation of the lungs, the heart is de-aired via the pulmonary artery and left ventricle. After defibrillation, the patient is weaned from CPB.

POSTOPERATIVE MANAGEMENT

Ventilation

In most cases, ventilatory management folllows standard criteria. The F_{IO_2} is adjusted to maintain a Pa_{O_2} greater than 65 mmHg. Standard volume ventilation is used, with a tidal volume of 12 to 15 ml/kg and PEEP of 5 to 7.5 cm H_2O. Significant barotrauma due to increased airway pressures is extremely uncommon after lung transplantation, and higher airway pressures may have a beneficial effect in minimizing postoperative pulmonary edema. Transition from volume ventilation to pressure ventilation before extubation may be useful to decrease the work of breathing

and serves to minimize differences in compliance between the native lung and allograft following SLT. Appropriate management of postoperative pain is also helpful in weaning these patients from the ventilator. Extubation is performed when the mental status of the patient is normal and the patient has achieved a reasonable rate of ventilation and spontaneous tidal volume, typically 48 to 72 h after the procedure. Maintaining good bronchopulmonary hygiene, with frequent endotracheal aspiration of secretions and physiotherapy, is important in achieving and maintaining extubation in these patients.

Patients with emphysema who undergo SLT are an exception to the above guidelines. These patients require particular attention to airway pressures and to the compliance difference between the allograft and the native lung. Hyperinflation of the native lung may not only result in compromise of cardiac filling but also interferes progressively with ventilation of the allograft. Efforts to control hyperinflation of the native lung include use of slightly lower tidal volumes (9 to 12 ml/kg) accompanied by higher respiratory rates to preserve minute ventilation and lower levels of PEEP (1 to 3 cm H_2O). Positioning

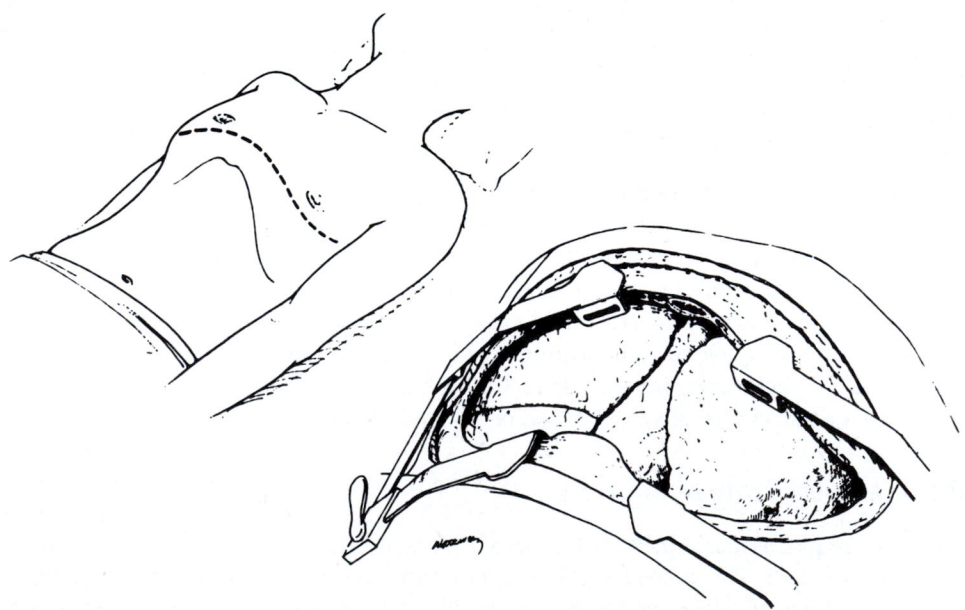

FIGURE 106-3   Approach to double-lung transplantation. The "clam shell" incision is used, consisting of bilateral anterior thoracotomy with transverse sternotomy, defined by the line of the inframammary crease. Entrance into the chest is through either the fourth or fifth intercostal space, followed by placement of bilateral rib retractors. *(From Shields: General Thoracic Surgery, Philadelphia, Lea & Febiger, 1994, with permission.)*

of the patient with the native lung down may further increase the impedance of that hemithorax and limit hyperinflation, although increased blood flow to the native lung induced by this maneuver may require adjustment of ventilatory parameters to maintain normocarbia. In rare circumstances, when significant edema has occurred in the allograft, independent lung ventilation using a double-lumen endotracheal tube may be needed.

In patients with significant pulmonary hypertension who undergo lung transplantation, the postoperative pulmonary hemodynamics are unique. In these patients, the right ventricle has been conditioned to generate peak systolic pressures against a markedly elevated pulmonary vascular resistance (PVR). Following lung transplantation, the PVR abruptly decreases to near-normal levels, accompanied by improved ventricular hemodynamics. Minimal catecholamine stimulation occurs when the patient awakes from anesthesia or is weaned from a ventilator, causing the right ventricle to respond by generating peak systolic pressures similar to those that existed preoperatively. The resultant abrupt increase in pulmonary artery pressure, in combination with increased capillary permeability due to ischemia and reperfusion injury and the absence of lymphatic continuity, causes fluid to accumulate rapidly in the donor lung. Typically, this pulmonary edema is very rapid in onset and results in hypoxia that elicits additional increase in pulmonary artery pressure. Preemptive treatment for this condition is necessary and requires maintenance of a high degree of sedation, or even of muscle paralysis, in the first 3 to 5 days after surgery. Following this period, patients can be awakened cautiously and weaned from the ventilator with standard methods while cardiac output, blood gases, and pulmonary artery pressures are closely monitored.

Fluid Management

The goal of fluid management after lung transplantation is to minimize the accumulation of edema fluid in the implanted lung while maintaining optimal cardiac function. As previously noted, the effects of ischemia, reperfusion injury, and lymphatic discontinuity all contribute to a tendency to develop pulmonary edema in the lung graft. Pulmonary artery pressures and pulmonary capillary wedge pressures need to be kept as low as possible after surgery without compromising ventricular preload. For most patients, a reduction in PVR almost immediately after lung transplantation results in improved right ventricular and, secondarily, left ventricular performance. However, some inotropic support may be required in patients who have preexisting right ventricular hypertrophy, particularly when pressure overload of the right ventricle occurs during the implantation procedure or following CPB.

Antimicrobial Therapy

Bacterial prophylaxis entails the use of vancomycin for prophylaxis against gram-positive organisms in combination with a broad-spectrum antibiotic to provide appropriate coverage for organisms identified preoperatively from the sputum of the recipient. Recipients who have been recently hospitalized, and therefore exposed to respiratory therapy equipment, or those with cystic fibrosis require coverage for *Pseudomonas* species, usually with ceftazidime. For cystic fibrosis patients, ongoing surveillance of sputum flora and determination of antibiotic sensitivities are important in the waiting period before transplantation so that an appropriate multidrug antimicrobial regimen can be developed for perioperative use. The addition of antimicrobial inhalation therapy, using either tobramycin or colistin, can have additive effects in the management of *Pseudomonas*. Postoperative antibacterial coverage should be modified if pathogens not already covered by the recipient-specific regimen are found in the sputum of the donor.

Routine prophylaxis for fungal organisms is useful when preoperative recipient sputum cultures have demonstrated the presence of *Aspergillus* species at any time before the transplant procedure, when there has been evidence of heavy overgrowth of yeast (e.g., *Candida*) in the donor sputum culture, or when cytolytic induction immunosuppression is used. In the case of *Aspergillus*, prophylactic therapy requires the use of amphotericin B; in the latter instances, fluconazole or low-dose ketoconazole therapy is effective.

The occurrence of herpes simplex infection, including mucosal ulceration and pneumonitis, has been eliminated by the routine use of acyclovir prophylaxis after lung transplantation. However, CMV infection remains a significant problem following lung transplantation. The incidence of CMV infection after lung transplantation is related to the preoperative CMV status of both the donor (D) and the recipient (R). A discordant CMV status between donor and recipient may result in either primary infection of the donor lungs by the recipient (in the case of D−/R+) or the more serious circumstance of primary systemic CMV infection (in the case of D+/R−). In either case, the incidence of acute and chronic rejection and mortality are higher than among patients in whom CMV status is concordant. For this reason, many centers prefer to match D and R status. However, the use of ganciclovir prophylaxis has been shown to eliminate the incidence of primary disease and to improve the outcome of CMV-disparate lung transplants.[1,3] *Pneumocystis carinii* infection in lung transplant patients has been eliminated by the routine use of trimethoprim-sulfamethoxazole beginning 1 week after surgery.

Nutrition

Maintaining optimal nutrition in the postoperative period is a useful adjunct for improving surgical outcome. When prolonged ventilatory support is required, the use of intravenous hyperalimentation or, preferably, enteral alimentation via a nasogastric feeding tube is mandatory. Patients with cystic fibrosis will have a malabsorptive syndrome, which will require resumption of preoperative pancreatic enzyme supplementation. These patients have difficulty absorbing medications such as cyclosporine—a circumstance that may be improved by the intake of bile salts (e.g., ursodeoxycholic acid 330 mg with each cyclosporine dose).

Immunosuppression

The induction of a state of relatively nonspecific immune suppression by pharmacologic means has been the key to successful clinical lung transplantation. While the ideal method would be to achieve specific, permanent tolerance of the allograft without the need for chronic medication, this is not possible at present. As a result, although the current regimens lead to satisfactory control of most acute rejection processes, the combined side effects of these medications and their incomplete ability to control chronic rejection in the lung account for the major long-term morbidity and mortality associated with lung transplantation.

The immunosuppressive regimens used for lung transplantation are based on the successful protocols that have evolved for renal and heart transplantation. Virtually all centers use a three-drug regimen for immunosuppression, with the hope of obtaining additive effects in terms of immune suppression while limiting drug toxicities. Although most centers use a combination of cyclosporine, azathioprine, and steroids for this purpose, a recent report of trials in which tacrolimus (FK-506) was substituted for cyclosporine has suggested a greater efficacy with this combination in the control of rejection.[23] Most lung transplant programs use steroids as part of the regimen for the induction of immunosuppression. However, some centers have used cytolytic therapies for this purpose, followed by a reduced incidence of episodes of acute rejection.[17]

Cyclosporine remains the mainstay of immunosuppression for lung transplantation. Intravenous administration is usually begun before the graft is implanted and continued postoperatively, provided renal function remains satisfactory. Subsequent conversion to oral dosing is completed when gastrointestinal function is normal. Blood levels of cyclosporine correlate with immunosuppressive effects and toxicity. Whole blood levels of 350 to 400 ng/ml or serum levels of 150 to 200 ng/ml are considered therapeutic. Nephrotoxicity, the major side effect of cyclosporine, results from vasoconstriction of the afferent glomerular arteriole.

Azathioprine, a purine analog, is converted to several purine metabolites, including 6-mercaptopurine, in red cells and hepatocytes. These purine metabolites have a variety of inhibitory effects on hematologic cell proliferation, with a somewhat greater effect on T cells than on B cells. Azathioprine is begun at a dosage of 2 to 2.5 mg/kg per day and adjusted downward to maintain a white blood cell count of more than 4000 cells/ml. The dosage is the same for both the intravenous and oral routes. If necessary, azathioprine may be omitted for several days without significant compromise of its immunosuppressive effect.

Corticosteroids have a variety of effects on the immune response, mediated by the interaction of the steroid with a high-affinity cytoplasmic receptor. Steroids affect both inflammation and immunity, and modulate lymphocyte-, mononuclear phagocyte–, and antigen-presenting cell functions. Prednisone, prednisolone, and methylprednisolone are all synthetic derivatives of cortisol that are used clinically for transplant patients. Intraoperatively, methylprednisolone is administered before reperfusion of the lung graft. Postoperatively, in the absence of cytolytic induction therapy, moderate-dose corticosteroid therapy is used in combination with cyclosporine and azathioprine for induction immunosuppression. An oral dose of prednisone (0.5 mg/kg per day) is usually begun on postoperative day 5 to 7. Although corticosteroids have profound inhibitory effects on wound healing, their use in this fashion in the immediate postoperative period has not adversely affected the outcomes of lung transplantation.[8]

Various antilymphocyte antibody preparations, so-called cy-

tolytic therapies, have been used in clinical lung transplantation. Both polyclonal preparations, such as antilymphocyte globulin and antithymocyte globulin (ATG), and a murine monoclonal antibody to the CD3 complex of human lymphocytes (OKT3) have been used. Initially, it was believed that strict avoidance of corticosteroids was needed in the early postoperative period to assure satisfactory healing of the bronchial anastomosis. As a result, cytolytic therapy was thought to be necessary to induce immunosuppression before the initiation of steroid therapy in the second postoperative week. The subsequent demonstration that moderate-dose corticosteroid therapy was well tolerated immediately after lung transplantation, as described above, as well as concerns regarding the risks of cytolytic therapy, resulted in most centers' reserving the use of these agents for the treatment of refractory acute rejection.

The two most significant concerns regarding the use of cytolytic therapy have been the increased incidence of CMV disease and the incidence of posttransplant lymphoproliferative disorder (PTLD). CMV disease can be effectively eliminated by several strategies, including matching of D/R CMV status and the use of prophylactic ganciclovir. The incidence of PTLD may also be minimized by the use of ganciclovir, which has additional effects against the Epstein-Barr virus (EBV), the likely cause of PTLD in most cases.[2,3]

Tacrolimus (FK-506) is a macrolide compound with a mechanism of action similar to that of cyclosporine through an immunophilin protein called the FK-binding protein (FKBP). Tacrolimus has been used for induction immunosuppression as part of a three-drug regimen with azathioprine and steroids and as a rescue therapy for patients with refractory rejection on a standard three-drug regimen (cyclosporine, azathioprine, steroids). Toxicity is similar to that of cyclosporine and includes reversible renal dysfunction, hypertension, and neurotoxicity. New-onset diabetes mellitus has also been reported. Hypertrichosis and gingival hyperplasia have not been seen with tacrolimus. In a randomized trial in lung transplant patients of three-drug regimens containing either cyclosporine or tacrolimus, the incidence of postoperative fungal infections was higher in patients receiving tacrolimus.[23]

Immunosuppressive drugs currently undergoing clinical trials include rapamycin and mycophenolic acid. Rapamycin is an analog of tacrolimus that also binds to FKBP. It inhibits the response of T lymphocytes to IL-2 and other cytokines but does not inhibit IL-2 production. Rapamycin has been shown to reverse ongoing rejection and to prolong graft survival in animal models. Although the drug does not cause nephrotoxicity, a major toxicity is necrotizing vasculitis of the gastrointestinal tract. Concurrent cyclosporine administration increases the potency of rapamycin, suggesting that it may be used as in combination with cyclosporine to lower the overall toxicity of a multidrug immunosuppressive regimen. Mycophenolic acid inhibits de novo purine synthesis by inhibiting the conversion of inosine monophosphate to xanthine monophosphate. Since lymphocytes depend almost exclusively on de novo purine synthesis, mycophenolic acid selectively inhibits their replication, including the formation of cytotoxic lymphocytes and both primary and secondary antibody formation. Mycophenolic acid has been shown to reverse acute rejection that is resistant to both corticosteroids and OKT3. It appears to have primarily gastrointestinal side effects, including nausea, gastritis, and ileus, without significant myelosuppressive toxicity.

Rejection

Lung grafts contain a large population of immunocompetent cells, including lymphocytes and macrophages within the parenchyma, hilar and pulmonary lymph nodes, and bronchus-associated lymphoid tissue (BALT). Most of these cells are memory T cells. A prominent interaction occurs between donor and recipient immune cells during the early period after implantation. Analysis of cells obtained by bronchoalveolar lavage (BAL) during the first month after transplant demonstrates donor-specific lymphocyte proliferation, suggesting in vivo mixed lymphocyte reactivity at a time when both donor and recipient immune-competent cells are present.[47] Subsequently, rapid replacement of donor lymphocytes and macrophages occurs. By 90 days after transplantation, most of the intraparenchymal cells are of recipient origin and BALT has been markedly depleted.[22]

In view of these rapid and profound changes in immune cell populations, it is not surprising that rejection is common in lung allografts and that, in the case of heart–lung grafts, lung rejection may occur more frequently than, and independent of, rejection of the heart. A protocol of routine transbronchial biopsy of the lung for identification of histologic evidence of lung rejection is usually recommended for both heart–lung and isolated-lung transplants because of the likelihood of rejection that may occur with minimal clinical symptoms. Typically, surveillance bronchoscopy is performed at 3 weeks, 6 weeks, 3 months, 6 months, 9 months, and 12 months after surgery. Bronchoscopy and biopsy are, of course, also performed for clinical symptoms or for changes in lung spirometry such as a decrease in FEV_1.[21]

Acute rejection (AR) is characterized by perivascular and subendothelial mononuclear cellular infiltrates (Fig. 106-4). Airway inflammation, a lymphocytic bronchitis or bronchiolitis, may also be seen as a component of AR. Clinically, the patients manifest dyspnea, low-grade fever, hypoxemia, and pulmonary infiltrates on chest radiograph. Flexible bronchoscopy with BAL and transbronchial biopsy are the most useful methods of differentiating AR from infection.[7] BAL is most useful in excluding infection and is not generally helpful in confirming rejection. The transbronchial biopsy is assessed with a standard histologic grading of AR based on the degree of perivascular infiltrate, with an additional category for assessing the degree of airway inflammation (Table 106-7). Although the severity of the perivascular process determines the "grade" of AR, the bronchial inflammation may be a significant factor in predicting the later development of chronic rejection that involves the airways.[49,50]

Because the incidence of AR in the first 3 weeks after lung transplantation exceeds 90 percent at most centers, antirejection therapy is usually administered empirically for transplant recipients with the appropriate clinical syndrome, even in the absence of confirmatory biopsy findings, if no infectious cause is found by BAL.[8] The initial treatment of AR is by the administration of a brief course of high-dose corticosteroids (e.g., methylprednisolone 500 mg intravenously every day for 3 days). Ganciclovir prophylaxis (5 mg/kg twice a day, tapered over 6 weeks)

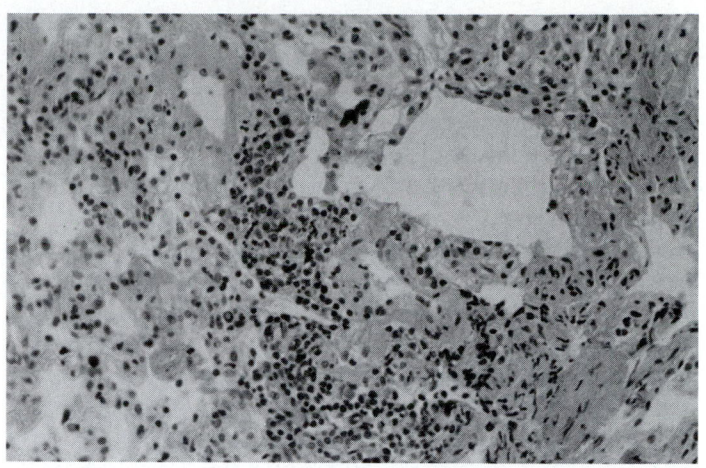

FIGURE 106-4   Lung allograft rejection—acute rejection, grade 2. Acute rejection is characterized by lymphocytic infiltration about pulmonary vessels. Grading of the rejection process is based on the extent of the lymphocytic infiltration into the surrounding lung parenchyma.

is necessary for all patients with CMV-disparate D/R status when antirejection therapy is initiated. In most patients, symptomatic and radiographic improvement is seen within 48 h. Thereafter, the maintenance dose of steroids is usually increased for several weeks and then slowly reduced to prerejection levels. As a rule, it is not necessary to repeat transbronchial biopsy to confirm resolution of the AR unless symptoms or radiographic abnormalities persist. Occasionally, some patients with persistent findings require a second course of steroids, either as previously administered or as a slightly longer course of oral therapy (e.g., "recycling" beginning with prednisone 200 mg a day and then a dosage reduced by 40 mg a day to return to a maintenance dose 10 mg a day higher than the dose on which rejection occurred). For the rare patient in whom these methods do not bring about resolution of the process, repeat bronchoscopy for BAL and transbronchial biopsy are recommended to confirm the diagnosis. If persistent AR is identified, cytolytic therapy with OKT3 or ATG should be considered.

Chronic rejection (CR) in the lung may affect either the pulmonary vasculature or the airway. Occasionally, accelerated sclerosis of the pulmonary arteries and veins may be encountered in lung allografts. These changes are analogous to the CR identified in many isolated cardiac allograft recipients. In fact, when this type of CR is identified in the lungs of HLT recipients, it appears to correlate with similar changes in the coronary arteries of these patients.[50]

More typically, CR in the lung is manifested by obstructive changes in the small airways. Clinically, progressive dyspnea occurs, although a gradual decline in FEV_1 or in expiratory flow rates often precedes symptoms. Histologically, this process is identified as bronchiolitis obliterans and consists of dense eosinophilic scarring of the membranous and respiratory bronchioles (Fig. 106-5). Further progression of this process leads to worsening dyspnea and bronchiectasis with secondary infection. Although this form of CR is uncommon in the first 3 months after lung transplantation, up to 50 percent of patients develop it within 2 years, and the mortality at 3 years after diagnosis is 40 percent or higher.[43,46] Risk factors for the development of this process include episodes of severe AR, three or more episodes of mild AR, and, in some centers, the occurrence of CMV disease. Some studies have suggested that the use of OKT3 for induction immunosuppression or the use of tacrolimus as part of a three-drug immunosuppressive regimen has been associated with a lower incidence of CR of the lung involving the airways.[4,23]

The term *bronchiolitis obliterans syndrome* (BOS) has been used to identify patients with CR of the lung involving the airways. Progressive symptoms and an unexplained fall in expiratory flow rates and are the hallmarks of this process. Because of sampling limitations of transbronchial biopsy, some patients with CR may not have histologic proof of bronchiolitis obliterans despite a course of progressive deterioration. Therefore, the diagnosis of BOS is based on symptoms and objective changes in pulmonary function and does not require histologic evidence of bronchioitis obliterans (Table 106-8). The clinical condition of patients with BOS is graded on a scale from 0 to 3. Although some patients with BOS will remain stable within a given grade, most demonstrate evidence of disease progression.[43] Some evidence suggests that augmented immunosuppression may stabilize the BOS process, particularly if initiated early in its evolution. Treatment is usually directed to patients with symptomatic BOS (grades 1 to 3). Augmented corticosteroid therapy, including the use of inhaled steroids, cytolytic agents, and tacrolimus, has been used for this purpose. Whether one type of therapy offers a specific advantage over another in the treatment of this syndrome is not yet clear.

Management of progressive BOS in its later stages is mostly palliative. At its most advanced stage, BOS is essentially an acquired form of septic lung disease, and management is similar to that required for other patients with septic lung disease awaiting lung transplantation. Retransplantation has been performed for some patients with BOS. The results demonstrate a significantly increased perioperative mortality for such patients. One-year survival is approximately 45 percent, less than half that for primary lung transplantation. Approximately 40 percent of patients surviving retransplantation develop recurrent BOS by 3 years—an incidence similar to that following primary lung transplantation.[31]

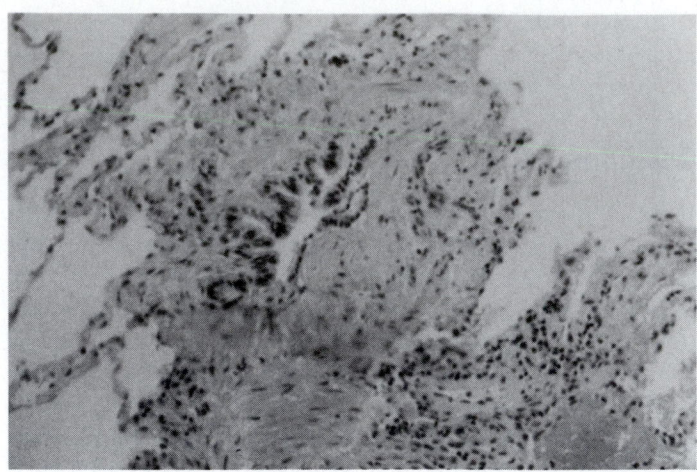

FIGURE 106-5 Lung allograft rejection—obliterative bronchiolitis. Chronic rejection in the lung most commonly involves the small airways, resulting in obliterative bronchiolitis. Dense submucosal scarring occurs and may completely obstruct the lumen of small airways. The process may be categorized as active or inactive, depending on the degree of associated inflammation.

Complications

SURGICAL COMPLICATIONS

Major technical complications following lung transplantation have become increasingly rare with improvements in surgical technique and perioperative management. *Postoperative hemorrhage* requiring reexploration is very uncommon with the use of the clam shell incision to improve operative exposure for patients requiring DLT or HLT and with the routine use of aprotonin infusions during CPB to diminish fibrinolysis. *Pulmonary artery obstruction* can occur as a result of anastomotic stenosis, kinking, or extrinsic compression. In these patients, persistent pulmonary hypertension and unexplained hypoxemia may be evident. Attention to anatomic factors, such as the length of donor and recipient pulmonary arteries and division of the pericardial attachments surrounding the donor pulmonary artery, as well as

---

TABLE 106-7

Proposed Classification of Lung Transplant Rejection

A. Acute rejection—perivascular inflammation
    Grade 0—None
    Grade 1—Minimal
    Grade 2—Mild
    Grade 3—Moderate
    Grade 4—Severe
B. Airway inflammation—lymphocytic bronchitis/bronchiolitis—documented with acute rejection
    Grade 0—None
    Grade 1—Minimal
    Grade 2—Mild
    Grade 3—Moderate
    Grade 4—Severe
C. Chronic airway rejection—bronchiolitis obliterans—active or inactive
D. Chronic vascular rejection—accelerated graft vascular sclerosis

TABLE 106-8

Staging Classification of Bronchiolitis Obliterans Syndrome

Stage	Severity	FEV_1 (%5 baseline)
0	No symptoms	>80%
1	Mild	66–80%
2	Moderate	51–65%
3	Severe	≤50%

All stages may be subcategorized according to the presence (subcategory a) or absence (subcategory b) of histologic evidence of bronchiolitis obliterans.

awareness of the potential for a flap wrapping the bronchial anastomosis to compress the adjacent anastomosis, helps to avoid these problems. *Left atrial anastomotic obstruction* can also occur because of faulty anastomotic technique or extrinsic compression by clot, pericardium, or an omental flap. This problem results in more severe abnormalities than pulmonary artery obstruction, including marked pulmonary hypertension and ipsilateral pulmonary edema. Diagnostic methods for these vascular anastomotic complications include routine intraoperative measurement of anastomotic gradients and transesophageal echocardiography, which is particularly helpful in assessing the left atrial anastomosis. Postoperatively, diagnostic measures include contrast angiography and ventilation/perfusion scanning. Reoperation and correction of the anastomosis are indicated if clinical compromise is apparent, which is particularly likely if there is significant left atrial anastomotic obstruction.

Some transplanted lungs demonstrate *acute graft dysfunction,* even without evidence of vascular anastomotic complications. As many as 20 percent of patients have severe early abnormalities of lung function, with rapidly progressive pulmonary edema, persistent pulmonary hypertension, and a markedly diminished pulmonary compliance that occurs rapidly after graft implantation. This process is to be differentiated from the "reimplantation response" that is seen in almost all patients 36 to 96 h after transplantation and consists of perihilar and peribronchiolar edema *without* significant abnormalities in gas exchange. In some patients, acute graft dysfunction is due to unsuspected abnormalities in the donor lung, such as aspiration or contusion, whereas in others it may be due to inadequate pulmonary preservation. However, no cause has been identified. Management includes evaluation of the vascular anastomoses, to rule out a potentially correctable technical complication, and maintenance of oxygenation using volume ventilation and PEEP. In most patients, regardless of the supportive measure required, the process resolves over several days, with satisfactory long-term graft function.[20]

Pleural space complications are not uncommon after lung transplantation, although they are usually of minor significance. *Pneumothorax* may occur on either the side of a lung graft or on the side of a native lung. Pneumothoraces that arise from the lung graft are of greatest concern because of the possibility that airway dehiscence will communicate with the pleural space. Fortunately, this is a rare occurrence. Nonetheless, flexible bronchoscopy is always indicated for diagnostic purposes in patients presenting with this problem. In most patients, placement of a chest tube with reexpansion of the lung limits the process acutely.

More commonly, pneumothorax is the result of rupture of a bullous lesion in an emphysematous native lung after SLT. Conservative management with intercostal tube drainage is indicated. Occasionally, pneumothoraces will be noted after DLT when a significant size discrepancy exists between the donor lungs and the recipient thorax. In these patients, the space resolves spontaneously in a short time and specific interventions are not required. *Pleural effusions* are common after lung transplantation, particularly when a significant size disparity exists between the donor lungs and the thorax. Continued chest tube drainage following the primary procedure is not indicated as a preventive measure for these effusions and may actually lead to secondary infection and empyema. Management of these effusions is best done conservatively, with diuretic therapy and dietary salt restriction. Invasive measures, such as thoracentesis and tube drainage, are indicated only for effusions complicated by a delayed pneumothorax, for enlarging effusions, or for large effusions that persist for more than 4 weeks after surgery.

Airway complications have been significantly less common in the recent experience with lung transplantation. Bronchial ischemia is the most common cause of postoperative airway complications. The most common methods of lung transplantation do not provide direct revascularization of the bronchial arterial circulation, and the donor bronchus must rely entirely on collateral perfusion from the pulmonary circulation in the initial postimplantation period. Airway ischemia at this time leads to mucosal ulceration, followed by progressive mural necrosis. Localized bronchomalacia is frequently present adjacent to this region. A spectrum of abnormalities, ranging from anastomotic dehiscence to submucosal fibrosis, may occur as a result. Most commonly, partial anastomotic dehiscence occurs, followed by formation of granulation tissue and eventually some degree of anastomotic stenosis.

The reduced incidence of these complications has been attributed to methods of anastomosis that limit the length of the donor bronchus, minimizing the amount of airway for which collateral perfusion is required. Most anastomotic techniques emphasize trimming the donor bronchus to within two rings of the upper-lobe orifice and the preservation of peribronchial tissues containing the collateral circulation. Telescoping the bronchi and covering the anastomosis with vascularized tissue are also useful adjunctive measures. The use of omentum does not appear to be a critical factor in most cases, although in patients who require prolonged mechanical ventilation because of graft dysfunction or in whom anastomotic dehiscence develops, the presence of an omental wrap helps to minimize the morbidity caused by these complications. The effect of improved methods of lung preservation and of more specific immunosuppression on the decrease in airway complications is difficult to quantitate, but these factors are probably of some importance in the reduced incidence of this problem.

The overall incidence of airway complications in all lung transplant patients is 15 to 20 percent. In approximately half of these patients, the diagnosis is made from endoscopic surveillance alone, and healing occurs without further treatment or secondary complication. In the rest, the airway complication requires more specific management and may lead to secondary complications. Of these patients, 70 percent will require anastomotic dilatation or stent placement and 20 percent develop a bronchopleural fistula that requires a chest tube and perhaps reoperation. Death due to extensive airway necrosis or secondary infectious complications occurs in 10 percent of patients who develop symptomatic airway complications.

Another complication following lung transplantation is *myocardial infarction,* which is usually due to pressure overload during the implantation procedure and can be prevented in most patients by prompt initiation of CPB. Postoperative management of these patients is similar to the routine management of patients with myocardial ischemia; it consists of the judicious use of nitrate therapy, reductions in preload and afterload, and observation for dysrhythmias. *Atrial dysrhythmias* are also common, as with other types of cardiothoracic surgery, and are managed in a similar fashion. Transplant patients are also prone to significant *gastrointestinal complications,* whose manifestations may be obscured by the anti-inflammatory effects of immunosuppressive therapy. Hepatobiliary and pancreatic complications are especially common after intrathoracic transplantation, particularly when CPB has been required. Preventive measures include laparoscopic cholecystectomy for patients with symptomatic biliary disease before transplantation. Postoperatively, continued surveillance of pancreatic exocrine function, bilirubin, and liver function tests is indicated to allow prompt diagnosis and intervention for specific abnormalities. In view of the surgical stress and use of corticosteroids in these patients, all patients should receive H_2-blocking agents and antacid therapy postoperatively to prevent upper gastrointestinal hemorrhage.

INFECTIOUS COMPLICATIONS

Lung transplant patients have several unique attributes that account for a rate of infectious complications that is higher than the rate for other transplant recipients. Before implantation, the donor lung may contain significant pathogens, owing to the changes in lung defense mechanisms that follow intubation and brain death. After the transplant, the lung allograft continues to be exposed both to the external environment and to sites in the upper respiratory tract, such as the sinuses, that may contain significant pulmonary pathogens. Finally, the lack of a cough reflex and a disturbed pattern of mucociliary clearance in the donor lung after the transplant predispose to pulmonary infection. An aggressive approach to the evaluation of all new pulmonary infiltrates, in either the lung graft or the native lung, is required in these patients. Flexible bronchoscopy with BAL or protected brushing is needed for proper diagnosis of pulmonary infections after lung transplantation. BAL specimens from both lungs should be routinely sent for Gram's stain, fungal smear, and acid-fast bacilli smear as well as for culture of these organisms. In addition, analysis of BAL for *P. carinii, Legionella* species, and viral assays is required.

Bacterial pneumonia is the most commonly acquired infection after lung transplantation. Pneumonia occurs most fre-

quently within 2 months of transplantation and is usually due to gram-negative bacilli. Diagnosis made with bronchoscopy and treatment with antibiotics administered intravenously lead to prompt resolution in most cases. Depending on the organism, aerosolized antimicrobial therapy, in addition to intravenous therapy, may be helpful. Potential native sources of contamination of the respiratory tract should be evaluated, particularly in patients with cystic fibrosis or recurrent pneumonias. Chronic sinusitis is common in cystic fibrosis patients and acts as a source of contamination of the lower respiratory tract. Careful otolaryngologic evaluation and sinus drainage are indicated in selected patients. Gastroesophageal reflux is common in both cystic fibrosis patients and patients with COPD and can lead to recurrent aspiration pneumonias in dependent regions of the lungs. In most patients, conservative treatment with elevation of the head of the bed and the administration of promotility agents, in addition to the H_2-blocking agents taken by most transplant recipients, will control the reflux. In patients who have undergone SLT, the native lung may occasionally be a site of graft contamination or, more commonly, may become the site of a pneumonia or a lung abscess. Standard therapy is recommended for such cases, although a localized area of anatomic abnormality in the native lung (e.g., focal bronchiectasis) may require surgical excision if it proves to be the source of recurrent infection.

Viral infections can be a major source of morbidity or mortality for lung transplant patients. Previously, *herpes simplex virus* infection was an occasional cause of tracheobronchitis or pneumonitis following lung transplantation. The use of prophylactic acyclovir or ganciclovir has eliminated these infections. *Respiratory syncytial virus* (RSV), which can cause pneumonitis and bronchiolitis in immunosuppressed patients, has been more frequently identified in lung transplant patients during the time of peak community infection (from November to March). Treatment of RSV requires the use of aerosolized ribavirin and RSV hyperimmune globulin. Although successful treatment of the acute disease has been reported, a major issue remains regarding the potential for later development of an obliterative bronchiolitis following RSV infection.

Cytomegalovirus, a member of the human herpesvirus family, is the second most frequent cause of infection in the lung transplant patient and the most important opportunistic infection that occurs in these patients. Following infection with CMV, the virus remains in a latent state in the body; evidence of the infection can be identified from a positive serologic assay. Approximately 80 percent of adults are seropositive for CMV. Immunosuppression can cause reactivation of the latent virus and shedding of CMV into both the urine and the sputum. Viremia may also be detected in more advanced cases of reactivation disease. CMV infection of a lung transplant recipient can occur either from reactivation of latent virus or from direct transmission to the patient. Direct transmission, which occurs by the transfusion of blood products obtained from seropositive donors into seronegative recipients, has been essentially eliminated by administration of blood products only from seronegative donors to seronegative recipients.

The incidence of CMV infection in the lung transplant recipient is related to the serologic status of both donor and recipient. Recipients who are seronegative for CMV and receive seronegative lungs should never develop CMV infection, provided they are protected from transmission of the virus by transfusion. CMV should never be found in their sputum. Alternatively, recipients who are seropositive for CMV and receive lungs from seropositive donors rarely develop CMV infection because of their preoperative immunity. These patients will, however, shed CMV in their sputum when the latent virus is reactivated by immunosuppression. When a seropositive recipient receives a lung from a seronegative donor, reactivation of the recipient's CMV can cause a CMV pneumonitis in the lung graft. This is an invasive infection, with evidence of viral-induced cytotrophic changes in the pulmonary parenchyma in addition to the presence of CMV in the sputum (Fig. 106-6). In these cases, CMV pneumonitis is generally well treated with a course of ganciclovir (5 mg/kg intravenously twice a day for 4 weeks). Conversely, when seronegative recipients receive lungs from a seropositive donor, reactivation of the CMV in the donor lung can cause a primary infection of the recipient. Primary CMV infection of an immunosuppressed host, such as the recipient of a lung transplant, is a potentially fatal systemic illness associated with viremia, pneumonitis, hepatitis, encephalitis, retinitis, and enterocolitis. Such patients require both ganciclovir (5 mg/kg intravenously twice a day) and CMV hyperimmune globulin (10 g intravenously every month) for prolonged courses of therapy until the disease is eradicated.

Although ganciclovir is effective therapy for CMV in patients with pneumonitis or primary infection, the occurrence of CMV infection in these patients can lead to significant morbidity. CMV infection seems to elicit acute graft rejection in many instances, requiring a complicated treatment plan to balance the need for augmented immunosuppression against adequate treatment of the infection. In addition, CMV disease in some series appears to be a risk factor for the subsequent development of BOS, the most common cause of late mortality following lung transplantation.[1,4] Many centers strive to match donor and recipient CMV status to minimize the potential for these problems. When precise donor–recipient matching is performed, the use of ganciclovir is reserved for cases of invasive CMV disease—i.e., CMV pneumonitis or primary infection with viremia. Other centers, how-

ever, have demonstrated the efficacy of a prophylactic regimen of ganciclovir (5 mg/kg intravenously twice a day, tapered over 6 weeks) in minimizing the incidence of CMV disease, even when donor–recipient CMV mismatching occurs. In these preemptive regimens, ganciclovir is used for all patients who are at risk for CMV disease during the induction of immunosuppression and whenever immunosuppression is augmented to treat acute rejection. This approach has led to an improvement in survival for patients with disparate donor–recipient CMV status. Relapse rates remain high, however, and the best approach to the management of the lung transplant patient with a mismatched donor–recipient CMV status remains to be determined.[3]

NEOPLASTIC COMPLICATIONS

Immunosuppression increases the risk of development of neoplasms after lung transplantation. The risk applies to a specific group of solid tumors, including squamous cell cancers of the lip and skin, Kaposi's sarcoma, soft tissue sarcomas, carcinomas of the vulva and perineum, and hepatobiliary tumors. Transplant recipients are not at increased risk for developing the more common cancers encountered in the general population, such as carcinoma of the lung, breast, colon, or prostate.

The most common malignancy seen after lung transplantation is a type of B-cell lymphoid proliferation known as *posttransplant lymphoproliferative disorder.* PTLD represents a morphologically diverse group of polyclonal lymphoid proliferations. The pathogenesis of PTLD appears to be related to EBV infection of B lymphocytes that are stimulated to proliferate by the recipient's immunosuppression. Clinically, a distinction can be made between patients presenting with PTLD within 1 year after transplantation and those presenting with PTLD at later times. The early patients tend to have localized disease that responds to a temporary reduction in immunosuppression; their long-term prognosis is excellent. Patients who present after 1 year usually have disseminated disease that does not respond to reduced immunosuppression and requires cytotoxic chemotherapy for treatment. The mortality from lymphoma in these patients is 70 percent.[2] Of interest is that the use of ganciclovir for prophylaxis against CMV disease in lung transplant patients may also help to control the incidence of PTLD, since ganciclovir also has significant activity against EBV. Future trials to assess the impact of ganciclovir therapy on the incidence of PTLD are planned.

RESULTS

Survival

Survival mortality following lung transplantation has decreased significantly over the past decade. The cause of this reduction is probably multifactorial—i.e., the result of technical improvements in the procedure, of improved recipient selection and preoperative management, and of increasing experience in perioperative management of these patients. In most recent series, surgical mortality following lung transplantation has been between 10 and 15 percent. The surgical mortality of DLT ranges from 15 to 20 percent as compared to that of SLT, which is usually 10 percent or less. This difference is attributable, in large

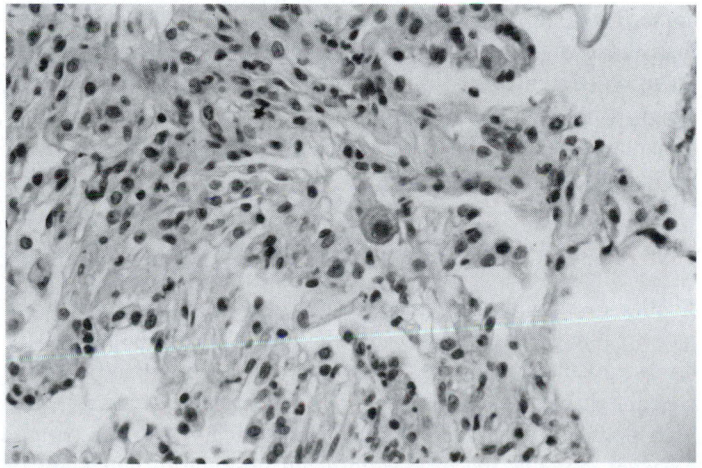

FIGURE 106-6   Cytomegalovirus (CMV) pneumonitis. A characteristic cytotrophic change in the pulmonary parenchyma is seen with invasive CMV infection.

part, to the increased likelihood of postoperative infectious complications in patients with septic lung disease who require DLT. Surgical mortality after HLT is usually slightly higher than for patients undergoing DLT, probably owing to the more advanced disease state of patients who require HLT. Most centers have not noted a marked difference in surgical mortality for patients undergoing SLT for different diseases, although preoperative pulmonary hypertension in these patients will usually increase the risk of perioperative morbidity.[3,8,40]

Infection is the major cause of early mortality in lung transplant recipients, accounting for 30 to 45 percent of deaths. The likelihood of pulmonary infection is greatest in the first 100 days after transplantation, before recipient defense mechanisms (e.g., cough) are restored. Risk factors for infection during this period include a positive sputum culture from the donor, a lower Pa_{O_2} in the donor lung (under 350 mmHg), a prolonged ischemic time (greater than 6 h), recipient age greater than 40 years, and CMV disease as the result of donor–recipient mismatching without ganciclovir prophylaxis. Postoperative graft failure with diffuse alveolar damage may also contribute to early mortality in as many as 15 percent of patients. Unfortunately, there do not appear to be any specific risk factors for acute graft failure. However, with newer methods of management (e.g., inhaled NO) and increased skill in treating these patients, mortality from this complication has been greatly reduced. Cardiovascular decompensation, termed "heart failure," is the third leading cause of early death. In most cases, this process occurs in the clinical setting of adult respiratory distress syndrome and persistent pulmonary hypertension with secondary cardiac dysfunction. Coronary artery disease or myocardial infarction is uncommon in these patients.[8]

Long-term survival data indicate a cumulative survival rate of 70 to 80 percent at 1 year. Survival curves can vary significantly beyond 1 year, depending on the disease for which transplantation was performed. Patients with emphysema and those with pulmonary vascular disease appear to have a survival advantage over patients with restrictive lung disease or septic lung disease, in whom infectious complications or recurrence of native disease in the lung graft is more common. By 3 years, survival ranges from 75 percent in the former group to 55 percent in the latter group. At this interval, BOS begins to have a significant impact on survival as well, leading to an overall survival rate of only 50 percent at 5 years. Causes of death in this period include infection, which has another peak of increased incidence throughout the second postoperative year, and BOS, which can be identified in half of the patients who survive to 3 years. Malignancy, usually PTLD, is the third most common cause of late mortality following lung transplantation.[3,8,43]

Functional Results

Most patients surviving lung transplantation experience a highly significant improvement in their functional capability over their preoperative state. Typically, patients can resume an exercise program without oxygen supplementation by 6 weeks after transplantation. However, in some patients who require muscular paralysis for management of postoperative graft failure, a demyelinating process may delay full recovery for 2 to 3 months.

Eventually, complete resolution is seen in most of these patients.

Improvements occur regardless of the native disease that led to transplantation. Unless BOS occurs, functional capacity based on the standards of reproducible exercise testing remains stable for at least 3 years. Controversy exists over the potential benefit of SLT as compared to DLT for younger patients with emphysema. Although the results of spirometry are obviously better in DLT recipients, exercise tolerance is similar initially in the two groups. Whether a significant later advantage exists for DLT recipients that would offset the increased perioperative risk of the procedure remains to be seen. Similarly, functional results following SLT or DLT for pulmonary vascular disease demonstrate little objective difference between the two approaches. However, DLT may provide a slight advantage in patients in whom preoperative pulmonary artery pressures approach systemic levels, because such an approach provides the maximum reduction of pulmonary vascular resistance. In addition, because the allograft receives up to 95 percent of the blood flow in these patients after SLT, the development of BOS, even at grade 1, has profound functional implications. The development of BOS in patients who have undergone DLT for pulmonary vascular disease causes less immediate hemodynamic compromise because the partition of blood flow between the two lungs is similar.[3,8,33]

Retransplantation

Pulmonary retransplantation has been undertaken with increasing frequency in recent years. Retransplantation is used either as a method to correct an acute complication, such as graft failure or diffuse airway necrosis, or as a treatment for a chronic process in the graft, such as BOS or airway stenosis. At the present time, BOS appears to be the most common indication. A variety of approaches have been used, including redo ipsilateral SLT, contralateral SLT, and DLT following either SLT or DLT. These are technically challenging procedures, with a surgical mortality of nearly 50 percent. Factors contributing to a more favorable outcome include an ambulatory status before retransplantation, the use of ABO-identical grafts, and prior institutional experience with retransplantation; notably, retransplantation with a CMV-seronegative donor has also been associated with a favorable outcome. The long-term results of retransplantation are much worse than those of initial lung transplantation. One-year survival is about 45 percent, and 2-year survival is about 35 percent. BOS occurs with a frequency similar to that seen with primary lung transplantation and can be identified in one-third of patients 2 years after retransplantation.[31]

SUMMARY

Significant progress has been made in the development of techniques of lung transplantation for all types of end-stage pulmonary diseases. Isolated lung transplantation has been applied with increasing success to the entire group of patients, including those with pulmonary vascular disease. A shortage of donor organs, however, remains the most significant obstacle to wider use of this method of treatment. Techniques of donor lung preservation and implantation allow ischemic intervals of 6 to 8 h for reasonable postoperative function. Surgical mortality is 10 to 15 percent, slightly lower for SLT and slightly higher for DLT and HLT. Functional results in survivors of the operation are excellent. Infection remains a significant source of morbidity and mortality in both the early and late postoperative periods. However, the most significant impediment to long-term survival is the development of chronic rejection in the lung allograft, manifested as BOS, in half of the patients by 3 years after transplantation. Further measures to prevent or treat this malady are critical to improving long-term survival rates following lung transplantation.

REFERENCES

1. Arbustini E, Morbini P, Grasso M, et al: Human cytomegalovirus: Early infection, acute rejection and major histocompatibility class II expression in transplanted lung. *Transplantation* 61:418–427, 1996.

2. Armitage JM, Kormos RL, Stuart SR, et al: Posttransplant lymphoproliferative disease in thoracic organ transplant patients: Ten years of cyclosporine-based immunosuppression. *J Heart Lung Transplant* 10:877–887, 1991.

3. Bando K, Paradis IL, Komatsu K, et al: Analysis of time-dependent risks for infection, rejection and death after pulmonary transplantation. *J Thorac Cardiovasc Surg* 109:49–57, 1995.

4. Bando K, Paradis IL, Similo S, et al: Obliterative bronchiolitis after lung and heart–lung transplantation: An analysis of risk factors and management. *J Thorac Cardiovasc Surg* 110:4–14, 1995.

5. Cahalin L, Pappagianopoulos P, Prevost S, et al: The relationship of the 6-minute walk test to maximal oxygen consumption in transplant candidates with end-stage lung disease. *Chest* 108:452–459, 1995.

6. Christie NA, Waddell TK: Lung preservation. *Chest Surg Clin North Am* 3:29–43, 1993.

7. Clelland CA, Higgenbottam TW, Stewart S, et al: Bronchoalveolar lavage and transbronchial lung biopsy during acute rejection and infection in heart–lung transplant patients. *Am Rev Respir Dis* 147:1386–1390, 1993.

8. Cooper JD, Patterson GA, Trulock EP, et al: Results of single and bilateral lung transplantation in 131 consecutive recipients. *J Thorac Cardiovasc Surg* 107:460–471, 1994.

9. Couraud L, Baudet E, Martigne C, et al: Bronchial revascularization in double lung transplantation: A series of 8 patients. *Ann Thorac Surg* 53:88–94, 1992.

10. D'Alonzo GE, Barst RJ, Ayres SM, et al: Survival in patients with primary pulmonary hypertension: Results from a national prospective registry. *Ann Intern Med* 115:343–349, 1991.

11. Date H, Matsamura A, Manchester JK, et al: Evaluation of lung metabolism during successful twenty-four hour canine lung preservation. *J Thorac Cardiovasc Surg* 105:480–491, 1993.

12. Demikhov VP: *Experimental Transplantation of Vital Organs.* New York, Consultants Bureau Enterprises, 1962.

13. Derome F, Barbier F, Ringoir S, et al: Ten month survival after lung homotransplantation in man. *J Thorac Cardiovasc Surg* 61:835–846, 1971.

14. Duncan SR, Paradis IL, Yousem SA, et al: Sequelae of cytomegalovirus pulmonary infections in lung allograft recipients. *Am Rev Respir Dis* 146:1419–1423, 1992.

15. Fremes SE, Patterson GA, Williams WG, et al: Single lung transplantation and closure of patent ductus arteriosus for Eisenmenger's syndrome. *J Thorac Cardiovasc Surg* 100:1–5, 1990.

16. Goldberg M, Lima O, Morgan E, et al: A comparison between cyclopsorine A and methylprednisolone plus azathioprine on bronchial healing following canine lung autotransplantation. *J Thorac Cardiovasc Surg* 85:821–826, 1983.

17. Griffith BP, Hardesty RL, Armitage JM, et al: Acute rejection of lung allografts with various immunosuppressive protocols. *Ann Thorac Surg* 54:846–851, 1992.

18. Hardin CA, Kittle CF: Experience with transplantation of the lung. *Science* 119:87–89, 1954.

19. Hardy JD: Lung homotransplantation in man. *JAMA* 186:1065–1066, 1963.

20. Haydock DA, Trulock EP, Kaiser LR, et al: Management of dysfunction in the transplanted lung: Experience with 7 clinical cases. *Ann Thorac Surg* 53:635–641, 1992.

21. Higgenbottam TW, Stewart S, Penketh AR, et al: Transbronchial lung biopsy for the diagnosis of rejection in heart–lung transplant patients. *Transplantation* 46:532–539, 1988.

22. Hruban RH, Beschorner WE, Baumgartner WA, et al: Depletion of bronchus-associated lymphoid tissue with lung allograft rejection. *Am J Pathol* 132:6–10, 1988.

23. Keenan RJ, Konishi H, Kawai A, et al: Clinical trial of tacrolimus versus cyclosporine in lung transplantation. *Ann Thorac Surg* 60:580–585, 1995.

24. Keenan RJ, Zeevi A, Banas R, et al: Microchimerism is associated with a lower incidence of chronic rejection after lung transplantation. *J Heart Lung Transplant* 13(Suppl):S32, 1994.

25. Kerem H, Reisman J, Corey M, et al: Prediction of mortality in patients with cystic fibrosis. *New Engl J Med* 326:1187–1191, 1992.

26. Low DE, Kaiser LR, Haydock D, et al: The donor lung: Infectious and pathologic factors affecting outcome in lung transplantation. *J Thorac Cardiovasc Surg* 106:614–620, 1993.

27. Mal H, Andreassian B, Pamela F, et al: Unilateral lung transplantation in end-stage pulmonary emphysema. *Am Rev Respir Dis* 140:797–802, 1989.

28. Mal H, Sleiman C, Jebrak G, et al: Functional results of single-lung transplantation for chronic obstructive lung disease. *Am J Respir Crit Care Med* 149:1476–1481, 1994.

29. Metras H: Note préliminaire sur la greffe totale du poumon chez le chien. *C R Acad Sci Paris* 231:1176–1178, 1950.

30. Novick RJ: New trends in lung preservation: A collective review. *J Heart Lung Transplant* 11:377–385, 1992.

31. Novick RJ, Kaye M, Patterson GA, et al: Pulmonary retransplantation. *J Heart Lung Transplant* 12:5–16, 1993.

32. Pasque MK, Cooper JD, Kaiser LR, et al: Improved technique for bilateral lung transplantation: Rationale and initial clinical experience. *Ann Thorac Surg* 49:785–791, 1990.

33. Pasque MK, Trulock EP, Kaiser LR, Cooper JD: Single lung transplantation for pulmonary hypertension: Three month hemodynamic follow-up. *Circulation* 84:2275–2279, 1991.

34. Patterson GA, Cooper JD, Goldman B, et al: Technique of successful clinical double-lung transplantation. *Ann Thorac Surg* 45:626–633, 1988.

35. Puskas JD, Winton TL, Miller JD, et al: Unilateral donor lung dysfunction does not preclude successful contralateral single-lung transplantation. *J Thorac Cardiovasc Surg* 103:1015–1018, 1992.

36. Ramirez JC, Patterson GA, Winton TL, et al: Bilateral lung transplantation for cystic fibrosis. *J Thorac Cardiovasc Surg* 103:287–294, 1992.

37. Reitz BA, Wallwork JL, Hunt SA, et al: heart–lung transplantation: Successful therapy for patients with pulmonary vascular disease. *New Engl J Med* 306:557–564, 1982.

38. Sharples L, Hathaway T, Dennis C, et al: Prognosis of patients with cystic fibrosis awaiting heart and lung transplantation. *J Heart Lung Transplant* 12:669–674, 1993.

39. Sommers KE, Griffith BP, Hardesty RL, Keenan RJ: Early lung allograft function in twin recipients from the same donor: Risk factor analysis. *Ann Thorac Surg* 62:784–790, 1996.

40. Spray TL, Mallory GB, Canter CB, Huddleston CB: Pediatric lung transplantation: Indications, techniques and early results. *J Thorac Cardiovasc Surg* 107:990–1000, 1994.

41. Starnes VA, Barr ML, Cohen RG: Lobar transplantation: Indications, technique and outcome. *J Thorac Cardiovasc Surg* 108:403–410, 1994.

42. Sundaresan S, Semenkovich J, Ochoa J, et al: Successful outcome of lung transplantation is not compromised by the use of marginal donor lungs. *J Thorac Cardiovasc Surg* 109:1075–1079, 1995.

43. Sundaresan S, Trulock EP, Mohanakumar T, et al: Prevalence and outcome of bronchiolitis obliterans syndrome after lung transplantation. *Ann Thorac Surg* 60:1341–1346, 1995.

44. Todd TRJ, Goldberg M, Koshal A, et al: Separate extraction of cardiac and pulmonary grafts from a single organ donor. *Ann Thorac Surg* 46:356–359, 1988.

45. Toronto Lung Transplant Group: Unilateral lung transplantation for pulmonary fibrosis. *New Engl J Med* 314:1140–1145, 1986.

46. Valentine VG, Robbins RC, Berry GJ, et al: Actuarial survival of heart–lung and bilateral sequential lung transplant recipients with obliterative bronchiolitis. *J Heart Lung Transplant* 15:371–383, 1995.

47. Westaby S: Aprotonin in perspective. *Ann Thorac Surg* 55:1033–1041, 1993.

48. Whitehead BF, Stoehr C, Wu CJ, et al: Cytokine gene expression in human lung transplant recipients. *Transplantation* 56:956–960, 1993.

49. Yousem SA: Lymphocytic bronchitis/bronchiolitis in lung allograft recipients. *Am J Surg Pathol* 17:491–495, 1993.

50. Yousem SA, Berry GJ, Cagle PT, et al: Revision of the 1990 working formulation for the classification of pulmonary allograft rejection: Lung rejection study group. *J Heart Lung Transplant* 15:1–15, 1996.

PART FIFTEEN

NEOPLASMS OF THE LUNGS

CHAPTER 107

GENETIC AND MOLECULAR CHANGES OF HUMAN LUNG CANCER

Jeffrey A. Kern / Geoffrey McLennan

GENETIC SUSCEPTIBILITY TO LUNG CANCER
  Acquired Genetic Changes

MOLECULAR CHANGES
  Cytogenetic Changes
  Dominant Oncogenes
  Tumor Suppressor Genes
  Other Proto-Oncogenes and Oncoproteins

THE PROGRESSION OF NORMAL AIRWAY EPITHELIUM TO MALIGNANT EPITHELIUM
  Colorectal Carcinogenesis

THE IMPACT OF MOLECULAR GENETIC CHANGES ON THE CELL CYCLE

Lung cancer is the phenotypic consequence of an accumulation of genetic changes in airway epithelial cells that result in unrestrained cellular proliferation. The genetic and molecular changes that typify lung cancer are complex and not yet fully understood. There continue to be advances in knowledge and, with this, a better understanding of how the changes might contribute to the cancer phenotype, with possible diagnostic and therapeutic measures arising from this understanding. Initial studies in the 1960s were performed using cytogenetics, and they allowed for developments in molecular biology to unravel some of the mystery of oncogenes. Although oncogenes were very much at the leading edge in the 1980s, in the early 1990s tumor suppressor genes (recessive oncogenes or antioncogenes) added

immensely to our understanding of tumorigenesis. Currently much interest is focused on the influence of these genetic factors on the cell cycle and on programmed cell death, or apoptosis. Underlying all this is the influence of environmental factors, especially cigarette smoke exposure, on any genetic susceptibility to lung cancer.

What is to be gained from understanding molecular and genetic changes in the development of lung cancer? We firmly believe that analysis of these factors will have a profound effect on diagnosis, histologic typing, the development of novel treatment strategies and therapeutic agents, prediction of response to therapy, and assessment of risk of relapse and long-term survival. Because of this, much effort has been expended translating newly discovered molecular and genetic changes into clinically useful information. Indeed, recent studies have begun to achieve this goal, with the realization that some genetic changes can identify patient subsets with differing prognoses and therapeutic responses, and with the design of novel therapeutic agents targeting the defect. In this chapter we review recent knowledge in molecular genetics as it relates to small cell lung cancer (SCLC) and non–small cell lung cancer (NSCLC).

GENETIC SUSCEPTIBILITY TO LUNG CANCER

Many epidemiologic studies have demonstrated that some cancers are clustered in families, suggesting that susceptibility to the cancer may be inherited. Lung cancer, however, is most commonly thought of as a cancer that is determined solely by the environment. Certainly, the risks of lung cancer associated with cigarette smoking and in certain occupations, such as uranium mining and shipbuilding, are well established. On the basis of clinical findings, however, differing susceptibilities for tumor formation due to these environmental agents have often been postulated.

Epidemiologic evidence for an increased familial risk of lung cancer was first noted in the early 1960s. In the largest study to date, a 2.4-fold increased risk of lung cancer was identified in relatives of lung cancer patients.[47] This familial risk is supported by recent data from the Utah Population Database.[5] More than one-third of all cancer cases in Utah were examined for a relationship with their genealogic record. These data also identified a familial clustering of lung cancer. Other studies have identified a gender disparity, with women at greater risk of developing lung cancer through familial factors than men. Epidemiologically, this is most likely to occur in women who do not have a history of heavy smoking, who have a younger age at onset of the disease, and who have squamous cell carcinoma.[1]

Modeling of the familial clustering data suggests a Mendelian pattern of codominant inheritance, the result of a rare autosomal gene. This model suggests that carriers of this gene have a young age at lung cancer onset, with a risk 2245-fold greater in non-smoking individuals homozygous for the affected gene. In this model, the putative lung cancer gene accounts for 69 and 47 percent of the cumulative incidence of lung cancer in patients up to 50 and 60 years old, respectively, and is involved in 22 percent of all lung cancers in persons up to age 70. Significantly, random environmental factors do not explain this familial clustering. Further segregation analysis of smoking-associated malignancies has demonstrated that 62 percent of the population appear to be genetically susceptible to smoking-associated lung cancers.[54] Though mathematically compelling, the physical existence of such a lung cancer susceptibility gene has not yet been demonstrated.

Acquired Genetic Changes

Not all lung cancers have a heritable basis. Thus, other explanations must exist for cancers that arise as sporadic or nonfamilial cases. These tumors are not due to germ line mutations or a cancer susceptibility gene that would result in a heritable cancer, but must be due to acquired somatic genetic alterations. The first persuasive evidence that cancer could be attributed to discrete, noninherited, genetic elements was the observation by Rous in 1911 that a cell free filtrate from a chicken sarcoma could induce sarcomas in other chickens. The cancer-causing element was ultimately found to be a virus, the Rous sarcoma virus, and its oncogenic potential was demonstrated to result from a specific gene called v-*src*, which was identified as a mutated cellular gene. Since the discovery of this oncogene, more than 50 different cellular oncogenes have been discovered and found to have critical roles in human cancer development.

There are two classes of oncogenes, *dominant oncogenes* and *recessive oncogenes,* or *tumor suppressor genes.* Oncogenes are derived from normal cellular genes called proto-oncogenes. The encoded protein product of a proto-oncogene often plays an important role in cell signaling, or cell growth regulation. These

genes can become activated by mutation, chromosomal translocation, amplification (gene duplication manyfold in the genome), or transcriptional dysregulation, resulting in the production of an abnormal protein or an overabundance of the normal protein. These activated proto-oncogenes are now called oncogenes, and their protein products are oncoproteins. Proto-oncogenes and oncogenes are named with a three-letter designation (e.g., *myc*). The same three-letter code, nonitalicized and starting with a capital letter, denotes the protein product (e.g., Myc). The prefix v, as in v-*src*, refers to an oncogene of viral origin. The corresponding cellular proto-oncogene is given the prefix c (c-*src*). In their activated form, the oncogenes provide a growth advantage for the expressing cell. Laboratory, clinical, and epidemiologic observations suggest that more than one genetic or biochemical event is needed to transform normal cells into malignant cells. Thus, the further accumulation of critical events in a cell population with a growth advantage results in tumorigenesis. Once a cell becomes transformed into a malignant cell (i.e., no growth restraint), other events are required for malignant cells to proliferate successfully, especially the provision of new blood vessels (angiogenesis) to create a favorable environment for growth. The interactions between the genetic changes in the cell nucleus and the changes necessary in the cell environment such as blood supply, nutrition, and extracellular matrix are only just beginning to be studied. However, these interactions are likely to be critical to conferring the various degrees of malignancy.

In practical terms, proto-oncogenes fall into five categories: growth factors, receptors for growth factors or hormones, intracellular signal transducers, nuclear transcription factors, and cell cycle control proteins. Thus, it is understandable that an oncogene, through the action of its corresponding oncoprotein, can have a profound effect on cell growth.

Dominant oncogenes are relatively easily identified, since they have a genetically dominant role in converting a nontransformed cell to a transformed (malignant) cell. In this instance, only one of the two alleles carrying a specific gene needs to be affected. The concept of dominant oncogenes and the resulting oncoproteins is illustrated in Fig. 107-1A. This figure also highlights oncogenes that have been noted so far in lung cancer.

Evidence for a second class of genes active in tumor formation—recessive oncogenes or tumor suppressor genes—has been much more difficult to establish. The earliest evidence for the existence of tumor suppressor genes in cancer genesis was from somatic cell genetic studies in which normal and tumor cells were fused. Surprisingly, the resultant hybrid cells were often not tumorigenic, an unexpected finding if a dominant oncogene was involved. If transformation was due to a dominant oncogene supplied by one member of the hybrid, the presence of normal genetic information supplied by the other member should have no effect on transformation. This led to the notion that the tumor cell had lost genetic information from both the maternal and paternal alleles of a critical genetic locus, which was replaced by the normal cell in the hybrid.

A second line of evidence for the existence of tumor suppressor genes was provided by studies of the genetics and natural history of pediatric tumors—in particular, retinoblastoma. It was proposed by Knudson that the development of retinoblastoma could be explained by the acquisition of two mutations (i.e.,

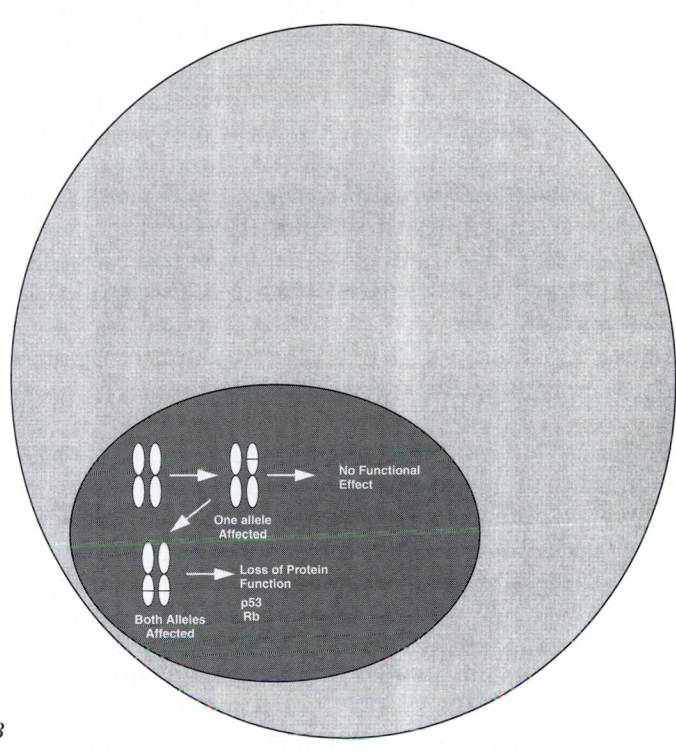

FIGURE 107-1   The role of dominant oncogenes and recessive oncogenes in human lung cancer. *A.* Dominant oncogenes require activation of only one allele. The resultant oncoprotein functions abnormally or is overproduced. Shown here are oncogenes and oncoproteins known to be active in lung cancer. *B.* Recessive oncogenes require two mutations, resulting in the actual loss or loss of function of the encoded protein. Shown here are recessive oncogenes known to be associated with lung cancer.

one mutation in both alleles of the same genetic locus). For each gene locus, the human genome has two gene copies, one maternal and one paternal. One mutation was proposed to be present in a parent's germ line and therefore abnormal in all somatic cells of the affected subject at birth. With the acquisition of a second mutation in the remaining normal allele, the protein product encoded by the affected gene became functionally inactive, and the retinoblast cell underwent malignant transformation. After elegant cytogenetic and molecular genetic analysis, it was determined that one allele of the retinoblastoma gene (*Rb*) was inactivated in the inherited form of retinoblastoma as hypothesized. On inactivation of the other retinoblastoma allele, a retinoblastoma developed. In the nonfamilial form of retinoblastoma, somatic mutations in both alleles of the retinoblastoma gene are acquired after birth. The acquisition of two events in the correct alleles is, of course, much less likely than the single event required for the heritable form of the disease, making sporadic retinoblastoma much rarer. Thus, for tumors to develop as a result of tumor suppressor oncogene abnormalities, both maternal and paternal alleles must be mutated/inactivated before the malignant phenotype is evident. Therefore, the name recessive oncogenes or tumor suppressor genes was developed. The concept of recessive oncogenes is shown in Fig. 107-1*B,* which also highlights recessive oncogenes found in lung cancer.

Many genetic regions containing suspected tumor suppressor genes have been discovered by examination of DNA obtained from malignant and normal cells from the same patient for loss of alleles, i.e., loss of heterozygosity (LOH). The two alleles of a gene locus, one maternal and one paternal, are often polymorphic and thus distinguishable through genetic techniques. However, the heterozygous pattern often found in normal tissue, due to alleles inherited from two parents, is not seen if one allele is lost or mutated. If a mutation is present in the remaining allele, the loss of the other allele unmasks the mutation, resulting in the outgrowth of cells that have lost the function of the affected gene, as in the example of retinoblastoma. In lung cancer, many such allelic losses in specific chromosomal regions have been identified. However, outside of the retinoblastoma and the *p53* gene, the presumed target of the losses (i.e., specific putative tumor suppressor genes) has not been identified.

MOLECULAR CHANGES

Cytogenetic Changes

Chromosomal changes are informative in tumors, as they point to a discrete area in the genome to examine for mutated or lost growth regulatory genetic information. Initially, chromosomal changes were discovered by examination of chromosomes in a dividing cell with microscopy. This tedious task, known as cytogenetics, began our genetic understanding of many malignant changes, beginning with the Philadelphia chromosome in 1960. In lung cancer, karyotypic or cytogenetic changes in SCLC have been repeatedly demonstrated, with consistent deletions of the short arm (p) of chromosome 3 (3p), especially 3p21-25, suggesting a tumor suppressor gene at that site. Also, losses cytogenetically of the long arm (q) of chromosomes 5, (5q21), 13 (13q14), and 17 (17q13) have been described cytogenetically. The last two sites contain the *Rb* and *p53* suppressor loci.[60] In addition, in NSCLC numerous chromosomal abnormalities are seen on cytogenetic study, most frequently (in descending order) in 3p14, 3q21, 19q13, 11p15, 1q11, 7q11, 1q21, 3p23, and 3p21. To date, the affected genes in these areas have not been described. However, these findings point out the many chromosomal defects in NSCLC that are likely to contribute to the pathogenesis of the disease, and new dominant and recessive oncogenes are likely to be discovered.[68]

Dominant Oncogenes

Myc family   The *myc* family of proto-oncogenes encode nuclear proteins that have DNA-binding properties and are thought to be active in the regulation of transcription. There are three members of this family, c-*myc* (chromosome 8q24), N-*myc* (chromosome 2p23-24), and L-*myc* (chromosome 1p32). Activation of this family of proto-oncogenes in lung cancer occurs by gene amplification and overproduction of the normal protein product. Amplification of all members of this family has been found in SCLC. In any single tumor, however, only one member of the family has been reported amplified at a time. Amplification of two or all three members simultaneously has not been found. The *myc* genes encode three related cell cycle–specific nuclear phosphoproteins. It is likely that the *myc* genes, which are highly conserved over large phylogenic distances, are important in normal cell growth and differentiation, in embryo genesis, and in apoptosis.[50] Clinically, c-*myc* gene amplification has been related to a more malignant course in SCLC. N-*myc* gene overexpression in SCLC has been correlated with a poor response to chemotherapy and a more aggressive clinical course. L-*myc* is also overexpressed in some patients with SCLC, but without apparent clinically significant effects. Understanding this abnormality has led to the possibility of targeting c-*myc* as a new form of therapy. Exposure of an SCLC cell line expressing L-*myc* to L-*myc* antisense DNA inhibited cell growth in a dose-dependent manner, perhaps suggesting a therapeutic opportunity as well as providing insight into function.[11] *Myc* gene amplification also occurs in NSCLC. In a recent study, c-*myc* amplification was found in 48 percent of NSCLC, but amplification of L-*myc* and N-*myc* was uncommon.[15] Unfortunately, the presence of c-*myc* amplification in NSCLC does not appear to have any clinical significance. It is emerging that there is clearly complex regulation of *myc* expression, and *myc* appears to regulate the expression of other proto-oncogenes. For example, c-*kit* expression may be regulated by c-*myc* when cells expressing c-*myc* do not express c-*kit*.[49]

Ras   There are three *ras* proto-oncogenes, H-*ras*, K-*ras*, and N-*ras*. These genes code for closely related 21-kDa guanosine triphosphate (GTP)–binding proteins, called p21ras, which are functionally related and have structural similarities to G proteins. These proteins are localized to the inner side of the cell membrane and participate in signal transduction. Specific K-*ras* point mutations are relatively common in NSCLC, especially in ade-

nocarcinomas. These mutations result in a single amino acid change in the protein, causing a marked reduction in its intrinsic GTPase activity, and the protein remains in an active GTP-bound state. Thus the protein is fixed in the "on" position and cannot turn off. Once acquired, these mutations appear stable, being present both in the primary tumor and in metastases, as is the case with most of the genetic mutations, although the *ras* abnormalities have been best studied in this regard. H-*ras* and N-*ras* mutations appear to be rare in human lung cancers. As the sensitivity of assays increases, the incidence of K-*ras* mutations continues to increase, occurring in up to 56 percent of lung cancers.[39] It is interesting that K-*ras* mutations have been noted in bronchial biopsies from smokers with no evidence of lung cancer,[6] and they can be found in sputum samples up to 1 year before the clinical diagnosis of lung cancer,[35] raising the question of their use as premalignant markers. Indeed, examination of the distribution of K-*ras* mutations in established tumors suggests that these changes occur at an early stage in the development of the malignancy.[34]

The carcinogen causing the K-*ras* mutation is not known, but K-*ras* mutations are closely associated with cigarette smoke exposure.[23] Whether this is a causative factor or only an association is unclear. Clinically, the presence of a K-*ras* mutation in an adenocarcinoma is an independent portent of poor survival.[30,56] The presence of this discrete molecular change has led to the design of a new treatment strategy. Tumor growth in cell lines containing a K-*ras* mutation is markedly reduced by a K-*ras* antisense RNA construct introduced by a retroviral vector.[69] Thus, a better understanding of this molecular change in lung cancer has led to the recognition of an important negative prognostic factor, a possible premalignant marker, and a novel therapeutic approach.

Ras Protein   The protein product of the *ras* gene (p21ras) has been demonstrated also to be an independent prognostic factor in defining survival in NSCLC.[41] Subjects whose tumors had a high level of p21ras expression had shorter survival than those whose tumors were p21ras negative. How this finding relates, if at all, to the known *ras* gene mutations in lung cancer and whether it provides information independent from them are unclear. Of great interest is the recent observation that inhibition of p21ras activity may be a viable treatment strategy by interfering with a posttranslational lipid modification of the molecule necessary for its function. With use of the farnesyltransferase inhibitor (FTI276), growth of a human lung cancer characterized by a K-*ras* mutation was inhibited in an animal host in a dose-dependent manner.[57]

Tumor Suppressor Genes

Retinoblastoma Gene   The retinoblastoma gene, located on 13q, was the first tumor suppressor gene to be identified, owing to its importance in the genesis of hereditary retinoblastoma. It encodes a 105,000-Da nuclear phosphoprotein (pRB) that is a regulator of cell division. pRB's phosphorylation status is key to a cell's progression through the cell cycle. pRB is underphosphorylated in G1, is heavily phosphorylated in late G1 just before S phase, but reverts to an unphosphorylated state just before G0.[67] pRB in its unphosphorylated state binds to the E2F family of transcription factors, not allowing the E2F-induced transcription of genes important to cell cycle progression. This results in a block of S phase entry, ultimately causing cell division to stop. pRB isolated from tumors is often mutated, resulting in a functionally inactive protein unable to bind E2F or to be regulated by phosphorylation. Thus, cellular proliferation becomes unregulated.[67] *Rb* gene inactivation may promote cell division by other measures as well, such as shortening telomere length.[21] In addition, differential regulation of the pRB protein may occur in SCLC versus NSCLC; pRB may be inhibited by p16 (a cyclin-dependent kinase inhibitor) in SCLC,[55] but not in NSCLC, indicating the complex relationships that exist in genetic abnormalities and are increasingly being demonstrated. However, the relationships between various common gene abnormalities have been assessed in lung cancer, and generally there is no clear or regular association of one gene defect with another.[26]

Defects in the *Rb* gene or in pRB are almost universal in SCLC but are seen in only 30 percent of NSCLC. No relationship to clinical survival has been found.[52] The central importance of pRB in growth regulation has been shown by reconstitution of the *Rb* gene into SCLC lines. This suppresses their growth, without the requirement for correction of other genetic abnormalities.[47] This finding perhaps points to another potential therapeutic strategy.

p53 Gene Initially, *p53* was thought to be a dominant oncogene, as the p53 protein was detected at very high levels in cancers. However, it is now realized that wild-type p53 is a regulator of cell growth, and mutations in the *p53* gene produce either a dysfunctional or no p53 protein. The mutant protein has a much longer half-life than the wild type, resulting in the high levels that are seen in transformed cells. The *p53* gene is located on chromosome 17p. *p53* gene abnormalities are common in lung cancer, usually as a point mutation. The encoded protein (p53) is probably a nuclear transcription factor, and it is a tumor suppressor factor by mechanisms that are not yet fully elucidated. p53 does regulate cell growth at the G1-S phase interface of the cell cycle, and it plays a role in inducing apoptosis, or programmed cell death, in cells with damaged DNA. Mutations in *p53* appear to be associated with exposures to environmental substances such as cigarette smoke.[66] Abnormalities in *p53* expression do not appear to be associated with prognosis in mixed lung tumors,[27] but they may confer a worse prognosis in patients with stage I adenocarcinomas.[24] It has been demonstrated in an animal model that wild-type *p53* can be transduced into lung cancer tumor spheroids with a retroviral vector. If the tumor cells were homozygous for a mutant *p53,* there was significant growth inhibition after transduction and expression of wild-type p53, with apoptosis induced in the cellular spheroids.[14] This raises the possibility of a novel therapeutic approach to lung cancers that have a *p53* gene mutation.

9p LOH on the short arm of chromosome 9 (9p) occurs in more than 50 percent of NSCLC,[37,43] and in SCLC there are abnormalities in the same region (9p21-22) in approximately 58 percent of cases.[38] Of interest is that 9p contains the interferon and the methylthioadenosine phosphorylase genes. These genes are deleted or rearranged in 36 to 43 percent of all lung tumor types and, while not themselves tumor suppressor genes, are probably

adjacent to a putative tumor suppressor gene.[45] This gene has recently been identified as the multiple tumor suppressor 1/cyclin-dependent kinase-4 inhibitor (*MTS 1/CDK4I*) gene and is inactivated in NSCLC.[18] When the *MTS1* gene encoding $p16^{INK4}$ is introduced into human lung cancer cell lines not expressing the gene, tumor proliferation is inhibited in vivo and in vitro. These tumor cells are growth arrested in G1 just before S phase.[25] This also raises the notion that such a gene may be a suitable gene therapy candidate in selected lung tumors.

5q Recently there have been further observations on the LOH involving 5q, which has been observed in 29 percent of NSCLC. 5q LOH correlates with tumor progression and poor survival.[12] In SCLC, 5q LOH is even more frequent, being found in more than 80 percent of cases.[8] This locus is in the region of the adenomatous polyposis coli (*APC*) gene associated with colorectal cancers, suggesting that a lung cancer tumor suppressor gene is present at this site and is associated with these lung carcinomas.

Other Proto-Oncogenes and Oncoproteins

Several other oncogenes in lung cancer appear to exert their effects through the overproduction of the normally encoded protein, not through a mutant gene or the production of an abnormal protein. The overproduction suggests a regulatory defect in transcription of the gene or gene amplification. The genes and protein products commonly affected in this manner are c-erbB-1 and c-erbB-2, both receptor tyrosine kinases; c-src, a nonreceptor tyrosine kinase; c-kit, c-met, and c-fms, also receptor tyrosine kinases; c-fos and c-jun, nuclear transcription factors; p40TAK, a protein kinase[9]; and RAF1, a serine kinase.[40] At least two of these oncoproteins—namely, c-kit in SCLC[53] and c-erbB-2 in NSCLC[29]—are increased without detectable gene amplification.

c-erbB-1 This membrane-bound proto-oncogene encodes a 170,000-Da tyrosine kinase growth receptor that is the epidermal growth factor receptor (EGFR). The proto-oncogene, through its protein product, functions in the normal lung to stimulate epithelial cell proliferation and to promote airway maturation during development. Overexpression of the proto-oncogene has been found in NSCLC, especially the squamous cell subtype, in 65 to 90 percent of reported cases. The mechanism for this is complex, as overexpression of c-erbB-1 alone does not result in transformation of cultured NIH3T3 cells. However, transformation of these cells does occur in the presence of the c-erbB-1 ligand (epidermal growth factor, transforming growth factor–α). Analysis of c-erbB-1's ability to transform airway epithelial cells has not been performed, so it is not clear whether c-erbB-1 overexpression is causative or simply associated with human lung cancer. The use of c-erbB-1 overexpression as a clinical prognostic marker is controversial, with some studies showing an association with poor survival while others do not.

c-erbB-2 This proto-oncogene is in the c-erbB-1 family of membrane-bound tyrosine kinase receptors; thus it is related to c-erbB-1 structurally and in amino acid sequence. The encoded protein, called p185c-erbB-2 or HER2, also is expressed in normal lung respiratory airway epithelial cells and may play a role in normal lung epithelium growth and differentiation. HER2 is coproduced with EGFR in many lung adenocarcinomas and almost certainly contributes to sustained cell growth.[51] This oncoprotein also co-localizes with integrin alpha 6 beta 4 at cell-cell junctions in a lung cancer cell line, suggesting one mechanism of action—namely, control of the tyrosine phosphorylation at these sites.[4] Overexpression of HER2 has been demonstrated in 34 percent of adenocarcinomas, and its presence is associated independently with a poor prognosis in this cell type.[30] This association of HER2 with prognosis has been independently confirmed, together with the finding that EGFR expression does not show any survival effect.[59] Of further interest is the recent demonstration of measurable serum levels of HER2 in 27 percent of adenocarcinomas, with an increased level in subjects with more advanced disease, suggesting a possible role as a systemic tumor marker.[48] Both of these c-erbB proteins have extracellular domains, making them attractive targets for specific antibodies, either for diagnosis or for therapy. However, therapeutic agents directed against this target may also interfere with normal epithelial turnover. Overexpression of c-erbB-2 in normal airway epithelial cells in vitro does not result in their transformation, suggesting that overexpression of c-erbB-2 alone does not result in tumor formation. With the recent identification that the receptor complex actually consists of a heterodimer consisting of HER2 and another member of the erbB family, HER3, transformation may require both to be present to form the correct heterodimeric receptor for the specific activating ligand, Heregulin.

fos   The c-*fos* gene encodes a transcription factor active in cell proliferation and differentiation. Increased expression of c-*fos* is seen in NSCLC, especially the squamous cell subtype.[64] In this study, c-Fos proteins were found in 41 percent of squamous cell lung tumors. c-Fos immunoreactivity has also been demonstrated in mucosal biopsies of the airways from asthmatic subjects, suggesting a role in normal inflammation.[10] Its role in lung cancer remains indeterminate.

jun   c-*jun* encodes an oncoprotein that functions as a transcriptional regulator. This product (c-Jun) associates with the c-*fos* product (c-Fos) to form a nucleoprotein transcription complex that interacts with AP-1 control elements. c-Jun is another oncogene product that is overexpressed in squamous cell lung cancer.[63] In this study, expression of c-*jun,* c-erbB-1, and c-*fos* were all associated with a poor prognosis. C-*myc* and c-erbB-2 overexpression did not have any survival effect. This study is one of the very few studies that has examined the co-expression of a variety of oncogenes; it is a demonstration that, in the future, clinical studies might be necessary to define the interaction of the various oncogenes and protein products, rather than just examining these aspects in isolation. The role of c-*jun* in the development of lung cancer is unclear, as apart from this study, very little other work on this oncogene has been performed.

src   The c-*src* protein (pp60) was identified as the Rous sarcoma virus transforming region *(src)*; it is expressed in both SCLC and NSCLC but not in histologically uninvolved lung tissue.[36] The importance of this remains uncertain.

THE PROGRESSION OF NORMAL AIRWAY EPITHELIUM TO MALIGNANT EPITHELIUM

As described thus far, many genetic alterations can be found in lung cancers. The current evidence suggests that many events, both genetic and epigenetic, are necessary for the transformation of normal cells to neoplastic cells. It is logical to postulate that with the accumulation of these events, the involved cell(s) would have characteristic genetic, biochemical, and morphologic changes. How many events are necessary for the malignant transformation of a lung epithelial cell and in what order they occur in lung cancer constitute an area of intense research. Colorectal carcinogenesis provides a useful paradigm for understanding this process. Further, it may be directly relevant to lung cancer, since embryologically the lung develops from the foregut, and both organs are constantly exposed to external carcinogens. In addition, the emerging association of lung cancer with known colorectal cancer genes is of great interest.

Colorectal Carcinogenesis

Morphologically, colorectal carcinomas arise from preexisting adenomas, which in turn arise from areas of hyperproliferative mucosa or from mucosa with abnormal tissue architecture. Thus, normal mucosa undergoes changes that result in proliferative or structural changes and forms microadenomas. With progression, the microadenoma becomes an early adenoma, an intermediate adenoma, a late adenoma, and finally a carcinoma. Through molecular genetic analysis of colorectal tissue at these defined morphologic stages, certain genetic alterations have been found to occur at a high frequency. These studies have become the basis for assigning a multistep pathway of genetic alterations that correspond to the mucosal phenotypic changes, summarized in Fig. 107-2.

Many studies have been performed on patients with familial adenomatous polyposis. These patients suffer from an autosomal dominant disorder resulting in diffuse colon polyp formation, and they are at increased risk for developing colorectal carcinoma. In this syndrome, germ line mutations (thus inherited) in the *APC* gene are believed to be responsible for the epithelial hyperproliferation found in the initial stage. In patients who do not have this inherited defect, LOH on chromosome 5q and/or somatic mutations of the *APC* gene may play a role in the early stages. LOH involving chromosomes 18q and 17p and mutations in the *DCC* (deleted in colorectal carcinoma) and *p53* genes occur more frequently at later stages of tumorigenesis and are infrequent in early-stage tumors. Mutations in the K-*ras* gene occur during the transition of early adenomas to intermediate adenomas. It should be made clear that the order of genetic changes is probably not invariant. It is the composite of changes rather than the specific sequence that is of importance. In addition, changes are likely to be carcinogen dependent, and therefore changes found in colorectal carcinomas may not be directly associated with pulmonary tumorigenesis. Finally, not all alterations may exist within a tumor. Thus the accumulation and interaction of numerous genetic events determine the histology and clinical phenotype of the tumor. This paradigm, while attractive, is a working model; it does not take into account quantitative alterations

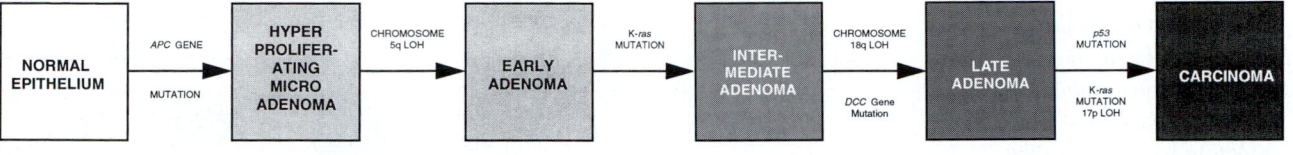

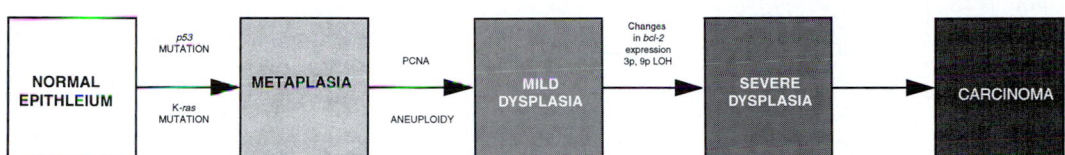

FIGURE 107-2   The multistage carcinogenesis model for colorectal cancer is shown in the top panel. This model has been reasonably validated for colorectal cancer and demonstrates a progressive series of genetic events. In contrast, the evolution of lung cancer (shown in the bottom panel) using the same multistage carcinogenesis approach is less well studied. Lung cancer, as indicated in the text, is more complex because of the different cell types and because peripheral lung tumors are not easily studied. Nevertheless, it is emerging that lung cancer also is likely to exhibit a series of defined genetic events that confer specific phenotype expression.

in levels of oncogene expression or the effect of growth factors, the surrounding connective tissue, tissue oxygenation, or angiogenesis factors. Although the model is logical and is supported by histologic and genetic studies, it is likely to be incomplete and perhaps simplistic.

Can this model be applied to the development of lung cancer? It probably can, with some similarities and many important differences. Lung cancer is also thought to develop through many stages of histologically defined epithelial changes. The earliest changes include squamous metaplasia, followed by dysplasia, carcinoma in situ, and microinvasive and invasive cancer.[2,61] While no longitudinal studies have definitely implicated the metaplastic and dysplastic lesions as premalignant, there is strong circumstantial evidence to support the notion that epithelial dysplasia represents an early stage in the development of bronchogenic carcinoma. In a study of 14,414 male smokers, the presence of atypical squamous metaplasia on cytologic examination of the sputum was considered an indicator of a modest elevation in the risk of bronchogenic carcinoma.[62] Perhaps the strongest factor making this link is the dose-response relationship between the number of cigarettes smoked per day and the frequency of dysplastic lesions in the bronchial epithelium. These changes are most evident in pulmonary squamous cell carcinomas, as has been assessed using serial sections around minute squamous cell carcinomas;[42] but they are not as clear in lung adenocarcinomas, owing to the inability to readily access, screen, and study areas of the peripheral lung from which these tumors usually arise. There is reasonable evidence, however, that a sequence of mor-

phologic changes occur in the bronchial mucosa, consistent with a multistage model of carcinogenesis for lung cancer development.

It is of great interest, therefore, to examine whether genetic changes occur in a stepwise fashion in the bronchial epithelium to correlate with the morphologic changes. This area is currently being defined, and extensive information is not yet available. However, the limited information that is available leads to the conclusion that stepwise accumulation of genetic changes also occurs in lung cancer. Not surprisingly, the events and their timing differ from the colorectal carcinoma paradigm, undoubtedly reflecting differences in the epithelium, the microenvironment, and the carcinogen exposure. The most studied molecular change has been in *p53* expression. In several analyses of preneoplastic lung lesions and lung neoplasms, alterations in the immunohistochemically defined levels of *p53* expression (which implies a mutation in *p53*) occur early, with *p53* abnormalities found in metaplastic and mild to moderate dysplastic lesions (10 to 30 percent of cases).[3,32,44,65] The frequency of *p53* alterations jumps to more than 60 percent in severe dysplasia and as high as 80 percent in carcinomas.[13,58] Further molecular changes have been the LOH of 3p and the LOH of chromosome 9p,[31] described at the severe-dysplasia stage.[22] Hyperproliferation is evident during early dysplasia, when proliferating cell nuclear antigen (PCNA), a marker of cell proliferation, is found in 33 percent of samples, as opposed to 25 percent of normal airway epithelium samples. This increases to 40 percent in severe dysplasia and to more than 85 percent at the carcinoma in situ stage.[20] This study suggests that hyperproliferation is quickly followed by DNA aneuploidy and then p53 immunoreactivity. Genetic instability is evident early in the natural history of bronchogenic cancer, with DNA aneuploidy found in 8 percent of samples with mild dysplasia, 33 percent with severe dysplasia, and 100 percent of samples with carcinoma in situ. K-*ras* mutations have not been studied as completely as *p53*, but they have been shown to occur early in the course of lung tumorigenesis, at least in adenocarcinomas.[34]

The information necessary to construct as complete a paradigm for pulmonary tumorigenesis as has been done for colorectal carcinogenesis is not available, though it is clearly being derived. Figure 107-2 provides a summary of our current understanding. It is clear that changes in specific oncogenes can be associated with specific phenotypes, giving credence to this paradigm. The ability to identify dysplastic airway lesions at bronchoscopy will create the opportunity to obtain a better collection of samples for analysis.[33] However, there is evidence of hyperproliferation in preneoplastic pulmonary epithelium, *p53* mutations, and genetic instability. The molecular paradigm for lung cancer is very complex because of the unclear familial genetics of the disease, the large number of carcinogens that may play a role in pulmonary tumorigenesis, and the variability in the malignant phenotypes that can be expressed (small cell versus large cell versus squamous cell). And unlike the situation with colon carcinoma, early events in the airway have not been as easily detected macroscopically, reducing the possibility of obtaining tissue. Also, surveillance bronchoscopies for early detection of lung cancer are not recommended, even in known at-risk patient groups.

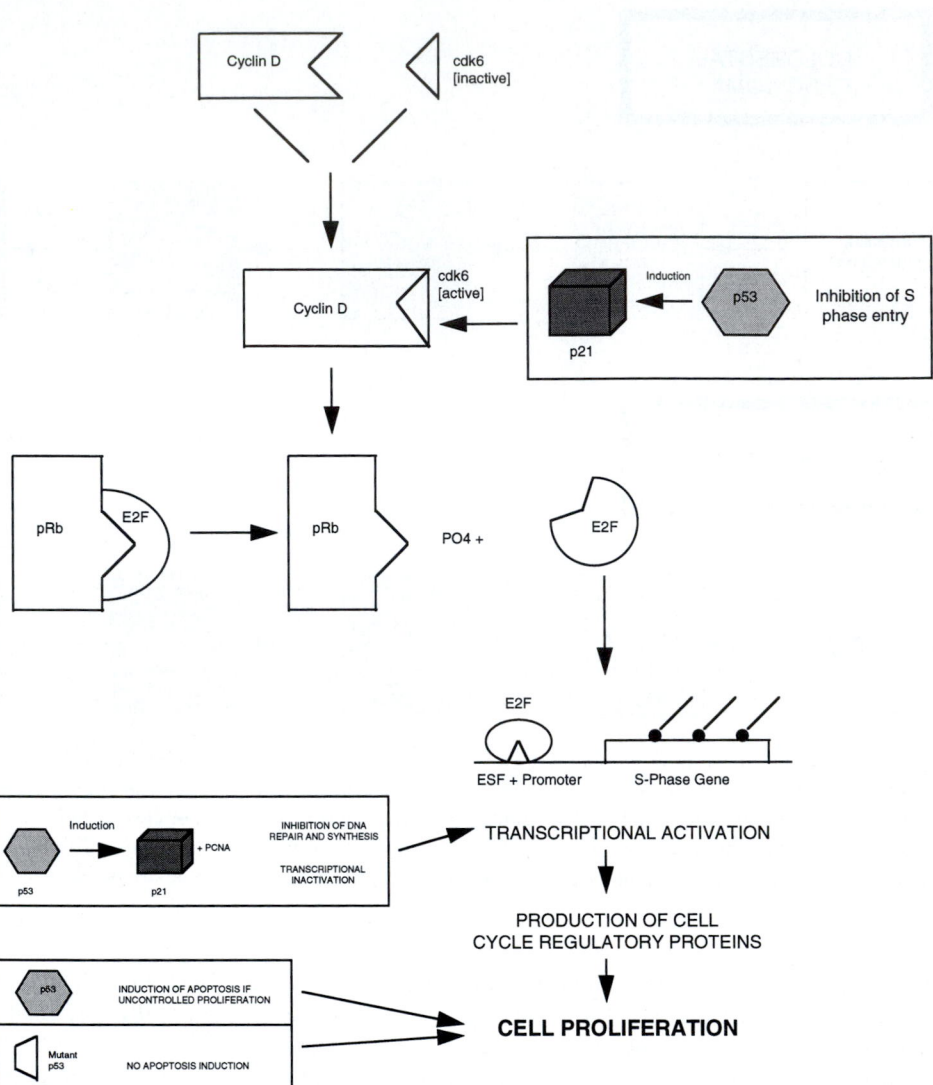

FIGURE 107-3 Tumor suppressor genes are thought to act on the cell cycle. Several different pathways of activity have been identified. The retinoblastoma protein (pRb) undergoes phosphorylation, allowing E2F to interact with its promoter, leading to transcriptional activation and the production of cell cycle regulatory proteins. p53 can act by inhibiting S phase entry through the induction of p21, by inhibition of DNA synthesis or repair through interaction with p21 and PCNA, or by inducing apoptosis.

THE IMPACT OF MOLECULAR GENETIC CHANGES ON THE CELL CYCLE

We have identified a number of genetic changes that have been found in lung cancer and proposed a multistep paradigm of lung cancer development. It is not clear, however, whether these molecular-genetic events are causative or simply associated with lung cancer. Are these events directly responsible for the genesis of lung cancer? The answer to this question is unknown, but there is evidence to suggest that some of these events may have a direct role in pulmonary tumorigenesis. At the simplest level, ma-

lignant transformation represents either the loss of regulated growth or the loss of programmed cell death (apoptosis). Therefore, if the genetic changes that occur in lung cancer affect growth regulation or apoptosis, a causative role may be implied.

Recently, much has been learned about events that regulate cell growth. In addition, all oncogenes and the genetic changes described in this chapter have an impact on cellular growth regulation. Within this framework, many of the genetic changes we have discussed affect the cell cycle. EGFR and HER2 are membrane-bound receptors that can initiate signaling and transmit a growth signal; p21 ras is also active in intracellular signaling pathways related to cell proliferation. Fos, Jun, and Myc are nuclear transcription factors that could control growth regulatory genes. The tumor suppressor genes provide the best examples of the effect of genetic changes on the cell cycle.

The cell cycle is divided into distinct periods—the G1 period (preparing for DNA synthesis), S phase (DNA synthesis), G2 period (postsynthesis), and M (mitosis). At various points in the cell cycle, there are checkpoints at which the cell has the ability to assess itself and determine whether it is ready to progress to the next phase of the cell cycle. These checkpoints are under the influence of both positive and negative regulators. If the function of a negative regulator is lost, or if a positive regulator is overexpressed, the cell may progress to the next portion of the cell cycle at an inappropriate time. Perhaps the most important checkpoint is the G1-to-S transition. At this time the cell must determine the integrity of its DNA before replication, so as not to replicate any DNA defects into the genetic code. If regulation of this checkpoint is lost, or a mutation inadvertently replicates in an important growth regulatory gene before it can be repaired, uncontrolled cell growth may result.

The Rb protein is a key regulator of the passage of cells through the G1 period. pRB function is regulated by its phosphorylation status. During the G1 period, pRB is primarily hypophosphorylated. Thus, the growth suppressive form of pRB is thought to be the hypophosphorylated form. In late G1, pRB goes through successive phosphorylations that inactivate its ability to suppress cell proliferation. The phosphorylation of pRB is regulated by a complex consisting of two subunits—a cyclin and a cyclin-dependent kinase (cdk). Specifically, the D type cyclins (D1, D2, D3) complex with and activate cdk4 and cdk6, which mediate the phosphorylation of pRB.[17] The cyclin/cdk complexes themselves are under regulation by a series of small protein inhibitors (p15, p16, p21, and p27). How is the phosphorylation of pRB important in regulation of the cell cycle? While this is still currently being defined,[7] it appears that in its unphosphorylated state, pRB binds and sequesters specific proteins necessary for cell cycle progression. The bound proteins include members of the E2F family of transcription factors, which are necessary for the expression of many genes active in DNA replication (DNA polymerase–α, PCNA). Thus, pRB binding to E2F prevents transcription from promoters containing E2F sites. Upon pRB phosphorylation, E2F is released, activating transcription. E2F DNA binding sites have been noted in a number of genes critical for cell entry into S phase. Thus, mutations of pRB that interfere with E2F binding, or affect pRB phosphorylation by cdk4 or cdk6, may result in unrestrained entry into S phase.

The G1-to-S transition is also a p53-regulated checkpoint. Structurally, p53 has hallmarks of a transcription factor; it has a sequence-specific DNA binding domain, and its amino terminus has a transcriptional activation domain. p53 has a role in DNA repair through one of its transcriptional targets, Gadd45.[19] In response to DNA damage, p53 levels rise, resulting in the transcriptional induction of the cdk inhibitor p21. p21 causes an accumulation of unphosphorylated pRB, which in turn causes G1 arrest; p53 levels also rise in response to hypoxia.[16] The p53 rise consequent on DNA damage not only seems to arrest the growth of the cell, thereby preventing transmission of the abnormal DNA, but under hypoxic conditions, it appears that the rise in p53 triggers apoptosis. In tumors that have a mutant *p53* gene, resulting in a functional loss of p53, control of cell cycle progression or apoptosis may be lost, leading to unrestrained cell growth.

Apoptosis is probably regulated by *p53* through a further mechanism. In the face of pRB inactivation or ectopic expression of E2F, entry into S phase is uncontrolled. In such cells, if

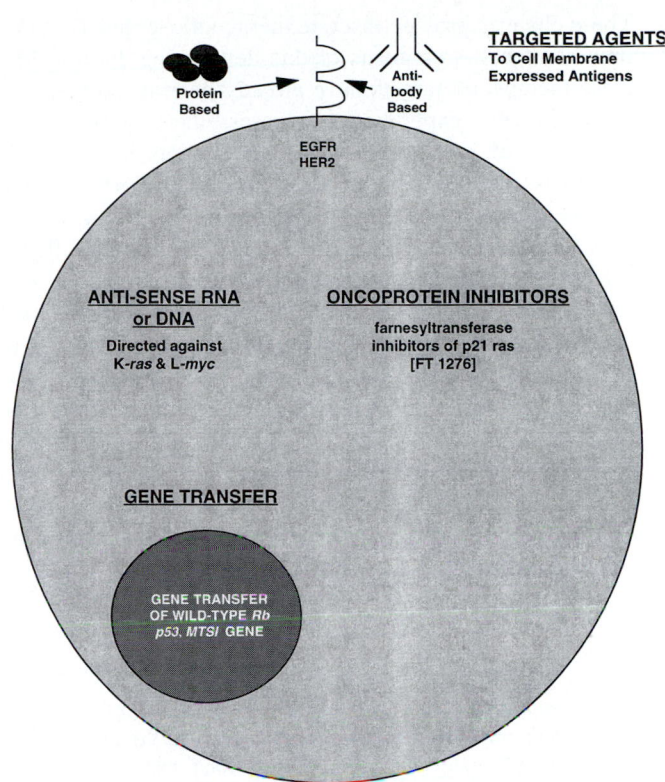

FIGURE 107-4 The potential sites for therapeutic targets are shown. Opportunities exist to target the extra cellular domain of EGFR and HER2, by either proteins or specific antibodies. Antisense RNA and DNA are currently being directed against K-*ras* and L-*myc* in cell culture studies, and specific oncoprotein inhibitors are also being tested for antitumor activity. Finally, gene transfer of several tumor suppressor genes is undergoing laboratory study, especially the transfer of the wild-type *Rb* and *p53* gene.

there is a wild-type p53 background, apoptosis ensues. In a mutant p53 background, apoptosis does not occur; uncontrolled cell proliferation ensues, with the ultimate result being neoplastic transformation. Thus, p53 regulates both cell cycle progression and apoptosis with a key role in protecting cells from duplicating damaged DNA.[28] These interactions are summarized in Fig. 107-3.

These two genes and the effects their mutations have on cell growth regulation illustrate how genetic events may play a direct role in tumor formation through deregulating cell growth. p53 and Rb have a clear impact on cell cycle regulation; however, many other genetic events found in lung cancer potentially have an impact on cell growth. p21 ras plays a role in signaling and in its mutant form may provide an unregulated growth stimulus signal; the *myc* family of oncogenes are believed to be transcriptional activators and in a mutated form perhaps provide unregulated transcription of genes important in the cell cycle; mutant or high-level expression of growth factor receptors or their ligands may result in a continuous growth stimulatory signal. Clearly, when more is understood about the function of these genetic events in lung cancer, it is likely that they will be found to have an effect on the cell cycle. In addition, many currently undescribed changes will be identified in known cell cycle genes and their encoded proteins, leading to a further understanding of genetic events occurring in pulmonary tumorigenesis.

These changes provide discrete therapeutic targets for the development of new treatments of this devastating disease. Many of these therapeutic targets have already been the subject of in vivo and in vitro experiments to assess the effects on tumor growth and differentiation. These experiments have been described in association with the description of the particular oncogene or oncoprotein and are summarized in Fig. 107-4. In all instances so far reported, there has been a measurable effect on tumor growth. It is therefore possible that major changes in the therapy of lung cancer will occur in the future with the use of these approaches either as single agents or, more likely, as part of a combined-modality therapy. This molecular approach to therapy will probably be combined with a molecular evaluation of the population most at risk, so that effective screening programs can be established. This, together with increasing efforts to reduce environmental exposures such as those from tobacco smoke, should help to bring the epidemic of deaths from lung cancer under control.

REFERENCES

1. Ambrosone CB, Rao U, Michalek AM, et al: Lung cancer histologic types and family history of cancer: Analysis of histologic subtypes of 872 patients with primary lung cancer. *Cancer* 72:1192–1198, 1993.
2. Auerbach O, Saccomanno G, Kuschner M, et al: Histologic findings in the tracheobronchial tree of uranium miners and non-miners with lung cancer. *Cancer* 42:483–489, 1978.
3. Bennett WP, Colby TV, Travis WD, et al: p53 protein accumulates frequently in early bronchial neoplasia. *Cancer Res* 53:4817–4822, 1993.
4. Campiglio M, Tagliabue E, Srinivas U, et al: Colocalization of the p185HER2 oncoprotein and integrin alpha 6 beta 4 in Calu-3 lung carcinoma cells. *J Cell Biochem* 55:409–418, 1994.
5. Cannon-Albright LA, Thomas A, Goldgar DE, et al: Familiality of cancer in Utah. *Cancer Res* 54:2378–2385, 1994.
6. Clements NC Jr, Nelson MA, Wymer JA, et al: Analysis of K-*ras* gene mutations in malignant and nonmalignant endobronchial tissue obtained by fiberoptic bronchoscopy. *Am J Respir Crit Care Med* 152:1374–1378, 1995.
7. Cordon-Cardo C: Mutations of cell cycle regulators. Biological and clinical implications for human neoplasia. *Am J Pathol* 147:545–560, 1995.
8. D'Amico D, Carbone DP, Johnson BE, et al: Polymorphic sites within the MCC and APC loci reveal very frequent loss of heterozygosity in human small cell lung cancer. *Cancer Res* 52:1996–1999, 1992.
9. Daya-Makin M, Sanghera JS, Mogentale TL, et al: Activation of a tumor-associated protein kinase (p40TAK) and casein kinase 2 in human squamous cell carcinomas and adenocarcinomas of the lung. *Cancer Res* 54:2262–2268, 1994.
10. Demoly P, Chanez P, Pujol JL, et al: Fos immunoreactivity assessment on human normal and pathological bronchial biopsies. *Respir Med* 89:329–335, 1995.
11. Dooley S, Wundrack I, Blin N, Welter C: Coexpression pattern of c-myc associated genes in a small cell lung cancer cell line with high steady state c-myc transcription. *Biochem Biophys Res Commun* 213:789–795, 1995.
12. Fong KM, Zimmerman PV, Smith PJ: Tumor progression and loss of heterozygosity at 5q and 18q in non–small cell lung cancer. *Cancer Res* 55:220–223, 1995.
13. Fontanini G, Vignati S, Bigini D, et al: Human non–small cell lung cancer: p53 protein accumulation is an early event and persists during metastatic progression. *J Pathol* 174:23–31, 1994.
14. Fujiwara T, Grimm EA, Mukhopadhyay T, et al: A retroviral wild-type p53 expression vector penetrates human lung cancer spheroids and inhibits growth by inducing apoptosis. *Cancer Res* 53:4129–4133, 1993.
15. Gazzeri S, Brambilla E, Caron de Fromentel C, et al: p53 genetic abnormalities and myc activation in human lung carcinoma. *Int J Cancer* 58:24–32, 1994.
16. Graeber TG, Peterson JF, Tsai M, et al: Hypoxia induces accumulation of p53 protein, but activation of a G1-phase checkpoint by low-oxygen conditions is independent of p53 status. *Mol Cell Biol* 14:6264–6277, 1994.
17. Grana X, Reddy EP: Cell cycle control in mammalian cells: Role of cyclins, cyclin-dependent kinases (CDKs), growth suppressor genes, and cyclin-dependent kinase inhibitors (CKIs). *Oncogene* 11:211–219, 1995.
18. Hayashi N, Sugimoto Y, Tsuchiya E, et al: Somatic mutations of the MTS (multiple tumor suppressor) 1/CDK4I (cyclin-dependent kinase–4 inhibitor) gene in human primary non–small cell lung carcinomas. *Biochem Biophys Res Commun* 202:1426–1430, 1994.
19. Hirama T, Koeffler HP: Role of the cyclin-dependent kinase inhibitors in the development of cancer. *Blood* 86:841–854, 1995.
20. Hirano T, Franzen B, Kato H, et al: Genesis of squamous cell lung carcinoma: Sequential changes of proliferation, DNA ploidy, and p53 expression. *Am J Pathol* 144:296–302, 1994.
21. Hiyama K, Ishioka S, Shirotani Y, et al: Alterations in telomeric repeat length in lung cancer are associated with loss of heterozygosity in p53 and Rb. *Oncogene* 10:937–944, 1995.
22. Hung J, Kishimoto Y, Sugio K, et al: Allele-specific chromosome 3p deletions occur at an early stage in the pathogenesis of lung carcinoma [published erratum appears in *JAMA* 273:1908, 1995]. *JAMA* 273:558–563, 1995.
23. Husgafvel-Pursiainen K, Hackman P, Ridanpää M, et al: K-ras mutations in human adenocarcinoma of the lung: Association with smoking and occupational exposure to asbestos. *Int J Cancer* 53:250–256, 1993.
24. Isobe T, Hiyama K, Yoshida Y, et al: Prognostic significance of p53 and ras gene abnormalities in lung adenocarcinoma patients with stage I disease after curative resection. *Jpn J Cancer Res* 85:1240–1246, 1994.
25. Jin X, Nguyen D, Zhang WW, et al: Cell cycle arrest and inhibition of tumor cell proliferation by the p16INK4 gene mediated by an adenovirus vector. *Cancer Res* 55:3250–3253, 1995.
26. Kashii T, Mizushima Y, Lima CE, et al: Studies on clinicopathological features of lung cancer patients with K-ras/p53 gene alterations: Comparison between younger and older groups. *Oncology* 52:219–225, 1995.
27. Kashii T, Mizushima Y, Monno S, et al: Gene analysis of K-, H-ras, p53, and retinoblastoma susceptibility genes in human lung cancer cell lines by the polymerase chain reaction/single-strand conformation polymorphism method. *J Cancer Res Clin Oncol* 120:143–148, 1994.
28. Kastan MB, Canman CE, Leonard CJ: P53, cell cycle control and apoptosis: Implications for cancer. *Cancer Metastasis Rev* 14:3–15, 1995.
29. Kern JA, Robinson RA, Gazdar A, et al: Mechanisms of p185HER2 expression in human non–small cell lung cancer cell lines. *Am J Respir Cell Mol Biol* 6:359–363, 1992.
30. Kern JA, Slebos RJC, Top B, et al: C-*erb*B-2 expression and codon 12 K-*ras* mutations both predict shortened survival for patients with pulmonary adenocarcinomas. *J Clin Invest* 93:516–520, 1994.

31. Kishimoto Y, Sugio K, Hung JY, et al: Allele-specific loss in chromosome 9p loci in preneoplastic lesions accompanying non–small-cell lung cancers [see comments]. *J Natl Cancer Inst* 87:1224–1229, 1995.

32. Klein N, Vignaud JM, Sadmi M, et al: Squamous metaplasia expression of proto-oncogenes and P 53 in lung cancer patients. *Lab Invest* 68:26–32, 1993.

33. Lam S, MacAulay C, Hung J, et al: Detection of dysplasia and carcinoma in situ with a lung imaging fluorescence endoscope device. *J Thorac Cardiovasc Surg* 105:1035–1040, 1993.

34. Li ZH, Zheng J, Weiss LM, Shibata D: c-k-ras and p53 mutations occur very early in adenocarcinoma of the lung. *Am J Pathol* 144:303–309, 1994.

35. Mao L, Hruban RH, Boyle JO, et al: Detection of oncogene mutations in sputum precedes diagnosis of lung cancer. *Cancer Res* 54:1634–1637, 1994.

36. Mazurenko NN, Kogan EA, Zborovskaya IB, Kisseljov FL: Expression of pp60c-src in human small cell and non–small cell lung carcinomas. *Eur J Cancer* 28:372–377, 1992.

37. Merlo A, Gabrielson E, Askin F, Sidransky D: Frequent loss of chromosome 9 in human primary non–small cell lung cancer. *Cancer Res* 54:640–642, 1994.

38. Merlo A, Gabrielson E, Mabry M, et al: Homozygous deletion on chromosome 9p and loss of heterozygosity on 9q, 6p, and 6q in primary human small cell lung cancer. *Cancer Res* 54:2322–2326, 1994.

39. Mills NE, Fishman CL, Rom WN, et al: Increased prevalence of K-ras oncogene mutations in lung adenocarcinoma. *Cancer Res* 55:1444–1447, 1995.

40. Miwa W, Yasuda J, Yashima K, et al: Absence of activating mutations of the RAF1 protooncogene in human lung cancer. *Biol Chem Hoppe Seyler* 375:705–709, 1994.

41. Miyamoto H, Harada M, Isobe H, et al: Prognostic value of nuclear DNA content and expression of the ras oncogene product in lung cancer. *Cancer Res* 51:6346–6350, 1991.

42. Nagamoto N, Saito Y, Sato M, et al: Lesions preceding squamous cell carcinoma of the bronchus and multicentricity of canceration—Serial slicing of minute lung cancers smaller than 1 mm. *Tohoku J Exp Med* 170:11–23, 1993.

43. Neville EM, Stewart M, Myskow M, et al: Loss of heterozygosity at 9p23 defines a novel locus in non–small cell lung cancer. *Oncogene* 11:581–585, 1995.

44. Nuorva K, Soini Y, Kamel D, et al: Concurrent p53 expression in bronchial dysplasias and squamous cell lung carcinomas. *Am J Pathol* 142:725–732, 1993.

45. Olopade OI, Buchhagen DL, Malik K, et al: Homozygous loss of the interferon genes defines the critical region on 9p that is deleted in lung cancers. *Cancer Res* 53:2410–2415, 1993.

46. Ooi WL, Elston RC, Chen VW, Bailey-Wilson JE, Rothschild H: Increased familial risk for lung cancer. *J Natl Cancer Inst* 76:217–222, 1986.

47. Ookawa K, Shiseki M, Takahashi R, et al: Reconstitution of the RB gene suppresses the growth of small-cell lung carcinoma cells carrying multiple genetic alterations. *Oncogene* 8:2175–2181, 1993.

48. Osaki T, Mitsudomi T, Oyama T, et al: Serum level and tissue expression of c-*erb*B-2 protein in lung adenocarcinoma. *Chest* 108:157–162, 1995.

49. Plummer H III, Catlett J, Leftwich J, et al: c-*myc* expression correlates with suppression of c-*kit* protooncogene expression in small cell lung cancer cell lines. *Cancer Res* 53:4337–4342, 1993.

50. Prins J, De Vries EG, Mulder NH: The myc family of oncogenes and their presence and importance in small-cell lung carcinoma and other tumour types. *Anticancer Res* 13:1373–1385, 1993.

51. Rachwal WJ, Bongiorno PF, Orringer MB, et al: Expression and activation of erbB-2 and epidermal growth factor receptor in lung adenocarcinomas. *Br J Cancer* 72:56–64, 1995.

52. Reissmann PT, Koga H, Takahashi R, et al: Inactivation of the retinoblastoma susceptibility gene in non–small-cell lung cancer. The Lung Cancer Study Group. *Oncogene* 8:1913–1919, 1993.

53. Sekido Y, Obata Y, Ueda R, et al: Preferential expression of c-kit protooncogene transcripts in small cell lung cancer. *Cancer Res* 51:2416–2419, 1991.

54. Sellers TA, Bailey-Wilson JE, Elston RC, et al: Evidence for mendelian inheritance in the pathogenesis of lung cancer. *J Natl Cancer Inst* 82:1272–1279, 1990.

55. Shapiro GI, Edwards CD, Kobzik L, et al: Reciprocal Rb inactivation and p16^{INK4} expression in primary lung cancers and cell lines. *Cancer Res* 55:505–509, 1995.

56. Silini EM, Bosi F, Pellegata NS, et al: K-ras gene mutations: An unfavorable prognostic marker in stage I lung adenocarcinoma. *Virchows Archiv* 424:367–373, 1994.

57. Sun J, Qian Y, Hamilton AD, Sebti SM: Ras CAAX peptidomimetic FTI 276 selectively blocks tumor growth in nude mice of a human lung carcinoma with K-Ras mutation and p53 deletion. *Cancer Res* 55:4243–4247, 1995.

58. Sundaresan V, Ganly P, Hasleton P, et al: p53 and chromosome 3 abnormalities, characteristic of malignant lung tumours, are detectable in preinvasive lesions of the bronchus. *Oncogene* 7:1989–1997, 1992.

59. Tateishi M, Ishida T, Kohdono S, et al: Prognostic influence of the co-expression of epidermal growth factor receptor and c-erbB-2 protein in human lung adenocarcinoma. *Surg Oncol* 3:109–113, 1994.

60. Testa JR, Graziano SL: Molecular implications of recurrent cytogenetic alterations in human small cell lung cancer. *Cancer Detect Prev* 17:267–277, 1993.

61. Trump BF, McDowell EM, Glavin F, et al: The respiratory epithelium: III. Histogenesis of epidermoid metaplasia and carcinoma in situ in the human. *J Natl Cancer Inst* 61:563–575, 1978.

62. Vine MF, Schoenbach VJ, Hulka BS, et al: Atypical metaplasia and incidence of bronchogenic carcinoma. *Am J Epidemiol* 131:781–793, 1990.

63. Volm M, Drings P, Woodrich W: Prognostic significance of the expression of c-fos, c-jun and c-erbB-1 oncogene products in human squamous cell lung carcinomas. *J Cancer Res Clin Oncol* 119:507–510, 1993.

64. Volm M, Efferth T, Mattern J: Oncoprotein (c-myc, c-erbB1, c-erbB2, c-fos) and suppressor gene product (p53) expression in squamous cell carcinomas of the lung: Clinical and biological correlations. *Anticancer Res* 12:11–20, 1992.

65. Walker C, Robertson LJ, Myskow MW, et al: p53 expression in normal and dysplastic bronchial epithelium and in lung carcinomas. *Br J Cancer* 70:297–303, 1994.

66. Wang X, Christiani DC, Wiencke JK, et al: Mutations in the p53 gene in lung cancer are associated with cigarette smoking and asbestos exposure. *Cancer Epidemiol Biomarkers Prev* 4:543–548, 1995.

67. Weinberg RA: Tumor suppressor genes. *Science* 254:1138–1146, 1991.

68. Whang-Peng J, Knutsen T, Gazdar A, et al: Nonrandom structural and numerical chromosome changes in non–small-cell lung cancer. *Genes Chromosom Cancer* 3:168–188, 1991.

69. Zhang Y, Mukhopadhyay T, Donehower LA, et al: Retroviral vector-mediated transduction of K-ras antisense RNA into human lung cancer cells inhibits expression of the malignant phenotype. *Hum Gene Ther* 4:451–460, 1993.

EPIDEMIOLOGY OF LUNG CANCER

Pieter E. Postmus

In the beginning of the twentieth century, lung cancer was a rare disease. Now, it has become the leading cause of cancer death in males in the industrialized world. For females the incidence is still increasing, and in some countries, it is already the most frequent cause of cancer death. The number of new cases is increasing rapidly in most countries in Eastern Europe and in most developing countries. For most other cancers, the death rates are either improving or, at least, leveling off. Worldwide, there is an epidemic, progress in therapy is minimal, and with the increasing use of tobacco, the prospects for a decrease in incidence or mortality appear dismal.

SMOKING AND LUNG CANCER

The lung cancer epidemic was first noted in males in the United States and a number of European countries during the 1940s.[49] By the early 1950s, epidemiologic studies using case control approaches had provided strong evidence that cigarette smoking was the predominant cause of the disease.[48] During the 1950s and 1960s, prospective cohort studies confirmed the findings of the case control studies, and epidemiologic and toxicologic evidence supported the conclusion that smoking was the major cause of lung cancer.[43]

In 1912, when cigarette smoking was rather uncommon, the incidence of primary lung cancer at autopsy in major hospitals in the United States and Western Europe was less than 0.5 percent.[1] In industrialized countries, incidence increased markedly in the following decades, first in men and later in both men and women. In 1930, the age-adjusted lung cancer death rate among United States males was about five per 1 million per year. This increased to 22.2 in 1950, 55.9 in 1970, and 74.9 in 1987. Among women in the United States, the corresponding lung cancer death rates were 3.0, 5.06, 12.2, and 28.5, respectively. Since 1987, lung cancer death rates among American men have reached a plateau and, in fact, have declined in younger men (under 45 years of age); among American women, lung cancer death rates continue to increase, except among the very young. Similar trends in lung cancer incidence have been observed in other developed countries. The incidence of 97 per 100,000 per year among males in the United Kingdom in 1980 is the highest reported anywhere.[5]

The consumption of cigarettes in the United States increased tremendously between World War I and the 1960s; but from 1976 to the present, the use of cigarettes has declined. Similar trends have been observed in other Western nations.[2,28] In 1950, 0.56 percent of the cigarettes smoked in the United States had filter tips. Since that time, the market share of filter-tipped cigarettes has increased to 19 percent in 1955, 51 percent in 1960, 80 percent in 1970, 92 percent in 1980, and more than 97 percent in 1992. Thirty to 50 percent of all cigarettes sold in the United States have perforated filter tips. In Japan, the United Kingdom, and Italy, the production of filter-tipped cigarettes began about 10 years later than in the United States. Today, at least 90 percent of all cigarettes sold in industrialized countries have filter tips—except France, where filter cigarettes make up only 70 percent of the market. In North America and Europe, only a small percentage of the cigarettes sold feature charcoal-containing filter tips. However, filter tips containing charcoal make up more than 70 percent of the cigarettes currently sold in Japan—a fact that may have implications on the development of lung cancer, which will be discussed below.[42]

Factors that influence the risk of developing lung cancer in cigarette smokers include the duration of smoking, the number of cigarettes smoked—usually quantified as the number of pack-years (1 pack-year is 20 cigarettes a day for 1 year)—the type of cigarettes smoked, and the age at initiation of cigarette smoking. Analysis of data from a study of British doctors indicated that the risk increased approximately with the fourth power of duration of smoking and with the square of the number of cigarettes smoked daily.[11] This relationship indicates that interpretation of age-specific trends of lung cancer rates should be based on both age-related patterns of the time at onset of smoking and amount of cigarettes smoked (Table 108-1).

Despite the overwhelming epidemiologic evidence of a causal relation between exposure to tobacco smoke and lung cancer, a number of unresolved issues remain to be discussed.

CIGARETTE SMOKING AND THE HISTOLOGY OF LUNG CANCER

The first large-scale case control study from the United States linking cigarette smoking and lung cancer was published in 1950. In this study, 597 of the 605 male lung cancer patients had a smoking history, and the ratio of squamous cell lung cancer to adenocarcinoma was 16:1.[48] Later studies from the United States demonstrated a significant change in the relative frequency of adenocarcinoma versus other histologic types in males (Table 108-2). From the ratio of 1:2.3 observed between 1969 and 1975, an increase in the number of adenocarcinomas changes this ratio to 1:1.4 observed between 1981 and 1988. While the number of adenocarcinomas increased, the frequency of squamous cell carcinoma remained stable.[10,51] Likewise, in women the number of adenocarcinomas increased faster than squamous cell lung cancer, also resulting in a change in the ratio.[47] Since 90 percent of men and approximately 80 percent of women who develop lung cancer have a smoking history, it is not unreasonable

TABLE 108-2

Histology Distribution for Three Time Intervals*

Period	Squamous	Adeno	Small Cell	Large Cell
1973–77	13.4	10.5	5.9	—
1978–82	15.1	14.2	8.2	3.9
1983–87	15.3	16.7	9.4	4.9

*Rate per 100,000 person-years.

to postulate that a change in incidence of lung cancer types may be related to the consumption of cigarettes.

From 1955 to the present, average cigarette smoke yields in the United States declined from 38 mg tar and 2.7 mg nicotine per cigarette to 13.5 mg and 1.0 mg, respectively.[20] These values were established under "standardized smoking conditions," which is the way a smoker smoked high-nicotine, nonfilter cigarettes in the 1930s: one puff per minute with a volume of 35 ml over 2 s.[6] Clearly, the most important factor for the way in which tobacco products are used is the dependency on nicotine. The amount of nicotine per puff is much lower in the low-yield filter cigarette than it was in the unfiltered, high-nicotine cigarette common in 1930. For most smokers, this has resulted in a much more intensive way of smoking modern-day cigarettes, which averages five puffs per minute with up to 55 ml per puff and a puff duration of almost 2 s.[24] When a smoking machine is set in this way, the yield of tar, nicotine, carbon monoxide, and most of the known carcinogens is two to three times higher than for "standardized conditions." With the higher volume per puff, it is likely that the smoke will be inhaled more deeply, resulting in exposure of the smaller bronchi and at the bronchoalveolar level to much higher amounts of certain smoke constituents, including carcinogenic, volatile aldehydes, polynuclear aromatic hydrocarbons, aromatic amines, and tobacco-specific N-nitrosamines (TSNA).[14]

In France, squamous cell lung cancer remains much more common than adenocarcinoma—a fact that may be related to the continued high-level use of unfiltered cigarettes, 87.8 percent in 1972 and 81.4 percent in 1992. Furthermore, black tobacco remains much more popular in France.[3] The smoke of black tobacco is slightly alkaline and results in a substantially higher amount of nicotine in free form, which makes deep inhalation unnecessary in comparison to cigarettes made of blended or bright tobaccos.

Another important factor is the relative increase of some carcinogens and the relative decrease of others in cigarette smoke. Carcinogenic polycyclic hydrocarbons cause squamous cell carcinoma in rodents, while TSNA in these animals is a strong inducer of an adenocarcinoma that resembles adenocarcinoma and bronchoalveolar carcinoma in humans. The topical carcinogenic effect of nitrosamines is weak. When they are metabolically activated, however, they can be converted to potent carcinogens. In the lung, such metabolic activation occurs when nitrosamines are applied in areas of rich vascularity.[21] One of the TSNAs, 4-(methylnitrosamino)-1-(3-pyridyl)-1-butanone (NNK), is a procarcinogen and is activated by cytochrome P_{450} which is present in human lung. Accordingly, the dose of the alkylating species

TABLE 108-1

Number of Cigarettes Smoked and Relative Risks of Death from Lung Cancer Among Male Smokers

No. per Day	U.S. Veterans	British Doctors
None	1.0	1.0
Current smokers	12.1	14.0
1–9	5.5	7.8
10–19	9.9	17.4
20–39	17.4	25.1
≥40	23.9	—

formed by α-hydroxylation of NNK (4-oxo-4-[3-pyridyl]butane diazohydroxide) is much greater in the richly vascularized bronchioles and alveoli than in the larger bronchi. These react with DNA to form methylated bases that may be responsible for the mutations frequently found on codon 12, the activated proto-oncogene K-*ras*, in lung adenocarcinomas developing in smokers. The K-*ras* mutations are also present in adenocarcinomas developing in ex-smokers; thus, this damage seems to be irreversible.[31] This may help to explain why ex-smokers, even those who quit many years ago, still have a higher risk of developing lung cancer than those who never smoked cigarettes (Table 108-3).

The amount of NNK in cigarette smoke increased by 45 percent between 1978 and 1992, and the most important hydrocarbon in cigarette smoke of nonfilter cigarettes in the United States has decreased by about 60 percent since 1965.[21] Both of these factors—together with the use of filter cigarettes, other tobaccos, and a different smoking pattern of low-yield cigarettes—may help to explain the relative decrease of squamous carcinoma and the absolute increase of adenocarcinoma.

PREDISPOSITION FOR LUNG CANCER

Data from a number of studies implicate host-specific factors in the pathogenesis of lung cancer. Indirect evidence is provided by the observation that less than 20 percent of heavy smokers develop the disease.[28] Case control studies and case control family studies consistently demonstrate that lung cancer clusters in families even after the effects of measured environmental factors are considered.[32] While the mechanisms underlying familial aggregation remain unknown, a number of biologically plausible hypotheses can be advanced. Tobacco smoke carcinogens are activated enzymatically to electrophiles that form carcinogen-DNA adducts. Detoxifying enzymes compete with the activating enzymes in the metabolism of the procarcinogenic smoke components. Variations from person to person are known to exist in these two types of enzymatic reactions, as well as in the repair rates of DNA damage caused by tobacco carcinogens. These interindividual differences in metabolic activation and DNA repair reflect the acquired and inherited host factors that may influence the risk for a smoker of developing lung cancer or cancer at other sites.

Several studies have indicated that the metabolism of the antihypertensive drug debrisoquine is under autosomal genetic control and that smokers who are extensive metabolizers of debrisoquine are at significantly greater risk for lung cancer than

those who are poor or intermediate metabolizers.[10] However, other studies have not confirmed this. The mechanism of such a predisposition is not clearly understood, but most studies have pointed to the likely involvement of phase 1 and 2 enzymes, which can play an important role in the activation of lung carcinogens. Among these are several isoforms of the cytochrome P_{450} monooxygenase system. For example, mutations in the *CYP2D6* debrisoquine hydroxylase locus, which result in severely impaired metabolism of more than 25 known drugs, were found in 8 to 10 percent of the Caucasian population.[7] Of interest is that among 361 lung cancer patients, no statistically significant change in the proportion of poor metabolizers relative to controls was identified. In a large twin study, no significant differences were found to support the possible inheritance of lung cancer.[7] This suggests that there might be small subgroups with a genetic predisposition to develop lung cancer, but for most patients, exogenous factors are far more important than the combination of exogenous and endogenous influences.

INFLUENCE OF GENDER

Several studies have shown that the relative incidence of adenocarcinoma is higher among females than males—especially in nonsmoking females, in whom adenocarcinoma was found in 50 to 80 percent of the affected patients.[23] The relative incidence of adenocarcinoma is higher in women, especially in nonsmoking women, than in men. It appears that the lungs of women may be more susceptible than those of men to the carcinogenic effects of cigarette smoke. For a given level of smoking, the relative risk for females to develop lung cancer is clearly higher (1.9).[19] Laboratory studies as well as clinical findings provide evidence that hormonal factors may play a role in causing lung cancer. In one study, estrogen replacement therapy significantly increased the risk of developing adenocarcinoma.[38]

INFLUENCE OF DIAGNOSTIC TECHNIQUES

During the 1970s, the fiberoptic bronchoscope became widely available for use in examining the tracheobronchial tree in suspected cases of lung cancer. This makes possible a more complete examination of the lungs. In addition, fine-needle aspiration has increasingly been used to establish a diagnosis with little risk to the patient. As a result of such advances in diagnostic techniques, it is likely that more people with suspected lung cancer have received a histologic or cytologic diagnosis and that elderly patients, in particular, are more likely to have a histologically confirmed diagnosis than in the past, when obtaining tissue subjected the patient to a major procedure. Furthermore, the introduction of computed tomography made it possible to determine the extent and spread of lung cancer within the thorax and has contributed to reducing misclassification of benign lesions as lung cancer.[16]

Data from the Surveillance, Epidemiology, and End Results (SEER) program of the U.S. National Cancer Institute confirm these speculations about diagnostic practice. As a result, the incidence of cases classified as "other and unspecified histology" declined in males from 1969 until 1986. Another factor that might

TABLE 108-3

Years After Quitting Smoking and Relative Risks of Lung Cancer in Males

Years after Cessation	U.S. Veterans	British Doctors
0	11.3	15.8
1–4	18.8	16.0
5–9	7.5	5.9
10–14	5.0	5.3
15–19	5.0	2.0
≥20	2.1	

play a role in the change in histologic patterns is the increasing use of mucin stains, since mucin-containing tumors are classified as adenocarcinomas. The classification of tumors by individual pathologists might also have influenced the classification. In a study reviewing histologic and cytologic diagnoses from tumors identified during the early 1970s and early 1980s, a lower number of adenocarcinomas were found in women, along with an increase in small-cell lung cancer—a pattern similarly noted in men.[9a]

INCIDENCE OF LUNG CANCER WORLDWIDE

Detailed information on smoking patterns and incidence and mortality trends remains unavailable from many areas of the world. Where data exist, we can conclude that in most of the developed countries, age-adjusted mortality in males increased steadily until the mid-1980s, when it plateaued and then started to decline. This is in contrast to data available for women, for whom the incidence is still increasing in most countries. The declining rates in younger males may be a reflection of the change in cigarette tar content during the past several years. Overall, the global incidence of lung cancer is increasing at a rate of 0.5 percent per year. In most parts of the world, the incidence is higher in urban than in rural areas, with a ratio of 1.2 to 2.[25] Lung cancer is a rapidly increasing problem in developing countries, especially in males. In females, except those of Chinese origin, the relative rate is low. For Chinese women these higher rates have been attributed to exposure to environmental pollutants, such as fossil fuel combustion products and cooking oils in the home.

When one is evaluating the incidence of lung cancer in developing countries, it is important to note that certain of these countries, most notably China and the nations of Eastern Europe, either lack regulations or are far less strict in regulating nicotine and tar content of cigarettes. In these parts of the world, the average tar yield is higher than in the United States, Western Europe, and Japan.

Additionally, an unexplained observation might be of importance for the future incidence of lung cancer, especially among African smokers. In the United States, there is a significant difference in mortality between African-Americans and white Americans, with a lower mortality among white males even though they smoke 25 percent more than blacks.[4] These differences may be attributable to differences in the way major constituents of cigarette smoke are metabolized. An example of these differences might be the metabolism of nicotine. In a biomarker study, the amount of urinary metabolites of one of the lung cancer carcinogens in cigarette smoke, NNK, was much higher in white smokers than in African-Americans, lending support to the concept of a difference in metabolism of tobacco smoke carcinogens.[44]

The role of smoking as the most important cause of lung cancer is undeniable. Other factors, however, are also implicated in lung cancer causation. In the early 1920s, the consumption of cigarettes increased rapidly. In the United States it reached a maximum in 1974, with 3800 cigarettes per adult; in the United Kingdom, this maximum was reached in 1970 with a consumption of 3300 cigarettes per adult. In Japan the increase of cigarette consumption started after World War II and reached a maximum in 1981 with 3400 cigarettes per adult. Since 1955 a higher proportion of men in Japan than in the United States have smoked. Since 1955 the percentage of smokers in the United States declined from 54.2 to 27.2 percent in 1985, whereas in Japan it declined from an all-time high of 82.3 percent in 1965 to 60 percent in 1985. The consumption of cigarettes by smokers in the two countries was comparable during these periods; therefore, one would expect comparable rates of lung cancer mortality in the two countries.[5] However, the age-adjusted death rates per 100,000 for the years 1986–88 were 60.9 for the United Kingdom, compared to 56.9 for the United States and only 28.6 for Japan. Except for smokers with a very high cigarette consumption (more than 40 a day), the relative risks of dying from smoking-related lung cancer remain far lower in Japan than in the United States or the United Kingdom.

Several factors might account for this difference, including age at start of smoking, personal smoking behavior, content of cigarettes, and dietary factors. The earlier the age at start of smoking, the greater the risk of developing lung cancer. Early start of smoking is also associated with higher cigarette consumption later in life. In Japan, less than 1 percent of all men start smoking before the age of 15, and 60 percent start between 20 and 24. In the United States, 16 to 20 percent of men start before the age of 15 and 49 to 56 percent became regular smokers between 15 and 19. However, even if one compares groups in Japan and the United States who started smoking at comparable ages, the risk of developing lung cancer in Japan is significantly lower. The cigarettes smoked in the two countries are made of similar tobacco blends, and contents of nicotine and tar have been comparable during recent decades. However, the yields of some toxic volatile agents in the smoke of Japanese cigarettes are expected to be significantly lower because more than 70 percent of all cigarettes sold in Japan have charcoal-containing filters. These filters selectively remove from smoke volatile constituents such as hydrogen cyanide and certain volatile aldehydes that inhibit lung clearance; they also retain a considerable amount of carcinogenic volatile N-nitrosamines.[9]

International ecologic studies have indicated that the fat content of the diet may play a key role in the risk of developing lung cancer among cigarette smokers. Several case control studies support these observations, noting a higher risk for the development of lung cancer for cigarette smokers with high-fat diets. In the United States, the average percentage of total caloric intake of fat ranged between 50 and 43.5 percent between 1950 and 1985. In Japan, it increased during the same period from 7.9 to 24.5 percent. An adequate intake of green-yellow vegetables and of fruits also reduces the risk of developing cancer among smokers; however, the intake of these vegetables is inversely related to the intake of fat.[51] From laboratory studies it is known that tea preparations may inhibit tumorigenesis, probably by antioxidative effects of some of the polyphenols in tea. In Japan, a population study demonstrated a protective effect of tea (primarily green tea) consumption. The per-capita consumption of green tea in Japan is much higher than the consumption of tea (primarily black tea) in the United States. In the United Kingdom, the significantly higher consumption of black tea does not seem to correlate with either cancer incidence or mortality.[17]

OTHER FACTORS RELATED TO LUNG CANCER

Environmental Tobacco Smoke

There is little doubt that tobacco smoke is by far the most important carcinogenic factor for the development of lung cancer. However, lung cancer is also seen in nonsmokers, especially in females: 20 percent of women who develop lung cancer are nonsmokers. Much attention has been given to environmental exposure to cigarette smoke. This so-called sidestream or secondhand smoke has been found to contain virtually all the carcinogens identified in the smoke inhaled directly by smokers.[8] Since sidestream smoke does not pass through the filters of the cigarettes, it contains around 100 times the weight of carcinogens of mainstream smoke. Consequently, elevated levels of carcinogens are found in the blood and urine of those passively exposed to cigarette smoke.

It is, therefore, biologically plausible that passive smoke exposure may cause lung cancer, since there is no established threshold level of exposure to carcinogens for the development of lung cancer. In an autopsy study of nonsmoking women who had been married to smokers, significantly more epithelial, possibly precancerous lesions were found in bronchi and pulmonary parenchyma than in wives of nonsmokers. In many homes and workplaces, environmental exposure to cigarette smoke has been common and remains so. It is only recently that in the developed countries smoking in public buildings, schools, and hospitals has been subject to governmental regulations to diminish involuntary exposure. The magnitude of the effect of environmental tobacco smoke on causation of lung cancer in different populations remains under study and debate. The percentage of cases in Western countries in nonsmokers attributed to environmental exposure has been estimated to be about 20 to 30 percent.[41]

Air Pollution

Pollutants in the urban air, other than tobacco smoke, have been investigated as potential causative agents that might be partly responsible for the epidemic increase of lung cancer. The products of fossil fuel combustion, principally polycyclic hydrocarbons, have been of particular concern. Other sources of ambient air pollution are motor vehicle and diesel engine exhausts, power plants, and industrial and residential emissions. Evidence to support the possible association of air pollution and lung cancer comes from the higher incidence of lung cancer in workers exposed to combustion products from fossil fuels. Also, roofers exposed to coal-tar fumes have a 50 percent higher risk of lung cancer after 20 years of exposure.[18]

Socioeconomic Status

Several studies have reported an inverse relationship between lung cancer mortality and socioeconomic status. A twofold gradient in mortality was observed between low and high social class, as measured by occupation, income, and education. Smoking patterns accounted for part of the risk differential, but other explanations could be a difference in risk factors such as occupation, diet, and exposure to other ambient air pollutants.

Radon Exposure

Exposure to radon gas, a decay product of uranium, at levels and under conditions found in underground mines can cause lung cancer. Radon can enter homes from subsoils and, in rare instances, accumulate to levels that exceed occupational standards in mines. This might have an impact on the incidence of lung cancer and especially increase the already considerable risk to smokers of developing lung cancer. The combination of radon exposure with smoking seems multiplicative and not just additive.[34]

Asbestos

Despite extensive measures in recent years to ban asbestos from the environment, there are many people who have been exposed to asbestos. Certain persons—in particular, shipyard workers and those who work with insulation materials—may have had considerable exposure. The most important malignancy related to asbestos exposure is malignant mesothelioma of the pleura and peritoneum. Furthermore, exposure to asbestos also causes a number of other abnormalities, such as pleural plaques and interstitial pulmonary fibrosis (asbestosis). When these are combined with cigarette smoking, the risk of developing lung cancer is extremely high. However, asbestos exposure alone also is associated with a higher risk of developing lung cancer.[45]

Other Occupational Factors

Besides tobacco smoke, a number of industrial processes and byproducts may increase the risk of lung cancer, especially in smokers (Table 108-4). Included in this group are arsenic, bischloromethyl ether, cloromethyl, methyl ether, chromium, nickel, polycyclic aromatic hydrocarbons, vinylchloride, and ionizing radiation.

Previous Lung Disease

Lung cancer incidence has been reported to be higher in patients with other diseases of the lung, such as tuberculosis, chronic bronchitis, or silicosis. Chronic cigarette smoking retards mucociliary clearance of foreign particles and respiratory tract secretions, evokes an inflammatory response accompanied by fibrosis and thickening in the membranous and respiratory bronchioles, and causes mucous gland hypertrophy, hyperplasia, and dysplasia in proximal airways. This structural bronchopulmonary and functional damage results in a sustained exposure of the mucosa to the carcinogenic products of tobacco combustion.

DETECTION OF LUNG CANCER

Attempts to reduce cigarette smoking generally have been met with resistance in a few segments of the population. Accordingly, a large increase in lung cancer incidence can be expected in countries where smoking has become a common habit, and the num-

TABLE 108-4

Lung Cancer Risk Factors

Agent	Source/Epidemiology
Arsenic	Byproduct of copper, lead, zinc, tin, or smelting In organic trivalent arsenic-containing pesticides
Asbestos	In several industries: miners, millers, textile, insulation, shipyard, cement
Bis-chloromethyl ether Chloromethyl, methyl either	Industries producing ion exchange resins, polymers, plastics
Chromium	Used in metal alloys, electroplating, lithography, magnetic tapes, paint pigments, cement, rubber, photo-engraving, floor covering
Nickel	Used in electroplating, manufacturing of steel and other alloys, ceramics, storage batteries, electric circuits, petroleum refinement, oil hydrogenation
Polycyclic aromatic hydrocarbons	Result from ferrochromium production, smelting of nickel-containing ores, aluminum production, iron and steel founding, coke production, coal gasification, coal tars, coal tar pitches, untreated mineral oils, soots from combustion, diesel engine exhausts
Radon	Underground miners
Vinylchloride	Used in production of plastics, packaging materials, vinyl asbestos floor tiles

ber of patients should remain high in the developed countries. It is perhaps more realistic to accept this fact and act accordingly than just deny it by noting that lung cancer should be a preventable disease. Therefore, attempts to improve the results of therapy should be a major priority.

One approach is to try to identify patients at an earlier stage after the detrimental effects of the usually prolonged exposure to carcinogens have taken place. Unfortunately, most patients with lung cancer present with metastatic disease; for these patients, the most important goal of therapy is palliation. However, the results of therapy for early-stage lung cancer are significantly better, and overall disease-free survival has improved during recent decades.[30] The identification of localized disease enhances the likelihood of long-term survival for those patients. This supports further research into methods to improve the early detection of lung cancer and to intervene at early stages.

Even more striking are the excellent results of endobronchial therapy for radiographically occult cancers, and attempts to detect lung cancer at this very early stage might be even more rewarding than detection of radiographically visible stage I disease.[36]

Historically, neoplastic diseases have been studied from the more advanced stages backward, which has encouraged our ways of thinking about cancer. It is uncertain when the critical neoplastic change is reached or when the change is no longer reversible. It is generally believed that development of the malignant phenotype follows a sequence from hyperplasia through dysplasia to carcinoma in situ (Fig. 108-1).

The development of most cancers is a multistep process comprising a series of genetic, molecular, and histopathologic changes. Lung cancer is the end result of an accumulated series of molecular, biochemical, and epigenetic changes involving the activation of dominant-acting cellular proto-oncogenes and the inactivation (chromosomal deletion) of recessive or "tumor suppressor genes." Considering cancer only when clinically evident disease is present confers a limited perspective.

Health professionals need to consider the carcinogenesis as a protracted process in which the progressive dysregulation of gene function in response to cell injury from exposure to genotoxic agents occurs over a period of several years. The preclinical phase of epithelial carcinogenesis may provide opportunities for more effective cancer control measures. An understanding of the process of genetic control of cell functions, especially with regard to genetic factors controlling cell growth, such as oncogenes and suppressor genes, may help to define the earliest events in the process of transformation. Attempts to block this process should be based on rationally derived prevention measures.

The existence of a preneoplastic state of lung cancer was recognized several decades ago. Precancerous conditions represent clinical states that are associated with a higher risk of cancer than is seen on average in the population. A premalignant lesion does not imply that cancer is inevitable. The term, at best, refers to certain well-defined histologic changes that increase the probability of risk of developing a malignancy. It has been found that not all early lesions progress to carcinoma but frequently disappear "spontaneously."[37] Identifying mechanisms that lead to spontaneous regression might be helpful in developing strategies designed to reverse the process of carcinogenesis. This approach of trying to intervene at an early, noninvasive stage of clonal expansion on the epithelial surface may improve cancer control because the earlier cancer cells may not yet possess the genetic plasticity of advanced cancer.

Approaches for Early Detection

The concept of carcinogenesis as a field effect comes from the observation that oral tumors often arise as multicentric lesions. The carcinogen-exposed epithelium is preconditioned to develop various premalignant and malignant foci. From many reports, it is known that patients with an upper respiratory tract malignancy are at high risk of developing other primary aerodirective malignancies. This group of patients is, therefore, ideal not only for early detection studies but also for studies of chemoprevention. The beneficial effect of retinoids with regard to development of

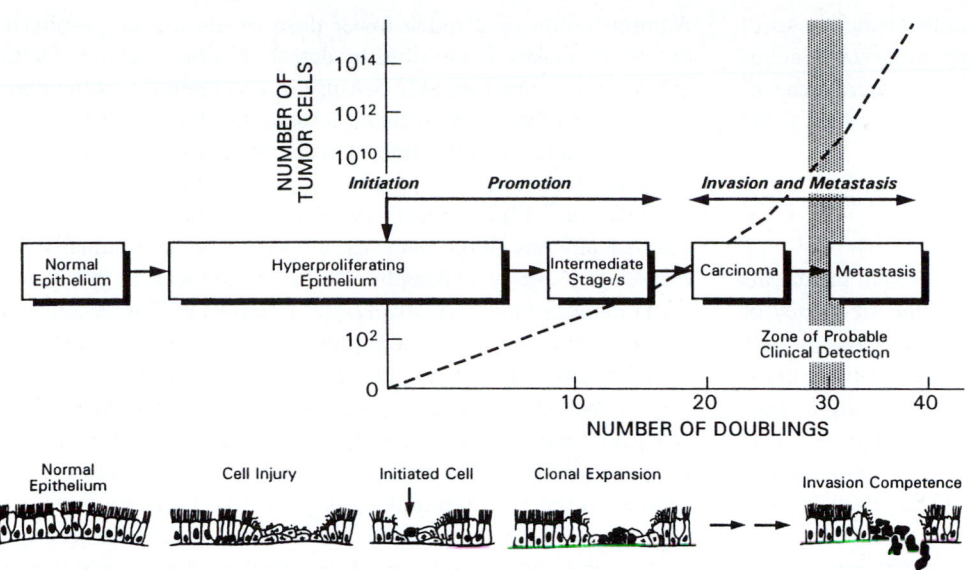

FIGURE 108-1   Estimated tumor burden at varying stages of invasive lung cancer. *(From Mulshine et al,[28a] with permission.)*

second primary tumors in head-and-neck cancer patients is a good example of the latter application.[22]

Genetic Predisposition

The detrimental effects of tobacco smoke are known, but other factors obviously play a role, since only about 20 percent of heavy smokers develop lung cancer. People differ in their ability to activate potential carcinogens; thus, the extent of biologic effects of carcinogens may vary from person to person. Metabolic phenotypes such as aryl hydrocarbon hydroxylase, debrisoquine hydroxylation, and glutathione-S-transferase activity have been considered possible markers of genetic susceptibility to lung cancer. Because, in all these studies, metabolic phenotypes and genotypes were used, it is not easy to apply this for screening as long as the specific marker for the genotype has not been identified.

Another type of susceptibility marker is the DNA repair capacity, which is known to vary significantly among people. A commonly used assay measures DNA repair in lymphocytes exposed in vitro to a mutagen or a carcinogen. It is now possible to measure the expression of a DNA repair gene in human tissues. These measurements may provide useful information on inherited predisposition of a host to cancer and the ability to face environmental challenges.[47] Not enough is yet known, however, for this assay to be used in screening subjects with risk factors for lung cancer, since the specificity of the assay remains to be determined.

Molecular Markers

Changes in genes, gene products, and chromosomal abnormalities have been advocated as biomarkers of premalignancy or early cancer. Overexpression of genes or structural abnormalities in genes are frequently found in established lung tumors.[33] Genes of the *ras* family are commonly identified as abnormal in lung cancer. K-*ras* mutations are associated with a somewhat less ag-

gressive course of non–small-cell lung cancer, whereas changes in H-*ras* are associated with a more aggressive course. *Her-2/neu* is overexpressed in a number of non–small-cell lung cancers, and detection of the gene in preneoplastic, metaplastic, or dysplastic shed cells in sputum by an antibody assay may help identify patients with precancerous lesions. Other candidate genes for detection by antisera or polymerasechain reaction amplification are *p53* and *rb*. The tumor suppressor gene *p53* especially is a good candidate because it is frequently found in non–small-cell lung cancers.

Chromosomal abnormalities potentially may also be used as biomarkers of susceptibility. Abnormalities have been reported in chromosome numbers 3, 11, 13, and 17, most often associated with tumor suppressor genes such as *p53* at chromosome 17 and *rb* on chromosome 13.

However, before changes in genes or gene products resulting from these genetic changes can be adopted as biomarkers of premalignant or early cancer, their use for this purpose needs to be validated. Ideally, this should be done in a randomized study comparing screening with and without a molecular marker.

Sputum Immunostaining

In a retrospective study from the Johns Hopkins Lung Project,[39] using monoclonal antibody staining of sputum cells collected as part of a randomized screening study of routine cytology, some encouraging results were found. Monoclonal antibodies that recognized small-cell and non–small-cell lung cancer determinants were used to immunostain 69 specimens randomly selected from the archived sputum specimens. This method detected neoplastic antigens in sputum with 91 percent sensitivity and 88 percent specificity an average of 24 months before the clinical diagnosis of lung cancer. Although moderate atypia was seen in only one-third of the patients who eventually developed cancer, a cell surface marker on the exfoliated cells in sputum could be detected at least 2 years before diagnosis in more than 90 percent of those who developed cancer. All specimens diagnostic of malignancy were excluded from this analysis. Twenty-six of the 69 participants randomly selected for the sputum staining with monoclonal antibodies subsequently developed lung cancer. The dual immunostaining had high overall sensitivity and specificity, but the precision to detect the different histologic types suffered from the small numbers available for the study.

The potential to exploit this method of cellular characterization at the epithelial surface provides the opportunity for the early detection of lung cancer when it is still confined to the bronchial mucosa if these markers are found to be expressed early in the process of carcinogenesis.

A major challenge remains the development of an automated method to detect malignancy-associated early changes. An automated morphometric analysis of atypical cells in sputum specimens represents a crucial step in developing a marker of cellular atypia that may be correlated with the stage of carcinogenesis. This would also make it possible to screen samples from many patients within a realistic time period.

New Investigations

The Lung Cancer Study Group has demonstrated that in patients after resection of a pathologic stage I tumor, the frequency of new lung tumors remains 1 to 3 percent per year, and this rate increases with increasing recurrence-free survival. Consequently, methods to detect second primary lung tumors as early as possible and to intervene with lung-conserving measures are of particular importance for this group. Immunostaining currently is being prospectively evaluated in a group of 900 to 1000 of these patients for a period of 3 years. Sputum specimens will be stained for standard cytopathology, as well as monoclonal antibody staining to detect neoplastic antigen expression. The specimens collected from this study will be used to evaluate other potential biomarkers, including growth factors such as GRP and others.

Lung-Imaging Fluorescence Endoscope

Tumors detected by sputum cytology or immunostaining of sputum need to be localized either by radiologic investigation (plain radiograph or CT) or by enhanced methods of bronchoscopy. Localization of lung cancer at this early stage generally can be accomplished by direct visual examination of the tracheobronchial tree using the flexible fiberoptic bronchoscope. Occasionally, a tumor is difficult to see at an early stage; therefore, methods to improve visibility of tumors at this stage have been developed.

One of the approaches uses laser-induced fluorescence after administration of photosensitizers such as hematoporphyrin derivatives. Chemical fluorescence from small superficial tumors is not seen with the conventional flexible fiber bronchoscope because of the combination of a low concentration of chemical in the tumor, a low fluorescence yield, and high optical losses in the fiberoptic bundles. Therefore, special instrumentation systems have been developed to overcome these technical problems. These systems rely on amplification of a fluorescence signal, which is then displayed as either an audio signal or a visual image. The overall experience using these detection systems demonstrates that they may be helpful in localizing tumors that are both radiographically and bronchoscopically occult.

The detection of fluorescence, however, is not specific for carcinoma. Areas of cellular atypia ranging in degree from moderate to marked have also been sites of low-level fluorescence. Therefore, the bronchoscopist must rely on diagnostic biopsies to confirm the localization of a cancer to a specific site. One of the problems that remains is to distinguish the difference between fluorescence from cancer foci and nonspecific autofluorescence of the normal bronchial mucosa. Autofluorescence has a peak at 580 nm, with some degree of fluorescence extending to 630 nm (red). This is superimposed on the main peak of hematoporphyrin fluorescence, which is in the red region. This explains why it is difficult to distinguish tumor from normal tissue in cases of the earliest in situ squamous cell carcinoma.

Administration of a much lower dose of the hematoporphyrin derivative makes it possible to detect in situ carcinoma with greater sensitivity, probably because of less retention of the photosensitizer in the normal mucosa than after a higher dose.

A different approach employs in vivo spectroscopy. The in vivo autofluorescence spectra of normal tissue and carcinoma in situ are different.[26] Fluorescence spectroscopy for normal tissue characteristically has a high intensity at 500 nm, which gradually decreases at longer wavelengths. On the other hand, in situ carcinoma demonstrates a relatively low intensity of fluorescence at 500 nm and remains low throughout the longer wavelengths. The lung-imaging fluorescence endoscope (LIFE) employs two-image intensifying cameras as well as a color video camera. This produces simultaneous, precisely matched and aligned images of tissue autofluorescence at different spectral bands. A xenon light source is used to obtain color images of the bronchoscopic appearance with a video camera. The autofluorescence image and the bronchoscopic image are combined on a color video monitor. The resultant pseudoimage is further corrected by determining the ratio of the fluorescence signals obtained by two light sources, standard white light and 442-nm laser light. The ratio fluorometric technique is a mathematical correction of the fluorescence signal based on the distance, angle, and intensity of the excitation light. Reports using the LIFE system have shown spectral differences between precancerous, cancerous, and normal bronchial mucosa. In experienced hands, the LIFE system detects at least 50 percent more abnormalities than a bronchoscopist can detect with a conventional fiberoptic bronchoscope. The system is commercially available, and several clinical trials are under way.[26]

Chest Radiographic Screening

It is widely accepted that screening for the detection of asymptomatic lung cancer using chest radiographs is not indicated.[13] However, it is also well accepted that the best results of therapy are achieved in patients with early-stage disease. Detection of lung cancer that is visible on chest radiograph is detecting malignancy relatively late in its natural course. The current views regarding screening for lung cancer are based on the early detection trials performed in the 1970s. The studies were designed to detect a major difference in disease-specific mortality—which would be difficult under the best of circumstances, since radiographically detectable lung cancer is far beyond the stage of early disease and could have already metastasized to distant sites. Furthermore, one might question whether the conclusions of these studies are still valid, given recent insights into the biology of the disease.

There has been a marked increase in the relative incidence of adenocarcinoma and a decrease in squamous cell carcinoma and small-cell lung cancer. This might have consequences for the detection rate with chest radiographs on the one hand and survival on the other, since adenocarcinoma tends to disseminate at an earlier stage than squamous cell lung cancer.

In four randomized trials, the role of chest radiographs was evaluated. These trials collectively included 37,724 participants. During the time the trials were performed, the epidemic of lung cancer in females had not yet become apparent; therefore, eligibility was restricted to male smokers. A problem with each of the four trials is that none had a true unscreened control group. In the Memorial Sloan-Kettering Lung Project and the Johns Hopkins Lung Project, participants were randomized at study entry to a dual-screen group (annual chest radiograph and sputum cytology every 4 months) or to a single-screen group (annual chest radiograph). In the Mayo Lung Project, all participants first underwent a prevalence screen, consisting of chest radiograph and sputum cytology. Those free of cancer were randomized to a study group, of which half underwent 4-monthly screening by chest radiography and sputum cytology; the others were advised to have an annual chest radiograph and sputum cytology. No effort was made to enforce compliance.

In the Sloan-Kettering and Johns Hopkins studies, the total number of cancers, the number of late-stage cancers, the number of resectable cancers, and the number of cancer deaths were almost identical in the two groups, with a 35 percent 5-year survival and a 76 percent 5-year survival for stage I disease. These results are significantly better than those observed during the same period in the National Cancer Institute's SEER program.[30] The addition of sputum cytology conferred no advantage in survival over chest radiograph alone.

The Mayo Lung Project and the study performed in the former Czechoslovakia actually compared regular rescreening by chest radiography to a control group with infrequent, sporadic, or, in some cases, no rescreening. The Mayo Lung Project is probably the most important of all four screening studies performed. At every point at which data were evaluated, the incidence of lung cancer was higher in the experimental group than in the control group. At the study's end, there were more cases of lung cancer detected, more were found to be resectable, and lung cancer-specific 5-year survival was more than double. Despite this survival advantage, however, there were slightly more lung cancer deaths in the experimental group than in the control group. Accordingly, there was a nonsignificant mortality advantage favoring the control group (Table 108-5A). In the Czechoslovak study, likewise, more tumors were detected, and resectability and 5-year survival rates were significantly better in the experimental group. However, mortality was higher in the experimental group, although the difference did not reach statistical significance (Table 108-5B).

Overall, the incidence of lung cancer was higher in both experimental groups than in the control groups—an observation that remains unexplained.[35] The question is, Why was this disparity observed? Overdiagnosis bias has been widely accepted as the most likely explanation for the observed incidence differences. However, it is highly questionable whether this hypothesis is biologically plausible. A malignancy as clinically virulent as lung cancer would not be a very likely candidate for overdiagnosis through screening. This is supported by the observation that resection was of major importance in patients in the Mayo, Memorial, and Hopkins with stage I non–small-cell lung cancer. Patients who were not operated on for a variety of reasons, including refusal or medical contraindications, had a cancer-specific survival of only 10 percent. This is much lower than the 70 percent 5-year survival of those who were treated by resection.[15] In both the Mayo lung study and the Czechoslovak study, follow-up data were available for several years after the trials were stopped; thus, it is highly unlikely that lead-time bias

or length bias was responsible for the differences. Since both studies were randomized, selection bias is not a likely explanation. The only remaining possible explanation is the influence of screening by itself, but the low dose of radiation of chest radiographs makes this impossible. In fact there is no good explanation available.

In the end, one may conclude that the screening studies of the 1970s did not result in an overall reduction in mortality, leading to the current recommendations against routine screening chest radiographs even in high-risk patients. However, if one looks at other end points that are of more importance for the clinician— such as stage of disease, resectability, and survival—screening may be worthwhile. If the improved 5-year survival rate is translated to the current situation, it may result in huge numbers of surviving patients. Therefore, the "screening debate" should not be closed despite the relatively unsophisticated techniques available for screening. Currently, a much larger and better-designed study comparing screening and standard medical care is ongoing, the results of which, it is hoped, will resolve the screening controversy.

Screening in Daily Practice?

The issue of screening for lung cancer entails not only the rather low yield of currently available techniques but also public health and economic consequences. Of all who smoke, only a small percentage develop lung cancer—which means that millions of smokers and ex-smokers need to be screened at regular intervals to detect a relatively small number of lung cancers at an earlier stage. An efficacious screening technique should, therefore, be cost-effective and efficient to use. Currently, no such technique is available, and the physician has to use available guidelines and judgment with regard to screening of patients who either smoke or formerly smoked.

There is a very close relationship between airflow obstruction and the development of lung cancer in smokers and nonsmokers, but particularly in smokers. Therefore, airflow obstruction, as judged with simple spirometry, increases the likelihood of finding a lung cancer by six- to sevenfold. This association exists also in both smoking and nonsmoking patients with asthma (or reversible airway obstruction). Therefore, the primary care physician should look closely for lung cancer in smokers who have symptoms and signs of airflow obstruction. In addition to smoking, other risk factors are a family history of lung cancer, exposure to environmental tobacco smoke, asbestos exposure, uranium mining, and occupational exposure to carcinogenic substances (Table 108-4).

The likelihood of developing lung cancer is directly related to the number of cigarettes smoked over time. Onset of smoking at a young age is a particularly strong risk factor. Twenty to 30 pack-years is considered the threshold for an increased risk of developing lung cancer. If the age plus the number of pack-years smoked results in a number greater than 70, the person may be at a significantly greater risk for developing lung cancer.[29]

Smoking cessation remains the best way of decreasing overall mortality from lung cancer. (Table 108-1).[12] Chest radiographs performed routinely in those who smoke will occasionally identify the person with an asymptomatic lung cancer.

Improved screening and detection of occult lung cancers or the predisposition to develop lung cancer awaits the further identification, development, and validation of specific molecular markers. Identification of genes associated with a predisposition to develop lung cancer in the person who smokes cigarettes would be of great benefit, but such a candidate gene or genes are not yet known. Until then, we should continue to look at better ways of treating established disease and stimulate and support those who want to stop smoking.

REFERENCES

1. Adler I: *Primary Malignant Growths of the Lung and Bronchi. A Pathological and Clinical Study.* New York, Longmans, Green, 1912.
2. Anon: Production of cigarettes: Import and export of cigarettes, 1992. *Tobacco J Int* 6:60–62, 1992; 1:40–42, 1993.
3. Anon: S.E.I.T.A. in the black again. *Tobacco J Int* 1:15–16, 1974; 1:26–27, 1984; 4:23–24, 1992.
4. Baquet CR, Horm JW, Gibbs T, Greenwald P: Socioeconomic factors and cancer incidence among blacks and whites. *J Natl Cancer Inst* 83:551–557, 1991.
5. Boring CC, Squires TS, Tong T: Cancer statistics, 1993. *CA Cancer J Clin* 43:7–26, 1993.
6. Bradford JA, Harlan WR, Hamner HR: Nature of cigarette smoke: Technic of experimental smoking. *Inc Eng Chem* 28:836–839, 1936.
7. Braun MM, Caporaso NE, Page WF, et al: Genetic component of lung cancer: Cohort study of twins. *Lancet* 334:440–443, 1994.
8. Brunnemann KD, Cos JE, Hoffmann D: Analysis of tobacco-specific *N*-nitrosamines in indoor air. *Carcinogenesis* 18:1957–1960, 1992.
9. Brunnemann KD, Yu L, Hoffmann D: Assessment of carcinogenic volatile *N*-nitrosamines in tobacco and in mainstream and sidestream smoke from cigarettes. *Cancer Res* 37:3218–3222, 1977.
9a. Butler C, Sam JM, Humble CG, Sweeney ES: Histopathology of lung cancer in New Mexico 1970–72 and 1980–81. *J Natl Cancer Inst* 8:85–90, 1987.
10. Caporaso NE, Tucker MA, Hoover RN, et al: Lung cancer and debrisoquine metabolic phenotype. *J Natl Cancer Inst* 82:1264–1272, 1990.
11. Doll R, Peto R: Cigarette smoking and bronchial carcinoma: Dose and time relationships among regular smokers and lifelong non-smokers. *J Epidemiol Community Health* 32:303–313, 1978.
12. Doll R, Peto R, Wheatley K, et al: Mortality in relation to smoking: 40 years' observations on male British doctors. *BMJ* 309:901–911, 1994.
13. Eddy D: Screening for lung cancer. *Ann Intern Med* 111:232–237, 1989.
14. Fischer S, Speigelhalder B, Preussmann R: Influence of smoking parameters on the delivery of tobacco-specific nitrosamines in cigarette smoke: A contribution to relative risk evaluation. *Carcinogenesis* 10:1059–1066, 1989.
15. Flehinger BJ, Kimmel M, Melamed MR: The effect of surgical treatment on survival from early lung cancer: Implications for screening. *Chest* 101:1013–1018, 1992.
16. Gilliland FD, Samet JM: Lung cancer. *Cancer Surv* 19-20:175–195, 1994.
17. Graham ILN: Green tea composition, consumption and polyphenol chemistry. *Prev Med* 21:334–350, 1992.
18. Hammond EC, Selikoff IJ, Lawther PL, et al: Inhalation of benzpyrene and cancer in man. *Ann NY Acad Sci* 271:116–124, 1976.
19. Harris RE, Zang EA, Anderson JI, Wynder EL: Race and sex differences in lung cancer risk associated with cigarette smoking. *Int J Epidemiol* 22:592–599, 1993.
20. Hoffmann D, Hoffmann I, Wynder EL: Lung cancer and the changing cigarette. *IARC Sci Publ* 105:449–459, 1991.
21. Hoffmann D, Rivenson A, Murphy SE, et al: Cigarette smoking and adenocarcinoma of the lung: The relevance of nicotine-derived *N*-nitrosamines. *J Smoking Rel Disord* 4:165–190, 1993.
22. Hong WK, Lippman SM, Itri LM, et al: Prevention of second primary tumors with isotretinoin in squamous-cell carcinoma of the head and neck. *New Engl J Med* 232:795–801, 1990.
23. Koo LC, Ho JHC: Worldwide epidemiological patterns of lung cancer in nonsmokers. *Int J Epidemiol* 19(Suppl 1):514–523, 1990.
24. Kozlowski LT, Rickert WS, Pope MA, et al: Estimating the yields to smokers of tar, nicotine and carbon monoxide from the lowest yield ventilated filter cigarettes. *Br J Addict* 77:159–165, 1982.
25. Kurihara M, Aoki K, Hisamichi S: *Cancer Mortality Statistics in the World, 1950–1985.* Nagoya, Japan, Nagoya University Press, 1989.
26. Lam S, MacAulay C, Hung J, et al: Detection of dysplasia and carcinoma in situ with lung imaging fluorescence endoscope device. *J Thorac Cardiovasc Surg* 105:1035–1040, 1993.
27. Lee PN: *Tobacco Consumption in Various Countries,* 4th ed. London, Tobacco Research Council, 1975.
28. Mattson ME, Pollack ES, Cullen JS: What are the odds that smoking will kill you? *Am J Publ Health* 77:425–428, 1987.
28a. Mulshine JL, Treston AM, Scott FM, et al: Lung cancer: Rational strategies for early detection and intervention. *Oncology* 5:25–32, 1991.
29. Petty TL: Lung cancer screening comp. *Therapy* 21:432–437, 1995.
30. Ries LAQ, Miller BA, Hankey BV, et al (eds), *SEER Cancer Statistics Review,* 1973–1991: NIH Pub No 94-2789, Bethesda, MD, Natl Cancer Institute, 1994.
31. Rodenhuis S, Slebos RJC: Clinical significance of ras oncogene activation in human lung cancer. *Cancer Res* 52(Suppl):2665s–2669s, 1992.
32. Selles RA, Chen PL, Potter CJD, et al: Segregation analysis of smoking-associated malignancies: Evidence for mendelian inheritance. *Am J Med Genet* 52:308–314, 1994.
33. Srivastava S, Kramer BS: Genetics of lung cancer: Implications for early detection and prevention. *Cancer Treat Res* 72:91–110, 1995.
34. Steindorf K, Lubin J, Wichmann HE, Becher H: Lung cancer deaths attributable to indoor radon exposure in West Germany. *Int J Epidemiol* 24:485–492, 1995.
35. Strauss GM, Gleason RE, Sugarbaker DJ: Chest x-ray screening improves outcome in lung cancer. *Chest* 107:270S–279S, 1995.
36. Sutedja G, Postmus PE: Bronchoscopy treatment of lung tumors. *Lung Cancer* 11:1–17, 1994.
37. Symposium on early lesions and the development of epithelial cancer. *Cancer Res* 36:2475–2706, 1976.
38. Taioli E, Wynder EL: Endocrine factors and adenocarcinoma of the lung in women. *J Natl Cancer Inst* 86:869–870, 1994.
39. Tockman MS, Gupta PK, Myers JD, et al: Sensitive and specific monoclonal antibody recognition of human lung cancer antigen on preserved sputum cells: A new approach to early lung cancer detection. *J Clin Oncol* 6:1685–1693, 1988.
40. Travis WD, Travis LB, Percy C, Devesa SS: Lung cancer incidence and survival by histologic type. *Cancer* 75:191–202, 1995.
41. Tredaniel J, Boffetta P, Saracci R, Hirsch A: Exposure to environmental tobacco smoke and risk of lung cancer: The epidemiological evidence. *Eur Respir J* 7:1887–1888, 1994.
42. US Department of Agriculture: Percent of total cigarette production which are filter-tipped cigarettes. *US Dep Agric Foreign Tobacco* 8:40–41, 1993.

43. US Department of Health, Education, and Welfare: *Smoking and Health: A Report of the Advisory Committee to the Surgeon General,* Washington, DC, US Government Printing Office, 1964.
44. Wagenknecht LE, Cutter GR, Haley NJ, et al: Racial differences in serum cotinine levels among smokers in the coronary artery risk development in (young) adults study. *Am J Publ Health* 80:1053–1056, 1990.
45. Wilkinson P, Hansell DM, Janssen J, et al: Is lung cancer associated with asbestos exposure when there are no small opacities on the chest radiograph? *Lancet* 345:1074–1078, 1995.
46. Wu A. II, Henderson BE, Thomas DC, Mack TM: Secular trends in histologic types of lung cancer. *J Natl Cancer Inst* 77:53–56, 1986.

47. Wu X, Hsu TC, Annegers JF, et al: A case-control study of nonrandom distribution of bleomycin-induced chromatid breaks in lymphocytes of lung cancer cases. *Cancer Res* 55:557–561, 1995.
48. Wynder EL, Graham EA: Tobacco smoking as a possible etiologic factor in bronchiogenic carcinoma. *J Am Med Assoc* 143:329–336, 1950.
49. Wynder EL, Hoffmann D: Smoking and lung cancer: Scientific challenges and opportunities. *Cancer Res* 54:5284–5295, 1994.
50. Wynder EL, Stellman SD: Comparative epidemiology of tobacco-related cancers. *Cancer Res* 37:4608–4622, 1977.
51. Wynder EL, Taioli E, Fujita Y: Ecologic study of lung cancer risk factors in the U.S. and Japan, with special reference to smoking and diet. *Jpn J Cancer Res* 83:418–423, 1992.

CHAPTER 109

CIGARETTE SMOKING AND HEALTH POLICY

Alfred P. Fishman

Physicians of all persuasions have a vital interest in preventing the use of tobacco products. Chest physicians have a particularly evident vested interest. In the United States, in 1990, cigarette smoking was implicated in more than 84,000 deaths from pulmonary disease, primarily pneumonia, chronic obstructive pulmonary disease, and influenza. Cigarette smoking is also the major cause of lung cancers as well as cancers of the mouth, pharynx, larynx, and esophagus. In addition to its harmful effects on the lungs, smoking increases the risk of cardiovascular disease, including stroke, myocardial infarction, and peripheral vascular disease. It is responsible for a variety of hematologic disorders, including leukemias, and is the cause of about 30 percent of all deaths from cancer.[7]

The relationship between lung cancer and cigarette smoking was pointed out in the 1940s. For a long while thereafter, however, this finding was not generally accepted. In the 1960s, awareness of this association heightened. In 1964, a report from the Office of the United States Surgeon General underscored the health hazards of cigarette smoking. Since then, cigarette smoking has been repeatedly identified as the leading cause of preventable morbidity in this country.[11,12,23,39,40]

In the United States, more than 400,000 people die prematurely from diseases attributable to the use of tobacco. Worldwide, more than 2 million deaths were predicted for 1995 and about 21 million for the decade 1990–99.[32] More than 50 percent of the deaths attributed to cigarette smoking are expected to occur in the 35- to 69-year age group.[42] Not only does tobacco smoking play a prominent role in causing death and disability, but it is also associated with other addictive behaviors—i.e., alcoholism and the illicit use of drugs.[27]

In the past few years, the frequency of tobacco smoking by adults has leveled off. Thus, in the early 1960s, more than 40 percent of all adults in the United States smoked, including more than 50 percent of adult men,[39] but by 1990, adult smoking prevalence had declined to 25.5 percent (28.4 percent in men and 22.8 percent in women) (Fig. 109-1).[11,34] Among white men, cigarette smoking fell from 52 percent in 1965 to 28 percent in 1990. The corresponding values for African-American men were 61 percent in 1965 and 33 percent in 1990. African-American women exhibited a trend similar to that of white women—i.e., a decrease from 35 percent in 1965 to 21 percent in 1990. Trend data are not available for the U.S. Hispanic population, but the 1990 National Health Interview Surveys reported a smoking prevalence rate of 31 percent for men and 16 percent for women.[11,29,39]

MORTALITY AND MORBIDITY

There is no doubt that cigarette smoking is a major contributor to cardiovascular-pulmonary diseases. Even smokers who have no complaints suffer from chronic inflammation of the lower airways and, over the years, experience a greater decrease in pulmonary function than do nonsmokers. Cigarette smoking has been implicated as the main cause of almost 90 percent of deaths from lung cancer, about 80 percent of deaths from chronic obstructive pulmonary disease, and about 20 percent of deaths from chronic heart disease.[30,31,35,39] Tobacco is harmful by every route in which it is used, including nasal and oral snuff and chewing tobacco. Women who used snuff chronically, but did not smoke, had a risk for oral cancer 50 times greater than nonusers.[44] Tobacco chewing, recently popularized by star athletes, holds promise of an associated increase in oropharyngeal cancers.

The list of illnesses in which cigarette smoking has been implicated, either as a risk factor or as an aggravating influence, is quite extensive. Aside from pulmonary and cardiac disease, cigarette smoking relates harmfully to peripheral vascular disease, the healing process in bones, macular degeneration, cataracts, fertility in women, and breast cancer.[2]

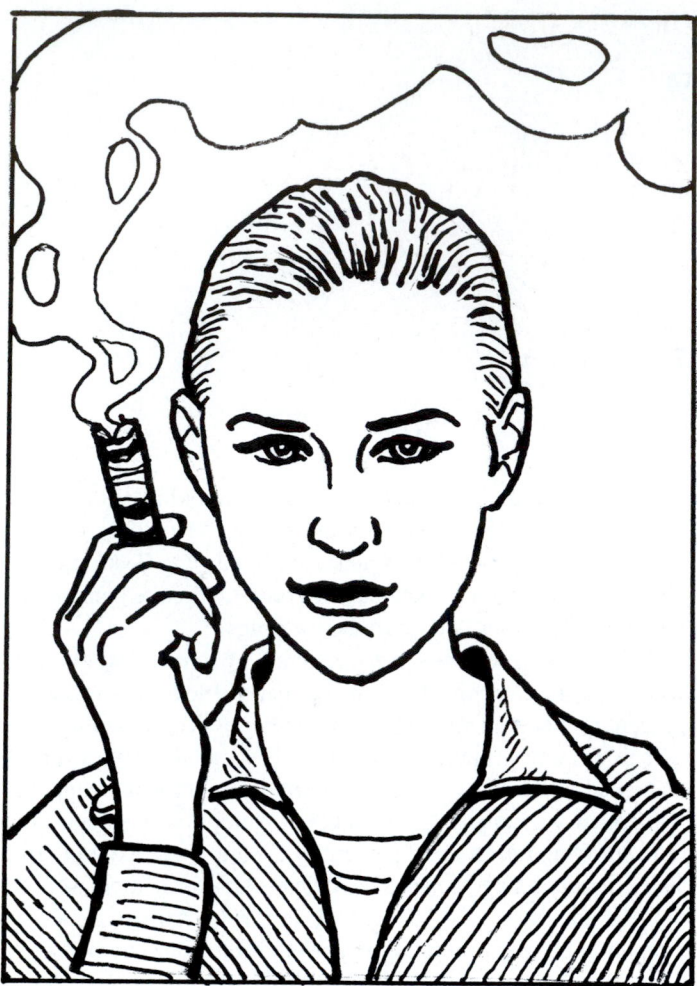

FIGURE 109-1   Women have picked up the slack.

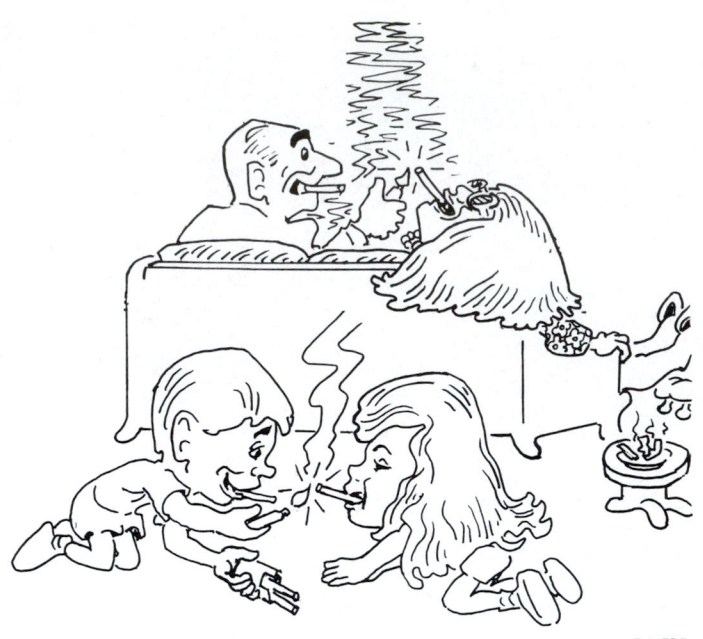

FIGURE 109-2   Side-stream smoke counts.

Not only the smoker but also the nonsmoker is at risk from cigarette smoke in the environment.[16,41] Those in the vicinity of a smoker are subjected not only to exhaled smoke but also to side-stream smoke—i.e., smoke released by the burning tobacco between puffs. Side-stream smoke contains more particles of smaller size and is considered by the Environmental Protection Agency to be in the same class of carcinogens as radon and asbestos. In the United States, about 3000 cases of lung cancer per year are attributed to environmental tobacco smoke.[19,40] Exposed nonsmokers experience more respiratory symptoms and more days lost from work than do nonexposed adults. Spouses of smokers are at considerable risk of developing lung cancers. Finally, infants and children are deleteriously affected by cigarette-smoking parents, who release cigarette smoke into their surroundings (Fig. 109-2).[41]

The more prolonged the exposure to cigarette smoke, the greater the likelihood of developing fatal cancers and cardiovascular accidents and, in women, of harming the reproductive structures and functions. The ill effects of tobacco on women have become a source of growing concern, since women younger than 25 represent the fastest-growing group of smokers. Women who smoke run the risk of reduced fertility, increased incidence of spontaneous abortions, and stillbirths. Moreover, cigarette smoking features prominently as a cause of cardiovascular diseases and lung cancer in women and has now surpassed breast cancer as the primary cause of death from cancer among women.[24]

ECONOMIC IMPACT

No matter how it is calculated, the cost of smoking is high. Estimates of the cost, based on direct health expenditures and loss of productivity due to smoking-related disability and death, run into the billions even if savings in Social Security and health-care costs due to premature deaths are taken into account. For 1990, the Office of Technology Assessment estimated this human cost of disease at $68 billion. However, such calculations have no way of putting a dollar value on the suffering of patients and their families. Another approach to estimating the social cost of smoking is based on the expectation that more than 1 million youths will continue to become regular smokers each year. These calculations suggest that these new smokers will cost the health-care system about $8.2 billion in extra medical expenditures before they die.[31]

WHY THE EPIDEMIC CONTINUES

The use of tobacco can be traced back to ancient civilizations. As indicated in Chapter 45, Columbus's discovery of the Americas introduced Europeans to tobacco and presaged its modern use. The Indians not only enjoyed its stimulatory affects but also believed that it had medicinal properties. Until the late 1880s, cigarette smoking was less frequent than other forms of tobacco usage (e.g., snuff). But the invention in the 1880s of the cigarette-rolling machine, followed by the development of safety matches, tilted the balance in favor of cigarette smoking. By 1945, cigarette smoking had largely replaced chewing snuff and cigar smoking. Currently, cigar smoking is once again on the rise, presumably as a symbol of affluence and power (Fig. 109-1).

The tobacco industry's drive for profits is the root cause of why cigarette smoking continues to thrive in the United States despite towering and irrefutable evidence that it is a health hazard and a form of drug addiction. This drive for profits, which began in Colonial days, has continued to the present, consistently outmaneuvering and outflanking all sorts of attempts to persuade the public that "cigarette smoking is dangerous to your health."[26] Social forces such as poverty, cultural and environmental influences, and peer pressure, provide firm footing for the marketers of cigarettes. In some countries, such as France, intellectuals and celebrities, by example, encourage smoking (Fig. 109-3).

Legislative initiatives to control cigarette smoking in the United States have not met with great success. The tobacco industry has successfully used a variety of clever strategies to neutralize attempts at legislative control and public education. Its primary tactics have been advertising, promotion, and lobbying. More than $10 million is spent every day in tobacco advertising. Advertising departments flood the marketplace with pictures of vigorous, handsome athletic men and women, posing with a particular cigarette in mouth or hand. These capture the attention and the imagination of people of all ages, including the young and the impressionable (Fig. 109-4). Movie heroes and heroines are featured on billboards. Picturesque animals are seen smoking. The Marlboro Man and smoking camels catch the eye on buses and billboards, in stadiums, and on racing cars. Smokers are reminded of their rights on the Internet, unaware that the convincing displays have been underwritten by secret contributions from cigarette manufacturers. Over the years, men and women took turns as targets; adolescents have tagged along: Virginia Slims were directed at women, Joe Camel primarily at men; both were attractive to youngsters.

Lobbying is a powerful instrument of the tobacco industry. Also, action committees sponsored by the tobacco interests contribute heavily to the coffers of the political parties and of individual politicians. For example, in 1996, 124 members of the House of Representatives signed a letter to the Food and Drug Administration opposing plans to restrict tobacco advertising that encouraged teenagers to smoke; oppositely, 103 representatives voted for the proposals. The average amount of money received by the 124 who opposed the measure to restrict advertising was

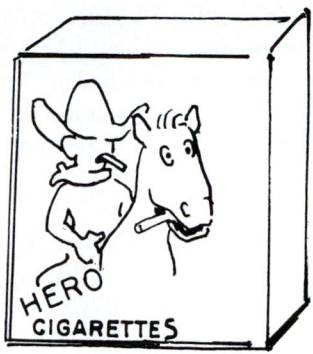

R. WEBB

FIGURE 109-4   Luring them on.

nearly 30 times the average received by the 103 who favored curtailment of advertising.[26]

An increase in cigarette excise tax has been associated with a decrease in consumption. However, the tobacco industry has successfully staved off, or minimized, such increases, thereby keeping the price of cigarettes within the affordable range of many who would otherwise be obliged to kick the habit. In Canada and California, considerable increments in the excise tax on cigarettes were accompanied by a decrease in consumption.

Not only do teams of lawyers argue against legislation that would limit access to cigarettes, but some even participate in the review of scientific projects to be funded by the industry.[7] The tobacco industry is currently in gear to resist implementation of legislation, sponsored by the Food and Drug Administration, that is designed to restrict access of minors to tobacco and to curtail the marketing of tobacco products to youngsters.

The United States military contributes significantly to the prevalence of cigarette smoking.[21] At military commissaries around the world, cigarettes and other tobacco products are sold at prices that are 30 to 60 percent lower than those charged by commercial grocery stores. It is therefore no wonder that the 1.4 million military personnel on active duty have a smoking rate that is greater than that of the general population (32 percent as compared to 25 percent). However, the Department of Defense, recognizing the high cost of cigarette smoking in health-care costs and lost productivity, is considering withdrawal of its subsidy to cigarette smoking—a proposal that, not surprisingly, is being resisted by the tobacco lobby and some members of Congress.

A ban on smoking in the workplace, announced $2\frac{1}{2}$ years ago by the Occupational Safety and Health Administration, has been stalled by strong opposition from tobacco and restaurant interests, coupled with reluctance on the part of governmental agencies to offend federal legislators. In response to the Congressional inertia, however,

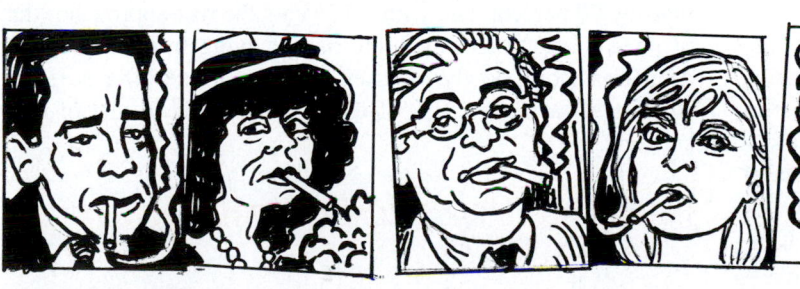

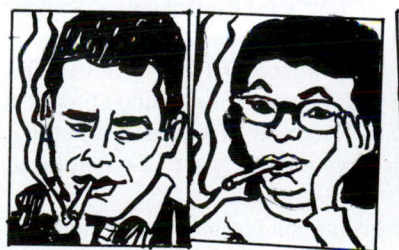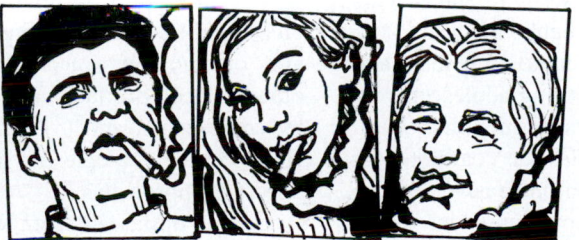

FIGURE 109-3   Intellectuals as role models.

state and local legislators have taken such initiatives as creating smoke-free job sites.[5] Volunteer agencies, such as the American Lung Association and the American Heart Association, are pressing hard for cessation of smoking. The newspapers and public interest groups are also urging that the habit be broken or, better still, that measures be taken to prevent the start of the habit.

NICOTINE ADDICTION

Nicotine from tobacco smoke rapidly enters the systemic circulation and is carried to organs throughout the body, including the brain. Smokeless tobacco—i.e., snuff and chewing tobacco—produces equivalent blood concentrations of nicotine. During the course of each day, tolerance increases. As the day progresses, more smoking is necessary to achieve the pleasurable and stimulatory effects. The increasing tolerance that develops as a result of repetitive use, qualifies nicotine for classification as an addictive drug. Smoked tobacco and smokeless tobacco can be equally addictive. Considerable individual variety exists in susceptibility to nicotine addiction and in the ability to stop the use of tobacco products once a person is addicted. Nicotine addiction is associated with addiction to alcohol and drugs.[28]

ENTRAPPING THE ADOLESCENT

Since the Surgeon General's 1964 report, which alerted the nation to the health hazards of cigarettes, the prevalence of smoking among adults has decreased considerably, from about 40 percent of the adult population in 1965 to about 26 percent in 1990; since then, the rate of smoking among adults has plateaued. This leveling off, reflecting a balance between those who quit smoking or turn to smokeless tobacco, and new smokers, is attributed to the continuing entry of young people into the rank of regular smokers at a rate virtually unchanged from that of the 1980s.[31] The estimated 3000 children and youths who become regular smokers each year suffice to ensure an enduring supply of adult smokers (Fig. 109-5).

SMOKING PREVENTION AND CESSATION

Interrupting the continuing inflow of adolescent smokers has become a central target of antismoking programs. Unfortunately, there is no broad public support or national policy to assist in this effort.[25] Nonetheless, an increasing number of agencies—federal, state, local, and voluntary—have initiated programs of their own. The American Stop Smoking Intervention Study for Cancer Prevention is a collaborative effort of the National Cancer Institute, the American Cancer Society, state health departments, and various public and private organizations to develop programs directed at controlling tobacco use in 17 states. This study has set two primary goals for this project by the year 2000: to reduce the prevalence of smoking in adults to 15 percent and to reduce the rates of smoking initiation among adolescents by 50 percent.[15] Statewide initiatives have been taken with the support of private foundations to promote statewide coalitions for the development and implementation of comprehensive tobacco control strategies, to launch public education campaigns to decrease the demand for tobacco, to improve the capacity of states

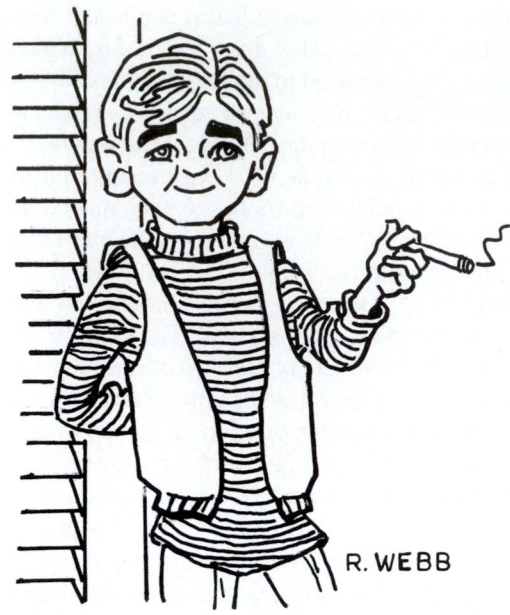

R. WEBB

FIGURE 109-5   Getting hooked.

to enhance tobacco prevention and treatment, and to develop policy plans to reduce the use of tobacco by the young.

Psychosocial factors play a key role in handicapping efforts in smoking prevention and cessation. Many different approaches have been taken to deal with these factors, not only with respect to tobacco use but also with respect to preventing and arresting diseases related to the use of tobacco products (e.g., chronic pulmonary diseases). However, success of such programs, notably those concerned with behavior modification, have proved difficult to assess.[29]

Smoking cessation affords immediate benefits.[4,14,37] It rapidly improves pulmonary function, especially in young persons, and slows the age-related decline in pulmonary function. Smoking cessation also decreases the risk of most smoking-related diseases: some risks decrease rapidly; others more slowly.[32,33] Thus, within 1 year of quitting, the risk of coronary heart disease plummets by 50 percent, and within 15 years the risk approaches that of nonsmokers.[40] However, the risk of dying from lung cancer decreases more slowly: it takes 10 to 14 years after stopping smoking to achieve a risk of dying comparable to that of nonsmokers.

INITIATIVES FOR SMOKING PREVENTION AND CESSATION

As a rule, initiatives to promote smoking prevention and cessation seem to rely on relatively few guiding principles: (1) increase public education and information about the health hazards of smoking, (2) regulate the marketing of cigarettes and other tobacco products, (3) preclude access to tobacco products by adolescents, and (4) limit promotion of cigarette smoking. However, the strategies for achieving these goals have employed different approaches.

Certain initiatives seem to be gaining ground: (1) community-wide programs to forbid the sale of tobacco products to children and adolescents;[1,8,13,15,20,25] (2) public advocacy of smoking cessation and of the use of other tobacco products;[6] (3) legislation to increase the federal excise tax on cigarettes by a considerable amount and to direct income produced by the tax at smoking prevention and cessation programs, especially if the programs are directed at young people;[5,38] (4) legislation to enable regulatory agencies to assume jurisdiction over tobacco products in order to reduce the harmful constituents in tobacco and enforce the use of strong and prominent package warnings;[15] (5) interventions to protect nonsmokers by expanding the number, nature, and extent of smoke-free public places and workplaces;[19] (6) legislation to curb the advertising and promotion of tobacco products, including cigarette vending machines;[10] (7) education in the schools and public;[36] (8) medical coverage of smoking cessation services; (9) continued research into the disease-promoting effects of tobacco and its constituents;[10,23] (10) assessment of the outcomes of interventions designed to limit tobacco use;[17] (11) ending financial assistance by the federal government to the tobacco-growing industry; and (12) repeal of federal law that impedes state and local initiatives directed at regulating tobacco promotion and advertising.[31] Tobacco control advocates generally believe that the best chance of success lies in a multifaceted integrated attack that will pull together many of these individual initiatives (e.g., higher taxes, more stringent laws for clean indoor air, stronger antiadvertising campaigns, and more intense educational programs in the schools and in public arenas).[9,10]

DOUBLE-DEALING BY THE TOBACCO INDUSTRY

Lawsuits against tobacco companies have become a public health strategy. Until 1994, lawsuits failed consistently on three accounts: (1) smoking is a free choice; (2) the courts were not swayed by the evidence that tobacco causes disease; and (3) the tobacco industry supported research on the effects of tobacco on health.[3]

The tide began to turn against the tobacco industry in 1994. A trove of secret documents showed that, despite its protestations, the industry knew not only that tobacco was harmful but also that it is addictive. Indeed, it turned its knowledge of the addictive properties to advantage in attracting smokers. Moreover, it not only knew of the harmful and addictive properties of tobacco but also went to considerable pains to conceal and obfuscate. Added to this evidence of duplicity by the industry and in keeping with the results of a plethora of epidemiologic studies came the direct evidence that one of the many ingredients of tobacco smoke, benzo[a]pyrene, can cause cancer by inducing a mutation in the p53 gene.[18]

The evidence of double-dealing by the tobacco industry and the mounting scientific proofs that cigarette smoking is harmful have become front-page news. Moreover, not only are more individuals taking the tobacco industry to court but also class actions and state-sponsored lawsuits have brought more resources into play to counter the wealth of the tobacco industry. A final touch was added recently by the settlement of five state suits by the Liggett Group of tobacco companies.

CALL TO ARMS

During the past few years, the public has become increasingly vocal in its call for tobacco controls. This call to action has led to a variety of initiatives. One such was the 1988 tax initiative in California (Proposition 99), which was brought about by cooperative aggressive policy that involved coalitions, community-based organizations, and counteradvertising strategies. Largely as a result of these activities, more than 15 percent of California's 471 cities now have a 100 percent smoke-free workplace and/or a 100 percent smoke-free restaurant ordinance. Nearly 300 of the cities have ordinances that limit smoking pollution and/or access of the young to cigarette vending machines. Paradoxically, although the legislation was directed primarily at decreasing the start of tobacco use by the young, the program has had its major impact on smoking cessation in adults, especially people more than 50 years old.[6] Another new initiative has been taken by women's health programs, prompted by the increase in the prevalence of lung cancer in women that accompanied an increase in cigarette smoking.

In the last 2 years, public sentiment against the tobacco companies reached its peak. The mounting rebellion emboldened political opposition to the industry, especially at state and local levels. As a result, by mid-1977, 25 state attorneys had filed lawsuits against the tobacco industry, i.e., tobacco companies, three trade associations, and a public relations firm, accusing it of conspiring to sell tobacco products to minors and fraudulently concealing and misrepresenting the dangers of these products to the public. The suit sought to recoup taxpayer money spent on treating tobacco-related illness.

Regulations promulgated by the Food and Drug Administration (FDA) concerning the sale of cigarettes to children went into effect in February 1997. The authority of the FDA to do so was immediately challenged by the tobacco industry. On April 25, 1997, a federal district judge, William L. Osteen, Sr., ruled against the industry by indicating that cigarettes can be regulated by the FDA. However, while indicating that the FDA did have the power to regulate tobacco as a drug, he denied the agency the power to control advertising aimed at youths. In the landmark decision favoring the FDA, he rejected every argument from the industry that would have denied the agency jurisdiction over nicotine as a drug and cigarettes as devises for delivery of the drug. Both sides are expected to appeal the bifid decision: The tobacco industry will challenge the power of the FDA and President Clinton will challenge the ruling on advertising.

At present, the tobacco firms and the state attorneys are negotiating to end the civil lawsuits. The tobacco companies are offering to pay $300 billion, to submit to FDA regulation, and to stop considerable cigarette advertising. In return, the companies are seeking to place the industry under stronger federal control and obtain blanket protection by Congress against future civil lawsuits.

The recognition of nicotine in tobacco as a drug and cigarettes as devices for delivering the drug to the body has broad implications. For example, it affords the FDA the opportunity to regulate the amount of nicotine per cigarette. Moreover, the FDA can investigate the composition of cigarettes with respect to minimizing the concentrations of inhaled pollutants. On a broader scale, should the ruling have its desired effects in the United States, globalization of cigarette smoking is apt to become more widespread in areas where legislation is less restrictive.

THE ROLE OF THE SOLO PHYSICIAN

Clearly, the physician has to play an active role in the control of smoking.[1,43] Each physician has the responsibility of explaining to the patient who smokes the medical risks associated with smoking and the benefits from smoking cessation. Even in smokers who do not develop chronic obstructive disease of the airways, a chronic bronchitis is inevitable (Fig. 109-6). In addition to encouraging abstinence, the physician should be familiar with counseling and therapeutic programs, strategies, and interventions that promote cessation. For example, behavior modification, as an approach to smoking prevention and cessation, may require the intervention and support of specially trained health professionals. Physicians should also participate in the public debate not only individually but also through medical societies and organizations.

Pharmacologic approaches to smoking cessation currently rely heavily on nicotine replacement. Nicotine replacement during early abstinence helps to relieve symptoms of withdrawal and can increase quit rates.[22] Although nicotine used as a medication may be addictive, nicotine-delivering transdermal and polacrilex gum medications appear to be of minimal addictive potential. Other systems under development, such as nasal sprays and vapor inhalers, may be of greater addictive potential but are expected to be lower in addictiveness and toxicity than are tobacco products. However, no matter how effective the therapeutic techniques directed at smoking cessation, the greater reward seems to reside in smoking cessation, especially in children and adolescents.[23]

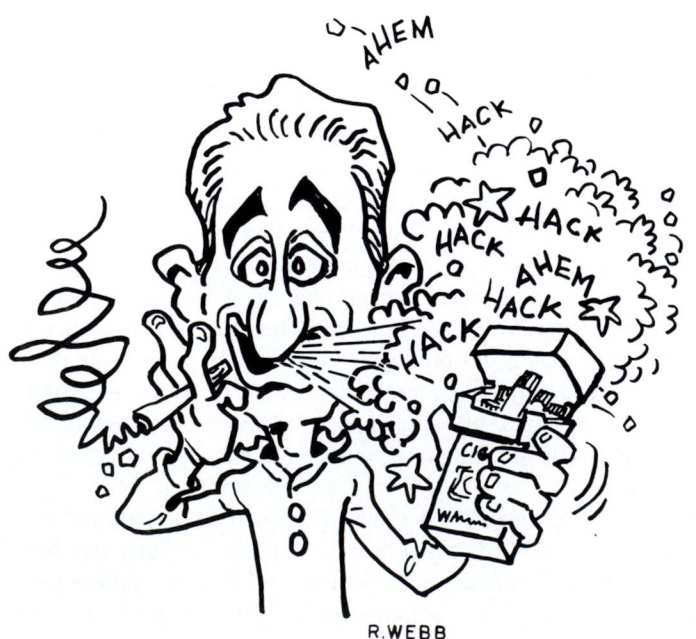

R. WEBB

FIGURE 109-6   "Smoker's cough."

CLINICAL PRACTICE GUIDELINE

The Agency for Health Care Policy and Research recently released a Clinical Practice Guideline that provides recommendations for three groups of health professionals: primary care clinicians, smoking cessation specialists, and others concerned with smoking cessation (health-care administrators, insurers, and purchasers). The major recommendations for the three audiences are as follows: (1) primary care clinicians are to use office-wide systems to identify smokers, treat every smoker with a cessation or motivational intervention, offer nicotine replacement except in special circumstances, and schedule follow-up contact to occur after cessation; (2) smoking cessation specialists are to use various individual or group counseling sessions lasting at least 20 minutes each, with sessions spanning several weeks, to offer nicotine replacement, and to provide problem-solving and social support counseling; and (3) health-care administrators, insurers, and purchasers are to use tobacco user identification systems in all clinics, and smoking cessation treatment is to be supported through staff education and training, dedicated staff, changes in hospital policies, and the provision of reimbursement for tobacco dependence treatment.[1] The feasibility of implementing such a comprehensive program remains to be established.

REFERENCES

1. The Agency for Health Care Policy and Research: Smoking cessation clinical practice guideline. *JAMA* 275:1270–1280, 1996.
2. Ambrosone CB, Freudenheim JL, Graham S, et al: Cigarette smoking, *N*-acetyltransferase 2 genetic polymorphisms, and breast cancer risk. *JAMA* 276:1494–1501, 1996.
3. Annas GJ: Tobacco litigation as cancer prevention: Dealing with the Devil. *New Eng J Med* 336:304–308, 1997.
4. Anthonisen NR, Connett JE, Kiley JP, et al: The Lung Health Study: Effects of smoking intervention and the use of an inhaled anticholinergic bronchodilator on the rate of decline of FEV_1. *JAMA* 272:1497–1505, 1994.
5. Bal DG, Kizer KW, Felten PG, et al: Reducing tobacco consumption in California: Development of a statewide anti–tobacco use campaign. *JAMA* 264:1570–1574, 1990.
6. Bal DG, Lloyd J: Advocacy and government action for cancer prevention in older persons. *Cancer* 74:2067–2070, 1994.
7. Bartecchi CE, MacKenzie TD, Schrier RW: The global tobacco epidemic. *Sci Am* 272(5):44–51, 1995.
8. Bero L, Barnes DE, Hanauer P, et al: Lawyer control of the tobacco industry's external research program: The Brown and Williamson documents. *JAMA* 274:241–247, 1995.
9. Brownson RC, Koffman DM, Novotny TE, et al: Environmental and policy interventions to control tobacco use and prevent cardiovascular disease. *Health Educ Q* 22:478–498, 1995.
10. Burns D, Pierce JP: *Tobacco Use in California, 1990–1991.* Sacramento, California Department of Health Services, 1992.
11. Carr-Gregg M: Interaction of public policy advocacy and research in the passage of New Zealand's Smoke-Free Environments Act, 1990. *Addiction* 88(Suppl):35S–41S, 1993.
12. Centers for Disease Control: Cigarette smoking among adults. *MMWR* 41:354–362, 1990.
13. Centers for Disease Control: Cigarette smoking among adults. *MMWR* 42:230–233, 1991.

14. Centers for Disease Control and Prevention, Office on Smoking and Health: Preventing tobacco use among young people. DHHS Publication No. 017-001-00491-0, 1994.

15. Coultas DB, Samet JM: Smoking cessation and pulmonary rehabilitation, in Fishman AP (ed), *Pulmonary Rehabilitation*. New York, Dekker, 1996, pp 401–420.

16. Cummings KM: Involving older Americans in the war on tobacco: The American Stop Smoking Intervention Study for Cancer Prevention. *Cancer* 74:2062–2066, 1994.

17. Dayal HH, Khuder S, Sharrar R, Trieff N: Passive smoking in obstructive respiratory disease in an industrialized urban population. *Environ Res* 65:161–171, 1994.

18. Denissenko MF, Pao A, Tang M-s, Pfeifer GP: Preferential formation of benzo[*a*]pyrene adducts at lung cancer mutational hotspots in *P53*. *Science* 274:430–432, 1996.

19. Emont SL, Zahniser SC, Marcus EE, et al: Evaluation of the 1990 Centers for Disease Control and Prevention smoke-free policy. *Am J Health Promot* 9:456–461, 1995.

20. Environmental Protection Agency: *Respiratory Health Effects of Passive Smoking: Lung Cancer and Other Disorders*. 1992.

21. Epps RP, Manley MW, Glynn TJ: Tobacco use among adolescents: Strategies for prevention. *Pediatr Clin North Am* 42:389–402, 1995.

22. Feigelman W: Cigarette smoking among former military service personnel: A neglected social issue. *Prev Med* 23:235–241, 1994.

23. Fiore MC, Jorenby DE, Baker TB: Tobacco dependence and the nicotine patch: Clinical guidelines for effective use. *JAMA* 268:2687–2694, 1992.

24. Giovino GA, Henningfield J, Tomar SL, et al: Epidemiology of tobacco use and dependence. *Epidemiol Rev* 17:48–65, 1995.

25. Gritz ER: Lung cancer: Now, more than ever, a feminist issue. *Cancer* 43:197–199, 1993.

26. Gritz ER: Reaching toward and beyond the year 2000 goals for cigarette smoking. *Cancer* 74(Suppl):1423–1432, 1994.

27. Herbert B: In America. *The New York Times*, October 25, 1996.

28. Henningfield JE, Clayton R, Pollin W: Involvement of tobacco in alcoholism and illicit drug use. *Br J Addict* 85:279–292, 1990.

29. Henningfield JE, Stapleton JM, Benowitz NL, et al: Higher levels of nicotine in arterial than in venous blood after cigarette smoking. *Drug Alcohol Depend* 33:23–29, 1993.

30. Kawachi I, Colditz GA, Stampfer MJ: Smoking cessation in relation to total mortality rates in women. *Ann Intern Med* 119:992–1000, 1993.

31. Lynch BS, Bonnie JR: *Growing Up Tobacco Free: Preventing Nicotine Addiction in Children and Youths*. Washington, National Academy Press, 1994.

32. McSweeny AJ, Czajkowski SM, Labuhn KT: Psychosocial factors in the rehabilitation of patients with chronic respiratory disease, in Fishman AP (ed), *Pulmonary Rehabilitation*. New York, Dekker, 1996, pp 443–479.

33. Ockene JK, Kuller LH, Svedsen KH, Meilahn E: The relationship of smoking cessation to coronary heart disease and lung cancer in the multiple risk factor intervention trial (MRFIT). *Am J Public Health* 80:954–958, 1990.

34. Peto R, Lopez AD, Boreham J, et al: Mortality from tobacco in developed countries: Indirect estimation from national vital statistics. *Lancet* 339:1268–1278, 1992.

35. Pierce JP, Fiore MC, Novotny TE, et al: Trends in cigarette smoking in the United States: Projections to the year 2000. *JAMA* 261:61–65, 1989.

36. Samet JM: *Epidemiology of Lung Cancer*. New York, Dekker, 1994.

37. Schaffler HH, Parkinson MD: Health insurance coverage for smoking cessation services. *Health Educ Q* 20:185–206, 1993.

38. Sherrill DL, Holberg CJ, Emright PL, et al: Longitudinal analysis of the effects of smoking onset and cessation on pulmonary function. *Am J Respir Crit Care Med* 149:591–597, 1994.

39. Townsend J, Roderick P, Cooper J: Cigarette smoking by socioeconomic group, sex and age: Effects of price, income and health publicity. *BMJ* 309:923–927, 1994.

40. U.S. Department of Health and Human Services (DHHS): Reducing the health consequences of smoking: 25 years of progress. A report of the Surgeon General. Rockville, MD: US DHHS, Public Health Service, DHHS Publication No. (CDC) 89-8411, 1989.

41. U.S. Department of Health and Human Services: Health benefits of smoking cessation. A report of the Surgeon General, Washington, DHHS Publication No. (CDC) 90-8416, 1990.

42. White JR, Froeb HF, Kulik JA: Respiratory illness in non-smokers chronically exposed to tobacco smoke in the workplace. *Chest* 100:39–43, 1991.

43. Williams M: Smoking and health: A physician's responsibility. *Monaldi Arch Chest Dis* 50:394–397, 1995.

44. Winn DM, Blot WJ, Shy CM, et al: Snuff dipping and oral cancer among women in the Southern U.S. *New Engl J Med* 304:745–749, 1981.

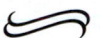

THE SOLITARY PULMONARY NODULE: A SYSTEMIC APPROACH

Alan M. Fein / Steven H. Feinsilver / Carlos A. Ares

The radiographic finding of a solitary pulmonary nodule, formerly known as a *coin lesion,* has long challenged the clinician. At the heart of the dilemma, the question has remained unchanged: "Is it malignant or benign?" Bronchogenic carcinoma is the most common malignancy found in solitary pulmonary nodules, and it remains the leading cause of cancer death in the United States. When faced with a solitary pulmonary nodule, the clinician and the patient usually have one of four choices: (1) remove it, (2) biopsy it, (3) observe it with serial radiographs, or (4) ignore it. This choice depends largely on radiographic appearance and epidemiology. Surgical resection of an early solitary lesion still represents the best chance for a cure. On the other hand, resection of a benign nodule exposes the patient to the morbidity and mortality of a surgical procedure.

The aim of this chapter is to review what we know about the solitary pulmonary nodule and to formulate a diagnostic approach to this often controversial problem.

DEFINITION

A solitary pulmonary nodule is defined as a single discrete pulmonary opacity that is surrounded by normal lung tissue and is not associated with adenopathy or atelectasis. There is some difference of opinion on the upper size limit for a nodule. Some early series included lesions up to 6 cm.[14] At present, most authors consider a nodule to be a lesion less than 3 cm in diameter.[20] A lesion 3 cm or larger is more likely to be malignant and is called a mass.

INCIDENCE AND PREVALENCE

The frequency with which a solitary pulmonary nodule is identified on chest radiography is on the order of 1 to 2 per thousand chest radiographs.[20] Most of these are clinically silent, and about 90 percent are noted as an incidental finding on radiographic examination. The prevalence of malignancy in nodules varies widely, depending on the patient population; thus, many case series may not be directly comparable. Surgical series in the era before computed tomography (CT), including both calcified and noncalcified nodules, reported an overall malignancy rate of 10 to 68 percent.[33] A Veterans Administration Armed Forces Cooperative Study in 1963 reported an overall 35 percent malignancy rate in a cohort that included a significant number of young military recruits (about half of them under age 50).[33] Infectious granulomas were found in 53 percent. When those over the age of 50 were studied, a 56 percent malignancy rate was noted, with a 30 percent incidence of granulomas. Of those under the age of 35, only three patients had a malignancy, one of which was a primary lung carcinoma. Series that have used chest CT to screen out benign-appearing calcified nodules show much higher overall malignancy rates: 56 to 100 percent.[20,28] A recent series of 360 patients from the Minneapolis Veterans Administration Medical Center, which utilized CT scan to exclude benign nodules, showed an increase in the percentage of malignant diagnoses at surgery.[28] The overall malignancy rate was 79 percent, with an increase from about 60 percent in the early 1980s to 100 percent from 1990 to 1994. This population included mostly male smokers aged about 65. A smaller series (40 patients), referred to the outpatient practice of a pulmonologist in an urban university hospital from 1990 to 1993, had a 53 percent malignancy rate.[19] The mean age was 65, 83 percent were smokers, and sex distribution was almost equal.

Younger patients from areas where granulomatous diseases such as tuberculosis, histoplasmosis, and coccidioidomycosis are endemic can be expected to have a lower malignancy rate. In an Air Force Medical Center study from Illinois of 137 patients, only 22 (16 percent) had a malignancy.[38] Granulomas were diagnosed in 103 patients (75 percent); 53 of them were attributable to histoplasmosis endemic to the area. Most of these patients (77 percent) were under age 45, and no malignant nodules were diagnosed in patients less than 35 years of age. This series predated the use of chest CT.

MALIGNANT SOLITARY PULMONARY NODULES

Risk factors for malignancy have been identified from studies of large series of solitary pulmonary nodules and include patient age, smoking history, nodule size, and prior history of malignancy. Risk of malignancy increases with age. In a series of 370 indeterminate solitary pulmonary nodules, the incidence of malignancy increased from 63 percent for patients between the ages of 45 and 54 to 74 percent for ages 54 to 64 and continued to rise with age to 96 percent for those above the age of 75.[28] These findings correlate with those of previous studies, which also show that malignancy is very rarely found in patients under the age of 35.[33,36,38]

Smoking is closely correlated with the development of lung cancer, particularly squamous and small cell carcinoma. The Surgeon General's report of 1964 and subsequent studies have demonstrated that the risk of lung cancer increases with the duration of smoking and the number of cigarettes smoked. Average smokers have about a 10-fold risk and heavy smokers a 20-fold risk of developing lung cancer when compared to nonsmokers. Smoking is responsible for about 85 percent of the cases of bronchogenic carcinoma. Cessation of smoking will reduce this risk after 10 to 20 years, but it now appears that former smokers have a slightly higher risk of cancer throughout their lifetimes.[25]

Nodule size is closely correlated to risk of malignancy. Several series have demonstrated an increased incidence of malignancy with increasing nodule size. Nodules larger than 3 cm will be malignant 80 to 99 percent of the time, while those under 2 cm in size will be malignant in 20 to 66 percent of cases.[19,26,28,38,44]

A history of current or prior extrapulmonary malignancy will greatly increase the probability that a nodule is malignant. Depending on the series, 33 to 95 percent of such nodules have proved to be malignant[2,3,24]—most representing metastases but some second primaries.[2] The most common histologic types of metastatic nodules are adenocarcinomas of colon, breast, kidney, head and neck tumors, sarcoma, and melanoma.

Primary bronchogenic carcinoma is the most common malignant tumor that presents as a solitary pulmonary nodule. In two recent large series that together looked at 1298 patients, 1041 (80 percent) had the diagnosis of malignancy; 940 of these (90 percent) were bronchogenic carcinomas.[19,28] Histologically, adenocarcinoma and squamous cell carcinoma make up the majority; of the two, adenocarcinoma is slightly more common. Less frequent as a solitary pulmonary nodule is the bronchioloalveolar cell carcinoma. Small cell carcinoma that presents as a solitary pulmonary nodule is rare. Other rare primary lung tumors that may present as solitary pulmonary nodules are bronchial carcinoids (1 to 5 percent), which are usually peripherally located; lymphomas; hemangioendotheliomas; and sarcomas.

Metastases may present as solitary pulmonary nodules in patients who have known primary malignancies or in whom the presence of primary malignancy is unknown. In up to 40 percent of such patients, who manifest only a single nodule on chest radiograph, CT scan may show other nodules that are not disclosed by plain chest radiograph.[23,29] Even though the lesion is solitary, in patients with an established diagnosis of cancer, up to 95 percent of these nodules will be malignant upon resection. Because of this high likelihood of malignancy, a nodule in a patient with an established diagnosis of cancer should be treated differently from other solitary nodules. Assuming no other obvious metastatic spread, one should consider proceeding directly to biopsy. Even in the presence of a known malignancy, some of these nodules may represent a second primary pulmonary malignancy that is similar in histologic appearance. Immunohistologic and other confirmatory marker studies may be indicated to determine the nature of the nodule. A solitary pulmonary nodule in a patient with a history of malignant disease should be removed as long as there is no other evidence of recurrent or metastatic disease.

BENIGN SOLITARY PULMONARY NODULES

Benign solitary pulmonary nodules are more common in the young and in nonsmokers. They include both infectious and noninfectious granulomas, benign tumors such as hamartomas, vascular lesions, and rare miscellaneous conditions (Table 110-1).

Hamartomas are the most common benign tumors presenting as solitary pulmonary nodules. They are believed to be developmental malformations composed mainly of cartilage, fibromyxoid stroma, and adipose tissue. Our review of six series of resected solitary pulmonary nodules since 1974 shows that 192 of 3802 nodules (5 percent) were histologically proven hamartomas.[8,16,27,28,36,38] In a series of 215 hamartomas resected at the Mayo Clinic, the peak incidence was in the seventh decade of life; male-to-female ratio was 1:1; and the average size was 1.5 cm, although some were as big as 6 cm.[12] Most hamartomas were asymptomatic (97 percent), and 17 percent were noted to grow slowly on serial radiographic examination. They may be identified radiographically by a pattern of "popcorn" calcification, which is often intermixed with areas of low attenuation on CT scan representing fat deposits within the nodule. CT appearance will be diagnostic in about 50 percent of hamartomas.[32]

Infectious granulomas make up more than 90 percent of all benign nodules. They arise as a result of healing after infection from a variety of organisms. The offending agents will vary, depending on geographic location. Among the most common causes are histoplasmosis, coccidioidomycosis, and tuberculosis.

Differential Diagnosis of Solitary Pulmonary Nodules

Malignant Tumors
Bronchogenic carcinoma (adenocarcinoma, large cell, squamous, small cell)
Carcinoid
Pulmonary lymphoma
Pulmonary sarcoma
Plasmocytoma
Solitary metastases (colon, breast, kidney, head and neck, germ cell, sarcoma, thyroid, melanoma, others)

Benign Tumors
Hamartoma
Adenoma
Lipoma

Infectious Granulomas
Tuberculosis
Histoplasmosis
Coccidioidomycosis
Mycetoma
Ascaris
Echinococcal cyst
Dirofilariasis (dog heartworm)

Noninfectious Granulomas
Rheumatoid arthritis
Wegener's granulomatosis
Sarcoidosis
Paraffinoma
Others

Miscellaneous
BOOP
Abscess
Silicosis
Fibrosis/scar
Hematoma
Pseudotumor
Spherical pneumonia
Pulmonary infarction
Arteriovenous malformation
Bronchogenic cyst
Amyloidoma

Other, less common causes are dirofilariasis (dog heartworm), mycetoma, echinococcal cyst, and ascariasis. A history of exposure is important in establishing a possible infectious origin. Clues such as prior travel history, places of residence, occupation, and pets may be invaluable in some instances.

Noninfectious granulomas sometimes occur as solitary pulmonary nodules in systemic diseases such as sarcoidosis, in which nodules are not invariably accompanied by hilar adenopathy; rheumatoid arthritis, usually in patients with active disease who will often have subcutaneous nodules; and Wegener's granulomatosis.

Miscellaneous causes of solitary pulmonary nodules have been described. Some of the more common conditions are lung abscess; rounded or spherical pneumonia; pseudotumor (Fig. 110-1), which represents fluid in an intralobar fissure; hematomas after thoracic trauma or surgery; and fibrosis or scars resulting from the resolution of infectious or inflammatory process. Rarer conditions presenting as solitary pulmonary nodules include silicosis, bronchogenic cyst, amyloidosis, pulmonary infarct, and vascular anomalies. Arteriovenous malformations may present as solitary pulmonary nodule. They may grow slowly and have a characteristic appearance on contrast-enhanced CT scan.

RADIOLOGIC TECHNIQUES

Plain Chest Radiography

Most solitary pulmonary nodules are discovered on routine plain chest radiograph while asymptomatic. Malignant nodules are usually identifiable on chest radiograph by the time they are 0.8 to 1 cm in diameter, although nodules 0.5 to 0.6 cm can occasionally be seen.[20] Most will be identified on posteroanterior (PA) projection, but some will be seen only on lateral projection, so standard PA and lateral chest radiography should be obtained whenever possible. When a nodule can be seen only on one projection, the clinician should question whether it is truly in the lung parenchyma. Structures overlying the skin of the chest wall—such as leads used for cardiac monitoring, nipple shadows, skin lesions, bone lesions, and pulmonary vessels on end—can all mimic pulmonary nodules. Once it has been ascertained that a true nodule exists, the first step is to make every effort to obtain previous radiographs for comparison. A nodule that has remained stable, with no increase in size, for 2 years, is very probably benign and warrants no further investigation. Conversely, a nodule that was not present on a comparable radiograph within the past 2 months is unlikely, having grown so rapidly, to be a malignancy. On rare occasions, small cell carcinoma may present as a solitary pulmonary nodule with a doubling time of less than 30 days.

Newer techniques, such as digital chest radiography,[4] which uses computerized postprocessing to enhance radiographic images, can improve the detection of nodules over normally radiopaque areas of the thorax, such as the mediastinum and the diaphragm. This is accomplished by means of computerized algorithms (e.g., adaptive spatial filtering) that selectively change

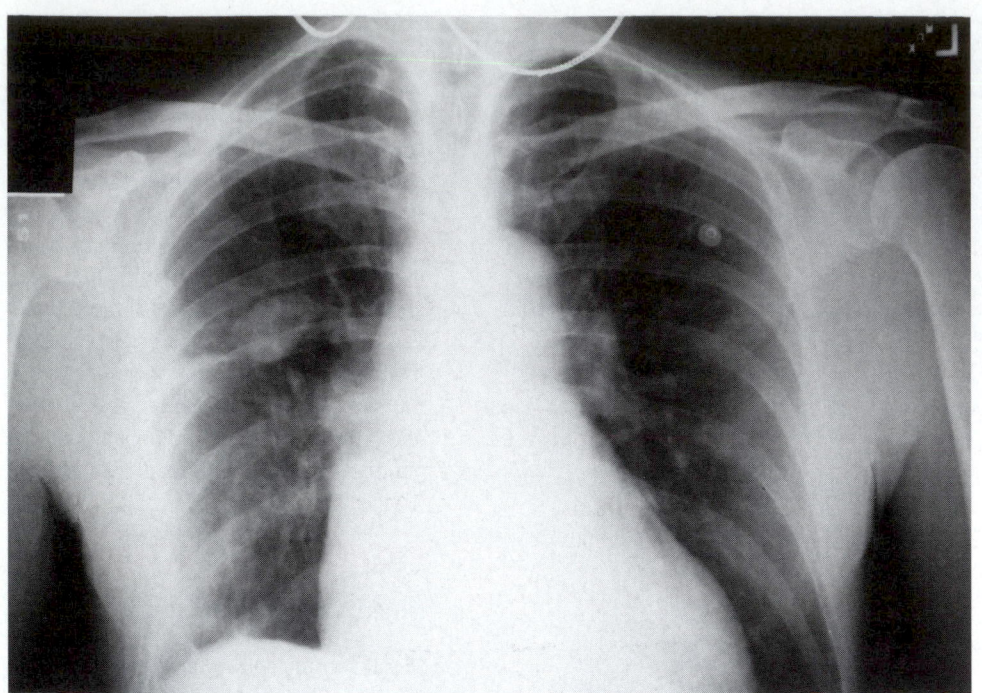

FIGURE 110-1   Pseudotumor. Fluid in a fissure, the result of both pleural disease and fluid overload, has the appearance of a pulmonary mass.

enhancement patterns over the areas of interest, making previously unseen nodules visible.

Standard and Computed Tomography

Standard tomography was once used extensively in the evaluation of solitary pulmonary nodules, and it can be very useful in determining their exact location and characteristics. With the advent of CT, however, this technique is now seldom used, and few radiologists are being trained to use the technique.

CT has replaced plain tomography as a more sensitive tool in the evaluation of solitary pulmonary nodules. CT is indicated when one is assessing indeterminate nodules less than 3 cm in diameter or in staging of larger lesions. It can pinpoint the exact location of the nodule and provide three-dimensional images of the lesion. Thin-section high-resolution CT (HRCT) can better define the borders and the nodule's relation to adjacent structures, such as vessels and the pleura.[41,45] It is more sensitive than standard tomography in detecting calcification patterns, and it can detect fat within a nodule—which, when coupled with calcification, is highly suggestive of a benign hamartoma. In up to 40 percent of cases, previously unseen synchronous lesions can be seen. CT may be useful in looking for hilar or mediastinal

adenopathy, and in evaluating accessibility of nodules for biopsy or resection.

HRCT[17,44] can quantify calcification in nodules even when they are not readily visible to the naked eye. Nodules with higher radiographic density are more likely to be benign (Fig. 110-2). This technique has been suggested for indeterminate nodules smaller than 3 cm in diameter.[31] Nodules that are bigger than 3 cm or that have suspect characteristics in the right clinical setting (e.g., an older smoker, spiculated borders) should be considered for biopsy or resection. Because it is difficult to standardize radiographic density on CT when a nodule is being examined for occult calcification, a phantom model is constructed to mimic the patient's chest, nodule size, and location. Benign nodules usually have a density greater than 164 Hounsfield units. Therefore, the reference nodule is created with a known density greater than this—at about 185 Hounsfield units. The patient's nodule density is measured with HRCT and is compared to the reference phantom. If the patient's nodule is denser than the phantom, it is very probably benign and can be observed with sequential conventional radiographs. If it is less dense than the reference phantom, it remains indeterminate and further workup is indicated. It should be noted that in a study of 85 nodules that were classified as having a high probability of benignity by the means of the 185 Hounsfield units cutoff, eight of them (9 percent) proved to be malignant on biopsy

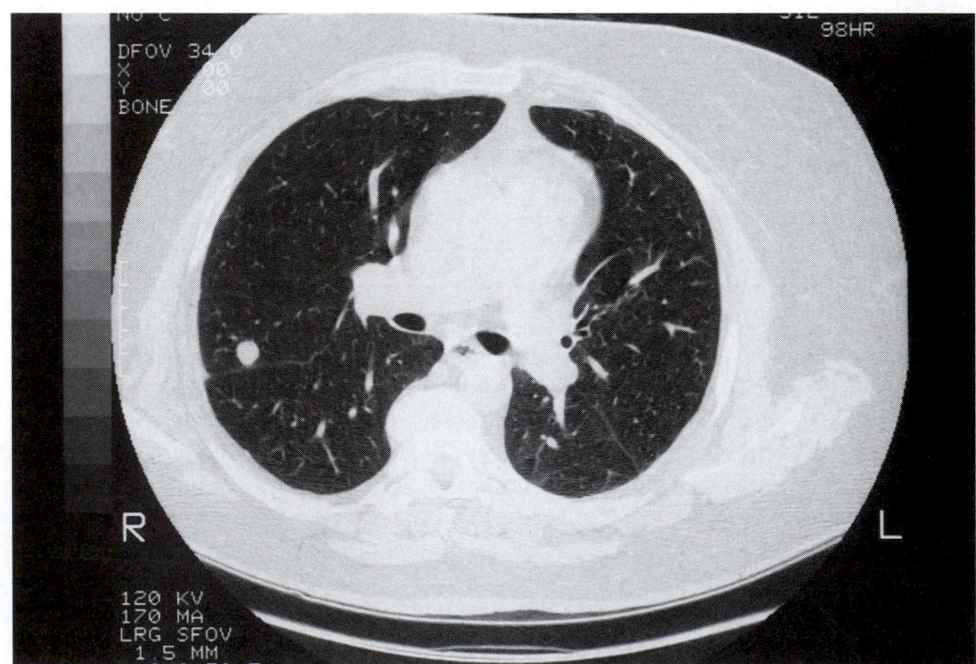

FIGURE 110-2   Noncontrast CT shows a round 1-cm nodule, with relatively high radiographic density, proven on resection to be a granuloma.

or resection.[34] The CT reference phantom technique can be a helpful adjunct in the evaluation of the solitary pulmonary nodule, but it is helpful in only about 30 percent of cases, with 70 percent of nodules evaluated remaining indeterminate.[17,40,44] CT densitometry has not achieved widespread clinical use.

Another CT technique that may be helpful is incremental dynamic CT, which uses serially increasing doses of iodinated IV contrast to look for enhancement of nodules.[43] Although malignant nodules enhance more than benign ones, benign lesions, such as hamartomas and tuberculomas, may also enhance. Further experience with this method is needed to determine its role in the evaluation of solitary pulmonary nodules. Spiral or helical CT may be useful in the evaluation of small nodules and to look for synchronous lesions.[1] It has the advantage of scanning a large area during a single breath hold, thereby eliminating respiratory artifact. Its ability to reconstruct images at different intervals and thicknesses also permits better detection of smaller nodules.

Other Radiologic Techniques

Newer imaging methods, such as positron emission tomography (PET), hold promise of helping to differentiate noninvasively between malignant and benign nodules. PET takes advantage of the fact that tumor cells have an increased glucose uptake and metabolism. A D-glucose analog labeled with a positron-emitting fluorine-18 radioisotope (FDG) is injected into the patient, and uptake by the nodule is then measured. Malignant nodules have a higher uptake of FDG, with a sensitivity of 95 percent and specificity of 80 percent.[6] This technique is not yet widely available, and more work needs to be done to define its role in the evaluation of solitary pulmonary nodules.

NODULE GROWTH RATE

Determination of nodule growth is based on the assumption that nodules are more or less spherical. Growth of a sphere must be considered in three-dimensional volume, not in two-dimensional diameter. The formula for volume of a sphere is $4/3(\text{Pi})r^3$, or $1/6(\text{Pi})D^3$, where r = radius and D = diameter. A nodule originally 1 cm in diameter whose diameter is now 1.3 cm has actually more than doubled in volume. Similarly, a 2-cm nodule has doubled in volume by the time its diameter reaches 2.5 cm. A nodule that has doubled in diameter has undergone an eightfold increase in volume. When old radiographs are available, growth rate and nodule *doubling time* (i.e., the time for a nodule to double in volume) can be estimated. Accepting the assumption that a tumor arises from serial doublings of a single cancerous cell, we can estimate that it will take 27 doublings for it to reach 0.5 cm, the smallest lesion detectable on chest radiography. By the time a nodule is 1 cm in diameter, it represents 30 doubling times and about 1 billion tumor cells. Depending on the exact growth rate, this theoretical 1-cm nod-

ule has probably existed for years before it is detected, as malignant bronchogenic tumors have doubling times estimated at between 20 and 400 days. The natural history of a tumor usually spans about 40 doublings, whereupon the tumor is 10 cm in diameter and the patient has usually died.[9] Squamous and large cell tumors have an average doubling time of 60 to 80 days. Adenocarcinomas double at about 120 days, and the rare small cell carcinoma that presents as a solitary pulmonary nodule can have a doubling time of less than 30 days.[2] A nodule that has doubled in weeks to months is probably malignant and should be removed when possible.

Benign nodules have doubling times of less than 20 days or more than 400 days. A nodule that doubles in size in less than 20 days is invariably the result of an acute infectious process, while those that grow very slowly are usually chronic granulomatous reactions or hamartomas. Such nodules can be observed with serial radiographs.

The question often arises whether observing a solitary pulmonary nodule (less than 3 cm that probably has been growing for years) for 3 to 6 months increases the likelihood of metastatic disease. There is no convincing evidence to support this hypothesis. In fact, early detection of lung cancer by screening has not been shown to improve overall survival significantly.

Nodule Shape and Calcification Patterns

Certain shapes make a nodule more likely to be malignant. Although nodules may appear to be spherical on plain chest radiograph, further study by CT may disclose irregular borders and shapes. The borders of benign nodules are often well circumscribed, with a rounded appearance. On the other hand, malignant nodules tend to have irregular, lobulated, or spiculated borders (Fig. 110-3).[31] A malignant nodule may have pleural tags or tails extending from its body (Fig. 110-4), or a notch may be present in the border of the nodule (Rigler's sign). None of these radiographic signs is entirely specific for malignancy.

Calcification is generally an indication of benignity in a solitary pulmonary nodule. Infectious granulomas tend to calcify with central, diffuse, or stippled patterns (Fig. 110-5). Laminar or concentric calcification is characteristic of granulomas caused by histoplasmosis. Popcorn calcification, when present, is suggestive of a hamartoma. Eccentric calcification patterns should

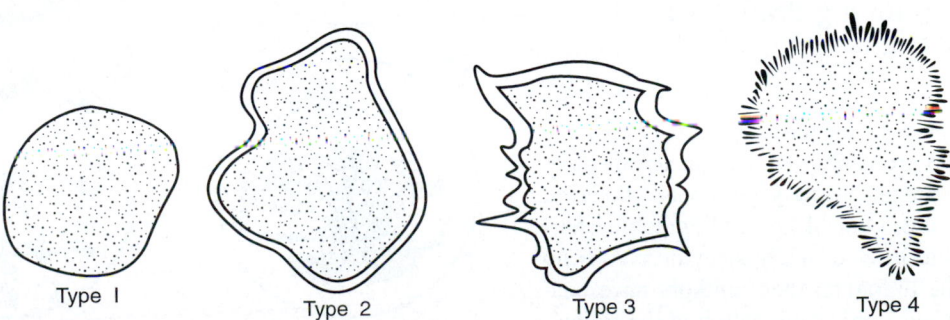

FIGURE 110-3 Characteristic appearance of nodule IV is edges. Type I is sharp and smooth, type II is lobulated, type III has irregular undulations, and type IV is grossly irregular with many spiculations. *(Based on data of Siegelman et al,[31] with permission.)*

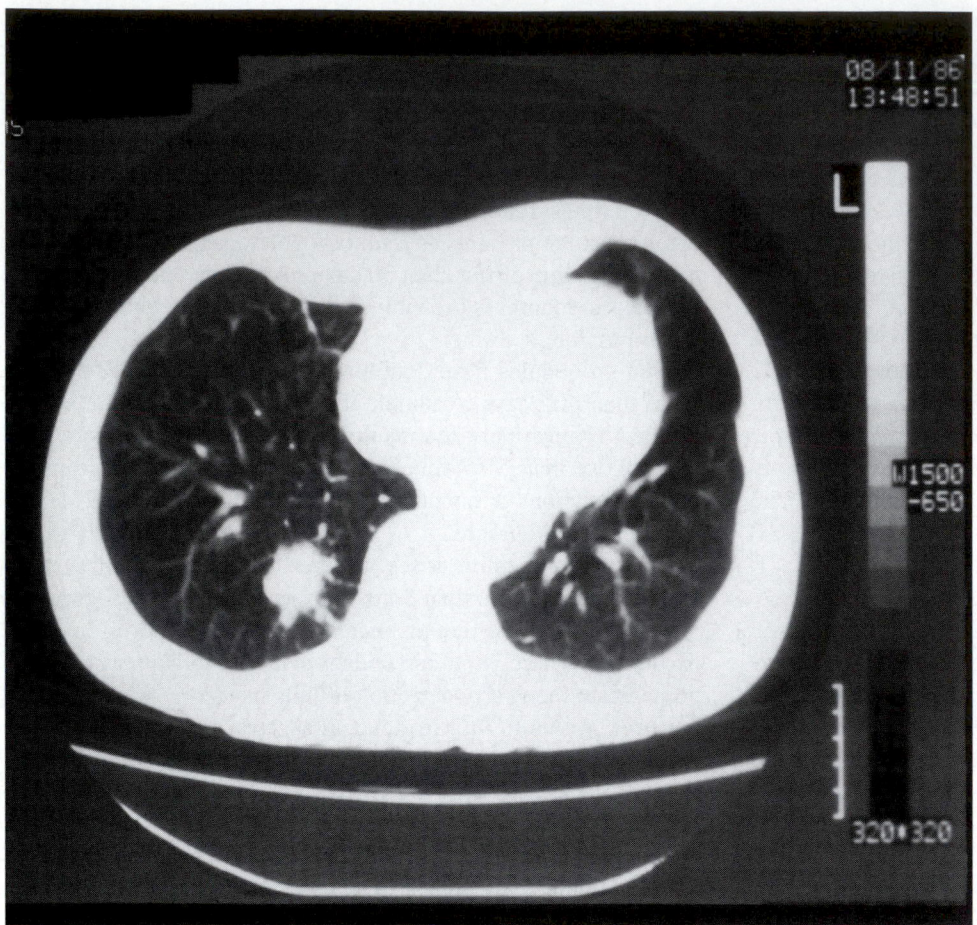

FIGURE 110-4   Three-centimeter mass with irregular borders and pleural tag highly suggestive of malignancy—proven adenocarcinoma.

make one suspicious for malignancy. It should be noted that, in general, 6 to 14 percent of malignant nodules exhibit calcification. When present, calcifications are usually eccentric and few. Benign patterns of calcification (central, diffuse, laminar, or popcorn) are very rare in malignant nodules. In one study of 1267 solitary pulmonary nodules, only seven malignant nodules (0.6 percent) had a benign calcification pattern.[35] Most nodules with a benign calcification pattern can be observed with serial radiographs.

Estimating Probability of Malignancy

Several authors have attempted to develop mathematical models to estimate the probability of malignancy of indeterminate solitary pulmonary nodules. Using clinical and radiographic characteristics of malignancy derived from the literature, these authors have analyzed some combination of the following malignant risk factors by Bayesian, neural network, and other methods to obtain a mathematical estimate of the

probability of malignancy: nodule size, location, growth rate, margin characteristics, age of the patient, smoking history, prevalence of malignancy in the community, and occult calcification on CT densitometry.

For example, in the Bayesian approach, each risk factor for a particular patient and nodule is assigned a likelihood ratio of malignancy derived from published data. In one model, overall prevalence of malignancy, diameter of the nodule, patient's age, and smoking history were considered.[5] The likelihood ratios for malignancy of each of these factors were then multiplied to provide odds of malignancy, which are then converted into a percent probability of cancer (pCa). Three different management strategies are followed, depending on the calculated pCa. If the pCa is under 5 percent, prospective observation is recommended; if the pCa is more than 60 percent, immediate resection of the nodule is warranted; if the pCa is between 5 and 60 percent, percutaneous needle aspiration biopsy is equal to or slightly preferable to resection. In a computerized neural network model that utilizes nonlinear mathematics to analyze input data, risk factors for malignancy were used and compared to the results of Bayesian analysis.[16] The authors found that their neural network was not as accurate as Bayesian analysis in predicting malignancy.

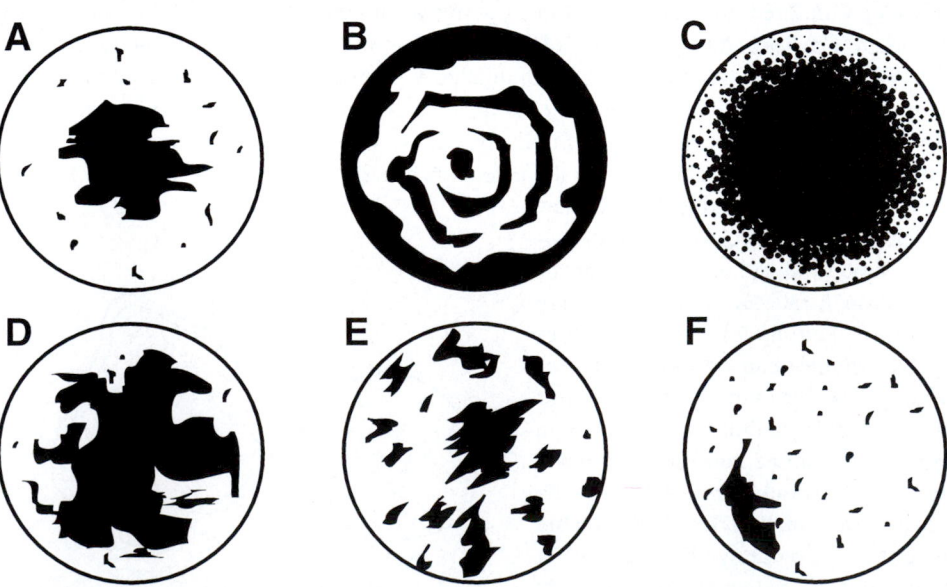

FIGURE 110-5   Patterns of calcification in nodules. *A.* Central. *B.* Laminated. *C.* Diffuse. *D.* Popcorn. *E.* Eccentric. Patterns A, B, C, and D generally indicate a benign process; E and F suggest malignancy. *(Based on data of Lillington,[20] with permission.)*

One of the problems with both of these and with other methods is the quality of the input data (i.e., the likelihood ratios), which may not be representative of all patient populations. In addition, Bayesian analysis presupposes that the likelihood ratios for a particular risk factor are not affected by the presence or absence of any other factor. It is not clear that this is true of the likelihood ratios. Therefore, although mathematical models to predict probability of malignancy may seem attractive, the complexity of the issue once again leaves us with an uncertain answer. This may explain why the above-described methods are not in widespread clinical use.

BIOPSY TECHNIQUES

The issues of whether it is at all useful to biopsy an indeterminate solitary pulmonary nodule and, if so, how to do it remain controversial. Most experts agree that in certain clinical circumstances, a biopsy procedure is warranted. For example, in a patient who is at high surgical risk, it may be useful in establishing a diagnosis and in guiding decision making. If the biopsy reveals malignancy, it may convince a patient who is wary of surgery to undergo thoracotomy or thoracoscopic resection of a potentially curable lesion. Another indication for biopsy may be anxiety to establish a specific diagnosis in a patient in whom the nodule seems to be benign. Some chest physicians argue that all indeterminate nodules should be resected if the results of history, physical examination, and laboratory and radiographic staging methods are negative for metastases. Others argue that this last approach exposes patients with benign nodules to the risks of needless surgery. In such cases, a biopsy procedure sometimes provides a specific diagnosis of a benign lesion and obviates surgery.

Once it has been decided to biopsy a solitary pulmonary nodule, the choice of procedure is a matter of debate but includes fiberoptic bronchoscopy, percutaneous needle aspiration, thoracoscopic biopsy (usually with video assistance), and open thoracotomy.

Bronchoscopy

Traditionally, bronchoscopy has been regarded as a procedure of limited usefulness in the evaluation of solitary pulmonary nodules. Various studies have shown variable success rates, with an overall diagnostic yield of 36 to 68 percent,[7,30] in nodules greater than 2 cm with bronchoscopic biopsy, brushings, and washings. In general, the yield for specific benign diagnoses has ranged from 12 percent to 41 percent.[7,8]

Bronchoscopic transbronchial biopsy is generally well tolerated, with few major complications. In prospective studies of transbronchial biopsies, pneumothorax has been reported in up to 4 percent, significant bleeding (more than 50 ml) in 2.1 percent, and death in 0.1 percent.[7]

A recent review of the role of bronchoscopy in the evaluation of the solitary pulmonary nodule concluded that the wide disparity of results among published studies was due to the different methods used in these studies.[22] The two main factors influencing diagnostic yield were nodule characteristics and the procedural approach.

After a review of the various studies, it was concluded that bronchoscopy can play a significant role in the evaluation of the solitary pulmonary nodule under certain circumstances. For example, it was found that nodules larger than 2 cm in diameter yielded the best results: Sensitivity, as high as 68 percent (average 55 percent), dropped to 11 percent for nodules smaller than 2 cm. The location of the nodule was important: Nodules located in the inner or middle one-third of the lung fields had the best diagnostic yield; nodules in the outer one-third of the lung are best approached with percutaneous needle aspiration.

Another useful characteristic of a solitary pulmonary nodule is its relation to a neighboring bronchus (Fig. 110-6).[39] Tsuboi and colleagues described four types of tumor–bronchus relationships: (1) the bronchial lumen is patent up to the tumor; (2) the bronchus is contained in the tumor mass; (3) the bronchus is compressed and narrowed by the tumor, but the bronchial mucosa is intact; and (4) the proximal bronchial tree is narrowed by peribronchial or submucosal spread of the tumor or by enlarged lymph nodes. The presence of types I and II, a bronchus leading to or contained within the body of a nodule or mass on HRCT, has subsequently been termed a *positive bronchus sign*. When a bronchus sign is present on HRCT, the diagnostic yield of fiberoptic bronchoscopy can be as high as 60 to 90 percent. With a negative bronchus sign, the yield drops to 14 to 30 percent. Signs and symptoms of airway involvement (cough, hemoptysis, localized wheezing), although rare in solitary pulmonary nodules, will increase diagnostic yield when present.

The issue of determining the optimal bronchoscopic procedural approach is a complicated one and depends largely on the skill and experience of the individual bronchoscopist. Fluoroscopic localization of the nodule improves diagnostic yield and should be used when possible. Most authorities agree that bronchoscopic forceps biopsy, brush cytology, and bronchial washings are complementary and are routinely performed by most. Other techniques, such as bronchoscopic needle aspiration

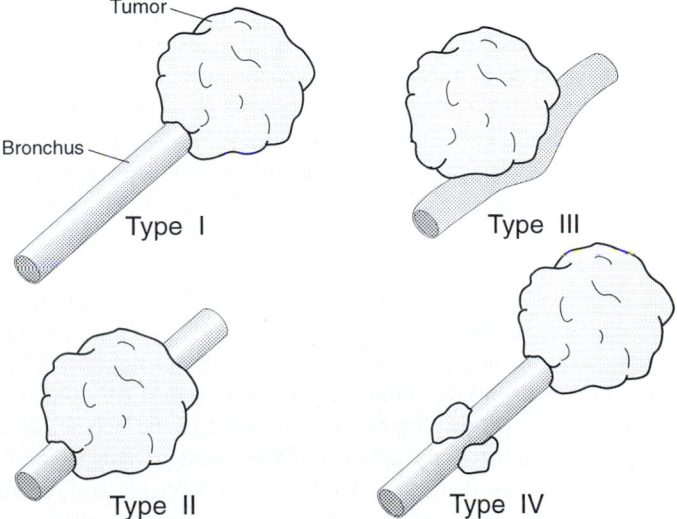

FIGURE 110-6   Schematic illustration of tumor–bronchus relationships (see text). (*Based on data of Tsuboi et al,[39] with permission.*)

(BNA) and needle brush and double-hinged curettage, may be useful, depending on the operator and the particular nodule characteristics. For example, BNA can be useful in types III and IV Tsuboi lesions that are bigger than 2 cm in diameter. Gasparini and colleagues reported an overall diagnostic yield for malignancy of 69 percent for BNA, 54 percent for transbronchial biopsy, and 75 percent for both combined in a series of 1027 consecutive cases.[8] When bronchoscopic biopsy failed to provide a diagnosis, percutaneous needle aspiration was performed immediately, with a pulmonologist, radiologist, and cytopathologist present in all cases. The combined overall yield for all three procedures was 95 percent for malignant and 60 percent for benign lesions. In this study, the average nodule size was 3.5 cm (95 percent were less than 6 cm). Unfortunately, breakdown of the results for nodules of greater than 3 cm was not provided. Future tech-

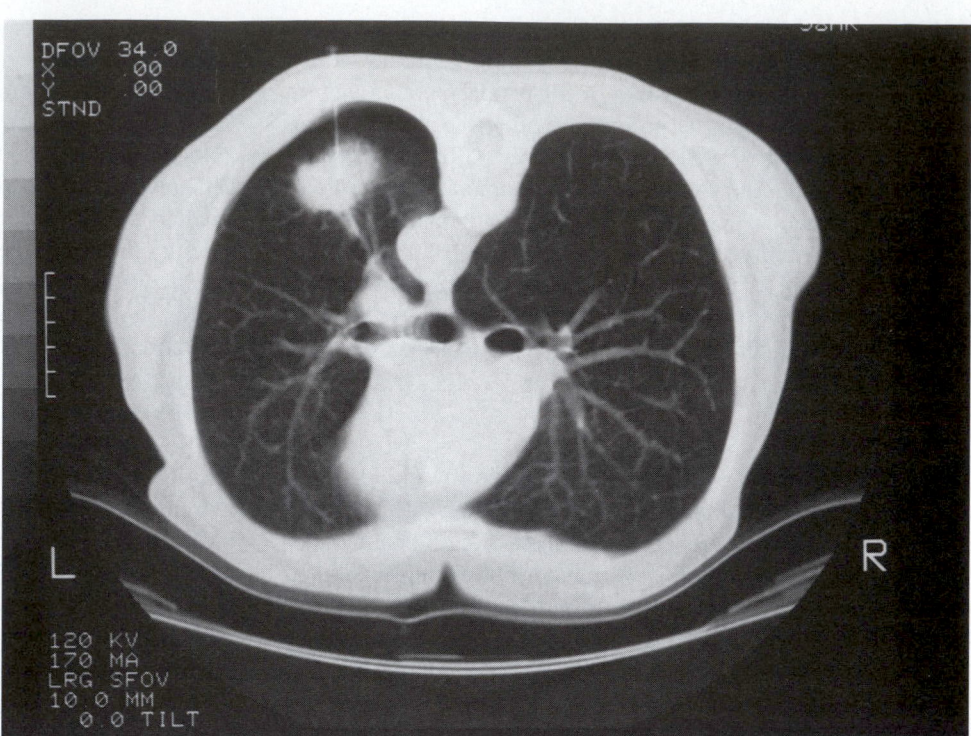

FIGURE 110-7   Malignant nodule during CT-guided aspiration showing development of pneumothorax.

niques, such as endoscopically guided bronchoscopic biopsy, may prove to be of use. It should be mentioned that routine preoperative staging bronchoscopy is of no value in asymptomatic patients with a solitary pulmonary nodule smaller than 3 cm because it has not been shown to alter management decisions.[13,37]

Percutaneous Needle Aspiration

Percutaneous needle aspiration can be performed under fluoroscopic or CT guidance, the choice often depending on the availability and the experience of the operator. It is most useful as the initial procedure in peripheral lesions, in the outer third of the lung, and in lesions under 2 cm in diameter. It can establish the diagnosis of malignancy in up to 95 percent of cases and can establish specific benign diagnosis (granuloma, hamartoma, infarct) in up to 68 percent of patients.[17] The use of larger-bore biopsy needles—such as 19 gauge, which provides a core specimen in addition to cytology—improves the yield for both malignant and benign lesions. The major limitation of percutaneous needle aspiration is its high rate of pneumothorax (10 to 35 percent overall);[42] pneumothorax is more likely when lung parenchyma lies in the path of the needle (Fig. 110-7). Of these pneumothoraxes, 5 to 10 percent require drainage with a chest tube. Because of the high rate of pneumothorax and its possible complications, the following patients should not undergo percutaneous needle aspiration: those with limited pulmonary reserve (e.g., FEV_1 under 1 L); those with bullous emphysema or blebs in the needle path; and postpneumonectomy patients. Other general contraindications are: bleeding diathesis, inability to hold breath, and severe pulmonary hypertension. Bronchoscopy can sometimes be used when percutaneous needle aspiration is contraindicated. The two procedures can be used successfully in a complementary fashion.

Thoracotomy and Thoracoscopy

Open thoracotomy and lobectomy with anatomic lymph node resection and staging remain the standard of care for stage I bronchogenic carcinoma, the most common malignancy among solitary pulmonary nodules. Nodules greater than 3 cm in diameter have a greater than 90 percent chance of being malignant, and in the face of a negative metastatic workup and adequate pulmonary reserve, indeterminate nodules of this size should be resected. Smaller nodules that remain indeterminate after appropriate radiographic evaluation and biopsy (bronchoscopic and/or percutaneous needle aspiration where indicated) either can be resected with open thoracotomy or thoracoscopy or can be observed with close serial radiographic follow-up. The decision will depend on the patient and on the physician, who must educate the patient on the alternatives and possible consequences. Thoracotomy has a reported mortality of 3 to 7 percent. It is higher in patients over age 70 and in patients with malignancy. These patients will usually have other coexisting illness, such as chronic obstructive pulmonary disease (COPD), coronary artery disease, etc. The mortality risk increases with the extent of the procedure. In one series by Ginsberg and coworkers, the mortality was 1.4 percent for wedge resection, 2.9 percent for lobectomy, and 6.2 percent for pneumonectomy.[10]

With the aid of fiberoptic telescopes and miniaturized video cameras, thoracoscopy has reemerged in the form of video-assisted thoracic surgery. This approach still requires general anesthesia but does not require a full thoracotomy incision or spreading of the ribs. The thoracoscope can be invaluable in the diagnosis and treatment of pleural disease and of late has become a useful tool in the management of solitary pulmonary nodules. Video-assisted thoracic surgery allows the experienced surgeon to identify and wedge out peripheral nodules in most cases with minimal morbidity and mortality. In a series by Mack and colleagues, 242 nodules were resected with no mortality and minimal morbidity. Average hospital stay was 2.4 days. Other groups have reported hospital stays of 4.6 days for video-assisted thoracic surgery, as against 7.8 days for standard open lateral thoracotomy. Video-assisted thoracic surgery can spare patients with benign nodules the risks of open thoracotomy and can be useful for wedging out nodules in patients who have limited pulmonary reserve and cannot otherwise tolerate a lobectomy. Lobectomy is preferable to wedge excision or segmental resection. The role of such limited pulmonary resections was studied by the Lung Cancer Study Group.[11] In this study, 276 patients with T1 N0 lesions were strictly staged to prove N0 status and randomized to lobectomy or limited resection.

In 247 patients, there was a 75 percent increase in recurrence rate and a 30 percent increase in overall death rate at 5 years after limited resection (wedge or segment). Therefore, if a diagnosis of malignancy is made on frozen section at the time of video-assisted thoracic surgery, and no contraindication exists, the procedure is usually converted to a formal thoracotomy and an anatomic resection is carried out. Video-assisted thoracic surgery is not indicated for lesions greater than 3 cm, as they are likely to be malignant and should be removed by open thoracotomy if the pulmonary reserve permits. Nor is the surgical technique indicated for centrally located lesions. Video-assisted thoracic surgery may be the initial procedure of choice for lesions that are not amenable to bronchoscopic or percutaneous needle aspiration biopsy because of the location—i.e., small peripheral lesions (outer third of lung), lesions located under ribs or the scapula, or lesions near areas of emphysema or bullous disease.

DIAGNOSTIC APPROACH

As is often the case in medicine, it is unwise to presume that an infallible algorithm can be provided for the evaluation of the solitary pulmonary nodule. Since no consensus can be reached on the basis of available data, the best that can be done is to offer recommendations. The pathway to be taken and final decision will rest on the individual clinician and patient. A 30-year-old nonsmoker, the mother of two children, with an indeterminate lesion, may not be willing to "observe serial radiographs" and demand a resection; in contrast, a 75-year-old smoker with

mild COPD and a lesion that seems to be a malignancy may decide to leave well enough alone and ignore it. The following recommendations represent one possible approach to a complex clinical problem (Fig. 110-8).

1. On discovering a solitary pulmonary nodule, the clinician should determine whether it is a true solitary nodule, spherical, and located within the lung fields. Standard PA and lateral radiographs often suffice. A lateral radiograph may show the lesion to be superficial or may show other lesions hidden behind the diaphragm or the mediastinum. If the existence of the lesion remains in question, CT is indicated. A thorough history and physical may provide clues about the nodule's possible cause (a history of tuberculosis in an asymptomatic patient will suggest granuloma, while weight loss and adenopathy will point toward malignancy). Most of the time, solitary pulmonary nodules are asymptomatic.

2. Once it has been established that the nodule is truly solitary,

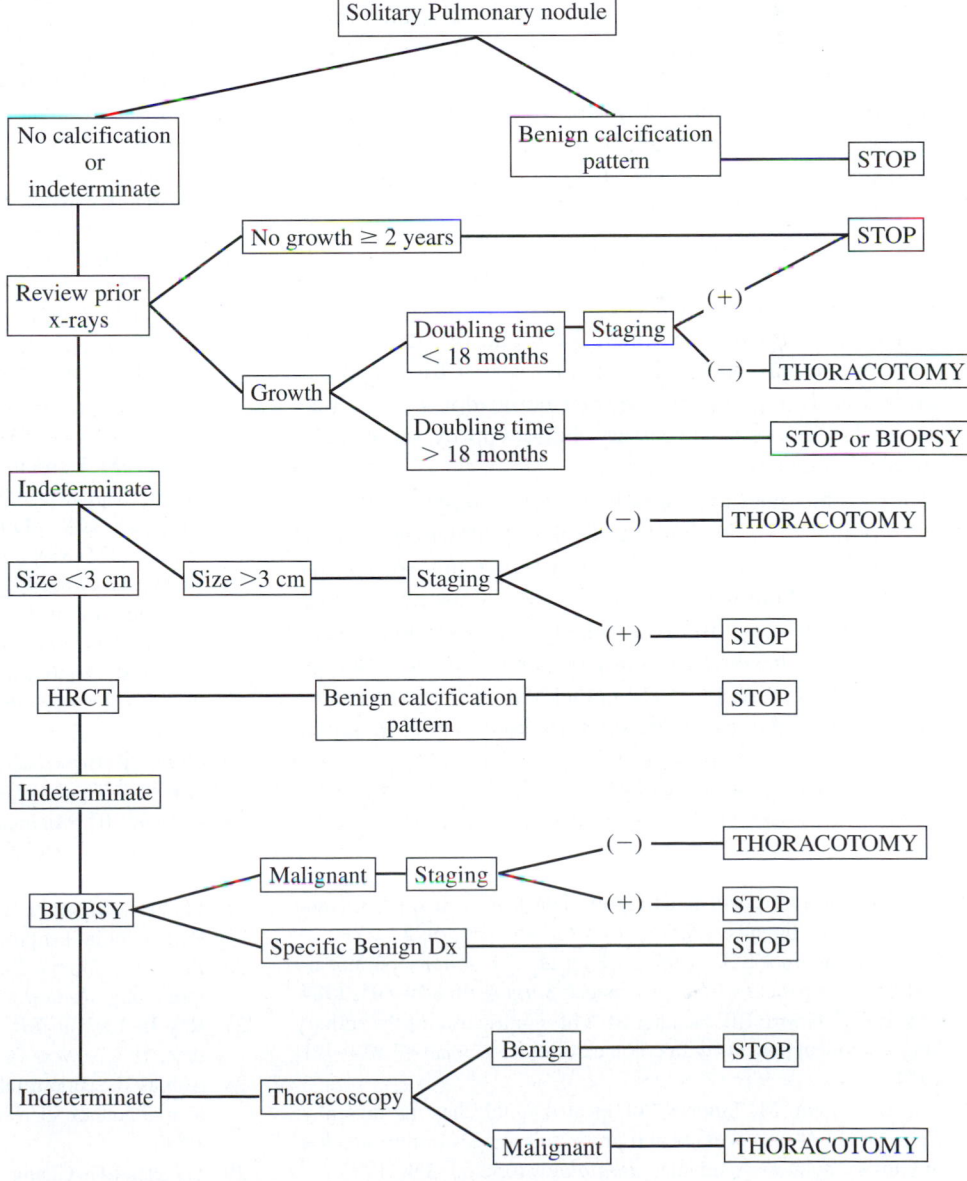

FIGURE 110-8   An approach to the solitary pulmonary nodule.

and a benign pattern of calcification is present, the nodule is considered benign and no further workup is necessary. Follow-up by serial radiographs is recommended every 6 months for a period of 2 years.

3. If prior chest radiographs are available, and the nodule remains unchanged for 2 years or longer, no further workup is necessary. Follow-up with serial radiographs is recommended every 6 months to a year for 2 years.

4. If the nodule has grown and the doubling time is more than 20 days but less than 18 months, it is considered malignant and should be resected. If the doubling time is more than 18 months, the nodule is presumed to be benign and close serial radiographic follow-up is warranted, perhaps every 2 to 3 months for the first year and every 6 months for the next year. Alternatively, depending on the patient, a biopsy procedure may be useful to provide further reassurance to the physician and the patient. If the nodule was not present on prior radiographs, an upper-limit doubling time is calculated. The assumption is made that a 0.8-cm nodule was present but not yet detectable in the last available radiograph, and the doubling time is then calculated. If the doubling time is again less than 18 months, it is considered to be malignant and resected. If the doubling time is more than 18 months, the nodule remains indeterminate. Nodules on which previous radiographs are unavailable are also indeterminate.

5. Noncalcified nodules greater than 3 cm and of indeterminate stability are likely to be malignant and should be resected if adequate pulmonary reserve is present and if staging CT shows resectability. Mediastinoscopy may be required for staging if CT is equivocal.

6. Noncalcified nodules less than 3 cm and of indeterminate stability should undergo HRCT, in a search for occult calcification. If a benign pattern of calcification is identified, no further workup is necessary. Follow-up by serial radiographs is recommended.

7. If no visible calcification is identified, a biopsy procedure is recommended. The initial procedure will depend on local availability, but either bronchoscopy or percutaneous needle aspiration or both will yield good results in the right setting. If no definite diagnosis is obtained or if the lesion is inaccessible to either bronchoscopy or percutaneous needle aspiration, thoracoscopy is recommended. If the lesion is inaccessible to thoracoscopy, open thoracotomy is required.

REFERENCES

1. Buckley JA, Scott WW, Siegelman SS, et al: Pulmonary nodules: Effect of increased data sampling on detection with spiral CT and confidence in diagnosis. *Radiology* 196:395–400, 1995.
2. Casey JJ, Stempel BG, Scanlon EF, et al: The solitary pulmonary nodule in the patient with breast cancer. *Surgery* 96:801–805, 1984.
3. Chang WG, Castro EB, Headier SI: The significance of the solitary lung shadow in patients with colon carcinoma. *Cancer* 33:414–421, 1974.
4. Correa J, Souto M, Tahoces PG, et al: Digital chest radiography: Comparison of unprocessed and processed images in the detection of solitary pulmonary nodules. *Radiology* 195:253–258, 1995.
5. Cummings SR, Lillington GA, Richard RJ: Estimating the proba-
bility of malignancy in solitary pulmonary nodules. *Am Rev Respir Dis* 134:449–452, 1986.
6. Dewan NA, Gupta NC, Redepenning LS, et al: Diagnostic efficacy of PET-FDG imaging in solitary pulmonary nodules. *Chest* 104:997–1002, 1993.
7. Fletcher EC, Levin DC: Flexible fiberoptic bronchoscopy and fluoroscopically guided transbronchial biopsy of solitary pulmonary nodules. *West J Med* 136:477–483, 1982.
8. Gasparini S, Ferretti M, Bichi Secchi E, et al: Integration of transbronchial and percutaneous approach in the diagnosis of peripheral pulmonary nodules or masses. *Chest* 108:131–137, 1995.
9. Geddes DM: The natural history of lung cancer: A review based on rates of tumor growth. *J Dis Chest* 73:1–17, 1979.
10. Ginsberg RJ, Hill LD, Eagan RT, et al: Modern thirty-day operative mortality for surgical resections in lung cancer. *J Thorac Cardiovasc Surg* 86:654–658, 1983.
11. Ginsberg RJ, Rubinstein LV: Randomized trial of lobectomy vs. limited resection for T1 N0 non–small cell lung cancer. *Ann Thorac Surg* 60:615–623, 1995.
12. Gjevre JA, Myers JL, Prakash UBS: Pulmonary hamartomas. *Mayo Clin Proc* 71:14–20, 1996.
13. Goldberg SK, Walkenstein MD, Steinbach A, et al: The role of staging bronchoscopy in the perioperative assessment of a solitary pulmonary nodule. *Chest* 104:94–97, 1993.
14. Good CA, Wilson TW: The solitary circumscribed pulmonary nodule: Study of seven hundred five cases encountered roentgenologically in a period of three and one-half years. *JAMA* 166:210–215, 1958.
15. Guerney JW, Swensen SJ: Solitary pulmonary nodules: Determining the likelihood of malignancy with neural network analysis. *Radiology* 196:823–829, 1995.
16. Higgins GA, Thomas WS, Keehn RJ: The solitary pulmonary nodule. *Arch Surg* 110:570–575, 1975.
17. Huston J III, Muhm JR: Solitary pulmonary nodules: Evaluation with a CT reference phantom. *Radiology* 170:653–656, 1989.
18. Khouri NF, Stitik FP, Erozan YS, et al: Transthoracic needle aspiration biopsy of benign and malignant lung lesions. *Am J Roentgenol* 144:281–288, 1985.
19. Libby DM, Henschke CI, Yankelevitz DF: The solitary pulmonary nodule: Update 1995. *Am J Med* 99:491–496, 1995.
20. Lillington GA: Management of solitary pulmonary nodules. *Dis Mon* 37:271–318, 1991.
21. Mack MJ, Hazelrigg SR, Landreneau RJ, et al: Thoracoscopy for the diagnosis of the indeterminate solitary pulmonary nodule. *Ann Thorac Surg* 56:825–832, 1993.
22. Metha AC, Kathawalla SA, Chan C, et al: Role of bronchoscopy in the evaluation of solitary pulmonary nodule. *J Bronchol* 2:315–322, 1995.
23. Muhm JR, Brown LR, Crowe JK: Use of computed tomography in the detection of pulmonary nodules. *Mayo Clin Proc* 52:345–348, 1977.
24. Neifield JP, Michaelis LL, Doppman JL: Suspected pulmonary metastases: Correlation of chest x-ray, whole lung tomograms, and operative findings. *Cancer* 39:383–387, 1977.
25. Pass HL, Mitchell JB, et al: *Lung Cancer Principles and Practice.* Philadelphia, Lippincott-Raven, 1996, p 310.
26. Proto AV, Thomas SR: Pulmonary nodules studied by computed tomography. *Radiology* 156:149–153, 1985.
27. Ray JF, Lawton BR, Magnin GE, et al: The coin lesion story: Update, 1976. *Chest* 70:332–336, 1976.
28. Rubins JB, Bloomfield Rubins H: Temporal trends in the prevalence of malignancy in resected pulmonary lesions. *Chest* 109:100–103, 1996.
29. Schaner EG, Chang AE, Doppman JL, et al: Comparison of computed and conventional whole lung tomography in detecting pul-

monary nodules: A prospective radiologic-pathologic study. *Am J Roentgenol* 131:51–54, 1978.

30. Shiner RJ, Roseman J, Katz I, et al: Bronchoscopic evaluation of peripheral lung tumors. *Thorax* 43:887–889, 1988.

31. Siegelman SS, Khouri NF, Leo FP, et al: Solitary pulmonary nodules: CT assessment. *Radiology* 160:307–312, 1986.

32. Siegelman SS, Khouri NF, Scott WW Jr, et al: Pulmonary hamartoma: CT findings. *Radiology* 160:313–317, 1986.

33. Steele JD: The solitary pulmonary nodule. *J Thorac Cardiovasc Surg* 46:21–39, 1963.

34. Swensen SJ, Harms GF, Morin RL, et al: CT evaluation of solitary pulmonary nodules: Value of 185-H reference phantom. *Am J Roentgenol* 156:925–929, 1991.

35. Theros EG: Varying manifestations of peripheral pulmonary neoplasms: A radiologic-pathologic correlative study. *Am J Roentgenol* 128:893–914, 1977.

36. Toomes H, Delphendahl A, Manke H, et al: The coin lesion of the lung. *Cancer* 51:534–537, 1983.

37. Torrington KG, Kern JD: The utility of fiberoptic bronchoscopy in the evaluation of the solitary pulmonary nodule. *Chest* 104:1021–1024, 1993.

38. Trunk G, Gracey DR, Byrd RB: The management and evaluation of the solitary pulmonary nodule. *Chest* 66:236–239, 1974.

39. Tsuboi E, Ikeda S, Tajima M, et al: Transbronchial biopsy smear for the diagnosis of peripheral pulmonary carcinomas. *Cancer* 20:687–698, 1967.

40. Ward HB, Pliego M, Diefenthal H, et al: The impact of phantom CT scanning on surgery for the pulmonary nodule. *Surgery* 106:734–739, 1989.

41. Webb WR: Radiologic evaluation of the solitary pulmonary nodule. *Am J Roentgenol* 154:701–708, 1990.

42. Westcott JL: Percutaneous transthoracic needle biopsy. *Radiology* 169:593–601, 1988.

43. Yamashita K, Matsunobe S, Tsuda T, et al: Solitary pulmonary nodule: Preliminary study of evaluation with incremental dynamic CT. *Radiology* 194:399–405, 1995.

44. Zerhouni EA, Stitik FP, Siegelman SS, et al: CT of the pulmonary nodule: A cooperative study. *Radiology* 160:319–327, 1986.

45. Zwirewich CV, Vedal S, Miller RR, et al: Solitary pulmonary nodule: High-resolution CT and radiologic-pathologic correlation. *Radiology* 179:469–476, 1991.

C H A P T E R 1 1 1

THE PATHOLOGY OF NON–SMALL CELL LUNG CARCINOMA

Leslie A. Litzky

The revised World Health Organization (WHO) classification, formulated in 1981, is the most frequently used scheme for categorizing lung tumors. Within this classification, there are six major types of malignant epithelial non–small cell lung tumors (Table 111-1). As a broad diagnostic category, non–small cell lung cancer (NSCLC) constitutes about 70 percent of all lung cancers. Squamous cell carcinoma, adenocarcinoma, and large cell carcinoma are often grouped as NSCLC for research studies and treatment purposes. This chapter deals with these major histologic subtypes and some other epithelial tumors, such as bronchial gland carcinomas, which are less common. Carcinoid tumors are discussed within the general context of neuroendocrine tumors. Other unusual tumors, both benign and malignant, are covered in a separate chapter (see Chapter 115).

HISTOLOGIC CLASSIFICATION AND NOMENCLATURE

Pathologic assessments are continually refined to reflect changes in surgical and medical management, as well as to incorporate an improved understanding of basic tumor biology. Once the diagnosis of malignancy has been made, the pathologic evaluation of NSCLC has traditionally focused on histologic subtyping and determining the extent of disease. Histologic classification is essentially predicated on the assumption that the quantitative predominance of a particular histologic pattern reflects distinctive biologic characteristics. There remains great expectation that developments in other disciplines, such as molecular biology, ultimately may have a profound impact on tumor characterization. Whether basic research in molecular genetics and other fields will substantiate or modify currently accepted histologic classification is currently an open and actively debated question.

Tumor classification and associated generalizations pertaining to tumor type are often made to seem much more straightforward than they are in reality. It is always a challenge for any proposed scheme of histopathologic classification to ensure the reproducible recognition of tumor subtypes. This is even true for distinction between small cell and non–small cell carcinoma and may be unsettling for the clinician faced with a choice between different therapeutic interventions and prognoses. In order to understand some of the difficulties in tumor subclassification, it is worth recalling that all the epithelial tissues in the lung are derived from an endodermal outpouching lined by a single layer

TABLE 111

WHO Classification of Malignant Epithelial Non–Small Cell Lung Tumors

Major Subtype	Variants
Squamous cell carcinoma	Spindle (squamous) cell carcinoma
Adenocarcinoma	Acinar adenocarcinoma
	Papillary adenocarcinoma
	Bronchioloalveolar carcinoma
	Solid carcinoma with mucus formation
Large cell carcinoma	Giant cell carcinoma
	Clear cell carcinoma
Adenosquamous carcinoma	
Carcinoid tumor	
Bronchial gland carcinoma	Adenoid cystic carcinoma
	Mucoepidermoid carcinoma
	Others
Others	

of cuboidal cells—which, in turn, differentiate to form the many different cell types that make up the epithelial lining and the secretory cells. Moreover, lung carcinomas are derived from pluripotential epithelial cells, which are capable of the same phenotypic variation. Therefore, it is not surprising that many epithelial tumors show a mixture of different cell types at both the light microscopic and ultrastructural levels. They also overlap with respect to their antigenic properties and the elaboration of hormones.

The WHO histologic criteria have proved to be relatively reproducible and therefore useful for predicting prognosis.[44] This classification is based on the dominant histologic type as exemplified by recognizable architectural patterns and individual cellular features that can be appreciated with light microscopy of a section stained with hematoxylin and eosin. Other histochemical stains, such as those used to determine the mucin production characteristic of an adenocarcinoma or silver stains for neuroendocrine tumors, are also referred to in the WHO descriptions, but quantitative criteria for categorization are not specified. Data from other ancillary studies, such as immunohistochemistry or molecular genetics, are not incorporated. As a result, some investigators have wondered if it is time to consider whether additional information gained by using these special studies would improve the subclassification of lung tumors.[42] This has been particularly true of studies on neuroendocrine differentiation (see subsequent section). However, such suggestions have broad implications, such as the cost of the laboratory tests, special equipment and technical expertise, and the definition of criteria for the interpretation of these tests. Prospective clinical trials will be needed to classify the diagnostic and therapeutic values of the special studies.

Pathologists usually assess the degree of differentiation of tumors, such as squamous cell carcinoma and adenocarcinoma, that show differentiation. This histologic grading is an attempt to quantify the extent to which phenotypically the tumor cells resemble normal cell types, such as a squamous cell or a glandular cell. Histologic grading is not histogenetic determination—i.e., that a tumor is derived from a specific cell of origin, such

as a squamous cell, or that the tumor cell has "dedifferentiated" from a particular cell of origin.

There are three histologic degrees of differentiation—well differentiated, moderately differentiated, and poorly differentiated. Few studies, based on current staging protocols, have specifically addressed the significance of differentiation as a prognostic variable. Nonetheless, the pathologic literature overall has acknowledged the importance of differentiation even though this is not formally part of the TNM staging system. This is due in part to the intuitive opinions of many pathologists who are accustomed to providing degree of differentiation for malignancies in other organ systems, such as the breast, where its prognostic value has been conclusively demonstrated. As a group, lung cancers tend to be poorly differentiated. It may be even more accurate to give the percentage of tumor showing well, moderate, and poor differentiation.[15]

As in any classification scheme, distinctions can be somewhat arbitrary. Before proceeding to a general discussion of histologic subtypes, it seems appropriate to consider the factors that lead to variability or lack of specificity in the classification of tumors.[3,37] Two aspects of variability have been singled out for special consideration: histopathologic variability within a particular tumor due to divergent pathways of differentiation and interobserver or intraobserver variation in applying a particular histopathologic classification scheme.[33]

Factors that affect inter- and intraobserver variability, both in published studies and in general practice, include the extent of tumor sampling, the source of the material (i.e., biopsy versus surgical versus autopsy), the number of observers, the number of cases studied, and the manner in which the tissue is evaluated. Keehn and colleagues reported an overall interobserver agreement in diagnosis of 76 percent.[20] Consensus concerning histologic diagnosis was best for small cell carcinomas (72 percent), intermediate for adenocarcinomas (56 percent) and squamous cell carcinomas (48 percent), and very poor for large cell carcinomas (4.8 percent). Roggli and coworkers reported a better overall consensus (94 percent), but instead of relying on agreement among six of eight, as was done by Keehn, Roggli's study required only three of five pathologists to agree.[34] Agreement was considerably poorer for further tumor subtyping and abysmal for bronchioloalveolar carcinoma (1.5 percent).

The practical impact of tumor heterogeneity is the occasional discrepancy between the cytologic and surgical pathologic diagnoses on the one hand and the final findings at autopsy on the other. Recognition of histologic heterogeneity depends to a great extent on sampling techniques. In one study of lung cancer heterogeneity in which differences in stage were taken into account, there was no significant difference in survival between patients with homogeneous and with heterogeneous tumors.[13] Keehn's interobserver agreement of 72 percent for small cell carcinoma is particularly troublesome and underscores the fact that lung tumor heterogeneity may confound a clear-cut pathologic distinction between non–small cell and small cell carcinoma.

ANCILLARY STUDIES

The lung is a common site for both primary tumors and metastases. Ancillary studies typically are used to narrow the differential diagnosis or to demonstrate differentiation. It is a general principle of laboratory diagnosis that the sensitivity and specificity of any test depend on the pretest prevalence of the disease. The appropriate use of ancillary studies is grounded in a well-formulated differential diagnosis that is based on the tumor's histologic appearance. The clinician contributes greatly by providing a comprehensive clinical history that helps direct the diagnostic workup, thereby avoiding unnecessary tests.

Histologic/Histochemical Stains

The histologic/histochemical stains that are used most commonly to identify adenocarcinomas by demonstrating their intracellular neutral mucins are the periodic acid–Schiff stain after diastase and the mucicarmine stain. As discussed in the chapter on the pleura (Chapter 88), stains for neutral mucins are often used to distinguish adenocarcinoma from epithelial mesothelioma. Alcian blue staining after hyaluronidase treatment has been used to distinguish the acid mucin of mesothelial cells from the neutral epithelial mucin associated with adenocarcinomas. Mucin stains are also typically performed on large cell carcinomas, which appear as solid carcinomas that lack glandular differentiation. These sometimes have mucin-containing vacuoles within many tumor cells and, on electron microscopy, prove to be poorly differentiated adenocarcinomas. At present, specialized stains for neuroendocrine tumors based on silver precipitation are rarely used.

Immunohistochemistry

Immunohistochemistry is based on a primary antigen-antibody reaction and a secondary antibody-enzyme complex that interacts with a chromogen to produce a microscopically visible color reaction. Since its introduction into diagnostic pathology in the early 1980s, immunohistochemistry has become an integral part of tumor diagnosis. Unfortunately, there are very few antibodies that approach 100 percent sensitivity and specificity. As experts in immunohistochemistry have emphasized, it is irrelevant for diagnostic purposes to speak of overall sensitivity and specificity for a particular antibody. Instead, it is more appropriate to speak of relative sensitivity and specificity within a particular differential diagnosis. This requires interaction between the clinician and the pathologist in generating a differential diagnosis. For example, the use of immunochemistry can be helpful in the workup of an undifferentiated large cell carcinoma—usually to exclude melanoma and lymphoma, which can mimic a highly pleomorphic epithelial tumor. Within this differential diagnosis of an undifferentiated tumor that is composed of large cells, cytokeratin antibodies (such as AE1/3 and CAM 5.2) are used to support the diagnosis of carcinoma. In another context, cytokeratin antibodies focally stain most non–small cell lung carcinomas of all histologic subtypes, in addition to a wide variety of carcinomas from other primary sites.

There are, however, potential pitfalls in the use of immunochemistry. Cytokeratin antibodies illustrate possible nonspecificity. Cytokeratin antibodies stain benign bronchial and alveolar epithelia entrapped within tumors and may lead to a false interpretation of malignancy. Reactive mesothelial cells as well as malignant mesothelioma cells are also cytokeratin positive. Finally, cytokeratin positivity, usually focal, has also been demonstrated in sarcomas and melanomas.

As discussed in the section on malignant mesothelioma, antibodies to glycoproteins—such as CEA, B72.3, LeuM1, and BerEP4—stain a high percentage of adenocarcinomas, including adenocarcinomas of the lung. Different staining patterns of epithelial membrane antigen (EMA) immunoreactivity have been reported as a means of distinguishing malignant mesothelioma from adenocarcinoma, but the utility of EMA for this purpose has been disputed. Wick and coworkers demonstrated EMA staining in 100 percent of peripheral pulmonary adenocarcinoma; however, nearly 85 percent of malignant epithelioid mesotheliomas were positive as well.[46]

S100 and HMB45 are considered markers of melanocytic differentiation, and often both stains are used. Although sensitive, S100 is less specific for melanoma and stains other tumors, including those of neural origin and some adenocarcinomas of both primary pulmonary and extrapulmonary origin, such as those in the breast. Leukocyte common antigen, CD30 (for Ki-1–positive large cell lymphomas), and B- and T-cell markers are the immunostains most frequently used to exclude lymphoma.

In only a limited number of instances are immunohistochemical stains useful in differentiating a primary lung carcinoma from a metastatic carcinoma. Besides thyroglobulin for thyroid tumors and prostate-specific antigen, most other antibodies have too much overlap in specificity to be conclusive. Staining with a panel of antibodies to bolster diagnostic certainty—as in the differential diagnosis of primary lung carcinoma and metastatic breast carcinoma—may enhance diagnostic accuracy. Fundamentally, however, this type of immunohistochemical analysis remains an exercise in probabilities and may not suffice in individual clinical circumstances.

SQUAMOUS CELL CARCINOMA

In the United States, about 30 percent of all lung cancers are squamous cell carcinomas.[41] This histologic subtype is strongly correlated with cigarette smoking. It also has a male predominance, although the incidence among females has increased along with the increase in the number of female smokers. About two-thirds of squamous cell carcinomas occur centrally and may involve a mainstream, lobar, or segmental bronchus (Fig. 111-1A). As expected from its endobronchial growth pattern, squamous cell carcinoma is frequently accompanied by bronchial obstruction and postobstructive pneumonia. In up to one-third of patients with squamous cell carcinomas, the tumors cavitate as the size increases (Fig. 111-1B). This feature also occurs with other histologic types, but less often.[8] Although most squamous cell carcinomas are centrally located, some also present as peripheral nodules (Fig. 111-1C).

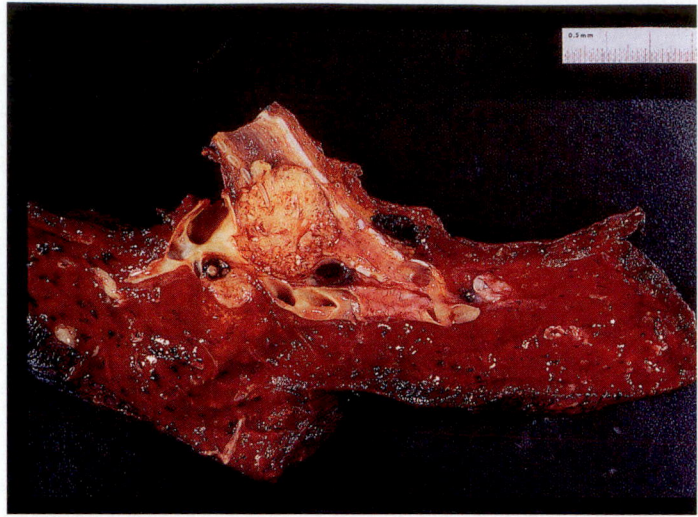

A

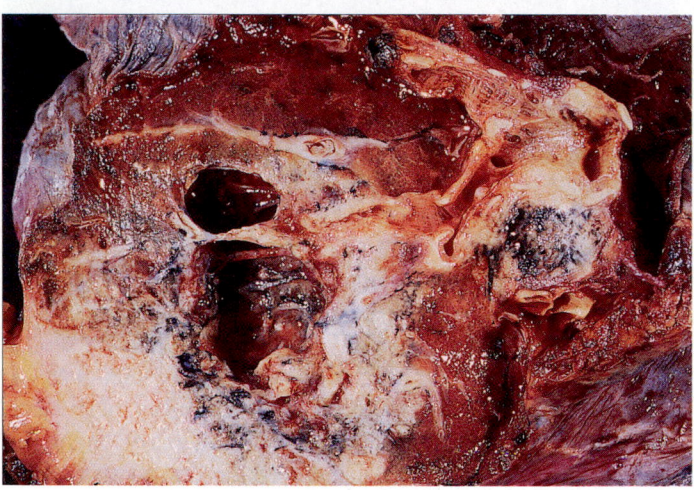

B

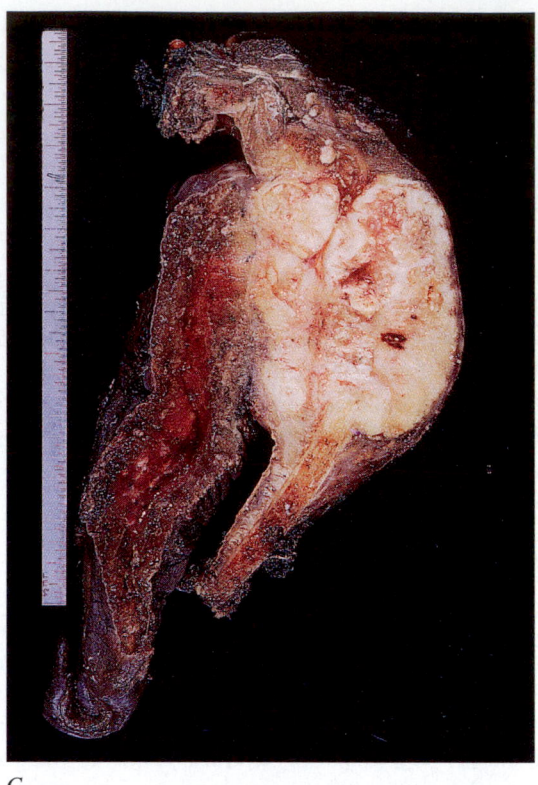

C

FIGURE 111-1   *A.* Large endobronchial squamous cell carcinoma with atelectasis and obstructive pneumonitis. *B.* Cavitation within a squamous cell carcinoma. *C.* Right upper lobectomy with chest wall resection for squamous cell carcinoma.

A fibrotic (desmoplastic) response is usually associated with the invasive nests of tumor cells (Fig. 111-2*A*). The tumor cells of a squamous cell carcinoma are large and polygonal with eosinophilic cytoplasm. Squamous differentiation is defined by keratinization or the presence of intercellular "bridges," (Figs. 111-2*B* and 111-2*C*). Intercellular "bridges" are seen in paraffin sections owing to cell shrinkage caused by fixation and correspond to the desmosomal attachments, which are visible ultrastructurally. Like the other histologic types of lung carcinomas, squamous cell carcinomas often show significant areas of histologic heterogeneity. Spindled cells, without conspicuous keratinization, or cells with clear cell cytoplasm, can be seen (Figs. 111-2*D* and 111-2*E*).

As a rule, it is easier to trace a trend in tumor progression in a squamous cell carcinoma than in other histologic types of lung carcinoma. Sampling of a resected specimen typically shows changes in the adjacent bronchial mucosa that range from squamous metaplasia to dysplasia to carcinoma in situ. The presence of an in situ component helps to differentiate a primary squamous cell carcinoma from a metastatic lesion. At present, there is no other conclusive means of differentiating a primary pulmonary squamous cell carcinoma from a metastasis. However,

metastatic tumors from the head and neck do tend to be better differentiated (i.e., show more extensive keratinization) than their primary pulmonary counterparts.

Electron microscopy demonstrates the presence of tonofilaments and desmosomes in squamous cell carcinomas. These findings are nonspecific, however, and may also be present in adenocarcinomas. There are currently no commercially available antibodies to distinguish a primary squamous cell carcinoma of the lung from those arising in other sites, such as the head and neck. It is common for squamous cell carcinomas to be immunoreactive with high-molecular-weight cytokeratin antibodies, but similar positivity also may be demonstrated in adenocarcinomas.

Basal Cell (Basaloid) Carcinoma of the Lung

Basaloid cells are typically described as small cells with moderately hyperchromatic nuclei, scant cytoplasm, a high mitotic rate, and peripheral palisading. Primary carcinomas of the lung with basaloid features have been reported and are considered by some to be a rare variant of squamous cell carcinoma.[10] The basaloid histologic features in lung carcinomas (Fig. 111-3) are similar to those seen in other extrapulmonary sites, such as the head and neck or cervix. Although Brambilla and coworkers acknowledge that basaloid carcinomas can be found in association with other histologic subtypes of non–small cell carcinoma, they argue that basaloid carcinoma is a distinct subtype that is histo-

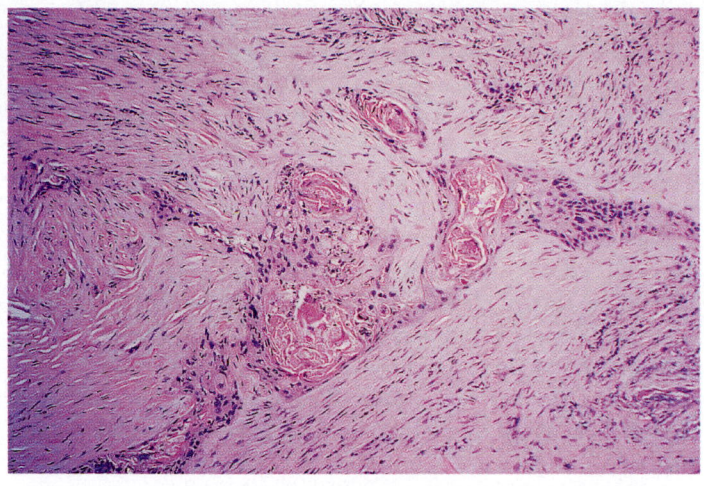

A

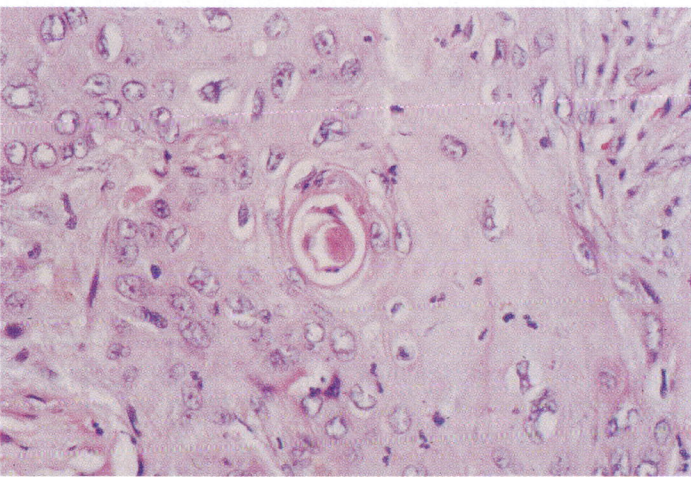

B

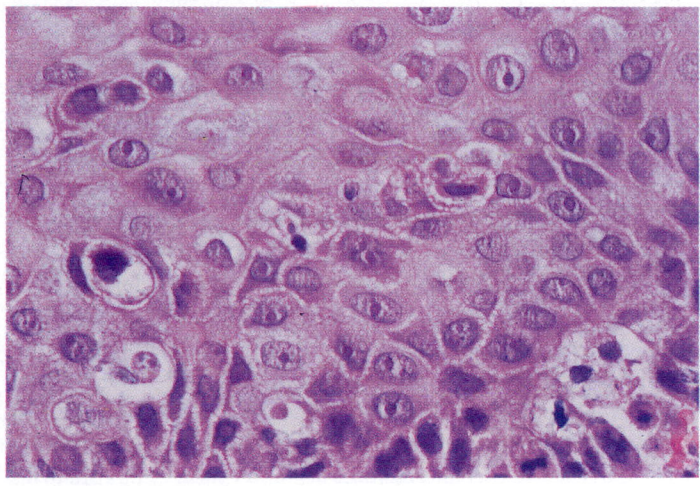

C

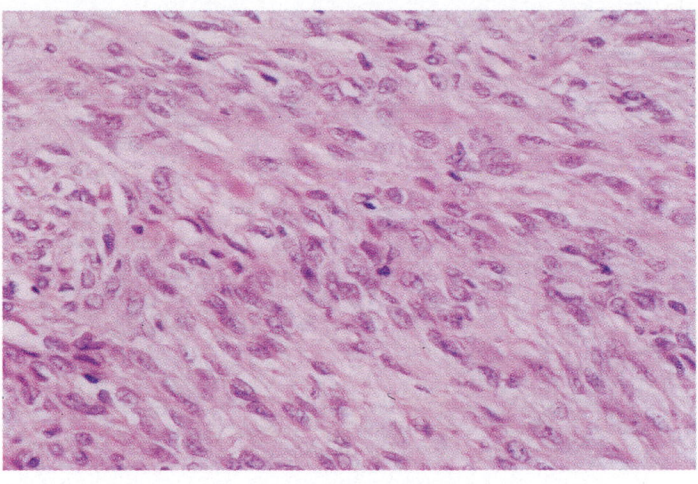

D

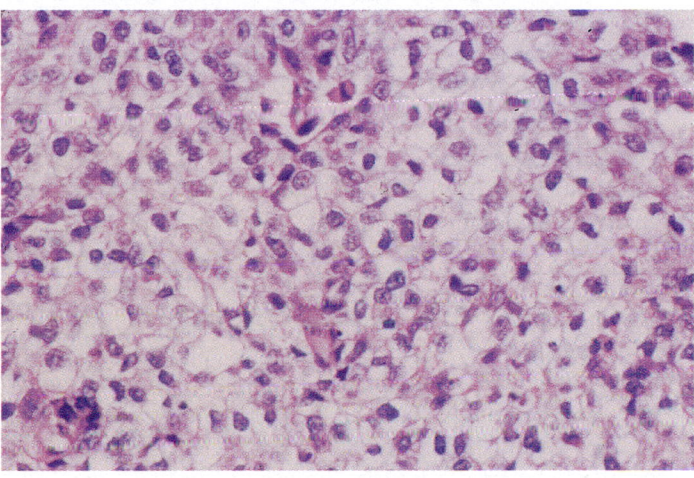

E

FIGURE 111-2 *A.* Desmosplastic response with nests of infiltrating squamous cell carcinoma. *B.* Squamous cell carcinoma with keratin "pearl" in center. *C.* Intercellular bridges between malignant squamous cells. *D.* Malignant spindled cells within a squamous cell carcinoma. *E.* Tumor cells with clear cytoplasm from a squamous cell carcinoma. H&E stains, ×400.

ADENOCARCINOMA, INCLUDING BRONCHIOLOALVEOLAR CARCINOMA

In the United States, adenocarcinoma is the most frequently diagnosed histologic type of lung cancer.[41] This represents a shift from 30 years ago, when the predominant histologic subtype was squamous cell carcinoma. Adenocarcinoma is the most frequently diagnosed subtype in women. Although most patients with adenocarcinoma are smokers, this histologic type also occurs in nonsmokers.[15]

Most adenocarcinomas arise in the periphery of the lung and are typically associated with puckering of the overlying pleura or with parenchymal scarring (Fig. 111-4). At one time, it was assumed that all these lesions represented a tumor arising in an area of preexisting fibrosis. However, a number of more recent studies have challenged this view, presenting evidence to support the hypothesis that the scarring represents a desmoplastic response to the tumor.[4,22,24] It is likely that both observations are

logically distinguishable from other tumors by light microscopy, immunohistochemistry, and electron microscopy.[5] In their series of 21 patients with stage I or stage II basaloid carcinomas (pure and mixed), the median survival was 22 months, with a 5-year survival probability of 10 percent.

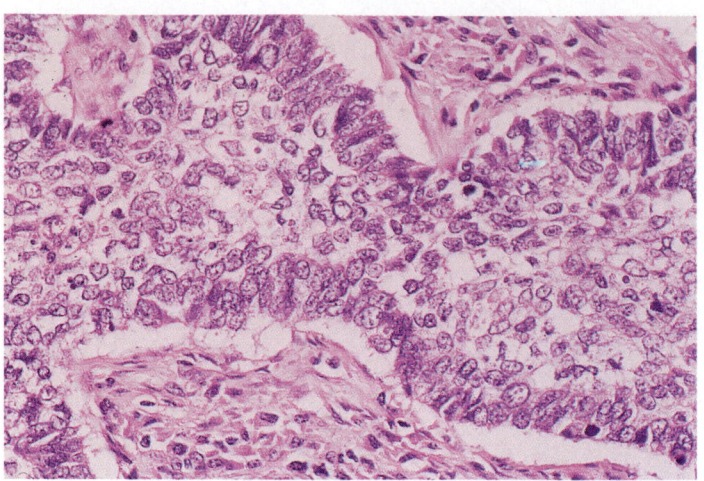

FIGURE 111-3 Basal cell carcinoma of the lung. The tumor cells are relatively small with hyperchromatic nuclei and scant cytoplasm. Note the tendency of the tumor cells to palisade at the periphery of the tumor nest. H&E, ×400.

correct and that the cause of the tumor-associated fibrosis depends on the clinical circumstances. Well-documented cases of adenocarcinoma have occurred in patients with diffuse pulmonary fibrosis, remote infarcts, and tuberculomas and within emphysematous bullae.

The histologic appearance of adenocarcinomas is extremely diverse. This histologic heterogeneity poses a significant problem when the differential diagnosis has to be made from metastasis or malignant mesothelioma. The WHO histologic classification recognizes four different histologic patterns of pulmonary adenocarcinoma—acinar, papillary, bronchioloalveolar, and solid. These subtypes depend on predominance of a particular histologic pattern. However, histologic variation within some tumors may make this distinction somewhat arbitrary. Acinar adenocarcinomas consist of irregularly contoured, but nonetheless recognizable, glandular structures and are often associated with a desmoplastic stroma (Figs. 111-5A and 111-5B). The papillary variant is illustrated in Fig. 111-5C. The presence of cytoplasmic vacuoles suggests the solid variant of adenocarcinoma, which is

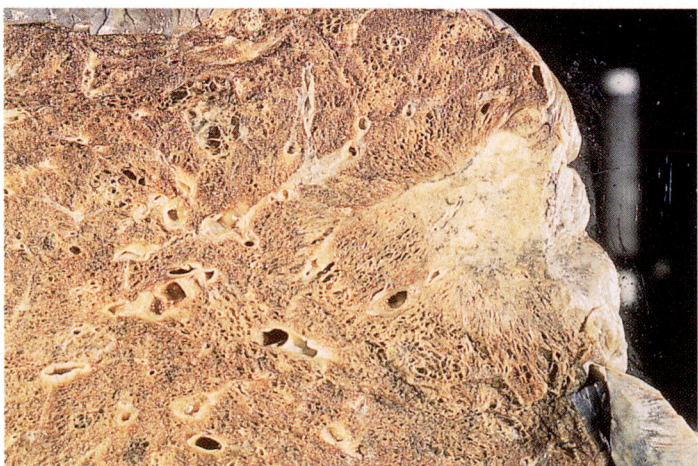

FIGURE 111-4 Peripheral adenocarcinoma of the lung with pleural puckering.

typically confirmed by a special stain for mucin (Fig. 111-5D). There are also rare variants, such as signet-ring carcinomas and cystic mucinous tumors, that resemble malignancies of other solid organs and may be very difficult to identify as primary lung lesions.

Distinction between peripheral adenocarcinomas with extensive pleural involvement and malignant mesothelioma may be problematic. The growth of some adenocarcinomas is in a manner that is virtually identical to that of malignant mesothelioma—i.e., with extensive pleural involvement and limited parenchymal invasion. Clinically, radiographically, and macroscopically, such malignancies are indistinguishable from malignant pleural mesothelioma. The histologic appearance may be equally confusing, requiring the use of immunohistochemical stains and electron microscopy.

It is common for bronchioloalveolar carcinoma (BAC) to be considered a distinct clinicopathologic entity. As outlined in Liebow's 1960 review of these tumors, the histologic features characteristic of BAC include a very peripheral origin, well-differentiated tumor cells, and the "tendency to spread chiefly within the confines of the lung by aerogenous and lymphatic routes," with "the walls of the distal airspaces often acting as supporting stroma for the neoplastic cells."[23]

As acknowledged in Liebow's original description, a clear-cut distinction between BAC and an "ordinary" pulmonary adenocarcinoma cannot always be made. Pathologists differ in their application of these criteria, some allowing for more histologic variability. It is common to see adenocarcinomas with a central, more poorly differentiated glandular component along with peripheral bronchioloalveolar features. These tumors should not be classified as the bronchioloalveolar subtype.

Classic BACs, consisting exclusively of malignant cells lining alveolar walls, tend to be small, well differentiated (by definition), and very peripheral. Stage and differentiation determine prognosis—e.g., greater than 90 percent 5-year survival for T1N0M0 tumors, as compared to 55 percent 5-year survival for T2N0M0 lesions.[9] Most BACs present as solitary peripheral nodules; some of them are slow-growing, but others may rapidly develop satellite lesions. Multicentric tumors and the diffuse pneumonic form carry a worse prognosis than the solitary lesions, even though the cytologic appearance of their tumor cells may suggest a low-grade malignancy.[7] Histologically, BACs are divided into two major subtypes, nonmucinous and mucinous. The nonmucinous type is more common and consists of cuboidal, columnar, or so-called hobnail cells with apical nuclei (Fig. 111-6A). The mucinous type consists of tall columnar cells with abundant apical mucinous cytoplasm and basally located nuclei (Fig. 111-6B). It is important to bear in mind that other mucinous carcinomas—particularly those of pancreatic or colonic origin—may metastasize to the lung and grow in a bronchioloalveolar pattern.

The ultrastructural appearance of adenocarcinomas can be quite heterogeneous. In contrast to malignant mesotheliomas, which have long microvilli, the cells have short, uniform microvilli and prominent rootlets with a fuzzy glycocalyx. The nuclei of nonmucinous BACs are more centrally located within the cell than the nuclei of malignant mesothelioma cells and contain varying numbers of granules, which range in size from 500 to 1500 nm. Some of these granules resemble lamellar bodies, while

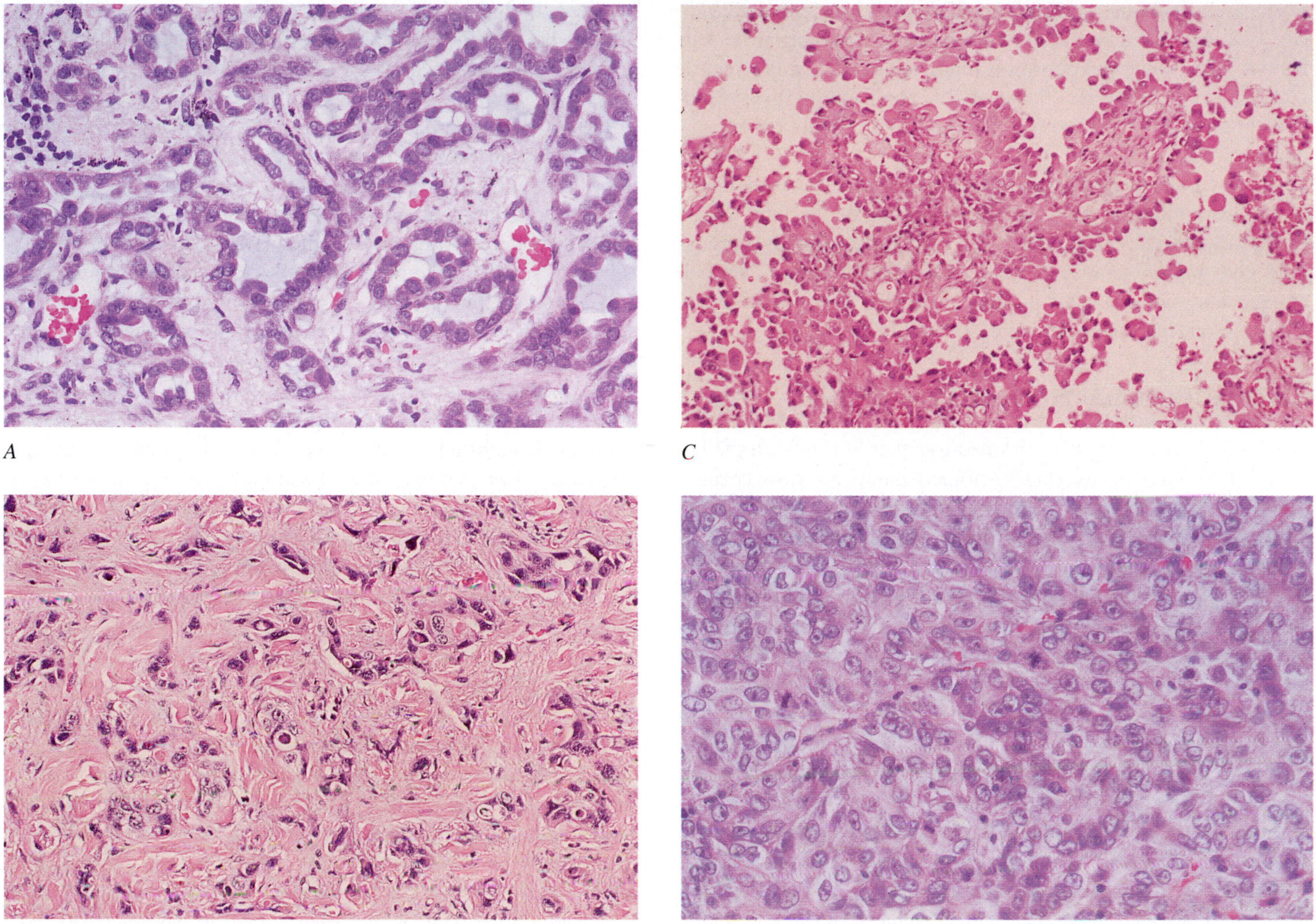

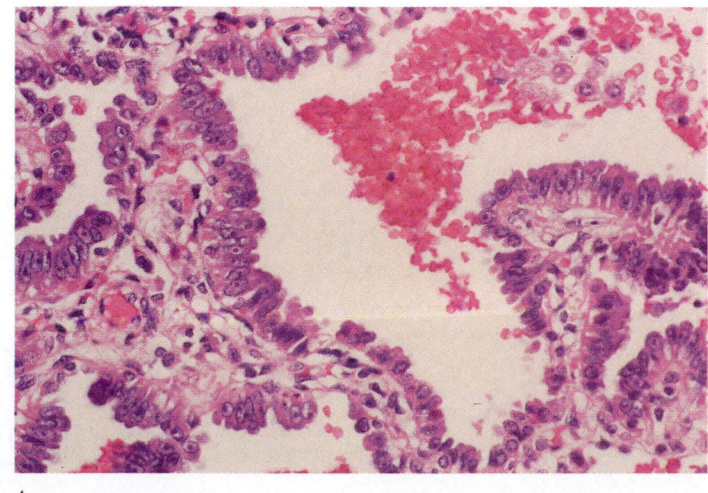

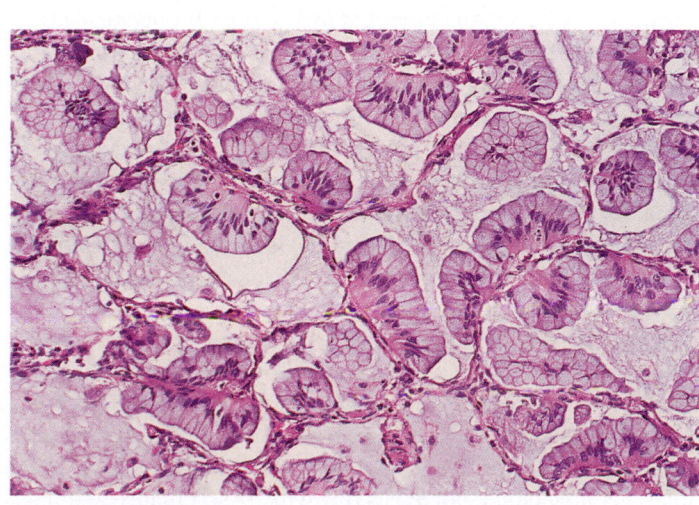

FIGURE 111-5 *A*. Moderately differentiated adenocarcinoma with recognizable gland formation. *B*. Poorly differentiated adenocarcinoma. Within the desmoplastic stroma, the tumor nests form occasional small, irregularly shaped glands with mucin vacuoles, *C*. Papillary adenocarcinoma. Malignant cells are arranged on the surface of fibrovascular cores. H&E stains, ×200. *D*. Adenocarcinoma with a solid growth pattern. This tumor is actually from the same patient illustrated in Fig. 111-5*A*. The two figures demonstrate the extreme range of histologic variation possible within a single tumor. H&E stain, ×400.

FIGURE 111-6 *A*. Bronchioloalveolar carcinoma, nonmucinous variant. Malignant cells uniformly line thickened alveolar septa. *B*. Mucinous bronchioloalveolar carcinoma. Tall columnar cells with abundant mucinous cytoplasm line the alveolar septa. H&E stains, ×400.

others are amorphous and electron dense. Intranuclear tubular inclusions, which immunostain for the apoprotein portion of surfactant, also occur, supporting a relationship to alveolar type II cells. Although often less conspicuous, short microvilli and mucous granules will also be found in less differentiated adenocarcinomas.

As discussed in the general section on immunohistochemistry, numerous antibodies stain adenocarcinomas of the lung. Many of these antibodies (CEA, B72.3, LeuM1, and BerEP4) recognize glycoproteins and are not specific for the lung. Clara cell antigen and surfactant apoprotein antibodies are commercially available but have limited diagnostic utility.

Alveolar Pneumocyte-Type Proliferations

A variety of lesions can be grouped together not only on the basis of the confusing overlap in nomenclature but also because these lesions may best be considered alveolar pneumocyte–type proliferations. In some of these lesions, the assumption of benignity is debatable, but it has proved difficult to demonstrate malignant potential. These tumors are typically discovered incidentally, either after pulmonary resection or in asymptomatic patients, without opportunity for long-term follow-up.

Atypical Adenomatous (Bronchioloalveolar) Hyperplasia and Bronchioloalveolar Adenoma   Atypical proliferations of alveolar lining cells long have been noted as an incidental finding in specimens resected for lung carcinoma. In 1988, Miller and colleagues reported a high incidence of such nodules in association with adenocarcinoma, terming these small (1- to 2-mm) lesions "atypical bronchioloalveolar hyperplasia."[28] The designation "bronchioloalveolar adenoma" was introduced into the literature in 1990 by Miller, who reported on other series of these nodules, which were found incidentally in 9.3 percent of consecutive specimens resected because of other histologic types of lung cancer.[27] Microscopically, these nodules are composed of alveolar lining cells, with a variable degree of cytologic atypia, growing in a so-called "lepidic" pattern along alveolar septa. Usually, some slight interstitial thickening accompanies the epithelial proliferation. Ultrastructurally, the cells have features of type II pneumocytes. In Miller's series, nodules greater than 5 mm were arbitrarily considered carcinomas and were believed to represent multicentric premalignant lesions analogous to adenomatous colonic polyps.[28]

Shimosato's team has argued in favor of Miller's concept by detailing a progression of increasing cytologic and architectural atypia from the periphery to the center of nonmucinous BAC.[36] This increased atypia is paralleled by abnormal ploidy, increased immunostaining with proliferating cell nuclear antigen, and increased immunostaining for the tumor-suppressor gene *p53*. As a practical matter, however, some degree of alveolar type II proliferation and atypia can be seen in many reactive processes. Although there is some evidence to support the hypothesis of premalignant change, atypical adenomatous nodules also occur as incidental findings in patients who do not have carcinoma of the lung. Unlike colonic polyposis, for which surveillance and intervention are easily accomplished, a conservative approach to considering the malignant potential of these lesions is recommended. Most authors would agree that a lesion larger than 5 mm with in-

termediate to marked cytologic atypia, prominent goblet cell metaplasia with intra-alveolar mucin, or conspicuous papillary architecture should be classified as a bronchioloalveolar carcinoma.

Alveolar Adenoma   This designation is applied to a rare group of well-circumscribed pulmonary lesions that consist of a benign proliferation of alveolar epithelium and septal mesenchyme.[47] In six asymptomatic patients, the lesion presented as a solitary peripheral nodule on the chest radiograph. Histologically, the lesions are sharply circumscribed, multicystic tumors consisting of large central dilated spaces formed by variably thick septa, with progression to smaller cystic spaces at the periphery. On ultrastructural examination the cysts are lined by alveolar pneumocytes, while the interstitium is composed of a proliferation of myxoid non–smooth muscle spindle-shaped cells mixed with mononuclear inflammatory cells. Follow-up of the six patients for up to 10 years demonstrated benign behavior. Four of the six patients had undergone lobectomy. The authors distinguished between this entity and sclerosing hemangioma, another unusual tumor, because of the lack of interstitial proliferation of distinct round cells within the stroma, which are characteristic of sclerosing hemangioma.

Sclerosing Hemangiomas of the Lung   These tumors were initially believed to be of endothelial origin. On the basis of ultrastructural and immunohistochemical analyses, most authors now believe that the neoplastic cells are epithelial, with the phenotype of a primitive airway cell.[49] These tumors typically present as a well-circumscribed, solitary subpleural mass in middle-aged women (Fig. 111-7). Grossly, the nodule usually has a hemorrhagic center, with a peripheral rim of compressed lung tissue. There is a great deal of histologic variation, with sclerotic, cellular, and vascular zones. However, the associated proliferation of uniform, bland round tumor cells in solid and papillary patterns is distinctive. These rare benign pulmonary epithelial tumors can be mistaken for BACs—particularly on frozen section, where cytologic detail and subtleties of architectural pattern can be obscured.

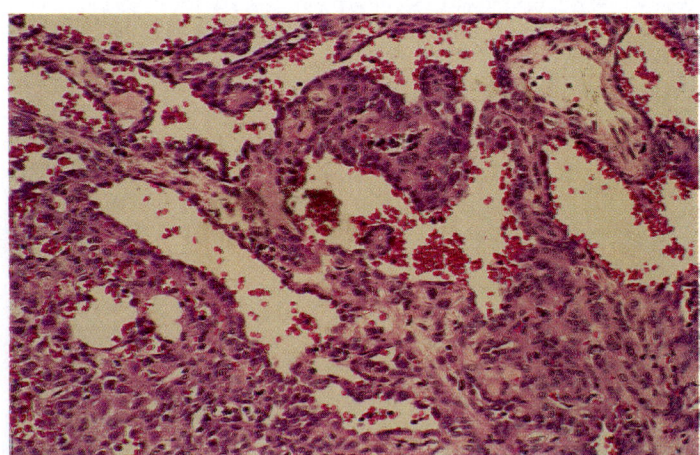

FIGURE 111-7   Sclerosing hemangioma. The tumor cells are uniform and cytologically bland with vascular and solid growth patterns. H&E stain, ×200.

LARGE CELL CARCINOMA

Large cell undifferentiated carcinoma is defined in the WHO classification as "a malignant epithelial tumor with large nuclei, prominent nucleoli, and usually well-defined cell borders, without the characteristic features of squamous cell carcinoma, small cell carcinoma, or adenocarcinoma" (Fig. 111-8).[44] As is evident from this description, the tumor is defined more by what it is not than by what it is. Therefore, for all practical purposes, this description makes it a diagnosis of exclusion. However, the WHO criteria are based on conventional microscopy and the use of a stain for mucin. On electron microscopy, many of these tumors show ultrastructural features consistent with adenocarcinoma. Other tumors prove to be poorly differentiated squamous cell carcinomas or to have neuroendocrine differentiation. Melanoma and malignant large cell lymphomas also can mimic large cell carcinoma, requiring the use of immunohistochemistry or electron microscopy to establish the diagnosis. Although the diagnosis of melanoma or lymphoma may have prognostic or therapeutic implications, the significance of differentiation that is not obvious on light microscopy is questionable. When mucin-positive cells are numerous, the designation is made of solid adenocarcinoma with mucin production. At present, there appears to be no clinical significance to a finding of focal mucin positivity within a solid tumor that is otherwise undifferentiated.

Giant Cell Carcinoma

The WHO classification recognizes giant cell carcinoma to be a variant of large cell carcinoma. Before this 1981 classification, "giant cell lung carcinoma" was used as a descriptive term but was not considered to be a discrete entity. According to the WHO criteria, giant cell carcinoma is a "large cell carcinoma containing a prominent component of highly pleomorphic multinucleated cells" (Fig. 111-9).[44] Despite the WHO criteria, which define this tumor as a variant of large cell carcinoma, giant cells can be seen in squamous cell carcinomas, adenocarcinomas, and small cell carcinomas. The reported incidence of the tumor varies between 0.8 and 4 percent. By current convention, 40 percent of

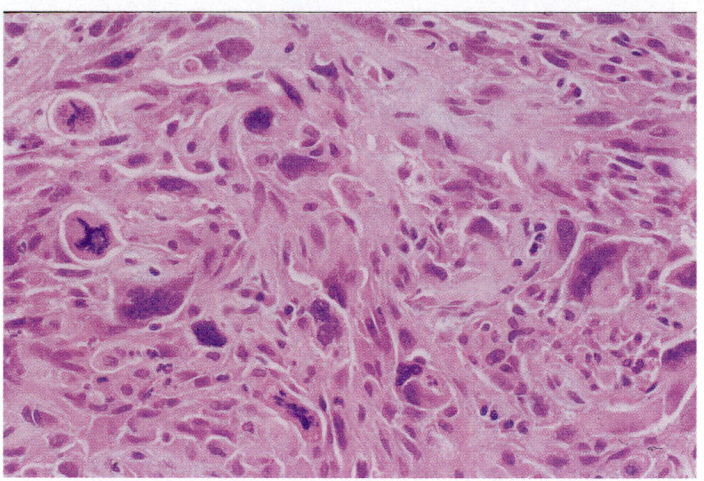

FIGURE 111-9   Giant cell carcinoma of the lung. H&E stain, ×400.

the tumor must consist of giant cells in order to be classified as a giant cell carcinoma.[15] Giant cell carcinoma was first described in 1958 by Nash and Stout as an aggressive tumor characterized by extensive local and distant spread, with extremely short patient survival (5 days to 7 months).[30] In a series of 16 patients with giant cell carcinoma, although attention was called to the high incidence of gastrointestinal metastases, the overall prognosis was similar to that for patients with other non–small cell histologic types of lung carcinoma.[14]

Clear Cell Carcinoma

The WHO classification considered clear cell carcinoma to be a rare variant of large cell carcinoma. The WHO classification described it as a carcinoma composed of elements with clear or foamy cytoplasm, without mucin, that may or may not contain glycogen.[44] This category excludes adenocarcinomas or squamous cell carcinomas with clear cells.

Despite the description suggesting that clear cell carcinoma is a discrete entity, it does not appear that the prognosis for this tumor is any worse than that for other types of non–small cell carcinoma of similar stage. In a review of 348 consecutive cases of lung carcinoma, Katzenstein and coworkers found only one case that strictly fulfilled the WHO criteria for clear cell carcinoma.[19] There were 14 other tumors (4 percent) that contained more than 50 percent clear cells, including 10 with predominant squamous differentiation and four with glandular differentiation. The clear cytoplasm in most cases stained strongly for glycogen. The authors concluded that these clear cell tumors should be classified according to the major WHO categories and not designated as a distinct clinicopathologic entity. For practical purposes, it is important to be aware of the fact that clear cell cytoplasm is a feature of some metastatic lesions—renal cell carcinoma in particular.

ADENOSQUAMOUS CARCINOMA

This tumor consists of well-defined squamous carcinoma and adenocarcinoma components. The tumor's behavior is, in general,

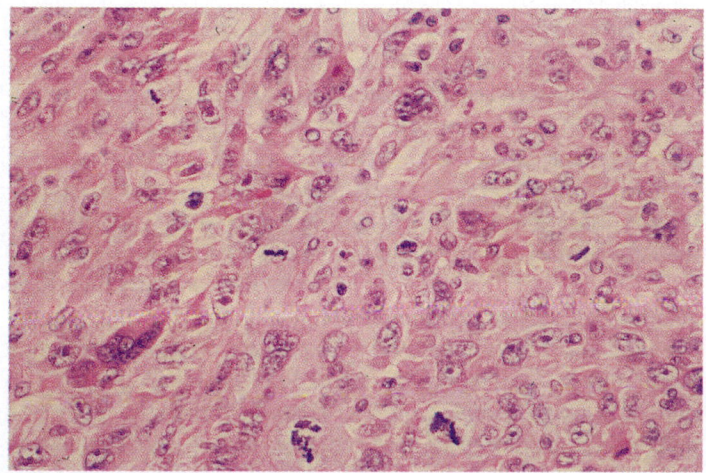

FIGURE 111-8   Large cell carcinoma of the lung. There is no obvious squamous differentiation in the form of keratinization or intercellular bridges. A mucin stain is negative. H&E stain, ×400.

similar to that of adenocarcinomas. The areas of glandular and squamous differentiation may be located in different areas of the tumor or may be intimately admixed. Different criteria have been used for this histologic subtype, and these differences in definition make it extremely difficult to compare survival rates. Takamori and colleagues, who defined the designation of adenosquamous carcinoma by indicating that each component should occupy at least 5 percent of the tumor area that was evaluated, reported a frequency of 2.6 percent and a shorter survival rate than with either squamous carcinomas or adenocarcinomas.[38] Ishida's group, which defined this subtype as a 20 percent squamous and an 80 percent adenocarcinoma mixture, noted a survival similar to that from other non–small cell lung carcinomas.[18]

SPINDLE CELL CARCINOMA (SARCOMATOID CARCINOMA, "CARCINOSARCOMA")

Tumors that are composed either exclusively or predominantly of malignant spindle cells have been noted in many primary organ sites, including the lung. There are a number of terms in the literature that refer to pulmonary tumors with this histologic appearance, and some authors have claimed that these tumors represent a unique clinicopathologic entity. The various terms in the literature include spindle cell carcinoma, sarcomatoid carcinoma, and pulmonary blastoma.

The WHO classification identifies *spindle cell carcinoma* as a biphasic variant of squamous cell carcinoma that includes one component identifiable as squamous cell carcinoma and another, consisting of spindle cells, that has a sarcomalike pattern.[44] *Carcinosarcoma* is defined as a malignant tumor with an admixture of carcinoma and sarcoma, which usually grow as polypoid structures in large bronchi.[44] The WHO classification acknowledges that carcinosarcomas are difficult to distinguish from spindle cell carcinomas "unless differentiation into specific tissues such as neoplastic bone, cartilage, and striated muscle is seen." In the pathology literature, tumors such as these, which contain cells with a neoplastic but differentiated connective-tissue phenotype, are said to have heterologous elements.

Pulmonary blastoma contains spindle cell elements that are histologically distinct from other spindle cell lesions because of a more embryonic appearance that resembles fetal lung, with distinctive "endometrioid"-type glands and a primitive cellular stroma (Figs. 111-10A and 111-10B). Although they have been seen in all age groups, Manivel and coworkers argue that the childhood intrathoracic tumor is a distinct clinicopathologic entity that differs from the adult type, particularly because of the absence of a carcinomatous component and its variable anatomic location.[25] They have proposed the alternative designation of *pleuropulmonary blastoma* for these pediatric tumors. The prognosis for the predominantly cystic variant of pleuropulmonary blastoma is reported to be favorable. Two cases have been reported of pediatric tumors that contained foci of primitive endometrioid glands as well as malignant stroma.[21] Whether the distinctive primitive histologic appearance of pulmonary blastomas makes a prognostic difference is unclear. Although about two-thirds of patients reported have died of their disease within 2 years after diagnosis, the staging information for these patients has not always been complete.

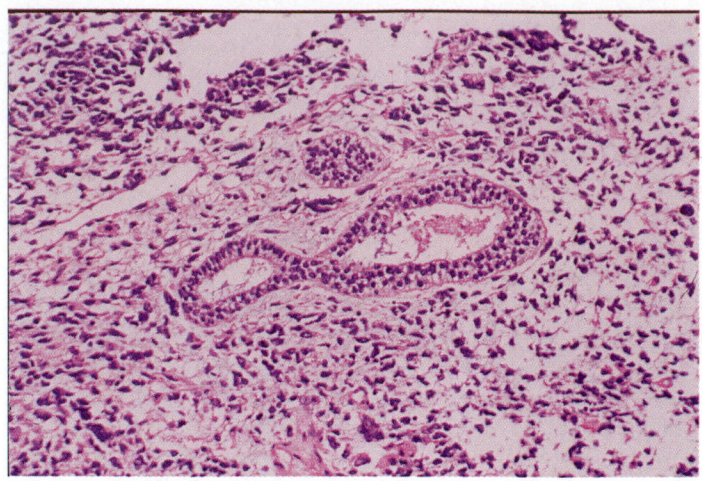

A

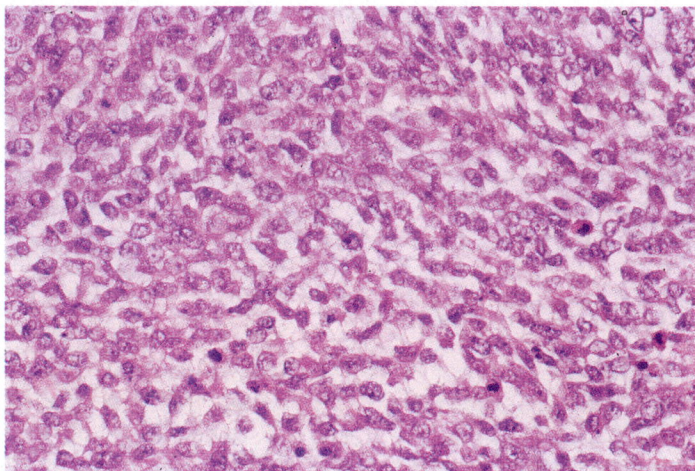

B

FIGURE 111-10   *A.* Pulmonary blastoma, showing a characteristic endometrioid-type gland, composed of cells with clear cytoplasm and basally oriented nuclei. H&E stain, ×200. *B.* Malignant stroma in a pulmonary blastoma. H&E stain, ×400.

In the practice of adult thoracic pathology, most of these tumors tend to fall into two groups: those that exclusively consist of spindle cells with or without an identifiable epithelial component (Fig. 111-11A) and those that have recognizably heterologous elements such as rhabdomyosarcoma, osteosarcoma, or chondrosarcoma (Fig. 111-11B). Although less common, pulmonary blastomas, composed exclusively of embryonic-type epithelial and mesenchymal elements, do occur. Adult tumors consisting entirely of malignant primitive glandular epithelium have also been described and termed "well-differentiated fetal adenocarcinomas."[21] Pathologists have tried to use electron microscopy or immunohistochemistry as a means of defining epithelial or mesenchymal differentiation. The lack of cytokeratin expression and the demonstration of mesenchymal markers, such as desmin and muscle-specific actin, have been used as evidence for a distinct clinicopathologic entity. Conversely, sarcomatoid carcinoma and carcinosarcoma may be merely phenotypic variations within the spectrum of lung tumors whose basic nature is epithelial.[17]

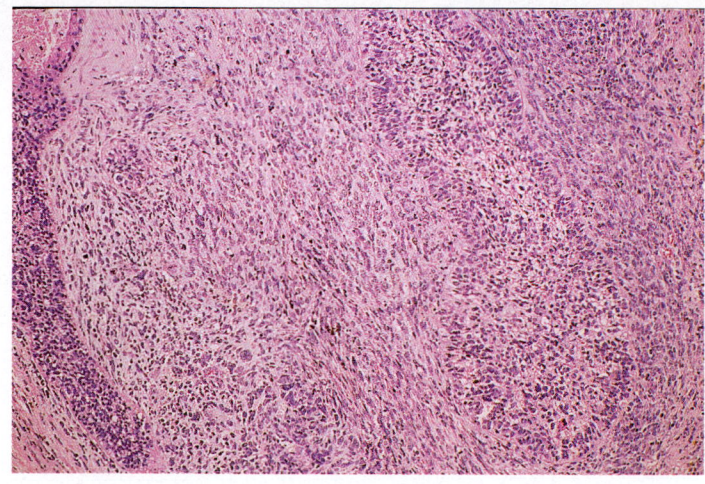

A

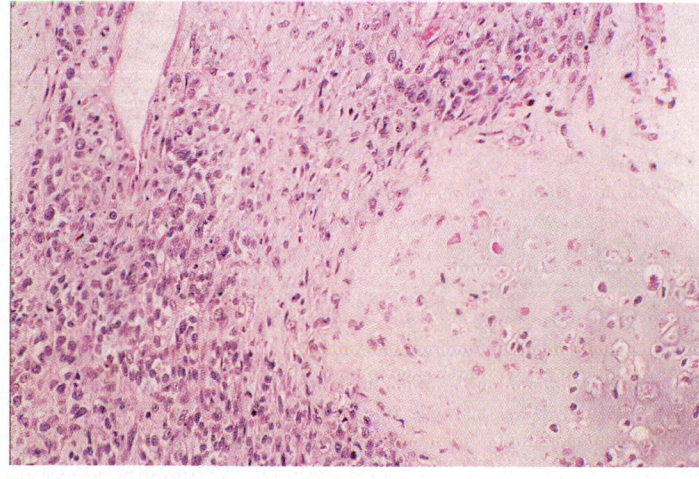

B

FIGURE 111-11   *A.* Biphasic sarcomatoid carcinoma showing a sarcomatous growth pattern (center) and epithelial differentiation at the peripheries H&E stain, ×100. *B.* Cartilagenous differentiation with a biphasic sarcomatoid carcinoma. H&E stain, ×200.

Four arguments have been outlined in favor of the hypothesis that sarcomatoid carcinomas and "carcinosarcomas" are part of a single clinicopathologic continuum: (1) the frequency of obviously epithelial foci merging imperceptibly with sarcomatoid areas in tumors that are well sampled; (2) the positive immunohistochemical reactivity with markers of epithelial differentiation in the sarcomatoid tumor cells; (3) the speciousness of arguing that a tumor that is not cytokeratin positive is not an epithelial tumor, since the immunohistochemical staining of poorly differentiated carcinomas may be negative for epithelial markers such as cytokeratin; and (4) the apparent lack of difference in the biologic behavior of sarcomatoid carcinomas and carcinosarcomas within the lung or within other organs.[30] The alternative terms *monophasic sarcomatoid carcinoma* has been suggested for tumors that have spindle cells and *biphasic sarcomatoid carcinoma* for tumors with obvious mesenchymal elements, such as cartilage, mixed in with the spindle cells.[30]

NEUROENDOCRINE TUMORS

The proliferation of terminology and proposed classifications of these lesions over the past 25 years has baffled clinicians and frustrated pathologists. In the past several years, a reasonably practical approach to the diagnosis of neuroendocrine tumors has evolved. Nevertheless, significant conceptual controversies remain and debate continues. There is still no consensus, but there is a growing recognition that some type of alternative classification system is needed, particularly if potential adjuvant therapies for neuroendocrine tumors are to be evaluated.

Neuroendocrine Differentiation

Recognition of neuroendocrine differentiation can be accomplished in a variety of ways. Some neuroendocrine tumors are recognized with simple light microscopy, on the basis of cytologic features and architecture alone. For example, bronchial carcinoids are typically composed of polygonal cells and regular oval nuclei with a stippled nuclear chromatin pattern described as "salt and pepper." These cytologic features are also shared by other neuroendocrine tumors that occur outside the lung, such as gastrointestinal carcinoids. Classic cases of small cell carcinoma similarly are recognized from morphologic criteria alone.

Ancillary tests for neuroendocrine differentiation are generally used when the morphologic findings are suggestive or inconclusive. Before the widespread use of immunohistochemistry, the earliest techniques for neuroendocrine differentiation were histochemical, based on the reduction of silver to form precipitates. Although time-consuming and expensive, electron microscopy can also be used to identify neurosecretory granules. Neuroendocrine (or dense core) granules are cytoplasmic structures, ranging in size from 30 to 200 nm, and are abundant in a variety of normal neuroendocrine cells. These granules have a central dense core, a pale halo, and a single delimiting outer membrane. Neuroendocrine granules may be rare in poorly differentiated tumors, necessitating a laborious, though frequently successful, search through many sections.

Unlike electron microscopy, which requires special preparation of sections, immunohistochemistry can be performed on standard formalin-fixed, paraffin-embedded tissue. Neuron-specific enolase (NSE), chromogranin, and synaptophysin are the antibodies most frequently used. Despite the promise of its name, NSE is a sensitive but not very specific marker for neuroendocrine differentiation. NSE immunoreactivity is usually not considered diagnostic in the absence of other, supporting immunohistochemical markers. Chromogranins are a family of proteins present in neurosecretory granules and their identification within tumor cells correlates with the presence of dense core granules by electron microscopy. Synaptophysin is a 38-kd protein present in the presynaptic vesicles of neurons. It is also expressed in a wide variety of neuroendocrine neoplasms inside and outside the lung. Other, less commonly used immunostains are Leu 7, N-CAM, and polypeptide hormones such as ACTH.

It is important to remember that no firm criteria have been established to define the limits of sensitivity and specificity for all these methods. Put in a different way, how many tumor cells have to be chromogranin positive to have "neuroendocrine differentiation"? Do rare neuroendocrine cells have clinical significance? The clinical issue fueling the neuroendocrine differentiation debate is the traditional dichotomy of non–small cell carcinoma versus small cell carcinoma and the different therapeutic implications. It has become increasingly apparent to pathologists that this distinction is not always neatly achieved. Resection is the treatment of choice for the rare small cell carcinoma that presents without evidence of lymph node involvement. There is also a suggestion that neuroendocrine differentiation in a non–small cell carcinoma is associated with a better response to chemotherapy but may signal a poorer prognosis. Attention has focused on neuroendocrine markers because of a general acknowledgment that histologic typing alone may not be adequate for determining prognosis or predicting a therapeutic response.

The currently accepted classification scheme includes minute pulmonary lesions such as tumorlets or neuroendocrine bodies, tumors with a neuroendocrine appearance (originally described on light microscopy without the use of special studies), and recently characterized non–small cell carcinomas with neuroendocrine features (as detected with immunohistochemistry or electron microscopy). It should be emphasized that in addition to conceptual controversies that have not been resolved, it has been difficult for pathologists to interpret and to apply reproducibly the morphologic criteria that have been set forth by numerous authors. This is true even for small cell carcinoma, for which the interobserver agreement has been reported to vary from 72 to 93 percent.[20,34] It is sobering to realize that the pathologic distinction is not always as neatly achieved in an area that many clinicians have traditionally viewed as straightforward. Also underappreciated are studies, such as Roggli's, in which 4 of the 11 cases (36 percent), despite a consensus diagnosis of small cell carcinoma, showed major heterogeneity—i.e., a non–small cell component.[34] It is fair to say that other lesions, such as "atypical carcinoids" or large cell neuroendocrine carcinomas, are even less reproducibly diagnosed. The literature on these relatively new entities is based on small numbers of tumors, and the staging and treatment have not always been uniform.

Neuroepithelial Bodies/Tumorlets

The smallest lesions with neuroendocrine differentiation are the *neuroepithelial bodies* and tumorlets (Fig. 111-12). These lesions usually are an incidental finding in lung parenchyma removed for other reasons. Although it was originally proposed that tumorlets were associated with other lesions, such as bronchiectasis or pulmonary fibrosis, tumorlets in otherwise normal lungs have been demonstrated at autopsy. Rare reports of tumorlets with lymph node metastases support the concept of tumorlets as neoplastic. Immunohistochemically and ultrastructurally, the cells of a tumorlet are identical to those of a carcinoid. An arbitrary size of 4 mm or less has been proposed as a cutoff point for a tumorlet. The question of whether these tumorlets are true neoplasms or represent hyperplasia of neuroendocrine cells normally present in the lung has long been debated.

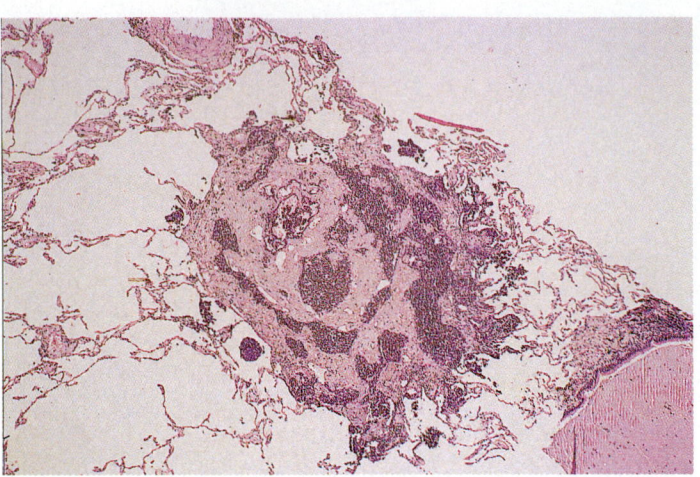

FIGURE 111-12   Tumorlet. H&E stain, ×40.

Carcinoid Tumors

Carcinoid tumors can be divided into central and peripheral variants. Both variants can be asymptomatic, but central carcinoids, which characteristically grow as an endobronchial mass, may present clinically with recurrent pneumonias or hemoptysis. The incidence among males and females is roughly equal, with an average age of 55 years, although carcinoids do occur in the very young and the elderly.[26]

Central carcinoids grossly appear as yellow or fleshy, polypoid masses (Figs. 111-13A and 111-13B). The tumor usually has a significant exophytic endobronchial component, but it can infiltrate between cartilaginous rings to invade the bronchial submucosa extensively. The tumor cells have a low nuclear-cytoplasmic ratio, with round to oval nuclei. As mentioned previously, the chromatin pattern is described as "salt and pepper," with the growth pattern described as organoid. The tumor cells form orderly arrangements such as nest, trabeculae, rosettes, or ribbons (Figs. 111-14A, 111-14B, and 111-14C). Mitoses should be extremely rare, and areas of necrosis are absent.

Peripheral carcinoids are frequently subpleural (Fig. 111-15A) and sometimes associated with a scar. They may be multiple. Unlike the cells of central tumors, which tend to be round or polygonal, the tumor cells of peripheral carcinoids tend to have prominent spindle cell features (Fig. 111-15B). These fusiform cells have less cytoplasm than central tumors, but this feature is not a sign of atypia. As with central carcinoids, mitoses should be very rare and there is no necrosis.

Although patients with carcinoid tumors have an excellent prognosis, with reported 5-year survival rates of 95 to 100 percent, carcinoids are potentially malignant tumors. There are currently no histologic characteristics that reliably predict which tumors will behave aggressively, although some correlation with large tumor size has been noted. Hilar and mediastinal lymph node metastases occur in 5 to 10 percent of cases but do not necessarily indicate a poor prognosis.

Other Pulmonary Neuroendocrine Tumors

The term *atypical carcinoid* was first introduced by Arrigoni and colleagues in 1972.[1] Twenty-three tumors were described that

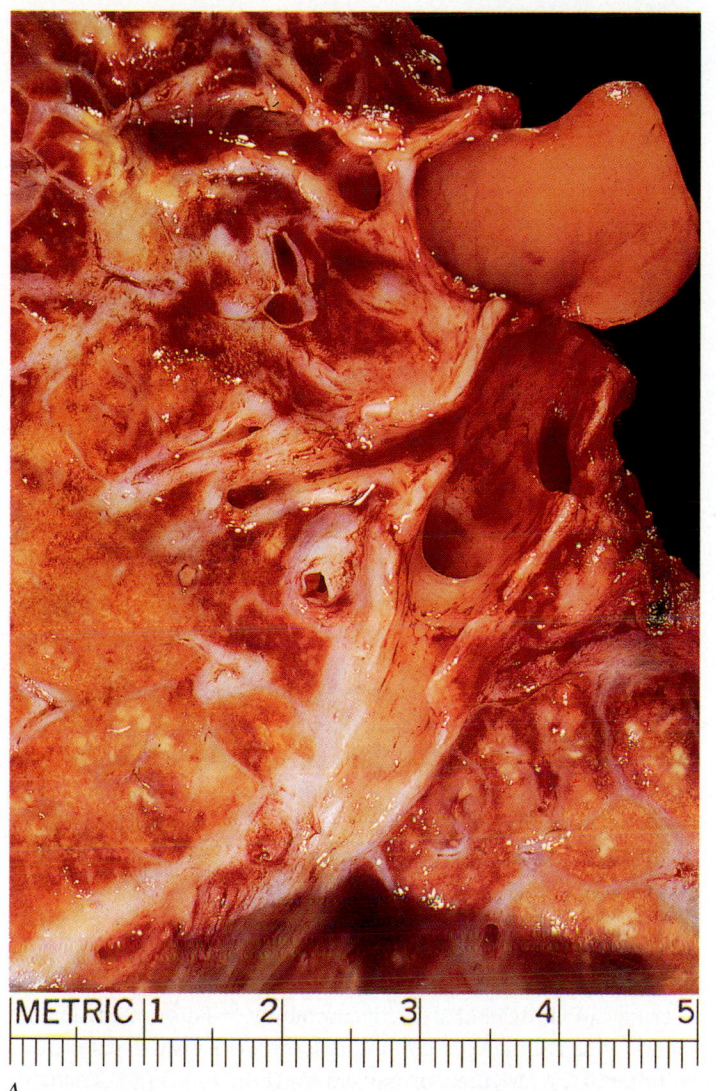

A

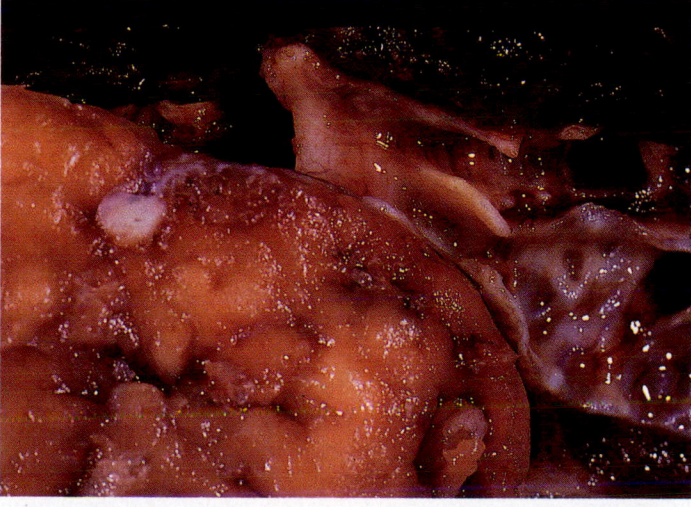

B

FIGURE 111-13   *A.* Large endobronchial carcinoid. *B.* Endobronchial carcinoid. Grossly, the tumor is yellow, fleshy, and vascular.

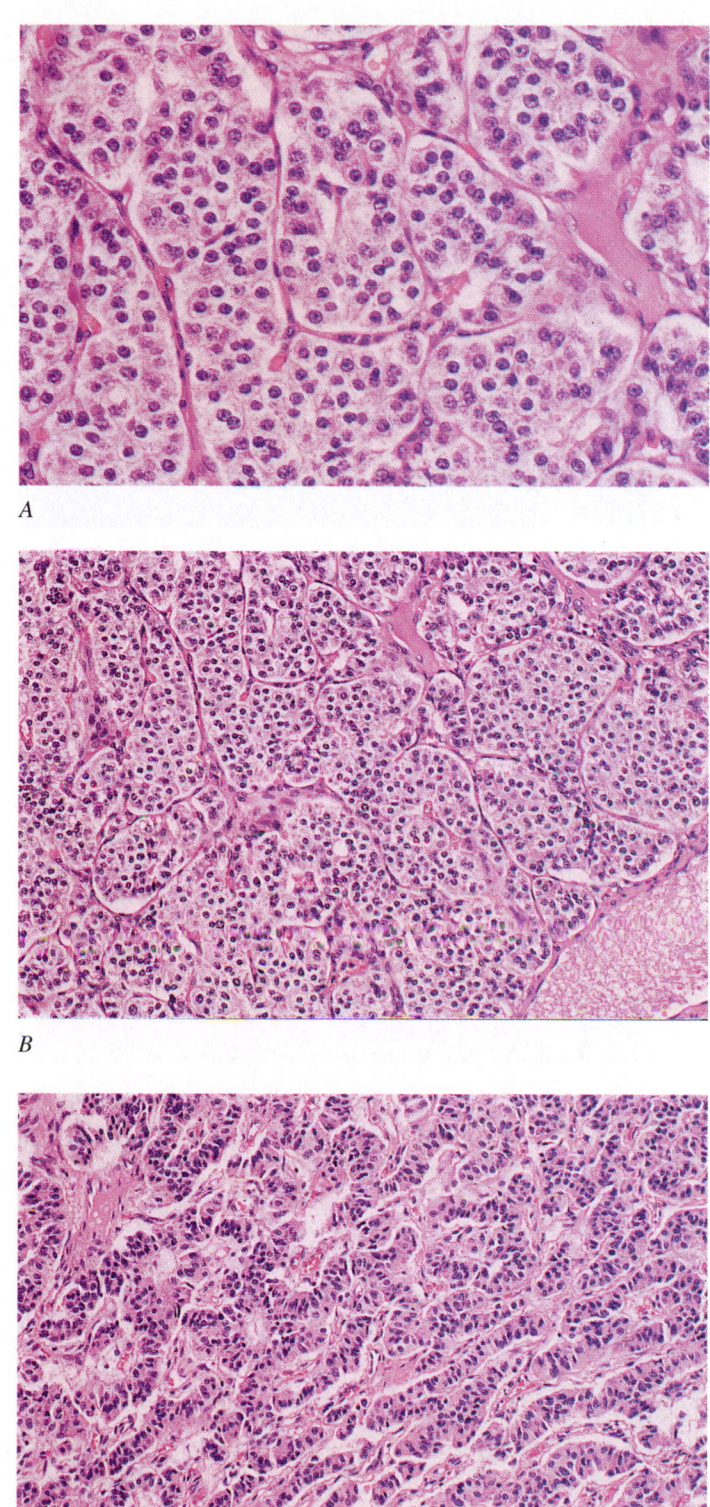

A

B

C

FIGURE 111-14   *A.* Cytologic features of carcinoid tumor with small, uniform cells. The nuclei are round to oval with a "salt and pepper" chromatin pattern. H&E stain, ×400. *B.* Carcinoid tumor, nested pattern. *C.* Carcinoid tumor, ribboned pattern. H&E stains, ×200.

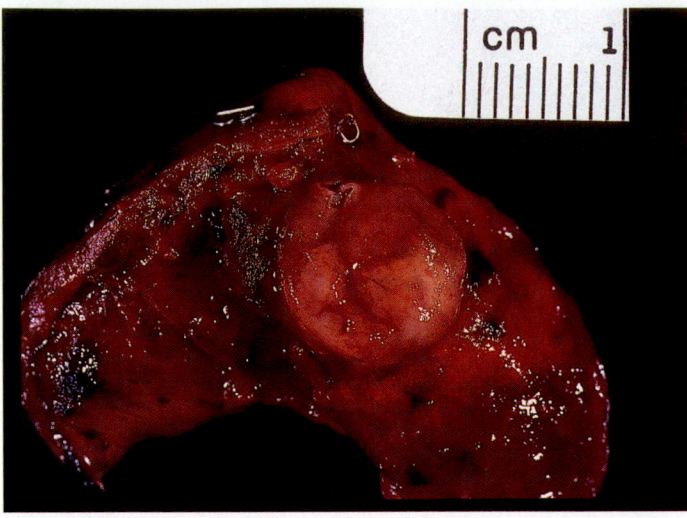

A

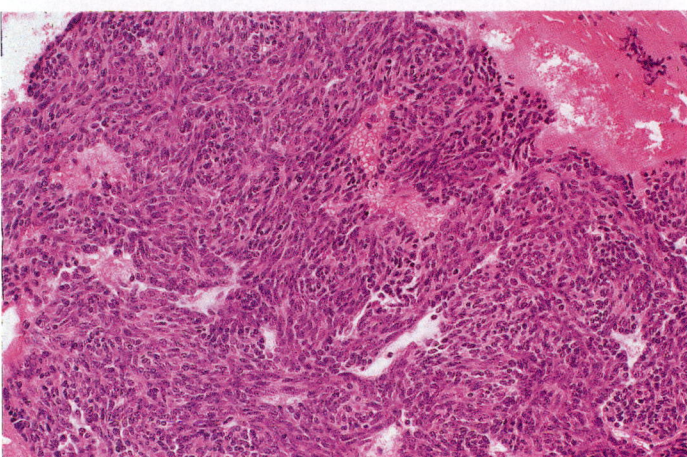

B

FIGURE 111-15   *A.* Peripheral carcinoid. *B.* Peripheral carcinoid with prominent spindle cell features. ×200.

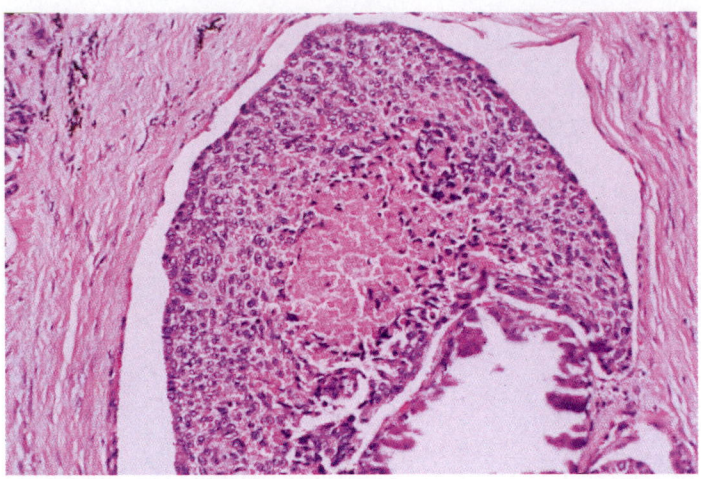

FIGURE 111-16   Central necrosis in an atypical carcinoid tumor. H&E stain, ×200.

appeared to have a general resemblance to carcinoid tumors but also had a focally disorganized growth pattern, areas of tumor necrosis, increased mitoses, and cellular pleomorphism (Fig. 111-16). Dissension was immediately generated by the use of the word "atypical"—given the aggressive biologic behavior in their series, with 30 percent of patients dead of disease at 3 years, a 70 percent incidence of metastases, and a mean survival of 27 months. For this reason, many pathologists now prefer the designation *well-differentiated neuroendocrine carcinoma* for the same entity, in order to avoid any confusion with carcinoid tumors and their considerably better prognosis.

Many other terms were introduced into the literature in the 1980s as more published reports detailing this entity appeared. Other terms used are *malignant carcinoid, well-differentiated neuroendocrine carcinoma, peripheral small cell carcinoma of lung resembling carcinoid tumor,* and *Kulchitsky cell carcinoma II.*[32,43] The tumors described in these reports have been a heterogeneous group. This is, in part, due to the subjective interpretation of features such as "architectural distortion." In defending atypical carcinoids as a distinct clinicopathologic entity,

Travis and colleagues emphasized that the overall architecture should be that of a recognizable carcinoid with a predominantly organoid growth pattern.[40] In published reports of this entity, men predominate and the age incidence overlaps that of other neuroendocrine tumors. The location of the tumor can be central or peripheral, and the patients present at various stages of tumor growth. Prognosis has been related to size, nodal disease, and vascular invasion. Chemotherapy and radiation have not been effective in therapy.

In 1991, Travis and coworkers proposed criteria for an entity termed *large cell neuroendocrine carcinoma,* which was considered histologically distinct from well-differentiated neuroendocrine carcinoma and atypical carcinoids.[40] This tumor has neuroendocrine features on light microscopy. The growth pattern can be organoid, trabecular, or palisading (Fig. 111-17*A*). The cells are relatively large and polygonal, with a low nuclear-cytoplasmic ratio. The nuclear chromatin is coarsely granular or vesicular with frequent nucleoli and finely granular eosinophilic cytoplasm (Fig. 111-17*B*). This coarse quality of the chromatin is to be contrasted with the more finely granular chromatin of an atypical carcinoid. The mitotic rate is high (greater than 10 per 10 high-power fields), and there is frequent necrosis. Neuroendocrine differentiation is evident on immunohistochemistry or electron microscopy. In this series, the patients were predominantly smokers and men of middle age. There was a mix of central and peripheral tumors, with a size range of 1.5 to 8 cm in diameter. Even low-stage tumors carried a poor prognosis, but the authors suggested that there was some responsiveness to chemotherapy. At 2-year follow-up, four of six patients with atypical carcinoid were dead of disease (survival range 0.33 to 10 years), one was alive with disease, and one had no evidence of disease. Of those with large cell neuroendocrine carcinoma, two were dead of disease at 15 and 25 months and three were alive with disease.

It is easy to confuse the designation *large cell neuroendocrine carcinoma* with the designation *large cell carcinoma of the lung with neuroendocrine differentiation* (Fig. 111-18).[45] The latter term has been proposed for tumors that are *not* obviously neuroendocrine tumors on light microscopy but do show neuroendocrine differentiation with immunohistochemistry or electron microscopy. The histologic features are essentially identical to those of the WHO classification for the diagnosis of large cell carcinoma. The cell size approximates that of other non–small cell carcinoma subtypes and is at least twice that of small cell carcinoma. The tumor cells have a monomorphic nuclear appearance and dispersed or vesicular chromatin with discernible nucleoli, without evident squamous or glandular differentiation. Although special studies to identify neuroendocrine differentiation are now frequently performed on large cell undifferentiated carcinomas, there are currently no uniform criteria for labeling a tumor as neuroendocrine on the basis of these special studies. Some authors have suggested that 20 percent of the tumor cells should mark as neuroendocrine before the designation is applied.

To make classification even more complex, an *intermediate variant of small cell carcinoma* with a slightly larger cell size, a more vesicular nucleus, and prominent nucleoli has also been described in the WHO subclassification of small cell carcinomas.[44] Subsequent studies using this WHO subclassification were not able to demonstrate a correlation between survival and histologic subtype. In 1988 the International Association for the Study of Lung Cancer proposed an alternative classification scheme that recognizes so-called *mixed carcinomas,* which consist of large cell undifferentiated carcinoma with small cell carcinoma, and *"combined" carcinoma,* which is small cell carcinoma with squamous cell carcinoma or adenocarcinoma.[16]

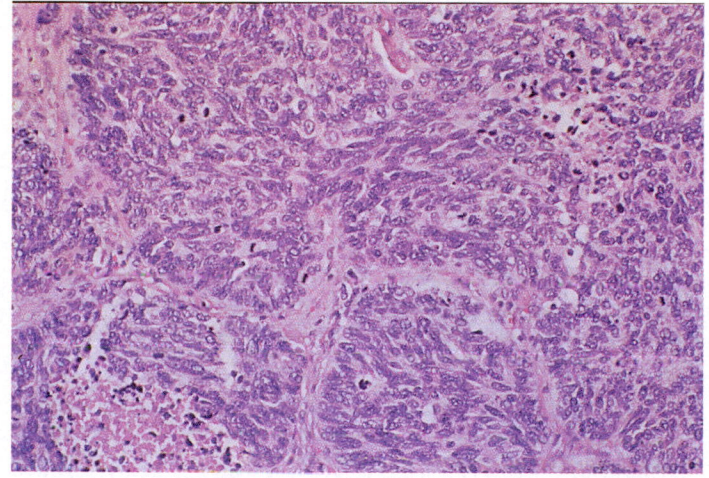

A

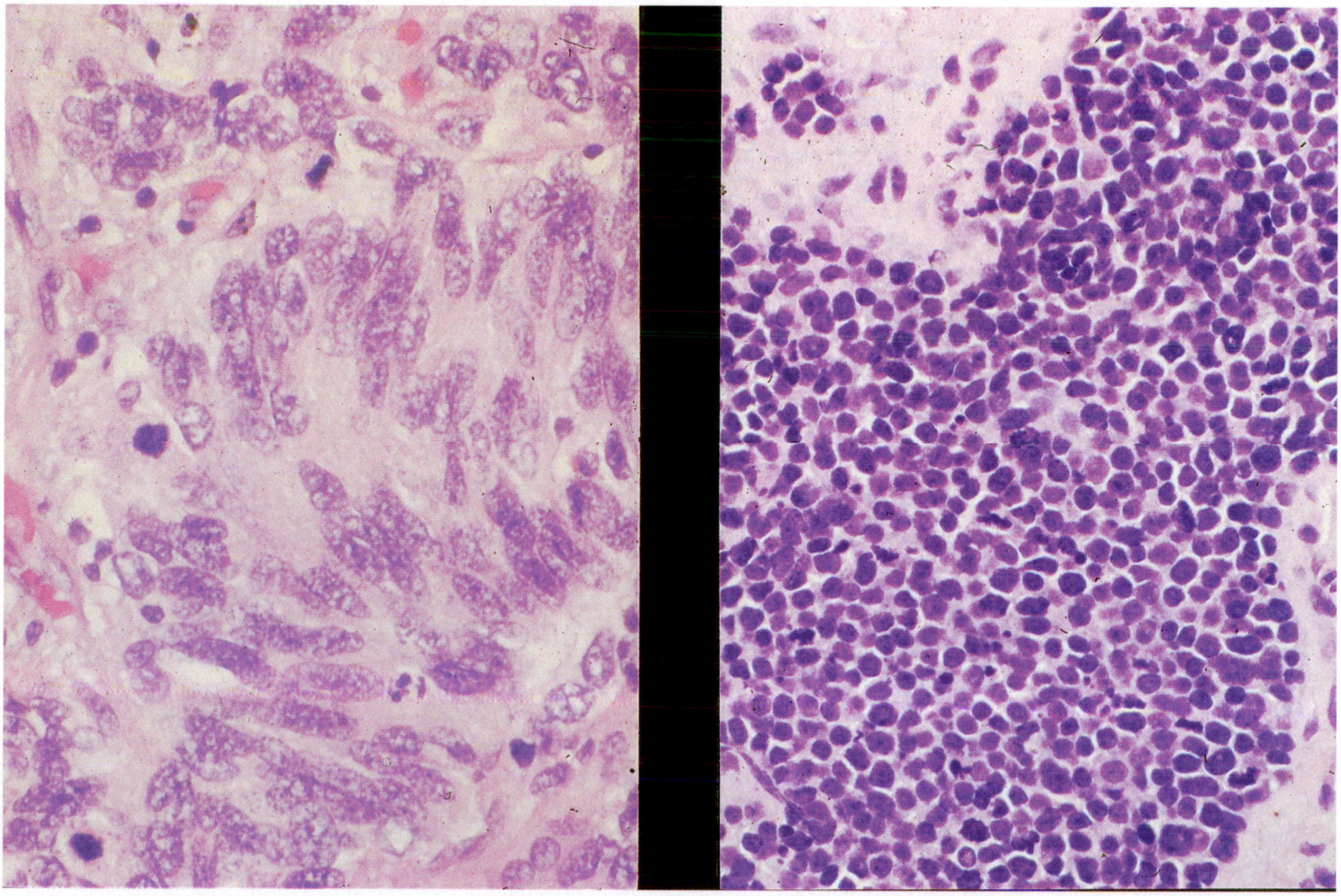

B

FIGURE 111-17 *A.* Large cell neuroendocrine carcinoma. The tumor cells are arranged in large organoid nests with numerous mitoses and necrosis. H&E stain, ×200. *B.* Comparison of large cell neuroendocrine carcinoma (left) with small-cell carcinoma (right) at same magnification. The large cell neuroendocrine cells are larger, with a lower nuclear-cytoplasm ratio, and the chromatin is coarsely granular. H&E stain, ×400.

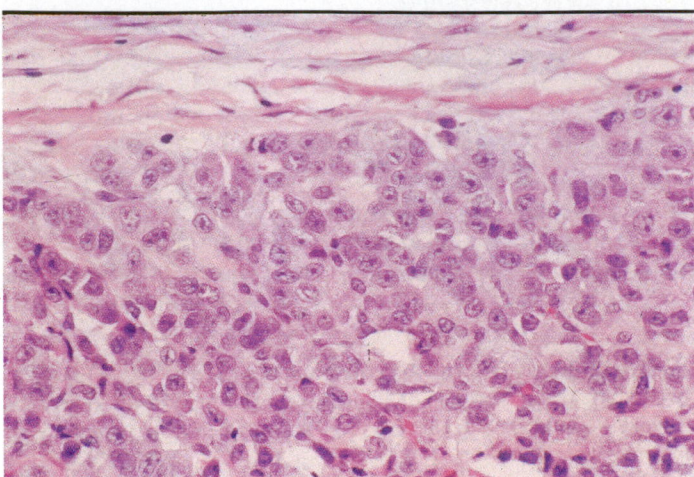

FIGURE 111-18 Undifferentiated large cell tumor with a vesicular nuclear chromatin pattern and prominent nucleoli. Immunohistochemical stains for neuorendocrine differentiation were focally positive. H&E stain, ×400.

Not all experts have accepted this new classification, and in practice, the heterogeneity of small cell carcinoma and the histologic continuum with other types of lung cancer continue to make it difficult for pathologists to separate these entities reproducibly. Estimations of cell size continue to be more subjective than the literature would suggest, and classic small cell features such as crush artifact or molding are often less conspicuous in larger surgical samples. In addition, the accurate subclassification of neuroendocrine tumors can be compromised by poor tissue fixation or small, crushed samples. In some instances, this has led to the unfortunate misdiagnosis of a typical carcinoid or atypical carcinoid as small cell carcinoma. It is generally accepted that the distinction between the original WHO subtypes of oat cell and intermediate variants is not biologically significant. One study has demonstrated no significant difference in survival for the mixed small- and large cell carcinomas.[12] A large controlled study of appropriately staged neuroendocrine tumors that looked at outcome correlated with relevant and reproducible histologic features could resolve this confusion within the rational context of prognostic significance and therapeutic response.

BRONCHIAL GLAND TUMORS

Mixed seromucinous glands are found in the tracheal and large bronchial submucosa. They are believed to give rise to a variety of tumors that are histologically indistinguishable from tumors of the major salivary glands. This category of neoplasms includes mucoepidermoid carcinoma, adenoid cystic carcinoma, pleomorphic adenoma, acinic cell carcinoma, oncocytoma, and mucous gland adenoma. Although they are less common, their distinctive morphology, growth pattern, and clinical presentation make salivary gland–type tumors of the lung an important subgroup of non–small cell carcinoma. This section considers two salivary gland–like tumors, adenoid cystic carcinoma and mucoepidermoid carcinoma.

Adenoid Cystic Carcinoma

Adenoid cystic carcinoma is the most common of the tracheobronchial gland tumors, accounting for between 20 and 35 percent of all tracheal tumors and 80 percent of all tracheobronchial gland tumors.[15] When first seen, the patients range in age from 18 to 82. The incidence is equal among men and women. The typical presenting symptoms—such as wheezing, progressive dyspnea, stridor, cough, and hemoptysis—are those of an intraluminal tumor of the airway. Unlike carcinoid tumors and mucoepidermoid carcinomas, which usually present as intraluminal endophytic masses, adenoid cystic carcinomas have a variable growth pattern. Some adenoid cystic carcinomas are nodular, with minimal invasion of the bronchus, whereas in others the growth pattern is mixed nodular and infiltrative or predominantly infiltrative (Figs. 111-19A and 111-19B). The more infiltrative tumors either appear as small nodules within the airway or cause a generalized constriction of the airway. Local lymph nodes may be affected, usually by direct extension; higher-grade tumors tend to spread radially into the adjacent parenchyma rather than along the airways.

The level of invasion seen microscopically is nearly always greater than what is grossly apparent. Complete resection may be quite difficult to achieve, and many frozen sections may be required before clear surgical margins are confirmed. The tumor cells are small, with a relatively high nuclear-cytoplasmic ratio, but nuclear pleomorphism and mitoses are rare. Characteristic mucinous cysts of varying size are present within the tubular and cribriform patterns (Fig. 111-19C). In poorly differentiated tumors, solid tumor nests are a significant component. As in the case of their salivary gland counterparts, adenoid cystic carcinomas are notorious for perineural spread. Adequate resection can achieve long-term survival, but local recurrence may occur long (more than 10 years) after resection. The most common site of disseminated disease is the lung parenchyma, but extrathoracic metastases also occur.

Mucoepidermoid Carcinoma

Mucoepidermoid carcinomas account for approximately 0.1 to 0.2 percent of lung cancers. Although patients with this tumor may be asymptomatic, it is common for patients to present with symptoms of bronchial obstruction caused by the endobronchial location of the tumor: wheezing, cough, and hemoptysis; some patients present with postobstructive pneumonia. The age at presentation varies, but approximately 60 percent of patients are between 45 and 70 years of age. A chest radiograph often reveals a solitary, centrally located mass with distal pneumonia or atelectasis.

Mucoepidermoid carcinomas usually affect the proximal bronchi but can invade the trachea as well. They range in size from a few millimeters to 6 cm in diameter; they grow as polypoid masses with a tan or gray surface (Figs. 111-20A and 111-20B). On cross section, the tumor may appear more mucoid or cystic than the non–small cell carcinomas of the lung.

Histologically, mucoepidermoid tumors are separable into low- and high-grade tumors. The tumors are composed of a mix of mucin-secreting cells, squamous cells, and so-called intermediate cells (Fig. 111-20C). The intermediate cells have a poly-

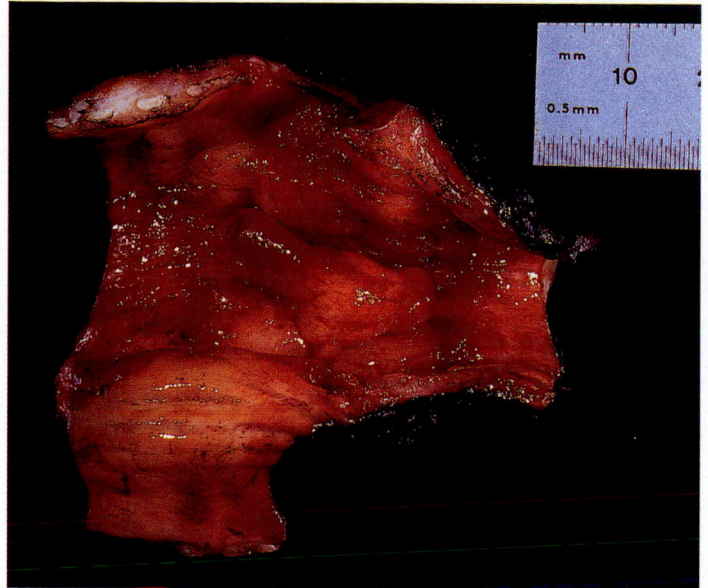

A

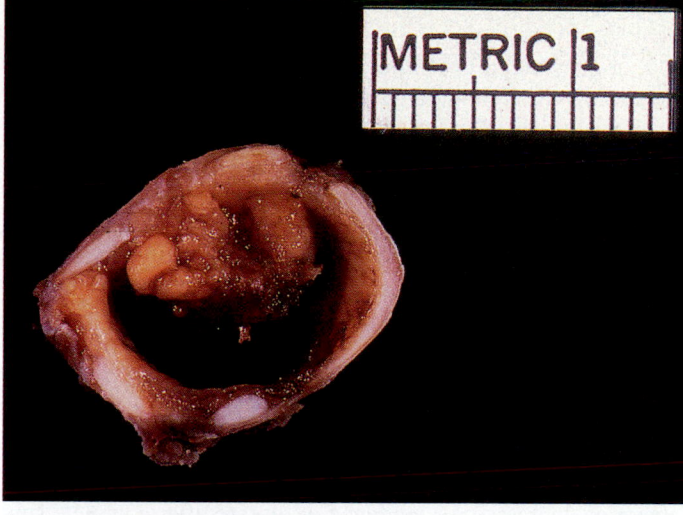

A

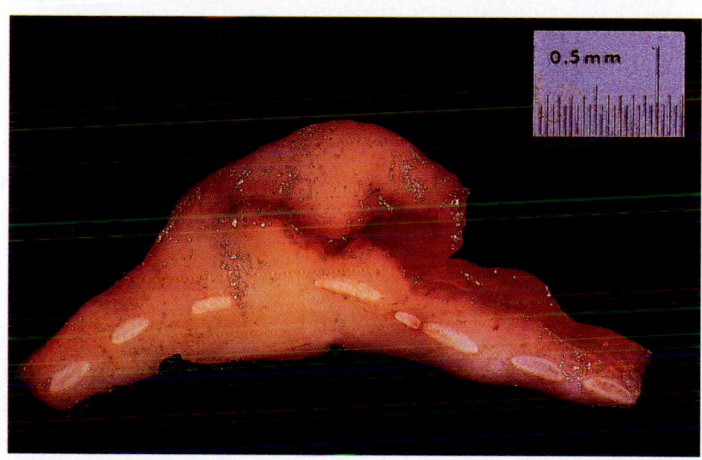

B

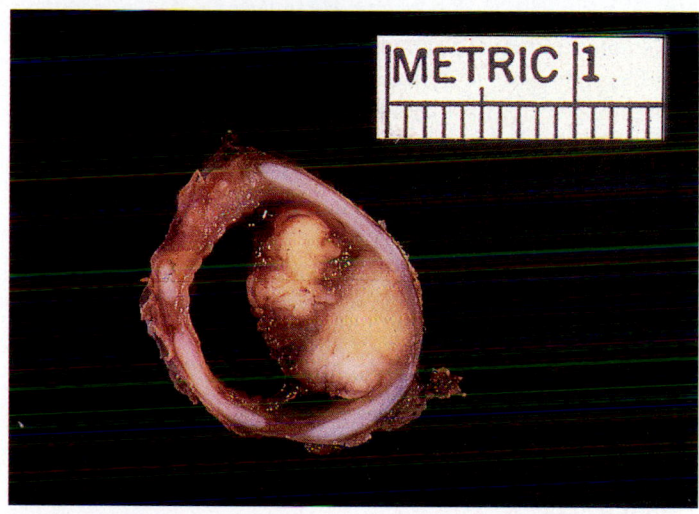

B

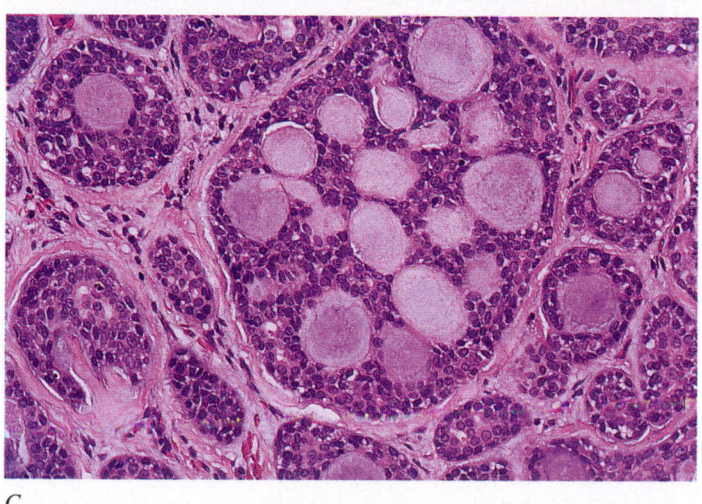

C

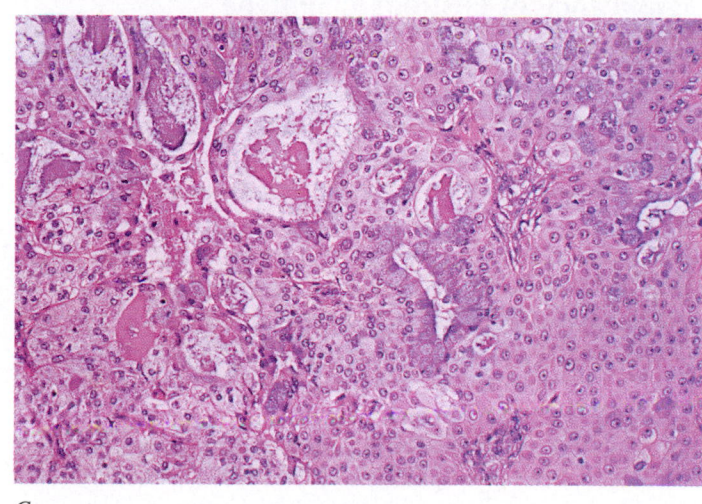

C

FIGURE 111-19 *A.* Carinal resection for adenoid cystic carcinoma with a mixed infiltrative and nodular growth within the submucosa. *B.* Same adenoid cystic carcinoma in cross section, illustratrating the extensive diffuse involvement of the submucosa with infiltration beyond the cartilage. *C.* Cribriform growth pattern of adenoid cystic carcinoma. H&E stain, ×200.

FIGURE 111-20 *A.* Left main-stem bronchus resection for an endobronchial mucoepidermoid carcinoma. *B.* Same mucoepidermoid carcinoma tumor in cross section, demonstrating an attachment to the bronchus, but invasion is limited to the superfical portion of the submucosa. *C.* Mucoepidermoid carcinoma. There are both well-differentiated mucinous glands (left) and intermediate cells (right), which have a polygonal shape and abundant eosinophilic cytoplasm. H&E stain, ×200.

gonal shape and eosinophilic cytoplasm but lack obvious squamous or glandular differentiation. The mucinous component consists of well-differentiated glands, with both intracellular and extracellular mucin. The squamous cells should not form keratin pearls—a feature that, if present, suggests the diagnosis of squamous or adenosquamous carcinoma. In low-grade tumors, the cells have minimal pleomorphism, rare mitoses, and minimal necrosis. Suggested criteria for high-grade tumors include an increased mitotic rate (average of 4 per 10 high-power fields), necrosis, and nuclear pleomorphism.

The clinical behavior of these neoplasms remains controversial, mainly because of ambiguities about the definition of high-grade mucoepidermoid carcinomas and their distinction from adenosquamous carcinomas. In a study of 58 cases in which the mucoepidermoid tumors were separated into low- and high-grade categories, there was no evidence of disease after complete surgical excision for 41 patients with low-grade tumors who were followed, on average, for 4 years.[48] Of the 13 patients with high-grade mucoepidermoid carcinomas, three died of metastatic disease but eight were still alive, without evidence of disease, at a median follow-up of 31 months.

Almost all of the mucoepidermoid tumors in patients younger than 30 years have been low-grade and mostly endobronchial. The prognosis for patients with such tumors is excellent. The incidence of lymph node metastases is low (about 2 percent). Local recurrence has followed incomplete excision, and adequate excision may require lobectomy, bronchoplastic procedure (sleeve lobectomy), or pneumonectomy. High-grade tumors, which tend to invade the adjacent lung parenchyma, generally affect older people and carry a worse prognosis.

PROGNOSTIC VARIABLES OTHER THAN STAGE

Significance of Histologic Subtype

One of the largest studies to consider the relationship of disease extent and cell type to survival was published in 1987 by Mountain and colleagues.[29] It should be noted that the nomenclature of the Working Party for the Study of Lung Cancer and the Lung Cancer Study Group for histologic classification expanded the WHO classification system to include the categories of poorly differentiated carcinoma as well as bi- and multicomponent or multidifferentiated carcinoma. Therefore, their analysis of survival differences between 549 patients with squamous cell carcinomas and 572 patients with adenocarcinoma is based on tumors that fit well into differentiated histologic categories. And in keeping with the previous discussion of intra- and interobserver variability, the *final* histologic classification was assigned by a single pathologist agreed on by the study's pathology committee. Discrepancies between the initial submitting pathologist's diagnosis and reviewer's final histologic classification were reviewed annually by a pathology committee. Thus, the study design provided a higher level of consistency than would be expected from a random sampling of pathologists.

In the 1121 patients, the cumulative proportion of those surviving 5 years according to cell type was significantly higher for those with squamous cell carcinoma than for those with adenocarcinoma—65 and 55 percent, respectively. However, when an-

alyzed according to stage and stage subsets, the significance of histologic type as a prognostic factor was variable: within the subsets of T1N0 and T1N1, patients with squamous cell carcinoma did significantly better than those with adenocarcinoma—83 percent versus 69 percent for T1N0 and 75 percent versus 52 percent for T1N1, respectively. No statistically significant difference for cell type was found in T2N0 tumors, suggesting the stronger influence of large tumor size, pleural invasion, or both on prognosis. Histologic type was significant in the survival of patients with T2N1 disease (53 percent for patients with squamous cell carcinoma versus 25 percent for patients with adenocarcinoma), although, as the authors point out, adenocarcinoma is infrequently diagnosed within this subgroup. There was no significant difference in survival by histologic cell type in stage IIIa patients, but this patient subgroup was heterogeneous with respect to tumor size and the presence or absence of N2 disease. In general, survival rates of patients with large cell undifferentiated carcinoma and adenosquamous carcinoma are similar to those of patients with adenocarcinoma.

Evaluation of Other Proposed Prognostic Variables

The study by Mountain and colleagues of histologic subtype demonstrates that the outcome evaluation of different therapeutic protocols depends greatly on accurate TNM staging and histologic classification.[29] The study also illustrates the need to evaluate the significance of any pathologic feature within the context of accurate TNM classification. There are numerous studies reporting new prognostic variables, but most of them fail the test of rigorous statistical analysis within the current staging system. In addition, all too often insufficient attention is directed to issues of technical or interobserver reproducibility. In an effort to determine which histologic features were predictive of survival, Elson and colleagues evaluated 47 stage I non–small cell lung carcinomas.[11] The histologic variables included vascular or lymphatic invasion, mitotic rate, anaplasia, inflammatory host response, the presence or absence of necrosis, tumor giant cells, a central scar, mucin production, benign giant cell reaction, or desmoplasia. The only significant indicator of survival, as well as the only histologic feature with acceptable interobserver agreement, was the extent of tumor necrosis. The authors emphasized that studies using histologic parameters should include several observers and interobserver comparison.

Tumor size has not proved to be as good a predictive factor for adenocarcinoma as for squamous cell carcinoma. It may be that more detailed analysis of larger patient subgroups within a uniform histologic subtype will clarify some issues related to histopathologic variables and prognosis. Takise's team retrospectively studied 75 patients with peripheral adenocarcinomas of less than 2 cm that were staged according to the TNM staging system.[39] Pathologic stage, lymph node involvement, and pleural involvement were found to be major determinants of prognosis. Other single proposed prognostic factors—such as tumor differentiation, vascular invasion, the degree of collagenization in foci of fibrosis, the standard deviation of nuclear areas, dense histocytic infiltration, and mitotic index—correlated significantly with prognosis in a univariate analysis. In a multivariate analysis, however, histologic differentiation and vascular invasion were eliminated as prognostic factors. The authors speculated that the elimination of histologic differentiation and vascular invasion as prognostic variables in their multivariate analysis might be related to the higher frequency of lymph node metastasis. The importance and frequency of vascular invasion have been emphasized by a number of groups. In this study, the incidence of vascular invasion was 60 percent, but approximately 50 percent of the patients were long-term survivors.

Flow Cytometry

Quality control is an ongoing problem in the flow cytometric evaluation of lung tumors. Differences in methods and data analysis also complicate comparisons. Most published reports have looked at flow cytometric parameters as a prognostic variable in retrospective studies using univariate analysis. Some of these studies have included stratification by staging and have considered the potential influence of histologic subtype.[35] Carey and colleagues examined intratumoral heterogeneity of DNA content in 208 resections for non–small cell lung carcinoma and found that more than half of the tumors would have been labeled diploid if not extensively sampled.[6] Although this degree of DNA heterogeneity is not surprising when one considers the degree of histologic heterogeneity, caution is appropriate in applying flow cytometric results to clinical practice and predicting outcome.

Molecular Markers

Although molecular markers in lung cancer are reviewed in a separate chapter (see Chapter 107), a few comments may be in order about the role of the pathologist in the ongoing evaluation of these markers for diagnosis, prognosis, and therapy. At present, the sequence-based technology that is available to identify genetic alterations requires identification of tumor cells and, in the case of allelic loss analysis, samples that are highly enriched for tumor cells. Therefore, the pathologist is in the pivotal position of determining the tissue sample for processing, as well as correlating the findings with standard histologic evaluation. Fresh or frozen tissue usually is preferred, but in some instances, formalin-fixed tissue may be used for analysis. When fresh or frozen tissue is used for analysis, cooperation among the pathologist, surgeon, bronchoscopist, and interventional radiologist is required. Immunochemistry, which is available in some hospitals, may be useful in determining the distribution of an oncogene product or to identify overexpression. For certain genetic abnormalities such as *p53* overexpression, commercially available antibodies with known specificity are available. As suggested by studies of flow cytometry, tumor heterogeneity may confound genetic analyses. Although it is likely that advances in molecular biology will influence standards of tumor diagnosis in the near future, from the practical perspective of patient management and currently available therapeutic methods, the utility of these tests outside a research setting and within the context of large prospective studies has yet to be established.

RECOMMENDATIONS FOR REPORTING

Recommendations for the reporting of resected primary lung carcinomas have been recently approved and issued by the Association of Directors of Anatomic and Surgical Pathology.[2] The recommendations are intended to provide an informative report for the clinician and to comment on specific features that are generally accepted as being of prognostic importance. Features that are required for staging or therapy are included.

The gross description should specify the location of the specimen (e.g., right upper lobe, left lung) and a description of attached structures, such as parietal pleura or hilar lymph nodes. Tumor size and location in relation to the lobar or main-stem bronchus should also be noted. The report should contain a description of the nontumorous lung, including the presence or absence of postobstructive changes and atelectasis. All these features are directly relevant to appropriate staging by the international TNM staging system. The histologic assessment should specify the histologic type (e.g., squamous cell) and histologic grade (e.g., well, moderately, or poorly differentiated), as well as the surgical margins and pleural involvement. In consultation with the thoracic surgeon, nodal groups should be specifically identified according to the American Joint Commission (AJCC) intraoperative staging system for regional lymph nodes, and the diagnosis for each numbered nodal group should appear on the final pathology report. Nodal involvement by direct extension should also be noted, if present.

Angiolymphatic invasion, perineural invasion, the presence of perinodal tumor extension (extracapsular), and the result of ancillary studies (flow cytometry, immunohistochemistry, or electron microscopy) all may be commented on in the final report but must be considered inconclusive with regard to prognostic significance.

CONCLUSION

In addition to the clinicopathologic features and histologic subtyping of non–small cell carcinoma, current controversies and unresolved issues in tumor classification have been reviewed. The pathologist makes a critical contribution to the management and treatment of lung carcinoma, but the final pathologic interpretation should not be rendered in a clinical vacuum. It is incumbent on the clinician caring for the patient to be sure that the pathologist has the benefit of complete clinical information. This should include symptoms at presentation, radiographic findings, and medical history, particularly as it relates to prior malignancies. The inclusion of the pathologist as an integral part of a multidisciplinary evaluation for a thoracic malignancy enhances the quality of care for the individual patient, as well as refining the general practice of thoracic oncology.

REFERENCES

1. Arrigoni MG, Woolner LB, Bernatz PE: Atypical carcinoid tumors of the lung. *J Thorac Cardiovasc Surg* 64:413–421, 1972.
2. Association of Directors of Anatomic and Surgical Pathology: Recommendations for the reporting of resected primary lung carcinomas. *Am J Clin Pathol* 104:371–374, 1995.
3. Auerbach O, Frasca JM, Parks VR, Carter HW: A comparison of World Health Organization classification of lung tumors by light and electron microscopy. *Cancer* 50:2079–2088, 1982.
4. Barsky SH, Huang SJ, Ghuta S: The extracellular matrix of pulmonary scar carcinomas is suggestive of a desmoplastic origin. *Am J Pathol* 124:412–419, 1986.

5. Brambilla E, Moro D, Veale D, et al: Basal cell (basaloid) carcinoma of the lung: A new morphologic and phenotypic entity with separate prognostic significance. *Hum Pathol* 23:993–1003, 1992.

6. Carey FA, Lamb B, Bird CC: Intratumoral heterogeneity of DNA content in lung cancer. *Cancer* 64:2266–2269, 1991.

7. Clayton F: Bronchioloalveolar carcinomas: Cell types, patterns of growth, and prognostic correlates. *Cancer* 57:1555–1564, 1986.

8. Colby TV, Koss MN, Travis WD (eds): *Atlas of Tumor Pathology: Tumors of the Lower Respiratory Tract.* Washington, DC, Armed Forces Institute of Pathology, 1995.

9. Daly RC, Trastek VF, Pairolero PC: Bronchioloalveolar carcinoma: Factors affecting survival. *Ann Thorac Surg* 51:368–377, 1991.

10. Daroca PJ, Robishaux WH: Basaloid carcinoma of the bronchus. *Surg Pathol* 2:339–344, 1989.

11. Elson CE, Roggli VL, Vollmer RT, et al: Prognostic indicators for survival in stage I carcinoma of the lung: A histologic study of 47 surgically resected cases. *Mod Pathol* 1:288–291, 1988.

12. Fraire AE, Johnson EH, Yesner R, et al: Prognostic significance of histopathologic subtype and stage in small cell lung cancer. *Hum Pathol* 23:520–528, 1992.

13. Fraire AE, Roggli VL, Vollmer RT, et al: Lung cancer heterogeneity: Prognostic implications. *Cancer* 60:370–375, 1987.

14. Ginsberg SS, Buzaid AC, Stern H, Carter D: Giant cell carcinoma of the lung. *Cancer* 70:606–610, 1992.

15. Hammar SP: Common neoplasms, in Dail DH, Hammar SP (eds), *Pulmonary Pathology.* New York, Springer-Verlag, 1994, pp 1123–1278.

16. Hirsch FR, Matthews MJ, Aisner S, et al: Histopatholgoic classification of small cell lung cancer: Changing concepts and terminology. *Cancer* 62:973–977, 1988.

17. Humphrey PA, Scroggs MW, Roggli VL, Shelburne JD: Pulmonary carcinoma with a sarcomatoid element. *Hum Pathol* 19:155–165, 1988.

18. Ishida T, Kaneko S, Yokoyama H, et al: Adenosquamous carcinoma of the lung: Clinicopathologic and immunohistochemical features. *Am J Clin Pathol* 97:678–685, 1992.

19. Katzenstein A-LA, Prioleau PG, Askin FB: The histologic spectrum and significance of clear cell change in lung carcinoma. *Cancer* 45:943–947, 1980.

20. Keehn R, Auerbach O, Nambu S, et al: Reproducibility of major diagnoses in a binational study of lung cancer in uranium miners and atomic bomb survivors. *Am J Clin Pathol* 101:478–482, 1994.

21. Koss MN, Hochholzer L, O'Leary T: Pulmonary blastomas. *Cancer* 67:2368–2381, 1991.

22. Kung ITM, Lui IOL, Loke SL, et al: Pulmonary scar cancer: A pathologic reappraisal. *Am J Surg Pathol* 9:391–400, 1985.

23. Liebow AA: Bronchiolo-alveolar carcinoma. *Adv Intern Med* 10:329–358, 1960.

24. Madri JA, Carter D: Scar cancers of the lung: Origin and significance. *Hum Pathol* 15:625–631, 1984.

25. Manivel JC, Priest JR, Watterson J, et al: Pleuropulmonary blastoma: The so-called pulmonary blastoma of childhood. *Cancer* 62:1516–1526, 1988.

26. McCaughan BC, Martini N, Bains MS: Bronchial carcinoids: Review of 124 cases. *J Thorac Cardiovasc Surg* 89:8–17, 1985.

27. Miller RR: Bronchioloalveolar cell adenomas. *Am J Surg Pathol* 14:904–912, 1990.

28. Miller RR, Nelems B, Evans KG, et al: Glandular neoplasia of the lung: A proposed analogy to colonic tumors. *Cancer* 61:1009–1014, 1988.

29. Mountain CF, Lukeman JM, Hammar SP, et al, and the Lung Cancer Study Group Committee: Lung cancer classification: The relationship of disease extent and cell type to survival in a clinical trials population. *J Surg Oncol* 35:147–156, 1987.

30. Nappi O, Glasner SD, Swanson PE, Wick MR: Biphasic and monophasic sarcomatoid carcinomas of the lung: A reappraisal of "carcinosarcomas" and "spindle-cell carcinomas." *Am J Clin Pathol* 102:331–340, 1994.

31. Nash AD, Stout AP: Giant cell carcinoma of the lung: Report of 5 cases. *Cancer* 11:369–376, 1958.

32. Paladugu RR, Benfield JR, Pack HY, et al: Bronchopulmonary Kulchitzky cell carcinomas: A new classification for typical and atypical carcinoids. *Cancer* 55:1303–1311, 1985.

33. Roggli VL: Histologic classification of lung cancers: Factors affecting its variability. *Am J Clin Pathol* 101:411–412, 1994.

34. Roggli VL, Vollmer RT, Greenberg SD, et al: Lung cancer heterogeneity: A blinded and randomized study of 100 consecutive cases. *Hum Pathol* 16:569–579, 1985.

35. Sahin AA, Ro JY, el-Naggar AK, et al: Flow cytometric analysis of the DNA content of non-small cell lung cancer: Ploidy as a significant prognostic indicator in squamous cell carcinoma of the lung. *Cancer* 65:530–537, 1990.

36. Shimosato Y, Noguchi M, Matsuo Y, Yamada T: Adenoma-carcinoma sequence in non-mucus producing bronchioloalveolar carcinoma of the lung. *Lung Cancer* 11:98–99, 1994.

37. Stanley KE, Matthews MJ: Analysis of a pathology review of patients with lung tumors. *J Natl Cancer Inst* 66:989–992, 1981.

38. Takamori S, Noguchi M, Morinaga S, et al: Clinicopathologic characteristics of adenosquamous carcinoma of the lung. *Cancer* 67:649–654, 1991.

39. Takise A, Kodama T, Shimosato Y, et al: Histopathologic prognostic factors in adenocarcinomas of the peripheral lung less than 2 cm in diameter. *Cancer* 61:2083–2088, 1988.

40. Travis WD, Linoila RI, Tsokos MG, et al: Neuroendocrine tumors of the lung with proposed criteria for large cell neuroendocrine carcinoma: An ultrastructural, immunohistochemical, and flow cytometric study of 35 cases. *Am J Surg Pathol* 15:529–553, 1991.

41. Travis WD, Travis LB, Devesa SS: Lung cancer. *Cancer* 75:191–202, 1995.

42. Wagenaar SS, Tazelaar HD: Ten years after the WHO classification for lung cancer: Where are we? *Lung Cancer* 11(Suppl 3):S39–S43, 1994.

43. Warren WH, Memoli VA, Gould VE: Immunohistochemical and ultrasturctural analysis of bronchopulmonary neuroendocrine neoplasms: II. Well-differentiated neuroendocrine carcinomas. *Ultrastruct Pathol* 7:185–199, 1984.

44. WHO: The World Health Organization histological typing of lung tumours, second edition: *Am J Clin Pathol* 77:123–136, 1982.

45. Wick MR, Berg LC, Hertz MI: Large cell carcinoma of the lung with neuroendocrine differentiation: A comparison with large cell "undifferentiated" pulmonary tumors. *Am J Clin Pathol* 97:796–805, 1992.

46. Wick MR, Loy T, Mills SE, et al: Malignant epithelioid pleural mesothelioma versus peripheral pulmonary adenocarcinoma: A histochemical, ultrastructural, and immunohistologic study of 103 cases. *Hum Pathol* 21:759–766, 1990.

47. Yousem SA, Hochholzer L: Alveolar adenoma. *Hum Pathol* 17:1066–1071, 1986.

48. Yousem SA, Hochholzer L: Mucoepidermoid tumors of the lung. *Cancer* 60:1346–1352, 1987.

49. Yousem SA, Wick MR, Singh G, et al: So-called sclerosing hemangiomas of the lung: An immunohistochemical study supporting a respiratory epithelial origin. *Am J Surg Pathol* 12:582–590, 1988.

NON–SMALL CELL LUNG CANCER—CLINICAL ASPECTS, DIAGNOSIS, STAGING, AND NATURAL HISTORY

Mitchell L. Margolis

CLINICAL ASPECTS

Clinical Assessment

HISTORY

Cough

The most common initial symptom of non–small cell lung cancer is cough, which is noted in 35 to 75 percent of cases. Since cough is also present, by definition, in all patients with chronic bronchitis, the mere presence of cough is seldom a helpful diagnostic clue. Indeed, many patients readily dismiss the symptom as a "smoker's cough." However, careful questioning may reveal a change in the character of cough, which may warrant investigation. Cough in non–small cell lung cancer is associated with ulcerative mucosal changes from the tumor itself, postobstructive pneumonitis, pleural effusion, atelectasis, and many other intrathoracic complications. Cough immediately after swallowing suggests a tracheo- or bronchoesophageal fistula. Severe cough may interfere with sleep or result in rib fractures or syncope. Unfortunately, no historical features of cough or sputum production are specific for non–small cell lung cancer. Even bronchorrhea, a dreaded complication of diffuse alveolar cell carcinoma, may be seen in rare cases of asthma, tuberculosis, and a few other diseases. Cough in non–small cell lung cancer is usually accompanied by other symptoms or significant roentgenographic abnormalities. Among patients with isolated cough and a normal chest film, non–small cell lung cancer is quite rare. In one series only 1 of 109 such cases could be attributed to non–small cell lung cancer.[28]

Dyspnea

Dyspnea has been reported in 26 to 60 percent of patients presenting with non–small cell lung cancer and is often an ominous development, signifying intrathoracic extension or dissemination. Among the thoracic complications of non–small cell lung cancer giving rise to dyspnea are pleural effusion, atelectasis, postobstructive pneumonia, lymphangitic carcinoma, tumor microembolism, upper airway obstruction, and pneumothorax. Occasionally patients with chest wall involvement or mediastinal extension report dyspnea from pain-induced restriction of respiration. Usually the chest radiograph in dyspneic patients demonstrates a sizable effusion, atelectasis of a lobe or entire lung, or clear evidence of intrapulmonary dissemination. A normal chest film in a dyspneic patient with non–small cell lung cancer suggests pulmonary tumor microembolism, occult lymphangitic spread, upper airway obstruction, or "conventional" pulmonary embolism. Dyspnea also frequently arises from important comorbid diseases, such as severe chronic obstructive pulmonary disease (COPD), which is strongly associated with non–small cell lung cancer independent of their common derivation from cigarette smoking. Finally, profound dyspnea may be seen in disseminated diffuse bronchoalveolar cell carcinoma with bronchorrhea. In such cases, palliation of dyspnea becomes the central clinical issue.

Chest Pain

Chest pain is reported at presentation in 20 to 45 percent of cases of non–small cell lung cancer and usually arises via direct invasion or metastatic involvement of pain-sensitive intrathoracic structures. Most commonly, a peripheral tumor invades the costal parietal pleura and chest wall, giving rise to sharp, intermittent pleuritic pain. With further progression, a steady, boring pain evolves, which can be extremely debilitating. It is important to distinguish the chest pain that accompanies direct contiguous chest wall extension from painful rib metastases that are anatomically remote from the primary lesion. Other patients with non–small cell lung cancer report a poorly localized, vague, persistent discomfort sometimes associated with central tumors with mediastinal extension and possible involvement of perivascular and peribronchial nerves. Finally, a dull, achy chest pain has been described in about 25 percent of cases with a malignant pleural effusion. The chest film in non–small cell lung cancer patients with chest pain usually discloses a conspicuous mass density or effusion that correlates with the clinical picture.

Hemoptysis

Hemoptysis is the sole presenting complaint in 5 to 10 percent of cases of non–small cell lung cancer but may be one of the initial symptoms in up to 50 percent of new cases. Typically hemoptysis consists only of blood-streaked sputum, which is sometimes erroneously attributed to chronic bronchitis. It is believed that local necrosis and inflammation of blood vessels within the tumor is responsible for this symptom. At this point, the chest radiograph may be normal, but it more commonly demonstrates a mass lesion or other suspicious findings. Among patients with hemoptysis and a normal chest radiograph, the frequency of occult non–small cell lung cancer demonstrated by bronchoscopy is only about 3 percent. In this setting, hemoptysis for several days in a row in a smoker over the age of 40 is particularly worrisome. If ignored, hemoptysis due to non–small cell lung cancer may increase but rarely results in asphyxia due to massive hemoptysis and clot formation. This horrific complication is associated with central squamous cell carcinoma, extensive cavitation, and sometimes direct erosion into a bronchial or pulmonary vessel. In one series, 23 of 29 cases of massive hemoptysis due to non–small cell lung cancer occurred after a clinical history of submassive hemoptysis for days to weeks.[21]

Hoarseness

Hoarseness is an initial complaint in 5 to 18 percent of cases of non–small cell lung cancer and is often accompanied by cough. It usually indicates direct mediastinal extension or adenopathy that involves the left recurrent laryngeal nerve, thereby causing unilateral left vocal cord paralysis. A paralyzed cord often produces a variable extrathoracic upper airway obstruction and is readily diagnosed by laryngoscopy. In patients with non–small cell lung cancer, the left vocal cord is far more likely to become paralyzed, owing to the lengthy course of the left recurrent laryngeal nerve as it loops around the ligamentum arteriosum at the level of the aortopulmonary window, a common site for lymph node involvement. Occasionally, hoarseness in a patient with non–small cell lung cancer is caused by an unrelated vocal cord polyp or tumor, but tumor–related recurrent laryngeal nerve involvement should always be at the top of the list until proven otherwise.

Less Common Thoracic Symptoms

Wheezing is a prominent initial symptom in 2 to 10 percent of patients and suggests partial obstruction of the trachea or mainstem bronchus by intraluminal tumor or extrinsic compression. Dysphagia is a presenting complaint in about 2 percent of cases, usually reflecting esophageal compression by metastatic mediastinal lymph node masses. Occasionally, however, recurrent laryngeal nerve involvement causes dysphagia and an increased risk of aspiration by interfering with cricoid and upper esophageal function[38] as well as producing incomplete glottic closure. A few non–small cell lung cancer patients present with fever, chills, and purulent sputum, resulting from postobstructive pneumonia or necrosis in a large cavitary tumor mass.

Extrathoracic Symptoms

Up to one-third of patients with non–small cell lung cancer present with symptoms due to metastatic disease. The most common symptom is bone pain, which usually signifies metastatic involvement of a specific skeletal site. Symptoms reflective of central nervous system (CNS) metastases are next most common, especially those resulting from increased intracranial pressure, such as headache, nausea, and vomiting. Focal brain lesions and diffuse leptomeningeal involvement may also produce symptoms, which vary according to the exact site of metastatic implantation. Back pain is a particularly important symptom, since it may result from metastatic involvement of vertebral bodies and potentially lead to cord compression. It is vital that this complication be recognized and treated at once—prior to the development of leg numbness, weakness, or incontinence—if there is to be a chance of reversibility. Rarely the chief complaint relates to other metastatic sites, such as abdominal pain from massive adrenal or hepatic involvement.

Systemic Factors

Though advanced age in itself does not preclude the usual diagnostic, staging, and therapeutic measures in non–small cell lung cancer, many authors have suggested that age significantly affects the clinical presentation. Tumors that are discovered in patients under the age of 40 probably select for an especially malignant subset, and at least one group of investigators has found quantitative cytochemical DNA differences that may account for this virulence.[18] On the other hand, non–small cell lung cancer presenting in elderly subjects may be relatively indolent, less likely to metastasize, and more likely to remain clinically occult. Still, the elderly are more likely to be afflicted with severe comorbid diseases such as COPD, coronary artery disease, and stroke that may profoundly affect non–small cell lung cancer management. A careful assessment of the severity and prognosis of these comorbid conditions is essential.

Significant weight loss in non–small cell lung cancer is deemed to have occurred when the patient has lost more than 10 lb or 5 percent of body weight. Weight loss reflects a complex interplay of factors that vary from patient to patient, including depression, anorexia, metabolic derangements, increased work of breathing, pain, and cough. Circulating tumor necrosis factor, interleukins, and other cellular mediators are likely involved; thus, weight loss can be considered in part a paraneoplastic syndrome. Nevertheless, it remains an important historical element and prognostic factor in non–small cell lung cancer.

Performance status—a clinical index that reflects the global effect of the patient's comorbid diseases, age, weight loss, and tumor burden—is a vital consideration. Whether scored by the 10-point Karnovsky scale (Table 112-1), the 5-point Eastern Cooperative Oncology Group scale, or a dichotomous ambulatory/nonambulatory system, performance status consistently ranks among the most important prognostic variables in non–small cell lung cancer.

Asymptomatic Non–Small Cell Lung Cancer

It has been estimated that only about 5 to 15 percent of patients are completely asymptomatic at the time of diagnosis. In most of these cases a chest radiograph performed as a routine upon hospital admission or as part of a "checkup" discloses an abnormality

TABLE 112-1

The Karnofsky Performance Scale

Definition	Percent	Criteria
Able to carry on normal activity and to work; no special care is needed.	100	Normal; no complaints; no evidence of disease.
	90	Able to carry on normal activity; minor signs or symptoms of disease.
	80	Normal activity with effort; some signs or symptoms of disease.
Unable to work; able to live at home; care for most personal needs; a varying amount of assistance is needed.	70	Cares for self; unable to carry on normal activity or to do active work.
	60	Requires occasional assistance but is able to care for most of needs.
	50	Requires considerable assistance and frequent medical care.
Unable to care for self; requires equivalent of institutional or hospital care; disease may be progressing rapidly.	40	Disabled; requires special care and assistance.
	30	Severely disabled; hospitalization is indicated, although death may not be imminent.
	20	Very sick; hospitalization necessary; active supportive treatment necessary.
	10	Moribund; fatal processes progressing rapidly.

that proves to be a non–small cell lung cancer. Sometimes more detailed questioning reveals that the patient was not truly asymptomatic; rather, the checkup was patient-initiated in response to the recent onset of insidious malaise, depression, weight loss, or mild chest symptoms. The main importance of asymptomatic non–small cell lung cancer is that these cases, by coming to clinical attention earlier in their natural history, often have the best chance of cure. Furthermore, the usual preoperative diagnostic and staging workup can often be omitted or curtailed in favor of prompt surgical intervention.

Screening   An important issue relating to asymptomatic presentations of non–small cell lung cancer is that of screening. The concept that lung cancer could be detected at an early, more curable stage is attractive; yet screening tends to disclose relatively indolent cancers that might have remained clinically inapparent. In 1984, a thorough, prospective multicenter trial was published that employed both sputum cytologies and chest radiographs to screen for early non–small cell lung cancer among male smokers over the age of 45.[3] The study demonstrated that chest roentgenography was a sensitive technique for detecting early-stage peripheral tumors, while sputum cytology, though less sensitive, permitted early recognition of many radiographically oc-

cult, central squamous cell carcinomas. Although a large proportion of early-stage tumors were detected and resected, it was extremely disappointing to find no change overall in lung cancer mortality in the screened population compared to a control population. Whether this result reflects lead-time bias, overdiagnosis, a statistical quirk, a host of putative shortcomings of the study (such as the absence of women in the cohort), or a real inability of the screening tests to alter the natural history of non–small cell lung cancer remains among the most contentious issues in thoracic oncology. A related nagging question is whether surgery truly alters the natural history of early non–small cell lung cancer or merely selects out a population of lesions with better prognoses. Since screening large at-risk populations is expensive and abnormal findings on screening tests may prompt needless biopsies, with their attendant complications, most authorities do not currently recommend screening for non–small cell lung cancer in the absence of a clear impact on mortality.[9] The effectiveness of screening more select at-risk populations, such as patients with severe COPD or previous lung cancer, awaits further inquiry. The introduction of more sensitive, molecular biology–based screening tools may also alter current clinical dogma.

PHYSICAL EXAMINATION

General

The general appearance of the patient with non–small cell lung cancer may be revealing. One may immediately perceive evidence of weight loss, depression, anxiety, dyspnea, jaundice, pallor, pain, or the superior vena cava syndrome, with its characteristic facial swelling and dilated collateral veins. Performance status is readily surmised from the history and the patient's ability to cooperate with the examination.

Thoracic

Examination of the thorax must be meticulous. Stridor, a distinctly unusual presenting sign, must be recognized at once, since upper airway obstruction may progress with surprising rapidity once a critical airway diameter is reached. A localized wheeze must be distinguished from the generalized wheezing of chronic airflow obstruction. A disparity between the intensity of normally transmitted voice sounds compared with diminished breath sounds suggests an endobronchial tumor causing partial occlusion of a lobar or main-stem bronchus. Dullness and the absence of breath sounds over one lung may be accompanied by ipsilateral tracheal deviation in the case of atelectasis and a contralateral shift in the case of massive pleural effusion. Mediastinal extension or lymph node metastases may also induce hoarseness due to recurrent laryngeal nerve involvement or elevation and paralysis of either hemidiaphragm due to phrenic nerve entrapment. Absent breaths sounds and a hyperresonant percussion note suggest the rare presentation with pneumothorax. Chest wall invasion is seldom appreciated on physical exam except for the rare instance of a palpable mass, when the lesion has invaded completely through an intercostal space. Localized pain as described by the patient is often the best clue to chest wall involvement. Signs of pulmonary hypertension usually reflect underlying lung disease but occasionally result from pulmonary tumor microembolism or carcinomatous lymphangitis. Classic signs of consolidation may result from postobstructive pneumonia or atelectatic lung, while pericardial or myocardial involvement may produce a full range of signs including arrhythmias, rubs, and pericardial tamponade due to effusion. Finally, it must be emphasized that most of the foregoing signs reflect intrathoracic extension or dissemination; in early-stage disease, the thoracic examination is usually normal.

Extrathoracic

When present, physical findings suggesting metastatic disease are valuable for planning the diagnostic and staging workup of non–small cell lung cancer. Nodular skin and subcutaneous lesions, though rare, should be sought, especially over the chest, back, and abdomen. Supraclavicular adenopathy is a common presenting feature of metastatic disease and should be sought as a routine. Bone tenderness often corresponds to focal skeletal metastases, while liver metastases occasionally produce hepatic nodularity, hepatomegaly, or—rarely—jaundice. Great care must be exercised during the examination of the CNS, particularly in the presence of symptoms such as back pain or headache. In such patients, appreciation of subtle sensory changes in the legs or early papilledema dictate the rapid performance of imaging and treatment measures to prevent catastrophic neurologic complications.

CHEST IMAGING

Plain Radiography

As a widely available, inexpensive, and safe test that can simultaneously suggest the diagnosis and localize non–small cell lung cancer, the standard chest radiograph remains the primary means for radiographic assessment. However, several important limitations pertaining to chest radiographs must be mentioned. First, up to 12 to 30 percent of lung cancers are missed on chest radiography; indeed, missed lung tumors are a leading cause for malpractice claims against radiologists.[22] Missed tumors can sometimes be attributed to the chest radiographic resolution limit of 2 to 3 mm for nodules, to overlapping soft tissue densities that obscure central endobronchial abnormalities or apical masses, or to human error. Second, chest radiographs cannot predict histologic subtype within the domain of non–small cell lung cancer or even reliably separate small cell from non–small cell lung cancer. Finally, a major problem resides with the low specificity of chest radiographic abnormalities. Even chest radiographic findings highly suspicious for non–small cell lung cancer, such as atelectasis of an entire lung, could alternatively result from benign tumors, metastases from extrapulmonary cancers, or foreign bodies. Another example is the solitary pulmonary nodule, since the average prevalence of malignancy for such lesions is only about 40 percent, at least in many older studies. Moreover, in the appropriate context, almost any chest radiographic abnormality can be related to non–small cell lung cancer. Thus, chest radiographs may initiate fruitless diagnostic workups, with their attendant expense and morbidity. A comparison of current chest radiographs with prior films remains perhaps the best means for identifying lesions of importance.

In view of the above, attempting to describe or classify the chest radiographic manifestations of non–small cell lung cancer is a daunting task. Most commonly the primary lesion is perceived as a localized opacity (Fig. 112-1). Slight predilections for the upper lobes, right lung, and anterior segment have been noted. Unfortunately, size, shape, and other radiographic features of non–small cell lung cancer—including presence of cavitation, calcification, spiculation, etc.—are highly variable and overlap with benign entities (Fig. 112-2). In general, large or uncalcified lesions are worrisome, and squamous cell tumors are more likely to cavitate. In addition, non–small cell lung cancer may generate a wide spectrum of chest radiographic changes via extension to major airways and other contiguous structures. These are described and illustrated separately in the section on thoracic presentations.

Computed Tomography

A rush of enthusiasm initially attended the introduction of computed tomography (CT) scans for imaging non–small cell lung cancer. The superior spatial resolution, enhanced ability to detect calcium, and cross-sectional detail provided by CT scans address many of the shortcomings of chest radiographs. Such scans provide a clearer image of the primary lesion and its anatomic

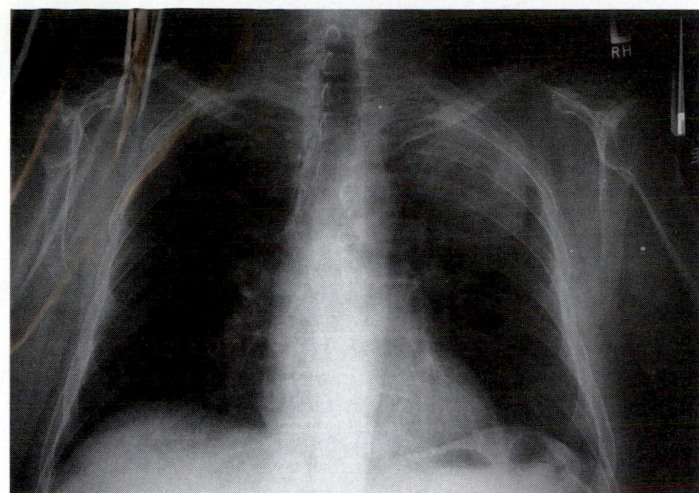

FIGURE 112-1 Chest radiograph showing typical large LUL mass lesion due to non–small cell lung cancer.

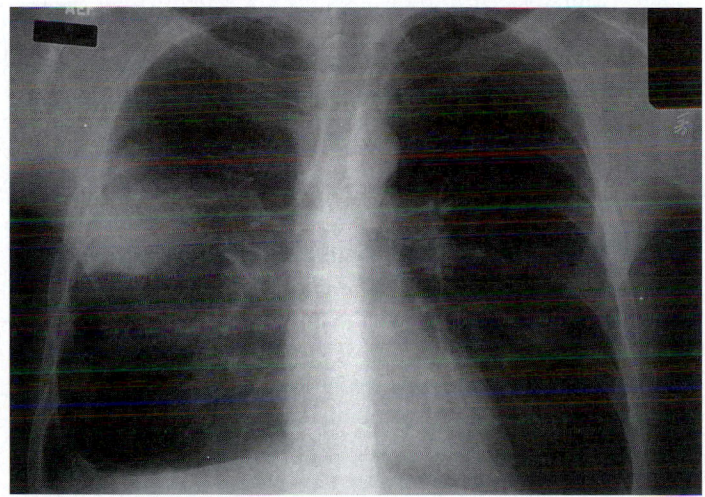

FIGURE 112-2 Chest radiograph showing large RUL mass suspicious for non–small cell lung cancer but proven to represent an inflammatory pseudotumor in this case.

relationship to nearby chest structures. They also allow an evaluation of extrabronchial tumor, which aids in planning surgical or laser resection. Often, CT scans can accurately predict malignancy, especially when a given lesion demonstrates contrast enhancement, and they can elucidate important intrathoracic complications of non–small cell lung cancer. These include distinguishing tumor from adjacent atelectatic lung or demonstrating superior vena cava compression, pericardial effusion, lymphangitic dissemination, and other conditions.

With further experience, some limitations of CT scanning have become apparent. To differentiate benign from malignant nodules (detailed elsewhere in this text), CT densitometry has proven definitive only for a minority of indeterminant lesions. Also, CT has severe limitations in distinguishing invasion of adjacent structures from simple abutment. Finally, many shortcomings apply to CT scans as a staging technique; these are discussed later in this chapter.

Magnetic Resonance Imaging and Other Tests

Magnetic resonance imaging (MRI) generally affords few advantages over CT in imaging primary non–small cell lung cancer. It is helpful in imaging apical lung tumors (see below); also, the increased intensity of recurrent lung cancer on T2-weighted images occasionally can be distinguished from the decreased signal of fibrotic lung. Nevertheless, MRI is typically reserved for specific staging problems in non–small cell lung cancer (see below).

Many other imaging techniques—including ultrasound, fluoroscopy, bronchography, superior venography, and lordotic, oblique, and lateral decubitus films—are occasionally of value in answering specific questions relating to non–small cell lung cancer and its intrathoracic complications. Also, positron emission tomography with fluoro-2-deoxyglucose has recently emerged as a potentially useful means of exploiting the high metabolic activity of non–small cell lung cancer to demonstrate primary tumor and metastatic lesions.[4]

PULMONARY FUNCTION TESTS

Pulmonary function tests are usually obtained as part of the initial clinical assessment of patients with non–small cell lung cancer. The severity of associated chronic airflow obstruction and adequacy of pulmonary reserve are paramount in planning treatment. These issues are covered elsewhere in this text. In addition, the tumor itself, directly or indirectly, may influence pulmonary function; these effects constitute another set of clinical manifestations of non–small cell lung cancer.

Perhaps the most common spirometric abnormality related to non–small cell lung cancer itself is a restrictive impairment. This may reflect chest pain, massive pleural fluid accumulation, atelectasis, respiratory muscle weakness, phrenic nerve paralysis, or the presence of a malignant main-stem bronchial obstruction. The latter may sometimes produce a characteristic biphasic flow-volume loop due to asynchronous emptying of the nonobstructed lung followed by the obstructed one. Of greater concern is the appearance of a true upper airway obstruction pattern, resulting either from tracheal involvement or vocal cord paralysis.

Other functional effects of note include a low diffusion capacity due to pulmonary tumor microembolism or lymphangitic metastases and shunting secondary to atelectasis, postobstructive pneumonia, or diffuse bronchoalveolar carcinoma.

ROUTINE LABORATORY TESTS

Complete blood counts, urinalyses, serum electrolytes and liver function tests are of limited usefulness in evaluating patients with non–small cell lung cancer.[3] Some abnormalities, including hypoalbuminemia and thrombocytosis, are common in non–small cell lung cancer but extremely nonspecific. Others, such as hyponatremia and proteinuria, may reflect paraneoplastic syndromes discussed elsewhere in this text. Another group of abnormalities—including anemia, hypercalcemia, and elevated levels of alkaline phosphatase—are often associated with disseminated disease and should prompt a search for distant disease. One should also recognize that disseminated intravascular coagulation, marked leukemoid reactions, eosinophilia, lactic acidosis, and other atypical laboratory features may rarely be associated with non–small cell lung cancer.

Clinical Presentations

THORACIC

Mediastinal Involvement

In roughly 40 percent of cases of non–small cell lung cancer, the mediastinum is involved either by the presence of lymph node metastases (Fig. 112-3) or by direct extension (Fig. 112-4), posing a critical clinical dilemma. The controversy over which of these patients should be referred for surgical resection reflects an important deficiency in our current clinical understanding of non–small cell lung cancer. Further uncertainty results from the tendency for mediastinal lymph node metastases to skip nodal stations in up to 30 percent of cases, thereby necessitating complete lymph node dissection to definitively exclude mediastinal spread.[43] Although nodal metastases are more common with central or undifferentiated tumors, verifiable mediastinal involvement remains somewhat unpredictable.

Patients with mediastinal spread from non–small cell lung cancer may be completely asymptomatic, but many complain of cough or vague chest pain and may exhibit symptoms and signs that reflect involvement of contiguous mediastinal structures. These include the phrenic nerve, left recurrent laryngeal nerve, pericardium and heart, pulmonary veins and arteries, aorta, superior vena cava, and esophagus. Massive adenopathy may also produce lymphatic blockade, resulting in pleural effusions or diffuse lymphangitic dissemination. These specific clinical scenarios are described separately below. Chest radiographs, CT scans, and MRI may clearly demonstrate mediastinal involvement but often "miss" normal-sized tumor-bearing nodes or fail to separate resectable from unresectable mediastinal incursion; they may also be misleading if nodal enlargement is due to hyperplasia or inflammation. Ultimately an invasive procedure—such as mediastinoscopy, mediastinotomy or thoracotomy—is necessary to reliably define the mediastinum in non–small cell lung cancer.

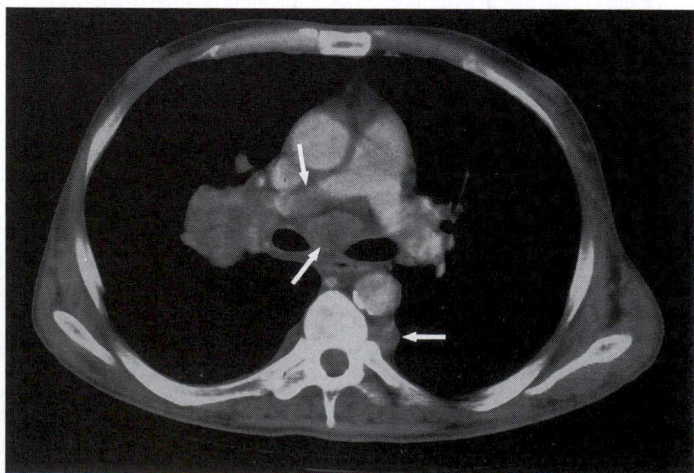

FIGURE 112-3 Computed tomography showing several enlarged mediastinal lymph nodes (arrows) due to metastatic non–small cell lung cancer.

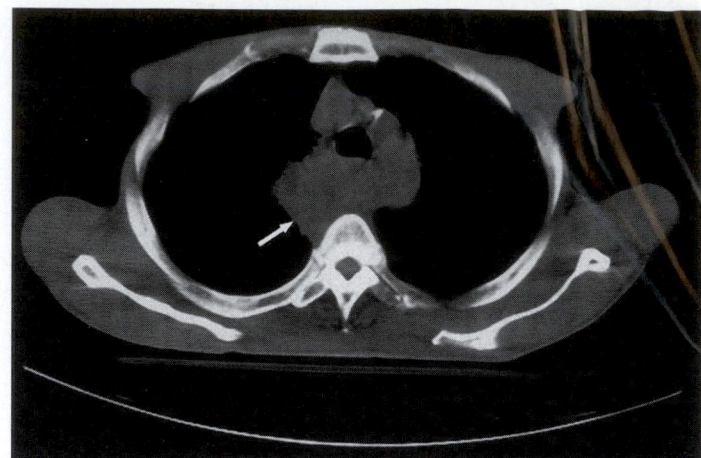

FIGURE 112-4 Computed tomography showing direct retrotracheal mediastinal invasion by non–small cell lung cancer (arrow).

Pneumonia, Obstructive Pneumonitis, and Atelectasis

Patients with alveolar infiltrates on the chest radiograph are frequently referred to the pulmonary clinician because of concern for underlying non–small cell lung cancer. Such patients may be asymptomatic or may suffer from typical symptoms of pneumonia, including fever, chills, and a productive cough with streaky hemoptysis. Serial chest films may show chronic, recurrent, or slowly resolving infiltrates. One obvious concern in this setting is that the chronic infiltrate itself represents the diffuse form of bronchoalveolar cell carcinoma. Alternatively, a hilar mass or radiographically occult endobronchial lesion may cause a true obstructive pneumonitis. Symptoms in obstructive pneumonitis correlate with the presence of heterogeneous, often polymicrobial bacterial infection, whereas asymptomatic pneumonitis probably reflects a combination of atelectasis, bronchiectasis with mucus plugging, and inflammation.[20] The timing of bronchoscopy to search for an underlying non–small cell lung cancer in patients with atypical resolution of pneumonia by chest radiography remains a matter of debate and varies with the patient population and nature of the infective episode. Though several older studies found that delayed resolution could not be linked to non–small cell lung cancer in a single case, a recent clinical profile of chronic bacterial pneumonia disclosed newly diagnosed non–small cell lung cancer in 14 percent of cases.[19] Furthermore, collected series suggest that lung carcinoma is associated with about one-fourth of cases of the right middle lobe syndrome.

Atelectasis is frequently the predominant feature of obstructing non–small cell lung cancer, particularly in the absence of infection. Atelectasis may vary from subsegmental to collapse of an entire lung (Fig. 112-5). When airway obstruction is complete, the key radiographic feature is the absence of an air bronchogram. Fissural shifts and the amount of distal volume loss are variable, and lobar and segmental collapse due to non–small cell lung cancer can be surprisingly difficult to recognize on chest radiography. For example, sometimes an entire lobe is "pancaked" against the mediastinal silhouette (Fig. 112-6). Symptoms, signs, and pulmonary function may or may not reflect the radiographic changes; while some patients with lobar collapse are dyspneic and hypoxemic, others remain asymptomatic.

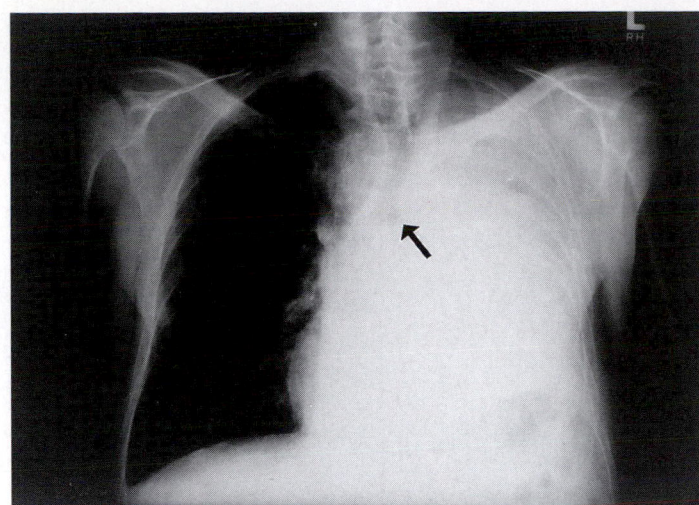

FIGURE 112-5   Chest radiograph showing left lung atelectasis due to non–small cell lung cancer. Note abrupt cutoff of left main-stem bronchus *(arrow)*.

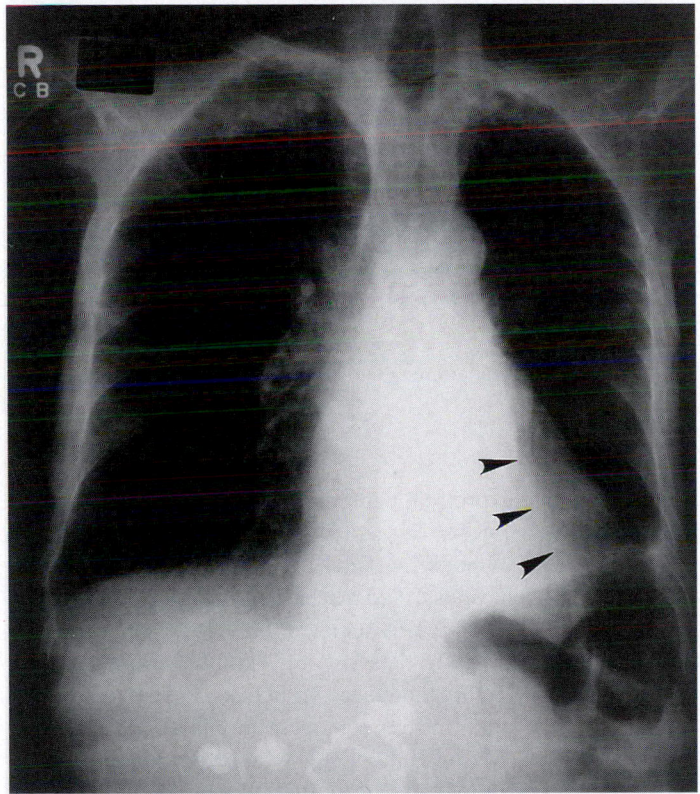

FIGURE 112-6   Chest radiograph showing LLL collapse due to non–small cell lung cancer. The border of the atelectatic lobe is visible medially *(arrowheads)*.

Chest Wall Involvement

In up to 5 percent of cases, non–small cell lung cancer invades the parietal pleura and chest wall. The most common presenting symptom in such cases is chest pain, which is initially described as an intermittent dull ache. Chest films clearly show a peripheral mass, but the presence and extent of chest wall invasion can be difficult to discern, even on CT scan or MRI. Squamous cell carcinoma formerly was the most frequent histologic subtype to present in this fashion, but adenocarcinoma and large cell tumors are also well represented. It is especially important to stage the mediastinum accurately in these cases, since the prognosis is relatively good with en bloc resection in the absence of nodal disease but quite poor if mediastinal nodal metastases are present.

Pleural Effusion

Pleural effusion can be detected in 7 to 24 percent of lung cancer cases at presentation and is a common cause of dyspnea in patients with non–small cell lung cancer. Effusion may also be associated with chest pain and cough or give rise to no symptoms at all. The pathogenesis of malignant effusions in non–small cell lung cancer is believed to begin with seeding of the visceral pleura via pulmonary arterial invasion and embolization, with subsequent shedding into the pleural space and migration to involve the parietal pleura.[30] A second important mechanism relates to lymphatic blockade at any point from the stomata of the parietal pleura to the mediastinal lymph nodes. The fluid itself may be serous, serosanguinous, or grossly bloody and is exudative in the vast majority of cases. Typically the effusion is ipsilateral to the main tumor and of moderate to large volume. Malignant cells can be demonstrated on a single large-volume thoracentesis in about 60 percent of cases, depending on histologic type, with closed pleural biopsy adding to the yield. The finding of malignant cells in the fluid confirms stage IIIb disease and a relatively poor prognosis.

One must not assume, however, that the presence of a pleural effusion in non–small cell lung cancer necessarily implies advanced disease. Occasionally fluid formation is only indirectly related to the tumor, via obstructive pneumonia or atelectasis. Alternatively, the effusion may be caused by an unrelated nonmalignant condition, such as congestive heart failure. In one series, 4 of 73 non–small cell lung cancer patients with pleural effusion had surgically resectable tumors and survived for intervals ranging from 3 to 14 years.[7]

Superior Vena Cava Syndrome

Though superior vena cava syndrome may result from small cell carcinoma, lymphoma, metastatic carcinoma, and a host of benign causes, it remains an important presentation of non–small cell lung cancer. The mechanism of superior vena cava obstruction is usually extrinsic compression by a large primary tumor or its mediastinal lymph node metastases, along with associated intraluminal thrombosis (Fig. 112-7). Patients characteristically complain of headache, swelling of the face, neck, and upper extremities, or a host of thoracic symptoms such as dyspnea, cough, chest pain, and dysphagia. Syncope or dizziness associated with bending is also mentioned frequently. Physical examination may show facial edema, neck vein distension, and striking collateral venous engorgement over the anterior chest wall and upper abdomen. The degree of collateral formation reflects the time over which superior vena cava obstruction developed and the relative anatomic site of blockade, since obstruction above the azygos vein is better tolerated. The chest radiograph typically shows a large right-sided central mass extending into the mediastinum. Contrary to prior clinical wisdom, it has been convincingly demonstrated that the superior vena cava syndrome does not con-

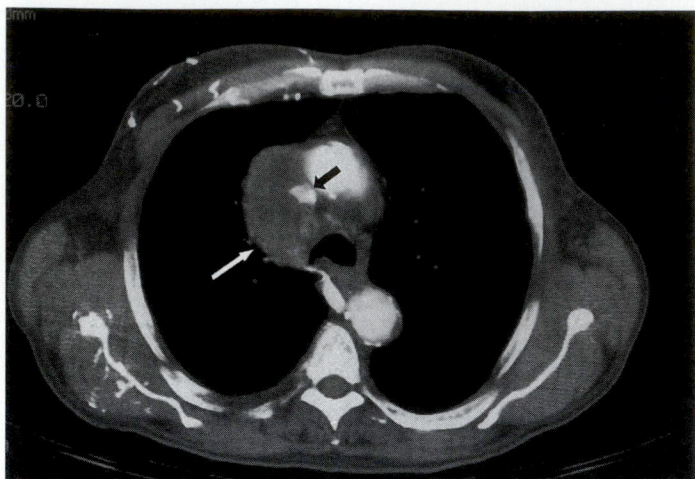

FIGURE 112-7　Computed tomography showing severe compression of superior vena cava *(black arrow)* by non–small cell lung cancer *(white arrow)*. Note contrast-filled collaterals in soft tissues of chest wall.

stitute a true medical emergency requiring urgent treatment without a tissue diagnosis.[1] An accurate diagnosis is especially important in view of the diverse etiologic considerations mentioned above. Moreover, it has been shown that sputum cytology, fiberoptic bronchoscopy, transthoracic needle biopsy, and mediastinoscopy, among other measures, can be employed safely and effectively to diagnose non–small cell lung cancer in this setting. While unrelieved superior vena cava obstruction itself is seldom if ever fatal, rapid diagnosis and institution of radiotherapy or chemotherapy for distressing symptoms is desirable.[1]

Pancoast (Superior Sulcus) Tumors

A characteristic clinical syndrome of arm and shoulder pain, Horner's syndrome, and atrophy of the small muscles of the hand is associated with tumors located in the extreme apex of the lung. This entity, described initially by Hare in 1838, was more fully detailed independently by Tobias and Pancoast in 1932. The manifestations of this syndrome are related to local invasion of the brachial plexus, sympathetic ganglion, and adjacent ribs. The pain is often severe and unrelenting; while initially confined to the shoulder and scapula, it later radiates down the arm following an ulnar distribution, reflecting involvement of the C8 and T1 nerve roots. There are many variants of this classic picture depending on the structures invaded. Pulmonary symptoms and signs are conspicuously absent, while arm weakness signifies advanced brachial plexus invasion. The chest radiograph may show an obvious apical mass, but frequently only a subtle increase in density is visible at the apex, which is often missed. Indeed, MRI has become the imaging modality of choice, because of the ability to reconstruct the images in the coronal and sagittal planes. Also, the better delineation of vascular structures by MRI makes it the better imaging modality for these lesions (Fig. 112-8). The vast majority of Pancoast tumors are due to non–small cell lung cancer, but small cell carcinoma, metastatic lesions from a wide variety of nonpulmonary cancers, and even some inflammatory processes may produce an identical clinical picture. Although Paulson originally accumulated a large personal experience treating these tumors with preoperative radiotherapy followed by

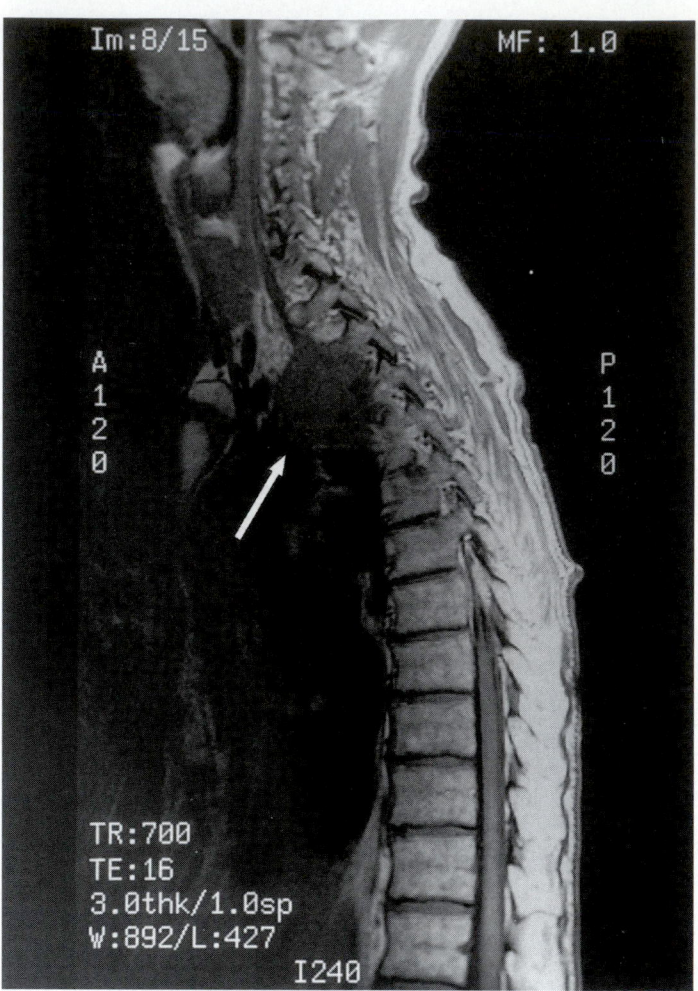

FIGURE 112-8　Sagittal T1-weighted MRI showing superior sulcus tumor *(arrow)* and its anatomic relationship to contiguous thoracic structures.

surgery without a pretreatment tissue diagnosis, transthoracic needle aspiration biopsy is a safe and efficient means for obtaining an initial diagnosis.

Some authors have ascribed a relatively indolent biologic behavior to Pancoast tumors, associated with a favorable prognosis. However more recent data suggest that non–small cell lung cancer at this site retains its usual propensity for nodal and distant metastatic spread. Indeed, Pancoast tumors are by definition stage IIIa lesions. Mediastinal or supraclavicular lymph node involvement can be demonstrated in up to 55 percent of cases and confers a very poor prognosis. Superior sulcus tumors may simply be recognized somewhat earlier than other non–small cell lung cancers, owing to the close proximity and thus early involvement of several pain-sensitive structures within the very confined site of origin, the thoracic inlet.

Phrenic Nerve Entrapment

Occasionally non–small cell lung cancer may involve either the left or right phrenic nerve via mediastinal extension, resulting in a paralyzed hemidiaphragm. Affected patients may be asymptomatic or complain of dyspnea, related in part to the decrements in FEV_1 and FVC resulting from hemidiaphragmatic paralysis.

Physical examination discloses unilateral basilar dullness and absence of the usual hemidiaphragmatic descent with inspiration. Chest radiographs demonstrate a lung mass, central in location, with obvious elevation of the hemidiaphragm. Since this latter feature may also result, to a lesser extent, from atelectasis or subpulmonic effusion, fluoroscopic sniff testing and demonstration of paradoxical motion is required to diagnose true diaphragm paralysis. Interestingly, the primary tumor may be radiographically occult. In one study of 142 cases of unexplained hemidiaphragmatic paralysis with otherwise normal chest films, 3 percent eventually demonstrated lung cancer with phrenic nerve involvement over the next 30 months.[27] Phrenic nerve involvement is staged as T3 disease (stage IIIa); if this is the only mediastinal structure invaded, it is not a contraindication to surgical resection. Involvement of other mediastinal structures often may only be evident at the time of operation; thus, patients with phrenic nerve involvement should not, as a matter of course, be denied the option of surgery.

Lung Metastases

Although pulmonary metastases are sometimes described in terms of three distinct clinical syndromes, considerable overlap exists, and multiple types of lung metastases are often present in patients with disseminated non–small cell lung cancer.

Pulmonary tumor microembolism is a rare complication of non–small cell lung cancer, reflecting diffuse tumor cell obstruction of the pulmonary arterial microvasculature, ranging from the alveolar septal capillaries to the pulmonary arterioles. The cardinal symptom is dyspnea and the clinical picture resembles that of subacute progressive pulmonary hypertension. The chest radiograph, perfusion lung scan, and pulmonary arteriogram are usually normal or nonspecific, and the diagnosis of this lethal entity is seldom made during life.[34]

Another important cause of dyspnea in late non–small cell lung cancer is carcinomatous lymphangitic spread, which may arise from retrograde lymphatic flow from metastatic mediastinal disease or from late mixed lymphohematogenous dissemination.[15] In several series, non–small cell lung cancer was the most common primary tumor giving rise to this syndrome. The chest radiograph may be normal but classically shows diffuse reticular or reticulonodular infiltrates with or without central adenopathy, Kerley B lines, and pleural effusions. High-resolution CT scans show a characteristic uneven nodular thickening of the interlobular septa and bronchovascular bundles (Fig. 112-9). Often the diagnosis rests on the clinical findings alone, but bronchoalveolar lavage, transbronchial biopsies, or microvascular cytology specimens from a wedged pulmonary artery catheter can provide histologic confirmation if necessary.

Non–small cell lung cancer may also give rise to single or multiple nodular metastases in the ipsilateral or contralateral lung. The presence of innumerable miliary nodules is associated with advanced bone metastases, while multiple "cannonball" metastases also clearly imply widespread metastases and a dire prognosis. A more vexing problem in terms of staging and treatment is posed by the patient with a large primary non–small cell lung cancer and one or two separate, small, noncalcified lesions on chest radiograph or CT scan. These nodules could represent clearly benign lesions, such as granulomas, lesions of uncertain

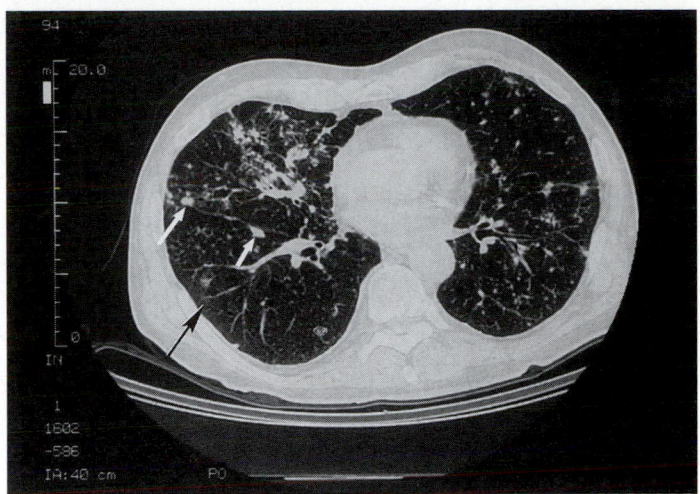

FIGURE 112-9   High-resolution CT scan showing lymphangitic spread of non–small cell lung cancer. Note characteristic spiculated septal thickening *(white arrows)* and "polygonal arcade" *(black arrow).*

malignant potential such as bronchoalveolar cell adenomas, metastases or satellite lesions from the dominant tumor, or synchronous primary lung cancers. The distinction between a solitary metastasis and a second primary may be particularly troublesome, even when detailed histologic comparison is possible. In such cases the physician must consider the therapeutic options in view of other staging tests and the overall clinical context. In the absence of other evidence of distant disease, the patient is treated under the assumption that he has two primary tumors— the most optimistic situation.

Bronchoalveolar Carcinoma

This fascinating tumor with a propensity for growth along alveolar walls has recently emerged as a common and important form of non–small cell lung cancer with a distinct dual clinical profile.[2] The more common subtype usually presents as a well-circumscribed peripheral opacity in an asymptomatic individual. This form, thought to arise from type II pneumocytes or nonciliated bronchiolar (Clara) cells, carries an excellent prognosis with surgical resection. The less common diffuse infiltrative form presents with cough and dyspnea and demonstrates poorly or sharply circumscribed coalescent alveolar consolidation or a reticulonodular pattern on the chest radiograph (Fig. 112-10). This subtype, believed to arise from bronchiolar goblet cells, is often multicentric, tends to recur after attempts at surgical extirpation, and may evolve into a lethal syndrome of progressive dyspnea, hypoxemia, and bronchorrhea. Most authorities consider the two subtypes distinct, although transition from a circumscribed to a diffuse tumor has been reported.

The diffuse form bears a close resemblance histologically to a contagious retroviral disease of sheep called "jaagsiekte," raising the possibility of a viral origin for human bronchoalveolar carcinoma.[10] Whether it is disseminated within the lung via endobronchial aspiration or arises from a widespread clone is unsettled. Though bronchoalveolar carcinoma is usually classified as a thoracic form of non–small cell lung cancer, distant metastases are well described, especially with the diffuse infiltrative subtype.

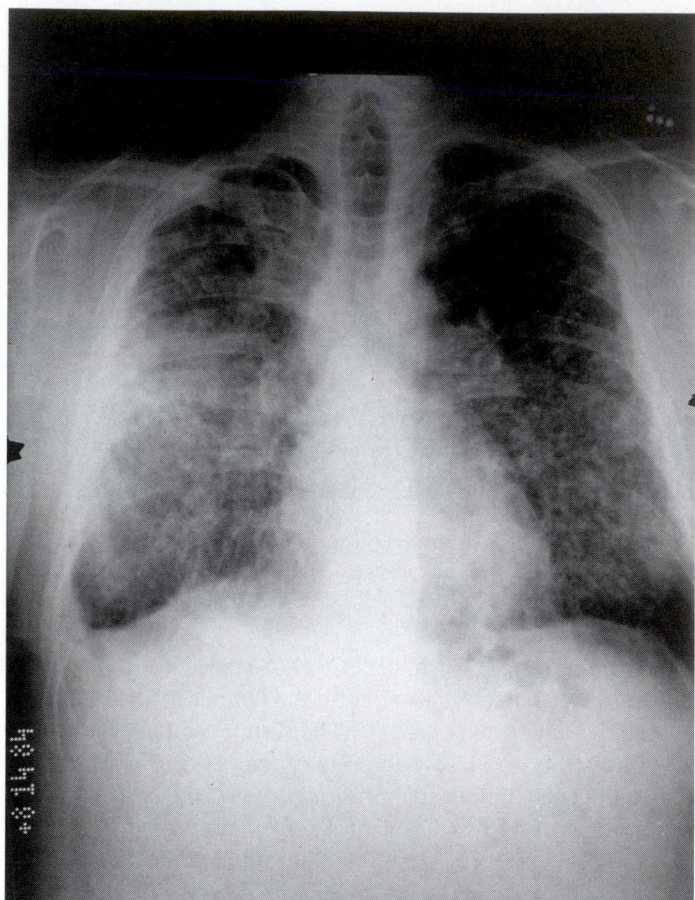

FIGURE 112-10 Chest radiograph showing diffuse infiltrates due to bronchoalveolar carcinoma.

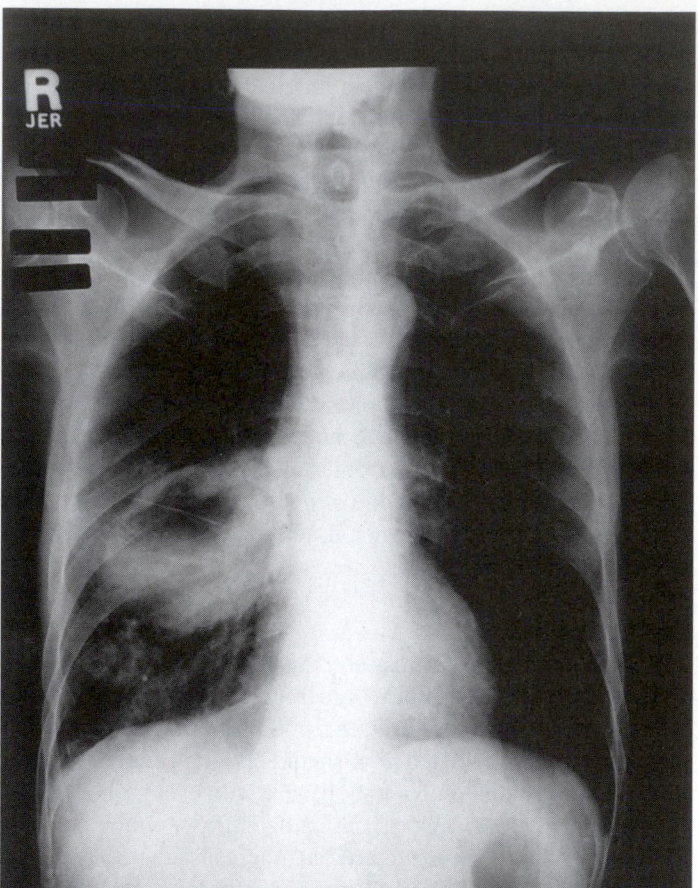

FIGURE 112-11 Chest radiograph showing large carcinomatous abscess due to squamous cell carcinoma.

Carcinomatous Lung Abscess

Non–small cell lung cancer, particularly squamous cell carcinoma, may present with a shaggy cavitary density indistinguishable from a conventional anaerobic lung abscess on chest radiograph (Fig. 112-11). Extensive central necrosis is responsible for the cavitary appearance. Several clinical clues may suggest the presence of cancer, including persistent hemoptysis, relative absence of fever and leukocytosis, and radiographic location in a nondependent region of the lung with minimal surrounding pneumonitis.

Scar Carcinoma

Some authors define a "scar cancer" as a peripherally located tumor with no evidence of bronchial origin, occurring around true hyalinized scar tissue. Others include tumors superimposed on chronic regional or diffuse interstitial fibrosis. Scar carcinomas tend to arise in the upper lobes, frequently present with extrapulmonary symptoms and signs, and may account for 5 to 40 percent of lung cancers. Scar cancers are almost all of the non–small cell type, with a preponderance of adenocarcinomas. Clinical concern for this entity is usually prompted by a careful comparison of current and old chest radiographs. There remains some controversy among pathologists as to whether scar carcinoma represents a distinct clinical entity or simply a carcinoma that is accompanied by an exuberant fibrous response.

Multiple Primary Lung Cancers

Multiple primary non–small cell lung cancers in the same patient are more often metachronous than synchronous. In either case the most frequent finding is two early-stage squamous cell carcinomas (Fig. 112-12). Synchronous primary tumors are dif-

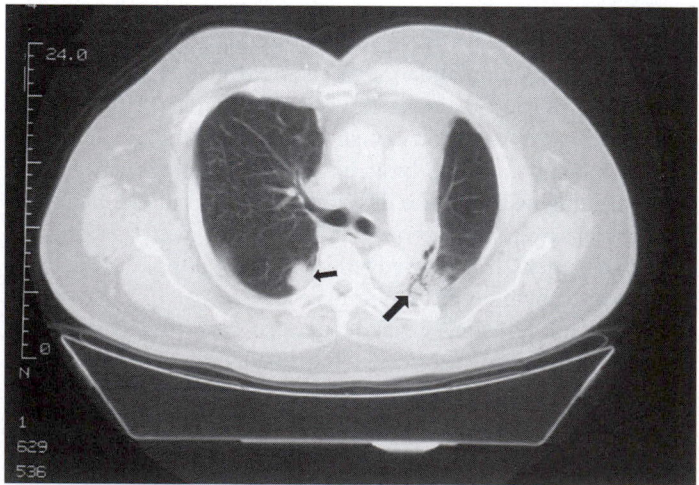

FIGURE 112-12 Computed tomography showing small metachronous squamous cell cancer in posteromedial RUL *(small arrow)*. Note posterior LUL scarring *(large arrow)* from radiotherapy for prior squamous cell cancer.

ficult to distinguish from metastatic disease, especially "satellite" metastases. Synchronous non–small cell lung cancers occur in only 0.5 percent of cases and are most reliably diagnosed when the masses in question represent different histologic subtypes or clearly arise from distinct endobronchial foci.[11] Flow cytometry, by identifying divergent DNA ploidy patterns in separate masses, can confirm the presence of truly independent tumors.

Pulmonary Vascular Involvement

Non–small cell lung cancer may invade or compress segmental, lobar, or main pulmonary arteries. This complication is often asymptomatic, but sometimes dyspnea, chest pain, and cough arise, suggesting associated pulmonary infarction. The chest film usually shows only the main tumor mass, but rarely a distal adjacent area of infarction is noted. Lung radionuclide scanning and pulmonary angiography may heighten concern for pulmonary embolism by

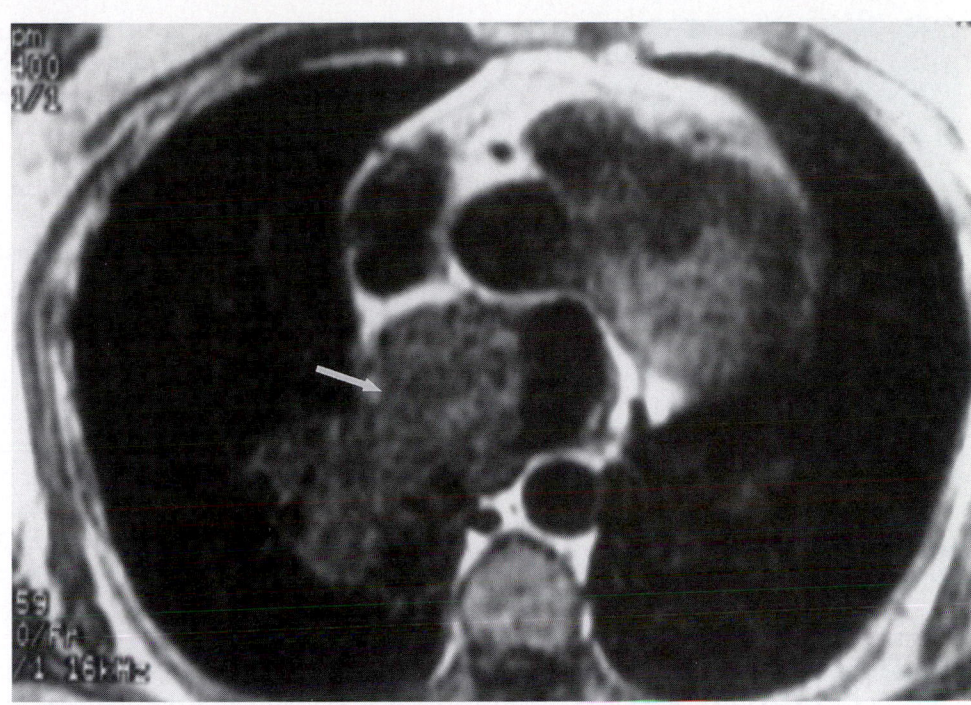

FIGURE 112-13   Left atrial invasion by non–small cell lung cancer *(arrow)* shown by T1-weighted MRI.

demonstrating greatly reduced or absent perfusion and vascular "cutoff" respectively. In this setting, chest MRI often provides the clearest assessment of the pulmonary artery. Frequently the involved artery is resected along with the tumor and the affected lobe or lung, but if the right ventricular outflow tract or proximal main pulmonary artery is encased or invaded, resection is not possible.

Pulmonary venous thrombosis with or without infarction is rare in non–small cell lung cancer and may be associated with nonspecific clinical features such as cough, chest pain, dyspnea, hemoptysis, or a systolic murmur. Transesophageal echocardiography may be helpful in delineating this complication. Anticoagulation and/or resection have been proposed for affected patients.

Pericardial, Cardiac, and Aortic Involvement

Pericardial involvement with non–small cell lung cancer, observed in about one-third of cases at autopsy, is frequently overlooked during life. Pericardial metastases may arise from direct extension, via retrograde lymphatic flow through epicardial lymphatics, or via hematogenous dissemination. The two most common presentations are the sudden onset of sinus tachycardia or atrial fibrillation or the asymptomatic detection of an enlarged cardiac silhouette on chest radiography or pericardial fluid layer on CT scan. Cardiac tamponade can occur with surprising rapidity, unaccompanied by neck vein distension and other classic physical signs. True cardiac involvement (Fig. 112-13), a rare but lethal complication arising from direct extension or hematogenous metastases, is sometimes appreciated only at the time of thoracotomy. When non–small cell lung cancer abuts the ascending aorta, the aortic arch, or the descending aorta, the main clinical issue is whether the vessel is truly invaded or can be surgically freed from neoplastic infiltration. Sometimes, MRI scans can demonstrate encasement, but often this question can be answered with confidence only at thoracotomy. Aortic involvement indicates a T4 primary tumor (stage IIIb) and is not usually considered a resectable situation.

Pneumothorax

Non–small cell lung cancer rarely presents as an ipsilateral spontaneous pneumothorax. This complication can arise from direct invasion of the pleura by a peripheral tumor with creation of an air leak and resultant lung collapse. Another mechanism is obstructive emphysema with rupture of a distal bleb. The most common underlying tumor is squamous cell carcinoma, and the prognosis is very poor.[36]

EXTRATHORACIC METASTASES

Non–small cell lung cancer frequently metastasizes to distant organs. Though the metastatic potential of non–small cell lung cancer is less than that of small cell carcinoma, distant spread is demonstrable at presentation in over one-third of cases, particularly with the large cell undifferentiated and adenocarcinoma subtypes. The usual sites of distant metastatic disease include the adrenals, brain, liver, lung, and bone, though virtually any organ can be affected. Metastases may present at the same time as the primary tumor or occur much later, and they may be single or multiple, clinically silent or demanding of emergent diagnosis and treatment.

Adrenal Metastases

Adrenal metastases are present in roughly 35 percent of patients dying of non–small cell lung cancer and are the most common

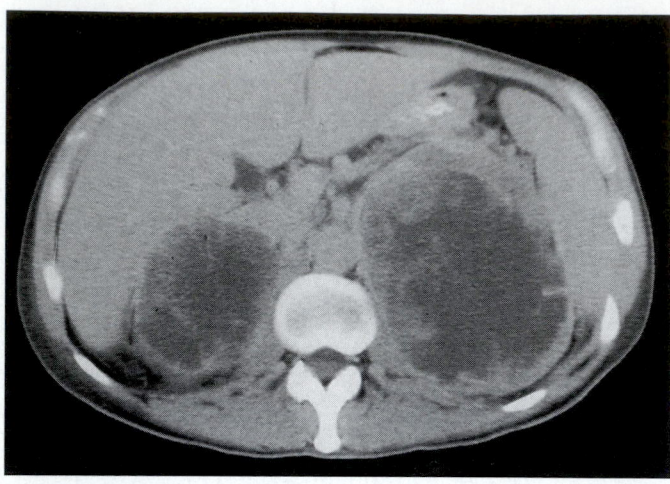

FIGURE 112-14 Computed tomography showing massive bilateral adrenal metastases from non–small cell lung cancer.

metastatic site in patients dying of lung cancer within 1 month of surgical resection with curative intent. Moreover, adrenal abnormalities represent the *only* site of metastatic involvement in up to 5 percent of cases. Adrenal metastases are usually silent clinically. However, on occasion massive lesions produce severe abdominal pain (Fig. 112-14); rarely, bilateral replacement of over 90 percent of all adrenal tissue may eventuate in adrenal insufficiency. Although patients with large tumor burdens and clinical indicators of widespread disease (such as weight loss and anemia) are more likely to harbor adrenal metastases,[32] the separation of adrenal metastases from benign adrenal masses remains problematic. This issue is discussed in the section on staging.

Central Nervous System Metastases

Metastases to the CNS are particularly important because of their frequency, wide spectrum, and often devastating impact. Any part of the CNS can be affected, and the prevalence is about 10 percent at presentation and 50 to 60 percent at autopsy. It is imperative that metastatic CNS involvement be distinguished from the numerous CNS paraneoplastic syndromes related to non–small cell lung cancer. In general, metastases produce asymmetrical, solitary neurologic deficits accompanied by focal radiographic abnormalities, while normal CNS imaging usually attends the symmetrical and multiple deficits classically associated with paraneoplastic syndromes.

Brain metastases are seen more frequently with the adenocarcinoma histologic subtype as compared with squamous carcinoma and carry a poor prognosis. Lung cancer is by far the most common cause for brain metastases, which are usually multiple but occasionally occur as solitary lesions (i.e., no other metastases present). The most frequent symptom is headache, and neurologic features most often suggest increased intracranial pressure. Seizures, cranial nerve deficits, hemiparesis, and other focal features may also appear, with the distribution of the middle cerebral artery most commonly affected. Infrequently, brain metastases may be asymptomatic, being found only with brain imaging. Leptomeningeal involvement is rare, but epidural spinal cord metastases probably represent the most frequent true emergency related to metastatic non–small cell lung cancer. Neu-

rologic deficits resulting from this complication tend to be irreversible and progressive, with sequential sensory, reflex, and motor impairment that eventuates in incontinence and paraplegia.

Liver Metastases

Liver metastases are found in 30 to 45 percent of cases of non–small cell lung cancer coming to autopsy. Unfortunately, the history, physical examination, and routine biochemical tests of hepatic function are unreliable indicators of liver metastases, though a general correlation with organ-specific and non–organ-specific clinical abnormalities has been repeatedly demonstrated. Thoracic CT scans are most frequently used to show hepatic metastases but are subject to numerous limitations, as described in the section on extrathoracic staging. When liver metastases become very extensive, anorexia, weight loss, elevated serum levels of alkaline phosphatase, and evidence of other distant metastases are typically present. Rarely, a large metastatic deposit in the porta hepatis produces jaundice.

Skeletal Metastases

Bone metastases in non–small cell lung cancer tend to develop in trabecular bone and are usually osteolytic, but osteoblastic metastases are occasionally associated with adenocarcinoma. Though demonstrable at autopsy in 25 to 40 percent of cases, osseous metastases must reach 1.0 to 1.5 cm in diameter and cause a 50 to 75 percent decrease in bone density to be demonstrable radiologically.[38] In fact, use of plain skeletal films, radionuclide scans, and MRI to delineate bone metastases is fraught with interpretive problems; this issue is further explored in the section on staging.

Bone metastases may be asymptomatic or produce pain and tenderness. The favored sites are the ribs, vertebrae, and long bones of the legs and arms. Metastases to the femoral neck are of special concern in that they prevent weight bearing and often demand urgent treatment. Hypercalcemia may accompany bone metastases but often instead represents a paraneoplastic syndrome due to elaboration of a parathyroid hormone–like substance. Rarely metastases to juxtaarticular bone or synovial tissue results in a monoarticular arthritis, most frequently involving the knee.

Lymphatic Metastases

The initial lymph node stations involved by metastatic non–small cell lung cancer are intrathoracic and include 13 intrapulmonary, hilar, and mediastinal sites designated in the American Joint Committee on Cancer (AJCC) system (Fig. 112-15). However, further lymphatic spread may occur in up to 42 percent of cases at presentation, especially to supraclavicular nodes, which are considered an N3 (stage IIIb) site. The right-sided supraclavicular space is particularly vulnerable, owing to greater traffic of lung lymphatic pathways to this site. Still more advanced lymphatic dissemination may result in cervical, axillary, inguinal, or abdominal adenopathy, classified as M1 (stage IV) disease. Extrathoracic metastatic adenopathy in non–small cell lung cancer is usually painless, with variable tenderness, size, fixation, etc. Its chief importance lies in providing an accessible, easy site for simultaneous diagnosis and staging via percutaneous or surgical biopsy.

a clinical problem. Renal metastases may appear as asymptomatic nodules on CT scan and rarely cause pain and hematuria. Gastric, small bowel, or colon metastases can cause perforation, ulceration, and obstruction, while pancreatic deposits may induce clinical pancreatitis. Clinical disease due to metastases to eye, skeletal muscle, placenta, and other sites has also been described.

DIAGNOSIS

Sputum Cytology

Sputum cytology, first used to diagnose lung cancer in 1887, remains the principal noninvasive means for diagnosing non–small cell lung cancer (Fig. 112-16), with a sensitivity ranging from 20 to 77 percent, depending on patient selection and numerous technical factors. The yield is significantly higher with central versus peripheral, lower lobe versus upper lobe, and large versus small tumors. The optimal number of specimens remains a matter of debate; most authorities recommend five separate deep-coughed fresh early morning samples, but a few studies show little increase in sensitivity beyond three samples. In addition to its relatively low diagnostic yield, sputum cytology lacks the localizing value of a bronchoscopic or transthoracic needle-derived diagnosis of non–small cell lung cancer. For example, a positive sputum cytology for squamous cell cancer in a patient with a peripheral nodule may arise from the peripheral lesion itself, from an unsuspected remote second lesion, or a head and neck primary tumor. Sometimes a sputum cytology specimen is diagnostic of non–small cell lung cancer but no abnormality is apparent on the chest radiograph or upper airway examination. In such cases a meticulous bronchoscopy with segmental sampling may be required to identify an early peripheral lesion. Unfortunately, an advanced tumor is sometimes found in spite of the negative chest film.

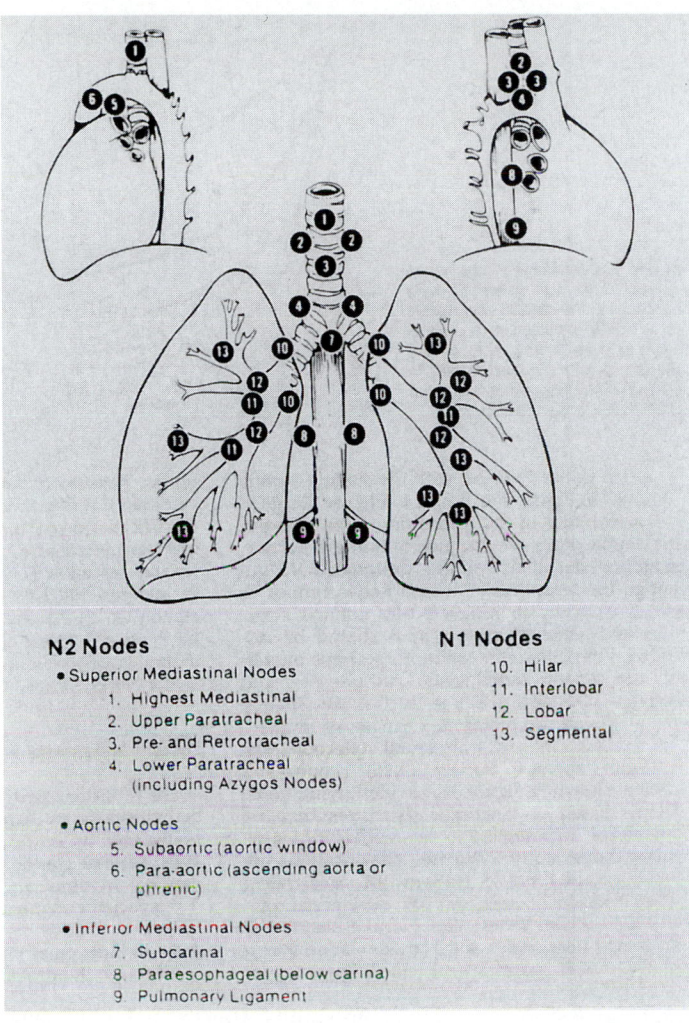

N2 Nodes

- Superior Mediastinal Nodes
  1. Highest Mediastinal
  2. Upper Paratracheal
  3. Pre- and Retrotracheal
  4. Lower Paratracheal (including Azygos Nodes)

- Aortic Nodes
  5. Subaortic (aortic window)
  6. Para-aortic (ascending aorta or phrenic)

- Inferior Mediastinal Nodes
  7. Subcarinal
  8. Paraesophageal (below carina)
  9. Pulmonary Ligament

N1 Nodes

10. Hilar
11. Interlobar
12. Lobar
13. Segmental

FIGURE 112-15   Thoracic lymph node map of the American Joint Committee on Cancer.

Skin and Subcutaneous Metastases

Skin and subcutaneous metastases usually consist of discrete, round, painless nodules with a firm or rubbery consistency. The lesions may be single or multiple, white or discolored, smooth or ulcerated. The most common locations are the chest, back, abdomen, scalp, and neck. The lower extremities are rarely affected, despite their relatively large surface area. Most series suggest a preponderance of undifferentiated cancers, but adenocarcinomas and squamous cell tumors are also well represented. Cutaneous metastases are rarely the first clinical manifestation of non–small cell lung cancer; usually other metastases are evident and the prognosis is extremely poor.[39]

Other Metastatic Sites

Less common metastatic sites for non–small cell lung cancer occasionally pose

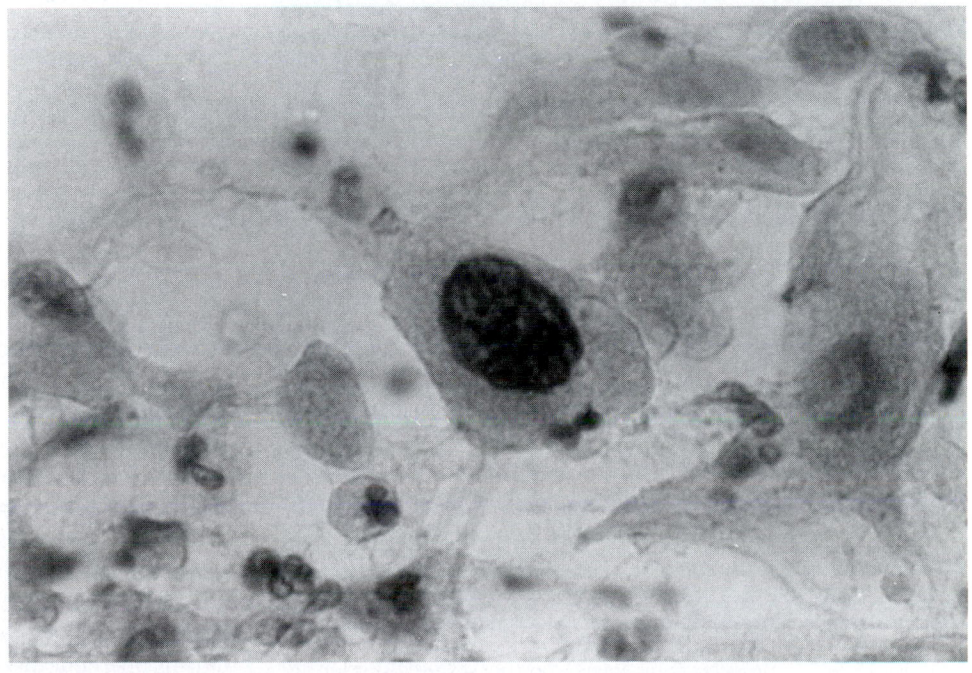

FIGURE 112-16   Sputum cytology diagnostic for non–small cell lung cancer. Note high nucleus-to-cytoplasm ratio, clumped chromatin, and irregular nuclear contour in central malignant cell.

Despite its limitations, sputum cytology may be helpful in diagnosis. Some patients refuse invasive procedures such as bronchoscopy or transthoracic needle biopsy, which have a higher diagnostic yield for non–small cell lung cancer but may prove uncomfortable. Also, patients with suspected non–small cell lung cancer often have important comorbidities, such as ongoing ischemic heart disease or severe COPD with large bullae or marginal ventilation, that render invasive procedures somewhat hazardous. For these subsets of patients, sputum cytology may provide an acceptable, well-tolerated alternative means of diagnosis.

Recently monoclonal antibodies directed against tumor antigens, flow cytometry and quantitative microscopy systems have been developed. These techniques can identify immunologic or DNA alterations ("malignancy-associated changes") in exfoliated bronchial epithelial cells, which may eventually improve the sensitivity of sputum cytology and the prospects for early noninvasive diagnosis of non–small cell lung cancer.

Fiberoptic Bronchoscopy

Fiberoptic bronchoscopy is probably the most frequently utilized and important test for diagnosing non–small cell lung cancer. With its extended visual range, excellent patient acceptance, low complication rate, and high diagnostic yield, fiberoptic bronchoscopy provides a safe and effective means for making the diagnosis. Non–small cell lung cancer may present the endoscopist with a normal endoscopic exam, evidence of distortion and extrinsic compression of a bronchus (Fig. 112-17), or a recognizable true endobronchial lesion (Fig. 112-18). Suspicious endobronchial areas are usually sampled with a series of techniques, including washings, brushings, and forceps biopsy. Many experts perform washings after the brushings and biopsies to increase

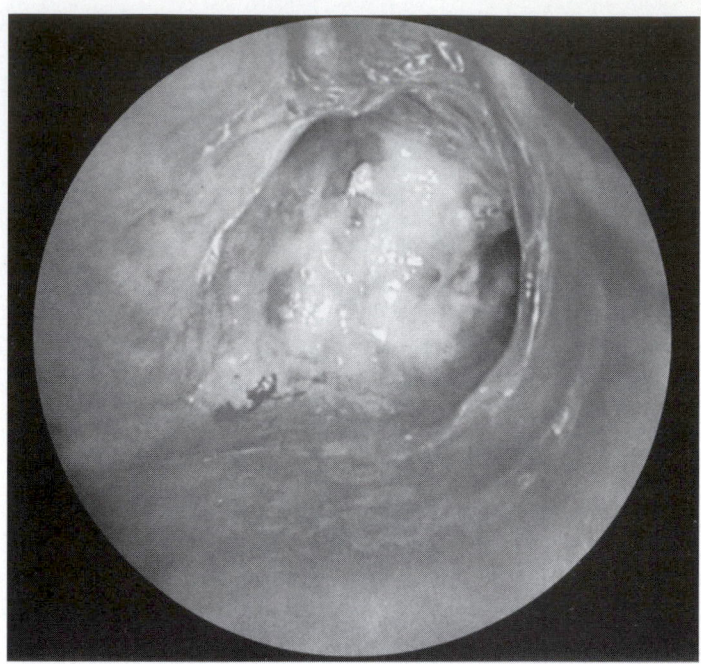

FIGURE 112-18 Bronchoscopic image showing endobronchial component of non–small cell lung cancer. (*From Stradling,*[37] *with permission.*)

cellular yield, while brush biopsy usually precedes forceps biopsy to prevent sheets of red cells from coating the brush. Each of these modalities has an average yield of 50 to 85 percent. Transbronchial needle aspiration is an additional technique of particular value when the tumor is infiltrating deeply beneath intact mucosa or causing bronchial compression. If no endobronchial lesion is apparent, brushings, transbronchial forceps biopsy, and transbronchial needle aspiration contribute to the diagnostic yield, particularly if C-arm or biplanar fluoroscopy is employed. Recently cytologic analysis of bronchoalveolar lavage (BAL) specimens has also been shown to improve the diagnostic yield for peripheral lesions,[8] though the specificity of elevated levels of tumor markers in BAL remains too low for most clinical purposes. Even postbronchoscopy sputum cytology specimens may be uniquely positive in an occasional patient.

The exact diagnostic yield of fiberoptic bronchoscopy in non–small cell lung cancer varies with the skill and persistence of the endoscopist, the cooperation of the patient, the presence of hemoptysis, and myriad technical details. These include the number of passes, availability of fluoroscopy, CT scan demonstration of an adjacent bronchus ("bronchus sign"), and care and expertise in processing, sectioning, and interpreting the bronchoscopic samples. The use of multiple sampling techniques maximized the diagnostic yield in some but not all studies. However, it is agreed that bronchoscopic yield is highly dependent on the size of the tumor. In one series, the yield was only 25 percent for malignant lesions under 2 cm, 40 percent for lesions between 2.0 and 3.0 cm, and 56 percent for those between 3.0 and 4.0 cm.[41] Ironically, very large lesions occasionally displace nearby bronchi, thereby posing unexpected technical difficulties during fiberoptic bronchoscopy. Location is also a prime determinant; for central endobronchial lesions, the overall yield approximates 90 percent, while peripheral lesions are diagnosed in

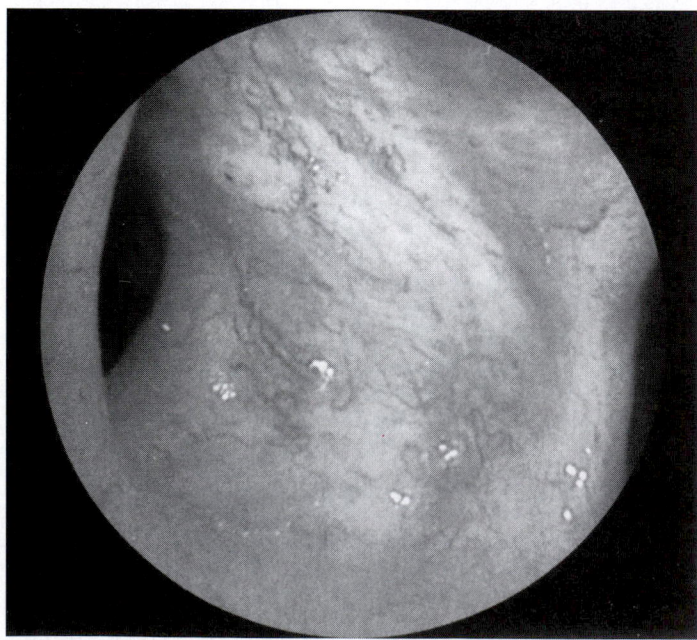

FIGURE 112-17 Bronchoscopic image showing severe distortion and compression of bronchus by submucosal non–small cell lung cancer. (*From Stradling,*[37] *with permission.*)

50 to 60 percent of cases. The optimal number of biopsies probably ranges from three to five for the former, while up to ten biopsies under fluoroscopic guidance have been advocated for the latter.[29,31] Histologic subtype may also affect yield and accuracy. Squamous cell carcinoma is the non–small cell lung cancer most likely to present with a central accessible mass. Adenocarcinomas and large cell cancers are more likely to present with peripheral masses that imply a somewhat lesser bronchoscopic yield. Although fiberoptic bronchoscopy specimens in non–small cell lung cancer are histologically concordant with definitive thoracotomy or autopsy specimens in about 80 percent of cases, small biopsy fragments suggesting undifferentiated large cell carcinoma often pose interpretive problems, including confusion with small cell carcinoma.

In recent years, interest has grown in the use of specialized fiberoptic bronchoscopy techniques to diagnose occult, very early endobronchial non–small cell lung cancer likely to be overlooked during conventional bronchoscopy. Fluorescent drugs such as hematoporphyrin derivative, which are concentrated with greater avidity in malignant versus nonmalignant tissue, have been developed for this purpose. A few days after intravenous injection of the photosensitizing agent, fluorescent bronchoscopy is performed, which allows for identification and biopsy of suspicious areas. Significant drawbacks to this technique, in addition to its limited applicability and availability, include false-positive and false-negative results and photosensitivity for the patient.

Despite its attractive features, fiberoptic bronchoscopy should not be performed in every patient with suspected non–small cell lung cancer. For patients with a small undiagnosed but growing lesion on the chest radiograph, fiberoptic bronchoscopy contributes little in terms of diagnostic yield or staging (see below); such patients can frequently be referred directly to the surgeon for definitive diagnosis and treatment via a single procedure (resection). In addition, patients with inoperable tumors and those with unmistakable clinical evidence of metastatic disease are often best diagnosed via sputum cytology, transthoracic needle biopsy, or other techniques.

Transthoracic Needle Aspiration Biopsy

Transthoracic needle aspiration biopsy (TTNA) is another effective and safe means for diagnosing non–small cell lung cancer. Unlike fiberoptic bronchoscopy, transthoracic needle aspiration is better suited for peripheral cancers, for which the diagnostic yield is maximized and incidence of transthoracic needle aspiration–related pneumothorax is minimized. As with fiberoptic bronchoscopy, the yield is clearly dependent on the size of the tumor. Though overall yields of up to 94

to 100 percent have been reported in selected series, it can be as low as 15 percent for lesions less than 2 cm and about 50 percent for lesions between 2.0 and 3.0 cm. The number of passes, gauge of the needle, and experience of the operator and cytopathologist are also major determinants of success. Cell-type agreement between transthoracic needle aspiration and surgical specimens ranges from 60 to 90 percent, but discordant subtyping within the histologic spectrum of non–small cell lung cancer currently carries little clinical import.

Transthoracic needle aspiration is perhaps most useful for patients with suspected non–small cell lung cancer who cannot tolerate or refuse fiberoptic bronchoscopy and for inoperable patients who require a tissue diagnosis prior to embarking on a course of radiotherapy (Fig. 112-19). Another appropriate subset includes patients who insist on the demonstration of pulmonary malignancy prior to consenting to definitive surgical treatment.

Transthoracic needle aspiration must not be employed indiscriminantly. For a small, peripheral growing lesion in a heavy smoker, it is often prudent to proceed directly to operation rather than attempting a needle biopsy. In such cases a negative biopsy is seldom fully reassuring and surgical excision is still warranted. A positive transthoracic needle aspiration for non–small cell lung cancer also mandates surgery, assuming the patient meets the usual operative criteria. Thus, patient management is not altered by transthoracic needle aspiration and it can be omitted in this setting.

The most important problem with transthoracic needle aspiration for non–small cell lung cancer diagnosis is false-negative results, which occur in up to 30 percent of cases, often related to tumor necrosis and surrounding inflammation. Rare but significant complications that relate to non–small cell lung cancer include false-positive results in 1 to 3 percent of cases and anecdotal reports of chest wall implantation metastases.

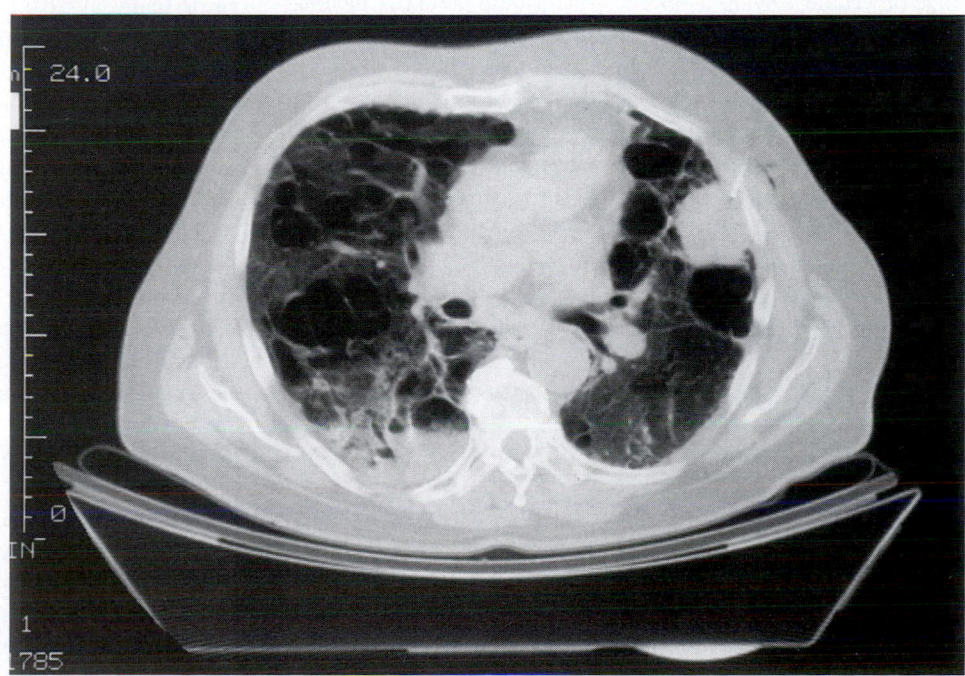

FIGURE 112-19 CT scan showing transthoracic needle aspiration biopsy of peripheral left-sided non–small cell lung cancer in a patient with advanced pulmonary fibrosis.

Thoracic Surgical Procedures

Invasive surgical procedures are sometimes necessary and appropriate to diagnose non–small cell lung cancer. For example, a highly suspicious growing nodule can be approached via thoracoscopy for simultaneous diagnosis and treatment. If a frozen section of the initial thoracoscopic wedge biopsy indicates that the nodule indeed represents non–small cell lung cancer, further surgery can proceed immediately via a variety of techniques. Thoracoscopy is also ideal to diagnose malignant effusions or pleural tumor studding that has eluded diagnosis via thoracentesis and closed pleural biopsy. Also, occasionally an obvious lesion is present, but sputum cytology, bronchoscopy with transbronchial needle aspiration, and/or transthoracic needle biopsy are nondiagnostic, and there is no convenient distant metastatic site for biopsy. If mediastinal involvement is suggested on radiographs, mediastinoscopy, mediastinotomy, or scalene node biopsy may provide the diagnosis with minimal surgical morbidity.[25] Formal thoracotomy with open lung biopsy is rarely required to diagnose non–small cell lung cancer owing to increasing expertise with bronchoscopic and thoracoscopic techniques.

Biopsy of Metastatic Sites

Occasionally the primary lung tumor is small and relatively inaccessible to fiberoptic bronchoscopy and transthoracic needle aspiration, but there is radiographic or clinical evidence of distant metastases. In this setting a tissue diagnosis is usually still required to distinguish non–small cell lung cancer from small cell cancer, provide a firm rationale for radiation therapy or chemotherapy, or yield definitive diagnostic and prognostic information for the patient and his or her family. A direct approach to an accessible metastatic site then becomes a convenient means for establishing the diagnosis and stage (M_1, or stage IV) with a single procedure. Owing to the vast metastatic potential of non–small cell lung cancer, virtually any organ can provide an appropriate target for this approach in a given case. For example, in one study, a 21-gauge needle was used to obtain cytologic material via peripheral lymph node aspiration biopsy with a diagnostic rate of 84 percent.[26] Another convenient target is the skin, since 1 to 12 percent of patients with lung cancer develop cutaneous metastases. Other metastatic sites—including the pleural space, adrenals, bones, brain and liver—may be approached via a variety of percutaneous or operative biopsy techniques to provide definitive evidence of metastatic disease.

Clinical Diagnosis without Biopsy

A small subset of patients refuse all biopsy procedures, and a few others have such advanced non–small cell lung cancer or comorbidities that biopsy procedures pose an excessive or inappropriate risk. In these rare cases, the physician may opt to provide palliative care without a definitive diagnosis. This strategy requires careful consideration of the clinical and radiologic data to ensure that a treatable alternative diagnosis is not being missed. Nevertheless, in one series, objective and subjective palliation was achieved in more than 70 percent of cases treated without a tissue diagnosis.[16]

STAGING

General Considerations

The clinical staging of non–small cell lung cancer is one of the most complex and important topics in thoracic oncology. The stage of non–small cell lung cancer is not only among the most powerful predictors of prognosis (along with weight loss and performance status) but also allows for meaningful comparisons among subsets of patients in terms of clinical characteristics and responses to treatment. Furthermore, the stage of non–small cell lung cancer is a critical determinant upon which individual treatment decisions are predicated.

In 1986, the AJCC substantially revised the TNM system for non–small cell lung cancer to reflect newly appreciated differences in prognostic groups and recent progress in thoracic surgery that enabled curative resection for several localized tumors previously considered unresectable. The new system, reproduced in its entirety in Table 112-2, is the foundation upon which rests much of the current preoperative evaluation of patients with non–small cell lung cancer.[23]

Despite widespread acceptance of the new staging system, several important limitations and controversies should be borne in mind. First, the radiographic tests most commonly used to stage patients clinically are subject to false-positive and false-negative results. For example, nuclear bone scans frequently show areas of increased uptake in ribs and lower vertebral bodies from old rib fractures and osteoarthritis, respectively. These "false-positive" areas must then be pursued with additional studies, such as spot films or MRI exams, to clarify the nature of the underlying abnormality. In addition, most widely utilized imaging modalities are incapable of detecting micrometastatic deposits that do not alter the normal size and shape of a given structure. For example, normal-sized mediastinal nodes, read as "negative" on thoracic CT scans, may harbor tiny metastatic foci in as many as 20 percent of cases, as proven at thoracotomy. Third, while the staging system provides a clinical-anatomic assessment of the extent of disease, it does not take into account other vital patient variables, such as weight loss, performance status, and comorbid diseases that may prove even more important than stage in determining prognosis or treatment options. Fourth, a long-standing controversy continues to rage over the proper utilization of noninvasive staging tests. For instance, should a CT or MRI scan of the head be ordered in all patients being considered for curative surgery for non–small cell lung cancer, or should these be restricted to those with headaches, focal neurologic signs, or other organ-specific clinical features suggesting CNS involvement? Some authors advocate ordering complete metastatic workups for patients with organ-specific or non–organ-specific clinical factors while omitting all scans if these features are absent.[33] Finally, our current staging system makes no allowance for the vast intrinsic biologic variability among non–small cell lung cancers, as detailed elsewhere in this text. It seems likely that "biologic staging" of tumors via their genetic characteristics will assume great importance in the near future.

A difficult question for the clinician is how thoroughly to pursue radiographic abnormalities demonstrated in the course of a staging workup. An otherwise healthy 40-year-old patient with a T1 N0 M0 lesion and a 3-cm unilateral adrenal mass on CT scan might warrant additional adrenal scans, percutaneous adrenal biopsy, or even exploratory abdominal surgery, if necessary, to establish the nature of the adrenal abnormality. Whether the adrenal lesion turns out to be an adenoma or a non–small cell lung cancer metastasis would have a profound impact on stage and treatment. On the other hand, a debilitated 85-year-old patient with a T3 N0 M0 lesion, a Karnovsky score of 60, a 20-kg weight loss, and five defects on liver scan should not be subject to liver biopsy to "prove" that the liver lesions indeed represent metastases; in this setting, characteristic radiographic evidence is considered sufficient to establish the presence of M1 (stage IV) disease. Unfortunately, actual clinical scenarios are rarely so clear-cut; the physician must assemble the available historical, physical exam, laboratory, and radiographic staging data and apply them to the unique personal, philosophical, and medical circumstances of the individual patient and his or her family. The clinician's judgment becomes a critical element in such cases.

Thoracic Staging

COMPUTED TOMOGRAPHY OF THE CHEST

Computed tomography of the chest is perhaps the most frequently ordered and informative radiographic staging tool in non–small cell lung cancer. In addition to a detailed image of the primary tumor and its anatomic relationship to other intrathoracic structures, the CT scan provides important information regarding the size of the mediastinal lymph nodes, the presence of other parenchymal lesions, and the status of the pleural space, thereby greatly facilitating the clinical staging of a given patient. When an intravenous contrast bolus is used in conjunction with the CT scan, differentiation of mediastinal adenopathy from normal vascular structures may be further clarified. Also, CT scans allow more accurate mediastinal lymph node sampling during subsequent transbronchial needle aspiration or mediastinoscopy.

TABLE 112-2

Staging of Lung Cancer: 1986 American Joint Committee on Cancer System

Primary tumor (T)

TX   Tumor proven by the presence of malignant cells in bronchopulmonary secretions but not visualized roentgenographically or bronchoscopically, or any tumor that cannot be assessed, as in a retreatment staging.

TO   No evidence of primary tumor.

TIS   Carcinoma in situ.

T1   A tumor that is 3.0 cm or less in greatest dimension surrounded by lung or visceral pleura, and without evidence of invasion proximal to a lobar bronchus at bronchoscopy.[a]

T2   A tumor more than 3.0 cm in greatest dimension; or a tumor of any size that either invades the visceral pleura or has associated atelectasis or obstructive pneumonitis extending to the hilar region. At bronchoscopy, the proximal extent of demonstrable tumor must be within a lobar bronchus or at least 2.0 cm distal to the carina. Any associated atelectasis or obstructive pneumonitis must involve less than an entire lung.

T3   A tumor of any size with direct extension into the chest wall (including superior sulcus tumors), diaphragm, or the mediastinal pleura or pericardium without involving the heart, great vessels, trachea, esophagus, or vertebral bodies; or a tumor in the main bronchus within 2 cm of the carina without involving the carina.

T4   A tumor of any size with invasion of the mediastinum or involving heart, great vessels, trachea, esophagus, vertebral bodies or carina; or with the presence of malignant pleural effusion.[b]

Nodal involvement (N)

N0   No demonstrable metastasis to regional lymph nodes.

N1   Metastasis to lymph nodes in the peribronchial or the ipsilateral hilar region, or both, including direct extension.

N2   Metastasis to ipsilateral mediastinal lymph nodes and subcarinal lymph nodes.

N3   Metastasis to contralateral mediastinal lymph nodes, contralateral hilar lymph nodes, ipsilateral or contralateral scalene or supraclavicular lymph nodes.

Distant metastasis (M)

M0   No (known) distant metastasis.

M1   Distant metastasis present; specify site(s).

Stage Grouping

Occult carcinoma	TX	N0	M0
Stage 0	TIS	Carcinoma in situ	
Stage I	T1	N0	M0
	T2	N0	M0
Stage II	T1	N1	M0
	T2	N1	M0
Stage IIIa	T3	N0	M0
	T3	N1	M0
	T1–3	N2	M0
Stage IIIb	Any T	N3	M0
	T4	Any N	M0
Stage IV	Any T	Any N	M1

[a]The uncommon superficial tumor of any size with its invasive component limited to the bronchial wall, which may extend proximal to the main bronchus, is classified as T1.

[b]Most pleural effusions associated with lung cancer are due to tumor. There are, however, some few patients in whom cytopathologic examination of pleural fluid (on more than one specimen) is negative for tumor, and the fluid is not bloody and is not an exudate. In such cases where these elements and clinical judgement dictate that the effusion is not related to the tumor, the patients should be staged T1, T2, or T3, excluding effusion as a staging element.

However, despite its safety and utility, a number of limitations pertain to the use of CT scanning as a staging test in non–small cell lung cancer. The accuracy of CT scanning of the mediastinum depends on the site of the lymph node involvement, the extent of lymph node dissection at the time of thoracotomy, technical details such as the type of scanner and spacing interval between cuts, and the patient population being studied. The inability of the CT scan to detect micrometastases has already been alluded to; it is equally important to note that enlarged inflammatory nodes are erroneously categorized as "positive" in as many as 20 percent of cases. Thus, the specificity and sensitivity of CT sans in detecting metastatic involvement of mediastinal nodes are probably in the range of 70 to 80 percent. Furthermore, the CT scan does not always clearly differentiate stage IIIa from stage IIIb nodes and probably contributes no useful staging information in T1 N0 M0 cases as assessed by clinical exam and chest radiograph. The CT scan is inferior to the MRI in staging apical lung tumors and inferior to fiberoptic bronchoscopy in identifying the extent of endobronchial abnormalities, though the newer helical scanners and software allowing 3D reconstruction and "virtual" bronchoscopy may change that. Finally, CT cannot reliably identify chest wall invasion, or distinguish resectable from unresectable invasion of the mediastinum or vertebral body except in advanced cases. A few experts even advocate a complete abandonment of CT scanning as a staging modality in non–small cell lung cancer, preferring to proceed directly from the chest radiograph to invasive procedures to definitively stage the mediastinum.[5]

MAGNETIC RESONANCE IMAGING OF THE CHEST

Initially it was hoped that MRI, by demonstrating divergent T1- and T2-weighted images for tumor-involved lymph nodes versus fat and fibrosis, would allow a clear separation of tumor-bearing nodes from benign mediastinal nodes. Unfortunately, signal characteristics overlap extensively, and size remains the sole criterion for MRI-defined mediastinal nodal involvement. Thus, MRI is subject to many of the same limitations described for CT scans, especially the tendency to miss small tumor-bearing nodes, in addition to its poorer spatial resolution characteristics. In fact, several studies have shown that MRI and CT scans are roughly equivalent for detecting mediastinal nodal involvement.[14] Therefore, MRI cannot be endorsed for routine use for thoracic staging of non–small cell lung cancer.

Most prospective studies comparing thoracic CT scans and MRI in terms of other staging applications have also failed to reveal a clear advantage for either study. However, MRI can sometimes provide useful staging data and is the imaging modality of choice for apical (superior sulcus) lung tumors. For these lesions, the coronal and sagittal planar images obtainable by MRI more clearly delineate invasion into chest wall, vertebral body, subclavian vessels, and brachial plexus. Vertebral body involvement and invasion of neural foramina is much more clearly delineated on MRI than on CT, and MRI should always be performed when a primary tumor is in close proximity to vertebral body on CT scan.

BRONCHOSCOPY

A thorough inspection of the upper airway, vocal cords, trachea, and bronchi down to the subsegmental level is warranted in all patients for whom curative surgery is planned. Bronchoscopic staging is usually performed via fiberoptic bronchoscopy as a separate preoperative procedure along with attempts at diagnosis, but it can also be performed by the thoracic surgeon in the operating room just prior to beginning the actual resection. The discovery of a paralyzed vocal cord, unsuspected remote second neoplastic focus, main carinal involvement, or proximal extension may radically alter the stage or therapeutic approach to a given patient. Such findings are associated with the presence of a sizable proximal primary lesion; in one recent study the yield for fiberoptic bronchoscopy staging was nil if the primary lesion was a small, asymptomatic, solitary nodule.[15]

Another important component of bronchoscopic staging of non–small cell lung cancer has emerged in recent years—the use of transbronchial needle aspiration to stage the mediastinum. This remarkably safe modality is easily performed during the course of a diagnostic fiberoptic bronchoscopy when the question of mediastinal spread of tumor is raised. Transbronchial needle aspiration in this setting should be performed prior to other sampling modalities to avoid contamination of a purported mediastinal sample with sloughed endobronchial tumor cells. In the hands of a few experts who helped to develop and promulgate this technique, the sensitivity of transbronchial needle aspiration for mediastinal tumor has been reported to approach 75 to 90 percent, especially when a prebronchoscopy CT scan is used to guide the procedure.[42] Others have cited yields of 21 to 48 percent, depending on attention to several technical details. Problems with this staging technique include limited applicability to lesions within 1.3 to 1.5 cm of the tracheobronchial tree, frequent false negatives due to technical factors, and rare false positives, which could erroneously and tragically misclassify a curable patient as incurable. Most practitioners opine that a positive transbronchial needle aspiration implies sufficient mediastinal disease to exclude a patient from aggressive surgical therapy. Thus, transbronchial needle aspiration may spare unnecessary mediastinoscopies and thoracotomies in roughly half of those eventually found to be inoperable due to mediastinal spread.

TRANSTHORACIC NEEDLE ASPIRATION BIOPSY

On occasion, transthoracic needle aspiration is useful as a staging procedure to document the presence of mediastinal metastases in non–small cell lung cancer. This clinical strategy is most appropriate for poor or borderline surgical candidates with suggestive evidence of mediastinal spread on radiographs but a negative transbronchial needle aspiration. In others, mediastinoscopy might pose a substantial risk due to active comorbid diseases or prior mediastinal surgery or scarring. In such patients, transthoracic needle aspiration provides a better-tolerated and less costly means of establishing the presence of mediastinal spread, which may effectively exclude a borderline patient from an aggressive surgical approach. Transthoracic needle aspiration can be applied to lesions in all three mediastinal compartments (including the problematic AJCC areas 5 and 6) or the hilus and has been reported to achieve a diagnostic yield of up to 94 percent in this setting. However, transthoracic needle aspiration cannot be used for staging when there is no radiographic evidence of mediastinal spread.

SURGICAL STAGING

Perhaps no topic related to non–small cell lung cancer engenders more controversy or a greater variation in clinical practice than the use of surgical procedures to invasively stage intrathoracic tumor, especially with regard to mediastinal involvement. In general, invasive staging is reserved for cases in which definitive assessment of mediastinal lymph node involvement will affect management, specifically whether to proceed with thoracotomy. Thus, the decision to employ surgical staging usually implies that the patient is free of distant metastases and consents to thoracotomy if surgical staging procedures are negative.

A variety of techniques may be utilized, including mediastinoscopy, anterior mediastinotomy, thoracoscopy, and thoracotomy, depending on local expertise and the exact anatomic sites to be sampled. Mediastinoscopy entails a small cervical incision that provides access to superior mediastinal nodes at levels 2, 4, 7 and 10. For left-upper-lobe tumors, levels 5 and 6 can be assessed via an extended cervical mediastinoscopy, or, more commonly, via a small anterior left parasternal mediastinotomy incision.[25] Video thoracoscopy may also be used to sample lymph nodes in the aortopulmonary window (levels 5 and 6) and posterior subcarinal location. Finally, thoracotomy itself can be viewed as a final staging modality that allows maximum access to mediastinal lymph node stations and definitive assessment of contiguous intrathoracic extension.

Variability in utilizing surgical staging procedures relates to the tendency of non–small cell lung cancer to skip nodal areas, and the superiority of complete lymph node dissection compared to visual assessment and selective lymph node sampling. Also, there are divergent opinions as to whether surgical staging should be performed as a preliminary, separate procedure, or, if negative frozen sections are reported, combined with thoracotomy. More profound discrepancies in surgical practice derive from continuing uncertainty regarding the prognostic implications of mediastinal node involvement. For example, those who regard *any* mediastinal nodal involvement as a contraindication to surgical cure frequently employ mediastinoscopy to document incurability, particularly with central lesions or poorly differentiated adenocarcinomas. Others believe that selected patients with certain single-station, intracapsular, or radiologically inapparent mediastinal metastases have significant long-term survival when complete resection is achieved. These practitioners may omit mediastinoscopy and proceed directly to thoracotomy if preoperative chest radiographs or CT scans do not suggest mediastinal nodal enlargement. Invasive staging of the mediastinum is also valuable in identifying patients for entry into clinical studies investigating the role of neoadjuvant therapy for non–small cell lung cancer with mediastinal lymph node involvement.

Extrathoracic Staging

ADRENAL GLANDS AND LIVER

Because of frequent occult metastases to the adrenal glands, thoracic CT scans, when ordered to stage non–small cell lung cancer, are routinely extended caudally to include them. Since 2 to 9 percent of the general population harbors incidental adrenal adenomas, the appearance of a unilateral adrenal mass on a staging CT scan for non–small cell lung cancer poses a common and thorny problem. Still, a few guidelines may be helpful in such cases. First, adrenal metastases are associated with organ-specific and non–organ-specific clinical findings that correlate with metastatic disease in general.[32] Second, although the shape and homogeneity of adrenal lesions may be nonspecific, size does have some predictive value, in that lesions greater than 3 cm are more likely to represent metastatic disease. Third, additional scanning techniques, such as MRI or ^{131}I-6-betaiodomethylnorcholesterol scintigraphy, may clarify the issue by demonstrating fat or cholesterol accumulation in benign adenomas.[17] Even a repeat CT scan after a few weeks to evaluate a given lesion for growth may be helpful. However, in the final analysis, needle or open biopsy may be necessary to resolve difficult cases.

Liver imaging is also a standard component of extrathoracic staging of non–small cell lung cancer, and CT scans, ultrasonography, and MRI may be employed for this purpose. Computed tomography, currently the favored modality, suggest metastatic foci in liver in a highly variable percentage of patients, depending on the presence or absence of clinical indicators suggesting metastatic disease. In one series of non–small cell lung cancer patients lacking clinical signs or symptoms, only 3 percent demonstrated evidence of hepatic metastases on CT scanning. Unfortunately, single or multiple liver defects on CT scans may also result from cysts, abscesses, hemangiomas, etc. Hepatic CT scans can also be falsely negative in the case of diffuse "isodense" metastatic involvement. Though difficult cases may be resolved with additional ultrasound or MRI studies, percutaneous or peritoneoscopic liver biopsy is sometimes necessary.

CENTRAL NERVOUS SYSTEM (BRAIN)

Computed tomography, particularly when combined with contrast enhancement, has emerged as the most widely utilized means for demonstrating metastatic CNS deposits (Fig. 112-20). Clinical findings specific to the CNS, such as headache and focal neurologic signs, were associated with an abnormal CT scan of the brain in 56 percent of cases in one series, while 15.5 percent of the scans were positive if only non–organ-specific features were present. Other investigators have found that up to 10 percent of patients harbor brain metastases in the absence of all clinical factors.[12] This finding, coupled with the usual futility of attempting curative thoracic surgery in the presence of brain metastases (with few exceptions), has led some clinicians to obtain a brain CT scan in virtually all patients with non–small cell lung cancer. Notable limitations of CT scanning of the brain include relatively poor visualization of the brainstem and occasional false-positive results, especially when only a single lesion

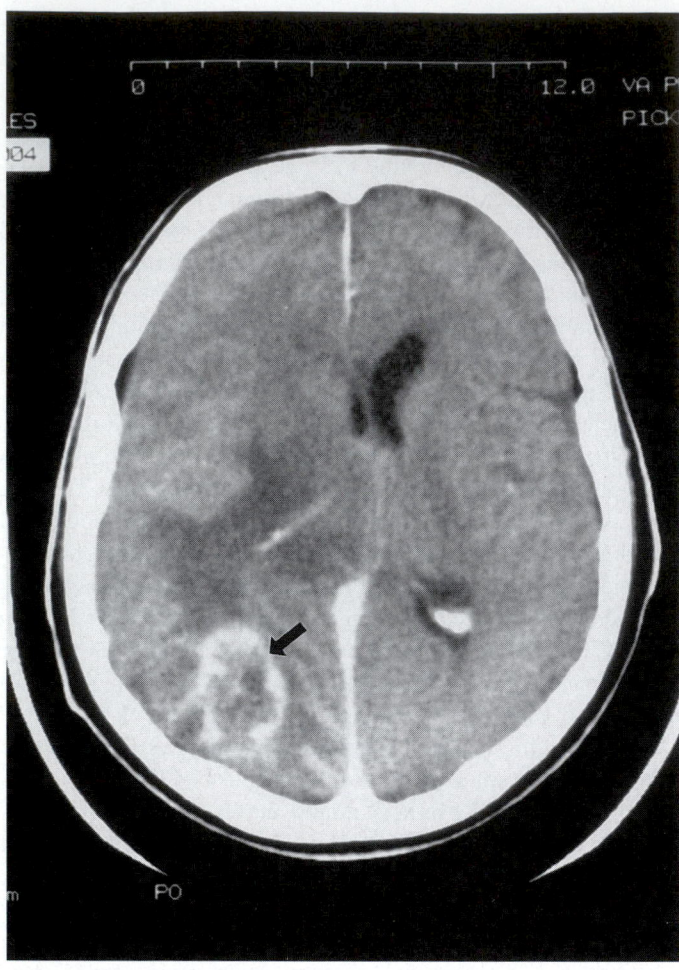

FIGURE 112-20   CT scan of brain showing solitary posterior metastasis *(arrow)* from non–small cell lung cancer. Note rim enhancement and adjacent low attenuation edema.

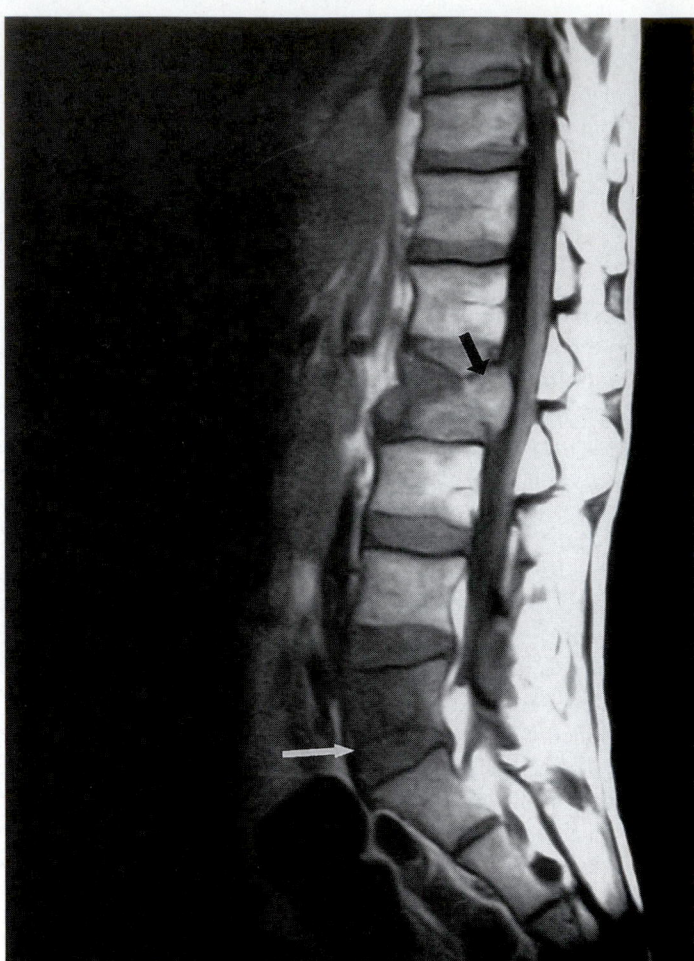

FIGURE 112-21   Metastatic non–small cell lung cancer replacing L5 vertebral body *(white arrow)* and compressing spinal cord at L2 level *(black arrow)* shown by T1-weighted MRI.

is found. In one well-publicized study of mostly non–small cell lung cancer patients with solitary lesions on brain CT, 11 percent were shown at craniotomy to harbor a variety of inflammatory or infectious lesions or primary brain tumors.[24] A CT scan showing multiple ring-enhancing lesions has a higher positive predictive value and provides a more reliable basis for establishing clinical M1 status.

There are excellent data to suggest that MRI of the brain, especially when combined with gadolinium-based contrast infusion, is more sensitive than CT for the detection of metastatic disease, particularly in delineating small lesions.[6] Whether these improvements translate into worthwhile patient benefit in terms of outcome is not known. Nevertheless, some centers routinely employ MRI for CNS staging, while others utilize MRI mainly as a problem-solving technique when the CT scan is equivocal. Also, MRI has rapidly become the imaging modality of choice for epidural spinal metastases (Fig. 112-21).

SKELETAL SYSTEM

The staging of the skeletal system is probably least satisfactory among the major extrathoracic sites in non–small cell lung cancer. The standard test is currently the technetium-99m radionuclide scan. Unfortunately, as alluded to previously, skeletal uptake of this isotope is quite nonspecific, and degenerative vertebral changes and old traumatic rib foci produce false-positive scans in up to 40 percent of cases. A second problem lies in correlating the bone scan with clinical features suggesting metastases. Most authors advocate bone scans only when organ-specific or non–organ-specific features suggesting metastases are present; this view was supported by a recent meta-analysis showing an 89 percent negative predictive value for the usual clinical survey in terms of bone metastases.[33] However, a few studies have demonstrated true-positive bone scans in up to 15 percent of cases with completely negative clinical profiles, suggesting that bone scans should be ordered in nearly all cases. A third difficulty is derived from the need for radiographic or histologic proof that a given area of radionuclide uptake truly represents a metastatic deposit. Depending on the clinical scenario, spot skeletal films, MRI, or an open biopsy may be appropriate. Alternatively, the case for metastatic disease may rest solely on the bone scan, especially in poor surgical candidates with multiple characteristic scan abnormalities (Fig. 112-22).

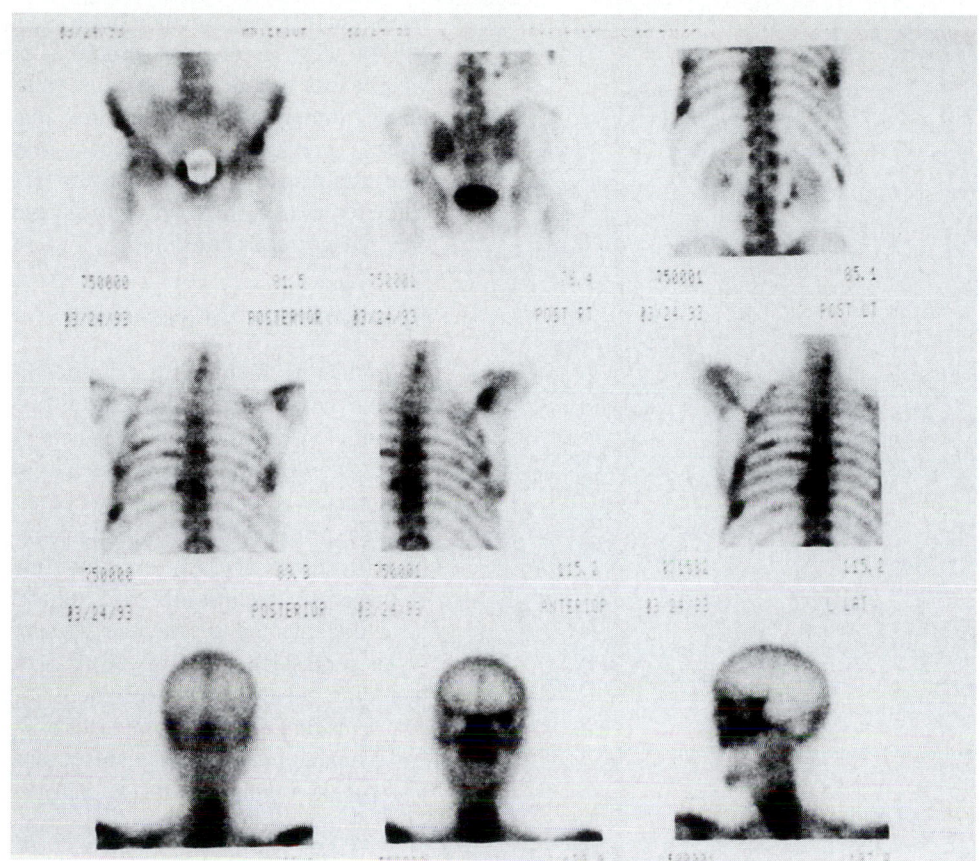

FIGURE 112-22   Radionuclide bone scan showing numerous characteristic areas of abnormal uptake in ribs, spine, skull, and other sites due to metastatic lung cancer.

NATURAL HISTORY

The natural history of non–small cell lung cancer is especially important to consider for the occasional patient who desires no treatment for lung cancer once a diagnosis is made. It is helpful to know the patient's feelings regarding treatment prior to pursuing a diagnostic procedure; if the patient early on expresses a desire for no treatment, how far one should proceed in establishing a tissue diagnosis is questionable. If only a simple procedure with minimal risk of morbidity is required, it should be done, since this allows for a discussion with the patient regarding expectations and prognosis. The patient must be informed that even though there may be no symptoms currently, with time, symptoms usually develop. The nature of the symptoms and the amount of time that elapses before they become apparent are dependent on the location and size of the primary tumor as well as involvement of mediastinal lymph nodes. Local effects of concern include pain from chest wall involvement, postobstructive pneumonitis from tumor obstructing an airway, hoarseness with difficulty swallowing due to recurrent laryngeal nerve involvement, superior vena cava syndrome with resultant facial edema, and dyspnea from either parenchymal consolidation or pleural effusion. Metastatic disease may warrant palliative measures, such as radiotherapy for bone pain, which must be considered in light of an even greater curtailment in life expectancy. Patients who opt for no treatment should be followed closely so that in-

tervention to relieve symptoms may begin promptly if the patient wishes to confine treatment only to symptom management.

Growth of the Primary Tumor

The primary tumor mass in non–small cell lung cancer is thought to comprise a heterogeneous, dynamic aggregate of rapidly dividing neoplastic cells, resting cells, necrotic areas, and stromal elements. Some tumors appear to grow at an exponential rate throughout most or all of their natural history, beginning with a single cell measuring 10 to 25 μm. This model predicts that 30 doublings are required to form a 1-cm nodule detectable on the chest radiograph, while 40 doublings would constitute a lethal burden of 10^{12} cells.[13] The exponential model, coupled with observed volumetric doubling times that range widely from 30 to 490 days, implies that most tumors have been present for years, even decades prior to clinical diagnosis. Further analyses suggest the presence of two subsets of lung cancer, one showing very rapid and the other much slower doubling times.

However, other data conflict with the uniform exponential growth model. Some untreated tumors seem to change growth rates when multiple serial radiographs are compared. Often the pattern corresponds to Gompertzian kinetics (i.e., an exponential growth rate that progressively decreases). The latter phase reflects a decrease in growth fraction and an increase in spontaneous cell death, perhaps secondary to an outstripped blood supply. The Gompertzian curve predicts that most cancers originate within 2 years or less of detection.

From a histologic standpoint, primary non–small cell lung cancer is believed to evolve from initial hyperplasia and disorganization of the basal cell layer of bronchial epithelium. This is followed by progressive squamous metaplasia with increasing cellular atypia, carcinoma in situ, microinvasion, and finally frank invasive carcinoma. The exact point when histologic changes result in an irreversible, progressive tumor is unclear. However, many authorities recommend resection of in situ carcinomas, even though tumors are thought incapable of metastasizing during this phase (Fig. 112-23). Once the tumor becomes locally invasive, it can displace, compress, and destroy adjacent lung tissue and contiguous thoracic structures.

Tumor Dissemination

Non–small cell lung cancer appears to disseminate via several routes, the mechanisms of which remain poorly understood. Pre-

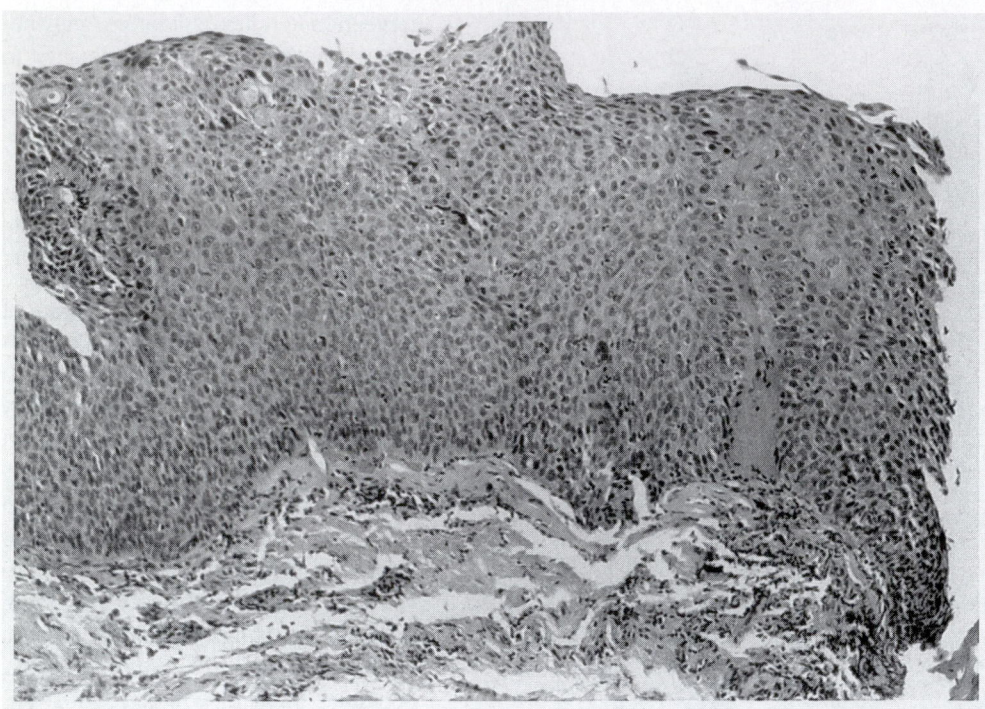

FIGURE 112-23 Endobronchial biopsy showing carcinoma in situ. Note intact basement membrane and maturation arrest.

factors such as performance status, age, and the presence of chest symptoms or weight loss are also of obvious prognostic importance; these were discussed previously. Additional, less well-established host influences include female sex (better prognosis) and anergy (worse prognosis).

Spontaneous Regression

A fascinating footnote that further illustrates variability in the natural history of non–small cell lung cancer is the extraordinarily rare occurrence of spontaneous regression. In some cases, modest shrinkage is noted, perhaps related to tumor necrosis or infarction. However, a handful of case reports have documented spectacular spontaneous regression of advanced tumors, including cases with proven mediastinal invasion or adrenal metastases.[35] Unfortunately, the mechanism of this phenomenon is unknown.

sumably multiple genetic changes accrue, and new clones of malignant cells arise with enhanced metastatic potential. Interestingly, metastases often seem to grow even faster than the primary tumor. Tumor cells invade the interstitial space and thereby gain access to submucosal lymphatics and eventually the systemic circulation. Alternatively, the tumor directly invades arterial and venous channels or disseminates in accordance with its own microvessel density. Peribronchial lymphatic involvement can proceed centrally to the hilar and mediastinal nodes or peripherally to the pleura. Also, diffuse bronchoalveolar cell carcinoma may spread endobronchially to seed remote areas of lung.

Other Influences

A vast array of intrinsic genetic and molecular biologic tumor characteristics influences the natural history of non–small cell lung cancer; these are discussed in Chapter 107. Significant impact on natural history and prognosis can be ascribed to a multitude of other tumor characteristics. For example, squamous cell tumors are more often localized to the thorax compared with adenocarcinomas and large cell tumors. The TNM stage correlates well with prognosis, though this is somewhat circular reasoning, since the TNM criteria evolved from follow-up studies. In one study of untreated patients with non–small cell lung cancer, the presence of lymph node metastases was the single best prognostic determinant.[40] Also, rapid doubling times, elevated serum tumor markers, the presence of giant cells, tumor cells in pulmonary venous blood, and high histologic grade have been correlated to a variable extent with a poor prognosis. Major host

REFERENCES

1. Ahmann FR: A reassessment of the clinical implications of the superior vena cava syndrome. *J Clin Oncol* 2:961–969, 1984.
2. Barsky SH, Cameron R, Osann KE, et al: Rising incidence of bronchioloalveolar lung carcinoma and its unique clinicopathologic features. *Cancer* 73:1163–1170, 1994.
3. Berlin NI, Buncher CR, Fontana RS, et al: The National Cancer Institute cooperative early lung cancer detection program: Results of the initial screen. *Am Rev Resp Dis* 130:545–549, 1984.
4. Chin R Jr, Ward K, Keyes JW Jr, et al: Mediastinal staging of non–small lung cancer with positron emission tomography. *Am J Respir Crit Care Med* 152:2090–2096, 1995.
5. Colice GL: Chest CT for known or suspected lung cancer. *Chest* 106:1538–1550, 1994.
6. Davis PC, Hudgins PA, Peterman SB, Hoffman JC Jr: Diagnosis of cerebral metastases: Double-dose delayed CT vs. contrast-enhanced MR imaging. *AJR* 156:1039–1046, 1991.
7. Decker DA, Dines DE, Payne WS, et al: The significance of a cytologically negative pleural effusion in bronchogenic carcinoma. *Chest* 74:640–642, 1978.
8. DeGracia J, Bravo C, Miravitlles M, et al: Diagnostic value of bronchoalveolar lavage in peripheral lung cancer. *Am Rev Respir Dis* 147:649–652, 1993.
9. Eddy DM: Screening for lung cancer. *Ann Intern Med* 111:232–237, 1989.
10. Edwards CW: Alveolar carcinoma: A review. *Thorax* 39:166–174, 1984.
11. Ferguson MK: Synchronous primary lung cancers. *Chest* 103:398S–400S, 1993.
12. Ferrigno D, Buccheri G: Cranial computed tomography as a part of the initial staging procedures for patients with non–small cell lung cancer. *Chest* 106:1025–1029, 1994.

13. Geddes DM: The natural history of lung cancer: A review based on rates of tumour growth. *Br J Dis Chest* 73:1–17, 1979.

14. Glover FL: The role of CT and MRI in staging of the mediastinum. *Chest* 106:391S–396S, 1994.

15. Goldberg SK, Walkenstein MD, Steinbach A, Aranson R: The role of bronchoscopy in the preoperative assessment of a solitary pulmonary nodule. *Chest* 104:94–97, 1993.

16. Green N, Melbye RW, Kern W: Radiotherapy for suspected lung cancer not proved by tissue diagnosis. *Chest* 64:476–479, 1973.

17. Gross MD, Shapiro B, Bouffard JA, et al: Distinguishing benign from malignant euadrenal masses. *Ann Intern Med* 109:613–618, 1988.

18. Huang M-S, Kato H, Konaka C, et al: Quantitative cytochemical differences between young and old patients with lung cancer. *Chest* 88:864–869, 1985.

19. Kirtland SH, Winterbauer RH, Dreis DF, et al: A clinical profile of chronic bacterial pneumonia—A report of 115 cases. *Chest* 106:15–22, 1994.

20. Liaw Y-S, Yang P-C, Wu Z-G, et al: The bacteriology of obstructive pneumonitis: A prospective study using ultrasound guided transthoracic needle aspiration. *Am J Respir Crit Care Med* 149:1648–1653, 1994.

21. Miller RR, McGregor DH: Hemorrhage from carcinoma of the lung. *Cancer* 46:200–205, 1980.

22. Miller WT, Wiot JF (ed): Carcinoma of the lung. *Semin Roentgenol* 25:1–124, 1990.

23. Mountain C: The new international staging system for lung cancer. *Surg Clin North Am* 67:925–935, 1987.

24. Patchell RA, Tibbs PA, Walsh JW, et al: A randomized trial of surgery in the treatment of single metastases to the brain. *New Engl J Med* 322:494–500, 1990.

25. Patterson GA: Surgical techniques in the diagnosis of lung cancer. *Chest* 101:523–526, 1991.

26. Phillips MS, Barker V: Extrathoracic lymph node aspiration in bronchial carcinoma. *Thorax* 40:398, 1985.

27. Piehler JM, Pairolero PC, Gracey DR, Bernatz PE: Unexplained diaphragmatic paralysis: A harbinger of malignant disease? *J Thorac Cardiovasc Surg* 84:861–864, 1982.

28. Poe RH, Israel RH, Utell MJ, Hall WJ: Chronic cough: Bronchoscopy or pulmonary function testing? *Am Rev Respir Dis* 128:160–162, 1982.

29. Popovich J Jr, Kvale PA, Eichenhorn MS, et al: Diagnostic accuracy of multiple biopsies from flexible fiberoptic bronchoscopy: A comparison of central versus peripheral carcinoma. *Am Rev Respir Dis* 125:521–523, 1982.

30. Sahn SA: The pleura: State of the art. *Am Rev Respir Dis* 138:184–234, 1988.

31. Shure D, Astarita RW: Bronchogenic carcinoma presenting as an endobronchial mass: Optimal number of biopsy specimens for diagnosis. *Chest* 83:865–867, 1983.

32. Silvestri GA, Lenz JE, Harper SN, et al: The relationship of clinical findings to CT scan evidence of adrenal gland metastases in the staging of bronchogenic carcinoma. *Chest* 102:1748–1751, 1992.

33. Silvestri GA, Littenberg B, Colice GL: The clinical evaluation for detecting lung cancer—A meta-analysis. *Am J Respir Crit Care Med* 152:225–230, 1995.

34. Soares FA, Pinto APFE, Landell GAM, de Oliveira JAM: Pulmonary tumor embolism to arterial vessels and carcinomatous lymphangitis: A comparative clinicopathological study. *Arch Pathol Lab Med* 117:827–831, 1993.

35. Sperduto P, Vaezy A, Bridgman A, Wilkie L: Spontaneous regression of squamous cell lung carcinoma with adrenal metastases. *Chest* 94:887–889, 1988.

36. Steinhauslin CA, Cuttat JF: Spontaneous pneumothorax—A complication of lung cancer. *Chest* 88:709–713, 1985.

37. Stradling P: *Diagnostic Bronchoscopy—A Teaching Manual,* 6th ed. Edinburgh, Churchill Livingstone, 1991.

38. Straus MJ (ed): *Lung Cancer—Clinical Diagnosis and Treatment,* 2d ed. New York, Grune & Stratton, 1983.

39. Terashima T, Kanazawa M: Lung cancer with skin metastases. *Chest* 106:1448–1450, 1994.

40. Vrdoljak E, Mise K, Sapunar D, et al: Survival analysis of untreated patients with non–small cell lung cancer. *Chest* 106:1797–1800, 1994.

41. Wallace JM, Deutsch AL: Flexible fiberoptic bronchoscopy and percutaneous needle lung aspiration for evaluating the solitary pulmonary nodule. *Chest* 81:665–671, 1982.

42. Wang K-P, Terry PB: Transbronchial needle aspiration in the diagnosis and staging of bronchogenic carcinoma. *Am Rev Respir Dis* 127:344–347, 1983.

43. Watanabe Y, Shimizu J, Tsubota M, Iwa T: Mediastinal spread of metastatic lymph nodes in bronchogenic carcinoma: Mediastinal nodal metastases in lung cancer. *Chest* 97:1059–1065, 1990.

PART I: TREATMENT OF NON–SMALL CELL LUNG CANCER: SURGICAL

Larry R. Kaiser

Lung cancer is a clinical problem of the twentieth century, having been virtually unrecognized until the early part of this century. It is a disease for which the cause is known in the majority of cases yet despite that knowledge the incidence in women continues to rise while it has leveled off for men. Thus it is both a travesty and an indictment against us as a society that lung cancer is the leading cause of death from cancer in both men and women despite our knowing that cigarette smoking causes the disease. The treatment of lung cancer has evolved from a single modality, surgery, to a multimodality approach that calls upon the skills of numerous specialists. Not many years ago an operation was all that could be offered to a patient, and it has taken a considerable amount of time to recognize that not only is an operation not for everyone but that it may be contraindicated in many situations. It has remained for students of the disease—surgeons, medical and radiation oncologists—to define the role that surgery should play in the modern management of lung cancer. Surgery was and is the cornerstone of management in this disease, and surgeons continue to assume a lead role in the diagnosis and treatment of patients with lung cancer.

DIAGNOSIS

It is illustrative to consider the route taken by most patients prior to being referred to a surgeon and the qualifications that the surgeon should ideally possess to contribute optimally to the management of the patient with lung cancer. Patients with lung cancer either present with symptoms or are found inadvertently to have an abnormal chest radiograph when the film has been done for some other reason. The symptomatic patient sees his or her primary care physician who may initiate further evaluation or more likely refer the patient to a pulmonary physician. Rarely is a patient referred directly to the surgical specialist for evaluation of an abnormal chest radiograph, although this does occur with greater frequency in certain communities. From the surgeon's viewpoint how should a patient with a presumed lung cancer be evaluated? How likely is it for a given patient to have a lung cancer? We look at smokers differently than we look at nonsmokers when evaluating an abnormal chest radiograph. Certainly lung cancer is seen in nonsmokers, but we are much less suspicious in this group than in smokers where an abnormal chest radiograph is lung cancer until proven otherwise. If a previous chest radiograph is available, the first move should be to compare it with the current film. A lesion present on a previous film markedly diminishes, though does not eliminate, the probability that the current finding represents a lung cancer.

The Symptomatic Patient

Patients present with symptoms either referable to the chest or related to the presence of metastatic disease. The initial evaluation should be directed toward an explanation of the symptoms. A complete discussion of the clinical presentation is available in Chapter 112. Patients with evidence of metastatic disease still require a tissue diagnosis. The method employed to obtain the tissue diagnosis should have the highest probability of success. Whereas bronchoscopy has a high likelihood of yielding a diagnosis in the patient who presents with cough or hemoptysis, it is less likely to be successful where the lung findings are confined to multiple small nodules. Often transthoracic needle biopsy may have the highest yield, and bronchoscopy is not required. Where a patient presents with presumed metastatic disease that is accessible, such as a palpable supraclavicular lymph node, a needle aspirate, done in the office, likely will be all that is required both to diagnose and to stage the patient. Again there is no need to bronchoscope such a patient unless specifically indicated. A percutaneous biopsy of an adrenal lesion may also provide both a diagnosis and stage. Too often extra procedures are performed which add no useful information to the subsequent management of the patient. Unfortunately the only question of significance in the patient with metastatic disease is the differentiation between small cell and non-small cell carcinoma, and this difference, though intuitively of great importance, is actually of minimal significance, since the chemotherapy, if indicated, is quite similar for both diseases.[4] Yet it seems important to know the histology if for no other reason than to be able to discuss prognosis with the patient. What is important in this early phase of the management of a patient with presumed metastatic lung cancer is to select a procedure that is likely to yield the most information with regard to both histologic type and stage and avoid unnecessary procedures in these individuals who have a limited life expectancy. Rarely is it necessary in the patient with metastatic disease to subject them to a procedure any more invasive than a needle biopsy or bronchoscopy. Occasionally mediastinoscopy may be required to obtain enough tissue and very rarely video thoracoscopic excision of a lung nodule, but a so-called exploratory thoracotomy really has no place in the management of these patients.[47]

The Asymptomatic Patient with Abnormal Chest Radiograph

Usually patients who are asymptomatic present with a solitary pulmonary nodule since those with an infiltrate or consolidation of a lobe rarely are without some symptom or sign of disease. The real question in this situation comes down to whether the nodule is malignant. A chest computed tomographic scan should be performed to determine if the nodule is solitary as well as to assess the status of the mediastinum, liver, and adrenals. The role of percutaneous needle biopsy of the solitary pulmonary nodule remains controversial. Bronchoscopy in this situation adds little and is probably not indicated.[50] One approach in certain patients, namely nonsmokers with a small nodule, is to follow the lesion over a period of time. A repeat chest radiograph in 4 to 6 weeks to assess a change in size of the nodule is a reasonable alternative as long as the patient can tolerate the uncertainty that the nodule may prove to be a carcinoma. If the lesion has increased in size, then excision is carried out. No change in size warrants continued observation with repeated chest radiographs. Conversely, in a smoker, where there is a high probability that the nodule is malignant, excision is justified in most cases no matter the result of a needle biopsy. A negative biopsy does not negate the fact that a suspicious nodule remains; if the biopsy is positive it only confirms what we already suspected, but the patient has been exposed to the risk of the needle biopsy namely, a 30 percent incidence of pneumothorax with a need for a chest tube in one-half of these.[9] The problem remains that a negative needle biopsy is of little help. Some positive information has to

be obtained, such as cartilage or fungal elements, for the biopsy to be definitive in order to prevent an operation. To really understand and use a negative needle biopsy to guide therapy we need to know not just what percentage of patients with negative needle biopsies prove to have cancers but what percentage of needle biopsies performed in patients where there is a high suspicion of cancer are negative. A recent study from the University of Toronto where essentially all patients with pulmonary nodules undergo needle biopsy shows that 6 percent of patients with a negative needle biopsy prove ultimately to have a cancer (T. Todd, personal communication).

The role of needle biopsy has been further diminished by the development of video thoracoscopy, which, in a relatively minimally invasive fashion, allows for the excision of a pulmonary nodule and a definitive diagnosis.[23] If the nodule proves to be benign, video thoracoscopic excision both makes the diagnosis and treats the problem. If the nodule is malignant, the procedure may be immediately converted to the appropriate anatomic pulmonary resection, most commonly lobectomy. Needle biopsy is useful for the patient who insists on having a diagnosis of malignancy prior to going to the operating room. The argument that needle biopsy should be performed to rule out small cell carcinoma is weak, since in the absence of mediastinal adenopathy, extremely rare for a small cell, a solitary nodule should be excised even if the needle biopsy suggests the diagnosis of small cell carcinoma by histology.[19] All the above notwithstanding, needle biopsies continue to be performed almost as a routine despite the current concern regarding costs.

STAGING

A discussion of noninvasive staging is beyond the scope of this chapter and is dealt with in a separate chapter. The role of invasive staging and the specific procedures utilized deserve mention. In discussing stage, distinction must be made between *clinical stage* and *pathologic stage.* The former is based solely on noninvasive imaging studies, whereas the latter depends on actual histologic material obtained either by invasive staging studies or at the time of the surgical resection.[28] A clinical stage is no more or no less than an assumption which is only as good as the noninvasive studies employed. A chest computed tomographic (CT) scan provides excellent visualization of the contents of the superior mediastinum. However, size of the lymph nodes remains the only criterion on which to base a judgment as to whether tumor is present in these nodes.[5] There are no other specific criteria either on CT or magnetic resonance imaging (MRI) on which to make such a judgment.[13,31] The sensitivity and specificity of CT depends on the size cutoff arbitrarily determined to separate a positive finding from a negative one. The smaller the size chosen, the greater the specificity but at the expense of the sensitivity. A larger size increases the sensitivity but decreases the specificity.[37] In this clinic, 1.5 cm is used as the threshold for determining whether a patient should have a mediastinoscopy performed. It has to be realized, however, that even though a size criterion has been determined, problems remain both in the subjectivity in measuring 1.5 cm on CT and the thickness of the slices utilized in performing the scan.

Mediastinoscopy provides a great deal of information about

the lymph node status of the superior mediastinum and is the gold standard for the assessment of the mediastinal lymph nodes.[21] The procedure has a false negative rate of less than 10 percent, far better than CT, but has the disadvantage of being an invasive procedure.[33,46] As the resolution of CT scans has improved, performing routine mediastinoscopy on all patients with lung cancer must be questioned when the procedure may be applied selectively based on the size of the lymph nodes seen on the CT. This avoids a needless operation in over 80 percent of patients.[16] There are nodal stations which cannot be accessed by standard cervical mediastinoscopy. These include the aortopulmonary window (level 5), a common site for lymph node involvement in left upper lobe tumors, and the posterior subcarinal space (level 7). However the anterior subcarinal space, usually representative of the contents of the posterior subcarinal space, is accessible to mediastinoscopic biopsy, and involved lymph nodes in the aortopulmonary window in the absence of other lymph node disease carries a prognosis equivalent to N1 (hilar) disease.[32]

Mediastinoscopy is performed through a small (2 cm) incision made in the neck 1 cm above the sternal notch. The area explored by mediastinoscopy, the superior mediastinum, is palpated first by inserting a finger along the anterior aspect of the trachea which also serves to develop the space and facilitate insertion of the mediastinoscope (see Fig. 113-I-1). Obviously involved lymph nodes often may be palpated, but palpation alone is insufficient, since intranodal disease may be present which can only be identified if representative biopsies of the important nodal stations are taken following insertion of the mediastinoscope.[12] Of major importance are the ipsilateral nodes, but just as important is the status of the contralateral lymph nodes especially in left lower lobe lesions, where right paratracheal lymph nodes are commonly involved. Despite notions to the contrary, left-sided lymph nodes are readily accessible at mediastinoscopy but are somewhat more difficult to identify. In fact the left paratracheal lymph nodes are much more easily sampled at mediastinoscopy than at left thoracotomy because of the location of the aortic arch relative to the left mainstem bronchus. Because of this we have a much lower threshold for performing mediastinoscopy for left-sided lesions.

Nodal stations most frequently sampled include levels 2 (upper paratracheal) and 4 (lower paratracheal) on the right, level 3 (pretracheal), level 7 (subcarinal), and level 4 on the left (see Fig. 113-I-2). Because the left level-4 lymph nodes occur at a slightly higher location, it is identifying separate level 2 nodes on the left can be difficult. It is not necessary always to sample all nodal stations; if there are nodes obviously involved, these, along with contralateral nodes, are all that is necessary to adequately stage the patient. This all makes it sound very simple to carry out this procedure, but in fact mediastinoscopy is a technically demanding procedure that is performed correctly and thoroughly only by those who have been well grounded in the techniques. It is a difficult procedure to teach, and the close proximity of a number of major vascular structures makes the procedure daunting even to the experienced practitioner. The vessels include the inominate artery, the aortic arch, the superior vena cava, the azygous vein, and the right main pulmonary artery. Unfortunately none of these structures are easily seen, and success requires that the operator know where they are located to avoid injury (see Fig. 113-I-3). The left recurrent laryngeal nerve and the esophagus are also subject to injury. Many surgeons have had disastrous experiences with mediastinoscopy and have great hesitation about performing it despite the wealth of information obtained when it is performed properly. These are usually the same clinicians who downplay the importance of the procedure in staging lung cancer and seek to avoid it. A surgeon attempting to practice thoracic surgery without the ability to perform a complete and thorough mediastinoscopy is at a great disadvantage which unfortunately is passed on to patients. This inability usually results in the performance of many thoracotomies that otherwise could be avoided.

Though mediastinoscopy is the mainstay of invasive staging for lung cancer, other procedures provide additional information that often complements that obtained at mediastinoscopy. The aortopulmonary window, a common site of nodal spread from tumors of the left upper lobe, may be reached with a parasternal mediastinotomy, or so-called Chamberlain procedure.[39] An incision is made over the left second costal cartilage, the cartilage is excised, and the pleural reflection is swept laterally to access the aortopulmonary window in an extrapleural plane. The involvement of lymph nodes at this level (level 5) in the absence of other nodal disease is associated with a 5-year survival that approaches 50 percent if the disease can be completely resected at thoracotomy, a survival that is almost identical to that seen with N1

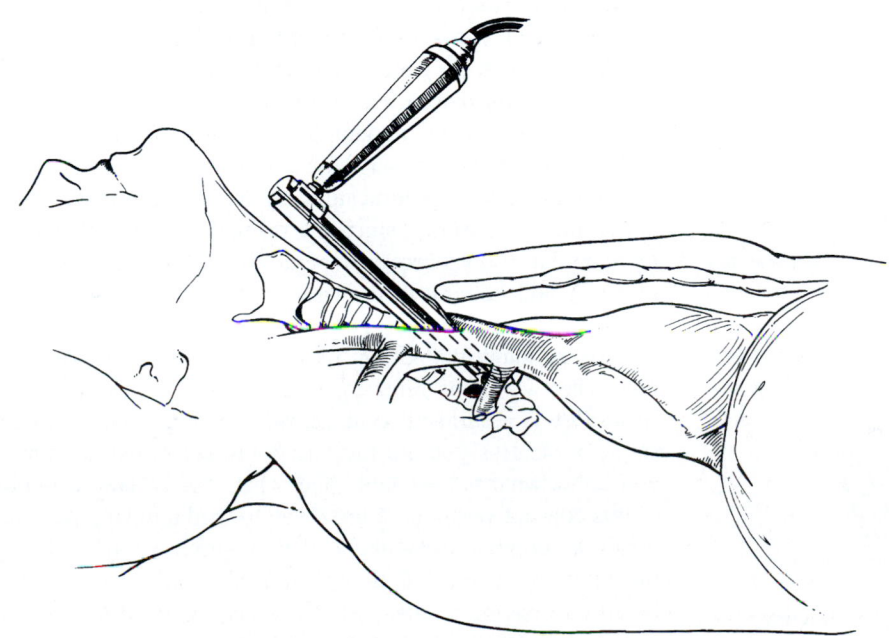

FIGURE 113-I-1   Mediastinoscope in place demonstrating the superior mediastinal plane.

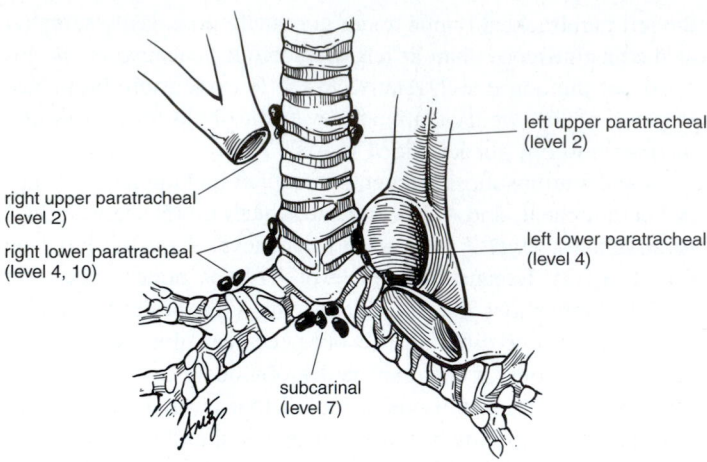

FIGURE 113-I-2 Lymph node stations accessible by cervical mediastinoscopy. For consistency the levels should be labeled with the appropriate number when submitted to surgical pathology.

(hilar) disease.[32] The rationale, then, behind performing parasternal mediastinotomy either is to assess resectability or document mediastinal nodal disease to justify placing the patient into an experimental protocol of neoadjuvant chemotherapy, radiation therapy, or both.

Similarly, video thoracoscopy aids in the staging of lung cancer, although not in lieu of mediastinoscopy, which offers an opportunity to sample nodes on the right and left through one incision, but as an adjunct.[48] Nodes inaccessible by mediastinoscopy, including the aortopulmonary window (level 5), sub-

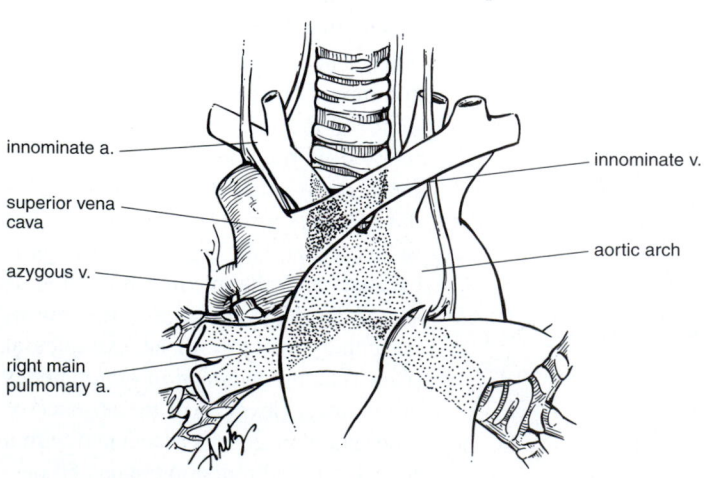

FIGURE 113-I-3 The relationship of major vascular structures potentially encountered during mediastinoscopy to the trachea and main bronchi.

carinal (level 7), and inferior pulmonary ligament (level 9) are easily sampled utilizing video thoracoscopy.[43] This technique also visualizes the pleural space, especially useful in the patient with a pleural effusion and negative fluid cytology, so as to rule out diffuse pleural involvement and prevent an unnecessary thoracotomy.[52] Other nodules seen on CT scan which may have an impact on treatment planning also may be excised and defined histologically prior to formal thoracotomy. Video thoracoscopic examination has not proven particularly useful in assessing resectability of a tumor where there is a question because of presumed invasion of an adjacent mediastinal structure. Usually the ultimate decision regarding resectability of a locally invasive lesion must be made at the time of thoracotomy when the lesion itself may be palpated and the dissection conducted under greater control. A logical progression from the less invasive to the more invasive procedures guided by the imaging studies often results in the patient being spared a procedure from which there will be no significant benefit.

Any discussion of staging presupposes that the information obtained will be used in the decision regarding therapy. It is of no use obtaining information, and subjecting the patient to the risk of an additional procedure, unless the information obtained in utilized. Discovering at mediastinoscopy that there is N2 disease and still proceeding on to thoracotomy makes little sense. Why bother with the mediastinoscopy? This introduces the concepts of operability and resectability, two terms which are *not* synonymous although used, mistakenly, as such. Any staging study or procedure, be it invasive or noninvasive, contributes to the decision regarding operability but usually has no bearing whatsoever on resectability. A patient who has bone metastases is *inoperable,* by definition, since the local control achieved by removing the primary tumor has no effect at all on the fact that the patient already has disseminated disease. Removing the primary tumor, though an extremely difficult concept to convey to the patient and family, offers nothing in terms of survival and only subjects the patient to the morbidity of the operation. This same patient, though *inoperable,* may have an eminently *resectable* lesion. *Resectability* is a surgical determination made by the surgeon at the time of the operation. Staging studies have little to do with determining resectability, the exception being the finding of gross extranodal disease at mediastinoscopy which both defines operability and, for the most part, precludes resection. Finding diffuse pleural studding at video thoracoscopy does not define resectability, since the primary tumor easily may be resected, but it does prove inoperability, since removing the tumor will add nothing to the overall outcome. Operability may also be determined by coexisting medical problems such as heart disease, although the patient may have a resectable primary tumor. The two terms refer to decidedly different concepts; *resectability* is a surgical term whose use should be confined to surgeons. Unless you are the one doing the resecting, how can you know what is resectable and what is not? The recognition of this concept would go a long way toward allowing patients to obtain a complete assessment of their disease followed by the institution of appropriate treatment. For a nonsurgeon to decide, based on imaging studies, what is *resectable* and then institute treatment without referring the patient to a thoracic surgeon at least for consultation does a disservice to the patient.

SURGICAL TREATMENT OF LUNG CANCER

Many patients undergo very little in the way of a staging evaluation prior to operation. The type and extent of the staging evaluation depends on a number of clinical factors. At a minimum patients should have a recent chest radiograph and CT scan of the chest. Most, but not all, should have a recent set of pulmonary function studies. The decision to search for disseminated disease with a bone scan and brain CT or MRI is a difficult one, and precise criteria to define when they should be obtained do not exist.[15] A complete discussion of this issue may be found in Chapter 112. The practice in this clinic is to obtain a complete evaluation of the extent of disease if there is any reason at all to do so. This would include any organ-specific or nonspecific signs or symptoms.[14,54] Nonspecific signs include weight loss, easy fatigueability, or anemia, and organ-specific signs include bone pain, elevated liver enzymes, or localizing neurologic findings. If any of these findings are present, a complete evaluation is obtained, not just the study pointed to by the organ-specific complaint. Any patient with a history of malignancy should have a complete extent of disease workup as should the patient who is at a higher risk for operation, such as an individual with multiple medical problems or borderline pulmonary function. As well, any patient with locally advanced disease in whom the indications for operation are being extended (i.e., N2 disease) or the nonsmoker with a lung mass should have disseminated disease ruled out. The aim is to avoid operating on a patient who proceeds to manifest disseminated disease within 1 year of operation, a finding which ideally should have been identified preoperatively.

Recognizing that operation is the best treatment for early-stage disease, it is important that the appropriate procedure be performed. Lobectomy remains the definitive resection for most lung cancers, since it is an anatomic resection which removes the regional lymph nodes that are located along the lobar bronchus. Doing less than a lobectomy must be considered a compromise, although a nonanatomic wedge excision is tempting for small primary tumors.[55] Not only does a wedge excision not include the lobar bronchus, precluding evaluation of lobar lymph nodes, but it provides only a minimal parenchymal margin. The Lung Cancer Study Group (LCSG) addressed the question of lobectomy versus limited resection for T1N0 lesions (tumor < 3 cm, negative lymph nodes) in a prospective randomized trial.[11] The early analysis of the data demonstrated an increased incidence of local recurrence in the limited resection group but no difference in survival. The final analysis revealed superior survival for patients in the lobectomy group. Other studies have looked retrospectively at patients undergoing limited resection, which includes segmental resection, and have demonstrated long-term survivors, but the LCSG study stands alone as the only randomized trial.[38,53]

For patients in whom lobectomy is not feasible, a lesser resection offers the best alternative, although admittedly it is a compromise.[6] Patients in this category are those with borderline pulmonary function or those who have had previous pulmonary resections. Whenever possible the lesser resection should be an anatomic segmental resection, which takes the segmental artery and vein as well as the segmental bronchus with its accompanying lymph nodes (see Fig. 113-I-4). A classic segmental resection is a relatively difficult operation, and many surgeons do not possess a significant amount of experience in performing this procedure. The prototype segmental resections include the lingular resection and resection of the superior segment of the lower lobe, but any lung segment may be removed anatomically.[8] The key to segmental resection is the identification of the segmental artery which, once ligated and divided, reveals the location of the segmental bronchus which is taken next. The segmental vein is divided last, and the parenchyma is divided with a stapler or "stripped" as was originally described.

With the development of video thoracoscopic techniques and the simplicity of wedge resection via this approach, there has been renewed interest in utilizing this technique for T1N0 lung cancers.[45] Based on the LCSG data this should be avoided, and patients who are found to have a cancer should be offered the best possible procedure, which, to the best of present knowledge, is a lobectomy. Wedge resection is, at best, a compromise, and patients who otherwise could tolerate an anatomic resection are not well served by having less done. There have also been several reports of tumor growing in thoracoscopic incision sites when lung cancers have been pulled through these small incisions.[10]

Depending mainly on the location of the tumor, more extensive and complex resections than lobectomy may be required.

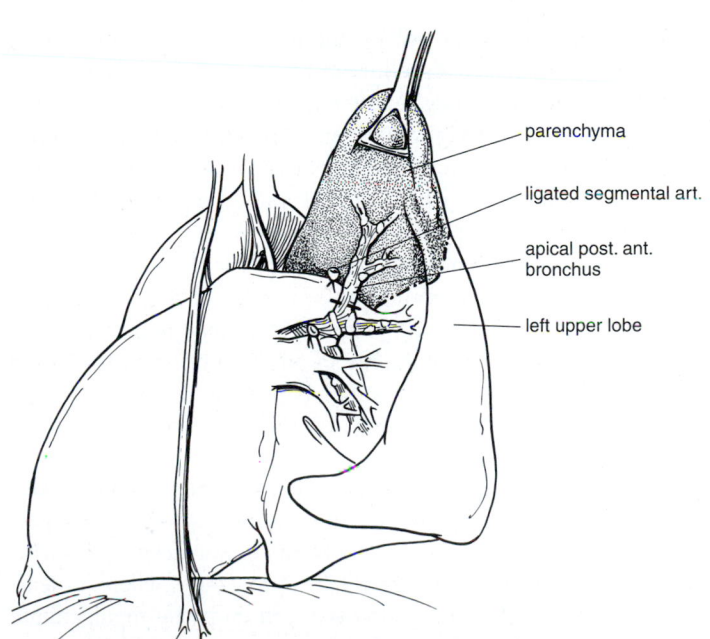

parenchyma

ligated segmental art.

apical post. ant. bronchus

left upper lobe

FIGURE 113-I-4 Segmental resection. The example shown here is the resection of the apical-posterior segment of the left upper lobe. The segmental pulmonary arterial branch is shown ligated and divided. The segmental bronchus has been dissected out and is the next structure to be divided.

The determination as to when to perform pneumonectomy is made at the time of operation, rarely preoperatively. Recognizing that even today pneumonectomy carries a perioperative mortality of at least 5 percent, we do everything possible to avoid removing an entire lung.[7] There are only a few absolute indications for performing pneumonectomy for the experienced surgeon. These include such proximal involvement of the main pulmonary artery that it is difficult to place a clamp on the artery, endobronchial tumor so extensive as to preclude sleeve resection, and involvement of the confluence of the pulmonary veins or of the left atrium. There is reason for concern if a surgeon is performing an abundance of pneumonectomies. A "difficult" fissure, unless tumor involves the artery in the fissure, is not an indication for pneumonectomy, nor is tumor crossing a fissure an absolute indication. Pneumonectomy, technically, is an easier operation to perform than lobectomy, requiring very little dissection and only several applications of the stapler. Sleeve resections, or bronchoplastic procedures, are technically more demanding procedures which result in the same bronchial resection as a pneumonectomy, yet preserve lung tissue.[17] The prototypical bronchoplastic procedure is the right upper lobe sleeve resection, where the main bronchus is divided just proximal to the right upper lobe takeoff and the bronchus intermedius is divided just distal to the upper lobe bronchus (see Fig. 113-I-5). The right upper lobe, with tumor present at the lobar orifice, is thus removed with a portion of the mainstem bronchus, and the bronchus intermedius is anastamosed to the mainstem bronchus. Thus the proximal bronchial division occurs essentially at the same site as if a pneumonectomy had been performed. Other sleeve resections are possible on both the right and left side, all result in lung conservation and are associated with long-term survival equivalent to pneumonectomy, depending on the indications.[18]

Even with proximal involvement of the pulmonary artery, partial resection or sleeve resection of the artery is possible to avoid removal of the entire lung. A patch angioplasty with pericardium may be utilized if a significant enough portion of the anterior wall of the artery is taken so as to narrow it. Alternatively a segment of the artery may be removed and an end-to-end anastamosis completed. Sometimes a pneumonectomy must be done, but the complete thoracic surgeon always looks to see if alternatives exist while preserving the principles of the cancer operation and not compromising margins. With any lung-conserving procedure, the margins of the resection should be sent for frozen section confirmation that no tumor is present.

A complete pulmonary resection requires more than simply excision of the tumor and the surrounding lung parenchyma be it lobe or entire lung. The operation is incomplete without excision of lymph nodes to complete the staging assessment. We perform a mediastinal lymph node dissection even if mediastinoscopy has been performed. This procedure, where, at least on the right side, the entire contents of the superior mediastinum are removed, is the only one that assures complete lymph nodes staging.[2] The hilar and peribronchial lymph nodes are removed with the lobectomy or pneumonectomy specimen but must be specifically searched for by the pathologist. Any sampling procedure of mediastinal lymph nodes depends on how the nodes to be sampled are chosen. The failure to include mediastinal

lymph nodes as part of a resection results in incomplete information. Not only must the mediastinal lymph nodes be removed as part of the resection but they should be labeled according to their location in the mediastinum.[30]

Having removed the mediastinal lymph nodes, it is not uncommon to find microscopic disease in a node that grossly appears normal. Finding tumor in mediastinal lymph nodes portends a significantly worse prognosis and at least prompts thought regarding postoperative treatment. Postoperative adjuvant therapy, usually radiation therapy, has not improved survival.[22,35] Currently patients with disease found in mediastinal lymph nodes (25 to 30 percent, 5-year survival) following a complete resection may be entered into a national randomized protocol which compares postoperative radiation therapy alone with concurrent chemotherapy and radiation therapy (ECOG 3509).The drugs employed, cis-Platinum and VP-16, are both active agents in non-small cell lung cancer and are reasonable well tolerated. Patients with N1 disease (hilar, peribronchial, and segmental nodes) are also eligible for treatment on this adjuvant protocol.

The designation *locally advanced* includes a wide variety of lesions which extend outside of the lung parenchyma whether by direct extension or nodal involvement to involve other struc-

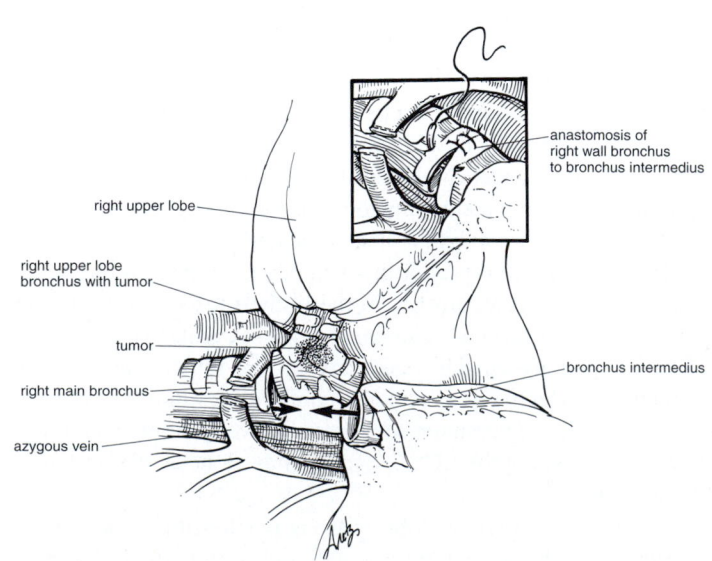

FIGURE 113-I-5   Right upper lobe sleeve resection. The right main bronchus has been divided just proximal to the right upper lobe takeoff where the tumor is located. The bronchus intermedius has been divided just distal to the right upper lobe bronchus. The bronchus intermedius is anastamosed to the right main bronchus (inset).

tures within the hemithorax. Certain criteria need to be fulfilled before considering extending the indications for resection, since the intent is to maximize survival. The most obvious criterion is the exclusion of disseminated disease, and thus it is key to complete an extent of disease evaluation before embarking upon a complex resection where the indications for resection have been extended.

N2 Disease

Classically the involvement of mediastinal lymph nodes with tumor precluded any attempt at surgical resection, since most of these patients died within 2 years due to the development of disseminated disease. Utilizing mediastinoscopy, mediastinal lymph node involvement may be detected prior to thoracotomy, saving the patient a needless operation. Contralateral nodal disease, which carries a significantly worse prognosis than ipsilateral disease, may also be detected at mediastinoscopy and if found usually takes the patient out of the realm of operative intervention even if combined with neoadjuvant therapy. Perhaps the first recognition that a subset of patients with mediastinal lymph node involvement could benefit from surgery came from the work of Martini, who was able to completely resect 151 patients out of approximately 500 with N2 disease.[24] Many of these patients, but not all, were treated with postoperative radiation therapy. For the group of completely resected patients he found a 28 percent 5-year actuarial survival and subsequently a 26 percent absolute survival. All the patients with N2 disease, resected or not, were identified at the time of thoracotomy, as mediastinoscopy was not performed. Breaking the patients down into two groups yields those staged as N0 or N1 preoperatively, and those with bulky disease, so-called clinical N2, noted either on preoperative chest radiograph or at bronchoscopy when carinal splaying was noted. Those patients thought to have N0 or N1 disease preoperatively had a 35 percent 5-year survival, and those with clinical N2 disease had 0 percent 5-year survival. Fewer than 10 percent of patients with clinical N2 disease could be completely resected.

In recognition that patients with bulky N2 disease not only had a low rate of resectability but a poor long-term outlook, an attempt was made to improve the resectability rate and, it was hoped, survival in this patient group by employing preoperative chemotherapy.[25] There was a 77 percent response rate to the chemotherapy regimen of velban and cis-Platinum with 10 percent complete responders. Sixty-five percent of patients who underwent operation were able to have a complete resection, a significant improvement over the rate able to be resected when no preoperative therapy was employed. Keep in mind that patients entered into this trial were those with bulky mediastinal disease. The overall survival was 28 percent at 3 years and 17 percent at 5 years with a median survival of 19 months. Patients who were able to undergo a complete resection had a mean survival of 27 months and 3- and 5-year survival of 44 percent and 26 percent, respectively. Multiple other nonrandomized phase II trials of preoperative therapy have been carried out in patients with N2 disease utilizing chemotherapy alone or chemotherapy combined with radiation therapy.[44]

Resections following preoperative therapy can be extremely difficult and hazardous because of the fibrosis that often results

TABLE 113-I-1

Summary from Randomized Trial of Chemotherapy plus Surgery versus Surgery Alone for Stage IIIa Disease

	Chemo + Surgery	Surgery Alone
Median survival (est)	64 months	11 months (p < .008)
2-year survival (est)	60%	25%
3-year survival (est)	56%	15%

SOURCE: From Roth et al.[42]

as a response to the therapy. This is especially significant when there has been a response in involved lymph nodes, since the nodes are intimately associated with the pulmonary artery and its branches, often making resection quite tricky. It is particularly important to have proximal control of the pulmonary artery prior to undertaking a resection in a patient with N2 disease who has received preoperative therapy, and resections of this type should ideally only be undertaken by a surgeon with experience in dealing with complex resections.

Two prospective, randomized trials have been completed demonstrating the superiority of preoperative neoadjuvant therapy followed by operation compared to operation alone in patients with N2 disease. Unfortunately neither of these trials dealt solely with a population of patients with N2 disease, as they both included patients with T3 disease. Roth and colleagues randomized 28 patients to a combined therapy group who received three cycles of preoperative chemotherapy with cyclophosphamide, etoposide, and cis-Platinum followed by operation, and 32 patients underwent operation without preoperative therapy.[42] Results of the trial are summarized in Table 113-I-1. Significant survival advantage was conferred upon those who received preoperative therapy (see Fig. 113-I-6). Median survival in the surgery-only group was 11 months versus 64 months in the combined therapy group (p > .008). This is all the more interesting considering that fewer than 40 percent of the patients in each

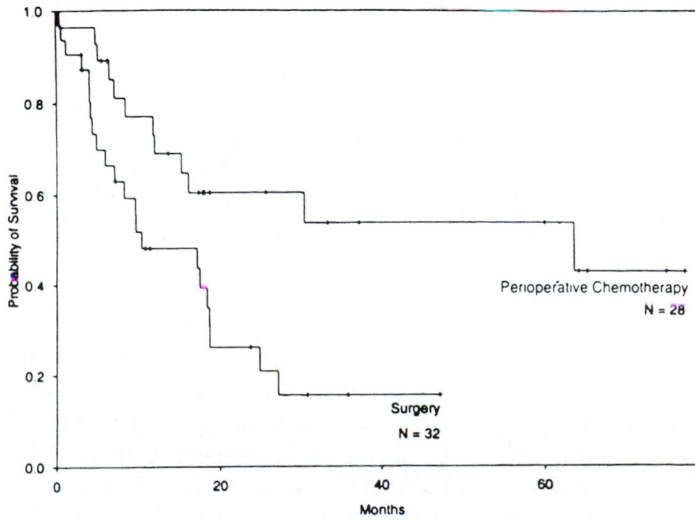

FIGURE 113-I-6 Time to death for all patients by treatment group, surgery alone versus chemotherapy plus surgery from the Roth trial. (From Roth et al,[42] with permission.)

group were able to have a complete resection. (39 percent versus 31 percent, combined versus surgery alone) This trial is notable for several reasons. It clearly demonstrates an advantage to neoadjuvant therapy in a group of patients with locally advanced disease. Survival in the surgery-only group was significantly shorter than expected, making the survival difference between the groups more striking. Excluded from the trial were patients with left lung tumors and left paratracheal disease, as these patients were felt to be unresectable, so there is some selection bias to the study population. However one must be impressed by the significant difference in survival observed in this randomized trial.

Likewise, Rosell randomized 60 patients with stage IIIa disease, 25 of whom had N2 disease who received chemotherapy followed by an operation.[41] Nineteen patients with N2 disease underwent operation as their only therapy. As in the Roth trial there was a significant survival benefit in the group which received combination therapy (median, 26 months versus 8 months, $p < .001$).

There is a suggestion that a preoperative regimen incorporating radiation therapy and chemotherapy may be more efficacious than either modality alone. In a phase II trial the Southwest Oncology Group studied concurrent induction chemotherapy with cis-Platinum and etoposide in both stage IIIa and IIIb patients.[1] Complete resection was accomplished in 74 percent of patients. Though there was an 8 percent incidence of postoperative death, no tumor was able to be found in 22 percent of the resections. Median survival was 13 months, and 2-year and 3-year survival was 37 percent and 27 percent, respectively. Patients with a pathologic complete response in the lymph nodes had a 30-month median survival compared to 10 months for those with persistent lymph node disease ($p < .0005$).

Despite the numerous studies addressing preoperative therapy, whether chemotherapy alone or combined with radiation therapy, the question as to what role surgical resection plays in the outcome of patients with N2 disease remains unanswered. To date no conclusive studies have proved that operation is superior to radiation therapy in controlling local disease in these patients. One reason for this is the difficulty in accruing patients on a study where the randomization chooses between a surgical and a nonsurgical arm. A study addressing this question, Radiation Therapy Oncology Group (RTOG) 89-01, accrued fewer than 80 patients in the 4 years it was open. Currently there is an ongoing intergroup phase III randomized trial (RTOG 9309) for patients with N2 disease comparing concurrent chemotherapy (cis-Platinum, vinblastine) and radiation therapy followed by surgical excision or additional radiation (total 61 Gy over 6 weeks).

Thus, although there is a suggestion that neoadjuvant therapy results in improved survival when compared to surgery alone, this has not been confirmed in a phase III randomized, large multi-institutional trial. There is evidence, however, that 60 to 75 percent of patients with lymph node disease as the only site of spread respond to the preoperative regimens, a significantly greater response than when the same regimens are used in patients with disseminated disease, and over half of these patients will go on to resection. Between 10 and 20 percent of patients resected have no evidence of disease found on histologic examination of the resected material.[36] The activity of the neoadju-

vant regimen in this patient population cannot be denied. Whether surgical excision is required or radiation is an acceptable modality for local control remains to be determined. Of great importance is the consideration of quality of life in patients undergoing these combined regimens, an area that has not been adequately addressed. The quality of life measurement tools are available to incorporate into future studies so that additional information should be forthcoming. Toxicity from these preoperative regimens can be substantial, especially if there is an element of postobstructive pneumonia. In the SWOG trial, two deaths resulted from the preoperative regimen, and 13 percent of patients experienced grade 4 or greater acute toxicity.[1] The overall treatment-related mortality was 15 percent in the neoadjuvant study from Toronto.[3] This further underscores the importance of confining multimodality therapy for N2 disease to controlled trials as opposed to routine community use, despite the current enthusiasm.

Chest Wall Resection

Approximately 5 percent of lung cancers involve the chest wall by direct extension. This involvement may be limited to the parietal pleura or may invade the endothoracic fascia, intercostal muscle, or ribs. Chest wall involvement by direct extension is *not* a contraindication to resection unless vertebral bodies are invaded, and even then, under some circumstances, resection may still be completed. Chest wall pain is the most sensitive predictor of chest wall involvement in a patient with a peripheral lung lesion where there is a question of chest wall invasion. Neither the CT scan nor the MRI can distinguish between abuttment and invasion unless there is gross invasion of bone. The radionuclide bone scan may be negative with chest wall involvement especially if only the parietal pleura and muscle are involved. Lesions involving parietal pleura or other chest wall structures are staged as T3 primary tumors, but often definitive staging cannot be accomplished until the time of operation.

As with any lung cancer it is important to rule out disseminated disease prior to considering operation in a patient with chest wall involvement. It is particularly important to assess the mediastinum in these patients, since mediastinal lymph node involvement is the single best prognostic indicator.[27] Three-year survival approaches zero in patients with chest wall and mediastinal lymph node involvement, underscoring the importance of invasive mediastinal lymph node staging, usually with mediastinoscopy, prior to considering thoracotomy in this patient group. Conversely, greater than 50 percent 5-year survival can be expected in patients with chest wall involvement with negative mediastinal lymph nodes as long as the resection margins are negative.[27]

The operation performed in a patient with suspected chest wall involvement begins by assessing the pleural space to rule out diffuse pleural disease and then defining whether the chest wall is invaded. Prior to beginning the chest wall resection it is important to assess the hilum of the lung to ensure that the findings do not preclude resection. It is disconcerting to resect a large chunk of chest wall only to find that there is such extensive disease at the pulmonary hilum as to preclude parenchymal resection. Often one finds only adherence with no evidence of invasion, and this is established by beginning the resection in the extrapleural plane, thus separating the parietal pleura from the endothoracic fascia in the area of the lesion. If this plane is easily developed, something that is very clear to the experienced surgeon, it may be that the parietal pleura are not invaded. If there is any question at all about invasion when attempting to develop the extrapleural plane, then chest wall resection is performed (see Fig. 113-I-7). Ideally the chest wall resection is performed in continuity with the parenchymal resection, that is the portion of chest wall resected remains attached to the underlying lung. The chest wall resection should include at least 1 rib and preferably 2 above and below the area of chest wall invaded. Three- to five-cm margins should also be taken anteriorly and posteriorly. The intent is to achieve negative margins so the resection should be wide; there is little if any additional morbidity to taking a somewhat larger piece of chest wall.

Once the chest wall block is totally mobilized, the lobectomy and mediastinal lymph node dissection are completed. A mediastinoscopy should have been performed earlier, but a lymph node dissection should be done for complete staging. A posterior chest wall defect is reconstructed with polypropylene mesh, and a defect in the anterior chest wall should be reconstructed with a sandwich of methylmethacrylate cement and polypropylene mesh. Posteriorly the defect is covered additionally by the scapula, but anteriorly the rigid fixation provided by the methyl methacrylate and mesh eliminates any paradoxical motion that might interfere with mechanics of breathing. Interference with the mechanics of breathing is much less likely to occur with posterior defects.

Chest wall resection adds little if any additional morbidity to a pulmonary resection. Patients tend to have the chest tubes in a few days longer following chest wall resection because of increased fluid drainage. Pain in the early postoperative period is best controlled with a thoracic epidural catheter which allows patients to be comfortable enough to maintain a good cough for clearance of secretions. There is no evidence that patient's undergoing chest wall resection are subject to more pain than those who have a simple lobectomy. If the cough is ineffective, then secretion retention is aggressively managed with periodic bronchoscopies.

Postoperative treatment for patients who have undergone chest wall resection with pulmonary resection remains controversial. The most important consideration is the attainment of negative resection margins at the time of operation. The surgeon should never think that a few close margins or even a small amount of gross disease left behind can be "cleaned up" by the radiation oncologist. Anything less than a complete resection is associated with poor long-term survival.[27] With negative surgical margins is there a role for radiation therapy? Currently no evidence exists that postoperative radiation therapy prolongs survival in this patient group, but local recurrence may be problematic.[44] Thus there may be a role for radiation therapy in some of these patients—in particular those with disease close to the spine, where local recurrence presents major management problems.

Tumors Involving the Mediastinum by Direct Extension

Some centrally located primary tumors may involve structures in the mediastinum by direct extension (see Fig. 113-I-8). The assessment of this involvement, whether there is true invasion or just abutment and adherence, cannot be determined until the findings are seen intraoperatively and then often only as the dissection proceeds. The presence of a central tumor that appears on CT scan to be close to the mediastinum is not justification for making a judgment of unresectability, especially if the judgment is being made by someone other than a surgeon. This is a judgment that can only be made intraoperatively, since no imaging modality readily distinguishes abutment from invasion. There may be other reasons why the patient should not be operated on, but it is dangerous to simply assume that a lesion is unresectable. The distinction between a T3

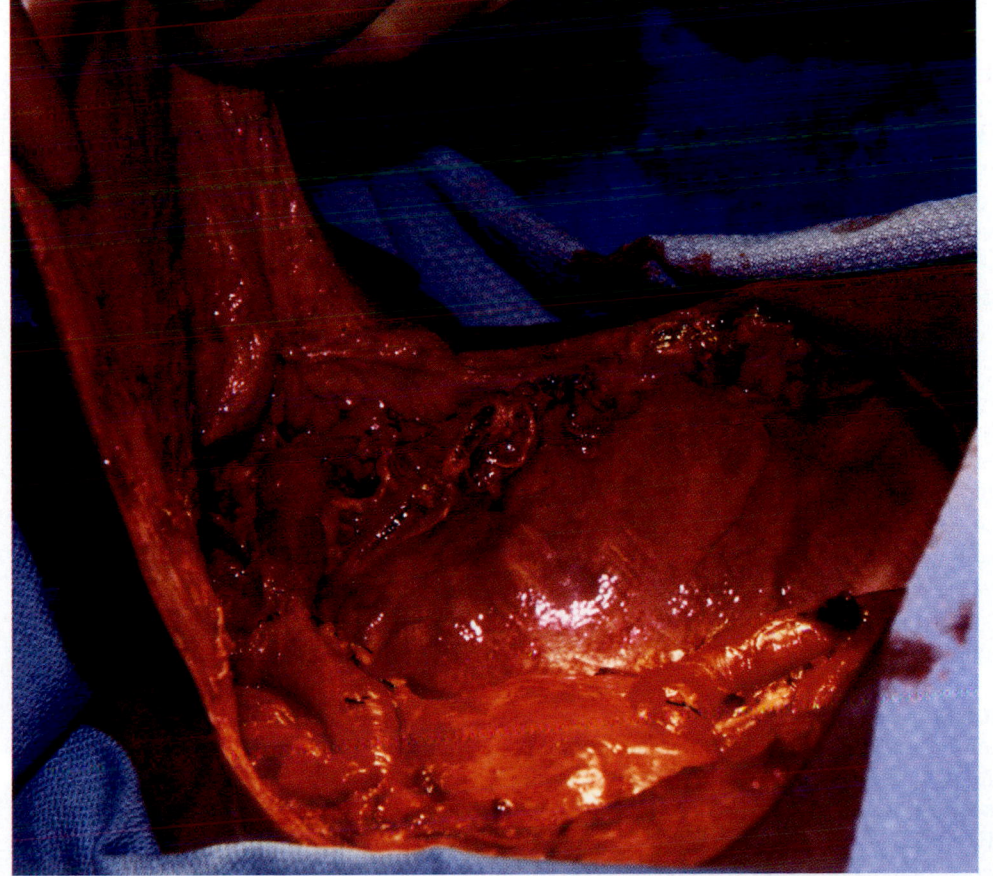

FIGURE 113-I-7 Operative photograph showing the defect left after resection of the left upper lobe in continuity with the anterior chest wall. This anterior defect requires reconstruction with prosthetic mesh and methylmethacrylate cement.

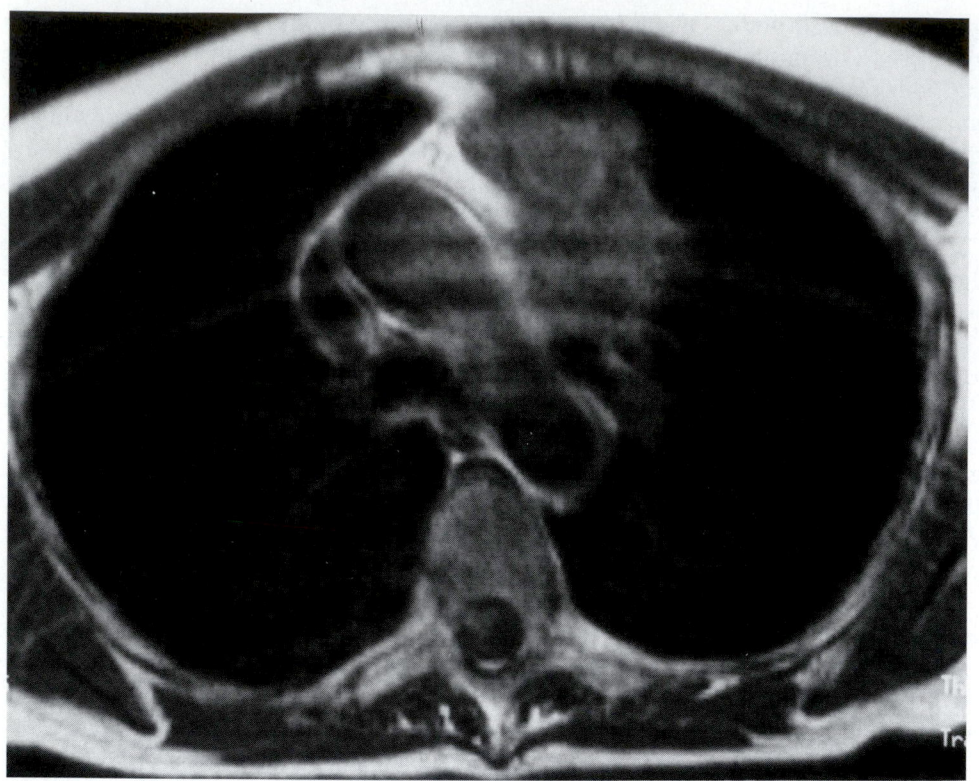

FIGURE 113-I-8 MRI scan showing a primary lung tumor involving the aorta by direct extension (T4 primary). The distinction between abuttment and invasion often cannot be made until the findings are seen at operation. MRI is no better at delineating invasion than CT.

tumor involving the mediastinum and a T4 tumor depends on the mediastinal structure invaded. Tumors invading structures such as the phrenic nerve, mediastinal pleura or fat, the pericardium, or the diaphragm that may be readily removed are classified as T3 primary tumors and as such are in the stage IIIa group which also includes mediastinal lymph node involvement and tumors involving chest wall. T4 primary tumors involve those structures which usually are not considered to be resectable such as aorta, left atrium, superior vena cava, trachea esophagus, or vertebral bodies. There are occasions when tumors involving these structures are resected, most commonly with lesions involving the vena cava or left atrium. Rarely, if ever, is a portion of aorta resected for excision of a lung tumor, but a lesion may involve only the muscular coat of the esophagus and thus may be amenable to resection. What is important to recognize, however, is despite the seeming ability to remove some of these invasive lesions, the prognosis for long-term survival is dismal.[26] For T4 lesions fewer than 10 percent of patients are alive at 5 years. From the viewpoint of the surgeon, though certainly recognizing the poor long-term survival with these tumors, in the absence of mediastinal lymph node involvement it is difficult to simply back out and leave the tumor in place when it is possible to resect the lesion with minimal morbidity. Such would be the situation where a portion of vena cava or a piece of left atrium is all that is necessary to complete a resection. Extensive involvement of one of these structures is an absolute contraindication to resection.

It is illustrative to discuss the situation of a patient who presents with the new onset of hoarseness and is found to have a paralysis of the left vocal cord. Almost always a tumor will be found in the left chest, usually the left upper lobe. In fact the acute onset of left vocal cord paralysis should be assumed to be from a cancer of the lung until proved otherwise. A benign problem causing a left vocal cord paralysis would be distinctly unusual. Rarely, if ever, is hoarseness due to right vocal cord paralysis because of the position of the right recurrent laryngeal nerve which "recurs" around the right subclavian artery above the apex of the chest. Conversely the left recurrent nerve is in a position of great vulnerability, since it arises after the vagus nerve crosses the aortic arch and recurs around the ligamentum arteriosum (see Fig. 113-I-9). The left recurrent nerve may be involved either by a primary tumor which encases the vagus nerve as it crosses the aortic arch or more commonly by lymph node disease in the aortopulmonary window. Because of the depth of the aortopulmonary window, there can be gross mediastinal lymph node involvement and a sheet of tumor with minimal plain radiographic evidence, since tumor underneath the aortic arch is not easily seen. CT scan usually confirms extensive involvement. Involvement of the left recurrent laryngeal nerve represents a contraindication to operation, since rarely are these lesions able to be completely resected. Left recurrent laryngeal nerve involvement should exclude patients from participating in neoadjuvant trials as well. The only exception is the occasional situation where the primary tumor involves the vagus nerve as it crosses the aortic arch, a situation which may prove to be resectable and justifies exploration.

Palliative Resections

There is essentially no role for palliative resections in the modern management of non-small cell lung cancer. Morbidity resulting from the primary tumor usually may be managed using modalities other than operation. There probably is no justification for operation if less than a complete resection is anticipated. At the present time there is no role for surgical "debulking" in the management of the patient with unresectable disease. With the newer treatment planning modalities available, radiation therapy can be given accurately and in high doses to patients who are inoperable or unresectable. Patients with hemoptysis or postobstructive pneumonia may benefit from laser excision of the endobronchial disease combined with external beam radiation therapy and endobronchial placement of radioactive sources.[49] Laser excision may be combined with stent placement to maintain open an obstructed bronchus or trachea. Chest wall pain usually is readily controlled by a course of radiation therapy.

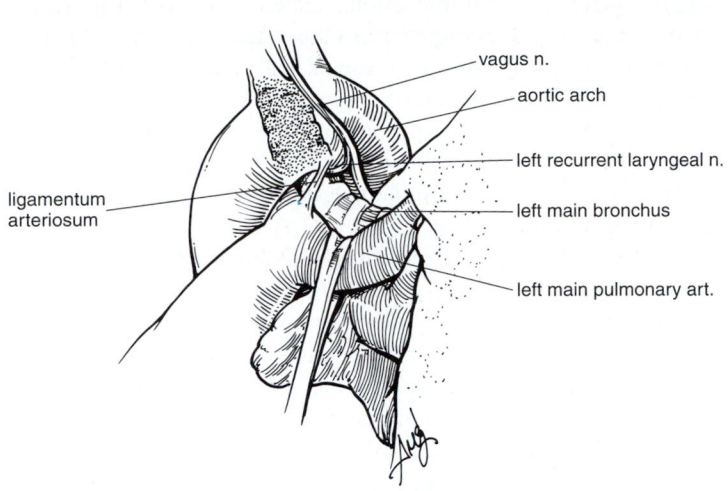

FIGURE 113-I-9   The anatomy of the aortopulmonary window showing the relationship of the left recurrent laryngeal nerve to the aortic arch and ligamentum arteriosum. The nerve is easily damaged in this location. Hoarseness may result from tumor involvement of the nerve in this location or from involvement of the vagus nerve at the level of the aortic arch proximal to the location where the recurrent laryngeal nerve originates.

RESULTS OF TREATMENT

Postoperative Complications

Major improvements in perioperative care of patients undergoing thoracic surgical procedures have led to decreased morbidity and mortality when compared to only 10 to 20 years ago.[7,40] Improved preoperative evaluation of patients has allowed us to identify risk factors associated with morbidity and to address these early. Experience with lung transplantation has shown that deconditioned patients benefit from at least a 6-week period of pulmonary rehabilitation, and selected patients with otherwise operable disease may be placed in a rehabilitation program prior to undergoing operation. Quantitative perfusion lung scans have allowed us to better select borderline patients for pulmonary resection, especially where pneumonectomy is a possibility. This information has all but eliminated the "pulmonary cripple" as a result of a lung resection. Recent experience with bilateral lung volume reduction surgery demonstrates that patients with severe emphysema and hyperinflation actually benefit from the resection of nonfunctional pulmonary parenchyma and has fueled the realization that no matter how poor the pulmonary function studies, many of these patients may be candidates for resection. The further refinement of lung-conserving procedures and the use of minimally invasive techniques such as video thoracoscopy along with better perioperative pain management provided by continuous epidural administration of narcotic have provided the incentive for us to operate on many patients previously thought not to be candidates because of poor pulmonary function. A greater recognition of the importance of preoperative teaching of postoperative maneuvers such as coughing and the use of chest phys-

iotherapy given by expertly trained individuals also has contributed to decreasing respiratory complications. With the ascent of a class of formally trained cardiothoracic surgeons who confine their practice to general thoracic surgery, as distinct from cardiac surgery, have come dedicated inpatient units to care for patients undergoing pulmonary resections.

Postoperative Mortality

Recent analyses identify that modern 30-day operative mortality from pulmonary resections should be less than 4 percent.[7] Lobectomies and lesser resections should have a mortality between 1 and 2 percent, and pneumonectomies still carry a mortality of 6 to 7 percent.[51] The mortality rate is directly proportional to increased age, associated diseases, and the extent of resection. Respiratory complications, not surprisingly, are the most common cause of postoperative mortality in patients undergoing pulmonary resection.[34] Cardiac complications also account for a significant percentage of mortality, and technical problems such as hemorrhage, bronchopleural fistula, and empyema account for a small but significant percentage of complications leading to death.

Postoperative Morbidity

Approximately 30 percent of patients undergoing pulmonary resection will sustain a postoperative complication of which approximately two-thirds are minor and the other one-third nonfatal major complications.[7] The most common complication is supraventricular arrhythmia, which occurs in up to 20 percent of patients, depending on how closely patients are monitored. Most of these respond to simple pharmacologic manipulation and rarely are hemodynamically significant at onset. With appropriate treatment the rhythm reverts to sinus rhythm quickly, and patients may be taken off the antiarrhythmic drugs usually after 1 month. Other minor complications include postoperative air leaks lasting greater than 7 days and atelectasis. Major nonfatal events most commonly are respiratory related, with patients developing significant infiltrates and pneumonitis. A small percentage of patients require reintubation in the postoperative period for respiratory failure usually related to the development of an infiltrate. There are no definitive predictors for postoperative pulmonary complications, although significant risk factors for major complications include age > 60 years, FEV_1 < 2 L, weight loss > 10 percent, associated systemic disease, and extent of disease.[34] Pulmonary complications can be minimized with meticulous attention to postoperative respiratory maneuvers including chest physiotherapy and preoperative teaching.

Other complications of pulmonary resection include wound infections and disturbances in mental status, especially in older patients. Postpneumonectomy complications, fortunately, are unusual, but the most common one is empyema with or without a bronchial stump leak.[51]

Prognosis Following Resection

Prognosis following pulmonary resection has been well analyzed, and results are summarized in Table 113-I-2. Prognosis depends mainly on TNM stage, a classification which was re-

TABLE 113-1-2

Five-Year Postoperative Survival by TNM Stage Based on Data from Lung Cancer Study Group Trials

Stage	Squamous Cell (n = 549), %	Adenocarcinoma (n = 572), %
Stage I		
T1N0	83	69 (p = .02)
T2N0	64	57
Stage II		
T1N1	75	52 (p = .04)
T2N1	53	25 (p < .01)
Stage IIIa		
T1-2N2	46	35
T3N0	37	21

vised as recently as 1986.[29] Short of disseminated disease, prognosis mainly depends on the status of the regional lymph nodes. Prognostic data are only as good as the sampling done at the time of operation, and lymph node dissection is the only sure way to ascertain definitively the status of the lymph nodes. Histologic type also has some prognostic significance but to a lesser extent, and histologic grade, according to present knowledge, has little prognostic significance. The presence of neuroendocrine features in what is otherwise a non-small cell carcinoma, however, may have prognostic significance.[20]

Sites of Recurrence

Patients with lung cancer die of disseminated disease, and it is a distant site that most commonly is the first site of recurrent disease. Over 30 percent of patients with adenocarcinomas will develop brain metastases, a percentage significantly higher than for patients with squamous carcinoma. Other common sites of metastatic disease include bone, lung, liver, and adrenals. Patients with higher-stage disease have a significantly greater likelihood of developing disseminated disease. This recognition has led to the neoadjuvant treatment regimens in patients with N2 disease. Local recurrence does occur most commonly associated with distant disease. Isolated local recurrence is a rare phenomenon but is sometimes amenable to resection. This underscores the importance of a complete resection at the time of the initial operative procedure. Sites of local recurrence which may cause problems include the chest wall (pain), superior vena cava (SVC syndrome), and involvement of the left recurrent laryngeal nerve (hoarseness and swallowing problems). Symptomatic local recurrence often is treated with radiation therapy, and chemotherapy is employed for some patients who develop disseminated disease, while recognizing that cure is usually not possible in patients who have developed distant disease.

Postsurgical Follow-up

Recognizing that essentially no patient is cured once distant disease is present might raise the question of why patients should be followed at all following pulmonary resection. Is there an ad-

vantage to recognizing the development of distant disease early rather than late? Actually there may be some advantage, especially when it comes to preventing some of the morbidity which may accompany disseminated disease if treatment begins early. Also the occasional patient presents with an isolated local recurrence which may be amenable to surgery. Perhaps most important is the sense of comfort patients derive from knowing that they are being closely followed by their physician or surgeon. Especially if the follow-up is done in a cost-efficient manner it is difficult to fault.

Since most local recurrences occur within the first 2 years following resection, patients should be seen every 3 months with a chest radiograph as the only diagnostic study. There is absolutely no need to obtain a CT scan as a follow-up study, and no blood tests are of any use in following these patients. Further studies are ordered based on patient complaints or findings elicited by a careful history and physical examination in addition to the chest radiograph. Between years 2 and 5 patients are seen every 6 months and after 5 years on a yearly basis. Usually the development of disseminated disease is obvious as the patients relate the history of problems since their last visit. Imaging studies tend only to confirm the clinical impression, and then a decision regarding further treatment needs to be made.

Future Directions

The role of surgery in the management of non-small cell lung cancer has been well defined and remains the standard therapy for patients with localized disease. The challenge for all who deal with lung cancer is the problem of disseminated disease. Perhaps the better way to deal with the problem is to identify causes of the disease in addition to the already well-defined risk of cigarette smoking. Thus far a "lung cancer susceptibility" gene has not been demonstrated, but, based on the recent explosion of knowledge related to breast cancer, the identification of one or more genes involved in the genesis of certain lung cancers is at hand. Cigarette smoking has been identified as a major risk factor, yet only a small percentage of patients who smoke develop lung cancers. Efforts to identify such susceptibility genes have been hampered by the relative lack of families with a genetic predisposition. The issue of smoking as a risk factor only serves to confound the search.

Molecular markers to identify patients at increased risk of developing recurrent disease are also desperately needed. Once identified these patients would begin adjuvant therapy designed to prevent recurrence in this high-risk group, sparing those patients who are at lower risk. This further underscores the need for better adjuvant therapy, since none exists at present. Targeting specific factors that control lung cancer development or specific receptors on lung cancer cells seems a more sensible strategy than that utilized by currently available antineoplastic agents. Major strides have been and continue to be made in the molecular biology and genetics of tumors, and we can expect lung cancer to be the beneficiary of some of these developments.

In the meantime refinements in surgical techniques and perioperative management of patients with lung cancer have allowed greater numbers of patients with localized and locally advanced disease to benefit from operative intervention. Many patients with mediastinal lymph node disease previously thought not to be operative candidates now are able to be operated upon with improved survival after a course of neoadjuvant therapy. Other patients with pulmonary function so compromised that it precluded resection now are often considered for resection using the minimally invasive techniques developed within the previous few years aided by better pain management and postoperative chest physiotherapy. It's safe to say that surgery will continue to play a major role in the management of patients with non-small lung cancer.

REFERENCES

1. Albain KS, Rusch VW, Crowley JJ, et al: Concurrent cisplatin/etoposide plus chest radiotherapy followed by surgery for stages IIIA (N2) and IIIB non-small-cell lung cancer: Mature results of Southwest Oncology Group phase II study 8805. *J Clin Oncol* 18:1330–1892, 1995.

2. Bollen EC, van Duin CJ, Theunissen PH, et al: Mediastinal lymph node dissection in resected lung cancer: Morbidity and accuracy of staging. *Ann Thorac Surg* 55: 961–966, 1993.

3. Burkes RL, Ginsberg RJ, Shepherd FA, et al: Induction chemotherapy with mitomycin, vindesine, and cisplatin for stage III unresectable non-small-cell lung cancer: Results of the Toronto Phase II Trial. *J Clin Oncol* 10:580–586, 1992.

4. Ihde DC: Chemotherapy of lung cancer. *New Engl J Med* 327:1434–1441, 1992.

5. Baly BD Jr, Faling LJ, Bite G, et al: Mediastinal lymph node evaluation by computed tomography in lung cancer. An analysis of 345 patients grouped by TNM staging, tumor size, and tumor location. *J Thorac Cardiovasc Surg* 94:664–672, 1987.

6. Date H, Andou A, Shimizu N: The value of limited resection for "clinical" stage I peripheral non-small cell lung cancer in poor-risk patients: Comparison of limited resection and lobectomy by a computer-assisted matched study. *Tumori* 30:422–426, 1994.

7. Deslauriers J, Ginsberg RJ, Piantadosi S, Fournier B: Prospective assessment of 3-day operative morbidity for surgical resections in lung cancer. *Chest* 106:329S–330S, 1994.

8. Fell SC: Segmental resection. *Chest Surg Clin North Am* 5:205–221, 1995.

9. Fish GD, Stanley JH, Miller KS, et al: Post-biopsy pneumothorax: Estimating the risk by chest radiography and pulmonary function tests. *AJR* 150:71–74, 1988.

10. Fry WA, Sidiqui A, Pensler JM, Mostafavi H: Thoracoscopic implantation of cancer with a fatal outcome. *Ann Thorac Surg* 59:42–45, 1995.

11. Ginsberg RJ, Rubinstein LV: Randomized trial of lobectomy versus limited resection for T1 N0 non-small cell lung cancer. Lung Cancer Study Group. *Ann Thorac Surg* 60:615–622, 1995.

12. Gross BH, Glazer GM, Orringer MB, et al: Bronchogenic carcinoma metastatic to normal-sized lymph nodes: frequency and significance. *Radiology* 166:71–74, 1988.

13. Grover FL: The role of CT and MRI in staging of the mediastinum. *Chest* 106:391S–396S, 1994.

14. Hatter J, Kohman LJ, Mosca RS, et al: Preoperative evaluation of stage I and stage II non-small cell lung cancer. *Ann Thorac Surg* 58:1738–1741, 1994.

15. Ichinose Y, Hara N, Ohta M, et al: Preoperative examination to detect distant metastasis is not advocated for asymptomatic patients with stages 2 and 2 non-small cell lung cancer. *Chest* 96:1104–1109, 1989.

16. Jolly PC, Hutchinson CH, Detterbeck F, et al: Routine computed tomographic scans, selective mediastinoscopy, and other factors in evaluation of lung cancer. *J Thorac Cardiovasc Surg* 102:266–270, 1991.

17. Kawahara K, Akamine S, Tsuji H, et al: Bronchoplastic procedures for lung cancer: Clinical study in 136 patients. *World J Surg* 18:822–825, 1994.

18. Kittle CF: Atypical resections of the lung: Bronchoplasties, sleeve resections, and segmentectomies—their evolution and present status. *Curr Probl Surg* 26:57–132, 1989.

19. Kreisman H, Wolkove N, Quoix E: Small cell lung cancer presenting as a solitary pulmonary nodule. *Chest* 101:225–231, 1992.

20. Lequaglie C, Patriarca C, Cataldo I, et al: Prognosis of resected well-differentiated neuroendocrine carcinoma of the lung. *Chest* 100:1053–1056, 1991.

21. Luke WP, Pearson FG, Todd TR, et al: Prospective evaluation of mediastinoscopy for assessment of carcinoma of the lung. *J Thorac Cardiovasc Surg* 91:53–56, 1986.

22. Lung Cancer Study Group: Effects of postoperative mediastinal radiation on completely resected stage II and stage III epidermoid cancer of the lung. *New Engl J Med* 315:1377–1381, 1986.

23. Mack MJ, Hazelrigg SR, Landreneau RJ, Acuff TE: Thoracoscopy for the diagnosis of the indeterminate solitary pulmonary nodule. *Ann Thorac Surg* 56:825–830, 1993.

24. Martini N, Flehinger BJ: The role of surgery in N2 lung cancer. *Surg Clin North Am* 67:1037–1049, 1987.

25. Martini N, Kris MG, Flehinger BJ, et al: Preoperative chemotherapy for stage IIIa(N2) lung cancer: The Sloan-Kettering experience with 136 patients. *Ann Thorac Surg* 55:1365–1373, 1993.

26. Martini N, Yellin A, Ginsberg RJ, et al: Management of non-small cell lung cancer with direct mediastinal involvement. *Ann Thorac Surg* 58:1447–1451, 1994.

27. McCaughan BC: Primary lung cancer invading the chest wall. *Chest Surg Clin North Am* 4:17–28, 1994.

28. Miller JD, Gorenstein LA, Patterson GA: Staging: The key to rational management of lung cancer. *Ann Thorac Surg* 53:170–178, 1992.

29. Mountain CF: A new international staging system for lung cancer. *Chest* 89:225S–233S, 1986.

30. Nakahara K, Fujii Y, Matsumura A, et al: Role of systematic mediastinal dissection in N2 non-small cell lung cancer patients. *Ann Thorac Surg* 56:331–335, 1993.

31. Patterson FA, Ginsberg RJ, Poon PY, et al: A prospective evaluation of magnetic resonance imaging, computed tomography, and mediastinoscopy in the preoperative assessment of mediastinal node status in bronchogenic carcinoma. *J Thorac Cardiovasc Surg* 97:679–684, 1987.

32. Patterson GA, Piazza D, Pearson FG, et al: Significance of metastatic disease in subaortic lymph nodes. *Ann Thorac Surg* 43:155–159, 1987.

33. Pearson FG: Staging of the mediastinum. Role of mediastinoscopy and computed tomography. *Chest* 103:346S–348S, 1993.

34. Pierce RJ, Copland JM, Sharpe K, Barter CE: Preoperative risk evaluation for lung cancer resection: Predicted postoperative product as a predictor of surgical mortality. *Am J Respir Crit Care Med* 150:945–955, 1994.

35. Pisters KM, Kris MG, Gralla RJ, et al: Randomized trial comparing postoperative chemotherapy with vindesine and cisplatin plus thoracic irradiation with irradiation alone in stage III (N2) non-small cell lung cancer. *J Surg Oncol* 56:236–241, 1994.

36. Pisters KM, Kris MG, Gralla RJ, et al: Pathologic complete response in advanced non-small-cell lung cancer following preoperative chemotherapy: Implications for the design of future non-small-cell lung cancer combined modality trials. *J Clin Oncol* 11:1757–1762, 1993.

37. Ratto GB, Frola C, Cantoni S, Motta G: Improving clinical efficacy of computed tomographic scan in the preoperative assessment of patients with non-small cell lung cancer. *J Thorac Cardiovasc Surg* 99:416–425, 1990.

38. Read RC, Yoder G, Schaeffer RC: Survival after conservative resection for T1 N0 M0 non-small cell lung cancer. *Ann Thorac Surg* 49:391–398, 1990.

39. Rendina EA, Venuta F, DeGiacomo T, et al: Comparative merits of thoracoscopy, mediastinoscopy, and mediastinotomy for mediastinal biopsy. *Ann Thorac Surg* 56:992–995, 1994.

40. Romano PS, Mark DH: Patient and hospital characteristics related to in-hospital mortality after lung cancer resection. *Chest* 101:1332–1337, 1992.

41. Rosell R, Gomez-Codina J, Camps C, et al: A randomized trial comparing preoperative chemotherapy plus surgery with surgery alone in patients with non-small-cell lung cancer. *New Engl J Med* 330:153–158, 1994.

42. Roth JA, Fossella F, Komaki R, et al: A randomized trial comparing perioperative chemotherapy and surgery with surgery along in resectable stage IIIA non-small-cell lung cancer. *J Natl Cancer Inst* 86:673–680, 1994.

43. Roviaro G, Varoli F, Rebuffat C, et al: Videothoracoscopic staging and treatment of lung cancer. *Ann Thorac Surg* 59:971–974, 1995.

44. Rusch VW: Adjuvant and neoadjuvant therapy for stages I through III non-small cell lung cancer. *Ann Thorac Surg* 58:899–900, 1994.

45. Shennib HA, Landreneau R, Mulder DS, Mack M: Video-assisted thoracoscopic wedge resection of T1 lung cancer in high-risk patients. *Ann Surg* 218:555–558, 1993.

46. Staples CA, Muller NL, Miller RR, et al: Mediastinal nodes in bronchogenic carcinoma: comparison between CT and mediastinoscopy. *Radiology* 167:367–372, 1988.

47. Steinbaum SS, Uretzky ID McAdams HP, et al: Exploratory thoracotomy for nonresectable lung cancer. *Chest* 107:1058–1061, 1995.

48. Sugarbaker DJ, Strauss GM: Advances in surgical staging and therapy of non-small-cell lung cancer. *Semin Oncol* 20:163–172, 1993.

49. Suh JH, Dass KK, Pagliaccio L, et al: Endobronchial radiation therapy with or without neodymium yttrium aluminum garnet laser resection for managing malignant airway obstruction. *Cancer* 73:2583–2588, 1994.

50. Torrington KG, Kern JD: The utility of fiberoptic bronchoscopy in the evaluation of the solitary pulmonary nodule. *Chest* 104:1021–1024, 1993.

51. Wahi R, McMurtrey MJ, De Caro LF, et al: Determinants of perioperative morbidity and mortality after pneumonectomy. *Ann Thorac Surg* 48:33–37, 1989.

52. Wain JC: Video-assisted thoracoscopy and the staging of lung cancer. *Ann Thorac Surg* 56:776–778, 1993.

53. Warren WH, Faber LP: Segmentectomy versus lobectomy in patients with stage I pulmonary carcinoma. Five-year survival and patterns of intrathoracic recurrence. *J Thorac Cardiovasc Surg* 104:1087–1093, 1994.

54. Winton TL: Staging for M disease. *World J Surg* 17:960–693, 1993.

55. Yano T, Yokoyama H, Yoshino I, et al: Results of a limited resection for compromised or poor-risk patients with clinical stage I non-small cell carcinoma of the lung. *J Am Coll Surg* 181:33–37, 1995.

PART II: TREATMENT OF NON–SMALL CELL LUNG CANCER: CHEMOTHERAPY

Joseph Treat

Approximately 60 percent of patients with non–small cell lung cancer (NSCLC) have evidence of disseminated disease when first seen by a physician. Such data have led to the assumption that NSCLC is generally a systemic disease and that relatively few patients have localized disease that is amenable to a surgical approach. Unfortunately, patients with disseminated disease are rarely cured despite our best efforts. Therefore, because even patients with localized disease are likely to develop disseminated disease, systemic therapy is an important component of therapy. In the most favorable prognostic group, those with T1N0 disease (i.e., up to 25 percent) are destined to fail within 5 years after surgery.

Historically, single chemotherapeutic agents have achieved only minimal response rates in NSCLC, so regimens that entail combinations of drugs have evolved as standard therapy—if any therapy can be designated as "standard" in this disease. Definition of the role of chemotherapy in the treatment of this disease continues to evolve. For example, controversy exists over the role and benefit of systemic chemotherapy in advanced-stage NSCLC. On the other hand, clinical trials during the past few years have shown the value of chemotherapy in treating localized disease.

CRITERIA FOR REPORTING RESULTS

Several criteria are used in the reporting of the results of chemotherapy. One of these is response rate. Response rate is the percent chance of decreasing tumor size; the decrease is measured in terms of complete (total disappearance by radiologic or physical examination) or partial (50 percent reduction in the product of the largest dimensions of the lesion without any new lesions). Responses are almost always partial in NSCLC.

Although response rates are important in the assessment of new agents or combinations, response rates that are reported by a single institution on the basis of a nonrandomized trial (without a "standard" comparison arm) should be interpreted with caution. A high response rate determined in this way may call attention to an active new agent or combination, but in the last analysis, efficacy can be demonstrated only by larger randomized trials. Many factors influence the response rate in single-arm phase II trials. These include patient selection in terms of performance status, extent of disease, weight loss, and symptoms. Sicker patients, with extensive disease, tend to be left out of these trials.

Once a new active drug or combination has been identified, a randomized trial is necessary to determine whether it offers advantages over a previously established regimen. Although response rates are still being reported, survival is the major end point in treating NSCLC by chemotherapy. Small improvements in survival (e.g., additional 10 weeks), although statistically significant, are of dubious biologic and clinical significance. In addition, quality-of-life indices that are standardized and reproducible are now available as part of the evaluation of clinical benefit. It seems likely that future clinical trials will include quality of life and cost analysis as measurable end points.

It is also important at this point to distinguish between *efficacy* and *effectiveness*. A particular regimen may demonstrate *efficacy* within the confines of a limited clinical trial conducted at academic institutions by interested and committed investigators who have a large cohort of patients from which to choose for the study. The extent to which the results of such a trial, based on a selected group of patients, is applicable is often unpredictable. An *efficacious* regimen administered within the confines of a limited clinical trial by dedicated investigators may prove not to be *effective* when applied to a larger population and administered by a multitude of clinicians. This dichotomy between *efficacy* and *effectiveness* needs to be kept in mind when one is evaluating results of any clinical trial. It is especially important, however, when one is looking at results of trials of therapeutic methods in advanced malignant disease, in which the response rates are modest at best.

LOCALIZED NON-SMALL CELL LUNG CANCER

Surgery remains the best option for patients with localized disease who do not have overwhelming medical contraindications to surgical resection. Staging is central to the therapeutic approach to NSCLC. This entails determination of the extent of invasion of the mediastinal lymph nodes. Mediastinoscopy is the procedure of choice for sampling mediastinal lymph nodes before thoracotomy. As for all surgical interventions for thoracic malignancy, complete nodal sampling or lymph node dissection is an integral part of the procedure. Staging of a patient with lung cancer is feasible only if the status of the mediastinal lymph nodes is ascertained. Reliance on noninvasive imaging is inadequate for accurate assessment of the mediastinum (Figs. 113-II-1 and 113-II-2).

If a patient has stage I disease, there is no role for chemotherapy or radiation therapy after resection. Patients with stage II disease (N1 lymph node involvasion) should be considered for inclusion in a postoperative adjuvant study. Although there are currently no data that demonstrate a survival advantage for postoperative adjuvant therapy in patients with completely resected stage II disease—regardless of whether the patient receives radiation therapy alone or radiation therapy and chemotherapy—most of these patients are treated with postoperative radiation therapy in order to decrease local recurrence. Unfortunately, prevention of local recurrence has not been shown to translate into survival benefit.[14]

LOCALLY ADVANCED NSCLC

The term *locally advanced,* includes several different presentations of primary lung cancer, but all have in common the absence

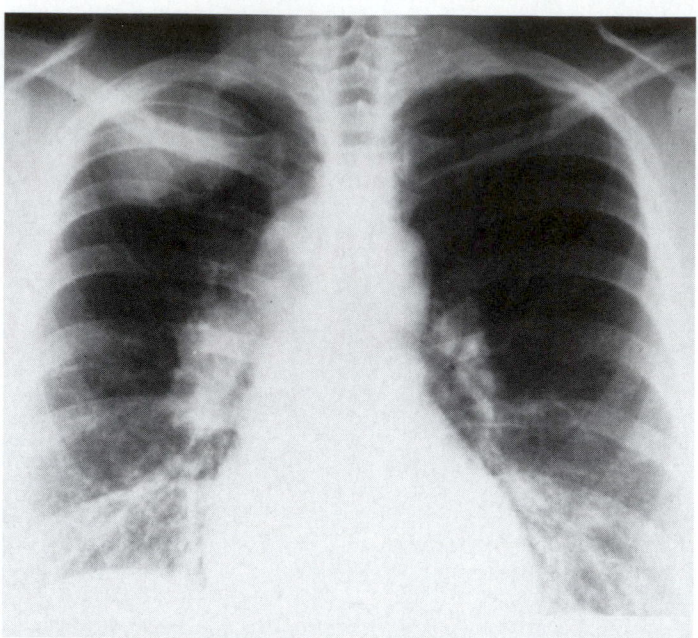

FIGURE 113-II-1 Chest radiograph of a 60-year-old female smoker who presented with increasing cough. The film shows a large right upper-lobe mass with obvious mediastinal and hilar adenopathy. Ipsilateral mediastinal lymph node involvement was confirmed by mediastinoscopy. An extent-of-disease evaluation failed to demonstrate any evidence of disseminated disease. The patient was treated in a protocol setting with preoperative chemotherapy.

of disease outside of the chest. Some of these lesions are eminently resectable, others marginally resectable, and others out of the realm of resectability. Included in this group of lesions (stage IIA) are those with mediastinal lymph node impairment (N2 dis-

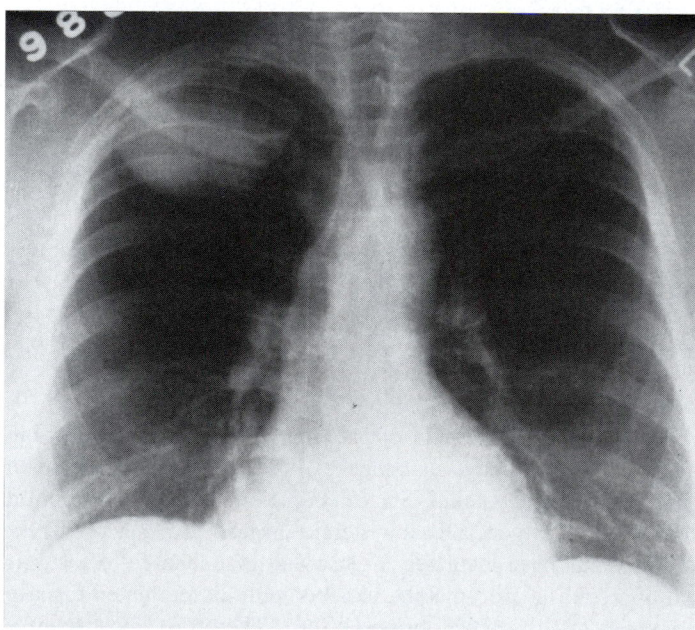

FIGURE 113-II-2 Chest radiograph of the same patient as in Fig. 113-II-1 following two cycles of chemotherapy. Note the minimal effect on the primary tumor but the considerable decrease in size of the nodal metastatic disease. The patient subsequently went to surgery and was able to have a complete resection.

ease), direct extension into certain mediastinal structures (T3), direct extension into the chest wall (T3), and certain endobronchial lesions.

Lesions that directly invade the mediastinum but affect structures that are not usually considered resectable (e.g., aorta, esophagus, and vertebral bodies) are classified as T4 and are considered to be stage IIIB. The distinction between IIIA and IIIB lesions is important, since prognosis is significantly worse for the latter lesions. The distinction between a T3 and a T4 primary often cannot be made on the basis of preoperative imaging and depends on a determination made at thoracotomy. As indicated above, mediastinal lymph node invasion can be determined before thoracotomy by way of mediastinoscopy, which also allows contralateral mediastinal lymph nodes to be sampled. Contralateral nodal invasion indicates N3 disease, which also falls within the stage IIIB classification.

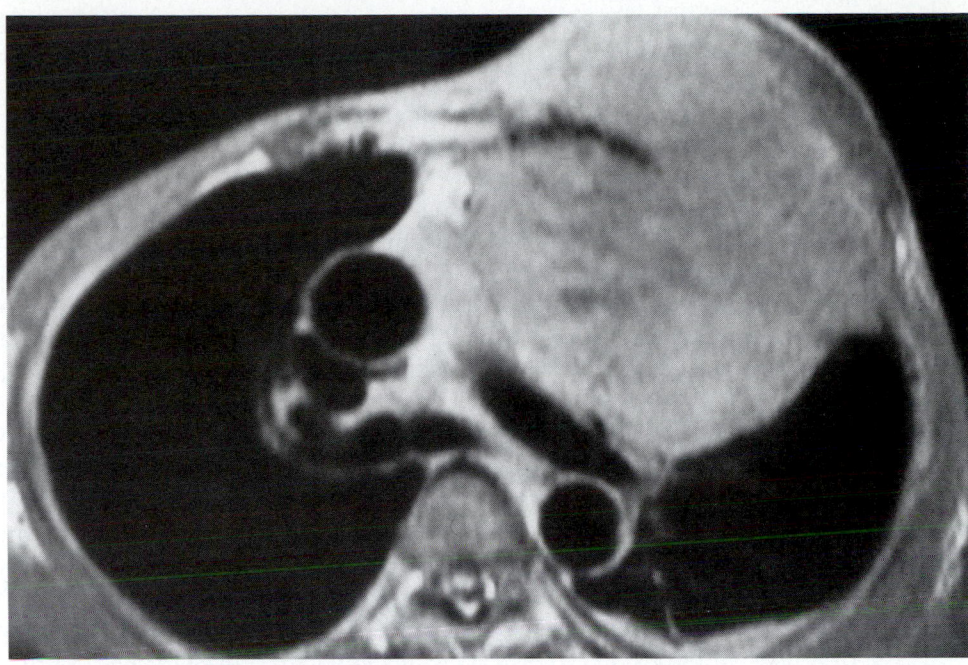

FIGURE 113-II-3   MRI scan of a patient with locally advanced disease invading the chest wall and at least abutting the mediastinum. At exploration, the lesion was found not to be invading the mediastinum and was completely removed with a lobectomy and chest wall resection.

To date, most studies in which patients with locally advanced disease were treated with chemotherapy, radiotherapy, or a combination of the two have relied on noninvasive determination of the extent of the disease. Thus, on the basis of enlarged mediastinal lymph nodes seen on a computed tomographic (CT) scan, patients were assumed to have N2 disease and were treated without histologic documentation of mediastinal lymph node impairment. Such studies are seriously flawed. For meaningful interpretation, accurate histologic staging has to be included as an entry criterion for any study of locally advanced disease.

About 40,000 cases of stage IIIA and IIIB disease occur per year in the United States. The best treatment approach to locally advanced disease has not yet been determined. A wide array of combined modality approaches have been used in stage IIIA patients (particularly those with N2 nodes). These include chemotherapy with surgery, radiation with surgery, chemotherapy with radiation (both sequentially and simultaneously), and chemotherapy with radiation and surgery. Unfortunately, some T3 patients have been included in many of these trials—again complicating interpretation of the results (Fig. 113-II-3).

Nonetheless, this trial did demonstrate responsiveness at the higher levels of radiation and improved survival at 3 years for the 6000-cGy-arm. At 5 years, all treatment arms were associated with a 5 percent survival. Today, after accurate staging, many of these patients would be eligible for combined modality studies that consisted of chemotherapy and radiation therapy, with or without surgery.

Another large study, conducted by the Southeastern Oncology Group, randomized patients to radiation alone (6000 cGy), single-agent chemotherapy with vindesine, or concurrent vindesine and radiation therapy.[11] The median survival and percentage of patients alive at 5 years were 8.6 months (3 percent), 10.1 months (1 percent), and 9.4 months (3 percent), respectively. These studies underscore the lack of effect of radiation as a single modality as well as the lack of improvement when a single drug is added to radiation therapy. Since combination chemotherapy that included a cisplatin-based drug regimen provided longer survival than did any single agent, combination chemotherapy was utilized in addition to radiation therapy in the attempt to improve results.

RADIATION THERAPY ALONE

Until recently, radiation therapy alone was the standard therapy for patients with N2 disease. This practice resulted in a 5-year survival of about 5 percent. This form of treatment was based largely on a clinical begun in 1973 by the Radiation Therapy Oncology Group (RTOG 73-01). This study looked at different doses of radiation (4000, 5000, or 6000 cGy) and split-course versus continuous therapy at 4000 cGy.[22] Interpretation of this study is difficult because of the relatively poor quality of the CT scan images available at that time and the lack of documentation of histologic evidence of N2 disease before entry into the study.

CHEMOTHERAPY FOLLOWED BY RADIATION THERAPY: RANDOMIZED TRIALS

Several prospective, randomized studies have compared radiation therapy alone and radiation therapy plus chemotherapy. Mattson's team reported a series of "inoperable" patients randomized to receive either radiation alone (5500 cGy) or chemotherapy (cyclophosphamide [Cytoxan], doxorubicin [Adriamycin], and cisplatin) followed by radiation.[18] Patients were entered into the trial if they had disease confined to the hemithorax or mediastinal lymph nodes. Thus, patients with N1 disease and presumed T3 disease were included and analyzed together. There was no statistically significant difference in median survival times (10.2 versus 10.9 months) or in long-term survival for the study groups as a whole. The study was flawed because of the inclusion of patients with different disease stages, a lack of histologic documentation of the stage of disease, and the use of a smaller than usual dose of cisplatin.

The North Central Cancer Treatment Group randomized patients to radiation alone (6000 cGy) versus chemotherapy followed by radiation and additional chemotherapy.[20] Again, no difference in median survival or long-term outcome could be demonstrated between the two treatment groups. Failure to find a difference may be due to the absence of cisplatin from the chemotherapy regimen.

In contrast, reports of cisplatin-based regimens do indicate an advantage for combined chemotherapy and radiation. Le Chevalier and associates randomized 353 patients to radiation alone (6500 cGy) or to cisplatin-based chemotherapy followed by radiation.[13] Using repeat biopsies, the study found a 17 percent incidence of local control in the radiation arm and a 15 percent incidence in the chemotherapy and radiation arm. One-, 2-, and 3-year survival rates all favored the combined therapy arm (51, 21, and 12 percent versus 41, 14, and 4 percent, respectively).

In a trial conducted by the Cancer and Leukemia Group B (CALGB), 155 patients were randomized to either radiation alone (6000 cGy) or a cisplatin-based regimen followed by radiation.[6] The median survival favored the combined arm (13.8 versus 9.7 months). The results at 1 and 2 years were so striking for the combined therapy group that the study was terminated early—a decision that subsequently prompted considerable criticism. The 3- and 5-year survival rates also favored the combination therapy (25 and 19 percent) over radiation therapy alone (11 and 7 percent). The intrathoracic failure rate was very high. Unfortunately, the study was limited to patients with a high performance status and less than 5 percent weight loss in the 6 months before enrollment in the trial. Limiting a study to the most favorable patients begs the question of the applicability of the results to the general group of patients with locally advanced lung cancer, many of whom have a decrease in their performance status and have lost considerable weight.

A study seeking to confirm the CALGB report was initiated by the RTOG, which randomized patients to the same two arms, in addition to a third arm using hyperfractionation radiation (69.6 cGy twice daily) as the single agent.[28] This study, RTOG-88-08, demonstrated that chemotherapy combined with radiation was indeed superior in the patients with good performance status (i.e., loss of weight of less than 5 percent in the previous 3 months). Analysis at 1 year showed median survival to be statistically longer for those in the combined chemotherapy and radiation arm. At 3 years' follow-up, however, no difference in survival (14 percent) was found

between the chemotherapy and radiation arm and the hyperfractionated arm. Both of these treatment regimens were better than standard radiation alone.

CONCURRENT CHEMOTHERAPY AND RADIATION THERAPY

The rationale for concurrent therapy (i.e., chemotherapy given during a course of radiation therapy) is based on the concept that some drugs or drug combinations (notably cisplatin) may act synergistically with radiation. The trade-off, however, may be an increase in toxicity and a regimen that is not well tolerated by all potentially eligible patients.

Several studies have tested the concept of concurrent therapy by combining frequent dosing of cisplatin with radiation. The largest, conducted by the European Organization for Research and Treatment of Cancer (EORTC), randomized 309 patients to radiation alone or to radiation with cisplatin given on either a daily or weekly schedule.[29] At 2 years, 26 percent of patients treated with concurrent radiation and daily cisplatin were alive, in contrast to only 13 percent survival in the group receiving radiation alone. When given on a weekly basis with radiation, the cisplatin did not confer any advantage over radiation alone. However, several other studies have failed to demonstrate an advantage for concurrent therapy in locally advanced disease (Table 113-II-1). The greatest advantage with combined chemotherapy and radiation therapy is seen at the 2- and 3-year marks. At present, concurrent therapy probably should be limited to clinical trials, since the benefit is modest and the toxicity is somewhat greater than that from sequential therapy or use of a single modality.

CHEMOTHERAPY FOLLOWED BY SURGERY

Neoadjuvant therapy, also referred to as *induction therapy,* has been applied to the treatment of NSCLC as well as to treatment of many other solid tumors. It entails treating patients with

TABLE 113-II-1

Randomized Trials in Stage II Disease: Radiation Alone vs. Radiation and Chemotherapy

Number of Patients	Therapy	Median Survival	Survival 1yr	2yrs	3yrs	Reference
155	RT	9.6	40	13	11	6
	RT/CT	13.8	55	26	23	
353	RT	10	41	14	4	13
	RT/CT	12	51	21	12	
238	RT	10.2	41	17		17
	RT/CT	10.9	42	19		
114	RT	10.3	45	16	7	18
	RT/CT	10.4	45	21	5	
95	RT	11				29
	RT/CT	16				
309	RT		46	13	2	28
	RT/CT		54	26	16	
			44	19	13	
183	RT	41	9			2
	RT/CT	35	15			

chemotherapy even though there is no clinical evidence that the primary cancer has spread. Lung cancers are particularly attractive targets for neoadjuvant therapy because even though many present as locally advanced disease confined to the chest, patients run a considerable risk of developing distant disease within a short time. Neoadjuvant therapy affords a unique opportunity to assess the sensitivity of the cancer to the drug regimen. This information may be useful in the postoperative period when the possibility of adjuvant therapy is under consideration. Moreover, preoperative neoadjuvant therapy may render resectable a tumor that would otherwise be regarded as unresectable.

The possibility exists that delaying surgery may be disadvantageous. However, in patients with localized advanced disease who are at high risk for developing disseminated disease, the delay imposed by the administration of chemotherapy provides an additional period of observation during which a nonresponder may manifest distant disease, thereby precluding surgery. Another consideration is that the required dose-intensive regimens are apt to be tolerated better before than after surgery, and chemotherapy may slow growth after the primary tumor is removed. Finally, neoadjuvant therapy may preserve the vasculature of the tumor for drug delivery and decrease the prospect of developing drug resistance.

There have been two phase III randomized trials of neoadjuvant chemotherapy in patients with locally advanced lung cancer (stage IIIA). Patients had N2 disease alone; others had T3N0 disease.[25,26] In contrast to results in patients with disseminated NSCLC in whom the response to chemotherapy at best approaches 30 percent, 60 to 70 percent of patients with locally advanced disease responded favorably. The explanation for this difference in responsiveness may be the better overall status of patients who are regarded as candidates for surgery and the smaller tumor burden that these patients bear. Alternatively, qualities inherent in the primary tumor that differ from those in tumor that has metastasized may contribute to a better response to chemotherapy. Currently, there is no way of assessing the response of micrometastatic disease other than the disease-free interval after resection and survival.

The largest experience with neoadjuvant chemotherapy for NSCLC was reported from the Memorial Sloan-Kettering Cancer Center.[16] The study was prospective but nonrandomized. It included 136 patients with "clinical N2" disease defined as bulky mediastinal adenopathy that could be seen on the conventional chest radiograph or was manifested at bronchoscopy by widening of the carina. Mediastinoscopy for documentation of N2 disease was performed in 122 of the patients. Patients received a cisplatin-based regimen (two or three cycles per day for 3 days) plus mitomycin. The overall response rate was 77 percent; 19 of the patients achieved a complete response that was confirmed by histologic examination. Seventy-five percent of patients were able to undergo resection even though resectability based on previous experience would have been anticipated to be about 10 percent. It must be emphasized that these patients had bulky mediastinal lymph node disease, not lymph nodes that appeared grossly normal but in whom disease was subsequently detected. The authors concluded that the results obtained paralleled those noted in neoadjuvant studies with other solid tumors in that response rates to chemotherapy were high, and complete resection rates were high after response to

chemotherapy. They identified response to chemotherapy as a significant prognostic indicator for survival: complete response was associated with prolonged survival.

CHEMOTHERAPY AND RADIATION FOLLOWED BY SURGERY

Various theoretical considerations have led to trials of chemotherapy and radiation followed by surgery: (1) tumor cell subpopulations in locally advanced NSCLC may respond differently to radiation and chemotherapy, and cells resistant to one treatment method may be sensitive to the other; (2) chemotherapy may promote the emergence of radiosensitive cells, thereby increasing the total number of cells killed by continued radiation treatments; and (3) induction of cell cycle synchronization by certain drugs may increase cell killing by radiation and induce recruitment of tumor cells in G_0.[33,35]

The Southwest Oncology Group conducted a trial using a cisplatin-based regimen with concurrent radiotherapy; the trial included both stage IIIA and IIIB patients.[27] All patients underwent mediastinoscopy for histologic evaluation of mediastinal lymph nodes. The response rate to the preoperative therapy was 69 percent, with a 73 percent resection rate. In 11 of the 53 who responded, histologic examination postoperatively yielded no evidence of cancer. The median survival for the group was 17 months. Somewhat surprising was the lack of difference in median survival between patients with stage IIIA and those with IIIB disease.

It remains to be proved that surgery is a necessary part of the treatment of these patients. The high response rate to chemotherapy in the high-performance patients entered into these clinical trials raises the question of whether radiation might be able to achieve a similar end point with regard to local control. A large intergroup study is currently addressing this question.

In summary, major issues remain concerning the sequence and number of treatment methods. A key issue is whether simultaneous chemotherapy and radiation are superior to sequential chemotherapy followed by radiation therapy. This is important in that toxicity is generally greater with simultaneous chemotherapy. Further complicating the issue is the question of how the newer chemotherapy agents and combinations will fit into combined modality approaches.

ADJUVANT THERAPY

It is well recognized that despite complete resection, most patients with locally advanced NSCLC will, at some time, develop disseminated disease. As noted above, the risk of developing disseminated disease can be predicted, with some accuracy, on the basis of the stage of the disease determined at the time of the initial resection. However, the value of the staging information depends on the completeness of the staging procedures carried out at the time of resection. Even with stage I disease, as many as 20 percent of patients will die of disseminated disease within 5 years. With stage II disease, less than 50 percent of patients will be alive at 5 years; with stage IIIA N2 disease, at best 30 percent of patients will be alive at 5 years. These numbers make clear the need for some additional therapy to improve on the overall survival achieved by surgery.

Despite numerous studies of adjuvant therapy in patients with locally advanced NSCLC administered while there is no evidence of disseminated disease, no prospective randomized trial has shown that any regimen improves survival. The concept is attractive (i.e., treat patients who have no evidence of disseminated disease but are deemed to be at high risk for dissemination of disease in the hope of eliminating micrometastatic disease). Although research conducted by the Lung Cancer Study Group on patients with either stage II or IIIA, who had undergone resection of a squamous cell carcinoma, showed that those who received postoperative radiation therapy had a significantly lower incidence of local recurrence than those receiving no postoperative radiation, there was no difference in survival between the treated and untreated groups.[14] Thus, the ability to decrease the incidence of local recurrence did not translate into survival benefit. This result should not be surprising, since patients with lung cancer die of disseminated disease and it is difficult to imagine how treating with postoperative radiation therapy—like surgery, a local modality—could prevent the development of disseminated disease. Nor has systemic chemotherapy in these patients improved survival.

Currently, there is no generally accepted postoperative therapy for patients who have undergone complete resection whose disease has been well staged. This does not mean that patients are not treated postoperatively. Quite the contrary. There is general belief, despite the lack of data for support, that patients with nodal disease found at the time of surgery should receive postoperative radiation therapy. This belief is so strongly held that it is currently impossible in the United States to mount a trial comparing postoperative treatment with no treatment. There is in progress a large national study, involving all of the cooperative oncology groups, in which patients are randomized following a complete resection to receive either radiation therapy alone or radiation therapy combined with cisplatin and VP-16. The control group in this trial is the group receiving radiation therapy alone. It was impossible to initiate this trial with a no-therapy arm even as a three-arm trial. Based on the evidence available, it seems questionable to subject a patient to postoperative adjuvant therapy outside of a protocol setting.

ADVANCED-STAGE NSCLC

The goal of chemotherapy in advanced-stage disease is palliation, since, with few exceptions, disseminated lung cancer, like most other solid tumors, is essentially impossible to cure. Among the issues that have been raised with respect to the relative value of chemotherapy in patients with disseminated disease are the response rate, survival data, cost-effectiveness, and the quality of life.

Prognostic criteria play an important role in analyzing and constructing clinical trials. For example, patients with a poor performance status (spending more than 50 percent of time in bed, significant weight loss) are much less likely to respond to chemotherapy than those with better performance status. In patients with poor prognosis, it is important to assess the effect of treatment-related toxicity on overall quality of life and the cost-effectiveness of therapy.

Several studies have randomized patients with disseminated disease to receive either best supportive care or systemic chemotherapy.[3,8,12,24,36] In addition, four meta-analyses have reviewed studies that randomized patients to best supportive care or chemotherapy.[9,16,31,32] In one meta-analysis, a median survival of 6.7 months followed chemotherapy, as compared with 3.9 months with best supportive care; the absolute difference in survival at 6 months was 20 percent.[16] These data can be used to make the case for or against systemic chemotherapy (i.e., that the patients did live longer when treated or that the three additional months of survival had little biologic significance). In general, meta-analyses have shown a 10 percent increase in survival at 1 year, but an increase in median survival of only 2 months.

A significant question is the issue of cost. If it is more expensive to treat patients with disseminated disease with chemotherapy, does the additional few months of survival warrant it? Some of the uncertainty depends on how *best supportive care* is defined. Most commonly, this does not imply only pharmacologic pain management and psychosocial support or hospice care. Usually it includes palliative radiotherapy and, at times, limited chemotherapy. In one study, the cost was found to be less in the group treated with chemotherapy, since patients in the best supportive care group required more frequent hospitalizations and had a greater need for palliative radiotherapy.[10]

Interpretation of the meta-analyses that deal with the survival advantages of chemotherapy has been challenged on the basis of clinical relevance.[5] At issue are concerns about how the quality-of-life assessments have been made and the balance between the toxicity of therapy and the modest survival advantage.[35] Most of the studies have included only the higher performance status patients—which calls into question the general applicability of the results. Whether to treat a patient with disseminated disease using chemotherapy or to treat symptoms as they arise often comes down to the judgment of the medical oncologist balanced against the wishes of the patient. Patients with poor performance status can be expected to have a poorer response to chemotherapy than those with relatively good performance status; therefore, they would not usually be offered chemotherapy. Adding to this uncertainty is the fact that experimental drugs are often advocated as first-line therapy in advanced-stage NSCLC based on the overall outcome from standard therapy—which, as noted above, is generally limited to those with relatively preserved performance status.

NEW DEVELOPMENTS

The past few years have been marked by the appearance of several new antineoplastic agents, several of which have novel mechanisms of action. These new agents have led to renewed enthusiasm for the role of chemotherapy in NSCLC. These agents include docetaxel,[4,7] camptothecins such as topotecan[15,23] and irinotecan,[19,21] gemcitabine,[1] and tirapazamine.[10a] It remains to be determined whether some of these agents will be associated with higher response rates either alone or in combination with more conventional agents in NSCLC patients with localized or disseminated disease.

CONCLUSION

Chemotherapy has an established role in the therapy of stage IIIA and IIIB NSCLC. Randomized clinical trial data demonstrate improved median and long-term survival when antineo-plastic agents are used as part of a multimodality approach. Response rates to chemotherapy are higher in patients with localized disease than in patients with disseminated disease. Some of these differences may be related to tumor burden or overall performance status. Questions that need to be addressed in future and ongoing trials include the optimal sequence for various modalities and the best modalities for each situation. The best chemotherapy regimen for use in a multimodality setting remains to be defined. There remains a need to test as part of combined modality therapy the newer classes of drugs (taxanes), as well as some of the drugs (tirapazamine, gemcitabine, camptothecins) that are currently investigational.

For advanced-stage NSCLC, difficult issues remain to be addressed. While statistical tools such as meta-analysis have shown an advantage with respect to survival in patients undergoing chemotherapy, there has not yet been a definitive prospective study that takes into account the issues of quality of life and cost-effectiveness. Moreover, the earlier studies utilized the older cisplatin-based combination chemotherapy regimens. Currently, there are ongoing studies with newer regimens employing cisplatin—in particular with Navelbine—as well as studies with combinations that do not include cisplatin. The newer, more effective regimens may improve upon the modest gains in survival or decreased toxicity reported in the meta-analyses, which were based on data derived from studies utilizing older cisplatin containing regimens. Some of the new agents have engendered cautious optimism; the need continues for identification of new compounds that will be effective in treating NSCLC.

REFERENCES

1. Anderson H, Thatcher N, Walling J, Hansen H: A phase I study of a 24-hour infusion of gemcitabine in previously untreated patients with inoperable non–small cell lung cancer. *Br J Cancer* 74:460–462, 1996.

2. Blanke C, Ansari R, Mantravadi R, et al: Phase III trial of thoracic irradiation with or without cisplatin for locally advanced unresectable non–small cell-lung cancer: A Hoosier Oncology Group protocol. *J Clin Oncol* 13:1425–1429, 1995.

3. Cellerino R, Tummarello D, Guidi F, et al: A randomized trial of alternating chemotherapy versus best supportive care in advanced non–small-lung cancer. *J Clin Oncol* 9:1453–1461, 1991.

4. Cerny T, Kaplan S, Pavlidis N, et al: Docetaxel (Taxotere) is active in non–small-cell lung cancer: A phase II trial of the EORTC Early Clinical Trials Group (ECTG). *Br J Cancer* 70:384–387, 1994.

5. Coates A, Forbes J: Is chemotherapy for non–small cell lung cancer worthwhile? *Lancet* 342:4, 1993.

6. Dillman RO, Seagren SL, Propert KJ, et al: A randomized trial of induction chemotherapy plus high-dose radiation versus radiation along in stage III non–small-cell lung cancer. *New Engl J Med* 323:940–945, 1990.

7. Fossella FV, Lee JS, Murphy WK, et al: Phase II study of docetaxel for recurrent or metastatic non–small-cell lung cancer. *J Clin Oncol* 12:1238–1244, 1994.

8. Ganz PA, Figlin RA, Haskell CM, et al: Supportive care versus supportive care and combination chemotherapy in metastatic non–small cell lung cancer: Does chemotherapy make a difference? *Cancer* 63:1271–1278, 1989.

9. Grilli R, Oxman AD, Julian JA: Chemotherapy for advanced non–small-cell lung cancer: How much benefit is enough? *J Clin Oncol* 11:1866–1872, 1993.

10. Jaakkimainen L, Goodwin PJ, Pater J, et al: Counting the costs of chemotherapy in a National Cancer Institute of Canada randomized trial in non-small-cell lung cancer. *J Clin Oncol* 8:1301–1309, 1990.

10a. Johnson CA, Kilpatrick D, van Roemeling R, et al: Phase I trial of tirapazamine in combination with cisplatin in a single dose every 3 weeks in patients with solid tumors. *J Clin Oncol* 15:773–780, 1997.

11. Johnson DH, Einhorn LH, Bertolucci A, et al: Thoracic radiotherapy does not prolong survival in patients with locally advanced, unresectable non-small cell lung cancer. *Ann Intern Med* 113:33–38, 1990.

12. Kassa S, Lund E, Thorud E, et al: Symptomatic treatment versus combination chemotherapy for patients with extensive non-small cell lung cancer. *Cancer* 67:2443–2447, 1991.

13. Le Chevalier T, Arriagada R, Quoix E, et al: Radiotherapy alone versus combined chemotherapy and radiotherapy in nonresectable non–small-cell lung cancer: First analysis of a randomized trial in 353 patients. *J Natl Cancer Inst* 83:417–423, 1991.

14. Lung Cancer Study Group: Effects of postoperative mediastinal radiation on completely resected stage II and stage III epidermoid cancer of the lung. *New Engl J Med* 315:1377–1381, 1986.

15. Lynch TJ Jr, Kalish L, Strauss G, et al: Phase II study of topotecan in metastatic non-small-cell lung cancer. *J Clin Oncol* 12:347–352, 1994.

16. Marino P, Pampallona S, Preatoni A, et al: Chemotherapy vs supportive care in advanced non-small-cell lung cancer: Results of a meta-analysis of the literature. *Chest* 106:861–865, 1994.

17. Martini N, Kris MG, Gralla RJ, et al: The effects of preoperative chemotherapy on the resectability of non-small cell lung carcinoma with mediastinal lymph node metastases (N2 M0). *Ann Thorac Surg* 45:370–379, 1988.

18. Mattson K, Holsti LR, Holsti P, et al: Inoperable non-small cell lung cancer: Radiation with or without chemotherapy. *Eur J Cancer Clin Oncol* 24:477–482, 1988.

19. Mori K, Ohnishi T, Yokoyajma K, Tominaga K: A phase I study of irinotecan and infusional cisplatin for advanced non–small cell lung cancer. *Cancer Chemother Pharmacol* 39:327–332, 1997.

20. Morton RF, Jett JR, McGinnis WL, et al: Thoracic radiation therapy alone compared with combined chemoradiotherapy for locally unresectable non-small cell lung cancer: A randomized, phase III trial. *Ann Intern Med* 115:681–686, 1991.

21. Negoro S, Fukuoka M, Masuda N, et al: Phase I study of weekly intravenous infusions of CPT-11, a new derivative of camptothecin, in the treatment of advanced non–small-cell lung cancer. *J Natl Cancer Inst* 83:1164–1168, 1991.

22. Perez CA, Stanley K, Rubin P, et al: A prospective randomized study of various irradiation doses and fractionation schedules in the treatment of inoperable non-oat-cell carcinoma of the lung. *Cancer* 45:2744–2753, 1980.

23. Perez Soler R, Fossella FV, Glisson BS, et al: Phase II study of topotecan in patients with advanced non–small cell lung cancer previously untreated with chemotherapy. *J Clin Oncol* 14:503–513, 1996.

24. Rapp E, Pater J, Wilan A, et al: Chemotherapy can prolong survival in patients with advanced non-small-cell lung cancer: Report of a Canadian multicenter randomized trial. *J Clin Oncol* 6:633–641, 1988.

25. Rosell R, Gómez-Codina J, Camps C, et al: A randomized trial comparing preoperative chemotherapy plus surgery with surgery alone in patients with non–small-cell lung cancer. *New Engl J Med* 330:153–158, 1994.

26. Roth JA, Fossella F, Komaki R, et al: A randomized trial comparing perioperative chemotherapy and surgery with surgery along in resectable stage IIIA non–small-cell lung cancer. *J Natl Cancer Inst* 86:673–680, 1994.

27. Rusch VW, Albain KS, Crowley JJ, et al: Surgical resection of stage IIIA and stage IIIB non-small-cell lung cancer after concurrent induction chemotherapy: A Southwest Oncology Group trial. *J Thor Cardiovasc Surg* 105:97–104, 1993.

28. Sause WR, Scott C, Taylor S, et al: Radiation Therapy Oncology Group (RTOG) 88-08 and Eastern Cooperative Oncology Group (ECOG) 4588: Preliminary results of a phase III trial in regionally advanced, unresectable non–small-cell lung cancer. *J Natl Cancer Inst* 87:198–205, 1995.

29. Schaake-Koning C, van den Bogaert W, Dalesio O, et al: Effects of concomitant cisplatin and radiotherapy on inoperable non–small-cell lung cancer. *New Engl J Med* 326:524–530, 1992.

30. Soresi E, Clerici M, Grilli R, et al: A randomized clinical trial comparing radiation therapy versus radiation therapy plus cis-dichlorodiamine platinum (II) in the treatment of locally advanced non-small cell lung cancer. *Semin Oncol* 15(Suppl 7):20–25, 1988.

31. Souquet PJ, Chauvin F, Boissel JP, et al: Polychemotherapy in advanced non small cell lung cancer: A meta-analysis. *Lancet* 342:19–21, 1993.

32. Stewart LA, Pignon JP, Parmar AKB, et al, and the NSCLC Collaborators Group: A meta-analysis using individual patient data from randomised clinical trials of chemotherapy in non-small cell lung cancer: Survival in the supportive care setting (abstract). *Proc Am Soc Clin Oncol* 13:337, 1994.

33. Strauss GM, Herndon JE, Sherman DD, et al: Neoadjuvant chemotherapy and radiotherapy followed by surgery in stage IIIA non-small-cell carcinoma of the lung: Report of a Cancer and Leukemia Group B phase II study. *J Clin Oncol* 10:1237–1244, 1992.

34. Vokes EE, Bitran JD: Non-small-cell lung cancer: Toward the next plateau. *Chest* 106:659–660, 1994.

35. Weiden PL, Piantadosi S, for the Lung Cancer Study Group: Preoperative chemotherapy (cisplatin and fluorouracil) and radiation therapy in stage III non–small-cell lung cancer: A phase II study of the Lung Cancer Study Group. *J Natl Cancer Inst* 83:266–273, 1991.

36. Woods RL, Williams CJ, Levi J, et al: A randomised trial of cisplatin and vindesine versus supportive care only in advanced non-small cell lung cancer. *Br J Cancer* 61:608–611, 1990.

PART III: TREATMENT OF NON–SMALL CELL LUNG CANCER: RADIATION THERAPY

William T. Sause/Mitchell Machtay

In 1995 lung cancer was the second most common cancer in males (behind prostate cancer) and the third most common cancer in females (behind breast and colorectal cancers). Of the estimated 170,000 new cases of lung cancer, 100,000 are expected to occur in men and 70,000 in women. Despite the increase in the number of new cases, the cure rates for lung cancer in 1995 remained stable at 10 to 13 percent. This translates into 157,000 deaths in 1995, making lung cancer the leading cause of cancer deaths in males and females. Since lung cancer represents a major health hazard not only in the United States but also worldwide, and the overall picture is discouraging, the magnitude of this health problem is such that even small improvements in treatment can affect large numbers of patients.

Most patients with lung cancer receive radiotherapy as part of their treatment, either as initial management or later in the course of their disease. This may include thoracic radiotherapy and/or irradiation of sites of metastatic disease.

Thoracic radiotherapy (RT) for non-small cell lung carcinoma is usually categorized as follows:

neoadjuvant = preoperative
adjuvant = postoperative
definitive = cure without surgery as treatment goal; with or without chemotherapy
palliative = directed at relief of thoracic symptoms

There is some overlap in these categories with respect to the goals of treatment. For example, most patients treated with definitive intent are not cured but do achieve palliation of intrathoracic symptoms. Similarly, a few patients originally considered to be technically unresectable may have a dramatic response to irradiation and/or chemotherapy, and the goal of treatment may then change from palliative to neoadjuvant. The size of the primary lesion and total dose of radiation are important factors in determining local control. A summary of radiotherapy for lung cancer is provided in Table 113-III-1.

Utilization of thoracic radiotherapy as part of the therapeutic regimen and the therapeutic goal of the therapy depends not only on tumor related-factors such as stage but also on patient-related factors such as pulmonary reserve and performance status. All these factors need to be considered when deciding whether to irradiate. Although radiotherapy might be appropriate for a patient with a postoperative forced expiratory volume (FEV_1) of 2.0 l and pathologic stage T2N2M0 disease with a close margin, the same treatment would be problematic in a patient with pathologic stage T1N1 disease and a postlobectomy FEV_1 of 1.1 l who has had a series of postoperative complications. Of course, such clearcut cases usually are the exception rather than the rule in clinical oncology. Table 113-III-2 lists the relative contraindications to thoracic radiation for lung cancer.

Finally, it must be remembered that the prognosis for most patients with non–small cell lung carcinoma is poor with stan-

TABLE 113-III-1

Summary of Radiotherapy for Lung Cancer: Indications and Treatment

Type	Indications	Fields	Dose (180–200 cGy* Daily Fractions)
Preoperative (with chemotherapy)	Pancoast tumor clinical N2	Large: primary with safety margin and hilum/mediastinum	4500 cGy
Postoperative	N+ disease T3 tumors Incomplete resection	Moderate: nodes/ stump; primary bed only if T3 or residual disease	5000–6500 cGy (depends on surg- path findings)
Definitive medically inoperable	T1-2N0-1 not surgical candidate or refuses surgery	Small: primary with safety margin with or without hilum	6000–7000 cGy
Definitive unresectable (with or without chemotherapy)	Selected stage III patients; performance status high	Large**	6000–7000 cGy
Palliative unresectable	Other stage III and IV patients with local symptoms	Small to moderate: areas of symptomatic disease	2000–5000 cGy in moderate to large fractions (250–400 cGy)
Small cell (with chemotherapy)	Limited stage	Large: primary with safety margin, and hilum/mediastinum	4500–5500 cGy

*1 cGy (centigray) = 1 rad = the basic unit dose of radiotherapy.
**In general, the fields used for the definitive treatment of unresectable non-small cell lung carcinoma are large, encompassing the primary tumor with a "safety" margin and multiple lymph node areas. However, smaller fields, including only gross disease based on CT scan, with or without the hilum, are becoming more acceptable.

dard therapy, and a concerted effort should be made to enter patients into clinical trials that are investigating new treatments or combinations of treatments for this disease.

MANAGEMENT OF NON–SMALL CELL LUNG CANCER (NSCLC)

Surgery, irradiation, and chemotherapy are all used in the treatment of lung cancer. Surgical resection remains the primary curative modality and may be the only treatment required in early-stage disease if all the cancer is removed. Most patients with stage I disease are cured by surgical resection and do not need

TABLE 113-III-2

Relative Contraindications to Thoracic Radiotherapy (RT) for Lung Cancer

Prior high dose thoracic radiotherapy
Connective tissue disease
$FEV_1 < 800$ cc
Tracheobronchial-esophageal fistula
Projected RT field to include > 40 percent of normal lung volume
Projected RT field to include > 50 percent of heart volume
Patient expected to be noncompliant with treatment or follow-up visits

postoperative irradiation if they have been completely resected and accurately staged.

The local failure rate in stage I patients after surgery alone is approximately 10 percent. With such a low incidence of local failure the addition of postoperative irradiation is unnecessary. Supporting this view is a prospective randomized trial that showed no benefit to the addition of postoperative irradiation to stage I (T1N0, T2N0) patients.[45] Unfortunately, most patients present with unresectable or marginally resectable disease. The addition of radiation and chemotherapy is aimed at decreasing the unacceptably high frequency of failure due to local and distant spread that occur with surgery alone. However, progress has been slow, and the overall survival of all patients with non-small cell lung cancer has remained essentially unchanged for the past 20 years.

Neoadjuvant Therapy

The current use of preoperative radiotherapy in the management of non-small cell lung carcinoma falls into two categories: (1) as part of neoadjuvant chemoradiotherapy for N2 (IIIA) disease, and (2) preoperative radiotherapy (with or without chemotherapy) for superior sulcus (Pancoast) tumors. For patients who are otherwise surgical candidates but are found at mediastinoscopy to have positive mediastinal lymph nodes (N2 disease), it is not clear whether neoadjuvant chemoradiotherapy is superior to neoadjuvant chemotherapy. In most institutions, preoperative radiotherapy for superior sulcus tumors, with or without chemotherapy, remains standard management. However, based on the surgical-pathologic findings, modern imaging techniques, including MRI of the spine and brachial plexus, have made it possible for selected patients to undergo surgery first followed by adjuvant treatment.

Conceptually, it has become attractive to attempt to convert patients with bulky mediastinal nodal disease to patients with microscopic mediastinal nodal disease, thereby rendering them candidates for surgical resection. A large number of phase II clinical trials have been conducted utilizing induction chemotherapy or induction radiation and chemotherapy in patients with bulky mediastinal adenopathy ("clinical" stage N2 disease). A major study conducted at the Memorial Sloan-Kettering Cancer Center, where patients were preoperatively treated with combination chemotherapy followed by surgical resection, found longer survival in the group receiving the neoadjuvant treatment than in a group of historical controls.[28] A large phase II cooperative trial conducted by the Southwest Oncology Group[56] also suggested that in patients with bulky mediastinal disease, improvement in median survival could be achieved with induction chemotherapy and radiation followed by surgical resection.[36,56] However, even though median and short-term survival seem to be improved in these patients who were treated preoperatively with combination chemotherapy, the data are far from convincing. Several phase II trials of nonsurgical treatment in patients with stage IIIA disease have resulted median survivals similar to those treated with induction therapy followed by surgery.[38] Moreover, in certain subsets of patients, particularly in those with postobstructive pneumonia, increased toxicity has accompanied the induction of chemotherapy followed by surgical resection.

A current trial sponsored by the National Cancer Institute (NCI) randomizes patients with stage IIIA disease to two categories: nonsurgical treatment or induction (neoadjuvant) chemotherapy and radiation therapy followed by surgery [Radiation Therapy Oncology Group (RTOG) 93-09]. Within the next 5 to 10 years, the role of induction therapy followed by surgery will be better defined.

Chemoradiotherapy followed by thoracotomy is an intensive treatment with considerable morbidity and mortality. Its use should be limited to patients with excellent cardiac and pulmonary reserve and a high performance status. Preferably this combination should be used in the context of a prospective clinical trial. Only patients with reasonable expectation of benefit should receive this form of aggressive management; thorough staging workups for metastatic disease (CT scans of the chest, abdomen, and brain, and bone scan) should be performed prior to the start of preoperative treatment and in the "window" period (i.e., after this therapy has been administered and before surgery). Lesions that are suspected of being distant metastases should be investigated by tissue biopsy.

Neoadjuvant irradiation requires a moderate dose, i.e., approximately 4500 cGy (see glossary at end of chapter) in standard daily fractions (180 to 200 cGy). Higher doses increase complications, particularly if pneumonectomy is ultimately required.[21] A slightly lower total dose using a larger daily fraction (3000 cGy in ten fractions of 300 cGy) completes treatment more rapidly. Because of improvements in the current use of concur-

rent chemotherapy and the recent knowledge that the occurrence of late radiotherapy complications are strongly related to the use of large fractions, daily fractions greater than 200 cGy are not often used as preoperative or postoperative therapy. Different regimens of fractionation (e.g., radiotherapy administered twice daily) has not been extensively tested in the preoperative setting for lung cancer and are not recommended unless done within the setting of a clinical trial.

Regardless of the dose fractionation scheme used, an interval of approximately 3 to 4 weeks between completion of irradiation and surgery is advised to minimize the risk of difficulties in wound healing. This time period also allows for maximal tumor response to the preoperative treatment and a chance to perform a restaging workup. However, it is not long enough for fibrosis, which would complicate the surgical resection, to occur.

Preoperative radiotherapy carries with it the potential disadvantage of limiting the ability to give additional radiotherapy if tumor proves to be unresectable or if residual disease remains after resection. After 4000 to 5000 cGy preoperatively, only about 3000 cGy of additional irradiation can be safely administered postoperatively; this is unlikely to sterilize aggressive residual disease and should probably only be given if indicated for palliation of local symptoms. A few medical centers have investigated the use of interstitial brachytherapy implants. Intraoperative radiotherapy, which is available in some institutions, is another possibility. However, in general, the patient left with residual or unresectable disease after preoperative chemoradiotherapy has a poor chance for permanent local control, and treatment goals at that point should be palliative.

Adjuvant Therapy

The primary tumor-related factors in considering postoperative radiotherapy are the pathologic stage and the completeness of the surgery. Based on its proven efficacy in decreasing the risk of local-regional recurrences, postoperative radiotherapy is generally considered to be the standard of care for patients with resected node-positive (N1 or N2) non–small cell lung carcinoma. Based on the Lung Cancer Study Group Trial in patients with N2 disease, which suggested a longer relapse-free survival in this subgroup, the presence of N2 disease would seem to favor postoperative radiotherapy.[25] There is no role for postoperative radiotherapy for T1-2N0 tumors completely resected by lobectomy or pneumonectomy. In fact, there is the suggestion of a slight detrimental effect of postoperative radiotherapy on overall survival.[45] It is less clear whether radiotherapy should be administered after a wedge resection, although in selected patients, the high local failure rate after this procedure suggests a possible role for postoperative treatment.[15]

Whether postoperative irradiation has any impact on survival is debatable. Many retrospective studies have shown a survival benefit when postoperative irradiation is added. In a retrospective report on 61 patients with completely resected stage II and stage III adenocarcinoma of the lung who were treated either by surgery alone or by surgery plus radiotherapy, the 5-year survival rates were 8 percent with surgery and 43 percent with surgery plus RT (p < 0.01).[6] Seventy-five patients with squamous cell cancer were also reviewed. In those with no evidence of disease (NED), survival at 4 years was 42 percent for surgery plus radiotherapy and 33 percent for surgery alone. This difference did not reach statistical significance. However, it should be noted that the majority of patients (52 percent) in the surgery plus radiotherapy group had N2 disease whereas 27 percent in the surgery only group had N2 disease.

Another review of survival rates of N2 patients after curative surgery reported that postoperative radiotherapy afforded a significant survival benefit.[19] Twenty-six percent of the patients treated with surgery and radiotherapy were alive at 5 years, whereas none of the patients treated with surgery alone survived for 5 years.

The only prospective, randomized trial evaluating the role of postoperative radiotherapy on completely resected stage II and stage III epidermoid lung cancers failed to find a survival benefit from the addition of postoperative radiotherapy even though the rate of local recurrence decreased in those who did receive radiation therapy: The 5-year survival rate was 38 percent for both groups (i.e., surgery plus radiotherapy and surgery alone).[25] However, a number of problems exist in the Lung Cancer Study Group trial. One major argument against the conclusion that postoperative radiotherapy does not prolong survival is that the study combined pathological N1 and N2 patients. If N1 and N2 patients are looked at separately, the number of patients in each group would be too small for valid conclusions to be made regarding the efficacy of postoperative radiotherapy.

Future studies should stratify patients according to documented N1 versus N2 disease. Furthermore, distinction should be made between patients with clinical N2 disease (bulky) and those with clinical N0/N1 disease. In a report of treatment of 706 patients with pathologic N2 disease, 151 (21 percent) were completely resected; of these 119 (79 percent) were clinical N0/N1, and 32 (21 percent) were clinical N2.[27] The clinical N2 patients had bulky nodal disease that could be detected on preoperative chest radiograph or by splaying of the carina seen at bronchoscopy. All but 10 percent of patients received postoperative radiotherapy. The 5-year survival rates were 34 percent for the clinical N0/N1 patients and 9 percent for the clinical N2 patients.

Currently, arguments against postoperative RT are based on the view that distant disease is the major problem and that increasing local control is a hollow victory. Others believe that overall survival can be improved by increasing local control. The truth probably lies somewhere between these two views. Since the time interval to distant disease is similar to that for local failure, an increase in local control may not lead to a significant increase in survival. If more effective therapy for distant disease is developed, then the improvement in local control may lead to consistent significant increases in survival.

Patients with chest wall invasion are an unusual subset of stage IIIa and have limited, but definite, curability. In 35 patients with chest wall invasion who were treated with either surgery alone or surgery plus irradiation, chest wall recurrences developed in 6 of 22 patients (27 percent) who were not irradiated compared to no recurrences in 13 patients who were irradiated.[31] The role of postoperative radiation following resection of a lesion which involves the chest wall remains controversial.

Postoperative radiotherapy for patients with node-positive disease who have undergone lobectomy with complete mediastinal lymph node dissection should consist of relatively modest field size encompassing the mediastinum, hilum, and bronchial stump with a margin of approximately 1.5 to 2 cm. If resection margins are negative and if there is no chest wall invasion, there is no reason to irradiate the "tumor bed"; doing so would only increase toxicity by irradiating that portion of remaining lung that has filled into the space left by the lobectomy. A radiation dose of 5000 to 5500 cGy using a standard fractionation schedule (180 to 200 cGy) should provide excellent local and regional control. Higher doses (6000 to 6500 cGy) may be indicated if resection margins are close (less than 3 mm), if there is evidence of extracapsular spread of tumor outside of lymph nodes, or if a complete mediastinal lymph node dissection was not done.

Patients whose tumors cannot be completely resected have a poor prognosis, although radiation is usually used in an attempt to maximize local control. What defines an incomplete resection varies from leaving gross disease behind to finding microscopic disease in the highest lymph node removed to tumor cells present in the peribronchial soft tissue of the resected specimen. There is almost no use for a so-called palliative resection when dealing with a primary lung cancer. If a tumor cannot be completely removed, there is no sense in removing part of it.

There is no evidence to suggest that incomplete removal of tumor at the time of operation can be "cleaned up" by radiation therapy. The Lung Cancer Study Group randomized patients with incompletely resected non-small cell lung cancer to receive either postoperative radiotherapy alone or radiotherapy plus chemotherapy.[24] Incomplete resection was defined as a positive margin or tumor in the highest mediastinal node sampled. Local-only failure occurred in 14 percent of patients in each group. The median time to recurrence was 8 months in the radiotherapy alone group versus 14 months in the combination group. Corresponding 1-year survival rates were 54 percent and 68 percent, respectively. There was no difference in long-term survival between the two groups.

In a retrospective study of 221 patients with incomplete resections after attempted curative surgery,[16] the results of postoperative therapy—whether radiation, chemotherapy, or both—were inconsistent; only 26 percent of patients were alive at 1 year and all but 4 percent of patients were dead by 5 years.

Locally recurrent disease following a complete resection must be treated on an individual basis. Rarely does local disease recur as an isolated phenomenon; most commonly it is associated with disseminated disease. Radiation therapy is used to treat symptoms related to the locally recurrent disease, the regimen differing somewhat depending on the presence or absence of disseminated disease. An occasional patient with a local parenchymal or chest wall recurrence may be a candidate for further resection. A thorough evaluation to rule out distant disease must be undertaken prior to any surgical intervention. Regional lymph nodes are a common site of local recurrence, and rarely can this type of recurrence be managed surgically. Most of these patients are treated with radiation while recognizing that the impact on long-term survival will be minimal.[10]

Certain areas of loco-regional recurrence engender more concern than others. Specifically recurrence in the region of the superior vena cava is noteworthy, since it is best to avoid obstruction of this vessel. A particularly concerning area of local recurrence is the aortopulmonary window in the left chest, where involvement of the left recurrent laryngeal nerve has a significant impact on the quality of life. Patients with a paralyzed left vocal cord are not only hoarse but have difficulty caused by aspiration. Unfortunately, once the nerve is involved, function of the vocal cord does not return even if radiation therapy is employed for the recurrent disease. Over time the voice improves as the contralateral vocal cord moves across the midline to appose with the paralyzed cord. The avoidance of local recurrence in certain areas is far preferable to attempts to treat it.

Definitive Therapy

Patients who do not have demonstrable distant metastases but are not candidates for surgery because of locally advanced stage and/or medical inoperability are often referred for radiation therapy, with or without concurrent or sequential chemotherapy. Patients with malignant pleural or pericardial effusions, while technically still having stage IIIB disease, should not be considered candidates for curative treatment and should be offered appropriate palliative measures, which may include surgical intervention (pericardial window or thoracoscopic sclerosis), chemotherapy, or moderate-dose palliative radiotherapy to bulky central disease. Combined chemotherapy and radiotherapy has not been tested in patients with medically inoperable stage I disease. Definitive radiotherapy alone remains the standard treatment for these patients in whom tumors often respond quite well to radiotherapy alone (Figs. 113-III-1 and 113-III-2).

For other nonoperable stage IIIA and IIIB patients, combined chemotherapy and radiation therapy is often considered an alternative to radiotherapy or supportive care alone. The most important factor to consider in selecting patients for combined modality therapy, which has considerable toxicity and a high level of patient time, commitment, and expense, is their performance status. In general, intensive chemoradiotherapy should be limited to patients whose Karnofsky scores are 70 percent or greater. Significant weight loss, defined in most cooperative group trials as greater than 5 percent, is also a relative contraindication to aggressive combined modality therapy. Although age itself is not a contraindication to combination therapy, intensive regimens should be applied cautiously in patients more than 70 years old. Of note is that in most of the trials utilizing chemoradiotherapy, the median age averaged 60 years. Although large tumor size is not a contraindication to definitive treatment, larger tumors generally result in a larger portion of normal tissue (lung, heart, and esophagus) being included in a radiotherapy portal, and the resultant high-dose irradiation may carry an unacceptable risk of complications. The location of the tumor (e.g., proximity to the heart) and the patient's pulmonary reserve may also influence the decision regarding definitive irradiation. Supraclavicular adenopathy (N3 disease) is not an absolute contraindication for definitive therapy, although its presence is a poor prognostic indicator.

There is no clear answer as to whether chemotherapy and irradiation should be given concurrently or sequentially (i.e., two cycles of chemotherapy followed by irradiation). However, sequential treatment seems to be less toxic and, except as part of a clinical trial, should probably be regarded as standard management for most patients. However, if threatening local problems, such as the superior vena caval syndrome, hemoptysis, or

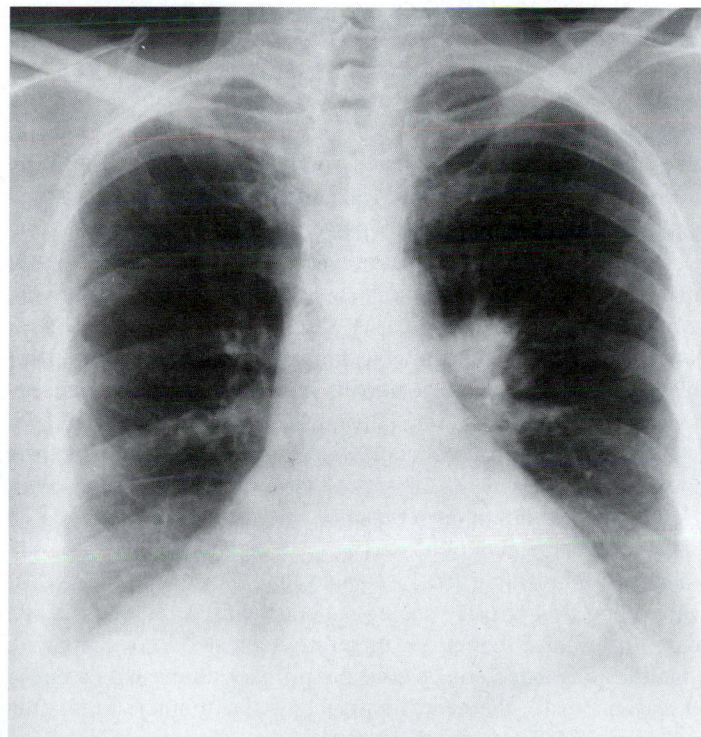

FIGURE 113-III-1   Pre-radiotherapy chest radiograph of a patient with a medically inoperable T2N0M0 non–small cell lung carcinoma of the left hilar region.

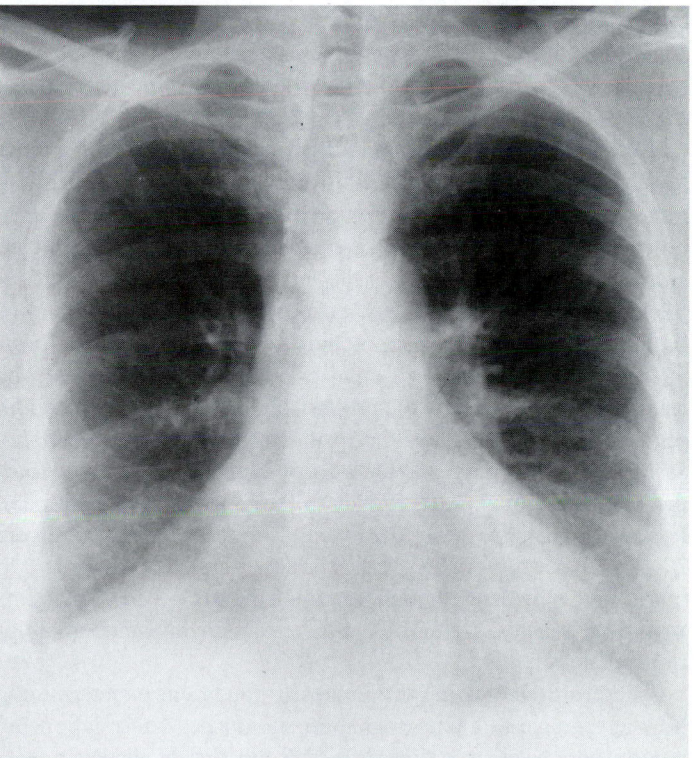

FIGURE 113-III-2   Chest radiograph 1 month after definitive radiotherapy for the patient shown in Figure 113-III-1.

high-grade mainstem bronchial obstruction, are impending, concurrent chemoradiotherapy may be in order in selected patients since the response rate would be expected to be higher than with chemotherapy alone.

The conventional dose fractionation schedule used for definitive irradiation is 6000 to 6400 cGy over a 6-week period using standard fractionation (180 to 200 cGy per day). Higher doses (6500 to 7000 cGy) may be given to small tumors in which the amount of normal tissue in the field is minimal. Hyperfractionation, using 120 cGy bid to a dose of 6960 cGy, has been tested extensively by the Radiation Therapy Oncology Group (RTOG) and may offer increased loco-regional control. However, no survival benefit for hyperfractionation has been demonstrated, and toxicity may be greater than standard dose-and-fractionation schedules. Therefore, the use of hyperfractionation for non-small cell lung carcinoma outside of clinical trials is generally not recommended.

For many years, the fields to be treated in the definitive therapy of non-small cell lung carcinoma have followed the Halsted principle of "radical en bloc" loco-regional therapy. The typical radiotherapy field, as defined in RTOG protocols, encompasses the primary tumor (with 2-cm margin), both the ipsilateral and contralateral hila, and the entire mediastinum from the thoracic inlet to a point 5 cm below the carina for upper lobe lesions and to the diaphragmatic insertion for lower lobe lesions (Fig. 113-III-3). In addition the supraclavicular fossae are irradiated for upper lobe lesions or in the presence of high mediastinal adenopathy. This usually results in a field size measuring approximately 16 by 20 cm.

Although a "conedown" to a smaller field size that encompasses only the gross disease is usually performed after 4500 cGy has been administered, the potential for toxicity is fairly high. Using "standard" fields, it has been estimated that greater than 30 percent of a patient's normal lung tissue is exposed to a dose of irradiation expected to cause permanent fibrosis and nonfunction.[12] In addition, despite these large fields, most patients treated with definitive irradiation to the chest fail, generally at the site of the original gross disease.

Because of these issues, in recent years, there has been a trend toward smaller field size in definitive radiotherapy, encompassing gross disease with an appropriate margin and fewer areas of "prophylactic" nodal stations. However, in most patients, it is still considered appropriate to include the ipsilateral hilar, bilateral paratracheal, and subcarinal areas. Of course, in patients with very limited pulmonary function, including most patients with medically inoperable stage I disease, even smaller fields should be used, encompassing only the primary tumor with a margin and, in selected patients, possibly the ipsilateral hilum (Fig. 113-III-4).

Many studies have shown a correlation between the size of the primary tumor and survival following radiation treatment. For example, in one study, the 3-year actuarial survival rates were 30 percent for tumors less than 3 cm, 17 percent for tumors 3 to 6 cm, and 0 percent for tumors larger than 6 cm in 77 patients with clinical stage I NSCLC who were medically inoperable or refused surgery.[37]

Therefore, one of the difficulties in treatment is determining how aggressive thoracic irradiation should be. The relationship among tumor size, local control, and the risk of distant metastases underscores the increasing potential of extrathoracic (systemic) failure in patients with extensive disease. The frequency

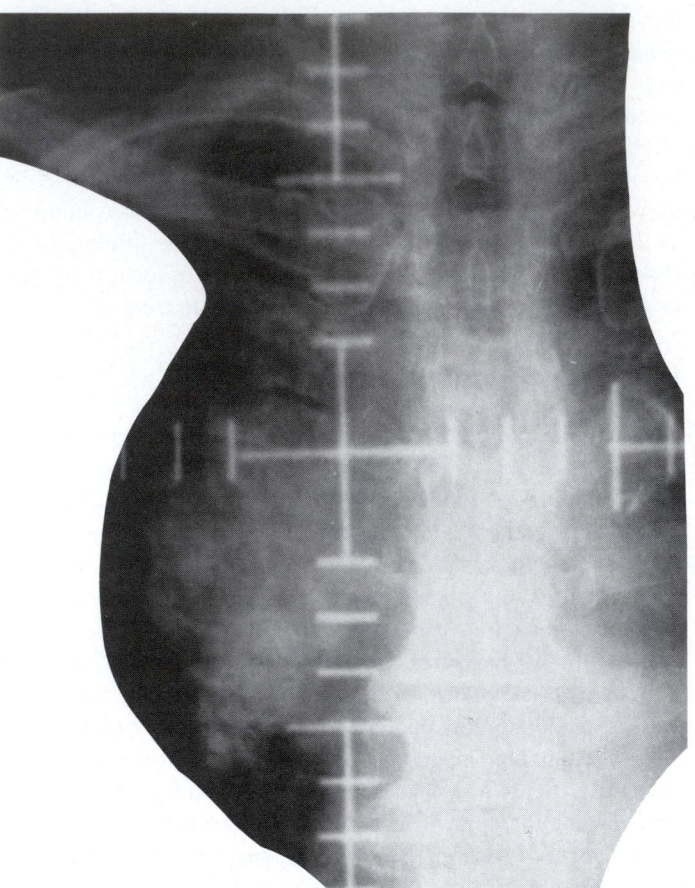

FIGURE 113-III-3 Simulation (radiation planning) film for "radical en bloc" radiotherapy for a patient with T4N2M0 non–small cell lung carcinoma of the right hilar region. The actual area being irradiated is inside the yellow boundaries. All other areas are shielded by customized leadlike blocks.

of nodal metastases in patients who underwent so-called curative surgery was found to depend on the extent of local disease: 79 percent of patients with T1 lesions were N0 compared to 59 percent for T2 lesions and 45 percent for T3/T4 lesions.[47]

In keeping with this observation are other data which suggest that local control has a diminishing effect on survival as the size of the primary tumor increases.[13] In 152 patients with a non-small cell lung cancer that is technically resectable but inoperable for medical reasons ("medically inoperable"), the median survival was 20 months for T2 and T3 lesions, irrespective of whether local control was achieved. For T1 lesions, however, the median survival was 30 months if the primary tumor was controlled and 17 months if it was not.

In summary, radiation therapy is of benefit in patients with medically inoperable but resectable lung cancer with a significant proportion of early-staged patients being cured of their disease. Aggressive therapy is, therefore, indicated in patients with small lesions, but as the size of the primary tumor and extent of disease increase, the necessity of aggressive thoracic irradiation is less well defined.

As a general rule, patients with clinical T4 and/or N3 disease usually are not considered to be surgical candidates. With supportive care consisting of antibiotics, expectorants, and oxygen, it

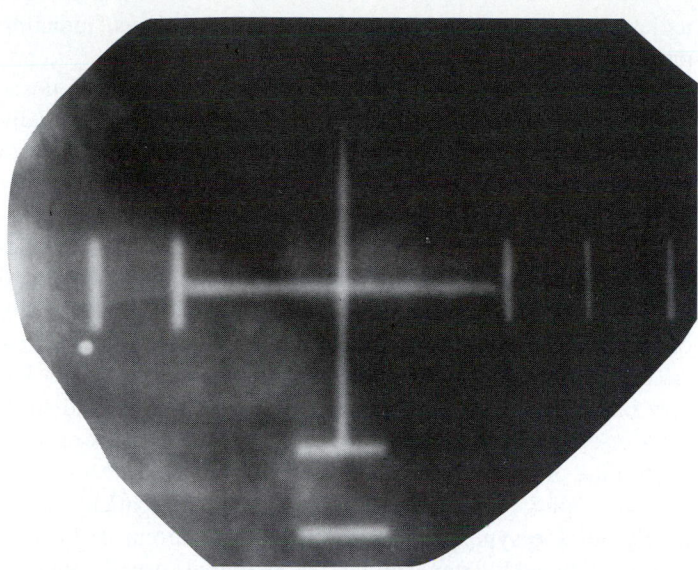

FIGURE 113-III-4   Radiotherapy simulation film (highly magnified, compared with Fig. 113-III-3) for the patient with medically inoperable NSCLC shown in Figs. 113-III-1 and 113-III-2. The area being irradiated is inside the yellow boundaries. CT-assisted radiation dosimetry revealed the amount of normal lung tissue in the treated field to be under 15 percent.

has been shown that only 4 percent are alive at 2 years.[9] Conversely, a number of trials have suggested that the addition of thoracic irradiation conveys a survival benefit. Median survival approximates 9 months with less than 10 percent of patients alive at 5 years.[39]

Not all patients with unresectable disease have the same prognosis. A recent analysis of 1592 patients in four studies conducted by the Radiation Therapy Oncology Group showed the following prognostic factors to be predicters of a poorer outcome: performance score less than 80, weight loss greater than 5 percent, age greater than 60, pleural effusion, and higher T and N stage.[39] Based on univariate analysis, not grade, radiation dose, nor histology were significant prognostic factors. However, *recursive partitioning* analysis showed that radiation dose is prognostically important for survival.

Other studies have shown that patients who have their local tumor controlled do better than patients who do not. Reviews of the failure pattern in locally advanced (T2-3, N0-2, M0) non-small cell lung cancer treated with irradiation alone indicated that the median survival increased from 6 to 12 months when the local tumor was controlled.[8] Approximately 75 percent of the patients with squamous cell cancer in this series died of complications of intrathoracic tumor compared to about 40 percent of patients with adenocarcinoma or large cell carcinoma. In the latter group, the majority of patients (55 percent) died from distant disease.

Some data suggest a dose-response relationship to improve the control of

intrathoracic tumors. The Radiation Therapy Oncology Group (RTOG) analyzed patients with medically inoperable stage I and stage II or unresectable stage III disease who were treated by irradiation alone.[32] Table 113-III-3 shows the various treatment schedules used and the corresponding response rates. Complete responders had a better 5-year survival rate than did partial or nonresponders; more patients treated with doses greater than 50 Gy were complete responders. Local and distant failures were a major problem in all treatment groups.

Because of the high incidence of intrathoracic failures with conventional radiotherapy, altered fractionation schedules have been developed in an attempt to improve local control. The RTOG conducted a series of prospective, randomized trials of altered irradiation schedules for patients with unresectable N2 disease.[7] Multiple 1.2 Gy bid hyperfractionation schedules have been used. Total doses of 60.9 Gy, 64.8 Gy, 69.6 Gy, 74.4 Gy, and 79.2 Gy were compared. Favorable patients (Karnofsky performance score 70 to 100 and weight loss less than 5 percent) had a better survival rate than did unfavorable patients. Also, survival rates were significantly better in favorable patients in the 69.6 Gy-total-dose arm than in the patients in the other total-dose arms, with a 3-year survival of 20 percent.

The RTOG has accepted the premise that in good performance patients, specifically in patients with minimal weight loss and high-performance status, aggressive therapy can alter the natural course of the disease and at least improve the median and 2-year survival of this group.[39] Radiation oncologists have attempted to increase the biologically effective dose of irradiation using a variety of techniques. This has included hypoxic sensitizers, immunotherapy, and cytotoxic chemotherapy with radiation.

In general, the most promising avenue of clinical investigation in the past 10 years has been the use of cytotoxic chemotherapy in combination with radiation. Approximately ten phase III trials have been conducted in recent years utilizing radiation therapy alone and radiation therapy with cytotoxic chemotherapy. The results have been contradictory. However, the last three large national trials including the Cancer and Leukemia Group B trial, and RTOG/Eastern Cancer Oncology Group trial, the French National trial have reported a statistically significant improvement

TABLE 113-III-3

RTOG Protocol 73-01

	40 Gy Split	40 Gy Continuous	50 Gy Continuous	60 Gy Continuous	3-Year Survival
Response					
Complete response, %	10.3	18.4	23.1	24.7	23
Partial response, %	36.1	29.1	42.8	40.0	10
No change, %	46.4	41.8	28.6	27.1	5
Failures					
Local failures only, %	24.7	33.0	22.0	13.0	—
Distant failures only, %	14.5	13.6	19.8	23.5	—
Local and distant failures, %	19.6	18.5	19.8	20.0	—

SOURCE: From Perez et al,[32] with permission.

in median and short-term survival in patients with locally advanced, presumed unresectable disease undergoing aggressive combined modality therapy.[38,40]

It must be stressed that the trials in which the outcomes were positive involved patients with the best performance status and minimal weight loss. Not all patients with presumed unresectable disease would benefit from this type of aggressive treatment.

Palliative Therapy

The goal of treatment in patients with advanced malignancies is to preserve the quality of life. This may require intervention with a potentially morbid treatment in order to relieve the patient of an unpleasant complication of the disease.

Palliative radiation therapy is most often used in situations where the patient's quality of life is, or could be, substantially compromised. Situations where treatment is commonly applied include locally advanced disease with hemoptysis, dyspnea, or obstructive pneumonia and metastatic disease.

Although response rates to chemotherapy have improved, radiotherapy remains the mainstay of palliative therapy for distressing local symptoms of lung cancer. The selection of patients for palliative radiotherapy is often more difficult than is the selection for adjuvant or definitive treatment, since the goals may be less well defined. The presence of a large lung cancer in and of itself is not an indication for palliative radiotherapy, particularly when a patient has been shown to have distant metastases with minimal, or no, local symptoms. Fairly clear situations which call for palliative thoracic radiotherapy include the superior vena caval syndrome, hemoptysis, and significant pain. Cough, often due to partial bronchial obstruction, is frequently palliated by radiotherapy. Atelectasis is rarely reversed by radiotherapy, although consideration should be given to irradiation in order to prevent refractory postobstructive atelectasis and pneumonia when impending obstruction of a mainstem or lobar bronchus is identified by bronchoscopy. A summary of the response rate (partial relief) of symptoms is shown in Table 113-III-4.

The palliative role of external irradiation in endobronchial disease has been evaluated in patients with inoperable non-small cell lung cancer.[41] Hemoptysis was relieved in 76 percent of patients, obstructive pneumonia in 59 percent, cough in 55 percent, chest pain in 50 percent, and dyspnea in 37 percent. Significant

TABLE 113-III-4

Response Rate to Palliative Radiotherapy (RT)

Symptom	Response Rate, %
Atelectasis	20
Cough	35–65
Dyspnea	35–50
Hemoptysis	75–85
Pain	50–75
SVC syndrome	60–80
Weight loss/anorexia	30–50
Vocal cord paralysis	5
Overall symptomatic response	60–75

SVC = superior vena cava.

toxicity occurred in less than 6 percent of patients; radiation pneumonitis was the most common adverse reaction.

Palliative radiotherapy generally involves lower total doses and smaller fields than does definitive radiotherapy. Larger daily fraction size is used (250 to 400 cGy per day) in the attempt to achieve relatively rapid palliation and to minimize the number of trips to the radiotherapy department. In addition, late radiotherapy complications (which are related to larger fraction size) are less relevant in this patient population. There is no standard palliation regimen, and treatments have ranged from 1000 cGy once to a full course of 6000 cGy in 200-cGy fractions. A typical compromise palliative radiotherapy schema is to deliver 300 cGy in 10 fractions, which may be followed by a second similar course of treatment, either after a 1- to 2-week break or later, at the time of local progression.

After full-course external beam irradiation, patients commonly develop symptoms associated with recurrent disease. In this situation, additional external radiotherapy is usually not possible, and endobronchial irradiation may be used.[42] Endobronchial irradiation has the advantage over external irradiation in that it is given over a relatively short period, the tumor most responsible for the symptoms receives the highest dose of radiation, and normal tissues, only a few centimeters away, are relatively spared.

In addition to being convenient for patients, excellent results have been reported from the use of endobronchial brachytherapy for symptomatic lung cancer. However, even though response rates are high, the mean survival following palliative treatment was approximately 6 months.[43] Complications were also more common (i.e., 12 percent of patients developed bronchial stenosis, and 7.3 percent experienced fatal hemoptysis).

Finally, radiotherapy plays an important role in the palliation of metastatic sites, including brain and bone metastases. Whole-brain irradiation, to a dose of 3000 cGy in 10 fractions, is appropriate therapy for multiple brain metastases. In addition to palliating neurologic symptoms in many patients, it appears to improve survival marginally more than can be achieved by steroids alone.[17] In addition, patients with solitary brain metastases appear to benefit from a combination of whole-brain irradiation and surgical resection.[30] Patients with solitary brain metastases who are not candidates for craniotomy may similarly benefit from high-dose focal stereotactic irradiation of metastases. For bony metastases, most patients will achieve at least partial pain relief from 2000 to 3000 cGy in 5 to 10 fractions. The appearance caused by disfiguring skin and subcutaneous metastases can be improved by similar modest dosages of irradiation. Occasionally, pain from adrenal metastases can be palliated with radiotherapy in patients in whom the radiotherapy field would not include an excessive amount of liver, kidney, or bowel.

LIMITED-STAGE SMALL CELL LUNG CARCINOMA

Thoracic Radiation

It is now generally accepted, based on the results of two meta-analyses, that combined chemotherapy and thoracic radiotherapy is superior to chemotherapy alone in the treatment of limited-stage small cell lung carcinoma.[33,46] However, the best way to combine these treatments remains controversial. Concurrent chemoradiation at the start of therapy appears to be superior to "consolidative" radiotherapy at the end of all chemotherapy,[29] although this comes at the expense of increased toxicity. A possible advantage of delayed radiotherapy is that chemotherapy usually shrinks bulky hilar/mediastinal tumor, allowing smaller and potentially less toxic radiotherapy portals to be used.[22]

In general, for patients with high performance status and good cardiopulmonary function, concurrent chemoradiotherapy (with etoposide and cisplatin) at the start of treatment represents the standard of care in the United States at this time. Although low doses of radiotherapy (less than 4000 cGy) appear to be less effective in local control, it is unclear whether increasing the dose above 4500 cGy improves outcome. Fractionation of 180 cGy once daily (standard fractionation) or 150 cGy bid (accelerated hyperfractionation) give similar survival; although local control is better with the latter regimen, esophageal toxicity is significantly increased.

In patients with limited-stage small cell lung carcinoma, the local control at 2 years was shown in one study to be increased from 61 percent to 82 percent by increasing the radiation dose from 45 Gy to 55 Gy.[3] Median overall survival was also increased in the patients treated with 55 Gy (20 months) as compared to 45 Gy (14 months).

Alternating radiotherapy and chemotherapy schedules were developed in an attempt to improve local control. Concurrent thoracic irradiation produced consistently better 2-year survival rates than did sequential irradiation.[23]

Prophylactic Cranial Irradiation

The role of prophylactic cranial irradiation (PCI) remains controversial. Its use should be considered only for patients in complete remission after chemotherapy and thoracic irradiation. PCI dramatically reduces the risk of brain metastases, but, to date, has not been shown to improve survival.[4]

The primary argument against the use of PCI is the high incidence of neurocognitive deficits in long-term survivors after PCI. These deficits may range from subtle abnormalities that are demonstrable only by sophisticated neuropsychologic testing to progressive dementia. Many studies critical of PCI have included patients who received relatively high doses of PCI and/or received PCI with concurrent chemotherapy. Moreover, recent neurocognitive studies of patients with newly diagnosed small cell lung cancer have shown deficits before any treatment was administered, suggesting that at least some of the problem with neurocognitive deficits is due to a paraneoplastic syndrome.[20]

When given, PCI should be delivered at least 2 to 3 weeks after all chemotherapy has been completed. In order to minimize the risk and severity of late sequelae, a whole-brain dose of 250 cGy in 10 fractions (2500 cGy) or 200 cGy in 15 fractions (3000 cGy) is recommended. Aside from alopecia and fatigue, acute toxicity from this treatment is minimal. Steroids are not usually needed for PCI (in contrast to their use when treating brain metastases). If steroids are required, however, extreme care must be taken in tapering them, since rebound radiation pneumonitis may develop (from the patient's prior thoracic radiotherapy).

TOXICITY OF THORACIC RADIOTHERAPY

Toxicity from radiotherapy occurs both as *acute* side effects, generally defined as those occurring during or within 90 days after the completion of a course of irradiation, and *late* effects, which do not develop until at least 90 days after the completion of irradiation. Although some of the same factors that predict acute effects also increase the likelihood of late effects, the acute effects themselves do not necessarily lead to the late, long-term complications. In general, most injuries from irradiation are a consequence of localized damage to tissue within the irradiated portal. However, some effects are more generalized [e.g., fatigue, immunosuppression, and the rare complication of diffuse adult respiratory distress syndrome (ARDS)]. The *grade* of radiation toxicity is generally reported on a 1 to 5 scale, with grade 1 toxicity representing mild effects (e.g., dyspnea on exertion) and grade 5 representing fatal toxicity.

In the treatment of thoracic malignancies, where high irradiation doses and large fields are often used, the organs of greatest concern for both acute and late complications are the lung, the esophagus, and the heart. Significant dermatologic toxicity has been virtually eliminated by the use of megavoltage equipment. Likewise, with modern treatment planning techniques, spinal cord complications should be extremely rare. Other structures at risk for injury by thoracic irradiation include the brachial plexus, the tracheobronchial tree, the great vessels, the ribs, and the sternum. Although many complications of thoracic irradiation are manageable, the most important prospect is prevention through sophisticated treatment planning and appropriate selection of patients for treatment.

Lungs: Acute Complications

Radiation pneumonitis and pulmonary fibrosis are the most common serious complications of thoracic irradiation. Radiation pneumonitis represents acute lung injury. It usually occurs from 1 to 4 months after irradiation, although rarely it occurs during a course of particularly intensive radiotherapy, often when it is combined with chemotherapy. Dyspnea is the most characteristic symptom, although cough, low-grade fever, and pleuritic chest pain often are also present (Figs. 113-III-5 to 113-III-7).

Although infiltrates outside of the radiation portal do not completely rule out radiation pneumonitis, they make the diagnosis less likely. Regardless of the radiographic appearance, community-acquired pneumonia and opportunistic infections as well as progressive malignancy can mimic radiation pneumonitis. Therefore, appropriate testing and consultation with the patient's radiation oncologist are indicated before empiric corticosteroids are begun. Mild cases should be treated supportively, reserving steroids for more severe symptoms. For severe radiation pneumonitis, prednisone 20 mg, 3 times per day, for approximately 2 weeks is used; tapering is done slowly (i.e., during the subsequent 2 to 4 weeks). Whether antibiotics should be used in addition to corticosteroids is controversial.

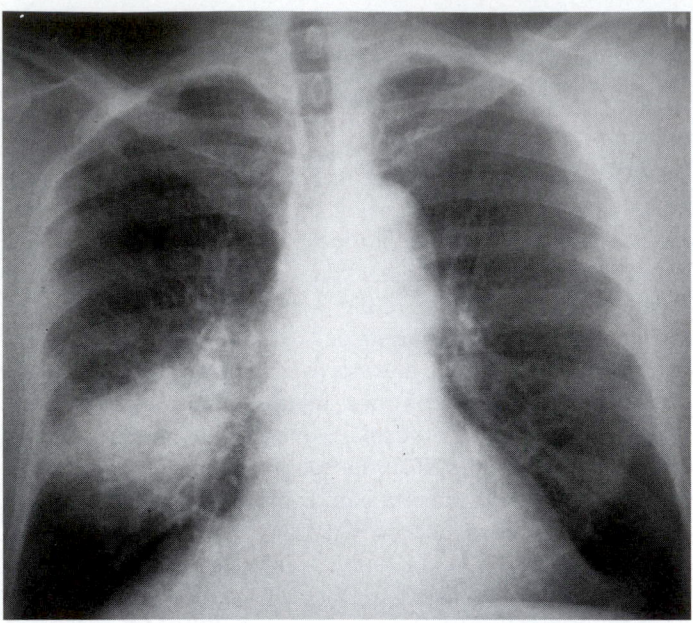

FIGURE 113-III-5   Preradiotherapy chest radiograph of a patient with limited-stage small cell carcinoma of the right lower lobe.

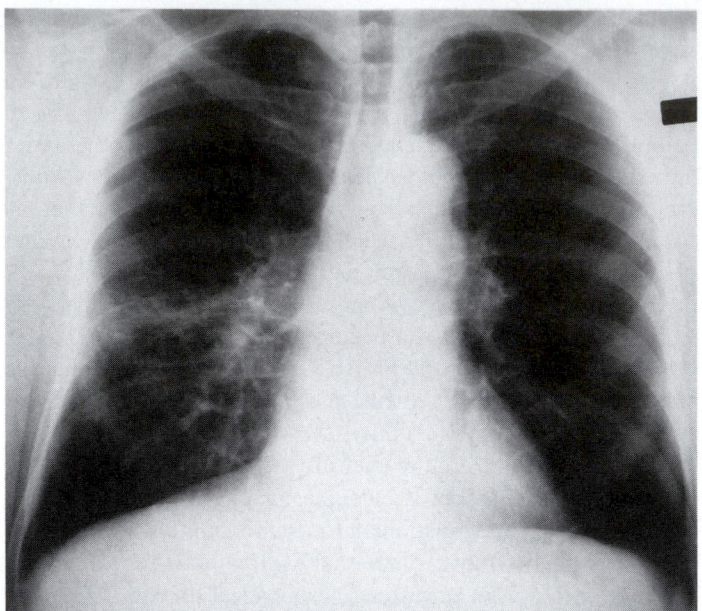

FIGURE 113-III-6   Chest radiograph 1 month after definitive radiotherapy and chemotherapy for the patient shown in Fig. 113-III-5.

The incidence of serious (greater than or equal to grade 3) radiation pneumonitis ranges from 5 to 15 percent, and the risk depends on several variables. The most important factor appears to be the field size: Studies using sophisticated CT-based radiation dosimetry have demonstrated that the risk increases dramatically with the percentage of increase in volume of the ipsilateral lung in the irradiated field.[26] Total radiotherapy dose appears to be somewhat less important, since virtually any dose used for the definitive or palliative treatment of lung cancer devitalizes the lung tissue within the treated portal. Other factors that appear to increase the risk of radiation pneumonitis include radiation dose per fraction (i.e., larger fraction size increases the risk) and tumor location (i.e., lower lobe lesions have a higher risk).[34] The use of chemotherapy (particularly the anthracyclines, methotrexate, bleomycin, and mitomycin) and poor pulmonary function before treatment also increase the risks of serious damage to the lungs by radiation.

On rare occasion, a patient develops an adult respiratory distress syndrome shortly after irradiation. The chest radiographs reveal diffuse infiltrates both within and outside of the radiotherapy portal. It has been hypothesized that a severe autoimmune response may be involved: Whereas mild and moderate radiation injury become manifest only in the irradiated portion of lung, a severe autoimmune response results in generalized bilateral lung injury.[35]

Lungs: Late Complications

The *late complication* of radiation fibrosis develops from 3 to 18 months after radiotherapy. Essentially 100 percent of patients irradiated for lung carcinoma with high doses of radiation develop radiologic evidence of radiation fibrosis (Fig. 113-III-8). The major difficulty is in distinguishing between fibrosis and residual, or recurrent, tumor. In radiation fibrosis, there is usually, but not always, a decrease in forced expiratory volume (FEV_1), and the predicted percentage decline in FEV_1 can be roughly estimated

by a formula that correlates a preradiotherapy lung perfusion scan with the radiation treatment field: post-RT FEV_1 = 1 − percent of perfusion in treated portal × pre-RT FEV_1.

Patients rarely experience a greater decline in FEV_1 than predicted by this formula.[11] However, pulmonary function tests may reveal a decrease in DLCO out of proportion to the spirometry changes, reflecting the primarily restrictive nature of long-term radiation fibrosis.[1]

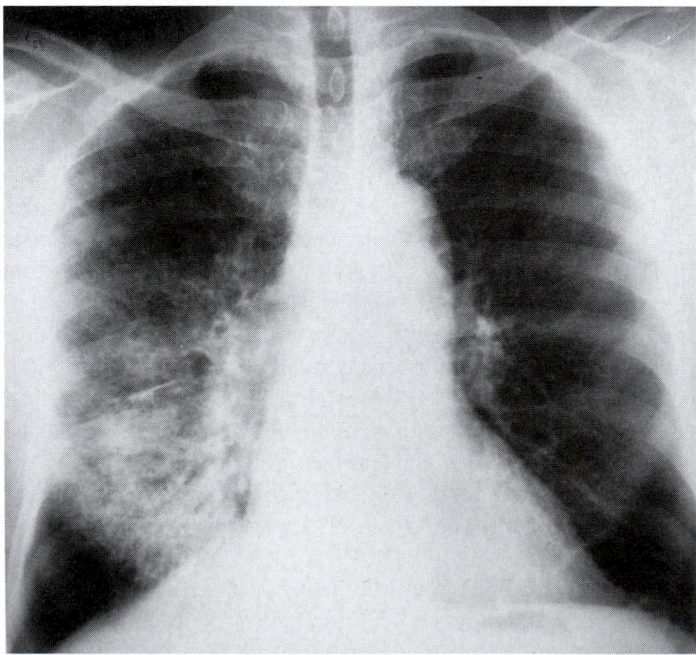

FIGURE 113-III-7   Chest radiograph 4 months after completion of radiotherapy for the patient shown in Figs. 113-III-5 and 113-III-6. He presented with severe dyspnea on exertion. Radiographic infiltrates conform to the shape of his radiation portal. He responded promptly to steroids but soon developed fatal brain metastases.

Severe symptoms from radiation fibrosis are uncommon. Established fibrosis does not respond to corticosteroids or any other therapy. Longitudinal studies in Hodgkin's disease patients suggest some recovery of lung function at approximately 3 years, after treatment.[16] It is less clear if lung cancer patients, who are far older and more chronically ill than most lymphoma patients, can expect appreciable recovery.

Esophagus

Most patients receiving moderate- to high-dose radiotherapy for lung cancer experience an acute mucositis of the esophagus that is similar to that seen on other epithelial surfaces after radiation therapy. With standard radiotherapy (6000 cGy), this mucositis is almost always self-limited and usually responds to topical agents, such as sucralfate slurry or "magic mouthwash" combinations (e.g., antacid, viscous lidocaine, and diphenhydramine); occasionally, narcotics may be needed. However, with more intensive radiotherapy or with concurrent chemotherapy, the incidence of grade 3 esophagitis is higher, and the recovery period is generally prolonged by several weeks to months.[18]

Esophageal stricture is a late complication and is increasing in frequency. The risk of esophageal stricture appears to be strongly dose-related, approximating 1 percent with 5000 cGy, 10 percent with 6000 cGy, and the risk may be as high as 50 percent with 7000 cGy (radiotherapy alone).[14] It is likely that the concurrent use of chemotherapy potentiates this effect. Most cases of radiation esophageal stricture respond well to endoscopic dilatation although the procedure may have to be repeated. More severe complications, such as esophageal fistula or perforation, fortunately, are rare.

Heart

Acute effects of radiotherapy on the heart during treatment are extremely uncommon. Radiation pericarditis may occasionally occur during a course of treatment but, in general, this is a subacute or late complication, developing several months to years after irradiation. The presentation is similar to that for other causes of pericarditis, and, as in the case of radiation pneumonitis, distinguishing between radiation pericarditis and tumor progression can be difficult. Most cases are self-limited and are treated supportively with antipyretics, analgesics, and occasionally with antiarrhythmic agents. Pericardiocentesis for tamponade is rarely required. Occasionally, severe constrictive changes may develop, leading to signs and symptoms of heart failure and necessitating pericardiectomy.

The risk of symptomatic radiation pericarditis is approximately 5 percent when doses of 6000 cGy are administered to one-third of the heart.[14] However, considerably lower doses (4000 cGy) can induce this disorder when a large part of the heart is in the treatment field (e.g., radiation therapy for Hodgkin's disease or for tumors in the left lower lobe). In addition to the risk of radiation pericarditis, irradiation has increased long-term morbidity and mortality from heart disease in patients cured of Hodgkin's disease, seminoma, and breast cancer, presumably due to accelerated coronary artery disease.[44]

Long-term cardiac complications of radiotherapy are rarely encountered in patients with lung cancer, since few patients survive long enough to manifest these effects. Furthermore, it can be difficult or impossible to distinguish between a cardiac event due to prior mediastinal irradiation and a cardiac event that is unrelated to radiation, since the risk of coronary artery disease is high in the older, heavy smoker who develops lung cancer.

ADVANCES IN RADIOTHERAPY

Biologic Advances

As the understanding of the relationship between radiation and cellular kinetics has grown, mathematical models have been developed that allow us to predict the responses of both normal tissue and tumor to radiation. This capability has led to many creative new fractionation schemes designed to maximize the destruction of tumor while minimizing damage to normal tissue. The difference in cellular kinetics between tumor cells and normal cells makes these new schemes possible and attractive. Both tumor cells and normal cells are injured by radiation; however, normal cells usually have a greater ability to repair this damage than do the tumor cells and can repopulate more between fractions.

Hyperfractionation utilizes multiple daily fractions in an effort to reduce the late effects in normal tissue without decreas-

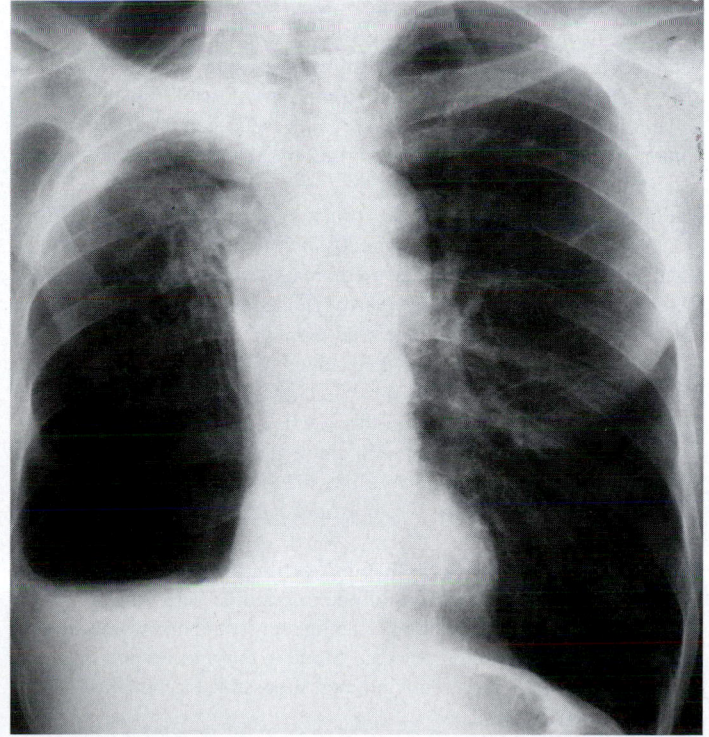

FIGURE 113-III-8 Chest radiograph of a patient 6 years after definitive radiotherapy for stage III unresectable non-small cell lung carcinoma. Radiation fibrosis in the right upper lobe with mediastinal shift to the treated side and an ipsilateral pleural effusion and thickening is evident. Patient remained asymptomatic.

ing tumor control. The overall treatment time is the same as conventional schedules, but multiple smaller fractions are given each day, and total doses are increased. By giving multiple smaller fractions, the normal tissues are able to repair a greater percentage of the damage during the course of treatment.

Tumor cells, however, are less able to repair the damage and therefore do not benefit as much from the smaller fractions. In general, hyperfractionation works well in situations where there is a large discrepancy in repair capabilities between tumor cells and normal tissue.

Accelerated treatment administers multiple fractions per day but also decreases the overall treatment time. Total dose and dose per fraction are similar to conventional treatment. It is designed to reduce the amount of repopulation that occurs during treatment of rapidly dividing tumors and, therefore, improve local control.

Much of the data on modified patterns of fractionation come from patients treated for cancers of the head and neck. In patients with epithelial neoplasms, both accelerated fractionation and hyperfractionation increase local-regional control. Non-small cell lung cancer may also benefit from altered fractionation. A phase III RTOG trial that is currently underway randomizes patients with stage II, IIIa, or IIIb and good performance status to conventional or hyperfractionated radiation therapy.

Technical Advances

Another method of increasing local control is through three-dimensional conformal radiation therapy. Utilizing three-dimensional planning of both the tumor and surrounding normal tissue, the radiation field can be *conformed* to the tumor as the field moves around the patient. The advantage of this approach is that the radiation can be delivered in a more precise fashion allowing the tumor dose to be raised and the normal tissue dose to be lowered. In a comparison of three-dimensional and two-dimensional planning in nine patients with non-small cell lung cancer, three-dimensional planning decreased the radiation dose to the ipselateral lung by 11 percent and by 51 percent to the contralateral lung.[2] Thus, three-dimensional planning allowed the tumor dose to be increased by 20 to 30 percent. Dose-escalation studies are currently under way to establish the maximum tolerable dose of radiation that can be delivered with conformal techniques to patients with non-small cell lung cancer.

SUMMARY

External beam radiotherapy plays a major role in the treatment of lung cancer. It improves local control and enhances curability in patients with marginally resectable non-small cell lung cancer. In patients with unresectable non-small cell lung cancer, such therapy generally affords palliation and, only occasionally, a cure.

APPENDIX

Glossary of Terms Related to Radiation Therapy

Adjuvant: Generally refers to postoperative therapy. However, chemotherapy given after definitive radiotherapy would also be considered adjuvant.

Blocks: Thick shields made of a leadlike alloy which can be shaped for each patient to block portions of their anatomy that would otherwise fall into the radiation field. In the treatment of lung cancer every attempt is made to block as much normal lung tissue as possible, as long as the tumor is not blocked.

Brachytherapy: Radiotherapy given in the form of radioactive sources placed directly into or around a patient's tumor. This may be given interstitially (sources imbedded directly into tissue) or intracavitary (sources laid into a cavity such as a bronchus).

cGy (centigray): A modern basic unit of radiotherapy in which the source of radiation is not x-rays but gamma rays emitted from a machine containing radioactive Cobalt-60.

Conedown: Shrinking the field size sometime during the course of radiotherapy, to take advantage of the decreasing size of tumor during treatment and to minimize the amount of toxicity of treatment. For example, a patient may begin radiotherapy with a 15- by 15-cm field and then have a conedown midway through treatment to a 10- by 10-cm field.

Conformal radiotherapy: The use of extremely sophisticated imaging studies and dosimetry to design radiation fields that *conform* precisely to the shape of a patient's tumor. Conformal radiotherapy usually uses smaller safety margins around a patient's tumor, a larger number of fields, and less prophylactic radiotherapy of clinically uninvolved lymph node areas.

Consolidative: Refers to radiotherapy given after a maximal or complete response to chemotherapy.

Course: A series or program of radiation treatments or fractions with a specific goal in mind for a patient (e.g., a 7-week course of daily radiotherapy to the lung for attempted cure).

Definitive: Refers to radiotherapy given with the intention of cure without surgery. May be given with other nonsurgical treatment such as chemotherapy.

Dosimetry: The process of optimizing the radiotherapy fields and dose by calculating the radiation dose to be received by a tumor and/or normal tissues in a radiation field. Physicists and "dosimetrists" work with the radiation oncologist in comparing possible radiation treatment plans with the goal of maximizing the radiation dose to the tumor while minimizing dose to normal tissue, often requiring sophisticated computer programs.

Endobronchial irradiation: A form of brachytherapy in which radioactive sources are placed directly into a bronchus using a hollow catheter threaded into the diseased area via bronchoscopy.

External beam radiotherapy (x-ray therapy): Radiotherapy given from a machine (usually a linear accelerator) which produces a high-energy x-ray beam which is then aimed at a patient's tumor and/or suspected tumor areas.

Field: An area at which a radiotherapy beam is directed, usually described as a rectangular shape, in cm (e.g., 10 by 14 cm). Blocks are often used to further customize the shape of a field. A single fraction of radiotherapy may include multiple fields, typically two to four.

Fraction: A single radiation therapy session, usually given over 1 to 3 min. A fraction may consist of one or multiple fields, and any dose, as prescribed by the radiation oncologist. Most courses of radiotherapy involve one fraction per day, Monday through Friday, over 1 to 7 weeks, although an infinite number of possible fractionation schedules are possible.

Gy (Gray): The SI modern basic unit of radiotherapy dose; 1 Gy = 100 cGy = 100 rad. One Gy = 1 joule per kilogram of absorbed energy.

Hyperfractionation (see also *fraction*): The delivery of two or more radiation fractions per day, generally given with a 4- or more hour interval between fractions.

Karnofsky score: A performance status scale commonly used in oncology to measure a patient's level of independent function. Scores range from 10 (moribund) to 100 (asymptomatic, able to work full-time). Karnofsky score has been shown to be highly predictive of survival in lung cancer.

Neoadjuvant: Generally refers to preoperative therapy. However, chemotherapy prior to definitive radiotherapy would also be considered neoadjuvant.

Palliative: Refers to therapy given with the goal of relieving distressing symptoms, without any anticipated effect on survival.

Prophylactic: Refers to radiotherapy given to a site at which there is no known tumor but which is considered to be at high risk for harboring occult "microscopic" disease, such as lymph node areas.

Rad: Basic unit of radiotherapy dose; terminology not changed to the SI units (cGy and Gy).

Radiation Therapy Oncology Group (RTOG): A National Cancer Institute–sponsored multicenter clinical trials cooperative group which performs studies related to radiation therapy, including many lung cancer studies.

Radiosensitizers: Drugs or other treatments which increase the cellular response to radiotherapy. Many chemotherapy drugs have radiosensitizing properties.

Safety margin: A margin of "normal-appearing" tissue which is added onto the visible tumor area for the purposes of radiation planning. Typically 1.5 to 2 cm in all dimensions is added, to account for microscopic extension of tumor cells and the possibility of slight patient motion during treatment.

Simulation: A detailed planning session for radiation therapy which simulates but does not actually deliver a radiation treatment. Simulation consists of immobilization of the patient in an appropriate position for radiation therapy, marking the patient's skin, localizing the area to be treated under fluoroscopy, taking radiographs of the area to be treated, and taking measurements of the patient's contour for dosimetry purposes.

REFERENCES

1. Abratt RP, Wilcox PA: The effect of irradiation on lung function and perfusion in patients with lung cancer. *Int J Radiat Oncol Biol Phys* 31:915–919, 1995.
2. Armstrong JG, Burman C, Leibel SA, et al: Conformal three-dimensional treatment planning may improve the therapeutic ration of high dose radiation therapy for lung cancer. *Int J Radiat Oncol Biol Phys* 21:146, 1991.
3. Arrigada R, Chevalier TL, Baldeyrou P, et al: Alternating radiotherapy and chemotherapy schedules in small cell lung cancer, limited disease. *Int J Radiat Oncol Biol Phys* 11:1461–1467, 1985.
4. Arriagada R, Le Chevalier T, Borie F, et al: Prophylactic cranial irradiation for patients with small-cell lung cancer in complete remission. *J Nat Can Inst* 87:183–190, 1995.
5. Byhardt RW: The evolution of radiation therapy oncology group (RTOG) protocols for nonsmall cell lung cancer. *Int J Radiat Oncol Biol Phys* 32:1513–1525, 1995.
6. Choi NCH, Grillo HC, Gardiello M, et al: Basis for new strategies in postoperative radiotherapy of bronchogenic carcinoma. *Int J Radiat Oncol Biol Phys* 6:31–35, 1980.
7. Cox JD, Azarnia N, Byhardt RW, et al: A randomized phase I/II trial of hyperfractionated radiation therapy with total doses of 60.0 to 79.2 Gy: Possible survival benefit with greater than or equal to 69.6 Gy in favorable patients with Radiation Therapy Oncology Group stage III non-small cell lung carcinoma: report of Radiation Therapy Oncology Group 83–11. *J Clin Oncol* 8:1543–1555, 1990.
8. Cox JD, Yesner R, Mietlowski W, Petrovich Z: Influence of cell type on local failure pattern after irradiation for locally advanced carcinoma of the lung. *Cancer* 44:94–98, 1979.
9. Cox JD, Komaki R, Byhardt RW: Is immediate chest radiotherapy obligatory for any or all patients with limited-stage non-small cell carcinoma of the lung? Yes. *Cancer Treat Rep* 67:327–331, 1983.
10. Curran WJ, Herbert SH, Stafford PM, et al: Should patients with post-resection locoregional recurrence of lung cancer receive aggressive therapy? *Int J Radiat Oncol Biol Phys* 24:25–30, 1991.
11. Curran WJ, Moldofsky PJ, Solin LJ: Observations on the predictive value of perfusion lung scans on post-irradiation pulmonary function among 210 patients with bronchogenic carcinoma. *Int J Radiat Oncol Biol Phys* 24:31–36, 1992.
12. Curran WJ Jr, Moldofsky PJ, Solin LJ: Analysis of the influence of elective nodal irradiation on postirradiation pulmonary function. *Cancer* 65:2488–2493, 1990.
13. Dosoretz DE, Galmarini D, Rubenstein JH, et al: Local control in medically inoperable lung cancer: An analysis of its importance in outcome and factors determining the probability of tumor eradication. *Int J Radiat Oncol Biol Phys* 27:507–516, 1993.
14. Emami B, Lyman J, Brown A, et al: Tolerance of normal tissue to therapeutic irradiation. *Int J Radiat Oncol Biol Phys* 21:109–122, 1991.
15. Ginsberg RJ, Rubinstein LV: Randomized trial of lobectomy versus limited resection for T1N0 non-small cell lung cancer. Lung Cancer Study Group. *Ann Thorac Surg* 60:615–622, 1995.
16. Horning SJ, Adhikari A, Rizk N, et al: Effect of treatment for Hodgkin's disease on pulmonary function: results of a prospective study. *J Clin Oncol* 12:297–305, 1994.
17. Horton J, Baxter DH, Olson DB, et al: The management of metastases to the brain by irradiation and corticosteroids. *AJR* 111:334–336, 1971.
18. Johnson DH, Kim K, Turrisi AT, et al: Cisplatin (P) and etoposide (E) + concurrent thoracic radiotherapy (TRT) administered once vs twice daily for limited-stage (LS) small cell lung cancer (SCLC): Preliminary results of an intergroup trial (meeting abstract). *Proc Am Soc Clin Oncol* 13:A1105, 1994.
19. Kirsh MM, Sloan H: Mediastinal metastases in bronchogenic carcinoma: influence of postoperative irradiation, cell type and location. *Ann Thorac Surg* 33:459–463, 1982.
20. Komaki R, Meyers CA, Shin DM, et al: Evaluation of cognitive function in patients with limited small cell lung cancer prior to and shortly following prophylactic cranial irradiation. *Int J Radiat Oncol Biol Phys* 33:179–182, 1995.
21. Langer CJ, Curran WJ, Keller SM, et al: Report of a phase II trial of concurrent chemoradiotherapy with radical thoracic irradiation (60 Gy), infusional fluorouracil, bolus cisplatin and etoposide for clinical stage IIIB and bulky IIIA non-small cell lung cancer. *Int J Radiat Oncol Biol Phys* 26:469–478, 1993.
22. Liengswangwong V, Bonner JA, Shaw EG, et al: Limited-stage small-cell lung cancer: patterns of intrathoracic recurrence and the implications for thoracic radiotherapy. *J Clin Oncol* 12:496–502, 1994
23. Livingston RB: Radiation-chemotherapy interactions in limited small cell lung cancer in Meyer JL, Vaeth JM (eds), *Frontiers in Radiation Therapy and Oncology,* vol 26. Basel, Karger, 1992, pp 72–82.
24. Lung Cancer Study Group: The benefit of adjuvant treatment for resected locally advanced non-small-cell lung cancer. *J Clin Oncol* 6:9–17, 1988.
25. Lung Cancer Study Group: Effects of postoperative mediastinal radiation on completely resected stage II and stage III epidermoid cancer of the lung. *New Engl J Med* 315:1377–1381, 1986.

26. Martel MK, Ten Haken RK, Hazuka MB, et al: Dose-volume histogram and 3-D treatment planning evaluation of patients with pneumonitis. *Int J Radiat Oncol Biol Phys* 28:777–779, 1994.

27. Martini N, Flehinger BJ: The role of surgery in N2 lung cancer. *Surg Clin North Am* 67:1037–1049, 1987.

28. Martini N, Kris MG, Gralla RJ, et al: The effects of preoperative chemotherapy on the resectability of non-small cell lung carcinoma with mediastinal lymph node metastases (N2M0). *Ann Thorac Surg* 45:370–379, 1988.

29. Murray N, Coy P, Pater JL, et al: Importance of timing for thoracic irradiation in the combined modality treatment of limited-stage small-cell lung cancer. The National Cancer Institute of Canada Clinical Trials Group. *J Clin Oncol* 11:336–344, 1993.

30. Patchell RA, Tibbs PA, Walsh JW, et al: A randomized trial of surgery in the treatment of single metastases to the brain. *New Engl J Med* 322:494–500, 1990.

31. Patterson GA, Ilves R, Ginsberg RJ, et al: The value of adjuvant radiotherapy in pulmonary and chest wall resection for bronchogenic carcinoma. *Ann Thorac Surg* 34:692–697, 1982.

32. Perez CA, Bauer M, Edelstein S, et al: Impact of tumor control on survival in carcinoma of the lung treated with irradiation. *Int J Radiat Oncol Biol Phys* 12:539–547, 1986.

33. Pignon JP, Arriagada R, Ihde DC, et al: A meta-analysis of thoracic radiotherapy for small-cell lung cancer. *New Engl J Med* 327:1618–1624, 1992.

34. Roach M, Gandara DR, Yuo HS, et al: Radiation pneumonitis following combined modality therapy for lung cancer: analysis of prognostic factors. *J Clin Oncol* 13:2606–2612, 1995.

35. Roberts CM, Foulcher, E, Zaunders JJ, et al: Radiation pneumonitis: a possible lymphocyte-mediated hypersensitivity reaction. *Ann Int Med* 118:696–700, 1993.

36. Rusch VW, Albain KS, Crowley JJ, et al: Surgical resection of stage IIIA and stage IIIB non-small-cell lung cancer after concurrent induction chemoradiotherapy: A Southwest Oncology Group trial. *J Thorac Cardiovasc Surg* 105:97–106, 1993.

37. Sandler HM, Curran WJ, Turrisi AT: The influence of tumor size and pretreatment staging on outcome following radiation therapy alone for stage I non-small cell lung cancer. *Int J Radiat Oncol Biol Phys* 19:9–13, 1990.

38. Sause W: Combination chemotherapy and radiation therapy in lung cancer. *Semin Oncol* 21:72–78, 1994.

39. Sause WT, Scott C, Byhardt R, et al: Recursive partitioning analysis of 1592 patients on four RTOG studies in non-small cell lung cancer. *Proc ASCO* 12:336, 1993.

40. Sause WR, Scott C, Taylor S, et al: RTOG 88-08, ECOG, preliminary results of a phase III trial in regionally advanced unresectable non-small cell lung cancer. *J Natl Cancer Inst* 87:198–204, 1995.

41. Simpson JR, Francis ME, Perez-Tamayo R, et al: Palliative radiotherapy for inoperable carcinoma of the lung: Final report of a RTOG multi-institutional trial. *Int J Radiat Oncol Biol Phys* 11:751–758, 1985.

42. Speiser BL, Spratling L: Remote afterloading brachytherapy for the local control of endobronchial carcinoma. *Int J Radiat Oncol Biol Phys* 25:579–587, 1993.

43. Speiser BL, Spratling L: Radiation bronchitis and stenosis secondary to high dose rate endobronchial-irradiation. *Int J Radiat Oncol Biol Phys* 25:589–597, 1993.

44. Stewart, JR, Fajardo LF, Gillette, SM, Constine LS: Radiation injury to the heart. *Int J Radiat Oncol Biol Phys* 31:1205–1211, 1995.

45. Van Houtte P, Rocmans P, Smets P, et al: Postoperative radiation therapy in lung cancer: A controlled trial after resection of curative design. *Int J Radiat Oncol Biol Phys* 6:983–986, 1980.

46. Warde P, Payne D: Does thoracic irradiation improve survival and local control in limited-stage small-cell carcinoma of the lung? A meta-analysis. *J Clin Oncol* 10:890–895, 1992

47. Watanabe Y, Shimizu J, Tsubota M, Iwa T: Mediastinal spread of metastatic lymph nodes in bronchogenic carcinoma. *Chest* 97:1059–1065, 1990.

CHAPTER 114

SMALL CELL LUNG CANCER: DIAGNOSIS, TREATMENT, AND NATURAL HISTORY

David H. Johnson / Charles D. Blanke

Small cell lung cancer (SCLC) is a paradox among neoplastic diseases. Untreated, it is a highly virulent malignancy, killing its victims in a matter of weeks. On the other hand, it is one of the most chemotherapy responsive of cancers in that, with proper treatment, partial or complete remissions occur in the vast majority of cases. Unfortunately, although many patients can be rendered free of clinical evidence of disease, most eventually relapse and die from this malignancy. This chapter reviews several aspects of the diagnosis, natural history, and best current therapies for SCLC.

EPIDEMIOLOGY

Lung cancer is the most common cause of neoplastic death for American men and women, and its incidence has risen for at least the past 50 years. Five-year survival rates have not improved substantially for either non–small cell lung cancer (NSCLC) or small cell carcinoma, with the latter demonstrating the worst 5-year survival rates, stage for stage, of all histologic subtypes of lung cancer (Table 114-1): 1995 estimates called for 169,900 cases of newly diagnosed lung cancer and 157,400 deaths from this disease. The latest Surveillance, Epidemiology, and End Results reported for all lung cancers from the years 1973–87 demonstrated that small cell carcinoma made up 16.8 percent of cases.[35] Among Caucasian women, the frequency of small cell carcinoma was higher than that of squamous cell cancer, the most common type of lung cancer in men. SCLC represents the most rapidly increasing histologic type of lung cancer.

Like all other lung cancers, SCLC is linked to a variety of environmental risk factors. By far the strongest association is with the use of tobacco: up to 98 percent of patients with small cell cancer have a history of smoking. In most populations, the incidence of SCLC rises with increasing tobacco exposure in a dose-dependent fashion, making the overall risk for smokers approximately 15-fold higher than for nonsmokers. Occupational risks for small cell carcinoma include exposure to bischloromethyl ethers, nickel, vinyl chloride, asbestos, cadmium, and radon daughters (in uranium miners). Other types of radiation exposure also appear to be significant risk factors, with an increased incidence of small cell carcinoma being reported in atomic bomb survivors and a higher incidence of the disease being noted in those exposed to therapeutic irradiation (patients treated for Hodgkin's disease or breast cancer). Industrial nations in general have an increased incidence of small cell carcinoma, possibly from higher levels of air pollutants.

HISTOPATHOLOGIC CLASSIFICATION

A vast array of different histologic classification schemes for SCLC have been proposed over the past 30 years. The initial report of this tumor's being an epithelial malignancy was published 7 decades ago.[4] "The Nature of the 'Oat-Celled Sarcoma,'" by

TABLE 114-1

Lung Cancer: 5-Year Relative Survival Rates by Histology and Stage for All Races and Both Sexes (1978–1986)

Histologic Type	No. of Cases	All Stages	Local	Regional	Distant
All carcinomas (CA)	87,128	13.9	39.6	14.4	1.5
Squamous cell CA	26,407	15.4	34.3	14.9	1.5
Adenocarcinoma	20,991	16.6	49.9	16.1	1.5
Adenoid cystic CA	33	47.8†	*	*	*
Mucoepidermoid CA	47	38.5†	*	*	*
Bronchioloalveolar CA	2382	42.1	65.1	31.8	4.2
Papillary adenocarcinoma	568	23.7	57.4†	25.8	5.4
Adenosquamous CA	1056	21.6	49.6	19.1	2.2
Giant cell/spindle cell CA	295	11.8	33.0†	12.3	1.6
Small cell CA	15,656	4.6	12.3	7.5	1.4
Carcinoid	689	83.2	—	76.5	15.5*
Large cell CA	7592	11.4	34.8	13.2	1.6
Soft-tissue tumors	111	29.7	58.0†	16.0†	0
Carcinosarcoma	59	20.8†	*	*	*

*Either <25 cases or standard error >10%, insufficient for calculation of survival.
†Standard error >5% and ≤ 10%.
SOURCE: Data from Travis et al.[35]

W. G. Barnard, was a four-subtype morphologic classification. Although the first World Health Organization (WHO) small cell carcinoma classification included only two subtypes (oat cell and polygonal), the first categorization published by WHO, in 1967, returned to the original four: fusiform, polygonal, lymphocyte-like, and "other." Subsequent modifications were suggested by pathologists in the Working Party for Therapy of Lung Cancer, and in 1981, WHO changed the lymphocytelike subtype to the oat cell classification and combined fusiform and polygonal cell types into the intermediate cell type classification. In 1988, citing lack of differences in biologic behavior among the various subtypes within the WHO classification scheme, the Pathology Committee of the International Association for the Study of Lung Cancer recommended discarding the terms "oat cell" and "intermediate" and substituting the terms "pure small cell carcinoma" (more than 90 percent of small cell cancers) and "variant" histology. The latter contains large cell elements (including *mixed,* a combination of generic small and large cells, and *combined,* an admixture of small cells with defined non–small cell adenocarcinoma or squamous cell cancer elements).[16] The clinical significance of dividing small cell cancer into these histologic subtypes is controversial (see "Prognosis," below). Regardless, pathologists must be cautious in making their diagnosis, since poor fixation can make small cell components appear to be large cells, and crush artifact can give large cells a small cell appearance.

TUMOR BIOLOGY

Most cancers arise as a consequence of genetic abnormalities caused by exposure to environmental carcinogens.[26] *Activation* of a dominant oncogene or *inactivation* of a tumor suppressor gene can also result in the development of a malignant phenotype. In SCLC, the most common genetic abnormalities identified include loss of chromosomal material associated with inactivation of specific tumor suppressor genes. This frees the cells from the normal growth constraint imposed by the gene products and results in unrestrained growth of the cancer cell.

The chromosomal abnormalities most commonly associated with SCLC include loss of a portion of the short arm of chromosomes 3, 9, 11, and 17.[34] Deletions in 3p are found in nearly all SCLC tumors and cell lines. The area most consistently affected resides within region 3p14-25.[19] The exact tumor suppressor gene has not been identified but may be a gene responsible for the retinoid receptor. Up to 70 percent of small cell cancers lack the retinoblastoma (*Rb*) gene located on chromosome 13. Transfection of a normal *Rb* gene into tumor cell lines with defective retinoblastoma genes causes normal Rb protein production in the tumor cells and reverses the malignant phenotype. Abnormalities of chromosome 17p, the location of the p53 gene, are found in about 80 percent of SCLC patients.[18]

Dominant oncogene abnormalities are less common in SCLC. For example, amplification of the *myc* oncogene is seen in approximately 25 percent of SCLC patients.[5] The *myc* gene family—*myc, n-myc,* and *l-myc*—are closely related nuclear DNA–binding phosphoproteins involved in gene regulation. In two retrospective studies, the presence of *myc* DNA amplification in tumor cell lines and *myc* family DNA amplification was associated with shortened survival in SCLC patients. In laboratory studies, transfection of *myc* into an SCLC cell line was found to be associated with faster growth, a greater cloning efficiency in soft agarose, altered cell structure, and altered histology in athymic nude mice. These findings connote a more aggressive form of SCLC in association with *myc* amplification. Mutations in *ras* are mainly observed in NSCLC and rarely in SCLC. It is interesting to note that the mutation is most commonly seen in adenocarcinomas and primarily in subjects with a smoking history. Like *myc* amplification, *ras* mutation in NSCLC is associated with a more aggressive tumor and worse prognosis.

SCLC has long been recognized as capable of producing numerous peptides, including ADH, ACTH, and calcitonin (see "Paraneoplastic Phenomena," below).[30] The autocrine growth promotion potential of these peptides was first proposed 15 years ago. Among the more recently identified and characterized autocrine growth factors are gastrin-releasing peptide (GRP), arginine vasopressin, insulinlike growth factor–1 (IGF-1), and transforming growth factor–β (TGF-β). The most extensively studied peptide in SCLC is GRP, a mammalian analog of the amphibian hormone bombesin. GRP is produced in SCLC cells, which have functional surface receptors for the peptide. GRP stimulates the growth of SCLC in vitro as well as in vivo in the nude mouse. Antibodies directed toward the growth factor or against the surface receptor may result in growth inhibition. A murine antibombesin monoclonal antibody directed against GRP inhibits the growth of SCLC and is currently in clinical trial.[21] Elevated levels of IGF-1 have been detected in more than 90 percent of SCLC tumors and cell lines, and receptors for IGF-1 are found on SCLC cell lines, suggesting a possible autocrine growth regulatory activity.

NATURAL HISTORY

The natural history of untreated SCLC is early dissemination and death. Unlike NSCLC, it is always considered a systemic disease at diagnosis, even if it appears clinically confined to the chest. Postmortem exams performed on patients who died from other causes shortly after the complete surgical resection of their SCLC have demonstrated identifiable metastases in up to 70 percent. Evidence of distant spread can be found in virtually any organ system. The most common sites of involvement, however, are the liver, bone and bone marrow, and central nervous system (Table 114-2). This pattern of spread dictates how the search for metastatic disease is made (see "Staging," below).

Patients with SCLC have short lifespans if therapy is not instigated in a timely fashion. The median survival for untreated patients is 4 to 6 months if they have disease that is apparently confined to the chest and 5 to 9 *weeks* if they present with distant disease. With therapy, survival improves significantly (see "Treatment," below). Chemotherapy with or without irradiation can extend median survival to an average of 14 to 20 months for those with thorax-confined disease and 7 to 10 months for those with more extensive spread. At 2 to 3 years, a consistent 10 to 25 percent of limited-stage patients will still be alive, although cure is not guaranteed even in these relatively long-term survivors (see "Late Complications," below). Recent trials indicate that 2-year survival rates may be as high as 40 percent for aggressively treated limited-stage patients.

TABLE 114-2

Involvement of Extrathoracic Sites at Diagnosis after Pretreatment Staging Studies in Small Cell Lung Cancer

Extrathoracic Site	Patients with Finding (%)
Final stage	
Limited stage	30–40
Extensive stage	60–70
Bone	19–38
Liver	17–34
Bone marrow	17–23
Brain	0–14
Lymph nodes	7–25
Soft tissue	3–11

SOURCE: Ihde DC: Small cell lung cancer, in DeVita VT et al (eds), *Cancer: Principles and Practice of Oncology*. New York, Churchill Livingstone, 1993, p 728.

Two- to 3-year survival remains a dismal 1 to 2 percent for those with metastases.

DIAGNOSIS

The diagnosis of SCLC is usually not difficult (see also "Histopathologic Classification," above). The gross specimen often reflects a central lesion arising from a major bronchus and extending into nearby pulmonary parenchyma.[25] Necrosis and hemorrhage are often present. The classic oat cell form of small cell cancer consists of sheets of heavily staining cells with scant cytoplasm, hyperchromatic nuclei, and nonprominent nucleoli. In general, any subtype or description of "small cell carcinoma"

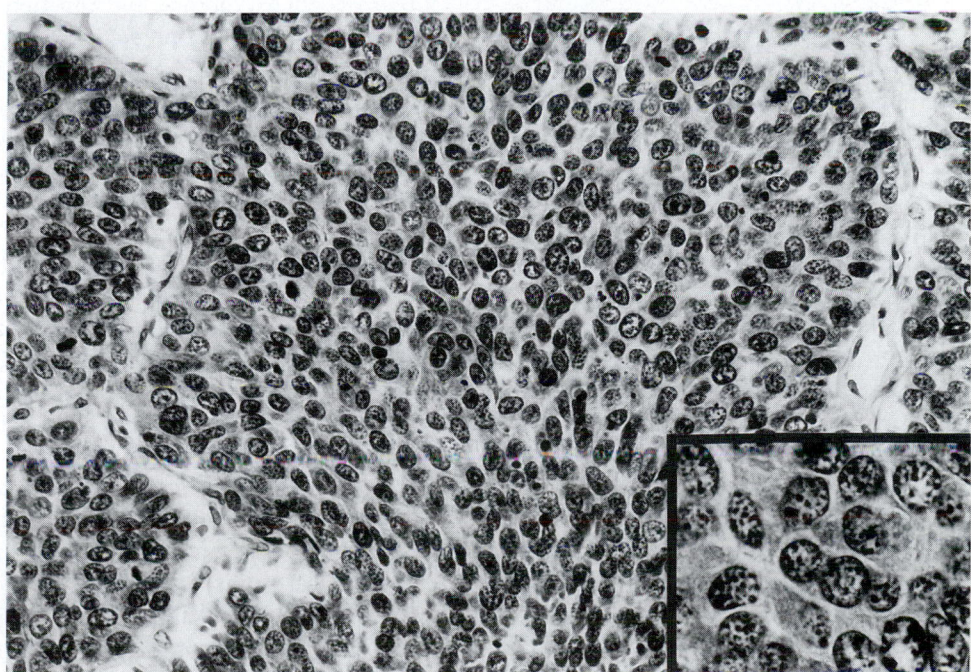

FIGURE 114-1 Photomicrograph of pure small cell carcinoma, demonstrating a homogeneous cell population with salt and pepper chromatin and moderately prominent nucleoli. H&E, ×250; inset ×400. (*Courtesy of Dr. Michael T. Lomis, Vanderbilt University.*)

includes cells double the size of a small lymphocyte, with salt-and-pepper chromatin, nuclear molding, and areas of necrosis (Fig. 114-1).[24] Inflammatory response and desmoplastic reactions are usually absent. Although biopsy specimens are ideal, cytologic specimens alone are often sufficient for diagnosis, with a sensitivity of 60 to 90 percent and a specificity of greater than 95 percent.[25]

Difficulty occasionally arises in distinguishing small cell carcinomas from lymphomas, other neuroendocrine tumors (e.g., atypical carcinoids), and poorly differentiated non–small cell cancers. The presence of "crush artifact" is more common in SCLC than in NSCLC, but it can also be present in lymphomas. If additional review fails to reveal subtle glandular or epidermoid differentiation, tests beyond routine light microscopy may be necessary to establish the diagnosis. Electron microscopy is often useful in this setting, revealing dense neurosecretory granules.

Although a detailed description of available antibodies is beyond the scope of this text, immunocytochemistry can be helpful in ruling in or out the diagnosis of small cell carcinomas. Antibodies reacting against the common leukocyte antigen would suggest the alternative identification of non-Hodgkin's lymphoma, while markers suggesting neural differentiation (e.g., chromogranin A) point toward the diagnosis of small cell carcinoma.

A variety of molecular biology techniques, including fluorescent in situ hybridization and utilization of the polymerase chain reaction, are currently available for the diagnosis of small cell cancers (see also "Tumor Biology," above). Abnormalities in the short arm of chromosome 3, overexpression or mutations of the *myc* proto-oncogene, or an altered p53 site on chromosome 17 is not specific for the diagnosis of small cell carcinoma, but changes in these loci can be strongly suggestive.

STAGING

Staging a cancer defines the anatomic extent of the tumor, helps determine prognosis, and guides treatment options. Although the TNM staging system can be used for small cell carcinoma, most authorities prefer a simpler two-stage system, which reflects not only the systemic nature of the disease at diagnosis but also the beneficial role of radiotherapy in early-stage cancer. This two-stage system has been found to have independent prognostic implications for patients with SCLC.

As originally proposed by the Veterans Administration Lung Cancer Study Group and still used today, the system places patients with disease that can be confined in a tolerable radiation portal in the limited-stage category (30 percent of all patients with small cell cancer); *all others* are defined as extensive stage (70 percent). Controversy still exists over whether an ipsilateral malignant pleural effusion (which technically could be confined within a radiation portal) represents limited or extensive disease, although most authorities would place it into the "extensive" category. Similar controversy exists for contralateral supraclavicular adenopathy. Clinical conditions, such as the superior vena cava (SVC) syndrome, are not strictly encompassed by this two-stage system. Many authorities do not believe SVC syndrome automatically places a patient into the "extensive" category, because it does not significantly change the prognosis of those

treated with combination chemotherapy. Some authors have even proposed a "very limited" stage, which purports to define a group of patients, without any mediastinal adenopathy (18.5 percent of limited-stage patients and approximately 6 percent of all small cell patients), who have long-term survival much beyond that normally seen for those who are "conventionally limited."[31]

A full history and physical examination, complete blood count with platelet analysis, blood chemistries (especially liver function tests and bone enzymes), and routine PA and lateral view chest radiography should be performed on all patients with SCLC. Tests such as mediastinoscopy, which may or may not be necessary for initial diagnosis, are not required for staging once the diagnosis has been made.

Further testing might be guided by a staging algorithm Figure 114-2 represents a modification of a proposed set of sequential steps that accurately stages patients with small cell carcinoma in an extremely cost-effective manner. Each sequential step, including radiographic testing and bone marrow assessment, is considered only if the history and physical exam or preceding steps do not direct the physician to the diagnosis of extensive disease. Note that on a clinical trial, however, extensive testing may be performed to strictly define *all* sites of metastatic disease and help decide whether different treatment groups consist of comparable patients.

Specifically, assessment of bony sites, believed by many authorities to be necessary, can be made with radionuclide bone scan or plain-film skeletal survey. One-third of patients with bone metastases will not have elevations in serum alkaline phosphatase, and most patients who would have positive bone scans do not have symptoms related to the metastases.

The remaining tests on the algorithm are considered controversial. Computed tomography (CT) scans of the upper abdomen (assessing primarily for hepatic metastases) rarely contradict normal liver function tests. They do, however, have a strong positive predictive value if any serum tests are abnormal.

CNS metastases from small cell carcinoma are usually intraparenchymal (brain) and are rarely asymptomatic. Using radionuclide brain scans, older studies found less than a 5 percent incidence of metastases in neurologically intact asymptomatic patients, and CT of the head has not truly improved on that number. Thus, CT of the head is not routinely recommended in asymptomatic patients.

Histologic bone marrow examination has historically been deemed to be of value in the initial evaluation of patients with otherwise limited SCLC. Unless significantly low, hematologic variables do not reliably presage bone marrow metastases, and leukoerythroblastic changes on peripheral smear are usually seen only with extensive marrow replacement. However, fewer than 5 percent of patients have bone marrow involvement as their only metastatic disease, and stage is rarely altered (less than 2 percent) on the basis of a bone marrow result alone. Thus, this test is not required if other staging studies are normal. The true incidence of marrow metastases is probably much higher than that reported from series utilizing histologic examination alone.[36] There is no proof, however, that immunostaining with monoclonal antibodies or doing cell cultures to detect microscopic bone marrow involvement will meaningfully change treatment planning.

CT scans of the chest generally do not add to information garnered from standard radiography, except in patients with pericardial disease, and routine use at the time of diagnosis is controversial.[13]

New technology may affect staging of SCLC. Bone marrow can noninvasively be assessed with magnetic resonance imaging, though the false-positive rate from this method of analysis may be unacceptably high. Thoracic ultrasonography is more specific than CT scanning for assessing possible malignant involvement of enlarged mediastinal nodes. Finally, "whole-body" single-modality assessments may someday be made with tests such as positron-emission tomography or with gallium citrate or octreotide scans. Although promising, these tests have not yet proved useful or become standard.

CLINICAL PRESENTATION

No aspect of the clinical presentation of SCLC distinguishes it from NSCLC or even neoplasms metastatic to the lungs. However, the duration of symptoms of small cell cancer tends to be very short, because of the rapid dissemination of the disease. Typically patients are middle-aged or elderly smokers with symptoms attributable to their pulmonary and mediastinal disease: cough, dyspnea, chest pain, hoarseness, and/or hemoptysis. Because of the endobronchial location of the tumor, patients often have an accompanying postobstructive pneumonia.

Constitutional symptoms may include weakness, anorexia, weight loss, and, rarely, fever. Symptoms may also arise from distant metastases, including headache or seizures in patients with CNS disease, and abdominal or bone pain with hepatic or osseous metastases, or from regional disease with attendant superior vena cava obstruction, manifesting as facial fullness, upper-extremity swelling, headache, and dysphagia. In rare instances, patients present with symptoms from a paraneoplastic syndrome.

Physical exam may yield only the stigmas of chronic obstructive pulmonary disease, or it may demonstrate affected lymph nodes, hepatomegaly, bone tenderness, or neurologic findings. Signs of the superior vena cava syndrome include venous distention of the neck and chest wall, cyanosis, facial plethora, and upper-extremity edema.

A chest radiograph typically demonstrates a central mass (75 percent of patients), with or without hilar nodal involvement (Fig. 114-3). Cavitation on chest radiograph would suggest the alternative diagnosis of squamous cell lung cancer, but postobstructive atelectasis and pneumonia are very common with small cell carcinoma.

Laboratory evaluation will reveal mild abnormalities of liver function (usually elevated alkaline phosphatase and, less commonly, SGOT or bilirubin) and/or serum lactate dehydrogenase in about 50 percent of patients, but low white blood cell or platelet counts are unusual and are hardly ever seen in the absence of widespread disease at a number of sites beside the bone marrow.

Two special situations warrant brief discussion. Organ involvement from small cell carcinoma can obviously lead directly

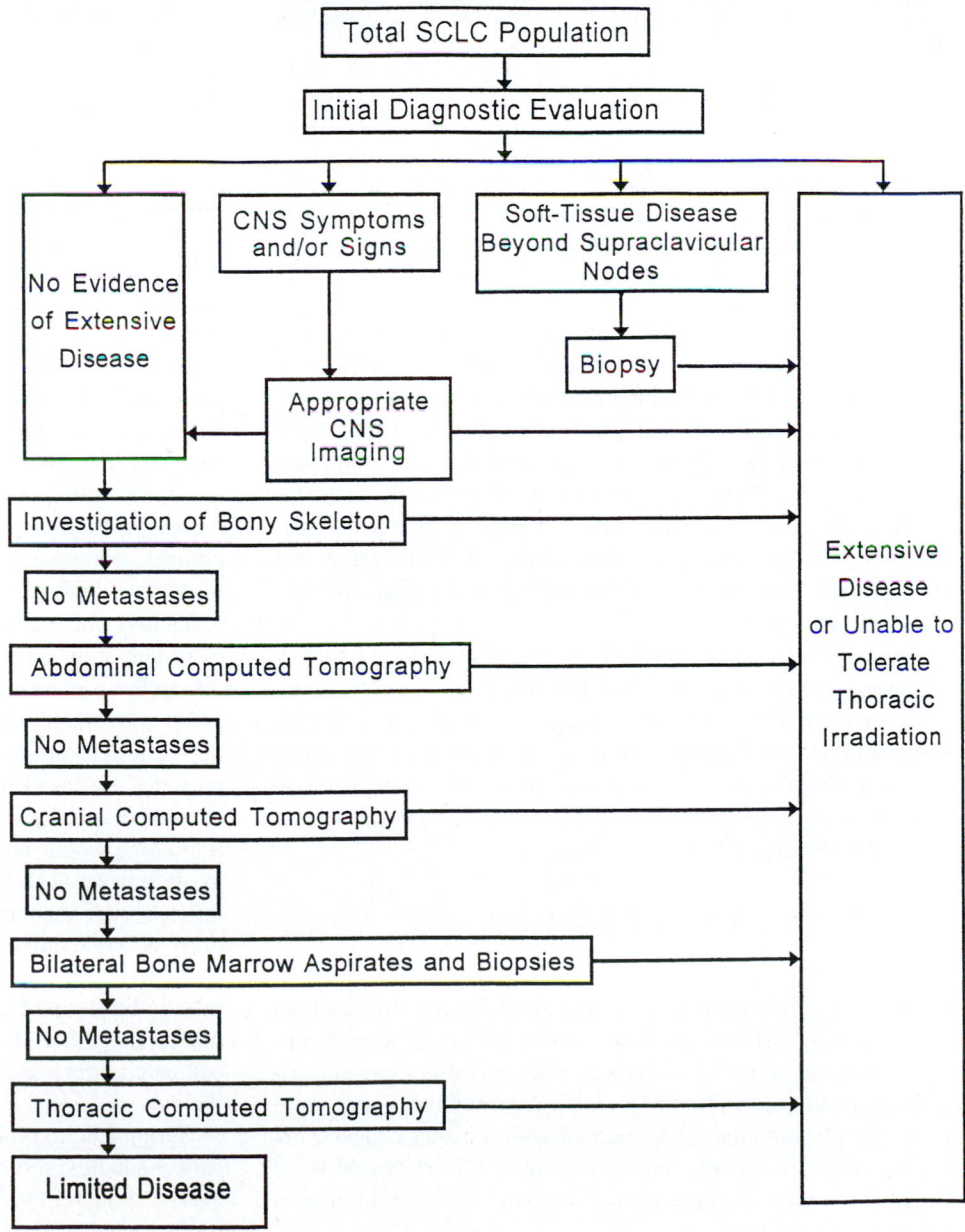

FIGURE 114-2 Proposed algorithm for staging small cell lung cancer. (*From Richardson: Arch Intern Med 153:329–337, 1993.*)

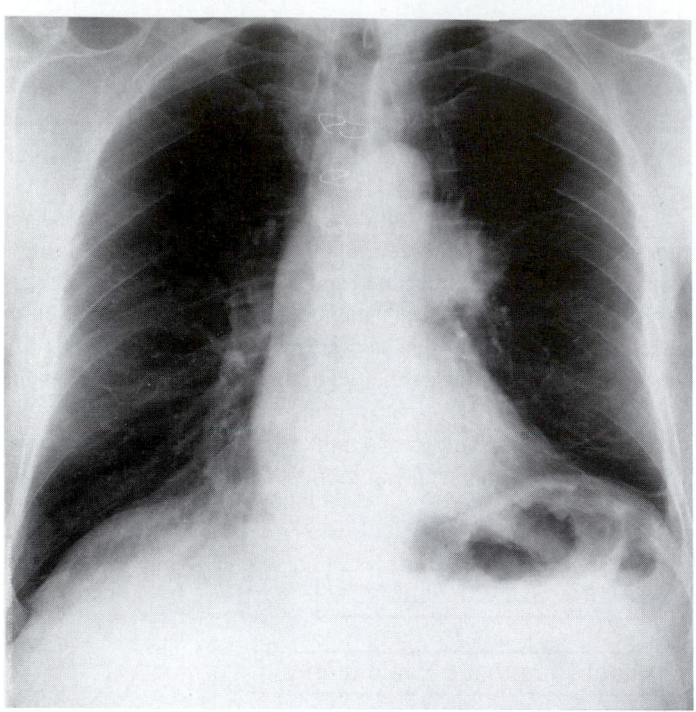

FIGURE 114-3 Chest radiograph of a patient with small cell lung cancer, demonstrating a left hilar mass extending into the (anterior) upper lobe. (*Courtesy of Dr. Russell DeVore, Vanderbilt University.*)

to failure of that organ, but this neoplasm can also cause problems in an indirect fashion. For example, hepatic insufficiency from frank neoplastic involvement (suspected because of abnormal blood work or the patient's becoming jaundiced) is a well-known phenomenon to those who treat small cell carcinoma and usually signals an extremely poor outcome. Other mechanisms for the dysfunction exist, however. Extrahepatic biliary obstruction from nodal metastases is well described in the literature and probably has a better prognosis than diffuse liver replacement by small cell carcinoma.

Pancoast's syndrome, with ptosis, anhydrosis, facial edema, and sensory neuropathic pain and functional loss, is more commonly thought of as being associated with squamous cell lung cancers or adenocarcinomas, but it has also been seen in patients with small cell disease. Obtaining a tissue diagnosis from an apical pulmonary mass is thus mandatory before radiotherapy or other treatment is started.

PARANEOPLASTIC PHENOMENA

Tumor cells in general cause symptoms because of mass effect and direct impingement on vital organs. However, they can act at a distance by virtue of production of antibodies, leading to immune reactions against host tissue, and by elaboration of various biologically active hormones and other proteins. These paraneoplastic phenomena are associated with all lung cancers, but they are most commonly noted with small cell tumors. Most of the paraneoplastic phenomena can be placed into endocrine or neurologic categories.

Ectopic adrenocorticotropic hormone (ACTH) production by small cell carcinoma has been a well-recognized phenomenon

for decades. Small cell carcinoma is the most common cancer associated with Cushing's syndrome, being responsible for more than 50 percent of cases in most series detailing an underlying malignancy. Clinical Cushing's syndrome is actually rare, occurring in only 5 percent of patients with small cell disease, but biochemical evidence of increased ACTH production is present in more than 50 percent. Cushing's syndrome from small cell carcinoma differs from Cushing's disease (the same syndrome produced by a pituitary adenoma) in that the onset of symptoms in the former is usually abrupt. When signs and symptoms do occur, they thus tend to be those associated with *acute* hypercortisolism-hypokalemic alkalosis, hypertension, hyperglycemia, and, rarely, edema and muscle weakness. The features of chronic exposure to steroids (e.g., the "buffalo hump" and moon facies) are usually absent. The effect of Cushing's syndrome on duration of survival of patients with small cell carcinoma is unclear, although some investigators believe that its onset heralds more aggressive tumor behavior. Also, lethal infections, including fungal disorders, often complicate the clinical course of these patients' disease. Treatment with standard medications, such as metyrapone and ketoconazole, is largely ineffective because of the extremely high levels of cortisol, and some patients have required bilateral adrenalectomy. The most effective treatment, however, is therapy for the underlying small cell cancer.

The syndrome of inappropriate antidiuretic hormone (SIADH), with its resultant refractory hyponatremia, is frequently associated with SCLC. Indeed, small cell carcinoma is by far the most common cause of acute or chronic SIADH in cancer patients. Clinically, SIADH is diagnosed in about 10 percent of patients with small cell cancer, though asymptomatic increased ADH levels are more common; up to 76 percent of small cell cancer tissue samples will stain for ADH. Also, some patients have the syndrome despite having normal ADH levels. Elevated atrial natriuretic peptide levels have also been found in patients with the clinical syndrome of excessive ADH production, although this protein's role as a contributor is unclear. As with the other paraneoplastic phenomena, the best therapy for SIADH is effective treatment of the cancer with chemotherapy. Vanderbilt University researchers demonstrated resolution of SIADH in 16 of 17 patients with small cell cancer treated with chemotherapy 8 to 26 days after the drugs were started.[14] The authors discussed temporizing measures for the hyponatremia while the effect of chemotherapy is awaited; they suggested that strict fluid restriction alone would maintain the serum sodium above 128 meq/L in all patients. The use of demeclocycline, an agent that blocks the action of vasopressin at the level of the renal tubule, is another possible adjunctive measure. The starting dose is 150 mg orally four times a day (600 mg total), but the daily dosage may need to be elevated to 1200 mg. Despite previous suggestions to the contrary, SIADH does not worsen the prognosis for small cell carcinoma patients, especially in the age of modern chemotherapy.

Serum calcitonin levels are elevated in up to half of small cell cancer patients; serum calcium levels are invariably normal, however. Although hypercalcemia is common with NSCLC patients, it is extremely unusual for those with small cell carcinoma. The rare patients who do have elevated calcium levels have been found to have inappropriately normal (i.e., not suppressed) levels of parathormone. The precise mechanism for the hypercalcemia is not clear, although these patients almost always have extensive bone or marrow involvement. Local destruction of bone alone is not a satisfying hypothesis, however, as the vast majority of small cell cancer patients with bone disease have normal calcium levels.

Neurologic paraneoplastic syndromes are frequently reported.[8] These are often the result of production of antibodies that react both with the small cell cancer cells and with normal host tissues. Well-described syndromes include the Eaton-Lambert myasthenic syndrome and cerebellar degeneration. Less frequent abnormalities include subacute sensory neuropathy, autonomic disturbances, myelopathies, progressive encephalopathy, and a visual paraneoplastic syndrome. Nonspecific neurologic findings that may be related to ectopic hormone or antibody production include weakness and anal sphincter disturbances.

Eaton-Lambert myasthenic syndrome is characterized by impaired release of acetylcholine from peripheral nerves. Clinically, the syndrome manifests with weakness, decreased reflexes, and occasional autonomic dysfunction. As contrasted to patients with myasthenia gravis, those with the myasthenic syndrome actually have improved strength with serial effort. The syndrome is thought to be caused by the blocking of calcium channels by IgG antibodies, and subsequent acetylcholine release, or by release of excess acetylcholinesterase. Immunosuppressive therapy, acetylcholinesterase inhibitors, and 3,4-diaminopyridine (an agent that enhances acetylcholine release from the nerve terminal) have been used to treat the syndrome, with limited success. Some patients who respond to combination chemotherapy will have resolution of the neurologic abnormalities, and this is the initial therapy of choice.

Subacute cerebellar degeneration—manifesting with ataxia, dysarthria, and dementia—is also commonly associated with SCLC. It has also been seen with female genitourinary carcinomas and other malignancies. Antibodies that react against Purkinje cells and other neurons are often found in these patients. One such antibody, anti-Yo, attacks a DNA binding protein thought to be important in gene expression. Treatment may include steroids, plasmapheresis, and chemotherapy.

Finally, elevations of gonadotropins, gastrin, β-melanocyte–stimulating hormone, and prostaglandins have all been described in SCLC patients. None has contributed significantly to a defined clinical syndrome.

EXTRAPULMONARY SMALL CELL CARCINOMA

The knowledge that small cell cancers can arise from tissues other than the lungs has existed for more than 6 decades. Extrapulmonary small cell cancer (EPSCC) remains relatively rare, however, with only about 1000 cases being diagnosed each year in the United States. EPSCC has been described as arising in the head and neck, esophagus, gastrointestinal tract, uterine cervix, prostate, ovaries, urinary bladder, and a host of other tissues. The cell of origin of the extrapulmonary cancer is thought to be a totipotent stem cell that can differentiate into either epithelial cells or neuroendocrine (and, thus, small cell cancer) elements.

EPSCC can be diagnostically distinguished from metastatic SCLC without a clear pulmonary parenchymal primary by the lack of deletion of chromosome 3p in the former.

EPSCC differs from the pulmonary form in other ways. Ectopic hormone production from EPSCC is extremely rare, and not all patients with EPSCC have a history of tobacco abuse, although the two are still associated. Staging, however, is similar for the two varieties. "Limited" disease is still defined as that confined to a small anatomic compartment, and extensive disease as that extending beyond locoregional lymph nodes. Most authorities would perform the same staging tests on these patients as on those with SCLC.

Treatment of EPSCC has not been rigorously studied. Tumors tend to be clinically aggressive and disseminate early. Thus, many clinicians offer combination chemotherapy with or without some form of local control (radiotherapy or surgery) as primary treatment. These tumors are chemosensitive, and some patients achieve long-term survival with this form of therapy.

PROGNOSTIC FACTORS

A variety of pretreatment factors have been reported as having value in predicting therapeutic outcomes for patients with small cell carcinoma. Since the aggressiveness of therapy may depend on this perceived outcome, it is important to determine before treatment how a patient is *likely* to do. The strongest and most consistent prognosticators from nearly all studies have been stage of disease (limited versus extensive) and performance status at presentation. The importance of stage has already been alluded to. In general, extensive-stage patients have a lower chance of achieving a complete response to chemotherapy, have shorter median survival times, and have a much smaller chance of being cured. Patients with extensive-stage disease, by virtue of having a *single* site of metastasis (especially in soft tissue, bone, or brain), often behave more like limited-stage patients, however, and should be treated accordingly. Within the extensive-stage group, having an increasing number of affected sites, especially if these include bone marrow or abdominal disease, carries a worse outlook.

The performance status, or ability of the patient to carry out normal daily activities, has a profound effect on the ability to tolerate chemotherapy and the chance that treatment will be effective. In general, patients with poor performance status have a lower chance of response to chemotherapy and a higher chance of having clinical toxicity. However, poor performance status (unlike non–small cell cancer) does not automatically exclude patients from receiving aggressive treatment, since an occasional bedridden patient can still experience improvement and even be cured with chemotherapy. Similar to performance status, substantial weight loss at the time of diagnosis (the definition of *substantial* varies, but most investigators believe it to be at least 10 percent of total body weight) is an independent prognostic factor for an adverse outcome. As would seem logical, achieving complete remission with chemotherapy in general portends a better outcome than being nonresponsive or having only a partial response. Similarly, relapse from remission clearly heralds short survival.

Most but not all epidemiologic studies suggest that women with small cell carcinoma have a significantly better chance of both responding to chemotherapy and obtaining a complete response. Their overall survival is also better than that of male patients. Variance in other epidemiologic factors, such as age (in the absence of poor performance status) and race, does not seem to be of consistent importance.

The continued use of tobacco is an adverse prognostic factor. Second malignancies, usually tobacco related, are a significant cause of death in long-term survivors of SCLC. Chronic obstructive pulmonary disease and ischemic heart disease, worsened by continuing exposure to tobacco, also remain sources of morbidity and mortality in patients with small cell cancer.

Abnormalities in various laboratory parameters have long been held to have prognostic value.[33] A high serum lactate dehydrogenase, suggesting more bulky disease, is an independent predictor of poor outcome for extensive-stage patients. Hypoalbuminemia and hyponatremia have also been found to presage poor outcomes in multivariate analyses. Finally, the serum tumor marker neuron-specific enolase is more often elevated at diagnosis in extensive-stage than in limited-stage patients, and the baseline value increases in proportion to the number of metastatic sites. The baseline value and value after chemotherapy significantly correlate with overall survival.

Histologic classification can also be of significance. Whereas some investigators report longer survival with the oat cell subtype than with tumors in the non–oat cell classification, most believe that there is not much biologic or prognostic difference among the subtypes of pure small cell carcinoma. The import if mixed elements, including a large cell component, are present is not clear. In a study of intensive treatment of 375 patients with small cell carcinoma, Hirsch and colleagues noted a median survival of 168 days for those with pure SCLC (of various non–large cell subtypes) versus 280 days for those with tumors with any large cell features.[15] This presumably reflects the inherent insensitivity to chemotherapy of NSCLC, which arguably makes up the majority of large cell components of mixed tumors. Data from an Eastern Cooperative Oncology Group publication, however, point to a different conclusion.[1] Investigators examined all patients with the diagnosis of variant histology (small cell with large cell elements) placed on an ECOG chemotherapy protocol. They found the variant histology actually was rare (fewer than 10 percent of cases) and did not lead to patients' having lower response rates or shorter median survival.

Finally, Albain and colleagues analyzed prognostic factors in the 2580-patient Southwest Oncology Group Small Cell Cancer Data Base.[2] For limited-stage patients, good performance status, female sex, younger age (under 70), white race, and normal serum lactate dehydrogenase were independent predictors for better survival. In extensive-disease patients, normal serum lactate dehydrogenase was the best predictor, followed by having a single metastatic focus of disease and receiving intensive combination chemotherapy.

TREATMENT

As previously stated, with extremely rare exceptions, the therapy for SCLC always includes chemotherapy. Chemotherapy can markedly prolong survival for patients with both stages of small cell carcinoma and can effect a cure in a significant number of those with limited disease. Early studies from the 1940s and 1950s showed nitrogen mustard had activity against anaplastic lung cancer (presumably including cases of SCLC). In the late 1960s, a large VA Lung Cancer Study Group trial established that cyclophosphamide, an alkylating agent, improved the survival of small cell cancer patients when tested against a placebo. Subsequent trials have elucidated a number of agents with activity against small cell carcinoma (Table 114-3). Complete responses to single agents remain relatively rare, however, and remissions induced by them are brief.

In the 1970s, combinations of drugs, each with independent activity against small cell cancer and with nonoverlapping toxicities, were employed. The drugs, given in combination, were often noted to have synergistic activity. Another advantage of using more than one drug at a time is the lower statistical likelihood of complete tumor resistance. A popular combination consisting of cyclophosphamide, doxorubicin (Adriamycin), and vincristine (CAV) and similar regimens with only minor modifications became the standard therapy until the mid-1980s, demonstrating response rates of 55 to 65 percent in those with extensive-stage cancer and rates up to 85 percent in limited-stage disease. From the mid-1980s till now, platinum-based regimens—especially etoposide-cisplatin (EP)—with or without CAV have become the therapy of choice in North America. Though not clearly superior (in terms of higher response rates) to CAV alone in randomized trials, EP is less toxic than CAV in extensive-stage patients. It has advantages that become even more apparent when it is used to treat limited-stage disease, as it is much easier to give in conjunction with chest irradiation.

Numerous manipulations to boost the efficacy of chemotherapy have been attempted. Increasing the number of cycles of induction given (i.e., maintenance chemotherapy) may prolong the time to progressive disease but does not improve overall survival, since patients not receiving maintenance therapy ultimately respond better to salvage therapy. There is no evidence to support giving more than four to six cycles of induction.[12] Escalating the doses of the chemotherapeutic agents for extensive-stage patients (dose intensification) may induce more complete remissions but does not affect overall survival and is much more toxic. Dose es-

TABLE 114-3

Single-Agent Chemotherapy Effective against Small Cell Lung Cancer

Carboplatin	Irinotecan
Lomustine (CCNU)	Methotrexate
Cisplatin	Mustard
Cyclophosphamide	Nitrogen
Docetaxel	Paclitaxel
Doxorubicin (Adriamycin)	Teniposide
Epirubicin	Topotecan
Etoposide	Vincristine
Gemcitabine	Vindesine
Hexamethylmelamine	Vinorelbine
Ifosfamide	

calation may be more important in limited-stage disease, but that concept still needs to be validated. A logical extension of the dose escalation principle—giving extremely high-dose chemotherapy with stem cell or autologous bone marrow support—has also been attempted, with mixed results. The only randomized study reported failed to show a survival advantage.[17] However, nonrandomized studies have shown that patients treated aggressively with high-dose chemotherapy, thoracic radiation therapy, and autologous bone marrow rescue can achieve excellent overall survival.

Alternating cycles with drugs that do not share common mechanisms of resistance ("non–cross-resistant") has theoretical appeal but is difficult to do in practice. Assuming at least one of the included regimens is highly effective against small cell carcinoma (e.g., EP), using alternating regimens appears to offer no advantage clinically over using the effective one consistently throughout. Also, to date, none of the studies has used completely non–cross-resistant regimens, so future trials testing this strategy with brand-new agents still have appeal. Pilot studies looking at weekly intense short-duration chemotherapy have found very encouraging results in terms of achieving high rates of complete remission and long-term survival.[27] Randomized trials will help define the role of this mode of delivering chemotherapy.

Single-Agent Drug Therapy

Recently attention toward single-drug treatment of SCLC has resurfaced, because of the interesting pharmacology of drugs like etoposide and teniposide. They are the most active single agents against small cell cancer, and protracted administration (even orally, over several days or weeks) achieves prolonged, fairly stable blood concentrations. Trials with these two agents alone have yielded response rates and long-term survival rates equaling those with the best combination regimens, with much less toxicity. The precise role and timing of the drugs (i.e., whether to use them up front in poor-risk patients or in the salvage setting) remain to be defined in randomized trials.

Salvage Chemotherapy

Most SCLC patients treated with chemotherapy will eventually relapse. Patients are more likely to respond to salvage chemotherapy if they had a good initial response to chemotherapy and if the interval between last treatment and relapse is a long one (6 months to 1 year).[11] The choice of agents is difficult. EP can generally induce a response in nearly 50 percent of CAV failures, but those failing EP and subsequently given CAV achieve remission in fewer than 10 percent of cases. Oral etoposide is becoming more popular in the salvage setting, because of its excellent efficacy and relatively low toxicity. Remissions to salvage chemotherapy, regardless of the agent(s) used, tend to be of short duration.

New Drugs

A number of new drugs have been shown to be active in small cell carcinoma.[9] These include the microtubule assembly-promoting taxanes paclitaxel and docetaxel, the topoisomerase-I–inhibiting camptothecin derivatives CPT-11 and topotecan, and the nucleoside analog-antimetabolite gemcitabine. Additional studies are needed to define more precisely the role of these agents in combination therapy or possibly as single agents in the salvage setting.

In summary, chemotherapy has profoundly changed the natural history of small cell cancer. Though the best regimen is still not defined, the most important lesson in chemotherapy for SCLC is that one must give full-course treatment on the originally selected schedule. Arbitrary dose reductions or delays may decrease the overall cure rate.

Radiation Therapy

SCLC is clearly sensitive to irradiation. All patients with small cell cancer are believed to have systemic disease; however, investigators have explored whether chest irradiation, in addition to chemotherapy, can improve local tumor control and, in turn, lead to improved survival for limited-stage patients. Multiple randomized studies have addressed this issue. Unfortunately, results have been mixed, with most chemotherapy plus irradiation trials showing a decrease in the incidence of local recurrence of disease but with differing results regarding survival benefit. This issue has also been dealt with in at least two meta-analyses, statistical tools in which researchers pool the data from a number of trials that do not in themselves have the power to prove an advantage to a particular therapy, to pick up small but statistically meaningful improvements. Both meta-analyses showed a clear improvement in survival with the addition of irradiation, with the magnitude of the difference being approximately 5 percent at 2 or 3 years. Although seemingly modest, this survival improvement rivals that gained through adjuvant chemotherapy for breast cancer, and almost all authorities agree thoracic radiation therapy should be used in the initial management of limited-stage SCLC. Also, because the study showing an advantage at 3 years based analysis on the "intent-to-treat" principle (all patients on a given study arm were analyzed regardless of whether or not they actually got the prescribed therapy), an even larger benefit might be possible if all patients were to comply assiduously with the prescribed radiotherapy.[29]

Questions remain regarding how best to add irradiation to combination chemotherapy. None of the randomized trials or the meta-analyses established the best *sequence* of chemoradiotherapy. The preponderance of evidence suggests that close administration of the two methods is superior, albeit with more toxicity. Early administration of irradiation may eliminate clones of tumor cells that are resistant to chemotherapy and thus boost the cure rate. However, it is apparent that giving concurrent chemotherapy and irradiation increases side effects and makes it more difficult to administer full-course chemotherapy on time. A Canadian study suggested that if therapy is given concurrently, early administration of irradiation (with cycle 2 versus cycle 6 of chemotherapy) strongly improves survival.[28] There are still no trials comparing any schedule of concurrent chemoradiotherapy with sequential (radiation after completion of chemotherapy) or alternating cycles (radiation and chemotherapy administered on a nonoverlapping, alternating schedule).

Although the optimal dose of radiotherapy is not known, low-dose irradiation (less than 40 Gy) leads to local failure rates as high as 80 percent. Increasing the standard dose to at least 45 Gy clearly improves local control, but it is not known whether further escalation would be beneficial. Fractionation issues are also still being explored. Laboratory data suggest an advantage to giving radiation treatment more than once daily, and this concept has been tested on humans with encouraging results.

Chest irradiation for extensive disease may improve local control, but it does not alter overall response rate, median survival, or cure rate. Its use should be limited to patients with symptomatic chest disease that requires radiation for palliation.

Prophylactic Cranial Irradiation

The need for prophylactic cranial irradiation (PCI) is one of the most controversial areas in the treatment of SCLC. The brain has long been considered a sanctuary site from chemotherapeutic agents, and it is also an area to which small cell carcinoma commonly metastasizes. The recommendation for PCI is generally limited to those whose disease has been put into a complete remission, since the vast majority of long-term survivors (those most likely to benefit from PCI) come from this group.

The risk of brain metastasis is significant for all patients with SCLC. Approximately 10 percent of patients have brain metastasis at the time of diagnosis, and 20 percent or more will develop CNS disease during systemic therapy. The cumulative risk by 2 years after diagnosis is somewhere between 50 and 80 percent. Brain relapse is often sensitive to chemotherapy or radiotherapy, but the brain is rarely the sole site of recurrence.

Numerous randomized trials have assessed the utility of PCI in small cell cancer. Unfortunately, not all trials required patients to be in complete remission before study entry, so their survival may already have been limited by disease outside the CNS. A recently reported French trial was more methodologically sound.[3] Researchers at the Gustave-Roussy Institute prospectively randomized nearly 300 patients with small cell carcinoma in complete remission to PCI or to a control group. Concomitant neuropsychological testing was performed. In this trial, PCI decreased the risk of brain metastases three-fold without increasing the neuropsychological complication rate, but there was no significant effect on overall survival. No trial has demonstrated a significant survival advantage for prophylactic radiation therapy, although most have found a decrease in CNS metastasis and possibly improved duration of survival without CNS disease. However, since fewer than 5 percent of patients have disease recurrence only in the brain, the maximum survival improvement one could reasonably demonstrate in controlled trials would be on the order of only 5 to 10 percent.

PCI remains controversial, despite its tendency to decrease brain metastasis, for several reasons. First, some studies show that relapsed patients with brain metastases still are highly responsive to therapy. Second, the benefit on overall survival and quality of life is still not clear. Third, PCI adds a significant financial cost to the treatment of small cell carcinoma. Finally, and most important, PCI is not without side effects. Acute toxicity can manifest as nausea and vomiting. Subacute problems, which are usually self-limited, include memory loss and confusion. Late sequelae are more ominous and can include severe permanent short-term memory loss, gait difficulties, CT scan abnormalities (cortical atrophy and ventricular dilation), and leukoencephalopathy.

Additional studies are needed before PCI can be routinely recommended when not part of a clinical trial, but at this point it is prudent to withhold PCI from any patient not achieving a complete remission with chemotherapy, and then to apply the technique only after the entire course of drug therapy is finished (since neurotoxicity may be worse with concomitant chemoradiotherapy).

Surgery

The role of surgery for SCLC has come full circle in the past 4 decades. The disease has been thought of as systemic from the outset, and chemotherapeutic treatment has long been standard. In the 1950s and '60s, however, the British Research Medical Council actually randomized patients with small cell carcinoma to one of two local therapies: surgery or thoracic radiation therapy.[10] The patients on the surgical arm actually had worse survival, but neither arm did particularly well, with a number of patients dying of distant disease. Subsequently, the VA Surgical Oncology Group entered more than 2000 patients in a study looking at the role of adjuvant chemotherapy after resection of NSCLC. One hundred forty-eight patients with small cell cancer were incidentally included in the study, and early-stage patients enjoyed superior survival.[32]

Surgery for low-stage small cell carcinoma, specifically that presenting as a single pulmonary nodule (5 percent of all small cell cancers), may be more appropriate, since it may be biologically different from more advanced disease. The Roswell Park Cancer Institute carried out a retrospective radiographic review of patients with "isolated" small cell carcinoma.[37] The patients studied did not receive "prompt" diagnosis or treatment of their cancers. Extremely slow growth of the tumors, over periods ranging from 14 to 40 months, was documented. No lymph node or systemic metastasis was found. Several other studies of resection for patients with T1N0M0 (small tumors without nodal or distant spread) have suggested a 50 to 80 percent 5-year survival rate, but it is the rare small cell cancer patient who falls into this category.

There is reason for *combining* surgery with other treatment in selected patients. First, small cell cancer treated with radiotherapy and chemotherapy still has a high local recurrence rate. Surgery for other thoracic malignancies, especially esophageal cancer, affords significant improvement in local control, even when added to radiotherapy. Second, surgery immediately puts the patient into a "no clinical evidence of disease" category, and both chemotherapy and radiotherapy work better on small-volume (microscopic) disease. Finally, as discussed above, many mixed-histology SCLCs contain large cell elements that may be less responsive to chemotherapy or irradiation. NSCLC is notoriously resistant to chemotherapy, and surgery remains the best curative option for this disease. Therefore, an argument could be made for resection of residual disease after chemotherapy, especially if the remaining element represents a non–small cell or a large cell fraction.

There has been one randomized study testing this role for surgery for SCLC. The Lung Cancer Study Group gave limited-stage patients standard chemotherapy for five cycles, followed by PCI and thoracic radiation; the patients were also randomized to receive or not receive definitive surgery.[22] It is interesting to note that 9 percent of patients who did undergo surgery had residual non–small cell elements. Actuarial 2-year survival was identical on the two arms at 20 percent; thus, no survival advantage was demonstrated for surgery. However, the study excluded patients who would have fallen into the extremely limited T1N0M0 or T2N0M0 non–small cell staging schema—the ones who had shown the most benefit in earlier studies from surgery. Thus, this trial is not helpful in promoting or excluding the role of surgery in small cell cancer.

Biologic Therapy

A host of immune function and biologic response modifiers have been used to treat small cell carcinoma. Nonspecific immune stimulants such as bacille Calmette-Guérin (BCG) do not improve response rate or survival when added to chemoradiotherapy. Results from trials using interferon have been mixed. Low-dose interferon does not seem to be effective by itself, but it may have a role in prolonging remission (i.e., as maintenance therapy) in patients responding to initial chemoradiotherapy. Monoclonal antibodies bound to cytotoxic agents ("immunotoxins") have been found to be relatively safe in early-phase testing, but it is too early to comment on their efficacy.[23]

Anticoagulant Therapy

Evidence exists that SCLC cells induce fibrin deposition in the stroma adjacent to the tumor, which may actually shield the cells from chemotherapeutic agents and aid in their ability to metastasize. Thrombin and subsequent fibrin generation can also directly affect tumor growth kinetics. Other tumor-produced procoagulants are also postulated to contribute to both growth and distant spread. One novel therapeutic strategy for small cell cancer has been to inhibit components of the coagulation cascade. An early randomized VA trial in small cell carcinoma showed a doubling of survival in patients treated with warfarin in addition to chemoradiotherapy over those given the latter alone.[38] The group given the anticoagulant also showed a significantly prolonged time to evidence of disease *progression,* again suggesting that the coagulation mechanism is important for cancer metastases. Pilot studies have also been done successfully testing the addition of urokinase and urokinase with warfarin to standard chemotherapy. Therapy with anticoagulants remains investigational, since at least one *randomized* trial testing the addition of warfarin to chemotherapy showed a higher response rate with the anticoagulant but led only to borderline statistical improvement in failure-free and overall survival.[6]

TREATMENT OF SMALL CELL CARCINOMA IN THE ELDERLY

Both the incidence of SCLC and the percentage of the population over 65 years old are growing rapidly. Historically, oncologists have been taught that because of poor bone marrow, renal, and hepatic reserve, elderly cancer patients tolerate aggressive chemotherapy less well than their younger counterparts. Curative chemotherapy is often not even attempted in the elderly for other malignant diseases, such as acute myelogenous leukemia.

However, treatment for small cell carcinoma need not merely be palliative in these patients.

In general, age alone is not an adverse prognostic factor in patients with SCLC if essential organ function is preserved. Retrospective reviews suggest that survival is based mostly on the treatment received. It is true that elderly patients are, as a group, less able to tolerate chemotherapy; but for those who do receive full-course treatment, survival is equal to comparable-stage younger patients. Those with good performance status and limited-stage disease should be offered potentially curative combination therapy (chemotherapy and radiation). Given the excellent response of patients to oral etoposide (see "Single-Agent Drug Therapy," above) and the essentially incurable nature of extensive disease, this agent also seems to be an excellent *starting* choice for elderly patients with disease beyond the hemithorax.[20] It is also an appropriate drug for limited-stage elderly patients with compromised organ function or poor performance status. A cooperative group trial attempting to compare aggressive intravenous chemotherapy (with cisplatin and etoposide) with oral etoposide unfortunately closed prematurely because of poor accrual.

LATE COMPLICATIONS

The treatment of SCLC can cause more morbidity than the neoplasm itself. Both radiotherapy and chemotherapy cause side effects specific to the agent used. Irradiation can have early (esophagitis, pneumonitis, superficial skin burns) and late (pulmonary fibrosis, late cardiac disease, myelitis) toxicities. Chemotherapy toxicities depend on the specific regimen used, but they generically include alopecia, nausea and vomiting, and myelosuppression. Bone marrow depression can lead to life-threatening bleeding episodes (from thrombocytopenia), but more commonly it is associated with (neutropenic) fever and occasionally fatal infection. Series have demonstrated that febrile episodes occur in approximately 30 percent of treated patients, documented infections in 5 to 15 percent, and fatal infections in up to 7 percent. Prevention of infection in patients treated with chemotherapy with or without irradiation has received significant attention: measures have included prophylactic use of nonabsorbable oral antibiotics to decontaminate the GI tract, as well as oral administration of quinolones and co-trimoxazole. Recently, a large randomized trial showed that granulocyte colony-stimulating factor in addition to chemotherapy led to a reduction in the number of episodes of neutropenic fever and in the number of documented infections.[7] Many oncologists do not agree that this is a cost-effective measure, however.

SCLC shares a number of risk factors with other pathologic conditions. Thus, a large portion of long-term small cell cancer survivors succumb to these other diseases. Cardiovascular and cerebrovascular diseases are extremely common in this population, related to the older age of these patients in general and to their tobacco abuse. Up to one-third of all long-term surviving patients, especially those who continue to smoke, have recurrence of their small cell cancer or, more rarely, develop new small cell lung tumors. Other aerodigestive cancers, especially NSCLC, are also extremely common, leading some investigators to propose trials of chemoprevention agents (retinoids) in long-term survivors of small cell cancer. Finally, patients with small cell carcinoma have an increased risk of developing hematologic malignancy. Secondary leukemias are believed to be related to treatment, especially if chemotherapy with alkylating agents was employed. Some of these leukemias that occur after small cell cancer therapy have also shown a deletion of chromosome 3, suggesting an underlying predisposition or common ancestor cell to both cancers, instead of a secondary leukemia arising from alkylating chemotherapy-induced genetic damage. Overall, the risk of a second cancer in 2-year SCLC survivors is probably as high as 50 percent, making long-term surveillance mandatory in these otherwise cured patients.

CONCLUSION

SCLC is distinct from the other three major histologic varieties of pulmonary neoplasms, which tend to behave similarly and be lumped together in classification schemes under the generic rubric "non–small cell lung cancer." It is biologically more active, secreting multiple hormones and neural markers and giving rise to a number of paraneoplastic syndromes. It is always thought of as a systemic disease, and therapy nearly always includes some form of drug treatment. Though it is highly responsive to chemotherapy, and survival is markedly prolonged with this kind of treatment, the complete eradication of small cell carcinoma in individual patients remains a relatively rare event. Long-term survivors are still subject to a host of morbid cardiopulmonary conditions, as well as secondary malignancies and recurrence of their small cell cancer. A number of questions remain regarding optimal chemotherapy drugs and combinations, dose and timing of irradiation, and the role of PCI.

REFERENCES

1. Aisner SC, Finkelstein DM, Ettinger DS, et al: The clinical significance of variant-morphology small-cell carcinoma of the lung. *J Clin Oncol* 8:402–408, 1990.
2. Albain KS, Crowley JJ, LeBlanc M, et al: Determinants of improved outcome in small-cell lung cancer: An analysis of the 2,580-patient Southwest Oncology Group Data Base. *J Clin Oncol* 8:1563–1574, 1990.
3. Arriagada R, Le Chevalier T, Borie F, et al: Prophylactic cranial irradiation for patients with small-cell lung cancer in complete remission. *J Natl Cancer Inst* 87:183–190, 1995.
4. Barnard WG: The nature of the "oat-celled sarcoma" of the mediastinum. *J Pathol Bacteriol* 29:241–244, 1926.
5. Brennan J, O'Connor T, Makuch RW, et al: *Myc* family DNA amplification in 107 tumors and tumor cell lines from patients with small cell lung cancer treated with different combination chemotherapy regimens. *Cancer Res* 51:1708–1712, 1991.
6. Chahinian AP, Propert KJ, Ware JH, et al: A randomized trial of anticoagulation with warfarin and of alternating chemotherapy in extensive-stage small-cell lung cancer by the Cancer and Leukemia Group B. *J Clin Oncol* 7:993–1002, 1989.
7. Crawford J, Ozer H, Stoller R, et al: Reduction by granulocyte colony–stimulating factor of fever and neutropenia induced by chemotherapy in patients with small-cell lung cancer. *New Engl J Med* 325:164–170, 1991.
8. Elrington GM, Murray NM, Spiro SG, et al: Neurological paraneoplastic syndromes in patients with small cell lung cancer: A prospective survey of 150 patients. *J Neurol Neurosurg Psychiatry* 54:764–767, 1991.
9. Ettinger DS: New drugs for treating small cell lung cancer. *Lung Cancer* 12 (suppl 3):53–61, 1995.
10. Fox W, Scadding JG: Medical Research Council comparative trial of surgery and radiotherapy for primary treatment of small-celled or oat-celled carcinoma of bronchus. *Lancet* 2:63–65, 1973.
11. Giaccone G, Dalesio O, McVie G, et al: Maintenance chemotherapy in small cell lung cancer: Long-term results of a randomized trial. *J Clin Oncol* 11:1230–1240, 1993.
12. Giaccone G, Ferrati P, Donadio M, et al: Reinduction chemotherapy in small cell lung cancer. *Eur J Cancer Clin Oncol* 23:1697–1699, 1987.
13. Griffin CA, Lu C, Fishman EK, et al: The role of computed tomography of the chest in the management of small-cell lung cancer. *J Clin Oncol* 2:1359–1365, 1984.
14. Hainsworth JD, Workman R, Greco FA: Management of the syndrome of inappropriate antidiuretic hormone secretion in small cell lung cancer. *Cancer* 51:161–165, 1983.
15. Hirsch FR, Osterlind K, Hansen HH: The prognostic significance of histopathologic subtyping of small cell carcinoma of the lung according to the classification of the World Health Organization. *Cancer* 52:2144–2150, 1983.
16. Hirsch FR, Matthews MJ, Aisner S, et al: Histopathologic classification of small cell lung cancer. *Cancer* 62:973–977, 1988.
17. Humblet Y, Symann M, Bosly A, et al: Late intensification chemotherapy with autologous bone marrow transplantation in selected small-cell carcinoma of the lung: A randomized study. *J Clin Oncol* 5:1864–1873, 1987.
18. Johnson BE: Biology of lung cancer, in Johnson BE, Johnson DH (eds), *Lung Cancer.* New York, Wiley-Liss, 1995, pp 15–40.
19. Johnson BE, Kelley MJ: Overview of genetic and molecular events in the pathogenesis of lung cancer. *Chest* 103:1S–3S, 1993.
20. Johnson DH: Treatment of the elderly patient with small-cell lung cancer. *Chest* 103:72S–74S, 1993.
21. Kelley MJ, Avis RI, Linnoila RI, et al: Complete response in a patient with small cell lung cancer treated on a phase II trial using a murine monoclonal antibody (2A11) directed against gastrin releasing peptide (GRP). *Proc Am Soc Clin Oncol* 12:339, 1993.
22. Lad T, Piantadosi S, Thomas P, et al: A prospective randomized trial to determine the benefit of surgical resection following response of small cell lung cancer to combination chemotherapy. *Chest* 106:320S–323S, 1994.
23. Lynch TJ: Immunotoxin therapy of small-cell lung cancer. *Chest* 103:436S–439S, 1993.
24. Matthews MJ, Gordon PR: Morphology of pulmonary and pleural malignancies, in Straus MJ (ed), *Lung Cancer: Clinical Diagnosis and Treatment.* New York, Grune & Stratton, 1977, pp 49–69.
25. McCue PA, Finkel GC: Small-cell lung carcinoma: An evolving histopathologic spectrum. *Semin Oncol* 20:153–162, 1993.
26. Minna JD: The molecular biology of lung cancer pathogenesis. *Chest* 103:449S–456S, 1993.
27. Murray N, Coy P, Pater JL, et al: Importance of timing for thoracic irradiation in the combined modality treatment of limited-stage small-cell lung cancer. *J Clin Oncol* 11:336–344, 1993.
28. Murray N, Shah A, Osoba D, et al: Intensive weekly chemotherapy for the treatment of extensive-stage small-cell lung cancer. *J Clin Oncol* 9:1632–1638, 1991.
29. Pignon J-P, Arriagada R, Ihde DC, et al: A meta-analysis of thoracic radiotherapy for small-cell lung cancer. *New Engl J Med* 327:1618–1624, 1992.
30. Russell PJ, O'Mara SM, Raghavan D: Ectopic hormone production by small cell undifferentiated carcinomas. *Mol Cell Endocrinol* 71:1–12, 1990.

31. Sheperd FA, Ginsberg RJ, Haddad R, et al: Importance of clinical staging in limited small-cell lung cancer: A valuable system to separate prognostic subgroups. *J Clin Oncol* 11:1592–1597, 1993.

32. Shields TW, Higgins GA, Matthews MJ, et al: Surgical resection in the management of small cell carcinoma of the lung. *J Thorac Cardiovasc Surg* 84:481–486, 1982.

33. Souhami RL, Bradbury I, Geddes DM, et al: Prognostic significance of laboratory parameters measured at diagnosis in small cell carcinoma of the lung. *Cancer Res* 45:2878–2882, 1985.

34. Testa JR: Chromosomal alterations in human lung cancer, in Pass HI, Mitchell JB, Johnson DH, Turrisi AT (eds), *Lung Cancer: Principles and Practice.* Philadelphia, Lippincott-Raven, 1995, pp 55–71.

35. Travis WD, Travis LB, Devesa SS: Lung cancer. *Cancer* 75:191–202, 1995.

36. Trillet-Lenoir VN, Arpin D, Brune J: Bone marrow metastases detection in small cell lung cancer: A review. *Anticancer Res* 14:2795–2797, 1994.

37. Urschel J: Pretreatment natural history of small cell lung cancer presenting as a solitary pulmonary nodule. *J Cardiovasc Surg* (Torino) 35:273–275, 1994.

38. Zacharski LR, Henerson WG, Rickles FR, et al: Effect of warfarin on survival in small cell carcinoma of the lung. *JAMA* 245:831–835, 1981.

PRIMARY LUNG TUMORS OTHER THAN BRONCHOGENIC CARCINOMA: BENIGN AND MALIGNANT

S t e v e n   M.   K e l l e r   /   K u s h a g r a   K a t a r i y a

BENIGN TUMORS
  Mucous Gland Adenoma
  Squamous Papilloma
  Cavernous Hemangioma
  Chondroma
  Intrapulmonary Fibroma/Fibrous Tumor
  Inflammatory Pseudotumor (Plasma Cell Granuloma)
  Granular Cell Myoblastoma
  Hamartoma
  Leiomyoma

MALIGNANT TUMORS
  Pulmonary Blastoma
  Carcinoid
  Carcinosarcoma
  Epithelioid Hemangioendothelioma
  Lymphomas
  Plasmacytoma
  Malignant Melanoma
  Malignant Germ Cell Tumors
  Salivary Gland-Type Tumors
  Sarcomas

Although bronchogenic carcinoma represents the overwhelming majority of primary pulmonary neoplasms, a great variety of tumors originate in the lung. Benign neoplasms of the lung (Table 115-1) comprise fewer than 1 percent of all resected lung tumors,[28] and nonbronchogenic primary pulmonary malignancies (Table 115-2) account for 3 to 5 percent of all lung tumors.[5] With the exceptions of carcinoid tumors and hamartomas, fewer than 100 cases of many of these unusual neoplasms have been reported. Numerous classifications of these rare tumors have been devised, although none has become widely accepted. Due to the disparate histogenesis of these varied tumors, it is best to discuss them individually.

BENIGN TUMORS

Mucous Gland Adenoma

Mucous gland adenoma, also known as *bronchial cyst adenoma,* originates in the bronchial mucous glands and usually occurs as an endobronchial mass with intact overlying epithelium.[8] The tumor is more common in women, and symptoms are usually related to obstruction or hemorrhage. Histologic examination reveals mucus-filled glands protruding into the bronchial lumen. Excision with conservation of lung tissue is the optimal treatment.

Squamous Papilloma

Bronchial papilloma is usually associated with childhood laryngeal papillomatosis. Solitary bronchial papillomas are much less common and usually affect adults in their fifth to seventh decade. These tumors protrude into the bronchial lumen and cause obstructive symptoms associated with distal bronchiectasis.[3] Malignant degeneration has been reported.[15] Once a firm diagnosis has been established the tumor may be resected endoscopically. Alternatively, a bronchotomy or sleeve resection may be performed to preserve normal lung parenchyma. Resection of distally destroyed lung is occasionally necessary.

Cavernous Hemangioma

Cavernous hemangiomas are a subset of pulmonary arteriovenous malformations that can be found in both endobronchial and parenchymal locations. Although usually described in adults, these tumors have been reported in infants with congestive heart failure.[16] Microscopic examination demonstrates a large thin-walled vascular space. Hereditary hemorrhagic telangiectasia, Rendu-Osler-Weber syndrome, should be considered if inspec-

TABLE 115-1

Benign Tumors of the Lung

Solitary Tumors	Other Solitary Tumors	Multiple Tumors
Epithelial tumors	Alveolar adenoma	Benign metastasizing leiomyoma
Clara cell adenoma	Pulmonary paraganglioma—chemodectoma	Lymphangioleiomyomatosis
Mucous gland adenoma	Glomus tumor	Cystic fibrohistiocytic tumors
Oncocytoma	Nodular amyloid	
Squamous papilloma	Pleomorphic adenoma—mixed tumor	
Soft tissue tumors	Pulmonary meningioma	
Cavernous hemangioma	Sclerosing hemangioma—pneumocytoma	
Chondroma	Sugar tumor—benign clear cell tumor	
Fibroma/fibrous polyp	Teratoma	
Fibromyxoma		

Inflammatory pseudotumor—
    fibrous histiocytoma,
    fibroxanthoma, plasma cell
    granuloma		

Granular cell myoblastoma		
Hamartoma		
Leiomyoma		
Lipoma		
Neurilemoma—schwannoma		
Neurofibroma		
Pulmonary hyalinizing granuloma		

tion of the resected specimen demonstrates evidence of arterial-venous malformations.

Chondroma

Chondromas of the lung may occur in the parenchyma or airways. The former are usually asymptomatic, and the latter are associated with obstructive symptoms. Many of these tumors have occurred in association with multiple gastric smooth muscle tumors and extra adrenal paraganglionomas,[7] the Carney triad. Microscopy of solitary chondromas reveals benign cartilaginous tissue, although those associated with the Carney triad may contain metaplastic bone, mature cartilage, and myxoid stroma. A lung-sparing resection should be performed whenever possible.

Intrapulmonary Fibroma/Fibrous Tumor

Intrapulmonary fibrous tumors are contiguous with the visceral pleura and are histologically identical to localized fibrous mesotheliomas. The lung is the most common location of these extrapleural fibrous tumors, but they may also be found in the retroperitoneum, mediastinum, and the parietal surfaces of the intra-abdominal viscera.[12] The diagnosis is usually established following resection of an asymptomatic lung mass found on routine chest radiographs. The operative procedure should spare as much parenchyma as possible without compromising complete tumor removal.

TABLE 115-2

Rare Primary Malignant Neoplasms of the Lung

Blastoma
Carcinoid tumors
Carcinosarcoma
Epithelioid hemangioendothelioma (IVBAT)
Malignant lymphoreticular disorders
  Hodgkin's disease
  Non-Hodgkin's lymphoma
  Plasmacytoma
Malignant melanoma
Malignant germ cell tumors
  Malignant teratoma
  Choriocarcinoma
Salivary gland-type tumors
  Adenoid cystic carcinoma
  Mucoepidermoid carcinoma
  Acinic cell tumor
Sarcoma
  Chondrosarcoma
  Osteosarcoma
  Soft tissue sarcoma
Miscellaneous
  Ependymoma, malignant
  Ewing's sarcoma
  Lymphoepithelioma
Pseudomesotheliomatous carcinoma

Inflammatory Pseudotumor (Plasma Cell Granuloma)

Inflammatory pseudotumors are usually asymptomatic solitary, well-circumscribed masses found on routine chest radiographs.[4] The tumors occur most commonly in adults but represent the most common benign lung tumor in children.[2] Serial radiologic examinations rarely demonstrate enlargement, and may even reveal a decrease in size. The diagnosis is infrequently made prior to resection. Microscopic examination demonstrates a mixture of inflammatory cells, including plasma cells, lymphocytes, and macrophages. The predominance of one of these cell types has caused some confusion regarding the true nature of this neoplasm, which may also be referred to as a *plasma cell granuloma, histiocytoma,* and *xanthoma.* Cultures are routinely negative. Lung-conserving surgical procedures are indicated, although intrathoracic recurrences may occur if wide margins are not obtained.[4]

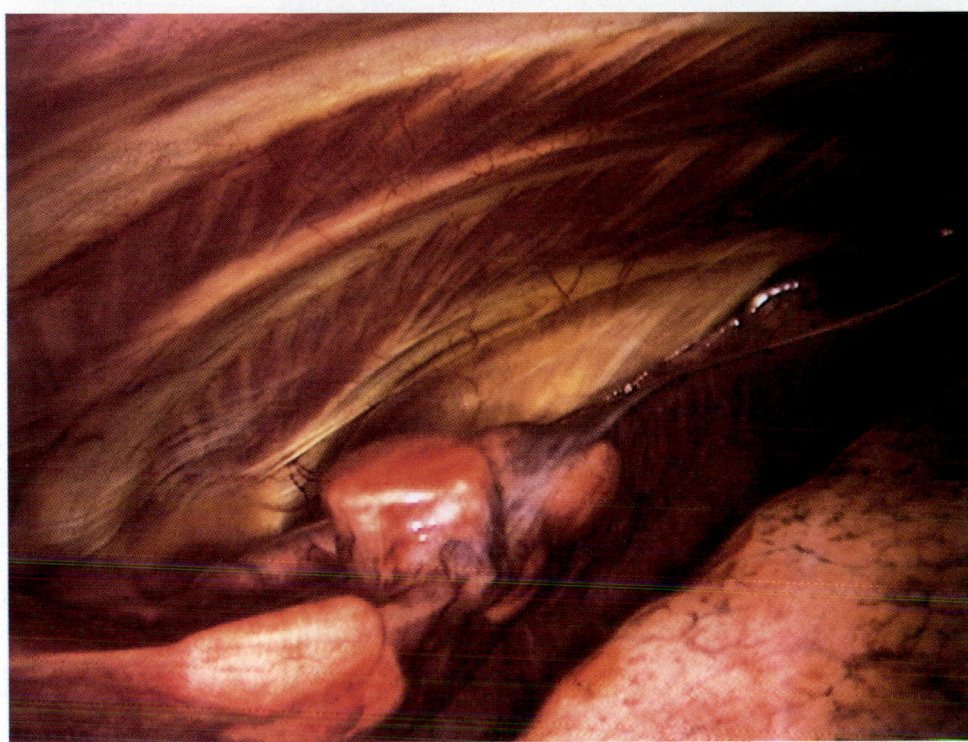

FIGURE 115-1   Pulmonary hamartoma seen at thoracoscopy. The tumor is easily visualized in a subpleural location. Incising the overlying pleura allows the lesion to be "popped" out.

Granular Cell Myoblastoma

Granular cell myoblastomas are thought to arise from Schwann cells and are most commonly found in the tongue, skin, and breast. The tumor occurs in the lung with equal frequency in men and women at a median age of 38 years.[38] Although the majority are endobronchial, they are usually discovered on a routine chest radiograph. Symptoms, when present, are related to bronchial obstruction. Appropriate treatment is complete excision with sparing of lung tissue. However, lung compromised by postobstructive bronchiectasis or abscess should be removed with the specimen.

Hamartoma

Hamartomas are the most common benign lung neoplasms and consist of cartilage, connective tissue, fat, smooth muscle, and respiratory epithelium.[8] Most tumors present as a solitary asymptomatic parenchymal lung nodule that may gradually increase in size (see Fig. 115-1). Approximately 10 percent of hamartomas are endobronchial and cause obstructive symptoms. The diagnostic radiograph finding of popcorn pattern of calcification occurs in fewer than 30 percent of patients. Percutaneous transthoracic needle biopsy yields diagnostic information in as many as 85 percent of patients.[17] The patient with a known peripheral hamartoma may be safely observed, as malignant transformation is rare. Excision is indicated if the diagnosis is in doubt or there are associated sequela of obstruction. Minimal amounts of normal lung tissue should be removed. Recurrences after complete excision are unusual, although a second primary hamartoma may occur.

Leiomyoma

Primary solitary leiomyoma accounts for approximately 2 percent of all benign lung tumors.[39] The tumor occurs with almost equal incidence in the proximal bronchi and parenchyma. Symptoms of obstruction are associated with the former, whereas the latter are found on routine radiograph. Patients are typically in their fourth decade. The tumor is slightly more common in women. Surgical resection is the treatment of choice, although laser resection of endobronchial tumors may afford prolonged palliation.

MALIGNANT TUMORS

Pulmonary Blastoma

This biphasic tumor is composed of both malignant mesenchymal and epithelial components that resemble the pseudoglandular stage of the 3-month fetal lung (Fig. 115-2). Koss and colleagues[22] reviewed 52 of the approximately 150 published cases of pulmonary blastomas and divided the tumors into two categories based on histologic features: well-differentiated fetal adenocarcinoma (WDFA) and biphasic blastoma. WDFA is a pulmonary blastoma with a malignant epithelial component but without a malignant stroma. The biphasic blastoma is composed of malignant mesenchyme without the malignant epithelium. An asymptomatic tumor was discovered on a routine chest radiograph in 21 of the 52 patients (41 percent), and the remainder presented with nonspecific complaints of cough, hemoptysis, or dyspnea. Twenty-eight tumors (54 percent) were classified as WDFA and 24 as biphasic blastomas. All patients underwent resection of the tumor, and a few received adjuvant chemotherapy.

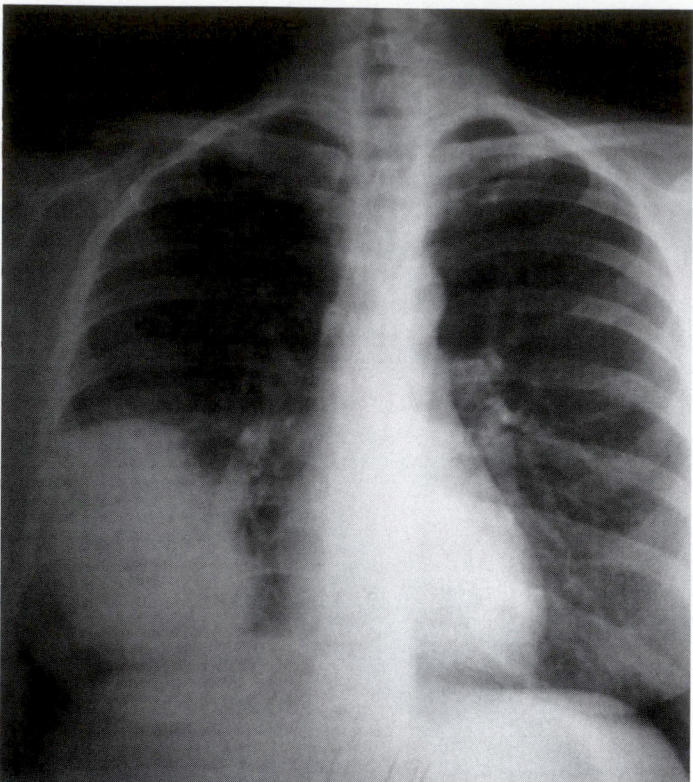

FIGURE 115-2 Chest radiograph demonstrating a pulmonary blastoma. The lesion presented as a large mass in the right lower lobe of a 25-year-old nonsmoking female.

Patients with the WDFA histologic subtype had a better survival than those whose tumors were of the biphasic blastoma type. The tumor-associated mortality was 14 percent for patients with the WDFA type, and 81 percent were alive and disease-free (median

follow-up 95 months). With a median follow-up of 13 months, 52 percent of patients with the biphasic subtype had died of tumor, and only 39 percent were disease-free. Additional poor prognostic factors include a tumor diameter larger than 5 cm, regional lymph node metastases, and tumor recurrence.

Carcinoid

Neuroendocrine or Kultschitzsky cells are the precursors of these low-grade malignant neoplasms that represent the second most common tumors arising in the tracheobronchial tree and 0.5 to 1.0 percent of all bronchial tumors (Fig. 115-3). Carcinoid tumors may be divided into typical and atypical subtypes with the latter accounting for 11 to 24 percent of all carcinoids and having more malignant histologic and clinical features.[1,8,29]

Approximately half the patients with carcinoid tumors are asymptomatic at presentation, and as many as 9 percent of tumors may be incidental findings at surgery or autopsy.[35] The most common clinical manifestations include hemoptysis, postobstructive pneumonitis, and dyspnea. Occasionally a case of atypical carcinoid may present with metastatic disease. A variety of paraneoplastic syndromes occurs with carcinoid tumors, including carcinoid syndrome, Cushing's syndrome—due to ectopic adrenocorticotropic hormone (ACTH) production, and acromegaly—due to ectopic growth hormone–releasing hormone (GHRH) production. Occasionally bronchial carcinoids may be

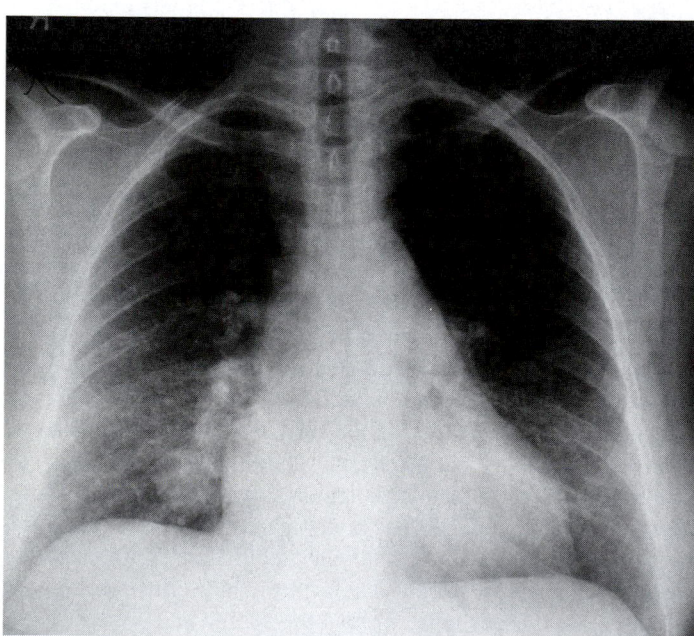

A

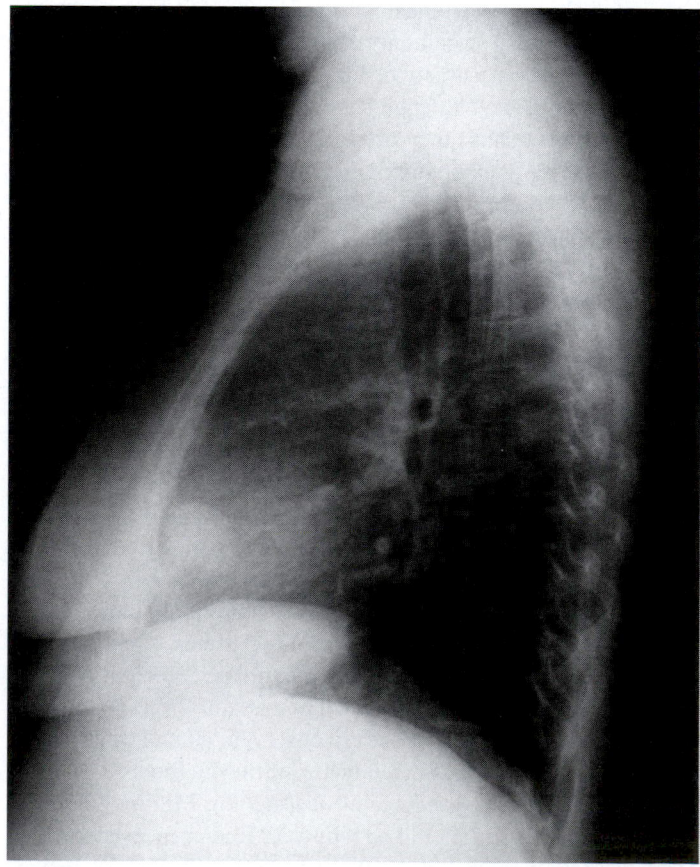

B

FIGURE 115-3 Solitary nodule presenting in a young asymptomatic woman. *A.* PA chest radiograph. *B.* Lateral film. The lesion was excised and found to be a typical carcinoid tumor with no evidence of mitoses or necrosis.

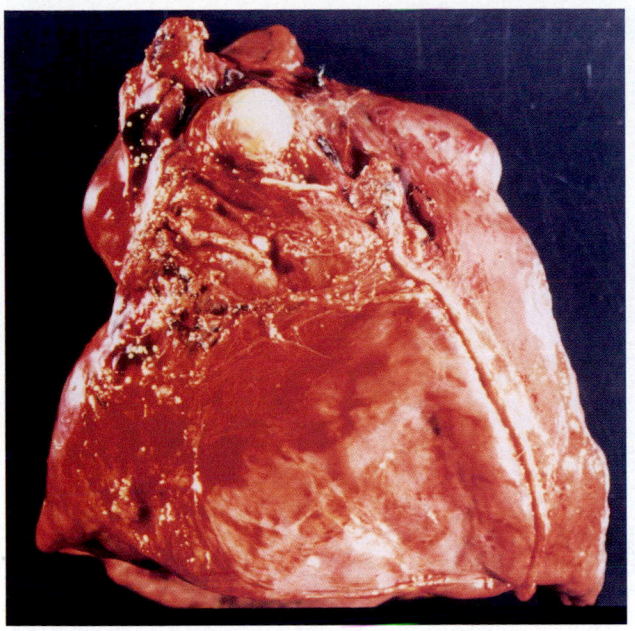

A

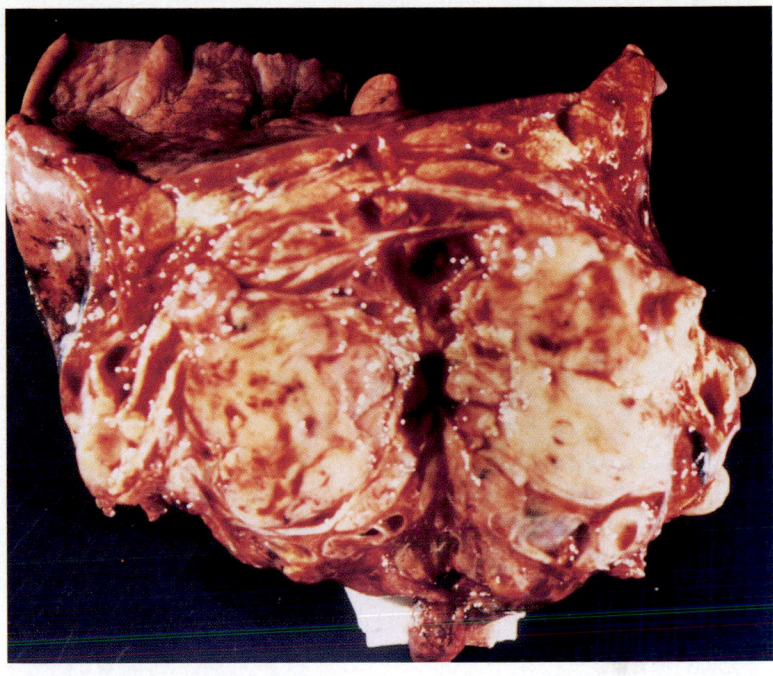

B

FIGURE 115-4   Carcinosarcoma. *A*. Endobronchial component of a carcinosarcoma. *B*. The parenchymal component of the same tumor bisected.

seen in patients with multiple endocrine neoplasia type I. Bronchial carcinoids are the most common malignant lung tumor of childhood.[24] Diffuse or punctate calcifications in the lesion are identified in approximately 30 percent of computed tomography studies. Homogenous contrast enhancement of typical carcinoids may be observed after the intravenous administration of a contrast bolus.[26] Sputum cytology is rarely helpful in the evaluation of carcinoid tumors, as few cells are shed into the bronchi. Fine-needle aspiration cytology is distinctive.[37] Almost 75 percent of all carcinoid tumors are visible bronchoscopically, and a bronchoscopic biopsy is usually diagnostic.

Treatment of both typical and atypical carcinoids localized to the lung consists of excision of the primary lesion and mediastinal lymph node dissection. This usually entails a lobectomy. A pneumonectomy is rarely required, although occasionally a centrally located tumor necessitates a "sleeve lobectomy" in order to avoid removal of an entire lung. Subtotal transbronchoscopic removal of the tumor may be accomplished in patients in whom a thoracotomy is contraindicated. Postoperative radiation therapy has been recommended for patients with atypical carcinoids or with lymph node metastasis. Combination chemotherapy, similar to that used for small cell carcinoma, may produce a response in 50 percent of patients. Five-year survival rates are greater than 90 percent for patients with typical carcinoid tumors,[13,18,27,35] and those with atypical carcinoids have a 5-year survival of less than 60 percent.

"Carcinoid tumorlets" were described by Whitwell in 1955[40] as isolated foci of atypical hyperplastic bronchial epithelium. They are now thought to represent hyperplasia of neuroendocrine cells, although one case of peribronchial lymph node metastasis has been recorded.[10]

Carcinosarcoma

Carcinosarcoma accounts for 0.3 percent of all pulmonary tumors and is three times more common in men. The majority occur in the upper lobes and are found in either central or peripheral locations (Fig. 115-4). A slow growth rate is characteristic, although metastases to the regional lymph nodes and distant organs may occur. Chest pain, cough, and hemoptysis are typical symptoms. Diagnosis of this rare lung tumor depends on the unequivocal presence of malignant epithelial and mesenchymal components. Cabarcos and associates reviewed 48 published reports in 1985.[6] The epithelial element was most commonly squamous cell carcinoma and the mesenchymal component a fibrosarcoma. Surgery is the treatment of choice, and 90 percent of tumors are resectable when first discovered. However, the median survival is 12 months, and 5-year survival rates range from 6 to 16 percent.[6,31]

Epithelioid Hemangioendothelioma

Originally named *intravascular bronchoalveolar tumor* (IVBAT),[11] this neoplasm has since been demonstrated to be of vascular endothelial origin rather than alveolar cell. The tumor is categorized as a low-grade sarcoma and is usually multifocal. Burt and Zakowski identified 33 published reports of epithelioid hemangioendotheliomas and found that 85 percent of patients were female, one-half of whom were asymptomatic and presented with bilateral pulmonary involvement.[5] No specific therapy is known, although excision of the rare solitary tumor is recommended. Chemotherapy and radiation therapy have proven ineffective. The 5- and 10-year survival rates are 61 and 55 percent, respectively.

Lymphomas

All the various elements of the lymphoreticular system are present within the lung and may undergo malignant degeneration. Non-Hodgkin's lymphoma, Hodgkin's disease, and plasmacytoma of the lung together comprise approximately 0.5 percent of all primary lung tumors. Secondary involvement of the lung by these processes is much more common.

The low-grade small lymphocyte lymphomas comprise 50 to 90 percent of all primary pulmonary lymphomas.[8] The majority are B-cell lymphomas arising in the bronchus-associated lymphoid tissue (BALT) (Fig. 115-5). Patients are typically in their sixth decade and approximately half are asymptomatic. The chest radiograph may demonstrate either a localized process or diffuse disease. As many as 20 percent of patients present with bone marrow involvement and a monoclonal serum protein. Resection is the treatment of choice for localized tumors. Long-term survival is excellent, although relapse may occur in the lung or other lymphoid tissue. Rarely these tumors evolve into an aggressive systemic lymphoma.

The angiocentric immunoproliferative lesion or angiocentric lymphomas (AIL/LYG) comprise the second most common group of pulmonary lymphomas.[23] The diagnostic microscopic findings are those of lymphoid cells forming nodules and infiltrates in proximity to lymphatics. Although thought to be a neoplasm of T-cell origin, B cells infected with the Epstein-Barr virus have been identified. The tumors are conveniently divided by histologic criteria into low-grade (uncommon) and high-grade categories. AIL/LYG occurs most commonly in men in their fifth decade. Approximately 10 percent of patients are symptomatic. Other organs such as the skin and central nervous system are frequently involved. The majority of patients have bilateral pulmonary nodules when first diagnosed. Despite aggressive treatment with multiple chemotherapeutic agents, the disease may ultimately involve other organs.

Large cell lymphomas are the least common of the pulmonary lymphomas and may be difficult to distinguish from AIL/LYG.[8] Patients generally present with a solitary nodule, and the diagnosis is made following resection. Treatment consists of adjuvant radiochemotherapy.

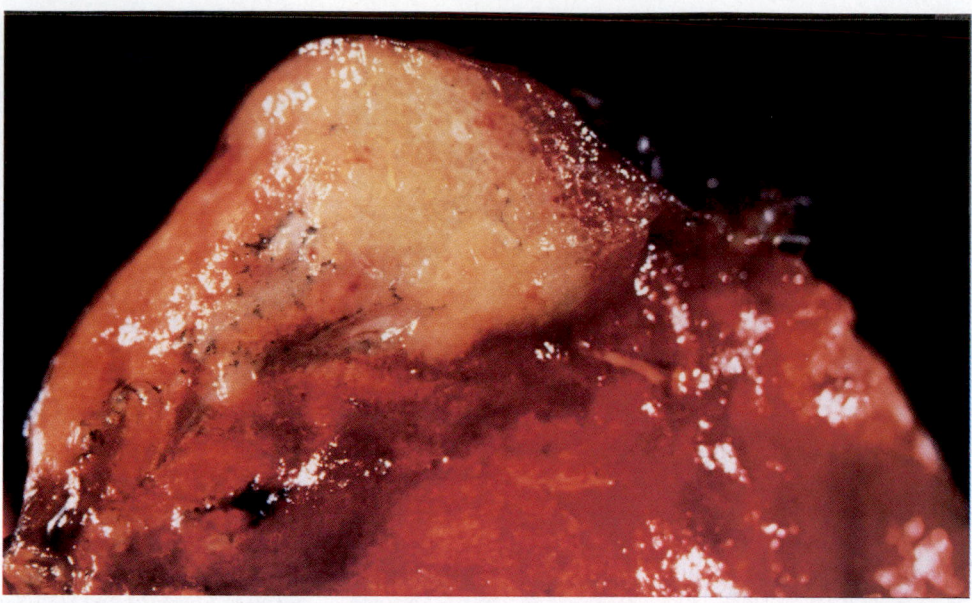

A

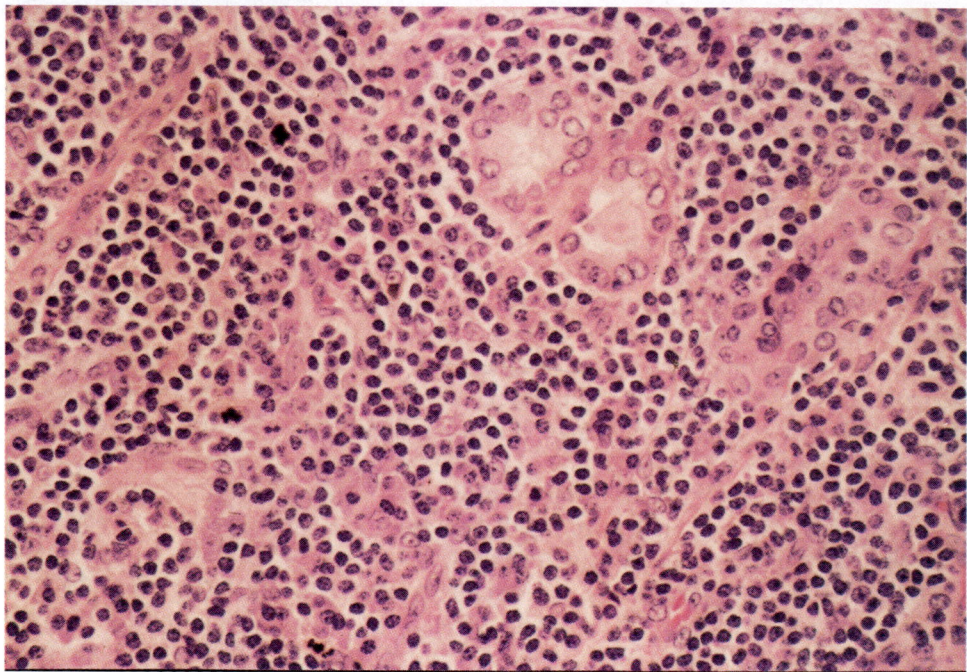

B

FIGURE 115-5 Pulmonary lymphoma (BALT). *A.* Gross appearance of a BALT following wedge excision. *B.* Microscopic appearance of the same BALT lesion showing the lymphoid cells along with some residual epithelial elements.

In order to diagnose primary Hodgkin's disease of the lung, the typical histologic features must be present within the lung substance but absent from regional lymph nodes and other common extrathoracic sites.[34] Most patients are female and present with systemic (type B) complaints such as weight loss, fever, malaise, and night sweats. The chest radiographs demonstrate either unilateral (more common) or bilateral abnormalities. The most frequent histologic subtype is the nodular sclerosing variety. The diagnosis is usually established following either resection or open biopsy. Combination chemotherapy and radiotherapy appear to be associated with the best survival.

Plasmacytoma

Primary plasmacytomas of the lung may present as parenchymal, endobronchial, or endotracheal tumors.[21] An extrathoracic primary site must be assiduously sought. Patients whose neoplasms are identified following resection require no further treatment, but those tumors identified prior to surgery may be treated with radiotherapy. Patients require careful monitoring as they may develop multiple myeloma.

Malignant Melanoma

Several theories have been postulated to explain pulmonary melanomas, including benign melanocytes that migrate with the pulmonary anlage during fetal life, melanocytic metaplasia of bronchial epithelial cells, and origin from neuroendocrine cells that can show melanocytic differentiation.[20] Potential sites of extrathoracic primary melanoma must be carefully evaluated prior to entertaining the diagnosis of primary pulmonary melanoma. The tumors generally occur within the lung parenchyma, although they may be found in the trachea. Men and women are affected equally. Resection of the tumor is the treatment of choice. Distant metastases are the most common cause of death.

Malignant Germ Cell Tumors

Malignant teratoma and choriocarcinoma constitute the histologically documented malignant germ cell tumors that arise in the lung.[8,33] Teratomas may harbor tissue remnants of all three germ cell layers. Patients present most commonly with cough, hemoptysis, and chest pain. The most specific symptom, trichoptysis, is rarely present. Radiologically, the mass may show calcification with peripheral radiolucency. Approximately 35 percent of teratomas are malignant, as demonstrated by the histologic presence of a carcinoma or sarcoma. Pulmonary resection is the preferred treatment.

Primary choriocarcinoma of the lung is extraordinarily rare and must be distinguished from a non–small cell lung cancer that can also produce human chorionic gonadotropin (HCG). The tumor is composed of syncytiotrophoblasts and cytotrophoblasts and is frequently necrotic and hemorrhagic. Resection and adjuvant therapy have been recommended.

Salivary Gland-Type Tumors

Adenoid cystic carcinoma is the most common salivary gland neoplasm found in the lung.[32] These tumors most frequently occur in the trachea or mainstem bronchi and cause symptoms of obstruction. Men and women are affected equally. The diagnosis is usually established with a bronchoscopic biopsy. Three histologic subtypes have been described: cribriform, tubular, and solid. Complete resection is the most effective treatment, although radiotherapy may be utilized for inoperable cancers and may benefit patients who have had incomplete resections. Metastases to intraparenchymal and mediastinal lymph nodes do not preclude long-term survival, which approximates 55 percent.[9,14]

Mucoepidermoid carcinomas occur most frequently in the mainstem bronchi but can arise peripherally.[41] Patients commonly present with symptoms of obstruction. Bronchoscopic biopsy may be accomplished without fear of hemorrhage and is usually diagnostic. The majority of tumors are low grade, as demonstrated by few mitoses and little nuclear pleomorphism and necrosis. Complete resection is the treatment of choice, although a lung-sparing procedure (sleeve resection) is preferred in this usually indolent, centrally occurring cancer. A nodal dissection should be performed to identify the occasional patients with regional metastatic disease. Radiation therapy is not believed to alter the course of the disease,[19] although one investigator[25] reported sufficient regression of an endobronchial tumor to allow resection. The use and efficacy of combination chemotherapy is not well defined. Patients with low-grade tumors that are completely resected may be considered to be cured. High-grade tumors are much more aggressive, with 100 percent mortality rates between 11 and 28 months.[19,25]

Acinic cell tumors (Fechner tumors) are usually found in the salivary glands, and hence a diligent search for an extrathoracic primary is mandatory.[32] Symptoms vary and are determined by whether the neoplasm is located in an endobronchial or peripheral position. Microscopy frequently demonstrates a pattern resembling a neuroendocrine tumor, and special stains may be necessary to differentiate from the more common carcinoid tumor. These tumors grow slowly, and recurrence or metastases after complete excision have not been reported.

Sarcomas

Primary pulmonary sarcomas arise from the mesenchymal cells found in the bronchial or vascular walls and interstices of the lung parenchyma.[36] Chondrosarcomas of the lung are usually slow-growing tumors that metastasize infrequently. They may occur either in the main bronchi or lung parenchyma and cause symptoms of obstruction. Complete resection is associated with cure in the majority of patients. Patients with primary osteosarcomas of the lung generally present with cough or hemoptysis. Tumors are solitary and frequently have a diameter greater than 4 cm. Pulmonary resection is the treatment of choice, although the prognosis is very poor. The majority of patients succumb from metastases to the mediastinal lymph nodes, lung, liver, and heart.

The variety of primary soft tissue pulmonary sarcomas reflects the range of mesenchymal tissue found in the lung (Table 115-3). Most of these lesions cause symptoms of cough, he-

TABLE 115-3

Primary Soft Tissue Sarcomas of the Lung

Leiomyosarcoma

Spindle cell sarcoma

Rhabdomyosarcoma

Malignant fibrous histiocytoma

Angiosarcoma

Fibrosarcoma

Malignant hemangiopericytoma

Neurogenic sarcoma

Synovial sarcoma

Kaposi's sarcoma

Liposarcoma

moptysis, dyspnea, and chest pain, although up to 25 percent may be asymptomatic and are detected on a routine chest radiograph.[5] The largest single report contains 43 patients of whom 29 underwent resection, 6 received radiation therapy, 2 received radiation and chemotherapy, and 6 received no therapy.[30] The overall 1-, 3- and 5-year survival rates were 55 percent, 31 percent, and 25 percent respectively with a median of 13 months. Tumor diameter less than 5 cm correlated with longer survival. Patients who underwent resection of their tumors lived significantly longer than those who received radiation therapy and/or chemotherapy or no therapy.

REFERENCES

1. Arrigoni MG, Woolner LB, Bernatz PE: Atypical carcinoid tumors of the lung. *J Thorac Cardiovasc Surg* 64:413–421, 1972.

2. Bahadori M, Liebow AA: Plasma cell granuloma of the lung. *Cancer* 31:191–208, 1973.

3. Basheda S, Gephardt GN, Stoller JK: Columnar papilloma of the bronchus: Case report and literature review. *Am Rev Respir Dis* 144:1400–1402, 1991.

4. Berardi RS, Lee SS, Chen HP, Stines GJ: Inflammatory pseudotumors of the lung. *Surg Gynecol Obstet* 156:89–96, 1983.

5. Burt M, Zakowski M: Rare primary malignant neoplasms, in Pearson FG, Deslauriers J, Ginsberg RJ, et al (eds), *Thoracic Surgery,* sect. 3, *Lung.* New York, Churchill Livingstone, 1995, pp 807–826.

6. Cabarcos A, Gomez Dorronsoro M, Lobo Beristain JL: Pulmonary carcinosarcoma: A case study and review of the literature. *Br J Dis Chest* 79:83–94, 1985.

7. Carney JA: The triad of gastric epitheliod leiomyosarcoma, pulmonary chondroma, and functioning extra-adrenal paraganglioma: A five year review. *Medicine* (Baltimore) 62:159–169, 1983.

8. Colby TV, Koss MN, Travis WD: Tumors of the lower respiratory tract, in *Atlas of Tumor Pathology*, 3d series. Washington, DC, Armed Forces Institute of Pathology, 1995.

9. Conlan AA, Payne WS, Woolner LB, Sanderson DR: Adenoid cystic carcinoma (cylindroma) and mucoepidermoid carcinoma of the bronchus. *J Thorac Cardiovasc Surg* 76:369–377, 1978.

10. D'Agati VD, Perzin KH: Carcinoid tumourlets of the lung with metastases to a peribronchial lymph node: Report of a case and review of the literature. *Cancer* 55:2472–2476, 1985.

11. Dail DH, Liebow AA, Gmelich JT, et al: Intravascular, bronchiolar, and alveolar tumor of the lung (IVBAT): An analysis of twenty cases of a peculiar sclerosing endothelial tumor. *Cancer* 51:452–464, 1983.

12. Dalton W, Zolliker A, McCaughey W, et al: Localized primary tumors of the pleura. *Cancer* 44:1465–1475, 1979.

13. Deschamps CR, Jex R, Fetsch J, et al: Bronchial carcinoid: Effect of staging on late survival. *Chest* 102:103s, 1992.

14. Diaz-Jimenez JP, Canela-Cardona M, Maestre-Alcacer J: Nd:YAG laser photoresection of low grade tumors of the tracheobronchial tree. *Chest* 97:920–922, 1990.

15. DiMarco AF, Montenegro H, Payne CB Jr, Kwon KH: Papillomas of the tracheobronchial tree with malignant degeneration. *Chest* 74:464–465, 1978.

16. Galliani CA, Beatty JF, Grosfeld JL: Cavernous hemangioma of the lung in an infant. *Pediatr Pathol* 12:105–111, 1992.

17. Hamper UM, Khouri NF, Stitik FP, Siegelman SS: Pulmonary hamartoma: Diagnosis by transthoracic needle-aspiration biopsy. *Radiology* 155:15–18, 1985.

18. Harpole DH Jr, Feldman JM, Buchanan S, et al: Bronchial carcinoid tumours: A retrospective analysis of 126 patients. *Ann Thorac Surg* 54:50–55, 1992.

19. Heitmiller RF, Mathisen DJ, Ferry JA, et al: Mucoepidermoid lung tumors. *Ann Thorac Surg* 47:394–399, 1989.

20. Jennings TA, Axiotis CA, Kress Y, Carter D: Primary malignant melanoma of the lower respiratory tract. Report of a case and literature review. *Am J Clin Pathol* 94:649–655, 1990.

21. Joseph G, Pandit M, Korfhage L: Primary pulmonary plasmocytoma. *Cancer* 71:721–724, 1993.

22. Koss M, Hochholzer L, O'Leary T: Pulmonary blastomas. *Cancer* 67:2368–2381, 1991.

23. Koss M: Pulmonary lymphoproliferative disorders, in Churg A, Katzenstein AL (eds), *The Lung.* Philadelphia, Williams & Wilkins, 1993.

24. Lack EE, Harris GBC, Eraklis AJ, Vawter GF: Primary bronchial tumors in childhood. A clinicopathologic study of six cases. *Cancer* 52:492–497, 1983.

25. Leonardi HK, Jung-Legg Y, Legg MA, Neptune WB: Tracheobronchial mucoepidermoid carcinoma: Clinicopathological features and results of treatment. *J Thorac Cardiovasc Surg* 76:431–438, 1978.

26. Magid D, Siegelman SS, Eggleston JC, et al: Pulmonary carcinoid tumors: CT assessment. *J Comput Assist Tomogr* 13:244–247, 1989.

27. Martensson H, Bottchwe G, Hambraeus G, et al: Bronchial carcinoids: An analysis of 91 cases. *World J Surg* 11:356–364, 1984.

28. Martini N, Beattie EJ: Less common tumors of the lung, in Shields TW (ed), *General Thoracic Surgery,* 2d ed. Philadelphia, Lea and Febiger, 1983, pp 770–779.

29. McCaughan BC, Martini N, Bains MS: Bronchial carcinoids: Review of 124 cases. *J Thorac Cardiovasc Surg* 89:8–17, 1985.

30. McCormack PM, Martini N: Primary sarcomas and lymphomas of the lung, in Martini N, Vogt-Moykopf I (eds), *Thoracic Surgery: Frontiers and Uncommon Neoplasms,* part 3, *Uncommon Pulmonary Neoplasms,* vol 5. St. Louis, Mosby, 1989, pp 269–274.

31. Miller DL, Allen MS: Rare pulmonary neoplasms. *Mayo Clin Proc* 68:492–498, 1993.

32. Moran CA: Primary salivary gland-type tumors of the lung. *Sem Diag Pathol* 12:106–122, 1995.

33. Morgan DE, Sanders C, McElvein RB, et al: Intrapulmonary teratoma: A case report and review of the literature. *J Thorac Imaging* 7:70–77, 1992.

34. Radin AI: Primary pulmonary Hodgkin's disease. *Cancer* 65:550–563, 1990.

35. Rea F, Binda R, Spreafico G, et al: Bronchial carcinoids: A review of 60 patients. *Ann Thorac Surg* 47:412–414, 1989.

36. Suster S: Primary sarcomas of the lung. *Semin Diag Path* 12:140–157, 1995.

37. Szyfelbein WK, Ross JS: Carcinoids, atypical carcinoids and small cell carcinomas of the lung: Differential diagnosis of fine needle aspiration biopsy specimens. *Diagn Cytopathol* 4:1–8, 1988.

38. Valenstein SL, Thurer RJ: Granular cell myoblastoma of the bronchus. *J Thorac Cardiovasc Surg* 76:465–468, 1978.

39. Vera-Roman JM, Sobonya RE, Gomez-Garcia JL, et al: Leiomyoma of the lung: Literature review and case report. *Cancer* 52:936–941, 1983.

40. Whitwell F: Tumourlets of the lung. *J Pathol Bacteriol* 70:529–541, 1955.

41. Yousem SA, Hochholzer I: Mucoepidermoid tumors of the lung. *Cancer* 60:1346–1352, 1987.

CHAPTER 116

EXTRAPULMONARY SYNDROMES ASSOCIATED WITH LUNG TUMORS

Bruce E. Johnson / John P. Chute

Lung cancers are the most common tumors associated with paraneoplastic syndromes. The paraneoplastic syndromes can be classified into endocrine, hematologic, and neurologic syndromes. Endocrine and hematologic syndromes associated with lung tumors are listed in Table 116-1.

The endocrine syndromes are characterized by the ectopic production of biologically active peptide hormones by tumor cells that bind to receptors in adjacent or distant organs, giving rise to a clinical syndrome.[7] The ectopic adrenocorticotropic hormone (ACTH) syndrome, the hyponatremia of malignancy, and hypercalcemia of malignancy are examples of this model. In order to establish the diagnosis of an endocrine paraneoplastic syndrome, the following criteria should be met: (1) a decrease in the level of the hormone after treatment of the tumor, (2) demonstration of hormone synthesis and secretion by tumor cells in vitro, (3) high concentrations of the hormone in the tumor, and (4) an arteriovenous gradient in hormone levels across the tumor bed.

Lung cancers also produce extrapulmonary syndromes by other mechanisms. Hematologic syndromes develop in patients with lung cancer through the production of cytokines by tumor cells that activate progenitor cells in the bone marrow. Neurologic syndromes, such as encephalomyelitis and subacute sensory neuropathy, are caused by the induction of antibodies directed against proteins expressed by the lung cancer cells and against antigens present on cells in the nervous system.

Although lung cancers produce and express various hormones, many (e.g., the gastrin-releasing peptide) do not cause a clinically evident syndrome. Other peptide hormones, such as ACTH precursors, are translated into prohormones, which are not processed into mature peptides. As a result, levels of the immunoreactive proteins in plasma are increased without a clinical syndrome.

This chapter focuses on the extrapulmonary syndromes that are encountered in clinical practice. An understanding of the extrapulmonary syndromes is important for several reasons: (1) the syndrome is often the presenting feature of the underlying cancer; (2) the course of the endocrine and hematologic syndromes

NOTE: The opinions and assertions contained herein are the private views of the authors and are not to be construed as official or as reflecting the views of the Department of the Navy or the Department of Defense.

usually parallels the course of the lung cancer, although the neurologic syndromes frequently do not; and (3) appropriate treatment of the extrapulmonary syndrome often reduces the patient's morbidity and may allow definitive treatment of the cancer. In general, definitive treatment of the underlying tumor by surgical resection, radiotherapy, or chemotherapy is the most effective form of therapy for the paraneoplastic syndrome.

HYPERCALCEMIA OF MALIGNANCY

Hypercalcemia is the most common paraneoplastic syndrome.[5] Approximately 1 percent of patients with lung cancer have hypercalcemia when first seen, but 10 to 20 percent of patients develop hypercalcemia during the course of their disease. Lung cancer is the most common solid tumor associated with hypercalcemia, accounting for 30 to 40 percent of all paraneoplastic cases.[31] Hypercalcemia is commonly seen in patients with squamous cell carcinoma of the lung, uncommonly in patients with adenocarcinoma, and very rarely in patients with small-cell lung cancer.

Hypercalcemia in patients with lung cancer is usually not caused by local osteolytic effects of bony metastases. Most cases of hypercalcemia in patients with lung cancer are caused by the ectopic production of parathyroid hormone–related peptide (PTHrP) by tumor cells (humoral hypercalcemia of malignancy).[8]

Biology

Ectopic production of PTHrP accounts for 80 to 90 percent of humoral hypercalcemia of malignancy in patients with lung cancer.[25] The PTHrP gene expresses three messenger RNAs (mRNAs); these encode for three distinct peptides, which differ at the COOH-terminal region (Fig. 116-1). Eight of the first 13 amino acids in PTHrP are homologous with PTH, so similar functional activity is shared between the two peptides.[8] PTHrP messenger RNA and peptides have been demonstrated in cancer cells from

TABLE 116-1

Endocrine and Hematologic Syndromes Associated with Lung Tumors

Syndrome	Tumor	Proteins/Cytokines
Hypercalcemia of malignancy	Non–small cell	Parathyroid hormone–related peptide Parathormone
Hyponatremia of malignancy	Small cell Non–small cell	Arginine vasopressin Atrial natriuretic peptide
Ectopic ACTH syndrome	Small cell Carcinoid tumors	Adrenocorticotropic hormone Corticotropin-releasing hormone
Acromegaly	Carcinoid tumors Small cell	Growth hormone–releasing hormone Growth Hormone
Granulocytosis	Non–small cell	G-CSF GM-CSF IL-6
Thrombocytosis	Non–small cell Small cell	IL-6
Thromboembolism	Non–small cell Small cell	Unknown

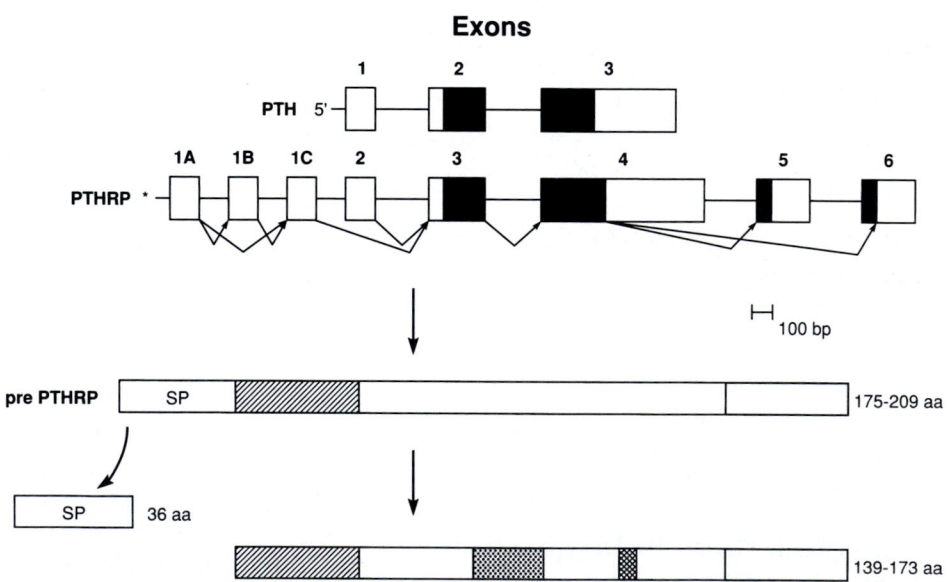

FIGURE 116-1   Parathyroid hormone and parathyroid hormone–related peptide. The human PTH gene has three exons, which constitute the protein-coding segments. The protein coding segments are represented by the black boxes. The PTHrP gene is more complex, with eight exons. Through alternative splicing, three different isoforms of mRNA can be produced. These isoform mRNAs encode the pre-PTHrP proteins, which vary in size from 175 to 209 amino acids (aa). Thirty-six amino acids are removed from the amino terminal end as the signal peptide. Three different PTHrP molecules are produced, with 139 to 173 amino acids. The rectangular region at the carboxy terminal represents the different lengths of PTHrP. The N-terminal region (aa 1–34) mimics the classic PTH-like function (hatched box). The midregion (aa 67–86) of the peptide stimulates placental calcium transport (shaded box). The C-terminal region (aa 107–111) inhibits osteoclastic bone resorption (double hatched box).

patients with lung cancer and hypercalcemia.[24] PTHrP has been shown to bind to PTH receptors in the bone and kidney, causing increased osteoclastic bone resorption, decreased bone formation, and decreased calciuria, leading to hypercalcemia. Levels of 1,25-dihydroxyvitamin D_3 are suppressed in patients with PTHrP-induced hypercalcemia but are raised in patients with primary hyperparathyroidism. This difference occurs because renal α-hydroxylase activity is low in PTHrP-induced hypercalcemia, unlike primary hyperparathyroidism. PTH production by lung cancer cells has also been described, but it is a very rare cause of humoral hypercalcemia.

Other factors that cause bone resorption have been identified in the plasma of patients with lung cancer, including transforming growth factor–α and a vitamin D metabolite. These are very rare, however, and their causative role in hypercalcemia has not been conclusively shown.

Diagnosis

The early symptoms of hypercalcemia include thirst, malaise, fatigue, anorexia, polyuria, constipation, nausea, and vomiting. As the hypercalcemia becomes increasingly severe, confusion, lethargy, coma, and death can occur.[23] The demonstration of an increased concentration (greater than 10.5 mg/dl) of calcium in the serum of a patient with non–small-cell lung cancer should suggest this paraneoplastic syndrome.

When hypercalcemia is identified in a patient with lung cancer, other potential causes of elevated serum calcium should be excluded. Thiazide diuretics, vitamin D or lithium administration, hyperthyroidism, and sarcoidosis are potential causes. A PTH radioimmunoassay should be performed because up to 10 percent of hypercalcemia in patients with cancer is caused by primary hyperparathyroidism. Bone scintiscan should be obtained to exclude bone metastases, and a PTHrP level should be determined. An elevated PTHrP level in the absence of bone metastases establishes the diagnosis of humoral hypercalcemia of malignancy caused by ectopic PTHrP.[5]

Treatment

As with other paraneoplastic syndromes, treatment of the underlying cancer is the most effective method of treating the humoral hypercalcemia associated with lung cancer. Patients in whom lung cancer cannot be eradicated can be treated with intravenous saline plus furosemide diuresis. Subcutaneous calcitonin has a rapid onset of action and is most useful in severe cases. Mithramycin and long-acting biphosphonates, such as pamidronate, are effective for long-term control of hypercalcemia. Corticosteroids exert their effect through inhibition of dihydroxyvitamin D_3 synthesis and therefore have less effect in patients with elevated PTHrP.

This syndrome usually develops in patients with advanced progressive cancer. Therefore, reversal of hypercalcemia should be undertaken only when there is some hope for control of the underlying cancer. It may be inappropriate to treat hypercalcemia in patients with far-advanced lung cancer, having them regain consciousness only to die of their underlying disease.

HYPONATREMIA OF MALIGNANCY

Hyponatremia is a frequent complication in patients with cancer. More than 90 percent of cases occur in patients with small-cell lung cancer. Ten to 15 percent of patients with small-cell lung cancer and 1 percent of patients with non–small-cell lung cancer present with hyponatremia. Most of these cases are caused by the ectopic production of arginine vasopressin (AVP).[7] This subset of hyponatremia is recognized as the *syndrome of inappropriate antidiuretic hormone* (SIADH). Ectopic production of atrial natriuretic peptide (ANP) may also play a role in the hyponatremia of malignancy, but the exact contribution of this hormone remains to be defined.[28]

Biology

AVP is a 9–amino acid peptide normally produced by the neurohypophysis. The peptide binds to receptors in the kidney to reduce the excretion of free water. When plasma osmolality exceeds 280 mosmol/kg, the release of arginine vasopressin from the pituitary increases, causing the kidney to retain more free water and maintain fluid and osmolar balance. In patients with small-cell lung cancer, ectopic production of AVP causes hyponatremia by inhibiting free-water excretion in the distal tubule of the kidney. Arginine vasopressin mRNA is expressed in small-cell lung cancer cells, and the peptide is translated and secreted (Fig. 116-2). Levels of AVP in plasma are increased.

A subgroup of patients with small-cell lung cancer and hyponatremia have been identified in whom the cancer and the cancer cell lines do not produce ectopic arginine vasopressin. The tumors from these patients express ANP mRNA, secrete the peptide, and have high levels of ANP in their plasma.[14] ANP is the leading candidate to be the natriuretic factor that Bartter and Schwartz proposed in their original description of SIADH.[3] Further investigation into the precise role of ANP in patients with small-cell lung cancer and hyponatremia of malignancy is ongoing.

Diagnosis

In patients with lung cancer, hyponatremia is most frequently diagnosed as a laboratory abnormality in the absence of significant symptoms. The symptoms associated with acute hyponatremia do not typically occur because the syndrome develops over a prolonged period in concert with the growth of the lung cancer. The symptoms of mild hyponatremia (more than 120 meq/ml) include headache, difficulty concentrating, nausea, weakness, and fatigue. Patients who develop a more acute hyponatremia may manifest confusion, lethargy, seizures, coma, and death.

In patients with lung cancer, nonmalignant causes of hyponatremia—including diuretic use, renal disease, cardiac dysfunction, hypoadrenalism, thyroid disease, and dilutional hyponatremia—should be considered in the initial evaluation. Medications that can induce SIADH include the chemotherapeutic agents cisplatin, vincristine, cyclophosphamide, and melphalan, along with narcotics, which are commonly used in

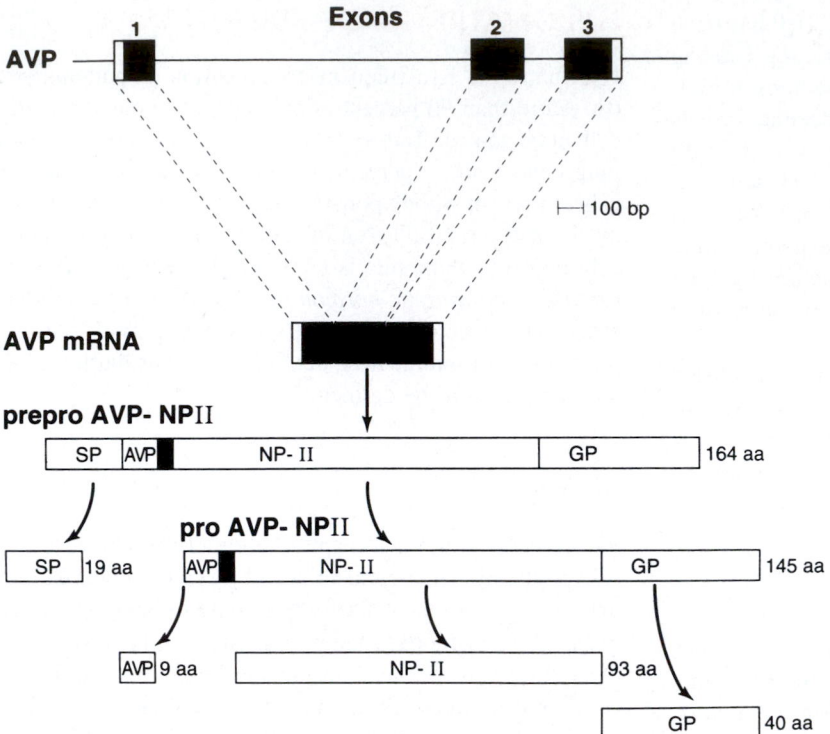

FIGURE 116-2 Arginine vasopressin. The three exons of the human AVP gene rise to a 700-base arginine vasopressin mRNA. The mRNA is translated into a 164-amino acid (aa) preprohormone with a 19–amino acid amino terminal signal peptide (SP). The signal peptide is cleaved, giving rise to a 145–amino acid prohormone. This prohormone is processed into the AVP nonapeptide (AVP), a 93–amino acid neurophysin (NP), and a 40–amino acid glycoprotein (GP). The black portions of the boxes represent the protein-coding portion of the gene and mRNA.

patients with lung cancer. The subgroup of hyponatremic patients with the diagnosis of SIADH should satisfy the following criteria: (1) plasma hypo-osmolality (under 280 mosmol/kg); (2) osmolality of urine greater than serum (usually over 500 mosmol/kg); (3) persistent urinary excretion of sodium in the absence of diuretics (more than 20 meq/l); (4) absent signs of volume depletion; and (5) normal renal, adrenal, and thyroid function.

Treatment

The initial therapy for hyponatremia caused by lung cancer is treatment of the underlying malignancy. This requires chemotherapy and/or radiotherapy for patients with small-cell lung cancer and surgery for non–small-cell lung cancers. In many patients, despite an initial tumor response to chemotherapy, the syndrome of hyponatremia persists or recurs after the cancer regrows. In these patients, the short-term treatment for mild hyponatremia is fluid restriction of 500 ml per day. Many patients with cancer cannot tolerate this level of fluid restriction for extended periods, so other treatments are usually required. Demeclocycline is the medication of choice for chronic management of SIADH in patients with small-cell lung cancer. When given in doses of 600 to 1200 mg orally per day, demeclocycline blocks the action of AVP on the renal tubule, inducing a diabetes insipidus that will correct the hyponatremia in most patients. Lithium and phenytoin also can be used to inhibit the effects of

AVP on the renal tubule, but administration of these agents is limited by their neurologic side effects.

In patients who present with severe, symptomatic hyponatremia, the intravenous administration of 3 percent hypertonic saline, along with the intravenous administration of furosemide, is recommended. The intravenous administration of furosemide rapidly causes an increase in the net free-water clearance. This method has been used successfully in patients with small-cell lung cancer. It can increase the concentration of sodium in serum from 120 to 133 meq/l in 6 to 8 h. Overly rapid correction of the level of sodium in serum (more than 2 meq/h) in patients with hyponatremia has been associated with a central pontine myelinolysis. Therefore, frequent measurements of serum sodium during treatment with hypertonic saline are required to avoid this complication.

ECTOPIC ACTH SYNDROME

Cushing's syndrome was first recognized in a patient with lung cancer caused by the ectopic production of ACTH. Twenty to 30 percent of Cushing's syndrome is caused by biologically active ACTH, which is produced by nonpituitary neoplasms.[7] Lung cancers are the most common neoplasms that cause ectopic ACTH production and Cushing's syndrome, accounting for 50 percent of all cases. Small-cell carcinoma accounts for 80 to 90 percent of cases associated with lung cancers, but carcinoid tumors (10 percent) and bronchial adenocarcinomas (5 percent) have also been reported to produce biologically active ACTH.[19] Although one-half of all cases of ectopic ACTH production are caused by small-cell carcinoma, fewer than 3 percent of patients with small-cell lung cancer have Cushing's syndrome at the time of diagnosis.[4]

Biology

Most cases of ectopic ACTH syndrome associated with lung cancers are caused by ectopic production of ACTH by the tumor.[11] The precursor gene, pro-opiomelanocortin (POMC), is expressed in the cancer cells, and a 241–amino acid prohormone is translated and then cleaved into ACTH (39 amino acids), melanocyte-stimulating hormone, and opiatelike hormones (Fig. 116-3).[6] The ACTH binds to receptors in the adrenal gland, causing them to produce excessive glucocorticoid and mineralocorticoid hormones.

A small number of patients with small-cell lung cancer or bronchial carcinoids have been reported to produce corticotropin-releasing hormone (CRH), thereby causing a Cushing's syndrome.[4] CRH is a 41–amino acid normally produced in the paraventricular nuclei of the hypothalamus, which stimulates the release of ACTH from the pituitary. In patients with small-cell carcinoma or bronchial carcinoid, CRH is produced by the cancer cells, thereby stimulating ACTH production by the pituitary gland and causing Cushing's syndrome.

Diagnosis

Ectopic ACTH production occurs with equal frequency in males and females—unlike Cushing's disease, which has an 8:1 female preponderance. Patients who have slow-growing tumors (carcinoids) often present with the clinical features of Cushing's syndrome: truncal obesity, moon facies, striae, polyuria, and polydipsia. In contrast, patients with small-cell lung cancer often present with other signs of mineralocorticoid and glucocorticoid excess due to the rapidity of tumor growth: edema, weakness, hypertension, and hypokalemic alkalosis.

The diagnosis of ectopic ACTH syndrome is established by the demonstration of increased 24-h excretion of urinary free cortisol (more than 400 nmol a day), increased plasma cortisol level (more than 600 nmol/l), and increased plasma ACTH level (over 22 pmol/l), which do not decrease in response to the administration of high-dose dexamethasone. Bronchial carcinoids are an exception because, in some tumors, ACTH and cortisol levels have been suppressed by dexamethasone. In patients in whom the dexamethasone suppression test does not establish the diagnosis of ectopic ACTH production, a CRH stimulation test or bilateral inferior petrosal vein sampling will provide the definitive diagnosis. After CRH infusion, pituitary tumors release increased amounts of ACTH, whereas pituitary-independent lung tumors should not. Similarly, in pituitary-dependent Cushing's syndrome, petrosal vein sampling will reveal a gradient between the level of ACTH in the petrosal vein and the peripheral concentration. In contrast, patients in whom ACTH is ectopically produced demonstrate no gradient between the petrosal vein and the peripheral blood.

Treatment

Management of a patient with lung cancer and ectopic ACTH syndrome requires therapy directed at both the underlying tumor and the hypercortisolism. The treatment for a patient with ectopic ACTH production is to remove the source of the ACTH. This requires combination chemotherapy, with or without irradiation, for patients with small-cell lung cancer and surgical resection and/or radiation for patients with carcinoid tumors. Chemotherapy for patients with small-cell lung cancer and ectopic ACTH syndrome has been only minimally successful. Pa-

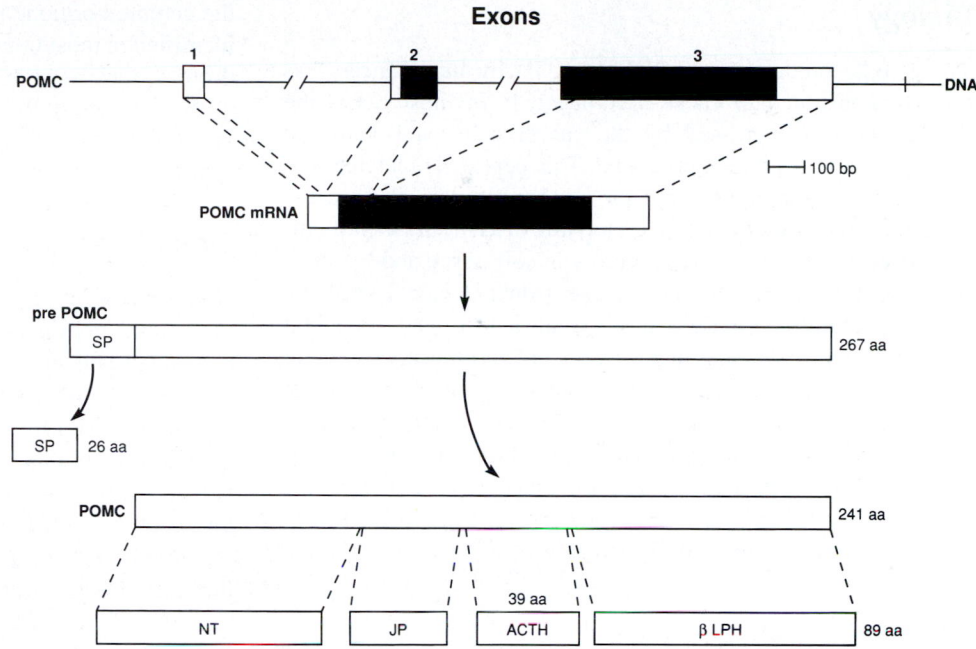

FIGURE 116-3 Pro-opiomelanocortin. The three exons of the POMC gene give rise to a 1072-base POMC mRNA. The mRNA is translated into a 267-amino acid pre-POMC with a 26–amino acid amino terminal signal peptide (SP). The signal peptide is cleaved, creating the 241–amino acid POMC. The POMC peptide is cleaved into many products, including the N-terminal peptide (NT), the joining peptide (JP), a 39–amino acid mature ACTH, and β-lipotropin (BLPH). The molecules can also undergo further processing. The black portions of the exons represent the protein-coding portion of the gene and mRNA.

tients often have a poor response to chemotherapy and are susceptible to early infection and death. Early control of a patient's glucocorticoid excess is beneficial and may reduce the morbidity of treatment.

When removal of the ectopic source of ACTH is not possible, medical therapy directed at decreasing adrenal secretion may be successful. Ketoconazole is an imidazole derivative that inhibits steroidogenesis at both adrenal and gonadal sites. A recent review of medical therapy for ectopic ACTH syndrome suggests that ketoconazole may be the most effective and least toxic agent available.[32] Metapyrone and aminoglutethimide also have shown limited success by inhibiting adrenal steroid synthesis. Octreotide, a somatostatin analogue, can suppress ectopic ACTH production and has been reported to be useful in some of these patients.

In some patients, the clinical signs and symptoms of ectopic ACTH production develop before the development of a clinically obvious lung cancer. In these cases, symptomatic management of hypercortisolism is undertaken and periodic imaging studies are performed because these patients may have a slow-growing carcinoid tumor that will be amenable to surgical resection.

ACROMEGALY

Carcinoid tumors of the lung and intestine are responsible for 70 percent of cases of ectopic acromegaly. Ectopic production of growth hormone–releasing hormone (GHRH) by tumor cells can be demonstrated in most patients, whereas a minority of tumors produce growth hormone.

Biology

The ectopic production of GHRH or GH by lung cancers has been demonstrated to cause acromegaly.[12] In most cases, the GHRH gene is expressed by the cancer cells, and a 40– or 44–amino acid peptide is produced. This peptide is secreted into the circulation and binds to receptors in the pituitary gland, causing the production of excessive amounts of GH. GH then mediates its effects through GH receptors in soft tissue and by stimulating the production of insulinlike growth factor–1 (IGF-1).

Immunoreactive GHRH can be identified in many bronchial carcinoids and small-cell lung cancers, but acromegaly occurs in a minority of these patients. Ectopic GHRH production may not cause clinically evident acromegaly because (1) the tumor produces inadequate amounts of GHRH to cause the clinical syndrome, (2) the hormone is synthesized but not secreted, or (3) the rapid progress of the malignancy prevents the full development of clinical features of acromegaly.

Diagnosis

The earliest features of GH excess are hypertrophy of the extremities and face (forcing increased glove, shoe, and ring size), thickened leathery skin, prominent skin folds, increased skin pigmentation, and hair growth. Bony changes, hypertension, and diabetes mellitus are later, less common findings.

The presentation of a patient with a lung mass and signs of acromegaly should raise suspicion of the paraneoplastic syndrome of acromegaly. This is particularly true if the lung tumor is a carcinoid. The diagnosis is established by the presence of increased levels of GHRH and IGF-1 in the patient's plasma, the absence of a pituitary tumor, and the demonstration of GHRH or GH in tumor tissue by immunohistochemistry or mRNA expression studies. Because coincidental pituitary tumors and solid tumors have been described, patients who have lung cancer in association with low GHRH levels and high GH and IGF-1 levels should undergo magnetic resonance imaging (MRI) to exclude a pituitary tumor.

Treatment

The treatment of choice for ectopic acromegaly is removal of the GHRH- or GH-secreting tumor. This can often be achieved in patients with lung carcinoid tumors. Radiation therapy has also been effective. Patients with ectopic acromegaly whose tumors cannot be removed or irradiated should undergo medical therapy using the somatostatin analogue octreotide or bromocriptine. Bromocriptine acts by inhibiting GH release by the pituitary; octreotide lowers both GH and IGF-1 levels in plasma and also appears to inhibit GHRH release by tumors. Clinical abatement of acromegalic features has been reported in patients treated with octreotide.

HEMATOLOGIC SYNDROMES

Most hematologic syndromes associated with lung tumors are not as well characterized as the endocrine syndromes, because the ectopic hormone responsible for the syndrome has not been identified in most tumor tissues. In many of the hematologic syndromes, such as granulocytosis and thrombocytosis, clinical sequelae are often absent. As with the endocrine paraneoplastic syndromes, the most appropriate therapy for the hematologic syndromes is the treatment of the underlying neoplasm.

Granulocytosis

Non–small-cell lung cancer is the most common cancer associated with granulocytosis. Twenty percent of patients with non–small-cell lung cancer have granulocytosis, with absolute white blood counts ranging from 10,100 to 25,000 (normal range is 4000 to 10,000).[2]

Although granulocyte colony–stimulating activity can be demonstrated in serum and/or urine in 80 percent of the patients, the specific peptide hormone causing the syndrome has not been identified. Tumor production of granulocyte colony–stimulating factor (G-CSF), granulocyte-monocyte colony–stimulating factor (GM-CSF), and interleukin-6 (IL-6) has been shown in a minority of patients.

Virtually all patients with lung cancer who present with tumor-associated granulocytosis are asymptomatic. The diagnosis is suggested by the presence of an increased white blood count in which neutrophils predominate without immature forms, in the absence of nonneoplastic causes. An increased leukocyte alkaline phosphatase score and a normal bone marrow are consistent with this diagnosis.

Thrombocytosis

Thrombocytosis is common in patients with lung cancer, afflicting 40 percent of patients with both non–small-cell and small-cell tumors.[9]

The pathogenesis of thrombocytosis in patients with lung cancer has not been definitively elucidated. IL-6, which is a cytokine for megakaryocytes, has been demonstrated in cell lines from patients with lung cancer and thrombocytosis, and increased levels of IL-6 have been demonstrated in the plasma of such patients. The recent identification of the thrombopoietin gene should lead to a better understanding of the role of this protein in paraneoplastic thrombocytosis.

Patients with thrombocytosis are nearly always asymptomatic and do not have an increased incidence of thromboembolism. The diagnosis of cancer-associated thrombocytosis is suggested by an increased platelet count (above 500,000 per cubic millimeter) in a patient with newly diagnosed lung cancer. A primary myeloproliferative disorder can be excluded only by a bone marrow biopsy.

Thromboembolism

Twenty percent of patients with lung cancer develop venous thromboembolism during the course of their disease.[18] Twenty percent of patients who present with recurrent idiopathic venous thrombosis are found to have an underlying diagnosis of cancer.[22] The spectrum of causes of thrombosis in patients with lung cancer is broad, including disseminated intravascular coagulation (DIC), Trousseau's syndrome (recurrent migratory venous thrombophlebitis), nonbacterial thrombotic endocarditis, and obstruction of great vessels. Surgical procedures and chemotherapy have also been demonstrated to increase cancer patients' risk of thrombotic complications.[26]

The treatment for venous thrombosis in patients with lung cancer depends on the underlying hematologic diagnosis. If the patient has an isolated venous thrombosis in the absence of DIC or Trousseau's syndrome, oral warfarin therapy is appropriate with the aim of an international normalized ratio two to three times normal. If there are recurrent thromboses, long-term subcutaneous heparin is more efficacious than warfarin.

NEUROLOGIC SYNDROMES

Neurologic dysfunction as a paraneoplastic manifestation of lung cancer was first described more than 30 years ago. Encephalomyelitis, cerebellar degeneration, retinopathy, opsoclonus/myoclonus, and the Lambert-Eaton syndrome have all been associated with lung tumors, most commonly small-cell lung cancer. Most of these neurologic paraneoplastic syndromes appear to be caused by an autoimmune response directed at antigens that are shared by the cancer cells and normal neural tissue. Unlike that of the endocrine and hematologic syndromes associated with lung cancer, the clinical course of the neurologic syndromes are typically independent of the course of the underlying disease. The autoantibodies associated with each neurologic syndrome are listed in Table 116-2.

Encephalomyelitis/Subacute Sensory Neuropathy

The paraneoplastic syndrome of encephalomyelitis/subacute sensory neuropathy was initially discovered in a patient with small-cell lung cancer. Currently, more than 70 percent of cases of paraneoplastic encephalomyelitis are diagnosed in patients with small-cell lung cancer. A specific antibody, anti-Hu, which reacts with the HuD antigen expressed by lung cancer cells and neuronal tissues, has been associated with the development of this syndrome.[1]

Biology

The anti-Hu antibody is an IgG antibody found in the sera of patients with sensory neuropathy and encephalomyelitis. This antibody reacts with 35- to 40-kD neuronal nuclear antigens in the cerebral cortex, brain stem, cerebellum, spinal cord, and dorsal root ganglia, and it reacts with surface proteins on some small-cell lung cancer cells. The HuD gene has been mapped to the chromosome 1p region and appears to be a marker of neuroendocrine differentiation in these cells.[27]

Diagnosis

The clinical features of this syndrome are diverse.[10] One-half of patients undergo progressive sensory loss in the hands and feet. Others present with a limbic encephalopathy characterized by memory loss, behavioral changes, and seizures. Focal myelopathy with weakness, brain-stem signs (nystagmus, dysarthria), and autonomic nervous system dysfunction also occur in patients with this syndrome. These clinical signs and symptoms can antedate the diagnosis of lung cancer, so a full evaluation for occult cancer in patients who present with encephalomyelitis or subacute sensory neuropathy is warranted. CT scans are typically normal in these patients, but MRI studies may show increased T2 signal in affected areas of the brain. Pathologic examination of brain biopsies show inflammatory infiltrates and neuronal destruction in the brain stem, hippocampus, spinal cord, and dorsal root ganglia. The demonstration of anti-Hu antibodies in a patient with encephalomyelitis and a diagnosis of small-cell lung cancer establishes the diagnosis.

Treatment

Treatment of the encephalomyelitis/subacute sensory neuropathy syndrome associated with lung cancer is treatment of the primary tumor. Immunosuppressive therapy with corticosteroids and plasmapheresis directed at removal of the offending immunoglobulin from the patient's serum have been shown to be effective in only 10 to 20 percent of patients.[13] Patients who are severely affected by the anti-Hu syndrome can die from neurologic sequelae (e.g., cardiovascular collapse) rather than from the underlying lung cancer.

Paraneoplastic Cerebellar Degeneration

A syndrome of cerebellar degeneration has also been noted in patients with small-cell lung cancer. This is believed to be a variant of the paraneoplastic cerebellar degeneration (PCD) observed in patients with gynecologic and breast tumors. In patients with gynecologic tumors and PCD, a specific anti-Purkinje cell antibody called anti-Yo has been identified that binds to 34- to 38-

TABLE 116-2

Neurologic Syndromes Associated with Lung Cancer			
Syndrome	*Tumor*	*Antibody*	*Antigen*
Encephalomyelitis/ subacute sensory neuropathy	Small cell	Anti-Hu	Hu-D antigen: 35–40-kD neuronal nuclear protein
Cancer-associated retinopathy	Small cell	Antirecoverin	23-kD protein specific to photoreceptor cells (recoverin)
Lambert-Eaton syndrome	Small cell	Anti-P//Q channel	P/Q-type calcium channel

kD and 62- to 64-kD proteins in the cytoplasm of Purkinje cells.[13] Patients with small-cell lung cancer and cerebellar degeneration have anti-Hu antibodies in their sera and do not have the anti-Yo antibody. These patients are considered to have the anti-Hu syndrome and frequently go on to develop encephalitis or sensory neuropathy.

Opsoclonus and Myoclonus

Opsoclonus is a disorder consisting of involuntary rapid conjugate eye movements in vertical and horizontal directions. It is often associated with myoclonus in patients with solid tumors. This syndrome of opsoclonus/myoclonus has been associated with both small-cell and non–small-cell lung cancer in numerous case reports, but less is known about this syndrome than about the syndrome of paraneoplastic encephalomyelitis/subacute sensory neuropathy.

A specific antibody called anti-Ri has been identified that binds to 55-kD nuclear proteins expressed in the dentate nucleus. Although this antibody is considered to be the cause of the opsoclonus/myoclonus syndrome in patients with gynecologic tumors, the antibody has not been demonstrated in patients with lung cancer.

The anti-Hu antibody has been identified in some patients with small-cell lung cancer and opsoclonus/myoclonus. As in patients with the anti-Hu antibody and cerebellar degeneration, patients who have opsoclonus and the anti-Hu antibody may have a variant of the encephalomyelitis/subacute sensory neuropathy syndrome. Patients who present with lung cancer and opsoclonus should be evaluated for the anti-Hu antibody.

CANCER-ASSOCIATED RETINOPATHY

Cancer-associated retinopathy is a rare paraneoplastic syndrome that occurs predominantly in patients with small-cell lung cancer.[15] Many autoantibodies have been identified in patients with this disorder; they bind to a photoreceptor-specific protein called recoverin.[29,30]

Biology

Retinal ganglion cells and their processes are characteristically lost in this disorder because of the autoantibodies that bind to recoverin, a 23-kD photoreceptor-specific protein found in rods and cones as well as in small-cell lung cancer cells.[21] The autoantibodies that cause the cancer-associated retinopathy specifically bind to the recoverin protein and do not recognize other retinal proteins.

Diagnosis

The clinical triad of photosensitivity, ring-scotomata visual field loss, and attenuation of retinal arteriole caliber is considered highly suggestive of cancer-associated retinopathy. The typical patient presents with symptoms of rapid visual loss, with night blindness and color loss. On physical examination, most patients show visual field deficits, disk pallor, and cells in the vitreous body, along with arteriolar narrowing.

Demonstration of the antirecoverin antibody in a patient with signs of retinopathy establishes the diagnosis.[30] As with paraneoplastic cerebellar degeneration, cancer-associated retinopathy is often the first sign of an occult carcinoma. Therefore, an evaluation for lung cancer should be performed in all patients who present with this syndrome.

Treatment

In contrast to those with the other paraneoplastic neurologic syndromes, more than half of patients with cancer-associated retinopathy have been reported to respond with visual improvement after systemic steroid therapy.[15] Treatment of the primary tumor without immunosuppressive therapy has not been shown to cause visual improvement in patients with cancer-associated retinopathy. Most of these patients develop progressive visual loss and blindness within 18 months.

LAMBERT-EATON SYNDROME

The Lambert-Eaton syndrome afflicts fewer than 2 percent of lung cancer patients but has been reported in up to 5 percent of patients with small-cell lung cancer. Sixty percent of all patients who present with the Lambert-Eaton syndrome have small-cell lung cancer.[7]

Biology

In patients with Lambert-Eaton syndrome and small-cell lung cancer, an IgG autoantibody has been identified that binds to calcium channels in motor and autonomic nerve terminals, thereby inhibiting acetylcholine release. This antibody also binds to the 58-kD synaptic vesicle protein synaptotagmin, which is present in small-cell lung cancer cells.[17] Recent evidence suggests that the P/Q calcium channel is the specific target of these antibodies.[16] The antibody binding of the P/Q calcium channel weakens the neuromuscular signal, and neurologic dysfunction follows. It has also been postulated that these autoantibodies induce the production of acetylcholinesterase, which would also diminish the neuromuscular signal.

Diagnosis

Clinical features include weakness of the pelvic girdle and thigh, fatigue, dry mouth, dysarthria, dysphagia, blurred vision, and muscle pain. Unlike the situation with myasthenia gravis, muscle strength improves with exercise and does not improve significantly with the administration of anticholinesterases (e.g., edrophonium). Electromyography performed in these patients demonstrates increased muscle action potential with repeated nerve stimulation. In patients with the Lambert-Eaton syndrome, IgG autoantibodies should be demonstrable in serum.

Treatment

Treatment of the underlying small-cell lung cancer with chemotherapy can effectively treat the associated Lambert-Eaton syndrome. For patients whose neuromuscular status does not improve with chemotherapy, immune modulation with azathioprine (2.5 mg/kg per day), plasma exchange, or intravenous γ-globulin (400 mg/kg per day for 5 days) has been shown to induce remissions. 3,4-Diaminopyridine in doses of 10 to 100 mg a day has also been used successfully to bring about short-term control of this syndrome.[20]

CONCLUSION

The paraneoplastic syndromes have long fascinated and perplexed oncologists, and only in recent years have the molecular bases for these syndromes been appreciated. Not only has this new knowledge led to more effective palliation of symptoms, but it may offer new clues to the pathogenesis of malignancy. The presence of signs and symptoms that suggest a paraneoplastic syndrome should prompt a search for malignancy.

REFERENCES

1. Anderson NE, Rosenblum MK, Graus F, et al: Autoantibodies in paraneoplastic syndrome associated with small-cell lung cancer. *Neurology* 38:1391–1398, 1988.
2. Ascensao JL, Oken MM, Ewing SL, et al: Leukocytosis and large cell lung cancer: A frequent association. *Cancer* 60:903–905, 1987.
3. Bartter F, Schwartz W: The syndrome of inappropriate secretion of antidiuretic hormone. *Am J Med* 42:790–806, 1967.
4. Becker M, Aron DC: Ectopic ACTH syndrome and CRH-mediated Cushing's syndrome. *Endocrinol Metab Clin North Am* 23:585–606, 1994.
5. Bender RA, Hansen H: Hypercalcemia in bronchogenic carcinoma: A prospective study of 200 patients. *Ann Intern Med* 80:205–208, 1974.
6. Bertanga X: Proopiomelanocortin-derived peptides, in Aron DC, Tyrrell JB (eds), *Cushing's Syndrome, Endocrinology and Metabolism Clinics of North America*. Philadelphia, WB Saunders, 1994, pp 467–485.
7. Block JB: Paraneoplastic syndromes, in Haskell CM (ed), *Cancer Treatment,* 4th ed. Philadelphia, WB Saunders, 1995, pp 245–246.
8. Burtis WJ: Parathyroid hormone-related protein: Structure, function, and measurement. *Clin Chem* 38:2171–2183, 1992.
9. Constantini V, Zacharski LR, Moritz TE, Edwards RL: The platelet count in carcinoma of the lung and colon. *Thromb Haemost* 64:501–505, 1990.
10. Dalmau J, Graus F, Rosenblum MK, Posner JB: Anti-Hu–associated paraneoplastic encephalomyelitis/sensory neuropathy: A clinical study of 71 patients. *Medicine (Baltimore)* 71:59–72, 1992.
11. Delisle L, Boyer MJ, Warr D, et al: Ectopic corticotropin syndrome and small-cell carcinoma of the lung. *Arch Intern Med* 153:746–752, 1993.
12. Faglia G, Arosio M, Bazzoni N: Ectopic acromegaly. *Endocrinol Metab Clin North Am* 21:575–595, 1992.
13. Furneaux HF, Reich L, Posner JB: Autoantibody synthesis in the central nervous system of patients with paraneoplastic syndromes. *Neurology* 40:1085–1091, 1990.
14. Gross AJ, Steinberg SM, Reilly JG, et al: Atrial natriuretic factor and arginine vasopressin production in tumor cell lines from patients with lung cancer and their relationship to serum sodium. *Cancer Res* 53:67–74, 1993.
15. Keltner JL, Thirkill CE, Tyler NK, Roth AM: Management and monitoring of cancer-associated retinopathy. *Arch Ophthalmol* 110:48–53, 1992.
16. Lennon VA, Kryzer TJ, Griesmann GE, et al: Calcium-channel antibodies in the Lambert–Eaton syndrome and other paraneoplastic syndromes. *New Engl J Med* 332:1467–1474, 1995.
17. Leveque C, Hoshino T, David P, et al: The synaptic vesicle protein synaptotagmin associates with calcium channels and is a putative Lambert-Eaton myasthenic syndrome antigen. *Proc Natl Acad Sci USA* 89:3625–3629, 1992.
18. Levine M, Hirsh J: The diagnosis and treatment of thrombosis in the cancer patient. *Semin Oncol* 17:160–171, 1990.
19. Limper AH, Carpenter PC, Scheithauer B, Staats BA: The Cushing syndrome induced by bronchial carcinoid tumors. *Ann Intern Med* 117:209–214, 1992.
20. McEvoy KM, Windebank AJ, Daube JR, Low PA: 3,4-Diaminopyridine in the treatment of Lambert–Eaton myasthenic syndrome. *New Engl J Med* 321:1567–1571, 1989.
21. Polans AS, Witkowska D, Haley TL, et al: Recoverin, a photoreceptor-specific calcium-binding protein, is expressed by the tumor of a patient with cancer-associated retinopathy. *Proc Natl Acad Sci USA* 92:9176–9180, 1995.
22. Prandoni P, Lensing AWA, Buller HR, et al: Deep-vein thrombosis and the incidence of subsequent symptomatic cancer. *New Engl J Med* 327:1128–1133, 1992.
23. Ralson SH, Gallacher SJ, Patel U, et al: Cancer-associated hypercalcemia: Morbidity and mortality. Clinical experience in 126 treated patients. *Ann Intern Med* 112:499–504, 1990.
24. Ralston SH, Danks J, Hayman J, et al: Parathyroid hormone–related protein of malignancy: Immunohistochemical and biochemical studies in normocalcemic and hypercalcemic patients with cancer. *J Clin Pathol* 44:472–476, 1991.
25. Ratcliffe WA, Hutchesson ACJ, Bundred NJ, Ratcliffe JG: Role of assays for parathyroid-hormone-related protein in investigation of hypercalcaemia. *Lancet* 339:164–167, 1992.
26. Saphner T, Tormey DC, Gray R: Venous and arterial thrombosis in patients who received adjuvant therapy for breast cancer. *J Clin Oncol* 9:286–294, 1991.
27. Sekido Y, Bader SA, Carbone DP, et al: Molecular analysis of the HuD gene encoding a paraneoplastic encephalomyelitis antigen in human lung cancer cell lines. *Cancer Res* 54:4988–4992, 1994.
28. Sorenson JB, Anderson MK, Hansen HH: Syndrome of inappropriate secretion of antidiuretic hormone (SIADH) in malignant disease. *J Intern Med* 238:97–110, 1995.
29. Thirkill CE, FitzGerald P, Sergott RC, et al: Cancer-associated retinopathy (CAR syndrome) with antibodies reacting with retinal, optic-nerve, and cancer cells. *New Engl J Med* 321:1589–1594, 1989.
30. Thirkill CE, Keltner JL, Tyler NK, Roth AM: Antibody reactions with retina and cancer-associated antigens in 10 patients with cancer-associated retinopathy. *Arch Ophthalmol* 111:931–937, 1993.
31. Vassilopoulou-Sellin R, Newman B, Taylor S, Guinee V: Incidence of hypercalcemia in patients with malignancy referred to a comprehensive cancer center. *Cancer* 71:1309–1312, 1993.
32. Winquist EW, Laskey J, Crump M, et al: Ketoconazole in the management of paraneoplastic Cushing's syndrome secondary to ectopic adrenocorticotropin production. *J Clin Oncol* 13:157–164, 1995.

CHAPTER 117

PULMONARY METASTASES

Michael Burt

Prior to the 1970s, the development of pulmonary metastases had been considered a grave prognostic sign, with the patient deemed incurable and death ensuing usually within the first year of diagnosis. Since that time advances have been made in the safe conduct of thoracic surgery, and resection of pulmonary metastases in selected patients has lead to gratifying results.

HISTORY

In 1939, Barney and Churchill reported a patient with a left renal cell carcinoma with a solitary metastasis to the left upper lobe.[4] The patient had undergone left nephrectomy in April 1932. The patient subsequently received 800 rads of radiation therapy to the left upper lobe mass. Four months later the nodule in the left upper lobe had increased in size by a factor of 2. It was then decided to resect this nodule, and on July 18, 1933, the patient had a wedge resection of the lingula. This patient survived for 23 years, finally succumbing to coronary disease. The authors concluded from the outcome of this patient that "if a metastasis is apparently solitary and accessible to surgical removal, it is definitely worthwhile to undertake removal of the metastasis as well as the primary growth."

   The first "series" of resection of metastatic tumor to lung was published by Alexander and Haight in 1947.[1] These authors reported six patients with sarcoma or carcinoma metastatic to lung. At the time of the report, three of the patients were alive without evidence of disease, two were alive with disease, and one had died of disease. During the ensuing 20 years, a number of small series were published suggesting benefit from pulmonary resection of metastatic tumors to the lung. Initially, resection of pulmonary metastases was reserved for patients with solitary metastases. However, the 10-year period from 1965 to 1975 witnessed an expanding role for resection of multiple and bilateral pulmonary metastases in selected patients. Similar survival rates for patients with multiple and bilateral pulmonary metastases and patients with a solitary metastasis were demonstrated as long as complete resection was carried out. Since the mid-1970s, there has been tremendous growth in the number of papers suggesting benefit from pulmonary metastatectomy in patients with various solid tumors. The literature now contains data on well over 5000 patients who have undergone resection of pulmonary metastases.

INCIDENCE

It is well known that the lung is a common site of metastatic disease. Approximately 30 percent of patients with malignant disease will, at some point in the natural history of the disease, develop pulmonary metastases. Importantly, 20 percent of patients dying of pulmonary metastases will have no other detectable sites of disease. In some primary tumors, such as renal cell carcinoma, choriocarcinoma, Wilms tumor, and osteosarcoma, there is a high incidence of synchronous pulmonary metastases at the time of the initial presentation (Table 117-1). In addition, at autopsy, the incidence of pulmonary metastases is greater than 25 percent in patients with melanoma, choriocarcinoma, renal cell carcinoma, Ewing's sarcoma, osteosarcoma, and testicular (germ cell) carcinoma. Therefore, pulmonary metastatic disease is a relatively common event, and the treatment of patients with pulmonary metastases, particularly those who present with isolated pulmonary metastases, becomes extremely important in attempts to prolong survival.

PRESENTATION

Symptoms

In the absence of involvement of major bronchi, visceral, or parietal pleura, or other contiguous structures, parenchymal pulmonary metastases for the most part are asymptomatic. Occasionally, patients will develop such extensive parenchymal

TABLE 117-1

Incidence of Pulmonary Metastases from Extrathoracic Tumors

Primary Lesion	Presentation	Autopsy
Melanoma	5%	80%
Thyroid	5–10	65
Breast	5	60
Colorectal	5	40
Head and neck	5	40
Bladder	5–10	30
Prostate	5	53
Choriocarcinoma	60	70–100
Kidney	5–30	50–75
Rhabdomyosarcoma	21	55
Wilm's tumor	20	60
Ewing's sarcoma	18	77
Osteosarcoma	15	75
Testicular (germinal)	12	70–80

SOURCE: Adapted from Gilbert and Hagan.[15]

involvement that they exhibit dyspnea on exertion or shortness of breath, but this is unusual and usually confined to rapidly growing tumors such as choriocarcinoma in women or metastatic germ cell carcinoma in men.

Most pulmonary metastases are discovered by routine chest radiograph either as a synchronous event with a primary tumor or as a metachronous event in a routine follow-up examination. Occasionally, patients will present with hemoptysis either due to primary endobronchial metastases or more commonly due to tumor arising in parenchyma but invading the major bronchi. Some patients may present with fever secondary to the neoplastic process or, rarely, with hypertrophic osteoarthropathy.

TABLE 117-2

Radiographic Patterns of Pulmonary Metastatic Lesions

Radiographic Pattern	Most Common Histology
Multiple nodules	
Calcified	Osteogenic sarcoma, chondrosarcoma, thyroid, ovarian, breast
Miliary	Thyroid, melanoma, renal cell, ovarian
Cannonball	Sarcoma, colorectal, renal cell, melanoma
Slow growing	Adenoid cystic (salivary gland), thyroid
Cavitary	Squamous cell, melanoma, sarcoma, germ cell, transitional cell (bladder)
Poorly defined	Choriocarcinoma, liposarcoma, laryngeal, pancreatic
Solitary nodules	Nonspecific
Lymphangitic features	Adenoca of breast, lung, prostate, stomach, pancreas
Hilar or mediastinal adenopathy	GU, head and neck, melanoma, seminoma, renal cell
Endobronchial disease	Breast, colorectal, pancreas, renal cell

SOURCE: Adapted from Whitesell and Peters.[49]

Distribution and Appearance

Pulmonary metastases can present with a myriad of radiologic findings (Table 117-2). They are most commonly bilateral, well-defined with smooth edges and located primarily in the periphery of the lung (Fig. 117-1). Although some autopsy reports demonstrate a predilection for metastatic involvement of the lower lung zones rather than the apices, evaluation of 100 patients with 344 surgically resected pulmonary metastases revealed the upper lobes to be involved in 41 percent, the lower lobes in 41 percent, and the middle lobe in 6 percent.[28] Whereas primary bronchogenic carcinoma usually displays spiculated and irregular radiologic appearance, metastatic lesions often show no specific radiologic signs of lung invasion. In one autopsy series where the location, size, and appearance of metastases were studied, 82 percent of lesions were peripheral, 59 percent were pleural or subpleural, and 59 percent were less than 5 mm in diameter.[11]

Although calcification of a pulmonary nodule often indicates that the lesion may be benign (granuloma or hamartoma), calcification is often noted in pulmonary metastases from osteosarcoma and, less frequently, in synovial cell sarcoma, chondrosarcoma, and carcinomas of the thyroid, breast, and colon. Calcifications may also be seen in metastatic or primary Hodgkin's disease in the lung. Although uncommon, pulmonary metastases may cavitate and, if subpleurally based, may lead to pneumothorax. Cavitation has also been reported, most commonly with metastatic squamous cell carcinoma from the head and neck region as well as genitourinary tract primary tumors.

Pulmonary lymphangitic metastatic disease also occurs, usually with adenocarcinomas of the breast, lung, prostate, stomach, or pancreas. Most commonly, lymphangitic metastases result from hematogenous spread with extension from the capillaries to lymphatics. Lymphangitic metastases also can result from retrograde lymphatic spread from mediastinal and hilar nodes into the lung parenchyma. The radiologic appearance may be quite subtle, and patients usually present with dyspnea out of proportion to the radiologic findings. Lymphangitic spread appears radiographically as an interstitial process with fine septal lines noted predominantly in the lower lobes.

Pulmonary metastases to lung parenchyma may occasionally metastasize

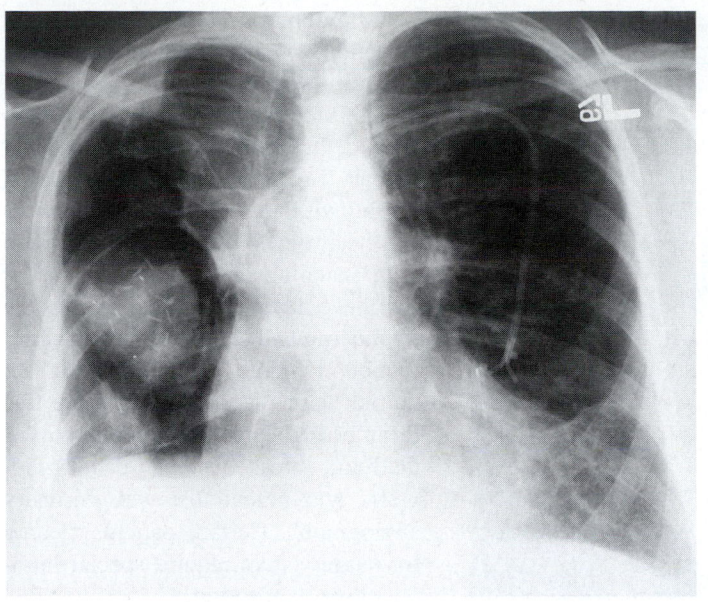

FIGURE 117-1   Chest radiograph of a young woman with a history of soft-tissue sarcoma and pulmonary metastases. She had previously undergone resection of multiple pulmonary nodules and now presents with recurrent disease. Several nodules, including a large one, are easily seen in the right lung. No nodules are seen in the left lung, but the CT scan demonstrated at least four nodules.

to hilar or mediastinal lymph nodes, but this is an infrequent event for most solid tumors. However, involvement of hilar or mediastinal nodes with pulmonary metastases from melanoma, seminoma, and breast carcinoma is more frequently reported than with other solid tumors.

Endobronchial metastases occur but are extremely uncommon. The most common primary tumors presenting with involvement of the mucosa of the bronchus are those of carcinomas of the breast, pancreas, colon, and kidney.[18] Patients with these tumors may present with hemoptysis and/or segmental or lobar atelectasis and dyspnea.

Visceral and parietal pleura may be involved in metastases from solid malignancies. This involvement usually presents as a pleural effusion, with breast carcinoma as the most common tumor causing pleural fluid. Occasionally, an effusion may result from impaired lymphatic drainage, and in this situation the pleural effusion may be cytologically negative. In this setting, thoracentesis is the diagnostic procedure of choice. If, however, the thoracentesis reveals a cytologically negative effusion, video-assisted thoracoscopy with biopsy is an integral part of the evaluation.

For the patient with a known primary tumor who subsequently presents with multiple pulmonary lesions, more than likely the patient has metastatic disease and not a benign process. A diagnostic problem may arise with a patient with a known prior malignancy who presents either synchronously or metachronously with a solitary nodule. In a study of 800 patients with previously diagnosed malignancies who presented with a solitary pulmonary nodule, 63 percent of these nodules proved to be a new primary lung carcinoma, 24 percent were solitary metastases, and 1 percent were benign lesions.[7] The probability that a solitary pulmonary nodule in a patient with a previously known cancer is a metastasis depends on the histology and site of the primary tumor (Table 117-3). In contrast, a study of 955 patients who underwent resection of a solitary pulmonary lesion without a previous history of malignancy, 49 percent of all lesions were malignant (38 percent were bronchogenic carcinoma and 9 percent were metastatic carcinoma), and 51 percent were benign.[46]

EVALUATION OF PULMONARY METASTASES

The radiologic methods available to detect pulmonary metastases include conventional chest radiography, whole lung tomography (LT), computer tomography (CT), and magnetic resonance imaging (MRI). Although a chest radiograph is the least sensitive imaging modality, with a limiting resolution of approximately 9 mm, it is the most specific, with 90 percent of nodules determined to be true metastases at the time of resection. Prior to the advent of computed tomographic scanning, linear tomography was the standard by which surgical decisions were based. Linear tomography is intermediate in both sensitivity and specificity between the plain chest radiograph and CT with the ability to detect nodules smaller than 6 mm with 78 percent of specificity. Since the late 1970s, linear tomography has been virtually replaced by CT for evaluation of pulmonary metastases. Computed tomography currently is accepted as the gold standard for the evaluation of pulmonary metastases, both allowing assessment for operative intervention and allowing evaluation of response to chemotherapy[31] (Fig. 117-2). High-resolution scanners now can detect nodules as small as 2 to 3 mm with anywhere from 60 to 90 percent specificity. This specificity is highly dependent on histology. In a group of patients with osteosarcoma or soft-tissue sarcoma, 95 percent of the nodules discovered by CT were true metastases.[31]

If there is a question of malignancy, serial CT scanning may be helpful. Enlarging masses on serial exam usually indicate malignancy. However, stability of a lesion on CT scanning even 2 to 3 months apart cannot be accepted as definitive evidence of a benign lesion. If there is a question concerning the histologic nature of a pulmonary nodule or nodules on CT scan in patients with no previous malignancy, fine-needle aspiration biopsy is warranted to confirm diagnosis prior to any planned procedure or therapy. Fine-needle aspiration biopsy can be performed safely and easily under flouroscopic guidance for lesions 1 cm or

TABLE 117-3

Diagnostic Probability of a Solitary Lesion in Patients with Known Cancer

Primary Cancer	New Primary Lung Cancer	Metastasis
Sarcoma	1	10
Melanoma	1	10
Head and neck, breast	2	1
Genitourinary, gastrointestinal, gynecologic	1	1

SOURCE: Adapted from Cahan et al.[7]

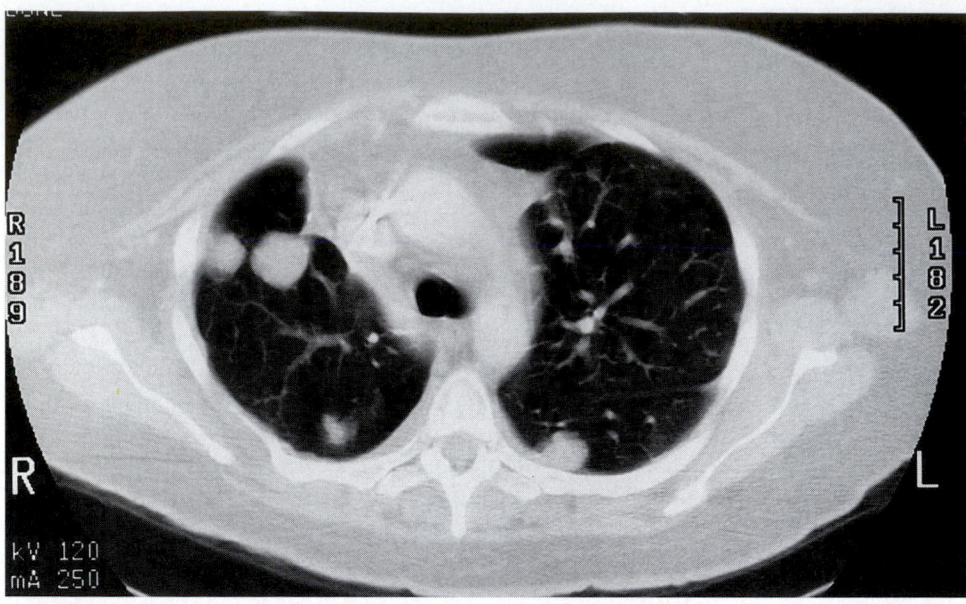

FIGURE 117-2 CT scan showing multiple bilateral nodules in a patient with metastatic sarcoma with lung as the only site of metastatic disease. The primary tumor is well controlled.

greater, and certainly CT scan can be utilized for smaller lesions. Overall, fine-needle aspiration biopsy carries an 80 percent sensitivity with almost 100 percent specificity.

Although flexible fiberoptic bronchoscopy has been extremely successful in obtaining tissue diagnosis in a patient with bronchogenic carcinoma, it has not been very useful for peripheral small multiple lesions.[32] The lower diagnostic yield may be secondary to the hematogenous origin of the metastases and a lack of continuity with bronchial epithelium and their peripheral location. However, some clinical findings suggest endobronchial disease, in which case, bronchoscopy results in higher diagnostic yields.[32]

Magnetic resonance imaging has been utilized to evaluate patients with pulmonary metastases. However, the spatial resolution of MRI is inferior to that of computer tomography. MRI, however, is superior to CT scanning in evaluating peripheral masses where a question exists as to whether the spine or a major vascular structure has been invaded.

TREATMENT

In general, patients with pulmonary metastases from a solid tumor are considered for resection only if the lung is the sole site of metastasis. Therefore, the primary goal of the preoperative evaluation of patients is to determine the extent of disease and to ensure that the lungs are the only site of metastases. Since the majority of solid tumors that have metastasized to the lung can also metastasize to brain, bone, and liver, the preoperative assessment of the patient being considered for surgical resection of metastatic disease should include a CT scan of the chest, a bone scan, and either CT or MRI of the brain. If indeed the lung is the only site of disease, the patient is potentially eligible for surgical resection. Two groups of patients with pulmonary metastases are not considered for resection: (1) those with metastases to other organs, and (2) those whose physiological status would

not allow them to tolerate the planned resection. The preoperative assessment includes the overall evaluation of the patient's medical condition with specific detail paid to cardiac and pulmonary function. Pulmonary function testing with arterial blood-gas analysis and, at times, ventilation-perfusion lung scanning ensure that the patient will have adequate pulmonary reserve to undergo and survive the planned resection. Patients with underlying acquired heart disease may require further testing, including adenosine or thallium stress testing, echocardiogram, and potentially even coronary angiography. Certain patients cleared for surgery may require special intraoperative monitoring.

Remember that some patients who have been treated with prior systemic chemotherapy may have a decreased pulmonary or cardiac reserve secondary to specific toxicity of those agents. In particular, bleomycin and mitomycin are both associated with a decrease in pulmonary diffusing capacity. Also, patients previously treated with doxorubicin may have a decrease in their cardiac reserve.

Patient Selection

It is absolutely essential that patients for resection of pulmonary metastatic disease be carefully selected. The following are the minimum criteria for resection of metastatic diseases:

1. The primary tumor has been controlled.
2. There are no extrathoracic metastases.
3. The radiologic features are consistent with pulmonary metastases.
4. The pulmonary metastases are deemed completely resectable.
5. There is adequate pulmonary reserve to allow for complete resection of all metastatic pulmonary disease.
6. The patient's general medical condition permits the planned operation.
7. Effective systemic therapy is not available.

Prognostic Factors

Although numerous factors in patients undergoing pulmonary resection of metastatic disease have been evaluated to predict prognosis, no consistent factor, or combination of factors, can be applied to individual patients in a meaningful manner, except for complete resection. In all studies evaluating the results of pulmonary resection for metastatic disease, the ability to completely resect all disease has consistently emerged as the single most important factor associated with long-term survival. Only those patients undergoing complete resection of disease are long-term survivors, and those undergoing incomplete or no resection show a marked decrease in survival. Therefore, it is essential that in the preoperative evaluation of the CT scan only those patients who are deemed resectable be selected for operation. Other factors that have been evaluated include disease free interval, tumor doubling time, and number of metastases.

Disease free interval is defined as the period of time from resection of the primary tumor to the time of diagnosis of pulmonary metastases. Some previous studies have demonstrated a correlation between long-term survival and disease free interval greater than 1 year, although some others have not corroborated this finding.[23,38] A recent review failed to demonstrate a correlation between disease free interval and survival in 716 patients with soft-tissue sarcoma.[14] Therefore, we believe that disease free interval should not be used as an absolute criterion on which to include or exclude patients from consideration of resection of their pulmonary metastases.

Several authors have shown that a longer tumor doubling time is associated with a better prognosis, others have been unable to demonstrate such a correlation.[9,21,37] Tumor doubling time is calculated by measuring the size of a nodule between two different time points and plotting the curve on semilogarithmic paper. Currently, utilizing the tumor doubling time to select patients for pulmonary resection for metastatic disease is rare.

In the past, pulmonary metastatectomy was reserved for those patients with solitary lesions; however, patients with bilateral and multiple lesions now are routinely accepted as surgical candidates.[5,14,24] The number of metastases may or may not be a prognostic indicator. Note, however, that most studies which attempt to correlate the number of pulmonary metastases resected with prognosis are based on patients who are completely resected, thus introducing some bias into the conclusion. Therefore, again, patients should be selected utilizing the CT scan to aid in predicting in which patients it should be possible to completely resect all disease. In those patients who undergo complete resection of pulmonary metastases, the number of metastases does not predict survival, but the ability to completely resect the disease is the one prognostic factor which independently predicts survival, and the number of metastases may influence the ability to resect completely all disease.

Recently, an International Registry of Lung Metastases was established. This registry includes 6207 cases of resection of pulmonary metastases in which 88 percent were complete resections and includes carcinomas, sarcomas, and melanomas (unpublished data). A multivariate analysis of this large group of patients showed that primary tumor type, disease free interval, and number of metastases were significant prognostic indicators. Further analysis of this valuable accumulation of data is underway with the goal of defining a system of classification for the various primary tumor types to better predict which patients will benefit from resection of metastatic pulmonary disease.

Operative Approach

All operative approaches for patients with metastatic pulmonary disease must attempt to achieve complete resection of all disease with maximal conservation of pulmonary parenchyma. The majority of pulmonary metastases are located at the periphery of the lung, which in most cases allows excision by wedge resection with only a small amount of surrounding normal lung tissue. A 1- to 2-cm margin appears to be adequate for resection, and this can be carried out with mechanical stapling devices or the electrocautery. Occasionally, more extensive anatomic resections are required because of the central location of the metastasis, and segmentectomy and lobectomy are both acceptable procedures. It is extremely uncommon that a pneumonectomy would be required for a patient with a central metastases, but if this is a possibility, it is crucial to evaluate the contralateral lung for other metastases and, more important, to make sure that the patient can tolerate a pneumonectomy.

There continues to be controversy over the best operative approach for patients with unilateral metastases as detected by CT scan. Traditionally, patients have been offered unilateral thoracotomy with resection of the known disease and then observed for recurrence either in the operated or the contralateral unoperated lung. In 13 patients with unilateral disease seen on CT scan, Roth and colleagues found that 38 percent had bilateral disease when median sternotomy was done and the "unaffected" lung evaluated.[41] This study has not been corroborated by other investigators, perhaps because it was completed prior to the current generation of CT scanners whose resolution capability is significantly better.

For patients with bilateral metastases there are three possible operative approaches: (1) bilateral staged thoracotomies, (2) median sternotomy, and (3) bilateral thoracosternotomy ("clamshell" incision). Historically, median sternotomy has been utilized for this group of patients.[41] However, metastases in the lower lobes and particularly in the posterior aspect of the left lower lobe can be quite difficult to resect through this approach. In the past, for these patients, particularly those with central lesions requiring lobectomy, staged bilateral thoracotomies performed approximately 1 week apart have been used. Although a median sternotomy may result in less postoperative pain and the entire procedure can be completed under one anesthetic, the overall complication rate of a median sternotomy versus staged bilateral thoracotomies is comparable.

Recently, the bilateral thoracosternotomy incision has been used in patients with bilateral disease.[6] This technique involves bilateral anterolateral thoracotomies with entry into the chest via the fourth intercostal spaces, transection of both internal mammary pedicles, and a transverse sternotomy. This approach results in excellent exposure of all areas of either lung, and any pulmonary resection—whether wedge resection, segmentectomy, lobectomy, or pneumonectomy—can be performed expeditiously and safely.

Whether a posterolateral thoracotomy, sternotomy, or bilateral thoracosternotomy incision is used to resect bilateral pulmonary metastases, the operative morbidity and mortality following any of these procedures remains consistently quite low. Reported mortality rates are less than 1 percent, with operative complications approximating 10 percent.[10,25,40,41]

The role of video thoracoscopy (VATS) in patients with pulmonary metastases has not yet been completely defined. Some would advocate that for patients with minimal pulmonary disease, VATS is an adequate approach both for diagnosis and therapy. It is clear, however, that additional lesions not seen on the preoperative CT scan often are found by palpation carried out at the time of thoracotomy or sternotomy, and this ability to thoroughly palpate the lung is lost when VATS is performed. A recent prospective study evaluated the role of VATS in patients with metastatic disease.[27] Patients with one or two lesions in one lung were registered and at the time of operation underwent an initial VATS procedure with presumed resection of all disease and then under the same anesthetic had a thoracotomy performed to determine if any further disease could be found on open exploration. In the 18 patients studied, 56 percent had additional lesions found at thoracotomy that were not identified at the time of the VATS procedure. Even taking into account the potential bias that exists in such a study, one cannot ignore that a VATS procedure would have resulted in incomplete resection of disease in the majority of patients in this series, and thus VATS is an excellent modality for making a diagnosis of pulmonary metastatic disease but is likely inadequate as definitive therapy in this group of patients. A prospective randomized trial would be required to determine if this discrepancy in the ability of VATS to resect all disease compared to thoracotomy translates into a difference in long-term survival. However, variables such as the amount of time that a patient with metastatic pulmonary nodules is followed prior to operation and bias on the part of the surgeon could easily influence the outcome of such a trial.

Recurrence and Patterns of Failure

After a complete resection of either unilateral or bilateral pulmonary metastases, the most common cause of death is recurrent disease in lung. Recurrence following complete initial pulmonary metastasectomy for soft-tissue sarcoma occurs in 67 to 86 percent of patients.[37] Of those patients who recur following an initial complete resection, 49 to 77 percent will have resectable disease again limited to the lungs. On subsequent recurrence, approximately 70 percent will have resectable disease limited to the lungs.

Patients who undergo repeated pulmonary resections for metastatic sarcoma can achieve prolonged survival.[34,40] In a series from the National Cancer Institute, the actuarial 5-year survival for 29 patients undergoing re-resection for soft-tissue sarcoma was 20 percent.[40] There was no significant difference in those patients undergoing one, two, or even three operations

for pulmonary metastases. Therefore, repeated resections of recurrent pulmonary metastases may be beneficial in those patients who have recurrences in the lung, in the absence of other disease.

Results of Resection of Pulmonary Metastases

The long-term survival in patients undergoing pulmonary resection for metastatic disease varies by the histology of the primary tumor. However, for most patients with completely resected pulmonary metastases, the 5-year survival approximates 25 to 30 percent. In a series of 891 patients who underwent complete resection of all pulmonary metastases from multiple sites, the overall survival was 36 percent (Fig. 117-3).

SOFT-TISSUE SARCOMA

In patients with primary soft-tissue sarcomas, the lungs are the most common site of distant disease, accounting for approximately 88 percent of all metastases in most series. Pulmonary metastases remain the major cause of death in these patients. Approximately 20 percent of patients with extremity soft-tissue sarcomas will present with isolated pulmonary metastases at some point in the natural history of their disease.[14] For patients who develop pulmonary metastases after treatment of the primary soft-tissue sarcoma, 80 percent will do so within the first two years of treatment.[36] Since systemic chemotherapy holds little chance for long-term survival, resection of pulmonary metastases remains the standard treatment for patients with metastatic soft-tissue sarcoma to lung who are deemed resectable. The overall 5-year survival after resection of pulmonary metastases approximates 25 percent in several series.[9,14,47]

The survival of 485 patients who underwent complete resection of metastatic sarcoma to lung is shown in Fig. 117-4. The figure includes patients with soft-tissue sarcoma, osteosarcoma, and chondrosarcoma. The 5-year survival of those with soft-tissue sarcoma was 32 percent.

Although surgical resection of pulmonary metastases salvages approximately one-third of patients, the majority will develop recurrent pulmonary metastases and, if unresectable, succumb to the disease. Although prognostic factors such as disease free in-

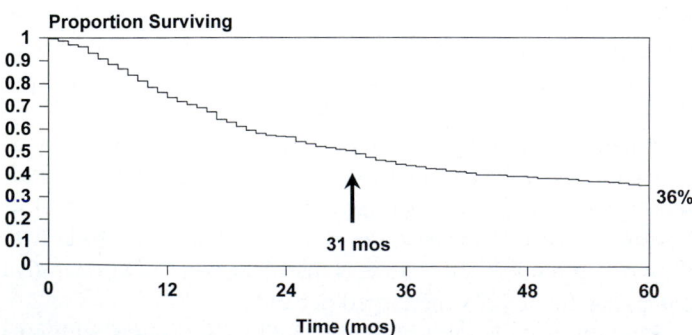

FIGURE 117-3 Survival for 891 patients with metastatic disease to the lungs undergoing complete resection from 1950 to 1990. The median survival for the entire group was 31 months. Many of these patients have undergone multiple operative procedures. (*Data from Memorial Sloan-Kettering Cancer Center.*)

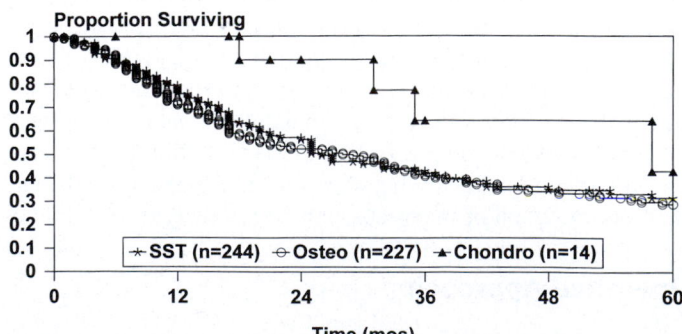

FIGURE 117-4 Survival for 465 patients with metastatic sarcoma to the lung who underwent complete resection of the pulmonary metastases. SST = soft tissue sarcoma, Osteo = osteosarcoma, Chondro = chondrosarcoma (*Data from Memorial Sloan-Kettering Cancer Center.*)

terval and tumor doubling time have been associated with a prolonged survival, the only factor which consistently predicts long-term survival is the ability to achieve a complete resection.[9,37]

OSTEOGENIC SARCOMA

The natural history of untreated pulmonary metastases from osteogenic sarcoma is well known. In patients who had the primary lesion treated by amputation, 83 percent developed pulmonary metastases. Of those patients who developed pulmonary metastases, 50 percent died within the first year, 88 percent within 2 years, 95 percent in 3 years, and no patients survived for 5 years. Since that time, the treatment of osteogenic sarcoma has been constantly evolving. Currently, multimodality therapy including adjuvant and neoadjuvant chemotherapy, limb-sparing surgery, and salvage therapy after relapse has translated into an improved survival.[5,8,38] The development of multidrug chemotherapy has improved survival.[44] It has been noted often that patients who have died from pulmonary metastases often had no evidence of extrathoracic disease.

Currently, patients with pulmonary metastases who have been treated with a combination of systemic chemotherapy and resection have an overall survival at 5 years that approximates 40 percent. For example, in 227 patients with osteogenic sarcoma and pulmonary metastases that were completely resected, the overall survival was approximately 33 percent (Fig. 117-4). Although this figure includes patients treated prior to the advent of effective systemic therapy, the overall results approximates those reported by others.

COLORECTAL METASTASES

There are approximately 100,000 cases of colorectal carcinoma in the United States yearly. Approximately one-third of patients with colorectal carcinoma develop pulmonary metastases. However, in only 2 to 4 percent of these patients are the metastases confined to the lung; the majority have metastases to other sites, usually to the liver. Systemic chemotherapy for metastatic colorectal carcinoma has not significantly improved long-term survival. In patients with isolated pulmonary metastases from colorectal carcinoma, pulmonary resection has been associated with an improved 5-year survival.[16,25,26] In 151 patients with isolated

pulmonary metastases from colorectal carcinoma who underwent complete resection (Fig. 117-5), the 5-year survival was 40 percent; the 10-year survival was 30 percent.[26] Patients with a history of colorectal carcinoma who present with a solitary pulmonary nodule have an equal chance of the nodule being a primary lung cancer or a metastasis from their previous cancer.

URINARY TRACT CANCER

For patients with renal cell carcinoma, the lung is the most common site of distant metastases, and approximately 50 percent of patients with renal cell carcinoma will develop pulmonary metastases.[33] In patients with unresected pulmonary metastases, the 5-year survival is less than 5 percent.[10] Since chemotherapy and immunotherapy have not improved long-term survival, resection of pulmonary metastases has been utilized in selected patients. The overall survival of 62 patients who underwent complete resection of renal cell carcinoma metastatic to lung at Memorial Sloan-Kettering Cancer Center is shown in Fig. 117-6. The 5-year survival approximated 40 percent. These data have been corroborated at other institutions where 5-year survival following resection of pulmonary metastases has been reported to range from 21 to 54 percent.[10,33]

The data to support resection of transitional cell carcinoma of bladder with metastases to lung are sparse. However, at Memorial Sloan-Kettering Cancer Center, 24 patients with transitional cell carcinoma of the bladder metastatic to lung have undergone complete resection of their metastatic pulmonary disease with a 5-year survival in the range of 25 percent (Fig. 117-6). For patients with transitional cell carcinoma of the bladder in whom metastases are confined to the lung, resection of the metastatic lesion in the lung should be considered.

TESTICULAR CARCINOMA

For patients with metastatic germ cell carcinoma, multimodality therapy has become the standard of care.[2] Cisplatin-based chemotherapy has dramatically improved the survival of patients with disseminated germ cell tumors.[19] At present approximately 80 percent of patients with disseminated germ cell carcinoma are cured of their disease.

In patients with metastatic germ cell carcinoma to the thorax (whether it be mediastinal or pulmonary metastases), chemotherapy is the mainstay of treatment. If residual mass is present af-

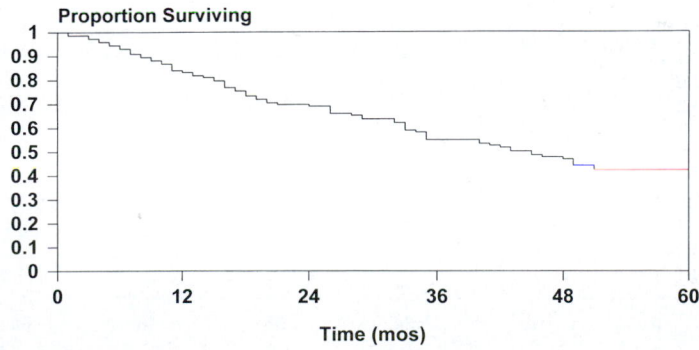

FIGURE 117-5 Survival for 151 patients with adenocarcinoma of either the colon or rectum following complete resection of isolated pulmonary metastases. *(Based, in part, on data from McCormack et al.* [26]*)*

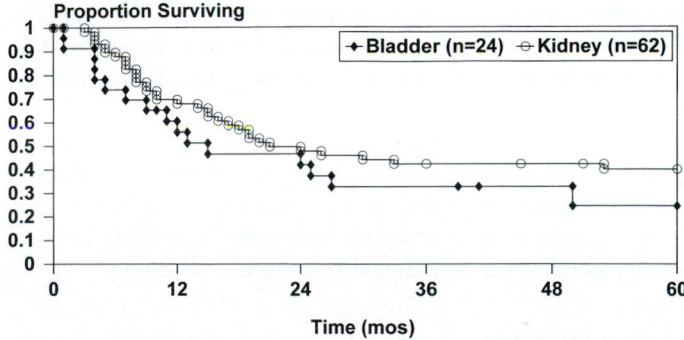

FIGURE 117-6 Survival for patients with malignancies of the genitourinary tract and isolated pulmonary metastases following complete resection. *(Data from Memorial Sloan-Kettering Cancer Center.)*

ter completion of chemotherapy, and if the tumor markers (α-fetoprotein and β-human chorionic gonadotropin) are normal, the residual mass should be resected.[2,51] In resected specimens, approximately 40 percent reveal only necrotic or fibrotic tissue, and another 40 percent show mature teratoma; however, in 20 percent viable germ cell carcinoma are found. The prognosis for patients with either necrosis or mature teratoma is excellent; i.e., approximately 90 percent of patients survive long-term. In patients who have been treated with first-line chemotherapy but in whom residual viable carcinoma is found in the resected specimen, the results of salvage chemotherapy are poor, and only about 20 to 30 percent of the patients are long-term survivors.

MELANOMA

In patients with malignant melanoma, the lungs are one of the most common sites for the development of metastatic disease.[43] From autopsy data, approximately 80 percent of patients have metastatic melanoma to the lung. Although most patients with metastatic malignant melanoma have diffuse metastases involving multiple organs, a small group of patients present with pulmonary metastases only, and resection occasionally has translated into long-term survival.[45,50] In a study of 200 patients with distant metastases, Balch and colleagues noted that the first evidence of disseminated disease was an asymptomatic pulmonary nodule in almost 40 percent of patients.[3] Of all the solid tumors in which pulmonary metastases develop and where resection of metastases is part of the treatment plan, melanoma is consistently associated with the lowest 5-year survivals despite a complete resection.[17,22,35] Harpole and colleagues analyzed 945 cases of melanoma metastatic to the lung and found that survival correlated with complete resection, a limited number of pulmonary nodules (one or two), and no involvement of hilar or mediastinal lymph nodes.[17]

HEAD AND NECK CANCER

Approximately 40 percent of patients with squamous cell carcinoma of the head and neck present with distant metastases at some point during their course. In the majority of these patients the metastases are to the lung. Resection of pulmonary metastatic disease has resulted in 5-year survival in the range of 29 to 43 percent.[12] In 65 patients with head and neck carcinomas who underwent complete resection of pulmonary metastatic disease, the 5-year survival was approximately 60 percent (Fig. 117-7).

Thus for patients with head and neck primary carcinomas who develop pulmonary metastases as the only site of disseminated disease, resection appears to be associated with improved survival. One should also keep in mind the markedly increased incidence of other aerodigestive malignancies in patients with head and neck cancers. Thus a solitary pulmonary nodule cannot simply be assumed to be a metastatic lesion but more likely is a new primary lung cancer and should be treated accordingly.

BREAST CARCINOMA

Breast carcinoma is the second most common cause of death from cancer in women in United States and accounts for ap-

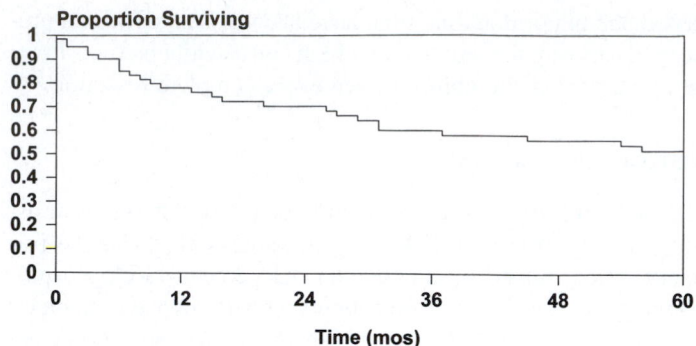

FIGURE 117-7   Survival for patients with malignancies of the head and neck following complete resection of isolated pulmonary metastases. In most, but not all, histologic examination showed squamous cell carcinoma. *(Data from Memorial Sloan-Kettering Cancer Center.)*

proximately 30,000 deaths per year. Approximately 20 percent of patients succumb to the disease with only isolated pulmonary metastases. In a series of 24 patients with breast carcinoma that was metastatic to the lung, complete resection of the pulmonary disease was associated with a 5-year survival in the range of 40 percent (Fig. 117-8). Similar results have been reported from other institutions.[23] Currently, with high-dose multidrug chemotherapy and bone marrow rescue, relatively few patients with metastatic breast cancer are referred to the thoracic surgeon for resection of pulmonary metastases. However, resection may play a role in selected patients who fail chemotherapy but have isolated pulmonary metastases.

GYNECOLOGIC MALIGNANCIES

Resection of pulmonary metastases from uterine or cervical carcinoma has been associated with 5-year survival rates ranging from 24 to 52 percent.[42] For choriocarcinoma metastatic to lung, the standard treatment is multidrug chemotherapy. However, occasionally the metastases become resistant to chemotherapy, and resection should be considered. Xu and colleagues resected pulmonary metastases from choriocarcinoma in 43 women who had become chemoresistant and noted a 5-year survival of approximately 50 percent.[52]

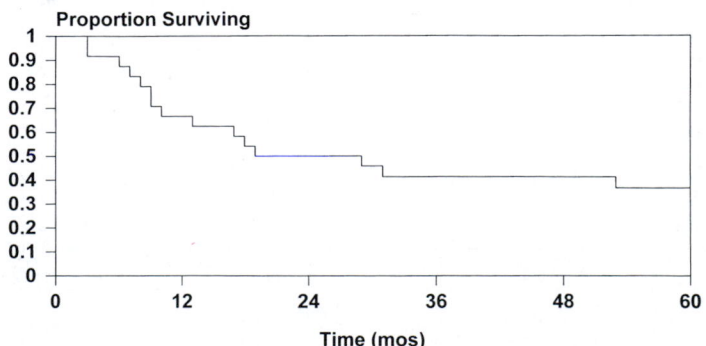

FIGURE 117-8   Survival following complete resection of isolated metastases from carcinoma of the breast. *(Data from Memorial Sloan-Kettering Cancer Center.)*

ENDOCRINE TUMORS

Metastatic endocrine carcinomas may lead to symptoms secondary to the production of excess hormone. Alleviation of symptoms with resection of metastases has been reported in patients with adrenocortical and parathyroid carcinoma metastatic to lung.[13,20] Therefore, in patients with metastatic adrenocortical or metastatic parathyroid carcinoma to lung, operation is indicated not only to rid the patient of the mass effect of the tumor but to decrease the hormone production of these tumors and thus palliate the symptoms related to excess steroid or parathormone production.

CONCLUSION

For most solid tumors metastatic to lung, effective chemotherapy that translates into prolonged survival is lacking. Therefore, in the very select group of patients with pulmonary metastases as the only site of metastatic disease, surgical resection is currently the accepted and best treatment available. However, resection of metastatic disease does have its obvious limitations, and the majority of patients will recur with disease, usually within 2 years of the initial resection. As more effective chemotherapy is developed, a multimodality approach to pulmonary metastases from solid tumors which includes resection in some cases may result in further improvements in survival for these unfortunate individuals.

REFERENCES

1. Alexander J, Haight C: Pulmonary resection for solitary metastatic sarcoma and carcinomas. *Surg Gynecol Obstet* 85:129–139, 1947.
2. Bajorin D, Herr H, Motzer R, Bosl G: Current perspectives on the role of adjunctive surgery in combined modality treatment for patients with germ cell tumors. *Sem Oncol* 19:148–158, 1992.
3. Balch C, Soong S, Murad T: A multifactorial analysis of melanoma: prognostic factors in 200 melanoma patients with distant metastases. *J Clin Oncol* 1:126–133, 1983.
4. Barney J, Churchill E: Adenocarcinoma of the kidney with metastasis to the lung. *J Urol* 42:269–278, 1939.
5. Beattie E, Harvey J, Marcove R, Martini N: Results of multiple pulmonary resections for metastatic osteogenic sarcoma after two decades. *J Surg Oncol* 46:154–160, 1991.
6. Bains MS, Ginsberg RJ, Jones WG II, et al: The clamshell incision: An improved approach to bilateral pulmonary and mediastinal tumor. *Ann Thorac Surg* 58:30–33, 1994.
7. Cahan W, Shah J, Castro E: Benign solitary lesions in patients with cancer. *Ann Surg* 187:241–249, 1978.
8. Carter S, Grimer R, Sneath R, Matthews H: Results of thoracotomy in osteogenic sarcoma with pulmonary metastases. *Thorax* 46:727–731, 1991.
9. Casson A, Putnam J, Natarajan G, et al: Five-year survival after pulmonary metastasectomy for adult soft tissue sarcoma. *Cancer* 69:662–669, 1992.
10. Cerfolio R, Allen M, Deschamps C, et al: Pulmonary resection of metastatic renal cell carcinoma. *Ann Thorac Surg* 57:339–344, 1994.
11. Crow J, Slavin G, Kreel L: Pulmonary metastasis: A pathologic and radiologic study. *Cancer* 47:2595–2601, 1981.
12. Finley R III, Verazin G, Driscoll D, et al: Results of surgical resection of pulmonary metastases of squamous cell carcinoma of the head and neck. *Am J Surg* 164:594–602, 1992.
13. Flye MW, Brennan MR: Surgical resection of metastatic parathyroid carcinoma. *Ann Surg* 193:425–435, 1981.
14. Gadd M, Casper E, Woodruff J, et al: Development and treatment of pulmonary metastases in adult patients with extremity soft tissue sarcoma. *Ann Surg* 218:705–712, 1993.
15. Gilbert HA, Hagan AR: Metastases: Incidence, detection, and evaluation without histologic confirmation, in Weiss L (ed), *Fundamental Aspects of Metastasis*. Amsterdam, North-Holland, 1976, pp. 385–405.
16. Girard P, Ducreux M, Baldeyrou P, et al: Surgery for lung metastases from colorectal cancer: Analysis of prognostic factors. *J Clin Oncol* 14:2047–2053, 1996.
17. Harpole DH, Johnson DM, Wolfe WG, et al: Analysis of 945 cases of pulmonary metastatic melanoma. *J Thorac Cardiovasc Surg* 103:743–750, 1992.
18. Heitmiller RF, Marasco WJ, Hruban RH, Marsh BR: Endobronchial metastasis. *J Thorac Cardiovasc Surg* 106:537–542, 1993.
19. Israel A, Bosl G, Golbey R, et al: The results of chemotherapy for extragonadal germ-cell tumors in the cisplatin era: The Memorial Sloan-Kettering Cancer Center experience (1975 to 1982). *J Clin Oncol* 3:1073–1079, 1985.
20. Jensen JC, Pass HI, Sindelar WF, Norton JA: Recurrent or metastatic disease in select patients with adrenocortical carcinoma. *Arch Surg* 126:457–461, 1991.
21. Joseph WL, Morton DL, Adkins PC: Prognostic significance of tumor doubling time in evaluating operability in pulmonary metastatic disease. *J Thorac Cardiovasc Surg* 61:23–32, 1971.
22. Karakousis C, Velez A, Driscoll D, Takita H: Metastasectomy in malignant melanoma. *Surgery* 115:295–301, 1994.
23. Lanza L, Natarajan G, Roth J, Putnam J: Long-term survival after resection of pulmonary metastases from carcinoma of the breast. *Ann Thorac Surg* 54:244–248, 1992.
24. Mark J: Surgical treatment of pulmonary metastases, where do we stand? *Ann Surg* 218:703–709, 1993.
25. McAfee M, Allen M, Trastek V, et al: Colorectal lung metastases: Results of surgical excision. *Ann Thorac Surg* 53:780–786, 1992.
26. McCormack P, Burt M, Bains M, et al: Lung resections for colorectal metastases. *Arch Surg* 127:1403–1406, 1992.
27. McCormack P, Bains MS, Begg CB, et al: Role of video-assisted thoracic surgery in the treatment of pulmonary metastases: Results of a prospective trial. *Ann Thorac Surg* 62:213–217, 1996.
28. Muller K, Respondek M: Pulmonary metastases: pathologic anatomy. *Lung* 168:1137–1144, 1990.
29. Murphy B, Breeden E, Donohue J, et al: Surgical salvage of chemorefractory germ cell tumors. *J Clin Oncol* 11:324–330, 1993.
30. Nordenstrom B: Technical aspects of obtaining cellular material from lesions deep in the lung. *Acta Cytologica* 28:233, 1984.
31. Pass H, Dwyer A, Makuch R, Roth J: Detection of pulmonary metastases in patients with osteogenic and soft-tissue sarcomas: The superiority of CT scans compared with conventional linear tomograms using dynamic analysis. *J Clin Oncol* 3:1261–1265, 1985.
32. Poe R, Ortiz C, Israel R, et al: Sensitivity, specificity, and predictive values of bronchoscopy in neoplasm metastatic to lung. *Chest* 88:84–91, 1985.
33. Pogrebniak H, Haas G, Linehan W, et al: Renal cell carcinoma: Resection of solitary and multiple metastases. *Ann Thorac Surg* 54:33–38, 1992.
34. Pogrebniak H, Roth J, Steinberg S, et al: Reoperative pulmonary resection in patients with metastatic soft tissue sarcoma. *Ann Thorac Surg* 52:197–203, 1991.
35. Pogrebniak H, Stovroff M, Roth J, Pass H: Resection of pulmonary metastases from malignant melanoma: Results of a 16-year experience. *Ann Thorac Surg* 46:20–23, 1988.

36. Potter D, Glenn J, Kinsella T, et al: Patterns of recurrence in patients with high-grade soft-tissue sarcomas. *J Clin Oncol* 3:353–366, 1985.

37. Putnam J, Roth J, Wesley M, et al: Analysis of prognostic factors in patients undergoing resection of pulmonary metastases from soft tissue sarcomas. *J Thorac Cardiovasc Surg* 87: 260–268, 1984.

38. Putnam J Jr, Roth J, Wesley M, et al: Survival following aggressive resection of pulmonary metastases from osteogenic sarcoma: Analysis of prognostic factors. *Ann Thorac Surg* 36:516–522, 1983.

39. Regnard JF, Marzello J, Silbert D, et al: Surgical management of pulmonary metastases of carcinoma of the breast. *Dev Oncol* 49:393–401, 1986.

40. Rizzoni W, Pass H, Wesley M, et al: Resection of recurrent pulmonary metastases in patients with soft-tissue sarcomas. *Arch Surg* 121:1248–1252, 1986.

41. Roth J, Pass H, Wesley M, et al: Comparison of median sternotomy and thoracotomy for resection of pulmonary metastases in patients with adult soft tissue sarcomas. *Ann Thorac Surg* 42:134–138, 1986.

42. Seki M, Nakagawa K, Tsuchiya S, et al: Surgical treatment of pulmonary metastases from uterine cervical cancer. *J Thorac Cardiovasc Surg* 104:876–881, 1992.

43. Sirott M, Bajorin D, Wong G, et al: Prognostic factors in patients with metastatic malignant melanoma. *Cancer* 72:3091–3097, 1993.

44. Skinner K, Eilber F, Holmes E, et al: Surgical treatment and chemotherapy for pulmonary metastases from osteosarcoma. *Arch Surg* 127:1065–1071, 1992.

45. Tafra L, Dale PS, Wanek LA, et al: Resection and adjuvant immunotherapy for melanoma metastatic to the lung and thorax. *J Thorac Cardiovasc Surg* 110:119–129, 1995.

46. Toomes H, Delphendahl A, Manke H, Vogt-Moykopf I: The coin lesion of the lung. *Cancer* 51:534–539, 1983.

47. Van Geel A, Van Coevorden F, Blankentsteijn J, et al: Surgical treatment of pulmonary metastases from soft tissue sarcomas: A retrospective study in the Netherlands. *J Surg Oncol* 56:172–179, 1994.

48. Van Geel AN, Pastorino V, Jarich KW, et al: Surgical treatment of lung metastases. *Cancer* 77:675–682, 1996.

49. Whitesell P, Peters S: Pulmonary manifestations of extrathoracic malignant lesions. *Mayo Clin Proc* 68:483–492, 1993.

50. Wong J, Euhus D, Morton D: Surgical resection for metastatic melanoma to the lung. *Arch Surg* 123:1091–1095, 1988.

51. Wood D, Herr H, Motzer R, et al: Surgical resection of solitary metastases after chemotherapy in patients with nonseminomatous germ cell tumors and elevated serum tumor markers. *Cancer* 70:2354–2359, 1992.

52. Xu LT, Sun CF, Wang YE, Song HZ: Resection of pulmonary metastatic choriocarcinoma in 43 drug-resistant patients. *Ann Thorac Surg* 39:257–259, 1985.

CHAPTER 118

LYMPHOPROLIFERATIVE AND HEMATOLOGIC DISEASES INVOLVING THE LUNG

Giuseppe G. Pietra / Kevin E. Salhany

MICROANATOMY OF THE PULMONARY LYMPHOID SYSTEM

BENIGN LYMPHOID PROLIFERATIONS
  Diffuse Lymphoproliferative Processes
  Localized Lymphoid Proliferations

MALIGNANT LYMPHOMAS
  Diagnosis and Workup
  Primary Pulmonary Non-Hodgkin's Lymphomas
  High-Grade Large B-Cell Lymphomas
  Pulmonary Hodgkin's Disease
  Other Lymphoproliferative and Hematologic Disorders
    Involving the Lung

The diagnosis of lymphoproliferative disorders in the lung is often difficult because of their rarity and their frequent overlap with infections and other reactive processes. Moreover, advances in immunohistochemistry and molecular biology have revolutionized traditional morphologic concepts. Thus, lymphoproliferative lesions that were once considered inflammatory in nature are now recognized to be low-grade neoplasms. To understand the rapidly evolving classification of lymphoproliferative disorders in the lung, it is necessary to review the normal microanatomy of the pulmonary lymphoid system.

MICROANATOMY OF THE PULMONARY LYMPHOID SYSTEM

Both nodal and extranodal organized aggregates of lymphoid tissue are present in the lung. The nodal tissue includes the peribronchial and hilar lymph nodes, which are always present, and small intrapulmonary lymph nodes, which may occur in proximity of the pleura or interlobar septa. The extranodal tissue comprises lymphoid aggregates located along the airways and the lymphatic routes of the lung. Within lymph nodes, B and T lymphocytes are organized into zones, which are best appreciated in reactive nodes after antigenic stimulation. B lymphocytes are located predominantly in the cortical follicles and medullary cords, plasma cells in the medullary cords, and T lymphocytes in the paracortical areas between the follicles. In reactive lymph nodes, the primary follicles expand and develop germinal centers composed of actively proliferating small and large noncleaved cells admixed with small and large cleaved follicular center cells. The germinal centers are surrounded by a peripheral rim, or mantle zone, composed of small lymphocytes.

The extranodal lymphoid tissue has been designated as the bronchus-associated lymphoid tissue, or BALT,[5] which includes B- and T-cell lymphoid aggregates located within the submucosa and adventitia of the airways and along the lymphatic channels (lymphatic routes) in the interlobular septa and pleura. The BALT is thought to be a branch of a specialized extranodal lymphoid tissue associated with mucosal epithelia throughout the body. The general term for this mucosa-associated lymphoid tissue is MALT.[5] The function of MALT is to provide specific immunity to epithelial surfaces exposed to exogenous antigens. This is accomplished by synthesis and secretion of IgA and other immunoglobulins in response to mucosal surface antigens. The MALT B lymphocytes circulate and "home" to other mucosal surfaces. They can transfer to another epithelium immunity-specific to epithelial pathogens acquired elsewhere.

BENIGN LYMPHOID PROLIFERATIONS

This category includes polymorphous lymphoid proliferations, either reactive or postinflammatory, which can present either as diffuse infiltrates or as space-occupying lesions. Diffuse infiltrates are caused by diffuse lymphoid hyperplasia, follicular bronchitis and bronchiolitis, or lymphoid interstitial pneumonitis. Space-occupying processes include the inflammatory myofibroblastic tumor (plasma cell granuloma), hyalinizing granuloma, and Castleman's disease.

Diffuse Lymphoproliferative Processes

LYMPHOID HYPERPLASIA, FOLLICULAR BRONCHITIS, AND BRONCHIOLITIS

Pathology

Diffuse lymphoid hyperplasia of the BALT system is characterized by expansion of the lymphatic routes by nodular aggregates of small lymphocytes (Fig. 118-1).[34,45] Reactive germinal centers are often prominent. The lymphoid nodules compress adjacent alveolar spaces but do not extend into the alveolar septa, which remain of normal width.

Lymphoid hyperplasia limited to the airways has been also designated follicular bronchitis or bronchiolitis.[34,45] Lymphoid aggregates with prominent germinal centers are located in the bronchial or bronchiolar submucosa and the peribronchial connective tissue.

Diffuse lymphoid hyperplasia and follicular bronchitis/bronchiolitis are nonspecific proliferative responses of the BALT to a variety of injuries. According to the nature and intensity of the injury and to the host immune state, the response involves proliferation of B and/or T cells. Large germinal centers and accumulation of plasma cells are hallmarks of B-cell proliferation, usually a response to bacterial antigens and some inanimate antigens. Viral antigens and drugs stimulate T-cell proliferation, characterized by infiltration of the lymphatic routes with small lymphocytes and large "transformed" lymphocytes. This is a general rule with many exceptions because the repertoire of immune responses to antigenic stimuli is limited and the interactions between B and T cells are complex. Thus, the specific etiology of lymphoid hyperplasia in an individual case cannot be established by morphology alone.

Clinical Features

Diffuse lymphoid hyperplasia and follicular bronchitis/bronchiolitis are most often secondary to chronic airway infections, bronchial obstruction, asthma, chronic obstructive pulmonary disease, and cystic fibrosis. In the absence of pulmonary disease, lymphoid hyperplasia and follicular bronchitis/bronchiolitis are seen in association with connective tissue diseases and autoimmune disorders (particularly rheumatoid arthritis, juvenile rheumatoid arthritis, and Sjögren's syndrome), congenital or acquired immunodeficiency syndromes—including human immunodeficiency virus (HIV) infection—and systemic hypersensitivity reactions.[45]

Symptoms are nonspecific and include progressive shortness of breath, cough, and fever. Chest radiographs show diffuse bilateral reticulonodular infiltrates.

LYMPHOCYTIC INTERSTITIAL PNEUMONIA

Pathology

Lymphocytic interstitial pneumonia (LIP) is an uncommon condition in which the alveolar septa and extra-alveolar interstitial space are markedly expanded by small lymphocytes, plasma cells, and histiocytes (Fig. 118-2). In some cases, germinal centers and nonnecrotizing giant cell granulomas are also present. In these cases, diffuse involvement of the alveolar septa is the feature that distinguishes between LIP and lymphoid hyperpla-

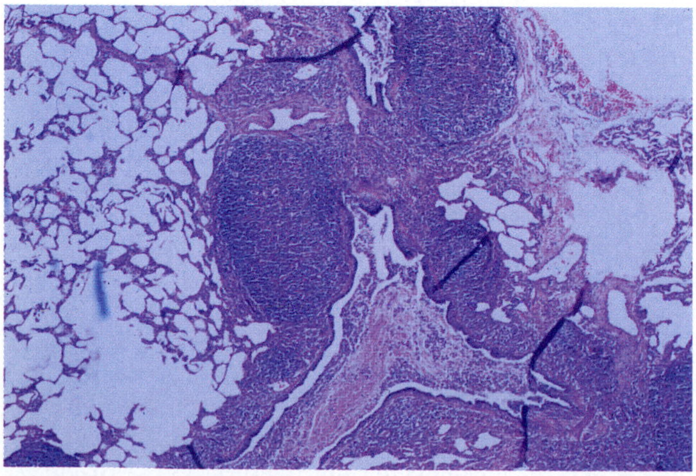

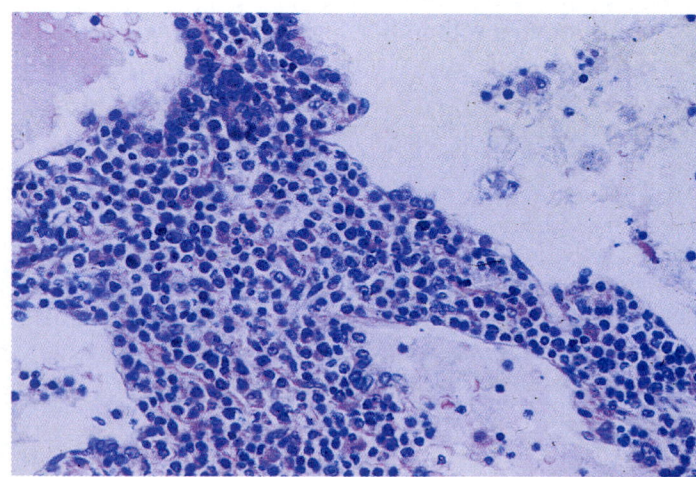

FIGURE 118-1 Diffuse lymphoid hyperplasia. The lymphatic routes in the peribronchial–perivascular interstitial spaces are expanded by nodular aggregates of lymphoid cells. The alveolar septa are not involved. Hematoxylin-eosin, ×40.

FIGURE 118-2 Lymphoid interstitial pneumonia (LIP). The alveolar interstitium is diffusely widened with an inflammatory infiltrate composed of small lymphocytes and plasma cells. Hematoxylin-eosin, ×120.

sia. The lymphocytes are small, with minimal atypia and modest mitotic activity. Immunohistochemistry reveals a polyclonal B-cell infiltrate associated with T cells, particularly CD4[+] T-helper cells. Progression to interstitial fibrosis and honeycomb lung may occur. Coexistence of LIP with nodular pulmonary amyloidosis has also been reported.

Clinical Features

Lymphocytic interstitial pneumonia occurs predominantly in adults, with a female predominance, but children may also be affected. Dyspnea and cough are the most frequent complaints. Cyanosis and clubbing of the fingers may be present.

Chest radiographs show nonspecific patterns; therefore LIP can be confused with lymphangitic metastases of carcinoma or with a pneumonia, depending on the extent of the pulmonary involvement and the acuteness of the clinical onset. The most common pattern shows bibasilar reticular or reticulonodular infiltrates (Fig. 118-3).[6] In advanced disease, encroachment on the airspaces by the expanded interstitium may result in air bronchogram or multiple poorly defined nodules. Hilar or mediastinal adenopathy and pleural effusions are usually absent.

Lymphocytic interstitial pneumonia represents a heterogeneous group of conditions. It may be idiopathic or associated with acquired or congenital abnormal immunologic responses, connective tissue diseases, allogeneic bone marrow transplantation, primary biliary cirrhosis, Hashimoto thyroiditis, or myasthenia gravis.[21] Some patients have been reported to have an associated monoclonal gammopathy, usually IgM but occasionally

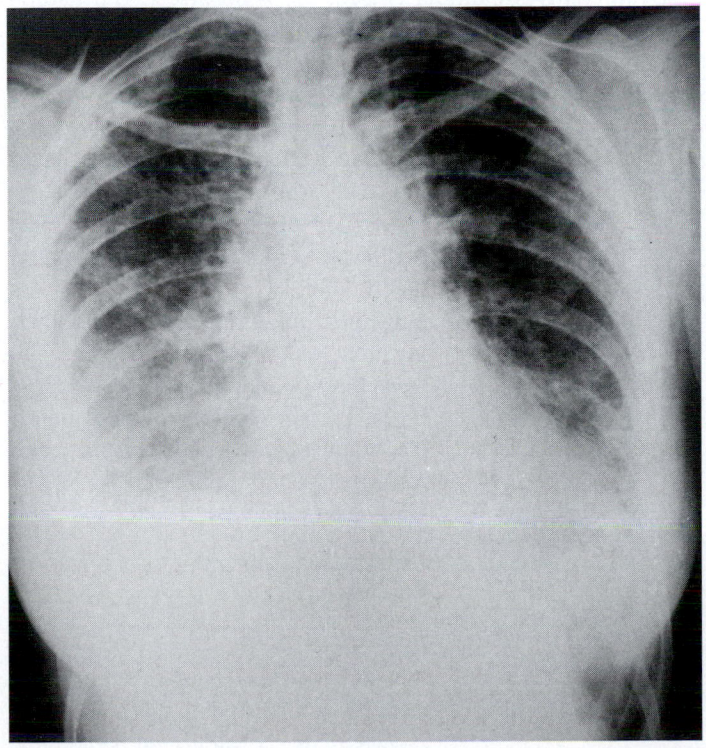

FIGURE 118-3   Lymphoid interstitial pneumonia (LIP). Posteroanterior chest radiograph showing bilateral reticulonodular opacities. *(Courtesy of Dr. W. T. Miller, Sr.)*

IgG in type. However, these individuals are probably suffering from lymphomas rather than from LIP.[1,34] Thus, the progression of LIP is extremely variable, depending on the associated conditions.[21]

Lymphocytic interstitial pneumonia has been reported in patients with AIDS, particularly among children.[20] In these patients it may be associated with reactive lymph node hyperplasia, hepatomegaly, and reduced ratio of T-helper to suppressor cells in bronchoalveolar lavage fluid. Response to steroid treatment has been irregular but occasionally excellent.[20]

Localized Lymphoid Proliferations

INFLAMMATORY MYOFIBROBLASTIC TUMOR

Pathology

This lesion is known by a variety of terms (plasma cell granuloma, lymphoid inflammatory pseudotumor, histiocytoma, xanthoma, fibroxanthoma, mast cell granuloma), reflecting the controversial views on its histogenesis and natural history. Although not a lymphoproliferative lesion in a strict sense, this entity is discussed here because it has been reported in the literature as "plasma cell granuloma" and may be confused with "pseudolymphoma" and pulmonary plasmacytoma, which are true lymphoid neoplasms. The term *plasma cell granuloma*[4] is well entrenched in the medical literature, but it should be abandoned, since this lesion is neither a granuloma nor a predominantly plasmacytic proliferation. The term *inflammatory myofibroblastic tumor* (IMT) is currently preferred because these lesions have been shown to be a nodular proliferation of fibroblasts and myofibroblasts[2,42] associated with a variable polyclonal population of plasma cells and lymphocytes.

Macroscopically, IMT forms a well-circumscribed but not encapsulated white-yellow mass, more frequently located in a lower lobe. It may grow to a large size, extending into the mediastinum or pleura.[42] Bronchial obstruction may result from external compression or from endobronchial growth.[2] Although lung is the most common site, IMTs have been reported in the trachea and major bronchi,[2] mesentery, spleen, liver, and soft tissues. Microscopically, IMTs are composed of interlacing bundles of myofibroblasts with a storiform configuration and a variable admixture of plasma cells, lymphocytes, foamy histiocytes, and multinucleated giant cells (Fig. 118-4). Germinal centers, amyloid deposits, or microcalcifications may be present.

The etiology and natural history of the IMT are still controversial. Originally considered to be a benign inflammatory reaction to unknown infectious agents,[4] it is now generally considered to be a locally invasive, low-grade neoplasm of myofibroblasts with the potential to recur if incompletely resected.[2]

Clinical Features

Although most of the cases have been reported in young individuals with a median age of 25, IMTs can occur in any age group. The incidence is slightly higher in females. The clinical presentation varies with the location and size of the lesion. Many patients are asymptomatic, the lesion being discovered during routine chest radiographic examination. Others present with

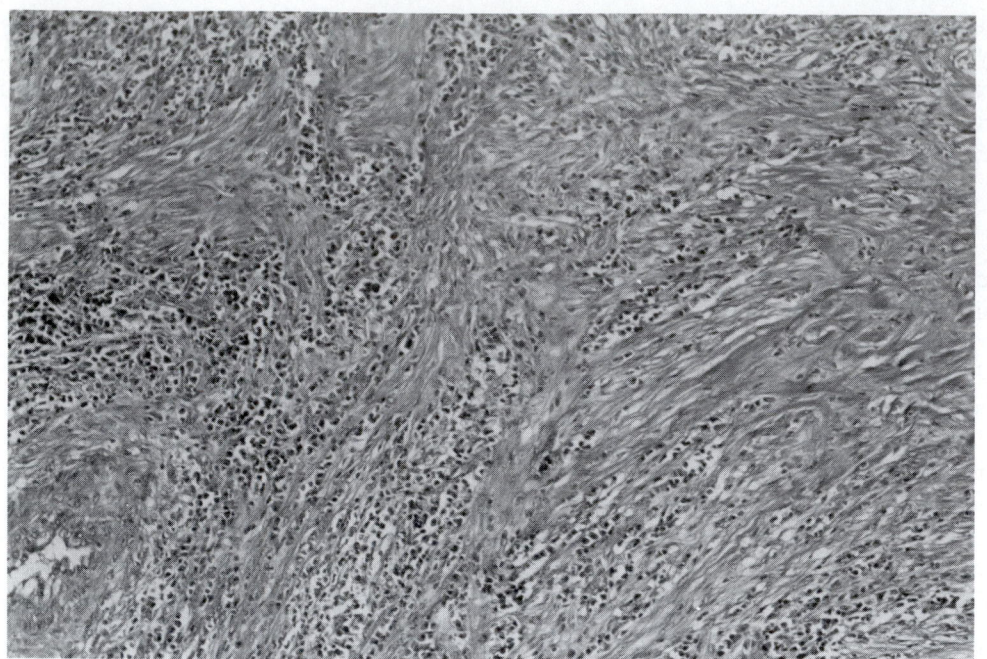

FIGURE 118-4 Inflammatory myofibroblastic tumor (plasma cell granuloma). The tumor is composed of a haphazard proliferation of plump spindle cells interspersed with lymphocytes and plasma cells. Hematoxylin-eosin, ×160.

cough, shortness of breath, and hemoptysis, the latter often resulting from intrabronchial lesions.[2] Chest pain, cyanosis, clubbing of the digits, and a history of recent acute respiratory illness may prompt the radiographic studies that lead to discovery of the lesion.

Serial chest radiographs reveal a solitary mass that slowly increases in size, mimicking a neoplasm or obstructive pneumonia due to endobronchial tumors. Rarely, multiple nodules may be present.

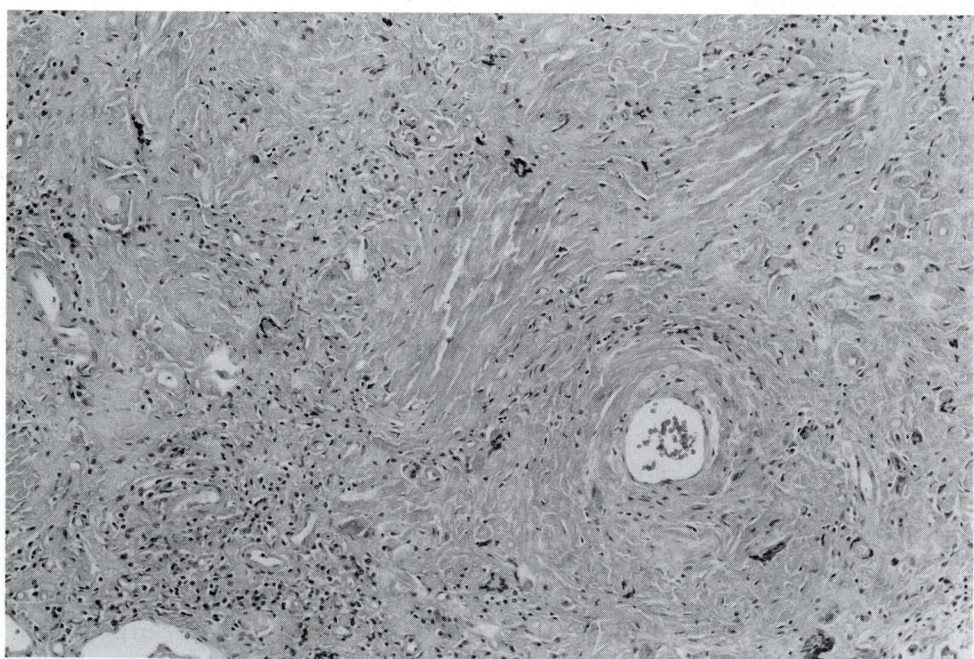

FIGURE 118-5 Pulmonary hyalinizing granuloma. Dense lamellar collagen is deposited in concentric layers around small blood vessels. Lymphocytes, plasma cells, and multinucleated giant cells are scattered within the collagen deposits. Hematoxylin-eosin, ×80.

HYALINIZING GRANULOMA

Pathology

This entity is not a true granuloma but a localized accumulation of layers of hyaline collagen surrounded by a rim of lymphocytes and plasma cells. Macroscopically, hyalinizing granuloma appears as a sharply circumscribed white-tan rubbery mass. The hyalinized collagen is frequently deposited in concentric layers around medium-sized blood vessels (Fig. 118-5). This material may stain positive with Congo red but does not have the ultrastructural characteristics of amyloid.[46] Calcifications, ossification, and multinucleated giant cells may be present.

Clinical Features

Both sexes are equally affected, their ages ranging from the second to the eighth decades. Most often patients are asymptomatic and the lesions are discovered during routine chest radiographs. However, chest pain, cough, and hemoptysis can occur.

Chest radiographs show homogeneous round nodules, 2 to 4 cm in diameter, but in rare instances they can be much larger. The nodules are often multiple and bilateral. Occasionally calcification or cavitation is present.

Hyalinizing granuloma is rare; its pathogenesis and natural history are not defined. Hyperimmunity to infection, particularly fungal, has been proposed,[46] but skin tests, cultures, and histochemical stains for fungal or mycobacterial microorganisms have been negative. The association with sclerosing mediastinitis or retroperitoneal fibrosis and other immunologic abnormalities in a number of cases suggests the possibility of an underlying derangement in autoimmunity. Hyalinizing granuloma is benign and solitary lesions have not recurred after resection. However, progressive growth of multiple nodules may cause dyspnea and respiratory compromise.[46]

CASTLEMAN'S DISEASE (ANGIOFOLLICULAR HYPERPLASIA)

Pathology

Castleman's disease is an uncommon form of reactive lymphoid hyperplasia known under a variety of synonyms (giant lymph node hyperplasia, angiofollicular lymph node hyperplasia, or lymph node hamartoma). These reflect the initial confusion surrounding its nature and histogenesis. Originally described as a localized mass in the middle mediastinum, it has subsequently been found in a variety of extranodal sites, including the lung. In the mediastinum and lung, Castleman's disease forms a solitary, well-circumscribed mass with a soft, smooth, gray-red surface.

Histologically, Castleman's disease is subdivided into hyaline-vascular, plasma cell, and mixed variants.[14] The hyaline-vascular variant is the most common histologic subtype and accounts for essentially all cases of pulmonary Castleman's disease. It is characterized by small atrophic or "burnt-out" germinal centers that are frequently penetrated by small hyalinized venules and prominent interfollicular proliferation of branching venules lined by plump endothelial cells. In the atrophic germinal centers, the number of follicular center cells is decreased and the dendritic reticulum cells are increased. The germinal centers are surrounded by expanded mantle zones with concentric rings of small lymphocytes and follicular center cells that impart an "onionskin" appearance (Fig. 118-6). The plasma cell variant, characterized by hyperplastic germinal centers and sheets of interfollicular plasma cells, accounts for 10 percent of localized Castleman's disease; it usually involves lymph nodes and not the lung. The mixed subtype has histologic features of both hyaline-vascular and plasma cell variants and the disease is usually multicentric.

Clinical Features

Castleman's disease may present as either localized or multicentric disease. Localized Castleman's disease characteristically presents as a mediastinal mass in young to middle-aged individuals of either sex. Occasionally it presents as a pulmonary mass. Localized Castleman's disease is generally asymptomatic and usually discovered during a routine chest radiographic examination. The lesions may be present for many years without changing size. The plasma cell variant is often associated with fever, anemia, and polyclonal hypergammaglobulinemia. Surgi-

cal resection of localized Castleman's disease provides permanent cure and disappearance of systemic symptoms.[14]

Multicentric Castleman's disease frequently presents with systemic symptoms and tends to involve peripheral lymph nodes rather than lung or mediastinum. Histologically, multicentric Castleman's disease has features of either the plasma cell or mixed variants and is associated with an increased incidence of multiple myeloma, other B-cell neoplasms, and Kaposi's sarcoma. Systemic chemotherapy and/or steroids, alone or in combination, usually result in resolution of symptoms and often induce sustained remissions in multicentric Castleman's disease.[35] Surgical management is not indicated for this form of Castleman's disease.

MALIGNANT LYMPHOMAS

Pulmonary lymphomas are uncommon, representing less than 1 percent of primary lung cancers.[29] Malignant lymphomas are traditionally divided into Hodgkin's disease and non-Hodgkin's lymphomas. The classification of lymphoid neoplasms is continuously evolving and expanding as new information on lymphocyte biology progresses. The current diagnosis and classification of lymphomas are highly dependent on the close integration of histopathology with immunophenotyping, cytogenetics, molecular genetics, and clinical features. The International Lymphoma Study Group has recently proposed a new classification of lymphoid neoplasms that recognizes distinct clinicopathologic entities based on these multiparameter studies (Table 118-1).[16] This classification defines several categories of lymphoma that are not included in previous lymphoma classifications, including lymphomas of the mucosa- or bronchus-associated lymphoid tissue (MALT/BALT) and angiocentric lymphomas. Most primary pulmonary lymphomas are included within these categories (Table 118-2).

Diagnosis and Workup

The traditional histologic criteria of monomorphic growth, cytologic atypia, and infiltrative or destructive growth remain the mainstay for the general diagnosis of pulmonary lymphomas; however, some low-grade lymphomas lack cytologic atypia and other lymphomas have polymorphous cellular composition. Multiparameter studies—including immunophenotyping as well as cytogenetic and molecular genetic studies—are often required to separate low-grade lymphoid neoplasms from reactive processes and to identify distinct lymphoma entities. The routine application of these new methods of pathologic diagnosis has led to the recognition that pulmonary "pseudolymphomas"—lesions previously considered to be reactive because of their indolent clinical course, polymorphous cellular composition, and lack of cytologic atypia—are actually clonal, low-grade B-cell lymphomas.[1,33]

Routine application of multiparameter studies to the diagnosis of lymphomas has become a reality with the widespread availability of these techniques in many community hospitals, regional medical centers, or commercial laboratories. The basic workup of pulmonary lymphomas includes histologic examination and immunophenotyping.[39] Immunohistochemical studies

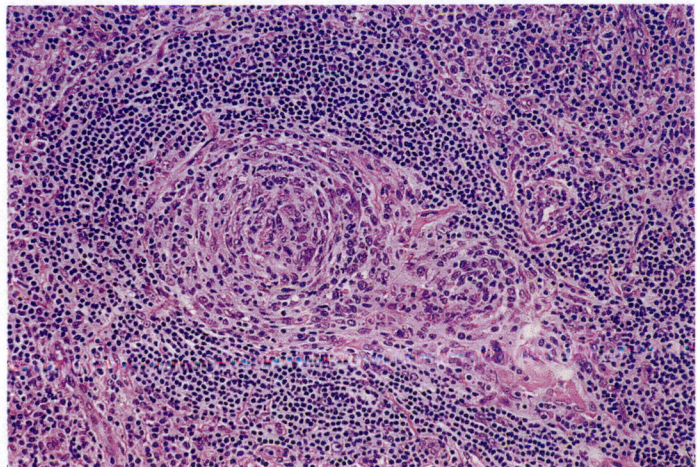

FIGURE 118-6 Angiofollicular hyperplasia, hyaline-vascular variant (Castleman's disease). Each atrophic or burnt-out germinal center is surrounded by an expanded mantle zone. The mantle zone and follicular center cells are organized into concentric "onionskin" arrangements. Vascularity is increased within the interfollicular area, mantle zone, and germinal center. Hematoxylin-eosin, ×100.

TABLE 118-1

International Lymphoma Study Group Classification of Lymphoid Neoplasms

B-cell neoplasms
  Acute lymphoblastic leukemia/lymphoblastic lymphoma, precursor B cell
  Chronic lymphocytic leukemia/small lymphocytic lymphoma
  Lymphoplasmacytoid lymphoma (Waldenström's macroglobulinemia)
  Mantle cell lymphoma (intermediate lymphocytic)
  Follicular lymphoma (follicular center cell; small cleaved, mixed, or large cell)
  Marginal zone B-cell lymphoma (splenic, nodal, or extranodal MALT/BALT)
  Hairy cell leukemia
  Multiple myeloma/plasmacytoma
  Diffuse large B-cell lymphoma (including immunoblastic, mediastinal, intravascular)
  Burkitt's lymphoma (small noncleaved cell)
  High-grade B-cell lymphoma, Burkitt-like

T- and NK-cell neoplasms
  Chronic lymphocytic/prolymphocytic leukemia, $CD4^+$ T cell
  Large granular lymphocytic leukemia ($CD8^+$ T cell, or NK cell)
  Mycosis fungoides/Sezary syndrome
  Peripheral T-cell lymphoma (small cell, mixed, or large cell)
  Hepatosplenic $\gamma\delta$ T-cell lymphoma
  Subcutaneous panniculitic T-cell lymphoma
  Angioimmunoblastic T-cell lymphoma (AILD)
  Angiocentric lymphoma (lymphomatoid granulomatosis, lethal midline granuloma)
  Intestinal T-cell lymphoma (enteropathy associated)
  Adult T-cell leukemia/lymphoma (HTLV-1 associated)
  Anaplastic large cell lymphoma, $CD30^+$ (T cell, or null cell)

Hodgkin's disease
  Lymphocyte predominance
  Nodular sclerosis
  Mixed cellularity
  Lymphocyte depletion

SOURCE: Modified from Harris et al,[16] with permission.

TABLE 118-2

Primary Pulmonary Lymphomas and Lymphoproliferative Disorders

A. BALT lymphoma
   1. Low-grade, small B-cell
   2. High-grade, large B-cell
B. Large B-cell lymphoma (not otherwise specified)
C. Angiocentric lymphoma (lymphomatoid granulomatosis)
D. Primary pulmonary Hodgkin's disease
E. Posttransplant lymphoproliferative disorders
F. HIV-related lymphomas
G. Extramedullary plasmacytoma
H. Primary pulmonary Langerhans' cell histiocytosis (eosinophilic granuloma)

on formalin-fixed, paraffin-embedded tissue can be used to determine the basic B- or T-cell phenotype and to distinguish Hodgkin's disease from non-Hodgkin's lymphoma or lymphoma from nonlymphoid malignancies. However, flow cytometry or frozen-section immunohistochemistry is usually required to demonstrate light-chain restriction or detailed immunopheno-types. Immunoglobulin and T-cell receptor gene rearrangements may be necessary to prove clonality of pulmonary lymphoproliferations when immunophenotyping is inconclusive or suggests a T-cell phenotype. Cytogenetic studies can also provide evidence of clonal lymphoid proliferations. Although cytogenetic and molecular genetic abnormalities characteristic for primary pulmonary lymphomas have not yet been identified, demonstration of abnormalities characteristic of other non-Hodgkin's lymphoma may be found, i.e., t(14;18) translocation and bcl-2 gene rearrangement in follicular lymphoma or t(11;14) translocation and cyclin D1 (bcl-1) gene rearrangement in mantle cell lymphoma.[38] Electron microscopy can be helpful in differentiating hematopoietic/lymphoid neoplasms from other poorly differentiated malignant neoplasms.

Wedge excision of a suspected lymphoma by open lung biopsy or video-assisted thoracoscopy is preferable to bronchoscopic or needle biopsy in order to ensure that adequate tissue is available for all necessary diagnostic studies. Multiple samples should be obtained with the aspiration needle in order to provide the material needed for ancillary immunophenotyping, cytogenetics, and molecular diagnostic studies; this material should be placed in normal saline or tissue culture media. Endobronchial or transbronchial biopsies may be diagnostic for lymphoma in some cases. But in general, these are less likely than wedge resection to provide adequate material for ancillary studies. Immunophenotyping and gene rearrangement studies can also be used to diagnose lymphoma on bronchial lavage samples containing large numbers of lymphocytes.

Proper handling of biopsies for possible lymphoma or leukemia requires that the pathologist and the physician performing the biopsy be alerted to this possibility.[39] These biopsies must immediately be sent to pathology, either fresh in saline or in saline-moistened gauze to allow tissue to be procured for immunophenotyping studies, cytogenetic analysis, and molecular genetic studies. Fixation of representative sections in B5 solution is recommended for optimal morphologic evaluation. Formalin-fixed sections are also useful for immunophenotyping, in situ hybridization, and molecular studies on paraffin-embedded tissue. Glutaraldehyde fixation is used for electron microscopy. Air-dried touch imprints of fresh tumor can be used for cytochemical stains such as myeloperoxidase or to evaluate Wright's-stained morphology. Fresh tumor snap-frozen in liquid nitrogen or isopentane cooled in liquid nitrogen and stored at –70°C is useful for immunophenotyping and molecular studies. Tissue can be frozen in a cryostat and stored at –20°C if necessary. Cell suspensions made from excess fresh tumor can be used for immunophenotyping by flow cytometry, cytogenetic analysis, and molecular studies; this material can be transported in normal saline or in an appropriate tissue culture medium.

Primary Pulmonary Non-Hodgkin's Lymphomas

Primary pulmonary lymphomas are those in which the lung is the major site of disease at the time of clinical presentation. In most studies, primary pulmonary lymphomas have been confined to the lung radiographically; however, histologic involvement of contiguous hilar or mediastinal lymph nodes has been documented in up to 20 percent of these cases.[45] Primary pulmonary lymphomas represent less than 10 percent of all extranodal lymphomas; secondary lung involvement by systemic or mediastinal lymphoma is much more common, occuring in up to 50 percent of cases during the course of the disease.[12,45] Most primary pulmonary lymphomas are B-cell, non-Hodgkin's lymphomas of BALT origin; primary Hodgkin's disease of the lung is rare. For

practical purposes, primary pulmonary non-Hodgkin's lymphomas can be subdivided into three major clinicopathologic groups: (1) low-grade, small B-cell lymphomas of BALT origin, (2) high-grade, large B-cell lymphomas, and (3) angiocentric lymphomas.

LOW GRADE, SMALL B-CELL LYMPHOMA OF BALT ORIGIN

Pathology

The majority (75 to 90 percent) of primary pulmonary non-Hodgkin's lymphomas are low-grade, small B-cell lymphomas. Most of them are thought to originate from the BALT[12,24] and are frequently associated with preexisting chronic immune system stimulation, including Sjögren's syndrome.

Low-grade BALT lymphomas are slowly progressive neoplasms, some of which were originally designated as "pseudolymphoma" by Saltzstein on the basis of apparently benign clinicopathologic features.[40] Histologically, the presence of reactive germinal centers and a polymorphous infiltrate of plasma cells and small lymphocytes without significant cytologic atypia were considered markers of nonneoplastic reactive lymphoid proliferations. Clinically, pseudolymphomas had an indolent clinical course and were thought to be completely cured by surgical resection alone. However, longer follow-up of patients with this condition has shown recurrence of some lesions and progression to overt lymphoma.[24] Moreover, immunohistochemical and immunogenetic techniques have shown the presence of monoclonal B cells within pseudolymphomas. The significance of these occult B-cell clonal proliferations has been debated, but there is a growing consensus that patients with pseudolymphoma are at increased risk for development of overt pulmonary or extrapulmonary lymphomas and that most pseudolymphomas are actually low-grade BALT lymphomas.[1,12,38]

Low-grade BALT lymphomas typically present as a solitary, well-delineated, white-tan, fleshy mass (Fig. 118-7) but sometimes as multiple unilateral or bilateral nodules. Less frequently,

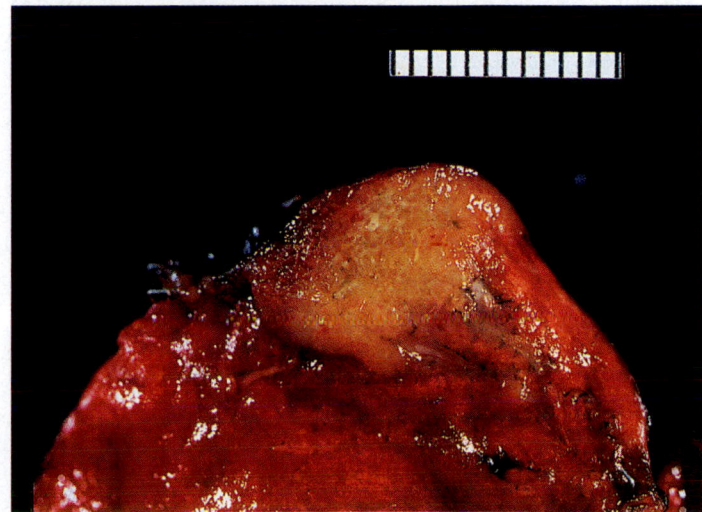

FIGURE 118-7 Low-grade BALT lymphoma. The gross appearance is that of a solitary, well-defined, peripheral lung mass. The cut surface has a solid white-tan fleshy appearance with slightly irregular peripheral borders. *(From Salhany,[38] with permission.)*

they may appear as more or less diffuse infiltrates along the bronchovascular bundles and the interlobular septa or as extensive lobar infiltrates. Histologically, low-grade BALT lymphomas are characterized by a dense proliferation of minimally atypical, small, "centrocytelike" lymphocytes with slightly cleaved nuclei or monocytoid B cells with abundant pale cytoplasm. These surround reactive follicular centers and infiltrate bronchial or bronchiolar epithelium to form lymphoepithelial lesions. Plasma cells and plasmacytoid lymphocytes, which may be polyclonal or monoclonal, are often associated with the lymphoma (Fig. 118-8).[1,12,24,38,45] Other low-grade BALT lymphomas are relatively monomorphic, with inconspicuous or absent germinal centers and plasma cells. Nodular interstitial infiltration of lymphoma along lymphatic routes near bronchovascular bundles is typically found at the periphery of the tumor. Infiltration of the bronchial mucosa may cause luminal narrowing with associated obstructive pneumonia or atelectasis.

Centrocytelike cells of low-grade BALT lymphomas can have varied cytologic appearances, including small round lymphocytes, small cleaved cells, plasmacytoid lymphocytes, or monocytoid B cells (Fig. 118-8).[1,12,24,38,45] This has led to varied histologic classification of low-grade BALT lymphomas in the Working Formulation as well as the Rappaport and Kiel classifications as small (well-differentiated) lymphocytic lymphoma, mantle cell (intermediate lymphocytic) lymphoma, small cleaved cell lymphoma, lymphoplasmacytoid lymphoma (Waldenström's), and monocytoid B-cell lymphoma.

Lymphomas of the BALT type are invariably B-cell lymphomas. Demonstration of light-chain restriction or clonal immunoglobulin gene rearrangements is helpful in the diagnosis of low-grade BALT lymphomas with histologic features of "pseudolymphoma."[1,33,38] Immunophenotyping and molecular studies are also helpful in differentiating monomorphic low-grade BALT lymphomas from other small B-cell lymphomas.[38]

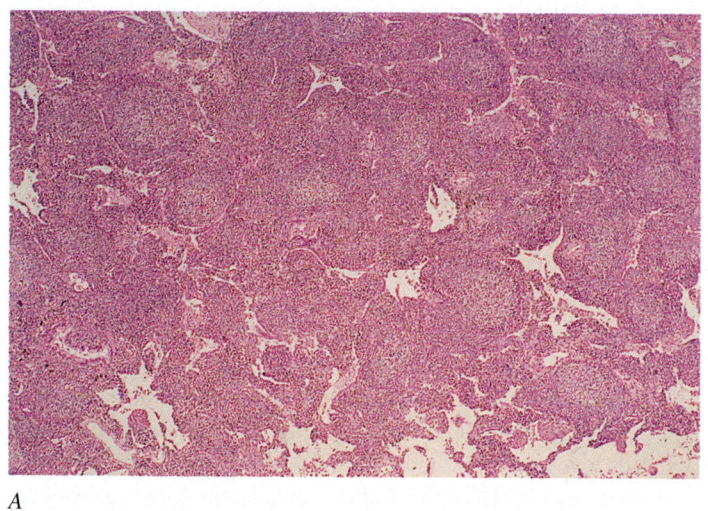

A

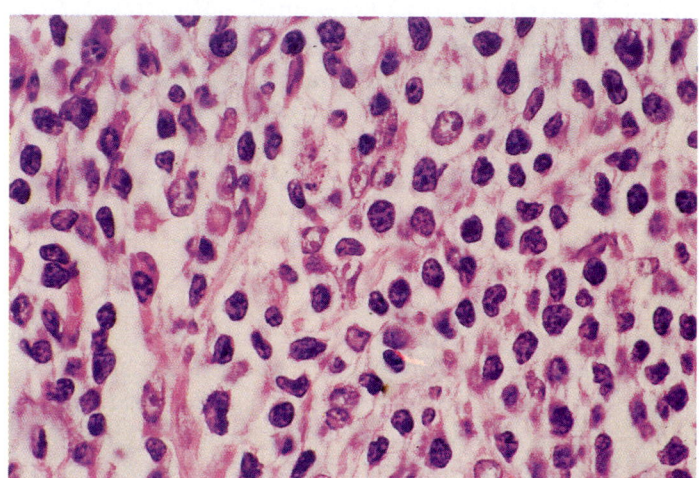

B

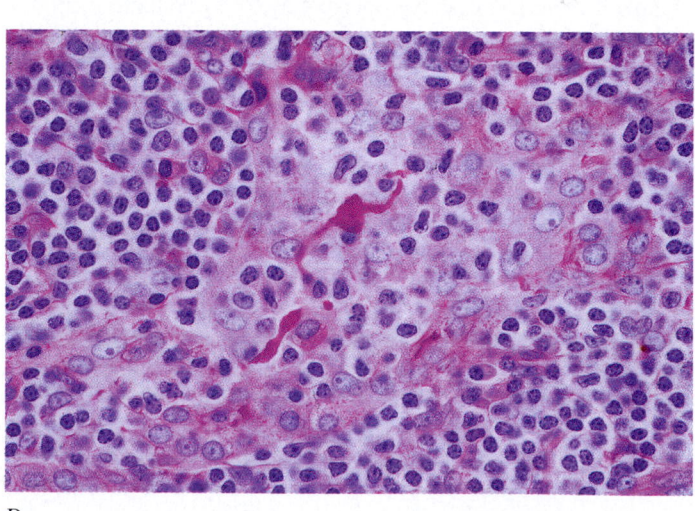

C

D

FIGURE 118-8 Low-grade BALT lymphoma. *A.* This low-grade BALT lymphoma with prominent reactive germinal centers would have previously been classified as "pseudolymphoma." Hematoxylin-eosin, ×20. *B.* Higher magnification reveals the typical dense interfollicular infiltrate of small, round to irregular "centrocytelike" cells with scattered plasma cells. Plasma cells in this case were monoclonal, indicating plasmacytic differentiation; in other cases, they may be polyclonal and reactive. Hematoxylin-eosin, ×500. *C.* Small B cells, found in some cases, have increased pale cytoplasm resembling monocytoid B cells *(left)* with a parafollicular or "marginal zone" distribution (* identifies a reactive germinal center). Hematoxylin-eosin, ×300. *D.* Infiltration of bronchial or bronchiolar epithelium gives rise to characteristic "lymphoepithelial lesions." Hematoxylin-eosin, ×300. (A and D *from Salhany,[38] with permission.*)

The neoplastic small B cells in BALT lymphomas express monotypic immunoglobulin and B-cell–associated antigens but do not express CD5, as seen in small lymphocytic or mantle cell lymphoma, or CD10, as seen in small cleaved follicular lymphoma. Furthermore, BALT lymphomas do not have bcl-1 or bcl-2 gene rearrangements, which are characteristic of mantle cell and small cleaved follicular lymphomas, respectively.[16,38] At the present time there are no markers that specifically define cells of BALT origin. Consistent cytogenetic abnormalities have not been described in BALT lymphomas; trisomy 3, found in some gastrointestinal MALT lymphomas, has not been associated with BALT lymphomas.

Hilar and mediastinal lymph nodes are usually not involved by BALT lymphomas, but when they are involved, the lymphomatous infiltration preferentially involves the parafollicular or marginal zone, similar to monocytoid B-cell lymphomas. Bone marrow biopsies are typically negative in low-grade BALT lymphomas.

Low-grade, small T-cell lymphomas are extremely rare, constituting only 1.5 percent of primary pulmonary lymphomas in one large series.[24] It is uncertain whether these rare cases are derived from the T-cell component of the BALT.

Radiographic Features

The results of radiographic imaging studies are quite variable. The densities may be homogeneous and sometimes quite large, located centrally or peripherally; the lesions may be either single (Fig. 118-9) or multiple. Radiographic differentiation from

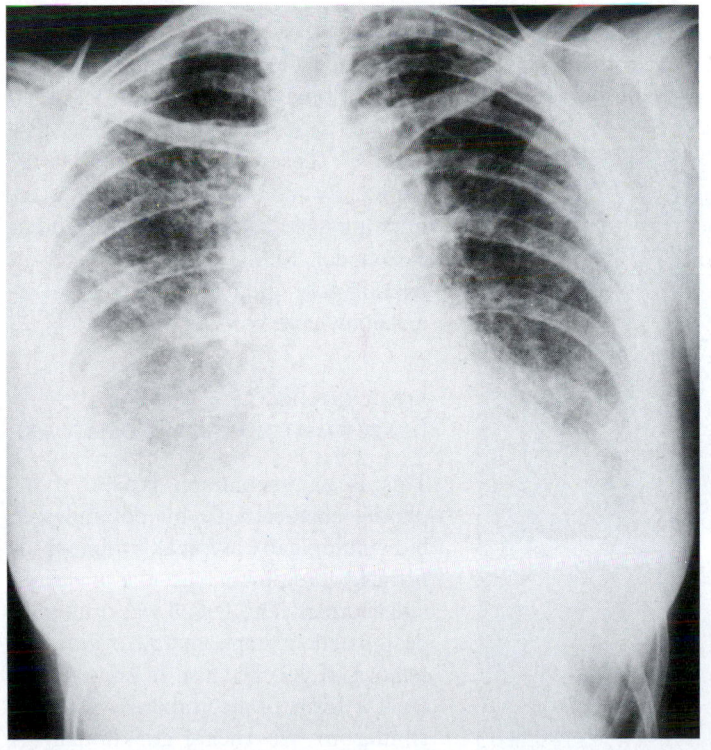

FIGURE 118-9 Low-grade BALT lymphoma. Posteroanterior radiograph showing an area of airspace consolidation in the right lower lobe. The hilum and mediastinum are normal. *(Courtesy of Dr. W. T. Miller, Sr.)*

lung carcinoma is often not possible. Alternatively, there is a reticulonodular infiltrate simulating lymphangitic spread of metastatic carcinoma or pneumonic consolidation, which may involve one or several lobes. Air bronchograms are usually present but cavitation and hilar adenopathy are usually absent. In one large series, atelectasis and pleural effusion were reported in about 3 percent of patients.[9]

Clinical Presentation

Patients with low-grade lymphomas at presentation range in age from 25 to 85 years, with a peak incidence in the sixth decade of life.[9,24] Both sexes are equally affected. Nearly half of the patients are asymptomatic and the disease is discovered on a routine chest radiograph. In some patients, abnormal chest radiographs are present for several years before biopsy and definitive histopathologic diagnosis.[9] Symptoms are nonspecific, consisting of cough, mild dyspnea, hemoptysis, and crackles over the involved areas. The presence of constitutional symptoms such as fever, weight loss, and night sweats suggests extrathoracic involvement.

Lung function studies may reveal an obstructive ventilatory defect. Serologic studies show a monoclonal gammopathy, most often IgM, in about 25 percent of cases; in some cases free kappa or lambda light chains can be demonstrated.

In half of the patients, fiberoptic bronchoscopy reveals bronchial stenosis or inflammation. Transbronchial biopsy may show lymphomatous infiltration of the bronchial wall. In some instances, bronchoalveolar lavage has been successful in demonstrating monoclonal populations of small lymphocytes.

Prognosis

The prognosis of BALT lymphomas depends on the predominant cell type and stage of the disease. The vast majority of low-grade BALT lymphomas are indolent, localized tumors that are usually cured by surgery alone. Chemotherapy and radiation may be indicated if the patient is symptomatic and surgery is not feasible. Extrapulmonary involvement should be ruled out by bone marrow examination and appropriate imaging studies. Careful follow-up is essential, since BALT lymphomas may recur locally or in other extrapulmonary MALT sites. Most patients who experience a relapse in their disease have prolonged disease-free intervals between recurrences. An important reason for careful follow-up is that some cases can transform from low-grade, small-cell to high-grade, large B-cell lymphoma, which is associated with more aggressive behavior.[12,24]

High-Grade Large B-Cell Lymphomas

Pathology

High-grade large cell lymphomas represent 6 to 20 percent of primary pulmonary lymphomas.[12,24] The vast majority are B-cell lymphomas subclassified as either diffuse large noncleaved cell or immunoblastic large cell types. Some of these lymphomas have developed on a background of low-grade BALT lymphoma, suggesting that many primary pulmonary large cell lymphomas are of BALT origin. However, specific markers are not available to confirm BALT origin for most pulmonary large cell lymphomas.

Grossly, most primary large cell lymphomas of the lung are solitary masses larger than 3 cm in diameter, but sometimes they appear as diffuse infiltrates or multiple nodules along lymphatic routes (Fig. 118-10). The cut surfaces reveal white-tan fleshy tumors, often with foci of necrosis or cavitation. Histologically, the tumors are composed of sheets of large transformed lymphocytes with large noncleaved cell or immunoblastic morphology (Fig. 118-11). The histologic appearance of large cell BALT lymphomas usually cannot be distinguished from that of other large cell non-Hodgkin's lymphomas unless a residual low-grade BALT component is present. Mitotic activity is usually prominent, and foci of tumor necrosis are often seen. Lymphatic tracking of lymphoma along bronchovascular bundles, interlobular septa, and visceral pleura may be present at the periphery of tumors, or benign lymphoid hyperplasia along lymphatic routes may be found.

Except for angiocentric lymphomas, other primary high-grade T-cell lymphomas of lung are rare.[12,24] Most are either diffuse large cell or mixed medium and large pleomorphic cell types. Most high-grade T-cell lymphomas in the lung represent secondary involvement by extrapulmonary peripheral T-cell lymphomas.

Clinical Presentation

In contrast to the low-grade lymphoma, patients with high-grade lymphoma usually present with pulmonary and constitutional symptoms: cough, dyspnea, hemoptysis, loss of weight, and fever.[9,24] Pulmonary function studies often show a restrictive pattern. Bronchoscopy may show mucosal inflammation or stenosis due to lymphomatous infiltration.

Radiographic Features

Chest radiographs or computed tomography (CT) scans reveal nodular masses or diffuse pneumonic infiltrates with air bron-

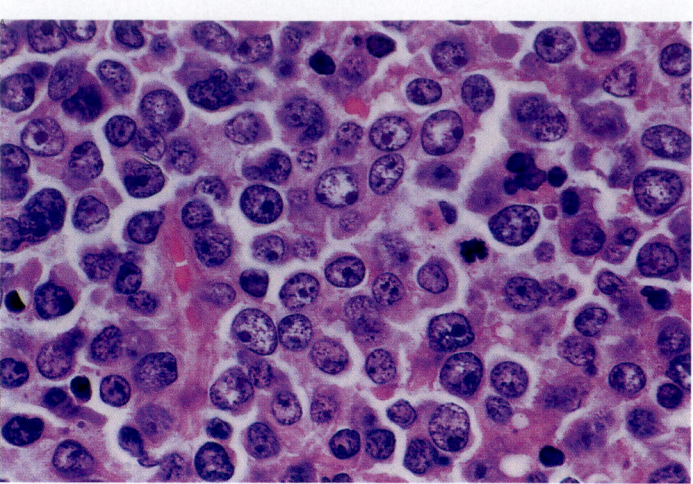

FIGURE 118-11   High-grade large B-cell lymphoma, BALT-derived. This lymphoma has a diffuse proliferation of monomorphic large transformed lymphocytes with vesicular chromatin and prominent nucleoli. Apoptotic cells indicate areas of focal necrosis. Pulmonary large cell lymphomas may arise de novo or secondary to transformation of low-grade BALT lymphoma. Hematoxylin-eosin, ×500.

chograms. The nodules may be multiple and may cavitate secondary to necrosis (Fig. 118-12);[17] nodules and infiltrates may also develop rapidly, suggesting an infectious process or vasculitis. The hilar and mediastinal lymph nodes are usually not enlarged radiographically but may be involved on microscopic examination. Pleural effusions, with or without lymphoma cells, may be present.

Prognosis

Even with aggressive chemotherapy, the survival rate of patients with high-grade pulmonary lymphomas is significantly less than that of patients with low-grade disease.[9,24] These tumors are prone to recur locally and often disseminate to extrapulmonary sites, usually to other extranodal MALT sites. Despite an overall poor prognosis, long-term remissions have been reported.[24]

ANGIOCENTRIC LYMPHOMA (LYMPHOMATOID GRANULOMATOSIS)

This is an uncommon type of lymphoma characterized by polymorphic but cytologically atypical lymphoid infiltrates, prominent vascular invasion, and necrosis. This lesion was originally designated lymphomatoid granulomatosis (LyG) because it was considered a form of necrotizing vasculitis similar to Wegener's granulomatosis but with a propensity to progress to malignant lymphoma.[25] It has also been designated polymorphic reticulosis, malignant angiitis, and granulomatosis.

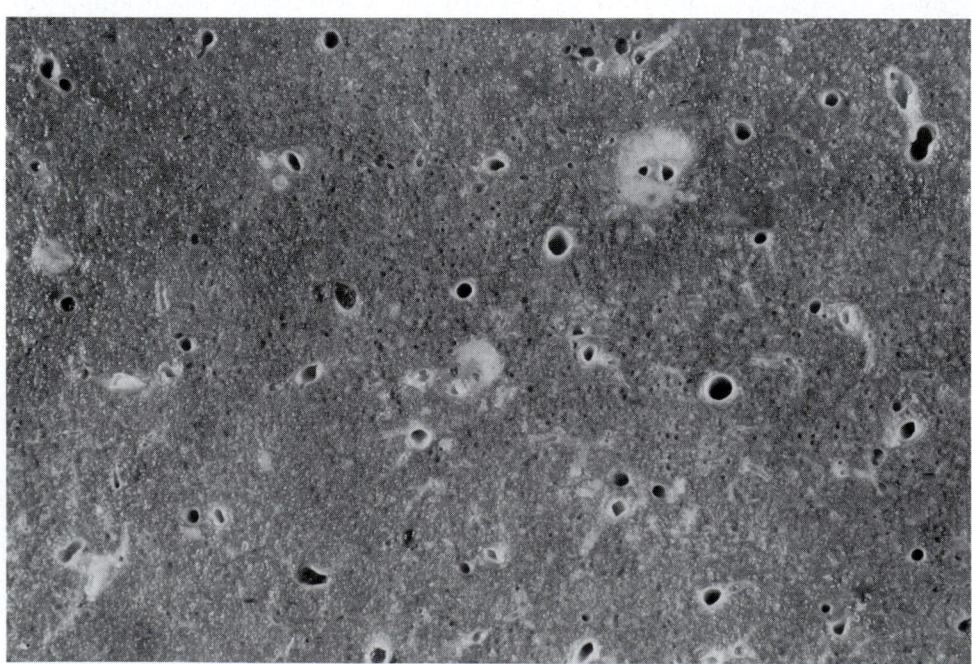

FIGURE 118-10   Primary high-grade pulmonary lymphoma. Multiple well-demarcated tumor nodules (*white*) of variable size are located along lymphatic routes.

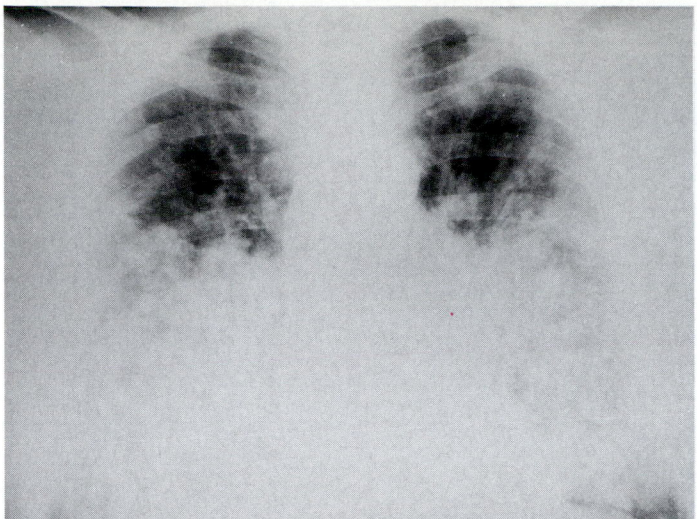

FIGURE 118-12 Primary high-grade pulmonary lymphoma. Posteroanterior radiograph revealing extensive involvement of both lungs, with multiple nodular opacities of homogeneous density. *(Courtesy of Dr. W. T. Miller, Sr.)*

Pathology

The macroscopic appearance of angiocentric lymphoma is that of multiple gray-white nodules with a variable degree of necrosis. Microscopically, the nodules contain angiocentric, polymorphic infiltrates with foci of necrosis centered around vessels. The vessel walls are infiltrated transmurally by a polymorphic infiltrate of small lymphocytes, plasma cells, histiocytes, variable numbers of atypical large transformed lymphocytes, and immunoblasts with prominent nucleoli (Fig. 118-13). Transmural infiltration, particularly of intimal regions, can be so severe as to totally obliterate the vascular lumen, resulting in ischemic necrosis of the surrounding tumor and lung parenchyma.

The current consensus is that LyG is a distinctive polymorphic form of angiocentric lymphoma.[16,31,45] The polymerase chain reaction (PCR) and in situ hybridization studies have strongly implicated the Epstein-Barr virus (EBV) in the pathogenesis of pulmonary angiocentric lymphomas (Fig. 118-14).[15,31] These lesions were initially thought to be peripheral T-cell lymphomas because immunophenotyping studies demonstrated a predominance of atypical cells expressing T-cell–associated antigens.[26] However, T-cell receptor gene re-

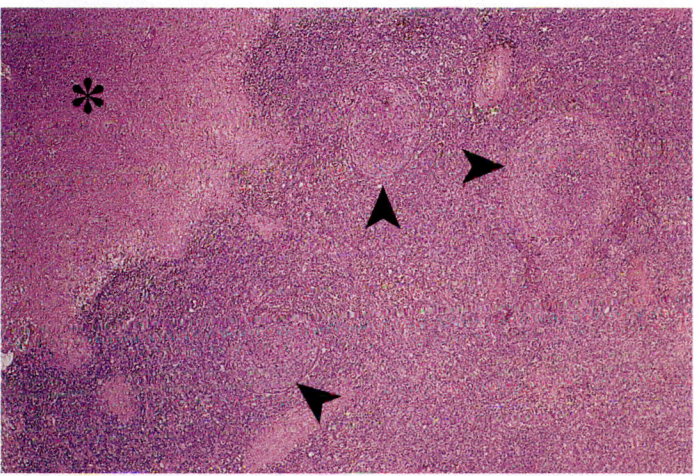

A

B

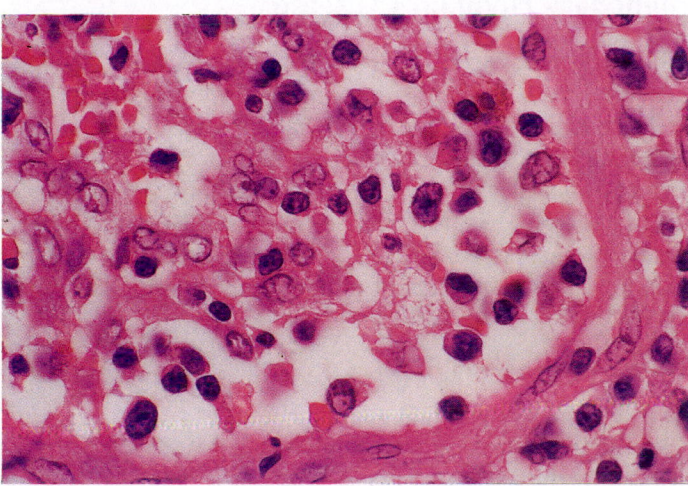

C

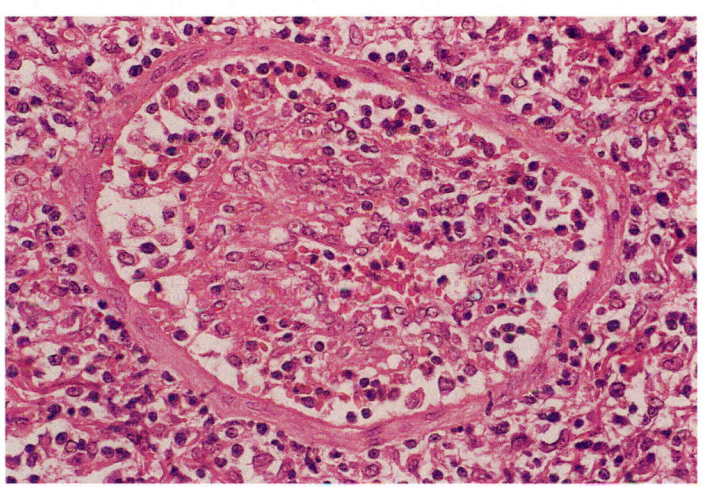

D

FIGURE 118-13 Angiocentric lymphoma (LyG, AIL). *A.* Lymphoma with extensive vascular infiltration and severe luminal narrowing *(arrows)*, resulting in a large focus of necrosis (*). Hematoxylin-eosin, ×40. *B.* Severe vascular occlusion by an extensive polymorphic intimal and transmural infiltrate typical of classic LyG (angiocentric lymphoma, mixed small and large cell; AIL grade 2). Hematoxylin-eosin, ×200. *C.* Higher magnification showing the mixed intimal infiltrate of small lymphocytes, histiocytes, eosinophils, and atypical large transformed lymphocytes. Hematoxylin-eosin, ×500. *D.* Angiocentric large cell lymphoma (AIL grade 3) showing a relatively monomorphic intimal infiltrate of large transformed lymphocytes. A residual band of smooth muscle from the vessel wall media is present *(arrow)*. Hematoxylin-eosin, ×300.

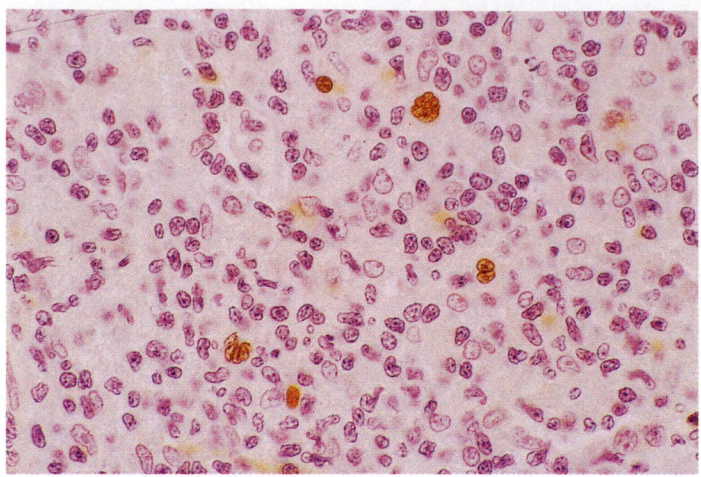

FIGURE 118-14 Angiocentric lymphoma, in situ hybridization for EBV. Scattered nuclei of large atypical lymphocytes are positive for EBER-1 RNA *(brown).* DAB-hematoxylin, ×300. *(Case provided by Dr. Betsy Schloo, Deborah Heart and Lung Center, Brown Mills, NJ.)*

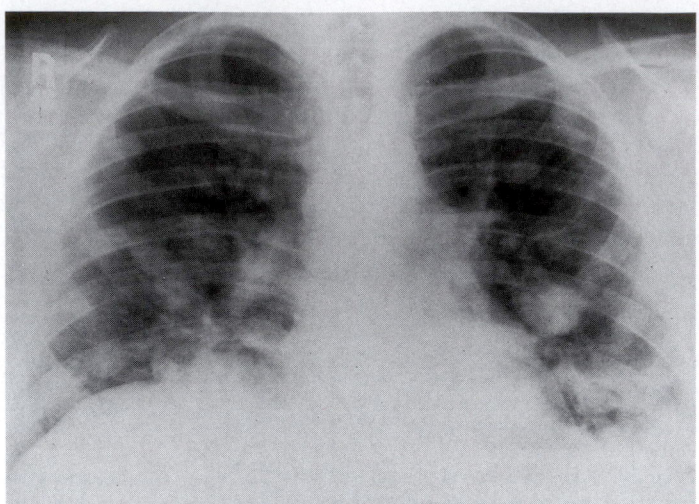

FIGURE 118-15 Angiocentric lymphoma. Posteroanterior roentgenogram showing multiple bilateral isolated and confluent nodular opacities. *(Courtesy of Dr. W. T. Miller, Sr.)*

arrangement studies have usually been germline. Recently, PCR and immunohistochemistry studies have demonstrated small, monoclonal populations of large, atypical, EBV-positive B cells, indicating that many angiocentric lymphomas of LyG type are actually EBV-positive B-cell lymphomas with a high content of reactive T cells.[15,31] However, some lesions appear to be peripheral T-cell lymphomas; these tumors are EBV-negative.[31]

Clinical Presentation

Since the spectrum of pulmonary lymphomas has broadened, there is considerable overlap in the clinical presentation of patients with LyG (angiocentric lymphoma) and other forms of pulmonary lymphomas. Series of cases defined on the basis of strict morphologic criteria have shown a distinct male preponderance and a peak incidence in the fifth decade of life. Respiratory symptoms, cough, dyspnea, and chest pain are present in the majority of patients at the time of diagnosis and are frequently associated with systemic symptoms—i.e., fever, malaise, and weight loss. Extrathoracic manifestations are common, most often due to involvement of the skin, kidneys, central nervous system, or peripheral nerves. Occasionally, respiratory symptoms are the initial manifestations of the disease.

Radiographic Features

The radiographic findings are variable, depending on the stage of evolution of the disease. Typically, there are bilateral nodules (Fig. 118-15) that may contain cavities with thick walls.[17] Radiographic findings are occasionally limited to nonspecific reticulonodular infiltrates.[6] The nodules may rapidly increase or decrease in size and may even disappear completely. Hilar adenopathy is rare. Pleural effusion is present in one-third of the patients.

Prognosis

Lymphomatoid granulomatosis is an aggressive angiocentric lymphoma. The prognosis is related to the extent of involvement of the lung and extrathoracic sites and to the histologic grade. In general, the prognosis is inversely related to the percentage of large atypical lymphocytes. The grading system devised by Lipford and colleagues[26] identified histologic grades of "angiocentric immunoproliferative lesions" (AIL). Grade 1 AIL corresponds to benign lymphocytic vasculitis and responds to chlorambucil. Grades 2 and 3 represent angiocentric lymphomas. Grade 2 AIL corresponds to classic LyG or mixed small and large cell angiocentric lymphoma (Fig 118-13*B* and *C*). Grade 3 AIL represents large cell angiocentric lymphoma (Fig. 118-13*D*). Until recently, nearly two-thirds of the patients with grade 2 or 3 angiocentric lymphomas were dead within a year of diagnosis. Advances in chemotherapy have improved the prognosis somewhat.

Pulmonary Hodgkin's Disease

Pulmonary involvement with Hodgkin's disease is usually by direct extension from intrathoracic nodal sites. Primary pulmonary Hodgkin's disease is rare.[36,47] Pulmonary involvement with Hodgkin's disease has been found at first encounter in 12 percent of patients with mediastinal or extrathoracic disease; it sometimes represents the major site of initial disease.[47] Over 50 percent of patients with Hodgkin's disease have lung involvement at autopsy. Lung and pleura are also common sites of relapse.

Pathology

Hodgkin's disease, regardless of its primary or secondary origin, forms tumor nodules along the lymphatic routes in the bronchovascular bundles, the interlobular septa, and the visceral pleura. Coalescence of tumor nodules along the lymphatic routes gives rise to masses that may cavitate or compress adjacent alveolar spaces. Infiltration of bronchial mucosa from tumor along bronchovascular bundles can result in diffuse thickening or endobronchial polypoid masses. Disseminated Hodgkin's disease often gives rise to a miliary pattern of lung involvement due to numerous small tumor nodules along lymphatic routes.

The microscopic appearance of pulmonary Hodgkin's disease can resemble all of the histologic variants seen in lymph nodes, but most have features of nodular sclerosis. The diagnostic elements are Reed-Sternberg cells and variants in an appropriate reactive background of small lymphocytes, plasma cells, eosinophils, histiocytes, and variable amounts of collagen fibrosis (Fig. 118-16). Occasionally lesions are necrotic, with or without large numbers of eosinophils and neutrophils, which may mimic infectious abscesses or other forms of necrotizing inflammation (Fig. 118-17). Nonnecrotizing giant cell granulomas may also be present but usually represent a reaction to noninfectious antigenic stimuli.

Clinical Manifestations

Most patients with Hodgkin's disease present with enlarged lymph nodes or with constitutional symptoms such as fever, night sweats, pruritus, weight loss, and fatigue. Those with pulmonary involvement may also have cough and dyspnea. A mediastinal mass or hilar lymphadenopathy usually accompanies pulmonary

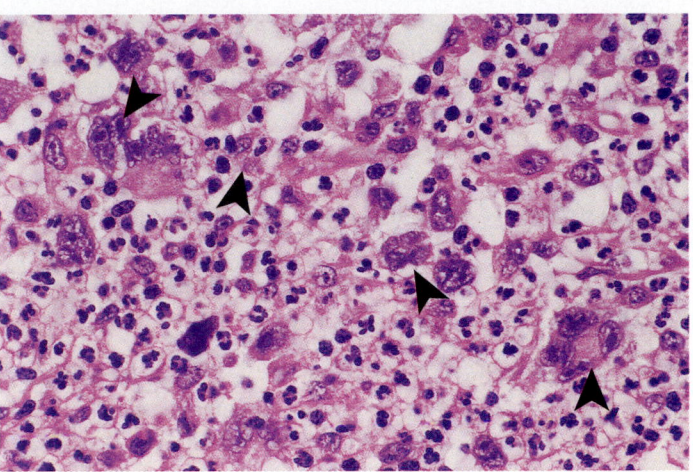

FIGURE 118-17 Pulmonary Hodgkin's disease mimicking an abscess. Numerous neutrophils and eosinophils in the inflammatory reaction to Hodgkin's disease can lead to confusion with an infectious pulmonary abscess. Identification of Reed-Sternberg cells and variants *(arrows)* among the inflammatory cells establishes the correct diagnosis. Hematoxylin-eosin, ×300.

involvement. Pleural effusion occurs in about one-third of patients, probably secondary to extensive lymphatic obstruction. Patients with primary pulmonary Hodgkin's disease have the same bimodal age distribution and symptoms as those with pulmonary involvement secondary to nodal disease, but females predominate.[36,47] The most common sites of relapse following mediastinal radiation therapy are the lungs, pleura, upper mediastinal lymph nodes, and diaphragm.

Radiographic Features

The most common radiographic appearance in Hodgkin's disease is a coarse reticulonodular and linear pattern reflecting the anatomic distribution along the lymphatic routes of the bronchovascular bundles, interlobular septa, and pleura. Confluent nodules may form large opacities with central cavitation. Lymph nodes at bronchial bifurcations may be enlarged. Bronchial obstruction by extrinsic compression or endobronchial polypoid lesions can result in lobar or segmental atelectasis.

Prognosis and Staging

Patients with Hodgkin's disease have an overall 5-year survival of approximately 75 percent with current radiation and chemotherapy regimens. Stage is the single most important prognostic factor and is the primary factor that dictates the type of therapy given.[41] Patients with primary pulmonary Hodgkin's disease are clinical stage I$_E$ (extranodal). An "E" designation is also given to secondary pulmonary involvement due to contiguous spread from mediastinal or hilar nodal Hodgkin's disease to distinguish these patients from those with pulmonary involvement secondary to disseminated stage IV Hodgkin's disease.[27] Contiguous lung involvement is considered equivalent to a contiguous lymph node group for assigment of the principal stage. Thus, a patient with stage II Hodgkin's disease with a mediastinal mass and contiguous lung involvement is designated stage II$_E$ rather than stage IV.

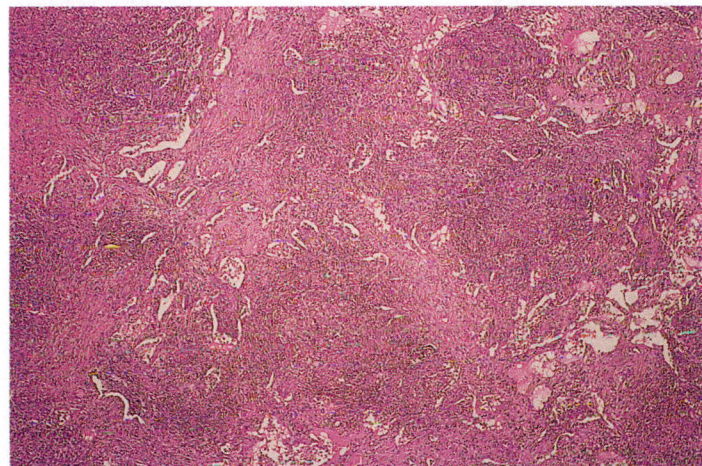

A

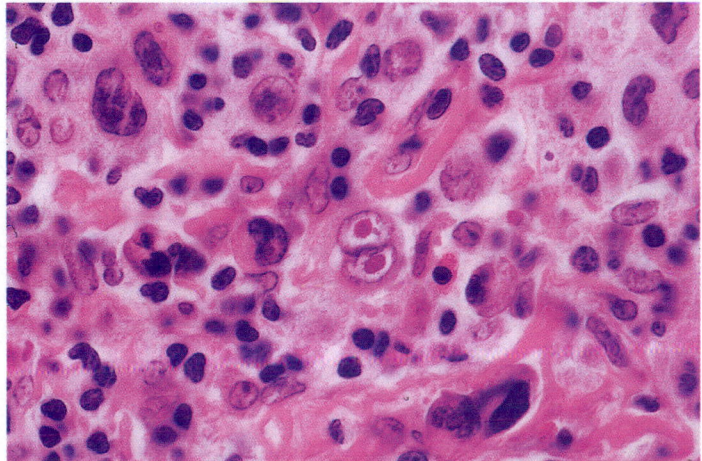

B

FIGURE 118-16 Pulmonary Hodgkin's disease. *A.* Low magnification shows several ill-defined tumor nodules with intervening fibrosis in a nodular sclerosis pattern. Hematoxylin-eosin, ×20. *B.* Binucleate Reed-Sternberg cell in a reactive background of small lymphocytes, scattered plasma cells, and eosinophils. Hematoxylin-eosin, ×500.

Other important prognostic variables for patients with Hodgkin's disease include age, bulky mediastinal disease, and histologic subtype; however, the independent significance of histologic subclassification has greatly diminished with current therapeutic regimens.[10] Patients with Hodgkin's disease are also at increased risk for the development of non-Hodgkin's lymphoma and therapy-related acute leukemia and myelodysplasia.

Other Lymphoproliferative and Hematologic Disorders Involving the Lung

Secondary involvement of lung by disseminated lymphoma is much more common than primary pulmonary lymphoma. Pulmonary involvement can be documented in up to 50 percent of common nodal lymphomas at some time during their course; lung is one of the most frequently involved organs at autopsy. The pattern of lung involvement tends to follow lymphatic routes along bronchovascular bundles, interlobular septa, and visceral pleura. Disseminated lymphoma usually presents as multiple pulmonary nodules or with a miliary pattern.

Systemic lymphoma, lymphoproliferative disorders, and hematologic diseases that may present with prominent lung involvement include posttransplant lymphoproliferative disorders, HIV-related lymphomas, intravascular lymphoma, multiple myeloma and extramedullary plasmacytoma, Langerhans' cell histiocytosis, leukemia, and graft-versus-host disease. Pulmonary manifestations of these diseases are discussed below.

POSTTRANSPLANT LYMPHOPROLIFERATIVE DISORDER AND HIV-RELATED LYMPHOMA

Lymphoid proliferations morphologically indistinguishable from malignant lymphoma occur with greater frequency in organ transplant recipients than in the general population; but, unlike malignant lymphomas in immunocompetent patients, these lesions often regress if immunosuppression is sufficiently reduced.[19,32] Epstein-Barr virus infection, either preexisting in the recipient or acquired from the donor, is strongly implicated in the pathogenesis of posttransplant lymphoproliferative disorder (PTLD).[30,37] Immunosuppression is thought to permit uncontrolled proliferation of EBV-stimulated B cells by inhibition of suppressor T cells. Initial polymorphic, polyclonal proliferations progress to monomorphic, monoclonal proliferations. Monoclonal proliferations can subsequently acquire mutations of oncogenes or tumor suppressor genes, leading to fully malignant behavior and loss of responsiveness to restored immune regulation. Mutations of c-*myc*, N-*ras,* and p53 genes have recently been implicated in terminal progression of PTLD.[19,28]

This condition frequently involves extranodal sites, including lung. Lung involvement by PTLD may present as nodular or diffuse reticulonodular infiltrates, as solitary or multiple lung masses, or with hilar and mediastinal lymphadenopathy.[6] Pulmonary nodules often have foci of necrosis. Histologically, PTLD can range from polymorphic B-cell hyperplasia to monomorphic B-cell proliferations indistinguishable from diffuse large cell or immunoblastic lymphoma.[19,32] Polymorphic B-cell hyperplasia has a mixture of small lymphocytes, plasma

cells, and immunoblasts without significant cytologic atypia. These cases are usually polyclonal and respond to reduction in immunosuppression. Monomorphic PTLD has sheets of monoclonal large transformed cells or immunoblasts (Fig. 118-18). In spite of their frankly malignant appearance, some monomorphic tumors will regress after reduction of immunosuppression; nonresponders require chemotherapy but usually succumb to progressive disease. Neither histologic appearance nor clonality studies can accurately predict response of an individual patient to reduction in immunosuppression.

The incidence of PTLD is greatest among heart (2 to 13 percent), lung (12 percent) and heart/lung (5 to 9 percent) transplant recepients; PTLD is reported less frequently in liver (2 percent), renal (1 to 3 percent), and bone marrow (1 to 2 percent) transplants.[7,19,30] These differences in incidence of PTLD may be partly attributed to higher doses of cyclosporine A or anti-OKT3

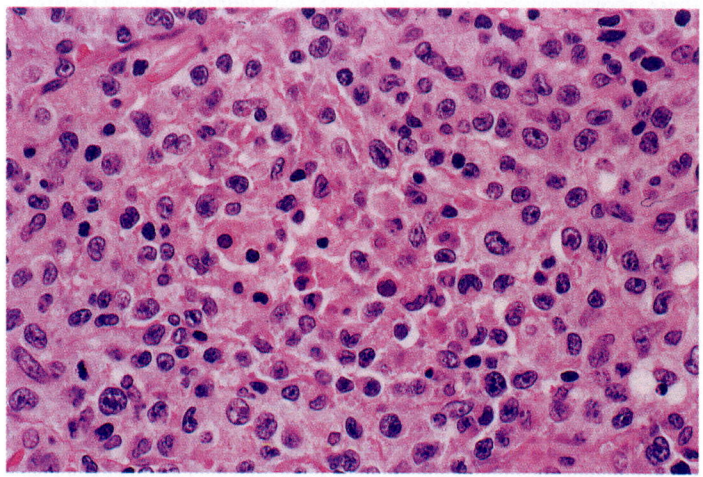

A

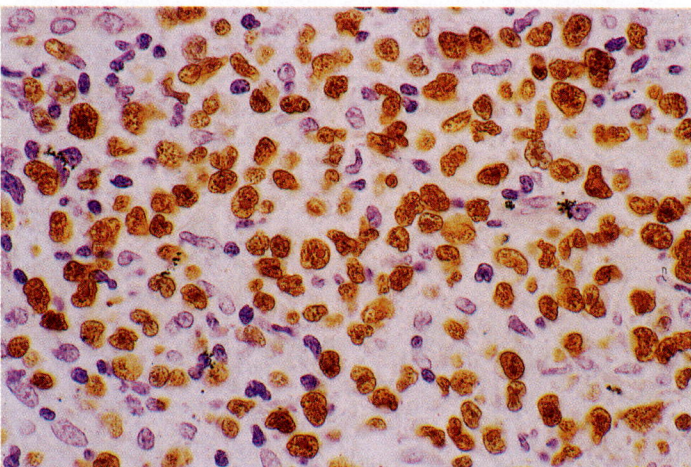

B

FIGURE 118-18   Pulmonary PTLD in a cardiac transplant patient. *A.* This PTLD composed of monomorphic large immunoblastic cells would be diagnosed as immunoblastic large cell lymphoma in an immunocompetent patient; it was proven to be monoclonal. However, a second pulmonary nodule regressed following reduction in immunosuppression. Hematoxylin-eosin, ×300. *B.* In situ hybridization for EBV RNA is strongly positive in nuclei of most large atypical cells *(brown)*. Biotinylated EBER-1 probe, DAB-hematoxylin, ×300.

in immunosuppressive regimens for heart and lung transplantation. Another possible contributing factor may be transplantation of BALT and nodal tissue harboring EBV in the donor transplant. This is supported by studies from our lung transplantation program that have demonstrated EBV genome in 14 percent of the peribronchial lymph nodes from donor lungs.[30] In lung transplant recipients, PTLD may develop in the allograft lung, lymph nodes, or other MALT sites. The peak incidence of PTLD is 3 to 4 months after transplantation, but it may develop as early as 6 days after transplantation. Patients with early onset of PTLD within the first year have a better prognosis than those developing disease later.[3] Treatment of PTLD is most effective in early stages, before progression to monomorphic, monoclonal proliferations occurs.

Immunosuppressed patients with HIV infection also have an increased incidence of pulmonary lymphomas.[7,23] These lymphomas are generally high grade with diffuse large cell, immunoblastic, or small noncleaved cell (Burkitt or Burkitt-like) morphology. Like PTLD, HIV-related lymphomas are usually EBV-positive B-cell proliferations; however, unlike PTLD, these lymphomas respond poorly to therapy because immunocompetence cannot be restored.

INTRAVASCULAR (ANGIOTROPIC) LARGE CELL LYMPHOMA

This rare neoplastic disorder is a large B-cell lymphoma characterized by multifocal intravascular proliferation of atypical, large transformed lymphocytes (Fig. 118-19).[43] These lymphomas differ from angiocentric lymphomas in that lymphoma is confined within the lumens of blood vessels without infiltration of the vessel walls or surrounding tissue. Despite plugging of vascular lumens by lymphoma, necrosis of surrounding tissue and peripheral blood involvement are not seen.

Intravascular lymphoma most commonly affects the central nervous system and the skin, but also frequently involves the lungs and other organs.[43,45] Rarely, clinical manifestations initially present in the lungs with progressive exertional dyspnea, cough, fever, hypoxemia, fine bilateral linear infiltrates on chest radiographs, and reduced diffusion capacity on pulmonary function tests.[45] Prognosis is extremely poor, largely due to difficulty in reaching the diagnosis. Many cases escape detection until autopsy because clinical symptoms are nonspecific and ill defined. Early diagnosis and aggressive chemotherapy may lead to improved survival.[11]

PULMONARY PLASMACYTOMA AND MULTIPLE MYELOMA

Pulmonary involvement in multiple myeloma is common at some time during its course, but solitary plasmacytoma originating in the lung is very rare.[18] Pulmonary plasmacytoma presents as a nodule or lobulated mass composed of a pure population of plasma cells with varying degrees of atypia. Amyloid or immunoglobulin deposits may be present around blood vessels or within the tumor. In small biopsies, immunohistochemistry may be useful in distinguishing plasmacytoma from plasma cell granuloma (see "Inflammatory Myofibroblastic Tumor," above). Primary pulmonary plasmacytoma is usually not associated with serum or urine paraproteins. Plasmacytomas in general are cured by surgical resection, but progression to disseminated multiple myeloma can occur.[18]

LANGERHANS' CELL HISTIOCYTOSIS (HISTIOCYTOSIS X, EOSINOPHILIC GRANULOMA)

Pulmonary eosinophilic granuloma is a proliferation of Langerhans' histiocytes previously included under the term *histiocytosis X. Langerhans' cell histiocytosis (LCH)* is now the preferred term for these disorders, because they have recently been shown to be clonal proliferations of Langerhans' histiocytes.[44] This condition may present as disseminated acute disease in infants and young children (Letterer-Siwe syndrome), chronic multifocal disease (Hand-Schüller-Christian disease), or indolent, localized disease (eosinophilic granuloma).

Pulmonary LCH may be part of multisystem disease or limited to the lungs (eosinophilic granuloma, primary pulmonary

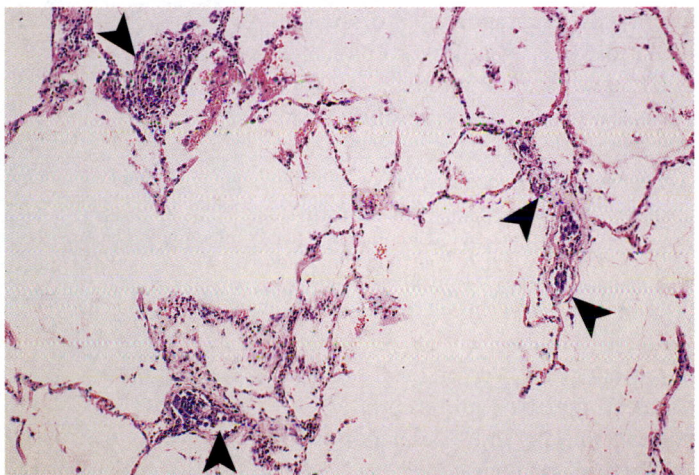

A

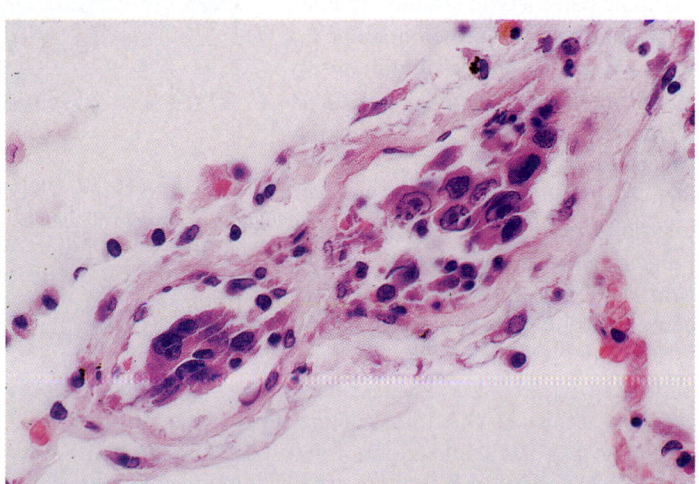

B

FIGURE 118-19   Intravascular large B-cell lymphoma involving lung. Autopsy specimen. *A.* Multiple vascular lumens are filled and distended by intravascular lymphoma *(arrows).* Lymphoma does not infiltrate the surrounding pulmonary parenchyma. Hematoxylin-eosin, ×50. *B.* Higher magnification of a vascular lumen shows large cell lymphoma. Hematoxylin-eosin, ×500.

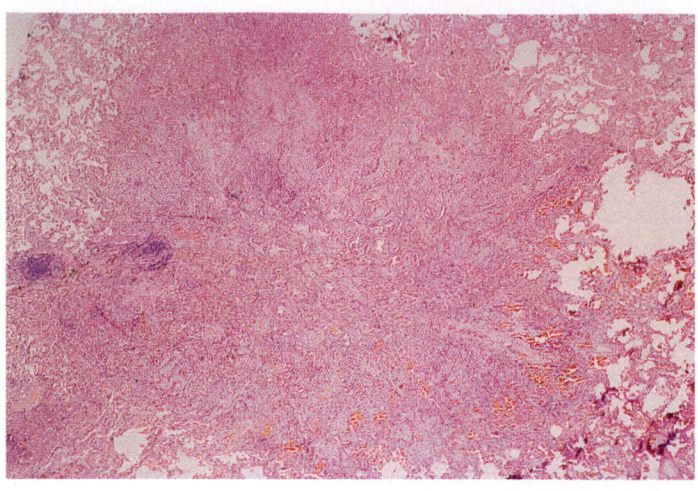

A

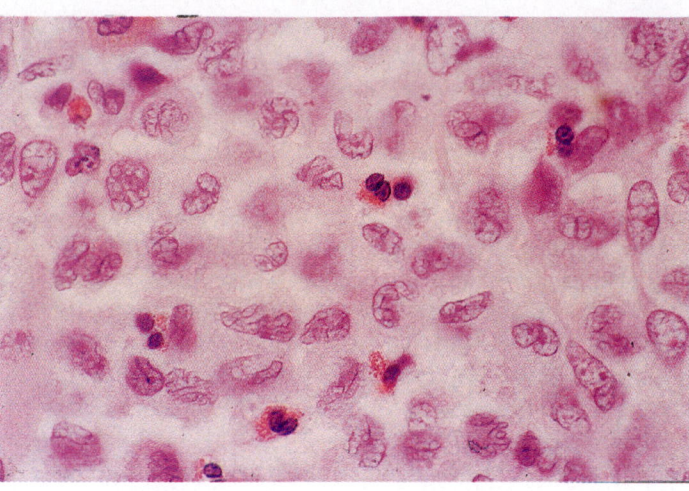

B

LCH).[8,13] Most patients with pulmonary LCH do not have disseminated disease. Primary pulmonary LCH tends to occur in younger adults and may be asymptomatic or present with dyspnea, cough, fatigue, fever, or weight loss. Pulmonary function tests may demonstrate decreased diffusing capacity and vital capacity. Radiographically, pulmonary LCH may present as solitary nodules or as bilateral, reticulonodular, interstitial infiltrates or densities, preferentially involving middle and basilar regions.

The gross appearance of pulmonary LCH resembles the radiographic pattern with solitary nodules or widespread, ill-defined nodular infiltrates. Early infiltrates within the interstitium of alveolar septa as well as the peribronchial and perivascular tissue progress to form interstitial nodules (Fig. 118-20*A*). The defining histologic feature is proliferation of Langerhans' histiocytes with prominent nuclear folds and grooves accompanied by a variable background of eosinophils, giant cells, and lymphocytes (Fig. 118-20*B*). Langerhans' cells are defined by the ultrastructural presence of Birbeck granules (Fig. 118-20*C*), and expression of CD1 antigen, S-100 protein, and a variety of histiocyte-associated antigens. Large nodules may undergo central necrosis and cavitation. Late lesions in chronic progressive disease develop fibrosis, which may lead to emphysema, bronchiectasis, and honeycomb lung.[8]

The prognosis in pulmonary LCH is generally favorable.[8,13] Most solitary lung lesions are cured with surgical resection; multifocal lung disease will often regress or stabilize, but some cases progress to chronic fibrosis, emphysema, and bronchiectasis.

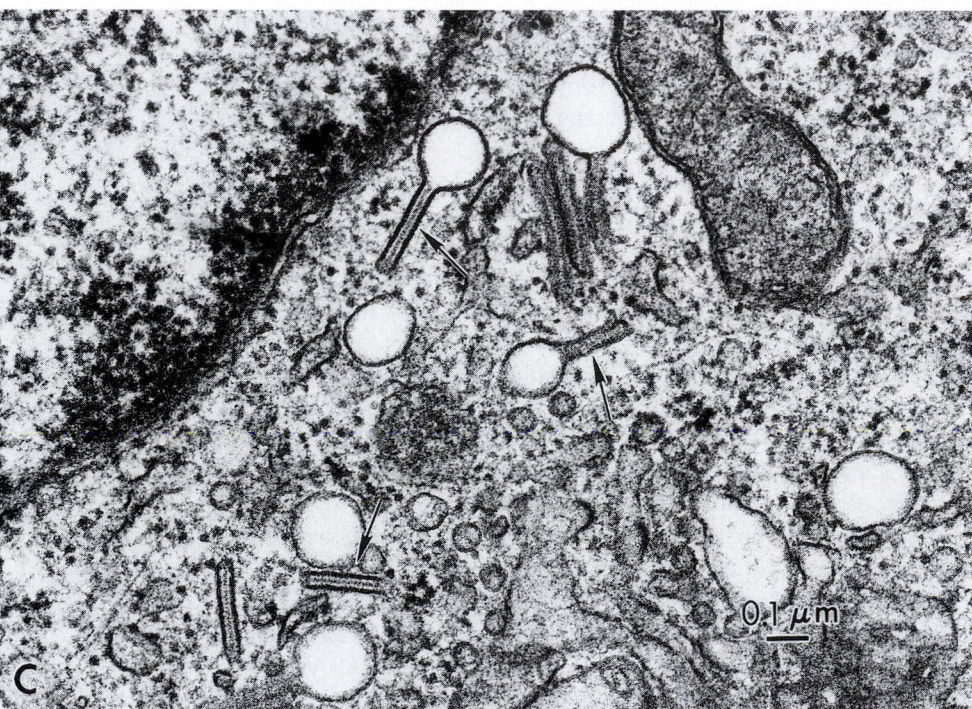

C

FIGURE 118-20   Pulmonary Langerhans' cell histiocytosis (eosinophilic granuloma, histiocytosis X). *A.* A consolidated nodule shows interstitial extension of the infiltrate at the periphery. Hematoxylin-eosin, ×20. *B.* The nodule contains a proliferation of Langerhans' histiocytes with characteristic nuclear folding and grooves along with scattered eosinophils and small lymphocytes. Hematoxylin-eosin, ×500. *C.* Electron microscopy of Langerhans' histiocytes demonstrates the characteristic racquet- and rod-shaped Birbeck granules within their cytoplasm. Uranyl acetate–lead citrate, ×75,000.

Progressive pulmonary disease may respond to radiation or chemotherapy.[13]

LEUKEMIA

Pulmonary complications occur in nearly 80 percent of patients with leukemia. Microscopic pulmonary and pleural infiltrates are commonly found at autopsy; however, the clinical and radiographic abnormalities seen during life are usually due to opportunistic infections, hemorrhage, alveolar proteinosis, or chemotherapy. Pulmonary symptoms directly related to leukemic infiltration—including cough, dyspnea, fever, and hemoptysis—usually result from interstitial infiltrates or leukostasis in poorly controlled acute myeloid or lymphoblastic leukemia with blast cell counts above 100,000/mm³.[22] Pulmonary involvement by chronic lymphocytic leukemia is usually asymptomatic but occasionally may present with marked dyspnea. Leukemic lung involvement should be considered in all symptomatic patients with negative cultures, particularly in acute leukemia with a high blast count.

Microscopically, leukemic cells infiltrate the peribronchial and perivascular interstitium, alveolar septa (Fig. 118-21), and pleura, appearing radiographically as diffuse, bilateral, interstitial, or reticulonodular infiltrates. Occasionally leukemic infiltrates are localized to one or two lobes, mimicking a bacterial pneumonia.[22] Leukostasis is characterized by plugging of the alveolar capillaries and small blood vessels with blast cells and microthrombi. Leukostasis may be associated with interstitial

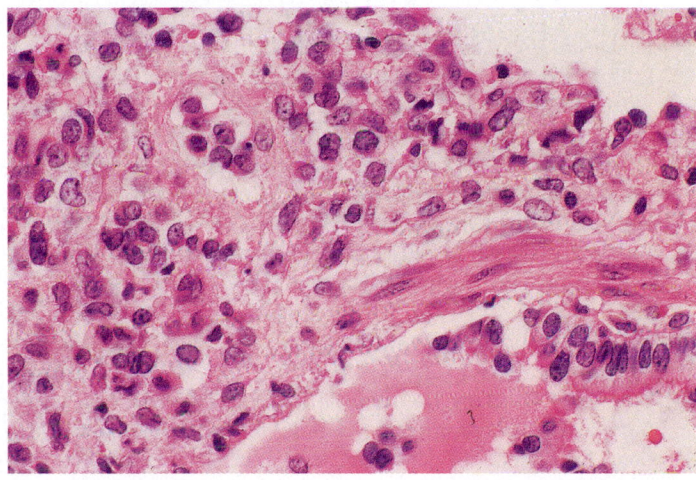

A

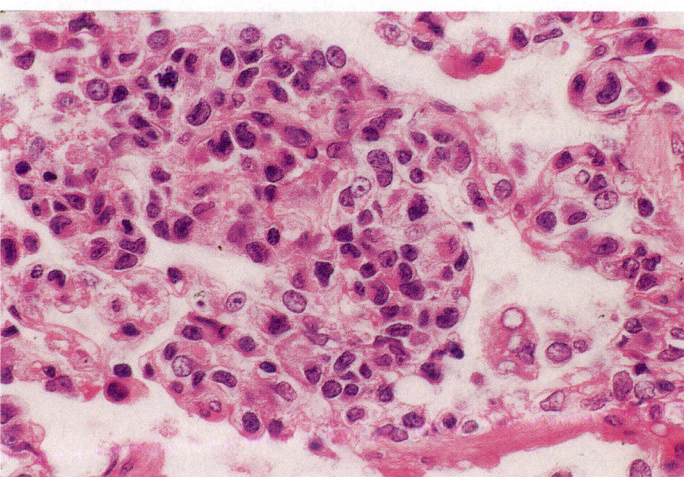

B

FIGURE 118-21   Acute myeloid leukemia involving lung. *A.* Infiltration of the bronchial submucosa by leukemic blast cells. Hematoxylin-eosin, ×300. *B.* Leukostasis of alveolar capillaries and infiltration of alveolar septa by blast cells in a patient with 130,000/mm³ blast cells in the peripheral blood. Hematoxylin-eosin, ×300.

edema and diffuse alveolar damage, possibly due to local ischemia or from the release of toxic byproducts from the leukemic cells.

PULMONARY GRAFT-VERSUS-HOST DISEASE

Allogeneic, autologous, and syngeneic bone marrow transplantation is now the treatment of choice in children and adults with certain hematologic, neoplastic, or genetic disorders. Pulmonary complications related to pretransplantation chemotherapy or radiation therapy, posttransplant immunosuppression, and graft-versus-host disease (GVHD) occur in a high percentage of syngeneic and allogeneic bone marrow transplant patients. Pneumonia, pulmonary GVHD, diffuse alveolar damage, lymphocytic interstitial pneumonitis, lymphocytic bronchitis, or proliferative and obstructive bronchiolitis may occur.

Pneumonias caused by encapsulated gram-negative rods and gram-positive cocci are by far the most common pulmonary complications, occurring in 60 to 80 percent of bone marrow transplant recipients within the first month posttransplant. Invasive aspergillosis and candidal pneumonia depend on the length of neutropenia after transplant, whereas cytomegalovirus (CMV) infection is related to recipient seropositivity and GVHD.

Graft-versus-host disease may present as acute or chronic pulmonary disease, and occurs in a significantly higher percentage of allogeneic bone marrow transplant recipients than in those with syngeneic or autologous bone marrow transplants, resulting from minor histocompatibility differences between donor and recipient in HLA-matched transplants. Pulmonary GVHD may manifest as diffuse alveolar damage, lymphocytic interstitial pneumonitis, lymphocytic bronchitis, and bronchiolitis. The pathogenesis of these different forms of GVHD is not well established; distinction from lung injury secondary to CMV or pretransplant chemotherapy is often difficult.

Diffuse alveolar damage, which is characterized by interstitial mononuclear infiltrates, pulmonary edema, and hyaline membranes, may occur early during the first 2 weeks after transplantation or several months later. The early form is believed to be a consequence of pretransplantation chemotherapy and radiation and is usually self-limited, with improvement or resolution occurring within a few weeks.[48] The late-onset diffuse alveolar damage is either due to GVHD or occult infections, particularly with CMV and herpes. Mortality is high for patients with progressive interstitial fibrosis.

Lymphocytic interstitial pneumonia (LIP) is a late manifestation of GVHD that involves the pulmonary interstitial space and airways.[48] LIP presents with diffuse interstitial infiltrates, fever, increasing dyspnea, and hypoxemia. Progression to interstitial fibrosis can occur.

Lymphocytic bronchitis is characterized by focal epithelial necrosis, reparative epithelial hyperplasia, and lymphoplasmacytic infiltration of the mucosa and submucosa. The airway infiltrates may be associated with varying degrees of interstitial lymphocytic pneumonitis. Clinical symptoms are nonspecific, with subacute onset of a dry, nonproductive cough and dyspnea, often associated with evidence of GVHD in the skin, intestine, and liver. Chest roentgenograms may be normal or may show mild hyperinflation or bilateral interstitial infiltrates.

Proliferative and obstructive bronchiolitis, with or without organizing pneumonia, may occur as either an early or a late complication of bone marrow transplantation and can be rapidly progressive. Patients with chronic GVHD and low immunoglobulin levels are at particular risk for bronchiolitis, which may progress to severe respiratory insufficiency and require treatment by lung transplant.

Other pulmonary complications of allogeneic bone marrow transplantation include diffuse alveolar hemorrhages, with and without microangiopathy and veno-occlusive disease. These serious complications are believed to be induced by pretransplantation chemotherapy.

REFERENCES

1. Addis B, Hyjek E, Isaacson PG: Primary pulmonary lymphoma: A reappraisal of its histogenesis and its relationship to pseudolymphoma and interstitial pneumonia. *Histopathology* 13:1–17, 1988.
2. Altman H, Pietra GG, LiVolsi VA, et al: Tracheobronchial inflammatory myofibroblastoma: A locally invasive, potentially recurrent neoplasm. *Int J Surg Pathol* 2: 93–98, 1994.
3. Armitage JM, Kormos RL, Stuart S, et al: Posttransplant lymphoproliferative disease in thoracic organ transplant patients: Ten years of cyclosporine-based immunosuppression. *J Heart Lung Transplant* 10:877–887, 1991.
4. Bahadori H, Liebow AA: Plasma cell granulomas of the lung. *Cancer* 31:191–208, 1973.
5. Bienenstock J, Befus AD: Gut- and bronchus-associated lymphoid tissue. *Am J Anat* 170:437–445, 1984.
6. Bragg DG, Chor PJ, Murray KA, et al: Lymphoproliferative disorders of the lung: Histopathology, clinical manifestations, and imaging features. *Am J Roentgenol* 163:273–281, 1994.
7. Cohen JI: Epstein-Barr virus lymphoproliferative disease associated with acquired immunodeficiency. *Medicine* 70:137–160, 1991.
8. Colby TV, Lombard C: Histiocytosis X presenting in the lung. *Hum Pathol* 14:847–856, 1983.
9. Cordier JF, Chailleux E, Lauque D, et al: Primary pulmonary lymphomas. A clinical study of 70 cases in non-immunocompromised patients. *Chest* 103:201–208, 1993.
10. Culine S, Henry-Amar M, Diebold J, et al: Relationship of histological subtypes to prognosis in early stage Hodgkin's disease: A review of 312 cases in a controlled clinical trial. *Eur J Cancer Clin Oncol* 25:551–556, 1989.
11. DiGiuseppe JA, Nelson WG, Seifter EJ, et al: Intravascular lymphomatosis: A clinicopathologic study of 10 cases and assessment of response to chemotherapy. *J Clin Oncol* 12:2573–2579, 1994.
12. Fiche M, Capron F, Berger F, et al: Primary pulmonary non-Hodgkin's lymphomas. *Histopathology* 26:529–537, 1995.
13. Friedman PJ, Liebow AA, Sokoloff J: Eosinophilic granuloma of lung: Clinical aspects of histiocytosis in adults. *Medicine* 60:385–396, 1981.
14. Frizzera G: Castleman's disease and related disorders. *Semin Diagn Pathol* 5:346–364, 1988.
15. Guinee D, Jaffe E, Kingma D, et al: Pulmonary lymphomatoid granulomatosis: Evidence for a proliferation of Epstein-Barr virus infected B-lymphocytes with a prominent T-cell component and vasculitis. *Am J Surg Pathol* 18:753–764, 1994.
16. Harris NL, Jaffe ES, Stein H, et al: A revised European-American classification of lymphoid neoplasms: A proposal from the International Lymphoma Study Group. *Blood* 84:1361–1392, 1994.
17. Jackson SA, Tung KT, Mead GM: Multiple cavitating pulmonary lesions in non-Hodgkin's lymphoma. *Clin Radiol* 49:883–885, 1994.
18. Joseph G, Pandit M, Korfhage L: Primary pulmonary plasmacytoma. *Cancer* 71:721–724, 1993.
19. Knowles DM, Cesarman E, Chadburn A, et al: Correlative morphologic and molecular genetic analysis demonstrates three distinct categories of posttransplantation lymphoproliferative disorders. *Blood* 85:552–565, 1995.
20. Kornstein MJ, Pietra GG, Hoxie JA, et al: The pathology and treatment of interstitial pneumonitis in two infants with AIDS. *Am Rev Respir Dis* 133:1196, 1986.
21. Koss MN, Hochholzer L, Langloss JM, et al: Lymphoid interstitial pneumonia: Clinicopathological and immunopathological findings in 18 cases. *Pathology* 19:178–185, 1987.
22. Kovalski R, Hansen-Flaschen J, Lodato RF, Pietra GG: Localized leukemic pulmonary infiltrates: Diagnosis by bronchoscopy and resolution with therapy. *Chest* 97:674–678, 1990.
23. Levine AM: AIDS-associated malignant lymphoma. *Med Clin North Am* 76:253–268, 1992.
24. Li G, Hansmann ML, Zwingers T, Lennert K: Primary lymphomas of the lung: Morphological, immunohistochemical and clinical features. *Histopathology* 16:519–531, 1990.
25. Liebow AA, Carrington CB, Friedman PJ: Lymphomatoid granulomatosis. *Hum Pathol* 3:457–558, 1972.
26. Lipford EH Jr, Margolick JB, Longo DL, et al: Angiocentric immunoproliferative lesions: A clinicopathologic spectrum of postthymic T-cell proliferations. *Blood* 72:1674–1681, 1988.
27. Lister TA, Crowther D, Sutcliffe SB, et al: Report of a committee convened to discuss the evaluation and staging of patients with Hodgkin's disease: Cotswolds meeting. *J Clin Oncol* 7:1630–1636, 1989.
28. Locker J, Nalesnik M: Molecular genetic analysis of lymphoid tumors arising after organ transplantation. *Am J Pathol* 135:977–987, 1989.
29. Miller DL, Allen MS: Rare pulmonary neoplasms. *Mayo Clin Proc* 68:492–498, 1993.
30. Montone KT, Litzky LA, Wurster A, et al: EBV-associated posttransplant lymphoproliferative disorder following lung transplantation: Experience of a single lung transplant center. *Surgery* 119:544–551, 1996.
31. Myers JL, Kurtin PJ, Katzenstein ALA, et al: Lymphomatoid granulomatosis: Evidence of immunophenotypic diversity and relationship to Epstein-Barr virus infection. *Am J Surg Pathol* 19:1300–1312, 1995.
32. Nalesnik MA, Jaffe R, Starzl TE, et al: The pathology of posttransplant lymphoproliferative disorders occuring in the setting of cyclosporine A–prednisone immunosuppression. *Am J Pathol* 133:173–192, 1988.
33. Nicholson AG, Wotherspoon AC, Diss TC, et al: Pulmonary B-cell non-Hodgkin's lymphomas; The value of immunohistochemistry and gene analysis in diagnosis. *Histopathology* 26:395–403, 1995.
34. Nicholson AG, Wotherspoon AC, Diss TC, et al: Reactive pulmonary lymphoid disorders. *Histopathology* 26:405–412, 1995.
35. Peterson BA, Frizzera G: Multicentric Castleman's disease. *Semin Oncol* 20:636–647, 1993.
36. Radin AI: Primary pulmonary Hodgkin's disease. *Cancer* 65:289–292, 1990.
37. Randhawa PS, Jaffe R, Demetris AJ, et al: The systemic distribution of Epstein-Barr virus genomes in fatal posttransplantation lymphoproliferative disorders: An in situ hybridization study. *Am J Pathol* 138:1027–1033, 1991.
38. Salhany KE, Pietra GG: Extranodal lymphoid disorders. *Am J Clin Pathol* 99:472–485, 1993.

39. Salhany KE: Lymph node biopsy, in Macdonald JS, Haller DG, Mayer RJ (eds): *Manual of Oncologic Therapeutics*. Philadelphia, Lippincott, 1995, pp 8–9.

40. Saltzstein SL: Pulmonary malignant lymphomas and pseudolymphomas: Classification, therapy and prognosis. *Cancer* 16:928–955, 1963.

41. Straus DJ, Gaynor JJ, Myers J, et al: Prognostic factors among 185 adults with newly diagnosed advanced Hodgkin's disease treated with alternating potentially noncross-resistant chemotherapy and intermediate-dose radiation therapy. *J Clin Oncol* 8:1173–1186, 1990.

42. Tan Liu N, Matsubara O, Grillo H, Mark E: Invasive fibrous tumor of the tracheobronchial tree. *Hum Pathol* 20:180–184, 1989.

43. Wick MR, Mills SE: Intravascular lymphomatosis: Clinicopathologic features and differential diagnosis. *Semin Diagn Pathol* 8:91–101, 1991.

44. Willman CL, Busque L, Griffith BB, et al: Langerhans'-cell histiocytosis (histiocytosis X): A clonal proliferative disease. *New Engl J Med* 331:154–160, 1994.

45. Yousem SA, Colby TV: Pulmonary lymphomas and lymphoid hyperplasias, in Knowles DM (ed): *Neoplastic Hematopathology*. Baltimore, Williams & Wilkins, 1992, pp 979–1007.

46. Yousem SA, Hochholzer L: Pulmonary hyalinizing granuloma. *Am J Clin Pathol* 87:1–6, 1987.

47. Yousem SA, Weiss LM, Colby TV: Primary pulmonary Hodgkin's disease: A clinicopathologic study of 15 cases. *Cancer* 57:1217–1224, 1986.

48. Yousem SA: The histological spectrum of pulmonary graft-versus-host disease in bone marrow transplant recipients. *Hum Pathol* 26:668–675, 1995.

PART SIXTEEN

INFECTIOUS DISEASES OF THE LUNGS

CHAPTER 119

MICROBIAL FLORA AND COLONIZATION OF THE RESPIRATORY TRACT

Waldemar G. Johanson, Jr. / Lisa L. Dever

It is important that physicians who treat patients with respiratory diseases understand the concept of *colonization* and can differentiate between colonization and infection when it is possible to do so. Surprisingly, that distinction is often difficult to make. The term *colonization* implies the persistence of microorganisms at a particular site. Some sites within the respiratory tract, such as the oropharynx, are normally colonized by many bacteria, including pathogenic species. Colonization is considered abnormal when bacteria are present that are highly likely to cause disease or when normally sterile regions are colonized. Abnormal colonization generally is the result of a major disruption of host defenses, especially those that protect the epithelial surface.

DEFINITIONS

Colonization can be defined as the persistence of microorganisms at a body site without evidence of a host response. Infection implies either a host response or evidence of injury to host tissues. Presence and persistence of microorganisms are easy to demonstrate. The problem with these definitions lies in the assessment of the host response. For example, normal persons may have local or circulating antibody against bacteria that have colonized their oropharynx, representing evidence of a host response. Patients who have been endotracheally intubated for respiratory failure often demonstrate bacteria persistently in tracheal secretions in the presence of neutrophils. It is unclear whether the presence of local inflammation is due to local infection or mechanical trauma with colonization. The term *persistence* in this context means continual presence over some undefined period. It is known that some persons may harbor pathogenic strains of *Streptococcus pneumoniae*—especially type 3—in their upper respiratory tract for years in the absence of infection and that some normal persons appear to be lifelong nasal carriers of *Staphylococcus aureus.* On the other hand, acquisition and persistence of these organisms for even a brief time by immunocompromised persons may pose a substantial risk of infection.

As a practical matter, clinical medicine is usually concerned with colonization over brief periods; colonization is considered to have occurred if the same bacterial strains are identified at a site in two cultures, or even in a single culture if one can reasonably expect continual presence in a subsequent culture. Recovery of the same species from two or more cultures does not necessarily mean persistence of the same microorganism. For epidemiologic research studies, both antibiotic susceptibility assays and molecular techniques are available that allow an accurate determination of the relatedness of strains recovered.[1]

SITES OF COLONIZATION AND THE NORMAL MICROBIAL FLORA

Microorganisms that infect the lungs often enter the body through the mouth and oropharynx. Therefore, for the purposes of this chapter, the mouth and oropharynx are considered to be part of the upper respiratory tract. The mouth and oropharynx are heavily colonized by certain species of bacteria. *Candida* species may be present as well. The level of contamination can be easily demonstrated by quantitative cultures of saliva, which typically contains 10^8 to 10^9 aerobic bacteria per milliliter and about equal numbers of anaerobic species. The anterior nares and nasal passages are less heavily contaminated but are universally colonized with bacteria. Microorganisms that are commonly isolated from these sites are listed in Table 119-1. Despite their contiguity with the nasal passages, the paranasal sinuses are normally sterile. Bacteria are infrequently found distal to the vocal cords in normal subjects, and the airways and lung distal to the carina are considered to be normally sterile. That epithelial surfaces exposed to millions of microorganisms remain free of continuous infections is extraordinary. The sterility of these regions is maintained by the host defenses, which play a critical role in maintaining the complex microflora of the human respiratory tract while protecting epithelial surfaces (reviewed in detail in Chapter 120).

Studies of the distribution of colonization are hampered by artifacts caused by the sampling techniques. In the case of the respiratory tract, the possibility for contamination of samples obtained from distal airways or lung by proximal secretions is great,

since most samples are obtained with instruments that pass through the nose or mouth. Collection of these samples generally requires topical anesthesia; anesthesia-related aspiration of oropharyngeal contents may produce positive cultures from sites that were sterile before the sampling procedure. On the other hand, small numbers of bacteria are present in ambient air and are inhaled into the lung. Oropharyngeal secretions are regularly aspirated into the tracheobronchial tree by healthy persons, at least during sleep. However, lung antibacterial defenses are highly efficient, and viable bacteria that are introduced into the lungs tend to be swiftly inactivated or removed, so the number of viable organisms diminishes rapidly. Thus, the results of one sample at one point in time represent the interplay of all these factors: artifacts induced by sampling, ongoing inoculation by inhalation or aspiration, and bacterial clearance processes. These considerations explain the occasional recovery of bacteria from aseptically resected lung tissue or aseptically sampled distal airways in healthy persons. The bulk of the evidence suggests that these regions are usually sterile in normal subjects; bacteria that are present are those of the upper respiratory tract representing recent contamination, and they do not persist.

CHARACTERISTICS OF THE NORMAL MICROBIAL FLORA

The initial bacterial flora of the upper respiratory tract is acquired within the first few days of life from the infant's environment, including his or her attendants.[3] Thereafter, the bacterial flora tend to demonstrate the characteristics listed in Table 119-2. Despite the diversity of bacteria in nature, only a few species are commonly found in the human respiratory tract. Humans show a high degree of similarity for broad groups of organisms. The specific strains and relative proportions of various strains differ widely among healthy people, but they tend to remain quite constant over time for a single individual. Certain organisms, such as *Hemophilus influenzae*, are readily acquired by most members of a family after introduction by one family member. Some organisms, such as β-hemolytic streptococci, are much less likely to be shared; others, such as gram-negative bacilli, are almost never found in other family members when one individual is colonized. In addition, in one person, marked differences in the bacterial flora can exist between anatomic regions of the upper respiratory tract. For example, *Streptococcus mutans* is regularly present in dental plaque but absent from the dorsum of the tongue, while the reverse pattern is characteristic of *S. salivarius*.[16] These observations suggest that maintenance of the normal flora is determined by selective processes that determine both the composition and the distribution of the normal micro-

TABLE 119-1

Microorganisms That Colonize the Normal Upper Respiratory Tract

Viridans streptococci
Streptococcus pyogenes
Streptococcus pneumoniae
Staphylococci, including *S. aureus*
Micrococcus spp.
Neisseria spp.
Moraxella (Branhamella) catarrhalis
Hemophilus spp., including *H. influenzae*
Lactobacillus spp.
Corynebacterium spp.
Obligate anaerobes
Candida spp.

TABLE 119-2

Characteristics of the Normal Respiratory Flora

Restricted variety of organisms present
Composition resistant to change in an individual
Varies among regions of the upper respiratory tract
Excluded from some contiguous sites, e.g., paranasal sinuses, airways

bial flora in the respiratory tract. Alterations in these factors cause the abnormal patterns of colonization that are often associated with disease.

DETERMINANTS OF THE NORMAL MICROBIAL FLORA

A variety of hypotheses have been advanced in attempts to explain the composition of normal microbial flora (Table 119-3). The physiochemical milieu of the oropharynx may explain why a number of bacterial species fail to colonize human hosts. These considerations are of importance in the establishment of anaerobic bacteria in the gingival crevices but not on exposed mucosal surfaces. On the other hand, they do not explain individual differences in nasal carriage of *S. aureus* or the persistence of certain species of aerobic bacteria in one human host versus another. Physiochemical properties such as pH, redox potential, electrostatic charge, steric properties, and availability of certain nutrients explain a small but important number of the observations in question.

Bacterial interference refers to the laboratory, and possibly clinical, phenomenon in which one bacterial species inhibits the growth of another.[20,37] Known mechanisms underlying this observation include the preferential consumption of essential nutrients and the elaboration of a variety of antibacterial substances by certain species. *S. mutans,* for example, produces an antimicrobial peptide, or bacteriocin, termed *mutacin,* which inhibits the growth of other streptococci and many other gram-positive bacteria. Recent characterization of a mutacin produced by group II *S. mutans* suggests that this substance is bactericidal and that it exerts its activity by inhibiting essential enzyme functions, thus interfering with the capacity of cells to generate metabolic energy.[7] Such substances provide the microorganisms with a competitive advantage and are likely to play a role in primary colonization.

Even though bacterial interference has been studied in vitro for more than 100 years, its significance in vivo remains largely speculative. Some years ago it was noted that intentional colonization of newborn infants with an avirulent strain of *S. aureus,* 502A, tended to diminish colonization and infection by highly pathogenic strains of *S. aureus.* However, infections due to the "avirulent" strain began to occur, and the procedure was abandoned.[15] Attempts to prevent postoperative oropharyngeal colonization with gram-negative bacilli after antimicrobial therapy by manipulation of the normal flora have been reported.[30] Many organisms contained in the normal flora are capable of inhibiting the growth of gram-negative bacilli in vitro. Penicillin therapy markedly reduced the number of these inhibitory organisms and was associated with gram-negative colonization in vivo. Penicillin resistance was induced in the normal flora by small doses of penicillin administered preoperatively; these penicillin-resistant and gram-negative inhibitory organisms persisted despite high doses of penicillin postoperatively, and colonization by gram-negative bacilli was diminished. Neither follow-up nor confirmatory studies of these observations have been reported. If bacterial interference is important in vivo, one would expect that alteration of the existing flora by antimicrobial therapy would lead to long-lasting changes in the normal flora; such are not observed. The role of this phenomenon in regulating the normal flora remains unclear.

The concept that the normal flora may be determined by selective adherence of only certain bacteria to regional epithelial cells is relatively recent but is supported by a variety of observations.[5] Organisms that are part of the normal oropharyngeal flora adhere in large numbers to oropharyngeal cells during incubation in vitro, whereas other bacteria do not. Further, cells recovered from various regions of the mouth and oropharynx bind organisms in vitro in similar proportions to those observed in cultures obtained from the same regions in vivo. Alterations of the host that induce increased in vitro adherence of certain organisms such as gram-negative bacilli are associated with a markedly increased risk of colonization with the same organisms in vivo.[21] Figure 119-1 demonstrates avid adherence of numerous bacilli to a buccal epithelial cell of a patient colonized with *Pseudomonas aeruginosa.* Finally, studies of the gut and urinary tract strongly suggest that epithelial cell adherence of bacteria is an essential step in the establishment of a new microbial flora.

Bacterial adherence to mammalian epithelial cells appears to occur through a variety of binding mechanisms.[4] Bacteria have developed specialized surface molecules or structures, termed adhesins, that bind firmly to specific sites on host cells. These adhesins are associated with surface fibrillae in gram-positive organisms and with fimbriae in gram-negative bacilli.[5] However, binding mechanisms differ for most of the species that have been studied, and numerous mechanisms may coexist in some bacteria. A single adhesin may have more than one host receptor, or ligand, and the receptor may be recognized by many adhesins. For example, type I fimbriated *Escherichia coli* bind to cells via mannose-sensitive and mannose-resistant ligands found on host cell membranes and by other adhesins not associated with fimbriae.[5,26] *S. pneumoniae* appears to bind to specific carbohydrate sequences found on epithelial cells. A proteinlike adhesin molecule has been described that acts to bridge the pneumococcal cell wall component and the cell surface receptor.[2] *Candida albicans* binds by a mannan adhesin that is also the antigen most influential in the host lymphocyte response.[14] Microbial adherence may be species specific. Capsid proteins of rhinoviruses adhere to human cell receptors but not to those of mice. This species specificity has led to the identification of ICAM-1, a member of the immunoglobulin superfamily, as the major human receptor for rhinoviruses.[17]

TABLE 119-3

Factors That Maintain the Normal Flora of the Upper Respiratory Tract

Mechanical factors (aerodynamic filtration, salivary and mucociliary flow, cough)

Selective epithelial cell adherence

Physiochemical milieu (pH, redox potential, nutrients)

Immunoglobulins, especially secretory IgA

Epithelial-derived antimicrobial peptides (LAP, TAP)

Bacterial (interbacterial) interference

Local cytokine response

Other (lysozyme, iron-binding proteins)

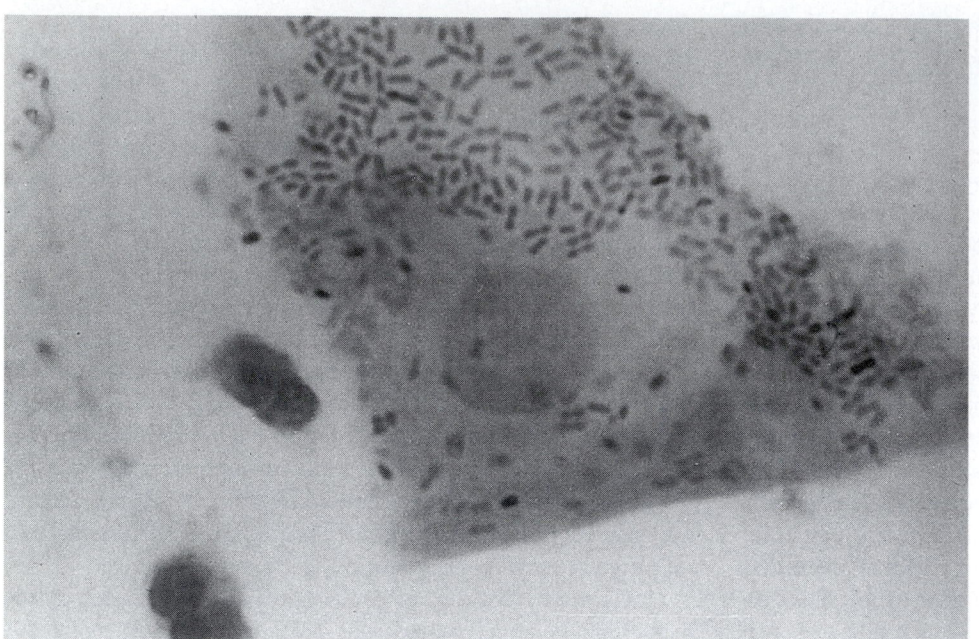

FIGURE 119-1   Buccal epithelial cell from a patient colonized with *Pseudomonas aeruginosa* showing abundant attachment of bacteria.

bind selectively to ciliated respiratory cells.[19,42] *S. pneumoniae* produces two cytoplasmic enzymes, neuraminidase and pneumolysin, that may facilitate colonization and pathogenesis.[27] Neuraminidase cleaves sialic acid from glycolipids and gangliosides, exposing receptors for pneumococcal attachment. Pneumolysin has been shown to inhibit beating of respiratory cilia and in this fashion may facilitate attachment and colonization. Such observations suggest that the interactions between bacterial adhesins and respiratory cell surface receptors are both highly specific and widely variable among organisms that may inhabit the respiratory tract.

Recent investigations have identified locally produced antimicrobial peptides that may be important in protecting epithelial surfaces.[12,34] Lingual antimicrobial peptide (LAP) and tracheal antimicrobial peptide (TAP) are members of the β-defensin class and possess antifungal and antibacterial activity. These peptides are abundant on the epithelial surface, and their concentrations can markedly increase in response to injury. Increased expression of LAP and TAP may result from direct stimulation by bacteria or from production of cytokines, such as tumor necrosis factor. Secretory IgA also contributes to respiratory tract host defenses. Nasopharyngeal secretions containing high concentrations of IgA have been shown to significantly reduce adherence of *S. pneumoniae* and *H. influenzae* to nasopharyngeal epithelial cells in vitro.[24] Host defenses are discussed further elsewhere in this text (see Chapter 134).

BACTERIAL COLONIZATION AND INFECTION

Bacterial infections of the respiratory tract may follow inoculation by bloodborne or airborne bacteria. In these situations, prior colonization of the upper respiratory tract is unimportant, if it occurs at all. However, the great majority of bacterial infections are preceded by colonization by the offending bacterium before the onset of invasive disease. Two patterns of colonization are important to consider: (1) colonization of usually contaminated sites in previously healthy persons by highly virulent organisms and (2) colonization of persons with underlying disease by any of a variety of organisms, not necessarily those possessing great native virulence. In the latter circumstance, the extent of colonization often includes normally sterile sites.

Colonization of Normal Persons by Highly Virulent Organisms

Several common organisms serve as examples of this interaction: *N. meningitidis, S. pyogenes,* and probably *S. pneumoniae.* Although long-term colonization of healthy subjects with each of these organisms is known to occur, outbreaks of acute disease

In some situations, there appears to be a reciprocal relationship between the adherence of two differing bacterial species; cells that bind many of one species will bind few of the other.[1,38] This appears to be especially true of streptococci and *E. coli.* Streptococci bind via a lipoteichoic acid adhesin expressed on fibrillae to fibronectin, a glycoprotein present on the epithelial surface. *E. coli* do not bind to fibronectin and, if this protein is present on the cell surface, adherence of *E. coli* is prevented. If cell-surface fibronectin is absent or diminished, streptococci do not adhere, but *E. coli* is able to bind directly to the cell surface. Because of the multiplicity of binding mechanisms, it seems unlikely that attempts to block or manipulate this interaction will be successful, although some promising results have been reported. For example, intranasal instillation of purified lipoteichoic acid has been shown to block colonization by group A streptococci and prevent death in mice after intranasal challenge with these microorganisms.[9] In the GI and urinary tracts, and perhaps at other sites where a limited variety of organisms are important, immunization with bacterial adhesins may provide protection against colonization and infection.[31,32] Successful GI immunization may also extend to protection of other mucosal surfaces via mucosal IgA, including the lungs.

Bacterial binding to the various cell types that may be present in the normal upper respiratory tract has received relatively little attention but may prove to be of fundamental importance in understanding these complex interactions. Fibronectin accumulates on the surface of squamous cells as the latter mature and become keratinized. Bacteria that bind to cell surface fibronectin become more numerous as a consequence of cell age, whereas other bacterial species may predominate if epithelial cell turnover is high. *Neisseria meningitidis* binds only to nonciliated cells in the nasopharynx, although colonization with these organisms produces a marked toxic effect on ciliated cells as well.[40] In contrast, *Bordetella pertussis* and *Mycoplasma pneumoniae* also occur and can be traced to person-to-person transmission of organisms. The role of adherence in colonization by such organisms is controversial. Highly virulent respiratory pathogens are typically encapsulated, and the presence of an extracellular capsule markedly diminishes adherence to epithelial cells in vitro. Several investigators have found that avirulent, nonencapsulated mutants adhere more readily to respiratory epithelial cells than do encapsulated strains associated with infections.[38] Further, using labeled antibody against capsular antigens, pneumococci were rarely found on the surface of regional epithelial cells, even in patients who were demonstrably colonized by usual culture techniques.[36] These observations have been used to suggest that epithelial cell adherence is not an important factor in colonization by these organisms. Recent evidence shows that the production of extracellular appendages and capsular material can be turned on and off with incredible rapidity.[38] Loss of the capsule and production of fibrillae or fimbriae facilitate mucosal adherence. On the other hand, regeneration of the capsule confers resistance against host defenses, especially phagocytes, and facilitates tissue invasion.

An interesting series of experiments with *N. meningitidis* supports this sequence of events. Although encapsulated strains adhere poorly to nasopharyngeal cells in vitro, organisms incubated with small explants of nasopharyngeal mucosa adhere to and penetrate the epithelium.[29] Such organ culture models of the mucosa that do not immerse the cultures in liquid medium, but rather attempt to simulate the air-mucosal interface, more realistically simulate the complex environment of the human respiratory tract. The interaction of unencapsulated *H. influenzae* with respiratory mucosa has also been studied in this model.[43] These studies showed that more than 24 h was required before bacteria were seen adhering to epithelial cells and that they adhered only to structurally damaged cells. Fimbriation of nontypable strains increased adherence to buccal cells but did not increase adherence or epithelial damage in the organ culture model. In infected preparations, bacteria were able to invade nonciliated cells and were found in membrane-bound vacuoles within cells. These findings suggest that adhesins other than fimbriae may be involved in the interaction between nontypable *H. influenzae* strains and the respiratory epithelium.

COLONIZATION OF PERSONS WITH UNDERLYING DISEASE

In this situation, the properties of the responsible organism are of less importance than the underlying condition of the host. Abnormal colonization patterns are commonly observed in the presence of a variety of acute or chronic diseases, and may be manifested by the abnormal presence or absence of organisms in the respiratory tract. The propensity of bacterial infections to develop on the background of a respiratory viral infection may, in part, be related to such phenomena. Infection of cells in tissue culture with influenza A virus markedly increases their adherence of *S. aureus*.[10] Disruption of the airway epithelium by influenza infection in vivo exposes novel sites to which bacteria adhere readily, in contrast to the resistance of the normal epithelium. Gram-negative enteric bacilli infrequently colonize the upper respiratory tract of healthy persons but are found most

often in patients with serious, life-threatening illnesses.[22] The frequency of colonization of elderly people parallels their degree of chronic disability. Colonization by gram-negative bacilli correlates well with the degree to which these organisms adhere to respiratory epithelial cells in vitro: cells obtained from colonized subjects bind large numbers of organisms, while cells from noncolonized people do not.

Binding sites for gram-negative bacilli appear to be present on normal respiratory squamous cells, since enzymatic treatment of such cells in vitro markedly increases bacillary adherence. It appears that fibronectin, a large protein molecule that is normally present on the surface of these cells, may block these binding sites. Cells from colonized persons are deficient in fibronectin— a finding that may be related to the proteolytic activity of secretions.[44]

Patients with chronic bronchitis may demonstrate persistence of bacterial flora in the distal airways. The mechanisms underlying this observation have received little attention. It seems likely that adherence of the responsible organisms to sites in the distal airways is implicated, but this is unproven. Increased adherence could be related to the development of islands of squamous epithelium, loss of ciliary activity, or alterations in bronchial secretions. A similar occurrence of chronic colonization of a normally sterile site is often present in patients with chronic sinusitis. In this situation, as in chronic bronchitis, it is difficult to distinguish between cause and effect. Chronic inflammation is associated with a number of mucosal changes, one of which is bacterial colonization. These abnormalities lead to impaired mucociliary function, reduced drainage, and retention of secretions—all of which promote bacterial infection.

Colonization of the lower airways is common in patients with cystic fibrosis and may persist for extended periods, leading to pulmonary injury and subsequent infection. Unlike chronic bronchitis, in which the colonizing microorganisms are most often *H. influenzae*, *S. pneumoniae*, and *M. catarrhalis*, the airways of cystic fibrosis patients are most frequently colonized with *S. aureus* or *P. aeruginosa*. Molecular typing techniques have demonstrated that the colonizing strains usually remain constant over time, rather than acquiring new or genetically different strains. The pathophysiological basis for selective colonization with these microorganisms in cystic fibrosis is not well understood. Some of this colonization undoubtedly reflects the selection of relatively antibiotic-resistant bacterial strains over time. However, *S. aureus* isolates from cystic fibrosis patients demonstrate markedly increased adherence to bronchial epithelial cell lines, ciliated and squamous nasal cells, and buccal epithelial cells compared to isolates from healthy subjects.[35] Adherence does not appear to be affected by age, severity of pulmonary disease, or presence of other bacteria in the airways. Prior proteinase treatment of *S. aureus* isolates prevents their binding to epithelial cells, suggesting that one or more peptide adhesin mediates attachment.

Conflicting data have been reported on the differential adherence of *P. aeruginosa* to respiratory epithelial cells from cystic fibrosis patients versus cells from normal subjects. Differences in techniques and strains of *P. aeruginosa* used in these experiments may account for the differences in results. Cystic fibrosis airway epithelial cells have higher than normal concentrations of asialylated glycolipids, receptor sites for *P. aeruginosa* fimbriae.[33] Recent studies suggest that the binding of *P. aeruginosa* to these receptors stimulates the production of inflammatory cytokines, such as IL-8, by the respiratory epithelium.[13] Mucin glycoproteins have also been implicated as potential binding sites for *P. aeruginosa* in the airways; however, specific receptors have not been identified. Aggregation of *P. aeruginosa* cells is induced by salivary mucin and may be induced by secretory products from respiratory epithelial cells. This bacterial aggregation may facilitate colonization by preventing clearance and allowing greater contact between bacterial cells and host receptors. Recent data suggest a role for the cystic fibrosis transmembrane conductance receptor (CFTR) in host defense against *P. aeruginosa*.[28] Mutant CFTR is unable to mediate ingestion of *Pseudomonas* organisms by human airway epithelial cells in vitro.

Clinical Distinctions Between Colonization and Infection

The importance of colonization lies in two areas: (1) since it is the initiating pathogenic step for many infections, colonization may represent a significant risk factor for infection in some circumstances; and (2) confusion with infection may lead to a failure to treat infections due to pathogenic organisms, on the one hand, or may cause antimicrobial treatment of incidental colonization, on the other. Clinical decision making, in the first instance, requires an analysis of risk versus benefit. The analysis of risk must include the likelihood of infection, the severity of the resultant illness, and the potential harm associated with prophylactic therapy. Each of these factors varies widely in specific clinical circumstances. For example, asymptomatic nasal colonization with *S. aureus* does not require treatment in most subjects, but treatment may be beneficial for a patient with recurrent furunculosis or in a surgeon whose patients are experiencing staphylococcal wound infections.

By far the most common problems with colonization in clinical chest disease entail colonization of the airways in patients with acute or chronic underlying disease. Gram-negative bacilli appear in tracheobronchial secretions in at least 50 percent of patients who are intubated for ventilatory support. Similarly, colonization of the respiratory tract by new pathogens, usually gram-negative bacilli, occurs in at least 20 percent of patients undergoing treatment for pneumococcal pneumonia or other specific infections. In these circumstances, the clinician must decide whether the appearance of new organisms represents a significant superinfection or merely colonization. Well-validated criteria for this decision making are not available. As a general rule, it is wise to remember the axiom that patients, not laboratory results, are being treated; if the patient is doing well without unusual susceptibility to significant disease, the new culture findings should be examined critically. Some clinicians recommend performing serial microscopic examinations of tracheobronchial secretions, believing that an increase in neutrophils, along with increasing numbers of gram-negative bacilli, is a more reliable criterion of superinfection than culture results alone. Others recommend quantitative cultures of secretions; increasing colony counts or absolute values greater than 10^6 per milliliter have been said to identify patients with new infections.

Invasive sampling procedures, including transtracheal aspiration, transthoracic needle aspiration, and, lately, fiberoptic bronchoscopy with distal lung samples obtained by a protected specimen brush technique, have been recommended. Each of these approaches has advocates and advantages in some circumstances. Each adds substantially to the cost of patient care, and none can be recommended as a routine procedure. Our approach has been to limit concern to patients who seem likely to have superinfections on clinical grounds and to investigate those patients by bronchoscopy and selective sampling if further microbiologic data or specific antimicrobial therapy based on those data will significantly alter clinical management.

EFFECTS OF ANTIBIOTICS ON COLONIZATION

Antimicrobial therapy causes major disruptions in the natural balances previously described, and has been used in attempts to prevent colonization of the respiratory tract and prevent infection. The technique that has received the most attention is termed *selective decontamination of the digestive tract* (SDD), which includes application of topical antimicrobial agents to the buccal mucosa and instilled into the stomach.[11] The rationale for this approach is that colonization precedes infection in critically ill patients and that high concentrations of antimicrobial agents at the mucosal surface will eliminate existing microorganisms and prevent the acquisition of new microorganisms. A number of studies have demonstrated that this technique is, in fact, effective in reducing respiratory infections in seriously ill patients.[18,23] However, despite the reductions of infection, mortality was not reduced in most of these studies. Perhaps the greatest risk associated with attempts at manipulating the flora with topical antimicrobials is the selection for colonization and infection by antibiotic-resistant bacteria. Increased rates of colonization and infection by enterococci and methicillin-resistant *S. aureus* have occurred in some ICUs in which SDD has been used.[6,8] It is unlikely that any antimicrobial regimen will ever be completely successful in preventing colonization with unwanted microorganisms and in preventing subsequent infection.

Antimicrobial agents have profound effects on the ability of bacteria to adhere to epithelial cells. Although both increased and decreased adherence have been described, bacterial adherence is generally decreased by subinhibitory concentrations of antibiotics—that is, concentrations that do not kill or significantly inhibit growth of the organism.[25] Although the mechanisms by which adherence is altered have not been well defined, presumably there are alterations of bacterial surface properties and structures that interfere with attachment. The clinical applicability of this phenomenon in the prevention of colonization, particularly given the propensity of bacteria to develop resistance, seems limited.

SUMMARY

Colonization of the respiratory tract represents a dynamic balance between microbes and host defenses, especially those operative on the epithelial surface. In health, these defenses determine the composition and extent of the normal microbial flora.

In the presence of acute or chronic illness, defenses are altered, allowing colonization by new microorganisms or allowing normally sterile regions to become colonized—either of which can lead to invasive infection. Understanding colonization is key to understanding respiratory infection.

REFERENCES

1. Abraham SN, Beachey EH, Simpson WA: Adherence of *Streptococcus pyogenes, Escherichia coli* and *Pseudomonas aeruginosa* to fibronectin-coated and uncoated epithelial cells. *Infect Immun* 41: 1261–1268, 1983.

2. Andersson B, Beachey EH, Tomasz A, et al: A sandwich adhesin on *Streptococcus pneumoniae* attaching to human oropharyngeal epithelial cells in vitro. *Microb Pathog* 4:267–278, 1988.

3. Aniansson G, Alm B, Andersson B, et al: Nasopharyngeal colonization during the first year of life. *J Infect Dis* 165(Suppl 1): S38–S42, 1992.

4. Beachey ED: Bacterial adherence: Adhesion-receptor interactions mediating the attachment of bacteria to mucosal surfaces. *J Infect Dis* 143:325–345, 1981.

5. Beachey ED, Eisenstein BI, Ofek I: Bacterial adherence in infectious diseases. *Current Concepts.* Kalamazoo, Michigan, Upjohn, 1982.

6. Bonten MJM, Gaillard CA, van Tiel FH, et al: Colonization and infection with *Enterococcus faecalis* in intensive care units: The role of antimicrobial agents. *Antimicrob Agents Chemother* 39:2783–2786, 1995.

7. Chikindas MD, Novak J, Driessen AJM, et al: Mutacin II, a bactericidal antibiotic from *Streptococcus mutans. Antimicrob Agents Chemother* 39:2656–2660, 1995.

8. Daeschner F: Emergence of resistance during selective decontamination of the digestive tract. *Eur J Clin Microbiol Infect Dis* 11:1–3, 1992.

9. Dale JB, Baird RW, Courtney HS, et al: Passive protection of mice against group A streptococcal pharyngeal infection by lipoteichoic acid. *J Infect Dis* 169:319–323, 1994.

10. Davison VE, Sanford BA: Factors influencing adherence of *Staphylococcus aureus* to influenza A virus–infected cell cultures. *Infect Immun* 37:946–955, 1982.

11. Dever LL, Johanson WG Jr: An update on selective decontamination of the digestive tract. *Curr Opin Infect Dis* 6:744–750, 1993.

12. Diamond G, Zasloff M, Eck H, et al: Tracheal antimicrobial peptide, a cysteine-rich peptide from mammalian tracheal mucosa: Peptide isolation and cloning of a cDNA. *Proc Natl Acad Sci USA* 88: 3952–3956, 1991.

13. DiMangio E, Zar HJ, Bryan R, Prince A: Diverse *Pseudomonas aeruginosa* gene products stimulate respiratory epithelial cells to produce interleukin-8. *J Clin Invest* 96:2204–2210, 1995.

14. Domer JE, Garner RE: Immunomodulation in response to Candida. *Immunol Ser* 47:293–317, 1989.

15. Drutz DJ, Van Way MH, Schaffner W, Koenig MG: Bacterial interference in the therapy of recurrent staphylococcal infections: Multiple abscesses due to the implantation of the 502A strain of staphylococcus. *New Engl J Med* 275:1161–1165, 1966.

16. Gibbons RJ, van Houte J: Bacterial adherence in oral microbial ecology. *Annu Rev Microbiol* 29:19–44, 1975.

17. Greve JM, Davis G, Meyer AM, et al: The major human rhinovirus receptor is ICAM-1. *Cell* 56:839–847, 1989.

18. Hamer DH, Barza M: Prevention of hospital-acquired pneumonia in critically ill patients. *Antimicrob Agents Chemother* 37:931–938, 1993.

19. Hu PC, Collier AM, Baseman JB: Surface parasitism by Mycoplasma pneumoniae of respiratory epithelium. *J Exp Med* 145: 1328–1343, 1977.

20. Johanson WG Jr, Blackstock R, Pierce AK, Sanford JP: The role of bacterial antagonism in pneumococcal colonization of the human pharynx. *J Lab Clin Med* 75:946–952, 1970.

21. Johanson WG Jr, Higuchi JH, Chaudhuri TR, Woods DE: Bacterial adherence to epithelial cells in bacillary colonization of the respiratory tract. *Am Rev Respir Dis* 121:55–63, 1980.

22. Johanson WG Jr, Pierce AK, Sanford JP: Changing pharyngeal bacterial flora of hospitalized patients. *New Engl J Med* 281:1137–1140, 1969.

23. Kollef MH: The role of selective digestive tract decontamination on mortality and respiratory tract infections: A meta-analysis. *Chest* 105:1101–1108, 1994.

24. Kurono Y, Shimamura K, Shigemi H, Mogi G: Inhibition of bacterial adherence by nasopharyngeal secretions. *Ann Otol Rhinol Laryngol* 100:455–458, 1991.

25. Ofek I, Beachey EH: Suppression of bacterial adherence by subminimal inhibitory concentrations of beta-lactam and aminoglycoside antibiotics. *Rev Infect Dis* 1:832–837, 1979.

26. Ofek I, Beachey EH, Sharon N: Surface sugars of animal cells as determinants of recognition in bacterial adherence. *Trends Biochem Sci* 3:159–160, 1978.

27. Paton JC, Andrew PW, Boulnois GJ, Mitchell TJ: Molecular analysis of the pathogenicity of *Streptococcus pneumoniae:* The role of pneumococcal proteins. *Annu Rev Microbiol* 47:89–115, 1993.

28. Pier GB, Grout M, Zaidi TS, et al: Role of mutant CFTR in hypersusceptibility of cystic fibrosis patients to lung infections. *Science* 271:64–67, 1996.

29. Rayner CFJ, Dewar A, Moxon ER, et al: The effect of variations in the expression of pili on the interaction of *Neisseria meningitidis* with human nasopharyngeal epithelium. *J Infect Dis* 171:113–121, 1994.

30. Redman LR, Lockey E: Colonization of the upper respiratory tract with gram-negative bacilli after operation, endotracheal intubation, and prophylactic antibiotic therapy. *Anesthesia* 22:220–227, 1967.

31. Roberts J, Hardaway K, Kaack B, et al: Prevention of pyelonephritis by immunization with P-fimbriae. *J Urol* 131:602–607, 1984.

32. Rutter JM, Jones GW: Protection against enteric disease caused by *Escherichia coli:* A model for vaccination with a virulence determinant. *Nature* 242:531–532, 1973.

33. Saiman L, Prince A: *Pseudomonas aeruginosa* pili bind to asialoGM1 which is increased on the surface of cystic fibrosis epithelial cells. *J Clin Invest* 92:1875–1880, 1993.

34. Schonwetter BS, Stolzenberg ED, Zasloff MA: Epithelial antibiotics induced at sites of inflammation. *Science* 267:1645–1647, 1995.

35. Schwab UE, Wold AE, Carson JL, et al: Increased adherence of *Staphylococcus aureus* from cystic fibrosis lungs to airway epithelial cells. *Am Rev Respir Dis* 148:365–369, 1993.

36. Selinger DS, Reed WP: Pneumococcal adherence to human epithelial cells. *Infect Immun* 23:545–548, 1979.

37. Sprunt K, Redman W: Evidence suggesting importance of role of interbacterial inhibition in maintaining balance of normal flora. *Ann Intern Med* 68:579–590, 1968.

38. St. Geme JW III, Falkow S: Loss of capsule expression by *Haemophilus influenzae* type b results in enhanced adherence to and invasion of human cells. *Infect Immun* 59:1325–1333, 1991.

39. Stanislawski L, Simpson WA, Hasty D, et al: Role of fibronectin in attachment of *Streptococcus pyogenes* and *Escherichia coli* to human cell lines and isolated oral epithelial cells. *Infect Immun* 48:257–259, 1985.

40. Stephens DS, Hoffman LH, McGee ZA: Interaction of *Neisseria meningitidis* with human nasopharyngeal mucosa: Attachment and entry into columnar epithelial cells. *J Infect Dis* 148:369–376, 1983.

41. Tenover FC, Arbeit RD, Goering RV, et al: Interpreting chromosomal DNA restriction patterns produced by pulsed-field gel electrophoresis: criteria for bacterial strain typing. *J Clin Microb* 33: 2233–2239, 1995.

42. Tuomanen EI, Hendley JO: Adherence of *Bordetella pertussis* to human respiratory epithelial cells. *J Infect Dis* 148:125–130, 1983.

43. Wilson R, Read R, Cole P: Interaction of *Haemophilus influenzae* with mucus, cilia, and respiratory epithelium. *J Infect Dis* 165 (Suppl 1):S100–S101, 1992.

44. Woods DE, Straus DC, Johanson WG Jr, Bass JA: Role of salivary protease activity in adherence of gram-negative bacilli to mammalian buccal epithelial cells in vitro. *J Clin Invest* 68:1435–1440, 1981.

CHAPTER 120

PULMONARY CLEARANCE OF INFECTIOUS AGENTS

Galen B. Toews

MECHANICAL DEFENSES
   Nasopharyngeal Airways
   Conducting Airways

INNATE IMMUNITY
   Alveolar Macrophages
   NK Cells
   Complement
   Surfactant

INFLAMMATORY RESPONSES

SPECIFIC IMMUNE RESPONSES
   Initiation of Specific Immune Responses to Pulmonary
      Antigens
   T Lymphocyte–Mediated Immune Responses in the
      Lower Respiratory Tract
   B Lymphocyte–Mediated Immune Responses in the
      Lung

CONCLUSION

The lung is an immense surface for interaction of the host with the external environment. The primary function of the lungs is the exchange of gases at a rate required to support tissue metabolism. While the delicate respiratory apparatus of the lung allows diffusion of oxygen from the environment into the blood and elimination of carbon dioxide, its continuous contact with ambient air and its enormous vascular bed cause the lung to be exposed to a varied burden of foreign materials, including infectious agents. Additionally, the lung is repeatedly exposed to microbes via aspiration of secretions from the upper respiratory tract, particularly during sleep. To perform gas exchange adequately, the lung must defend itself against a potentially hostile environment. This group of nonrespiratory functions has been collectively termed *pulmonary host defenses.*[44]

The various components of the pulmonary host defense system are distributed throughout the respiratory tract. The function of these components is to recognize and eliminate microorganisms before their multiplication leads to clinical disease. Most of the defense functions require a coordinated interaction of cells or cells and soluble factors. Pulmonary host defenses can be divided into four major parts. 1. Mechanical defenses include anatomic barriers, aerodynamics, epithelial cell barriers, mucus, and the mucociliary escalator. In certain circumstances, microbes overwhelm these mechanical defenses. Fortunately, the lung possesses three additional defenses against microbes (Fig. 120-1).

2. Cells of the innate immune system are present both in the airways and on the alveolar surface. The alveolar macrophage is one of the primary resident phagocytic cells in the lung that effectively remove certain microbes. If the microbial burden is large or more virulent, the ability to generate an acute inflammatory response is crucial. 3. An inflammatory response recruits numerous polymorphonuclear neutrophils (PMN), complement factors, and soluble humoral immune effector molecules from the systemic vasculature. 4. Host responses to viruses, fungi, and mycobacteria require more complex specific immune responses for their elimination. During such pulmonary infections, antigens are processed by intraepithelial or interstitial dendritic cells that enter the lymphatics and draining hilar lymph nodes. Central processing occurs as dendritic cells present antigen to T lymphocytes. Upon arrival at the initial site of antigen deposition, activated T lymphocytes are stimulated by resident antigen-presenting cells to release cytokines that generate an inflammatory response by recruiting effector cells such as monocytes and activating them to kill microorganisms. CD4 T lymphocytes also stimulate the differentiation of B cells into antibody-producing plasma cells. Specific antibodies that enter the lung during inflammatory responses enhance phagocytosis, promote microbial killing, and neutralize toxins. Finally, CD8 T lymphocytes mediate cellular toxicity that is crucial to effective host defenses against viral agents.

MECHANICAL DEFENSES

Specialized mechanical defenses exist along the entire respiratory tract from the nares to the alveolar surfaces. Mechanical defenses are remarkably efficient in removing the bulk of potentially harmful agents from the lung.

Nasopharyngeal Airways

Inhaled air is humidified as it moves through the upper respiratory tract. Particulates and microbes are enveloped in droplets of water. During this process, particulates assume the aerodynamic characteristics that determine if and where they will be deposited in the respiratory tract. Nasal hairs remove most particulates bigger than 10 μm. Rapid airflow and rapid changes in direction of the airstream in the nose favor inertial deposition of additional large particulates. Following this inertial impaction on the mucus-covered nasopharyngeal epithelium, these particulates are cleared primarily by swallowing, sneezing, or coughing.[41,42]

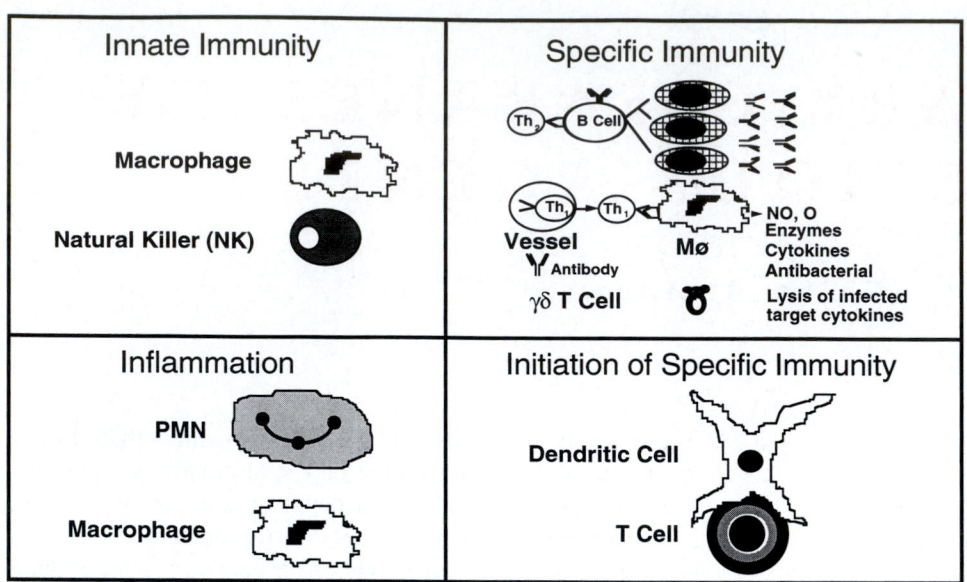

FIGURE 120-1   Pulmonary immune defenses. Three immune defense systems protect the airways and lower respiratory tract. Alveolar macrophages and pulmonary natural killer cells effectively remove certain microbes. Inflammatory responses, which lead to the recruitment of polymorphonuclear (PMN) leukocytes and monocytes, are crucial for the pulmonary clearance of most microbes. Specific immune responses are required for effective pulmonary clearance of viruses, encapsulated bacteria, fungi and mycobacteria. The initiation of specific immune responses requires dendritic cell–T lymphocyte interactions. The expression of immune responses requires the interaction of Th1 lymphocytes and macrophages and Th2 lymphocytes and B cells.

Mucociliary clearance participates in the removal of particulates from the nasaopharynx. Ciliated mucosa is present on the nasal septum and turbinates; mucociliary action sweeps mucus toward the posterior pharynx, where secretions are either swallowed or cleared from the throat.

Conducting Airways

MUCOCILIARY ESCALATOR

Conducting airways constitute the segment of the respiratory tract between the upper airway (larynx) and the gas-exchanging portion of the lung (terminal bronchioles, alveoli). Most particulates larger than 2 μm in diameter impact in the conducting airways, while 2-μm particles reach the alveolar surface. Mucociliary clearance and coughing are the principal means of mechanical defense (Fig. 120-2).[6] The mucosa of the conducting airways is lined with mucus secreted by goblet cells, bronchial glands, and Clara cells. The mucous blanket is composed of two distinct layers: a watery sublayer, in which most ciliary movement takes place, and an upper viscous layer that is just penetrated by the ciliary tip. Not all of the epithelium is covered with mucus; droplets form preferentially around impacted particulates.

Mucus is propelled up the respiratory tract by the pseudostratified ciliated epithelium that lines the conducting airways. Approximately 200 cilia are present on each ciliated cell. Ciliary length is approximately 5 to 6 μm, and ciliary frequency is 12 to 14 beats per second. Particulates can be cleared from the trachea with a half-time of 30 minutes and from distal airways with a half time of hours.

The movement of mucus requires groups of cilia to beat synchronously in a coordinated fashion. The cilia are coupled to the overlying mucous blanket. Each ciliary beat cycle includes an effective stroke and a recovery stroke. Cilia are fully extended perpendicular to the cell surface during the effective stroke and sweep the mucous cephalad. Cilia bend and flex near the cell surface in the watery sublayer and return to their resting position. The recovery stroke takes twice as long as the effective stroke. The mucociliary escalator entraps and removes most inhaled particulates, noxious gases, and vapors. Tight cellular junctions between epithelial cells also prevent the passage of macromolecules into the submucosa.

Several clinically relevant circumstances alter conducting airway defenses. Cigarette smoke disrupts epithelial junctions and allows passage of substances into the submucosa. Cigarette smoke also adversely affects cells that produce mucus; mucus production is increased, and its biochemical and biophysical characteristics are altered. Poor nutrition also alters the integrity of mucosal epithelial cells. This alteration allows the adherence of pathogenic microbes to the epithelium.

IRON-BINDING PROTEINS

Iron is an essential ingredient for survival of many microbes, including bacteria. Iron is generally sequestered in cells or firmly complexes to transport proteins. Microbes compete for this iron with their own transport proteins, known as siderophores. Iron transport proteins are present in airway mucosal secretions and in alveolar lining fluid. Lactoferrin, found predominantly in the airways, and transferrin, found predominantly in the alveolar spaces, effectively complex any free iron in mucosal secretions, suppressing bacterial growth by making iron difficult for bacteria to obtain.

INNATE IMMUNITY

Microbes or particulates of a certain size (0.5 to 3 μm in diameter) are deposited on the alveolar surface. Clearance of microbes from the alveoli depends entirely on cellular and humoral factors (Fig. 120-2). These include alveolar macrophages, natural killer (NK) cells, complement factors, defensins, and phospholipid surfactant.

Alveolar Macrophages

Alveolar macrophages are a heterogeneous population of phagocytes that constitute the first line of defense against microbes that

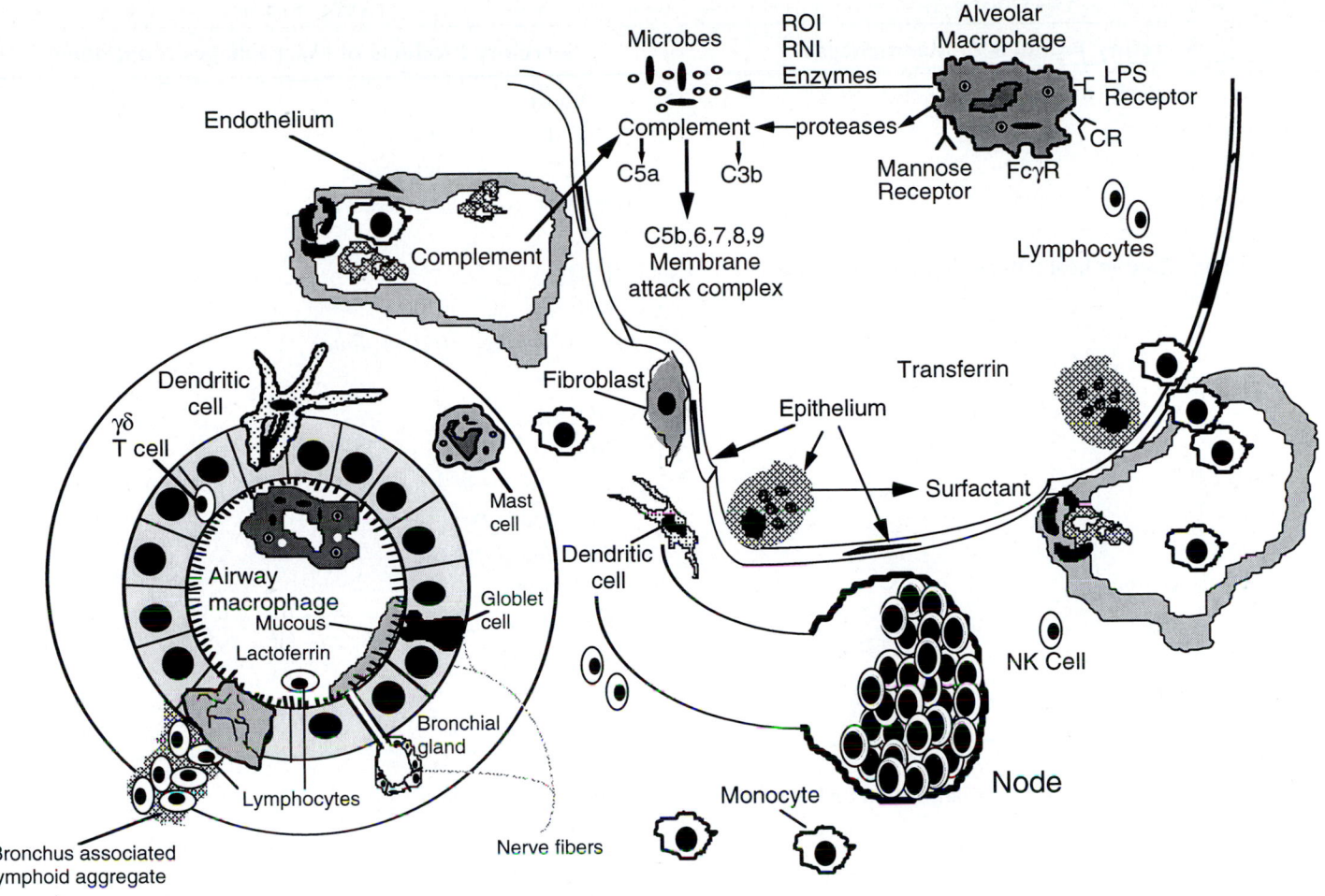

FIGURE 120-2 Resident defenses of conducting airways and alveoli. Conducting airways are lined by ciliated epithelium, which moves mucus generated by bronchial glands and goblet cells cephalad, where it is expectorated or swallowed. Airway macrophages ingest and kill small inocula of most aspirated and airborne bacteria. The alveolar spaces rely on innate immunity for the clearance of microbes that reach the alveolar surface. Alveolar macrophages are the first line of defense against microbes. Complement, surfactant, and iron-binding proteins are important humoral microbicidal factors.

reach the alveolar surface. Alveolar macrophages are derived from monocytes and proliferating macrophage precursors in the interstitium of the lung. Alveolar macrophages undergo differentiation within the lung. Alveolar macrophages have a life span of months to years. The signals and ligands that modulate monocyte traffic into the normal lung have not been defined.

The microbicidal function of alveolar macrophage is dependent on four critical attributes. Macrophages recognize signals, ingest particulates, secrete mediators, and migrate in response to stimuli (Table 120-1). Macrophages recognize signals in their microenvironment via surface receptors capable of binding specific ligands, including complement proteins, immunoglobulins, cytokines, lipids, polysaccharides, and toxins. Receptor-ligand interactions allow macrophages to ingest microorganisms and respond to cytokines and proteins. Complement receptors, receptors for the Fc fragment of immunoglobulin G, and mannose receptors have been studied most comprehensively (Fig. 120-2).[3,30]

Macrophages express two distinct receptors for the third component of complement.[3] Complement receptor 1 (CR1) preferentially binds C3b but also binds C3bi and C4b. Complement receptor 3 (CR3, Mo-1, MAC-1, CD11b/18) is a member of β2 integrin family. CR3 is a receptor for C3bi but also recognizes a sequence in the gamma chain of fibrinogen and lipopolysaccharide (LPS). CR3 also binds directly to *Histoplasma capsulatum*. The ability of CR3 to bind directly to microbes might represent an important recognition mechanism of microbes before the onset of specific immunity. CR3 is also essential for migration of leukocytes from the vasculature into tissues. CR3 functions in cell-cell and cell-substrate adhesion. Patients with a genetic deficiency in the CD18 complex have recurrent life-threatening infections, documenting the crucial role of CR3 in defense against infectious agents.

Three Fcγ receptors recognize the Fc domain of immunoglobulin G (IgG).[30] All classes of FcγR have at least two transcripts. All transcripts have closely related extracellular and transmembrane regions but differ in their cytoplasmic domains. All FcRs function as signal-transducing molecules. FcγRI is expressed on monocytes and macrophages. FcγRI triggers both phagocytosis and cytolytic responses. FcγRII binds monomeric IgG with relatively low affinity, but it effectively mediates the phagocytosis of IgG-coated particles and cytotoxic reactions. FcγRIII is expressed on mature macrophages but not on mono-

TABLE 120-1

Secretory Products of Macrophages

Cytokines, Growth Factors, and Hormones

  Growth factors

    GM-CSF

    M-CSF

    G-CSF

  Proteins involved in host defense and inflammation

    C1

    C4

    C2

    C3

    C5

    Factor B

    Factor D

    Properdin

    C3b inactivation

    βIH

    Lysozyme

    Interferon-γ

    Fibronectin

    Lactoferrin

  Cytokines that promote acute inflammation and regulate lymphocytes

    TNF

    IL-1α/β

    IL-6

    IL-8

    IL-12

    GROα/β/γ

    CTAPIII

    β-Thromboglobulin

    IP-10

    MCP-1

    MIP-1α

    MIP-1β

  Cytokines that inhibit acute inflammation and lymphocyte responses

TABLE 120-1

Secretory Products of Macrophages (*continued*)

    IL-10

    TGF-β_1, -β_2, -β_3

    IL-1 receptor antagonist

Reactive Oxygen Intermediates

    O_2^-

    H_2O_2

    OH·

Reactive Nitrogen Intermediates

    NO·

    NO_2

    NO_3

Enzymes Active in Microbicidal Activity and Inflammation

    Acid hydrolases

    Acid phosphatases

    Cathepsins

    Cytolytic proteinase

    Hyaluronidase

    Lysozyme

    Phospholipase A_2

    Plasminogen activator

Inhibitors of Enzymes

    α_1-Antiprotease

    α_2-Macroglobulin

    Inhibitors of plasminogen

    Inhibitors of plasminogen activator

    Lipomodulin

Lipids Active in Host Defense and Inflammation

    PGE_2

    $PGF_{2\alpha}$

    Prostacylin

    Thromboxane A_2

    Leukotrienes B, C, D, and E

    Mono-HETES

    Di-HETES

    PAF

    Lysophospholipids

---

cytes. FcγRIII mediates phagocytosis and cytotoxicity. The redundancy of the three FcγRs may confer a selective advantage; patients who lack FcγRI have no increased susceptibility to infection.

Macrophages are also capable of ingesting microbes in the absence of complement or immunoglobulin. The ability to recognize surface oligosaccharides on microorganisms is probably a primitive mechanism of host defense. The mannose receptor, a 162-kDa membrane glycoprotein, binds mannose and fucose-bovine serum albumin (BSA) with high affinity. The mannose

receptor is effective in mediating phagocytosis of yeasts, zymosan particles, and *Pneumocystis carinii* (Fig. 120-2).

Phagocytosis follows recognition of the microbe. The intracellular signal(s) that mediate the movement of pseudopods around ligand-coated microbes is poorly defined. Ligated surface receptors apparently generate binding sites for cytoskeletal proteins. Particle engulfment requires engagement of specific receptors and the generation of transmembrane signals. Movement of the phagocyte plasma membrane over a ligand-coated particle is governed by the availability of unbound receptors on the surface of the phagocyte and of ligands on the surface of the particle (zipper hypothesis). Phagocytosis requires sequential, circumferential interaction of phagocyte surface receptors with complementary ligands on the surface of the particle.

Alveolar macrophages (AM) use both oxidative and nonoxidative processes to kill ingested microbes (Table 120-1). Differentiation of monocytes to macrophages in vitro results in a marked decline in antimicrobial activity against intracellular pathogens such as *Cryptococcus neoformans* and *Toxoplasma gondii*. A decrease in the magnitude of the respiratory burst and the loss of granule peroxidase accounts for the decline in antimicrobial activity. Because resident AM contain minimal myeloperoxidase (MPO), their MPO-H_2O_2-halide system is deficient. AM kill *Staphylococcus aureas* but are ineffective in killing many gram-negative microbes, *C. neoformans*, *T. gondii*, and *Leishmania donovani*.

Microbes can also be killed by macrophage-dependent nonoxidative mechanisms, including proteases, lysozyme, and defensins. Defensins are a multiple-member family of broad-spectrum cytotoxic peptides that kill many gram-positive organisms (*S. aureus*, *S. epidermidis*, *Streptococcus*) and gram-negative species (*Escherichia coli*, *Pseudomonas aeruginosa*, *Klebsiella pneumoniae*). Defensins also kill fungi and inactivate certain viruses. Defensins are present in the alveolar macrophages of some species.

NK Cells

NK cells are present within the lung. Active NK cells are located primarily in the interstitium of the lung. Pulmonary NK cells play a protective role in influenza infections and in fungal infections. NK cells play a role in early resistance against *C. neoformans* if the organism is delivered intravenously, but NK cells are not important determinants of survival or resistance to infection if *C. neoformans* is delivered to the alveolus.[27]

Complement

Normal alveolar lavage fluids contain a functional alternative complement pathway. Complement activation generates C3b, which has opsonic activity and promotes receptor-mediated phagocytosis of microbes by macrophages. Complement activation also generates C5a, an important chemoattractant for PMNs. Activation of the entire complement pathway in the presence of a microbe could result in its lysis and killing. The importance of the complement system to pulmonary host defenses has been documented in animal models; experimental depletion of the complement system impairs the pulmonary clearance of certain bacteria.[13]

Surfactant

The alveolar epithelium is more than a mere physical barrier to microbial invasion. Microbes that enter the alveolar space encounter alveolar epithelial cell–derived substances that might inactivate them. Surfactant, secreted by type II pneumocytes, has

antibacterial activity against staphylococci, rough colony strains of gram-negative bacteria, and some fungi.[7]

INFLAMMATORY RESPONSES

While resident alveolar macrophages are the first line of defense against microbes in the lower respiratory tract, in most instances, pulmonary antibacterial defenses are dependent on a dual phagocytic system that involves both alveolar macrophages and polymorphonuclear leukocytes.[37,43] In murine pulmonary infection models, small doses of aerosolized *S. aureus* are contained solely by macrophages. *K. pneumoniae*, *P. aeruginosa*, and *Streptococcus pneumoniae* invoke a PMN exudate in the alveoli. When selectively granulocytopenic animals were challenged, *K. pneumoniae*, *P. aeruginosa*, and *S. pneumoniae* were all cleared suboptimally—demonstrating that circulating PMN must be available for recruitment to the lung to effectively clear most bacterial pathogens. The mechanism(s) whereby the host senses that resident defenses are overwhelmed is unknown. Microbial characteristics such as inoculum size and virulence are important determinants of the magnitude of the pulmonary inflammatory response.[37] Phagocytic cell numbers and their state of activation as well as the availability of specific antibody may also be monitored in some fashion by the host. Whether macrophages, lymphocytes, or parenchymal cells sense that the resident defenses are overwhelmed is unknown.

Enormous strides have been made in understanding the molecular basis for recruitment of cells to sites of inflammation (Fig. 120-3).[1,45] PMN recruitment into the alveoli is initiated within the alveolar space. On arrival within the alveolus, bacteria directly activate the alternative complement pathway. C3b,Bb complexes form on the surface of microorganisms and function as active C3/C5 convertases. Binding of properdin is favored by the absence of complement regulatory proteins on bacterial surfaces; binding of properdin stabilizes the C3b,Bb convertase activity. This convertase initiates the conversion of free C3 molecules found in alveolar lining fluid to C3b, which coats the surface of the microbe. The membrane-bound complex also binds C5 and induces its cleavage to C5a. The C5 molecule and its fragments are important PMN chemotaxins in murine lungs after bacterial challenges. C5-deficient mice have reduced chemotactic activity in bronchoalveolar lavage and diminished PMN recruitment to the lung after intratracheal inoculation with *S. pneumoniae*, *P. aeruginosa*, and *Hemophilus influenzae* when compared to congenic C5-sufficient mice.[50]

Subsequently, bacterial products activate alveolar macrophages. Macrophages are highly secretory cells that rapidly release cytokines after the uptake of microbes (Table 120-1). Cytokines released early following the ingestion of microbes include IL-1, TNFα, C-C, and C-X-C chemokines. These cytokines are crucially active in the generation of acute inflammatory responses.

The process of cellular recruitment can be divided into four steps: adhesion to endothelial cells, transmigration through the endothelial layer, penetration through the vascular basement membrane, and migration through the extracellular matrix along a chemotactic gradient.[1,45] Each of these steps requires the sequential interaction of cytokine/chemokines, cell adhesion mol-

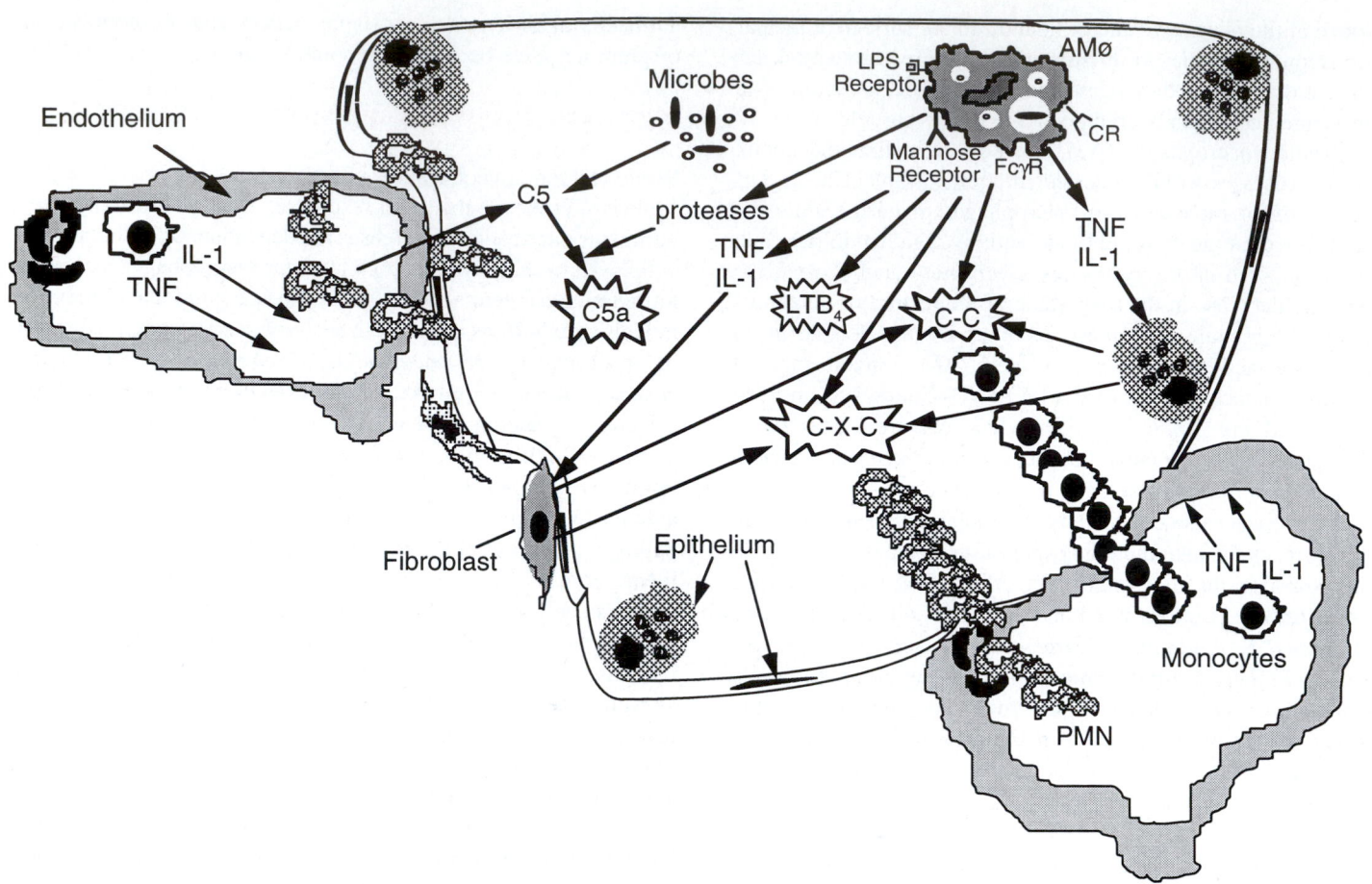

FIGURE 120-3 Initiation of inflammatory responses in the lower respiratory tract. Chemotaxins are generated sequentially following the entry of bacteria or bacterial products into the alveolus. Complement activation occurs early via the alternative pathway, generating C5a. LPS stimulates alveolar macrophages to produce TNFα, IL-1β, IL-8, and leukotriene B4. TNFα and IL-1β induce gene expression and production of chemokines by epithelial cells and fibroblasts present in the alveolar-capillary wall and induce the expression of adherence molecules on inflammatory cells and endothelial cells.

ecules, and proteases. Adhesion molecule expression on endothelial cells is normally low; adhesion molecule expression increases rapidly when proinflammatory cytokines (IL-1, TNFα) or microbial products (LPS) activate endothelial cells. Selectins, integrins, and members of the immunoglobulin supergene family all play crucial roles in inflammatory cell adhesion. L-selectin, differentially expressed on leukocytes, binds to CD34 and an unidentified adhesion molecule on the surface of the endothelial cells. L-selectin mediates leukocyte rolling on vascular endothelium at sites of tissue inflammation. P-selectin and E-selectin are rapidly expressed on the endothelium after activation with inflammatory cytokines and bind inflammatory cells via interaction with the ligands sialyl Lewis A and sialyl Lewis X. While these bonds are relatively weak, selectin-ligand binding slows rapidly moving inflammatory cells in the blood vessel. Integrins (VLA-4, LFA-1, MAC-1, and p150,95) are heterodimeric proteins that bind to members of the immunoglobulin superfamily (VCAM-1, ICAM-1, ICAM-2, and PECAM). Under the influence of cytokines, β_2 integrins of the PMN surface (LFA-1, Mo-1/MAC-1) are converted to a high affinity state. IL-1 and TNFα induce ICAM expression on endothelial cells. Binding of leukocyte integrins to endothelial cell ICAM leads to firm adhesion of the inflammatory cells to the endothelium.

Subsequent transmigration of the inflammatory cells through endothelial cell junctions is mediated by PECAM-1 (CD31) via interaction of leukocyte PECAM-1 with endothelial cell PECAM-1 (homotypic binding).

Directed migration into the alveolar space is dependent on cytokines and chemokines. Two closely related families of chemotactic cytokines, C-C and C-X-C chemokine families, are important mediators of pulmonary inflammation.[31,38] The C-X-C chemokine family, which includes IL-8, MIP-2 (the functional murine homologue of IL-8), platelet factor 4, GRO, ENA-78, and interferonγ-inducible protein, is composed of homologous 8 to 10-kD peptides. Members of this chemokine family have predominant neutrophil stimulatory and chemotactic activities. Bacterial products stimulate AM production of C-X-C chemokines. Additionally, bacterial products stimulate the production of TNFα and IL-1, both of which induce gene expression and secretion of chemokines from endothelial cells, fibroblasts, and pulmonary epithelial cells.[46,47] Macrophages also generate leukotriene B4, which is a potent chemotactic substance. Thus, the recruitment of inflammatory cells to the lung entails a cell-cell network, where the function of each cell is dependent on mediators synthesized by neighboring cells. The entire alveolar capillary wall is engaged in the recruitment of inflammatory cells.

A role for C-X-C chemokines in pulmonary host defenses has been demonstrated in both patients and animal models. Interleukin-8 is detected in increased amounts in respiratory secretions from patients with acute pulmonary bacterial infections. TNFα and MIP-2 are rapidly induced in murine lungs following *K. pneumoniae* pulmonary infections. Treatment of infected mice with anti–MIP-2 antibodies results in decreased clearance of *K. pneumoniae* and early dissemination of *K. pneumoniae* to the blood. C-X-C chemokines also enhance phagocytic and bactericidal activity of PMNs in vitro. IL-8 and MIP-2 have both been shown to increase phagocytosis and enhance killing of *E. coli*.

SPECIFIC IMMUNE RESPONSES

Specific pulmonary immune responses are of importance in the defense of the lung against certain pathogens, particularly intracellular organisms that survive in normal macrophages (mycobacteria, fungi, virulent encapsulated bacteria, and viruses).[28] Microbial infections that elude the innate defense mechanisms and inflammatory responses generate a threshold dose of antigen, which is needed to trigger antigen-specific immune responses. Antigen-specific immune responses require at least 7 to 10 days for their development; this time is required for the proliferation and differentiation of antigen-specific T and B lymphocytes. During the development of specific immune responses, pathogens may continue to grow in the host or be held in check by innate and inflammatory mechanisms. The generation of specific immune responses to infectious antigens can be divided into three phases: the afferent phase, the central control/processing phase, and the efferent phase.

Initiation of Specific Immune Responses to Pulmonary Antigens

The activation of T lymphocytes is a crucial early event in all immune responses.[9] Activation of T lymphocytes requires a cognate interaction between T lymphocytes and an antigen-presenting cell. The interaction between the antigenic epitope presented in association with the MHC molecule on the surface of the antigen-presenting cell and the T-lymphocyte receptor/CD3 complex is a central event in T-lymphocyte activation. This event provides specificity for T-lymphocyte activation. However, three additional molecular interactions are required: adhesion molecules that promote binding of APC to T lymphocytes, costimulatory molecules that promote growth and differentiation of T lymphocytes, and soluble cytokines (TNFα, IL-1). Cell-cell contact and transmembrane signaling are promoted by the interaction of lymphocyte function–associated antigen (LFA) molecules on T lymphocytes with ICAM molecules on APC. CD2 interacts with LFA-3, and CD4 interacts with MHC class II molecules. Costimulatory molecules are required to activate T lymphocytes to produce cytokines. B7 molecules (B7-1, B7-2) are important costimulatory molecules expressed on APC.[24] B7 molecules are members of the immunoglobulin supergene family. CD28 expressed on T lymphocytes is an important ligand for B7 costimulation. Both B7-1 and B7-2 bind CD28. Engagement of CD28 by B7 enhances transcription of cytokine genes through the expression of an enhancer protein that binds to the IL-2 gene.

Soluble cytokines are also released during antigen presentation. IL-1 production by antigen-presenting cells is profoundly increased during antigen presentation. Although IL-1 was originally believed to be a major costimulatory molecule, its role in T-lymphocyte activation is more limited than was initially proposed.

Antigen-presenting cells are present both in the lower respiratory tract and in airway epithelium (Fig. 120-4). Extensive studies in experimental animals and humans suggest that dendritic cells are the major antigen-presenting cells in the lung.[18,36,39] Dendritic cells—found in the interstitium, in alveolar septi, and throughout the columnar epithelium of the bronchi—are ideally situated to function as sentinel antigen detection cells.[48] Dendritic cells constitutively express high levels of MHC class II molecules and both B7-1 and B7-2. Initiation of an immune response requires maturation of pulmonary dendritic cells to potent antigen-presenting immunostimulatory cells. GM-CSF, TNFα, IL-4, and IL-1, produced by interstitial macrophages and epithelial cells, are required for this differentiative step.[2,5] Antigens that breech the epithelial barrier probably injure/stimulate epithelial cells and macrophages to secrete the required cytokines to induce maturation of dendritic cells and initiate their migration from the lung to hilar lymph nodes. Dendritic cells activate antigen-reactive lymphocytes within the hilar node.

Alveolar macrophages are ineffective antigen-presenting cells. Alveolar macrophages are less effective than monocytes in inducing proliferation of blood T lymphocytes to recall antigens. Alveolar macrophages effectively stimulate proliferation of T lymphocyte lines and clones. Thus, alveolar macrophages are ineffective stimulators of naïve T lymphocytes or resting memory cells but can restimulate recently activated T lymphocytes. Alveolar macrophages fail to effectively activate CD4 T lymphocytes because they bind resting T lymphocytes poorly and do not express B7 costimulatory cell surface molecules. Antigen presentation by alveolar macrophages can be restored by the addition of a CD28 stimulant (anti-CD28mAb). The mechanism by which alveolar macrophages limit expression of B7-1 and B7-2 is unknown.

Resident pulmonary alveolar macrophages not only function poorly as antigen-presenting cells, but alveolar macrophages actively suppress T-lymphocyte proliferation induced by antigen. Compelling evidence for the presence of active alveolar macrophage suppression in vivo exists; selective depletion of murine alveolar macrophages by intratracheal administration of a lyposome-encapsulated macrophage cytotoxic drug induced gross hyperresponsiveness to pulmonary antigen administration.[19] The potential value of such a steady-state down-regulatory control mechanism within the lung is self-evident. While the lung is frequently exposed to antigens, immune responses must be restricted and down-regulated within the pulmonary parenchyma. Since immune reactions inevitably result in significant damage to gas exchange surfaces, alveolar macrophage suppressive activity can be reversed. GM-CSF and TNFα both significantly lessen alveolar macrophage suppressive activity. Thus, microbial stimuli (LPS) lessen the down-regulatory tone of alveolar macrophages by inducing GM-CSF production by macrophages and/or alveolar and airway epithelial cells and TNFα production by macrophages to allow local T-cell activation in the face of microbial challenges.[17]

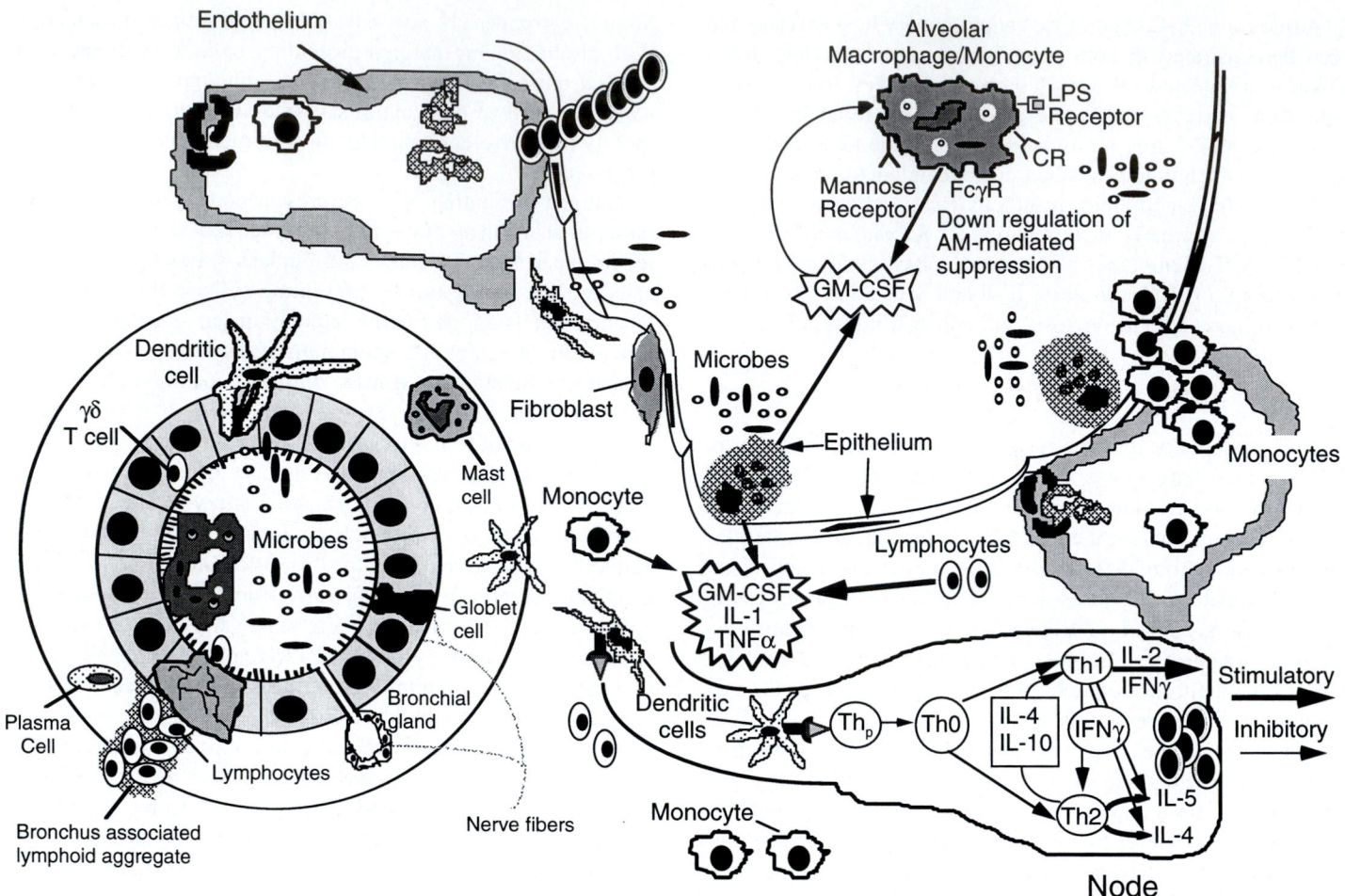

FIGURE 120-4 Initiation of specific immune responses in the lung. Dendritic cells located in the interstitium of the lung and in the airway epithelium function as sentinel antigen-presenting cells. Dendritic cells reside in close contact to airway epithelial cells, alveolar epithelial cells, and interstitial macrophages. Following exposure to microbial antigens, DC differentiation occurs as a result of exposure to cytokines produced by cells of the innate immune system (macrophages) and cytokines pro-duced as a result of injury to epithelial cells. Differentiated DC migrate to local nodes and present antigen to naive T lymphocytes. The control of CD4 T-lymphocyte subset differentiation occurs via complex, cross-regulatory interactions mediated by lymphokines. The development of CD8 effector cells and plasma cells usually requires cognate interac-tions with CD4 regulatory T lymphocytes.

T lymphocytes can be separated into three subsets according to their use of T-cell receptors and accessory molecules, which interact with MHC gene products on target cells. T-lymphocyte subsets include CD4α/β T lymphocytes, which recognize anti-genic peptides in the context of MHC class II molecules; CD8α/β T lymphocytes, which recognize antigenic peptides in the context of MHC class I molecules; and γ/δ T lymphocytes, which lack both CD4 and CD8 molecules. Two subsets of CD4 T lymphocytes have been defined on the basis of their lym-phokine secretion patterns.[35,40] Th1 cells secrete IL-2, IFN-γ, TNFα, and GM-CSF and mediate delayed-type hypersensitiv-ity responses. Th2 cells produced IL-4, IL-5, IL-6, and IL-10 and are largely responsible for B-lymphocyte maturation and immunoglobulin isotype switching. CD8 lymphocytes secrete IL-2 and IFN-γ. Cytokines control the development of Th1 and Th2 CD4 cells. IFN-γ produced by Th1 cells suppresses the de-velopment of Th2 cells. IL-10 and IL-4 produced by Th2 cells suppress the development of Th1 cells. Innate immune cells play a crucial role in the development of Th1 and Th2 cells.[20,35] Af-ter the ingestion of microbes, macrophages produce IL-12. IL-12 powerfully induces the development of Th1 cells following the interaction of naïve CD4 cells with antigen-bearing dendritic cells. IL-12 is also a powerful inducer of IFN-γ secretion by NK cells. γ/δ T lymphocytes also secrete IFN-γ following their interaction with microbes. IL-4 is required for the development of Th2 cells following the interaction of naïve CD4 cells with antigen-bearing dendritic cells. Basophils and mast cells pro-duce IL-4 following exposure to certain antigens. γ/δ T lym-phocytes secrete IL-4 following interaction with certain mi-crobes. An NK 1.1$^+$, CD4$^+$, CD8$^-$ T lymphocyte found in lymphoid tissues also produces IL-4. The interaction of cy-tokines produced by innate immune cells and cytokines pro-duced by developing Th1 and Th2 cells determines whether Th1 or Th2 cells develop as a result of antigen exposure. Chronic exposure to antigen is required to produce highly segregated Th1 or Th2 responses.

T Lymphocyte–Mediated Immune Responses in the Lower Respiratory Tract

T lymphocyte–mediated immune responses are required for the clearance of intracellular microbes. Intracellular microbes represent an extremely heterogeneous group of pathogens. The kinetics of T lymphocyte–mediated immune responses in the lung parenchyma and the lymphocyte subsets involved in pulmonary host defenses have been defined almost exclusively from serial studies of experimental models of mycobacterial, fungal, and viral infections. T lymphocytes are critical to microbial clearance of each of these infections (Fig. 120-5).

CD4 T lymphocytes play a central role in host defenses against mycobacteria and fungi.[23,25,32] Antigen-specific CD4 T lymphocytes isolated from *M. tuberculosis*–infected mice pro-

duce IL-2, IFN-γ and small amounts of IL-4. Thus, Th0 and Th1 cells appear to be importantly involved in pulmonary host responses to *Mycobacterium tuberculosis*. T lymphocytes isolated from *C. neoformans*–infected mice also produce both Th1 and Th2 cytokines. Either a combination of Th1 and Th2 cells and/or Th0 cells are present in the lung during protective immune responses to *C. neoformans*. Class I restricted CD8 lymphocytes also participate in the immune response to mycobacterial and fungal pathogens.[25] CD8 T lymphocytes express specific cytolytic activities and produce IFN-γ. CD8 lymphocytes are present in the outer mantle of many granulomatous lesions. CD8 lymphocytes are necessary during the afferent and challenge phases, as well as for the expression of delayed-type hypersensitivity to *C. neoformans*.[33] The relative roles of these lymphocyte subsets can be investigated by selective in vivo elim-

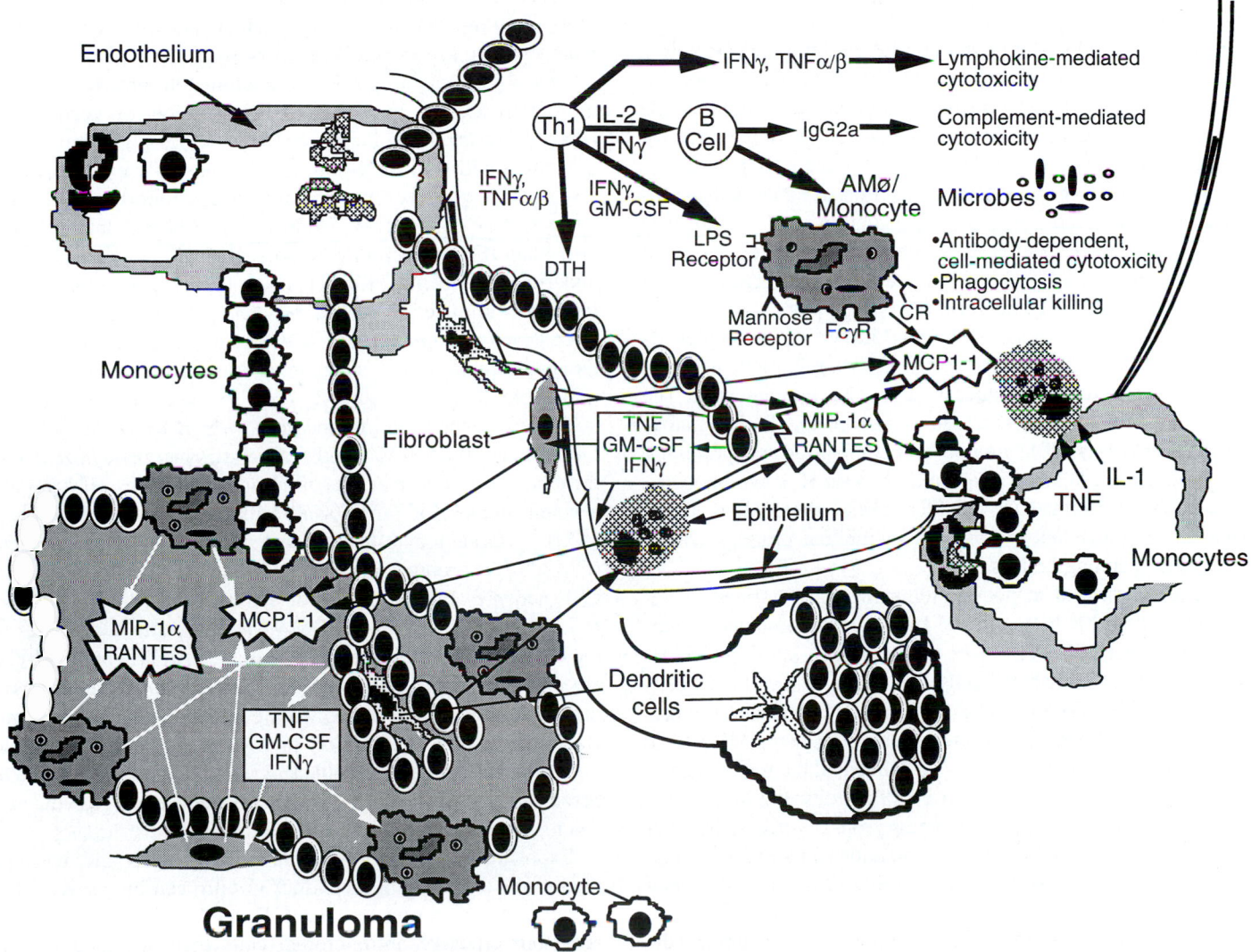

FIGURE 120-5   Expression of specific immune responses in the lower respiratory tract. Activated T lymphocytes recirculate from draining regional lymph nodes and enter sites of microbial multiplication via a series of highly regulated events involving cytokines and adherence molecules expressed on both lymphocytes and endothelial cells. Activated Th0 or Th1 lymphocytes are stimulated by resident antigen-presenting cells to produce high levels of IFN-γ, GM-CSF, and TNF, which recruit and activate monocytes from the circulation. Adherence receptor ligand interactions between monocytes and endothelial cells are important in their recruitment. A unique subset of mononuclear cell chemotaxins (MIP-1α, MCP-1) are probably active in recruitment of mononuclear phagocytes. Recruited, activated mononuclear phagocytes are crucial to the clearance of certain pathogens.

ination of T-lymphocyte subsets in both murine tuberculosis and fungal infections. This approach has revealed a dominant role for CD4 lymphocytes, with an important contribution by CD8 T cells.[23,25,32]

γ/δ T lymphocytes are also significant to antimicrobial granulomas.[25] Three lines of experimental evidence indicate an important role for these cells: (1) mice immunized with *M. tuberculosis* contain γ/δ T lymphocytes, which respond vigorously to *M. tuberculosis* antigens in vitro; (2) an extraordinarily high percentage of murine γ/δ T-cell hybridomas react with purified protein derivative; (3) γ/δ T lymphocytes can be readily expanded by in vitro stimulation of peripheral blood cells from normal human volunteers with *M. tuberculosis*. γ/δ T lymphocytes appear prior to α/β T lymphocytes in most animal models. Mycobacteria-stimulated γ/δ T lymphocytes express various biologic functions relevant to defense against intracellular microbes, including lysis of microbacterial infected target cells and secretion of IFN-γ and TNF-α.

Cytokines produced by CD4 and CD8 T lymphocytes play a central role in two closely related but different events in the generation of T lymphocyte–mediated immune responses in the lower respiratory tract. Cytokines are of central importance for the early infiltration of inflammatory mononuclear phagocytes and the activation of microbicidal function in macrophages. Inflammatory cell recruitment after inoculation of *C. neoformans* is dependent upon specific T lymphocytes, since depletion of both CD4 and CD8 T lymphocytes ablates the recruitment of monocytes following *C. neoformans*.[23]

Chemokines are crucial to the recruitment of monocytes after inoculation of *C. neoformans*. The C-C family of chemokines is chemotactic for mononuclear cells and lymphocytes. The C-C chemokine family includes macrophage inflammatory protein–1 (MIP-1-α/β), monocyte chemoattractant protein–1 (MCP-1), and regulated on activation, normal T lymphocyte–expressed and secreted (RANTES). These chemokines signal cells via receptors that are integral membrane proteins with 7 membrane spanning helices.

The recruitment of monocytes following *C. neoformans* is dependent on both MCP-1 and MIP-1α.[22] Specific immune T lymphocytes generate GM-CSF, IFN-γ, and TNFα—all of which activate monocytes, endothelial cells, fibroblasts, and epithelial cells to produce MCP-1. Additionally, activated T lymphocytes produce MIP-1α and RANTES. Studies with neutralizing anti–MCP-1– or anti–MIP-1α–specific antisera have documented the importance of these two molecules in mononuclear cell recruitment. MCP-1 and MIP-1α appear to share overlapping roles, since either antichemokine alone can decrease inflammation by more than 50 percent. Neither antichemokine treatment achieves the same degree of inhibition of leukocyte recruitment as can be achieved by treatment with anti–T-lymphocyte antibodies. Few studies have addressed the role of chemokines in mycobacterial infections in vivo. Antibodies to MIP-1 and MIP-2 were effective in reducing neutrophilia in mice during a peritoneal infection. Both MIP-1α and MCP-1 are produced during schistosoma granuloma formation.

Monocyte recruitment to the lung requires monocytes to traverse numerous tissue planes before eventually entering the alveolar space. Expression of proteases by monocytes is crucial for their migration to inflammatory sites. Urokinase-type plasmino-

gen activator (uPA) is required for protective cellular recruitment and host defenses against *C. neoformans*.[14,15] Mice with specific targeted disruption of the uPA gene have had markedly diminished recruitment of inflammatory cells in response to pulmonary *C. neoformans* infection.[14] The recruitment of both neutrophils and macrophages as well as CD4 lymphocytes is blunted. In the absence of uPA, pulmonary *C. neoformans* is not adequately cleared; the infection disseminates to spleen and brain. While all uPA+/+ mice survive, uPA−/− mice did not survive infection with *C. neoformans*.

Many microbes, including bacteria (*Legionella pneumophila, M. tuberculosis*), fungi (*H. capsulatum, C. neoformans, Candida albicans, Blastomyces dermatiditis*), protozoa (*T. gondii*), and chlamydiae continue to grow within resident pulmonary macrophages. Cytokines secreted by Th1 CD4 lymphocytes and CD8 lymphocytes are required to activate pulmonary macrophages after exposure to certain cytokines. The antimicrobial activity of pulmonary macrophages can be increased to allow these phagocytes to kill intracellular microbes.

IFN-γ plays a central role in granulomatous protection against most intracellular microbes. Administration of recombinant IFN-γ protects mice against lethal *M. tuberculosis* infection; neutralization with anti–IFN-γ antibodies markedly exacerbates the disease. IFN-γ is also a potent stimulator of fungistasis in murine mononuclear phagocytes. Studies with IFN-γ deletion (IFN-γ −/−) and IFN-γ receptor deletions (IFN-γR−/−) mutants have underlined the central role of this cytokine in immunity to tuberculosis in mice.[8,11,12,21] *M. tuberculosis*–infected IFN-γ−/− mice developed granulomas with caseous necrosis, widespread tissue destruction, and widespread dissemination of the infection. Both IFN-γ−/− and IFN-γR−/− animals failed to produce reactive nitrogen intermediates, which are essential for antimicrobial killing. IFN-γ and TNF-α are synergistic in activating the tuberculostatic capacities of murine phagocytes. IFN-γ is also a potent inducer of fungistasis in murine alveolar macrophage (AM).[34] Granulocyte-macrophage colony–stimulating factor (GM-CSF) is produced by Th0, Th1, and Th2 CD4 subsets. GM-CSF activates macrophages for killing of *C. neoformans* and *C. albicans*.[4] GM-CSF and IFN-γ have cooperative activities for the induction of anticryptococcal killing.[4,34] IFN-γ and GM-CSF are not effective as an activation scheme in mycobacterial systems; however, TNFα and GM-CSF cooperate to induce significant intracellular destruction of mycobacteria. Th2 cytokines have important roles in granulomatous diseases. IL-4 induces tuberculostatic activity and reduces mycobacterial growth, even when given after infection of the animals.

Exposure of resident alveolar macrophages and recruited monocytes to activating cytokines in vitro causes a several-fold increase in their respiratory burst. Recently recruited monocytes are more effective antimicrobial cells than activated resident macrophages. The increase in microbicidal activity is due to the formation of H_2O_2, hydroxyl radical, and/or nitrogen oxides. Nitrite (NO_2), nitrate (NO_3), and nitric oxide (NO·) are formed by activated macrophages via the oxidation of the guanidine nitrogen L-arginine. Nitric oxide formation by murine macrophages contributes to fungal stasis and killing, antiparasitic activity, and bacterial killing. Nitric oxides produce injurious effects by causing iron loss from the target cell and by inhibition of DNA synthesis and mitochondrial respiration. Activated macrophages also release increased amounts of proteases and lysozyme.

Antigen-specific CD8 cytotoxic T lymphocyte responses are crucial in the defense against pulmonary viral infections. Specific CD8 cytotoxic T lymphocytes appear in large numbers in the lung parenchyma within 1 week after pulmonary viral infections. Following replication of viral particles in the cytosol of infected cells, viral antigens are presented on the surface of infected cells in conjunction with MHC class I molecules. Eradication of viral infections is accomplished when cytotoxic CD8 cells recognize MHC class I–associated viral antigens on the surface of infected cells and effect the lysis of these infected cells.[44]

B Lymphocyte–Mediated Immune Responses in the Lung

Immunoglobulins are a major protein constituent of the mucus that lines the luminal surface of conducting airways and alveolar lining fluid. IgA is the predominant immunoglobulin in secretions of the trachea and major bronchi while both IgG and IgE are present as well. IgG is the predominant immunoglobulin in alveolar lining fluid.

The secretory IgA found in external secretions consists of two molecules of IgA that are held together by a joining chain and by a secretory component, a glycoprotein produced by epithelial cells. The secretory component is required for transporting IgA through epithelial cells and bronchial glands. Accordingly, secretory IgA is the product of both plasma cells and epithelial cells. The role of IgA in pulmonary defenses remains enigmatic. The usual specificity of IgA antibodies is antiviral. Specific IgA antibodies against hemagglutinating antigen have been isolated from patients infected with influenza A. IgA may also be important in inhibiting bacterial adherence to the respiratory epithelium; it may also serve as an antitoxin, since specific IgA against *Bordetella pertussis* toxin has been isolated from the respiratory secretions of patients with pertussis. While IgA is believed to fix complement poorly, IgA1 antibodies from volunteers vaccinated with meningococcal polysaccharide vaccine induced classic complement pathway–mediated killing of group C *Neisseria meningitis*. Finally, IgA may also have a role as an opsonin, since human alveolar macrophages bear Fc receptors that bind either IgA1 or IgA2. Certain bacteria elaborate proteases that digest IgA; these proteases may provide a selective colonization advantage to the microbes.[44]

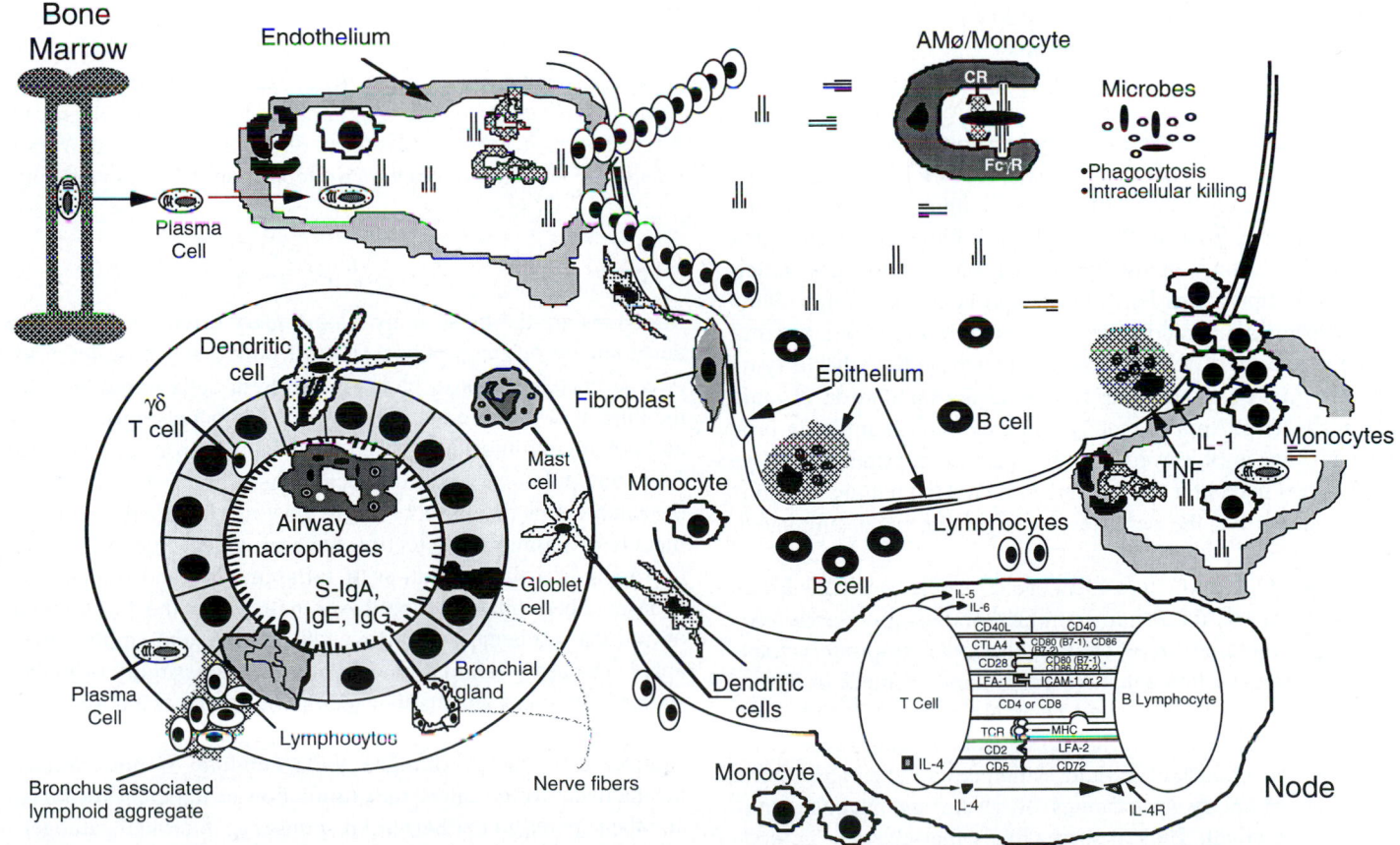

FIGURE 120-6 Expression of B lymphocyte–mediated immune responses in the lower respiratory tract. Initial events in B-lymphocyte proliferation and differentiation occur in T lymphocyte–dependent areas of regional lymph nodes. Proliferation, somatic hypermutation, and selection occur within the lymphoid follicle. B lymphocytes then migrate to bone marrow and to the lung, where they undergo differentiation to mature antibody-producing plasma cells. Serum antibody that gains access to the alveolar spaces of uninflamed lungs is present in large amounts during intra-alveolar infectious processes. Antibodies neutralize pathogens and their toxins, activate complement, and function as opsonins to enhance macrophage recognition and ingestion of extracellular pathogens.

The availability of specific antibody is an important ingredient in lower respiratory tract defenses against extracellular microbes (Fig. 120-6). Most extracellular bacteria possess polysaccharide capsules that allow them to evade phagocytic cells. Antibodies have three important host defense functions: they are the principal opsonins that allow phagocytes to recognize and ingest microbes via the involvement of Fc receptors; they activate complement, which enhances opsonization and can directly lyse some bacteria; and they neutralize pathogens or their toxins by binding to microbes or their products, thereby preventing injury to cells.

Studies of experimental animal models have defined the mechanisms of accumulation of antibody-forming cells in the lung and the production of immunoglobulins.[10] Humoral immune responses to most pathogens occur only after antigen-specific Th2 CD4 lymphocytes have been generated, since B cells specific for most protein microbial antigens cannot be activated until they encounter an activated helper CD4 T lymphocyte specific for the antigen. Accordingly, the initial phase of B-lymphocyte proliferation occurs in T-lymphocyte areas of lymphoid tissues. Primary foci of clonally expanded B lymphocytes appear approximately 5 days after primary immunization. B lymphocytes then migrate to the lymphoid follicle, where they undergo proliferation, somatic hypermutation, and selection. Once activated, lymphocytes leave the lymph node via efferent lymphatics. Some activated B lymphocytes migrate to bone marrow to complete their differentiation into plasma cells; other B lymphocytes migrate to the lung following the instillation of antigens in the lung. Approximately 90 percent of all antibody produced in vivo is produced by bone marrow plasma cells. The lymphocytes that enter the lung are attracted to the lung by spontaneous migration, the persistence of antigen, or inflammatory mediators.

The role of antibody in resident bacterial defenses in the lower respiratory tract is uncertain. Immunoglobulins are clearly present in the epithelial lining fluid of the lower respiratory tract. Systemic immunization enhances pulmonary clearance of *P. aeruginosa*, *Proteus mirabilis*, and *H. influenzae*.[16,29,50] Enhanced clearance correlates with the appearance of antibodies and serum and bronchoalveolar lavage fluid, which are directed against the organisms. Antibody specificities of serum and alveolar antibodies are identical. Thus, it seems likely that alveolar antibodies are derived in large part from serum.

Serum IgG can clearly gain access to the alveolar space in normal subjects and during inflammation when large changes in alveolar permeability occur. Serum IgG can clearly and directly enhance bacterial clearance from the lower respiratory tract, since intravenous injection of a murine IgG monoclonal

TABLE 120-2

Pulmonary Host Defense-Microbe Interactions

Host Mood	Defense Mechanism	Timing	Microbial Behavior
Content	Mechanical Epithelial barrier Mucociliary escalator	Continuous	Commensal
Irritated	Innate Immunity Macrophages, NK cells, γ/δ T lymphocytes	Hours–days	Replication in the airway and alveolar space
Interested	Inflammation Macrophages/PMN	Minutes–hours	Invasion
Angry	Antigen-specific immunity DC; CD4, CD8 T lymphocytes; B lymphocytes	3–7 days	Tissue invasion/ replication in phagocytes
Hysterical	Immunopathology Macrophages; CD4, CD8 T cells; NK cells, B cells		Dissemination to many tissues

antibody specific for a cell surface–exposed epitope of nontypable *H. influenzae* resulted in enhanced pulmonary clearance. Accordingly, it seems likely that direct airway immunization would not be required to obtain protective antibodies in the lung.

CONCLUSION

Infections are the most likely evolutionary driving force for the development of a complex system of pulmonary host defenses. A coordinated response of many different cells is required for the lung to clear pulmonary pathogens. An increasingly complex and potentially injurious cascade of host responses is mobilized following pulmonary microbial challenges (Table 120-2). While the interactions of microbes in the host are invariably complex, models of pulmonary infection have provided crucial information regarding the regulation of inflammatory and immune responses. These insights should eventually allow the development of rational strategies regarding vaccination and immunotherapy.[26] The use of animal models offers the possibility of understanding the mechanisms that regulate immune responses sufficiently well that the response to a specific antigen could be controlled. A more complete understanding of host defense mechanisms would allow the stimulation of deficient responses and the suppression of harmful responses to microbial pathogens and other antigens that enter the lung.

REFERENCES

1. Albelda SM, Smith CW, Ward PA: Adhesion molecules and inflammatory injury. *FASEB J* 8:504–512, 1994.

2. Armstrong LR, Christensen PJ, Paine R III, et al: Regulation of the immunostimulatory activity of rat pulmonary and interstitial dendritic cells by cell-cell interactions and cytokines. *Am J Respir Cell Mol Biol* 11:682–691, 1994.

3. Brown EJ: Complement receptors and phagocytosis. *Curr Opin Immunol* 3:76–82, 1991.

4. Chen G-H, Curtis JL, Mody CH, et al: Effect of granulocyte-macrophage colony–stimulating factor (GM-CSF) on rat alveolar macrophage anticryptococcal activity in vivo. *J Immunol* 152:724–734, 1994.

5. Christensen PJ, Armstrong LR, Chen G-H, et al: Modulation of rat pulmonary dendritic cell function by alveolar epithelial cells in vitro. *Am J Respir Cell Mol Biol* 13:426–433, 1995.

6. Clark SW, Pavia D: Mucociliary clearance, in Crystal RG, West JB (eds), *The Lung: Scientific Foundations*. New York, Raven, 1991, pp 1845–1859.

7. Coonrod JD, Lester RL, Hsu LC: Characterization of the extracellular bactericidal factors of rat alveolar lung material. *J Clin Invest* 74:1269–1279, 1984.

8. Cooper AM, Dalton DK, Stewart TA, et al: Disseminated tuberculosis in interferon-γ gene-disrupted mice. *J Exp Med* 178:2243–2247, 1993.

9. Croft M: Activation of naïve, memory and effector T cells. *Curr Opin Immunol* 5:431–437, 1994.

10. Curtis JL, Kaltreider HB: Characterization of bronchoalveolar lymphocytes during a specific antibody-forming cell response in the lungs of mice. *Am Rev Respir Dis* 139:393–400, 1989.

11. Dalton DK, Pitts-Meer S, Keshav S, et al: Multiple defects of immune cell function in mice with disrupted interferon-γ genes. *Science* 259:1739–1742, 1993.

12. Flynn JL, Chan J, Triebold KJ, et al: An essential role for interferon γ in resistance to *Mycobacterium tuberculosis* infection. *J Exp Med* 178:2249–2254, 1993.

13. Gross GN, Rehm SR, Pierce AK: The effect of complement depletion on lung clearance of bacteria. *J Clin Invest* 62:373–378, 1978.

14. Gyetko MR, Chen G-H, McDonald RA, et al: Urokinase is required for the pulmonary inflammatory response to *Cryptococcus neoformans*. *J Clin Invest* 97:1818–1826, 1996.

15. Gyetko MR, Todd RF III, Wilkinson CC, Sitrin RG: The urokinase receptor is required for human monocyte chemotaxis in vitro. *J Clin Invest* 93:1380–1387, 1996.

16. Hansen EJ, Hart DA, McGehee JL, Toews GB: Immune enhancement of pulmonary clearance of nontypable *Haemophilus influenzae*. *Infect Immun* 56:182–190, 1988.

17. Holt PG: Regulation of antigen-presenting cell function(s) in lung and airway tissues. *Eur Respir J* 6:120–129, 1993.

18. Holt PG, Haining S, Nelson DJ, Sedgwick JD: Origin and steady-state turnover of class II MHC-bearing dendritic cells in the epithelium of the conducting airways. *J Immunol* 153:256–261, 1994.

19. Holt PG, Oliver J, Bilyk N, et al: Downregulation of the antigen presenting cell function(s) of pulmonary dendritic cells in vivo by resident alveolar macrophages. *J Exp Med* 177:397–407, 1993.

20. Hsieh C-S, Macatonia SE, Tripp CS, et al: Development of TH1 CD4+ T cells through IL-12 produced by *Listeria*-induced macrophages. *Science* 260:547–549, 1993.

21. Huang S, Hendriks W, Athage A, et al: Immune responses in mice that lack the interferon-γ receptor. *Science* 259:1742–1745, 1993.

22. Huffnagle GB, Strieter RM, Standiford TJ, et al: The role of monocyte chemotactic proteins–1 (MCP-1) in the recruitment of monocytes and CD4+ T cells during a pulmonary *Cryptococcus neoformans* infection. *J Immunol* 155:4790–4797, 1995.

23. Huffnagle GB, Yates JL, Lipscomb MF: Immunity to a pulmonary *C. neoformans* infection requires both CD4+ and CD8+ T cells. *J Exp Med* 173:793–800, 1991.

24. June CH, Bluestone JA, Nadler LM, Thompson CB: The B7 and CD28 receptor families. *Immunol Today* 15:321–331, 1994.

25. Kaufmann SHE: Immunity to intracellular bacteria. *Annu Rev Immunol* 11:129–163, 1992.

26. Lambert PH: New vaccines for the world—Needs and prospects. *Immunologist* 1:50–55, 1993.

27. Lipscomb MF, Alvarellos T, Toews GB, et al: Role of natural killer cells in resistance to *Cryptococcus neoformans* infections in mice. *Am J Pathol* 128:354–361, 1987.

28. Lipscomb MF, Bice DE, Lyons CR, et al: The regulation of pulmonary immunity. *Adv Immunol* 59:369–454, 1995.

29. McGehee JL, Radolf JD, Toews GB, Hansen EJ: Effect of primary immunization on pulmonary clearance of nontypable *Haemophilus influenzae*. *Am J Respir Cell Mol Biol* 1:201–210, 1989.

30. Mellman I: Relationships between structure and function in the Fc receptor family. *Curr Opin Immunol* 1:16–25, 1988.

31. Miller MD, Krangel MS: Biology and biochemistry of the chemokines: A family of chemotactic and inflammatory cytokines. *Crit Rev Immunol* 12:17–46, 1992.

32. Mody CH, Lipscomb MF, Street NE, Toews GB: Depletion of CD4+ (L3T4+) lymphocytes in vivo impairs murine host defense to *Cryptococcus neoformans*. *J Immunol* 144:1472–1477, 1990.

33. Mody CH, Paine R III, Jackson C, et al: CD8 cells play a critical role in delayed type hypersensitivity to intact *Cryptococcus neoformans*. *J Immunol* 152:3970–3979, 1994.

34. Mody CH, Tyler CL, Sitrin RG, et al: Interferon-γ activates rat alveolar macrophages of anticryptococcal activity. *Am J Respir Cell Mol Biol* 5:19–26, 1991.

35. Mosmann TR, Coffman RL: TH1 and TH2 cells: Different patterns of lymphokine secretion lead to different functional properties. *Annu Rev Immunol* 7:145–173, 1989.

36. Nicod LP, Lipscomb MF, Weissler JC, et al: Mononuclear cells in human lung parenchyma: Characterization of a potent accessory cell not obtained by bronchoalveolar lavage. *Am Rev Respir Dis* 136:818–823, 1987.

37. Onofrio JM, Toews GB, Lipscomb MF, Pierce AK: Granulocytealveolar macrophage interactions in the pulmonary clearance of *Staphylococcus aureus*. *Am Rev Respir Dis* 127:335–341, 1983.

38. Oppenheim JJ, Zachariae LOL, Mukaida N, Matzushima K: Properties of the novel proinflammatory supergene intercrine cytokine family. *Annu Rev Immunol* 11:817–848, 1993.

39. Pollard AM, Lipscomb MF: Characterization of murine lung dendritic cells: Similarities to Langerhans cells and thymic dendritic cells. *J Exp Med* 172:159–167, 1990.

40. Powrie F, Coffman RL: Cytokine regulation of T cell function: Potential for therapeutic intervention. *Immunol Today* 14:270–274, 1993.

41. Proctor DF: The upper airways: I. Nasal physiology and defense of the lungs. *Am Rev Respir Dis* 115:97–129, 1977.

42. Proctor DF: The upper airways: II. The larynx and trachea. *Am Rev Respir Dis* 115:315–342, 1977.

43. Rehm SR, Gross GN, Pierce AK: Early bacterial clearance from murine lungs: Species-dependent phagocyte response. *J Clin Invest* 66:194–199, 1980.

44. Reynolds HY: Norman and defective respiratory host defenses, in Pennington JE (ed), *Respiratory Infections: Diagnosis and Management*. New York, Raven, 1994, pp 1–34.

45. Springer TA: Traffic signals for lymphocyte recirculation and leukocyte immigration: The multistep paradigm. *Cell* 76:301–314, 1994.

46. Standiford TJ, Kunkel SL, Basha MA, et al: Interleukin-8 gene expression by a pulmonary epithelial cell line: A model for cytokine networks in the lung. *J Clin Invest* 86:1945–1953, 1990.

47. Strieter RM, Phan SH, Showell HJ, et al: Monokine-induced neutrophil chemotactic factor gene expression in human fibroblasts. *J Biol Chem* 264:10621–10626, 1989.

48. Toews GB: Pulmonary dendritic cells: Sentinels of lung-associated lymphoid tissues. *Am J Respir Cell Mol Biol* 4:204–205, 1991.

49. Toews GB, Hart DA, Hansen EJ: Effect of systemic immunization on pulmonary clearance of *Haemophilus influenzae* type b. *Infect Immun* 48:343–349, 1985.

50. Toews GB, Vial WC: The role of C5 in polymorphonuclear leukocyte recruitment in response to *Streptococcus pneumoniae*. *Am Rev Respir Dis* 129:597–601, 1984.

CHAPTER 121

APPROACH TO THE PATIENT WITH PULMONARY INFECTIONS

Morton N. Swartz

NONINFECTIOUS PROCESSES TO BE CONSIDERED IN THE DIFFERENTIAL DIAGNOSIS OF PULMONARY INFECTIONS
Drug-Induced Pulmonary Disease
Extrinsic Allergic Alveolitis (Hypersensitivity Pneumonitis)
Injury Due to Inhaled Toxic Gases, Dusts, and Chemicals
Chronic Eosinophilic Pneumonia
Acute Eosinophilic Pneumonia
Pulmonary Infiltrate with Eosinophilia
Interstitial Lung Disease Associated with Connective Tissue Disorders and Pulmonary Vasculitis
Interstitial Lung Disease Associated with Pulmonary Airway Disease
Chronic Interstitial Pneumonias of Unknown Cause
Pulmonary Neoplasms
Sarcoidosis
Pulmonary Infarction
Lipoid Pneumonia
Radiation Pneumonitis
Miscellaneous Mimics of Pulmonary Infection
Acute Respiratory Distress Syndrome
Pulmonary Leukoagglutinin Transfusion Reactions

PULMONARY INFECTIONS: PATHOLOGIC AND PATHOGENETIC FEATURES
Bacterial Pneumonia
Lung Abscess
Bronchitis and Bronchiectasis
Chronic Cavitary Disease
Miliary Lesions

MICROBIAL CAUSES OF PNEUMONIA
Community-Acquired Pneumonia
Bacterial Pneumonia
Pneumonia in the Elderly
Prognosis of Community-Acquired Pneumonia
Nosocomial Pneumonia
Pneumonia in the Immunocompromised Host

RADIOGRAPHIC FEATURES OF PNEUMONIA
Alveolar Pneumonia
Bronchopneumonia
Interstitial Pneumonia (Peribronchovascular Infiltrate)
Nodular Infiltrates

NONINVASIVE DIAGNOSTIC STUDIES
Direct Examination of the Sputum
Serologic Tests
Molecular Diagnostic Testing
Skin Tests of Delayed Hypersensitivity
Gallium Scan

INITIAL ANTIMICROBIAL THERAPY

INVASIVE DIAGNOSTIC PROCEDURES
Flexible Fiberoptic Bronchoscopy with Lung Biopsy
Percutaneous Transthoracic Needle Lung Biopsy
Open Lung Biopsy

The clinical scenario of pulmonary infection characteristically consists of a patient with fever, pulmonary symptoms such as cough (with or without sputum production) or shortness of breath, and a pulmonary lesion on radiographic examination. Each of the specific categories of pulmonary infection and the pathogenesis commonly associated with pulmonary infection are considered in detail elsewhere in this text (see Chapter 20). Delineation of an infecting agent requires a sequence of steps. Since the pulmonary process may be noninfectious, an early step is the consideration of the categories and clinical features of any possible "mimics" of pulmonary infection. When one finds no clues to a noninfectious process, the next step is to define the gross pathologic and pathogenetic features of the pulmonary infection: frank pneumonia, focal infiltrate, lung abscess, chronic cavitary lesion, bronchiectasis, miliary lesions. As a corollary, since pulmonary infections are occasionally generated by the hematogenous rather than by the bronchogenic route, possible initiating factors in the pathogenesis of the pulmonary infection should be weighed.

The third step considers likely etiologic agents on the basis of frequency statistics. In this appraisal, it is helpful to resort to clinically meaningful groupings. For example, pneumonia can be divided into three major groupings: community-acquired, nosocomial, and pneumonia in the immunocompromised patient. Each group, in turn, would be considered either typical, in that direct sputum examination or culture provides the diagnosis and includes primarily the common bacterial pneumonias, or atypical, in that the sputum examination and culture fail to provide a diagnosis; this subset would consist primarily of viral or mycoplasmal pneumonia.

The fourth step in defining the etiologic agent entails a careful search for clinical clues. This is particularly important in the patient with atypical pneumonia. Epidemiologic information may be extremely important. For example, coccidioidomycosis becomes a consideration in a patient who develops atypical pneumonia in the San Joaquin Valley of California but not in a patient with atypical pneumonia who has spent his or her whole life in New York City.

Other sources of clinical clues may be provided by the patient's symptoms. A desultory onset of symptoms over a week or 10 days and a prominent headache might suggest *Mycoplasma pneumoniae* pneumonia. On the other hand, an abrupt onset of illness with recurrent (over several days) shaking chills after a prodromal period of 24 h or less, particularly if associated with mild diarrhea for 1 or 2 days, might suggest Legionnaires' disease. Further clinical clues may be provided by physical findings. Thus, a relative bradycardia in a patient with the clinical picture of pneumonia might suggest psittacosis or Legionnaires' disease, extensive periodontal disease and an absent gag reflex might indicate the likelihood of aspiration pneumonia, or the occurrence of bullous myringitis might suggest a mycoplasmal origin.

Other general clinical clues to the cause of atypical pneumonia may be provided by examination of the results of initial blood counts, urinalysis, and routine blood chemistries. For example, the presence of mild liver function abnormalities might suggest Q fever, tularemia, miliary tuberculosis, or Legionnaires' disease. A hemolytic anemia with a markedly elevated level of cold agglutinins would direct attention to the possibility of *M. pneumoniae* pneumonia; the presence of pigmented casts in the urine and markedly elevated serum levels of creatine phosphokinase might focus attention on the possibilities of influenza virus pneumonia, Legionnaires' disease, or a pulmonary infiltrate associated with intravenous drug abuse.

The fifth step entails categorization of the radiographic features. This step is particularly helpful in evaluating the immunocompromised patient, in whom the number of possible causes is particularly extensive. It is important to bear in mind, however, that no radiographic findings are specific enough to define the microbial origin of a given pneumonia or pulmonary infiltrate. The only definitive way to reach a specific etiologic diagnosis is through demonstration of the infecting organism—i.e., by examination of stained smears of sputum and pleural fluid or other biologic materials, by culture of respiratory secretions and blood, or by demonstrating an increase in antibody titer against the infecting microorganism. Nonetheless, the radiographic picture, taken along with other clinical information, can favor one or several etiologic agents. Accordingly, it is of value to define the radiographic pattern as lobar or segmental consolidation, patchy bronchopneumonia, nodules (large, small, or miliary), or an interstitial process. Many large round pulmonary densities in a renal transplant recipient suggest *Nocardia* infection rather than *Pneumocystis* pneumonia, whereas in a heroin addict with cough, fever, and pleuritic chest pain, such densities suggest acute right-sided endocarditis rather than pneumococcal pneumonia.

The sixth step, examination of an appropriately stained smear of sputum or pleural fluid (or occasionally a buffy coat of centrifuged blood), often provides a provisional diagnosis. Although given as the sixth step in progression to an etiologic diagnosis, in practice, examination of an appropriately stained smear of sputum is performed earlier in the evaluation process and can provide a shortcut to diagnosis if the findings are reasonably definitive. Gram-stained smear provides information not only concerning the morphology and the tinctorial properties of bacteria (and some fungi) but also, most important, concerning the presence of polymorphonuclear leukocytes and squamous cells, the latter indicating that the specimen originated in the upper, rather than the lower, respiratory tract. On occasion, when clinical features warrant, other special staining methods (e.g., Wright-Giemsa or one of its variants, such as Diff-Quik, or methenamine silver staining of an induced sputum for *Pneumocystis carinii* or direct fluorescent antibody for *Legionella pneumophila* on a specimen of pleural fluid) may provide a diagnosis. Culture of sputum (and blood) may be required for a specific etiologic diagnosis of some pneumonias when evaluation of a Gram-stained smear has not supplied a provisional diagnosis, either because the infecting agent cannot be distinguished from components of the normal upper-respiratory-tract flora incorporated in the specimen or because the particular microorganism is not visible on Gram-stained smear (e.g., *Aspergillus* species or *M. pneumoniae*). In some patients, an etiologic diagnosis cannot be made on the basis of examination of initial stained smears of sputum or the results of initial bacteriologic culture. In such circumstances, a definitive diagnosis can sometimes be made only retrospectively, by serologic means, as in psittacosis, Q fever, or adenovirus pneumonia.

The seventh step requires selection of initial antimicrobial therapy. If examination of the Gram-stained (or other) smear does not provide the necessary insights about cause, beginning therapy is empiric and based primarily on available clinical clues. Thus, for a community-acquired pneumonia in an otherwise healthy adult, therapy might start with a β-lactam antibiotic, such as penicillin or ampicillin, or a second-generation cephalosporin, such as cefuroxime. If, on the other hand, a patient with HIV infection and a lowered CD4 cell count develops fever, cough, and a bilateral pulmonary infiltrate that is consistent radiologically with *Pneumocystis* infection, empiric therapy with trimethoprim-sulfamethoxazole would be more appropriate. Clearly, the selection of drug(s) for empiric therapy depends on the clinical setting and on the gravity of the pulmonary process.

The eighth step in the approach to the patient with a pulmonary infection entails the performance of an invasive diagnostic procedure to obtain either uncontaminated lower-respiratory-tract secretions or pulmonary tissue for microbiologic and histologic analysis. This step becomes necessary in patients in whom the rate of progression of the illness precludes the initiation of a meaningful trial of empiric therapy or requires that such a trial be concluded prematurely. These restrictions apply particularly to the immunosuppressed patient, for whom the number of possible causes and therapeutic options is large: the rapid progression of the disease does not permit sequential trials of individual antimicrobial agents, and the hazard of potential side effects precludes the indiscriminate use of multiple-drug combinations. At this juncture, only specific etiologic diagnosis can direct meaningful therapeutic efforts.

Among the invasive procedures that are available are (1) protected specimen brushing (PSB), (2) plugged telescoping catheter (PTC) sampling, (3) standard bronchoalveolar lavage (BAL), (4) protected bronchoalveolar lavage (P-BAL or PTC-BAL), (5) transtracheal aspiration (now rarely done because of concern for complications), (6) fiberoptic bronchoscopy with transbronchial biopsy, (7) needle biopsy of the lung, and (8) open lung biopsy via limited thoracotomy. The choice of invasive diagnostic procedure should be individualized. Important considerations in this decision include the type and location of the pulmonary lesion, the ability of the patient to cooperate with the required manipulations, the presence of coagulopathies, and experience at the particular hospital in performing each of the procedures.

NONINFECTIOUS PROCESSES TO BE CONSIDERED IN THE DIFFERENTIAL DIAGNOSIS OF PULMONARY INFECTIONS

The list of noninfectious disorders that mimic pulmonary infections is extensive (Table 121-1). These are considered briefly in the course of taking the initial history and explored in greater detail should evaluation of the Gram-stained smear (and culture) of sputum be unrevealing, if the initial response to empiric antimicrobial therapy proves unsatisfactory, or if radiographic findings are atypical.

TABLE 121-1

Noninfectious Causes of Febrile Pneumonitis Syndrome (Mimics of Pulmonary Infection)

Drug-induced pulmonary disease
    Noncytotoxic drugs
    Cytotoxic drugs
Extrinsic allergic alveolitis
Injury due to inhaled toxic gases, dusts, chemicals
Acute eosinophilic pneumonia
Pulmonary infiltrate with eosinophilia (PIE syndrome)
Chronic eosinophilic pneumonia
Interstitial lung disease associated with connective-tissue disorders
    Systemic lupus erythematosus
    Polymyositis-dermatomyositis
    Mixed connective-tissue disease
Interstitial lung disease associated with pulmonary vasculitis
    Wegener's granulomatosis
    Lymphomatoid granulomatosis
    Churg-Strauss syndrome (allergic angiitis and granulomatosis)
    Polyangiitis overlap syndrome
Intersitital lung disease associated with pulmonary airway disease
    Allergic bronchopulmonary aspergillosis
    Bronchocentric granulomatosis
    Bronchiolitis obliterans and bronchiolitis obliterans with organizing pneumonia
Acute or subacute interstitial pulmonary fibrosis (IPF, Hamman-Rich syndrome)
Chronic interstitial pneumonias of unknown origin
    Usual interstitial pneumonia (UIP)
    Lymphocytic interstitial pneumonia (LIP)
    Desquamative interstitial pneumonia (DIP)
    Giant cell interstitial pneumonia (GIP)
Pulmonary neoplasms
    Carcinoma or lymphoma
    Kaposi's sarcoma in AIDS
Sarcoidosis
Pulmonary infarction
Acute chest syndrome in sickle cell crisis
Radiation pneumonitis
Lipoid pneumonia (exogenous or endogenous)
Acute respiratory distress syndrome (ARDS)
    Associated with extrapulmonary sepsis
    Associated with oxygen toxicity, chemical inhalation or aspiration, or aspiration of gastric contents
    Associated with pancreatitis
    Associated with fat embolization
    Associated with shock of various etiologies
    Associated with drug overdose
    Associated with chest trauma
Pulmonary leukoagglutinin transfusion reactions
Miscellaneous
    Pulmonary alveolar proteinosis
    Plasma cell granuloma
    Histiocytosis X
    Idiopathic pulmonary hemosiderosis
    Goodpasture's syndrome
    Rheumatic pneumonia (in acute rheumatic fever)

Drug-Induced Pulmonary Disease

Drugs producing pulmonary reactions are conveniently considered in two categories: noncytotoxic and cytotoxic drugs. Noncytotoxic drugs producing hypersensitivity pneumonitis include antimicrobials, anticonvulsants, diuretics, antiarrhythmics, tranquilizers, and antirheumatic agents (Table 121-2).[17,62]

NONCYTOTOXIC DRUGS

The commonly used antibacterial drug nitrofurantoin can produce two patterns of pulmonary reaction: (1) acute, which occurs within 2 weeks of starting therapy and consists of dyspnea, nonproductive cough, chills, fever, crackles, eosinophilia, and diffuse interstitial or patchy infiltrates (often with pleural effusion), and (2) chronic, which is less common and occurs after months to years of continuous treatment. The picture of the chronic form is one in which exertional dyspnea and nonproductive cough appear gradually and are unaccompanied by fever; the pattern is not that of an acute pulmonary infection but, rather, that of diffuse interstitial pneumonitis or pulmonary fibrosis.

Sulfasalazine (and other sulfonamides) can produce hypersensitivity lung disease that includes cough, fever, dyspnea, and peripheral hazy acinar or diffuse reticular infiltrates. Although

---

TABLE 121-2

Noncytotoxic Drugs Capable of Inducing a Picture Resembling Pulmonary Infection

Antimicrobial agents
　Nitrofurantoin
　Penicillins, cephalosporins
　Sulfasalazine, other salfonamides
　Minocycline, tetracycline
　Amphotericin B (acting with leukocyte transfusions)
　Para-aminosalicylic acid
Anticonvulsants
　Phenytoin
　Carbamazepine
Diuretics
　Hydrochlorothiazide
Antiarrhythmics
　Amiodarone
　Tocainide
Narcotics
　Heroin
　Methadone
　Propoxyphene
　Cocaine
Antirheumatic agents
　Gold salts
　Penicillamine
　Naproxen
Drugs that can induce a lupus erythematosuslike syndrome
　Hydralazine
　Procainamide
　Isoniazid
　Chlorpromazine

---

synergistic pulmonary toxicity between amphotericin B administered intravenously and leukocyte transfusions has been suggested, it has not been confirmed.

Phenytoin can produce hypersensitivity responses in the lung 3 to 6 weeks after initiation of therapy. Fever, cough, and dyspnea are accompanied by radiographic findings of bilateral acinar, nodular, or reticular infiltrates. The presence of a maculopapular skin rash, generalized lymphadenopathy, and peripheral eosinophilia direct attention toward hypersensitivity and away from the diagnosis of pulmonary infection.

Pulmonary reactions occasionally occur with the diuretic hydrochlorothiazide. The sudden onset of cough, dyspnea, fever, chest pain, and crackles after the agent is ingested, and after a finding of radiographic evidence that is suggestive of pulmonary edema, raises the prospect of a hypersensitivity mechanism.

Pulmonary side effects occasionally follow 5 to 6 months of therapy with the antiarrhythmic agent amiodarone. Exertional dyspnea, nonproductive cough, malaise, and fever (in about half the patients) are gradual in onset, over weeks to several months. The radiographic findings generally resemble those of chronic eosinophilic pneumonia, tuberculosis, or diffuse interstitial disease, and consist of peripheral areas of consolidation that affect primarily the upper lobes. In some instances, coarse reticular interstitial infiltrates are present. Withdrawal of the medication, coupled with the administration of corticosteroids, usually leads to complete resolution.

Patients receiving gold salts as treatment for rheumatoid arthritis occasionally develop a nonproductive cough, fever, and progressive dyspnea over the course of several weeks. The radiographic findings are primarily those of diffuse reticulonodular infiltrates. Hydralazine, procainamide, and isoniazid are capable of inducing a lupuslike syndrome; the clinical picture often includes pleuropulmonary involvement.

CYTOTOXIC DRUGS

Three clinicopathologic patterns characterize cytotoxic drug–induced pulmonary disease: chronic pneumonitis with pulmonary fibrosis, acute hypersensitivity lung disease, and noncardiogenic pulmonary edema (Table 121-3).[16] A variety of predisposing factors may contribute to the development of these reactions. The cumulative dose of certain drugs (e.g., bleomycin, busulfan, and carmustine) appears to be particularly important. Older age seems to be a risk factor for pulmonary toxicity from bleomycin.

Syndrome of Acute or Chronic Pneumonitis with Fibrosis

Essentially all types of cytotoxic drugs capable of inducing pulmonary disease can produce this kind of reaction. The clinical manifestations develop over weeks to months and include nonproductive cough, progressive dyspnea on exertion, fatigue, and malaise. End-inspiratory crackles are audible on examination. The radiographic findings are consistent with those of an interstitial inflammatory process and pulmonary fibrosis. Fever is not intrinsic to this process. An exception is the case of cyclophosphamide-induced pulmonary injury; more than 50 percent of these patients exhibit fever. However, since cytotoxic drugs are administered to patients whose underlying disease (or complications thereof) is often associated with fever, distinguishing be-

TABLE 121-3

Cytotoxic Drugs Capable of Inducing a Picture Resembling Pulmonary Infection

Acute or chronic pneumonitis with pulmonary fibrosis
  Antibiotics
    Bleomycin, mitomycin, neocarzinostatin
  Alkylating agents
    Busulfan, cyclophosphamide, chlorambucil, melphalan, chlorozotocin
  Nitrosoureas
    Carmustine (BCNU), semustine (methyl CCNU), lomustine (CCNU), chlorozotocin
  Antimetabolites
    Methotrexate, azathioprine, mercaptopurine, cytosine arabinoside, 6-thioguanine
  Miscellaneous
    Vinblastine, VM-26, vindescine
Hypersensitivity lung disease
  Antimetabolites
    Methotrexate
  Antibiotics
    Bleomycin
  Miscellaneous
    Procarbazine
Noncardiogenic pulmonary edema
  Antimetabolites
    Methotrexate, cytosine arabinoside
  Alkylating agents
    Cyclophosphamide
  Miscellaneous
    VM-26

tween chronic pneumonitis with pulmonary fibrosis and pulmonary infection becomes an important practical issue.

Syndrome of Hypersensitivity Lung Disease

Methotrexate, bleomycin, and procarbazine have each caused an acute syndrome of dyspnea, nonproductive cough, fever, and occasionally pleuritic chest pain. The presence of blood eosinophilia and a skin rash suggests a hypersensitivity reaction. The radiographic findings include a diffuse reticular pattern and, in some patients, bilateral acinar infiltrates.

Extrinsic Allergic Alveolitis (Hypersensitivity Pneumonitis)

Inhalation of organic dusts can produce chills, fever, nonproductive cough, dyspnea, and pulmonary crackles a few hours after exposure to an organic dust or vapor in a sensitive person. The chest radiograph usually shows bilateral patchy acinar infiltrates, completing a picture suggestive of pulmonary infection. The history of a specific exposure provides the clue to diagnosis, particularly when such episodes have been recurrent. More than two dozen such diseases have been described. Farmer's lung occurs with hypersensitivity to moldy hay containing *Thermoactinomyces* species and *Micropolyspora faeni*. "Air-conditioner" or "humidifier" lung is associated with exposure to similar moldy antigens stemming from occult microbial growth on these air-exchanging systems in offices and homes (Fig. 121-1).

In other hypersensitivity pneumonitides, the offending antigens may be of avian origin (pigeon breeder's disease) or from other environmental fungi contaminating natural products in industry (e.g., maple bark stripper's lung; moldy sugar cane in bagassosis).

Injury Due to Inhaled Toxic Gases, Dusts, Chemicals

An acute syndrome mimicking acute bacterial or viral pneumonia clinically and radiologically can follow exposure to nitrogen dioxide in silo-filler's disease. A degenerative interstitial pneumonitis–like picture may result from exposure to organic (e.g., wood, mycotoxin containing) and inorganic (e.g., silicates, tungsten carbide) dusts.[34] Severe interstitial disease and organizing pneumonia have occurred among workers exposed to aerosols of organic chemicals (designed to polymerize on mixing) used in textile dyeing.[38]

Chronic Eosinophilic Pneumonia

Chronic eosinophilic pneumonia usually has a course of weeks to months, characterized by fever, night sweats, nonproductive cough, and dyspnea.[13] Pulmonary crackles are variably present. Chest radiographs show a characteristic pattern of peripheral acinar infiltrates that usually involve the upper lobes; it resembles the appearance of butterfly pulmonary edema on the photographic negative. In contrast to the usual infectious pneumonias, peripheral blood eosinophilia is common. Occasionally, chronic eosinophilic pneumonia has an acute onset, and the diagnosis is made within 2 weeks of the initial symptoms. Even though the onset in such cases is acute, the course, if untreated (corticosteroids), is prolonged, just as in typical chronic eosinophilic pneumonia.

Acute Eosinophilic Pneumonia

Acute eosinophilic pneumonia was initially described as an acute febrile illness with severe hypoxemia, diffuse pulmonary infiltrates, increased numbers of eosinophils in BAL fluid, and prompt response to corticosteroid therapy without relapse.[2] Drug hypersensitivity may be the cause in some cases. More recently, a subset was described with the same acute onset with high fever, a radiologic picture of micronodular and diffuse ground-glass infiltrates, and spontaneous improvement without relapse.[32]

Pulmonary Infiltrate with Eosinophilia

The term *pulmonary infiltrates with eosinophilia* (PIE syndrome) may be used to encompass a wide range of definable clinical en-

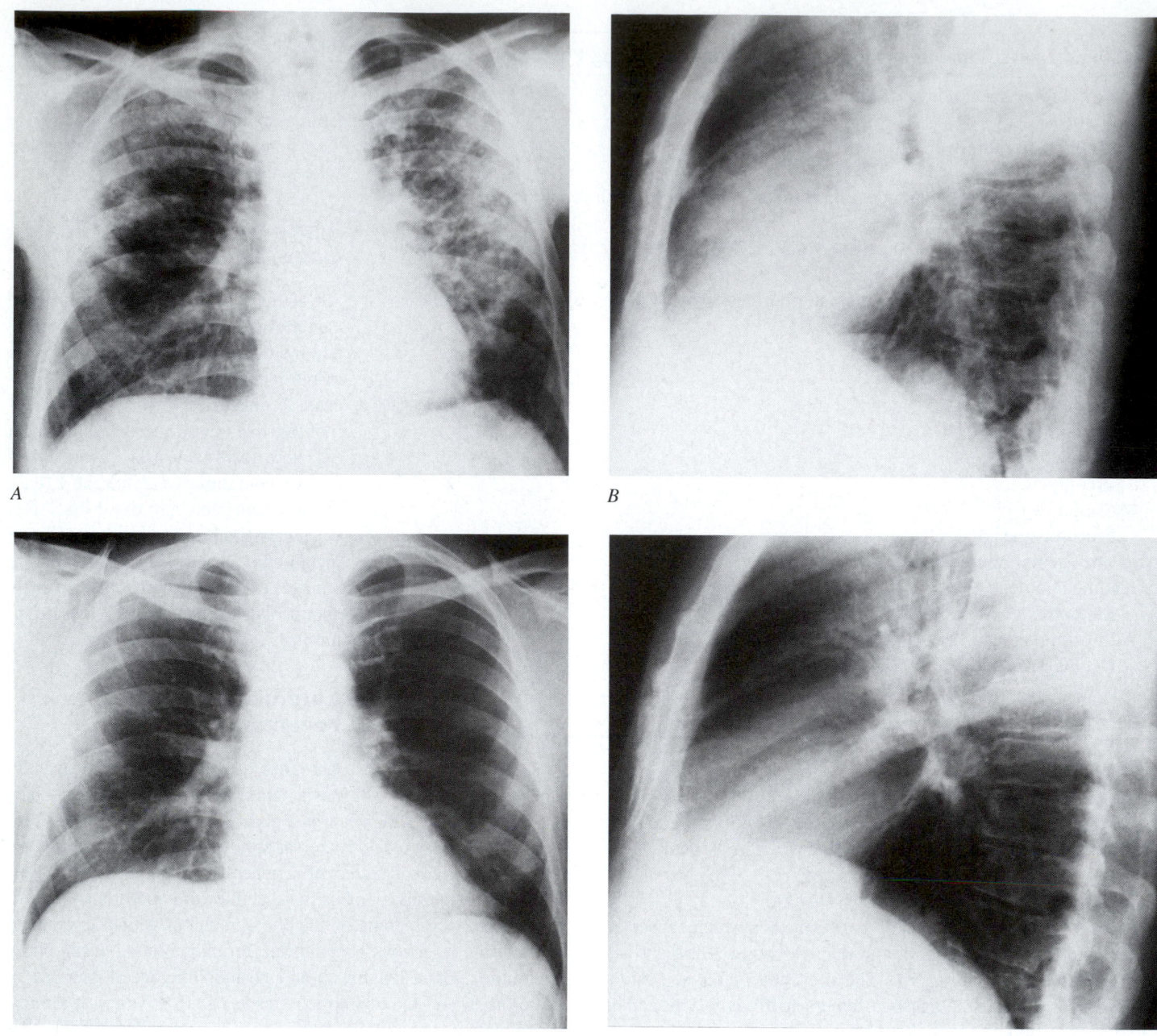

A

B

C

D

FIGURE 121-1 Hypersensitivity pneumonitis following introduction into the home of two humidifiers containing stagnant water. PA and lateral views in a 45-year-old man. *A* and *B*. Dense bilateral infiltrates as-sociated with acute onset of incapacitating dyspnea. *C* and *D*. Resolution of infiltrates and breathlessness while on large doses of steroids.

tities such as acute eosinophilic pneumonia, chronic eosinophilic pneumonia, allergic pulmonary aspergillosis, and Churg-Strauss vasculitis. For these purposes, they will be considered independently, and the term *PIE syndrome* will be used to refer to a syndrome consisting of fleeting pulmonary infiltrates, dry cough and mild wheezing, low-grade fever, and blood and pulmonary eosinophilia. Loeffler's syndrome, a form of PIE, may be associated with parasitic infestation (migration or hypersensitivity) with *Ascaris lumbricoides, Strongyloides stercoralis, Ancylostoma duodenale, Toxocara canis,* and others, or due to drug hypersensitivity. Tropical eosinophilia is a similar syndrome, en-

demic to India and southern Asia, Africa, and South America, and most likely due to filarial infection.

Interstitial Lung Disease Associated with Connective Tissue Disorders and Pulmonary Vasculitis

A variety of connective tissue disorders and vasculitides may mimic pulmonary infections (Table 121-1). Systemic lupus erythematosus may be associated with transitory infiltrates, interstitial disease, or frank consolidation of a noninfectious nature.

Interstitial pneumonitis occurs in 5 to 10 percent of patients with polymyositis and may be mistaken for a pulmonary infection, since pulmonary manifestations and fever may precede muscle weakness.

Three types of vasculitis in particular may mimic pulmonary infection. Wegener's granulomatosis involves the lung in approximately 95 percent of cases. The lesions radiologically ap-

pear as patchy infiltrates or as sizable nodular lesions, the latter suggesting a lung abscess or cavity due to mycobacterial or mycotic infection (Fig. 121-2). Allergic angiitis and granulomatosis (Churg-Strauss syndrome) occurs in the setting of asthma and peripheral eosinophilia; it characteristically involves the lung, producing pulmonary infiltrates associated with granulomatous and vasculitic lesions. The polyangiitis overlap syndrome com-

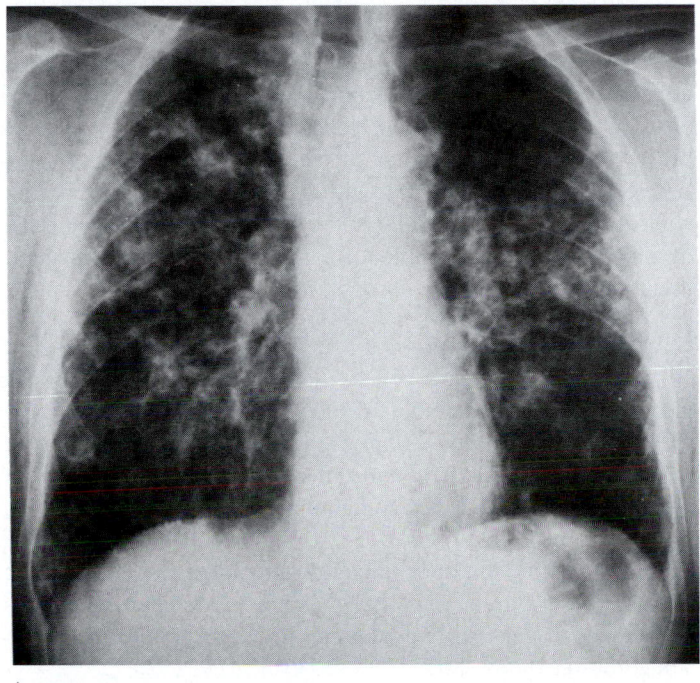

A

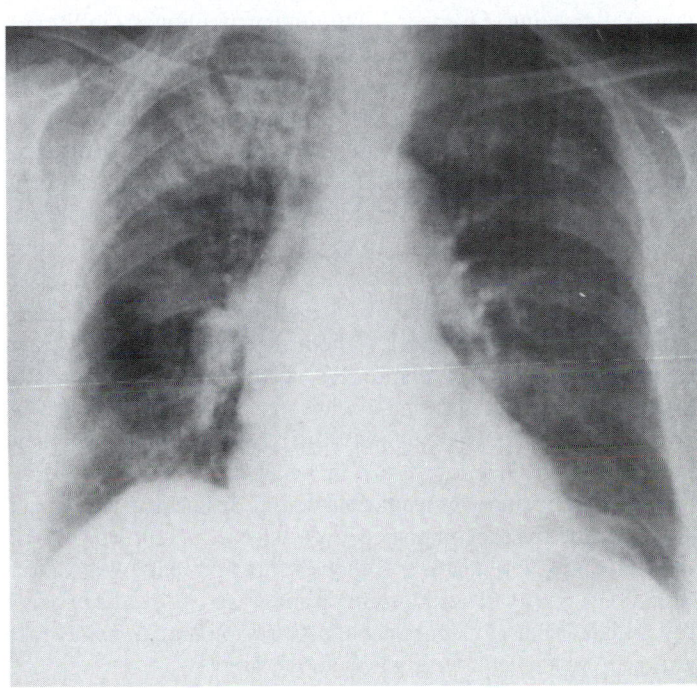

B

C

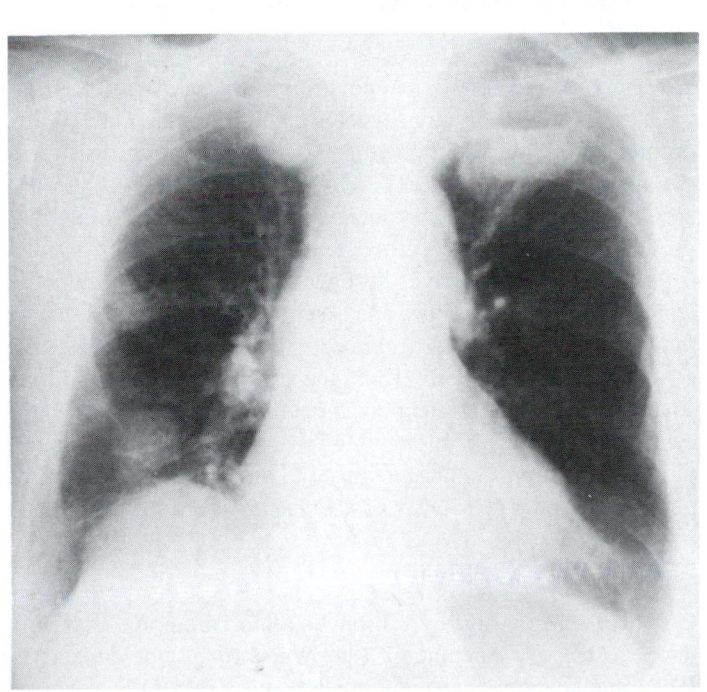

D

FIGURE 121-2 Wegener's granulomatosis. *A.* Onset with chills and fever in a previously healthy 64-year-old man. Lung biopsy was interpreted as Wegener's granulomatosis. Partial clearing in response to combined chemotherapy (cyclophosphamide and prednisone). *B.* Onset with malaise, headaches, and fever in a previously healthy 62-year-old woman. Bilateral maxillary sinusitis. Widespread nodular pulmonary infiltrates are most marked on the right. *C.* Same patient as *B* after 3 years of intermittent combined chemotherapy. Bilateral large masses. *D.* Same patient as *C,* 2 months later. Necrosis within mass in left upper lobe has produced a fluid level.

bines some of the characteristic features of classic polyarteritis nodosa and of allergic angiitis and granulomatosis, including prominent pulmonary impairment in some instances.

Interstitial Lung Disease Associated with Pulmonary Airway Disease

Allergic bronchopulmonary aspergillosis, characterized by cough, wheezing, fever, and intermittent pulmonary infiltrates, can suggest a pulmonary infection, although an accompanying eosinophilia provides a clue to the true nature of the process. Bronchocentric granulomatosis, a necrotizing process of unknown cause affecting small bronchi may, in some patients, produce an acute febrile illness. The pulmonary lesions vary from mucoid impaction to diffuse and nodular infiltrates.

Bronchiolitis obliterans, an occasional complication of pulmonary viral or bacterial infections, cocaine toxicity, drug hypersensitivity, connective tissue disease, and inhalation of chemical irritants, can also occur without apparent cause; the last is often associated with patchy areas of pneumonitis, necrosis of bronchiolar epithelium, and occlusion of terminal airways by granulation tissue. Bronchiolitis obliterans with organizing pneumonia (BOOP) refers to cases in which the presence of organizing inflammatory polypoid masses in distal bronchioles and alveolar ducts is accompanied by a chronic pneumonitis with lipid-laden macrophages.[22] Although most patients with BOOP respond promptly to corticosteroids and up to two-thirds undergo full clinical remission, occasional patients undergo a rapidly progressive course even with intensive therapy.[15]

Chronic Interstitial Pneumonias of Unknown Cause

A variety of interstitial pneumonias, known as usual interstitial pneumonia (UIP), lymphocytic interstitial pneumonia (LIP), desquamative interstitial pneumonia (DIP), and giant cell interstitial pneumonia (GIP), are conditions of unknown origin that are defined on histologic grounds (Fig. 121-1). Most often they present clinically as afebrile subacute or chronic processes characterized by progressive dyspnea, cyanosis, nonproductive cough, pulmonary crackles, and a radiographic picture of diffuse reticulonodular infiltrates (more prominent at the lung bases) or a "ground glass" pattern. Thus, the clinical picture would not suggest a pulmonary infection. In a minority of patients, however, the onset may be rapid, with fever suggesting an acute respiratory infection. A subacute onset in an immunocompromised person raises the possibility of a *Pneumocystis* infection.

Pulmonary Neoplasms

Bronchial obstruction by a bronchogenic carcinoma may produce obstructive pneumonia ("drowned lung") or atelectasis. Fever and signs of consolidation/atelectasis may fail to respond to antimicrobial therapy. Infection is common as a secondary feature. Recurrent pneumonia in the same portion of the lung should suggest this possibility. Hodgkin's disease and non-Hodgkin's lymphoma may present with fever, cough, dyspnea, and pulmonary lesions suggesting infection. In Hodgkin's disease, a single mass lesion may be present and cavitate, suggesting a lung abscess.

Sarcoidosis

In the patient with sarcoidosis and interstitial lung disease, fever is uncommon unless hilar adenopathy or other features, such as erythema nodosum, are present as well (Fig. 121-3). Thus, this process is usually not mistaken for a primary pulmonary infection.[54]

Pulmonary Infarction

Fever, dyspnea, pleuritic chest pain, leukocytosis, and segmental pleural-based infiltrates (and possibly accompanying pleural effusion) of pulmonary infarction might also suggest the diagnosis of pneumococcal pneumonia. The additional presence of blood-streaked sputum might suggest the possibility of *Streptococcus pyogenes* pneumonia, with its hemorrhagic tracheobronchitis. Occasionally, several round lesions in the lung of a febrile, dyspneic patient with pulmonary emboli might suggest aspirational or bacteremic lung abscesses.

Lipoid Pneumonia

Exogenous lipoid pneumonia results from inhaling or aspirating fatty materials (oily nose drops, mineral oil). Endogenous lipoid pneumonia (often called *cholesterol* pneumonia) consists of chronic inflammatory foci containing cholesterol and its esters, derived from destroyed alveolar walls located either behind a bronchial obstruction or in lung parenchyma at a site of chronic suppuration. Sputum, fine-needle aspirates, or BAL specimens may reveal macrophages containing lipoid vacuoles, as demonstrated by fat stains (Sudan, oil red O).[63]

Radiation Pneumonitis

The acute phase of radiation pneumonitis usually develops within 3 or 4 months of initiation of radiation therapy. It is characterized by fever, dyspnea, cough, and radiographic changes (infiltrates or ground-glass density) sharply demarcated geometrically to the portal of irradiation rather than to natural pulmonary anatomic divisions. This reaction might be mistaken for a bacterial pneumonia. The late phase of radiation pneumonia, characterized by pulmonary fibrosis, occurs 9 months or more after radiation therapy and is not accompanied by fever.

Miscellaneous Mimics of Pulmonary Infection

Pulmonary alveolar proteinosis usually begins slowly, with dyspnea as the principal symptom. Radiographic features are those of a bilateral diffuse, predominantly perihilar airspace disease. The radiographic, but not the clinical, manifestations might suggest pulmonary infection. Fever is ordinarily absent. However, since pulmonary alveolar proteinosis may occasionally be associated with hematologic malignancies (e.g., lymphoma and acute leukemias) that themselves cause fever, the mimicry of pulmonary infection might apply. In addition, pulmonary alveolar proteinosis is sometimes complicated by pulmonary infections—e.g., nocardiosis (most frequently), cryptococcosis, aspergillosis, tuberculosis, and histoplasmosis.

Plasma cell granuloma is a postinflammatory pseudotumor of the lung. The combination of cough, fever, and radiologic changes of atelectasis and consolidation suggests the diagnosis

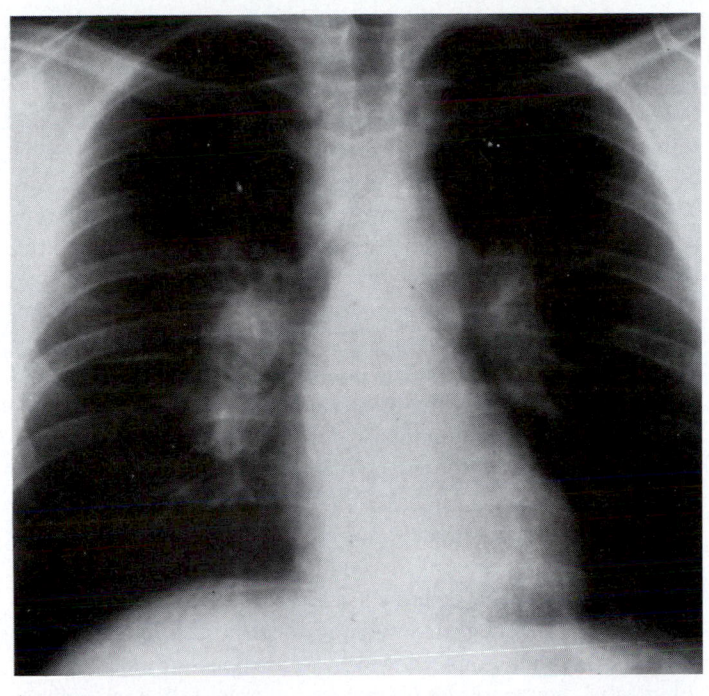

A

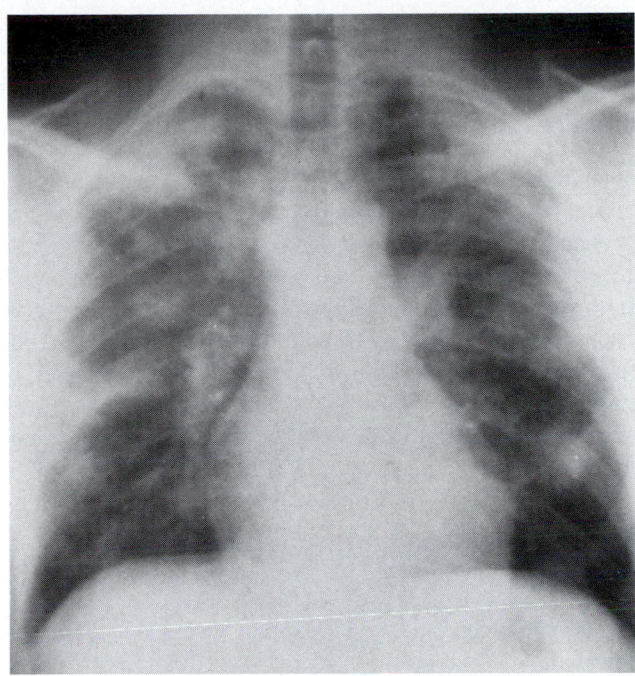

B

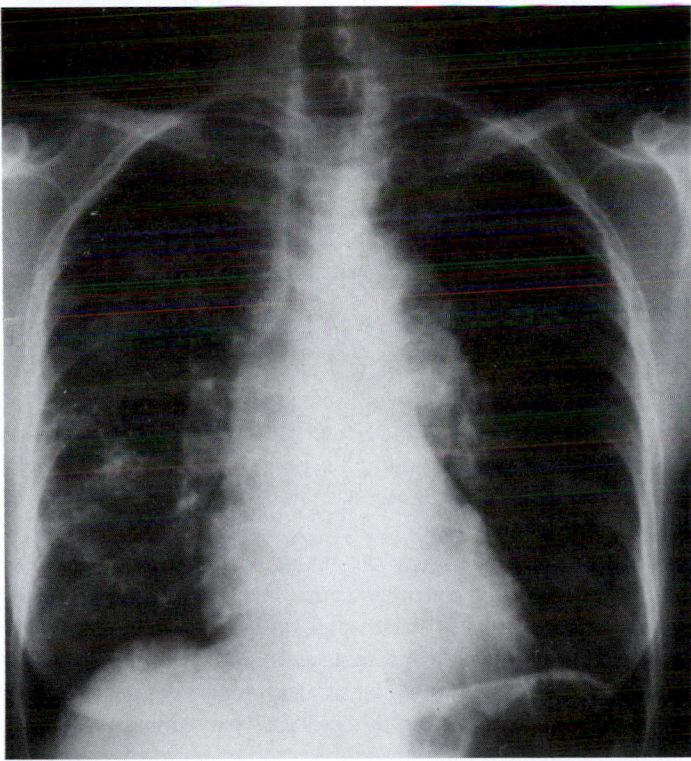

C

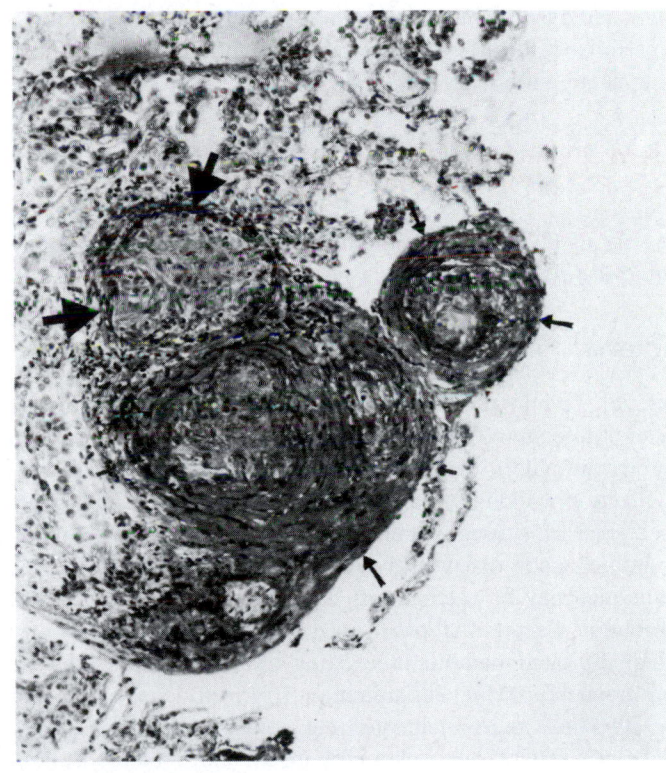

D

FIGURE 121-3 *A* to *C*. Chest radiographs illustrating the various stages of sarcoidosis. *A*. Stage I, bilateral hilar adenopathy. *B*. Stage II, bilateral hilar adenopathy with parenchymal infiltrates. *C*. Stage III, parenchymal infiltrates without hilar adenopathy. *D*. Transbronchial lung biopsy from a patient with sarcoidosis. Small arrows indicate granuloma with a surrounding rim of collagen (confirmed by positive trichrome staining). The large arrows indicate a granuloma without a surrounding rim of collagen. Original magnification ×10. *(From Rossman and Dauber,[54] with permission.)*

of pulmonary infection associated with bronchial obstruction. This process is very similar to the previously described cholesterol pneumonia.

Eosinophilic granuloma of the lung (pulmonary histiocytosis X) usually is manifested as a noninfectious interstitial pulmonary process with dyspnea and nonprogressive cough. In about 15 percent of patients, however, fever occurs, suggesting the possibility of pulmonary infection. The radiographic findings are those of small nodules and reticulation or honeycombing; these findings in the febrile patient might suggest the diagnosis of miliary tuberculosis, invasive mycotic infection, or viral disease (e.g., varicella-zoster).

Acute Respiratory Distress Syndrome

Many unrelated conditions (Table 121-1) involving the lungs primarily or having their initial impact elsewhere have in common the capacity to cause diffuse damage to the alveolar-capillary membrane and produce noncardiogenic pulmonary edema. The process progresses rapidly with inflammatory cell infiltration and pulmonary fibrosis. Extensive pulmonary infiltrates are evident on chest radiographs. Many of the underlying processes producing acute respiratory distress syndrome (ARDS) are associated with fever, and thus fulminant bacterial or viral pneumonia becomes a major diagnostic consideration.

Pulmonary Leukoagglutinin Transfusion Reactions

An acute pulmonary reaction may follow receipt of a blood transfusion with which there has been passive transfer of leukoagglutinins and antibodies cytotoxic to recipient lymphocytes. The clinical picture of an abrupt onset of chills, fever, tachycardia, cough, and dyspnea, accompanied by numerous fluffy and nodular perihilar infiltrates on radiograph, might easily be mistaken for an acute pulmonary infection.

PULMONARY INFECTIONS: PATHOLOGIC AND PATHOGENETIC FEATURES

The various pulmonary infections can be categorized according to their distinctive pathologic aspects and pathogenetic features.

Bacterial Pneumonia

Bacterial pneumonia commonly results from bronchogenic spread of infection following microaspiration of secretions. Such particles are able to reach terminal airways and alveoli to initiate infection, which has the anatomic distribution and radiologic appearance of subsegmental, segmental, or lobar pneumonia. Sometimes, particularly in the elderly or in debilitated patients, pneumonia may be patchy, with a peribronchial and multifocal distribution. Factors that predispose to these patchy pneumonias include aspirated material, preexisting chronic bronchitis, diffuse acute tracheobronchial inflammation (e.g., influenza), and specific infecting microorganisms (e.g., oral anaerobic bacteria).

The progression of a pulmonary infiltrate or lobar consolidation to parenchymal destruction (necrotizing pneumonia or lung abscess) usually is the consequence of one or two factors: the nature of the infecting organism(s) and the presence of bronchial obstruction by tumor or foreign body. Although *Streptococcus pneumoniae* is the most frequent cause of bacterial pneumonia, it almost never produces necrosis of the lung unless there is a complicating factor such as bronchial obstruction, mixed infection, or bacterial superinfection. In contrast, aspirational polymicrobial pneumonia is frequently a necrotizing process.[6] Pleural extension of such anaerobic pulmonary infections often results in putrid empyema.[5] *Klebsiella pneumoniae* sometimes causes a

necrotizing pneumonia, with progression to abscess or chronic cavity formation; in the upper lobe, the latter may mimic pulmonary tuberculosis.

Pneumonia may occasionally develop via the bacteremic rather than the bronchogenic route. The clinical setting and the radiographic pattern usually suggest this form of pathogenesis. The intravenous-drug abuser with fever, cough, purulent sputum, a murmur of tricuspid insufficiency, numerous irregular infiltrates and rounded densities on chest radiograph, and *Staphylococcus aureus* bacteremia undoubtedly has acute right-sided endocarditis rather than primary *S. aureus* pneumonia. Similarly, an extensively burned patient with secondary infection of affected skin surfaces, with *Pseudomonas aeruginosa* bacteremia and multiple nodular pulmonary densities, is likely to have bacteremic *Pseudomonas* pneumonia, with bacterial invasion of pulmonary arterial walls rather than pneumonia developing via the bronchogenic route. Frankly septic pulmonary emboli, arising from septic thrombosis of the jugular vein as a complication of postanginal sepsis, sometimes produce a clinical and radiographic picture suggestive of multifocal bronchopneumonia.[61] On the chest radiograph, however, the lesions are nodular; histologically, they represent pulmonary infarcts (following emboli) upon which are engrafted pyogenic infection and abscess formation.

Lung Abscess

Lung abscess is an area of pulmonary infection that has gone on to parenchymal necrosis (see Chapter 130). It is usually solitary but may occur as multiple discrete lesions. Most often it is secondary to aspiration of anaerobic organisms that are components of the normal flora of the upper respiratory tract and are associated with periodontal disease. If the process is subacute, the clinical features may be overlooked initially, so that the first evidence of illness appears only after breakdown of tissue has resulted in an abscess cavity. If there is some degree of ball-valve bronchial obstruction, air may enter while contained pus fails to drain, producing the radiographic picture of an air-fluid level. Alternatively, the initial process may be an aspirational (anaerobic) necrotizing pneumonia with extensive microscopic foci of abscess formation. Progression of this process with confluence of small necrotic foci can either cause one or more lung abscesses or lead to a grossly shrunken and destroyed lobe. *Pulmonary gangrene* is an unusual consequence of severe pulmonary infection characterized by sloughing of a pulmonary segment or lobe. The features distinguishing this process from ordinary necrotizing pneumonia and lung abscess are the extent of necrosis and pulmonary infarction of an entire segment or lobe secondary to thrombosis of both bronchial and pulmonary arteries. The most commonly implicated organism has been *K. pneumoniae*, but others have been *S. pneumoniae*, *Escherichia coli*, mixed anaerobes, *Hemophilus influenzae*, and *S. aureus*.[48]

Other causes of lung abscess are (1) progression of a bronchogenic pneumonia due to a pathogen with necrotizing potential (e.g., *K. pneumoniae*), or *Nocardia asteroides* in an immunocompromised patient,[69] (2) bacteremic spread of infection, and (3) septic pulmonary emboli. Lung abscesses complicating necrotizing pneumonia (Fig. 121-4) should be distinguished from

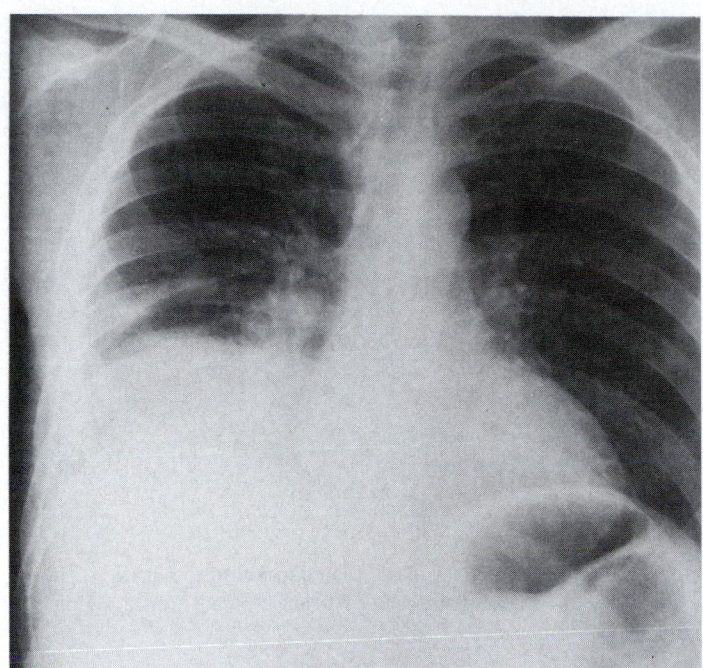

A

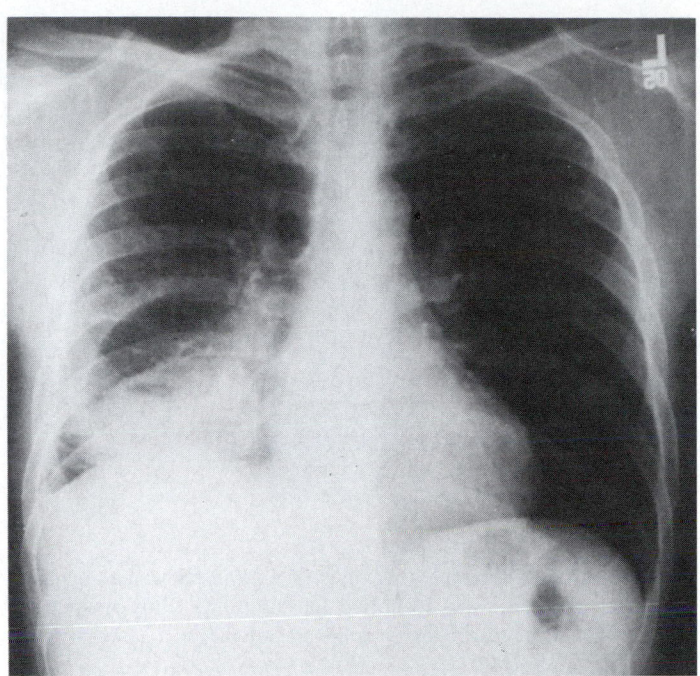

B

FIGURE 121-4   Necrotizing pneumonia, probably secondary to aspiration in a 39-year-old man, smoker and drinker, previously healthy. Onset with cough, shortness of breath, fever, and right-sided pleuritic pain. Despite antibiotics, signs and symptoms progressed to include high fevers, night sweats, greenish sputum, leukocytosis, and manifestations of hypertrophic osteoarthropathy. *A.* On admission, there was consolidation of right lower lobe, a right hilar mass (or adenopathy), and right pleural effusion. Mediastinoscopy and bronchoscopy revealed no tumor. *B.* Three months later, the process in the right lower lobe is more circumscribed. Right lower lobectomy revealed extensive necrotizing pneumonia, multiple abscesses, and "reactive" lymph nodes. Postoperatively, the patient was free of signs and symptoms, including hypertrophic osteoarthropathy.

pneumatoceles; the latter are thin-walled, air-filled structures that often develop early in the course of staphylococcal pneumonia, particularly in infants and young children, and usually disappear over the course of a few months.

Bronchitis and Bronchiectasis

Acute bronchitis is an inflammatory process, usually of viral origin, confined to the bronchi and bronchioles; it does not extend appreciably to surrounding pulmonary parenchyma and is not evident on radiographic examination (see Chapter 127). Purulent secretion is a common concomitant even though there is no discernible bacterial infection. Sometimes purulent secretions represent bacterial superinfection that is evident on examination of Gram-stained smears of sputum and sputum culture. The diagnosis of an acute exacerbation of chronic bronchitis is based solely on clinical grounds; the manifestations are increased cough, dyspnea, and enhanced production of purulent sputum, with or without fever, in a patient with chronic obstructive pulmonary disease. Bacteriologic examination generally reveals large numbers of pneumococci or nontypable *H. influenzae*, either as infecting organisms or as chronic colonizers of the bronchial tree (which is the site of a newly acquired viral infection).

Bronchiectasis is characterized by destruction of epithelial, elastic, and muscular elements of bronchi, resulting in their irreversible dilatation (see Chapter 132). The major proximate cause is repeated or chronic bacterial infection. However, predisposition to such infections may be a consequence of a variety of factors, including certain types of prior infection (pertussis, adenovirus, or rubeola infections, necrotizing pneumonia), bronchial obstruction, immunodeficiencies, congenital anatomic lung disease (e.g., congenital tracheobronchomegaly), and other hereditable disorders, such as ciliary dysfunctional states and α_1-antitrypsin deficiency.[66] Currently, cystic fibrosis is the most common predisposing factor for bronchiectasis in this country. As a result of repeated infections, stasis of secretions, and peribronchial fibrosis, bronchi are grossly distorted or completely destroyed. Although pneumonia or lung abscess may accompany recurrent acute infections, exacerbations are usually confined to bronchial and peribronchial tissues.

Chronic Cavitary Disease

Chronic cavitary pulmonary tuberculosis commonly begins with a focus of pneumonitis, usually in the subapical posterior portion of an upper lobe (Fig. 121-5). This patch of pneumonitis occurs at a latent site of earlier metastatic infection (Simon focus) produced by lymphohematogenous spread from primary pulmonary tuberculous lesions. Progressive caseation necrosis at this site, followed by drainage of caseous material through the bronchial tree, produces a cavity. The cavity is encased in a rigid wall of fibrous tissue.

In addition to pyogenic lung abscess and pulmonary tuberculosis, other pulmonary infections can produce chronic cavities.

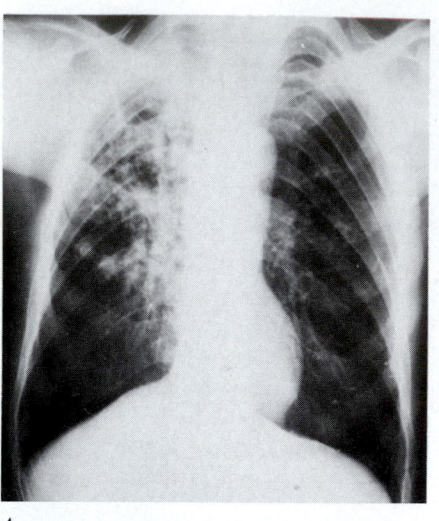
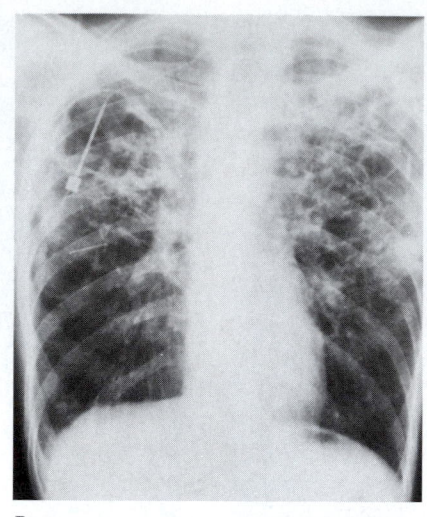
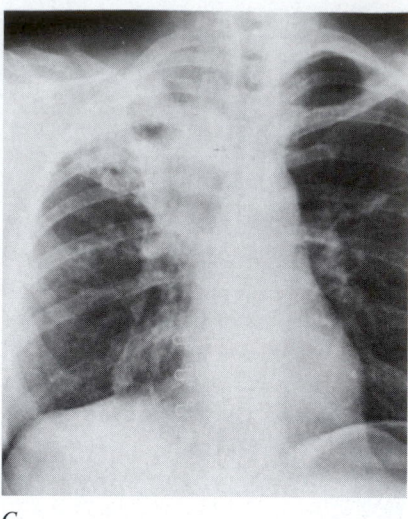

A   B   C

FIGURE 121-5 Tuberculous cavities. In each instance, the organisms were seen on smear and identified by culture. *A.* Fifty-six-year-old African-American man. Cavity amid consolidation. *B.* Seventy-two- year-old African-American man. Bilateral, multiple cavities. *C.* Forty-eight-year-old African-American woman. Spread from original involvement of right upper lobe.

These include nocardial infections, actinomycosis, and chronic primary pulmonary mycoses (particularly histoplasmosis, occasionally coccidioidomycosis, uncommonly blastomycosis). Sporotrichosis can affect the lung and produce cavities, usually thin walled. Rare parasitic infestation of the lung (paragonimiasis, echinococcosis) can take the form of cavitary disease as well.

Pulmonary cavities may also occur in noninfectious disorders (e.g., Wegener's granulomatosis, lymphoma or bronchogenic carcinoma, bland pulmonary infarcts, and intrapulmonary nodules of rheumatoid lung disease). Such cavitary lesions, as well as the cystic lesions that occur in chronic pulmonary sarcoidosis and in the markedly dilated bronchi of saccular bronchiectasis, can be sites of growth of *fungus balls.* These represent tangled masses of fungal hyphae and debris lying freely within pulmonary cavities as noninvasive saprophytic growths.[59] The mycotic agent responsible most commonly is an *Aspergillus* species (usually *A. fumigatus*), and the infection is known as an aspergilloma. Hemoptysis originating from the cavity wall is common and may be severe.

Miliary Lesions

Hematogenous dissemination of tuberculosis can follow initial infection in children or adults (Fig. 121-6). It also can result from breakdown of formerly quiescent sites of pulmonary or extrapulmonary infection.[10] Clinically, unexplained fever is accompanied by miliary lesions (very small and uniform in shape) on the chest radiograph;[40] histologically, these lesions are foci of granulomatous reaction. Similar radiographic lesions also occur in the course of hematogenously disseminated mycotic infections such as cryptococcosis and histoplasmosis.

MICROBIAL CAUSES OF PNEUMONIA

In dealing with a patient with pneumonia, it is helpful, while microbiologic data are being gathered, to consider the relative frequencies of various causes as an aid in selecting initial antimicrobial therapy. Categorization of pneumonias by clinical settings is a practical first step (Table 121-4).

Community-Acquired Pneumonia

An estimated 2 to 2.5 million cases of pneumonia occur annually in the United States. The largest category consists of community-acquired pneumonias (see Chapter 127). A global view of the relative frequencies of the major groupings can be seen in a compilation of data from five series reported for the years 1981 to 1991 (Table 121-5). These cases represent patients with pneumonia of sufficient severity to have warranted hospital admission. Clearly, not all patients with pneumonia require hospitalization. At one institution, as many as 50 percent of patients reporting to an emergency room with pneumonia were believed

---

TABLE 121-4

Practical Categorization of Pneumonia by Clinical Setting

Community-acquired pneumonia
   Typical (i.e., classic) pneumonia
   Atypical pneumonia
   Aspiration pneumonia
Pneumonia in the elderly
   Community acquired
   In nursing home residents
Nosocomial pneumonia
Pneumonia in immunocompromised hosts
   Pneumonia in patients with immunoglobulin and
      complement deficiencies
   Pneumonia in patients with granulocyte deficiency
   Pneumonia in patients with cellular immune deficiences
      Pneumonia in patients with neoplastic disease
      Pneumonia in transplant recipients
      Pneumonia in patients with AIDS
      Pneumonia in other immunocompromised patients

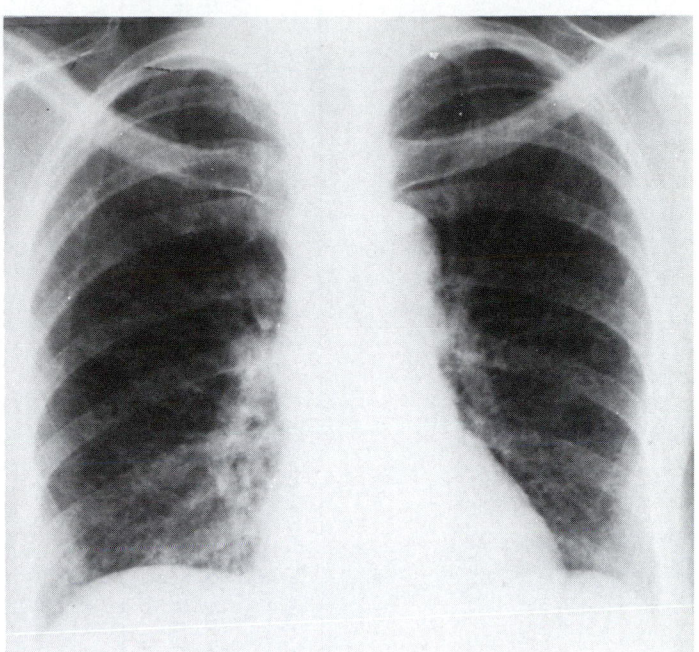

A

B

FIGURE 121-6 Miliary tuberculosis. A 64-year-old African-American woman complaining of urinary frequency and progressive weight loss for 1 year. *A.* On admission, close inspection reveals fine nodular lesions throughout both lung fields. *B.* Four weeks later, the lesions are larger and many have become confluent, especially on the right. Bronchoscopic washings, biopsy, and culture positive for *M. tuberculosis*. Urine culture strongly positive for *E. coli* but negative for *M. tuberculosis*.

not to require hospitalization. In a Seattle study in a large medical cooperative, 15 percent of all pneumonias were due to *M. pneumoniae* (Fig. 121-7), but only 2 percent of the patients with *M. pneumoniae* pneumonia were hospitalized. Thus, this cause is likely to be underrepresented in a compilation such as that shown in Table 121-5.

Bacterial causes are the most frequent (35 percent) in community-acquired pneumonias. Of the bacterial species implicated, *S. pneumoniae* is the predominant one, accounting for 33 percent of cases with a bacterial origin. Fifteen percent of patients have definable nonbacterial etiologies such as *Mycoplasma*, viruses, *Chlamydia*, and *Coxiella burnetii*. Certain uncommon causes may be endemic, in particular geographic niches, but are not evident more generally. Thus, *C. burnetii* was responsible for 3.1 percent of cases of community-acquired pneumonia reported from Nova Scotia;[35] and in Little Rock, Arkansas, *Francisella tularensis* was the cause in 3.2 percent.[9] In 46 percent of the cases of community-acquired pneumonia, the etiologic agent is not defined. Some of these cases undoubtedly represent viral and mycoplasmal pneumonias that have not been identified. It is also likely that others represent patients with pneumococcal pneumonia whose sputum cultures failed to grow this somewhat fastidious microorganism, patients with *Legionella* pneumonia, patients with aspirational pneumonia caused by oral anaerobes, or patients with undescribed etiologic agents.

BACTERIAL PNEUMONIA

S. pneumoniae is the preeminent bacterial cause of community-acquired pneumonia. *H. influenzae*, usually unencapsulated

strains, may produce pneumonia in patients with chronic bronchitis. It also may be the causative agent of pneumonia in the chronic alcoholic. Apart from *S. pneumoniae*, however, the most important pathogen in this type of patient, by virtue of its virulence and special antibiotic susceptibilities, is *K. pneumoniae*. During an outbreak of influenza viral infections, bacterial superinfections often occur, usually in the elderly or in pa-

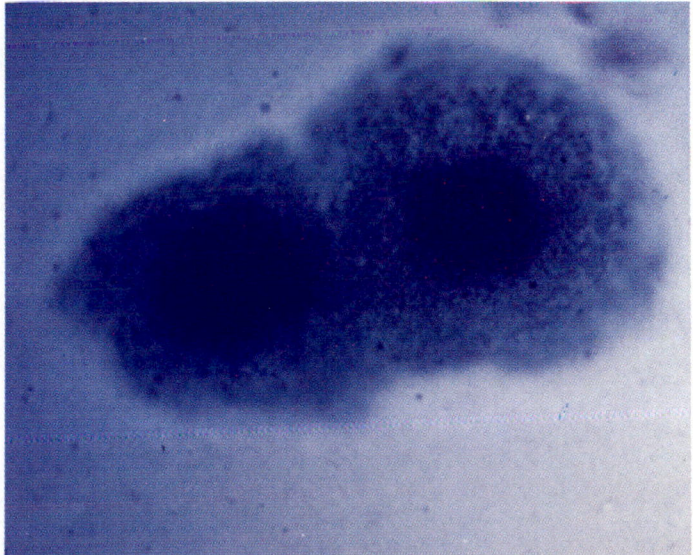

FIGURE 121-7 Subculture on mycoplasma agar of *Mycoplasma* isolated from sputum of a 22-year-old man with atypical pneumonia. The two colonies show the "fried egg" appearance that is more typical of *M. hominis* and other *Mycoplasma* species than of *M. pneumoniae* on primary isolation. Dienes stain, ×45.

TABLE 121-5

Relative Frequencies of Major Categories of Community-Acquired Pneumonia

Author (ref.), Location	Years	Total No. Patients	No. with Bact. Origin	% with Bact. Origin	S. Pneumoniae Cause: % of Total Bacterial	% of Total: Viral, Chlamydial, Mycoplasmal	% of Total with More Than 1 Pathogen	% of Total with Aspiration or Post-obstruction	% of Total with Unknown Origin
Marrie et al.[37] (Halifax, Nova Scotia)	1981–87	719	188	26	32	23	10	9	47
Fang et al.[23] (Pittsburgh)	1986–87	359	171	48	32	6	3	9	33
Bates et al.[9] (Little Rock)	1985	154	58	38	16	16	6.5	Not stated	51
Ostergaard & Andersen[47] (Aarhus, Denmark)	5-Year period including 1987–88	254	80	32	44	5	3	Not stated	63
Mundy et al.[39] (Baltimore)	1990–91	205	89	44	35	8	4	14 (aspiration)	32
TOTALS		1691	586	35	33	15	7	10	46

tients with chronic cardiopulmonary disease. Patients with secondary bacterial pneumonia often have up to 4 days of clinical improvement after the initial influenzal illness before the onset of overt pulmonary infection. The superinfecting microorganisms are the pathogens that would ordinarily colonize the upper airways but opportunistically invade a tracheobronchial tree that has been recently damaged. These organisms include *S. pneumoniae, H. influenzae, S. aureus, S. pyogenes, M. catarrhalis,* and *K. pneumoniae.* The use of antibiotics at the time of the initial respiratory infection not only is useless against viral influenza but also may selectively promote the emergence of a more resistant bacterial flora in the respiratory tract. *S. aureus* is a very uncommon cause of community-acquired pneumonia. Indeed, the occurrence of several cases of *S. aureus* pneumonia in the community during the winter months is usually a good indicator of the presence of an ambient influenza outbreak.

Pneumonia due to *S. pyogenes* is quite uncommon. Usually it occurs as a superinfection in a patient with influenza or as a primary pneumonia in the course of a regional outbreak of group A streptococcal infections (as still occurs from time to time when a new M-antigenic type appears in a community).

ATYPICAL PNEUMONIA SYNDROME

In the evaluation of patients with community-acquired pneumonia, it is often helpful to consider separately a group of patients whose illness is characterized by little, if any, sputum production and, if sputum is raised, examination on Gram-stained (and Ziehl-Neelsen–stained) smears and routine culture fails to reveal a microbial cause. Often, the clinical onset of illness is less acute than in the typical bacterial pneumonias, the radiologic picture is more likely to consist of patchy infiltrates or an interstitial pattern than a lobar consolidation, and a peripheral leukocytosis is less common. For convenience, this grouping has been designated *atypical pneumonia.*

The entities in the category of atypical pneumonia are highly heterogeneous (Table 121-6), and the syndrome accounts for about 60 percent of cases of community-acquired pneumonia. *M. pneumoniae* is the causative agent in about 25 percent of the cases of atypical pneumonia. Respiratory viruses are responsible for about another 30 percent.[9,23,35,39,47] However, the predominant etiologic agent varies considerably with the season and the prevalence of influenza A in the community. A viral respiratory illness becomes a major cause of atypical pneumonia during an outbreak of the latter. The recently described *Chlamydia pneumoniae* (formerly known as *Chlamydia* strain TWAR), an infectious agent that causes pneumonia and can be spread from person to person without an avian host, appears to be responsible for 12 to 21 percent of cases of atypical pneumonia. This form of pneumonia typically occurs in young adults as a sporadic mild pneumonia.[30,31] Occasional outbreaks have occurred.

The epidemiologic and clinical characteristics of certain types of atypical pneumonias may provide a basis for suspecting these causes before results of specific laboratory tests become available. In adults, *M. pneumoniae* pneumonia, in contrast to bacterial pneumonia, often begins insidiously with malaise, fever, and prominent headache. Sore throat is common, but coryza is minimal or absent. Nonproductive cough develops over the next few days and is the hallmark of this disease. Skin rash (erythema multiforme) and bullous myringitis, usually appearing late in the course of illness, are uncommon findings but, when present, do suggest the diagnosis. Mini-outbreaks of *M. pneumoniae* infection in households are frequently not appreciated because of the long incubation period (3 weeks) and the varied forms that the illness can assume. One characteristic sequence to illustrate the diversity of clinical presentations is as follows: the infection with *M. pneumoniae* is introduced by a grade-school child whose illness may be a sore throat and earache; 3 weeks later, a parent develops atypical pneumonia; and several weeks after that, a second child, of high-school age, develops a troublesome persistent dry cough with minimal fever. Outbreaks have occurred in military camps.

Infections with respiratory viruses occur predominantly in the winter and early spring. Influenza virus is the one agent that may be associated with sizable outbreaks or major epidemics of upper-respiratory infections. Primary influenza viral pneumonia usually occurs in the setting of an influenza A outbreak. It occurs primarily in patients with underlying heart disease, particularly mitral stenosis. Other risk factors are chronic pulmonary disease and pregnancy. Unlike secondary bacterial pneumonia after influenza—a complication that occurs after a period (1 to 4 days) of improvement following a typical influenzal upper-respiratory illness—primary influenza pneumonia immediately follows typical influenza. Very rarely, in the course of systemic infection with viruses whose principal impact is not ordinarily on the respiratory tract, viral pneumonia develops in an otherwise healthy person. Pulmonary infiltrates occur in 16 percent of young

TABLE 121-6

Causes of Community-Acquired Atypical Pneumonias

Mycoplasma
   M. pneumoniae
Respiratory tract viruses
   Influenza, adenovirus, respiratory syncytial virus (RSV), parainfluenza virus,
   pulmonary hantavirus
Other viral agents
   Varicella-zoster, measles, Epstein-Barr virus (EBV)
Rickettsia
   C. burnetii (Q fever)
Chlamydia
   C. psittaci (psittacosis), *C. pneumoniae* (formerly strain TWAR)
Bacteria
   Legionella, F. tularensis, Y. pestis, B. anthracis
Fungi
   Histoplasma, Blastomyces, Coccidioides

adults with varicella, but only 2 to 4 percent have clinical manifestations suggestive of pneumonia. Pneumonia in children with varicella is more likely to represent bacterial superinfection than primary viral pneumonia. On rare occasions, pulmonary infiltrates develop in patients with clinical infectious mononucleosis; the infiltrates represent atypical pneumonia due to Epstein-Barr virus.

In 1993, an acute illness associated with a novel Hantavirus, Sin Nombre virus, emerged in outbreak form in the Four Corners area of New Mexico, Arizona, Colorado, and Utah.[20] The principal host for Sin Nombre virus is the deer mouse, and infection is acquired through exposure to this rodent, rodent excreta, or contaminated dust. By late 1996, 145 cases had been reported, mainly in the West and Southwest, but occasional cases have occurred as far east as New York and Rhode Island. The Hantavirus pulmonary syndrome begins with a 3- to 6-day prodromal period consisting of myalgias and fever, sometimes accompanied by gastrointestinal symptoms. The prodrome is followed by progressive cough, dyspnea, tachycardia, and hypotension. Crackles are present on auscultation. Laboratory findings include hemoconcentration, leukocytosis, and thrombocytopenia; the radiologic findings are those of interstitial edema, peribronchial cuffing, and bilateral airspace (bibasilar and perihilar) disease.[11] The picture suggests pneumonia, but the microscopic findings are those of pulmonary edema (interstitial and alveolar) consistent with a diffuse pulmonary capillary leak syndrome. The case fatality rate for the Hantavirus pulmonary syndrome is 50 percent.

Q fever, due to *C. burnetii*, like many of the other causes of the atypical pneumonia syndrome, is suspected on the basis of epidemiologic clues. Transmission of this disease to humans occurs as a result of inhalation of aerosols from surroundings contaminated by placental and birth fluids of infected livestock (cattle, sheep, goats), wild rabbits, and domestic animals (cats). Veterinarians, ranchers, and medical investigators, such as those who use goats or sheep to produce antibodies, are at particular risk. Since the incubation period of Q fever is approximately 20 days, a source of exposure during foreign travel may easily be overlooked. Although the clinical picture resembles that of *M. pneumoniae* pneumonia, the onset may be more abrupt, with chills and high fever. Liver function abnormalities or clinical hepatitis in a patient with atypical pneumonia is suggestive of Q fever. In some geographic areas (Australia, France), hepatitis has been the most frequent clinical presentation of *C. burnetii* infection; in others (Spain, Nova Scotia), pneumonia has been the major presenting sign.[21]

Chlamydia trachomatis causes pneumonia in the newborn but has not been proved to be a cause of pneumonia in adults. *C. psittaci*, the causative agent of psittacosis, is spread to humans by avian species. Although psittacine birds (parakeets, parrots) are the major reservoir, human infection can be acquired from pigeons, sparrows, and turkeys. In a patient with atypical pneumonia, the clinical features that raise the possibility of this etiology are relative bradycardia, splenomegaly and hepatomegaly, and hepatic dysfunction. *C. pneumoniae* variant TWAR produces atypical pneumonia without the usual bird-to-human transmission of *C. psittaci* infection. The clinical picture of TWAR-strain infection is indistinguishable from that of *M. pneumoniae* pneumonia.

Legionella infections (due to *L. pneumophila* and other *Legionella* species) account for 2 to 4 percent of cases of atypical pneumonia (see Chapter 144). Although *Legionella* is an important nosocomial pathogen, it is also responsible for community-based sporadic cases and major outbreaks. The occurrence of summer outbreaks associated with the use of air conditioners and evaporative condensers should call attention to this possible cause of atypical pneumonia.[27] Various extrapulmonary manifestations have been attributed to Legionnaires' disease; among them are a relative bradycardia, diarrhea for 24 h at the onset of illness, confusion and obtundation, mild renal dysfunction (azotemia, microscopic hematuria, proteinuria), acute rhabdomyolysis, and mild hepatic dysfunction. Although many of these manifestations also occur with other pneumonias, the coincidence of several of these features should raise the possibility of *Legionella* infection. This is particularly important in view of the fact that the antibiotic treatment (erythromycin) for Legionnaires' disease differs from that for the more common bacterial pneumonias, and that the mortality from Legionnaires' disease, if inadequately treated, can be as high as 15 percent. Recurrent chills, which occur over several days in Legionnaires' disease, are rare in pneumococcal pneumonia unless septic complications (e.g., endocarditis and pericarditis) develop. Although the initial radiographic picture of *Legionella* pneumonia is often that of an interstitial, segmental, or bronchopneumonic pneumonia, if the disease is untreated, it progresses to lobar or multilobar consolidation, a picture that mimics pneumococcal or *Klebsiella* pneumonia.

The other noteworthy bacterial types of atypical pneumonia are those due to *F. tularensis* (tularemic pneumonia), *Yersinia pestis* (plague pneumonia), and *Bacillus anthracis* (anthrax pneumonia). These are all singularly uncommon causes of pneumonia, and the principal clues to diagnosis again derive from epidemiologic considerations. Exposure to *F. tularensis* comes through contact with tissues of an infected animal (rabbit), animal bites (coyote, cat), inhalation of infectious aerosols, tick or deerfly bites, or ingestion of contaminated water or poorly cooked meat from an infected animal. Ulceroglandular tularemia, or the typhoidal form of tularemia, may be complicated by patchy pulmonary infiltrates. Indeed, it is likely that typhoidal tularemia often represents infection initially acquired via the bronchogenic route. Plague is less common than tularemia in the United States and is strictly localized to southwestern states, including California. The diagnosis should be considered in a person from an endemic area who has a septic illness (septicemic plague) or painful localized lymphadenopathy with fever (bubonic plague) and a history of bites by rodent fleas or of handling tissues of infected animals, such as prairie dogs or coyotes. Pneumonia occurs as a complication in 10 to 15 percent of patients with bubonic or septicemic plague. Primary (inhalation) pneumonic plague is extremely rare and occurs only as a result of exposure to aerosolized particles from an infected animal or following close contact with cases of plague pneumonia. Anthrax pneumonia (inhalation anthrax) is also extremely rare in this country; it is a consequence of the inhalation of anthrax spores during the processing, or use, of goat hair or wool (usually imported from the Middle East, Asia, or Africa).

The principal clues that the cause of atypical pneumonia in a given patient might be a primary pulmonary mycosis are epidemiologic (see Chapter 148). For example, the principal endemic areas for histoplasmosis in this hemisphere are in the midwestern United States and Central America. The organism is present in high concentrations in soil sites where avian, chicken, or bat excrement has accumulated. Movement of soil in such endemic areas by cleaning chicken coops, knocking down old starling roosts, or cleaning out old attics or basements can expose people to high concentrations of airborne spores that, when inhaled, produce an acute pneumonia. Atypical pneumonia in a person with this type of geographic exposure, or in a spelunker, should automatically raise the possibility of histoplasmosis.

Blastomycosis occurs in most states in this country, but the endemic area is principally in the southeastern and south central areas. Rural exposure to soil contaminated with animal excrement appears to be a risk factor. Skin lesions, either verrucous or ulcerative, are the most common extrapulmonary manifestations of blastomycosis and afford a clinical clue to diagnosis.

Coccidioidomycosis is endemic in the southwestern United States (California, particularly the San Joaquin Valley, and Arizona) and in neighboring portions of Mexico. Infection is usually acquired in these areas by inhalation of highly infectious arthrospores. Occasionally, major dust storms carry the arthrospores considerable distances from their soil source and produce unexpected outbreaks of infection. Archeologic digs sometimes cause infection in those living elsewhere who receive an artifact uncovered in the explorations. Erythema nodosum may be associated with any of the primary pulmonary mycoses, but most often with coccidioidomycosis. The coincidence of this hypersensitivity skin lesion and an atypical pneumonia syndrome in a person from an endemic area suggests the possibility of one of these pulmonary mycoses.

Paracoccidioidomycosis (South American blastomycosis) is endemic to Brazil (mainly), Colombia, Venezuela, and Argentina; this disease is caused by *Paracoccidioides brasiliensis*. In adults, the manifestations of this disease are mainly pulmonary; radiographs show patchy or confluent areas of consolidation, often bilateral. Cases have occurred in North America and Europe, but in those instances, the patients had previously resided in endemic areas where initial infection presumably had been acquired.

ASPIRATION PNEUMONIA

Community-acquired aspiration pneumonia may occur after an overt episode of aspiration (e.g., of gastric contents) or of bronchial obstruction by a foreign body (see Chapter 129). More often the predisposing circumstances are less clear-cut (e.g., alcoholism, nocturnal esophageal reflux, pyorrhea, a prolonged session in the dental chair, epilepsy, or chronic sinusitis in a patient with absent gag reflex). In these circumstances, since the pneumonia may develop more insidiously than after overt aspiration, the relationship of the developing pneumonia to the predisposing circumstances may not be appreciated at the time. For this reason, specific questioning regarding such possible pathogenetic factors and evaluation of the gag reflex should be part of the examination of any patient with pneumonia.

If untreated, aspiration pneumonia may progress rapidly to a necrotizing process that is usually due to anaerobic organisms. The process may involve a pulmonary segment, a lobe, or an entire lung, with ultimate extension to the pleura ("putrid empyema"); in some patients, the necrotizing pneumonia culminates in lung abscesses. In others, aspiration produces an illness of several weeks' duration that is characterized by malaise, productive cough, and low-grade fever. If a chest radiograph is first taken after several weeks of untreated illness, it may show little, if any, evidence of pneumonia but will clearly identify a well-formed lung abscess.

In community-acquired aspiration pneumonia, insight into the etiologic agents has been obtained primarily from bacteriologic studies after transtracheal aspiration; these studies have provided a statistical basis for selecting the initial antimicrobial therapy. Anaerobic bacteria are etiologically implicated in about 90 percent of community-acquired aspiration pneumonias and lung abscesses. In 40 to 65 percent of these patients, anaerobic organisms are the sole infecting agents; in 40 to 45 percent, the cause is a mixture of anaerobes and aerobes. The most common anaerobes are *Prevotella melaninogenica*, *Bacteroides* species, *Porphyromonas* species, *Fusobacterium* species, peptostreptococci, peptococci, and microaerophilic streptococci. β-Lactamase–producing *Bacteroides* species, *P. melaninogenica*, and members of the *B. fragilis* group are present in about 15 percent of cases. *P. melaninogenica* may be the most important contributor in such mixed infections. The aerobic indigenous flora in mixed aerobic-anaerobic infections are *S. viridans*, *M. catarrhalis*, and *Eikenella corrodens*.[26] A rare form of anaerobic aspiration pneumonia (actinomycosis) that is community acquired is that due to *Actinomyces israelii*, part of the normal flora in the gingival crevice (Fig. 121-8). The direct extension of such a necrotizing pneumonia to the pleura and chest wall is a characteristic finding that strongly suggests the diagnosis of actinomycosis.

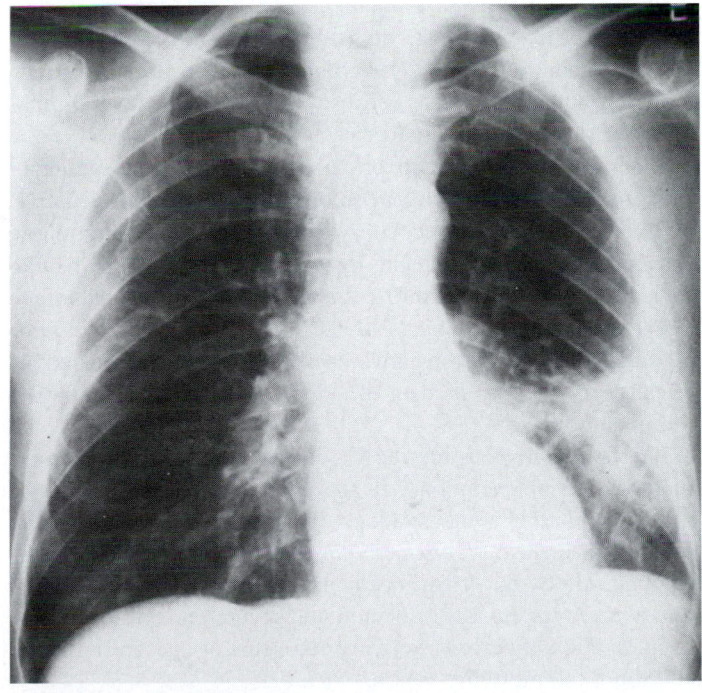

FIGURE 121-8   Actinomycosis in a 54-year-old chronic alcoholic man with pyorrheic gums who was admitted with signs of brain tumor. Chest radiograph shows mass in left lower lobe. Computed tomography is consistent with brain metastasis. Transthoracic needle aspirate revealed *A. israelii*.

Although anaerobic members of the oropharyngeal flora have a preeminent role in community-acquired aspiration pneumonia and lung abscess, occasionally gram-negative enteric bacilli such as *K. pneumoniae*, *E. coli*, and *Proteus* species may be the cause.

Persistence of a necrotizing pneumonia or lung abscess despite antimicrobial therapy that would be expected a priori to be effective raises the possibility of an underlying bronchogenic carcinoma, particularly if the patient is edentulous. In a prospective study of 1269 patients with community-acquired pneumonia, nine (0.7 percent) had the episode of pneumonia as the initial manifestation of carcinoma of the lung.[36]

Pneumonia in the Elderly

Community-acquired pneumonia in the elderly (over 60 years) primarily affects two groups: one population that lives at home and another that resides in nursing homes. The latter, from the point of view of oropharyngeal flora and the extent of exposure to antimicrobial agents, might be regarded as midway between community residents and patients in hospital. The clinical features of pneumonia in the elderly may differ in presentation from that in younger people. Infection has a more gradual onset, with less fever and cough, often with a decline in mental status or confusion and generalized weakness, but with less readily elicited signs of consolidation on examination.[67] Eliciting a deep breath from the patient may be helpful in demonstrating a localized wheeze or rales that might otherwise be undetectable. Among the bacterial causes of community-acquired pneumonia in the elderly, *S. pneumoniae* is the most frequent, accounting for 30 to 60 percent of cases.[49,67] *H. influenzae*, primarily nontypable strains, is the second most common cause (about 20 percent). *M. catarrhalis* is another cause of pneumonia in this age group, primarily in patients with chronic bronchitis. Aspiration pneumonia due to mixed aerobic-anaerobic flora occurs in this age group, particularly because of the presence of a diminished gag reflex or impaired pharyngeal motor function.

In nursing home residents or persons with recent hospitalizations, increased oropharyngeal colonization with gram-negative bacilli occurs, probably secondary to antibiotic administration in such institutions. Subsequent microaspirational events would predispose to pneumonia due to species such as *K. pneumoniae*, *E. coli* and other Enterobacteriaceae, and *P. aeruginosa*. In several studies, such gram-negative bacilli have been implicated as the cause in 25 to 40 percent of elderly nursing home residents with pneumonia.[28,49]

S. aureus is responsible for 2 to 10 percent of cases of community-acquired pneumonia in the elderly overall, more commonly in nursing home residents and during community outbreaks of influenza. *M. pneumoniae* pneumonia occurs primarily in young adults, but it can occur in the elderly. Among 64 patients with *M. pneumoniae* pneumonia severe enough to require hospitalization, 9 percent were over 65 years of age. Even in this age group, the mortality was low.[37]

Prognosis of Community-Acquired Pneumonia

The overall mortality in a summary of approximately 33,000 patients (reported between 1966 and 1995) with community-acquired pneumonia necessitating hospitalization was 13.7 percent.[25] The mortality was associated with microbial etiology and a variety of clinical prognostic factors. For example, the mortality for pneumococcal pneumonia was 12.3 percent; for *S. aureus* pneumonia, 31.8 percent; and for *M. pneumoniae*, 1.4 percent. Adverse clinical prognostic factors included co-morbid conditions (neurologic or neoplastic disease, alcoholism, congestive heart failure), bacteremia, multilobar involvement, and azotemia.

Nosocomial Pneumonia

Nosocomial pneumonia is the second most common nosocomial infection in the United States and occurs at a rate of 5 to 10 cases per 1000 hospital admissions (see Chapter 143).[3] The incidence increases 6- to 20-fold in patients receiving assisted ventilation. The strikingly different bacterial causes of nosocomial pneumonia from those of community-acquired pneumonia should serve to direct the clinician's thinking about etiology and therapeutic approach before results of cultures become available.

The cause of hospital-acquired pneumonia depends on the time of onset of the pneumonia, the type of hospital (community or university tertiary care), and whether the patient is intubated or in the intensive care unit. Thus, the "early onset" (first 4 days) bacterial pneumonia is more often due to *S. pneumoniae*, *H. influenzae*, and *M. catarrhalis*, whereas "late onset" (after 4 days) is more commonly (45 to 75 percent) due to aerobic gram-negative bacilli (*K. pneumonae*, other Enterobacteriaceae, *Acinetobacter* species, and *P. aeruginosa*.[18] In respiratory intensive care units, *Burkholdaria* (formerly *Pseudomonas*) *cepacia*, *Stenotrophomonas* (formerly *Xanthomonas*) *maltophilia*, and *Acinetobacter baumannii* (formerly *Acinetobacter calcoaceticus* variant *anitratus*) have been implicated in localized outbreaks of nosocomial pneumonia.[24] In a study by the National Nosocomial Infections Surveillance System of respiratory tract isolates from adults with nosocomial pneumonia, *P. aeruginosa* was the most common pathogen found, and *S. aureus* was the most common gram-positive organism, at a frequency about one-third that of *P. aeruginosa*.[58] Gram-negative bacilli rapidly colonize the oropharynx of ill, hospitalized patients, and they are the most common cause of aspiration pneumonia that occurs subsequently.

Nosocomial outbreaks of *Legionella* pneumonia have occurred in hospitals secondary to environmental problems related to potable water, air-conditioning systems, or water-cooling towers. Although in these circumstances immunocompromised patients have been particularly at risk, patients with alcoholism and chronic obstructive airway disease have also been particularly vulnerable.[45]

In previous years, attention focused on nosocomial pneumonias of bacterial origin. However, it is now appreciated that hospital-acquired viral pneumonias are also of considerable import.[29] During major influenza outbreaks, the incidence of nosocomial pneumonias increases and is accompanied by considerable mortality. These pneumonias represent primary influenza viral pneumonia or, more often, bacterial pneumonia complicating influenza.

Statistical information about the etiology of nosocomial pneumonia does provide some knowledge that is of general predictive value. In dealing with the individual patient, however, more useful information is provided by awareness of the bacterial species that is most often implicated in nosocomial pneumonia in the particular hospital and the antimicrobial susceptibilities of sputum isolates from patients in that institution. The hospital epidemiologist or the physicians working in an intensive care unit can often provide insights into the cause of outbreaks of nosocomial pneumonia either in the hospital or in their specific sector. With respect to treating a particular patient, examination of sputum (or an endotracheal or bronchoscopic aspirate) after Gram's staining is essential as a guide to the selection of initial antimicrobial therapy.

Pneumonia in the Immunocompromised Host

To utilize statistics in assessing the likely cause of a febrile pneumonitis syndrome in a patient who has an underlying disorder of host defenses, it is helpful to distinguish among several categories of abnormal defense mechanisms. Depending on the underlying defect, the types of pneumonia developing in these settings can differ (see Chapters 134 to 141).

HYPOGAMMAGLOBULINEMIA

Patients who have congenital or acquired deficiencies of the immunoglobulins are particularly susceptible to recurrent pneumonias caused by encapsulated bacterial species, particularly *S. pneumoniae* and *H. influenzae* type b.

GRANULOCYTE DEFICIENCY

This category includes patients who have deficiencies both in granulocyte function and in granulocyte numbers (see Chapters 136 and 139).

Defects in Granulocyte Function
Patients with the hyperimmunoglobulin E syndrome, characterized by chronic eczema, "cold" cutaneous abscesses, and mucocutaneous candidiasis, have a chemotactic defect for polymorphonuclear leukocytes.[19] As a result, they are subject to recurrent skin and sinopulmonary infections. The principal bacteria causing pneumonia in these patients are *S. aureus*, *H. influenzae*, and, to a lesser extent, *S. pneumoniae*.

Patients with chronic granulomatous disease of childhood suffer from an inherited disorder of oxidative microbicidal activity of polymorphonuclear leukocytes and monocytes. These patients are subject to suppurative lymphadenitis, soft-tissue and hepatic abscesses, and sometimes pneumonia. Pathogens producing infections in these patients are primarily *S. aureus*, Enterobacteriaceae (*K. pneumoniae, Serratia*), *Pseudomonas* species or *B. cepacia*, *Nocardia*, *Candida* species, and *Aspergillus* species.

Granulocytopenia
Granulocytopenia (fewer than 500 or 1000 granulocytes per microliter of blood) is an important risk factor for pulmonary infections, particularly those caused by gram-negative bacilli, *S. aureus*, and fungi such as *Aspergillus* and *Candida* species. The predisposing granulocytopenia usually develops in the course of treating leukemia to induce a remission; during leukemic relapse,

aplastic anemia, or cytotoxic drug therapy for neoplastic disease; or in association with organ transplantation. The pulmonary infections that occur in recipients of bone marrow transplants represent a special case because of the combination of profound granulocytopenia, severe combined immunodeficiency, and graft-versus-host disease produced by intense cytotoxic drug or radiation therapy that is used to ablate the bone marrow (see Chapter 137). As a result, an additional group of infecting agents (cytomegalovirus [CMV] and *P. carinii*) become likely on statistical grounds.

Pneumonias that affect granulocytopenic hospitalized patients occur most often via the microaspiration route. Although mixed anaerobic oral commensals may be responsible, gram-negative bacilli (particularly *P. aeruginosa*) are among the most frequent causative agents. In about 75 percent of patients with leukemia who develop gram-negative bacillary pneumonia, the responsible bacterial species has colonized the oropharynx within the preceding 3 days. Bacteremic spread of infection to the lung can also occur from an initiating site of infection in the perineum, intestinal tract, or urinary tract. However, although bacteremia occurs in 30 to 40 percent of patients with gram-negative bacillary pneumonia, the pulmonary infection usually precedes the bacteremia.

CELLULAR IMMUNE DEFICIENCY

The number of immunocompromised patients who have defects primarily in T-cell function and/or numbers has increased markedly in recent years on several accounts: (1) the prolonged survival of patients with neoplastic disease, (2) the increasing number of organ transplantations (and the attendant use of cytotoxic drugs), (3) the increasing number of patients with collagen vascular disease (which is responsive to drugs such as cyclophosphamide and corticosteroids), and (4) the current large number of patients in the United States with the acquired immunodeficiency syndrome (AIDS). These diverse entities share a common clinical picture of fever and a pulmonary infiltrate. The principal immunodeficiency in each of these situations is the lack of cell-mediated immunity. However, because the causes of the same clinical picture of fever and a pulmonary infiltrate are diverse among these entities, it is worthwhile to consider each of the groups separately as a basis for approaching diagnosis from a statistical viewpoint.

Pneumonia in Patients with Neoplastic Disease
Although patients with neoplastic diseases are considered a specific category of patients with deficient cell-mediated immunity for present purposes, the group is far from uniform (see Chapter 136). Variations in the nature of the neoplastic process (leukemia, lymphoma, carcinoma) and in the duration and type of therapy (cytotoxic drugs, radiation, corticosteroids) may evoke differing patterns of immunosuppression and pulmonary pathology. Until recently, in patients with leukemia and lymphoma, bacterial origins were two to 15 times as common as fungal causes of fatal pneumonias. But in recent years, the percentage of fatal fungal pneumonias appears to be increasing.

The diversity of infectious and noninfectious causes of the febrile pneumonitis syndrome in patients with neoplastic disease is shown in Table 121-7. In patients with neoplastic disease, and in patients who have undergone renal transplantation, important clues to narrow the field of etiologic possibilities are provided by two considerations: the rate of progression of the illness and the radiologic features of the pulmonary process (see "Radiographic Features of Pneumonia," below). An acute pulmonary process, developing in 24 to 36 h, should suggest (1) a bacterial cause (usual respiratory pathogens, nosocomial gram-negative bacilli, *S. aureus, Legionella* species), (2) pulmonary emboli, (3) pulmonary edema, (4) pulmonary hemorrhage, or (5) a leukoagglutinin (transfusion) reaction. A subacute to chronic process developing over several days to weeks suggests a different set of etiologic considerations: (1) fungal infection (*Aspergillus, Mucor, Cryptococcus, Candida*, etc.), (2) nocardial infection, (3) viral infection (common respiratory viruses causing pneumonia in healthy persons, CMV, varicella-zoster virus, herpes simplex virus, and adenoviruses), (4) *P. carinii* infection and disseminated strongyloidiasis, (5) mycobacterial infection (principally *M. tuberculosis* but also "atypical" mycobacteria), (6) radiation pneumonitis, (7) drug-induced pulmonary toxicity or hypersensitivity reaction, and (8) invasion of the lungs by tumor or leukemia.

Pneumonia in Transplant Recipients

Although the infecting agents that cause pneumonia in transplant recipients are common to the various types of organ transplantation, certain opportunistic infections are more common for certain organs (e.g., bone marrow) than for others (e.g., kidney) (see Chapter 138).

Another clue to the cause of pneumonia in transplant recipients is the time after transplantation at which the pulmonary process develops. In the renal transplant recipient, pulmonary infections during the first month after organ transfer are almost always due to conventional bacterial pathogens rather than to fungal, viral, or protozoal agents. Should an opportunistic infection occur during this interval, environmental contamination in the transplant unit becomes a serious consideration. The problem may be due to infection with *Legionella* spread via potable water or airflow systems, or the airborne spread of *Aspergillus* species, commonly associated with construction and renovation. A single instance of either of these types of infection in the early posttransplant period should prompt an immediate epidemiologic investigation to forestall a nosocomial outbreak in this highly vulnerable population.

In the 1 to 6 months after renal and other solid organ transplantation, serious opportunistic infections pose the greatest risk because of the cumulative effects of continuing immunosuppression, particularly if pulses of antirejection therapy have been administered. Viral pneumonias due to CMV, adenovirus, and herpes simplex can occur during this period. CMV infection, symptomatic and asymptomatic, is particularly noteworthy in transplant recipients because of its frequency and the possible additional element of immunosuppression it may add, per se. From 40 to 90 percent of renal transplant recipients and most cardiac transplant recipients develop evidence of CMV infection after transplantation. In the series reported by Ramsey and colleagues, CMV was the cause of 15 percent of 54 episodes of pulmonary disease that followed renal transplantation.[50] The clinical and radiographic picture is that of an interstitial pneumonia. The incidence of CMV infection (Fig. 121-9) in bone marrow transplantation (BMT) is considerably greater: about 50 percent of allogeneic BMT patients develop interstitial pneumonitis, and CMV is the cause in about half of these cases; in the other half, the cause is unclear. The recent use of suppressive and preemptive ganciclovir therapy in bone marrow and solid organ trans-

---

TABLE 121-7

Cause of Syndrome of Fever with Pulmonary Infiltrates in 100 Patients with Neoplastic Disease

Cause	No. of Patients
Infectious agents (73)	
Conventional bacterial species	26
Viruses	11
Fungi	10
N. asteroides	5
P. carinii	6
M. tuberculosis	1
Mixed infections	14
Noninfectious causes (27)	
Pulmonary emboli	3
Recurrent tumor	8
Radiation pneumonitis	7
Pulmonary edema	1
Drug-induced pneumonitis	5
Leukoagglutinin reaction	2
Pulmonary hemorrhage	1

SOURCE: Data from Rubin and Greene.[55]

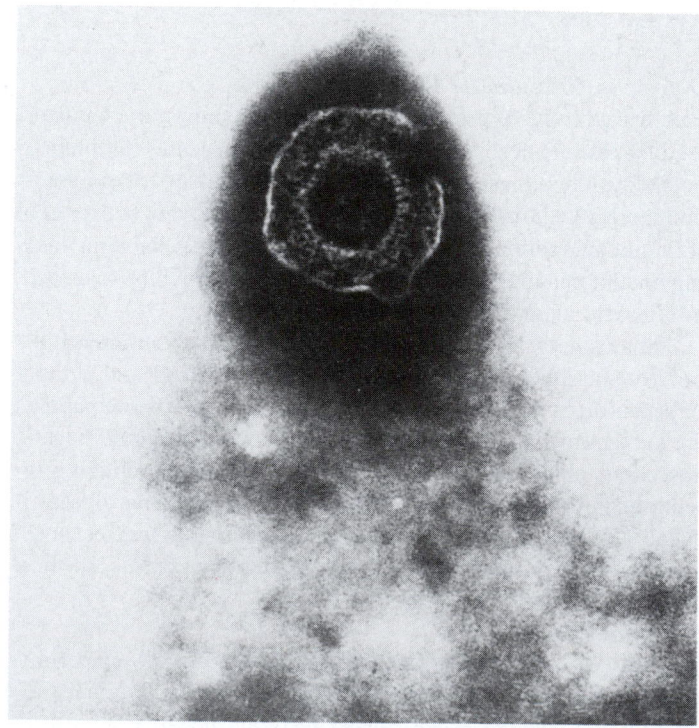

FIGURE 121-9   Electron micrograph of cytomegalovirus. (*Courtesy of Dr. S. Stagno and the Research Resources Information Center, National Institutes of Health.*)

plant recipients has reduced the incidence and severity of CMV disease in the population at risk.

During the same vulnerable period (1 to 6 months after transplantation), *Aspergillus* and *Nocardia* infections of the lung occur, usually complicating a preceding bacterial pneumonitis or CMV infection. Reactivation of latent pulmonary infection with *Coccidioides immitis*, *Blastomyces dermatitidis*, and *Histoplasma capsulatum* may also occur during this period of cumulative immunosuppressive effects. In this circumstance, a careful epidemiologic history is of paramount importance.

P. carinii pneumonia occurs during the same 1- to 6-month period of immunosuppression as that in which other opportunistic pulmonary infections usually become manifest. There appears to be a particularly close association between CMV and *Pneumocystis* infections. Fine pulmonary crackles, characteristic of an interstitial process, are common in *Pneumocystis* pneumonia. In one study of renal transplant recipients, *P. carinii* was identified as the cause of only 4 percent of pneumonias.[55] Many renal transplant programs now utilize prophylactic trimethoprim-sulfamethoxazole to prevent pyelonephritis in the renal graft and also to prevent *Pneumocystis* infection in patients with symptomatic CMV infection. This practice may further decrease the incidence of *Pneumocystis* infection in the renal transplant population.

Pulmonary infections with *Cryptococcus neoformans* tend to occur later in the posttransplant period (after 4 to 6 months). They may take the form of pneumonitis or miliary disease that may present simultaneously with cryptococcal meningitis.

Pneumonia in Patients with Acquired Immunodeficiency Syndrome

The relative frequencies of the various causes of pulmonary infiltrates in patients with AIDS show prominent differences from those observed in organ transplant recipients and patients with neoplastic disease (Table 121-8) (see Chapter 135). *P. carinii* is the preeminent cause of pneumonia in this setting. Pyogenic bacteria are less common causes of pneumonia in patients with AIDS than in transplant recipients and in patients with hematologic and other malignancies. Bacterial infections are increasing as a cause of pulmonary infections in patients with AIDS.[41,42] The use of trimethoprim-sulfamethoxazole as chemoprophylaxis for *P. carinii* infection may have lowered the incidence of pyogenic pneumonia, since this antimicrobial has been active against some strains of *H. influenzae* and *S. pneumoniae*, the principal causes of community-acquired pneumonia in patients with HIV infection. Less frequent bacterial causes of pneumonia in HIV-infected patients are *S. aureus*, *K. pneumoniae*, and *Rhodococcus equi*. Pulmonary infections with *Nocardia* and *Aspergillus* are remarkably infrequent among pulmonary infections in patients with AIDS until quite late in the course of disease (Table 121-8). About 30 percent of patients with AIDS have two or more coexisting pulmonary infections.

Noninfectious processes must also be considered as possible causes of pulmonary infiltrates in febrile patients with AIDS.[42] Unexplained interstitial pneumonias occur.

Lymphocytic interstitial pneumonias of unknown origin appear to be common in children with AIDS but rare in adults. Antecedent infection and replication of Epstein-Barr virus (EBV) was implicated as the cause of lymphocytic interstitial pneumonia (LIP).[41,42] Lung biopsy specimens from children with LIP contained EBV DNA, but biopsy specimens from children with other infections and adults with AIDS did not.[4] A possible direct role of HIV in LIP has been suggested by the detection by in situ hybridization of HIV RNA in the lung of one infant and the demonstration of both HIV antigen and specific IgG antibody in BAL fluid from two adults.[14,52]

About 8 percent of patients with AIDS and pulmonary processes have Kaposi's sarcoma (KS) in the lung.[41] Among patients with known KS presenting with pulmonary problems, pulmonary KS is found to be the cause of the respiratory symptoms in 21 to 40 percent.[68] In addition to the statistical evidence that shows a predominant role for *P. carinii*, certain clinical clues about the nature of the pulmonary process can be provided by epidemiologic considerations and physical findings. For example, tuberculosis is endemic in Haiti. Among Haitians with AIDS, tuberculosis is an important possible cause of a pulmonary infiltrate (see Chapter 163). The presence of extensive chorioretinitis (with the "melted cheese and catsup" appearance of the fundus) suggests widespread CMV infection that often also invades the lung. The presence of intraoral and pharyngeal lesions of KS raises the question of pulmonary impairment by the same process.

RADIOGRAPHIC FEATURES OF PNEUMONIA

The radiographic features of a pneumonia do not provide a specific etiologic diagnosis; this can come only from microbiologic information. However, the radiographic pattern, combined with clinical and epidemiologic information, can narrow the diagnostic considerations while microbiologic data are being obtained (see Chapter 32). This information will also aid in the selection of initial antimicrobial therapy. Several radiographic patterns can be helpful in categorizing infectious and noninfectious causes: (1) airspace or alveolar pneumonia, (2) broncho- or lobular pneumonia, (3) interstitial pneumonia, and (4) nodular infiltrates. Although the chest radiographs of a particular patient may not fit

TABLE 121-8

Cause of 778 Pulmonary Infections in Patients with AIDS

Infectious Agent	Percent
P. carinii	57
M. avium-intracellulare	14
Cytomegalovirus	13
M. tuberculosis	6
Pyogenic bacteria	3
Legionella species	3
Cryptococcus	2
Other fungi (*Candida, Histoplasma, Aspergillus*)	1
Herpes simplex	0.4
Nocardia	0.1
Toxoplasma	0.1
Miscellaneous other infectious agents	0.4
	100.0

SOURCE: Data from Murray et al.[41,42]

neatly into one or another of these categories, identification of a predominant pattern can be helpful in directing attention to certain causes.

Alveolar Pneumonia

This form of consolidation occurs when certain organisms, notably *S. pneumoniae*, induce inflammatory edema in peripheral alveoli. When the extent of the consolidation involves an entire lobe, this is the classic *lobar pneumonia*. But more often the process is not that extensive, although the pathogenesis is the same. An air bronchogram is characteristic. Loss of volume is absent or minimal during the acute stage of consolidation, but some atelectasis may develop owing to obstruction of bronchi by exudate during resolution of the process.

K. pneumoniae is another bacterial cause of community-acquired pneumonia, which, like pneumococcal pneumonia, shows homogeneous parenchymal consolidation containing air bronchograms. Although *K. pneumoniae* pneumonia classically affects the right upper lobe and produces a dense, homogeneous lobar consolidation with bulging of the fissure (Fig. 121-10A), these features are not pathognomonic and cannot be relied on for diagnosis without supportive bacteriologic data. The propensity for *K. pneumoniae* to produce tissue destruction and abscess formation (Fig. 121-10B) may, in fact, result in a shrunken, rather than an expanded, lobe. Pneumococcal pneumonia may also cause bulging of the fissure, albeit less commonly and less prominently. Extensive alveolar consolidation may occur with a variety of other bacterial causes of pneumonia, including mixed anaerobes of aspiration pneumonia and a variety of gram-negative bacilli implicated in nosocomial pneumonias (Fig. 121-11).

Occasionally, an unusual configuration of airspace consolidation, *spherical pneumonia*, occurs, particularly in children,

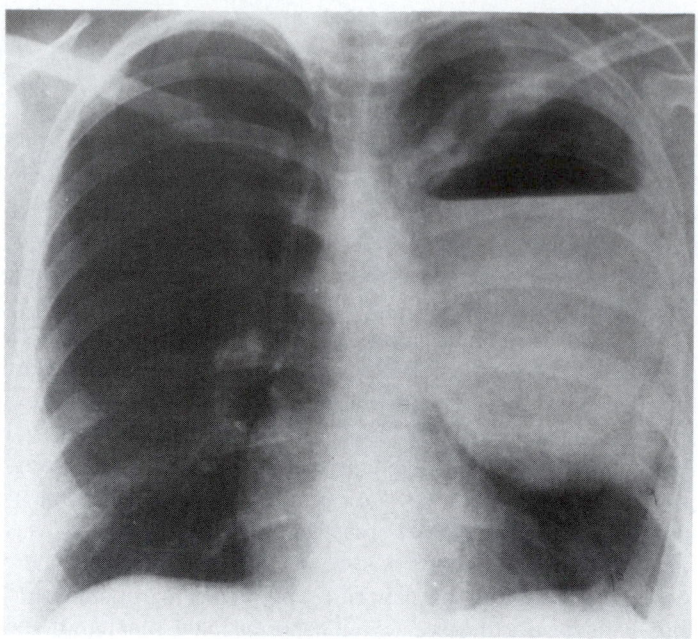

FIGURE 121-11   Left upper lobe pneumonia in a 17-year-old girl due to *S. aureus* that has progressed to formation of a huge lung abscess. Note air-fluid level. *(Courtesy of Dr. R. Greene.)*

with pneumococcal or *H. influenzae* pneumonia. It has also been reported with Q fever.

In the compromised host, alveolar consolidation on the chest radiograph suggests a variety of causes. Among the infectious causes, bacterial agents are a major consideration. If the consolidation is lobar or multilobar, *L. pneumophila* is an important possibility to consider. Other likely infectious agents are fungi (e.g., *Aspergillus*), *Nocardia*, and *M. tuberculosis*. Less often, viruses (e.g., CMV) elicit a predominantly alveolar pattern. Bi-

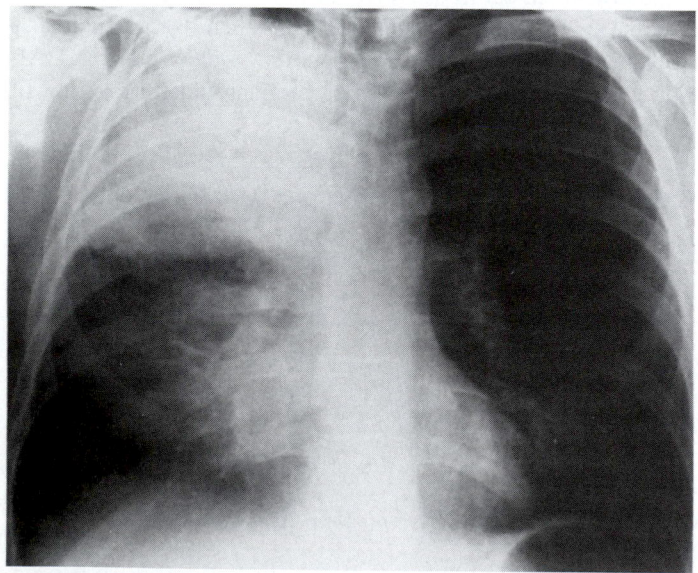

A

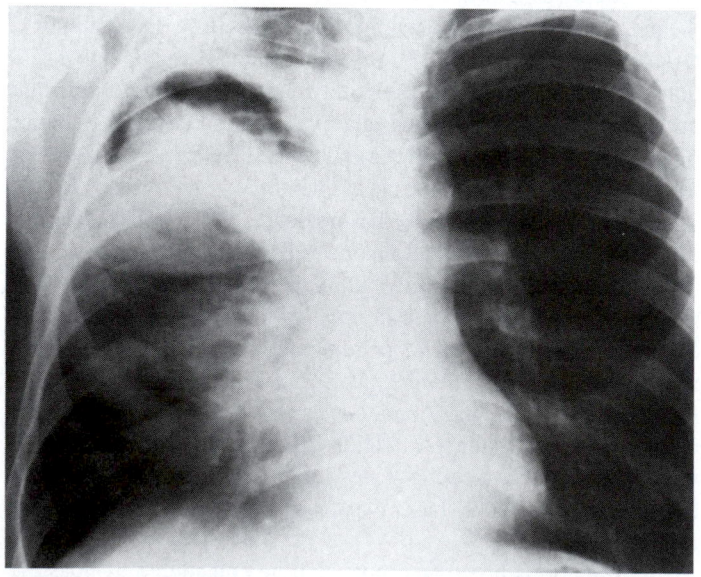

B

FIGURE 121-10   *A.* Dense lobar consolidation involving right upper lobe in an alcoholic patient with *Klebsiella pneumoniae* pneumonia. The minor fissure is bulging downward. There is also involvement of the right middle lobe. *(Courtesy of Dr. R. Greene.) B.* Same patient 7 days later. Despite antibiotic therapy, *K pneumoniae* pneumonia progressed to become a necrotic process with formation of multiple abscesses. *(Courtesy of Dr. R. Greene.)*

lateral diffuse involvement with an airspace pattern resembling pulmonary edema is not uncommonly a feature of *P. carinii* pneumonia.

Bronchopneumonia

In bronchopneumonia, the focus of infection and the inflammatory response is in the bronchi and surrounding parenchyma. Consolidation is segmental in distribution, and involvement is patchy; segmental involvement may become confluent to produce a more homogeneous pattern. Bronchopneumonic patterns are commonly observed in pulmonary infections due to *S. aureus* or nonencapsulated *H. influenzae*. With *S. aureus* infections, macro- and microabscess formation may occur rapidly. Also, pneumatoceles occur during the first week of lung impairment in about half the children with *S. aureus* pneumonia. These cystic spaces are believed to be the consequence of a check valve opening between a peribronchial abscess and an adjacent bronchus.

A bronchopneumonic pattern of consolidation is commonly observed when pneumonia is engrafted on underlying bronchiectasis or chronic bronchitis. In such predisposing circumstances, *S. pneumoniae* infection may produce a bronchopneumonic pattern rather than its usual lobar consolidation. In the presence of underlying emphysema, the radiographic pattern of pneumococcal pneumonia may also be altered from its usual homogeneous pattern to one that contains multiple radiolucencies (representing unconsolidated emphysematous areas) that may be misinterpreted for abscesses.

Segmental bronchopneumonia is the radiographic picture in pneumonia due to *C. pneumoniae* (strain TWAR) or *M. pneumoniae* and in many viral pneumonias (Fig. 121-12). Any of the bacterial species that cause nosocomial pneumonia can produce a radiographic pattern of bronchopneumonic consolidation.

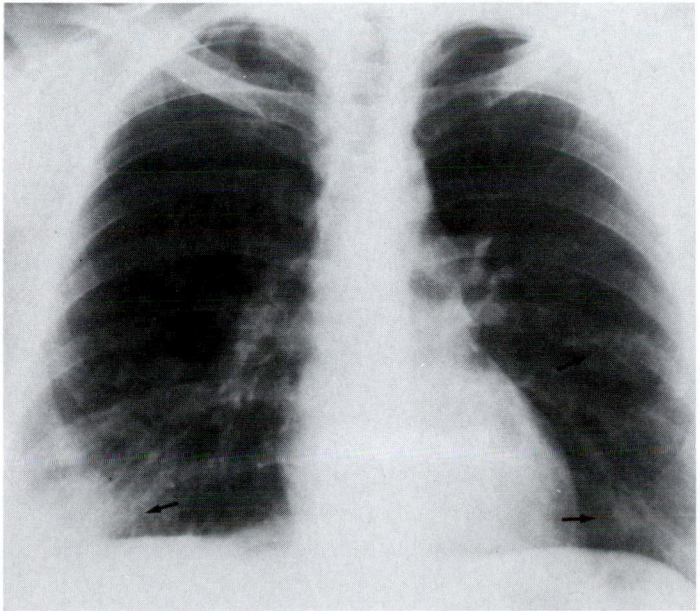

FIGURE 121-12   Multifocal (arrows) pneumonia in a patchy bronchopneumonic pattern in a 36-year-old female homemaker. Clinical course and laboratory findings were consistent with a viral origin, but viral isolation was not attempted.

Interstitial Pneumonia (Peribronchovascular Infiltrate)

A reticular or reticulonodular pattern of infiltration is the radiographic representation of interstitial inflammation—i.e., a peribronchovascular infiltrate. In otherwise healthy persons, *M. pneumoniae* is high on the list of community-acquired causes of a radiographic pattern of interstitial pneumonia. In some instances, interstitial infiltration progresses to produce patchy consolidation of airspaces, most often in the lower lobes. Pneumonias due to respiratory viruses sometimes have an interstitial pattern that progresses to patchy segmental consolidation or to diffuse airspace disease that resembles pulmonary edema. A variety of noninfectious causes of interstitial lung disease (e.g., hypersensitivity lung disease, collagen vascular disease, and sarcoidosis) may also produce a reticular pattern on the chest radiograph.

In immunocompromised patients, particularly in those with AIDS, the infectious causes of interstitial pneumonia are broadened to include early *P. carinii* pneumonia and additional opportunistic viral agents (CMV, varicella-zoster, herpes simplex, and probably EBV and possibly HIV). Noninfectious causes of a reticular pattern on chest radiography in an immunocompromised host include drug-induced (bleomycin, methotrexate, etc.) pneumonitis, early radiation pneumonitis, and pulmonary edema.

Nodular Infiltrates

Nodular infiltrates are considered here as well-defined large (greater than 1 cm^2 on the chest radiograph) round focal lesions. Such a lesion may represent an aspirational lung abscess (without telltale air-fluid level), a fungal or tuberculous granuloma, or a lesion of pulmonary nocardiosis. Multiple nodular infiltrates may also represent the necrotic lesions that develop in the lung secondary to the septic vasculitis produced by *P. aeruginosa* bacteremia or the consequences of fungemic spread of candidal infection from an infected intravascular catheter. Infected nodular pulmonary lesions are sometimes caused by septic pulmonary infarcts produced by infected emboli that originate from right-sided bacterial endocarditis, septic thrombophlebitis of pelvic veins, or septic jugular vein phlebitis. On rare occasions, similar nodular lesions are produced by necrotic (but not infected) pulmonary infarctions; primary or metastatic neoplastic lesions may have a similar appearance. Nodular lesions that undergo rapid necrosis with cavity formation can be a feature of Wegener's granulomatosis.

In the immunocompromised patient, nodular infiltrates may be due to bacteremic or fungemic spread of infection, most often as a nosocomial infection caused by an infected intravenous catheter. In this type of patient, nodular lesions should bring to mind the possibilities of pulmonary nocardial infection, aspergillosis, or other fungal infections. Tuberculous granulomas in the lungs may develop or enlarge in the immunosuppressed patient. Metastatic neoplasm or lymphoma sometimes presents a similar radiologic picture.

MILIARY PULMONARY DISEASE

Disseminated miliary lesions of infectious nature suggest miliary tuberculosis, histoplasmosis, or blastomycosis in either the normal or immunosuppressed host (Fig. 121-13). In the immunosuppressed patient, a miliary pattern may also be seen in disseminated cryptococcal infection.

SMALL NODULAR INFILTRATES

Multiple small nodules, larger than miliary lesions but smaller than the gross nodular lesions described above, raise the possibility, in the immunocompromised host, of varicella-zoster or CMV infection of the lung.

CT Scanning

CT scanning of the chest may be helpful in certain situations in patients with pulmonary infections: in determining whether a pneumonia is necrotizing, whether consolidation is secondary to bronchial obstruction (as by hilar lymphadenopathy or by endobronchial tumor), whether a pleural effusion or empyema accounts for part of the pulmonary density observed on chest radiograms, whether bronchiectasis is present, whether a circumscribed pulmonary density represents a fungus ball within a cavitary lesion, etc. When small granulomatous lesions are present, CT scanning can provide information on the extent of the process. When a single nodule is present, CT scanning can assist in determining whether needle aspiration is feasible and, if so, to direct the biopsy needle.

NONINVASIVE DIAGNOSTIC STUDIES

Noninvasive studies can provide information indicating the specific microbial cause of a pulmonary infection or can narrow the field of likely etiologic agents.

Direct Examination of the Sputum

CYTOLOGIC EXAMINATION

Examination of Gram-stained sputum smears can be of major value in pinpointing a bacterial cause of pneumonia and guiding initial therapy. The most valuable bacteriologic information from sputum examination is that in which the results from stained smears and cultures are mutually confirmatory. The quality of a sample of expectorated or induced sputum submitted for examination is the prime determinant of the results that can be expected. Culture of sputum that consists principally of saliva is valueless. What are sought are lower-respiratory secretions produced by a cough, not nasopharyngeal secretions. Cytologic examination provides an evaluation of the quality of the sample and its suitability for culture and interpretation of a Gram-stained smear made from it. Scanning of Gram-stained smears or application of specific quantitative criteria is helpful in selecting meaningful specimens for bacteriologic evaluation on smear and in culture. Squamous epithelial cells (normally exfoliated from the oropharynx), when present in numbers of 10 or more per low-power ($\times100$) magnification field (Fig. 121-14), indicate that the specimen is unsatisfactory; culture of such a specimen correlates poorly with results from culture of a transtracheal aspirate. The presence of numerous polymorphonuclear neutrophils on Gram-stained smear (10 to 25 or more per low-power microscopic field) in the absence of an excessive number of squamous cells (see above) is indicative of a good specimen for bacteriologic evaluation.

EXAMINATION OF GRAM-STAINED SMEARS FOR BACTERIA

The oil immersion fields examined, and the immediately adjacent fields, should not contain any squamous cells; each should

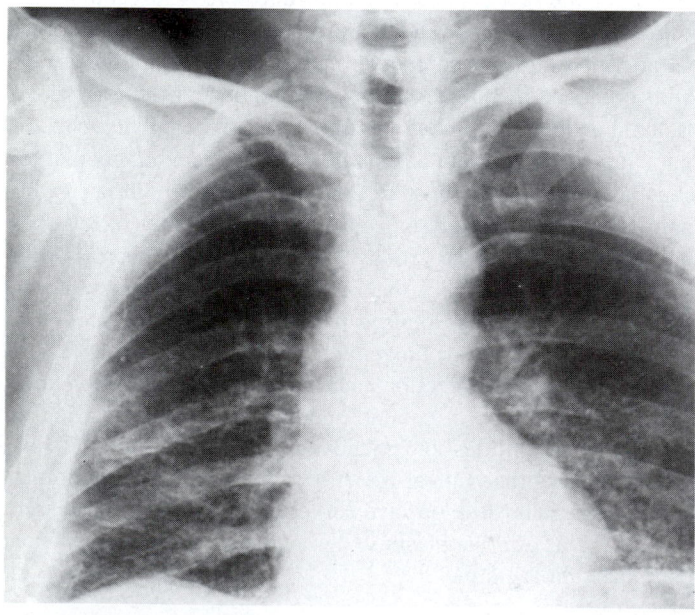

A

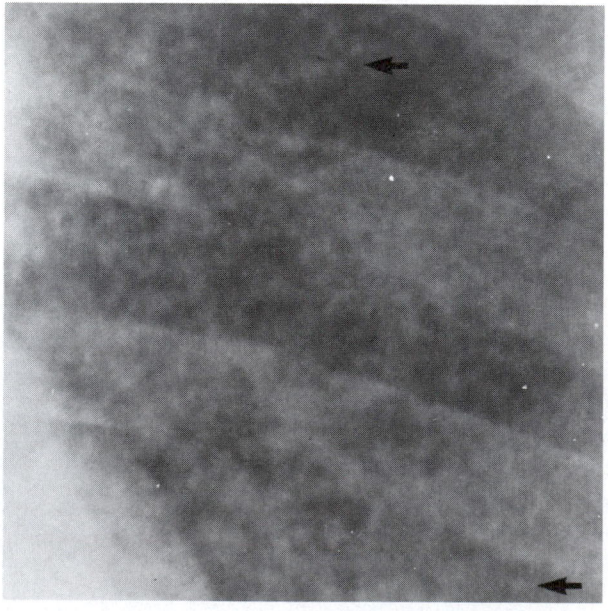

B

FIGURE 121-13 Miliary tuberculosis in a 45-year-old immigrant from Portugal with old calcified tuberculous empyema on the right. *A.* Fine nodularity present in both lungs. *B.* Arrows point to individual miliary lesions, which are more readily visible with added magnification. (*Courtesy of Dr. R. Greene.*)

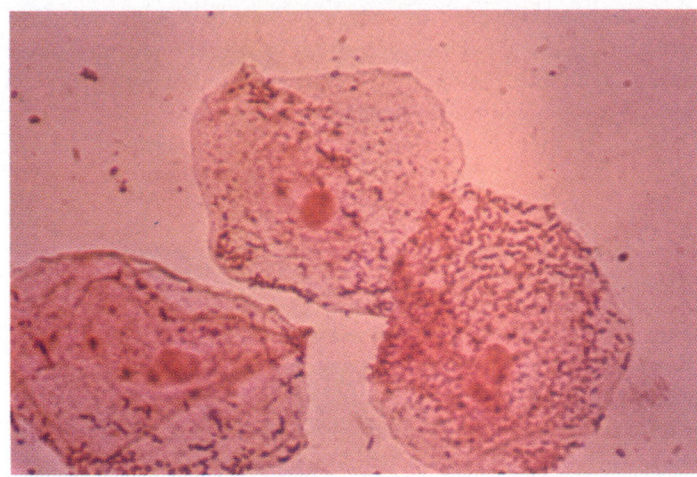

FIGURE 121-14   Three large oropharyngeal epithelial cells from a specimen of "sputum" that is inadequate for Gram's stain analysis and culture because of its origin in the upper respiratory tract. Note the large number of organisms agglutinated on the surface of the squamous epithelial cells. ×400.

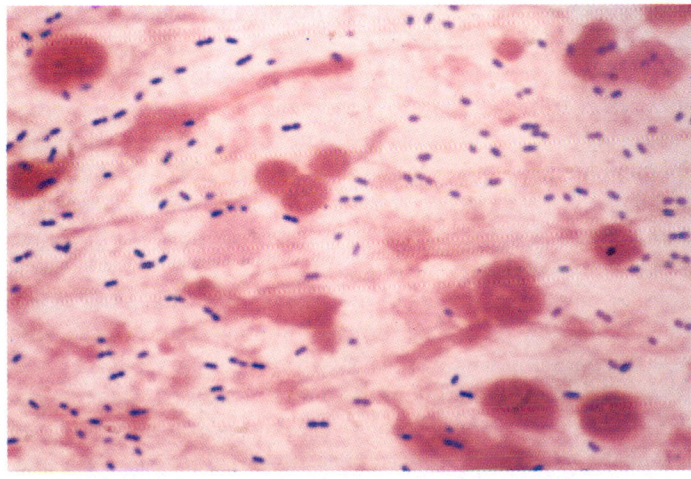

A

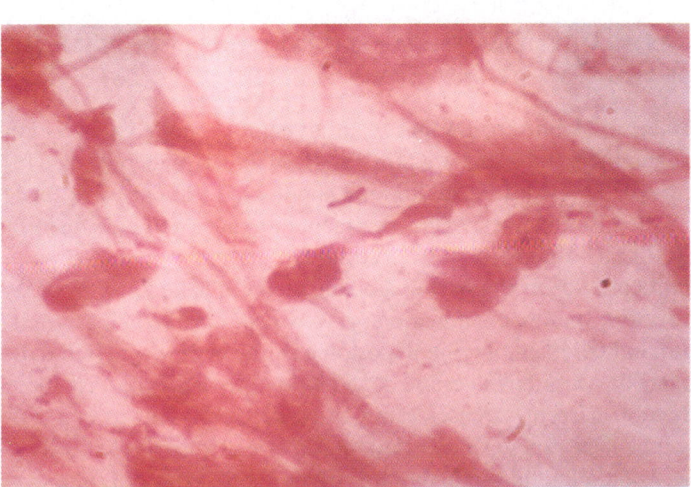

C

also contain at least three or four neutrophils. The presence of squamous cells not only indicates that the specimen is derived from the upper respiratory tract but also may be confusing to the uninitiated because of the large number of bacteria, often gram-positive diplococci, which might be mistaken for *S. pneumoniae*, adherent to the surface of these cells.

A variety of bacterial respiratory tract pathogens have rather characteristic morphologies and strongly suggest an etiologic role when present in considerable numbers in a suitable specimen of sputum (or in a transtracheal aspirate) that contains the proper numbers of inflammatory cells. Such organisms include *S. pneumoniae* (gram-positive oval or lancet-shaped diplococci), *H. influenzae* (small, pleomorphic gram-negative bacilli), *M. catarrhalis* (gram-negative, biscuit-shaped diplococci), or the similar-appearing *Neisseria meningitis*, enteric gram-negative bacilli (not distinguishable from one another with respect to species except for large encapsulated rods that are suggestive of *Klebsiella*), and *S. aureus* (large gram-positive cocci in small groups or clusters) (Fig. 121-15). Since normal oral flora include a variety of streptococcal species that are morphologically somewhat similar to *S. pneumoniae*, sputum smears may be misinterpreted. Thus, a definite predominance of gram-positive diplococci in multiple appropriate oil immersion fields needs to be observed to implicate *S. pneumoniae*. A quantitative aspect to the evaluation has been suggested: at least 10 gram-positive lancet-shaped diplococci per oil immersion field foretells the isolation of *S. pneumoniae* from sputum cultures. With use of the aforementioned criteria (numbers of PMNs, absence of epithelial cells, and numbers of gram-positive lancet-shaped diplococci), the

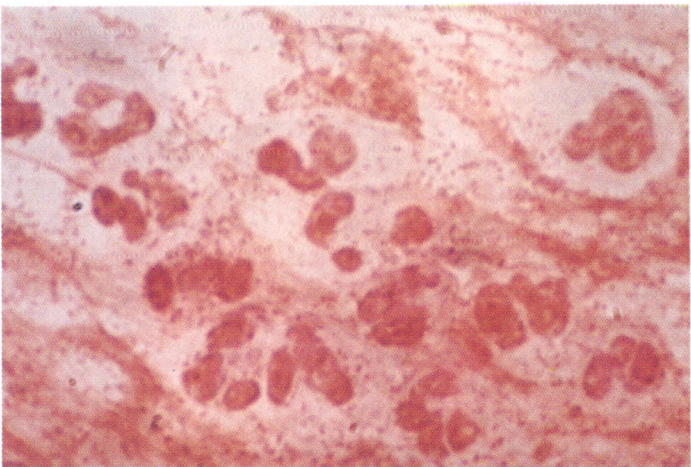

B

FIGURE 121-15   *A.* Gram-stained smear of sputum from patient with pneumococcal lobar pneumonia. ×1000. In this field there are numerous gram-positive lancet-shaped diplococci and polymorphonuclear leukocytes. *B.* Gram-stained smear of sputum from patient with bronchopneumonia superimposed on chronic bronchitis. This field (×1000) is teeming with gram-negative coccobacilli. Many polymorphonuclear leukocytes are present. *H. influenzae* was isolated from sputum as predominant organism. *C.* Gram-stained smear of sputum from patient with lobar pneumonia due to *K. pneumoniae*. In this field (×1000) there are moderate numbers of polymorphonuclear leukocytes and large, thick gram-negative bacilli. *(A to C Courtesy of H. Provine.)*

specificity of Gram's stain for identifying *S. pneumoniae* is 85 percent, with a sensitivity of 62 percent.[51]

Gram-stained smears can be helpful not only in the etiologic diagnosis of community-acquired bacterial pneumonia due to the usual respiratory pathogens but also in supporting a diagnosis of atypical pneumonia when sputum examinations repeatedly show neither neutrophils nor bacteria. Uncommon bacterial species may be implicated in a pulmonary infection on the basis of unusual morphology on Gram-stained smear: irregularly staining, beaded, delicate gram-positive branching filaments suggest either *Nocardia* or *Actinomyces*.

Several organisms, uncommon causes of pulmonary infection, have morphologic characteristics that may mimic other, more common respiratory pathogens. *Pasteurella multocida* and *Acinetobacter* species, both small gram-negative coccobacilli, have each been mistaken in sputum of patients with pulmonary infections for either *H. influenzae* or *M. catarrhalis*, or for a mixture of the two.

Sputum or pleural fluid with foul odor provides evidence of activity of anaerobic organisms in infective processes such as lung abscess, aspiration pneumonia, empyema, and, occasionally, bronchiectasis. In these settings, the findings on Gram-stained smear may corroborate the preliminary diagnosis. Organisms of the *P. melaninogenicus-asaccharolyticus* group are small gram-negative coccobacilli. *Fusobacterium nucleatum* is a long, tapering, pale-staining gram-negative bacillus with irregularly staining gram-positive internal granules. Purulent secretions or pus from such anaerobic infections contains numerous neutrophils and usually a mixture of bacterial species, including anaerobic and microaerophilic streptococci on stained smear.

EXAMINATION OF ZIEHL-NEELSEN OR FLUOROCHROME-STAINED SMEARS FOR MYCOBACTERIA

The number of new cases of tuberculosis in the United States steadily declined over past decades, reaching a nadir in 1995. During the period 1985 to 1991, the rate of development of new cases (often due to multidrug-resistant strains of *M. tuberculosis*) increased, primarily associated with microepidemics among the urban poor, racial and ethnic minorities, drug abusers, hospital and correctional facility populations, and patients with HIV infection (see Chapters 158 to 164). In the past several years, the number of new cases has once again leveled off. Pulmonary tuberculosis in the aforementioned settings may take the form of chronic cavitary tuberculosis or forms more likely to suggest pyogenic or atypical pneumonia—i.e., progressive primary tuberculosis and tuberculous pneumonia. Acid-fast smears of sputum can provide the very first evidence of this disease. Mycobacteria are seen on smears of about 50 percent of specimens that subsequently prove to contain *M. tuberculosis*. Most laboratories currently employ a fluorochrome stain with auramine-rhodamine (mycobacteria fluoresce orange-yellow) for initial examination of sputum or other body fluids. Atypical mycobacteria may be demonstrated on sputum smears of patients, usually older people with slowly progressive pulmonary disease. In patients with AIDS, disseminated *M. avium-intracellulare* infection is usually diagnosed by isolation of the organism from blood culture (lysis centrifugation method) or by histopathologic diagno-

sis on biopsy. However, the organism can be demonstrated on acid-fast smears and culture of respiratory secretions even though there may be little radiographic evidence of pulmonary infection directly attributable to its presence.

Modified Ziehl-Neelsen–stained smears are helpful in detecting Nocardia.

FUNGAL WET MOUNTS (POTASSIUM HYDROXIDE, KOH PREPARATIONS)

Fungal wet mounts, smears stained with Calcofluor white chemifluorescent agent or phase-contrast microscopy, are employed when epidemiologic considerations suggest community-acquired pulmonary mycoses (particularly coccidioidomycosis and blastomycosis). They should be a routine part of evaluation of respiratory secretions and lung biopsy materials from immunocompromised patients in whom additional fungal pathogens (e.g., *Aspergillus* and *Mucor*) may be active.

DIRECT IMMUNOFLUORESCENT MICROSCOPY

Direct fluorescent antibody (DFA) staining can be useful in rapid diagnosis of respiratory tract pathogens. DFA staining reagents for *L. pneumophila* are commercially available. Their use is not recommended in examination of sputum specimens because of the presence of cross-reacting species (*Bacteroides* species, *Pseudomonas* species, *Bordetella pertussis*) in the upper respiratory tract. However, biopsy specimens of lung (needle, bronchoscopic, or surgical), bronchoscopic aspirates, BAL washings, and pleural fluid samples are suitable for DFA staining for *L. pneumophila*. Although a variety of stains (toluidine blue O, methenamine silver, Wright-Giemsa, Diff-Quik, Calcofluor) are useful in identifying *P. carinii* in induced sputa or BAL specimens, or on imprint smears of tissue specimens, the most widely used diagnostic technique utilizes immunofluorescence with monoclonal antibodies against *P. carinii*. Rapid viral diagnosis (RSV, influenza, parainfluenza, adenovirus) by DFA can be applied to specimens from bronchial lavage or brushings or from nasopharyngeal swabs or washings. Anti–*B. pertussis* DFA may be used on nasopharyngeal aspirate smears in the presumptive diagnosis of pertussis.

GIEMSA AND OTHER SPECIAL STAINED SMEARS FOR DIAGNOSIS OF PNEUMOCYSTIS INFECTION

Since *P. carinii* pneumonia is an alveolar process, examination of routinely collected sputum for *P. carinii* is generally not regarded as rewarding in immunosuppressed patients with neoplastic disease or transplant recipients. In these patients, fiberoptic bronchoscopy and transbronchial biopsy, combined with BAL, provide the highest diagnostic yield. In patients with AIDS, however, sputum examination for *P. carinii* may be helpful. Sputum induction employing hypertonic saline is the usual initial diagnostic procedure attempted, and it provides a diagnosis in more than 80 percent of cases (after microscopy of stained cytocentrifuged specimens) at institutions experienced in its use.[60] Toluidine blue O and methenamine silver stains stain only the cyst and not the trophozoite forms of *P. carinii*. Giemsa and Diff-

Quik stain trophozoites and intracystic sporozoites. Immunofluorescent assays, with monoclonal antibodies to *P. carinii*, of induced sputum have a sensitivity of 69 to 92 percent, compared with that of 28 to 80 percent for tinctorial stains.[60] If results of examination of induced sputum are negative and clinical circumstances warrant further attempts at diagnosis, follow-up bronchoscopy with transbronchial biopsy or BAL is performed. The sensitivity of each of these procedures for diagnosis of *P carinii* pneumonia is more than 90 percent.

SPECIAL MICROSCOPIC EXAMINATIONS

Occasionally, in the setting of apparent pulmonary inflammation with features atypical for infection, microscopic examinations using stains other than Gram's stain may be indicated. For example, Wright-stained smears may show the presence of eosinophils in allergic pulmonary aspergillosis or other causes of pulmonary infiltrates that are accompanied by eosinophilia. Cytologic examination of exfoliated sputum using Papanicolaou's stain may reveal a pulmonary neoplasm. Birefringent calcium oxalate crystals (needlelike in rosettes or arranged like sheaves of wheat) in sputum cytologic specimens have been reported as suggesting pulmonary infection with *Aspergillus* (aspergilloma and, occasionally, invasive aspergillosis), a fungus that excretes oxalic acid as a metabolic product.[33]

In the intubated or tracheotomized patient, whose tracheobronchial secretions commonly contain neutrophils and often some bacteria on Gram-stained smears, it may be difficult at times to distinguish between colonization and nosocomial pneumonia. The presence on light microscopy ($\times400$) of characteristic elastin fibers with split ends (in a drop of tracheal aspirate to which a drop of 40 percent KOH has been added), in the appropriate clinical setting, is a strong indicator of a necrotizing pulmonary infection.[57]

Intense bacteremias sometimes accompany pulmonary infections, and the etiologic agent may be demonstrable on stained smears of the buffy coat of centrifuged blood: pneumococci have been identified in Gram-stained or Wright-Giemsa–stained smears of buffy coats from splenectomized patients; occasionally, *M. avium-intracellulare* has been found intracellularly in acid-fast stains of buffy coats from patients with AIDS.

Additional special microscopic examinations may be indicated for immunocompromised patients who have patchy pulmonary infiltrates on the chest radiograph. For example, the presence of the hyperinfection syndrome of strongyloidiasis (often accompanied by *E. coli* bacteremia) can be established by the finding of filariform larvae in the sputum and in the stool after the latter is suitably prepared by concentration techniques. Although eosinophilia is often present in patients with strongyloidiasis, it may be absent in the hyperinfection syndrome.

SPUTUM CULTURES

In most patients with the common types of community-acquired and nosocomial bacterial pneumonia, the etiologic diagnosis can be made on the basis of the combined results of a Gram-stained smear of sputum and of proper culture of a suitable exudative portion of a freshly obtained sputum specimen. The criteria for a proper sample of sputum have been noted above ("Cytologic Examination" of sputum). Culture entails streak dilution on blood agar and McConkey media. Reliance on "routine" sputum specimens of doubtful quality, collected by paramedical personnel and automatically cultured (often after prolonged transit times to the laboratory) without screening for suitability, is responsible for the unwarranted conclusion that sputum cultures are of very limited value in the diagnosis of pneumococcal pneumonia. Before strict attention began to be paid to the quality of sputum specimens, only about half of the patients with bacteremic pneumococcal pneumonia had positive sputum cultures. Subsequently, however, a comparative study of cultures of expectorated sputum, of sputum procured at bronchoscopy, and of sputum obtained by transtracheal aspiration showed that in 16 patients with acute bacterial pneumonia, the pneumonia was due to *S. pneumoniae* in 13 and that in these 13 patients, each of the three types of specimens obtained from each patient yielded almost pure cultures of *S. pneumoniae* (on the third and fourth quadrants of dilution-streaked blood agar plates).[65]

Expectorated sputum should not be cultured anaerobically, since contamination with oral anaerobes is inevitable and the results will be uninterpretable. Because patients with Legionnaires' disease often raise little if any sputum suitable for culture, most attempts to isolate *Legionella* resort to specimens obtained either by transtracheal aspiration, fiberoptic bronchoscopy, or lung biopsy or at thoracentesis. Cultures of such materials are plated on buffered charcoal-yeast extract (BCYE) agar. Occasionally, *Legionella* species can be isolated from sputum with the use of a semiselective medium, either BCYE or BCYE-containing cefamandole, polymyxin B, and anisomycin. Culture is the most definitive method for diagnosis of *Legionella* infection. Unfortunately, it may take 5 or more days for colonies to appear.

Cultures for mycobacteria are undertaken when clinical circumstances raise the possibility of pulmonary infections due to *M. tuberculosis* or atypical mycobacteria. Similarly, cultures of sputum for primary invasive mycotic agents (e.g., *H. capsulatum*, *B. dermatitidis*, and *C. immitis*) are dictated by clinical and epidemiologic circumstances. In immunosuppressed patients, cultures of sputum are also directed toward a variety of opportunistic fungi, including *C. neoformans*, *Aspergillus* species, and Mucoraceae.

Most hospitals do not have facilities for isolating viruses by tissue culture. This lack poses little problem in dealing with most community-acquired viral pneumonias, for which viral isolation is not necessary and the cost is prohibitive. However, viral isolation from throat washings is warranted in certain circumstances (e.g., to prove the presence of an outbreak of influenza), to establish that an outbreak among young children is due to respiratory syncytial virus, and to identify a specific viral agent, such as an adenovirus, as the cause of a serious pneumonia that is not responding to antibacterial therapy. In immunosuppressed patients with pneumonia, a variety of opportunistic viral infections (CMV, respiratory syncytial virus, varicella-zoster virus, herpes simplex) are diagnostic considerations. Cultures are grown in cell lines susceptible to the viral infections under consideration in either standard "tube cultures" or "shell vial" cultures (rapid culture achieved by centrifugation of specimens against the cultured cells). Viral replication in the tissue culture can be confirmed within 48 h after inoculation with use of fluorescent monoclonal antibodies. Because CMV and herpes simplex are frequently present in the oral secretions of immunosuppressed patients, isolation of these viruses is apt to be meaningful only if the materials used for the isolation procedure were obtained either by bronchoscopy with PSB or with BAL, lung biopsy, or transtracheal aspiration.

BLOOD CULTURES

Blood cultures should always be performed in patients with suspected bacterial pneumonia. Bacteremia occurs in approximately 30 percent of patients with pneumococcal pneumonia. Demonstration of bacteremia in other patients with pneumonia may indicate that the pulmonary infection is secondary to bacteremia originating from a focus of infection elsewhere (e.g., acute right-sided *S. aureus* endocarditis or *P. aeruginosa* infection of thermal burns). In patients with AIDS and disseminated *M. avium-intracellulare* infection, blood cultures are almost always positive. The lysis centrifugation technique permits ready and rapid isolation of the mycobacterium and quantifies the intensity of the bacteremia. *L. pneumophila* has been isolated with some frequency from automated radiometric blood culture bottles, but blind subculture onto BCYE agar is necessary because growth in the liquid medium does not achieve detectable levels.[53]

BACTERIAL ANTIGEN DETECTION IN SPUTUM AND URINE

The quellung reaction was extensively used in the preantibiotic era to identify *S. pneumoniae* in sputum. It entails the use of light microscopy to detect capsular swelling after pneumococcal antiserum has been added to a loopful of sputum. The occurrence of the quellung reaction was shown to correlate closely with the presence of *S. pneumoniae* in sputum culture—in about 90 percent of the patients. This procedure is no longer used.

Pneumococcal antigens may be detected in the sputum of patients with pneumococcal pneumonia by ELISA, latex particle agglutination, or counterimmunoelectrophoresis.[46] The first two are more readily available. ELISA is the most sensitive method. Antigen detection in sputum may have as high a sensitivity as 70 to 90 percent; but specificity is a problem, with about 20 percent false positives, probably due in part to the difficulty in distinguishing oropharyngeal contamination and colonization (e.g., in patients with chronic bronchitis without pneumonia). Antigen detection in the urine has been less sensitive, and the sensitivity of antigen detection in the serum has been even lower.

A radioimmunoassay and an enzyme-linked immunoassay for *L. pneumophila* antigenuria are commercially available and provide a means of rapid (under 24 h) diagnosis of *Legionella* pneumonia, particularly in patients without sputum production.[1] The sensitivity of the radioimmunoassay is 89 to 95 percent, and the specificity is very high (estimated at 99 percent). The test is positive despite antibiotic administration, and antigenuria may persist for weeks or months after recovery from pneumonia. It must be remembered that the assay is available only for *L. pneumophila* serogroup 1, and this serogroup is responsible for only 80 percent of *L. pneumophila* infections.

RAPID VIRAL DIAGNOSIS BY ANTIGEN DETECTION

The need for methods that can rapidly identify viruses stems from the recent introduction of effective chemotherapy for several viral agents that cause pulmonary infections and from the long time (3 to 10 days) required for viral isolation and identification by standard tube culture. As noted earlier ("Direct Immunofluorescent Microscopy"), DFA can be used to detect viral antigens (adenovirus, influenza, parainfluenza, and RSV, as well as CMV and HSV) in specimens of bronchial brushings, BAL, or nasopharyngeal washings. Enzyme immunoassay can also be used to detect viral antigens in respiratory secretions. The presence of CMV antigenemia can be detected with the use of peroxidase-labeled antibody staining of peripheral blood buffy coat. The demonstration (culture, antigen) of CMV in BAL fluids may be interpreted variously in different clinical settings. Strict criteria for CMV pneumonia include demonstration of the virus, typical cytologic changes, and absence of other evident pathogens. This would be applicable in patients with AIDS, in whom CMV is frequently isolated but in whom CMV rarely causes pneumonia. In contrast, isolation of CMV from BAL fluid in bone marrow transplant recipients with pneumonia is sufficient evidence to make the diagnosis and institute treatment, in view of the high frequency and mortality of CMV pneumonia in these patients.

Serologic Tests

Serologic tests are sometimes of considerable help in establishing the causes of a number of pulmonary infections when the causative agents are difficult to isolate. However, this approach, requiring the demonstration of a 4-fold or greater rise in titer between acute and convalescent samples, neither enables rapid diagnosis nor provides assistance in initial selection of antimicrobial therapy. Microimmunofluorescence serologic tests are of value in the diagnosis of psittacosis (*C. psittaci*). A 4-fold rise in IgG or the presence of IgM antibody indicates recent infection. The indirect immunofluorescent antibody test (4-fold titer rise to 1:128 or higher indicates recent infection) may provide a retrospective diagnosis of Legionnaires' disease, but the antibody rise occasionally may not be demonstrable for 4 to 6 weeks after the clinical onset. Antibodies may persist for months or up to a year or more. Thus, a single titer of 1:256 or higher may reflect a prior *Legionella* infection. Cold agglutinins develop in about half the patients with *M. pneumoniae* pneumonia, but such antibodies occur in other conditions; complement fixation testing is the preferred diagnostic procedure. The most sensitive and specific serologic test for infection with *C. pneumoniae* is the microimmunofluorescence test. A 4-fold rise in IgG titer or an IgM titer of 1:16 or more reflects an acute infection. The complement fixation test is usually used to confirm a diagnosis of Q-fever pneumonia, but microimmunofluorescence, microagglutination, and enzyme-linked immunosorbent assays have been used to diagnose acute *C. burnetii* pulmonary infection. Tularemic pneumonia can be diagnosed serologically with an agglutination test for *F. tularensis*.

Serologic tests are also helpful in the diagnosis of invasive infection due to the primary pulmonary mycotic pathogens. Serum

IgM precipitins (latex agglutination, immunodiffusion) appear with primary coccidioidomycosis. Abnormally high complement fixation titers (at least 1:32) are present in most patients who have disseminated infection due to *C. immitis*. A 4-fold increase in complement fixation titer to yeast and to mycelial phases of *H. capsulatum* (or possibly a single titer of 1:64 or higher) and the presence of H and M precipitin bands strongly suggest histoplasmosis. Complement fixation tests for blastomycosis lack sensitivity and specificity: titers of at least 1:8 suggest recent or active disease, particularly if precipitins to the A antigen are also present. Cryptococcal antigenemia is detectable from latex particle agglutination in patients with cryptococcal pneumonia or disseminated cryptococcal infection. Sporotrichosis can be diagnosed with a serologic agglutination test when the titer is 1:80 or greater.

Serologic tests (paired acute and convalescent sera) may be helpful for the retrospective diagnosis of infections due to influenza A and B, respiratory syncytial virus, adenoviruses, and parainfluenza viruses.

Molecular Diagnostic Testing

A variety of nucleic acid target amplification tests known as polymerase chain reactions (PCR) are available, or being developed as research tools, for the direct detection of pulmonary pathogens. PCR tests approved by the FDA can detect *M. tuberculosis* (as distinct from nontuberculosis mycobacteria) directly from sputum and BAL specimens. These tests have shown a sensitivity of 90 to 100 percent in specimens that are AFB smear positive but a sensitivity of only 65 to 85 percent for specimens that are smear negative. Consequently, these PCR assays have been approved for use only on acid-fast bacillus (AFB) smear–positive specimens. In some major medical centers, PCR assays for detection of *C. pneumoniae* and *M. pneumoniae* on nasopharyngeal or throat swab specimens are available to markedly shorten (by 1 to 2 days) the time required to isolate these organisms by culture (up to 3 weeks).

Other PCR tests that appear to increase detection of respiratory pathogens (*P. carinii*, *L. pneumophila*) are still at the stage of research tools. Although PCR tests for herpes simplex virus, cytomegalovirus, and adenovirus are available or in development, their detection by PCR of respiratory tract specimens might be difficult to interpret, since they might represent only upper-respiratory pathogens or reactivation of a prior infection and be unrelated to the process causing pneumonia.[60]

Skin Tests of Delayed Hypersensitivity

The tuberculin skin test is of great importance in the evaluation of a pulmonary infection of unknown origin (see Chapter 161). The intermediate (5 tuberculin unit) purified protein derivative (IPPD) test should be used if no information is available about previous testing. A positive test does not distinguish between prior and current infection, but in persons who are either less than 35 years old or members of high-risk groups (immigrant, HIV positive), a positive reaction carries considerable diagnostic weight.

A negative second-strength PPD skin test in a patient who is not anergic is strong evidence against a tuberculous origin of a pulmonary process. However, several caveats are noteworthy: since it may take 4 to 6 weeks for the skin test to become positive, the tuberculin skin test may be initially negative in progressive primary pulmonary tuberculosis, and in the patient who was infected long ago, cutaneous hypersensitivity may wane; in the elderly person, in whom waning has occurred, repeat testing several weeks later may show a positive result (booster effect) even if the original IPPD skin test was negative.

Fungal skin tests do not distinguish between current and past infection; indeed, active disease is often accompanied by a negative skin test. The coccidioidin skin test is the best of the available tests, but the diagnosis of coccidioidomycosis is not excluded by a negative test. Blastomycin and histoplasmin skin tests are of little value because of frequent false-negative results and cross reactions. Also, the performance of the histoplasmin skin test may falsely elevate antibody levels to the *H. capsulatum* mycelial antigen.

A negative skin test response to a specific antigen must be interpreted in the light of possible anergy related to underlying conditions such as malnutrition, immunosuppressive and corticosteroid therapy, and AIDS. A battery of control antigens (mumps, *Candida*, *Trichophyton*, streptokinase-streptodornase) serves to detect such anergy.

Gallium Scan

Increased gallium 67 uptake by the lungs can be found in patients with *P. carinii* pneumonia and essentially normal chest radiographs. With the greater awareness of the early changes of *P. carinii* pneumonia on the radiographs of patients with AIDS, this radionuclide study is of less value. It can only indicate a pulmonary inflammatory process and cannot pinpoint a specific cause.

INITIAL ANTIMICROBIAL THERAPY

Initial therapy of community-acquired pneumonia is based on the clues provided by clinical, epidemiologic, and radiologic information and by evaluation of Gram- and AFB-stained smears of sputum (see Chapter 122). In the case of a presumed bacterial pneumonia of which an etiologic agent is identified on the sputum smear, initial treatment is tailored to this organism. When initial clinical and laboratory evidence suggests *S. pneumoniae* as the cause, penicillin or amoxicillin is the preferred treatment. In view of the current frequency of penicillin resistance among pneumococci (about 25 percent in some areas of the United States), uncomplicated pneumonia due to such strains requires treatment with high doses of parenteral penicillin or a third-generation cephalosporin such as cefotaxime.

Modification of initial therapy is made on the basis of the results of sputum and blood cultures, urinary *L. pneumophila* antigen tests, or, if available, PCR for *M. pneumoniae*, *C. pneumoniae*, and *M. tuberculosis*. But if the causative agent cannot be identified in the sputum smear, initial therapy is directed at the likely agents. A variety of approaches for empiric therapy have been proposed when initial diagnostic tests have failed to provide guidance.[7,43] Pneumonia in young adults considered manageable as outpatients might reasonably be treated with an oral macrolide (erythromycin, clarithromycin, or azithromycin) active against *M. pneumoniae, C. pneumoniae,* and *L. pneumophila.* Oral amoxicillin or a second-generation cephalosporin is an alternative. If epidemiologic factors suggest Q fever or psittacosis, a tetracycline is indicated in initial therapy. Pneumonia in persons 60 years of age and older and in those with coexisting conditions (e.g., chronic obstructive lung disease, congestive heart failure, chronic alcoholism, asplenia) who can be treated as outpatients might be treated with an oral second-generation cephalosporin, active against *H. influenzae* and susceptible strains of *S. pneumoniae,* or amoxicillin. Alternatives for patients with penicillin allergy would include an oral macrolide and doxycycline.

For patients with severe community-acquired pneumonia requiring hospitalization, treatment should include a parenteral second-generation (cefuroxime) or third-generation (cefotaxime or ceftriaxone) cephalosporin, with erythromycin added if the clinical picture suggests the possibility of *L. pneumophila* pneumonia. In the special setting of an influenza viral outbreak, the possibility of a severe pneumonia being due to *S. aureus* superinfection should be considered, and therapy might include use of nafcillin or oxacillin. However, sputum production is frequently a feature of *S. aureus* pneumonia, and the organisms can usually be identified on Gram's stain of the sputum. In the alcoholic patient with a dense lobar consolidation and large gram-negative bacilli on stained smear of the sputum, *K. pneumoniae* is a likely cause, and treatment should include a second- or third-generation cephalosporin plus an aminoglycoside.

Initial treatment of community-acquired aspiration pneumonia or lung abscess would be directed at the normal aerobic and anaerobic bacterial flora of the upper-respiratory tract that are etiologic. Clindamycin or a combination of penicillin (or ampicillin) with metronidazole is the pharmacotherapy of choice for initial treatment.

For hospital-acquired pneumonia (HAP), the American Thoracic Society has proposed that consideration of time of onset, severity, and presence of specific risk factors can be used to suggest pathogens likely to be implicated and provide some initial guidance in selection of antimicrobial therapy while one is awaiting culture results (see Chapter 143).[3] In patients with mild to moderate HAP with onset anytime after hospitalization and without unusual risk factors, a core group of organisms (*H. influenzae, S. pneumoniae,* methicillin-susceptible *S. aureus,* and nonpseudomonal enteric gram-negative bacilli) are likely to be responsible. Monotherapy in this setting uses a second-generation cephalosporin (e.g, cefuroxime), a third-generation cephalosporin, or a β-lactam–β-lactamase inhibitor combination (e.g., ticarcillin-clavulanate, ampicillin-sulbactam). If the pathogen is likely to be an *Enterobacter* species, and a third-generation cephalosporin is used, addition of another agent (e.g., gentamicin or tobramycin) is indicated because of possible β-lactamase induction.

In patients with mild to moderate HAP associated with specific risk factors, additional antibiotics should be included along with those already indicated for the core group of pathogens. Thus, for example, if aspiration were a consideration, clindamycin might be added; if high-dose corticosteroids had been employed (and *Legionella* infection became a possibility), ery-

thromycin might be added; if the patient were granulocytopenic, antipseudomonal therapy should be included (see below). In patients with severe HAP of early onset and with specific risk factors, and in patients with severe HAP and onset late in hospitalization, other organisms (*P. aeruginosa, Acinetobacter* species) in addition to core pathogens should be considered possible causes. Such circumstances require initial combination therapy with an antipseudomonal penicillin or cephalosporin (or imipenem) or an antipseudomonal β-lactam–β-lactamase inhibitor combination plus an aminoglycoside (or fluoroquinolone). In some patients, methicillin-resistant *S. aureus* (MRSA) is also a consideration, and vancomycin may be added to the aforementioned combination therapies. Cognizance should always be taken of local epidemiologic data (e.g., in a given intensive care unit, clusters of cases of pneumonia that are due to organisms that are less common and more difficult to treat), such as *Acinetobacter* species or *B. cepacia,* and their antimicrobial susceptibility patterns.

In the febrile granulocytopenic patient who has been treated for 10 days or so with a cephalosporin and aminoglycoside for presumed sepsis of unknown origin, the development of a wedge-shaped pulmonary infiltrate might raise the question of a fungal infection (e.g., *Aspergillus*) that warrants the intravenous administration of amphotericin B.

Extrapulmonary findings sometimes suggest the cause of a pulmonary process and, thereby, direct initial therapy. Thus, acyclovir given intravenously would be indicated in the immunocompetent or immunosuppressed adult who has varicella-zoster and a diffuse pulmonary infiltrate that consists of small nodules.

The patient with AIDS whose chest radiograph shows a bilateral interstitial or airspace process that is compatible with *P. carinii* pneumonia is likely, on statistical grounds, to have *P. carinii* pneumonia. Initial therapy using trimethoprim-sulfamethoxazole is appropriate for the mildly ill patient; invasive diagnostic procedures are undertaken if a favorable response does not materialize in several days. In the patient whose illness is severe when first seen, whose course has progressed rapidly, whose radiographic picture is complex, and whose pulmonary infiltrates may represent several causes, not only is initial therapy begun with trimethoprim-sulfamethoxazole but also an invasive procedure is performed simultaneously in order to obtain a tissue diagnosis.

INVASIVE DIAGNOSTIC PROCEDURES

In certain circumstances, a more aggressive approach is required to uncover the cause of a pneumonia or other pulmonary infection. This approach entails either the forgoing of the initial empiric trial of antibiotics or the foreshortening of the duration of such a trial and resort to invasive diagnostic procedures. Such an approach may be required at the outset for the patient who has a severe, rapidly progressive community-acquired pneumonia or for a life-threatening community-acquired pneumonia that has caused the patient's condition to deteriorate despite empiric antimicrobial therapy. In the immunocompromised patient, early invasive diagnostic approaches are mandated by the large number of etiologic agents that may be responsible, the frequent involvement of many infectious or noninfectious agents in the pulmonary process, the multiplicity of antimicrobial choices available against different organisms (e.g., bacteria, viruses, fungi, protozoa, and *Chlamydia*), and the rapidity with which clinical deterioration may preclude further diagnostic and therapeutic actions. Among such invasive diagnostic procedures are bronchoscopy, BAL, open lung biopsy, and transthoracic needle aspiration.

Flexible Fiberoptic Bronchoscopy with Lung Biopsy

When the seriousness of the pulmonary process and lack of definable cause with noninvasive measures (e.g., sputum induction) indicate the necessity for biopsy in order to obtain histopathologic and cultural identification of the cause of the pulmonary lesions, a choice has to be made among one of several invasive procedures. The choice depends on the experience and skill with the different procedures at a given hospital. Also important in determining the proper procedure are location and radiographic appearance of the pulmonary lesions.

Fiberoptic bronchoscopy using specialized devices to shield against oropharyngeal contamination (PSB) is used at some institutions to obtain tracheobronchial secretions for culture in certain acute bacterial pneumonias. A peripheral nodule or cavity (more than 1 cm in diameter) that is readily visualized on conventional (posteroanterior and lateral) radiographs and fluoroscopy, and is in an accessible location, may be aspirated and biopsied by needle percutaneously. A nodule that is inaccessible to needle aspiration, or a process placed peripherally, where the need for histopathology is not apt to be met by needle aspiration and biopsy, is best approached by open lung biopsy.

Fiberoptic bronchoscopy in conjunction with transbronchial lung biopsy provides an etiologic diagnosis in about 50 percent of immunosuppressed patients who do not have AIDS and in 60 to 90 percent of patients who do have AIDS, in whom *P. carinii*, CMV, and *M. avium-intracellulare* infections are common.

Contraindications to transbronchial biopsy include inability of the patient to cooperate, marked hypoxemia, bleeding disorders (particularly those associated with hypoprothrombinemia, thrombocytopenia refractory to platelet transfusion, and uremia), and pulmonary hypertension.

Tissue specimens are processed for histopathologic examination (hematoxylin and eosin stain, tissue acid-fast stains, Gomori's methenamine-silver stain, periodic acid–Schiff stain, tissue Gram's stain, and Dieterle silver stain). Impression smears from tissues are made with sterile slides, which, after appropriate fixation, are stained with Giemsa, Gram, Ziehl-Neelsen, and methenamine silver (for *P. carinii*) stains, as previously described. As indicated, DFA staining for *Legionella* and monoclonal antibody staining for *P. carinii* are performed on separate impression smears. Appropriate cultures are made with tissue obtained either transbronchially or at open lung biopsy.

BRONCHOALVEOLAR LAVAGE

In patients with AIDS, fiberoptic bronchoscopy coupled with subsegmental BAL has proved particularly useful, providing a diagnosis in more than 95 percent of cases of *Pneumocystis* pneu-

monia (see Chapter 150). BAL alone, without transbronchial biopsy, is often substituted in patients who are thrombocytopenic, on mechanical ventilation, or severely hypoxemic. The material obtained by BAL is processed for smear and culture. As indicated earlier, a variety of stains are available for demonstrating the presence of *Pneumocystis* in the cytocentrifuged material.

Stained cytocentrifuged BAL specimens can also be helpful in establishing other diagnoses: Papanicolaou's stain is useful in detecting neoplastic cells and in identifying viral cytopathic effects in epithelial cells.

In at least two-thirds of immunosuppressed patients with CMV pneumonia, the diagnosis can be made from the finding of inclusion bodies in cytocentrifuged BAL specimens and with immunofluorescent monoclonal antibody staining. CMV is isolated more often on culture in these patients, but culture alone is not sufficient to establish the diagnosis, since viral isolation may represent only viral shedding in the presence of pulmonary disease due to other causes.

INVASIVE DIAGNOSTIC TESTING IN VENTILATOR-ASSOCIATED PNEUMONIA

PSB with quantitative culture and protected-catheter BAL, also with quantitative culture, have been employed to obtain bacteriologic information while minimizing opportunity for contamination from colonization of the upper airway in patients with ventilator-associated pneumonia (VAP).[8,12] The role of quantitative diagnostic techniques in the evaluation of patients with HAP and VAP remains controversial because of questions of accuracy of the results and what the threshold concentration of bacteria should be.[65] In one study, tracheal aspirate cultures correlated with PSB cultures in patients with VAP, suggesting no added value to use of such an invasive procedure to direct initial therapy.[56] At present, such invasive diagnostic testing is not considered a standard for routine management of patients with suspected VAP.[44]

Percutaneous Transthoracic Needle Lung Biopsy

Percutaneous needle biopsy is often the invasive diagnostic procedure of choice for a sizable (greater than 1.0 cm) pulmonary nodule or cavity that is located peripherally. The use of smaller-gauge needles has reduced the frequency of pneumothorax as a complication. Diagnostic yields of 60 to 80 percent have been obtained in immunocompromised patients with pneumonia. This procedure has also provided the diagnosis in 70 percent of patients in whom the underlying lesion was granulomatous. The small core of tissue and aspirated fluid is examined by stained smear and culture for various infectious agents (see "Flexible Fiberoptic Bronchoscopy with Lung Biopsy"). Cytologic examination should be done for neoplastic cells. Because of the nature of the specimen, however, histopathologic examination is generally fruitless.

Open Lung Biopsy

Open lung biopsy provides the most definitive procedure for histopathologic diagnosis in the immunocompromised host. It provides sufficient lung tissue for diagnosis and also makes it possible to sample several different sites. It is particularly suitable for evaluating processes that may not be infectious (e.g., neoplasm such as Kaposi's sarcoma, antineoplastic drug toxicity, drug hypersensitivity, and lymphocytic interstitial pneumonia). Open lung biopsy has provided a specific diagnosis in 60 to 90 percent of immunocompromised patients in whom it has been employed. Its major advantages include the ability to control bleeding, air leaks, and the airway. Its disadvantages relate to the thoracotomy: the need for general anesthesia, the inherent delay in preparing the patient for the surgical procedure, the need for intubation, the usual placement of a chest tube, and postoperative splinting due to incisional pain. The mortality from the procedure is about 1 percent. Bleeding is a complication in about 1 percent of patients and delayed pneumothorax in about 9 percent. Fiberoptic bronchoscopy combined with transbronchial biopsy and segmental BAL is the usual initial invasive diagnostic procedure in the immunocompromised patient with an undefined diffuse pulmonary process. If this fails to provide a diagnosis, open lung biopsy is indicated. For the patient in whom the pace of the illness does not allow this sequential approach, open lung biopsy may have to be the first choice. It is also preferred in the patient who is unable to cooperate with fiberoptic bronchoscopy or in whom thrombocytopenia or hypoxemia presents additional problems for transbronchial biopsy.

Processing of lung biopsy specimens should include special stained imprint smears for *P. carinii*, bacteria (including *Nocardia* and mycobacteria), fungi, and viral inclusion bodies; cultures for bacteria, viruses, fungi, and mycobacteria; and tissue sections stained for histology and for various infectious agents (see "Flexible Fiberoptic Bronchoscopy with Lung Biopsy").

REFERENCES

1. Aguero-Rosenfeld ME, Edelstein PH: Retrospective evaluation of the Du Pont radioimmunoassay kit for detection of *Legionella pneumophila* serogroup 1 antigenuria in humans. *J Clin Microbiol* 26: 1775–1778, 1988.

2. Allen JN, Pacht ER, Gadek JE, Davis WB: Acute eosinophilic pneumonia as a reversible cause of noninfectious respiratory failure. *New Engl J Med* 321:569–574, 1989.

3. American Thoracic Society Consensus Statement: Hospital-acquired pneumonia in adults: Diagnosis, assessment of severity, initial antimicrobrial therapy, and preventive strategies. *Am J Respir Crit Care Med* 153:1711–1725, 1995.

4. Andiman WA, Martin K, Rubinstein A, et al: Opportunistic lymphoproliferation associated with Epstein-Barr viral DNA in infants and children with AIDS. *Lancet* 2:1390–1393, 1985.

5. Bartlett JG, Finegold SM: Anaerobic infections of the lung and pleural space. *Am Rev Respir Dis* 110:56–77, 1974.

6. Bartlett JG, Gorbach SL, Finegold SM: The bacteriology of aspiration pneumonia. *Am J Med* 56:202–207, 1974.

7. Bartlett JG, Mundy LM: Community-acquired pneumonia. *New Engl J Med* 333:1618–1624, 1995.

8. Baselski VS, Wunderink RG: Bronchoscopic diagnosis of pneumonia. *Clin Microbiol Rev* 7:533–558, 1994.

9. Bates JH, Campbell GD, Barron AL, et al: Microbial etiology of acute pneumonia in hospitalized patients. *Chest* 101:1005–1012, 1992.

10. Biehl JP: Miliary tuberculosis: A review of sixty-eight adult patients admitted to a municipal general hospital. *Am Rev Tuberc* 77:605–622, 1958.

11. Butler JC, Peters CJ: Hantaviruses and hantavirus pulmonary syndrome. *Clin Infect Dis* 19:387–395, 1994.

12. Cantral DE, Tape TG, Reed EC, et al: *Am J Med* 95:601–607, 1993.

13. Carrington CB, Addington WW, Goff AM, et al: Chronic eosinophilic pneumonia. *New Engl J Med* 280:787–798, 1969.

14. Chayt KJ, Harper ME, Marselle LM, et al: Detection of HTLV-III RNA in lungs of patients with AIDS and pulmonary involvement. *JAMA* 256:2356–2359, 1986.

15. Cohen AJ, King TE Jr, Downey GP: Rapidly progressive bronchiolitis obliterans with organizing pneumonia. *Am J Respir Crit Care Med* 149:1670–1675, 1994.

16. Cooper JAD, White DA, Matthay RA: Drug-induced pulmonary disease. Part 1: Cytotoxic drugs. *Am Rev Respir Dis* 133:321–340, 1986.

17. Cooper JAD, White DA, Matthay RA: Drug induced pulmonary disease. Part 2: Noncytotoxic drugs. *Am Rev Respir Dis* 133:488–505, 1986.

18. Craven DE, Steger KA: Epidemiology of nosocomial pneumonia: New perspectives on an old disease. *Chest* 108(Suppl):S1–S16, 1995.

19. Curnutte JT, Boxer LA: Clinically significant phagocytic cell defects, in Remington JS, Swartz MN (eds), *Current Clinical Topics in Infectious Diseases*, vol 6. New York, McGraw-Hill, 1985, pp 103–155.

20. Duchin JS, Koster FT, Peters CJ, et al: Hantavirus pulmonary syndrome: A clinical description of 17 patients with a newly recognized disease. *New Engl J Med* 330:949–955, 1994.

21. Dupont HT, Raoult D, Brouqui P, et al: Epidemiologic features and clinical presentation of acute Q fever in hospitalized patients: 323 French cases. *Am J Med* 93:427–434, 1992.

22. Epler GR, Colby TV, McCloud TC, et al: Bronchiolitis obliterans organizing pneumonia. *New Engl J Med* 312:152–158, 1985.

23. Fang G-D, Fine M, Orloff J, et al: New and emerging etiologies for community-acquired pneumonia with implications for therapy. *Medicine* 69:307–316, 1990.

24. Fang FC, Madinger NE: Resistant nosocomial gram-negative bacillary pathogens: *Acinetobacter baumannii, Xanthomonas maltophilia,* and *Pseudomonas cepacia,* in Remington JS, Swartz MN (eds), *Current Clinical Topics in Infectious Diseases*, vol. 16. Cambridge, MA, Blackwell Science, 1996.

25. Fine MJ, Smith MA, Carson CA, et al: Prognosis and outcomes of patients with community-acquired pneumonia: A meta-analysis. *JAMA* 275:134–141, 1996

26. Finegold SM: Aspiration pneumonia. *Rev Infect Dis* 13(Suppl):S737–S742, 1991.

27. Fraser DW, Tsai T, Orenstein W, et al: Legionnaires' disease: Description of a epidemic of pneumonia. *New Engl J Med* 297:1189–1197, 1977.

28. Garb JL, Brown RB, Garb JR, Tuthill RW: Differences in etiology of pneumonias in nursing home and community patients. *JAMA* 240:2169–2172, 1978.

29. Graman PS, Hall CB: Nosocomial viral respiratory infections. *Semin Respir Infect* 4:253–260, 1991.

30. Grayston JT: Infections caused by *Chlamydia pneumoniae* strain TWAR. *Clin Infect Dis* 15:757–763, 1992.

31. Grayston JT, Kuo CC, Wang SP, Altman J: A new *Chlamydia psittaci* strain, TWAR, isolated in acute respiratory tract infections. *New Engl J Med* 315:161–168, 1986.

32. Hayakawa H, Sato A, Toyoshima M, et al: A clinical study of idiopathic eosinophilic pneumonia. *Chest* 105:1462–1466, 1994.

33. Lee SH, Barnes WG, Schaetzel WP: Pulmonary aspergillosis and the importance of oxalate crystal recognition in cytology specimens. *Arch Pathol Lab Med* 110:1176–1179, 1986.

34. Lougheed MD, Roos JO, Waddell WR, Munt PW: Desquamative interstitial pneumonitis and diffuse alveolar damage in textile workers. Potential role of mycotoxins. *Chest* 108:1196–1200, 1995.

35. Marrie TJ: *Mycoplasma pneumoniae* pneumonia requiring hospitalization, with emphasis on infection in the elderly. *Arch Intern Med* 153:488–494, 1993.

36. Marrie TJ: Pneumonia and carcinoma of the lung. *J Infect* 29:45–52, 1994.

37. Marrie TJ, Durant H, Yates L: Community-acquired pneumonia requiring hospitalization: 5-year prospective study. *Rev Infect Dis* 11:586–599, 1989.

38. Moya C, Antó JM, Taylor AJN, and the Collaborative Group for the Study of Toxicity in Textile Aerographic Factories: Outbreak of organizing pneumonia in textile printing sprayers. *Lancet* 343:498–502, 1994.

39. Mundy LM, Auwaerter PG, Oldach D, et al: Community-acquired pneumonia: Impact of immune status. *Am J Respir Crit Care Med* 152:1309–1315, 1995.

40. Munt PW: Miliary tuberculosis in the chemotherapy era: With a clinical review in 69 American adults. *Medicine* 51:139–155, 1972.

41. Murray JF, Felton CP, Garay SM, et al: Pulmonary complications of the acquired immune deficiency syndrome: Report of a National Heart, Lung, and Blood Institute Workshop. *New Engl J Med* 310:1682–1688, 1984.

42. Murray JF, Mills J: Pulmonary infectious complications of human immunodeficiency virus infection. *Am Rev Respir Dis* 141:1356–1372, 1582–1598, 1990.

43. Niederman MS, Bass JB Jr, Campbell GD, et al: Guidelines for the initial management of adults with community-acquired pneumonia: Diagnosis, assessment of severity, and initial antimicrobial therapy. *Am Rev Respir Dis* 148:1418–1426, 1993.

44. Niederman MS, Torres A, Summer W: Invasive diagnostic testing is not needed routinely to manage suspected ventilator-associated pneumonia. *Am J Respir Crit Care Med* 150:565–569, 1994.

45. Nguyen MH, Stout JE, Yu VL: Legionellosis. *Infect Dis Clin North Am* 5:561–584, 1991.

46. Örtquist A, Jonsson I, Kalin M, et al: Comparison of three methods for detection of pneumococcal antigen in sputum of patients with community-acquired pneumonia. *Eur J Clin Microbiol Infect Dis* 8:956–961, 1989.

47. Ostergaard L, Andersen PL: Etiology of community-acquired pneumonia. Evaluation by transtracheal aspiration, blood culture, or serology. *Chest* 104:1400–1407, 1993.

48. Penner C, Maycher B, Long R: Pulmonary gangrene: A complication of bacterial pneumonia. *Chest* 105:567–573, 1994.

49. Peterson PK, Stein S, Guay DRP, et al: Prospective study of lower respiratory tract infections in an extended-care nursing home program: Potential role of oral ciprofloxacin. *Am J Med* 85:164–171, 1988.

50. Ramsey PG, Rubin RR, Tolkoff-Rubin NE, et al: The renal transplant patient with fever and pulmonary infiltrates: Etiology, clinical manifestations and management. *Medicine* 59:206–222, 1980.

51. Rein MF, Gwaltney JM, O'Brien WM, et al: Accuracy of the Gram's stain in identifying pneumococci in sputum. *JAMA* 239:2671–2673, 1978.

52. Resnick L, Pitchenik AE, Fisher E, Croney R: Detection of HTLV-III/LAV-specific IgG and antigen in bronchoalveolar lavage fluid from two patients with lymphocytic interstitial pneumonitis associated with AIDS-related complex. *Am J Med* 82:553–556,1987.

53. Rihs JD, Yu VL, Zuravleff JJ, et al: Isolation of *Legionella pneumophila* from blood using the BACTEC: A prospective study yielding positive results. *J Clin Microbiol* 22:422–424, 1985.

54. Rossman MD, Dauber JH: Sarcoidosis: Assessment of inflammatory activity, in Fishman AP (ed), *Update: Pulmonary Diseases and Disorders*. New York, McGraw-Hill, 1982, pp 193–204.

55. Rubin RH, Greene R: Clinical approach to the compromised host with fever and pulmonary infiltrates, in Rubin RH, Young LS (eds), *Clinical Approach to Infection in the Compromised Host*, 3d ed. New York, Plenum, 1994, pp 121–161.

56. Rumbak MJ, Bass RL: Tracheal aspirate correlates with protected specimen brush in long-term ventilated patients who have clinical pneumonia. *Chest* 106:531–534, 1994.

57. Salata RA, Lederman MM, Shlaes DM, et al: Diagnosis of nosocomial pneumonia in intubated, intensive care unit patients. *Am Rev Respir Dis* 135:426–432, 1987.

58. Schaberg DR, Culver DH, Gaynes RP: Major trends in the microbial etiology of nosocomial infection. *Am J Med* 91 (Suppl):72S–75S, 1991.

59. Severo LC, Geyer GR, Porto PN: Pulmonary aspergillus intracavitary colonization (PAIC). *Mycopathologia* 112:93–104, 1990.

60. Shelhamer JH, Gill VJ, Quinn TC, et al: The laboratory evaluation of opportunistic pulmonary infections—An NIH conference. *Ann Intern Med* 124:585–599, 1996.

61. Sinave CP, Hardy GJ, Fardy PW: The Lemierre syndrome: Suppurative thrombophlebitis of the internal jugular vein secondary to oropharyngeal infection. *Medicine* (*Baltimore*) 68:85–94, 1989.

62. Sitbon O, Bidel N, Dussopt C, et al: Minocycline pneumonitis and eosinophilia. *Arch Intern Med* 154:1633–1640, 1994.

63. Spickard A III, Hirschmann JV: Exogenous lipoid pneumonia. *Arch Intern Med* 154:686–692, 1994.

64. Talavera WS, Mildvan D: Pulmonary infections in the acquired immunodeficiency syndrome. *Semin Respir Infect* 1:202–211, 1986.

65. Thorsteinsson SB, Musher DM, Fagan T: The diagnostic value of sputum culture in acute pneumonia. *JAMA* 233:894–895, 1975.

66. Trucksis M, Swartz MN: Bronchiectasis: A current view, in Remington JS, Swartz MN (eds), *Current Clinical Topics in Infectious Diseases*. Boston, Blackwell Scientific, 1991, pp 170–205.

67. Veghese A, Berk SL: Bacterial pneumonia in the elderly. *Medicine* 62:271–285, 1983.

68. White DA, Matthay RA: Noninfectious pulmonary complications of infection with the human immunodeficiency virus. *Am Rev Respir Dis* 140:1763–1787, 1989.

69. Wilson JP, Turner HR, Kirchner KA, et al: Nocardial infections in renal transplant recipients. *Medicine* 68:38–57, 1989.

CHAPTER 122

PRINCIPLES OF ANTIBIOTIC USE AND THE SELECTION OF EMPIRIC THERAPY FOR PNEUMONIA

Michael S. Niederman

Antibiotics are the foundation of therapy for respiratory infections, but the approach to their use varies with the type of pneumonia present (community acquired or nosocomial), as well as with the age of the affected patient, the presence of various comorbid illnesses, and the severity of the acute illness. Appropriate antimicrobial therapy that is initiated in a timely fashion has a number of proven benefits. For most patients, initial therapy is aimed at a broad spectrum of potential pathogens and is empiric because the infecting pathogen is not known. Therapy can be more specifically focused on the basis of results of diagnostic tests. In some cases, initial empiric therapy must be continued because no etiologic pathogen is identified, with appropriateness defined by the patient's clinical response to treatment.

Antibiotic therapy can improve survival in patients with community-acquired pneumonia (CAP) or hospital-acquired pneumonia (HAP), and the benefits are most evident in patients who are not otherwise terminally ill (see also Chapters 127 and 143).[6] In the setting of CAP, effective initial antibiotic therapy is associated with a marked improvement in survival, compared to ineffective initial therapy, particularly in patients with severe illness.[24] Data on patients with severe CAP provide the most convincing argument for the use of empiric therapy. In several stud-

ies, identification of the pathogens causing severe CAP did not lead to an improved survival rate, while the use of a broad-spectrum, empiric regimen directed at likely pathogens reduced mortality.[38,57] In patients with HAP, survival is improved with the use of antibiotics to which isolated pathogens are susceptible, compared to empiric, nonspecific therapy.

Even with the use of the correct agents, not all patients recover.[36] The fact that some HAP patients die in spite of microbiologically appropriate therapy is a reflection of the degree of antibiotic efficacy, as well as a reflection of the fact that not all deaths are the direct result of infection. In some HAP patients, death is the result of underlying serious illness; the percentage of deaths that occur because of infection, termed the "attributable mortality" of HAP, has been estimated to be about 50 percent.[15] Thus, since up to half of all the deaths of HAP patients occur regardless of the presence of infection, it is not surprising that reported survival rates for severe HAP are never near 100 percent, but typically are 70 to 80 percent, even with the use of an optimal therapeutic regimen.

In recent years, a number of paradigms for empiric therapy for both CAP and HAP have been developed, but several caveats should be remembered. First, a guideline must be viewed as nothing more than a hypothesis that must be validated, based on outcome data, to show its utility in a given clinical setting.[17] Second, guidelines must be reevaluated relative to local patterns of antibiotic susceptibility. In the case of CAP, the emergence of penicillin-resistant pneumococcus may affect the selection of initial therapy, particularly if resistance is prevalent in a community.[39] In the setting of HAP, each hospital has its own unique flora and antibiotic susceptibility patterns (see Chapter 143); a knowledge of such patterns is essential. Finally, guidelines for empiric therapy have often been developed on the basis of in vitro susceptibility patterns, because carefully controlled trials comparing specific agents have often not been conducted.

In this chapter, the principles underlying antibiotic use will be examined, followed by a discussion of the rationale for using empiric therapy to treat patients with both CAP and HAP. Then the principles underlying empiric therapy selection, along with suggested regimens, are presented.

PRINCIPLES OF ANTIBIOTIC USE

Mechanisms of Action

Antibiotics interfere with the growth of bacteria by undermining the integrity of their cell wall or by interfering with bacterial protein synthesis or common metabolic pathways. The terms *bactericidal* and *bacteriostatic* are broad categorizations, and may not apply for a given agent against all organisms, with certain antimicrobials being bactericidal for one bacterial pathogen but bacteriostatic for another. Bactericidal antibiotics kill bacteria, generally by inhibiting cell wall synthesis or by interrupting a key metabolic function of the organism. Bacteriostatic agents inhibit bacterial growth, do not interfere with cell wall synthesis, and rely on host defenses to eliminate bacteria. The use of specific agents is dictated by the susceptibility of the causative organism(s) in a given location to individual antibiotics. However, when neutropenia is present, or if there is accompanying endocarditis, meningitis, or osteomyelitis, the use of a bactericidal agent is preferred.

Antimicrobial activity is often described by the terms MIC and MBC. The term MIC defines the minimum concentration of an antibiotic that inhibits the growth of 90 percent of a standard sized innoculum, leading to no visible growth in a broth culture. The term MBC refers to the minimum concentration needed to cause a 3-logarithmic decrease (99.9 percent killing) in the size of the standard inoculum. These terms must be interpreted cautiously. For example, in the treatment of pneumonia, the clinician must consider MIC and MBC data in light of the penetration of an agent into lung tissues. The MIC is used to define the *sensitivity* of a pathogen to a specific antibiotic, under the assumption that the concentration required for killing can be reached in serum in vivo, although lung concentrations can be substantially lower than serum concentrations.

Penetration into the Lung

The concentration of an antibiotic in the lung depends on the permeability of the capillary bed at the site of infection (the bronchial circulation), the degree of protein binding of the drug, and the presence or absence of an active transport site for the antibiotic in the lung. In the lung, the relevant site to consider for antibiotic penetration is controversial and not clearly defined. Sputum and bronchial concentrations may be most relevant for bronchial infections, while concentrations in lung parenchyma, epithelial lining fluid, and cells such as macrophages and neutrophils are probably more important for parenchymal infections. The localization of the pathogen may also be

important, and intracellular organisms such as *Legionella pneumophila* and *Chlamydia pneumoniae* may be best eradicated by agents that achieve high concentrations in macrophages. Local concentrations of an antibiotic must be considered in light of the activity of the agent at the site of infection. For example, antibiotics can be inactivated by certain local conditions. Aminoglycosides have reduced activity at acidic pH's, which may be present in infected lung tissues.[3] Bacterial resistance to antimicrobial agents (e.g., β-lactamase enzymes), "permeation mutants" (requiring that higher concentrations than are possible to achieve be present in order to be killed) that become impermeable to antibiotic entry or modify an antibiotic binding site, will diminish efficacy.[19]

The concentration of an antibiotic in lung parenchyma depends on its penetration through the bronchial circulation capillaries.[21,27,56] The bronchial circulation has a fenestrated endothelium, so antibiotics penetrate in proportion to their molecular size and protein binding, with small molecules that are not highly protein bound passing readily into the lung parenchyma. When inflammation is present, penetration is further improved. For an antibiotic to reach the epithelial lining fluid, it must pass through the pulmonary vascular bed, which has a nonfenestrated endothelium. This presents an advantage for lipophilic agents, which are generally not inflammation dependent. Agents that are lipophilic and thus inflammation independent for their entry into the epithelial lining fluid include chloramphenicol, the macrolides, clindamycin, the tetracyclines, the quinolones, and trimethoprim-sulfamethoxazole. Agents that are poorly lipid soluble are inflammation dependent for their entry into the epithelial lining fluid and include the penicillins, cephalosporins, aminoglycosides, carbapenems, and monobactams.[21,27]

Active transport can facilitate antibiotic entry into lung tissue and phagocytes. Agents that are concentrated in phagocytes in this manner include the macrolides, clindamycin, and the fluoroquinolones. Antibiotics, such as the β-lactams, that are not concentrated in phagocytes by active transport remain in the extracellular space, which constitutes 40 percent of the weight of bronchial tissue; thus, penicillins achieve only about 40 percent

---

TABLE 122-1

Penetration of Antibiotics into Respiratory Secretions

Good Penetration: Lipid Soluble, Concentration Not Inflammation Dependent

Quinolones
New macrolides: azithromycin, clarithromycin
Tetracyclines
Clindamycin
Trimethoprim/sulfamethoxizole

Poor Penetration: Relatively Lipid Insoluble, Inflammation Dependent for Concentration in the Lung

Aminoglycosides
β-lactams
  Penicillins
  Cephalosporins
  Monobactams
  Carbapenems

of their serum level in lung tissue. Considering all of these factors, some general categories can be established (Table 122-1). Drugs that penetrate well into the sputum or bronchial tissue include the quinolones, the newer macrolides (azithromycin and clarithromycin), the tetracyclines, clindamycin, and trimethoprim-sulfamethoxazole. On the other hand, the aminoglycosides, and to some extent the β-lactams, penetrate less well into these sites.

Antibiotic Pharmacodynamics

The way in which an antibiotic reaches the site of infection, considering the frequency of administration and dose administered, can affect its ability to kill bacteria. Some agents are bactericidal in relation to how long they stay above the MIC of the target organism (time-dependent killing), while others are effective in relation to the peak concentration achieved (concentration-dependent killing).[11,45] If antibiotic killing is time dependent, dosing schedules should be chosen to achieve the maximal time above the MIC of the target organism. Antibiotics of this type include the β-lactams and vancomycin. The rate of killing is saturated once the antibiotic concentration exceeds four times the MIC of the target organism. Therefore, the optimal dosing strategy is to dose often and not let trough concentrations fall below the MIC of the target organism. With these considerations in mind, continuous infusion of β-lactams is under study to optimize treatment with β-lactam agents.

When killing is concentration dependent, activity is related to how high a concentration is achieved at the site of infection and how great is the "area under the curve" of drug concentration plotted versus time.[11] Agents of this type include the aminoglycosides and the fluoroquinolones. Optimal use of these agents would entail infrequent administration but high doses—the underlying principle behind the once-daily administration of aminoglycosides.[30,41] With once-daily dosing regimens, the patient achieves a high peak concentration (maximal killing), and a low trough concentration (minimal nephrotoxicity), relying on the "postantibiotic effect" (PAE) to maintain the efficacy of the antibiotic after the serum (or lung) concentrations fall below the MIC of the target organism.[11] If an antibiotic has a PAE, it is capable of suppressing bacterial growth even after its concentration falls below the MIC of the target organism. While most agents exhibit a PAE against gram-positive organisms, a prolonged PAE against gram-negative bacilli is achieved by the aminoglycosides, fluoroquinolones, tetracyclines, macrolides, and rifampin. Most of these agents also kill in a concentration-dependent fashion. Agents with little or no PAE against gram negatives are generally also agents that kill in a time-dependent fashion; thus they are given several times daily. The β-lactams (including the penicillins, cephalosporins, and monobactams) generally have little or no PAE against gram negatives; one notable exception is imipenem, which has a modest PAE against *Pseudomonas aeruginosa*. In clinical practice, the use of once-daily aminoglycoside dosing has had variable benefits in both efficacy and toxicity, but the advent of this type of dosing regimen follows from an understanding of pharmacodynamic principles.[30,41]

A phenomenon similar to PAE is termed *postantibiotic leukocyte enhancement* (PALE), which refers to the ability of functioning white blood cells to kill organisms while they are in the postantibiotic phase of growth. Thus, when the patient has functioning neutrophils, the PAE of some agents is extended by their PALE.[11]

Recently, some investigators have suggested that antibiotic therapy be chosen on the basis of another property of certain agents: their ability to stimulate inflammation and cytokine production in response to the presence of the bacterial cell wall lysis products that they generate. It has been known for many years that certain antibiotics liberate bacterial cell wall products that can interact with cytokine-producing cells, stimulating the production of high levels of cytokines such as tumor necrosis factor.[41] In theory, this could lead to the development, or worsening, of the sepsis syndrome in patients immediately after therapy for pneumonia is started (see Chapter 133). Whether these considerations should be used for antibiotic selection remains uncertain, but the cytokine release response of inflammatory cells to bacterial lysis products can be measured in vitro. In general, bactericidal antibiotics lead to more of a host inflammatory response than bacteriostatic agents; antibiotics that are cell wall active, and that kill slowly, have been associated with the greatest cytokine release. In particular, if an antibiotic has a high affinity for bacterial penicillin-binding protein 3, it may kill slowly and lead to filamentous cell wall products that are potent stimuli for cytokine release.[42,55] On the other hand, agents that kill rapidly and do not interact with penicillin-binding protein 3 are associated with lower levels of in vitro stimulation of cytokine production by host inflammatory cells.

RATIONALE FOR EMPIRIC ANTIBIOTIC THERAPY OF RESPIRATORY INFECTIONS

Community-Acquired Pneumonia

Although it may be intellectually unsatisfying to initiate antibiotic therapy without knowing exactly what organism is causing an infection, empiric therapy is essential for appropriate management of CAP. This follows from several observations: 1. Current diagnostic testing is of limited value, and thus a specific etiologic diagnosis is made in only about half of all patients.[2] 2. Empiric therapy is possible because the bacteriology of CAP is predictable, based on a knowledge of the severity of pneumonic illness, patient age, the presence of certain co-morbid illnesses, and local epidemiologic patterns, as reviewed in detail by Marrie (Chapter 127).[35] 3. In order to be effective, antibiotic therapy must be prompt.[4] 4. In studies of severe CAP, outcome has been improved with the timely initiation of effective broad-spectrum empiric therapy, while outcome has not been improved by identifying a specific etiologic pathogen.[24,31]

Limits of Current Diagnostic Testing   Several series of patients with CAP have shown that even with extensive diagnostic testing, an etiologic pathogen is often not identified. In one study of 154 patients at a VA hospital, all patients had a diagnostic workup that included sputum culture and Gram's stain; sputum studies for *Legionella* species and *C. pneumoniae;* serologic testing for viruses, *Legionella* species, *C. pneumoniae, Mycoplasma pneumoniae,* and other pathogens; and, in some cases, diagnostic bronchoscopy. With the provision that sputum culture and Gram's stain not be used, by themselves, to define bacteriology, an etiologic diagnosis was made in 51 percent of patients, often based on serologies, requiring the collection of acute and convalescent titers and the passage of many weeks.[2] This experience is typical of the reported efficacy of routine extensive diagnostic testing in CAP, and many other series have reported similar results.[33,35] Some experts have argued in favor of using the sputum Gram's stain to guide initial empiric therapy of CAP,[1] but this practice remains controversial and was not endorsed by the American Thoracic Society (ATS) in its guidelines for the treatment of CAP.[35] Concerns about the sputum Gram's stain include the fact that many patients are unable to provide a satisfactory sample, expert interpretation is often lacking, and the test can be either sensitive or specific but generally not both.[47]

Predictability of Etiologic Pathogens
One fundamental principle of empiric therapy is that the organism that is likely to be causing infection can be accurately predicted, and this prediction can be used to guide the selection of empiric therapy (see Chapter 122). The ATS has proposed that the pathogen for CAP can be predicted from a knowledge of the severity of illness (mild, moderate, or severe), the place of therapy (inpatient or outpatient), and the presence of advanced age (over 60 years) or co-morbid illness.[35] With this approach, each patient will fall into one of four categories, each with its own set of likely pathogens (Table 122-2). These four categories are (1) mild to moderate illness, treated out of the hospital in the absence of advanced age and co-morbid illness; (2) mild to moderate illness, treated out of the hospital with advanced age, co-morbid illness, or both being present; (3) hospitalized patients without severe pneumonia, regardless of age or the presence of co-morbid illness; and (4) patients with severe HAP, regardless of age or co-morbid illness. This paradigm leads to patient classifications and to empiric therapy regimens, and was developed on the basis of a number of studies of CAP bacteriology. The accuracy of the algorithm for predicting bacteriology and for guiding appropriate therapy still requires validation.

Several principles apply to predicting the bacteriology of patients with CAP. The most common etiologic organism, in any patient group, is *Streptococcus pneumoniae*. In the elderly and in cigarette smokers, *Hemophilus*

influenzae is common. Also in the elderly, aspiration (often silent) is common, and anaerobic organisms should be considered. Atypical pathogens and viruses are more common in young and otherwise healthy patients. In the elderly and chronically ill, gram negatives account for 20 to 40 percent of all pathogens, and in patients with severe CAP, *P. aeruginosa* may be responsible for 10 to 15 percent of all infections.[12,57] In general, the bacteriology of severe CAP is different from that of CAP, with an etiologic diagnosis often not made; the most commonly identified pathogens are pneumococcus, *L. pneumophila,* and enteric gram negatives (see Table 127-5, Chapter 127). Some series have found that *H. influenzae* and *Staphylococcus aureus* are also common.[31,49] Although debate continues about the actual prevalence of *Legionella* infection, recent studies have shown that the incidence of infection with this organism cannot be accurately esti-

TABLE 122-2

Categories of Patients with CAP and the Likely Pathogens for Each Group (in Descending Order of Frequency)

Outpatients, Mild to Moderate Illness, No Co-morbidity, Age <60

S. pneumoniae

M. pneumoniae

Respiratory viruses

C. pneumoniae

H. influenzae

Others: *Legionella* spp., *S. aureus, M. tuberculosis,* endemic fungi, enteric gram negatives

Outpatients, Mild to Moderate Illness, with Co-morbidity, Age >60, or Both

S. pneumoniae

Respiratory viruses

H. influenzae

Enteric gram negatives

S. aureus

Others: *M. catarrhalis, Legionella* spp., *M. tuberculosis,* endemic fungi

Hospitalized Patients, Moderately Ill, Any Age, with or without Co-morbidity

S. pneumoniae

H. influenzae

Polymicrobial, including anaerobes and enteric gram-negative bacilli

Legionella spp.

S. aureus

C. pneumoniae

Respiratory viruses

Others: *M. pneumoniae, Moraxella catarrhalis, M. tuberculosis,* endemic fungi

Severe Illness, Any Age, with or without Co-morbidity

S. pneumoniae

Legionella spp.

Enteric gram-negative bacilli

H. influenzae

M. pneumoniae

Respiratory viruses

Others: *M. tuberculosis,* endemic fungi

mated unless acute and convalescent serum titers are collected from patients, because a single acute titer is not a sensitive enough test to recognize most infected patients (see Chapter 144).[40] Although *S. aureus* is not a common CAP pathogen, it should be considered in patients with postinfluenza pneumonia and in those with diabetes or renal failure. While HIV-infected patients were not considered in the ATS CAP guidelines, they have a similar bacteriology when they develop CAP, with pneumococcus and *H. influenzae* being common. *Pneumocystis carinii* and *Mycobacterium tuberculosis* should always be considered in the differential diagnosis of CAP; infection by *P. aeruginosa* has also been reported.[20]

Recently, penicillin-resistant *S. pneumoniae* has become a concern. Most episodes of infection with this organism are with intermediately resistant strains (MIC >0.12 μg/ml but <2.0 μg/ml) and not with highly resistant strains (MIC ≥ 2.0 μg/ml), and therapy with high doses of penicillin or a third-generation cephalosporin is adequate.[39] In fact, in one recent study, the presence of penicillin resistance was not, independent of host factors, associated with an adverse outcome in CAP.[39] However, atypical infections (meningitis, sepsis, endovascular infections) due to *S. pneumoniae* should be treated with vancomycin and ceftriaxone until susceptibility data are available. Penicillin resistance should be considered a possibility, particularly if the patient has had β-lactam antibiotic therapy in the preceding 3 months or if the patient is debilitated with an immunosuppressive illness.[34]

Prompt Antibiotic Therapy   Few studies have looked at the timing of initiating antibiotic therapy for CAP. In general, initiation of therapy as soon as possible has been a stated goal in pneumonia management.[29] However, if antibiotics are initiated before the collection of respiratory tract cultures, diagnostic yield will suffer.[16] Thus the question arises, should empiric therapy, not based on extensive testing, be initiated in an effort to provide timely therapy, or is the information from diagnostic testing so vital that therapy should be delayed? The ATS guidelines for CAP have emphasized a limited initial diagnostic evaluation, reserving extensive testing for patients who have not responded to initial empiric therapy and for patients suspected of having infection with an unusual or resistant pathogen. If therapy is delayed for performance of diagnostic testing, outcome may suffer. In one study of 453 patients with CAP, 45 percent of the patients received antibiotic therapy before hospital admission. When pneumococcal pneumonia was present, no patient who received preadmission antibiotics died, whereas 6 percent of those without preadmission therapy and pneumococcal pneumonia died. A similar trend applied for other pathogens.[4]

Empiric Therapy with Broad-Spectrum Agents and Outcomes
The effort to define the etiologic pathogen is unsuccessful in over half of all patients with severe CAP, as in patients with milder forms of CAP.[31,38,57] On the other hand, the bacteriology of severe illness is predictable, and thus empiric therapy has generally entailed broad-spectrum treatment, usually with an intravenous macrolide and a second- or third-generation cephalosporin or another β-lactam agent (see Table 127-8, Chapter 127). In several studies, the use of such an empiric regimen, aimed at the predicted pathogens, has led to an improved outcome, while the

identification of a specific cause has not had substantial benefit. In one series of severe CAP, an etiologic diagnosis was established in 40 percent of survivors; and in 42 percent of nonsurvivors;[38] in another series, mortality was 31 percent when an etiologic diagnosis was made and only 8 percent when the cause remained unknown.[31] While diagnostic testing is of limited value, several investigators have shown that an optimal empiric regimen for severe CAP can lead to improved patient survival. In one study, of 286 patients with severe CAP, mortality was 11 percent when initial therapy was effective as defined by clinical response at 72 h; mortality reached 60 percent in the 92 patients given ineffective initial therapy.[24] In another series, the use of erythromycin plus either an aminoglycoside or cephalosporin was associated with an 85 percent survival rate, while the use of any other regimen was associated with a survival rate of 68 percent.[38] Thus, not only is effective empiric therapy, based on knowledge of the likely pathogens, an important determinant of outcome in severe CAP, but the identification of a specific etiologic pathogen has not been shown to be of value.

Hospital-Acquired Pneumonia

Tremendous controversy surrounds the diagnosis of HAP (see also Chapter 143). Some investigators advocate that antibiotic therapy be initiated only after a microbiologic diagnosis of pneumonia has been established, usually with invasive bronchoscopic methods and quantitative cultures.[9,14] However, others advocate the use of a clinical definition of pneumonia in the decision to initiate therapy.[37] If invasive methods are used, the results of respiratory tract secretion Gram's stain and culture are used to guide antibiotic therapy. If a clinical diagnosis is used to decide when to initiate therapy, initial antibiotic selection is empiric, based on specific algorithms, and therapy is adjusted when the results of sputum, tracheal aspirate, or blood cultures become available. Regardless of whether the decision to initiate antibiotic therapy for suspected HAP is ultimately based on clinical or microbiologic grounds or both, there is reason to believe that prompt empiric therapy, initiated after the clinical diagnosis of pneumonia, has distinct advantages.

The rationale for empiric, algorithm-based therapy of HAP is based on the following considerations: 1. Although the clinical definition of HAP may not be specific, it is extremely sensitive, and it should be relied on in making the decision when to initiate therapy. If only invasive bacteriologic methods are used, early forms of pneumonia may go unrecognized and therapy may be delayed.[37] 2. Algorithms have been developed that can guide initial antibiotic selection, based on readily available clinical assessments.[7,26,36] 3. Initial empiric therapy can be modified when tracheal aspirate culture results become available, and tracheal aspirates are reliable for defining the bacteriology in intubated patients.[52] 4. If invasive methods are used to manage HAP patients, information may become available at a time when it is unlikely to be of any clinical benefit.[25,32]

Clinical Criteria for Recognizing Early Cases of HAP   The clinical definition of HAP requires the presence of a new or progressive lung infiltrate plus usually two of the following: fever, leukocytosis, and purulent sputum. Other criteria for diagnosis are a positive blood culture, radiographic cavitation, and histologic evidence of pneumonia.[53] When clinical criteria are used, HAP can be overdiagnosed, especially in mechanically ventilated patients, but the magnitude of this error is debated. Some investigators have reported that this diagnosis can be confirmed microbiologically in only one in three cases that satisfy the clinical definition of pneumonia, while others have reported a good correlation between clinical and microbiologic criteria.[14,44] In one study, a clinical pulmonary infection score was developed using six criteria: fever, white blood cell count and differential, tracheal secretions, oxygenation status, radiographic pattern, and the nature of sputum pathogens.[44] Each clinical feature was scored on a scale from 0 to 2, and thus patients had a total score from 0 to 12. When the score was over 6, it was highly predictive of bronchoscopic confirmation of pneumonia, while none of patients with a score under 6 satisfied the microbiologic criteria for infection. Thus, a "weighted" clinical judgment can be a very potent tool for recognizing HAP.

On the other hand, bronchoscopy with quantitative cultures may miss early, and potentially treatable, forms of HAP. When invasive methods are used, a microbiologic threshold is defined. When results fall below this concentration, therapy is withheld, whereas if culture results exceed this concentration, therapy is administered. For the protected specimen brush (PSB), this threshold is usually 10^3 organisms per milliliter, for bronchoalveolar lavage it is 10^4 organisms per milliliter, and for quantitative endotracheal aspirates it is 10^5 organisms per milliliter. In one study, patients had repeat bronchoscopy after the initial results of PSB cultures showed a concentration between 10^2 and 10^3, a value below the diagnostic threshold.[13] When a repeat bronchoscopy was done within 72 h, one-third of the patients fell above the diagnostic threshold for pneumonia, implying that an early form of infection had been present in some patients when the first procedure was done. These data suggest that pneumonia is on a bacteriologic continuum, and that a strict threshold concentration for defining infection does not exist. This conclusion is also suggested by the finding from autopsy studies that histologic lung infection can begin as bronchiolitis and progress to confluent pneumonia and then to necrotizing infection.[51] In addition to all of these concerns, there are a number of methodologic problems associated with invasive diagnostic methods for pneumonia. For example, the data may not be readily reproducible from one institution to another—or even within a given patient when numerous samples are collected.[28,37]

Algorithms to Guide Initial Empiric Antibiotic Therapy   Once the decision to treat a patient for HAP has been made, empiric therapy can be initiated based on a knowledge of the likely etiologic pathogens for any given patient. All patients with HAP are at risk for infection with a *"core" group of organisms* that include nonpseudomonal enteric gram negatives, *H. influenzae*, pneumococcus, and methicillin-sensitive *S. aureus*. Among the enteric gram negatives composing this core group of bacteria are *Enterobacter* species, *Escherichia coli*, *Klebsiella* species, *Proteus* species, and *Serratia marcescens*.[7,26] In one study of mild to moderate HAP, the most common pathogens were *S. pneumoniae* and *H. influenzae*, which accounted for 31 percent of all episodes, while gram-negative bacilli were isolated in only 24 percent of patients, and *S. aureus* in 10 percent of patients.[54] Even in the setting of severe, ICU-acquired HAP, the same organisms predominate in patients who have no unusual risk factors for specific pathogens and whose pneumonia has begun within the first 5 days of hospitalization. In fact, in one study of patients with severe early-onset HAP (defined as occurring within 5 days of admission), 54 percent of all episodes were due to *S. pneumoniae*, *H. influenzae*, or *S. aureus*, while only 17 percent of cases were due to enteric gram-negative bacilli.[43] This pattern changes dramatically if risk factors for specific pathogens are present or if the pneumonia is of late onset.

In patients with mild to moderate illness, in the presence of specific risk factors, the core organisms remain a concern; but other pathogens must be considered, depending on the nature of the risk factor.[7,26] If the patient is witnessed to aspirate or has had recent thoracoabdominal surgery, anaerobes are a concern. If the patient has coma or head injury, early-onset infection with methicillin-sensitive *S. aureus* is especially likely. If the patient has received antibiotics or corticosteroids or has had a prolonged stay in the ICU, even if the pneumonia is not severe, drug-resistant pathogens, in addition to the core pathogens, should be considered and treated empirically. These may include *P. aeruginosa*, *Acinetobacter* species, and methicillin-resistant *S. aureus*, as well as any institution-specific pathogens known to be present on the basis of microbiologic data or surveillance cultures (see also Chapter 143).

When severe HAP is present, the pathogens vary with the presence of risk factors and the time of onset of pneumonia. As mentioned, if risk factors are absent and if pneumonia is of early onset, only the core pathogens are likely. However, if added risk factors are present or if the pneumonia begins on or after the fifth hospital day, additional nosocomial pathogens are also a concern, especially *P. aeruginosa*, *Acinetobacter* species, and methicillin-resistant *S. aureus*. The use of antibiotics before the onset of pneumonia is an important risk factor for infection with these organisms.[48] Other risk factors identified for *P. aeruginosa* pneumonia are prolonged mechanical ventilation, malnutrition, and corticosteroid use. In one recent study, many of these factors were also present in patients infected with methicillin-resistant *S. aureus*.[50]

Tracheal Aspirates to Define the Bacteriology of HAP in Ventilated Patients   Even though quantitative cultures of respiratory tract secretions cannot be relied on to determine when to initiate antibiotic therapy, cultures may be useful for focusing antibiotic therapy. In intubated patients, tracheal aspirate cultures are a sensitive, although not specific, tool for reliably identifying the organisms that are causing pneumonia. In one study of 52 episodes of pneumonia in patients ventilated long term, tracheal aspirate and PSB cultures were performed.[52] In 36 episodes, both methods identified the same pathogens, while in four episodes, no pathogen was found with either method. The tracheal aspirate was more sensitive than the PSB, showing organisms that were not recovered on the PSB in 11 episodes. However, it was very unusual for an organism to be identified on the PSB and not be recovered from the tracheal aspirate—a circumstance found in only one episode. Similar data emerged from another study, which showed that tracheal aspirate recovered 90 percent of the organisms that were found in PSB cultures.[22] These data indicate that although the tracheal aspirate can harbor an organism that is not causing pneumonia, the absence of a specific pathogen in a tracheal aspirate is strong evidence that the organism is not leading to pneumonia. Thus, the findings of tracheal aspirate cultures can be used to narrow initial empiric therapy choices, or to modify them, once antimicrobial sensitivity data become available.

Invasive Methods May Give Information of No Clinical Benefit   One of the strongest arguments for early empiric therapy of suspected HAP is that therapy is most likely to be effective if it is given early in the course of illness. Therapeutic decisions based on the data obtained by bronchoscopy may be delayed until the information becomes available too late to influence outcome. Data suggest that microbiologically appropriate or effective initial therapy for HAP leads to improved outcomes when compared with regimens to which the causative organisms are not susceptible.[8,25,36] However, timing of therapy is also important.

Montravers and colleagues studied 76 patients with nosocomial pneumonia who were being mechanically ventilated; all patients had their diagnosis confirmed by PSB sampling.[32] After 3 days of therapy, all patients had repeat bronchoscopy. A total of 76 patients were studied: 51 had sterile cultures on repeat bronchoscopy, 16 had organisms at concentrations under 10^3, and 9 had organisms at concentrations above 10^3. Thus, bronchoscopy defined nine patients as being therapeutic failures, on the basis of bacteriologic data. Unfortunately, awareness of this information had little effect on patient outcome. For the 67 patients with an initial good bacteriologic response, the clinical outcome was favorable in 92 percent; however, for the nine patients without initial bacteriologic control, clinical outcome was favorable in only 44 percent. Thus, if initial therapy is ineffective, altering that therapy on the basis of culture data is unlikely to be of clinical benefit. Similarly, in a study of 109 patients with suspected ventilator-associated pneumonia undergoing BAL, Luna and colleagues showed that adequate antibiotic therapy was effective in reducing mortality only if given early in the course of illness, as part of initial empiric therapy, but that the use of adequate therapy had no benefit if it was first given after culture data became available.[25]

SPECIFIC REGIMENS FOR EMPIRIC THERAPY OF RESPIRATORY INFECTIONS

Community-Acquired Pneumonia

Recommended Antibiotic Choices   As discussed above, and as shown in Table 122-2, each patient with CAP will fall into one of four groups, each with its own set of likely pathogens. The selection of antimicrobial therapy should be guided by a knowledge of the expected etiologic pathogens for a given patient, with more specific therapy being used if blood cultures, or other diagnostic testing, provide definitive information about the responsible pathogen. Although not every patient needs an extensive diagnostic evaluation, sputum culture and sensitivity testing should be performed if a drug resistant-pathogen is suspected,

as would be the case if the patient had completed a course of antibiotic therapy in the preceding 3 months.[34] In addition, if an unusual pathogen is suspected, or if the patient is known to be immune compromised, culture of respiratory tract secretions is recommended. Specific therapies are discussed in Chapter 127; however, general guidelines in designing an empiric regimen are discussed below.

For patients with mild to moderate CAP treated out of the hospital, in the absence of advanced age or co-morbidity, empiric therapy should be with a macrolide.[35] If the patient is intolerant of erythromycin or if *H. influenzae* is a concern, one of the extended-spectrum macrolides, azithromycin or clarithromycin, should be used. Tetracyclines are a second choice and have less activity against pneumococcus than macrolides. When a patient has mild to moderate CAP and is treated out of the hospital, but has advanced age, co-morbid illness, or both, the likely etiologic pathogens and the initial therapies are different (discussed above and in Chapter 133). Because of the presence of advanced age or co-morbidity, *H. influenzae,* enteric gram negatives, and anaerobes are more likely, but *S. pneumoniae* is still the most common pathogen. Monotherapy should be with a second-generation oral cephalosporin (such as cefuroxime), trimethoprim-sulfamethoxazole, or a β-lactam–β-lactamase inhibitor combination (amoxicillin-clavulanate). A macrolide can be used as a second agent in this situation if *M. pneumoniae* or *Legionella* species are suspected.[35]

For the hospitalized patient, not severely ill, regardless of age or the presence of co-morbid illness, initial therapy should be given intravenously with a second-generation or nonpseudomonal third-generation cephalosporin (such as cefuroxime, ceftriaxone, or cefotaxime) or a β-lactam–β-lactamase inhibitor combination (ampicillin-sulbactam or piperacillin-tazobactam). If penicillin-resistant pneumococcus is suspected, initial therapy with cefotaxime or ceftriaxone has been shown to be generally adequate until culture results become available.[39] If there is concern about *Legionella* species or *M. pneumoniae,* a macrolide can be added as a second agent. If the patient is not severely ill, the macrolide can be given orally, and the concomitant administration of an intravenous β-lactam agent should be adequate for any potentially bacteremic organisms.[17] If severe CAP is present, therapy must be intravenous and use several agents, including a macrolide and one or two antipseudomonal agents. While antipseudomonal therapy should be based on antimicrobial susceptibility data, possibly effective agents include the aminoglycosides; the third-generation cephalosporin ceftazidime; the fluoroquinolone ciprofloxacin; the monobactam aztreonam; the carbapenem imipenem; the antipseudomonal penicillins such as piperacillin, azlocillin, or mezlocillin; and the β-lactam–β-lactamase inhibitor combinations such as ticarcillin-clavulanate or piperacillin-tazobactam.

Response to Empiric Therapy   With appropriate therapy, clinical improvement should be seen in CAP patients within 48 to 72 h, and a response occurs in 80 to 90 percent of all patients.[35] If the patient's condition deteriorates or does not improve within this period, a careful diagnostic evaluation is necessary to look for alternative diagnoses or specific bacteriologic entities. To determine whether a patient is responding appropriately to empiric therapy, clinical features, not radiographic patterns, should be evaluated, since chest radiographic improvement may lag behind the clinical response. If clinical improvement is inadequate, respiratory secretions should be recultured, and bronchoscopy and CT scanning of the chest should be considered. Diagnostic testing should be directed at defining whether the lack of response to therapy is the result of a noninfectious process (inflammatory lung disease), a complication of infection or of therapy (metastatic infection, antibiotic-induced colitis), an unsuspected or unusual pathogen (tuberculosis or fungus), or the result of the wrong antibiotic having been used (because a pathogen was not susceptible to the agent selected).

If the initial clinical response is good, consideration should be given to an early switch from intravenous to oral therapy. Several recent studies have indicated that this switch can be made on day 3 of hospitalization for patients with uncomplicated disease.[46,58] Criteria for switch include the absence of severe illness, the absence of certain "high-risk" pathogens, and the absence of life-threatening complications in an immunologically normal host.[58] In one study, criteria for a switch to oral therapy included that the patient was afebrile on two occasions measured 8 h apart, that the white blood cell count was returning toward normal, that the symptoms of cough and shortness of breath were abating, and that the GI tract was functioning.[46] Many questions about the criteria for early oral step-down therapy remain, including at what time point bacteremic patients can make the transition to oral therapy and whether a successful combination intravenous regimen should be followed by a combination oral regimen.

Hospital-Acquired Pneumonia

Recommended Antibiotic Choices   As discussed above, patients with HAP can be categorized into one of three groups based on an assessment of severity of illness (mild to moderate or severe), the presence of risk factors for specific pathogens, and the time of onset of infection (Fig. 122-1). In making these distinctions, the ATS developed a definition for severe pneumonia, and this definition can be used for patients with either CAP or HAP. Severe pneumonia is defined by the presence of at least one of the following: respiratory rate above 35 per minute, hypoxemia defined as either a $Pa_{O_2}/F_{I_{O_2}}$ ratio under 250 or the need for more than 35 percent supplemental oxygen to maintain arterial oxygen saturation greater than 90 percent, need for mechanical ventilation, rapid radiographic worsening of pneumonia, shock, oliguria, or acute renal failure.[7] Risk factors that affect the likely etiologic pathogens and should be considered as being either present or absent in HAP patients are recent abdominal surgery, witnessed aspiration, diabetes, coma, head

trauma, renal failure, prolonged ICU stay, corticosteroid therapy, prior antibiotics, and structural lung disease. In terms of the time of onset of pneumonia, patients are categorized as having early onset (before day 5) or late onset (on or after day 5).

The first category is that of patients with no risk factors for unusual organisms and either mild to moderate HAP, beginning at any time in the hospital stay, or severe HAP of early onset. These patients are at risk only for the "core pathogens" (discussed above)[7,26,36] and should generally receive monotherapy with a second-generation (cefuroxime) or nonpseudomonal third-generation cephalosporin (ceftriaxone or cefotaxime) or a β-lactam–β-lactamase inhibitor combination (ampicillin-sulbactam, ticarcillin-clavulanate, or piperacillin-tazobactam). If the patient is penicillin allergic, alternative therapy would be with a fluoroquinolone (ciprofloxacin or ofloxacin) or the combination of clindamycin and aztreonam.

The second category is patients with mild to moderate pneumonia, of early or late onset, with specific risk factors for other pathogens in addition to the core organisms. Therapy is with one of the above-mentioned antibiotics with consideration of a second agent, depending on which risk factor is present.[7,26,36] Thus, if anaerobes are a concern because of possible aspiration, clindamycin can be added to a cephalosporin, or a β-lactam–β-lactamase inhibitor can be used alone. If *S. aureus* is a concern because of coma, head injury, or diabetes, the first agent selected should have good staphylococcal coverage, or vancomycin should be considered (especially if a methicillin-resistant organism is suspected). A macrolide may be added if the patient has received corticosteroids and nosocomial *Legionella* species are prevalent. If the patient has had a prolonged ICU hospitalization, recent antibiotics, or corticosteroids or if a potentially drug-resistant nosocomial organism is possible, the patient should be treated ac-

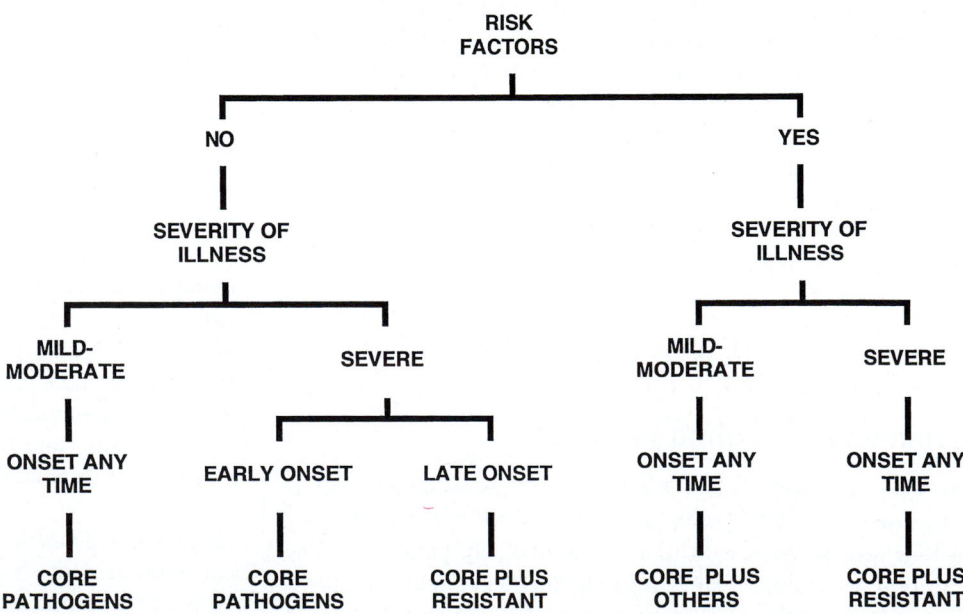

FIGURE 122-1 Patients with hospital-acquired pneumonia can be categorized by the presence or absence of specific risk factors for certain organisms, the severity of illness, and the time of onset of infection. Each patient is likely to be infected by one of three groups of organisms (defined in the text): the "core pathogens," the core pathogens plus others common to groups with certain risk factors, and the core pathogens plus potentially resistant, nosocomially acquired organisms.

cording to the algorithm for severe pneumonia even with only mild to moderate illness.

Patients with severe pneumonia of early onset in the presence of risk factors, or of late onset regardless of risk factors, fall into a third category.[7,26,36] These patients are at risk for infection with the core organisms and potentially resistant organisms, both gram-negative and gram-positive (e.g., methicillin-resistant *S. aureus*) bacteria, although the exact organisms will vary from one institution to another. These patients need to be treated initially with a combination of antimicrobial agents. Although monotherapy has been as successful as combination therapy for the treatment of HAP of mild to moderate severity, it is not recommended for patients with severe HAP. However, there have been few studies of monotherapy for patients with severe HAP.[10,18,23] There are several putative benefits of combination therapy, including the prevention of resistance by such organisms as *P. aeruginosa,* the opportunity of providing a broad spectrum of antimicrobial coverage, and the achievement of antibacterial synergy against certain organisms. Only in the setting of *P. aeruginosa* bacteremia, or with a neutropenic patient, is it likely that the synergistic activity of certain combination therapies will lead to a survival advantage.[36] Practically speaking, when combination therapy is used for patients with severe HAP, it is because of concerns about the possible emergence of resistance if monotherapy is used.[18,36]

Combination therapy should be used initially for patients with severe HAP. Synergy of antimicrobial activity has been documented only for antipseudomonal therapy with a β-lactam (such as piperacillin or ceftazidime) in combination with an aminoglycoside. Concerns about this approach include poor penetration of the aminogylcoside into respiratory secretions, aminoglycoside inactivity at the acidic tissue pH's associated with pneumonia, and the development of nephrotoxicity.[7,36] In one study, imipenem was compared to the combination of imipenem and netilmicin in 177 patients with HAP (97 of them mechanically ventilated). The use of combination therapy did not lead to any higher success than when monotherapy was used, although nephrotoxicity occurred as a complication of the aminoglycoside regimen.[10] In addition, eradication rates for *P. aeruginosa* were no higher when the combination regimen was used. This study raises the possibility that aminoglycosides add very little to the therapy of patients with severe HAP, and that other combination regimens should be considered. The use of a dual β-lactam combination is not likely to be useful, because of the concern that resistance to both agents could emerge simultaneously and because of the possibility that the two agents' effects are not additive or synergistic. A third approach to combination therapy is to use a quinolone (ciprofloxacin is the only currently available antipseudomonal quinolone) combined with a β-lactam—a regimen that may benefit from the excellent lung penetration characteristic of fluoroquinolones.

When a combination regimen is started, it should be continued until the results of tracheal aspirate cultures become available. If *P. aeruginosa, Acinetobacter* species, or other highly resistant organisms are not identified, and if the patient is having a good clinical response, streamlining to monotherapy should be done. In one recent study of monotherapy, with either ciprofloxacin or imipenem, in 405 patients with severe HAP, monotherapy was effective for the 70 percent of patients who did not have *P. aeru-*

ginosa infection.[18] The two monotherapy regimens had comparable bacteriologic eradication rates, but ciprofloxacin was associated with a significantly better clinical response and a better eradication rate for the Enterobacteriaceae group of organisms. If *P. aeruginosa* was isolated, both monotherapy regimens were associated with a high rate of resistance developing during therapy. The data in this study show the efficacy of monotherapy, even for severe HAP, provided that *P. aeruginosa* is not present. Thus, on the basis of this information, the conservative approach to the treatment of severe HAP is to start with a combination regimen; but in the absence of a highly resistant pathogen from respiratory tract cultures, therapy can be safely completed with selected single agents.

The optimal duration of therapy for HAP has not been defined, but therapy is usually continued for a minimum of 10 to 14 days, with longer courses being employed for patients with multilobar disease, cavitary infiltrates, malnutrition, severe debility, or highly resistant pathogens.[7] The switch to oral therapy can be made in responding patients, provided that intestinal absorption is adequate, although the exact timing of such a change in treatment has not been determined. If the patient is not responding to initial empiric therapy or the patient's condition deteriorates during therapy, a diagnostic evaluation with bronchoscopy, CT scanning, and, possibly, open lung biopsy is needed to look for noninfectious diagnoses or to identify drug-resistant or unsuspected infectious pathogens.

In severely ill patients, adjunctive topical antibiotic therapy, usually with an aminoglycoside, can be used. This approach assures high local levels of antibiotics, but there is no evidence that the routine addition of topical therapy to systemic antibiotics adds to the likelihood of a favorable clinical response (see Chapter 123).[5]

REFERENCES

1. Bartlett JG, Mundy LM: Community-acquired pneumonia. *New Engl J Med* 333:1618–1624, 1995.
2. Bates JH, Campbell GD, Barron AL, et al: Microbial etiology of acute pneumonia in hospitalized patients. *Chest* 101:1005–1012, 1992.
3. Bodem CR, Lampton LM, Miller DP, et al: Endobronchial pH: Relevance to aminoglycoside activity in gram-negative pneumonia. *Am Rev Respir Dis* 127:39–41, 1983.
4. British Thoracic Society: Community-acquired pneumonia in adults in British hospitals in 1982–1983: A survey of aetiology, mortality, prognostic factors and outcome. *Q J Med* 62:195–220, 1987.
5. Brown RB, Kruse JA, Counts GW, et al: Double-blind study of endotracheal tobramycin in the treatment of gram-negative bacterial pneumonia. *Antimicrob Agents Chemother* 34:269–272, 1990.
6. Bueno-Cavanillas A, Delgado-Rodríguez M, López-Luque A, et al: Influence of nosocomial infection on mortality rate in an intensive care unit. *Crit Care Med* 22: 55–60, 1994.
7. Campbell GD, Niederman MS, Broughton WA, et al: Hospital-acquired pneumonia in adults: Diagnosis, assessment of severity, initial antimicrobial therapy, and prevention strategies. A consensus statement. *Am J Respir Crit Care Med* 153:1711–1725, 1996.
8. Celis R, Torres A, Gatell J, et al: Nosocomial pneumonia a multivariate analysis of risk and prognosis. *Chest* 93:318–324, 1988.

9. Chastre J, Fagon JY: Invasive diagnostic testing should be routinely used to manage ventilated patients with suspected pneumonia. *Am J Respir Crit Care Med* 150:570–574, 1994.

10. Cometta A, Baumgartner JD, Lew D, et al: Prospective randomized comparison of imipenem monotherapy with imipenem plus netilmicin for treatment of severe infections in nonneutropenic patients. *Antimicrob Agents Chemother* 38:1309–1313, 1994.

11. Craig W: Pharmacodynamics of antimicrobial agents as a basis for determining dosage regimens. *Eur J Clin Microbiol Infect Dis* 12:6–8, 1993.

12. Dahmash NS, Chowdhury M: Re-evaluation of pneumonia requiring admission to an intensive care unit: A prospective study. *Thorax* 49:71–76, 1994.

13. Dreyfuss D, Mier L, Le Bourdelles G, et al: Clinical significance of borderline quantitative protected brush specimen culture results. *Am Rev Respir Dis* 147:941–951, 1993.

14. Fagon J-Y, Chastre J, Hance AJ, et al: Detection of nosocomial lung infection in ventilated patients: Use of a protected specimen brush and quantitative culture techniques in 147 patients. *Am Rev Respir Dis* 138:110–116, 1988.

15. Fagon J-Y, Chastre J, Hance A, et al: Nosocomial pneumonia in ventilated patients: A cohort study evaluation attributable mortality and hospital stay. *Am J Med* 94:281–288, 1993.

16. Fang GD, Fine M, Orloff J, et al: New and emerging etiologies for community-acquired pneumonia with implication for therapy: A prospective multicenter study of 359 cases. *Medicine* 69:307–316, 1990.

17. Fein AM, Niederman MS: Guidelines for the initial management of community-acquired pneumonia: Savory recipe or cookbook for disaster? *Am J Respir Crit Care Med* 152:1149–1153, 1995.

18. Fink MP, Snydman DR, Niederman MS, et al, and the Severe Pneumonia Study Group: Treatment of severe pneumonia in hospitalized patients: Results of a multicenter, randomized, double-blind trial comparing intravenous ciprofloxacin with imipenem-cilastatin. *Antimicrob Agents Chemother* 38:547–557, 1994.

19. Grayson ML, Eliopoulos GM: Antimicrobial resistance in the intensive care unit. *Semin Respir Infect* 5:204–214, 1990.

20. Hirschtick RE, Glassroth J, Jordan MC, et al: Bacterial pneumonia in persons infected with the human immunodeficiency virus. *New Engl J Med* 333:845–851, 1995.

21. Honeybourne D: Antibiotic penetration into lung tissues. *Thorax* 49:104–106, 1994.

22. Jourdain B, Novara A, Joly-Guillou M-L, et al: Role of quantitative cultures of endotracheal aspirates in the diagnosis of nosocomial pneumonia. *Am J Respir Crit Care Med* 152:241–246, 1995.

23. LaForce FM: Systemic antimicrobial therapy of nosocomial pneumonia: Monotherapy versus combination therapy. *Eur J Clin Microbiol Infect Dis* 8:61–68, 1989.

24. Leroy O, Santré C, Beuscart C, et al: A five-year study of severe community-acquired pneumonia with emphasis on prognosis in patients admitted to an intensive care unit. *Intensive Care Med* 21:24–31, 1995.

25. Luna CM, Vujacich P, Vay C, et al: Impact of BAL culture result on the therapy an outcome of ventilator associated pneumonia (VAP). *Chest* 108(Suppl):145S, 1995.

26. Mandell LA, Marrie TJ, Niederman MS: Initial antimicrobial treatment of hospital acquired pneumonia in adults: A conference report. *Can J Infect Dis* 4:317–321, 1993.

27. Mandell LA: Antibiotics for pneumonia therapy. *Med Clin North Am* 78:997–1014, 1994.

28. Marquette CH, Herengt F, Mathieu D, et al: Diagnosis of pneumonia in mechanically ventilated patients: Repeatability of the protected specimen brush. *Am Rev Respir Dis* 147:211–214, 1993.

29. Marrie TJ: Community-acquired pneumonia. *Clin Infect Dis* 18:501–505, 1994.

30. Miyagawa CI: Aminoglycosides in the intensive care unit: An old drug in a dynamic environment. *New Horizons* 1:172–180, 1993.

31. Moine P, Vercken J, Chevret S, et al, and the French Study Group for Community-Acquired Pneumonia in the ICU: Severe community-acquired pneumonia: Etiology, epidemiology, and prognosis factors. *Chest* 105:1487–1495, 1994.

32. Montravers P, Fagon J-Y, Chastre J, et al: Follow-up protected specimen brushes to assess treatment in nosocomial pneumonia. *Am Rev Respir Dis* 147:38–44, 1993.

33. Mundy LM, Auwaerter PG, Oldach D, et al: Community-acquired pneumonia: Impact of immune status. *Am J Respir Crit Care Med* 152:1309–1315, 1995.

34. Nava JM, Bella F, Garau J, et al: Predictive factors for invasive disease due to penicillin-resistant *Streptococcus pneumoniae*: A population-based study. *Clin Infect Dis* 19:884–890, 1994.

35. Niederman MS, Bass JB, Campbell GD, et al: Guidelines for the initial management of adults with community-acquired pneumonia: Diagnosis, assessment of severity, and initial antimicrobial therapy. *Am Rev Respir Dis* 148:1418–1426, 1993.

36. Niederman MS: An approach to empiric therapy of nosocomial pneumonia. *Med Clin North Am* 78:1123–1141, 1994.

37. Niederman MS, Torres A, Summer W: Invasive diagnostic testing is not needed routinely to manage suspected ventilator-associated pneumonia. *Am J Respir Crit Care Med* 150:565–569, 1994.

38. Pachon J, Prados MD, Capote F, et al: Severe community-acquired pneumonia: Etiology, prognosis, and treatment. *Am Rev Respir Dis* 142:369–373, 1990.

39. Pallares R, Linares J, Vadillo M, et al: Resistance to penicillin and cephalosporin and mortality from severe pneumococcal pneumonia in Barcelona, Spain. *New Engl J Med* 333:474–480, 1995.

40. Plouffe JF, File TM, Breiman RF, et al: Reevaluation of the definition of Legionnaires' disease: Use of the urinary antigen assay. *Clin Infect Dis* 20:1286–1291, 1995.

41. Prins JM, Buller HR, Kuijper EJ, et al: Once versus thrice daily gentamicin in patients with serious infections. Lancet 341:335–339, 1993.

42. Prins JM, Van Deventer S, Kuijper EJ, Speelman P: Clinical relevance of antibiotic-induced endotoxin release. *Antimicrob Agents Chemother* 38:1211–1218, 1994.

43. Prod'hom G, Leuenberger P, Koerfer J, et al: Nosocomial pneumonia in mechanically ventilated patients receiving antiacid, ranitidine, or sucralfate as prophylaxis for stress ulcer: A randomized controlled trial. *Ann Intern Med* 120:653–662, 1994.

44. Pugin J, Auckenthaler R, Mili N, et al: Diagnosis of ventilator-associated pneumonia by bacteriologic analysis of bronchoscopic and nonbronchoscopic "blind" bronchoalveolar lavage fluid. *Am Rev Respir Dis* 143:1121–1129, 1991.

45. Redington J, Craig WA: Pharmacology of antimicrobials in the elderly, in Niederman, MS (ed), *Respiratory Infections in the Elderly*. New York, Raven, 1991, pp 239–275.

46. Ramirez JA, Srinath L, Ahkee S, et al: Early switch from intravenous to oral cephalosporins in the treatment of hospitalized patients with community-acquired pneumonia. *Arch Intern Med* 155:1273–1276, 1995.

47. Rein MF, Gwaltney JM Jr, O'Brien WM, et al: Accuracy of Gram's stain in identifying pneumococci in sputum. *JAMA* 239:2671–2673, 1978.

48. Rello J, Ausina V, Ricart M, et al: Impact of previous antimicrobial therapy on the etiology and outcome of ventilator-associated pneumonia. *Chest* 104:1230–1235, 1993.

49. Rello J, Quintana E, Ausina V, et al: A three-year study of severe community-acquired pneumonia with emphasis on outcome. *Chest* 103:232–235, 1993.

50. Rello J, Ricart M, Valles J, et al: Ventilator-associated pneumonia by *Staphylococcus aureus:* Comparison of methicillin-resistant and methicillin-sensitive episodes. *Am J Respir Crit Care Med* 150:1545–1549, 1994.

51. Rouby J-J, de Lassale EM, Poete P, et al: Nosocomial bronchopneumonia in the critically ill: Histologic and bacteriologic aspects. *Am Rev Respir Dis* 146:1059–1066, 1992.

52. Rumback MJ, Bass RL: Tracheal aspirate correlates with protected specimen brush in long-term ventilated patients who have clinical pneumonia. *Chest* 106:531–534, 1994.

53. Salata RA, Lederman MM, Shlaes DM, et al: Diagnosis of nosocomial pneumonia in intubated, intensive care unit patients. *Am Rev Respir Dis* 135:426–432, 1987.

54. Schleupner CJ, Cobb DK: A study of the etiologies and treatment of nosocomial pneumonia in a community-based teaching hospital. *Infect Control Hosp Epidemiol* 13:515–525, 1992.

55. Simon DM, Koenig G, Trenholme GM: Differences in release of tumor necrosis factor from THP-1 cells stimulated by filtrates of antibiotic-killed *Escherichia coli. J Infect Dis* 164:800–802, 1991.

56. Sonnesyn SW, Gerding DN: Antimicrobials for the treatment of respiratory infection, in Niederman MS, Sarosa GA, Glassroth J (eds), *Respiratory Infections: A Scientific Basis for Management.* Philadelphia, WB Saunders, 1994, pp 511–537.

57. Torres A, Serra-Batlles J, Ferrer A, et al: Severe community-acquired pneumonia: Epidemiology and prognostic factors. *Am Rev Respir Dis* 144:312–318, 1991.

58. Weingarten SR, Riedinger MS, Varis G, et al: Identification of low-risk hospitalized patients with pneumonia: Implications for early conversion to oral antimicrobial therapy. *Chest* 105:1109–1115, 1994.

CHAPTER 123

LOCAL THERAPY AND PHARMACOKINETICS OF ANTIBIOTICS IN THE LUNGS

Jean A. Klastersky/Mickael Aoun

Among the factors that influence the efficacy of antibiotic therapy, the local concentration of the antimicrobial agent at the site of infection is among the most important.[44] Within the lungs, penetration of antibiotics to various locations will vary, and local concentrations may not be reflected by serum levels.[6] Microorganisms will be found in sputum or bronchial mucosa,[27] or in the epithelial lining fluid or alveolar macrophages.[61] The penetration of antibiotics depends on the ability of the antimicrobial agent to cross cell membranes and concentrate within cells. For example, the capillary endothelium is relatively permeable, with antimicrobial concentrations in interstitial fluid equivalent to that of the serum,[71] while connective tissue and the lining epithelium are relatively impermeable.[67]

The physicochemical properties of each class of antibiotics as well as the degree of inflammation or fibrosis of the lung tissue markedly influence the antibiotic penetration into lung tissue. If poor penetration by some antibiotics can be compensated by a higher systemic delivery dose, for agents with a low therapeutic index, such as the aminoglycosides, this compensation is hampered by potential toxicity. Furthermore, aminoglycosides may be partly inactivated in purulent bronchial secretions by the acidic pH environment and the large binding to nucleoproteins present at high concentrations in purulent bronchial secretions.[39] Similarly, some of the β-lactam antibiotics are inactivated by β-lactamases produced by Enterobacteriaciae colonizing the respiratory tract.[43]

Local antibiotic administration allows the delivery of high concentrations at the site of infection while reducing the risk of systemic toxicity. For the respiratory tract, two methods of local delivery have been developed: (1) direct injection in the tracheal lumen of intubated or tracheostomized patients of the antibiotic diluted in 2 to 5 ml of saline, either intermittently or continuously, and (2) aerosolization by administration with a nebulizer. The drug bioavailability following aerosol delivery depends markedly on the patient's ability to inhale in a controlled fashion and on the droplet size generated by the nebulizer. The optimal size of the particles is between 2 and 5μ. Below this size, particles will not deposit; conversely, beyond this size, particles will deposit in the upper respiratory tract.[57] The available agents for local antibiotic administration to the lungs have increased so as to be useful in a broader array of bacterial and some fungal, protozoal, and viral infections.

ANTIBACTERIAL THERAPY

Pharmacokinetics

Among the different classes of antibiotics, the aminoglycosides have been the most commonly used in local therapy in pulmonary infections. The aminoglycosides have high bactericidal activity against pulmonary pathogens, especially multiresistant gram-negative bacteria. However, the concentration levels in bronchial secretions are low, representing only 20 to 40 percent of corresponding plasma levels after systemic administration of amikacin and gentamicin respectively, and up to 60 percent for tobramycin.[6] Moreover, the narrow therapeutic index does not allow an increase in the systemic dosage. Thus, local aminoglycoside delivery to the lungs is potentially attractive, and has been studied extensively. It should be stressed that aerosolized or endotracheally injected drugs will not reach nonventilated areas because of bronchial obstruction, atelectasis, or consolidation, which may limit the access of inhaled drugs to infected tissue.

The pulmonary disposition of aerosolized gentamicin was evaluated in a study of patients with cystic fibrosis.[29] Only 10 percent of the gentamicin dose reached the lungs, with the deposition markedly influenced by the patient's pulmonary function. A significant fraction of the dose—up to 90 percent—is lost owing to impaction in the mouth or swallowing or leakage into the environment or is left as a residuum in the nebulizer. High gentamicin sputum levels correlate with central pulmonary deposition and severely compromised pulmonary function, while lower gentamicin sputum levels correspond to peripheral distribution in patients with conserved pulmonary function. The concentrations obtained in sputum and bronchial mucosa are generally above the MIC values of the main pulmonary pathogens. For a given dose, sputum drug levels are significantly higher after direct instillation than after aerosolization.[3] Because of methodologic difficulties with measurement of antibiotic levels in sputum and bronchial secretions, precise drug levels are not reliable and can be used only as a crude estimate of the concentration achieved by local therapy. For gentamicin, at the intratracheally injected dose of 2 mg/kg, a mean concentration as high as 480 μg/ml was measured 30 min after direct instillation in tracheotomized patients.[52] The clearance of instilled antibiotics from the lungs is slow, as attested by residual concentrations of 43 and 14 μg/ml after 4 and 6 h, respectively.

Aerosolization of the same dose of gentamicin (2 mg/kg) produces much lower concentrations in bronchial secretions, with a mean level of 22 μg/ml. Another study,[29] using a similar dose (160 mg) of aerosolized gentamicin in patients with cystic fibrosis, showed higher levels (up to 400 μg/ml in sputum). This difference may reflect central disposition of the aerosol in patients with compromised lung function. Aerosolization of 80 mg of tobramycin produces low concentrations (2 μg/ml) in the bronchoalveolar lavage (BAL) fluid,[4] while sisomicin instilled endotracheally at the dose of 0.7 mg/kg showed very high levels (up to 1300 μg/ml).[69] For netilmicin instilled endotracheally by continuous administration, doses higher than 8 mg/kg resulted in accumulation of the drug in the serum, without renal insufficiency.[1]

The pulmonary fate of inhaled or instilled aminoglycoside on tissue or cellular levels remains unclear. There is good evidence that deposition and removal kinetics are a function of droplet size. Binding of the aminoglycoside to nucleoproteins in purulent bronchial secretions decreases the pulmonary bioavailability of the drug. The proportion that is taken up by the alveolar macrophages and the epithelial lining cells is unknown. Mucociliary clearance seems to be the major route of elimination, although a small proportion of the administered dose is absorbed by the bronchial mucosa mainly through passive diffusion mechanism. Systemic absorption is higher after direct instillation than after aerosol delivery. In most studies, the serum levels of the aminoglycoside—gentamicin, tobramycin, or sisomycin—were less than 1 μg/ml after local administration.[3,12,52,69] In patients with decreased renal function, however, gentamicin serum levels as high as 4 μg/ml have been reported.[37] Measurements of urinary excretion of aminoglycosides administered endotracheally suggest that 15 to 17 percent of the aminoglycoside dose directly injected in the tracheal lumen is recovered from the 24-h collected urine and represents the amount of absorbed drug. By contrast, after aerosolization of 80 mg of gentamicin and 250 mg of kanamycin, the proportion recovered from urine was only 1 to 5 percent, indicating negligible systemic absorption.[40,56]

In addition to aminoglycosides, other antibiotics have been delivered locally to the lungs. These include polymyxin B,[18] chloramphenicol derivatives,[54] amoxycillin,[64] carbenicillin,[62] cephaloridine,[51] and ceftazidime.[62] All have been used mainly

with aerosol delivery. Only the pharmacokinetic parameters of ceftazidime have been well studied. Ceftazidime gave comparable bronchial concentrations after either direct insillation or aerosolization, with peak levels well above the MICs of most pulmonary pathogens and a prolonged lung residence time. After the direct instillation of 1 g of ceftazidime, the mean peak concentration obtained in bronchial mucosa was 1300 μg/ml and the mean residual concentration after 24 h was 57 μg/ml.[62]

Clinical Efficacy

PROPHYLAXIS

Intubated and tracheotomized patients admitted to the intensive care unit (ICU) are at high risk of nosocomial pneumonia. As a consequence of alterations of local defense mechanisms, the respiratory tract is frequently colonized by gram-negative bacilli. Local delivery of antibiotics to the respiratory tract by either direct instillation or aerosolization is aimed at reducing the rate of colonization and the prevention of nosocomial pneumonia. Three consecutive trials using aerosol of polymyxin B have addressed this issue.[18,22,33] In the first, tracheal colonization by gram-negative bacilli was significantly reduced by polymyxin B aerosol as compared to placebo (21 versus 68 percent). The two subsequent trials showed a reduction in the overall incidence of pneumonia in patients admitted to the ICU. However, they failed to demonstrate a reduction in mortality. Moreover, when polymyxin B aerosol was used over a 7-month period, emergence of polymyxin-resistant organisms was observed and associated with fatal pneumonias.

Another study, by Klastersky and colleagues,[32] used direct endotracheal instillation of 80 mg of gentamicin, three times daily, in a double-blind, controlled trial against placebo, in 85 tracheotomized neurosurgical patients. Tracheal colonization by gram-negative bacilli, pneumonia, and associated mortality were less frequent in the group receiving endotracheal gentamicin. A similar placebo-controlled trial, by Lode and associates,[41] used gentamicin 40 mg four times daily as direct endotracheal instillations in 162 intubated patients (85 patients received endotracheal gentamicin and 77 patients received placebo). The incidence of pneumonia during the 16 days after assisted ventilation was 34 and 32 percent, respectively. However, colonization by antibiotic-resistant *P. aeruginosa* was 2.7 percent and 7.8 percent respectively. Despite the reduction in the colonization rate, the incidence of pneumonia and the mortality were not decreased significantly by the endotracheal gentamicin. In some studies, prophylactic administration of antibiotics to the lungs has been coupled to selective digestive decontamination. These studies, like those described previously, are often difficult to evaluate and compare, given a lack of consensus for definition of clinical and microbiologic evaluations and endpoints.

CYSTIC FIBROSIS

Aerosolized antibiotics have also been given for prophylaxis in patients with cystic fibrosis. Pulmonary infection is responsible for 75 percent of hospitalizations and 72 percent of deaths in this disease. *Pseudomonas aeruginosa* is the predominant pathogen, accounting for 70 to 88 percent of episodes.[19] Many different antibiotics have been used as aerosol therapy in trials for prophylaxis in cystic fibrosis with different end points. In 1981, a controlled study by Hodson and coworkers[28] comparing a nebulized combination of carbenicillin (1 g) and gentamicin (80 mg), twice daily, with placebo showed a reduction in the rate of decline of pulmonary function and less frequent hospitalizations. Another nebulized combination, using ticarcillin (1 g) and tobramycin (80 mg), twice daily, also showed less frequent hospitalizations and increases in the body weight of the children; however, lung function tests remained unchanged when compared before and after therapy. Nebulized gentamicin alone, at 20 to 80 mg twice or thrice daily, did not show any benefit,[36,50] while nebulized tobramycin, 80 mg twice or thrice daily, demonstrated a slowing of the decline in respiratory function.[42,63]

Colistin, a polymyxin antibiotic with good activity against *P. aeruginosa,* has been administered by Jensen and colleagues[31] (nebulized colistin, 1 million units twice daily), in a randomized, double-blind, placebo-controlled study, to 29 patients with cystic fibrosis. Lung function, respiratory clinical scores, and inflammatory parameters were improved by colistin aerosol. By contrast, the study by Nolan's team,[51] which included the greatest number of patients (47 over 2 years), did not demonstrate any advantage of the cephaloridine aerosol as compared to a control group. All patients received oral cloxacillin. The lack of activity of the antibiotics used in this study against *P. aeruginosa* may explain the relative therapeutic failure.

In order to establish the benefits and risks of nebulized antipseudomonal therapy in cystic fibrosis, a meta-analysis combining the results of five controlled trials has been performed. This analysis showed a clear benefit for nebulized antipseudomonal antibiotic therapy, with no demonstrable adverse effect other than an increase in the in vitro antibiotic resistance of *P. aeruginosa.*[48] Some investigators have advocated aerosol antibiotic prophylaxis from the time of diagnosis of the cystic fibrosis. As a result, aminoglycoside aerosols are being delivered early in the course of disease in order to prevent colonization by *P. aeruginosa.* The long-term impact of this approach in regard to efficacy and changing microbiologic flora and resistance patterns remains to be established.

OTHER INFECTIONS

The use of local antibiotic administration in the treatment of pulmonary infection remains controversial. In experimental animal models, a single dose of kanamycin (5 mg/kg), delivered either by aerosol or intramuscularly, improved survival in mice infected by an aerosol of *Klebsiella pneumoniae.* Similar results were obtained with 10 mg/kg of kanamycin given over 3 days, or 24 to 48 h after infection.

Assessment of the clinical efficacy of local therapies is difficult, especially in mechanically ventilated patients. Pines and associates[55] treated 81 patients with chronic bronchiectasis with exacerbations, including purulent secretions; most were colonized by *P. aeruginosa.* The patients received a variety of regimens, including aerosolized gentamicin, colistin, or carbenicillin as adjunctive measures to parenteral antibiotics. No advantage could be demonstrated from the aerosol therapy in this study.

In clinical studies by Klastersky, local administration of gentamicin (80 mg every 8 h) or sisomicin (25 mg every 8 h) in in-

tubated patients in ICUs was found to significantly improve outcomes of patients with nosocomial pneumonia when combined with parenteral therapy. However, favorable responses were noted only for organisms *susceptible* to the locally administered agent. Subsequent studies have suggested, however, that clinical outcome may not be affected by local (tobramycin) administration *despite* improved clearance of pulmonary organisms.[7] Often, the observed clearance or reduction of pulmonary infection achieved with local therapy is transitory—reflecting the local kinetics of the antibiotic levels achieved. Bacterial resistance to the locally administered agent has emerged during the course of such treatments. Thus, it may be reasonable to reserve topical treatments, if any, for difficult-to-treat pulmonary infections to avoid progressive colonization with resistant, nosocomial organisms.

LOCAL TOLERANCE

Aerosol antibiotic therapy may cause irritation of the throat and bronchi, with reflex coughing and bronchospasm. Factors related to the aerosolized solution seem to play an important role in local toxicities. Impairment in respiratory function may be greater with hypertonic solutions such as ticarcillin (3080 mosmol/kg) than with isotonic saline or hypotonic tobramycin solution.[66] The molecule itself, in the case of polymyxin B, or the addition of preservatives, including bisulfites, can trigger severe bronchospasm. Dally and colleagues[14] demonstrated that the solvent for aerosolized gentamicin, when nebulized separately, induced bronchospasm in asthmatic patients. Thus, powder-base and lyophilized products may be preferred to commercially available solutions. Most factors, such as chronic bronchitis and bronchial hypersensitivity, have also been implicated in local toxicity. Gorski and coworkers[21] reported the occurrence of bronchospasm associated with elevated histaminemia in 85 percent of asthmatic patients who received polymyxin B aerosol. Dickie and DeGroot[16] showed significant decreases in the maximum expired volume per second in 17 patients with chronic bronchitis after kanamycin or polymyxin B aerosol.

Direct instillation of aminoglycosides—including gentamicin, sisomicin, amikacin, and tobramycin—has been well tolerated. However, it should be stressed that patients should be followed for deterioration in respiratory function on tests performed before and after aerosol therapy in order to detect bronchial hypersensitivity.

SYSTEMIC TOXICITY

No untoward systemic toxicity has been reported for aerosol and endotracheally instilled antibiotic therapy. In patients with renal impairment, however, potentially toxic levels may be achieved in the serum with the endotracheal instillation of aminoglycosides, especially when systemic aminoglycoside therapy is in use.[37] Therefore, monitoring of serum levels is mandatory in patients with renal failure.

EMERGENCE OF RESISTANT BACTERIA

Bacterial resistance resulting from exposure to inhaled or instilled antibiotic is a major concern. The occurrence of bacterial resistance has been reported mainly in prophylactic studies, and more frequently in hospitalized patients with tracheostomies or assisted ventilation, rather than in patients with chronic cystic fibrosis. In cystic fibrosis, resistant *P. aeruginosa* colonization has been observed following local therapy, but without clinical consequences. Emergence of polymyxin-resistant strains has been observed during sustained use of polymyxin B aerosol over a prolonged period; this resulted in an increased incidence of pneumonia, with high mortality.[18] Endotracheally instilled gentamicin has also been associated with the emergence of resistant pathogens, including *Providencia* and *Pseudomonas*.[32] Inhaled or instilled antibiotics may select for intrinsically resistant pathogens; this has been seen with the prophylactic use of colistin aerosol in cystic fibrosis. Superinfection by *Burkholderia* (formerly *Pseudomonas*) *cepacia,* which is intrinsically resistant to colistin, has been observed.[8] Therefore, the potential for selecting multiply resistant microorganisms has to be evaluated carefully. Surveillance cultures are mandatory in patients receiving endotracheal instillation of antibiotics, in order to detect the possible emergence of resistance.

EXPOSURE OF HEALTH-CARE WORKERS

Leakage of antibiotics in the environment, during nebulization or after exhalation, may theoretically expose the health-care workers to potentially noxious substances. Local irritation with allergic rhinitis, conjunctivitis, or bronchospasm should be considered, although few reports of such events exist. The use of aerosolized ribavirin for the treatment of respiratory syncytial virus (RSV), for example, has been implicated in bronchospasm, eye irritation, contact lens damage, and other upper respiratory symptoms in health-care workers. Infection due to *Mycobacterium tuberculosis* has been spread to health-care workers caring for AIDS patients receiving prophylaxis for *Pneumocystis* infection with aerosolized pentamidine. Many new nebulizers include filtration, scavengers, and valve systems to limit the release of antibiotics to the environment.[68]

Possible Impact of the AIDS Epidemic

Bacterial pneumonia is a major cause of morbidity and mortality in patients with advanced HIV disease. A substantial number of these patients develop recurrent pulmonary infections, with repeated hospitalizations, and chronic colonization by *P. aeruginosa.* The evolution in bronchiectasis and pulmonary damage in this subgroup of HIV patients is similar to that in cystic fibrosis patients, and may encourage the evaluation of new aerosol antibiotic therapies.

New Developments

The amount of drug delivered by aerosolization is often limited by the inhalation time. Alert patients usually complete therapy in 15 to 30 min. In order to increase the efficiency of drug delivery, micronized powders have been tested. Micronized gentamicin powder delivery induced bronchial gentamicin levels similar to those achieved after jet nebulizer delivery. However, irritation of the throat with reflex coughing occurred in 50 percent of the patients.[20] Nebulization of drug-containing liposomes

is a promising alternative. Liposomes can facilitate the nebulization of poorly water-soluble drugs. They can serve as pulmonary reservoir for the nebulized drug and may increase the pulmonary residence time. Liposomes may also serve as a targeting vehicle of the antibiotic to specific cells, such as the alveolar macrophages.[59] Liposomal amikacin demonstrated enhanced in vitro activity against *Mycobacterium aviumintracellulare* in alveolar macrophages.[70]

The cost-effectiveness of the inhaled or instilled antibiotics has not been assessed adequately. Defining the most cost-effective strategy may help in selecting between preventive or adjunctive local therapy. This is an important issue to be addressed in the next few years.

ANTIFUNGAL THERAPY

Two methods of local antifungal drug delivery to the lungs have been developed: intracavitary instillation and aerosol therapy. Experience with both is very limited. Intracavitary instillation of antifungal drugs was studied in patients with symptomatic and inoperable aspergilloma. In 1970, 23 patients with such disease were treated by direct intracavitary injections of a paste containing nystatin or amphotericin B, with encouraging results.[35] A more recent study,[26] reporting on six patients with symptomatic aspergilloma, demonstrated clinical and radiologic improvement in four after percutaneous intracavitary instillation of amphotericin B. Single daily instillations up to 50 mg were well tolerated, and cumulative doses up to 500 mg were achieved without any systemic toxicity. Thus, bronchoscopically directed instillation of antifungal therapy could be an alternative in central pulmonary lesions. It should be stressed that systemic antifungal therapy is often disappointing for treatment of aspergilloma.

Aerosolization of amphotericin B has been studied by Schmitt and colleagues[58] in an experimental rat model of pulmonary aspergillosis. They were able to show that inhaled amphotericin B was biologically available, with excellent activity in preventing the spread of infection as well as in curing established infection. In humans, inhaled amphotericin B has rarely been used for therapy. Eisenberg and Oatway[17] reported on four cases of coccidioidomycosis treated with 40 mg of aerosolized amphotericin B once daily. They observed a clinical abatement of the infection, without any significant toxicity.

More experience is available in the prevention of fungal infection by inhaled amphotericin B. In granulocytopenic patients, amphotericin B nasal spray was well tolerated, decreased the nasopharyngeal colonization by *Aspergillus,* and significantly reduced the incidence of invasive aspergillosis.[45] However, when *Aspergillus* spores have already colonized the lower respiratory tract, which is not reached by the nasal spray, efficacy is reduced.[13] Aerosolized amphotericin B, which can diffuse to the bronchioles and alveolar spaces, may eliminate the problem of inhaled spores. Conneally's team,[9] in a noncomparative study of aerosolized amphotericin B (10 mg once daily) delivered prophylactically to granulocytopenic patients, observed a marked reduction in the incidence of invasive aspergillosis in comparison to historical controls. The local tolerance of the aerosol was excellent, with the exception of mild nausea during the inhalation.

No systemic toxicity was observed, indicating that negligible systemic spillover of amphotericin B occurred. Another noncontrolled pilot study reported one case of invasive aspergillosis in 40 bone marrow transplant recipients receiving 10 mg of nebulized amphotericin B twice daily. However, further prospective randomized trials are needed to assess the role of inhaled amphotericin B in the prevention of pulmonary aspergillosis.

ANTIVIRAL THERAPY

Ribavirin has excellent in vitro activity against many viruses, including influenza A and B and RSV. Nebulized ribavirin, in a daily dose of 10 to 16 mg/kg, has been delivered safely over a period of 12 to 20 h a day for at least 3 to 6 days. Higher daily doses, up to three times the usual dose, have been delivered over a short period 2 h a day) for 5 days without increased toxicity. Higher concentrations in bronchial secretions were achieved secondary to this modification.[34] The efficacy of nebulized ribavirin has been studied mainly in children, with or without underlying diseases, who developed RSV bronchiolitis. Most of these studies were double-blind and placebo-controlled. They demonstrated a more rapid clinical improvement with the nebulized ribavirin than with the placebo, even for those with mechanical ventilation.[23,24] The effect on viral shedding was variably reported, with a more rapid clearance in favor of the nebulized ribavirin. Studies on clinical efficacy of ribavirin aerosol in adults are scarce. Anecdotal reports have shown clinical responses in healthy adult patients and in renal transplantation recipients with serious RSV pneumonia.[2,53]

ANTI-*PNEUMOCYSTIS* THERAPY

Local, pulmonary anti-*Pneumocystis* prophylaxis and therapy using aerosolized pentamidine (AP) are discussed in detail elsewhere (see Chapter 150). When given parenterally, pentamidine induces major side effects, such as hypotension, hypoglycemia, arrhythmia, and renal insufficiency, which are seen less often with aerosolized drug. AP also carries the potential for achieving sustained levels in the alveolar spaces, which are the primary site of *P. carinii* replication. The comparison of AP with intravenous administration, in experimental animal models, found higher concentrations in the alveolar space with AP, while systemic drug levels were negligible.[15] This has been confirmed in human studies. Higher concentrations of pentamidine in BAL fluid (705 ± 242 versus 9.3 ± 1.7 ng/ml) and lower systemic concentrations (5.9 ± 0.9 versus 60.5 ± 15 ng/ml) were obtained with AP than with intravenous therapy.[10,47,60] Throat irritation with reflex coughing occurs in 10 to 20 percent of patients and bronchospasm in 1 to 2 percent.[11] Parageusia was transient. However, hypoglycemia may occur in up to 27 percent of the patients during the administration of AP.[47] Several controlled trials with a variety of regimens have demonstrated *Pneumocystis* breakthrough rates of 9 percent for primary or secondary prophylaxis, compared with 27 to 50 percent for placebo.[38,46,49]

In the San Francisco dose comparison study,[38] patients were randomized to receive 30 mg bimonthly, 150 mg bimonthly, or 300 mg monthly. AP was delivered with the Respirgard II Nebulizer System. The mean duration of follow-up was 10 months. The lowest recurrence rate of infection (6.2 percent) was observed in the group receiving 300 mg monthly. Consequently, this regimen has been approved by the Food and Drug Administration for prophylaxis of *P. caninii* pneumonia (PCP). In two randomized trials including high-risk HIV patients treated with oral trimethoprim-sulfamethoxazole (TMP-SMX), in both primary and secondary PCP prophylaxis, a clear clinical superiority of oral TMP-SMX was noted, with greater cost-effectiveness.[25] In addition, TMP-SMX has the potential for protection against other major opportunistic infections, including toxoplasmosis. Moreover, some limitations to AP prophylaxis have appeared, including extrapulmonary infections, atypical presentations of PCP, and pneumothoraces. Therefore, TMP-SMX is recommended as the first-line choice for PCP prophylaxis. AP represents a reasonable alternative for patients who cannot tolerate TMP-SMX.

CONCLUSION

Local antibiotic therapy delivered to the lungs, either by direct endotracheal instillation or by aerosolization, carries the potential of achieving high concentrations in bronchial secretions and bronchial mucosa. Nebulized antipseudomonal antibiotic therapy has an established beneficial effect on pulmonary exacerbations, respiratory pseudomonal load, and spirometric lung function in cystic fibrosis. Endotracheal instillation of aminoglycosides may be useful as adjuvant to systemic treatment of nosocomial pneumonia in tracheotomized and ventilated patients. Aerosolized pentamidine for PCP prophylaxis constitutes a good alternative to TMP-SMX in case of allergy or intolerance. The role of nebulized ribavirin and amphotericin B should be assessed further.

REFERENCES

1. Aguilera D, Coupry A, Holzapfel L, et al: Etude des concentrations sériques et bronchiques au cours de l'administration continue de nétilmicine intratrachéale. *Pathol Biol (Paris)* 34:657–662, 1986.
2. Aylward RB, Burdge DR: Ribavirin therapy of adult respiratory syncytial virus pneumonitis. *Arch Intern Med* 151:2303–2304, 1991.
3. Baran D, Dachy A, Klastersky J: Concentration of gentamicin in bronchial secretions of children with cystic fibrosis or tracheotomy. *Int Clin Pharmacol* 12:336–341, 1975.
4. Baran D, de Vuyst P, Ooms HA: Concentration of tobramycin given by aerosol in the fluid obtained by bronchoalveolar lavage. *Respir Med* 84:203–204, 1990.
5. Berendt RF, Long GG, Walker JS: Treatment of respiratory *Klebsiella pneumoniae* infection in mice with aerosols of kanamycin. *Antimicrob Agents Chemother* 8:585–590, 1975.
6. Bergogne-Berezin E: Penetration of antibiotics into the respiratory tree. *J Antimicrob Chemother* 8:171–174, 1982.
7. Brown RB, Kruse JA, Counts GW, et al., and the Endotracheal Tobramycin Study Group: Double-blind study of endotracheal tobramycin in the treatment of gram-negative bacterial pneumonia. *Antimicrob Agents Chemother* 34:269–272, 1990.
8. Chua HL, Collis GG, Le Souëf PN: Bronchial response to nebulized antibiotics in children with cystic fibrosis. *Eur Respir J* 3:1114–1116, 1990.

9. Conneally E, Cafferkey MT, Daly PA, et al: Nebulized amphotericin B as prophylaxis against invasive aspergillosis in granulocytopenic patients. *Bone Marrow Transplant* 5:403–406, 1990.

10. Conte JE Jr, Hollander H, Golden JA: Inhaled or reduced-dose intravenous pentamidine for *Pneumocystis carinii* pneumonia. *Ann Intern Med* 107:495–498, 1987.

11. Corkery KJ, Luce JM, Montgomery AB: Aerosolized pentamidine for treatment and prophylaxis of *Pneumocystis carinii* pneumonia: An update. *Respir Care* 33:676–685, 1988.

12. Crosby SS, Edwards WA, Brennan C, et al: Systemic absorption of endotracheally administered aminoglycosides in seriously ill patients with pneumonia. *Antimicrob Agents Chemother* 31:850–853, 1987.

13. Cushing D, Bustamante C, Devlin C, et al: Aspergillus infection prophylaxis: Amphotericin-B (AB) nose spray, a double-blind trial. Program and Abstract of the 31st Interscience Conference on Antimicrobial Agents and Chemotherapy, American Society for Microbiology (eds), 737, 1991.

14. Dally MB, Kurrle S, Berslin ABX: Ventilatory effects of aerosol gentamicin. *Thorax* 33:54–56, 1978.

15. Debs RJ, Straubinger RM, Brunette EN, et al: Selective enhancement of pentamidine uptake in the lung by aerosolization and delivery in liposomes. *Am Rev Respir Dis* 135:731–737, 1987.

16. Dickie KJ, DeGroot WJ: Ventilatory effects of aerosolized kanamycin and polymyxin. *Chest* 63:694–697, 1973.

17. Eisenberg RS, Oatway WH: Nebulization of amphotericin B. *Am Rev Respir Dis* 103:289–292, 1971.

18. Feeley TW, Dumoulin GC, Hedley-Whyte J, et al: Aerosol polymyxin and pneumonia in seriously ill patients. *New Engl J Med* 293:471–475, 1975.

19. Galanternik L, Gubbay L, Lopez Holtmann G, Marcri CN: Microbiology of the pulmonary secretions in cystic fibrosis (CF). Program and abstract of the 36th Interscience Conference on Antimicrobial Agents and Chemotherapy, American Society for Microbiology (eds), K95, 267, 1996.

20. Goldman JM, Boyston SM, O'Connor S, Meigh RE: Inhaled micronized entamicin powder: A new delivery system. *Thorax* 45:939–940, 1990.

21. Gorski P, Rosniecki J, Szmidt M, Rychlicka I: Pulmonary function and histaminemia after polymyxin B. *Agents Actions* 11:74–75, 1981.

22. Greenfield S, Teres D, Bushnell LS, et al: Prevention of gram-negative bacillary pneumonia using aerosol polymyxin as prophylaxis. I: Effect on the colonization pattern of the upper respiratory tract of seriously ill patients. *J Clin Invest* 52:2935–2940, 1973.

23. Hall CB, McBride JT, Gala CL, et al: Ribavirin treatment of respiratory syncytial viral infection in infants with underlying cardiopulmonary disease. *JAMA* 254:3047–3051, 1985.

24. Hall CB, McBride JT, Walsh EE, et al: Aerosolized ribavirin treatments of infants with respiratory syncytial viral infection: A randomized double-blind study. *New Engl J Med* 308:1443–1447, 1983.

25. Hardy WD, Feinberg J, Finkelstein DM, et al: A controlled trial of trimethoprim–sulfamethoxazole or aerosolized pentamidine for secondary prophylaxis of *Pneumocystis carinii* pneumonia in patients with the acquired immunodeficiency syndrome. *New Engl J Med* 327:1842–1848, 1992.

26. Hargis JL, Bone RC, Stewart J, et al: Intracavitary amphotericin B in the treatment of symptomatic pulmonary aspergillomas. *Am J Med* 68:389–394, 1980.

27. Hers JG, Mulder J: The mucosal epithelium of the respiratory tract in mucopurulent bronchitis caused by *Haemophilus influenzae*. *J Pathol Bacteriol* 66:103–108, 1953.

28. Hodson ME, Penketh AR, Batten JC: Aerosol carbenicillin and gentamicin treatment of *Pseudomonas aeruginosa* infection in patients with cystic fibrosis. *Lancet* 2:1137–1139, 1981.

29. Ilowite JS, Gorvoy JD, Smaldone GC: Quantitative deposition of aerosolized gentamicin in cystic fibrosis. *Am Rev Respir Dis* 136:1445–1449, 1987.

30. Itoh H, Ishii Y, Maeda H, et al: Clinical observations of aerosol deposition in patients with airways obstruction. *Chest* 80:837–840, 1991.

31. Jensen T, Pederson SS, Garne S, et al: Colistin inhalation therapy in cystic fibrosis patients with chronic *Pseudomonas aeruginosa* lung infection. *J Antimicrob Chemother* 19:831–838, 1987.

32. Klastersky J, Huysmand E, Weerts D, et al: Endotracheally administered gentamicin for the prevention of infection of the respiratory tract in patients with tracheostomy: A double-blind study. *Chest* 65:650–654, 1974.

33. Klick JM, du Moulin GC, Hedley-Whyte J, et al: Prevention of gram-negative bacillary pneumonia using polymyxin aerosol as prophylaxis. II: Effect on the incidence of pneumonia in seriously ill patients. *J Clin Invest* 55:514–519, 1975.

34. Knight V, Wilson SZ, Quarles JM, et al: Ribavirin small-particle aerosol treatment of influenzae. *Lancet* 2:945–949, 1981.

35. Krakowska P, Traczyk K, Walczak J, et al: Local treatment of aspergilloma of the lung with a paste containing nystatin or amphotericin B. *Tubercle* 51:184–191, 1970.

36. Kun P, Landau LI, Phelan PD: Nebulized gentamicin in children and adolescents with cystic fibrosis. *Aust Paediatr J* 20:43–45, 1984.

37. Lake KB, Van Dijke JJ, Rumsfeld JA: Combined topical pulmonary and systemic gentamicin: The question of safety. *Chest* 68:62–64, 1975.

38. Leoung GS, Feigal DW Jr, Montgomery AB, et al, and the San Francisco County Community Consortium: Aerosolized pentamidine for prophylaxis against *Pneumocystis carinii* pneumonia. *New Engl J Med* 323:769–775, 1990.

39. Levy J: Antibiotic activity in sputum. *J Pediatr* 108:841–846, 1986.

40. Lifschitz MI, Denning CR: Safety of kanamycin aerosol. *Clin Pharmacol Ther* 12:91–95, 1971.

41. Lode H, Hoffken G, Kemmerich B, Schaberg T: Systemic and endotracheal antibiotic prophylaxis of nosocomial pneumonia in ICU. *Intensive Care Med* (Suppl 1) 18:S24–S27, 1992.

42. MacLushky IB, Gold R, Corey M, Levison H: Long-term effects of inhaled tobramycin in patients with cystic fibrosis colonized with *Pseudomonas aeruginosa*. *Pediatr Pulmonol* 7:42–48, 1989.

43. Maddocks JL, May FR: "Indirect pathogenicity" of penicillinase-producing enterobacteria in chronic bronchial infections. *Lancet* 1:793–795, 1969.

44. May JR: The laboratory background to the use of penicillin in chronic bronchitis and bronchiectasis. *Br J Tuberc Dis Chest* 49:166–173, 1955.

45. Meunier-Carpentier F, Snoeck R, Gerain J, et al: Amphotericin B nasal spray as prophylaxis against aspergillosis in patients with neutropenia (letter). *New Engl J Med* 311:1056, 1984.

46. Montaner JSG, Lawson LW, Gervais L, et al: Aerosol pentamidine for secondary prophylaxis of AIDS-related *Pneumocystis carinii* pneumonia: A randomized, placebo-controlled study. *Ann Intern Med* 114:948–953, 1991.

47. Montgomery AB, Debs RJ, Luce JM, et al: Aerosolized pentamidine as sole therapy for *Pneumocystis carinii* pneumonia in patients with the acquired immunodeficiency syndrome. *Lancet* 2:480–483, 1987.

48. Mukhopadhyay S, Singh M, Cater JI, et al: Neublized antipseudomonal antibiotic therapy in cystic fibrosis: A meta-analysis of benefits and risks. *Thorax* 51:364–368, 1996.

49. Murphy RL, Lavelle JP, Allan JD, et al: Aerosol pentamidine prophylaxis following *Pneumocystis carinii* pneumonia in AIDS patients: Results of a blinded dose-comparison study using an ultrasonic nebulizer. *Am J Med* 90:418–426, 1991.

50. Nathanson I, Cropp GJA, Li P: Effectiveness of aerosolized gentamicin in cystic fibrosis. *Cystic Fibrosis Club Abstracts* 26:145, 1985.

51. Nolan G, McIvor P, Levison H, et al: Antibiotic prophylaxis in cystic fibrosis: Inhaled cephaloridine as an adjunct to oral cloxacillin. *J Pediatr* 101:626–630, 1982.

52. Odio W, Van Laer E, Klastersky J: Concentrations of gentamicin in bronchial secretions after intramuscular and endotracheal administration. *J Clin Pharmacol* 15:518–524, 1975.

53. Peigue-Lafeuille H, Gazuy N, Mignot P, et al: Severe respiratory syncytial virus pneumonia in an adult renal transplant recipient: Successful treatment with ribavirin. *Scand J Infect Dis* 22:87–89, 1990.

54. Pines A, Bundi RS, Greenfield JSB: Chloramphenicol analogues in the intrabronchial treatment of severe chronic chest infections. *Br J Dis Chest* 59:81–89, 1965.

55. Pines A, Raafat H, Siddiqui GM, Greenfield JSB: Treatment of severe *Pseudomonas* infections of the bronchi. *Br Med J* 1:663–665, 1970.

56. Regula H, Wieser O, Naumann P, et al:. Pharmakokinetische Untersuchungen über Sputum-, Serum- und Urinkonzentration von Gentamycin nach Aerosol-Inhalation. *Int J Clin Pharmacol* 7:95–100, 1973.

57. Schleisinger RB: Comparative deposition of inhaled aerosols in experimental animals and humans: A review. *J Toxicol Environ Health* 15:197–214, 1985.

58. Schmitt HJ, Bernard EM, Hauser M, Armstrong D: Aerosol amphotericin B is effective for prophylaxis and therapy in a rat model of pulmonary aspergillosis. *Antimicrob Agents Chemother* 32:1676–1679, 1988.

59. Schreier H: Liposomes aerosols. *J Liposome Res* 2:145–184, 1992.

60. Soo Hoo GW, Mohsenifar Z, Meyer RD: Inhaled or intravenous pentamidine therapy for *Pneumocystis carinii* pneumonia in AIDS: A randomized trial. *Ann Intern Med* 113:195–202, 1990.

61. Spencer H: The bacterial pneumonias, in *Pathology of the Lung.* Elmsford, NY, Pergamon, 1985, pp 167–213.

62. Stead RJ, Hodson ME, Batten JC: Inhaled ceftazidime compared with gentamicin and carbenicillin in older patients with cystic fibrosis infected with *Pseudomonas aeruginosa. Br J Dis Chest* 81:272–279, 1987.

63. Steinkamp G, Tummler B, Gappa M, et al: Long-term tobramycin aerosol therapy in cystic fibrosis. *Pediatr Pulmonol* 6:91–98, 1989.

64. Stockley RA, Hill SL, Burnett D: Nebulized amoxicillin in chronic purulent bronchiectasis. *Clin Ther* 7:593–599, 1985.

65. Stoutenbeek CP, van Saene HKF, Miranda DR, Zandstra DF: The effect of selective decontamination of the digestive tract on colonization and infection rate in multiple trauma patients. *Intensive Care Med* 10:185–192, 1984.

66. Tablan OC, Martone WI, Doershuk CF, et al: Colonization of the respiratory tract with *Pseudomonas cepacia* in cystic fibrosis: Risk factors and outcomes. *Chest* 91:527–532, 1987.

67. Taylor AE, Guyton AC, Bishop US: Permeability of the alveolar membrane to solutes. *Circ Res* 16:535–561, 1965.

68. Thomas SHL, Langford JA, George RDG, Geddes DM: Improving the efficiency of drug administration with jet nebulisers (letter). *Lancet* 1:126, 1988.

69. Thys JP, Klastersky J: Concentrations of sisomicin in serum and in bronchial secretions after intratracheal administration, in Seingenthaler W, Luthey R (eds): Current Chemotherapy, American Society of Microbiology, Washington, DC, 920–921, 1978.

70. Wichert BV, Gonzalez-Rothi RJ, Straub LE, et al: Amikacin liposomes: Preparation, characterization and in vitro activity against *Mycobacterium avium-intracellulare* infection in alveolar macrophages. *Int J Pharmaceut* 78:227, 1992.

71. Wiebel ER: The ultrastructure of the alveolar-capillary barrier, in Fishman AP, Hecht HH (eds), *The Pulmonary Circulation and Interstitial Space.* Chicago, University of Chicago Press, 1969.

CHAPTER 124

VACCINATION FOR PULMONARY INFECTIONS

Michael S. Simberkoff

BACTERIAL VACCINES FOR PULMONARY PATHOGENS
 Pneumococcal Vaccine
 H. Influenzae Vaccine
 Pertussis Vaccine
 BCG Vaccine

VACCINES AGAINST VIRAL PULMONARY INFECTIONS
 Influenza Vaccine
 Measles Vaccine
 Varicella Vaccine
 Adenovirus Vaccine

CONCLUSIONS

Vaccines have been developed and are recommended to prevent pulmonary infections. There are several reasons to encourage their use:

1. Pulmonary infections, such as pneumonia, are associated with substantial morbidity. For example, a prospective study carried out in a region of Finland showed that community-acquired pneumonia (CAP) occurred at a rate of 11.6 cases per 1000 inhabitants per year.[39] The incidences of radiographically proven pneumonia were highest among children less than 5 years old and in adults over 60 years of age.

2. Pneumonia and influenza are the most common infections and, overall, the sixth leading reported cause of death in the United States, ranking below heart disease, cancer, stroke, unintentional injury, and chronic obstructive pulmonary disease. In 1994, the crude death rate for pneumonia and influenza in the United States was 31.8 per 100,000 population.[8]

3. Pulmonary pathogens tend to be more resistant to antibiotics, even when acquired in the community. This makes appropriate treatment of these infections increasingly difficult. Resistance has been observed among the bacterial, mycobacterial, and viral microorgansims that infect the lungs. For example, penicillin-resistance was recently found in 25 percent of the invasive *Streptococcus pneumoniae* isolates from patients living in Atlanta.[36] Seven percent of these isolates were highly resistant to penicillin (minimal inhibitory concentration [MIC] of at least 2 μg/ml), 9 percent were resistant to cefotaxime, and 25 percent were resistant to multiple antibiotics. Multidrug-resistant strains of *Mycobacterium tuberculosis* have been documented in diverse loca-

tions in the United States.[4,21,30] Drug resistance also has been detected among viral respiratory pathogens. Strains of influenza A resistant to amantadine hydrochloride were detected in nursing home residents at three facilities in Washington State during 1992.[37] One of these isolates was obtained from a patient before either amantadine or rimantadine was used in that facility.

4. Vaccines that are licensed for use in the United States are remarkably safe. Most produce transient local or, infrequently, mild systemic side effects (described below).

5. The licensed vaccines are effective in preventing pulmonary infections and their complications. However, efficacy may vary in different patient populations. Specific examples will be discussed under individual vaccines.

6. Vaccines are generally inexpensive, whereas the pulmonary infections they prevent are often expensive to diagnose and treat. Further, infected patients are often unable to work for extended periods. Thus, use of vaccines to prevent pulmonary infections is cost-effective for individual patients, employers, insurers, and society.

BACTERIAL VACCINES FOR PULMONARY PATHOGENS

A number of microorganisms infect the lungs, including a diverse group of bacteria, mycobacteria, mycoplasma, chlamydia, viruses, and some fungi. *S. pneumoniae* is the most common cause of CAP, occurring in 20 to 70 percent of cases, and *Hemophilus influenzae* is the second most common pathogen isolated, occurring in 3 to 10 percent of cases (see Chapter 127).[3,23,48,51,65]

Four vaccines against bacterial pulmonary pathogens are available (Table 124-1). These are the *S. pneumoniae* (pneumococcal) polysaccharide vaccine, the *H. influenzae* type b polysaccharide-protein conjugate vaccine, the *Bordetella pertussis* vaccines (whole cell and acellular), and the live bacille Calmette-Guérin (BCG) vaccine.

Pneumococcal Vaccine

The pneumococcal polysaccharide vaccine (PPV) is designed to elicit protective antibody against the strains of *S. pneumoniae*

TABLE 124-1

Vaccines for Bacterial Pulmonary Pathogens

Pathogen	Vaccine	Targeted Population	Frequency
S. pneumoniae	23-valent capsular polysaccharide	Elderly (≥65 years); asplenia; chronic pulmonary, cardiac, or renal diseases; diabetes; HIV	Administer once; may repeat in highest-risk patients after 6 years
H. influenzae type b	Protein-conjugated polysaccharide	Children (2 months to 5 years of age); elderly; chronic pulmonary disease; HIV	Children: 3 doses at 2-month intervals, boosters 12 months later and 4–6 years Adults: Single dose
B. pertussis	Whole-cell (P) and acellular(aP)	Infants and children	1st dose: P, at 2 months 2d dose: P, at 4 months 3d dose: P, at 6 months 4th dose: P or aP, at 15 months Booster dose: P or aP, at 4–6 years of age
M. tuberculosis	Live, attenuated BCG	Infants and children who are PPD negative and continuously exposed to patients with infectious tuberculosis	Children: 0.2–0.3 ml of reconstituted vaccine, percutaneously Infants (< 1 month): Half dose, repeat with full dose at 1 year

NOTE: P = Whole-cell pertussis vaccine; aP = Acellular pertussis vaccine.

that are commonly associated with invasive infection. At present, 83 pneumococcal serotypes are recognized by serologic reactions with their capsular polysaccharide. Included among these are 19 serogroups consisting of two to four antigenically related serotypes. A 14-valent vaccine against pneumococcal capsular polysaccharide was licensed in the United States in 1977, and the current 23-valent vaccine was licensed in 1983. The 23 capsular types included in the pneumococcal capsular polysaccharide vaccine cause 88 percent of the bacteremic pneumococcal disease in the United States.[9]

Efficacy of the PPV was evaluated in three recent studies. In the first of these, Shapiro and coworkers performed a case-control study in 11 hospitals in Connecticut between September 1984 and June 1990.[54] The cases were in adult patients (at least 18 years of age) with S. pneumoniae isolates from blood, pleural fluid, or cerebrospinal fluid and a recognized indication for use of PPV. For each case, a control subject was matched according to age, site of hospitalization, condition that constituted the indication for PPV in the case, and duration of the condition. A total of 1054 case-control pairs were established. Hospital, clinic, and private physician records of each case and control patient were reviewed to determine PPV exposure. Among the patients, 13 percent received PPV, whereas it was administered to 20 percent of the control subjects. The calculated efficacy against strains represented in the 14- or 23-valent pneumococcal vaccines was 61 percent (95 percent confidence intervals [CI], 47 to 72 percent) among immunocompetent case-control pairs, but it was only 21 percent (95 percent CI, 55 to 60 percent) among the immunocompromised case-control pairs.

Butler and colleagues determined the serotypes of 2837 S. pneumoniae isolates from blood or cerebrospinal fluid that were submitted to the Centers for Disease Control and Prevention (CDC) from patients older than 5 years of age between May 1978 and April 1992.[6] With the use of an indirect cohort analysis, the overall efficacy of vaccine for preventing infection by vaccine serotype S. pneumoniae strains was estimated to be 57 percent (95 percent CI, 50 to 95 percent). Efficacy was demonstrated for the subsets of patients with diabetes mellitus, coronary artery disease, congestive heart failure, chronic pulmonary disease, and anatomic asplenia. Efficacy for immunocompetent patients over 65 years of age was estimated to be 75 percent (95 percent CI, 57 to 85 percent). Not surprisingly, efficacy was not demostrated for several groups of immunocompromised patients, including those with immunoglobulin deficiency, multiple myeloma, Hodgkin's disease, non-Hodgkin's lymphoma, leukemia, chronic renal failure, and alcoholism or cirrhosis.

Fine's team performed a meta-analysis of nine randomized, controlled trials of PPV in adults published between 1966 and 1991.[29] The patients in these trials were divided into low- and high-risk groups. The low-risk patients were gold miners, subsistence farmers, mental health patients, and ambulatory patients belonging to a health maintenance program. The high-risk patients were hospice and nursing home patients; those with bronchogenic carcinoma; elderly patients (over 55 years of age); diabetics; those with chronic renal, hepatic, pulmonary, or cardiac diseases; or immunosuppressed patients. The meta-analysis showed that the PPV was effective in the low-risk patients in preventing definitive pneumococcal pneumonia (radiographically proven pneumonia with isolation of S. pneumoniae from blood, transthoracic lung puncture, or normally sterile body fluid); definite vaccine-type pneumococcal pneumonia; presumed pneumococcal pneumonia (radiographically proven pneumonia with isolation of S. pneumoniae from sputum or nasal swab only); and presumed vaccine-type pneumococcal pneumonia. It was not effective in preventing these infections in the high-risk patients.

Two conclusions can be drawn from review of these articles on PPV efficacy. First, the PPV is more effective in preventing invasive disease than uncomplicated pneumococcal pneumonia.

Second, PPV failures are more likely to occur in immunocompromised patients and those in whom chronic disease impairs immunologic function. Therefore, it may be better to immunize patients early in the course of chronic diseases in order to take advantage of their relatively intact immunologic systems.

PPV is recommended for immunocompetent adults at risk for pneumococcal disease or its complications because of chronic diseases (such as diabetes mellitus, alcoholism, cirrhosis, chronic cardiovascular disease, chronic pulmonary disease, and cerebrospinal fluid leak) and for those who are 65 years of age or older.[9] It is also recommended for immunocompromised persons (such as those with functional or anatomic asplenia, Hodgkin's disease, lymphoma, multiple myeloma, chronic renal failure or nephrotic syndrome, transplant recipients and patients receiving immunosuppression, and HIV-infected patients). However, its benefit is less certain in the latter groups.

PPV elicits a type 2, thymus-independent B cell response.[59] As a consequence, it generates few (if any) memory B cells. The lack of memory B cells results in an absence of an anamnestic response after PPV revaccination. Therefore, revaccination should be considered for only the highest-risk patients, and this should be done 6 or more years after initial vaccine administration.

Patients with HIV infection and AIDS have an increased incidence of pneumococcal infections.[52,53,56,64] The available data suggest that patients with AIDS have an impaired response to pneumococcal vaccine and that the response of patients with earlier HIV infection is variable.[2,38] Treatment with zidovudine (AZT) appears to improve the response to pneumococcal vaccine.[32] A protein-conjugated PPV (PCPPV) was used in a small number of HIV-infected patients.[1] The PCPPV elicited a significantly higher IgG response in non–HIV-infected adults than did the polysaccharide vaccine. However, responses to PPV and PCPPV did not differ in the HIV-infected patients.

H. Influenzae Vaccine

H. influenzae is the second most common bacterial pathogen isolated from patients with pneumonia and it is a common cause of bronchitis. Although many of the isolates from respiratory secretions are nontypable, *H. influenzae* type b (Hib) is frequently associated with bacteremic pneumonia. For example, Farley and colleagues found a total of 47 cases of invasive *H. influenzae* infection in patients 18 years of age or older in metropolitan Atlanta during the period from December 1, 1988 to May 31, 1990 and calculated that the annual incidence was 1.7 cases per 100,000 population.[25] Bacteremic pneumonia accounted for 70 percent of the cases, and 55 percent of the 29 pneumonia-associated blood isolates which were serotyped were Hib. The incidence of bacteremic Hib infection increased with age. Twenty-two of the cases reported by Farley et al. occurred in adults over 60 years of age (incidence 5.6 per 100,000 per year), and 21 of these 22 cases were bacteremic pneumonia. Patients with HIV infection are another group at particularly high risk for bacteremic Hib infection.[7]

Safe, immunogenic, protein-conjugated Hib vaccines (HbCV) exist, and these have proved to be remarkably effective in preventing invasive Hib infection in children. For example, in a randomized, controlled trial of 114,000 infants in Finland, there were only four cases of Hib bacteremia among vaccine recipients compared to 64 cases in placebo recipients.[22] In addition, provisional data for 1994 from the National Notifiable Diseases Surveillance System, the National Bacterial Meningitis and Bacteremia Reporting Service, and a multistate laboratory-based surveillance system showed a total of only 60 cases (incidence of 1.7 cases per 100,000) of invasive Hib disease among children less than 5 years of age in the United States.[10] In 1988, the rate of invasive Hib infections in children less than 5 years of age had been over 40 per 100,000. This dramatic decline is a consequence of intensive efforts to immunize young children throughout the United States. Although proof of efficacy of HbCV in adults is lacking, the vaccines are recommended for patients with functional or anatomic asplenia and those with leukemia and HIV infection.[11] In addition, HbCV should be considered for elderly people (over 65 years of age).

Pertussis Vaccine

B. pertussis causes severe whooping cough in infants and young children. In recent years, however, clinical infections have been observed commonly in adolescents and young adults. During the period from 1980 to 1989, 9.9 and 8.9 percent of the cases of pertussis reported to the CDC occurred in adolescents 10 to 19 and adults at least 20 years of age, respectively.[24] Studies of young adults with "persistent" cough reporting to a university student health or urban medical center clinic show evidence of recent *B. pertussis* infection in 20 to 25 percent of cases.[46,67] These data suggest that young adults both are susceptible to *B. pertussis* infection and can serve as a reservoir for its transmission. Indeed, a recent study showed that an adult had the index case in 15 percent of households with pertussis infection.[63]

The typical features of *B. pertussis* infection are a persistent cough, paroxysms of cough followed by inspiratory gasps (whoops), vomiting, cyanosis, and apnea. Complications (e.g., pneumonia, seizures, and encephalopathy) are most common in infants less than 1 year of age and are associated with inadequate vaccination.[24] Death occurs in 0.4 percent of cases.

Two pertussis vaccines are licensed for use in the United States, the whole-cell (P) and acellular (aP) vaccines. Whole-cell vaccines are prepared from disrupted or inactivated whole bacterial suspensions. Acellular vaccines are composed of purified components of the bacteria that are thought to elicit protective immunity. In the United States, the licensed acellular vaccines contain combinations of the filamentous hemagglutinin (FHA); pertussis toxin (PT); pertactin, an outer-membrane protein; and two agglutinogens, fimbriae types 2 and 3.

Pertussis vaccine is generally administered to infants and small children in combination with diphtheria (D) and tetanus (T) vaccines. In the United States, the whole-cell combination (DTP) is recommended for the first three doses at 2 months, 4 months, and 6 months of age.[12,13] A fourth dose, given at 15 months, and a booster dose, given at 4 to 6 years of age, may consist of either DTP or DTaP. While booster doses of DT are recommended at 10-year intervals for adolescents and adults, additional booster doses of P or aP are not recommended. However, the increased recognition of clinically significant pertussis infections in adolescents and adults may stimulate reconsideration of these recommendations.

Both whole-cell and acellular pertussis vaccines are effective. One large review showed that whole-cell vaccine efficacy has ranged from 50 to 90 percent in controlled trials, as high as 100 percent in cohort studies, 4 to 96 percent in secondary attack rate studies, and up to 94 percent in case control studies.[28] Several factors could explain the variation observed. First, most studies have used clinical criteria of whooping cough to determine efficacy. In general, the whole-cell vaccines have proved to be more effective when more severe manifestations of disease were required for case definition. Second, the vaccines used differed, and some P vaccines are clearly more effective than others. Third, the strains of *B. pertussis* that circulated in the communities have differed. This could result in differing antigenic relationships to the vaccines used. Fourth, dose schedules for vaccination varied. It is clear that multiple doses of vaccine are required to elicit protective antibodies. The first of these should be given after 1 month of age, when maternal antibodies have begun to wane. Finally, the duration between final vaccine dose and disease has varied. Pertussis immunity wanes with time.

Controlled trials also confirmed the efficacy of acellular pertussis vaccines. A randomized, double-blind trial conducted in Sweden assigned infants to receive either DT or a DTaP preparation.[61] The acellular pertussis vaccine consisted of a hydrogen peroxide–inactivated pertussis toxoid. The observed efficacy of the DTaP vaccine against confirmed pertussis was 62 percent (95 percent, CI 51 to 70 percent).

Pertussis vaccines may produce significant side effects.[12,13] Local reactions include pain, tenderness, erythema, and induration at the inoculation site. Mild systemic reactions to pertussis vaccines include low-grade fever, drowsiness, fretfulness, and vomiting. Moderate to severe systemic reactions include temperature above 105°F, persistent inconsolable crying lasting at least 3 h, and collapse (hypotonic-hyporesponsive episodes). Local and mild or moderate to severe systemic reactions occur more commonly with whole-cell than with acellular pertussis vaccine. Most severe reactions, such as prolonged convulsions or encephalopathy, have not been reported with the acellular vaccines in use in the United States.

BCG Vaccine

Derivatives of the attenuated bovine tubercle bacillus originally developed by Albert Calmette and Camille Guérin, BCG, are among the most widely studied and used vaccines to prevent pulmonary infection. Despite 60 years of use, there is still debate about the efficacy of BCG. A recently published meta-analysis of trials and case-control studies attempted to resolve some of the controversy.[19] In this meta-analysis, Colditz and coworkers combined data from 15 prospective trials and 10 case-control studies. The combined efficacy of BCG in preventing clinical tuberculosis in the trials was 51 percent (risk ratio 0.49; 95, CI 0.34 to 0.70). Its combined efficacy in preventing clinical tuberculosis in the case-control studies was 50 percent (odds ratio 0.50; 95, CI 0.39 to 0.64). In seven trials, tuberculosis-associated death was evaluated as an endpoint, and its combined efficacy was 71 percent (risk ratio 0.29; 95 percent, CI 0.16 to 0.53). Unfortunately, these data do not resolve all questions concerning BCG vaccine efficacy.

One problem with BCG vaccine is that its observed efficacy varied greatly in different studies, ranging from 0 to 80 percent. An explanation for the observed differences is not obvious. It has been suggested that the differences in efficacy could have been due to differences in the strains of BCG used. However, Brewer and Colditz failed to demonstrate a relationship between the strains of BCG used in specific trials and subsequent protection against clinical tuberculosis.[5] Further, they found that the same BCG strain provided vastly different levels of protection in different trials. Differing degrees of heterologous immunity in populations exposed to different environmental mycobacteria could explain some of the observed differences in BCG vaccine efficacy.[27] However, this hypothesis fails to account for the high prevalence of clinical *M. tuberculosis* infections in areas of the world where exposure to environmental mycobacteria—hence, heterologous immunity—would be most likely to occur.

In the United States, BCG vaccine is recommended to prevent tuberculosis for very limited patient populations.[14,58] It is strongly recommended for PPD-negative infants and children who are at high risk of prolonged exposure to untreated or ineffectively treated patients with infectious pulmonary tuberculosis who cannot be removed from this exposure or placed on long-term treatment. BCG vaccine is also recommended for PPD-negative children who are continuously exposed to persons with infectious tuberculosis known to be resistant to both isoniazid and rifampin, and for PPD-negative children in groups in which the annual rate of new infections exceeds 1 percent per year and for whom surveillance and treatment have been unsuccessfully attempted.

BCG vaccine is not recommended for health-care workers.[14] Instead, precautions are taken to rapidly identify, isolate, and appropriately treat patients, thereby limiting the risk of transmitting *M. tuberculosis* infection within the facility. In addition, early infections in health-care workers are monitored by periodic PPD skin tests and treated with isoniazid prophyaxis when skin-test conversion occurs.

BCG vaccine (Tice strain) is administered percutaneously to PPD-negative infants and children. Infants less than 1 month of age are given half the dose given to older children. A full dose can be given to these children if they remain PPD negative after they reach 1 year of age and other indications for use of the vaccine persist. BCG vaccine should not be given to infants and children with immunodeficiency from congenital disease, HIV infection, leukemia, or lymphoma, or those receiving treatment with immunosuppressants such as steroids, alkalating agents, or radiation treatment.

BCG side effects occur in 1 to 10 percent of vaccine recipients.[14] They include persistent ulcerations at the vaccination site, lymphadenitis, and lupus vulgaris. Osteomyelitis, disseminated infection, and death occur in 1 to 10 per million. These serious side effects generally occur in immunosuppressed patients.

Outside the United States, BCG vaccine is considered an adjunct to national tuberuclosis programs.[66] Rapid case detection and treatment are considered the highest priority for control of tuberculosis. In countries where the prevalence and incidence of *M. tuberculosis* are high, BCG vaccine is recommended for infants as soon after birth as possible and certainly within the first year of life. Revaccination with BCG is not recommended.

VACCINES AGAINST VIRAL PULMONARY INFECTIONS

Although most viral infections of the respiratory tract are transient and benign, some can be associated with serious complications. Vaccines have been developed to prevent infections or to limit the morbidity of some viral respiratory pathogens (Table 124-2). The most important of these are the vaccines against influenza, measles (rubeola), and chickenpox (varicella). An adenovirus vaccine is used exclusively by the military.

Influenza Vaccine

Influenza viruses cause significant morbidity in all groups, but they are a particularly important cause of serious illness among aged and debilitated patients, resulting in hospitalization and mortality. It has been estimated that annual attack rates of influenza are between 10 and 20 percent[43]; more than 20,000 influenza-associated deaths have occurred during epidemics, particularly among the elderly.[15]

Influenza type A viruses are classified into subtypes on the basis of two surface antigens: hemagglutinin, which has three subtypes (H1, H2, and H3), and neuraminidase, which has two subtypes (N1 and N2). Immunity to these antigens, especially the hemagglutinin, reduces the chance of infection and the severity of the disease if infection does occur. Influenza type A and type B undergo antigenic variation, although the latter has more antigenic stability.

Influenza virus infections can be prevented by annual vaccination or, for influenza type A virus, by chemoprophylaxis with amantadine hydrochloride or rimantadine hydrochloride. Influenza vaccines are made from inactivated, egg-grown viruses, which are highly purified. Every year, three virus strains, usually two type A and one type B, are included in the influenza vaccine preparation. These represent the influenza viruses that are anticipated to circulate in the United States during the influenza season. There are generally three types of vaccine preparations available: whole viruses, subvirions, and purified surface antigens. The last two preparations are prescribed for children to minimize febrile reactions. Placebo-controlled trials showed that most patients report mild and transient local reactions to the influenza vaccine (such as arm soreness at the injection site) and that there are no differences in the systemic symptoms reported by vaccine and placebo recipients.[33,44] Unlike the 1967 swine influenza vaccine, recent influenza vaccines have not been associated with Guillain-Barré syndrome.[15] However, a history of a severe allergic reaction to egg protein or other vaccine components is a contraindication to influenza vaccine use.

Influenza vaccines have been effective in preventing secondary bacterial pneumonia as well as influenza hospitalizations in elderly, high-risk populations, and their use reduced mortality from all causes. In a case-control study conducted among participants in an health maintenance organization (HMO) in Portland, Oregon, from 1980 to 1989, Mullooly and colleagues found that the use of the influenza vaccine reduced hospitalizations for influenza and pneumonia by 30 percent (95 percent, CI 17 to 42 percent) among high-risk patients and by 40 percent (95 percent, CI 1 to 64 percent) in non–high-risk, elderly patients.[47] In a nonrandomized study conducted in elderly adults enrolled in an HMO in Minneapolis–St. Paul during three consecutive seasons (1990–93), Nichol and coworkers found that influenza vaccination was associated with a 48 to 57 percent reduction in hospitalizations for influenza and pneumonia, a 27 to 39 percent reduction in hospitalizations for all acute and chronic respiratory disease, and a 39 to 54 percent reduction in mortality.[50] Both of these studies demonstrated that use of the influenza vaccine was cost-effective in the elderly. Even healthy, working adults may benefit from use of the influenza vaccine. A randomized, double-blind, placebo-controlled trial conducted during the 1994–95 season among working adults who were 18 to 64 years of age showed that influenza vaccine use resulted in fewer episodes of upper respiratory infections, fewer days of sick leave, and fewer physician visits.[49]

Influenza vaccines are indicated for persons at increased risk for complications of influenza, health-care workers, persons in close contact with people in high-risk groups, and persons who wish to lessen the likelihood of becoming infected with influenza.[15] Annual revaccination is necessary because antibody concentrations decline rapidly.

The United States Immunization Survey estimates that among elderly adults, influenza vaccination rates rose from 33 percent

---

TABLE 124-2

Vaccines for Viral Pulmonary Pathogens

Pathogen	Vaccine	Targeted Population	Frequency
Influenza viruses type A and B	Inactivated whole or split trivalent vaccines	Elderly; chronic pulmonary, cardiac, or renal diseases; diabetes	Administer annually
Measles (rubeola)	Live, attenuated virus, usually administered with live, attenuated mumps and rubella vaccines as MMR	All children, susceptible adolescents and adults	1st dose: 12–15 months 2d dose: 4–6 years of age or before entrance to high school or college
Varicella-zoster virus	Live attenuated virus	All children; susceptible adolescents and adults, particularly health-care workers	Children (1–12 years): 1 dose Adolescents and adults: 2 doses 6–8 weeks apart
Adenoviruses types 4 and 7	Live virus	Available only for U.S. Armed Forces	Single oral dose in enteric-coated capsule

in 1989 to 52 percent in 1993.[16] Several factors accounted for the increase: education, greater awareness among physicians and the public of both the benefits and lack of systemic side effects of the vaccine, reminders about vaccine availability, and direct mailings to patients and physicians.

Measles Vaccine

Measles was a major cause of morbidity and mortality in the United States, and it remains an important pathogen in some other parts of the world. Before 1963, the year that a measles vaccine was introduced, 500,000 cases of measles were reported in the United States annually, and there were 500 measles-associated deaths.[17] In 1994, only 963 cases of measles were reported in the United States.[18] Thirty-nine percent of these cases were in adolescents (10 to 19), and 24 percent were in adults at least 20 years of age. Despite the overall improvement, there is concern that the numbers of susceptible children, adolescents, and young adults is sufficient to allow resurgence of measles in the future. Indeed, a survey of recruits inducted into the U.S. Army in September and October 1989 showed that approximately 17 percent of these young adults lacked measles antibodies.[41]

Both measles and atypical measles can affect the lung. A study of 3220 Air Force recruits with measles showed pneumonia in 106 (3.3 percent) cases.[34] The patients with pneumonia had high fever and required prolonged hospitalization (mean 14.5 days) compared to those without pneumonia (mean 3.6 days). Atypical measles is the syndrome that occurs when persons who previously received either the killed measles vaccine or the killed followed closely by a live virus vaccine are exposed to wild measles virus. Cough and pulmonary infiltrates are very common in these patients.[45]

Live attenuated measles virus vaccine is recommended for all children, adolescents, and young adults born after 1957 without specific contraindication.[17] A dose of the measles vaccine, generally combined with attenuated mumps and rubella vaccines (MMR), is recommended for children 12 to 15 months of age. A second dose should be given to children 4 to 6 years of age before entry into kindergarten. Many colleges require documentation of two doses of measles vaccine before admission.

Measles vaccine should not be given to pregnant young women or to those with severe (anaphylactic type) reactions to eggs. In addition, it should not be given to patients with leukemia or lymphoma or to those who are immunosuppressed because of treatment with corticosteroids, alkalating agents, antimetabolites, or irradiation. Measles vaccine is recommended for children with HIV infection because infection with the wild type of virus is more severe and more likely to be fatal in these patients. For example, Kaplan and coworkers reported three cases and reviewed 27 cases of measles in HIV-infected patients and found that 69 to 78 percent developed pneumonitis and approximately 40 percent were fatal.[40] Similar or higher rates of pneumonitis and death were observed when measles occurred in patients with childhood malignancies such as acute lymphocytic leukemia.

Low-grade fever occurs in 5 to 15 percent of measles vaccine recipients and generally lasts 1 to 2 days. A transient rash occurs in 5 percent of vaccine recipients.

Varicella Vaccine

The varicella-zoster virus (VZV) causes chickenpox in susceptible children and adults and, as a result of a latent infection in sensory ganglia, zoster in those who have previously had chickenpox. Approximately 7 percent of healthy young adults lack antibodies to VZV.[41]

Primary VZV infection is considered to be a relatively benign disease in childhood. However, it is associated with greater morbidity and mortality in adults. For example, 16 percent of military personnel with primary VZV infection had radiographic evidence of pneumonia.[62] A number of factors increase the risk of developing pneumonia with primary varicella infection, including cigarette smoking, pregnancy, prolonged use of nasal or inhaled steroids, immunodeficiency, malignancy, and transplantation.[26] Untreated varicella pneumonia in adults is associated with a 10 percent mortality.[60]

Live attenuated varicella vaccine was approved for use in the United States in 1995. A double-blind, randomized, placebo-controlled trial in healthy children showed that the varicella vaccine was 100 percent effective in the first year, 96 percent effective in the second year, and 95 percent effective over 7 years of follow-up.[42] The 23 cases of varicella that occurred in vaccine recipients were milder than those observed in placebo recipients. Fifty percent of the vaccinated children who developed varicella reported a nonvesicular rash, and only 14 percent reported temperatures of at least 102°F. In the same study, the varicella vaccine was 92 percent effective in protecting against household exposure to infection, a stringent test of efficacy.

Controlled trials of varicella vaccine efficacy have not been done in adults. However, the vaccine is recommended for susceptible adolescents and adults because of the increased severity of primary VZV infection in these patients. Susceptible health-care workers are specifically targeted for identification by serologic screening and for vaccination because of their increased risk of exposure to VZV and because they can serve as a reservoir for transmission of infection to immunocompromised patients.

Varicella vaccine is lyophilized and must be stored in a freezer at −15° to −20°C until use. It must be given within 30 min of thawing and reconstitution. Healthy children 1 to 12 years of age should receive a single subcutaneous dose of the attenuated varicella vaccine. Susceptible older adolescents and adults should receive two subcutaneous doses 4 to 8 weeks apart.

Approximately 15 percent of children inoculated with the attenuated varicella vaccine develop low-grade temperature elevations, and 7 percent develop a transient, mild varicellalike rash.[31]

Adenovirus Vaccine

Adenoviruses cause respiratory infections in infants, children, adolescents, and young adults. They have been associated with pharyngitis, croup, bronchitis, and pneumonia. They are a particular problem in the military, where susceptible young men and women are brought together and where acute respiratory infections, caused by adenovirus types 4 and 7, are a leading cause of infirmary visits and hospitalization.

Inactivated vaccines, containing adenoviruses types 4 and 7 that were grown in monkey kidney tissue culture cells and then treated with formalin, were prepared and tested in military recruits in the 1950s and early '60s. Randomized, controlled studies showed the inactivated vaccines to be 90 to 98 percent effective in reducing confirmed adenovirus infection.[55,57]

Problems in production and contamination with simian viruses hampered further development of the inactivated adenovirus vaccine. An alternative, live adenovirus vaccine was prepared in human embryonic kidney tissue culture. Though not attenuated, the live virus vaccine containing adenoviruses types 4 and 7 elicited an antibody responses to both viruses and did not cause respiratory disease when selectively delivered to the GI tract by an enteric-coated capsule.[20] However, adenovirus was shed in the stools of all volunteers, and some developed transient conjunctivitis, possibly as a result of self-contamination.

Gutekunst and colleagues tested the live enteric type 4 adenovirus vaccine in a placebo-controlled trial among marine recruits.[35] The vaccine was 100 percent effective in preventing febrile respiratory diseases in which adenovirus type 4 was recovered, 67 percent effective in preventing all febrile respiratory infections requiring hospitalization, and 77 percent effective in preventing all febrile respiratory illnesses occurring during the observation period. These data demonstrate both the effectiveness of the live enteric adenovirus vaccine and the importance of preventing adenovirus respiratory tract infections for the military. At present, adenovirus vaccines are available for clinical use only in the U.S. Armed Forces.

CONCLUSIONS

Use of vaccines to prevent pulmonary infections has not been adequately emphasized in the past. Vaccines are a safe, effective, and relatively inexpensive means of preventing pulmonary infections that can be debilitating and, in some cases, lethal. A number of vaccines are available and should be used in appropriate patients. These include the 23-valent pneumococcal polysaccharide vaccine; *H. influenzae* type b protein-conjugate vaccine; whole-cell or acellular pertussis vaccine; trivalent inactivated whole, subvirion, or split influenza vaccine; live attenuated measles vaccine; and live attenuated varicella vaccine. BCG vaccine is recommended for a very limited patient population in the United States. A live enteric-coated adenovirus vaccine is available only for the U.S. Armed Forces.

REFERENCES

1. Ahmed F, Steinhoff MC, Rodriguez-Barradas MC, et al: Effect of human immunodeficiency virus type 1 infection on the antibody response to a glycoprotein conjugate pneumococcal vaccine: Results from a randomized trial. *J Infect Dis* 173:83–90, 1996.
2. Dallet JJ, Sulcebe G, Couderc LJ, et al: Impaired antipneumococcal antibody response in patients with AIDS-related persistent generalized lymphadenopathy. *Clin Exp Immunol* 68:479–487, 1987.
3. Bartlett JG, Mundy LM: Community-acquired pneumonia. *N Engl J Med* 333:1618–1624, 1995.
4. Beck-Sague C, Dooley SW, Hutton MD, et al: Hospital outbreak of multidrug-resistant *Mycobacterium tuberculosis* infections: Factors in transmission to staff and HIV-infected patients. *JAMA* 268:1280–1286, 1992.
5. Brewer TF, Colditz GA: Relationship between Bacille Calmette-Guérin (BCG) strains and the efficacy of BCG vaccine in the prevention of tuberculosis. *Clin Infect Dis* 20:126–136, 1995.
6. Butler JC, Breiman RF, Campbell JF, et al: Pneumococcal polysaccharide vaccine efficacy: An evaluation of current recommendations. *JAMA* 270:1826–1831, 1993.
7. Casadevall A, Dobroszycki J, Small C, Pirofski LA: *Haemophilus influenzae* type b bacteremia in adults with AIDS and at risk for AIDS. *Am J Med* 92:587–590, 1992.
8. Centers for Disease Control and Prevention: Pneumonia and influenza death rates—United States, 1979–1994. *MMWR* 44:535–537, 1995.
9. Centers for Disease Control: Update on adult immunization: Recommendations of the Immunization Practices Advisory Committee (ACIP): Pneumococcal disease. *MMWR* 40(No. RR-12):42–44, 1991.
10. Centers for Disease Control and Prevention: Progress toward elimination of *Haemophilus influenzae,* type b disease among infants and children—United States, 1993–1994. *MMWR* 44:545–550, 1995.
11. Centers for Disease Control and Prevention: Update on adult immunization: Recommendations of the Immunization Practices Advisory Committee (ACIP): *Haemophilus influenzae,* type b. *MMWR* 40(No. RR-12):40–41, 1991.
12. Centers for Disease Control and Prevention: Pertussis vaccination: Acellular pertussis vaccine for reinforcing and booster use—Supplementary ACIP statement. Recommendations of the Immunization Practices Advisory Committee (ACIP). *MMWR* 41(No.RR-1):1–10, 1992.
13. Centers for Disease Control and Prevention: Pertussis vaccination: Acellular pertussis vaccine for the fourth and fifth doses of the DTP series—Update to supplementary ACIP statement. Recommendations of the Immunization Practices Advisory Committee (ACIP). *MMWR* 41(No.RR-16):1–5, 1992.
14. Centers for Disease Control and Prevention: Use of BCG vaccines in the control of tuberculosis: A joint statement by the ACIP and the Advisory Committee for Elimination of Tuberculosis. *MMWR* 37:663–675, 1988.
15. Centers for Disease Control and Prevention: Prevention and control of influenza: Recommendations of the Advisory Committee on Immunization Practices (ACIP). *MMWR* 44(No.RR-3):1–22, 1995.
16. Centers for Disease Control and Prevention: Influenza and pneumococcal vaccine coverage levels among persons aged ≥65 years—United States. *MMWR* 44:506–515, 1995.
17. Centers for Disease Control and Prevention: Update on adult immunization: Recommendations of the Immunization Practices Advisory Committee (ACIP): Measles. *MMWR* 40(No. RR-12):19–22, 1991.
18. Centers for Disease Control and Prevention: Summary of notifiable diseases, United States, 1994. *MMWR* 43:1–80, 1994.
19. Colditz GA, Brewer TF, Berkey CS, et al: Efficacy of BCG vaccine in the prevention of tuberculosis: Meta-analysis of the published literature. *JAMA* 271:698–702, 1994.
20. Couch RB, Chanock RM, Cate TR, et al: Immunization with type 4 and 7 adenovirus by selective infection of the gastrointestinal tract. *Amer Rev Resp Dis* 88:394–403, 1963.
21. Edlin BR, Tokars JI, Grieco MH, et al: An outbreak of multidrug-resistant tuberculosis among hospitalized patients with the acquired immunodeficiency syndrome. *New Engl J Med* 326:1514–1521, 1992.
22. Eskola J, Kayhty H, Takala AK, et al: A randomized, prospective filed trial of a conjugate vaccine in the protection of infants and young children against invasive *Haemophilus influenzae,* type b disease. *New Engl J Med* 323:1381–1387, 1990.
23. Fang GD, Fine M, Orloff J, et al: New and emerging etiologies for community-acquired pneumonia with implications for therapy: A prospective multicenter study of 359 cases. *Medicine* 69:307–316, 1990.

24. Farizo KM, Cochi SL, Zell ER, et al: Epidemiological features of pertussis in the United States, 1980–1989. *Clin Infect Dis* 14: 708–719, 1992.

25. Farley MM, Stephens DS, Brachman PS, et al. Invasive *Haemophilus influenzae* disease in adults: A prospective, population-base surveillance. *Ann Intern Med* 116:806–812, 1992.

26. Feldman S: Varicella-zoster virus pneumonitis. *Chest* 106(Suppl): S22–S27, 1994.

27. Fine PEM: Variation in protection by BCG: Implications of and for heterologous immunity. *Lancet* 346:1339–1345, 1995.

28. Fine PEM, Clarkson JA: Reflections on the efficacy of pertussis vaccines. *Rev Infect Dis* 9:866–883, 1987.

29. Fine MJ, Smith MA, Carson CA, et al: Efficacy of pneumococcal vaccination in adults: A meta-analysis of randomized controlled trials. *Arch Intern Med* 154:2666–2677, 1994.

30. Fischl MA, Uttamchandani RB, Daikos GL, et al: An outbreak of tuberculosis caused by multiple-drug-resistant tubercle bacilli among patients with HIV infection. *Ann Intern Med* 117:177–183, 1992.

31. Gardner P, Eickhoff T, Poland GA, et al: Adult immunizations. *Ann Intern Med* 12:35–40, 1996.

32. Glaser JB, Volpe S, Aguirre A, et al: Zidovudine improves response to pneumococcal vaccine among persons with AIDS and AIDS-related complex. *J Infect Dis* 164:761–764, 1991.

33. Govaert TME, Dinant GJ, Aretz K, et al: Adverse reactions to influenza vaccine in elderly people: Randomised double blind placebo contolled trial. *BMJ* 307:988–990, 1993.

34. Gremillion DH, Crawford S: Measles pneumonia in young adults: An analysis of 106 cases. *Am J Med* 71:539–542, 1981.

35. Gutekunst RR, White RJ, Edmondson WP, Chanock RM: Immunization with live type 4 adenovirus: Determination of infectious dose and protective effect of enteric infection. *Am J Epidemiol* 86:341–349, 1967.

36. Hofmann J, Cetron MS, Farley MM, et al: Prevalence of drug-resistant *Streptococcus pneumoniae* in Atlanta. *New Engl J Med* 333: 481–486, 1995.

37. Houck P, Hemphill M, LaCroix S, et al: Amantadine-resistant influenza A in nursing homes: Identification of a resistant virus prior to drug use. *Arch Intern Med* 155:533–537, 1995.

38. Huang KL, Ruben FL, Rinaldo CR, et al: Antibody responses after influenza and pneumococcal immunization in HIV-infected homosexual men. *JAMA* 257:2047–2050, 1987.

39. Jokinen C, Heiskanen L, Juvonen H, et al: Incidence of community-acquired pneumonia in the population of four municipalities in eastern Finland. *Am J Epidemiol* 137:977–988, 1993.

40. Kaplan LJ, Daum RS, Smaron M, McCarthy CA: Severe measles in immunocompromised patients. *JAMA* 267:1237–1241, 1992.

41. Kelley PW, Petruccelli BP, Stehr-Green P, et al: The susceptibility of young adult Americans to vaccine-preventable infections: A national serosurvey of U.S. Army recruits. *JAMA* 266:2724–2729, 1991.

42. Kuter BJ, Weibel RE, Guess HA, et al: Oka/Merck varicella vaccine in healthy children: Final report of a 2-year efficacy study and 7-year follow-up studies. *Vaccine* 9:643–647, 1991.

43. LaForce FM, Nichol KI, Cox NJ: Influenza: Virology, epidemiology, disease, and prevention. *Am J Prev Med* 10(Suppl):31–44, 1994.

44. Margolis KL, Nichol KL, Poland GA, Pluhar RE: Frequency of adverse reactions to influenza vaccine in the elderly: A randomized, placebo-controlled trial. *JAMA* 264:1139–1141, 1990.

45. Martin DB, Weiner LB, Nieberg PI, Blair DC: Atypical measles in adolescents and young adults. *Ann Intern Med* 90:877–881, 1979.

46. Mink CAM, Cherry JD, Christenson P, et al: A search for *Bordetella pertussis* infection in university students. *Clin Infect Dis* 14:464–471, 1992.

47. Mullooly JP, Bennett MD, Hornbrook MC, et al: Influenza vaccination programs for elderly persons: Cost-effectiveness in a health maintenance organization. *Ann Intern Med* 121:947–952, 1994.

48. Mundy LM, Auwaerter PG, Oldach D, et al: Community-acquired pneumonia: Impact of immune status. *Am J Respir Crit Care Med* 152:1309–1315, 1995.

49. Nichol KL, Lind A, Margolis KL, et al: The effectiveness of vaccination against influenza in healthy, working adults. *New Engl J Med* 333:889–893, 1995.

50. Nichol KL, Margolis KL, Wuorenma J, von Sternberg T: The efficacy and cost effectiveness of vaccination against influenza among elderly persons living in the community. *New Engl J Med* 331: 778–784, 1994.

51. Ostergaard L, Andersen PL: Etiology of community-acquired pneumonia: Evaluation by transtracheal aspiration, blood culture, or serology. *Chest* 104:1400–1407, 1993.

52. Polsky B, Gold JWM, Whimbey E, et al: Bacterial pneumonia in patients with the acquired immunodeficiency syndrome. *Ann Intern Med* 104:38–41, 1985.

53. Redd SC, Rutherford GW, Sande MA, et al: The role of human immunodeficiency virus infection in pneumococcal bacteremia in San Francisco residents. *J Infect Dis* 162:1012–1017, 1990.

54. Shapiro ED, Berg AT, Austrian R, et al: The protective efficacy of polyvalent pneumococcal polysaccharide vaccine. *New Engl J Med* 325:1453–1460, 1991.

55. Sherwood RW, Buescher EL, Nitz RE, Couch JW: Effects of adenovirus vaccine on acute respiratory disease in U.S. Army recruits. *JAMA* 178:1125–1127, 1961.

56. Simberkoff MS, El Sadr W, Schiffman G, Rahal JJ Jr: *Streptococcus pneumoniae* infections and bacteremia in patients with acquired immune deficiency syndrome, with report of a pneumococcal vaccine failure. *Am Rev Resp Dis* 130:1174–1176, 1984.

57. Stallones RA, Hilleman MR, Gauld RL, et al: Adenovirus (RI-APC-ARD) vaccine for prevention of acute respiratory illness: 2. Field evaluation. *JAMA* 163:9–15, 1957.

58. Statement of the American Thoracic Society: Treatment of tuberculosis and tuberculosis infection in adults and children. *Am J Respir Crit Care Med* 1994; 149:1359–1374, 1994.

59. Stein KE: Thymus-independent and thymus-dependent responses to polysaccharide antigens. *J Infect Dis* 165(Suppl 1):S49–S52, 1992.

60. Triebwasser JH, Harris RE, Bryant RE, Rhoades ER: Varicella pneumonia in adults: Report of seven cases and a review of the literature. *Medicine* 46:409–423, 1967.

61. Trollfors B, Taranger J, Lagergård T, et al: A placebo-controlled trial of a pertussis-toxoid vaccine. *New Engl J Med* 333:1045–1050, 1995.

62. Weber DM, Pellecchia JA: Varicella pneumonia: Study of prevalence in adult men. *JAMA* 192:572–573, 1965.

63. Wirsing von König CH, Postels-Multani S, Bock HL, Schmitt HJ: Pertussis in adults: Frequency of transmission after household exposure. *Lancet* 346:1326–1329, 1995.

64. Witt DJ, Craven DE, McCabe WR: Bacterial infections in adult patients with the acquired immune deficiency syndrome (AIDS) and AIDS-related complex. *Am J Med* 82:900–906, 1987.

65. Woodhead MA, Macfarlane JT, McCracken JS, et al: Prospective study of the aetiology and outcome of pneumonia in the community. *Lancet* 1:671–674, 1987.

66. World Health Organization: Global tuberculosis programme and global programme on vaccines: Statement on BCG revaccination for the prevention of tuberculosis. *Wkly Epidemiol Rec* 70:229–231, 1995.

67. Wright SW, Edwards KM, Decker MD, Zeldin MH: Pertussis infection in adults with persistent cough. *JAMA* 273:1044–1046, 1995.

CHAPTER 125

MICROBIAL VIRULENCE FACTORS IN PULMONARY INFECTIONS

James L. Michel / Gerald B. Pier

GENERAL MECHANISMS OF INFECTIOUS PROCESSES IN THE RESPIRATORY TRACT

MOLECULAR FACTORS AND PROCESSES IN RESPIRATORY INFECTIONS

SPECIFIC VIRULENCE MECHANISMS OF MICROBIAL PATHOGENS

EXAMPLES OF THE MOLECULAR PATHOGENESIS OF ACUTE AND CHRONIC BACTERIAL RESPIRATORY INFECTIONS

Beginning at birth, organisms enter and leave the body, primarily on external or mucosal surfaces. Some of these largely commensal organisms become resident; others are transient, and still others establish latent foci. Over a lifetime, a person is the reservoir for hundreds of strains of viruses, thousands of bacterial species, and a scattering of fungi and parasites. When these organisms violate their niche, invade, or produce toxic products, virulent interactions take place and occasionally lead to disease. Organisms can cause disease without entering the parenchyma, particularly by releasing toxic products. However, many infections are preceded by attachment of organisms to surfaces, followed by their entry into cells or otherwise sterile spaces. These processes of invasion are complex and involve factors present in both the host and the organism. Most organisms are cleared by a variety of nonspecific and specific mechanisms; in some cases, however, organisms are able to propagate and produce clinical symptoms. A number of pathologic conditions in the host predispose to entry and survival of microbes, ranging from breaks in mucosal surfaces to defects in the immune system. Organisms become parasites when they express the requisite *virulence determinants* to gain entry and overcome or evade host defenses.

An important step in establishing infection occurs when the potential pathogen encounters the immune system. There are numerous mechanisms whereby the immune system detects and tries to limit the extent of microbial challenge, including inflammation (acute and chronic), phagocytosis (polymorphonuclear leukocytes and macrophages), complement, and humoral and cellular immune responses. The immune system also maintains surveillance for organisms that invade phagocytes, propagate, and resist killing, and for organisms that invade nonphagocytic cells. Means by which microbes can be controlled range from physical clearance mechanisms to nutritional depletion (e.g., sequestration of iron, which is an essential nutrient for bacterial growth).

Microbes have evolved a variety of strategies to overcome host defenses, evade the immune system, scavenge for nutrients, and survive to spread to other hosts. These processes can lead to tissue damage, even death of the host. However, ultimate survival of the microbe requires eventual spread to a new host. A new "generation" of microbes is established (by clonal division) approximately once an hour, whereas a new generation of humans occurs about once every 20 years. Thus the microbes have a clear genetic advantage in selecting properties that enhance virulence and survival. In response, the human immune system has developed to present a variety of defenses against a broad range of pathogenic mechanisms. Infections can occur at specific sites on surfaces or within the body or involve local, distal (metastatic), or systemic spread. Infection can occur without damaging cells, through direct cellular damage by microorganisms or their toxins, or as a consequence of the immune response. When physiological disruption or cellular damage occurs, the host needs to recover and repair. In addition, the immune system attempts to recognize the pathogen and prevent reinfection. Pathogens have also evolved a series of mechanisms to avoid immune detection, including local interference with immune processes, antigenic variation, and avoidance of inducing an immune response.

Organisms are constantly evolving to meet the demands and opportunities of modern society. Just as the cities of the Middle Ages brought together humans and rats and caused outbreaks of bubonic plague, the use of antibiotics, chemotherapy, and various medical devices has led to a number of new pathogenic interactions between microbes and humans. A key to understanding the pathophysiology of infectious diseases and appreciating the complexity of both the immune system and the microbial world is knowledge of the facts and processes of each; this knowledge base is necessary for an understanding of the ideas presented above and the conceptual basis of immunity and infection as related to respiratory tract infections.

GENERAL MECHANISMS OF INFECTIOUS PROCESSES IN THE RESPIRATORY TRACT

The pathogenesis of acute and chronic microbial infections of the lungs entails complex interactions between the microorganisms and a variety of host defense mechanisms. The host can mobilize both specific and nonspecific immune effectors that encompass local and generalized defense mechanisms. Although the alveolar spaces are generally sterile, low levels of microorganisms are continually inhaled into the lungs; inoculation of the lungs can occur from a variety of sources. Most commonly, inhaled organisms, either alone or in association with particles of mucus, gain access to the lower airways. They are generally either cleared by mucociliary flow or scavenged by phagocytes (see Chapter 120). Particulates greater than 10 μm in diameter are filtered in the upper airways unless there is a breakdown in normal defense mechanisms. Particles of less than 5 μm that are not cleared in the upper airways can be deposited in alveoli. Most particulate matter is not infectious, and only spores or organisms that remain viable can cause infection. Thus, the pathogenesis of microbial infection will initially depend on a microbe's ability to enter the respiratory system and avoid clearance by immune and inflammatory mechanisms.

Microorganisms can reach the lower airways from various sources. Organisms in ambient air can be inhaled as droplet nuclei—particularly in closed environments, where density is great and infected individuals can deposit organisms into the air. Another important source of organisms is the "normal" flora of the upper respiratory tract. A large ecosystem of microorganisms that includes both pathogenic and nonpathogenic bacteria and fungi normally resides in the upper airways (see Chapters 119 and 143). The quantity and species diversity of many of these organisms can be stable over long periods, but transient colonization with a variety of microbes also occurs with some frequency, and these changes are often correlated seasonally. For example, *Streptococcus pneumoniae* and *Neisseria meningitidis* are more frequently isolated from throats during the winter months. Organisms that make up the normal microbial flora in other parts of the body are transferred to the lung, where they can cause infection. In early-onset group B streptococcal pneumonia and sepsis in neonates, the *Streptococcus* is transferred during birth from the vaginal canal of the mother to the respiratory tract of the infant. Examples of the transfer of normal flora to the lung also include aspiration of gastric contents, often containing anaerobic oral flora—leading to aspiration pneumonia, which is both a bacterial infection and a chemical pneumonitis.

Organisms causing infections at other body sites can spread to the lungs. Although not common, hematogenous spread from the bloodstream to the lungs can occur. Parapneumonic infectious agents can gain access to the pulmonary parenchyma through direct contact with the infected tissues. The existence of heavy colonization or infection in the upper airways also increases the potential for infection in the lungs by a variety of mechanisms. Upper-airway infection or colonization increases

the likelihood of spread by a simple dose effect, whereby a large burden of potentially pathogenic organisms overwhelms the clearance mechanism of the lungs. Another mechanism for pneumonic infection can result from infections that perturb the specific and nonspecific defenses, leading to respiratory infection as a sequela of another pathogenic process. The most common examples of this process are bacterial infection secondary to influenza and respiratory infection resulting from immunodeficiency due to HIV infection. Finally, any process that disrupts the physiological and physical barriers between the upper and lower airways can lead to infection—for example, the placement of an endotracheal tube or changes in normal clearance mechanisms associated with cystic fibrosis.

Once a microorganism gains access to the lower respiratory tract, it must be able to attach to tissue factors, remain viable, and multiply. Usually organisms will either multiply locally, resisting local defenses, or spread to other body sites by traversing epithelial barriers that normally inhibit microbial spread. In order for extracellular organisms to multiply, they must scavenge for nutrients; of particular note is the universal requirement for iron, which must be extracted from iron-binding molecules such as transferrin. Many bacteria produce iron-binding substances known as siderophores that have an affinity for iron of greater than 10^{18} M and bind to high-affinity receptors on the bacterial surface. Organisms must also avoid or resist opsonophagocytosis or be able to survive and multiply within phagocytes. Subsequent to microbial growth and resistance of host defenses, damage to the host tissues occurs, aided by a variety of pathogenic factors and resulting in invasion and destruction of cells. Secreted toxins can act locally and be systemically spread to cause clinical symptoms. The potential for inflammation to cause tissue destruction is an ominous consequence of microbial growth in normally sterile lung sites. Finally, although not necessary for the pathologic process to take place, most organisms that successfully multiply will have mechanisms with which to leave the body and transmit disease, thereby propagating their species.

MOLECULAR FACTORS AND PROCESSES IN RESPIRATORY INFECTIONS

The study of pathogenic microorganisms has benefited greatly from the ability to identify microbial factors that are at work to elicit a particular pathologic process. Often these factors by themselves are responsible for a particular aspect of the infectious process, whereas at other times these factors act in consort to promote microbial colonization, growth, infection, and ultimately host responses and disease. As noted above, a general scenario for establishment of an infection can be divided into the following categories: establishment of colonization on (or in) a host tissue; microbial growth, which may or may not be followed by spread to other tissues; elaboration of microbial factors and the concomitant host response involving inflammatory mediators; frank disease that compromises and destroys tissue; and resolution of disease, usually followed by the development of an acquired immune response that can provide immunity against future infections caused by antigenically related strains of the same organism.

The success of the microorganism in establishing infection (the presence of a microorganism in a tissue where it is not normally found) and causing disease (the signs and symptoms of clinical illness) is therefore predicated on the organism's ability to elaborate specific molecular factors that allow it to progress from the colonization to the disease state. Factors that inhibit or neutralize the host's response to eliminate the organism are also critical for pathogenesis. The ability of specific microorganisms to produce virulence or pathogenic factors is highly variable and is doubtless a major reason for the differences in pathogenicity among closely related strains of bacteria. Host immunity obviously influences the disease process, and the ability of the host to prevent initial colonization, limit growth, neutralize soluble microbial factors, and eliminate microorganisms can be mediated by a variety of nonspecific and specific immune effectors. Most of the nonspecific immune effectors come into play early during infection and make up the classic components of the inflammatory response; in a nonimmune host, specific antibody and cell-mediated immunity develop over 1 to 2 weeks and are needed to eliminate the pathogen and reestablish tissue homeostasis.

Initially, most microbes that enter through the oral or respiratory route and establish themselves in the respiratory tract will bind to host tissues, often in a specific manner. Pathogens will produce specific molecules to promote this process. Some potentially pathogenic microorganisms, such as S. pneumoniae and N. meningitidis, can establish colonization in the throat without causing harmful effects. Almost everyone is colonized by these potential pathogens many times during life. Viruses and obligate intracellular parasites, such as Chlamydia and Rickettsia, usually must find their way to the lower respiratory tract and invade a specific cell in order to start growing. Bacterial pathogens, such as Legionella pneumophila and Mycobacterium tuberculosis, need to encounter alveolar macrophages where they are ingested but resist destruction within these cells.

Fungal pathogens, about which little is known in terms of molecular mechanisms of infection, probably bind to specific factors in the respiratory tract during their initial stage of colonization. In some cases, as long as a potential pathogen confines itself to a local site, no disease will ensue. Alternatively, as is seen with tuberculosis, tissue invasion leads not to disease but to either microbial containment or clearance. At other times, growth at the local site causes frank disease; this is the mechanism of group A streptococcal pharyngitis and whooping cough caused by Bordetella pertussis. If a pathogen grows heavily in a tissue in the upper respiratory tract, it can cause a disease such as epiglottitis due to Haemophilus influenzae. Microbial spread to a sinus can lead to sinusitis, which can be caused by many different pathogens. In general, the throat readily tolerates the presence of a dynamic bacterial population, comprising mostly nonpathogenic strains and potential pathogens that do not spread to other tissues. Overgrowth or spread of microbes to normally sterile sites of the respiratory tract is the cause of most infectious diseases in these tissues.

Most of the initial host response to pathogens in normally sterile sites, indicative of infection, involves the basic inflammatory response. The microbes generally initiate this response by activating complement, binding quasi-specific host molecules such as mannan-binding protein, and generating other tissue signals that lead to an influx of inflammatory cells and serum factors into the site of infection. Elaborating molecules that allow a microbe to avoid being destroyed by inflammatory mediators is crucial to progression of the pathogenic process. Inflammation leads to clinical symptoms in the form of a sore throat, sneezing, coughing, feeling of malaise, etc. Some particularly virulent microbes can produce much more serious disease rapidly as the organisms spread throughout the respiratory tract. This leads to increased inflammation in the tissues where the microbes are growing. Successful control of infection, with the resultant limitations in microbial spread, will begin to bring resolution of disease. Alternatively, failure to control microbial growth and sustained inflammation lead to pathologic tissue destruction. The balance between the host inflammatory response and microbial growth is the key factor in the disease process. As is often the case with microbial infection, inflammation is a double-edged sword, critically important for resolution of infection but also responsible for tissue damage.

SPECIFIC VIRULENCE MECHANISMS OF MICROBIAL PATHOGENS

Almost all of our knowledge in the area of molecular mechanisms that microbial pathogens use to establish and cause respiratory infections is derived from studies of bacteria. In the case of viruses, clear factors, such as the neuraminidase and hemagglutinin proteins on the coat of the influenzavirus, are needed to expose cellular receptors and promote viral binding, subsequent cellular invasion, viral replication, inflammation, and disease. All viruses causing respiratory infections must enter cells in some manner that includes binding of a specific viral factor to a specific host cellular receptor. Intracellular nonviral microbes such as Chlamydia are probably taken into cells nonspecifically by phagocytosis or endocytosis.

A fairly good understanding of the molecular basis for the pathogenesis of pertussis infection has been established. A summary of these features is given in Table 125-1. B. pertussis binds exclusively to the cilia on ciliated respiratory epithelium, using at least two bacterial cell-surface factors, designated pertactin and filamentous hemagglutinin (FHA). A fraction of the organism's cell wall, the muramyl dipetide, is then extensively produced and secreted, and this factor is toxic to the ciliated tracheal cells. These cells are extruded from the epithelial surface, perhaps in an attempt to clear the bacteria from the respiratory tract.[2] Secretion of pertussis toxin probably causes much of the pathology leading to whooping cough. Pertussis toxin is composed of two subunits, designated A and B; the B subunit binds to receptors on host cells, allowing the A subunit to enter the cell. The A subunit transfers the ADP-ribosyl part of NAD to a membrane-bound GTP-binding protein that normally inhibits the enzyme adenyl cyclase. This leads to increased synthesis of cAMP, which presumably affects normal tissue function and leads to whooping cough. As reported in early 1996, clinical trials of an acellular pertussis vaccine containing inactivated pertussis toxin, purified FHA, and pertactin had an 85 percent efficacy rate in prevention of pertussis. This vaccine will replace the currently licensed inactivated whole-cell vaccine, which, al-

TABLE 125-1

Steps and Molecular Factors for Infectious Microorganisms to Cause Lung Disease

Step	Molecular Factors	Result
Attachment to or entry into the body	Pili, flagella, surface proteins, LPS, specific ligands for receptors on host cells or mucins	Establishes organisms in a host
Multiplication	Iron-binding factors; control of host cell protein synthesis	Increase in microbial numbers; initiation of clinical symptoms
Local or general spread into the lungs	Capsular polysaccharides, antiphagocytic factors, toxins and tissue destructive enzymes	Evade defenses and the natural barriers to spread
Cause damage to lungs	Exotoxins, LPS, cytotoxins, immunosuppressive agents	Basic pathology due to the infectious agent
Shedding (exit) from the body	Not identified	Leave body at site and on a scale that ensures spread to a new host

though effective, has been perceived to have unacceptable levels of toxicity in infants receiving pertussis immunizations.

Other extracellular pathogens that cause lung infections establish themselves in tissues by binding to either cellular receptors or factors in the mucus, notably mucin. Krivan and colleagues[5] reported that numerous bacterial pathogens that frequently cause pneumonia—including *Pseudomonas aeruginosa, H. influenzae, Staphylococcus aureus, S. pneumoniae, Klebsiella pneumoniae,* and some *Escherichia coli*—bind specifically to terminal or internal GalNAc β_{1-4} Gal sequences lacking sialic acid residues commonly found on cellular glycolipids in the respiratory tract. *P. aeruginosa* itself has been prominently studied in regard to binding to respiratory mucins as a mechanism to establish and maintain infection in the lung.[11] Nontypable *H. influenzae* also appears to utilize mucins to establish chronic infections in the lung.[6]

Intracellular respiratory bacterial pathogens usually are ingested by alveolar macrophages and must resist phagocytic killing in order to establish infection and cause disease. *M. tuberculosis* enters these cells in the lower and middle airways with high airflow, as it is an obligate aerobic organism. Bacterial ligands and cellular receptors involved in this process are not characterized. Following inhalation, most individuals will effectively clear or contain the tubercle bacilli, while in a minority the bacteria escape from the macrophage phagolysosome, or prevent its formation in the first place, leading to bacterial growth and host inflammation and resulting in lesions typical of tuberculosis. A major outer-membrane porin protein of *L. pneumophila* is coated with fragments of the third component of complement when this organism enters a host, and the bacteria are ingested by macrophages owing to binding of the complement fragments to complement receptors.

Elaboration of additional bacterial virulence factors beyond those needed to establish infection in normally sterile tissues is not well characterized. Many respiratory pathogens are encapsulated—a critical factor in promoting bacterial resistance to phagocytic killing. Neutralization of this antiphagocytic property

by specific antibody results in high-level host immunity. Successful vaccines against *S. pneumoniae, H. influenzae* type b, and certain serogroups of *N. meningitidis* have been developed by engendering capsule-specific immunity via immunization, and comparable vaccines against *P. aeruginosa, K. pneumoniae,* group B streptococcus, and *S. aureus* are in various stages of development and testing in humans. Many studies support a role for the M protein capsulelike antigen of group A streptococcus in preventing phagocytosis of this organism, although recent studies suggest that the nonimmunogenic hyaluronic acid capsule plays a more prominent role as an antiphagocytic factor for group A streptococci.[13]

Although many of these pathogens, such as *P. aeruginosa, S. aureus,* and group A streptococci, elaborate some very potent extracellular toxins, none of them have been shown to have a major role in causing pneumonia or other respiratory disease, although it is likely that a role will be found in the future. The gram-negative endotoxin, also called lipopolysaccharide (LPS), can cause serious damage to lung tissues, although the lung seems relatively resistant to the effects of inhaled endotoxin when compared with the systemic response to circulating LPS. Thus, inhalation of fairly large doses of LPS (2 to 1000 μg) is required to elicit very modest decrements in FEV_1 in healthy adults, while injection of 1 to 5 μg into the blood will provoke a systemic shock–like disease. However, adult respiratory distress syndrome (ARDS) is highly associated with systemic infections due to gram-negative rods.[4] Given that endotoxin by itself can activate many of the inflammatory responses that underlie the genesis of ARDS, it is likely that endotoxin effects could directly contribute or even cause much of the pathology leading to ARDS.

EXAMPLES OF THE MOLECULAR PATHOGENESIS OF ACUTE AND CHRONIC BACTERIAL RESPIRATORY INFECTIONS

Two highly important pathogens causing different types of lung infection have been intensively studied to elucidate the mechanisms whereby these organisms cause pneumonia and sepsis. As important a pathogen as *S. pneumoniae* is in the respiratory tract, the understanding of how it causes pneumonia and sepsis is not extensive. The capsular polysaccharide is a critical virulence factor, but beyond this, the role of other bacterial entities in pathogenesis is not well elaborated. The cell-wall bacterial phosphorylcholine of virulent *S. pneumoniae* has been shown to bind to the G protein–coupled platelet-activating factor (PAF) receptor following inflammatory activation of human cells.[3] This leads to invasion of epithelial and endothelial cells, indicating a mechanism whereby *S. pneumoniae* could escape through the lung epithelium via the vascular endothelium into the circulation to cause sepsis. The fact that lung inflammation increases PAF receptor levels could underlie the hypersusceptibility of people with viral influenza to secondary infection with *S. pneumoniae*.

Chronic lung infections can be caused by a variety of bacterial pathogens, many of which occur in persons with underlying lung disease. Patients with chronic obstructive pulmonary disease are particularly susceptible to chronic infection with nontypable *H. influenzae,* although beyond the propensity of the organism to bind to respiratory mucins,[6] the molecular bases for infection and disease are unclear. The organism produces a variety of cell membrane proteins that elicit immune responses; one of them, designated P2, undergoes extensive antigenic variation during infection, indicating an important mechanism whereby this organism evades host defenses. Among patients with cystic fibrosis (CF), 80 to 90 percent will become chronically infected with *P. aeruginosa*. This infection is currently the major factor limiting their life expectancy to about 30 years and is probably the factor most amenable to therapy with new antimicrobial reagents. A large research effort has focused on understanding how this pathogen infects the vast majority of patients with a genetic defect that does not appear related to chronic bacterial lung infection. In patients with CF, mutations are found in the CF transmembrane conductance regulator (CFTR) protein, a large protein that regulates chloride ion secretions directly and also appears to affect the flow of other ions, such as sodium. Ninety percent of people carry at least one mutant CFTR allele that lacks the codon for the phenylalanine at position 508 (âF508 mutation), and about two-thirds of affected persons are homozygous for this mutation. The lack of phenylalanine at position 508 leads to an inability of the mature protein to get into the cell membrane. More than 600 mutations in CFTR have been found, and the protein defect arising from these mutations results in either no CFTR protein in the membrane or a nonfunctional protein in the cell membrane.

The relationship of mutant CFTR and hypersusceptibility to chronic *P. aeruginosa* infection is undergoing intensive study. Pier and colleagues have proposed that clearance of *P. aeruginosa* from the lung following inhalation of bacteria is critically dependent on CFTR-controlled internalization of the bacterium by lung epithelial cells.[9] This can lead to bacterial clearance due to shedding of cells with internalized bacteria, as well as initiation of additional inflammatory responses that promote clearance. In cultured cells from an individual homozygous for the ΔF508 mutation in CFTR, internalization of *P. aeruginosa* was defective. This could be corrected by transfecting the cells with DNA encoding a wild-type CFTR protein or by growing the cells at 26%C, a process that promotes appearance of mature and functional mutant ΔF508 CFTR protein in the epithelial cell membrane.

The CFTR protein has been identified as the actual cellular receptor for clearance of *P. aeruginosa* from the lung. In a neonatal mouse model of clearance of *P. aeruginosa* from the lungs after nasal inoculation of bacteria, it was found that blocking of CFTR-mediated epithelial cell ingestion of *P. aeruginosa* led to higher bacterial burdens in the lung. However, the binding of bacteria to lung cells is not initially mediated by CFTR; this protein is expressed at too low a level in the cells for a high amount of bacterial attachment. It is likely that *P. aeruginosa* initially binds to airway epithelial cells through a variety of bacterial ligands, including pili, LPS, possibly flagella, and a nonpilus adhesin encoded for by bacterial genes needed for flagella synthesis.[1,11] Following this binding, the cell membrane accumulates CFTR protein, which binds to only a small portion of the bacterial cell surface but nonetheless leads to bacterial internalization into cells. An additional finding suggests that airway epithelial cell fluid from CF patients inhibits the antimicrobial activity of a small, defensinlike material, preventing effective killing of inhaled bacteria that land on an airway epithelial cell surface.[12] Thus, the initial establishment of *P. aeruginosa* infections in the lungs of CF patients can be directly attributable to the lack of functional CFTR in cell membranes, which prevents efficient bacterial clearance from the lung.

The pathogenesis of chronic *P. aeruginosa* lung infections in CF patients is more extensive. After avoiding initial clearance, the bacteria probably adhere to mucins and within a short time (days to no more than a few months) undergo a phenotypic conversion wherein they lose both their ability to produce the long O polysaccharide side chains that are usually on the LPS and acquire the ability to elaborate copious quantities of a bacterial exopolysaccharide referred to as both mucoid exopolysaccharide (MEP) and alginate. MEP is unable to provoke a protective antibody response in the host[10] and encases the bacteria in microcolonies within the lung.[7] Within this protective coating, phagocytes such as PMN are unable to ingest and kill the microorganisms. This leads to a vicious cycle of additional but ineffective inflammation and bacterial growth, the result of which is tissue destruction subsequent to the chronic inflammatory process. For most of the patient's life, *P. aeruginosa* infection remains confined to endobronchial surfaces, which become plugged with mucus while the airway tissues are being destroyed. An average yearly decline of 2 to 3 percent in FEV_1 will occur in most subjects, although females usually have worse disease than males.[8] Therefore, the pathogenesis of chronic *P. aeruginosa* infection in CF involves at least two components: an initial phase of hypersusceptibility to infection that is predicated on an inability of CF patients to kill or clear inhaled *P. aeruginosa* cells and a subsequent phase directly related to the bacterium's ability to elaborate MEP, which allows the organism to resist host defenses while continuing to provoke inflammation that damages lung tissues.

From these two examples we garner some important insights into mechanisms whereby bacterial pathogens cause lung infections. Many of the principles apply to other types of pathogenic microbes that follow the basic scenario of entry, attachment, multiplication and survival, elicitation of inflammation, and ultimately tissue damage and compromise of respiratory function. Although each of these steps can often be characterized at a highly specific molecular level, usually using isolated factors such as toxins to elicit clinical symptoms of disease, the overall pathogenesis of disease requires that elaboration of molecular factors of pathogenesis be coordinated and that each step in the process occur under the proper circumstances and at the right time. Research in identification and understanding of the microbe's genetic and molecular factors that control and coordinate pathogenesis is in its infancy. Presumably, greater understanding of particular factors and the interactions among both the factors and host tissues will lead to development of better vaccines and other therapies that will minimize the occurrence of microbial infections in the lung.

REFERENCES

1. Arora SK, Ritchings BW, Almira EC, et al: Cloning and characterization of *Pseudomonas aeruginosa fli*F, necessary for flagellar assembly and bacterial adherence to mucin. *Infect Immun* 64:2130–2136, 1996.
2. Cookson BT, Cho H-L, Herwaldt LA, Goldman WE: Biological activities and chemical composition of purified tracheal cytotoxin from *Bordetella pertussis. Infect Immun* 57:2223–2229, 1989.
3. Cundell DR, Gerard NP, Gerard C, et al: *Streptococcus pneumoniae* anchor to activated human cells by the receptor for platelet-activating factor. *Nature* 377:435–438, 1995.
4. Hyers TM, Fowler AA: Adult respiratory distress syndrome: Causes, morbidity, and mortality. *Federation Proc* 45:25–29, 1986.
5. Krivan HC, Roberts DD, Ginsburg V: Many pulmonary pathogenic bacteria bind specifically to the carbohydrate sequence GalNAcβ1-4Gal found in some glycolipids. *Proc Natl Acad Sci USA* 85:s6157–6161, 1988.
6. Kubiet M, Ramphal R: Adhesion of nontypeable *Haemophilus influenzae* from blood and sputum to human tracheobronchial mucins and lactoferrin. *Infect Immun* 63:899–902, 1995.
7. Lam J, Chan R, Lam K, Costerton JW: Production of mucoid microcolonies by *Pseudomonas aeruginosa* within infected lungs in cystic fibrosis. *Infect Immun* 28:546–556, 1980.
8. Parad RB, Gerard C, Zurakowski D, et al: A model for predicting pulmonary outcome in cystic fibrosis from genotype, mucoid *Pseudomonas aeruginosa* (MAP) colonization status and the presence of antibody to MPA (abstract). *Pediatr Pulmonol* 19:64, 1995.
9. Pier GB, Grout M, Zaidi TS, et al: Role of mutant CFTR in hypersusceptibility of cystic fibrosis patients to lung infections. *Science* 271:64–67, 1996.
10. Pier GB, Saunders JM, Ames P, et al: Opsonophagocytic killing antibody to *Pseudomonas aeruginosa* mucoid exopolysaccharide in older noncolonized patients with cystic fibrosis. *New Engl J Med* 317:793–798, 1987.
11. Ritchings BW, Almira EC, Lory S, Ramphal R: Cloning and phenotypic characterization of *fle*S and *fle*R, new response regulators of *Pseudomonas aeruginosa* which regulate motility and adhesion to mucin. *Infect Immun* 63:4868–4876, 1995.
12. Smith JJ, Travis SM, Greenberg EP, Welsh MJ: Cystic fibrosis airway epithelia fail to kill bacteria because of abnormal airway surface fluid. *Cell* 85:229–236, 1996.
13. Wessels MR, Bronze MS: Critical role of the group A streptococcal capsule in pharyngeal colonization and infection in mice. *Proc Natl Acad Sci USA* 91:12238–12242, 1994.

CHAPTER 126

INFECTIONS OF THE UPPER RESPIRATORY TRACT

Marlene Durand / Saumil N. Merchant / Ann Sullivan Baker

Upper respiratory tract infections are the most common infections and the most frequent reasons for office visits in the United States.[3] Although most upper respiratory infections are mild and self-limiting, some—such as peritonsillar abscess, epiglottitis, Ludwig's angina, invasive fungal sinusitis, and invasive otitis externa—are potentially life-threatening.

THE COMMON COLD

The common cold is a mild, self-limited upper respiratory tract infection. Adults have an average of two to four colds and children six to eight colds per year.[22] Most colds are caused by rhinovirus, coronavirus, influenza virus, parainfluenza virus, respiratory syncytial virus, or adenovirus. Rhinovirus and coronavirus are most common, causing about 40 and 10 percent of colds in adults, respectively.[22] All these viruses have several immunotypes; rhinovirus has 100.

Peak incidence of colds occurs during the colder months in the United States. Young children are the main reservoir of respiratory viruses, and adults with children have more colds than those without. Transmission probably occurs either by inhalation of infectious droplets or by hand-to-nose "self-inoculation" after touching infectious secretions. The pathogenesis of rhinovirus infections is thought to include viral entry into the nose, followed by infection of the epithelial cells of the upper airway. Viral replication peaks at 48 h and lasts for up to 3 weeks.[23] Symptoms (sneezing, nasal discharge and congestion, and a "scratchy" throat) develop 16 to 72 h after inoculation, and last for 1 to 2 weeks.

Treatment is symptomatic. Few studies have been done in children; antihistamines, decongestants, ipratropium bromide nasal spray (Atrovent), and nonsteroidal anti-inflammatory drugs may be effective in relieving symptoms in adults. Efforts to produce vaccines against the major cold viruses have been undermined by the sheer number of viral immunotypes. Careful handwashing may be the most effective preventive measure.

PHARYNGITIS

Most cases of acute pharyngitis occur as part of the common cold and are caused by viruses such as rhinovirus, coronavirus, and parainfluenza virus. These cases are mild, nonexudative, and self-limiting. Patients with primary HIV syndrome may also have a nonexudative pharyngitis.[31] A severe, usually exudative pharyngitis occurs in about half of patients with either adenovirus infection or Epstein-Barr virus mononucleosis. The pharyngitis seen in herpangina, due to group A coxsackievirus, is characterized by a vesicular enantham. Lesions (usually only two to six) begin as papules on the soft palate between the uvula and tonsils. These vesiculate, then ulcerate. Primary herpes simplex virus may cause a severe vesicular or ulcerative pharyngitis; when there is an overlying exudate, it may mimic streptococcal pharyngitis.

Group A streptococcus (*Streptococcus pyogenes*) is the most important bacterial cause of pharyngitis because of its suppurative (e.g., peritonsillar abscess) and nonsuppurative complications (e.g., rheumatic fever, acute poststreptococcal glomerulonephritis). It causes about 15 percent of all cases of pharyngitis. Symptoms and signs vary; patients may have a severe exudative pharyngitis, accompanied by fever, leukocytosis, and cervical lymphadenopathy, or they may have a mild pharyngitis that mimics that of the common cold. Some patients with mild disease may have a viral pharyngitis but are colonized with group A streptococci. These patients must also be treated for presumed streptococcal disease. Diagnosis of streptococcal pharyngitis is made by culture or by rapid antigen test. The latter is as specific but not as sensitive as culture; therefore, a negative test requires culture confirmation, while a positive test is sufficient for the diagnosis. Oral penicillin (or erythromycin in penicillin-allergic patients) should be given for 10 days, as a shorter course may not eradicate the organism. Alternatively, a single intramuscular dose of benzathine penicillin may be used. Cephalosporins such as cefuroxime appear to be at least as efficacious as penicillin, and a recent prospective randomized trial of 4-day cefuroxime versus 10-day penicillin therapy found no difference in bacteriologic or clinical cure rates.[2]

Other bacteria may also cause pharyngitis. Group C and G streptococci may cause an exudative pharyngitis and may be endemic or related to foodborne outbreaks. *Arcanobacterium hemolyticum* may cause an exudative pharyngitis along with a maculopapular rash, and typically occurs in children and young adults. Diphtheria, caused by *Corynebacterium diphtheriae,* is rare in the United States. Sore throat is a common symptom (in 90 percent), and findings include mild pharyngeal injection and an overlying adherent gray membrane (especially over the tonsillar pillars) that bleeds if removal is attempted. *Yersinia enterocolitica* may cause an exudative pharyngitis, and adults may not have an associated enterocolitis.[9] *Neisseria gonorrhoeae* may cause a mild pharyngitis, although most cases are asymptomatic. *N. meningitidis* has rarely been noted as a cause of pharyngitis,

but it is often isolated from throat cultures of patients with (and without) pharyngitis because the meningococcal carrier state is common. In a 32-month study of families during a nonepidemic period, 18 percent of the population were carriers at some point, and carriage lasted for a median duration of about 10 months.[21] Carriers are not treated except in epidemic situations or if they have had close contact with a case of invasive meningococcal disease. *Chlamydia pneumoniae* and *Mycoplasma pneumoniae* are other causes of pharyngitis.

A *peritonsillar abscess (quinsy)* may follow untreated streptococcal pharyngitis or may be due primarily to mouth anaerobes. Patients have severe sore throat and trismus, and may speak with a "hot potato" voice. There is marked unilateral peritonsilar swelling and erythema, causing deviation of the uvula. The abscess should be aspirated[37] or incised and drained by an otolaryngologist, and antibiotics active against streptococci and mouth anaerobes (e.g., penicillin plus metronidazole or clindamycin) should be given for at least 10 days.

ORAL CAVITY INFECTIONS

The oral cavity extends from the lips to the circumvallate papillae of the tongue. Various streptococci (e.g., *S. mutans, S. mitis, S. salivarius*) and anaerobes (e.g., *Peptostreptococcus, Veillonella, Lactobacillus, Bacteroides, Prevotella*) heavily colonize this area, and are the main pathogens in dental and oral cavity infections. *S. mutans* is a major pathogen in dental cavities. Gingivitis and periodontitis are associated with anaerobic gram-negative rods such as *Prevotella intermedia* and *Porphyromonas gingivalis*. Mouth anaerobes are the major cause of Vincent's angina (acute necrotizing ulcerative gingivitis, or trench mouth). Patients have gingival pain, halitosis, cervical adenopathy, and ulcerations of the interdental papillae. Treatment is with oral clindamycin or penicillin plus metronidazole.

Ludwig's angina is a rapidly spreading cellulitis of the sublingual and submandibular spaces. It usually begins in the floor of the mouth from an infected mandibular molar tooth. The sublingual area becomes edematous, pushing the tongue to the roof of the mouth. The infection can cause acute airway obstruction. Patients present with fever, difficulty swallowing, drooling, and prominent submandibular and sublingual swelling. They should be admitted for airway monitoring (intubation or tracheostomy may be necessary) and for intravenous antibiotics active against streptococci and anaerobes (e.g., penicillin plus metronidazole, ampicillin-sulbactam, or clindamycin). Surgical incision of the infected soft tissue compartment may be necessary. Noma, or cancrum oris, is a rare infection caused by mouth anaerobes, especially fusospirochetal organisms such as *Fusobacterium nucleatum.* It occurs mainly in malnourished children, and begins as a gingival ulcer that rapidly spreads as a necrotizing cellulitis of the lips and cheeks. Therapy includes high-dose intravenous penicillin, débridement, and correction of dehydration and malnutrition.

Primary herpes simplex infection may cause painful vesicles on the buccal mucosa as well as the lips and tongue, and should be treated with hydration and acyclovir. The most common fungal infection of the oral cavity is thrush, usually due to *Candida* species. It occurs most often in immunocompromised patients but may occur in normal hosts after prolonged antibiotic therapy or in patients with asthma using inhaled steroids.[44] Treatment is with topical antifungal solutions (e.g., nystatin) or with oral fluconazole.

LARYNGITIS

Laryngitis, or inflammation of the larynx, is characterized by hoarseness. Acute laryngitis is usually caused by the same viruses that cause the common cold (e.g., rhinovirus, influenza virus, adenovirus, parainfluenza virus), and treatment is symptomatic. Streptococcal pharyngitis may be associated with laryngitis and should be treated with penicillin. Adults with laryngitis may have a higher rate of colonization with *Moraxella catarrhalis* than do controls, and a randomized study of patients with acute laryngitis found subjective but not objective evidence of improvement in the erythromycin-treated group compared with controls.[38] Patients with HIV infection may have unusual causes of hoarseness and stridor,[35] such as laryngeal lymphoma or fungal (e.g., cryptococcal) infection.

Patients with chronic hoarseness must be examined for laryngeal malignancies. In rare instances, fungi or mycobacteria may cause chronic laryngitis. In chronic progressive disseminated histoplasmosis, ulcers may occur on the larynx, as well as on the tongue, buccal mucosa, and gingiva. Blastomycosis may also produce laryngeal ulcers. Tuberculosis may cause laryngeal lesions that mimic a laryngeal neoplasm; the most common endoscopic findings in one study were mucosal hyperemia and thickening, granular nodular areas, and focal ulcerations.[43] Two of the 15 patients in this study had no evidence of active or prior tuberculosis on admission chest radiograph (eight had apical thickening and fibrosis), and only three patients had a history of fever and night sweats. Laryngeal tuberculosis is probably as contagious as pulmonary tuberculosis but not more so,[28] as was once believed.

CROUP

Croup, or acute laryngotracheobronchitis, is characterized by subglottic edema and occurs most often in 2- and 3-year-old children. It is rare in children over age 6, and has only relatively recently been reported in adults.[12] It is characterized by a low-grade fever, inspiratory and expiratory stridor, and a "seal's bark" cough. Croup usually follows the onset of upper respiratory tract infection symptoms by 1 to 2 days. The cause is nearly always viral, with parainfluenza viruses accounting for about half of all cases.[27] Other viruses that cause croup are influenza virus, respiratory syncytial virus, adenovirus, rhinovirus, and enterovirus. Measles may also be complicated by croup. Herpes simplex type 1 has been noted as a cause of prolonged croup in two immunocompetent toddlers.[29]

The diagnosis of croup is based primarily on clinical grounds, and may be supported by neck radiographs. The most important differential diagnosis is epiglottitis (see below). Children with epiglottitis usually appear more toxic, and their illness worsens more rapidly. In croup, the anteroposterior neck radiograph shows the "hourglass sign" from subglottic edema, and the lateral neck radiograph shows a normal epiglottis. In epiglottitis, the lateral neck film shows a thickened epiglottis.

Treatment of croup consists of nebulized racemic epinephrine, corticosteroids, and humidified air. Severely ill patients must be hospitalized and monitored with oximetry; airway obstruction may occur, requiring intubation. Nebulized racemic epinephrine has been shown to be effective in treating mild to moderately severe croup.[34] It may have a peak effect 1 h after administration, so children should be monitored for rebound edema for several hours after initiation of therapy. The value of corticosteroid therapy is controversial. A single intramuscular dose of dexamethasone (0.6 mg/kg) appears to reduce the duration and severity of illness in children hospitalized with croup, as well as in those treated as outpatients.[10] In children with mild to moderate croup, nebulized glucocorticoid therapy (budesonide) has also been shown to be helpful.[32]

EPIGLOTTITIS

Acute epiglottitis (supraglottitis) is a medical emergency, as it can rapidly lead to airway obstruction. It begins as a cellulitis between the base of the tongue and the epiglottis, pushing the epiglottis posteriorly. It then involves the epiglottis itself, with rapid swelling and airway compromise. The peak incidence occurs in 2- to 4-year-old children, but it may affect older children and even adults. The overall incidence has decreased markedly since the advent of vaccination against *Hemophilus influenzae* type b in 1985. This organism is isolated from blood or epiglottis cultures in nearly 100 percent of pediatric cases and in about one-fourth of adult cases.[41] Other pathogens isolated from throat cultures in adults with supraglottitis are *H. parainfluenzae, Streptococcus pneumoniae,* group A streptococcus, and *S. aureus,* although the correlation between throat and epiglottis cultures is unclear. Viral epiglottitis is very rare; isolated cases due to parainfluenza virus, influenza virus, and herpes simplex virus type 1 have been described.

The onset of symptoms of epiglottitis occurs rapidly, usually within 6 to 12 h. Patients are febrile and irritable and complain of sore throat and dysphagia. Children prefer to sit leaning forward, and may be drooling. Inspiratory stridor may occur, but the barking cough seen in croup is not characteristic here. Adolescents and adults may have a less fulminant presentation, and particularly complain of sore throat that developed over the previous 2 days. Adults may also present with dyspnea (in 25 percent), drooling (15 percent), and inspiratory stridor (10 percent). Lateral neck radiographs are helpful if they show the "thumb sign" of an edematous epiglottis (Fig. 126-1), but may be falsely negative. Obtaining these radiographs may cause a critical delay in securing the airway.

Children suspected of having epiglottitis should be transported, sitting up, to the operating room for direct endoscopic visualization of the epiglottis. An uncuffed endotracheal (or nasotracheal) tube should be immediately inserted (or, if necessary, a tracheostomy performed) if a "cherry red" edematous epiglottis is seen. Adults with suspected epiglottitis should also be examined by an otolaryngologist, although intubation is not necessary in most adults (unlike children), as the airway is larger and acute obstruction less common.

All patients with epiglottitis should be monitored in an intensive care unit. Intravenous antibiotics active against *H. in-*

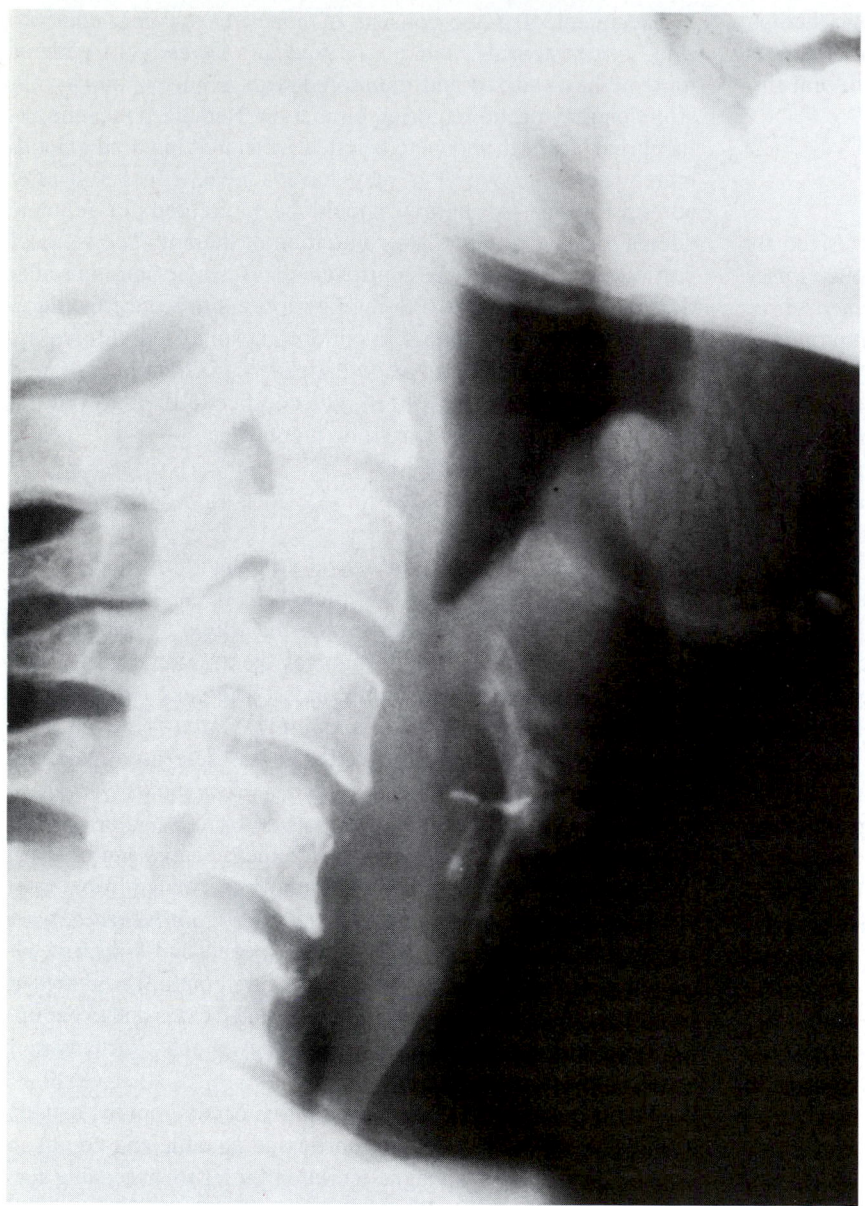

FIGURE 126-1   Lateral radiograph of the neck of a patient with epiglottitis.

fever, stridor, and worsening respiratory distress after a viral prodrome. They do not respond to racemic epinephrine.

Neck radiographs usually show subglottic narrowing; however, they should not be performed on a patient when there is risk of acute airway obstruction. On endoscopy, patients are usually found to have a normal epiglottis, but the subglottic trachea is covered with a thick exudate. Inspissated secretions may produce a pseudomembrane. Cultures of tracheal secretions yield various bacteria, but the major pathogens include *S. aureus* (51 percent), streptococci, including *S. pneumoniae* (18 percent), and *H. influenzae* (15 percent).[14] Gram-negative organisms other than *H. influenzae* (e.g., *Klebsiella, Pseudomonas,* and *Proteus*) are seldom found. Viral cultures usually yield parainfluenza virus and occasionally influenza virus.

Most patients require intubation; some require tracheostomy. Up to 60 percent will have concurrent pneumonia. Intravenous antibiotics active against *S. aureus* and *H. influenzae* (e.g., cefuroxime, or nafcillin plus ceftriaxone) should be given, along with airway humidification and aggressive pulmonary toilet. Inspissated or copious secretions may cause airway obstruction even in patients with an artificial airway; several patients have died because of this complication.

LARYNGEAL PAPILLOMATOSIS

Papillomas of the respiratory tract are benign tumors caused by human papillomaviruses, especially types 6 and 11. They are most often found on the larynx, and may occur in children or adults. Patients usually present with hoarseness. Papillomas may be solitary or multiple. Recurrent respiratory papillomatosis may occur and may extensively involve the upper airway. Typically, this disease is more aggressive in children than in adults. Treatment is with endoscopic laser surgery. Interferon-α may be beneficial.[36] In rare cases, the rapid growth of papillomas may cause airway obstruction, and tracheotomy may be necessary. Tracheotomy carries the risk of distal spread of the papillomas, however. A recent retrospective review concluded that most of this distal spread was limited to the tracheotomy site, and that spread to the bronchial tree was rare.[40]

SINUSITIS

The paranasal sinuses develop as outpouches of the nasal cavity. The maxillary and ethmoid sinuses are present at birth, the frontal sinus develops after age 2, the sphenoid sinus after age 7. The sinuses are lined with respiratory epithelium that includes ciliated cells and mucus-producing goblet cells. The cilia normally move the mucus blanket toward the sinus ostia (and then to the nasopharynx) at a speed of up to 1 cm per min.[1] In the

fluenzae (e.g., cefuroxime, ceftriaxone, ampicillin-sulbactam) should be given. In adults, an antistaphylococcal agent should be included (e.g., nafcillin plus ceftriaxone or cefuroxime alone) because of the role of *S. aureus* in some cases. If the patient with epiglottitis due to *H. influenzae* has household contacts that include an unvaccinated child under age 4, the patient and all members of the household should receive rifampin prophylaxis to eradicate carriage of the organism.

BACTERIAL TRACHEITIS

This rare disorder, sometimes called membranous croup, presents acutely like epiglottitis but primarily involves the subglottic region like croup. It may represent bacterial superinfection of a viral tracheitis. It usually affects children aged 3 weeks to 13 years, with a mean age of about $4\frac{1}{2}$.[14] It is uncommon in adults. Patients present with the acute onset of high presence of inflammation, the frequency of the cilia decrease from 700 to 300 beats per min.[20] In addition, inflammation causes mucosal congestion, which narrows the already small sinus ostia (e.g., ethmoid ostia are only 1 to 2 mm), impeding flow of the mucus blanket. Delay in the mucociliary transport time and obstruction of the ostia lead to sinusitis.

The most common cause of inflammation leading to sinusitis is a viral upper respiratory infection. Most adults with common colds have CT evidence of ostial obstruction and sinus abnormalities,[24] although only about 0.5 percent of all "colds" are complicated by acute sinusitis. Viral infections increase the amount of mucus produced and may damage ciliated cells; both factors decrease mucociliary transport time. Another predisposing factor for sinusitis is allergic rhinitis, which may cause ostial obstruction by mucosal edema or polyps. Dental infections, especially of the upper teeth that abut the maxillary sinus (second bicuspid, first and second molars), may cause 5 to 10 percent of cases of maxillary sinusitis. Anatomic obstruction of the sinus ostia due to a deviated septum, tumor, granulomatous disease (e.g., Wegener's granulomatosis or rhinoscleroma), or foreign body (e.g., nasotracheal tube) may also lead to sinusitis. Barotrauma from deep-sea diving or airplane travel, chemical irritants, and mucus abnormalities (e.g., cystic fibrosis) are other risk factors for sinusitis.

Acute Bacterial Sinusitis

Symptoms of acute bacterial sinusitis include purulent nasal or postnasal drainage, nasal congestion, and sinus pain or pressure. The location of this pain depends on the sinus affected. Patients usually complain of pain in their cheek or upper teeth in maxillary sinusitis, the sides of the bridge of the nose in ethmoid sinusitis, supraorbital or frontal pain in frontal sinusitis, and retroorbital, frontal, occipital, or vertex pain in sphenoid sinusitis. Fever occurs in about half of adults with acute sinusitis.

The diagnosis of acute bacterial sinusitis is often difficult on the basis of history and physical examination alone.[47] Identical symptoms may occur in patients with viral upper respiratory infections. The sensitivity and specificity of individual symptoms (e.g., pain at bending forward, purulent rhinorrhea, and sinus tenderness) are less than 70 percent, making these features of limited diagnostic usefulness.[47] However, several symptoms (maxillary toothache, history of colored nasal secretions, poor response to decongestants) and signs (abnormal transillumination, purulent secretion), taken together, are more highly predictive of the diagnosis.

In evaluating a patient for sinusitis, the routine physical examination may be augmented by sinus transillumination and nasal endoscopy. The usefulness of transillumination has been debated: It is helpful only in diagnosing maxillary and frontal sinusitis in adults, and then only if there is complete opacification. The sensitivity and specificity of nasal endoscopy have been incompletely evaluated. Since this procedure requires special skill and experience, it is performed by otolaryngologists but not by primary care providers. It is therefore unlikely to become widely used in evaluating routine cases of sinusitis.

Radiographic evaluation includes four-view sinus radiographs and sinus CT. Plain films of the sinus are helpful in evaluating patients suspected of having acute sinusitis if there is complete sinus opacification, an air–fluid level, or mucosal thickening of at least 4 mm. Sinus CT is much more sensitive than routine radiographs, particularly for ethmoid and sphenoid disease. CT should be reserved for complicated cases, however, as frequent use in routine cases would most likely lead to overdiagnosis of bacterial sinusitis. Acute, reversible sinus abnormalities are frequently seen on CT scanning of patients with the common cold.[24] Abnormalities are most common in the maxillary sinus (87 percent), followed by ethmoid (64 percent), sphenoid (39 percent), and frontal sinuses (34 percent).

The bacteriology of sinusitis has been well defined only for acute, community-acquired maxillary sinusitis. This disease in adults has been studied with direct sinus puncture and aspiration by Gwaltney and colleagues in Charlottesville. In 383 aspirates taken between 1975 and 1990, the most common isolates were *S. pneumoniae* (41 percent) and *H. influenzae* (35 percent).[25] The *H. influenzae* found are almost always unencapsulated (i.e., not group b). Streptococci (other than pneumococci) and anaerobes each accounted for 7 percent of isolates, while *S. aureus* accounted for only 3 percent. *Moraxella catarrhalis,* found in 4 percent of cultures of adults, was found in 15 percent of children with acute maxillary sinusitis.[45] Studies of sinuses other than the maxillary sinus are hindered by the difficulty of obtaining culture material that is not contaminated by nasal flora.

Treatment of acute community-acquired sinusitis should be empiric, directed against the bacterial pathogens noted above. Sinus puncture is not indicated in routine cases. Antibiotics used should be active against streptococci and β-lactamase–producing bacteria, such as *H. influenzae* and (in children) *M. catarrhalis.* Unfortunately, such antibiotics (e.g., amoxicillin–clavulinic acid and cefuroxime axetil) are expensive ($50 to $100 for 10 days). Trimethoprim-sulfamethoxazole is inexpensive but has a higher incidence of side effects (particularly rash). Adjunctive treatment with topical vasoconstrictors may be helpful, and these are widely used, although controlled trials of efficacy are not available.

Treatment of nosocomial sinusitis (e.g., in intubated patients in intensive care units) should be directed against *S. aureus* and gram-negative bacilli initially (e.g., with nafcillin and ceftriaxone), then simplified as results of sinus cultures become available.

Surgery for acute severe sinusitis, either nosocomial or community acquired, may be necessary to widen the sinus ostia and allow adequate drainage of thick secretions. This is especially true for frontal, ethmoid, and sphenoid disease that fails to respond to medical therapy, or in sinusitis complicated by orbital inflammation (see below).

Chronic Bacterial Sinusitis

Chronic sinusitis is characterized by symptoms that last for weeks to months. Patients complain of persistent dull pain, postnasal drainage, foul odor and taste, and fatigue. True fever is rare, although many patients complain of having temperatures around 99°F. Most patients have stable, low-grade symptoms punctuated by episodes of acute sinusitis. These episodes are signaled by a change to purulent secretions and increased sinus pressure. A sinus CT scan is indicated in almost all patients with chronic sinusitis to define the extent of disease and as part of an evaluation to exclude other diagnoses (e.g., obstructing tumor or granulomatous disease). Patients should be evaluated by an otolaryngologist, who may directly look for anatomic obstruction (e.g., deviated septum, polyps) with nasal endoscopy. Surgery, often done endoscopically, may be helpful to open narrow sinus ostia, particularly in the osteomeatal complex that drains the maxillary, frontal, and anterior ethmoidal cells. Intraoperative sinus cultures should be sent for study for anaerobes, aerobes, and fungi.

The bacteriology of chronic sinusitis is not well defined. Most patients with chronic disease will have sinus cultures positive for bacteria, but whether these are colonizers or pathogens is not always clear. Many of these patients will be colonized with *S. aureus* or gram-negative bacilli, especially if they have received several courses of antibiotics. Anaerobes have been shown by some investigators to play an important role in chronic sinusitis.[5] The need for antibiotic therapy must be determined on an individual basis, and antibiotic choice should be guided by the patient's recent culture results.

Complications of Bacterial Sinusitis

The most common complication of bacterial sinusitis is orbital inflammation. There are several types of orbital involvement, and Chandler's team has provided a classic diagram (Fig. 126-2) and description of these.[6] Most cases of orbital cellulitis and abscess are secondary to ethmoid sinusitis, since the ethmoid is separated from the orbit by only a very thin plate of bone, the lamina papyracea. Patients with preseptal cellulitis present with erythema and edema of the eyelids, but have no proptosis or limitation of ocular movement. Patients with orbital cellulitis present with fever, periorbital edema and erythema, proptosis, conjunctival injection and chemosis, and, occasionally, limitation of ocular movement. Patients with subperiosteal or orbital abscess frequently have limitation of eye movement: If the abscess is located medially (as is the case when it is secondary to ethmoid sinus disease), the eye looks "down and out." In patients with sinusitis and orbital findings, broad-spectrum antibiotics with activity against *S. aureus*, streptococci, and *H. influenzae* (e.g., cefuroxime, or nafcillin plus ceftriaxone) should be started immediately. A CT scan is helpful in determining extent of disease. The finding of a subperiosteal or orbital abscess usually immediate surgical drainage. In orbital cellulitis without abscess, treatment with intravenous antibiotics alone is usually successful, but if this does not produce improvement within 24 h, the affected sinus should be drained.

Frontal subperiosteal abscess ("Pott's puffy tumor") is another extracranial complication of sinusitis. This results from frontal sinusitis, and patients present with frontal pain and a tender, doughy swelling over the forehead. Treatment consists of 6 weeks of intravenous antibiotic therapy; surgical drainage of the abscess and the frontal sinus may be necessary. Intracranial complications of sinusitis usually result from frontal or sphenoid sinusitis. These include epidural abscess, subdural empyema, meningitis, cerebral abscess, and dural vein thrombophlebitis. Because of the proximity of the sphenoid sinus to the cavernous

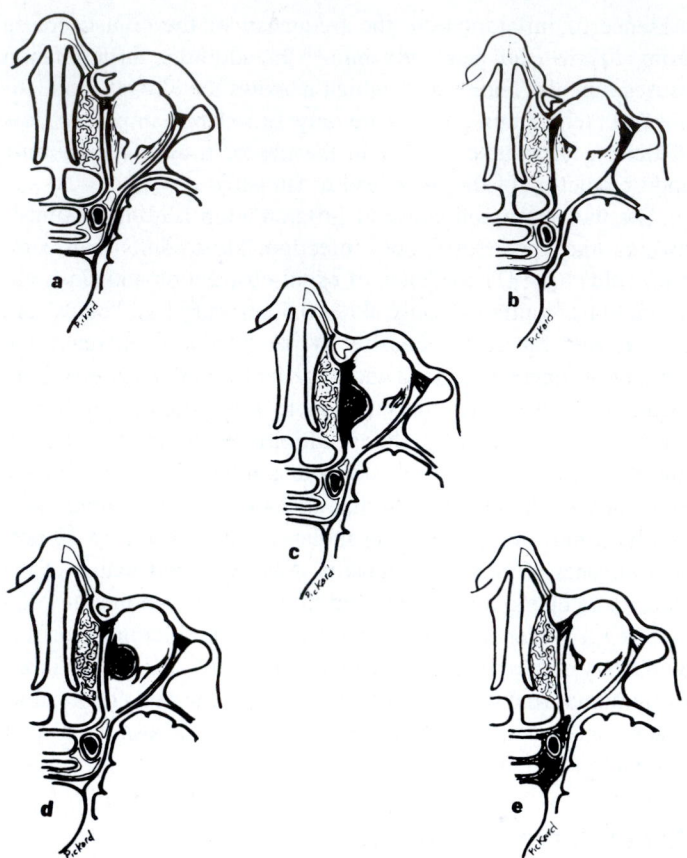

FIGURE 126-2 Orbital complications of sinusitis. *A.* Preseptal cellulitis. *B.* Orbital cellulitis. *C.* Subperiosteal abscess. *D.* Orbital abscess. *E.* Cavernous sinus thrombosis. *(From Chandler et al,[6] with permission.)*

sinus, sphenoid sinusitis is a major cause of cavernous sinus thrombophlebitis.

Fungal Sinusitis

There are three forms of fungal sinusitis: allergic fungal sinusitis, sinus aspergilloma, and invasive fungal sinusitis.

Allergic fungal sinusitis is defined by the presence of diagnostic "allergic mucin" in sinuses. The pathogenesis is thought to be similar to that of allergic bronchopulmonary aspergillosis, with fungi eliciting a local type I or type III hypersensitivity reaction. Patients with allergic fungal sinusitis often present with chronic sinusitis-type symptoms, with sinus pain and congestion being most common. Nearly all patients have nasal polyps; half also have asthma, and many have aspirin hypersensitivity. A review of the Mayo Clinic experience found that diagnostic allergic mucin occurred in 6.5 percent of patients who had undergone sinus exploration for chronic sinusitis between 1984 and 1992.[8]

The diagnosis of allergic fungal sinusitis is often suspected at surgery because allergic mucin is usually extremely tenacious, with the consistency of anchovy paste. It has histologic features similar to that of mucin found in bronchi of patients with allergic bronchopulmonary aspergillosis, with many eosinophils, Charcot-Leyden crystals, and rare fungal hyphae but no evidence of tissue invasion. About 40 percent of the Mayo Clinic patients with allergic mucin did not have hyphae on histopathology or positive fungal cultures. Cultures, when positive, grew *Bipolaris, Curvularia,* or *Alternaria* more often than *Aspergillus.*

The CT typically shows inhomogeneous opacification of one or more sinuses (often unilateral), and there may be evidence of bony erosion of the sinus. Erosion is due to pressure necrosis, not fungal invasion. On MRI, the affected sinus characteristically appears black on T2 ("T2-weighted signal void"). Surgical removal of the inspissated mucus may be curative. Prospective clinical trials of different treatment regimens have not been conducted, but in patients who have rapid recurrence, intranasal or systemic steroids may be indicated. Because of the lack of tissue invasion, antifungal agents have not been used.

Sinus aspergilloma is a noninvasive fungal disease that may cause symptoms of obstruction and chronic sinusitis. Usually only one sinus (most often maxillary) is affected, and symptoms are therefore unilateral. Surgical removal of the fungus ball is usually curative. Careful review of the pathologic slides is required to verify that there is no tissue invasion.

Invasive fungal sinusitis carries a significant risk of mortality, in contrast to the other two benign forms of fungal disease. Estimates of mortality depend on the sinus affected and the immune state of the patient. In immunocompromised hosts, fungal disease presents acutely. Rhinocerebral mucormycosis is a life-threatening infection due to fungi of the order Mucorales *(Rhizopus, Mucor, Absidia).* It usually affects diabetics who are in ketoacidosis, but may also affect leukemic patients with prolonged neutropenia, and has been noted in hemodialysis patients receiving deferoxamine chelation therapy.[48] Patients usually present with facial pain, headache, and fever. They may have signs of orbital or cavernous sinus involvement with proptosis, decreased eye movement, and loss of cranial nerve V_1 sensation. Involvement of cranial nerve VII is a poor prognostic sign. Patients in whom the diagnosis is suspected should undergo emergency endoscopy by an otolaryngologist in a search for a characteristic black eschar overlying necrotic tissue in the nasal passages. The eschar should be biopsied and the tissue immediately examined for fungus by a pathologist and an infectious-disease specialist. The finding of tissue invasion with broad-based, nonseptate hyphae warrants extensive surgical débridement and intravenous amphotericin therapy.

Aspergillus and other fungi may also cause invasive fungal sinusitis.[46] Immunocompromised patients, such as those who have received organ transplants, usually present acutely. Treatment is aggressive surgical débridement and intravenous amphotericin. Normal hosts, in contrast, have very slowly progressive disease. Typically, the diagnosis of invasive fungal sinusitis is not made for at least 6 months after the onset of symptoms. Fungi in the ethmoid and sphenoid sinuses may invade the orbital apex and cavernous sinus, affecting cranial nerves III, IV, V, and VI. Symptoms include headache, unilateral retroorbital pain, proptosis, ptosis, limitation of eye movement, decreased vision, and hypesthesia in the distribution of cranial nerve VI on the affected side. Symptoms of sinus congestion or drainage are often absent. Diagnosis is suggested by the clinical findings and CT and MRI scans showing sinus disease (sometimes just mucosal thickening) and inflammation in the orbital apex or cavernous sinus. Surgery should be done to débride the affected paranasal si-

nus. The tissue (not swabs) is sent to the microbiology lab as well as to pathology. On histopathology, special fungal stains show rare fungi with tissue invasion. Cultures may grow *Aspergillus, Bipolaris, Curvularia,* and *Exserohilum.* Unlike immunocompromised patients with invasive fungal disease, these patients may not require aggressive surgical débridement (such as exenteration for orbital involvement); the disease is slowly progressive, allowing time for assessment of antifungal therapy.

Treatment consists of amphotericin administered intravenously for a total of at least 2 g; the addition of flucytosine may be helpful. Patients should have close follow-up, with periodic MRI or CT scans to look for recurrence. After completion of amphotericin treatment, prolonged (e.g., 1 year) suppressive therapy with itraconazole should be given.

EAR AND MASTOID INFECTIONS

Auricular Cellulitis and Perichondritis

In auricular cellulitis, the ear is usually red, edematous, hot, and mildly tender. The lobule is especially swollen and red. There may be a history of minor ear trauma from earrings, scratching, Q-tips, etc. Treatment is with warm compresses and antibiotics (e.g., nafcillin) directed against *S. aureus* and streptococci.

Perichondritis is an infection of the perichondrium of the ear that is often accompanied by infection of the cartilage of the pinna (chondritis). It may lead to ear deformity due to necrosis of the cartilage. Patients present with a swollen, hot, red, and exquisitely tender pinna; the lobule is usually spared. Usual causes include significant trauma to the ear (e.g., boxing) and burns. The most common pathogens are *Pseudomonas aeruginosa* and *S. aureus.* Intravenous antibiotics active against these organisms, such as ticarcillin–clavulinic acid or nafcillin plus oral ciprofloxacin, should be given for at least 4 weeks. Improvement often occurs slowly. Incision and drainage may be helpful for culture and resolution of infection. This infection must be distinguished from relapsing polychondritis.

Otitis Externa

The external auditory canal is about 2.5 cm long. It is lined by a thin layer of skin, which covers cartilage in the lateral half of the canal, bone in the medial half. In the bony portion, the skin lacks a subcutaneous layer and is attached directly to the periosteum. This is an important feature in the pathogenesis of invasive otitis externa (see below). Glands secrete cerumen, which acidifies the canal and suppresses bacterial growth. Desquamated skin and retained moisture make the canal especially susceptible to *P. aeruginosa,* a hydrophilic organism.

Acute otitis externa, or swimmer's ear, occurs mostly in summer months and is often a result of exposure to water. It may be due to a decrease in canal acidity and the resulting bacterial overgrowth. The ear is pruritic and often extremely painful; the canal appears swollen and red. The usual pathogens are *P. aeruginosa, S. aureus,* and streptococci. Treatment consists of cleaning the ear (aural toilet) and topical antibiotic drops (e.g., polymyxin-neomycin 4 drops four times a day for 5 days). Analgesics may be needed, and patients should avoid getting the infected ear wet.

Herpes zoster oticus (Ramsay Hunt syndrome) is due to inflammation of the facial nerve by varicella-zoster virus. It is characterized by vesicles in the ear canal or concha, severe otalgia, loss of taste in the anterior two-thirds of the tongue, and ipsilateral facial nerve paralysis. Acyclovir has decreased the expected severity of the facial paralysis in some patients,[42] although controlled trials have not been published.

Invasive ("malignant") otitis externa is a potentially life-threatening osteomyelitis of the temporal bone and skull base. First described in 1959, it occurs primarily in elderly diabetics and is nearly always caused by *P. aeruginosa.* Some studies have reported a mortality of 14 percent in patients with no cranial nerve palsies, 53 percent for patients with isolated facial nerve paralysis, and 60 percent when other cranial nerves are affected or other CNS involvement is present.[15]

The infection begins in the external canal, then invades the adjacent soft tissues, mastoid, temporal bone, and eventually the base of the skull. In affected diabetic patients, their diabetes may be mild and is usually under good control (unlike the situation in sinoorbital mucormycosis infections). Many patients have had ear pain and drainage for weeks to months.

On examination, there is an edematous ear canal with granulation tissue in the inferior wall about halfway down the canal, in the region of the bony–cartilaginous junction. Some patients have trismus, partial facial paralysis (cranial nerve VII), neck pain, or dysphagia (cranial nerves IX and X). Fever is rare. The white blood cell count is usually normal, but the sedimentation rate is often high. A CT and an MRI scan are essential for defining the extent of involvement and for helping to determine a biopsy site. Bony involvement is best seen on CT, while soft tissue changes are best seen on MRI.[17]

Invasive otitis externa is a slowly progressive disease. Antibiotics should not be started until after a deep biopsy specimen has been obtained and sent for culture and pathology. Superficial cultures of the external canal may be unreliable. Nearly all cases are due to *P. aeruginosa;* indeed, one report noted that only seven exceptions had been published (due to *S. aureus, Proteus, Aspergillus,* and *S. epidermidis*).[4] Still, it is important to obtain tissue for culture because the antibiotic sensitivity of the *Pseudomonas* implicated in a particular case will guide the type of antibiotic therapy given. Antibiotics active against *Pseudomonas* (e.g., ticarcillin plus an aminoglycoside) are given intravenously for 6 weeks, or longer in severe cases. Adjuvant hyperbaric oxygen may be a consideration in some patients, especially in those who have had recurrences after conventional therapy

or who are unable to tolerate the optimal antibiotics because of side effects.[11]

Acute Otitis Media

The middle ear is connected to the nasopharynx by the eustachian tube. Acute otitis media (Fig. 126-3), or infection of the middle ear, is thought to result from bacterial entry into the middle ear via the eustachian tube. It is often initiated by a viral upper respiratory infection, and is consequently most common in fall, winter, and spring. The incidence of acute otitis media decreases with age. More than two-thirds of children under age 3 have had at least one episode of otitis media. The incidence in adults is only 0.25 percent.[39] The most common symptoms are ear pain and decreased hearing. Children often have fever, but this is less common in adults. The tympanic membrane is usually red, opaque, and bulging. Spontaneous perforation of the tympanic membrane may occur, resulting in otorrhea and, frequently, decreased pain.

The bacteriology has been best defined in pediatric patients with otitis media;[13] the most common pathogens in nonneonates are *S. pneumoniae* (35 percent), *H. influenzae* (25 percent), and *M. catarrhalis* (15 percent). About 10 percent of *H. influenzae* strains are type b, and these cases may develop bacteremia or

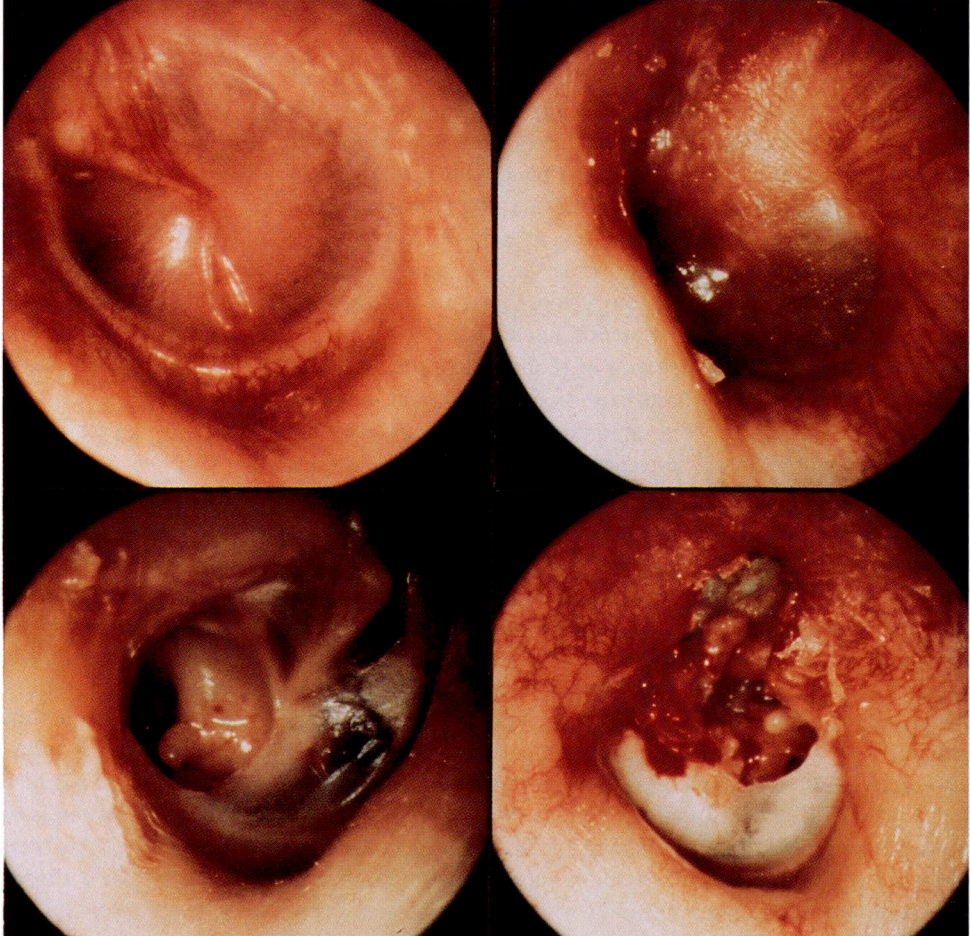

FIGURE 126-3 *Clockwise, from top left,* tympanic membranes: normal ear, resolving acute otitis media, CSOM (chronic suppurative otitis media) with cholesteatoma, CSOM without cholesteatoma. *(Courtesy of Steven D. Rauch, M.D.)*

meningitis. Group B streptococci and enteric gram-negative bacilli are important in neonates. Viruses are recovered, sometimes along with bacteria, in 25 percent of pediatric cases.[7] *H. influenzae* and *S. pneumoniae* are the most common isolates in adults.[39]

Treatment of acute otitis media is usually empiric. Tympanocentesis may be necessary for patients who appear toxic, who are immunocompromised, or whose infection is refractory to therapy. Although about 30 percent of *H. influenzae* strains and 75 percent of *M. catarrhalis* strains produce β-lactamase, amoxicillin is recommended as first-line therapy by some experts because of its cost-effectiveness.[33] Antibiotics active against β-lactamase–producing strains include amoxicillin-clavulinate, trimethoprim-sulfamethoxazole, erythromycin-sulfisoxazole, clarithromycin, and second-generation cephalosporins such as cefuroxime-axetil and loracarbef. An increasing problem is penicillin resistance in pneumococci. This is not β-lactamase mediated. Penicillin-resistant pneumococci may respond to erythromycin, clindamycin, or sulfa drugs, but serious infections require intravenous vancomycin or a third-generation cephalosporin such as ceftriaxone. Adjunctive therapy in acute otitis media with antihistamines has not been shown to be beneficial.

Recurrent episodes of acute otitis media in children are due to the same pathogens that cause initial episodes (*S. pneumoniae, H. influenzae, M. catarrhalis*). Approximately three-fourths of early recurrences are not relapses, but instead are due to different organisms or different strains of the organism that caused the initial episode. Treatment should be with antibiotics active against β-lactamase–producing organisms. Patients with frequent recurrences (e.g., three episodes within 6 months) may benefit from once-daily amoxicillin or sulfisoxazole prophylaxis during the winter months, or from placement of tympanostomy tubes.

Serous Otitis Media

Serous otitis media, also called otitis media with effusion, refers to the persistence of middle-ear fluid without other signs of infection. Diagnosis is made with otoscopy. It is associated with a 5- to 35-decibel hearing loss in the affected ear. Cultures of the middle-ear fluid are often negative, although several clinical trials have found that effusions resolve more quickly in antibiotic-treated children than in controls.[18] Adenoidectomy, myringotomy, or tympanostomy tubes have been shown to decrease the duration of effusion in some children.

Chronic Suppurative Otitis Media

Chronic suppurative otitis media (CSOM) is an inflammatory disease of the middle ear and mastoid. It is characterized by a perforation of the tympanic membrane, with intermittent or constant purulent drainage, and it is associated with irreversible pathologic changes of the mucosa of the middle ear and mastoid. There are two major subtypes of CSOM: CSOM with cholesteatoma and CSOM without cholesteatoma.

In *CSOM with cholesteatoma,* there is a perforation of the tympanic membrane, usually at the margin, which leads into a sac within the middle ear lined by keratinized squamous epithelium (i.e., skin). This sac constitutes a cholesteatoma. It contains desquamated keratin and invites bacterial overgrowth. This, in turn, results in purulent drainage via the perforation. An important feature of a cholesteatoma is its ability to enlarge by erosion of surrounding bone, which can result in serious intratemporal and intracranial complications.

In *CSOM without cholesteatoma,* there is a chronic central perforation of the tympanic membrane. Bacterial infection of the middle ear or mastoid can occur and leads to purulent drainage through the perforation ("active" chronic otitis media). Such drainage may be constant or episodic. The latter may be incited by an upper respiratory infection or by exposure of the ear canal to water.

The classic symptoms of both types of CSOM are painless otorrhea and hearing loss. Diagnosis is made with otoscopy. The appearance of the tympanic membrane varies with the type of CSOM (Fig. 126-3). Audiologic assessment usually reveals a conductive type of hearing loss. Cultures of ears with CSOM in both adults and children often yield *S. aureus, Pseudomonas* and other gram-negative bacilli, and anaerobes. A study in adults found that 50 percent had mixed aerobic and anaerobic infection.[16] The most common aerobes were *Pseudomonas* (37 percent), *S. aureus* (23 percent), and *Klebsiella pneumoniae* (21 percent), while the most common anaerobes were peptostreptococci and *Bacteroides* species.

Most cases of CSOM with cholesteatoma require a mastoidectomy and tympanoplasty operation to remove the cholesteatoma and reconstruct the middle-ear sound transmission mechanism. For cases of "active" CSOM without cholesteatoma, medical therapy is initiated to control the otorrhea. This includes ear cleansing (aural toilet), topical antibiotic drops (e.g., cortisporin), and oral antibiotics. The choice of antibiotics should be guided by culture results from the purulent middle-ear

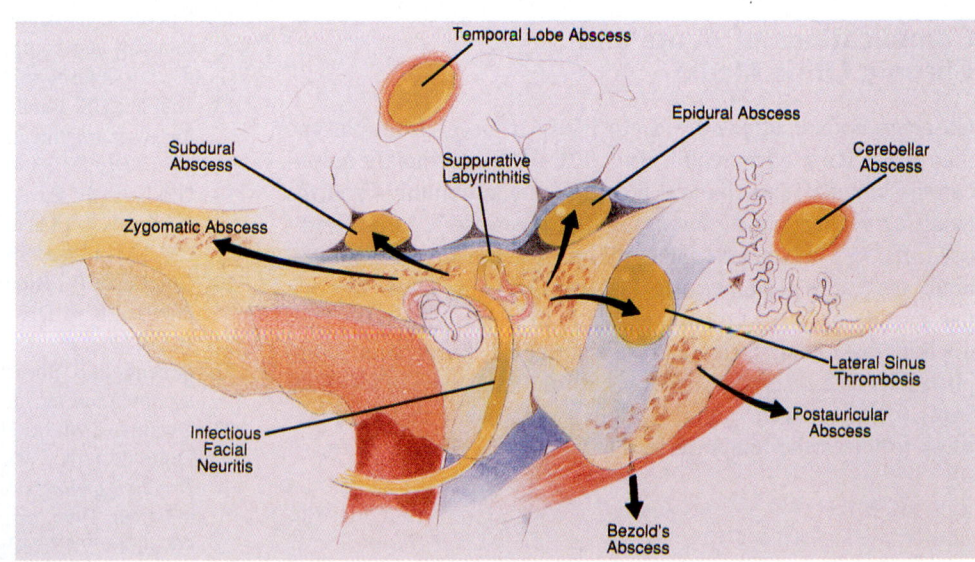

FIGURE 126-4   Complications of chronic otitis media. (*From Harris and Darrow,*[26] *with permission.*)

drainage. A report of using short-course (average 9 days) intravenous antibiotics to treat active CSOM without cholesteatoma in children who had failed oral and topical antibiotic therapy found that 78 percent had resolution of their otorrhea at long-term (mean 4.3 years) follow-up.[30] Surgery may be necessary if medical therapy fails to control otorrhea, or to reconstruct the middle-ear hearing mechanism.

Acute Mastoiditis

The mastoid is the portion of the temporal bone posterior to the middle ear that contains a honeycomb of air cells lined by low, cuboidal epithelium. These air cells connect with the middle ear. Some degree of mastoid mucosal inflammation invariably accompanies episodes of acute otitis media and is also present in many cases of chronic suppurative otitis media. The term *acute mastoiditis* refers to an acute bacterial infection of the mastoid that exceeds mere mucosal involvement. If left untreated, it will result in breakdown of the bony partitions between the mastoid air cells and extension beyond the mastoid compartment.

True acute mastoiditis has become rare in the antibiotic era, probably because of prompt treatment of acute otitis media. Patients with acute mastoiditis present with pain, tenderness, and swelling over the mastoid. The pinna is pushed out and forward when there is an overlying subperiosteal abscess or cellulitis. A CT scan may demonstrate bony destruction or a mastoid abscess. Most infections are due to a mixture of anaerobes and aerobes, with *S. pneumoniae,* group A streptococci, *S. aureus, Pseudomonas, H. influenzae,* and *Proteus* the aerobes most commonly isolated.[19] Ideally, middle-ear fluid should be obtained by tympanocentesis and sent for aerobic and anaerobic cultures before empiric treatment with broad-spectrum antibiotics is begun. Initial antibiotics should include antipseudomonal agents (e.g., ticarcillin–clavulinic acid plus gentamicin), and coverage should be narrowed once culture results are known. Surgical intervention (e.g., myringotomy, drainage of subperiosteal abscess, or simple mastoidectomy) is often required.

Complications of Acute and Chronic Otitis Media

Otogenic complications are more likely to occur from chronic than from acute otitis media (Fig. 126-4). Extracranial complications include sensorineural hearing loss, labyrinthitis and the resulting vertigo, facial nerve palsy, and petrositis. In mastoiditis, infection may track under the periosteum of the temporal bone and cause a subperiosteal abscess, or may break through the mastoid tip and cause an abscess in the neck deep to the sternocleidomastoid muscle (Bezold's abscess). Intracranial complications include epidural abscess, thrombophlebitis of the dural veins (most often the sigmoid sinus), meningitis, and brain abscess (often in the temporal lobe).

REFERENCES

1. Amedee RG: Sinus anatomy and function, in Bailey BJ (ed), *Head and Neck Surgery—Otolaryngology.* Philadelphia, JB Lippincott, 1993, pp 342–349.

2. Aujard Y, Boucot I, Brahimi N, et al: Comparative efficacy and safety of four-day cefuroxime axetil and ten-day penicillin treatment of group A beta-hemolytic streptococcal pharyngitis in children. *Pediatr Infect Dis J* 14:295–300, 1995.

3. Bamberger DM, Jackson MA: Introduction: Overview of upper respiratory infections. *Semin Respir Infect* 10:1–2, 1995.

4. Barrow HN, Levenson MJ: Necrotizing "malignant" external otitis caused by *Staphylococcus epidermidis. Arch Otolaryngol Head Neck Surg* 118:94–96, 1992.

5. Brook I: Bacteriology of chronic maxillary sinusitis in adults. *Ann Otol Rhinol Laryngol* 98:426–428, 1989.

6. Chandler JR, Langenbrunner DJ, Stevens FR: The pathogenesis of orbital complications in acute sinusitis. *Laryngoscope* 80:1414–1428, 1970.

7. Chonmaitree T, Hoowie VM, Truant AL: Presence of respiratory viruses in middle ear fluids and nasal wash specimens from children with acute otitis media. *Pediatrics* 77:698–702, 1986.

8. Cody DT, Neel B, Ferreiro JA, Roberts GD: Allergic fungal sinusitis: The Mayo Clinic experience. *Laryngoscope* 104:1074–1079, 1994.

9. Cover TL, Aber RC: *Yersinia enterocolitica. New Engl J Med* 321:16–24, 1989.

10. Cruz MN, Stewart G, Rosenberg N: Use of dexamethasone in the outpatient management of acute laryngotracheitis. *Pediatrics* 96:220–223, 1995.

11. Davis JC, Gates GA, Lerner C, et al: Adjuvant hyperbaric oxygen in malignant external otitis. *Arch Otolaryngol Head Neck Surg* 118:89–93, 1992.

12. Deeb ZE, Einhorn KH: Infectious adult croup. *Laryngoscope* 100:455–457, 1990.

13. Del Baccaro MA, Mendelman PM, Inglis AF, et al: Bacteriology of acute otitis media: A new perspective. *J Pediatr* 120:81–84, 1992.

14. Donnelly BW, McMillan JA, Weiner LB: Bacterial tracheitis: Report of eight new cases and review. *Rev Infect Dis* 12:729–735, 1990.

15. Doroghazi RM, Nadol JB, Hyslop NE, et al: Invasive external otitis: Report of 21 cases and review of the literature. *Am J Med* 71:603–614, 1981.

16. Erkan M, Sevuk E, Aslan T, Guney E: Bacteriology of chronic suppurative otitis media. *Ann Otol Rhinol Laryngol* 103:771–774, 1994.

17. Gherini SG, Brackmann DE, Bradley WG: Magnetic resonance imaging and computerized tomography in malignant external otitis. *Laryngoscope* 96:542–548, 1986.

18. Giebink GS, Batalden PB, Le CT, et al: A controlled trial comparing three treatments for chronic otitis media with effusion. *Pediatr Infect Dis J* 9:33–40, 1990.

19. Gliklich RE, Eavey RD, Iannuzzi RA, Camacho AE: A contemporary analysis of acute mastoiditis. *Arch Otolaryngol Head Neck Surg* 122:135–139, 1996.

20. Gluckman JL, Righi PD, Rice DH: Sinusitis, in Donald PJ, Gluckman JL, Rice DH (eds), *The Sinuses.* New York, Raven, 1995, pp 161–171.

21. Greenfield S, Sheede PR, Feldman HA: Meningococcal carriage in a population of "normal" families. *J Infect Dis* 123:67–73, 1971.

22. Gwaltney JM Jr: The common cold, in Mandell GL, Bennett JE, Dolin R (eds), *Mandell, Douglas and Bennett's Principles and Practice of Infectious Diseases,* 4th ed. New York, Churchill Livingstone, 1995, pp 561–566.

23. Gwaltney JM Jr: Rhinovirus infection of the normal human airway. *Am J Respir Crit Care Med* 152(Suppl):S36–S39, 1995.

24. Gwaltney JM Jr, Phillips CD, Miller RD, et al: Computed tomography study of the common cold. *New Engl J Med* 330:25–30, 1994.

25. Gwaltney JM Jr, Scheld WM, Sande MA, Sydnor A: The microbial etiology and antimicrobial therapy of adults with acute community-acquired sinusitis: A fifteen-year experience at the University of Virginia and review of other selected studies. *J Allergy Clin Immunol* 90:457–462, 1992.

26. Harris JP, Darrow DH: *Surgery of the Ear and Temporal Bone.* New York, Raven, 1993.

27. Henrickson KJ, Kuhn SM, Savatski LL: Epidemiology and cost of infection with human parainfluenza virus types 1 and 2 in young children. *Clin Infect Dis* 18:770–779, 1994.

28. Horowitz G, Kaslow R, Friedland G: Infectiousness of laryngeal tuberculosis. *Am Rev Respir Dis* 114:241–244, 1976.

29. Inglis AF Jr: Herpes simplex virus infection: A rare cause of prolonged croup. *Arch Otolaryngol Head Neck Surg* 119:551–552, 1993.

30. Kenna MA, Rosane BA, Bluestone CD: Medical management of chronic suppurative otitis media without cholesteatoma in children: Update 1992. *Am J Otol* 14:469–473, 1993.

31. Kessler HA, Blaauw B, Spear J, et al: Diagnosis of human immunodeficiency virus infection in seronegative homosexuals presenting with an acute viral syndrome. *JAMA* 258:1196–1199, 1987.

32. Klassen TP, Feldman ME, Watters LK, et al: Nebulized budesonide for children with mild-to-moderate croup. *New Engl J Med* 331:285–289, 1994.

33. Klein JO: Otitis externa, otitis media, mastoiditis, in Mandell GL, Bennett JE, Dolin R (eds), *Mandell, Douglas and Bennett's Principles and Practice of Infectious Diseases,* 4th ed. New York, Churchill Livingstone, 1995, pp 579–584.

34. Kristjansson S, Berg-Kelly K, Winso E: Inhalation of racemic adrenaline in the treatment of mild and moderately severe croup: Clinical symptom score and oxygen saturation measurements for evaluation of treatment effects. *Acta Paediatr Scand* 83:1156–1160, 1994.

35. Laing RB, Wardrop PJ, Welsby PD, Brettle RP: Stridor in patients with HIV infection. *J Laryngol Otol* 109:1197–1199, 1995.

36. Leventhal BG, Kashima HK, Mounts P, et al: Long-term response of recurrent respiratory papillomatosis to treatment with lymphoblastoid interferon alfa-n1. *New Engl J Med* 325:613–617, 1991.

37. Savolainen S, Jousimies-Somer HR, Mäkitie AA, Ylikoski JS: Peritonsillar abscess: Clinical and microbiologic aspects and treatment regimens. *Arch Otolaryngol Head Neck Surg* 119:521–524, 1993.

38. Schalén L, Eliasson I, Fex S, et al: Acute laryngitis in adults: Results of erythromycin treatment. *Acta Otolaryngol Suppl (Stockh)* 492:55–57, 1992.

39. Schwartz LE, Brown RB: Purulent otitis media in adults. *Arch Intern Med* 152:2301–2304, 1992.

40. Shapiro AM, Rimell FL, Pou A, et al: Tracheotomy in children with juvenile-onset recurrent respiratory papillomatosis: The Children's Hospital of Pittsburgh experience. *Ann Otol Rhinol Laryngol* 105:1–5, 1996.

41. Shapiro J, Eavey RD, Baker AS: Adult supraglottitis: A prospective analysis. *JAMA* 259:563–567, 1988.

42. Smith JT, Dickins JRE, Graham SS: Herpes zoster oticus: Treatment with intravenous acyclovir. *Laryngoscope* 98:776–779, 1988.

43. Thaller SR, Gross JR, Pilch BZ, Goodman ML: Laryngeal tuberculosis as manifested in the decades 1963–1983. *Laryngoscope* 97:848–850, 1987.

44. Vogt FC: The incidence of oral candidiasis with use of inhaled corticosteroids. *Ann Allergy* 43:205–210, 1979.

45. Wald ER, Reilly JS, Casselbrant M, et al: Treatment of acute maxillary sinusitis in childhood: A comparative study of amoxicillin and cefaclor. *J Pediatr* 104:297–302, 1984.

46. Washburn RG, Kennedy DW, Begley MG, et al: Chronic fungal sinusitis in apparently normal hosts. *Medicine* 67:231–247, 1988.

47. Williams JW, Simel DL: Does this patient have sinusitis? Diagnosing acute sinusitis by history and physical examination. *JAMA* 270:1242–1246, 1993.

48. Windus DW, Stokes TJ, Julian BA, et al: Fatal *Rhizopus* infections in hemodialysis patients receiving deferoxamine. *Ann Intern Med* 107:678–680, 1987.

ACUTE BRONCHITIS AND COMMUNITY-ACQUIRED PNEUMONIA

Thomas J. Marrie

ACUTE BRONCHITIS

Acute bronchitis is an inflammation of the tracheobronchial tree, usually in association with a generalized respiratory infection. It occurs most commonly during the winter months and is associated with respiratory viruses, including rhinovirus, coronavirus, influenza viruses, and adenovirus. *Mycoplasma pneumoniae, Chlamydia pneumoniae,* and *Bordetella pertussis* may also cause bronchitis. Secondary invasion with bacteria such as *Hemophilus influenzae* and *Streptococcus pneumoniae* may also play a role in acute bronchitis.

Cough is the most prominent manifestation of acute bronchitis. Initially the cough is nonproductive, but later mucoid sputum is produced. Still later in the course of the illness, purulent sputum is present. Many patients with acute bronchitis also have tracheitis. Symptoms of tracheal impairment include burning substernal pain associated with respiration and a very painful substernal sensation with coughing. Rhonchi and coarse crackles may be heard on examination of the chest; however, there are no signs of consolidation and the chest radiograph shows no opacity.

Most cases of acute bronchitis require measures directed only at relieving cough. For patients with fever or a predominant tracheitis component and purulent sputum, the sputum should be Gram stained and cultured. If there is a predominant microorganism seen in the presence of more than 25 polymorphonuclear neutrophils and under 10 squamous epithelial cells per low-power field, antibiotic therapy directed against *S. pneumoniae* and *H. influenzae* should be instituted. Most patients, however, do not require antibiotic therapy for acute bronchitis—it is a self-limited disease.

PNEUMONIA

Definition

Pneumonia is defined as inflammation and consolidation of lung tissue due to an infectious agent. Pneumonia that develops outside the hospital is considered community acquired. Pneumonia developing 72 h or more after admission to hospital is nosocomial, or hospital acquired. There is still some debate as to whether nursing home–acquired pneumonia should be considered community-acquired or nosocomial pneumonia. For this reason, it is perhaps best to divide pneumonia into community acquired and institution acquired. (The latter includes hospitals, nursing homes, extended-care facilities, psychiatric institutions, and rehabilitation facilities.)

Epidemiology

Pneumonia is a common disease. The overall attack rate is about 12 cases per 1000 persons per year. The attack rates are highest at the extremes of age. Pneumonia is the sixth leading cause of death in the United States.

The epidemiology of pneumonia has changed in recent years. This is due in part to changes in the population at risk and in part to the discovery of new microbial agents that cause pneumonia and changes in antimicrobial susceptibility of old microbial agents, such as *S. pneumoniae, H. influenzae,* and *Staphylococcus aureus.* Population changes include continued increase in the number and proportion of patients who are 65 years of age or older. The annual incidence of pneumonia requiring hospitalization among persons in the age group 75 years or older is 11.6 per 1000 persons, compared with a rate of 0.54 per 1000 among persons aged 35 to 44. Likewise, there has been a steady increase

TABLE 127-1

Clues to the Etiology of Pneumonia from the History and Physical Exam

Feature	Organism
Environmental	
Exposure to contaminated air-conditioning cooling towers, recent travel associated with a stay in a hotel, exposure to a grocery store mist machine, visit or recent stay in a hospital with contaminated (by *L. pneumophila*) potable water	*Legionella pneumophila*
Pneumonia after windstorm in an endemic area	*Coccidioides immitis*
Outbreak of pneumonia in shelters for homeless men, jails, military training camps	*Streptococcus pneumoniae* *Mycobacterium tuberculosis* *S. pneumoniae* *Chlamydia pneumoniae*
Exposure to contaminated bat caves, excavation in endemic areas	*Histoplasma capsulatum*
Animal contact	
Exposure to infected parturient cats, cattle, sheep, or goats	*Coxiella burnetii*
Exposure to turkeys, chickens, ducks, or psittacine birds	*C. psittaci*
Travel history	
Travel to Thailand or other countries in Southeast Asia	*Burkholderia (Pseudomonas) pseudomallei (melioidosis)*
Pneumonia in immigrants from Asia or India	*M. tuberculosis*
Occupational history	
Pneumonia in a health-care worker who works in a large city with patients infected with HIV	*M. tuberculosis*
Host factors	
Diabetic ketoacidosis	*S. pneumoniae* *Staphylococcus aureus*
Alcoholism	*S. pneumoniae* *Klebsiella pneumoniae* *S. aureus*
Chronic obstructive lung disease	*S. pneumoniae* *Hemophilus influenzae* *Moraxella catarrhalis*
Solid organ transplant recipient (pneumonia occurring > 3 months after transplant)	*S. pneumoniae* *H. influenzae* *Legionella* spp. *Pneumocystis carinii* *Cytomegalovirus* *Strongyloides stercoralis*
Sickle cell disease	*S. pneumoniae*
HIV infection	*P. carinii*
CD4 cell count < 200/μl	*S. pneumoniae* *H. influenzae* *Cryptococcus neoformans* *M. tuberculosis* *Rhodococcus equi*
Physical findings	
Periodontal disease with foul-smelling sputum	Anaerobes, may be mixed aerobic-anaerobic infection
Bullous myringitis	*Mycoplasma pneumoniae*

TABLE 127-1 *(Cont.)*

Feature	Organism
Absent gag reflex, altered level of consciousness, or a recent seizure	Polymicrobial (oral aerobic and anaerobic bacteria) can be macro- or microaspiration
Encephalitis	*M. pneumoniae* *C. burnetii* *L. pneumophila*
Cerebellar ataxia	*M. pneumoniae* *L. pneumophila*
Erythema multiforme	*M. pneumoniae*
Erythema nodosum	*C. pneumoniae* *M. tuberculosis*
Ecthyma gangrenosum	*P. aeruginosa* *Serratia marcescens*
Cutaneous nodules (abscesses) and CNS findings	*Nocardia* species

SOURCE: From *Clin Infect Dis* 18:501–515. 1994.

in the number of organ transplant recipients in the general population and the number of patients with HIV infection. This has created a subset of patients with community-acquired pneumonia who may be infected not only with the traditional pathogens that cause pneumonia but also with opportunistic pathogens; furthermore, they may have severe or atypical presentation of this infection. Newer pathogens recognized as causing pneumonia include *Chlamydia pneumoniae* and Hantavirus. *Pneumocystis carinii,* previously a rare cause of pneumonia in intentionally immunocompromised patients, is a common cause of pneumonia in HIV-infected patients.

Clinical Manifestations

Symptoms that are suggestive of pneumonia include fever, chills, pleuritic chest pain, and cough. The cough may be nonproductive (dry) or productive of mucoid or purulent sputum. It may be rusty in color and frankly bloody; in patients with a lung abscess (anerobic infection), it may have a foul odor. For some time it was held that typical pneumonia (due to pyogenic organisms such as pneumococcus, staphylococcus, or *H. influenzae*) could be distinguished from that due to *Mycoplasma, Legionella,* and *Chlamydia pneumoniae*—so-called atypical pneumonia. The latter is said to be characterized by a more indolent illness than that of typical pneumonia, with a cough that is nonproductive or productive of mucoid sputum only. Careful studies have shown that one cannot reliably distinguish between typical versus atypical pneumonia on clinical grounds. However, this is not to say that a careful history and physical examination are not helpful in suggesting a cause of the pneumonia. Table 127-1 gives a partial list of clues to the cause of pneumonia that may be obtained from the history and physical exam.

Nonrespiratory symptoms such as headache, nausea, vomiting, abdominal pain, diarrhea, myalgia, and arthralgia are also common symptoms in patients with pneumonia. It is wise to remember that the elderly complain of fewer symptoms with pneumonia than do younger patients.

Physical Examination

Fever is usually present, but some patients may be hypothermic (a poor prognostic sign), and some (20 percent) are afebrile at the time of presentation with their pneumonia. Crackles are heard on auscultation over the affected area of lung, and physical findings of consolidation (dullness to percussion, increased tactile, and vocal fremitus, whispering pectoriliquy, and bronchial breath sounds) are present in about 20 percent of patients with pneumonia. A pleural friction rub is heard in about 10 percent of cases.

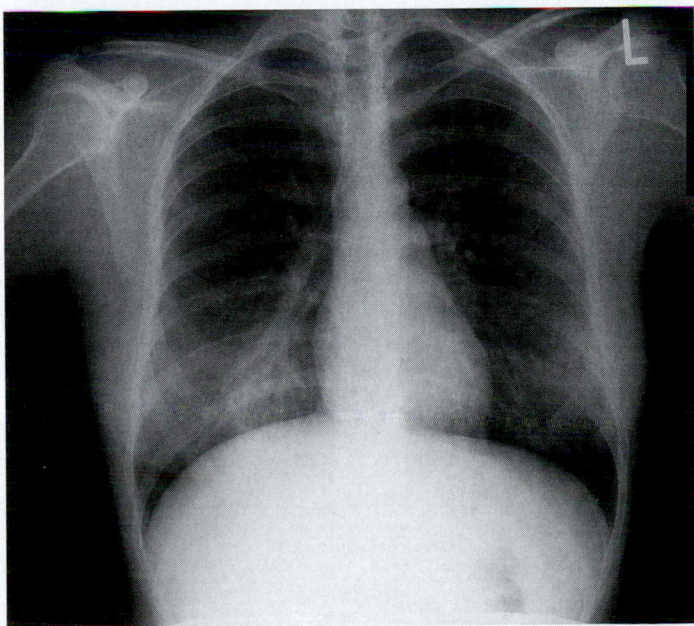

FIGURE 127-1   Right lower lobe pneumonia due to *Coxiella burnetii* (Q fever). This young woman developed pneumonia after exposure to the products of conception of her infected pet cat.

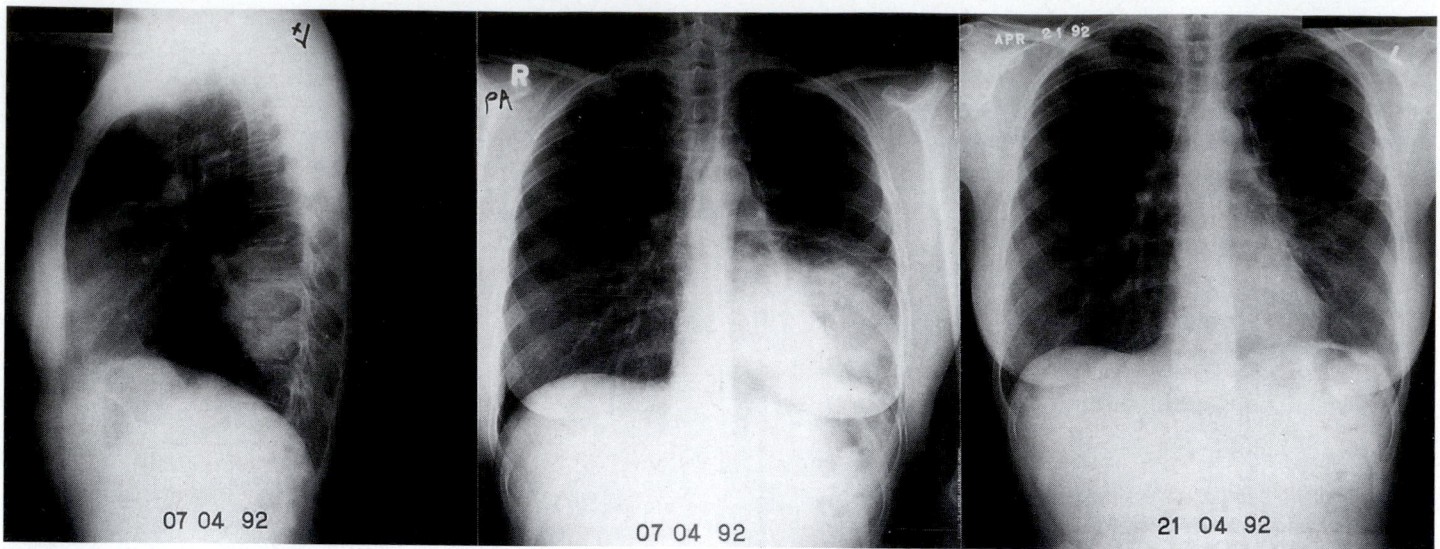

FIGURE 127-2 Serial chest radiographs of a 32-year-old nurse with *Chlamydia psittaci* pneumonia. She was severely ill with fever, chills, and headaches. She had severe fatigue for 8 months after this episode of pneumonia.

Radiographic Diagnosis

Clinical suspicion of pneumonia usually prompts a chest radiograph. An opacity on the chest radiograph is considered the "gold standard" for the diagnosis of pneumonia. However, this opacity may be due to infection, infarction, hemorrhage, edema fluid, malignancy, or inflammation caused by a variety of processes, such as vasculitis or adverse drug reactions. Several studies have shown that radiologists cannot differentiate bacterial from nonbacterial pneumonia on the basis of the radiograph. Certain radiographic patterns are more commonly associated with some microbial agents than with others. Table 127-2 gives such a list. Representative chest radiographs of patients with pneumonia are shown in Figs. 127-1–127-4.

Etiologic Diagnosis

Pneumonia represents a difficult challenge for the clinician, since the cause cannot be determined from the clinical presentation and data from microbiologic studies are not available for at least 48 h. Even then, in the case of microorganisms isolated from the sputum, one cannot be sure that this is

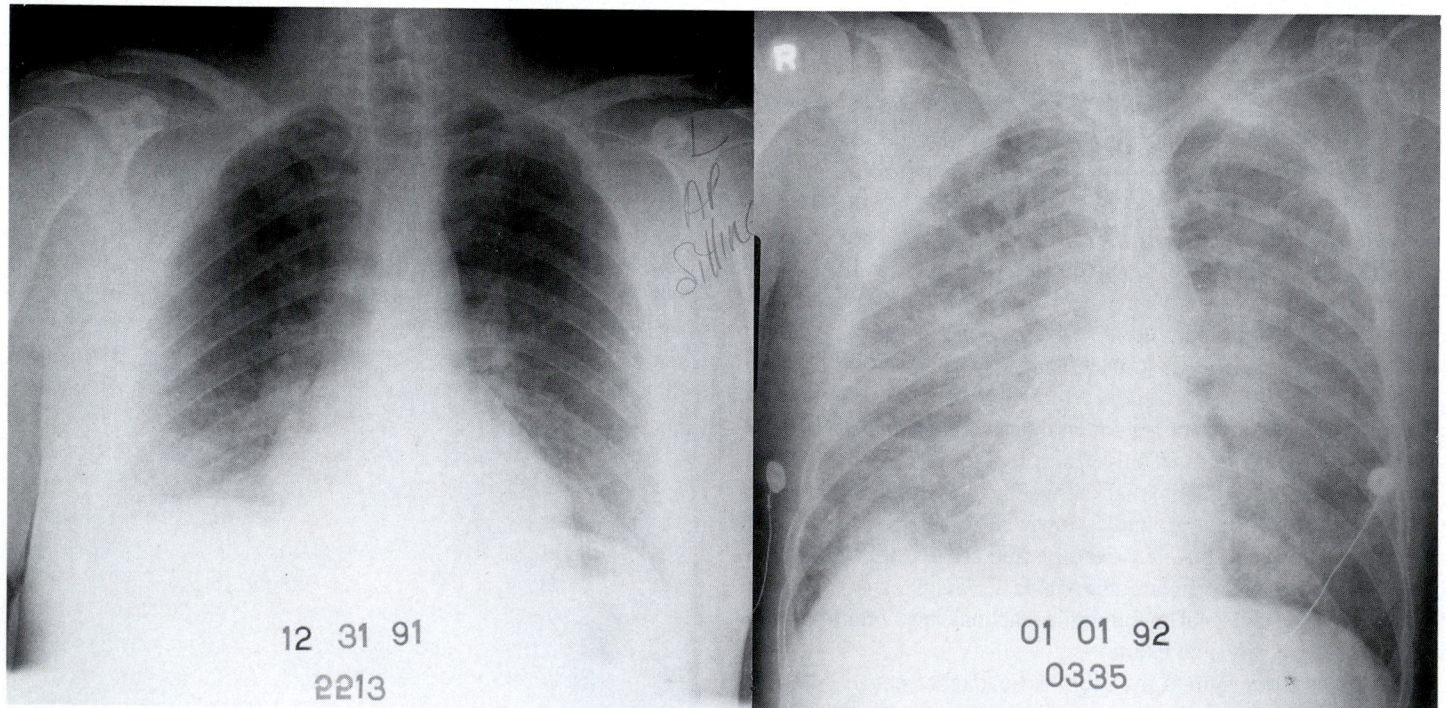

FIGURE 127-3 Chest radiographs showing rapidly progressive diffuse pulmonary opacities in a 22-year-old man with bacteremic *Streptococcus pneumoniae* pneumonia. This patient had had his spleen removed 6 years earlier. He rapidly developed septic shock and died about 8 h after admission.

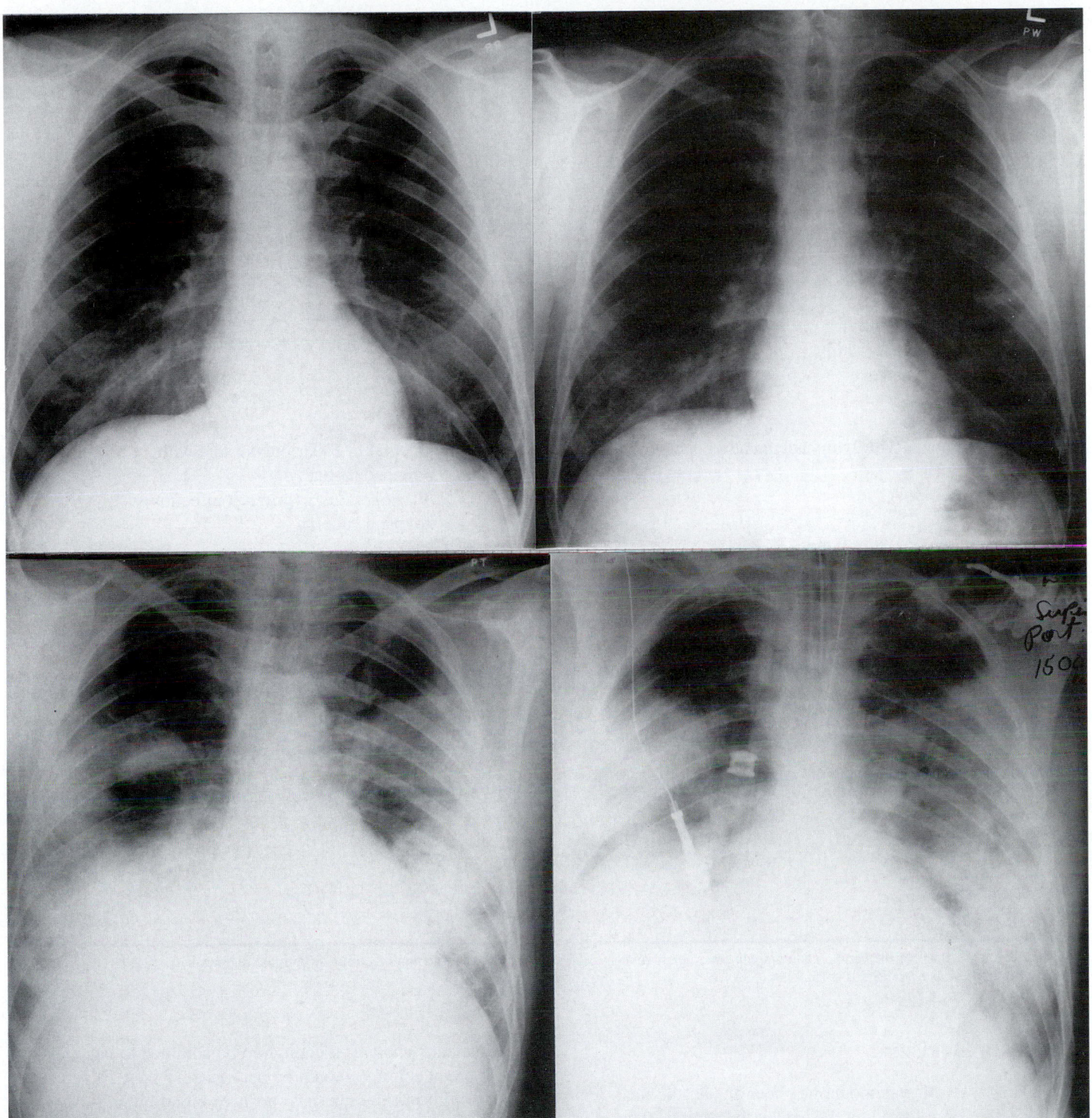

FIGURE 127-4   Serial chest radiographs of a 40-year-old man with pneumonia due to *Legionella pneumophila* serogroup 6.

the organism causing the pneumonia. For this reason, it is useful to categorize the etiology of pneumonia as definite or probable (Table 127-3).

The etiology of community-acquired pneumonia (CAP) as determined in prospective studies is given in Tables 127-4, 127-5, and 127-6. Table 127-5 shows data for patients with severe pneumonia requiring admission to intensive care units. Table 127-6 gives the etiologic data for bacterial pneumonia in patients with

HIV infection. Early in the course of the HIV epidemic, *P. carinii* accounted for most cases of pneumonia. Now, with widespread use of prophylaxis to prevent *Pneumocystis* pneumonia, it is evident that bacterial pneumonia is common in HIV disease (see Chapters 135 and 150). Indeed, the rates of pneumococcal pneumonia and *H. influenzae* pneumonia are 20 times higher among HIV-infected persons than in those of an age- and sex-matched population without HIV infection.

TABLE 127-2

Differential Diagnosis of Common Patterns on Chest Radiography in a Patient with a Clinical Picture of Pneumonia

Focal opacity
  Streptococcus pneumoniae
  Mycoplasma pneumoniae
  Legionella pneumophila
  Staphylococcus aureus
  Chlamydia pneumoniae
  Mycobacterium tuberculosis
  Blastomyces dermatitidis

Interstitial
  "Viruses"
  M. pneumoniae
  Pneumocystis carinii
  C. psittaci

Interstitial pneumonia with lymphadenopathy
  Epstein-Barr virus
  Francisella tularensis
  C. psittaci
  M. pneumoniae   Fungi

Cavitation
  Mixed aerobic anaerobic (lung abscess)
  Aerobic gram-negative bacilli
  M. tuberculosis
  L. pneumophila
  Cryptococcus neoformans
  Nocardia asteroides
  Actinomyces israelii
  Coccidioides immitis
  P. carinii

Bulging fissure
  Klebsiella pneumoniae
  L. pneumophila

Multifocal opacities
  S. aureus
  Coxiella burnetii
  L. pneumophila
  S. pneumoniae

Miliary
  M. tuberculosis
  Histoplasma capsulatum
  C. immitis
  B. dermatitidis
  Varicella zoster

Segmental or lobar pneumonia with lymphadenopathy
  M. tuberculosis (primary infection)
  Atypical rubeola

Pneumatoceles
  S. aureus
  S. pyogenes
  P. carinii

"Round" pneumonia
  C. burnetii
  S. pneumoniae
  L. pneumophila
  S. aureus

Only the microbial causes of the various radiographic patterns are given—each also has an extensive noninfectious differential diagnosis.
SOURCE: From *Clin Infect Dis* 18:501–515, 1994.

Admission Decision

Once a diagnosis of pneumonia has been made, the next decision is whether or not to admit the patient to hospital. Now, more than ever, there is considerable pressure to treat as many patients as possible at home. In order to do this, it is important to know the factors that are predictive of complicated course in pneumonia. Some of these factors are given in Table 127-7.

Diagnostic Workup

Patients who are well enough to be treated as outpatients need minimal diagnostic workup. This should include a chest radiograph, complete white blood count, electrolytes, creatinine, and oxygen saturation if pulse oximetry is available to the physician. Attempts should be made to obtain sputum for culture in patients with chronic obstructive pulmonary disease (COPD).

In patients who are ill enough to be admitted to hospital, two sets of blood cultures should be performed. About 10 percent of patients with pneumonia have positive blood cultures. *S. pneumoniae* is the most common cause of bacteremic pneumonia, accounting for 60 percent of all cases. Despite the controversy about the utility of sputum Gram's stain and culture, this is still a useful test. Take the time to obtain the specimen yourself. One of the chief reasons why this test has fallen into disrepute is that collecting the specimen is a task assigned to other members of a busy health-care team. A sample collected hours after antimicrobial therapy has been initiated is useless.

Sputum Gram's Stain and Culture

A sputum specimen should be cultured only if a smear of a representative portion shows more than 25 polymorphonuclear neutrophils and fewer than 10 squamous epithelial cells per low-

TABLE 127-3

Guidelines for Determining the Etiology of CAP

Definite

Blood cultures positive for a pathogen

Pleural fluid positive for a pathogen

Presence of *Pneumocystis carinii* in induced sputum or in bronchoalveolar lavage fluid

A fourfold or greater rise in antibody titer to *Mycoplasma pneumoniae, Chlamydia pneumoniae*

Isolation of *Legionella pneumophila* or a fourfold rise in antibody titer or positive urinary antigen test for *Legionella*

Positive direct fluorescence antibody test for *Legionella* plus an antibody titer of ≥ 1:256 for *Legionella*

Serum or urine positive for *Streptococcus pneumoniae* antigen

Isolation of *Mycobacterium tuberculosis* from sputum

Probable

Heavy or moderate growth of a predominant bacterial pathogen on sputum culture and a compatible Gram's stain

Light growth of a pathogen in which sputum Gram's stain reveals a bacterium compatible with the culture results

Aspiration pneumonia is diagnosed on clinical grounds.
SOURCE: Modified from Fang et al.[4]

power field. The Gram's stain on such a specimen is useful. If only one morphologic type of bacteria is seen in such a specimen, it is likely that this microorganism is causing the pneumonia. Indeed, in one study, when more than 10 g of positive lancet-shaped diplococci were seen, the sputum was considered positive for pneumococci. This criterion was met in 62 percent of specimens that were culture positive for *S. pneumoniae*.

In patients with HIV infection, sputum production may be induced by inhalation of hypertonic saline, which irritates the tracheobronchial tree and produces bronchorrhea. This results in a specimen that is useful for examination for *P. carinii*, thereby obviating bronchoscopy.

Patients who are ill enough to require admission to an intensive care unit for the treatment of their pneumonia should have an aggressive diagnostic workup. This will usually include at least a bronchoscopy, with use of a pro-

TABLE 127-4

Etiology of Community-Acquired Pneumonia Requiring Hospitalization—North America

Reference number	4	5	1
No. of patients studied	359	719	151 (154 episodes)
No. (%) patients with sputum cultured	336 (94)	257 (36)	None[†]
Location	Pittsburgh, Pa.	Halifax, N.S.	Little Rock, Ark.
Time period of study	Jul 1/86–Jun 30/87	Nov 1/81–Mar 18/87	1985
No. (%) with pneumonia of:			
Unknown cause	118 (32.9)	340 (47)	75 (48.7)
More than one cause	10 (2.8)	74 (10.3)	10 (6.4)
Streptococcus pneumoniae	39 (10.9)	61 (8.5)	9 (5.8)
Aspiration	12 (3.3)	52 (7.2)	Not stated
Mycoplasma pneumoniae	7 (2)	40 (5.6)	5 (3.2)
Influenza A virus	Not tested	40 (5.6)	7 (4.5)
Staphylococcus aureus	12 (3.3)	29 (4.0)	9 (5.8)
Hemophilus influenzae	39 (10.9)	27 (3.7)	2 (1.3)
Coxiella burnetii	Not tested	22 (3.1)	0
Influenza B virus	Not tested	17 (2.4)	0
Pneumocystis carinii	9 (2.5)	14 (1.9)	0
Legionella spp.	24 (6.7)	16 (2.2)	14 (9)
Mycobacterium tuberculosis	4 (1.1)	10 (1.4)	3 (1.9)
Chlamydia pneumoniae	22 (6.1)	18/301 (6)*	12 (7.8)
Postobstructive	19 (5.3)	13 (1.8)	Excluded
S. epidermidis	0	0	4 (2.6)
Aspergillus spp.	0	0	1 (0.6)
Nocardia spp.	0	0	1 (0.6)
Francisella tularensis	Not tested	Not tested	5 (3.2)
Streptococcus spp.	10 (2.8)	19 (2.6)	4 (2.6)
Anaerobic bacteria	0	4 (0.6)	2 (1.3)
Other aerobic gram-negative bacteria	21 (5.9)	22 (3.1)	8 (5.2)

*Only 301 patients had serum samples tested for antibodies to *Chlamydia pneumoniae*.
†This study did not use information from sputum cultures in determining cause. Some patients had a variety of invasive diagnostic procedures.

TABLE 127-5

Etiology of CAP in Patients Requiring Admission to an ICU

Reference	3	9	8	7
No. studied	60	92	67	53
Mean age (yr)	54	53	56.8	52
No. (%) died	29 (48)	18 (20)	14 (21)	13 (25)
No. (%) with pneumonia due to (six most common causes listed):				
Unknown	25 (42)	44 (48)	45 (67)	25 (47)
Streptococcus pneumoniae	11 (18)	13 (14)	12 (17)	15 (28)
Hemophilus influenzae	7 (12)			
Legionella pneumophila	7 (12)	13 (14)	7 (10)	
Mycoplasma pneumoniae	4 (7)	6 (7)		3 (5)
Influenza virus	3 (5)			2 (4)
Staphylococcus aureus	2 (3)	1		2 (4)
Streptococcus species		3 (3)		
Chlamydia psittaci				2 (4)
Other aerobic gram-negative bacilli	2 (3)	5 (5)	8 (12)	

tected brush to sample respiratory secretions and brochoalveolar lavage. If this is carried out before the initiation of antibiotic therapy, the diagnostic yield is up to 80 percent. When this procedure is performed after 72 h or more of antibiotic therapy, however, the microbiologic yield is much lower—18 percent.

Transthoracic needle aspiration can be used when the basal segment(s) of the lungs is (are) consolidated. A 20 gauge 3.5-inch needle is used to inject 2 to 3 ml of nonbacteriostatic saline into the lung. This is then aspirated and placed into a blood culture bottle. The diagnostic yield from this procedure ranges from 33 to 85 percent.

Occasionally, patients with CAP require an open lung biopsy. However, this is usually a last resort in a patient whose condition continues to deteriorate and there is no etiologic diagnosis

TABLE 127-6

Etiology of Bacterial CAP in Patients with HIV Infection

Reference	3
Location of study	San Francisco, CA
Period of study	May 1990–April 1991
No. of pneumonia episodes	216
Cause of pneumonia (no., %)	
Hemophilus influenzae	4 (1.9)
Streptococcus pneumoniae	66 (30.6)
Moraxella catarrhalis	1 (0.5)
Other streptococcus	15 (6.9)
Cause unknown	54 (25)
Mixed infections	13 (6)
Hemophilus spp.	42 (19.4)
Klebsiella pneumoniae	4 (1.9)
Staphylococcus aureus	10 (4.6)
Pseudomonas aeruginosa	5 (2.3)
Serratia marcescens	1 (0.5)
Neisseria meningitidis	1 (0.5)

despite the usual workup, including bronchoscopy.

An acute-phase serum sample should be obtained from all patients who are admitted to hospital with CAP. If the patient responds promptly to antibiotic therapy, there is no need to obtain a convalescent sample. If the patient responds poorly to therapy, however, a convalescent sample should be obtained 3 to 6 weeks after the acute-phase sample. The diagnostic battery ordered will depend on local epidemiologic conditions. In general, *M. pneumoniae, C. pneumoniae, Coxiella burnetti, Legionella pneumophila,* adenovirus, influenza A and B viruses, parainfluenza viruses 1, 2, and 3, and respiratory syncytial virus antibodies can be measured in most laboratories. Antibody titers to *S. pneumoniae* pneumolysin and detection of immune complexes to this antigen may be a tool for diagnosis of pneumococcal pneumonia in those who do not have sputum available for culture.

L. pneumophila serogroup 1 infection can be reliably diagnosed from detection of antigen in urine with a radioimmunoassay or an enzyme-linked imunosorbent assay.

TREATMENT

The initial therapeutic approach to pneumonia is empirical. Categorize the severity of the pneumonia as mild, moderate, or severe. It is then usually self-evident where the patient will be treated—at home, in hospital, or in an intensive care unit. Table 127-8 outlines the guidelines for initial antimicrobial therapy for community-acquired pneumonia as proposed by the American Thoracic Society.

Once the etiologic diagnosis has been made, treatment should be changed to employ the cheapest, narrowest-spectrum agent effective against that microorganism. For example, if *S. pneumoniae* is determined to be the cause of the pneumonia, penicillin therapy is still appropriate in most instances. The response of patients to treatment depends on the severity of the pneumonia and the presence of co-morbidities that may be made worse by the pneumonia. Outpatients with mild to moderate pneumonia do very well. Mortality is rare (less than 1 percent), and only about 4 percent of patients fail therapy and require hospitalization.

The overall mortality for those admitted to hospital for treatment of pneumonia is 20 percent. In patients with nursing home–acquired pneumonia, it may approach 40 percent. For many of these patients, pneumonia is the last straw.

A recent concept in therapy of pneumonia requiring hospitalization is early switch to oral antibiotics. Patients who are stable by hospital day 3 (as evidenced by temperature of 37.5°C or less for 16 h, white blood cell count returning toward normal, normal hemodynamics, no requirement for auxiliary oxygen, no complications of pneumonia such as empyema, and ability to

TABLE 127-7

Risk Factors for a Complicated Course or Mortality in Patients with CAP

Age >65 years

Co-morbid illnesses that are likely to be made worse by the pneumonia, especially chronic renal failure, ischemic heart disease, congestive heart failure, and severe COPD

Concurrent malignancy

Postsplenectomy state

Altered mental status

Alcoholism

Immunosuppressive therapy

Respiratory rate >30 breaths per minute

Diastolic blood pressure <60 mm Hg; systolic blood pressure <90 mm Hg

Hypothermia

Creatinine >150 mm/l or BUN >7 mm/l

Leukopenia <3,000/μl or leucocytosis >30,000/μl

O_2 <60 mm Hg or P_{CO_2} >48 mm Hg while breathing room air

Albumin <30 gm/l

Hemoglobin <9 gm/l

Pseudomonas aeruginosa or *Staphylococcus aureus* as the cause of the pneumonia

Bacteremic pneumonia

Multilobe involvement on chest radiograph

Rapid radiographic progression of the pneumonia defined as increase in the size of the pulmonary opacity of ≥50% within 36 h

take antibiotics by mouth) can be switched to antibiotics and discharged shortly thereafter. About one-third of patients qualify for this therapy.

Some patients see their condition fail to improve or indeed worsen during therapy. Table 127-9 gives the factors that should be considered in this setting.

Radiographic evidence of resolution of pneumonia lags behind clinical resolution and correlates with age and the presence of COPD. In general, those who are under 50 years of age and have no COPD show radiographic resolution of pneumonia within 4 weeks. In contrast, resolution requires 12 or more weeks for those with pneumonia who are older than 50 years and have coexistent COPD or alcoholism. In about 2 percent of patients, pneumonia will be the presenting manifestation of carcinoma of the lung (postobstructive pneumonia). It is important to demonstrate that the pneumonia has resolved radiographically for those who are at risk for carcinoma of the lung. In general, all tobacco smokers and those who are 50 years of age or older and have pneumonia should have a chest radiograph to determine whether or not the pneumonia has completely resolved.

PREVENTION

Influenza vaccination of the elderly results in reduction in the rate of hospitalization for pneumonia and influenza by 48 to 57 percent. The role of pneumococcal vaccine has not been as clearly defined as that of influenza vaccine; however, the Advisory Committee on Immunization Practice recommends pneumococcal vaccine for persons older than 65 years of age.

Specific Pathogens

STREPTOCOCCUS PNEUMONIA

S. pneumoniae is still a common cause of pneumonia. Patients with bacteremic pneumococcal pneumonia are more likely to have diabetes mellitus, COPD, or alcoholism than those who have other causes of CAP. Capsular polysaccharide types 14, 4, 1, 6A/6B, 3, 8, 7F, 23F, and 18C are the most frequent causes of pneumococcal disease. Currently, 10 to 15 percent of *S. pneumoniae* isolates in the United States are intermediately or highly resistant to penicillin. These isolates are usually also resistant to erythromycin, tetracycline, and trimethoprim-sulfamethoxazole. Types 19A, 6A, 23, 19, 11, 6, 16, 9, and 14 are most frequently associated with penicillin resistance. The minimal inhibitory concentration (MIC) of penicillin for susceptible strains is under 0.06 μg/ml; isolates with MICs of 0.1 to 1 μg/ml are of intermediate resistance, and those with MICs of at least 2 μg/ml are highly resistant. These levels were established for CNS infections, for which trough concentrations of penicillin at 10 times MIC are necessary for cure. Generally, with intravenous antibiotics high concentrations can be achieved in pulmonary tissue, so even resistant strains of *S. pneumoniae* will usually respond to treatment with high doses of penicillin or third-generation cephalosporin. If there is concomitant meningitis, however, both a third-generation cephalosporin and vancomycin should be given.

STAPHYLOCOCCUS AUREUS

Pneumonia due to this agent is usually of sudden onset, affects persons with co-morbid illnesses (except during influenza outbreaks, when healthy young adults may be infected), and is frequently complicated by cavitation (20 percent), pneumothorax (10 percent), jaundice (8 percent), empyema (5 percent), acute renal failure (5 percent), and pericarditis (2 percent).

Methicillin-resistant *S. aureus* (MRSA) is a rare cause of CAP. It does occur, however, and once established in a region, it can be a major problem. Vancomycin is used to treat MRSA, whereas cloxacillin or nafcillin is used to treat methicillin-susceptible strains. Surgical drainage is necessary for treatment of empyema. If multiple rounded opacities are seen in a patient with *S. aureus* pneumonia, suspect right-sided endocarditis. Toxic shock syndrome may complicate *S. aureus* pneumonia.

HEMOPHILUS INFLUENZAE

This cause of pneumonia is more common in older patients with COPD. Both type B and non-B strains can cause pneumonia. About 30 percent of all *H. influenzae* isolates now produce

TABLE 127-8

Initial Empiric Antimicrobial Therapy for CAP

1. Clinical presentation: not severe; *oral therapy*
   A. Previously well and/or <60 years old
      Macrolide or tetracycline
   B. Co-morbid illness and >60 years old
      Cephalosporin (second-generation)
      or
      Trimethoprim-sulfamethoxazole
      or
      Amoxicillin plus β-lactamase inhibitor
   If *Legionella* is a concern, add a macrolide
2. Clinical presentation: severe; intravenous therapy
   (i) Treatment site: hospital ward
   Cephalosporin (second or third generation) ± macrolide ± rifampin
   Penicillin-allergic patients: trimethoprim-sulfamethoxazole plus
      macrolide
   (ii) Treatment site: ICU
   Cephalosporin (third generation) with antipseudomonas activity
      and a macrolide ± rifampin
      or
      Imipenem-cilastatin
      or
      Ciprofloxacin + macrolide ± rifampin
3. Treatment site: nursing home
   (i) Clinical presentation: not severe
      Cephalosporin (second generation)
      or
      Trimethoprim-sulfamethoxazole
      or
      Amoxicillin–clavulinic acid
   Add a macrolide if *Legionella* is a concern
   (ii) Clinical presentation: severe
      Penicillin plus ciprofloxacin (oral)
      or
      Cephalosporin (second generation)*
      or
      Ceftriaxone (intramuscular)*
   Penicillin-allergic patients: ciprofloxacin + clindamycin (intramuscular)

*Add a macrolide if *Legionella* is a concern.
SOURCE: Modified from Neiderman et al[6] (see Chapter 122).

β-lactamase and hence are resistant to ampicillin and amoxicillin. Between 7 and 14 percent of *H. influenzae* isolates are resistant to trimethoprim-sulfamethoxazole. More than 90 percent of *H. Influenzae* isolates are resistant to erythromycin; 1 to 2 percent are resistant to tetracycline. Amoxycillin–clavulinic acid and a second- or third-generation cephalosporin will reliably treat *H. influenzae* pneumonia. Sir William Osler died from *H. influenzae* pneumonia.

STREPTOCOCCUS PYOGENES (GROUP A STREPTOCOCCUS)

This agent is uncommon as a cause of pneumonia. One of its presentations is pneumonia accompanied by explosive pleuritis. Cases of group A streptococcal pneumonia may be accompanied by "toxic strep syndrome." Clindamycin, 600 mg given intravenously every 8 h, is superior to penicillin for the treatment of serious group A streptococcal infections. Jim Henson, creator of the Muppets, died from group A streptococcal pneumonia.

MYCOPLASMA PNEUMONIAE

This agent accounts for up to 30 percent of pneumonias treated on an outpatient basis. The extrapulmonary manifestations of *M. pneumoniae* are many and include cold agglutinin–induced hemolytic anemia, thrombocytopenia, encephalitis, cerebellar ataxia, Guillain-Barré syndrome, Stevens-Johnson syndrome, and myocarditis. This is primarily a disease of younger patients, but it accounts for 5 percent of all cases of pneumonia in persons 65 years of age or older. Macrolides (erythromycin, clarithromycin, azithromycin) or tetracyclines are the treatment of choice.

LEGIONELLACEAE

This family, which includes 29 species and more than 49 serogroups, causes two clinical syndromes—legionnaires' disease and a self-limited flulike illness (Pontiac fever). *L. pneumophila* serogroup 1, the microorganism responsible for the 1976 outbreak in Philadelphia that gave this disease its name, accounts for 70 to 90 percent of the cases of Legionnaires' disease. Legionnaires' disease can be community or hospital acquired, and it can occur in sporadic, endemic, and epidemic forms. Exposure to contaminated water (showers, cooling towers, or even ingestion of such water and subsequent microaspiration) is the prime mode of acquisition of this illness. Older age, male sex, immunosuppression (especially with corticosteroids), nosocomial acquisition, end-stage renal disease, and infection with *L. pneumophila* serogroup 5 are risk factors for death from this infection. Erythromycin, 1 g given intravenously every 6 h, along with rifampin, 300 mg twice a day, is used to treat seriously ill patients with Legionnaires' disease. The disease may continue to progress for up to 4 days despite optimal therapy. Other options are doxycycline, 100 mg given twice intravenously in 24 h and then 100 mg OD intravenously, and ciprofloxacin, 400 mg every 12 h intra-

TABLE 127-9

Considerations When Pneumonia Fails to Resolve or Worsens During Therapy

Reconsider the pneumonia diagnosis: Could this be pulmonary infarction, malignancy, vasculitis, drug reaction, or eosinophilic pneumonia?

Reconsider the etiologic diagnosis: Are you treating the appropriate microorganism(s)? Remember that 10% of cases of community-acquired pneumonia are polymicrobial. Tuberculosis can mimic pyogenic pneumonia. Also consider unusual organisms such as *Actinomyces* or *Nocardia* species.

Are you dealing with a resistant microorganism? *Streptococcus pneumoniae* resistant to penicillin, erythromycin, and tetracycline is common in several European countries and in the United States.

Has your patient developed nosocomial pneumonia? Such an event is common, particularly in patients who require endotracheal intubation and assisted ventilation. Is your hospital's potable water supply contaminated by *Legionella* spp.? If so, consider nosocomial legionnaires' disease. Nosocomial legionnaires' disease should be a consideration anytime a patient with CAP is improving and develops nosocomial pneumonia.

Could this be postobstructive pneumonia (i.e., is endobronchial obstruction present)?

Have you considered empyema? Pus in the pleural space will continue to cause fever until it is drained.

Has metastatic infection occurred? Occasionally, patients who are bacteremic as a result of their pneumonia develop endocarditis, meningitis, septic arthritis, or a deep abscess such as splenic or renal abscess.

Always consider drug fever.

---

venously. Relapses have occurred with treatment courses of less than 21 days.

HANTAVIRUS

In May 1993, reports of deaths due to severe pulmonary disease were received by the New Mexico Department of Health. Many of the affected persons were residents of the Navajo reservation located near the Four Corners area of New Mexico, Arizona, Colorado, and Utah. Within a few months a new Hantavirus, Sin Nombre ("no name") virus, had been isolated and shown to be responsible for this outbreak, which had affected 17 persons. Hantavirus pulmonary syndrome (HPS) is characterized by a flulike prodromal illness, followed by rapidly progressive noncardiogenic pulmonary edema. Fever, myalgia, cough or dyspnea, nausea or vomiting, and diarrhea are the most common symptoms. Hypotension, tachypnea, and tachycardia are the usual findings on physical exam. Leukocytosis (often with a severe left shift), thrombocytopenia (median lowest platelet count 64,500 per mm^3), prolonged prothrombin and partial thromboplastin times, and elevated serum lactate dehydrogenase concentration are the most common laboratory findings. The mortality was high (88 percent) in the Four Corners outbreak. The initial chest radiograph showed infiltrates in 65 percent and no abnormality in 24 percent. Subsequently, 16 (94 percent) had rapidly evolving bilateral diffuse infiltrates. In the few months after identification of this new Hantavirus, two more new Hantaviruses were identified in the United States and cases of HPS continue to be reported. The deer mouse, *Peromyscus maniculatus*, is the primary rodent reservoir for this virus.

CHLAMYDIA PNEUMONIAE

This intracellular pathogen of humans is spread by aerosols. It causes sinusitis, pharyngitis, bronchitis, otitis media, and pneumonia. The last can be as a result of primary infection or as reactivation of latent infection. Primary infection affects mainly young adults and may be followed by reactive airway disease. Two weeks' treatment with doxycycline is adequate. Clarithromycin is very active in vitro against *C. pneumoniae,* but whether it is superior to doxycycline is not known.

The reactivation type of infection occurs in older adults, often as part of a polymicrobial infection. The rate of *C. pneumoniae* in this setting is unknown.

Diagnosis is by isolation of the organism from respiratory secretions or by serology. A greater than fourfold rise in IgM or IgG by microimmunofluorescence test or a single IgM titer of at least 1:16 or an IgG titer of at least 1:512 is considered diagnostic.

REFERENCES

1. Bates JH, Campbell GD, Barren AL, et al: Microbial etiology of acute pneumonia in hospitalized patients. *Chest* 101:1005–1112, 1992.
2. British Thoracic Society Research Committee and the Public Health Laboratory Service: The aetiology, management, and outcome of severe community-acquired pneumonia on the intensive care unit. *Respir Med* 86:7–13, 1992.
3. Burack JH, Hahn JA, Saint-Maurice D, et al: Microbiology of community-acquired bacterial pneumonia in persons with and at risk for human immunodeficiency virus type 1 infection: Implications for rationale empiric antibiotic therapy. *Arch Intern Med* 154:2589–2596, 1994.
4. Fang GD, Fine M, Orloff J, et al: New and emerging etiologies for community-acquired pneumonia with implications for therapy: A prospective multicenter study of 359 cases. *Medicine* 69:307–316, 1990.
5. Marrie TJ, Durant H, Yates L: Community-acquired pneumonia requiring hospitalization: 5-year prospective study. *Rev Infect Dis* 11:586–599, 1989.
6. Neiderman MS, Bass JB, Campbell GD, et al: Guidelines for the initial empiric therapy of community-acquired pneumonia: Diagnosis, assessment of severity, and initial antimicrobial treatment. *Am Rev Respir Dis* 148:1418–1426, 1993.
7. Örtqvist Å, Sterner G, Nilsson JA: Severe community-acquired pneumonia: Factors influencing need of intensive care treatment and prognosis. *Scand J Infect Dis* 17:377–386, 1985.
8. Pachon J, Prados MD, Capote F, et al: Severe community-acquired pneumonia: Etiology, prognosis and treatment. *Am Rev Respir Dis* 142:369–373, 1990.
9. Torres A, Serra-Battles J, Ferrer A, et al: Severe community-acquired pneumonia: Epidemiology and prognostic factors. *Am Rev Respir Dis* 144:312–318, 1991.

PNEUMONIA IN CHILDHOOD

Mark S. Pasternack

Lower respiratory tract infections in children may be organized as a collection of distinct clinical syndromes on the basis of the age of the child and the clinical setting. Pneumonia is a rather common problem for the practicing pediatrician, yet its management may be problematic because of a paucity of objective data. Historical information is often scant, especially in treatment of younger patients. The clinical and especially the radiologic features of pneumonia are often not closely correlated with particular etiologic agents. Furthermore, it is frequently difficult or impossible to obtain sputum for microscopic analysis and culture. In addition, pneumonia in early childhood may reflect a congenital anomaly or a genetic disorder associated with impaired host defense. Thus, the management of pneumonia in children often presents a greater challenge to the clinician than does that of similar illnesses in adults.

NEONATAL PNEUMONIA

Bacterial pneumonia in neonates generally follows acquisition of a pathogen during passage through the birth canal and is a common focus of early-onset neonatal sepsis. The incidence of neonatal bacterial infection is roughly 0.1 percent of all births, but it is much greater in "high risk" infants—those delivered before the 36th week of gestation, after prolonged rupture of maternal membranes, after maternal intrapartum fever, etc. At present, group B streptococcus *(S. agalactiae),* especially serogroup III, is the most common cause of neonatal sepsis, causing roughly 60 percent of episodes; enteric gram-negative bacilli (predominantly *Escherichia coli*) are responsible for roughly 25 percent of episodes.

Early-onset group B streptococcal infection is commonly acquired intrapartum, with clinical evidence of sepsis appearing within the first few hours of life. In contrast, meconium aspiration is more common among term infants and is generally apparent in the delivery room. Respiratory distress, with grunting, flaring, and intercostal retractions, is the most commonly encountered sign of neonatal pneumonia. Thus, infants with group B streptococcal pneumonia cannot be readily distinguished clinically from infants with hyaline membrane disease.[1,51] The presence of fever or hypothermia, irritability, or hypotonia points toward neonatal sepsis. The white blood cell count is frequently abnormal, with either marked leukocytosis and an associated "left shift" with bands and earlier myeloid forms or leukopenia, but it is not a reliable indicator of neonatal infection. Approximately half of the chest radiographs of infants with group B streptococcal pneumonia demonstrate symmetric ground-glass airspace infiltrates that are indistinguishable from the radiographic findings of hyaline membrane disease (Fig. 128-1). The remaining infants have asymmetric lobar or multilobar consolidations, which are typical of bacterial pneumonia.

The presence of a unilateral pleural effusion in a neonate with pulmonary infiltrates strongly suggests group B streptococcal pneumonia. Since the clinical features of group B streptococcal pneumonia overlap with those of hyaline membrane disease, all infants with respiratory distress should undergo a "septic workup," including blood, urine, and cerebrospinal fluid examination, followed by the empiric administration of ampicillin and gentamicin for 48 to 72 h, pending the results of the initial cultures. Infants requiring intubation and mechanical ventilation because of hypoxemia should also have endotracheally suctioned specimens sent for Gram's stain and culture. These infants must be monitored for

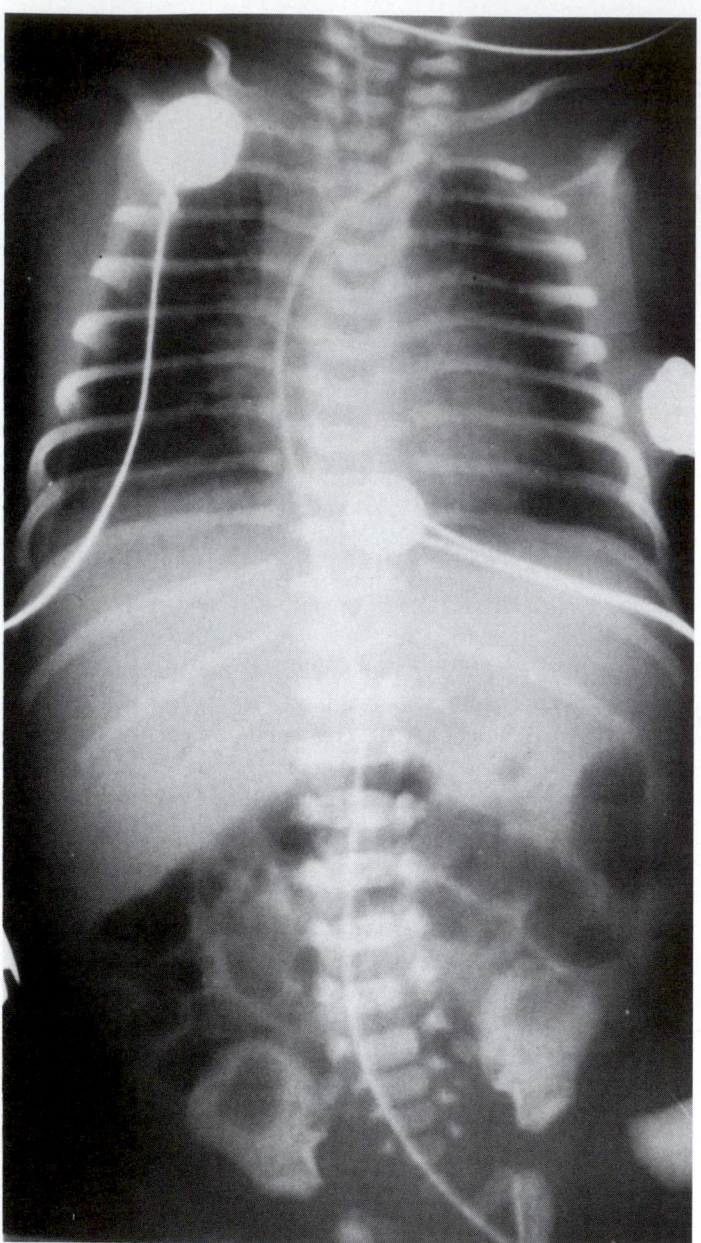

FIGURE 128-1   Early-onset group B streptococcal pneumonia. There are hazy symmetric "ground glass" infiltrates bilaterally obscuring the cardiac silhouette. Note the presence of a small right pleural effusion.

the development of enlarging pleural effusions, which may require drainage to improve ventilatory function, and for the development of metastatic skeletal infections or meningitis. The duration of therapy is determined, in part, by the presence of bacteremia and metastatic infection, since meningitis will require 3 weeks of therapy and skeletal infection, even longer treatment.

Infants with protracted stays in a neonatal intensive care unit are at risk for the late development of nosocomial pneumonia, particularly those requiring prolonged intubation because of severe prematurity and respiratory distress, or those with anatomic (e.g., tracheoesophageal fistulas, duodenal atresia) or neurologic defects resulting in aspiration. In such infants, the spectrum of potential pathogens causing pneumonia is broad. In addition to the conventional neonatal pathogens, nosocomial flora may in-

clude any multiply resistant organism, such as methicillin-resistant *Staphylococcus aureus*, Enterobacteriaceae *(Klebsiella, Enterobacter, Serratia)*, or nonenteric gram-negative bacilli such as *Pseudomonas aeruginosa* or *Acinetobacter.* Hence, broad-spectrum empiric antibiotic therapy such as treatment with vancomycin and gentamicin or amikacin, often with a third-generation cephalosporin such as ceftazidime, should be given until a specific pathogen can be identified; antibiotic therapy can be modified at that time. The particular nosocomial pathogens that pose the greatest risks to infants with nosocomial pneumonia reflect colonization patterns that may vary among different hospitals, so the empiric antibiotic therapy used in this situation is frequently hospital specific.

Congenital viral infections such as cytomegalovirus and rubella may be responsible for pneumonitis early in the neonatal period. Congenitally infected infants who have symptomatic tachypnea or hypoxemia in addition to the stigmas of congenital viral infection usually have extensive viral disease with hepatosplenomegaly, microcephaly, and/or jaundice. Despite the radiologic findings of diffuse interstitial infiltrates, the clinical picture of sytemic viral disease usually predominates, and respiratory failure is infrequent. In contrast, neonatal herpes simplex infections are the consequence of intrapartum acquisition of virus through the birth canal of a generally primarily infected mother rather than true congenital infections. Early-onset herpetic infection can occur despite the absence of typical perinatal risk factors for bacterial sepsis. Herpes simplex pneumonitis in this setting is usually seen in disseminated disease, in which the systemic features of fulminant herpetic infection with hepatitis, encephalitis, and myocarditis predominate. The prognosis in this setting is poor despite the availability of nucleoside antiviral agents such as acyclovir. Similarly, early postnatal viral infections, such as adenovirus, may also result in fulminant respiratory failure in previously healthy full-term infants.

PNEUMONIA IN EARLY INFANCY

The bacterial pathogens responsible for neonatal pneumonia are rarely encountered after the first month of life, since most episodes of bacterial pneumonia accompany the early-onset form of neonatal bacterial sepsis. By the second month of life, infants have an increasing risk of developing viral infection as well as chlamydial pneumonia (Fig. 128-2). Despite the broad range of potential pathogens, the lungs of young infants have a limited repertoire of response to illness. The combination of diminutive airways, compromised further by inflammatory mucosal edema or intraluminal secretions, results in characteristic airway obstruction. Infants may wheeze, and chest radiographs demonstrate hyperinflation and interstitial infiltrates, with or without atelectasis. Patchy asymmetric airspace disease may be present as well. Thus, the nonspecific chest radiographic findings are not helpful in narrowing the differential diagnosis, and clinical and epidemiologic features guide management and therapy.

Chlamydia Trachomatis Pneumonia

Chlamydial pneumonia accounts for up to one-third of pneumonias in infants during the first 4 months of life.[6,22,49] Infants gen-

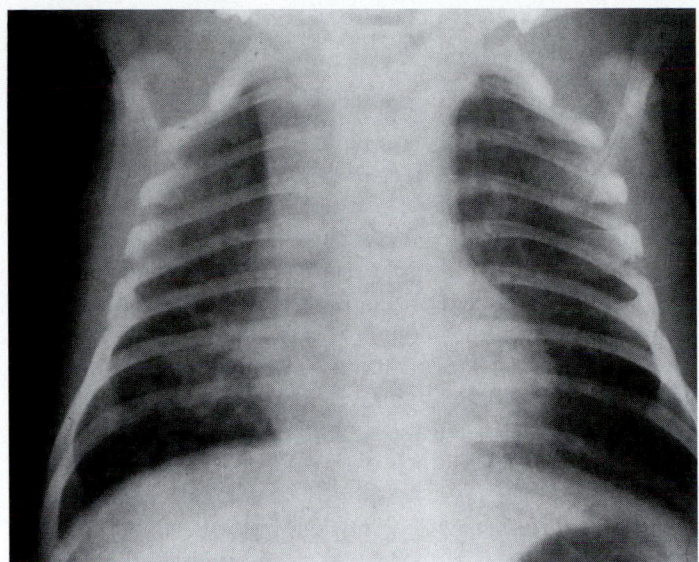

FIGURE 128-2   *Chlamydia trachomatis* pneumonitis. This 12-day-old infant had stereotypic findings of hyperinflation and asymmetric interstitial infiltrates.

erally acquire *C. trachomatis* during their passage through the birth canal from chronically (and usually asymptomatically) infected mothers, although horizontal infection in a nursery or at home due to inadequate handwashing is possible. Thus, the incidence of chlamydial infection is inversely proportional to the mother's age and proportional to the number of sexual partners. When infected secretions are aspirated intrapartum, symptomatic lower respiratory tract infection may develop during the first month of life. More commonly, the conjunctivae or upper respiratory tract mucosa is infected initally, with subsequent spread of infection following aspiration of infected upper respiratory secretions. The illness progresses insidiously, with the gradual development of cough and congestion over several days, with low-grade or no fever. Respiratory distress is generally only mild to moderate unless there is concomitant infection with a second pathogen, such as respiratory syncytial virus (RSV), or there is an underlying pulmonary process such as bronchopulmonary dysplasia. Chest auscultation generally reveals scattered rales, and chest radiograph shows the nonspecific patchy pneumonitis and hyperinflation pattern described above.[43] Infants often have mild leukocytosis, sometimes with modest eosinophilia. Hyperglobulinemia is common but nondiagnostic. Only one-half of infants with chlamydial pneumonitis have associated conjunctivitis. The laboratory diagnosis of chlamydial pneumonia can be confirmed by antigen detection in nasopharyngeal swab samples using monoclonal antibody kits or nucleic acid detection methods. Systemic therapy with erythromycin (40 mg/kg per day, given every 6 h) hastens resolution of symptoms. Infants with conjunctivitis should receive topical therapy with erythromycin ophthalmic ointment or tetracycline solution.

Acute Viral Pneumonia

Most episodes of pneumonia in infants more than 2 months of age present as acute febrile illnesses and are due to viral pathogens.

Respiratory Syncytial Virus

RSV is the most important cause of lower respiratory tract infection in infants.[7,30] Virtually all infections are symptomatic, although there is a spectrum from pure bronchiolitis, with wheezing and hyperinflation as the dominant clinical features, to pneumonia with true airspace disease. Most infants possess features of both processes. RSV circulates widely every winter, although in a given community the peak incidence may shift anywhere from early fall to early spring in a particular year. There are two RSV serotypes, and in a particular year a single RSV serotype may predominate;[24] however, the immune response following RSV infection in infants is not significantly protective against symptomatic lower respiratory tract disease after exposures during subsequent winters, regardless of the circulating serotype.[23] RSV pneumonia is not common until the second month of life, and it is believed that transplacentally acquired anti-RSV antibodies may be protective. As the titer of protective antibody wanes, infants are at risk for more severe illness.

RSV infection generally begins with a brief prodromal illness with low-grade fever and nasal congestion and/or rhinorrhea. Within a day or two, infants develop increased fever (101° to 103°F) and progressive respiratory distress, with tachypnea and intercostal retractions. Wheezing, which is prominent, is believed to reflect mechanical obstruction of the airways due to inflammation, edema, and associated secretions, as well as true IgE-mediated allergic wheezing. The presence of rales reflects atelectasis and areas of pneumonitis. In very young infants and in premature infants, the initial presentation of RSV disease may be atypical, with little or no fever or wheezing and with frequent episodes of apnea and bradycardia. High-risk infants—i.e., infants with severe immunodeficiency states and those with primary congenital heart disease, particularly those with left-to-right shunts with pulmonary hypervascularity, or pulmonary disease such as bronchopulmonary dysplasia—are at particular risk for prolonged and life-threatening infection.[20] In general, RSV infection in HIV-infected children is well tolerated, although prolonged viral replication and shedding may persist, with attendant risks of nosocomial spread.[30] Approximately 1 percent of infected infants develop respiratory distress requiring hospitalization.

The specific diagnosis of RSV infection can be confirmed in 85 to 90 percent of cases by rapid antigen detection techniques such as ELISA or direct immunofluorescence of nasopharyngeal wash specimens. Specimens that are negative according to rapid diagnostic methods can be cultured for RSV on HEp-2 cells, with diagnostic syncytia formation appearing after 3 to 6 days. The treatment of RSV infection with the aerosolized nucleoside ribavirin remains controversial. Ribavirin therapy was associated with mild clinical improvement when administered to normal infants based on a subjective clinical scoring system.[21] The response to ribavirin therapy was somewhat more dramatic when it was administered to high-risk infants.[20] Ribavirin has been administered to intubated infants requiring mechanical ventilation for severe RSV disease, with significant[47] or no[36] benefit reported. Aerosolized ribavirin has to be administered for up to 18 h a day in a hood or tent system equipped with a scavenger device to prevent dissemination of the drug into the environment, since there are concerns regarding possible teratogenicity among chronically exposed health-care workers. In many tertiary care centers, ribavirin therapy is administered to perhaps 10 percent of infants hospitalized with RSV. Hospitalized infants with RSV pneumonia should be isolated (and cohorted if necessary) and placed under contact and respiratory precautions, since the virus can spread by large droplet, fomite, and aerosol. The Food and Drug Administration has approved the use of monthly RSV immune globulin as a prophylactic agent to prevent RSV disease in premature and other high-risk infants.[19]

Other Respiratory Viral Pathogens in Infancy

The parainfluenza viruses (of which there are three serotypes) and the influenza viruses (of which there may be two type A strains and a type B strain circulating during a particular winter season) are also responsible for lower respiratory tract infections in infants.[14,15,25] Although parainfluenza virus 1 is commonly associated with croup (viral laryngotracheitis) and parainfluenza virus 3 frequently mimics RSV and is more commonly associated with bronchiolitis and viral pneumonitis, all three serotypes can produce any syndrome of upper or lower respiratory tract infection. Thus, bronchiolitis and viral pneumonia in infants mimicking RSV infection may be caused by a parainfluenza virus. Distinction among these possibilities is of some utility in severe cases, since aerosolized ribavirin has had only anecdotal usage in parainfluenza virus infection,[53] and is probably less active in these infections than in RSV disease.[44] Although these viral pathogens are ubiquitous and responsible for little morbidity among most infants, fulminant disease leading to respiratory failure and death can occur even in the absence of underlying immunodeficiency. Children with primary or acquired immunodeficiency are at increased risk for developing progressive and ultimately fatal infections with these respiratory viral pathogens, and efforts to establish a prompt etiologic diagnosis by viral culture or rapid diagnostic testing is crucial in order to institute prompt antiviral therapy. Similarly, influenza may cause lower respiratory tract disease in infancy. When suspicion of influenza is high, the diagnosis may be confirmed by rapid antigen detection testing and the illness treated by the administration of amantadine (8 mg/kg a day every 12 h). Adenoviruses are another important, but sporadic, cause of severe viral pneumonia in infants.

Acquired Cytomegalovirus Pneumonia

Occasionally, infants in the first 2 months of life have an indolent syndrome of interstitial pneumonitis that mimics chlamydial pneumonia but actually represents cytomegalovirus (CMV) pneumonia.[55] In contrast to infants with congenital CMV, in whom pulmonary disease is associated with severe congenital infection, otherwise healthy infants may develop mild to moderate respiratory distress as the result of peripartum or neonatal acquisition of CMV through breast milk or, in premature infants, through blood transfusion. A single culture for CMV obtained at the time of respiratory symptoms cannot readily distinguish between postnatal primary infection or asymptomatic shedding of congenitally acquired CMV. Otherwise uncomplicated postnatal

CMV pneumonia does not serve as an indicator of significant underlying immunodeficiency.

Additional Causes of Pneumonia in Infancy

Conventional diagnostic techniques for chlamydial and viral pathogens fail to identify a pathogen in roughly half of all cases of pneumonia in infants. More intensive microbiologic and serologic analyses have suggested that a significant number of infants may have neonatal pneumonia due to *P. carinii* and *Ureaplasma urealyticum* in addition to the conventional pathogens described above.[8] Pneumonitis cases associated with these pathogens were not readily distinguished from infections due to *C. trachomatis*. The short-term prognosis of these infections is presumably favorable, since diagnostic techniques to identify such infections are not employed in most centers, and infants with indolent pneumonia generally do well with supportive care. Long-term follow-up has suggested that recurrent wheezing and abnormalities in pulmonary function testing may be common in these children after neonatal pneumonia.

PNEUMONIA AFTER THE FIRST 6 MONTHS OF LIFE

After the first 4 to 6 months of life, *C. trachomatis* pneumonia is no longer observed. Several careful longitudinal studies of lower respiratory tract infections in infants and children have been performed during the past 20 years, utilizing both microbiologic and serologic techniques to determine the specific causes of pneumonia in infancy. Although roughly one-half of episodes never receive a specific diagnosis, most proven episodes of pneumonia are due to the same viral pathogens responsible for viral pneumonia in early infancy.[14,15] As noted above, recurrent symptomatic RSV disease in the second and third years of life is very common, and often results in clinically significant episodes of bronchiolitis or RSV pneumonia.[23] Since the related parainfluenza and influenza agents represent at least six immunologically distinct pathogens that circulate in epidemic fashion each year, it is not surprising that infants remain at risk of developing significant viral pneumonia.

Bacterial Pneumonia

Although far less common than viral pneumonia, bacterial pneumonia may be difficult to distinguish prospectively on a clinical basis from episodes of viral pneumonia. Both forms of pneumonia are common during the first 2 years of life after the neonatal period.[39] Since the pathogenesis of bacterial pneumonia generally represents aspiration of pharyngeal pathogens, often in the setting of inflammatory edema and increased secretions triggered by an upper respiratory tract infection, the two processes may have similar initial prodromal findings associated with a low-grade fever. As the lower respiratory process evolves, infants and toddlers will have similar features of significant fever, tachypnea, and possible respiratory distress with acral cyanosis and intercostal retractions regardless of the cause. A few physical findings are helpful: diffuse wheezing, when present, reflects bronchiolitis, making RSV or other viral pathogens (especially parainfluenza viruses and, to a lesser extent, influenza viruses) the likely cause of infection. Similarly, markedly asymmetric breath sounds, with unilateral percussive dullness or a unilateral pleural friction rub, strongly suggest bacterial infection, with spread of disease to the pleural space. Laboratory findings are also often nonspecifically abnormal, since the presence of moderate leukocytosis (e.g., to 15,000) and band forms may be seen in either type of pneumonitis. Extreme leukocytosis, with abundant early forms, usually suggests a bacterial process, often with bacteremia or spread of infection to the pleural space. Blood cultures should routinely be obtained in children with high fever, leukocytosis, or moderate respiratory distress, since such cultures may represent the only approach to recovering a bacterial pathogen. Chest radiographs are sensitive but surprisingly nonspecific in attempts to assess the cause of pneumonia in children.[25]

Although focal consolidation is usually caused by bacterial infection, viral pneumonia may present with a dense focal infiltrate (Fig. 128-3). Conversely, bacterial infection may be associated with patchy segmental infiltrates or even interstitial changes, particularly in younger children. Radiologic investigation is helpful in assessment of the extent of disease and the presence of intrathoracic complications, but it has a more limited role in determining the cause of pneumonia. Thus, the pediatrician is often forced to initiate antimicrobial therapy for possible bacterial pneumonia based on inconclusive clinical and laboratory findings. In the patient sufficiently ill to require hospitalization, nasotracheal suctioning should be considered in order to obtain material for Gram's stain and culture.

Even when these parameters point toward a bacterial process, identification of a specific pathogen remains problematic. Only the most severely ill infants and children have bacteremia accompanying pneumonia. Unless a bacterial pathogen is recovered from the blood or from a site of a secondary infection (joint fluid, cerebrospinal fluid, pleural fluid), the specific cause cannot be readily determined. It is not possible to obtain expectorated sputum, and invasive attempts at culture at the time of nasotracheal suctioning or bronchoscopy may be unrewarding because of the incidental recovery of pharyngeal flora or because prior antibiotic therapy has suppressed recovery of the true pathogen in the lung. In general, because of limited sensitivity, rapid bacterial antigen detection techniques have not been helpful in determining the cause of pneumonia in children. Recovery of the pathogen from a sterile site facilitates antimicrobial susceptibility testing, but most episodes require empiric therapy.

The microbiology of community-acquired pneumonia in infancy and early childhood reflects pharyngeal carriage of respiratory pathogens, and the spectrum of causative agents resembles that seen with otitis media. Although amoxicillin is inexpensive and well tolerated, it will be efficacious only in roughly 80 to 85 percent of cases. Since failure of initial oral therapy may lead to hospitalization and greatly enhanced expense, the use of a more potent initial oral agent—such as an oral second- or third-generation cephalosporin, the β-lactam–β-lactamase combination amoxicillin–clavulanic acid, or a newer macrolide—to decrease the risk of primary antibiotic failure can be justified. Among hospitalized infants, the use of second-generation cephalosporin agents, such as cefuroxime, has become increasingly attractive,

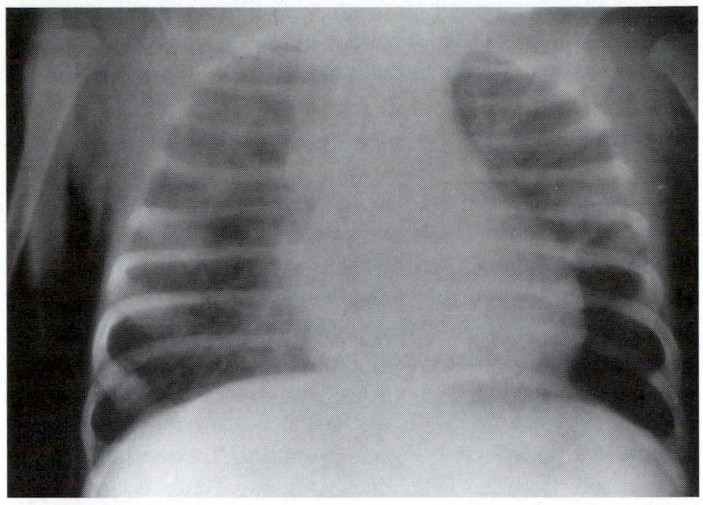

A

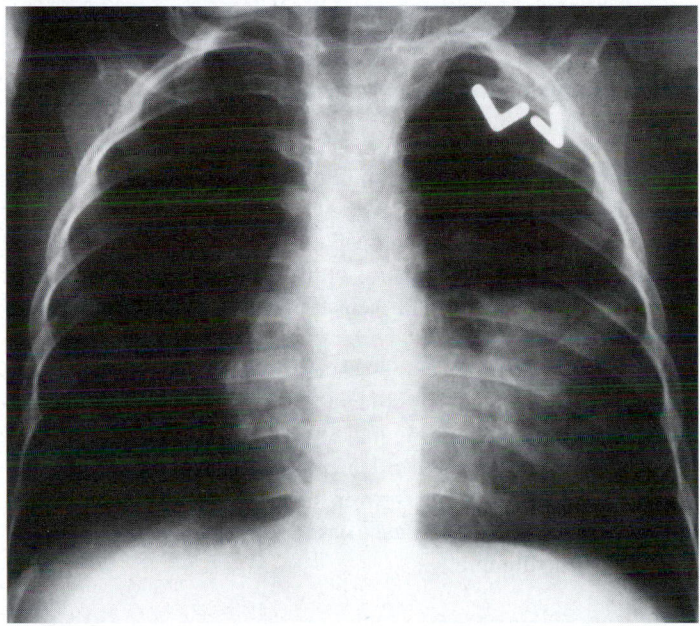

B

FIGURE 128-3   Viral pneumonia. *A.* This infant's chest radiograph is notable for hyperinflation and asymmetric interstitial infiltrates, representing a combination of atelectasis and pneumonitis. *B.* The presence of focal consolidation does not reliably distinguish between bacterial and viral infection in young children. This child did not respond to intravenous antibiotic therapy, and adenovirus was recovered in nasopharyngeal specimen.

since essentially all commonly encountered pathogens responsible for bacterial pneumonia in children are susceptible to this agent. The β-lactam–β-lactamase inhibitor combination agents, such as ampicillin-sulbactam, are also popular (although more costly) but are ineffective against penicillin-resistant pneumococci. Both agents are effective against *S. aureus* as well as the routinely encountered encapsulated pathogens, but not against pneumococci with reduced susceptibility to penicillin. As penicillin-resistant pneumococci become more prevalent, the routine use of third-generation cephalosporin agents, such as cefotaxime and ceftriaxone, provides effective treatment of moderately resistant pneumococci (those with penicillin minimal inhibitory concentrations of 0.1 to less than 1 μg/ml); highly resistant pneumococcal isolates will require the addition of vancomycin.

Pneumococcal Pneumonia

Pneumococci are the cause of most episodes of bacterial pneumonia in infants and children. The importance of polysaccharide-based serotype-specific opsonizing antibody, and the inability of children to mount antipolysaccharide antibody responses in the first 2 years of life, presumably explains why these encapsulated pathogens cause pneumonia so frequently. Pneumococci colonize the upper respiratory tract, and spread contiguously to cause otitis media and sinusitis as well as pneumonia, or invade the bloodstream primarily from the pharynx or secondarily from the initial sites of invasive infection. Children with sickle cell disease or other hemolytic anemias associated with splenic dysfunction are at particular risk of life-threatening infection.[10]

Hemophilus Influenzae Pneumonia

The routine use of conjugate *H. influenzae* type B (HIB) vaccines has led to a marked diminution in pharyngeal carriage of HIB and a virtual disappearance of invasive HIB disease. Upper respiratory carriage of nontypable *H. influenzae* persists, and these strains continue to cause otitis, sinusitis, and pneumonia. The risk of bacteremia and metastatic infection is very low following nontypable *H. influenzae* pneumonia, in contrast to the significant frequency of metastatic infections associated with HIB pneumonia.[4,17] A significant fraction of these strains produce β-lactamase, requiring therapy with a second- or third-generation cephalosporin or a β-lactam–β-lactamase inhibitor combination. If an infant has proven invasive HIB disease, family contacts (as well as the index case) should receive eradicative therapy with rifampin.

Staphylococcal Pneumonia

S. aureus pneumonia is associated with necrotizing infection in infants, just as in older patients. Nasal carriage may lead to the aspiration of staphylococci, particularly in an acute viral upper respiratory tract infection. Severe systemic toxicity, respiratory distress, and clinical or radiologic evidence of necrotizing pneumonitis are common. Chest radiographs characteristically demonstrate focal airspace disease, often with lobar consolidation, associated with cavitation or the development of smaller subpleural pneumatoceles. Pleural space invasion is also common, and patients with *S. aureus* pneumonia frequently present with dyspnea because of a giant pleural effusion. Depending on the duration of illness before evaluation, the pleural effusion may be small or large and free-flowing or loculated. Later diagnosis is associated with larger and more viscid or even loculated pleural effusions. Pneumothorax or pyopneumothorax may develop, depending on the extent of subpleural necrotizing infection. These abnormalities are not uniquely seen in staphylococcal pneumonia, but they are occasionally encountered in the course of other bacterial processes in children. Initial empiric antibiotic cover-

age with a second-generation cephalosporin such as cefuroxime or with ampicillin-sulbactam is reasonable. If staphylococcal disease is confirmed, antibiotic therapy with high doses of a semisynthetic penicillin (nafcillin, 200 mg/kg a day) or a first- or second-generation cephalosporin (cefazolin, 100 mg/kg a day, or cefuroxime, 150 mg/kg a day, respectively) should be administered. In patients who have immediate hypersensitivity to β-lactam agents, parenteral clindamycin (40 mg/kg a day) is far easier to administer than vancomycin (30 to 40 mg/kg a day).

The decision to perform a thoracentesis must be individualized. This invasive procedure has the potential of confirming the microbiologic diagnosis and establishing antimicrobial susceptibilities, reducing respiratory distress by facilitating enhanced expansion of the affected lung, and preventing the evolution of a thick, loculated empyema, which may be the source of continuing respiratory distress and ongoing infection.[28] The availability of experienced clinicians to perform the procedure, with suitable sedation or anesthesia, as well as radiologic guidance with computed tomography (CT) or ultrasound, has made thoracentesis in infants and young children a generally safe and successful procedure. When the fluid is thin, free-flowing, and not grossly purulent, the initial drainage procedure aimed at evacuating the pleural space is generally sufficient. If the initial fluid is turbid or viscous, thoracostomy drainage should be instituted. The clinical course is usually one of very slow improvement. Fever for a week or more is common. Unfortunately, many infants are referred to a tertiary care center after the the development of established empyemas, and they remain persistently febrile with a rising erythrocyte sedimentation rate despite placement of an initial chest tube. Sometimes, remaining loculated infection may be identified with chest CT scan and evacuated by additional drainage procedures, but often these persistently ill infants will require thoracotomy or thoracoscopy, with disruption of the loculated pleural space infection and placement of additional thoracostomy tubes.

Streptococcal Pneumonia

Pneumonia due to group A streptococcal infection is, like staphylococcal disease, commonly associated with the development of pleural effusions. In contrast to staphylococcal pneumonia, in which empyema is a complication of destructive subpleural infection, group A streptococcal pneumonia elicits a marked increase in lymphatic drainage. When the rate of inflammatory edema generation exceeds the fixed capacity of pulmonary lymphatic vessels to drain this fluid, the excess lymphatic drainage accumulates as a pleural effusion. These collections occur very frequently with group A streptococcal pneumonia, and may be considered a part of the process rather than a complication. These effusions are generally free-flowing, and are often sterile parapneumonic collections early in the course of infection. The collections may become infected as group A streptococci are carried to the pleural space by the lymphatic drainage, and they may become exudative, resulting in frank empyemas requiring surgical débridement. Once again, early intervention by percutaneous drainage may obviate more extensive surgical procedures late in the course of the infection. In addition to concerns regarding the local complications of group A streptococcal pneumonia, vigilance for the possible systemic sequelae following group A streptococcal infection should be shown. The expression of pyrogenic exotoxin A, particularly in M serotypes 1 and 3, has been associated with the development of streptococcal toxic shock syndrome, with scarlatiniform rash, shock, and multiple organ system dysfunction.[54]

PNEUMONIA IN OLDER CHILDREN

Bacterial Pathogens

MYCOPLASMA PNEUMONIAE

The incidence of pneumonia due to the encapsulated bacterial pathogens such as pneumococci and *H. influenzae* declines with increasing age, as do all invasive infections associated with these pathogens. Although serologic and microbiologic studies have confirmed that *M. pneumoniae* infection occurs in children of all ages, young children tend to have mild or nonlocalizing infections, whereas school-age children develop "atypical pneumonia" more frequently.[12,15] The syndrome of mycoplasmal pneumonia in school-age children, which is probably responsible for more than 50 percent of all episodes of pneumonia in this age group, closely resembles symptomatic infection in adults, with an indolent influenzal illness, fever, pharyngitis, myalgias, headache, and progressive hacking nonproductive cough or, in older children, a cough productive of mucoid or mucopurulent sputum. A variety of extrapulmonary features may be present, such as rash (including erythema multiforme), bullous myringitis, and meningoencephalitis; on occasions, these features overshadow any mild pulmonary symptoms that a child may have. Indolent intrafamilial secondary spread of infecton occurs regularly, with sequential illnesses occurring among siblings separated by intervals of 1 to 2 weeks.[16] Physical examination is notable for fever and tachypnea, but there is often a paucity of adventitial sounds on chest auscultation. The radiologic features of mycoplasmal pneumonia may range from patchy asymmetric bibasilar infiltrates with platelike atelectasis to dense focal airspace disease suggestive of bacterial pneumonia; pleural effusions and hilar adenopathy may occur but are infrequently seen.

Prompt laboratory diagnosis of *M. pneumoniae* infection is difficult. Direct cultivation of this organism requires special media and up to a 5-day incubation. Serologic confirmation of mycoplasmal infection requires paired acute and convalescent specimens. The development of cold agglutinins, IgM antibodies reactive with autologous erythrocytes, occurs in a minority of patients and is not truly specific for mycoplasmal disease. Thus, the diagnosis of *M. pneumoniae* is presumptive in children and is the most likely cause of pneumonia in school-age children. The differential diagnosis of atypical pneumonia includes adenoviral infection and *Chlamydia pneumoniae* (TWAR) infection.[18] Both mycoplasmal and chlamydial infections respond to macrolide therapy, as do most pneumococcal infections. Thus, erythromycin therapy is routinely administered for the treatment of pneumonia in school-age children. If children are intolerant of erythromycin, the newer macrolide agents clarithromycin or azithromycin may be given. Alternatively, tetracycline administration may be considered in children over the age of 8 years.

CHLAMYDIA PNEUMONIAE PNEUMONIA

A second rather common cause of atypical pneumonia has been identified and ascribed to a novel chlamydial species, *C. pneumoniae* strain TWAR.[18] *C. pneumoniae* infections have a spectrum of illness, like that of mycoplasmal infections, that ranges from isolated upper respiratory tract syndromes (pharyngitis or sinusitis) and bronchitis to clinically significant episodes of pneumonia. *C. pneumoniae* is thought to be responsible for more than 10 percent of cases of community-acquired pneumonia in children over the age of 5 as well as in adults. Pneumonia due to *C. pneumoniae* is rare in young children. Pharyngitis is more common with this agent than with *M. pneumoniae,* although in individual patients, differentiation of these two illnesses with clinical criteria is difficult and not really necessary, since both agents respond to macrolide or tetracycline therapy.

LEGIONNAIRES' DISEASE

Seroepidemiologic surveys of pediatric inpatients with pneumonia have documented that a very small percentage (under 2 percent) of children of all ages may develop acute *Legionella* pneumonia.[38,42] Although most children with *Legionella* infection are chronically ill with a variety of underlying diseases, no discrete pattern of underlying immunodeficiency has been specifically associated with the development of legionellosis. Environmental exposures, particularly to contaminated sources of warm water, remain the dominant risk factor for *Legionella* infection. Nosocomial infections, including nosocomial pneumonia in premature infants in neonatal intensive care units, remain an important problem. Although macrolide therapy is beneficial, an extremely high index of suspicion is required to pursue this diagnosis in pediatric patients. Rapid diagnosis by urinary antigen testing for *L. pneumophila* serogroup 1 and serologic diagnosis (attempting to document either a high-titered acute specimen or a conventional rise or fall in paired serum samples) are available. The presence of legionellosis among adults within a community due to an endemic source or an acute epidemic of legionellosis should alert pediatricians to the risk of *Legionella* pneumonia among children within the community.

TUBERCULOSIS

The prompt diagnosis of tuberculosis in children is particularly important, since the development of life-threatening complications, such as tuberculous meningitis and miliary tuberculosis (Fig. 128-4), can occur promptly after the clinical onset of primary tuberculous pneumonia in infants and young children, and since the development of tuberculosis in a child documents the presence of a contagious person within the patient's circle of family, neighbors, or day-care or school personnel. The pathogenesis of tuberculosis in young children is the same as for adults: one or a few *M. tuberculosis* bacilli are inhaled as small droplet aerosols and deposited within an alveolus (typically in a lower lobe). Unlike adults with primary tuberculous infection, children often have ineffective local and regional lymphatic barriers to mycobacterial dissemination, presumably because of subtle developmental deficiencies of T-lymphocyte activation or

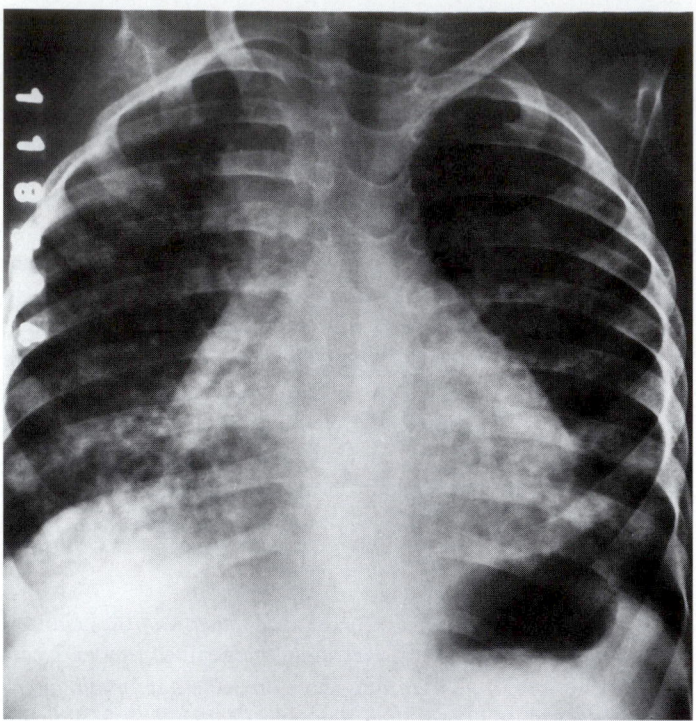

FIGURE 128-4 Miliary tuberculosis. The miliary pattern is quite prominent in this radiograph. Routine chest radiography may be normal in miliary tuberculosis.

macrophage mycobactericidal activity. As a result, mycobacterial proliferation at the site of primary infection may result in local spread of organisms, producing primary tuberculous pneumonia (Fig. 128-5) as well as spread through the regional lymph nodes (with early bacillary dissemination to extrapulmonary foci of infection).

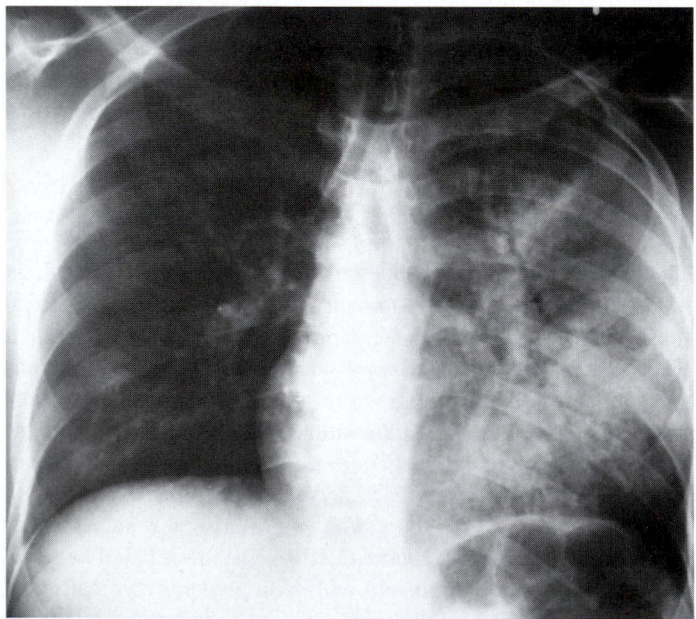

FIGURE 128-5 Acute tuberculous pneumonia. This 15-year-old Haitian boy had slowly progressive fatigue, cough, and low-grade fever for 1 month before evaluation.

Infants and children with primary tuberculous pneumonia are often only mildly ill, with persistent cough and little or no fever despite often repeated courses of conventional oral antibiotic therapy. Chest radiographs that demonstrate hilar adenopathy ipsilateral to the often patchy area of airspace consolidation strongly suggest possible mycobacterial infection. At times, atelectasis or lobar emphysema may be seen, owing to extrinsic compression of a bronchus by enlarged lymph nodes, and this may be accompanied by localized wheezing. The presence of pleural effusions or pulmonary cavitation is rare in children with primary tuberculosis. A positive tuberculin reaction usually develops within 4 to 6 weeks of initial infection, so that many children have a positive Mantoux test result when they are evaluated for persistent respiratory symptoms. The presence of a compatible clinical illness with a positive Mantoux test provides presumptive evidence for *M. tuberculosis* infection. Since young children do not have a productive cough, confirmation of the diagnosis can be achieved through the culture of gastric aspirates obtained by nasogastric suction each morning on 3 successive days, or by bronchoscopy, which is usually reserved for children in whom the differential diagnosis may be broader or airway compromise requires bronchoscopy to exclude the presence of an obstructing foreign body. It is highly desirable to recover each child's *M. tuberculosis* isolate in order to confirm the diagnosis and determine antibiotic susceptibility, although this information can be extrapolated from a newly diagnosed index case.

The treatment of tuberculosis in children utilizes the same principles used to treat adult tuberculosis.[48] Initial combination chemotherapeutic regimens should include isoniazid, rifampin, and pyrazinamide. In communities where there is heightened concern regarding drug-resistant tuberculosis, such as among immigrants and in children residing with adults who have failed conventional therapy for tuberculosis (including patients with HIV infection), ethambutol should be included as a fourth agent until a child's isolate has been studied for drug resistance. After a 2-month course of intensive therapy, in the absence of proven drug resistance, pyrazinamide may be omitted to complete a 6-month course of therapy. The incidence of isoniazid hepatotoxicity in children is considerably lower than that seen in adult patients, but monitoring for hepatotoxicity with these multidrug regimens is prudent. Although the ocular toxicities associated with ethambutol use cannot be elicited by history or color vision screening in young children, the incidence of this side effect is very low, particularly when ethambutol dosage is reduced to 15 mg/kg a day following an initial 4- to 6-week period of 25 mg/kg a day.

PNEUMONIA COMPLICATING CHILDHOOD VIRAL EXANTHEMS

Both varicella and measles may be complicated by the development of primary viral pneumonia as well as life-threatening bacterial superinfection. Pneumonia is a common complication requiring hospitalization among children with varicella (mean age 4 to 6 years) and measles (mean age 2 years), and it occurs among normal as well as immunocompromised children.

Varicella

Varicella pneumonia generally develops a few days after the onset of the typical bullous eruption, but it can occur before the onset of the rash. Symptoms of dyspnea, cough, and tachypnea are associated with an interstitial and fine nodular infiltrate, and they may be severe, requiring intubation and mechanical ventilation. The prognosis generally is favorable if the child can be supported adequately during the acute phase of the illness.[13,27] Symptomatic pneumonitis in this setting should lead to the prompt institution of parenteral acyclovir therapy (30 mg/kg a day, given every 8 h). Bacterial superinfection occurs in a large number of children with varicella pneumonia. This complication is associated with the development of typical focal consolidation and can be accompanied by the development of a pleural effusion or frank empyema. The common bacterial pathogens–*S. pneumoniae, S. pyogenes, S. aureus,* and *H. influenzae*—are the usual etiologic agents and require appropriate antibiotic coverage in addition to primary therapy with acyclovir. Although the risk of varicella pneumonia is extremely high in children receiving chemotherapy for hematologic malignancy, the risk of serious visceral complications is actually rather low in children with HIV infection. Neonates with peripartum exposure to maternal varicella are also at high risk of developing primary varicella pneumonia, and they should be given zoster immune globulin at birth and parenteral acyclovir if they develop varicella.

Measles

The epidemiology of measles pneumonia and its complications closely resemble the features of varicella pneumonia, although most cases of measles pneumonia are seen in younger children. In contrast to the low incidence of varicella pneumonia in children, radiologic evidence of pulmonary involvement is more frequently seen in measles (2.7 to 36 percent), although some children are minimally symptomatic and some develop a croup syndrome rather than pneumonitis. Primary measles pneumonia is associated with a diffuse interstitial infiltrate; it may also be associated with the development of bacterial pneumonia.[2,33] Fulminant respiratory failure may develop in association with diffuse interstitial pneumonia, diffuse airspace consolidation consistent with the adult respiratory distress syndrome, bacterial pneumonia, and/or spontaneous pneumothorax before intubation and mechanical ventilation. As with varicella pneumonia, typical community-acquired bacterial pathogens are generally responsible for bacterial pneumonia and may be associated with bacteremia. The acute mortality of measles pneumonia requiring intensive care support approaches 50 percent, and pulmonary fibrosis or bronchiolitis obliterans may develop during or after the acute phase of the illness.

Aspiration Pneumonia

Aspiration is commonly observed among children with strong clinical risk factors for this complication, so the diagnosis of aspiration pneumonia is usually rather straightforward.[5] Infants with neonatal asphyxia and other causes of profound neurologic impairment frequently have feeding difficulties and may aspirate food or saliva. In these infants, fundoplication and placement of a feeding gastrostomy tube may reduce the risk of aspiration of gastric contents but not of oral contents. However, aspiration pneumonia may occur in otherwise normal infants (Fig. 128-6). Aspiration during or shortly after feeding is most commonly due to gastroesophageal reflux and far less commonly to tracheoesophageal fistulas or vascular ring anomalies. Thus, the occurrence of aspiration pneumonia in infants necessitates a suitable diagnostic evaluation in addition to antibiotic therapy. Similarly, infants with recurrent pneumonia may be aspirating despite the absence of apparent feeding difficulty, and they should undergo a structural evaluation in addition to the screening studies for occult immunodeficiency.

Aspiration pneumonia is also a common complication of status epilepticus and of posttraumatic neurologic injury; it may be seen as a complication of general anesthesia, particularly after emergency procedures. Older children may develop aspiration pneumonia as the result of drug overdoses or from primary muscle disorders, such as muscular dystrophy and myasthenia gravis. The radiologic features of aspiration pneumonia usually demonstrate the expected airspace consolidation in the dependent portions of the lung—although, of course, infants and children may be supine at the time of aspiration. Cavitation or pleural disease is infrequently seen at the time of initial evaluation, since the interval between the aspirational event and presentation with pneu-

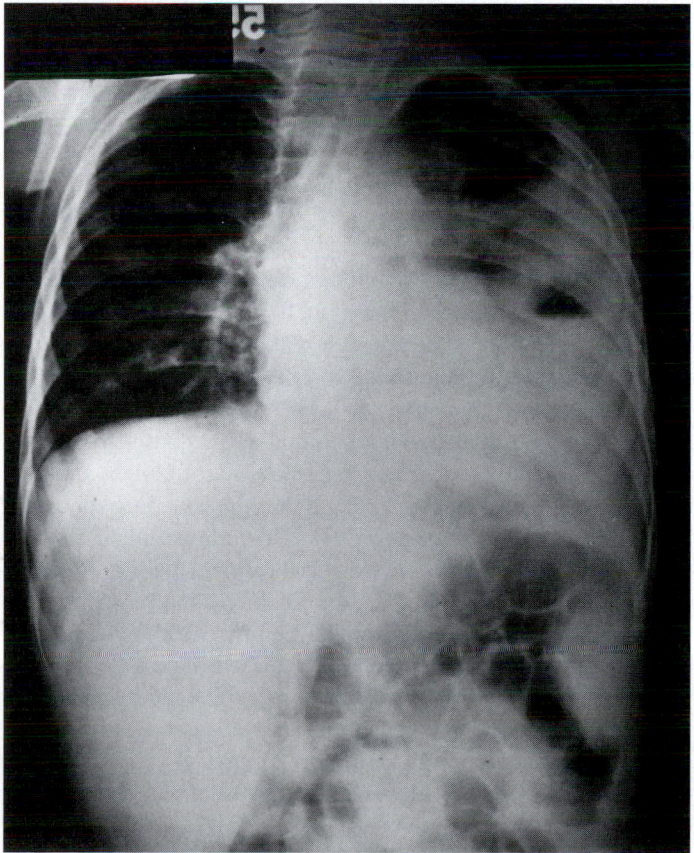

FIGURE 128-6   Aspiration pneumonia. This toddler presented with a loculated empyema (note multiple air-fluid levels) that grew mixed oropharyngeal flora in association with left lower-lobe pneumonitis.

monia is usually brief. The presence of a radiopaque foreign body is occasionally seen and requires prompt bronchoscopy.

The therapy for aspiration pneumonia depends on the child's age and overall clinical status. Neonates are usually given ampicillin and gentamicin to treat the conventional neonatal pathogens. Infants are not usually colonized by anerobic bacteria until the eruption of primary dentition. Colonization of the oropharynx by ampicillin-resistant encapsulated pathogens such as *H. influenzae* and *M. catarrhalis* offers a rationale for treating older infants and toddlers with a β-lactamase–resistant agent such as cefuroxime. In older children, penicillin, ampicillin, or clindamycin (in β-lactam–allergic patients) may be considered. A poor response to initial antibiotic therapy may be the result of inadequate antibiotic coverage or the presence of an obstructing endobronchial foreign body. Aspirated foreign bodies are particularly common in toddlers and preschool children, who often place small objects in their mouths. Bronchoscopy is indicated in children who respond poorly to therapy or develop cavitation or empyema, to exclude the presence of a foreign body as well as to obtain suitable endotracheal specimens for bacterial culture.

RECURRENT PNEUMONIA

The occurrence of more than one episode of focal consolidative pneumonia, especially within a 1-year interval, raises concerns that a child may be experiencing recurrent pneumonia on the basis of local or systemic risk factors.[52] The radiologic distribution of these infiltrates directs the subsequent evaluation: recurrent pneumonia in a single lobe or lung suggests local risk factors, and recurrent infections distributed throughout the lungs suggest systemic causes of heightened susceptibility to infection.

Recurrent Diffuse Pneumonia

PNEUMOCYSTIS CARINII

Symptomatic infections in children due to *P. carinii* generally occur in infants rendered immunodeficient by profound malnutrition and in children of any age with significant compromise of cell-mediated immunity due to underlying disease or to immunosuppressive chemotherapy (Fig. 128-7). A more benign form of *P. carinii* pneumonia in normal infants has also been reported.[8] The infantile form of *P. carinii* is an indolent and generally afebrile process manifested by progressive tachypnea and poor feeding over a period of weeks. In contrast, older children typically present with an acute febrile illness with nonproductive cough and tachypnea disproportionate to the bland physical examination and often mild symmetric interstitial and fine alveolar infiltrate present on chest radiograph. The course of *P. carinii* infection in HIV-infected children may be quite variable and may resemble either the indolent progressive course seen in malnourished infants or the more rapidly progressive illness seen in older children. The diagnosis of *P. carinii* pneumonia can be made noninvasively in older children by microscopic examination of induced sputum, but in infants and young children, bronchoscopy or lung biopsy is required. Trimethoprim-sulfamethoxazole therapy remains the mainstay of treatment, usually given in a dosage of 20 mg/kg a day of the trimethoprim

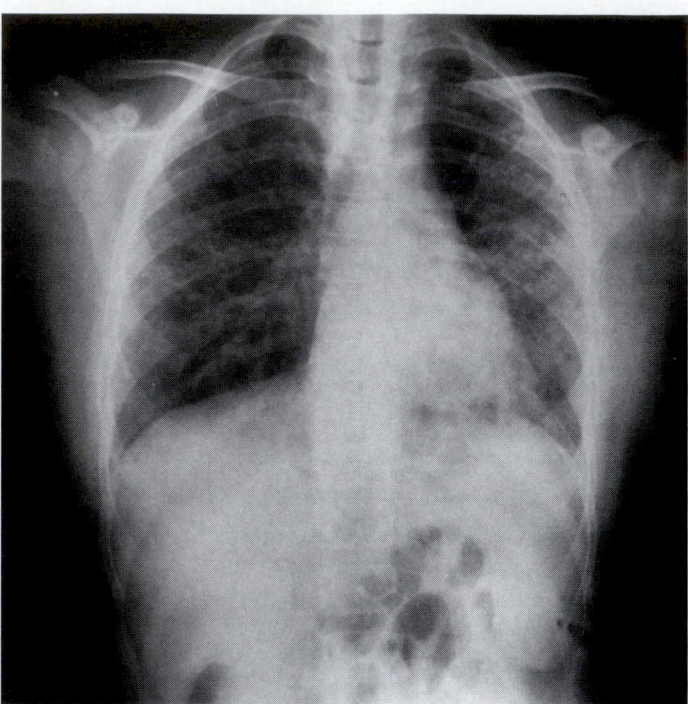

FIGURE 128-7   *Pneumocystis carinii* pneumonia in a teenager with acute leukemia. Depending on the extent of disease at the time of presentation, there may be predominance of interstitial or airspace disease. The radiographic findings are nonspecific and may mimic viral pneumonitis and noninfectious causes of interstitial and alvelolar lung disease, such as drug hypersensitivity reactions.

component every 6 h for 2 to 3 weeks. Children intolerant to sulfonamide therapy are usually given intravenous pentamidine, 4 mg/kg a day for 2 weeks. Short-term administration of methylprednisolone (1 mg/kg every 6 h for 7-days, followed by 7 day tapering course) has been associated with improved survival in HIV-infected patients.[46] Long-term prophylaxis (with trimethoprim-sulfamethoxazole or one of several alternative regimens) is essential to reduce the risk of relapse.

Recurrent Focal Pneumonia

Recurrent lobar pneumonia may be due to a variety of intraluminal lesions, particularly the presence of a foreign body, or to extraluminal compression due to enlargement of perihilar or regional lymph nodes due to granulomatous infection or malignancy (Fig. 128-8). In addition, a variety of pulmonary or bronchial lesions may be responsible for recurrent infection. Bronchial stenosis and bronchiectasis (especially in the right middle lobe bronchus) are the most common bronchial abnormalities responsible for recurrent focal pneumonia. Congenital lesions such as bronchogenic cysts and pulmonary sequestra may present as recurrent or nonresolving pneumonia.[33] Since these structures lack normal communications with functional bronchi, pneumonitis that develops in these regions as a result of contiguous spread of infection from normal lung is slow to resolve and frequently does not respond to conventional medical therapy. Aspiration should be considered in the patient with recurrent basilar pneumonia. Evaluation of children with recurrent

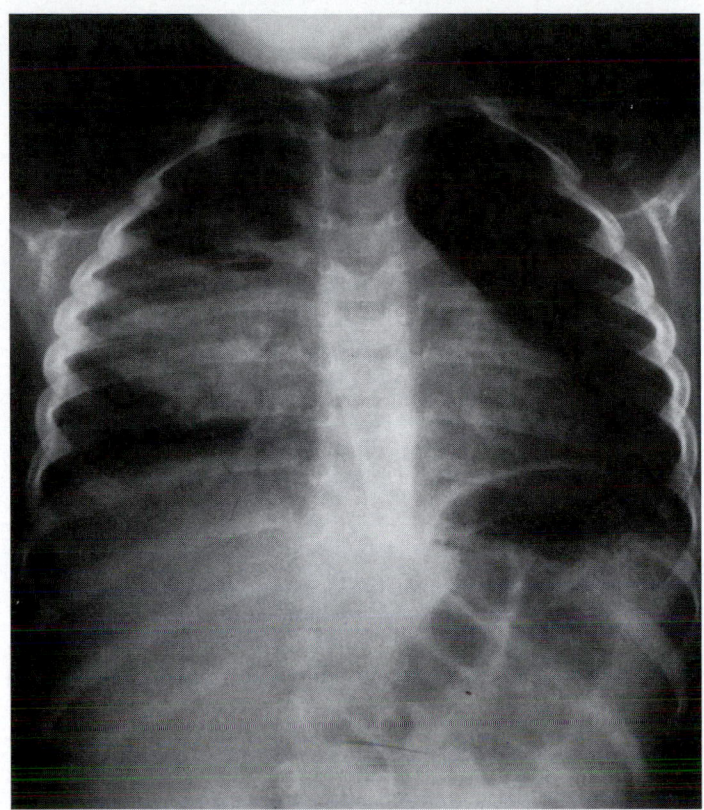

FIGURE 128-8 Recurrent pneumonia. This 5-year-old girl had three episodes of right lung consolidation, involving different lobes, shortly after immigrating to the United States from the Azores. At bronchoscopy, cellophane tape was recovered from the right main-stem bronchus.

focal pneumonia should begin with bronchoscopy, which identifies obstructing intraluminal lesions and intrinsic bronchial abnormalities, as well as extrinsic bronchial compression, and serves as the primary method for the removal of retained foreign material. When bronchoscopy is nondiagnostic, a chest CT scan may be helpful to identify a distal bronchial obstruction, bronchiectasis, or the presence of a bronchogenic cyst or pulmonary sequestration. When pulmonary sequestration is suspected, vascular imaging by conventional contrast or magnetic resonance angiography demonstrates the aberrant systemic vascular supply associated with these lesions.

Recurrent Pneumonia in Different Locations

Compromise of any of a variety of pulmonary or systemic host defense mechanisms may be associated with recurrent pneumonia; in the setting of a generalized impairment, recurrent infections may occur anywhere in the lungs.

Defects in Pulmonary Defenses

Abnormalities in the bronchial mucociliary transport system are important considerations. Children with cystic fibrosis (CF) first may become symptomatic beyond the neonatal period with recurrent bronchopneumonia rather than with a picture of steator-

rhea and failure to thrive, as is common in neonates. A large variety of distinct CF genotypes have been identified, and some are associated with a later and milder onset of respiratory symptoms; in fact, on occasion the diagnosis of CF may not become apparent until adulthood.[9] A family history of CF is often lacking among the families of children with CF. Initial episodes of pneumonia in these patients may be associated with conventional encapsulated bacterial pathogens or *S. aureus*; the development of chronic *P. aeruginosa* infection may be a relatively late event. The diagnosis should be explored with pilocarpine iontophoresis testing ("sweat test") at a center experienced in the diagnosis of CF.

In contrast, congenital abnormalities of the ciliary system are very rare. Kartagener's syndrome of bronchiectasis, sinusitis, and dextrocardia is a subset of the group of immotile ciliary disorders.[11] Such children often experience upper respiratory tract infections such as sinusitis and suppurative otitis media in addition to recurrent pneumonia. Ciliary disease can be assessed by analysis of ciliary beat frequency from nasal mucosal specimens. The classic method of diagnosing immotile cilia based on ciliary morphology requires electron microscopic analysis of a bronchial biopsy. This procedure should be performed some weeks after recovery from an acute episode of pneumonia, since ultrastructural abnormalities may be seen after infection in the absence of a heritable ciliary defect. Tracheomalacia and tracheobronchomegaly (Mounier-Kuhn syndrome) also impair clearance of mucus and are associated with recurrent pneumonia.

Defects in Systemic Host Defenses

HUMORAL IMMUNODEFICIENCY

Humoral immunodeficiency states are the most common host defects associated with recurrent bacterial pneumonia. A variety of different antibody deficiency syndromes have been identified. Bruton's (X-linked) agammaglobulinemia is the most extreme example, with a virtual absence of all circulating immunoglobulins. The hyper-IgM syndrome is due to the inability of T cells to activate B cell CD40, which is necessary to drive B-cell differentiation to produce normal quantities of IgG and IgA antibodies. In these children with profound hypogammaglobulinemia, recurrent pyogenic infections, including recurrent pneumonia, develop after transplacentally derived maternal antibody wanes after the first 6 months of life. Common variable hypogammaglobulinemia and transient hypogammaglobulinemia of infancy have moderate reductions in IgG and IgM levels, and may have little or no IgA. In contrast to these more dramatic conditions, IgG subclass deficiency states, particularly of IgG2 and IgG4, have been associated with recurrent respiratory tract infections.[50] Patients have occasionally been shown to have isolated qualitative defects, with an inability to mount IgG responses to the conventional encapsulated bacterial pathogens.[3]

Definitive therapy with intravenous immunoglobulin (IVIG) administration is both costly and somewhat cumbersome—especially in young children, in whom peripheral venous access is problematic and central venous catheters pose a significant rate of catheter-associated bacteremia. It is reasonable to offer a trial of chronic oral suppressive antibiotic therapy with a β-lactamase–resistant agent in patients with mild or moderate disease, and to reserve IVIG therapy for children who fail to improve on suppressive antibiotics. Complement deficiency states—particularly C3, C5, and properdin deficiencies—are rare heritable causes of recurrent bacterial infections. Patients have an increased incidence of a variety of soft-tissue and sytemic infections in addition to recurrent pnuemonia.

GRANULOCYTE DISORDERS

Quantitative and qualitative granulocyte abnormalities are rarely responsible for recurrent pneumonia. Routine differential white cell counts will identify children with agranulocytosis; serial monitoring and bone marrow examinations will distinguish among cyclic neutropenia, immune neutropenia, and congenital agranulocytosis. In these children, pneumonia is often due to *S. aureus* or gram-negative bacilli, including *Pseudomonas,* or to fungal pathogens such as *Aspergillus.* If no response is seen to initial empiric therapy, bronchoscopy or lung biopsy may be necessary to guide further antibiotic therapy. A trial of granulocyte colony–stimulating factor is reasonable in this setting, since the transient response in granulocyte number may hasten the resolution of the pneumonia. In contrast, children with chronic granulomatous disease have normal granulocyte number but impaired intracellular killing of bacteria. As in patients with complement deficiency, focal soft-tissue, skeletal, and lymph node infections may be seen in addition to recurrent pneumonia. The use of interferon-γ and long-term antibiotic suppressive therapy has greatly improved the long-term outlook for such patients.[26] Defects in granulocyte function may result in invasive pneumonia due to fungi as well as bacterial pathogens. As with neutropenic children, focal infiltrates that persist or progress (particularly with cavitation) despite reasonable initial empiric antibiotic therapy require vigorous investigation with chest CT scanning and biopsy.

CELL-MEDIATED IMMUNODEFICIENCY

Defects in T-cell function are asssociated with primary immunodeficiency diseases such as severe combined immunodeficiency and DiGeorge syndrome, lymphoid malignancies such as acute lymphoblastic leukemia, therapy with immunosuppressive agents for the treatment of a variety of inflammatory diseases and organ transplantation, and HIV infection. The immunodeficient state triggered by acute systemic viral infection is transient and rarely associated with opportunistic pulmonary infection. Regardless of the initial mechanism of T-cell immunosuppression, such children are at risk of developing life-threatening pneumonia due particularly to common viral pathogens such as RSV, measles, and parainfluenza virus; fungal infections such as cryptococcosis and infection with the endemic soil fungi; higher bacteria such as *Nocardia asteroides* and mycobacteria (both *M. tuberculosis* and atypical mycobacteria); and *P. carinii.* The radiologic features may point toward particular pathogens (e.g., focal infiltrates implicate fungal or bacterial pathogens, and diffuse infiltrates implicate viral pathogens or *P. carinii*), but the broad differential diagnosis, the possibility of polymicrobial infection and of noninfectious processes such as drug hypersensi-tivity reactions, and the complexities of therapy dictate an invasive approach to diagnosis with bronchoscopy or open lung biopsy.

HIV

HIV infection in children results not only in a heightened susceptibility to infection by *P. carinii* and other pathogens classically associated with T-cell immunodeficiency states but also in an increased susceptibility to bacterial infection, with an increased risk of bacterial pneumonia and bacteremia due to encapsulated pathogens such as *S. pneumoniae.*[32,41] In addition, lymphoid interstitial pneumonia, an infiltrative process possibly associated with Epstein-Barr virus infection, may be responsible for pulmonary infiltrates and respiratory distress in these children.[29,37] Unlike adult HIV-infected patients, children have a risk of *P. carinii* pneumonia that is not closely correlated with the CD4 count. Infants with vertically transmitted HIV have an increased risk of acquiring *P. carinii* pneumonia regardless of CD4 count during the first year of life.[45] All infants born of HIV-infected mothers should begin *P. carinii* prophylaxis at 4 weeks of life and continue treatment until it can be shown that HIV transmission has not occurred, or until 1 year of life. The need for continued prophylaxis thereafter among HIV-infected infants is based on the number of circulating CD4 cells present. The management of recurrent bacterial infections, including pneumonia, in these infants is controversial. Administration of IVIG every 4 weeks to HIV-infected infants has been shown to reduce the number of serious bacterial infections,[40] but maintaining long-term venous access frequently requires placement of a central venous catheter, which has its own risks of catheter-related bacteremia and candidemia. At present, IVIG is generally reserved for children who have had at least one episode of life-threatening bacterial infection. When HIV-infected children develop respiratory distress associated with diffuse interstitial and alveolar infiltrates, the broad differential diagnosis and the significant possibility of multiple concurrent processes warrant early consideration of an invasive biospy process. Depending on the severity and progress of illness, an empiric trial of therapy for *P. carinii* pneumonia may be given, with lung biopsy reserved for patients who fail to improve.

REFERENCES

1. Ablow R, Driscoll S, Effman E, et al: A comparison of early onset group B streptococcal neonatal infection and the respiratory distress syndrome of the newborn. *New Engl J Med* 294:65–70, 1976.
2. Abramson O, Dagan R, Tal A, Sofer S: Severe complications of measles requiring intensive care in infants and young children. *Arch Pediatr Adolesc Med* 149:1237–1240, 1995.
3. Ambrosino DM, Siber GR, Chilmonczyk BA, et al: An immunodeficiency characterized by impaired antibody responses to polysaccharides. *New Engl J Med* 316:790–793, 1987.
4. Asmar BI, Slovis TL, Reed JO, Dajani AS: *Hemophilus influenzae* type b pneumonia in 43 children. *J Pediatr* 93:389–393, 1978.
5. Bauer ML, Figueroa-Colon R, Georgeson K, Young DW: Chronic pulmonary aspiration in children. *South Med J* 86:789–795, 1993.

6. Beem MO, Saxon EM: Respiratory-tract colonization and a distinctive pneumonia syndrome in infants infected with *Chlamydia trachomatis. New Engl J Med* 296:306–310, 1977.

7. Brandt C, Kim H, Arrobio J, et al: Epidemiology of respiratory syncytial virus infection in Washington, DC. III: Composite analysis of eleven consecutive yearly epidemics. *Am J Epidemiol* 98:355–364, 1973.

8. Brasfield DM, Stagno S, Whitley RJ, et al: Infant pneumonitis associated with cytomegalovirus, *Chlamydia, Pneumocystis,* and *Ureaplasma:* Follow-up. *Pediatrics* 79:76–83, 1987.

9. Case Records of the Massachusetts General Hospital. *New Engl J Med* 309:375–383, 1984.

10. Castro O, Brambilla DM, Thorington B, et al: The acute chest syndrome in sickle cell disease: Incidence and risk factors. *Blood* 84:643–649, 1994.

11. Eliasson R, Mossberg B, Camner P, Afzelius BA: The immotile cilia syndrome: A congenital ciliary abnormality as an etiologic factor in chronic airway infections and male sterility. *New Engl J Med* 297:1–6, 1977.

12. Fernald G, Collier A, Clyde W: Respiratory infections due to *Mycoplasma pneumoniae* in infants and children. *Pediatrics* 55:327–335, 1973.

13. Fleisher G, Henry W, McSorley M, et al: Life-threatening complications of varicella. *Am J Dis Child* 135:896–899, 1981.

14. Foy H, Cooney M, Maletzky A, et al: Incidence and etiology of pneumonia, croup and bronchiolitis in preschool children belonging to a prepaid medical group over a four-year period. *Am J Epidemiol* 97:80–92, 1973.

15. Foy H, Cooney M, McMahan R, et al: Viral and mycoplasmal pneumonias in a prepaid medical care group during an eight-year period. *Am J Epidemiol* 97:93–102, 1973.

16. Foy HM: Infections caused by *Mycoplasma pneumoniae* and possible carrier state in different populations of patients. *Clin Infect Dis* (Suppl) 17:S37–S46, 1993.

17. Ginsburg CM, Howard JB, Nelson JD: Report of 65 cases of *Haemophilus influenzae* b pneumonia. *Pediatrics* 64:283–286, 1979.

18. Grayston JT, Campbell LA, Kuo CC, et al: A new respiratory tract pathogen: *Chlamydia pneumoniae* strain TWAR. *J Infect Dis* 161:618–625, 1990.

19. Groothuis JR, Simoes EAF, Levin MJ, et al: Prophylactic administration of respiratory syncytial virus immune globulin to high-risk infants and young children. *New Engl J Med* 329:1524–1530, 1993.

20. Hall CB, McBride JT, Gala CL, et al: Ribavirin treatment of respiratory syncytial viral infection in infants with underlying cardiopulmonary disease. *JAMA* 254:3047–3050, 1985.

21. Hall CB, McBride JT, Walsh EE, et al: Aerosolized ribavirin treatment of infants with respiratory syncytial viral infection. *New Engl J Med* 308:1443–1447, 1983.

22. Harrison H, English M, Lee C, et al: *Chlamydia trachomatis* infant pneumonitis. *New Engl J Med* 298:702–708, 1978.

23. Henderson F, Collier A, Clyde W, et al: Respiratory-syncytial virus infections, reinfections, and immunity. *New Engl J Med* 300:530–534, 1979.

24. Hendry RM, Talis AL, Godfrey E, et al: Concurrent circulation of antigenically distinct strains of respiratory syncytial virus during community outbreaks. *J Infect Dis* 153:291–297, 1986.

25. Henrickson KJ, Kuhn SM, Savatski LL: Epidemiology and cost of infection with human parainfluenza virus types 1 and 2 in young children. *Clin Infect Dis* 18:770–779, 1994.

26. International Chronic Granulomatous Disease Cooperative Study Group: A controlled trial of interferon gamma to prevent infection in chronic granulomatous disease. *New Engl J Med* 324:509–516, 1991.

27. Jackson MA, Burry VF, Olson LC: Complications of varicella requiring hospitalization in previously healthy children. *Pediatr Infect Dis J* 11:441–445, 1992.

28. Joosten KFM, Hazelzet JA, Tiddens HAWM, et al: Staphylococcal pneumonia in childhood: Will early surgical intervention lower mortality? *Pediatr Pulmonol* 20:83–88, 1995.

29. Joshi VV, Oleske JM, Minnefor AB, et al: Pathologic pulmonary findings in children with the acquired immunodeficiency syndrome: A study of ten cases. *Hum Pathol* 16:241–246, 1985.

30. Kim HW, Arrobio J, Brandt C, et al: Epidemiology of respiratory syncytial virus infection in Washington, DC. I: Importance of the virus in different respiratory tract disease syndromes and temporal distribution of infection. *Am J Epidemiol* 98:216–225, 1973.

31. King JC Jr, Burke AR, Clemens JD, et al: Respiratory syncytial virus illnesses in human immunodeficiency virus– and noninfected children. *Pediatr Infect Dis J* 12:733–739, 1993.

32. Krasinski K, Borkowsky W, Bonk S, et al: Bacterial infections in human immunodeficiency virus–infected children. *Pediatr Infect Dis J* 7:323–328, 1988.

33. Kravitz RM: Congenital malformations of the lung. *Pediatr Clin North Am* 41:453–472, 1994.

34. Mason WH, Ross LA, Lanson J, Wright HT: Epidemic measles in the postvaccine era: Evaluation of epidemiology, clinical presentation and complications during an urban outbreak. *Pediatr Infect Dis J* 12:42–48, 1993.

35. McCarthy P, Spiesl S, Stashwick C, et al: Radiographic findings and etiologic diagnosis in ambulatory childhood pneumonias. *Clin Pediatr* 20:686–691, 1981.

36. Meert KL, Sarnaik AP, Gelmini MJ, Lieh-Lai MW: Aerosolized ribavirin in mechanically ventilated children with respiratory syncytial virus lower respiratory tract disease: A prospective, double-blind, randomized trial. *Crit Care Med* 22:566–572, 1994.

37. Moran CA, Suster S, Pavlova Z, et al: The spectrum of pathological changes in the lung in children with the acquired immunodeficiency syndrome: An autopsy study of 36 cases. *Hum Pathol* 25:877–882, 1994.

38. Muldoon RL, Jaecker DL, Kiefer HK: Legionnaires' disease in children. *Pediatrics* 67:329–332, 1981.

39. Murphy TF, Henderson FW, Clyde WA Jr, et al: Pneumonia: an eleven-year study in a pediatric practice. *Am J Epidemiol* 113:12–21, 1981.

40. National Institute of Child Health and Human Development Intravenous Immunoglobulin Study Group: Intravenous immune globulin for the prevention of bacterial infections in children with symptomatic human immunodeficiency virus infection. *New Engl J Med* 325:73–80, 1991.

41. Nicholas SW: The opportunistic and bacterial infections associated with pediatric human immunodeficiency virus disease. *Acta Paediatr* (Suppl) 400:S46–S50, 1994.

42. Orenstein WA, Overturf GD, Leedom JM, et al: The frequency of *Legionella* infection prospectively determined in children hospitalized with pneumonia. *J Pediatr* 99:403–406, 1981.

43. Radkowski MA, Kranzler JK, Beem MO, Tipple MA: *Chlamydia* pneumonia in infants: Radiography in 125 cases. *Am J Roentgenol* 137:703–706, 1981.

44. Shigeta S, Mori S, Baba M, et al: Antiviral activities of ribavirin, 5-ethynyl-1-β-D ribofuranosylimidazole-4-carboxamide, and 6′-(R)-6′-C-methylneplanocin A against several ortho- and paramyxoviruses. *Antimicrob Agents Chemother* 36:435–439, 1992.

45. Simonds RJ, Lindgren ML, Thomas P, et al: Prophylaxis against *Pneumocystis carinii* pneumonia among children with perinatally acquired human immunodeficiency virus infection in the United States. *New Engl J Med* 332:786–790, 1995.

46. Sleasman JW, Hemenway C, Klein AS, Barrett DJ: Corticosteroids improve survival of children with AIDS and *Pneumocystis carinii* pneumonia. *Am J Dis Child* 147:30–34, 1993.

47. Smith DW, Frankel LR, Mathers LH, et al: A controlled trial of aerosolized ribavirin in infants receiving mechanical ventilation for severe respiratory syncytial virus infection. *New Engl J Med* 325:24–29, 1991.

48. Starke JR: Modern approach to the diagnosis and treatment of tuberculosis in children. *Pediatr Clin North Am* 35:441–464, 1988.

49. Tipple MA, Beem MO, Saxon EM: Clinical characteristics of the afebrile pneumonia assoicated with *Chlamydia trachomatis* infection in infants less than 6 months of age. *Pediatrics* 63:192–197, 1979.

50. Umetsu DT, Ambrosino DM, Quinti I, et al: Recurrent sinopulmonary infection and impaired antibody response to bacterial capsular polysaccharide antigen in children with selective IgG subclass deficiency. *New Engl J Med* 313:1247–1251, 1985.

51. Vollman J, Smith W, Ballard E, et al: Early onset group B streptococcal disease: Clinical, roentgenographic, and pathologic features. *J Pediatr* 89:199–203, 1976.

52. Wald ER: Recurrent and nonresolving pneumonia in children. *Semin Respir Infect* 8:46–58, 1993.

53. Wendt CH, Hertz MI: Respiratory syncytial virus and parainfluenza virus infections in the immunocompromised host. *Semin Respir Infect* 10:224–231, 1995.

54. Wheeler MC, Roe MH, Kaplan EL, et al: Outbreak of group A streptococcus septicemia in children: clinical, epidemiologic, and microbiological correlates. *JAMA* 266:533–537, 1991.

55. Whitley RJ, Brasfield D, Reynolds D, et al: Protracted pneumonitis in young infants associated with perinatally acquired cytomegaloviral infection. *J Pediatr* 89:16–22, 1976.

CHAPTER 129

ASPIRATION DISEASE AND ANAEROBIC INFECTION

John G. Bartlett

Aspiration pneumonia and anaerobic pleuropulmonary infections are distinctive but overlapping topics. Anaerobic bacteria are relatively common pulmonary pathogens and are well documented as the major agents of aspiration pneumonia and its suppurative complications, including lung abscess and empyema. *Aspiration pneumonia* refers to the pulmonary consequences that follow abnormal entry of fluid, particulate substances, or endogenous secretions from the upper airways or gastric contents into the lower airways. The usual predisposing conditions are twofold. First, there needs to be a compromise of the usual defenses that protect the lower airways, including glottic closure, cough reflex, or other clearing mechanisms. The second requirement is an inoculum that must be deleterious to the lower airways by direct toxic effect, a bacterial challenge sufficient to initiate an inflammatory process, or an adequate volume to cause obstruction. Aspiration pneumonia consequently comprises several syndromes based on the inoculum, and bacterial infection is simply one, but it is probably the most frequent that is clinically recognized. Anaerobic bacteria are the most common pathogens in this setting, reflecting both pathogenic potential and numeric dominance in the normal flora of the upper airways.

HISTORY

The clinical and bacteriologic features of anaerobic infections of the lung have been documented by extensive studies during two periods of investigation. The first was at the turn of the century, when anaerobic bacteria were initially reported as important causes of empyema.[45] This early work continued through the late 1920s, when David Smith conducted classic studies on the pathogenesis of lung abscess.[51] At that time, approximately one-third of patients with lung abscess died. Smith noted that the bacteria in the walls of the abscess at autopsy resembled the bacteria found in the gingival crevice, leading him to conclude that aspiration was the major mechanism in pathogenesis. He subsequently supported this hypothesis by inoculating the trachea of experimental animals with gingival crevice material to reproduce the sequence of events of pneumonitis, followed in 7 to 10 days by lung abscess formation. Bacteriologic studies of the inoculum showed that four bacterial species were critical, and all were anaerobic bacteria: a fusiform bacterium now recognized as *Fusobacterium nucleatum*, *Prevotella melaninogenica* (formerly *Bacteroides melaninogenicus*), Peptostreptococcus, and an anaerobic spirochete. This study is one of the first demonstrations of bacterial synergy; the demonstration of two or more bacterial species are required to produce a pathologic process that could not be reproduced by any single component of the inoculum.

There was a paradoxical neglect of this work in the first 2 or 3 decades of the antibiotic era. At that time, the role of anaerobic bacteria in this and other pathologic processes was largely ignored. It was paradoxical in the sense that bacteriology studies were neglected at the time when effective pathogen-directed treatment became available. At that time, patients with lung abscesses often had putrid sputum and no identifiable pathogen; these infections were frequently referred to as *nonspecific lung abscess*. Although the microbial cause was unknown, it was well established that these patients almost invariably responded to penicillin treatment.[58] The role of anaerobes in empyema was also largely ignored. Much of this neglect is ascribed to the paucity of laboratories capable of cultivating oxygen-sensitive bacteria.

The second period extended from the late 1960s through the late 1970s, when simultaneous developments spawned renewed interest in anaerobes: (1) cultivation of anaerobes became relatively easy for clinical laboratories with the introduction of Gas-Pak jars; (2) workers at the Virginia Polytechnic Institute and others finally placed a very confusing group of anaerobic bacteria into taxonomic order; (3) many studies, often sponsored by pharmaceutical support for study of new drugs (clindamycin, metronidazole, cefoxitin), showed relatively high rates of anaerobes in various settings. The introduction and widespread use of transtracheal aspiration (TTA) in the late 1960s made it realistic to collect uncontaminated specimens from the lower airways that were valid for anaerobic culture. This source of respiratory secretions for culture, combined with renewed interest in cultivation of anaerobes, permitted redefinition of clinical features, bacteriologic findings, and the therapeutic principles of anaerobic lung infections.[3] At the present time, TTAs are seldom performed, so anaerobic bacteria are rarely established pulmonary pathogens. Nevertheless, these organisms are often suspected on the basis of their documented importance in patients with clinical features suggesting aspiration pneumonia and its late complications, including necrotizing pneumonia, lung abscess, and empyema.

INCIDENCE

The establishment of anaerobic bacteria in pulmonary infections requires specimens of respiratory secretions that are devoid of contamination from the upper airways. The usual procedures satisfying this criterion are TTA, transthoracic aspiration, open lung biopsy, thoracentesis, and, most recently, bronchoscopy with quantitative cultures. In addition, there must be appropriate laboratory expertise for cultivation of anaerobic bacteria. The incidence of anaerobic lung infections reported in published studies from the antibiotic era that satisfy both requirements is summarized in Table 129-1.

Most published reports deal with the role of anaerobic bacteria in aspiration pneumonia or lung abscess, and these show recovery rates ranging from 62 to 100 percent.[11,15,29,38] The usual specimens in these studies are TTA and transthoracic aspiration. One of the best studies is by Beerens and Tahon-Castel,[12] who used transthoracic needle aspiration to characterize the flora in lung abscesses; this series showed recovery of anaerobic bacteria, usually in pure culture, in 22 of 26 cases (85 percent). A more recent report by Gudiol and colleagues[29] employed similar techniques and showed anaerobic bacteria in 37 of 41 cases (90 percent).

Empyema is more easily studied because of the relative ease of obtaining specimens appropriate for anaerobic culture—in this case, pleural fluid. In the preantibiotic era, *Streptococcus pneumoniae* accounted for 60 to 70 percent of cases; studies at that time indicated that empyema fluid was putrid (and thus implicated anaerobes) in about 5 to 7 percent of cases.[23] More recent studies of empyema have shown a sharp decrease in the frequency of empyema and a marked shift in the bacteriology, so that the pneumococcus accounts for only 5 to 10 percent of cases while anaerobes are found in 25 to 40 percent.[35] The highest yield reported in recent years is a collaborative study at Cook County Hospital in Chicago and two VA hospitals in Los Angeles. Anaerobes were recovered in 63 of 83 cases (76 percent).[5]

There have been few studies to identify the frequency of anaerobic bacteria in unselected cases of community-acquired pneumonia. One was by Ries and coworkers, who performed TTAs in patients hospitalized with a diagnosis of pneumonia and recovered anaerobic bacteria in 29 of 89 cases (33 percent).[46] A more recent study by Pollock and colleagues, using fiber-optic bronchoscopy with a protected catheter and quantitative cultures, showed recovery of anaerobes in 16 of 74 patients (22 percent).[44] These two reports suggest that anaerobic bacteria are actually relatively common pathogens among patients with community-acquired pneumonia and presumably account for a substantial proportion of cases that are now considered enigmatic.[6]

There have been few studies of nosocomial pneumonia using appropriate culture techniques to detect anaerobes. One study by our group utilized TTA in 159 consecutive patients and showed anaerobes in 56 (35 percent).[7] Nevertheless, most of these patients also showed the concurrent presence of aerobic gram-negative bacilli or *Staphylococcus aureus,* and our impression was that the latter organisms were probably more important in the pathologic events.

TABLE 129-1

Incidence of Anaerobic Infection of the Lung

With Anaerobes	Total	Percent	Reference
Number of Patients			
Lung abscess			
53	57	93	Bartlett JG et al[10,11,38]
22	26	85	Beerens H, Tahon-Castel M[12]
9	10	90	Brook I, Finegold SM[14]
37	41	90	Gudiol F et al[29]
Aspiration pneumonia			
61	70	87	Bartlett JG et al[10,11,38]
17	17	100	Gonzales-C CL, Calia FM[26]
29	47	62	Lorber B, Swenson RM[37]
69	74	93	Brook I, Finegold SM[15]
Empyema			
63	83	76	Bartlett JG et al[5]
23	45	51	Beerens H, Tahon-Castel M[12]
28	72	39	Sullivan KM et al[53]
25	100	25	Mavroudis C et al[39]
26	90	29	Grant DR, Finley RJ[27]
20	70	29	Lemmer J et al[35]
Community-acquired pneumonia			
28	89	33	Ries K et al[46]
16	74	22	Pollock HM et al[44]
Nosocomial pneumonia			
56	159	35	Bartlett JG et al[7]

PATHOPHYSIOLOGY

The bacteria implicated in anaerobic lung infections represent the normal flora of the oral cavity—primarily the gingival crevice, where anaerobic bacteria are found in concentrations that approach the geometric limits with which bacteria occupy space: 1012 per gram.[33] Compromised consciousness or dysphagia predisposes most frequently to clinically significant aspiration. Common conditions associated with clinically significant aspiration include alcoholism, general anesthesia, seizure disorder, drug abuse, esophageal lesions, and neurologic deficits.[3,10,11,38]

Numerous studies indicate that virtually all healthy persons aspirate, but that this is usually inconsequential. In one study, in which contrast material was placed in the mouths of sleeping patients, chest radiographs the following day showed contrast material in the lung in most of them, but there was no evidence of a disease process.[1] Similarly, dye markers placed in the stomach of postoperative patients can be aspirated from the tracheobronchial tree at the time of surgery, indicating aspiration of gastric contents during general anesthesia in 7 to 16 percent.[13,24] Scintigraphic methods have also been used to demonstrate frequent aspiration in patients with intubation of the airways or gastrointestinal tract.[19,49,52] None of these studies have demonstrated any clinical consequences from this type of occult aspiration. The conclusion is that aspiration is relatively common, but usually resolves spontaneously. The decisive factor for the development of lung complications depends on the frequency, volume, and character of the material in the inoculum. The conditions cited above as causing clinically significant disease are associated with more frequent aspiration or aspiration of large volumes—factors that define the populations at greatest risk.

Additional conditions that appear to predispose to anaerobic infections include pulmonary infarction, obstruction due to carcinoma or a foreign body, and bronchiectasis.[10,11,38] These conditions are associated with stasis or necrosis of tissue, which presumably accounts for the association with anaerobic infections.

A somewhat unique feature of anaerobic lung infections is the penchant for necrosis of tissue, resulting in abscess formation or a bronchopleural fistula associated with empyema. Virulence factors of anaerobic bacteria presumed to account for this association include the capsular polysaccharide of anaerobic gram-negative bacilli. The most extensively studied is the polysaccharide of *Bacteroides fragilis,* but the same observations appear to apply to *P. melaninogenica* and probably other anaerobic gram-negative bacilli as well.[41] The capsule consists of a family of polysaccharides composed of oligosaccharide repeating units with sugars containing positively charged free amino groups and negatively charged carboxyl or phosphorate groups. These positive and negative charges mediate the capacity to induce

abscess formation in experimental animals.[56] Another virulence factor possessed by most anaerobic bacteria is the production of short-chain fatty acids that inhibit phagocytic killing at low pH levels.[47] Short-chain volatile fatty acids are metabolic products of anaerobic bacteria that are used to classify these organisms taxonomically, and they appear to be responsible for the putrid odor that is often a characteristic feature of infections by these organisms.

CLINICAL FEATURES

Common clinical features of anaerobic pulmonary infections are summarized in Table 129-2,[11] which categorizes the patients with respect to pneumonitis, lung abscess, or empyema. Although these are distinctive clinical syndromes, there is no evidence of microbiologic distinctions in their etiology. Anaerobic lung infections may be acute, subacute, or chronic. The first stage in the infection is pneumonitis. One review of 46 patients with anaerobic bacterial pneumonitis showed clinical features that were similar to those of pneumococcal pneumonia.[9] The diagnosis was established by TTA, and the results in this group were compared with those in a second group of patients in whom TTAs yielded *S. pneumoniae.* The two groups were similar in terms of age, changes on the chest radiograph, peak temperature, and peripheral leukocyte count. Significant differences in the group with anaerobic infections were the lack of rigors, a somewhat longer duration of symptoms before presentation, and a more frequent association with predisposing conditions for aspiration. An important point to emphasize is that patients seen in this early stage of infection rarely have the features that are commonly associated with anaerobic lung infections, such as putrid sputum, tissue necrosis with abscess formation, and a chronic course. These infections presumably account for some and possibly many of the cases of community-acquired pneumonia in which no etiologic diagnosis is established despite extensive study; such cases account for 40 to 50 percent of cases in most series.

TABLE 129-2

Clinical Features of Anaerobic Pulmonary Infections*

	Lung Abscess (83 pts)	Empyema (51 pts)	Pneumonitis (only) (79 pts)	Total 193 (pts)
Age (median)	52 yrs	49 yrs	60 yrs	51 yrs
Peak temperature (mean, °F)	102.1	102.4	102.6	102.4
Peripheral leukocyte count (median/mm³)	15,000	21,600	13,700	15,000
History of weight loss	36 (43%)	28 (55%)	3 (4%)	57 (30%)
Putrid discharge	41 (49%)	32 (63%)	4 (5%)	62 (32%)
Lethal outcome	3 (4%)	3 (6%)	3 (4%)	8 (4%)

*Based on retrospective chart review of 193 cases established by recovery of anaerobes as dominant flora in TTA, pleural fluid, or blood culture.
SOURCE: From Bartlett[10,11] and Marina et al,[38] with permission.

The initial stage of pneumonitis is often more subtle or neglected, so that many patients do not seek medical attention until the infection has been present for weeks or even months. These cases are more analogous to tuberculosis than to most bacterial infections of the lung. As noted, many of these infections progress to suppurative complications, with presentation as lung abscess or empyema. The studies by David Smith cited above and sequential chest radiographs in patients who have a defined period of aspiration (as with seizure or general anesthesia) generally show that 7 to 14 days is required for cavity formation.[51] Occasionally, patients present with chronic pneumonitis.

Nearly all patients with anaerobic lung infections have the usual constitutional findings for patients with infection (Table 129-2). A review of 193 bacteriologically confirmed cases showed that the mean peak temperature for hospitalized patients was 39.1°C, and all but five patients were febrile.[11] The average peripheral leukocyte count was 15,000 per cubic millimeter. Patients who presented with the suppurative complications had a longer duration of symptoms before presentation; this was commonly associated with other evidence of chronic disease, including weight loss and anemia. Another common feature of patients with suppurative complications was putrid sputum or empyema fluid, which was noted in 40 to 60 percent. It should be emphasized that the putrid discharge in these cases is considered diagnostic of anaerobic infection, since aerobic bacteria are not capable of producing this characteristic odor either in vitro or in vivo.

Chest radiographs in patients with anaerobic lung infections show infiltrates, with or without cavitation, that most frequently involve dependent pulmonary segments. The favored locations are the superior segment of the lower lobes or posterior segments of the upper lobes; these are dependent in the recumbent position. The basilar segments of the lower lobes are favored in patients who aspirate in the upright position. The right lung is more frequently affected, owing to the more direct takeoff of the right main-stem bronchus.

These observations show that anaerobic bacteria may cause a diverse range of pulmonary infections, which may be acute, subacute, or chronic. The anaerobic etiology is rarely established or even suspected in patients with acute pneumonitis unless the appellation *aspiration pneumonia* is applied; in this case, anaerobes are the presumed pathogens in most community-acquired cases, and they may be contributing factors in many nosocomial infections. (It should be emphasized that other pathologic processes are operative in aspiration pneumonia, described below.) By contrast, anaerobic bacteria are readily recognized as probable pathogens in patients who have the late suppurative complications, such as lung abscess or empyema.

Features of anaerobic infections that are nearly unique are the association with conditions that predispose to aspiration and infection in the gingival crevice, putrid discharge, and a high frequency of suppurative complications in late stage-disease.

LABORATORY DIAGNOSIS

Establishment of anaerobic infections of the lower airways requires a specimen devoid of contamination by the flora of the upper airways or quantitative cultures that will distinguish pathogens from normal flora. Uncontaminated specimens that are considered valid for anaerobic culture include pleural fluid, transtracheal aspirates, transthoracic aspirates, and specimens obtained at thoracotomy.[10,11,38] The most common technique used in the early 1970s was TTA. It was critical to obtain the specimen before administration of antibiotics, since this treatment rapidly alters the cultivable flora.[8] TTA is now rarely used, and relatively few physicians are trained in the technique.

An alternative specimen source that is gaining popularity is quantitative cultures of specimens obtained at fiber-optic bronchoscopy, either by BAL or with the protected brush.[32,44,60] Anaerobic bacteriology, as conventionally done, should not be used for bronchoscopic aspirates. It should be noted that quantitative culture of lower-airway secretions improves diagnostic accuracy with virtually any specimen that is subject to contamination, including expectorated sputum and tracheostomy aspirates.[4] Most studies employing these techniques use them for detection of aerobic bacteria, and there are relatively few studies in which anaerobic cultures have been performed. Those in which anaerobic cultures were done tend to support the validity of this method.[4,32,44,60] Nevertheless, it is important to emphasize the importance of obtaining specimens before inception of antibiotic treatment and the need to adhere rigorously to techniques with established merits.

The second criterion for documenting anaerobic infections of the lower airways is proper attention to transport and processing of specimens. These specimens should be expeditiously transported to the laboratory for prompt microbiologic processing. Technical expertise for recovering and identifying anaerobic bacteria is highly variable. Most of these infections are polymicrobial, and many of the organisms grow slowly in vitro. Thus, it often takes several days to separate, identify, and report results of anaerobic cultures. There is also great variation in the quality of in vitro susceptibility tests, and many laboratories simply do not offer this service for anaerobic bacteria. These factors contribute to the necessity for empiric decisions regarding antibiotic selection.

The above comments account for limited information obtained from culture and sensitivity tests of anaerobes. It is important, however, to emphasize the simplicity and utility of Gram's stain. Most anaerobic gram-negative bacteria have unique morphologic features that make them relatively easy to identify or suspect on direct Gram's stain. Peptostreptococci appear like their aerobic counterparts. These are usually mixed infections involving multiple bacteria, and about half of the cases demonstrate mixtures of aerobic and anaerobic bacteria. Thus, the detection of polymicrobial flora or bacteria with the unique morphology of anaerobes on any specimen that is devoid of contamination by normal flora represents an important clue to the probable presence of anaerobic infection.

BACTERIOLOGY

The bacteriologic findings in anaerobic lung infections from two large series are summarized in Table 129-3.[10,11,38] Most of these infections involve multiple bacterial species, and approximately half of the patients have anaerobic bacteria combined with potentially pathogenic aerobic or facultative anaerobes. Analysis of

TABLE 129-3

Bacteriology of Anaerobic Lung Infections

	Bartlett[11]	Marina et al[38]
Period reviewed	1968–75	1976–91
Patients	193	110
Total anaerobic isolates	461	404
Major isolates		
Gram-negative bacilli		
Bacteroides fragilis group	38*	18
Pigmented Prevotella†	76	63
Nonpigmented Prevotella	—	40
B. ureolyticus	—	23
Fusobacterium nucleatum	56	34
Bacteroides species (other)	37	138
Peptostreptococcus/Peptococcus‡	126	39
Gram-positive bacilli		
Clostridium spp	18	12
Eubacterium spp	18	22
Actinomyces	5	19
Lactobacillus	8	22
Propionibacteria	10	9

*Numbers indicate the total number of isolates. Some of the differences are due to taxonomic changes.
†Pigmented Prevotella refers to organisms previously classified as *B. melaninogenicus.*
‡Most peptococci have been reclassified as Peptostreptococcus.

community-acquired infections involving only anaerobes versus those that are mixtures of aerobic and anaerobic bacteria shows common clinical features with no difference in terms of the frequency of suspected aspiration, indolent presentation, or the frequency of putrid discharge. The implication is that a putrid lung abscess with *E. coli* in expectorated sputum or anaerobic bacteria plus *E. coli* in a TTA should usually be considered an anaerobic infection.[3,10,11,38] Caution is advised in applying these conclusions to nosocomial pulmonary infections, since this is a setting in which the aerobic component of the infection is probably the most important.[7]

The major bacterial isolates in patients with anaerobic lung infections are Peptostreptococcus, *F. nucleatum,* and *P. melaninogenica.*[11] These are considered the "big three" anaerobic bacteria in oral and pulmonary infections involving the oral flora. Aerobic and microaerophilic streptococci are commonly present as well, and may be contributing factors in the pathogenic events. At least 15 to 25 percent of anaerobic bacteria responsible for lung infections are resistant to penicillin, almost always because of penicillinase production.[2] These sensitivity data are rarely available in individual cases: most patients with anaerobic pulmonary infection never have cultivation of the putative agent, and those who do are usually not subjected to susceptibility testing.

TREATMENT

The most important component of treatment is antibiotics—except empyemas, for which the mainstay of treatment is drainage. The standard drug historically for aspiration pneumonia and lung abscess involving anaerobic bacteria has been penicillin, usually given intravenously or with high-dose oral treatment.[57,58] Several trials performed from 1950 through 1975 showed that the great majority of patients responded. Occasionally, those who did not respond to penicillin responded to tetracycline. These recommendations have been confounded in recent years by the observations summarized above; penicillinase production has been noted in up to 40 to 60 percent of strains of fusobacteria and *P. melaninogenica,* as well as many other anaerobic gram-negative bacilli.[2]

There have been two therapeutic trials in patients with lung abscess involving anaerobic bacteria (Table 129-4). Both compared clindamycin to intravenous penicillin,[29,36] and in both series, clindamycin proved superior in terms of response rates and time to defervescence. Alternative regimens in which the anecdotal experience is favorable include amoxicillin-clavulanate (Augmentin) and penicillin combined with metronidazole. Metronidazole should not be used as a single agent in patients with anaerobic lung infections, since there is a poor response in about 50 percent.[43] The presumed explanation is the contributing role of aerobic and microaerophilic streptococci, which are resistant to this drug.

TABLE 129-4

Antibiotic Treatment of Anaerobic Lung Infections: Results of Two Randomized Trials

Source	Treatment	# Pts	Number of Patients with:			
			Failure	Relapse	Fever	Putrid Sputum
Levinson (1983)[36]	Penicillin (6 mil units/d)	21	5 (29%)	3 (19%)	7.7	7.8
	Clindamycin (1.8 g/d)	17	0*	0	4.7*	4.1*
Gudiol (1990)[29]	Penicillin (12 mil units/d)	18	7 (39%)	2 (11%)	7.2	7.3
	Clindamycin (2.4 g/d)	19	1 (5%)	0	6.4	3.9*

*Difference for treatment favoring clindamycin is statistically significant.

There are many other antibiotics that might be successful in anaerobic lung infections but have not been studied. These include any combination of a betalactam with a betalactamase inhibitor (ticarcillin-clavulanate, ampicillin-sulbactam, amoxicillin-clavulanate, piperacillin-tazobactam), chloramphenicol, imipenem, and selected cephalosporins such as cefoxitin or cefotetan. All these drugs have established merit in treating anaerobic infections at several anatomic sites.[2] Macrolides (erythromycin, clarithromycin, and azithromycin) have not been extensively studied for anaerobic pulmonary infections, but they show good in vitro activity against most strains except fusobacteria. Penicillin is not active against many strains; nevertheless, this drug may be adequate for most patients, especially those characterized by pneumonitis without suppurative complications. The same applies to other penicillins, especially when used in high doses, including ampicillin and antipseudomonad penicillins. Oxacillin and nafcillin are much less active. Tetracyclines show limited activity against many anaerobic bacteria in vitro; vancomycin is active only against gram-positive anaerobes. Drugs that have virtually no activity against anaerobes include aminoglycosides, currently available quinolones, aztreonam, and trimethoprim-sulfamethoxazole.

OTHER ASPIRATION SYNDROMES

Aspiration pneumonia refers to distinctive syndromes that are distinguished on the basis of the character of the inoculum, which dictates the pathogenesis of pulmonary complications, clinical presentation, and management strategies (Table 129-5). Although there may be overlap in individual cases and some are hard to classify, these distinctions provide a useful conceptual approach to a complex and common medical problem. Thus, aspiration pneumonia includes at least three different syndromes: chemical pneumonitis, bacterial infection, and airway obstruction. The discussion above has emphasized the role of anaerobic bacteria in bacterial infection, which is probably the most common of these syndromes.

Chemical Pneumonitis   This refers to the aspiration of an inoculum that is inherently toxic to the lungs. Examples include acid, animal fats such as milk and mineral oil, and volatile hydrocarbons. These substances are toxic to the lower airways, and they initiate an inflammatory reaction. The prototypic example based on extensive study is gastric acid pneumonitis as classically described by Mendelson and often referred to as Mendelson's syndrome.[40]

The classic study by Mendelson, published in 1946, included 61 obstetric patients who aspirated gastric contents during anesthesia. The onset of respiratory distress followed rapidly, usually within 2 h.[40] Common clinical features described by Mendelson were the abrupt onset of cyanosis, dyspnea, tachypnea, and tachycardia. Most patients had bronchospasm. Chest radiographs showed infiltrates that were located in one or both lower lobes. Despite the severity of the illness, all 61 patients recovered and most were actually stable within 24 to 36 h despite the lack of specific forms of treatment. Sequential radiographs showed infiltrates cleared within 4 to 7 days in most patients. Subsequent studies of this syndrome show a higher frequency of fever, reduced frequency of bronchospasm, but, most important, substantial mortality.[16,21] The presumed explanation for the difference is that the patients reported by Mendelson were young and

TABLE 129-5

Classification of Aspiration Pneumonia

Inoculum	Pulmonary Sequelae	Clinical Features	Therapy
Acid	Chemical pneumonitis	Acute dyspnea, tachypnea; tachycardia; ± cyanosis, bronchospasm, fever Sputum: pink, frothy Radiographic: infiltrates in one or both lower lobes Hypoxemia	Positive-pressure breathing Intravenous fluids Tracheal suction
Oropharyngeal bacteria	Bacterial infection	Usually insidious onset Cough, fever, purulent sputum Radiographic: infiltrate in dependent pulmonary segment or lobe ± cavitation	Antibiotics
Inert fluids	Mechanical obstruction Reflex airway closure	Acute dyspnea, cyanosis ± apnea Pulmonary edema	Tracheal suction Intermittent positive-pressure breathing with oxygen and isoproterenol
Particulate matter	Mechanical obstruction	Dependent on level of obstruction, ranging from acute apnea and rapid death to irritating chronic cough ± recurrent infections	Extraction of particulate matter Antibiotics for superimposed infection

previously healthy obstetric patients; by contrast, more recent reports often describe debilitated patients with many associated, often serious underlying medical conditions. Blood gas analysis, not available at the time of Mendelson's report, shows hypoxemia that is usually accompanied by a normal or low P_{CO_2} and a respiratory alkalosis. Factors that contribute to hypoxemia are pulmonary edema, reduced surfactant activity, reflex airway closure, hyaline membrane formation, and alveolar hemorrhage. These patients' pulmonary function tests show decreased compliance, abnormal ventilation-perfusion, and reduced diffusing capacity. Severe disease often progresses to the adult respiratory distress syndrome (ARDS). The second potential complication is a superimposed bacterial infection, which may occur later in the course of events.

The pathophysiology of gastric acid pneumonitis has been studied in experimental animals with intratracheal instillation of graded acid inocula.[28] This work shows that the pH must be 2.5 or less for the inflammatory process to be initiated. There must also be a relatively large inoculum, usually 1 to 4 ml/kg. It is possible that smaller volumes initiate a less dramatic presentation or may go undetected. Support for this hypothesis is the observation of frequent bouts of pneumonitis and otherwise unexplained pulmonary fibrosis in patients with gastric reflux or esophageal disease.

The pathologic changes in acid pneumonia occur rapidly in the experimental animal studies[28,42,54,55] and in patients as well.[16,21,40] Atelectasis occurs within seconds and is extensive by 3 min. There is also peribronchial hemorrhage, pulmonary edema, and bronchial epithelial cell degeneration. The alveolar spaces are filled with neutrophils by 4 h and hyaline membranes are seen within 48 h. Resolution begins by the third day and may be complete or may result in residual scarring of the pulmonary parenchyma.

The clinical features of Mendelson's syndrome, as classically described, support the observations in the animal model. Clinical findings that suggest chemical pneumonitis after aspiration include the abrupt onset of symptoms, dyspnea, cyanosis or arterial hypoxemia, low-grade fever, rales, and infiltrates on chest radiograph in dependent pulmonary segments. The course of the disease was examined in a retrospective review by Bynum and Pierce.[16] These investigators found three categories of patients: the first accounted for 12 percent and had a course characterized by fulminant progression with death shortly after aspiration, apparently due to ARDS; the second group accounted for 62 percent and had rapid improvement of the chest radiograph within a mean time of 4.5 days; the third group accounted for 26 percent and showed clinical improvement, followed by new infiltrates and fever ascribed to pulmonary superinfection. Long-term follow-up studies in patients who have gastric acid pneumonia show either complete recovery or radiographic evidence of pulmonary fibrosis with abnormal gas exchange.[50]

The diagnosis of acid pneumonia is usually presumed on the basis of clinical observations such as the abrupt onset of dyspnea in a patient who is aspiration prone and has radiographic evidence of infiltrates, usually in the lower lobes. Other characteristic clinical features are the rapid clearing of the infiltrates and progression to ARDS. Bronchoscopy demonstrates erythema of the bronchi, suggesting a "chemical burn." Confirmation of the acid inoculum is not possible because of rapid neutralization by pulmonary edema fluid and bronchial secretions within minutes after aspiration.

The treatment of gastric acid aspiration includes tracheal suction to clear fluids and particulate matter that may be aspirated concurrently. Supportive care consists primarily of intravenous fluids due to decreased intravascular volume with hypotension. Studies in animal models show benefit with positive-pressure ventilation, large-molecular-weight colloids given intravenously, and sodium nitroprusside.[42,55] It has been difficult to establish the role of these therapeutic interventions in patients with appropriate controlled trials, in part because of the relative infrequency of gastric acid pneumonia. There is a consensus that ventilatory support is mandatory, but other recommendations are controversial. With regard to corticosteroids, studies in animals have given variable results, but their use in patients has been uniformly unsuccessful.[17,61] The role of antimicrobial agents is also controversial. There is no evidence that bacteria play a role in the acute events either in the animal model or in patients; indeed, bacteria cannot survive at the pH of the inoculum necessary to initiate this process. Studies in experimental animals suggest that the acid-injured lung is highly susceptible to bacterial infection, and many patients develop pulmonary superinfections after initial clinical improvement.[16] Antibiotic administration to aspiration-prone patients has not proved useful.[30] Despite these comments, many or most of these patients will be treated with antibiotics because it is difficult or impossible to exclude a contributing role for infection even early in the course of events.

Mechanical Obstruction Aspiration pneumonia may involve fluid or particulate material. In this form of aspiration pneumonia, the inoculum is not toxic to the lung but may cause obstruction or reflux airway closure. In most cases there is only transient, self-limited hypoxemia due to rapid clearance. Some patients develop pulmonary edema, however, with hypoxemia and reduced compliance apparently due to an intrinsic pulmonary reflex closure.[20] Other patients suffer sequelae due to failure to clear relatively large volumes of the aspirate, as with near-drowning victims and patients with profound neurologic deficits or in coma. The obvious critical intervention is tracheal suction.

Aspiration with mechanical obstruction may also be associated with solid particles. Foreign-body aspiration is most frequent in children 1 to 3 years of age. The most common objects in the lower airways are vegetable particles, inorganic materials, and teeth. The severity of the obstruction depends on the relative size of the material aspirated and the caliber of the lower airways. Large objects may cause obstruction at the level of the larynx or trachea, leading to sudden respiratory distress, cyanosis, and, in some cases, aphonia. This is referred to as *café coronary syndrome* because it often involves meat aspiration during restaurant dining and may simulate an acute myocardial infarction.[31] Aspiration of smaller particles may result in complete obstruction of more distant components of the tracheobronchial tree or partial obstruction. Chest radiographs often show atelectasis or obstructive emphysema. An important clue in some cases is unilateral wheezing. Bacterial infection is not important in the early stages of obstruction, but is a common feature when obstruction has been present for more than 1 week. The most common pathogens are anaerobic bacteria from the upper airways.[34] These patients may respond well to antibiotics, but often have recurrent infections in the same pulmonary segment.

The most important therapeutic intervention is removal of the foreign body, usually with bronchoscopy.

PREVENTION

Methods to prevent aspiration have been most extensively studied in hospitalized patients, especially those who are aspiration prone. Most important is use of the semirecumbent or upright position.[25] Additional factors that have variable degrees of success are tracheostomies, reduction of the stomach volume with suction or metoclopramide, feeding via gastrostomy or nasogastric tube, and neutralization of gastric acid with H_2 blockers or antacids.[18,22] Many of these procedures actually predispose to aspiration or invite other sequelae. An example is the neutralization of gastric acid, which may reduce the risk of chemical pneumonia but may increase the risk of bacterial infection following aspiration of gastric contents.[22] Tracheostomy is useful in some patients with repeated aspiration, but inflation of the balloon may occlude the esophagus and promote aspiration of upper-airway contents. Patients who require nasogastric feedings are aspiration prone; percutaneous endoscopic gastroscopy is an attractive method to address this issue, but study results are quite variable. An alternative method sometimes favored is a feeding jejunostomy.[59] Surgery has been employed for preventing esophageal lesions due to Zenker's diverticula.[48] The use of surgery with gastroesophageal reflux has given variable results.

REFERENCES

1. Amberson JB Jr: Aspiration bronchopneumonia. *Internat Clin* 3:126–138, 1937.
2. Appelbaum PC, Spangler SK, Jacobs MR: Beta-lactamase production and susceptibilities to amoxicillin, amoxicillin-clavulanate, ticarcillin, ticarcillin-clavulanate, cefoxitin, imipenem, and metronidazole of 320 non–*Bacteroides fragilis Bacteroides* isolates and 129 fusobacteria from 28 U.S. centers. *Antimicrob Agents Chemother* 34:1546–1550, 1990.
3. Bartlett JG, Finegold SM: Anaerobic infections of the lung and pleural space. *Am Rev Respir Dis* 110:56–77, 1974.
4. Bartlett JG, Finegold SM: Bacteriology of expectorated sputum with quantitative culture and wash technique compared to transtracheal aspirates. *Am Rev Respir Dis* 117:1019–1027, 1978.
5. Bartlett JG, Gorbach SL, Thadepalli H, Finegold SM: Bacteriology of empyema. *Lancet* 1:338–340, 1974.
6. Bartlett JG, Mundy LM: Community-acquired pneumonia. *New Engl J Med* 333:1618–1624, 1995.
7. Bartlett JG, O'Keefe P, Tally FP, et al: Bacteriology of hospital-acquired pneumonia. *Arch Intern Med* 146:868–871, 1986.
8. Bartlett JG: Diagnostic accuracy of transtracheal aspiration bacteriologic studies. *Am Rev Respir Dis* 115:777–782, 1977.
9. Bartlett JG: Anaerobic bacterial pneumonitis. *Am Rev Respir Dis* 119:19–23, 1979.
10. Bartlett JG: Anaerobic bacterial infections of the lung. *Chest* 91:901–909, 1987.
11. Bartlett JG: Anaerobic bacterial infections of the lung and pleural space. *Clin Infect Dis* 16(Suppl 4):S248–S255, 1993.
12. Beerens H, Tahon-Castel M: *Infections humaines à bactéries anaérobies nontoxigènes.* Brussels, Presses Académiques Européenes, 1965, pp 91–114.
13. Berson W, Adriani J: Silent regurgitation and aspiration during anesthesia. *Anesthesiology* 15:644–649, 1954.
14. Brook I, Finegold SM: Bacteriology and therapy of lung abscess in children. *J Pediatr* 94:10–12, 1979.
15. Brook I, Finegold SM: Bacteriology of aspiration pneumonia in children. *Pediatrics* 65:1115–1120, 1980.
16. Bynum LJ, Pierce AK: Pulmonary aspiration of gastric contents. *Am Rev Respir Dis* 114:1129–1136, 1976.
17. Chapman RL Jr, Downs JB, Modell JH, Hook CI: The ineffectiveness of steroid therapy in treating aspiration of hydrochloric acid. *Arch Surg* 108:858–861, 1974.
18. Ciocon JO, Silverstone FA, Graver LM, Foley CJ: Tube feedings in elderly patients: Indications, benefits, and complications. *Arch Intern Med* 148:429–433, 1988.
19. Cole MJ, Smith JT, Molnar C, Shaffer EA: Aspiration after percutaneous gastrostomy: Assessment by Tc-99m labeling of the enteral feed. *J Clin Gastroenterol* 9:90–95, 1987.
20. Colebatch HJH, Halmagyi DFJ: Reflex airway reaction to fluid aspiration. *J Appl Physiol* 19:787, 1964.
21. DePaso WJ: Aspiration pneumonia. *Clin Chest Med* 12:269–284, 1991.
22. Driks MR, Craven DE, Celli BR, et al: Nosocomial pneumonia in intubated patients given sucralfate as compared with antacids or histamine type 2 blockers: The role of gastric colonization. *New Engl J Med* 317:1376–1382, 1987.
23. Ehler AA: Non-tuberculous thoracic empyema: Collective review of literature from 1934 to 1939. *Int Abst Surg* 72:17–38, 1941.
24. Gardner AMN: Aspiration of food and vomit. *Q J Med* 27:227–242, 1958.
25. Gipson SL, Stovall TG, Elkins TE, Crumrine RS: Pharmacologic reduction of the risk of aspiration. *South Med J* 79:1356–1358, 1986.
26. Gonzalez-C CL, Calia FM: Bacteriologic flora of aspiration-induced pulmonary infections. *Arch Intern Med* 135:711–714, 1975.
27. Grant DR, Finley RJ: Empyema: Analysis of treatment techniques. *Can J Surg* 28:449–451, 1985.
28. Greenfield LJ, Singleton RP, McCaffree DR, et al: Pulmonary effects of experimental graded aspiration of hydrochloric acid. *Ann Surg* 170:74–86, 1969.
29. Gudiol F, Manresa F, Pallares R, et al: Clindamycin vs. penicillin for anaerobic lung infections: High rate of penicillin failures associated with penicillin-resistant *Bacteroides melaninogenicus. Arch Intern Med* 150:2525–2529, 1990.
30. Hamelberg WV, Bosomworth PP: *Aspiration Pneumonitis.* Springfield, IL, Charles C Thomas, 1968.
31. Haugen RK: The café coronary: Sudden deaths in restaurants. *JAMA* 186:142–143, 1963.
32. Henriquez AH, Mendoza J, Gonzalez PC: Quantitative culture of bronchoalveolar lavage from patients with anaerobic lung abscesses. *J Infect Dis* 164:414–417, 1991.
33. Hirsch RS, Clarke NG: Infection and periodontal diseases. *Rev Infect Dis* 11:707–715, 1989.
34. Lansing AM, Jamieson WG: Mechanisms of fever in pulmonary atelectasis. *Arch Surg* 87:168–174, 1963.
35. Lemmer J, Botham MJ, Orringer MB: Modern management of adult thoracic empyema. *J Thorac Cardiovasc Surg* 90:849–855, 1985.
36. Levison ME, Mangura CT, Lorber B, et al: Clindamycin compared with penicillin for the treatment of anaerobic lung abscess. *Ann Intern Med* 98:466–471, 1983.

37. Lorber B, Swenson RM: Bacteriology of aspiration pneumonia: A prospective study of community- and hospital-acquired cases. *Ann Intern Med* 81:329–331, 1974.

38. Marina M, Strong CA, Civen R, et al: Bacteriology of anaerobic pleuropulmonary infections: Preliminary report. *Clin Infect Dis* 16(Suppl):S256–S262, 1993.

39. Mavroudis C, Symmonds JB, Minagi H, Thomas AN: Improved survival in management of empyema thoracis. *J Thorac Cardiovasc Surg* 82:49–57, 1981.

40. Mendelson CL: The aspiration of stomach contents into the lungs during obstetric anesthesia. *Am J Obstet Gynecol* 52:191–205, 1946.

41. Pantosti A, Tzianabos AO, Reinap BG, et al: *Bacteroides fragilis* strains express multiple capsular polysaccharides. *J Clin Microbiol* 31:1850–1855. 1993.

42. Peitzman AB, Shires GT III, Illner H, Shires GT: Pulmonary acid injury: Effects of positive end-expiratory pressure and crystalloid *vs* colloid fluid resuscitation. *Arch Surg* 117:662–668, 1982.

43. Perlino CA: Metronidazole vs clindamycin treatment of anaerobic pulmonary infection. *Arch Intern Med* 141:1424–1427, 1981.

44. Pollock HM, Hawkins EL, Bonner JR, et al: Diagnosis of bacterial pulmonary infections with quantitative protected catheter cultures obtained during bronchoscopy. *J Clin Microbiol* 17:255–259, 1983.

45. Rendu M, Rist E: Etude clinique et bactériologique de trois cas de pleurésie putride. *Bull Mém Soc Méd Hôp Paris* 16:133–150, 1899.

46. Ries K, Levison ME, Kaye D: Transtracheal aspiration in pulmonary infection. *Arch Intern Med* 133:453–458, 1974.

47. Rotstein OD, Vittorini T, Kao J, et al: A soluble *Bacteroides* by-product impairs phagocytic killing of *Escherichia coli* by neutrophils. *Infect Immun* 57:745–753, 1989.

48. Schmit PJ, Zuckerbraun L: Zenker's diverticula by cricopharyngeus myotomy under local anesthesia. *Am Surg* 58:710–716, 1992.

49. Silver KH, Van Nostrand D: The use of scintigraphy in the management of patients with pulmonary aspiration. *Dysphagia* 9:107–115, 1994.

50. Sladen A, Zanca P, Hadnott WH: Aspiration pneumonitis: The sequelae. *Chest* 59:448–450, 1971.

51. Smith DT: Experimental aspiratory abscess. *Arch Surg* 14:231–239, 1927.

52. Spray SB, Zuidema GD, Cameron JL: Aspiration pneumonia: Incidence of aspiration with endotracheal tubes. *Am J Surg* 131:701–703, 1976.

53. Sullivan KM, O'Toole RD, Fisher RH, Sullivan KN: Anaerobic empyema thoracis. *Arch Intern Med* 131:521–527, 1973.

54. Toung TJ, Bordos D, Benson DW, et al: Aspiration pneumonia: Experimental evaluation of albumin and steroid therapy. *Ann Surg* 183:179–184, 1976.

55. Toung TJ, Cameron JL, Kimura T, Permutt S: Aspiration pneumonia: Treatment with osmotically active agents. *Surgery* 89:588–593, 1981.

56. Tzianabos AO, Onderdonk AB, Zaleznik DF, et al: Structural characteristics of polysaccharides that induce protection against intraabdominal abscess formation. *Infect Immun* 62:4881–4886, 1994.

57. Weiss W: Oral antibiotic therapy of acute primary lung abscess: Comparison of penicillin G and tetracycline. *Curr Ther Res* 12:154–160, 1970.

58. Weiss W: Cavity behavior in acute, primary nonspecific lung abscess. *Am Rev Respir Dis* 108:1273–1275, 1973.

59. Weltz CR, Morris JB, Mullen JL: Surgical jejunostomy in aspiration risk patients. *Ann Surg* 215:140–145, 1992.

60. Wimberley NW, Bass JB Jr, Boyd BW, et al: Use of a bronchoscopic protected catheter brush for the diagnosis of pulmonary infections. *Chest* 81:556–562, 1982.

61. Wolfe JE, Bone RC, Ruth WE: Effects of corticosteroids in the treatment of patients with gastric aspiration. *Am J Med* 63:719–722, 1977.

CHAPTER 130

EMPYEMA AND LUNG ABSCESS

Sydney M. Finegold / Jay A. Fishman

The evaluation of empyemas and lung abscesses has been greatly facilitated by improvements in noninvasive and minimally invasive diagnostic techniques, including computerized tomography, radiologic drainage-catheter placement, and thoracoscopic surgery. *Empyema* refers to a purulent collection in any body site, but is commonly used to indicate infection of the pleural space. Empyema is commonly associated with underlying pulmonary parenchymal infection, but may also be associated with blood-borne infection, thoracic surgery, trauma, abdominal infection, or neoplasm.

Lung abscesses reflect infection with an unusual microbial burden (e.g., acute aspiration), a failure in microbial clearance mechanisms (e.g., bronchial obstruction; see Chapter 120), or both, with necrosis of pulmonary tissue and formation of cavities containing necrotic debris or fluid (Fig. 130-1). The formation of multiple smaller (less than 2 cm) abscesses in pulmonary tissue is occasionally referred to as *necrotizing pneumonia* or *lung gangrene*. Both lung abscess and necrotizing pneumonia are manifestations of the same pathologic processes, and the distinction is, therefore, arbitrary.

Failure to recognize and to treat either empyema or lung abscess is associated with a poor clinical outcome.[1,45,49] In the preantibiotic era, lung abscess was associated with a mortality approaching 40 percent. However, controversy exists over the best approaches to both processes in terms of antimicrobial selection and physical drainage.

EPIDEMIOLOGY AND MICROBIOLOGY

Etiology of Empyema

Empyema is often defined as the presence of pleural fluid with an excess of 25,000 cells per milliliter that are largely neutrophils *or* by the demonstration of microorganisms by examination of smears or by culture, *or* it may be inferred from the presence in pleural fluid of a pH less than 7.0, a lactic dehydrogenase of more than 1000 IU/L, glucose level of less than 40 mg/ml, or lactate level over 5 mmol/L or 45 mg/ml. Empyema is generally a complication of pneumonia, although only a small percentage of parapneumonic effusions develop the cellular, proteinaceous, and microbial contents associated with empyema (Fig. 130-2).[2,4,7,36,42,49] Empyema fluid is susceptible to infection because of the presence of protein, the suppression of leukocyte function by endotoxins and exotoxins, the absence of complement and other opsonins, and acidity. The presence of anaerobic infection is favored by the relative absence of oxygen and/or a low pH in these fluids. The size of the fluid collection is determined by physical constraints (i.e., pleural scar), the intensity of the host response, and the nature and persistence of the underlying cause of the pleural fluid (e.g., congestive heart failure).

Empyema is most often associated with pneumonia, particularly aspirational events with anaerobic microbiology (see Chapters 80 and 129) (Fig. 130-2). However, empyema is increasingly a complication of previous surgery, which now represents up to 30 percent of cases.[11] These infections most often reflect nosocomial transmission (*Staphylococcus aureus,* aerobic gram-negative bacteria), with or without underlying pneumonia. Serous pleural effusions can be infected with gram-negative bacteria in the absence of underlying tissue infection.[26] Following trauma or with pleural hematoma or free blood, the incidence of superinfection is high, particularly due to staphylococci and enterococci. Following lung surgery for the diagnosis of pulmonary infections, the infecting agents—particularly *Aspergillus,* the *Mucoraceae,* the mycobacteria, and *Coccidioides*—may disseminate to the pleural space. Leakage from a bronchial stump remaining after pulmonary resection is also associated with severe and persistent infection of the pleural space.

In the absence of trauma or surgery, the infecting organisms spread from primary infections in the blood or in any of the tho-

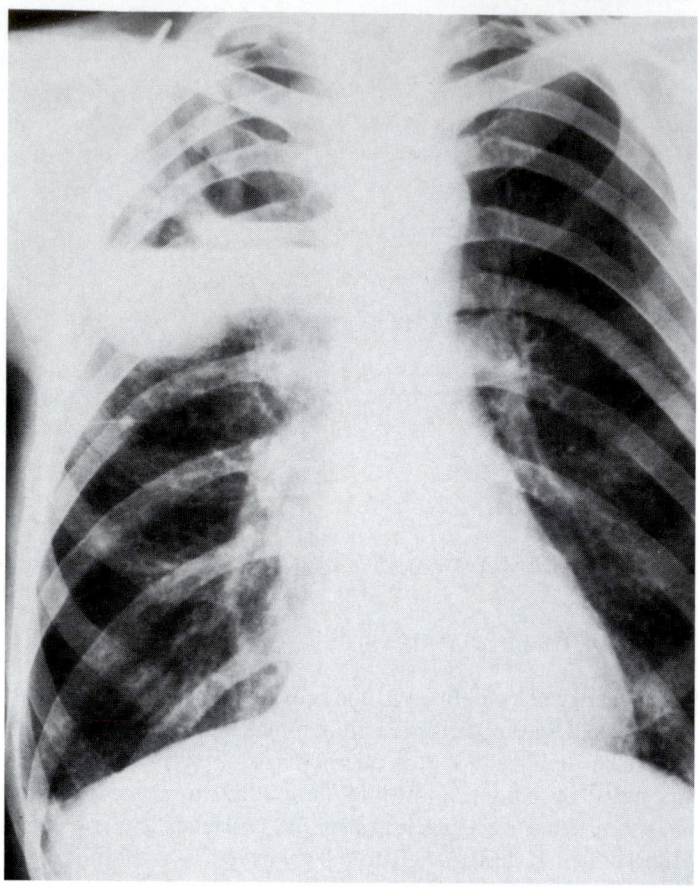

A

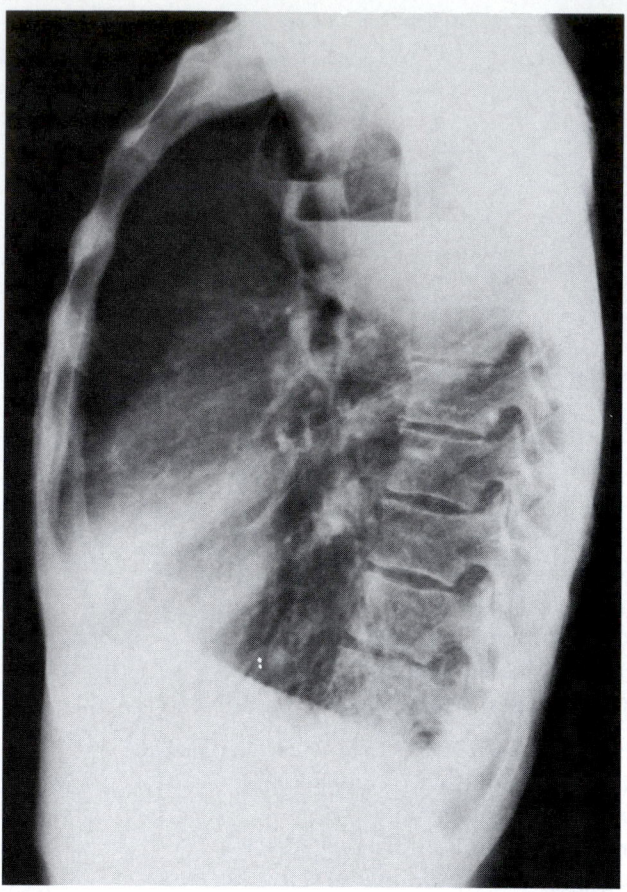

B

FIGURE 130-1 *A.* Anaerobic pneumonia with abscess formation in a 48-year-old alcoholic man. The abscesses are located in the posterior segment of right upper lobe, a dependent segment that is seen best on lateral view *B.*

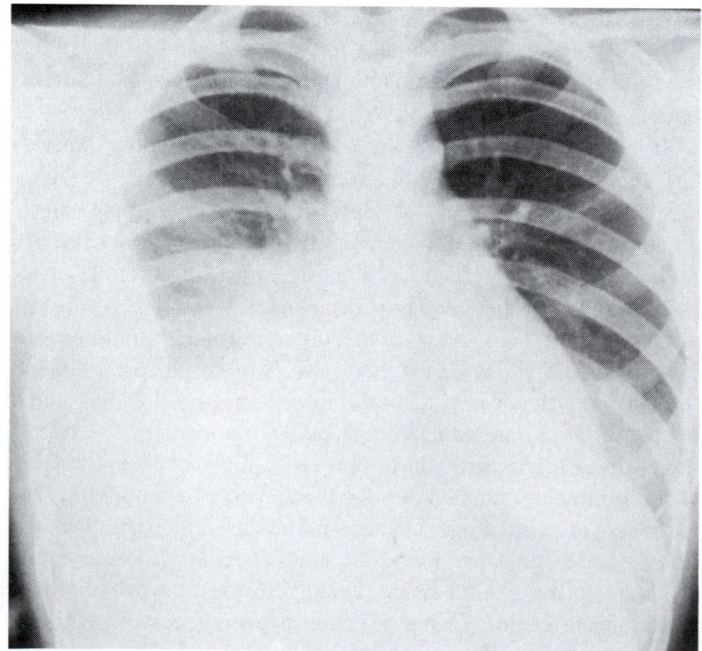

FIGURE 130-2 Large anaerobic empyema accompanying right middle-lobe pneumonia.

racic or abdominal organs, including pneumonia, mediastinitis, esophagitis, spinal epidural abscess and osteomyelitis, lymph node infection, pericarditis, cholangitis, and diverticulitis. Bronchopleural fistula is frequently associated with empyema and may adversely affect the success of therapy if it remains undetected or persists despite treatment.[3,11] Peritonsillar, perimandibular, or parapharyngeal abscess, odontogenic infection, or prevertebral neck space infection may also present with empyema that spreads via the "danger spaces" (see Chapter 126). These sources, or the spread of infection due to thoracentesis performed with inadequate sterile technique, following intravenous drug injection in the supraclavicular space, following esophageal rupture, or due to hematogenous spread, contribute up to 15 percent of cases of empyema.

Microbiology of Empyema

In the preantibiotic era, up to 11 percent of cases of pneumococcal pneumonia were associated with empyema; 64 percent of all cases of empyema were associated with *Streptococcus pneumoniae.*[12,15] β-Hemolytic streptococci (15 percent) and staphylococci (8 percent) were the other organisms most commonly isolated from empyema fluid. The relative absence of useful anaerobic culture systems in the 1950s prevented the routine isolation of these organisms. With the introduction of the sulfa drugs and penicillins, the expansion of thoracic surgery, and the emergence of antibiotic resistance in the staphylococci, the isolation of *S. pneumoniae* decreased and that of *S. aureus* and other nosocomial pathogens in empyema fluids increased.

ANAEROBIC BACTERIA

In the 1960s and 1970s, improvements in microbiological techniques increased the rate of isolation of anaerobic organisms in pleural fluid. Thus, one study found *only* anaerobic bacteria in pleural empyema fluid in 35 percent of cases, and a *mixture of* aerobic and anaerobic bacteria in 41 percent in a series of 83 medical patients who had not received antibiotics or surgical intervention (Tables 130-1 and 130-2) (Figs. 130-3 and 130-4).[7,9]

The frequency of anaerobic infection of the lung and pleural space is a function of the colonization pattern of the individual patient, including the presence of hospital-acquired pathogens and the role of aspiration in many of these infections (Table 130-2). The most frequent isolates are the anaerobes *Prevotella, Fusobacterium nucleatum,* and *Peptostreptococcus* and the streptococci (Figs. 130-5 and 130-6). In early studies, the *Bacteroides fragilis* group was isolated from 15 to 20 percent of patients with anaerobic pleuropulmonary infections. However, later studies employing newer techniques and utilizing newer taxonomic cri-

TABLE 130-1

Bacteriology of Anaerobic Empyema: Predominant Flora

Organism	No. Isolates
Anaerobic iolates	
Fusobacterium nucleatum	19
Prevotella denticola-melaninogenica group	10
Prevotella oris	9
Prevotella intermedia-nigrescens group	8
Prevotella oralis	4
Prevotella buccae	3
Bacteroides fragilis	5
Other *B. fragilis* group	6
Unidentifiable *Bacteroides* spp.	4
Bacteroides gracilis	3
Campylobacter spp.	3
Peptostreptococcus micros	9
Peptostreptococcus anaerobius	5
Peptostreptococcus spp.	4
Peptostreptococcus magnus	3
Streptococcus intermedius	5
Eubacterium spp.	7
Lactobacillus spp.	7
Actinomyces spp.	4
Actinomyces odontolyticus	3
Propionibacterium acnes	4
Clostridium perfringens	3
Clostridium spp.	3
Aerobic Isolates	
α-hemolytic streptococcus	21
Nonenterococcal group D streptococcus	4
Coagulase-negative staphylococci	4
Proteus spp.	3

SOURCE: Based on data of Civen et al.[9]

teria found *B. fragilis* group isolates in only 6.8 percent of 46 patients with pleural empyema specimens. The *B. fragilis* group is important because of resistance to penicillin G (a property shared by a number of common anaerobes) and other antimicrobial agents.[1,3,5,14] Subdiaphragmatic infection may extend to the lung or pleural space by way of lymphatics, directly through the diaphragm or defects in it, or by way of the bloodstream. Anaerobic pulmonary and pleural processes rarely extend to the chest wall unless associated with actinomycosis, tuberculosis, or tumor.[19]

NONANAEROBIC INFECTIONS

In immunologically normal adults, the aerobic organisms currently most often associated with empyema are *S. aureus,* β-hemolytic streptococci, and various gram-negative aerobic or facultatively anaerobic bacilli, particularly *Pseudomonas aeruginosa, Escherichia coli, Klebsiella* species, and other nosocomial enteric gram-negative organisms—reflecting infections associated with thoracic surgery. Mixed aerobic-anaerobic infections are often related to subdiaphragmatic processes. Increasingly, *Mycobacterium tuberculosis, Nocardia asteroides,* and fungi have been identified. In the immunocompromised host, the infecting organisms will more often be gram-negative bacteria (especially *Pseudomonas* and *Enterobacter*) or *Candida* or *Aspergillus* species, or will be due to reactivation of latent or subclinical infections due to *M. tuberculosis, Candida* species, or the less virulent streptococci.

The Etiology of Lung Abscess

Because the most important predisposing condition for lung abscess is *aspiration* (see Chapters 80 and 129), lung abscesses are most often located in the posterior segment of the right upper lobe, less often in the left upper lobe and the apical segments of the lower lobes (Fig. 130-1). Periodontal disease is highly associated with lung abscess formation; in edentulous people, lung abscesses are uncommon and may suggest the presence of an obstructing lesion of the bronchus, pulmonary embolus, septic embolus, or unsuspected pathogen.[4] Nosocomial aspiration (see Chapters 119 and 143) will often involve gram-negative bacteria, particularly organisms with hospital-acquired antibiotic resistance patterns.

Lung abscesses generally develop after inflammation produces tissue necrosis with cavitation. In the presence of preexisting cavitary disease (emphysema or old tuberculous lesions), infection may proceed without frank necrosis. The abscess cavity may become lined with regenerated epithelium. Local obstruction may produce bronchiectasis or emphysema in the surrounding lung.

The classification of lung abscesses is based on the duration and likely cause of the process. *Acute abscesses* are less than 4 to 6 weeks old, whereas *chronic abscesses* are of greater duration. *Primary abscesses* are infections due to aspiration or to pneumonia in the normal host; *secondary abscess* is due to preexisting conditions (obstruction, spread from an extrapulmonary site, bronchiectasis, immune compromise). Abscesses with foul odors associated with anaerobic organisms are often called *putrid abscesses*.

TABLE 130-2

Correlation of Infecting Organism and Conditions Underlying Anaerobic Pleuropulmonary Infection

Bacteria	Aspi-ration	Tonsil-litis, Tonsil-lectomy	Gingivitis, Dental Extraction, Pyorrhea	Bronchi-ectasis	Broncho-genic Carcinoma	Chest Trauma, Thora-cotomy	Peritoneal Infection or Source in Bowel	Pelvic Infection
Bacteroides fragilis group	11	1	0	3	1	3	16	1
Pigmented gram-negative anaerobic rods	13	0	7	2	0	0	2	0
Fusobacterium nucleatum	24	2	7	4	4	4	6	1
F. necrophorum	2	45	2	1	2	0	5	4
Peptostreptococcus	27	5	9	4	2	10	6	8
Microaerophilic streptococcus	17	0	5	0	4	0	5	1
Anaerobic, non–spore-forming, catalase-negative, gram-positive rods	6	1	0	1	2	1	3	0
Clostridium	6	3	1	0	0	15	7	1

SOURCE: Based on data of Finegold.[14]

Microbiology of Lung Abscess

In lung abscesses, anaerobes are recoverable from up to 89 percent of patients.[5,41,43] In some patients, anaerobic organisms of presumably greater virulence (e.g., *Fusobacterium nucleatum* or *Peptostreptococcus* species) may be found as the sole infecting organism. In studies by Bartlett and coworkers, 46 percent of patients with lung abscesses had *only* anaerobes isolated in cultures, while an additional 43 percent had a *mixture* of anaerobes and aerobic bacteria.[5] In addition to anaerobes, among the organisms often implicated in lung abscess formation or in necrotizing pneumonia are *S. aureus, Streptococcus pyogenes, Klebsiella pneumoniae,* and *P. aeruginosa.* Infrequently, other gram-negative bacilli, such as *E. coli* and *Haemophilus influenzae* type B, may cause pulmonary necrosis. Uncommon but important causes of cavitating pneumonia are *N. asteroides, Paragonimus westermani,*

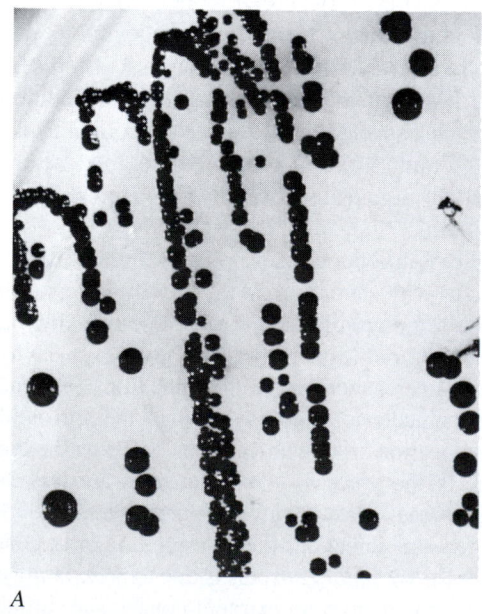

A

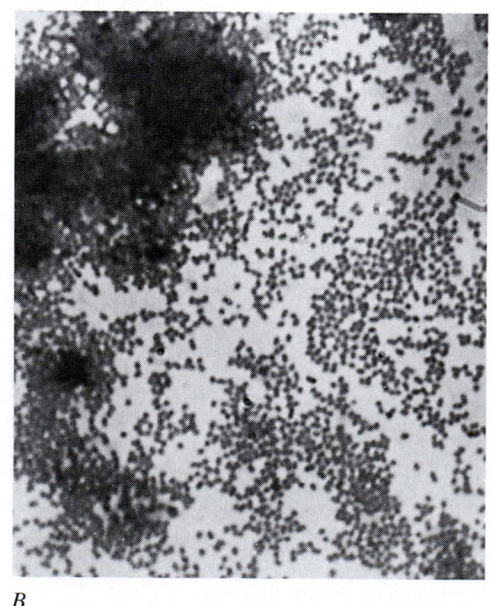

B

FIGURE 130-3   *Prevotella melaninogenica.* A. Distinctive black colonies (on blood-containing medium); pigment is hematin. B. Microscopically, the organism is a coccobacillus.

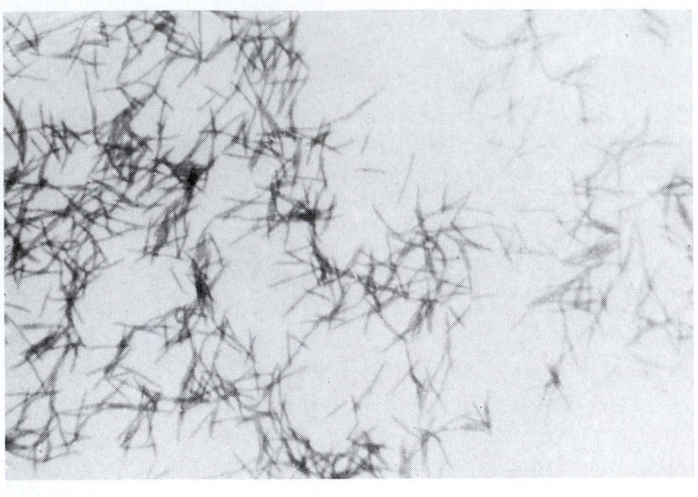

A

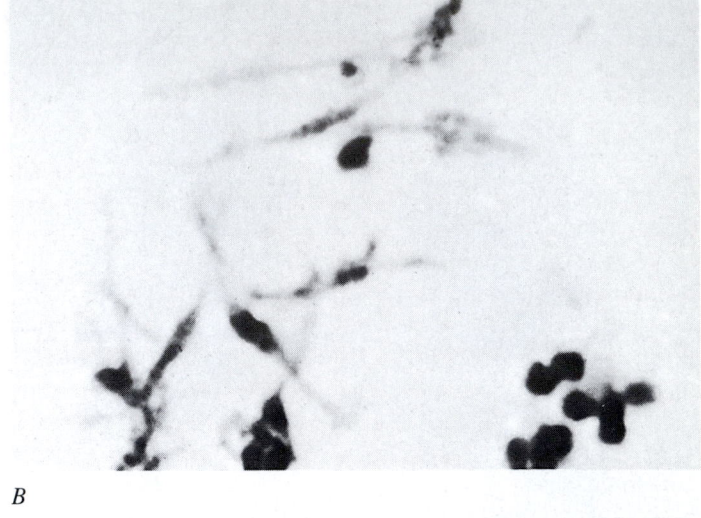

B

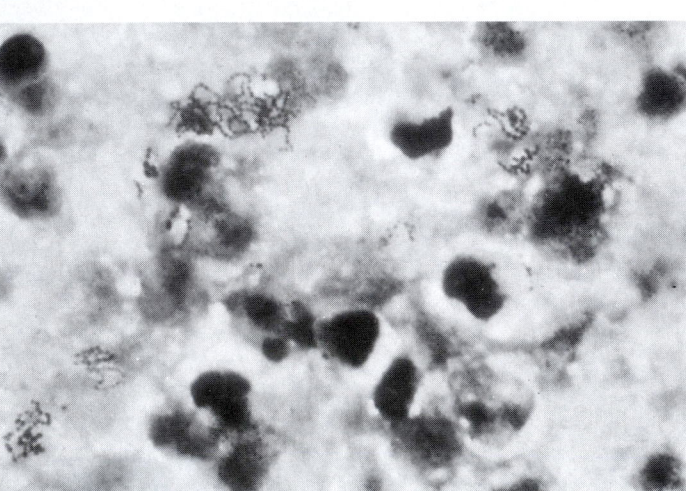

C

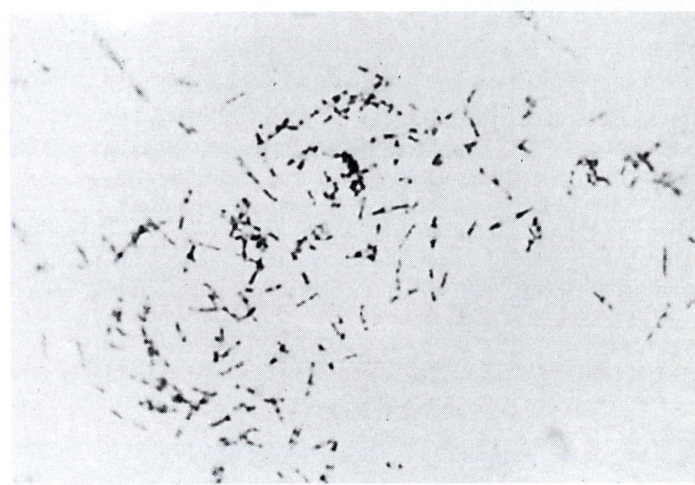

D

FIGURE 130-4   Bacteriology of empyema and lung abscess. *A. Fusobacterium nucleatum,* microscopic morphology. Organism is thin and delicate gram-negative bacillus with tapered ends (sometimes filamentous). *B.* Pleomorphic gram-negative bacillus with filaments containing swollen portions and with large round bodies. This appearance is seen with *F. necrophorum, F. mortiferum,* and *F. varium. C.* Pus showing microaerophilic streptococcus. *D.* Microscopic morphology of *Bacteroides fragilis.* Organism is an irregularly stained, gram-negative rod. Bipolar staining may be seen.

Legionella species, *Burkholdaria pseudomallei* and *B. mallei* (glanders), and tuberculosis. Certain fungal infections may cause cavitation in diabetic and immunocompromised hosts (e.g., the *Mucoraceae, Aspergillus* species).[31] *Entamoeba histolytica* is an important, but uncommon, cause of lung abscess, almost always in the basilar portion of the right lower lobe.

CLINICAL MANIFESTATIONS AND DIAGNOSIS

The pathogenesis and presentation of both pleural empyema and lung abscesses are often indistinguishable. Shared presentations of empyema and lung abscess include the indolent development of symptoms, most often fever, sweats, cough, dyspnea, weight loss, and pleurisy; an association with conditions predisposing to aspirational events (altered consciousness, dysphagia, and gingivitis); and foul odors of sputum or breath associated with anaerobic bacteriology. Lung abscesses and empyemas often coexist. Both are generally associated with primary pneumonias.

Clinical Presentation of Empyema

The clinical presentation of empyema is determined by the underlying cause of infection. Empyema associated with aspiration pneumonia may develop over 1 to 3 weeks, usually with associated symptoms of pneumonia. The patient may have high fever and leukocytosis. Physical examination reveals dullness to percussion and decreased breath sounds on auscultation. These changes may be quite localized in the setting of loculated fluid. The empyema fluid is generally purulent by the time of detection, but pleural infection may be noted only after treatment for pneumonitis has failed to resolve fever or pleurisy. Empyema associated with thoracic surgery may be radiologically "hidden" in areas of the chest undrained by chest tubes or behind relatively benign pleural effusions. The patient may appear minimally toxic or severely ill, depending on the extent of the infection and the organisms present. The presentation will be modified by "routine" prophylactic antibiotic use, sedation, intubation, and an-

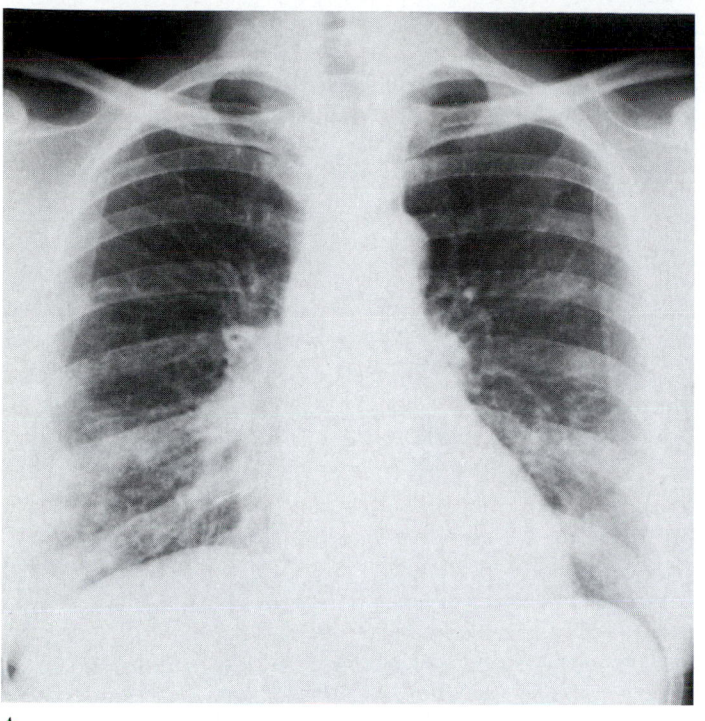

A

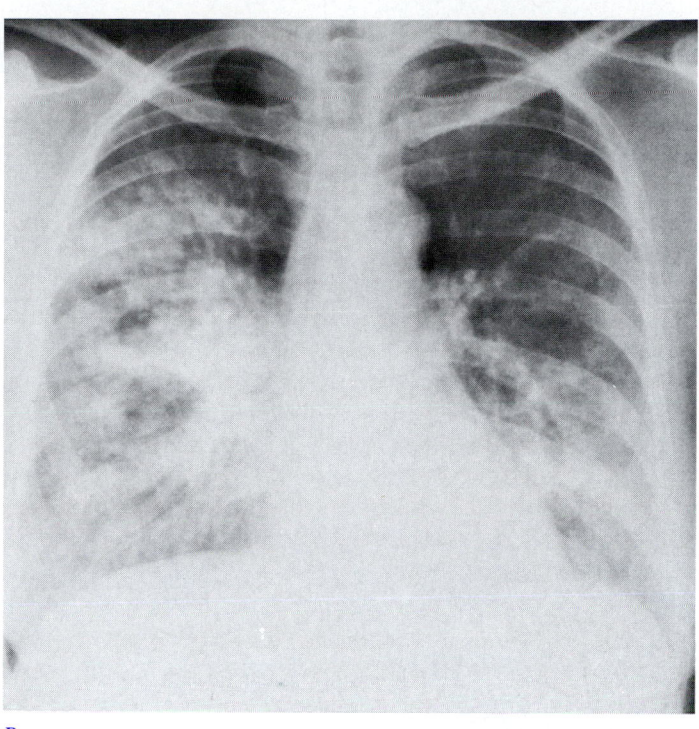

B

FIGURE 130-5 Fulminating anaerobic pneumonia in a 44-year-old woman with onset of pneumonia 6 days before admission. *A.* Day of admission. Patchy consolidation in right lower lung field and behind the cardiac silhouette. *B.* One day after admission: Extensive patchy alveolar infiltrates bilaterally with areas of rarefaction on right suggestive of cavitation. The patient died 2 days later.

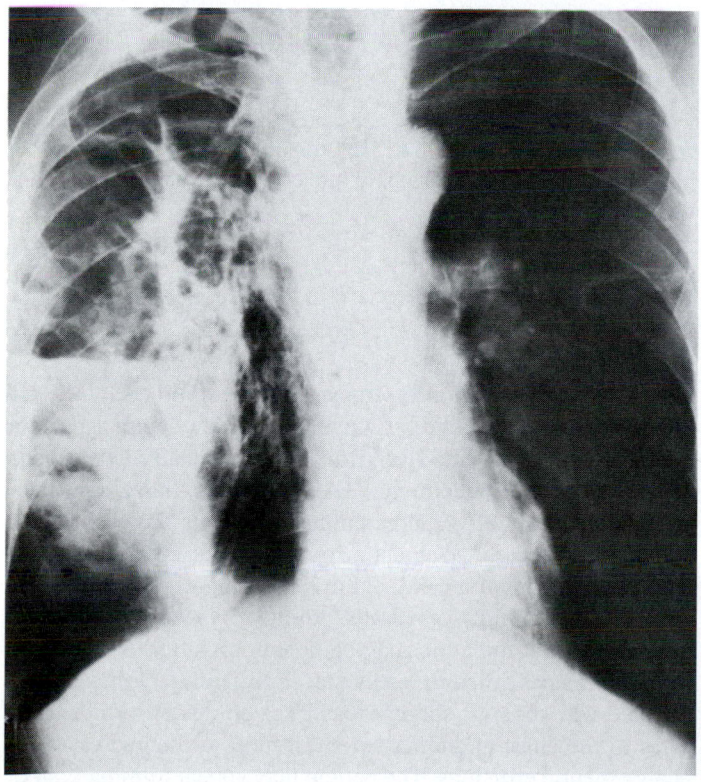

A

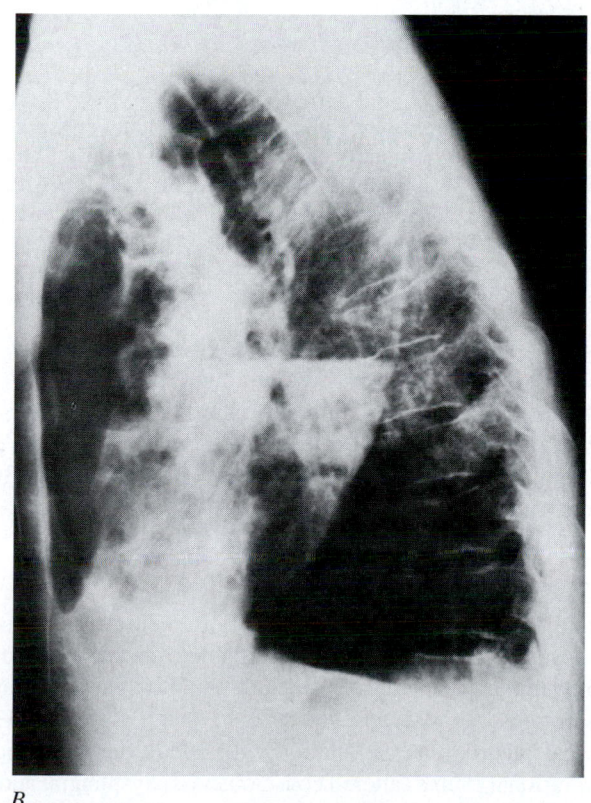

B

FIGURE 130-6 "Gangrene" of the lung after aspiration, anteroposterior *(A)* and lateral *(B)* views. Extensive cavitation following necrotizing pneumonia in a 65-year-old man.

tipyretics. Acute empyema may be seen in staphylococcal and streptococcal infections and following rupture of hepatic abscesses, especially those due to *E. histolytica*.

In general, chest radiographs will reveal fluid, most often in the costophrenic angles; free-flowing effusions will layer on lateral decubitus radiographs. Loculations and pleural disease are often best defined by computerized tomography of the chest, which should include the neck and diaphragms to rule out extrathoracic sites of infection. Spinal disease is better detected with magnetic resonance imaging (MRI). Before invasive diagnostic procedures, a careful history and physical examination may suggest a reason for the accumulation of pleural fluid. Noninfectious causes include bland pulmonary embolus, malignant effusion, benign postsurgical changes, pericardiotomy syndrome, collagen-vascular diseases (systemic lupus, rheumatoid arthritis), congestive heart disease, sympathetic effusion related to subdiaphragmatic disease (pancreatitis), leakage of ascites or peritoneal dialysis fluids, and hemorrhage (from venous access catheters or aortic tears). Infectious causes include extension of all classes of pulmonary infections from the lungs (parapneumonic), esophageal rupture, parapharyngeal space drainage, drainage or sympathetic effusion due to hepatic or subdiaphragmatic abscesses, septic metastasis, and direct infection via thoracic defects or chest tubes used for pleural drainage. Pyopneumothorax, in the absence of bronchopleural fistula, prior surgery, or prior thoracentesis, suggests the possibility of gas formation by bacteria implicated in the infection. Although nonspecific, pyopneumothorax suggests a component of anaerobic infection.

Diagnosis of Empyema

The diagnosis of empyema is based solely on the characteristics of thoracic fluid. The urgency to diagnosis is due to the development of pleural scar and of loculated effusions in the presence of undrained pus. Thus, diagnostic thoracentesis should be attempted unless the nature of the pleural fluid is clear or the clinical risk to the patient is too great. Pleural fluid should be prepared for Gram's stain and cultures (routine, anaerobic, mycobacterial, and fungal), parasitologic examination when appropriate, fluid cell count and differential, cytology, pH, lactic dehydrogenase, and glucose measurements. Purulent fluid requires drainage. Empyema (defined above) is diagnosed on the basis of the neutrophilic predominance in fluids with more than 25,000 white blood cells per milliliter. Parapneumonic effusions will generally have lower white blood counts, negative Gram's stains and cultures, a pH over 7.3, and glucose over 50 percent of serum glucose levels. Parapneumonic fluids may become infected over time.[28]

Clinical Presentation of Lung Abscess

The clinical presentation of lung abscess may be coincident with the initial presentation of a pneumonia or other underlying condition, or may occur later in the clinical course. Suspicion may be heightened by the presence of conditions predisposing to aspiration or to anaerobic pneumonia: alcoholism or other causes of altered consciousness, anaesthesia, dysphagia or pharyngeal dysfunction, gingivitis or pyorrhea, blunt or penetrating chest trauma or lung surgery, obstruction due to neoplasm, bronchiec-

tasis, or pulmonary embolism. "Bad breath" or putrid sputum may be noted. However, the absence of a foul odor does not exclude the possibility of anaerobic infection, since certain anaerobes do not generate the end products of metabolism responsible for this type of odor, and communication may be lacking between the lesion and the tracheobronchial tree. A change in sputum production, either increased or decreased, may be noted in patients with chronic bronchitis or bronchiectasis.

The patient with *primary lung abscess* will gradually develop fever, cough, pleurisy, chest heaviness, shoulder pain, and malaise. Pneumonia may be present or suspected from history for a period of 1 to 3 weeks before the recognition of the lung abscess. By contrast, *secondary lung abscesses*—due, for example, to septic pulmonary emboli with infarction—can evolve over 48 to 72 h (Fig. 130-7). Clinically, the distinction between primary and secondary abscesses may be inapparent at the time of presentation, but is important in the proper management of the patient. Thus, the patient with staphylococcal or streptococcal endocarditis may present with pneumonia, lung abscess, and empyema. The main clue to the presence of underlying endocarditis may be the development of new lung abscesses during the course of therapy. The patient with lung abscesses complicating subdiaphragmatic infection (amebic abscess of the liver or pancreatic phlegmon) may have abdominal signs in addition to acute pulmonary disease. Seizures due to brain abscesses are occasionally the presenting clinical manifestation of bacteremia due to lung abscesses.

Radiographic Appearance of Lung Abscess

The classic radiographic appearance of a lung abscess is an irregularly shaped cavity with an air-fluid level inside. Because the presentation is often indolent, numerous chest radiographs may be needed to follow the evolution of pneumonia into *necrotizing pneumonia* and then into a pulmonary cavity (Figs. 130-5 and 130-6). Anaerobic infection is suggested by rapid pulmonary cavitation within a dense segmental consolidation; there may be rapidly enlarging nodular lesions, with or without cavitation. Although anaerobic pulmonary infections may be acute and fulminating, almost two-thirds of them have a subacute or chronic presentation. Natural progression of virulent infection, delays in appropriate therapy, or tissue infarction may allow the underlying infection to progress into *pulmonary gangrene* (Fig. 130-4). Seeding of infection or rupture of a lung abscess into the pleural space may cause empyema (Fig. 130-7). Up to one-third of lung abscesses may be accompanied by empyema. Solitary cavities are generally observed with primary lung infections, whereas many smaller collections may be found in metastatic infection (see Chapter 133). Chest tomography will define the size and location of abscesses, and may distinguish between related processes (empyema, infarction) better than conventional radiographs.[18,34,42] The common organisms and conditions associated with lung abscesses are listed in Table 130-3.

Evaluation of the Patient with Lung Abscess

The microbiology of lung abscesses was generally limited to anaerobic bacteria in the preantibiotic and pre–thoracic surgery eras. Recently, the spectrum of organisms causing lung abscesses

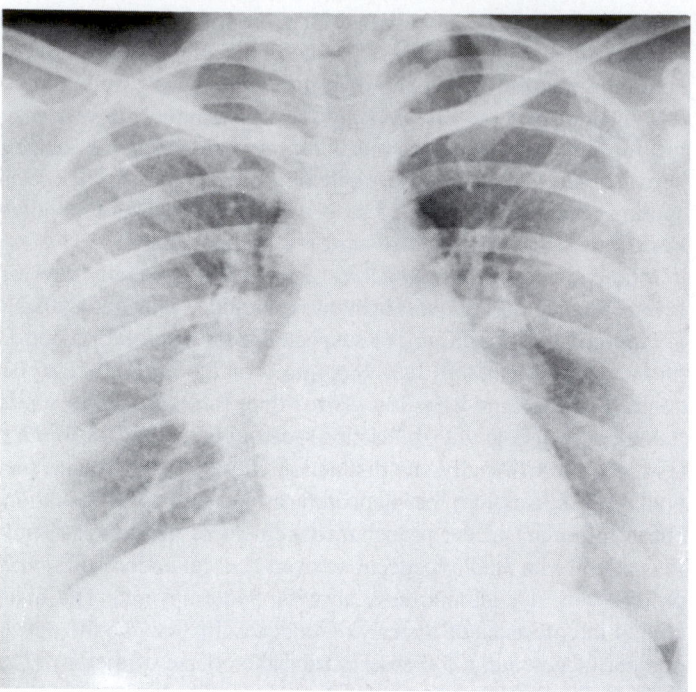

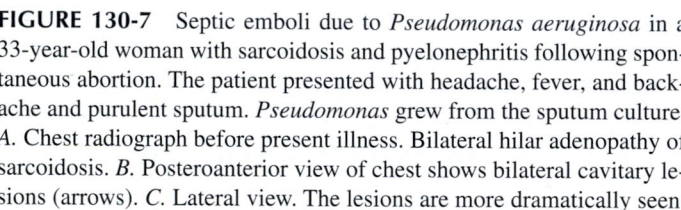

A

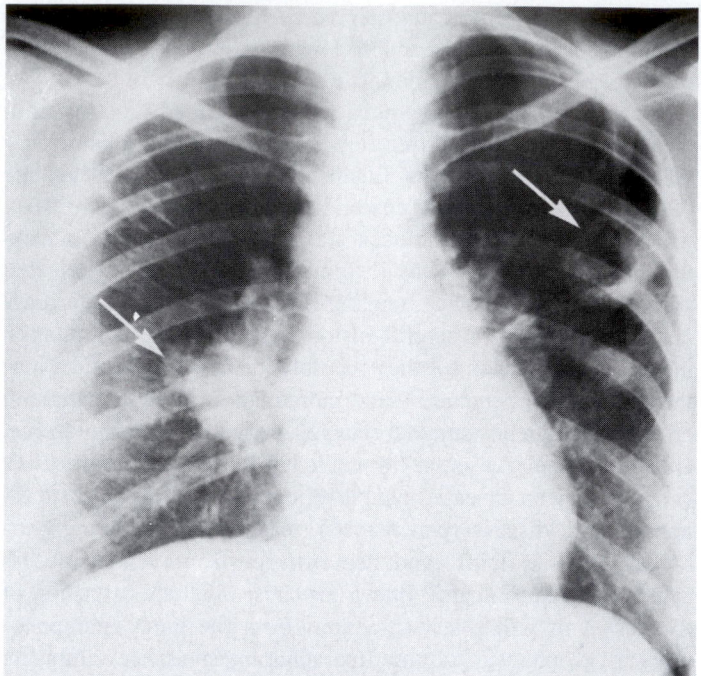

B

FIGURE 130-7 Septic emboli due to *Pseudomonas aeruginosa* in a 33-year-old woman with sarcoidosis and pyelonephritis following spontaneous abortion. The patient presented with headache, fever, and backache and purulent sputum. *Pseudomonas* grew from the sputum culture. *A*. Chest radiograph before present illness. Bilateral hilar adenopathy of sarcoidosis. *B*. Posteroanterior view of chest shows bilateral cavitary lesions (arrows). *C*. Lateral view. The lesions are more dramatically seen.

has widened as patients present with complex medical and surgical conditions, antibiotic resistance has emerged, and the size of the population of immunocompromised persons has increased. Thus, clinical specimens are increasingly needed to guide therapy. Microbiologic specimens from patients with lung abscesses should be obtained, if possible, without contamination by oral flora, especially after nosocomial colonization. Thus, invasive procedures are preferred to routine sputum samples. In particular, the diagnosis of anaerobic infection is complicated by the prevalence of large numbers of anaerobes as normal flora in the mouth and upper respiratory tract (Fig. 130-8). However, there may also be significant colonization with nosocomially acquired pathogens in hospitalized patients.

Blood cultures and sputum cultures should be obtained as adjunctive guides to therapy. When empyema or bacteremia complicates lung abscess, adequate specimens for microbiologic evaluation may be obtained from the blood or pleura. However, to obtain adequate specimens from the abscess itself, bronchoalveolar lavage, use of the Wimberly-Bartlett protected double-lumen catheter, percutaneous transtracheal aspiration (in experienced hands), or percutaneous transthoracic aspiration under radiographic guidance is recommended.[6,24,49] The specific procedure selected will depend on the location of the infection and the expertise of the institution. Specimens collected through a fiberoptic bronchoscope, using bronchoalveolar lavage or a plugged double-lumen sampling catheter with a protected sampling brush, are preferred; these require the use of quantitative cultures. Growth at a dilution of 10^{-3} from a protected brush represents approximately 10^5 to 10^6 or-

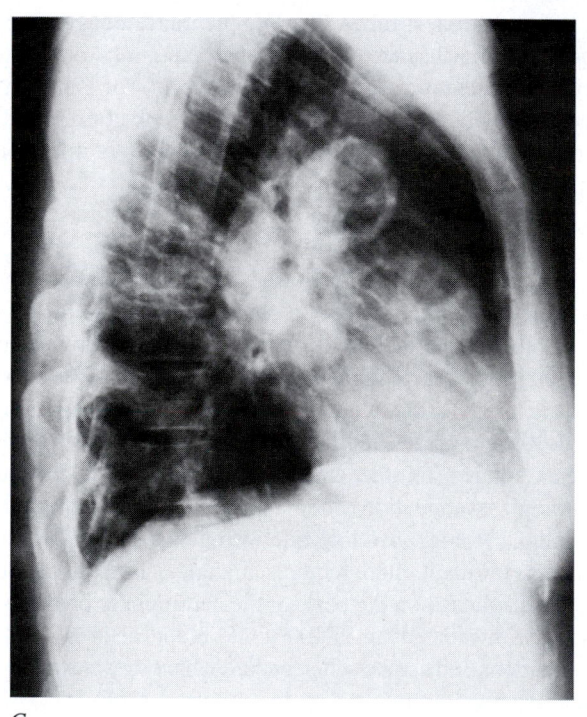

C

ganisms per milliliter in the lower respiratory tract. Recovery of nonbacterial and anaerobic bacteria from these specimens has not been well standardized. Specimens obtained from blind, deep suctioning via an endothracheal tube may also be useful if cultured quantitatively and examined microscopically.

It is essential that material obtained for culture be placed under anaerobic conditions promptly before transport to the laboratory. A sealed syringe provides the best container, with delivery of the specimen to the laboratory within 20 to 30 min for immediate plating. It is imperative that air bubbles be eliminated from the syringe and needle. Special anaerobic transport tubes

TABLE 130-3

Organisms and Conditions Associated with the Radiographic Appearance of Lung Abscess

Infectious	Noninfectious and Predisposing Conditions
Bacteria	Anatomic
Anaerobes; *Staphylococcus aureus*, Enterobacteriaceae, *Pseudomonas*	Fluid-filled cysts, bland infarction
aeruginosa, streptococci, *Legionella* spp, *Nocardia*	Bronchiectasis
asteroides, *Burkholdaria pseudomallei*	Vasculitis
Mycobacteria (often multifocal)	Goodpasture's syndrome, Wegener's
M. tuberculosis, *M. avium* complex,	granulomatosis, periarteritis
M. kansasii, other mycobacteria	Obstruction (neoplasm, foreign body)
Fungi	Pulmonary sequestration
Aspergillus spp, Mucoraceae, *Histoplasma capsulatum*,	Pulmonary contusion
Pneumocystis carinii, *Coccidioides immitis*, *Blastocystis*	Carcinoma
hominis	
Parasites	
Entamoeba histolytica, *Paragonimus westermani*,	
Strongyloides stercoralis (post-obstructive)	
Empyema (with air-fluid level)	
Septic embolism (endocarditis)	

are also available for brush or liquid specimens. It is important to obtain additional pulmonary specimens for culture and antibiotic susceptibility measurements from patients failing to respond to initial therapy (Fig. 130-9). Such data may demonstrate the presence of unrecognized or antibiotic-resistant organisms.

TREATMENT OF EMPYEMA AND LUNG ABSCESS

Management of Empyema

The management of empyema includes antimicrobial treatment, identification and treatment of any underlying or primary processes, and drainage of the infected fluid. The approach to a specific patient will be based on the clinical status of the patient as well as the microbiology of the infection. The initial choice of *antimicrobial agents* should be guided by the Gram's stain and the likely bacteriology of the infection, and then adjusted as culture data become available. The history and a review of old data may be useful in the selection of specific antibiotics. For example, patients with empyema following thoracic surgery and other hospitalized patients may have useful culture data available from chest tube drainage samples or sputum cultures to assist in the selection of antibiotics. The Gram's stain may indicate the predominant organism type. Mixed aerobic and anaerobic organisms may be the first suggestion of esophageal tear or parapharyngeal infection. Fastidious organisms (*S. pneumoniae*, anaerobes) may be seen on Gram's stain but not isolated in culture. Antibiotic susceptibility data should be used to guide therapy, especially in nosocomially acquired infection. Local administration of antibiotics (e.g., inhaled) is unnecessary and may be irritating; intrapleural injection of antibiotics should be reserved for pleural ablation (pleuradesis), as may be achieved with erythromycin.

Drainage of empyema fluid is recommended but controversial. Ten to 20 percent of empyemas will require external drainage or surgical intervention. Noninfected parapneumonic pleural fluids will resolve with appropriate treatment of the underlying infections. Drainage is *required* if infection or frank pus is present. In the presence of pleural fluid and unexplained fever, leukocytosis, or bacteremia, or in the postoperative patient, thoracentesis should be performed routinely. Diagnostic thoracentesis may be performed with a needle adequate for removal of all but the most viscous material. Highly viscous or purulent fluids and fluids with acid pH will require the insertion of a chest tube via thoracostomy or the thoracoscopic drainage of the fluid.[8,23,25,28,33,36,42]

In the *early* or *exudative* phase of parapneumonic effusion, the fluid will be thin and serous or serosanguineous. This may

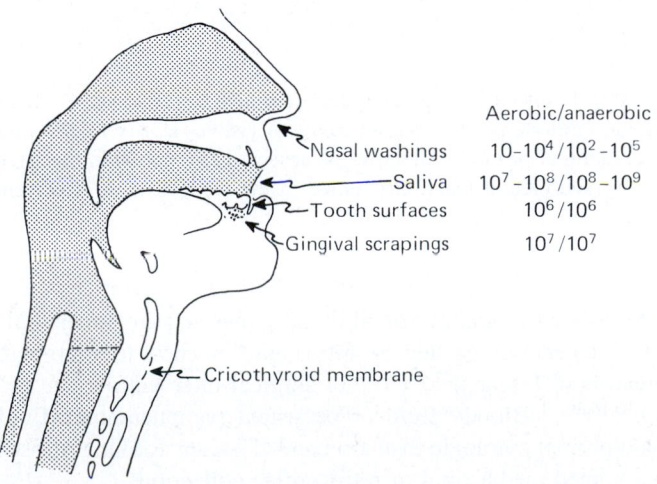

	Aerobic/anaerobic
Nasal washings	$10{-}10^4/10^2{-}10^5$
Saliva	$10^7{-}10^8/10^8{-}10^9$
Tooth surfaces	$10^6/10^6$
Gingival scrapings	$10^7/10^7$

Cricothyroid membrane

FIGURE 130-8 Sagittal section illustrating presence of large numbers of organisms, including anaerobes, as indigenous flora in upper respiratory tract. (Values given as number of aerobic/anaerobic organisms per milliliter.) *(Courtesy of P.D. Hoeprich.)*

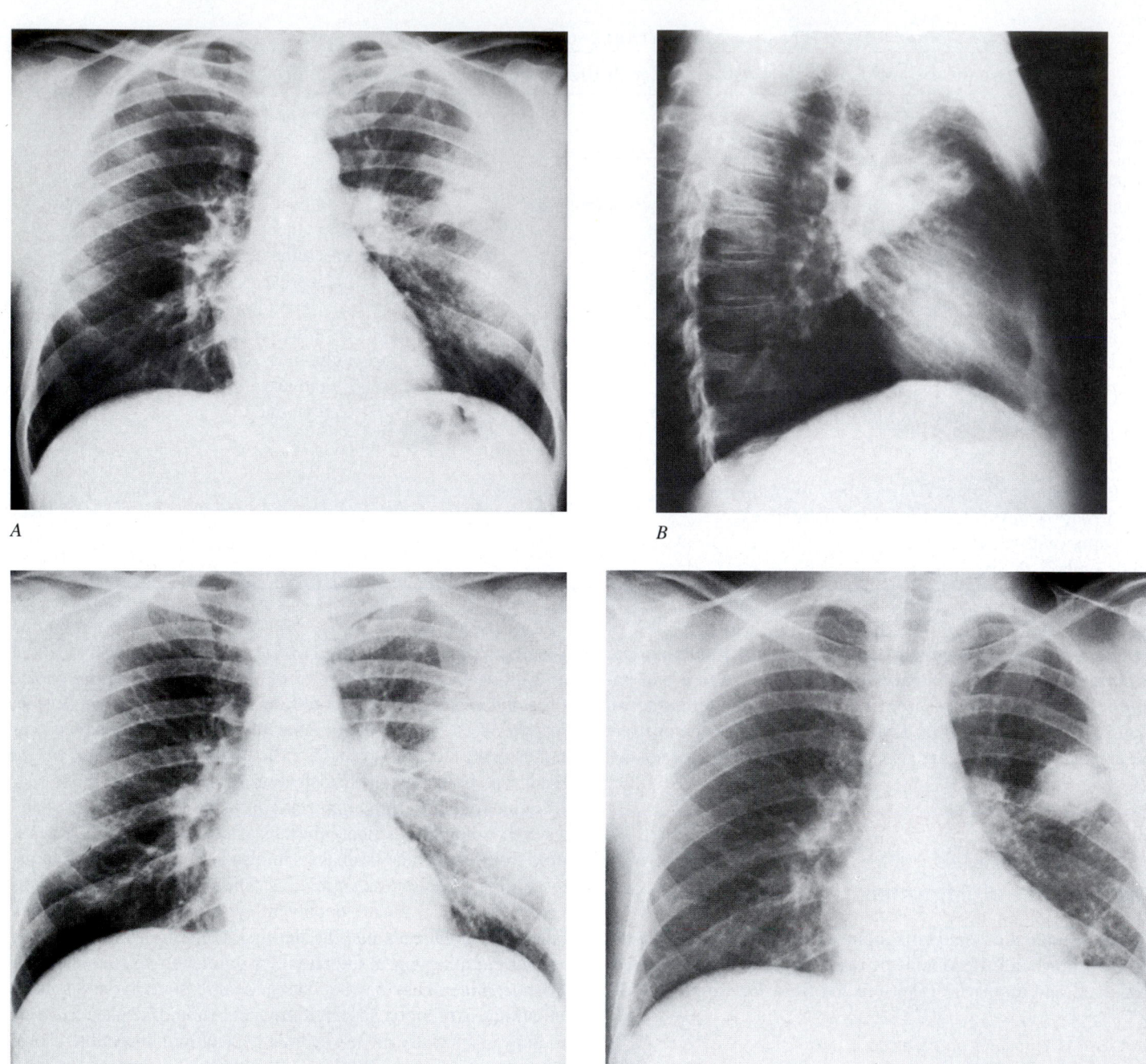

FIGURE 130-9 Failure of penicillin therapy for anaerobic lung abscess in a 29-year-old alcoholic man. *A*. Admission chest radiograph reveals a radiolucent area within a zone of consolidation in the left upper lung field. *B*. Lateral view demonstrates multiple cavities. The patient was treated for 5 days with penicillin (6 million units per day intravenously), followed by the same dosage orally for 10 days. *C*. Radiographic infiltrate persists but no cavity is visible. *D*. Six weeks after the cessation of penicillin therapy, the abscess has recurred in the same area. Marked pleural reaction is noted in the vicinity of the recurrent disease.

resolve during appropriate antibiotic therapy either without drainage or with multiple needle aspirations. If the pH is over 7.3, this method may be preferred. If the pH is less than 7.0, however, complete drainage should be performed, often requiring closed chest tube insertion.[32] If the pH is between 7.0 and 7.3, failure to demonstrate improvement of infection or inflammation on multiple thoracenteses over 3 to 4 days should lead to consideration of formal drainage, especially if the primary process is adequately treated. Loculation of pleural fluid or fail-

ure to respond to antimicrobial therapy may require either multiple thoracenteses guided by ultrasound or chest tomographic evaluation (CT scans)[21,24,35,46] or surgical intervention (see below).[10,16,20,49] Bloody fluid or persistent parapneumonic fluid should prompt cytologic evalation and CT-scans for lung masses or undrained mediastinal or retrocardiac collections.

Empyema diagnosed later in the course, persistently infected pleural fluid, viscous fluid, or fluids with acid pH may require large bore tube drainage.[32,39,47] This heavily proteinaceous fluid is characteristic of the *fibropurulent phase* of the evolving empyema. Indications for closed chest tube placement include bronchopleural fistula with empyema, loculated fluid unresponsive to thoracentesis and antibiotics, the presence of blood clots, and rapidly accumulating empyema not otherwise manageable. Under suction, and with removal of the gellike material, pus, and clots, the lung expands and obliterates the empyema space. Failure to expand the underlying lung, persistence of drainage beyond 7 days, inability to achieve drainage assessed radiologically, fever without change in 2 to 3 days, or pus formation with persistent infection (as opposed to colonization of the chest tubes) necessitates a search for undrained foci of infection, failure to close a bronchopleural fistula or esophageal tear, undetected rupture of a lung abscess, or antibiotic failure.[11,49] As the infection enters the *chronic phase,* open drainage with rib resection or pleurocutaneous fistula formation may be needed with or without decortication to achieve lung expansion and healing. Open drainage is obtained by making the pleura adherent to the chest wall during the insertion of chest tubes directly into the empyema cavities. Drainage achieved too late in the course of infection may result in the development of pleural scar and fibrous peel with restrictive pulmonary physiology. Decortication may be needed to achieve sterilization of the pleural space and to restore lung expansion. Thoracoscopic drainage of empyema has been used with excellent results at a number of institutions, particularly in children.[13,22,27,39,44] Often, thoracoscopic drainage of empyema is used as a temporizing maneuver (e.g., following acute rupture of a lung abscess into the pleural space). Patients achieving rapid reexpansion of the lungs may avoid open drainage procedures while achieving limited decortication and disruption of loculations. Alternatively, once a patient is stabilized and can better tolerate open drainage, or has demonstrated an inability to resolve the empyema without further drainage, surgical intervention may be needed. Early, aggressive treatment of empyema may reduce the duration of hospitalization and the risk of nosocomial superinfection.

Treatment of Lung Abscess

The treatment of lung abscess must be guided by the microbiology and knowledge of any underlying or associated conditions that may predispose to the development of severe pulmonary infection. A small abscess in an otherwise healthy person may respond to conservative management with antimicrobial therapy, chest physical therapy, and postural drainage. A rapidly expanding pulmonary abscess in an immunocompromised host (e.g., due to one of the *Mucoraceae*) requires urgent lung resection in addition to antimicrobials. Intermediate to these approaches would be the use of bronchoscopic or radiographically guided catheter drainage of any fluid and necrotic debris. In the absence of antibiotics, the mortality of lung abscess is approximately 33 percent.[1] However, up to half of patients surviving a lung abscess acutely in the preantibiotic era had significant pulmonary complications, including recurrent infections and abscesses, pleural empyema and adhesions, chronic bronchitis, and bronchiectasis. The introduction of penicillin, orally or parenterally administered, resulted in resolution or collapse of the abscess in up to 90 percent of patients (although long courses of treatment were often needed).[45,50] These patients could, therefore, avoid surgical resection. A subgroup of patients responded to tetracycline after incomplete resolution on penicillin.

At present, an increasing number of anaerobes (up to 35 percent of a variety of species of anaerobic gram-negative rods) are producing β-lactamases and demonstrate in vitro and clinical resistance to penicillin G (Fig. 130-9). These include members of *Prevotella* and *Bacteroides* species, and of the fusobacteria. However, some patients infected with such strains will respond clinically to treatment with penicillin G. Thus, while penicillin G may be useful, clindamycin has given superior clinical results based on the number of patients responding, the speed of resolution of fever, radiographic findings, and sputum infection, and in terms of the number of relapses after treatment.[5,17,37,48,49] When penicillin is used, it should be used in high dosage (12 to 18 million units per day intravenously in average-size adults with normal renal function) and in *combination* with metronidazole (2 g per day in four divided doses) to cover β-lactamase–producing organisms. Metronidazole alone is often ineffective, in part because of resistance of such organisms as aerobic and anaerobic streptococci. In certain locales, there is significant resistance of the *B. fragilis* group to clindamycin and cefoxitin.

Other alternatives include imipenem and combinations of β-lactam drugs with β-lactamase inhibitors (e.g., ticarcillin-clavulanate). For patients who have aspirated or developed a lung abscess in the hospital setting, therapy should also include antibiotics appropriate for the aerobic and facultative bacteria, either those known to be implicated in the initial pneumonia or the major nosocomial pathogens of the institution—including *S. aureus,* Enterobacteriaceae, and *Pseudomonas*—that may be encountered with the anaerobes. Failure to recover a likely pathogen on routine aerobic culture of appropriate material raises the probability of anaerobic involvement.

The appropriate duration of therapy is dependent on the clinical and radiographic response of the patient. Patients should be treated at least until fever, putrid sputum, and abscess fluid have resolved, and the abscess cavity is resolved or unchanged over 2 to 3 weeks. A *minimum* of 2 to 3 weeks of antibiotics is recomended. Longer courses are often necessary. Relapse is common and may involve organisms resistant to initial antibiotic agents (Fig. 130-9).

The role of drainage or surgery is based on serial clinical assessments of the patient. Bronchoscopic drainage may be most useful in the relief of abscesses without air-fluid levels, which indicate the possibility of persistent connection with the bronchi. However, experience dictates *caution* with the bronchoscopic drainage of closed cavities; spillage of cavity contents into other lung segments may produce catastrophic pulmonary dysfunction. Further, there are few data to suggest that bronchoscopic drainage offers a significant advantage in terms of rapidity of recovery in the immunologically normal host. In patients with coexistent empyema and lung abscess, it is often useful to address drainage of the empyema first, stabilizing the patient, and then considering further procedures for the lung abscess. In the critically ill patient, or those with bronchial obstruction related to the abscess cavity, bronchoscopic drainage should be considered.

Bronchoscopy or chest CT have major roles in the evaluation of the patient failing therapy. Persistence of bacteremia or high-grade fevers after 72 h, or the absence of change in sputum production or character or in the radiographic images over 7 to 10 days, suggests unappreciated anatomical or microbiologic problems. Obstruction or resistant organisms (including fungi, parasites, or mycobacteria) may be present.[19,31] Multiple loculations may be present or empyema, including drainage of the abscess into the pleural space, may develop. New sites of infection, including extrathoracic, may have developed in the bacteremic patient. Progression of pulmonary infiltrates may occur after the initiation of appropriate antibiotic therapy, reflecting the relatively poor activity of many antibiotics at the low pH levels of poorly ventilated and underperfused, infected lung tissues, as well as the delayed radiographic response to treatment.

Surgical resection of necrotic segments of lung is helpful if the response to antibiotics is poor, for large abscesses, or if ventilation-perfusion scans suggest little residual lung function in a limited necrotic region. Infarcted lung or rapidly progressive infection may force surgical resection of the affected tissue. Surgery is also indicated if airway obstruction limits drainage. Such presentations are seen in the presence of tumor or a foreign body. In patients thought to be poor surgical risks, percutaneous drainage via catheters may be a useful temporizing measure. However, leakage of the abscess contents into the pleural space in such patients may be disastrous and must be avoided.

Mortality in patients with lung abscesses reflects the quality of the host's inflammatory response and overall condition. Patients with large abscesses (over 5 to 6 cm), progressive pulmonary necrosis, obstructing lesions, aerobic bacteria, immune compromise, old age, or systemic debility, and those with major delays in seeking medical attention, have a significantly increased mortality.

REFERENCES

1. Abernathy RS: Antibiotic therapy of lung abscesses: Effectiveness of penicillin. *Dis Chest* 53:592–598, 1968.
2. Bartlett JG: Bacterial infections of the pleural space. *Semin Respir Infect* 3:309–319, 1988.
3. Bartlett JG: Anaerobic bacterial infections of the lung and pleural space. *Clin Infect Dis* 16(Suppl 4):S248–S255, 1993.
4. Bartlett JG, Finegold SM: Anaerobic infections of the lung and pleural space. *Am Rev Respir Dis* 110:56–77, 1974.
5. Bartlett JG, Gorbach SL, Tally FP, Finegold SM: Bacteriology and treatment of primary lung abscess. *Am Rev Respir Dis* 109:510–518, 1974.
6. Bartlett JG, Rosenblatt JE, Finegold SM: Percutaneous transtracheal aspiration in the diagnosis of anaerobic pulmonary infection. *Ann Intern Med* 79:535–540, 1973.
7. Benfield GF: Recent trends in empyema thoracis. *Br J Dis Chest* 75:358–366, 1981.
8. Cicero R, del Vecchyo C, Porter JK, Carreño J: Open window thoracostomy and plastic surgery with muscle flaps in the treatment of chronic empyema. *Chest* 89:374–377, 1986.
9. Civen R, Jousimies-Somer H, Marina M, et al: A retrospective review of cases of anaerobic empyema and update of bacteriology. *Clin Infect Dis* 20(Suppl 2):S224–S229, 1995.
10. Cohn LH, Blaisdell EW: Surgical treatment of nontuberculous empyema. *Arch Surg* 100:376–381, 1970.
11. Deschamps C, Allen MS, Trastek VF, Pairolero PC: Empyema following surgical resection. *Chest Surg Clin North Am* 4:583–592, 1994.
12. Ehler AA: Non-tuberculous thoracic empyema: Collective review of literature from 1934–1939. *Int Abstr Surg* 72:17–27, 1941.
13. Ferguson M: Thoracoscopy for empyema, bronchopleural fistula, and chylothorax. *Ann Thorac Surg* 56:644–645, 1993.
14. Finegold SM: *Anaerobic Bacteria in Human Disease.* New York, Academic, 1977.
15. Finland M: The significance of pneumococcal types in disease including types IV to XXXII (Cooper). *Ann Intern Med* 15:1531–1536, 1939.
16. Foglia RP, Randolph J: Current indications for decortication in the treatment of empyema in children. *J Pediatr Surg* 22:28–33, 1987.
17. Gudiol F, Manresa F, Pallares R, et al: Clindamycin vs penicillin for anaerobic lung infections: High rate of penicillin failures associated with penicillin-resistant *Bacteroides melaninogenicus. Arch Intern Med* 150:2525–2529, 1990.
18. Hochberg L, Kramer B: Acute empyema of the chest in children: A review of 300 cases. *Am J Dis Child* 57:310–319, 1939.
19. Hooker TP, Hammond M, Corral K: Empyema necessitatis: Review of the manifestations of thoracic actinomycosis. *Cleve Clin J Med* 59:542–548, 1992.
20. Hoover EL, Hsu HK, Ross MJ, et al: Reappraisal of empyema thoracis: Surgical intervention when the duration of illness is unknown. *Chest* 90:511–515, 1986.
21. Hunnam GR, Flower CD: Radiologically-guided percutaneous catheter drainage of empyemas. *Clin Radiol* 39:121–126, 1988.
22. Hutter J, Harari D, Braimbridge M: The management of empyema thoracis by thoracoscopy and irrigation. *Ann Thorac Surg* 39:517–520, 1985.
23. Iioka S, Sawamura K, Mori T, et al: Surgical treatment of chronic empyema: A new one-stage operation. *J Thorac Cardiovasc Surg* 90:179–185, 1985.
24. Klein JS, Schultz S, Heffner JE: Interventional radiology of the chest: Image-guided percutaneous drainage of pleural effusions, lung abscess, and pneumothorax. *AJR Am J Roentgenol* 164:581–588, 1995.
25. Le Roux BT, Mohlala ML, Odell JA, Whitton ID: Suppurative diseases of the lung and pleural space: Empyema thoracis and lung abscess. *Curr Probl Surg* 23:93–159, 1986.
26. LeBlanc KA, Tucker WY: Empyema of the thorax. *Surg Gynecol Obstet* 158:66–70, 1984.
27. Lewis R, Caccavale R: One hundred consecutive patients undergoing video-assisted thoracic operations. *Ann Thorac Surg* 54:403–409, 1992.
28. Light R: Parapneumonic effusions and empyema. *Clin Chest Med* 6:55–61, 1985.
29. Mayo P: Early thoracotomy and decortication for nontuberculous empyema in adults with and without underlying disease: A twenty-five year review. *Am Surg* 51:230–236, 1985.
30. McLaughlin FJ, Goldman DA, Rosenbaum DM, et al: Empyema in children: Clinical course and long-term follow-up. *Pediatrics* 73:587–593, 1984.
31. Mesnard R, Lamy T, Dauriac C, Le Prise PY: Lung abscess due to *Pseudallescheria boydii* in the course of acute leukaemia: Report of a case and review of the literature. *Acta Haematol* 87:78–82, 1992.
32. Moore DWO: Management of acute empyema. *Chest* 102:1316–1317, 1992.
33. Morgan JF: Surgical management of pleural space infections. *Semin Respir Infect* 3:383–394, 1988.
34. Nowak SJG: Empyema thoracis: An analytical study of 500 cases with general remarks. *Med Clin North Am* 23:1355–1369, 1939.
35. O'Moore PV, Mueller PR, Simeone JF, et al: Sonographic guidance in diagnostic and therapeutic interventions in the pleural space. *AJR Am J Roentgenol* 149:1–8, 1987.

36. Orringer MB: Thoracic empyema: Back to basics. *Chest* 93:901–902, 1988.
37. Panwalker AP: Failure of penicillin in anaerobic necrotizing pneumonia. *Chest* 82:500–501, 1982.
38. Poe RH, Marcus HR, Emerson GL: Lung abscess due to *Pseudomonas cepacia. Am Rev Respir Dis* 115:861–865, 1977.
39. Ridley PD, Braimbridge MV: Thoracoscopic debridement and pleural irrigation in the management of empyema thoracis. *Ann Thorac Surg* 51:461–464, 1991.
40. Savdie E, Pigott P, Jennis F: Lung abscess due to *Corynebacterium equi* in a renal transplant recipient. *Med J Aust* 1:817–819, 1977.
41. Schweppe HI, Knowles JH, Kane L: Lung abscess: An analysis of the Massachusetts General Hospital cases from 1943 through 1956. *New Engl J Med* 265:1039–1043, 1961.
42. Shank PJ: Empyema of the lung: Review of literature and analysis of 169 cases. *Am J Surg* 66:224–244, 1944.
43. Shoemaker EH, Yow EM, Byrd WC: Antibiotic therapy of primary pulmonary abscesses. *Arch Intern Med* 96:683–692, 1955.
44. Silen M, Weber T: Thoracoscopic debridement of loculated empyema thoracis in children. *Ann Thorac Surg* 59:1166–1168, 1995.
45. Smith DT: Medical treatment of acute and chronic pulmonary abscesses. *J Thorac Surg* 17:72–90, 1948.
46. Stavas J, van Sonnenberg E, Casola G, Wittich GR: Percutaneous drainage of infected and noninfected thoracic fluid collections. *J Thorac Imaging* 2:80–87, 1987.
47. Vanway C, Narrod J, Hopeman A: The role of early limited thoracotomy in the treatment of empyema. *J Thorac Cardiovascular Surg* 96:436–439, 1988.
48. Wexler HM, Finegold SM: Antimicrobial resistance in *Bacteroides. J Antimicrob Chemother* 19:143–146, 1987.
49. Wiedemann HP, Rice TW: Lung abscess and empyema. *Semin Thorac Cardiovasc Surg* 7:119–128, 1995.
50. Weiss W: Delayed cavity closure in acute nonspecific primary lung abscess. *Am J Med Sci* 255:313–319, 1968.

CHAPTER 131

MEDIASTINITIS

Mark E. Rupp

ANATOMICAL CONSIDERATIONS

ACUTE MEDIASTINITIS
  Epidemiology and Pathogenesis
  Bacteriology
  Clinical Manifestations and Diagnosis
  Treatment
  Antibiotic Prophylaxis
  Complications and Prognosis

CHRONIC MEDIASTINITIS

Mediastinitis can be conveniently organized into acute or chronic forms with etiologies, clinical presentations, and treatments which are strikingly different. *Acute mediastinitis* is a life-threatening infection that is increasingly recognized as a postoperative complication of cardiovascular surgery. Other less common causes of mediastinitis include esophageal perforation and contiguous spread from oropharyngeal foci. Regardless of the route of infection, a high index of suspicion must be maintained for this clinical entity so that aggressive, potentially life-saving measures can be promptly initiated.

Chronic mediastinitis, also known as *sclerosing mediastinitis, fibrosing mediastinitis,* or *granulomatous mediastinitis,* is a rare disorder that is most often due to *Histoplasma capsulatum.*

ANATOMICAL CONSIDERATIONS

Detailed descriptions of mediastinal anatomy are available, and a thorough review of this material is beyond the scope of this chapter. However, a few fundamental points will be emphasized. The mediastinum is the region within the thorax between the pleural sacs (Fig. 131-1). The mediastinum extends from the diaphragm inferiorly to the superior aperture of the thorax. The 12 thoracic vertebral bodies border the mediastinum posteriorly, and the sternum and costal cartilages make up the anterior boundary. The mediastinum is arbitrarily divided into four subdivisions: superior, posterior, anterior, and middle. Structures within the mediastinum include the heart and great vessels, the esophagus, the distal portion of the trachea and mainstem bronchi, vagus and phrenic nerves, the thymic remnant, and the thoracic duct. These structures are surrounded by adipose tissue, loose connective tissue, and lymph nodes. The mediastinum communicates with the structures of the head and neck via several fascial planes and potential spaces (Figs. 131-2 and 131-3). The three major routes by which infection spreads from the head and neck to the mediastinum are (1) the pretracheal space, (2) the long fascial planes of the posterior neck, and (3) the viscerovascular or lateral pharyngeal space. The long fascial planes of the posterior neck extend from the base of the skull to the diaphragm and are made up of the retropharyngeal or retrovisceral space, the prevertebral space, and the danger space. Pearse attempted to delineate the relative importance of each route in the pathogenesis of mediastinitis and found the retropharyngeal space to be involved in 71 percent of cases followed in frequency by the lateral pharyngeal space (21 percent) and the pretracheal space (8 percent).[48] Knowledge of these fascial planes and anatomic relationships helps one to understand the pathogenesis and potential complications of mediastinitis.

ACUTE MEDIASTINITIS

Epidemiology and Pathogenesis

Primary infection of the mediastinum is a rare event. Essentially all cases of mediastinitis are secondary to the spread of infection from other sites or direct inoculation due to trauma or surgery. The causes of mediastinitis are summarized in Table 131-1 and can be conveniently grouped into the following four categories: cardiothoracic surgery, esophageal perforation, head and neck infection, and infection originating at another site. The pathogenesis, clinical manifestations, and treatment vary due to the underlying cause of mediastinitis.

MEDIASTINITIS SECONDARY TO CARDIOTHORACIC SURGERY

Cardiothoracic operations are among the most common surgical procedures performed in larger hospitals. Coronary artery bypass grafting and cardiac valve replacement accounted for 11.4 percent of the procedures reported between 1987 and 1990 to the Center for Disease Control's National Nosocomial Infection Surveillance System.[13] Because of the large number of median sternotomies that are performed, mediastinitis has become largely a postsurgical infection. Numerous studies have documented the incidence of mediastinitis following cardiothoracic surgery and the risk factors for development of this serious complication. In 1984 Sar and colleagues reviewed the available literature and found the incidence of mediastinitis to range from 0.4 percent to 5 percent of patients undergoing median sternotomy.[55] Since that time studies documenting the experience in over 75,000 patients have been published with incidence rates

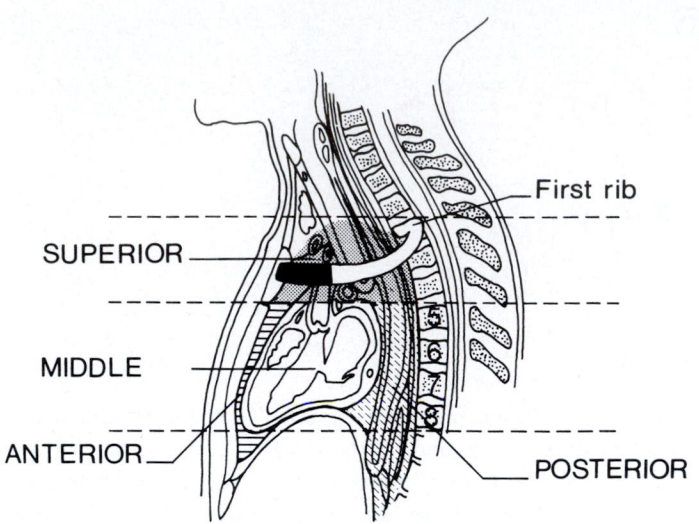

FIGURE 131-1 Anatomic boundaries and divisions of the mediastinum.

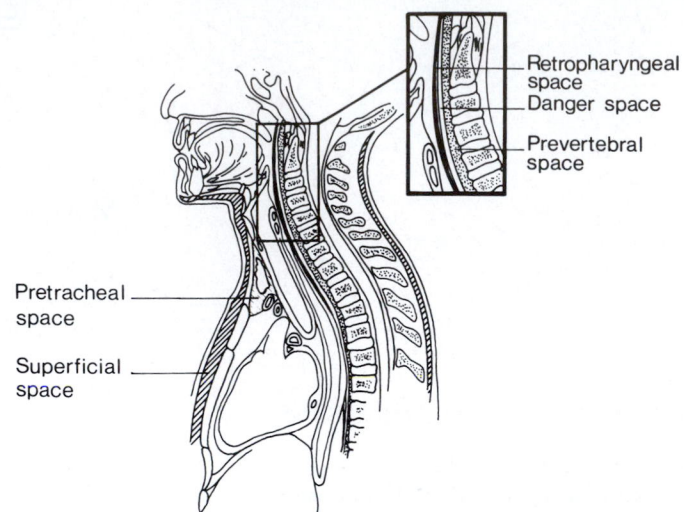

FIGURE 131-3 Cross-section of the neck at the level of the 7th cervical vertebrae demonstrating the potential spaces for spread of infection from the head and neck into the mediastinum.

ranging from 0.66 percent to 2.4 percent.[21,25,34,36,38,42,43,45] The incidence of mediastinitis during outbreaks has been as high as 5 percent to 23.7 percent. Patients undergoing heart transplantation are at higher risk of developing mediastinitis with incidences of 2.5 percent to 7.5 percent.[3,32,40] This risk of mediastinitis is further increased if a mechanical device, such as a left ventricular assist device or a total artificial heart, is used to support a patient while awaiting a suitable donor heart.[49] The incidence of mediastinitis in this situation ranges from 7.5 percent to 35.7 percent.

A number of factors have been implicated that place patients at higher risk of mediastinitis. The studies examining these risk factors are primarily retrospective case-control studies and, thus, are limited by the problems inherent in retrospective surveys. Risk factors can be divided into the following groups: preoperative, intraoperative, and postoperative. Risk factors that can be identified preoperatively include diabetes mellitus, obesity, previous sternotomy, chronic obstructive pulmonary disease, cigarette smoking, low cardiac output states, remote infection, history of endocarditis, method of hair removal, and prolonged preoperative

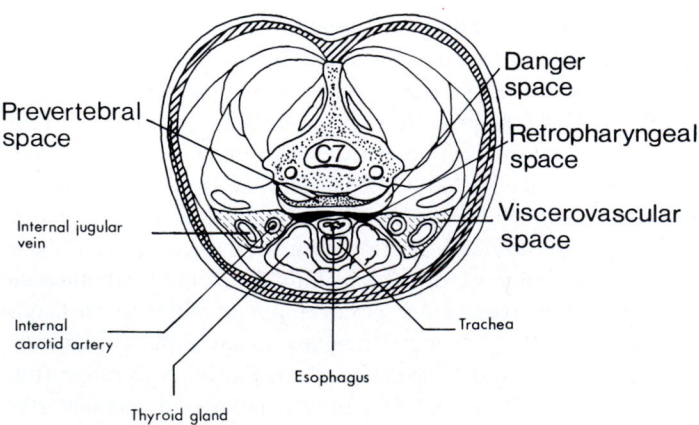

FIGURE 131-2 Sagittal section of the head and neck showing relationship of the fascial spaces to the mediastinum.

hospitalization.[7,21,25,27,33,36,42,43,45,55] Intraoperative and surgical factors include complexity of surgery, type of bone saw used, type of sternal closure, use of internal mammary arteries in coronary artery bypass grafting, use of bone wax, prolonged operative time, prolonged time on cardiopulmonary bypass, blood transfusions, indiscriminate use of electrocautery, and antibiotic prophylaxis.[12,16,21,23,25,27,28,33,36,38,43,45,53,55] Postoperatively patients at greater risk for mediastinitis have been found to require reexploration to control bleeding, prolonged length of stay in the intensive care unit, mechanical ventilation for greater than 24 to 48 h, need for tracheostomy, use of cardiopulmonary resuscitation, and low cardiac-output states.[7,12,21,27,36,38,43,45,52,53,55] Note that there is no universal agreement regarding any of these factors. For instance, despite over three decades of surgical experience, it is unclear whether the use of internal mammary artery (IMA) grafts in coronary artery bypass surgery predisposes patients to mediastinitis. In 1972 Arnold suggested that, based upon anatomical studies of sternal blood supply, the use of the IMA in coronary artery bypass procedures might lead to significant sternal ischemia and thus predispose patients to sternal osteomyelitis and mediastinitis.[2] This has been supported by several laboratory and clinical studies.[12,27] However, other investigators have observed no significant increase in sternal wound infections in patients undergoing coronary artery bypass grafting when the IMA is used.[28,36]

It is generally believed that the pathogenesis of post-cardiac-surgery mediastinitis is primarily due to the inoculation of organisms from the patient's endogenous bacterial flora or from the surgical field into the operative wound. Bacteria are able to propagate in the relatively protected avascular area of the surgical wound and cause infection. Thus, a number of the putative risk factors make intuitive sense, such as length of time of surgery, the complexity of surgery, and need for reexploration. In addition, outbreaks of mediastinitis have been epidemiologically linked to sources such as bacteria from a particular surgeon's hands or nares, lending support to the belief that intraoperative factors are important in the pathogenesis of me-

TABLE 131-1

Causes of Acute Mediastinitis

Esophageal perforation

Iatrogenic: Esophagogastroduodenoscopy, esophageal dilitation, esophageal variceal sclerotherapy, naso-gastric tube, Sengstaken-Blakemore tube, endotracheal intubation, esophageal surgery, paraesophageal surgery

Swallowed foreign bodies: Bones, coins, can pull-tabs, drug-filled condoms, swords

Trauma
Penetrating: gun shot wound, knife wound
Blunt: steering wheel injury, seat-belt injury, cardiopulmonary resuscitation, whiplash injury, barotrauma

Spontaneous/Other: emesis, cricoid pressure during anesthesia induction, heavy lifting, defecation, parturition,

Head and neck infections
Odontogenic, Ludwig's angina, pharyngitis, tonsillitis, parotitis, epiglottitis

Infection originating at another site
Pneumonia, pleural space infection/empyema; subphrenic abscess; pancreatitis; cellulitis/soft-tissue infection of the chest wall; osteomyelitis of sternum, clavicle, ribs, or vertebrae; hematogenous spread from distant foci

Cardiothoracic surgery
Coronary artery bypass grafting, cardiac valve replacement, repair of congenital heart defect, heart transplantation, heart-lung transplantation, cardiac assist devices, other types of cardiothoracic surgery

diastinitis. Ferrazzi and coworkers observed a significant decrease in the incidence of gram-negative mediastinitis, but no significant change in gram-positive infections, with changes in the operating room environment, supporting the belief that many of these infections arise from gram-positive organisms resident on the patient's skin.[23] Archer and Armstrong have demonstrated that patients are colonized by small numbers of antibiotic-resistant coagulase-negative staphylococci that become the predominant species when subjected to the selective pressure of prophylactic antibiotics.[1] In addition, various immunosuppressive effects of cardiopulmonary bypass have been elucidated that may contribute in the pathogenesis of post-cardiac-surgery mediastinitis. The importance of postoperative factors has also been emphasized by outbreaks of mediastinitis that have been linked to environmental sources and poor hand-washing technique in the postoperative care of cardiac surgery patients.[14,17] However, Kaiser has persuasively warned against taking a "make-a-change-and-see-what-happens" approach to the analysis of risk factors related to the pathogenesis of postoperative infection.[31] Controlled prospective studies are needed to better define the factors that influence post-cardiac-surgery mediastinitis.

MEDIASTINITIS SECONDARY TO ESOPHAGEAL PERFORATION

Prior to the development of cardiac surgery, perforation of the esophagus was the leading cause of mediastinitis, followed by suppurative infections of the oropharynx.[48] In 1724 Herman Boerhaave graphically described the first case of mediastinitis due to spontaneous rupture of the esophagus in a Dutch admiral who died $18\frac{1}{2}$ h after self-induced emesis.[4,6] Subsequently, this entity has been known as *Boerhaave's syndrome.* Currently, esophageal perforation is most frequently due to iatrogenic

events. Flexible fibrooptic endoscopy of the upper gastrointestinal tract is complicated by esophageal perforation in 0.074 percent to 0.4 percent of procedures.[11] This occurs more frequently when sclerotherapy or dilatation procedures are performed. Swallowed foreign bodies, esophageal carcinoma, and nonsurgical trauma may also result in perforation of the esophagus and mediastinitis.

Depending on where the esophageal perforation occurs, mediastinitis may result from migration into the mediastinum via the fascial planes of the neck or from direct spillage of esophageal contents into the posterior mediastinum. A necrotizing chemical mediastinitis ensues which is followed by an aerobic and anaerobic bacterial mediastinitis. Often a synergistic necrotizing form of mediastinitis is observed.[20] Spread of infection from the neck into the mediastinum is influenced by respiratory dynamics in which the negative intrathoracic pressure generated during respiration tends to force the infection into the mediastinum.[46]

MEDIASTINITIS SECONDARY TO HEAD AND NECK INFECTION OR FROM OTHER SITES

Before antibiotics were widely available odontogenic and pharyngeal infections caused from 10 percent to 31 percent of cases of mediastinitis.[48] Fortunately, these infections rarely cause mediastinitis today. The prototypic odontogenic infection leading to mediastinitis is Ludwig's angina. This generally arises from an infection of the second or third mandibular molar to involve the sublingual and submandibular spaces. From there, the infection can spread via the lateral pharyngeal space to involve the retropharyngeal space or carotid sheath and thus track into the mediastinum. During the antibiotic era approximately 3.5 percent of cases of Ludwig's angina have been complicated by mediastinitis.[41] Mediastinitis resulting from infections involving the lateral pharyngeal space may originate from a number of sources including the teeth, parotid glands, tonsils, or rarely from otitis or mastoiditis. Retropharyngeal space infections generally arise from perforation of the esophagus or extension from pharyngitis, epiglottitis, or tonsillitis. From the long fascial planes of the neck, these infections easily spread into the superior mediastinum, or, if the danger space is involved, the posterior mediastinum.[20,35] The pretracheal space descends into the anterior mediastinum and most often is involved in mediastinitis complicating surgery of the thyroid or trachea.[48]

Rarely, mediastinitis is due to spread from other sites. Cases have been described secondary to the following conditions: pneumonia, pleural space infection, osteomyelitis of the ribs, clavicle, sternum, or vertebrae, subphrenic abscess, pancreatitis, cellulitis, and hematogenous seeding from distant foci.[24]

Bacteriology

The bacteriology of mediastinitis complicating cardiovascular surgery and that secondary to odontogenic or other head and neck infections are strikingly different and are summarized in Table 131-2. Mediastinitis secondary to cardiothoracic surgery is primarily due to gram-positive cocci with lesser contributions by gram-negative bacilli. The bacteriology of mediastinitis secondary to extension from head and neck sources is somewhat more complicated. The majority of infections are polymicrobic. Often a synergistic infection made up of a number of oral anaerobes and gram-negative bacilli is evident. The most frequently isolated organisms include viridans streptococci, peptococci, peptostreptococci, *Bacteroides* spp., and *Fusobacterium* spp. The relative frequency with which these organisms are isolated is difficult to determine due to the difficulty of obtaining reliable anaerobic culture data.

Clinical Manifestations and Diagnosis

The clinical manifestations of mediastinitis also differ based on the underlying cause of disease. Patients experiencing mediastinitis from extension of odontogenic or pharyngeal infections generally have obvious primary infections with significant pain, fever, and swelling of the affected site. Esophageal perforation may be clinically obvious or inapparent. Early in the course of mediastinitis, signs and symptoms may be subtle, but as the condition progresses, patients note increasing chest pain, respiratory distress, and dysphagia. Chest pain is often the most prominent symptom and may localize depending upon which portion of the mediastinum is involved. In anterior mediastinitis, pain is often located in the cervical or substernal region.[24,46] Pain due to posterior mediastinitis may localize to the epigastric area with radiation to the interscapular region. Pleuritic chest pain may also be experienced due to the relatively frequent complication of pleural effusion. Retroperitoneal extension may be accompanied by acute abdominal signs and may prompt unnecessary exploratory laparotomy.[20] Examination may reveal fever, tachycardia, crepitus,

and edema of the chest or neck. *Hamman's sign,* a crunching rasping sound heard over the precordium synchronous with the cardiac rhythm, due to emphysema of the mediastinum, may be present in up to 50 percent of patients with pneumomediastinum.[30] The heart sounds may appear distant and dull. In the later stages of disease, signs of bacteremia and sepsis may predominate. The early diagnosis of mediastinitis in the infant or

TABLE 131-2

Microbiology of Mediastinitis

Organisms Frequently Recovered in Mediastinitis Secondary to Infection of the Head and Neck or Esophageal Perforation

Anaerobic	Aerobic or Facultative	Fungi
Gram-positive cocci	Gram-positive cocci	C. albicans
Peptococcus spp.	Streptococcal spp.	
Peptostreptococcus spp.	Staphylococci spp.	
Gram-positive bacilli	Gram-positive bacilli	
Actinomyces	Corynebacterium	
Eubacterium	Gram-negative cocci	
Lactobacillus	Branhamella	
Gram-negative cocci	Gram-negative bacilli	
Veillonella	Enterobacteriaceae	
Gram-negative bacilli	Pseudomonas spp.	
Bacteroides spp.	Eikenella corodans	
Fusobacterium spp.		

Organisms Frequently Recovered in Mediastinitis Secondary to Cardiothoracic Surgery

Organism	Range	Representative Rate
Gram-positive cocci		
S. aureus	7.1%–66.7%	25%
S. epidermidis	6%–45.5%	30%
Enterococcus spp.	8%–18.8%	10%
Streptococci spp.	0%–18.2%	2%
Gram-negative bacilli		
E. coli	0%–12.5%	5%
Enterobacter spp.	4%–21.4%	10%
Klebsiella spp.	0%–21.1%	3%
Proteus spp.	0%–7.1%	2%
Other Enterobacteriaceae	0%–20%	2%
Pseudomonas spp.	0%–54%	2%
Fungi		
C. albicans	0%–14.3%	<2%
Polymicrobial	0%–40%	10%
Other occasionally reported		
Acinetobacter		
Legionella spp.		
B. fragilis		
C. tropicalis		
Nocardia spp.		
Kluyvera		
M. fortuitum		
M. chelonei		
Rhodococcus bronchialis		

Other Unusual Causes of Mediastinitis

Anthrax, brucellosis, actinomycoses, paragonimiasis

neonate may be particularly challenging. A peculiar, interrupted, staccato type of inspiration has been described in a number of cases.[22] The signs and symptoms of mediastinitis in older children are similar to those observed in adults. Laboratory tests usually reveal a leukocytosis with a leftward shift evident on the differential. Radiographically, plain films of the chest may reveal mediastinal widening, air-fluid levels, and subcutaneous or mediastinal emphysema.[56] The lateral chest radiograph may be useful in demonstrating superior mediastinal gas not evident on upright films. Approximately 50 percent of cases of pneumomediastinum are not evident without lateral views. Examples of some of the radiographic manifestations of mediastinitis are shown in Figs. 131-4 and 131-5. Complications of mediastinitis, such as pleural effusion or pneumoperitoneum, may also be evident on the chest radiograph. Esophageal perforation is best demonstrated by contrast esophagography which reveals extravasation of dye in 59 percent to 100 percent of cases.[5,19,58] A water-soluble contrast agent should be used initially to detect gross extravasation due to the inflammation and granuloma formation evoked by barium. If extravasation is not observed, barium should be used to detect subtle defects, as it provides better definition of the anatomy. Computed tomography (CT) is often helpful in cases where the diagnosis is not evident clinically or on plain films.[10] Technetium-labeled white blood cell scans have been reported helpful in the diagnosis of mediastinitis in specialized circumstances when CT scan was not readily available. The role of magnetic resonance imaging (MRI) in the evaluation of mediastinitis has not been well established.

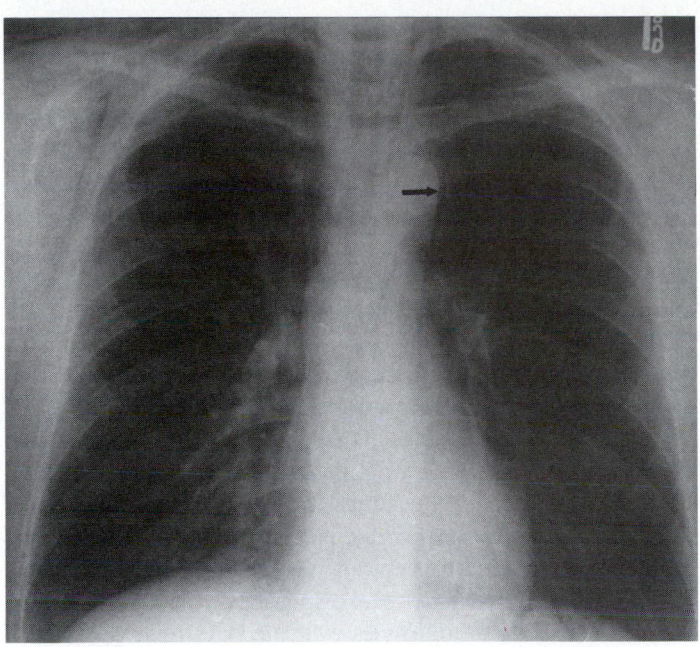

FIGURE 131-5 Chest radiograph demonstrating pneumomediastinum (arrow). (*Radiograph courtesy of Dr. J. Gurney, University of Nebraska Medical Center.*)

Post-cardiothoracic-surgery mediastinitis usually presents within the first 2 weeks following surgery.[7,34,55] However, rare cases have been described presenting over 1 year postoperatively.[7] Infections due to gram-negative organisms generally present earlier. One study found that all cases of mediastinitis presenting later than 2 weeks postoperatively were due to gram-positive organisms.[7] The presentation of mediastinitis may be fulminant or subtle. Some cases may present as sepsis without localizing signs. Patients may experience greater-than-normal postoperative pain which may be pleuritic in nature. Dys-

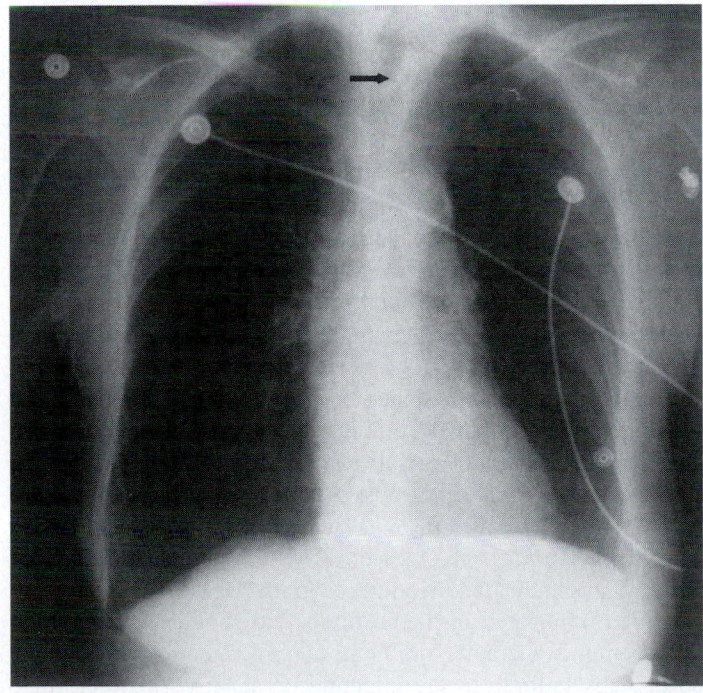

A

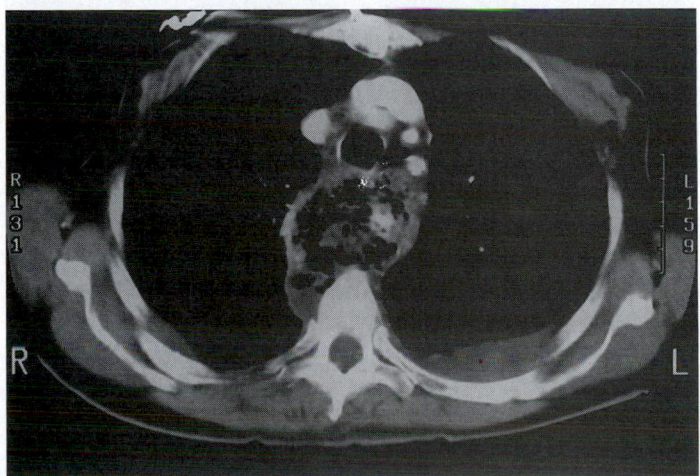

B

FIGURE 131-4 *A.* Chest radiograph of elderly woman with esophageal perforation and mediastinitis. The patient had senile dementia and had unknowingly swallowed a portion of a broken glass jar resulting in esophageal perforation. The chest radiograph reveals a foreign body within the esophagus (arrow) and widening of the mediastinum. *B.* Computed tomography of the chest at the level of the 6th thoracic vertebrae demonstrating a large abscess within the posterior mediastinum and a left-sided pleural effusion. (*Radiographs courtesy of Dr. J. Gurney, University of Nebraska Medical Center.*)

phagia is a rare complaint. Fever and an abnormal appearance of the surgical wound, characterized by erythema, cellulitis, or purulent discharge, are the most frequent signs of mediastinitis.[7,28,34,55] Sternal instability, dehiscence, or the observation of bubbles emanating from the sternal wound are less frequent findings. Occasionally chest wall emphysema is observed. Poststernotomy mediastinitis presenting as a deep neck abscess without abnormal findings on chest exam has been reported. Laboratory tests usually show a moderate leukocytosis with a leftward shift on the white blood cell differential. Radiographically, mediastinal widening is a rare finding on plain chest films and generally routine radiographs are of very little use in the diagnosis of mediastinitis following cardiothoracic surgery (Fig. 131-6).[7,55] CT scanning has proven helpful in many cases of postoperative mediastinitis, particularly in differentiating superficial wound infections from deeper retrosternal processes.[10] However, normal postoperative collections of fluid and gas are at times difficult to differentiate from early signs of mediastinitis. The diagnostic value of nuclear scans has been espoused by several investigators.[50] Browdie and colleagues evaluated the relative value of CT, indium-111-labeled leukocyte scanning, and epicardial pacer wire cultures in 24 patients being evaluated for possible mediastinitis.[8] They found CT had a sensitivity of 67 percent and specificity of 71 percent, indium-111-labeled leukocyte scan was 83 percent sensitive and 100 percent specific, and epicardial pacer wire cultures were reported to be 100 percent sensitive and 92 percent specific. Another investigator however found epicardial pacer wire cultures to be associated with an unacceptably high false-positive rate.[51] The role of magnetic resonance imaging is not well-delineated; MRI is contraindicated in instances where ferro-magnetic metals are used in sternal wires, artificial heart valves, cardiac pacemakers, or vascular clips. Several investigators have found mediastinal needle aspiration useful in the diagnosis of mediastinitis.[12,27,55,57] This method, which has been reported positive in 65.8 percent of patients, appears to be particularly useful in diagnosing mediastinitis before it becomes more clinically obvious.

Treatment

Therapy that includes both medical and surgical techniques should be promptly initiated once the diagnosis of mediastinitis is made. In all cases aggressive supportive and nutritional therapy is required. Barrett is credited with documenting the first successful treatment of mediastinitis due to esophageal perforation in 1946.[4] Since then, most authorities recommend aggressive surgical drainage, debridement, and repair in cases of mediastinitis secondary to esophageal perforation.[56,60] However, based on experience with eight patients, Cameron and coworkers identified a subset of patients that could be treated without surgical intervention.[9] These patients should have a well-contained disruption of the esophagus, the abscess should drain back into the esophagus, minimal symptoms should be present, and there should be minimal evidence of clinical toxicity. Shaffer and colleagues expanded upon these recommendations based on the recognition of patients with esophageal perforation due to instrumentation before major mediastinal contamination had occurred.[58] Santos and Frater have recommended transesophageal irrigation for patients in whom primary repair of the esophagus is not possible due to advanced local infection with extensive tissue necrosis.[54]

As in cases of mediastinitis due to esophageal perforation, cases secondary to descending odontogenic or pharyngeal infection require prompt surgical intervention. Because transcervical drainage is frequently inadequate, a transthoracic approach is generally necessary.[20,61]

Although the importance of supportive therapy and surgical intervention cannot be overemphasized, administration of appropriate antibiotics is also an essential component of therapy. Empiric regimens are based upon the underlying etiology and should cover the major pathogens listed in Table 131-2. Penicillin G has traditionally been the antibiotic of choice in the treatment of anaerobic infections arising above the diaphragm and continues to exhibit excellent activity against most oral anaerobic bacteria. Unfortunately, oral *Bacteroides spp.* are increasingly resistant to penicillin G and, therefore, when infection with *Bacteroides* is suspected, treatment with metronidazole, clindamycin, or broad spectrum β-lactam antibiotics with activity against *Bacteroides spp.*, as well as other oropharyngeal anaerobes, may be indicated. In addition, gram-negative enteric bacilli are often implicated in mediastinitis and should be covered in initial empiric therapy. Antibiotic therapy should then be more specifically tailored to the infecting organisms when definitive culture results are available, but therapy directed against anaerobic oropharyngeal organisms should probably be continued due to the difficulty in obtaining reliable anaerobic cultures. Duration of therapy, which may range from weeks to months, is determined by the virulence of the bacteria, host factors, and the patient's response to therapy.

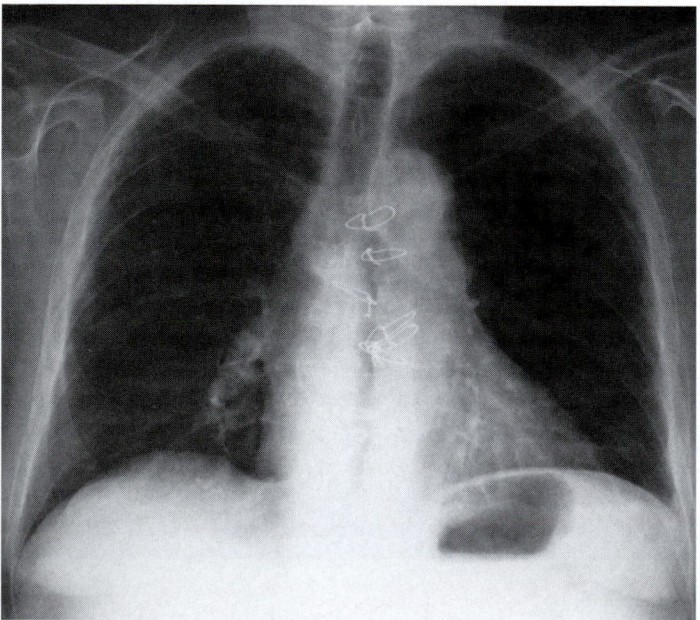

FIGURE 131-6   Chest radiograph of patient with mediastinitis following cardiac surgery. Dehiscence of median sternotomy is demonstrated by asymmetry of sternal wires. *(Radiograph courtesy of Dr. J. Gurney, University of Nebraska Medical Center.)*

The treatment of post-cardiac-surgery mediastinitis generally requires aggressive surgical drainage and debridement. A small number of patients have been successfully treated via percutaneous catheter drainage. Two approaches have been utilized in the surgical management of post-cardiac-surgery mediastinitis—an open technique and a closed technique. The open technique involves debridement of infected tissue and open packing of the wound with delayed closure.[12,27,36,55] Disadvantages of this technique include respiratory insufficiency due to lack of mechanical support for the thorax, delayed healing and closure of the surgical wound, and hemorrhage from exposed vessels.[55] The closed method involves debridement of affected tissues, closure of the sternum, and postoperative irrigation through drainage tubes within the mediastinum.[12,27,36,55] Irrigants have included a variety of antimicrobial and antiseptic solutions, such as neomycin, gentamicin, bacitracin, polymyxin B, saline, and Dakin's solution. These solutions have been associated with a variety of complications including emergence of resistant organisms, pericardial and tissue toxicity, and systemic absorption and toxicity. The most commonly employed irrigant is providone-iodine. Use of povidone-iodine has been associated with iodine toxicity, renal failure, metabolic acidosis, and seizures. Therefore, this agent must be used with caution, and serum iodine concentration should be measured to ensure that toxic levels are not reached. Durandy and colleagues reported a closed technique successfully utilizing Redon drainage devices in 11 patients who did not require postoperative irrigation.[18] A number of investigators have reported the successful use of muscle flaps and omental grafts, many times at the time of initial debridement, to close mediastinal wounds with or without postoperative irrigation.[27,39]

The use of parenteral antibiotics has remained a cornerstone of therapy. Generally, empiric therapy should be directed at staphylococci and gram-negative aerobic bacilli until definitive culture results are available. As with mediastinitis secondary to infection of the head and neck, the duration of therapy is determined by multiple factors and may be quite prolonged.

Antibiotic Prophylaxis

Although cardiothoracic surgical procedures are classified as clean procedures, and the risk of infection is low, the consequences of infection are devastating. Therefore, despite the lack of placebo-controlled studies documenting efficacy, antibiotic prophylaxis has become commonplace. Cefazolin has generally been regarded as the drug of choice for prophylaxis. The use of vancomycin or second-generation cephalosporins, such as cefamundole and cefuroxime, has also been considered. Studies regarding the relative efficacy of first- and second-generation cephalosporins are conflicting, and no agent has conclusively been shown superior to another. In a comparison among vancomycin, cefazolin, and cefamandole, Maki and coworkers demonstrated a significant reduction in postoperative wound infection in patients receiving vancomycin prophylaxis.[37] Vancomycin should be considered as a choice for prophylaxis in centers with a high prevalence of infections due to methicillin-resistant staphylococci. The major disadvantages associated with the use of vancomycin are the long infusion time

required and the small numbers of patients experiencing adverse events, such as hypotension and "redman syndrome." In addition, the emergence of vancomycin-resistant enterococci, due in part to the overuse of vancomycin in empiric therapy, must be considered as a long-term disadvantage to the use of vancomycin as a prophylactic agent.

Complications and Prognosis

Complications of mediastinitis include extension of the infection into a number of contiguous structures and spaces including the pericardial space, resulting in pericardial effusion and tamponade, the pleural space, and the peritoneum, resulting in peritonitis.[20] A major complication of post-cardiac-surgery mediastinitis is sternal osteomyelitis. Prior to the development of modern surgery and antibiotics, mediastinitis, due primarily to esopha-geal perforation, was regarded as uniformly fatal. Unfortunately, since the time of Barrett's first successful surgical repair of the esophagus, morbidity and mortality have remained high, with many studies recording mortality rates of 30 percent to 50 percent.[7,20,36,61] Survivors of mediastinitis usually have no permanent sequela. In examining the economic ramifications of mediastinitis, Loop and colleagues found that the hospital charges for coronary artery bypass surgery patients who experience mediastinitis were 280 percent greater than patients with uncomplicated bypass surgery, and the median length of stay ranged from 38 to 51 days.[36] The most important factor in determining outcome has been the length of time to diagnosis and initiation of definitive therapy. Other prognostic indicators have included BUN, white blood cell count, culture positivity, type of surgical repair, and cytomegalovirus shedding.

CHRONIC MEDIASTINITIS

Sclerosing, fibrosing, or *granulomatous mediastinitis* are terms for a chronic form of mediastinitis characterized by an invasive and compressive inflammatory infiltrate. The first report of this entity, which may cause up to 10 percent of all primary mediastinal masses, reportedly dates to a description by Ulmont in 1855. Although the etiology of up to 83 percent of cases of sclerosing mediastinitis remains obscure, many authorities believe that most cases are secondary to infection with *Histoplasma capsulatum.*[26,47] Gryboski and coworkers and Peabody and coworkers found that up to 73 percent of cases previously characterized as nonspecific granulomatous mediastinitis could be reclassified as secondary to *Histoplasma capsulatum* by restaining the tissue with fungal stains and thoroughly reviewing the pathological sections.[29,47] Other infectious etiologies that have been reported to cause this condition include tuberculosis, actinomycoses, nocardiosis, blastomycosis, coccidioidomycosis, aspergillosis, and infection with *Rhizopus spp.* Older literature often lists syphilis as a prominent cause of this condition. However, this was based upon seropositivity without other supporting evidence. Other conditions which closely mimic this entity include sarcoidosis, silicosis, lymphoma, mesothelioma, and mediastinal fibrosis associated with radiation therapy, idiopathic retroperitoneal fibrosis, Reidel's struma, or sclerosing cholangitis.

Approximately 40 percent of patients with sclerosing mediastinitis are asymptomatic and come to medical attention when a chest roentgenogram incidentally reveals a mediastinal mass. Symptomatic patients usually note symptoms related to invasion or obstruction of structures within or adjacent to the mediastinum. Sclerosing mediastinitis is the most common nonmalignant cause of superior vena cava syndrome, responsible for up to 23 percent of cases. These patients generally present with plethora and edema of the face, neck, and upper torso, neck vein distention, headache, and visual disturbances. Patients presenting with obstruction of the pulmonary arteries often note cough, dyspnea, and symptoms consistent with right-sided heart failure. Pulmonary infarction, although rare, has been reported to occur in patients with sclerosing mediastinitis. Pulmonary venous obstruction causes patients to experience cough, dyspnea, and hemoptysis. Patients with airway obstruction due to sclerosing mediastinitis usually present with wheezing, cough, hemoptysis, and recurrent episodes of bacterial bronchitis or pneumonia. Patients complaining of dysphagia may have esophageal obstruction due to posterior extension of the mediastinitis.

Sherrick and colleagues recently reviewed the radiographic findings in 33 patients with sclerosing mediastinitis. Findings included bronchial narrowing (33 percent), pulmonary artery narrowing (18 percent), esophageal narrowing (9 percent), and superior vena cava narrowing (39 percent).[59] Two distinctly different pulmonary infiltrate patterns were noted: localized with calcification (82 percent) and diffuse without calcification (18 percent). These authors felt that the localized pattern was most often secondary to histoplasmosis, whereas the diffuse pattern was more likely to be due to a noninfectious etiology. Patients with sclerosing mediastinitis will often be observed to have a mediastinal mass, most frequently located in the superior mediastinum at the level of the bifurcation of the trachea. Computed tomography often reveals calcification and delineates the extent of infiltration, whereas magnetic resonance imaging is superior in assessment of the vascular integrity. Ventilation-perfusion lung scans often reveal large perfusion deficits due to obstruction of the pulmonary vessels.

The diagnosis of sclerosing mediastinitis requires pathologic examination. There is a continuum of disease ranging from a predominantly granulomatous entity to an almost completely fibrosing process. Lesions described include caseating granuloma, dense hyalinized collagenous tissue, and infiltrations of lymphocytes, plasma cells, and giant cells. Specific stains for fungi often reveal organisms consistent with histoplasma, but cultures are usually negative.

The pathologic features of this disease suggest a marked inflammatory reaction. Several different mechanisms have been proposed to explain the pathology of fibrosing mediastinitis. Some investigators believe that a caseous lymph node from primary infection with histoplasma ruptures into the mediastinum invoking an intense inflammatory reaction. A second hypothesis is the development of a delayed hypersensitivity reaction due to the spread of soluble histoplasma antigens into the mediastinum. An alternative explanation proposes that fibrosing mediastinitis represents an abnormality of collagen production and organization similar to idiopathic retroperitoneal fibrosis or Riedel's struma. Noguchi and colleagues have incriminated the eosinophil

in the pathogenesis of fibrosing mediastinitis by demonstrating eosinophils or major basic protein in tissue specimens from 5 of 7 patients with fibrosing mediastinitis.[44]

No controlled trials of medical or surgical therapy in the treatment of fibrosing mediastinitis have been conducted. Although there is some anecdotal evidence of a beneficial effect of antifungal agents, most authorities believe that at the time of presentation there is little evidence of an active infection, and antifungal agents are not indicated. Because the natural history of this disease is variable, with some patients progressing to compression of vital structures while others seem to have self-limited disease, it is difficult to make recommendations regarding the timing of surgical intervention. It has been suggested that early surgical intervention and removal of granulomatous tissue may prevent the development of subsequent end-stage fibrosis and involvement of vital structures. Clearly, patients experiencing obstruction or invasion of mediastinal structures require intervention, even though such surgery is often difficult, and results are at times less than optimal. Superior vena cava syndrome due to fibrosing mediastinitis has been successfully alleviated through use of Palmaz stents.[15] Therapy with corticosteroids does not appear to have a role in the treatment of fibrosing mediastinitis.

REFERENCES

1. Archer GL, Armstrong BC: Alteration of staphylococcal flora in cardiac surgery patients receiving antibiotic prophylaxis. *J Infect Dis* 147:642–649, 1983.
2. Arnold M: The surgical anatomy of sternal blood supply. *J Thorac Cardiovasc Surg* 64:596–610, 1972.
3. Baldwin RT, Radovancevic B, Sweeney MS, et al: Bacterial mediastinitis after heart transplantation. *J Heart Lung Transplant* 11:545–549, 1992.
4. Barrett NR: Report of a case of spontaneous perforation of the oesophagus successfully treated by operation. *Br J Surg* 35:216–218, 1947.
5. Berry BE, Ochsner JL: Perforation of the esophagus: A 30 year review. *J Thorac Cardiovasc Surg* 65:1–7, 1973.
6. Boerhaave H: Artocis, nec descripti prius Morbi Historia, *Secundem Artis Leges Conscripta*, Lugdunis Batavorum Bouresteniana, 1724.
7. Bor DH, Rose RM, Modlin JF, et al: Mediastinitis after cardiovascular surgery. *Rev Infect Dis* 5:885–897, 1983.
8. Browdie DA, Bernstein RW, Agnew R, et al: Diagnosis of poststernotomy infection: Comparison of three means of assessment. *Ann Thorac Surg* 1:290–292, 1991.
9. Cameron JL, Kieffer RF, Hendrix TR, et al: Selective nonoperative management of contained intrathoracic esophageal disruptions. *Ann Thorac Surg* 27:404–408, 1979.
10. Carrol CL, Jeffrey B Jr, Federle MP, Vernacchia FS: CT evaluation of mediastinal infections. *J Comput Assist Tomogr* 11:449–454, 1987.
11. Chow AW: Life-threatening infections of the head and neck. *Clin Infect Dis* 14:991–1004, 1992.
12. Culliford AT, Cunningham JN, Zeff RH, et al: Sternal and costochondral infections following open-heart surgery. *J Thor Cardiovasc Surg* 72:714–726, 1976.
13. Culver DH, Horan TC, Gaynes RP, et al: Surgical wound infection rates by wound class operative procedure, and patient risk index. *Am J Med* 91 (Suppl 3B):152–157, 1991.

14. DeSilva MI, Rissing JP: Postoperative wound infections following cardiac surgery: significance of contaminated cases performed in the preceding 48 hours. *Infect Control* 5:371–377, 1984.

15. Dodds GA, Harrison JK, O'Laughlin MP, et al: Relief of superior vena cava syndrome due to fibrosing mediastinitis using the Palmaz stent. *Chest* 106:315–318, 1994.

16. Doebbeling BN, Pfaller MA, Kuhns KR, et al: Cardiovascular surgery prophylaxis. *J Thorac Cardiovasc Surg* 99:981–989, 1990.

17. Dandalides PC, Rutala WA, Sarubbi FA Jr: Postoperative infection following cardiac surgery: Association with an environmental reservoir in a cardiothoracic intensive card unit. *Infect Control* 5:378–384, 1984.

18. Durandy Y, Batisse A, Bourel P, et al: Mediastinal infection after cardiac operation: A simple closed technique. *J Thorac Cardiovasc Surg* 97:282–285, 1989.

19. Elleson DA, Rowley SD: Esophageal perforation: Its early diagnosis and treatment. *Laryngoscope* 92:678–680, 1982.

20. Estrera AS, Landay MJ, Grishom JM, et al: Descending necrotizing mediastinitis. *Surg Gyn Obstet* 157:545–552, 1983.

21. Farinas MC, Peralta FG, Bernal JM, et al: Suppurative mediastinitis after open-heart surgery: A case-control study covering a seven-year period in Santander, Spain. *Clin Infect Dis* 20:272–279, 1995.

22. Feldman R, Gromisch DS: Acute suppurative mediastinitis. *Am J Dis Child* 121:79–81, 1971.

23. Ferrazzi P, Allen R, Crupi G, et al: Reduction of infection after cardiac surgery. *Ann Thorac Surg* 42:321–325, 1986.

24. Freidman BC, Pickul DC: Acute mediastinitis: What to do when the cause is nonsurgical. *Postgrad Med* 87:273–285, 1990.

25. Gaynes R, Marosok R, Hanley JM, et al: Mediastinitis following coronary artery bypass surgery: A 3-year review. *J Infect Dis* 163:117–121, 1991.

26. Goodwin RA, Loyd JE, Des Prez RM: Histoplasmosis in normal hosts. *Medicine* 60:231–266, 1981.

27. Grossi EA, Culliford AT, Krieger KH, et al: A survey of 77 major infectious complications of median sternotomy: a review of 7949 consecutive operative procedures. *Ann Thoracic Surg* 40:214–223, 1985.

28. Grossi EA, Esposito R, Harris LJ, et al: Sternal wound infections and use of internal mammary artery grafts. *J Thorac Cardiovasc Surg* 102:342–347, 1991.

29. Gryboski WA, Crutcher RR, Holloway JB, et al: Surgical aspects of histoplasmosis. *Arch Surg* 87:590–599, 1963.

30. Hamman L: Spontaneous mediastinal emphysema. *Bull Johns Hopkins H* 64:1–21, 1939.

31. Kaiser AB: Risk factors for infection in cardiac surgery: Will the real culprit please stand up? *Infect Control* 5:369–370, 1984.

32. Karwande SV, Renlund DG, Olsen SL, et al: Mediastinitis in heart transplantation. *Ann Thorac Surg* 54:1039–1045, 1992.

33. Ko W, Lazenby D, Zelano JA, et al: Effects of shaving methods and intraoperative irrigation on suppurative mediastinitis after bypass operations. *Ann Thorac Surg* 53:301–305, 1992.

34. Kutsal A, Ibrisim E, Catav Z, et al: Mediastinitis after open heart surgery. *J Cardiovasc Surg* 32:38–41, 1991.

35. Levine TM, Wurster CF, Krespi YP: Mediastinitis occurring as a complication of odontogenic infections. *Laryngoscope* 96:747–750, 1986.

36. Loop FD, Lytle BW, Cosgrove DM, et al: Sternal wound complications after isolated coronary artery bypass grafting: Early and late mortality, morbidity, and cost of care. *Ann Thorac Surg* 49:179–187, 1990.

37. Maki DG, Bohn MJ, Stolz SM, et al: Comparative study of cefazolin, cefamandole, and vancomycin for surgical prophylaxis in cardiac and vascular operations. *J Thorac Cardiovasc Surg* 104:1423–1434, 1992.

38. Miholic J, Hudec M, Domanig E, et al: Risk factors for severe bacterial infections after valve replacement and aortocoronary bypass operations: analysis of 246 cases by logistic regression. *Ann Thorac Surg* 40:224–228, 1985.

39. Miller JI, Nahai F: Repair of the dehisced median sternotomy incision. *Surg Clin N Amer* 69:1091–1102, 1989.

40. Miller R, Rudler J, Karwande SV, Burton NA: Treatment of mediastinitis after heart transplantation. *J Heart Transplant* 5:477–479, 1986.

41. Moreland LW, Corey J, McKenzie R: Ludwigs angina: Report of a case and review of the literature. *Arch Intern Med* 148:461–466, 1988.

42. Nagachinta T, Stephens M, Reitz B, Polk BF: Risk factors for surgical-wound infection following cardiac surgery. *J Infect Dis* 156:967–973, 1987.

43. Newman LS, Szczukowski LC, Bain RP, Perlino CA: Suppurative mediastinitis after open heart surgery. *Chest* 94:546–553, 1988.

44. Noguchi H, Kephart GM, Colby TV, Gleich GJ: Tissue eosinophilia and eosinophil degranulation in syndromes associated with fibrosis. *Am J Pathol* 140:521–528, 1992.

45. Ottino G, De Paulis R, Pansini S, et al: Major sternal wound infection after open-heart surgery: A multivariate analysis of risk factors in 2579 consecutive operative procedures. *Ann Thorac Surg* 44:173–179, 1987.

46. Payne WS, Larson RH: Acute mediastinitis. *Surg Clin North Am* 49:999–1009, 1969.

47. Peabody JW, Brown RB, Sullivan MB, Cannon A: Mediastinal granulomas. *J Thorac Surg* 35:384–396, 1958.

48. Pearse HE Jr: Mediastinitis following cervical suppuration. *Ann Surgery* 108:588–611, 1938.

49. Phillips WS, Burton NA, Macmanus Q, Lefrak EA: Surgical complications in bridging to transplantation: The thermo cardiosystems LVAD. *Ann Thorac Surg* 53:482–486, 1992.

50. Quirce R, Serano J, Arnal C, et al: Detection of mediastinitis after heart transplantation by gallium-67 scintigraphy. *J Nucl Med* 32:860–861, 1991.

51. Robicsek F: Poststernotomy infections. *Ann Thorac Surg* 52:896–900, 1991.

52. Rutledge R, Applebaum RE, Kim BJ: Mediastinal infection after open heart surgery. *Surgery* 97:88–92, 1985.

53. Sanfelippo PM, Danielson GK: Complications associated with median sternotomy. *J Thorac Cardiovasc Surg* 63:419–423, 1972.

54. Santos GH, Frater WM: Transesophageal irrigation for the treatment of mediastinitis produced by esophageal rupture. *J Thorac Cardiovasc Surg* 91:57–62, 1986.

55. Sarr MG, Gott VL, Townsend TR: Mediastinal infection after cardiac surgery. *Ann Thorac Surg* 38:415–423, 1984.

56. Sarr MG, Pemberton JH, Payne WS: Management of instrumental perforations of the esophagus. *J Thorac Cardiovasc Surg* 84:211–218, 1982.

57. Sarr MG, Watkins L Jr, Stewart JR: Mediastinal tap as useful method for the early diagnosis of mediastinal infection. *Surg Gynecol Obstetr* 159:79–82, 1984.

58. Shaffer HA, Valenzuela G, Mittal RK: Esophageal perforation. *Arch Intern Med* 152:757–761, 1992.

59. Sherrick AD, Brown LR, Harms GF, Myers JL: The radiographic findings of fibrosing mediastinitis. *Chest* 106:484–489, 1994.

60. Trastek VF: Esophageal perforation: A reassessment of the criteria for choosing medical or surgical therapy. *Arch Intern Med* 152:693, 1992.

61. Wheatley MJ, Stirling MC, Kirsh MM, et al: Descending necrotizing mediastinitis: Transcervical drainage is not enough. *Ann Thorac Surg* 49:780–784, 1990.

C H A P T E R   1 3 2

BRONCHIECTASIS

Morton N. Swartz

Bronchiectasis is a chronic abnormal dilatation and distortion of bronchi caused by destruction of the elastic and muscular components of the bronchial walls. This is basically an anatomic definition. Usual clinical features include those of chronic or recurrent pulmonary infections: cough, copious mucopurulent sputum, and fetid breath. Dilatation of bronchi can also occur in chronic bronchitis. Distinction between the two processes is a matter of the degree and extent of the abnormality (milder and more generalized in chronic bronchitis). True bronchiectasis is permanent and should be distinguished from the reversible changes of pneumonia, tracheobronchitis, and atelectasis; these disorders may cause abnormalities on bronchography simulating bronchiectasis if this procedure is performed during or shortly after the acute pulmonary process.[42,44]

PREVALENCE

Bronchiectasis, a common disabling and often fatal illness in the preantibiotic era, has become a comparatively rare disease over the past 3 decades in developed countries.[3,4] This change stems, in large measure, from the greater availability of antibiotics for the treatment of respiratory tract infections and from the widespread use of immunization in childhood, particularly against pertussis and measles. For a group of children's hospitals in the United Kingdom, Field found that the admission rate for patients with bronchiectasis had decreased from about 48 per 10,000 admissions to about 10 per 10,000 admissions between 1952 and 1960.[16] At the Boston Children's Hospital, the number of new cases of bronchiectasis associated with infection (pneumonia, pertussis, measles, etc.) seen in a 5-year period (1946 to 1950) had declined from 47 to only 2 cases a decade later (1956 to 1960). At the Massachusetts General Hospital, the number of patients with bronchiectasis per 10,000 admissions declined from 45 in 1947 to about 9 in 1984; in the decade from 1979 to 1988, the number of annual admissions of patients with the diagnosis of bronchiectasis (all types other than those with underlying cystic fibrosis) remained relatively constant at 30 to 60 per year.[48]

PATHOLOGY

The abnormal bronchial dilatation in bronchiectasis principally affects the medium-sized bronchi but extends to the more distal bronchi and bronchioles as well.[36] The airways are markedly dilated, sometimes as much as four times their normal diameter. On gross examination, the bronchi and bronchioles are usually so prominent as to be visible all the way to the pleural surface (Fig. 132-1). This is in contrast to the normal lung, in which the bronchioles can be followed by gross dissection only to a point 2 to 3 cm from the pleura. Bronchiectatic segments commonly are filled with purulent secretions, and the mucosal surface is swollen, inflamed, and often ulcerated.[52] The bronchial epithelial lining may have a "polypoid" appearance as a result of prominent subjacent granulation tissue formation. Further distortion of

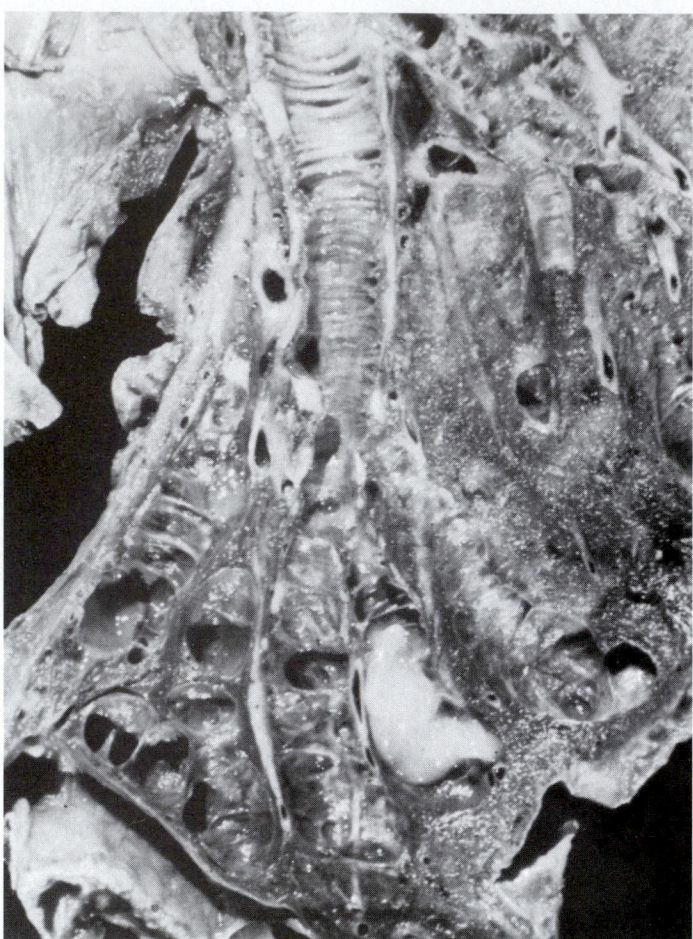

FIGURE 132-1   Severe saccular bronchiectasis with atelectasis and consolidation and cystic bronchi extending close to pleural surface.

the bronchial lumen is produced by exaggerated, transverse ridging of the encircling bronchial smooth muscle (Fig. 132-2) and by the pitted appearance caused by dilated bronchial mucous glands and ducts. With severe and extensive impairment, an almost cystic pattern is evident on the cut surface of the lungs (Figs. 132-1 and 132-3) and may be evident on chest radiograph. As infection continues and spreads in the bronchial wall, the epithelial lining is denuded and elastic tissue, smooth muscle, and

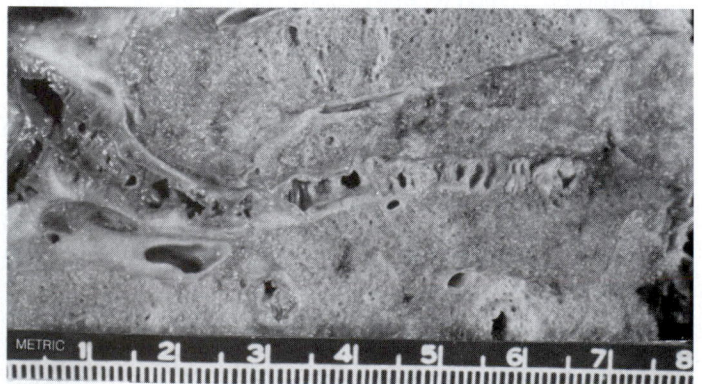

FIGURE 132-2   Gross section of lung showing cylindric bronchiectasis. The dilated bronchus with thick intraluminal secretions and thickened walls shows transverse ridging due to muscle and cartilage changes.

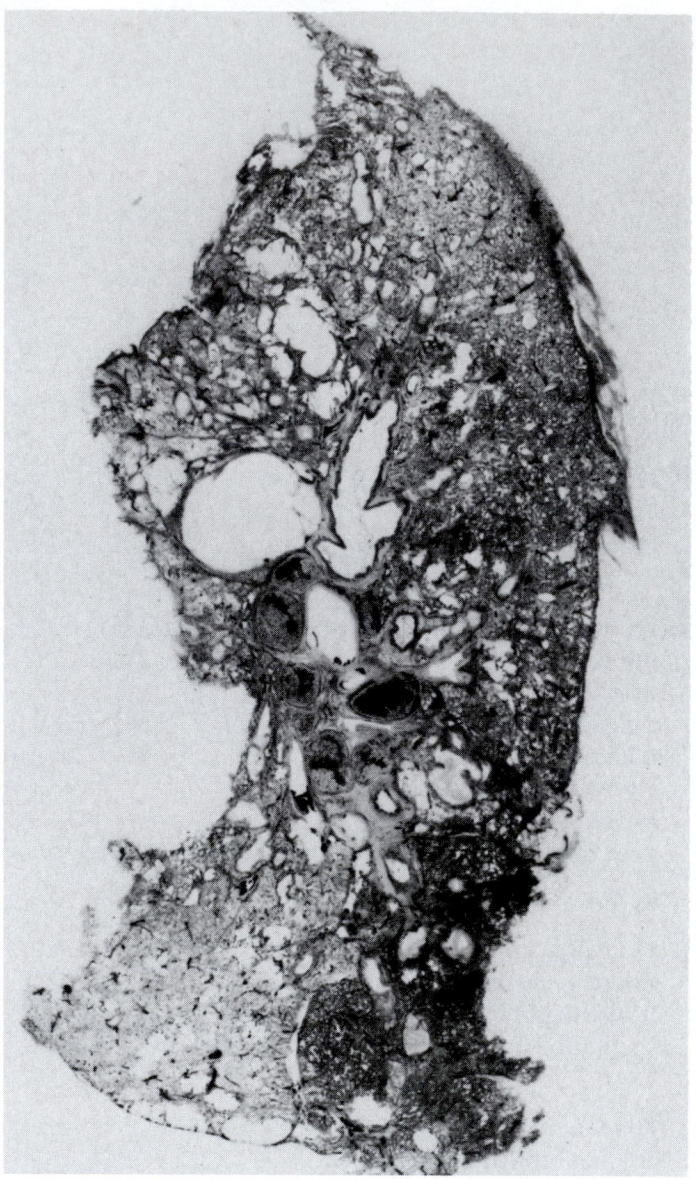

FIGURE 132-3   Gough section of lung of 59-year-old patient with a long history of recurrent pneumonias and chronic bronchiectasis who died with corpulmonale. Enlarged hilar nodes and severe bronchiectasis, particularly in the midlung fields, are evident. Large sacs, up to 4 cm in diameter, appear grossly to be continuous with the bronchi.

even surrounding cartilage are distorted and destroyed (Fig. 132-4).[37] Focal lung abscesses may develop as a result of the necrotic process beginning in the bronchial walls. In more chronic bronchiectasis, marked fibrosis occurs in and surrounding bronchial walls, replacing muscle, mucous glands, and cartilage.

Circulatory changes may develop in the lung as a consequence of bronchiectasis. Morphologically, bronchial arteries may be considerably enlarged (up to three times their normal caliber of 1.5 mm) and tortuous in patients with extensive bronchiectasis. This is believed due to the development of extensive anastomoses between the bronchial and pulmonary arterial circulations at the precapillary levels in the extensive granulation tissue in the walls of bronchiectatic airways. Evidence for such collateral circulation has been found on pathologic examination of bronchiectatic

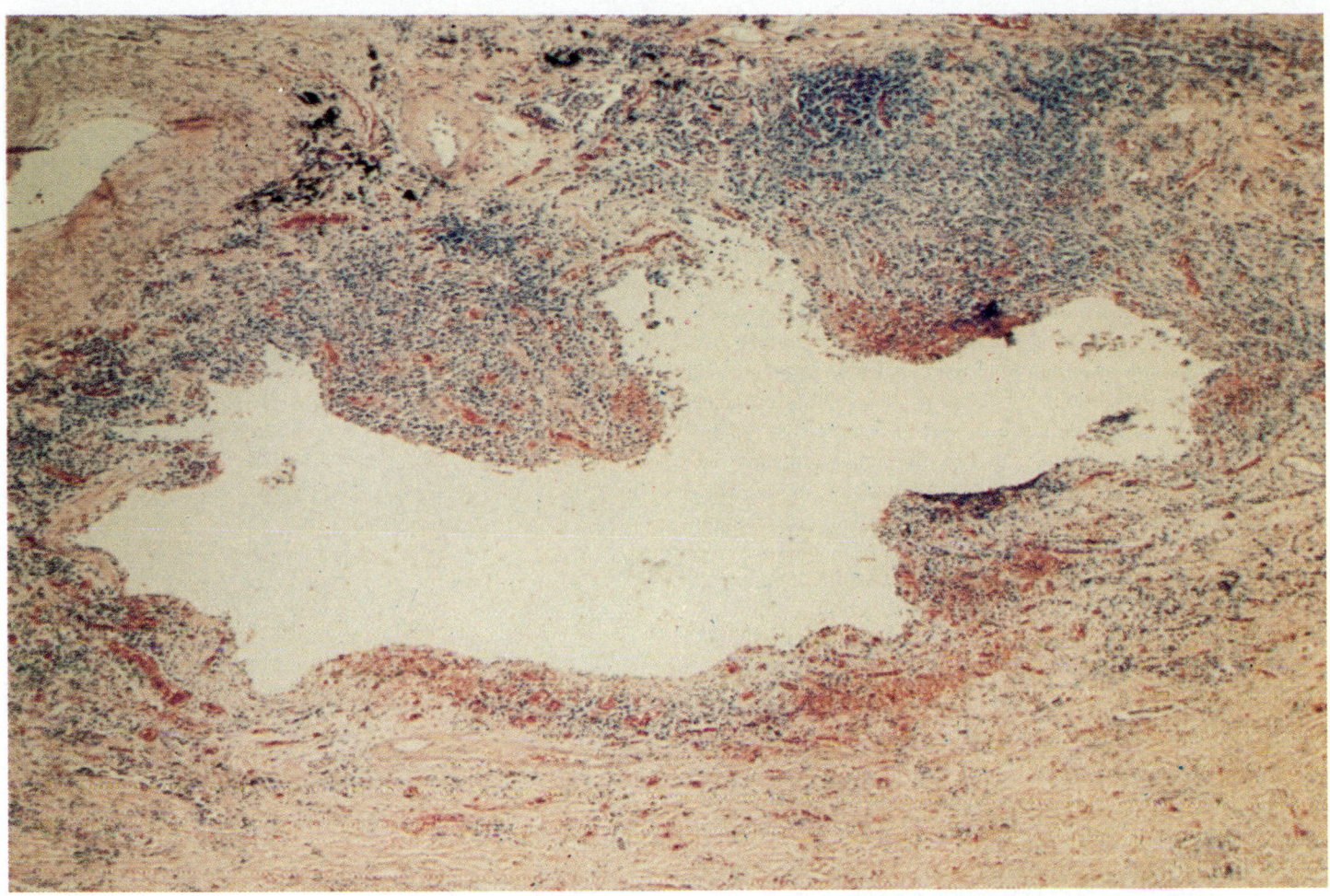

FIGURE 132-4 Microscopic section of lung of patient with bronchiectasis. Lining of small bronchus is totally denuded of surface epithelium. There is extensive surrounding inflammation with numerous capillaries and polypoid excrescences extending into the lumen. H&E, ×100.

lung and by angiographic demonstration of bronchopulmonary anastomoses.[30] Once such anastomotic channels are sufficiently enlarged, shunting of oxygenated blood from the higher-pressure systemic bronchial (or intercostal) arteries into the lower-pressure pulmonary circulation occurs. Measurement of such aortopulmonary collateral flow by dye dilution methods indicates that it may amount to 3 to 12 percent of pulmonary flow. The extent of collateral flow roughly correlates with the extent of bronchiectasis.

Bronchiectasis is bilateral in about 30 percent of patients (more frequently in patients with underlying cystic fibrosis). The lower lobes are most frequently invaded. The left lower lobe is affected more than three times as frequently as the right, particularly in children. This may be because the right bronchus is more readily drained by virtue of being a continuation of the trachea, there is slight compression of the left bronchus where it is crossed by the left pulmonary artery, and the left bronchus is narrower than the right. In 50 to 80 percent of patients with bronchiectasis of the left lower lobe severe enough to have warranted resection, the lingula was affected as well. In left lower-lobe bronchiectasis, the segmental impairment is unequal (i.e., the posterior basal segment is almost always diseased and the apical segment is spared in 75 percent of cases).

The particular lobes affected may sometimes bear a relationship to the underlying predisposition. For example, when bronchiectasis develops as a consequence of foreign-body aspiration, it is more likely to occur on the right and in the lower lobes or in the posterior segments of the upper lobe. Central (perihilar) bronchial impairment is a characteristic of bronchiectasis due to allergic pulmonary aspergillosis (APA). Invasion of the upper-lobe bronchi (along with others) may more often be a feature of bronchiectasis due to APA, cystic fibrosis in the adult, or tuberculosis than of usual bronchiectasis.

Classification

Bronchiectasis may be classified in a variety of ways: by pathogenetic mechanisms or predisposing factors, by bronchographic findings, and by gross and microscopic appearance on pathologic examination. All provide valuable information for the clinician and insights into pathogenesis and pathophysiological consequences. Since the investigations of Reid in 1950 provided a correlation between bronchographic findings and pathologic (gross and microscopic) changes in resected bronchiectatic lobes, it is described here.[36] It is the most widely used classification employed by pulmonologists, radiologists, and pathologists. Classification of bronchiectasis by predisposing factors is considered in a later section.

CYLINDRIC BRONCHIECTASIS

On bronchogram, the bronchi are regularly outlined (tubular) and not greatly increased in diameter; their walls are straight. The affected bronchi come to an abrupt, squared end instead of tapering (Fig. 132-5). The anatomic changes occurring in the bronchial tree can also be evaluated by examining the number of subdivisions of the bronchial tree in the bronchiectatic segment (e.g., posterior basal segment of the left lower lobe) extending down to the respiratory bronchioles leading to the costal surface. In the normal adult lung, the posterior basal bronchus has approximately 20 subdivisions, and this number is roughly the same in cylindric bronchiectasis of the same pulmonary segment. Although the number of subdivisions in cylindric bronchiectasis appears normal as viewed from dissection and microscopic examination of excised lobes, on bronchography before surgical resection the number of subdivisions is markedly reduced. This discrepancy stems from obstruction to filling by radiocontrast material caused by thick secretions, bronchial casts, and inflammatory edema of the bronchial walls of the peripheral bronchial tree.

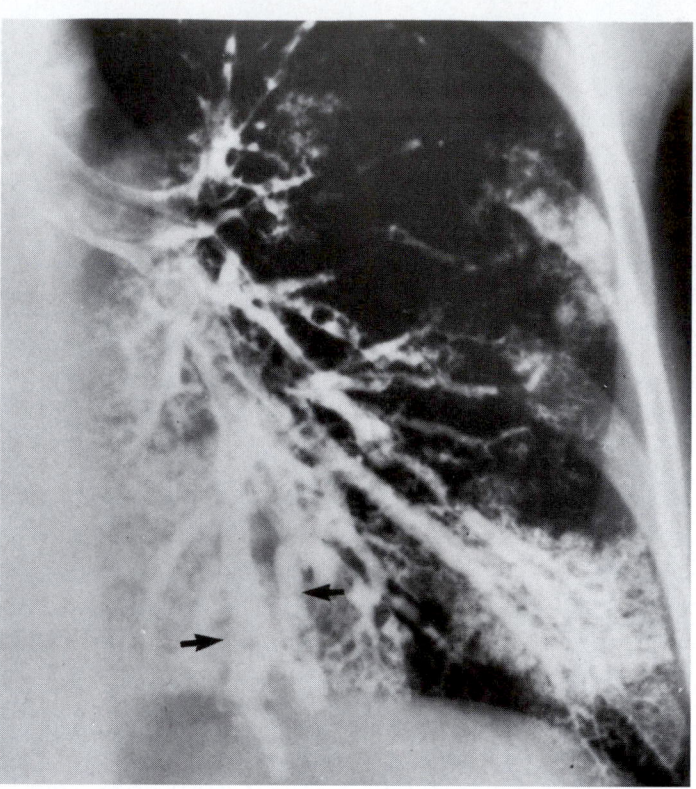

FIGURE 132-6 Bronchogram showing varicose bronchiectasis of basal segments of left lower-lobe (arrows). *(Courtesy of Dr. T. McLoud.)*

VARICOSE BRONCHIECTASIS

On bronchogram, the bronchi are generally dilated and irregular in form and size. Unlike normal bronchi, they do not taper in diameter as they extend peripherally. Their terminations are distorted and characteristically bulbous (Fig. 132-6). Their irregular bulging contour is highly reminiscent of the appearance of saphenous varicosities. The average number of bronchial divisions is reduced on microscopic examination to about half the number present in the normal lung. In many areas, the bronchial lumen is totally obliterated by fibrous tissue containing bundles of muscle fibers, elastic tissue, and even remnants of the cartilaginous plates of the former bronchial wall. This fibrotic replacement of bronchial lumen may extend for a short distance; farther on, the peripheral remnants of the bronchial tree may be distinguishable. Some of the distal bronchial remnants become epithelium-lined, fluid-filled cysts. In other areas, medium-sized bronchi terminate in dense fibrous tissue that extends cordlike along the route of the former bronchus.

SACCULAR (CYSTIC) BRONCHIECTASIS

On bronchogram, the bronchi are dilated, and this ballooning in outline (Fig. 132-7) increases as they progress to the lung periphery almost to the pleural surface. The examination is sharply reduced (one-fourth to one-fifth the number found normally). Saccular bronchiectasis was once thought to invade smaller bronchioles because of the location of the bronchiectatic pus-filled cavities (saccules) adjacent to the pleura. However, this view is

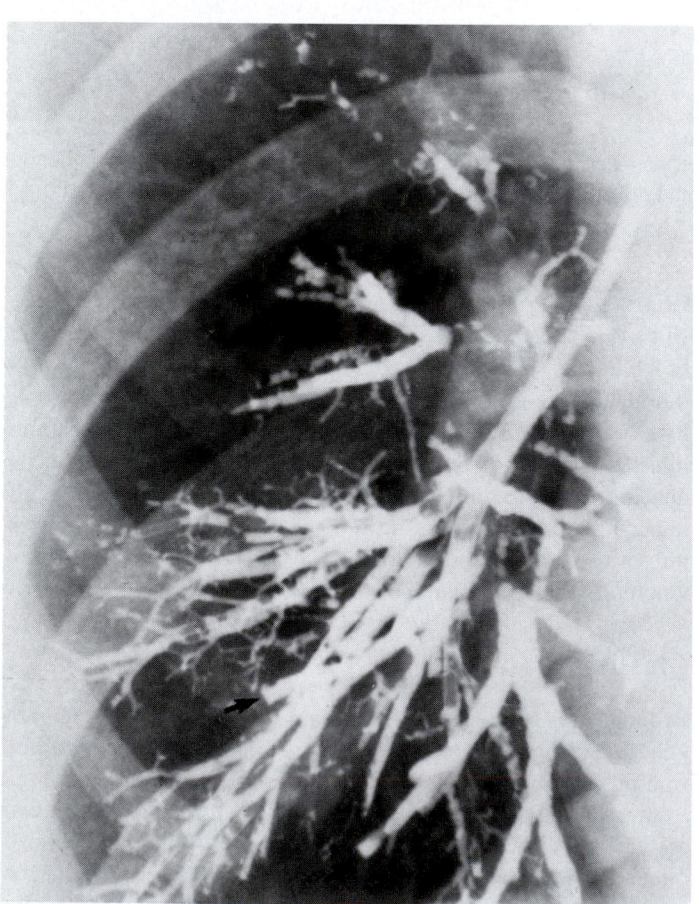

FIGURE 132-5 Bronchogram demonstrating cylindric bronchiectasis in some lower-lobe bronchi. Note the mild increase in diameter and blunt squared ends of bronchi (arrows). *(Courtesy of Dr. T. McLoud.)*

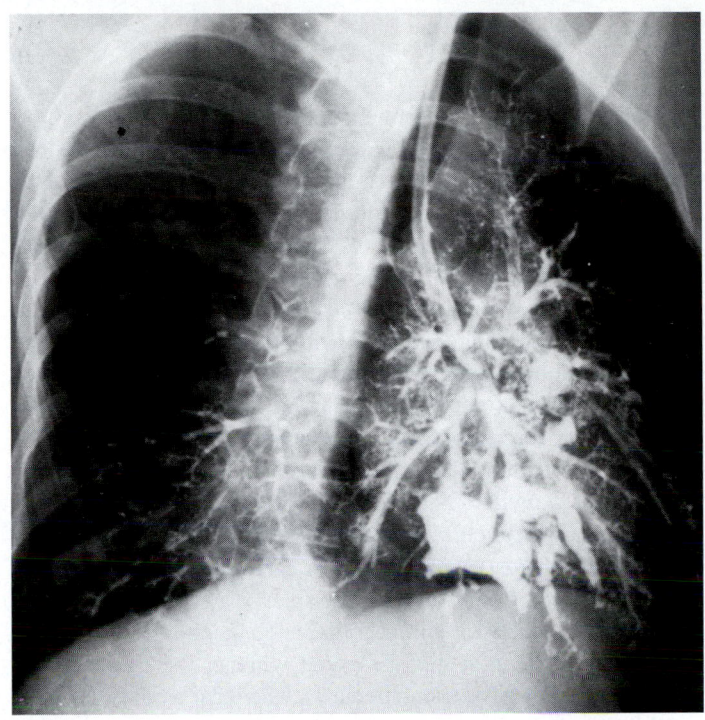

A

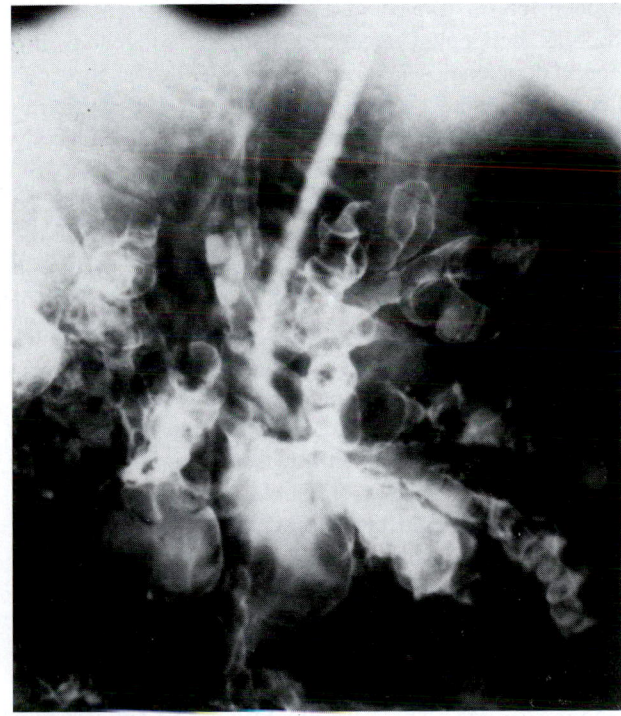

B

FIGURE 132-7   Bronchograms showing saccular (cystic) bronchiectasis. *A.* Saccular bronchiectasis of left lower lobe in a young man. *(Courtesy of Dr. C. Hales.) B.* Severe saccular bronchiectatic changes shown on this close-up were widespread in both lungs. *(Courtesy of Dr. T. McLoud.)*

not supported by the findings on pathologic examination of resected lobes, in which the fifth subdivision (there are 20 subdivisions in the normal lung) of the dilated bronchial tree is the terminal one, ending blindly immediately subjacent to the pleura.[10] The "saccules" are the terminations of the diseased segments of the bronchial tree, with all the more peripheral branches destroyed beyond recognition or totally fibrosed. The larger presaccular bronchi are not dilated despite marked inflammation in the bronchial walls. The most prominent change in these bronchi is polyposis of bronchial epithelium, with numerous large fronds often causing bronchial obstruction. The saccular shape of the bronchiectatic airways probably results from extension of the inflammation of the bronchial walls to supporting structures and surrounding pulmonary parenchyma, which are destroyed or undergo fibrosis, and partial obstruction of presaccular bronchi by polyposis of its mucosa, preventing drainage of the saccular bronchi, which become distended with pus. Squamous metaplasis is common in saccular bronchiectasis but uncommon in other forms of bronchiectasis.

Other Pathologically Defined Forms of Bronchiectasis or Pathologically Similar Conditions

FOLLICULAR BRONCHIECTASIS

Follicular bronchiectasis is defined from strictly histologic criteria rather than on clinical or radiographic grounds. The most prominent feature is the formation of lymphoid follicles and nodes in the walls of bronchi and bronchioles and in adjacent pulmonary parenchyma. Hilar lymph node enlargement is usually present. Involvement may be localized to a single bronchopulmonary segment or may include an entire lobe or several lobes. Associated with lymph follicle formation, elastic tissue is lost; with more extensive involvement, widespread destruction of smooth muscle and cartilage follows. Subepithelial lymph follicles produce partial obstruction of bronchial lumina and compress the openings of peripheral branches of diseased bronchi. The principal lesions develop in smaller bronchi, bronchioles, and adjacent alveoli. With more extensive inflammation, the distal bronchial tree is obliterated and the more proximal bronchi become involved, with destruction of surrounding supporting tissues. Mucous gland ducts enlarge as a result of this circumbronchial necrosis and form part of the weakened bronchial or bronchiolar wall. Interstitial pneumonia is very often present as well. The bronchographic picture can be that of any of the three types of bronchiectasis described above, depending on the severity of the process. Follicular bronchiectasis has been described primarily as a consequence of either a childhood viral infection (measles, adenovirus, or herpes simplex) or a bacterial infection (pertussis or a primary bronchopneumonia).

Follicular bronchiectasis may be accompanied by prominent lymphoid bronchiolectasis. The latter should be distinguished from another process, follicular bronchitis-bronchiolitis, which is characterized by abundant peribronchiolar lymph follicles compressing the bronchiolar lumen to a slitlike opening, acute purulent exudate in the bronchiolar lumen, and disruption of the reticular layer of the bronchiolar wall in the absence of chronic obstructive pulmonary disease or bronchiectasis. Follicular bronchitis-bronchiolitis occurs in the setting of collagen vascular disease (particularly rheumatoid arthritis and Sjögren's syndrome), immunodeficiency syndromes, and hypersensitivity states with eosinophilia.

TRACTION BRONCHIECTASIS

"Traction bronchiectasis" can occur in patients with diffuse pulmonary fibrosis of any cause as a result of strong retroactive forces from the fibrous tissue and elevated negative intrapleural pressure pulling on and dilating the airways. On CT imaging, the dilated bronchi have a characteristic corkscrew appearance. The other features of usual bronchiectasis are lacking. Since traction bronchiectasis has a different pathogenesis, one in which intrinsic airway disease is not implicated, it probably should be considered a separate entity apart from true bronchiectasis.

CONGENITAL BRONCHIAL CYSTS OR CONGENITAL (BRONCHIAL) CYSTIC DISEASE

These congenital cysts in the pulmonary parenchyma represent developmentally abnormal bronchial wall structures, partly or completely filled with mucus and lined by respiratory tract epithelium. Histologically, they may mimic bronchiectasis. They occur in two forms. The first is the *central congenital cyst*. These cysts are usually solitary, lack connection with their parent bronchus, and do not communicate with the distal alveolar parenchyma. The lumen is lined with respiratory epithelium, and the walls contain mucous glands, elastic tissue, muscle, and cartilage. If they become infected, communication with the proximal tracheobronchial tree may be established. Under these circumstances, the intraluminal mucus is replaced by pus, and the cysts may become distended with air as a result of a check-valve mechanism. The second type is the *peripheral congenital cyst*. These cysts are frequently multiple and represent a defect in bronchial maturation at a later stage in fetal development. They usually lack mucous glands, are lined by nonciliated columnar epithelium, and contain serous fluid; their walls contain much elastic tissue and a few abnormal cartilaginous plates. If infection occurs in these cysts, their congenital nature may be completely obscured, and the process resembles bronchiectasis by virtue of the inflammation, loss of respiratory epithelium, and apparent loss of much of the supporting cartilage.

INTRALOBAR BRONCHOPULMONARY SEQUESTRATION

This congenital malformation consists of a detached segment of pulmonary tissue, adjoining normal lung and covered by the same visceral pleura, which receives its blood supply from an anomalous artery taking origin from the aorta or one of its branches. Pneumonia in the sequestered segment is common in adults. The affected area contains cystic spaces that are lined by ciliated columnar or flattened epithelium and are filled with mucus or, when infected, pus. Ordinarily, since there is no normal bronchial connection with the sequestered lung, the latter does not contain air. With infection, communication often develops between the cystic, sequestered area of lung and the bronchial tree. Inflammatory cells are present in the cyst walls, which lack cartilage (a bronchial wall component often totally obliterated in bronchiectasis) and mucous glands.

PATHOGENESIS AND PREDISPOSING FACTORS

The proximate cause of bronchiectasis is almost universally a necrotizing infection (or a sequence of infections) in the tracheobronchial walls and surrounding pulmonary parenchyma. In years past, since its manifestations first appeared in childhood, bronchiectasis was considered to be predominantly a congenital disease due to some anatomic or functional abnormality of bronchi and bronchioles that predisposed to chronic infection. It now appears that "congenital" bronchiectasis is quite rare and due to definable abnormalities in tracheobronchial cartilage structure, defects in ciliary structure and function, alterations in the character of upper respiratory tract mucus, etc. (Table 132-1).[29] The sharp decline in the prevalence of bronchiectasis following the introduction of modern antimicrobial therapy and widespread use of immunization for childhood diseases strongly suggests that infection per se is responsible for most cases of this disease. Such a steep decline in frequency over the span of a few decades would be difficult to reconcile with a putative congenital defect.

The question might then be asked whether there exists such an entity as congenital bronchiectasis. The term would most reasonably be applied to the small number of cases of congenital or hereditary disorders in which there is a high incidence of secondary bronchiectasis (Table 132-1). Even with such predisposing factors as congenital anatomic defects, congenital immunoglobulin deficiencies, and respiratory tract dysfunction due to hereditary ciliary defects, cystic fibrosis, or α_1-antitrypsin deficiency, the associated bronchiectasis is thought to develop early in childhood rather than being present at birth.

The basic element in the development of ordinary acquired bronchiectasis appears to be inflammatory destruction of the components (elastic tissue, smooth muscle, cartilage) of the bronchial wall (see "Pathology," above).[52] As a consequence of this inflammatory reaction, alterations develop in the configuration of the affected bronchi secondary to pressure changes occurring on respiration and coughing as well as secondary to peribronchial fibrosis. The result is the distortion and ballooning of the diseased bronchi. A requirement for such a definition of acquired bronchiectasis is microscopic evidence of inflammatory destruction of the walls of ectatic bronchi. The term *congenital bronchiectasis* might reasonably apply, then, in infants and young children to regional clusters of ectatic bronchi whose walls show no significant evidence of inflammation. Culiner considered three congenital processes characterized by areas of dilated or cystic bronchi (*bronchial cysts, intralobar pulmonary sequestration,* and *congenital cystic bronchiectasis*) to be variants of a single group of anomalies.[10] In congenital cystic bronchiectasis, in contrast to the other two entities, the bronchial cysts are not usually isolated from the remainder of the bronchial tree but represent ectatic bronchial canalization in continuity with normal segmental bronchi. Lower lobes from children with such anomalies and lacking evidence of inflammation have occasionally been observed and might qualify for the designation *congenital bronchiectasis*. With time, infection develops in these areas, eliminating mural inflammation as a discriminant between acquired and congenital bronchiectasis.

TABLE 132-1

Predisposing Factors for Bronchiectasis

Categories	Specific Entities
Bronchopulmonary infections	
Childhood diseases	Pertussis; measles
Other bacterial infections	Infections due to *S. aureus, Klebsiella, M. tuberculosis, H. influenzae*
Other viral infections	Infections due to adenovirus (particularly types 7 and 21), influenza, herpes simplex; viral bronchiolitis; HIV
Miscellaneous infections	Mycotic infections (histoplasmosis); ? mycoplasmal infections; nontuberculous mycobacteria
Bronchial obstruction	
Foreign-body aspiration	Peanut; chicken bone; grass inflorescence, etc.
Neoplasms	Laryngeal papillomatosis; adenomas; bronchogenic carcinoma
Hilar adenopathy	Tuberculosis; histoplasmosis; sarcoid
Mucoid impaction	Allergic bronchopulmonary aspergillosis; bronchocentric granulomatosis; postoperative mucoid impaction
Chronic obstructive pulmonary disease	Chronic bronchitis; bronchial asthma
Acquired tracheobronchial disease	Relapsing polychondritis; tracheobronchial amyloidosis
Congenital anatomic defects	
Tracheobronchial	Bronchomalacia; bronchial cysts; cartilage deficiency (Williams-Campbell syndrome); tracheobronchomegaly (Mounier-Kuhn syndrome); ectopic bronchus; endobronchial teratoma; tracheoesophageal fistula
Vascular	Pulmonary (intralobar) sequestration; pulmonary artery aneurysm
Lymphatic	Yellow-nail syndrome
Immunodeficiency states	
IgG deficiency	Congenital (Bruton's type) agammaglobulinemia; selective deficiency of subclasses (IgG_2, IgG_4); acquired immune globulin deficiency; common variable hypogammaglobulinemia; Nezelof's syndrome; "bare lymphocyte" syndrome
IgA deficiency	Selective IgA deficiency ± ataxia-telangiectasia syndrome
Leukocyte dysfunction	Chronic granulomatous disease
Hereditary abnormalities	
Ciliary defects of respiratory mucosa	Kartagener's syndrome; immotile cilia syndrome; ciliary dyskinesis
α_1-Antitrypsin deficiency	Production of abnormal antitrypsin molecules; failure of gene transcription
Cystic fibrosis (mucoviscidosis)	Typical early childhood syndrome; adolescent presentation with solely pulmonary symptoms
Miscellaneous disorders	
Young's syndrome	Obstructive azoospermia with sinopulmonary infections
Recurrent aspiration pneumonias	Alcoholism; neurologic disorders; lipoid pneumonia
Inhalation of irritants	Ammonia, nitrogen dioxide, or other irritant gases; smoke; talc; silicates; detergents
Following combined heart-lung transplantation	Associated with obliterative bronchiolitis
Connective-tissue disease	Associated with rheumatoid arthritis and Sjögren's syndrome

A genetic predisposition to bronchiectasis has been suggested by its apparently greater incidence in certain racial groups.[11] In the United States, the prevalence of bronchiectasis is about 60 per 100,000 population. Among Polynesians in Western Samoa the incidence, based on detection of gross disease by radiologic screening, is an order of magnitude higher. Similarly, the annual incidence rate of bronchiectasis among native Alaska Indians and Inuits is high—6.8 cases per 10,000 children aged up to 10 years, compared to 1.06 per 10,000 children in Scotland. However, factors other than ethnic ones may play the primary role in these geographic areas: inadequate diet, crowded living conditions (contributing to increased numbers of respiratory infections), and lack of medical attention and antimicrobial therapy (allowing progression of acute bronchopulmonary infections to a chronic destructive state). At present, such issues preclude assigning any specific role of genetic factors to these cases of bronchiectasis. It is of interest to note, however, that abnormal cilia have been observed on electron microscopic examination of respiratory tract epithelium of a high percentage of Polynesians with bronchiectasis. Dextrocardia, however, is not associated with bronchiectasis in these patients.

Infections

In the first half of the century, before extensive immunization against pertussis and measles, a variety of pulmonary infections during childhood were associated with subsequent bronchiectasis (Table 132-1). Severe preceding lower respiratory infections have been reported in as many as 69 percent of cases of childhood bronchiectasis, whereas antecedent aspirational events occurred in 16 percent, and the predisposing factor in the remaining 15 percent was a congenital disorder. Studies by Ogilvie earlier in this century suggested that the initiating infection is not necessarily a severe one: in 66 percent of cases, the symptoms of bronchiectasis dated from the first 5 years of life, and in 43 percent of the cases the onset had been insidious and could not be related to any specific event.[34]

In a compilation of 10 series of cases of bronchiectasis in children and adults from this country and abroad published between 1935 and 1989, antecedent infections were the underlying predisposing causes in the majority—about 70 percent (pneumonia, 32 percent; pertussis, 10 percent; measles, 11 percent; tuberculosis, 16 percent).[7,42] Of the remainder, other predisposing conditions were hypogammaglobulinemia (6 percent), foreign-body and other aspirational events (5 percent), and Kartagener's syndrome (1 percent). Since this compilation included patients with bronchiectasis from the earlier part of this century and from abroad, there is a disproportionate representation of certain infections (e.g., tuberculosis, measles, pertussis) that would not now have so prominent a role in this country. Indeed, predisposing conditions in patients with bronchiectasis admitted to the Massachusetts General Hospital from 1979 to 1988, reviewed by Trucksis and Swartz, included a smaller percentage of infections (particularly tuberculosis), a lower incidence of hypogammaglobulinemia, and a far greater prominence of cystic fibrosis (Table 132-2).[48]

MEASLES

The association of measles with bronchiectasis is much less prominent now in the United States than formerly.[27] In the 1960s and 1970, 14 percent of cases of childhood bronchiectasis appeared to have been associated with antecedent measles. In underdeveloped countries, this association is currently much more prominent. Follicular bronchiectasis is generally considered to be a complication of measles, pertussis, or influenza viral pneumonia. The presence of extensive peribronchial inflammation as well as striking proliferation of bronchial and bronchiolar epithelium in fatal cases of measles pneumonia is consistent with the concept of acute bronchial damage that might progress to follicular bronchiectasis. In children dying within a month of onset of measles, other causes of complicating necrotizing bronchopneumonia have been observed. These include infections due to adenovirus, herpesvirus, and bacteria (*Staphylococcus aureus, Klebsiella, Pseudomonas*). In other children recovering from such infections, the bronchial damage is presumed to lead to varying de-

TABLE 132-2

Predisposing Conditions for Bronchiectasis: Massachusetts General Hospital (1979–88)

Categories	Specific Entities	Patients (%)
Infections		16
Childhood infections	Pertussis	4
Necrotizing pneumonia	*S. aureus*	1
	K. pneumoniae	1
	M. tuberculosis	8
Miscellaneous	Histoplasma	1
	P. carinii	1
Obstruction	Bronchogenic carcinoma	4
Immunodeficiency states	IgA deficiency	1
Hereditary abnormalities		33
Cystic fibrosis	31	
Ciliary defects; Kartagener's syndrome		1
α_1-antitrypsin deficiency		1
Miscellaneous	Young's syndrome	1
Unknown origin		45
		100

SOURCE: Modified from Trucksis and Swartz,[48] with permission.

grees of follicular bronchiectasis, accentuated by subsequent lower respiratory tract infections.

PERTUSSIS

Secondary necrotizing bacterial pneumonia is an important factor in the development of bronchiectasis following whooping cough. However, pertussis itself can produce a necrotizing bronchitis. In the course of pertussis, inspissated mucus and debris may produce resorptive atelectasis in infants and young children and serve as an additional contributing factor in postpertussis bronchiectasis.

OTHER BACTERIAL PULMONARY INFECTIONS

The bacterial pneumonias that appear to predispose to the development of subsequent bronchiectasis are usually necrotizing processes due to species such as *S. aureus, Klebsiella pneumoniae,* and *Pseudomonas aeruginosa.* Lobar pneumonia due to *Streptococcus pneumoniae,* which is not ordinarily destructive of tissue and heals without significant scarring, is not likely to render the bronchial tree susceptible to subsequent bronchiectasis. *S. pneumoniae,* however, may colonize the bronchial tree in some patients with bronchiectasis. *Hemophilus influenzae* type b can cause invasive pneumonias in infants and children but appears to play no important role in bronchiectasis. On the other hand, unencapsulated *H. influenzae* is very often present in the sputa of patients with bronchiectasis, as colonizers, and also as contributors to chronic progressive infection of the bronchial tree. *Moraxella (Branhamella) catarrhalis* may have a similar role as a colonizer in bronchiectasis.

Necrotizing Pneumonia due to Anaerobic Bacteria

Anaerobic necrotizing pneumonia is usually of aspirational origin or a consequence of bronchial obstruction. The necrotizing nature of the process is reflected by the frequent progression to parenchymal destruction (pulmonary gangrene), lung abscess, putrid empyema, and, in some instances, chronic bronchiectasis. The bacteria responsible consist of a mixture of facultative and obligately anaerobic species indigenous to the oral cavity.

Tuberculosis

The pathogenesis of so-called tuberculous bronchiectasis may take several forms.[39] 1. A marked degree of caseation necrosis of bronchial walls can occur, particularly when upper lobes are invaded. Tuberculous granulomatous inflammation can be observed at the distal end of some saccular lesions, suggesting that, at least in some cases, bronchiectasis represents extension of an initial tuberculous bronchitis. 2. Scarring of an initial tuberculous involvement of larger bronchi can produce bronchial stenosis. Mixed bacterial infection and retained purulent secretions can then produce bronchiectasis as might occur following any other type of bronchial obstruction. 3. Extraluminal obstruction of larger bronchi by tuberculous hilar lymphadenopathy can produce the same consequences as intraluminal obstruction and result in bronchiectasis. As with bronchostenotic tuberculosis, the inflammatory destruction of bronchial walls is in large measure related to bacterial infection (indigenous upper respiratory tract

flora or superimposed pyogens such as *S. aureus*) rather than to *Mycobacterium tuberculosis.* 4. A rare but important cause of bronchial obstruction is penetration by a calcified tuberculous node into the airway and broncholith formation. 5. Some or all of the bronchiectatic sacs in the upper lobes may represent healing or healed tuberculous cavities that have become partly relined with ciliated epithelium. Such cavities may or may not have established continuity with the bronchial tree. *Mycobacterium avium-intracellulare* (MAI) has recently been associated with bronchiectasis in apparently normal hosts or in persons with emphysema. In some patients, bronchiectasis appears to be a consequence of primary MAI infection; in other patients with pre-existing bronchiectasis, it seems to be a secondary invader, contributing to progressive disease; and in others it seems to be a "colonizer" in areas of bronchiectasis with little, if any, impact on furtherance of the process.

Mycotic Infections

Pulmonary histoplasmosis is probably the best example of a primary pulmonary mycotic infection that can predispose to bronchiectasis. The sequence here is that of hilar lymphadenopathy, bronchial obstruction, and secondary bacterial inflammation, with resultant ectasia of bronchial walls.

Bronchial Obstruction

A variety of mechanisms have been proposed for the development of *atelectatic bronchiectasis,* the form of bronchiectasis associated with bronchial obstruction. It has been suggested that collapse follows bronchial obstruction, and the bronchi proximal to the obstruction would then be subject to strong dilating forces caused by the difference between atmospheric pressure in the bronchi and negative pressure in the pleural space. It was also thought that traction on more distal airways due to the collapse of surrounding, normally cushioning alveoli would contribute to bronchial dilatation following obstruction of peripheral bronchi. Whitwell offered evidence against the latter pathogenetic mechanism from studies of follicular and saccular bronchiectasis in which obstruction of peripheral bronchi was almost uniformly present.[52] In the lung units affected, atelectasis was absent. Collateral air drift or ventilation, the passage of air to alveoli other than by direct airway connections, appeared to account for this. Adequate collateral air circulation is provided under these circumstances by a number of possible routes: Kohn's pores (circular openings in the walls between adjoining alveoli) and canals of Lambert (epithelium-lined tubules between preterminal bronchioles and surrounding alveoli—not only those in normal sequence to the particular preterminal bronchiole but also those normally aerated via other preterminal bronchioles).

Evidence indicates that bronchial obstruction per se does not cause bronchiectasis but, rather, facilitates its development by interfering with bronchial clearance and encouraging bacterial infection. Ligation of bronchi of rabbits, causing bronchi to fill with secretions, does not produce bronchiectasis unless infection occurs spontaneously or is intentionally introduced. Ligation of bronchi of rats, which have indigenous bronchial flora, commonly leads to bronchial infection and bronchiectasis unless infection is initially controlled by appropriate antibiotic administration.

In contrast to the frequency of bronchiectasis following atelectasis and infection secondary to bronchial obstruction, bronchiectasis has been a rarity after collapse of the lung due to hydrothorax or therapeutic pneumothorax. The explanation probably lies in the absence of bronchial infection in the latter.

FOREIGN-BODY BRONCHIECTASIS

Bronchiectasis may develop many years after unrecognized aspiration of a foreign body such as a chicken bone, pipe stem, or peanut. Such postobstructive bronchiectasis is a localized rather than a diffuse process. Bronchiectasis can be produced in animals 2 to 8 weeks after introduction of sterile foreign bodies into the bronchial tree. Obstructive emphysema, atelectasis, and infection precede the development of chronic inflammation and ensuing bronchiectasis.

A particularly difficult-to-diagnose type of foreign-body aspiration in children is that of a grass inflorescence (flowering head). By virtue of being relatively inert, it is less likely to cause immediate respiratory symptoms than is aspiration of an inorganic foreign body or a peanut. Also, the configuration of a grass inflorescence is less likely to completely occlude a bronchus or produce a ball valve obstruction. Such grass heads commonly migrate into segmental bronchi, where they are extremely difficult to visualize on bronchoscopy. Months later, chronic cough, recurrent pneumonias, and hemoptysis herald the development of localized progressive bronchiectasis.

NEOPLASMS

Various endobronchial tumors—such as adenomas, fibromas, chondromas, and carcinomas—can cause partial airway obstruction, leading to localized bronchiectasis. Laryngeal papillomas with papillomatosis of the lower respiratory tract also may produce bronchial obstruction and resultant bronchiectasis.

MUCOID IMPACTION

Allergic Bronchopulmonary Aspergillosis
The principal features of allergic bronchopulmonary aspergillosis (ABPA) are episodic wheezing and bronchial obstruction, recurrent febrile episodes, peripheral blood eosinophilia, intermittent pulmonary infiltrates, and expectoration of mucous plugs containing eosinophils and *Aspergillus* species (usually *A. fumigatus*).[22] Laboratory findings include elevated levels of IgG and serum precipitins against *Aspergillus* antigens, elevated total serum IgE and specific IgE antibodies to *Aspergillus,* and immediate wheal and flare and type III skin test reactivity. Invasive bronchopulmonary aspergillosis does not develop; the fungus remains within the bronchial lumen. The underlying pathogenesis of ABPA appears to be an allergic response to the presence of *Aspergillus* species in the bronchial tree. A type I hypersensitivity reaction, mediated by IgE, is responsible for bronchospasm; a type III (Arthus) reaction, mediated by immune complexes, is thought to be responsible for bronchial and peribronchial inflammation. The latter is manifest radiologically as acute patchy infiltrates, particularly in the upper lobes, and as the so-called tramline shadows, which are transitory and then parallel line densities, probably representing edema of bronchial walls. Cylindric bronchiectasis may complicate ABPA, developing in bronchial segments that have previously been sites of transient infiltrations and sites of *Aspergillus* antigen in mucous plugs (mucoid impaction). The bronchiectasis of ABPA is characteristically a proximal cylindric, segmental bronchiectasis; lesser bronchi and bronchioles are distally more normal than in the pattern generally seen with usual infectious bronchiectasis.

A clinical, serologic (IgG and IgE antibodies to the specific mold implicated), and radiologic picture similar to that of ABPA has been produced by other fungi (e.g., *Curvularia lunata, Helminthosporium, Drechslera hawaiiensis, Fusarium vasinfectum*) in a few instances. Rarely, mucoid impaction of the bronchus is produced not by an allergic reaction to a fungus but by processes such as bronchocentric granulomatosis or fibrinous bronchitis.

Chronic Obstructive Airway Disease
Bronchiectasis can complicate diffuse obstructive airway diseases such as asthma and chronic bronchitis. Hypertrophy of mucous glands and hypersecretion of mucus are characteristic of chronic bronchitis. In the early stages of this disorder, the bronchographic findings are those of incomplete peripheral filling, most likely representing partial or complete obstruction by mucus of the smallest peripheral bronchi. With continued infection and intermittent mucoid impaction, bronchial inflammation can sometimes gradually progress to bronchiectasis.

Congenital Anatomic Defects

Although a congenital basis for most cases of bronchiectasis was suggested by many in the first half of this century, current evidence does not sustain this concept. The congenital anatomic defect may be categorized as tracheobronchial, vascular, or lymphatic.

TRACHEOBRONCHIAL

Congenital Bronchial Cartilage Deficiency (Williams-Campbell Syndrome)
A small number of patients with bronchiectasis develop respiratory symptoms in the first year (or even first weeks) of life as a result of specific anatomic defects.[26,29] Children with the rare Williams-Campbell syndrome have the clinical features of bronchiectasis (persistent cough, sputum production, recurrent pulmonary infections, and clubbing); the bronchographic findings are those of airway dilatations, and radiologic findings are those of dilated air-filled bronchi along with lobar or segmental atelectasis; pulmonary function testing shows hyperinflation with obstruction to expiration on inspiration and almost complete airway collapse on expiration of the second- to eighth-order bronchi.[50] Wheezing (particularly on forced expiration) and dyspnea are more frequent than with other types of bronchiectasis.

Anatomic features of the Williams-Campbell syndrome include deficiency of bronchial cartilage extending proximally to the first and second segmental divisions, but presence of intact cartilaginous plates at bronchial bifurcations out to seventh-order divisions; absence of destruction of other (noncartilaginous) bronchial wall structures by inflammation; and uniform, bilateral distribution of the process. In addition to these anatomic features, which distinguish this process from the more common forms of bronchiectasis, bronchographic findings early in the course of the disease have been much more marked and extensive than would have been anticipated on the basis of the duration and severity of infection. Proximal extension of the bronchiectatic lesions to the second-order bronchi would be most unusual in acquired bronchiectasis and serves to distinguish this disease. Whether true bronchiectasis is present at birth or develops rapidly very early in life as a consequence of congenital bronchomalacia is not known.

Tracheobronchomegaly (Mounier-Kuhn Syndrome)

This very rare disorder of the lower respiratory tract consists of marked dilatation of the trachea and central bronchi, associated with repeated episodes of pulmonary infection.[21] Beyond the involved major bronchi the transition is abrupt to normal-caliber airways. Symmetric saccular bronchiectasis is frequently present. Widening of the tracheal air column is evident on posteroanterior radiographs of the chest. On bronchography, saccular outpouchings of the lumen between the cartilage rings of the dilated trachea and major bronchi are visible. They represent protrusions of redundant mucosa between the transverse bundles of trachealis muscle fibers, which connect the posterior ends of the U-shaped tracheal cartilages.

Limited pathologic study suggests that the underlying process is a primary atrophy of the elastic tissue and smooth muscle of the trachea and major bronchi.

Clinically, most patients with this syndrome present in adult life, but cases have sometimes been diagnosed in infants. The distinctive features are those of tracheobronchomegaly associated with symmetric impairment of the bronchial tree in varicose and saccular bronchiectasis. In addition, the marked pliability of the airways and redundancy of mucosa may produce obstructive airway disease as a consequence of airway collapse during expiration.

VASCULAR

Bronchopulmonary (Intralobar) Sequestration

This topic has been considered above (see "Intralobar Bronchopulmonary Sequestration").

LYMPHATIC

Yellow-Nail Syndrome

This very rare syndrome is a combination of lymphedema of the lower extremities, recurrent pneumonia and bronchiectasis, and yellow discoloration of the nails. No clear common thread has been uncovered to account for this bizarre combination of abnormalities, although some form of lymphatic obstruction has been suggested as contributory to an inability to adequately recover from pulmonary infections. Pathologic examination of excised lobes has shown only advanced stages of conventional bronchiectasis.

Immunodeficiency States

Bronchiectasis is more often associated with defects in humoral than cellular immunity.

IgG DEFICIENCY

Repeated infections with invasive pyogenic bacteria such as pneumococci, streptococci, and H. influenzae characterize X-linked agammaglobulinemia. Bruton's original patient had had 19 episodes of pneumococcal sepsis by 8 years of age. The most common types of infection in patients with this form of immunodeficiency are sinusitis, pneumonia, otitis, bacteremia, meningitis, and furunculosis. If untreated, recurrent episodes of pulmonary infection in boys with this condition often progress to chronic bronchiectasis. Replacement of gamma globulin prevents recurrent infection and the ultimate development of chronic pulmonary disease. Occasionally, children with normal levels of total IgG have selective deficiencies of IgG subclasses (IgG2, IgG4, IgG3) and are subject to recurrent sinopulmonary infection, sometimes progressing to chronic bronchiectasis. Such IgG subclass deficiency should be considered in any child or young adult with otherwise unexplained recurrent sinopulmonary infections and bronchiectasis. Similar problems or pulmonary infections and bronchiectasis occur in patients (male or female) at any age who develop common variable immunodeficiency.

OTHER IMMUNODEFICIENCIES

Recurrent sinopulmonary infections are frequent in patients with selective IgA deficiency. Occasionally, patients go on to develop bronchiectasis, particularly if levels of an IgG subclass (IgG2 or IgG3) are also reduced. The rarer isolated IgE and isolated IgM deficiencies have occasionally been complicated by chronic pulmonary infections and bronchiectasis. The so-called bare lymphocyte syndrome, a failure of lymphocytes to express cell surface histocompatibility antigens (HLA-A, HLA-B, etc.), may, in some patients, be associated with immunodeficiency and be manifest as recurrent sinopulmonary infections and progressive diffuse bronchiectasis.

Recurrent infections occurring in patients with chronic granulomatous disease, a group of disorders characterized by defects in oxygen-dependent neutrophil microbicidal activity, include pneumonia and lung abscess. Pulmonary fibrosis and bronchiectasis may follow a prolonged course of repeated infections. However, bronchiectasis appears to be a less common complication of this disorder than might be expected.

Bacterial pneumonia occurs at an increased frequency in patients with HIV infection, probably related to defects in B-lymphocyte function. In the past few years, bronchiectasis has been seen in adults and children with HIV infection, in the former as a consequence of recurrent episodes of pyogenic pulmonary infection (due to S. pneumoniae, H. influenzae, M. catarrhalis, S. aureus) and in the latter as a complication of lymphocytic interstitial pneumonia (LIP). Among children with LIP (in the setting of HIV infection) and subsequent bronchiectasis, recurrent bacterial superinfections do not appear to be a feature. With LIP the lungs are chronically consolidated with volume loss. Radiologically the picture is that of cylindric bronchiectasis. Pathogenetically, it has been suggested that lymphocytic infiltration into the mucosa and submucosa of the respiratory bronchioles, often as nodular aggregates, results in tissue damage, fibrosis, atelectasis, and ensuing bronchiolar and bronchial dilatation.

Hereditary Abnormalities

An impressive array of genetic defects are associated with clinical syndromes in which bronchiectasis is sometimes a striking feature.

CILIARY DEFECTS OF RESPIRATORY MUCOSA

Immotile Cilia Syndrome (Dyskinetic Cilia Syndrome)

In humans, ciliated epithelium lines the nasal cavity, paranasal sinuses, middle ear, respiratory tract down to the level of the respiratory bronchioles (see Chapter 2), cerebral ventricles, and oviducts; in addition, corneal cells lining the anterior chambers each bear a solitary cilium. In the respiratory tract, coordinated beating of the cilia mechanically assists clearance of the airways of aggregates of bacteria and phagocytic cells. On electron microscopy, cross-sectional structure of the central core (axoneme) of a respiratory tract cilium is highly ordered; nine peripheral pairs of microtubules surround a central microtubular doublet ("9+2 pattern") (Fig. 132-8). Each peripheral pair of microtubules is connected to adjacent doublets by nexin links. Appended symmetrically to the comparable microtubule of each peripheral doublet are two hooklike structures: inner and outer dynein arms. The dynein arms are made up of the protein dynein, which has ATPase activity, and are oriented in a clockwise direction. Surrounding the central pair of tubules is a sheath, and a series of radial spokes connect the central tubules to each of the outer doublets. The same anatomic features are evident in the tails of spermatozoa.

The rhythmic motion of cilia effecting mucociliary transport in the respiratory tract is produced by the linking by dynein arms of one pair of outer tubules to the adjacent doublet and the sliding of actin filaments of the microtubular pairs past each other, much as occurs with actin and myosin in muscle. The hydrolysis of adenosine triphosphate by the dynein ATPase powers this reaction. Since the outer filaments are tied together by nexin links and tied to the central sheath by radial spokes, the sliding of the microtubule pairs is converted to a bending motion of the ciliary shaft. The directing of bending is dictated by the relationship of the peripheral tubules vis-à-vis the central tubules. Coordinated bending of sheets of cilia on respiratory epithelial cells is necessary to move the overlying mucous blanket. This is made possible by orientation of central doublet pairs within 25° of each other.

The immotile cilia syndrome is a genetic disorder (frequently seen among siblings in areas where consanguinity is high) whose molecular lesion produces immotile or otherwise defective cilia.[1,13,40] As a result of the wide distribution of cilia, symptoms produced include sinusitis, otitis, chronic rhinitis, chronic or recurrent bronchitis, bronchiectasis, male sterility, corneal abnormalities (malformations), and impaired olfactory function. The concept of an immotile cilia syndrome stemmed from initial ob-

servations by Petersen and Afzelius in several infertile men of the production of spermatozoa that were living but whose tails were stiff, straight, and immotile.[1,24] The structure of the spermatozoa was relatively normal except for the absence of dynein arms. These patients had had frequent colds, otitis media, and pneumonias, as well as chronic sinusitis and bronchitis, since childhood. Bronchial cilia from such patients had a similar abnormal ultrastructure and absence of dynein arms, and they were immotile.

The criteria for diagnosis of the immotile cilia syndrome include (1) clinical manifestations of recurrent and chronic upper and lower respiratory tract infections such as rhinitis, sinusitis, otitis, bronchitis, and bronchiectasis; (2) absence or near absence of tracheobronchial or nasal mucociliary transport (Fig. 132-9); (3) total or near-total absence of dynein arms

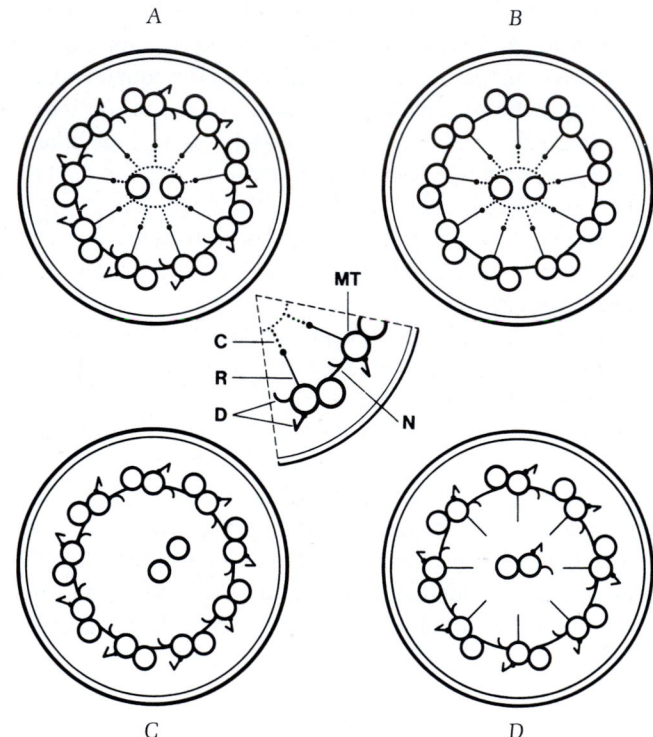

FIGURE 132-8 Schematic cross section views of cilia. *A.* Normal cilium with nine outer pairs of microtubules (MT) distributed symmetrically around a central pair, which is ringed by a central sheath (C). The outer pairs of microtubules are connected to each other by nexin links (N). Radial spokes (R) connect each of the outer pairs to the central sheath. As a consequence of this binding of the pairs of microtubules, their shortening is translated into bending motion. The driving energy for the shortening of the MT is provided by ATP hydrolysis catalyzed by the ATPase located in the dynein arms (outer and inner; designated D in inset). *B* to *D* represent various forms of congenital ciliary defects. *B.* Immotile cilia lacking dynein arms. *C.* Immotile cilia with missing radial spokes; central pair is eccentrically placed. *D.* Another type of cilia (immotile) defect in which the abnormality is a transposition of an outer microtubular pair to the central position. As a result, only eight pairs of microtubules are present in the peripherally placed array. At the more proximal portion of the cilium (near the cell surface), the appearance may be that of nine normal peripheral microtubular pairs without a central pair. Inset indicates various components (MT, C, R, D, N) of the cilial structure. (*Based on data of Davis et al,*[11] *with permission.*)

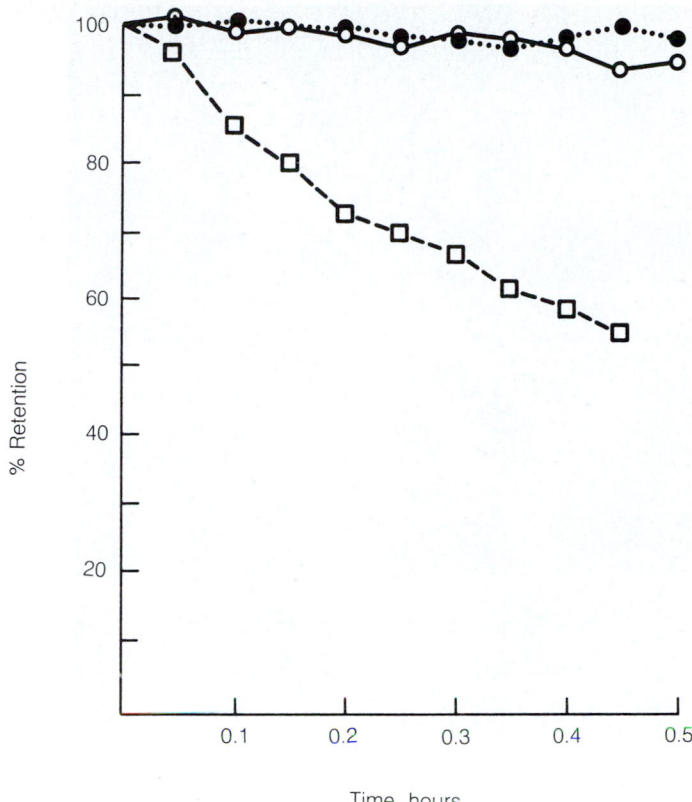

FIGURE 132-9 Nasal mucociliary transport as measured by removal of a 0.02-ml droplet of ^{99m}Tc-labeled albumin from the nasal cavity over 30 min. Clearance of radioactivity is calculated from the radioactivity (disintegrations per minute) retained in the nasal cavity as a percentage of the initial dpm measured (percent retention). ● = mean clearance curve for four patients with bronchiectasis and chronic sinusitis and immotile cilia (but without situs inversus); ○ = mean clearance curve for six patients with Kartagener's syndrome; □ = mean clearance curve for 13 normal subjects. Pulmonary mucociliary transport was similarly deficient in patients with the immotile cilia syndrome, both those with and those without Kartagener's syndrome. *(Based on data of Rossman et al,[40] with permission.)*

of the cilia in nasal or bronchial mucosa; rarely, ultrastructural axonemal defects other than absent dynein arms, such as absent or defective radial spokes or transposition of a peripheral microtubular doublet to the center of an axoneme; and (4) sterility in males associated with living but immotile spermatozoa with similar axonemal ultrastructural abnormalities. In women, reduced fertility is a feature as well. The term *immotile cilia syndrome* is generally used to describe this tetrad of clinical and laboratory findings associated with dynein-deficient cilia. However, the terms *ciliary dyskinesia syndrome* and *dyskinetic cilia syndrome* have been suggested as a result of the finding that the cilia in some patients with this syndrome, although anatomically abnormal, are in fact motile, albeit with abnormal motions. Such rare cases are seen in patients with isolated ciliary disorientation (mean deviation of direction of central tubule pairs greater than 30°), with resultant lack of coordination of ciliary beating and impairment of mucociliary clearance. It is important to distinguish this process from secondary ciliary disorientation, which may oc-

cur as a result of respiratory tract inflammation due to infection and be reversible with prolonged therapy with appropriate antimicrobials.

Bronchiectasis associated with abnormally long (but without structural abnormalities) bronchial mucosal cilia with markedly decreased beat frequency has been described in two children. Two siblings with Usher's syndrome type I (congenital sensorineural deafness, unintelligible speech, vestibular dysfunction, and early-onset retinitis pigmentosa) also had chronic sinusitis and bronchiectasis with reduced nasal mucociliary clearance (but no ultrastructural ciliary abnormalities). Since the three sensory systems affected (photoreceptors, auditory hair cells, vestibular hair cells) develop from ciliated precursor cells, the possibility of an underlying primary ciliary dyskinesia is suggested.

The frequency of bronchiectasis in the immotile cilia syndrome is high (about 30 percent), but the long-term prognosis for patients is relatively good, some of them living to an advanced age. Some patients over 35 years of age with this syndrome show only mild to moderate airway obstruction on pulmonary function testing. Exacerbations of infections tend to be more severe in late childhood and adolescence; in adult years, there may be resolution of symptoms.

Kartagener's Syndrome

The triad of bronchiectasis, sinusitis, and situs inversus (Kartagener's syndrome) (Fig. 132-10) is a subset of the immotile cilia syndrome and occurs in about 50 percent of patients with this cilial dysfunction syndrome.[25,40] How the situs inversus of Kartagener's syndrome fits into the cilial dysfunction syndrome is unclear. Afzelius has postulated that in normal embryos the cilia on epithelia have fixed positions and direction of beating.[1] As a result, in the normal course of development the cilia are presumed to cause the embryonic viscera to bend into a right-handed helical configuration, shifting the heart to the left. In the absence of ciliary function, whether the embryonic viscera would make a right-handed twist (to normal situs) or a left-handed twist or malrotation (to situs inversus) would be determined solely by chance. In keeping with this postulate is the fact that among siblings with the immotile cilia syndrome, about half have complete and half have partial (no situs inversus) Kartagener's syndrome.

Kartagener's syndrome affects about one person in 68,000 and appears to be inherited as an autosomal recessive trait. Of patients with bronchiectasis who have been studied, about 1.5 percent have Kartagener's triad. Of persons with situs inversus, about 15 percent have the complete Kartagener's syndrome. Essentially all patients with Kartagener's syndrome have immotile cilia with obvious ultrastructural defects (usually absent or defective dynein arms) in the ciliary axoneme. However, one patient with Kartagener's syndrome had no obvious ciliary abnormality on electron microscopy. It is very likely that the defect here is a functional abnormality in the cilia, perhaps in the dynein ATPase or other enzymatic constituent.

Among Polynesians, New Zealand Maoris, and Samoan islanders, bronchiectasis is a common problem. It is often associated with sinusitis, impaired mucociliary clearance, and immotile spermatozoa. On electron microscopy of bronchial or nasal ciliated epithelium, dynein arms are either absent or incomplete.

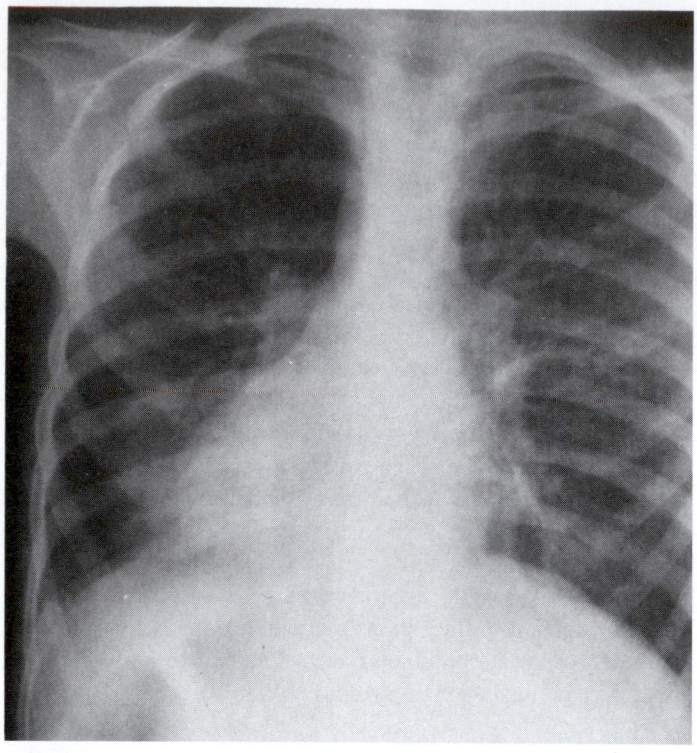

A

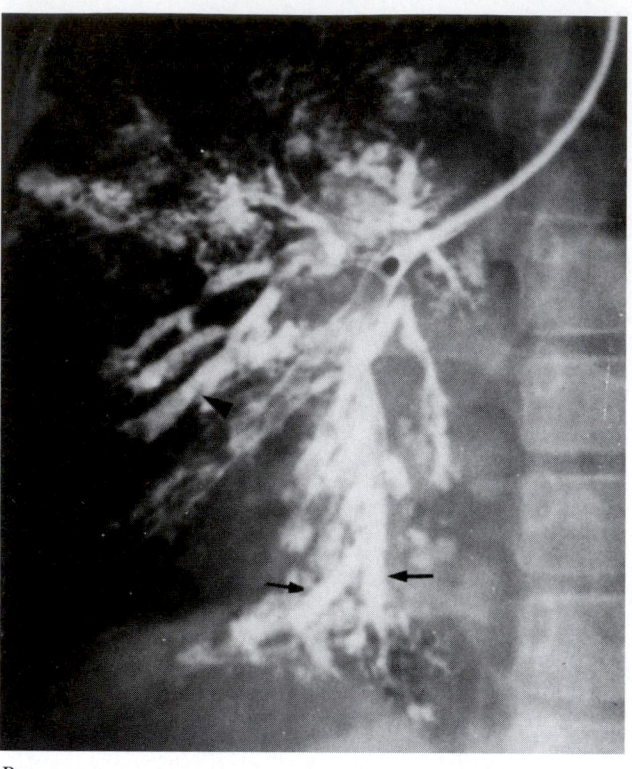

B

FIGURE 132-10 Young girl with Kartagener's syndrome. *A.* Chest radiograph at age 5 years shows dextrocardia, as part of situs inversus, and right lower-lung infiltrate. *B.* Bronchogram performed at age 8 years shows varicose bronchiectasis of bronchi to lower lobe (arrows) and of bronchi that represent lingular equivalents (arrowhead). *(Courtesy of Dr. D. Kushner.)*

Unlike the case in Europeans or Americans, however, these abnormalities are not associated with dextrocardia, and this fact is an argument against Afzelius's postulate. The ciliary microstructural abnormalities observed among Polynesians are more varied than those seen in Kartagener's syndrome. In addition to lack of dynein arms, these include cilia with missing, misplaced, or supernumerary tubules and compound cilia (containing several axonemes) (Fig. 132-11). Perhaps the mutation in the Polynesians is distinct from that in Europeans with Kartagener's syndrome.

In addition to anomalies of the bronchial ciliary apparatus that are congenital, acquired ones occur. The latter, by compromis-

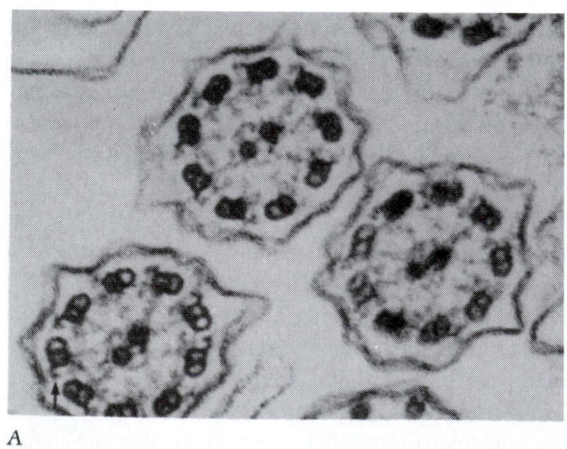

A

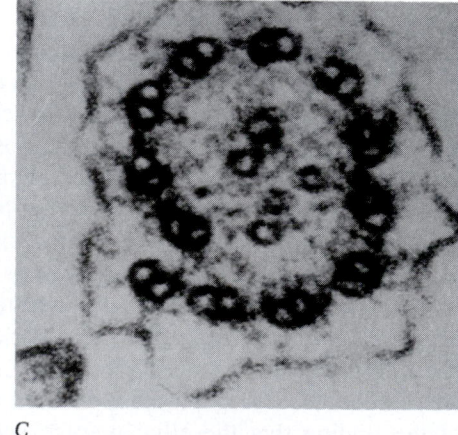

B   *C*

FIGURE 132-11 Electron micrographic cross sections of cilia from human conducting airways. *A.* Cross section of cilia from a healthy person showing the normal 9+2 microtubular pattern as well as the appropriate parallel alignment of the central pairs of microtubules of adjacent cilia. The small arrow points to the outer dynein arm of one of the peripheral microtubular pairs. *B.* A compound cilium, one of the many abnormalities observed in respiratory tract cilia of Polynesians with bronchiectasis or in normal subjects in association with acute viral respiratory tract infections. *C.* A cilium with marked configurational alterations, again consistent with the varied aberrations observed in Polynesians with bronchiectasis and normal subjects following acute viral respiratory tract infections. *A* and *B,* approximately ×100,000; *C,* ×216,000). *(Courtesy of Dr. G. R. Dickerson.)*

ing mucociliary clearance, may predispose to recurrent or prolonged pulmonary infections and, in this way, ultimately lead to bronchiectasis (an unproven hypothesis).[44] Dysmorphic changes in ciliary ultrastructure of respiratory epithelia, particularly microtubular additions or deletions in the 9+2 pattern, have been observed focally during viral illnesses (Fig. 132-11). These include infections due to influenza, parainfluenza, adenovirus, and respiratory syncytial virus. Similarly, in several young children with recurrent undefined lower respiratory infections or, in one instance, *Mycoplasma pneumoniae* infection, ciliary abnormalities such as megacilia, fused cilia, disorganized axonemes, and partial lack of dynein arms have been observed in bronchial epithelium. Such infection-related changes appear to operate at the level of microtubule assembly during the course of cilioneogenesis. Normal organization of epithelium and ultrastructure of cilia is restored by 10 weeks after infection.

α_1-ANTITRYPSIN DEFICIENCY

Patients with severe deficiency of the major serum protease inhibitor α_1-antitrypsin are particularly susceptible to the development of early-onset panlobular emphysema (see Chapter 55). Production of α_1-antitrypsin occurs in the liver and in mononuclear phagocytes. It functions by binding to and inhibiting leukocyte elastase and other proteases. When the serum α_1-antitrypsin level is below 35 percent of normal (150 to 350 mg/dl) as a result of mutation, the protease–antiprotease balance in the lung is disturbed. Approximately 2 percent of patients with emphysema have a hereditary deficiency of α_1-antitrypsin. Some patients with the deficiency develop the pulmonary complication of chronic bronchitis or, occasionally, bronchiectasis. Smoking accelerates the progression of pulmonary disease in patients with α_1-antitrypsin deficiency and may hasten death.

CYSTIC FIBROSIS (MUCOVISCIDOSIS)

Cystic fibrosis currently is the principal predisposing factor in at least half the cases of bronchiectasis identified in the first 2 decades of life (see Chapter 53). It is a heritable (autosomal recessive) disease of endocrine and exocrine glands characterized by unusually viscid mucous secretions that cause chronic pulmonary disease and pancreatic insufficiency as major organ dysfunctions, but other manifestations as well.[51] Almost 95 percent of the mortality is a consequence of infection and chronic obstructive pulmonary disease (see Chapters 42, 43, and 44).

The gene responsible for cystic fibrosis, the cystic fibrosis transmembrane conductance regulator on chromosome 7, encodes a cyclic AMP–activated cellular chloride channel. Mutations in this gene cause defective cyclic AMP–mediated regulation of chloride channels, with resulting increased transepithelial potential difference due to enhanced sodium absorption and decreased chloride permeability. In the airways, this defective regulation of apical membrane chloride channels of epithelial cells results in their failure to secrete chloride (and accompanying fluid) toward the lumina of the bronchial tree. As a consequence, airway secretions become thick and viscid, producing mucous plugging.[31] The most common mutation (ΔF 508), accounting for 70 percent of cases of cystic fibrosis, causes the deletion of a single amino acid in a highly conserved region of the first nucleotide-binding fold of the transmembrane channel. About 500 other mutations in the cystic fibrosis gene have been noted in patients with the disease. Occasionally, such mutations have been associated with a modified phenotype (usually mild course, lack of pancreatic insufficiency, normal sweat electrolyte concentrations, exceptional longevity, bronchiectasis with only late decline in pulmonary function).

Viscid secretions characterizing this disease produce extensive peripheral small-airway obstruction and air trapping.[5] Recurrent episodes of viral bronchiolitis and bacterial bronchitis increase the obstructive changes. Chronic infection takes over, with secretions and inflammatory exudate blocking larger bronchial subdivisions, and results in bronchiectasis. Thereafter, progressive disease is characterized by recurrent flare-ups of bronchitis and bronchopneumonia. Sinusitis and nasal polyps are common.

The changes of cystic bronchiectasis were noted radiographically in 64 percent of 200 adults with cystic fibrosis; another report, of 50 patients, indicated that 90 percent of the adults with cystic fibrosis had the specific radiologic features of bronchiectasis.[11] Bronchiectasis is found on pathologic examination of essentially all autopsied patients more than 6 months of age.[16] Peribronchial or focal pneumonia, sometimes with areas of abscess formation, is often present at autopsy. Bronchial lymph node enlargement is usually present.

Pulmonary function tests in patients with advanced cystic fibrosis show prominent findings of obstructive airway disease, or sometimes of a mixed obstructive-restrictive process reflecting the onset of fibrosis. An increased alveolar-to-arterial difference of P_{O_2} reflects uneven alveolar ventilation in the face of normal perfusion. With progression of pulmonary involvement and partial obstruction of large bronchi, expiratory flow rates decrease and both residual and total lung volumes increase. Arterial hypoxemia, pulmonary hypertension, and hypercapnia ensue. In more than 70 percent of patients, cor pulmonale develops eventually.

As patients with cystic fibrosis grow older, hemoptysis occurs with increasing frequency. Active bronchiectasis is the cause of the hemoptysis. The pathogenetic factors of the hemoptysis include destruction of lung tissue and erosion of blood vessels by active infection, increased tortuosity and size of bronchial arteries, increase in bronchial arterial circulation in the peribronchial granulation tissue, and pulmonary arterial hypertension. Most major bleeding originates in the bronchial circulation.

As a result of early diagnosis and effective treatment of pancreatic insufficiency with enzyme replacement, and of recurrent pulmonary infections with antimicrobials, patients with cystic fibrosis have had longer life expectancy, with median survival now approaching 30 years of age. Additional patients with chronic pulmonary infections developing only in their second or third decade have been found to have cystic fibrosis. In a limited number of patients with cystic fibrosis and extensive irreversible pulmonary damage, life expectancy has been extended by lung transplantation. By late 1994, 466 patients had undergone lung transplantation, with 57 percent survival at 3 years.

Radiographic Findings

The early radiographic changes of cystic fibrosis in childhood are usually secondary to mucous plugging of small airways and consist of hyperinflation and bronchial wall thickening. With recurrent infections, patchy pulmonary infiltrates, atelectasis, and further hyperinflation are observed. Lobar atelectasis occurs often during the initial episode of clinical pulmonary disease and is most common in the upper right lobe. Initially, some of the radiographic changes clear with antibiotic treatment of intercurrent infections. As the pulmonary disease advances, the typical radiographic changes seen with chronic bronchiectasis become more evident: mucous plugs, mucoid impaction, pus-filled bronchi, thickened bronchial walls, and dilated bronchial (ring) shadows (Fig. 132-12). Additional linear, nodular, or irregular densities, not readily identified as bronchi or bronchial walls, can be seen in otherwise clear parts of the lung. Large (2 cm or more in diameter) thin-walled air-filled cysts (bullae) may appear in the upper lobes over the course of several years. Pneumothorax and pneumomediastinum may occur as complications.

Bacteriology of Pulmonary Infections in Cystic Fibrosis

The pulmonary pathogens of clinical importance in cystic fibrosis have changed over time.[42] Before 1950, *S. aureus* was the predominant organism, isolated from the sputum or pharynx of 80 percent of children under 12 months of age with cystic fibrosis. Two decades later, this figure had declined to 30 percent; currently, *S. aureus* is isolated from the sputum of fewer than 20 percent of children and young adults with cystic fibrosis. Although *H. influenzae* type b is an important respiratory tract pathogen in children and unencapsulated *H. influenzae* is a common colonizer and potential pathogen in the lower respiratory tract of adults with

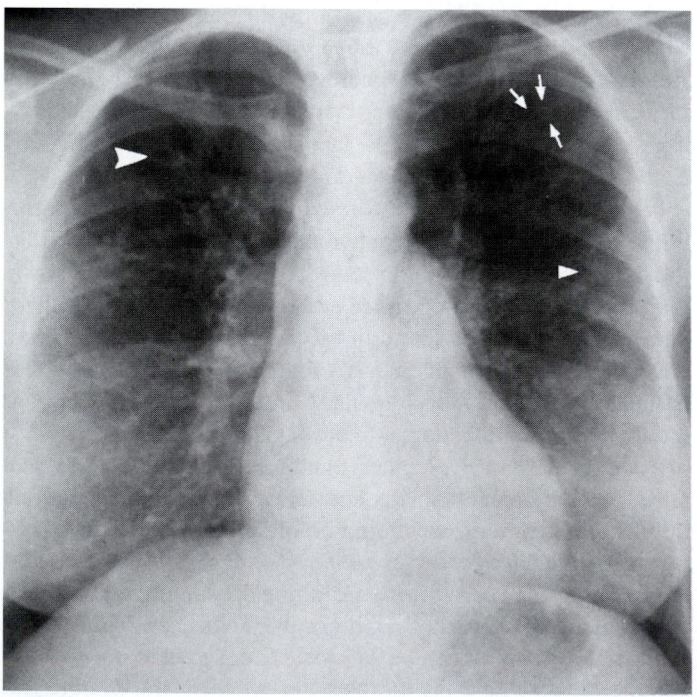

FIGURE 132-12 Chest radiograph of 17-year-old young girl with cystic fibrosis. The large arrowhead in right upper lobe indicates a ring shadow. In the left upper lobe, the two arrows pointing down indicate the upper aspect of a "tramline" (thickened bronchial walls displayed longitudinally); the arrow pointing up indicates the inferior wall of the same bronchus. The small arrowhead in the left midlung field indicates a nodular density, probably an area of mucoid impaction.

chronic bronchitis, their prevalence in sputum cultures of children with cystic fibrosis is less than 15 percent.

At present, the leading pulmonary pathogen in patients with cystic fibrosis who have chronic pulmonary disease (bronchitis, bronchiolitis, and bronchiectasis) is *P. aeruginosa*. Prevalence studies indicate colonization rates as high as 60 to 90 percent. Many factors appear to contribute to this frequency of colonization by *P. aeruginosa* (see Chapter 125). Among the most important are the ubiquity of this species in the environment and the selective pressure exerted by chronic antibiotic therapy with oral drugs with efficacy against the usual respiratory tract pathogens operative in the community but not against *P. aeruginosa*.

Initially, colonization of the lower respiratory tract of patients with cystic fibrosis by *P. aeruginosa* involves run-of-the-mill strains that exhibit nonmucoid colonial morphology. Ultimately, mucoid strains exhibiting a shiny appearance due to profuse production of an exopolysaccharide, alginate, appear and predominate.[38] Adherence of nonmucoid *P. aeruginosa* to respiratory epithelium is mediated by *Pseudomonas* pili; for this to occur, the cell surface layer of fibronectin must be depleted. The proteases in sputum of cystic fibrosis patients may facilitate initial adherence of *P. aeruginosa* by degrading fibronectin. On the other hand, adherence of mucoid *Pseudomonas* to respiratory tract epithelium appears to be mediated by the exopolysaccharide of the organism. The abundant alginate produced by the bacteria undoubtedly complicates mechanical clearance of secretions in the bronchial tree. In addition, it appears to impair polymorphonuclear leukocyte function and to act as a barrier to bactericidal antibodies.

P. aeruginosa, both mucoid and nonmucoid, produces a variety of toxins that undoubtedly contribute in varying degrees to the production of bronchiectasis and continuing damage to bronchopulmonary tissues. These toxins include exotoxin A, an inhibitor of protein synthesis with cytotoxic and necrotizing effects; exotoxin S, also an inhibitor of protein synthesis; and proteases, particularly an alkaline protease and elastase, which can cleave complement components (and thus inhibit opsonization and chemotaxis) and IgG and IgA, destroy connective-tissue components, and stimulate profuse mucin production. Additionally, pyocyanin, produced by *P. aeruginosa*, and one of its breakdown products, 1-hydroxyphenazine, inhibit the beating of human respiratory cilia in vitro.

Production of alginate by isolates of *P. aeruginosa* from patients with cystic fibrosis of long standing is common (more than 80 percent of isolates) in contrast to isolates of *P. aeruginosa* from other infections (2.5 percent). Isolation of mucoid strains of *P. aeruginosa* repeatedly from bronchial secretions of patients with a chronic pulmonary process indicates cystic fibrosis or bronchiectasis of some other causation.

In recent years, *Burkholderia cepacia* has emerged as a pathogen with an increasing prevalence (up to 40 percent in some centers) in patients with cystic fibrosis.[45] Some features of this organism in the setting of cystic fibrosis warrant concern: (1) its capacity to spread from patient to patient both in and out of the hospital (Sun's team has identified, by molecular methods, highly transmissible strains with unusual giant cablelike adhesin pili capable of binding to the mucin of cystic fibrosis and interfering with mucociliary transport); (2) its association with more severe lung disease and with accelerated clinical deterioration in some patients (accompanied by necrotizing pneumonia and even bacteremia, features not ordinarily observed with *P. aeruginosa* infections in cystic fibrosis); and (3) its resistance to aminoglycosides and to most β-lactam antipseudomonal antibiotics. (The only antibiotics to which *B. cepacia* has been susceptible have been trimethoprim-sulfamethoxazole and, occasionally, chloramphenicol; recently developed antibiotics, such as ceftazidime, imipenem, aztreonam, and ciprofloxacin, have shown some activity in vitro.)

Up to 50 percent of patients with cystic fibrosis carry Enterobacteriaceae (*Escherichia coli, Klebsiella,* etc.) in their sputum from time to time. In some patients, mucoid variants of *E. coli,* producing exopolysaccharide composed of colanic acid rather than the alginic acid characteristic of mucoid strains of *P. aeruginosa,* are isolated.

Miscellaneous Disorders

YOUNG'S SYNDROME

Young's syndrome consists of a combination of obstructive azoospermia (with normal spermatogenesis) and chronic sinopulmonary infections.[24] This syndrome is distinguished from the immotile cilia syndrome by its lack of ultrastructural ciliary abnormalities and from cystic fibrosis by its lack of family history and the presence of normal sweat electrolytes and pancreatic enzyme secretion. Young's syndrome appears to be more common than the immotile cilia syndrome. Thirty to 70 percent of patients with this syndrome have bronchiectasis; the other patients have clinical evidence of chronic bronchitis. The sinopulmonary infections appear in childhood, become milder in adult life, and do not attain the severity usually observed in cystic fibrosis or the immotile cilia syndrome. Respiratory function shows only mild impairment (increase in residual volume and decrease in FEV_1). Although a productive cough is usual, the raising of copious amounts of purulent sputum is uncommon. Rales are audible in a few patients, and manifestations of advanced chronic pulmonary disease—such as clubbing, cyanosis, and cor pulmonale—are usually lacking. Decreased tracheobronchial mucociliary clearance of inhaled particles has been reported in the few patients who have been studied.

Since the pulmonary manifestations of Young's syndrome are mild and nonspecific, the diagnosis is most often made when the patient seeks medical attention for infertility. Testicular function is normal. Anatomically normal spermatozoa are present in distended epididymal heads, and the middle region of the epididymis is obstructed by amorphous material; in contrast, in cystic fibrosis, male infertility is caused by congenital atresia of the vas deferens.

INFLAMMATORY PROCESSES

Bronchitis and bronchiectasis appear to occur with increased frequency in patients with rheumatoid arthritis as compared with matched controls. This relationship is more relevant in patients with long-standing severe rheumatoid arthritis in whom bronchiectasis has developed as a late feature. A possible association between ulcerative colitis and bronchiectasis has been reported in a few instances.

Role of Elastase and Proteases in Airway Damage

Proteolytic enzymes have been implicated in the pathogenesis of the destructive changes in several chronic lung diseases. Among these are diseases, such as bronchiectasis, in which pathologic changes occur in the bronchial epithelium exposed to purulent secretions potentially rich in such proteases, including elastase, collagenase, and cathepsin G. Polymorphonuclear leukocytes contain and release such neutral proteases, which are able to act on and destroy elastin, collagen, and proteoglycans—all important structural components of the lung and bronchial tree.[46] Purified granulocyte elastase can directly damage bronchial epithelium and inhibit normal ciliary action. In addition to their action on structural proteins of the lung, granulocyte proteases can inactivate complement component C3 and IgG and IgM immunoglobulins. Neutrophil proteases also act as stimulators of bronchial gland secretion in bronchiectasis.

In patients with bronchiectasis, elastolytic activity is an almost constant feature of purulent secretions. Purulent bronchial secretions from patients with cystic fibrosis and *P. aeruginosa* infection of the airways have markedly higher levels of granulocyte elastase activity than do bronchial secretions from patients with bronchiectasis and exacerbations of chronic bronchitis.[46] The latter two groups have more elastase activity in bronchial secretions than do patients without bronchial infection. Whether this strikingly higher level of granulocyte elastase activity in patients with cystic fibrosis is intrinsic to that disease or merely represents a measure of the severity of bronchiectasis and purulence of bronchopulmonary secretions in that disease is unclear. The presence of high levels of granulocyte elastase in the bronchial secretions of patients with cystic fibrosis indicates an imbalance between this protease and the antiproteases in the lung, such as α_1-antitrypsin. The α_1-antitrypsin in purulent bronchial secretions is present in an inactive form. Whether this is due to the action of oxidants released by granulocytes during phagocytosis or to cleavage by *P. aeruginosa* elastase is not known.

A "vicious cycle" hypothesis for the overall pathogenesis of bronchiectasis has been proposed by Cole that incorporates the previously noted concept of protease-mediated airway damage.[9] According to this model, an underlying disease (or damage to the bronchial tree) compromises mucociliary clearance, favoring microbial colonization of airways. Such bacteria (e.g., *P. aeruginosa*) release proteases that damage ciliated epithelium. The host's inflammatory response not only is unable to eliminate the colonizing bacteria but also contributes to further lung damage by release of neutrophil elastase and other proteases. Activation of macrophages and the cell-mediated immune response follows in the inflamed areas of bronchiectatic lung, probably contributing to furtherance of lung damage.

CLINICAL FEATURES

In the preantibiotic era, when bronchiectasis was much more common, symptoms began in the first decade of life; indeed, in 60 to 90 percent of patients, symptoms were evident by 5 years of age. The common initiating events were infections such as measles, pertussis, necrotizing pneumonia, and tuberculosis. Since the incidence of several of these infections has been sharply reduced by immunization and since progressive destruction of lung parenchyma in others has been almost eliminated by the use of antimicrobial agents, the clinical setting of the disease has changed. Currently, many children or young adults with bronchiectasis have some inherited anatomic or functional abnormality; about half have cystic fibrosis. Although most cases of cystic fibrosis present in early childhood, the diagnosis is not made in about 20 percent of the cases until after the age of 15 years, when significant chronic symptoms develop.

Cough, sometimes in paroxysms, is almost invariably present and may be the only symptom for years in childhood. Purulent sputum production—frequently worse in the morning, having accumulated during recumbency in sleep—is present in more than 90 percent of patients. Occasionally, expectoration is not a feature or is not persistent, and "dry phases" (periods when sputum is mucoid rather than purulent) occur. Sometimes, but by no means exclusively, these changes occur following antimicrobial therapy. The volume of sputum produced in older children and adults with advanced untreated disease, rarely seen nowadays, can be prodigious: up to 600 ml per day. In the preantibiotic era, fetid sputum and foul odor of the breath were observed in about 25 percent of patients, but that is unusual today. The classic characterization of bronchiectatic sputum entailed description of the separation of a 24-h collection of sputum into three layers: (1) an upper, colorless or slightly greenish brown one containing air bubbles, pus, and mucus; (2) a middle, thin mucoid layer similar to the first but containing less air; and (3) a lower layer comprising a thick greenish sediment made up of pus cells, debris, fibrin, bronchial plugs, and sometimes fatty acid crystals and elastic fibers. These findings are less commonly observed in the antibiotic era, as early antibiotic therapy and postural drainage reduce sputum volume, purulence, and secondary overgrowth of anaerobic bacteria.

Exacerbations of bronchiectasis, induced by intercurrent viral bronchiolitis, bacterial bronchitis, or bronchial plugging, may be accompanied by fever (in about one-third of cases), increased cough, sputum production, and shortness of breath. Multiple recurrent episodes are associated with anorexia and weight loss as well. Hemoptysis occurred in 40 to 70 percent of cases during the preantibiotic era; it occurs less commonly now that exacerbations of the disease can be treated by antimicrobials. So-called dry bronchiectasis is uncommon and may exhibit no symptoms other than occasional hemoptysis. Investigation may then reveal bronchiectatic changes on bronchography or computed tomography. Upper-lobe involvement is more common in this syndrome. Bronchostenosis, sometimes due to endobronchial tuberculosis, may underlie the bronchiectatic process. Wheezing and dyspnea are associated with exacerbations at first but become more persistent as the bronchiectasis progresses.

Sinusitis may be associated with bronchiectasis, particularly in congenital predisposing syndromes such as cystic fibrosis, Young's syndrome, Kartagener's syndrome, and various immunoglobulin deficiencies.

Involvement of many lobes is a feature of bronchiectasis complicating cystic fibrosis. Early and predominant involvement of upper lobes, particularly on the right, is more characteristic of this disease than of classic bronchiectasis of the preantibiotic era, when involvement was more frequent in the lower lobes (and middle lobe) and in the left lung particularly. In an occasional patient, "pleurisy" may be the presenting or most prominent symptom.

More patients with bronchiectasis have abnormalities on physical examination. The most important finding is the presence of persistent "moist" crackles over the affected lobes. The crackles are medium to coarse, start early in inspiration, continue to midinspiration, and fade out by the end of inspiration. In contrast, the crackles of fibrosing alveolitis may begin in either the early or middle phase of respiration, are fine and "close to the ear," and continue to the end of inspiration. Diffuse rhonchi and a prolonged expiratory phase of respiration may be present. Dullness and decreased breath sounds are sometimes present over extensively invaded lobes. With complicating pneumonia—or sometimes even in its absence—bronchovesicular or bronchial breath sounds may be a feature. Decreased respiratory expansion of the lungs is evident in patients with more advanced disease and with complicating emphysema. Hyperexpansion may be evident—particularly in children, who may develop barrel chest.

Clubbing of the fingers and cyanosis were common (40 percent of cases) in the preantibiotic era. By the 1960s, clubbing was observed in only 7 percent of cases. In advanced and ultimately fatal cases of bronchiectasis in the past, cor pulmonale occurred in 10 to 22 percent of cases. It is now less common a complication than in the past, except perhaps in patients with cystic fibrosis and extensive bronchopulmonary damage. Secondary amyloid disease is now very rare, even with long-standing bronchiectasis.

RADIOGRAPHIC FINDINGS

Chest Radiography

The routine chest radiograph commonly does not show distinctive changes; it may be totally unremarkable, particularly in early bronchiectasis.[18,19] The earliest change observed may be a nonspecific increase in peribronchial markings in specific segments of the lung. Of more diagnostic significance is the appearance of *tubular shadows*—paired parallel or slightly tapered line shadows, extending distally, sometimes branching, and following a bronchovascular distribution. These line shadows ("tramlines"), outlining the affected bronchial area, are produced by thickened bronchial walls, peribronchial fibrosis, and adjacent alveolar collapse. The same structures, when viewed in cross section, may appear as peripheral rounded or irregularly nodular densities or as ring shadows. As bronchiectasis becomes more chronic, associated atelectasis becomes more marked, resulting in crowding together of numerous tubular shadows, usually in the lower lobes. Loss in lung volume may be extensive enough to cause a shift in the position of a fissure or hemidiaphragm or deviation of the trachea. When thickened bronchiectatic segments become filled with retained secretions or pus, they form homogeneous radiodense bands, which have been referred to as *mucoid impaction* or, when branched, as *gloved finger shadows*.[18,19]

With advanced saccular bronchiectasis, large cystic air-containing areas (with or without fluid levels), representing dilated terminations of abnormal bronchi, can be seen (Fig. 132-13).[20] Since they communicate with the proximal airways, these cysts, unlike those in patients with emphysematous bullae, can enlarge on inspiration and diminish on expiration. In very severe disease, a coarse honeycomb pattern is observed. The rarefied areas here, in contrast to the cystic spaces representing dilated bronchial termini, do not fill with contrast on bronchography. These areas represent emphysematous regions surrounded by fibrosis rather than dilated bronchi.

Compensatory hyperinflation of the rest of the lung is common. This may be particularly prominent in patients with cystic fibrosis, in whom it may be evident relatively early. Patchy areas of bronchopneumonia may punctuate the course of bronchiectasis, particularly in patients with cystic fibrosis. Hilar lymphadenopathy may be visible, both in a causative role (producing bronchial obstruction and resulting bronchiectasis) and as a consequence of the chronic infection that characterizes established bronchiectasis.

Bronchography

The finding on plain film of structures representing the parallel walls of dilated bronchi provides presumptive evidence of bronchiectasis. In 7 to 20 percent of patients with established bronchiectasis, however, conventional radiographs show no such abnormalities. Although bronchography has been the gold standard for documenting the presence and extent of bronchiectasis in the past, because of its limitations (temporary impairment of ventilation, need for local anesthesia, patient discomfort) it has generally been replaced by chest CT as the optimal (noninvasive) means for diagnosis (see above).[43] However, bronchography is still performed, sometimes preoperatively, for evaluation of unilateral or segmental disease previously identified on CT or, postoperatively, to evaluate surgical airway complications such as dehiscence or fistula formation.[2,23]

Several technical considerations are important in evaluating bronchial shadows on bronchograms.[47] Tubular shadows outlining bronchial walls contain air in the lumen. If such shadows end abruptly, they usually suggest that air is passing freely to the periphery but that there is insufficient contrast to coat the more peripheral extent of the bronchus; this does not indicate bronchial obstruction. Solid shadows in the bronchi may be produced because of the presence of too much contrast medium and no air in the lumen, even though peripheral filling is complete. True nonfilling of peripheral bronchi may be due to bronchial obstruction or to focal areas of retained secretions. To minimize the latter, bronchography should be performed only after adequate postural drainage and antibiotic therapy. Fiberoptic bronchoscopy has made it possible to perform more selective segmental bronchography with less adverse effects and discomfort. This procedure may be of particular help in evaluating a patient with recurrent hemoptysis when bronchoscopy shows the bronchopulmonary segment that is the site of bleeding but no endobronchial lesion is observed ("dry bronchiectasis").

The bronchographic features of *cylindric bronchiectasis* (Fig. 132-5) include regularly outlined dilated bronchi with not greatly increased diameters peripherally, abrupt ending of bronchiectatic segments with little or no peripheral filling, and crowding of bronchiectatic segments. Obstructed bronchi in cylindric bronchiectasis (and other types) may show air bubbles in the in-

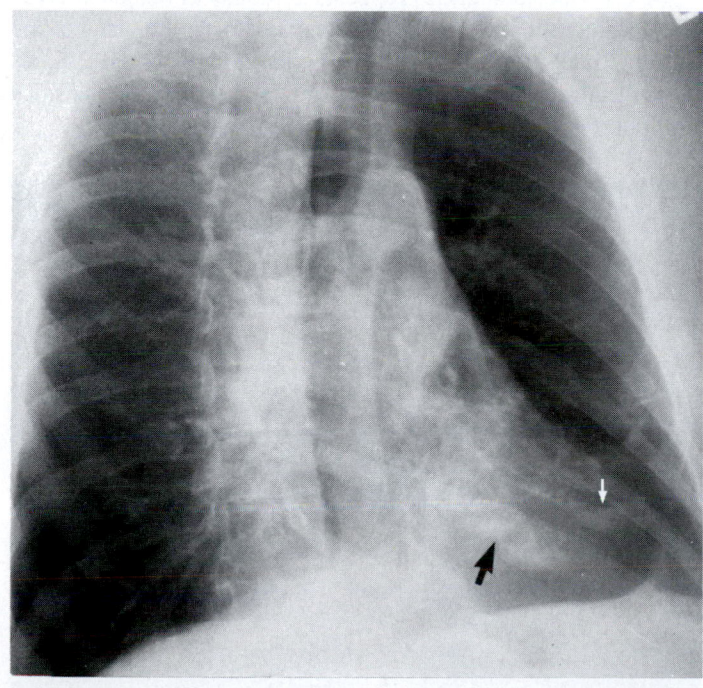

A

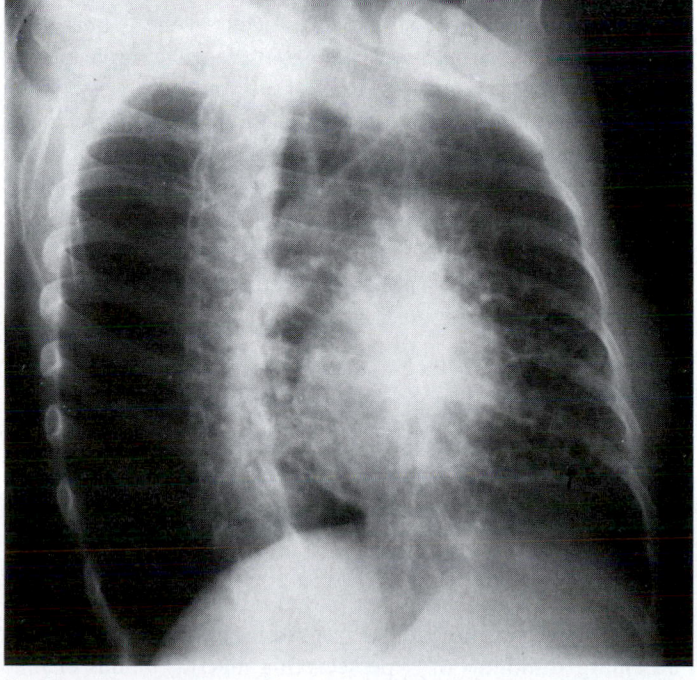

B

FIGURE 132-13   Plain chest radiographs of two patients with saccular bronchiectasis. *A.* Large fluid-filled cystic bronchial termini. Large arrow points to inferior edge of fluid-filled dilated bronchus. Smaller arrow points to air–fluid level in cystic bronchial terminus. *B.* Oblique view of chest radiograph demonstrating multiple cystic areas in the lower half of the lung beyond the heart border. The small arrow points to a cystic area with thickened walls, indicating active inflammation in the involved region.

traluminal contrast medium, since the air cannot enter the smaller bronchi. *Varicose bronchiectasis* is characterized by bronchial dilatation, which is somewhat greater than that of cylindric bronchiectasis. In addition, local constrictions cause irregularities in the outline of bronchi, giving an appearance akin to that of varicose veins (Fig. 132-6). Invaded bronchial segments show bulbous terminations, with failure of peripheral filling. In *saccular bronchiectasis,* bronchi exhibit a ballooned outline. Cystic spaces containing contrast material (Fig. 132-7) or exhibiting air-fluid levels may be present.

"PSEUDOBRONCHIECTASIS" (REVERSIBLE BRONCHIECTASIS)

Pneumonia may produce changes in the bronchial tree acutely, with subsequent resolution. Bachman and colleagues performed bronchograms on 60 young soldiers with radiographically proven pneumonia and no prior history of pulmonary disease.[2] Bronchography was performed after the acute illness (1 to 8 weeks after onset) but usually before resolution of the pulmonary infiltrate. Twenty-five of the patients showed bronchial abnormalities. Of 16 patients with initial bronchial abnormalities who were followed with repeated bronchograms (seven with considerable widening of bronchi considered to be radiographically consistent with bronchiectasis and nine with milder bronchial abnormalities), 10 showed return of the bronchogram to normal within 4 months. Thus, in a patient with a chronic productive cough and pneumonia who is suspected of having bronchiectasis, bronchography should be postponed for at least 4 months after the acute pneumonia; otherwise, reversible dilatation of segmental bronchi without destruction, a change that often occurs in acute pneumonia, may be erroneously attributed to irreversible cylindric bronchiectasis.

Reversible bronchiectasis also can occur in the patient with acute bronchial obstruction. Acute extensive cystic bronchiectasis has followed traumatic stenosis of a bronchus 4 weeks after closed-chest trauma. Resection of the stenotic segment produced nearly complete reversal of the bronchographic abnormalities in 8 days and total recovery in a month. Presumably, the initial changes were due to bronchial dilatation secondary to retained secretions and to atelectasis caused by the bronchostenosis. Since secondary infection was not introduced, the changes were reversible on relief of the obstruction.

BRONCHOGRAPHIC CHANGES IN CHRONIC BRONCHITIS

A variety of bronchographic changes can be observed in patients with chronic bronchitis and should be distinguished from the changes of bronchiectasis. These include lack of parallelism of the walls of medium-sized bronchi; lack of full delineation of distal parts of bronchial tree, probably because of mucus obstructing small peripheral airways; and mucosal pouches arising from sides of larger bronchi, representing either enlarged mouths of hypersecreting mucous glands or mucosal ridging. With advanced disease, "peripheral pools" (emphysematous spaces filled with contrast) and a concertina appearance (due to structural changes in the bronchial wall) can be observed.

Computed Tomography

Computed tomography is now the favored means of establishing the diagnosis of bronchiectasis and of determining its extent and severity.[32–34,43] Clinical correlations with CT findings have been extensively reviewed by McGuinness and Naidick.[32] The accuracy of diagnosis has been enhanced by the advent of high-resolution CT (HRCT). A sensitivity of 96 percent and a specificity of 93 percent have been attained with 1.5-mm-collimation CT at 10-mm intervals. Cylindric bronchiectasis, within the plane of a CT section, appears as uniformly dilated airways that fail to taper normally while progressing toward the lung periphery. The abnormally thickened bronchial walls are visible as "train tracks." In cross section, dilated bronchi appear as ring structures with internal diameters greater than those of their accompanying pulmonary artery branches. This size difference relationship forms the basis of the "signet ring" sign, with the wall of the dilated bronchus representing the band of the ring and the density due to the artery serving as the signet. In varicose bronchiectasis, the bronchi are more dilated than in cylindric bronchiectasis and exhibit a beaded appearance due to alternating focal areas of more and less dilation in an individual bronchus. The CT changes in cystic bronchiectasis include markedly dilated bronchi, air-fluid levels in bronchi, "strings of cysts" (linear arrays of consecutive cystic dilatations of a bronchus visualized in a horizontal course), and "cluster of cysts" (dilated bronchi in groups mimicking a cluster of grapes) (Fig. 132-14). Visualization of dilated bronchi with thickened walls in the lung periphery must be interpreted with caution as a feature of bronchiectasis on CT, since pneumonia or other causes of parenchymal consolidation can produce a similar picture without bronchiectasis.

On CT, mucoid impaction appears as tubular or branched structures, representing mucus-filled bronchi seen on the plane of the section. Small-airway disease may be identifiable on HRCT, because of thickening of bronchiolar walls, as 2- to 3-mm densities with poorly defined nodular or branching appearance.

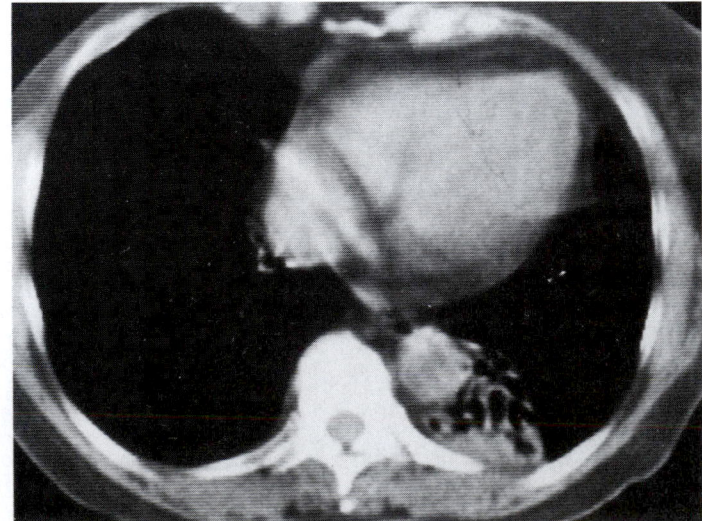

FIGURE 132-14 CT scan of chest showing a grapelike cluster of dilated bronchi characteristic of cystic bronchiectasis in an atelectatic left lower lobe. *(Courtesy of Dr. T. McLoud.)*

PATHOPHYSIOLOGICAL CHANGES

Pulmonary Function

Although there is no specific pattern of pulmonary function associated with bronchiectasis, a variety of abnormalities are commonly seen. The degree of impairment depends not only on the nature and extent of the morphologic abnormalities in the invaded areas but also on the presence or absence of associated disease (chronic bronchitis, emphysema) elsewhere in the smaller airways and lung parenchyma. Patients with very localized bronchiectasis without chronic bronchitis have little dysfunction. However, there is not always a direct correlation between the number of affected bronchial segments or the type of anatomic change (cylindric, etc.) and the dysfunction measured.

Patients with severe bronchiectasis show impaired airway dynamics similar to that of patients with chronic bronchitis and emphysema.[17] In normal persons, forced expiration or cough produces a proportionate narrowing throughout the bronchial tree. In patients with saccular and varicose bronchiectasis, cough produces a disproportionate, premature collapse of the large (usually lower-lobe) bronchi, causing obstruction to airflow and possibly contributing to air trapping. Inflammatory changes of chronic bronchitis are presumed responsible for the weakening of the proximal bronchi producing this phenomenon. As a consequence of airflow obstruction and reduced effectiveness of cough, bronchopulmonary toilet is impaired. Retained secretions predispose to further infection, and peribronchial inflammation extends.

In most patients with diffuse involvement, pulmonary function tests show a pattern of airways obstruction: reduced FVC, FEV_1, FEV_1/FVC, $FEF_{25-75\%}$, and increased residual volume. Abnormal maximum expiratory flow volume tracings at low lung volumes and other studies (closing volume, frequency dependence of dynamic compliance) can be helpful in detecting diffuse involvement of small airways. In some patients, particularly those with considerable associated atelectasis and fibrosis, abnormalities (e.g., decreased vital capacity and functional residual capacity, reduced specific compliance) are of a mixed obstructive-restrictive pattern or a largely restrictive one.

Reduced regional ventilation, a lesser degree of reduction in perfusion, and decreased ventilation–perfusion ratios are observed in areas of bronchiectatic involvement.[6] Additional evidence of ventilatory dysfunction includes increased dead-space ventilation and abnormal nitrogen washout studies. Generally, the disturbances in overall lung function are more dependent on the extent of involvement (and associated bronchitis) than on the anatomic type of bronchiectasis. With progressive or extensive bronchiectasis, arterial hypoxemia may develop secondary to abnormalities in gas exchange in adjacent areas. Carbon dioxide retention occurs only in patients in whom bronchiectasis is associated with severe obstructive airway disease, generally severe chronic bronchitis, and advanced emphysema.

Tracheobronchial Clearance

In patients with bronchiectasis, as in patients with chronic bronchitis, inhaled aerosol particles are deposited in more central bronchi than in the case of normal subjects. This has been ascribed to more turbulent airflow in obstructed large bronchial segments. In addition, particle clearance is impaired. A number of abnormalities can contribute to such impairment: loss of normal ciliated epithelium from the lining of involved bronchi, hereditary ciliary defects (immotile cilia syndrome, Kartagener's syndrome), and altered mucous blanket of the bronchial tree.

Mucociliary transport (MCT) can be accurately measured by monitoring over several hours the disappearance of ^{99m}Tc–human serum albumin aerosol deposited as a bolus in the large airways. Rapid loss of radioactivity from the lung occurs in normal persons, but marked retention of the radioactive particles is characteristic of patients with Kartagener's syndrome and bronchiectasis.

Several features of bronchiectasis alter the character and viscosity of the sputum produced. The purulent sputum is more viscid, particularly as a result of its deoxyribonucleic acid content and disulfide linkages of proteins, resulting in slower MCT.[5] This property is not specific for the purulent sputum of bronchiectasis. Patients with bronchiectasis also produce mucoid sputum. The submucosal glands of the bronchi are hyperactive and, unlike other hypersecretory states, the ratio of serous to mucous cells is not decreased. Purulent bronchial secretions from patients with cystic fibrosis (and accompanying bronchiectasis) contain granulocyte neutral proteases, which are able to cleave major structural proteins (collagen, elastin, proteoglycans) of the lung. Enhancing the proteolytic capability of the purulent bronchial secretions in cystic fibrosis is the *P. aeruginosa* elastase. This enzyme is capable of destroying the two principal inhibitors of granulocyte proteases in the lung (α_1-antitrypsin and bronchial mucosal protein inhibitor). Thus, the synergistic effect of this infecting organism and the proteolytic activity of polymorphonuclear leukocytes of the inflammatory response contribute in a major way to the progressive destruction of structural bronchial and parenchymal proteins and to the advance of the inflammatory process in bronchiectasis.

Hemodynamic Changes

Hemodynamic changes in bronchiectasis are of several types. Extensive systemic-to-pulmonary anastomoses occur at the precapillary level in the granulation tissue around bronchiectatic segments.[30] Such anastomoses can lead to bronchial artery enlargement and left-to-right shunts.[8] This is not an important contributor to the pulmonary hypertension and ultimate cor pulmonale that develop in a few patients with severe bronchiectasis. If pulmonary hypertension should develop, hypoxia—generally attributable to a severe underlying chronic bronchitis and emphysema—has a major etiologic role.

DIAGNOSIS

Diagnosis comprises two elements: the identification of bronchiectasis as the cause of suppurative bronchopulmonary disease and the ascertainment of any predisposing process. The history of chronic cough, purulent sputum, recurrent exacerbations of bronchitis, recurrent pneumonias, or recurrent hemoptyses in a patient with a chest radiograph showing increased and crowded pulmonary markings (including tramlines, ring densities, or cystic areas with fluid levels) effectively makes the clinical diagnosis of bronchiectasis. In less clear-cut cases or when definition of the extent of involvement is important, CT of the chest can be a helpful noninvasive means of diagnosis. The gold standard for diagnosis in patients in whom there is uncertainty about the presence of bronchiectasis, or when surgery is being considered, remains bronchography.

Bronchography

The role of bronchography in diagnosis has declined strikingly as a result of the better appreciation of the radiographic findings of this disease on plain chest films and the use of chest CT for diagnosis. Nonetheless, bronchography remains the procedure of choice before surgery to assess the extent of the process, to confirm the diagnosis in a doubtful case (e.g., dry bronchiectasis with recurrent hemoptysis), or to evaluate the bronchial tree when a congenital defect may be a predisposing factor.

Adverse effects may accompany bronchography. These include possible allergic reactions to the topical anesthetic or iodine-containing contrast material, impairment of ventilation due to the filling of bronchi with contrast, and segmental pulmonary collapse, particularly in children who have undergone general anesthesia with a readily diffusible gaseous agent. In patients with considerably impaired pulmonary function, bronchography should be avoided.

Bronchoscopy

Bronchoscopy is not of value in directly diagnosing bronchiectasis, but it may be of value in defining the presence of an obstructing lesion responsible for localized segmental bronchiectasis or in defining the bronchopulmonary segment that is the source of recurrent hemoptysis in a patient without a discernible endobronchial lesion but with bronchiectasis. Bronchography with fiberoptic bronchoscopy can be helpful in confirming the presence of localized bronchiectasis and has the advantages in this circumstance of selective instillation of contrast and less likelihood of inducing hypoxia in a patient with diminished respiratory reserve.

Computed Tomography

Chest CT provides a useful noninvasive means of establishing the diagnosis of bronchiectasis and defining its anatomic extent. It appears to be less reliable in detecting cylindric, or possibly varicose, changes. The ability to identify a bronchus on CT depends on its size and orientation. Horizontally oriented bronchi are more readily visualized and evaluable than bronchi with vertical courses. Since the basilar segmental bronchi, apical bronchi, bronchus intermedius, and lower-lobe bronchi are seen only on cross section, cylindric or mild varicose changes in these locations may be more readily overlooked than similar changes in the lingular or right middle-lobe bronchi.

Bacteriologic Findings

Definitive delineation of the bacteriology of bronchiectasis has not been accomplished. Many of the studies of bronchiectasis in the first half of this century, when the disease was more common, suffered from the fact that they were retrospective, that they antedated modern techniques for anaerobic bacteriology, and that their data were derived from culture of sputum (readily contaminated with oropharyngeal flora on passage through the oral cavity). Accurate information from transtracheal aspiration and culture of resected lung is not at hand. Available data indicate the frequent presence of *H. influenzae* (usually unencapsulated) and *S. pneumoniae* in the sputum of patients with bronchiectasis in addition to normal components of the oropharyngeal flora. Suppurative pneumonias following measles and predisposing to bronchiectasis have been due to *S. aureus, K. pneumoniae,* and *P. aeruginosa.* In bronchographically confirmed "pseudo-bronchiectasis" following pneumonia, the cause has been either *Streptococcus pyogenes* or "atypical pneumonia." In the antibiotic area, the organisms isolated from patients with bronchiectasis can show shifts in the resident bronchial species as a result of antibiotic selective pressure. Mucoid strains of *P. aeruginosa* have been isolated from patients with bronchiectasis who do not have cystic fibrosis. As noted earlier in this chapter, in cystic fibrosis patients initial sputum isolates are often *H. influenzae* or *S. aureus.* Later in the course of the disease, Enterobacteriaceae, mucoid strains of *P. aeruginosa,* or *B. cepacia* tends to predominate, in large measure influenced by antimicrobial selective pressure.

Anaerobic bacteria undoubtedly play an important primary or contributory role in some cases of bronchiectasis. Evidence for this includes (1) the foul, putrid odor of the sputum of some patients; (2) the fact that bronchiectasis has sometimes followed necrotizing aspiration pneumonias associated with oral anaerobes (*Bacteroides melaninogenicus, Fusobacterium necrophorum,* peptococci, peptostreptococci, etc.); (3) the finding at autopsy in the preantimicrobial era of fusiform bacteria and spirochetes in stained sections of bronchiectatic segments; (4) the isolation from bronchiectatic lobes removed at surgery during the preantibiotic era of fusobacteria, always in association with facultative cocci; and (5) the occasional complication of bronchiectasis by brain abscess due to mixed anaerobes.

Other Laboratory Studies

Gram-stained smear of sputum shows numerous polymorphonuclear leukocytes and mixed bacterial flora, often including fusiform bacteria as well as a variety of gram-negative rods and gram-positive cocci. In some, there may be no single predominating organism; in others, the predominating organism may vary. Leukocytosis is variable and may be associated with an exacerbation. Anemia of chronic infection is present with long-standing disease. Since cystic fibrosis may be manifest primarily as bronchiectasis appearing in late adolescence or early adult life, a sweat chloride test should be performed in patients of such an age in whom there is no evidence of antecedent pneumonia, obstructing lesion, or other evident predisposing cause of bronchiectasis. Serum immunoglobulins should be determined in a young patient, particularly a young male, with recurrent pneumonias and bronchiectasis. The electrocardiogram may show evidence of cor pulmonale in the presence of advanced disease.

DIFFERENTIAL DIAGNOSIS

There are two aspects of the differential diagnosis of bronchiectasis. The first relates to distinguishing this disease from other processes that may produce a similar constellation of symptoms, physical findings, and radiographic changes. The second relates to determination of whether any of the numerous predisposing conditions producing secondary bronchiectasis are present.

Chronic bronchitis is the most common disease that closely resembles bronchiectasis in symptoms, physical findings, and abnormal pulmonary function tests. Bronchiectasis may be accompanied by small-airway disease; reciprocally, localized bronchiectatic areas can develop in the setting of chronic bronchitis and emphysema. The presence of tramline and ring shadows on chest radiographs is more suggestive of bronchiectasis, but HRCT or bronchographic visualization may be the only means to distinguish between these processes. Allergic bronchopulmonary aspergillosis, a form of hypersensitivity lung disease, is characterized by episodic wheezing, expectoration of mucous plugs, intermittent pulmonary infiltrates, and irregularly dilated proximal bronchi that connect with normal bronchi and bronchioles peripherally. In contrast, in bronchiectasis the sputum is usually more abundant and purulent, and the involvement is in the more distal bronchial tree. The distinction between these two disorders may be blurred by the fact that cylindric bronchiectasis may complicate long-standing ABPA. Other entities that should be distinguished from bronchiectasis are bronchiolitis obliterans, recurrent episodes of pneumonia, and organized or unresolved pneumonia.

Productive cough, dyspnea, and occasional hemoptyses, clinical manifestations of bronchiectasis, occur also in a relatively rare pulmonary disease known as the unilateral hyperlucent lung (Swyer-James or Macleod's syndrome). The diagnosis is usually made on the basis of radiographic findings of hyperlucency of a lung or lobe resulting from air trapping (particularly during expiration) and decreased pulmonary vascular markings in the affected area. This syndrome appears to be a consequence of bronchiolitis obliterans resulting from viral or bacterial infection in childhood, eventuating in subsequent underdevelopment of the affected portion of lung. Decreased pulmonary artery size reflects decreased flow and is an effect rather than a cause of the findings in this disease. Decreased ventilation and perfusion are present in the affected area on radionuclide lung scans. Bronchograms show dilated and beaded-appearing smaller bronchi consistent with bronchiectasis.

Pulmonary sequestration is suspected in a patient with recurrent infiltrates around a single chronically invaded area containing cystic spaces in a basilar segment of a lower lobe. A clue to diagnosis may be provided by the presence of a continuous bruit over the chest or axilla on the affected side due to shunting of blood from systemic artery to pulmonary vein in the intralobar sequestration.

Numerous congenital abnormalities of the tracheobronchial tree, acquired obstructive bronchial lesions and destructive parenchymal processes, and various inherited disorders predisposing to bronchiectasis should be considered in the evaluation of a patient with this disease (see "Pathogenesis and Predisposing Factors," above) (Table 132-1).

COMPLICATIONS AND PROGNOSIS

The principal complications of bronchiectasis are progressive suppuration, hemoptysis and major pulmonary hemorrhage, obliteration of peripheral airways with associated extensive bronchitis and emphysema, and chronic respiratory insufficiency and cor pulmonale.[28,35] Continued active suppuration has been more readily controlled in the antibiotic area, but recurrent episodes of bronchopneumonia and exacerbations of chronic bronchial infections (often due to antibiotic-resistant organisms such as *B. aeruginosa* in patients with cystic fibrosis) are still frequent in some patients.[9] Metastatic brain abscess is now a rare complication because of better control of active pulmonary infection with antimicrobials. In rare instances, pulmonary hemorrhage can be major, requiring surgery, or can be massive, with death due to exsanguination or asphyxiation. The greatest disability stems from the combination of bronchiectasis and emphysema producing chronic respiratory failure. Now, with better control of its suppurative aspects, bronchiectasis is rarely complicated by amyloidosis.

Over time, despite repeated antibiotic administration, the process could advance in already affected bronchial segments.[14] In the preantibiotic area, spread of the process from infected segments or lobes to other pulmonary segments appeared to follow bronchopulmonary aspirational events that produced new foci of pneumonia. In the antibiotic era, such spread to previously normal segments is unusual, unless bronchiectasis has developed in the setting of a diffuse predisposing process such as cystic fibrosis or the immotile cilia syndrome. Even with such underlying disease, in which bronchiectasis may be extensive, appropriate use of antibiotics may control symptoms, slow progression, and render surgery unnecessary. Indeed, now about 50 percent of patients with cystic fibrosis survive to approach 30 years of age.

Patients with childhood bronchiectasis often tend to get better during their teens and 20s and may remain relatively stable thereafter.[16] Even in the preantibiotic era, cases of bronchiectasis did not deny longevity.[35] Laënnec's famous patient, a piano teacher with chronic productive cough since age 16, continued her occupation and died at age 82. At autopsy, she had gross bronchiectasis in four lobes.

TREATMENT

The aim of treatment is control of symptoms and prevention of progression. In addition to measures directed at specific predisposing conditions (removal of obstructing endobronchial lesions, gamma globulin replacement for immunoglobulin deficiency), treatment consists of control of infection and basic supportive measures to provide good pulmonary toilet and relief of bronchospasm and small-airway disease.

There are several elements in control of infection. Appropriate immunizations against potential pulmonary pathogens (influenza vaccine, pneumococcal vaccine) should be performed. In children, the basic immunizations against childhood diseases (*H. influenzae* type b, measles, pertussis) that can predispose to bronchiectasis should have been carried out. Prompt antimicrobial treatment of superimposed acute pneumonitis or acute febrile exacerbations of bronchitis is indicated. Guidance in antibiotic selection is provided by evaluation of Gram-stained smears of sputum and results of sputum culture. Based on the frequent isolation of *H. influenzae,* pneumococci, or mixed oral flora, initial treatment with ampicillin, amoxicillin, or trimethoprim-sulfamethoxazole may be sufficient. The presence of *S. aureus* warrants the use of a penicillinase-resistant penicillin, such as oral dicloxacillin or intravenous nafcillin, or a cephalosporin. For patients with cystic fibrosis in whom *B. aeruginosa* may be the dominant bacterial flora during an acute episode of clinical infection, treatment usually requires the use of ticarcillin (or one of the ureidopenicillins) in combination with an aminoglycoside. Third-generation cephalosporins with antipseudomonal activity (e.g., ceftazidime) may be of value in treating infections due to resistant *B. aeruginosa.* Although ceftazidime has been successfully as monotherapy, combination with an aminoglycoside is probably preferable, to avoid selection of resistant strains during acute pulmonary infections severe enough to require hospitalization.

In patients with bronchiectasis whose cough and sputum volume and purulence increase but whose illness does not require hospitalization, oral therapy with ampicillin, amoxicillin, amoxicillin-clavulanate, tetracycline, or trimethoprim-sulfamethoxazole is reasonable during the symptomatic exacerbation. (Ofloxacin orally for 10 to 15 days has been employed for treatment of infective exacerbations in bronchiectasis when gram-negative enteric bacteria or *B. aeruginosa* have been predominant.) Therapy may be initiated similarly at the onset of a viral upper respiratory infection or with symptomatic sinusitis. In some patients with bronchiectasis, as in some patients with chronic bronchitis, such exacerbations are frequent and debilitating. Suppressive prophylactic antimicrobial therapy with one of the aforementioned drugs during the winter may be warranted in selected patients. Patients with cystic fibrosis are often managed with periodic pulmonary "clean-outs," in which a course of parenteral antibiotics and intensive pulmonary physiotherapy are combined. Also, in a trial of clinically stable patients with cystic fibrosis, 4-week courses of high-dose aerosol tobramycin

were effective in improving pulmonary function and decreasing the numbers of *B. aeruginosa* in sputum, and may have reduced the frequency of courses of intravenous antibiotics needed.

Pulmonary toilet by postural drainage and chest percussion is of major importance in management, particularly in patients with sputum volumes greater than 30 to 50 ml per day. Bronchoscopy is not indicated to assist in removal of secretions, only for removal of a foreign body or bronchial plug. Hydration should be well maintained to avoid inspissation of secretions. Inhalation of a nebulized mist may sometimes be useful in loosening secretions. In view of the high content (10.2 percent of dry weight) of leukocyte-derived DNA, a major contributor to the viscosity of the sputum of patients with cystic fibrosis, attempts have been made to reduce the viscoelasticity of bronchial secretions by administration of recombinant human deoxyribonuclease I (rh DNase) by nebulizer (24-week outpatient treatment). Such treatment is well tolerated and has produced a modest reduction in exacerbations of respiratory symptoms requiring antibiotic therapy and a slight improvement in pulmonary function. The ultimate role of this form of therapy must await results of longer trials, longer follow-up, and assessment of cost-effectiveness.

Bronchodilators may be helpful because of the associated diffuse small-airway disease; improved mucociliary clearance and removal of pooled secretions may follow. In some patients, however, reduction in bronchomotor tone may inhibit the cough reflex and promote further pooling of secretions, with resultant deterioration of pulmonary function. Smoking should be proscribed. Medical management is satisfactory in most patients with bronchiectasis. Surgical resection is reserved primarily for young patients with troublesome symptoms (severe cough, recurrent pneumonias, profuse purulent sputum) that persist despite conservative management and interfere with normal life.[41] Such patients with localized disease can be cured by segmental resection or lobectomy; patients with extensive disease are less likely to benefit, although bilateral resections have been successful when the remaining lung is essentially unaffected.[12,41,53]

Another indication for surgical resection is major hemorrhage from an eroded vessel in a bronchiectatic segment. The principal

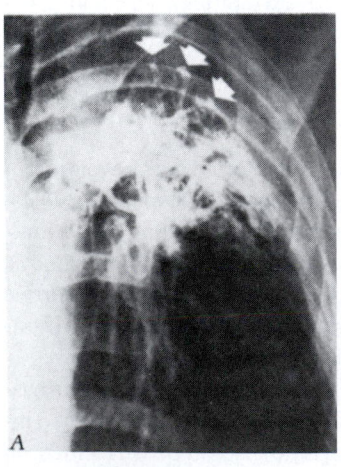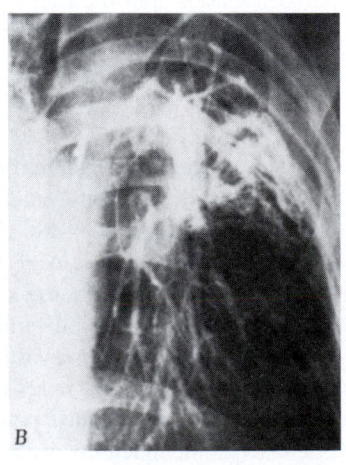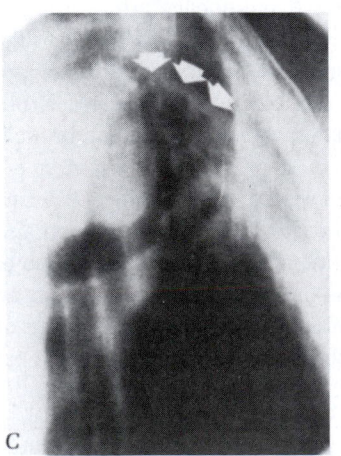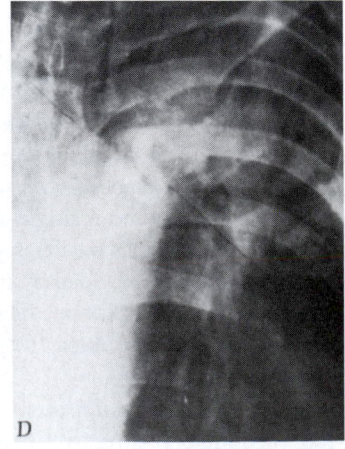

FIGURE 132-15 Hypervascularity around bronchiectatic lesions demonstrated on bronchial arteriography. *A.* Arterial tufts (arrows) in periphery of left upper-lobe bronchiectasis. *B.* Extensive bronchial to pulmonary arterial shunting with prominent opacifications of left pulmonary artery. *C.* Tomographic view of the cystic dilated left upper-lobe bronchi (arrows). *D.* Angiographic view showing occlusion of the left bronchial artery after embolization. *(Based on data of Uflacker et al,[49] with permission.)*

source of bleeding in patients with major hemoptyses—with the rare exception of the patient with a Rasmussen aneurysm of the pulmonary artery in a tuberculous cavity—is from a branch of a bronchial artery. Bronchial arteriography and embolization (Fig. 132-15) has been used to control massive or repeated hemoptysis in patients with bronchiectasis.[15,49] This procedure may be indicated for patients who are not surgical candidates by virtue of diffuse involvement of both lungs (e.g., patients with advanced cystic fibrosis) or as a temporizing measure for patients who require immediate stabilization in preparation for later elective surgery. Cessation of major bleeding has been achieved in patients with cystic fibrosis by this procedure, although minor hemoptyses later recurred in several. The presence of a spinal radicular artery arising from a bronchial artery is considered a contraindication to embolization because of risk of spinal cord injury.

REFERENCES

1. Afzelius BA: "Immotile-cilia" syndrome and ciliary abnormalities induced by infection and injury. *Am Rev Respir Dis* 124:107–109, 1981.
2. Bachman AL, Hewitt WR, Beekley HC: Bronchiectasis: A bronchographic study of 60 cases of pneumonia. *Arch Intern Med* 91:78–96, 1953.
3. Barker AF: Bronchiectasis. *Semin Thorac Cardiovasc Surg* 7:112–118, 1995.
4. Barker AF, Bardana EJ Jr: Bronchiectasis: Update of an orphan disease. *Am Rev Respir Dis* 137:969–978, 1988.
5. Barton AD, Lourenço RV: Bronchial secretions and mucociliary clearance: Biochemical characteristics. *Arch Intern Med* 131:140–144, 1973.
6. Bass H, Henderson JAM, Hecksher T, et al: Regional structure and function in bronchiectasis. *Am Rev Respir Dis* 97:598–609, 1968.
7. Carson JL, Collier AM, Hu SS: Acquired ciliary defects in nasal epithelium of children with acute viral upper respiratory infections. *New Engl J Med* 312:463–468, 1985.
8. Cherniack NS, Carton RW: Factors associated with respiratory insufficiency in bronchiectasis. *Am J Med* 41:562–571, 1966.
9. Cole PJ: A new look at the pathogenesis and management of persistent bronchial sepsis: A "vicious circle" hypothesis and its logical therapeutical connotations, in Davies RJ (ed), *Strategies for the Management of Chronic Bronchial Sepsis.* Oxford, The Medicine Publishing Foundation, 1984, pp 1–20.
10. Culiner MM: Intralobar bronchial cystic disease, the "sequestration complex" and cystic bronchiectasis. *Dis Chest* 53:462–469, 1968.
11. Davis PB, Hubbard VS, McCoy K, Taussig LM: Familial bronchiectasis. *J Pediatr* 102:177–184, 1983.
12. Drapanas T, Siewers R, Feist JH: Reversible poststenotic bronchiectasis. *New Engl J Med* 275:917–921, 1966.
13. Eliasson R, Mossberg B, Camner P, Afzelius BA: The immotilecilia syndrome: A congenital ciliary abnormality as an etiologic factor in chronic airway infections and male sterility. *New Engl J Med* 297:1–6, 1977.
14. Ellis DA, Thornley PE, Wightman AJ, et al: Present outlook in bronchiectasis: Clinical and social study and review of factors influencing prognosis. *Thorax* 36:659–664, 1981.
15. Fellows KE, Khaw KT, Schuster S, Shwachman H: Bronchial artery embolization in cystic fibrosis: Technique and long-term results. *J Pediatr* 95:959–963, 1979.
16. Field CE: Bronchiectasis: Third report on a follow-up study of medical and surgical cases from childhood. *Arch Dis Child* 45:551–561, 1969.
17. Fraser RG, Macklem PT, Brown WG: Airway dynamics in bronchiectasis: A combined cinefluorographic-manometric study. *Am J Roentgenol* 93:821–835, 1965.
18. Fraser RG, Pare JAP: Roentgenologic signs in the diagnosis of chest disease, in Fraser RG, Pare JAP (eds), *Diagnosis of Diseases of the Chest,* 2d ed. Philadelphia, Saunders, 1977, pp 518–525.
19. Fraser RG, Pare JAP: Diseases of the airways, in Fraser RG, Pare JAP (eds), *Diagnosis of Diseases of the Chest,* 2d ed. Philadelphia, Saunders, 1977, pp 1443–1456.
20. Friedman PJ, Harwood IR, Ellenbogen PH: Pulmonary cystic fibrosis in the adult: Early and late radiologic findings with pathologic correlation. *Am J Roentgenol* 136:1131–1144, 1981.
21. Gay S, Dee P: Tracheobronchomegaly—the Mounier-Kuhn syndrome. *Br J Radiol* 57:640–644, 1984.
22. Glimp RA, Bayer AS: Fungal pneumonias. Part 3: Allergic bronchopulmonary aspergillosis. *Chest* 80:85–94, 1981.
23. Gregg I, Trapnell DH: The bronchographic appearance of early chronic bronchitis. *Br J Radiol* 42:132–139, 1969.
24. Handelsman DJ, Conway AJ, Boylan LM, Turtle JR: Young's syndrome: Obstructive azoospermia and chronic sinopulmonary infections. *New Engl J Med* 310:3–9, 1984.
25. Holmes LB, Blennerhassett JB, Austen KF: A reappraisal of Kartagener's syndrome. *Am J Med Sci* 255:13–28, 1968.
26. Jederlinic PJ, Sicilian LS, Baigelman W, Gaensler EA: Congenital bronchial atresia: A report of 4 cases and a review of the literature. *Medicine (Baltimore)* 66:73–83, 1987.
27. Kaschula ROC, Druker J, Kipps A: Late morphologic consequences of measles: A lethal and debilitating lung disease among the poor. *Rev Infect Dis* 5:395–404, 1983.
28. Konietzko NFJ, Carton RW, Leroy EP: Causes of death in patients with bronchiectasis. *Am Rev Respir Dis* 100:852–858, 1969.
29. Lewiston NJ: Bronchiectasis in childhood. *Pediatr Clin North Am* 31:865–878, 1984.
30. Liebow AA, Hales MR, Lindskog GE: Enlargement of bronchial arteries, and their anastomoses with pulmonary arteries in bronchiectasis. *Am J Pathol* 25:211–231, 1949.
31. Lopez-Vidriero MT, Reid L: Chemical markers of mucous and serum glycoproteins and their relation to viscosity in mucoid and purulent sputum from various hypersecretory diseases. *Am Rev Respir Dis* 117:465–477, 1978.
32. McGuinness G, Naidich DP: Bronchiectasis: CT/clinical correlations. *Semin Ultrasound CT MRI* 16:395–419, 1995.
33. Muller NL, Bergin CJ, Ostrow DN, Nichols DM: Role of computed tomography in the recognition of bronchiectasis. *Am J Roentgenol* 143:971–976, 1984.
34. Ogilvie AG: The natural history of bronchiectasis—a clinical, roentgenologic and pathologic study. *Arch Intern Med* 68:395–465, 1941.
35. Perry KMA, King DS: Bronchiectasis: A study of prognosis based on a follow-up of 400 patients. *Am Rev Tuberc* 41:531–548, 1940.
36. Reid LM: Reduction in bronchial subdivision in bronchiectasis. *Thorax* 5:233–247, 1950.
37. Reid LM: The pathology of obstructive and inflammatory airway diseases. *Eur J Respir Dis* 147:26–37, 1986.
38. Rivera M. Nicotra MB: Pseudomonas aeruginosa mucoid strain: Its significance in adult chest disease. *Am Rev Respir Dis* 126:833–836, 1982.
39. Rosenzweig DY, Stead WW: The role of tuberculosis and other forms of bronchopulmonary necrosis in the pathogenesis of bronchiectasis. *Am Rev Respir Dis* 93:769–785, 1966.
40. Rossman CM, Forrest JB, Ruffin RE, Newhouse MT: Immotile cilia syndrome in persons with and without Kartagener's syndrome. *Am Rev Respir Dis* 121:1011–1016, 1980.

41. Sanderson JM, Kennedy MCS, Johnson MF, Manley DCE: Bronchiectasis: Results of surgical and conservative management: A review of 393 cases. *Thorax* 29:407–416, 1974.

42. Schreiber JR, Goldman DA: Infections complicating cystic fibrosis, in Remington JS, Swartz MN (eds), *Current Clinical Topics in Infectious Diseases,* vol 7. New York, McGraw-Hill, 1986, pp 51–81.

43. Silverman PM, Godwin JD: CT/bronchographic correlations in bronchiectasis. *J Comput Assist Tomogr* 11:52–56, 1987.

44. Similä S, Linna O, Lanning P, et al: Chronic lung damage caused by adenovirus type 7: A ten-year follow-up study. *Chest* 80:127–131, 1981.

45. Sun L, Jiang R-Z, Steinbach S, et al: The emergence of a highly transmissible lineage of cbl$^+$ *Pseudomonas (Burkholderia) cepacia* causing CF centre epidemics in North America and Britain. *Nature Medicine* 1:661–666, 1995.

46. Suter S, Schaad UB, Roux L, et al: Granulocyte neutral proteases and *Pseudomonas* elastase as possible causes of airway damage in patients with cystic fibrosis. *J Infect Dis* 149:523–531, 1984.

47. Trapnell DH, Gregg I: Some principles of interpretation of bronchograms. *Br J Radiol* 42:125–131, 1969.

48. Trucksis M, Swartz MN: Bronchiectasis: A current view, in Remington JS, Swartz MN (eds), *Current Clinical Topics in Infectious Diseases,* vol 11. Boston, Blackwell, 1991, pp 170–205.

49. Uflacker R, Kaemmerer A, Neves C, Picon PD: Management of massive hemoptysis by bronchial artery embolization. *Radiology* 146:627–634, 1983.

50. Wayne KS, Taussig LM: Probably familial congenital bronchiectasis due to cartilage deficiency (Williams-Campbell syndrome). *Am Rev Respir Dis* 114:15–22, 1976.

51. Wentworth P, Gough J, Wentworth JE: Pulmonary changes and cor pulmonale in mucoviscidosis. *Thorax* 23:582–589, 1968.

52. Whitwell F: A study of the pathology and pathogenesis of bronchiectasis. *Thorax* 7:213–239, 1952.

53. Wilson JF, Decker AM: The surgical management of childhood bronchiectasis: A review of 96 consecutive pulmonary resections in children with nontuberculous bronchiectasis. *Ann Surg* 195:354–363, 1982.

CHAPTER 133

SYSTEMIC INFECTION, THE SEPSIS SYNDROME, AND THE LUNGS

Richard Teplick / Jay A. Fishman

The relationship of extrapulmonary processes to the development of infection in the lungs is mediated by three main mechanisms: (1) as a part of the underlying disease process (e.g., direct extension of systemic infection to the lungs); (2) by altering the host so as to enhance the susceptibility of the lungs to injury (e.g., altered colonization patterns due to the use of antibiotics or H_2—histamine receptor—blockers); and (3) via the systemic release of mediators that directly or indirectly alter the susceptibility of the lungs to infection or parenchymal injury (e.g., cytokine mediators of the "sepsis syndrome" and the adult respiratory distress syndrome. The manifestations of such injuries are determined by the nature of the host response and by the location, intensity, and duration of the exposure to organisms capable of causing infection. This chapter is devoted to a discussion of extrapulmonary processes that may alter pulmonary susceptibility to infection and to the pulmonary effects of extrapulmonary infection and inflammation.

THE LUNGS IN EXTRAPULMONARY INFECTION

Extrapulmonary infection affects the lungs directly, via the spread of organisms in the bloodstream or lymphatics, airways, or contiguous structures into the lungs or pleural spaces, or indirectly, via the actions of systemic mediators of inflammation synthesized and released by cells either at the site of localized tissue injury or infection or by bacterial products or tissue debris released into the systemic circulation. The activation of systemic mediators results in the initiation of a pulmonary-specific response that includes aspects of inflammation and repair even in the absence of pulmonary infection. Failure to regulate these responses may cause transient or permanent pulmonary damage and enhance susceptibility to infection.

Terminology

The terminology to describe systemic infection is complicated by the use of terms such as *sepsis, bacteremia, septicemia,* and *septic shock.* A high percentage of patients dying with respiratory failure such as the acute respiratory distress syndrome (ARDS) die from multiple organ failure and systemic hemodynamic instability or the "sepsis syndrome" rather than respiratory failure with infection per se.[47] In one series, only one-third of trauma patients thought to be septic had definite infectious foci, and the presence of identifiable infection was unrelated to mortality.[26] In this retrospective series, the lungs were consistently the first organ system to fail. Thus, many septic-appearing patients are not infected; necrotic or inflamed tissue alone can produce the syndrome, and there is currently no way to differentiate among these causes on the basis of clinical criteria.[16] As a result, it is important to establish definitions of the terms used to discuss systemic infection, inflammation, and their sequelae. For purposes of this discussion, the following terms, adapted from the American College of Chest Physicians/Society of Critical Care Medicine Consensus Conference,[2] will be used.

1. *Infection*—the presence of organisms in any location where they are not normally present or an inflammatory response to microorganisms. Many authors would limit this definition to organisms in normally sterile sites. However, this precludes consideration of altered microbial flora in the gastrointestinal tract (e.g., infection in *Clostridium difficile* colitis).

2. *Bacteremia*—the presence of bacteria in the blood. Similarly, fungemia, viremia, and parasitemia imply the demonstration of these organisms in the bloodstream.

3. *Systemic inflammatory response syndrome*—the presence of two or more of the following criteria associated with a systemic inflammatory response: abnormal temperature (less than 36°C or greater than 38°C), tachycardia (heart rate above 90 beats/min), tachypnea (respiratory rate above 20 breaths/min or hyperventilation with P_{CO_2} below 32 mmHg), leukocytosis (white blood cell count greater than 12,000 cells/mm^3) or leukopenia (white blood cell count under 4000 cells/mm^3) or greater than 10 percent immature cells. All these changes should reflect a change from baseline.

4. *Sepsis*—the systemic inflammatory response syndrome occurring as a result of infection.

5. *Severe sepsis*—sepsis associated with organ dysfunction, hypoperfusion, or hypotension in the absence of other causes of hypotension, such as cardiac failure.

6. *Septic shock*—sepsis with hypotension and marked perfusion abnormalities despite fluid resuscitation, often dependent on pharmacologic support of blood pressure, heart rate, or perfusion.

7. *Multiple organ dysfunction syndrome*—progressive organ dysfunction in an acutely ill patient.

Pulmonary Infections Following Systemic Infection

GENERAL ISSUES

In general, the lungs are protected from the direct effects of toxins or of infection due to the filtration and metabolic functions of the liver, spleen, blood-borne phagocytes, and lymphatics. Most organisms reaching the lungs are cleared by phagocytic cells of the lungs and cells recruited from the blood into the pulmonary parenchyma. Thus, pulmonary infection is established only when these protective mechanisms are overwhelmed (e.g., persistent high-grade bacteremia) or inactivated (e.g., radiotherapy or chemotherapy for cancer) or preexisting conditions diminish the host response to infection (e.g., immune deficiency).[5,6] Consequently, the risk of pulmonary infection is a function of the net level of the host's susceptibility to infection balanced against the infectious burden. A variety of factors alter the net level of the host's susceptibility to infection. Intrinsic or host factors include alterations in the pulmonary parenchyma due to fibrosis, infarction, or edema, and diminished clearance, as is seen with ciliary defects or cystic fibrosis. Factors that increase the relative infectious burden include a decrease in the clearance of bacteria from the blood (as in cir-

rhosis with portal hypertension), high-level bacteremia (associated with right-sided endocarditis or loculated, undrained pus), or characteristics of the organisms that increase "virulence" (the ability to invade tissues, replicate, or survive host inflammatory responses), such as the ability of *Salmonella* species to adhere to vascular tissues (see Chapter 125).

Systemic infectious sources may seed the lung and pleural space from a contiguous focus or via the bloodstream or lymphatics. Contiguous spread often entails the decompression of an intra-abdominal or pharyngeal abscess along tissue planes into the thoracic cavity. These may be catastrophic clinical events, as in the rupture of a subphrenic or a hepatic abscess across the diaphragm due to *Entamoeba histolytica*, with the sudden development of amebic pneumonia. A more insidious picture occurs when a peritonsillar abscess (or infections of the parapharyngeal space) or submandibular infection (Ludwig's angina) decompresses into the retropharyngeal space. This potential space extends down to the level of thoracic vertebra 1 or 2, and may allow the drainage of pus directly into the mediastinum, causing mediastinitis.

Alternatively, embolic spread of infection to the lungs or pleura may result from the seeding of organisms into the parenchymal or pleural space, from septic embolization due to an infected thrombus (Fig. 133-1), or from the debris of a distant infection. Bacteremia tends to cause areas of pneumonia throughout the parenchyma. This is a pattern seen in miliary tuberculosis or in staphylococcal bacteremia due to endocarditis (Fig. 133-2). If multiple abscesses develop, they are usually peripheral. If pulmonary emboli develop as a complication of septic thrombophlebitis or of tricuspid valvular infective endocarditis, infarction may accompany infection. In this situation, abscess formation is rapid and unimpeded by appropriate host responses. Rarely do sterile emboli become secondarily infected. However, infarction may accompany pneumonia due to *Aspergillus* or *Pseudomonas aeruginosa* because of vascular tropism and due to the vasculitis that these organisms cause (Fig. 133-1).

Diffuse pulmonary injury may also be caused without infection by systemic inflammatory processes—mediated either indirectly by cytokines and other inflammatory mediators or directly by substances produced by the organisms (toxins).[7] The injuries produced by such systemic processes generally represent a significant predisposition to infection that may be further enhanced by failure of multiple organs. Thus, ARDS or multiple organ dysfunction should prompt a search for infectious foci. Such systemic syndromes as toxic shock syndrome (TSS), aspiration pneumonitis with bacteremia, gram-negative sepsis, and inflammation and necrosis without infection resulting from pancreatitis may be clinically indistinguishable.

PNEUMONIA IN THE POSTSURGICAL PATIENT

Fever is common in the postoperative setting, with surgery itself a major cause (for discussion, see Chapters 140 and 143). Up to 40 percent of post–thoracic surgery patients develop pneumonia, but the diagnosis is confused by the presence of other causes of radiologic pulmonary infiltrates, including congestive heart failure, atelectasis, pulmonary embolus, contusion, and pleural ef-

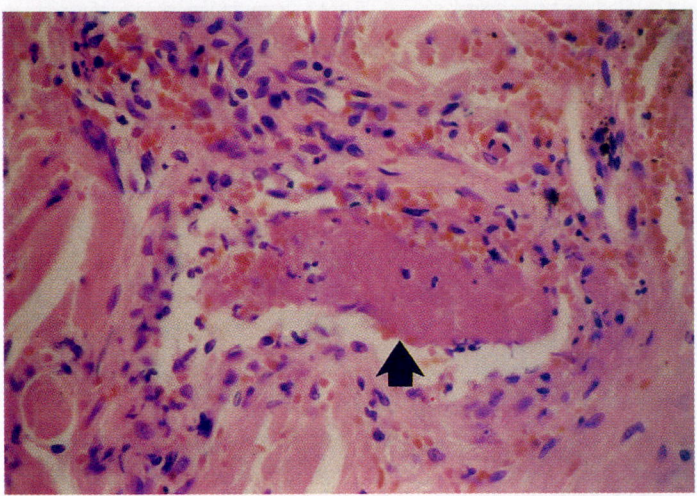

A

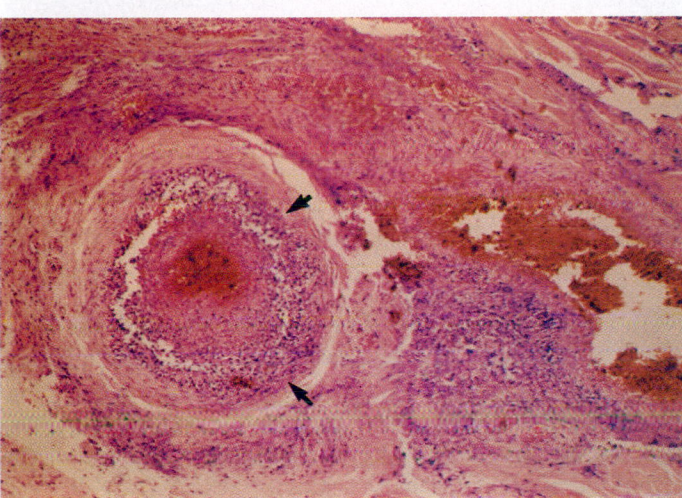

B

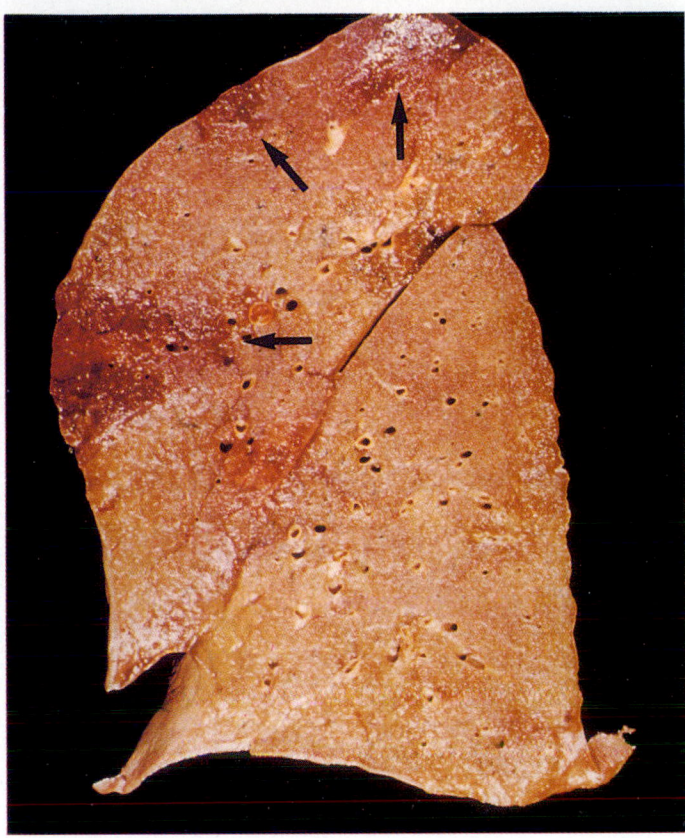

C

FIGURE 133-1 *Pseudomonas aeruginosa* bacteremia from an infected pelvic vein thrombus presenting as cutaneous vasculitis *(A)* with small arteries occluded by fibrin thrombi (arrow) and with bacterial and leukocytic infiltration of the vascular wall (arrows, *B*). The patient developed multiple septic pulmonary emboli with infarction (arrows, *C*)

with both organisms and leukocytes deep within the emboli. The pattern of microvascular thrombosis due to disseminated intravascular coagulation and ecthyma gangrenosum (arterial vasculitis due to infection) is characteristic of persistent high-grade bacteremia with *Pseudomonas* and other organisms.

fusions.[12,19,20,42] Hospital-acquired pneumonia has a high mortality (20 percent in community hospitals to 50 percent in teaching hospitals), although only a third is directly attributable to the pneumonia itself rather than to an array of postoperative complications. Nosocomial pneumonia may add little to the risk of dying in the already critically ill patient; patients may develop pneumonia because they are critically ill rather than vice versa. Bacteremia occurs in 2 to 6 percent of nosocomial pneumonia, with a resultant threefold increase in mortality. The incidence of nosocomial pneumonia in postoperative patients is approximately 17.5 percent, with mortality related largely to the causative organism. Mortality in patients with gram-negative pneumonia approaches 50 percent (up to 70 to 80 percent in those with *Pseudomonas* infection) and 5 to 24 percent in patients with gram-positive infections. Colonization by highly virulent or antibiotic resistant pathogens is the main determinant of the species isolated.

Pulmonary Effects of Systemic Inflammatory Processes

GENERAL MECHANISMS

The metabolic effects of systemic infection are part of the systemic inflammatory response (protein catabolism, acute-phase reactant synthesis, leukocytosis, proteinuria, cytokine release) that occurs in both localized and generalized infectious processes. The dissection of the pulmonary inflammatory response is complicated by the observations that many cytokines, including the interleukins (IL), tumor necrosis factor (TNF), and the chemokines, and other factors (e.g., growth factors) are active in the coordinated inflammatory response.[1,5] These factors have both specific and overlapping functions (described in detail in Chapters 24 and 25) and are synthesized by various components of the pulmonary architecture (including epithelia, endothelia, lymphocytes, macrophages, and neutrophils) that are

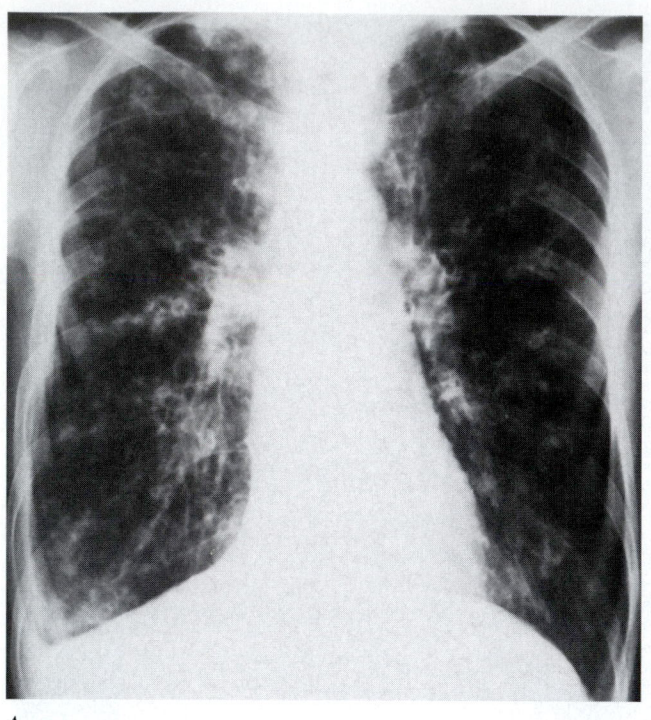
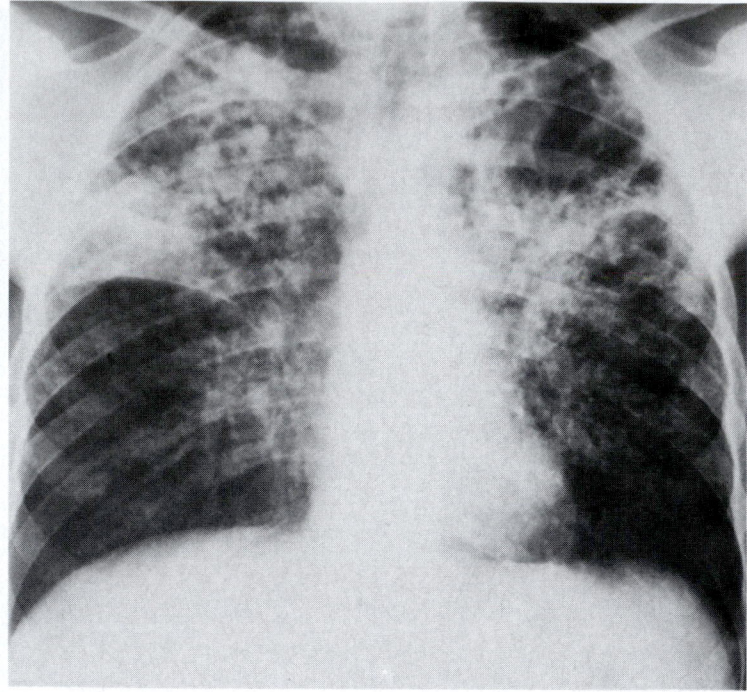

A   *B*

FIGURE 133-2   Right-sided *Staphylococcus aureus* endocarditis in a heroin abuser with multiple pulmonary abscesses due to septic emboli *(A)*. The distribution of lung involvement contrasts with the patchy pneumonic picture of miliary (i.e., bacteremic) tuberculosis *(B)*.

differentially regulated. Thus, when stimulated by TNF-α and IL-1 in the circulation, resident alveolar macrophages produce TNF, IL-6, IL-8 platelet activating factor (PAF), and additional IL-1. IL-8—in conjunction with TNF, IL-1, and other chemotactic factors—attracts neutrophils (see below) and initiates the pulmonary inflammatory response (see Chapter 120).

The systemic inflammatory response induced by infection or injury may induce inflammatory changes in the lung that persist long after the acute stimulus has dissipated. For example, following bacteremia or burn injury, TNF, γ-interferon, and IL-1β are released into the circulation, and induce local production of mRNA and proteins for TNFα, IL-6, and IL-8 in the lungs.[18,43,45,53] IL-6

and IL-8 levels are many times higher in the bronchial secretions than in the systemic circulation and persist at elevated levels for weeks.[51] This results in the local recruitment of inflammatory cells, fibroblast proliferation, and lymphocyte activation, which continue long after the initial insult has dissipated. Components of the arachidonic acid metabolism pathway (thromboxane B_2 and prostaglandins E and F) may contribute to the down-regulation of monocyte function.

Persistence of systemic stimulation (e.g., in burn injury, pancreatitis, or infection) results in the recruitment of blood monocytes into the lung, enhancing local IL-1α production. Persistently elevated levels of IL-1α and IL-1β and TNF-α up-regulate pro-

TABLE 133-1

Immunotherapies

Agent	Site of Action	Animal Studies	Human Trials
E5 antibody	Endotoxin	Variable results Species specific	Questionable benefit in subgroup without refractory shock
HA-1A	Endotoxin	Variable results (harmful in dogs)	No benefit and possibly harmful
Anti-TNF antibody	TNF	Variable results, depending on model of sepsis	No benefit (phase III trial to evaluate only in septic shock)
Soluble TNF receptor	TNF	Variable	No benefit and possibly harmful
IL-1ra	IL-1 receptor	Beneficial	Possible benefit in subgroup with high mortality risk (phase III follow-up pending)
IL-6 antibody	IL-6	Beneficial	Pending
IL-8 antibody	IL-8	Pending	Pending

SOURCE: Adapted from St John RC, Dorinsky PM: Immunologic therapy for ARDS, septic shock, and multi-organ failure. *Chest* 103:932, 1993.

duction of IL-6, IL-8, and IL-1 by fibroblasts and endothelial cells. This results in the local production of IL-2, IL-3, γ-interferon, IL-4, IL-5, IL-6, IL-7, and PAF. The complex inflammatory cascade will result in the recruitment of T cells, the proliferation of B cells, proliferation of fibroblasts with collagen synthesis, production of IgE, eosinophil growth and differentiation, endothelial injury, and platelet aggregation and degranulation.[13,51] This cascade is normally balanced, in part, by the downregulatory effects of IL-10 and the synergistic effect of IL-1α and TNF-α to inhibit fibroblast proliferation and collagen production.

The net result of the local response to the activation of the systemic inflammatory cascade is the amplification in the lungs of systemic changes induced by extrapulmonary injury. While the appropriate pulmonary inflammatory response is protective, and results in the clearance of infectious organisms or the repair of damaged tissues, a failure to regulate the intensity and duration of the pulmonary inflammatory response, or the presence of a second "hit" or injury to the lungs, may result in parenchymal injury and increased susceptibility to infection (see below). This unregulated response may be reflected in a variety of common clinical syndromes, including ARDS, fibrosis, and pulmonary edema, with increased susceptibility to infection. The cytokine cascade is accompanied by the systemic effects of the myriad products of bacterial (or fungal or parasitic) replication, including exotoxins (e.g., TSS toxin) and bacterial lipopolysaccharide (LPS or endotoxin), which may contribute directly to systemic toxicity.

The results of studies in which the systemic cytokine cascade has been interrupted have been variable. While some studies have demonstrated increased resistance to death due to hemorrhage, LPS, or bacterial sepsis—e.g., using tumor necrosis factor receptor,[13] especially if given before or during an LPS challenge—others have not demonstrated benefit or even shown worsened outcomes. Human studies of TNF-α antibodies in sepsis either have not shown any benefit or resulted in higher mortality (Table 133-1). Thus, although the prevention of pulmonary infection or injury is linked to the activation of the systemic inflammatory response, generalized inhibition has not proved beneficial.

EXOTOXINS

A few exotoxins merit individual mention. *Staphylococcus aureus* α-toxin mediates the formation of nonphysiological calcium channels in pulmonary endothelium in vitro and the initiation of the arachidonic acid cascade in isolated perfused rabbit lungs. These changes are accompanied by pulmonary hypertension, probably due to thromboxane A_2 release, though the vasodilator prostaglandin prostacyclin is also activated. The toxin may also be responsible for direct pulmonary endothelial cell injury. However, the in vivo role of these changes is unclear. Two additional staphylococcal exotoxins have been implicated in the development of TSS. This syndrome was recognized in 1978 in children with high fever, hypotension, diarrhea, confusion, renal failure, and erythroderma.

The menstrual form of TSS, described in 1979, consists of high fever, a diffuse macular erythroderma accompanied by desquamation that includes the palms and soles of the feet, hypotension, and involvement of at least three organ systems from among the following: mucous membranes (hyperemia); gastrointestinal tract (diarrhea or vomiting); muscles (myalgias or twice normal creatine phosphokinase levels); kidneys (pyuria without urinary tract infection or twice normal concentration in serum of creatinine or urea nitrogen); hepatic (twice normal concentration in serum of total bilirubin or transaminases); blood (thrombocytopenia, platelets less than 100,000/ml); central nervous system (altered mental status without focal neurologic signs when normotensive without fever); and the absence of evidence for other infections, including leptospirosis, Rocky Mountain spotted fever, and measles. These findings have been observed in many hosts, but they were initially described in the context of menstruating young women using hyperabsorbable tampons and without microbiologic evidence of infection. More than 98 percent of TSS patients have *S. aureus* isolated from vaginal cultures or other sites, with more than 75 percent of these isolates positive for TSST-1 and 25 percent for other toxin types. The lungs are often affected in TSS, with changes consistent with "shock lung" (Fig. 133-3); pulmonary hemorrhage, edema, atelectasis, hyaline membrane formation, and capillary thrombosis are prominent in the absence of pulmonary infection.

Staphylococci and streptococci produce more than 20 bacterial products—i.e., toxins, enzymes, and factors—which have unclear roles in the development of infections. Among these, the hyaluronidases, lipases, hemolysins, streptokinase, and streptolysins are believed to enhance the spread of infection along, or through, tissue planes and may account for the ability of these organisms to cause bacteremic infection. These toxins also serve as "superantigens," which stimulate T cells to release high levels of proinflammatory cytokines and enhance the systemic inflammatory response. These organisms are also among the most common oropharyngeal colonizers and nosocomial organisms in hospitals, so the frequency of infection with these agents may also reflect their preponderance in the environment.

Gram-negative organisms also produce a variety of toxins, proteases, and immunologically active factors. Like *S. aureus*, *P. aeruginosa* produces a nonenzymatic protein, cytotoxin, which also induces prostacyclin production and creates discrete nonphysiological transmembrane channels in cultured pulmonary artery endothelial cells similar to those described for staphylococcal toxin. These channels allow the influx of calcium, which may modulate arachidonic acid metabolism in the cell. However, this organism also appears to have some unique characteristics that allow it to cause lung injury. *P. aeruginosa* is frequently associated with the development of ARDS during bacteremia or pneumonia (Fig. 133-4). In this setting it is associated with microvascular lung injury, which appears to be related to the pulmonary vascular sequestration of stimulated blood neutrophils even without infection of the pulmonary parenchyma. This pattern is similar to that seen in systemic inflammation. Even in the absence of granulocytes, however, *Pseudomonas* cytotoxin has been shown to mimic the presentation of ARDS in sheep and pigs. *Pseudomonas* also causes ARDS in the neutropenic patient. This effect is due to a marked and irreversible increase in pulmonary vascular permeability, which is distinct from the reversible, prostaglandin-mediated increase in pulmonary vascular resistance described above. This effect is also separable from the effects of bacterial endotoxin (see below), which has an over-

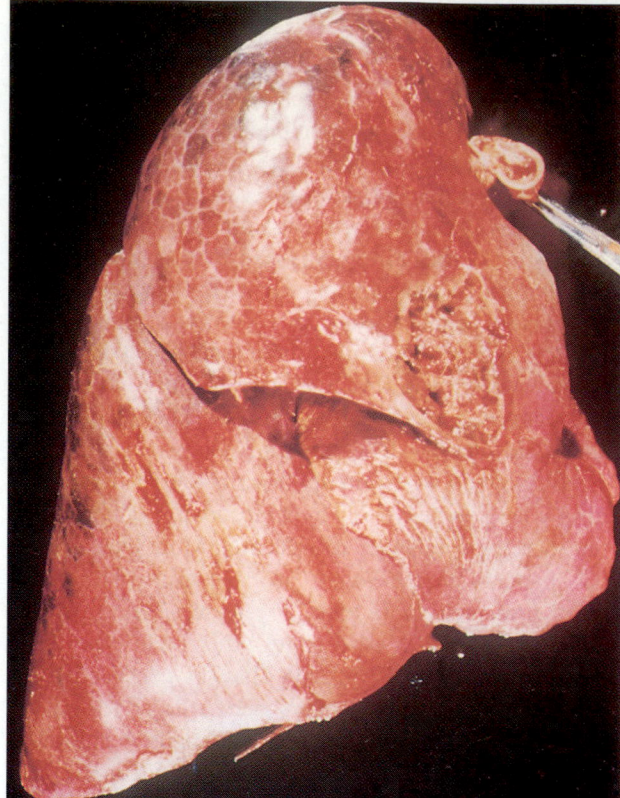

A

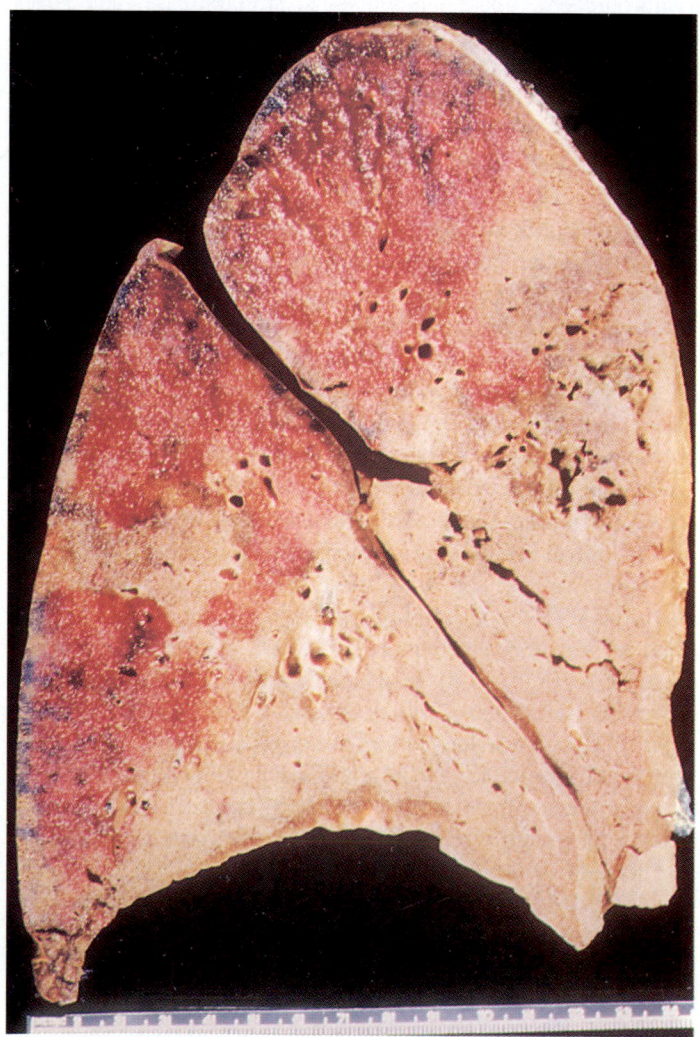

B

C

FIGURE 133-3 Toxic shock syndrome due to *S. aureus* bacteremia in a 20-year-old man following knee joint arthroscopy. Pleural hyperemia and inflammation *(A)* accompany the parenchymal hemorrhage and consolidation of staphylococcal pneumonitis *(B)*. Cavitation with abscess formation progressed despite appropriate antibiotics *(C)*.

lapping array of pulmonary manifestations. It is also a major pulmonary pathogen that can adhere to pulmonary endothelium, cause capillary thrombosis and inflammation, and invade the pulmonary interstitium (Fig. 133-1). *Pseudomonas* may mimic pulmonary thromboembolism with infarction during high-level bacteremia associated with bacterial invasion of pulmonary vessel walls. These many manifestations of *Pseudomonas* infection illustrate a variety of mechanisms by which systemic infection may cause significant pulmonary injury.

THE NEUTROPHIL

Neutrophil activation, which is manifest as enhanced production of products such as inflammatory mediators and oxygen radicals, can play a primary role in damaging the lungs during infection, but it is not essential to the development of such injuries. ARDS and bacteremic pneumonia are often seen in the neutropenic, bacteremic patient. Neutrophils have been recognized not only as effector cells but also as immunoregulatory cells capable of communicating with other inflammatory and structural cells. During infection or after exposure to LPS, IL-1, or TNF-

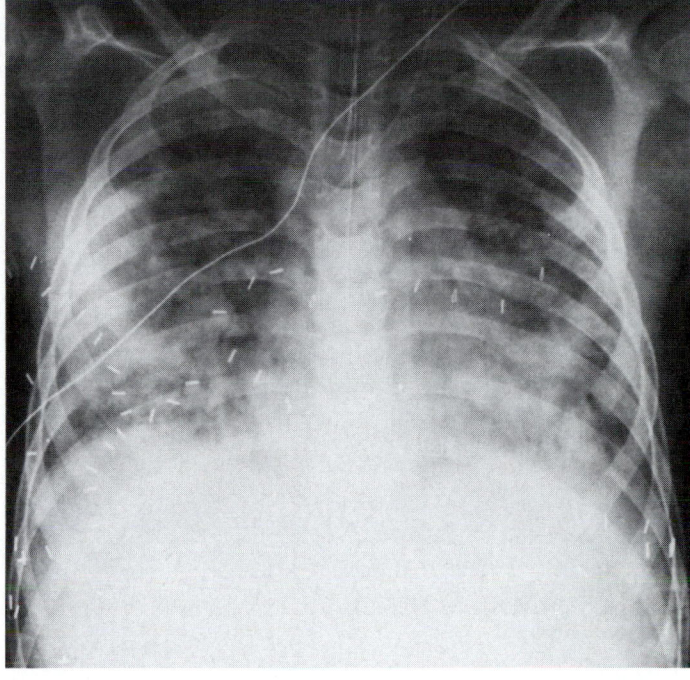

A

B

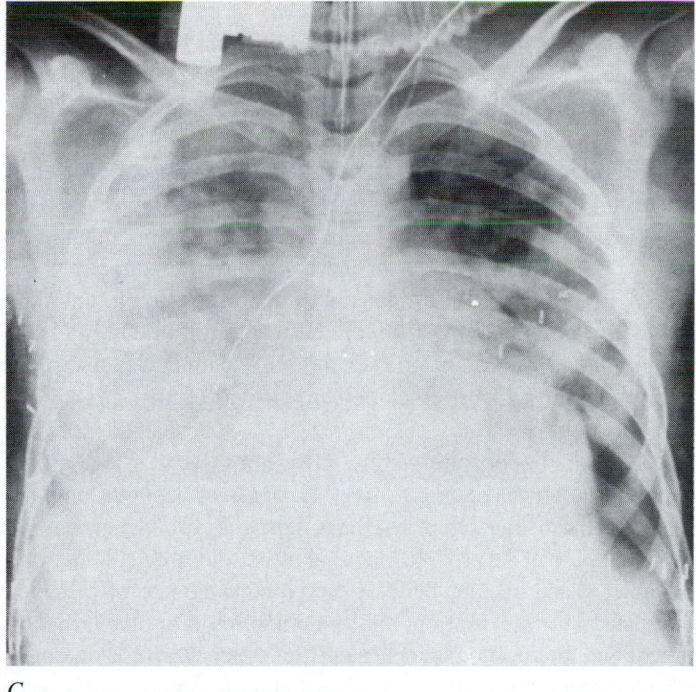

C

FIGURE 133-4   A child was admitted with a clear chest radiograph *(A)* after 55 percent body burns. After 2 weeks and numerous skin grafting procedures, the patient developed a mild cough. Sputum contained no inflammatory cells and sheets of gram-negative rods on Gram-stained smear. Therapy was initiated for *P. aeruginosa* empirically, despite an unchanged chest radiograph. Forty-eight h into therapy, bronchopneumonia developed on chest radiograph *(B)* and progressed rapidly (72 h, *C*), requiring intubation. The patient survived. Cultures of sputum grew *P. aeruginosa.*

leukotriene B_4, lipoxin A, and platelet-activating factor. Phagocytosis of bacteria (opsonized or not) and binding of endothelial adhesion molecules (ELAM-1 and ICAM-1) also stimulate neutrophil activation.

Once activated, neutrophils release a large variety of mediators that may be proinflammatory (IL-1α and β, TNF-α, IL-6 and 8) as well as anti-inflammatory (IL-1 receptor antagonist and TGF-β) and antiviral (IFN-α) (Table 133-2). Growth factors and IL-3 stimulate hematopoiesis and prime inflammatory cells for secondary stimuli. Neutrophil activation can be modified by alterations in signal transduction pathways, mediator binding, or synthesis. The effects of activation can be modified by antagonism of neutrophil-derived mediators and by inhibition of their binding to endothelium.

As discussed, the lung will amplify and prolong cytokine synthesis and release following a systemic inflammatory response. In the setting of pneumonia, neutrophil accumulation and activation are rapid and persistent. Within 1 h of the initial insult, neutrophils may cause pulmonary capillary endothelial injury, with edema and interstitial accumulation of protein and cells. The release of proteolytic enzymes, oxygen free radicals, and arachidonic acid metabolites from neutrophils will continue to injure the pulmonary parenchyma for as long as the stimulus persists. Pulmonary injury is potentiated by both hypoxia and hyperoxia and by conditions associated with chronic inflammation,

α, neutrophils marginate, adhering to the pulmonary endothelium, and consequently accumulate rapidly in the alveolar capillaries. Neutrophils also accumulate in other organs damaged during infection. Depletion of neutrophils attenuates these injuries to some degree. IL-8 has been identified as a potent chemoattractant chemokine whose local concentration appears to correlate with the level of histologic inflammation and the likelihood of developing ARDS. Many factors "activate" neutrophils, including IL-1, TNF-α, LPS (via an acute-phase protein-LPS–binding factor), complement fragments (C5a), f-met-leu-phe, IL-8, growth factors (G- and GM-CSF), IFN-γ,

TABLE 133-2

Neutrophil-Derived Mediators

Oxygen metabolites
  OH
  O_2^-
  H_2O_2
Granular enzymes
  Neutral serine proteases
  Metalloproteinases
  Myeloperoxidase
  Acid protease
Bioactive lipids
  Leukotriene B_4
  Platelet-activating factor
Cytokines
  IL-1α, β*
  TNF-α*
  IFN-α
  GM-CSF, G-CSF, M-CSF, IL-3
  IL-8*
  IL-6*
  IL-1 receptor antagonist
  TGF-β
  MIP-1α

*Known to be stimulated by LPS, infection, or phagocytosis; others under study.

such as bronchiectasis, bronchitis, chronic interstitial disease, and radiation or chemotherapy injury.

Neutrophils entering the lung parenchyma during the acute inflammatory response are thought to be committed to programmed cell death (apoptosis). This is a lung-protective response, during which DNA degradation is accompanied by neutrophil membrane stabilization, decreased enzyme leakage, and improved uptake by macrophages of dying neutrophils with diminished lung injury. In contrast, necrosis, or nonprogrammed cell death, results in the uncontrolled release of neutrophil enzymes, increased local acidosis, and diminished macrophage and monocyte function, which might aid in bacterial clearance. The progression to apoptosis or necrosis is controlled locally; the process can be interrupted by unknown factors secreted, most likely, by lung monocytes. LPS, granulocyte colony–stimulating factor, and monocyte-conditioned medium may delay neutrophil apoptosis and macrophage ingestion, increasing lung injury. Thus, normal neutrophil apoptosis plays a role in the curtailment of the inflammatory response, removing neutrophils before the release of histotoxic contents.

BACTEREMIA AND SEPTIC SHOCK

Bacterial, viral, and fungal organisms are often present in the circulation. Leakage of organisms into the bloodstream is common: across the colonic mucosa; from tooth brushing; from in-hospital procedures (e.g., bronchoscopy, liver biopsy, sigmoidoscopy); and in the course of localized infections of the urinary tract, lungs, gallbladder, or sinuses. Usually, this leakage is nonthreatening to the immunologically normal host. "High-grade"

bacteremia or persistent infection of the blood elicits distinctive systemic effects. Whether an infection will become high-grade depends on the location of infection, the defense mechanisms of the infected host, and the organism(s) responsible. Infection that causes "pus under pressure" (e.g., obstruction of drainage from a viscus, the biliary tree, or the urinary tract) or a large or perivascular abscess is likely to cause continuous leakage of organisms into the bloodstream. Bacteremia is detected in 6 to 10 percent of infections that do not originate in the bloodstream. However, the true incidence is probably significantly greater. Similarly, intravascular infection (e.g., endocarditis), infected vascular grafts, and central venous catheters have immediate access to the circulation. The increasing incidence of fungal, mycobacterial, and anaerobic bacteremia reflects technologic advances in culturing of the blood and, to an even greater extent, the increased survival of immunocompromised patients, use of broad-spectrum antibiotics, and the increase of a wide variety of surgical and mechanical interventions.

Bacteremia occurs in 4 to 10 out of every 1000 patients and in approximately 7.5 percent of all infections. Of all blood culture isolates at the Massachusetts General Hospital, approximately 35 to 40 percent are aerobic gram-positive species (largely *Staphylococcus* and *Streptococcus*), 35 to 40 percent are aerobic gram-negative species (largely *Escherichia coli, Klebsiella,* and *Pseudomonas*), 10 to 15 percent are anaerobic bacteria, and 5 to 10 percent are *Candida* and other fungi. Up to 25 percent of all blood isolates represent duplicate positive cultures, or organisms of unknown pathogenic importance, including *Propionibacterium, S. epidermidis,* and diphtheroids. Fungi and mycobacterial species are becoming of greater importance as immunocompromised patients represent an increasing segment of the total population.

The organisms responsible for bacteremia are largely those colonizing the gastrointestinal tract, respiratory tract, and skin. Thus, bacteremia arising from the GI tract is often due to *E. coli* and to the anaerobic bacteria. Community-acquired bacteremias in immunologically normal persons are generally gram positive—usually *S. aureus* or *Streptococcus* species. As more patients leave the hospital with indwelling vascular or urinary catheters and more people with AIDS, organ transplants, and malignancies are managed as outpatients, a broader range of pathogens are observed. Nosocomial infections are generally predictable, based on the status of the patient, the site of infection or of surgical intervention, and the epidemiology of the institution. Thus, in an intensive care unit in which *Serratia* or *Enterobacter* species predominate, *Pseudomonas* sepsis should suggest a unique predisposition to infection with this organism. In burn patients, organisms colonizing the skin commonly include *P. aeruginosa, Candida* species, or *S. aureus,* and bacteremia generally involves these pathogens.

Mortality from known bacteremia ranges from 20 to 40 percent. Antibiotic therapy has not significantly reduced this mortality. Circulatory collapse or shock may occur in the presence or absence of documented blood-borne infection. Bacteremia is demonstrated in only half of patients with "septic shock." Up to half of patients with gram-negative bacteremia (and fewer with gram-positive organisms) develop signs (e.g., hypotension) of severe sepsis. The presence of septic shock doubles the mortality from bacteremia.

ETIOLOGY OF THE "SEPSIS SYNDROME"

The Structure and Activities of LPS

The activation of systemic mediators of inflammation is often, but not exclusively, due to the effects of endotoxin (bacterial lipopolysaccharide, LPS) (Table 133-3). The importance of endotoxin's association with gram-negative infection is emphasized by the mortality from gram-negative bacteremia (20 to 30 percent) and gram-negative septic shock (50 percent). In the setting of ARDS, the mortality from gram-negative sepsis may approach 80 to 90 percent. Although endotoxemia is usually associated with gram-negative infections, it also occurs in association with almost all bacterial, fungal, and viral species. Endotoxin has also been isolated from *Rickettsia,* spirochetes, and some fungi (including *Candida*). In both gram-negative and gram-positive bacteremias, the level of bacteremia is correlated with hypotension and mortality.

Comparison of gram-positive and -negative sepsis suggests that the hemodynamic consequences encountered clinically are generally more dramatic with gram-negative bacteremia. The decrease in systemic vascular resistance and the drop in central venous pressure are more rapid and profound than those in gram-positive infection, as are oliguria and metabolic acidosis. The decrease in blood pressure is also more protracted and refractory to therapy. Cardiac output is normal or high in both types of sepsis even though a myocardial depressant factor appears in the circulation. In time, this "high-output" state is usually described as being succeeded by heart failure, although this seems more common in animal models than in humans. Nonetheless, the change to a "low-output" state is predictive of high mortality in all infections. Similarly, advancing age, immune compromise, cardiac disease, hepatic dysfunction, fluid loss, renal failure, and delayed or incorrect choice of initial antibiotics or supportive therapies are associated with increased mortality.

Bacterial endotoxins are mixtures of numerous components of the bacterial outer membrane, including lipids, proteins, and polysaccharides. Most of the biologic effects of endotoxin are mimicked by the "core glycolipid," which is lipid A (lipoidal acylated glucosamine disaccharide) attached to an acidic hetero-oligosaccharide (called KDO). The roles played by the protein and sugar moieties in the in vivo syndrome are poorly defined. It is also unclear whether the "active" endotoxin is free or bound to intact bacteria. Cellular stimulation (and activation of the systemic inflammatory response) may occur through an interaction with the CD14 surface molecule, facilitated by an acute-phase protein-LPS–binding factor called lipopolysaccharide-binding protein. Other receptors and plasma factors may also be engaged in this interaction. The ability to block the effects of administered endotoxin using diverse blocking agents—i.e., antibodies or receptor antagonists for tumor necrosis factor, CD14, or IL-1, opiate antagonists (e.g., naloxone), prostaglandin or protease inhibitors and platelet inhibitors—suggests that a variety of mechanisms as well as a complex cascade of mediators cause the systemic effects currently ascribed to endotoxin.

Endotoxin is cleared from the circulation in two phases: a rapid hepatic clearance that accounts for more than 50 percent and a gradual second phase. Less than 5 percent of circulating endotoxin is deposited in the lungs. However, within the lungs the effects of small amounts of endotoxin are greatly amplified. Endotoxin is deactivated by a variety of metabolic mechanisms, including deacylation and dephosphorylation. Some of this activity may be carried out by circulating leukocytes. The binding of endotoxin to high-density lipoproteins, acute-phase reactants, or antibodies decreases its toxicity. The elimination of LPS from the body is slow (days), and there is no evidence of degradation. In general, the structure of lipid A is preserved among the Enterobacteriaceae. However, minor changes in the structure of lipid A cause considerable changes in the biologic activity of the bacterial endotoxins. Support for the role of endotoxin in the pathogenesis of sepsis stems from the reproduction of the manifestations of this disorder by administration of purified bacterial cell wall extracts and chemically synthesized LPS to experimental animals. These manifestations include activation of the complement cascades, the cytokine cascades, the coagulation and fibrinolytic systems, the kallikrein and bradykinin systems, platelet-activating factor, and the induction of the physiological alterations associated with gram-negative sepsis (Table 133-3). Further evidence comes from the ability of antibodies to core glycolipid to block many of the effects of sepsis due to gram-negative organisms (Table 133-1).

Acute infusion of endotoxin in animals causes a biphasic physiological response similar to that seen clinically in bacteremic shock. Within 5 min, a stage of hypoperfusion and hypotension develops. This initial phase is not clearly related to the serum level of endotoxin. It appears to entail the pooling of blood in the splanchnic bed and peripherally; cardiac function appears to be unaffected. The initial phase is

---

TABLE 133-3

Effects of Bacterial Endotoxins

Activation of complement (C3 and alternative pathway, inflammation)

Hageman factor activation (fibrinolysis)

Plasma thromboplastin antecedent (coagulation)

Interleukin 1 release (fever, catabolic state, leukocyte activation)

Cachectin/TNF synthesis (fever, IL-1β, hypotension, cachexia)

Prostaglandin activation (pulmonary hypertension, platelet activation, vasoconstriction, leukocyte activation)

Kinin activation (edema, hypotension)

Endothelial injury (leukocyte margination, TNF, clotting)

Decreased surfactant function

Immunogenicity (mitogen and adjuvant); nonspecific stimulation

Thrombocytopenia

Neutropenia

Shwartzman phenomenon

followed by a progressive fall in arterial blood pressure, associated with a loss in vascular tone and an increase in vascular permeability. Endotoxin prompts the release of a broad spectrum of vasoactive substances into the circulation: serotonin, histamine, catecholamines, thromboxane, prostaglandins, endorphins, adrenal corticosteroids, lysozymes, lipases, proteases, elastases, kallikrein, and bradykinin (Table 133-3). Some are released from neutrophils at the site of localized infection (Table 133-2); others are parts of the systemic response to infection and to endotoxin. The relative contribution of each of these factors, as with the contributions of the organisms themselves, is controversial.

The depletion of some serum complement components caused by endotoxin is associated with the release of chemotactic factors, notably those of the alternative pathway, via the cleavage of C3. These factors mediate the release of kinins and histamine, chemotaxis and activation of neutrophils and monocytes, B-lymphocyte proliferation, bacterial opsonization, and vascular permeability. Activation of serum complement is not necessary for the development of hypotension in this syndrome, but it may account for some of the alveolar-capillary leakage.

Disseminated Intravascular Coagulation, Vascular Injury, and Shock Lung

In endotoxemia, activation of Hageman factor, resulting in the simultaneous initiation of both fibrinolysis and coagulation (owing to the cleavage of preplasmathromboplastin antecedent), may be responsible for the syndrome of disseminated intravascular coagulation (DIC) or consumptive coagulopathy with dysfunctional coagulation and bleeding diathesis. DIC should be suspected when unexplained bleeding, thrombocytopenia, prolongation of coagulation parameters, fibrin split products, or systemic microemboli occur in the absence of liver disease or other explanations for coagulopathy. DIC will result in the thrombosis of small systemic blood vessels due to the deposition of fibrin at sites of injury to the vascular endothelium (see below) and to trapping of microemboli in small vessels (Fig. 133-1). The syndrome of DIC is not unique to gram-negative bacteria; it is seen in a wide variety of gram-positive fungal and, occasionally, viral infections; it is also a prominent feature of some carcinomas and may occur with trauma or prolonged hypotension. DIC is a clinical concern in only 5 to 10 percent of patients with a major infection.

In addition to systemic activation of neutrophils and monocytes that adhere to the injured cells or are trapped in the pulmonary capillaries, endotoxin causes direct vascular endothelial injury and intense pulmonary vascular vasoconstriction.[11] One marker of pulmonary endothelial injury is the leakage of endothelial angiotensin-converting enzyme into blood flowing through the lungs. The principal direct actions of endotoxin are on small blood vessels that are innervated by the sympathetic nervous system. Local release of prostaglandins also contributes to the endotoxin-induced vasoconstriction and can be reversed by prostaglandin inhibitors. Consequently, pulmonary hypertension may develop in the face of systemic hypotension. The development of pulmonary hemorrhages or pulmonary vascular microthrombi from endotoxin therefore relates to the induction of DIC and to derangements produced in the endothelial surface and vasculature. Sludging of blood in areas of increased pulmonary vascular resistance and alveolar-capillary leakage predispose to vascular thrombosis in small vessels. The resultant derangements in the ventilation-perfusion relationships interfere with the oxygenation of the blood leaving the lungs.

Much of the histopathology of "shock lung" is nonspecific. Though it is leaky, pulmonary capillary endothelium remains grossly intact. The loss of alveolar epithelial type I cells occurs acutely, however, and is accompanied by hyaline membrane formation, hemorrhagic edema, and type II alveolar cell proliferation. As this injury becomes chronic, interstitial fibrosis may occur and is reflected in decreasing lung compliance. Large leaks across the capillary endothelium are rapidly repaired. Leakage of serum proteins into the alveolar spaces affects the concentration, and the surface activity, of pulmonary surfactant, thereby predisposing to the development of atelectasis during bacteremia and shock. Endotoxin also forms complexes with surfactant that alter the morphology, surface charges, and surface tension properties of this material. Complexes of endotoxin with pulmonary surfactant appear to be more toxic in mice than is endotoxin alone. Thus, the interaction of bacteria, or bacterial products, with the lungs may increase the toxicity of systemic infection.

Cytokines and Endotoxin

Serum levels of TNF-α peak in 90 to 120 min following endotoxemia. It is cleared rapidly, becoming undetectable in 4 to 6 h. Persistence of systemic effects, therefore, is due to continuous production or to a series of second mediators, including IL-1 and local chemokines. TNF-α plays a role in the anorexia and the weight loss that accompanies chronic infections, such as that seen in trypanosomiasis or in the acquired immunodeficiency syndrome (AIDS). Administration of TNF-α induces a syndrome essentially identical to severe sepsis: fever, hypotension, acidosis, and DIC. TNF-α causes activation of neutrophil adherence, degranulation, and phagocytosis, suppresses endothelial anticoagulant activity, and enhances procoagulant activity—changes that correlate with the tendency to thrombosis during gram-negative bacteremia. TNF-α is also a pyrogen. Antibodies or passive immunization to TNF-α protects against the lethal effects of administered endotoxin and can attenuate the resultant lung injury in some animal models even if administered 1 h after LPS (Table 133-1). However, other studies have failed to demonstrate beneficial effects, and even showed increased mortality reversed by infusion of TNF-α. IL-1β, also known as endogenous pyrogen, lymphocyte-activating factor, or the leukocytic endogenous mediator, and TNF mediate many of the same inflammatory reactions, including fever, neutrophilia, and systemic metabolic changes, and appear to be the major systemic mediators of many of the effects of endotoxin. These effects are augmented by many other factors released in the process of the host response to infection, and are themselves amplified by other lymphokines—e.g., γ-interferon, IL-2, and IL-6—and by cellular activities.

Although corticosteroids can block the production and translation of TNF messenger ribonucleic acid (mRNA) as well as suppress IL-1β release, steroids administered to patients in septic shock have not been demonstrated to increase survival and may predispose to superinfection. Corticosteroids have proved beneficial in animal models only if administered *before* the administration of the endotoxin. Thus, even though much remains to be learned about how the corticosteroids exert their effects, it appears that there is no therapeutic role for corticosteroids once bacterial sepsis has developed.

Septic Shock Without Endotoxin

Although the mechanisms responsible for gram-positive, viral, and fungal shock are more elusive than those considered above for gram-negative bacterial shock, it is likely that the same mediators of inflammation are important in producing septic shock both with and without initiation by endotoxin. The apparent lack of specificity of the hypotensive effects of inflammation is demonstrated by early studies on the equal ability of tissue necrosis, turpentine-induced sterile abscesses, or localized intraoperative infection to produce hypotension in experimental animals.

Many of the gram-positive organisms produce exotoxins (discussed above) and enzymes that may injure infected tissues and elicit inflammation. Common organisms have been popularized in the lay press for toxin-mediated activities, including the "flesh-eating bacteria" (generally toxin-secreting streptococcal infection), gas gangrene (due to *Clostridia* species), and common pulmonary agents such as pneumococcus (*Streptococcus pneumoniae*). Unique toxins from diphtheria (myocarditis), *Shigella* and *Cholera* species (intestinal fluid loss), and anthrax (systemic edema) can all produce hypotension or shock, but this is not usually associated with high cardiac output and low vascular resistance. Thus, the choice of antibiotic therapy should be guided by the isolation of the causative organism *before therapy is begun,* because of the broad spectrum of organisms that can cause septic shock.

THE "SECOND-HIT PHENOMENON"

Sequences of events that alone do not cause serious organ damage seem to act synergistically when they occur within a short time of each other. This has been shown both at the cellular and at the whole-organ level. For example, neutrophils can be primed by platelet-activating factor so that a second stimulus induces them to cause endothelial damage, whereas neither stimulus alone would result in tissue damage.[5,59] Anderson and colleagues[3,4] demonstrated that the transient accumulation of neutrophils in rat lungs induced by the administration of endotoxin caused neutrophil activation and a protein leak only if a subsequent dose of N-formylneoleucylphenylalanine (FNLP), which activates neutrophils, was administered within 12 h. FNLP alone did not cause damage. Similarly, the "second-hit phenomenon" may explain why small doses of endotoxin may induce pulmonary injury following intestinal translocation of both bacteria and endotoxin after ischemia-reperfusion or thermal injury.[29–31,49,55] LPS alone and ischemia-reperfusion alone induce neutrophil sequestration in the lung accompanied by minimal histologic changes, whereas the combination produces major changes in histopathology and permeability. Repeated stresses may also prevent or delay a beneficial acute-phase response such as the heat-shock response. Pepe and coworkers[48] described major clinical conditions related to the development of respiratory failure, including the sepsis syndrome, gastric contents aspiration, pulmonary contusion, multiple emergency transfusions (greater than 22 units), and major long-bone fractures. However, the incidence

of respiratory failure increased with each additional condition. Although the authors did not perform a multivariate analysis, these data suggest that one condition might be sufficient to "prime" the patient with the second or third condition, resulting in activation and pulmonary damage.

ALTERATIONS IN THE HOST PREDISPOSING TO LUNG INJURY

Many interventions and disease states change the flora in the nasopharynx, from community-acquired gram-positive and anaerobic organisms to nosocomial, antibiotic-resistant, and predominantly gram-negative bacteria. These events are discussed in detail by Weber and colleagues (see Chapter 143) and Johanson and Dever (see Chapter 119). In addition, the likelihood of aspiration may be increased by many conditions, such as acute alcoholism, obtundation, and prolonged tracheal intubation (see Chapter 129). Primary and acquired immune deficiencies are also discussed in individual chapters in this text (see Chapters 134–141). For purposes of this discussion, therefore, these will be mentioned only briefly. The primary organisms responsible for pulmonary infection are those colonizing the airways. The most virulent respiratory pathogens are typically encapsulated, which tends to diminish adherence. Loss of capsule and production of fibrillae or fimbriae facilitate mucosal adherence but also increase susceptibility to host defenses (see Chapter 125). Experimental addition of fimbriae does not increase adherence in nonvirulent strains. Thus, the balance of bacterial virulence and host defenses is emphasized.

Malnutrition and GI Function

Protein malnutrition seems to blunt the inflammatory response to cytokine stimulation and could account for an increased susceptibility to infection of protein-malnourished persons. Protein malnutrition plus endotoxin produces translocation of aerobic organisms into mesenteric lymph nodes, spleen, and liver in mice. Animal data suggest that gut mucosal atrophy occurs when enteral feeding is withheld[32] and that dietary fiber is important in maintaining the gut barrier to bacteria and preventing mucosal atrophy.[41] This barrier can also be compromised by prolonged gut immotility. For example, culture-positive mesenteric lymph nodes were found in 10 of 17 patients with bacterial overgrowth secondary to small-bowel obstruction, in contrast to 1 of 25 patients undergoing elective surgery.[15] Enteral feeding may also affect the response to endotoxin. For example, endotoxin administration to normal subjects fed enterally produced higher levels of epinephrine, glucagon, and TNF-α than when administered to subjects fed parenterally for 7 days.[38,39]

Gastric pH and Alimentary Tract Flora

The organisms in 30 to 40 percent of nosocomial pneumonias are also present in the stomach. Because gastric bacterial growth is inhibited by an acid milieu, there has been considerable interest in using a form of stress ulcer prophylaxis that does not raise gastric pH. Although studies have produced conflicting results,[58] it does appear that if the gastric pH is reduced, regardless of the method used, the incidence of nosocomial pneumonia in patients receiving prolonged mechanical ventilation (more than 4 days) can be reduced. However, data from various studies are difficult to compare because of methodologic differences, particularly in the definition of pneumonia and the use of concomitant antibiotics. In a review of the role of gastric pH and nosocomial pneumonia, Tryba[58] makes convincing arguments for the following points: (1) colonization of the stomach is inhibited by low gastric pH; (2) when the stomach does become colonized, the source of bacteria is, at least in part, from duodenal reflux rather than the oropharynx; (3) gastric colonization can result in colonization of the oropharynx with the same organisms within a few days; and (4) oropharyngeal aspiration is the source of some of the nosocomial pneumonias. It seems likely, therefore, that in patients at risk for gastric colonization, such as those with impaired motility or reflux, the maintenance of an acid milieu in the stomach can reduce the incidence of nosocomial pneumonia.

There has been considerable interest in eliminating fungi and the aerobic gram-negative bacteria from the alimentary tract in an effort to reduce the incidence of nosocomial pneumonia and improve survival in patients who are intubated for a period long enough for pulmonary contamination from oropharyngeal flora (usually more than 4 days). This process, termed selective digestive decontamination (SDD), utilizes nonabsorbable enteral antibiotics to suppress gut aerobic gram-positive and -negative flora without inhibiting anaerobic flora. Theoretically, SDD should both decrease gut bacterial translocation that may occur with shock and eliminate gram-negative oropharyngeal flora, thereby protecting against lung injury and nosocomial infection.[60] Interpretation of the studies of SDD is hampered by numerous methodologic problems.[14] Paramount among these are the difficulties and inconsistencies in defining pneumonia, especially since tracheal aspirates, Gram's stains, and culture results may be altered by pulmonary contamination from the antibiotics used for SDD. Comparisons among studies of SDD are also difficult because of differences in the regimens used for SDD, the use of concomitant parenteral antibiotics, the methods used to diagnose pneumonia, the patient populations, the enormous variation in the incidence of pneumonia, and the use and type of stress ulcer prophylaxis.

As of 1993, there were over 100 publications describing the use of SDD in such patients. The results are inconsistent. Although a meta-analysis of 16 trials indicated that the incidence of nosocomial pneumonia may be reduced by SDD, there was a reduction in mortality in only one study.[34] Two more-recent studies do not show a reduction in either nosocomial pneumonias or mortality with SDD.[23,61] SDD is considerably more expensive than conventional management. Despite the data suggesting that SDD may reduce the incidence of nosocomial pneumonia, Silver and Bone[57] recommend avoiding SDD because "it appears that selective digestive decontamination does too little for patients and probably costs too much for the benefit it may provide. It is too early to tell if subsets of critically ill patients may benefit. . . ."

Endotracheal Devices

The risk of nosocomial pneumonia has been shown to increase with the duration of mechanical ventilation. For example, Langer's team[37] found the risk increased almost 5 percent per day for the first 10 days. The epidemiology of nosocomial pneumonia in intensive care units has been reviewed[24] and is discussed further in Chapter 143. Although concomitant diseases leading to intubation may contribute to nosocomial pneumonia, the presence of an endotracheal device may itself increase the risk of nosocomial pneumonia for numerous reasons. The cuff does not completely protect against aspiration, which may occur even with a properly sealed endotracheal tube. Moreover, because the glottis cannot be closed, an effective cough is lost. The endotracheal tube also colonizes with bacteria usually embedded in an amorphous matrix that may be dislodged with manipulation, thus serving as a source of bacterial inoculation. Endotracheal tubes may also cause increases in tracheal mucus secretion, thereby providing a better milieu for bacteria. The endotracheal tube itself, as well as the low-pressure cuff, leads to tracheal damage, especially ciliary denudation but also mucosal ulceration, inflammation, and submucosal hemorrhage. If the position of the tube changes, which is likely, or when it is removed, these areas of denudation presumably interfere with bacterial expulsion via the cilia.

Diabetes

There is no convincing clinical evidence that diabetes increases the incidence of pulmonary disease. Granulocytic chemotaxis does seem to be impaired independently of ketoacidosis, although it can be restored with antioxidants. Gram-negative oropharyngeal colonization is more common in diabetics. In addition, other systemic diseases, such as renal failure and derangements in gastrointestinal motility, may predispose the diabetic patient to pulmonary infections.

Age

Advancing age has been associated with an increase in the incidence of pneumonia.[10] Although it is well documented that older patients have a higher risk for nosocomial pneumonia,[28] it is not clear whether this is a direct consequence of age or reflects a greater prevalence of underlying diseases and longer hospital stays. For example, Hanson and coworkers[28] found that patients over the age of 65 had a relative risk of 2.1 for nosocomial pneumonia compared with patients aged 25 to 50. These authors did not find any differences in the risk factors between these two age groups. However, patients over 65 who developed pneumonia were more commonly malnourished and had a higher incidence of neuromuscular diseases than age-matched patients without pneumonia. Moreover, elderly patients developed pneumonia later in their hospital stay than did younger patients. The available data suggest that the underlying diseases and state of health are more important in increasing the risk of pneumonia in the elderly than is age itself. Nonetheless, changes in the immune system and in mechanical function may increase the risk of pneumonia with age. These changes[27] include mostly impaired T-cell proliferation with exposure to an antigenic stimulus, although decreases in serum IgG have also been found. This impairment, due both to a decreased number of responding T cells and to a decreased proliferation of T cells that do respond, may be related to age-dependent changes in lung function and clearance mechanisms.

Ischemia and Reperfusion Injuries

Pulmonary changes similar to those found in ARDS with intestinal ischemia and reperfusion have been induced in many animal models. This effect is related, in part, to the wide variety of inflammatory mediators released from the gut. Plasma from an ischemia-reperfusion model has been shown to directly decrease adenosine triphosphate (ATP) in cultured rat pulmonary endothelial cells.[25] This occurred without any effect on ATP metabolites or cell structure, suggesting an increase in metabolic rate rather than inhibition of synthesis. It is also possible that ARDS associated with hypotension is related to bacterial translocation from the gut.[35] Koziol and colleagues[35] showed in a rat model that within 2 h of hemorrhage to a mean pressure of 30 mmHg, positive blood cultures for gut bacteria were found in one-third of the animals; by 5 h, all blood cultures were positive. Rats subjected to 30 to 90 min of severe hemorrhagic shock to 30 mmHg also showed a progressive increase in bacterial translocation to both mesenteric lymph nodes and other organs, especially liver and spleen.[6] The significance of this finding is unclear, however, as these bacteria might be cleared by the liver and spleen. Nonetheless, other rat models of gut ischemia and reperfusion have shown that pulmonary injury is clearly produced by this process.[34,59] Notably, the combination of endotoxin and reperfusion injury caused marked histopathologic changes in the lung,[34] consistent with the multiple-hit hypothesis described above.

Although animal data documenting bacterial translocation are consistent, the relevance to the human pulmonary dysfunction following periods of hypotension is unclear. There are data relating transfusion requirements to infection risk in trauma patients independently of shock;[17] a study of portal vein and systemic blood cultures following major torso trauma found few patients with positive blood cultures.[46] However, 4 out of 12 patients had culture-positive ileocolic lymph nodes. Three of these 4 patients were in shock on arrival. Moreover, in a second group of 31 patients, none had positive blood cultures if their admission systolic blood pressure was greater than 90 mmHg, whereas 3 of 11 with pressures less than 90 mmHg had positive cultures. By contrast, Rush and coworkers[54] found that 26 percent of patients admitted to a trauma service had positive blood cultures within 3 h of admission. Moreover, 55 percent of these patients with admission blood pressures less than 80 mmHg had positive cultures, 33 percent for gram-positive bacteria. Taken together, these results suggest that hypotension can cause systemic translocation of gut bacteria.[29–31,49,55] The risk seems to be related to the degree and duration of hypotension. Moreover, the route of spread may be lymphatic rather than via the portal circulation. In either case, the high incidence of respiratory failure associated with hypotension may be related to intestinal ischemia and reperfusion. This effect may be amplified by hepatic or lymphatic release of inflammatory mediators.

Alcoholism and Hepatic Disease

Alcoholism has been cited as a predisposing factor in a high percentage of patients with community-acquired pneumonia.[10,22] However, it has been difficult to establish whether it is the consumption of alcohol itself or the presence of coexisting diseases, particularly liver injury, that increases the risk of pneumonia.[8,9,44] In a case control study, acute alcohol ingestion was the only identifiable risk factor for pneumonia in a multivariate analysis, although cirrhosis was also a univariate risk factor.[22] Of interest is that pharyngeal colonization with gram-negative bacteria is more common in alcoholics but has no relationship to the pathogen causing the pneumonia. However, such studies are generally confounded by the prior use of antibiotics and the difficulties of using expectorated sputum to identify the causative agent of the pneumonia. Nonetheless, oropharyngeal carriage of gram-negative bacteria is increased among ambulatory alcoholics, as is the number of colony-forming units.[22] Moreover, alcoholics are more prone to aspiration and often have depressed cough reflexes and mucociliary clearance. Trauma is common in these patients, and secondary infection of hematomas surrounding clavicular and rib fractures may occur.

The alcoholic, particularly if cirrhotic, suffers from a series of immune deficits. The presence of portal venous hypertension predisposes to intermittent bacteremias, presumably because of colonic flora leaking across the edematous bowel wall. These bacteremias are poorly cleared, owing to systemically diminished phagocytic function. Should endotoxemia occur, it is likely to persist as a consequence of the compromised metabolic functions of the liver. A serum inhibitor of neutrophil chemotaxis, the acute neutrophil dysfunction seen in the presence of alcohol, a mild chronic neutropenia, and a decreased ability to mobilize immune responses to new antigens combine to reduce the efficacy of the alcoholic's inflammatory response. The alcoholic tends to seek medical help later than do other patients and, thus, tends to have more advanced infection at the time of presentation to the hospital. *Klebsiella* or *E. coli* is more often responsible for bacteremia in these patients than are gram-positive bacteria.

The Kupffer cells of the liver constitute 80 percent of the total reticuloendothelial mass, and normally almost all splanchnic venous flow passes through the liver before entering the systemic circulation. Moreover, the liver is the major source of newly synthesized proteins and an important source of, and responder to, cytokines and other inflammatory mediators in the acute phase response. As the liver is also important in clearing cytokines (TNF-α) and other inflammatory mediators (eicosanoid lipoxygenation products), especially those produced by the gut, hepatic dysfunction may increase the exposure of the lungs to these mediators. Consistent with this supposition, patients with shock and cirrhosis have been found to have a greater likelihood of developing multiple organ failure, including respiratory failure, than similar patients without cirrhosis.[44] Patients who developed multiple organ failure had persistently higher serum TNF levels. Similarly, in animal models with reduced hepatic blood flow, levels of TNF-α, neutrophils in bronchoalveolar lavage (BAL) fluid, and mortality are significantly increased. Patients with cirrhosis without infection also have higher levels of TNF and IL-6 than noncirrhotic controls. Thus, it seems likely that alcoholic intake, both chronic and acute, contributes directly and indirectly to the risk of pneumonia.

Liver failure is associated with changes in the lung ranging from hypoxia with a normal chest radiograph to ARDS. In one retrospective study of 29 patients with nonalcoholic end-stage liver failure awaiting liver transplantation, 23 developed ARDS and none survived.[43] The most common associated factor was sepsis syndrome, for which a bacterial or fungal source could not be identified in 39 percent. Both chronic and acute liver disease are associated with reduced Pa_{O_2} which is often accompanied by diffuse dilatation of the pulmonary arterial system. Although spider nevi may be present in the pleura, true arteriovenous anastomoses are very rare.

The syndrome of liver disease, reduced Pa_{O_2}, and intrapulmonary vascular dilatation is often referred to as the hepatopulmonary syndrome.[36] This syndrome is also often associated with digital clubbing, cyanosis, dyspnea, and orthodeoxia (a decrease in Pa_{O_2} with upright posture). There is some suggestion that spider nevi may be a systemic marker for the intrapulmonary vascular dilatation defining this syndrome. Hyperventilation is common in this syndrome; typically, cardiac output is elevated while systemic and pulmonary arterial pressures are normal or low. Although anatomically abnormal pulmonary arterial to pulmonary venous anastamoses have been reported, their demonstration by echocardiography or ^{99m}Tc-labeled macroaggregated albumin scanning may actually reflect dilated alveolar vessels. The importance of true shunts, if they exist, in reducing Pa_{O_2} in this syndrome is questionable; some of these patients have marked improvement in Pa_{O_2} with high Fi_{O_2}, a phenomenon not expected with true pulmonary shunt. Such improvement is more characteristic of low V/Q regions of the lung. Moreover, using the multiple inert gas method, relatively high flow to low V/Q areas has been documented both with minimal or no true shunt (V/Q < 0.005)[52] and with 4 to 28 percent true shunt. However, baseline Pa_{O_2} was normal in the study of cirrhotics when true shunt was negligible.[52] The authors of this study found differences in patients with spider nevi that they interpreted as indicating a reduced response to hypoxic vasoconstriction. Unfortunately, confidence limits and therefore statistical comparisons cannot be obtained from the multiple inert gas method because of limitations in the mathematical model.[57] Possibly the diffuse dilation of the arterial tree leads to increased low V/Q regions and accounts for the relatively low Pa_{O_2} often seen in these patients.

Hepatic disease is also rarely associated with pulmonary hypertension. Portal hypertension rather than liver disease itself may link these two entities. Noncardiogenic pulmonary edema may occur in acute hepatic failure.

PANCREATITIS

A low Pa_{O_2} is a relatively common finding in pancreatitis. In a study of 84 patients with pancreatitis, 45 percent had a Pa_{O_2} below 60 mmHg, with chest radiograph findings varying from normal to pleural effusions to bilateral diffuse infiltrates.[33] In contrast, hypoxia occurred in only 19 percent of 68 patients in a control group with acute abdominal disease from other causes. In a rat model of acute edematous pancreatitis, the initial pulmonary injury was preceded by the accumulation of neutrophils.[63] This occurred before inflammatory infiltration in the pancreas. Pulmonary interstitial edema and changes in endothelial cells became apparent later, although the alveolus itself was unchanged. Hypoxic vasoconstriction was shown to be attenu-

ated in this model, although the response to angiotensin II was preserved.[21] Moreover, pulmonary vascular permeability was increased. Other models of more severe pancreatitis have shown progressive destruction of the capillary endothelium. These changes seem to mimic those found in humans with acute pancreatitis and demonstrate that the pancreatic injury itself can cause pulmonary injury. Exudative pleural effusions with very high amylase values are found in as many as a third of patients with acute or chronic pancreatitis.

RENAL FAILURE

Although infection has been found to be the leading cause of death in patients undergoing chronic dialysis,[40] as with diabetes, it is difficult to determine a direct causal relationship while excluding coexistent diseases and conditions, dialysis, or hospitalizations. There are no convincing clinical data to indicate that renal failure per se directly enhances the risk of pulmonary disease. However, there are some effects of uremia that may predispose to pulmonary disease. For example, altered colonization of the nasopharynx with *Staphylococcus* species may occur, and activation of neutrophils is depressed in uremic patients; this depression is not related to dialysis, although it can be exacerbated with cuprophane dialysis membranes. There are also metabolic changes in patients with renal failure that might cause a predisposition to infection. For example, the alterations in iron, zinc, and calcium stores that occur in these patients can depress neutrophil function and enhance bacterial growth.

There is clinical evidence that patients with abdominal sepsis, including those with infected peritoneal dialysates, have a higher than expected incidence of pneumonia. Such patients tend to be intubated or prone to postoperative aspiration, however, and they may have low lung volumes and atelectasis. In animal models, intra-abdominal infection increases the retention of bacteria in the lungs without altering either macrophage recruitment or viability,[50] although macrophage killing of pulmonary bacteria was decreased in animals with intra-abdominal sepsis. The specific bacteria and inoculum size are critical to the outcome of such studies. For example, *P. aeruginosa* may replicate in the lungs more rapidly than *S. aureus* during *E. coli* abdominal infection.[62] The combination of the clinical data and such experimental models suggests that intra-abdominal infection increases the risk for pneumonia rather than the need for dialysis per se.

THERMAL INJURY

Pulmonary injury and infection cause significant morbidity in burn patients despite improvements in their management and surgical care. Pulmonary infections and dysfunction are greater impediments to the recovery of burn patients than wound infections, owing to improvements in burn wound care. The advent of improved broad-spectrum antibiotics has shifted the distribution of pathogens associated with postburn pneumonias from gram-positive organisms to relatively antibiotic-resistant gram-negative organisms, including *P. aeruginosa,* and fungi, including *Candida* species. Bacterial translocation from the gut following burns has been related to activation of cytokines, prostaglandins, and neutrophils, with microvascular permeability and edema. A number of studies have demonstrated that thermal injury causes activation of neutrophils and transient sequestration of neutrophils in the lungs (and other tissues), largely in the vascular tree.

Systemic levels of γ-interferon, IL-1β, and IL-6 are elevated following burn injury in rats and in patients. In the absence of infection, elevated levels of IL-1β, TNF, and IL-6 are detectable for more than 6 weeks after thermal injury, with levels of IL-1 correlating with burn size; low serum levels of IL-1β in the immediate postburn period are an indicator of poor prognosis. The serum IL-6 level has an inverse relationship to the survival of the patient.[18,43,45,51,53] IL-2 secretion (T-cell growth factor) and IL-2 mRNA synthesis are consistently suppressed in lymphocytes from mice with thermal injuries. IL-6 and TNF-α levels are further elevated in patients with infections following thermal injuries when compared to those with thermal injuries alone. However, serum IL-1β, IL-6, and TNF-α levels are not predictive of the risk of infection in burn patients.

In the absence of endotoxemia, thermal injury to skin or muscle in animals produces transient elevations in IL-1β levels in lung and liver but not in skin, spleen, ilium, thymus, kidney, or plasma from the same animals. By contrast, endotoxin challenge causes elevation of IL-1β in all these organs. In studies of patients with thermal skin injury, both protein synthesis and mRNA for TNF-α, IL-6, and IL-8 were significantly elevated in the lung, normal (uninjured) skin, blood, and thermally injured skin.[45,51,53] The TNF, IL-6, and IL-8 proteins present in the bronchial secretions and skin are generated locally and do not originate in the systemic cytokine pool. IL-6 and IL-8 levels are many times higher in the lung than in the blood. The local production of IL-8 is associated with the occurrence of pulmonary physiological dysfunction and nosocomial pulmonary infection.[18] These effects are independent of the presence of sepsis or endotoxemia. Both in burns and in models of endotoxic shock, a significant oxidant injury may occur in the lungs, with increased levels of pulmonary malondialdehyde due to the circulation of unreduced peroxides released by circulating neutrophils.

Patients with full-thickness burns generally receive one prophylactic dose of penicillin at the time of admission, to prevent acute streptococcal infection of the skin and bloodstream. Antibiotics are also administered prophylactically before manipulation of burned skin, débridement, or skin-grafting procedures to deal with anticipated bacteremia. Healing and reversal of the systemic inflammatory state are reliant upon excision of injured skin and avoidance of superinfection. The antibiotics used tend to reflect the common flora of burns at a given medical center; they also determine which antibiotic-resistant organisms will become the colonizing agents of the injured skin. Before the advent of topical antibacterial therapy and artificial burn coverings, local infection was responsible for the progression of a partial-thickness burn to a fully necrotic dermis. Topical therapies are aimed at the reduction of the bacterial burden of the injured skin: silver sulfadiazine is more effective against gram-negative organisms, whereas mafenide acetate is better against the gram-positive bacteria. The best method for reducing infection is to cover the burned area with skin autografts or allografts as soon as possible after the patient has been stabilized hemodynamically. The mortality from burns relates to the level of infection

of the viable tissues that surround the burn site. Quantitative bacterial cultures of biopsies taken of burned tissues have demonstrated a correlation between the type and the number of organisms isolated from the skin and those that ultimately cause death.

Because patients with body surface area burns over 40 percent do not adequately mobilize neutrophils, either locally or systemically, they are effectively immunosuppressed. Bacteremia and hematogenous infection, notably of the lungs, are common. Because of the poor neutrophil response, bronchopneumonia can occur without infiltrates on the chest radiographs. An example of the development of pneumonia in the absence of an appropriate local leukocyte response is shown in Fig. 133-4. In these patients, subtle changes in either the skin wounds (i.e., discoloration, weeping, and hemorrhage) or the hematologic parameters (i.e., new coagulation defects, abnormal white blood cell counts in the peripheral blood, abnormal liver function tests) or abnormalities in the chest radiograph are a basis for concern. Because fungal growth in blood cultures from these patients is often slow and only intermittently positive, it may progress unnoticed (Fig. 133-5).

Inhalational burn injury of the lungs, resulting in atelectasis, edema, decreased mucociliary function, necrosis, and ARDS, promotes the rapid development of pneumonia. Necrotic muscle caused by burns is often infected. If so, the infected muscle or fascia must be resected to save viable tissues and to prevent dissemination of infection.

INTRAVASCULAR INFECTIONS

Disseminated infection and high-grade bacteremias are most often associated with infection in, or adjacent to, the bloodstream. The best-described entity of this type is infective endocarditis (IE). The terms *acute* and *subacute endocarditis* were descriptive names applied to heart valve infections in the preantibiotic era; the infections were largely staphylococcal and streptococcal. Most of the criteria for infections that might invade the lungs apply to infective endocarditis. For a given organism to cause IE, it must adhere to a heart valve, replicate, and produce infection that is relatively resistant to host defenses. In principle, these qualifications should limit the number of species that can produce the syndrome. Even though streptococci and staphylococci account for more than 80 percent of all instances of IE, however, the frequency of gram-negative, anaerobic, and fungal infections as the cause of IE is increasing. Many of the latter organisms gain access to the circulation by way of invasive therapies, including central venous catheters and pacemakers; some of the increased incidence is also due to the prolonged survival of patients after severe trauma or with immune compromise.

The development of IE depends on the preexistence of an irregular or damaged heart valve or endocardial surface onto which fibrin or platelets have been deposited. Turbulence of blood flow or the erosion caused by a cardiac catheter may suffice to cause injury, even though the "classic" disruption is the scarring of the mitral and aortic valves as a result of rheumatic carditis. Nonbacterial, thrombotic endocarditis is then superinfected by a strain of bacteria that can adhere to the fibrin mesh. Transient bacteremia is sufficient to infect the endocardial surface. The ability of the bacteria to secrete enzymes that allow deeper pen-

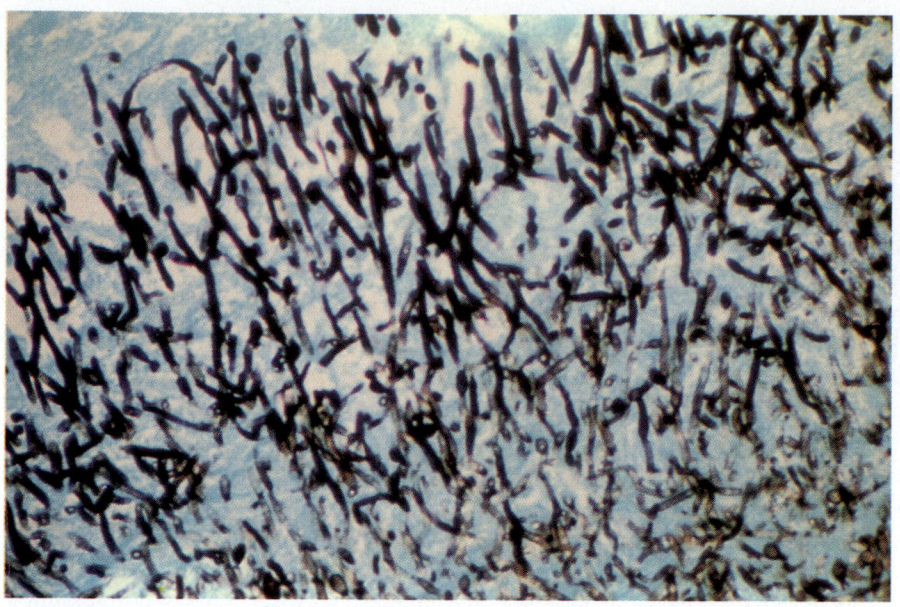

A

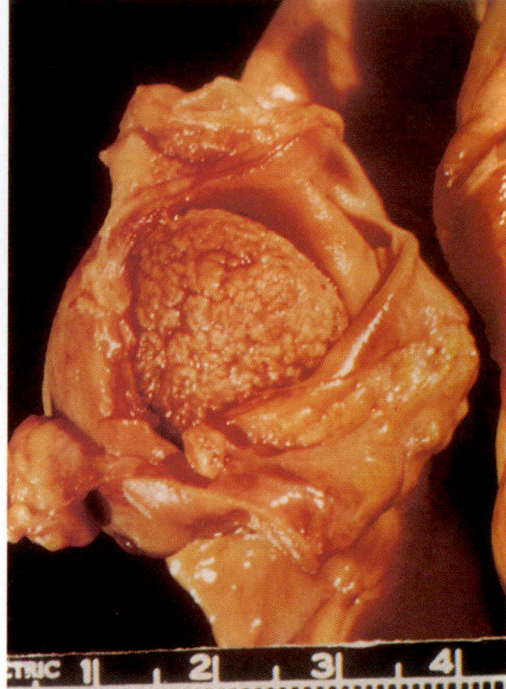

B

FIGURE 133-5 Fungal right-sided endocarditis (IE) in a patient with 50 percent total body burns resulted in embolization of *Candida albicans* from the infected valve *(A)* to the bifurcation of the pulmonary artery *(B)*. Pleural involvement with fungal seeding of the pleural surface is a common complication of right-sided IE (C).

C

etration into the fibrin or cardiac tissue renders the infection impervious to host defenses. The growth of the fibrin/platelet/bacterial thrombus on the valve ("vegetation") prevents the penetration of neutrophils to the main nidus of infection. The systemic effects of infective endocarditis are diverse; weight loss, malaise, fevers, and dyspnea are common. On the one hand, the clinical manifestations may reflect the role of cachectin/TNF, interleukin 1β, and recurrent bacteremias; on the other, they may represent the hemodynamic consequences of bacteremia, which may be aggravated by valvular damage. Systemic emboli, both infected and sterile, are often accompanied by splenomegaly, heart murmurs, and multiorgan dysfunction. Clubbing is present in up to 20 percent of cases, and cutaneous manifestations of embolic infection in up to 50 percent. Major emboli and congestive heart failure occur in up to a third of patients. Pulmonary involvement in infective endocarditis is usually secondary to elevated left

atrial end pressures caused by aortic or mitral valve dysfunction or myocarditis. In addition, tachycardia, fever, and hypotensive episodes contribute to the cardiac abnormalities. Direct pulmonary involvement is common in right-sided (e.g., tricuspid valve) disease or in congenital cardiac anomalies with left-to-right shunting (e.g., tetralogy of Fallot). In this setting, pulmonary emboli, followed by acute pneumonia or lung abscess, are common. Pleural embolic seeding is also frequent, with the subsequent development of pleural effusions and empyema (Fig. 133-5).

Intravenous drug abusers are most often affected by the pulmonary complications of IE. Tricuspid valvular involvement occurs in over half of the patients, with or without infection of other heart valves. The clinical presentation is often that of a young person with dyspnea of sudden onset, pleurisy, fever, or occasionally hemoptysis. Cutaneous manifestations of sepsis and infected injection sites are common. The patient generally develops radiographic evidence of septic embolic involvement of the lung (pneumonia, pulmonary infarction, pleural effusion) during the early period of hospitalization (Fig. 133-6). Tricuspid insufficiency can be demonstrated only in a minority of these subjects, but transesophageal echocardiography is the diagnostic test of choice after blood cultures. Pulmonary impairment can be worsened by the presence of talc, cotton fibers, or other impurities in the intravenous drug mixture (Fig. 133-7). "Skin poppers" who inject narcotics subcutaneously are also subject to right-sided IE. All injectable illicit drugs are potentially contaminated; local infection of the skin (abscesses) or veins (thrombophlebitis) is common and may require surgical intervention for cure.

Therapy is guided by the results of blood cultures drawn under sterile conditions during the first 24 h of hospitalization. In the gravely ill patient, however, the empiric intravenous administration of broad-spectrum bactericidal antibiotics directed at both gram-negative and gram-positive bacteria is acutely necessary. Even in these patients, blood cultures should be drawn before antibiotics are started parenterally. Peripheral sites of infection (e.g., skin lesions, infected veins) often yield organisms, and a Gram's stain of the blood buffy coat may be helpful in directing therapy. In the addict, the organisms responsible for IE include *S. aureus, P. aeruginosa, Candida albicans,* other gram-negative aerobes and anaerobes. Occasionally, several organisms are isolated. The spectrum of organisms seen in infections in the intravenous drug user has been greatly expanded owing to the susceptibility of this population to the development of opportunistic infection (e.g., *Bartonella* or mycobacteria) due to AIDS. Fungal endocarditis is common not only in the drug addict population but also in patients who have recently undergone cardiac surgery, in immunocompromised patients, in patients infected with the *Mucor* agents or with *Trichosporon beigelii,* and in those who have had prolonged exposure to intravenous central catheters for monitoring, therapy, or parenteral nutrition (Figs. 133-5 and 133-8). The development of fever and systemic signs may be quite insidious in these patients; until embolic phenomena occur, fungal blood isolates are often disregarded as contaminants of the cultures.

The development of fungal pneumonia in the addict is probably related to the presence of fungal contaminants in inhaled marijuana and cocaine preparations. In these persons, direct inhalation or sinusitis may be the source of a bacteremic infection. Intravascular infection of the venous circulation, followed by pulmonary embolization, occurs in association with thrombosis of the deep veins of the pelvis or legs, or in the presence of vein grafts and intravascular prosthetic devices (Fig. 133-1). Septic thrombophlebitis is a major cause of secondary lung abscess—usually presenting as a single area of pneumonitis, in contrast to the multiple peripheral lesions seen in bacteremic disease. Possibly because of the tendency of emboli to lodge distally in the pulmonary circulation, approximately one-third are complicated by empyema and occasionally by bronchopleural fistula. Invasive organisms—*Staphylococcus, Streptococcus, Klebsiella,* and *E. coli*—, tend to invade the pleural space in the course of bacteremic pneumonia. Embolic infection is also a complication of prolonged intravenous therapy. Contamination of vascular catheters occurs in up to 10 percent of patients; this contamina-

tion is accompanied by bacteremia or fungemia in about three patients per 1000 catheter-use days. The initial therapy for catheter-related infection is to remove the device.

TREATMENT OF SYSTEMIC INFECTIONS OF THE LUNGS

General Principles

The patient with systemic infection and pulmonary disease is often critically ill. Treatment of the illness is greatly simplified if, rather than starting antibiotic therapy empirically, the source is identified and the antibiotic sensitivities of the organisms responsible for the infection can be determined. If the source is suspected to be a localized abscess or a collection of infected fluid but organisms have not been identified, initial empiric therapy is usually directed at the bacteremia, with coverage of the likely pathogens based on the suspected source. If the patient can be stabilized in less than a few hours by medical therapy alone or if the putative source is amenable to percutaneous drainage, surgical intervention may be avoided. The reversibility of septic shock falls with time. Rehydration of the patient in septic shock is essential and may be guided by a central venous or pulmonary artery pressure monitoring. Oxygen demands must be minimized and O_2 delivery optimized. Empiric antibiotic therapy, using antistaphylococcal and anti–gram-negative bacterial coverage, suffices unless a suspected source exists for anaerobic (e.g., abdominal), resistant gram-negative fungal organisms or CNS infection. It cannot be overemphasized that therapy can be tailored to the patient's needs only if the proper cultures are obtained *before* antibiotic therapy is initiated. Occasionally, lung abscesses or empyema develops despite appropriate therapy and requires a drainage procedure to ensure resolution (see Chapter 130).

A few infections that involve the respiratory system should be considered life-threatening emergencies. These infections merit consideration in any patient with deterioration of respiratory function without a clear reason (e.g., pneumothorax or cardiac disease) and include mediastinitis, Ludwig's angina, strongyloidiasis in the immune-compromised host, toxic shock syndrome, tetanus, epiglottitis, peritonsillar abscess, diphtheria, amebic bronchopleural fistula, and *P. falciparum* malaria. The recognition of these entities may be lifesaving in unstable patients, most notably those with head and neck infections, paralytic disease, or underlying immune compromise. However, pulmonary function may be as severely impaired in patients with sepsis without pulmonary infection as in those with infection.

There are few prospective, randomized clinical trials of initial, empiric antibiotic regimens for sepsis in the immunologically normal host. In patients with an identifiable site or type of infection, the choice of antimicrobial agents is simplified—e.g., gram-negative rods seen in pyelonephritis (Table 133-4). Familiarity with individual patients may also suggest appropriate therapies (e.g., the patient with recurrent staphylococcal or streptococcal infections). In general, however, a combination of antibiotics is used until definitive microbiologic data are available. Ideally, synergistic combinations should be used whenever possible. Synergy suggests that the antimicrobial effect of two agents together is greater than the sum of the activities of each

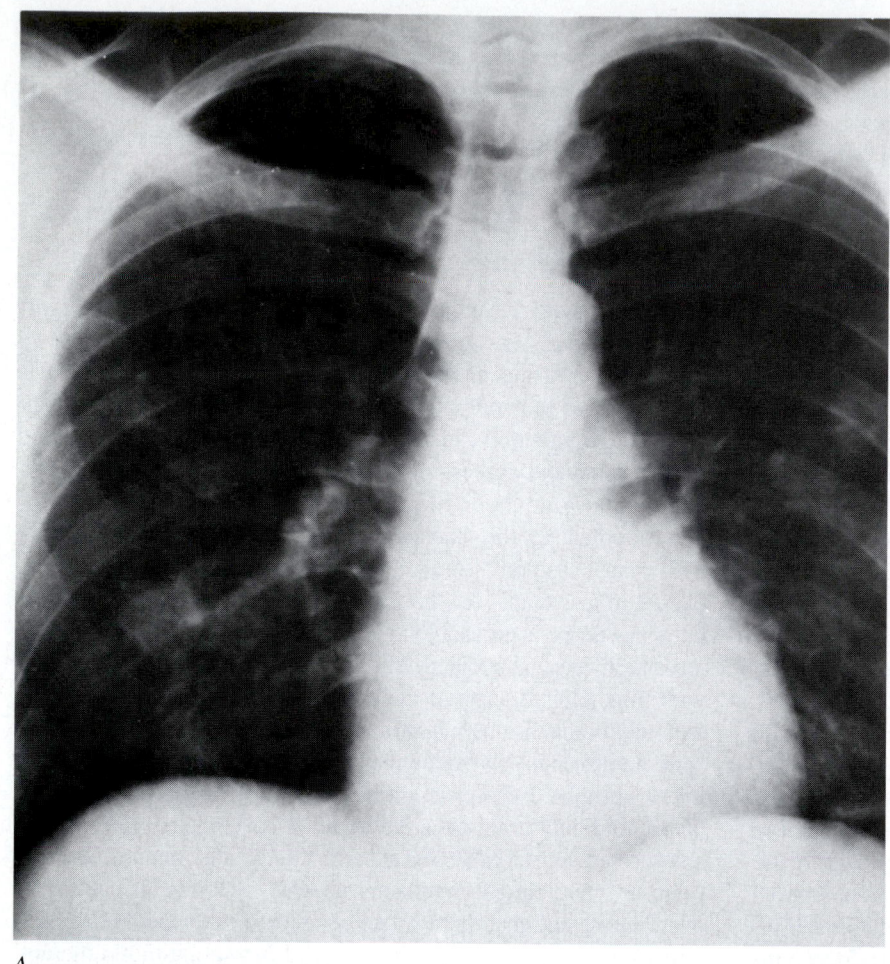

A

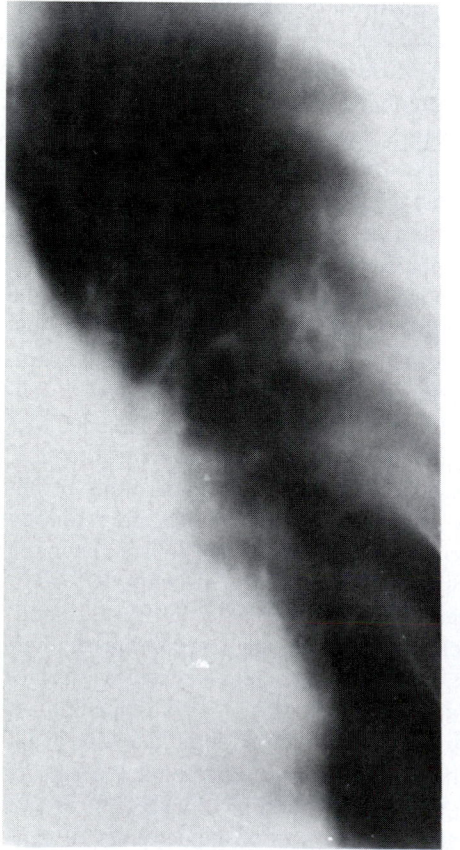

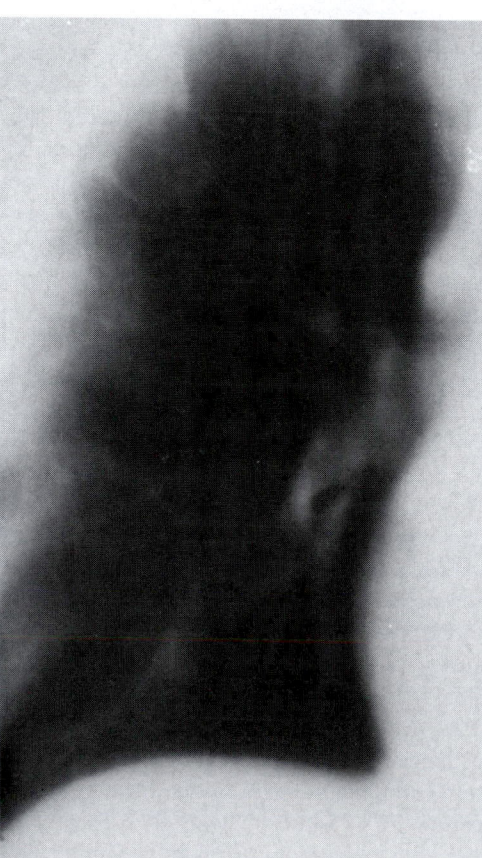

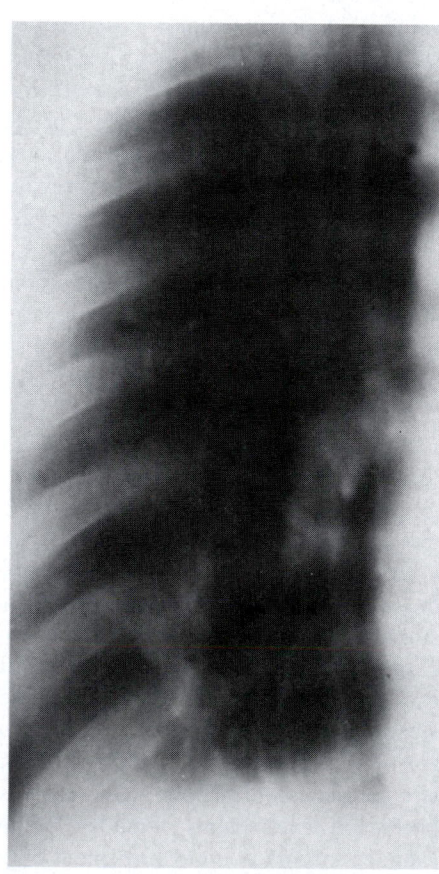

B

FIGURE 133-6 Septic pulmonary emboli. *A.* Many areas of infiltration and cavitation in a 38-year-old drug addict with bacteremia. *B.* Cavitary lesions are more evident on tomographic chest radiographs.

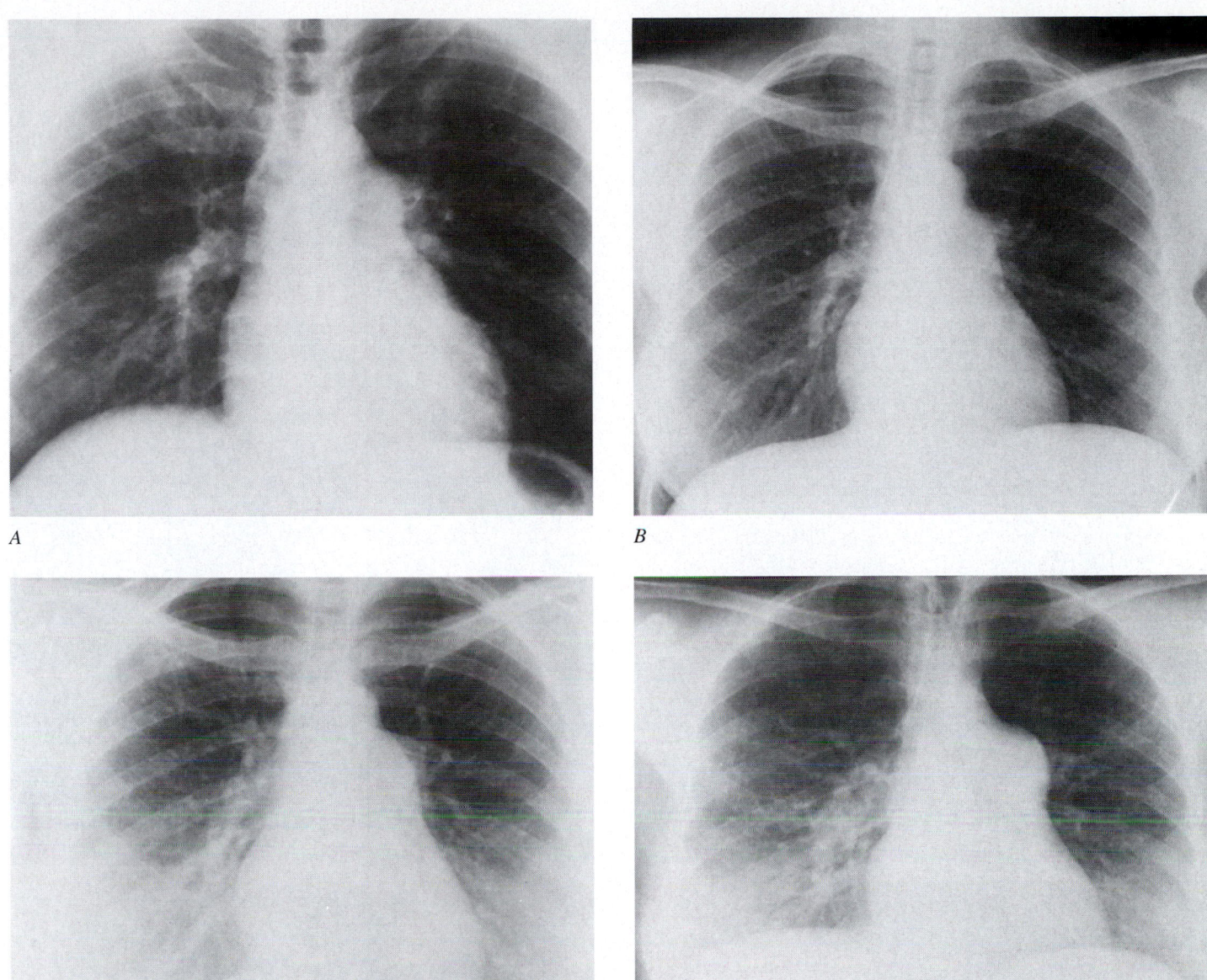

A   *B*

C   *D*

FIGURE 133-7   Pulmonary hypertension and radiographic infiltrates due to use of intravenous drugs. *A.* A 39-year-old male heroin user with progressive pulmonary hypertension (pulmonary artery pressures increased from 57/34 to 85/40 mmHg). Open lung biopsy revealed intimal proliferation and medial hypertrophy. Birefringent talc crystals were found free and in foreign-body–type giant cells. *(Courtesy of Dr. D. Murphy.)* *B–D.* Chest radiographs of a 30-year-old woman with a 15-year history of intravenous and subcutaneous injection of heroin, methylphenidate (Ritalin), and pentazocine (Talwin), with progressive pulmonary infiltrates and pulmonary hypertension. *B.* Enlargement of the cardiac silhouette and pulmonary arteries is observed on the initial chest radiograph. *C.* At 30 months, the patient has progression of pulmonary hypertension and a new right-sided pulmonary infiltrate. *D.* At 6 years, bilateral pulmonary infiltrates are observed with nodular reticular infiltrates throughout both lung fields.

agent alone. In practice, however, purportedly synergistic combinations have not improved outcome in patients with gram-negative bacterial infections, with the possible exception of neutropenic patients, nor have they decreased the emergence of resistant organisms. Moreover, the methods for demonstrating antibiotic synergy are problematic and often yield conflicting results, even in vitro. Nonetheless, combination therapy may avoid "missing" coverage in polymicrobial infection.

Given the relative lack of antistaphylococcal and antistreptococcal activities of third-generation cephalosporins, some preference exists for combinations that include first- or second-generation cephalosporins, clindamycin, penicillinase-resistant synthetic penicillins, imipenem, vancomycin, or combination β-lactam–β-lactamase inhibitor agents. Cost-effective therapies are available to meet these recommendations (Table 133-4). Generally, combinations of bactericidal and bacteriostatic agents are

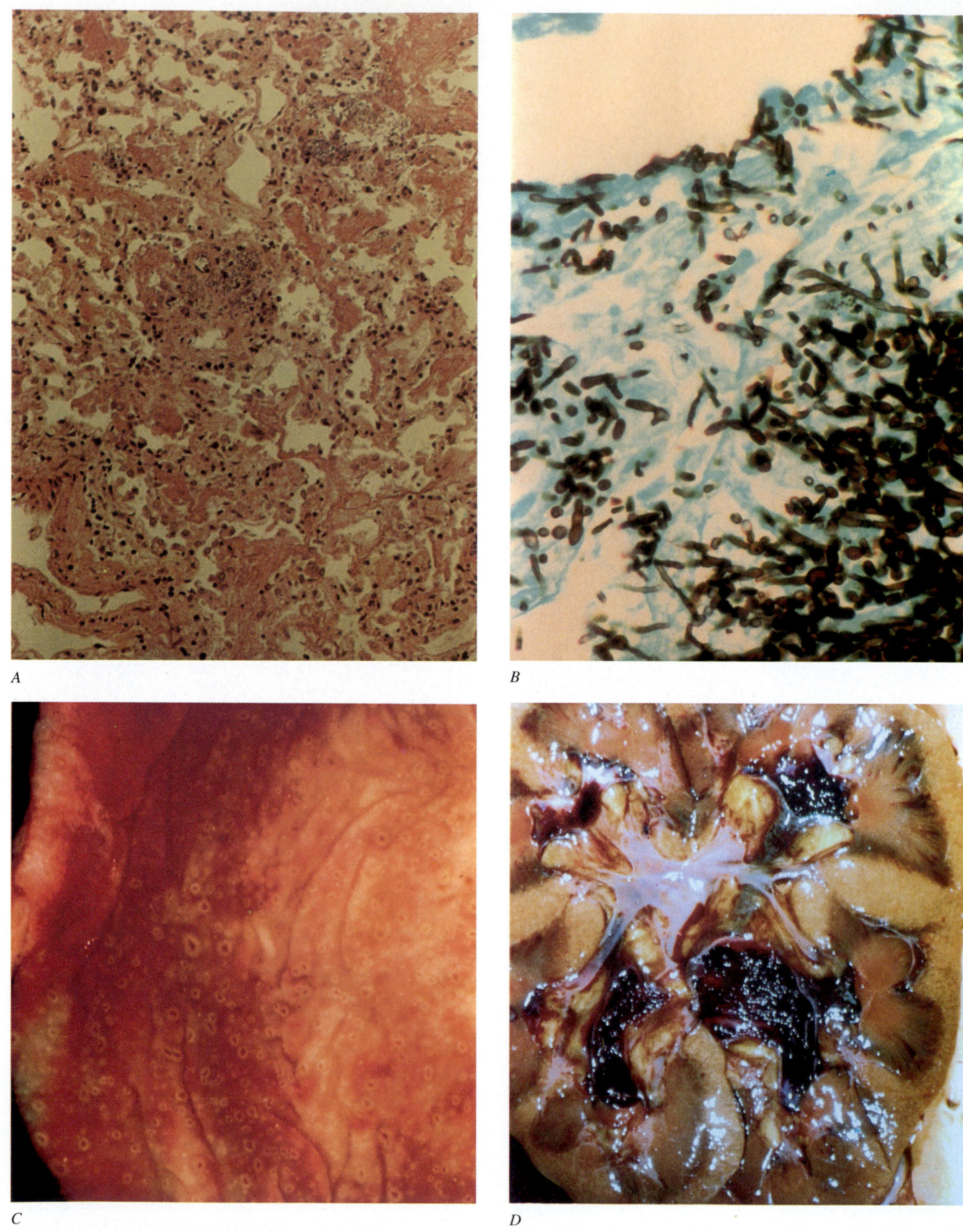

A

B

C

D

FIGURE 133-8

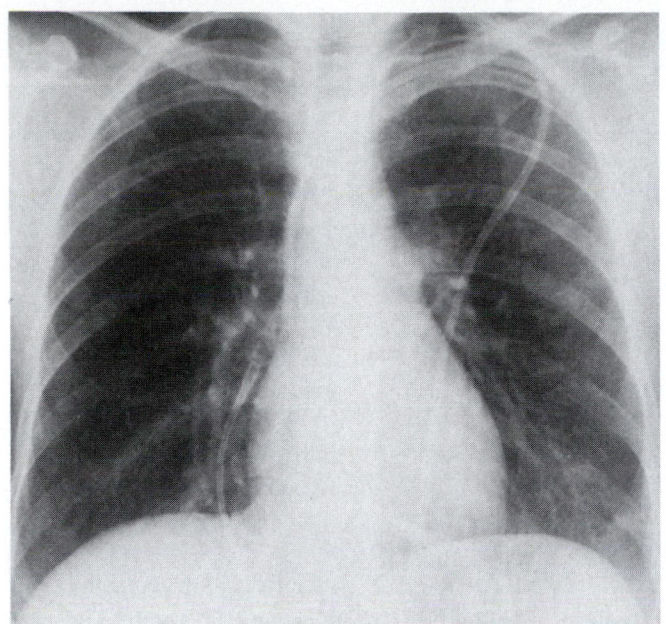

E

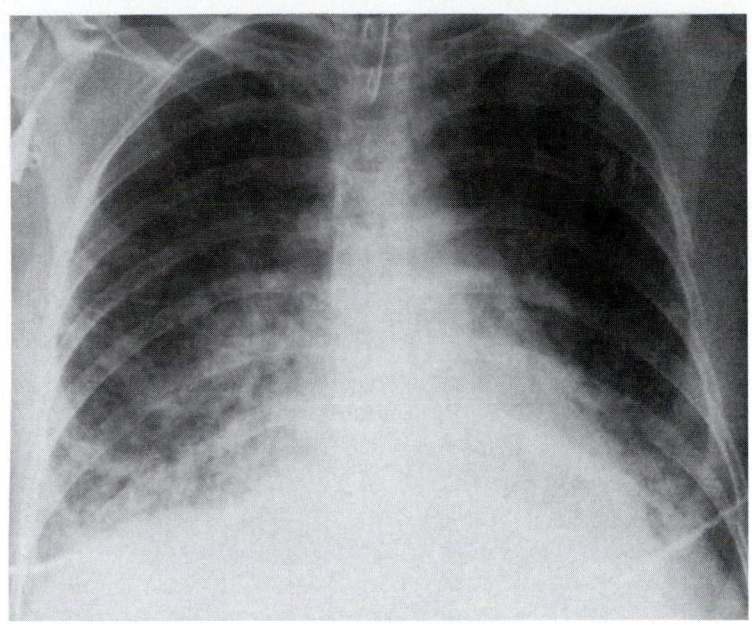

F

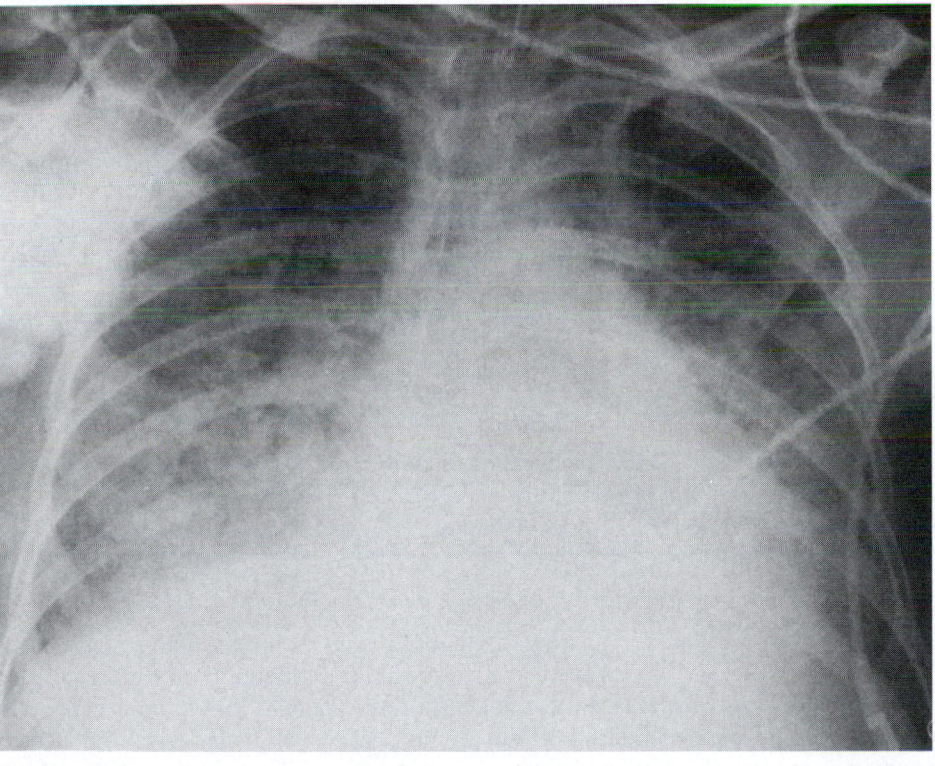

G

FIGURE 133-8 *(Cont.)* Catheter-related fungal pneumonia and hemorrhage. A 46-year-old woman with acute myelogenous leukemia developed fungemia with Trichosporon beigelii related to an infected Hickman catheter site (A–D). Metastatic bronchopneumonia (A) was due to the fungus (B). Ulceration of the gastric mucosa (C) and disseminated intravascular coagulation with renal hemorrhage (D) occurred. Over a period of 7 days, the chest radiograph progressed from essentially clear (E) to patchy bronchopneumonia (F) and finally to a picture of diffuse infiltrates and the adult respiratory distress syndrome (G).

avoided because of potential antagonism. Aminoglycosides and vancomycin are generally used with monitoring of blood levels to assure therapeutic levels and to minimize the potential for toxicity. Such monitoring has not been shown to either increase efficacy or reduce toxicity, however, and probably has no role in once daily aminoglycoside dosing. In animal models, aminoglycoside toxicity has been shown to be greatly potentiated in the presence of hypotension or endotoxin. Moreover, aminoglycosides are inactivated by low pH and a variety of enzymes found in abscesses or necrotic tissue.

TABLE 133-4

Empiric Therapies for the Adult Sepsis Syndrome

Clinical Syndrome	Preferred Regimen	Alternative Regimen
Intra-abdominal/pelvic source	Ampicillin + metronidazole + gentamicin	Vancomycin + metronidazole + gentamicin *or* ampicillin/sulbactam + gentamicin *or* imipenem
Urinary source	Ampicillin +/− gentamicin	Vancomycin + gentamicin *or* third-generation cephalosporin (ceftriaxone) +/− gentamicin *or* quinoline +/− gentamicin
Unknown source and injection drug users	Gentamicin + metronidazole + *either* nafcillin *or* vancomycin	Vancomycin + ceftriaxone metronidazole
Neutropenic host with fever	Gentamicin + *either* cefazolin *or* ticarcillin *or* ceftazidime	Gentamicin + vancomycin + *either* ticarcillin *or* ceftazidime
Splenectomized	Cefotaxime or ceftriaxome + vancomycin	Ampicillin/sulbactam (or other β-lactam–β-lactamase inhibitor combination) *or* fluoroquinolone +/− gentamicin
Streptococcal toxic shock	Penicillin + clindamycin +/− gentamicin	Erythromycin or ceftriaxone + clindamycin
Endocarditis—native value	Ampicillin or penicillin + nafcillin + aminoglycoside	Vancomycin + gentamicin

Adjunctive Therapies

The inability to improve outcomes markedly in patients with septic shock has lead to a large variety of therapeutic trials of antibacterial and anti-inflammatory agents. There are no convincing data that corticosteroids either accelerate the rate of recovery or lessen mortality in critically ill patients with sepsis. While some of the manifestations of sepsis (fever, some hypotension) may be blocked in individual patients, large clinical trials have failed to demonstrate the utility of steroid therapy in the adrenally sufficient patient. Similarly, no clear benefit of anticoagulation therapy has been demonstrated. Many other agents are under study. Particular interest has centered around the use of antisera directed against bacteria, bacterial products, and cytokines in sepsis (Tables 133-1, 133-2, and 133-3). Antiserum prepared by immunization of normal persons with the J5 mutant of *E. coli* was infused into patients with sepsis syndrome with a reduction in mortality (39 to 22 percent) and reversal of shock in some patients with gram-negative infections. However, careful analysis of larger trials did not confirm clinical efficacy (HA1A and E5 antibody trials) outside of small, retrospectively identified, subgroups of septic patients. Antibodies and binding proteins for endotoxin, TNF-α, and IL-1β, and use of IL-1 receptor and receptor antagonist, IL-10 administration, anti-CD14, anti-LBP, and PAF receptor antagonist are under evaluation.

REFERENCES

1. Abraham E, Jesmok G, Tuder R, et al: Contribution of tumor necrosis factor–α to pulmonary cytokine expression and lung injury after hemorrhage and resuscitation. *Crit Care Med* 23:1319–1326, 1995.

2. American College of Chest Physicians/Society of Critical Care Medicine Consensus Conference Committee: Definitions for sepsis and organ failure and guidelines for the use of innovative therapies in sepsis. *Crit Care Med* 20:864–874, 1992.

3. Anderson BO, Brown JM, Bensard DD, et al: Reversible lung neutrophil accumulation can cause lung injury by elastase-mediated mechanisms. *Surgery* 108:262–268, 1990.

4. Anderson BO, Harken AH: Multiple organ failure: Inflammatory priming and activation sequences promote autologous organ injury. *J Trauma* 30(Suppl):S44–S49, 1990.

5. Anderson BO, Poggetti RS, Shanley PF, et al: Primed neutrophils injure rat lung through a platelet activating factor dependent mechanism. *J Surg Res* 50:510–514, 1991.

6. Baker JW, Deitch EA, Berg RD, Specian RD: Hemorrhagic shock induces bacterial translocation from the gut. *J Trauma* 28:896–906, 1988.

7. Bernard GR, Artigas A, Brigham KL, et al, and the Consensus Committee: The American-European consensus conference on ARDS. *Am J Resp Crit Care Med* 149:818–824, 1994.

8. Bermudez L, Young LS: Ethanol augments intracellular survival of *Mycobacterium avium* and impairs macrophage response to cytokines. *J Infect Dis* 163:1286–1292, 1991.

9. Blussé van Oud A, Janssens AR, Leijh PCJ, van Furth R: Functions of granulocytes and monocytes in primary biliary and alcoholic cirrhosis. *Clin Exp Immunol* 62:724–731, 1985.

10. British Thoracic Society Research Committee: Community-acquired pneumonia in adults in British hospitals in 1982–1983: A survey of aetiology, mortality, prognostic factors and outcome. *Q J Med* 62:195–220, 1987.

11. Buchman TG, Abello PA, Smith EH, Bulkley GB: Induction of heat shock response leads to apoptosis in endothelial cells previously exposed to endotoxin. *Am J Physiol* 265:H165–H170, 1993.

12. Cabanes LR, Weber SN, Matran R, et al: Bronchial hyperresponsiveness to methacholine in patients with impaired left ventricular function. *New Engl J Med* 320:1317–1322, 1989.

13. Chollet MS, Montravers P, Gilbert C, et al: Subpopulation of hyperreactive polymorphonuclear neutrophils in patients with adult respiratory distress syndrome. *Am Rev Resp Dis* 146:990–996, 1992.

14. Crouser ED, Dorinsky PM: Gastrointestinal tract dysfunction in critical illness: Pathophysiology and interaction with acute lung injury in adult respiratory distress syndrome/multiple organ dysfunction syndrome. *New Horizons* 2:476–487, 1994.

15. Deitch EA: Simple intestinal obstruction causes bacterial translocation in man. *Arch Surg* 124:669–701, 1989.

16. Deitch EA: Multiple organ failure: Pathophysiology and potential future therapy. *Ann Surg* 216:117–134, 1992.

17. Dellinger EP, Oreskovich MR, Wertz MJ, et al: Risk of infection following laparatomy for penetrating abdominal injury. *Arch Surg* 119:20–27, 1984.

18. Drost AC, Burleson DG, Cioffi, WG Jr, et al: Plasma cytokines following thermal injury and their relationship with patient mortality, burn size, and time postburn. *J Trauma* 35:335–339, 1993.

19. Faggiano P: Abnormalities of pulmonary function in congestive heart failure. *Int J Cardiol* 44:1–8, 1994.

20. Faggiano P, Lombardi C, Sorgato A, et al: Pulmonary function tests in patients with congestive heart failure: Effects of medical therapy. *Cardiology* 83:30–35, 1993.

21. Feddersen CO, Willemer S, Karges W, et al: Lung injury in acute experimental pancreatitis in rats: II. Functional studies. *Int J Pancreatol* 8:323–331, 1991.

22. Fernández-Solá J, Junqué A, Estruch R, et al: High alcohol intake as a risk and prognostic factor for community-acquired pneumonia. *Arch Intern Med* 155:1649–1654, 1995.

23. Ferrer M, Torres A, González J, et al: Utility of selective digestive decontamination in mechanically ventilated patients. *Ann Intern Med* 120:389–395, 1994.

24. George DL: Epidemology of nosocomial pneumonia in intensive care unit patients. *Clin Chest Med* 16:29–44, 1995.

25. Gerkin TM, Oldham KT, Guice KS, et al: Intestinal reperfusion-ischemia injury causes pulmonary endothelial cell ATP depletion. *Ann Surg* 217:48–56, 1993.

26. Goris RJ, Boekhorst PA, Nuytinck KS: Multiple organ failure: Generalized autodestructive inflammation. *Arch Surg* 120:1109–1115, 1985.

27. Gyetko MR, Toews GB: Immunology of the aging lung. *Clin Chest Med* 14:379–391, 1993.

28. Hanson LC, Weber DJ, Rutala WA: Risk factors for nosocomial pneumonia in the elderly. *Am J Med* 92:161–166, 1992.

29. Hechtman HB: Mediators of local and remote injury following gut ischemia. *J Vasc Surg* 18:134–135, 1993.

30. Hershman MJ, Polk HC Jr, Pietsch JD, et al: Modulation of infection by gamma interferon treatment following trauma. *Infect Immun* 56:2412–2416, 1988.

31. Hill J, Lindsay T, Valeri CR, et al: A CD18 antibody prevents lung injury but not hypotension following intestinal ischemia-reperfusion. *J Appl Physiol* 74:659–664, 1993.

32. Hosoda N, Nishi M, Nakagawa, et al: Structural and functional alterations in the gut of parenterally or enterally fed rats. *J Surg Res* 47:129–133, 1989.

33. Imrie CW, Ferguson JC, Murphy D, Blumgart LH: Arterial hypoxia in acute pancreatitis. *Br J Surg* 64:185–188, 1977.

34. Kollef MH: The role of selective digestive tract decontamination on mortality and respiratory tract infections: A meta-analysis. *Chest* 105:1101–1108, 1994.

35. Koziol JM, Rush BF Jr, Smith SM, Machiedo GW: Occurrence of bacteremia during and after hemorrhagic shock. *J Trauma* 28:10–16, 1988.

36. Krowka MJ, Cortese DA: Hepatopulmonary syndrome: Current concepts in diagnostic and therapeutic considerations. *Chest* 105:1528–1537, 1994.

37. Langer M, Mosconi P, Cigada M, Mandelli M, and the Intensive Care Unit Group of Infection Control: Long-term respiratory support and risk of pneumonia in critically ill patients. *Am Rev Respir Dis* 140:302–305, 1989.

38. Lowry SF: The route of feeding influences injury responses. *J Trauma* 30(suppl):S10–S15, 1990.

39. Lowry SF: Modulating the metabolic response to injury and infection. *Proc Nutr Soc* 51:267–277, 1992.

40. Mailloux LU, Bellucci AG, Wilkes BM, et al: Mortality in dialysis patients: Analysis of the causes of death. *Am J Kidney Dis* 18:326–335, 1991.

41. Mainous MR, Block EFJ, Deitch EA: Nutritional support of the gut: How and why. *New Horizons* 2:193–201, 1994.

42. Mancini D, Henson D, LaManca J, Levine S: Respiratory muscle function and dyspnea in patients with chronic congestive heart failure. *Circulation* 86:909–918, 1992.

43. Marano MA, Moldawer LL, Fong Y, et al: Cachectin/TNF production in experimental burns and *Pseudomonas* infection. *Arch Surg* 123:1383–1388, 1988.

44. Matuschak GM, Martin DJ: Influence of end-stage liver failure on survival during multiple systems organ failure. *Transplant Proc* 19(4 Suppl 3):40–46, 1987.

45. Mester M, Carter EA, Tompkins RG, et al: Thermal injury induces very early production of interleukin-1α in the rat by mechanisms other than endotoxemia. *Surgery* 115:588–596, 1994.

46. Moore FA, Moore EE, Poggetti R, et al: Gut bacterial translocation via the portal vein: A clinical perspective with major torso trauma. *J Trauma* 31:629–638, 1991.

47. Montgomery AB, Stager MA, Carrico CJ, Hudson LD: Causes of mortality in patients with the adult respiratory distress syndrome. *Am Rev Respir Dis* 132:485–489, 1985.

48. Pepe PE, Potkin RT, Reus DH, et al: Clinical predictors of the adult respiratory distress syndrome. *Am J Surg* 144:124–130, 1982.

49. Redan JA, Rush BF, Lysz TW, et al: Organ distribution of gut-derived bacteria translocation caused by bowel manipulation or ischemia. *Am J Surg* 159:85–90, 1990.

50. Richardson JD, DeCamp MM, Garrison RN, Fry DE: Pulmonary infection complicating intra-abdominal sepsis. *Ann Surg* 195:732–738, 1982.

51. Rodriguez JL, Miller CG, Garner WFL, et al: Correlation of the local and systemic cytokine response with clinical outcome following thermal injury. *J Trauma* 34:684–695, 1993.

52. Rodriguez-Roisin R, Roca J, Agusti AG, et al: Gas exchange and pulmonary vascular reactivity in patients with liver cirrhosis. *Am Rev Respir Dis* 135:1085–1092, 1987.

53. Roumen RM, Hendriks T, van der Ven-Jongekrijg J, et al: Cytokine patterns in patients after major vascular surgery, hemorrhagic shock, and severe blunt trauma: Relation with subsequent adult respiratory distress syndrome and multiple organ failure. *Ann Surg* 218:769–776, 1993.

54. Rush BF, Sori AJ, Murphy TF, et al: Endotoxemia and bacteremia during hemorrhagic shock. *Ann Surg* 207:549–554, 1988.

55. Schmeling DJ, Caty MG, Oldham KT, et al: Evidence for neutrophil-related acute lung injury after intestinal ischemia-reperfusion. *Surgery* 106:195–202, 1989.

56. Shelhamer JH, Toews GB, Masur H, et al: Respiratory disease in the immunosuppressed patient. *Ann Intern Med* 117:415–431, 1992.

57. Silver MR, Bone RC: Selective digestive decontamination in critically ill patients. *Crit Care Med* 21:1418–1424, 1993.

58. Tryba M: The gastropulmonary route of infection: Fact or fiction? *Am J Med* 91:135–146, 1991.

59. Vercellotti GM, Yin HQ, Gustafson KS, et al: Platelet activating factor primes neutrophil responses to agonists: Role in promoting neutrophil mediated endothelial cell damage. *Blood* 71:1100–1107, 1988.

60. Wells CL: Editorial response to "A decade of experience with selective decontamination of the digestive tract as prophylaxis for infections in the intensive care unit: What have we learned?" *Clin Infect Dis* 17:1055–1057, 1993.

61. Weiner J, Itokazu G, Nathan C, et al: A randomized, double-blind, placebo controlled trial of selective digestive decontamination in a medical surgical intensive care unit. *Clin Infect Dis* 20:861–867, 1995.

62. White JC, Nelson S, Winkelstein JA, et al: Impairment of antibacterial defense mechanisms of the lung by extrapulmonary infection. *J Infect Dis* 153:202–208, 1986.

63. Willemer S, Feddersen CO, Karges W, Adler G: Lung injury in acute experimental pancreatitis in rats: I. Morphological studies. *Int J Pancreatol* 8:305–321, 1991.

CHAPTER 134

INTRODUCTION: PULMONARY INFECTION IN SPECIAL HOSTS

Jay A. Fishman

THE CONTINUUM OF SPECIAL HOSTS

THE EPIDEMIOLOGY OF INFECTION

NEWER CONCEPTS OF VIRULENCE

PROTECTING THE PATIENT FROM INFECTION

THE TIME COURSE OF INFECTION

RECOGNITION OF NEW SYNDROMES

MULTIPLE SIMULTANEOUS PROCESSES

PATIENT MANAGEMENT

AIDS, and advances in medical technology that include solid organ and bone marrow transplantation, ablative chemotherapeutic regimens for cancer, and prolonged survival of immnuosuppressed patients with "connective tissue diseases," have greatly expanded the pool of "immunocompromised hosts." These patients are defined by their susceptibility to infection with organisms that have little native virulence for the normal host. The detection of underlying immune compromise has been facilitated by improvements in microbiologic techniques and assays for various aspects of immune function. Survival has also been improved by the availability of new antimicrobial agents, including azole antifungal agents, macrolides, antiviral (ganciclovir, foscarnet, oral agents) and antiretroviral (for HIV) agents. The

clinical use of cytokines and growth factors has also strengthened approaches to the compromised host.

With the changing health-care scene, medical care of immunocompromised individuals is increasingly managed outside of academic centers. Therefore, information about the clinical management of these patients has become increasingly important to the entire spectrum of medical practitioners. Discussions following this chapter (Chapters 135 to 141) of the important infectious syndromes associated with specific types of immune deficits are encompassed by several common themes: the epidemiology and prevention of infection; the types and presentations of common infections; the time course of infections seen in each type of host; and common difficulties in the recognition and diagnosis of infection in these complicated patients. The main goal of this section is to address the issues in infectious disease associated with the care of immunocompromised patients in a practical manner that is in keeping with the complexity of these patients.

THE CONTINUUM OF SPECIAL HOSTS

Traditional discussions of infectious diseases have grouped patients either by specific pathogens or, in the immunocompromised host, by the primary immune defect. Thus, infections in the neutropenic host and the transplant recipient have customarily been considered separately from infections of the foot in a patient with diabetes or infections in a postsurgical patient who has been rendered susceptible to infection by the presence of incisions, drains and catheters, devitalized tissues, mechanical ventilation, or compromised vascular and/or neuronal supplies. This approach continues to be useful in assessing the types of organisms, the time course of infection, and the common presentations of infections in highly susceptible individuals. Each of the major classes of immunocompromised hosts is discussed in Chapters 135 to 141.

However, such divisions are arbitrary and do not consider the complexity of the immunocompromised patient. For example, in the alcoholic patient with hepatitis C and cirrhosis who has undergone liver transplantation, the so-called net state of immune suppression is the sum total of all the factors that place the patient at increased risk for infection. Among these are the immunologic and inflammatory effects of infection by hepatitis C virus and of cirrhosis; exposure to, and colonization with, community-acquired and nosocomial organisms; and any new infections (e.g., spontaneous peritonitis) that may occur during the prolonged waiting period for a compatible organ. When the organ for transplantation does become available, it may arrive contaminated by organisms acquired by the donor during hospitalization. For the patient to receive the organ, the present allocation scheme requires that he or she be the most severely decompensated. This gravely ill patient is then subjected to a major surgical procedure. After the operation, the lungs are apt to be compromised, recovery of function in the allograft is apt to be subnormal, immune-suppressive drugs are initiated, biliary (T-tube), intravenous, and urinary catheters are placed, and major incisions have to heal. Drug toxicities at this stage are common, resulting in neutropenia and hepatitis. Biliary function and anastomotic integrity are assessed by injecting contrast dye into ducts and tubes (e.g., T-tube cholangiogram) that are colonized by native and nosocomial organisms. The sum of the underlying, operative, and transplant-related factors is the *net state of immune suppression*. Thus, the "spectrum" of susceptibility to infection is a *continuum* from individual deficits (e.g., viral upper respiratory infection that paves the way for bacterial superinfection) to multiple simultaneous deficits (e.g., the transplant recipient).

THE EPIDEMIOLOGY OF INFECTION

The level of exposure of the individual to potential pathogens will determine which organisms will "take advantage" of immune deficiencies. *Opportunistic infections* are those infections that are due to relatively benign organisms or with degrees of severity out of proportion to the native virulence of the offending organism. *Infections that "should not occur" in the normal host suggest the presence of an immune defect.* Thus, relatively benign organisms in the normal host (e.g., *Pneumocystis carinii,* anaerobic bacteria, cytomegalovirus) cause life-threatening disease in compromised hosts with AIDS or diabetes and after transplantation of bone marrow or a solid organ. Similarly, "benign" organisms in the wrong location (e.g., empyema, meningitis) or in an obstructed viscus in an otherwise normal host are no less threatening. Thus, all infections are "opportunistic" in nature (i.e., the right place for the organism at the wrong time for the patient).

NEWER CONCEPTS OF VIRULENCE

The risk of infection in any individual patient depends not only on the sum of the immune deficits and the nature, duration, and intensity of the exposures to potential pathogens but also on the *virulence* of the organism (Chapter 125). Recent data suggest that the *specific host–pathogen interactions* are a critical factor in the development of infection. Host cells may *enhance* the virulence of the invading organism by the *induction of genes in that organism* that contribute to bacterial persistence or invasion.[1,8,16] Thus, resistance to phagocytosis is induced by target cells in *Yersinia* infections. Also, the survival of uropathogenic *E. coli* in urine and the growth of pili for attachment are induced by contact with the targeted uroepithelial cells. Another example of the host–pathogen interaction is the role of cytomegalovirus (CMV) in transplantation.[12] CMV is the cause of common clinical syndromes that frequently occur in immunocompromised patients. Among these are pneumonitis, hepatitis, glomerulonephritis, gastritis, colitis, retinitis, and mononucleosislike syndromes. CMV also induces an array of host responses (i.e., neutropenia, immune suppression, up-regulation of histocompatibility antigens and other cell surface antigens, TNFα secretion, possibly cardiac allograft atherogenesis, and graft rejection) that contribute to the host's susceptibility to infection. Thus, the concept of "immune status" balanced against "epidemiologic exposure" may be incomplete: The immunoregulatory effects of some pathogens and the interaction of the organisms with the "correct" target cells of the host are best regarded as only part of the response to opportunistic infection.

Physical defects may also contribute to virulence. Foreign materials (vascular grafts, sutures, eye or limb prostheses) may provide a nidus for infection by an organism which would not be capable of causing infection under normal conditions. Local immune defects coupled to physical factors may predispose to life-threatening infection. Thus, corticosteroid eye drops used for inflammation due to prosthetic lens implants may lead to eye infections with *Streptomyces, Bartonella, Sporothrix,* and *Fusarium* species. *Salmonella* infection in the organ transplant recipient "homes" to vascular anastomoses and may persist despite appropriate therapy, causing mycotic aneurysms.

PROTECTING THE PATIENT FROM INFECTION

Although the clinical care of the compromised host has improved, flaws in the armamentarium against infection have been highlighted by the emergence of bacteria and fungi that are resistant to common antimicrobial agents. For example, increasingly *Streptococcus pneumoniae* and *Neisseria gonorrhoeae* are detected that are resistant to penicillins; enterococci that are resistant to penicillin, tetracycline, vancomycin, teichoplainin, streptomycin, and gentamycin; *Pseudomonas* and the enteric gram-negative bacteria that are resistant to broad-spectrum β-lactamases; and the azole-resistant yeasts, all of which are routinely isolated both in the community and in hospitalized patients. Moreover, decreases in the aquisition of infection by compromised hosts can only be accomplished by *complete* reverse precautions that entail the use of laminar airflow rooms and access to the patient only via glove-ports or the use of gowns, gloves, masks, caps, and shoe covers.[2,6,13] This practice reduces the incidence of hospital-acquired infection (as distinguished from spread of endogenous infection) by up to 50 percent, to the approximate rate of such infections in granulocytopenic patients.

However, the practice of *complete* reverse precautions is very costly. Consequently, protection against both acquired and endogenous infections has fallen onto the broad use of prophylactic antibiotics. Such oral agents as trimethoprim-sulfamethoxazole, quinolones, acyclovir (and related agents), and azole antifungal drugs now have widespread use in the management of both inpatients and outpatients. Oral decontamination regimens (i.e., nonabsorbable antibiotics), although useful for limited periods of time, are poorly tolerated because of taste, consistency, malabsorption of glucose and xylose bases, and cost.[5,15] Moreover, the use of such prophylactic agents may contribute to the emergence of antibiotic-resistant organisms. Occasionally, cessation of the use of oral decontamination regimens has been associated with the reemergence of resistant bacteria in the alimentary tract and systemic dissemination. Alternatives that are helpful adjuncts to practice include restriction of diets to cooked foods, cleaning without the use of aerosols, the use of phenolic cleaning agents, and the use of leukocyte filters for blood product transfusions.

The development of vaccines for use in the compromised host has been slowed by the inability of many such hosts to mount a protective immune response, by the identification of antigenic variation in some organisms (e.g., *Pneumocystis carinii*), and by the reluctance of pharmaceutical companies to invest in the development of vaccines because of the associated costs, issues related to liability, and the relatively small market for such vaccines.

The high costs of care for the prolonged survival of cancer, transplant, AIDS, and other immunocompromised hosts are in direct conflict with attempts to minimize expenditures for patient care, particularly those directed at limiting the use of newer drugs and referrals to medical specialists for management. New antiviral, antibacterial, and immune-suppressive agents are extremely costly. Monitoring of patients (e.g., determination of viral loads for HIV and hepatitis C, CD4+ lymphocyte counts, routine radiographs and blood tests, drug levels) is equally costly. Thus, primary care physicians are under pressure to minimize the use of drugs and to curtail hospitalization costs at the same time that the population of such patients and the maintenance costs for each patient are growing.

THE TIME COURSE OF INFECTION

In each of the major conditions that predispose to opportunistic infection, there exists a time course of susceptibility to specific agents.[11,14] The risks of infection may be *relatively stable* over time, as in the diabetic with vasculopathy and neuropathy who is prone to skin and soft tissue infections caused by trauma to insensate limbs with diminished tissue integrity and neutrophil function. The risks of infection may be *time limited,* as in the postsurgical patient without complications or in the autologous bone marrow transplantation recipient with engraftment. The risk of infection may be *cumulative and progressive,* as in the AIDS

patient, in whom infection is a function of declining immunity (without therapy), falling CD4+ lymphocyte counts, rising viral loads, and the effects of other persistent infections (CMV, *Cryptosporidium*). In these individuals the occurrence of new infections suggests the progression of immune compromise. The risks may also be *progressive but not cumulative.* Thus, the risks of infection in the recipient of allogeneic bone marrow or of a solid organ *change predictably with time* as a function of the changing condition of the patient. For example (Fig. 134-1), in the early phase after bone marrow transplantation, infection is a result of nosocomial exposures and neutropenia. Subsequently, with engraftment, viral pneumonitis (CMV) and hepatic veno-occlusive disease may occur. Finally, during the development of, and treatment for, acute and chronic graft-versus-host disease, susceptibility to infection is largely a function of immune suppression and mucosal injuries. In the organ transplant recipient, *changing risk factors* (i.e., surgery, immune suppression, chronic immune suppression, acute and chronic rejection, reemergence of underlying diseases, viral infections) are similarly associated with changing opportunistic pathogens (Fig. 134-1). The pulmonary pathogens to which the bone marrow and solid organ transplantation recipients are susceptible at various times after transplantation are diagrammed in Fig. 134-2.

Because each risk factor renders the patient susceptible to infection by new groups of pathogens, *infections occurring with the "wrong" pathogen or at the wrong time suggest an undiscovered immune deficit or an unusual epidemiologic exposure.* The occurrence of specific infections can be prevented by the use of antibiotic prophylaxis, vaccines, and behavioral modifications (e.g., no raw vegetables or digging in gardens without masks). This will result in a "shift to the right" of the infection time line—infections generally observed later in the course of disease or therapy will be observed at the appropriate time *in the absence of infections that tend to occur earlier* but have been prevented by a variety of preventative measures.

RECOGNITION OF NEW SYNDROMES

The identification of *new* infectious disease syndromes has often occurred in individuals with immune deficits. Thus, the cluster of cases of *Pneumocystis carinii* pneumonia in homosexual males was the first indicator of a new viral pathogen (HIV-1), and the role of *Cryptosporidium* as a common cause of diarrhea in both normal and compromised individuals was elucidated as a result of diarrheal disease in AIDS patients in the 1980s. Similarly, many uncommon viruses (Kaposi's-associated herpes virus 8), fungi (*Penicillium*), and parasites (*Microsporidia*) have been identified or characterized in immunocompromised patients. Thus, a continuing lookout for new pathogens or novel presentations of known pathogens is essential for the care of the immunocompromised patient (Fig. 134-3). Often, infection in immunocompromised hosts presents without the expected signs and symptoms of infection. This lack of clinical manifestations may delay identification of the critically ill patient. In the outpatient setting, the practitioner must have a low threshold for performing tests (e.g., blood counts, cultures, radiographs) on patients with minimal complaints. For example, when an organ transplant patient telephoned to complain of low-grade fever

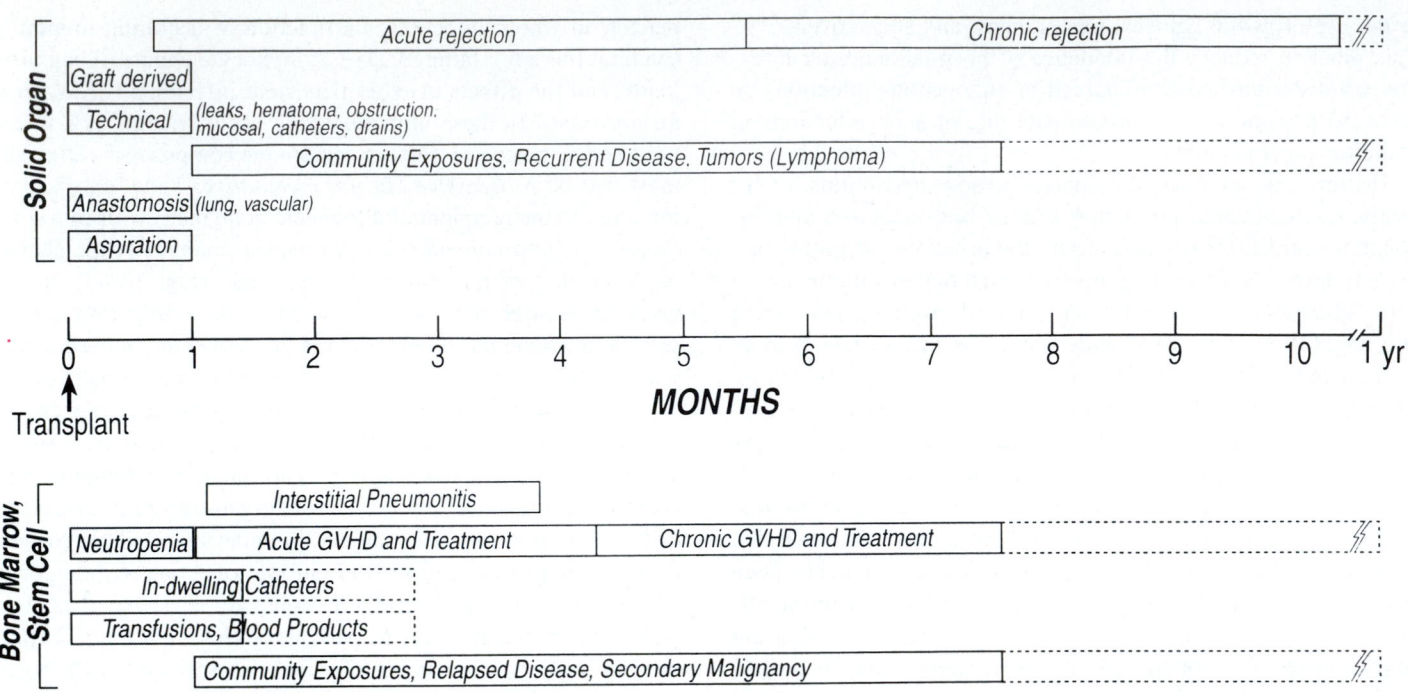

FIGURE 134-1   The timeline of conditions predisposing to infection in solid organ transplantation (above the timeline) and in bone marrow and stem cell transplantation (below the timeline). Patients will vary in individual susceptibility patterns.

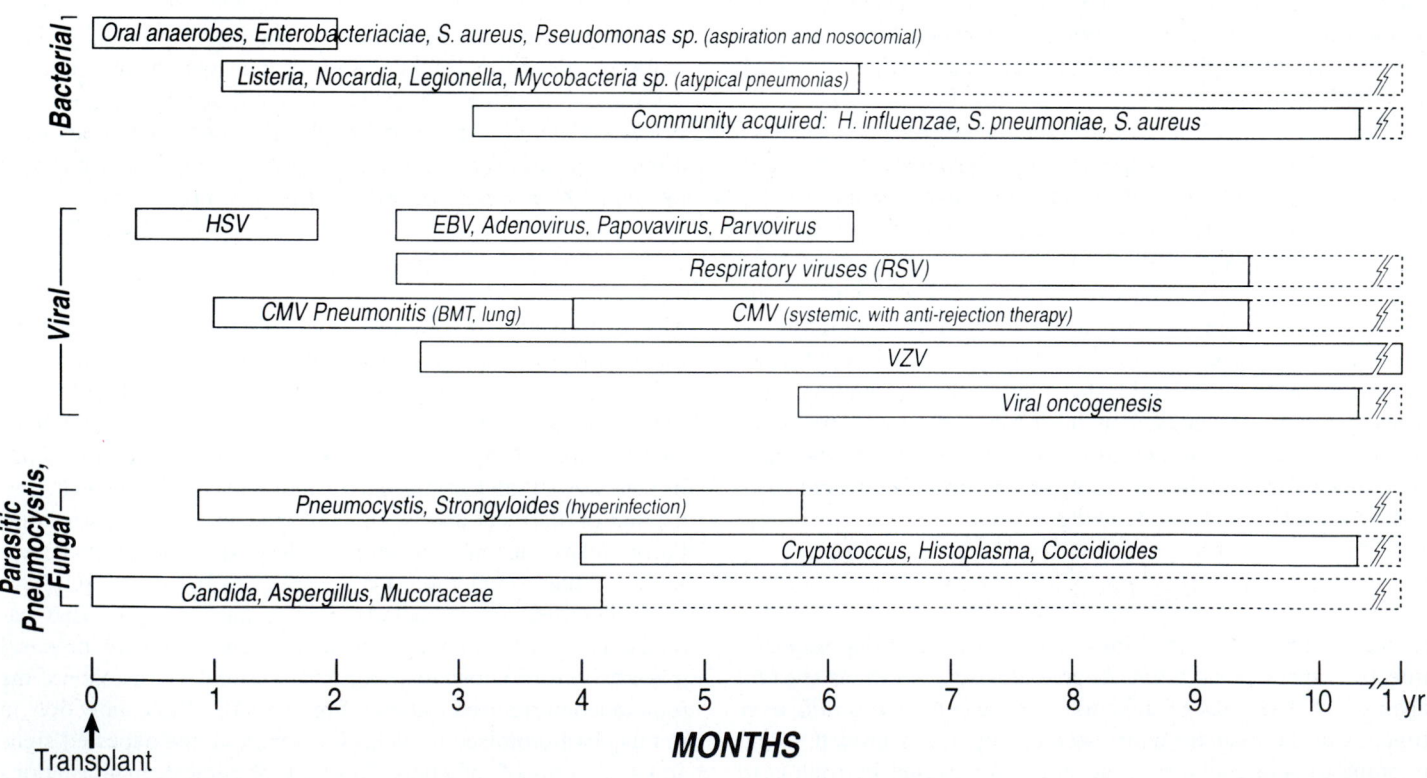

FIGURE 134-2   The timeline of infections commonly observed following solid organ transplantation and in bone marrow and stem cell transplantation. Although the specific factors contributing to the net state of immune deficiency differ between individuals and various forms of immune suppression, the general temporal presentation of infection is similar in the two groups. Individual patients may deviate from the predicted pattern based on specific predisposing conditions. Infections occurring out of sequence should suggest the presence of an excessive epidemiological exposure or an undetected immunosuppressive condition.

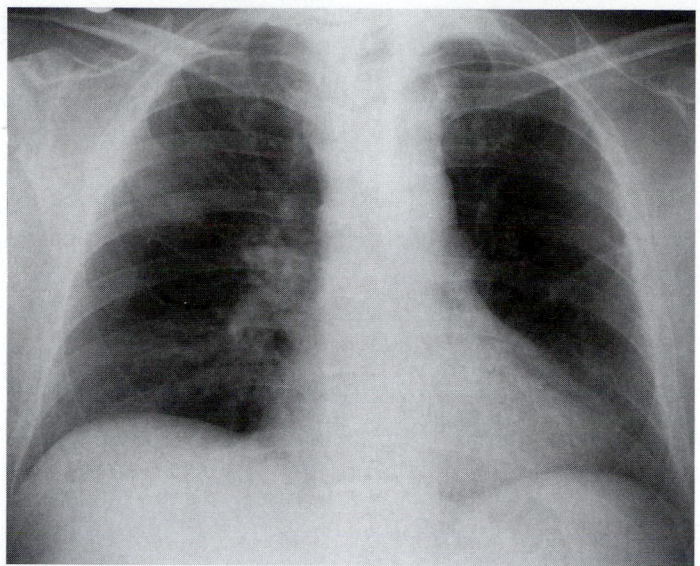

A

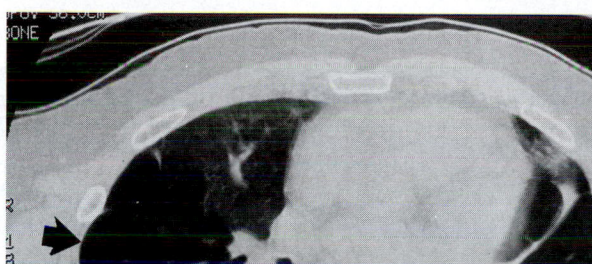

B

FIGURE 134-3   A 39-year-old man with progressive Wegener's granulomatosis complained of dyspnea developing over 2 weeks. He was maintained on oral predisone with intermittent cytotoxic therapies for acute exacerbations of pulmonary disease. Routine chest radiographs (*A*) revealed diffuse interstitial haziness without focality. Computed tomography (*B*) demonstrated nodular densities (white arrow) and large peripheral pulmomary infarcts (black arrow), which were present previously, and new, dense interstitial infiltrates throughout the remaining lung parenchyma. Cultures obtained from bronchoscopic lavage were negative. Bronchoscopic biopsy of the lung was positive by culture and immunoperoxidase stains for cytomegalovirus. Blood antigenemia assay for CMV was also strongly positive. The patient improved rapidly on monotherapy with ganciclovir over 7 days.

(100° F) and minimal cough, the chest radiograph revealed opacification of the left lung due to *M. tuberculosis* (Fig. 134-4); the patient was anergic to control and to PPD skin testing.

MULTIPLE SIMULTANEOUS PROCESSES

Early and aggressive therapy of infection is required in the immunocompromised patient. Thus, most febrile or possibly infected patients are treated empirically while awaiting data that

identify specific pathogens. The occurrence of multiple simultaneous infections or conditions may complicate and delay appropriate therapy. Thus, CMV infection may complicate the treatment of graft rejection or veno-occlusive disease and contribute to the pathogenesis of *Pneumocystis* or *Toxoplasma* pneumonia.

In the lungs, standard radiographic techniques may not detect the presence of multiple patterns of infection. Similarly, radiographic patterns may change during the care of the patient (e.g., cavitation of pulmonary nodules after the resolution of neutropenia). It is commonly necessary to repeat tests, to utilize computed tomography (CT), or to use invasive diagnostic modalities (biopsy) in the evaluation of the patient who is unresponsive to therapy (Fig. 134-5). In the compromised host with fever and pneumonitis, chest radiographs may be difficult to interpret.[3,9,10,14] Noninfectious causes of pulmonary infiltrates may coexist with infection, and atypical patterns predominate. Drug toxicities (bleomycin, cytoxan, sulfa drugs), leukoagglutinin reactions, radiation injury, pulmonary emboli, and lesions of metastatic cancer may coexist with opportunistic infection. The "typical" evolution of pulmonary infection may be altered by the presence of underlying (e.g., interstitial) pulmonary disease as well as by diminished inflammatory responses.

Complications of therapy may contribute to the development of new infections: Trimethoprim-sulfamethoxazole can cause pneumonitis, hepatitis, or Stevens-Johnson syndrome; ganciclovir can cause renal failure and neutropenia; transfusion reac-

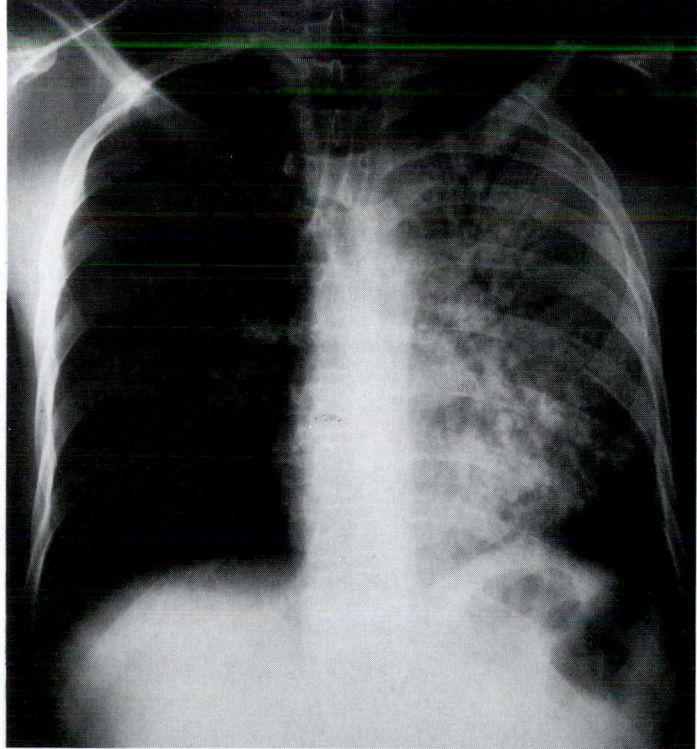

FIGURE 134-4   Chest radiograph of a 53-year-old man 3 years after successful liver transplantation. The patient called following a stay of 6 months in Brazil and complained of low-grade fever (100° F), nonproductive cough, and mild dyspnea while playing tennis. He was anergic to skin testing. Induced sputum examination revealed acid-fast bacilli, and cultures grew *Mycobacterium tuberculosis*.

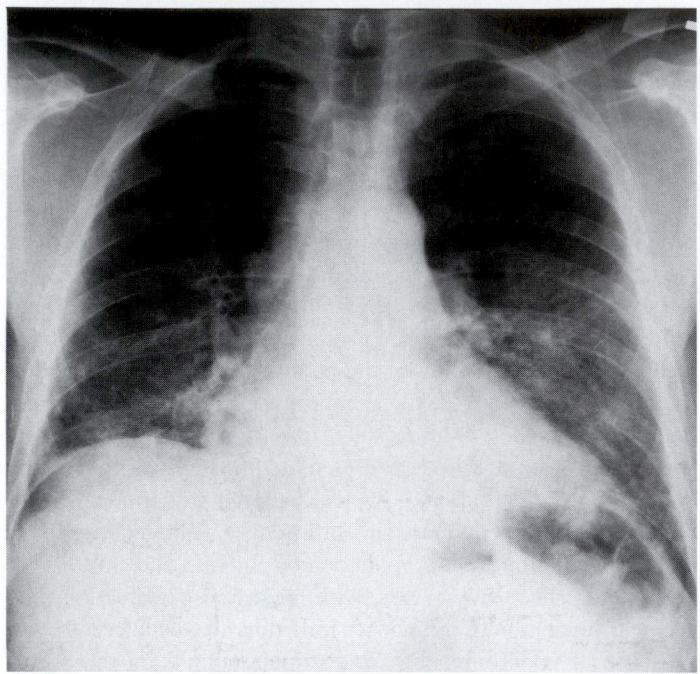

A

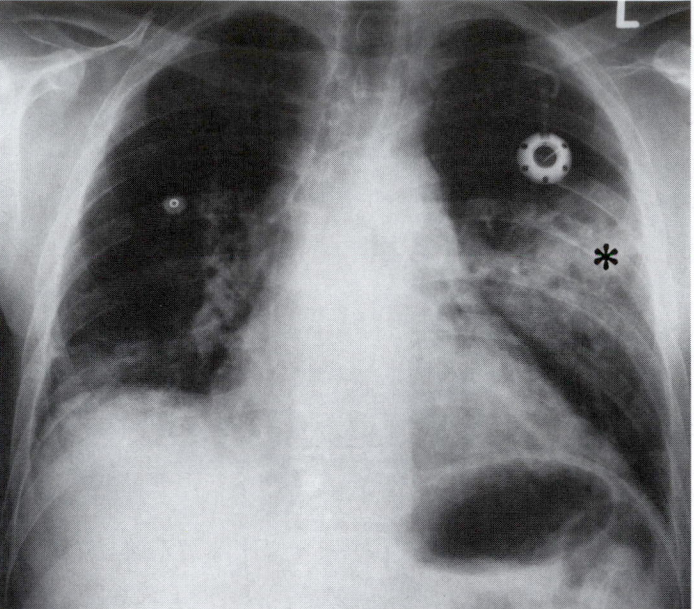

B

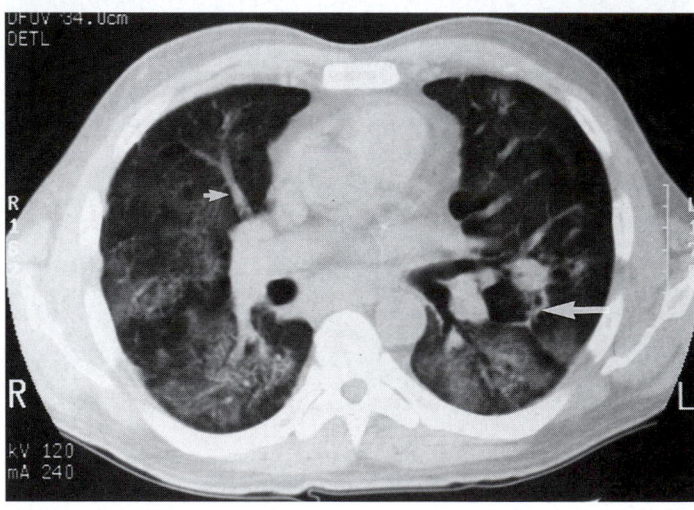

C

FIGURE 134-5 Chest radiographs of a 33-year-old man following chemotherapy for acute myelogenous leukemia. *A.* The patient presented with acute onset of cough and dyspnea, with induced sputum examination demonstrating *Pneumocystis carinii.* He is sulfa drug–allergic. Despite appropriate therapy with intravenous pentamidine isethionate and improving dyspnea, the patient remained febrile, clinically ill, with persistent cough. *B.* Repeat chest radiographs demonstrated a new infiltrate in the left lung field (asterisk). *C.* Computed tomography revealed a new left-sided abscess cavity (large arrow), bronchiectasis (small arrow), and dense parenchymal infiltrates. Samples examined from percutaneous needle aspiration contained thin, beaded, branched gram-positive filaments that stained by modified acid-fast technique and grew *Nocardia asteroides* in culture.

tions can cause pulmonary infiltrates and hemolysis; cyclosporine can cause hemolytic-uremic syndrome; antibiotics can cause thrush or *C. difficile* colitis.

PATIENT MANAGEMENT

Antibiotics alone may not suffice in the treatment of infection in the immunocompromised host. Many major infections require improvement in the immune responses of the host in order to clear ongoing infection. Infections may respond to a decrease in exogenous immune suppression, to correction of neutropenia by growth factors, or to treatment of simultaneous infections that predispose to superinfection (e.g., respiratory syncytial virus, CMV). Drainage of collections of infected fluid such as a hematoma or a lymphocele or removal of drains or catheters enhances the treatment of infection. Identification of metastatic sites of infection (e.g., infections of the central nervous system due to *Nocardia* or *Cryptococcus* species) may facilitate management. Synergistic antibiotic therapy must be used when available. Compromises often must be made. The loss of renal function due to antibiotics used in the treatment of fungal infections

significantly hinders patient management. However, progression of a fungal infection while on inadequate doses of amphotericin must be avoided.

Infection must be prevented in the susceptible host, since antibiotics are often ineffective during acute infection. If proper vaccines are available, vaccination should be used before immune suppression and, with nonlive vaccines, should be used during immune suppression to prevent or ameliorate infections due to common pathogens. Repletion of immunoglobulin deficiencies and the use of specific hyperimmune globulins (i.e., for exposure to varicella or for CMV) may help to prevent infection. Similarly, in patients susceptible to infection, the use of antibiotics to prevent common infections is cost-effective. The use of preemptive therapies based on tests that demonstrate the presence of infection (e.g., the administration of ganciclovir in patients with evidence of CMV infection by antigenemia assays or polymerase chain reaction studies) allows the interruption of infection before disease becomes manifest clinically. Similarly, routine surveillance cultures have been useful to detect specific pathogens in subgroups of patients (e.g., neutropenic patients with *Aspergillus* colonization) or in specific geographic regions.[7] Routine chest radiographs and blood tests, albeit expensive, are often valuable in the detection of unsuspected processes (infection or malignancy) in these patients.

The clinical *evaluation of the patient prior to immune suppression,* if elective, may be very helpful in preventing disease. Patients with cystic fibrosis or chronic bacterial sinusitis may become colonized in the airways or sinuses with *Pseudomonas* or *Aspergillus* species (Fig. 134-6). These colonizing organisms may reactivate during immune suppression. Careful evaluation by radiography and invasive cultures may prevent major infection. Similarly, patients who are not immune to varicella zoster *may* benefit from vaccination. Patients seronegative for *Toxoplasma gondii* or CMV are at high risk of reactivation in the presence of an organ transplant from a seropositive donor. Similarly, seropositive patients with AIDS or before seronegative bone marrow transplantation are at high risk for reactivation disease due to *Leishmania,* CMV, or *Toxoplasma.* In endemic areas, transfusions and transplants may provide entry of *T. gondii, Trypanosoma cruzi* (Chagas' disease), *Leishmania* species, *Acanthamoeba, Naeglaria, Strongyloides stercoralis, Taenia*

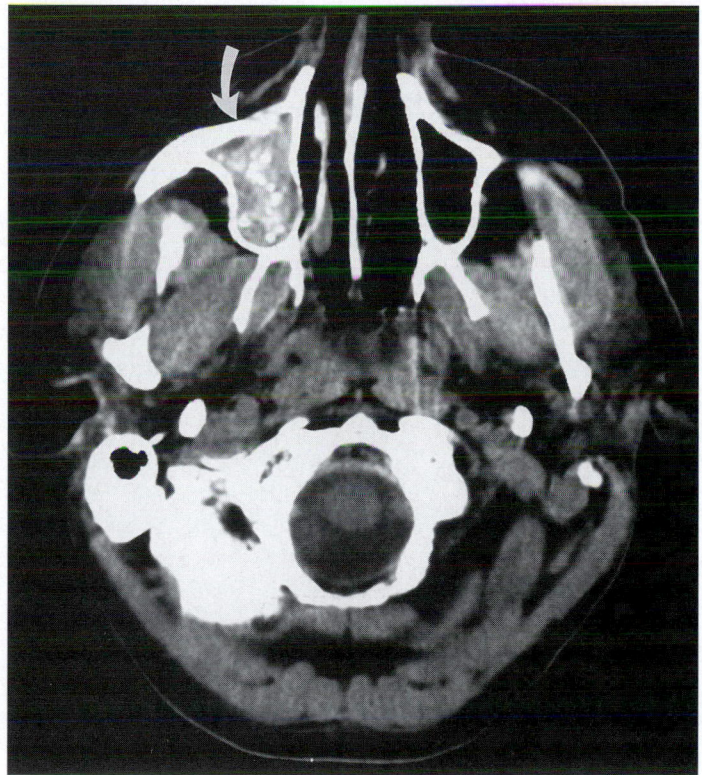

FIGURE 134-6 Computed tomography of the head in a 39-year-old man with chronic sinusitis prior to liver transplantation. Right maxillary sinus was opacified (arrow) and contained calcifications consistent with chronic infection due to *Aspergillus* species. Cultures of material aspirated from the sinus grew *Staphylococcus aureus* and *Aspergillus fumigatus.*

species, or *Echinococcus* species with exacerbation of infection by immune suppression. A careful clinical history and pretreatment of known infections or specific antibiotic prophylaxis may prevent such complications of immune deficiency.

REFERENCES

1. Cotter PA, Miller JF: Triggering bacterial virulence. *Science* 273:1183–1184, 1996.
2. Dietrich M, Gaus W, Vosen J, et al: Protective isolation and antimicrobial decontamination in patients with high susceptibility to infection: A prospective cooperative study of gnotobiotic care in acute leukemia patients. I. Clinical results. *Infection* 5:3–10, 1977.
3. Ettinger NA, Trulock EP: Pulmonary considerations of organ transplantation: Parts 1–3. *Am Rev Resp Dis* 143:1386–1405, 1991; 144:213–223, 433–451, 1991.
4. Fishman JA: *Pneumocystis carinii* and parasitic infections in the immunocompromised host, in Rubin RH, Young LS (eds), *Clinical Approach to Infection in the Compromised Host,* 3d ed. New York, Plenum, 1994, pp 275–334.
5. Klastersky J, Debusscher L, Weerts D, et al: Use of oral antibiotics in protected units environment: Clinical effectiveness and role in the emergence of antibiotic-resistant strains. *Pathol Biol* 22:5–12, 1973.
6. Levine AS, Siegel SE, Schreiber AD, et al: Protected environments and prophylactic antibiotics: A prospective controlled study of their utility in the therapy of acute leukemia. *New Engl J Med* 288:477–483, 1973.
7. Newman KA, Schimpff SC, Young VM, et al: Lessons learned from surveillance cultures from patients with acute non-lymphocytic leukemia: Usefulness for epidemiologic prevention and therapeutic research. *Am J Med* 70:423–431, 1982.
8. Pettersson J, Nordfelth R, Dubinina E, et al: Modulation of virulence factor expression by pathogen target cell contact. *Science* 273:1231–1233, 1996.
9. Rosenow EC III, Wilson WR, Cockerill FR III: Pulmonary disease in the immunocompromised host. *Mayo Clin Proc* 60:473–487, 610–631, 1985.
10. Rubin RH, Greene R: Clinical approach to the compromised host with fever and pulmonary infiltrates, in Rubin RH, Young LS (eds), *Clinical Approach to Infection in the Compromised Host,* 3d ed. New York, Plenum, 1994, pp 121–161.
11. Rubin RH: Infection in the organ transplant recipient, in Rubin RH, Young LS (eds), *Clinical Approach to Infection in the Compromised Host,* 3d ed. New York, Plenum, 1994, pp 629–705.
12. Rubin RH: The indirect effects of cytomegalovirus infection on the outcome of organ transplantation. *JAMA* 261:3607–3609, 1989.
13. Wade JC: Epidemiology and prevention of infection in the compromised host, in Rubin RH, Young LS (eds), *Clinical Approach to Infection in the Compromised Host,* 3d ed. New York, Plenum, 1994, pp 5–32.
14. Williams DM, Krick JA, Remington JS: Pulmonary infection in the compromised host. *Am Rev Resp Dis* 114:359–394, 593–627, 1976.
15. Yates JW, Holland JF: A controlled study of isolation and endogenous microbial suppression in acute myelocytic leukemia patients. *Cancer* 32:1490–1498, 1973.
16. Zhang JP, Normark S: Induction of gene expression in *Escherichia coli* after pilus-mediated adherence. *Science* 273:1234–1236, 1996.

CHAPTER 135

HIV INFECTION AND OPPORTUNISTIC PULMONARY INFECTIONS IN AIDS

Jay A. Fishman

More than 300,000 people have died from infection with human immunodeficiency viruses (HIV) and acquired immunodeficiency syndrome (AIDS) since the first report of unexplained immunodeficiency disease in homosexual men with *Pneumocystis carinii* pneumonia in 1981. In general, the cause of death was opportunistic infection or malignancy related to the progressive immune deficiency caused by retroviral infection (see Table 135-1). Over time, with improved understanding and therapeutics, the pattern of opportunistic processes in these hosts has shifted; this "frame shift" reflects the role of appropriate prophylactic regimens for the prevention of infections, particularly those due to *P. carinii, Candida* species, and the mycobacteria.[17,29,38] As a result, infections have "shifted" to pathogens with greater virulence (e.g., *Aspergillus* species), with novel antimicrobial resistance patterns (multidrug-resistant tuberculosis and cytomegalovirus),[15,19,29] or that are more difficult to recognize (e.g., *Bartonella*-associated infections). Perhaps more ominous, the frequency of AIDS in developing regions, especially in Africa and Southeast Asia, has grown dramatically.

HIV disease refers to the chronic viral infection and the progressive decline in immune function that predispose to opportunistic infection or neoplasm (Fig. 135-1). *AIDS* is the syndrome caused by infection with HIV characterized by immune deficiency and with one or more associated opportunistic infections, neoplasms, or conditions consistent with an acquired defect in cell-mediated immunity. Many HIV-infected patients are clinically stable and receive outpatient care for the bulk of the clinical course of their disease.

HIV EPIDEMIOLOGY

HIV-1, first isolated in 1983, is a human lymphotropic retrovirus that is generally cytopathic for infected cells. HIV-2, a retrovirus closely related to HIV-1, was originally isolated in West Africa and induces an AIDS-like disorder indistinguishable from that caused by HIV-1; however, HIV-2 generally has a longer clinical latency (up to 19 years).[3,11] The risk of heterosexual transmission of HIV-2 also appears to be significantly less than that of HIV-1 (by up to 11-fold), and disease progression may be slower. Although so far geographically restricted, HIV-2 has also been identified as a cause of heterosexually transmitted AIDS in India. A third virus, HIV-3, has been seen in areas of high prevalence of heterosexually transmitted AIDS, particularly in Southeast Asia.

Each of the HIV agents is related to simian immunodeficiency virus (SIV), which induces an AIDS-like condition in captive macaque monkeys and appears to be endemic but nonpathogenic

TABLE 135-1

Infectious Agents Commonly Associated with AIDS

Viral (with HIV-1, HIV-2)
 Cytomegalovirus
 Herpes simplex
 Herpes zoster
 Epstein-Barr virus
 Parvovirus B19
 HHV-6, HHV-8
 HTLV-1, HTLV-2
Protozoan
 Toxoplasma gondii
 Cryptosporidium
 Isospora belli
 Microsporidium
 Cyclospora
Fungal
 Candida species
 Cryptococcus neoformans
 Histoplasma capsulatum
 Blastomyces dermatidis
 Aspergillus species
 Petriellidium boydii
 Coccidioides immitis
 Pneumocystis carinii
 Sporothrix schenckii
Bacterial
 Mycobacterium avium-intracellulare complex
 M. tuberculosis
 Legionella species
 Nocardia asteroides
 Encapsulated gram–positive bacteria
 Salmonella species
 Rhodococcus equi
 Bartonella species
 Campylobacter species

TABLE 135-2

Prevalence of HIV Infection in Selected Populations in the United States

Population	Estimated HIV Seroprevalence (%)
Homosexual men	30–50
Injection drug users	2–60
Prostitutes	0–57
Hemophiliacs, factor VIII	75
Hemophiliacs, factor IX	35
Blood donors	0.02
Patients with tuberculosis	2–29
Patients with sexually transmitted disease	1–5
Pregnant women	0–1.5
Hospitalized adults without AIDS	0.2–1.4
College students	0.2
Military applicants	0.13

in wild African green monkeys (Fig. 135-2). These viruses are closely related to the "transforming retroviruses," including the human T-cell leukemia/lymphotropic viruses (HTLV-1 and -2), which cause malignant transformation in infected cells. HTLV-1 is endemic to Japan and the Caribbean, and is associated with tropical spastic paraparesis, adult T-cell leukemia, and lymphoma. HTLV-2 is associated with hairy-cell leukemia (although direct causation remains unclear) and is commonly detected in intravenous drug abusers.

The World Health Organization currently estimates that almost 20 million people are infected with one of the HIV strains. The relative restriction of AIDS to homosexual men that was noted early in the epidemic has been replaced by an increasing incidence of transmission in heterosexual men, women, and children. This shift is due to bisexual contacts, transmission with blood products in hemophiliacs and transfusion recipients, sexual promiscuity in association with other sexually transmitted diseases, and identification of HIV strains better adapted to heterosexual spread (Table 135-2). In particular, maternal–fetal transmission rates (estimated at 12 to 48 percent) have caused

an increasing incidence in children worldwide, with more than 1 million already infected.

Transmission occurs by three routes: bidirectionally with sexual contacts, with blood or blood products, and vertically in the perinatal period. The risk of transmission from an isolated needle stick from an HIV-infected person is about one in 250 to 300; heterosexual transmission occurs in about one in 1500 contacts; receptive anal intercourse causes transmission in one in 100 contacts; and maternal–fetal transmission is implicated in up to one in three cases. Infants may be infected by breast-feeding from an HIV-seropositive mother. In developing countries, the risks of HIV transmission via breast-feeding by women not known to be HIV infected may be outweighed by the benefits of protection against diarrheal and other diseases in the general population. Zidovudine therapy for HIV-infected pregnant women during the second and third trimesters and for the infant during the first 6 weeks of life significantly reduces the risk of maternal transmission. Up to 90 percent of persons receiving transfusions from HIV-infected persons will acquire infection; thus, more than 70 percent of people with hemophilia A in the United States have HIV infection. The risk of infection from screened blood products is approximately one in 100,000.

HIV PATHOGENESIS

HIV-1 is a 100-nm retrovirus with a lipid envelope surrounded by an electron-dense cylindric core (Fig. 135-3). The virus consists of at least nine different transcribed genes, which are relevant to diagnostic testing methods and are detected with Western blot or molecular methods.

1. *Gag:* group antigen gene that encodes structural proteins, including p55, p15 (single-stranded genomic RNA associated), p17, and p24, a viral antigen detectable in the serum of HIV-infected persons early and late in the course of disease.
2. *Pol:* polymerase gene that includes p66/51 (reverse transcriptase) and p31 (integrase/endonuclease), which partici-

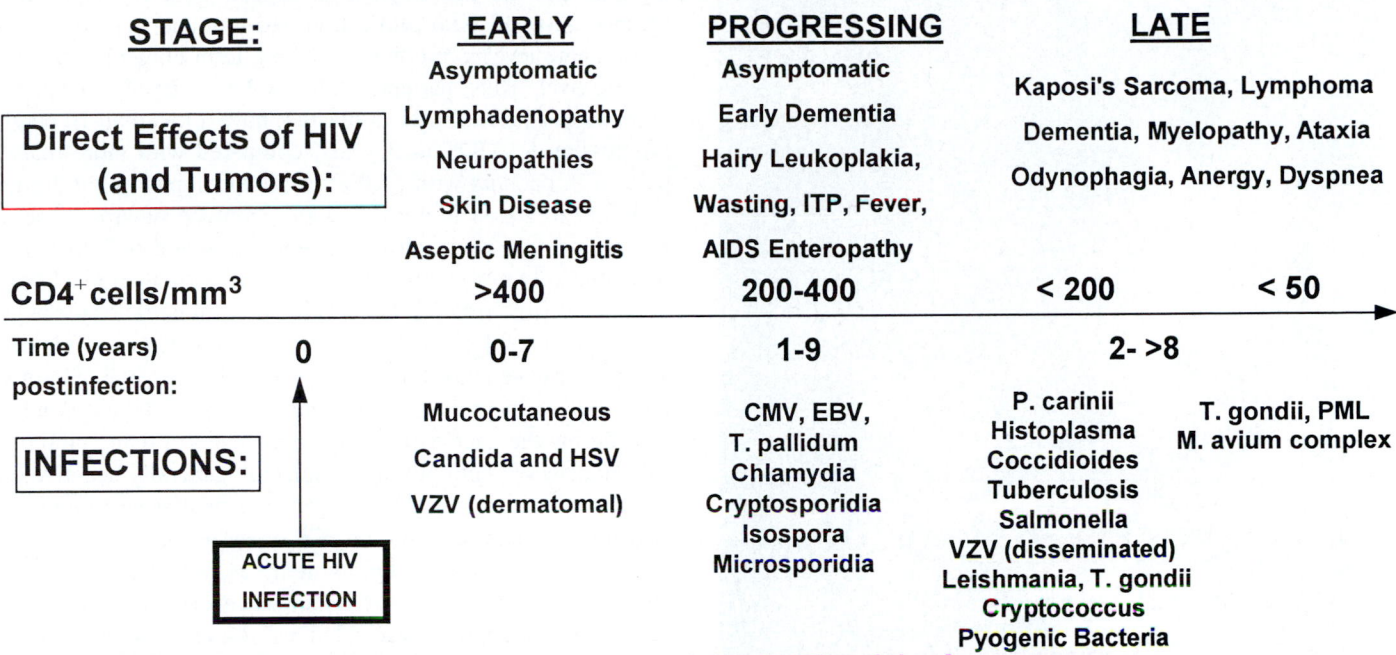

FIGURE 135-1   The progression of AIDS-associated conditions.

pate in replication. *Pol* is a major target for antiretroviral therapies.

3. *Env:* envelope gene that encodes the envelope glycoproteins, including gp160 (*env* precursor), gp120 (exterior glycoprotein), and gp41 (transmembrane glycoprotein). This region is highly variable between isolates and includes the V3 loop, a region that carries the principal neutralization determinant, a target for antiviral immune therapies.

4. *Tat:* transactivator gene encodes regulatory functions of replication.

5. *Rev:* regulator of virion protein that encodes regulatory functions of replication.

6. *Vpr:* function not known.

7. *Vpu:* function not known.

8. *Vif:* virion infectivity factor; function not known.

9. *Nef:* negative regulatory factor, function not known, but *nef* appears to play a role in the virulence of viral isolates, and *nef*-deleted strains may be used in the development of attenuated viral vaccines.

The HIV replication cycle is susceptible to interruption at a variety of virus-specific steps (see Chapter 152). HIV begins replication by binding the envelope glycoprotein to cell surface receptors (and the fusin protein) on the surface of CD4+ target cells. The virus then fuses with the cell membrane, penetrates the cytoplasm, and uncoats to release viral RNA into the cell. The RNA is transcribed into DNA by virally encoded reverse

transcriptase, the DNA is circularized, and some of this DNA is integrated into the host genome. This creates the latent, or "proviral," form of the viral genome. When viral activation occurs (the in vivo mechanism is unclear), the DNA copy is transcribed into viral messenger RNA, which is processed, binds to ribosomes, and initiates translation of virus-specific proteins. Some of these proteins are cleaved and glycosylated in the cellular endoplasmic reticulum and transported by the Golgi apparatus to the cellular plasma membrane, where new virus buds off into the extracellular environment.

NATURAL HISTORY OF HIV INFECTION

The pathogenesis of infection due to HIV-1 is related to tropism for specific cells of the immune system, particularly the CD4 antigen–expressing T lymphocytes (CD4+, T4+), but also for macrophage/monocyte cells, follicular dentritic cells, neurons, and glial cells. Tropism or specificity for specific cell types is determined by the interaction of gp120 components (V1/V2 and V3) with the CD4 molecule and with the specific coreceptors expressed on a given cell type. Thus, HIV has the ability to adapt to replicate in different cells based on variation in the gp120 molecule. The details of these infections as related to pulmonary disease are discussed in Chapter 152. However, the pathogenesis of opportunistic infections and other processes is closely linked to the loss of coordinate immune function in each host. The specific manifestations of disease will depend on the indi-

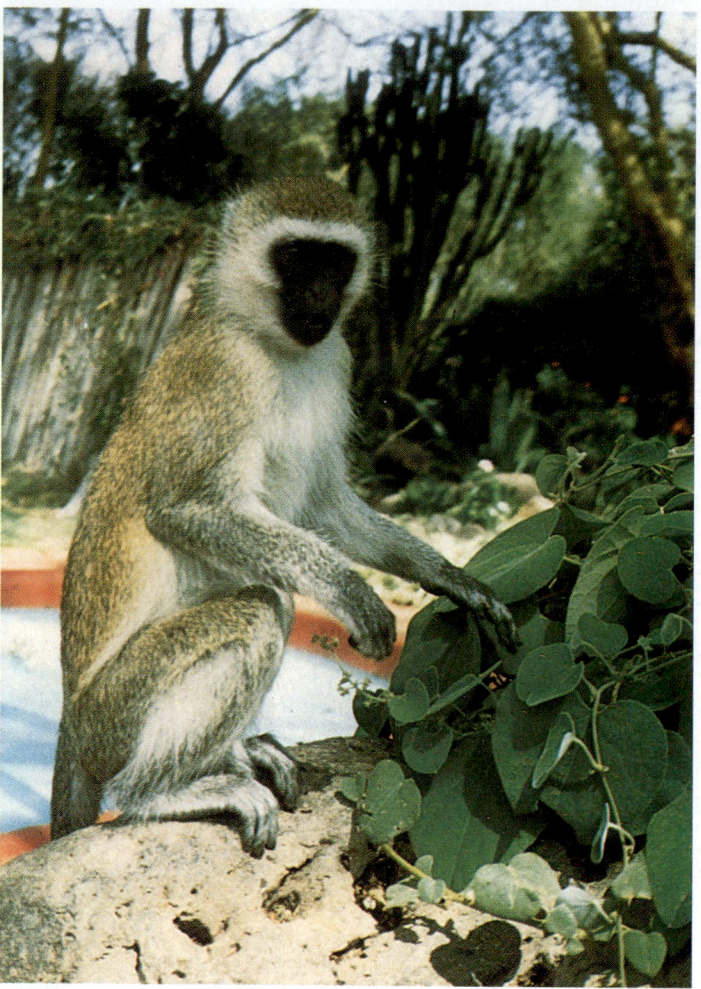

FIGURE 135-2 African green monkey (*Cercopithecus aethiops*), a species found throughout sub-Saharan Africa that is naturally infected with simian immunodeficiency virus (SIV), a virus closely related to the human immunodeficiency viruses (HIV). (*Courtesy of Dr. P. J. Kanki.*)

vidual infected, the rate of viral replication, the rate of lymphocyte loss, possibly the level of production of antiviral immunity and inflammatory factors (chemokines) and of proviral growth factors (macrophage colony–stimulating factor), and the specific isolate of virus responsible for infection—tropism for different cell types or anatomic compartments. Thus, certain strains are more tropic for macrophage/monocyte cells, while others are lymphocytotropic.

Primary HIV infection results in a mononucleosis-type syndrome with fever, myalgias, chills, diarrhea, nausea, vomiting, headache, lymphadenopathy, pharyngitis, and, occasionally, meningitis or encephalitis. Symptoms may occur as early as 1 week after exposure, but the incubation period is generally in the 3- to 6-week period, with 30 to 70 percent being symptomatic. In heterosexual infection, HIV probably enters Langerhans or dendritic cells in the vagina. Viral spread to the draining lymph nodes allows productive infection of CD4$^+$ T lymphocytes. The mode of transmission may, therefore, participate in the pattern of infection (which cells in which location) due to HIV-1. Primary infection is accompanied by high-level viremia (more than 1 million virions per milliliter of plasma) with seeding of lym-

phoid organs. A rapid drop-off in viral levels is associated with the development of a cellular immune response. The subsequent level of HIV in the blood is a reflection of the equilibrium reached between viral replication and immune function.[18] This steady-state level is predictive of long-term clinical outcome— i.e., survival. Thus, patients with low-level viremia (fewer than 5000 copies per milliliter of plasma) have a less than 10 percent progression to AIDS in 5 years, compared with more than 60 percent in patients with 35,000 to 50,000 copies per milliliter.[6]

Initial infection is with a *single* genotype of virus. The apparent latent phase in viral infection—a period of 7 to 8 years with relatively low serum virus levels and without clinical symptoms—probably reflects the trapping of viral particles in the germinal centers of the lymphoid organs by follicular dendritic cells. Trapped virus remains infectious even in the presence of humoral immunity to the virus. Degeneration of the infected dendritic cells during the course of disease contributes to rising viral titers later in disease. Antibody test results are generally negative during this period, while p24 antigenemia or plasma viremia (by polymerase chain reaction, or PCR) may be detected early.

Current data suggest that as many as one in 100 peripheral blood mononuclear cells are infected with HIV-1. The half-life of the virus is approximately 2 days. Rapid viral turnover contributes to the development of mutant virus, allowing the *rapid emergence of viral resistance* to antiviral agents. As a result, the entire population of virus may convert to a resistant phenotype in 28 days. Thus, each patient harbors many different subtypes of mutant strains, or "quasispecies," of HIV.

As many as 1 billion CD4 cells turn over each day during infection. The development of combination antiviral therapies was aimed, in part, at overcoming the ability of the virus to develop resistance to multiple agents simultaneously (by accumulation of multiple resistance mutations) without significantly impairing the viability of the virus. Synergistic therapy might reduce the amount of each agent required for treatment (and the associated toxicities) and might be necessary to target different viral subtypes harbored in different cell types (lymphocytes, macrophages, neurons). Similarly, the antigenic variability of virus within an individual is a major impediment to vaccine development. Sequenced HIV isolates from different geographic regions differ by up to 50 percent in certain viral proteins; six major subtypes of HIV-1 have been described. *Quantitative measures of viral load* have a strong predictive value for the course of the disease and have become the basis for measuring antiviral treatment efficacy.

The binding of HIV-1 to cells expressing the CD4 cell surface antigen occurs by binding of the HIV envelope glycoprotein (gp120) to the CD4 molecule in the presence of a fusion coreceptor called LESTR or "fusin." Fusin is a G protein with homology to the interleukin-8 β-chemokine receptor. Alternative routes of cell entry have been described, including galactosyl ceramide on neurons and Fc-receptor–mediated uptake. Infection results in viral integration and viral RNA production in infected cells as well as in syncytium formation and cell death in vitro. Cell death may be due to a variety of mechanisms, including viral replication, toxic viral products, virus-specific immune responses, viral infection of stem cells, superantigens, apoptosis, and in vivo syncytium formation.

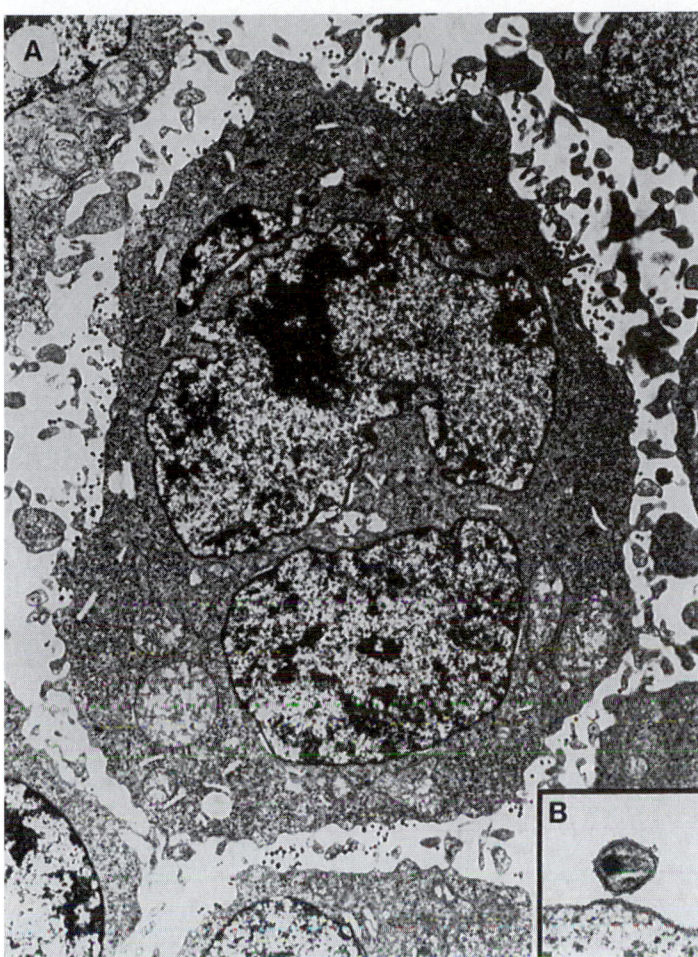

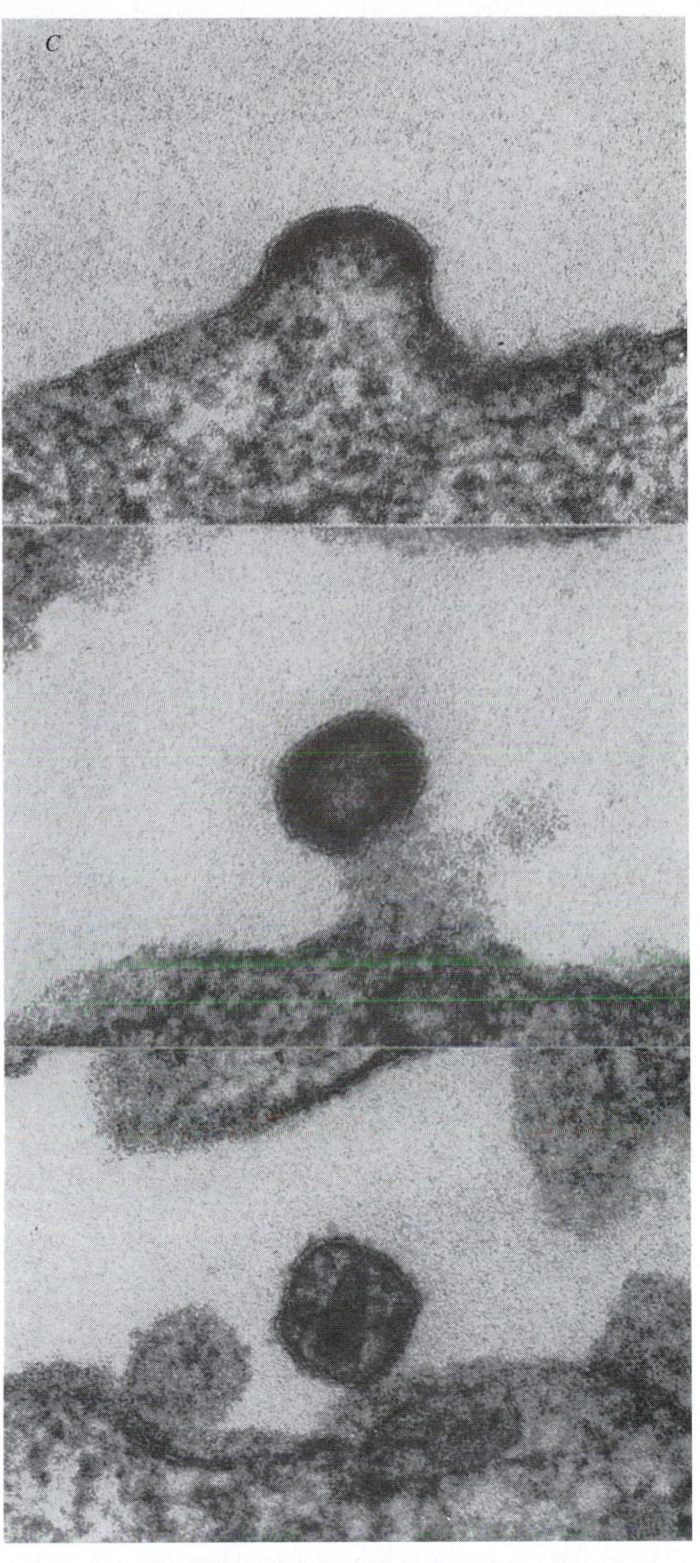

FIGURE 135-3   Electron microscopy of HIV-1. *A.* A multinucleated leukocyte producing particles of the AIDS retrovirus. Large numbers of virus particles can be seen budding off along the margin of the cell. *B.* A mature virus particle with the characteristic cylindric core. *C. Top:* Viral budding, the earliest visible stage of virus replication, with accumulation of viral glycoproteins at the host cell surface. *Middle:* Budding-off of the virus, with a membrane-encapsulated sphere with a dense center or viral nucleoid. *Bottom:* Free extracellular infectious HIV-1. Condensation of the viral nucleoid into an elongate bar may distinguish HIV from other retroviruses. (*Courtesy of Dr. M. A. Gonda.*)

The progression of HIV disease depends on the infection of CD4 lymphocytes, which normally serve to orchestrate much of the host immune response. A switch in the predominant cytokine profile reflecting diminished activation (the "TH1-to-TH2 switch") has also been postulated as a contributor to the progressive immune decline.[12]

DEVELOPMENT OF AIDS

The median time between acute viral exposure and an immune response is approximately 2 months. Many infected persons are unaware of infection. The risk of progression to AIDS (Table 135-3) is described as a function of the progressive fall in the CD4 lymphocyte count but may ultimately be correlated better with "viral load" and with more specific measures of declining systemic immune functions.[14] Clinical disease is often initiated by constitutional symptoms or development of opportunistic infection as the plasma viremia rises and the CD4+ lymphocyte counts fall. More than 50 percent of people with CD4+ lymphocyte counts of under 150 per cubic millimeter develop AIDS within 18 months. With the rising viral titers, immune "activation" is reflected in rising levels of β_2-microglobulin, neopterin, and proinflammatory cytokines coincident with declining immune function.

TABLE 135-3

Revised CDC Classification System for HIV Infection and Expanded AIDS Surveillance Case Definition for Adolescents and Adults

CD4 Cell Count	Clinical Categories		
Categories	A	B	C
≥500 µl or greater	A1	B1	C1
200–400 µl	A2	B2	C2
<200 µl (AIDS indicator, T-cell count)	A3	B3	C3
	Asymptomatic HIV infection	Symptomatic, non-A or -C conditions (formerly AIDS related-complex)	AIDS indicator (opportunistic conditions)
	Acute (primary) HIV infection	Bacillary angiomatosis	Candidiasis, pulmonary or esophageal
	Persistent generalized lymphadenopathy	Candidiasis, oral or recurrent vaginal	Cervical cancer (invasive)
	Acute retroviral syndrome	Cervical dysplasia	Coccidioidomycosis
		Constitutional symptoms (such as fever or diarrhea) >1 month	Cryptococcosis, extrapulmonary
		Hairy leukoplakia, oral	Cryptosporidiosis >1 month
		Herpes zoster infection (>1 episode or >1 dermatome shingles)	Cytomegalovirus, chronic (>1 month) or esophageal
		Idiopathic thrombocytopenic purpura	Histoplasmosis
		Listeriosis	Isosporiasis
		Pelvic inflammatory disease	Kaposi's sarcoma
		Peripheral neuropathy	Lymphoma
			Mycobacterium avium complex
			M. kansasii
			M. tuberculosis
			Pneumocystis carinii
			Pneumonia, recurrent
			Progressive multifocal leukoencephalopathy
			Salmonellosis
			Toxoplasmosis (CNS)
			Wasting due to HIV
			Encephalopathy

SOURCE: Modified from CDC 1993 revised classification system.[8]

Variation in the rate of progression may reflect viral subtypes or a variety of immunologic factors. A group of "long-term non-progressors"—persons infected with HIV but who have not developed AIDS—has been identified. The basis of protection in these people is unknown. Humoral immunity, cellular immunity, "CD8 suppressor factor" (soluble factors secreted by activated $CD8^+$ lymphocytes, including β-chemokines and interleukin-16), and intrinsic (genetic) resistance to infection by HIV have all been demonstrated. Thus far, despite promising studies of viral immunization, efforts aimed at the development of protective or therapeutic HIV vaccines have been unrewarding.

HIV TESTING

HIV testing should be considered for all persons in high-risk groups [intravenous drug users, sexually active homosexual or bisexual men, hemophiliacs, persons with sexually transmitted diseases (especially syphilis), pregnant women, health-care workers with exposure to body fluids or needle stick injury, and all patients with conditions commonly associated with AIDS] (Table 135-4).

Testing for HIV infection is generally divided into viral culture assays, antibody tests, and specific viral tests. Issues of confidentiality, informed consent, and counseling need to be addressed regarding HIV testing. Culture systems for HIV are nonstandardized and are not available in most nonacademic centers. Most patients produce antibodies to HIV within 6 to 8 weeks, and almost 100 percent will have detectable antibodies by 6 months after exposure. These tests are well standardized, easy to perform, and less expensive than culture; however, antibody tests may have false positives (cross-reacting antibodies) and false negatives (e.g., in the early period). The ELISA and

TABLE 135-4

When to Suspect HIV Infection

History

High-risk behaviors or exposures

Unsafe or promiscuous sex

Sex with prostitutes

Sex with person at risk for HIV

Injection drug use

Blood or blood product transfusion between 1975 and 1985 (especially in high-prevalence areas)

Blood clotting concentrate transfusion before January 1985

Sexually transmitted disease

Tuberculosis, especially extrapulmonary

Racial and ethnic minority populations in high-prevalence areas of HIV disease

Homeless persons in high-prevalence areas of HIV disease

Individuals from high-prevalence areas for heterosexual transmission

Symptoms and Signs

Acute retroviral syndrome (see text)

Unexplained constitutional symptoms

Fatigue, malaise, fever, diarrhea, night sweats, anorexia, weight loss

Lymphatic

Persistent generalized lymphadenopathy

Dermatologic manifestations

Infectious

Severe herpes simplex (oral, anogenital), oral or genital candidiasis, staphylococcal skin infections, herpes zoster (especially recurrent), superficial dermatophytoses (tinea nail infection), molluscum contagiosum, warts, condyloma acuminata, oral hairy leukoplakia (EBV), necrotizing gingivitis or periodontitis

Noninfectious

Kaposi's sarcoma, petechiae (ITP), seborrheic dermatitis, psoriasis (new or worsening), eosinophilic folliculitis, severe drug eruptions, aphthous ulcers, intraepithelial neoplasia

Neurologic conditions

Cranial neuropathy, Guillian-Barré syndrome, aseptic meningitis, peripheral neuropathy, myopathy, cognitive impairment

Laboratory Findings

Unexplained anemia, leukopenia, lymphocytopenia, atypical lymphocytosis, thrombocytopenia

CD4 lymphocytopenia

Polyclonal hyperglobulinemia

Elevated blood urea nitrogen or serum creatinine, proteinuria, hypoalbuminemia

Elevated lactate dehydrogenase

Hypocholesterolemia and hypertriglyceridemia

Western blot tests are in this group. The ELISA test has a sensitivity of 99.7 percent and specificity of 98.5 percent; if results are negative, no further testing is performed unless new, acute infection is suspected. If results are positive, confirmation by Western blot is performed. Between 4 and 20 percent of Western blot tests are *indeterminate* because of seroconversion in progress, loss of antibody in advanced HIV disease, cross-reacting antibodies in pregnancy, blood transfusions, autoantibodies from collagen vascular disease, infection with HIV-2, recent influenza vaccination, or in recipients of trial HIV vaccines. These subjects should be retested at 2 to 3 and 6 months, and inconclusive assays resolved with specific viral (molecular, p24 antigen, or culture) testing. Western blot test results are considered positive if *two bands* are present from the gp41, gp160/120, or p24 group, indeterminate with a single band, and negative with no bands.

Specific viral tests include the p24 antigen detection, molecular amplification by PCR, and culture-based assays. These are positive earlier than the antibody tests and therefore may be useful in primary infection before the development of antibody; they have high sensitivity (95 to 99 percent) and are often useful when the Western blot is indeterminate. Quantitative techniques are very useful in assessing the response to antiviral therapy and disease progression. These tests tend to be expensive, may require working with infected sera and live virus, are operator dependent, and are not yet fully standardized between laboratories. The limits of viral detection of the available molecular assays are approximately 500 copies per milliliter for the branched-chain assays (second-generation bDNA) and 50 to 200 copies per milliliter for the PCR tests. P24 assays may be negative in infected persons.

Measures of HIV viral RNA in plasma do not correlate exactly with the CD4$^+$ lymphocyte count. The CD4 count provides a surrogate marker for the response to antiviral therapy and the risk of infection and death. At present, the best predictive value of testing is the combination of viral load with CD4$^+$ lymphocyte enumeration. Viral RNA levels in long-term nonprogressors are consistently under 10,000 copies per milliliter, while progression and immunologic deterioration are often associated with loads over 50,000 to 100,000 copies. Patients with viral loads of 10,000 to 50,000 are considered at intermediate risk. Viral load changes generally precede CD4 count changes. Immune alterations due to infection (e.g., cytomegalovirus) or immune modulation therapy (interferons) are not yet interpretable.

AIDS PATIENT MANAGEMENT

Details of patient management are beyond the scope of this discussion. However, a number of general caveats are useful in considering the risks of opportunistic infection or neoplasia in a person infected with HIV. Laboratory tests are notoriously variable within individual patients and between laboratories. Thus, any important test merits being repeated before being acted on. This is especially valid for blood counts (white blood cells, CD4 cell counts, differential counts). Baseline knowledge of the patient's HIV viral load, blood counts, chemistries, CD4 count, PPD status with controls, Pap smear, VDRL, serologies for *Toxoplasma gondii,* cytomegalovirus, hepatitis B, varicella zoster virus, hepatitis C, and chest radiograph will be very valuable for future management. Careful attention to the patient's nutritional status and unique epidemiologic exposures is important in AIDS as for all immunocompromised patients. PPD testing (see Chapter 161) is often misleading in this population; special attention must be paid to any special exposures or risk groups.[31]

Immunization is a part of the routine management of AIDS.[13] In general, HIV-infected persons are susceptible to the same community-acquired respiratory pathogens (with additions) as the normal host but with a greater severity of disease.[4,23] Thus, patients should be vaccinated early in the course of disease when they are clinically stable. Live vaccines are generally contraindicated, but measles vaccine is generally well tolerated in children, and MMR is recommended for unvaccinated adults born after 1957 or vaccinated between 1963 and 1967. The efficacy of vaccination in this population is not clear; HIV viral loads may temporarily increase after vaccination. However, general practice suggests that pneumococcal, influenza (inactivated whole virus and split virus vaccines), *Hemophilus influenzae,* hepatitis B recombinant vaccine, and MMR be given as indicated. Prophylactic antibiotics and vaccinations are presented in Tables 135-5 and 135-6.

Underlying lung disease is common in HIV-infected patients even before the development of opportunistic infection.[35] While FEV_1 and FVC are nearly normal, 11 to 13 percent of patients with $CD4^+$ lymphocyte counts below 200 per mm^3 or with a history of AIDS-associated extrapulmonary diseases (including thrush and varicella zoster infections) and weight loss have decreased D_{LCO} measurements. Intravenous drug users have a higher incidence of abnormal FVC, FEV_1, and D_{LCO} measurements (33.3 percent), consistent with patterns of cigarette smoking and racial distribution. Thus, susceptibility to pulmonary infection is further exacerbated in this population and the importance of vaccination increased.

THE MANAGEMENT OF VIRAL INFECTION DUE TO HIV

A number of virus-specific replication steps have been identified as targets for antiviral therapies:

Reverse Transcriptase Inhibitors Two classes of agents have been developed in this category—the *nucleoside* and *nonnucle-*

oside inhibitors. The nucleoside inhibitors compete with natural 2'-deoxynucleotides for binding to the reverse transcriptase and cause chain termination when incorporated into the nascent DNA strands. This group includes zidovudine (AZT, ZDV), didanosine (dideoxyinosine, ddl), zalcitabine (dideoxycytidine, ddC), stavudine (d4T), lamivudine (3TC), adefovir, dipivoxil, and 1592U89. The nonnucleoside inhibitors (nevirapine, delavridine, loviride) include compounds that bind directly to the enzyme complex (viral RNA-DNA-nucleotide-enzyme) to inhibit polymerization. These compounds are HIV-1 specific, with HIV-2 lacking the amino acid residues of the binding site for this class of drug. Resistance to the nonnucleoside agents emerges rapidly, but they may prove useful in combination therapy.

Protease Inhibitors These compounds bind to the catalytic site of the viral protease, which is responsible for cleavage of the larger proteins of immature virus as it buds off from the host cell and becomes infectious. This class of compounds includes indinavir, ritonavir, saquinavir, and a variety of trial compounds not yet available for routine clinical use.

Antisense Compounds and Ribozymes Antisense DNA oligomers bind to specific segments of the viral mRNA.

Gene Therapy RNA decoys and transdominant mutant proteins are under development.

Castanospermine This compound inhibits the enzyme glucosidase I and modifies the glycosylation of gp120.

Tat, Rev, and Nef Inhibitors Direct binding to the regulatory proteins to inhibit viral replication is not yet of documented efficacy (Ro24-7429, ALX40-4C).

Immune Modulators Interleukins 12 and 2 and γ-interferon remain of unclear clinical significance. The role of cytokines, particularly the chemokines, may be central to host protection and susceptibility to HIV infection and progression.

Inhibitors of Viral Binding to $CD4^+$ Cells These are recombinant soluble CD4 and related proteins.

Vaccines These inhibit viral infection of target cells.

Early studies with the first nucleoside analog for treatment of HIV-1 infection (zidovudine) demonstrated a survival benefit from antiviral therapy and a 50 percent reduction in the incidence of opportunistic infection with this agent for the duration of the effective antiviral effects. Significant toxicities have been demonstrated with each of the nucleoside antiviral agents and are often limiting: zidovudine (anemia, leukopenia, myopathy); didanosine (peripheral neuropathy, pancreatitis, gout, headache, diarrhea); and zalcitabine (peripheral neuropathy, rash, stomatitis, pancreatitis). The nonnucleoside agents have different toxicities, including diarrhea (saquinavir, ritonavir), increased hepatic amino transaminase levels and triglyceride levels (ritonavir), and indirect bilirubinemia and nephrolitiasis (indinavir).

Experience with the use of zidovudine demonstrated the equivalent efficacy of lower-dose therapy (600 mg maintenance per day versus 1500 mg) with a significant reduction in toxicity. However, resistance to zidovudine emerges in 89 percent of HIV-infected patients with advanced disease by 12 months on therapy, compared with 39 percent of those with less severe disease. *High-level resistance* occurs within 6 to 18 months in patients

TABLE 135-5

Recommended Antibiotic Prophylaxis for First Episode Opportunistic Infections in HIV-Infected Adults*

Pathogen	Indication	Preventive Regimens	
		First Choice	Alternatives
Pneumocystis carinii	CD4$^+$ <200 cells/mm^3 or <14% Unexplained fever for ≥2 weeks Oropharyngeal candidiasis	TMP-SMX 1SS or DS PO qd or DS tiw	Dapsone 50 mg PO qd, *plus* pyrimethamine 50 mg PO qw, *plus* leucovorin 25 mg PO qw Dapsone 100 mg PO qd Aerosolized pentamidine 300 mg q 3–4 wk
Mycobacterium tuberculosis Isoniazid-sensitive	Skin test reaction ≥5 mm or prior positive TST result without treatment or contact with active tuberculosis	Isoniazid 300 mg PO, *plus* pyridoxine 50 mg PO qd × 12 months Isoniazid 900 mg PO, *plus* pyridoxine 50 mg PO biw × 12 months	Rifampin 600 mg PO qd × 12 months
Isoniazid-resistant only	High probability of exposure to isoniazid-resistant tuberculosis	Rifampin 600 mg PO qd × 12 months	Rifabutin 300 mg PO qd × 12 months
Multidrug-resistant (isoniazid and rifampin)	High probability of exposure to multidrug-resistant tuberculosis	Choice of drugs requires consultation with infectious disease experts	None
Toxoplasma gondii	IgG antibody positive to *Toxoplasma* and CD4$^+$ <200 cells/mm^3	TMP-SMX 1 DS PO qd	TMP-SMX 1 SS PO qd or 1 DS PO tiw Dapsone 50 mg PO qd *plus* pyrimethamine 50 mg PO qw, *plus* leucovorin 25 mg PO qw Atovaquone 1500–3000 mg suspension PO qd (investigational)
Streptococcus pneumoniae[†]	All patients	Pneumococcal vaccine 0.5 ml IM × 1	None
Mycobacterium avium complex[†]	CD4$^+$ <75 cells/mm^3	Clarithromycin 500 mg PO bid Azithromycin 1200 mg PO weekly	Rifabutin 300 mg PO qd (A1)

*Not all agents F.D.A. approved for all indications.

[†]Recommended for consideration. Proven survival advantage to prophylaxis of MAC with clarithromycin (*not* to exceed 1 G *total* per day).[9]

with advanced disease.[34] The mutations responsible for this resistance have been well characterized.

The strategy of combining antiviral agents has allowed the use of lower doses of each agent in some cases, but it has also unmasked new toxicities.[42] Great excitement has developed regarding the use of combination antiviral therapies, especially combinations including the newer HIV protease inhibitors, because of dramatic and long-standing reductions in viral loads in the persons in whom these therapies have been used. Because of the high viral replication rate and the generation of viral quasispecies during the course of viral infection, resistance to antiviral therapy has generally been the rule with new antiviral agents.[34] The tropism of viral isolates for different compartments within the body (lymphocytes, macrophages, neurons) and potential variation in the rate of replication in different sites and

accessibility to antiviral agents in these locations (e.g., lymphocytes in the blood versus lymph nodes) make interpretation of early survival data difficult. Even if all new acute infection of cells could be prevented by aggressive antiviral therapy, it would take more than 3 years before all infected cells could be cleared, given the turnover of latently and persistently infected cells. This "cure" scenario also assumes that there are no "sanctuary" sites in the infected person that are not treated by antiviral agents (such as the central nervous system). These suppositions have yet to be demonstrated.

OPPORTUNISTIC INFECTIONS

The problem of opportunistic infection in the AIDS patient is unique because of the *progressive decline* in immune function

TABLE 135-6

Suggested Prophylaxis of Opportunistic Infections in HIV-Infected Adults

Pathogen	Indication	Preventive Regimens	
		First Choice	Alternatives
Bacteria	Neutropenia, recurrent infection	Granulocyte colony–stimulating factor (G-CSF) (with oral TMP-SMX or quinolone)	Granulocyte-macrophage colony–stimulating factor (GM-CSF)*
Candida species	CD4$^+$ <50 cells/mm^3	Fluconazole 100–200 mg PO qd	Ketoconazole 200 mg PO qd
Cryptococcus neoformans	CD4$^+$ <50 cells/mm^3	Fluconazole 100–200 mg PO qd	Itraconazole 200 mg PO qd
Histoplasma capsulatum	CD4$^+$ <50 cells/mm^3, endemic area	Itraconazole 200 mg PO qd	Fluconazole 200 mg PO qd
Coccidioides immitis	CD4$^+$ <50 cells/mm^3, endemic area	Fluconazole 100–200 mg PO qd	Itraconazole 200 mg PO qd
CMV	CD4$^+$ <50 cells/mm^3, CMV antibody$^{(+)}$	Ganciclovir 1 G PO tid	(Under study)
Hepatitis B virus	All susceptible patients	Energix-B, 20 μg IM × 3 Recombivax HB, 10 μg IM × 3	None
Influenza virus	All patients (annually)	Whole or split virus, 0.5 ml IM/y	Rimantadine 200 mg PO bid
Herpes simplex virus	Any CD4$^+$ cell count History of recurrences	Acyclovir 400–800 mg PO bid	Valaciclovir, famciclovir

*M-CSF or GM-CSF *may* stimulate HIV replication.

when compared with the intermittent compromise seen after chemotherapy or the relatively stable immunosuppression utilized after solid organ transplantation. The specific opportunistic infections that occur depend on the nature and duration of immune suppression as well as on the infectious exposures of the patient (Table 135-1).[27] As a result of the progressive and cumulative risks, the incidence of opportunistic infections *increases* over time. A "time line" exists for the common infections and noninfectious manifestations seen in AIDS, relating to the total CD4$^+$ lymphocyte count as a measure of susceptibility (Fig. 135-1). It is assumed that the time line is also related to the patient's viral load, but the exact correlation between these measures of HIV infection is not yet known. The specific pattern of opportunistic syndromes will change for individual patients, but it reflects the overall progressive immunological deterioration of AIDS.

Many opportunistic pulmonary infections in AIDS patients were initially assumed to be reactivation of latent infection. However, some of these processes—including *P. carinii, T. gondii,* tuberculosis, and histoplasmosis—represent a mix of both new exposures and old disease. For example, by genetic analysis, a number of patients treated for primary infection due to *P. carinii* have been shown to develop "recurrent infection," which has been demonstrated to be due to organisms of a different genotype than the organisms isolated from the initial infection. Similar observations have been made in terms of the drug susceptibility of mycobacterial isolates in recurrent disease. This observation may have implications for the development of prophylactic therapies.

The clinical manifestations of opportunistic infections in AIDS are altered by prophylactic and therapeutic regimens, adverse drug reactions, and drug interactions. The clinical appearance of these infections is also altered by the underlying immune deficiencies and by the nutritional status of the host. The specific immune deficiencies reflect not only the CD4 count or viral load but also the impact of the specific HIV viral isolate on immune function. That is, patients with monocytotropic strains of HIV would be assumed to have increased susceptibility to intracellular pathogens. Diagnosis is further complicated by the recognition of new infectious agents (Table 135-1), the presence of multiple simultaneous infections (Fig. 135-4), and the interpretation of new diagnostic tests (e.g., PCR). Opportunistic infections may also contribute to the "net state of immune suppression"; cytomegalovirus and *Leishmania* are globally immunosuppressive organisms that contribute to susceptibility to other opportunistic pathogens.

The "maturation" of the AIDS epidemic has been accompanied by changes in the spectrum of opportunistic infections.[29] This change reflects factors including the successful use of anti-*Pneumocystis* prophylaxis, the prolonged survival of patients on antiviral therapies, generally improved clinical care, the recognition of new or drug-resistant opportunistic organisms, and improved maintenance therapies including nutritional support.[17,19,29,39] Thus, as the incidence of *Pneumocystis* pneumonia has declined, infections due to *Mycobacterium avium* complex, tuberculosis, cytomegalovirus (CMV), and bacteria and the incidence of lymphoma have increased. For example, AIDS patients with low CD4 counts who have previously received sev-

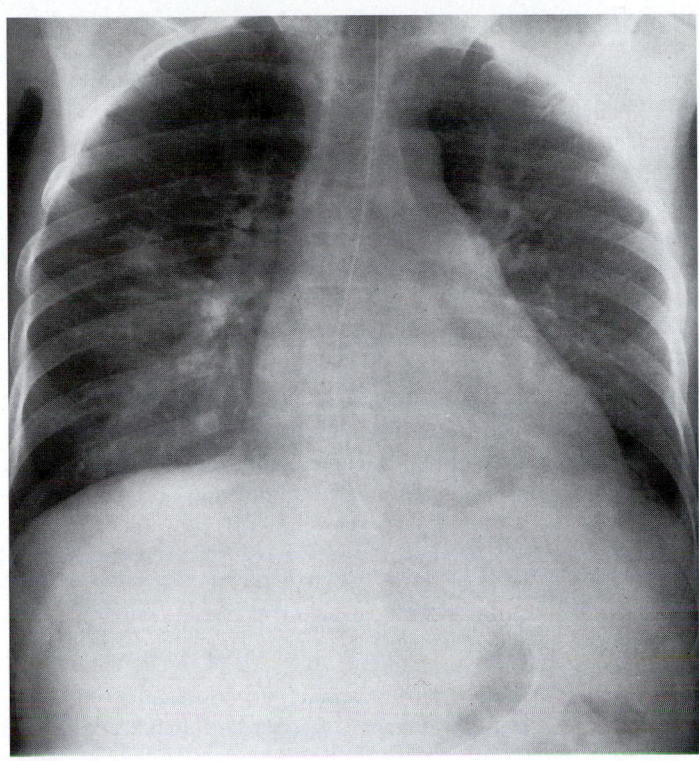

FIGURE 135-4   Chest radiograph of a 48-year-old heterosexual man with community-acquired pneumonia unresponsive to therapy. The patient was diagnosed as having AIDS on the basis of HIV seropositivity, CD4$^+$ lymphocyte count of 113 per milliliter, and *Pneumocystis carinii* and *Mycobacterium avium-intracellulare* complex pneumonia.

eral courses of antibiotics, and some with indwelling catheters, have developed *Aspergillus* and *Pseudomonas* infections. Although the clinical response to therapy is often delayed, more therapeutic options are available for the treatment of these infections than in the past.

Toxicities of both prophylactic and therapeutic drug regimens (particularly rash, marrow suppression, and hepatic toxicities) are much more frequent in HIV-infected patients and are exacerbated by the simultaneous need for antiviral therapies. Given the large number of drugs that patients with advanced HIV disease may be asked to ingest, compliance issues must be addressed realistically with each patient. New strategies for prophylaxis that are under study combine the properties of individual regimens aimed at preventing common infections, including those due to *P. carinii*, mycobacteria, *Histoplasma*, *Candida* species, and CMV. This approach is especially important in the care of HIV-infected children.

SPECIFIC AGENTS OF OPPORTUNISTIC INFECTION IN AIDS

Each of the specific pathogens encountered in AIDS are addressed in detail in other chapters of this text. Thus, specific comments are limited to unusual presentations and alterations in the patterns of pulmonary opportunistic infections in AIDS patients. A general approach to the prophylaxis of infection in AIDS is presented in Tables 135-5 and 135-6. The need for continued primary prophylaxis in AIDS patients who have CD4$^+$ lymphocyte

counts that rise from below 200/mm^3 to above this level in response to antiviral therapies has not been resolved.

Up to 15 to 20 percent of AIDS patients have more than one opportunistic infection at one time. The spectrum of clinical diagnoses in pulmonary disease in AIDS includes bacterial infection (45.5 percent), *P. carinii* pneumonia (27 percent), Kaposi's sarcoma (7 percent), bronchitis (5 percent), *M. tuberculosis* (4.3 percent), other mycobacteria (4 percent), lymphoma (2.1 percent), and a variety of other processes.[26,39] Common community-acquired upper respiratory infections, manageable on an ambulatory basis, constitute more than 50 percent of respiratory illnesses in HIV-infected persons.[4,23] The incidence of fungal infections varies by geographic region, while the rate of demonstration of viral pulmonary infection is closely related to the diagnostic testing techniques used at each center and to seasonal variation.

Pneumocystis carinii Infections

The incidence of *P. carinii* as a cause of pneumonia in AIDS patients remains high. In patients not receiving prophylactic antibiotics, the incidence of infection is probably more than 80 percent during the course of disease. *P. carinii* causes more than 25 percent of community-acquired pneumonias in HIV-infected persons. The incidence of *P. carinii* pneumonia as the AIDS-defining event dropped from 47 percent in 1988 to 25 percent in 1991, while the use of prophylaxis increased to 55.4 percent, according to the Multicenter AIDS Cohort Study.[29] Similar changes were observed in European studies.[38] The first-choice agent for prophylaxis and therapy is trimethoprim-sulfamethoxazole (TMP-SMX). The rate of death due to *P. carinii* has also declined, with a drop from 32.7 to 13.3 percent of AIDS-related deaths due to this infection. The severity of infection and response to therapy are greatly altered by coinfection with CMV. The relative proportion of extrapulmonary pneumocystosis appears to have increased, but this observation is confounded by a heightened sensitivity to this manifestation of infection.[16] More than half of these cases are in persons *not* receiving aerosolized pentamidine prophylaxis.

Pyogenic Bacterial Infections

Pyogenic bacterial infections are increasingly recognized in AIDS patients.[26] Such infections are reduced by the use of TMP-SMX prophylaxis. The role of intravenous immune globulin in preventing such infections, especially in children, remains to be established. Community-acquired pneumonias have the same general distribution as for normal hosts—with the exception of *P. carinii* pneumonia.[4] These infections are often due to *Streptococcus pneumoniae*, *Hemophilus influenzae*, and other streptococci.[4,20,23,26] Sinusitis is often recurrent or persistent, may be asymptomatic, and is generally due to common bacterial agents. Chronic infections of the sinuses are increasingly associated with *Pseudomonas* species and occasionally with *Aspergillus* and a variety of unusual fungi. In intravenous drug users, major pyogenic infections are often a harbinger of progression to AIDS. Right-sided endocarditis, including fungal endocarditis and *Salmonella* infections, is seen in this population, and morbidity and mortality due to bacterial infections are greater than in the general population. *Salmonella* infections merit treatment with quinolones, ampicillin, chloramphenicol, or TMP-SMX. Antibiotic resistance is not uncommon. Syphilis (neurosyphilis) is also a major problem. False-positive serologic testing may persist because of polyclonal B-cell activation. False-negative test results seldom occur.

Bartonella (formerly *Rochalimaea*) *henselae* and *B. quintana* have been associated with bacillary angiomatosis, peliosis hepatis, and bacteremias in AIDS patients.[22] Bacillary angiomatosis nodules may be found throughout the body, including the lungs. Infection can be demonstrated by Warthin-Starry silver stain, in culture, by PCR, and by serologic testing. This infection is generally responsive to erythromycin, the newer macrolides, or doxycycline. Rifampin and gentamicin may be effective.

Rhodococcus species, particularly *R. equi* (formerly *Corynebacterium equi*), have been isolated from the lungs and occasionally other sites in a variety of immunocompromised hosts, including patients with AIDS. *R. equi* is a soil-derived organism originally associated with respiratory disease of horses and other animals. Relapsing disease associated with right-sided endocarditis has been observed at our institution. The presentation of infection is systemic, with fever, malaise, and cough progressing to necrotizing pneumonia with upper-lobe nodules and cavitation—similar to the clinical presentations of tuberculosis or *Nocardia* infections. Surgical resection has often been needed for cure in association with prolonged courses of antibiotics. The organism is susceptible to erythromycin in combination with rifampin, or to vancomycin, aminoglycosides, or chloramphenicol. In vitro susceptibility to β-lactam antibiotics may be misleading. *N. asteroides* and *Actinomyces* have been identified in the lungs of small numbers of AIDS patients.

Among the bacteria, the *mycobacteria* have posed one of the most difficult challenges of AIDS care (see Chapter 163). Alterations in the response to tuberculin skin testing and the emergence of multidrug-resistant *M. tuberculosis* have combined to make preemptive and acute therapy less effective (see Chapter 161). Worldwide, *M. tuberculosis* is the major opportunistic pathogen associated with AIDS. Reactivation of tuberculosis occurs earlier in the course of AIDS (i.e., at higher CD4 counts) than do infections due to other intracellular pathogens. The risk of latent infection progressing to active disease is 8 to 10 percent per year, and it increases as immune function declines. The latent period of disease also declines with AIDS progression. Up to 50 to 80 percent of HIV-infected persons without an AIDS-defining illness will be PPD positive. Exposure of an HIV-infected person to active tuberculosis should prompt initiation of a full course of prophylactic therapy regardless of the results of skin testing. Many patients are *anergic* to skin test antigens; these patients should receive prophylaxis if they belong to a high-prevalence group and have a CD4$^+$ count under 200 per mm^3. The presentations of active infection are often altered; up to 10 percent of HIV-infected patients with positive sputum samples have normal chest radiographs (Fig. 135-8). Extrapulmonary disease is frequent. Therapy has been altered by the emergence of multidrug resistance. To be successful, therapy must take place in the setting of the overall clinical management of HIV infection and of social and nutritional deficiencies; this often requires directly observed therapy.

Mycobacterium avium Complex

M. avium complex (MAC) produces a systemic syndrome in AIDS patients, with fever, night sweats, weakness, anorexia, diarrhea, hepatosplenomegaly, and bone marrow suppression.[30,31] In these patients, the pulmonary symptoms are generally muted by comparison. Among patients with AIDS, 43 percent will develop MAC bacteremia within 2 years.[30] Disseminated MAC infection is uncommon with CD4$^+$ lymphocyte counts above 50 per milliliter. Positive sputum or stool cultures may represent colonization rather than invasive disease. Diagnosis of infection is important, however, owing to the availability of improved antibiotics for treatment. Treatment includes at least two effective drugs, one of which is usually clarithromycin or azithromycin. Ethambutol is the second-choice agent; clofazamine, rifabutin, rifampin, amikacin, imipenem, and ciprofloxacin are also useful.

Fungal Pathogens

Fungal pathogens were largely restricted to mucosal infections with *Candida* species early in the AIDS epidemic. Oral, esophageal, vaginal, gastrointestinal, and skin infections are commonly seen in AIDS patients. Oropharyngeal and esophageal candidiasis (thrush) may present as pseudomembranous plaques, angular chelitis, erythematous (atrophic) lesions, or more erosive infections. All of the mucosal infections may become resistant to therapy, either because of intrinsic resistance to topical or systemic (azole) therapies as with *C. kreusei, C. glabrata,* or some *C. albicans,* or because of advanced AIDS (CD4$^+$ count under 11) or coinfection with herpes simplex, CMV or other pathogens.[25]

Cryptococcus neoformans enters the body via the lungs but is generally recognized as a pathogen of the central nervous system (80 percent of patients have headache), bone, and bloodstream in 5 to 10 percent of AIDS patients in the United States and in up to 40 percent of African patients in Europe. Most of these infections (more than 95 percent) are due to *C. neoformans* variety *neoformans,* which causes only 60 percent of cryptococcal infections in other hosts.[5,10] Pulmonary disease may present as nodules, as lobar or interstitial pneumonitis, or with pleural effusion (Fig. 135-5). Skin lesions, lymphadenopathy, and "sepsis" may also be observed. Antigen detection systems and cultures are valuable for diagnosis and for following responses to treatment.

Endemic fungi (*Histoplasma capsulatum, Coccidioides immitis, Blastomyces dermatidis*) cause disease largely in the geographic areas of greatest prevalence (see Chapters 148 and 149).[1] Atypical presentations are common; most patients present with nonspecific complaints, including fever and dyspnea. Interstitial pneumonitis, granulomas, skin ulcers, anemia, hepatosplenomegaly, or gastrointestinal infection is seen with *Histoplasma* infections; 43 percent of patients have normal chest radiographs.[41] Serologies are useful epidemiologically, while urine antigen detection tests are highly sensitive and specific. Positive cultures for *Histoplasma* may be obtained from blood, bone marrow, liver, lungs, lymph nodes, urine, and cerebrospinal fluid. Reticulonodular (45 percent, with a mean CD4 count of 44) or focal (35 percent, with a mean CD4 count of 143) pulmonary radiographic infiltrates are common with *Coccidioides*

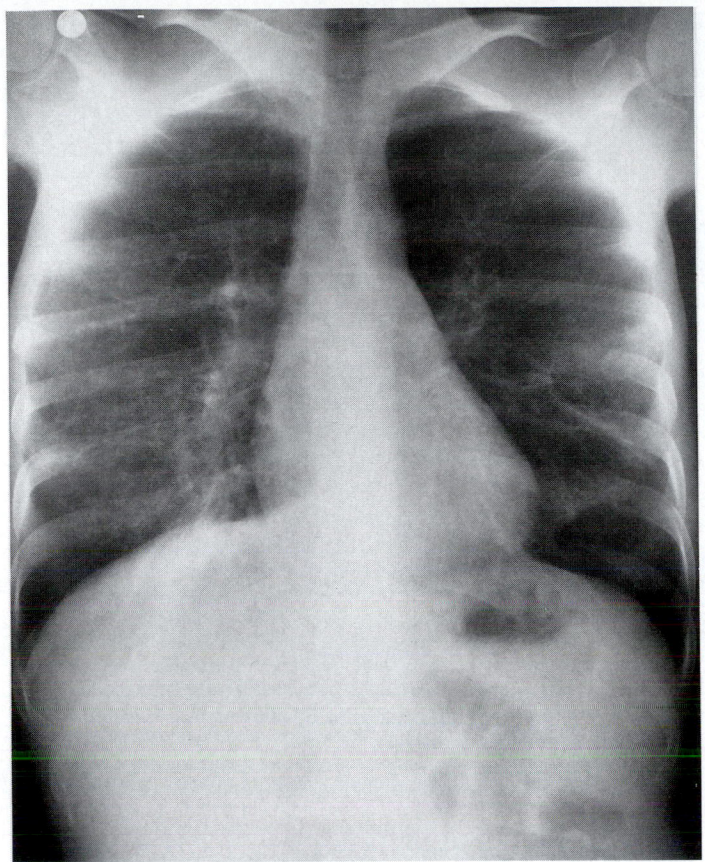

FIGURE 135-5   Chest radiograph of an AIDS patient with atypical cryptococcal pneumonia. Diffuse interstitial infiltrates may be observed in fungemic patients with primary or secondary pulmonary infection.

ties) and coexisting neutropenia. Pulmonary infections due to *Sporothrix schenckii* have been noted.

Protozoan Infections

Parasitic infestations occur in patients with appropriate epidemiologic exposures. Unusual infections have been identified in this population, including those due to the intestinal parasites *Isospora belli, Microsporida* and *Cryptosporidium,* and the blue-green alga-like *Cyclospora cayetanensis.*[24,32,40] All will cause gastrointestinal and biliary infection. Of these, the microsporidians *Encephalitozoon cuniculi* and *E. hellem* and *Septata intestinalis* have been identified in the sinuses; *E. hellem* has also been associated with bronchiolitis. Leishmaniasis has been identified in AIDS patients in Spain and Portugal. Toxoplasmosis occurs in proportion to the seropositivity of a given population (10 to 15 percent in the United States and up to 85 percent in Africa and the Caribbean). Toxoplasmic encephalitis remains the most common manifestation of infection due to *Toxoplasma gondii,* presenting with multiple ring-enhancing lesions on contrast CT or MRI scans of the head. Pulmonary disease, the second most common form of this infection,[33] presents with dyspnea, cough, fever, and hypotension. Diffuse nodules and interstitial infiltrates are seen on chest radiograph, and organisms may be identified on bronchoalveolar lavage samples. This infection is usually prevented by daily TMP-SMX in seropositive subjects.[7] In addition to the sulfa drugs, clindamycin, and pyrimethamine, atovaquone, trimetrexate, azithromycin, and the tetracyclines are active against *T. gondii.* The clinical utility of these agents remains under investigation.

Viral Infections

Of the viral infections, CMV is a major pathogen in all compromised hosts. Up to 50 percent of all people in the United States are seropositive for CMV and therefore capable of reactivating infection with immune suppression. In AIDS, the presentation is typically retinitis, colitis, peripheral nerve involvement (occasionally encephalitis), or adrenalitis. CMV is uncommon as a primary pathogen of the lungs, but it is an im-

(15 percent present with extrapulmonary disease), generally in the setting of nonspecific systemic complaints and a $CD4^+$ count of under 100 per milliliter. As with other populations of immunocompromised hosts, a broad range of fungal infections may be observed (Table 135-7). *Aspergillus fumigatus* colonizes 3 to 5 percent of AIDS patients, with some series showing a 1 to 9 percent incidence of invasive disease. This infection is generally seen in patients with end-stage disease (CD4 count under 50), particularly those with preexisting lung disease (e.g., cavi-

TABLE 135-7

Roentgenographic Findings in Opportunistic Pulmonary Diseases in AIDS

Diffuse Infiltrates	Cavitary Lesions	Hilar Adenopathy	Focal Infiltrates	Nodular Lesions	Pleural Effusions
Pneumocystis carinii	Tuberculosis	Tuberculosis	*Legionella* sp.	*C. neoformans*	Tuberculosis
Tuberculosis	Pyogenic bacteria	Lymphoma	Tuberculosis	*H. capsulatum*	Fungal
Toxoplasma gondii	Aspergillosis	Kaposi's sarcoma	*P. carinii*	Tuberculosis	Pyogenic
Histoplasma capsulatum	*Cryptococcus neoformans*	*Cryptococcus neoformans*	*Streptococcus pneumoniae*	*P. carinii*	Lymphoma
P. carinii and other agents	*P. carinii*	HIV acute	Kaposi's sarcoma	Kaposi's sarcoma	Kaposi's sarcoma
Lymphocytic interstitial pneumonitis	*Rhodococcus equi*	EBV acute	*Nocardia asteroides*	Lymphoma	
	Septic emboli (addicts)		*C. neoformans*	Septic emboli	

portant cofactor with infections due to *Pneumocystis* and *T. gondii*. The role of CMV in the activation of disease due to other viruses (HIV, EBV, hepatitis B) is under investigation. Because this virus is globally immunosuppressive, treatment may be required during therapy for other infections. Viremia due to CMV is not quantitatively uniform. Retinitis may occur at the lowest levels of detectable viremia, but clinical progression will not occur without advanced immune deficiency. Newer detection systems, including the antigenemia assays, and PCR amplification systems are highly sensitive. In the presence of visceral disease, the amount of CMV detected in peripheral blood monocytes or neutrophils increases by up to 30-fold over baseline levels in the HIV-infected and CMV-seropositive subject. Thus far, detection of viremia (by PCR or culture) in the presence of lung disease is highly efficient; these tests are often negative in the presence of severe, isolated gastrointestinal disease.

Papovavirus infection of the central nervous system presents as progressive multifocal leukoencephalopathy. *Fifth disease* (parvovirus B19) causes profound anemia in AIDS by infection of erythroid precursors.

Tumor Viruses and Malignancies

Cancers are often metastatic in the AIDS patient at the time of diagnosis. Common tumors include those due to human papillomavirus, which causes epithelial neoplasia in men (anus) and women (cervix); hepatitis B, with a possibly increased incidence of hepatocellular carcinoma; and Epstein-Barr virus, which causes oral hairy leukoplakia (irregular hairy white lesions on the side of the tongue) and contributes to many of the lymphomas observed in AIDS patients. *Lymphoma* in AIDS patients is generally intermediate or high-grade non-Hodgkin's lymphoma (B cell origin), primary CNS lymphoma of the high-grade non-Hodgkin's type, and Hodgkin's type lymphoma. The presentation is generally with advanced extranodal disease, with rapid progression.

Kaposi's Sarcoma

Kaposi's sarcoma (KS) is the most commonly diagnosed malignancy in AIDS patients.[21] While the incidence of new KS in AIDS patients appears to be declining, deaths due to this tumor are increasing. These highly vascular tumors present as red to purple nodules or plaques, often with surrounding edema, that can occur in many new sites simultaneously. Skin involvement is most common, with lymph node, oral, and gastrointestinal disease also common. Pulmonary disease occurs late in the course of disease, may cause hemoptysis or obstruction, and carries a poor prognosis (Figs. 135-6 and 135-7). The natural course of disease is quite variable. KS has been associated with infection due to a new herpesvirus, human herpesvirus 8, also termed the Kaposi's sarcoma herpesvirus. This association has been used as a basis for therapeutic trials with foscarnet. Antitumor therapy with recombinant human α-interferon is approved for patients with CD4$^+$ counts greater than 200 per milliliter, while traditional therapy with doxorubicin, liposomal daunorubicin, bleomycin, vinblastine, and vincristine is available. Combination therapies and therapy with paclitaxel (Taxol), interferon, and a variety of other agents are in clinical trials.

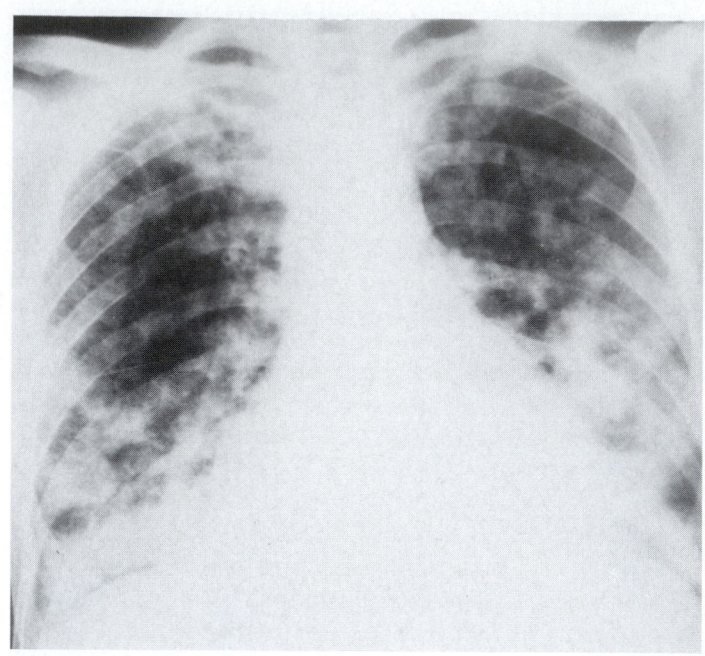

FIGURE 135-6 Chest radiograph of a 36-year-old homosexual man not known to be HIV-1 infected, with bilateral nodular infiltrates due to pulmonary Kaposi's sarcoma.

APPROACHES TO THE DIAGNOSIS OF OPPORTUNISTIC PULMONARY INFECTIONS IN AIDS

With the wide array of potential pathogens causing disease in HIV-infected patients, the frequency of atypical and multiple infections, and the urgency to diagnosis of infection in the immunocompromised host, a systematic approach to lung disease in these hosts is imperative. A few general rules are useful.

1. *Prophylaxis is generally effective.* When failure of prophylaxis occurs, it is usually due to noncompliance, malabsorption of drugs, emerging antibiotic resistance, or coinfection or tumor that alters the local environment. For example, it is often impossible to eradicate *Candida* esophagitis unless erosive esophageal herpes simplex virus infection is also treated. *Pneumocystis* is difficult to treat in the presence of CMV infection or bronchial obstruction.

2. Specific therapies for individual infections have a *high incidence of adverse reactions in the HIV-infected patient.* Thus, presumptive or empiric therapy without microbiologic confirmation, though often appropriate, has a greater risk in this population than in the normal host.

3. The *utilization of newer diagnostic tests* has improved the care of AIDS patients. The interpretation of some tests (e.g., PCR for CMV or *P. carinii*) is unclear, and the availability of some tests (urinary *Histoplasma* antigen or immunoperoxidase stains for *T. gondii*) is not universal. The *induced sputum examination* has been very useful in the early, noninvasive diagnosis of *Pneumocystis* infection, and for mycobacterial disease in the absence of spontaneous sputum production. The sensitivity of sputum induction for *Pneumocystis* infection approaches 90 percent, but the negative predictive value of the test is only 50 percent. The cost and sensitivity of this procedure cannot be justified for the rou-

tine diagnosis of bacterial infections, particularly in persons capable of producing sputum samples.

The use of *more invasive tests,* such as bronchoscopy, with the obvious limitations of cost and risk to the patient, has the advantage of providing subglottic specimens and the potential for diagnosis of a broader range of pathogens. The interpretation of positive cultures for CMV or for MAC may be uncertain without tissue histopathology for confirmation. In patients with a rapidly deteriorating clinical condition or a failure to respond to initial therapy, bronchoscopy with biopsy or needle aspiration may be preferable to bronchoalveolar lavage or sputum induction as an initial procedure. In general, noninvasive, nuclear isotope–based radiologic tests are rarely useful in the diagnostic evaluation of pulmonary disease in AIDS patients. Diffuse pulmonary disease causing hypoxemia will alter physiological testing, measures of diffusion capacity, and gallium scintigraphy. "Gallium scans" are abnormal in most diffuse pulmonary processes and are useful only if *normal* in excluding infections in AIDS.

4. The *rate of progression of infection* is often a clue to the type of disease. Thus, community-acquired pneumonia develops rapidly (in 2 to 5 days), while the initial episode of *P. carinii* pneumonia generally evolves more slowly (over 7 to 12 days). Fungal infection and mycobacterial infection are generally preceded by systemic complaints. Pyogenic pulmonary infection is generally associated with sputum production, while the "atypical" infections may have little or no sputum despite cough and dyspnea.

5. The *radiographic pattern* is often suggestive of the diagnosis (Table 135-7). All "typical" patterns are altered by progressive immune deficits and coexisting or prior lung disease (Fig. 135-4).

Diffuse infiltrates (alveolar or interstitial) may be seen with a homogeneous distribution, as in *P. carinii, T. gondii,* CMV, mycobacterial species, *Histoplasma,* or *Coccidioides.* Drug toxicity may also cause pulmonary infiltrates. Inhomogeneity with these pathogens reflects altered pulmonary parenchyma from previous disease, obstruction (e.g., with tumor, *Strongyloides stercoralis*), or upper-zone disease or

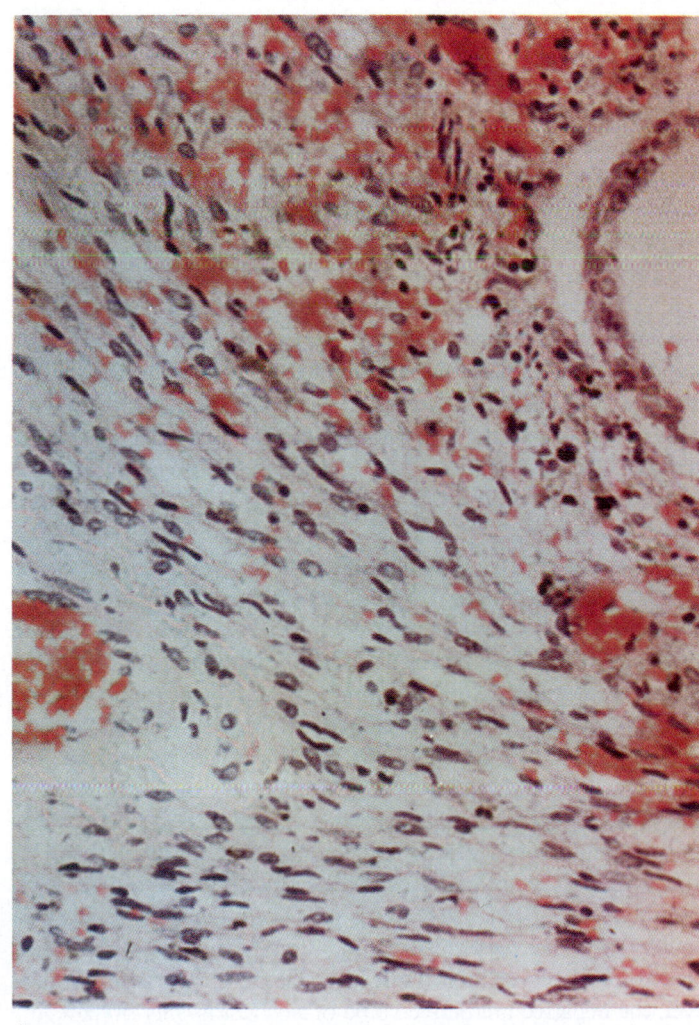

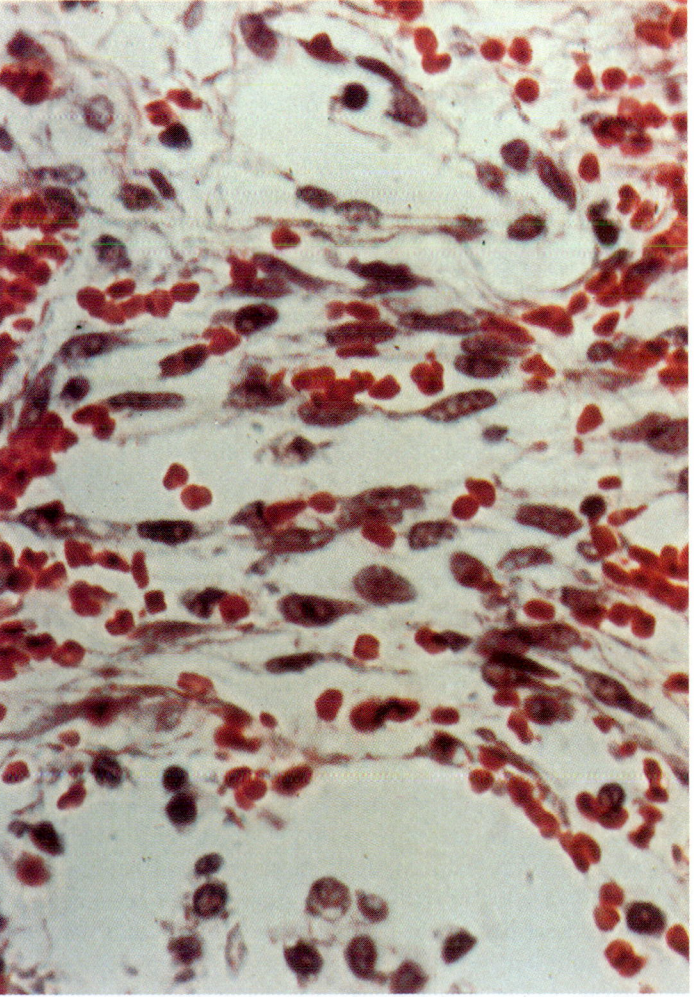

A

FIGURE 135-7 Histologic appearance of Kaposi's sarcoma. *A.* Loosely aggregated spindle cells surround a small bronchus and pulmonary arteriole and extend into the interstitium. H&E stain, ×30.

B

B. Atypical and mitotically active spindle cells with irregular cleftlike spaces and extravasated erythrocytes. H&E stain, ×188.

pneumothorax in *Pneumocystis* pneumonia. Tumors may appear with interstitial radiographic patterns in HIV disease. Lymphoid interstitial pneumonitis is an interstitial process of unknown origin that is seen in AIDS patients. Diffuse interstitial infiltrates are often due to *P. carinii,* but not in patients receiving TMP-SMX prophylaxis and rarely without hypoxemia. Thus, the presence of a sepsislike picture with a diffuse interstitial infiltrate in a patient receiving anti-*Pneumocystis* prophylaxis might suggest mycobacterial disease, *Legionella* infection, or *C. neoformans.*

Focal airspace disease is most often seen with bacterial infections (pyogenic, mycobacteria, *Legionella* species), *Mycoplasma pneumoniae* (viral influenza, adenovirus, CMV), and mixed infections (e.g., CMV and *P. carinii*). Occasionally, primary cryptococcal pneumonia, *Aspergillus* infection, or obstructive disease will present with focal infiltrates. Each of these processes may evolve to frank *cavitation,* particularly infections due to pyogenic bacteria (*Staphylococcus, Klebsiella, S. pneumoniae*) or *M. tuberculosis.* Small cavities are seen with *P. carinii,* the mycobacteria, and metastatic tumors. Large cavities are uncommon; *M. tuberculosis* or aspergilloma is most often present.

Nodular lesions can be seen with any of the metastatic tumors or hematogenous infections. Endocarditis, KS, toxoplasmosis, tuberculosis, MAC, and *Cryptococcus* may all progress from nodules to small cavities. In particular, unusual bacterial pathogens (*Bartonella, Rhodococcus, Candida, Salmonella*) have been observed as pulmonary nodules associated with right-sided endocarditis in AIDS patients.

Intrathoracic adenopathy is common in AIDS patients, most often with infections earlier in the course of disease (CD4$^+$ count greater than 400 per milliliter) and with tumors late in disease. Fungal infections (*Cryptococcus, Histoplasma, Coccidioides*), CMV, and mycobacterial infections may also cause adenopathy. Adenopathy should prompt invasive diagnosis in the absence of a clear etiology in AIDS.

Pleural effusions are common with tuberculosis, other pyogenic bacterial infections, and tumors.

6. The *CD4$^+$ lymphocyte count* is a good indicator of susceptibility to specific infections, while the viral load is most closely associated with overall disease prognosis (Fig. 135-1).[28] Often, community-acquired pneumonia due to *S. pneumoniae, H. influenzae, Mycoplasma,* or *Legionella* species may be the sentinel infection of HIV disease. As host immunity declines, other opportunistic infections will occur. *M. tuberculosis,* an organism of high virulence, will cause infections at *any* CD4$^+$ lymphocyte count but will occur increasingly as the CD4$^+$ lymphocyte count falls below 500 per milliliter. In contrast, less virulent organisms will cause disease only with greater degrees of immune compromise. Thus, MAC is more common below CD4$^+$ counts of 200 per milliliter. *P. carinii* causes pneumonia in less than 1 percent of persons with CD4$^+$ counts over 200 per milliliter but in 18 percent per year with CD4$^+$ counts below 200.

7. *Chronic or recurrent sinus infection* may provide a source of *Pseudomonas* or *Aspergillus* for pulmonary infection. Such pathogens as *Microsporida* and *Pneumocystis* and metastatic Kaposi's lesions with obstruction have also contributed to

chronic sinus infections and, probably, to subsequent pulmonary infections with organisms found in the sinuses.

8. The *spectrum of pulmonary disease varies by geographic region* and by HIV transmission category. This reflects both the heightened risk of certain infections in inner-city areas and in intravenous drug users (tuberculosis, *Bartonella* species, endocarditis), in areas with endemic fungal or parasitic infections (*Histoplasma, Coccidioides, Leishmania*), and in developing countries (tuberculosis is increased with a lower rate of diagnosis of *Pneumocystis*). Similarly, KS tends to be more common in homosexual and bisexual men than in intravenous drug users.

9. *Physical findings* are often useful in establishing a differential for pulmonary disease. The presence of lymphadenopathy or cutaneous lesions of KS may increase the likelihood of pulmonary malignancy. Diffuse rales or rhonchi are more often found in *Pneumocystis,* cryptococcal, or MAC-related infections than with pyogenic infections.

INVASIVE AND NONINVASIVE DIAGNOSIS OF PULMONARY DISEASE IN AIDS

The clinical manifestations of pulmonary processes in AIDS often belie the severity of disease. As with all immunocompromised hosts, early therapy is essential to a good outcome. Further, the frequency of dual processes mitigates toward early, invasive diagnostic procedures.[36,37] In contrast, the chronicity of AIDS has pushed most care into the outpatient setting. For this reason, experience with compromised hosts is helpful in deciding when to commit to more invasive approaches.

Initial evaluation of pulmonary disease in AIDS should include standard tests: physical and radiologic examinations; blood and urine cultures; sputum for Gram's stain, fungal, bacterial, and mycobacterial smears and cultures; blood for cultures for bacteria, fungi, and mycobacteria; CD4$^+$ lymphocyte count; and HIV viral load. In the appropriate settings, serum cryptococcal antigen, lumbar puncture, and additional radiologic (head CT) or minimally invasive (flexible sigmoidoscopy) procedures may be advisable.

Following the initial evaluation, a decision must be made as to "how sick the patient is" and what the likely pathogens might be. Any HIV-infected patient with diffuse pulmonary radiographic infiltrates or hypoxemia merits evaluation for *P. carinii* with an induced sputum examination (unless he or she is receiving TMP-SMX prophylaxis). To be useful, this test depends on the methods of procurement and specimen evaluation. Patients must be hydrated, with clean teeth and mouth. Contamination with oral *Candida,* mycobacteria, and bacteria is common. Nebulized hypertonic (3 percent) saline is inhaled for 15 to 20 min. Expectorated specimens with chest percussions are liquefied (acetylcysteine) and smeared. Giemsa (for trophozoites) and silver (for cyst walls) stains have been largely displaced by direct immunofluorescent stains for *P. carinii.* However, the negative predictive value of this test is only 50 percent. The induced sputum examination is also of use in the diagnosis of *M. tuberculosis* infection, although progressive pulmonary disease in the setting of a negative induced sputum sample should prompt more invasive testing (Fig. 135-8).

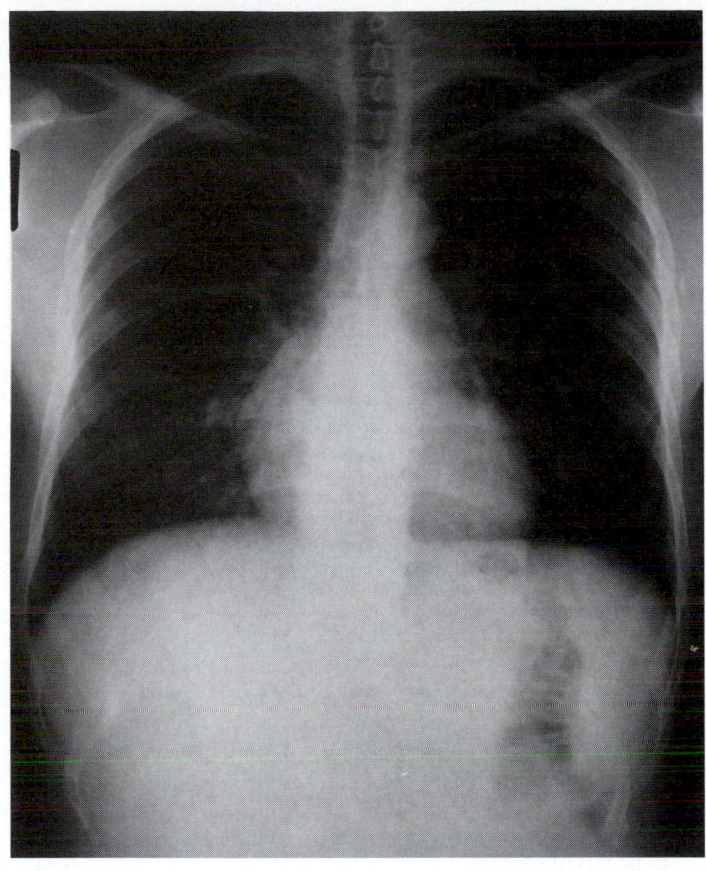

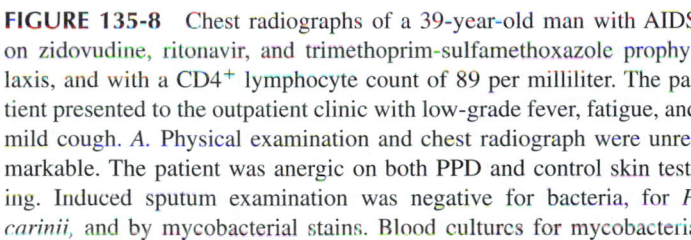

A

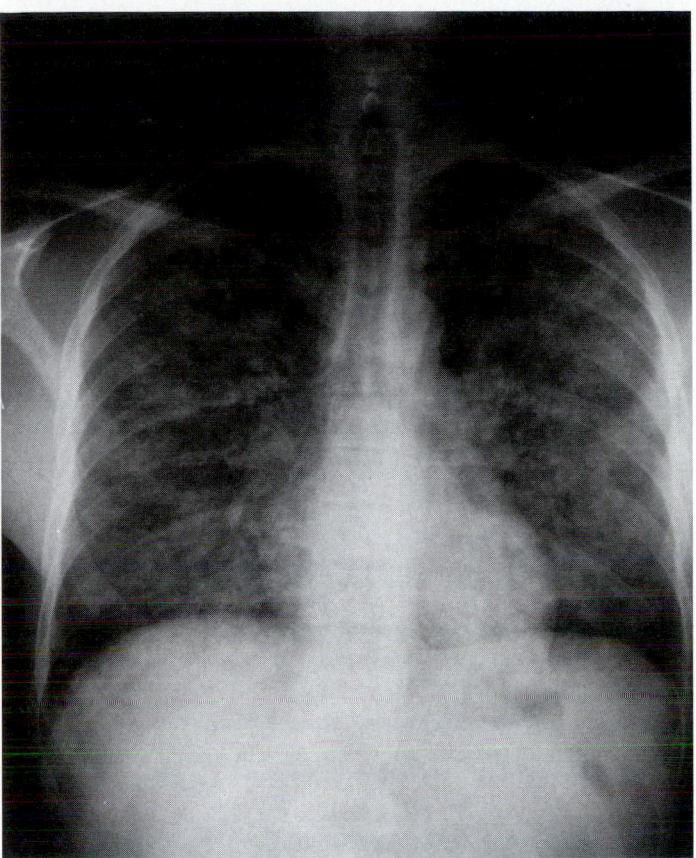

B

FIGURE 135-8   Chest radiographs of a 39-year-old man with AIDS on zidovudine, ritonavir, and trimethoprim-sulfamethoxazole prophylaxis, and with a CD4+ lymphocyte count of 89 per milliliter. The patient presented to the outpatient clinic with low-grade fever, fatigue, and mild cough. *A.* Physical examination and chest radiograph were unremarkable. The patient was anergic on both PPD and control skin testing. Induced sputum examination was negative for bacteria, for *P. carinii,* and by mycobacterial stains. Blood cultures for mycobacteria were obtained. *B.* Ten days after initial presentation, the patient was admitted to the hospital with minimal dyspnea and cough; chest radiograph was remarkable for bilateral pulmonary reticulonodular infiltrates. Bronchoalveolar lavage samples were positive for mycobacteria. The organisms were subsequently identified from cultures of both blood and sputum as *M. tuberculosis,* resistant to both isoniazid and ethambutol. Induced sputum sample cultures remained negative for mycobacteria.

Bronchoscopy and lung biopsy are used to evaluate pulmonary processes not diagnosed by noninvasive approaches.[2,36] Diagnosis is often made by other means (e.g., blood cultures) by the time invasive testing is selected. Often, empiric antibiotic therapy has been initiated (e.g., TMP-SMX and a macrolide) and may alter the yield of microbiologic testing. Thus, the risk of delay in invasive diagnosis may be significant. Bronchoalveolar lavage (wedged, terminal) increases the yield to 85 to 90 percent for *P. carinii.* Bronchoscopic transbronchial biopsy has a yield of 97 percent for *P. carinii* and more than 50 percent for all other organisms. Lavage with multiple biopsies and appropriate histology and cultures have nearly a 100 percent yield for *P. carinii* and 95 percent for all other pathogens in the hands of experienced bronchoscopists. The diagnosis of *P. carinii* pneumonia is, therefore, rarely at issue. In patients with a high risk of other pathogens, early biopsy is recommended. However, endobronchial Kaposi's lesions (Fig. 135-7) and, occasionally, lymphomas may be sources of significant bleeding after biopsy or minimal trauma. The yield of lung lavage is higher in experienced hands; otherwise, open or thoracoscopic biopsies may be preferred.[37] Standard protocols should be established at each institution to assure the proper handling of valuable specimens from invasive procedures.

REFERENCES

1. Ampel NM, Dols CL, Galgiani JN: Coccidioidomycosis during HIV infection: Results of a prospective study in a coccidioided endemic area. *Am J Med* 94:235–240, 1993.

2. Baughman RP, Dohn MN, Frame PT: The continuing utility of bronchoalveolar lavage to diagnose opportunistic infection in AIDS patients. *Am J Med* 97:515–522, 1994.

3. Berry N, Ariyoshi K, Jobe O, et al: HIV type 2 proviral load measured by quantitative polymerase chain reaction correlates with CD4+ lymphopenia in HIV type 2–infected individuals. *AIDS Res Hum Retroviruses* 10:1031–1037, 1994.

4. Burack JH, Hahn JA, Saint-Maurice D, Jacobson MA: Microbiology of community-acquired bacterial pneumonia in persons with and at risk for human immunodeficiency virus type 1 infection. *Arch Intern Med* 154:2589–2596, 1994.

5. Cameron ML, Bartlett JA, Gallis HA, Waskin HA: Manifestations of pulmonary cryptococcosis in patients with acquired immunodeficiency syndrome. *Rev Infect Dis* 13:64–87, 1991.

6. Cao Y, Qin I, Zhang L, et al: Virologic and immunologic characterization of long-term survivors of human immunodeficiency virus type 1 infection. *New Engl J Med* 332:201–208, 1995.

7. Carr A, Tindall B, Brew BJ, et al: Low-dose trimethoprim-sulfamethoxazole prophylaxis for toxoplasmic encephalitis in patients with AIDS. *Ann Intern Med* 117:106–111, 1992.

8. Centers for Disease Control and Prevention: 1993 revised classification system for HIV infection and expanded surveillance case definition for AIDS among adolescents and adults. *MMWR* 41(RR-17):1–19, 1992.

9. Centers for Disease Control and Prevention: Prevention of opportunistic infections in persons infected with human immunodeficiency virus. *Clin Infect Dis* 21(Suppl 1):S1–S141, 1995.

10. Clark RA, Greer DL, Valainis GT, Hyslop NE: *Cryptococcus neoformans* pulmonary infection in HIV-1–infected patients. *J Acquired Immune Defic Syndr* 3:480–484, 1990.

11. Clavel F, Guetard D, Brun-Vezinet F, et al: Isolation of a new human retrovirus from West African patients with AIDS. *Science* 233:343–346, 1986.

12. Clerici M, Shearer GM: A TH1 → TH2 switch is a critical step in the etiology of HIV infection. *Immunol Today* 14:107–111, 1993.

13. Craven DE, Fuller JD, Barber TW, Pelton SI: Immunization of adults and children with human immunodeficiency virus. *Infect Dis Clin Pract* 1:330–337, 409–423, 1992.

14. Crowe SM, Carlin JB, Stewart KI, et al: Predictive value of CD4 lymphocyte numbers for the development of opportunistic infections and malignancies in HIV-infected persons. *J Acquired Immune Defic Syndr Hum Retrovirol* 4:770–776, 1991.

15. Cunliffe N, Denning D: Uncommon invasive mycoses in AIDS. *AIDS* 9:411–420, 1995.

16. Fishman JA: Case records of the Massachusetts General Hospital. *New Engl J Med* 332:249–257, 1995.

17. Gradon JD, Timpone JG, Schnittman SM: Emergence of unusual opportunistic pathogens in AIDS: A review. *Clin Infect Dis* 15:134–157, 1992.

18. Haynes BF, Pantaleo G, Fauci AS: Toward an understanding of the correlates of protective immunity to HIV infection. *Science* 271:324–328, 1996.

19. Hoover DR, Saah AJ, Bacellar H: Multicenter AIDS Cohort Study: Clinical manifestations of AIDS in the era of pneumocystis prophylaxis. *New Engl J Med* 329:1922–1926, 1993.

20. Janoff EN, Breiman RF, Daley CL, et al: Pneumococcal disease during HIV infection: Epidemiologic, clinical, and immunologic perspectives. *Ann Intern Med* 117:314–324, 1992.

21. Kaplan LD, Hopewell PC, Jaffe H, et al: Kaposi's sarcoma involving the lung in patients with the acquired immunodeficiency syndrome. *J Acquired Immune Defic Syndr Hum Retrovirol* 1:23–30, 1988.

22. Koehler JE, Tappero JW: Bacillary angiomatosis and bacillary peliosis in patients infected with human immunodeficiency virus. *Clin Infect Dis* 17:612–624, 1993.

23. Kvale PA, Hansen NI, Markowitz N, et al: Routine analysis of induced sputum is not an effective strategy for screening persons infected with human immunodeficiency virus for *Mycobacterium tuberculosis* or *Pneumocystis carinii*. *Clin Infect Dis* 19:410–416, 1996.

24. Lacey CJN, Clarke AMT, Fraser P, et al: Chronic microsporidian infection of the nasal mucosae, sinuses and conjunctivae in HIV disease. *Genitourin Med* 68:179–181, 1992.

25. Maenza JR, Keruly JC, Moore RD, et al: Risk factors for fluconazole-resistant candidiasis in human immunodeficiency virus–infected patients. *J Infect Dis* 173:219–225, 1996.

26. Magnenat J, Micod LP, Auckenuthaler R, et al: Mode of presentation and diagnosis of bacterial pneumonia in human immunodeficiency virus in infected patients. *Am Rev Respir Dis* 144:917–922, 1991.

27. Marchevsky A, Rosen MJ, Chrystal G, Kleinerman J: Pulmonary complications of the acquired immunodeficiency syndrome: A clinicopathologic study of 70 cases. *Hum Pathol* 16:659–670, 1985.

28. Masur H, Ognibene FP, Yarchoan R, et al: CD4 counts as predictors of opportunistic pneumonias in human immunodeficiency virus (HIV) infection. *Ann Intern Med* 111:223–231, 1989.

29. Muñoz A, Schrager LK, Bacellar H, et al: Trends in the incidence of outcomes defining acquired immunodeficiency syndrome (AIDS) in the Multicenter AIDS Cohort Study: 1985–1991. *Am J Epidemiol* 137:423–438, 1993.

30. Nightingale SD, Byrd LT, Southern P, et al: Incidence of *Mycobacterium avium-intracellulare* complex bacteremia in human immunodeficiency virus–positive patients. *J Infect Dis* 1165:1082–1085, 1992.

31. Packer SJ, Cesario T, Williams JHJ: *Mycobacterium avium* complex infection presenting as endobronchial lesions in immunosuppressed patients. *Ann Intern Med* 109:389–393, 1988.

32. Pape JW, Verdier RI, Boncy M, et al: Cyclospora infection in adults infected with HIV: Clinical manifestations, treatment and prophylaxis. *Ann Intern Med* 121:654–657, 1994.

33. Pomeroy C, Filice GA: Pulmonary toxoplasmosis: A review. *Clin Infect Dis* 14:863–870, 1992.

34. Richman DD: Resistance of clinical isolates of human immunodeficiency virus to antiretroviral agents. *Antimicrob Agents Chemother* 37:1207–1213, 1993.

35. Rosen MJ, Lou Y, Kvale PA, et al: Pulmonary function tests in HIV-infected patients without AIDS. *Am J Respir Crit Care Med* 152(2):738–745, 1995.

36. Stover DE, White DA, Romano PA, Gellene RA: Diagnosis of pulmonary disease in acquired immunodeficiency syndrome (AIDS): Role of bronchoscopy and bronchoalveolar lavage. *Am Rev Respir Dis* 130:659–662, 1984.

37. Stulbarg MS, Golden JA: Open lung biopsy in the acquired immunodeficiency syndrome (AIDS). *Chest* 91:639–640, 1987.

38. Wall PG, Porter K, Noone A, Goldberg DJ: Changing incidence of *Pneumocystis carinii* pneumonia as initial AIDS defining disease in the United Kingdom. *AIDS* 7:1523–1525, 1993.

39. Wallace JM, Rao AV, Glassroth J, et al: Respiratory illness in persons with human immunodeficiency virus infection. *Am Rev Respir Dis* 148:1523–1529, 1993.

40. Weber R, Kuster H, Keller R: Pulmonary and intestinal microsporidiosis in a patient with the acquired immunodeficiency syndrome. *Am Rev Respir Dis* 146:1603–1605, 1992.

41. Wheat LJ, Slama TG, Zeckel ML: Histoplasmosis in the acquired immune deficiency syndrome. *Am J Med* 78:203–210, 1985.

42. Wilson CC, Hirsch MS: Combination antiretroviral therapy for the treatment of human immunodeficiency virus type-1 infection. *Proc Assoc Am Phys* 107:19–27, 1995.

CHAPTER 136

PULMONARY INFECTIONS IN NEUTROPENIA AND CANCER

Jay A. Fishman

The number of people with cancer and/or neutropenia has increased with increases in the life spans of such people due to advances in diagnosis, supportive care, bone marrow transplantation, the use of intensive chemotherapeutic regimens, and the availability of new antibiotics. More than 1.3 million new cases of cancer will be diagnosed in the United States in 1997.

One of the most challenging problems in the practice of infectious disease is the care of the immunocompromised host, particularly the cancer patient with increased susceptibility to infection due to chemotherapy. This patient population is similar to organ transplant recipients in that there is a predictable pattern of susceptibility to various infections due to the effects of exogenous immune suppression. Specific acquired or congenital immune defects predispose to a predictable array of pathogens to which the host is rendered susceptible (see Chapter 139) (Table 136-1). For example, staphylococcal infections are of great importance in chronic granulomatous disease. In contrast, most cancer patients have mixed immune defects, and the relative risk of infection is related to the *severity and duration of cumulative deficits*. Thus, risks of infection are associated with the tumor type itself, chemotherapy, acquired immune deficits (e.g., splenectomy, mucositis), nosocomial exposures, and the neutropenia associated with cancer chemotherapy.

Prophylactic strategies for cancer patients are generally aimed at common community-acquired infections, organisms common for the specific tumor type or for any suspected immune defects, nosocomial exposures, and the treatment of immunomodulating viral infections (e.g., cytomegalovirus [CMV]) while minimizing the total amount and duration of immunosuppressive therapies. Many vaccines for common infections (from *S. pneumoniae*, *H. influenzae*, influenza virus, varicella zoster, or hepatitis B) are not approved for use in immunocompromised patients or are ineffective in these hosts. While some prophylactic strategies are very successful [e.g., the use of trimethoprim-sulfamethoxazole (TMP-SMX) for the prevention of *Pneumocystis carinii* and bacterial infections], improved patient survival and the prolonged use of prophylactic antibiotics have contributed to the emergence of, and colonization by, antibiotic-resistant organisms, including the fluconazole-resistant yeasts, TMP-SMX–resistant pneumococci, and vancomycin-resistant enterococci. Ultimately, therefore, prevention of infection may be best achieved by *reconstitution of the systemic immune response* rather than by focusing on the use of antibiotics or vaccines for the prevention of infection. This chapter concentrates on pulmonary infections in the neutropenic patient and in the cancer patient, and on some of the newer approaches to repairing defects in the inflammatory and immune response mechanisms.

TABLE 136-1

Infections Associated with Specific Immune Defects

Defect	Common Causes	Associated Infections
Granulocytopenia	Leukemia, cytotoxic chemotherapy, AIDS, drug toxicity, Felty syndrome	Enterobacteriaceae, *Pseudomonas*, *S. aureus*, *S. epidermidis*, streptococci, *Aspergillus*, *Candida*, other fungi
Neutrophil chemotaxis	Diabetes, alcoholism, uremia, Hodgkin's disease, trauma (burns), lazy leukocyte syndrome, CT disease	*S. aureus*, *Candida*, streptococci
Neutrophil killing	Chronic granulomatous disease, myeloperoxidase deficiency	*S. aureus*, *E. coli*, *Candida* spp. (*C. kreusei*, *C. albicans*, *C. glabrata*), *Aspergillus*
T-cell defects	AIDS, congenital, lymphoma, sarcoidosis, viral infection, organ transplants, steroids	Intracellular bacteria (*Legionella*, *Listeria*, mycobacteria), HSV, VZV, CMV, EBV, parasites (*Strongyloides*, *Toxoplasma*), fungi (*P. carinii*, *Candida*, *Cryptococcus*)
B-cell defects	Congenital or acquired agammaglobulinemia, burns, enteropathies, splenic dysfunction, myeloma, ALL	*S. pneumoniae*, *H. influenzae*, *Salmonella* and *Campylobacter* spp., *G. lamblia*
Splenectomy	Surgery, sickle cell, cirrhosis	*S. pneumoniae*, *H. influenzae*, *Salmonella* spp., *Capnocytophaga*
Complement	Congenital and acquired defects	*S. aureus*, *Neisseria* spp., *H. influenzae*, *S. pneumoniae*
Anatomic	Vascular or Foley catheters, incisions, anastomotic leaks, mucosal ulceration, tumor obstruction, vascular insufficiency	Colonizing organisms, antibiotic-resistant nosocomial organisms

DEFECTS IN HOST RESPONSES TO INFECTION IN NEUTROPENIA AND CANCER

Infection is the main obstacle to the successful treatment of cancer. First, patients with malignancy are at increased risk of infection due to physical factors related to tumor growth (mucosal injury, obstruction of airways, mass effects, tumor ulceration, surgery, bleeding) and the replacement of normal cells by cancer cells with diminished immune function, as in leukemia or lymphoma. Second, treatment generally produces injury (chemotherapy or radiation) to both cancerous and normal cells, particularly to the rapidly replicating cells of hematopoietic origin and in the gastrointestinal mucosa. The ability to target therapy to specific cancer cells (e.g., via hormonal therapies or using nucleic acid or antibody-based targeting of toxins) is a response, in part, to the systemic toxicities of many current therapeutic regimens. The level of susceptibility to infection depends on the *sum* of the impact of the underlying disease and treatments on the number and function of immune, inflammatory, and phagocytic cells. Thus, in multiple myeloma, overproduction of a monoclonal immunoglobulin decreases the relative amount of organism-specific antibody and increases the turnover of all immunoglobulins nonspecifically, making the host effectively *specific* immunoglobulin deficient.

Chemotherapy for myeloma decreases the number of malignant cells, as well as the number and function of circulating leukocytes, further compromising immune function. Mucosal injury (gastrointestinal, urinary) resulting from the chemotherapy, and colonization with hospital-derived flora, predisposes to the entry of potential pathogens. Recovery of the marrow is associated with return of the immune responses, but the *time course to complete recovery of normal immunity* has not been well characterized. Thus, when cells are normal in terms of numbers or in vitro functions, the patient may continue to lack specific immune responses, may fail to heal injured tissues, and may not produce the "factors" (cytokines, chemokines, interferons, growth factors, immunoglobulins) responsible for an *optimal and coordinated host response.*

THE RISK OF INFECTION IN CANCER PATIENTS

Defects Due to Tumors and Chemotherapy

The incidence of infection in cancer patients is determined partly by the nature of the underlying neoplasm. Many studies of infection in cancer have focused on patients with leukemia and lymphoma, owing to the severe and predictable nature of the immune deficiencies developed by these people. In a series conducted by Bodey and colleagues, fatal infections in acute leukemics were caused by bacteria in 66 percent, fungi in 33 percent, viruses in 0.2 percent, and protozoa (including *P. carinii*, now considered a fungus) in 0.1 percent. In contrast, fatal infection in lymphoma patients (86 percent) and solid-tumor patients (94 percent) were more often bacterial.[9,13,22,30,52] A study of the incidence of gram-negative bacteremia in cancer patients supports these differences.[66] Among 76 patients with leukemia, including chronic lymphocytic leukemia, 33 (43 percent) died of gram-negative sepsis, whereas only 18 of 377 patients (5 percent) with either solid tumors or lymphoma died of gram-negative sepsis.

In studies of cryptococcal infection in cancer patients, the rate of cryptococcal infection in chronic lymphocytic leukemia was more than double that in Hodgkin's disease (24.3 versus 10.9 per thousand), and the rate in breast cancer was only 0.159 per thousand. Other tumors are also associated with specific infections. For example, lung cancer is associated with tuberculosis at a rate of 92 per 1000, second only to the rate in patients with Hodgkin's disease (96 per 1000), who have a known cellular immune defect.[15,34] Without therapy, the degree of depression in cellular immunity (delayed-type hypersensitivity) is more prominent in lymphoma, whereas humoral immunity is impaired to a greater degree in diseases affecting B-lymphocyte function, such as multiple myeloma and chronic lymphocytic lymphoma. Thus, the lymphoma patient is particularly susceptible to intracellular organisms including *Listeria monocytogenes*, *Mycobacterium tuberculosis*, viruses, and fungi, whereas the myeloma patient is more apt to develop pneumonia or bacteremia due to *Hemophilus influenzae*, *Streptococcus pneumoniae*, and a variety of other acute bacterial infections.[34] In lymphoma, the mobilization (chemotaxis) of leukocytes may be impaired to a greater degree than the phagocytosis and killing of potential pathogens.[35,51,54] Defects in the uptake and killing of bacteria may reflect toxicities of chemotherapy rather than intrinsic defects associated with the underlying disease.[35,54] Acute leukemia is associated with a depression in the number and function of circulating granulocytes and is associated with severe pyogenic, bacterial infections. Patients with acute and relapsed leukemia have demonstrated impaired phagocytosis and killing of fungi and bacteria by these cells, which may appear morphologically normal.[15,38] These defects may persist well into periods of remission and may progress along with progression of the underlying disease.[35,66]

The impact of the various forms of chemotherapy on host defenses must be added to those caused by the cancer itself. A variety of immune functions are impaired by chemotherapy, including the phagocytosis and killing of bacteria by neutrophils (corticosteroids, carmustine, radiation); antibody production (methotrexate, cyclophosphamide, L-asparaginase, 6-mercaptopurine); uptake and processing of antigen by macrophages (corticosteroids, cyclophosphamide, dactinomycin); recognition of antigens by T and B lymphocytes (corticosteroids, cyclophosphamide); and antigen-driven lymphocyte proliferation (methotrexate, 5-fluorouracil, fludarabine, cytarabine, L-asparaginase, dactinomycin, 6-mercaptopurine, hydroxyurea). Predisposition to infection induced by chemotherapy may mask more subtle defects due to underlying disease; e.g., the effects of granulocytopenia due to intensive chemotherapy will generally predominate over the effects of underlying lymphoma or myeloma.

Neutropenia

The most common predisposing condition for infection in the cancer patient is granulocytopenia, often due to chemotherapy. However, the function of inflammatory cells and of other immune (e.g., mucosal) barriers are of equal importance to the *number* of granulocytes. In neutropenia, the risk of infection increases as granulocyte counts decrease. Thus, the risk of infection in the patient with neutropenia (under 1000 total granulocytes per mm^3) increases when granulocyte numbers fall further, to below 500 per mm^3; the risk is greatest when counts are lower than 100 per mm^3.[8,50] The many causes of neutropenia differ qualitatively (Table 136-2). They include iatrogenic neutropenias (chemotherapy, drug toxicities), aplastic anemia and other immune neutropenias, the hereditary and acquired cyclic neutropenias, and malignancy-associated (especially acute leukemias) and infection-induced neutropenias.

The rate of decline in white blood cell numbers and the duration of neutropenia influence the risk of infection. Thus, the patient with acute leukemia and rapidly falling neutrophil counts is at greater risk than the person in whom counts are falling slowly or are stable. Infection in neutropenia is generally (more than 80 percent of the time) due to endogenous organisms from the host, including those from remote exposures *(Strongyloides)* or infections (herpes simplex or herpes-zoster virus), as well as gastrointestinal and oral flora; the risk of nosocomial colonization with gram-negative bacteria or fungi is greatest in this population, but may also relate to the degree of mucosal injury. Prophylactic programs that leave the anaerobic flora intact are helpful (e.g., oral TMP-SMX, quinolines, and/or antifungals).

TABLE 136-2

Causes of Neutropenia

Iatrogenic
  Cancer chemotherapy
  Drug toxities (TMP-SMX, chloramphenicol, ganciclovir, AZT)
Infection
  Viral (cytomegalovirus, HIV, Epstein-Barr virus, hepatitis B)
  Parasitic *(Leishmania)*
  Bacteria *(Clostridium)*
  Acute neutropenia of sepsis/endotoxemia (gram-negative sepsis)
  Bone marrow failure of neonatal sepsis
Immune
  Drug-induced autoimmunity (haptenic: penicillins, sulfa drugs)
  Aplastic anemia (includes idiosyncratic reactions: phenothiazines, chloramohenicol)
  Alloimmune neonatal neutropenia (maternal-fetal incompatibility)
  Congenital autoimmune neutropenia
  Primary autoimmune (systemic lupus erythematosus, Felty's syndrome, rheumatoid
    arthritis)
  Transfusion induced
  Antineutrophil antibody mediated
  Cyclic neutropenia (CD57 lymphocyte expansion)
Hereditary
  Infantile genetic agranulocytosis
  Familial neutropenia
  Cyclic neutropenia (autosomal dominant)
  Old age

THE MICROBIOLOGY OF INFECTION IN NEUTROPENIA AND CANCER

Pulmonary infections in patients with functional or quantitative defects in neutrophils can reach the lungs via inhalation, microaspiration of colonizing organisms, and bacteremia after non-respiratory penetration and bacteremia (e.g., from vascular catheters or disrupted mucosal surfaces). Decisions about the management of these patients are often made without microbiologic data because of the urgency of therapy in the immunocompromised host. Distinctions between pulmonary and extrapulmonary infections often become blurred in the attempt to treat most of the likely pathogens in a febrile neutropenic cancer patient. Often a specific, unsuspected pulmonary pathogen is detected on routine blood or urine culture or from a biopsy of an extrapulmonary infected site.

Common Infections in Neutropenic Patients

Common infections in the neutropenic host and the cancer patient are most often the result of colonization with, and infection by, pyogenic bacteria, including *S. pneumoniae*, *Staphylococcus aureus*, the Enterobacteriaceae, *Pseudomonas aeruginosa*, *H. influenzae*, and *Stenotrophomonas* (formerly *Xanthomonas*) *maltophilia*. Common fungal pathogens include *Candida albicans*, *Aspergillus* species, *C. kreusei*, *C. glabrata*, *Mucor*, *Absidia*, and *Rhizopus* species (Fig. 136-1). The emergence of antibiotic-resistant strains of bacteria and fungi takes on special importance in the neutropenic host because empiric therapy must be started before the results of microbiologic culture and susceptibility testing of clinical specimens obtained from the patients become available. The common "resistant" organisms include vancomycin- and ampicillin-resistant *Enterococcus faecium* and *faecalis*, methicillin-resistant *S. aureus*, inducible chromosomal and acquired plasmids encoding β-lactamases in gram-negative bacteria, and azole (i.e. fluconazole) resistance to *C. kreusei* and *C. glabrata*.

In a series of bacteremic patients with leukemia and lymphoma from 1977, *Escherichia coli* was detected in 24 percent, *P. aeruginosa* in 15 percent, *Klebsiella* or *Enterobacter* in 11 percent, *S. aureus* in 9 percent, *Candida* species in 5 percent, streptococcal species in 3 percent, polymicrobial bacteremia in 17 percent, and other organisms in 15 percent.[52] Over time, the organisms identified as causing infection in febrile neutropenic cancer patients have shifted to include more gram-positive bacteria and fungi and more highly antibiotic-resistant gram-negative bacteria. This shift may reflect the increased use of broad-spectrum antibiotics aimed at gram-negative bacteria, indwelling central venous catheters, and increasing antibiotic resistance in gram-positive organisms and yeasts.

In individual patients, the spectrum of colonizing organisms also changes over time, especially with antibiotic use (and abuse). Accordingly, the importance of *S. aureus* and *S. epidermidis*, enterococci, β-hemolytic streptococci, *L. monocytogenes*, *Clostridium difficile*, and *Corynebacterium jeikeum*, and of multiply-antibiotic-resistant *P. aeruginosa*, *Burkholdaria* (formerly *Pseudomonas*) *cepacia*, and *S. maltophilia* has increased. The development of microbiologic culture methods for the *Legionella* species and the iden-

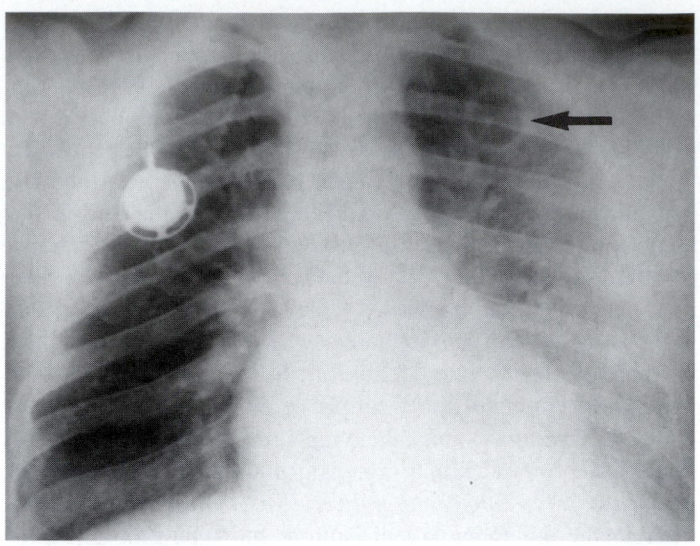

FIGURE 136-1 Lung abscess (arrow) in a febrile patient following intensive chemotherapy for relapsed acute myelogenous leukemia. Patient developed fever while granulocytopenic (< 50 neutrophils/mm^3 for 8 days) without localizing symptoms and a clear chest radiograph. When the neutrophil count exceeded 200/mm^3, a lung abscess was detected in the left upper lobe. *Aspergillus fumigatus* was detected in fluid obtained from the abscess via CT-guided percutaneous needle aspiration. The infection responded well to amphotericin B treatment.

tification of these organisms in cooling systems and in potable water supplies have similarly contributed to the "growth" in the incidence of the common respiratory pathogens.

Seeding from blood-borne infection (e.g., due to vascular access catheters or localized infection) occurs most often with the organisms described above; other organisms are *Candida* and *Aspergillus* and, occasionally, mycobacteria. Patients with solid lung tumors may develop obstructive pneumonia or pulmonary hemorrhage, followed by superinfection with the flora of the upper respiratory tract and oropharynx (Fig. 136-2).

Fungi and Less Common Pathogens

Combined cellular and granulocytic deficiencies are often present after chemotherapy. As a result, in addition to the common pathogens described above, pathogens normally controlled by cellular immune mechanisms (especially intracellular pathogens) can be detected; among these are *M. tuberculosis*, *Brucella* species, the geographic fungi, *Cryptococcus neoformans*, *Strongyloides stercoralis*, *Salmonella*, and *Pneumocystis carinii*. Thus, while *Aspergillus* infection can be expected to occur along with neutropenia early in the course of cancer therapy, it is likely to occur later in AIDS as T-cell defects are joined by neutropenia. Similarly, because of the pathogenetic role of cellular dysfunction in setting the stage for certain infections, *P. carinii* is apt to be manifest early in the course of AIDS and at variable times in the course of cancer therapy. Also, *P. carinii* infection is more frequent in Hodgkin's disease than in patients with solid tumors, because of the differing levels of underlying cellular immune deficits.

Unusual pathogens have been identified in increasing numbers of cancer patients with neutropenia. The classic presenta-

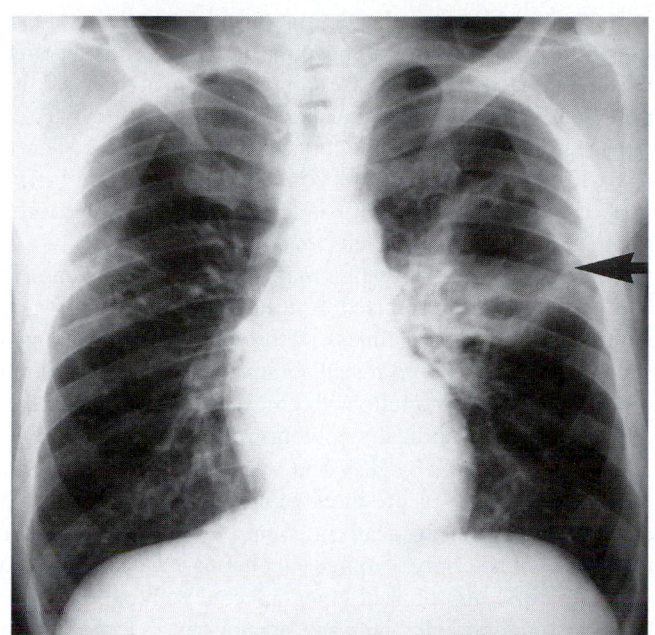

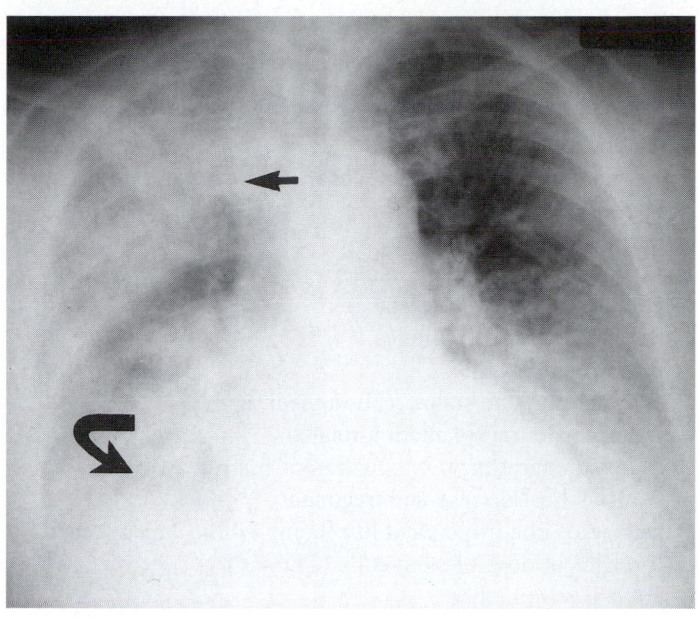

A

FIGURE 136-2 Postobstructive pneumonia and lung abscess (arrow) in a 45-year-old man with adenocarcinoma of the lung in the right hilum. The abscess was drained via a bronchoscopic approach. Cultures of the abscess fluid grew common oral bacterial flora, including *Prevotella melaninogenica* and *Bacteroides* species.

tions of pneumonia, inflammation and perforation of the cecum (often with *Pseudomonas* and anaerobes), and typhlitis (often *Clostridium septicum*) may be the first signs of life-threatening infection in a neutropenic patient. Atypical presentations of infection may be from a portal of entry other than the gastrointestinal tract or the lungs. Thus, the first clinical signs of infection may be "spontaneous" or line-associated bacteremia (*S. aureus, S. epidermidis, Clostridia, Bacillus, C. jeikeum, S. maltophilia, Candida* species, *Fusarium*), skin lesions (gram-negative sepsis, *Candida* species, *Nocardia asteroides, C. neoformans*, herpes simplex or varicella zoster), gingivitis (anaerobes), hepatic dysfunction (hepatosplenic candidiasis), or seizures (*N. asteroides* in brain abscess associated with slowly progressive pneumonia) (Fig. 136-3).

Because of the widespread use of antibacterial agents, mucosal injury, use of intravenous catheters and bone marrow transplantation, fungal infections have occurred with increasing frequency, most often in acute leukemia patients (see Table 136-3). *C. glabrata* and *C. kreusei* that are resistant to fluconazole develop during antibiotic treatment. Although Mucoraceae (*Rhizopus, Mucor, Absidia*), like the *Aspergillus* species, may present with invasive disease of the sinuses and periorbital and frontal cortex, they can also cause rapidly progressive hemorrhagic pneumonia with infarction and fungemia. Invasive disease of the sinuses and periorbital and frontal cortex is especially prevalent in neutropenic diabetics and in patients treated with desferoxamine, with prolonged corticosteroid therapy, or with broad-spectrum antibiotics. The treatment of this invasive disease is surgical débridement in addition to antifungal therapy. In patients with neutropenia or acute leukemia, a group of "benign" dermatophytes—including *Trichosporon beigelii, Au-*

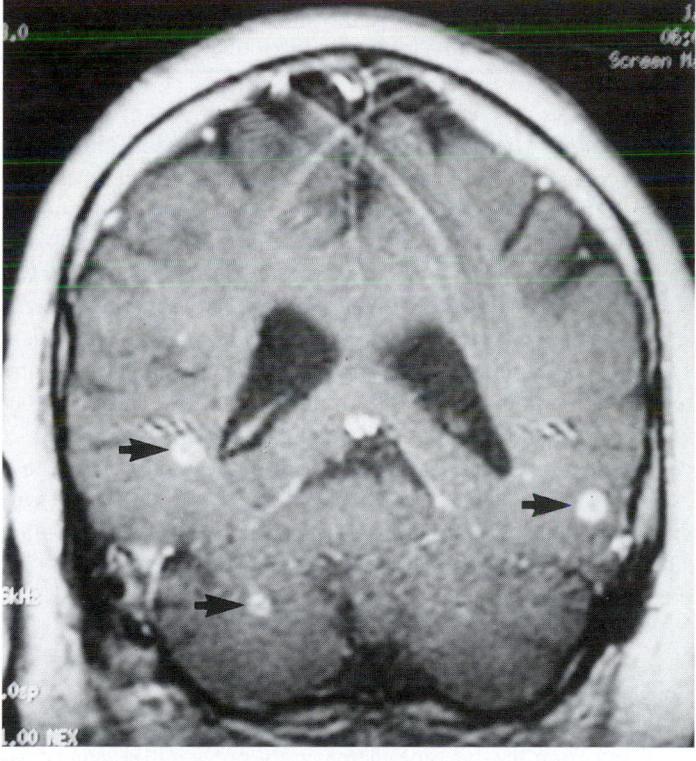

B

FIGURE 136-3 Many simultaneous infections in a 46-year-old man with Wegener's granulomatosis. The patient was treated with cyclophosphamide and prednisone for deteriorating pulmonary function and developed progressive pneumonia and neutropenia. Sputum cultures were unrevealing. *A.* Bronchoalveolar lavage revealed *Nocardia asteroides* (curved arrow), but the patient's condition failed to improve with therapy. Bronchoscopic biopsy of a small abscess in the upper lobe (small arrow) revealed *Fusarium* species. *B.* Magnetic resonance imaging (MRI) of the head revealed numerous (more than 30) small abscesses (arrows) diffusely distributed throughout the brain. These were initially thought to be consistent with infection due to *Toxoplasma gondii*. Brain biopsy revealed *Nocardia asteroides*.

TABLE 136-3

Factors in the Development of Fungal Infections in Cancer Patients

Age/performance status
Prior chemotherapy or radiotherapy: Dose and duration
  Steroids
  Purine analogues
Prior infections (specific isolates)
Recent antibiotic use (resistance)
  Broad spectrum antibiotics
  Prophylactic agents
Functional immune status (cell number, activity)
Hematopoietic transplantation-related
  Delayed engraftment or function of marrow
  Graft-vs-host-disease and treatment
  Degree of donor-recipient histocompatibility mismatch
  Insufficient dose of stem cells (CD34+)
  Total T-cell number
Integrity of mucosal barriers (catheters, gastrointestinal)
Neutropenia (severity, duration $\geq$ 2 weeks)
Hospital environment
Nonhematopoietic organ failure (e.g., dialysis)
Other simultaneous infections (e.g., cytomegalovirus)

---

reobasidium, *Alternaria, Curvularia, Phialophora, Wangiella,* and *Cladosporium*—have been associated both with disease of the skin and with invasive infection of the lungs, the sinuses, and the central nervous system. Ocasionally infections are caused by "atypical fungi" (e.g., *Saccharomyces cerevisiae, Pseudallescheria boydii, Cunninghamella bertholletiae, Drechslera, Fusarium* species, *Geotrichum candidum,* and *Penicillium* species). *Fusarium* causes infection of the bloodstream and lungs that is indistinguishable from that due to *Aspergillus,* but with greater tendency to cutaneous involvement (Fig. 136-3). *P. carinii* infection occurs most often during the period of recovery from neutropenia (see Chapter 150); it presents as a syndrome of febrile pneumonitis (discussed below). The cardinal sign of *Pneumocystis* pneumonia is the presence of arterial hypoxemia out of proportion to physical or radiologic signs.

Viral Infections

Viral infection has become increasingly prevalent in cancer patients. Herpes simplex virus (HSV) and varicella zoster virus (VZV) are frequently reactivated during periods of neutropenia. Patients who are undergoing chemotherapy for Hodgkin's disease or who have received bone marrow transplants are at greater risk than other immunocompromised hosts (35 to 50 percent in the first year). Specific antiviral prophylaxis is effective in reducing the incidence and severity of these relapses. Most often, these viruses cause painful, but relatively benign, skin or mucosal (especially esophageal, gastrointestinal, and perianal) lesions. These lesions may progress in up to 50 percent of neutropenic cancer chemotherapy patients, and the skin rash may become more diffuse, with hemorrhagic or nonhemorrhagic le-

sions extending beyond the dermatomal limits. Systemic dissemination to visceral organs occurs in 10 percent of patients with disseminated skin disease commonly involving the liver, lungs, brain, or gastrointestinal tract. Nasal, oropharyngeal, or esophageal HSV or VZV infections may spread directly to the lungs with the development of vesicular lesions in the trachea, or may cause viral pneumonitis in the parenchyma as a result of viremia secondary to cutaneous reactivation.

Primary varicella pneumonia may accompany chickenpox in adults and in the compromised host. Pulmonary invasion occurs within the first 7 days of illness, with mortality approaching 18 percent. Chest radiographs reveal nodular or interstitial infiltrates in up to 16 percent of adults with chickenpox, whereas only 10 to 25 of these have clinical symptoms.[24,44,58,62]

Pulmonary invasion by HSV and VZV in the neutropenic host should be considered a life-threatening emergency. Among the most common causes of death in compromised hosts with viral pneumonia is bacterial (or fungal, including *Pneumocystis*) superinfection of compromised lungs infected with pathogens, including respiratory syncytial virus, adenovirus, cylomegalovirus (CMV), and influenza. These patients may have high fevers despite the absence of neutrophils. Viral skin lesions may also provide a portal for the entry of other pathogens in the compromised host. Dissemination of cutaneous infection suggests the presence of severe immune deficiency.

In bone marrow transplantation (BMT) recipients, pulmonary infection due to CMV occurs in the CMV-seropositive recipient of CMV-seronegative marrow (see Chapter 137). Because much of the lung injury is due to immune responses to CMV antigens, the full pneumonitis develops not during lymphopenia but, rather, with the engraftment of the marrow and with the reemergence of immune function. Viral replication is not needed for CMV pneumonitis to occur. CMV infection in lymphocytic leukemias generally takes the form of asymptomatic viral shedding. In the BMT recipient, interruption of viral replication by ganciclovir after CMV antigens are expressed on lung cell surfaces does not reduce the severity of the disease. In the granulocytopenic host, pulmonary CMV infection may be fatal.

Parasitic Infection

The predominant parasitic infection enhanced by immune compromise is that due to *S. stercoralis,* a nematode that infects more than 100 million people worldwide, producing lifelong infection (see Chapter 156). *Strongyloides* is distinguished by its *ability to complete the replicative cycle within the human host.* Malnutrition is a major cofactor; neutropenia and corticosteroids are common coinducers of parasite replication. In the normal pattern of infection, the filariform larvae penetrate the skin, follow the veins to the lungs, and are then swallowed, entering the small intestine. The "hyperinfection syndrome" is the result of activation in the gastrointestinal tract by immune suppression, which causes penetration or transudation of worms across the wall, carrying gastrointestinal organisms with them. Peritonitis, bacteremia, and gram-negative, eosinophilic meningitis may result. Pneumonia may result from bacteremia or from obstruction of small airways and pneumonitis; the pulmonary infection fails to resolve without therapy directed at eliminating the nematode.

CLINICAL APPROACHES TO INFECTION IN THE CANCER PATIENT

Prevention of Infection in Cancer Patients

The neutropenic patient should be managed either in a single hospital room with strict handwashing precautions or at home. Although the relative gain from the use of single rooms is small, separation of the neutropenic patient from other patients seems advisable because of increasing colonization in hospital patients and in the community by resistant organisms, particularly gram-positive bacteria, and the persistence and spread of such organisms on surfaces. Because infections may be communicated by minimal contacts from asymptomatic persons, visitors should be limited in number and the use of masks and gloves encouraged. Fresh fruits and vegetables should be eliminated from the diet. The patient should not be allowed to become constipated or dehydrated, and attention should be paid to maintenance of skin integrity. Intravenous lines and blood drawing should be minimized. Bathtubs should not be shared.

While complete precautions (laminar airflow and gowns and gloves) are useful in reducing the transmission of respiratory infections, these are hard to justify other than for the most highly immunosuppressed hosts (e.g., after chemotherapy and before bone marrow transplantation) because of their limited benefits and high costs. At institutions in which the incidence of infection due to *Aspergillus* (e.g., associated with building construction) is high and fixed, complete precautions may be helpful. Further, patients in such restrictive environments may be exposed to other sources of infection (e.g., *Legionella* in potable water) and diagnosis may be delayed, since such patients are apt to be examined less often than comparable patients without such restrictive environments. Supportive measures may include fluid and electrolyte replacement and nutritional support.

Some prophylactic measures *may* be useful (e.g., the administration of immune globulin in hypogammaglobulinemic patients, the use of hyperimmunoglobulins to prevent CMV infection, and the use of pneumococcal and *H. influenzae* vaccines in patients who will be splenectomized, who will undergo plasmapheresis, or who are predictably neutropenic (but not during chemotherapy). Loculated infection must be sought and drained; antibiotics alone will be ineffective in the presence of pus under pressure (e.g., biliary disease, appendiceal abscess). TMP-SMX prophylaxis reduces the incidence of *P. carinii* (as well as *Listeria* and *Nocardia*) to nearly zero. The use of nystatin, clotrimazole, or oral amphotericin B, especially in patients receiving broad-spectrum antibacterial therapy, has been useful in preventing oral and esophageal yeast infections. Similarly, the use of oral antifungal agents (fluconazole) has reduced the incidence of superficial *C. albicans* infections, has appeared to prevent some deep yeast infections, and has reduced the need for amphotericin therapy at some centers. As fluconazole resistance has become more prevalent, however, infections due to yeasts have increased in frequency.[64,65] Although nonabsorbable antibiotic regimens, administered by mouth, have some efficacy in preventing nosocomial pneumonias and bacteremia, their use has been associated with the emergence of resistance in bacteria and fungi of the gastrointestinal tract; moreover, they are generally unpalatable.

The quinoline antibiotics have little impact on the anaerobic component of the intestinal flora. In clinical trials and in animal models of neutropenia and immune suppression, these antibiotics have been reported to decrease the incidence of infections due to susceptible gram-negative organisms.[12] Interpretation of this decrease is difficult, however, since gram-negative infections in immunocompromised cancer patients have decreased overall. Gram-positive bacterial prophylaxis (e.g., with macrolides) is under study.[37] However, none of these regimens has been shown to increase patient survival.

Clinical Signs of Infection

Identification of the presence of infection is often delayed in the neutropenic or cancer patient because the inflammatory response is diminished (decreased numbers or mobilization of granulocytes) and the usual signs of infection are absent.[55] Thus, in neutropenic patients, pneumonia may not be associated with sputum production and radiologic changes (Fig. 136-1).[63] In one series of cancer patients with pneumonia, only 8 percent of neutropenic patients produced purulent sputum, while 84 percent of patients without neutropenia had purulent sputum.[55,59] In the febrile neutropenic patient with leukemia, the source of obscure infection is often the perineal and perirectal areas; less common are infections of the urinary tract, skin (including venous lines and wounds), and the lungs. In non-hematopoietic cancer patients, however, pulmonary infections predominate. A site of origin for a febrile episode is undetermined in 20 to 50 percent of patients. Many sites of infection are detected only at autopsy, notably in patients with disseminated fungal or combined fungal and bacterial infections (Fig. 136-4).[16] Mortality in the febrile neutropenic population is 30 to 50 percent. Noninfectious causes of fever are common; among them are pulmonary thromboembolism, tumor, radiation pneumonitis, atelectasis with pulmonary edema, drug allergy or toxicity, and pulmonary hemorrhage. Often, the resolution of fever in response to a trial of antibiotics is the only evidence of infection.

Initial Management of the Cancer Patient with Fever: Stratification of Risk

Each patient presenting with signs of infection must be evaluated in terms of the perceived risks of infection and noninfectious causes of fever and for the presence of neutropenia or other immune dysfunctions. Attempts to manage patients with greater efficiency and to shorten hospital stays have led to the development of *critical pathways*, which include standard patterns of evaluation and treatment for many patients, including those with cancer.[40] Such uniform approaches are useful in establishing a *minimal standard* of care, but they do not address concerns about the pitfalls of failing to individualize therapy.

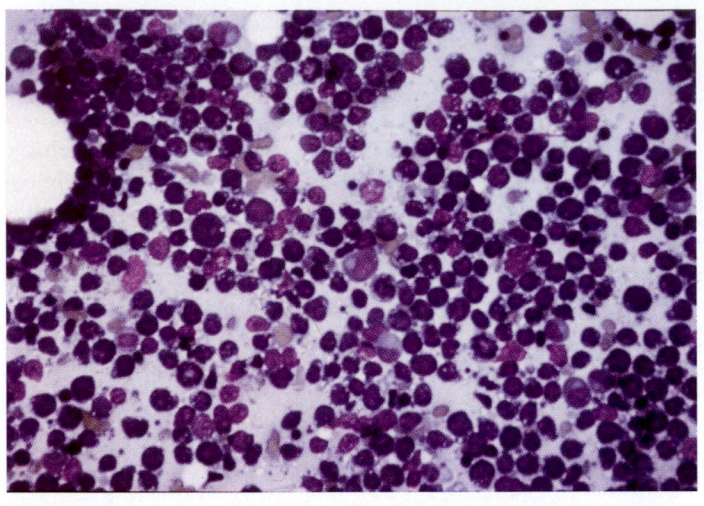

A

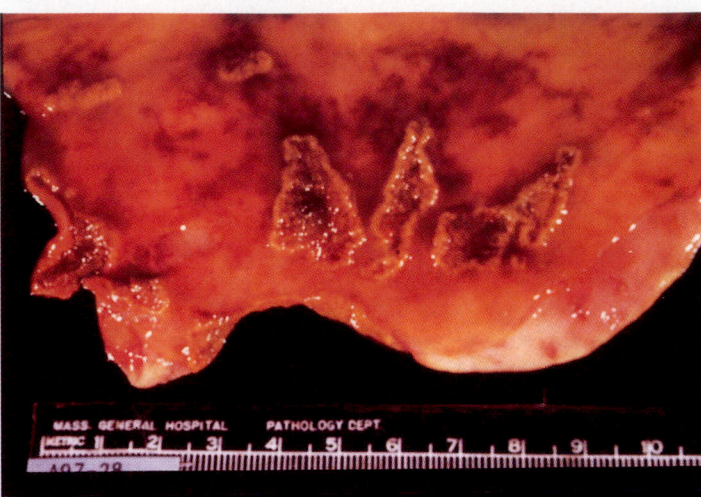

D

B

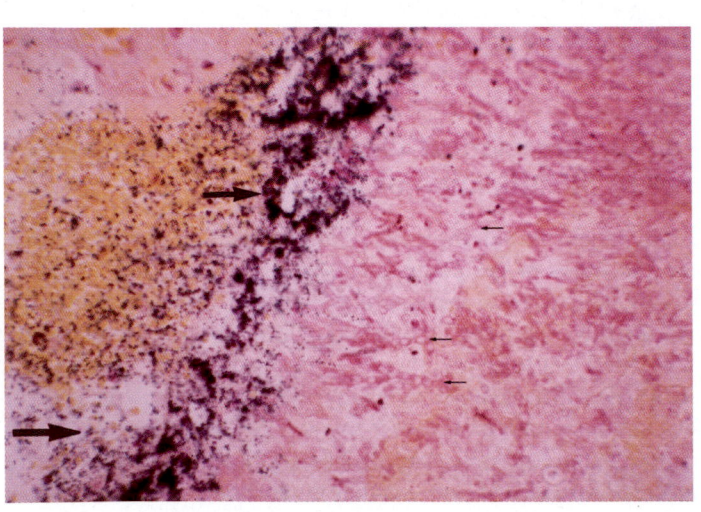

C

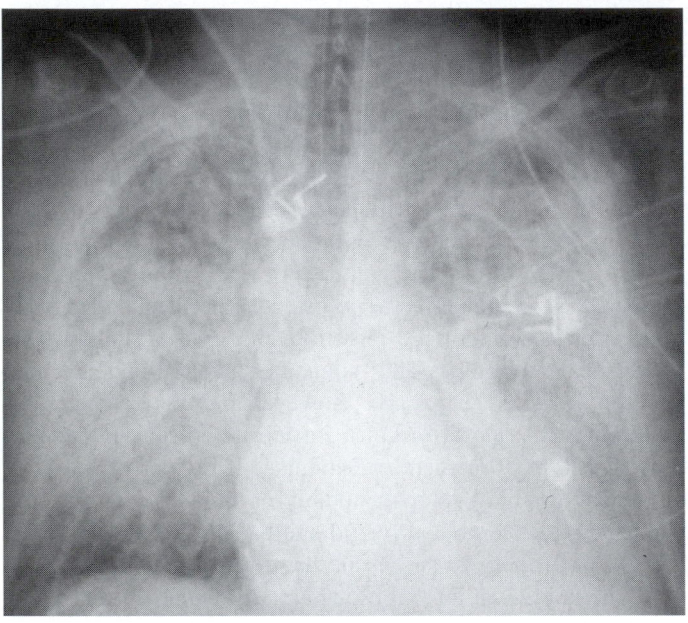

E

FIGURE 136-4 Unsuspected infection in a neutropenic patient. A 53-year-old man developed malignant Burkitt's type lymphoma *(A)* 5 years after liver transplantation. *B.* Tumor lysis following chemotherapy was acompanied by persistent neutropenia and diffuse pulmonary infiltrates. Sputum cultures revealed *E. coli. C.* Open lung biopsy revealed bacteria of a variety of morphologies *(large arrows)*, including *E. coli, Serratia marcescens*, and vancomycin-resistant *Enterococcus fecalis* by culture, and diffuse infiltration by fungi with narrow, acute-angle branched, septate hyphae *(small arrows)*, *Aspergillus fumigatus* on culture, Brown and Hopps stain). At autopsy, gastric ulcerations and serpiginous, raised plaques *(D)* were also found to contain *A. fumigatus* (*E*, methenamine silver stain).

The safe application of critical pathways for the outpatient management of neutropenic patients necessitates careful stratification of these compromised patients by experienced clinicians in terms of their risk for infectious complications. *Any sign of infection* requires at least a brief hospitalization (1 to 3 days), with careful evaluation. However, many experienced oncologists now manage most febrile neutropenic patients *routinely* as outpatients. Any febrile neutropenic patient—or patient in whom absolute neutrophil count (ANC) is expected to fall below 1000 per mm³—with localizing signs (headache, altered mental status, rash, dyspnea, chest pain, pain over an indwelling catheter site, pulmonary infiltrates) should be considered for emergency admission. In particular, patients with leukemia or lymphoma, uncontrolled metastatic cancer, recent need for antibiotics, or ANC under 100 (or expected to fall below 100) are generally considered "higher-risk" patients and are best managed as inpatients until clinically stable. Patients with a history of frank rigors or hypotension merit admission. Any febrile cancer patient needs an assessment of vital signs, oxygen saturation, complete blood count with differential, electrolytes and blood urea nitrogen and creatinine (for obstruction by tumor or acute drug toxicity), blood cultures (at least one peripheral and one from any indwelling catheter), urine sediment examination and culture, sputum Gram's-stain examination and culture, and chest radiograph. After a careful physical examination, the threshold for lumbar puncture and the determination of serum or spinal cryptococcal antigen should be low. The patient's history and medical record should be reviewed, with attention to current drugs, recent chemotherapy (especially corticosteroids), recent microbiologic data and antibiotic use, allergies, and exposures.

Empiric Use of Antibiotics in Fever and Neutropenia

After appropriate smears and cultures have been obtained, empiric antimicrobial therapy in the febrile neutropenic patient is essential, preferably within 1 to 2 h of arrival, because infection disseminates rapidly in these hosts. Awareness of the pathogens commonly encountered in different diseases and of the pathogens that are most prevalent in the particular institution are central to the proper selection of empiric therapies. Every attempt should be made to obtain specimens that will provide a microbiologic diagnosis prior to antibiotic therapy. This will minimize avoidable drug toxicities and allow the optimal selection of antibiotics. Invasive diagnosis, when clinically practical (i.e., in the absence of bleeding diathesis), should be considered *early*, since adequate specimens may not be available after the first dose of antibiotics has been administered.

The specific antibiotics selected for "routine use" in the febrile neutropenic patient remain controversial.[4,11,25,33] Ultimately, this is because many combinations appear to work equally well, and because there are few studies of various combinations in identical patient populations using the same entry and end-point criteria. The antibiotics selected must "cover" previously documented infections or surveillance culture data, physical findings, known hospital flora, and potential community exposures.

Initial therapy should assume that the organisms causing infection are likely to be resistant to prophylactic antibiotics currently in use by the patient. Many infections are loculated and require drainage (sinusitis, postobstructive pneumonitis). Patients thought to be at *low risk* for infection or other complications (nonleukemic, underlying cancer not progressing, no serious coexisting illness, no recent infections or courses of antibiotics, expected ANC to remain above 100) may be *considered* for home management after 24 h (to await blood culture data), based on the clinical assessment.[11,49,56] In these patients, empiric antibiotics might include ticarcillin (or ticarcillin-clavulanate, piperacillin with or without tazobactam, or ceftriaxone) plus gentamicin (or tobramycin or amikacin).[6,7,10,17] In medical centers in which the rate of infections with *P. aeruginosa* is minimal, a common empiric combination is cefazolin and gentamicin. However, this combination offers little coverage for *Pseudomonas*, especially in pulmonary infection;[17] therefore, it cannot be generally recommended at medical centers that have a high level of resistance of gram-negative organisms to aminoglycosides.

Patients at *high risk* for complications or progression of disease (see above) are treated with ticarcillin and gentamicin (with or without cefazolin) *or* ceftazidime and gentamicin (with or without cefazolin). Monotherapy with ceftazidime or imipenem has also been found to be effective in medical centers that do not have nosocomial flora resistant to these agents. Optimal antibiotic therapy should include synergistic therapy for *Pseudomonas* infection in medical centers in which this organism is prevalent or if the patient is profoundly neutropenic.[19] Although double coverage without synergy (e.g., two antibiotics for gram-negative organisms) does provide some insurance against possible resistance to one of the selected antibiotics, this approach affords no advantage over monotherapy with an agent to which the organism is susceptible. The routine use of quinolones or aztreonam for initial therapy in high-risk patients has not been well studied and is not recommended.[39]

In the critically ill patient, or if infection due to *S. epidermidis* or methicillin-resistant *S. aureus* is suspected, vancomycin should be added or used to replace cefazolin.[61] Such patients might include those with skin wounds, decubitus ulcers, or indwelling vascular access catheters. Gram-positive bacterial infections generally progress more slowly than do the gram-negative infections. Therefore, the *routine use* of vancomycin in these patients does not appear to be justified, because of the increased risk of vancomycin-resistant enterococci.

If an abdominal or anaerobic bacterial source is suspected, clindamycin or metronidazole can be added. Anaerobic infections other than those due to *Bacteroides fragilis* are uncommon as a source of major morbidity in these patients. Restrictions on the use of clindamycin have been instituted at many centers because of outbreaks of *C. difficile* colitis. Topical oral antifungal therapy (clotrimazole, nystatin) is commonly administered with parenteral antibiotics. Antibiotics may be adjusted on the basis of microbiologic data or if the patient is afebrile for 7 to 10 days with the ANC over 500 and increasing.

FEVER AND PULMONARY INFILTRATES

Pulmonary disease in the cancer patient is clinically challenging, owing to the large array of processes that may cause radiologic infiltrates (Table 136-4). Noninfectious causes of pulmonary infiltrates and fever (edema, cancer, radiation injury, drug toxicity, leukoagglutinin transfusion reaction, pulmonary embolus, hemorrhage, alveolar proteinosis) are common (up to 25 percent) and may closely mimic infection.[14,45] Conversely, the absence of inflammatory cells or mobilization may mask the signs of significant infection (Fig. 136-1). In the patient undergoing chemotherapy or in the neutropenic host, cough, sputum, radiologic infiltrates or cavitation, and fever may all be absent. Infection may spread to the chest from contiguous structures (e.g., per-

TABLE 136-4

Common Causes of Pneumonia in Cancer Patients Based on Radiographic Abnormalities and Disease Progression

Abnormality on Chest Radiograph	Common Cause by Rate of Disease Progression*	
	Acute (<24 h)	*Subacute-Chronic*
Consolidation	Bacteria (include *Legionella*) pulmonary embolus, hemorrhage, pulmonary edema	Fungi, *Nocardia*, tuberculosis (drug, virus [RSV], *P. carinii*, radiation)
Interstitial infiltrate	Pulmonary edema (include drug) Leukoagglutinin reaction (bacterial)	Viral, *Pneumocystis*, radiation, drug (fungi, *Nocardia*, tuberculosis, tumor)
Nodular infiltrate	Bacteria, edema (CMV, VZV)	Tumor, fungal, *Nocardia*, TB *Pneumocystis* (CMV)

*Common causes (and less common in parentheses) in the absence of specific epidemiologic exposures or past history.

foration of the esophagus due to *Aspergillus*) or may complicate anatomic changes (e.g., bronchial obstruction in lung cancer).

The consequences of pneumonia may also differ in the neutropenic host from those in the normal host: the incidence of bacteremia in children with leukemia and pneumonia is around 64 percent, whereas the frequency in normal hosts is nearly zero.[8,43,63] Up to 58 percent of patients with cancer and neutropenia have *unsuspected pulmonary infection* (i.e., untreated pneumonia) at the time of autopsy (Fig. 136-4).[8,43] Superinfection of noninfectious lung processes is common, especially in intubated patients. Mortality approaches 100 percent in patients who are receiving corticosteroids as a part of cancer therapy, and who present with arterial hypoxemia (Pa_{O_2} under 50 mmHg) and require assisted mechanical ventilation.[43]

Microbiology of Pneumonia

The etiology of infectious pneumonitis in cancer patients is diverse.[45] The isolated organisms include conventional bacteria (37 percent), fungi (14 percent), viruses (15 percent), *P. carinii* (8 percent), *N. asteroides* (7 percent), *M. tuberculosis* (1 percent), and mixed infections (20 percent). The incidence and severity of pneumonia change, depending on the geographic area and nosocomial exposures, the types of cancer and intensity of chemotherapy, the duration of neutropenia, and previous infections and antibiotic use. Aspiration remains an important source of pulmonary infection in cancer patients (Fig. 136-2). Nosocomial pneumonias in the neutropenic host often occur because of microaspiration of colonizing organisms from the oropharynx. These include oral anaerobic flora and nosocomial gram-negative organisms that have colonized the patient only recently (within 3 to 5 days of hospitalization). Among these are *Pseudomonas* and the Enterobacteriaceae. H_2-blocking antacids and enteral feedings favor gastric colonization with nosocomial gram-negative organisms; these may extend to the trachea and contribute to nosocomial pneumonia. Bacterial and fungal

superinfection can occur during or following infection with community acquired viruses, including influenza, parainfluenza, pertussis, adenovirus, and respiratory syncytial virus.

Arterial hypoxemia, with minimal radiographic findings (accompanied by an increase in serum), is common in *P. carinii* infection. By contrast, arterial hypoxemia (until late in the disease) in conjunction with pulmonary consolidation is uncommon in nocardiosis, tuberculosis, and fungal infections. Metastases of pulmonary infections are sometimes diagnosed more readily than the original pulmonary infections. For example, skin lesions or cerebrospinal fluid often demonstrates *Nocardia* or *Cryptococcus* before sputum or lung biopsy specimens are available. Hematogenous spread from elsewhere in the body (line sepsis, hepatosplenic candidiasis) can produce peripheral lesions in the lungs (*S. aureus, Candida tropicalis, C. albicans, Aspergillus*) as a signal of important extrapulmonary disease.

Radiologic Clues to Diagnosis

A number of clues are available to assist in the differential diagnosis of pulmonary infiltrates in cancer patients. For example, the clinical and radiographic appearance and progression of disease may suggest a diagnosis based on the time course and nature of the infiltrate (Table 136-4). In general, acute processes include both bacterial infections and noninfectious injuries, such as pulmonary embolus or edema. Subacute processes include *P. carinii*, viral, *Mycoplasma*, or *Nocardia* or *Aspergillus* infections. More chronic processes include drug-induced, radiation-induced, mycobacterial, nocardial, or malignant invasion of the lungs.

In particular, bronchial obstruction by tumor or enlarged lymph nodes may cause atelectasis or postobstructive pneumonia. The underlying process may be suggested by a pneumonia that either fails to respond to antibiotic therapy or recurs in the same location after successful treatment. Tumor masses, especially those due to lymphoma, may cavitate, giving the appearance of a lung abscess. Finally, it is important to bear in mind that a chronic process may be superinfected by an acute bacterial, viral, or drug-induced lung injury.

The clinical assessment coupled with the radiologic pattern of lung disease is usually the basis for forming a differential diagnosis for the patient with fever and pneumonitis. Computed tomography (CT scans) has greatly improved differentiation of some processes. For example, in patients with simultaneous processes affecting the lung (e.g., aspiration and tumor), CT scans may disclose distinctive patterns of parenchymal involvement (consolidation and infiltrative lesions with associated adenopathy) better than do conventional chest radiographs. Intrathoracic complications of bone marrow transplantation are found by CT scans in 57 percent of patients in whom routine radiographs are negative.[26] Subtle interstitial infiltrates (*P. carinii*) or nodules (*Cryptococcus*) are better detected by CT scans than by conventional radiographs. Similarly, the response of infection to therapy is better assessed by CT scans than by conventional chest radiographs.

Noninfectious Pneumonitis

After a dose of radiation greater than 2000 rads, radiation injury is common. The injury may become evident either acutely or more than 6 months after the initial exposure. The acute form of radiation pneumonitis may present as a bronchitis or esophagitis with dry cough, fever, fatigue, hypoxemia, and dyspnea that develop over 6 to 12 weeks. The histologic picture reveals vascular damage, mononuclear infiltrates, and edema. The severity of lung injury due to radiation appears to correlate with the rapidity of the withdrawal of steroid therapy, but it may also reflect the emergence of the underlying inflammatory response. Radiation fibrosis usually occurs in 6 to 9 months, and pulmonary function may take up to 2 years to plateau.

Acute, drug-induced lung disease may reflect hypersensitivity to chemotherapeutic agents or to sulfonamide agents. Methotrexate, bleomycin, and procarbazine can cause a syndrome of nonproductive cough, fever, dyspnea, and pleurisy with skin rash and blood eosinophilia. Chest radiographs demonstrate diffuse reticular infiltrates. Cytoxan may cause a syndrome of subacute pulmonary disease with interstitial inflammation and pulmonary fibrosis. Fever, as well as dyspnea, fatigue, and cough, are common in cytoxan lung. Other common drugs causing lung injury are cytarabine and azathioprine (Table 121-3). Drug toxicity for agents such as bleomycin, BCNU, and CCNU may be related to the cumulative dose (for bleomycin, over 450 mg) and to the age of the patient. Synergistic toxicity for the lung occurs between radiation and a variety of chemotherapeutic agents (e.g., bleomycin, mitomycin, busulfan) and supplemental oxygen use.

A variety of noninfectious processes may mimic infection. Alveolar proteinosis may be associated with hematologic malignancies or accompany infection due to *Nocardia* or, less often, *Cryptococcus*, *Aspergillus*, *M. tuberculosis*, and *Histoplasma*. Pulmonary infarction may mimic infections by causing hemoptysis, leukocytosis, pleuritic chest pain, and segmental pleural-based infiltrates on the chest radiograph. Primary connective-tissue–collagen vascular diseases may present in the same way (i.e., fever, dyspnea, pulmonary infiltrates). They may also coexist with infectious diseases of the lungs. These patients often receive immunosuppressive therapies and are susceptible to the same infections (though generally less severe) as cancer chemotherapy patients. In particular, the infections include aspiration pneumonia, *P. carinii* pneumonia, Legionnaires' disease, CMV, and colonization or superinfection of devitalized lung tissues with *Aspergillus* and *Candida* species. Systemic lupus erythematosis is associated with parenchymal lesions that range from transient infiltrates to interstitial infiltrates or frank consolidation. The pulmonary-renal syndromes (e.g., Goodpasture's syndrome and Wegener's granulomatosis) may manifest pulmonary hemorrhage, consolidation, nodular lesions, and patchy infiltrates that may progress to cavitation. Sarcoidosis is generally associated with hilar lymph node enlargement and intersti-

tial infiltrates, but nodular disease and superinfection are common. Treatment of rheumatic disease with penicillamine, gold salts, or anti-inflammatory agents may cause acute or chronic reticulonodular pulmonary infiltrates that are associated with fever, dyspnea, and cough.

Adult respiratory distress syndrome is usually the result of severe pneumonia or may complicate extrapulmonary infectious or inflammatory processes. Although transfusion-associated leukoagglutinin reactions are uncommon, minor, transient pulmonary infiltrates often occur after transfusions or globulin infusions.

Microbiologic Evaluation of the Cancer Patient with Fever and Pneumonitis

In general, sputum examination is a necessary first step in the initial evaluation of the cancer patient who presents with fever and pneumonitis. Whether induced sputum is more informative than routine sputum specimens is still unsettled other than for *P. carinii* or mycobacterial infections.[23] In essence, although empiric therapy is appropriate in the absence of known causes of fever, pulmonary samples must be obtained in the febrile neutropenic cancer patient. Tissues for microbiology and histopathology are best obtained early, when the patient is most likely to tolerate these procedures. Peripheral lesions can be approached through needle aspirates or thoracoscopic biopsies, whereas more central lesions can be sampled with the bronchoscope or by mediastinoscopy (Fig. 136-4). Few histologic patterns are pathognomonic for given infectious agents. For example, granulomatous lesions, with or without "caseation" or necrosis, may be seen in many disorders, including tuberculosis, cryptococcosis, histoplasmosis, coccidioidomycosis, blastomycosis, Wegener's disease, sarcoidosis, syphilis, and cat-scratch disease. The mix of acute and granulomatous responses will vary with the level of immune function of the host. Similarly, necrotizing pneumonia may be seen in any of the common bacterial (*S. aureus*, *S. pneumoniae*, *Legionella* species, *P. aeruginosa*, *Klebsiella pneumoniae*), fungal (*Aspergillus*, Mucoraceae), or viral (CMV, adenovirus) pneumonias. Histologic clues to the identity of the pathogen may include the presence of infected macrophages (*Legionella* and CMV) in the inflammatory exudates.

Empiric Antibiotics for Pneumonia

The greatest unknown factor in the care of the patient with cancer or neutropenia is the timing of the return of immune function to "normal." At that time, the patient is at greatest risk for common community-acquired pathogens (see Chapter 127). Empiric therapy is then aimed at treating the infections that are likely to have high morbidity in the first 24 h of illness. Any of the regimens discussed previously would be appropriate for most of the common bacterial causes of pulmonary infection.

In acute pulmonary infections in the neutropenic host, in addition to the empiric regimens discussed above, suspicion of *P. carinii* or *Nocardia* should prompt the addition of TMP-SMX. Suspicion of infection due to mycoplasma, *Legionella*, *Chlamydia pneumoniae* (formerly strain TWAR), or pertussis merits empiric therapy with a macrolide while evaluation is under way (blood and sputum cultures including plating on buffered charcoal-yeast extract, urinary antigen for *L. pneumophila* type I, direct fluorescent antigen [DFA]). Evaluation for primary viral pneumonia (influenza A and respiratory syncytial viruses by DFA, HSV and CMV cultures, rarely infectious mononucleosis) or bacterial superinfection of viral pneumonia may be performed concurrently.

Infections in the central nervous system should raise the prospect of treating with either ampicillin (*Listeria monocytogenes*) or acyclovir (HSV or VZV). *Aspergillus, Mucor, Nocardia,* tuberculosis, and *Legionella* may present with neurologic symptoms (headache, seizures, cranial nerve deficits, tremors, focal deficits) in addition to rapidly progressive pneumonia with metastatic infection (Fig. 136-3). *Aspergillus* or *Mucor* infections, and any sinus infections, may require radical surgical débridement and drainage for cure. *Strongyloides* is associated with gram-negative meningitis and postobstructive pneumonia.

In patients known to be at risk for CMV infection, ganciclovir therapy may be initiated while cultures or blood antigenemia or PCR assays are pending. Granulocyte-macrophage colony–stimulating factor has been used with ganciclovir in the successful management of cancer, bone marrow transplantation, and neutropenic patients with CMV infections. The increasing incidence of tuberculosis may suggest antituberculous therapy in patients with epidemiologic risk for this infection.

APPROACH TO PATIENTS ON EMPIRIC THERAPY

Cancer patients with fever or documented infection need frequent physical examinations (e.g., twice each day). Particular attention must be paid to the presence of injury to mucosal surfaces and to gingivitis, perirectal tenderness, abdominal pain, oral or vaginal HSV, shingles, and cellulitis (especially abdominal wall or extremity crepitance). *C. difficile* colitis must be considered in the differential diagnosis of immunocompromised patients who have received any antibiotics. Fever unresponsive to antibacterial therapy may be due to drug toxicity or to resistant organisms, particularly fungal infection. All skin lesions should be biopsied for histology and cultures, with particular concern about such pulmonary pathogens as *Cryptococcus, Aspergillus,* and *Nocardia.* Daily blood cultures may be helpful in assessing persistent fevers. Pathogens identified after the initiation of empiric antibiotic therapy may represent either the progression of the original infection or colonization and superinfection during antibiotic therapy. Antibiotic coverage may need to be broadened (see below). The need to change venous access lines should be assessed daily. Precautions (other than mask and handwashing) are not useful without a fully protected laminar airflow environment. Patients with negative cultures and lysis of fever by 48 h after admission may qualify for home therapy if there is no evidence of pneumonia or other focal infection, if the ANC is greater than 100 and rising, and if a mechanism exists for close follow-up care by a physician.

The duration of empiric therapy must be individualized.[20,57] In a patient receiving empiric therapy who becomes afebrile on antibiotics by 72 h and with a neutrophil count above 500 per mm³, the antibiotics may be stopped after 7 days and the patient reevaluated if no localizing source is found or untreated pathogens

detected. Patients who are clinically well and who become afebrile with neutrophil counts of 100 to 500 per mm³ should be afebrile for 5 to 7 days before antibiotics are stopped in order to reevaluate sources of infection. If the patient is not clinically well (e.g., has mucositis, fewer than 100 neutrophils per mm³, or unstable vital signs), the antibiotics should be continued until the patient is stable and afebrile for 48 to 72 h.

Unless a specific source of infection is located and the pathogen(s) identified, patients with persistent fever and neutropenia should have antibiotics broadened 48 to 72 h after the start of therapy. The options include (1) addition of vancomycin (or other gram-positive agent); (2) addition of antianaerobic therapy for oral mucositis or gingivitis, abdominal pain, or perirectal tenderness; (3) expansion of gram-negative bacterial coverage (generally adding a second agent from a different class of antibiotics); (4) consideration of antiviral therapy in patients with esophagitis or a history of HSV or VZV infections; and (5) addition of fluconazole or amphotericin B for symptoms of esophagitis or for documented or suspected fungal infection.[21,31] In general, the first dose of amphotericin B should be a full dose (0.6 to 0.8 mg/kg for yeasts, 1.0 to 1.5 mg/kg for suspected *Aspergillus* or *Mucor* infections) diluted in at least 250-ml solution and given slowly (4 h minimum) with premedication with acetaminophen. The patient must be well hydrated, and attention must be paid to magnesium and potassium maintenance. Premedication may include corticosteroids (25 to 50 mg of hydrocortisone intravenously or in the bottle) for patients who develop chills or fever. Slowly advancing doses of this drug (e.g., from a starting dose of 10 to 20 mg) have been advocated without much supporting data and entail the disadvantage of *days of delay* in achieving tissue levels of the drug.

Hepatosplenic candidiasis or endocarditis may require prolonged courses of treatment. The duration of therapy can be determined only after complete resolution of the clinical disease. In some centers, antifungal therapy is initiated with fluconazole early in the course of treatment (3 to 4 days), especially for known esophageal candidiasis or oral thrush, with the accepted risk of infection by fungi that are resistant to this agent. Itraconazole is useful in some *Aspergillus* infections, but it is not the preferred agent for management of the acutely ill patient with underlying immune deficits.

Studies and anecdotal reports of therapy using the liposomal preparations of amphotericin have demonstrated "complete responses to therapy" (needed in compromised hosts) in only 10 to 20 percent of patients not previously treated with standard amphotericin B. Available pharmacokinetic data do not address the extent to which the liposomal preparations penetrate the orbit, central nervous system, sinuses, peritoneal dialysis fluid, or bone, although the apparent penetration into the liver, spleen, and lungs is good. Clinical responses appear to be slower with liposomal preparations than with the parent drug. Fluconazole can be used for susceptible yeasts (starting doses of 400 to 800 mg may be needed), and itraconazole or liposomal amphotericin may replace amphotericin B after a clinical response is obtained ("mopping up") or significant renal dysfunction (e.g., creatinine over 3.0) occurs. Thus, after cultures of all possible sites are obtained, amphotericin B is started in the persistently febrile neutropenic patient (often days 5 to 7).

Special attention must be paid to any symptoms of pulmonary disease, the presence of new pulmonary infiltrates on chest radiographs, or the presence of sinus symptoms in patients with persistent fevers. New infiltrates should prompt examinations of sputum and procurement of specimens (open biopsy, thoracoscopic biopsy, or bronchoscopy, preferably with biopsies, or needle aspirates under tomographic guidance) for histologic and microbiologic evaluation.

CYTOKINES IN CANCER AND NEUTROPENIA

The immune system includes a diverse population of cells that communicate with each other via a series of soluble protein mediators called cytokines. These proteins include growth factors or colony-stimulating factors, interleukins, interferons, and chemokines. The effects of the individual factors are local (autocrine and paracrine) as well as systemic (endocrine). These factors mediate normal processes and beneficial responses to injury, as well as many of the detrimental effects of infection and injury that may be seen in sepsis leading to multiorgan system dysfunction and adult respiratory distress syndrome.

Because many of the effects of the various factors are overlapping and competitive, and many factors induce the synthesis and release of further mediators, the therapeutic use of these factors, or of inhibitors of these factors, is complex. Many of the receptors and intracellular mediators of cytokine activity are incompletely characterized. However, the use of recombinant growth factors in the repopulation of hematopoietic cells in neutropenic patients (e.g., after chemotherapy) has become routine, if excessive.[1,1a] Use of the same factors in the activation of cells of the immune system to enhance the host response to infection appears promising.

The Cytokines

Interferon-gamma (IFN-γ) is produced by type I CD4 cells, natural killer (NK) cells, and some CD8 cells. The biologic action of IFN-γ is the activation of macrophages with enhanced killing of intracellular pathogens, increased NK cell activity, increased expression of Fc receptors on monocytes and neutrophils and of MHC antigens, and increased antibody-mediated cytotoxicity. IFN-γ has been useful in enhancing immune responses to infections due to *P. carinii, Candida, Histoplasma, Cryptococcus, Blastomyces,* and *L. monocytogenes* in in vitro and some in vivo studies. Side effects include fever, chills, myalgias, headache, and some skin rashes. IFN-γ is used in the treatment of hepatitis B and C, with limited success in subgroups of patients. *IFN-α* and *IFN-β* have been used in the treatment of malignancies, but they were first recognized as inhibitors of viral proliferation. IFN-α is produced by leukocytes (monocytes, NK cells, lymphocytes), and IFN-β is produced by fibroblasts. Binding of these molecules to a cell surface receptor results in the production of many molecules that have antimicrobial (antiviral), antiproliferative, and immunomodulatory properties, including the up-regulation of class I and II major histocompatibility antigens on the cell surface. These molecules may produce elevations in hepatic enzymes, neutropenia, and flulike symptoms, including fever and chills, which decrease over time. Cardiac arrhythmias and seizures have also been observed.

Granulocyte colony–stimulating factor (G-CSF), granulocyte-macrophage colony–stimulating factor (GM-CSF), and monocyte-macrophage colony–stimulating factor (M-CSF) are hematopoietic growth factors that are critical for the growth and differentiation of granulocytic and monocytic cell lineages. G-CSF is produced by monocyte/macrophage cells, endothelial cells, and fibroblasts; it stimulates the proliferation, differentiation, and activation of granulocyte precursors. Endotoxin (lipopolysaccharide) and inflammatory cytokines (TNF-α, IFN-γ, interleukins 1, 3, and 4, and GM-CSF) induce secretion of G-CSF. After a brief (up to 1 h) drop in the white blood cell count, G-CSF causes rapid (within 36 h) increase in neutrophil counts due to the demargination of cells and the release of cells from the marrow reserves, followed by a shortening of the maturation time in the production of new hematopoietic cells. G-CSF increases the activation of neutrophils (phagocytosis, endocytosis, O_2 generation, LAP production, IgG receptor expression, increased adhesion factor affinity) and peripheral blood progenitor cells.[47] The drug is well tolerated and seldom produces bone pain, Sweet's syndrome, or allograft rejection.

GM-CSF is produced by activated T lymphocytes, monocytes, fibroblasts, and endothelial cells after exposure to endotoxin, inflammatory cytokines, and lectins. GM-CSF is an earlier factor than G-CSF in the stimulation of proliferation, differentiation, and activation of both monocyte and neutrophil cell lineages. In addition to the effects of G-CSF, the effects of GM-CSF on monocytes and eosinophils include increased survival, shortened maturation time, decreased migration and motility, and improved destruction of intracellular organisms (*T. cruzi, Mycobacterium avium* complex, influenza A, *Candida*).

GM-CSF (available for subcutaneous, intravenous, and oral use) is often associated with mild to moderate bone pain and fever and myalgias, skin rashes, hepatic transaminase elevation, and decreased cholesterol levels, and uncommonly with thrombotic events and capillary leak syndrome (over 30 µg/kg per day). GM-CSF is also associated with increased production of TNF-α, increased replication of HIV-1, and growth of Kaposi's sarcoma cells in vitro.[29] Of note, recombinant preparations made in yeast and *E. coli* hosts may not be equivalent in terms of efficicy or side effects.

M-CSF is synthesized by monocytes, fibroblasts, and endothelial cells and acts to increase the proliferation, differentiation, and activation of monocytes and macrophages. Limited experience with M-CSF demonstrates some myalgias and fevers as for GM-CSF, but the factor is well tolerated in general.

Interleukin 2 (IL-2) is produced by T cells and activates T cells, NK cells, and macrophages (the last via TNF-α and IFN-γ). This cytokine has been used in the treatment of malignancy, but dosage is limited by the occurrence of fevers, chills, neutropenia, thrombocytopenia, anemia, and a high incidence of intravenous catheter–related bacterial infections, which appear to be due to an *IL-2–induced neutrophil chemotaxis defect.*[28,36] This defect may be TNF mediated and may be *reduced* by corticosteroids or by the administration of IL-2 covalently linked to polyethylene glycol 80. While receiving IL-2 therapy, some patients develop fluffy pulmonary infiltrates, which may progress to severe pulmonary edema. This complication is due to a systemic capillary leak syndrome that can be fatal if unrecognized.

Interleukin 3 (IL-3) is produced by T lymphocytes and NK cells in response to endotoxin, TNF-α, and IL-1. IL-3 stimulates many hematopoietic cell types, including pleuripotent marrow progenitors (stem cells), resulting in the production of the full range of hematopoietic cells. Of note, this factor may be useful in enhancing the engraftment of transplanted bone marrow and may be central to the induction of tolerance to allogeneic transplants.

Some Clinical Applications of the Cytokines

IFN-α has been used in the treatment of hepatitis B and hepatitis C, and results in increased numbers of CD8$^+$ cells in the liver and up-regulation of HLA class I expression. Trials of IFN-α and IL-2 in HIV infection have suggested synergy with zidovudine. IFN-α and IFN-β have been used to prevent the activation and dissemination of VZV infection in neutropenic patients and hematopoietic malignancies. They have also been used in infections due to HSV, but have not been fully compared with current antiviral agents (acyclovir, ganciclovir). IFN-β has qualitatively similar effects to IFN-α, but definitive studies are not available. IFN-γ has been used successfully in the treatment of chronic granulomatous disease and leprosy. Some cytokines (IL-12, MCSF, IFN-α) have some degree of synergy with antifungal agents for fungal infections.

Immune Prophylaxis in Neutropenia

Cytokines have come into routine use in the management of patients with neutropenia and in enhancing the maturation of cells following recovery or engraftment of bone marrow.[1,1a,62] The early-activating cytokines (IL-3, GM-CSF, and stem cell factor) are lineage nonspecific and act locally, so circulating levels are not of great importance for efficacy. The later-acting factors (G-CSF, M-CSF, and thrombopoietin and erythropoietin) affect the later stages of maturation of cells and the release of cells from the marrow, are lineage specific, prevent cellular apoptosis, and act systemically, with circulating levels important for efficacy. All these factors work at very low concentrations via specific cell surface receptors. Under normal conditions, a feedback loop will increase the level of the growth factors in response to cellular deficiency. Acute infection increases the production of GM-CSF and G-CSF.

GM-CSF amd G-CSF have come into routine use in the prevention of infections due to neutropenia. In cancer chemotherapy–induced neutropenia, these factors reduce the duration of neutropenia, may raise the nadir of white blood cell counts after chemotherapy, and may reduce the number of febrile days, the number of days of hospitalization, the incidence of mucositis, the use of antibiotics, and the number of documented infections.[1,3,18,27,32,42,53] An effect on improving mucosal barrier integrity may be central to the efficacy of these factors. In patients with acute myelogenous leukemia who are over 55 years old, GM-CSF decreases the numbers of deaths and infections.[48] IFN-α, G-CSF, and GM-CSF have been useful in the reversal of immune suppression and neutropenia due to CMV and ganciclovir therapy. Benefits other than the reversal of antibiotic-induced neutropenia treatment in CMV infection are not yet documented.

Similar benefits of the growth factors have been seen in the treatment of the cyclic neutropenias, myelodysplastic syndromes, drug-induced neutropenias, and aplastic anemias. IL-3 has also been shown to induce production of neutrophils, platelets, and reticulocytes, but the onset of action is more delayed. A fusion protein of GM-CSF and IL-3 has been made that mimics the effects of both agents (PIXY 321). These factors also appear to be useful in the treatment of established infections due to bacteria and fungi.[2,5] In particular, M-CSF has been used with beneficial results in the treatment of fungal infections (*Candida* and *Aspergillus* species and *P. carinii*) in vitro, and in cancer chemotherapy and neutropenic patients. IL-10 also modulates monocyte activity in *Aspergillus* infection in vitro,[46] whereas IL-12 has been proposed for use in the treatment of tuberculosis with multidrug-resistant strains of *M. tuberculosis*.[41]

Concern has been expressed about the observed activation of HIV replication by GM-CSF and M-CSF, the increased growth of some leukemic cell clones, and the expansion of some clones of cancer cells in patients with myelodysplastic syndromes.

FRONTIERS OF IMMUNE RECONSTITUTION

The limited availability of marrow donors has hindered the development of bone marrow transplantation (BMT) to reverse neutropenia and to establish normal immune function in the cancer chemotherapy patient after ablative therapies. The use of BMT in patients infected with viruses (HIV, hepatitis, CMV) has been used to induce virus-specific immune responses (via CD8$^+$ lymphocytes activated in vitro with target antigens) for the treatment and prevention of infection. Further interest has developed in the use of xenotransplantation, or transplantation across species lines (e.g., from swine or nonhuman primates), in the treatment of chronic viral infections to provide immunocompetent cells (neutrophils and lymphocytes) that cannot be infected by the viruses because of the absence of the receptors or intracellular mechanisms needed to infect these cells and to propagate—i.e., resistance to infection at the cellular level.[23a] The critical feature of such disparate transplants, whether across human histocompatibility barriers or between species, is the *ability to regain normal immune function* without developing graft-versus-host disease or the need for excessive exogenous immune suppression.

Barriers to the multilineage engraftment of donor marrow, especially for mismatched or cross-species donors, include the need for the appropriate thymic environment to "educate" the new cells, the creation of "space" (e.g., marrow irradiation or high doses of donor cells) for the engraftment of long-lived, pleuripotent stem cells, the species-appropriate cytokines (growth factors), and adhesion molecules for the growth of donor cells versus those of the recipient and the appropriate tests for the immune competence of engrafted cells. In particular, it is unclear whether donor lymphocytes will function in the MHC-mismatched environment in which the carbohydrate antigens of the MHC groups are disparate. Although these barriers remain to be overcome, significant progress has been made in the development of BMT as a potential therapy for cancer, neutropenia, and viral infections that are currently unresponsive to more traditional forms of treatment.

REFERENCES

1. American Society of Clinical Oncology: Recommendations for the use of hematopoietic colony–stimulating factors: Evidence-based, clinical practice guidelines. *J Clin Oncol* 12:2471–2508, 1994.

1a. American Society of Clinical Oncology: Update of recommendations for the use of hematopoietic colony-stimulating factors: Evidence-based, clinical practice guidelines. *J Clin Oncol* 14(6): 1957–1960, 1996.

2. Anaissie E, Bodey G, O'Brien S, et al: Effects of granulocyte macrophage colony–stimulating factor on myelopoiesis and disseminated mycoses in neutropenic patients with hematologic malignancies (abstract). *Blood* 74:15A, 1989.

3. Antman K, Gale RP: Advanced breast cancer: High-dose chemotherapy and bone marrow auto-transplants. *Ann Intern Med* 108:570–574, 1988.

4. Armstrong D: Empiric therapy for the immunocompromised host. *Rev Infect Dis* 13(Suppl 9):S763–S769, 1991.

5. Biesma B, deVries E, Willemse P, et al: Efficacy and tolerability of recombinant human granulocyte macrophage colony–stimulating factor in patients with chemotherapy-related leukopenia and fever. *Eur J Cancer* 26:932–936, 1990.

6. Blanch C, Pollet J, Bauters F: Ceftriaxone plus amikacin in neutropenic patients: A report on 100 cases. *Chemotherapy* 37: 382–388, 1991.

7. Bodey G, Alvarez M, Jones P, et al: Imipenem-cilastatin as initial therapy for febrile cancer patients. *Antimicrob Agents Chemother* 30:211–214, 1986.

8. Bodey G, Buckley M, Sathe Y, et al: Quantitative relationships between circulating leukocytes and infection in patients with acute leukemia. *Ann Intern Med* 64:328–340, 1966.

9. Bodey G, Rodriguez V, Chang H, et al: Fever and infection in leukemic patients: A study of 494 consecutive patients. *Cancer* 41:1610–1622, 1978.

10. Bolton-Maggs PH, van Saene HK, McDowell HP, Martin J: Clinical evaluation of ticarcillin, with clavulanic acid, and gentamicin in the treatment of febrile episodes in neutropenic children. *J Antimicrob Chemother* 27:669–676, 1991.

11. Buchanan GR: Approach to treatment of the febrile cancer patient with low-risk neutropenia. *Hematol Oncol Clin North Am* 7: 919–935, 1993.

12. Carratalá J, Fernández-Sevilla A, Tubau F, et al: Emergence of quinolone-resistant *Escherichia coli* bacteremia in neutropenic patients with cancer who have received prophylactic norfloxacin. *Clin Infect Dis* 20:557–560, 1995.

13. Casazza A, Duvall C, Carbone P: Infection in lymphoma: Histology, treatment and duration in relation to incidence and survival. *JAMA* 197:710–716, 1966.

14. Chanock S: Evolving risk factors for infectious complications of cancer therapy. *Hematol Oncol Clin North Am* 7:771–795, 1993.

15. Cline MJ: Defective mononuclear phagocyte function in myelomonocytic leukemia and in some patients with lymphoma. *J Clin Invest* 52:2815–2819, 1973.

16. Coker DD, Morris DM, Coleman JJ, et al: Infection among 210 patients with surgically staged Hodgkin's disease. *Am J Med* 97:109–115, 1983.

17. Cornelissen J, Graeff A, Dekker A, et al: Imipenem versus gentamicin combined with either cefuroxime or cephalothin as initial therapy for febrile neutropenic patients. *Antimicrob Agents Chemother* 36:801–807, 1992.

18. Crawford J, Ozer H, Stoller R, et al: Reduction by granulocyte colony-stimulating factor of fever and neutropenia induced by chemotherapy in patients with small-cell lung cancer. *New Engl J Med* 325:164–170, 1991.

19. de Jongh C, Joshi J, Newman K, et al: Antibiotic synergism and response in gram-negative bacteremia in granulocytopenic patients with fever and neutropenia. *Amer J Med* 80:96–100, 1986.

20. DiNubile M: Stopping antibiotic therapy in neutropenic patients. *Ann Intern Med* 108:289–292, 1988.

21. Ellis M, Halim M, Spence D, Ernst P: Systemic amphotericin B versus fluconazole in the management of antibiotic resistant neutropenic fever—Preliminary observations from a pilot, exploratory study. *J Infect* 30:141–146, 1995.

22. Feld R, Bodey G, Rodriguez V, et al: Causes of death in patients with malignant lymphoma. *Am J Med Sci* 268:97–106, 1974.

23. Fishman JA, Roth RS, Zanzot E, et al: The use of induced sputum specimens for the microbiologic diagnosis of infection due to organisms other than *Pneumocystis carinii*. *J Clin Microbiol* 32: 131–134, 1994.

23a. Fishman JA: Xenosis and xenotransplantation: Addressing the infectious risks posed by an emerging technology. *Kidney Int* 51(Suppl 58): 41–45, 1997.

24. Fleisher G, Henry W, McSorley M, et al: Life-threatening complications of varicella. *Am J Dis Child* 135:896–899, 1981.

25. Giamarellou H: Empiric therapy for infectious in the febrile, neutropenic, compromised host. *Med Clin North Am* 79:559–580, 1995.

26. Graham N, Muller N, Miller R, et al: Intrathoracic complications following allogeneic bone marrow transplantation: CT findings. *Radiology* 181:153–156, 1991.

27. Grosh W, Quesenberry P: Recombinant human hematopoietic growth factors in the treatment of cytopenias. *Clin Immunol Immunopathol* 62(Suppl):S25–S38, 1992.

28. Hardy J, Moore J, Lorentzos A, et al: Infectious complications of interleukin 2 therapy (letter). *Cytokine* 2:311, 1990.

29. Hermans P, Gori A, Lemone M, et al: Possible role of granulocyte–macrophage colony stimulating factor (GM–CSF) on the rapid progression of AIDS-related Kaposi's sarcoma lesions in vivo. *Br J Haematol* 87:413–414, 1994.

30. Hersh E, Bodey G, Nies B, et al: Causes of death in acute leukemia: A ten-year study of 414 patients from 1954–1963. *JAMA* 193: 105–109, 1965.

31. Holleran W, Wilbur J, DeGregorio W: Empiric amphotericin B therapy in patients with acute leukemia. *Rev Infect Dis* 7:619–624, 1989.

32. Hollingshead L, Goa K: Recombinant granulocyte colony–stimulating factor: A review of its pharmacological properties and prospective role in neutropenic conditions. *Drugs* 42:300–330, 1991.

33. Hughes W: Guidelines for the use of antimicrobial agent in neutropenic patients with unexplained fever. *J Infect Dis* 161:381–396, 1995.

34. Kaplan MH, Armstrong D, Rosen PP: Tuberculosis complicating neoplastic disease: A review of 201 cases. *Cancer* 33:850–858, 1974.

35. King GW, Yanes B, Hurtubise PE, et al: Immune function of successfully treated lymphoma patients. *J Clin Invest* 57:1451–1460, 1976.

36. Klempner M, Noring R, Mier J, Atkins M: An acquired chemotactic defect in neutrophils from patients receiving interleukin-2 immunotherapy. *New Engl J Med* 322:959–965, 1990.

37. Kotilainen P, Nikoskelainen J, Huovinen P: Emergence of ciprofloxacin-resistant coagulase-negative staphylococcal skin flora in immunocompromised patients receiving ciprofloxacin. *J Infect Dis* 161:41–44, 1990.

38. Lehrer RI, Cline MJ: Leukocyte candicidal activity and resistance to systemic candidiasis in patients with cancer. *Cancer* 27: 1211–1217, 1972.

39. Malik I, Abbas Z, Karim M: Randomized comparison of oral ofloxacin along with combination of parenteral antibiotics in neutropenic febrile patients. *Lancet* 339:1092–1096, 1992.

40. Malik I, Khan W, Karim M, et al: Feasibility of outpatient management of fever in cancer patients with low-risk neutropenia: Results of a prospective randomized trial. *Am J Med* 98:224–231, 1995.

41. McDyer J, Hackley M, Walsh T, et al: Patients with multidrug-resistant tuberculosis with low CD4+ T cell counts have impaired Th1 responses. *J Immunol* 158:492–500, 1997.

42. Nemunaitis M, Rosenfeld CS, Ash R, et al: Phase III randomized, double-blind placebo controlled trial of rhGM-CSF following allogeneic bone marrow transplantation. *Bone Marrow Transplant* 15:949–954, 1995.

43. Poe R, Wahl G, Qazi R, et al: Predictors of mortality in the immunocompromised patient with pulmonary infiltrates. *Arch Intern Med* 146:1304–1308, 1986.

44. Preblud S: Varicella: Complications and costs. *Pediatrics* 78: 728–735, 1986.

45. Ramsey P, Rubin R, Tolkoff-Rubin N, et al: The renal transplant patient with fever and pulmonary infiltrates: Etiology, clinical manifestations, and management. *Medicine (Baltimore)* 59:206–222, 1980.

46. Roilides E, Dimitriadou A, Kadiltsoglou I, et al: IL-10 exerts suppressive and enhancing effects on antifungal activity of mononuclear phagocytes against aspergillus fumigatus. *J Immunol* 158: 322–329, 1997.

47. Roilides E, Walsh T, Pizzo P, Rubin M: Granulocyte colony–stimulating factor enhances the phagocytic and bactericidal activity of normal and defective neutrophils. *J Infect Dis* 163:579–583, 1991.

48. Rowe J: A randomized placebo-controlled phase III study of granulocyte macrophage colony–stimulating factor in adult patients (> 55 to 70 years of age) with acute myelogenous leukemia: A study of the Eastern Cooperative Oncology Group (E1490). *Blood* 86:457–462, 1995.

49. Rubenstein E, Rolston K: Outpatient treatment of febrile neutropenic patients with cancer. *Eur J Cancer* 31A:2–4, 1995.

50. Schimpff S: Therapy of infection in patients with granulocytopenia. *Med Clin North Am* 61:1101–1118, 1977.

51. Sheagren NJ, Block JB, Wolff SM: Reticuloendothelial system phagocytic function in patients with Hodgkin's disease. *J Clin Invest* 46:855–862, 1967.

52. Singer C, Kaplan M, Armstrong D: Bacteremia and fungemia complicating neoplastic disease: A study of 364 cases. *Am J Med* 62:731–742, 1977.

53. Smith W, Sumnicht GE, Sharpe RW, et al: Granulocyte colony–stimulating factor versus placebo in addition to penicillin G in a randomized blinded study of gram-negative pneumonia sepsis: Analysis of survival and multisystem organ failure. *Blood* 86: 1301–1309, 1995.

54. Steigbigel RT, Lambert LH, Remington J: Polymorphonuclear leukocyte, monocyte, and macrophage bactericidal function in patients with Hodgkin's disease. *J Lab Clin Med* 88:54–62, 1976.

55. Suckles E, Greene W, Wiernik P, et al: Clinical presentation of infection in granulocytopenic patients. *Arch Intern Med* 135:715–719, 1975.

56. Talcott J, Finberg R, Mayer R, Goldman L: The medical course of cancer patients with fever and neutropenia: Clinical identification of a low-risk subgroup at presentation. *Arch Intern Med* 148: 2561–2568, 1988.

57. Tomiak A, Yau J, Stewart D, et al: Duration of intravenous antibiotics for patients with neutropenic fever. *Ann Oncol* 5:441–445, 1994.

58. Triebwasser J, Harrie R, Bryant R, et al: Varicella pneumonia in adults: Report of seven cases and a review of literature. *Medicine (Baltimore)* 46:409–423, 1967.

59. Valdivieso M, Gil-Extremera B, Zornoza J, et al: Gram-negative bacillary pneumonia in the compromised host. *Medicine (Baltimore)* 56:241–254, 1977.

60. Vose J, Armitage J: Clinical application of hematopoietic growth factors. *J Clin Oncol* 13:1023–1033, 1995.

61. Wade J, Schimpff S, Newman K, et al: *Staphylococcus epidermidis:* An increasing cause of infection in patients with granulocytopenia. *Ann Intern Med* 97:503–508, 1987.

62. Weber D, Pellechia J: Varicella pneumonia: Study of prevalence in adult men. *JAMA* 192:572–573, 1965.

63. Williams D, Krick J, Remington J: Pulmonary infection in the compromised host. *Am Rev Respir Dis* 114:359–394, 1976.

64. Wingard JR, Merz WG, Rinaldi MG, et al: Increase in *Candida krusei* infection among patients with bone marrow transplantation and neutropenia treated prophylactically with fluconazole. *New Engl J Med* 325:1274–1277, 1991.

65. Winston DJ, Chandrasekar PH, Lazarus HM, et al: Fluconazole prophylaxis of fungal infections in patients with acute leukemia: Results of a randomized placebo-controlled, double-blind, multicenter trial. *Ann Intern Med* 118:495–503, 1993.

66. Young LS, Martin WJ, Meyer RD, et al: Gram-negative rod bacteremia: Microbiologic, immunologic, and therapeutic considerations. *Ann Intern Med* 86:456–471, 1977.

RESPIRATORY DISEASE IN BONE MARROW AND HEMATOPOIETIC STEM CELL TRANSPLANTATION

Stephen W. Crawford

PULMONARY COMPLICATIONS AFTER BONE MARROW AND HEMATOPOIETIC STEM CELL TRANSPLANTATION

Incidence and Significance of Pulmonary Complications

Significant advances have been made in the techniques of hematopoietic stem cell transplantation, and the indications for the procedures continue to broaden. Sources of donor stem cells to serve as a marrow graft have expanded from autologous and sibling (allogeneic) bone marrow to include a pool of unrelated marrow donors, fetal cord blood, and growth factor–stimulated peripheral blood (Table 137-1). As a result, the number of transplants and the centers performing them have increased. It is advisable to refer to the procedures as *hematopoietic stem cell transplantation*, rather than bone marrow transplantation, in view of the widening sources of these precursors. Many of the data available relate specifically to the procedure of marrow transplantation and are no doubt applicable to other stem cell transplantation procedures.

Pulmonary disease occurs in 40 to 60 percent of patients after marrow transplantation.[31] The incidence is higher among recipients of specific transplants, such as allogeneic (compared to syngeneic or autologous) transplants, those receiving total-body irradiation or high-dose chemotherapy, those with malignancy (especially lymphoma) rather than aplastic anemia, and those of older age. The incidence of pulmonary complications associated with peripheral stem cell transplantation appears comparable with that in marrow transplantation when the intensity of radiochemotherapy and graft-versus-host disease (GVHD) are considered. A shorter duration of neutropenia associated with peripheral stem cell transplantation may decrease fungal infections. Pneumonia as a clinical syndrome is the leading infectious cause of death. Until the advent of effective prophylaxis and treatment, cytomegalovirus was the most common cause of pulmonary infection with a case fatality rate exceeding 85 percent, but the incidence of this infection appears to be declining. Diffuse noninfectious pulmonary injury, putatively due to intensive cytoreductive chemotherapy and irradiation, remains common; these "idiopathic interstitial" pneumonias have case fatality rates exceeding 60 percent (Table 137-2).[8]

A large proportion of transplant recipients develop significant pulmonary dysfunction months to years after successful transplantation. Airflow obstructive defects occur in at least 10 percent of allogeneic marrow recipients with chronic GVHD. The obstruction, often due to obliterative bronchiolitis, may progress to profound respiratory insufficiency and death. Additionally, up to 20 percent of recipients develop restrictive lung disease months to years after transplantation.

TABLE 137-1

Sources of Donor Marrow Stem Cells for Transplantation

Autologous & Syngeneic
Bone marrow
Peripheral blood

Allogeneic (Related or Unrelated Donors)
Bone marrow
Peripheral blood
Fetal cord blood

RESPIRATORY FAILURE

Respiratory failure is a dramatic outcome of pulmonary disease after transplantation. Studies of intensive care for respiratory failure of patients with cancer, hematologic malignancies, and marrow transplantation all have reported low survival rates. In most centers, approximately 3 percent of marrow recipients receiving mechanical ventilation survived to 6 months after transplantation, and the same poor prognosis is reported in pediatric marrow transplant recipients as noted among adults.[15,19] Age over 40 and respiratory failure within 90 days after transplantation have been noted as indicators of poor outcome in some studies.[19] In addition, intensive care for marrow recipients with respiratory failure utilizes inordinate medical resources.

Long-term survival is possible for some transplant recipients, but at a significant financial and emotional cost. In an attempt to identify patients destined to die despite life support without compromising the chances of potential survivors, the Fred Hutchinson Cancer Research Center identified specific predictors of mortality in mechanically ventilated marrow transplant recipients (Fig. 137-1).[43] In a nested case control study of 865 consecutive mechanically ventilated marrow transplant recipients, survival (defined as being alive 30 days after extubation and discharge from hospital) was statistically associated with

TABLE 137-2

Pulmonary Complications

Early Complications (<100 days)	Approx. Incidence (%)
Pulmonary edema syndromes	0–50
Infectious pneumonia	20–30
Bacterial	2–30
Fungal	4–13
Viral	4–10
Protozoa	<5
Idiopathic pneumonia	7–12
Oral mucositis	50–70
Pulmonary veno-occlusive disease	Rare
Late Complications (>100 days)	
Bronchopneumonia	20–30
Idiopathic pneumonia	10–20
Viral pneumonia	0–10
Airflow obstruction (obliterative bronchiolitis)	2–11*

*Obstructive airflow among marrow recipients with chronic GVHD.

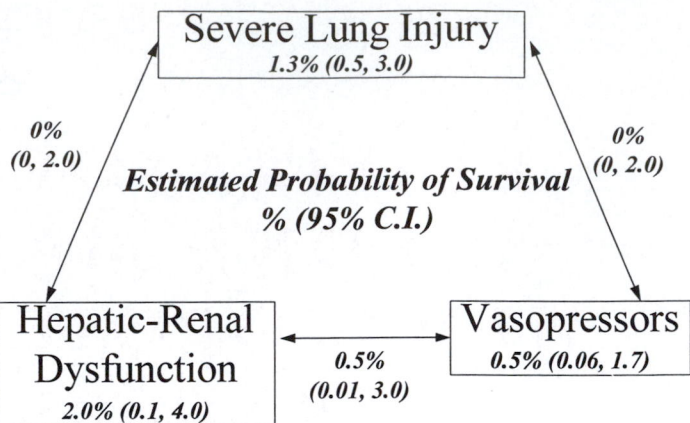

FIGURE 137-1 Clinical factors associated with mortality in marrow transplant recipients receiving mechanical ventilation. Survival is defined as being alive 30 days after extubation and discharged from the hospital. "Severe lung injury": requirement for F_{IO_2} >0.6 or PEEP >5 cm H_2O after the first 24 h of ventilatory support; "hepatorenal dysfunction": bilirubin >4 mg/dl and creatinine >2 mg/dl at any time during ventilatory support; "vasopressors": requirement for dopamine >5 μg/kg/min at any time during ventilatory support.

younger age, lower APACHE III score, and a shorter time from transplant to intubation; but these lacked sensitivity for clinical use. However, there were *no* survivors among an estimated 398 patients who had severe lung injury (F_{IO_2} greater than 0.6 or PEEP greater than 5 cm H_2O) and who also required more than 4 h of vasopressor support or sustained combined hepatic and renal insufficiency. With use of these factors, an accurate prediction of death could be made within 4 days of mechanical ventilation in 90 percent of nonsurvivors.

These data suggest that severe lung injury, combined with hemodynamic instability or hepatic–renal insufficiency, is a sensitive and highly specific predictor of nonsurvival in mechanically ventilated marrow transplant recipients. These scenarios are probably more common among older patients and those early after transplantation. The overwhelmingly negative results justify a standard of care for certain mechanically ventilated hematopoietic stem cell transplant patients that restricts prolonged intensive care. Patients and families should be counseled regarding the expected outcomes of such situations, and life support should be withdrawn when there is no precedence for survival, as with severe respiratory failure in the presence of multiorgan failure.

TEMPORAL SEQUENCE OF PULMONARY DISEASE SYNDROMES

Specific pulmonary complications may be grouped according to the time of presentation relative to the day of transplantation. "Early" events occur within the first 100 days after transplant, and "late" events occur beyond day 100. The classification in part reflects the fact that chronic GVHD occurs beyond day 100 after allogeneic transplantation. The early period can be further subdivided into the period of profound neutropenia, which exists for a variable period after transplantation, and the period of acute GVHD, which begins 2 to 3 weeks after allogeneic transplantation and extends approximately to day 100. Although this division is clinically useful, overlap occurs in the timing of spe-

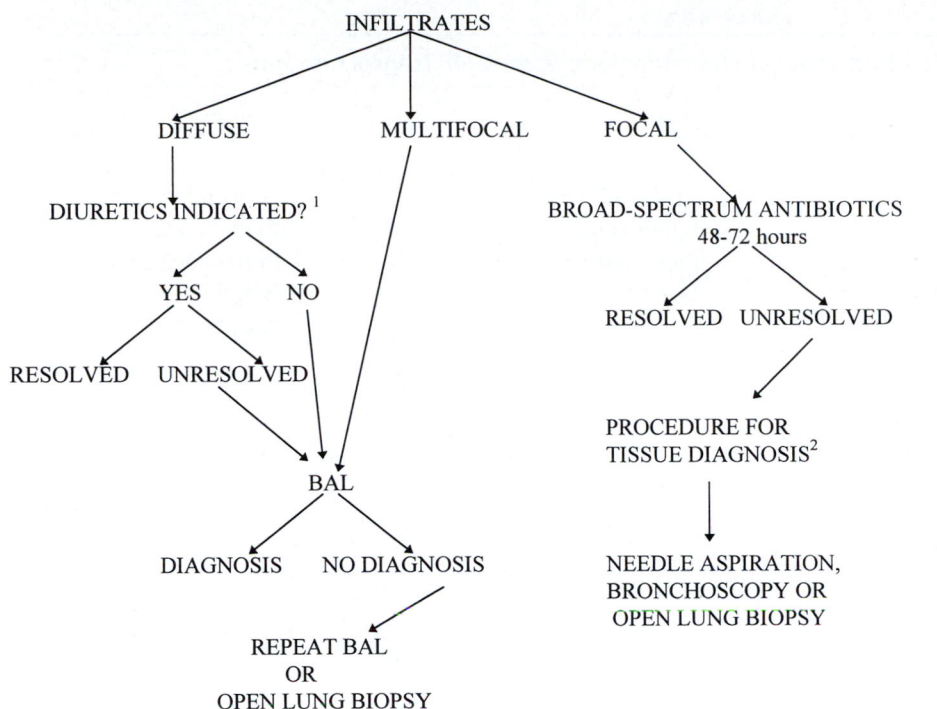

FIGURE 137-2 Diagnostic approach to pulmonary infiltrates after hematopoietic stem cell transplantation.

[1]Diuretics often indicated in the first 30 days after transplantation.
[2]Choice of procedure often influenced by results of CT scan of thorax.

cific complications, and the categorization of pulmonary complications is often arbitrary, since the cause of many respiratory abnormalities is uncertain.

The most important characteristic that separates patients receiving allografts from those receiving syngeneic or autologous marrow or stem cells is the occurrence of GVHD in the former group. Syngeneic and autograft recipients share early risk factors such as neutropenia with patients receiving allogeneic transplants, and are at risk of early pulmonary complications, such as bacterial or fungal pneumonia and noninfectious treatment-related pulmonary injury. Transplant recipients who have delayed engraftment or subsequent marrow failure are at continued risk of bacterial or fungal infection. Allogeneic marrow recipients with GVHD have continued abnormalities in immune function that increase the risk of opportunistic infections by mechanisms that are incompletely understood but include suppressive agents to treat the condition (cyclosporine and corticosteroids). Among patients with chronic GVHD, infection and pneumonia due to encapsulated organisms (e.g., *Streptococcus pneumoniae, Hemophilus influenzae,* and *Staphylococcus aureus*) appear related to deficiencies in specific antibody production or perhaps to continued defects in macrophage function.

COMMON CLINICAL PRESENTATIONS

Signs and symptoms of pulmonary disorders related to marrow and hematopoietic stem cell transplantation are often nonspecific. Tachypnea is common, as are fever, cough, and rales. However, any or all of these may be absent at the time of presentation of pulmonary complications. Routine chest radiographs are obtained frequently during the first weeks of neutropenia and often provide the first indication of pulmonary impairment. The strategy for evaluating pulmonary disorders is based on the timing after marrow infusion and the pattern of radiographic abnormalities (Fig. 137-2 and Table 137-3).

Diffuse Infiltrates
Diffuse infiltrates are common radiographic abnormalities noted in marrow recipients. However, these infiltrates are most often nonspecific. Infectious causes for diffuse infiltrates have been documented in fewer than 20 percent of marrow recipients undergoing open lung biopsy within 30 days after marrow transplantation.[13] Within this early period, pulmonary edema syndromes predominate. The edema may be associated with cardiac decompensation or intravascular volume excess, or with acute respiratory distress syndrome (ARDS) and pulmonary capillary leak due to treatment-related toxicities or sepsis syndrome. Infections presenting with diffuse infiltrates within the first weeks after transplantation include respiratory viral causes, such as respiratory syncytial virus, whereas cytomegalovirus is uncommon. Alveolar hemorrhage may contribute to the radiographic infiltrates in the presence of thrombocytopenia, regardless of the cause of the lung injury.

Between 30 days and 180 days after marrow transplantation, infections are a major reason for diffuse radiographic abnormalities.[13,38] Cytomegalovirus was common, but it is now unusual in patients receiving appropriate prophylaxis. Diffuse pneumonia due to bacterial infections also is unusual; however, diffuse involvement with fungus may occur in as many as 20 percent of diffuse infiltrates and may be extremely difficult to detect.

Focal Lesions
Focal parenchymal infiltrates are frequently due to infection regardless of the time of presentation after transplant. Focal consolidations or masses are related to local fungal infection in 80 percent of marrow transplant recipients receiving broad-spectrum antibiotics. Other causes are *Legionella* species, *Nocardia,* relapse of lymphoma in patients transplanted for that disorder, bronchiolitis obliterans with organizing pneumonia (BOOP), and, rarely, infarct due to thromboembolic disease.

Aspiration
Desquamation of the oropharyngeal mucosa is a frequent complication after intensive chemotherapy, and the stomatitis is often referred to as "mucositis." It develops within the first week after radiotherapy and reaches its greatest severity after 10 to 14 days,[49] and impaired mucociliary clearance is common.[50] Recurrent aspiration of oropharyngeal contents is common among

TABLE 137-3

Causes of Radiographic Infiltrates in Hematopoietic Stem Cell Transplantation

	Diffuse	*Focal*	*Multifocal*

Noninfectious	Idiopathic
	  IPS
	  ARDS
	  Alveolar hemorrhage
	Edema
	  Heart failure
	  Volume excess
	  Capillary leak syndromes
	    ARDS
	    Acute GVHD
	Leukemic infiltrate
	Fat emboli syndrome
		Leukemic infiltrate
		Lymphoma
		Pulmonary embolus
		BOOP
			Leukemic infiltrate
			Lymphoma
			Pulmonary emboli
			BOOP
			Aspiration

Infectious	Viral
	  CMV
	  RSV
	  Parainfluenza
	  Influenza
	  Adenovirus
	  HSV
	  VZV
	  HHV-6 (?)
	Fungal
	  Mycelial fungi
	Pneumocystis carinii
	Protozoan
	  Toxoplasmosis
		Fungal
		  Mycelial fungi
		
		Bronchopneumonia
		  Gram-positive bacteria
		  Gram-negative bacteria
		  Legionella species
		Nocardia
		Mycobacteria
			Viral
			  HSV
			  VZV
			Fungal
			  Mycelial fungi
			  Yeasts
			Bronchopneumonia
			  Gram-positive bacteria
			  Gram-negative bacteria
			  Legionella species
			Nocardia
			Mycobacteria
			Toxoplasmosis
			Septic emboli

transplant recipients with oral mucositis due to sedation, poor cough reflex, and dysphagia. These patients may present with basilar infiltrates or consolidation.

A history of recurrent aspiration can be obtained in many of these cases. Typically, cough is induced by attempts at swallowing, or there are nocturnal paroxysms of cough in the setting of severe mucositis. The appropriate approach to such patients is conservative: moderating the administration of sedatives, encouraging pulmonary toilet, and avoidance of mucosal bleeding by adequate platelet support. Most patients receive broad-spectrum antibiotics. Tracheal intubation may be required to avoid massive aspiration in a profoundly obtunded patient or acute airway obstruction in the presence of severe upper-airway bleeding.

Pleural Effusions

Pleural effusions are common in the first weeks after marrow transplantation and are rarely related to an identifiable infectious source. Pleural effusions may be associated with fluid retention of any cause, especially with ascites secondary to hepatic veno-occlusive disease (HVOD). HVOD may occur in as many as 60 percent of patients after total-body irradiation.[35] Characteristics include weight gain within the first weeks after transplantation and elevation of the serum bilirubin, which usually precede the development of pleural effusions. The effusions are frequently bilateral. Bilateral pleural effusions in the presence of weight gain can be approached conservatively without diagnostic thoracentesis. Cautious diuresis often produces satisfactory results. Small effusions are common and may be associated with treatment-related pleuropericarditis or thromboembolic events, but a specific cause is seldom determined. A large unilateral or rapidly accumulating effusion in the presence of fever or ipsilateral chest pain may represent hemorrhage or infection and should be evaluated promptly by thoracentesis.

NONINFECTIOUS ETIOLOGY

Noninfectious causes of lung injury after marrow and hematopoietic stem cell transplantation include a spectrum of syndromes:

idiopathic pneumonia, alveolar hemorrhage, pulmonary edema, obliterative bronchiolitis, and BOOP.

Idiopathic pneumonia is characterized as a syndrome of hypoxemia and radiographic nonlobar infiltrates in the absence of congestive heart failure and without evidence of an infectious origin.[58] It is included as a form of "interstitial" pneumonia. The term *interstitial pneumonia* in marrow transplant recipients refers to the syndrome of diffuse inflammatory pulmonary disease presenting with fever and tachypnea. This term includes noninfectious causes, as well as infectious pneumonia due to viruses or protozoa. The interstitium of the lung denotes the parenchymal fibrocellular structures surrounding the alveolar capillaries in the alveolar septa, at the alveolar junctions, and in the bronchovascular sheaths. Therefore, the term *interstitial pneumonia* should be reserved as a strictly histopathologic description. To avoid the ambiguity of the term *interstitial* in relation to inflammatory disorders of the lung, it is preferable to classify the clinical conditions as *diffuse* pneumonia on the basis of the radiographic presentation. However, the term *interstitial pneumonia* is firmly entrenched in the literature.

Most noninfectious causes of lung injury are attributed to treatment-related toxicities. Alkylating chemotherapy agents and ionizing irradiation are likely contributors; however, ARDS secondary to sepsis syndrome also may occur. While pneumonia is associated with the presence of GVHD, whether GVHD causes a direct lung injury is unproved. The role of unrecognized infections remains a concern.

Idiopathic Pneumonia Syndrome

INCIDENCE AND EPIDEMIOLOGY

The largest studies of idiopathic pneumonia after allogeneic marrow transplantation estimate the incidence at 12 to 17 percent.[37,58] Although similar rates have been found between allogeneic (12 percent) and syngeneic transplants (11 percent),[37] others have reported a lower incidence of idiopathic pneumonia after autologous marrow transplantation (7 to 8 percent).[58,60] In these studies, the diagnosis of idiopathic pneumonia largely relied on the results of lung biopsy and autopsy. Virologic evaluation most often was limited to histochemical staining and conventional culture, and frequently lacked recently developed techniques, such as immunocytochemistry for the sensitive detection of cytomegalovirus and respiratory viruses (respiratory syncytial virus and parainfluenza).

The spectrum of idiopathic lung injury was referred to as a "syndrome" (idiopathic pneumonia syndrome, or IPS) by a National Institutes of Health–sponsored workshop on idiopathic lung injury after marrow transplantation[8] in recognition of the probability of multiple causes and varied clinical presentation (Table 137-4). The diagnosis of IPS is defined by a bronchoalveolar lavage (BAL) that does not reveal an infection in the presence of nonlobar radiographic infiltrates and physiological changes consistent with pneumonia. A common series of laboratory evaluations is presented in Table 137-5. Many clinicians use IPS only to describe noninfectious lung injury occurring within the first 3 to 4 months after transplantation.

Recent findings from the Fred Hutchinson Cancer Research Center in Seattle suggest that the incidence within 3 months of transplantation of IPS as currently defined was 7 percent.[30] No significant difference in incidence between allogeneic and autologous marrow recipients was noted. Median onset of IPS was earlier than previously noted—3 weeks after transplant. Seventy percent of patients progressed rapidly to respiratory failure.

PATHOGENESIS

The causes of diffuse idiopathic pneumonia are probably multiple, and include treatment-related toxicities due to radiation or chemotherapeutic agents. However, sepsis-related pulmonary toxicity may account for a proportion of cases of diffuse idiopathic pneumonia with histology consistent with ARDS. While GVHD is associated with an increased incidence of idiopathic lung injury, it is unclear whether this is a cell-mediated immune response to the lung or related to an increased incidence of sepsis in these immunosuppressed patients. Also, administration of large volumes of blood products during the transplantation procedure may lead to pulmonary vascular injury through leukoagglutination reactions. Other unusual causes of noninfectious diffuse pneumonia after marrow transplantation are leukemic infiltration due to relapse of primary malignancy, injection of malignant cells with reinfused autologous marrow, and fat embolization due to marrow infusion. Several cases of fat embolizationwere associated with pulmonary hemorrhage and steroid administration.

CLINICAL PRESENTATION

The clinical presentation of IPS is nonspecific. Most patients develop a syndrome of fever, nonproductive cough, and tachypnea. Hypoxemia with hyperventilation is common. The onset is

---

TABLE 137-4

Criteria for Diagnosis of Idiopathic Pneumonia Syndrome

Evidence of widespread alveolar injury
  Multilobar infiltrates on chest radiograph or computed tomography
  Symptoms and signs of pneumonia
  Evidence of abnormal physiology

and

Absence of active lower respiratory tract infection documented by
  Negative bronchoalveolar lavage
Lung biopsy or autopsy with examination of stains and cultures for bacteria, fungi and viruses, including cytomegalovirus (CMV) centrifugation culture, cytology for viral inclusions and *Pneumocystis carinii,* and immunofluorescence monoclonal antibody staining for CMV, respiratory syncytial virus, influenza virus, parainfluenza virus, and adenovirus

TABLE 137-5

Routine Laboratory Evaluation of Bronchoalveolar Lavage Specimens in Marrow and Stem Cell Transplant Recipients

Pathology*

Wright-Giemsa stain
Papanicolaou stain
Silver stain
Modified Jimenez stain (or other suitable for detecting *Legionella*)
Consider: monoclonal fluorescent antibody stain for *Pneumocystis*

Microbiology

Stains:
  Gram's
  Wet mount KOH or calcofluor white
  Modified acid-fast
  Fluorescent antibody stain for *Legionella*
Culture:
  Bacterial (aerobic), semiquantitative method
  Fungal
  Legionella (chocolate yeast extract)
  Acid-fast

Virology

Fluorescent antibody stains†:
  CMV
  HSV
  RSV, parainfluenza and influenza
    viruses pooled antibodies‡,¶
Culture (rapid centrifugation technique preferred)#:
  CMV
  HSV
  Adenovirus
  RSV, parainfluenza, and influenzaviruses (in appropriate clinical setting)

*Studies usually reviewed by a pathologist.
†Studies may be performed in virology or pathology laboratory.
‡Separate studies for each virus should be performed if the study with pooled antibodies is positive.
¶Fluorescent antibody stains may be supplemented or replaced by enzyme immunoassays (EIA) as available.
#If available. Culture may be replaced with fluorescent antibody stains or EIA alone if culture facilities are unavailable.

most often rapid, occurring over a few days. Occasionally, insidious onset similar to that of idiopathic pulmonary fibrosis is seen. Median onset is within the first 3 weeks of transplantation, but it may occur up to months later. The chest radiograph shows diffuse intra-alveolar and/or interstitial infiltrates. The presentation is not sufficiently distinct to be readily differentiated from that of pulmonary edema syndromes or diffuse infectious pneumonia. Marked tachypnea in the absence of radiographic infiltrates should raise the suspicion of obstructive airway disease or pulmonary veno-occlusive disease rather than idiopathic pneumonia.

PATHOLOGY

IPS after marrow transplantation represents a histologic spectrum ranging from a primarily interstitial reaction with diffuse or focal widening of the alveolar septa and interstitial spaces with mononuclear inflammatory cells and edema to diffuse alveolar damage (DAD) with alveolar epithelial necrosis, intra-alveolar hyaline membranes, edema and hemorrhage, and type 2 cell hyperplasia.[24,51] The predominantly interstitial presentation has been referred to as *idiopathic interstitial pneumonia,* whereas the pathology of diffuse alveolar damage is identical to that of ARDS. Variable degrees of alveolar hemorrhage may be seen with either of these presentations. Elements of both histologic pictures may be seen in any pathologic specimen. Recent experience from Seattle found that the interstitial pattern predominated in more than 50 percent and DAD in one-third of lung biopsies from marrow recipients with idiopathic pneumonia. By definition, all microbiologic and histologic evaluations for infectious agents (viral, protozoal, fungal, and bacterial) are negative in idiopathic pneumonia. The importance of a thorough microbiologic examination lies in the fact that these histologic presentations are similar to those of infectious pneumonia, especially cytomegalovirus pneumonia.

COURSE OF DISEASE

The mortality from idiopathic lung injury after marrow transplantation remains over 70 percent. There are few descriptions of the clinical course of idiopathic pneumonia other than those of mortality. In a series of 41 marrow recipients with idiopathic pneumonia diagnosed by lung biopsy between 1983 and 1988, overall in-hospital mortality was 71 percent and the case fatality rate was 59 percent, with 32 percent dying with progressive respiratory failure.[12] Infection was present at autopsy in 69 percent of cases. More recent experience with patients diagnosed by BAL and meeting the diagnostic criteria of IPS revealed similar mortality. Respiratory failure generally developed within 2 days of onset of radiographic infiltrates, and two-thirds of all deaths were associated with progressive respiratory failure. In one-quarter of cases, the pneumonia resolved. This suggests that although the mortality associated with idiopathic lung injury is high, there are competing causes for mortality, specifically subsequent (or undetected) infection.

The diagnosis of idiopathic lung injury rests largely on the results of BAL. Lung biopsy (transbronchial or open) appears to add little to the diagnostic sensitivity of BAL for infection in the presence of diffuse parenchymal infiltrates. At present, histopathology does not help to direct therapy in idiopathic lung injury after hematopoietic stem cell transplantation. Lung biopsy should be considered in cases with patchy or multifocal infiltrates because of the higher incidence of infection and concern for false-negative results from BAL (Fig. 137-2).

Recently, BOOP was reported in three children 2 to 3 months after marrow transplantation that either was mismatched with respect to the major histocompatibility gene complex (HLA) or from an unrelated donor.[33] The onset was associated with fever, cough, and patchy radiographic infiltrates. The syndrome resolved over 1 to 2 months in two of the three children after treatment with corticosteroids. Confirmation of the diagnosis requires lung biopsy.

TREATMENT

There are no randomized studies of treatment of idiopathic lung injury after marrow transplantation. High-dose corticosteroids (ranging from 1 to 16 mg/kg per day of methylprednisolone) are commonly used, and anecdotal reports suggest successful outcomes. However, not all retrospective analyses have supported a beneficial effect. Corticosteroid administration has been reported effective in diffuse lung injury in treatment protocols containing bis-chloroethyl-1-nitrosourea (BCNU, or carmustine).

Pulmonary Hemorrhage

INCIDENCE AND CLINICAL SYNDROME

Robbins and colleagues[42] described a potentially specific form of idiopathic pneumonia: diffuse alveolar hemorrhage (DAH). The syndrome consisted of progressive dyspnea, hypoxemia, cough, and a progressively bloodier return from BAL in autologous marrow recipients, usually within 2 weeks of transplant.

The incidence of DAH was 20.5 percent and was associated with age over 40 years, high fever, transplantation for a solid tumor, severe mucositis, white blood cell recovery, and renal insufficiency. Thrombocytopenia was a common finding, and patients with (DAH) received more platelet transfusions than patients without DAH. Memorial Sloan-Kettering Cancer Center[29] reported an 8 percent incidence of noninfectious DAH in 77 consecutive lymphoma patients treated with high-dose therapy and autologous marrow transplant. There was an association between DAH and prior booster doses of thoracic irradiation. It is unclear whether this hemorrhagic pneumonia represents a unique syndrome or represents severe lung injury in the presence of a bleeding diathesis.

Most episodes of alveolar hemorrhage occur with or after periods of profound thrombocytopenia. Platelet counts below 20,000 per cubic millimeter are the rule among these patients, as in patients with leukemia. Onset of IPS within several weeks of allogeneic transplantation is associated with a higher incidence of alveolar hemorrhage than later onset.[13] Rapid development of radiographic pulmonary densities in the absence of overt clinical change in a thrombocytopenic marrow recipient should raise the clinical suspicion of alveolar hemorrhage. Although such presentations are common, especially in the presence of ecchymosis in other soft tissues (such as sclerae), proof of alveolar hemorrhage in these cases is rare. Hemoptysis is rare. The clinical diagnosis of hemorrhage is often difficult to substantiate. There is little that distinguishes patients with alveolar hemorrhage associated with idiopathic pneumonia clinically from other marrow recipients with diffuse lung injuries. The course of disease in alveolar hemorrhage appears similar to that of IPS.

TREATMENT

High-dose corticosteroid administration is commonly used to treat alveolar hemorrhage after marrow transplantation. Chao's team[6] reported four patients undergoing autologous marrow transplant for leukemia with DAH who recovered after receiving methylprednisolone in initial doses of 1 g per day. In a retrospective study, Metcalf and coworkers[36] reported that the mortality of DAH declined from 92 to 67 percent at the University of Nebraska when patients were given a dosage of methylprednisolone of at least 30 mg per day. The effectiveness of this treatment remains unproved, however. Supportive care—including correction of coagulation disorders, platelet support, supplemental oxygen, and careful fluid management—is indicated.

Pulmonary Edema Syndromes

Biventricular failure after transplantation is often iatrogenic and associated with excessive fluid administration and an increase in total body weight. Radiographic evidence of pulmonary edema after marrow transplantation has been reported in up to 50 percent of patients,[17] most occurring in the second week. Close attention to the total amount of sodium and fluids administered can lead to dramatic reduction in the incidence of pulmonary edema. Also, pulmonary edema may be associated with left ventricular decompensation related to cardiotoxic cytoreductive regimens, including anthracyclines in excess of 500 mg/m^2 and high-dose cyclophosphamide. Posttransplantation cardiac and pericardial toxicity occur in 4 to 10 percent of cases, usually associated with total-body irradiation and cyclophosphamide, often in the setting of prior anthracycline administration. The utility of cardiac imaging studies before transplantation to predict heart failure is limited.

The most frequent noncardiac association with pulmonary edema states is HVOD.[34] The syndrome is often associated with interstitial pulmonary edema, the formation of pleural effusions, and renal failure. Noncardiac pulmonary edema also develops in association with acute GVHD and may be due, in part, to DAD and capillary leak.

The presentation of pulmonary edema is nonspecific and usually occurs within 30 days after marrow infusion. Marrow recipients are often febrile and tachypneic at this time in the transplant course, and recipients of allogeneic marrow may display evidence suggestive of acute GVHD. Thus, the distinction between pulmonary edema and idiopathic pneumonia often cannot be made with certainty without pulmonary artery catheterization. However, recent increase in total body weight appears to correlate well with total-body fluid accumulation and should prompt a trial of diuretic therapy before consideration of invasive diagnostic procedures. Noninvasive assessment of cardiac function with ultrasonographic or radionuclide techniques is often warranted to guide treatment.

New-Onset Airflow Obstruction and Obliterative Bronchiolitis

EPIDEMIOLOGY AND INCIDENCE

About 10 percent of allogeneic marrow recipients with chronic GVHD are likely to develop airflow obstruction consistent with obliterative bronchiolitis.[11] However, the reported incidence of obliterative bronchiolitis varies, in part, with the method used to identify the presence of the disease. Retrospective review of samples obtained by biopsy or at autopsy identified the histopathology of obliterative bronchiolitis in approximately 2 percent of all allogeneic marrow transplant recipients and in approximately 6 percent of patients with chronic GVHD.[27] On the other hand, pulmonary function tests detected an obstructive airflow defect (i.e., FEV$_1$/FVC under 70 percent) in 14 percent of patients 1 year after transplantation.[52] Specifically, among recipients of allogeneic grafts who develop chronic GVHD, at least 11 percent have a significant decrease in airflow (i.e., a decrease in FEV$_1$/FVC of more than 15 percent) compared to pretransplantation values.[7] Since few of these patients underwent histologic examination, the incidence of the specific pathologic entity known as *obliterative bronchiolitis* may be overestimated. The incidence of airflow obstruction may be higher in children after transplantation, possibly because of decreased airway diameter.

PATHOGENESIS

The onset of progressive airflow disease more than 100 days after allogeneic marrow transplantation is strongly related to the development of chronic GVHD.[5] Factors associated with the in-

creased risk of GVHD, such as increasing age and HLA-nonidentical marrow grafts, are not independent risk factors for the development of obliterative bronchiolitis. However, the administration of methotrexate after transplantation for the prophylaxis of GVHD is associated with airflow obstruction.[27] Also, there is a higher incidence of decreased levels of IgG among patients with obliterative bronchiolitis than in other marrow recipients.[27] This hypogammaglobulinemia may be a manifestation of the immunologic lesion responsible for the airway disease or may merely be related to the presence of chronic GVHD.

The cause of obliterative bronchiolitis after marrow transplantation is unknown. Possible causes include those recognized in otherwise normal hosts, including recurrent aspiration; viral infection with influenza, adenovirus, or measles; and bacterial or mycoplasmal infection. None of these factors has been found consistently in affected marrow recipients. The strong association between chronic GVHD and the development of airflow obstruction suggests an immunologic mechanism including bronchial epithelial injury.[7] The lung epithelium may be the target of immune-mediated injury in chronic GVHD through the expression of Ia antigen and subsequent activation of donor cytotoxic T cell. This hypothesis is unproved, however. The association with the administration of methotrexate also raises the possibility of direct drug-related injury to the pulmonary bronchial epithelium.

CLINICAL PRESENTATION

The usual clinical manifestation of new-onset airflow obstruction is the insidious onset of tachypnea, dyspnea on exertion, and dry, nonproductive cough. Fever is uncommon. Although the chest radiograph is commonly interpreted as normal, high-resolution chest CT often reveals parenchymal hypoattenuation and segmental bronchial dilatation.[44] Auscultation of the chest may reveal scattered expiratory wheezing and occasionally diffuse inspiratory crackles, but results are sometimes normal. Arterial blood-gas analysis reveals moderate hypoxemia and, in the later stages, hypercarbia. When the presentation is beyond 150 days after marrow grafting, evidence of chronic GVHD is usually present. However, the disorder may occur at any time after transplantation, and some cases are recognized only after several years. The major differential diagnoses of the gradual onset of nonspecific respiratory symptoms in the presence of a normal chest radiograph include pulmonary veno-occlusive disease and pulmonary embolism. Obliterative bronchiolitis is characterized by reduction in expiratory airflow on spirometry and increases in residual lung volumes not found in the other two diseases.

COURSE OF DISEASE

Prospective evaluation of pulmonary functions after marrow transplantation identified marrow recipients with variable courses of disease progression.[7] Patients with onset of airflow obstruction within the first 150 days after marrow transplantation tend to have a rapid decline in pulmonary function and a fatal outcome. These patients may not survive long enough to develop manifestations of chronic GVHD but usually display acute GVHD after marrow grafting. It is possible that infection plays a role in the development of the airflow obstruction in some of these patients. Marrow recipients with the onset of airflow obstruction beyond 150 days after transplantation tend to have a more gradual decline in lung function. Airflow may stabilize in 50 percent of these patients. Since up to 50 percent of patients have a respiratory infection noted at the time of diagnosis of airflow obstruction,[5] evaluation including BAL may be warranted before initiation of treatment.

TREATMENT

There are no prospective trials of treatment for new-onset airflow obstruction. At present, the accepted approach to these patients is to aggressively control with immunomodulating agents the chronic GVHD that most often accompanies the airflow obstruction. Treatment usually consists of increased immunosuppression with corticosteroids, often with the addition of cyclosporine and azathioprine in severe or progressive cases. Reversal of the airflow obstruction is reported in only 8 percent of cases.[5] The usual goal of management is stabilization of the obstruction. For this reason, prompt recognition and treatment for this progressive process are critical. Supportive measures include prophylaxis against *Pneumocystis carinii* pneumonia and *S. pneumoniae* infection, inhaled bronchodilators, supplemental immunoglobulin administration to maintain normal serum levels, and prompt treatment of intercurrent infections.

Pulmonary Veno-Occlusive Disease

Pulmonary veno-occlusive disease (PVOD) is a rare complication of treatment with chemotherapeutic regimens, and as a solitary pulmonary complication, PVOD is a very uncommon complication after marrow grafting.[25,54] The primary histologic lesion of PVOD—obstruction of the pulmonary veins and venules by loose intimal fibrosis proliferation—may be difficult to detect with hematoxylin and eosin stains alone, and specific stains for elastic tissues, such as Verhoff–van Gieson stain, are required to demonstrate the fibrotic reaction in the veins. Three cases of PVOD were reported after marrow transplantation in children with acute lymphocytic leukemia. Two of the three had received BCNU, VP-16 (etoposide), and cyclophosphamide without total-body irradiation as cytoreductive preparation before transplantation.[25] An association between histologic evidence of PVOD and HVOD has been reported, but not confirmed elsewhere.[59]

The typical presentation of PVOD is that of insidious dyspnea on exertion and resting tachypnea within 3 to 4 months after transplantation. Significant hypoxemia may occur along with hyperventilation. The chest radiograph is often unrevealing. On cardiac exam, there is evidence of pulmonary hypertension. Auscultation of the lungs is often normal, although scattered inspiratory crackles may be heard. Noninvasive examinations, echocardiography, perfusion–ventilation nucleotide scans, and electrocardiograms are nondiagnostic. Pulmonary function testing may be consistent with mild restrictive defect, but airflow obstruction, suggesting obliterative bronchiolitis, is absent. BAL has failed to demonstrate pathogens or inflammatory cells. The diagnostic procedure of choice is a pulmonary angiogram. Right

heart catheterization reveals elevated pulmonary artery pressure, with normal pulmonary artery wedge pressures. Angiography excludes the presence of thrombi as a cause of the pulmonary hypertension.

In most cases presenting after treatment for malignancy, the disease has followed an insidious course, with progressive hypoxemia and dyspnea on exertion due to pulmonary hypertension. The high mortality reported may, in part, be related to the initial recognition of the disease at autopsy. However, in two of the three cases that occurred after marrow transplantation, the patients recovered from their pulmonary symptoms with high-dose corticosteroid therapy (methylprednisolone, 2.0 mg/kg per day).[25]

INFECTIOUS ETIOLOGY

Viral Pneumonia: Cytomegalovirus

INCIDENCE AND EPIDEMIOLOGY

The incidence of cytomegalovirus (CMV) pneumonia has declined significantly in recent years. The rates now appear to be approximately 4 percent for both allogeneic and autologous transplantation. The decline is attributable to effective prophylaxis and preemptive treatment. It is presumed that most, if not all, CMV infection occurring in seropositive patients is due to reactivation of latent infection. The risk of infection in seronegative patients with seronegative marrow donors is attributable to blood product exposure, and this risk can be virtually eliminated by use of screened seronegative or filtered blood products.[3]

PATHOGENESIS

The pathogenesis of CMV pneumonia is not completely understood. The occurrence of active CMV infection is obviously crucial to pathogenesis of pneumonia. The association of CMV pneumonia with allogeneic transplantation and with the occurrence of acute GVHD suggests that the immune response, either absent or disordered, plays an important role. The acquisition of CMV-specific immune responses appears essential for limiting primary infection and maintaining the clinical state of latency. Host immunity induced by CMV infection includes both cellular and humoral responses. Cell-mediated responses by both $CD4^+$ (T helper) and $CD8^+$ cytotoxic T-lymphocytes (CTL) are detected in CMV-seropositive subjects.[41] Additionally, it has been hypothesized that the immune response contributes to the pathogenesis or clinical expression of CMV pneumonia. Natural killer activity in the lung, as sampled by BAL, is demonstrably increased in patients with CMV pneumonia compared to patients with other forms of pneumonia after marrow transplantation.[3] Cause and effect remain to be sorted out. Abnormalities in immune responses are not restricted to allograft recipients with GVHD, presumably explaining the occasional occurrence of CMV pneumonia in twin or allograft recipients. The effect of increased patient age and intensity of conditioning regimen on the incidence of CMV pneumonia suggests that previous or underlying damage to the lung increases the risk. The high incidence of CMV pneumonia after marrow transplant, contrasted with the paucity of cases after renal transplant, for example, may suggest that the pulmonary toxicity of transplant conditioning increases the tropism of CMV for the lung.

CLINICAL PRESENTATION

The clinical presentation of CMV pneumonia is not distinct from that of other entities that cause diffuse pneumonia. Patients with CMV pneumonia may have nonproductive cough, dyspnea, hypoxemia, or fever, with a median onset of 60 days after marrow transplant. Onset within the first 2 weeks is unusual. The period of risk of CMV pneumonia generally ends by approximately the fourth or fifth month after transplant, although later cases occur among patients with chronic GVHD or after autologous transplant. Chest radiograph generally shows bilateral infiltrates; in later stages, diffuse consolidation occurs. Unilateral, focal, and even nodular infiltrates have been seen in the early stages.

PATHOLOGY

The hallmark of CMV pneumonia is the Cowdry type A intracytoplasmic inclusion bodies within the areas of inflammation. The presence of these eosinophilic bodies appears related to the duration of infection and may be absent early in the process. Immunohistologic probes may detect CMV-specific DNA and antigen in these cases of "histologically occult" CMV pneumonia. The pneumonia may be primarily a mononuclear interstitial disease, or it may be associated with diffuse alveolar epithelial desquamation with hyaline membrane formation. Both diffuse parenchymal and multifocal patterns have been described.

COURSE OF DISEASE

Historically, CMV pneumonia was an inexorable process leading to death within 2 to 4 weeks (usually less) in 85 percent of patients with biopsy-proven disease. Treatment with a variety of antiviral agents, including ganciclovir, did not change the course. At present, survival of 30 to 70 percent can be expected with the combination of ganciclovir and intravenous immunoglobulins.[18,40,45] While improved survival rates are encouraging, it remains possible that this change is in part due to treatment earlier in the disease course. Survival of patients with respiratory failure at time of initial treatment remains uncommon.

TREATMENT AND PREVENTION

Recent studies suggest that the combination of ganciclovir and intravenous human immunoglobulins substantially improves survival from CMV pneumonia compared to experience with a variety of antiviral agents, including vidarabine, acyclovir, and leukocyte or lymphoblastoid interferons, given alone or in various combinations.[18,40,45] The present approach to the ganciclovir component of the regimen is to initiate treatment at a dose of 5.0 mg/kg every 12 h, with appropriate adjustments for renal function for a period of 14 days—referred to as "induction" treatment. If the patient's condition has improved at that time, the dosage is reduced to 5.0 mg/kg, given once daily for 30 days or more—referred to as "maintenance." Induction treatment is continued beyond 14 days if patients have not responded, with response defined as improved oxygenation and decreased respiratory rate. Maintenance may continue for more than 30 days, depending on individual patient characteristics.

Recommendations for the immunoglobulin regimen are more varied, since different immunoglobulins were used in different studies. In studies in Seattle, a high-titer CMV intravenous immunoglobulin was given at the dose of 400 mg/kg on days 1, 2, and 7 of treatment, followed by a dose of 200 mg/kg on days 14 and 21. Immunoglobulin was then discontinued. A 50 percent response rate has been observed with this regimen.[40] In studies from other centers, available "unscreened" intravenous immunoglobulin was given at a dose of 500 mg/kg every other day for 10 doses, and then once weekly for as long as maintenance ganciclovir was continued. A 75 percent response has been reported with this regimen.[18,45] Whether this apparently better response reflects differences attributable to the regimen or to differences in the patient group is unknown.

The major toxicity observed with this regimen is marrow suppression, attributed to ganciclovir. Between 25 and 50 percent of treated patients experience a decrease in leukocyte counts, usually occurring after the first 2 weeks of treatment and often during maintenance therapy. Neutropenia may be profound and prolonged, and superinfection remains a hazard.

Efforts to prevent CMV pneumonia have been directed primarily at preventing CMV infection and preemptively treating patients at highest risk of pneumonia. Among allograft recipients who are seronegative before transplant and have seronegative marrow donors, CMV infection and therefore pneumonia can be eliminated by use of screened seronegative blood products.[3] This approach is less successful among seronegative patients with seropositive marrow donors, since the marrow itself serves as a source of infection. High-dose acyclovir delays reactivation of latent virus and reduces the probability of CMV pneumonia by approximately 50 percent in seropositive allogeneic but not autologous transplant recipients.

CMV pneumonia can be virtually prevented in all cases with the prophylactic administration of ganciclovir to all seropositive recipients. This approach, however, did not lead to improved overall survival, owing to an increase in sepsis related to the ganciclovir-induced neutropenia.[23] An additional theoretical concern with this approach is a delay in reestablishing CMV-specific CTL and, thus, an increased risk for CMV pneumonia at a later time. Most seropositive patients who are at the highest risk of developing CMV pneumonia can be prospectively identified by routine cultures of body fluids. Patients with positive blood, throat, urine, or BAL cultures have a significantly increased probability of developing CMV pneumonia. Treatment of patients at the time of viral excretion significantly decreases the incidence of CMV pneumonia and improves survival, but 30 percent of marrow recipients develop CMV pneumonia without recognized excretion and are missed by this approach.[23,46]

Detection of CMV antigens in blood leukocytes (using peroxidase-labeled monoclonal antibodies) or CMV DNA in plasma or blood leukocytes (using polymerase chain reaction) are sensitive and specific in the identification of patients at highest risk for CMV pneumonia. The negative predictive value of such testing approaches 100 percent. Prospective use of these techniques after allogeneic transplantation permits preemptive treatment with ganciclovir, which appears to eliminate the incidence of CMV pneumonia.

Other Viral Infections: RSV, Parainfluenza, Adenovirus, HSV, HHV-6

INCIDENCE AND EPIDEMIOLOGY

Viral pneumonias other than CMV may occur after marrow transplantation at an incidence that is lower and usually poorly defined. The most common of these is due to adenovirus. Adenovirus infection occurs in 5 percent of patients within the first 3 months after transplantation, attributable in almost all cases to reactivation of latent virus. Approximately 20 percent of marrow transplant patients with adenovirus infection develop pneumonia.[48]

Pneumonia due to herpes simplex virus (HSV) or varicella-zoster virus (VZV) occurs uncommonly. HSV pneumonia is generally due to contiguous spread of virus to the trachea or aspiration from the oropharynx, although it may be due to generalized infection with viremia.[39] Pneumonia due to VZV occurs among patients with disseminated infection and viremia. Both situations have become exceedingly uncommon with the advent of acyclovir treatment and, in the case of HSV, acyclovir prophylaxis.

Pneumonia due to "typical" respiratory viruses—including parainfluenza types 1 and 3, influenza A and B, and respiratory syncytial virus (RSV)—occurs sporadically as in other immunocompromised patients and in normal persons and is (except with parainfluenza type 1) more common during the winter months. Nosocomial transmission from infected health-care workers has been documented. The incidence of respiratory virus infection may be higher than previously appreciated. An incidence of 15 percent was observed over two winter periods in marrow transplant patients in Seattle, occurring predominantly before transplantation.[32] Several epidemics of respiratory viral infections have been reported in transplant recipients when infection was noted in the community.[26] Most patients developed upper respiratory infections with fever, coryza, and cough. Approximately one-half of these progressed to lower respiratory tract disease with radiographic infiltrates and hypoxemia. Mortality approached 80 percent despite treatment with aerosolized ribavirin. Although seemingly less common, similar experiences with parainfluenza infections have been reported.[55]

Recently described members of the herpesvirus family have been noted in lung tissues of patients with pneumonia and blood of febrile recipients after transplantation. Human herpesvirus 6, the cause of childhood roseola (exanthema subitum), has been detected in the lungs of some patients with idiopathic pneumonia.[9] It is unclear whether this virus is a cause of pneumonia or merely latently reactivated, since virtually all adults are seropositive for the virus.

COURSE OF DISEASE, PREVENTION, AND TREATMENT

Most patients with adenovirus pneumonia have a progressive course leading to death over days to weeks, usually with multisystem disease. Usually the diagnosis is made only at postmortem examination. There is no proven treatment for adenovirus infection, although interferon remains a theoretical possibility and intravenous ribavirin has been tried.

The mortality for patients with RSV pneumonia is 50 to 80 percent even after treatment with aerosolized ribavirin, but survival may be better in patients with onset later after transplantation. Patients with parainfluenza may have a lower mortality. Finally, the course of VZV and, presumably, HSV pneumonia should be similar to the other manifestations of these infections, with response to acyclovir treatment expected over several days to a week and ultimate survival expected.

With the exception of acyclovir treatment for HSV or VZV infection, proven effective therapy for other viral pneumonia is not available. Intravenous acyclovir should be given at the dose of 500 mg/m^2 every 8 h, with appropriate adjustment for renal function. Treatment should be continued for a minimum of 7 days, and longer courses may be necessary if new lesions continue to form among patients with VZV infection and depending on the clinical response of the patient. Both ribavirin and leukocyte interferon use has been attempted for adenovirus infection, with unclear results.

Aerosolized ribavirin has been given for parainfluenza and RSV pneumonia. Patients with RSV pneumonia who have survived tended to develop disease after marrow engraftment and were treated before the onset of respiratory failure. A recent report of combined treatment with aerosolized ribavirin and intravenous immunoglobulin (IV-Ig, 500 mg every other day) was associated with survival in eight of nine patients who were treated before the onset of respiratory failure.[56] Clearly, early detection of infection and treatment with ribavirin (and possibly IV-Ig) are crucial to improved outcome. Prompt screening of nasal and throat specimens (rapid culture and viral detection method, such as fluorescence antibody stains or ELISA) from patients with upper respiratory tract symptoms is critical to identifying infected patients. Those with signs or symptoms of lower respiratory tract disease should be aggressively evaluated with BAL and treated before the development of significant hypoxemia. Hand-washing and segregation of infected patients and staff are important measures to stem the spread of infection.

Fungal Infections

INCIDENCE AND EPIDEMIOLOGY

Fungal infections have emerged as a major clinical problem after marrow transplantation and may be found in as many as 30 percent of all patients at autopsy. These infections are discussed in detail in Chapter 147. *Aspergillus* infection is documented in 4 to 13 percent of marrow recipients; also seen are *Mucormycosis, Fusarium, Rhizopus,* and *Petriellidium* (also known as *Pseudoallescheria).*[57] Disseminated yeast infection, especially with *Candida albicans* or *tropicalis,* is reported in over 20 percent of patients receiving therapy for hematologic malignancies, and in our center approximately 50 percent of patients with invasive *Candida* infection have pulmonary involvement.[22] In contrast, pulmonary involvement by filamentous fungi is the rule in infected patients. Many of these diagnoses are made at autopsy, as the premortem diagnosis may be difficult to establish.

Major risk factors for invasive fungal infections are the level and duration of neutropenia, age of the patient, the presence of GVHD, total number of other infections, and corticosteroid administration after marrow grafting.[57] The frequency of *Aspergillus* infections is similar in recipients of allogeneic and autologous transplants, but they occur during periods of neutropenia before engraftment among autologous marrow recipients and after engraftment among allogeneic recipients. Autologous recipients have less *Candida,* but not *Aspergillus,* infection than allograft recipients.

CLINICAL PRESENTATION

Most marrow recipients with clinical evidence of *Aspergillus* infections have been described as having fever that is unresponsive to antibiotics. However, a more specific finding is the presence of a focal parenchymal lesion on chest radiograph. Of 23 marrow transplant patients with such lesions, 78 percent were found to have fungal infections, regardless of absence of fever.[14] Although the radiographic presentation of pulmonary fungal disease was unilateral in 52 percent of pediatric marrow recipients at the University of Minnesota, bilateral changes were frequent because of concurrent or mixed infections.[1] In addition, *Aspergillus* infection may manifest with metastatic foci, such as seizure activity due to cerebral spread. Detection of filamentous fungi in respiratory secretions (sputum or BAL) in immunosuppressed patients is highly suggestive of active infection. Such findings should prompt early treatment. Detection of yeast in such specimens often represents colonization, rather than pneumonia. Establishing yeast, such as *Candida* species, as the cause of pneumonia is difficult, often requiring biopsy and/or empiric therapy.

COURSE OF DISEASE AND TREATMENT

The mortality from pulmonary infection with filamentous fungi among marrow transplant recipients is estimated at 80 percent.[31] Among 20 cases of *Aspergillus* infection detected premortem by Wingard and colleagues,[57] only one patient recovered. Early diagnosis and treatment, however, may improve survival rates. Favorable outcome with pulmonary filamentous fungal infection has followed treatment with amphotericin at 1 mg/kg per day to a total dose of 2 g or more.[1,14,57] The optimal therapy and dosing for invasive aspergillosis have not been established, but the regimen should probably include amphotericin. Some centers administer the drug at doses up to 1.5 mg/kg per day and add 5-fluorouracil to the course of therapy. Although most successful treatment of these pulmonary fungal infections after marrow transplantation has also included surgical resection, the precise role of surgery is not clear. Recovery by marrow recipients without complete surgical resection has been noted. Adjunctive therapy with granulocyte transfusions and/or granulocyte colony-stimulating factors (G-CSF) remains investigational.

Treatment for invasive *Candida* infection is largely empiric. Amphotericin in doses of at least 0.5 mg/kg per day until clinical response occurs is commonly employed.

PREVENTION

Respiratory colonization with fungal spores or organisms is a putative step in the pathogenesis of pulmonary fungal infection with agents such as *Aspergillus.* Some centers have experienced outbreaks of fungal pneumonia associated with environmental exposure—during a period of construction, for instance—and the use of HEPA filtered air may be effective in this circumstance. This has not been a universal observation, however, and in our center we have not seen a decrease in the incidence of *Aspergillus* infection associated with the use of protective environment. Prophylactic administration of oral fluconazole decreases the incidence of *C. albicans* infection, but other *Candida* species persist as a problem.[21]

Bacterial Infections

Pathologic specimens rarely confirm bacterial bronchopneumonia after marrow transplantation.[13,14,24] However, this may represent a selection bias of patients undergoing biopsy, since bacterial pneumonia has been reported in as many as 28 percent of autopsies of marrow recipients in some centers.[51] The distribution of bacteria responsible for pulmonary infections during the neutropenic period is unknown. Aerobic gram-negative organisms are frequently detected during episodes of bacterial pulmonary infection.[10] Half of the cases of bacteremia after marrow transplantation are due to gram-positive organisms, especially coagulase-negative *Staphylococcus,* with the rest due primarily to aerobic gram-negative Enterobacteriaceae.

There is little to distinguish the presentation of bacterial pneumonia from that in other neutropenic hosts. Fevers occur frequently after transplantation, as do pulmonary infiltrates. Bronchopneumonia after marrow transplantation may appear as patchy or confluent bilateral alveolar consolidation that progresses rapidly. During the early posttransplantation period, the difficulty lies more in the similarities in presentation of bacterial and nonbacterial pulmonary diseases, such as oral aspiration. Sputum production is rare among profoundly neutropenic patients, and diagnosis relies on the clinical response to empiric therapy, blood cultures, or invasive diagnostic procedures, such as bronchoscopy or lung biopsy.

Although infection with *Legionella* species among marrow recipients has been an uncommon finding, the presentation appears to have characteristics similar to those in other patient groups (see Chapter 144). Focal infiltrates and spiking fevers unresponsive to broad-spectrum antibiotics are often reported. Pulmonary infection with *Legionella micdadei* has been reported to present as focal radiographic lesions, occasionally with few systemic symptoms.[47] This clinical appearance should also prompt consideration of invasive pulmonary fungal disease or pulmonary infarct due to embolus.

Uncommon Nonbacterial Infections

PNEUMOCYSTIS

Pneumocystis carinii pneumonia occurs in as many as 10 percent of marrow transplant recipients without the use of trimethoprim-sulfamethoxazole prophylaxis, although regional and center-to-center variations exist (see Chapter 150). As in children with acute leukemia, routine prophylaxis has markedly reduced the occurrence of *P. carinii* pneumonia. At this time the predominant, if not exclusive, occurrence of *P. carinii* is among patients who fail to receive any prophylaxis after transplant because of either poor ngraftment or documented allergy to trimethoprim-sulfamethoxazole. Thus, *P. carinii* pneumonia should be considered in the differential diagnosis of diffuse pneumonia among patients who have not received prophylaxis. *P. carinii* pneumonia also occurs among recipients of autologous and twin transplants.

Except for patients being treated for chronic GVHD (who remain at risk and who should continue to receive prophylaxis), the risk period for *P. carinii* pneumonia ends approximately 120 days after transplantation. Because it is highly effective, trimethoprim-sulfamethoxazole is the prophylactic regimen of choice. Various trimethoprim-sulfamethoxazole regimens for the prevention of *P. carinii* pneumonia have been employed, starting from twice-weekly use at high dose (240 mg) of the trimethoprim. Although not studied in comparative trials, the dose of 5 mg/kg (trimethoprim component) given as half of the dose twice daily on 2 days of the week (i.e., one double-strength tablet twice daily in most adults) has provided effective prophylaxis. This dose was originally instituted because of gastrointestinal intolerance and concerns about marrow toxicity when prophylaxis was given daily, although the latter concern remains poorly documented.

Prophylaxis is initiated before transplantation and discontinued 48 h before marrow infusion. It is then reinstituted after engraftment, i.e., as a circulating neutrophil count of at least 0.5×10^9/L. In patients without chronic GVHD, this regimen is discontinued approximately 120 days after transplantation. However, *P. carinii* remains a risk among patients with chronic GVHD, and prophylaxis is continued for as long as treatment for chronic GVHD is necessary. An additional benefit of the daily trimethoprim-sulfamethoxazole dose among patients with chronic GVHD appeared to be reduction in bacterial infections, including infection with *S. pneumoniae*. Prophylaxis is also given until day 120 after transplantation to recipients of autologous and twin transplants. Patients with allergies to sulfa may undergo desensitization so that prophylaxis with trimethoprim-sulfamethoxazole can be administered. Alternatives include dapsone and pentamidine. We do not favor pentamidine, having experienced cases of fatal *P. carinii* pneumonia during courses of both oral and aerosolized drug.

The median onset of *P. carinii* pneumonia is 60 days after transplantation. The clinical signs and symptoms are not distinct from those of other causes of diffuse pneumonia that occur in immunocompromised patients. Treatment for *P. carinii* pneumonia after marrow transplant is similar to that in other patients. Best results have been achieved with intravenous trimethoprim-sulfamethoxazole at a dose of 15 to 20 mg/kg per day of the

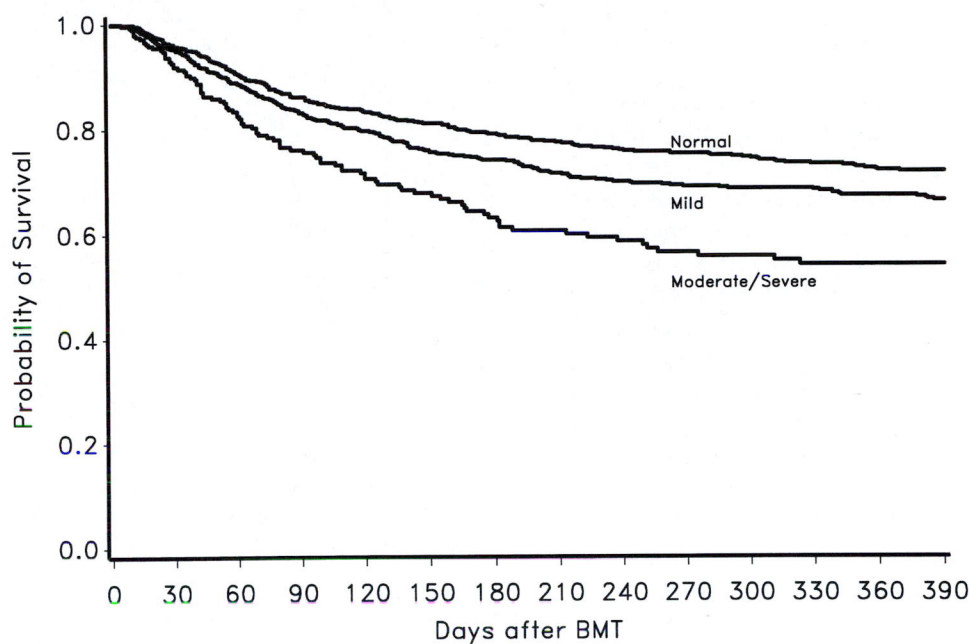

A

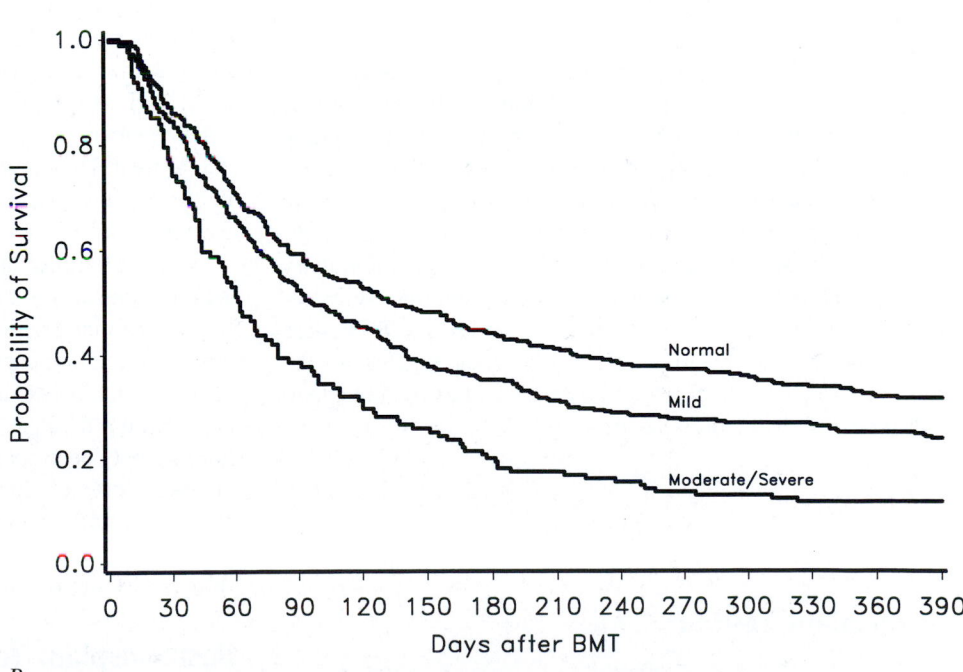

B

FIGURE 137-3 Kaplan-Meier survival plots estimated from the Cox proportional hazards regression model for "low-risk" patients compared to those for "high-risk" patients for various degrees of $D_{L}CO_{sb}$ abnormality. *A.* "Low-risk" patients were less than 21 years old with malignancy in remission and received HLA-identical marrow grafts. *B.* "High-risk" patients were more than 21 years old with malignancy in relapse and received HLA-nonidentical marrow grafts. *(Based on data of Crawford and Fisher,[11] with permission.)*

trimethoprim component, given in divided doses every 6 to 8 h for 14 to 21 days. Oral administration may be used after clinical response is observed. Intravenous pentamidine at recommended doses is the major alternative in patients with documented severe allergy to trimethoprim-sulfamethoxazole.

TOXOPLASMA

Most marrow transplant patients with *Toxoplasma gondii* infection have had only central nervous system disease diagnosed and treated during life, or involvement of heart and brain documented at postmortem. However, several have had more generalized disease, diagnosed only at autopsy, in the myocardium, lungs, and brain. Chest radiographs in these patients showed diffuse, patchy involvement. These patients also had concomitant bacterial or viral infection, and the contribution of *Toxoplasma* to either the signs or symptoms of pulmonary disease is uncertain. Most infections have been fatal. Treatment is similar to that for other immunocompromised patients.

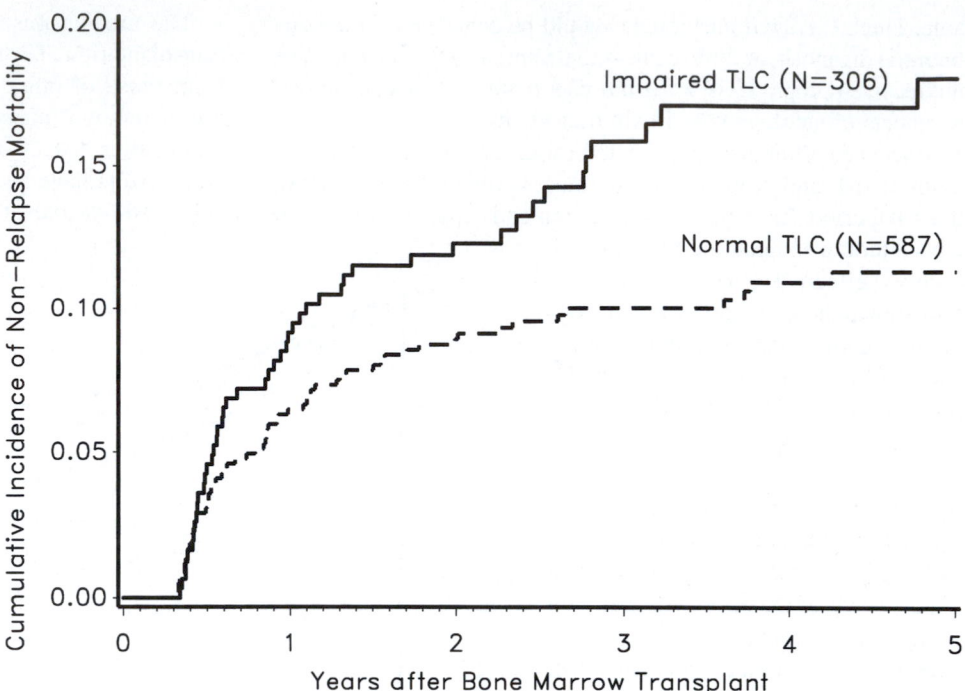

FIGURE 137-4   Estimates of the cumulative probabilities of nonrelapse death as a function of total lung capacity (p = 0.004, log rank). The solid curve corresponds to marrow recipients with pulmonary function test result impairment and the dashed curve to those with normal pulmonary function test results. *(Based on data of Crawford et al,[16] with permission.)*

MYCOBACTERIA

Both typical and atypical mycobacterial infection has been reported in a small number of patients. Although infection with *M. avium-intracellulare* has been reported in patients undergoing transplantation in Texas, this organism has otherwise been uncommon. Clinical signs and symptoms have been similar to those in other immunocompromised patients. Of interest, we have observed several patients with development of single pulmonary nodules in the first several months after transplant that were presumed to be fungal. Biopsy revealed *M. tuberculosis*. Both were known to be skin test positive before transplant. Because of the paucity of cases of typical tuberculosis after marrow transplant, a high index of suspicion is needed.

PULMONARY FUNCTION TESTING IN HEMATOPOIETIC STEM CELL TRANSPLANTATION

Pretransplant Testing

Pulmonary function testing (PFT) is a standard part of the pretransplant evaluation at many centers. The results form baseline data for comparison with later testing, and have been used as an indication to exclude a candidate for transplantation. Abnormalities in the measures of airflow, lung volume, and diffusing capacity have been associated with increased risk of pulmonary complications after transplantation.[4,11,20] After accounting for

other clinical characteristics associated with death after transplantation (age, relapsed malignancy, HLA-mismatched graft), restrictive lung defect (decreased total lung capacity), hypoxemia, and reduced diffusing capacity are associated with statistically increased risk of death, especially within the first few months after transplant (Fig. 137-3). The risks associated with these PFT results are applicable to autologous as well as allogeneic marrow recipients, suggesting that they predict mortality due to treatment-related toxicities. Hypoxemia and reduced diffusing capacity were independently associated with death, each carrying risk.

While pretransplant PFT results are statistically associated with complications and death, there are no absolute values for these tests that predict these outcomes with specificity. On average, a total lung capacity or diffusing capacity value (corrected for hemoglobin content) below the lower limits of normal, or an A-a gradient for P_{O_2} ($P[A-a]O_2$) that exceeds the upper limits of normal, may be associated with a probability of a 20 percent decrease in survival. Such information should not be used as an absolute contraindication to transplantation, but rather in combination with other known risks for transplant-related mortality to fully assess the risks.

Posttransplant Testing

PFT performed after marrow transplantation has consistently revealed reductions in lung volumes and diffusing capacities associated with total-body irradiation and intensive chemotherapy. PFT abnormalities have been reported to include declines in lung volume, gas diffusion, and airflow. Losses of lung volume are more pronounced among patients who survive pneumonia after transplant.[52] The reductions are not significantly different between autologous and allogeneic transplants when acute GVHD is accounted for.[53] Reductions in lung volumes, diffusing capacity, and exercise tolerance were documented after treatment for leukemia in children as well, and were thought to be largely secondary to chemotherapy.[28] The declines in lung volume may be at least partly reversible within 2 years after transplantation, while the low diffusing capacity reportedly persists for several years. Development of airflow obstruction has been seen in approximately 10 percent of allogeneic marrow recipients in the presence of chronic GVHD and most often is related to obliterative bronchiolitis. Such PFT results strongly suggest that lung parenchymal and vascular injury are common features of marrow transplant, even in the absence of recognized infection or idiopathic pneumonia.

Few reports have examined abnormalities in other PFT results for association with increased mortality. Badier and colleagues[2] noted that both relapse of malignancy and overall mortality correlated with falls in lung volumes and diffusion 1 year after marrow transplantation. Recently, PFT results at 3 months after transplant were shown to be associated with nonrelapse mortality.[16] At 3 months after transplantation, a restrictive lung defect or a significant decline (at least 15 percent) in total lung capacity from baseline despite remaining within the normal range is associated with a twofold increased risk of nonrelapse mortality (Fig. 137-4). Neither airflow obstruction nor impairment in diffusing capacity is associated with an increased risk. Abnormalities of total lung capacity 3 months after transplant are associated with death from respiratory failure, but not with an increased risk of chronic GVHD. On the basis of these results, we routinely evaluate lung function 3 months and yearly after marrow transplantation.

REFERENCES

1. Allan BT, Patton D, Ramsay NKC, et al: Pulmonary fungal infections after bone marrow transplantation. *Pediatr Radiol* 18:118–122, 1988.

2. Badier M, Guillot C, Delpierre S, et al: Pulmonary function changes 100 days and one year after bone marrow transplantation. *Bone Marrow Transplant* 12:457–461, 1993.

3. Bowden RA, Sayers M, Flournoy N, et al: Cytomegalovirus immune globulin and seronegative blood products to prevent primary cytomegalovirus infection after marrow transplantation. *New Engl J Med* 314:1006–1010, 1986.

4. Carlson K, Backlund L, Smedmyr B, et al: Pulmonary function and complications subsequent to autologous bone marrow transplantation. *Bone Marrow Transplant* 14:805–811, 1994.

5. Chan CK, Hyland RH, Hutcheon MA, et al: Small-airways disease in recipients of allogeneic bone marrow transplants. *Medicine* 66:327–340, 1987.

6. Chao NJ, Duncan SR, Long GD, et al: Corticosteroid therapy for diffuse alveolar hemorrhage in autologous bone marrow transplant recipients. *Ann Intern Med* 114:145–146, 1991.

7. Clark JG, Crawford SW, Madtes DK, Sullivan KM: Obstructive lung disease after allogeneic marrow transplantation: Clinical presentation and course. *Ann Intern Med* 111:368–376, 1989.

8. Clark JG, Hansen JA, Hertz MI, et al: NHLBI Workshop Summary: Idiopathic pneumonia syndrome following bone marrow transplantation. *Am Rev Respir Dis* 147:1601–1606, 1992.

9. Cone RW, Hackman RC, Huang M-LW, et al: Human herpesvirus-6 in lung tissue from patients with pneumonitis after bone marrow transplantation. *New Engl J Med* 329:156–161, 1993.

10. Cordonnier C, Bernaudin JF, Beirling P, et al: Pulmonary complications occurring after allogeneic bone marrow transplantation. *Cancer* 58:1047–1054, 1986.

11. Crawford SW, Fisher L: Predictive value of pulmonary function tests before marrow transplantation. *Chest* 101:1257–1264, 1992.

12. Crawford SW, Hackman RC: Clinical course of idiopathic pneumonia after marrow transplantation. *Am Rev Respir Dis* 147:1393–1400, 1993.

13. Crawford SW, Hackman RC, Clark JG: Open lung biopsy diagnosis of diffuse pulmonary infiltrates after marrow transplantation. *Chest* 94:949–953, 1988.

14. Crawford SW, Hackman RC, Clark JG: Biopsy diagnosis and clinical outcome of focal pulmonary lesions after marrow transplantation. *Transplantation* 48:266–271, 1989.

15. Crawford SW, Petersen FB: Long-term survival from respiratory failure after marrow transplantation. *Am Rev Respir Dis* 145:510–514, 1992.

16. Crawford SW, Pepe M, Lin D, et al: Abnormalities of pulmonary function tests after marrow transplantation predict nonrelapse mortality. *Am J Respir Crit Care Med* 152:690–695, 1995.

17. Dickout WJ, Chan CK, Hyland RH, et al: Prevention of acute pulmonary edema after bone marrow transplantation. *Chest* 92:303–309, 1987.

18. Emanuel D, Cunningham I, Jules-Elysee K, et al: Cytomegalovirus pneumonia after bone marrow transplantation successfully treated with the combination of ganciclovir and high-dose intravenous immune globulin. *Ann Intern Med* 109:777–782, 1988.

19. Faber-Langendoen K, Caplan AL, McGlave PB: Survival of adult bone marrow transplant patients receiving mechanical ventilation: A case for restricted use. *Bone Marrow Transplant* 12:501–507, 1993.

20. Ghalie R, Szidon JP, Thompson L, et al: Evaluation of pulmonary complications after bone marrow transplantation: The role of pretransplant pulmonary function tests. *Bone Marrow Transplant* 10:359–365, 1992.

21. Goodman JL, Winston DJ, Greenfield RA, et al: A controlled trial of fluconazole to prevent fungal infections in patients undergoing bone marrow transplantation. *New Engl J Med* 326:845–851, 1992.

22. Goodrich JM, Reed EC, Mori M, et al: Clinical features and analysis of risk factors for invasive candidal infection after marrow transplantation. *J Infect Dis* 164:731–740, 1991.

23. Goodrich JM, Bowden RA, Fisher L, et al: Ganciclovir prophylaxis to prevent cytomegalovirus disease after allogeneic marrow transplant. *Ann Intern Med* 118:173–178, 1993.

24. Hackman RC: Lower respiratory tract, in Sale GE, Shulman HM (eds), *The Pathology of Bone Marrow Transplantation*. New York, Masson, 1984, pp 156–170.

25. Hackman RC, Madtes DK, Petersen FB, Clark JG: Pulmonary veno-occlusive disease following bone marrow transplantation. *Transplantation* 47:989–992, 1989.

26. Harrington RD, Hooton TM, Hackman RC, et al: An outbreak of respiratory syncytial virus in a bone marrow transplant center. *J Infect Dis* 165:987–993, 1992.

27. Holland HK, Wingard JR, Beschorner WE, et al: Bronchiolitis obliterans in bone marrow transplantation and its relationship to chronic graft-v-host disease and low serum IgG. *Blood* 72:621–627, 1988.

28. Jenney ME, Faragher EB, Jones PH, Woodcock A: Lung function and exercise in survivors of childhood leukemia. *Med Pediatr Oncol* 24:222–230, 1995.

29. Jules-Elysee K, Stover DE, Yahalom J, et al: Pulmonary complications in lymphoma patients treated with high-dose therapy and autologous bone marrow transplantation. *Am Rev Respir Dis* 146:485–491, 1992.

30. Kantrow SP, Hackman RC, Boeckh M, et al: Idiopathic pneumonia syndrome after marrow transplantation: The changing spectrum of lung injury. *Transplantation*. In press.

31. Krowka MJ, Rosenow EC, Hoagland HC: Pulmonary complications of bone marrow transplantation. *Chest* 87:237–246, 1985.

32. Ljungman P, Gleaves CA, Meyers JD: Respiratory virus infections in immunocompromised patients. *Bone Marrow Transplant* 4:35–40, 1989.

33. Mathew P, Bozeman P, Krance RA, et al: Bronchiolitis obliterans organizing pneumonia (BOOP) in children after allogeneic bone marrow transplantation. *Bone Marrow Transplant* 13:221–223, 1994.

34. McDonald GB, Sharma P, Matthews DE, et al: Venocclusive disease of the liver after bone marrow transplantation: Diagnosis, incidence, and predisposing factors. *Hepatology* 4:116–122, 1984.

35. McDonald GB, Shulman HM, Wolford JL, Spencer GD: Liver disease after human marrow transplantation. *Semin Liver Dis* 7:210–229, 1987.

36. Metcalf JP, Rennard SI, Reed EC, et al: Corticosteroids as adjunctive therapy for diffuse alveolar hemorrhage associated with bone marrow transplantation. *Am J Med* 96:327–334, 1994.

37. Meyers JD, Flournoy N, Thomas ED: Nonbacterial pneumonia after allogeneic marrow transplantation: A review of ten years' experience. *Rev Infect Dis* 4:1119–1132, 1982.

38. Meyers JD, Flournoy N, Thomas ED: Risk factors for cytomegalovirus infection after human marrow transplantation. *J Infect Dis* 153:478–488, 1986.

39. Ramsey PG, Fife KH, Hackman RC, et al: Herpes simplex virus pneumonia. *Ann Intern Med* 97:813–820, 1982.

40. Reed EC, Bowden RA, Dandliker PS, et al: Treatment of cytomegalovirus pneumonia with ganciclovir and intravenous cytomegalovirus immunoglobulin in patients with bone marrow transplants. *Ann Intern Med* 109:783–788, 1988.

41. Riddell SR: Pathogenesis of cytomegalovirus pneumonia in immunocompromised hosts. *Semin Respir Infect* 10:199–208, 1995.

42. Robbins RA, Linder J, Stahl MG, et al: Diffuse alveolar hemorrhage in autologous bone marrow transplant recipients. *Am J Med* 87:511–518, 1989.

43. Rubenfeld GD, Crawford SW: Withdrawing life support from mechanically ventilated bone marrow transplant patients: A case for evidence-based guidelines. *Ann Intern Med* 125:625–633, 1996.

44. Sargent MA, Cairns RA, Murdoch MJ, et al: Obstructive lung disease in children after allogeneic bone marrow transplantation: Evaluation with high-resolution CT. *AJR Am J Roentgenol* 164:693–696, 1995.

45. Schmidt GM, Kovacs A, Zaia JA, et al: Ganciclovir/immunoglobulin combination therapy for the treatment of human cytomegalovirus-associated interstitial pneumonia in bone marrow allograft recipients. *Transplantation* 46:905–907, 1988.

46. Schmidt GM, Horak DA, Niland JC, et al: A randomized, controlled trial of prophylactic ganciclovir for cytomegalovirus pulmonary infection in recipients of allogeneic bone marrow transplantation. *New Engl J Med* 324:1005–1011, 1991.

47. Schwebke JR, Hackman R, Bowden R: *Legionella micdadei* in bone marrow transplant recipients. *Rev Infect Dis* 12:824–828, 1990.

48. Shields AF, Hackman RC, Fife KH, et al: Adenovirus infections in patients undergoing bone-marrow transplantation. *New Engl J Med* 312:529–533, 1985.

49. Schubert MM, Williams BE, Lloid Me, et al: Clinical assessment scale for the rating of oral mucosal changes associated with bone marrow transplantation. *Cancer* 69:2469–2477, 1992.

50. Sisson JH, Reed EC, Robbins RA, et al: Impairment of nasal mucociliary clearance during bone marrow transplantation. University of Nebraska Medical Center Bone Marrow Transplantation Pulmonary Study Group. *Bone Marrow Transplant* 13:631–633, 1994.

51. Sloane JP, Depledge MH, Powles RL, et al: Histopathology of the lung after bone marrow transplantation. *J Clin Pathol* 36:546–554, 1983.

52. Springmeyer SC, Flournoy N, Sullivan KM, et al: Pulmonary function changes in long-term survivors of allogeneic marrow transplantation, in Gale RP (ed), *Recent Advances in Bone Marrow Transplantation*. New York, Alan R Liss, 1983, pp 343–353.

53. Tait RC, Burnett AK, Robertson AG, et al: Subclinical pulmonary function defects following autologous and allogeneic bone marrow transplantation: Relationship to total body irradiation and graft-versus-host disease. *Int J Radiat Oncol Biol Phys* 20:1219–1227, 1991.

54. Troussard X, Bernaudin JF, Cordonnier C, et al: Pulmonary veno-occlusive disease after bone marrow transplantation. *Thorax* 39:956–957, 1984.

55. Wendt CH, Weisdorf DJ, Jordan MC, et al: Parainfluenza virus respiratory infection after bone marrow transplantation. *New Engl J Med* 326:921–926, 1992.

56. Whimbey E, Champlin RE, Englund JA, et al: Combination therapy with aerosolized ribavirin and intravenous immunoglobulin for respiratory syncytial virus disease in adult bone marrow transplant recipients. *Bone Marrow Transplant* 16:393–399, 1995.

57. Wingard JR, Beals SU, Santos GW, et al: Aspergillus infections in bone marrow transplant recipients. *Bone Marrow Transplant* 2:175–181, 1987.

58. Wingard JR, Mellits ED, Sostrin MB, et al: Interstitial pneumonia after allogeneic marrow transplantation. *Medicine (Baltimore)* 67:175–186, 1988.

59. Wingard JR, Mellits ED, Jones RJ, et al: Association of hepatic veno-occlusive disease with interstitial pneumonitis in bone marrow transplant recipients. *Bone Marrow Transplant* 4:685–689, 1989.

60. Valteau D, Hartmann O, Benhamou E, et al: Nonbacterial nonfungal interstitial pneumonitis following autologous bone marrow transplantation in children treated with high-dose chemotherapy without total-body irradiation. *Transplantation* 45:737–740, 1988.

PNEUMONIA IN THE ORGAN TRANSPLANT PATIENT

Jay A. Fishman / Robert H. Rubin

The challenge of pulmonary infection in the organ transplant patient is a daunting one for the transplant clinician. Pneumonia is the most common cause of potentially fatal infection in these patients. The possible etiologies of pulmonary infection are diverse, ranging from common bacterial and viral pathogens that affect the entire community (although the impact of such pathogens may be considerably greater in these patients) to opportunistic pathogens that cause invasive disease only in immunocompromised hosts. The impaired inflammatory response induced by the immunosuppressive therapy required to prevent and treat allograft rejection will often suppress the clinical and radiologic findings usually engendered by microbial invasion, rendering early diagnosis, the key to successful therapy, difficult. The antimicrobial therapy required to treat established infection is far more complex than that necessary in the normal host due to the need for extended courses of potentially toxic drugs (e.g., amphotericin B) and the propensity for drug interactions with the mainstays of modern immunosuppressive therapy for transplant recipients, cyclosporine and tacrolimus (FK506).[29,33] The purpose of this chapter is to provide a practical approach to the challenge of preventing and treating pulmonary infection in the organ transplant patient, with a particular emphasis on the link between the nature and intensity of the immunosuppressive therapy and the pathogenesis of important forms of pulmonary infection.

RISK OF INFECTION

The risk of serious infections including pneumonia in the organ transplant patient is largely determined by the interaction between two factors: the patient's *epidemiologic exposures* and the patient's *net state of immunosuppression*. The relationship between these two factors should be regarded as a semiquantitative one. For example, the occurrence of opportunistic infection when the immune status of the patient is near normal is *prima facie* evidence that an excessive environmental exposure has occurred; conversely, even minimal environmental exposures can cause invasive infection in an individual who is maximally immunosuppressed.[29]

Epidemiologic Exposures

The epidemiologic exposures of importance to the transplant patient can be divided into two general categories: those occurring within the community and those occurring within the hospital. Within the community, the major concerns are *Mycobacterium tuberculosis,* the geographically restricted systemic mycoses (blastomycosis, coccidioidomycosis, and histoplasmosis), *Strongyloides stercoralis, Pneumocystis carinii, Legionella* species, and community-acquired respiratory viral infections (e.g., influenza, respiratory syncytial virus, and parainfluenza) (see Fig. 138-1). For *M. tuberculosis* and the systemic mycoses, three patterns of disease are observed: reactivation of an old dormant focus with secondary dissemination; progressive primary disease, with postprimary dissemination; and, perhaps most interesting, superinfection in which a previously immune individual is rendered susceptible by posttransplant immune suppression and becomes reinfected following fresh exposure, with the potential for systemic spread. Clinical syndromes that suggest the possibility of one of these processes in individuals with a recent or remote history of possible exposure to one of these agents,

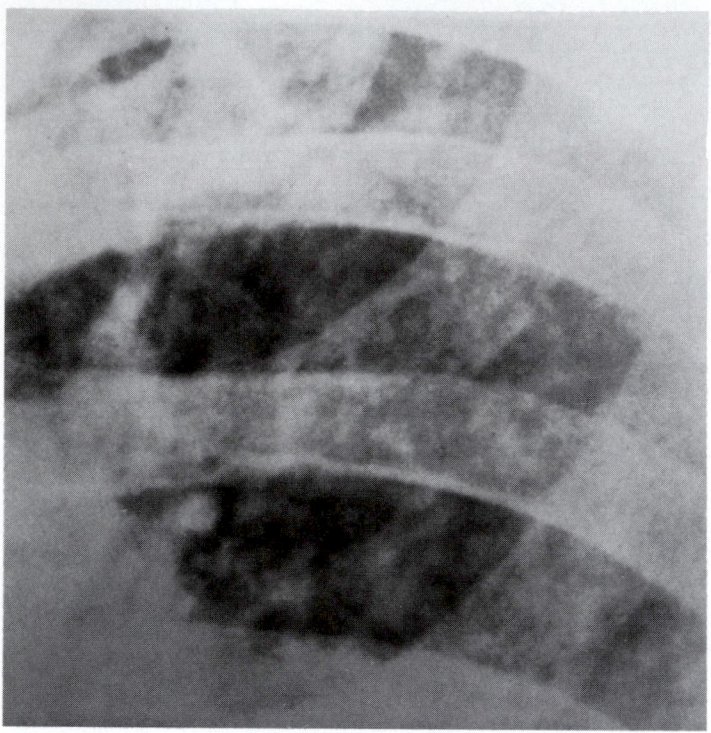

A

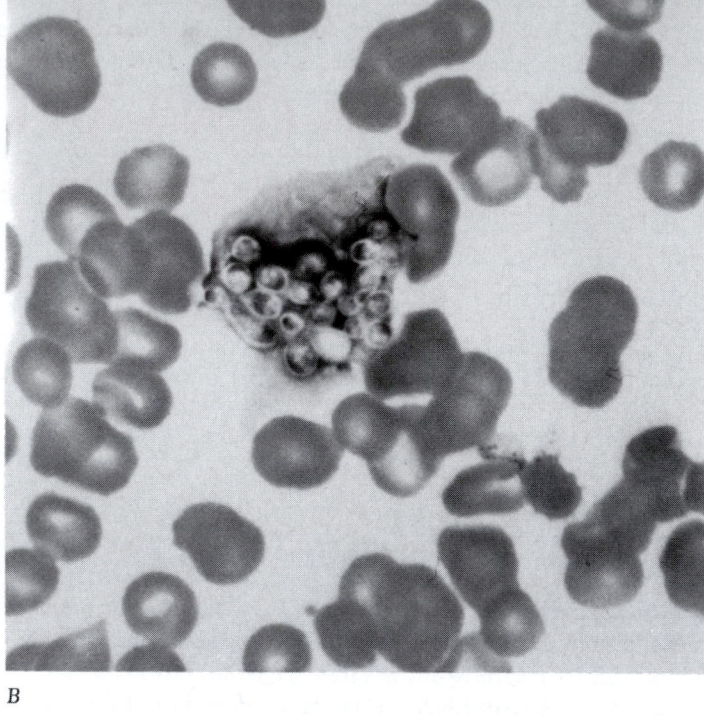

B

FIGURE 138-1 *Histoplasma capsulatum.* A 56-year-old man, lifelong resident of Kansas, presented $2\frac{1}{2}$ years after a renal transplant with fever, nonproductive cough, and 3-month weight loss. The chest radiograph was diffusely abnormal. *A.* Close-up reveals extensive micronodular dis-

ease. *B.* Peripheral blood smear on which the diagnosis of disseminated histoplasmosis was made shows a macrophage laden with *Histoplasma capsulatum.* Treatment with a total of 2.5 g of amphotericin B resulted in total clearing of the radiograph and blood and cure of the infection.

include the occurrence of fever of unknown origin, subacute pulmonary infection, or disseminated infection to the skin, liver, brain, skeletal system, or other sites.[29]

Strongyloides stercoralis is the one protozoan infection affecting the lungs that is an important potential pathogen in this patient population because of its unique autoinfection cycle. Once acquired, this organism can remain dormant in the gastrointestinal tract for decades. Although in the normal host the rhabditiform larvae complete development into infectious filariform larvae outside the body, in the immunocompromised host the change to infective larvae can be completed within the body. The clinical consequences of reactivation in the transplant patient result from hyperinfection, with hemorrhagic enterocolitis and pneumonitis reflecting the normal sites of replication, and systemic dissemination as filariform larvae penetrate the bowel wall and invade surrounding tissues, accompanied by gut microbial flora. The clinical presentations of these events include asthma; gram-negative sepsis with the acquired respiratory distress syndrome (ARDS), and/or gram-negative meningitis; postobstructive pneumonitis with cavitation and hemorrhage due to pulmonary filariform larvae; or other syndromes of overwhelming infection. Eosinophilia is often absent. Treatment of acute *Strongyloides* pulmonary infection with antihelminthic therapies is often ineffective; therapy is effective only for the mature intestinal parasites. Because of the excessive mortality of strongyloidiasis when it occurs after a transplant (greater than 50 percent), prevention by screening of transplant candidates with a history of residence in such endemic areas as Southeast Asia or South or Central America is indicated. Screening entails the examination

of material obtained at either duodenal intubation or after purging. Serologic testing is available (with limited cross-reactivity) and may be used as presumptive evidence of infection unless treatment has been received. Unlike the desperate situation after a transplant, asymptomatic infection is easily treated with thiabendazole (see Chapter 156).[6,7,20,36]

As increasing numbers of organ transplant patients are successfully rehabilitated and returned to their communities, the occurrence of community-acquired respiratory viral infections has become an important problem. Influenza and respiratory syncytial virus (RSV) infections have become especially important, with a rate of clinical pneumonia, due to both the virus and to bacterial superinfection, being far higher than for the general population. Unfortunately, the efficacy of influenza immunization in the transplant patient is far less than for the normal host and the efficacy of other prophylactic interventions (e.g., amantadine or RSV immune globulin) remains to be demonstrated in transplant recipients. These issues appear to be especially important in the lung and heart–lung transplant patients, who appear to be particularly susceptible to respiratory viral infection.[34]

Within the hospital, excessive environmental exposures can be divided into two general categories: *domiciliary* and *nondomiciliary*. Domiciliary exposures occur on the hospital unit where the patient is housed, when the air supply or potable water is contaminated with such pathogens as *Aspergillus* species, *Legionella* species, and such gram-negative bacilli as *Pseudomonas aeruginosa*. Nondomiciliary exposures occur when the patient is transported to operating rooms, radiology suites, or catheterization laboratories for essential procedures, and these environments are contaminated. Whereas domiciliary outbreaks are usually detected quite readily because of clustering of cases in time and space, nondomiciliary outbreaks, although possibly more common, are often more difficult to detect because of the lack of clustering on a particular hospital unit. The leading clue to the occurrence of a possible nosocomial hazard is the occurrence of opportunistic infection in a patient whose net state of immunosuppression would not normally lead to such an event.[29]

Net State of Immunosuppression

The net state of immunosuppression is a complex function determined by the interaction of several factors: the dose, duration, and temporal sequence in which immunosuppressive drugs are deployed (the most important); the presence of foreign bodies or injuries to the primary mucocutaneous barrier to infection (in this context, the endotracheal tube or bronchial anastomotic problems in the lung allograft recipient); neutropenia; metabolic problems including protein-calorie malnutrition, uremia, and, perhaps, hyperglycemia; the presence of devitalized tissues, hematoma, effusions, or adhesions following surgery; and infection with immunomodulating viruses that are particularly common in the transplant patient population—cytomegalovirus (CMV); Epstein-Barr virus (EBV); hepatitis B and C (HBV and HCV); and the human immunodeficiency virus (HIV). Although the immunosuppressive therapy is the major determinant of the risk of infection, the contribution of other factors is illustrated by the following observations from the Massachusetts General Hospital: There is a tenfold greater incidence in life-threatening infection in those patients with significant hypoalbuminemia (serum albumen less than 2.8); more than 90 percent of opportunistic infections of the lung occur in the setting of immunomodulating viral infection, with virtually all the exceptions being traceable to excessive environmental exposures. In general, more than one factor is present in the infected host; the identification of all the relevant factors is central to the prevention and treatment of infection in these hosts.[29]

TIMETABLE OF INFECTION

As immunosuppressive regimens have become standardized in recent years, it has become apparent that *different infectious processes occur at different points in the posttransplant course.* That is, although pneumonia can occur at any point in the posttransplant course, the etiology of pneumonia will vary depending on the amount of time that has passed since transplantation. As delineated in Fig. 138-2, the posttransplant course for all organ trans-

plant patients can be effectively divided into three time periods— the first month after transplant, the period 1 to 6 months after transplant, and the late period more than 6 months after transplant. The timetable is useful in three ways: in defining the differential diagnosis in the patient with pulmonary infection; as a clue to the presence of an excessive environmental hazard, particularly one within the hospital, since exceptions to the timetable are usually due to such exposures; and as a guide for designing preventative antimicrobial strategies that are most cost-effective.[29]

Infections in the First Month after Transplantation

In the first month after transplant, two major causes of pulmonary infection apply to all forms of organ transplantation. The first is the recurrence of pneumonia that was present prior to transplantation (in the lung allograft donor or in the recipient) but was incompletely treated, and which may be exacerbated after transplant due to superinfection with nosocomially acquired gram-negative bacilli and fungal species. This is most commonly seen in patients with end-stage liver or cardiac disease who require critical care support prior to transplant. Second, infection due to aspiration of nosocomial flora is often the result of postoperative vomiting (because of gastric distention or metabolic dysfunction) or due to a technical problem with the endotracheal tube in the perioperative period. The risk of antibiotic-resistant pneumonia will increase with the duration of the pretransplant hospitalization as well as with the duration of posttransplant intubation or ventilatory restriction (following the transplant operation).[12,29]

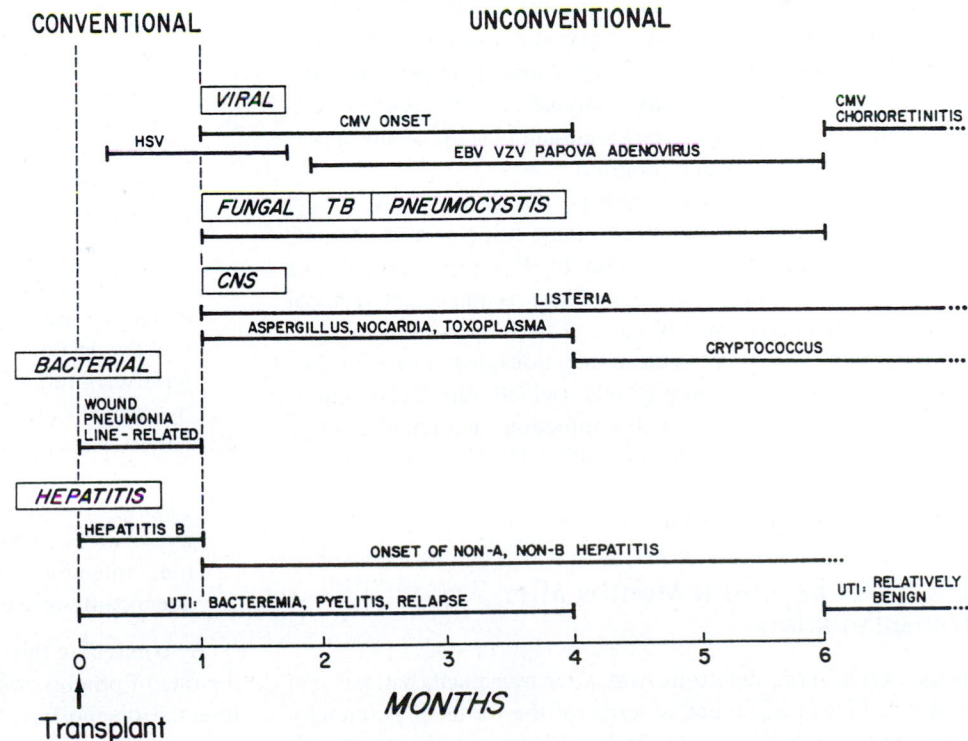

FIGURE 138-2   Timetable for the occurrence of infection following solid organ transplantation. *(From Rubin.[32])*

Extensive pulmonary injury before transplant places the patient at high risk for postoperative pneumonia that is poorly responsive to therapy. In the special case of the lung transplant patient who may require prolonged intubation, bacterial pneumonia and infection that threatens the bronchial anastomosis, particularly with fungi, are special concerns. These patients require exquisite attention to the technical aspects of the transplant procedure, to the management of the endotracheal tube, and the maintenance of pulmonary toilet (including, on occasion, repeated therapeutic bronchoscopy). Notable by their absence in the first posttransplant month are the opportunistic infections, despite the fact that the highest daily doses of immunosuppression are administered during this first month. This emphasizes that it is the *sustained exposure to immunosuppressive therapy,* "the area under the curve," that is the major determinant of the net state of immunosuppression.[29]

Infections 1 to 6 Months after Transplantation

In the period 1 to 6 months after transplant, the nature of pulmonary infection changes markedly. During this time period the immunomodulating viruses, particularly CMV, exert the maximal effects. Thus, CMV can directly cause pneumonia itself; CMV may contribute to the incidence of graft rejection necessitating increased exogenous immune suppression and increasing the risk of opportunistic infection; or CMV (and the other immunomodulating viruses) are globally immunosuppressive and can enhance the likelihood of pulmonary infections due to *Pneumocystis carinii, Aspergillus* species, and *Nocardia asteroides* in the *absence* of an unusual epidemiologic exposure. Unlike the bone marrow transplant recipient (see Chapter 137), the risk of active CMV *disease* (as compared with viral secretion) in the solid organ transplant recipient is greatest in the CMV-seronegative recipient of an organ from a seropositive donor. Thus, CMV prevention and the utilization of diagnostic techniques for CMV viremia (e.g., antigenemia assays, polymerase chain reaction testing, shell vial cultures with early antigen detection) are important parts of the therapeutic program.[29]

During this period, *in the absence of specific prophylaxis,* significant nonviral pulmonary infections are common at most transplant centers including those due to *P. carinii, Aspergillus* species, and *Nocardia asteroides.* There is important regional variation in the occurrence of each of these pathogens. At centers with high endemicity of these infections, low dose trimethoprim-sulfamethoxazole prophylaxis (which effectively eliminates *Pneumocystis* and nocardial infection) and epidemiologic protection against *Aspergillus* (as with a HEPA filtered air supply within the hospital) are effective, particularly in the context of effective CMV prevention.[29]

Infections beyond 6 Months after Transplantation

In the period more than 6 months after transplant, patients can be divided into two groups in terms of the forms of pulmonary infection that can develop. More than 85 percent of patients will have had a good result from their transplant and will have good allograft function and receive relatively modest levels of maintenance immunosuppression. These patients are subject to community-acquired respiratory virus infection, particularly influenza, and RSV and pneumococcal pneumonia. The remaining patients have had a less positive outcome from their transplant; these individuals have less satisfactory graft function and require far more intensive acute and chronic immunosuppressive therapies to manage rejection. These patients, often termed "chronic ne'er do wells," are the subgroup of transplant patients at highest risk for pulmonary infection with such organisms as *Pneumocystis carinii, Cryptococcus neoformans, Nocardia asteroides,* and *Aspergillus* species. For this subgroup of patients, prolonged trimethoprim-sulfamethoxazole prophylaxis, epidemiologic protection, and a consideration of fluconazole prophylaxis are indicated.[12,29]

RADIOLOGIC CLUES TO THE DIAGNOSIS OF PNEUMONIA IN THE ORGAN TRANSPLANT PATIENT

The presentation and evolution of the chest radiograph provide important clues to both the differential diagnosis of pulmonary infection in the transplant patient and the appropriate diagnostic workup that should be undertaken. The following radiologic parameters are useful in developing clinical-radiologic-pathologic correlations:[32]

1. Time of appearance, rate of progression, and time to resolution of pulmonary roentgenographic abnormalities in relation to clinical events.
2. Distribution of radiologic abnormalities. An abnormality confined to one anatomic area is considered *focal,* whereas widespread lesions are considered *diffuse.* Abnormalities that are present in more than one area, but are countable, are termed *multifocal.* As visualized particularly on computed tomographic scanning (CT), abnormalities may be located *centrally* or *peripherally* or both.
3. Which of three types of pulmonary infiltrate is present. The first type is a *consolidation,* in which there is substantial replacement of alveolar air by material of tissue density, typically with air bronchograms and a peripheral location of the abnormality. The second type is *peribronchovascular* (or *interstitial*), in which the infiltrate is predominantly oriented along the peribronchial or perivascular bundles. Finally, *nodular* lesions are space-occupying, nonanatomic lesions with well-defined, more or less rounded edges surrounded by aerated lung.
4. Other characteristics. These include pleural fluid, atelectasis, cavitation, lymphadenopathy, and cardiac enlargement. Pleural fluid is a clue to congestive heart failure and fluid overload when bilateral, and to necrotizing or granulomatous infection, especially when associated with lymphadenopathy or cavitation, when unilateral.

By combining this classification with information concerning the rate of progression of the illness (Table 138-1), a useful differential diagnosis is then generated. Thus, focal or multifocal consolidation of acute onset will quite likely be caused by bacterial infection. Similar multifocal lesions with subacute to chronic progression are more likely secondary to fungal, tuber-

TABLE 138-1

Differential Diagnosis of Fever and Pulmonary Infiltrates in the Organ Transplant Recipient According to Roentgenographic Abnormality and the Rate of Progression of the Symptoms

Chest Radiographic Abnormality	Etiology According to the Rate of Progression of the Illness	
	Acute*	*Subacute-Chronic**
Consolidation	Bacterial (including Legionnaires' disease) Thromboembolic	Fungal Nocardial Tuberculous Viral,
	Hemorrhage (Pulmonary edema)	(Drug-induced, radiation, *Pneumocystis* tumor)
Peribronchovascular	Pulmonary edema (Leukoagglutinin, reaction bacterial)	Viral *Pneumocystis* (Fungal, nocardial, tuberculous, tumor)
Nodular infiltrate†	(Bacterial, pulmonary edema)	Fungal Nocardial Tuberculous (*Pneumocystis*)

*An acute illness develops and requires medical attention in a matter of relatively few hours (<24). A subacute-chronic process develops over several days to weeks. Note that unusual causes of a process are in parentheses.
†A nodular infiltrate is defined as one or more large (>1 cm² on chest radiography) focal defects with well-defined, more or less rounded edges, surrounded by aerated lung. Multiple tiny nodules of smaller size, as sometimes caused by such an agent as CMV or varicella-zoster virus, are not included here.
SOURCE: Modified from Rubin and Greene.[30]

culous, or nocardial infections. Large nodules are usually a sign of fungal or nocardial infection in this patient population, particularly if they are subacute to chronic in onset. Subacute disease with diffuse abnormalities, either of the peribronchovascular type or miliary micronodules, are usually caused by viruses (especially CMV) or *Pneumocystis carinii* (or, in the lung transplant patient, rejection). Additional clues can be found by examining the pulmonary lesion for the development of cavitation, with cavitation suggesting such necrotizing infections as those caused by fungi, *Nocardia,* and certain gram-negative bacilli (most commonly with *Klebsiella pneumoniae* and *Pseudomonas aeruginosa*).[5,32,40]

The depressed inflammatory response of the immunocompromised transplant patient may greatly modify or delay the appearance of a pulmonary lesion on radiograph, particularly if neutropenia is complicating the effects of the antirejection therapy. In particular, radiologic evidence of fungal invasion, which excites a less exuberant inflammatory response than does bacterial invasion, will often be very slow to appear on conventional chest radiograph. CT of the chest has revolutionized the evaluation of these immunocompromised patients, and CT is particularly useful when the chest radiograph is negative or when the radiologic findings are subtle or nonspecific. An additional important application of CT in this patient population is defining the extent of the disease process. Particularly with opportunistic fungal and nocardial infection, precise knowledge of the extent of the infection at diagnosis, and the response of all sites to therapy, will lead to the best therapeutic outcome, as therapy should

be continued until all evidence of infection is eliminated, not just the primary site.[5,32,40]

The morphology of the abnormalities found on CT scan can be very useful in developing a differential diagnosis in the individual patient. Thus, cavitary CT lesions are suggestive of infections with *Nocardia, Cryptococcus,* and *Aspergillus*. Rapidly expanding pulmonary lesions with cavitation and/or hemorrhage are associated with the Mucoraciae, especially in the diabetic. Opacified secondary pulmonary lobules in the lung periphery are suggestive of bland pulmonary infarcts, and if cavitated, of septic or hemorrhagic *Aspergillus* infarcts (Fig. 138-3). Peribronchial distribution of CT opacities is suggestive of fluid overload, viral or *Pneumocystis* infection, and, in the lung transplant recipient, allograft rejection. In contrast, dense regional or lobar consolidation on CT is most suggestive of bacterial pneumonia. Lymphadenopathy is variably observed due to immune suppression; mycobacterial, CMV, *Legionella* and cryptococcal infections, drug (e.g., trimethoprim-sulfamethoxazole) reactions, and posttransplant lymphoproliferative disease (PTLD, generally lymphoma) associated with EBV may be causative. Finally, CT scans will detect multiple simultaneous patterns that may be undetected by conventional radiographs. Such atypical CT findings may suggest the presence of dual or sequential infection of the lungs—not uncommon in transplant patients. For example, in a patient under treatment for *Pneumocystis* infection, the appearance of acinar, macronodular, or cavitary lesions is highly suggestive of the presence of a second process, often secondary *Aspergillus* invasion of lung tissue compromised by the primary process.[5,23,26,32,40]

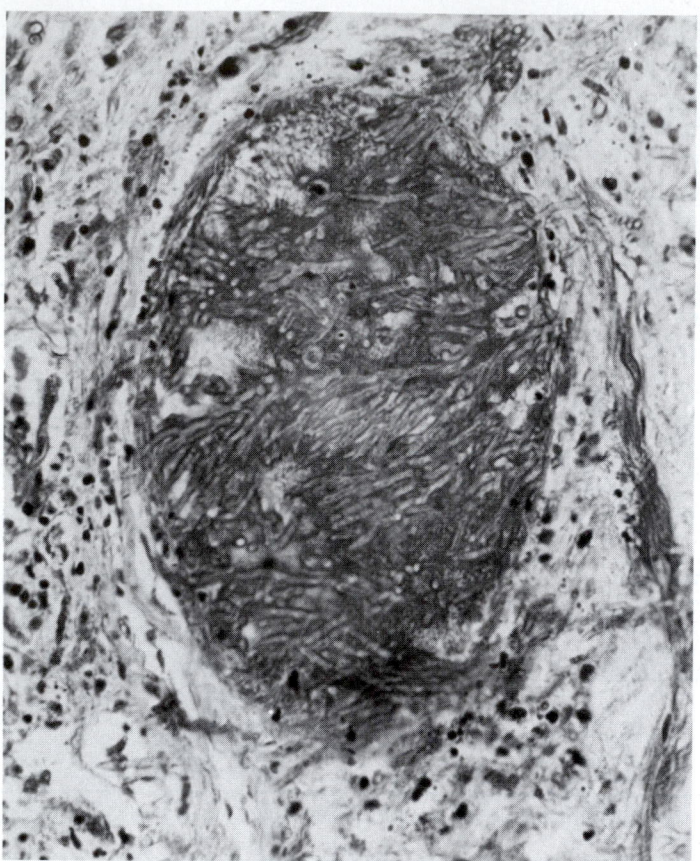

FIGURE 138-3 *Aspergillus fumigatus.* The fungus is invading the wall and filling the lumen of a pulmonary blood vessel of a leukemic patient with invasive pulmonary aspergillosis. Note the characteristic hyphal form that branches dichotomously at a 45° angle. H&E, ×520.

CT findings are also quite useful in defining which invasive diagnostic procedure should be utilized to obtain diagnostic samples and in identifying the anatomic site at which sampling should be directed to optimize the diagnostic yield. Thus, CT can provide precise guidance for needle biopsy or for thoracoscopic or open-lung excision in the case of peripheral lung nodules. CT is also the best means of predicting whether bronchoscopy is likely to be the most appropriate diagnostic procedure for a particular patient. For example, in patients with pulmonary nodules, CT demonstration of the feeding bronchus correlates with a 60 percent diagnostic yield with bronchoscopy, as opposed to a 30 percent yield if this finding is not present. If CT demonstrates centrally located diffuse opacifications, a bronchoscopic approach is the procedure of choice.[14,22,24,32]

SPECIFIC DIAGNOSIS OF PULMONARY INFECTION IN THE ORGAN TRANSPLANT RECIPIENT

The organ transplant patient with pulmonary infection differs from other immunocompromised hosts in one important respect: In other patient groups such as the patient with advanced AIDS, leukemia, or metastatic cancer, a limited life span is expected even if recovery from infection occurs; in the organ transplant patient, if recovery from the pulmonary infection occurs, then an

extended life span and the potential for full rehabilitation are to be expected. Given this difference, invasive biopsy procedures for specific diagnosis are indicated more often in the transplant patient, in contrast to the use of more empiric therapies in some of the other types of immunosuppressed patients. Thus, the general rule in transplant patients with possible pulmonary infection is to *be aggressive in pursuing early diagnosis and specific therapy.*[32]

The techniques available for specific diagnosis include immunologic techniques (serologic assays and skin testing); antigen detection systems; molecular assays (polymerase chain reaction), coupled to sputum examination and invasive techniques including bronchoscopy; and aspiration-needle biopsy, thoracoscopic biopsy, and open-lung biopsy. Immunologic techniques are generally of little use in the diagnosis of active infection in the transplant recipient for two reasons: Immune responses to microbial invasion may be greatly attenuated or delayed in organ transplant patients because of their immunocompromised state; conversely, many individuals may have positive immunologic tests in the absence of clinical disease. Finally, appropriate serologic or skin tests are not available for many of the disease processes that should be considered. The major use of such tests is prior to transplant, when a positive tuberculin skin test and knowledge of the CMV and *Toxoplasma gondii* serologies of both donor and recipient can define the risk of active infection after transplantation and will assist in the design of preventive strategies. Similarly, consideration is being given to the development of prophylactic strategies for Epstein-Barr virus infections to prevent EBV-associated lymphomas. Newer, molecular-based screening tests may enhance the sensitivity of pre- and post transplantation diagnosis, facilitating both prophylaxis and early treatment of infections.[32]

The Sputum Examination

Microscopic examination of an expectorated sputum specimen (following Gram's stain, fungal wet mount, or acid-fast smear) and culture can be useful in the diagnosis of pneumonia in the transplant patient. However, strict criteria should be employed when carrying out the microscopic examination before trusting the validity of the procedure: few squamous epithelial cells (fewer than 10 per low-power field) and many polymorphonuclear leukocytes (greater than 25 per high-power field in the nonneutropenic host). If such criteria are not met, then the significance of culture results should be questioned. The yield of this standard approach to diagnosis is considerably less in the transplant patient with pneumonia than it is in the nonimmunocompromised patient for several reasons: Sputum production may be minimal because of the impaired inflammatory response; the upper respiratory tract is frequently colonized with a large number of potential pathogens under normal conditions (particularly gram-negative bacilli and fungi), so that the culture of an expectorated sputum specimen may be contaminated and yield misleading information; and, finally, infection due to fungi and viruses, common causes of pneumonia in this patient population, cannot be diagnosed with this approach. Induced sputum examinations have improved the quality of the specimens obtained for this diagnostic approach and have largely replaced transtracheal aspiration in the early evaluation of these patients. However, at the Massachusetts General Hospital the yield of cultures and examination of induced sputum specimens is superior to routine samples (when available) only for the diagnosis of mycobacterial infection and *P. carinii*. If a diagnosis is not clearly made with these noninvasive modalities, rapid deployment of more invasive procedures for the direct sampling of lower respiratory secretions, pulmonary tissue, or both should be accomplished.[16,21,32]

Invasive Procedures

The cornerstone of invasive diagnostic studies for the evaluation of the organ transplant patient with pneumonia is fiberoptic bronchoscopy. This procedure provides the opportunity for bronchoalveolar lavage, transbronchial biopsy, bronchial brushing, and inspection of the anatomy of the tracheobronchial tree. Whereas bronchoalveolar lavage, which has the lowest rate of complications of bronchoscopic interventions, is the procedure of choice in AIDS patients, the smaller organism burden in the transplant patient with pneumonia often requires biopsy. In particular, rather than bronchoalveolar lavage alone, bronchoscopy with multiple transbronchial biopsies should be obtained initially when clinically feasible to avoid a delay in diagnosis and the need for multiple procedures. Thus, whereas in the AIDS patient with cryptococcal or *Pneumocystis* infection bronchoalveolar lavage has a diagnostic yield of better than 90 percent than in the organ transplant patient, the yield for *Pneumocystis* is 10 to 20 percent less and for cryptococcal infection, 50 to 80 percent less, with transbronchial biopsy adding significantly to the diagnostic value of the bronchoscopic procedure.[23,26,27,28,32]

The yield from transbronchial biopsies is clearly operator- and institution-dependent, and at many centers, including our own, thoracoscopic biopsy has come into extensive use in the diagnosis of diffuse lung disease not immediately delineated by bronchoscopic procedures and in the diagnosis of focal disease in the periphery of the lungs or for pleural-based disease. Thoracoscopic biopsy provides a better specimen for cultural and pathologic assessment than transbronchial biopsy and is better tolerated than open-lung biopsy in terms of morbidity and complications.[3,32]

Aspiration-needle biopsy is the initial procedure of choice for the invasive diagnosis of focal pulmonary processes in this patient population. It is particularly well suited for diagnosing focal peripheral lung lesions, such as those due to *Nocardia,* fungi, or tuberculosis, with a sensitivity of better than 80 percent at most institutions. Our own experience has been that we have been able to diagnose more than 90 percent of fungal or nocardial infections not diagnosed by induced sputum examination, with the diagnostic yield being particularly high if cavitation is present in the lesion. In contrast, the diagnostic yield of this procedure in patients with diffuse lung disease is quite low, and transthoracic needle aspiration should not be carried out in such individuals.[8,24,32,35,39] The complication rate of this procedure is relatively low, as long as certain precautions are taken: With modern 22- or 23-gauge thin-wall needles in patients with adequate clotting parameters (platelet count greater than or equal to $75,000/mm^3$, normal prothrombin and partial thromboplastin times), the incidence of significant hemoptysis is less than 1 per-

cent[24]; similarly, if the procedure is carried out appropriately with cooperative patients who do not have advanced chronic obstructive lung disease (single pleural puncture at biopsy, placement of the patient with the puncture site down for at least 1 h after procedure, and restriction of coughing, talking, and activity for this period), the need for a chest tube to treat pneumothoraces is also less than 1 percent.[18,19,24,39]

The definitive diagnostic procedure in the organ transplant patient with pneumonia remains open-lung biopsy, which should be seriously considered if arterial hypoxemia is intensifying, the pulmonary infiltrates are spreading rapidly, and the case is generally regarded as a "therapeutic emergency." Alternatively, open-lung biopsy remains an important option for the diagnosis of patients in whom bronchoscopy and/or aspiration-needle biopsy has failed to yield the diagnosis (a "diagnostic dilemma"). It should be pointed out, however, that thoracoscopic biopsies have increasingly become the procedure of choice for both these categories of patient when the area of lung involvement is peripheral and pleural-based. Open-lung biopsies remain the approach for more central lesions. A specific diagnosis is made in 80 to 90 percent of transplant patients who come to open-lung biopsy, with a false negative rate of less than 5 percent (these instances presumably being related to sampling error or inappropriate handling of specimens).[1,13,17,32,37]

IMPORTANT CAUSES OF PNEUMONIA IN THE ORGAN TRANSPLANT RECIPIENT

Detailed discussion of each of these forms of infection is available in other chapters of this text; the following comments are meant to emphasize the specific aspects of these infections in the transplant recipient.

Bacterial Pneumonia

The bacterial pneumonias that occur in the organ transplant patient may be divided into four general categories:[5,12,26,32]

1. Superinfection, usually with relatively resistant gram-negative bacilli, of areas of lung injured prior to transplant or in the postoperative period. This is a particular problem in the patient with end-stage liver disease who is subject to extensive aspirational lung injury because of hepatic encephalopathy and inability to protect the airway, and patients with end-stage cardiac or pulmonary disease who require ventilatory support while awaiting an allograft. The general rule is that the airway must be protected, the endotracheal tube expertly managed, and any pulmonary injury/infection aggressively treated prior to transplantation. As far as postoperative bacterial infection, lung transplant patients are at greatest risk, because of several factors: Their lower respiratory tracts are frequently colonized with gram-negative infection; the bronchial anastomosis is particularly at risk for suture line infection, disruption, and the need for a prosthetic device—all factors increasing the risk for infection; mechanical factors such as ciliary function, cough reflex, and the presence of an endotracheal tube for extended periods all increase the risk of pneumonia. Further, the transplanted lung, which has been physically traumatized as well as subjected to possible immunologic injury, is far more susceptible to invasive infection than are the lungs of other organ transplant recipients.

2. Pulmonary infection resulting from environmental exposures, usually contaminated air or potable water. Thus, epidemic gram-negative pneumonia (often due to such organisms as *Pseudomonas aeruginosa* or *Klebsiella pneumoniae*) have occurred in transplant patients due to a contaminated air supply, and several epidemics of *Legionella pneumophila* infection, usually due to contaminated potable water, have also been noted in this patient population.

3. Bacterial pneumonia akin to that seen in the general community, usually following community-acquired respiratory virus infection or following an aspirational episode.

4. Nocardial or tuberculous infection. Nocardial infection is easily prevented with low-dose trimethoprim-sulfamethoxazole prophylaxis; the prevention of active tuberculosis is somewhat more challenging. The key issue is the management of the patient with a known positive tuberculin test after transplant, in the face of a 5 to 15 percent incidence of hepatic dysfunction due to chronic viral hepatitis (both hepatitis B and C). Isoniazid prophylaxis is recommended for transplant patients with positive tuberculin tests and at least one additional risk factor. Risk factors of importance include non-Caucasian racial background; the presence of other immunosuppressing illnesses, particularly protein-calorie malnutrition; history of active, clinical tuberculosis; known, intimate, recent exposure to active tuberculosis; and the presence of significant abnormalities on chest radiograph. For those patients without one of these risk factors who are reliable in terms of follow-up, close observation appears to be the best approach. The patient with nocardial infection should be assumed to have disseminated infection at the time of diagnosis. Sampling of the cerebrospinal fluid and careful bone examination (e.g., bone scan) are mandatory for the detection of metastatic infection and the assessment of the efficacy of therapy.

Viral Pneumonia

The most important cause of viral pneumonia in the transplant patient is cytomegalovirus. This usually occurs 1 to 4 months after transplant, is most common in those patients at risk for primary CMV infection (donor seropositive and recipient seronegative) and who are treated most intensively with immunosuppressive therapy. In general, CMV disease is similar in all forms of organ transplantation, with one notable exception: The attack rate and severity of pneumonia are far higher in recipients of lung allografts than in the other transplant groups.[32] The special impact of CMV on the lung allograft patient is probably due to the interaction of several factors; most notably cytokines elaborated in response to CMV infection probably increase the occurrence of allograft injury from rejection conversely, cytokines elaborated in the course of rejection actively stimulate the replication of CMV via NFκB (a "bidirectional trafficking" in cytokines, between rejection and CMV infection).[4,30]

As with most viral infections, CMV usually begins insidiously with constitutional symptoms. In about one-third of patients with fever, a dry, nonproductive cough develops within a few days of the onset of these symptoms, with about one-fourth of these developing varying degrees of tachypnea and dyspnea, with hy-

poxemia proportional to the degree of respiratory embarrassment being noted. If acute respiratory deterioration over less than 12 h occurs, superinfection with bacterial or fungal agents should be considered rather than attributing such a deterioration to an exacerbation of the CMV infection.[29] The radiologic manifestations of CMV pneumonia can take many forms: most commonly, a bilateral, symmetrical, peribronchovascular and alveolar process that affects predominantly the lower lobes. Less common is a focal consolidation more suggestive of bacterial or fungal infection, or even a solitary pulmonary nodule caused by CMV.[29,31] Mixed patterns may suggest dual infection of which CMV and *P. carinii* are the most commonly associated. Treatment is with high-dose intravenous ganciclovir, with some centers also adding anti-CMV hyperimmune globulin to the therapeutic program. Foscarnet or combinations of foscarnet with ganciclovir are also useful for therapy of CMV infection with the limitation of increased nephrotoxicity with this agent.[33] A recent report of ganciclovir-resistant infection in a lung transplant recipient is of great importance and underlines the importance of active surveillance for such resistance, particularly in patients with persistent or relapsing infection. Preventive strategies, as outlined in Table 138-2, are improving but need further refinement.

The transplant patient, as previously noted, is at greater risk for pneumonia than the normal host in the setting of community-acquired respiratory infection, with influenza, RSV, and adenovirus infection having a particular impact on this group of individuals. This impact includes both viral pneumonia and a significantly higher rate of bacterial pneumonia occurring as superinfection of a previous respiratory viral infection.[34]

Fungal Pneumonia

The three most important causes of fungal pulmonary infection are *Pneumocystis carinii*, *Aspergillus* species (especially *A. fumigatus*), and *Cryptococcus neoformans*. In patients not receiving trimethoprim-sulfamethoxazole (or alternative drugs) as prophylaxis, transplant centers report an incidence of *Pneumocystis carinii* pneumonia of 5 to 15 percent in the first 6 months after transplant, with a continuing risk in the "chronic ne'er do wells," the patients with a poor outcome from the transplant.[6] The occurrence of *Pneumocystis* infection is highly associated with the occurrence of CMV infection, possibly because of the inhibitory effect of CMV on alveolar macrophages and, systemically, on CD4 lymphocyte function. The importance of *preventing Pneumocystis* infection is underlined by the following observation: Whereas low-dose trimethoprim-sulfamethoxazole or other prophylactic programs are well tolerated in this patient population, treatment doses of trimethoprim-sulfamethoxazole or pentamidine are associated with a high rate of toxicities, particularly renal and hepatic, due primarily to interactions with the immunosuppressive drugs. The clinical and radiologic manifestations of *P. carinii* pneumonia are virtually identical to those of CMV. Indeed, the clinical challenge is to determine which pathogen is present, or whether both are present, requiring treatment.[29,33]

Invasive pulmonary aspergillosis has two forms in this patient population—primary infection, when it is the first invader of the lung, and secondary infection, when it invades lung al-

TABLE 138-2

Estimated Efficacies of Prophylactic Antiviral Strategies against CMV Infection in Different Forms of Organ Transplantation

Type of Transplant	Form of CMV Infection	Antimicrobial Strategy Used*	Estimated Efficacy
Kidney	Primary†	CMV hyperimmune globulin	2+
		High-dose acyclovir	2+
		CMV hyperimmune globulin + moderate-dose acyclovir	3+
	Secondary†	High-dose acyclovir	3+
		CMV hyperimmune globulin + moderate-dose acyclovir	3+
Heart and/or lung	Primary	High-dose ganciclovir (1 month)	0
	Secondary*	High-dose ganciclovir (1 month)	4+
Liver	Primary	CMV hyperimmune globulin	0
	Secondary*	CMV hyperimmune globulin	3+

*Unless otherwise noted, the regimens outlined were administered for a minimum of 3 months. Semiquantitative assessments of efficacy during the period of greatest risk (1–6 months after transplant) are given, because of the recognition that the type of immunosuppression used will have a major effect on the efficacy of each of these regimens.
†Primary infection: infection developing as a result of transplantation (or transfusion) from a CMV-seropositive donor to a seronegative recipient; Secondary infection: CMV infection developing in a seropositive recipient. Risk of infection is enhanced by antirejection therapy, especially with antilymphocyte antibody preparations.
SOURCE: Modified from Rubin et al.[31]

ready damaged by a previous process. Whereas primary infection is virtually always focal and macronodular on radiograph, the radiograph picture in secondary cases can be obscured by the manifestations of the primary process. Secondary invasion by *Aspergillus* should be suspected when there is new evidence of focal, nodular disease, particularly when the previous process was diffuse in nature (Fig. 138-4). The risk of invasive pulmonary aspergillosis appears to be greater than 50 percent once the respiratory tract is colonized, either before or after transplant. Because of this risk, we advocate a course of "preemptive" antifungal therapy, usually amphotericin B, when such colonization is noted. The clinical presentation is usually one of fever and toxicity, with a variable occurrence of such respiratory systems as cough, dyspnea, tachypnea, and pleurisy. The clinical course is determined by the pathologic features of this infection—a necrotizing bronchopneumonia with vascular invasion, leading to the three cardinal features of invasive pulmonary aspergillosis—tissue infarction, hemorrhage, and metastases. As many as 50 percent of patients already have metastatic disease at the time of diagnosis, with the brain and skin being relatively common sites for metastatic infection (Fig. 138-5). Amphotericin B remains the cornerstone of therapy, with liposomal amphotericin and itraconazole, at present, reserved for "wrap-up therapy" after initial control of the process has been gained. In the lung transplant recipient, invasion of the broncheal anastomosis is generally catastrophic and requires resection of the affected tissue in addition to antifungal therapy for cure.[2,9,10,11,23,29,32,38]

Cryptococcal infection of the lungs in transplant patients is usually asymptomatic or minimally symptomatic, with the most common presentation being that of an asymptomatic pulmonary nodule on routine chest radiograph (Fig. 138-6). Occasionally, a subacute consolidation with influenzalike symptoms may be noted. The major importance of cryptococcal pulmonary infec-

tion is not that the lung infection is a source of significant morbidity and mortality; rather, the lung is the portal of entry for disseminated infection, particularly to the central nervous system. It is for this reason that all such asymptomatic nodules are aggressively pursued, with preemptive fluconazole or ampho-

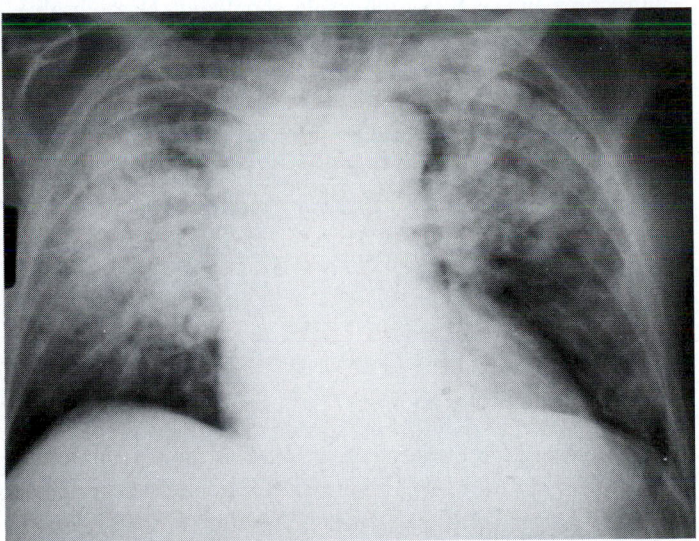

FIGURE 138-4 Invasive pulmonary aspergillosis after liver transplantation. A diffuse *Klebsiella* pneumonia had been treated with cephalothin and gentamicin, and the initial clinical response was favorable. However, after 2 days of no fever, fever returned and was accompanied by increasing shortness of breath, although the chest radiograph remained unchanged. One day after this radiograph was taken, the patient died. Autopsy revealed two processes in the lungs: a diffuse gram-negative pneumonia and focal areas of invasive aspergillosis restricted to the right lower and middle lobes. This figure illustrates the difficulty in differentiating the focal areas of *Aspergillus* superinfection from the primary bacterial process.

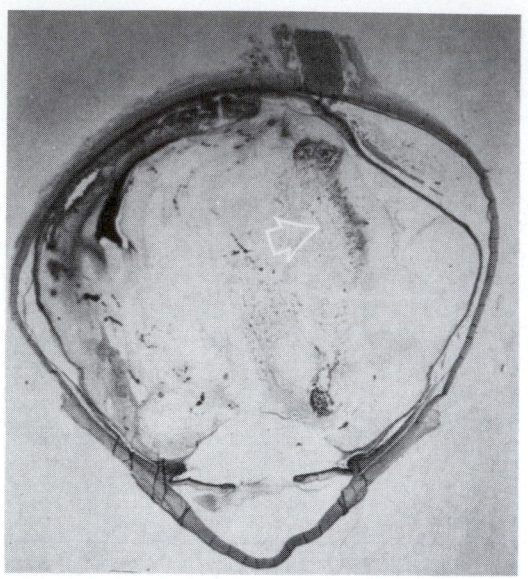

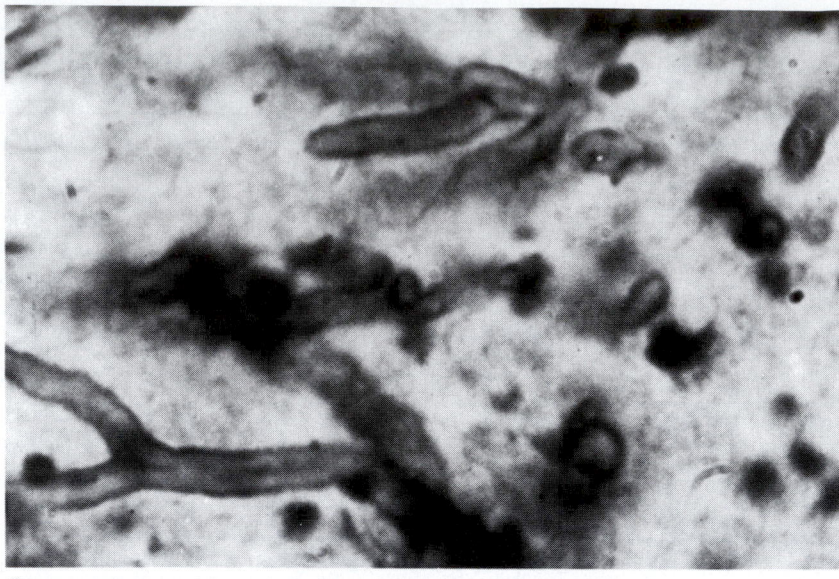

A   B

FIGURE 138-5 Metastatic infection with *Aspergillus fumigatus* involving the eye. The removed eye of a 32-year-old woman, 3 months after renal transplant, who presented with fever, nonproductive cough, and normal chest radiograph accompanied by increasing pain and loss of vision in one eye. All vision was lost in that eye during the next 3 days. The eye was removed for relief of pain and for diagnosis. *A.* Low-power photomicrograph (×7) of the eye reveals areas of increased inflammation (arrow). *B.* High-power photomicrograph (×425) of the area of inflammation reveals the metastatic invasive *Aspergillus* infection.

tericin therapy administered to prevent subsequent systemic or neurologic disease.[9]

Notable by its absence from this discussion is pulmonary infection due to *Candida* species. Although candidal isolation from sputum cultures is common, cases of pulmonary invasion are vanishingly rare, and such cultural results should not, by themselves, lead to either therapy or an aggressive diagnostic program.[29]

SUMMARY AND CONCLUSIONS

Pulmonary infection is the most common form of tissue-invasive infection observed in organ transplant patients. The risk of pulmonary infection, particularly opportunistic infection of the lungs, is primarily determined by the interaction of two factors—the epidemiologic exposures encountered and the patient's net state of immunosuppression. Although pneumonia may occur at any time in the posttransplant course, the etiologies are very different at different times, and these etiologies can be delineated

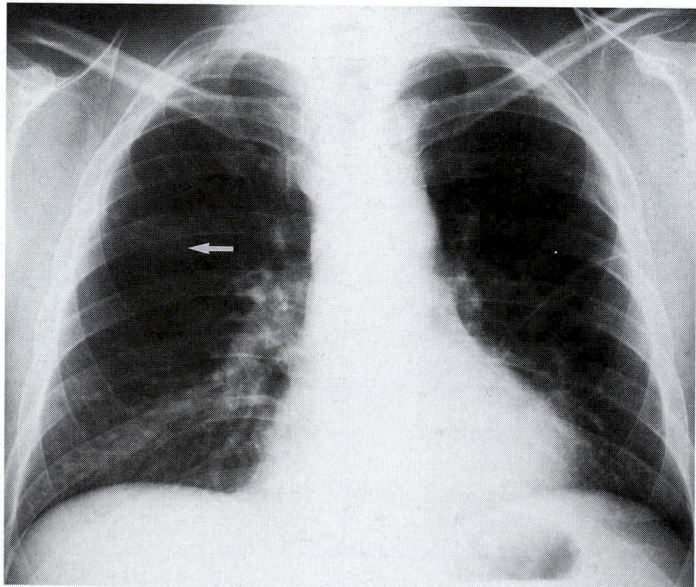

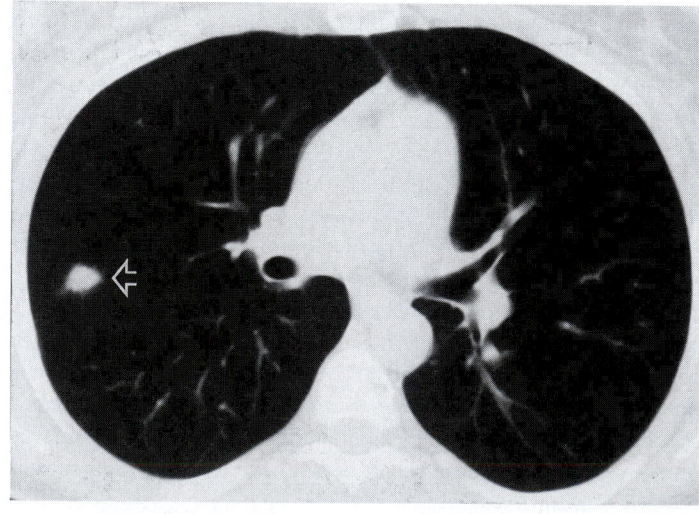

A   B

FIGURE 138-6 *Cryptococcus neoformans* in an asymptomatic renal transplant patient. The patient presented with minimal complaint of nonproductive cough of a few weeks' duration. *A.* The chest radiograph was essentially clear other than a shadow in the right midlung field (arrow). *B.* Chest tomography revealed a nodular lesion in the right midlung field (arrow). Percutaneous needle aspiration of this lesion yielded *Cryptococcus neoformans* on fungal culture.

by a timetable. Exceptions to this timetable usually are due to unusually intense epidemiologic exposures. A logical diagnostic approach can be constructed on the basis of the timetable, the radiologic appearance (especially on CT scan) of the infection, and the rate of progression of the process. These lead to the appropriate deployment of diagnostic techniques, including not only the examination of sputum, but, commonly, bronchoscopy, needle aspiration, thoroscopic biopsy, and open-lung biopsy. The important principle that dominates the clinical approach to pulmonary infection in this immunocompromised patient population is that if cure is achieved, the patient has a reasonable chance for full rehabilitation. Therefore, invasive diagnostic techniques are perhaps more justifiable in this immunocompromised patient population than in others. Early diagnosis and specific therapy remain the cornerstones of cure.

REFERENCES

1. Cockerill FR III, Wilson WR, Carpenter HA, et al: Open lung biopsy in immunocompromised patients. *Arch Intern Med* 145:1398–1404, 1985.

2. Dauber JH, Paradis IL, Dummer JS: Infectious complications in preliminary allograft recipients. *Clin Chest Med* 11:291–308, 1990.

3. Dijkman JH, van der Meer JWM, Bakker W, et al: Transpleural lung biopsy by the thoracoscopic route in patients with diffuse interstitial pulmonary disease. *Chest* 82:76–83, 1982.

4. Docke WD, Prosch S, Fietze E, et al: Cytomegalovirus reactivation and tumour necrosis factor. *Lancet* 343:268–269, 1994.

5. Ettinger NA, Trulock EP: Pulmonary considerations of organ transplantation: Parts 1–3. *Am Rev Resp Dis* 143:1386–1405, 1991; 144:213–223, 433–451, 1991.

6. Fishman JA: *Pneumocystis carinii* and parasitic infections in the immunocompromised host, in Rubin RH, Young LS (eds), *Clinical Approach to Infection in the Compromised Host,* 3d ed. New York, Plenum, 1994, pp 275–334.

7. Genta RM: Global prevalence of strongyloidiasis: Critical review with epidemiologic insight into the prevention of disseminated disease. *Rev Infect Dis* 11:755–767, 1989.

8. Greene R: Transthoracic needle aspiration biopsy, in Athanazoulis C, Pfister R, Greene R, et al (eds), *International Radiology.* Philadelphia, Saunders, 1981, pp 587–634.

9. Hadley S, Karchmer AW: Fungal infections in solid organ transplant recipients. *Infect Dis Clin North Am* 9:1045–1074, 1995.

10. Hibberd PL, Rubin RH: Clinical aspects of fungal infection in organ transplant recipients. *Clin Infect Dis* 19(suppl 1):533–536, 1994.

11. Hofflin JM, Potasman I, Baldwin JC, et al: Infectious complications in heart transplant recipients receiving cyclosporine and corticosteroids. *Ann Intern Med* 106:209–216, 1987.

12. Houston SH, Sinnott JT: Management of the transplant recipient with pulmonary infection. *Infect Dis Clin North Am* 9:965–986, 1995.

13. Jaffe JP, Maki DG: Lung biopsy in immunocompromised patients: One institution's experience and an approach to management of pulmonary disease in the compromised host. *Cancer* 48:1144–1153, 1981.

14. Jamzen DL, Adler BD, Padley SPG, et al: Diagnostic success of bronchoscopic biopsy in immunocompromised patients with acute pulmonary disease: Predictive value of disease distribution as shown on CT. *Am J Roentgenol* 160:21–24, 1993.

15. Lurain NS, Ammons HC, Kapell KS, et al: Molecular analysis of human cytomegalovirus strains from two lung transplant recipients with the same donor. *Transplantation* 62:497–501, 1996.

16. Masur H, Shelhamer J, Parrillo JE: The management of pneumonias in immunocompromised patients. *JAMA* 253:1769–1773, 1985.

17. McKenna RJ Jr, Mountain CF, McMurtey MJ: Open lung biopsy in immunocompromised patients. *Chest* 86:671–674, 1984.

18. Miller KS, Fish GB, Stamley JH, et al: Prediction of pneumothorax rate in percutaneous needle aspiration of the lung. *Chest* 93:742–745, 1988.

19. Moore EH, Shepard JO, McLoud TC, et al: Positional precautions in needle aspiration lung biopsy. *Radiology* 175:733–735, 1990.

20. Morgan JS, Schaffner W, Stone WJ: Opportunistic strongyloidiasis in renal transplant recipients. *Transplantation* 42:518–524, 1986.

21. Murrary PR, Washington JA II: Microscopic and bacteriologic analysis of expectorated sputum. *Mayo Clin Proc* 50:339–344, 1975.

22. Naidich DP, Sussman R, Kutcher WL, et al: Solitary pulmonary nodules: CT-bronchoscopic correlation. *Chest* 3:595–598, 1988.

23. Paya CV: Fungal Infections in solid organ transplantation. *Clin Infect Dis* 16:677–688, 1993.

24. Perlmutt LM, Johnston WW, Dunnick NR: Percutaneous transthoracic needle aspiration: A review. *Am J Roentgenol* 152:451–455, 1989.

25. Plunkett MB, Peterson MS, Landercneau RJ, et al: Peripheal pulmonary nodules: Preoperative percutaneous needle localization with CT guidance. *Radiology* 185:274–276, 1992.

26. Ramsey PG, Rubin RH, Tolkoff-Rubin NE, et al: The renal transplant patient with fever and pulmonary infiltrates: Etiology, clinical manifestations, and management. *Medicine* 59:206–222, 1980.

27. Rosenow EC III, Wilson WR, Cockerill FR III: Pulmonary disease in the immunocompromised host. *Mayo Clin Proc* 60:473–487, 610–631, 1985.

28. Rosenow EC III: Diffuse pulmonary infiltrates in the immunocompromised host. *Clin Chest Med* 11:55–64, 1990.

29. Rubin RH: Infection in the organ transplant recipient, in Rubin RH, Young LS (eds), *Clinical Approach to Infection in the Compromised Host,* 3d ed. New York, Plenum, 1994, pp 629–705.

30. Rubin RH: The indirect effects of cytomegalovirus infection on the outcome of organ transplantation. *JAMA* 261:3607–3609, 1989.

31. Rubin RH, Cosimi AB, Tolkoff-Rubin NE, et al: Infectious disease syndromes attributable to cytomegalovirus and their significance among renal transplant recipients. *Transplantation* 24:458–464, 1977.

32. Rubin RH, Greene R: Clinical approach to the compromised host with fever and pulmonary infiltrates, in Rubin RH, Young LS (eds), *Clinical Approach to Infection in the Compromised Host,* 3d ed. New York, Plenum, 1994, pp 121–161.

33. Rubin RH, Tolkoff-Rubin NE: Antimicrobial strategies in the care of organ transplant recipients. *Antimicrob Agents Chemother* 37:619–624, 1993.

34. Sable CA, Hayden FG: Orthomyxoviral and paramyxoviral infections in transplant patients. *Infect Dis Clin North Am* 9:987–1003, 1995.

35. Scott WW, Kuhlman JE: Focal pulmonary lesions in patients with AIDS: Percutaneous transthoracic needle biopsy. *Radiology* 180:419–421, 1991.

36. Scowden EB, Schaffner W, Stone WJ: Overwhelming strongyloidiasis: An unappreciated opportunistic infection. *Medicine* 57:527–544, 1978.

37. Toledo-Pereyra LH, DeMeester TR, Kineuley A, et al: The benefit of open lung biopsy in patients with previous non-diagnostic transbronchial lung biopsy: A guide to appropriate therapy. *Chest* 77:647–650, 1980.

38. Weiland D, Ferguson RM, Peterson PK, et al: Aspergillosis in 25 renal transplant patients: Epidemiology, clinical presentation, diagnosis, and management. *Ann Surg* 198:622–629, 1983.

39. Westcott JL: Percutaneous transthoracic needle biopsy: State of the art. *Radiology* 169:593–601, 1988.

40. Williams DM, Krick JA, Remington JS: Pulmonary infection in the compromised host. *Am Rev Resp Dis* 114:359–394, 593–627, 1976.

CHAPTER 139

PULMONARY INFECTIONS IN PATIENTS WITH PRIMARY IMMUNE DEFECTS

Harry R. Hill / Kathleen D. Pfeffer

ANTIBODY (B-CELL) DEFICIENCY
X-Linked Agammaglobulinemia
Common Variable Immunodeficiency
Selective IgG Subclass Deficiencies
Selective IgA Deficiency
Hyper-IgM Deficiency

COMPLEMENT DISORDERS

CELL-MEDIATED IMMUNITY
DiGeorge's Syndrome
Severe Combined Immunodeficiency Disease
Purine Nucleoside Phosphorylase
Wiskott-Aldrich Syndrome
Ataxia-Telangiectasia

PHAGOCYTIC DEFECTS
Disorders of Phagocyte Numbers
Defects of Phagocyte Function
Leukocyte Adhesion Deficiency
Hyperimmunoglobulin E Syndrome

SUMMARY

Pulmonary immune responses are critical for defense of the lung. In the normal host, inhaled foreign material encounters a highly efficient system of pulmonary defense that prevents injury, infection, or antigenic stimulation of lung tissue by relying on the nonspecific mechanisms of mechanical barriers and phagocytosis, and the specific mechanisms provided by immune reactions. Impairment of certain aspects of both of these mechanisms can occur in primary immune system dysfunction, resulting in serious infectious disorders of the lungs and upper airways.

Primary immunodeficiencies are defined as alterations in the immune system that are congenital, as opposed to those related to chemotherapy, autoimmune disease, organ transplant, or chronic systemic disease.

This chapter describes the major primary immunodeficiencies and discusses in detail the pulmonary infections associated with each immunodeficiency state, and the therapies, both established and experimental, that are available.

Immune reactions that occur in the respiratory tract do not differ fundamentally from those that occur systemically. As represented in Fig. 139-1, after tissue invasion, antigen-presenting cells (APCs) such as macrophages or dendritic cells, abundant in the airways and parenchyma of the lung, engulf and process antigen by partial degradation. These cells subsequently display relevant antigenic determinants on cell-surface membranes, in association with class II macromolecular gene products of the major histocompatibility complex (MHC), and secrete cytokines. As the antigen-reactive cells of the immune system, lymphocytes recognize both antigen and class II MHC determinants on the APC. In addition, interleukin-1 (IL-1) released from the APCs bind to IL-1 receptors expressed on the surface of helper T cells, leading to activation and up-regulation of IL-2 receptors on these cells. After activation, the helper T cells produce lymphokines and express CD40 ligand. These T cells can then bind to CD40 on B cells and drive B cells to proliferate and differentiate into plasmablasts and plasma cells, which secrete specific antibody, and into memory B cells for secondary immune responses. Immune responses initiated by interaction of APCs with CD4$^+$ cells (helper/inducer T cells) result in cellular enlargement and elaboration of IL-2. The binding of IL-2 to T-cell IL-2 receptors results in further T-cell activation and lymphokine production. These factors amplify and modulate the immune response in cooperation with other cells and cytokines of the immune system. CD8$^+$ cytotoxic T cells also interact with IL-2, proliferating and reacting with viral antigens associated with human leukocyte class I antigen molecules on infected cells. Activated CD4$^+$ cells also interact with the MHC determinants and antigen complexed on B-lymphocyte surfaces, providing help in the form of cytokines, such as IL-2, -4, -5, -6, and interferon-gamma (IFN-γ), which cause B-cell activation, growth, and differentiation.

Elaborated cytokines, such as IL-1, tumor necrosis factor (TNF-α), and IFN-γ, activate endothelial cells and leukocytes, including polymorphonuclear neutrophils (PMNs), to increase expression of adhesion molecules and facilitate leukocyte binding and transmural migration, providing a mechanism for local accumulation of effector cells. IFN-γ also activates macrophages, which play a central role in maintaining normal lung structure and function through their many capacities and secretory products.

This scenario occurs throughout the respiratory tree, wherever antigens have escaped removal or suppression through mechanical clearance mechanisms (filtration, impaction, coughing, sneezing, epithelial barriers, mucociliary transport), iron-binding proteins, antibody activity of secretory immunoglobulins (par-

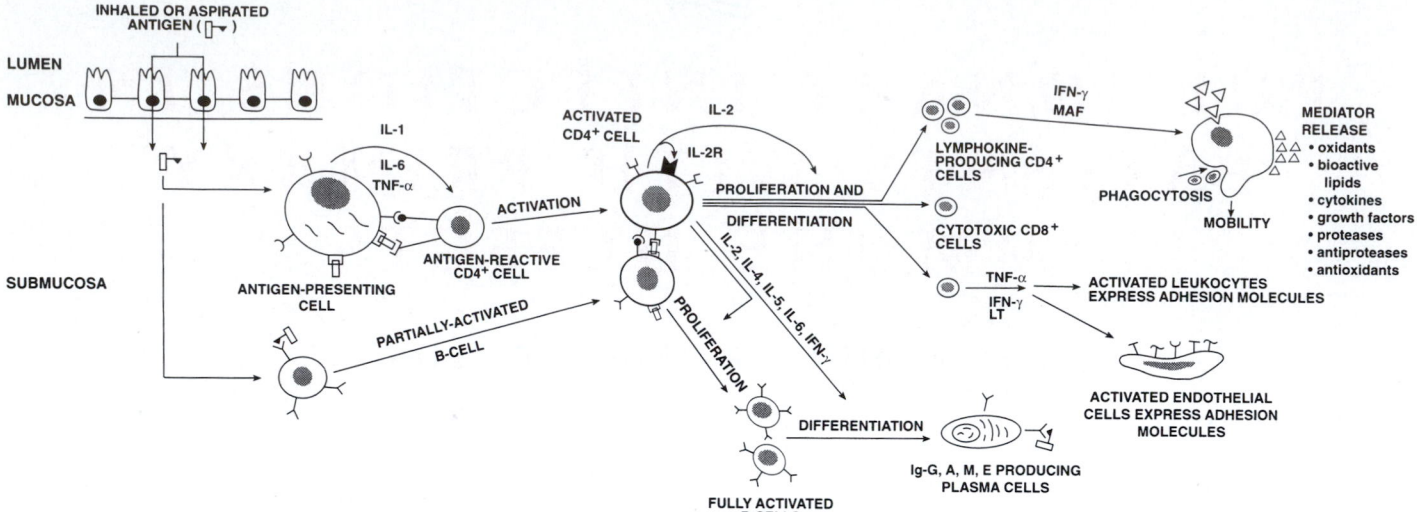

FIGURE 139-1 Schematic representation showing the cellular interactions between T cells, B cells, PMNs, and macrophages during an immune response to a complex antigen. Antigen-presenting cells uptake, process, and display an antigenic epitope (▯) that, in association with class II MHC determinants, binds to specific clones of CD4$^+$ T cells (—●). B cells may also bind epitopes (—▼) present on intact antigen, internalize it, and present appropriate epitopes associated with class II MHC determinants (●—) to the activated T cells. As a result of autocrine (IL-2) and paracrine (IL-1 and IL-6) stimulation, CD4$^+$ T cells proliferate and differentiate into clones of T effector cells. IL-2, IL-4, IL-5, IL-6, and IFN-γ promote growth, differentiation, and activation of CD8$^+$ cytotoxic T cells, B cells, and natural killer (NK) cells. TNF, lymphotoxin (LT), and IFN-γ activate and induce adhesion molecule expression on endothelial cells and leukocytes, including PMNs, promoting their recruitment into inflammatory sites.

ticularly IgA), or surface phagocytosis. Antigens that penetrate these barriers may be taken up by APCs associated with submucosal lymphoid tissue, may be distributed systemically by the bloodstream, or may reach regional lymph nodes via lymphatic drainage. Immune responses expressed at mucosal surfaces of the conducting airways result in the synthesis and secretion of specific antibody by lymphoid cells that are primarily resident in the mucosa. Immune reactions expressed in the interstitium of gas exchange units of the parenchyma depend on local recruitment of previously sensitized memory lymphocytes from the circulation that proliferate and differentiate in response to antigen in the lung. The regional hilar and tracheobronchial lymph nodes initially generate both B- and T-cell–mediated immune responses against antigens absorbed from various regions of the lung. Previously activated memory cells are then available for recruitment from the circulation into lung tissue.

Clinical problems that require evaluation of the immune system include chronic or recurrent bacterial or fungal infections of the skin, sinuses, and respiratory and digestive tracts and repeated infections with unusual viruses. Other suggestive signs and symptoms are persistent atypical rashes, chronic diarrhea, failure to thrive, paucity of lymphoid tissue, lymphadenopathy, chronic conjunctivitis, and unusual reactions to live virus vaccines.

The evaluation of recurrent infections should analyze all compartments of the host defense system, including anatomic structures, mucociliary function, B- and T-cell activity, phagocytic cell function, and complement activity. Table 139-1 outlines both initial and confirmatory screening tests available to most clinicians.

Most of the primary immunodeficiencies are diagnosed during infancy or childhood on the basis of the above-mentioned signs, symptoms, and results of laboratory data. Early recognition and aggressive management of the pulmonary problems associated with immunodeficiency are vital to the long-term health and well-being of these patients, who quite often die as a result of progressive respiratory failure due to recurrent infection resulting in bronchiectasis and/or pulmonary fibrosis.

Although the major components and associated defects of the pulmonary host defense will be discussed in separate sections, the immune system, as vividly illustrated in Figure 139-1, is notable for its high degree of complex synergies and intricate regulatory interactions. More often than not, many of these primary immunodeficiencies result in numerous dysfunctions of the immune system.

ANTIBODY (B-CELL) DEFICIENCY

Antibody deficiency states are among the most common of the primary immunodeficiency diseases. Although the defect in immunoglobulin production can occur at any point in B-cell maturation/activation or secretion of antibody, or even in T- and B-cell interaction, the end result is a decrease in serum antibody levels or the inability to respond to antigens with specific antibody. Patients typically present with recurrent sinopulmonary infections caused by encapsulated bacteria such as *Streptococcus pneumoniae, Hemophilus influenzae* (both type b and nontypable), and *Staphylococcus aureus.* Diseases caused by mycoplasma, enteroviruses, and intestinal parasites are also occasionally seen. The incidence of autoimmune abnormalities and hematologic malignancies is also significant in patients with these defects.

Treatment for most of these defects relies on the administration of gammaglobulin. Immunoglobulin replacement therapy is

TABLE 139-1

Immunologic Workup

Suspected Abnormality	Screening Tests	Confirmatory Tests
Antibody deficiency	Serum IgM, IgG, IgA levels IgG antibody response to protein (diphtheria, tetanus, influenza) and polysaccharide (pneumococcus, *Hemophilus influenzae*) antigens Isohemagglutinin titers for IgM antibody response Serum IgG subclass levels	B-cell enumeration (total B [CD20] and surface IgM-, IgG-, IgA-, IgD-bearing B cells) In vitro immunoglobulin synthesis
Cell-mediated immunodeficiency	Total lymphocyte count Delayed hypersensitivity skin tests (diphtheria, tetanus, *Candida*, PPD, SK/SD for T cell function) Tests for HIV antibodies	Enumerate total T cells and T-cell subsets (CD3, CD4, CD8) Measure T-cell function with mitogenic, antigenic, and allogeneic (mixed lymphocyte reaction) responses, lymphokine production, cytotoxic assay Assays for Th and Ts activity Enzyme assay (ADA, PNP) for ADA or PNP deficiency
Complement deficiency	CH_{50} or CH_{100} for classical pathway activity APH_{50} for alternative pathway activity Serum C2, C3, C4, C5, and factor B levels	Other specific component levels C1 esterase inhibition levels C1 esterase functional component
Phagocyte defects	NBT test for respiratory burst activity (defect in CGD) Serum IgE levels for HIE	Leukocyte adhesive protein analysis: (CD11a/CD18, CD11b/CD18, and CD11c/CD18) Adherence and aggregation Chemotaxis and random motility Phagocytosis Assays for respiratory burst activity (chemiluminescence, oxygen radical production) Bacterial killing test Enzyme assay (MPO, glucose-6-phosphate dehydrogenase) for phagocyte enzyme defects Cytochrome *b* or cytosolic protein measurement for CGD

typically given as an intravenous infusion, even though it can be given intramuscularly. Intravenous administration of γ-globulin (IVIG) results in higher serum and tissue concentrations, fewer overall adverse side effects, and usually a significant reduction in infectious incidences as well as chronic complications, such as pulmonary disease.[19] Acute and chronic administration of antibiotics and aggressive, routine chest physiotherapy are concomitant and mandatory with immunoglobulin administration. Table 139-2 lists both recognized and experimental therapeutic options from which hypogammaglobulinemic patients may benefit. Annual chest radiographs and pulmonary function tests are especially helpful, given that the lung disease in patients with hypogammaglobulinemia may be insidious in onset and progression.

X-Linked Agammaglobulinemia

X-linked agammaglobulinemia (XLA or Bruton's Agammaglobulinemia) is a relatively common inborn error of immunity, occurring in 1 per 50,000 live births. A block in the normal maturation of immunoglobulin-producing B cells (block in V_HDJ_H recombination) results in the absence or severe reduction of serum immunoglobulin, absence of circulating mature B cells, and absence of plasma cells in all lymphoid tissue.[13] T-cell number and function are intact. Inheritance is sex-linked recessive, although a clinically indistinguishable syndrome with autosomal recessive inheritance has been observed in some patients. Recent studies have localized the defect to a protein tyrosine kinase gene

TABLE 139-2

Treatment Options in Hypogammaglobulinemic States

I. Intravenous Immunoglobulin or Intramuscular Gamma Globulin

Indications

Intravenous immune globulin is indicated in the treatment of primary immunodeficiency
states in which severe impairment of antibody-forming capacity has been shown.

IM gammaglobulin may also be used in some patients, primarily because of financial
considerations.

Dose

IVIG: 400–700 mg/kg q 3–4 weeks to maintain trough levels greater than 500 mg/dl.

IMIG: 100 mg/kg q 3 weeks *or* 1/3 of this dose q week.

II. Antibiotics

A. IV antibiotics

Length of treatment should be dictated by patient's clinical exam and pulmonary function
data, in conjunction with sputum culture results and microbial sensitivites. Home IV
therapy has proved helpful in patients requiring courses longer than 2–3 weeks.

B. Inhaled antibiotics[2]

Although almost all antibiotics available in IV form can be nebulized, cephalosporins
are particularly amenable to aerosolization and are typically the antibiotic of choice
in these patients. 1–3-month treatment plans can be used to extend the benefits of an
IV antibiotic course or to treat a mild respiratory exacerbation in conjunction with
oral antibiotics.

C. Oral antibiotics

Routine, daily antibiotic therapy in patients with proven chest radiographic and/or
pulmonary function abnormalities, a history of recurrent sinopulmonary infections,
chronic cough, or dyspnea may be beneficial in preventing further pulmonary
compromise or the onset of clinically relevant disease. "Rotating" combinations of
two or three antibiotics given monthly in recurrent cycles have anecdotal success.

III. Chest Physiotherapy

A. Percussion and postural drainage

Should be taught by a respiratory therapist to assure correct technique and positions

B. Positive expiratory pressure mask or valve with Huff cough technique[3]

C. Percussion vests[4]

IV. DNase[5]

To enhance mobility, clearance, and expectoration of viscous retained secretions.

V. Cimetidine—experimental

VI. IL-2, IFN-γ—experimental

(Bruton's tyrosine kinase, *btk*) on the proximal region
(q21.3–q22) of the X chromosome.[61] After maternal antibody is
consumed (usually after the first 4 to 6 months of life), patients
develop sinopulmonary infections, bacteremia, and meningitis
with encapsulated gram-positive and gram-negative bacteria,
such as *H. influenzae, S. pneumoniae, S. aureus, Pseudomonas
aeruginosa,* and *Mycoplasma pneumoniae.* Respiratory disease
due to *Pneumocystis carinii* or gastrointestinal infection with *Giardia lamblia* is also commonly observed. Although viral infections are not typical, enterovirus (polio and echo) and hepatitis
viruses may cause severe or fatal disease. Autoimmune diseases,
such as rheumatoid arthritis, occur in up to 20 percent of patients, while lymphomas and other lymphoreticular malignancies
occur in approximately 5 percent of cases.[51]

IgG levels are very low (less than 100 mg/dl), and IgA and
IgM are often undetectable. Treatment consists of IVIG given
every 3 to 4 weeks to maintain trough
levels at 500 mg/dl. IVIG preparations
containing low levels of IgA should be
used in patients with no IgA to decrease the possibility of anaphylactic
reactions mediated by IgE or IgG4 antibodies directed against the IgA.[20] A
low threshold for antibiotic use and aggressive pulmonary toilet are mandatory adjuncts to IVIG in slowing the
progression of bronchiectasis, fibrosis,
and ultimate cardiopulmonary failure.[19] Vaccinations with live attenuated
viruses must be avoided. Recently, it
has been possible to disrupt *btk* in
mice, providing a potential model for
experimental gene therapy.

Common Variable Immunodeficiency

Common variable immunodeficiency
(CVI) is a not uncommon defect due,
in general, to various B-cell activation
or differentiation defects, resulting in
low serum levels of IgG and depressed
levels of IgA or IgM. B cells may be
normal, high, or low, and T-cell number and function, although usually normal at diagnosis, deteriorate with time.
Putative mechanisms of CVI include
defective receptors for T_H-elaborated
cytokines, intrinsic block(s) of isotype
switching, and autoantibodies directed
against either B or T lymphocytes.[58,28]
T_H cytokine production has also been
shown to be dysregulated in some patients with the syndrome, who may
have deficits of cell-mediated immunity.[57]

Although the disease is familial, it
is not strictly X-linked or autosomally
inherited. In some patients, the genomic defects of both CVI and
isolated IgA deficiency appear to be localized to the major histocompatibility complex region of chromosome 6.[55] The disease
is characterized by the development of recurrent sinopulmonary
infections or chronic bronchiectasis in childhood or adulthood.
Chest radiograph findings consistent with atelectasis, bronchiectasis, and/or interstitial markings, along with pulmonary function tests revealing mild to severe obstruction and restrictive disease, are seen in 60 to 80 percent of CVI patients (Fig. 139-2).
This contrasts with the 30 to 40 percent of XLA patients with
similar chest radiographic and pulmonary function test abnormalities. These differences suggest that T-cell defects that occur
in patients with CVI, but not in patients with XLA, may predispose them to a wider spectrum of infectious diseases, although
persistent enterovirus infections of the central nervous system
are less frequent in CVI. A few patients with CVI present with

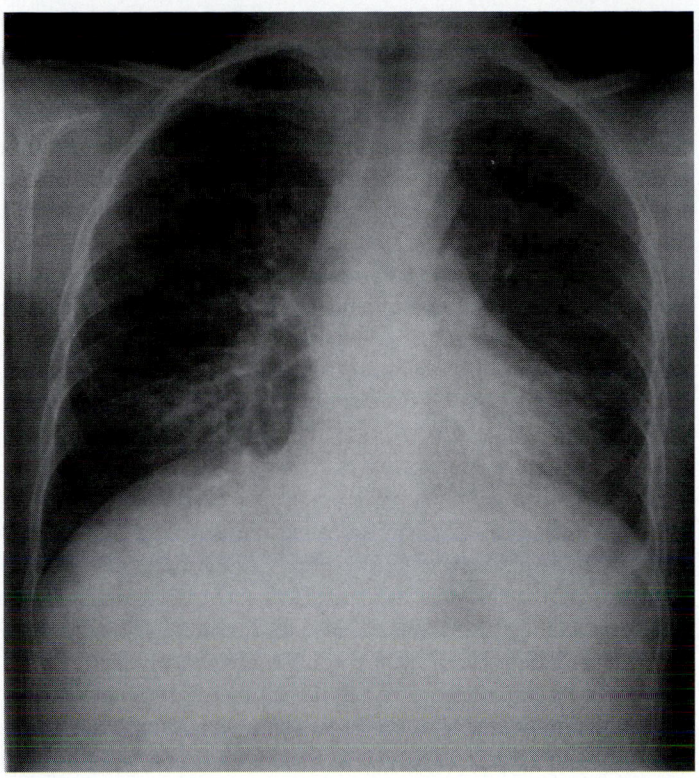

A

LUNG MECHANICS		Actual	Pred.	%Pred.
FVC	(L)	1.03	2.92	35
FEV1	(L)	0.97	2.56	38
FEV1/FVC	(%)	94	88	
FEF 25%	(L/sec)	7.10	4.82	147
FEF 50%	(L/sec)	2.98	3.51	85
FEF 75%	(L/sec)	0.80	1.89	43
FEF MAX	(L/sec)	7.34	6.46	114
FEF 25-75%	(L/sec)	2.29	2.95	78

B

FIGURE 139-2 *A.* PA chest radiograph of an adolescent boy with common variable immunodeficiency demonstrating marked bibasilar opacification, atelectasis, and infiltrative changes. Sputum culture grew only *H. influenzae* (nontypable). *B.* Pulmonary function tests from the same patient demonstrate significant restrictive, obstructive disease, supported by RV/TLC measurements. Marked improvement in radiographs and pulmonary function tests occurred with the use of continuous, rotating ciprofloxacin, ceclor, and biaxin, in conjunction with aggressive chest percussion via a percussor vest and inhaled DNase.

infections with unusual organisms, such as *P. carinii,* mycobacteria, or fungi. Recurrent attacks of both herpes simplex and zoster are not uncommon.

Some patients with CVI have developed unusual pulmonary parenchymal lymphocytic infiltrations or sarcoid granulomas.[16] CVI is also associated with pernicious anemia (30 percent), polyarthritis, systemic lupus erythematosus (SLE), idiopathic thrombocytopenic purpura, leukemia, lymphoma (particularly in affected women), GI tumors (gastric carcinoma), and malignant thymomas (10 percent). In fact, the overall frequency of cancer

in CVI patients is approximately 10 times greater than among normal persons.[18]

Accepted treatment is similar to that for XLA. We have had particular success in severely affected patients, using either inhaled antibiotics or a combination of oral antibiotics given on a monthly cycle, with *aggressive* chest physiotherapy, in conjunction with IVIG therapy, in preventing acute exacerbations and obviating intravenous antibiotics (see Table 139-2).

Experimental therapies based on advances in lymphocyte biology include retinoic acid analogs to promote B-lymphocyte differentiation[1] and histamine receptor antagonists, such as cimetidine, to override histamine receptor modulation of T-cell inhibition and increase production of immunoglobulins.[56] Of recent interest is the monthly subcutaneous administration of polyethylene glycol–conjugated IL-2. Administration of this cytokine is based on the finding that more than 50 percent of CVI patients also have abnormalities of T-cell activation and evidence of deficient IFN-γ, IL-2, I-4, IL-6, and IL-10 secretion and/or activity. It has been hypothesized that B cells from CVI patients may be defective because of a lack of these essential cytokines. Preliminary results show that prolonged (more than 3 months) subcutaneous administration of IL-2 markedly improved cellular immune functions, including increased T-cell proliferation in response to mitogens and antigens and restoration of lymphocyte secretion of IL-2, IL-6, and a novel B-cell differentiation factor.[17]

Selective IgG Subclass Deficiencies

Patients with selective IgG subclass deficiencies have recurrent sinopulmonary infections associated with normal or decreased total concentrations of serum IgG, but with selective deficiencies of IgG subclass 1, 2, 3, or 4. Patients with IgG2 subclass deficiency can make antibody, but the spectrum of the response is decreased, resulting in recurrent infection. Recent studies suggest a critical role for IL-6 and IFN-γ in enhancing IgG subclass production.[37,38] Titers to bacterial polysaccharide antigens are low even after immunization, since antibody responses to polysaccharides reside predominantly in the IgG2 subclass. Titers to protein antigens such as tetanus or diphtheria toxoids may be normal. IgG2 subclass deficiency may be associated with IgG4 subclass deficiency, IgA deficiency, Wiskott-Aldrich syndrome, and ataxia-telangiectasia. Persons with low or absent IgG2 or IgG4 appear to be particularly predisposed to recurrent or severe pneumonias and middle ear infections. Selective IgG3 deficiency is also associated with recurrent sinopulmonary infections, but the mechanism is not clear. These IgG3-deficient patients have normal responses to both common protein (Dt) and polysaccharide antigens; however, responses to influenza or rubella vaccine may be abnormal.

The wide spectrum of manifestations of IgG subclass defects—in normal subjects as well as those afflicted with severe, recurrent pneumonias—suggests that treatment be based on clinical findings of recurrent infections, rather than isolated laboratory abnormalities. Acute or chronic antibiotics, pulmonary toilet, and (in severe cases, with a documented inability to respond to specific antigens) IVIG replacement are the mainstays of therapy. It is important to document not only a low concentration of a subclass but also failure to make specific antibody when immunized, before immunoglobulin therapy is contemplated.

Selective IgA Deficiency

This most common of all the inborn defects of humoral immunity, occurring in 1 per 700 persons, accounts for more than 1 percent of recurrent infections in children.[46] The defect is assumed to be a differentiation block affecting IgA-committed B cells. Typically, peripheral counts of patients with IgA deficiency show normal numbers of mature B lymphocytes, as well as normal numbers and proportions of CD4$^+$ and CD8$^+$ cells. Selective IgA deficiency has been defined as serum IgA less than 5 mg/dl in severe deficiency and greater than 5 mg/dl but less than 2 SD below the age normal mean in partial IgA deficiency. As with IgG subclass deficiencies, there is considerable heterogeneity within this syndrome. While some patients are asymptomatic, at least 20 to 50 percent suffer from recurrent sinopulmonary infections. Approximately 50 percent of the patients with IgA deficiency and recurrent sinopulmonary infections also have IgG2 subclass deficiency or other IgG subclass deficiencies.[24] Recent studies have shown that infection susceptibility is more closely related to concomitant deficiency of IgG2 with or without deficiency of IgG4, as well as to low basal serum concentrations of pneumococcal polysaccharide antibodies and poor responses to the pneumococcal vaccine, rather than the degree of IgA deficiency. In fact, patients have been described with normal IgA and IgG subclasses whose only detectable defect appears to be an inability to respond to certain polysaccharide antigens. There is a report, however, of an adolescent with selective IgA deficiency and no other immunologic abnormality or secondary illness with bronchiectasis.[30] Thus, the diagnosis and treatment of IgA deficiency depend not only on the serum level of IgA but also on the history and results of related diagnostic studies, particularly the immune workup. In general, treatment relies on the administration of appropriate antibiotics for acute infection or chronic suppressive therapy for chronic infection. When IgA deficiency is associated with IgG2 deficiency, IVIG depleted of IgA may be indicated.

Hyper-IgM Immunodeficiency

The block in this disease resides in the normal ontogeny of B lymphocytes occurring during the differentiation of IgM$^+$ B cells into IgG- and IgA-secreting cells. Thus, patients have absent or markedly reduced IgA, IgE, and IgG levels, elevated levels of IgM, circulating mature B lymphocytes bearing IgM or IgD and plasma cells, as well as hyperplastic lymphoid tissue.[47] Recurrent neutropenia, probably secondary to autoimmune phenomena, may coexist with the humoral defect. Recent data indicate that the defect in hyper-IgM is the result of abnormal expression or function of the T-cell ligand for B lymphocyte CD40, a costimulatory receptor that mediates isotype switching. Both X-linked and autosomal recessive inheritance have been described. X-linked cases are due to abnormalities of the T-cell molecule CD40 ligand, which has been mapped to Xq26.3–27.1,[40] while autosomal recessive forms appear to be due to signal transduction abnormalities associated with CD40 on the B cells.[14]

Because antibody protection for the gastrointestinal and respiratory tracts is normally provided by IgA and IgG isotypes, patients with this syndrome are especially prone to respiratory and GI infections with pyogenic organisms. They are also predisposed to *P. carinii* pneumonia. As with other immunoglobulin deficiencies, patients with the hyper-IgM syndrome have very high rates of autoimmune (involving the formed elements of the blood) and lymphoproliferative disorders.

Treatment centers on IVIG replacement, with simultaneously aggressive use of antibiotics and chest physiotherapy. As with CVI, the use of cimetidine to ameliorate aberrant T-cell regulatory functions has been reported.[11]

COMPLEMENT DISORDERS

Disorders due to primary deficiencies of complement components are rare causes of pulmonary infections. Complement function can be assessed by determining the total hemolytic activity in serum (CH50), which measures the ability of serum to lyse antibody-coated sheep cells. A low to absent CH50 suggests a deficiency in a classic pathway complement component. Levels of specific complement components can then be determined. Although C2 deficiency is the most common complement deficiency, occurring in 1 in 30,000 to 1 in 10,000 people, it is mostly associated with a propensity toward collagen vascular–like diseases, particularly SLE, with an increased susceptibility for pyogenic bacterial infections of the sinopulmonary tract or bloodstream due to pneumococci. Twenty-five percent of persons with C2 deficiency are apparently healthy.

Because of the importance of C3 in the enhancement of phagocytosis (opsonization), congenital absence of C3 or consumption of C3 due to deficiency of factor I (C3b inactivator) results in a clinical picture like that seen in deficiency of the critical antibody opsonins, including surface and bacteremic infections primarily due to pyogenic bacteria. Patients with homozygous C3 deficiency have been encountered with severe and recurrent pneumonias due to *S. pneumoniae, H. influenzae,* and Enterobacteriaceae that are as severe as those in agammaglobulinemic patients. It was recently found that levels of IgG4 are markedly reduced in patients with hereditary deficiency of the classic pathway proteins (C1q, C1r/C1s, C4, C2) and C3.[6]

The terminal complement components, C5–9, form the cytolytic membrane attack complex (MAC), and deficiency of any one of these will block MAC formation. MAC plays an important role in lysing *Neisseria* species. C5–9 deficiencies therefore predispose to disseminated infection with *N. meningococci* and *N. gonococci.* Deficient subjects typically present after age 10 with recurrent episodes of meningococcal meningitis or systemic gonoccocal infections.

C1 esterase inhibitor deficiency results in persistent consumption of C2 and C4 by the C1 esterases, resulting in release of vasoactive kinins and the development of nonpruritic angioedema. Although angioedema can occur in any tissue, including the GI tract, edema of the upper airway can be life-threatening. Diagnosis is suggested by family history (autosomal dominant state), edema without pruritus, and chronically decreased C4 and C2 levels, especially during the 24 to 72 h of the episode. Patients with the familial form of the disease will have low to absent C1 esterase inhibitor concentrations. Angioedema with later onset, without a familial pattern, may be due to the absence of the functional component of the inhibitor, which may be associated with malignancy. Treatment is with danazol, a semisynthetic androgen that increases serum levels of C1 inhibitor and is used prophylactically, or purified C1 inhibitor for acute attacks.

CELL-MEDIATED IMMUNITY

Cellular immunity is defined as those responses that can be transferred to naïve hosts by transfusion or transplantation of T lymphocytes. Effector T cells either lack the specific responses to peptide MHC complexes, resulting in the inability of CD8$^+$ cells to lyse cells bearing particular viral antigens, or lack the ability to secrete cytokines and other products that typically result in activation and recruitment of macrophages, natural killer cells, and other inflammatory cells. In a sense, T lymphocytes coordinate most effector limbs of the immune system, including proliferation and differentiation of antibody-producing B cells, synthesis of complement components, as well as phagocyte recruitment and activation. Thus, although the most characteristic infections in these patients are those caused by opportunistic intracellular pathogens, including protozoa (*P. carini* and *Toxoplasma gondii*), fungi (*Candida* and *Aspergillus* species), viruses (particularly those of the herpesvirus family), and some intracellular bacteria (including *Listeria* and *Mycobacteria species*), defects in humoral or phagocyte defense mechanisms can also be seen.

DiGeorge's Syndrome

DiGeorge's syndrome (DGS) is a constellation of abnormalities resulting from dysmorphogenesis of the third and fourth pharyngeal pouches. Patients have hypoplasia or aplasia of the thymus and the parathyroid glands, complex cardiac malformations, esophageal atresia, bifid uvulas, cleft palate, short philtrums, mandibular hypoplasia, hypertelorism, and low-set notched ears. Most of the mortality attributable to this syndrome among afflicted infants is the result of either cardiovascular abnormalities or neonatal hypocalcemic tetany. DGS is considered to be a developmental field defect that may have more than one cause. It is now well established that most cases of DGS are due to haploinsufficiency of the chromosome 22q11 region (monosomy 22q11).[9]

The severity of immunologic manifestations varies from severe forms with complete thymic aplasia, resembling severe combined immunodeficiency disease (SCID), to only latent hypoparathyroidism, which may also be seen in relatives of patients with DGS. Most patients have partial T-cell function, which may improve with age, presumably due to the adaptation of functional extrathymic sites for T-lymphocyte maturation. T-cell numbers are typically reduced, with reduced percentages of CD3$^+$ and CD4$^+$ cells, but CD8$^+$ cells may be normal or even elevated. Patients with more significant CD4$^+$ T-cell deficiency seem to have more frequent and severe infections requiring hospitalization. B-lymphocyte counts are usually normal; antibody production is also usually normal, but of poor biologic quality. Some patients may have low IgA or elevated serum IgE levels. Surviving infants often have the tendency to acquire parathyroid function, cell-mediated immunity, and functional T cells.

Patients are prone to severe viral pneumonias, particularly those of the herpes and measles family. Pneumonias due to fungal and gram-negative bacilli and *P. carinii* also occur.

Treatment consists of transplantation of HLA-identical marrow.[42] Transplants of fetal thymus or thymic epithelial cells have not resulted in long-term correction. Treatment with thymosin fractions has also been reported and is associated with a decline in CD8$^+$ T-cell percentage and an increased response to IL-2.[5]

Severe Combined Immunodeficiency Disease

SCID is a syndrome of heterogeneous lymphocyte stem cell defects that affect both T- and B-cell function, resulting in profound hypogammaglobulinemia and absence of T-cell function. Laboratory analysis may reveal lymphopenia (10 to 20 percent) and normal or increased numbers of circulating B cells, but severely reduced IgG levels. Several genetic defects resulting in the SCID syndrome have been described. Approximately 50 percent of patients have the X-linked recessive variant, which has been localized to the gene controlling the development of the gamma chain of the IL-2 receptor in the Xq13–13.3 region.[49] The gamma chain of IL-2R is also a common component for receptors of IL-4 and IL-7, which, with IL-2, are important in the growth and development of both T and B cells.

The other 50 percent of SCID syndrome patients have an autosomal recessive variant, of whom about 50 percent have an associated adenosine deaminase (ADA) deficiency—resulting in an accumulation of adenosine and deoxyadenosine, which is preferentially toxic to T lymphoblasts. The gene for ADA deficiency has been mapped to chromosome 20q13-ter, where different types of mutations have been identified.[33] Diagnosis is made by examination of red or white blood cells for ADA content.

Another cause of autosomal recessive SCID is ZAP-70 deficiency. The absence of ZAP-70 (as a result of mutations in the ZAP-70 gene), a non-Src protein tyrosine kinase localized to chromosome 2q12, is associated with defects in T-cell antigen receptor (TCR) signal transduction.[10]

Another form of the SCID syndrome is referred to as the *bare lymphocyte syndrome,* reflecting the lack of MHC class I or class II antigens on B cells, macrophages, and dendritic cells, resulting in the inability to present antigen to T and B cells.[29]

In general, SCID syndrome patients present with a triad of mucocutaneous candidiasis, intractable diarrhea, and *P. carinii* pneumonia, evident shortly after birth or within 6 to 9 months of life and progressing to severe failure to thrive. Within a few days after birth, patients may also develop a morbilliform rash that is probably a manifestation of graft-versus-host disease (GVHD) from passively transferred maternal lymphocytes. Infections with a wide range of microbes occur in all forms of SCID, including viral pathogens, particularly herpesviruses (herpes, cytomegalovirus, varicella), adenovirus, measles, influenza, and *Legionella.* Fatal giant-cell pneumonia has resulted from measles infection and live measles vaccination, and progressive vaccinia has occurred after smallpox vaccination.

Enzyme replacement using frozen, irradiated erythrocyte transfusions, polyethylene glycol–modified bovine ADA,[41] and bone marrow transplantation have been used successfully in the management of ADA-deficient patients.[34] In addition, patients with ADA deficiency have been treated with autologous lymphocytes or stem cells corrected in vitro with retroviral vector–inserted normal human DNA. Blaese and coworkers recently reported on the encouraging 4-year follow-up of the initial trial of T-lymphocyte–directed gene therapy for ADA-deficient SCID.[7]

Purine Nucleoside Phosphorylase

Absence of the enzyme purine nucleoside phosphorylase (PNP) is associated with marked cell-mediated immunodeficiency but intact humoral immunity. The gene encoding the enzyme is localized to chromosome 14q13.1.[45] Although the thymuses of these patients are hypoplastic, other defects associated with DGS are absent. The accumulation of purine metabolites, such as deoxyguanosine triphosphate, has toxic effects on cellular division of T lymphocytes, resulting in marked and progressive lymphopenia, but normal $CD4^+ : CD8^+$ ratios and normal immunoglobulin levels. Diagnosis is made by measurement of PNP in hemolyzed red blood cells. Heterozygotes have half the normal level of this enzyme. Serum uric acid levels are low because of the absence of the enzyme: A normal uric acid level can help rule out this disease. Patients are prone to disseminated viral infections, P. carinii infection, mucocutaneous candidiasis, and chronic diarrhea. Neurologic disorders afflict more than 50 percent of patients, and more than a third of PNP patients develop autoimmune diseases. Enzyme replacement therapy using normal, irradiated erythrocyte transfusions may lead to partial correction. Bone marrow transplantation is the only successful therapy at present. An in vitro model of retroviral transfer of the gene into mouse lymphoma T cells has been described, suggesting that gene therapy may be a promising possibility in the near future.

Wiskott-Aldrich Syndrome

Wiskott-Aldrich syndrome (WAS) is caused by a defect localized to the short arm of the X chromosome (Xp11.22–11.3),[53] resulting in severely impaired production of antibodies to polysaccharide antigens, as well as variable reductions of T-cell numbers and impaired mitogen responses that tend to worsen with age. In several kindreds, isolated X-linked thrombocytopenia maps to the same gene locus and is probably a variant of this syndrome. Both T-cell numbers and function progressively decrease, and profound lymphopenia becomes apparent at approximately 6 years of age. Most patients have abnormalities of serum immunoglobulin levels, with low IgM and isohemagglutinin concentrations, a tendency toward elevated IgA and IgE levels, and normal or slightly depressed IgG levels. WAS is associated with deficiencies of various cell surface glycoproteins—most notably CD43, a leukocyte marker localized to chromosome 16 that may be active in T-cell activation.[21] Recently, Derry and colleagues isolated a novel gene, WASP, that was not expressed in four patients with WAS because of point mutations or single base deletions. This gene encodes a proline-rich protein that may be an important regulator of lymphocyte and platelet function.[26] Males afflicted with this syndrome suffer from a triad of recurrent infections, thrombocytopenia, and a skin disease indistinguishable from atopic dermatitis. Because of the serious complications observed in this disorder, including hemorrhage, the mean age of survival before management with splenectomy, IVIG, and bone marrow transplant was 6 years, with death often due to infection. Typical infections include pyoderma or cellulitis associated with eczematoid eruptions, chronic otitis media with persistent otorrhea and/or mastoiditis, and chronic pneumonitis. Encapsulated pyogenic bacteria, such as S. pneumoniae, H. influenzae, herpesvirus, and P. carinii, are the most frequently identified pathogens. Bone marrow transplantation may correct both the platelet and the immunologic abnormalities.

Ataxia-Telangiectasia

This syndrome (AT) is characterized by profound deficiencies of cellular immunity, (including lymphopenia, defects in cutaneous anergy, decreases in Th : Ts ratios, decreases in cytotoxic T cells, and an increase in immature T cells with increased gamma/delta TCR expression), impaired humoral responses (thymic hypoplasia associated with IgA deficiency, IgE deficiency, and IgG2 and IgG4 subclass deficiency), and a constellation of progressive cerebellar ataxia with degeneration of Purkinje cells. The defective genes of the two most common AT variants map to chromosome 11q22.3, which may result in a recombination defect that interferes with the rearrangement of T-cell and B-cell genes, an inability to repair damaged DNA, and a failure of normal organ maturation.[62] Savitsky and coworkers have identified a single telangiectasia gene in this autosomal recessive disorder by positional cloning on chromosome 11q22.23. A cDNA clone of this gene encodes a protein that is similar to mammalian phosphatidylinositol-3 kinases, which are operative in mitogenic signal transduction, meiotic recombination, and cell cycle control. Telangiectasias, particularly ocular and cutaneous, and a high incidence of malignancies, particularly non-Hodgkin's lymphoma, and breast cancer (in heterozygous female carries of the AT allele) are also seen. AT is also associated with insulin-resistant diabetes mellitus, gonadal agenesis, premature aging, elevated levels of serum α_1-fetoprotein and carcinoembryonic antigen, and hypersensitivity of fibroblasts and lymphocytes to ionizing radiation, reflecting an inability to repair damaged DNA.

Patients suffer from an increased incidence of bacterial and viral sinopulmonary infections, and many eventually develop chronic bronchiectasis. The most frequent pulmonary pathogens are S. aureus and other encapsulated bacteria. Concurrent IgG2 (50 percent), IgG4, and IgA deficiencies (70 percent) may be associated with the tendency toward recurrent infections of the respiratory tract. Approximately 80 percent of patients have depressed IgE levels.

Treatment with synthetic serum thymic factor has been reported to improve antibody production, particularly both serum and salivary IgA, and decrease the incidence of chronic bronchial infections among this population.[8] This effect on humoral immunity is associated with an increase in the peripheral T-cell level and the return to normal of deficient responses to mitogens in vitro. Plasma infusions[2] and IL-2 administration[23] have also yielded some evidence of clinical improvement in afflicted persons. IVIG therapy may also be helpful, in light of the IgG subclass deficiencies. Kodama's team[39] reported an in vitro study showing the suppression of radiographically induced chromosome aberrations in AT cells by introduction of a normal human chromosome 11. Thus, gene therapy for AT may become possible in the future.

PHAGOCYTIC DEFECTS

Phagocytosis is a critical component of the respiratory defense against extracellular bacteria. The functional activity of phagocytic cells includes adherence to vascular endothelium, recognition of and migration toward a chemical stimulus (chemotaxis), phagocytosis, and killing of ingested microorganisms. Defects in the process of phagocytic defense can occur as a consequence of a defect in any of these functions. Most of these defects have been identified in neutrophils, monocytes, and macrophages, as well as eosinophils—all considered to be phagocytic cells. The most frequently encountered primary deficiencies of phagocytes are the result of absolute reductions in number or function (migration, adherence/aggregation, or killing) of granulocytes.

Disorders of Phagocyte Numbers

These disorders include cyclic neutropenia, Kostmann's syndrome, Shwachman-Diamond syndrome, and autoimmune neutropenia. They are characterized by absolute PMN counts as low as 50 to 200/mm³ but typically lower than 1000/mm³. Owing to the presence of a compensatory monocytosis, these disorders are associated with a low incidence of severe respiratory infections, although pneumonia is seen—as are furunculosis, subcutaneous abscess, and otitis media. Typical pathogens include *S. aureus, P. aeruginosa,* and enteric bacteria. Traditional treatment has relied on antibiotics; however, the use of recombinant granulocyte colony stimulating factor (rGCSF) has been very promising, particularly in patients with Felty's syndrome and severe chronic neutropenia of congenital cyclic, or idiopathic origin.

Defects of Phagocyte Function

CHRONIC GRANULOMATOUS DISEASE

CGD is caused by a defect in a membrane-associated nicotinamide adenine dinucleotide phosphate (NADPH) oxidase in phagocytic cells, resulting in the failure of phagocytic cells to produce superoxide, hydrogen peroxide, and other reduction products of oxygen that are necessary for killing certain microbial species. The larger subunit of a phagocyte-specific cytochrome, which is part of the oxidase complex heterodimer, is abnormal in these patients. In the X-linked form, the gene for the 91kD cytochrome *b* subunit, which is located in band p21 of the X chromosome, is absent, truncated, or mutated,[52] whereas in the autosomal recessive form of CGD, other components of the NADPH oxidase system are affected, including the 22kD light chain[22] of this cytochrome, or 47kD or 67kD cytosolic factors.[12] Diagnosis is made by the inability of neutrophils to re-

duce nitroblue tetrazolium (NBT) from yellow to blue-black formazan and by the inability of neutrophils to kill staphylococci or other catalase-positive microorganisms. Fifty percent of stimulated PMNs from female carriers of CGD reduce NBT, as against less than 5 percent in males with CGD. NBT is reduced by 70 to 90 percent in PMNs from normal persons of both sexes after stimulation. Additional laboratory findings suggestive of CGD include leukocytosis, elevation of erythrocyte sedimentation rate, abnormal chest radiographs, and hypergammaglobulinemia.

Onset is typically in infancy, childhood or, less commonly, early adolescence, with a male-to-female ratio of 6:1. All forms of CGD are characterized by abscess formation at sites of bacterial tissue invasion and in lymph nodes, liver, and lung. Patients present with severe recurrent lymphadenitis and infections of the sinopulmonary and GI tracts, as well as of the skin. Severe and recurrent pulmonary infections occur in almost all patients with CGD, including bronchopneumonia, empyema, lung abscess, and hilar adenopathy syndromes. Among CGD patients followed at the University of Minnesota Hospital from 1954, pneumonia represented the most common presenting illness and the most common cause of morbidity.[50] Complications of recurrent pneumonia represent the reported cause of death in 15 to 50 percent of CGD patients. Pulmonary infections are protracted and refractory or slow to respond to therapy. Persistent fever and cough (often nonproductive) are typical clinical presentations. Chest radiographs may demonstrate segmental, lobar, or diffuse infiltrates or diffuse reticulonodular or miliary densities that represent areas of granuloma formation.

Approximately 20 percent of CGD patients develop pulmonary abscesses and/or empyema. Some patients develop areas of diffuse pneumonitis that resolve into discrete areas of consolidation referred to as *encapsulating pneumonias,* which typically measure 2 to 6 cm in diameter and are often homogeneous and round. Most young adult patients demonstrate chronic bilateral infiltrates, pulmonary fibrosis, or pulmonary calcifications associated with restrictive/obstructive disease (Fig. 139-3). Aggregates of granulomas, leading to mechanical obstruction, may form as a response of activated macrophages to microbial persistence and chronic antigenic stimulation. These are particularly troublesome when associated with the gastrointestinal or genitourinary tract, but they can also be seen within the respiratory system. Pathogens associated with CGD are either hydrogen peroxide producers, which also make catalase (neutralizing any hydrogen peroxide produced as a byproduct of microbial metabolism), or organisms that do not intrinsically synthesize hydrogen peroxide. *S. aureus* represents by far the most common cause of infections in CGD, accounting for 30 to 55 percent of clinical isolates overall. Other catalase-positive and non–H_2O_2-producing organisms—including *Escherichia coli, Klebsiella,* and *Enterobacter* species, *Serratia marcescens, Salmonella* and *Pseudomonas* species—account for approximately 30 percent of infections. Less commonly, pneumonias in CGD patients may be caused by *Mycobacterium tuberculosis,* atypical mycobacteria, and *P. carinii.* In specific geographic locations, such as the southeastern United States, *Chromobacterium violaceum* has been recognized as the cause of infection in several CGD patients.[44] *Nocardia* infection, particularly of the respiratory sys-

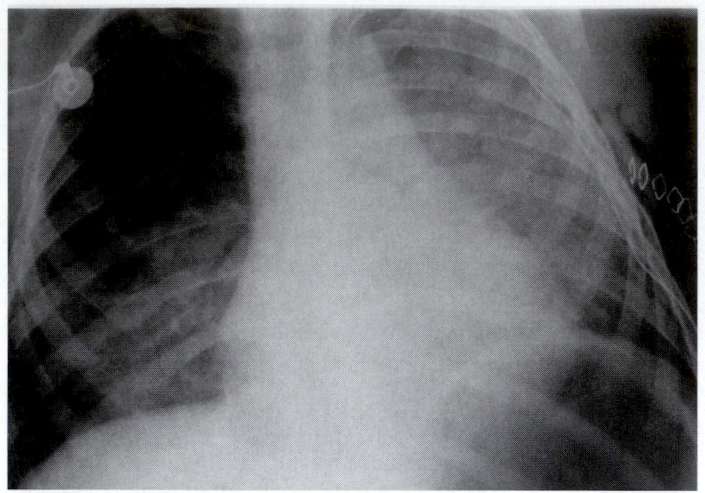

A

LUNG MECHANICS		Actual	Pred.	%Pred.
FVC	(L)	1.03	2.92	35
FEV1	(L)	0.97	2.56	38
FEV1/FVC	(%)	94	88	
FEF 25%	(L/sec)	7.10	4.82	147
FEF 50%	(L/sec)	2.98	3.51	85
FEF 75%	(L/sec)	0.80	1.89	43
FEF MAX	(L/sec)	7.34	6.46	114
FEF 25-75%	(L/sec)	2.29	2.95	78

B

FIGURE 139-3 *A.* PA chest radiograph of a child with CGD who originally presented as an infant with recurrent pneumonia in the right upper lobe diagnosed radiographically as cystic adenomatoid malformation. Subsequent histologic examination and culture revealed this to be nocardial pneumonia. This radiograph reveals recurrent diffuse nocardial pneumonia. *B.* Pulmonary function tests from the same patient showing mild restrictive disease, probably secondary to right upper lobectomy and recurrent airspace disease.

tem, is also relatively common, as are fungal infections (Fig. 139-4). Particularly problematic are pneumonias due to invasive aspergillus, which may be lethal in up to 50 percent of cases. *Candida albicans* and species of *Torulopsis* account for most of the other fungal agents.

Attempts to culture potential pathogens from CGD patients are difficult, with reports of only a 50 percent success rate, despite extensive cultural surveillance of infected tissue sites or body fluids. Treatment classically has relied on antibiotic prophylaxis, particularly with trimethoprim-sulfamethoxasole and surgical incision and drainage of abscesses. Antibiotic treatment is justified for weeks or even months in light of the high incidence of relapsing infection due to the internal sequestration, rather than the killing of microorganisms by CGD phagocytes. Although the ubiquity and nature of the infecting agents in CGD patients preclude attempts to define and eliminate exposure to potential pathogens, marijuana smoking is an identified risk that should be avoided, since marijuana may be heavily contaminated with *Aspergillus* or *Salmonella* organisms. Treatment with subcutaneous rIFN-γ, which has been reported to enhance the

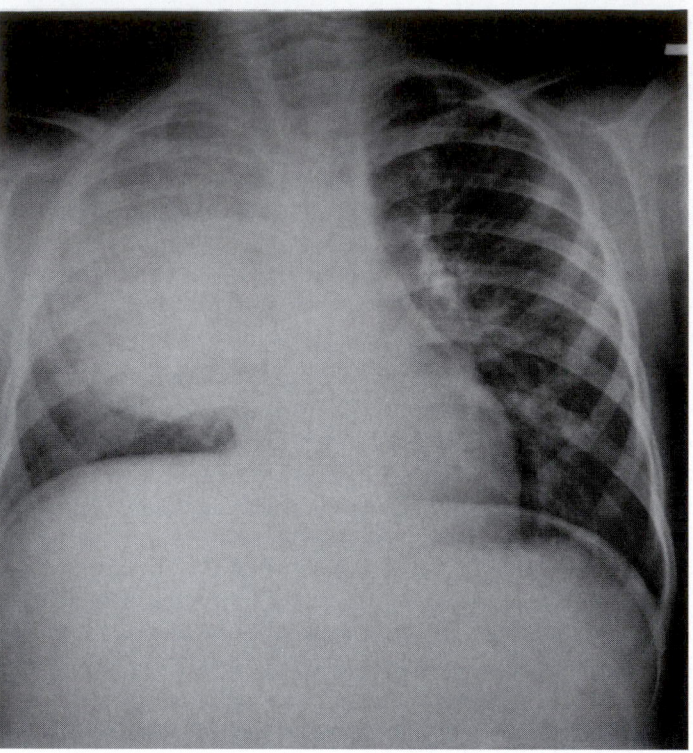

FIGURE 139-4   PA chest radiograph in a patient with CGD demonstrating nocardial abscess of right upper lobe, extending into the anterior chest wall.

macrophage oxidative burst activity by increasing transcription of cytochrome *b,* has been shown to decrease the frequency of infections.[24] Although no statistical improvement in neutrophil staphylococcal killing or superoxide production was demonstrated in CGD patients receiving IFN-γ in the recent International CGD Cooperative Study, a significant clinical benefit was noted, with an approximate 70 percent reduction in infectious complications.[35] Thus, the ameliorative effects of IFN-γ may not result solely from enhancement of the neutrophil NADPH oxidase system, but may also involve nonoxidative immunologic processes. Bone marrow transplantation, while curative in a few patients, exchanges the immunodeficiency of CGD for the need to be on immunosuppressive agents to prevent GVHD, which may not be an advantageous tradeoff.

GLUCOSE-6-PHOSPHATE DEHYDROGENASE DEFICIENCY

This variant of CGD, in which G6PD levels are less than 1 percent, results in an inability to generate oxygen by-products, leading to a slightly milder form of disease than that in most patients with CGD.[15] The defect is thought to result from a deficiency of NADPH, which is needed as substrate for the initiating oxidase, resulting in diminished intracellular killing of catalase-positive organisms and failure to reduce NBT or generate chemiluminescence, O_2^-, or H_2O_2. Unlike CGD, methylene blue does not normalize hexose monophosphate shunt activation by G6PD-deficient leukocytes. As would be expected, patients with severe variants of G6PD deficiency are susceptible to a spectrum of infectious agents and complications similar to that seen in persons with CGD. Although most mild to moderate variants of G6PD deficiency do not demonstrate host defense deficits related to leukocyte dysfunction, almost all are characterized clinically by chronic nonspherocytic hemolytic anemia. Treatment is similar to that for CGD.

CHEDIAK-HIGASHI SYNDROME

CHS is a rare autosomal recessive defect characterized by abnormal fusion of azurophilic lysosomes of neutrophils and cytoplasmic granules of monocytes and lymphocytes. This defect results in impaired microbicidal activity of phagocytes due to the presence of giant lysosomal granules, which have abnormal postphagocytic phagolysosomal fusion and degranulation. In addition, neutrophil counts tend to be low, secondary to their rapid turnover. Chemotactic defects and impaired natural killer cell activity have also been noted.

Patients present with recurrent skin and upper and lower respiratory tract infections, including recurrent or chronic otitis media, sinusitis, and pharyngitis, in addition to lower respiratory tract infections, including bronchopneumonia. Segmental or lobar lung involvement can account for up to 30 percent of documented infections. Most infections are due to *S. aureus, H. influenzae,* group A streptococcus, and gram-negative enteric organisms (*Klebsiella, Proteus, Shigella, Pseudomonas*). *Aspergillus* and *Candida* represent less common etiologic agents. Respiratory failure can occur with extensive histiocytic infiltration of the lungs during an accelerated lymphomalike proliferative phase marked by widespread tissue infiltrates of lymphoid and histiocytic cells, usually without malignant histologic characteristics. Anemia, hypersplenism, and platelet dysfunction, associated with the accelerated phase, and albinism or hypopigmentation, due to abnormal fusion of melanocyte pigment organelles, are also seen. Attempts to alter the biochemical abnormalities of CHS with cholinergic agents or cyclic GMP and ascorbic acid have not been successful in changing the clinical course of these patients.

Treatment, aside from antibiotic therapy and chest physiotherapy, is allogeneic bone marrow transplantation.

Leukocyte Adhesion Deficiency

Patients with this autosomal recessive disease lack or have markedly reduced β_2 integrins, essential glycoprotein constituents of the CD11/CD18 receptor complex that mediates leukocyte adhesion. These defects are due to deficiency of the 95kD beta chain (CD18), which, when noncovalently associated with an alpha subunit, forms the CD11/18 family of adhesion receptors on nearly all bone marrow–derived cells.[12] Complete and partial forms of the deficiency have been identified.

Recurrent necrotic and indolent infections of soft tissues, primarily in skin, mucous membranes, and the intestinal tract, are the clinical hallmarks of this disease. Superficial infections of body surfaces may invade locally or systemically. Typical small, erythematous, nonpustular skin lesions may lead to large, well-demarcated, ulcerative craters or pyoderma gangrenosa, which heals slowly or with dysplastic eschars. Septicemia progressing from omphalitis associated with delayed umbilical cord separa-

tion has been observed. Perirectal abscesses, cellulitis leading to peritonitis and/or septicemia, and ulcerative mucous membrane lesions of the oral cavity, resulting in facial or deep cervical cellulitis, have been observed. Recurrent invasive *Candida* esophagitis, erosive gastritis, acute appendicitis, and necrotizing enterocolitis have been reported. Severe gingivitis or periodontitis is a major feature among all patients who survive infancy. Upper respiratory infections, including recurrent otitis media with progression to mastoiditis and facial nerve paralysis, have been seen, as have severe bacterial sinusitis, laryngotracheitis, and recurrent pneumonitis.

The recurrent infections reflect a profound impairment of leukocyte mobilization into extravascular inflammatory sites, despite peripheral blood granulocyte counts of 15,000 to 161,000/mm³. A wide spectrum of gram-positive or -negative bacteria (*S. aureus* and gram-negative enteric bacteria) and fungal microorganisms (*Candida* and *Aspergillus*) infect LAD patients, similar to those with neutropenia syndromes (Fig. 139-5). Deep-seated granulomatous infections typical of CGD have not been observed. Purulent discharge containing leukocytes is absent at the site of infections because of abnormal adherence and chemotaxis of the cells. Although the predominance of recurrent bacterial (as opposed to viral or fungal) infections in LAD patients suggests that the functions of neutrophils or monocytes are more profoundly affected than those of lymphocytes, deficits of the LFA-1–dependent function of lymphocytes have also been observed.

The diagnosis of this syndrome can be made by assessing the expression of the MAC-1 (CD11b) on the patient's neutrophils using monoclonal MAC-1 and flow cytometry. Further confirmation can be made by assessing expression of these glycoproteins after exposure to a degranulating stimulus, such as calcium ionophore A23187.

Treatment relies on acute and prophylactic use of antibiotics. Trimethoprim-sulfamethoxazole is a useful agent because of its wide spectrum of antimicrobial activity. Generally, the use of in-

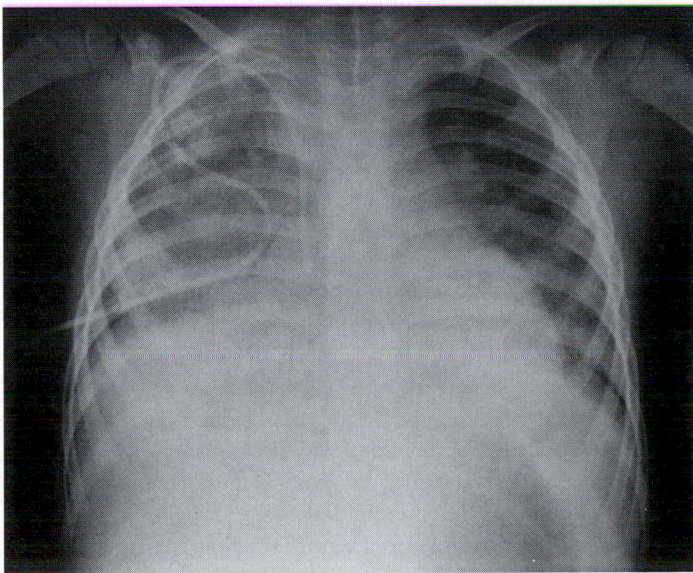

FIGURE 139-5   PA chest radiograph in a child with CD18 neutrophil receptor deficiency demonstrating extensive airspace disease due to probable candidal and pyogenic bacterial pneumonia.

travenous antibiotics results in resolution of recognized infections. Transfusion of granulocytes has been associated with enhancement of inflammatory function and clinical resolution of selected infections, with a concomitant decrease in the absolute peripheral blood leukocyte count. Bone marrow transplantation remains the definitive treatment and should be considered for patients with the severe phenotype. Additionally, methods for successful transfection of normal CD18 cDNA into LAD lymphoblasts have resulted in the normal expression and function of LFA-1 alpha-beta complexes on cell surfaces. Thus, there is a real possibility for gene therapy in the future.[63]

Hyperimmunoglobulin E Syndrome

Also known as the hyper-IgE recurrent infection or Job's syndrome, this unusual disorder, which appears to be autosomal dominant with incomplete penetrance, is lacking an exact immunologic defect. It is most often attributed to deficiencies of PMN and monocyte chemotaxis, which may be intrinsic or the result of abnormal lymphocyte regulation, with dysregulation of subsets of IFN-γ– and IL-4–producing CD4$^+$ T cells.[27,31,32] Although lymphocyte numbers and phenotype ratios are usually normal, primary and secondary antibody responses, as well as in vitro cellular immune responses, may on occasion be abnormal. Serum levels of polyclonal IgE are markedly elevated (above 2000 IU/ml), but immunoglobulins other than IgE are normal. Complete blood counts and differentials are mildly abnormal, with occasional borderline neutropenia. Most patients have mild to moderate eosinophilia, despite lacking a significant history of classic allergic diseases. All patients have chronically elevated erythrocyte sedimentation rates, usually between 30 and 60 mm/h.

A strict definition of this syndrome is necessary because of the number of patients with clinical features suggestive of the HIE syndrome, such as those with atopic eczema colonized by S. aureus at cutaneous sites or those with prominent allergic histories and recurrent sinopulmonary infections but without "cold abscesses" or extremely high levels of serum IgE. "Cold abscesses" are not seen in all HIE patients, but they are rare in other immunodeficiency states. They can present in any part of the body as fluctuant masses, with little evidence of inflammation and often without fever. Drainage of these abscesses usually reveals large volumes of purulent material, which almost always grow S. aureus.

Otitis externa and chronic otitis media, occasionally complicated by mastoiditis, are common in HIE patients. Recurrent bronchitis represents the most common pulmonary manifestation of HIE. Patients often suffer several days a month of productive cough, rarely associated with fever. Less commonly, pneumonia, with or without associated complications—including bronchiectasis, lung abscess, empyema, pneumatocele formation, and bronchopleural fistula formation—may represent serious and potentially devastating features in HIE patients (Fig. 139-6A). S. aureus and H. influenzae are the most frequent causes of pneumonias in HIE. Complications frequently require chest tube drainage of purulent collections, or segmental or lobar lung resections to attenuate progression of bronchiectasis, particularly when associated with recurrent hemoptysis. As a result of in-

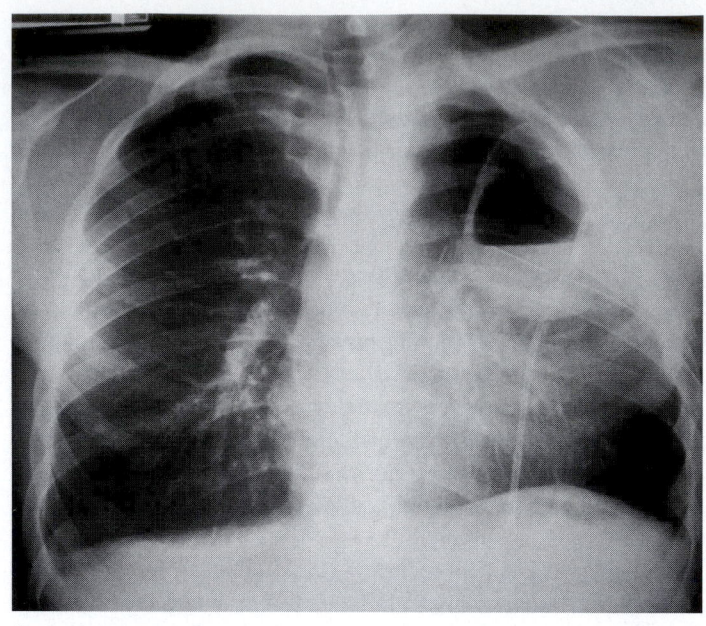

A

		Actual	**Pred.**	**%Pred.**
LUNG MECHANICS				
FVC	(L)	3.14	3.90	81
FEV1	(L)	2.66	3.66	73
FEV1/FVC	(%)	85	94	
FEF 25%	(L/sec)	6.08	5.08	120
FEF 50%	(L/sec)	3.05	3.69	83
FEF 75%	(L/sec)	1.29	1.99	65
FEF MAX	(L/sec)	6.95	6.22	112
FEF 25-75%	(L/sec)	2.86	3.24	88

B

FIGURE 139-6 *A.* PA chest radiograph in a patient with Job's syndrome, after left upper lobectomy for bronchiectasis due to *Aspergillus fumigatus,* resulting in recurrent, severe hemoptysis. Chest radiograph shows residual bronchopleural fistula with loculated air collection in the left upper lobe, extensive airspace disease in the left lower lobe, and pleural thickening. *B.* Pulmonary function tests from the same patient showing mild restrictive and obstructive disease despite his extensive left-sided pulmonary disease.

fection and surgical intervention, pulmonary function tests can reveal both obstructive and restrictive defects (Fig. 139-6B).

As stated, the overwhelmingly predominant pathogen is *S. aureus,* with pneumonias and other infections occasionally due to *H. influenzae,* streptococcal species, and *P. aeruginosa.* Candidal infections of the skin and mucous membranes are also frequently seen.

Diagnosis of HIE can be established in patients (usually during infancy) with a history of staphylococcal infections of the skin and sinopulmonary tract, and IgE levels at least 10 times normal. Coarse facies, chronic eczematoid eruptions, cold cutaneous or subcutaneous abscesses, eosinophilia, and mucocutaneous candidiasis are also seen, as are recurrent bone fractures and osteopenia.

Management relies on the use of narrow-spectrum antistaphylococcal prophylaxis, such as cloxacillin or dicloxacillin. Trimethoprim-sulfamethoxazole may also be employed as a prophylactic agent. Serious infections require treatment with intravenous antibiotics, which should continue for 2 to 6 weeks or more to assure satisfactory clinical resolution. Surgical intervention or drainage of abscesses in HIE should be considered early and encouraged. Conservative courses of antibiotics and observation usually result in progression of cold abscesses, with greater morbidity and prolonged recuperation time. H$_2$ histamine receptor blockade therapy has been reported to result in a decreased frequency of infections by increasing the neutrophil chemotactic response.[60] Ascorbic acid has also been reported to improve the chemotactic responsiveness of neutrophils in patients with recurrent infections and high IgE, but it has been studied only in patients not meeting the strict definition of HIE. More recently, very limited studies with subcutaneous IFN-γ, administered as in chronic granulomatous disease, have resulted in subjective improvement in three out of four patients, especially with regard to decreasing the amount of mucus production.[36]

SUMMARY

Pulmonary disease is a major problem in most primary immunodeficiency diseases, particularly those resulting in deficient antibody production or function and impaired phagocytic activity. Early recognition of a primary immunodeficiency and aggressive treatment and management of secondary pulmonary complications can result in substantial improvement in a patient's overall health and well-being and decrease the risk of future cardiopulmonary insufficiency and death. Although advances in gene therapy may allow correction of most of these defects, the reality of the morbidity and mortality associated with immunodeficiency disease–mediated pulmonary complications must be acknowledged and aggressively addressed.

REFERENCES

 1. Adelman DC, Yen TY, Cumberland WG, et al: 13-Cis retinoic acid enhances in vivo B-lymphocyte differentiation in patients with common variable immunodeficiency. *J Allergy Clin Immunol* 88:705–712, 1991.

 2. Ammann AJ, Good RA, Bier D, et al: Long-term plasma infusions in a patient with ataxia-telangiectasia and deficient IgA and IgE. *Pediatrics* 44:672–676, 1969.

 3. Anderson DC, Smith CW, Springer TA: Leukocyte adhesion deficiency and other disorders of leukocyte motility, in Scriver CR, Beaudet AL, Sly WS, Valle P (eds), *The Metabolic Basis of Inherited Disease.* New York, McGraw-Hill, 1989, pp 2751–2777.

 4. Arens R, Gozal D, Omlin KJ, et al: Comparison of high frequency chest compression and conventional chest physiotherapy in hospitalized patients with cystic fibrosis. *Am J Respir Crit Care Med* 150:1154–1157, 1994.

 5. Barrett DJ, Wara DW, Ammann AG, et al: Thymosin therapy in the DiGeorge syndrome. *J Pediatr* 97:66–71, 1980.

 6. Bird P, Lachmann PJ: The regulation of IgG subclass production in man: Low serum IgG4 in inherited deficiencies of the classical pathway of C3 activation. *Eur J Immunol* 18:1217–1222, 1988.

 7. Blaese RM, Culver KW, Miller AD, et al: T-lymphocyte–directed gene therapy for ADA-SCID: Initial trial results after 4 years. *Science* 270:475–480, 1995.

 8. Bordigoni P, Faure G, Bene MC, et al: Improvement of cellular immunity and IgA production in immunodeficient children after treatment with synthetic serum thymic factor (FTS). *Lancet* 2:293–297, 1982.

 9. Borzy MS, Ridgway D, Nowa FJ, et al: Successful bone marrow transplantation with split lymphoid chimerism in DiGeorge syndrome. *J Clin Immunol* 9:386–392, 1989.

10. Chan AC, Kadlecek TA, Elder ME, et al: ZAP-70 deficiency in an autosomal recessive form of severe combined immunodeficiency. *Science* 264:1599–1601, 1994.

11. Ciboddo G, Crosti F, Di Lucca G, Bellone M: Cimetidine treatment in hyper-IgM hypogammaglobulinemia (letter). *JAMA* 258:1892, 1987.

12. Clark RA, Malech HL, Gallin JI, et al: Genetic variants of chronic granulomatous disease: Prevalence of deficiencies of two cystolic components of the NADPH oxidase. *New Engl J Med* 321:647–652, 1989.

13. Conley M: B cells in patients with X-linked agammaglobulinemia. *J Immunol* 134:3070–3074, 1985.

14. Conley ME, Larche M, Bonagura VR, et al: Hyper-IgM syndrome associated with defective CD40-mediated B cell activation. *J Clin Invest* 94:1404–1409, 1994.

15. Cooper MR, DeChatelet LR, McCall CE: Complete deficiency of leukocyte glucose-6-phosphate dehydrogenase with defective bactericidal activity. *J Clin Invest* 51:769–778, 1972.

16. Cunningham-Rundles C: Clinical and immunologic analyses of 103 patients with common variable immunodeficiency. *J Clin Immunol* 9:22–23, 1989.

17. Cunningham-Rundles C, Kazbay K, Hassett J, et al: Brief Report: Enhanced humoral immunity in common variable immunodeficiency after long-term treatment with polyethylene glycol-conjugated interleukin-2. *New Engl J Med* 331:918–921, 1994.

18. Cunningham-Rundles C, Siegal FP, Cunningham-Rundles S, et al: Incidence of cancer in 98 patients with common variable immunodeficiency. *J Clin Immunol* 7:294–299, 1987.

19. Cunningham-Rundles C, Siegal F, Smithwick E, et al: Efficacy of intravenous immunoglobulin in primary human immunodeficiency disease. *Ann Intern Med* 101:435–439, 1984.

20. Cunningham-Rundles C, Zhuo Z, Mankarious S, Courter S: Long-term use of IgA-depleted intravenous immunoglobulin in immunodeficient subjects with anti-IgA antibodies. *J Clin Immunol* 13:272–278, 1993.

21. Derry JMJ, Ochs HD, Francke U: Isolation of a novel gene mutated in Wiskott-Alrich syndrome. *Cell* 78:635–664, 1994.

22. Dinauer MC, Pierce EA, Bruns GAP, et al: Human neutrophil cytochrome *b* light chain (p22-*phox*): Gene structure, chromosomal location, and mutations in cytochrome-negative autosomal recessive chronic granulomatous disease. *J Clin Invest* 86:1729–1737, 1990.

23. Doi S, Saiki O, Hara T, et al: Administration of recombinant IL-2 augments the level of serum IgM in an IL-2 deficient patient. *Eur J Pediatr* 148:630–633, 1989.

24. Ezekowitz RAB, Dinauer MC, Jaffe HS, et al: Partial correction of the phagocyte defect in patients with X-linked chronic granulomatous disease by subcutaneous interferon gamma. *New Engl J Med* 319:146–151, 1988.

25. Fuchs HJ, Borowitz DS, Wohl ME, et al: Effect of aerosolized recombinant human DNase on exacerbations of respiratory symptoms and on pulmonary function in patients with cystic fibrosis. *New Engl J Med* 331:637–642, 1994.

26. Gatti RA, Boder E, Vinters HV, et al: Ataxia-telangiectasia: An interdisciplinary approach to pathogenesis. *Medicine* 70:99–117, 1991.

27. Geha RS, Leung DY: Hyperimmunoglobulinemia E syndrome. *Immunodefic Rev* 1:155–172, 1989.

28. Geha RS, Schereebeyer E, Merler E, et al: Heterogeneity of "acquired" or common variable agammaglobulinemia. *New Engl J Med* 291:1–6, 1974.

29. Griscelli C, Lisowska-Grospierre B, Mach B: Combined immunodeficiency with defective expression in MHC class II genes. *Immunodef Rev* 1:135–153, 1989.

30. Gómez-Carrasco JA, Barrera-Gómez MJ, García-Mouriño V, et al: Selective and partial IgA deficiency in an adolescent male with bronchiectasis. *Allergol Immunopathol (Madr)* 22:261–263, 1994.

31. Hill HR: Clinical disorders of leukocyte functions. *Curr Top Immunol* 14:345–393, 1984.

32. Hill HR, Quie PG, Pabst HF, et al: Defect in neutrophil granulocyte chemotaxis in Job's syndrome of recurrent "cold" staphylococcal abscesses. *Lancet* 2:617–619, 1974.

33. Hirschhorn R: Adenosine deaminase deficiency. *Immunodef Rev* 2:175–198, 1990.

34. Hyodo Y, Itoh R, Kurozumi H, et al: Immunological and metabolic reconstitution following successful bone marrow transplantation from a HLA-identical sibling in an infant with adenosine deaminase deficiency and severe combined immunodeficiency: Partial restoration of purine metabolism. *Adv Exp Med Biol* 253A:543–547, 1989.

35. The International Chronic Granulomatous Disease Cooperative Study Group: A controlled trial of interferon gamma to prevent infection in chronic granulomatous disease. *New Engl J Med* 324:509–516, 1991.

36. Jeppson JD, Jaffe HS, Hill HR: Use of recombinant human interferon gamma to enhance neutrophil chemotactic responses in Job's syndrome of hyperimmunoglobulinemia E and recurrent infections. *J Pediatr* 118:383–387, 1991.

37. Kawano Y, Noma T, Kou K, et al: Regulation of human IgG subclass production by cytokines: Human IgG subclass production enhanced differentially by IL-6. *Immunology* 84:278–284, 1995.

38. Kawano Y, Noma T, Yata J: Regulation of human IgG subclass production by cytokines: Interferon-gamma and IL-6 act antagonistically in the induction of human IgG1, but additively in the induction of IgG2. *J Immunol* 153:4948–4958, 1994.

39. Kodama S, Komatsu K, Okumura Y, Oshimura M: Suppression of X-ray–induced chromosome aberrations in ataxia-telangiectasia cells by introduction of a normal human chromosome 11. *Mutation Res* 293:31–37, 1992.

40. Korthauer U, Graf D, Mages HW, et al: Defective expression of T-cell CD40 ligand causes X-linked immunodeficiency with hyper-IgM. *Nature* 361:539–541, 1993.

41. Levi Y, Hershfield MS, Fernandez-Mejia C, et al: Adenosine deaminase deficiency with late onset of recurrent infections: Response to treatment with polyethylene glycol–modified adenosine deaminase. *J Pediatr* 113:312–317, 1988.

42. Levy-Mozziconacci A, Wernert F, Scambler P, et al: Clinical and molecular study of DiGeorge sequence. *Eur J Pediatr* 153:813–820, 1994.

43. Littlewood JM, Smye SW, Cunliffe H: Aerosol antibiotic treatment in cystic fibrosis. *Arch Dis Child* 68:788–792, 1993.

44. Macher AM, Casale TB, Fauci AS: Chronic granulomatous disease of childhood and *Chromobacterium violaceum* infections in the Southeastern United States. *Ann Intern Med* 97:51–55, 1982.

45. Markert ML: Purine nucleoside phosphorylase deficiency. *Immunodef Rev* 3:45–81, 1991.

46. Mastecky J, Russel MW, Jackson S, et al: The human IgA system: A reassessment. *Clin Immunol Immunopathol* 40:105–114, 1986.

47. Notarangelo LD, Duse M, Ugazio AG: Immunodeficiency with hyper-IgM. *Immunodefic Rev* 3:101–121, 1992.

48. Oxelius VA, Laurell AB, Lindquist B, et al: IgG subclasses in selective IgA deficiency: Importance of IgG2-IgA deficiency. *New Engl J Med* 304:1476–1477, 1981.

49. Puck JM, Nussbaum RL, Smead DL, Conley ME: X-linked severe combined immunodeficiency: Localization within the region Xq13.1-21.1 by linkage and deletion analysis. *Am J Hum Genet* 44:724–730, 1989.

50. Regelmann W, Hays N, Quie PG: Chronic granulomatous disease: Historical perspective and clinical experience at the University of Minnesota Hospitals, in Gallin JI, Fauci AS (eds), *Advances in Host Defense Mechanisms,* vol 3. New York, Raven, 1983, pp 3–23.

51. Rosen FS, Cooper MD, Wedgwood RJP: The primary immunodeficiencies. *N Engl J Med* 311:235–242, 1984.

52. Royer-Pokora B, Kunkel LM, Monaco AP, et al: Cloning the gene for an inherited human disorder—chronic granulomatous disease—on the basis of its chromosomal location. *Nature* 322:32–38, 1986.

53. Saint-Basile G de, Arveiler B, Fraser NJ, et al: Close linkage of hypervariable marker DXS255 to disease locus of Wiskott-Aldrich syndrome. *Lancet* 2:1319–1320, 1989.

54. Savitsky K, Bar-Shira A, Giland S, et al: A single ataxia-telangiectasia gene with a product similar to PI-3 kinase. *Science* 268:1749–1753, 1995.

55. Schaffer FM, Palermos J, Zhu ZB, et al: Individuals with IgA deficiency and common variable immunodeficiency share polymorphisms of major histocompatibility complex class III genes. *Proc Natl Acad Sci USA* 86:8015–8019, 1989.

56. Segal R, Dayan M, Epstein N, et al: Common variable immunodeficiency: A family study and therapeutic trial with cimetidine. *J Allergy Clin Immunol* 84:753–761, 1989.

57. Siegal FP, Siegal MA, Good RA: Role of helper, suppressor and B cell defects in the pathogenesis of the hypogammaglobulinemias. *N Engl J Med* 299:172–178, 1978.

58. Spickett GP, Webster AD, Farrant J: Cellular abnormalities in common variable immunodeficiency. *Immunodefic Rev* 2:199–219, 1990.

59. Steen HJ, Redmond AOB, O'Neill D, Beattie F: Evaluation of the PEP mask in cystic fibrosis. *Acta Paediatr Scand* 80:51–56, 1991.

60. Thompson RA, Kummararatne DS: Hyper-IgE syndrome and H_2-receptor blockade (letter). *Lancet* 2:630, 1989.

61. Vetrie D, Vovechovský I, Sideras P, et al: The gene involved in X-linked agammaglobulinemia is a member of the *src* family protein-tyrosine kinases. *Nature* 361:226–233, 1993.

62. Walmann TA: Immunodeficiency diseases: Primary and acquired, in Samter M, Frank MM (eds), *Immunological Disease,* 4th ed. Boston/Toronto: Little, Brown, 1988, pp 411–465.

63. Wilson JA, Ping AJ, Krauss JC, et al: Correction of CD18-deficient lymphocytes by retroviral-mediated gene therapy. *Science* 248:1413–1416, 1990.

CHAPTER 140

POSTOPERATIVE PNEUMONIA

Ronald Lee Nichols / William D. Hardin, Jr.

Pneumonia remains the single greatest threat to survival that exists in the surgical patient.[6] In this patient population, postoperative pulmonary complications outnumber surgical wound infections, and pneumonia contributes significantly to postoperative mortality.[29] The diagnosis of pneumonia is now made in 5 to 19 percent of surgical patients, and it carries a mortality risk of 40 to 50 percent.[12,26] It is estimated that pneumonia is the proximate cause of death in 30 to 60 percent of surgical patients who succumb, depending on the population studied. In an aging population, with increasingly complicated medical problems and the use of increasingly sophisticated surgical techniques, it is likely that pneumonia will remain a significant problem and require increasing vigilance to control morbidity, mortality, and cost.

As with all infections, the individual risk of developing postoperative pneumonia is based on complex interactions between pathogens, the host, and the environment. The surgical suite is a dangerous environment. Intubation, mechanical ventilation, and the induction of general anesthesia all affect underlying pulmonary physiology, putting the patient at risk for the development of postoperative pneumonia. Host factors include the patient's age, medical condition, nutritional status, smoking history, immune status, and underlying pulmonary health. The pathogens responsible for postoperative pneumonia span the microbial spectrum. Gram-positive and -negative aerobic and anaerobic bacteria have been isolated, while in the immunocompromised patient, opportunistic infections caused by fungi or viruses are also encountered.

The approach to managing pneumonia in the surgical patient has to begin with a preoperative risk assessment and a focus on prevention.[7] The early identification of risk factors can be used to guide surgical care in all phases of the care continuum. Modification of risk factors is an option preoperatively if the planned surgery is elective. It may influence the timing of surgery and is essential for optimizing postoperative care. Pneumonia is insidious in onset, and the diagnosis is made difficult by the requisite delay in culture and sensitivity data. Pneumonia remains a clinical diagnosis based on physical findings and laboratory and radiologic criteria. Treatment of patients with postoperative pneumonia is based on supportive care and antimicrobials. The choice of antibiotics is initially an empiric decision dictated by the clinical situation. Definitive care is determined by the culture results and the initial response to empiric therapy.

PATHOGENESIS

The surgical patient is especially vulnerable to infection in the immediate postoperative period (see Chapter 143). Patients are often debilitated by the effects of the disease process requiring surgical intervention. Intravenous lines, bladder catheters, and endotracheal tubes are but a few of the medical interventions that predispose the patient to nosocomial infection. In traumatic wounds, including surgical wounds, the natural skin barrier is breached, and there is increased risk of invasive infection. In the 1985 study on the efficacy of nosocomial infection control project, conducted by the Centers for Disease Control and Prevention (CDC), it was estimated that more than 2 million nosocomial infections occur in acute-care hospitals in the United States. Urinary tract infections accounted for 42 percent of infections, 24 percent were surgical wound infections, and 10 percent were pneumonia.[18]

Host immunity is compromised in the surgical patient. There is a general down-regulation of the immune system in response to acute injury or the presence of serious disease.[24,25,28] The surgical patients who are at highest risk for compromise of the host immune response are burn and trauma patients. Shortly after injury, the ratio of suppressor to helper T cells is increased and remains so for 1 to 2 weeks after injury.[2] Levels of interleukin 1 (IL-1) increase, and there is increased circulation of immune inhibitory factors such as endotoxin, prostaglandin E, and cutaneous burn toxin.[37] These suppressive factors inhibit the cell-mediated immune response. Increased levels of thromboxane B_2 and prostaglandins E and F further compromise mononuclear cell function and complement production.[21]

The response to tissue injury is a complex process engaging various molecular cascades, feedback systems, and cellular processes that are discussed in detail elsewhere.[33] For simplicity's sake, the response can be viewed in three phases. The first phase is inflammation, produced locally by activation of the coagulation and complement systems. Activated platelets and inflammatory cells release systemic mediators, which further activate lymphocytes, polymorphonuclear cells, and monocytes and initiate a variety of organ-specific inflammatory responses. Migration and proliferation of connective-tissue cells and blood vessels constitute the second phase of the response. Finally, there is the deposition of new connective-tissue matrix. The inflammatory response is a delicate balance between repair and destruction. An excessive host response threatens function in tissues beyond the site of injury. This is believed to be the underlying mechanism of multisystem organ failure (see Chapters 24 and 133).[17]

Postoperative pulmonary complications are the leading cause of morbidity and death in the surgical patient. They are common, often inconsequential, and occasionally persistent, but they may lead to lethal sequelae.[6] Pneumonia is statistically the most significant of these. The pulmonary complications found in the postoperative surgical patient are listed in Table 140-1. Atelectasis, defined as the collapse of alveoli, is the most common postoperative pulmonary complication, occurring in up to 90 percent of patients.[30] Microatelectasis or miliary atelectasis is usually undetectable both clinically and radiologically. It may produce fever on the first postoperative day and is a common postoperative complication. In most instances, the atelectasis resolves within 48 to 72 h of surgery with resumption of ambulation. Atelectasis, which is visible on plain films of the chest, affects more lung and produces more serious lung volume changes. Larger segments of collapsed lung, combined with bacterial contamination from retained secretions, may be the basic underlying pathophysiological mechanism in the start of pneumonia.

While the causative role of atelectasis in the onset of pneumonia is an attractive theory, it has yet to be proved. Other routes of infection are possible, with the bloodstream and lymphatic systems serving as the primary routes for distant spread. Sepsis and pneumonia are often caused by the enteric gram-negative bacteria. These organisms may derive from pharyngeal colonization and aspiration, but bacterial translocation from the intestines may be of greater importance. Sepsis and hypotension are both capable of producing bacterial translocation, mesenteric lymph node infection, and, presumably, bacteremia and bacterial seeding of distant sites.

The organisms responsible for postoperative pneumonia span the microbial spectrum. More than 90 percent of nosocomial pneumonia is bacterial, and in 50 to 70 percent of cases the organisms responsible are gram-negative bacilli.[9] The most important causative gram-negative enteric organisms include *Klebsiella* species, *Escherichia coli*, and *Pseudomonas aeruginosa*. In patients who are being ventilated, *Hemophilus influenzae* and *Serratia* species have also emerged as significant pathogens.[5,13] The mortality in patients with gram-negative pneumonia is 50 percent—unless *P. aeruginosa* is the causative organism, in which case the mortality approaches 80 percent. Gram-positive pneumonia due to *Staphylococcus aureus* or the *Streptococcal* species is responsible for 15 to 30 percent of postoperative pneumonia. Outbreaks of *Streptococcus pneumoniae* infections are common on military installations and in schools. Pneumonia caused by anaerobic bacteria and those that are polymicrobial are among the most difficult to treat.

RISK FACTORS

In terms of expense, morbidity, and mortality, pulmonary complications represent one of the most costly problems that exist in the surgical patient. The identification of risk factors for this problem is important. These factors can be categorized as preoperative, intraoperative, or postoperative and, perhaps more important, as modifiable or not. The cumulative effects of these factors determine the risk of developing a postoperative pulmonary complication. A customized plan that encompasses all phases of the surgical care can then be devised.

Age

Age is frequently cited as an independent risk factor for postoperative pulmonary complications.[35] Starting at age 20, a gradual deterioration occurs in the pulmonary function of all people. The slope of that curve and the time at which pulmonary function becomes a critical issue are determined not just by the chronologic age but more by the physiological age of the lungs. The additive effects of smoking, obesity, and chronic heart disease all affect the quality of pulmonary function. Nonetheless, the effects of aging alone on pulmonary physiology are important to consider. Aging is associated with four basic effects on the lungs: (1) decreased pulmonary elasticity, (2) increased stiffness of the chest wall, (3) decreased motor power, and (4) decreased size of the intervertebral disk space (see Chapter 19).

With age, there appears to be a remodeling of the cross linkages between collagen fibrils and elastin in the pulmonary parenchyma.[31] There is no loss in either the amount of collagen or the tensile strength of the lung. Remodeling explains the loss of elastic recoil and a tendency to increased resting lung volumes at resting transpulmonary pressures. In the absence of other changes, this increased static compliance of the lung would lead

---

TABLE 140-1

Postoperative Pulmonary Complications

Atelectasis
Pneumonitis
Pleural effusion
Pneumonia
Pulmonary edema
Pulmonary emboli
Pneumothorax
ARDS
Multisystem organ failure

to an increased functional residual capacity (FRC). This tendency is counteracted, however, by the increased stiffness of the chest wall, which results from ossification of the costal cartilages and stiffening of the ribs.

Total lung capacity (TLC) decreases approximately 10 percent between the ages of 20 and 70.[16] This loss may be due more to shrinkage of the intervertebral disks and loss in height than to any intrinsic lung factors.[35] The components of TLC, vital capacity (VC) and residual volume (RV), also change with age. Starting at age 20, there is a loss in VC of 20 to 30 ml per year, with a progressive increase in RV of 10 to 20 ml per year. In terms of the ratio between RV and TLC, there is an increase from 25 percent at 20 years of age to 40 percent at 70 years of age. Dynamic lung volumes and capacities also deteriorate with age. Both the forced expiratory flow rate (FEV_1) and the maximal midexpiratory flow rate (FEV_{25-75}) decrease with age. In men the decrease in FEV_1 is estimated at 27 ml per year, whereas in women the deterioration occurs at 22 ml per year. Most of this loss in dynamic lung function is the result of reductions in motor power in the accessory muscles of respiration and to decreased expansion of the stiffer chest wall.

Obesity

The relationship between obesity and medical or surgical complications is well established.[23] Chronic hypertension, congestive heart failure, diabetes mellitus, and renal insufficiency are all more common in the obese. Postoperative pulmonary complications are also more common, with specific increases in the frequency of atelectasis, pulmonary emboli, and pulmonary edema. Obesity also compromises pulmonary physiology. Additional factors in the obese patient are increased duration of surgery, prolonged intubation and mechanical ventilation, and greater immobilization, which pose additional threats to normalization of respiratory function following surgery. The cumulative effect is that the obese patient is at high risk for developing postoperative pulmonary complications. The relationship between obesity and postoperative pneumonia is less well established, although it appears to be a significant risk factor.

The effects of obesity on pulmonary physiology have been studied, and significant changes occur. FRC, VC, and expiratory reserve volume are all decreased in the obese patient.[4] In addition, both lung and chest wall compliance are reduced. Dynamic flow measures such as FEV_1 and FEV_{25-75} are also reduced. Gas exchange is impaired, with increased alveolar dead space and ventilation-perfusion mismatch. In the extreme, these effects may produce hypoxia. The negative effects of obesity on the status of pulmonary health are significant and greatly increase the risks of developing postoperative pulmonary complications.

Smoking History

The deleterious effects of smoking are well established and are now accepted as fact by all but the tobacco companies. The physiological effects of smoking on lung volumes and capacities are significant.[1] There are marked decreases in VC, FEV_1, FEV_{25-75}, and FEV/VC%. Residual volume is increased, as is the ratio of RV/TLC. It has been estimated that the reductions in VC associated with age may be accelerated up to ninefold in smokers,

although not all smokers exhibit this rate of deterioration. Closing volumes increase disproportionately to age, leading to further ventilation-perfusion mismatch. Gas exchange is also impaired. The oxyhemoglobin dissociation curve is shifted to the left, owing to increased levels of carboxyhemoglobin. In addition to the physiological effects of smoking, the clinical effects must be examined. Smokers are at increased risk for tracheobronchitis, increased tracheobronchial secretions, impaired mucociliary clearance, altered bronchial reactivity, and chronic obstructive pulmonary disease. The risk of postoperative pulmonary complications in smokers is estimated at 12 to 100 percent and the threshold of smoking that places the patient at increased risk appears to be clear at 20 pack-years.[34]

While the dangers of smoking are well known and increased attention is directed toward smoking cessation in patients being prepared for elective surgery,[1] the physiological benefits of smoking cessation are less clear. Carboxyhemoglobin levels begin to normalize with as little as 12 h of smoking cessation. The return of the oxyhemoglobin dissociation curve to normal has obvious benefits to gas exchange. Warner and colleagues have demonstrated that the risk of postoperative pulmonary complications is four times higher in smokers and those who have quit smoking for less than 2 months than in those who have quit for more than 2 months. Patients who have not smoked in more than 6 months have postoperative pulmonary complication rates equal to those who have never smoked.

Preexisting Lung Disease

The presence of acute or chronic lung disease is associated with abnormal pulmonary function and an increased frequency of postoperative pulmonary complications. The most significant risk is found in those with chronic obstructive pulmonary disease (COPD). Acute respiratory infections or chronic restrictive disease may also increase the risk of postoperative pulmonary complications, but to a lesser degree than does COPD. COPD is a diagnosis based on pulmonary function testing. Using criteria proposed by Gold (Table 140-2), COPD is stratified into three classifications: severe, mild to moderate, and none.[15] Patients with an FEV_1 that is more than 80 percent of predicted are considered normal and without evidence of obstructive disease. In mild to moderate disease the FEV_1 ranges between 79 and 50 percent of predicted values, while those with FEV_1 less than 50 percent of predicted represent severe cases. In a 1993 study by Kroenke, the effects of COPD on the incidence of postoperative pulmonary complications were established.[20] Serious postoperative pulmonary complications (those that included pneumonia, respiratory failure, and adult respiratory distress syndrome (ARDS)) occurred in 23 percent of patients with severe COPD, 10 percent in those with mild to moderate COPD, and 4 percent of those without COPD. The death rates in the three groups were 19, 4, and 2 percent, respectively, although most of the deaths were attributable to nonrespiratory causes.

Nutritional Status

There is now clear evidence that protein depletion is an independent variable associated with increased risk of postoperative

TABLE 140-2

CDC Criteria for Diagnosis of Adult Pneumonia

Rales or dullness to percussion *plus* any of the following:
New-onset purulent sputum or change in character of sputum
Organism isolated from blood culture
Organism isolated from sputum obtained by:
    Transtracheal aspirate
    Bronchial brushings
    Biopsy
New chest radiograph showing progressive infiltrate,
    consolidation, cavitation, or effusion *plus* any of the
    following:
New-onset purulent sputum or change in character of sputum
Organism isolated from blood culture
Organism isolated from sputum obtained by:
    Transtracheal aspirate
    Bronchial brushings
    Biopsy
Isolation of virus or viral antigen in respiratory secretions
Diagnostic single antibody titer (IgM) or fourfold increase in
    paired serum samples (IgG) for pathogen
Histologic evidence of pneumonia

---

pulmonary complications, in particular postoperative pneumonia. In a study reported by Windsor and Hill, the effects of protein depletion on postoperative pulmonary complications were determined by prospectively following 80 patients who had undergone a preoperative nutritional assessment.[36] In the patients who were adequately nourished, the incidence of postoperative pulmonary complications was 15 percent and there were no deaths. In the protein-depleted group, the incidence of postoperative pulmonary complications was 50 percent and there was a 15 percent mortality. The findings were statistically significant.

There are many reasons why protein depletion is harmful to the host and increases the risk of pulmonary infection postoperatively. Malnutrition results in loss of skeletal and diaphragmatic muscle mass, thereby reducing the strength of the accessory muscles and their contribution to ventilation. Muscle wasting or weakness diminishes the patient's capacity to ambulate and impedes restoration of normal lung volumes after surgery. Maximal minute ventilation is reduced, and the ability to cough is diminished. Protein deprivation also diminishes the quality of the host's immune response.

Emergency Versus Elective Surgery

While most of the studies that have evaluated the risks of postoperative pulmonary complications have focused on the elective patient, Seymour and Vaz compared the risks in patients undergoing emergency versus elective surgical procedures.[32] In their study, the incidence of postoperative pulmonary complications was 46 percent in patients undergoing emergency surgical procedures and 17 percent in patients undergoing elective surgery. The reasons for this are multifactorial, but are probably related most to the underlying health of the patient and the status of the immune system.

Duration of Anesthesia

During the intraoperative period, one of the risk factors cited as placing the patient at increased risk for postoperative pulmonary complications is the duration of anesthesia. In general, the longer the anesthetic and surgical procedure, the higher the incidence of postoperative pulmonary complications.[14] The changes in lung volumes that occur, the inhibitory effects of the anesthetic on normal pulmonary clearance mechanisms, and the physiological changes associated with more complicated surgical procedures are all likely mechanisms that contribute to these findings. The exact time at which increased risk occurs is less clear. Some authors have suggested 3 to 5 hours. It may be that time is related more to the underlying procedure than to any absolute time frame.

Site and Type of Surgery

The risk of postoperative pulmonary complications is related to the surgical site and the type of surgery performed.[19] Thoracic procedures are associated with the highest risk. In general, these patients have the most serious underlying pathophysiological changes, and these are often exacerbated in the postoperative period. Cardiac and pulmonary operations frequently entail the use of chest tubes, prolonged intubation, and mechanical ventilation, and all these factors contribute to the risk of postoperative pulmonary complications.

Upper abdominal operations, particularly those in which a vertical incision is employed, are also associated with increased risk of postoperative pulmonary complications. These incisions are used in a large number of complex abdominal procedures and may be associated with postoperative impairment of diaphragmatic function. Transverse incisions are less painful and do not have the same morbidity as vertical incisions. Lower abdominal incisions or operations performed on extremities present the lowest risk of postoperative pulmonary complications.

While much is made of the site of surgery and the type of incision used, it is likely that the type of surgery performed is also correlated with the risk of postoperative pulmonary complications. Coronary artery bypass grafts, pancreatic procedures, liver resections, and pulmonary resections are associated with higher risks of complication than are other procedures. The important fact is that the more serious the operation, the higher the risk of pulmonary complications, including postoperative pneumonia.

Duration of Mechanical Ventilation

Prolonged intubation is a proven risk factor in the development of postoperative pneumonia. Endotracheal tubes compromise pulmonary clearance mechanisms and are associated with an increased risk of aspiration of oropharyngeal secretions. Aspiration is an important mechanism in pulmonary contamination and is common in the mechanically ventilated patient. Gastric distention, increased gastroesophageal reflux, compromise of the epiglottic protection of the airway, impaired mucociliary function, and an inability to cough all contribute to the aspiration load in the airways.

Also of significance is the bacterial overgrowth that occurs in the stomach of patients receiving stress ulcer prophylaxis. Antacids and H_2 blockers both significantly lower gastric pH, one of the primary host defense mechanisms responsible for controlling bacterial overgrowth in the gastrointestinal tract. In a recent study by Driks and colleagues, bacterial overgrowth was far more common in patients with an increased gastric pH.[10] The use of sucralfate provided equal protection against stress ulceration, without the effect of increasing gastric pH. Bacterial overgrowth was inhibited in the sucralfate-treated group, and—more important to the issue at hand—the incidence of postoperative pneumonia was significantly decreased in the sucralfate-treated group.

Immobilization and Supine Positioning

The critically ill postoperative patient receiving intensive cardiopulmonary and hemodynamic support is more likely to require mechanical ventilation, use of paralytic agents, and prolonged immobilization. Most of these patients are maintained in a supine position. Intraoperatively, the length of surgery and maintenance of a single position for the duration of the procedure contribute to the harmful effects of immobilization.

The physiological effects of immobilization include prolonged impairment of resting and dynamic lung volumes. FRC is increased, while VC and flow rates are decreased. Secretions tend to pool, and the ability to mobilize secretions is impaired. Ventilation-perfusion mismatch leads to impaired oxygenation, and the tachypnea that ensues increases the work of breathing. Gastric distention, splinting, the use of mechanical binders or casts, pain, and excessive narcotic use may exacerbate the pulmonary compromise.

Inappropriate Pain Management

Pain management must be tailored to the individual patient's needs. Both underuse and overuse of narcotic analgesics may have deleterious effects on pulmonary function. With too little pain relief, there is increased splinting, less spontaneous movement, reduced depth of breathing, and a weakened cough; with too much pain relief, the patient may have a reduced level of consciousness, inability to participate in postoperative care, and reduced depth of breathing. The goal of pain management should be blunting of postoperative pain with facilitation of early restoration of ambulatory function.

While the narcotic analgesics still provide optimal pain relief, newer nonnarcotic analgesics and synthetic analgesics do provide pharmacologic options. Early intraoperative loading with nonnarcotic analgesics may facilitate their efficacy in the postoperative period. The injection of long-acting local anesthetics into the surgical incision, regional nerve blocks, epidural catheters and analgesia, caudal anesthetics, and patient-controlled delivery mechanisms all provide therapeutic options to achieve pain relief. The choice of technique employed is an important issue in the postoperative management of the patient and does affect the occurrence of postoperative pulmonary complications.

CLINICAL PRESENTATION AND DIAGNOSIS

Pneumonia is classically viewed as a disease that occurs in two distinct clinical settings. The first and generally less virulent form is community-acquired pneumonia. Patients are frequently healthy and present with the usual nonspecific signs of infection: fever, leukocytosis, and tachycardia. In addition, patients are frequently tachypneic, have increased sputum production, and may have parenchymal lung consolidation on chest radiograph. The most common pathogens responsible for community-acquired pneumonia include *Mycoplasma pneumoniae,* viruses, *S. pneumoniae,* and *Legionella* species (Chapter 127).

In contrast to community-acquired pneumonia, hospital-acquired pneumonia occurs in the intensive care unit, in patients with complicated medical problems in whom the clinical diagnosis is far more difficult to prove (Table 140-2) (see Chapter 143). Postoperative pneumonia is one subset of hospital-acquired pneumonia. In these patients, the causative organisms are quite different from the community-acquired pathogens. Gram-negative bacilli are much more common in the hospital setting. Table 140-3 presents a list of the most common hospital-acquired pathogens responsible for postoperative pneumonia.[30] *P. aeruginosa* is the most common pathogen, and gram negatives are responsible for nearly 60 percent of hospital-acquired cases. The mortality from postoperative pneumonia in patients infected with gram-negative bacilli approaches 50 percent; in patients with *P. aeruginosa* pneumonia, the mortality is 70 to 80 percent.[29]

The early diagnosis of pneumonia in the postoperative patient is based on clinical criteria. These criteria have been formalized by the CDC and are listed in Table 140-2. Presumptive diagnosis is based on the clinical findings of rales or reduced breath sounds in the presence of increased purulent sputum production, culture-proven infection, or consolidation of the lung on plain films of the chest. The interpretation of clinical findings is difficult in the critically ill postoperative patient because confounding variables are present. Yet it is these patients who are at greatest risk and in whom early empiric therapy has the highest potential for improving survival.

The examination and culturing of expectorated sputum represent the time-honored technique for isolating the offending pathogen in cases of pneumonia. Unfortunately, the sensitivity

TABLE 140-3

Pathogenic Bacteria in Postoperative Pneumonia

Pathogen	Frequency
P. aeruginosa	15.1
Klebsiella species	12.8
S. aureus	12.8
Enterobacter species	10.0
E. coli	7.1
S. marcescens	5.6
Proteus	4.4

SOURCE: Adapted from National Nosocomial Infection Study Report and Annual Summary, 1983.[29]

of sputum Gram's stains is only 40 to 60 percent, and reliance on this technique can sometimes be misleading or even harmful to the patient. Criteria have been established to verify the quality of the sputum sample obtained by expectoration. When more than 25 polymorphonuclear neutrophils (PMNs) per high-power field are present and there are fewer than 10 squamous cells per high-power field, the sample is considered to be of acceptable quality.[27] When these criteria are applied, however, less than 25 percent of specimens meet the quality test. The most serious problem in obtaining quality sputum samples for culture and sensitivity is oropharyngeal contamination.

In addition to the problems of specimen contamination, isolation of some bacterial species can be difficult. Fastidious organisms such as *M. pneumoniae, H. influenzae, Neisseria meningitidis,* and the anaerobic species may not be identified on culture. Overgrowth with gram-positive cocci may also confuse the clinician with false positive results.

The limitations imposed by sputum Gram's stain are important because empiric antibiotic therapy is based on these findings. Because of the broad variability in microbial pathogens in postoperative pneumonia, obtaining quality specimens *before* the start of empiric therapy is vitally important. Transtracheal aspiration, bronchoalveolar lavage, protected brush specimens obtained bronchoscopically, or cultures of lung tissue obtained through biopsy improve the culture reliability and sensitivity.

TREATMENT

Supportive Care

Postoperative pulmonary care has become far more sophisticated than the simple "turn, cough, and deep breath" approach that has been practiced for most of the past 100 years.[6] Yet despite this sophistication, the principles embodied by the practice are the foundation for modern pulmonary care. Responsibility for providing that care remains one of the primary functions of the nursing staff, although respiratory therapists are now more likely to be engaged in care as well.[22] The intensive care unit is usually reserved for patients who go into respiratory failure and require mechanical ventilation. Early ambulation, use of incentive spirometers, frequent coughing, and deep-breathing exercises should be aggressively pursued to avoid pulmonary deterioration and the need for mechanical ventilation.

Over the years, many devices and practices have been introduced for the purpose of improving postoperative ventilation. Further study of these devices has frequently led to the discovery of flaws in design, with an absence of physiological benefit. Examples of this include the use of blow bottles, surgical gloves and balloons, and the practice of CO_2 rebreathing. Blow bottles were used to produce positive-pressure expiration, thereby producing an artificial Valsalva maneuver. The rationale for this treatment was the unproven belief that positive-pressure expiration leads to reexpansion of collapsed alveoli. Subsequent studies, however, have shown this not to be true. In the postoperative patient, the most important respiratory maneuver is a sustained maximal inspiration.

Another important practice in the early postoperative period is frequent turning of the patient. The supine position reduces FRC and leads to pooling of endobronchial secretions. Frequent turning leads to faster resolution of postoperative shunting and ventilation-perfusion (V/Q) mismatch. In addition, the mobilization and control of secretions are improved. Turning should begin immediately after surgery and be continued at least through the return to independent ambulation. Timing of turning is dependent on the needs of the patient. In the fresh postoperative patient who has undergone major surgery, turning should be performed at least every 2 h. In a patient who is being mechanically ventilated or when multiple intravenous drips are in use, routine turning is cumbersome and frequently forgotten.

Nearly all surgical patients are encouraged to resume early progressive ambulation in the immediate postoperative period. Ambulation corrects many of the physiological imbalances imposed by surgery and general anesthesia. Ventilation is stimulated, perfusion is increased, airway secretions are more effectively mobilized, and gas exchange is improved. Early ambulation also improves cardiopulmonary function. Venous pooling is discouraged, and deep vein thrombosis and pulmonary emboli less likely. In a study reported by Dull and Dull, the beneficial effects of early ambulation were enhanced little by either the addition of deep-breathing exercises or the use of incentive spirometry.[11]

The importance of deep breathing, in particular, in creating a sustained maximal inspiration is attributed to a 1973 study reported on by Bartlett and colleagues.[3] In that report, the creation of a negative 30- to 50-cm H_2O intrathoracic pressure and a 5- to 15-s pause on maximal inspiration were the standards recommended. This level of effort can be achieved voluntarily with support of the nursing personnel or through the use of a graduated incentive spirometer. The latter device is best used when introduced in the preoperative period and combined with a strong preoperative education session. A baseline is established, and the patient has a goal to achieve in the postoperative period. Use of the incentive spirometer should be encouraged every 1 to 2 h, with 8 to 10 breaths taken in each set of exercises.

Chest physiotherapy and postural drainage are often utilized in high-risk patients or those unable to adequately move or take deep breaths. Patients with chronic bronchitis, smokers, and those with COPD are at increased risk for the production and pooling of mucus in the tracheobronchial tree and in the smaller airways. Despite these efforts, some patients develop postoperative atelectasis that is refractory to routine pulmonary support. In these patients, a short controlled trial with intermittent positive pressure breathing (IPPB) or positive airway pressure in the form of constant positive airway pressure (CPAP) or positive end-expiratory pressure may be of benefit and may obviate reintubation. The use of chest tubes, mechanical ventilation, nasogastric decompression, or whole-body casts further complicates management in the early postoperative period.

Antibiotic Therapy

Because of the high mortality associated with postoperative pneumonia, antibiotic therapy should begin empirically before culture results are available if the clinical criteria for diagnosis are met. The sputum Gram's stain is used to guide the initial choice of antibiotic therapy. An abundance of gram-positive or

-negative organisms in the presence of PMNs is an important finding and can be used to aid in the initial choice of antimicrobial therapy. The choice of antibiotics in patients who have a predominantly gram-positive flora depends on the incidence of methicillin resistance in the hospital. In hospitals in which methicillin resistance is a major problem, vancomycin is the agent of choice for empiric therapy; in hospitals in which methicillin resistance is not a major problem, methicillin, oxacillin, or first- or second-generation cephalosporin antibiotics are good choices for initial therapy.

For patients with an abundance of gram-negative organisms present on Gram's stain, therapy is usually guided by the clinical situation. If the patient is not intubated and on mechanical ventilation, a single-agent third-generation cephalosporin is appropriate.[8] These agents provide good coverage in patients infected with *E. coli, Hemophilus,* or *Klebsiella* species. In the intubated patient, the possibility of infection with *P. aeruginosa* or *Serratia* species warrants broader coverage with combination therapy. While aminoglycosides are limited in their ability to penetrate lung infections, the combination of an aminoglycoside and a β-lactamase inhibitor or semisynthetic penicillin represents effective therapy. Other agents with efficacy are the quinolines, imipenam-cilastin, third-generation cephalosporins, and the β-lactamase inhibitors.

Patients who develop pneumonia following aspiration are frequently infected with gram-positive bacteria or anaerobic organisms. In these patients, clindamycin is a very effective agent and may be considered a first-line drug.[8] Clindamycin may also be of value in patients who are not responding to antimicrobial therapy as expected. In many of these patients, anaerobic bacteria may play a significant role in pathogenesis, but not be isolated on culture.

Antimicrobial therapy in patients with postoperative pneumonia should be guided by culture results and the response to therapy. The use of newer antimicrobial agents that are not associated with nephrotoxicity should be considered. Culture and sensitivity results can be a useful guide to antibiotic selection, but the true test of in vivo sensitivity is the response to therapy. In patients who are not responding to therapy as expected, polymicrobial or resistant infection must be suspected. Sputum should be recultured and Gram stained. The addition of anaerobic coverage or broader gram-negative coverage is warranted in patients who are not responding to antibiotics.

The length of therapy is also guided by the clinical response. In general, antimicrobial therapy should be maintained for a minimum of 5 to 7 days in patients infected with gram-positive organisms. The exception to this rule occurs in patients infected with a methicillin-resistant organism. In these patients, vancomycin should be continued for, in general, at least 3 weeks. In patients infected by one of the gram-negative organisms, antibiotics should be continued for a minimum of 7 to 10 days. If aminoglycosides are necessary as a part of the combination, a 14-day course of treatment seems prudent. It may be preferable, however, to omit aminoglycosides in many surgical patients (hypotension, renal dysfunction), and penetration in the lungs is generally poor. One way to establish the adequacy of the length of antimicrobial therapy is to perform a repeat bronchoscopy, obtain a sputum sample, and reexamine it on Gram's stain. An abundance of PMNs or organisms would suggest that inflammation or infection is still present, and additional antimicrobial therapy, often directed at newly isolated pathogens, may be required.

In recent years, additional therapeutic modalities have emerged and show promise for the future. Selective gut decontamination is yet to be proven efficacious, although the importance of translocation of gastrointestinal flora in the pathogenesis of postoperative pneumonia would seem to make this an appealing option. New specific vaccines against *Pseudomonas* may become available and hold promise in high-risk patients. Finally, a number of immunomodulators, antiendotoxin antibodies, and monoclonal antibodies are undergoing clinical evaluation. While these agents hold great promise in providing additional therapeutic options to reduce the morbidity and mortality associated with postoperative pneumonia, their clinical utility has not yet been established.

REFERENCES

1. Anderson ME: Short-term preoperative smoking abstinence. *Am Fam Physician* 41:1191–1194, 1990.
2. Antonacci AC, Good RA, Gupta S: T-cell populations following thermal injury. *Surg Gynecol Obstet* 155:1–8, 1982.
3. Bartlett RH, Gazzaniga AB, Geraghty TR: Respiratory maneuvers to prevent postoperative pulmonary complications. *JAMA* 224:1017–1021, 1973.
4. Bedell GN, Wilson WR, Seebohm PM: Pulmonary function in obese persons. *J Clin Invest* 37:1049–1060, 1958.
5. Berk SL, Verghese A: Emerging pathogens in nosocomial pneumonia. *Eur J Clin Microbiol Infect Dis* 8:11–14, 1989.
6. Brooks-Brunn JA: Postoperative atelectasis and pneumonia. *Heart Lung* 24:94–115, 1995.
7. Brooks-Brunn JA: Postoperative atelectasis and pneumonia: Risk factors. *Am J Crit Care* 4:340–351, 1995.
8. Clevenger F: Postoperative pneumonia, in Fry DE (ed), *Surgical Infections.* Boston, Little, Brown, 1995, pp 327–337.
9. Craven DE, Barber TW, Steger KA, Montecalvo MA: Nosocomial pneumonia in the 1990s: Update of epidemiology and risk factors. *Semin Respir Infect* 5:157–172, 1990.
10. Driks MR, Craven DE, Celli BR, et al: Nosocomial pneumonia in intubated patients given sucralfate as compared with antacids or histamine type 2 blockers. *New Engl J Med* 317:1376–1382, 1987.
11. Dull JL, Dull WL: Are maximal inspiratory breathing exercises or incentive spirometry better than early mobilization after cardiopulmonary bypass? *Phys Ther* 63:655–659, 1983.
12. Ephgrave KS, Kleiman-Wexler R, Pfaller M, et al: Postoperative pneumonia: A prospective study of risk factors and morbidity. *Surgery* 114:815–821, 1993.
13. Fry DE, Fry RV, Shlaes DM: Serratial bacteremia in the surgical patient. *Am Surg* 53:438–441, 1987.
14. Garibaldi RA, Coleman ML, Reading JC, Pace NL: Risk factors for postoperative pneumonia. *Am J Med* 70:677–680, 1981.
15. Gold WM: Pulmonary function testing, in Murray JF, Nadel JA (ed), *Textbook of Respiratory Medicine.* Philadelphia, WB Saunders. 1993, chap 28, pp 798–900.
16. Goldman HI, Becklake MR: Respiratory function tests: Normal values at median altitudes and the prediction of normal results. *Am Rev Tuberc Pulmon Dis* 79:457–467, 1959.
17. Goris RJA, Boekhorst TP, Nuytinck JK, Gimbrere JK: Multiple-organ failure: Generalized autodestructive inflammation? *Arch Surg* 120:1109–1115, 1985.

18. Haley RW, Culver DH, White JW, et al: The nationwide nosocomial infection rate: A new need for vital statistics. *Am J Epidemiol* 121:159–167, 1985.

19. Hall JC, Hall JL, Mander J: A multivariate analysis of the risk of pulmonary complications after laparotomy. *Chest* 99:923–927, 1991.

20. Kroenke K: Postoperative complications after thoracic and major abdominal surgery in patients with and without obstructive lung disease. *Chest* 104:1445–1451, 1993.

21. Lappin DF, Whaley K: Prostaglandins and prostaglandin synthetase inhibitors regulate the synthesis of complement components by human monocytes. *Clin Exp Immunol* 49:623–630, 1982.

22. Lennon BB: Nursing care of surgical patients: Before and after anesthesia. *Am J Nurs* 41:534–537, 1941.

23. Luce JM: Respiratory complications of obesity. *Chest* 78:626–631, 1980.

24. MacLean LD, Meakins JL, Taguchi K, et al: Host resistance in sepsis and trauma. *Ann Surg* 182:207–217, 1975.

25. Marshall J, Sweeney D: Microbial infection and the septic response in critical surgical illness. *Arch Surg* 125:17–23, 1990.

26. Martin LF, Asher EF, Casey JM, Fry DE: Postoperative pneumonia. *Arch Surg* 119:379–383, 1984.

27. Martin RS, Sumarah RK, Robart EM: Assessment of expectorated sputum for bacteriological analysis based on polymorphs and squamous epithelial cells. *J Clin Microbiol* 8:635–637, 1978.

28. Meakins JL: Clinical importance of host resistance to infection in surgical patients. *Adv Surg* 15:225–229, 1981.

29. National Nosocomial Infection Study Report and Annual Summary, 1983. *MMWR* 33:1SS, 1985.

30. Peper EA: Respiratory complications of surgery and thoracic trauma, in George R et al (eds), *Chest Medicine: Essentials of Pulmonary and Critical Care.* Baltimore, Williams & Wilkins, 1990, pp 453–473.

31. Pierce JA: Tensile strength of the human lung. *J Clin Invest* 66:652–658, 1965.

32. Seymour DG, Vaz FG: A prospective study of elderly general surgical patients: II. Postoperative complications. *Age Ageing* 18:316–326, 1989.

33. Tchervenkov JI, Meakins JL: Altered host defense mechanisms in septic patients, in Fry DE (ed), *Surgical Infections.* New York, Little, Brown, 1995, pp 19–41.

34. Tobin MJ: Short-term effects of smoking cessation. *Respir Care* 29:641–651, 1984.

35. Wahba WM: Influence of aging on lung function—Clinical significance of changes from age twenty. *Anesth Analg* 62:764–776, 1983.

36. Windsor JA, Hill GL: Risk factors for postoperative pneumonia: The importance of protein depletion. *Ann Surg* 208:209–214, 1988.

37. Wood JJ, Rodrick ML, O'Mahony JB, et al: Inadequate interleukin 2 production: A fundamental immunological deficiency in patients with major burns. *Ann Surg* 200:311–320, 1984.

CHAPTER 141

RESPIRATORY INFECTIONS IN THE ECONOMICALLY DISADVANTAGED

Edward A. Nardell / David Kent

That the poor are sicker than the rich is perhaps the most consistent observation in the public health literature. This holds true for every society studied—capitalist, communist, or socialist—in eras as far back as the twelfth century, no matter what measure of social status is employed (income, education, or occupation), and for virtually every disease examined. Traditional accounts of disease pathogenesis fail to incorporate the complex interactions between host, society, and environment that contribute to profound health disparities among diverse populations. The dramatic decline in mortality due to tuberculosis before the introduction of effective pharmacotherapy is cited as an example of the relative importance of social determinants of health (Fig. 141-1). It has been estimated that chemotherapy accounts for only 3 percent of this decline.[44] Similar trends have been noted for other infectious diseases, such as diphtheria, pertussis, scarlet fever, rheumatic fever, and measles.[37] René Dubos considered tuberculosis "a social disease, with some important medical aspects."

All respiratory infections are diseases not just of individuals but of communities. The risk of becoming sick depends not only on the virulence of organisms and the resistance of individuals but also on the transmission dynamics of the infection in the community. Transmission dynamics are determined by a number of factors, including the prevalence of the infectious cases, the size, growth, or decline of the population, the general and specific resistance of the population to infection and disease, exposure conditions, the effectiveness of preventive measures, and access to and compliance with effective medical therapy for those who fall ill. Complex interactions of these and other parameters determine the propagation cycle of infectious diseases. Such cycles create threshold phenomena, whereby small changes in one or more of the determining parameters can have dramatic long-term effects on disease prevalence, for better or worse. Poverty potentially influences several parameters, thereby having profound consequences on the health of individuals and of communities.

Tuberculosis, again, is an apt example. Under endemic conditions, most people exposed to tuberculosis do not become infected, and most infected do not develop active communicable disease. The average number of secondary infectious cases that are produced from an infectious individual is termed the *effective reproductive rate* (R). In order for tuberculosis to remain endemic in a community, each person with active disease must, on average, infect enough people so that at least one other person eventually develops active disease and becomes infectious (i.e., R must be greater than 1).

Two extreme patterns of propagation occur simultaneously in different areas of the country and within a given area in different subpopulations (Fig. 141-2).[47] In most American communities, tuberculosis is an uncommon disease, the diagnosis of new cases is not long delayed, cure is nearly certain with appropriate therapy, and most of the relatively few infected contacts can be identified and placed on preventive therapy. Under these circumstances, R is less than 1 and the disease has been declining steadily, albeit slowly, over the past century. In subpopulations including the inner-city poor, the homeless, and recent immigrants from high-prevalence countries, an R of much greater than 1 is due to crowding, impaired immunity, and delays in diagno-

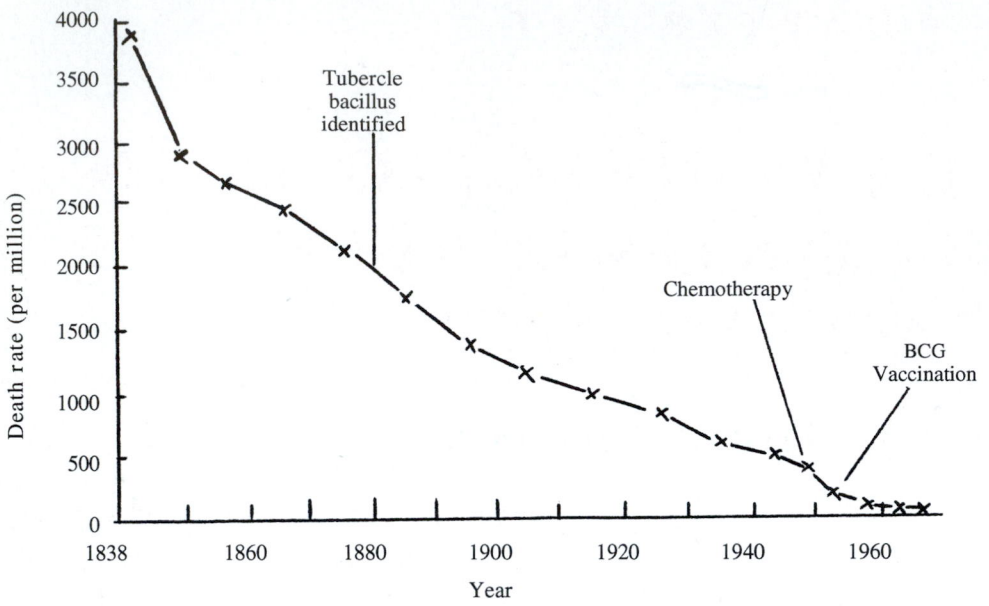

FIGURE 141-1   Respiratory tuberculosis: Mean annual death rates (standardized to 1901 population) in England and Wales. *(From McKeown,[44] with permission.)*

determinants into three broad categories: (1) exposure to respiratory pathogens, (2) immunity of individuals to respiratory pathogens, and (3) access and compliance to efficacious medical treatment. Respiratory infections in selected groups of the disadvantaged—refugees and immigrants, prisoners, and the homeless—will be considered with reference to public health issues, as well as clinical issues relevant for physicians who treat these populations.

EXPOSURE

From the perspective of the respiratory pathogen, successful propagation in the absence of a suitable animal reservoir depends on encountering and infecting a series of susceptible human hosts. The task of the pathogen is made easier when humans live and work in close proximity to one another. Thus, in the early part of this century, crowded living and working conditions among immigrants in the garment district of New York City facilitated transmission of tuberculosis, just as crowded shelters and prisons have facilitated transmission among homeless persons in recent years.

Such concepts have been formalized. The cornerstones of mathematical epidemiology are the mass action principle and the threshold theory. According to the mass action principle, the rate of spread, or force of infection, is proportional to the density of infectious individuals and the density of susceptible individuals. The threshold theory adds that the introduction of a few infectious individuals into a population of susceptible individuals will not give rise to an epidemic unless the density of susceptible individuals exceeds a certain critical value. The importance of these principles can be demonstrated when one examines the effects of family size or population density on infectious disease. The incidence of rheumatic heart disease, for example, was found to be linearly related to the number of people per bedroom (Fig. 141-3),[37] and Black demonstrated earlier serologic conversion for measles in children from large families,[6] just as median age of measles infection has been demonstrated to be much lower in African urban areas than in rural areas.[59] Such mathematical modeling indicates that a higher rate of vaccination is needed to attain herd immunity in densely populated areas than that needed in sparsely populated areas. Spatial inhomogeneity within areas, such as cities with prisons, will make disease eradication more difficult.

Whether in shelters, tenements, welfare offices, buses, or prisons, the poor are more likely to spend time in close quarters with one another than are people of means. This is not an absolute distinction between rich and poor, however, as airliners and cruise ships have also been associated with outbreaks of respiratory pathogens. Whatever the congregate setting, however, the probability that an infectious source is present and of the vulnerability of those exposed are generally

sis and effective treatment. These circumstances have contributed to the resurgence of tuberculosis and to the increase in multidrug-resistant strains.

The introduction of HIV infection into a population acts as a catalyst for the spread of tuberculosis, so that *accelerated epidemic propagation* is observed. Whereas typically 90 percent of active cases in the United States had been thought to arise from the reactivation of foci of infection acquired years or decades earlier, recent transmission now plays an important role in spread.

The rest of this chapter expands on the model of tuberculosis to discuss the determinants of accelerated propagation of respiratory infections among the impoverished, dividing those

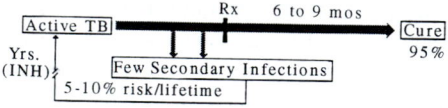

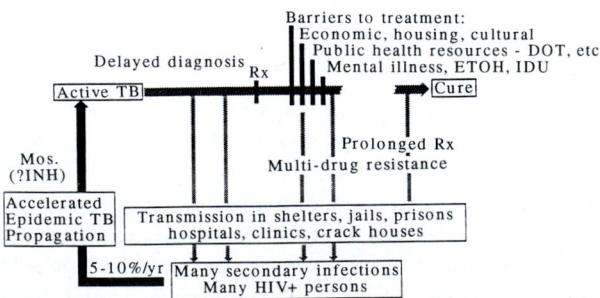

FIGURE 141-2   The tuberculosis propagation cycle. *Top panel:* Tuberculosis propagation under ideal conditions. *Bottom panel:* Tuberculosis propagation cycle under conditions associated with the current resurgence, and with the emergence and transmission of multidrug-resistant organisms. *(From Nardell,[47] with permission.)*

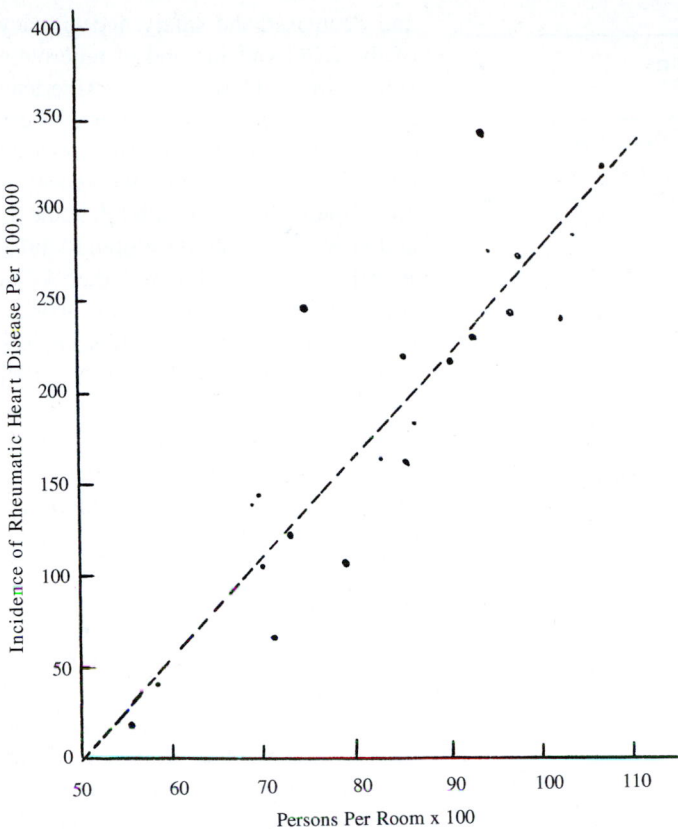

FIGURE 141-3   The correlation between the incidence of rheumatic heart disease per 100,000 and the number of persons per room (×100) in various districts of Bristol, England, in 1927–30. (The size of the dots indicates roughly the comparative population size of the districts.) *(From Kass,[36] with permission.)*

higher among the poor. Thus, an outbreak of pneumococcal pneumonia, usually viewed as a sporadic illness, was reported in a Boston shelter that was also the site of ongoing tuberculosis transmission.[18]

While persons with respiratory infections are rarely officially quarantined, a consequence of the social barriers between economic classes is a "social quarantine" that may effectively limit transmission to certain high-risk groups, such as the poor. Although shelter workers, hospital staff, and prison staff are regularly exposed to persons with tuberculosis in congregate settings, and transmission has occurred, outbreaks of drug-resistant tuberculosis that have occurred in these settings appear not to have spread to the general population to any large extent. The effect of social quarantine has been demonstrated. In the United States, the prevalence of tuberculosis in a given zip-code area correlates with the degree of poverty in that district (Fig. 141-4). The concept of social quarantine can be extended to a more global level: in de-

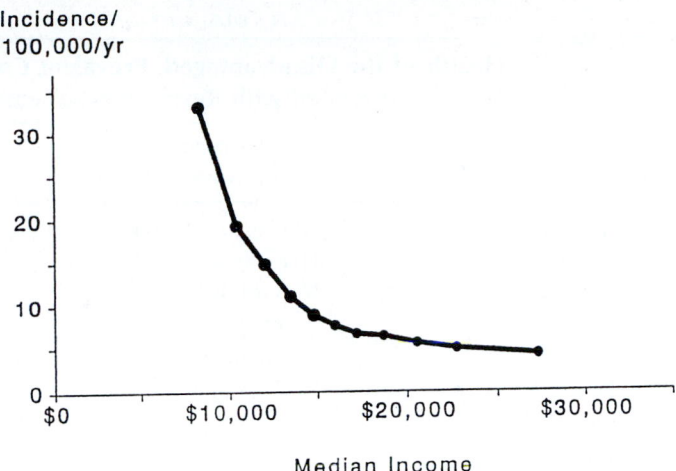

FIGURE 141-4   Tuberculosis incidence by income in each zip code area of residence. *(Courtesy of the Centers for Disease Control and Prevention.)*

veloping countries, tuberculosis accounts for 7 percent of all deaths and 19 percent of deaths among adults 19 to 59 years of age.[42]

INDIVIDUAL IMMUNITY

Many conditions associated with poverty impair pulmonary defenses. Table 141-1 provides a brief summary of the mechanisms by which the poor become more vulnerable to infection. Table 141-2 reviews some data on the prevalence of such predisposing conditions among disadvantaged populations. Notably absent from this chart is alcoholism, which is equally prevalent among social classes in the United States. However, Schmidt and De Lint[53] found that alcoholics from lower social classes have a far higher mortality as a result of their drinking. Clearly, it is only by considering the interactions between risk factors, both social and physiological, that we can begin to account for the magnitude of the observed differences in health between the rich and poor.

TABLE 141-1

Impairments of Pulmonary Defenses Under Conditions of Poverty

	Mechanical	Phagocytic	T Cell	B Cell	Nonspecific
Cigarette use	+	+	+	+	+
Protein energy malnutrition	+	+	+	+/−	+
Micronutrient deficiencies					
Vitamin A	+	−	−	−	−
Vitamin D	−	+	+	−	−
Iron	+	−	+	−	−
Zinc	+	−	+	−	−
Copper	−	−	−	+	−
Alcoholism	+	+	+	+	+
AIDS	+	+	+	+	+
Stress	−	+	+	+	+
Pollutants	+	+	+	+	+
Coinfection	+	+	+	+	+

SOURCE: Adapted from Bor and Epstein.[7]

TABLE 141-2

Health of the Disadvantaged: Prevalent Conditions Associated with Respiratory Disease

Health Condition	Prevalence in Disadvantaged (%)		Prevalence in General Population (%)
Cigarette smoking	Blacks	34	29
	Hispanics	33	
	Non–high school graduates	34	
Secondary exposure to cigarettes (children <6 years)	Low income	66	36
Asthma hospitalization	Blacks	0.334	0.188
Breast-feeding			
Early postpartum	Low income	32	54
At 5–6 months	Low income	9	21
Iron deficiency			
Children 1–2 years	Low income	21	9
Childbearing women	Low income	8	5
Obesity			
Women >20 years	Low income	37	26
Diabetes			
Prevalence	Blacks	3.6	2.8
Deaths	Blacks	65	30
Low birthweight (1987)	Blacks	12.7	7
Smokers	Low income	9.9	6.5
Oral health			
Gingivitis	Low income	50	42
AIDS incidence in 1989	Hispanics	40.3	17.7
(cases per 100,000)	Blacks	48.9	

SOURCE: From Bor and Epstein,[7] with permission.

HIV Infection

HIV is more prevalent among economically disadvantaged persons and among economically disadvantaged nations. Risk can be defined individually (e.g., among male homosexuals, intravenous drug users and their sexual consorts, commercial sex workers), as well as collectively. A theoretical index of collective vulnerability can be used to assess communal and national risk of the HIV epidemic, based on measures such as level of education, health expenditures, and access to health care. In the United States and Europe, areas of low collective vulnerability, individual risk factors are most important to vulnerability; a growing proportion of cases are being seen among IV drug users. In impoverished sub-Saharan Africa and Southeast Asia, where heterosexual sex remains the dominant mode of transmission, factors affecting collective vulnerability are of greatest importance.

The impact of HIV coinfection on the propagation cycle of tuberculosis is discussed above. HIV has increased the effective "infectiousness" of tuberculosis and increased the morbidity and mortality associated with infection, played an important role in the emergence of multidrug-resistant tuberculosis (MDR-TB),

and decreased the safety and efficacy of the BCG vaccine and of tuberculin skin testing. Outbreaks in American prisons and homeless shelters, where coinfection is not a rarity, are discussed below. However, roughly 95 percent of all people coinfected with tuberculosis and HIV live in the developing world. As HIV rises in India and other Asian countries, where poverty and tuberculosis have long been established, the morbidity of tuberculosis and AIDS will soon surpass that of Africa. As in Africa, there are few prospects for effective intervention in Asia with currently available resources, technology, and political will.

Alcoholism

The association between alcoholism and respiratory infections is well grounded in clinical experience, and yet, because alcoholism is so typically associated with other risk factors for pneumonia—malnutrition, COPD, liver disease, pancreatitis, depressed consciousness, frequent emesis, periodontal disease, and other hygienic and lifestyle factors—distinguishing the direct effects of alcohol per se may be quite difficult. Further, alcohol can cause immune dysfunction through various mechanisms not only in the setting of chronic abuse but also acutely— as seen, for example, in the demonstrated depression of serum bactericidal activity of normal subjects after ethanol infusion.[35] In their review, Bor and Epstein[7] emphasized abnormalities of suppressor T cells, which increase in proportion, leading to faulty control of antibody production, increased immunoglobulin levels, and autoantibodies.

Among infections, the combination of defense impairments seen in the alcoholic creates a particular vulnerability to those of the respiratory tract. Alcohol has been shown to increase the frequency, alter the etiology, worsen the severity, and increase the mortality of pneumonia.[23,48] In a series of hospital admissions studied by Nolan,[48] 17 percent of alcoholics had an admission diagnosis of pneumonia, compared to 6.5 percent of nonalcoholic patients admitted. Moreover, the course of their pneumonia was affected by their alcoholism; in 60 percent of patients, there was a significant delay in seeking medical attention, and in 60 percent, their alcohol dependence interfered with their management in hospital. This experience is reinforced by other studies. In an autopsy series of 37 fatal cases of lobar pneumonia reported by Chomet and Gach,[15] fully 30 persons were found to have been alcoholic (22 of whom died within 1 day of presentation), leading the author to suggest delay in presentation as a significant cause of increased mortality. In a recent study comparing alcoholic patients with pneumonia to nonalcoholic patients,[23] investigators found that alcoholic patients presented with worse symptoms (more dyspnea, chest pain, and purulent sputum) and more frequent multilobar involvement. The patients tended to have longer fevers, required longer hospital stays and longer IV antibiotic treatment, and had lingering pulmonary infiltrates. They also found that patients admitted to the hospital with pneumonia were about twice as likely to be alcoholic as those admitted with other medical diagnoses.

In treating patients with pneumonia, it is important to have a high clinical suspicion for underlying alcoholism. Prophylaxis of withdrawal and aggressive treatment of early withdrawal not only help prevent dangerous complications but also are necessary to ensure compliance with inpatient therapy. Alcoholic patients who progress to delirium tremens frequently require intubation not for their pneumonia but for adequate treatment of their withdrawal.

Although, as in the general population, pneumococcal pneumonia is the most common type in alcoholics, there is a well-recognized association between anaerobic infections and alcohol abuse, due to the high incidence of significant gingivodental disease among alcoholics and their proclivity for aspiration. Whereas normal subjects will aspirate radioactive tracer from the pharynx while asleep, the amount aspirated dramatically increases in a drunken stupor, in turn increasing the likelihood that infection will result.[33] Aspiration of anaerobic material leads to a number of clinical syndromes, including anaerobic pneumonia, necrotizing pneumonitis, empyema, and lung abscess. Organisms frequently isolated include *Fusobacterium, Bacteroides,* and anaerobic cocci.

The susceptibility to gram-negative infections is also believed to be especially high in alcoholics. The oropharynx of alcoholics is commonly colonized with gram-negative organisms—particularly from the *Klebsiella-Enterobacter* group. In one study, gram-negative organisms were isolated from 59 percent of alcoholics, as compared to only 14 percent of controls.[26] Traditionally, the unique predisposition to *Klebsiella* pneumonia, with its characteristic tenacious bloody sputum, has been emphasized. However, a review of cases from Pittsburgh demonstrated that alcohol had been a predisposing factor in only a third of the cases of *Klebsiella* pneumonia.[21]

Alcoholism has been shown to be a major risk factor for tuberculosis; estimates of relative risk in alcoholics compared to that in the general population vary greatly, in some studies exceeding 50.[1] Although studies generally do not control for associated risk factors, an attempt to do so could not account for a large proportion of the observed difference.[39] Aside from increasing prevalence, alcoholism complicates the prolonged therapy. Many studies have demonstrated high rates of incomplete or erratic treatment. However, a study that followed alcoholics after ensuring 18 months of treatment found no increase in the relapse rate, suggesting that alcohol per se does not alter the prognosis of treated tuberculosis.[30]

Malnutrition

Malnutrition impairs both thoracopulmonary function and immune defenses to respiratory infections. When severe, it can compromise respiratory muscle function, decrease ventilatory drive, and alter pulmonary immune defense mechanisms. This may render the malnourished more vulnerable to respiratory infections and alter the course of the disease, typically making the presentation more subtle and the course more prolonged, more severe, and more often fatal.

The particular sensitivity of cell-mediated immunity has been emphasized by some authors.[7] In severely malnourished patients, thymus and peripheral T-cell lymphoid tissue atrophy is observed, T-cell differentiation and maturation cease, and CD4 counts are especially depressed. The vulnerablility of cell-mediated immunity was evidenced interestingly by Martin's anecdotal review[41] of the Warsaw ghetto experience during 1942, noting reports of diminished response to tuberculin skin testing with worsening malnutrition, increased severity of tuberculosis in malnourished children, and, ironically, the spontaneous abatement of allergic phenomena such as asthma and urticaria. These changes in cellular immunity, when severe, can mimic AIDS, as exemplified by epidemics of *Pneumocystis carinii* pneumonia (PCP) in European orphanages during and after World War II and, since then, in orphanages in the Middle East.

Malnourished states increase susceptibility to microbial colonization, invasion, and infections, which, in turn, worsen malnutrition by increasing metabolic demands for calories, proteins, and micronutrients, even as nutritional supplies diminish, secondary to concomitant anorexia, malabsorption, and diarrhea. Recovery depends not only on treatment of infection but also on nutritional support well in excess of baseline needs.

The effect of malnutrition on the frequency and course of respiratory infections has been well documented. More than 12 million children in developing nations die annually, most with malnutrition, a third from pneumonia. In a study of hospitalized children with severe malnutrition in Bangladesh, Brown and colleagues[9] found 50 percent of these children to have pneumonia and noted that mortality was higher in the malnourished than nonmalnourished patients. Similarly, Tupasi and coworkers,[57] studying children hospitalized with pneumonia in Manila, found a proportionate relationship between nutritional status and mortality. Similar results were noted by Kielman's team[38] in a prospective nutritional supplementation study of Punjabi children, in whom mortality doubled with each 10 percent decline below 80 percent of weight for age. Further, the benefit of supplementation was shown, with villages receiving nutritional supplementation having only half the mortality of control villages.

Apart from protein-calorie malnutrition, deficiencies of certain vitamins and micronutrients may impair host defenses against respiratory infections. Vitamin A deficiency has been shown to be related to mortality among persons with respiratory infections, and supplementation of vitamin A has been demonstrated to decrease respiratory complications and mortality in African children hospitalized with measles.[32] This effect is thought to be mediated through vitamin A's effect on epithelial integrity and repair, although other mechanisms have been postulated.

Deficiency of vitamin D, which activates macrophages and increases the synthesis of interleukin-1 and tumor necrosis factor, has been associated epidemiologically and in vitro with impaired host responses to tuberculosis.[52] Before chemotherapy, the beneficial effects attributed to sunlight exposure among sanitarium patients may have been mediated by vitamin D metabolism. And Davies[17] has implicated diminished levels of vitamin D in the high incidence of tuberculosis in Asian immigrants who went to cloudy Great Britain from their sunny lands.

Among the micronutrients, iron, zinc, and copper have an important role in healthy immunologic functioning. The role of deficiency in infectious states and the role of supplementation in such states remain to be fully elucidated.

Tobacco

As the antismoking campaigns have begun to cause a dramatic decline in smoking in the United States, particularly among educated consumers, marketing strategies have shifted to more vulnerable markets. In the United States, the single greatest determinant of tobacco use is level of education. Worldwide, tobacco consumption remains on the rise. Cigarettes often become a principal currency in prison, among the homeless, and during wartime. For example, the standard monthly salary of a municipal worker in Sarajevo during the recent war was two cartons of cigarettes.

Cigarette smoking alters defenses against respiratory infections. As respiratory tract impairment increases, so does the probability that a respiratory infection will be caused by a more virulent organism, such as *H. influenzae, S. pneumoniae,* or *M. catarrhalis.* Patients with advanced chronic bronchitis and obstructive airway disease are, of course, at the highest risk. In these conditions, the normally sterile airways are colonized by bacteria, and during exacerbations the profile of colonizing bacteria shifts to more virulent organisms, particularly *H. influenzae.*

The degree to which tobacco consumption impairs defenses of otherwise healthy young smokers remains controversial. Studies on the frequency and severity of acute respiratory infections in this population have yielded mixed results. Generally, acute bronchitis in healthy young smokers tends to be viral or mycoplasmal, and the treatment and course do not differ dramatically from those of nonsmokers. In the Centers for Disease Control Tuberculosis Trial 21, a field trial of 9 months of chemotherapy, smokers had a poorer outcome than nonsmokers, independent of other variables. Obstructive lung disease also predisposes to infection with environmental lung disease and chronic histoplasmosis.[40a]

Stress

The nervous and immune systems are richly interconnected. The stress response, in general, is accompanied by suppression of immune function, mediated both through the autonomic nervous system (via connections to primary and secondary lymphoid tissue) and through the effects of stress hormones, principally cortisol. The clinical significance of this interaction remains controversial. In controlled studies, greater severity of symptoms has been observed both in worried students challenged with infected nasal secretions[34] and in healthy volunteers with recent life stresses challenged with rhinovirus. Other studies have shown grieving persons to have more frequent pneumonias[51] and divorced persons to have increased mortality from pneumonia and tuberculosis.[55] The degree to which the economically disadvantaged carry a larger burden of psychologic stress is difficult to assess. In a series of studies, Dohrenwend[19a] found that lower-income respondents were exposed to more stressful life events, and these events were more frequently beyond their control, than higher-income respondents. In a Canadian community sample,[45] the prevalence of major depression was 1.9 percent, 4.5 percent, and 12.4 percent in high, average and low socioeconomic groups, respectively.

Incomplete Vaccination

In developing countries, vaccine-preventable diseases remain an important cause of morbidity and mortality. Measles, for example, causes an estimated 2 million deaths annually, many from pneumonitis with or without secondary bacterial pneumonia. In more developed countries, it is again the poor who are vulnerable to these diseases. In Glasgow, for example, it has been found that hospitalization rates for pertussis and measles correlate with degree of deprivation.[40] In the United States, disadvantaged preschool children often have low rates of vaccination; data indicate that only 11 percent of the 2-year-olds in Houston were fully immunized. For comparison, WHO data indicate that more than 50 percent of children in developing countries have received a primary series of DPT immunizations by their first birthday.[63] Adult vaccines are still more neglected. Less than 30 percent of persons at risk for pneumococcus have received the vaccine, with lowest coverage in blacks, Hispanics, and persons living below the poverty level.[14] Outbreaks have been reported in nursing homes and homeless shelters. Influenza causes approximately 20,000 deaths annually in the United States, with vaccination of the highly susceptible elderly, poor minorities being inadequate.[14]

Environmental Factors

Around the world, the most socioeconomically disadvantaged segments of populations often live in the most polluted areas of cities and work at the most hazardous of jobs. Exposure to air pollution, both outdoors and indoors, in the workplace and at home, has been associated with a wide variety of lung disorders, some of which may predispose to respiratory infections.[5]

Notorious examples of low-level laborers suffering from job-associated lung injury have included immigrant coalminers in Pennsylvania, young women recovering beryllium from fluorescent bulbs in Massachusetts, cotton workers in the South, silo-fillers in the Plains states, and asbestos workers worldwide. Although respiratory infections may complicate many environmental and occupational lung injuries, such as silicotuberculosis among hard-coal workers, they are usually not directly related. Specific occupational lung diseases are discussed elsewhere in this text.

Whereas hazardous occupational exposures are usually job associated, affecting primarily those directly engaged in specific activities, outdoor air pollutants have the potential to adversely affect the health of broader segments of the population.

HEALTH CARE: ACCESS AND COMPLIANCE

Public policy debate on socioeconomic disparities in health tends to focus on access to medical care, with much attention paid to the 40 million uninsured and the need for universal health insurance as a remedy. Some have argued, however, that universal insurance would do little to change the socioeconomic gradient in health, citing as evidence countries with both universal insurance and similar disparities.[2] It is well established that persons lacking insurance have reduced access to care, particularly primary and preventive care, and more often delay or forgo treatment for serious medical symptoms.[29,62] The short- and long-term consequences of this have been demonstrated: the uninsured are more likely to have potentially avoidable hospitalizations, be sicker at the time of admission, and have a higher inhospital mortality.[60,61,63] Once in hospital, they are less likely to receive invasive procedures and are at greater risk of suffering a medical injury due to substandard care.[12,60]

A prospective study of close to 5000 patients followed for more than 20 years found that uninsured patients had virtually twice the mortality during that period (18.4 percent versus 9.6 percent).[24] Moreover, a difference persisted—with a hazard ratio of 1.25 for those lacking insurance—when the analysis was adjusted for sex, race, baseline age, education, income, employment status, the presence of morbidity on examination, self-reported health, smoking status, leisure, exercise, alcohol consumption, and obesity. The ill effects of being uninsured were seen in all socioeconomic groups.

Type of insurance also plays a role in services rendered and clinical outcomes. For example, among critically ill patients with PCP, patients with Medicaid are less likely to receive diagnostic bronchoscopy, more likely to be treated empirically, and more likely to die in hospital than privately insured patients.[28] Further, with adjustment for confirmation of PCP, Medicaid patients no longer had a significantly higher inhospital mortality, leading the study's author to infer a causal relationship between the limited access to invasive diagnostic procedures and increased mortality.

From the above discussion, it is clear that access is not a simple, binary variable. Also confounding discussions of access is the degree to which the concept overlaps that of compliance. For the insured, for example, requiring a copayment has been shown to have clinically important adverse outcomes.[8] Another example of the blurred borders between access and compliance has been discussed in the previous section: vaccines may be freely available, but not obtained because of inadequate public health programs. Similarly, in the treatment of tuberculosis, issues traditionally understood as patient compliance problems might be more usefully understood as system problems or failures of access to appropriate case management.

A series of clinical trials of shorter tuberculosis treatments has culminated in regimens of 6 months' duration for smear-positive disease caused by drug-susceptible organisms. Still, even when care is provided free, completion of this shortened course of therapy has proved difficult for some patients. Barriers to care may be cultural, economic, social, legal, or psychiatric. Although obvious to those with experience in working with the very poor, it is often unappreciated by others that some are so impoverished that they lack the means to tend to their medical needs, even when medication and visits are provided at no charge.

In Brudney and Dobkin's study of tuberculosis cases admitted to Harlem Hospital in 1988,[11] 89 percent of 178 patients discharged on antituberculous therapy failed to complete the therapy. Within 12 months of discharge, 48 of 178 patients (27 percent) were readmitted with confirmed active tuberculosis at least once, and nearly all of them were again lost to discharge. In another provocative article,[10] they contrasted this abysmal failure to the relative success of the tuberculosis control program in impoverished, war-torn Nicaragua, which achieved a better than 75 percent cure rate in Managua. Important aspects of the program, lacking in New York, include concentrating resources on active cases and not on prophylactic therapy, on-site microscopy for rapid diagnosis, a proactive educational campaign, and a combination of directly observed therapy and close supervision with aggressive outreach programs.

Farmer and colleagues[22] reported data comparing tuberculosis treatment programs in two sectors in a community-based research project in rural Haiti. Sector one received free medication, financial aid, incentives to attend a monthly clinic, and aggressive home follow-up. Sector two, acting as a "control group," received free medication only. Those receiving financial aid and other services had fewer missed appointments, a higher sputum conversion rate, quicker weight gain, faster return to work, and a cure rate of 100 percent, compared with 56.7 percent in those who received free medicines but fewer support services. The authors challenge the conventional notion that cultural health beliefs are the most important determinants of compliance with therapy and assert the primacy of economic barriers to completion. Travel to distant clinics in rural areas to obtain medication often means losing valuable income for the family. After the symptoms respond to treatment, the economic price of continued therapy—even "free" therapy—may be too great for disadvantaged persons to sustain.

Similarly, in developed countries, especially where free clinics may be chaotic and alienating, the demands of work and child care or difficulty with transportation may deter some patients from completing treatment. For the homeless in particular, tuberculosis treatment often competes with other demands, such as personal safety, shelter, care for acute ailments, the demands of substance abuse, and obstacles such as incarceration and mental illness.

A more recent report on the tuberculosis control program in New York City showed some progress,[25] with a greater than 20 percent decrease in the number of new cases between 1992 and 1994, following a dramatic reexpansion of the services of the city's Bureau of Tuberculosis Control. Greater use of directly observed therapy—with outreach workers traveling not only to patients' homes and workplaces but also to street corners, bridges, subway stations, park benches, and even "crack dens"—increased treatment completion from 50 percent in 1989 to 90 percent in 1994. In addition to directly observed therapy and intensive case management, involuntary hospital confinement was instituted for the approximately 1 percent of patients who failed all other treatment approaches. The threat of detention, as a strategy of last resort, was believed to have a salutary effect on patient compliance. Financial or other incentives (e.g., food

TABLE 141-3

A Progressive, Stepwise Case Management Approach to Tuberculosis Treatment

Least restrictive	1. Self-administered daily short-course therapy with monthly clinic visits.
	2. Directly observed therapy, twice or thrice weekly, fully supervised in clinic, home, or alternative site.
	3. Voluntary long-term hospitalization in a specialized tuberculosis treatment unit.
Most restrictive	4. Compulsory, court-ordered long-term hospitalization in a secure tuberculosis treatment unit.

SOURCE: From Nardell,[47] with permission.

coupons) have also been found to increase compliance and are believed to be more cost-effective for some patients than incarceration. A progressive, stepwise case management approach is illustrated in Table 141-3, and Table 141-4 summarizes the benefits of long-term hospitalization.

SPECIAL GROUPS

Prisoners

The United States currently imprisons well over 1 million people, making it the country with the highest known rate of incarceration in the world. Prisons are charged with both the care and the custody of their inmates. In practice, the functions of rehabilitation are subordinated to the more central functions of security, deterrence, and punishment. Correspondingly, the central concern of a prisoner typically is not health and illness but imprisonment and freedom. Prisoners often seek medical attention to mitigate the terms of their incarceration (to gain extra meals, extra mattresses, special housing, trips to the hospital). The doctor may be caught between the conflicting demands of patients and the punitive environment of the work. The primary care physician, in the role as gatekeeper, must be constantly vigilant against exploitation, but also against becoming cynical, callous, or apathetic. Although prisoners are the only group in the United States with a Constitutionally guaranteed right to health care, sick inmates in such an environment are often subject to substandard care. The challenges of primary care in the prisons are heightened by the fact that in these institutions, peculiarly unsuited for screening, many inmates arrive with undiagnosed (and

sometimes communicable) chronic diseases and may not seek care when they become ill.

During the 1980s, the population of U.S. prisons and jails more than doubled, causing prisons to operate with censuses far exceeding their capacities. Most of the prisoners come from ethnic and socioeconomic groups with a relatively high incidence of tuberculosis infection. The incidence of AIDS in state and federal prisons is approximately 14-fold higher than that in the general population (202 versus 14.6 per 100,000).[36] The prevalence of HIV infection in the nation's entire prison system is unknown and varies greatly from state to state. In many Midwestern states, where testing is mandatory, seroprevalence is less than 1 percent. In New York, authorities estimate seroprevalence to be approximately 30 percent. Particularly in states with high prevalence, seropositivity correlates closely with a history of intravenous drug use. As of June 1990, 94 percent of AIDS patients in New York State prisons had such a history. In contrast to the situation in the general population, seropositivity is significantly higher in the minority of inmates who are female, due to the high rates of prostitution, intravenous drug use, and sex with male addicts. Time between diagnosis and death is approximately half that for those diagnosed outside the system. In one study, the first episode of PCP was found to carry an in-prison mortality of 22 percent, compared to 8 percent outside the prison.[54] The few studies that have investigated the potential for transmission of the human immunodeficiency virus in prisons have found very low rates of transmission.[36]

Against this background, an epidemic of tuberculosis has taken root in focal areas of the country's prison system. Nationwide, the incidence of tuberculosis among inmates is estimated to be four times that in the general population, and in some states as much as 15 times that in the general population.[58] More worrisome still have been the outbreaks of MDR-TB. In the New York State prison system, through 1991, 39 inmates were identified with MDR-TB; some characteristics of these patients are reviewed in Table 141-5. These 39 inmates lived in 23 different prisons. Twelve inmates were transferred a total of 20 times while potentially infectious, including transfer of inmates with known MDR-TB. A single index case was identified for 31 of these 39 inmates. And through the first 8 months of 1992, nine additional

TABLE 141-4

Advantages of Long-Term Hospitalization for Hard-to-Treat TB Patients

Achieves cures not otherwise possible due to patient noncompliance

Definitively interrupts transmission in institutions

Cost-effective in terms of cases prevented

Allows concurrent medical, behavioral, psychiatric, social, and economic issues to be addressed more effectively than in the outpatient setting

Fewer treatment interruptions due to concurrent alcohol or drug use; lower risk of treatment complications

Permits effective use of compulsory treatment under court order for uncooperative patients considered public health threats

SOURCE: From Etkind et al,[20a] with permission.

TABLE 141-5

Characteristics of Early-Stage Outbreak of MDR-TB in New York State Prison (1991–92)

Number of identified cases	39	100%
HIV+ (CD4 0-80)	38	97%
Died by 12/92	34	87%
Received no treatment	30	77%
Epidemiologically linked by RFLP	31	80%

SOURCE: Adapted from Valway et al.[58]

inmates (all HIV positive) had been diagnosed with MDR-TB, with the same susceptibilities and restriction fragment length polymorphism (RFLP) pattern. As data were collected only on inmates with proven active MDR-TB, the full scope of the outbreak is not known and is potentially much greater.

The potential for such outbreaks exists in prisons worldwide, since penal systems have concentrated a population at high risk for both tuberculosis infection and immunosuppression. For example, in a Barcelona penitentiary, 56 percent of the prisoners examined had *M. tuberculosis* infection and 43 percent of the intravenous drug users were coinfected with both *M. tuberculosis* and HIV.[20] In Madrid penitentiaries, the incidence rate of tuberculosis was 1170 per 100,000 in 1991–92. Of the 138 prisoners with tuberculosis, 84 percent were intravenous drug users and 84 percent were coinfected with HIV.

If one wished to design a system for the efficient dissemination of a respiratory pathogen, the example of MDR-TB in prisons would provide a reasonable blueprint. The rapid spread of this resistant organism was facilitated by the *high turnover of inmates,* the *high rate of noncompliance,* and various institutional failures, including *poor record keeping, delay in diagnosis* of symptomatic disease, *poor follow-up, treatment of active cases in an infirmary or hospital setting with susceptible HIV patients, poor ventilation,* and *lack of ultraviolet room disinfection.*

Refugees and Immigrants

The United States and other developed countries have long attracted immigrants and refugees from economically depressed regions of the world. These immigrants bring with them a high rate of latent, prepatent, and chronic infections, many of which are not familiar to Western clinicians. They also come with more typical pathogens, but these may have unusual resistance patterns, such as penicillin-resistant streptococci from Papua–New Guinea, Spain, or South Africa. Further, because of varying exposures and immunization policies and vaccine availabilities, immigrants arrive with different specific immunities. Lastly, they bring their own language and culture, which include explanatory models frequently incongruent with medical science, affecting communication, symptom expression, and compliance with therapy.

From 1986 through 1993, more than 8 million immigrants were legally granted permanent residence.[43] Approximately 85 percent of these legal immigrants came from Latin America, Asia, and the Caribbean. There were an additional 3 to 4 million illegal foreign-born residents by the early 1990s. Although im-

migrants are screened for active tuberculosis, HIV infection, narcotics addiction, and alcohol abuse, these screening procedures are imperfect. No screening procedures are done on illegal immigrants or the 20 million nonimmigrant visitors and foreign students. Among the top five countries of origin (Mexico, the Philippines, Vietnam, China, and South Korea), the tuberculosis incidence rates are 10 to 30 times greater than the rate in the United States.[43] The shifting demographics of immigration have led inevitably to a progressive increase in the proportion of persons in this country reported to have tuberculosis who were foreign born. This has led some tuberculosis authorities to emphasize the need to curtail immigration in order to control tuberculosis. In California, Proposition 187, which requires publicly funded health-care facilities to deny care to illegal immigrants and to report them to government officials, is intended as one such deterrent to illegal immigration. Such approaches have the potential to worsen the incidence of any endemic infection by raising barriers to diagnosis and treatment. As an alternative approach, some officials have advocated greater efforts by the developed countries, coordinated through international organizations, to improve infection control programs in developing nations.

Clinicians who treat immigrants have become increasingly sensitive to the possibility that foreign-born patients presenting with respiratory or systemic symptoms may have tuberculosis. The injunction to "think tuberculosis" in such patients with pulmonary infiltrates, however, may be too well heeded. There is evidence in Massachusetts of overdiagnosis of tuberculosis among foreign-born tuberculin-positive children, based on clinical findings without culture confirmation. Several unusual diseases can reactivate years after immigration, with or without immunosuppression.[43] These include melioidosis, paracoccidioidomycosis, coccidioidomycosis, histoplasmosis, visceral leishmaniasis, strongyloidiasis, and toxoplasmosis. Some of these can be easily confused with tuberculosis, presenting as they do with suggestive symptoms in patients who frequently have positive tuberculin skin tests (Table 141-6).

TABLE 141-6

Special Considerations in the Diagnosis of Pulmonary Infections in Immigrants

Infections That May Resemble TB	Parasitic Infections with Peripheral Blood Eosinophilia	Latent Infections That Can Become Active after Immigration
Melioidosis	Ascariasis	TB
Paracoccidio- idomycosis	Hookworm infection	Melioidosis
Histoplasmosis	Strongyloidiasis	Paracoccidio- idomycosis
Coccidioidomycosis	Tropical pulmonary eosinophilia	Histoplasmosis
Paragonimiasis	Visceral larva migrans	Coccidioidomycosis
	Trichinosis	Stronglyoidiasis
	Schistosomiasis	Amebiasis
	Echinococcosis	
	Paragonimiasis	

SOURCE: Iralu and Maguire.[33a]

One example of such infection is melioidosis, a bacterial infection caused by *Burkholderia* (formerly *Pseudomonas*) *pseudomallei,* which can reactivate more than a decade after exposure and presents with a highly variable clinical picture that may resemble chronic tuberculosis, with fever, weight loss, hemoptysis, and cavitary upper-lobe disease as seen on chest radiograph. Its prevalence in Southeast Asia has earned it the name *Vietnam tuberculosis,* but it is present in other tropical regions as well. Serologic studies have found elevated titers in as many as 29 percent of Southeast Asian immigrants.[4] Asymptomatic persons with elevated antibody titers to *B. pseudomallei* are not treated, as the risk of reactivation is low. Diagnosis of active disease requires a high degree of suspicion, as the clinical picture is so variable and the organism—easily cultured from sputum, pleural fluid, or other body fluid or tissues—frequently discounted as a contaminant. High antibody titers are also helpful. Treatment of active disease is at least a 2-month course of conventional antibiotics, guided by susceptibility tests.

Among parasitic infections, paragonimiasis is also frequently misdiagnosed as tuberculosis. The disease is endemic throughout much of Southeast Asia and other tropical areas, and its clinical features include pleural effusions, pleural thickening, lung infiltrates, calcifications, nodular densities, and cavitary pulmonary disease. Approximately 1 percent of patients with pulmonary paragonimiasis will also have cerebral involvement. The causative agent is a lung fluke, most often ingested in the larval stage in raw or undercooked crabs. Eosinophilia in the context of a tuberculosislike illness should raise the suspicion of paragonimiasis in the appropriate patient, but the diagnosis is based on stool examination. Serologic tests are also useful. Treatment is a 2-day course of praziquantel, even in asymptomatic cases. Other helminthic infections that can present with pulmonary infiltrates and peripheral eosinophilia are listed in Table 141-6 and discussed in Chapter 156. It is important to bear in mind that such a patient from an area endemic with parasites is more likely to have a common bacterial or viral pneumonia with a coincidental intestinal parasite than to have a parasitic pneumonia.

Loeffler's syndrome should be considered in recent immigrants presenting with new onset of asthmatic symptoms. It occurs within weeks of infection with *Ascaris,* hookworm, or *Strongyloides,* as the larvae migrate through the lungs en route to the gut, where they mature into adult worms. Patients present with cough, wheeze, and "fleecy" peripheral infiltrates but no fever. The stools are negative for ova and parasites. Diagnosis is made from detection of the larvae in sputum or gastric aspirate. Among helminths, only *Strongyloides* can complete its life cycle in humans. This allows for chronic infections, person-to-person transmission, and, when host cell–mediated immunity becomes impaired, a hyperinfection syndrome, in which larvae migrate outside the gut, commonly in the lungs. Patients can present with fever, cough, wheeze, and radiographic lesions that may be reticulonodular, consolidated, or cavitary. As many as 11.5 percent of recent immigrants may be infected.[26] It is prudent to check the stool of immigrants before starting any corticosteroid treatment (e.g., for asthma) or other immunosuppressant therapies.

Evaluation of an immigrant with a pulmonary infiltrate should include a thorough travel history (including intermediate sites), immunization history, a tuberculin skin test, smears and culture for mycobacteria and fungi, a blood smear for eosinophils, and examination of the stool for ova and parasites.

Homeless

Homeless men and women in the United States are heterogeneous in age, race, and ethnicity. Smoking, however, is a habit many of them share, and the respiratory complications of smoking—lung cancer, emphysema, and respiratory infections—account for about 40 percent of their medical complaints, according to a review by O'Connell, and for about 20 percent of all deaths in this population.[49] The effects of smoking on host defenses are compounded by various forms of substance abuse, by increased exposure to respiratory pathogens inherent in congregate living, and increasingly by the devastating consequences of HIV infection.

In contrast to tuberculosis, relatively little has been written about bacterial and viral respiratory infections among the homeless. It is likely that only a minority of homeless persons suffering from severe upper respiratory tract infections or from acute and chronic infections seek medical attention. Yet from nearly 15,000 medical encounters in 1990, the Boston Health Care for the Homeless Project reported that respiratory illness was the primary or secondary diagnosis in more than 10 percent, and more than 50 percent of those were acute respiratory infections.[49]

Transmission of type 1 capsular pneumococcal pneumonia within a large Boston shelter has been characterized.[49] Nose and throat cultures from regular residents of the shelter yielded an unusually high carriage rate—a precondition to the aspiration of pneumococci, which are droplet-borne rather than airborne organisms. The efficacy of immunization against pneumonia and influenza infections among the homeless is unknown and difficult to assess. Outbreaks of infection due to invasive type b *H. influenzae* have also been associated with shelters, and increased pharyngeal carriage has been found.

Shelters for the homeless have long been associated with tuberculosis. In 1983, the first of an ongoing outbreak of epidemiologically and bacteriologically linked cases of tuberculosis was diagnosed at a Boston homeless shelter.[46] Similar outbreaks were soon reported from New York and other large cities. The index case in the Boston outbreak was subsequently identified as an alcoholic man with a 10-year history of previously treated isoniazid- and streptomycin-resistant tuberculosis. He had resided at the shelter for 11 months before the first of the secondary cases was diagnosed. Over the next several years, the tuberculosis rate among the homeless of Boston soared, with roughly half of the cases caused by organisms resistant to isoniazid and streptomycin. Through phage typing, almost 50 cases of active tuberculosis originating from this single source were identified. Closer scrutiny of the linked cases led to insights into the pathogenesis and transmission of tuberculosis among the homeless in shelters.

Many of the epidemiologically linked shelter cases presented with upper-lobe cavitary disease—a pattern usually associated with disease reactivation, long believed to be the predominant pathogenic mechanism for cavitary tuberculosis in low-prevalence countries. However, the epidemic pattern and the bacteriologic markers strongly favored recent transmission rather than coincidental, spontaneous reactivation of old tuberculosis foci. Exogenous reinfection of previously infected persons is one mechanism that resolved this apparent contradiction—a mechanism that had been postulated as an important cause of cavitary tuberculosis in high-prevalence countries. When reinfection does occur, liquefaction necrosis and cavitation are accelerated because of preexisting hypersensitivity to tuberculoproteins in these patients. Rapid lung cavitation, a pathologic event associated with greater infectivity, then leads to accelerated epidemic transmission in the shelter.

An increasing proportion of patients with shelter-related tuberculosis are coinfected with HIV. As with exogenous reinfection among immunocompetent hosts, HIV coinfection has been linked to an accelerated pattern of epidemic transmission observed in shelters, drug treatment facilities, and hospitals.[13,16,19] This pattern of accelerated transmission has profound implications for the use of congregate housing for HIV-infected persons, for the safety of shelter and health-care workers, and for the feasibility of conventional contact tracing and preventive strategies for tuberculosis. Small-group living arrangements are preferable to large shelters, because they should be less conducive to widespread transmission. Secondary cases may develop so rapidly after an index case as to leave no time for skin testing and prophylaxis. Additionally, HIV patients may be anergic. Therefore, preventive therapy may need to be based on group risk rather than on evidence of individual infection, and the use of screening chest radiographs should be considered for some populations. Air disinfection may be necessary to help reduce transmission among residents and staff.

SUMMARY

"The world's most ruthless killer and the greatest cause of suffering on earth is . . . extreme poverty," according to WHO's *World Health Report*, published in 1995.[63] The effect of economics on health is profound. Researchers have consistently found that about two-thirds of the variation in mortality in both developed and developing nations is related to the distribution of income in each nation's population.[31] The gap in mortality between the relatively advantaged and the disadvantaged is very large—larger than the gap due to many other well-known risk factors, including smoking.[3] Pappas[50] found that the inverse relation between mortality and socioeconomic status that was present in 1960 persisted in 1986 and was stronger than in 1960, which he relates to increasing inequalities in income, education, housing, and standard of living. Poverty and poor health may be seen as being linked by a web of despair, drugs, alcohol, poor nutrition, stress, medical noncompliance, crowding, and poor health care, creating a tenaciously stable dynamic system, self-organizing and autocatalytic.

The past several decades have witnessed a spectacular growth in the health-care industry and spectacular advances in the medical sciences, but relatively modest gains in the major measures of public health. Technical advances, even those of demonstrable clinical utility, have not been as tightly linked to improvements in our health as we would have liked to believe. Further, there exists a body of research suggesting that improving social conditions for the poor may have more profound consequences on their health than simply the adequate delivery of health care.

The passion and curiosity of medical scientists are more engaged in the pursuit of new pharmaceuticals and biotechnologic advances than in innovations in effective public health interventions. More than a quarter century ago, Kass posed this challenge to medicine: Can we find drives in social welfare that will direct and harness our productive and creative energies?[37] If not, the gap between the state of medical science and the health of the world will only continue to widen.

REFERENCES

1. Adams H, Jordan C: Infections in the alcohol. *Med Clin North Am* 68:179–200, 1984.
2. Adler N, Boyce T, Chessey M, et al: Socioeconomic status and health: The challenge of the gradient. *Am Psychol* 49:15–24, 1994.
3. Angell M: Privilege and health—What's the connection? *New Engl J Med* 329:126–127, 1993.
4. Ashdown L, Guard R: The presence of human melioidosis in Northern Queensland. *Am J Trop Med Hyg* 33:474–478, 1984.
5. Bascom R, Bromberg PA, Costa DA et al: State of the art: Health effects of outdoor air pollution. *Am J Respir Crit Care Med* 153:3–50, 477–498, 1996.
6. Black F: Measles antibodies in the population of New Haven, Connecticut. *J Immunol* 82:74–83, 1959.
7. Bor D, Epstein P: Pathogenesis of respiratory infection in the disadvantaged. *Semin Respir Infect* 6:194–203, 1991.
8. Brook R, Ware JE Jr, Rogers WH, et al: Does free care improve adults' health? Results from a randomized controlled trial. *New Engl J Med* 309:1426–1434, 1983.
9. Brown K, Gilman RH, Gaffar A, et al: Infections associated with severe protein-calorie malnutrition in hospitalized infants and children. *Nutr Res* 1:33–46, 1981.
10. Brudney K, Dobkin J: A tale of two cities: Tuberculosis control in Nicaragua and New York City. *Semin Resp Infect* 6:261–272, 1991.
11. Brudney K, Dobkin J: Resurgent tuberculosis in New York City. *Am Rev Respir Dis* 144:745–749, 1991.
12. Burstin H, Lipsitz S, Brenen T: Socioeconomic status and risk for substandard care. *JAMA* 268:2383–2387, 1992.
13. Centers for Disease Control: Nosocomial transmission of multidrug-resistant tuberculosis to health-care workers and HIV-infected patients in an urban hospital—Florida. *MMWR* 39:718–722, 1990.
14. Centers for Disease Control: Influenza and pneumococcal vaccination coverage levels among persons aged greater than 65—United States, 1973–93. *MMWR* 506–515, 1995.
15. Chomet B, Gach BM: Lobar pneumonia and alcoholism: An analysis of thirty-seven cases. *Am J Med Sci* 253:300–304, 1967.
16. Daley C, Small PM, Schecter GF, et al: An outbreak of tuberculosis with accelerated progression among persons infected with the immunodeficiency virus. *New Engl J Med* 326:231–235, 1992.
17. Davies P: A possible link between vitamin D deficiency and impaired host defence to *Mycobacterium* tuberculosis. *Tubercle* 66:301–306, 1985.
18. De Maria A Jr, Browne K, Berk SL, et al: An outbreak of type 1 pneumococcal pneumonia in a men's shelter. *JAMA* 244:1446–1449, 1980.
19. Di Perri G et al: Nosocomial epidemic of active tuberculosis among HIV-infected patients. *Lancet* 2:1502–1504, 1989.
19a. Dohrenwend BS: Social status and stressful life events. *J Pers Soc Psycho* 28:225–235, 1973.

20. Drobniewski F: Tuberculosis in prisons—forgotten plague. *Lancet* 346:948–949, 1995.

20a. Etkind S et al: Treating hard-to-treat tuberculosis patients in Massachusetts. *Semin Respir Infect* 6:273–282, 1991.

21. Fang G, Fine M, Orloff J, et al: New and emerging etiologies for community acquired pneumonia with implication for therapy: A prospective multicenter study of 359 cases. *Medicine* 62:271–285, 1990.

22. Farmer P, Robin S, Ramilus SL, et al: Tuberculosis, poverty, and "compliance": Lessons from rural Haiti. *Semin Respir Infect* 6:254–260, 1991.

23. Fernandez-Sola J et al: Alcohol intake as a risk and prognostic factor for community-acquired pneumonia. *Arch Intern Med* 155:1649–1654, 1995.

24. Franks P, Clancy C, Gold M: Health insurance and mortality: Evidence from a national cohort. *JAMA* 270:737–741, 1993.

25. Frieden TR, Fujiwara PI, Washko RM, et al: Tuberculosis in New York City—Turning the tide. *New Engl J Med* 333:229–233, 1995.

26. Fuxench-López Z, Ramínez-Ronda CH: Pharyngeal flora in ambulatory alcoholic patients. Prevalence of gram-negative bacilli. *Arch Intern Med* 138:1815–1816, 1978.

27. Genta R: Global prevalence of strongyloidiasis: Critical review of epidemiologic insights into the prevention of disseminated disease. *Rev Infect Dis* 11:755–765, 1989.

28. Glassroth J: Empiric diagnosis of *Pneumocystis carinii* pneumonia. *Am J Respir Crit Care Med* 152:1433–1434, 1995.

29. Hafner-Eaton C: Physician utilization disparities between the uninsured and insured: Comparisons of the chronically ill, acutely ill, and well non-elderly populations. *JAMA* 262:787–792, 1993.

30. Hudson LD, Sbarbaro JA: Twice weekly tuberculosis chemotherapy. *JAMA* 223:139–143, 1978.

31. Hurowitz J: Sounding board: Toward a social policy for health. *New Engl J Med* 329:130–133, 1993.

32. Hussey G, Klein M: A randomized controlled trial of vitamin A in children with severe measles. *New Engl J Med* 323:160–164, 1990.

33. Huxley E, Viroslav J, Gray W: Pharyngeal aspiration in normal adults and patients with depressed consciousness. *Am J Med* 64:564–568, 1978.

33a. Iralu JV, Maguire JH: Pulmonary infections in immigrants and refugees. *Semin Respir Infect* 6:235–246, 1991.

34. Jackson G, Darling HF, Anderson TO, et al: Susceptibility and immunity to common upper respiratory viral infection—The common cold. *Ann Intern Med* 53:719–738, 1960.

35. Johnson WD, Stokes P, Kaye D: The effect of intravenous ethanol on the bactericidal activity of human serum. *Yale J Biol Med* 42:71–89, 1969.

36. Kantor E: AIDS and HIV infection in prisoners, in Cohen P, Sande M, Volberding P (eds): *The AIDS Knowledge Base.* Waltham, MA, The Medical Publishing Group, 1995, pp 1.8–1.9.

37. Kass EH: Infectious diseases and social change. *J Infect Dis* 123:110–114, 1971.

38. Kielman A, Taylor C, Parker R: The Narangwal nutrition study: A summary review. *Am J Clin Nutr* 31:2040–2057, 1978.

39. Lewis J, Chamberlain D: Alcohol consumption and smoking habits in male patients with pulmonary tuberculosis. *Br J Prev Soc Med* 17:149–152, 1963.

40. Maclure A, Stewar G: Admission of children to hospitals in Glasgow: A summary review. *Lancet* 2:682–685, 1984.

40a. Marcy T, Merrill W: Cigarette smoking and respiratory tract infection. *Clin Chest Med* 8:381–391, 1987.

41. Martin T: The relationship between malnutrition and lung infections. *Clin Chest Med* 8:359–372, 1987.

42. May RM: The rise and fall and rise of tuberculosis. *Nature Med* 1:752, 1995.

43. McKenna MT, McCray E, Onorato I: The epidemiology of tuberculosis among foreign-born persons in the United States, 1986 to 1993. *New Engl J Med* 332:1071–1076, 1995.

44. McKeown T: *The Origins of Human Disease.* Oxford, Basil Blackwell, 1988.

45. Murphy J, Olivier DC, Monson RR, et al: Depression and anxiety in relation to social status: A prospective epidemiologic study. *Arch Gen Psychiatry* 48:223–229, 1991.

46. Nardell E, McInnis B, Thomas B, et al: Exogenous reinfection with tuberculosis in a shelter for the homeless. *New Engl J Med* 315:1570–1575, 1986.

47. Nardell EA: Beyond four drugs: Public health policy and the treatment of the individual patient with tuberculosis. *Am Rev Respir Dis* 148:2–5, 1993.

48. Nolan J: Alcohol as a factor in the illness of university service patients. *Am J Med Sci* 249:135–142, 1965.

49. O'Connel J: Nontuberculous respiratory infections among the homeless. *Semin Respir Infect* 6:247–253, 1991.

50. Pappas G, Queen S, Hadden W, et al: The increasing disparity in mortality between socioeconomic groups in the United States, 1960 and 1986. *New Engl J Med* 329:103–109, 1993.

51. Parkes C, Brown R: Health and bereavement: A controlled study of young Boston widows and widowers. *Psychosom Med* 34:449–461, 1972.

52. Rook G: The role of vitamin D in tuberculosis. *Am Rev Respir Dis* 138:768–770, 1988.

53. Schmidt W, De Lint J: Social class and the mortality of clinically treated alcoholics. *Br J Addict* 64:327–331, 1970.

54. Sharp V: Comparison of first episode of PCP in community patients and inmates (abstract pbp18), vol 5, p289. IV International Conference on AIDS, Montreal, 1989.

55. Somers A: Marital status, health and use of health services: An old relationship revisited. *Ann Intern Med* 241:1818–1822, 1979.

56. Totman R, Kiff J, Reed SE, et al: Predicting experimental colds in volunteers from different measures of recent life stress. *J Psychosom Res* 24:155–163, 1980.

57. Tupasi T, Mangubat NV, Sunico MES, et al: Malnutrition and acute respiratory infections in Filipino children. *Rev Infect Dis* 12(Suppl 8):S1047–S1054, 1990.

58. Valway SE, Greifinger RB, Papania M, et al: Multidrug-resistant tuberculosis in the New York State prison system, 1990–1991. *J Infect Dis* 170:151–156, 1994.

59. Walsh J: Selective primary health care: Strategies for control of disease in the developing world. IV. Measles. *Rev Infect Dis* 5:330–340, 1983.

60. Weissman J, Epstein A: Case mix and resource utilization by uninsured hospital patients in the Boston metropolitan area. *JAMA* 261:3572–3576, 1989.

61. Weissman J, Gatsonis C, Epstein A: Rates of avoidable hospitalization in Massachusetts and Maryland. *JAMA* 268:2388–2394, 1992.

62. Weissman J, Stern R, Fielding SL, et al: Delayed access to health care: Risk factors, reasons and consequences. *Ann Intern Med* 114:325–331, 1991.

63. World Health Organization: *The World Health Report.* Geneva, Switzerland, World Health Organization, 1995.

64. Yergan J, Flood AB, Diehr P, et al: Relationship between patient source of payment and the intensity of hospital services. *Med Care* 26:255–262, 1988.

CHAPTER 142

PNEUMONIAS CAUSED BY GRAM-POSITIVE BACTERIA

Alan L. Bisno / Gordon M. Dickinson / David S. McKinsey

A variety of gram-positive organisms are associated with human pneumonia. Some, such as *Mycobacterium tuberculosis* and *Nocardia asteroides*, are considered elsewhere in this book. Among the gram-positive cocci, *Streptococcus pneumoniae*, *Staphylococcus aureus*, *S. pyogenes,* and *Rhodococcus equi* have been singled out for consideration in this chapter; the gram-positive anaerobic cocci are considered in Chapters 129 and 130. Among the bacilli, *Bacillus anthracis* is also considered in this chapter.

STREPTOCOCCUS PNEUMONIAE

S. pneumoniae (the "pneumococcus") is the most common cause of community-acquired bacterial pneumonia.[27,40] On occasion, the organism may also be a cause of nosocomial pneumonia, especially in elderly, debilitated patients.[28] Despite major advances in the diagnosis, treatment, and prophylaxis of pneumococcal pneumonia, this entity has been estimated to account for up to 40,000 deaths annually in the United States and is a major source of morbidity and mortality throughout the world.

Historical Perspective

S. pneumoniae was simultaneously identified by Pasteur and by Sternberg in 1881. Two years later, Friedlander noted the association of this organism with lobar pneumonia. In the early 1900s, Neufeld discovered the presence of distinct pneumococcal serotypes. This finding led to the development of type-specific antisera, the first specific form of therapy for the disease. The work of Griffith demonstrating transformation of rough strains of type II pneumococcus into type III smooth strains in the 1920s laid the groundwork for the demonstration by Avery, Macleod, and McCarty in 1944 that DNA contains the genetic code of living cells. Following the purification of pneumococcal capsular polysaccharide in the early 1940s, a polyvalent vaccine was developed, but its use was discontinued when penicillin became available for civilian use and was found to be extremely effective in the treatment of pneumococcal infections. A vaccine was reintroduced in the 1970s after clinical studies demonstrated that the morbidity and mortality of bacteremic pneumococcal infections remained high despite the availability of seemingly effective antibiotics. In 1967, penicillin-resistant pneumococci were identified in Australia, and in 1978 multiply-antibiotic-resistant strains of *S. pneumoniae* were reported from South Africa. Highly resistant strains are now present in many parts of the world.

Microbiology

S. pneumoniae is the causative agent of pneumococcal pneumonia. This organism is an encapsulated gram-positive coccus that measures 0.5 to 1.25 μm in diameter and is characteristically lancet-shaped. The composition of the organism's polysaccharide capsule varies among the different serotypes. Pneumococci typically associate in pairs, but they may occur singly or in short chains.

Pneumococci are facultative anaerobes. When cultivated on blood agar plates at 37°C, young colonies are circular and glistening and measure approximately 1 mm in diameter. If incubated under aerobic conditions, they are surrounded by a zone of hemolysis. Pneumococci can be differentiated from other α-hemolytic streptococci by their susceptibility to optochin (ethylhydrocupreine), their solubility in bile, and their high degree of virulence in mice. When type-specific antipneumococcal serum is added to specimens containing pneumococci of the homologous serotype, the optical density of the organisms' capsules is altered, causing them to appear swollen and distinct. This test, known as the quellung or Neufeld's reaction, not only enables the differentiation of pneumococci from other streptococci but also allows the separation of pneumococci into distinct serotypes, of which 84 are currently recognized.

Epidemiology

Because pneumococcal pneumonia is not a reportable disease in the United States, exact incidence figures are unavailable. It is estimated that *S. pneumoniae* causes approximately 500,000 cases of pneumonia and approximately 3000 cases of meningitis each year. The incidence of pneumococcal pneumonia increases with advancing age. As discussed below, a variety of medical illnesses, including HIV infection, predispose to pneumococcal pneumonia. There is seasonal variation in the incidence of the disease; most cases occur in the winter or early spring.

CARRIAGE

S. pneumoniae often constitutes part of the microbial flora of the upper respiratory tract. Asymptomatic carriage rates in the general population are highly variable and depend on such factors as age and environment. In general, carriage rates diminish with advancing age and are highest during the winter months. A study in Charlottesville, Virginia, demonstrated that carriage rates ranged from 6 percent in childless adults to 38 percent in preschool children.[22] Even higher rates have been reported in certain closed populations, such as those in military training camps. Interpatient transmission may occur within health-care facilities,[28] and patients with pneumonia were isolated in the pre-antibiotic era. The rapid response of pneumococcal pneumonia to antibiotics, however, is such that nosocomial transmission is not currently viewed as a threat once appropriate therapy has been instituted.

RISK FACTORS

Several conditions are associated with an increased risk of pneumococcal pneumonia. Viral upper respiratory infections are reported as an antecedent event in a high percentage of cases. Conditions that are conducive to the aspiration of nasopharyngeal contents into the lungs—e.g., alcoholism and chilling—are common concomitants of pneumococcal pneumonia. Because fluid-filled alveoli are more susceptible to infection, there is an increased risk of pneumonia in persons with congestive heart failure, viral pneumonia, or noxious gas exposure. An association of increased risk for pneumococcal infections is well established for patients with multiple myeloma, sickle cell disease, congenital or acquired hyposplenism, and chronic pulmonary disease. The emergence of the HIV pandemic, however, arguably has become the foremost predisposing factor for pneumococcal infection. *S. pneumoniae* is now recognized as one of the major bacterial pathogens causing pneumonia in persons with HIV infection.[24] In the United States, two or more episodes within one year of bacterial pneumonia—of which *S. pneumoniae* is the leading cause—in a person with HIV infection establishes a diagnosis of AIDS.

PNEUMOCOCCAL SEROTYPES

Only a limited number of the 84 serotypes account for most infections. Approximately 80 percent of cases of pneumococcal pneumonia in adults are caused by serotypes 1, 3, 4, 6, 7, 8, 9, 12, 14, 18, 19, and 23. The mortality from infections caused by the different serotypes is highly variable. For example, in one major study, bacteremic type III infections were found to carry a mortality of 55 percent, compared to an overall rate of 24.8 percent for all bacteremic pneumococcal infections.[6]

Pathophysiology

Pharyngeal colonization by pneumococci appears to be mediated by a ligand on the bacterial surface that binds to the disaccharide N-acetylglucosamine β1-3 galactose on oral epithelial cells.[15] Patients who develop pneumococcal pneumonia are usually colonized with a virulent strain of the organism. The capsule, a polysaccharide substance of varied composition, is the major established virulence factor of *S. pneumoniae*. The primary role of the capsule is to inhibit opsonin-mediated phagocytosis by polymorphonuclear leukocytes. The glycopeptide components of the pneumococcal cell wall, however, provoke an intense inflammatory reaction: some of the known actions are recruitment of leukocytes into the site of infection, attachment to endothelial and epithelial cells with separation of contiguous cells, induction of cytokine production, initiation of the procoagulant cascade, and stimulation of platelet-activating factor production.[41] A number of surface proteins, not yet fully defined and with incompletely understood biologic activities, including pneumococcal surface protein A, pneumolysin, and several peptide permeases, may contribute to pneumococcal virulence.[11,41]

Patients with pneumococcal pneumonia generally have impaired local host defense mechanisms, due to either transient derangements or chronic medical illnesses. Under these circumstances, virulent pneumococci can be aspirated from the nasopharynx into the alveoli, after which pneumococcal pneumonia develops in a characteristic fashion. The presence of bacteria in the alveoli elicits an outpouring of serous fluid, which supports replication of the organisms and, in addition, transports them outward via the pores of Kohn to adjacent alveoli. The spread of edema fluid continues until it is halted by anatomic barriers such as the visceral pleura or the pericardium. Within a few hours, alveoli become consolidated with polymorphonuclear leukocytes and erythrocytes. In the later stages of infection, macrophages migrate into the alveoli and ingest the remaining debris. Because the alveolar walls are not destroyed, the pulmonary parenchyma is usually normal after resolution of the infection.

As with other forms of aspiration pneumonia, pneumococcal pneumonia typically affects the dependent portions of the lungs. In most cases, the infection is confined to a single lobe. Interlobar spread, however, can occur if infected edema fluid flows from the bronchus of an affected lobe into that of an unaffected lobe. Multilobar impairment occurs in approximately 20 to 30 percent of cases. Pneumococci can gain access to the pleural or pericardial spaces via direct spread from the pulmonary parenchyma, resulting in empyema or purulent pericarditis.

Lymphatic drainage of organisms occurs early in the course of the illness. If regional lymph nodes are unable to contain the infection, organisms enter the bloodstream. Bacteremia occurs in about 25 to 30 percent of patients and is usually associated with the more virulent serotypes. Bacteremia sometimes results in metastatic infection, such as meningitis, septic arthritis, endocarditis, endophthalmitis, and, rarely, peritonitis.

In the early stages of infection, phagocytosis is dependent on activation of the alternative complement pathway by components of the pneumococcal cell wall. Type-specific anticapsular antibodies appear 5 to 10 days after the onset of infection. The appearance of such opsonic antibodies, which markedly enhance phagocytosis of pneumococci, correlates temporally with the clinical "crisis" observed in the preantibiotic era, during which the patient undergoes an abrupt and striking improvement.

Clinical Manifestations

Few diseases have a clinical course that is as dramatic and as highly characteristic as that of pneumococcal pneumonia in its classic form. The illness often occurs shortly after an upper respiratory infection. Its onset is abrupt and is frequently manifested by a severe shaking chill (the "herald chill"), which lasts for up to an hour. Shortly thereafter, the patient develops fever of 39.4 to 41.1°C, marked tachycardia and tachypnea, a dry cough, and severe pleuritic chest pain. Nausea and vomiting occur in about a third of patients. By the second or third day of the disease, the patient is acutely ill, with prominent malaise, weakness, and prostration. Marked respiratory distress is occasionally present, in part because of severe chest pain, which leads to splinting of the chest wall. The cough, which is initially dry, becomes productive of thick, tenacious sputum, which is "rusty" because of intra-alveolar hemorrhage.

On examination, the patient appears toxic and is in moderate to severe respiratory distress. The temperature, pulse rate, and respiratory rate are elevated, often markedly so. There is prominent diaphoresis. Many patients have herpes labialis. Respirations are shallow, and expiratory grunting is present.

In established cases of pneumococcal pneumonia, examination of the chest often reveals evidence of voluntary splinting of the muscles of the chest wall and consolidation of the affected area of the lung. Movement of the afflicted hemithorax is restricted to varying degrees. On palpation, there is increased tactile fremitus and occasionally a palpable rub over the area of impairment. Dullness to percussion can be detected in cases in which there is extensive consolidation. Auscultation over the impaired area of lung may reveal coarse inspiratory rales, increased vocal fremitus, bronchial breath sounds, egophony, and a localized pleural friction rub. These auscultatory findings may be obscured, however, in the presence of a sizable pleural effusion or empyema.

Although the preceding paragraphs describe the "classic" presentation of pneumococcal pneumonia, in many patients the signs and symptoms of the disease are much more muted.[31] A minority of hospitalized patients describe chills or pleuritic chest pain, and even such cardinal manifestations as fever and sputum production are not invariably present. In elderly or debilitated patients, localizing signs of infection are sometimes absent, and mental status abnormalities may be the most striking finding.

Clinical Course

In an untreated case of pneumococcal pneumonia, the patient is acutely ill for 5 to 10 days, after which in surviving patients the infection either resolves promptly by "crisis" or subsides more gradually by "lysis." Patients who receive penicillin therapy usually improve quickly. Defervescence often occurs within 24 to 36 h. However, even in appropriately treated, uncomplicated cases due to penicillin-susceptible pneumococci, fever may take several days to resolve completely. It is unnecessary to alter therapy in such cases. More worrisome is the recurrence of fever after an initial response to therapy. Among the causes of recurrent fever are extrapulmonary foci of infection (see "Complications," below), bronchial obstruction by tumor or foreign body, drug fever, thrombophlebitis at sites of intravenous infusion, misidentification of the original infecting organism, and superinfection.

Complications

Patients with pneumococcal pneumonia may develop a wide variety of local or distant complications. Pleural effusions are the most common local complications. Such effusions are exudative and are usually small and self-limited. Although most effusions are sterile, empyema develops on occasion, usually in cases in which antimicrobial therapy is delayed or inadequate. Empyema should be suspected in patients with pleural effusions who have persistent fever and leukocytosis, and thoracentesis should be performed in all such patients. Pneumococcal pericarditis, once the most common form of bacterial pericarditis, is now a rare complication. Suggestive clinical features include persistent fever, tachycardia, chest pain, a pericardial friction rub, and radiographic evidence of an enlarging cardiac silhouette.

Pneumococcal meningitis results from bacteremic spread of organisms to the meninges. A high index of suspicion must be maintained for this life-threatening disease—particularly in elderly or debilitated patients, in whom the clinical features may not be clear-cut and confusion or agitation may be attributed to other causes. Less common metastatic complications of pneumonia include infective endocarditis, septic arthritis, and endophthalmitis.

A variety of nonsuppurative complications have been reported. Jaundice has been noted in up to 26 percent of patients with lobar pneumonia in some series. When the right lower lobe is affected, tenderness in the right upper quadrant of the abdomen and hepatomegaly may be prominent findings, occasionally to such a degree that the pneumonia is overlooked while diagnosis of acute cholecystitis, hepatitis, or cholangitis is entertained. The pathophysiology of jaundice associated with pneumococcal pneumonia is unclear. There is often evidence of intrahepatic cholestasis, perhaps related to impaired bile transport, and mild hepatocellular injury. In some cases, hemolysis due to glucose-6-phosphate dehydrogenase deficiency may be a contributing cause. Other complications that have been reported are acute respiratory distress syndrome, rhabdomyolysis, and the syndrome of inappropriate secretion of antidiuretic hormone.

Prognosis

In the preantibiotic era, pneumococcal pneumonia was a dreaded disease with a mortality approaching 30 percent. Since the introduction of penicillin, overall mortality has fallen to approximately 5 percent in nonbacteremic cases and 17 percent in bacteremic cases.[6] There is considerable variation in prognosis among different patient subgroups. Death rates are higher in infants, the elderly, alcoholics, women in late pregnancy, and persons with chronic underlying medical illnesses. Cases associated with leukopenia, multilobar impairment, or extrapulmonary complications carry a considerably increased mortality.

Diagnosis

Although the diagnosis of pneumococcal pneumonia may be strongly suggested by the clinical picture, a variety of laboratory tests are helpful in confirming the diagnosis. Although the diagnosis can be confirmed only by the isolation of *S. pneumoniae* from blood, pleural fluid, or lung tissue, a positive sputum Gram's stain can rapidly provide strong presumptive evidence of pneumococcal pneumonia. To be accepted as adequate, the expectorated sputum specimen must contain numerous polymorphonuclear leukocytes (unless the patient is neutropenic) and few epithelial cells, to assure that one is not simply examining oropharyngeal contents. The presence of lancet-shaped, gram-positive diplococci in close association with leukocytes (Fig. 142-1) is highly suggestive of pneumococcal infection and correlates with a favorable clinical response to antipneumococcal therapy.[10] A nondiagnostic Gram's stain does not exclude the possibility of pneumococcal pneumonia. The sputum culture is of much less value than the Gram's stain in the diagnosis of pneumonia. False-negativity rates of up to 50 percent have been reported. Moreover, in one series of patients with bacteremic pneumococcal pneumonia, more than one-quarter of sputum cultures grew potential pathogens other than *S. pneumoniae*.[7]

Unfortunately, adequate sputum specimens are difficult to obtain in many patients, particularly those who are elderly, debilitated, or dehydrated. In selected patients in whom the differential diagnosis is particularly challenging, sputum specimens may be obtained via invasive techniques such as bronchoscopy (using a protected catheter tip to avoid oropharyngeal contamination) or, rarely, transtracheal aspiration. The decision to employ the latter technique, however, must be individualized and must take into account the experience of the operator in performing the procedure and the risk of potentially serious complications.

There has been recent investigative interest in employing the polymerase chain reaction (PCR) for rapid identification of *S.*

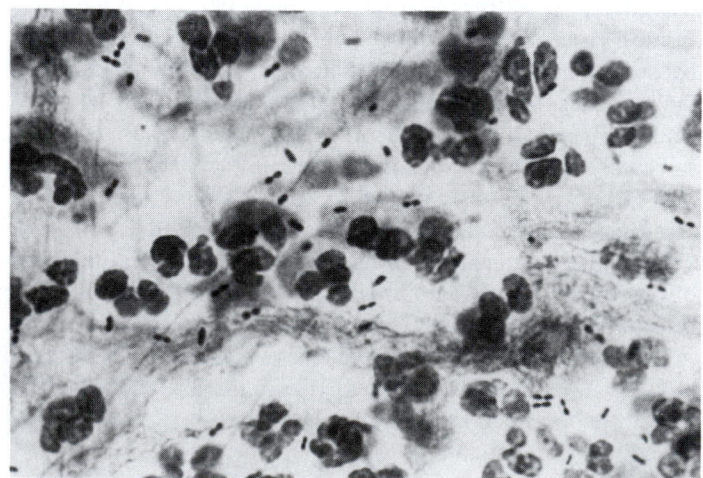

FIGURE 142-1 Sputum Gram's stain from patient with pneumococcal pneumonia. Numerous lancet-shaped diplococci are seen in association with polymorphonuclear leukocytes. ×565.

pneumoniae DNA in acutely infected patients.[18,35,36,44] Various primers have been used to successfully detect *S. pneumoniae* DNA in blood and even sputum, although the application of this promising technique has yet to be rigorously evaluated in large clinical trials, and for the present PCR remains a research tool. The high rate of pneumococcal throat carriage in the general population suggests that the specificity of PCR for testing sputum will be low.

A variety of nonspecific laboratory abnormalities are observed in patients with pneumococcal pneumonia. These include leukocytosis, often with a shift to the left; elevation of the erythrocyte sedimentation rate; and either hypernatremia or hyponatremia, reflecting varying degrees of dehydration, sodium depletion related to fever, vomiting, ileus, or inappropriate secretion of antidiuretic hormone. Arterial blood gases reveal varying degrees of hypoxemia. Leukopenia is sometimes observed in patients with overwhelming infections. Liver function tests are occasionally abnormal, usually in a mixed cholestatic and hepatocellular pattern.

Chest radiographic findings are variable. In patients with full-blown lobar pneumonia, there is opacification of the affected area, and air bronchograms are present (Fig. 142-2). In recent years, lobar pneumonia has been seen less frequently; bronchopneumonia, manifested by multiple patchy infiltrates, has been a common radiographic finding.[31] Pleural effusions are detected in about 10 percent of cases. Necrotizing or cavitating lesions occur only rarely in pneumococcal pneumonia.

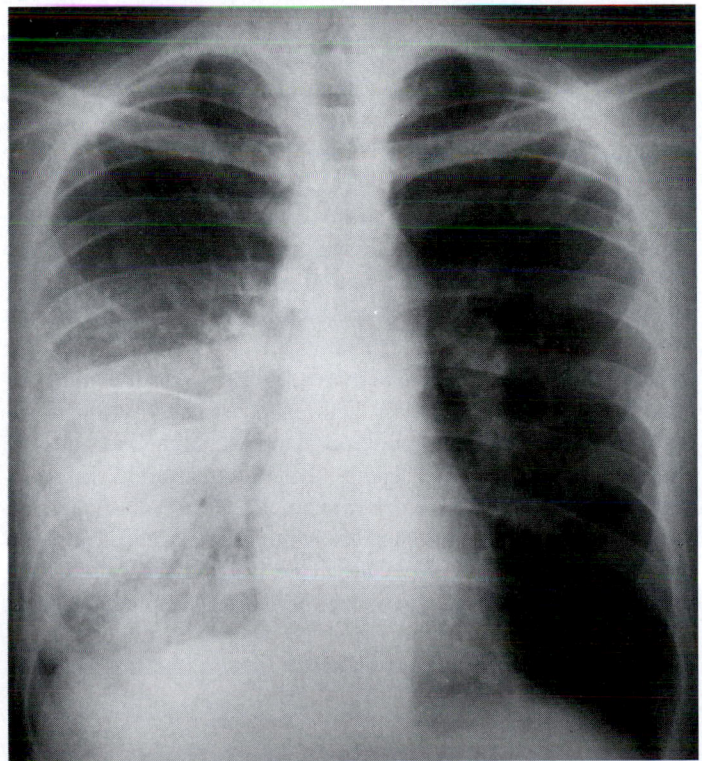

FIGURE 142-2 Chest radiograph from 38-year-old man with bacteremic pneumococcal pneumonia. There is extensive consolidation of right lower lobe with air bronchograms and partial obscuration of the right hemidiaphragm. *(Courtesy of Dr. Cynthia Cofer.)*

Pulmonary infiltrates are often masked in patients who are dehydrated and may not become apparent until the patient receives fluid replacement. Therefore, the absence of an infiltrate on initial chest radiograph does not unequivocally exclude the possibility of pneumonia. Radiographic resolution of pneumococcal pneumonia is often delayed, even when there is prompt clinical improvement.[25] More than one-half of patients have persistent radiographic abnormalities 4 weeks after the episode of pneumonia has resolved. However, if infiltrates persist for more than 8 weeks, the patient should be investigated for specific causes of treatment failure, such as malignancy, empyema, or bronchopleural fistula.

Differential Diagnosis

Pneumonia due to *S. pneumoniae* must be differentiated from that due to other agents that commonly cause community-acquired pulmonary infection, such as *Legionella pneumophila*, *Mycoplasma pneumoniae*, and *Chlamydia pneumoniae* (see Chapters 127 and 145). There are many overlapping features among these diseases.[21,43] Pneumococcal infection characteristically presents with lobar or segmental consolidation. Legionnaires' disease tends to cause patchy, bilateral infiltrates, but severe extrapulmonary manifestations once considered typical of legionnaires' disease clearly are typical only of the more advanced cases and do not distinguish legionnaires' from pneumococcal pneumonia (see Chapter 144). Mycoplasmal and chlamydial pneumonias are usually more indolent illnesses that rarely cause lobar consolidation and occur year-round without any distinct seasonality (see Chapter 145). In some cases, however, *C. pneumoniae* and even *M. pneumoniae* may cause an acute and severe pneumonia.

Several other microorganisms can cause pulmonary infections that simulate pneumococcal pneumonia. *Klebsiella pneumoniae* causes necrotizing lobar pneumonia, often involving the upper lobes; patients may produce an extremely mucoid "currant jelly" type of sputum. *H. influenzae* type b and *Neisseria meningitidis* are less common causes of pneumonia, but pulmonary infections caused by these organisms are clinically indistinguishable from pneumococcal pneumonia. Infections due to *S. aureus*, *S. pyogenes*, or *M. tuberculosis* can at times also mimic pneumococcal pneumonia. In certain hosts, pneumonia due to a variety of gram-negative bacilli, nontypable strains of *H. influenzae*, or anaerobes may also mimic pneumococcal pneumonia. This broad differential diagnosis underscores the importance of obtaining adequate bacteriologic studies in patients with pneumonia.

In addition, several noninfectious diseases must be considered. Pulmonary infarction can cause fever, pleuritic chest pain, dyspnea, and hemoptysis, but the degree of systemic toxicity (chills, high fever, striking leukocytosis) is generally less than in classic pneumococcal lobar pneumonia. Although lung scanning may be helpful in assessing the probability of pulmonary embolism, occasionally pulmonary angiography is necessary to differentiate between pneumonia and infarction. Pneumococcal pneumonia can also be mimicked by pulmonary manifestations of atelectasis, malignancy, systemic lupus erythematosus, congestive heart failure, uremia, or sickle cell disease, and by intra-abdominal infections in the subdiaphragmatic spaces.

Treatment

Pneumococcal pneumonia is a potentially life-threatening illness that requires careful monitoring and appropriate treatment to assure optimal outcome. Most patients require hospitalization, although young, otherwise healthy persons with mild infections can be managed as outpatients. Attention to fluid balance and electrolyte status in those with severe infection is often critical for successful management, especially in the elderly or patients with significant underlying organ system disease, as dehydration and electrolyte imbalance can evolve rapidly, with lethal consequences. For any patient in whom oxygenation is in question, arterial blood gases should be checked and, if significantly impaired, monitored until the patient is clinically improved and out of danger. Supplemental oxygen should be administered as needed.

Pleuritic chest pain can be quite severe, and potent analgesic agents are often necessary to control it. Codeine may suffice in milder cases, but parenteral meperidine or morphine sulfate may be required. In such instances, care should be taken to avoid significant respiratory depression, especially in elderly persons.

Because the indiscriminate use of antipyretics masks the fever curve and subjects the patient to frequent uncomfortable temperature swings, their use should generally be minimized. Certain patients with high and prolonged fever will clearly require judicious use of antipyretics. Otherwise, the primary indication for antipyretics is for the prevention of fever-induced tachycardia in patients who tolerate tachycardia poorly because of cardiac disease or advanced age.

Patients in whom pneumonia is complicated by empyema require drainage procedures in addition to antimicrobial therapy. Thin, free-flowing empyemas may be successfully drained by the traditional chest tube thoracostomy. "Pigtail" catheters placed under radiographic guidance can be used for loculated collections, although multiloculated or thick empyemas often require video-assisted thoracostomy or open drainage procedures.

Strains of *S. pneumoniae* were exquisitely susceptible to penicillin for more than 2 decades after the drug was introduced. Concentrations of less than 0.06 μg/ml were bactericidal, and penicillin was the drug of choice for pneumococcal infections. Strains were typically susceptible to cephalosporins, erythromycin, tetracyclines, clindamycin, and chloramphenicol. As noted above, the antimicrobial susceptibility of *S. pneumoniae* isolates can no longer be taken for granted. The medical literature is replete with descriptions of the increasing numbers of pneumococcal infections caused by antibiotic-resistant strains, and it appears that the trend will continue. Penicillin resistance is defined as relative or intermediate if the minimum inhibitory concentration is 0.1 to 1.0 μg/ml and highly resistant if the MIC is 2.0 μg/ml or greater. The mechanisms of resistance include point mutation in genes for penicillin-binding proteins (PBP), horizontal spread of penicillin-resistant mosaic PBP genes, and acquisition of DNA sequences from heterologous DNA donors that encode for alterations in PBP. Most resistant strains have belonged to serotypes 6, 14, 15, 19, and 23.

In most instances, the initial treatment will be empiric, although clinical and epidemiologic data may suggest the diagnosis of pneumococcal pneumonia. Therapeutic recommendations for initial empiric therapy of etiologically undefined pulmonary infections are discussed in Chapter 122 and elsewhere.[4,8] Penicillin G is the drug of choice for non penicillin-allergic patients whose infection is due to fully penicillin-susceptible strains of *S. pneumoniae*. Such infections may be successfully treated with modest doses of penicillin (e.g., 600,000 units of procaine penicillin intramuscularly every 12 h), and dosages of 1 million units intravenously every 4 to 6 h are adequate even for most relatively penicillin-resistant strains (but see below).[32] Newer penicillins—such as ampicillin-sulbactam, ticarcillin-clavulanate, and piperacillin-tazobactam—offer no advantage over penicillin in the treatment of pneumococcal pneumonia. Cephalosporins such as cefazolin are also effective. Macrolides—popular agents because of their oral bioavailability and their activity against *Mycoplasma*, *Chlamydia*, and *Legionella*—are often effective for treatment of pneumococcal pneumonia, but emerging resistance may limit their use.

For the penicillin-allergic patient, intravenous erythromycin or vancomycin is an appropriate alternative. Oral erythromycin or one of the new macrolides, clarithromycin and azithromycin, can be given to patients who are less acutely ill provided the organism is susceptible. In persons whose allergic history is that of a mild and delayed skin rash, a first-generation cephalosporin may be administered. Cephalosporins should not, however, be used in patients with a history of immediate-type hypersensitivity reaction to β-lactam antibiotics.

Pneumonia caused by relatively resistant strains of *S. pneumoniae* (minimum inhibitory concentration [MIC] of 0.1 to 1 μg/ml) responds to high doses of penicillin G,[32] but if the causative strain is highly resistant (MIC of at least 2 μg/ml), a third-generation cephalosporin, such as cefotaxime or ceftriaxone, imipenem, or vancomycin should be administered.[17] In all cases, the antimicrobial susceptibility of the infecting organism to these alternative agents should be ascertained.[17,19] Certain multiply-resistant strains may be susceptible only to vancomycin. Because of increasing pneumococcal resistance to tetracycline, macrolides, and trimethoprim-sulfamethoxazole, agents often used for empiric therapy of pneumonia because of their broad spectrum of activity, therapy with these agents is not recommended. Currently available quinolines possess limited activity against *S. pneumoniae*, although members of this class with enhanced activity are in development. A new class of antibiotics, the oxazolidinones, possess excellent in vitro activity against penicillin-resistant *S. pneumoniae*, but clinical trials are not yet complete.

In view of the apparent increase in the prevalence of antibiotic-resistant strains of *S. pneumoniae* in the United States, physicians must continue to monitor new developments. As noted, agents in early clinical trials may soon provide alternatives to the armamentarium now available to clinicians treating severe pneumococcal infections.

Pneumococcal Vaccine

Efforts to produce an effective vaccine against *S. pneumoniae* commenced in 1911 and culminated in the licensing of a six-valent vaccine in 1945. Interest in the vaccine waned after penicillin became widely available, and the manufacturer ceased production of the vaccine 2 years later.

Landmark studies conducted between 1952 and 1962 by Austrian and associates led to reconsideration of the role of a pneumococcal vaccine.[5] These studies demonstrated that despite the widespread use of penicillin, the prevalence and case fatality rate of bacteremic pneumococcal infections remained high, particularly among certain high-risk populations. Furthermore, the majority of cases were caused by a limited number of serotypes. New vaccine trials, initiated in the 1970s, demonstrated efficacy rates of up to 92 percent among South African gold miners, and a 14-valent vaccine was licensed in 1977. This was replaced in 1983 by the 23-valent vaccine currently available. The 23 polysaccharide antigens (Danish types 1, 2, 3, 4, 5, 6B, 7F, 8, 9N, 9V, 10A, 11A, 12F, 14, 15B, 17F, 18C, 19A, 19F, 20, 22F, 23F, 33F) represent the serotypes accounting for 85 to 90 percent of cases of pneumococcal bacteremia in the United States.[34]

In recent years, however, new questions have been raised about the efficacy of the pneumococcal vaccine, particularly in the high-risk groups who would benefit most from an effective vaccine. Although the vaccine has been demonstrated to be highly immunogenic and protective in healthy young men, it is less effective in young children, immunocompromised patients, and the elderly. Children under the age of 2 years do not mount an adequate antibody response to polysaccharide antigens, so it is not surprising that the vaccine has been ineffective in this patient population. Studies of vaccine immunogenicity in immunocompromised adults have demonstrated impaired antibody response to pneumococcal polysaccharide in patients with chronic renal failure, multiple myeloma, nephrotic syndrome, renal allografts, and Hodgkin's disease. Moreover, a large cooperative study demonstrated that most "high-risk" persons over the age of 55 (i.e., those with chronic pulmonary, cardiac, hepatic, or renal dysfunction, diabetes mellitus, or alcoholism) who subsequently developed pneumococcal infections had not mounted an adequate antibody response to the vaccine.[38] A meta-analysis of randomized, controlled trials of the efficacy of pneumococcal vaccination in adults has concluded that vaccination of healthy adults reduces both the overall rate of pneumococcal pneumonia and that of infections due to vaccine-containing pneumococcal antigen types, but it has no demonstrable protection for high-risk adults.[16] The authors suggest that the current recommendations to vaccinate high-risk adults but not low-risk adults should be reconsidered.

Despite the vaccine's limited efficacy in high-risk groups, most authorities, including the Immunization Practices Advisory Committee of the Centers for Disease Control and Prevention and the American College of Physicians, continue to recommend its use in patients at increased risk of pneumococcal infection.[1-3] The vaccine is safe, inexpensive, and potentially effective against the vast majority of strains causing bacteremic pneumococcal infections in the United States. Current recommendations call for the immunization of persons over 2 years of age who have sickle cell disease, anatomic or functional asplenia, cerebrospinal fluid leaks, or nephrotic syndrome. Additional indications for immunization in adults include alcoholism, multiple myeloma, Hodgkin's disease, renal failure, chronic cardiac or pulmonary disease, and HIV infection. Despite the theoretical concern that vaccination may stimulate HIV replication, the substantial increase in risk of pneumococcal infections in AIDS patients would seem to outweigh such considerations. To assure an optimal response, it is advisable to immunize HIV-infected patients as early as possible in the course of their infection.[2,26] In addition, it is recommended that all adults over age 65 receive the vaccine.

In view of the difficulty in achieving protective immunity in the populations most at risk, consideration in future may well be given to immunizing healthy adults at an even earlier age than 65. Although the cost-benefit of vaccinating low-risk persons might be questioned, such a strategy would more likely assure the presence of protective immunity in the substantial number of persons who later develop risk factors for invasive pneumococcal infection. Moreover, the worldwide spread of penicillin-resistant *S. pneumoniae* has probably changed the cost-benefit equation in favor of wider use of pneumococcal vaccine.

The vaccine is given as a single intramuscular injection. In about half of vaccine recipients, local tenderness occurs; fewer than 5 percent develop transient fever or myalgias. Adverse effects on the fetus have not been reported in women receiving pneumococcal vaccine during pregnancy. Thus, unimmunized pregnant women with conditions placing them at high risk for pneumococcal infection may be vaccinated, although it is preferable to do so after the first trimester.[3] Because detectable antibody responses to pneumococcal polysaccharide gradually decline, reimmunization after 6 years is recommended by the American College of Physicians[3] for adults at highest risk of serious or fatal infection (e.g., surgical or functional hyposplenism) and for patients suffering from conditions in which rapid decreases in pneumococcal antibody levels have been shown (e.g., nephrotic syndrome, renal failure, and organ transplantation).

Vaccines based on conjugates of pneumococcal polysaccharide covalently linked to a protein carrier, similar to the successful *H. influenzae* b conjugate vaccine, are under development. It is hoped that such a vaccine will soon be available, making possible the routine vaccination of infants under 2 years, an age group at high risk of pneumococcal infection.

STAPHYLOCOCCUS AUREUS

Staphylococcal pneumonia is a relatively uncommon disease that nevertheless occurs in a wide variety of clinical settings and has protean clinical manifestations. In its most severe form, it is a fulminating, devastating illness that is associated with high mortality rate.

Microbiology

S. aureus is a gram-positive coccus that measures 0.8 to 1.0 μm in diameter and often occurs in grapelike clusters. When grown on blood agar plates, colonies appear smooth and round, measure 1 to 4 mm in diameter, and are usually golden yellow. Staphylococci produce a variety of toxins and extracellular enzymes; the presence of the extracellular enzyme coagulase enables the rapid differentiation of *S. aureus* from other species of staphylococci.

Epidemiology

S. aureus is a ubiquitous microorganism that frequently colonizes human skin and mucous membranes. Approximately 15 percent of adults are persistent nasal carriers, and transient carriage is common among the rest of the population. Most cases of staphylococcal pneumonia are presumed to occur in previously colonized subjects. Several studies have emphasized the role of *S. aureus* as a cause of nosocomial pneumonia, particularly among intubated neurosurgical patients. In such cases, spread from colonized hospital personnel to patients is likely. In previously healthy children or adults, staphylococcal pneumonia occurs as a complication of influenza A infection. There have been rare reports of transmission of *S. aureus* via droplet spread of the organisms from colonized infants who developed concomitant viral upper respiratory infections.

Pathophysiology

Staphylococcal infection can be established in the lower respiratory tract via either of two mechanisms. Bronchogenic spread of organisms results from aspiration of infected nasopharyngeal secretions into the lungs and is the basis of postinfluenza pneumonia. Persons with anatomic abnormalities of the respiratory tract and those who are immunosuppressed because of underlying diseases or immunosuppressive medications are also predisposed to infection by the bronchogenic route.

Hematogenous spread results from the release of staphylococci into the bloodstream from an intravascular focus. Organisms are transported via the pulmonary circulation to one or more areas of the lung, where infection is established. Persons at high risk for hematogenous staphylococcal pneumonia include intravenous drug abusers, hemodialysis patients, persons with infected intravascular devices, and patients with suppurative thrombophlebitis or tricuspid endocarditis.

Regardless of the route of entry, *S. aureus* elicits an intense inflammatory response in the lung, manifested by polymorphonuclear leukocytic infiltration, local edema, and hemorrhage. In severe infections, there is extensive tissue necrosis with destruction of alveolar walls. Because inhaled air can enter these damaged alveoli but cannot escape, air-filled cavities are sometimes created. Thin-walled air-filled cavities called *pneumatoceles* are highly characteristic of staphylococcal pneumonia, particularly in children. In adults, thick-walled abscess cavities are a more common finding.

Clinical Manifestations

The clinical presentation of staphylococcal pneumonia is highly variable, depending on the age and previous health of the patient. Because there are no unique manifestations of staphylococcal pneumonia to differentiate it from other bacterial pneumonias, correct diagnosis requires a high index of suspicion.

In children less than 1 year old, staphylococcal pneumonia is almost always related to an antecedent episode of influenza or measles and is manifested by an unexpected deterioration in the infant's condition shortly after an upper respiratory infection.

Typical findings include high fever, tachypnea, grunting respirations, and cough. Examination usually reveals diminished breath sounds and localized rales over the area of involvement. Pleural effusions occur in most cases, and empyema and pneumothorax are not uncommon.

Similarly, staphylococcal pneumonia in previously healthy adults almost always occurs as a complication of influenza A. In a classic monograph published in 1919, Chickering and Park were the first to provide a detailed description of the clinical features of postinfluenza staphylococcal pneumonia. Their observations, quoted below, remain pertinent today.

> The onset of *S. aureus* pneumonia is almost always insidious and rarely accompanied by the chill and localized pain of a typical lobar pneumonia, though the course of the disease is extremely rapid. The facies, the anxious expression, and deep cyanosis suggest a grave prognosis from the onset, at a period when physical signs of pulmonary involvement are but scanty. Herpetic eruptions on the lips are scarcely ever noted, nor is delirium present except rarely. Usually the mind is clear almost to the end. Occasionally pleuritic pain is complained of, but this is not usual. It is the picture of a general septicemia. The fever on the whole is high, ranging between 104 and 106, with frequent remissions to 101. These patients rarely have the painful and labored breathing seen in pneumococcus infections.
>
> Clinical examination of the chest of the average case reveals a very atypical type of pneumonic involvement. Signs of congestion of both lower lobes are found frequently, though in the majority of cases a diffuse process in all the lobes may be present. At the onset, only slightly diminished resonance to percussion may be elicited, with diminished breath sounds and many coarse and fine moist rales. But rarely are there signs of pure consolidation of one or more lobes, and then only late in the disease. Frequently there is an abundance of coarse moist rales heard throughout the chest.[14]

Staphylococcal pneumonia is not always associated with an antecedent viral infection. It may occur, apparently de novo, in chronically ill or immunocompromised patients, and it is one of the leading causes of pneumonia among intubated patients in intensive care units.[30] The clinical picture in such patients ranges from a subacute, smoldering infection to an acute, life-threatening illness as described above. In all forms of staphylococcal pneumonia, pleural effusion and empyema are common complications. Bacteremia has been reported in approximately 20 percent of cases.

Patients who acquire staphylococcal pneumonia by the hematogenous route typically have a subacute pulmonary illness manifested by fever, cough, and dyspnea. They occasionally develop hemoptysis or pleuritic chest pain. The illness tends to be milder than bronchogenic pneumonia.

Diagnosis

Initial presumptive diagnosis hinges on the epidemiologic and clinical features of the case and on accurate interpretation of the sputum Gram's stain. The latter characteristically reveals gram-positive cocci in clusters or tetrads in close association with polymorphonuclear leukocytes (Fig. 142-3). Because the organisms often remain viable for several hours after phagocytosis, intracellular bacteria are occasionally observed.

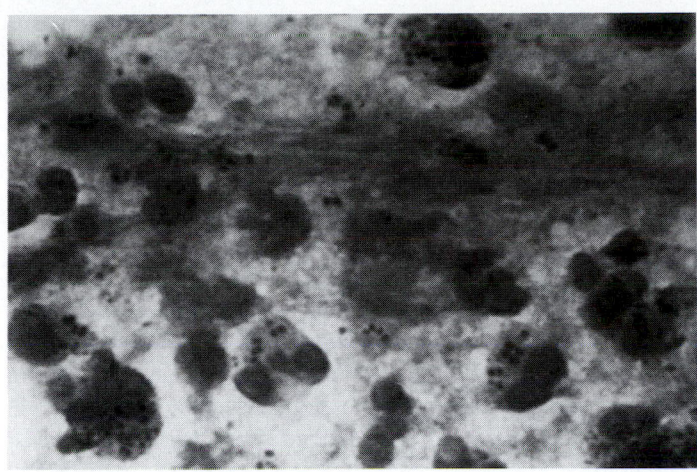

FIGURE 142-3 Sputum Gram's stain from a patient with staphylococcal pneumonia, demonstrating numerous intracellular cocci in tetrads and clusters. ×565.

Confirmation of the diagnosis of staphylococcal pneumonia requires isolation of the organism from blood, pleural fluid, or lung tissue, although such evidence is frequently lacking.

Radiographic abnormalities are variable. Most commonly, single or multiple patchy areas of bronchopneumonia appear; they rapidly enlarge, cavitate, and form air-filled cavities (either pneumatoceles or thick-walled abscess cavities) (Figs. 142-4 and 142-5). Localized areas of consolidation are relatively unusual. Pleural effusions are common, particularly in infants.

Treatment

Patients with staphylococcal pneumonia are usually critically ill. Even with appropriate therapy, the death rate can be as high as 50 percent. As with pneumococcal pneumonia, successful management requires both intensive supportive care and appropriate antimicrobial therapy.

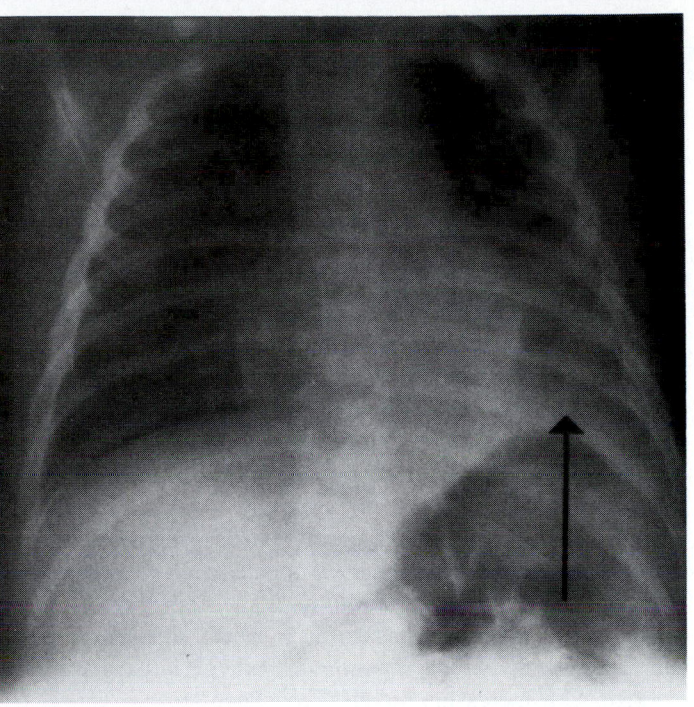

FIGURE 142-5 Chest radiograph from 1-month-old boy with staphylococcal pneumonia in the left lower lobe. A large pneumatocele is present (arrow), with two superimposed smaller pneumatoceles. *(Courtesy of Dr. Sarah Fitch.)*

Despite the availability of a variety of effective antimicrobial agents, treatment of staphylococcal pneumonia is often challenging, in part because of variable antibiotic resistance patterns. Although penicillin is the agent of choice against susceptible strains, almost all strains of *S. aureus* are now highly penicillin-resistant owing to plasmid-mediated penicillinase production. Therefore, initial therapy of staphylococcal pneumonia should always include a penicillinase-resistant penicillin (nafcillin or oxacillin), a cephalosporin such as cefazolin (but see caveat be-

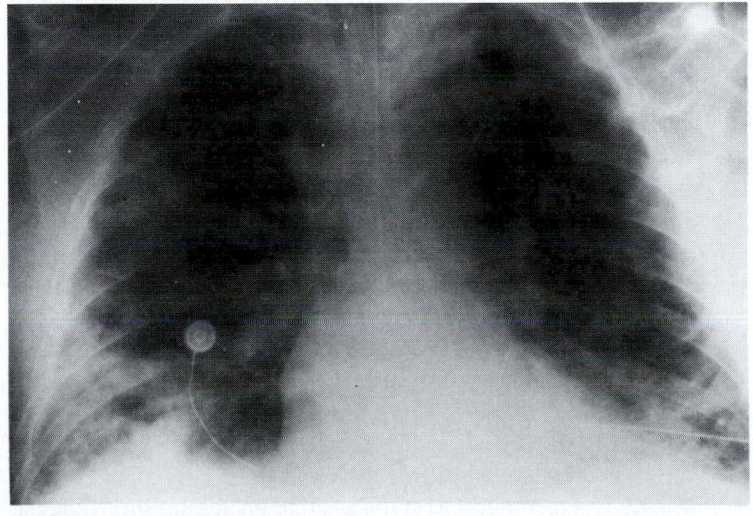

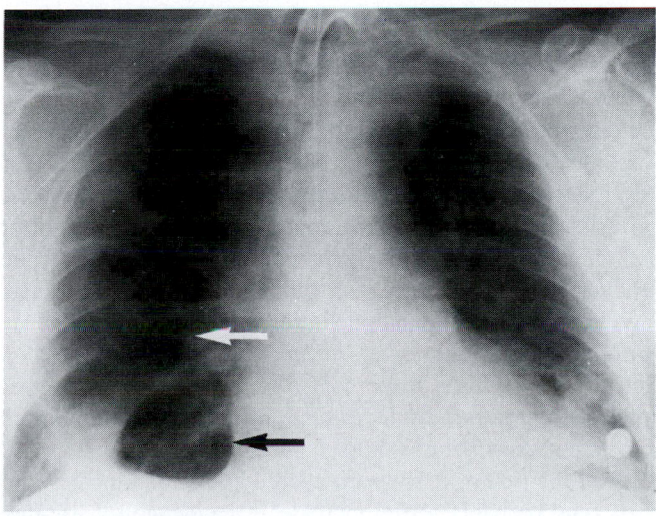

A

B

FIGURE 142-4 Serial chest radiographs from 58-year-old man with bronchogenic staphylococcal pneumonia superimposed on chemical pneumonitis secondary to inhalation of ammonia and chlorine gas. *A.*

Infiltrates in both lower lobes and right midlung field with early cavitation in right lower lobe. *B.* Same patient 18 days later. Note two large pneumatoceles.

low regarding methicillin-resistant strains), or vancomycin, any of which is highly active against *S. aureus*. Specific therapy can then be instituted once the results of antimicrobial susceptibility testing are available. The recommended dose of the penicillinase-resistant penicillins is 1.5 to 2 g intravenously every 4 h and of cefazolin, 1 to 2 g intravenously every 8 h. Vancomycin may be given to adults with normal renal function at a dose of 500 mg intravenously every 6 h or 1 g every 12 h. The optimum duration of antimicrobial therapy has not been established. Because staphylococcal pneumonia tends to be a serious, deep-seated infection that is slow to respond to therapy, a 4-week course of antibiotics may be required. If the patient's condition improves promptly, treatment can be completed with dicloxacillin, an oral agent that is well absorbed and attains high blood levels.

Penicillin-allergic patients can be treated cautiously with a first-generation cephalosporin, using the guidelines set forth above. If there is a history of an immediate hypersensitivity reaction, vancomycin is the agent of choice.

The emergence of methicillin-resistant strains of *S. aureus* (MRSA) in recent years has posed a special therapeutic problem. They are important nosocomial pathogens that have been reported with increasing frequency.[23] Such strains represent a small but possibly increasing proportion of isolates in the community. MRSA are resistant to all penicillins and cephalosporins. The agent of choice for the treatment of MRSA infections is vancomycin, to which such organisms have been universally susceptible.

Adding gentamicin to the treatment regimen has been shown to enhance bactericidal activity against *S. aureus* in the laboratory and hasten the clinical response of bacteremic infections. Although combination therapy for severe pneumonia is intuitively attractive, there are no data to support this approach. Rifampin, which is active against staphylococci, penetrates well into leukocytes and tissues, and has been used at times as ancillary therapy for staphylococcal infections. Its role, if any, in treatment of life-threatening cases of staphylococcal pneumonia remains undefined.

STREPTOCOCCUS PYOGENES

Pneumonia due to *S. pyogenes* was once a common epidemic infection among military recruits,[9] but it has become a rare entity since the advent of penicillin. Streptococcal pneumonia is usually related to an antecedent episode of influenza, measles, or varicella. The illness is characterized by the abrupt onset of fever and chills, followed by dyspnea, cough, blood-streaked sputum production, and pleuritic chest pain. Chest radiographs generally reveal evidence of bronchopneumonia; lobar consolidation is uncommon. Bacteremia is present in approximately 10 to 15 percent of cases. Up to 40 percent of patients develop empyema, which is manifested by large pleural effusions containing thin, serosanguineous pleural fluid.

Over the past 5 to 10 years, there has been an increase in reports (and probably a true increase in incidence) of life-threatening invasive group A streptococcal infections in many parts of the world. Although such infections usually affect skin and soft tissues, there have been reported instances of streptococcal pneumonia as well. For example, during the first 6 months of 1988,

group A streptococcal pneumonia, a previously very rare entity, was diagnosed in 20 patients in Norway.[29] Many pneumonia cases have also been reported in nursing homes in the United States.[13]

Fortunately, in sharp contrast to pneumococci and staphylococci, all strains of *S. pyogenes* remain exquisitely susceptible to penicillin. Appropriate therapy of streptococcal pneumonia includes administration of aqueous penicillin G, 6 to 12 million units per day divided into four to six intravenous injections, and chest tube drainage of empyema fluid as needed. In patients manifesting the hypotension and multiorgan failure characteristic of the streptococcal toxic shock syndrome, intravenous clindamycin should be added.[39] Therapeutic options in the penicillin-allergic patient are identical to those described above for pneumococcal pneumonia.

Group B streptococcus *(S. agalactiae)* is a well-recognized cause of infections, including pneumonia, in neonates and of puerperal sepsis in mothers. This organism also causes invasive infections in nonpregnant adults. Group B streptococcus has occasionally been reported to cause nosocomial pneumonia in elderly patients, sometimes in association with concomitant *S. aureus* pulmonary infection.[42] The organism is uniformly susceptible to penicillin, although MICs are four- to 10-fold higher (range 0.01 to 0.04 μg/ml) than for group A streptococcus.

RHODOCOCCUS EQUI

The AIDS epidemic has raised *R. equi* from relative obscurity as a rare cause of pneumonia among immunosuppressed persons to a well-recognized opportunistic pathogen that will be encountered from time to time in most medical centers throughout the world. It is a well-known cause of bronchopneumonia in foals and of serious infections in other livestock. Formerly known as *Corynebacterium equi*, the genus was changed to *Rhodococcus*, meaning "red-pigmented coccus."[33] Several other *Rhodococcus* species have been identified as a cause of human infection, although collectively they remain rarely recognized pathogens.

Historical Review

Magnusson first identified *R. equi* as a pathogen when he isolated the organism from the lungs of 10 foals. Not until 1967 was infection in a human reported. Relatively few cases were reported until AIDS became prevalent in the 1980s; it is no longer considered a rare pathogen in patients with this disease. Nearly all reported infections have been in immunosuppressed persons. There are a handful of reports of extrapulmonary infection: endophthalmitis, mycetoma, and osteomyelitis have occurred in the absence of pulmonary disease.

Microbiology

R. equi is a pleomorphic gram-positive bacterium that varies in morphology from a long, curved, clublike rod to a coccus. It is an aerobic, nonmotile, non–spore-forming organism that grows well on standard media such as blood agar or brain-heart infusion to produce irregularly shaped, salmon-colored mucoid colonies. Infection is often associated with bacteremia, and *R. equi* is readily detected in blood culture systems. It also can be isolated from sputum of patients with pneumonia, although the colonies may be misinterpreted as normal flora if the laboratory is not alerted to screen for *R. equi*. Lack of carbohydrate fermentation and liquefaction of gelatin distinguish *R. equi* from other corynebacteria. It is acid-fast with both Kinyoun and modified Kinyoun staining methods when grown on Löwenstein-Jensen medium, whereas organisms grown on blood agar and other nutrient media are often not acid-fast. Capsular antigens can be used to differentiate most isolates into one of seven types, although little is known about the correlation of serotyping with virulence properties. Many clinical isolates possess plasmids that express cell surface antigens associated with virulence in murine infection and, presumably, humans.

Epidemiology

There is controversy over the natural ecology of *R. equi*. It has been isolated from soil, especially from animal runs, and less frequently from soil not in contact with animals, throughout the world, but also from the intestinal contents of horses, cattle, pigs, and other mammals; it has even been isolated from the intestinal tract of humans. Foals less than 6 months of age are at particular risk for lethal bronchopneumonia. *R. equi* is a major cause of morbidity and mortality in these animals; it may also cause urogenital and lymphatic infections in older horses as well as cattle, swine, and sheep. Many humans with infection report contact with farm animals or soil frequented by animals, although a history of such contact is not invariable.

Pathophysiology

R. equi infects macrophage and polymorphonuclear cells, a trophism attributed to binding of the third component of complement to Mac-1, a receptor expressed mainly by these two cells. Most infections with *R. equi* involve the lung, and it is presumed that the process starts with inhalation of organisms that lodge in alveoli or small bronchioles. Replication takes place within macrophages and leukocytes. The fact that nearly all human infections have occurred among persons with severe deficiency of cellular immune function suggests that cellular rather than humoral host defenses are critical in the control of *R. equi*. The infection is characterized by an extensive influx of polymorphonuclear leukocytes, necrosis, and abscess formation.[37] Elements of granulomatous reaction, including giant-cell formation, may be present adjacent to the acute inflammation.

Clinical Manifestations

The onset of *R. equi* pneumonia is typically gradual; fever, fatigue, cough, and slowly progressive dyspnea are the characteristic but nonspecific symptoms. The temperature curve varies widely from patient to patient, and even for an individual patient the curve may range from low-grade to a hectic pattern with spikes of more than 39°C. The cough may be either dry or productive; the sputum is often purulent and may be frankly bloody. Chest pain is not uncommon. Symptoms in many of the cases

reported have been present for several weeks before the diagnosis is established. Any lobe may be affected; extension to adjacent lobes occurs with time if the disease is not treated. Extension to the pleura, with secondary effusions and/or empyema, is common in untreated infection. Secondary bacteremia and metastatic infection elsewhere may also occur.

The chest radiographic findings evolve from a localized, solid infiltrate to several areas of consolidation, which may invade adjacent lung tissue or other lobes. Cavitation develops in approximately 50 percent of cases, and pleural effusions are common. The appearance of *R. equi* pneumonia is often reminiscent of tuberculosis or nocardiosis.

An indolent and progressive course, with a tendency to persist in spite of intense, prolonged antibiotic therapy, is characteristic of *R. equi* infection. Necrosis, with destruction of lung tissue and cavity formation, is typical. As noted above, the infection may spread locally to the pleural space, and metastases to the brain and bone have been observed.

Diagnosis

Culture of *R. equi* from sputum, blood, or other specimens—such as lung tissue, pleural fluid, and abscesses in other organs—is the mainstay of diagnosis. Although *R. equi* has been isolated from human feces, it is not a recognized constituent of normal human flora. Identification of *R. equi* in clinical specimens from any patient with pneumonia is indicative of its causative role. Occasionally it may be confused with nonpathogenic diphtheroids, and any report of *Corynebacterium* species or diphtheroids in clinical specimens from an immunosuppressed patient with pneumonia should prompt a request to the laboratory for definitive identification.

Treatment

Erythromycin, vancomycin, aminoglycosides, doxycycline, clindamycin, rifampin, and sulfamethoxazole are active against *R. equi* in vitro. Isolates from soil but not from humans are also susceptible to penicillins and cephalosporins. The poor response of many infections has prompted experimentation with combinations of antibiotics. Although a combination such as rifampin and erythromycin is frequently recommended, an optimal regimen has not been determined.

Azithromycin and clarithromycin, two macrolide antimicrobials that are concentrated within white blood cells, are theoretically attractive agents for treatment of *R. equi*, but experience is limited. The response to treatment is slow and frequently incomplete. Because of incomplete clearing of pneumonia with weeks of antibiotic treatment, surgical resection of the affected lobe has been performed in many cases.[20]

BACILLUS ANTHRACIS

Inhalation anthrax (woolsorters' disease) is a rare entity that is primarily of historical interest.[12] Fewer than 20 cases have been reported in the United States in the 20th century. The disease occurs sporadically (or, rarely, in epidemics) as a result of inhalation of *B. anthracis* spores from imported goat hair. It primarily afflicts textile mill workers, tannery employees, or laboratory personnel.

Following inhalation of *B. anthracis* spores into the alveoli, the spores are ingested by alveolar macrophages and transported to the mediastinal lymph nodes. Organisms rapidly multiply and produce toxin, which causes extensive mediastinal edema, hemorrhage, and necrosis. The organisms then enter the bloodstream and are widely disseminated; meningeal involvement occurs in approximately 50 percent of cases.

Inhalation anthrax is a biphasic illness. The initial phase consists of nonspecific flulike symptoms, including low-grade fever, malaise, myalgias, nonproductive cough, and occasionally a sensation of chest pressure. After a few days, the patient's condition spontaneously improves, only to enter the second phase of the illness and deteriorate abruptly. At this stage of the disease, there is prominent dyspnea and occasionally stridor due to tracheal compression by enlarged mediastinal nodes. Vasomotor collapse often ensues rapidly. Chest radiographs almost always reveal prominent widening of the mediastinum.

Because of the rarity of this disease, there have been no controlled trials to guide treatment decisions. Recommended therapy consists of intravenous aqueous penicillin G, 2 million units every 2 h. Even with aggressive treatment, however, few patients survive.

REFERENCES

1. Advisory Committee on Immunization Practices of the Centers for Disease Control and Prevention: Pneumococcal polysaccharide vaccine. *MMWR* 38:64–68, 73–76, 1989.

2. Advisory Committee on Immunization Practices of the Centers for Disease Control and Prevention: Use of vaccines and immune globulins for persons with altered immunocompetence. *MMWR* 42:1–18, 1993.

3. American College of Physicians Task Force on Adult Immunizations and Infectious Disease Society of America. *Guide for Adult Immunization.* Philadelphia: American College of Physicians, 1994.

4. American Thoracic Society: Guidelines for the initial management of adults with community-acquired pneumonia: Diagnosis, assessment of severity, and initial antimicrobial therapy. *Am Rev Respir Dis* 148:1418–1426, 1993.

5. Austrian R: Pneumococcal pneumonia: Diagnostic, epidemiologic, therapeutic and prophylactic considerations. *Chest* 90:738–743, 1986.

6. Austrian R, Gold J: Pneumococcal bacteremia with especial reference to bacteremic pneumococcal pneumonia. *Ann Intern Med* 60:759–776, 1964.

7. Barrett-Connor E: The non-value of sputum culture in the diagnosis of pneumococcal pneumonia. *Am Rev Respir Dis* 103:845–848, 1971.

8. Bartlett JG, Mundy LM: Community-acquired pneumonia. *New Engl J Med* 333:1618–1624, 1995.

9. Basiliere IL, Bistrong HW, Spence WF: Streptococcal pneumonia: Recent outbreaks in military recruit populations. *Am J Med* 44:580–589, 1968.

10. Boerner DF, Zwadyk P: The value of the sputum Gram's stain in community-acquired pneumonia. *JAMA* 247:642–645, 1982.

11. Boulnois GJ: Pneumococcal proteins and the pathogenesis of disease caused by *Streptococcus pneumoniae. J Gen Microbiol* 138: 249–259, 1992.

12. Brachman PS: Inhalation anthrax. *Ann NY Acad Sci* 353:83–93, 1980.

13. Centers for Disease Control and Prevention: Nursing home outbreaks of invasive group A streptococcal infections—Illinois, Kansas, North Carolina, and Texas. *MMWR* 29:577–579, 1990.

14. Chickering HT, Park JH: *Staphylococcus aureus* pneumonia. *JAMA* 72:617–626, 1919.

15. Cundell D, Masure HR: The molecular basis of pneumococcal infection: A hypothesis. *Clin Infect Dis* 21:S204–S212, 1995.

16. Fine MJ, Smith MA, Carson CA, et al: Efficacy of pneumococcal vaccination in adults: A meta-analysis of randomized controlled trials. *Arch Intern Med* 154:2666–2677, 1994.

17. Friedland IR, McCracken GH Jr: Management of infections caused by antibiotic-resistant *Streptococcus pneumoniae. New Engl J Med* 331:377–382, 1994.

18. Gillespie SH, Ullman C, Smith MD, Emery V: Detection of *Streptococcus pneumoniae* in sputum samples by PCR. *J Clin Microbiol* 32:1308–1311, 1994.

19. Haas DW, Stratton CW, Griffin JP, et al: Diminished activity of ceftizoxime in comparison to cefotaxime and ceftriaxone against *Streptococcus pneumoniae. Clin Infect Dis* 20:671–676, 1995.

20. Harvey RL, Sunstrum JC: *Rhodococcus equi* infection in patients with and without human immunodeficiency virus infection. *Rev Infect Dis* 13:139–145, 1991.

21. Helms CM, Viner JP, Sturm RH, et al: Comparative features of pneumococcal, mycoplasmal, and Legionnaires' disease pneumonias. *Ann Intern Med* 90:543–547, 1979.

22. Hendley JO, Sande MA, Stewart PM, Gwaltney JM: Spread of *Streptococcus pneumoniae* in families: I. Carriage rates and distribution of types. *J Infect Dis* 132:55–61, 1975.

23. Iwahara T, Ichiyama S, Nada T, et al: Clinical and epidemiologic investigations of nosocomial pulmonary infections caused by methicillin-resistant *Staphylococcus aureus. Chest* 105:826–831, 1994.

24. Janoff EN, Breiman RF, Daley CL, Hopewell PC: Pneumococcal disease during HIV infection: Epidemiologic, clinical, and immunologic perspectives. *Ann Intern Med* 117:314–324, 1992.

25. Jay SJ, Johanson WG, Pierce AK: The radiographic resolution of *Streptococcus pneumoniae* pneumonia. *New Engl J Med* 293: 798–801, 1975.

26. Kaplan JE, Masur H, Holmes KK, et al, and USPHS/IDSA Prevention of Opportunistic Infections Working Group: USPHS/IDSA guidelines for the prevention of opportunistic infections in persons infected with human immunodeficiency virus: An overview. *Clin Infect Dis* 21:S12–S31, 1995.

27. Macfarlane JT, Finch RG, Ward MJ, Macrae AD: Hospital study of adult community-acquired pneumonia. *Lancet* 2:255–258, 1982.

28. Mandigers CM, Diepersloot RJ, Dessens M, et al: A hospital outbreak of penicillin-resistant pneumococci in the Netherlands. *Eur Respir J* 7:1635–1639, 1994.

29. Martin PR, Hoiby EA: Streptococcal serogroup A epidemic in Norway, 1987–88. *Scand J Infect Dis* 22:421–429, 1990.

30. Musher DM, Lamm N, Darouiche RO, et al: The current spectrum of *Staphylococcus aureus* infection in a tertiary care hospital. *Medicine* 73:186–208, 1994.

31. Ort S, Ryan JL, Barden G, D'Esopo N: Pneumococcal pneumonia in hospitalized patients: Clinical and radiological presentations. *JAMA* 249:214–218, 1983.

32. Pallares R, Linares J, Vadillo M, et al: Resistance to penicillin and cephalosporin and mortality from severe pneumococcal pneumonia in Barcelona, Spain. *New Engl J Med* 333:474–480, 1995.

33. Prescott JF: *Rhodococcus equi:* An animal and human pathogen. *Clin Microbiol Rev* 4:20–34, 1991.

34. Robbins JB, Austrian R, Lee CJ, et al: Considerations for formulating the second-generation pneumococcal capsular polysaccharide vaccine with emphasis on the cross-reactive types within groups. *J Infect Dis* 148:1136–1159, 1983.

35. Rudolph KM, Parkinson AJ, Black CM, Mayer LW: Evaluation of polymerase chain reaction for diagnosis of pneumococcal pneumonia. *J Clin Microbiol* 31:2661–2666, 1993.

36. Salo P, Ortqvist A, Leinonen M: Diagnosis of bacteremic pneumococcal pneumonia by amplification of pneumolysin gene fragment in serum. *J Infect Dis* 171:479–482, 1995.

37. Scott MA, Graham BS, Verrall R, et al: *Rhodococcus equi*—An increasingly recognized opportunistic pathogen: Report of 12 cases and review of 65 cases in the literature. *Am J Clin Pathol* 103:649–655, 1995.

38. Simberkoff MS, Cross AP, al-Ibrahim M, et al: Efficacy of pneumococcal vaccine in high-risk patients: Results of a Veterans' Administration Cooperative Study. *New Engl J Med* 315:1318–1327, 1986.

39. Stevens DL, Gibbons AE, Bergstrom R, Winn V: The Eagle effect revisited: Efficacy of clindamycin, erythromycin, and penicillin in the treatment of streptococcal myositis. *J Infect Dis* 158:23–28, 1988.

40. The British Thoracic Society and the Public Health Laboratory Service: Community-acquired pneumonia in adults in British hospitals in 1982–83: A survey of aetiology, mortality, prognostic factors and outcome. *Q J Med* 62:195–220, 1987.

41. Tuomanen EI, Austrian R, Masure HR: Pathogenesis of pneumococcal infection. *New Engl J Med* 332:1280–1284, 1995.

42. Verghese A, Berk SL, Boelen LJ, Smith JK: Group B streptococcal pneumonia in the elderly. *Arch Intern Med* 142:1642–1645, 1982.

43. Woodhead MA, Macfarlane JT: Comparative clinical and laboratory features of legionella with pneumococcal and mycoplasma pneumonias. *Br J Dis Chest* 81:133–139, 1987.

44. Zhang Y, Isaacman DJ, Wadowsky RM, et al: Detection of *Streptococcus pneumoniae* in whole blood by PCR. *J Clin Microbiol* 33:596–601, 1995.

CHAPTER 143

NOSOCOMIAL RESPIRATORY TRACT INFECTIONS AND GRAM-NEGATIVE PNEUMONIA

David J. Weber / William A. Rutala / C. Glen Mayhall

Nosocomial pneumonia is the second leading cause of hospital-acquired infection and accounts for approximately 19 percent of all nosocomial infections in the United States.[7] It has been estimated that there are 150,000 to 200,000 nosocomial respiratory tract infections per year in the United States. Nosocomial pneumonia results in an average of 5.9 extra hospital days at a cost of $5683 in 1992 dollars.[22] Overall, nosocomial pneumonia results in an estimated 7087 deaths and contributes to 22,983 deaths per year in the United States.[22]

Nosocomial pneumonia has been defined as an infection of the lung parenchyma that was neither present nor incubating at the time of hospital admission. This chapter will review the epidemi-ology, pathophysiology, etiology, and treatment of nosocomial pneumonia and strategies to prevent it. Clinicians will need to adapt the treatment recommendations and preventive strategies to their own institutions, as the routes of infection and agents causing pneumonia vary considerably among health-care facilities.

PATHOGENESIS

The pathogenesis of nosocomial pneumonia has been extensively reviewed.[5,6,9,15,16] Bacteria may invade the lower respiratory tract by three major routes: aspiration of oropharyngeal flora, inhalation of infected aerosols, and, less frequently, hematogenous spread from a remote focus of infection (Fig. 143-1). Recently, investigators have proposed bacterial translocation from the gastrointestinal tract as an additional mechanism of infection.[6]

The major cause of nosocomial pneumonia is believed to be colonization of the oropharynx and gastrointestinal tract by pathogenic microorganisms, followed by aspiration of these pathogens, and the development of pneumonia in the setting of impaired host defenses (see Chapter 119). Aspiration of oropharyngeal secretions has been noted in approximately 45 percent of normal subjects during sleep. In normal subjects, however, the volumes of aspirate are small and the aspirated flora are generally nonpathogenic. Several factors that commonly occur in hospitalized patients are associated with an increased frequency or volume of aspiration: altered consciousness, abnormal swallowing, depressed gag reflexes, delayed gastric emptying, and decreased gastrointestinal motility (see Chapter 129).[15] Oropharyngeal colonization with aerobic gram-negative bacilli is favored by coma, hypotension, acidosis, azotemia, alcoholism, diabetes mellitus, leukocytosis, leukopenia, pulmonary disease, use of nasogastric or endotracheal tubes, and antibiotic use.[57] Thus, hospitalized patients, especially those in intensive care units, have an increased frequency of oropharyngeal colonization by more pathogenic aerobic gram-negative bacilli and are often at increased risk for aspirating this more pathogenic flora.

The importance of oropharyngeal colonization in nosocomial pneumonia was elegantly demonstrated by Johanson and colleagues, who showed that pneumonia occurred in 23 percent of

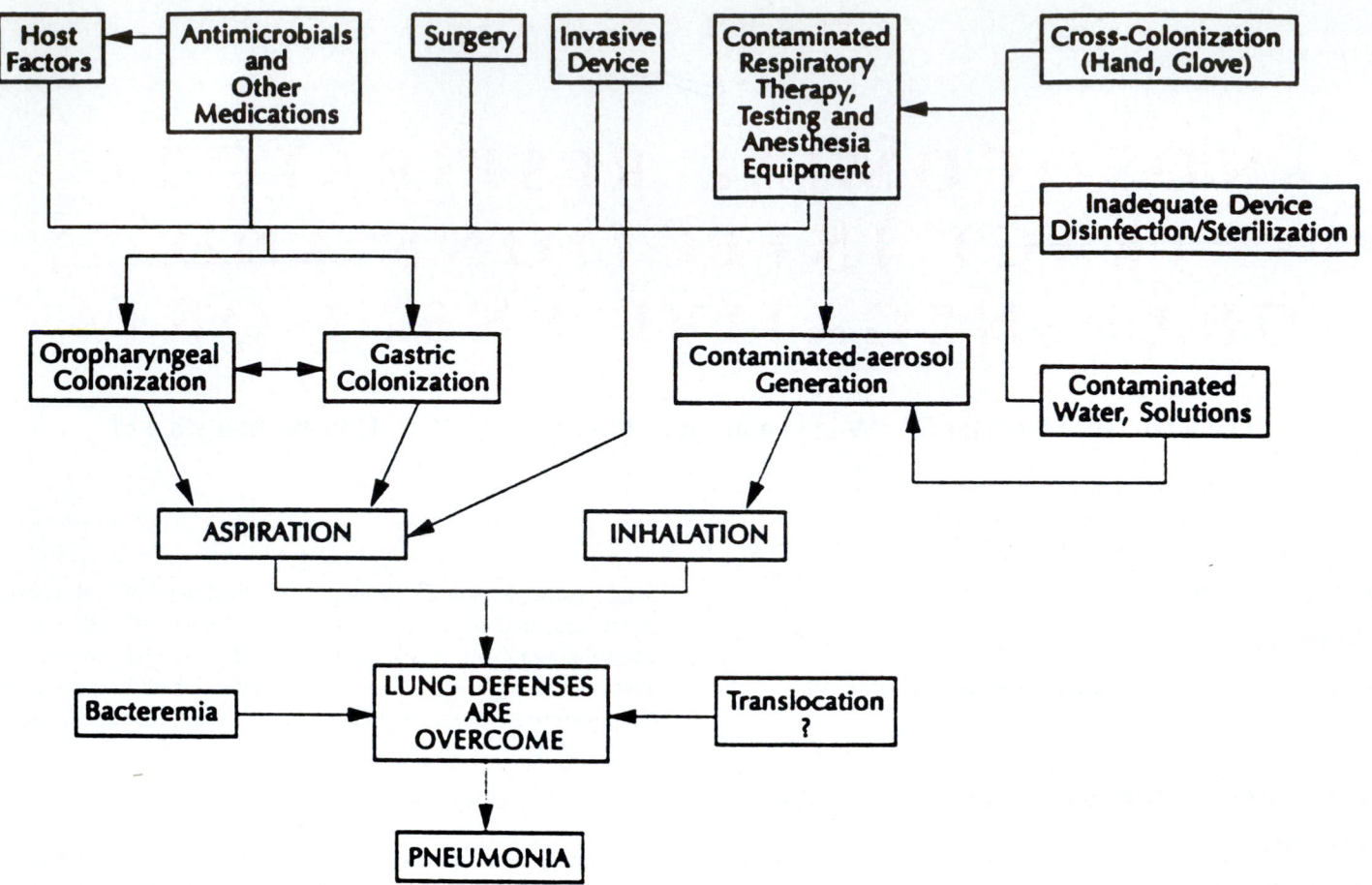

FIGURE 143-1   Pathogenesis of nosocomial bacterial pneumonia. *(Based on data of Tablan et al,[57] with permission.)*

patients colonized with aerobic gram-negative bacilli but only 3 percent of noncolonized patients.[37] More recently, the stomach has been postulated as an important reservoir of organisms capable of causing nosocomial pneumonia. Normally, the stomach is rendered sterile by hydrochloric acid; however, elevations of gastric pH from normal levels to levels at or above 4 allow microorganisms to multiply to high concentrations. Elevated gastric pH may occur in patients with advanced age, achlorhydria, ileus, or upper gastrointestinal disease, and in patients receiving enteral feeding, antacids, or histamine$_2$ (H$_2$) antagonists.[57]

Intubation for respiratory support is the most important risk factor for subsequent nosocomial pneumonia. Nasotracheal or orotracheal intubation predisposes patients to bacterial colonization and nosocomial pneumonia by a variety of pathophysiological alterations: (1) sinusitis and trauma to the nasopharynx (nasotracheal tube), (2) impaired swallowing of secretion, (3) acting as a reservoir for bacterial proliferation, (4) increased bacterial adherence and colonization of airways, (5) ischemia secondary to cuff pressure, (6) impaired ciliary clearance and cough, (7) leakage of secretions around the cuff, and (8) suctioning often required to remove secretions.[43] Contaminated respiratory care equipment may lead to nosocomial pneumonia by two routes.[62] First, respiratory care equipment may serve as a reservoir for microorganisms, especially gram-negative bacilli. Fluid-containing devices such as nebulizers and humidifiers may become heavily contaminated by bacteria capable of multiplying

in water. Pathogens may then be spread to the patient by hospital personnel or by aerosolization into room air. Second, contaminated equipment may lead to direct airway inoculation of microorganisms if it is directly linked to the ventilatory system or if contaminated medications are instilled by aerosolization. The role of contaminated respiratory equipment as a source or reservoir for nosocomial pneumonia has recently been reviewed.[57,62]

Hospital personnel and the hospital environment also play an important role in nosocomial pneumonia. Cross-transmission between patients may occur when the hands of medical personnel become transiently colonized with pathogenic organisms. Such pathogens may be acquired from direct patient care or from contact with contaminated equipment or hospital surfaces. For this reason, it is crucial that health-care providers carefully wash their hands before and after each patient contact. Patients may acquire respiratory infections—including influenza, respiratory syncytial virus, pertussis, group A streptococcus, diphtheria, and *M. tuberculosis*—transmitted by the droplet or airborne routes from infected health-care personnel, other patients, or visitors.

The hospital environment may serve as a reservoir for *Aspergillus, Zygomycetes,* and *Legionella.* Nosocomial pneumonia may result when these pathogens are inhaled, especially if the patient is immunocompromised. The recovery of *Aspergillus* or *Zygomycetes* within hospitals has been variable, but commonly at least small numbers can be isolated from the air, accumulated dust, and environmental surfaces. More than 25 outbreaks of nosocomial fungal pneumonia have been reported. Sources of airborne fungi in hospitals have been reported to include (1) dust associated with hospital renovations; (2) outside construction, with an inadequate or malfunctioning hospital ventilation system; (3) contaminated cellulose fireproofing material; (4) contamination of the hospital air supply by pigeon droppings, helicopter flights from a roof helipad, or contaminated air filters and air-conditioning coils; and (5) an inadequate filtration system, coupled with location of the outside air intake vent near a refuse container.[55]

Nosocomial acquisition of *Legionella pneumophila* and *L. bozemanii* have been linked to contamination of hospital water supplies, and the association has been strengthened by use of molecular epidemiologic typing methods (e.g., DNA fingerprinting by pulsed field gel electrophoresis) and clinical and environmental strains (see Chapter 144).[63] *Legionella* can be isolated from more than 50 percent of the potable water supplies and more than 10 percent of the distilled water supplies in hospitals. The subjects of *Legionella* in hospitals[33] and disinfection of water distribution systems for *Legionella*[47] have been reviewed.

INCIDENCE

The incidence of nosocomial pneumonia reported in the literature varies tremendously among hospitals for a variety of reasons, including the sensitivity and specificity of the surveillance definition, the vigor with which the diagnosis is sought, and the frequency of intrinsic (e.g., patient age) and hospitalization-specific (e.g., intubation) factors among patients that alter their risk for nosocomial pneumonia. The most representative data regarding the incidence of nosocomial pneumonia have been provided by the National Nosocomial Infections Surveillance (NNIS) system, a Centers for Disease Control and Prevention (CDC) surveillance system of more than 150 hospitals. In 1984, the overall incidence of nosocomial pneumonia was 6.0 per 1000 discharged patients.[34] The incidence varied by hospital type, being 4.2 in nonteaching hospitals, 5.4 in small teaching hospitals, and 7.7 in large teaching hospitals.

The incidence of ventilator-associated pneumonia has ranged from 11 to 54 cases per 100 patients, depending on the population studied (Table 143-1). Intubation and mechanical ventilation represent the most important risk factor for nosocomial pneumonia, with a 6- to 21-fold increased risk. For this reason, the CDC and other investigators now report the incidence of nosocomial pneumonia as cases per 1000 days of mechanical ventilation. This serves to adjust the rates to take into account the presence and duration of mechanical ventilation. Ventilator-associated pneumonia rates (cases per 1000 ventilator days) reported by the NNIS system vary by hospital, type of intensive care unit (ICU), and, for neonatal intensive care units, patient birthweight.[7] Rates among ICUs ranged from 6.0 in the pediatric ICU to 22.2 in the burn ICU. Rates reported from individual hospitals exhibit considerable variation; for medical-surgical ICUs, the lowest 10 percent of reporting hospitals had a rate of 3.8, while the upper 10 percent had a rate of 20.0.

Several investigators have described the actuarial risk of pneumonia as a function of the duration of mechanical ventilation.

Langer and associates showed that the rate of pneumonia was constant through the first 8 to 10 days of respiratory assistance and then decreased.[40] While the rate of nosocomial pneumonia per day decreases, the cumulative incidence increases, so by day 30 of mechanical ventilation, an episode of nosocomial pneumonia will have developed in more than 60 percent of patients. Fagon and coworkers reported the actuarial risk of pneumonia during mechanical ventilation as 6.5 percent at 10 days, 19 percent at 20 days, and 28 percent at 30 days.[23] Ruiz-Santana and colleagues reported actuarial risks for pneumonia as 8.5 percent at day 3, 21.1 percent at day 7, 32.4 percent at day 14, and 45.6 percent for ventilation after 14 days.[53]

RISK FACTORS FOR NOSOCOMIAL PNEUMONIA

Many risk factors have been demonstrated to be associated with nosocomial pneumonia (Table 143-2).[15,16,29,57] In general, these factors can be divided into several broad categories: (1) intrinsic host factors such as age, underlying medical disorders such as pulmonary disease, and nutritional status; (2) hospital factors such as abdominal or thoracic operations, antibiotic use, immunosuppression, and treatment in an ICU; (3) equipment and device use, especially intubation with mechanical ventilation; and (4) factors that increase the risk of aspiration such as depressed consciousness.

Intrinsic Factors

The incidence of nosocomial pneumonia is increased at the extremes of life. However, a case control study by Hanson and colleagues, using regression analysis, demonstrated that age was not an independent risk factor for nosocomial pneumonia.[32] Rather, the increased incidence of pneumonia in the elderly was a function of an increased frequency of both intrinsic and hospital risk factors, such as poor nutrition, neuromuscular disease, and endotracheal intubation.

Intrinsic risk factors reported in the literature have included chronic lung disease, poor nutrition, and immunosuppression.

Hospital Factors

Management in an ICU has been reported as an important risk factor for the development of nosocomial pneumonia. The incidence (number per 100 patients) in various intensive care patients is as follows: ICUs, all patients, 0.5 to 31.5 (median 9.5); intensive care patients, no ventilation, 0.4 to 6.9; adult medical and surgical intensive care patients, mechanical ventilation, 8 to 54 (median 24); and pediatric intensive care patients, mechanical ventilation, 1.5 to 8.[29]

Other important hospital factors reported in the literature are intracranial pressure monitor, chest and abdominal surgery, large-volume gastric aspiration, reintubation, tracheostomy, prior antibiotic use, organ failure, and use of H_2-blocker therapy.

Many studies have documented that the administration of antacids and H_2 blockers—used to prevent stress bleeding in critically ill, intensive care patients—has been associated with gastric bacterial overgrowth. Several studies and three meta-analy-

TABLE 143-1

Incidence and Mortality of Ventilator-Associated Pneumonia in Recent Studies

Reference	Year	Study Years	Patient Population	Diagnostic Criteria	Ratio*	Rate†	Case Fatality Ratio
Craven et al.	1986	1983–84	MSICU, MV >48 h	Clinical	21	~21	55
Rashkin and Davis	1986	1983–84	MICU, TI >72 h	Clinical	11	—	—
Ruiz-Santana et al.	1987	—	MSICU, any MV	Clinical	31	~30	—
Daschner et al.	1987	—	MSICU	Clinical	31 (any MV)	—	—
					43 (MV >24 h)	—	—
Daschner et al.	1988	1983–?	MSICU, any MV	Clinical	48	—	—
Fagon et al.	1989	1981–85	MSICU, MV >72 h	PSB	9	~10	71
Jiminez et al.	1989	1986	MSICU, MV >48 h	Clinical & PSB	27	~16	28
Klein et al.	1989	1984–87	PICU, any MV	Clinical	8	15, 21	—
Langer et al.	1989	1983–84	MSICU, MV >24 h	Clinical	23	~35	44
Reusser et al.	1989	1984–86	NSICU, MV >48 h, TI >96 h	Clinical	38	—	13
Deppe et al.	1990	1986–87	MSICU, TI >48 h	Clinical	27	—	—
Jacobs et al.	1990	—	MSICU, EF, MV >72 h	Clinical	54	—	—
Torres et al.	1990	1987–88	MSICU, MV >48 h	Clinical & PSB	24	—	23
Dreyfuss et al.	1991	—	MSICU, MV >96 h	PSB	30	—	23
Rello et al.	1991	1988–89	MSICU, MV >48 h	Clinical & PSB	22	—	21
Kollef	1993	1992–93	MICU/SICU/CTICU, MV >24 h	Clinical	16	—	37
CDC	1995	1990–95	CCU	Clinical	—	9.8	—
	1995	1990–95	MICU	Clinical	—	9.6	—
	1995	1990–95	MSICU	Clinical	—	12.7	—
	1995	1990–95	NSICU	Clinical	—	20.7	—
	1995	1990–95	PICU	Clinical	—	6.0	—
	1995	1990–95	SICU	Clinical	—	15.4	—
	1995	1990–95	BICU	Clinical	—	22.2	—
	1995	1990–95	RICU	Clinical	—	6.3	—
	1995	1990–95	TICU	Clinical	—	16.6	—
	1995	1992–95	Neonates, ≤1000 g	Clinical	—	4.8	—
	1995	1992–95	Neonates, 1001–1500 g	Clinical	—	4.6	—
	1995	1992–95	Neonates, 1501–2500 g	Clinical	—	3.9	—
	1995	1992–95	Neonates, >2500 g	Clinical	—	3.0	—

*Ratio: Number of cases per 100 patients.
†Rate: Number of cases per 1000 ventilator days.

NOTE: BICU = burn intensive care unit; CCU = coronary care unit; MICU = medical intensive care unit; MSICU = medical/surgical intensive care unit; MV = mechanical ventilation; NSICU = neurosurgical intensive care unit; PICU = pediatric intensive care unit; PSB = protected specimen brush; RICU = respiratory intensive care unit; SICU = surgical intensive care unit; TI = tracheal intubation; TICU = trauma intensive care unit; CTICU = cardiothoracic intensive care unit; EF = emergency floor.

TABLE 143-2

Risk Factors for Nosocomial Pneumonia

Ventilator-Associated Pneumonia	Ventilator and Nonventilated Patients
Independent Risk Factors	**Univariate Risk Factors for Pneumonia**
Age >60 years	Age >60 years
COPD/PEEP/pulmonary disease	Male sex
Coma/impaired consciousness	Smoking
Therapeutic interventions*	Underling disease, rapidly fatal vs nonfatal/ultimately fatal
Intracranial pressure monitoring	Simplified acute physiological score >9
Organ failure	ASA class IV
Large volume gastric aspiration	Inspired O_2 >0.50
Prior antibiotics	Prior care facility
H_2 blocker +/– antacids	Alcohol intake
Gastric colonization and pH	Renal failure/dialysis
Season: fall, winter	Intra-aortic balloon pump
Ventilator circuit changes 24 vs 48 h	Chronic obstructive pulmonary disease
Reintubation	Chemical paralysis
Mechanical ventilation ≥2 days	Airway instrumentation
Tracheostomy	Aspiration before intubation
Supine head position	Mechanical ventilation >2 days
	No prior surgery
Ventilated and Nonventilated Patients	H_2 blockers or antacids vs sucralfate
Independent Risk Factors	Coma
Age >60 years	Head trauma
APACHE II >16	Cascade humidifier vs heat moisture exchanger
Trauma/head injury	Tracheostomy
Impaired airway reflexes	Continuous enteral feeding
Coma	Prior antibiotics
Bronchoscopy	Nosocomial maxillary sinusitis
Nasogastric tube	Type of intensive care unit
Endotracheal intubation	Repeat intensive care unit admission
Upper abdominal/thoracic surgery	APACHE II score
Low serum albumin	Emergency surgery
Neuromuscular disease	Nasotracheal tube
	Nasogastric tube
	Subglottic secretions

*Interventions were markers of severe underlying disease and included dopamine, dobutamine ≥5 μg/min, barbiturate therapy for increased intracranial pressure and continuous intravenous antiarrhythmic or artihypertensive therapy.
NOTE: APACHE = acute physiological score and chronic health evaluation; ASA = American Society of Anesthesiology; COPD = chronic obstructive pulmonary disease; PEEP = positive end-expiratory pressure.
SOURCE: Adapted from Craven and Steger.[16]

ses[10,11,59] have demonstrated a lower rate of pneumonia in patients treated with sucralfate, a cytoprotective agent, than in those treated with antacids or H_2 blockers. In their review, Craven and Steger note that most current data using a clinical diagnosis of ventilator-associated pneumonia suggest that sucralfate provides similar protection against stress bleeding but poses a lower risk of nosocomial pneumonia.[16] For this reason, they recommend that if stress bleeding prophylaxis is prescribed and there is no contraindication, the risk–benefit ratio for reducing ventilator-associated pneumonia appears to favor the use of sucralfate over antacid or H_2 blockers for patients who require a gastric tube.[16]

The use of a nasogastric tube is increasingly recognized as a risk factor for nosocomial pneumonia. Nasogastric tubes may increase the risk of nosocomial sinusitis, oropharyngeal colonization, reflux, and bacterial migration.

RISKS ASSOCIATED WITH RESPIRATORY DEVICES

Intubation with mechanical ventilation is the single most important risk factor for the development of nosocomial pneumonia. For this reason, intubation should be used only when medically necessary, and strict adherence to equipment maintenance is critical.

Fluid-containing respiratory devices are the major environment-associated reservoirs for nosocomial pneumonia.[63] However, most or all phases of respiratory support have been linked to nosocomial respiratory infections or suggested as potential environmental reservoirs. These include mechanical ventilation bags, ventilators, aerosolized medications, bronchoscopy, suction catheters, and respiratory support personnel. Evidence suggests that alterations in infection control practices during the 1960s decreased the number of cases of nosocomial pneumonia from environmental sources.

Flexible bronchoscopy has proved to be an invaluable diagnostic and therapeutic procedure. In general, the incidence of postprocedure fever or pneumonia has been reported to be less than 1 percent.[63] However, the use of contaminated bronchoscopes has led to both pseudoepidemics and clinical infection.[56,63] Pseudoepidemics with clusters of positive cultures of bronchoscopic washings have been linked to the use of contaminated bronchoscopes, contaminated tubing or suction devices, cocaine for topical use, and green dye added to the topical anesthetic. Microorganisms isolated in these cases included *Trichosporon cutaneum* and *Penicillium* species, *Pseudomonas aeruginosa, P. fluorescens-putida, Bacillus* species, *Mycobacterium* species, and *Rodotorula rubra*. Cross-transmission of respiratory pathogens has led to clinical infections with *M. tuberculosis, P. aeruginosa,* and *Serratia marcescens*. Factors leading to the use of contaminated bronchoscopes have included postdisinfection rinsing in tap water and disinfection with an iodophor, cetrimide-chlorhexidine, and 70 percent alcohol. Failure to sterilize damaged bronchoscopes or bronchoscope suction valves contaminated by *Mycobacteria* has been noted with both ethylene oxide and immersion in 2 percent glutaraldehyde for 30 min. Prevention of nosocomial infection related to contaminated bronchoscopes requires adherence to guidelines that delineate proper techniques of cleaning and disinfection of bronchoscopes.

MORTALITY

Nosocomial pneumonia is an important cause of mortality in hospitalized patients. Nosocomial pneumonia has been reported to contribute to 60 percent of all infection-related hospital deaths.[31] Daschner and colleagues reviewed 1000 autopsy reports and noted that pneumonia was associated with 7.5 percent of deaths and was the most common nosocomial infection contributing to death.[17] Intensive care patients with nosocomial pneumonia have a 2- to 10-fold increased risk of mortality compared to patients without pneumonia.[29] Independent risk factors for mortality in nonventilated patients include infection with *P. aeruginosa,* bilateral infiltrates on chest radiography, and respiratory failure.[29]

The crude mortality for ventilator-associated nosocomial pneumonia has ranged from 13 to 70 percent, but most investigators have reported rates in the range of 20 to 40 percent. Many risk factors have been associated with mortality in ventilated patients (Table 143-3). Several studies using a matched cohort design have evaluated the attributable mortality from nosocomial pneumonia.[12,24,25,42] In these studies, in which patients were matched by demographic factors and comorbidity, the attributable mortality was reported to be 13.7, 33.3, 27.1, and 35.8 percent, respectively.

ETIOLOGIC AGENTS

The common etiologic agents of nosocomial pneumonia reported from the NNIS hospitals from 1990 to 1992 were *Staphylococ-*

TABLE 143-3

Risk Factors for Mortality in Patients with Nosocomial Pneumonia

Aerobic gram-negative bacilli as pathogen(s), especially *P. aeruginosa*

Severity of underlying illness

Inappropriate antibiotic therapy

Advanced age

Shock

Bilateral infiltrates

Prior antibiotic therapy

Neoplastic disease

Duration of prior hospitalization

Supine head position in patients receiving mechanical ventilation

SOURCE: Adapted from George.[29]

---

cus aureus (20 percent), *P. aeruginosa* (16 percent), *Enterobacter* species (11 percent), *Klebsiella pneumoniae* (7 percent), *Candida albicans* (5 percent), *Hemophilus influenzae* (4 percent), *Escherichia coli* (5 percent), *Acinetobacter* species (4 percent), and *S. marcescens* (3 percent) (Table 143-4). As a group, aerobic enteric gram-negative bacilli accounted for approximately one-third of all pathogens responsible for pneumonia. In ventilated patients, gram-negative bacilli have accounted for 58 to 83 percent of infections, gram-positive cocci for 14 to 38 percent, and anaerobes for only 1 to 3 percent. Polymicrobial infections were common, being noted in 26 to 53 percent of cases (median 40 percent). The importance of viral diseases such as cytomegalovirus, influenza, and respiratory syncytial virus is unknown, but they have clearly been underascertained and underreported.

The relevance of the NNIS data is called into question by reports that document the inability of clinical criteria to accurately identify cases of nosocomial pneumonia and the failure of expectorated sputum or tracheal aspirates to reliably identify pathogens in the distal areas of the lung (Table 143-5). Combining reports in which the diagnosis of pneumonia was made by an invasive procedure and more specific microbiologic criteria were used, the etiologic agents of pneumonia were *P. aeruginosa* (16 percent), *S. aureus* (20 percent), *Acinetobacter* species (14 percent), *H. influenzae* (10 percent), *S. pneumoniae* (4 percent), and other streptococci (4 percent). Enteric gram-negative bacilli (*E. coli, Enterobacter, Proteus, Serratia, Klebsiella,* and *Citrobacter*) accounted for only 13 percent of isolates. Thus, generalizing from the NNIS data would overestimate the importance of enteric gram-negative bacilli and underestimate the importance of *Acinetobacter* species as causes of pneumonia in ventilated patients. One must stress that the specific etiologic agents isolated in an individual institution may vary from these summary statistics depending on many factors, including patient demographics, patterns of antimicrobial use, environmental reservoirs for pathogens such as *Legionella* and *Aspergillus,* and the mix of host defects in the patient population.

TABLE 143-4

Common Pathogens Currently Associated with Nosocomial Pneumonia

Pathogen	Frequency (%)*	Source of Organism
Early-onset bacterial pneumonia		
S. pneumoniae	5–20	Endogenous; other patients
H. influenzae	<5–15	Respiratory droplet
Late-onset bacterial pneumonia	≥ 20–60	
Aerobic gram-negative bacilli		Endogenous; other patients, environment, enteral feeding; health-care workers; equipment, devices
P. aeruginosa		
Enterobacter spp.		
Acinetobacter spp.		
K. pneumoniae		
S. marcescens		
E. coli		
Gram-positive cocci		
S. aureus	20–40	Endogenous; health-care workers; environment
Early- and late-onset pneumonia		
Anaerobic bacteria	0–35	Endogenous
Legionella spp.	0–10	Potable water; showers, faucets; cooling towers
M. tuberculosis	<1	Endogenous; other patients, staff
Viruses		
Influenza A and B	<1	Other patients, staff
Respiratory syncytial virus	<1	Other patients, staff; fomites
Fungi/protozoa		
Aspergillus spp.	<1	Air; construction
Candida spp.	<1	Endogenous; other patients, staff
P. carinii	<1	Endogenous; other patients (?)

*Crude rates of pneumonia may vary by hospital, patient population, and method of diagnosis.
SOURCE: Adapted from Craven and Steger.[15]

DIAGNOSIS

In recent years, it has become increasingly apparent that it is difficult to accurately diagnose nosocomial pneumonia. Clinicians have traditionally relied on the presence of clinical findings (i.e., fever, cough, the development of purulent sputum, and evidence of consolidation on physical examination), radiographic evidence of new or progressing pulmonary infiltrate, and laboratory findings (Gram's stain of sputum and cultures of sputum, blood, tracheal aspirate, and pleural fluid). Many studies have demonstrated that clinical criteria with appropriate cultures of tracheal specimens may be sensitive for bacterial pathogens but are highly nonspecific, especially in intubated patients on mechanical ventilation. Blood cultures have been reported to yield the etiologic pathogen in approximately 10 to 20 percent of patients with nosocomial pneumonia. Among patients with severe nosocomial pneumonia, however, an additional source of infection has been present in up to 50 percent of those with positive blood cultures.[57]

Several new techniques are now available for diagnosing nosocomial pneumonia or providing specimens for culture, including quantitative cultures of bronchoalveolar lavage (BAL) and quantitative culture of protected specimen brushing (PSB).[3]

The reported sensitivity and specificity of these methods have ranged from 70 to 100 percent and 60 to 100 percent, respectively. In the absence of a "gold standard", however, the sensitivity and specificity of these measures cannot be definitely determined. False-positive results using PSB have been attributed to prior antibiotic therapy or bacterial colonization of the lower airway. False-negative results may also occur in significant numbers. Invasive procedures used to diagnose pneumonia may lead to clinically important complications, including hypoxemia, bleeding, and arrhythmia.[57] A consensus conference has formulated recommendations for the standardization of methods to diagnose pneumonia in clinical research studies of ventilator-associated pneumonia.[45] The diagnosis of nosocomial pneumonia has been the subject of several recent reviews.[1,9,27,44]

Diagnostic strategies recommended in the literature for the diagnosis of nosocomial pneumonia range from a clinical approach to routine use of invasive techniques to obtain lower respiratory cultures.[8,48] Controversy exists as to which invasive approach is most effective. For this reason, a definitive algorithm cannot be provided for the diagnosis of nosocomial pneumonia. However, the following approach to nosocomial pneumonia is suggested (Table 143-6). Patients with suspected nosocomial pneumonia should undergo a careful history and physical exam-

TABLE 143-5

Microorganisms Isolated from Respiratory Tract Specimens Obtained by Various Representative Methods from Adult Patients with a Diagnosis of Nosocomial Pneumonia

	Emori, 1993	Barlett, 1986	Fagon, 1989	Torres, 1990
Hospital type	NNIS	Veterans	General	General
Patients studied				
Ventilated or nonventilated	Mixed	Mixed	Ventilated	Ventilated
Number	N/A	159	49	78
Number of episodes of pneumonia	N/A	159	52	78
Specimen culture	Sputum, tracheal aspirate	Transtracheal aspirate, blood, pleural fluid	Protected specimen brush	Protected specimen brush, lung aspirate, pleural fluid, blood
Culture results				
No organisms isolated	N/A	0	0	54%*
Polymicrobial	N/A	54%*	40%*	13%*
Number of isolates	8891	314	111	N/A
Aerobic bacteria				
Gram-negative bacilli	59%†	46%‡	75%‡	16%§
Pseudomonas aeruginosa	16%†	9%‡	31%‡	5%§
Enterobacter spp.	11%	4%	2%	0%
Klebsiella spp.	9	23	4	0
Escherichia coli	4	14	8	0
Serratia spp.	3	0	0	1
Proteus spp.	2	11	15	1
Citrobacter spp.	1	0	2	0
Acinetobacter calcoaceticus	4	0	15	9
Others	5	0	10	0
Hemophilus influenzae	5	17%‡	10%‡	0%§
Legionella spp.	N/A	N/A	2%‡	2%§
Gram-positive cocci	26%†	56%‡	52%‡	4%§
Staphylococcus aureus	20%†	25%‡	33%‡	2%§
Streptococcus spp.	2	31	21	2
Others	4	0	8	0
Anaerobes	0	35%‡	2%‡	0
Peptostreptococcus	N/A	14%‡	N/A	0
Fusobacterium spp.	N/A	10	N/A	0
Peptococcus spp.	N/A	11	N/A	0
Bacteroides melaninogenicus	N/A	9	N/A	0
B. fragilis	0	8	N/A	0
Fungi	7%†	N/A	0	1%§
Aspergillus spp.	N/A	N/A	0	1%§
Candida spp.	6%†	N/A	0	0
Viruses	1	N/A	N/A	N/A

*Percent episodes.
†Percent isolates.
‡Percent episodes (percentages not additive owing to polymicrobial origin in some episodes).
§Percent patients with pure cultures.
NOTE: NNIS = National Nosocomial Infection Surveillance System; N/A = Not applicable: not tested or reported.
SOURCE: Adapted from Tablan et al.[57]

ination to define the severity of pneumonia. An arterial blood gas or pulse oximetry should be performed both to aid in defining the severity of infection and to determine the need for supplemental oxygen. Mechanical ventilation should be considered for patients with hypoxia not correctable by supplemental oxygena-

tion, hypercapnia, or inability to protect their airway. If the patient is suspected to have a communicable disease transmitted by the droplet or airborne route (e.g., respiratory syncytial virus, tuberculosis, influenza), appropriate respiratory precautions (droplet precautions or airborne precautions; see below) should

TABLE 143-6

Evaluation of Patients with Suspected Nosocomial Pneumonia

Routine Evaluation

  History

    Recent exposure to possible pulmonary infectious agents (e.g., influenza, tuberculosis)
    Travel
    Occupational exposures
    Animal exposure
    Immunocompromising conditions (e.g., steroids, risk factors for HIV)

  Physical evaluation

  Chest radiograph

  Measure of oxygen saturation (arterial blood gas or pulse oximetry)

  Obtain expectorated sputum in nonventilated patients and a tracheal aspirate in patients who have been intubated or have a tracheostomy. Send the specimen for Gram's stain and bacterial cultures. Consider additional diagnostic tests, depending on the clinical findings and epidemiologic circumstances: viral culture, direct antigen testing for respiratory syncytial virus, *Legionella* DFA and culture, smear and culture for *Mycobacteria,* smear and culture for fungi, stain for *P. carinii*

Evaluation to Exclude Extrapulmonary Sources of Infections

  Routine evaluation

    Blood cultures from two different sites
    Urine analysis and culture
    Examination of wounds, if present

  Additional tests directed by history, physical examination, and laboratory findings

    Consider removal of central and arterial vascular catheters, with semiquantitative culture of the subcutaneous portion and tip of the catheter in patients with positive blood cultures and/or evidence of sepsis
    Consider lumbar puncture following head CT or MRI in patients at high risk (e.g., after neurosurgery) or with unexplained change in mental status
    Consider radiographic imaging of the abdomen (CT or MRI) in patients with rigid abdomen, ileus, or localized or diffuse tenderness or at high risk for abdominal sepsis (i.e., after abdominal surgery, with pancreatitis, gastrointestinal bleeding, or carcinoma, or receiving high-dose corticosteroids)
    Consider abdominal ultrasound in patients with right upper-quadrant tenderness or abnormal liver function tests, or who are too unstable for transfer to CT
    Obtain stools for *C. difficile* toxin assay in patients with more than two watery stools per day. If fever persists with a discernible cause, consider CT scan of sinuses to exclude sinusitis, with aspiration of the maxillary sinus in patients with air–fluid levels or opacification, and/or consider nucleotide scan (gallium 67 scintigraphy, tagged white cell scan)

Additional Pulmonary Evaluation

  If pleural effusion is suspected, obtain decubitus films, ultrasound, or CT. If pleural effusion is present, consider diagnostic thorocentesis
  Consider need to exclude thromboembolic disease: impedance plethysmography or Doppler ultrasound evaluation of the lower extremities; ventilation-perfusion scan of the lung; pulmonary arteriogram
  Consider need for invasive diagnosis in patients with rapidly progressive pneumonia, severe pneumonia in intubated patients on mechanical ventilation, immunocompromised patients, and patients who have failed to respond to empiric therapy or have progressed on empiric therapy: bronchoscopy with protected specimen brush and bronchoalveolar lavage or protected bronchoalveolar lavage
  Evaluation to rule out atelectasis

    Inhalation of bronchodilators every 2 h for 4 treatments, then every 4 h
    Percussion or vibration over the area of the chest with new densities on chest radiography
    Repeat chest radiograph in 48 h

Consider Other Sources of Fever

  Incorrect antibiotic administration: incorrect dose, route, frequency
  Drug fever
  Noninfectious source of fever and pulmonary infiltrate (e.g., aspiration, hemorrhage)
  Foreign body
  Superinfection
  Overgrowth
  Development of drug-resistant pathogen

SOURCE: Adapted from Meduri.[44]

be instituted. All patients should undergo chest radiography and two sets of blood cultures. The chest radiograph will aid in identifying the presence of pneumonia, the extent and location of infiltrates, and the presence of a pleural effusion. The radiographic appearance may provide clues to the cause of the respiratory failure. Other laboratory studies (complete blood count, electrolytes, liver function tests, tests of renal function, etc.) may be useful in patient management.

When a pleural effusion is present, consideration should be given to obtaining a diagnostic thoracentesis, especially if the patient is toxic or a large effusion (greater than 10 mm on a lateral decubitus film) is present. The pleural fluid should be sent for complete blood cell count and differential, protein, glucose, LDH, pH, Gram's stain, and aerobic and anaerobic bacterial cultures. Consideration should also be given to fungal and mycobacterial stains and appropriate fungal and mycobacterial cultures.

In nonintubated patients, an expectorated sputum should be obtained for Gram's stain and bacterial culture. Epidemiologic or clinical findings should be reviewed, and consideration should be given to obtaining appropriate stains and cultures for viruses, fungi, mycobacteria, *Legionella,* and *P. carinii.* It is important, however, to remember that an expectorated sputum is neither sensitive nor specific for the diagnosis of nosocomial pneumonia. Its major value is to identify the antibiotic susceptibilities of the organisms present and thereby aid in the proper choice of therapy.

In intubated patients, a tracheal aspirate should be obtained. The Gram's stain may reveal a predominant pathogen. The culture has been shown to have both poor sensitivity and specificity in identifying the etiologic agents of nosocomial pneumonia. Cultures obtained by tracheal aspiration may be of most use in excluding certain potential pathogens (e.g., methicillin-resistant *S. aureus*) and providing information about the antimicrobial susceptibility spectrum of isolated pathogens.

Consideration should be given to performing an invasive procedure to better assess the diagnosis of pneumonia and potential pathogens in the following circumstances: an immuno-compromised patient with a broad range of potential pathogens (e.g., heart or lung transplant patient), a critically ill patient with severe hospital-acquired pneumonia (see below), and a patient whose condition does not improve with empiric antimicrobial therapy.

Clinicians should always consider other potential causes of fever and pulmonary infiltrate in the hospitalized patient—including atelectasis, acute radiation pneumonitis, large-volume gastric aspiration, pulmonary embolus with infarction, lung contusion (in trauma patients), pulmonary hemorrhage, and acute respiratory distress syndrome with diffuse alveolar damage.

THERAPY

General Considerations

Despite the development of broad-spectrum antibiotic agents, nosocomial pneumonia continues to carry an unacceptably high mortality. A recently published consensus statement provides broad guidelines for the treatment of nosocomial pneumonia.[1] However, these recommendations should be considered only general guidelines, for the following reasons: (1) new antibiotics continue to be approved for the treatment of nosocomial pneumonia (e.g., cefepime); (2) the spectrum of pathogens causing nosocomial pneumonia varies among hospitals (e.g., frequency of *Legionella*); (3) the antimicrobial susceptibility spectrum of nosocomial pathogens varies among hospitals (e.g., frequency of methicillin-resistant *S. aureus*); and (4) the role of invasive techniques to diagnose nosocomial pneumonia remains incompletely defined.

Initial empiric therapy of presumed nosocomial pneumonia may be guided by an assessment of disease severity, the presence of risk factors for specific organisms, and time of onset of nosocomial pneumonia (Fig. 143-2; Tables 143-7, 143-8, and 143-9). The choice of a specific agent will depend on several factors. The first is the spectrum of antimicrobial susceptibility of respiratory pathogens causing nosocomial pneumonia at one's health-care facility. It is important for all health-care facilities to periodically review the pathogens causing nosocomial pneumonia and their susceptibility patterns and disseminate this information to clinicians. Second, a history of allergic reactions to antimicrobials should be obtained from all patients. Because of the possibility of cross reactivity between β-lactam antibiotics, the use of a cephalosporin in a penicillin-allergic patient should be considered only if the ben-

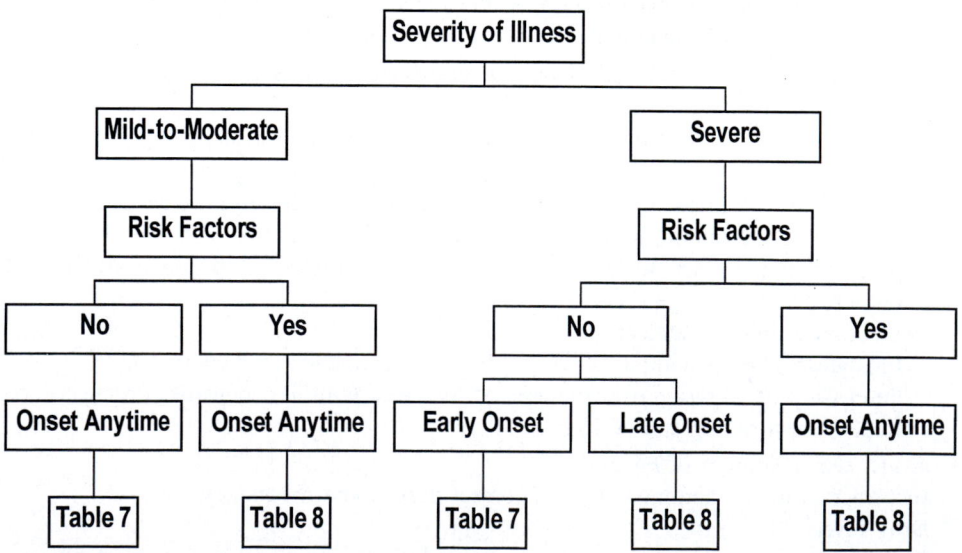

FIGURE 143-2   Algorithm for classifying patients with nosocomial pneumonia. Specific drugs and doses, recommended in Tables 143-7, 143-8, and 143-9, are adapted from the American Thoracic Society Consensus Statement and represent the views of the authors. Doses provided are for an adult of average weight and normal renal and hepatic function. Doses may need to be adjusted depending on the patient's weight, age, renal function, hepatic function, use of interacting agents, and other factors. Physicians should be thoroughly familiar with the guidelines in individual drug manufacturers' inserts regarding dosing, drug interaction, contraindications, precautions, and administration.

TABLE 143-7

Patients with Mild to Moderate Nosocomial Pneumonia, No Unusual Risk Factors, Onset Anytime, or Patients with Severe Nosocomial Pneumonia with Early Onset*†

Core Organisms	Core Antibiotics
Enteric gram-negative bacilli (non-*Pseudomonas*)	Piperacillin-tazobactam 3.375 g IV Q 4 h *or*
Enterobacter spp.	Piperacillin-tazobactam‡ 4.5 g IV Q 6 h *or*
Escherichia coli	Cefotaxime 1–2 gm IV Q 8 h *or*
Klebsiella spp.	Ceftriaxone 1 gm IV Q 12 h *or*
Proteus spp.	if allergic to penicillins/cephalosporins
Serratia marcescens	Clindamycin *or* vancomycin *plus*
Hemophilus influenzae	Ciprofloxacin IV *or* aztreonam
Methicillin-sensitive *S. aureus*	
Streptococcus pneumoniae	

*Excludes patients with immunosuppression.
†Early-onset pneumonia, ≤4 days after hospitalization.
‡Not an FDA-approved indication or dose.
SOURCE: Adapted from the American Thoracic Society.[1]

antibiotics exhibit a prolonged post-antibiotic effect in which bacterial replication is suppressed for a period after antibiotic levels have fallen below inhibitory concentrations. These pharmacologic features may lead to specific dosing recommendations such as the use of single daily dosing of aminoglycosides.

A controversial area in the treatment of respiratory infections is the importance of antibiotic penetration into lung tissue. It remains unclear whether concentrations in bronchial secretions or in epithelial lining fluid are relevant for predicting efficacy in patients with pneumonia. Also controversial is the role, if any, of inhaled antibiotics in seriously ill patients with nosocomial pneumonia.

efit exceeds the risk. Third, antimicrobial therapy should be chosen to minimize drug interactions. Fourth, in patients with renal or hepatic dysfunction, specific drugs may be chosen to minimize the need for dose adjustment. Fifth, potential drug toxicities may provide relative contraindications to use in specific patients (e.g., avoidance of aminoglycosides in patients with neuromuscular disorders or avoidance of aminoglycosides in patients predisposed to renal dysfunction). Sixth, intrinsic patient factors—including age, pregnancy, and breast-feeding—may limit the choice of antibiotics. Finally, if several equally efficacious and safe choices exist, the least costly regimen should be instituted.

The mechanism of bacterial action may be relevant in antibiotic selection and dosing. In general, bactericidal rather than bacteristatic antibiotics are preferred. β-Lactam antibiotics (penicillins, cephalosporins, carbapenems, monobactams) and vancomycin are bactericidal in a time-dependent fashion. Quinolones and aminoglycosides, which are bactericidal in a concentration-dependent fashion, exhibit killing more rapidly at high concentrations. In general, bactericidal

Specific Regimens

Initial empiric therapy for nosocomial pneumonia may be guided by severity, presence or absence of risk factors for specific pathogens, and length of hospital stay before the development of nosocomial pneumonia (Tables 143-7, 143-8, and 143-9). In the absence of specific risk factors, the most common pathogens of early-onset nosocomial pneumonia are *S. pneumoniae*, *H. influenzae*, enteric gram-negative bacilli (*E. coli*, *Enterobacter* species, *Klebsiella* species, *Proteus* species, *S. marcescens*), and *S. aureus*. For these patients, a nonpseudomonal third-generation cephalosporin or β-lactam–β-lactamase inhibitor combination should be adequate.

In the presence of certain risk factors, initiation of broader coverage may be warranted. Anaerobic bacteria are frequently isolated from the respiratory tract of patients with witnessed gastric aspiration, recent thoracoabdominal surgery, or the presence of an obstructing foreign body in the airway. The significance of these anaerobes is unclear, however, since the aerobic bacteria are generally more pathogenic. Nevertheless, patients with wit-

TABLE 143-8

Patients with Mild to Moderate Nosocomial Pneumonia with Risk Factors, Onset Anytime*

Core Organisms Plus:	Core Antibiotics Plus:
Anaerobes (recent abdominal surgery, witnessed aspiration)	Clindamycin 600 mg IV Q 8 h *or* Piperacillin-tazobactam 3.375 g IV Q 4 h (alone)
Staphylococcus aureus (coma, head trauma, diabetes mellitus, renal failure)	+/– Vancomycin (until methicillin-resistant *S. aureus* excluded)
Legionella spp.	Erythromycin 1 gm IV Q 6 hours +/– rifampin†
P. aeruginosa (prolonged ICU stay, steroids, antibiotics, structural lung disease)	Treat as severe nosocomial pneumonia (Table 143-6)

*Excludes patients with immunosuppression.
†Rifampin may be added if *Legionella* spp. are documented.

TABLE 143-9

Patients with Severe Nosocomial Pneumonia with Risk Factors, Early Onset, or Patients with Severe Nosocomial Pneumonia, Late Onset*†

Core Organisms Plus:	Therapy
P. aeruginosa Acinetobacter spp. Consider methicillin-resistant S. aureus	Aminoglycoside (gentamicin, tobramycin, amikacin)‡ *or* 　Ciprofloxacin 400 mg IV Q 12 h *plus* one of the following: 　Piperacillin-tazobactam 3.375 g IV Q 4 h *or* 　Piperacillin-tazobactam§ 4.5 g IV Q 6 h *or* 　Imipenem 500 mg IV Q 6 h *or* 　Meropenem§ 1.0 g IV Q 8 h *or* 　Ceftazidime 2.0 g IV Q 8 h *or* 　Cefepime 1–2 g IV Q 12 h *or* 　Cefpirome¶ 2.0 g Q 12 h 　+/− Vancomycin 1 g IV Q 12 h

*Excludes patients with immunosuppression.
†Late-onset pneumonia, ≥5 days after hospitalization.
‡Consider single daily dosing.
§Not an FDA-approved indication or dose.
¶Not an FDA-approved drug.
SOURCE: Adapted from the American Thoracic Society.[1]

nessed gastric aspiration should be treated with a broad-spectrum agent with anaerobic coverage (e.g., piperacillin-tazobactam, imipenem, meropenem) or have a specific anaerobic agent added (e.g., clindamycin). Prolonged hospitalization, prior antibiotic therapy, and mechanical ventilation in an ICU increase the likelihood of infection with more resistant bacteria, including methicillin-resistant S. aureus, P. aeruginosa, Enterobacter species, and Acinetobacter species. In such patients, initial empiric therapy should include broad coverage.

The American Thoracic Society has provided a definition of severe hospital-acquired pneumonia (Table 143-10). Although few studies have evaluated severe nosocomial pneumonia, it is reasonable to initiate very broad empiric antibiotic coverage in patients meeting this definition. As with mild to moderate nosocomial pneumonia, additional antibiotics will be necessary to treat methicillin-resistant S. aureus and Legionella species.

Immunocompromised Patients

The above guidelines were not designed to provide recommendations for the treatment of patients with immunocompromising conditions such as HIV infection, organ transplantation, neutropenia, hematologic malignancies, or high-dose steroid use. The presentation and etiology of respiratory infection in immunocompromised patients depend on several factors: (1) the nature of specific host defense abnormalities, (2) the duration of immunosuppressing conditions, (3) the presence or absence of latent infections (e.g., cytomegalovirus), and (4) epidemiologic exposures. The patient's overall susceptibility to infection will reflect the net sum of all fac-

tors that alter host defenses, including underlying medical conditions, immunosuppressive therapy, and hospital-related interventions (e.g., indwelling lines). Although consensus guidelines have not been published to aid the clinician in the treatment of nosocomial infections in immunocompromised patients, this subject has been reviewed.[52]

PREVENTION

General Preventive Interventions

Prevention of nosocomial pneumonia begins with strict adherence to standard infection control guidelines (Table 143-11). Among the most important infection control guidelines are proper handwashing,[41] institution of isolation precautions,[26] and proper disinfection and sterilization of equipment.[55] Patients with potentially communicable diseases should be rapidly evaluated and placed on appropriate isolation precautions. "Standard precautions" synthesize the major features of universal precautions (blood and body fluid precautions) and body substance

TABLE 143-10

Definitions of Severe Nosocomial Pneumonia

Admission to the intensive care unit

Respiratory failure, defined as the need for mechanical ventilation or the need for >35% oxygen to maintain an arterial saturation >90%

Rapid radiographic progression, multilobar pneumonia, or cavitation of a lung infiltrate

Evidence of severe sepsis with hypotension and/or end-organ dysfunction:
　Shock (systolic blood pressure <90 mmHg or diastolic blood pressure <60 mmHg)
　Requirement for vasopressors for more than 4 h
　Urine output <20 ml/h or total urine output <80 ml in 4 h (unless another explanation is available)
　Acute renal failure requiring dialysis

SOURCE: Adapted from the American Thoracic Society.[1]

TABLE 143-11

General Methods to Reduce the Frequency of Nosocomial Pneumonia in Mechanically Ventilated Patients

General Methods
  Aggressive treatment of patient's underlying disease
  Review need and avoid antacids + histamine$_2$ blockers for stress ulcer prophylaxis
  Keep patient elevated at ≥30°
  Review nutrition regimen and tube feeding procedures
  Extubate and remove nasogastric tube as clinically indicated
  Controlled use of antibiotics
Respiratory Care Equipment
  Discriminate between equipment with nebulizers and humidifiers
  ≥48-h circuit changes (tubing and humidifier) for mechanical ventilators with humidifiers; no changes for circuits with heat-moisture exchangers
  Proper removal of tubing condensate and education of staff to prevent washing contaminated condensate into the patient's trachea
  No transfer of equipment or devices between patients
  Review use and care of in-line medication nebulizers
Infection Control
  Surveillance in the ICU
  Education and awareness programs on nosocomial infection
  Handwashing and/or barrier precautions
  Review technique for suctioning patients; type of catheter used
  Review method of condensate disposal
  Use effective methods of disinfection of devices and equipment
  Consider selective decontamination of the digestive tract with oral nonabsorbable antibiotics to prevent nosocomial infections

SOURCE: Adapted from Craven and Steger.[14]

isolation and apply them to all patients receiving care in hospitals, regardless of their diagnosis or presumed infection status. Standard precautions apply to blood; all body fluids, secretions, and excretions except sweat, regardless of whether or not they contain visible blood; nonintact skin; and mucous membranes. Standard precautions are designed to reduce the risk of transmission of microorganisms from both recognized and unrecognized sources of infection in hospitals. Standard precautions include handwashing before and after patient contact, whether or not gloves are worn; wearing gloves when touching blood, body fluids, secretions or excretions, and contaminated items; wearing a mask and eye protection or a face shield during procedures and patient-care activities that are likely to generate splashes or sprays of blood, body fluids, secretions, or excretions (e.g., bronchoscopy, arterial line placement); and wearing a gown during procedures and patient-care activities that are likely to generate splashes or sprays of blood, body fluids, secretions, or excretions.

Airborne precautions are used for patients with a communicable disease transmitted by the airborne route, such as tuberculosis, varicella-zoster virus infections (with the exception of dermatomal zoster in the nonimmunocompromised host), and measles. Patients with these diseases should be placed in rooms with the following air-handling characteristics: private room, room at negative pressure with respect to the corridor, air directly exhausted to the outside or monitored high-efficiency filtration before the air is circulated to other areas of

the hospital, and 6 to 12 air exchanges per hour. Personnel caring for patients with known or suspected tuberculosis should don an N-95 respirator before entering into the room. Droplet precautions are used for patients with diseases transmitted by the droplet route, such as pertussis, meningococcal pneumonia, pharyngeal diphtheria, rubella, measles, *H. influenzae* epiglottitis, mycoplasmal pneumonia, and group A streptococcal infections (in infants and young children). Droplet precautions consist of private room and limiting patient transport. Personnel should don a surgical mask when working within 3 feet of the patient. Contact precautions are used for patients infected or colonized by direct contact, transient colonization of the hands of caregivers, or contamination of an inanimate object such as a medical instrument. Diseases requiring contact precautions include varicella-zoster infection, *C. difficile* infection, rotavirus, shigellosis, herpes simplex, methicillin-resistant *S. aureus,* and infection by multidrug-resistant pathogens.

Many reports attest to the ability of contaminated bronchoscopes to transmit pathogens leading to outbreaks or pseudo-outbreaks. For this reason, all endoscopic equipment should be rigorously cleaned immediately after use and then appropriately disinfected or sterilized.[54]

Selective Decontamination with Antibiotics

In recent years, many studies have tried to determine whether selective decontamination of the digestive tract (SDD) is associated with a decreased incidence of nosocomial pneumonia. The SDD regimens have usually included a combination of nonabsorbable local antibiotics (e.g., an aminoglycoside, polymyxin B, and amphotericin) and intravenously administered drugs (e.g., cefotaxime, trimethoprim, or a quinolone). The local antibiotics have been applied as a paste in the oropharynx, and often also provided orally or through the nasogastric tube.

Craven and Steger recently summarized all trials employing SDD to prevent lower respiratory tract infection.[16] They noted that despite several favorable reports, two large double-blind, placebo-controlled trials were unable to demonstrate that SDD was beneficial. Concerns have been expressed that the use of SDD may lead to the emergence of antibiotic-resistant pathogens and the lack of effect on the duration of mechanical ventilation or hospital stay and cost-effectiveness. For these reasons, many experts and the CDC do not support the routine use of SDD for all medical and surgical intensive care

TABLE 143-12

Infection Control Measures for Prevention of Nosocomial Pneumonia Depending on the Presence of Specific Risk Factors

Risk Factor	Infection Control Measures Suggested to Prevent Nosocomial Pneumonia
Bacterial Pneumonia	
Host related: age >65 years	
Underlying illness:	
Chronic obstructive pulmonary disease	Perform incentive spirometry, positive end-expiratory pressure, or continuous positive airway pressure by face mask.
Immunosuppression	Avoid exposure to potential nosocomial pathogens; decrease duration of immunosuppression, such as by granulocyte-macrophage colony–stimulating factor (GM-CSF).
Depressed consciousness	Administer CNS depressants cautiously.
Surgery (abdominal/thoracic)	Properly position patient; promote early ambulation; appropriately control pain.
Device related	Properly clean, sterilize or disinfect, and handle devices; remove devices as soon as the indication for their use ceases.
Endotracheal intubation and mechanical ventilation	Gently suction secretions; place patient in semirecumbent position (30° to 45° head elevation); use nonalkalinizing gastric cytoprotective agent on patients at risk for stress bleeding; do not routinely change ventilation circuits more often than every 48 h; drain and discard inspiratory tubing condensate, or use heat-moisture exchanger if indicated.
Nasogastric tube (NGT) placement and enteral feeding	Routinely verify appropriate tube placement; promptly remove NGT when no longer needed; drain residual; place patient in semirecumbent position as described above.
Personnel or procedure related	
Cross-contamination by hands	Educate and train personnel; wash hands adequately and wear gloves appropriately; conduct surveillance for cases of pneumonia, and give feedback to personnel.
Antibiotic administration	Use antibiotics prudently, especially on high-risk intensive care patients.
Legionnaires' Disease	
Host related	
Immunosuppression	Decrease duration of immunosuppression.
Device related	
Contaminated aerosol from devices	Sterilize or disinfect aerosol-producing devices before use; use only sterile water for respiratory humidifying devices; do not use cool-mist room-air "humidifiers" without adequate sterilization or disinfection.

patients. Additional data will be needed regarding the benefits of SDD in special patient populations, such as those with trauma.

Infection Control Guidelines to Prevent Nosocomial Pneumonia

Measures to prevent nosocomial pneumonia are based on an understanding of the risk factors associated with pneumonia (Table 143-12). Despite the use of these guidelines, however, the frequency of nosocomial pneumonia and subsequent morbidity is unacceptably high. Additional research to validate current preventive practices and innovative strategies to further reduce nosocomial pneumonia are sorely needed.

GRAM-NEGATIVE PNEUMONIA

Gram-negative pneumonias may be divided into several groups: community-acquired pathogens (*H. influenzae, Klebsiella, Bordetella pertussis*), hospital-acquired pathogens (enteric gram-negative rods, especially *E. coli, Enterobacter, Proteus,* and *Serratia*), and zoonotic pathogens (*Francisella tularensis, Yersinia pestis,* and *P. multocida*). The separation of gram-negative pathogens into community-acquired and hospital-acquired groups is only relative, as any of these pathogens may cause pneumonia in either setting.

A large number of bacterial pathogens are gram negative. Only the clinically most important species are discussed below.

TABLE 143-12

continued

Risk Factor	Infection Control Measures Suggested to Prevent Nosocomial Pneumonia
Environment related	
Aerosols from contaminated water supply	Hyperchlorinate or superheat hospital water system; routinely maintain water supply; consider use of sterile water for drinking by immunocompromised patients.
Cooling-tower draft	Properly design, place, and maintain cooling towers.
Aspergillosis	
Host related	
Severe granulocytopenia	Decrease duration of immunosuppression, such as by administration of GM-CSF; place patients with severe and prolonged granulocytopenia in protected environment.
Environment related	
Construction activity	Remove granulocytopenic patients from vicinity of construction; if not already done, place severe granulocytopenic patients in protected environment; make severely granulocytopenic patients wear a mask when they leave their protected environment.
Other environmental sources of *Aspergillus*	Routinely maintain air-handling system and rooms of immunocompromised patients.
Respiratory Syncytial Virus Infection	
Host related	
Age <2 years; congenital pulmonary/ cardiac disease, immunosuppression	Consider routine readmission screening of patients at high risk for severe RSV infection, followed by cohorting of patients and nursing personnel during hospital outbreaks of RSV infection; consider prophylactic administration of RSV immunoglobulin (hyperimmune preparation).
Personnel or procedure related	
Cross-contamination by hands	Educate personnel; wash hands, wear gloves; wear a gown; during outbreaks, use private rooms or cohort patients and nursing personnel, and limit visitors.
Influenza	
Host related	
Age >65 years; immunosuppression	Vaccinate high-risk patients before the influenza season each year; use amantadine or rimantadine for chemoprophylaxis during an outbreak.
Personnel related	
Infected personnel	Before the influenza season each year, vaccinate personnel caring for high-risk patients; use amantadine or rimantadine for prophylaxis during an outbreak.

SOURCE: Adapted from Tablan.[57]

Common Community-Acquired Pneumonias

HEMOPHILUS INFLUENZAE

Microbiology and Epidemiology

H. influenzae is a small, nonmotile, non–spore-forming bacillus that is often part of the normal flora of the human respiratory tree. Aerobic growth requires two supplements, called X and V factor. Because of these growth requirements *H. influenzae* must be cultured on chocolate agar or around a streak of *S. aureus* (a source of V factor) on a blood agar plate. In the latter method, *H. influenzae* will revolve around the *S. aureus* streak—a finding that allows presumptive identification.

H. influenzae is found only in humans; no animal or environmental reservoirs exist. At any given time, up to 80 percent of the population carries the organism. Most adults are colonized with nonencapsulated strains, but in 3 to 5 percent the isolates have a capsule (usually type b). Nonencapsulated strains are principally associated with chronic bronchitis, otitis media, sinusitis, and conjunctivitis. Encapsulated strains more commonly cause epiglottitis, meningitis, pneumonia and empyema, and bone and joint infections.

Transmission between people is via the large-droplet route or by direct contact. With the widespread use of *H. influenzae* vaccine, the incidence of invasive disease has dropped dramatically.

Clinical Features and Diagnosis

H. influenzae type b is an unusual cause of pneumonia in children between 4 months and 4 years of age. The clinical findings are similar to those of bacterial pneumonia due to *S. aureus* or *S. pneumoniae*, except that the onset is more often insidious. Primary pneumonia in children is frequently associated with evidence of infection at other sites, including meningitis, epiglottitis, and bone and joint infection.

In adults, pneumonia may also be caused by nonencapsulated strains. Overall, *H. influenzae* is responsible for approximately 10 to 15 percent of adult pneumonias requiring hospital admission. Risk factors include alcoholism, underlying lung disease, and older age.

The onset of symptoms is generally abrupt. Common symptoms consist of fever, shaking chills, cough productive of purulent sputum, dyspnea, and pleuritic pain. Physical examination usually reveals acute illness with fever, tachypnea, lower-lobe rales, and consolidation. Irrespective of age, the chest radiograph usually reveals a segmented, lobar, bronchopneumonic, or interstitial pattern. Pleural effusions are common, but empyema is rare.

Diagnosis is made from smear and culture on chocolate media. Sputum cultures are positive in about 70 percent of cases and blood cultures in 20 percent.

Treatment and Prevention

H. influenzae strains increasingly produce β-lactamase and therefore exhibit resistance to penicillin or ampicillin. The most active drugs include third-generation cephalosporins (cefotaxime, ceftriaxone) and combinations of penicillins with a β-lactamase inhibitor (piperacillin-tazobactam, ampicillin-sulbactam, amoxicillin-clavulanate). Most strains are susceptible to trimethoprim-sulfamethoxazole, second-generation cephalosporins, and quinolones. The newer macrolides, azithromycin and clarithromycin, may also be used to provide oral therapy. Most patients respond to therapy within 24 h.

All children should be immunized according to current recommendations of the Advisory Committee on Immunization Practices and the American Academy of Pediatrics "Red Book" against *H. influenzae* type b.

MORAXELLA CATARRHALIS

Microbiology and Epidemiology

Moraxella catarrhalis is a nonmotile, strictly aerobic, oxidase-positive gram-negative bacillus. The organism is part of the normal flora of the upper respiratory tract. *M. catarrhalis* may cause otitis media, sinusitis, bronchitis, and pneumonia.

Clinical Features and Diagnosis

M. catarrhalis may cause pneumonia indistinguishable from that caused by *H. influenzae*. Sepsis is unusual.

Treatment and Prevention

M. catarrhalis strains often produce β-lactamases. The organism's susceptibility profile is similar to that of *H. influenzae*.

BORDETELLA PERTUSSIS

Microbiology and Epidemiology

Bordetella pertussis is the causative agent of pertussis or whooping cough. The *Bordetellae* are tiny (0.2 to 0.5 by 0.5 to 2.0 μm) coccobacillary organisms that appear singly or in pairs and often have a bipolar appearance.[61] The organism is a strict aerobe that exhibits optimal growth at 35°C. *B. pertussis* produces a number of biologically active substances that may play a role in disease, including filamentous hemagglutinin, adenylate cyclase toxin, dermonecrotic toxin, pertussis toxin, tracheal cytotoxin, and α-hemolysin. Occasionally, *B. parapertussis* and *B. bronchiseptica* may produce a clinical illness similar to that caused by *B. pertussis*.

More than 4500 cases of pertussis were reported to the CDC in 1994. However, CDC surveillance may detect as few as 10 percent of cases. Pertussis incidence is usually characterized by a cyclic pattern, with peaks occurring at 3- to 4-year intervals. The current levels of pertussis are considerably higher than levels reported between 1976 and 1980. Reasons for the resurgence of pertussis are unclear, but according to the CDC, the higher levels reported in recent years are not related to a decrease in vaccine coverage (about 70 percent for children aged 2) or to a substantive reduction in efficacy of diphtheria, pertussis, tetanus (DPT) vaccine.

Adolescents and young adults play an important role in transmitting pertussis to susceptible infants because immunization-induced immunity to pertussis wanes with increasing age. Furthermore, because booster immunizations are not given after the age of 6, immunity in adults is boosted only through inadvertent exposure to the organism. It has been estimated that approximately 50 million adults in the United States are susceptible to pertussis, and this number will continue to increase.[4] Adults and adolescents are also an important vector in the transmission of pertussis to children because pertussis in adults is mild or "atypical" and frequently not diagnosed.

Humans are the only reservoir of *B. pertussis*. Transmission occurs by close contact via large aerosol droplets from the respiratory tract of symptomatic persons. Fomites play no role in transmission. The attack rate among immunized household contacts of children with pertussis may exceed 80 percent.

Clinical Features and Diagnosis

The incubation period for pertussis ranges from less than 1 week to more than 3 weeks (average, 7 to 10 days). Classically, the early phase (catarrhal) is characterized by rhinorrhea, lacrimation, mild conjunctival injection, malaise, and low-grade fever. The later phase (paroxysmal) is characterized by cough paroxysms (the "whoop"), especially in children. Patients often exhibit leukolymphocytosis, and pulmonary consolidation may occur.

Pertussis in adults is characterized most commonly by upper respiratory tract symptoms or prolonged cough. Classic disease, including the whoop, can occur; however, 20 percent of infected adults may remain asymptomatic. Because the signs and symptoms in adults usually are nonspecific, pertussis is rarely considered in adults until a child contact develops classic disease.

Pertussis may be diagnosed with culture, direct fluorescent antibody (DFA) techniques performed on smears, serology, and polymerase chain reaction. Cultures must be obtained by the nasopharyngeal method and plated on either Bordet-Gengou or Regan-Lowe (preferred because of longer shelf life). Detection often requires 3 to 6 days of growth. Although culture is the gold-standard method, newer serologic methods have demonstrated that culture is not a sensitive method of diagnosis. In addition, the ability to isolate *B. pertussis* in culture declines significantly when patients reach the paroxysmal phase of disease. Unfortunately, the currently available DFA lacks sensitivity and is subject to interobserver variability. Newer serologic tests are highly sensitive and specific, but are generally not clinically available.

Treatment and Prevention

B. pertussis continues to be highly susceptible in vitro to erythromycin, although there have been several isolated reports of erythromycin-resistant strains. Chloramphenicol, ampicillin, and oxytetracycline have moderate activity. Most strains of *B. pertussis* are resistant to clindamycin, methicillin, and first- and second-generation cephalosporins. Erythromycin has been shown to decrease the duration of illness when administered early in the course of pertussis. Treatment of infected persons with erythromycin has been shown to eliminate pertussis organisms in a few days. For these reasons, erythromycin is the drug of choice for treatment and prophylaxis of pertussis. Some investigators prefer the use of the estolate preparation because it produces higher blood levels than the ethylsuccinate or stearate preparations. However, the use of a higher dose of erythromycin base (50 to 60 mg/kg a day) also has been reported to be effective. Treatment or prophylaxis requires a 14-day course of therapy. The newer macrolides, clarithromycin and azithromycin, are active in vitro against *B. pertussis*. Preliminary data from Japan suggest that they are clinically effective. However, they are not FDA approved for the prophylaxis or treatment of *B. pertussis*.

Immunization with DPT vaccine should be part of a routine childhood immunization program. Acellular pertussis vaccines are now FDA approved for use in children of all ages. As they demonstrate similar or improved efficacy and reduced toxicity, they should replace whole-cell pertussis vaccine.

KLEBSIELLA

Microbiology and Epidemiology

The family Enterobacteriaceae consists of a heterogeneous group of gram-negative bacteria, including *E. coli, Klebsiella, Shigella, Edwardsiella, Citrobacter, Enterobacter, Serratia, Hafnia, Proteus, Morganella, Providencia, Yersinia,* and *Erwinia*. Although many of these bacilli may cause pneumonia, *Klebsiella* is the most common enteric gram-negative rod that causes community-acquired pneumonia. However, it accounts for only about 1 to 5 percent of community-acquired pneumonias.

Although *Klebsiella* is a community-acquired pathogen, most patients who develop pneumonia have underlying medical ailments. Risk factors include alcoholism, chronic obstructive pulmonary disease, and diabetes mellitus.

Clinical Features and Diagnosis

K. pneumoniae is an important cause of community-acquired lobar pneumonia. Classically, *Klebsiella* pneumonia has an acute onset and leads to a severe destructive lung infection. Symptoms include rigors (in about 60 percent of patients), high fever, productive cough, and pleuritic chest pain (in about 80 percent). The sputum has been described as "currant jelly" in quality. The classic radiographic picture is of a swollen infiltrated lobe. (This may produce the "bowed fissure" radiographic sign.) Complications are common and include abscess formation, cavitation, and empyema. Mortality is high because many patients have underlying illnesses and because of the destructive nature of the pneumonic process. *Klebsiella* may also cause less severe respiratory tract infections, such as bronchitis or bronchopneumonia.

A Gram's stain of the sputum may reveal short, plump, gram-negative bacilli. In many patients, however, the sputum is not revealing. Blood cultures are positive in up to 25 percent of patients. The mortality ranges from 20 to 50 percent in appropriately treated patients.

Treatment and Prevention

Klebsiella strains are often sensitive to cephalosporins, the most active being the third- (ceftriaxone, cefotaxime) and fourth-generation cephalosporins (cefepime). Resistance due to expanded-spectrum β-lactamases is an increasing problem, most notably in nosocomial cases. Therapy should be based on susceptibility testing. Other drugs with potential are piperacillin-tazobactam, carbapenems (imipenem, meropenem), and quinolones. No vaccine is currently available.

Unusual Community-Acquired Pneumonias

TULAREMIA

Microbiology and Epidemiology

The etiologic agent of tularemia ("rabbit-skinner's disease") is *Francisella tularensis,* a small, gram-negative, nonmotile coccobacillus. Tularemia is a vector-borne disease. The tick vectors in the United States include *A. americanum* in the southeastern and south central states, *D. andersoni* in the West, and *D. variabilis,* which has the widest distribution of the three tick vectors. Tularemia may also be transmitted by the bite of the deerfly, *Chysops discalis*. The reservoirs of *F. tularensis* include numerous small animals—especially rabbits, hares, muskrats, and beavers—and some domestic animals, as well as various hard ticks.

Approximately 100 cases of tularemia were reported to the CDC in 1994. The disease is widespread throughout the United States, but the greatest number of cases have been reported from Arkansas, Missouri, and Oklahoma. Cases occur in all months of the year; the incidence may be higher in adults in early winter during rabbit-hunting season and in children during summer, when ticks and deerflies are abundant.

In patients with pneumonia, tularemia may be transmitted from person to person. Patients with known or suspected tularemic pneumonia should be placed on droplet precautions.

Clinical Features and Diagnosis

The incubation period of tularemia averages 3 to 5 days (range, 1 to 21 days). Tularemia usually starts abruptly, with onset of fevers, chills, headache, anorexia, malaise, and fatigue. Symptoms may also include myalgias, cough, vomiting, pharyngitis, abdominal pain, and diarrhea. Fever typically lasts for several days, remits for a brief period, and then recurs.

The clinical presentation largely depends on the route of inoculation. Clinical syndromes include ulceroglandular fever (in 21 to 87 percent of cases), which follows tick bites and animal contact; it is characterized by enlarged and tender local adenopathy and an ulcer at the inoculation site. Glandular tularemia (in 3 to 20 percent) occurs when patients present with tender regional adenopathy without evidence of a local cutaneous lesion. Oculoglandular tularemia (in up to 5 percent) is characterized by photophobia and lacrimation. Pharyngeal tularemia (in up to 12 percent) is acquired from contaminated foods or water and is characterized by exudative pharyngitis or tonsillitis. Typhoidal tularemia (5 to 30 percent) may result from any mode of transmission. Symptoms suggest multiorgan involvement and include fever, headache, chills, myalgias, nausea, vomiting, abdominal pain, and cough. Secondary pneumonitis may occur in up to 45 percent of patients.

Finally, tularemic pneumonia (in 7 to 20 percent of cases) may occur following inhalation of the organism.[46] Symptoms include fever, cough, minimal or no sputum production, substernal chest tightness, and occasionally pleuritic chest pain. Physical examination is frequently nonspecific but may reveal rales, consolidation, or a pleural rub. Suggestive findings on physical exam include a cutaneous eschar, a tender enlarged lymph node, and pharyngeal exudate with tender cervical adenopathy.

The various clinical presentations of tularemia frequently lead to misdiagnosis. Pneumonic tularemia is in the differential diagnosis of atypical pneumonia, viruses, *Mycoplasma* and *Legionella* infections, plague, anthrax, Q fever, and psittacosis. The key to proper diagnosis is obtaining a history of potential exposure to *F. tularensis;* routine laboratory tests are nonspecific. *F. tularensis* may be recovered from the blood, lymph nodes, wounds, sputum, and pleural fluid when processed on special media. Tularemia presents a special hazard to laboratory personnel, and they should always be informed if tularemia is considered. The diagnosis is usually confirmed with serologic studies. ELISA is the preferred diagnostic test. Acute and convalescent sera are usually required.

Treatment and Prevention

The drug of choice for treatment is streptomycin, administered at a dosage of 7.5 to 10 mg/kg intramuscularly every 12 h for 7 to 14 days. (The alternative is gentamicin.) The pediatric dose is 30 to 40 mg/kg per day intramuscularly in two divided doses for 7 days. Tetracycline and chloramphenicol have been used orally for therapy, but both are bacteriostatic and a high rate of relapse has been noted. Many other drugs (erythromycin, rifampin, cefoxitin, cefotaxime, ceftriaxone, quinolones) have demonstrated activity in vitro, but clinical studies of in vivo effectiveness are, in general, unavailable.

Prevention requires careful handling of animal skins and carcasses. Tick prevention includes the use of tick repellents, long pants, and high socks outdoors in the summer and a careful search for ticks at least twice per day with removal if any are found.

PASTEURELLOSIS

Microbiology and Epidemiology

Pasteurellosis is caused by *Pasteurella multocida,* a small, nonmotile, non–spore-forming gram-negative coccobacillus. On Gram's smear, the organisms generally appear as a single bacillus but may occur in pairs or chains. They frequently show bipolar staining. The organisms are aerobic and facultatively anaerobic and grow well at 37°C on blood, chocolate, and Mueller-Hinton agar but not on MacConkey's agar. Growth is facilitated by enriched media and increased carbon dioxide tension.

P. multocida has been isolated from the digestive system or respiratory tract of many animals, including domestic cats and dogs, large cats (e.g., lions), rodents, rabbits, cattle, swine, and horses. Carriage rates of *P. multocida* in oral or nasal secretions have been reported to be 70 to 90 percent in cats and 50 to 66 percent in dogs. Most human infections result from direct inoculation by bites or scratches. Infections following animal exposure in the absence of bites or scratches probably stem from contact with animal secretions. Human-to-human spread of infection has not been documented, and contaminated food and water have not been implicated as sources of infection.

Clinical Features and Diagnosis

Infections with *P. multocida* may be divided into three categories: (1) soft tissue infections following animal bites or scratches, (2) oral and respiratory infections, and (3) serious invasive infection unrelated to animal bites, such as meningitis, intra-abdominal infections, or ocular infection. The respiratory tract is second to animal bite wounds as a source of *P. multocida* isolates from humans. *P. multocida* may cause sinusitis, otitis media, tonsillitis, bronchitis, pneumonia, or empyema. Most patients who have *P. multocida* respiratory tract infections also have underlying pulmonary disorders such as bronchiectasis, carcinoma of the lung, obstructive pulmonary disease, or chronic sinusitis. In such patients, *P. multocida* may colonize the respiratory tree for long periods.

P. multocida may be diagnosed from culture of sputum with standard techniques.

Treatment and Prevention

P. multocida is highly susceptible to many antibiotics, including penicillin G, ampicillin, piperacillin, second- and third-generation cephalosporins, chloramphenicol, and quinolones. Penicillin is the drug of choice. Less active agents include first-generation cephalosporins, aminoglycosides, vancomycin, erythromycin, and clindamycin.

YERSINIA PESTIS

Microbiology and Epidemiology

The genus *Yersinia* includes *Y. pestis, Y. enterocolitica,* and *Y. pseudotuberculosis. Y. pestis,* the cause of plague, is a gram-negative bipolar-staining bacillus. It grows aerobically on most culture media, including blood and MacConkey's agar, after 24-h incubation at 35°C.

Plague occurs worldwide, but most cases are reported from the less developed countries in Africa and Asia. In the United States, most cases are reported from the Southwest and occur between May and October. Man is an accidental host; the reservoir for *Y. pestis* includes rodents (especially rats), pigs, and birds. Plague is transmitted by flea bites, by ingestion of contaminated animal tissues, or by inhalation. In rare instances, pneumonic plague may be transmitted from person to person. Risk factors for acquisition include direct contact with rodents, the presence of shelter or food for wild rodents in the vicinity of the home, and inadequate protection against fleas for domestic cats and dogs.

Clinical Features and Diagnosis

The major clinical syndromes of plague include bubonic plague, septicemic plague, and pneumonic plague. The incubation for bubonic plague is 2 to 8 days following the bite of an infected flea. Characteristically, patients suddenly develop fever, chills, weakness, headache, and then intense pain, with swelling of a regional lymph node (the "bubo"). Some patients develop septicemic plague, characterized by overwhelming sepsis. Secondary pneumonia may develop with hematogenous spread of bacteria during sepsis. Pneumonic plague is highly contagious and has a high mortality. Clinical findings, in addition to fever and lymphadenopathy, include cough, chest pain, and frequently hemoptysis. The chest radiograph most commonly reveals patchy bronchopneumonia, cavities, or consolidation.

As with other zoonotic disease, an epidemiologic exposure in the setting of an appropriate clinical syndrome should lead one to suspect plague. A bacteriologic diagnosis is easily made in most patients from smear and culture of a bubo aspirate. The smear should be processed for both Gram's and Wayson's stains. In pneumonic plague, the organism is readily isolated from sputum. Cultures may be sent to the CDC for identification, but all cultures should be handled with extreme caution, as they represent a significant risk to laboratory personnel. Serology can also be used to confirm the diagnosis.

Treatment and Prevention

Streptomycin is the drug of choice for plague. It should be administered intramuscularly at a daily dose of 30 mg/kg in two divided doses for 10 days. In allergic patients, tetracycline is an acceptable alternative in a dose of 2 to 4 g a day in four divided doses for 10 days.

Prevention consists of avoidance of areas of the world with endemic or epidemic plague and extreme care when handling animal carcasses.

Nosocomial Pneumonias

ENTEROBACTERIACEAE

Microbiology and Epidemiology

Enteric gram-negative bacilli are an important cause of nosocomial pneumonia. In certain patients, such as those in chronic care facilities, immunocompromised patients, or those with underlying lung disease, they are also an important cause of community-acquired pneumonia. Of the enteric pathogens, the most common agents in pneumonia are *Klebsiella, E. coli, Enterobacter, Proteus,* and *Serratia.* All these pathogens grow readily on blood or MacConkey's agar. These bacteria are normal flora of the gastrointestinal tract. As previously noted, hospitalization and other host factors (e.g., alcoholism) favor colonization of the oral cavity.

Clinical Features and Diagnosis

The enteric bacteria are opportunistic pathogens that cause pneumonia in the setting of impaired host defenses. All may produce a destructive pneumonia. Characteristically, patients with pneumonia due to enteric pathogens have fever, chills, cough with production of sputum, shortness of breath, and pleuritic pain. The clinical features are not specific enough for one to be able to distinguish among the many enteric bacteria capable of causing pneumonia. In some patients—including immunosuppressed persons, the elderly, and patients with hematogenously spread pneumonia—the signs and symptoms of pneumonia may be reduced or absent. Blood cultures have been reported to be positive in 10 to 50 percent of patients, depending on the etiologic agent and the patient population. The radiographic findings do not allow microbiologic diagnosis, although they may be suggestive. As previously noted, the presence of a bulging fissure suggests pneumonia with *K. pneumoniae.* Gram-negative pneumonia is suggested by early necrosis and abscess formation, although it may also be seen with *S. pneumoniae, S. aureus,* and *Legionella.*

Treatment and Prevention

The most active agents against gram-negative enteric pathogens are the third- and fourth-generation cephalosporins (cefotaxime, ceftriaxone, ceftazidime, cefepime), a penicillin combined with a β-lactamase inhibitor (piperacillin-tazobactam), carbapenems (imipenem, meropenem), monobactams (aztreonam), and quinolones (ciprofloxacin). Aminoglycosides are also active but are rarely used as primary therapy. Some strains of *Klebsiella, Enterobacter,* and *Serratia* may be resistant to a number of antibiotics. Definitive therapy should be guided by in vitro susceptibility results and clinical response.

PSEUDOMONAS AERUGINOSA

Microbiology and Epidemiology

The family Pseudomonadaceae contains more than 150 species. However, the most important member of this family is *P. aeruginosa. P. aeruginosa* is an obligate, motile, rod-shaped (0.5 to 0.8 by 1.5 to 3.0 μm) gram-negative bacillus with a single flagellum. It may produce a variety of pigments, including pyocyanin (a pigment produced by approximately 50 percent of clinical strains), which causes colonies to appear blue or green. *P. aeruginosa* is capable of utilizing more than 30 organic compounds for growth. It grows optimally at 37°C.

P. aeruginosa can be isolated from soil, water, plants, and animals. Its minimal nutritional requirements allow it to reproduce in many ecologic niches in the hospital. Reservoirs discovered during outbreaks have included many moist devices and surfaces found in hospitals, including endoscopes, endoscope washers, disinfectants, food mixers, and enteral foods. *P. aeruginosa* may also be part of the normal flora of humans. *P. aeruginosa* is primarily a nosocomial pathogen and is the most common gram-negative bacillus causing hospital-acquired pneumonia. Within the hospital, *P. aeruginosa* acts as opportunistic pathogen. Particularly vulnerable are patients with skin or mucous membrane disruption, intravenous catheters, urinary tract catheters, neutropenia, immunosuppressive medication, cystic fibrosis, and diabetes mellitus.

The pathogenesis of *P. aeruginosa* infections is very complex and includes many virulence factors. Key factors include the pili or fimbriae, which mediate adherence to respiratory epithelial cells; the mucoid capsule, which aids in anchoring the organism to its environment; cell-associated factors, which protect the organism from host phagocytes and complement; and extracellular enzymes and toxins, which promote penetration and impair host defenses.

Clinical Features and Diagnosis

P. aeruginosa causes respiratory infection almost exclusively in patients with impaired respiratory host defenses. Only occasionally does *P. aeruginosa* cause community-acquired pneumonia, and then usually in patients cared for in extended care facilities or with chronic lung disease or other serious underlying illness. *P. aeruginosa* and *S. aureus* are the most important pathogens in patients with cystic fibrosis. Pneumonia due to *P. aeruginosa* is usually a fulminant infection and is characterized by fever, rigors, severe dyspnea, cough productive of sputum, cyanosis, and systemic shock. The chest radiograph commonly reveals a diffuse bilateral bronchopulmonary pneumonia with distinctive nodular infiltrates and small areas of radiolucency. Although pleural effusions are common, empyema is rare.

Bacteremic pneumonia may occur in severely neutropenic patients. Patients with bacteremic pneumonia characteristically have ill-defined hemorrhagic, nodular areas that are frequently subpleural. Central necrosis of these areas may occur.

Treatment and Prevention

P. aeruginosa is typically treated with an aminoglycoside and an antipseudomonal penicillin (piperacillin), cephalosporin (ceftazidime, cefepime), carbapenem (imipenem, meropenem), or monobactam (aztreonam). The quinolones are also active, but only ciprofloxacin is currently available as an intravenous preparation. Despite therapy, the mortality from hospital-acquired pseudomonal pneumonia is approximately 70 percent. Unfortunately, there are no specific measures to prevent nosocomial pseudomonal infections available at the present time.

REFERENCES

1. American Thoracic Society: Hospital-acquired pneumonia in adults: Diagnosis, assessment of severity, initial antimicrobial therapy, and preventive strategies. *Am J Respir Crit Care Med* 153:1711–1725, 1996.
2. Bartlett JC, O'Keefe P, Tally FP: Bacteriology of hospital-acquired pneumonia. *Arch Intern Med* 146:868–871, 1991.
3. Baselski VS, el-Torkey M, Coalson JJ, Griffin JP: The standardization of criteria for processing and interpreting laboratory specimens in patients with suspected ventilator-associated pneumonia. *Chest* 102(Suppl 1):571S–579S, 1992.
4. Bass JW, Stephenson SR: The return of pertussis. *Pediatr Infect Dis* 6:141–144, 1987.
5. Cassiere HA, Niederman MS: New etiopathogenic concepts of ventilator-associated pneumonia. *Semin Respir Infect* 11:12–23, 1996.
6. Centers for Disease Control and Prevention: Draft guidelines for prevention of nosocomial pneumonia. *Federal Register* 59:4980–5022, 1994.
7. Centers for Disease Control and Prevention: National Nosocomial Infections Surveillance (NNIS) Semiannual Report, May 1995. *Am J Infect Control* 23:377–385, 1995.
8. Chastre J, Fagon J-Y: Invasive diagnostic testing should be routinely used to manage ventilated patients with suspected pneumonia. *Am J Respir Crit Care Med* 150:570–574, 1994.
9. Chastre J, Trouillet J-L, Fagon J-Y: Diagnosis of pulmonary infections in mechanically ventilated patients. *Semin Respir Infect* 11:65–76, 1996.
10. Cook DJ, Laine LA, Guyatt GH: Nosocomial pneumonia and the role of gastric pH. *Chest* 100:7–13, 1996.
11. Cook DJ, Reeve BK, Scholes LC: Histamine H-2-receptor antagonists and antacids in the critically ill population: Stress ulceration versus nosocomial pneumonia. *Infect Control Hosp Epidemiol* 15:437–442, 1994.
12. Craig CP, Connelly S: Effect of intensive care unit nosocomial pneumonia on duration of stay and mortality. *Am J Infect Control* 12:233–238, 1984.
13. Craven DE, Kunches LM, Kilinsky V, et al: Risk factors for pneumonia and fatality in patients receiving continuous mechanical ventilation. *Am Rev Respir Dis* 133:792–796, 1986.
14. Craven DE, Steger KA: Nosocomial pneumonia in the intubated patient: New concepts on pathogenesis and prevention. *Infect Dis Clin North Am* 3:843–866, 1989.
15. Craven DE, Steger KA: Epidemiology of nosocomial pneumonia: New perspectives on an old disease. *Chest* 108(Suppl):1S–16S, 1995.
16. Craven DE, Steger KA: Nosocomial pneumonia in mechanically ventilated adult patients: Epidemiology and prevention in 1996. *Semin Respir Infect* 11:32–53, 1996.
17. Daschner F, Nadjem H, Langmaack H, Sandritter W: Surveillance, prevention and control of hospital-acquired infections: III. Nosocomial infections as cause of death: Retrospective analysis of 1000 autopsy reports. *Infection* 6:261–265, 1978.
18. Daschner F, Kappstein I, Schuster F, et al: Influence of disposable ("Conchapak") and reusable humidifying systems on the incidence of ventilation pneumonia. *J Hosp Infect* 11:161–168, 1988.
19. Daschner F, Kappstein I, Engels I, et al: Stress ulcer prophylaxis and ventilation pneumonia: Prevention by antibacterial cytoprotective agents? *Infect Control Hosp Epidemiol* 9:59–65, 1988.
20. Deppe SA, Kelly JW, Thoi LL, et al: Incidence of colonization, nosocomial pneumonia, and mortality in critically ill patients using a Trach Care closed-suction system versus an open-suction system: Prospective, randomized study. *Crit Care Med* 18:1389–1393, 1990.
21. Dreyfuss D, Djedaini K, Weber P, et al: Prospective study of nosocomial pneumonia and of patient and circuit colonization during mechanical ventilation with circuit changes every 48 hours versus no change. *Am Rev Respir Dis* 143:738–743, 1991.
22. Emori TG, Gaynes RP: An overview of nosocomial infections, including the role of the microbiology laboratory. *Clin Microbiol Rev* 6:428–442, 1993.

23. Fagon J-Y, Chastre J, Domart Y, et al: Nosocomial pneumonia in patients receiving continuous mechanical ventilation. *Am Rev Respir Dis* 139:877–884, 1989.

24. Fagon J-Y, Chastre J, Hance AJ, et al: Nosocomial pneumonia in ventilated patients: A cohort study evaluating attributable mortality and hospital stay. *Am J Med* 94:282–288, 1993.

25. Fagon J-Y, Chastre J, Vuagnat A, et al: Nosocomial pneumonia and mortality among patients in intensive care units. *JAMA* 275:866–869, 1996.

26. Garner JS: Guideline for isolation precautions in hospitals. *Infect Control Hosp Epidemiol* 17:53–80, 1996.

27. Garrard CS, A'Court CD: The diagnosis of pneumonia in the critically ill. *Chest* 108(Suppl):17S–25S, 1995.

28. George DL: Epidemiology of nosocomial ventilator-associated pneumonia. *Infect Control Hosp Epidemiol* 14:163–169, 1993.

29. George DL: Epidemiology of nosocomial pneumonia in intensive care patients. *Clin Chest Med* 16:29–44, 1995.

30. Gómez J, Esquinas A, Agudo MD, et al: Retrospective analysis of risk factors and prognosis in non-ventilated patients with nosocomial pneumonia. *Eur J Clin Microbiol Infect Dis* 14:176–181, 1995.

31. Gross PA, Neu HC, Aswapokee P, et al: Deaths from nosocomial infections: Experience in a university hospital and a community hospital. *Am J Med* 68:219–223, 1980.

32. Hanson LC, Weber DJ, Rutala WA: Risk factors for nosocomial pneumonia in the elderly. *Am J Med* 92:161–166, 1992.

33. Hart CA, Makin T: *Legionella* in hospitals: A review. *J Hosp Infect* 18(Suppl A):481–489, 1991.

34. Horan TC, White JW, Jarvis WR, et al: Nosocomial Infection Surveillance, 1984. *MMWR CDC Surveill Summ* 35:15–29, 1986.

35. Jacobs S, Chang RWS, Lee B, Bartlett FW: Continuous enteral feeding: A major cause of pneumonia among ventilated intensive care unit patients. *J Parenter Enter Nutr* 14:353–356, 1990.

36. Jiménez P, Torres A, Rodríguez-Roisin R, et al: Incidence and etiology of pneumonia acquired during mechanical ventilation. *Crit Care Med* 17:882–885, 1989.

37. Johanson WG, Pierce AK, Sanford JP, Thomas GD: Nosocomial respiratory infections with gram-negative bacilli: The significance of colonization of the respiratory tract. *Ann Intern Med* 77:701–706, 1972.

38. Klein BS, Perloff WH, Maki DG: Reduction of nosocomial infection during pediatric intensive care by protective isolation. *N Engl J Med* 320:1714–1721, 1989.

39. Kollef MH: Ventilator-associated pneumonia: A multivariate analysis. *JAMA* 270:1965–1970, 1993.

40. Langer M, Mosconi P, Cigada M, Mandelli M, and the Intensive Care Unit Group of Infection Control: Long-term respiratory support and risk of pneumonia in critically ill patients. *Am Rev Respir Dis* 140:302–305, 1989.

41. Larson EL: APIC guidelines for handwashing and hand antisepsis in health care settings. *Am J Infect Control* 23:251–269, 1995.

42. Leu H-S, Kaiser DL, Mori M, et al: Hospital-acquired pneumonia: Attributable mortality and morbidity. *Am J Epidemiol* 129:1258–1267, 1989.

43. Levine SA, Niederman MS: The impact of tracheal intubation on host defenses and risks for nosocomial pneumonia. *Clin Chest Med* 12:523–543, 1991.

44. Meduri GU: Diagnosis and differential diagnosis of ventilator-associated pneumonia. *Clin Chest Med* 16:61–91, 1995.

45. Meduri GU, Johanson WG: Introduction to the consensus conference. *Infect Control Hosp Epidemiol* 13:633–634, 1992.

46. Miller RP, Bases JH: Pleuropulmonary tularemia: A review of 29 patients. *Am Rev Respir Dis* 99:31–41, 1969.

47. Muraca PW, Yu VL, Goetz A: Disinfection of water distribution systems for *Legionella*: A review of application procedures and methodologies. *Infect Control Hosp Epidemiol* 11:79–88, 1990.

48. Niederman MS, Torres A, Summer W: Invasive diagnostic testing is not needed routinely to manage suspected ventilator-associated pneumonia. *Am J Respir Crit Care Med* 150:565–569, 1994.

49. Rashkin MC, Davis T: Acute complications of endotracheal intubation. *Chest* 89:165–167, 1986.

50. Rello J, Quintana E, Ausina V, et al: Incidence, etiology, and outcome of nosocomial pneumonia in mechanically ventilated patients. *Chest* 100:439–444, 1991.

51. Reusser P, Zimmerli W, Scheidegger D, et al: Role of gastric colonization in nosocomial infections and endotoxemia: A prospective study in neurosurgical patients on mechanical ventilation. *J Infect Dis* 160:414–421, 1989.

52. Rubin HH, Green R: Clinical approach to the compromised host with fever and pulmonary infiltrate, in Rubin RH, Young LS (eds), *Clinical Approach to Infection in the Compromised Host.* New York, Plenum, 1994.

53. Ruiz-Santana S, García Jimenez A, Esteban A, et al: ICU pneumonias: A multi-institutional study. *Crit Care Med* 15:930–932, 1987.

54. Rutala WA: APIC guidelines for selection and use of disinfectants. *Am J Infect Control* 18:99–118, 1990.

55. Rutala WA, Weber DJ: Environmental issues and nosocomial infections, in Farber BF (ed), *Infection Control in Intensive Care.* New York, Churchill Livingstone, 1987, pp 131–171.

56. Spach DH, Silverstein FE, Stamm WE: Transmission of infection by gastrointestinal endoscopy and bronchoscopy. *Ann Intern Med* 118:117–128, 1993.

57. Tablan OC, Anderson LJ, Arden NH, et al, and the Hospital Infection Control Practices Advisory Committee: Guideline for prevention of nosocomial pneumonia. *Infect Control Hosp Epidemiol* 15:587–627, 1994.

58. Torres A, Aznar R, Gatell JM, et al: Incidence, risk and prognosis factors of nosocomial pneumonia in mechanically ventilated patients. *Am Rev Respir Dis* 142:523–526, 1990.

59. Tryba M: Sucralfate versus antacids or H2-antagonists for stress ulcer prophylaxis: A meta-analysis on efficacy and pneumonia rate. *Crit Care Med* 19:942–949, 1991.

60. Weber DJ, Rutala WA: Infection control in critical care units, in Moylan J (ed), *Surgical Critical Care.* St. Louis, CV Mosby, 1994.

61. Weber DJ, Rutala WA: Management of healthcare workers exposed to pertussis. *Infect Control Hosp Epidemiol* 15:411–415, 1994.

62. Weber DJ, Rutala WA: Nosocomial infections associated with respiratory therapy, in Mayhall CG (ed), *Hospital Epidemiology and Infection Control.* Baltimore, Williams & Wilkins, 1996, pp 748–758.

63. Weber DJ, Rutala WA: Environmental issues and nosocomial infections, in Wenzal R (ed), *Prevention and Control of Nosocomial Infections,* 3d ed. Baltimore, Williams & Wilkins. In press.

CHAPTER 144

LEGIONELLOSIS

Victor L. Yu / Emanuel N. Vergis

Legionnaires' disease was named after the outbreak of severe pneumonia afflicting 182 people attending the American Legion Convention in Philadelphia in 1976. In the several months after the outbreak, investigators from the Centers for Disease Control (CDC) identified a previously unknown microbial agent from postmortem lung tissue. The organism was named *Legionella pneumophila* (Greek for "lung loving").

Analysis of sera isolated from patients from a number of prior unexplained pneumonia outbreaks also implicated *L. pneumophila* as the causative agent. For example, in 1957, an outbreak of an unexplained pneumonia occurred at a meat-packing plant in Austin, Minnesota.[49] A retrospective serologic case control survey suggested that *L. pneumophila* was the pathogen.

Legionellosis describes the collective clinical syndromes produced by members of the Legionellaceae family. Legionnaires' disease is pneumonia due to *L. pneumophila*, whereas the nonpneumonic acute febrile illness known as Pontiac fever is serologically linked to *L. pneumophila* and other *Legionella* species.

MICROBIOLOGY

Legionellaceae is the family, and the genus is *Legionella*. Forty species have been described. *L. pneumophila* is the species most frequently implicated in infection, but 20 other species have also been implicated in human infection; the most common are *L. micdadei* (Pittsburgh pneumonia agent), *L. bozemanii*, *L. dumoffii*, and *L. longbeachae*.[15] In addition, there are more than 50 serogroups within the individual species. Of the 14 serogroups of *L. pneumophila*, serogroups 1, 4, and 6 account for the vast majority of strains implicated in human disease. Molecular and biochemical techniques are used to distinguish *L. pneumophila* from other members of the family.

Legionella are gram-negative aerobic, unencapsulated bacilli. Visualization of the organism by Gram's stain is difficult in clinical specimens. Gimenez staining gives better results than Gram's stain. Silver staining techniques such as Dieterle and Warthin-Starry stains are used for visualizing *Legionella* in paraffin-fixed tissues.

Legionella are nutritionally fastidious and require special bacteriologic media for growth. Charcoal yeast extract buffered to pH 6.9 is the primary medium used for isolation of these organisms. Most strains of *Legionella* show a single flagellum and multiple fimbriae or pili. Other ultrastructural features are an inner trilaminar cytoplasmic membrane, a peptidoglycan layer, and an outer trilaminar membrane, typical of gram-negative bacilli. The major outer membrane protein of *L. pneumophila* forms nonpermeable channels within lipid membranes, as is characteristic for porins. The lipopolysaccharide of *L. pneumophila* serogroup 1 is tightly bound to this protein. Immunofluorescent techniques detect antibodies that are directed primarily at the lipopolysaccharide.

L. pneumophila produces a variety of extracellular products, including hemolysins, esterases, phosphatases, aminopeptidases, endonucleases, and a major secretory metalloprotease. Despite numerous laboratory investigations, none of these products have been linked to virulence.

EPIDEMIOLOGY

Ecology

Aquatic bodies—including rivers, lakes, streams, and thermally polluted waters—appear to be the natural habitat for *L. pneumophila*, although *L. longbeachae* has been grown from potting soil. However, the organism can be found only in minute numbers in these aquatic habitats. Man-made reservoirs serve as amplifiers for the organism. Water distribution systems, cooling towers, evaporative condensers, and water-containing respiratory devices have been shown to be sources of infection in humans.

L. pneumophila exhibits remarkable survivability under a wide range of environmental conditions. The optimal temperature for growth in water is 40° to 45°C, but it can survive at temperatures ranging from 0° to 63°C. Water samples stored at 2° to 8°C have been found to contain viable organisms after many years. Since *Legionella* species are chlorine tolerant, the organisms can survive water treatment processing and pass into the water distribution system.

L. pneumophila requires the presence of symbiotic microorganisms such as algae, amebas, and water bacteria for optimal growth. In natural aquatic bodies, free-living protozoa, including amebas and ciliated protozoa, support the intracellular growth of *Legionella*.

Hospital water tanks colonized with *L. pneumophila* were significantly more likely to have lower temperatures (under 140°F or 60°C). Vertically oriented tanks also are more likely to be colonized than horizontally oriented tanks because of the thicker sediment accumulation at the bottom with greater temperature strata. Water temperature and the presence of commensal microflora as well as sediment accumulation are factors important for the colonization of water distribution systems by *Legionella*.

Mode of Transmission

Many modes of transmission of *Legionella* to humans are likely. There is evidence for aerosolization, aspiration, and even direct instillation into the lungs during respiratory tract manipulation. Strong evidence for aerosolization and airborne dissemination was obtained from the investigation of the 1968 Pontiac fever outbreak. The central air-conditioning unit may have been contaminated by aerosols from an evaporating condenser.[29] Sentinel guinea pigs exposed to the air at the facility were subsequently found to have *L. pneumophila* in their lungs.

We have challenged the role of cooling towers as a reservoir for nosocomial Legionnaires' disease,[46,67] but this is highly controversial.[2] Outbreaks have been linked to cooling towers in a few studies, but most of these studies were conducted in the era before the knowledge that potable water could be the source. Nosocomial outbreaks of Legionnaires' disease attributed to cooling towers all but disappeared once it was recognized that potable water distribution systems could be a source. For example, in the United Kingdom, 19 of 20 hospital outbreaks of Legionnaires' disease investigated by the British Communicable Diseases Surveillance Center were attributed to hospital potable water distribution systems. Water distribution systems in homes and workplaces have now been implicated in community-acquired cases.[6,47,51,59]

The major mode of transmission from a water source to humans is aspiration. Preceding surgical procedures were more common in the patients with Legionnaires' disease than in patients with pneumonias of other origins.[68] General anesthesia with endotracheal intubation may be the predisposing factor for aspiration. Similarly, an outbreak of nosocomial legionellosis at Stanford University Hospital occurred mainly in patients undergoing cardiothoracic surgery; pneumonia usually occurred in the early postoperative period.[37,61] Patients with Legionnaires' disease have also been shown to be significantly more likely to have undergone endotracheal intubation[44] and to have experienced longer duration of intubation.[37]

In a prospective study performed in patients with head and neck cancer, 30 percent of the postoperative pneumonias were attributed to *Legionella*—one of the highest incidences ever recorded for nosocomial legionellosis.[25] These patients have an almost universal propensity for aspiration, since the site of tumor and surgical resection is the oropharynx. In addition, most of these patients have a history of heavy cigarette smoking—a risk factor not only for head and neck cancer but also for Legionnaires' disease. Microaspiration of contaminated water used to irrigate nasogastric tubes has been linked to Legionnaires' disease in anecdotal cases[9,24,40] and epidemiologic investigations.[3,38]

The initial isolation of *L. pneumophila* in a hospital was from a showerhead; since then, it has been widely assumed that shower aerosols are a mode of dissemination. Only a small amount of *Legionella* is aerosolized, however, and only for short periods when simulation studies were conducted. Furthermore, prospective studies have failed to show an epidemiologic association between showers and disease.[55,68]

Respiratory equipment and aerosol-generating devices have been linked to Legionnaires' disease. Table 144-1 summarizes nosocomial and community-acquired disease outbreaks and cases associated with such devices.

Humidifiers Humidifiers mechanically add water vapor to air, oxygen, or other gases without the production of particulate water. The water reservoir within the humidifier may be filled with tap water colonized with *Legionella*. Demonstration experiments have shown that guinea pigs exposed to a room humidifier contaminated with *Legionella* experience subclinical infection as demonstrated by seroconversion.[69] Furthermore, recovery of aerosolized *Legionella* increased with proximity to the humidifier, and seroconversion of exposed animals was directly proportional to concentration of *Legionella* in humidifier water. In a hospital setting, a portable room humidifier filled with *Legionella*-contaminated tap water disseminated the organism up to distances of 300 cm.[64]

Humidifiers have been implicated in transmission of Legionnaires' disease in humans. Patients with nosocomial Legionnaires' disease in one hospital had been exposed to bubble diffuser humidifiers filled with water containing *L. pneumophila*.[43] An immunosuppressed patient in another hospital exposed to a room humidifier filled with contaminated tap water for 15 days subsequently acquired Legionnaires' disease.[1] Use of a room humidifier was also associated with 18 cases of nosocomial Legionnaires' disease in a 2-year period in a retrospective study.[27] In all three of the above-mentioned studies, the humidifiers had been filled with tap water. A postlaryngectomy patient died from pneumonia following exposure to a room humidifier. *L. pneumophila*, serogroups 4 and 5, were isolated from the patient's lung and from tap water and a jerry can used to fill the humidifier reservoir.[28] One patient with *L. dumoffi* pneumonia was exposed to a room humidifier presumably filled with contaminated distilled water.[26]

TABLE 144-1

Legionellosis Associated with Respiratory Equipment

Device	Setting	No. of Patients	Immuno-suppressed (%)	Lung Disease (%)	Surgery/ Transplant (%)	Days Before Disease*	Infecting Organism	Epid Link†	Reference
Nebulizer	University	4 1	100	0	20	>7	Lp 1, 6 Lp 6	No	1
Tracheostomy	Home	1	100	0	0	5	Lp 6	Yes	4
Nebulizer, face masks	Pediatric hospital	7	70	70	0	>12	Lp	No	5
Nebulizer humidifier	University hospital	5	80	>20	>20	<10	*L. dumoffii*	Yes	26
Nebulizer humidifier, IPPB	Community hospital	18	44	NA	NA	<10	Lp 1, 4, 5	No	7
Humidifier	Hospital	1	0	0	100	<9	Lp 6 Lp 4, 5	Yes	28
Mist machine	Grocery store	28	7	0	NA	<2 h	Lp 1	Yes	35
Nebulizer	Community hospital	13	77	92	NA (0?)	<15	Lp 3	Yes	39
Humidifier, chest drain	Hospital	5 3	0	0	60	>10	Lp 1	No	43
Humidifier	Home	1	NA	NA	100	14	Lp 1	Yes	51

*Days before disease represent the number of days of exposure to the device before clinical symptoms of Legionnaires' disease.
†Epid link stands for *epidemiologic links;* infecting organism type matched environment organism type (see text).
NOTE: Lp = *L. pneumophila.* NA = Not available.
SOURCE: Data from Woo et al.[63]

Nebulizers   Nebulizers generate aerosols of uniform particulate size. These water particles, if less than 1 μm, can bypass upper-airway protective mechanisms and directly enter the alveoli. Medication jet nebulizers have been shown to aerosolize respirable-size droplets (less than 5 μm) containing *L. pneumophila* when 1 ml of nebulizer water was seeded with 500 colony-forming units of the organism.[39] Jet nebulizers have been linked to nosocomial Legionnaires' disease.[1] Inhalation of contaminated tap-water aerosols from jet nebulizers was a highly significant risk factor for four patients who acquired nosocomial Legionnaires' disease. *L. micdadei* was isolated from the couplant reservoirs of ultrasonic nebulizers in a hospital with endemic Pittsburgh pneumonia, although a causal relationship to nosocomial disease was not documented.[20] A significant association between nebulizer use and nosocomial Legionnaires' disease was also seen in the previously cited study that implicated humidifiers; the authors noted that the nebulizers had been rinsed with tap water.[27]

In addition to the filling of nebulizers with tap water, rinsing the chambers of handheld medication nebulizers has been suggested as a source of contamination. In a study of 13 patients with nosocomial Legionnaires' disease due to *L. pneumophila*, serogroup 3, there was found to be a trend toward more frequent use of nebulizer medications by patients with Legionnaires' disease. It was subsequently established that jet nebulizers were often rinsed with tap water.[39] Medication nebulizers have also been implicated in one of the few reports of pediatric nosocomial Legionnaires' disease. Two children with Legionnaires' disease received nebulizer treatments employing equipment likely to have been rinsed under tap water.[5]

Community-acquired Legionnaires' disease has also been associated with such devices. One patient developed Legionnaires' disease 3 days after cardiac transplantation. Hospital water sites failed to yield the organism, but the ultrasonic nebulizer in the patient's home showed heavy colonization by *L. pneumophila* and had been in use almost continuously for the 2 weeks before admission for Legionnaires' disease.[51] Monoclonal antibody subtyping of the patient's isolate of *L. pneumophila* matched that of the nebulizer isolate (Yu VL, unpublished data, 1988). Twenty-eight persons exposed to an ultrasonic mist machine in a grocery store contracted Legionnaires' disease.[35] This machine continuously generated a mist over the produce section. A higher incidence of Legionnaires' disease was associated with longer duration of shopping at the store and proximity to the mist machine. *L. pneumophila*, serogroup 1, isolated from the lung specimens of two patients matched the *L. pneumophila* isolated from the reservoir of the mist machine. Test aerosol experiments showed that the machine was capable of aerosolizing 1- to 5-μm water droplets containing *L. pneumophila*.

Other Respiratory Care Devices   Hand-powered resuscitation bags and intermittent positive-pressure breathing (IPPB) ventilators have also been implicated. Although these respiratory devices are not filled with water, simple rinsing of tubing components with contaminated tap water may seed a secondary reservoir. Resuscitation bags are frequently dismantled and rinsed with tap water to remove debris and secretions. After a resuscitation bag or its tubing was rinsed with contaminated tap water and the bag was squeezed, *L. pneumophila* could be recovered on culture plates 20 cm away.[64] In such a scenario, aerosols containing *Legionella* could be propelled directly into the respiratory tract. In fact, an immunosuppressed patient developed Legionnaires' disease after cleaning his tracheostomy cannula with contaminated tap water at home.[4] In two separate investigations, patients contracting nosocomial Legionnaires' disease were significantly more likely to have undergone endotracheal tube placement and to have longer duration of intubation than patients with pneumonias of other origins.[37,44]

IPPB ventilators have been associated with nosocomial legionellosis or, more likely, their tubing attachment components. The use of IPPB was epidemiologically linked to Legionnaires' disease in 18 hospital patients over a 2-year period;[27] again, it was noted that the IPPB equipment was rinsed with tap water between treatments.

Incidence

The incidence of Legionnaires' disease depends on the extent of contamination of the aquatic reservoir by the organism and the susceptibility of the population exposed to the water reservoir. Additionally, the expertise of the testing laboratory and availability of specialized testing are critical to the correct identification of the disease's origin.

L. pneumophila has been consistently shown to be among the three most common bacterial causes of community-acquired pneumonia if *Legionella* laboratory diagnostic tests are routinely applied. The incidence of community-acquired pneumonia in various studies ranges from 1 to 16 percent, with a median of about 5 percent. The incidence of nosocomial disease has been reported to be from 10 to 50 percent of nosocomial pneumonia cases in hospitals with a contaminated water supply.

The major risk factors are cigarette smoking and chronic pulmonary disease. Immunosuppressive therapy, especially with corticosteroids, is a major predisposing factor. Surgery is a risk factor for nosocomial disease. Organ transplant recipients appear to be at highest risk for contacting Legionnaires' disease. Legionnaires' disease may be seen within several weeks after transplantation and may be associated with episodes of rejection and increased immunosuppressive treatment. *Legionella* infection is increasingly seen in patients with AIDS. Extrapulmonary manifestations, bacteremia, and lung abscesses, uncommon in most patients, occur frequently in AIDS patients. Finally, infection in immunosuppressed children is now being reported; virtually all such infection has been hospital acquired, usually in neonatal or pediatric intensive care units.[52,58]

PATHOLOGY

Multifocal fibrinopurulent pneumonia is typical in the lungs of patients with Legionnaires' disease. The pneumonitis is characterized by acute alveolitis and bronchiolitis. Longer-standing lesions appear nodular and are composed of a central area containing both cell types, surrounded predominantly by macro-phages. Severe cases often lead to destruction of the lung parenchyma. Macroscopically visible abscess formations were seen in 20 percent of autopsies in one series. A prominent finding is the presence of fibrin-rich exudate in alveoli with polymorphonuclear cells and alveolar macrophages. A striking lysis of the exudate has been reported. Pulmonary fibrosis was noted as a sequela in one report. Extrapulmonary involvement of the spleen, liver, kidney, myocardium, brain, prostate, thyroid, and muscle has been observed.

PATHOGENESIS AND VIRULENCE

L. pneumophila is considered a facultative intracellular pathogen of mononuclear phagocytes, principally monocytes and alveolar macrophages. Mononuclear phagocytes ingest the bacteria through a process mediated by monocyte complement receptors, complement component C3, and the major outer membrane protein on the surface of *L. pneumophila*. Once phagocytized, *L. pneumophila* evades destruction by inhibiting phagosome-lipsome fusion.[22] Activated monocytes inhibit intracellular replication of *L. pneumophila* rather than killing the organism. Polymorphonuclear leukocytes appear to act in concert with monocytes in killing *L. pneumophila*.

The primary host defense mechanism is cell-mediated immunity. Inhibition of intracellular replication is effected by interferon-activated mononuclear phagocytes. Polymorphonuclear leukocytes activated by interferon and tumor necrosis factor enhance the killing of the organism.

Humoral immunity is a secondary line of host defense. Antibody does not promote killing of *L. pneumophila* by complement, promotes only modest activity of mononuclear phagocytes against *L. pneumophila*, and is not inhibitory to intracellular replication. However, type-specific antibody—usually IgM at first, followed by IgG—is assayable in the first weeks of infection.

Pathogens that are capable of surviving in their environment for extended periods tend to be relatively virulent. And *Legionella* appears to be more virulent than many other pulmonary pathogens. For example, severe community-acquired pneumonia is more often due to *L. pneumophila* than to most common bacterial pathogens. *L. pneumophila* is the second most common cause of community-acquired pneumonia in patients admitted to intensive care units.[13,14,50,53,56,62,65]

L. pneumophila, serogroup 1 can be subtyped with molecular methods, including monoclonal antibodies (MABs). It is interesting that subtypes of *L. pneumophila* differ in ability to cause disease. For example, the overwhelming majority of isolates recovered from patients react with MAB-2, whereas environmental strains do not. This observation has led to speculation that the MAB-2 epitope is a virulence marker. This monoclonal antibody recognizes a lipopolysaccharide (LPS) antigenic determinant in the outer membrane of *L. pneumophila*, serogroup 1. *L. pneumophila* LPS has also been shown to activate the classic complement pathway. Serum resistance has been linked to expression of the MAB-2 epitope. Virulent strains are resistant to the bactericidal activity of normal human serum and fail to bind complement components on the

TABLE 144-2

Reported Outbreaks of Pontiac Fever

Location	Year	Organism	Source	No. of Patients	Attack Rate (%)	Reference
County Health Department Pontiac, Michigan	1968	*L. pneumophila,* serogroup 1	Air conditioning	144	95	18
James River, Virginia	1973	*L. pneumophila*	Compressed air used to clean a steam turbine engine	10	90	16
Hotel Vermont	1981	*L. pneumophila,* serogroup 6	Whirlpool spa	34	92	57
Automobile plant Windsor, Ontario	1981	*L. feeleii*	Water-based coolant	317	5–100*	21
Racquet Club, Michigan	1982	*L. pneumophila,* serogroup 6	Whirlpool spa	14	100	36
Office building, New York	1984	*L. pneumophila,* serogroup 1	Cooling tower	86	78	17
Gloucester, England	1986	*L. pneumophila,* serogroup 1	Cooling tower	3	?	23
Lochgoilhead Hotel, Scotland	1988	*L. micdadei*	Whirlpool spa	170	91	19
Resort, Vermont	1991	*L. pneumophila*	Whirlpool spa	5		60
Resort, Colorado	1992	*L. pneumophila,* serogroup 6	Whirlpool spa	13	100	42
Office building, Tokyo	1994	*L. pneumophila,* serogroup 7	Cooling tower	45	100	66

*Location of departments within the plant, duration of exposure, and direction of prevailing winds accounted for the gradient in attack rates. Overall, the attack rate exceeded 94%.

cell surface. Avirulent strains are serum sensitive, and complement components C3 and C9 are deposited on the surface.

L. pneumophila can infect and replicate within various protozoa species found in soil and water. *L. pneumophila* grown in amebas are more invasive for macrophages and epithelial cells than *L. pneumophila* on agar. Expression of a 24-kDa immunoreactive protein is necessary for optimal intracellular infectivity.[12] The protein was designated Mip, for macrophage infectivity potentiator. Mutants lacking the Mip protein were impaired in ability to infect human alveolar macrophages and U937 cells. However, the mutant was still capable of intracellular multiplication.

A zinc metalloprotease, termed the major secretory protein, induces cell-mediated immune responses and protective immunity against lethal aerosol challenge with *L. pneumophila* in a guinea pig model of Legionnaires' disease.

CLINICAL MANIFESTATIONS

There are two very different forms of *Legionella* infection: Pontiac fever and pneumonia or Legionnaires' disease. It is not known why two different forms occur, though it is speculated that inocula of the organisms, differing modes of transmission, and host factors are important in explaining this discrepancy.

Pontiac Fever

The first documented outbreak of Pontiac fever occurred at a health department building in Pontiac, Michigan, in 1968.[18] *L. pneumophila,* serogroup 1, was eventually determined by indirect immunofluorescence to be the causative agent.[29] Other *Legionella* species—including *L. pneumophila* serogroup 6,[36] *L. feeleii,*[21] and *L. micdadei*[19]—have likewise been implicated in outbreaks of Pontiac fever. Documented outbreaks of Pontiac fever are listed in Table 144-2. Unlike the situation for Legionnaires' disease, aerosolization has been convincingly documented as the mode of transmission. These outbreaks are characterized by an attack rate in excess of 90 percent and an incubation period of 1 to 2 days after exposure to an environmental source.

Malaise, fatigue, and myalgias are the most frequent symptoms, occurring in 97 percent of patients. Fever usually with chills occurs in about 80 to 90 percent of patients. Headache is seen in 80 percent. Although pneumonia has never been seen on chest radiograph, a nonproductive cough and chest pain are common. A dry, nonproductive cough is reported in 30 to 60 percent of cases. Chest pain or constrictive sensations occur in about 40 percent of cases. Other symptoms seen in less than 50 percent are arthralgias, nausea, abdominal pain, and diarrhea. A modest leukocytosis with a neutrophilic predominance may be present.

TABLE 144-3

Chest Radiograph in Legionnaires' Disease at Presentation: Literature Review

Radiographic Finding	Domingo et al,[8] 1991	MacFarlane et al,[34] 1984	Muder et al,[45] 1987*	Kroboth et al,[32] 1983	Dietrich et al,[7] 1978
Patchy alveolar infiltrate	—	—	100% (17/17)	76% (26/34)	—
Unilobar involvement	49% (35/71)	61% (30/49)	65% (11/17)	59% (20/34)	—
Multilobar involvement	51% (36/71)	39% (19/49)	35% (6/17)	50% (17/34)	—
Lower-lobe involvement	—	—	—	79% (27/34)	—
Upper-lobe involvement	—	—	—	65% (22/34)	—
Unilateral involvement	75% (53/78)	—	—	50% (17/34)	—
Bilateral involvement	25% (18/71)	—	—	—	—
Ground-glass infiltrate	—	—	—	—	100% (24/24)
Pleural effusion	34% (24/71)	24% (12/49)	35% (6/17)	35% (12/34)	38% (9/24)
Cavitation	3% (2/71)†	2% (1/49)	—	3% (1/34)	—
Pulmonary collapse/ atelectasis	—	37% (8/49)	—	—	—

L. micdadei and *L. pneumophila*.
†On presentation. However, by 8–10 days, 10% showed presence of cavitation.

The illness is self-limited, and full recovery occurs within 1 week without sequelae.[18] Treatment is primarily symptomatic. The diagnosis is made from documentation of antibody seroconversion.

Legionnaires' Disease

Pneumonia is the predominant clinical syndrome in Legionnaires' disease. As the disease has become increasingly recognized, less severely ill patients are seen earlier in the course of the disease. Severe clinical manifestations of disseminated disease, once considered distinctive for Legionnaires' disease, are now known to be nonspecific. The incubation period ranges from 2 to 10 days. The onset can be gradual, with features of flulike syndrome including malaise, myalgias, anorexia, and headache. Coryza, however, is uncommon. Fever is universally present and can exceed 40°C. The onset may be abrupt, especially in immunosuppressed patients. Many patients appear quite toxic and near prostration.

The cough initially is mild and nonproductive or minimally productive of nonpurulent sputum, which may be blood streaked. Paroxysms of cough and breathlessness are seen. Chest pain, often pleuritic, can be a prominent feature in some patients. Gastrointestinal symptoms have been reported in 13 to 54 percent of cases, with diarrhea predominating. The diarrhea is watery rather than bloody. Other GI complaints are nausea, vomiting, and abdominal pain.

Examination of the chest early in the course of illness shows scattered rales, rhonchi, or evidence of small pleural effusion. Findings of consolidation are present as disease progresses. Pulse-temperature dissociation has been overemphasized as a useful clinical finding, but it can occasionally be seen in elderly patients with severe pneumonia. Hypotension was reported in 17 percent of patients with severe cases of community-acquired *Legionella* pneumonia.[14] Nonspecific abdominal findings or tenderness is seen in a few patients.

Hyponatremia (serum sodium 130 meq/L or less) appears to occur significantly more frequently in Legionnaires' disease than in pneumonias of other causes.[31,41,68] Laboratory data in Legionnaires' disease otherwise tends to be nonspecific. Frequently, there is a polymorphonuclear leukocytosis on presentation. Elevated serum trasminases, hypophosphatemia, elevated creatinine phosphokinase, thrombocytopenia, and hematuria are seen in more severely ill patients, but do not occur significantly more often in Legionnaires' disease than in other bacterial diseases.

A variety of other miscellaneous findings have been reported, including disseminated intravascular coagulation, glomerulitis, rhabdomyolysis, various rashes, neuropathies, and hepatic failure. These findings may be nonspecific and related to the severity of the infection, type of underlying disease, and perhaps side effects of drug therapy.

Thus, the presentation of Legionnaires' disease can be nonspecific. However, several clues should heighten clinical suspicion: (1) persistent fever exceeding 40°C; (2) Gram's stain of sputum in which neutrophils predominate but few, if any, organisms are seen; (3) hyponatremia (serum sodium 130 meq/L or less); (4) failure of a therapeutic response to β-lactam (penicillin or cephalosporin) or aminoglycoside antimicrobial; and (5) occurrence in a setting in which the potable water supply is known to be contaminated with *Legionella*.

L. pneumophila is often considered an "atypical" pathogen with *Chlamydia pneumoniae*, *Mycoplasma pneumoniae*, and viruses. The clinical similarities include the fact that the cough is relatively nonproductive and that grossly purulent sputum is uncommon. Gram's stain for the "atypical" pathogens show numerous leukocytes, with no organisms visualized. And the atypical pathogens (excluding viruses) respond to macrolides, tetracyclines, and quinolones, but not to β-lactam or aminoglycoside agents. On the other hand, the clinical manifestations of Legionnaires' disease are usually more severe than those of most

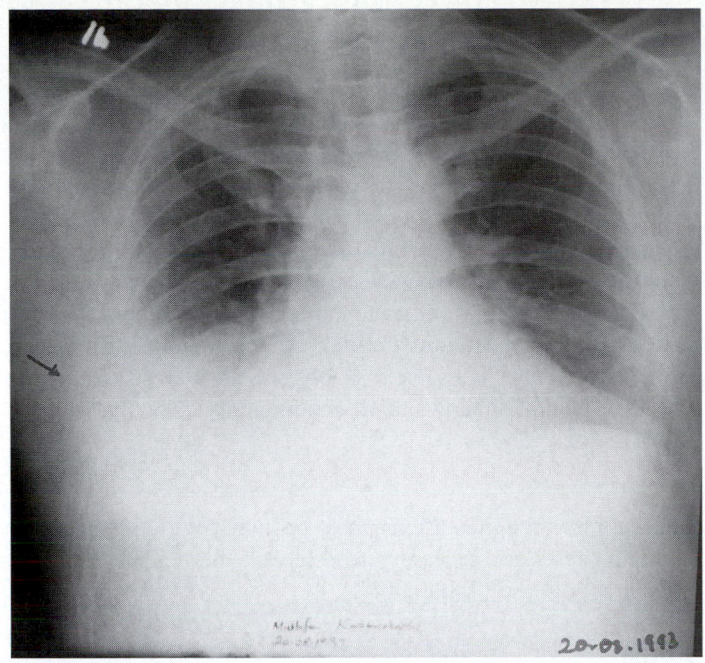

A

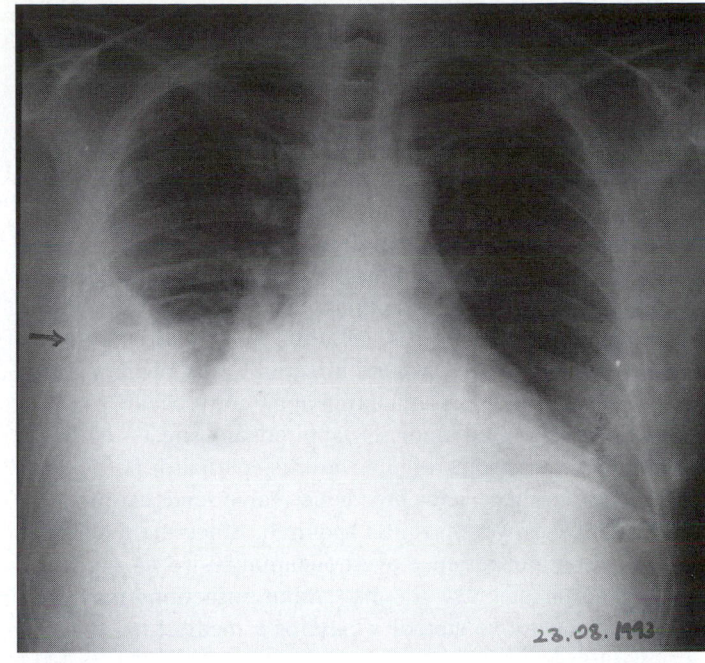

B

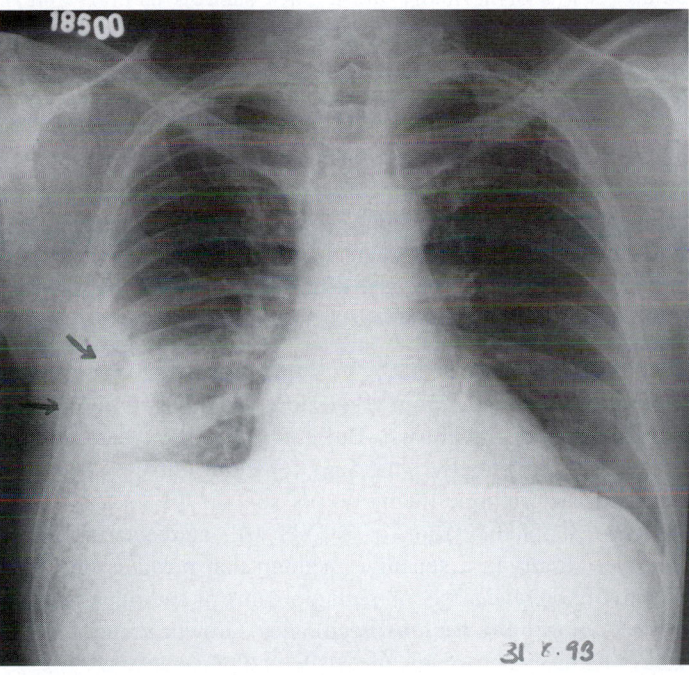

C

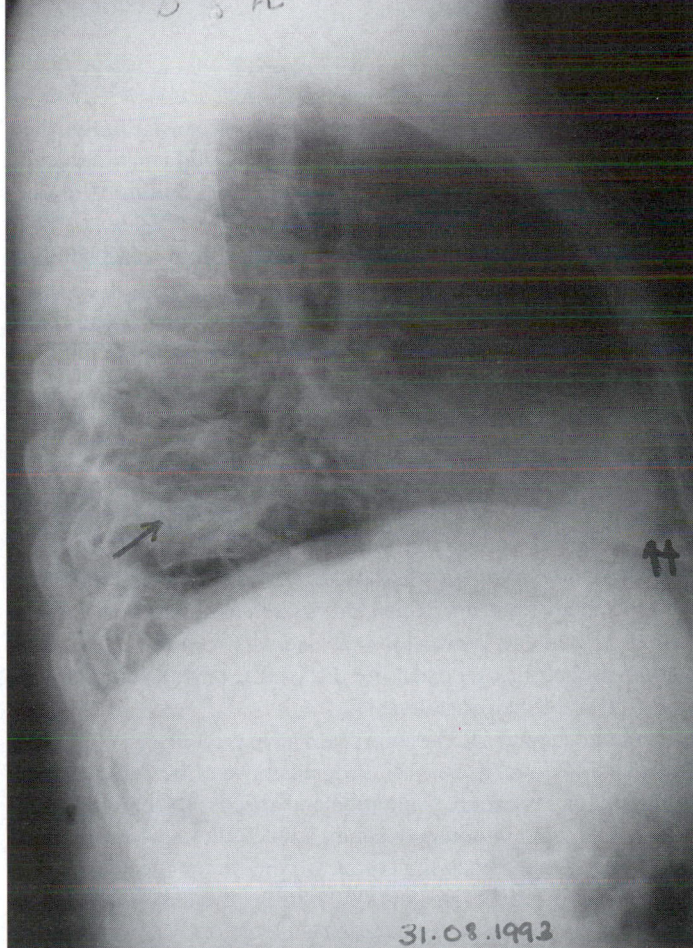

D

FIGURE 144-1 The patient was a 43-year-old male cigarette smoker who presented with a 15-day history of cough, dyspnea, fever, and right-sided pleuritic chest pain. *(Courtesy of Lutfiye Mulazimoglu, M.D.)* A. A right-sided pleural effusion is seen on this admission chest radiograph. Azithromycin plus rifampin was initiated. *B.* Three days after admission, consolidation and increase of pleural effusion are seen. Cavity development can be seen with air fluid level (arrow). *C.* Eight days after admission, pleural thickness with abscess formation is clearly seen on posterior anterior view. Symptoms of pneumonia had resolved. *D.* Lateral view shows air fluid level (arrow) and pleural effusion (double arrows). The chest radiograph 20 days after onset of pneumonia showed pleural thickness with a residual cavity. The patient was clinically well at this time. He ultimately had an uneventful recovery. Cultures of sputum and pleural fluid were unrevealing. The serology showed seroconversion to *L. pneumophila* at 1:1024. He refused any follow-up chest radiographs.

atypical pneumonias, and the course and prognosis are more akin to those of pneumococcal pneumonia with bacteremia than the other atypical pathogens. For example, patients with community-acquired Legionnaires' disease are significantly more likely to be admitted to an intensive care unit upon presentation than patients with pneumonia of other origin.

Extrapulmonary legionellosis is rare.[33] Since the index of suspicion is low, these infections can be easily overlooked. Anecdotal cases of sinusitis, cellulitis, pancreatitis, peritonitis, perirectal abscesses, wound infections, and pyelonephritis have been reported. Dissemination apparently occurs via bacteremia. The most common extrapulmonary site is the heart, with numerous reports of myocarditis, pericarditis, postcardiotomy syndrome, and prosthetic valve endocarditis.[48,61] Most such cases were hospital acquired. Since many of these patients did not experience overt pneumonia, it was suggested that the portal of entry for the cardiac infections may have been a postoperative sternal wound or a mediastinal tube insertion site.[33]

Chest Radiography

Several radiographic features are somewhat characteristic of Legionnaires' disease in the appropriate clinical setting.[45] These include progressive infiltrates despite appropriate antibiotic therapy, pleural effusions, pleural-based infiltrates that clinically mimic pulmonary embolism, and circumscribed peripheral densities. A summary of the chest radiographic findings is shown in Table 144-3: however, it must be conceded that these findings are not highly specific.

Most patients have abnormal chest radiographs on presentation with a unilateral infiltrate. Virtually all patients exhibit abnormalities by the second or third day of the illness. The initial infiltrates are typically alveolar and may be segmental or lobar. In some instances, patchy and diffuse infiltrates are seen on presentation. Domingo and colleagues examined the radiographic appearance of nosocomially acquired Legionnaires' disease in patients treated with erythromycin either at the onset of illness or shortly thereafter.[8] A clear predominance of unilateral shadowing was apparent in 75 percent of the cases and bilateral disease in 25 percent. Lower-lobe disease was seen in 72 percent—similar to the rates reported in other studies. Multilobar disease was seen in 50 percent of cases.

Immunosuppressed patients often have circumscribed peripheral densities and nodules.[45] Progression can be rapid, with a tendency for cavitation. Cavitation and abscess formation are uncommon in the immunocompetent patient with Legionnaires' disease.[45] In patients receiving corticosteroid therapy, however, cavitation can often be striking.[10] Multiple bilateral cavities are usually peripheral or in a pleural-based location.[7,10,45] Cavity formation may occur up to 14 days after presentation despite administration of appropriate antibiotics.

Pleural effusions are seen in one-third of patients and may precede the radiographic infiltrate.[8,32,45,54] Empyema can occur.[45] Pericardial effusion can be seen in some cases.[8,33,48]

The extent of radiographic abnormalities does not correlate well with the clinical severity or outcome.[45] In one study, the degree of radiographic severity did correlate significantly with the

amount of *L. pneumophila* visualized in the sputum with direct fluorescent antibody staining.[32] Radiographic clearance or improvement in patients with Legionnaires' disease tends to lag behind clinical improvement for several days.[30,32] Progression of infiltrates to invade other lobes during appropriate antibiotic therapy has been noted in several studies (Fig. 144-1). In one study of nosocomial pneumonia, 29 percent of patients showed progression of a unilateral infiltrate that extended to other lobes despite erythromycin administration.[8] At follow-up of 12 weeks, about 50 percent of chest radiographs still showed scarring, volume loss, pleural shadows, and, uncommonly, a cavity.[8]

LABORATORY DIAGNOSIS

Since clinical manifestations may be nonspecific, specialized laboratory tests are necessary to establish the diagnosis of Legionnaires' disease (Table 144-4).

Stains

Gram's stains of normally sterile sites such as pleural fluid or lung tissue can occasionally suggest the diagnosis: *Legionella* is not easily visualized in sputum. The organism appears as small, pleomorphic, faint gram-negative bacilli. *L. micdadei* can appear as weakly or partly acid-fast bacilli in clinical specimens. The modified acid-fact stain substitutes 1 percent sulfuric acid for the traditional 3 percent hydrochloric acid; the less aggressive decolorizer increases the yield of *L. micdadei* visualized by this stain. Patients have often been empirically treated with antituberculosis medications because of false-positive acid-fast smears.

Culture

Culture of *Legionella* from respiratory secretions is the definitive method of diagnosis. Buffered charcoal yeast extract (BCYE) is the preferred medium for culturing the organism. Standard bacteriologic media do not support the growth of *Legionella*. Supplementation of BCYE with antibacterial agents and dyes results in a sensitive medium that prevents the overgrowth of *Legionella* by competing organisms and imparts a distinctive color to the *Legionella* colonies. Growth occurs for 3 to 5 days before macroscopically visible colonies appear.

TABLE 144-4

Specialized Laboratory Tests for Diagnosis of Legionnaires' Disease

Test	Sensitivity (%)	Specificity (%)
Culture		
Sputum*	80	100
Transtracheal aspirate	90	100
DFA stain of sputum	50–70	96–99
Urinary antigen†	70	100
Antibody serology‡	40–60	96–99

*Use of multiple selective media with dyes.
†Serogroup 1 only.
‡IgG and IgM testing for both acute and convalescent sera. A single titer ≥1:128 is considered presumptive, while a single titer ≥1:256 or fourfold seroconversion is considered definitive.

The sensitivity of bronchoscopy specimens is approximately the same as that for sputum; however, if sputa are not available, bronchoscopy specimens may yield the organism. Bronchoalveolar lavage gives higher yields than bronchial wash specimens.

Direct Fluorescent Antibody Stain

Direct fluorescent antibody (DFA) staining is a rapid diagnostic test that allows direct visualization of *Legionella* in clinical specimens. Positive results with DFA staining depend on the presence of a large number of organisms and is more likely to be positive if there is multilobar disease present on chest radiograph.[32] Although cross reactivity with other gram-negative bacilli has been reported, false-positive results are usually due to laboratory technique or contamination. Results using the monoclonal antibody reagents (Genetic Systems, Seattle) are easier to interpret; however, they are more expensive than the polyclonal reagent and have the same sensitivity. DFA reagents for non-*pneumophila* species and serogroups are not commercially available. We do not recommend the routine use of DFA for sputum samples, but we do endorse its routine use in specimens obtained by bronchoscopy, open lung biopsy, and autopsy specimens.

Antibody Detection

Serology techniques have become less useful with the advent of culture and specialized tests. The indirect fluorescent antibody (IFA) and enzyme-linked immunoabsorbent assay (ELISA) give comparable results. A fourfold rise in antibody titer to 1:128 is diagnostic. Both acute and convalescent sera are required because 4 to 12 weeks is required for detection of an antibody response. A single elevated titer 1:128 in a patient with pneumonia is presumptive evidence of disease, while a single titer to 1:256 is considered definitive. Elevated titers may be seen in 25 to 40 percent of patients in the first week of disease. The specificity of serologic testing is estimated to be about 95 percent in the diagnosis of *L. pneumophila* infection; however, false-positive results can occur with the other *Legionella* species. So definitive diagnosis of the non-*pneumophila* species (e.g., *L. micdadei*) resides in isolation of the organisms on culture.

Polymerase Chain Reaction

Polymerase chain reaction amplification coupled with DNA probe is more sensitive for the non-*pneumophila* species than culture and DFA; however, it appears to be less sensitive than culture for detecting *L. pneumophila* in sputum. The advantage is its ability to detect the organism rapidly. Test kits are undergoing evaluation and will soon be commercially available.

Urinary Antigen

Detection of *Legionella*-soluble antigen in urine (Binax, South Portland, Maine) is a rapid diagnostic test that is relatively easy to perform. We recommend its use in every clinical laboratory. The sensitivity is second only to culture, and it is highly specific. The test is available only for *L. pneumophila*, serogroup 1, although this serogroup causes about 80 percent of *Legionella* infection. Antigen in urine is detectable 3 days after the onset of the clinical disease, even if specific therapy is started and it persists for several weeks. Ironically, it is often easier to obtain a urine specimen than an adequate sputum for laboratory evaluation.

TREATMENT

Until recently, erythromycin was the antibiotic of choice. However, the newer macrolides (azithromycin, clarithromycin, roxithromycin) and quinolones (ciprofloxacin, ofloxacin, levofloxacin, pefloxacin) demonstrate superior in vitro activity and improved pharmacokinetics over erythromycin.

When the intravenous formulations become available, it is likely that one of the newer macrolides will displace erythromycin as the antibiotic of choice for Legionnaires' disease. The 4-g-a-day intravenous dosage of erythromycin recommended specifically for Legionnaires' disease poses numerous management problems, including the necessity for a large fluid volume, which is problematic because so many cases of Legionnaires' disease have underlying cardiac disease. Symptomatic ototoxicity confirmed by audiograms was seen in 21 percent of patients receiving the 4-g dose as empiric therapy for community-acquired pneumonia; ototoxicity was reversible when the erythromycin was discontinued.

Numerous anecdotal successes with the quinolones (ciprofloxacin, ofloxacin, pefloxacin) have been reported.[11] Given the pharmacologic interaction of the macrolides and rifampin with transplant immunosuppressive medications, we recommend ciprofloxacin as the antibiotic of choice for transplant recipients with Legionnaires' disease.

Rifampin is highly active in vitro and in vivo against *Legionella* and is recommended as part of combination therapy

TABLE 144-5

Antibiotic Therapy for *Legionella* Infection

Antimicrobial Agent	Dose	Route	Frequency
Azithromycin	500 mg*	PO, IV	q 24 h
Clarithromycin	500 mg	PO, IV†	q 12 h
Roxithromycin	300 mg†	PO	q 12 h
Erythromycin	1 g	IV	q 6 h
	500 mg	PO	q 6 h
Ciprofloxacin	400 mg	IV	q 8 h
	750 mg	PO	q 12 h
Ofloxacin	400 mg	PO, IV	q 12 h
Doxycycline	100 mg*	PO, IV	q 12 h
Minocycline	100 mg*	PO, IV	q 12 h
Tetracycline	500 mg	PO, IV	q 6 h
Trimethoprim-sulfamethoxazole	160/800 mg	IV	q 8 h
	160/800 mg	PO	q 12 h
Rifampin	600 mg	PO, IV	q 12 h

*Consider doubling first dose.
†Investigational in U.S.

(with a macrolide or a quinolone) for severe pneumonias. Tetracycline proved efficacious in the original American Legion outbreak, and successes with minocycline and doxycycline have been documented. Imipenem, trimethoprim-sulfamethoxazole, and clindamycin have proved efficacious in a few cases.[11]

Parenteral therapy should be given until objective clinical response has occurred; most patients become afebrile within 3 days. Then oral therapy can be substituted. Dosages are given in Table 144-5. It should be noted that these doses are based on anecdotal experience and not on clinical trials. Duration of therapy is 10 to 14 days; however, longer treatment is appropriate for the immunosuppressed host. Relapse has been reported, although many of these cases may be due to reinfection as a result of continued exposure to contaminated water.

The mortality from Legionnaires' disease in immunocompetent patients is low with appropriate antibiotic therapy. The rate may approach 50 percent in nosocomial disease, especially if antibiotics were started late. The most common cause of death is progressive respiratory failure. The chest radiograph is not helpful for monitoring clinical response. Delayed diagnosis and subsequent delay in initiation of appropriate antibiotics remain the crucial factor in outcome determination.

PREVENTION

Theoretically, prevention of Legionnaires' disease is possible because the environmental reservoir for this illness has been discovered. *Legionella* contamination of water distribution systems was not found to be associated with appearance, degree of cleanliness, or regular preventive maintenance measures, so it is unlikely that newer engineering codes and guidelines will affect colonization of water distribution systems.

Nosocomial legionellosis could easily exist undiagnosed, especially in hospitals that lack specialized testing. The presence of *L. pneumophila* in the hospital water supply has led investigators in Pittsburgh to suggest environmental culturing of hospitals, including those that have never experienced Legionnaires' disease. Clinical surveillance for Legionnaires' disease stimulated by positive results of water distribution cultures has uncovered cases of unsuspected Legionnaires' disease. Sterile water should be used for filling and rinsing humidifiers, nebulizers, and all other respiratory devices.

The ultimate preventive measure for hospital-acquired legionellosis is disinfection of the hospital water distribution system. Numerous methods have been tried, but only two have emerged as being cost-effective. Superheating of the water to 60 to 77°C (140 to 170°F) and flushing of the distal sites with hot water for 30 min are especially useful in urgent or outbreak situations. Following the flushings, the hot-water temperature should be maintained at 60°C or higher to minimize recolonization. The drawbacks are the logistic difficulties of flushing distal sites and the need for periodic disinfection. The second method is installation of copper-silver ionization units on the hot-water recirculating ions (LiquiTech, Burr Ridge, Illinois; Tarn-Pure, High Wycombe, England). Efficacy has been documented in numerous hospitals, and disinfection is readily sustained with low-maintenance concentrations of the ions. Hyperchlorination is no longer recommended. Not only is this method the most expensive but it is also the least efficacious. Corrosion of the piping has wrought extensive damage to many hospital water systems over time. Furthermore, chlorine byproducts are now known to be carcinogenic.

REFERENCES

1. Arnow PM, Chou T, Weil D, et al: Nosocomial Legionnaires' disease caused by aerosolized tap water from respiratory devices. *J Infect Dis* 146:460–467, 1982.
2. Bhopal R: Source of infection for sporadic Legionnaires' disease: A review. *J Infect* 30:9–12, 1995.
3. Blatt SP, Parkinson MD, Pace E, et al: Nosocomial Legionnaires' disease: Aspiration as a primary mode of transmission. *Am J Med* 95:16–22, 1993.
4. Bouvet A, de Fenoyl O, Desplaces N: Maladie des légionnaires due au sérogroup 6 de *Legionella pneumophila*: Contamination à domicile par canule de trachéostomie. *Presse Med* 15:15–35, 1986.
5. Brady M: Nosocomial legionnaires disease in a children's hospital. *J Pediatr* 115:46–50, 1989.
6. Castellani Pastoris M, Vigano EF, Passi C: A family cluster of *Legionella pneumophila* infections. *Scand J Infect Dis* 20:489–493, 1988.
7. Dietrich P, Johnson R, Fairbank J, Walke J: The chest radiograph in Legionnaires' disease. *Radiology* 127:577–582, 1978.
8. Domingo C, Roig J, Planas F, et al: Radiographic appearance of nosocomial legionnaires' disease after erythromycin treatment. *Thorax* 46:633–666, 1991.
9. Dournon E, Bure A, Desplaces N, et al: Legionnaires' disease related to gastric lavage with tap water (letter). *Lancet* 1:797–798, 1982.
10. Ebright J, Tarakji E, Brown W, Sunstrum J: Multiple bilateral lung cavities caused by *Legionella pneumophila*: Case report and review. *Infect Dis Clin Prac* 2:195–199, 1993.
11. Edelstein PH: Antimicrobial chemotherapy for Legionnaires' disease: A review. *Clin Infect Dis* 21 (Suppl 3): S265–S276, 1995.
12. Engleberg CN: Genetic studies of *Legionella* pathogenesis, in Barbaree JM, Breiman RF, Dufour AP (eds), *Legionella—Current Status and Emerging Perspectives.* Washington, DC, American Society of Microbiology, 1993, p 63.
13. Falcó V, Fernández de Sevilla T, Alegre J, et al: *Legionella pneumophila*: A cause of severe community-acquired pneumonia. *Chest* 100:1007–1011, 1991.
14. Fang GD, Fine M, Orloff J, et al: New and emerging etiologies for community-acquired pneumonia with implications for therapy: A prospective multicenter study of 359 cases. *Medicine* 69:307–316, 1990.
15. Fang GD, Yu VL, Vickers RM: Disease due to Legionellaceae (other than *Legionella pneumophila*): Historical, microbiological, clinical, and epidemiological review. *Medicine* 68:116–132, 1989.
16. Fraser DW, Deubner DC, Hill DL, Gillian DK: Nonpneumonic, short-incubation-period legionellosis (Pontiac fever) in men who cleaned a steam turbine condenser. *Science* 205:690–691, 1979.
17. Friedman S, Spitalny K, Barbaree J, et al: Pontiac fever outbreak associated with a cooling tower. *Am J Public Health* 77:568–571, 1987.
18. Glick TH, Gregg MB, Berman B, et al: Pontiac fever: An epidemic of unknown etiology in a health department: I. Clinical and epidemiologic aspects. *Am J Epidemiol* 107:149–160, 1978.
19. Goldberg DJ, Wrench JG, Collier PW, et al: Lochgoilhead fever: Outbreak of non-pneumonic legionellosis due to *Legionella micdadei.* *Lancet* 1:316–318, 1989.

20. Gorman GW, Yu VL, Brown A, et al: Isolation of Pittsburgh pneumonia agent from nebulizers used in respiratory therapy. *Ann Intern Med* 93:572–573, 1980.

21. Herwaldt LA, Gorman GW, McGrath T, et al: A new *Legionella* species, *Legionella feeleii* species nova, causes Pontiac fever in an automobile plant. *Ann Intern Med* 100:333–338, 1984.

22. Horwitz MA: Toward an understanding of host and bacterial molecules mediating *L. pneumophila* pathogenesis, in Barbaree JM, Breiman RF, Dufour AP (eds), *Legionella—Current Status and Emerging Perspectives.* Washington, DC, American Society of Microbiology, 1993, p 55.

23. Hunt DA, Cartwright KA, Smith MC, et al: An outbreak of Legionnaires' disease in Gloucester. *Epidemiol Infect* 107:133–141, 1991.

24. Ivashkin VT, Sinopal'nikov AI: [The diagnosis of primary atypical pneumonias]. *Voen Med Zh* 80:18–22, 1994.

25. Johnson JT, Yu VL, Best M, et al: Nosocomial legionellosis uncovered in surgical patients with head and neck cancer: Implications for epidemiologic reservoir and mode of transmission. *Lancet* 2:298–300, 1985.

26. Joly JR, Diery P, Gauvrau L, et al: Legionnaires' disease caused by *Legionella dumoffi* in distilled water. *Can Med Assoc J* 135:1273–1277, 1986.

27. Jones E, Checko P, Dalton A, et al: Nosocomial legionnaires' disease associated with exposure to respiratory therapy equipment, Connecticut, in Thornsberry C, Balonos A, Feeley JC, Jakubowski W (eds), *Proceedings of the 2d International Symposium.* Washington, DC, American Society Microbiology, 1984, p 225.

28. Kaan JA, Simoons-Smit AM, MacLaren DM: Another source of aerosol causing nosocomial Legionnaires' disease. *J Infect* 11:145–148, 1985.

29. Kaufman AF, McDade J, Patton C, et al: Pontiac fever: Isolation of the etiologic agent *(Legionella pneumophila)* and demonstration of its mode of transmission. *Am J Epidemiol* 114:337–347, 1981.

30. Kirby BD, Peck H, Meyer RD: Radiographic features of Legionnaires' disease. *Chest* 76:562–565, 1979.

31. Kirby BD, Snyder K, Meyer R, Finegold SM: Legionnaires' disease: Report of 65 nosocomially acquired cases and a review of the literature. *Medicine* 59:188–205, 1980.

32. Kroboth FJ, Yu VL, Reddy S, Yu AC: Clinicoradiographic correlations with the extent of Legionnaires' disease. *AJR* 141:263–268, 1983.

33. Lowry PW, Tompkins LS: Nosocomial legionellosis: A review of pulmonary and extrapulmonary syndromes. *Am J Infect Control* 21:21–27, 1993.

34. MacFarlane JT, Miller AC, RoderickSmith WH, et al: Comparative radiographic features of community acquired Legionnaires' disease, pneumococcal pneumonia, mycoplasma pneumonia, and psittacosis. *Thorax* 39:28–33, 1984.

35. Mahoney FJ, Hoge CW, Farley TA, et al: Community-wide outbreak of legionnaires' disease associated with a grocery store mist machine. *J Infect Dis* 165:736–739, 1992.

36. Mangione EJ, Remis RS, Tait KA, et al: An outbreak of Pontiac fever related to whirlpool use, Michigan 1982. *JAMA* 253:535–539, 1985.

37. Markowitz L, Tompkins L, Wilkinson H, et al: Transmission of nosocomial Legionnaires' disease in heart transplant patients. Program and Abstracts of the 24th Interscience Conference of Antimicrobial Agents and Chemotherapy. Washington, DC, American Society of Microbiology, 1984.

38. Marrie TJ, Haldane D, MacDonald S, et al: Control of endemic nosocomial legionnaires' disease by using sterile potable water for high risk patients. *Epidemiol Infect* 107:591–605, 1991.

39. Mastro TD, Fields BS, Breiman RF, et al: Nosocomial legionnaires' disease and use of medication nebulizers. *J Infect Dis* 163:667–671, 1991.

40. Mermel LA, Josephson SL, Girogio CH, et al: Association of Legionnaires' disease with construction: Contamination of potable water? *Infect Control Hosp Epidemiol* 16:76–81, 1995.

41. Miller AC: Hyponatremia in Legionnaires' disease. *Br Med J* 284:558–559, 1982.

42. Miller L, Beebe J, Butler J, et al: Use of polymerase chain reaction in an epidemiologic investigation of pontiac fever. *J Infect Dis* 168:769–772, 1993.

43. Moriaghi A, Castellani Pastoris M, Barral C, et al: Nosocomial legionellosis associated with use of oxygen bubble humidifiers and underwater chest drain. *J Hosp Infect* 10:47–50, 1987.

44. Muder RR, Yu VL, McClure JK, et al: Nosocomial legionnaires' disease uncovered in a prospective pneumonia study: Implications for underdiagnosis. *JAMA* 249:3184–3188, 1983.

45. Muder RR, Yu VL, Parry M: Radiology of *Legionella* pneumonia. *Semin Respir Infect* 2:242–254, 1987.

46. Muder RR, Yu VL, Woo A: Mode of transmission of *L. pneumophila:* A critical review. *Ann Intern Med* 146:1607–1612, 1986.

47. Muraca PW, Stout JE, Yu VL, et al: Legionnaires' disease in the work environment: Implications for environmental health. *Am Ind Hyg Assoc J* 49:584–590, 1988.

48. Nelson DP, Rensimer ER, Raffin TA: *Legionella pneumophila* pericarditis without pneumonia. *Arch Intern Med* 145:926, 1985.

49. Osterholm MT, Chin TDY, Osborne DO, et al: A 1957 outbreak of Legionnaires' disease associated with a meat packing plant. *J Epidemiol* 117:60–67, 1983.

50. Pachon J, Prados MD, Capote F, et al: Severe community-acquired pneumonia—Biology, prognosis, and treatment. *Am Rev Respir Dis* 142:369–373, 1990.

51. Phillips SJ, Zeff RH, Gervich D: Legionnaires' disease (letter). *Ann Thorac Surg* 44:564, 1987.

52. Quaresima T, Castellani Pastoris M: Infezioni da *Legionella* sp. nel bambino. *Riv Ital Pediatr* 18:125–136, 1992.

53. Rello J, Quintana E, Ausina V, et al: A three-year study of severe community-acquired pneumonia with emphasis on outcome. *Chest* 103:232–235, 1993.

54. Roig J, Aguilar X, Ruiz J, et al: Comparative study of *Legionella pneumophila* and other nosocomial-acquired pneumonias. *Chest* 99:344–350, 1991.

55. Shands KN, Ho JL, Meyer RD, et al: Potable water as a source of legionnaires' disease. *JAMA* 253:1412–1416, 1985.

56. Sorensen J, Forsberg P, Hakanson E, et al: A new diagnostic approach to a patient with severe pneumonia. *Scand J Infect Dis* 21:33–41, 1989.

57. Spitalny KC, Vogt RL, Orciarl L, et al: Pontiac fever associated with a whirlpool spa. *Am J Epidemiol* 120:809–817, 1984.

58. Stout JE, Yu VL: Current concepts: Legionellosis. *New Engl J Med,* 1997.

59. Stout JE, Yu VL, Muraca P, et al: Potable water as a cause of sporadic cases of community-acquired legionnaires' disease. *New Engl J Med* 326:151–155, 1992.

60. Thomas D, Mundy L, Tucker P: Hot tub legionellosis: Legionnaires' disease and Pontiac fever after a point-source exposure to *Legionella pneumophila.* *Arch Intern Med* 153:2597–2599, 1993.

61. Tompkins LS, Roessler BJ, Redd SC, et al: Legionella prosthetic-valve endocarditis. *New Engl J Med* 318:530–535, 1988.

62. Torres A, Sera-Batilles J, Ferrer A, et al: Severe community acquired pneumonia: Epidemiology and prognostic factors. *Am Rev Respir Dis* 144:312–318, 1991.

63. Woo AH, Goetz A, Yu VL: Transmission of *Legionella* by respiratory equipment and aerosol generating devices. *Chest* 102:1586–1590, 1992.

64. Woo AH, Yu VL, Goetz A: A potential in-hospital mode of transmission for *Legionella pneumophila:* Demonstration experiments for dissemination by showers, humidifiers, and rinsing of ventilation bag apparatus. *Am J Med* 80:567–573, 1986.

65. Woodhead MD, MacFarlane JT, Rodgers FG, et al: Aetiology and outcome of severe community-acquired pneumonia. *J Infect* 10:204–210, 1985.

66. Yabuuchi E, Mori M: An outbreak of Pontiac fever due to *Legionella pneumophila* serogroup 7 in Tokyo. Proceedings of the European Working Group on *Legionella* infections, Istanbul, 1995.

67. Yu VL: Could aspiration be the major mode of transmission for *Legionella? Am J Med* 95:13–15, 1993.

68. Yu VL, Kroboth FJ, Shonnard J, et al: Legionnaires' disease: New clinical perspective from a prospective pneumonia study. *Am J Med* 73:357–361, 1982.

69. Zuravleff JJ, Yu VL, Shonnard J, et al: *Legionella pneumophila* contamination of a hospital humidifier: Demonstration of aerosol transmission and subsequent subclinical infection in exposed guinea pigs. *Am Rev Respir Dis* 128:657–661, 1983.

MYCOPLASMA, CHLAMYDIA, AND "ATYPICAL PNEUMONIAS"

Maurice A. Mufson

Atypical pneumonia encompasses a grouping of pneumonias that exhibit similar clinical and radiographic features and respond to treatment with antibiotics. It is characterized by a gradual onset of illness, mostly nonproductive cough, infrequent hemoptysis, few auscultatory signs, and mainly an interstitial infiltrate on chest radiographs. The pathogens of atypical pneumonia include *Mycoplasma pneumoniae, Chlamydia pneumoniae, C. psittaci,* and *Coxiella burnetii* (Q fever). Of these pathogens, *M. pneumoniae* and *C. pneumoniae* predominate, accounting for about one-third of the 500,000 community-acquired pneumonias (CAP) among adults admitted to hospital annually (see also Chapter 127); the other pathogens occur uncommonly. Unlike the viral pneumonias, the atypical pneumonias due to *M. pneumoniae, C. pneumoniae, C. psittaci,* and *C. burnetii* can be effectively treated with broad-spectrum antibiotics, mainly of the tetracycline and macrolide classes.

The term *atypical pneumonia* or *primary atypical pneumonia* (PAP), introduced in the late 1930s, indicated the opposite of a *typical pneumonia.* Lobar pneumonia, the typical pneumonia, is caused by bacteria, most commonly pneumococci. It begins acutely with clinical and radiographic evidence of pulmonary consolidation and associated high case fatality rate. In contradistinction, atypical pneumonia is characterized by an insidious onset and interstitial inflammation of the lung, demonstrating a patchy infiltrate on chest radiographs. Atypical pneumonias, as a group, pursue a much less virulent course, and very few patients succumbed. The primary pathogens of atypical pneumonia were identified 10 years later.

Antibiotic treatment trials of atypical pneumonia conducted in the early 1950s mainly investigated the efficacy of tetracycline. Although flawed by inappropriate controls and a paucity of diagnostic procedures, they provided marginal evidence that at least some of the group of atypical pneumonias responded to such treatment and supported the concept that nonviral pathogens caused atypical pneumonia. In the 1960s, *M. pneumoniae* (referred to in the literature of the 1940s and 1950s as the "organism of primary atypical pneumonia" and later as the "Eaton agent") was shown conclusively by Chanock and coworkers to be a major pathogen of atypical pneumonia.[5a,5b,24] Subsequently, other microorganisms were recognized as pathogens of atypical pneumonia—especially *C. pneumoniae,* which was identified in the 1980s as a respiratory pathogen through the detailed studies of Grayston and colleagues.[12,13]

M. PNEUMONIAE PNEUMONIA

History

M. pneumoniae pneumonia—often abbreviated as mycoplasmal pneumonia—is the archetypal atypical pneumonia. Five decades ago, when the term *atypical pneumonia* was defined but its origin undetermined, the search for "the" cause of atypical pneumonia (or PAP) lead to the discovery of M. pneumoniae as the etiologic agent of cold agglutinin–positive atypical pneumonia. The microbiologic and epidemiologic studies that provided the basis for this discovery represent a classic exposition of Koch's postulates. In pioneering experiments during the 1940s, Eaton isolated a filterable agent, which he called the organism of PAP, in respiratory secretions from adults ill with atypical pneumonia. When these secretions were administered to cotton rats, they produced pneumonia. Eaton's attempts to isolate the agent in embryonic chicken eggs were unsuccessful. However, in the 1950s, Eaton and Liu experimentally infected bronchial epithelium of embryonated chicken eggs with the Eaton agent. They devised an indirect immunofluorescent antibody assay employing frozen sections of the lung and convalescent sera from adults recovering from cold agglutinin–positive atypical pneumonia.[20a,20b,21]

Subsequently, in detailed epidemiologic studies, Chanock and colleagues confirmed that the Eaton agent was associated with cold agglutinin–positive atypical pneumonia.[5a,5b,24] Chanock proved that the Eaton agent was a mycoplasma by isolating it on cell-free medium that supported the growth of mycoplasmas. It was named M. pneumoniae to connote its role as a pathogen of pneumonia. Finally, volunteers who were given a pure culture of M. pneumoniae developed atypical pneumonia and responded to treatment with antibiotics. Chanock's comprehensive and insightful studies provided unequivocal evidence that M. pneumoniae is the etiologic agent of cold agglutinin–positive atypical pneumonia.

Epidemiology

M. pneumoniae is an ubiquitous infection that is transmitted by infectious droplets by means of the respiratory tract; close contact encourages its spread. It exhibits a propensity to move slowly among susceptible persons in families and semiclosed populations.[4] Usually, 8 to 10 weeks elapse before all household members become infected, with a median of 23 days between person-to-person spread; about one-half of household members develop pneumonia. The incubation period is 16 to 32 days. M. pneumoniae occurs throughout all seasons, with annual cycles of 4 to 7 years. Attack rates are highest among adolescents and adults in their 20s and 30s; however, 5 percent of M. pneumoniae pneumonias occur in persons older than 65 years. Immunity to M. pneumoniae increases with age. Overall, about 1 in 30 persons who become infected develop pneumonia.

Microbiology and Pathogenesis

Mycoplasmas constitute a group of the smallest microorganisms and have several distinct features: they can replicate on enriched cell-free medium; they require cholesterol, as they are unable to synthesize it; and they lack a cell wall but possess a limiting membrane. M. pneumoniae belongs to the class Mollicutes, order I Mycoplasmatales, family I Mycoplasmataceae, genus I *Mycoplasma,* which includes several human and animal mycoplasmas. It possesses one of the smallest genomes, approximately 800 to 840 kb, of which 6 percent consist of gene sequences for the adhesin, an attachment organelle.[29] Two adhesins, P1, a 176-kDa component, and a second adhesin (unnamed), mediate virulence and attachment of M. pneumoniae to cells through sulfated glycolipids on α_{2-3}–linked sialyloligosaccharides (glycoproteins).[9,20] The P1 gene shows two differing, but highly conserved sequences, types 1 and 2. The two types exhibit varying epidemiologic patterns. M. pneumoniae produces a soluble hemolysin, hydrogen peroxide, which causes hemolysis and alters the I antigen of erythrocytes. Cold agglutinins, a nonspecific anti-I antibody that reversibly agglutinates erythrocytes at 4°C, arise during some severe M. pneumoniae infections.

Clinical Manifestations

M. pneumoniae pneumonia begins insidiously with fever, nonproductive cough, and anterior nonpleuritic chest pain intensified by coughing.[6] A few patients develop pleural effusion, malaise, headache, and anorexia. Other common symptoms are pharyngitis, dyspnea, diaphoresis, and tachycardia. Hemoptysis rarely occurs. Cervical lymphadenopathy and sinusitis occur uncommonly and tympanitis or a bullous myringitis very rarely. As the illness progresses, sputum production begins; it is usually white and mucoid, rarely purulent.

Clinically, examination of the lungs reveals few rales. As the pneumonia progresses, however, rales appear. A chest radiograph taken early in the course of the pneumonia may show more extensive lung involvement than is suspected from the scarcity of rales (Figs. 145-1, 145-2, and 145-3). Auscultation several days later may detect increased rales, and the radiograph may show some progression.

M. pneumoniae pneumonia progresses slowly. The usual course of untreated illness is 10 to 14 days. Antibiotic treatment hastens resolution of signs and symptoms and of the abnormalities on chest radiographs. Most pneumonias occur in one lung; usually they appear interstitial or reticulonodular (Figs. 145-1 and 145-2). About one-fourth of pneumonias are bilateral, mostly in the lower lobes, but occasionally they show a symmetric involvement extending from the hila, suggesting a "butterflylike" pattern (Fig. 145-3). Pleural effusions occur in about one-fourth of pneumonias. They are exudates, characteristically clear, with relatively small numbers of polymorphonuclear leukocytes and mononuclear cells and an elevated protein. Some persons recover extremely slowly, so radiographic evidence of resolving pneumonia or residual pleural effusion may remain as long as 4 months in up to one-fourth of pneumonia illnesses. Cough may persist for several weeks or months. Most patients with M. pneumoniae pneumonia recover without residual abnormalities or complications.

Death occurs in very few persons who develop complications. Rarely, M. pneumoniae pneumonia progresses to a fulminant pneumonia, complicated by respiratory failure, which is sometimes fatal.[5] Other scarce pulmonary complications are residual

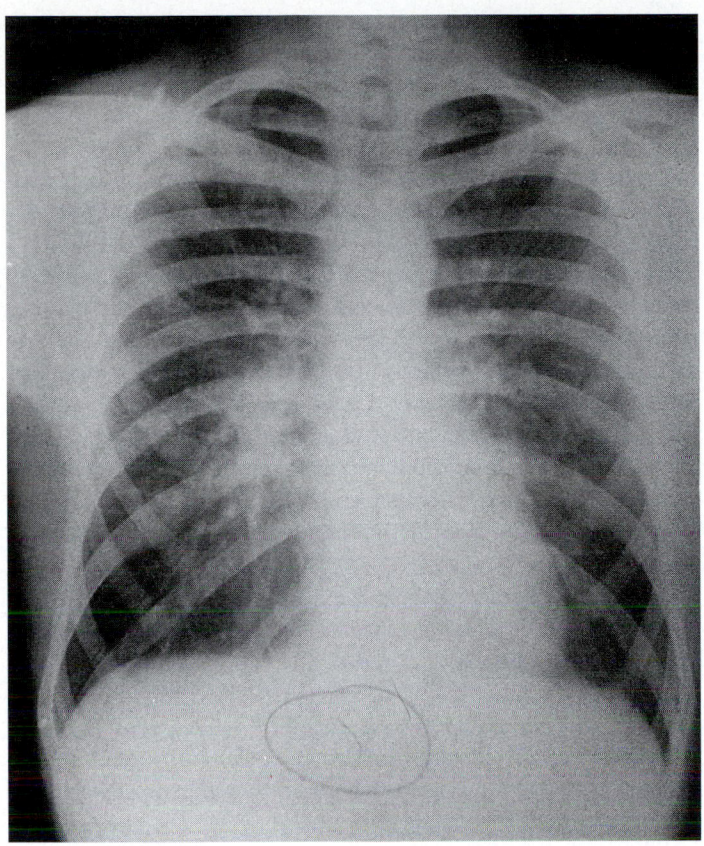

FIGURE 145-1   Chest radiograph of a young man with proven *M. pneumoniae* pneumonia confirmed by a demonstration of diagnostic rise in antibody measured by indirect immunofluorescence during convalescence. The right hilum shows an extensive infiltrate. Both costophrenic angles are clear.

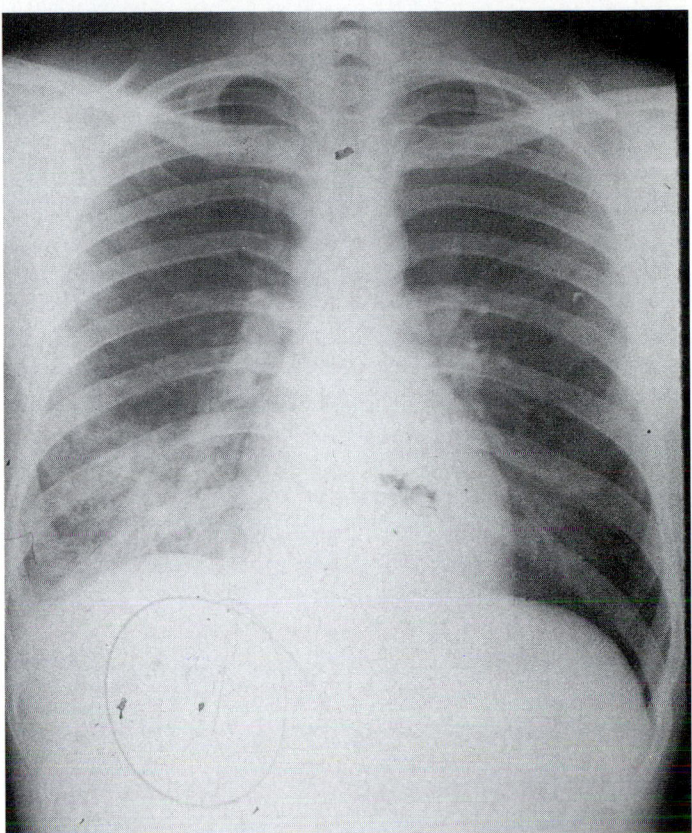

FIGURE 145-2   Chest radiograph of a young man with proven *M. pneumoniae* pneumonia confirmed by a demonstration of diagnostic rise in antibody measured by indirect immunofluorescence during convalescence. The right lower lung field shows a patchy infiltrate streaking from the right hilum. Both costophrenic angles are clear.

pleural abnormalities, lung abscess, adult respiratory distress syndrome, and lobar consolidation. Nonpulmonary complications occur infrequently in *M. pneumoniae* pneumonia, including cold hemagglutinin–mediated hemolytic anemia, Stevens-Johnson syndrome, pericarditis, erythema nodosum, and myriad nervous system diseases (encephalitis, meningitis, meningoencephalitis, transverse myelitis, polyradiculitis, acute cerebellar ataxia, Guillain-Barré syndrome, Fisher syndrome, polyneuritis cranialis, and bilateral optic neuritis). CNS complications occur about once in 1000 *M. pneumoniae* infections.[19,26]

The results of routine laboratory tests are usually normal, including a complete blood count, liver function studies, electrolytes, glucose, and renal function studies. About one-fourth of patients with *M. pneumoniae* pneumonia develop elevated leukocyte counts or an elevated erythrocyte sedimentation rate, but neither finding contributes to a diagnosis of the infection.

Laboratory Diagnosis

A specific diagnosis of *M. pneumoniae* infection can be established by isolation of the organism from respiratory tract secretions, identification of antigen in respiratory tract secretions or fluids from usually sterile sites, and detection of an early immune response by IgM antibody elevation or fourfold or greater rise in (IgG) antibody during convalescence. Isolation from throat swabs nominally serves as the "gold standard" for the diagnosis of in-

fection because isolation of the organism represents definitive evidence of infection, but it is not sufficiently sensitive. Typically, a throat swab specimen contains only 200 to 600 colony-forming units (CFU). Moreover, the organism grows slowly on agar and in broth specially formulated to support its growth and its isolation may take 1 to 3 weeks.[18] On agar, the colonies of *M. pneumoniae* lack the characteristic "bull's-eye" or "fried egg" appearance of the typical mycoplasma colony; this feature suggests, but does not confirm, its identity. A disk inhibition procedure, using antibody-impregnated disks, can identify the colony of *M. pneumoniae*. Antibiotic treatment of *M. pneumoniae* pneumonia does not immediately eradicate the organism from respiratory secretions, so it can be isolated soon after the start of therapy.

Isolation of *M. pneumoniae* as a routine procedure for laboratory diagnosis of infection has been replaced, for the most part, by rapid diagnostic procedures—primarily antigen detection in respiratory tract secretions by indirect immunofluorescence, enzyme immunoassay, DNA-RNA probe, polymerase chain reaction (PCR), and early immune response by IgM antibody determination.[15,17,18] These procedures provide quick and reliable results of high specificity but of differing levels of sensitivity, varying from 25 to 100 percent. All of these tests, except PCR, have been developed commercially for routine use. However, PCR may prove to be the most sensitive assay, as selected primer pairs from the P1 gene can detect less than 1 CFU/μl.[25]

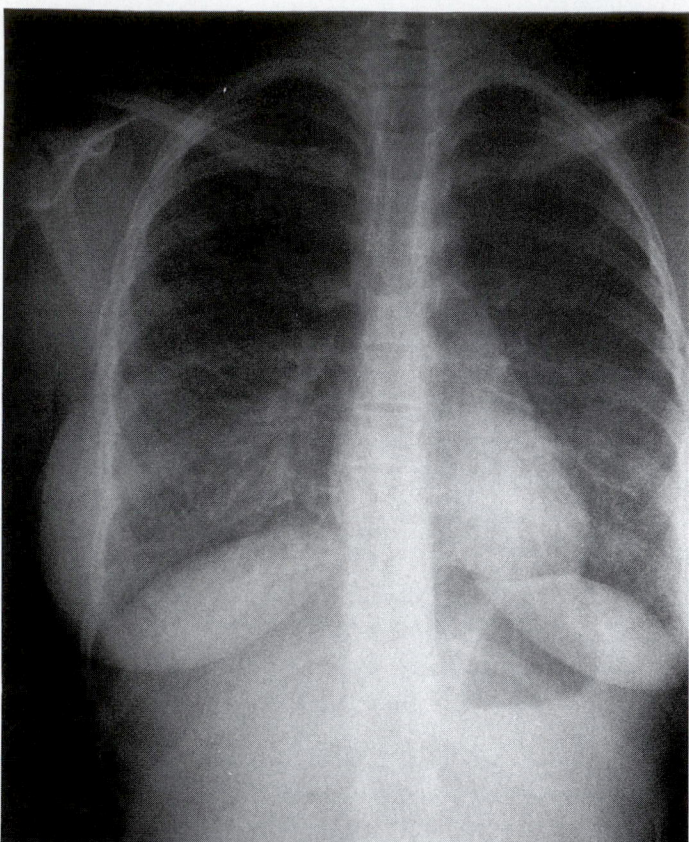

FIGURE 145-3   Chest radiograph of a 14-year-old girl with *M. pneumoniae* pneumonia confirmed serologically. A patchy interstitial infiltrate involves both lower lobes. The costophrenic angles are clear.

The diagnosis of *M. pneumoniae* infection can also be made by the detection of a fourfold or greater (diagnostic) rise in antibody during convalescence. Until rapid procedures were developed, the demonstration of a diagnostic rise in antibody had been the principal means of establishing a laboratory diagnosis of *M. pneumoniae* infection. It remains the mainstay of epidemiologic studies, and lacking a positive culture or antigen detection test, it can demonstrate a high proportion of infections. Of necessity, it provides retrospective information, because of the requirement for obtaining a second serum specimen during convalescence. The various methods for measuring antibody include complement fixation (CF), immunofluorescence (IMF), enzyme immunoassay (EIA), metabolic inhibition, and passive agglutination (employing antigen-coated high-density particles). IgM-specific *M. pneumoniae* antibody, which occurs as early as 1 week after the onset of illness, confirms infection. In reinfection, the demonstration of IgG antibody between acute and convalescent serum specimens is required.

Prevention and Treatment

M. pneumoniae pneumonia can be effectively treated with broad-spectrum antibiotics belonging to the macrolide and the tetracycline classes (Table 145-1).[23] *M. pneumoniae* is sensitive in vitro to tetracyclines and the macrolides, and in clinical trials these drugs have proved successful in its treatment.[3,16] Erythromycin

remains the drug of choice. Tetracycline is less often used, mainly because it is contraindicated in children and women of child-bearing age as it stains the teeth enamel. Minocycline is preferred for treatment of the CNS complications of *M. pneumoniae* because of higher solubility in lipids.

Prompt differentiation and treatment of *M. pneumoniae* pneumonia are important not only because appropriate antibiotic treatment speeds recovery in mild or moderately severe cases but also because it may be lifesaving in the rare instances of life-threatening *M. pneumoniae* pneumonia. On the basis of clinical and radiographic features, *M. pneumoniae* pneumonia cannot be differentiated with any certainty from the typical pneumonias that constitute most CAP. Bacterial pneumonias due to the common pathogens may present with radiographic findings substantially the same as those from an atypical pneumonia. A macrolide or tetracycline antibiotic should be added to empiric treatment of CAP when *M. pneumoniae* cannot be ruled out as the infecting microorganism.

No *M. pneumoniae* vaccine is available. Although various approaches to developing an effective and safe vaccine have been employed, including inactivated whole organism and live attenuated vaccines, none has been successful. Recently, purified or acellular vaccines composed of several *M. pneumoniae* proteins, especially the P1 adhesin protein, have shown promise by inducing protective antibody when administered to primates.[10]

Special Considerations

CAP represents a continuing challenge because of its frequent occurrence, and because initial clinical and laboratory examinations often fail to provide definitive information for the physician to identify with a high degree of certainty the specific infecting pathogen. The physician needs to assess the likelihood that the patient may have *M. pneumoniae* pneumonia, especially because the clinical presentation may not allow a clear differentiation between an atypical and typical pneumonia. Faced with the necessity to begin antibiotic treatment promptly, most physicians choose empiric therapy, and currently this means a β-lactam antibiotic, which will not cover *M. pneumoniae*. If *M. pneumoniae* pneumonia appears a possible consideration, it behooves the physician to include an antibiotic effective against it in the treatment regimen, at least long enough to confirm whether or not it is the infecting organism.

C. PNEUMONIAE PNEUMONIA

History

The prototype strain of *C. pneumoniae*, designated TWAR, was recognized as a respiratory tract pathogen in the 1980s through the detailed studies of Grayston and colleagues. Grayston applied the name TWAR to signify the TW from strain TW-183 and the AR from strain AR-39; TW was recovered from the eye of a child with trachoma in the 1960s, and AR was recovered from the pharynx of an adult with upper respiratory tract disease.[27] The worldwide isolation of *C. pneumoniae* from persons with pneumonia during the past 20 years provided the epidemiologic evidence of its etiologic role in CAP.[12,13] Today, in the

United States, it accounts for 10 to 20 percent of CAP, depending on the community and time period(s), and remains an important pathogen of atypical pneumonia. It is associated also with pharyngitis, sinusitis, and bronchitis.

Epidemiology

C. pneumoniae occurs worldwide through all seasons of the year, with an epidemic cycle of 4 to 6 years.[27] It spreads effectively in semiclosed populations, such as military groups, and in families, usually infecting all family members (excluding children under 3 years of age) and causing lower respiratory tract disease in most of them.[1,2,7] Person-to-person spread occurs quickly over 1 to 3 weeks. Attack rates in young children are low—about 5 percent—and increase markedly among adolescents to about 20 percent, based on the geographic location of the population. Among adults, *C. pneumoniae* can account for as much as one-fifth of CAP. *C. pneumoniae* is most likely transmitted by infectious droplets from the respiratory tract and possibly also by fomites. The incubation period is about 15 to 23 days. At a minimum, about one in 10 persons develop pneumonia during primary infection. Persons who become reinfected experience milder respiratory tract illness, and they are less predisposed to develop pneumonia. By age 50 years, more than one-half of persons have been infected with *C. pneumoniae*. No reservoirs for the organism in nature have been identified.

Microbiology and Pathogenesis

C. pneumoniae, an obligate intracellular bacterial parasite, belongs to the Chlamydiaceae family. It is a distinct species, and its 16S ribosomal DNA sequence differs significantly from those of *C. psittaci* and *C. trachomatis,* which exhibit only about 96 and 94 percent homology, respectively. Moreover, oligonucleotide primers constructed for sequences of the 16S rRNA homologous to *C. pneumoniae,* as compared with *C. psittaci* and *C. trachomatis,* amplified only *C. pneumoniae* and not the other chlamydias. These experiments demonstrate evidence that *C. pneumoniae* is a distinct species and provide a basis for its identification in clinical specimens. Only a single serovar (serologic variant) has been identified. During the growth cycle, *C. pneumoniae,* like the other chlamydia species, manifests two morphologic forms—a metabolic reticulate body (RB), which differentiates to an infectious extracellular "pear-shaped" elementary body (EB). When infected cells rupture, the EB releases to the extracellular environment and maintains the cycle of transmission.

The EB of *C. pneumoniae* is dense and spherical; its diameter is about 0.2 to 0.4 μm. Two cysteine-containing envelope proteins integral to the growth cycle are expressed during this process, one 9 kDa and the other 60 kDa. The outer membrane of the EB embraces lipopolysaccharide and the major outer membrane protein (MOMP), about 40 kDa. MOMP induces antibody during infection, but it is not available to binding by antibody. The sequence of the MOMP gene shows four variable domains of marked dissimilarity with other chlamydia species and five conserved domains.

Clinical Manifestations

C. pneumoniae pneumonia begins gradually with symptoms and signs indistinguishable from other atypical pneumonias, especially *M. pneumoniae* pneumonia: hoarseness, pharyngitis, fever, nonproductive cough, nonpleuritic chest pain, headache, malaise, and fatigue. Hemoptysis rarely occurs; rales occasionally occur. As the pneumonia progresses, more rales become evident.

On the chest radiograph, *C. pneumoniae* pneumonia begins predominantly as a unilateral alveolar infiltrate.[22] Small to medium-size pleural effusions, not unlike those in *M. pneumoniae* pneumonia, occur commonly, and most are present early in the course of illness. In some persons they develop later, during their hospital course. *C. pneumoniae* pneumonia often progresses to bilateral involvement, with a mixed pattern of interstitial and alveolar infiltrates, before resolving during the next several weeks. Persons undergoing primary infection with *C. pneumoniae* more often present with an alveolar pattern on chest radiographs, and those experiencing reinfection more often show a mixed picture. The differing radiographic patterns do not distinguish primary from recurrent infections.

Extrapulmonary manifestations and death rarely occur. Recurrences occur relatively often, however, and the organism can be shed for months. Antibiotic treatment of *C. pneumoniae* pneumonia often fails to eradicate it from the pharynx, so persistent infection can ensue. If eradication can be achieved, antibiotics must be administered in sufficiently high dose and for a prolonged period.[14]

The routine laboratory tests are usually normal. An elevation of the peripheral leukocyte count occurs in a small proportion of patients.

Laboratory Diagnosis

The diagnosis of *C. pneumoniae* infection can be established by isolation of the organism from respiratory tract secretions; amplification of antigen by PCR in respiratory tract specimens; and, in primary infections, detection of an IgM immune response in a serum obtained early in the course of illness, specifically an IgM antibody titer of at least 1:16 in acute-phase serum specimen or detection of a fourfold or greater (diagnostic) rise in IgM or IgG antibody in paired serum specimens obtained during the acute and convalescent phases of illness.[8,11] In reinfection, a serologic diagnosis can be made by demonstration of stable IgG titer of at least 1:512 or a fourfold or greater rise in IgG antibody during convalescence, in the absence of complement-fixing antibody. Isolation of *C. pneumoniae* from throat swabs serves as the "gold standard" for the diagnosis of infection. PCR and IgM antibody detection provide more rapid and highly sensitive and specific means of identifying infection and are coming into greater use.

Because it is an extremely fastidious organism, the isolation of *C. pneumoniae* is substantially influenced by the type of cell cultures used. Isolation of *C. pneumoniae* from nasopharyngeal or throat swab specimens can be carried out with a high degree of success employing as a substrate HL or HEp-2 cell cultures for inoculation. Growth of *C. pneumoniae* in these cells can be seen 72 h after inoculation by immunofluorescent procedures using a species-specific monoclonal antibody. Even so, the organism is not isolated from all patients.

The method for measuring IgM and IgG antibodies to *C. pneumoniae* is micro-IMF, using whole organism as antigen, EIA, and CF. The results of CF antibody determinations done in parallel assist in classifying primary infections from reinfections.

Prevention and Treatment

C. pneumoniae is sensitive to the tetracyclines and macrolides. However, unlike the regimen for treatment of *M. pneumoniae* pneumonia, the duration of treatment for *C. pneumoniae* pneumonia should be prolonged to prevent recurrences of signs and symptoms and eradicate the organism from the respiratory tract. Erythromycin or one of the tetracyclines—for example, doxycycline—is the recommended antibiotic (Table 145-1).[27] *C. pneumoniae* is sensitive to other macrolides, such as clarithromycin and azithromycin; however, few clinical trials with these antibiotics have been done.[3] Treatment of children with *C. pneumoniae* pneumonia with erythromycin or clarithromycin eradicated the organism in four-fifths of instances. The organism is also sensitive to quinolones. Ofloxacin represents an alternative choice for treatment of adults; however, the quinolones are not recommended for children. Empiric therapy of CAP with a β-lactam antibiotic will not cover *C. pneumoniae*. No vaccine is available for *C. pneumoniae*.

Special Considerations

Of the chlamydia organisms that cause pneumonia, *C. pneumoniae* dominates. Although the appropriate serologic tests can differentiate this infection from those of other chlamydias, serologic cross-reactions occasionally obscure the diagnosis. The important point is that *C. pneumoniae* infection is a common infection; all other chlamydias associated with respiratory tract infections occur very seldom. Except for a clearly documented recent exposure to psittacine birds in a person with atypical pneumonia, any positive serologic tests for chlamydia should be considered indicative of *C. pneumoniae* infection, and appropriate treatment regimens started.

Other Pathogens of Atypical Pneumonia

Two other nonviral pathogens that also cause atypical pneumonia, albeit very infrequently, are *C. psittaci* and *C. burnetii* (Q fever). Both infections occur only after exposure to the infected animal reservoir—psittacine birds and poultry in the case of *C. psittaci* and cattle, sheep, and goats in the case of *C. burnetii*. Both pathogens respond to treatment with the appropriate antibiotics (Table 145-1).

C. PSITTACI PNEUMONIA

History

By comparison with *M. pneumoniae* and *C. pneumoniae*, *C. psittaci* is an old organism, as the first recognized cases of infection date from the last decades of the 1800s. At that time, par-

rots and parakeets were identified as reservoirs of the organism, and the name *psittacosis* (or *ornithosis*) was coined. In 1930, the organism was isolated for the first time in studies among infected zoo animals. Its classification as an intracellular obligate bacterial parasite and its designation of genus and species were assigned in the mid-1900s.

Epidemiology

C. psittaci is endemic to psittacine birds and many other species of birds. It spreads to humans who inhale the dried excreta from infected birds. *C. psittaci* pneumonia or psittacosis occurs uncommonly; annually about 200 cases are reported to the Centers for Disease Control and Prevention (CDC). Today, birds imported through controlled sources are treated to ensure that they are disease-free, accounting for a decreased reservoir of infection and a very low annual incidence of infection in humans. Birds acquired through underground sources have a high likelihood of being infected. Infection with *C. psittaci* represents a unique occupational disease of persons who work with psittacine birds or species of birds (for example, poultry) that harbor the organism.

Microbiology and Pathogenesis

C. psittaci, like all other chlamydias, possesses both DNA and RNA. An obligate intracellular parasite belonging to the Chlamydiaceae family, it is a distinct species, whose 16S ribosomal DNA sequence differs significantly from that of *C. pneumoniae*. The 16S ribosomal DNA of *C. psittaci* and that of *C. trachomatis* differ little, by about 5 percent. The structural characteristics of the EB form and cycle of infection are similar for all chlamydias. Replication entails cell attachment and penetration by the EB form and its change to the RB form in the infected cell phagosome; the RB grows and divides by binary fission and subsequently evolves into the EB form for release from ruptured cells. Several distinct serovars of *C. psittaci* exist.

Clinical Manifestations

The clinical characteristics of *C. psittaci* pneumonia mimic those of *C. pneumoniae* pneumonia. These two pneumonias cannot be differentiated on the basis of clinical and routine laboratory findings. Patients suspected of having psittacosis must be queried about exposure(s) to psittacine birds: whether they keep a bird as a pet, whether a friend or neighbor does, whether they have visited a household in another geographic location, or whether the possibility of an occupational exposure exists.

The illness begins with fever, chills, headache, diaphoresis, and myriad other common systemic and respiratory tract symptoms, including malaise, arthralgia, myalgias, hemoptysis, and pharyngitis. The severity of psittacosis can vary from mild upper respiratory tract illness to severe pneumonia, with a small percentage of deaths in the most serious cases. Few physical findings in the lungs may be audible. Splenomegaly occurs commonly; the diagnosis of psittacosis should be considered when splenomegaly is found in a patient with an atypical pneumonia. Subclinical *C. psittaci* infection also occurs commonly.

TABLE 145-1

Antibiotics Recommended in the Treatment of Atypical Pneumonia

Pathogen	Recommended Therapy	Alternative Therapy	Comment
Mycoplasma pneumoniae	Erythromycin, 0.5 g, qid, PO, for 10–14 days	Clarithromycin, 0.5 g, bid, PO, for 10–14 days	In vitro sensitivity very good; few clinical trials of these two macrolides
		Azithromycin, 0.5 g day 1 and 0.25 g, bid, PO, for 5 days	
		Minocycline, 0.100 g, bid, PO, for 14–21 days	Use if there is CNS impairment
		Tetracycline, 0.25–0.5 g, qid, PO, for 10–14 days	Avoid in women of childbearing age and in children
Chlamydia pneumoniae	Erythromycin, 0.5 g qid, PO, for 21 days	Doxycycline, 0.2 g on day 1 and 0.1 g, bid, PO, for 21 days	
		Tetracycline, 0.25–0.5 g, qid, PO, for 21 days	Avoid tetracycline in women of child-bearing age and in children
		Clarithromycin, 0.5 g, bid, PO, for 21 days	In vitro very good; few clinical trials of these two macrolides
		Azithromycin, 0.5 g on day 1 and 0.25 g, bid, PO, for 5 days	
Chlamydia psittaci	Tetracycline, 0.25–0.5 g, qid, PO, for 10–14 days	Chloramphenicol, 0.5 g, qid, PO, for 10–14 days	Avoid tetracycline in women of child-bearing age and in children
Coxiella burnetii	Doxycycline, 0.2 g on day 1 and 0.1 g, od, PO, for 10–14 days (at least 1 week after fever abates)	Chloramphenicol, 0.5 g qid, PO, for 10–14 days	Fluoroquinolones not recommended for children
	Tetracycline, 0.25–0.5 g, qid, PO, for 10–14 days (at least 1 week after fever abates)	Ciprofloxacin, 1.0 g, bid, PO, for 10–14 days	Fluoroquinolones not recommended for children
		Ofloxacin, 0.4 g, bid, PO, for 10–14 days	Avoid tetracycline in women of child-bearing age and in children

The radiographic features of *C. psittaci* pneumonia include predominantly unilateral reticular infiltrates, often appearing as streaks from the hilum to the bases, small pleural effusions, and sometimes bilateral lung involvement; consolidation is rare. The pneumonia usually resolves within a few weeks.

Laboratory Diagnosis

The diagnosis of *C. psittaci* infection can be established by isolation of the organism from respiratory tract secretions, detection of an IgM immune response in a serum obtained early in the course of illness, and demonstration of a fourfold or greater rise in IgM or IgG antibody during convalescence.[8,11]

The serologic diagnosis of *C. psittaci* infection can be made from detection of immune response by demonstration of an IgM antibody titer of at least 1:16 in an acute-phase serum specimen or a diagnostic rise in IgM or IgG antibody in paired serum specimens obtained during the acute and convalescent phases of illness.[8] EIA and CF are the methods for measuring IgM and IgG antibodies to *C. psittaci*.

Prevention and Treatment

Psittacosis pneumonia can be treated effectively with tetracyclines or chloramphenicol (Table 145-1). However, tetracyclines should be avoided in women of childbearing age and in children. No vaccine is available for *C. psittaci*. Avoiding exposure to infected psittacine birds and poultry obviously prevents infection. Workers in the poultry industry need to be especially vigilant to avoid occupational exposure. Empiric therapy of CAP with a β-lactam antibiotic will not cover *C. psittaci*.

Special Considerations

Unless the physician asks the pertinent questions about a possible exposure, the diagnosis of *C. psittaci* will probably be missed or at least will be delayed until a succession of antibody tests are completed in the search for clues to the diagnosis. Many exposed persons will deny or at least fail to remember an exposure. Physician awareness to the possibility of the diagnosis remains paramount. To this end, a physician must maintain vigilance to identify the source of the infection when presented with several patients with common situations or exposures.

C. BURNETII (Q FEVER) PNEUMONIA

History

Query fever (Q fever) was initially described in the mid-1930s. A few years later, the pathogen was found and categorized by Burnet and Freeman as a rickettsia, and subsequently it was designated as *C. burnetii*. It is an uncommon cause of atypical pneumonia, is rarely fatal, and is usually self-limited.

Epidemiology

Highly contagious, *C. burnetii* infection occurs after exposure to infected animals, mainly ruminants (including cattle, goats, and sheep), which serve as a reservoir, and pregnant cats and ticks.

The incubation period is about 2 weeks. Ticks are not engaged in transmission of the infection to humans from animals. Humans become infected, and can develop undifferentiated respiratory tract illness or an atypical pneumonia, by inhalation of infected aerosols of only a few organisms. The illness is often complicated by hepatic impairment.

Microbiology and Pathogenesis

C. burnetii is an intracellular obligate bacteria that exists in two variations, designated phase I and phase II, reflecting differing antigenic characteristics. Phase I forms occur naturally, and phase II forms emerge on multiple passage in embryonated eggs. In its spore stage, the organism survives harsh conditions, such as chemical and physical agents, that might otherwise destroy it. It persists many months in meat, wool, and tick feces. Lipopolysaccharide and three plasmids account for virulence factors.

Clinical Manifestations

Usually characterized by an acute onset, *C. burnetii* infection begins with fever, signs of respiratory tract illness, mainly nonproductive cough, headache, malaise, and myalgia; rash rarely occurs.[28] Few auscultatory findings develop. Chest radiographic findings show patchy bronchopneumonic infiltrates. These usually lack distinguishing features, although they sometimes occur as segmental opacities that become round during resolution; multiple lesions may develop. Slow resolution of the radiographic findings seems to occur, and this offers a slim clue to the diagnosis.

The concomitant occurrence of hepatitis also suggests *C. burnetii* infection. Many persons undergoing *C. burnetii* infection develop evidence of abnormal liver function, mainly elevated liver cell enzymes and enlargement of the liver, and uncommonly jaundice. Very rarely, neurologic complications or endocarditis complicates Q fever.

Laboratory Diagnosis

The laboratory diagnosis of *C. burnetii* infection is made by serologic procedures. Unlike the other pathogens of atypical pneumonia, isolation of *C. burnetii* poses the risk of spread to laboratory workers and so it is not performed. Moreover, antibodies to it fail to agglutinate in the Weil-Felix test.

The serologic diagnosis of *C. burnetii* infection can be made by detection using IMF of elevated IgM (1:25) or IgG (>1:20) antibodies to phase II antigen in a single serum specimen and demonstration by CF, IMF, or IgM-ELISA of a fourfold or greater rise in antibody to phase II antigen during convalescence. Persistence of antibody to *C. burnetii* can be determined by assaying IgM employing an IMF procedure.

Prevention and Treatment

Although mainly a self-limited illness, *C. burnetii* pneumonia responds to treatment with doxycycline or tetracycline, chloramphenicol, ciprofloxacin, and ofloxacin with a shortened duration of fever (Table 145-1). However, tetracycline and the fluoroquinolones are not recommended for children, and the tetracyclines should be avoided in women of childbearing age. Vaccines composed of phase I or phase II organisms have been shown to be effective in experimental studies. No vaccine is available for general use; vaccine can be obtained for persons in occupational settings of high risk to *C. burnetii* infection. These workers need to be alert to avoid occupational exposure.

Special Considerations

As with psittacosis, the physician needs to ask appropriate questions about possible exposure during overseas and occupational exposures. Otherwise, the diagnosis of *C. burnetii* may be missed or, at least, it will be delayed until the results of laboratory tests suggest the diagnosis.

REFERENCES

1. Almirall J, Morató I, Riera F, et al: Incidence of community-acquired pneumonia and *Chlamydia pneumoniae* infection: A prospective multicentre study. *Eur Respir J* 6:14–18, 1993.
2. Berdal BP, Scheel O, Ogaard AR, et al: Spread of subclinical *Chlamydia pneumoniae* infection in a closed community. *Scand J Infect Dis* 24:431–436, 1992.
3. Block S, Hedrick J, Hammerschlag MR, et al: *Mycoplasma pneumoniae* and *Chlamydia pneumoniae* in pediatric community-acquired pneumonia: Comparative efficacy and safety of clarithromycin vs. erythromycin ethylsuccinate. *Pediatr Infect Dis J* 14:471–477, 1995.
4. Anonymous: Outbreaks of *Mycoplasma pneumoniae* respiratory infection—Ohio, Texas, and New York. *MMWR Morb Mortal Wkly Rep* 42:931, 937–939, 1993.
5. Chan ED, Welsh CH: Fulminant *Mycoplasma pneumoniae* pneumonia (clinical conference). *West J Med* 162:133–142, 1995.
5a. Chanock RM, Hayflick L, Barile MF: Growth on artificial medium of an agent associated with atypcal pneumonia and its identification as a PPLO. *Proc Natl Acad Sci USA* 48:41–49, 1962.
5b. Chanock RM, Mufson MA, Bloom B, et al: Eaton agent pneumonia. I. Etiology of infection in a military recruit population. J *Am Med Assoc* 175:213–220, 1961.
6. Clyde WA Jr: Clinical overview of typical *Mycoplasma pneumoniae* infections. *Clin Infect Dis* 17 (Suppl 1):S32–S36, 1993.
7. Ekman MR, Grayston JT, Visakorpi R, et al: An epidemic of infections due to *Chlamydia pneumoniae* in military conscripts. *Clin Infect Dis* 17:420–425, 1993.
8. Ekman MR, Leinonen M, Syrjala H, et al: Evaluation of serological methods in the diagnosis of *Chlamydia pneumoniae* pneumonia during an epidemic in Finland. *Eur J Clin Microbiol Infect Dis* 12:756–760, 1993.
9. Franzoso G, Hu PC, Meloni GA, Barile MF: The immunodominant 90-kilodalton protein is localized on the terminal tip structure of *Mycoplasma pneumoniae*. *Infect Immun* 61:1523–1530, 1993.
10. Franzoso G, Hu PC, Meloni GA, Barile MF: Immunoblot analyses of chimpanzee sera after infection and after immunization and challenge with *Mycoplasma pneumoniae*. *Infect Immun* 62:1008–1014, 1994.
11. Gaydos CA, Eiden JJ, Oldach D, et al: Diagnosis of *Chlamydia pneumoniae* infection in patients with community-acquired pneumonia by polymerase chain reaction enzyme immunoassay. *Clin Infect Dis* 19:157–160, 1994.
12. Grayston JT: *Chlamydia pneumoniae,* strain TWAR pneumonia. *Ann Rev Med* 43:317–323, 1992.
13. Grayston JT, Aldous MB, Easton A, et al: Evidence that *Chlamydia pneumoniae* causes pneumonia and bronchitis. *J Infect Dis* 168:1231–1235, 1993.
14. Hammerschlag MR, Chirgwin K, Roblin PM, et al: Persistent infection with *Chlamydia pneumoniae* following acute respiratory illness. *Clin Infect Dis* 14:178–182, 1992.
15. Hirai Y, Shiode J, Masayoshi T, Kanemasa Y: Application of an indirect immunofluorescence test for detection of *Mycoplasma pneumoniae* in respiratory exudates. *J Clin Microbiol* 29:2007–2012, 1991.
16. Ishida K, Kaku M, Irifune K, et al: In vitro and in vivo activities of macrolides against *Mycoplasma pneumoniae*. *Antimicrob Agents Chemother* 38:790–798, 1994.
17. Kai M, Kamiya S, Yabe H, et al: Rapid detection of *Mycoplasma pneumoniae* in clinical samples by the polymerase chain reaction. *J Med Microbiol* 38:166–170, 1993.
18. Kenny GE, Kaiser GG, Cooney MK, Foy HM: Diagnosis of *Mycoplasma pneumoniae* pneumonia: Sensitivities and specificities of serology with lipid antigen and isolation of the organism on soy peptone medium for identification of infections. *J Clin Microbiol* 28:2087–2093, 1990.
19. Koskiniemi M: CNS manifestations associated with *Mycoplasma pneumoniae* infections: Summary of cases at the University of Helsinki and review. *Clin Infect Dis* 17 (Suppl 1):S52–S57, 1993.
20. Layh-Schmitt G, Herrmann R: Spatial arrangement of gene products of the P1 operon in the membrane of *Mycoplasma pneumoniae*. *Infect Immun* 62:974–979, 1994.
20a. Liu C: Studies on primary atypical pneumonia—I. Localization, isolation, and cultivation of a virus in chick embryos. *J Exp Med* 106:455–466, 1957.
20b. Liu C, Eaton MD, Heyl JT: Studies on primary atypical pneumonia—II. Observations concerning development and immunological characteristics of antibody in patients. *J Exp Med* 109:545–566, 1959.
21. Marmion BP: Eaton agent—Science and scientific acceptance: A historical commentary. *Rev Infect Dis* 12:338–353, 1990.
22. McConnell CT, Jr, Plouffe JF, File TM, et al: Radiographic appearance of *Chlamydia pneumoniae* (TWAR strain) respiratory infections. *Radiology* 192:819–824, 1994.
23. McCormack WM: Susceptibility of mycoplasmas to antimicrobial agents: Clinical implications. *Clin Infect Dis* 17 (Suppl 1): S200–S201, 1993.
24. Mufson MA: *Mycoplasma pneumoniae* (editorial). *West J Med* 125:66–67, 1976.
25. Reznikov M, Blackmore TK, Finlay-Jones JJ, Gordon DL: Comparison of nasopharyngeal aspirates and throat swab specimens in a polymerase chain reaction-based test for *Mycoplasma pneumoniae*. *Eur J Clin Microbiol Infect Dis* 14:58–61, 1995.
26. Saitoh A, Ohya T, Yoshida S, et al: A case report of Stevens-Johnson syndrome with *Mycoplasma pneumoniae* infection. *Acta Paediatr Jpn* 37:113–115, 1995.
27. Thom DH, Grayston JT: Infections with *Chlamydia pneumoniae* strain TWAR. *Clin Chest Med* 12:245–256, 1991.
28. Tselentis Y, Gikas A, Kofteridis D, et al: Q fever in the Greek Island of Crete: Epidemiologic, clinical, and therapeutic data from 98 cases. *Clin Inf Dis* 20:1311–1316, 1995.
29. Wenzel R, Pirkl E, Herrmann R: Construction of an EcoRI restriction map of *Mycoplasma pneumoniae* and localization of selected genes. *J Bacteriol* 174:7289–7296, 1992.

CHAPTER 146

ACTINOMYCOSIS AND NOCARDIOSIS

Gregory A. Filice / Donald Armstrong

ACTINOMYCOSIS

Actinomycosis is an indolent, infectious disease characterized by a pyogenic response and necrosis, followed by intense fibrosis. Occasionally, the pus contains minute yellow granules consisting of clumps of *Actinomyces* filaments. Actinomycosis is usually caused by *Actinomyces israelii,* but other species of *Actinomyces* and *Propionibacterium propionicum* (formerly *Arachnia propionica*) are occasionally responsible. Since the different species are associated with similar disease, they will be considered together. Several syndromes have been associated with *Actinomyces* infection, including cervicofacial, pulmonary, abdominal, female genital, and disseminated actinomycosis and lacrimal canaliculitis. Only pulmonary actinomycosis will be considered in detail in this chapter.

Epidemiology and Pathogenesis

Pathogenic species of *Actinomyces (A. israelii, A. naeslundii, A. viscosus, A. meyeri, A. gerencseriae)* and *P. propionicum* are strict or facultative anaerobic bacteria that normally inhabit anaerobic niches in the human oral cavity. Thoracic actinomycosis often occurs in people with carious teeth and periodontal disease, in which numbers of these bacteria are increased. Aspiration of infective material is the probable inciting event. Spread to the mediastinum is usually from pulmonary or, less commonly, cervicofacial disease. Actinomycosis occurs throughout the world. Males are affected more often than females, and the disease affects people of all ages.

The typical lesion consists of abscesses filled with neutrophils and surrounded by dense fibrous tissue. Macrophages, plasma cells, and lymphocytes are abundant in the periphery of lesions. Giant cells are uncommon, and epithelioid granulomas are exceedingly rare. In the lung, consolidation can occur without macroscopic abscess formation. Sputum is usually white or yellow and has no distinctive odor. Malodorous sputum should suggest the presence of another anaerobic organism, possibly in combination with *Actinomyces* or *P. propionicum.*

In tissue, *Actinomyces* organisms tend to grow in dense microcolonies or granules that may reach 4 mm in size. These are often called sulfur granules because they are usually yellow, although they do not contain much sulfur. The bacteria are embedded in a mucopolysaccharide matrix containing substantial amounts of $Ca_3(PO_4)_2$. Host cells are excluded from the granules, but neutrophils surround them. At the periphery, tips of hyphae are often widened and are referred to as "clubs." These clubs are considered highly suggestive of *Actinomyces.*

Actinomycosis often spreads without regard for anatomic tissue planes. Disease extends to nearby structures, and fistulae or abscesses may appear at unexpected sites far from primary lesions. Skin, subcutaneous tissue, and bone are frequently invaded.

Lesions of actinomycosis often contain other bacteria, sometimes referred to as "concomitant bacteria," which may contribute to the pathogenesis. Generally, the concomitant bacteria are from the same oral mucosal niches as the *Actinomyces* organisms. The relationship between one such bacterium, *Actinobacillus actinomycetemcomitans,* and actinomycosis is so close that isolation of *A. actinomycetemcomitans* should always lead to a careful search for *Actinomyces.* Although concomitant bacteria are often present, the presence of *Actinomyces* species or *P. propionicum* is clearly necessary and often sufficient for the pathogenesis of this disease.

Clinical Manifestations

Pulmonary disease begins insidiously with cough, sputum, fever, and weight loss.[3,6] Hemoptysis and pleuritic pain occur in a minority of cases. Masses of inflammatory tissue may occur within bronchi and may cause partial obstruction.[7] Leukocytosis, neutrophilia, and moderate anemia are common. Symptoms are often surprisingly mild for the extent of disease.[15] In advanced cases, clubbing, pulmonary osteoarthopathy, or amyloidosis may occur.

Mediastinal impairment is common, and pericarditis and the superior vena cava syndrome have been reported.[3,6] Empyema is common. Pulmonary lesions may burrow through the chest wall to drain or to invade other chest wall structures; this should strongly suggest the diagnosis. Rib involvement typically produces a characteristic "wavy periostitis." Other adjacent structures that may be affected are the shoulder girdle, sternum, and thoracic vertebrae. Afflicted vertebrae characteristically appear mottled because of parallel processes of resorption and new bone formation.[6] Spread from one vertebra to another and intervertebral disk space narrowing are distinctly unusual, whereas they are common with pyogenic and tuberculous osteomyelitis. A few cases of endocarditis with *Actinomyces* species have been reported.[13]

On radiographs, infiltrates are often dense and well circumscribed (Fig. 146-1).[3,5,9,15] Since symptoms are often mild, the radiographic appearance often suggests a diagnosis of lung cancer (Fig. 146-2). Cavities, observed in about half of the cases, tend to be small (Fig. 146-3). Because of the lack of regard for anatomic barriers, actinomycosis may affect many lobes by spread through interlobar fissures. Other patterns that may occur are fibronodular and alveolar infiltrates (Fig. 146-4). Occasionally, erosion of a blood vessel results in miliary disease. Computed tomography scans sometimes add information about cavities, spread through fissures, or involvement of the chest wall that is not apparent on standard radiographs.[12]

Diagnosis

Since the organisms are part of the normal respiratory flora, a positive sputum culture is of little clinical significance. The presence of granules in sputum is suggestive of the diagnosis, but

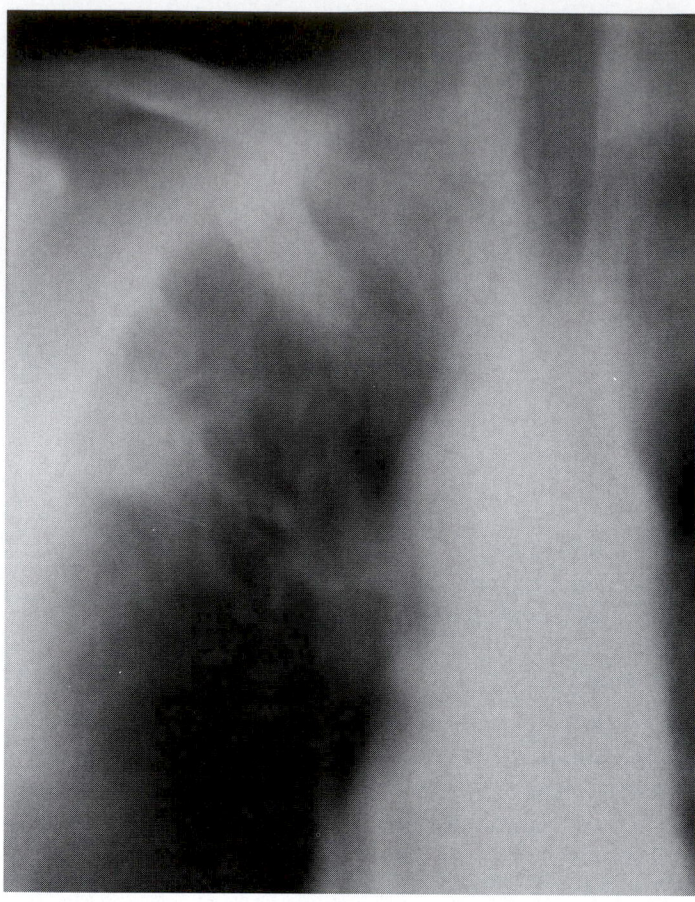

FIGURE 146-2 A tomogram showing a nodular density in the right upper lobe that suggested carcinoma but proved to be due to actinomycosis.

they are seldom found. A search should be made in suspected cases. If the diagnosis cannot be made by simpler means, transthoracic needle aspiration, transbronchial biopsy, or open lung biopsy should be performed. Cultures of bronchoscopy specimens may be contaminated by upper respiratory secretions, and reliance must be placed on histologic examination of tissue.

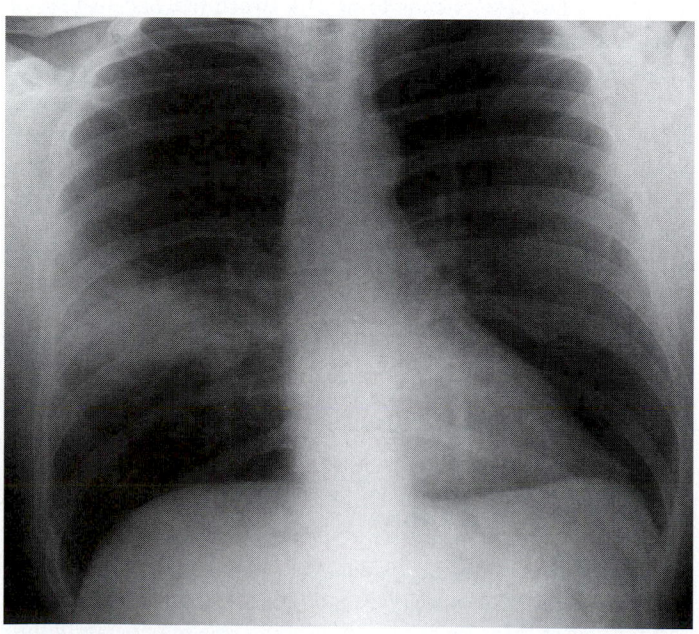

FIGURE 146-1 A dense infiltrate in the right lung, characteristic of pulmonary actinomycosis.

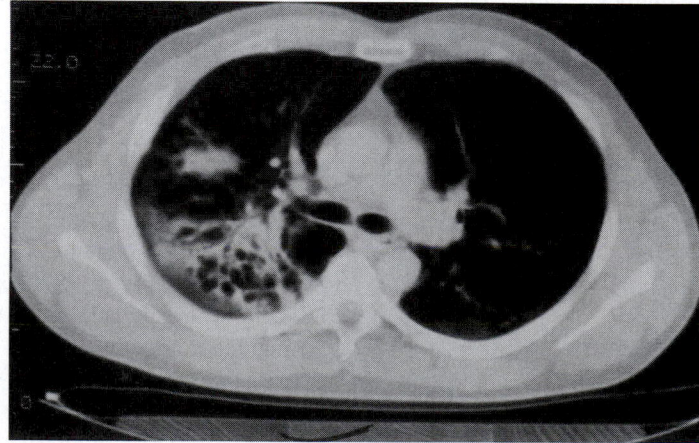

FIGURE 146-3 CT scan showing a dense infiltrate with several small cavities posteriorly in the right lung and a nodular density anterior to it.

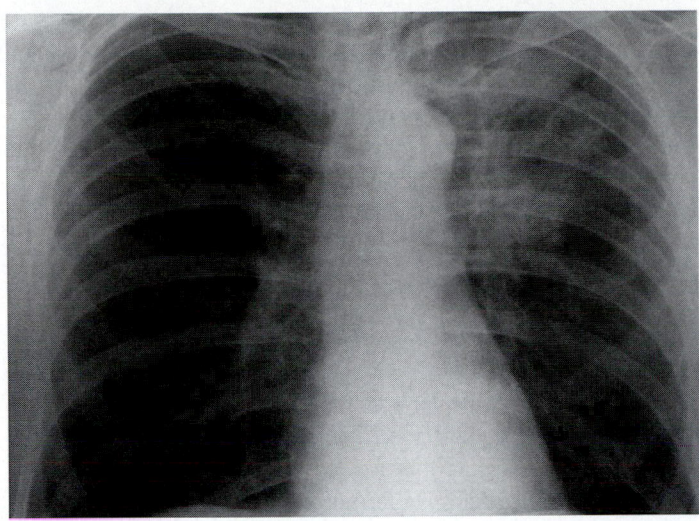

FIGURE 146-4 Left upper lobe fibronodular infiltrate due to pulmonary actinomycosis.

If there is a fistula, the presence of granules in secretions is a strong clue to the diagnosis. If granules are not immediately apparent in discharge from a wound, they can often be trapped in a gauze dressing. Suspect granules should be placed in water or KOH or Gram stained and then should be examined for the presence of typical branching filaments. The bacteria can be cultured from a granule if they have not succumbed to oxygen exposure.

In tissues, secretions, or granules, *Actinomyces* and *P. propionicum* are long, branching, beaded gram-positive filaments 0.2 to 0.5 μm in width and up to 50 μm in length. They are indistinguishable from *Nocardia* on Gram stain (Fig. 146-5). With age or under adverse conditions, the organisms may break up into coccobacillary forms, and they may appear gram negative. The beaded appearance and the occurrence of gram-positive segments interspersed with gram-negative ones may give the impression of many bacilli and cocci lined up end to end. *Actinomyces* fil-

aments can also be seen in KOH preparations. They are rarely acid fast; the presence of acid-fast organisms should suggest *Mycobacteria* or *Nocardia*. *Actinomyces* stain with methenamine silver and periodic acid–Schiff stains.

Cultures should be made from diseased tissue or normally sterile body secretions under strictly anaerobic conditions and inoculated promptly. If a specimen cannot be delivered to a laboratory immediately, a microbiologist should be consulted concerning use of a transport medium or inoculation at the bedside. Media known to support the growth of *Actinomyces* must be used. Prior antimicrobial therapy often makes cultures negative, and specimens should be obtained before such therapy is given.

Therapy

Penicillin is the drug of choice. In most cases, the drug should be given orally in maximal tolerated doses. In severe or rapidly progressive cases, penicillin should initially be given intravenously in high doses—10 to 20 million units per day. Tetracycline and clindamycin have also been used with good results.

In vitro tests of susceptibility of *Actinomyces* to antimicrobials are of uncertain clinical relevance. Penicillin, erythromycin, cephaloridine, minocycline, rifampin, and clindamycin are very active. Organisms are inhibited by achievable concentrations of cephalothin, ampicillin, tetracycline, doxycycline, and chloramphenicol. A few strains are susceptible to sulfamethoxazole. Metronidazole is ineffective.

Other bacteria frequently accompany *Actinomyces* in tissue and may contribute to the pathogenesis of the disease. The antimicrobial susceptibilities of these organisms often differ from those of *Actinomyces*. It is usually not necessary to use additional antimicrobial drugs to treat these associated organisms. They may contribute to the pathogenesis, but *Actinomyces* are essential, and successful treatment of *Actinomyces*—along with surgical drainage when appropriate—usually cures the disease.

Surgery should be used as it is for bacterial diseases of the chest in general. Empyemas should be drained. Surgery is sometimes required to relieve obstruction of mediastinal structures.

Actinomycosis has a marked tendency to relapse, and therapy should be continued for from 6 to 12 months. The exact duration should depend on the extent of the disease within and outside the chest and the response to treatment. With prompt diagnosis and appropriate treatment, approximately 90 percent of patients are cured.

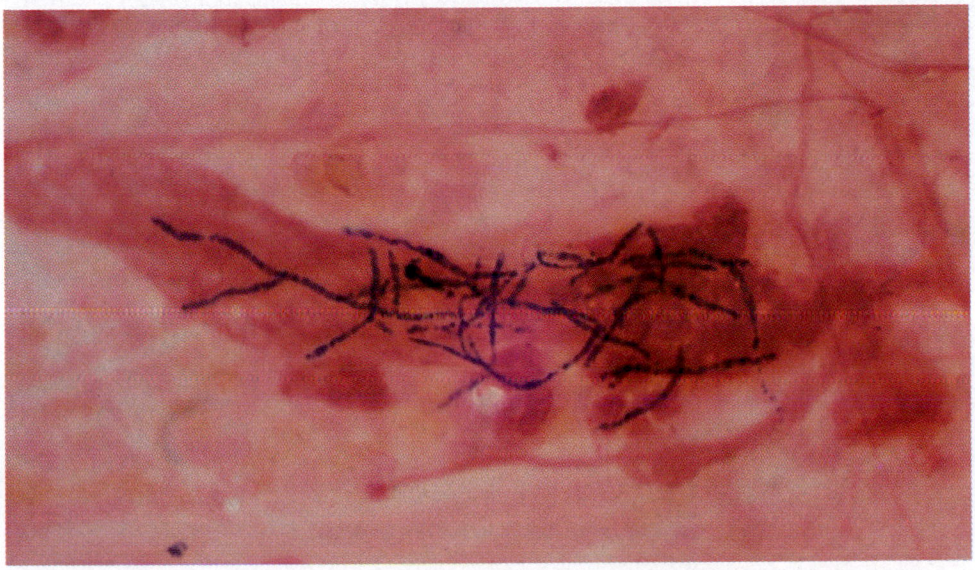

NOCARDIOSIS

Pulmonary nocardiosis is a subacute or chronic pneumonia caused by aerobic actinomycetes of the genus *Nocardia*. *Nocardia asteroides* is the most common pathogen, but *N. brasiliensis*,[19] *N. otitidis-caviarum* (formerly *N. caviae*),[2] *N. farcinica*,[25] *N. nova*,[23] *N.*

FIGURE 146-5 *Nocardia asteroides* in a Gram-stained smear of sputum. The neutrophils give an indication of the scale.

transvalensis,[14] and *N. pseudobrasiliensis*[22] have all been associated with pulmonary disease. *N. asteroides* frequently disseminates to other sites or is associated with mycetoma or skin and connective-tissue infection after transcutaneous inoculation or keratitis, but these diseases are beyond the scope of this chapter.

Epidemiology

Nocardiae are common, worldwide inhabitants of soil, where they contribute to decay of organic matter. In the soil, nocardiae form aerial mycelia, and it is thought that pneumonia follows inhalation of fragmented mycelia. The disease occurs worldwide. On the order of 1000 cases of nocardial infection are diagnosed each year in the United States, 85 percent of them pulmonary and/or systemic. The disease usually occurs in adults, and males are affected twice as often as females. There is no recognized seasonality.

Pathogenesis

A substantial number of reported cases occur in otherwise healthy people, but the incidence is greater in people with deficient host defenses. The risk is increased in people with impaired cell-mediated immunity, especially in those with lymphoma, transplanted organs, or AIDS.[1,4,18,21,26] Nocardiosis has also been associated with pulmonary alveolar proteinosis (Fig. 146-6), tuberculosis, and chronic granulomatous disease.

The typical lesions of nocardiosis are abscesses extensively infiltrated with neutrophils. There is usually extensive necrosis. Granulation tissue often surrounds the lesions, but extensive fibrosis or encapsulation is rare. Microcolonies (granules) are occasionally observed in histologic preparations but are almost never discharged from lesions. In rare cases, epithelioid granulomas are observed in the central nervous system.

Nocardiae have a number of properties that enable them to survive within phagocytes, including neutralization of oxidants, prevention of phagosome-lysosome fusion, and prevention of phagosome acidification. Neutrophils phagocytose the organisms and limit their growth but do not kill them. Cell-mediated immunity is important for definitive control of infection and eventual elimination of the bacteria from the body.

Clinical Manifestations

Pulmonary nocardiosis may be either subacute or chronic.[1,10,16,18,19,21,26] Patients typically present after symptoms have been present for many days or weeks. Remissions and exacerbations over periods of several weeks are frequent. The disease may be more acute in severely immunosuppressed patients. Cough is prominent and is often productive of small amounts of thick, purulent sputum, which is not malodorous. Fever, anorexia, weight loss, and malaise are common; dyspnea, pleuritic pain, and hemoptysis are not. Tracheitis, bronchitis, bronchial masses, mediastinitis, pericarditis, and endocarditis have been reported in some cases. Direct spread through the chest wall is rare. *Nocardia* species sometimes colonize patients without producing disease. Most of the time, such patients have abnormal airways or lung parenchyma.[10]

On radiographs,[11] infiltrates may be of any size and are usually of at least moderate density (Figs. 146-6, 146-7, and 146-8). Nodules are common (Fig. 146-9). Empyema is present in one-third of cases (Fig. 146-9). Cavitation is common (Figs. 146-7 and 146-8), and the radiographic appearance may suggest anaerobic lung abscess or a tumor. The radiographic appearance and clinical picture may suggest pulmonary tuberculosis or fungal

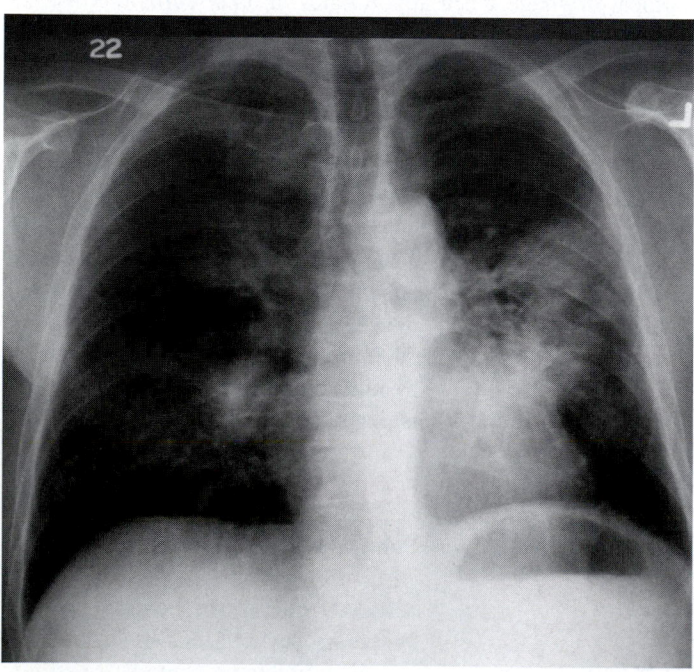

FIGURE 146-6   Nocardial pneumonia in a patient with multiple infiltrates due to pulmonary alveolar proteinosis.

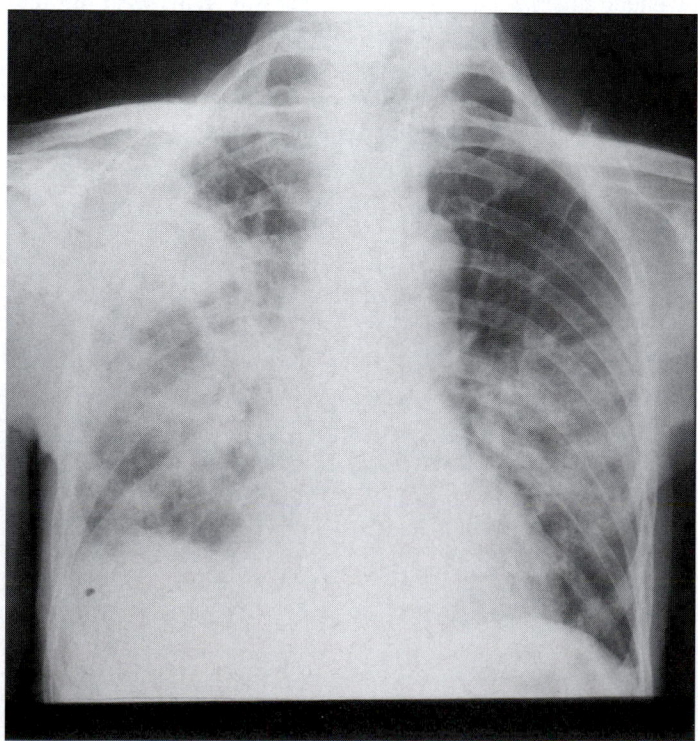

FIGURE 146-7   Bilateral nocardial pneumonia with a cavity in the right upper lobe.

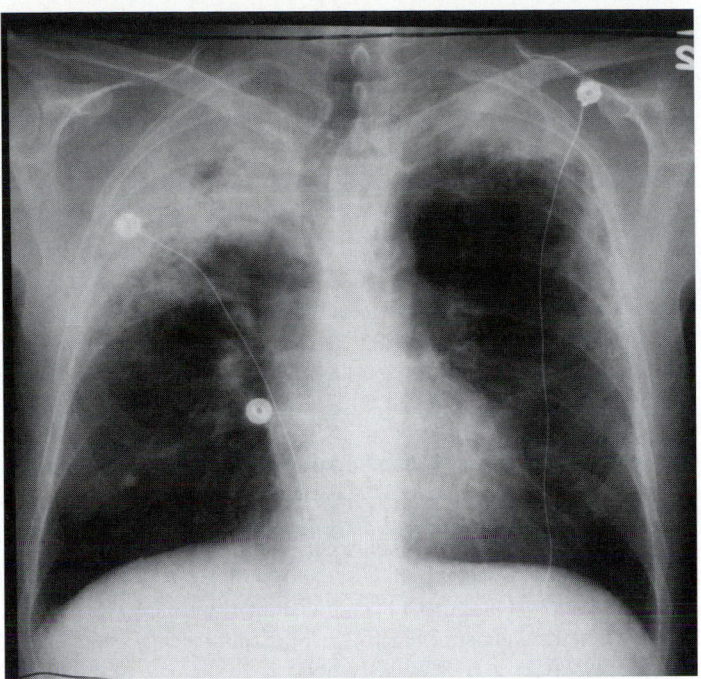

FIGURE 146-8 Nocardial pneumonia in the upper lobes, with a cavity in the right upper lobe.

pneumonia, but volume loss and fibrosis are usually less prominent with nocardiosis.

Disseminated disease occurs in one-half of cases of pulmonary nocardiosis.[16] The central nervous system is the most common location of disseminated disease and occurs in one-fourth of cases of pulmonary nocardiosis, typically as supratentorial brain abscesses. Other common locations are the skin and subcutaneous tissues, kidneys, bone, and muscle. Local infection from transcutaneous inoculation is common, but the physician should be aware that a lesion in skin or soft tissue may simply be the most obvious manifestation of pulmonary nocardiosis.

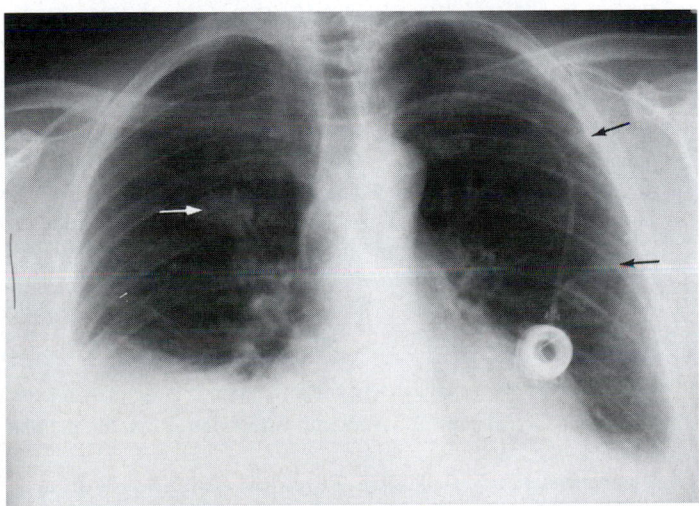

FIGURE 146-9 Multiple nodules (arrows) and empyema due to nocardial pneumonia.

Diagnosis

Examination of sputum after Gram and modified acid-fast stains is the first step when pulmonary nocardiosis is suspected. Sputum smears are often negative. Sputum cultures are positive more often, but colonies may not be apparent for days or weeks. If sputum examinations do not yield the diagnosis in a suspected case and the diagnosis cannot be made easily from lesions elsewhere in the body, more invasive diagnostic procedures should be performed. Bronchoscopy, needle aspiration, and open lung biopsy are all useful. Nocardiae are commonly associated with cellulitis in the tissues overlying the cricothyroid membrane after transtracheal aspiration, and transtracheal aspiration should be avoided if nocardiosis is suspected.

Nocardiae are thin, crooked, branching filaments that are weakly to strongly gram positive and appear beaded (Fig. 146-5). Most nocardiae in clinical specimens are acid fast if a weak acid is used for decolorization as with the modified Kinyoun, Ziehl-Neelsen, and Fite-Faraco methods. They usually lose their acid fastness in laboratory culture. With these methods, actinomyces and streptomyces are not acid fast. Nocardiae may stain with silver stains, but other common clinical stains are not helpful.

Nocardiae grow readily on most nonselective laboratory media, but they grow more slowly than most bacterial pathogens. The laboratory should always be alerted when nocardiae are suspected so that the likelihood of isolating nocardiae will be maximized. Nocardiae grow on nonselective mycobacterial and fungal media, but they often do not survive harsh sputum digestion procedures. Routine blood cultures are usually negative, but if biphasic cultures are incubated aerobically for up to 30 days, nocardiae can be isolated in some cases.[10]

Factors that should influence the interpretation of a positive sputum culture in the absence of obvious nocardial disease are the clinical presentation, the presence or absence of nocardiae on Gram stain, and the ability to isolate nocardiae in multiple cultures. A positive sputum culture in the absence of symptoms and signs of pulmonary infection is indicative only of colonization, but if symptoms and signs consistent with nocardial infection are present, the patient should be treated. A positive sputum culture in an immunosuppressed patient usually reflects disease and not colonization.

Therapy

Sulfonamides are the antimicrobials of choice.[8] Six to 8 g of sulfisoxazole or sulfadiazine should be given daily in four to six divided doses. In difficult cases, sulfonamide levels should be measured and dosages should be adjusted to keep serum levels between 100 and 150 μg/ml. Many patients have been treated with the combination of sulfamethoxazole and trimethoprim,[20] but it is unclear whether the combination is superior to the use of sulfonamides alone. If the combination is selected, 5 to 20 mg of trimethoprim and 25 to 100 mg/kg per day of sulfamethoxazole should be given in two or three divided doses. After the disease is brought under control, doses can be reduced to approximately 4 g per day of sulfonamides alone or to 5 mg of trimethoprim and 25 mg/kg per day of sulfamethoxazole for the remainder of therapy.

There is less experience with other antimicrobials. Minocycline (100 to 200 mg twice a day) appears to be the most effective orally administered alternative to sulfonamides. Other tetracyclines are less effective or inadequately tested. *N. nova* infections can be treated with erythromycin (500 to 750 mg four times a day) or ampicillin (1 g four times a day) alone or in combination, but other *Nocardia* species are usually resistant to ampicillin and erythromycin. The combination of amoxicillin (500 mg) and clavulanate (125 mg), given three times a day, can be used except for cases with *N. nova* where the clavulanate induces β-lactamase production. Ofloxacin (400 mg twice a day) and clarithromycin (500 mg twice a day) have each been used successfully in a few cases.

Amikacin (15 mg/kg per day in single or divided doses) appears to be the most reliable parental drug. Serum levels should be monitored with prolonged therapy, in the face of diminished renal function, or in the elderly. Newer β-lactam antibiotics—including cefotaxime, ceftizoxime, ceftriaxone, and imipenem—are usually effective except in cases with *N. farcinica.*

In most cases, isolates of *Nocardia* should be sent to an experienced reference laboratory for speciation and for susceptibility tests. The various pathogenic species differ in their susceptibility to second-line drugs.[22–25] While susceptibility testing is not as well established as with more common bacterial pathogens, the information may be helpful in cases in which standard drugs fail or cannot be used. Most nocardiae are susceptible to sulfonamides, minocycline, amikacin, cefotaxime, ceftizoxime, ceftriaxone, and imipenem and resistant to ampicillin and erythromycin. Invasive strains of *N. brasiliensis,* recently grouped into the new species *N. pseudobrasiliensis,*[17] appear to be resistant to minocycline and amoxicillin–clavulanic acid but susceptible to ciprofloxacin and clarithromycin.[22] *N. farcinica* strains differ in that they are usually resistant to cephalosporins, and one-fifth are resistant to imipenem.[25] *N. nova* strains are usually susceptible to erythromycin or ampicillin alone or in combination,[23] but other species are not.

Surgery is used as it is for other infectious diseases of the chest. Empyemas should be drained. Abscesses usually respond to antimicrobial therapy alone.

Immunosuppressive therapy increases the risk of nocardiosis, but patients can be treated successfully for nocardiosis even if immunosuppressive therapy is continued. When necessary to protect a transplanted organ or to treat an underlying disease, immunosuppressive therapy should be continued. In other cases, such therapy should be reduced or eliminated if possible.

Long courses of antimicrobial therapy are necessary to prevent relapse.[8] For nonimmunosuppressed patients, treatment of pulmonary nocardiosis should be continued for 6 to 12 months. CNS disease requires treatment for 1 year unless all apparent disease has been excised, in which case 6 months would be sufficient. Immunosuppressed patients with pulmonary nocardiosis should be treated for 1 year. In some patients, including a few with advanced AIDS, much longer treatment is necessary.[21] Patients should be carefully followed during therapy and for at least 6 months after therapy is stopped for signs of relapse. With prompt diagnosis and appropriate treatment, more than 95 percent of patients should be cured.

Nocardiosis is rare in an otherwise healthy child, and its occurrence in this setting may be a clue to the presence of chronic granulomatous disease. The phagocytes of such a child should be tested for the adequacy of their respiratory burst.

REFERENCES

1. Arduino RC, Johnson PC, Miranda AG: Nocardiosis in renal transplant recipients undergoing immunosuppression with cyclosporine. *Clin Infect Dis* 16:505–512, 1993.
2. Arroyo JC, Nichols S, Carroll GF: Disseminated *Nocardia caviae* infection. *Am J Med* 62:409–412, 1977.
3. Bates M, Cruickshank G: Thoracic actinomycosis. *Thorax* 12:99–124, 1957.
4. Berkey P, Bodey GP: Nocardial infection in patients with neoplastic disease. *Rev Infect Dis* 11:407–412, 1989.
5. Brock DW, Georg LK, Brown JM, Hicklin MD: Actinomycosis caused by *Arachnia propionica:* Report of 11 cases. *Am J Clin Pathol* 59:66–77, 1973.
6. Cope Z: *Actinomycosis.* London, Oxford University Press, 1938.
7. Dahlhoff K, Wallner S, Finck C, et al: Endobronchial actinomycosis. *Eur Respir J* 7:1189–1191, 1994.
8. Filice GA, Simpson GL: Management of nocardia infections, in Remington JS, Swartz MN (eds), *Current Clinical Topics in Infectious Diseases.* New York, McGraw-Hill, 1984, pp 49–64.
9. Flynn MW, Felson F: The roentgen manifestations of thoracic actinomycosis. *Am J Roentgenol* 110:707–716, 1970.
10. Frazier AR, Rosenow EC III, Roberts GD: Nocardiosis: A review of 25 cases occurring during 24 months. *Mayo Clin Proc* 50:657–663, 1975.
11. Grossman CB, Bragg DG, Armstrong D: Roentgen manifestations of pulmonary nocardiosis. *Radiology* 96:325–330, 1970.
12. Kwong JS, Müller NL, Godwin JD, et al: Thoracic actinomycosis: CT findings in eight patients. *Radiology* 183:189–192, 1992.
13. Lam S, Samraj J, Rahman S, Hilton E: Primary actinomycotic endocarditis: Case report and review. *Clin Infect Dis* 16:481–485, 1993.
14. McNeil MM, Brown JM, Georghiou PR, et al: Infections due to *Nocardia transvalensis:* Clinical spectrum and antimicrobial therapy. *Clin Infect Dis* 15:453–463, 1992.
15. McQuarrie DG, Hall WH: Actinomycosis of the lung and chest wall. *Surgery* 64:905–911, 1968.
16. Palmer DL, Harvey RL, Wheeler JK: Diagnostic and therapeutic considerations in *Nocardia asteroides* infection. *Medicine* 53:391–401, 1974.
17. Ruimy R, Riegel P, Carlotti A, et al: *Nocardia pseudobrasiliensis* sp. nov., a new species of *Nocardia* which groups bacterial strains previously identified as *Nocardia brasiliensis* and associated with invasive diseases. *Int J Syst Bacteriol* 46:259–264, 1996
18. Simpson GL, Stinson EB, Egger MJ, Remington JS: Nocardial infections in the immunocompromised host: A detailed study in a defined population. *Rev Infect Dis* 3:492–507, 1981.
19. Smego RA, Gallis HA: The clinical spectrum of *Nocardia brasiliensis* infection in the United States. *Rev Infect Dis* 6:164–180, 1984.
20. Smego RA Jr, Moeller MB, Gallis HA: Trimethoprim-sulfamethoxazole therapy for *Nocardia* infections. *Arch Intern Med* 143:711–718, 1983.
21. Uttamchandani RB, Daikos GL, Reyes RR, et al: Nocardiosis in 30 patients with advanced human immunodeficiency virus infection: Clinical features and outcome. *Clin Infect Dis* 18:348–353, 1994.

22. Wallace RJ Jr, Brown BA, Blacklock Z, et al: New *Nocardia* taxon among isolates of *Nocardia brasiliensis* associated with invasive disease. *J Clin Microbiol* 33:1528–1533, 1995.

23. Wallace RJ Jr, Brown BA, Tsukamura M, et al: Clinical and laboratory features of *Nocardia nova. J Clin Microbiol* 29:2407–2411, 1991.

24. Wallace RJ Jr, Steele LC, Sumter G, Smith JM: Antimicrobial susceptibility patterns of *Nocardia asteroides. Antimicrob Agents Chemother* 32:1776–1779, 1988.

25. Wallace RJ Jr, Tsukamura M, Brown BA, et al: Cefotaxime-resistant *Nocardia asteroides* strains are isolates of the controversial species *Nocardia farcinica. J Clin Microbiol* 28:2726–2732, 1990.

26. Young LS, Armstrong D, Blevins A, Leiberman P: *Nocardia asteroides* infection complicating neoplastic disease. *Am J Med* 50:356-366, 1970.

CHAPTER 147

ASPERGILLUS SYNDROMES, MUCORMYCOSIS, AND PULMONARY CANDIDIASIS

Alan M. Sugar / Elizabeth A. Olek

PULMONARY ASPERGILLOSIS

Pulmonary aspergillosis is a general term for the lung disease caused by the genus *Aspergillus*. The three commonly described categories are allergic aspergillosis, colonizing aspergillosis, and invasive diseases. The spectrum of pulmonary aspergillosis is described in Table 147-1. There is overlap among these categories, and patients may exhibit characteristics of more than one process or progress from one category to another. *Aspergillus* species are ubiquitous molds that reproduce by formation of conidia that are readily airborne and reach the airways following inhalation. Germination of conidia results in production of hyphae, which are the forms associated with disease. Sputum from nonimmunocompromised individuals following inhalation of *Aspergillus* conidia may contain the fungus for many days afterward in the absence of disease. Conversely, invasive pulmonary aspergillosis occurs in patients with prolonged and profound granulocytopenia, leading to relentless destruction of the lung. Host immune status, rather than the intensity of exposure, is usually the most important determinant of the disease process.

History

Human disease due to *Aspergillus* was first described in 1847 by *Sluyter*. In 1856, *Virchow* described four autopsy-proved cases of aspergillosis in which secondary invasion of preexisting lung lesions had occurred. The hazards of occupations exposing individuals to large numbers of *Aspergillus* spores, such as wig cleaning and pigeon feeding, gained attention, and a causal relationship for pulmonary aspergillosis was accepted during the early twentieth century.[64] Rénon in 1897 referred to *primary* and *secondary* aspergillosis, the latter category being associated with carcinoma, bronchopneumonia, or tuberculosis. Pulmonary aspergilloma was defined by *Deve* in 1938, and allergic bronchopulmonary aspergillosis was described in 1952 by Hinson.[30]

The emergence of invasive aspergillosis as an increasingly important opportunist was described by Young and coworkers in 1970.[64] Patients with leukemia, lymphoma, and other malignant diseases along with organ transplant recipients are important populations at risk (see Chapter 136). Aspergillosis associated with immunosuppressant therapy for the collagen vascular diseases and sarcoidosis is an important complication.

Epidemiology

Aspergillus species are ubiquitous and occur worldwide. The fungi grow well in many habitats and are commonly found on stored hay or grain, decaying vegetation, soil, dung, and various organic debris. Inhalation of conidia probably occurs regularly, although disease is uncommon. A seasonal variation in the prevalence of outdoor spore levels may influence the development of extrinsic hypersensitivity disease, although no seasonal variation in the incidence of invasive pulmonary aspergillosis has been shown. Outbreaks of invasive pulmonary aspergillosis in oncology and transplant wards have been described in association with hospital construction, renovation, or suboptimal maintenance of ventilation systems.[36] Pathogenic *Aspergillus* species have been isolated in the soil of indoor potted plants and have been suggested as a source of infection. Air sampling demonstrates increased levels of *Aspergillus,* but the link to infection has been difficult to prove. Environmental investigation of these cases

TABLE 147-1

Spectrum of Pulmonary Aspergillosis

Clinical Manifestation	Immune Status	Underlying Lung Architecture	Degree of Tissue Invasion
Simple colonization	Normal	Chronic obstructive airway disease	None
Hypersensitivity reactions			
Allergic bronchial asthma	↑ *	Normal	None
Allergic bronchopulmonary aspergillosis	↑	Excess airway mucus	None
Bronchocentric granulomatosis	↑	Excess airway mucus	None
Extrinsic allergic alveolitis	↑	Normal	None
Colonization			
Aspergilloma†	Normal	Preexisting cavity	None
Invasive disease			
Bronchial stump aspergillosis	Normal	Pneumonectomy	+
Chronic necrotizing pulmonary aspergillosis	↓ ‡	Normal	+
Invasive pulmonary aspergillosis	↓ ↓ ↓ §	Normal	+++

* ↑ = Hyperactive humoral response.
† May have features of invasive disease surrounding the cavity.
‡ ↓ = Suppressed immune response.
§ ↓ ↓ ↓ = Severely depressed immune response, neutropenia.

failed to reveal a single source for the cases of aspergillosis. Molecular epidemiologic methods utilizing DNA fingerprinting are useful for the investigation of the association between environmental sources of *Aspergillus* and infection.[22]

Mycology and Host Defenses

Human infection has been caused by only 19 species of the nearly 700 species described. The commonly isolated species include *A. fumigatus, A. flavus, A. niger,* and *A. terreus. A. fumigatus* is the most common cause of allergic pulmonary and invasive disease. *Aspergillus* species are rapidly growing, hardy molds, identified by the appearance of the colony and by microscopic examination of the spore-bearing structures. Microscopically, *Aspergillus* species are characterized by the production of uniform, 4- to 6-μm wide hyphae, with parallel walls and distinct septa. Dichotomous branching occurs at 45° angles. A wide range of microscopic appearances may be observed in clinical specimens. Other fungi such as *Fusarium* and *Pseudallescheria boydii* share the same microscopic appearance as *Aspergillus.*

Patient sputum specimens examined by direct mount or with KOH and ink may reveal the typical 45° branching hyphal fragments, often associated with eosinophils and Charcot-Leyden crystals in patients with allergic bronchopulmonary aspergillosis (ABPA). Stained tissue sections reveal regular hyaline septate hyphae best observed with periodic acid-Schiff (PAS) and Gomori's methenamine-silver (GMS) stains. Fungus ball specimens from cavities connected to open bronchi have hyphae that often appear lifeless and stain poorly, and,

although seldom seen, the fruiting heads and conidia may appear well formed.

Aspergillus produce airborne spores, termed *conidia,* that are small enough (2.5 to 3.0 μm) to reach the alveoli when inhaled. Pulmonary macrophages may kill the fungus under certain conditions in vitro, a function that is inhibited by corticosteroids. When first-line host defense mechanisms fail, germination of conidia results in production of hyphae. These hyphae may activate the complement cascade in serum, increase the generation of phagocytic chemotactic factors, and increase neutrophil degranulation. Once hyphae have formed, neutrophils can attach to and damage the fungal cells. Symptomatic pulmonary aspergillosis is reported among individuals with late-stage AIDS; because HIV-infected individuals have multiple immune defects, including defective neutrophil function, the role of T cell immunity in host defense against *Aspergillus* remains unclear.[42]

A. fumigatus produces several unique virulence factors, including a complement inhibitor and phagocytosis inhibitors including gliotoxin and aflatoxin.[44] Gliotoxin impairs macrophage phagocytosis and the induction of cytotoxic T cells in vitro. The surface of resting conidia is coated by rodlike structures of a hydrophobic protein called *hydrophobin,* the significance of which is not clear. The production of different proteolytic enzymes (elastases, collagenases, trypsine) by *A. fumigatus* may play a role in breaching the mucosal–epithelial barrier and in degradation of host defense factors.[34] Oxalic acid is produced by some species, especially *A. niger,* and presumably contributes to the inflammatory reaction around a fungus ball or *mycetoma* of the lung. Calcium oxalate forms in tissue and appears as birefringent crystals that may appear in the sputum.

Clinical Manifestations

HYPERSENSITIVITY REACTIONS

Aspergillus species are important fungi that are involved in several distinct pulmonary syndromes. Clinical manifestations of *Aspergillus* infection are largely determined by the immunologic status of the individual and any underlying lung pathology. For example, atopic individuals represent a unique subset of patients in whom the fungal antigen can cause various responses, including allergic asthma, ABPA, or bronchocentric granulomatosis. In nonatopic individuals, airway colonization or extrinsic allergic alveolitis can occur as a result of massive or repeated inhalation of conidia. Early recognition of these syndromes is important so that appropriate treatment can be started early to prevent progression to permanent lung damage. Table 147-2 summarizes the hypersensitivity reactions to *Aspergillus*.

SIMPLE COLONIZATION

Aspergillus can exist on body surfaces and in bronchi without eliciting a pathologic response. Patients suffering from underlying chronic obstructive pulmonary disease (COPD) frequently require corticosteroids or antibiotic therapy for management of exacerbations and are consequently at increased risk for fungal colonization. Tissue invasion is not a feature of saprophytic colonization, although pulmonary aspergillosis may develop with the alteration of host defenses. Patients may show immunologic responses including increased IgE antibody, increased precipitins, and immediate or delayed skin reactivity to *Aspergillus* antigen. However, specific *Aspergillus* IgE or IgG antibody levels are not elevated.

ALLERGIC BRONCHIAL ASTHMA

Asthmatic patients may become sensitized to *Aspergillus* conidia as a consequence of thick bronchial secretions that trap fungal spores. The conidia seldom germinate in the bronchial airways. The syndrome develops in patients who are atopic and is perpetuated by inhalation of *Aspergillus* antigens, which typically cause acute bronchospasm. Transient infiltrates have been described during the immediate reaction but are not usual. As is typical in asthma of other etiologies, serum eosinophils and IgE antibody are increased. Immediate skin reactions to *Aspergillus* antigens are positive, but specific precipitating antibodies (IgG) are usually negative. Attenuation of spore exposure can diminish the frequency and severity of bronchospasm in this group of patients.

ALLERGIC BRONCHOPULMONARY ASPERGILLOSIS

Clinical Features

Allergic bronchopulmonary aspergillosis is discussed in detail in Chapter 51. Here, certain aspects are highlighted or amplified. The disease occurs in atopic individuals with asthma or cystic fibrosis. The symptoms of ABPA include recurrent wheezing, malaise with low-grade fever, cough, sputum production (blood-streaked), chest pain, and pulmonary infiltrates. Patients may have a history of recurrent pneumonia and frequent antibiotic therapy. Chronic ABPA is characterized by cough and sputum

TABLE 147-2

Hypersensitivity Reactions to *Aspergillus*

	Asthma	Allergic Bronchopulmonary Aspergillosis	Extrinsic Allergic Alveolitis
Pathology	Hypertrophied mucus glands	Colonization of airways, viscid mucoid impaction, tissue eosinophilia	Lymphocytic infiltration of interstitium, non-caseating granuloma
Radiographic features			
Early	Normal, hyperinflation	Migratory peripheral infiltrates, atelectasis, bronchiectasis	Diffuse alveolar-interstitial infiltrates
Late	Normal, hyperinflation	Fibrosis	Reticulonodular interstitial opacities
Skin test reactions to *Aspergillus* antigens			
Immediate	Positive	Positive	Positive
Delayed	Negative	Positive	Positive
Peripheral eosinophilia	Negative	Positive	Negative
IgG precipitins	Positive (up to 25%)	Positive	Positive
Serum IgE levels	Normal or mildly elevated	Marked elevation	Normal

production with superimposed acute exacerbations. Bronchiectasis becomes dominant with the development of clubbing and fixed radiographic abnormalities.[63] Occasionally patients may present without symptoms or physical findings despite radiographic abnormalities.

The events involved in the development of ABPA occur when patients with asthma or cystic fibrosis develop bronchial allergic reactions to inhaled *Aspergillus* conidia. Mucous plugs form in the proximal bronchi and can progress to mucoid impaction resulting in atelectasis with transient pulmonary infiltrates. Mucous plugs often yield *Aspergillus* on culture (Figs. 147-1 and 147-2). Repeated allergic reactions in the bronchi cause bronchiectasis in the proximal bronchi, where characteristic circular or oblong radiodensities are formed—these "ring signs" and "tram shadows" are observable on chest radiograph and represent small rims of chronic peribronchial inflammation around dilated bronchi.

Radiographic Findings

Pulmonary infiltrates may be transient or permanent. Transient abnormalities may be the result of parenchymal infiltrates, mucoid impactions, or secretions in damaged bronchi.[43] "Toothpaste" shadows result from mucoid impactions in damaged bronchi. "Gloved finger" shadows result from distally occluded bronchi filled with secretions (Fig. 147-3). "Tramline" shadows are two parallel hairline shadows extending out from the hilum.

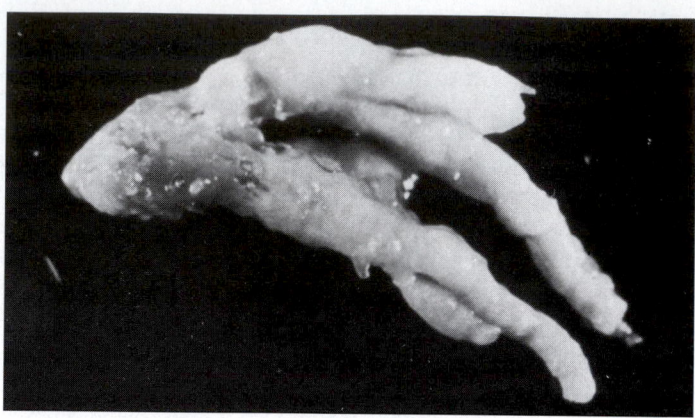

FIGURE 147-1   Mucous plug expectorated by a patient with ABPA. Note the tapering, cylindrical shape with branching characteristic of the parent bronchi. *(Courtesy of Dr. Frederic Askin, Chapel Hill, NC.)*

Permanent radiographic findings include proximal bronchiectasis, characterized by normal filling of bronchi distal to the saccular bronchial lesion (Figs. 147-3 and 147-4). This finding is considered a strong diagnostic feature of ABPA, especially on computed tomograms which have greater sensitivity.[4] Parallel-line or tramline shadows result from bronchiectasis with bronchial dilation; ring shadows are dilated bronchi *en face*. Late

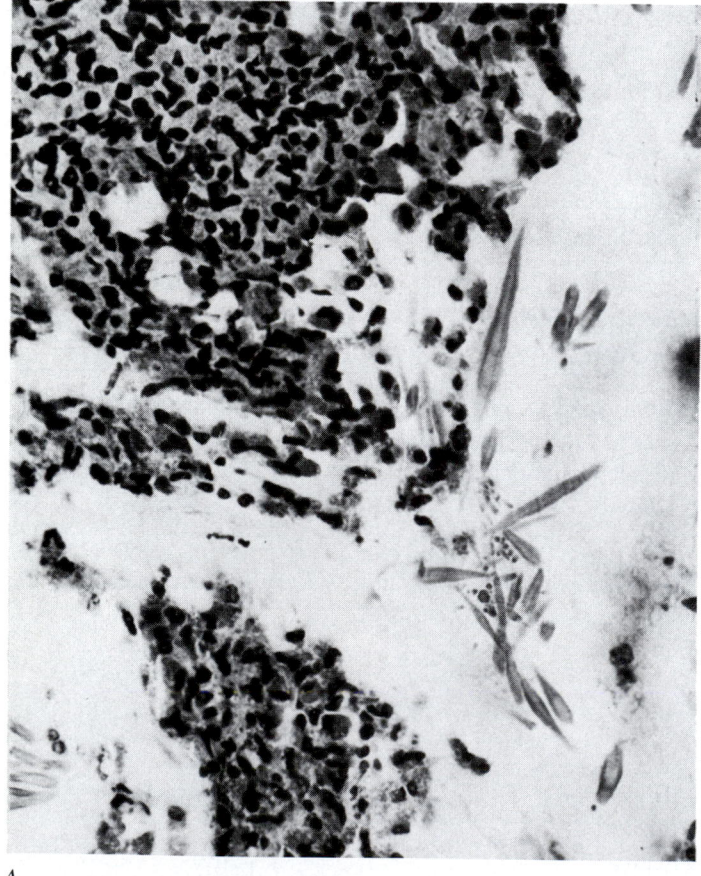

A

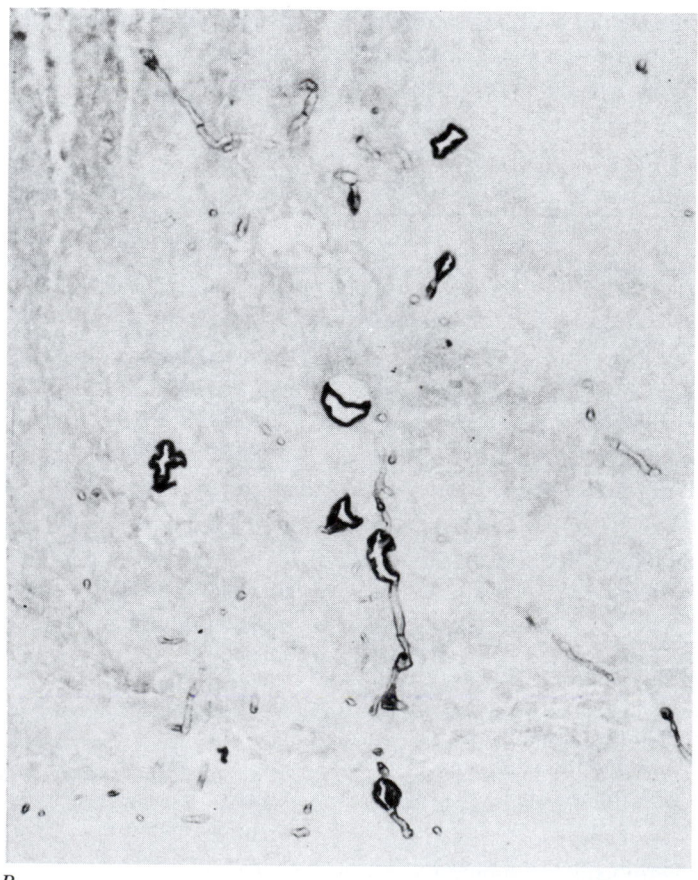

B

FIGURE 147-2   High-magnification photomicrograph of inspissated mucus in mucoid impaction of the bronchus. *A.* Groups of Charcot-Leyden crystals adjacent to clusters of necrotic eosinophils. H&E ×520.

B. Aspergillus hyphae. Note transition from regular, thin septate hyphae to dilated, often folded degenerating forms. H&E ×354. *(Courtesy of Dr. S. Albelda and Dr. G.H. Talbot.)*

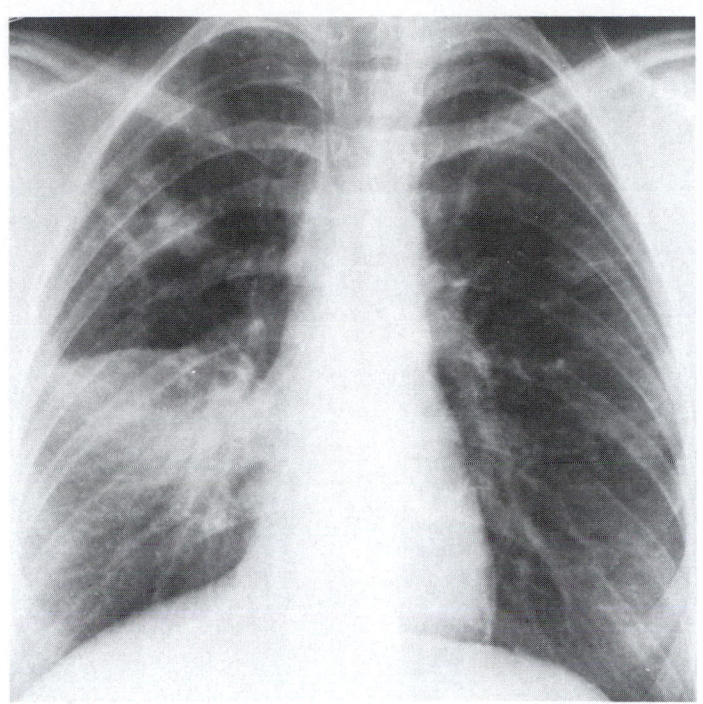

A

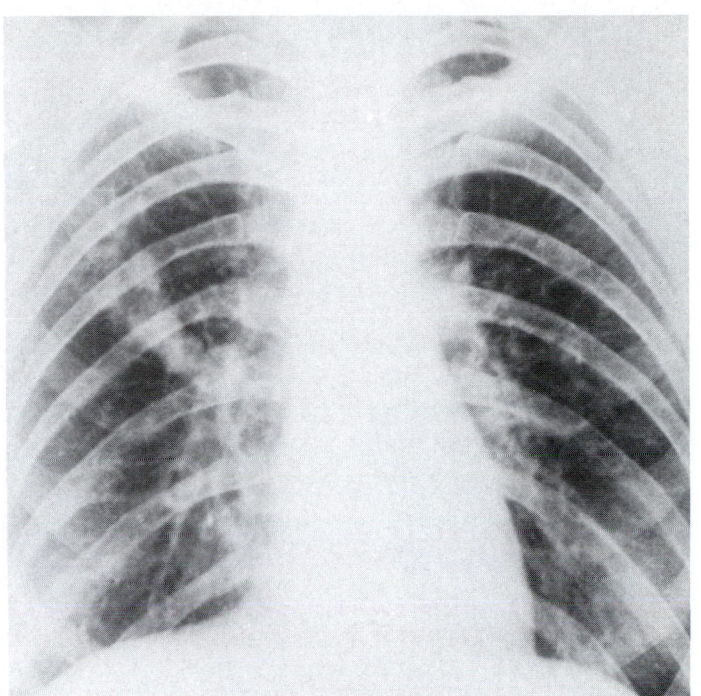

B

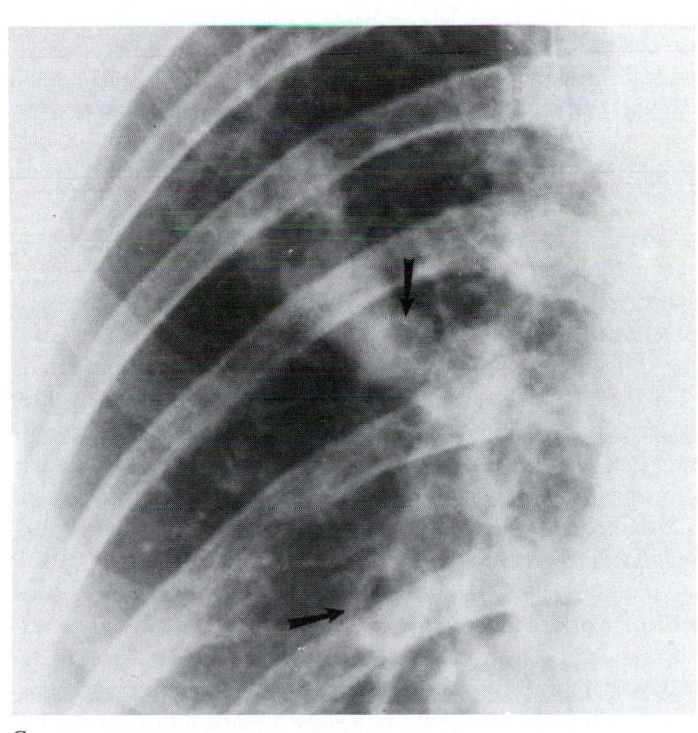

C

FIGURE 147-3   A 23-year-old female with documented allergic bronchopulmonary aspergillosis. *A.* Chest radiograph shows mucoid impaction in right upper lobe and alveolar consolidation in right middle lobe. *B.* Eight months later, alveolar consolidation has resolved, and appearance of mucoid impaction in right upper lobe has changed. *C.* Closeup of right lung from *B* shows "gloved finger" appearance of mucoid impaction as well as ring shadows (arrows) characteristic of bronchiectasis. *(Courtesy of Dr. S. Albelda and Dr. G.H. Talbot.)*

findings in ABPA include cavitation, local emphysema, contracted upper lobes, and honeycomb fibrosis.[43] A normal chest radiograph does not rule out a diagnosis of ABPA, and bronchiectasis may be better demonstrated by narrow-section (3-mm) computed tomograms.

Diagnosis

Patterson and coworkers have defined eight criteria (Table 51-1 of Chapter 51) for the diagnosis of ABPA. These are summarized in Table 147-3. Individuals meeting seven of eight criteria make the diagnosis of ABPA highly likely, and the presence of all eight criteria confirm the diagnosis. Brown mucous plugs containing eosinophils and hyphae may be present in expectorated sputum in up to 50 percent of patients with acute ABPA (Fig. 147-2). Asthma, eosinophilia, and a history of unexplained pulmonary infiltrates should alert clinicians to the possibility of ABPA .

Patients with ABPA demonstrate a hypersensitivity reaction to *A. fumigatus* in the bronchial tree without tissue invasion.[63] Type I and type III reactions are involved in and around bronchial walls, where fungal antigens are released. Type I, IgE-mediated, immediate hypersensitivity reactions are thought to mediate the bronchospastic component of the syndrome, via the release of cytokines (chemokines) by mast cells, leading to eosinophilia and increased vascular permeability. The immediate type skin reaction is manifested by a wheal and flare (within 20 min) to skin-prick testing with *Aspergillus* antigens and is positive in nearly all ABPA patients.[63] Immediate hypersensitivity to *A. fumigatus* is a useful screening test, since ABPA is very unlikely with a negative reaction. Difficulty with antigen standardization used in skin testing and serologic assays has been encountered and may account on occasion for failure to detect hypersensitivity. A recombinant antigen preparation has shown reproducible skin test results that correlate with serologic data and offers promise for standardization of antigen–allergen preparations.[44]

Type III, Arthus or immune complex–mediated reactions, may account for the bronchial and peribronchial inflammation re-

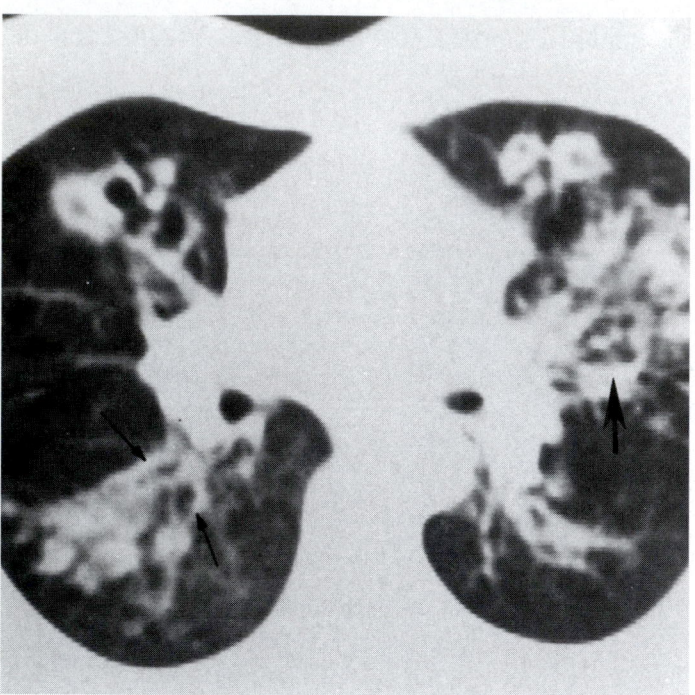

A

FIGURE 147-4   Proximal saccular bronchiectasis characteristic of allergic bronchopulmonary aspergillosis. *A.* Computed tomography reveals multiple rounded, dilated bronchi (small arrows); note air-fluid level (large arrow). *B* and *C.* Bronchography, viewed from lateral position, from two different patients shows both normally tapering bronchi and bronchi with saccular widening (arrows). *(Courtesy of Dr. S. Albelda and Dr. G.H. Talbot.)*

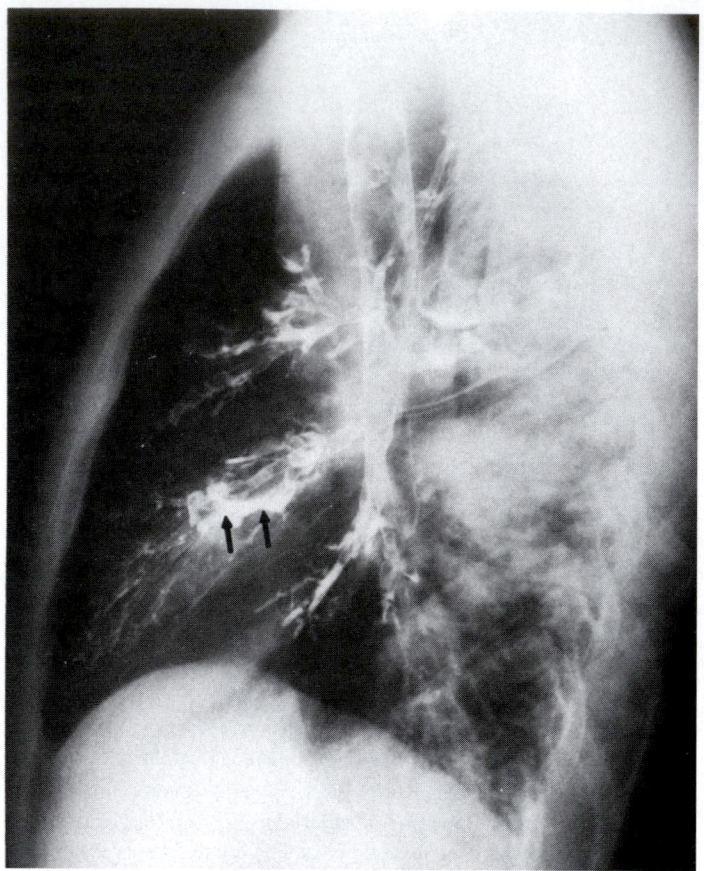

B

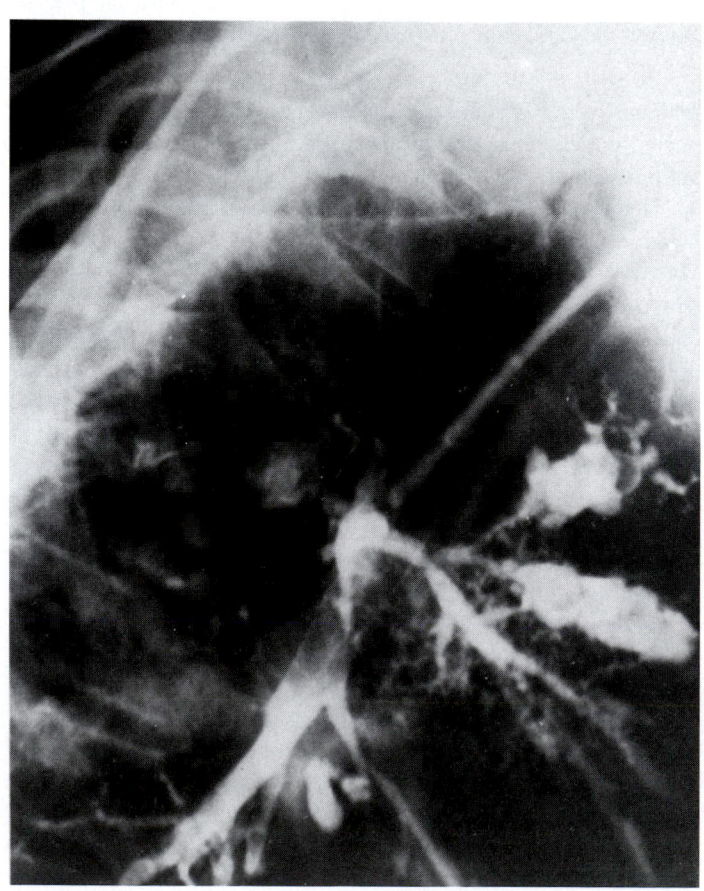

C

sponsible for the radiographic pulmonary infiltrates. The IgG-precipitating antibodies form an antigen–antibody complex leading to the delayed skin reaction (hemorrhagic cutaneous lesion at 4 to 10 h). These precipitating antibody complexes subsequently fix complement and liberate additional inflammatory factors that lead to chronic inflammation of bronchi resulting in bronchiectasis and pulmonary fibrosis. Granulomatous lesions and lymphocyte-mediated responses suggest that type IV immunopathogenic mechanisms may also have a role in ABPA.[53]

Total IgE increases during acute flares of ABPA and is a good indicator of disease activity even in the absence of clinical exacerbation.[62] However, elevated total IgE is not specific for ABPA and may be present in patients with other pulmonary diseases such as asthma. Approximately 5 percent of the total IgE is a specific component of IgE against *A. fumigatus* antigen and will also be elevated in ABPA. High titers of specific IgE antibodies reactive with *Aspergillus* may be more specific for ABPA. The level of IgE and IgG antibody in patients with ABPA to *A. fumigatus* is at least twice that of mold-sensitive asthmatic patients who demonstrate immediate skin reactivity to *A. fumigatus.*[62] Specific IgG antibodies have been found to be elevated in most patients but do not correlate with disease activity.

Sputum cultures are positive for *Aspergillus* species in approximately two-thirds of all cases of ABPA. Because *Aspergillus* can colonize bronchi without producing disease, sputum cultures may be suggestive but are not diagnostic of this

TABLE 147-3

Criteria for the Diagnosis of Allergic Bronchopulmonary Aspergillosis

Primary
  Episodic bronchial obstruction (asthma)
  Peripheral blood eosinophilia ($>1000/mm^3$)
  Immediate type skin reactivity to *Aspergillus* antigen
  Precipitating serum antibodies (precipitins) against *Aspergillus* antigen
  Elevated serum IgE concentrations (>1000 ng/ml)
  Elevated serum IgE and IgG antibodies specific to *Aspergillus fumigatus*
  History of pulmonary infiltrates (transient or fixed)
  Central bronchiectasis
Secondary
  Aspergillus fumigatus in sputum (by repeated culture or microscopic examination)
  History of expectoration of brown plugs or flecks
  Arthus reactivity (late skin reactivity) to *Aspergillus* antigen

SOURCE: Adapted with permission from Rosenberg et al.[54]

syndrome. Multiple positive cultures in a patient presenting with symptoms suggestive of ABPA support the diagnosis. Pulmonary function testing reveals reversible airway obstruction initially, followed by progressive fixed obstructive changes and hyperinflation. Restrictive airflow pattern and diminished carbon monoxide diffusing capacity become dominant in the chronic fibrotic stage of the disease. Patients studied chronically for ABPA demonstrated marked variability in pulmonary function measurements, and these measurements did not correlate with duration of ABPA or asthma.

No single clinical or immunologic feature is diagnostic of ABPA, and, although understanding and awareness has increased, ABPA remains an underdiagnosed disease. Asymptomatic pulmonary involvement occurs in ABPA and may lead to a delayed diagnosis and irreversible damage. Corticosteroid therapy for asthma may mask the signs of ABPA, allowing progressive decline in pulmonary function. Cystic fibrosis may also complicate the diagnosis of ABPA, since many of the clinical and laboratory features are similar.

Histopathology

The presentations of the hypersensitivity syndrome associated with the fungi are discussed in detail in Chapter 51. Some of the histopathologic presentations associated with ABPA overlap with those of infectious presentations of disease. Thus, eosinophilic infiltrates may be present in invasive disease as well as in Loeffler's syndrome and in chronic eosinophilic pneumonia. These syndromes, as well as tropical eosinophilic pneumonia, may also be seen in the presence of parasitic infection with pulmonary migratory cycles, particularly filariasis and strongyloidiasis (see Chapter 156). Mucoid impaction associated with ABPA or other fungi may predispose to superinfection (see Figs. 147-1 and 147-2). Necrotizing granulomata in association with *Aspergillus* species in asthmatic patients may be observed and considered part of the ABPA syndrome. The distinction between ABPA, with fungal elements restricted to the airways, and invasive aspergillosis may be obscured by tissue necrosis or in immunocompromised individuals by poor granuloma formation. These presentations are discussed further below and in Chapter 51.

Treatment

The five stages of disease activity proposed by Patterson and colleagues[48] and Mendelson and coworkers[40] are summarized in Table 147-4. No certain prognostic indicators for progression or regression of the disease have been identified.[40] Aggressive treatment of the early stages may halt progression to the final debilitating stage.[48] (Management problems and unanswered questions in the stages of ABPA are presented in Table 147-4.[48])

Corticosteroid therapy is recognized as the treatment of choice. Prednisone is administered in a daily dose of 1 mg/kg or greater in order to see resolution of the chest radiographic changes. Prednisone 0.5 mg/kg per day is continued for 2 weeks and then decreased to an alternate-day dosage schedule. Maintenance corticosteroid therapy is continued for a minimum of 3 to 6 months and then gradually tapered no faster than 5 mg per month. Monthly IgE levels may be measured, and if there is a twofold increase in the total serum IgE, a chest radiograph should be obtained to rule out exacerbation of ABPA.[48]

Itraconazole is an orally active triazole antifungal with low toxicity that often has excellent activity against *Aspergillus*. Preliminary studies suggest that itraconazole may be a useful adjunctive therapy in ABPA to aid in clearing the airway of *Aspergillus* and to offer a steroid-sparing effect. Improvements in clinical, serologic, and pulmonary functional status were noted. However, larger randomized trials are needed to better define the role of antifungal therapy in ABPA.

Inhaled corticosteroids may help to control the symptoms of asthma but do not prevent episodes of eosinophilic infiltration and mucous impaction and are generally not thought to have any influence on progressive lung damage.[63] Inhaled antifungal agents such as nystatin or amphotericin B may offer temporary suppression of colonization, but penetration into plugged bronchi is limited, and recolonization occurs once therapy is ended. Meticulous bronchial toilet is important for clearance of *A. fumigatus* from the airway. Bronchodilators and physiotherapy with postural drainage are important adjunctive treatments. Increased oral fluids, use of expectorants, and in selected patients bronchial lavage may aid in viscid mucous clearance. Avoidance of environmental reservoirs of *Aspergillus* such as compost heaps, grain silos, or decayed organic matter may help prevent exacerbations.

BRONCHOCENTRIC GRANULOMATOSIS

Bronchocentric granulomatosis is characterized histologically by necrotizing granulomatous replacement of bronchial mucosa with eosinophilic infiltration of bronchioles (Figs. 147-5 and 147-6). Blood vessels are not primarily affected.[11] *Aspergillus* hyphae have been demonstrated within the lesions of approximately half of the patients described, but tissue invasion does not occur. First de-

TABLE 147-4

Staging System for Allergic Bronchopulmonary Aspergillosis

Stage	Symptoms	Radiographic Features	Laboratory Features	Management
I. Acute	Fever, productive cough, wheezing	Pulmonary infiltrates, mucoid impaction	Blood eosinophilia, elevated serum IgE, positive skin test	Corticosteroids to achieve remission
II. Remission	Asymptomatic	Normal	Decrease in IgE and blood eosinophilia	Careful follow-up
III. Exacerbation	All or some of acute stage symptoms	All or some of acute stage findings	At least a doubling of IgE in asymptomatic patients and an increase in IgE in symptomatic patients	Retreat with steroids to induce remission
IV. Corticosteroid dependent	Symptomatic steroid requiring asthma	Variable	Usually continued elevation of Ige	Long-term steroids to control asthmatic symtoms and keep IgE levels at baseline
V. Fibrotic	Severe dyspnea fibrotic lung disease as well as bronchospasm	Pulmonary fibrosis	Restrictive plus reversible and irreversible obstructive function tests; may have continued increased IgE	Long-term corticosteroids

SOURCE: Adapted with permission from Mendelson et al.[40] and Patterson et al.[48]

scribed in 1973 by Liebow, patients presented with chronic symptoms, malaise, cough, fever, dyspnea, chest pain, and hemoptysis associated with a focal lesion on chest radiograph, often in an upper lobe.[38] The syndrome is associated with asthma in about half of the patients described and likely represents a severe manifestation of ABPA revealed as a localized pathologic reaction rather than the more generalized pulmonary pathology evident in ABPA.[63] Diagnosis is made by biopsy or often retrospectively after removal of the lesion, which is curative, although some patients may require corticosteroid therapy for ABPA or if multiple lesions are present.

EXTRINSIC ALLERGIC ALVEOLITIS

Heavy or repeated exposure to *Aspergillus* conidia and mycelia may result in a hypersensitivity reaction affecting the alveoli in nonatopic individuals known as *extrinsic allergic alveolitis*. Malt workers, distillers, brewers, and others exposed to moldy straw or grain have suffered attacks producing cough, dyspnea, fever, chills, myalgias, and malaise 4 to 8 h after exposure to the antigen.[17] Repeated exposure may lead to "malt worker's lung" or "farmer's lung" and to the development of granulomatous disease or interstitial fibrosis. The immunopathogenesis involves cell-mediated immunity (type IV response) and immune complex deposition (type III response) and likely involves an intricate interaction between these mechanisms.

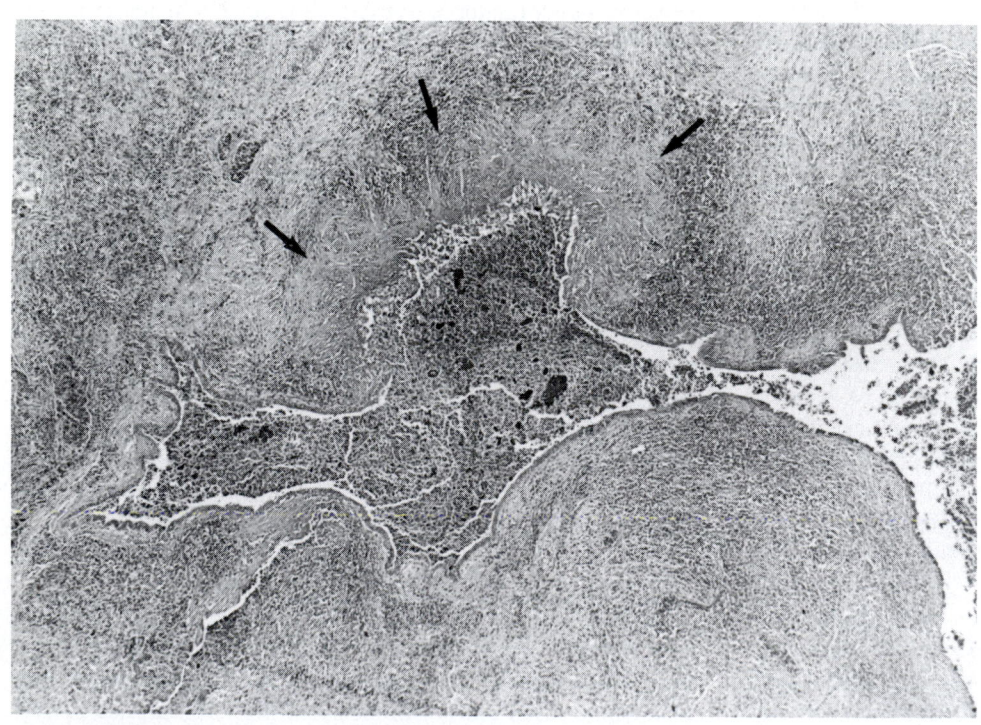

FIGURE 147-5 Low-magnification photomicrograph of bronchocentric granulomatosis showing partial replacement of bronchiolar mucosa by palisading histiocytes (arrows). H&E ×55. (*Courtesy of Dr. S. Albelda and Dr. G.H. Talbot.*)

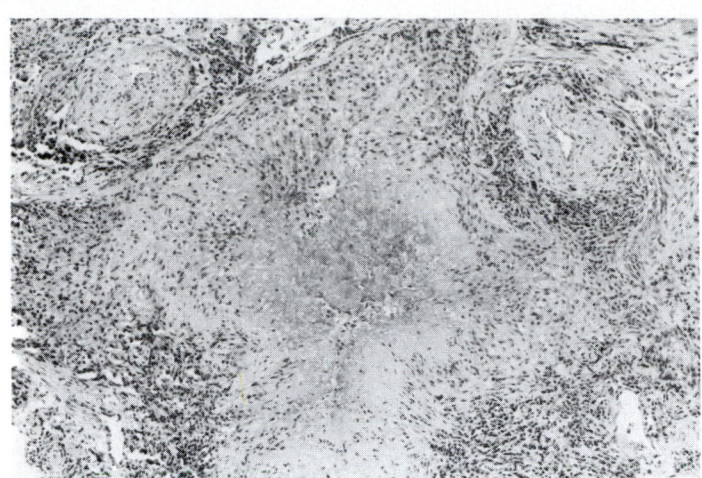

FIGURE 147-6 Necrotizing bronchocentric granuloma (center) in bronchocentric granulomatosis that has totally destroyed the bronchiole wall. The granuloma is inferred to be bronchocentric because of its location adjacent to branches of a pulmonary artery (top right and top left). H&E ×68.

Radiographic changes in the acute syndrome include diffuse alveolar-interstitial infiltrates that may resolve with removal of the inciting antigen. The chronic syndrome may reveal a fine reticulonodular interstitial infiltrate that may progress to pulmonary fibrosis with honeycombing.[17] Serum IgG antibody (precipitins) against *Aspergillus* antigen are present; however, serum IgE concentration is normal. Skin tests usually demonstrate an Arthus' reaction at 4 to 8 h and occasionally may be preceded by an immediate wheal and flare reaction and followed by a delayed reaction (36 to 48 h later). The management of extrinsic allergic alveolitis involves removal or avoidance of the source of antigen exposure. Spontaneous recovery may occur once exposure has ended. Corticosteroids are helpful in aiding the resolution of acute symptoms and reduce the likelihood of structural damage. However, corticosteroids are not helpful once fibrosis has developed.

ASPERGILLOMA

Saprophytic colonization of a parenchymal cavity by *Aspergillus* is referred to as *aspergilloma, mycetoma,* or *fungus ball.* A fungus ball consists of dead and living mycelial elements, fibrin, mucus, amorphous debris, inflammatory cells, and degenerating blood and epithelial elements.[24] The mycelia mass may lie free within the cavity or be attached to the cavity wall by granulation tissue. Spontaneous lysis has been reported in 7 to 10 percent of cases, more often associated with bacterial superinfection.[28] Bronchial epithelium or vascular granulation tissue may line the cavity, and surrounding lung may show pneumonitis. The usual species isolated is *A. fumigatus,* although others have been reported.

Pathophysiology

The pathogenesis of aspergilloma usually involves the colonization and proliferation of the fungus in a preexisting pulmonary cavity (secondary aspergilloma). Many factors may act to predispose an individual to development of a fungus ball. Tuberculous cavitary disease is the most common, with other cavitary pulmonary disorders such as sarcoid, cavitary neo-

plasm, pulmonary fibrosis, lung abscess, bronchial cyst, asbestosis, histoplasmosis, blastomycosis, ankylosing spondylitis, brochiectasis, pneumonia, cyanotic heart disease, pulmonary infarction, ABPA, and invasive aspergillosis also associated.[24] Per report by the British Thoracic and Tuberculosis Association, 11 to 17 percent of patients with posttuberculous cavities have radiographic changes consistent with aspergilloma.[7]

Primary aspergilloma, arising within the bronchial tree with a proliferation of *Aspergillus* causing a pulmonary cavity to develop, is far less common. The clinical conditions leading to the initiation of a cavitary process and fungus ball formation include: (1) invasive pulmonary aspergillosis (IPA); (2) chronic necrotizing pulmonary aspergillosis (CNPA); and (3) ABPA.[24] IPA may lead to primary aspergilloma during the period of bone marrow recovery as the host is able to mount an inflammatory response and wall off the fungus.[3] Pneumothorax may be a severe complication of pulmonary mycetoma that is reported as a rare occurrence in patients with hematologic malignancies. ABPA may cause bronchiectasis in the chronic phase of disease and result in aspergilloma secondary to growth of fungus distal to a plugged bronchus.[24] Aspergilloma has been found in 7 percent of one group of patients with ABPA and may provide a stimulus for the perpetuation of ABPA.

Clinical Features

Many patients remain asymptomatic, although cough (productive if the lesion communicates with bronchial passages), dyspnea, malaise, and weight loss can be present. Hemoptysis is the most frequent symptom and can be fatal, occurring in 74 percent of patients according to the results of a review of nine separate series.[24] Other associated symptoms include wheezing, chest pain, and, rarely, fever, more likely a consequence of underlying pulmonary pathology rather than due to the aspergilloma itself.

Chest radiograph reveals a solid round mass within a cavity (3 to 5 cm diameter) partially surrounded by a radiolucent crescent (Monod's sign)[25] (Fig. 147-7). Movement of the fungus ball may be appreciated within the cavity when comparing upright and decubitus films. Upper lung fields more frequently demonstrate aspergillomas, most frequently in preexisting cavities secondary to tuberculosis and as a solitary lesion, but they can be bilateral and multiple.[25] Chronic lung disease or local pneumonitis may obscure chest radiograph findings, and tomography may offer insight. Computed tomographic scanning may easily demonstrate characteristic lesions and may be desirable in difficult cases.[24] The only indicator of early disease may be thickening of a cavity wall or increased pleural thickening.

Sputum cultures are often not helpful, since communication with the bronchus may not be present and specimen contamination with colonizing *Aspergillus* cannot be excluded. Multiple positive sputum cultures are more suggestive. However, in a review of several series, 114 of 196 (58 percent) patients with aspergilloma had sputum cultures positive for *Aspergillus.*[24] Precipitating antibodies to *Aspergillus* antigens are present in the sera of most patients with aspergilloma. Eosinophilia, IgE, and skin-test reactivity may be seen in individuals who are allergic to the fungus, but are not consistent findings.

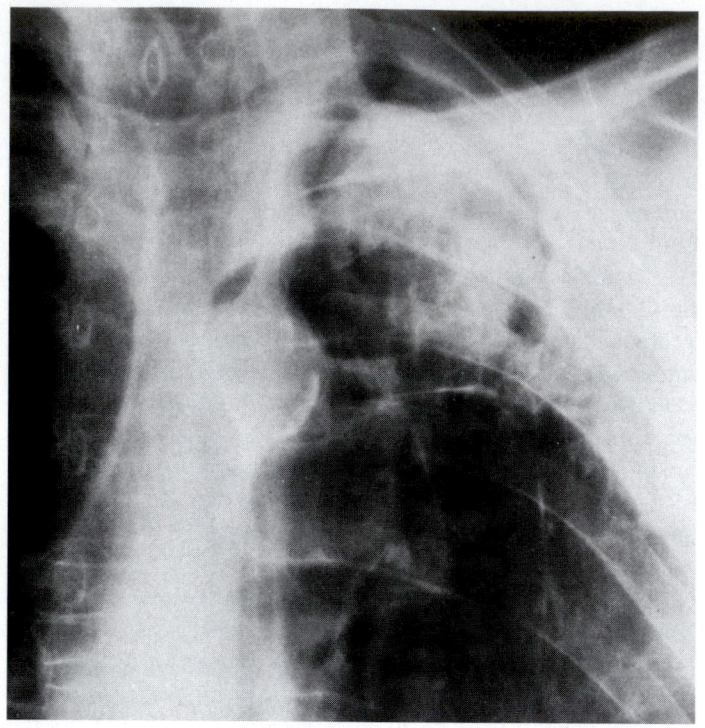
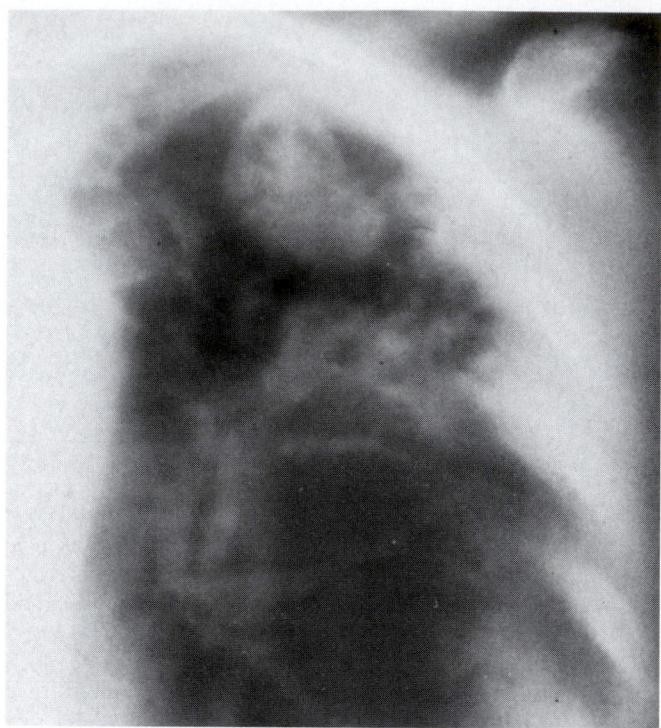

A
B

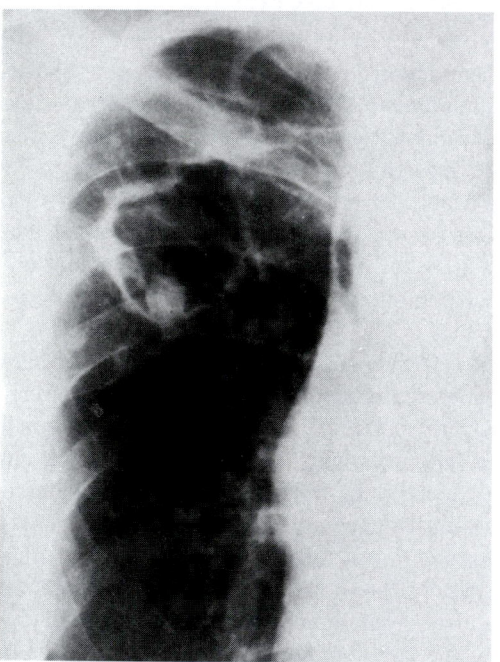
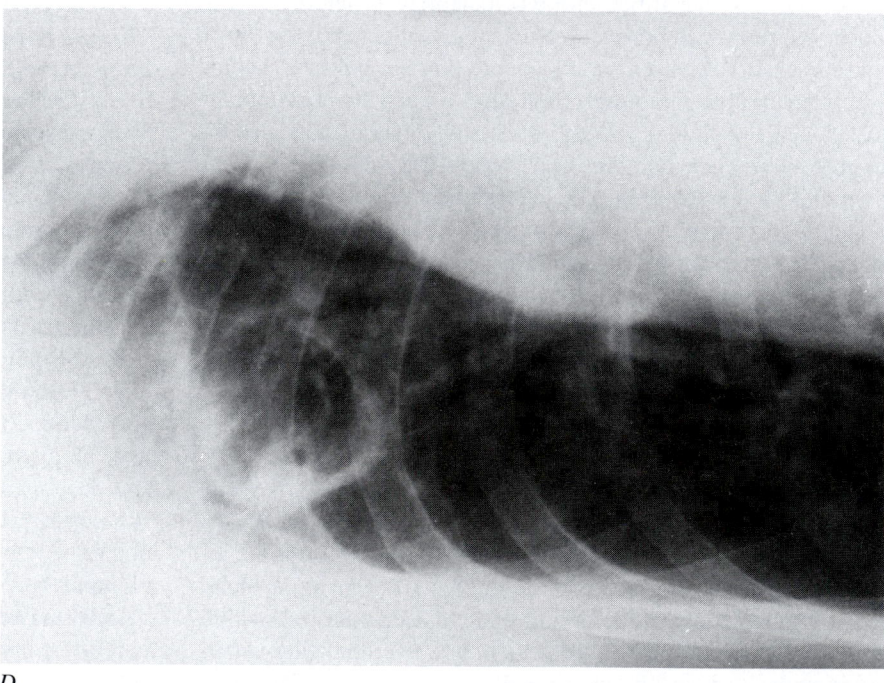

C
D

FIGURE 147-7 Radiographic appearances of pulmonary aspergillomas. *A.* A 51-year-old male with a history of tuberculosis shows the classic crescent-shaped patch of air (Monod's sign), as well as marked pleural thickening. *B.* Tomogram shows well-defined fungus within a thick-walled upper lobe cavity. *C.* A 49-year-old male with ankylosing spondylitis who developed an aspergilloma inside a thin-walled cavity. *D.* Decubitus film from same patient shows fungus ball moving when the patient changes position. *(Courtesy of Dr. S. Albelda and Dr. G.H. Talbot.)*

Treatment

Therapeutic options currently include systemic or local antifungal agents, surgical resection, or conservative management with careful follow-up, without specific medical or surgical intervention. Optimal management of patients with aspergilloma remains difficult and controversial. The major clinical concern is hemoptysis (Fig. 147-8). The risk of severe recurrent events in patients with aspergilloma may not be as high as has been estimated.[24] Often, the best management for asymptomatic patients is periodic chest radiographs without surgical intervention. Therapeutic considerations need to include the individual patient's health status with attention to the potential risks of treatment.

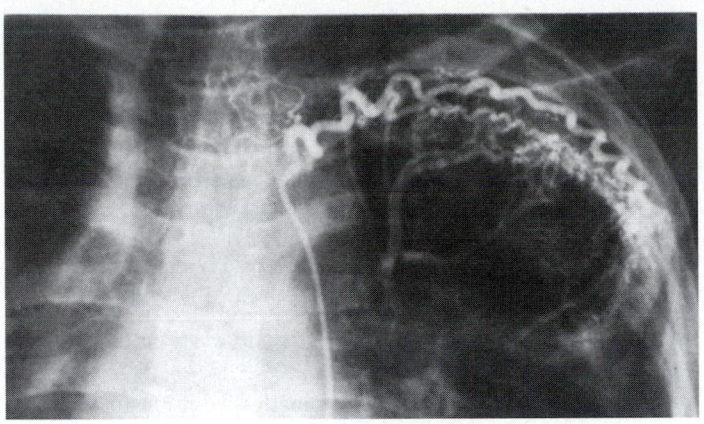

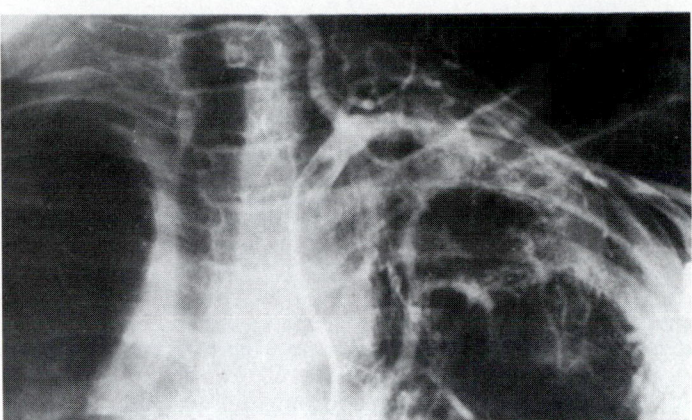

A

B

FIGURE 147-8   Arteriography was performed in a 43-year-old female with cystic sarcoidosis and a large left upper lobe aspergilloma because of massive hemoptysis. *A.* Injection of bronchial artery shows that much of the blood supply of the superior portion of the aspergilloma was sup-plied by this vessel. *B.* Injection of the left subclavian artery demonstrated additional extensive collateral blood flow through the chest wall via the long thoracic artery. *(Courtesy of Dr. S. Albelda and Dr. G.H. Talbot.)*

Surgical resection is indicated for patients with severe life-threatening hemoptysis, and some reviews have suggested surgical resection as a prophylactic therapeutic measure for all patients with aspergilloma, since resection is potentially curative.[24] Patients in this category frequently have severe underlying pulmonary disease, leaving them poor surgical candidates and with a substantial postoperative complication rate. Patients suffering major hemoptysis and who are poor surgical candidates may alternatively undergo arterial embolization or cavernoscopic evacuation of aspergilloma as a palliative measure.

Systemic antifungals offer little benefit in treating aspergilloma, possibly because of inadequate penetration into the cavity.[32] However, systemic antifungal therapy may help a subset of patients with systemic symptoms and locally invasive disease surrounding the aspergilloma (CNPA).

Direct intracavitary instillation of antifungal agents (amphotericin B, sodium iodide, natamycin, miconazole, ketoconazole, and 5-FC) has shown promise in symptomatic patients with aspergilloma.[32] Palliation of hemoptysis and sputum production and diminishment or disappearance of serum preciptins occurred in one study using glycerin and amphotericin B paste in 15 patients.[23] Optimal dose and length of treatment remain to be determined. Complications can include mild hemoptysis, hypersensitivity to the antifungal agent, invasion of a hypervascular area resulting in hemorrhage, and recurrence of aspergilloma.

Oral antifungal therapy would be particularly useful in the inoperable group of patients with aspergilloma. Itraconazole offers the advantages of oral availability, good activity against *A. fumigatus*, low toxicity, and good tissue penetration.[55] Response rates to itraconazole have been variable. Although recovery or improvement may be seen symptomatically, immunologically, or radiographically in patients treated with itraconzole, caution in attributing these findings to therapy is warranted. Findings in one study of nine patients with aspergilloma receiving 200 mg per day of itraconazole revealed a late response in two patients treated for 1 year, suggesting that prolonged therapy or higher dosages may be required.[7] However, long-term therapy is generally needed to prevent relapse.

BRONCHIAL STUMP ASPERGILLOSIS

Bronchial stump aspergillosis (BSA) is an unusual sequela of lung resection first reported in 1969 by Sawasaki and coworkers.[56] Patients may present with a productive cough and hemoptysis, sputum that may be putrid, and, occasionally, expectoration of fungal material or suture thread. The cause is secondary infection of silk suture material used to close the bronchus after pulmonary resection. A single line of suture penetrating the total layer of the bronchus from the mucosa to the serosa is most often used and is referred to as *Sweet's method*. Part of the suture thread protrudes into the bronchial lumen and may cause inflammation or infection. Incidence of BSA was found to be 1.5 percent when silk suture was used, and was eliminated with the institution of nylon monofilament suture.[56] Local inflammation, compromised tissue viability, and the high capillarity of silk thread favor *Aspergillus* infection.[52]

The period from surgery to onset of disease usually ranges from 6 to 12 months, although one case was noted to occur after 3 years.[56] One patient has been reported with mild hemoptysis and cough commencing 4 years after surgery, after an uneventful postoperative period.[52] Fiber-optic bronchoscopy may reveal the silk thread and inflammatory changes such as hyperemia, swelling, granulation, and purulence.[56] Biopsy of the bronchial mucosa shows necrotic areas and hyphae, and cultures are usually positive for *Aspergillus*. There are no characteristic radiographic findings.

Nylon monofilament substituted for silk suture at surgery eliminates this infectious complication.[56] Simple removal of the suture during bronchoscopy with forceps is also curative.[52] Oral itraconazole was able to suppress the infection and alleviate symptoms in three cases where sutures were not removed. Optimal dose and duration of therapy are not known, and a controlled study is needed to validate these preliminary findings.

A related syndrome occurs at the site of bronchial anastomosis in lung transplantation recipients. At this relatively avascular site with mucosal and epithelial disruption, *Aspergillus* infection may become established. Such disease may present with persistent bronchial secretions, fever, or anastomotic leak. Eradication of such infection without surgical resection in these immunocompromised individuals is often impossible. This infection may also progress to invasive aspergillosis (discussed below).

CHRONIC NECROTIZING PULMONARY ASPERGILLOSIS

Individuals with systemic immunocompromise as a result of corticosteroids, diabetes mellitus, alcoholism, or poor nutritional status, or who have underlying pulmonary disease such as COPD, sarcoidosis, inactive tuberculosis, pneumoconiosis, or radiation fibrosis, may develop a slowly progressive form of aspergillosis. Patients are frequently chronically ill with complaints of fever, weight loss, productive cough, and hemoptysis. Chronic infiltrates may be evident on chest radiographs, which may progress to form an aspergilloma.[5] A lesion may also begin as an aspergilloma and become locally invasive.

Sputum cultures and serum *Aspergillus* precipitins are often positive, and leukocytosis may be present. Tissue invasion of the cavity wall by *Aspergillus* hyphae, fibrosis, and a granulomatous reaction is evident by direct examination.[5] Extent and progression of the disease appear to depend on the ability of a host to contain the fungus. Disseminated spread is uncommon.

Intravenous amphotericin B with or without oral 5-FC has resulted in occasional dramatic responses.[5] Overall results with chemotherapy are, however, poor, and alternative agents, such as itraconazole or intracavitary amphotericin B, may be tried. Host defenses should be bolstered and immunosuppressive factors removed if possible. Surgical or percutaneous drainage may be necessary in patients with large necrotic cavities that do not drain via the tracheobronchial tree.[5] Surgical resection should be reserved for patients who have failed antifungal therapy or who have clearly localized disease and who are able to tolerate surgery.

INVASIVE ASPERGILLOSIS

Invasive pulmonary aspergillosis occurs in the immunocompromised host following inhalation of *Aspergillus* conidia most often, although hematogenous dissemination from cutaneous or gastrointestinal source can occur.[64] Patients with acute lymphocytic and acute myelogenous leukemia with prolonged granulocytopenia during treatment are particularly prone to developing this form of disease.[21] High-dose corticosteroids, especially when combined with other immunosuppressive agents in recipients of organ transplants, or chronic granulomatous disease, can cause immune dysfunction, predisposing such individuals to IPA. Patients usually die within 2 to 3 weeks unless immunosuppression is rapidly decreased. Invasive aspergillosis has been reported in apparently normal hosts, and heavy environmental exposure to *Aspergillus* spores has been linked to disease in both hospital epidemics and individual cases.[36]

Once germination of conidia occurs, endobronchial proliferation of hyphae, occasionally with ulcerative tracheobronchitis (discussed below), leads to invasion of pulmonary arterioles and lung parenchyma and, finally, to ischemic necrosis (Figs. 147-9 and 147-10). Hematogenous dissemination with thrombosis, hemorrhagic infarction, and invasion of distant organs may result from *Aspergillus* hyphae invading arterioles and occur in approximately one-third of cases.[64] Thus, invasive aspergillosis can present with a similar clinical picture to other thrombotic and embolic diseases such as pulmonary embolism, cerebral vascular accidents, Budd-Chiari syndrome, and renal papillary necrosis. Invasive aspergillosis can spread to contiguous structures, across the diaphragm to the stomach, or from the lung to the heart or superior vena cava.[64] The morphology of *Aspergillus* hyphae in tissue specimens is indistinguishable from that of several other fungi, such as *Pseudallescheria boydii* and *Fusarium* species, so that clinical correlation of the syndrome and culture identification are very important.

Clinical Features

Symptoms begin with fever, which may be followed by a mild nonproductive cough suggestive of bronchitis. Pleuritic chest pain and progression to pneumonia occur within 1 to 2 days. The appearance of lesions by chest radiograph may be delayed

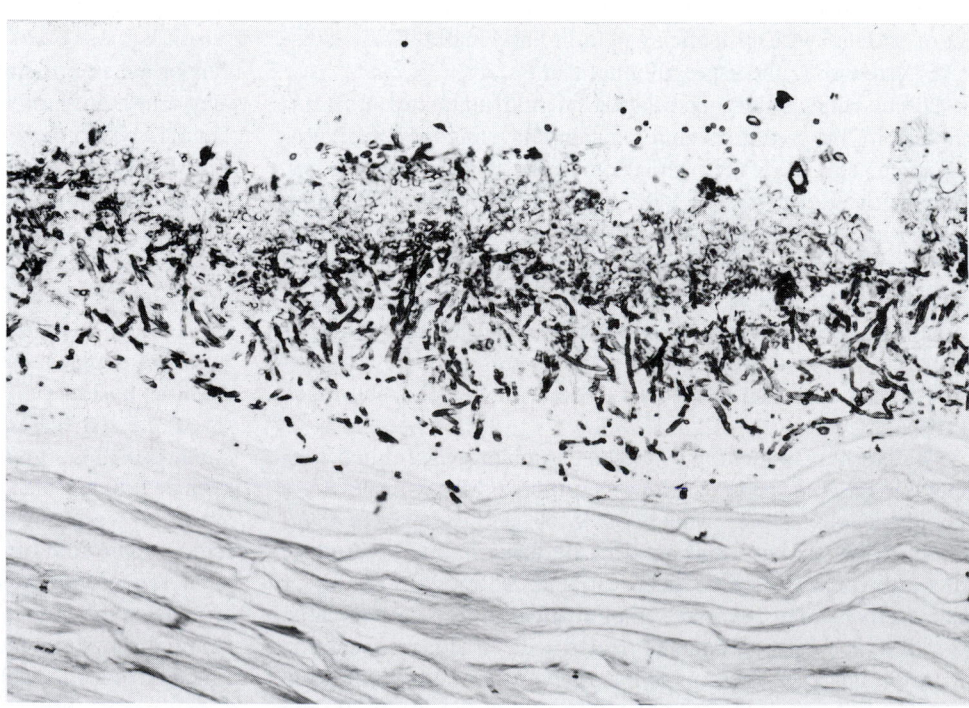

FIGURE 147-9   The characteristic appearance of *Aspergillus* in tissue. *(Courtesy of Dr. S.T. Nikulasson.)*

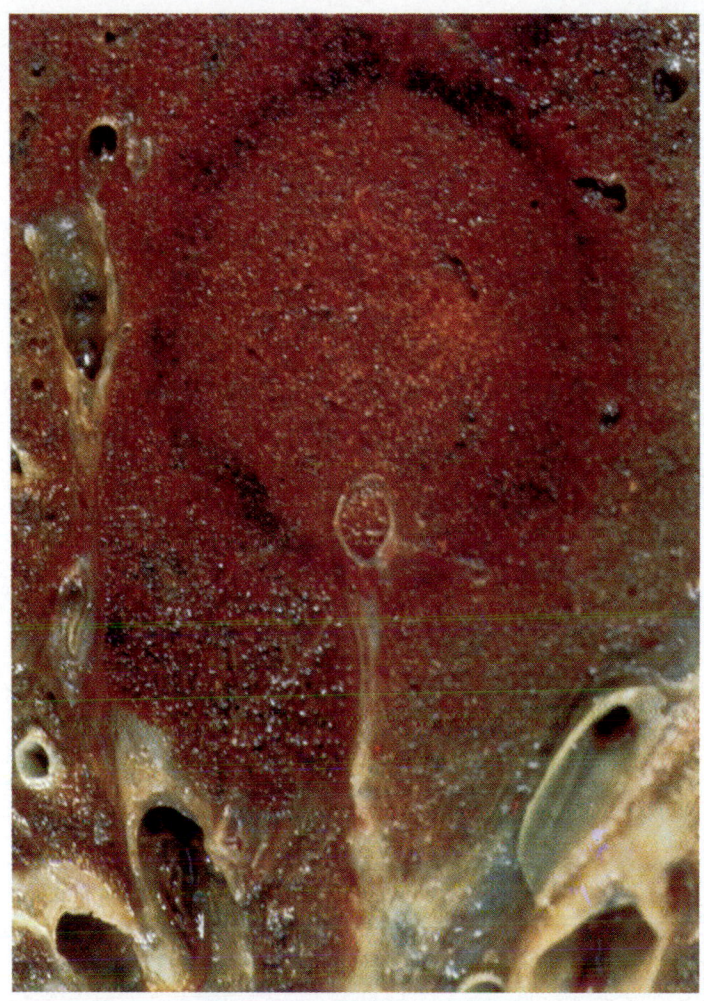

A

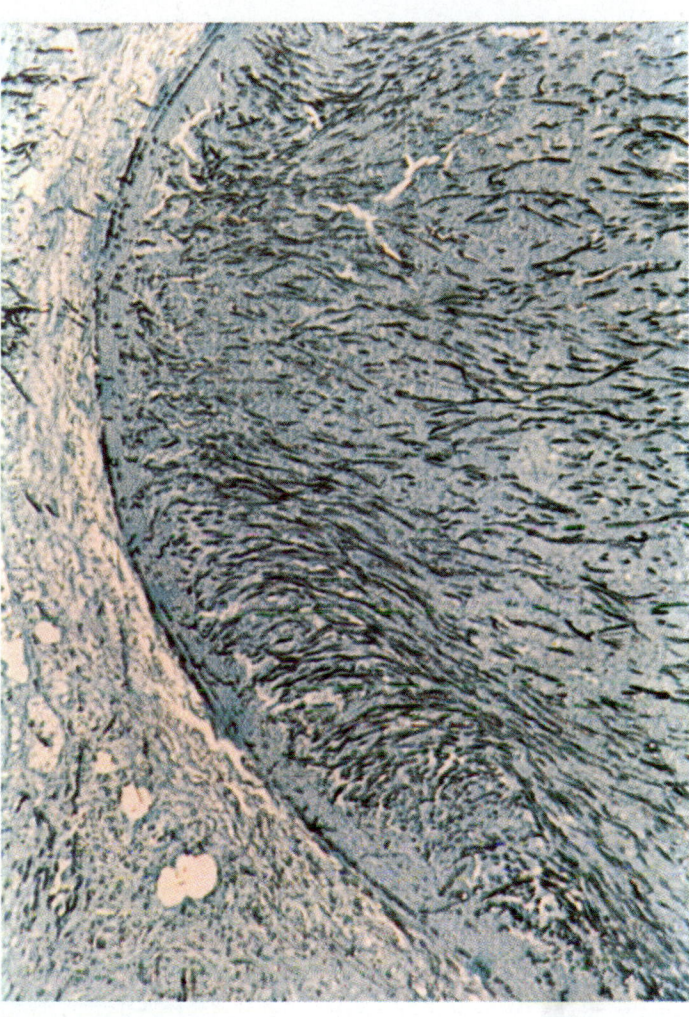

B

FIGURE 147-10   A 62-year-old male with acute leukemia who developed invasive pulmonary aspergillosis. *A.* Gross appearance of fungal lesion. A central necrotic area is surrounded by a lining of hemor-rhagic infarction. *B.* Grocott's stain shows characteristic appearance of aspergilli in tissue. *(Courtesy of Dr. G.G. Pietra.)*

in the leukopenic patient because of the impaired inflammatory response. The typical presenting finding may be one or more well-defined nodules or a patchy density (Fig. 147-11). The lesions then progress to diffuse consolidation or cavitation. Cavitation tends to occur in patients if immunosuppression is decreased, such as in leukemic patients during the period of recovering bone marrow function or when steroid therapy is reduced significantly, and on occasion gives rise to massive hemoptysis (Fig. 147-12).[3]

Pleuritic pain and slight hemoptysis may suggest pulmonary infarction. Patients may expectorate necrotic tissue filled with hyphae. Cough, sputum production, and pleural effusion are either absent or minimal.[3] Invasive aspergillosis must be strongly considered in susceptible patients who fail broad-spectrum antibiotics.[49]

Extrapulmonary sites may be involved, including the highly vascular organs such as the kidney, liver, spleen, and central nervous system. Invasive disease of the nose and paranasal sinuses occurs in immunocompromised patients, and contiguous invasive spread into the orbit or into the cranial vault can result in a syndrome similar to rhinocerebral mucormycosis.[64] Concomi-tant nasal ulceration and pulmonary infiltrate in the profoundly neutropenic host are suggestive of aspergillosis. *Aspergillus* is the most common fungal pathogen associated with sinusitis in the immunocompetent patient, but invasion into contiguous tissue rarely occurs.

Diagnosis

Tissue biopsy provides a definitive diagnosis. Histopathologic findings must demonstrate tissue or vascular invasion by hyphae that are morphologically consistent with *Aspergillus* (Fig. 147-9). Early clinical, laboratory, and radiographic findings of invasive aspergillosis are often not present, making the diagnosis difficult (Fig. 147-10). Invasive biopsy procedures in these patients are often precluded by severe illness and bleeding diatheses, and unfortunately the diagnosis is often not made until postmortem examination.[64] However, recognition of invasive fungal disease and early institution of therapy reduces the high mortality associated with IPA.[49]

Computed tomographic scanning may play a role in the early diagnosis of nonspecific pulmonary infiltrates in immunocom-promised hosts (Fig. 147-11) (see Chapter 138). In the appro-

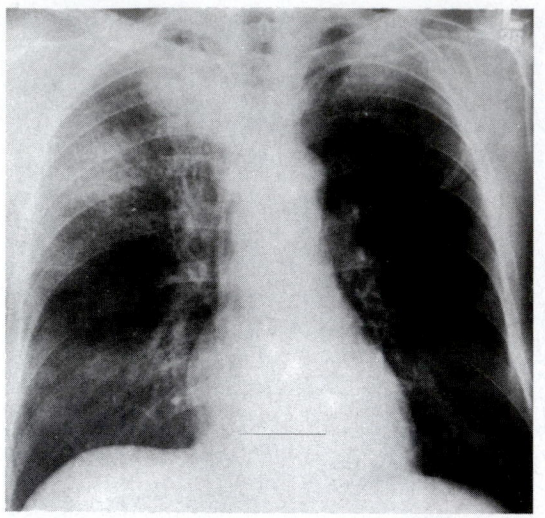

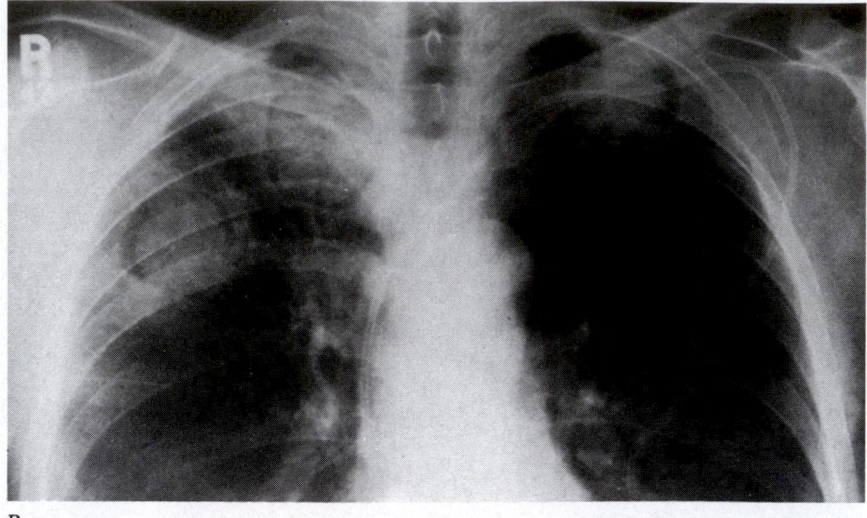

A

B

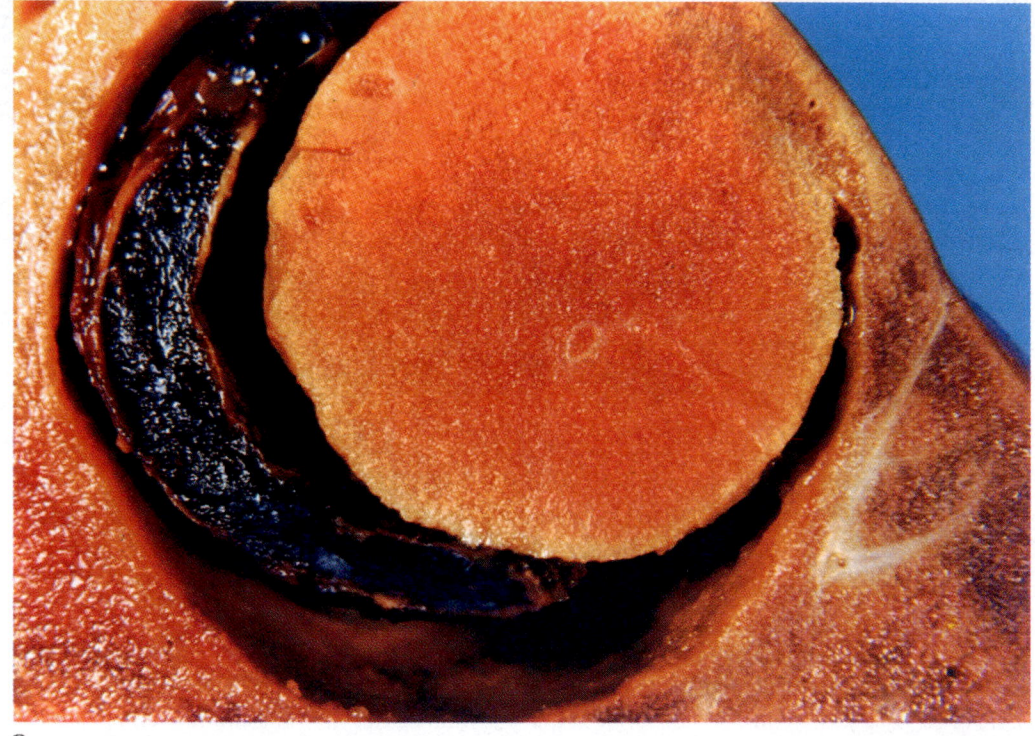

FIGURE 147-11 The characteristic pathologic and radiographic features of invasive pulmonary aspergillosis are illustrated in this 56-year-old man with acute leukemia. *A.* Multiple hazy nodular infiltrates appear after 2 weeks of chemotherapy-induced neutropenia. *B.* As the neutrophil count begins to rise, the lesions become more discrete and nodular in appearance. Two days after the neutrophil count exceeded 500 cells per mm^3, all the lesions have cavitated, creating "air crescents." *C.* Gross appearance of one of the lesions shows the necrotic "lung ball" surrounded by hemorrhage and a crescent of air. *(With permission of Gefter WB et al: Radiology 157:607, 1985.)*   C

priate clinical setting, the CT "halo sign" of a zone of low attenuation surrounding a nonspecific pulmonary mass or infiltrate may prove to be helpful in the early diagnosis of IPA in patients with leukemia. Magnetic resonance imaging may contribute to the early diagnosis of IPA by revealing the hemorrhagic content of pulmonary lesions typical in IPA.[29] Positive blood cultures are rare, since fungemia is not sustained, although clumps of broken hyphae may sporadically embolize to end organs.[64] In a highly susceptible patient, positive cultures of sputum, bronchoalveolar lavage fluid, or bronchial brushings are predictive of invasive aspergillosis, whereas negative cultures do not rule out disease. Sputum cultures positive for *Aspergillus* in less compromised patients with pneumonia should not be automatically dismissed as contaminant.

Detection of *Aspergillus* antigens in sera or other body fluids may offer an early noninvasive method for the diagnosis of IPA. A radioimmunoassay for circulating galactomannan *Aspergillus* antigens was 74 percent sensitive and 90 percent specific in 79 hematology patients at high risk for IPA.[59] Such an antigen detection test may prove useful for the rapid diagnosis of invasive aspergillosis. Antibody testing in IPA is usually not helpful, since patients with invasive aspergillosis often have greatly diminished or absent antibody production.

Treatment

The prognosis of patients with IPA is ultimately linked with the severity and outcome of the underlying disease.[64] Although antifungal therapy may delay progression of IPA, bone marrow re-

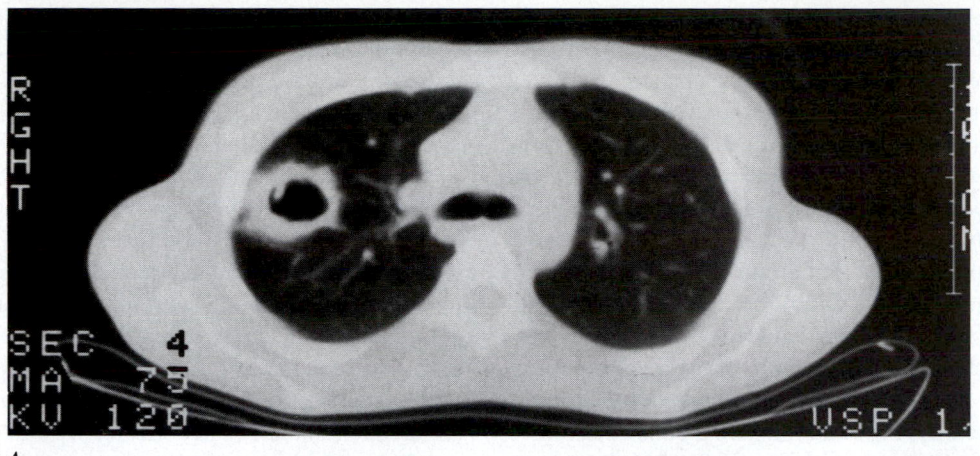

A

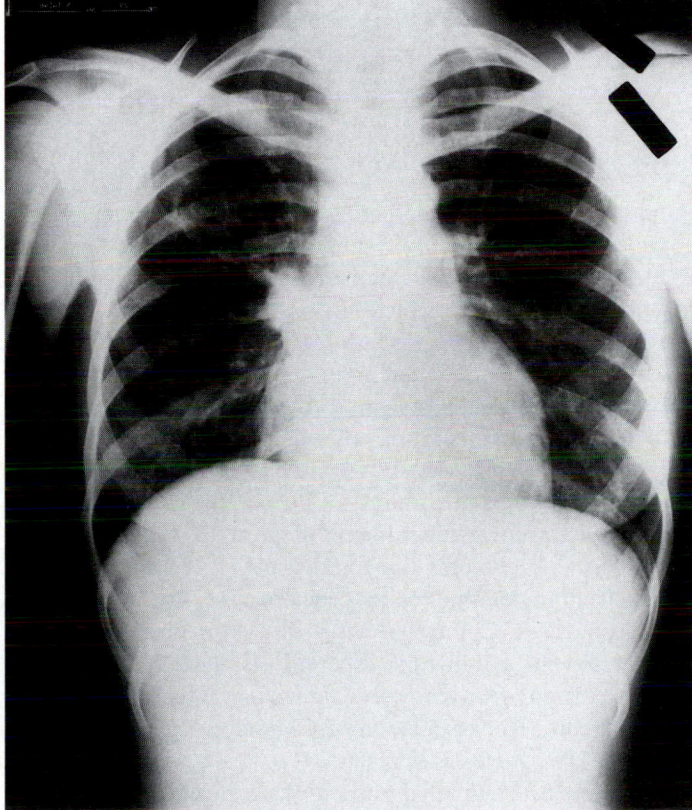

B

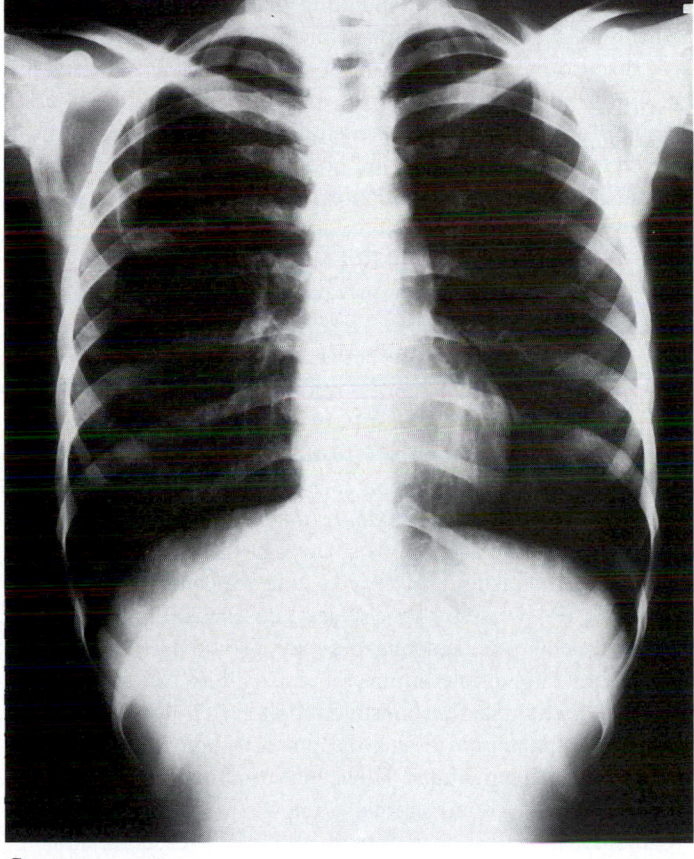

C

FIGURE 147-12 Sequential views of invasive Aspergillosis showing the progressive enlargement of a right upper lobe cavity. Note the early surrounding infiltrate followed by thinning of the cavity wall. *A.* Computed tomography of chest at presentation. *B.* Chest radiograph 4 months later. *C.* Chest radiograph 6 months after initial presentation.

covery in neutropenic patients is essential for cure.[20] Even with restored immune function, progressive invasive aspergillosis is devastating and may result in death, emphasizing the need for early diagnosis and treatment.

Amphotericin B remains the major intravenous agent available. In patients with persistent fever and unexplained pulmonary infiltrates who cannot tolerate invasive procedures, empiric amphotericin B therapy should be commenced.[49] A daily dose of up to 1.0 mg/kg of amphotericin B may be administered. Higher initial doses of amphotericin B (up to 1.5 mg/kg) have often been used. The dose may then be decreased to 0.6 to 0.8 mg/kg per day after the patient's condition improves or if dose-limiting toxicity occurs. Nephrotoxicity, phlebitis, hypokalemia, hypomagnesemia, and anemia are adverse effects of amphotericin B that must be monitored. Available data do not clearly indicate the exact dose of amphotericin B; results of therapy indicate that in neutropenic patients, high-dose amphotericin B (*at least* 1.0 mg/kg per day) is appropriate, since invasive aspergillosis has developed in patients *during treatment* with 0.5 mg/kg per day.[14] The duration of therapy is likely best individualized according to patient response, severity of disease, and immune status.

Amphotericin B in combination with flucytosine is often synergistic in animal models of aspergillosis and has been useful in the cases reported with an overall response rate of 68 percent, although early treatment failures were eliminated from the review.[14] No controlled data are available to prove the benefit of this combination. Rifampin is sometimes added empirically when a patient is declining in the face of maximal amphotericin B therapy. Rifampin induces liver enzymes and may adversely affect transplant patients on cyclosporine and steroid therapy and therefore should be avoided for empiric treatment of IPA when drug interactions are a consideration.[14] Liposomal amphotericin B offers the potential of a less toxic intravenous alternative and can be administered in higher doses (up to 5 mg/kg per day) depending on the formulation.[14] The efficacy of this type of preparation for initial therapy of invasive disease in immunocompromised individuals remains uncertain. Liposomal preparations may provide an alternative to standard amphotericin B following the development of drug-related toxicities that limit amphotericin dosing. Amphotericin B lipid complex is now available and approved for second-line therapy of aspergillosis. Ketoconazole is not recommended for addition to amphotericin B for the treatment of aspergillosis and has been shown in vitro and in animal models to be antagonistic.[14]

Itraconazole is an orally active triazole antifungal that has been effective therapy for aspergillosis. Variable absorption and interpatient variation of serum levels have been problems.[14] Itraconazole has been used in the treatment of IPA with reasonable success when adequate serum levels were attained.[55] The role for itraconazole in prophylaxis, primary treatment, and salvage therapy of invasive aspergillosis needs further controlled studies but appears promising.[14] However, some transplant patients have developed IPA while on prophylactic doses (200 to 400 mg per day) of itraconazole. Itraconazole may also be used to complete therapy for susceptible strains of *Aspergillus* following initial treatment and clinical response to amphotericin B. Concomitant use with amphotericin B has the potential for antagonism and adverse drug interactions. However, combination therapy has shown promise in some animal studies.

Another modality of treatment is surgical resection alone or in combination with antifungal therapy in selected patients with localized lesions. Surgery may be indicated in patients with leukemia who develop pulmonary aspergillosis and require further chemotherapy or transplantation or when failure of medical therapy alone has occurred.[14] Systemic therapy should be initiated *prior* to surgical manipulation of infected lung tissue to prevent systemic dissemination. In the nonimmunocompromised host sinusitis and BSA are the only two types of invasive aspergillosis that may be handled with surgery alone.

Mucosal colonization may be reduced by administration of antifungals either orally or locally. In a retrospective study of invasive aspergillosis, intranasal aerosolized amphotericin B was found effective in prophylaxis in neutropenic patients.[33] Although positive nose cultures for *Aspergillus* have been shown to have predictive value for subsequent invasive disease,[1] the ob-

servations in that study were uncontrolled. Itraconazole may also be useful for prophylaxis in neutropenic patients, and further controlled studies are needed.[14] Success in reducing the rate of *Aspergillus* colonization and infection has also been attributed to effective mechanical air filtering systems.[33]

Empiric treatment for aspergillosis with amphotericin B in neutropenic patients with fever and no response to antibacterial therapy is a reasonable and recommended approach. Early empiric therapy with amphotericin B appears to decrease morbidity and mortality among neutropenic patients at high risk for fungal infection.[49] Four to seven days of fever while the patient is receiving broad-spectrum antibiotic therapy is a generally accepted course. Careful evaluation to exclude secondary bacterial infection not adequately treated by the antimicrobial regimen should occur prior to the commencement of antifungal therapy.[49] Once fever resolves and bone marrow recovery is underway, antifungal therapy can be stopped, provided that aspergillosis has been ruled out. Patients may suffer relapse if chemotherapy is resumed and neutropenia recurs.

PULMONARY ASPERGILLOSIS IN AIDS

Pulmonary aspergillosis in patients with AIDS is relatively uncommon but increasing in frequency with prolonged survival of HIV-infected persons. Qualitative defects of neutrophils and alveolar macrophages, which are the major cells for host defense against *Aspergillus,* may be involved. All such patients have very low helper T cell counts, cells not known to be involved in the host defense against *Aspergillus.* Neutropenia and corticosteroid administration were associated in 54 percent of reported cases.[42] Previously described cases have associated smoking of marijuana with invasive aspergillosis; in one recent review, such use was identified in 4 out of 13 patients with aspergillosis.[13] Pneumonia due to other pathogens and the use of broad-spectrum antibiotics precede many of the invasive aspergillosis cases. Cytomegalovirus disease is prevalent among the reported cases of invasive aspergillosis in AIDS and has been also associated with increased pulmonary infections in transplant patients. The association of CMV and *Aspergillus* infection in AIDS patients is unclear.[13]

Symptoms of pulmonary aspergillosis in AIDS are nonspecific. AIDS patients may develop the whole spectrum of aspergillosis-related pulmonary disorders, including chronic cavitary, invasive, and bronchial forms of aspergillosis.[42] Two patterns of aspergillosis that have been reported are possibly AIDS-specific. Termed *obstructing bronchial aspergillosis* and *pseudomembranous bronchial aspergillosis,* they resemble ABPA in many ways.[42]

Another form of airway aspergillosis is ulcerative tracheobronchitis, which appears as inflammatory ulcers or nodules involving the main-stem and segmental bronchi on bronchoscopy. *Aspergillus* can be isolated on biopsy specimens, and the clinical and histologic features of the AIDS patients described were similar to those reviewed without AIDS. Patients may present with fever, cough, dyspnea, or hemoptysis. Varying degrees of bronchial mucosal invasion occur, and subsequent disseminated aspergillosis occurred in two patients. *Aspergillus* ulcerative tracheobronchitis may therefore progress to IPA in the susceptible individual and warrants prompt investigation and treatment.

The mortality from pulmonary aspergillosis in AIDS patients was 56 percent in one series, to widespread pulmonary or systemic infection or to fatal hemoptysis.[42] Risk factors and clinical and radiographic features resemble those of non-HIV-infected patients with aspergillosis. AIDS patients are susceptible to the range of *Aspergillus*-associated disorders, a feature not seen in other risk groups.[42]

PULMONARY MUCORMYCOSIS

Mucormycosis refers to the acute and rapidly developing infection caused by fungi of the order Mucorales. Other names for this disease have been used in the past, such as, *phycomycosis* and *zygomycosis*. *Phycomycosis* is an outdated term derived from an earlier classification scheme, and *zygomycosis* is too vague since all Zygomycetes do not cause the same clinical syndrome.[58] The term *mucormycosis* is most useful to clinicians and will be used herein to describe this infection. Table 147-5 describes the taxonomic relationship of the pathogenic Zygomycetes.

History

Mucormycosis was first described in animals, including dogs, pigs, horses, and cows. In 1855, Kurchenmeister described the first human case of mucormycosis in a cancerous lung, and Furbinger expanded on the work in 1876 by clearly demonstrating pulmonary pathology due to Mucor. In 1885, Paltauf first documented a disseminated case of mucormycosis originating in the larynx and pharynx with subsequent gastric involvement, likely a case of rhinocerebral mucormycosis with dissemination. A description in 1895, by Herla, of a woman with pulmonary cavity mucormycosis who died of cancer of the liver, helped to establish the link between cancer and mucormycosis.

Rhinocerebral mucormycosis went largely unreported until 1943, when Gregory and colleagues published their classic description of the syndrome and its relation to diabetes and acidosis. Pulmonary mucormycosis was also rarely reported until recently and is becoming more commonly identified as the number of immunocompromised patients increases.

Epidemiology

The Zygomycetes are ubiquitous fungi found throughout the world and are thermotolerant inhabitants of decaying organic matter. Species of Mucorales pathogenic to humans grow rapidly on any carbohydrate substrate and produce sporangiospores in large numbers. Spores become airborne, and inhalation of conidia occurs on a daily basis. Even though these fungi grow in many ecologic niches, the infrequency of disease due to these organisms attests to their low virulence potential in the human host. Patients with severe immune compromise, diabetes mellitus, or trauma are the most commonly affected, but mucormycosis is a rather rare development in any of these patient groups.

Rhinocerebral disease is most often associated with diabetic ketoacidosis, and the most commonly encountered genera is *Rhizopus*. Central nervous system mucormycosis is rare, occurring in severely debilitated patients usually as a result of the fungus

Classification of the Agents of Mucormycosis and Related Diseases

I. Zygomycotina
  A. Zygomycetes
    a. Mucorales
      1. Mucoraceae
        i. *Absidia*
          (a) *A. corymbifera*
          (b) *A. ramosa*
        ii. *Mucor*
          (a) *M. circinelloides*
        iii. *Rhizomucor*
          (a) *R. pusillus*
        iv. *Rhizopus*
          (a) *R. oryzae (R. arrhyziae)**
          (b) *R. arrhizus*
          (c) *R. rhizopodiformis*
      2. Cunninghamellaceae
        i. *Cunninghalella*
          (a) *C. bertholletiae*
      3. Mortierellaceae
        i. *Mortierella*
          (a) *M. wolfii*
      4. Saksenaeaceae
        i. *Saksenaea*
          (a) *S. vasiformis*
      5. Syncephalastrum
        i. *Syncephalastrum*
      6. Apophysomyceae
        i. *Apophysomyces*
          (a) *A. elegans*
      7. Thamnidiaceae
        i. *Cokeromyces*
          (a) *C. recurvatus*
    b. Entomophthorales
      1. *Conidiobolus*
        i. *C. coronatus (Entomophthora coronata)**
        ii. *C. incongruans*
      2. *Basidiobolus*
        i. *B. haptosporus (B. meristosporus; B. ranarum)**

*Obsolete synonyms.

spreading from the initial site of invasion through the nose, paranasal sinuses, or from intravenous drug use. Rhinocerebral infection may also occur in organ transplant patients or as a complication of severe cutaneous burn injury.[50]

Pulmonary infection is associated with leukemia and lymphoma and other malignancies when patients are neutropenic, have decreased neutrophil function, and are receiving broad-spectrum antibiotics.[41] It has also been observed in organ transplant recipients, particularly in diabetics (see Chapters 136 and 138) (Fig. 147-12). Steroid administration and hyperglycemia were also prevalent in leukemic patients in one series.[41] Less commonly, diabetes without underlying malignancy occurs.[45] Increased risk for mucormycosis occurs in renal failure patients receiving the drug deferoxamine, as an iron- or aluminum-chelating agent.[6] There have been only seven reports of HIV-1-positive patients with mucormycosis, one each of cutaneoarticular, renal invasion, and pulmonary disease, and four cases of rhinocerebral mucormycosis.[57] Gastric involvement is encountered in children with kwashiorkor and immunosuppressed patients. Disseminated disease may progress from one of the primary anatomic locations and occurs in patients with profound immunocompromise, such as patients with acute leukemia or bone marrow transplants.[41]

Mycology and Pathogenesis

Zygomycetes are molds characterized by growth of hyphae in the environment and in tissue. They grow quickly, within 2 to 5 days on most media, as fluffy gray or brownish colonies. As the colony matures the mycelium may darken and show a black pepperlike effect as large numbers of sporangia are formed. Cyclohexamide inhibits the growth of these fungi, and media that contain this compound, such as Mycosel and Mycobiotic agar, should not be used. All pathologic species grow at 37°C.

Microscopic examination for the presence and location of rhizoids, apophyses, and the morphology of the columellae differentiates the genera. Isolating and speciating the organism is important for treatment considerations. Issues of potential species-specific responses to antifungal drugs, determining the efficacy of therapy in eradicating the pathogen, or of whether a subsequent clinical isolate is the same, new, or contaminating are compelling reasons to identify the strain involved in an infection. The most commonly isolated genus is *Rhizopus,* followed by *Rhizomucor.*

The pathogenesis of mucormycosis begins with the inhalation of spores into the respiratory tract, where they are deposited in the nasal turbinates and may be inhaled into the pulmonary alveoli. In the normal lung, the spores are unable to germinate, as bronchoalveolar macrophages harvested from normal mice phagocytose *Rhizopus* spores and prevent their growth but do not kill them.[60] Animals with diabetes mellitus or corticosteroid pretreatment experience a rapidly progressive pulmonary infection with hematogenous dissemination and death after inhalation of Mucorales spores. Macrophages recovered from the bronchial trees of the impaired animals reveal decreased ability to inhibit spore germination.[60]

Neutrophils are the major host effector cell responsible for blocking growth of the Mucorales. Fungus-derived chemotactic factors, and the products of activation of the alternate complement pathway, recruit neutrophils into the site of infection.[8] Oxidative metabolites generated by the phagocyte respiratory burst are fungicidal to *R. oryzae* hyphae.[15] Cationic proteins obtained from mammalian phagocytic cells, termed *defensins,* also have significant ability to kill *R. oryzae* spores and hyphae.[37] The exact roles of oxidative and nonoxidative fungicidal mechanisms in normal and altered immune states associated with mucormycosis have yet to be worked out.

There is no doubt that undefined defects of macrophages and neutrophils are involved in allowing the propagation of mucormycosis in a suitable host. Immunologically healthy individuals are not susceptible to mucormycosis and demonstrate the ability to clear spores from their lungs. The relative infrequency of reported cases of mucormycosis in AIDS underscores the importance of the neutrophil. However, more cases are being recognized in AIDS patients and may be attributable to prolonged longevity and the multiple immune defects that occur during later stages of disease, likely affecting neutrophils.[57]

The final phase in pathogenesis involves tissue invasion by hyphae and the progression toward blood vessels. Histopathologic characteristics include thrombosis and tissue necrosis after vascular penetration occurs.[41]

Clinical Manifestations

Patient factors influence the particular mucormycotic syndrome exhibited. Mucormycosis arises from the inhalation of airborne organisms that invade the nasal, tracheal, or gastrointestinal mucosa. Infection may remain localized in the lung or disseminate hematogenously.

Patients with pulmonary mucormycosis often present with fever and may have other symptoms similar to a bacterial infection such as cough, dyspnea, or pleuritic chest pain. Hemoptysis may develop secondary to continued tissue necrosis and blood vessel invasion, and bronchopleural fistula and fatal pulmonary hemorrhage may result. Radiographic findings include infiltrate or a mass and, less commonly, pulmonary consolidation, cavitation, or an effusion. Radiographic pulmonary lesions due to Mucorales may expand very rapidly, particularly in the immunocompromised host (Fig. 147-13). There is no specific lobar predilection, and a chest film is rarely suggestive of a fungal etiology. Spread to contiguous areas of the lung and to the mediastinum occurs.

Nosocomial mucormycosis in critically ill patients is an important, though rare, consequence of acute multiple-organ failure and invasive resuscitative measures. Corticosteroids, acidosis, parenteral alimentation, and broad-spectrum antibiotic therapy act in concert to provide suitable conditions for Mucorales to invade and proliferate. Assisted ventilation may promote the inhalation of spores or the aspiration of upper respiratory tract flora.

Some atypical presentations of pulmonary mucormycosis include disease in the absence of underlying systemic disease or predisposing factors,[39] solitary nodules in a diabetic, multiple mycotic pulmonary artery aneurysms and pseudoaneurysms,[12] bronchial obstruction, or in patients with a normal chest radiograph. A less fulminant, subacute clinical course is occasionally described in patients with diabetes mellitus, suggesting the need for aggressive diagnostic and therapeutic measures in patients who are at risk for this infection. Allergic *Rhizomucor* sinusitis affects immunocompetent individuals with or without nasal polyposis and is similar to the syndrome associated with *Aspergillus* sinusitis.[26]

Diagnosis

The diagnosis of mucormycosis requires a high index of suspicion and depends on demonstrating the organism in tissue. Routine laboratory studies are likely to be of low yield, and many specimens including blood, sputum, gastric fluid, and nose swabs are difficult to culture and often offer no diagnostic value. Spu-

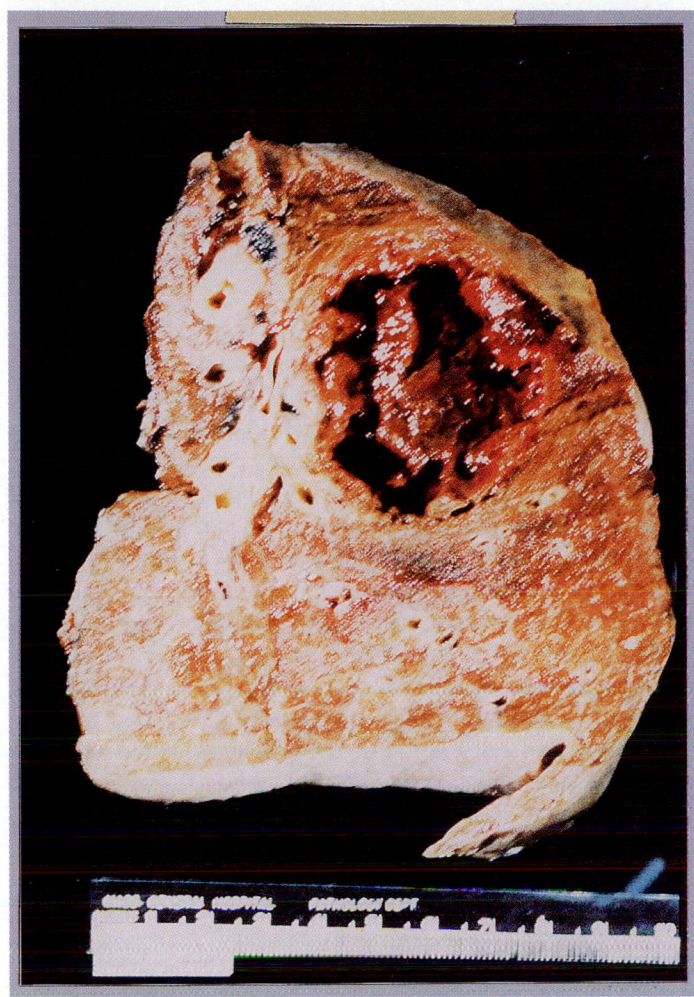

FIGURE 147-13 Pulmonary mucormycosis in 63-year-old diabetic renal transplant recipient with rapidly expanding pulmonary mass. *(Courtesy of Jay A. Fishman, Massachusetts General Hospital.)*

tum cultures are not reliable indicators of infection, since some species of Mucorales may occasionally be found in the sputum of individuals without clinical disease, and Gram's stain is not likely to be helpful.

In order to provide histopathologic evidence of invasive disease, bronchoscopy with transbronchial biopsy, percutaneous needle biopsy of the lung, or open lung biopsy must be employed. Touch slides prepared from the biopsy specimen with potassium hydroxide may reveal fungal hyphae. Hematoxylin-and-eosin-stained tissue sections will show the typical hyphae in infected tissue. These fungi stain poorly with the PAS and Gram's stains but very well by the Grocott's rapid silver stain. The use of lectin-binding stains on histologic preparations has been reported for the confirmation of the diagnosis of mucormycosis, but these are not widely available.

The fungi appear as broad (10 to 20 μm in diameter) nonseptate hyphae with branches occurring at right angles. Rarely, occasional septae can be visualized. During the handling of tissues hyphae may collapse and fold, giving the characteristic ribbon appearance. It is recommended not to grind tissue for culturing. The differentiation of *Aspergillus*, *Fusarium*, and

Pseudallescheria sub-species from Mucorales hyphae in tissue involves visualizing thinner, more regularly shaped fungal elements with more frequent acute angle branching and the presence of septae in the former group. Culture and identification of the fungi will provide the specific genus and species. Agents of mucormycosis are relatively difficult to isolate from infected tissue and are very rarely recovered from blood cultures.[41]

Tissue histology of Mucorales infection reveals a neutrophil infiltrate (in the nonneutropenic host), necrosis, and invasion of blood vessels with thrombosis. An inflammatory vasculitis involves arteries and veins, and in chronic cases mononuclear cell infiltration is observed with occasional giant cells. Serologic diagnosis by fungal antigen detection remains investigational, and no assay of sufficient sensitivity or specificity has been identified.

Mucormycosis, although a rarely encountered pathogen, is increasing in incidence and is potentially treatable. Aggressive diagnostic procedures including biopsy with histologic confirmation and culture may lead to earlier diagnosis and institution of treatment.

Treatment

Respiratory tract mucormycosis is an opportunistic infection that is virtually nonexistent in the immune-competent patient. Aggressive elimination of the compromising factors is the first and potentially most important therapeutic intervention. Rapid tapering of immunosuppressive drugs and corticosteroids should be carried out. Hyperglycemia and acidosis should be corrected, and neutropenia reversed if possible. The ultimate outcome of mucormycosis depends on the prognosis of the underlying disease.[41]

Amphotericin B is the standard therapy for mucormycosis, and high doses are recommended. Dosage range in this illness is 1.0 to 1.5 mg/kg per day in most patients. Alternate-day amphotericin B may be considered once the patient has stabilized. Liposomal formulations allow higher doses of amphotericin to be given, and reports indicate that successful outcomes were obtained in several patients with rhinocerebral mucormycosis treated with different liposomal amphotericin B preparations.[19] Further work to determine safety and efficacy of liposomal amphotericin B formulations in comparison to the standard preparation of amphotericin B needs to be completed, but at present it seems reasonable to use a liposomal preparation in patients not tolerating conventional amphotericin B.

Although a single case report of a cure of rhinocerebral mucormycosis with ketoconazole and rare case reports of response to fluconazole exist, Mucorales subspecies are generally resistant to the azole class of antifungals. The addition of other agents such as rifampin to amphotericin B in an attempt to obtain synergistic antifungal activity is controversial and cannot be recommended as standard therapy.[9] The application of in vitro susceptibility data for fungi to in vivo conditions of infection is difficult because the minimum inhibitory concentration for the organism depends on the specific conditions selected for the assay. Interpretation of in vitro susceptibility tests for single drugs is problematic for all filamentous fungi and often not useful in clinical decision making.[18]

Aggressive surgical debridement of necrotic tissue is an important intervention in the treatment of pulmonary mucormycosis. Removal of as much of the infected or devitalized tissue as possible while the infection is localized is of most benefit. Lobectomy is often required, and pneumonectomy may be necessary for proximal or extensive involvement. Repeated procedures may be needed. There is diminished benefit from pulmonary resection as dissemination occurs. The optimal combination and timing of therapy and surgery have not been resolved. Early diagnosis and institution of amphotericin B with surgical debridement has been successful in some patients, although most patients suffer a devastating downhill course with systemic deterioration regardless of interventions. Overall mortality was 80 percent in one study; in patients with disease confined to the lungs, the mortality was lower (65 percent), revealing a slight survival advantage with combined surgical intervention and medical therapy.

There is no recognized method for the prevention of systemic mucormycosis. High-efficiency particulate air filters have been shown to reduce the risks of aspergillosis and mucormycosis in neutropenic patients; however, overall mortality is unchanged and cost is prohibitive.

PULMONARY CANDIDIASIS

Candida albicans is a very common skin, oral, and gastrointestinal saprophyte that frequently invades the compromised host. *Candida glabrata,* formerly *Torulopsis glabrata,* is an opportunistic yeast that has many characteristics in common with *C. albicans* infection in the compromised host. *C. glabrata* pneumonia often accompanies fungemia and disseminated disease and is a particularly common secondary invader. Radiographic signs are indistinguishable from those found in infection with *C. albicans.*

C. tropicalis has been associated with disseminated infection in neutropenic patients and may be more pathogenic than other *Candida* species. *C. parapsilosis* seems to be the least pathogenic of the common types of *Candida* that cause fungemia. The virulence factors involved in the pathogenesis of *Candida* infections remain unclear.

Pulmonary *Candida* infections may present as a manifestation of disseminated candidiasis by hematogenous spread or as a primary bronchial or pulmonary process from the airway.[46] The latter condition appears to be rare, although the true incidence is unknown because there are no established and reliable methods for making the diagnosis.[10] Histopathologic findings from biopsy or autopsy material provide a definitive diagnosis.[46]

Epidemiology

Candida is widespread in the environment and a human commensal. The fungus is found in the human gastrointestinal tract, in the female genital tract, and on the skin. Alterations of the usual distribution and low colony counts of yeasts occur when the normal microbial flora is diminished by antibiotic therapy or when host defenses are impaired (see Chapter 119). A patient's own normal flora may therefore become the source of the *Candida* species that becomes invasive. Intravenous catheters and indwelling bladder catheters are common portals of entry. Indwelling intravenous catheters in place for total parenteral nutrition are particularly associated with the hematogenous spread of *Candida.*

Multiple immune defects observed in some premature neonates and in the elderly may also predispose to invasion by *Candida.* Normal hosts have only rarely been reported to develop *Candida* pneumonia, and most reported cases are in immunocompromised individuals.[53] The incidence of primary pulmonary candidiasis acquired by the endobronchial route is difficult to estimate, since the portal of entry for infection is often unclear.[46]

Pathogenesis

Defense against *Candida* requires an intact immune system, particularly polymorphonuclear leukocytes (PMNs). *Candida* pulmonary infection occurs in chemotherapy-induced neutropenia, chronic granulomatous disease with myeloperoxidase deficiency, corticosteroid therapy, and diabetes mellitus. Maintenence of bacterial flora is an important defense that is frequently affected by antibiotic therapy as well as by other host factors such as nutrition and systemic illness. An immunocompromised state may be produced by the disruption of normal barriers, such as a surgical wound site or by gastrointestinal tract disuse or blind loops (Roux en Y) allowing fungi to penetrate the mucosa.[10] Drugs for induction of immunosuppression for organ or bone marrow transplantation specifically diminish lymphocyte function and have been associated with *Candida* pulmonary infection. Table 147-6 lists some of the predisposing factors for *Candida* infection.

Experimental pulmonary candidiasis in the rabbit model reveals that PMNs play the initial role in the host response, followed by macrophages and granuloma formation. The addition of corticosteroids results in the proliferation of *Candida,* with the production of greater numbers of pseudohyphae. Within the infected lungs a less cellular and more necrotic response is noted in corticosteroid-treated animals.[46]

Clinical Manifestations

Persistent fever is the most common clinical feature of *Candida* pulmonary disease. Patients may present without symptoms but subsequently develop symptoms of pneumonia (cough, sputum production, chest pain, and dyspnea). Physical exam and routine laboratory studies are often unremarkable. Chest radiographs may demonstrate a local or diffuse infiltrate involving

---

TABLE 147-6

Predisposing Factors for *Candida* Pneumonia

Abdominal surgery, trauma, mucosal erosion, or peptic ulceration with perforation of the gastrointestinal tract

Indwelling catheters for intravenous alimentation, peritoneal dialysis, urinary tract drainage

Intravenous drug use

High-dose, prolonged corticosteroid administration

Broad-spectrum antibiotic therapy

Neutropenia or hematologic malignancy

Diabetes mellitus

Colonization of multiple sites with *Candida*

one or both lungs, more often associated with infection acquired by the endobronchial route. A miliary–nodular pattern is more often associated with hematogenous seeding of the lung in disseminated candidiasis and often appears late in the clinical course of disease.[46]

Extrapulmonary manifestations such as skin lesions, myositis, or endophthalmitis may be the first signs of *Candida* fungemia. Multiple organ involvement prior to or concurrent with pulmonary findings, particularly kidney and myocardial failure, may indicate hematogenous seeding that warrants investigation.

Lung transplant patients may manifest an early (within 2 weeks) and fulminant *Candida* pneumonia. The association is probably due to occult aspiration in the donor followed by invasive pulmonary *Candida* infection after transplantation when immunosuppression is most intense.[65]

A number of other forms of pulmonary disease have been described, including acute or chronic bronchitis and allergic asthma.[35] Allergic bronchopulmonary candidiasis is a syndrome with a course and immunologic findings consistent with APBA, presenting with asthma, positive sputum culture for *C. albicans*, fleeting pulmonary infiltrates, immediate skin reactivity to *C. albicans* antigen, precipitating antibody against *C. albicans* antigen, elevated serum IgE concentration, and elevated serum IgE and IgG antibody against *C. albicans*.[2] A significant decrease was observed in serum IgE levels and IgE antibody against *C. albicans* after corticosteroid treatment for 3 months. Allergic bronchopulmonary candidiasis should be considered in patients with this syndrome and negative serologic and skin tests to *Aspergillus*. Early diagnosis and treatment may prevent late fibrosis.

Diagnosis

The diagnosis of pulmonary candidiasis depends on convincing evidence that tissue invasion is present. Accordingly, *Candida* infections of the bronchi and the lungs are difficult to diagnose definitively.[46] The isolation of yeast from sputum does not prove the presence of yeast in the respiratory tract, due to contamination with commensals from the oropharynx—*Candida* is present in the oropharynx of approximately 20 percent of all patients with chronic lung disease. In the case of hematogenous spread of *Candida*, the sputum often does not show yeast on Gram's stain. Chest radiograph findings are nonspecific and occasionally normal. Serology to detect *Candida* antigen or metabolites of *Candida* in serum or other body fluids is currently not helpful. Isolation of *Candida* from the blood may be helpful in disseminated disease. Lysis centrifugation blood cultures are the most sensitive and rapid way to recover *Candida* from blood. CT scans of the abdomen may suggest invasive hepatosplenic candidiasis in compromised hosts with an unrevealing microbiologic evaluation.

Bronchial washings or bronchoalveolar lavage provide a more representative picture of the respiratory pathology; however, they can still be contaminated with mouth flora. Aspirates through tracheostomies often reveal colonization with yeast and may be misleading. However, if other organisms are absent and abundant *Candida* pseudohyphae are present, clinical suspicion of invasive candidiasis should be high. In neutropenic patients, typi-

cal bronchial epithelial cells and the absence of normal pharyngeal flora are suggestive but not diagnostic.[10]

Tissue invasion by *Candida* demonstrated on open lung biopsy histopathology is definitive, although such biopsy is difficult to perform in neutropenic patients with pneumonia. Gram's stain, KOH smear, and culture of lung tissue are only supportive of the diagnosis. Transbronchial biopsy revealing tissue invasion by *Candida* is an indication for treatment. Percutaneous needle biopsy and aspirate can be used to provide direct microscopic evidence for infection, although sampling for culture has been of little value.[46]

Treatment

The mainstay of treatment has been amphotericin B, and like other opportunistic infections, reversal of the factors affecting the immune status of the individual is crucial. Removal of indwelling intravenous lines or urinary catheters, in the setting of hematogenous spread, is also very important.

Amphotericin B in doses from 0.5 mg/kg per day may be given; total dosage and duration of therapy are unclear. However, 1.5 to 3.0 gm over 2 to 4 weeks is a general guideline. In one study, patients with candidemia, of whom some had pneumonia, benefited by the addition of flucytosine to amphotericin B.[31] The known adverse affects of flucytosine may limit its use in critically ill immunosuppressed patients. The combination of rifampin with amphotericin B has shown synergy in vitro, but controlled studies have not been done to demonstrate increased efficacy of the addition of rifampin.[16]

Fluconazole has been shown effective for cryptococcal meningitis in AIDS patients, oropharyngeal candidiasis in patients with malignancy, hepatosplenic candidiasis, and candidemia.[51] Fluconazole offers many advantages, and studies in fungemic patients are ongoing to evaluate its efficacy. However, its use in *Candida* pulmonary disease has not been well studied. A decision to use fluconazole for this indication should be made on a case-by-case basis. Initiation of therapy with amphotericin B rather than fluconazole may be appropriate in the debilitated or critically ill patient with disseminated infection due to *Candida* subspecies.

Extensive studies are underway with various preparations of liposome-encapsulated amphotericin B. These preparations (AmBisome, Amphotericin B lipid complex, amphotericin B colloidal dispersion) are better tolerated than conventional amphotericin B, even in much higher daily doses (up to 5 mg/kg per day), but randomized, controlled studies of efficacy and pharmacokinetics of these agents are needed. These new amphotericin formulations should be useful in patients who cannot tolerate conventional amphotericin B.

Prophylaxis of *Candida* pulmonary infection is not well studied. Ketoconazole and fluconazole have been efficacious in preventing oral *Candida* infections in cancer patients and AIDS patients and have lowered the incidence of deep fungal infections in patients undergoing bone marrow transplants.[27] Routine use of these agents have, however, enhanced the emergence of azole-resistant *Candida* species. Prophylaxis of pulmonary candidiasis is best achieved by eliminating or limiting those factors that predispose patients to *Candida* colonization and aspiration.

REFERENCES

1. Aisner J, Murillo J, Schimpff SC, et al: Invasive aspergillosis in acute leukemia: Correlation with nose cultures and antibiotic use. *Ann Intern Med* 90:4–9, 1979.

2. Akiyama K, Mathison DA, Riker JB, et al: Allergic bronchopulmonary candidiasis. *Chest* 85:699–701, 1984.

3. Albelda SM, Talbot GH, Gerson SL, et al: Pulmonary cavitation and massive hemoptysis in invasive pulmonary aspergillosis. *Am Rev Respir Dis* 131:115–120, 1985.

4. Angus RM, Davies M-L, Cowan MD, et al: Computed tomographic scanning of the lung in patients with allergic bronchopulmonary aspergillosis and in asthmatic patients with a positive skin test to *Aspergillus fumigatus. Thorax* 49:586–589, 1994.

5. Binder RE, Faling LJ, Pugatch RD, et al: Chronic necrotizing pulmonary aspergillosis: A discrete clinical entity. *Medicine* 61:109–124, 1982.

6. Boelaert JE, de Locht M, Van Cutsem J, et al: Mucormycosis during deferoxamine therapy is a siderophore-mediated infection. In vitro and in vivo animal studies. *J Clin Invest* 91:1979–1986, 1993.

7. British Thoracic and Tuberculosis Association Report: Aspergilloma and residual tuberculosis cavities: The result of a resurvey. *Tubercle* 51:227–245, 1970.

8. Chinn RYW, Diamond RD: Generation of chemotactic factors by *Rhizopus oryzae* in the presence and absence of serum: Relationship to hyphal damage mediated by human neutrophils and effects of hyperglycemia and ketoacidosis. *Infect Immun* 38:1123–1129, 1982.

9. Christenson JC, Shalit I, Welch DF, et al: Synergistic action of amphotericin B and rifampin against *Rhizopus* species. *Antimicrob Agents Chemother* 31:1775–1778, 1987.

10. Chu FE, Armstrong D: *Candida* species pneumonia, in Sarosi GA, Davies SF (eds), *Fungal Diseases of the Lung,* 2d ed. New York, Raven Press, 1993, pp 125–131.

11. Clee MD, Lamb D, Clark RA: Bronchocentric granulomatosis: A review and thoughts on pathogenesis. *Br J Dis Chest* 77:227–234, 1983.

12. Coffey MJ, Fantone J, Stirling MC, Lynch JP: Pseudoaneurysm of pulmonary artery in mucormycosis. Radiographic characteristics and management. *Am Rev Respir Dis* 145:1487–1490, 1992.

13. Denning DW, Follansbee SE, Scolaro M, et al: Pulmonary aspergillosis in the acquired immunodeficiency syndrome. *New Engl J Med* 324:654–662, 1991.

14. Denning DW, Stevens DA: Antifungal and surgical treatment of invasive aspergillosis: Review of 2,121 published cases. *Rev Infect Dis* 12:1147–1201, 1990.

15. Diamond RD, Haudenschild CC, Erickson NF III: Monocyte-mediated damage to *Rhizopus oryzae* hyphae in vitro. *Infect Immun* 38:292–297, 1982.

16. Edwards JE, Morrison J, Henderson DK, et al: Combined effect of amphotericin B and rifampin on *Candida* species. *Antimicrob Agents Chemother* 14:484–488, 1980.

17. Ellis M, Friend J: Progressive lung disease in a maltworker. *Thorax* 36:552–553, 1981.

18. Eng RHK, Person A, Mangura C, et al: Susceptibility of zygomycetes to amphotericin B, miconazole, and ketoconazole. *Antimicrob Agents Chemother* 20:688–690, 1981.

19. Ericsson M, Anniko M, Gustafsson H, et al: A case of chronic progressive rhinocerebral mucormycosis treated with liposomal amphotericin B and surgery. *Clin Infect Dis* 16:585–586, 1993.

20. Fisher BD, Armstrong D, Yu B, Gold JWM: Invasive aspergillosis. Progress in early diagnosis and treatment. *Am J Med* 71:571–577, 1981.

21. Gerson SE, Talbot GH, Hurwitz S, et al: Prolonged granulocytopenia: The major risk factor for invasive pulmonary aspergillosis in patients with acute leukemia. *Ann Intern Med* 100:345–351, 1984.

22. Girardin H, Sarfati J, Traore F, et al: Molecular epidemiology of nosocomial invasive aspergillosis. *J Clin Micro* 32:684–690, 1994.

23. Giron JM, Poey CG, Fajadet PP, et al: Inoperable pulmonary aspergilloma: Percutaneous CT-guided injection with glycerin and amphotericin B paste in 15 cases. *Radiology* 188:825–827, 1993.

24. Glimp RA, Bayer AS: Pulmonary aspergilloma. Diagnostic and therapeutic considerations. *Arch Intern Med* 143:303–308, 1983.

25. Goldberg B: Radiologic appearances in pulmonary aspergillosis. *Clin Radiol* 13:106, 1962.

26. Goldstein MF, Dvorin DJ, Dunsky EH, et al: Allergic *Rhizomucor* sinusitis. *J Allergy Clin Immunol* 90:394–404, 1992.

27. Goodman JL, Winston DJ, Greenfield RA, et al: A controlled trial of fluconazole to prevent fungal infections in patients undergoing bone marrow transplant. *New Engl J Med* 326:845–851, 1992.

28. Hammerman KJ, Christianson CS, Huntington I, et al: Spontaneous lysis of aspergillomata. *Chest* 64:697–699, 1973.

29. Herold CJ, Kramer J, Sertl K, et al: Invasive pulmonary aspergillosis: Evaluation with MR imaging. *Radiology* 173:717–721, 1989.

30. Hinson KFW, Moon AJ, Plummer NS: Broncho-pulmonary aspergillosis. A review and a report of eight new cases. *Thorax* 7:317–333, 1952.

31. Horn R, Wong B, Kiehn TE, Armstrong D: Fungemia in a cancer hospital: Changing frequency, earlier onset, and results of therapy. *Rev Infect Dis* 7:646–655, 1985.

32. Jackson M, Flower CDR, Shneerson JM: Treatment of symptomatic pulmonary aspergillomas with intracavitary instillation of amphotericin B through an indwelling catheter. *Thorax* 48:928–930, 1993.

33. Jeffery GM, Beard MEJ, Ikram RB, et al: Intranasal amphotericin B reduces the frequency of invasive aspergillosis in neutropenic patients. *Am J Med* 90:685–692, 1991.

34. Kauffman HF, Tomee JFC, van der Werf TS, et al: Review of fungus-induced asthmatic reactions. *Am J Respir Crit Care Med* 151:2109–2116, 1995.

35. Keeney EL: *Candida* asthma. *Ann Intern Med* 34:223, 1951.

36. Lentino JR, Rosenkranz MA, Michaels JA, et al: Nosocomial aspergillosis. A retrospective review of airborne disease secondary to road construction and contaminated air conditioners. *Am J Epidemiol* 116:430–437, 1982.

37. Levitz SM, Selsted ME, Ganz T, et al: In vitro killing of spores and hyphae of *Aspergillus fumigatus* and *Rhizopus oryzae* by rabbit neutrophil cationic peptides and bronchoalveolar macrophages. *J Infect Dis* 154:483–489, 1986.

38. Liebow AA: The J Burns Amberson Lecture—pulmonary angiitis and granulomatosis. *Am Rev Respir Dis* 108:1–18, 1973.

39. Matsushima T, Soejima R, Nakashima T: Solitary pulmonary nodule caused by phycomycosis in a patient without obvious predisposing factors. *Thorax* 35:877–878, 1980.

40. Mendelson EB, Fisher MR, Mintzer RA, et al: Radiographic and clinical staging of allergic bronchopulmonary aspergillosis. *Chest* 87:334–339, 1985.

41. Meyer RD, Rosen P, Armstrong D: Phycomycosis complicating leukemia and lymphoma. *Ann Intern Med* 77:871–879, 1972.

42. Miller WT Jr, Sais GJ, Frank I, et al: Pulmonary aspergillosis in patients with AIDS. *Chest* 105:37–44, 1994.

43. Mintzer RA, Rogers LF, Kruglik GD, et al: The spectrum of radiologic findings in allergic bronchopulmonary aspergillosis. *Radiology* 127:301–307, 1978.

44. Moser M, Crameri R, Brust E, et al: Clinical aspects of allergic disease. Diagnostic value of recombinant Aspergillus fumigatus allergen I/a for skin testing and serology. *J Allergy Clin Immunol* 93:1–11, 1994.

45. Murray HW: Pulmonary mucormycosis with massive fatal hemoptysis. *Chest* 68:65–68, 1975.

46. Odds FC: Candida *and Candidosis. A Review and Bibliography,* 2d ed. London, Bailliere Tindall, 1988.

47. Orr DP, Myerowitz RL, Dubois PJ: Patho-radiologic correlation of invasive pulmonary aspergillosis in the compromised host. *Cancer* 41:2028, 1978.

48. Patterson R, Greenberger PA, Radin RC, Roberts M: Allergic bronchopulmonary aspergillosis: Staging as an aid to management. *Ann Intern Med* 96:286–291, 1982.

49. Pizzo PA, Robichaud KJ, Gill FA, et al: Empiric antibiotic and antifungal therapy for cancer patients with prolonged fever and granulocytopenia. *Am J Med* 72:101, 1982.

50. Rabin ER, Lundberg GD, Mitchell ET: Mucormycosis in severely burned patients. *New Engl J Med* 264:1286–1289, 1961.

51. Rex JH, Bennett JE, Sugar AM, et al: A randomized trial comparing fluconazole with amphotericin B for the treatment of candidemia in patients without neutropenia. *New Engl J Med* 331:1325–1330, 1994.

52. Roig J, Ruiz J, Puig X, et al: Bronchial stump aspergillosis four years after lobectomy. *Chest* 104:295–296, 1993.

53. Rosenbaum RB, Barber JV, Stevens DA: *Candida albicans* pneumonia. Diagnosis by pulmonary aspiration, recovery without treatment. *Am Rev Respir Dis* 109:373–378, 1974.

54. Rosenberg M, Patterson R, Roberts M, Wang J: The assessment of immunologic and clinical changes occurring during corticosteroid therapy for allergic bronchopulmonary aspergillosis. *Am J Med* 64:599–606, 1978.

55. St. Georgiev V: Treatment and developmental therapeutics in aspergillosis: 2. Azoles and other antifungal drugs. *Respiration* 59:303–313, 1992.

56. Sawasaki H, Horie K, Yamada M, et al: Bronchial stump aspergillosis: Experimental and clinical study. *J Thorac Cardiovasc Surg* 58:198–208, 1969.

57. Smith AG, Bustamante CI, Gilmor GD: Zygomycosis (absidiomycosis) in an AIDS patient. *Mycopathologia* 105:7–10, 1989.

58. Sugar AM: Agents of mucormycosis and related species, in Mandell GL, Bennett JE, Dolin R (eds), *Mandell, Douglas and Bennett's Principles and Practice of Infectious Diseases,* sec. G, *Mycoses,* vol 2. New York, Churchill Livingstone, 1995, pp 2311–2321.

59. Talbot GH, Weiner MH, Gerson SL, et al: Serodiagnosis of invasive aspergillosis in patients with hematologic malignancy: Validation of the *Aspergillus fumigatus* antigen radioimmunoassay. *J Infect Dis* 155:12–27, 1987.

60. Waldorf AR, Levitz SM, Diamond RD: In vivo bronchoalveolar macrophage defense against *Rhizopus oryzae* and *Aspergillus fumigatus. J Infect Dis* 150:752, 1984.

61. Waldorf AR, Ruderman N, Diamond RD: Specific susceptibility to mucormycosis in murine diabetes and bronchoalveolar macrophage defense against *Rhizopus. J Clin Invest* 74:150–160, 1984.

62. Wang JLF, Patterson R, Rosenberg M, et al: Serum IgE and IgG antibody activity against *Aspergillus fumigatus* as a diagnostic aid in allergic bronchopulmonary aspergillosis. *Am Rev Respir Dis* 117:917–927, 1978.

63. Wardlaw A, Geddes DM: Allergic bronchopulmonary aspergillosis: A review. *J Royal Soc Med* 85:747–751, 1992.

64. Young RC, Bennett JE, Vogel CL, et al: Aspergillosis. The spectrum of disease in 98 patients. *Medicine* 49:147–173, 1970.

65. Zenati M, Dowling RD, Dummer JS, et al: Influence of the donor lung on development of early infections in lung transplant recipients. *J Heart Transplant* 9:502–509, 1990.

CHAPTER 148

ENDEMIC MYCOSES OF NORTH AMERICA: HISTOPLASMOSIS, COCCIDIOIDOMYCOSIS, AND BLASTOMYCOSIS

L. Joseph Wheat

The endemic mycoses are restricted geographically, based on environmental and other factors that favor the growth of these organisms in the soil. Histoplasmosis and blastomycosis mostly afflict patients in the Mississippi and Ohio river valleys, while coccidioidomycosis occurs primarily in the desert of the southwestern United States. These mycoses are increasing in importance as causes for opportunistic disease in immunocompromised patients, including those with AIDS. Advances in diagnosis and treatment provide opportunities to improve the outcome of these patients. Preventive strategies are under investigation.

HISTOPLASMOSIS

Histoplasmosis is the most common of the endemic mycoses and a major cause of morbidity in patients who live in endemic areas. It has emerged as an important complication of AIDS. Understanding of the clinical syndromes and untreated course of the infections is essential in the diagnosis of histoplasmosis and the management of patients with the disease. Improved laboratory tests have made it possible to diagnose severe cases more rapidly. Expanded treatment options are available with triazole antifungal agents and liposomal formulations of amphotericin B.

Mycology

Histoplasma capsulatum grows as a mold (Fig. 148-1) in the soil and is found primarily in microfoci containing large amounts of rotted bird or bat guano. Microconidia measuring 2 to 5 μm in diameter are the infectious particles in the mold phase of the organism. At temperatures above 35°C, *H. capsulatum* grows as a yeast, which is the pathogenic form that infects tissues (Fig. 148-1).

Epidemiology

H. capsulatum is endemic in areas of North and Latin America (Fig. 148-2),[11] but it can be found throughout the world. Factors accounting for its geographic distribution include humid environmental conditions and acidic, permeable soil characteristics.

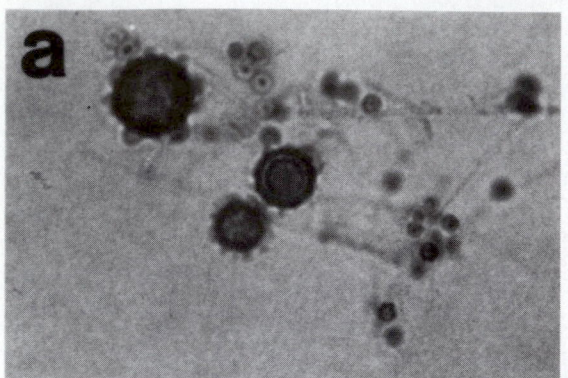

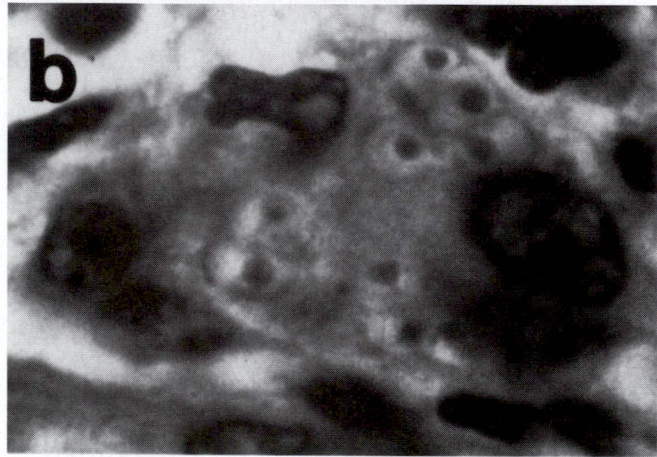

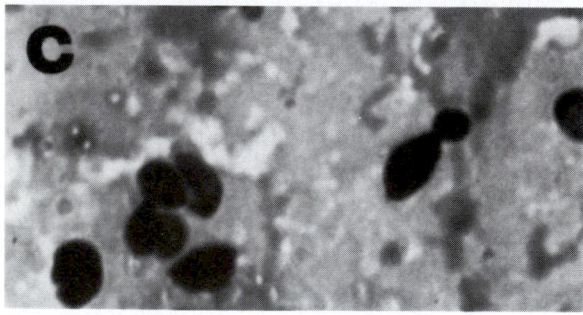

FIGURE 148-1 Fungal stains showing mold by lactol phenol cotton blue stain (A) and yeast by H&E stain (B) and by methenamine-silver stain (C). *(From Wheat,[50] with permission.)*

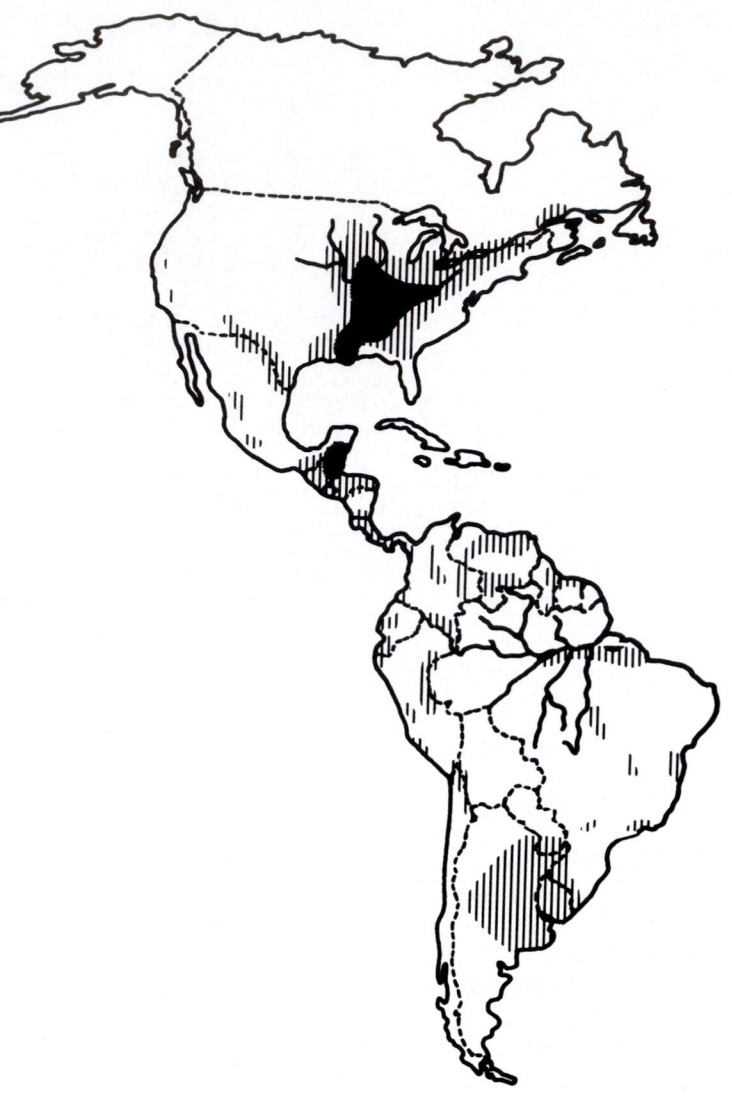

FIGURE 148-2 Endemic distribution of histoplasmosis in the Americas. The highest incidence is in the finely stippled area of North and Central America. *(From Rippon,[36] with permission.)*

Bird and bat excrement enhance growth of the organism in soil by accelerating sporulation. Reactivation of latent infection may account for some cases in persons with previous histoplasmosis who become immunocompromised.

Pathogenesis

Infection develops when conidia are inhaled and germinate into yeasts or when old foci of infection reactivate. Cellular immunity plays the key role in defense against *H. capsulatum*. With development of specific T-cell–mediated immunity, cytokines, including γ-interferon and interleukin-12, activate macrophages to kill the fungus and halt progression of the disease. These defense mechanisms are sufficient to control the

infection in immunocompetent subjects, explaining the subclinical or self-limited course characteristic of acute histoplasmosis.

Clinical Manifestations

Most clinically recognized infections are self-limited.[39,60] The common self-limited presentations include acute pulmonary histoplasmosis, pericarditis,[59] and rheumatologic syndromes (Fig. 148-3).[37]

ACUTE PULMONARY HISTOPLASMOSIS

Most patients present with symptoms of fever, cough, and retrosternal or pleuritic chest pain. Chest radiographs show mediastinal lymphadenopathy with patchy infiltrates (Fig. 148-4). In rare instances, cavitation occurs in acute pulmonary histoplasmosis. Patients recover in a few weeks but may experience fatigue for months.

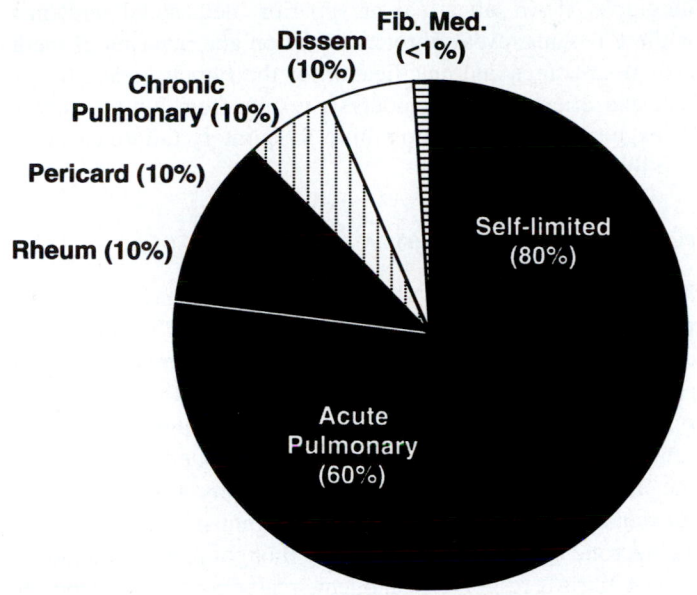

FIGURE 148-3   Distribution of clinical manifestations of histoplasmosis based on analysis of symptomatic cases identified during recurrent outbreaks in Indianapolis. *(From Wheat et al.,[58] with permission.)*

Following heavy exposure, patients present with diffuse pulmonary impairment, which often causes respiratory insufficiency (Fig. 148-5).[23] Patients may present with obstructive symptoms resulting from enlarged mediastinal lymph nodes.[25]

RHEUMATOLOGIC SYNDROMES

Patients with acute histoplasmosis may experience arthritis or arthralgia accompanied by erythema nodosum.[37] Chest radiographs usually show findings typical of acute pulmonary histoplasmosis, but they may be normal. Symptoms are best managed by treatment with anti-inflammatory agents but may recur when treatment is stopped.

PERICARDITIS

Pericarditis is another inflammatory complication of acute self-limited histoplasmosis, occurring in less than 10 percent of cases.[59] Chest radiographs usually show mediastinal lymphadenopathy and an increase in the cardiac silhouette (Fig. 148-4). Patients typically respond to anti-inflammatory treatment, but up to one-fourth of them exhibit pericardial tamponade. Late constriction is rare.

CHRONIC PULMONARY HISTOPLASMOSIS

Chronic pulmonary histoplasmosis occurs in patients with underlying lung disease and is characterized by recurrent symptoms, progressive lung infiltrates, fibrosis, and cavitation.[19,60] Upper-lobe infiltrates are present in nearly all cases, and cavities are found in most (Fig. 148-6). Progression is manifested by cavity enlargement, formation of new cavities, spread to new ar-

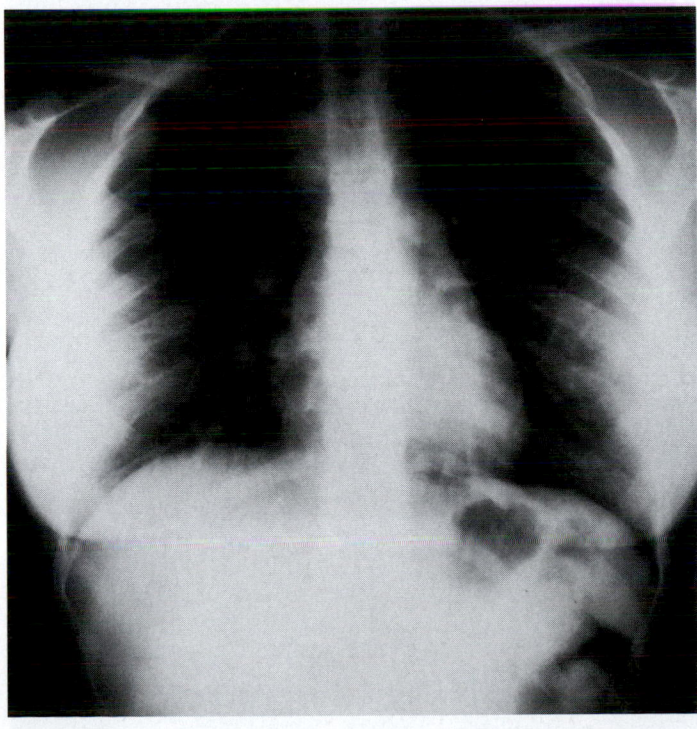

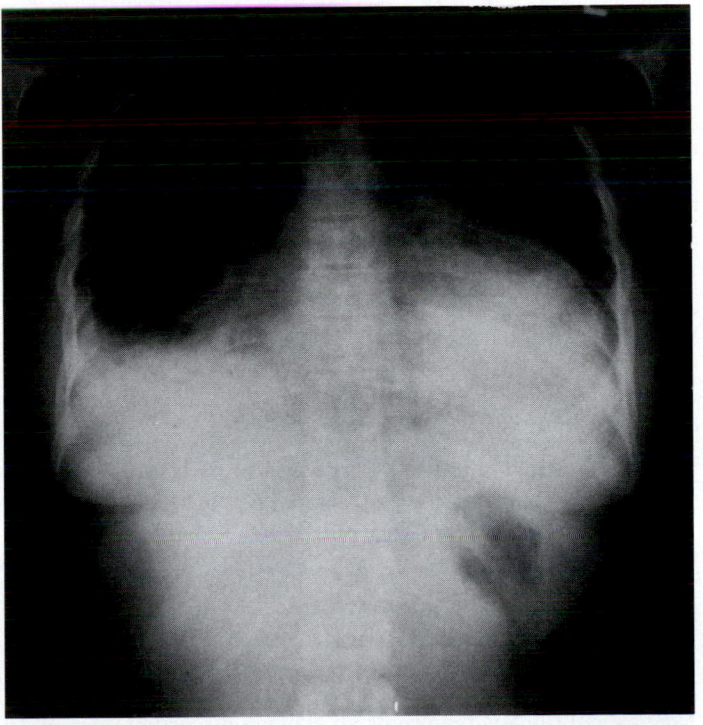

A

B

FIGURE 148-4   Chest radiogram showing right paratracheal lymphadenopathy (left) in a patient with chest pain and cough who 2 weeks later presented with pericardial tamponade caused by *Histoplasma* pericarditis. *(From Wheat,[51] with permission.)*

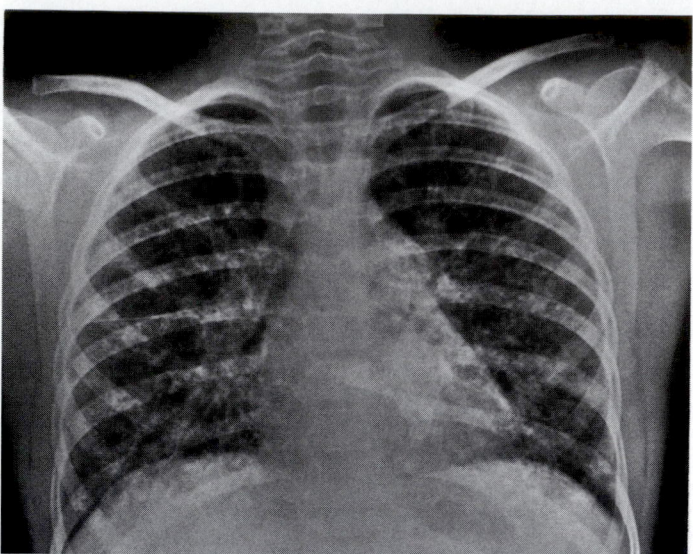

FIGURE 148-5 Chest radiograms showing miliary reticulonodular pattern characteristic of disseminated or heavy-inoculum pulmonary histoplasmosis.

eas of the lungs, and bronchopleural fistulas. Aspergilloma, bacterial infection, and malignancy also must be considered in evaluation of new masses or infiltrates in patients with chronic pulmonary histoplasmosis.

DISSEMINATED HISTOPLASMOSIS

Progressive disseminated histoplasmosis occurs in about one in 2000 acute infections,[39] usually in patients who are immunosuppressed or at the extremes of age. Fever and weight loss are the most common symptoms. Examination reveals hepatomegaly or splenomegaly in about half of cases and lymphadenopathy in a third. A sepsis presentation with shock, respiratory, hepatic, and renal failure, and coagulopathy may complicate severe cases.[54] Meningitis or focal brain lesions occur in 10 to 20 percent of cases.[53] Other common sites of dissemination are the oral mucosa, skin, and adrenal glands, seen in 5 to 10 percent of cases. Chest radiographs are abnormal in 70 percent of patients, usually showing diffuse interstitial or reticulonodular infiltrates (Fig. 148-5).

BRONCHOLITHIASIS

Lymph nodes and pulmonary granulomas calcify and may erode into adjacent bronchi, causing hemoptysis or obstruction.[2] Patients may expectorate rocklike particles of tissue and experience recurrent and severe hemoptysis, bronchial obstruction, or tracheoesophageal fistula.

MEDIASTINAL FIBROSIS

Mediastinal fibrosis represents an exuberant scarring reaction to prior histoplasmosis.[18,25] Mediastinal structures commonly affected are the superior vena cava, airways, pulmonary arteries or veins, and esophagus.[18,25] Fibrosis may invade the thoracic duct, recurrent laryngeal nerve, or, in rare cases, the atrium. Chest ra-

diographs show subcarinal or superior mediastinal widening, while CT scans reveal fibrotic restriction and invasion of mediastinal structures and calcification of the lymph nodes. Recurrent and often serious hemoptysis results from lung or airway damage and vascular compromise. Respiratory failure ensues in one-third of cases.

PULMONARY HISTOPLASMOMA

Patients may develop a slowly enlarging pulmonary nodule, which has been called "enlarging histoplasmoma."[20] These range in diameter from 8 to 35 mm and enlarge an average of 2 mm per year. Although these lesions are not associated with clinical symptoms, they may lead to concern about malignancy. Calcification occurs in the necrotic central and surrounding fibrous tissue. Histologically, they are characterized by a necrotic center surrounded by a fibrouslike capsule. Organisms may be seen in the necrotic center. These lesions are thought to represent an excessive fibrosis response to antigenic materials released from the central core into the surrounding tissue rather than progressive infection, a similar mechanism to that postulated for fibrosing mediastinitis. Results of serologic tests or cultures were not presented, but they probably would be negative in most cases on the basis of experience in patients with fibrosing mediastinitis or solitary coin lesions.[20] Antifungal treatment would not be expected to alter the course of enlarging histoplasmomas and probably is not indicated.

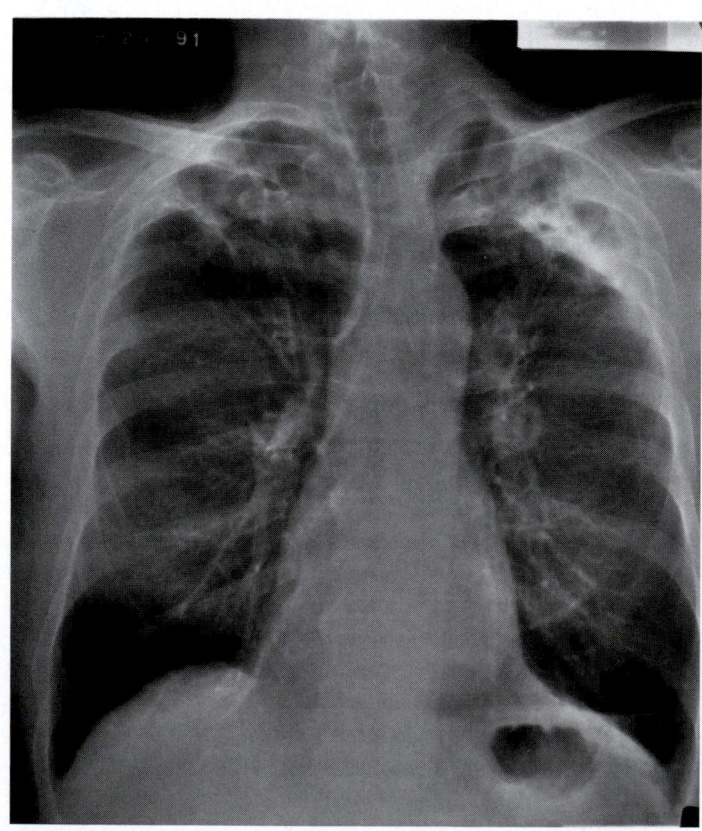

FIGURE 148-6 Chest radiogram showing fibronodular upper-lobe infiltrates in a patient with emphysema complicated by chronic pulmonary histoplasmosis. (*From Wheat,[52] with permission.*)

Diagnosis

Diagnostic modalities include cultures, fungal stains of tissue or body fluids, and tests for antibodies and antigens. The role of each test varies with the severity of the infection.[61] Serologic tests for antibodies form the basis for diagnosis in most patients with mild infections, whereas use of a battery of tests is needed in patients with more severe disease. Diagnosis can be established from culture or serologic testing for antibodies in most patients with chronic pulmonary histoplasmosis.

ANTIGEN DETECTION

Detection of antigen in the body fluids offers a valuable approach to diagnosis in severe cases, including those with disseminated and extensive pulmonary histoplasmosis,[57,61] providing results within 24 to 48 h. Antigen is found in the blood, urine, and bronchoalveolar lavage fluid of most patients with disseminated histoplasmosis and in up to 75 percent of those with diffuse lung invasion during acute pulmonary histoplasmosis. Antigen may be found in CSF of 25 to 50 percent of patients with chronic meningitis caused by histoplasmosis.

Positive results caused by cross-reacting antigens occur in patients with African histoplasmosis, blastomycosis, paracoccidioidomycosis, and *Penicillium marneffii* infection. Cross reactions have not been recognized in patients with more common fungal infections, such as candidiasis, cryptococcosis, aspergillosis, or coccidioidomycosis.

Antigen levels decline during the first year after treatment or spontaneously in patients with self-limited histoplasmosis and increase with relapse,[55] providing a tool for monitoring therapy.[55] Antigen testing is available only at the Histoplasmosis Reference Laboratory.

FUNGAL STAIN

Fungal staining permits rapid diagnosis but with a lower sensitivity than culture or antigen detection. The highest yield is from bone marrow.[39,54] *H. capsulatum* may be seen in peripheral blood smears in patients with severe disease. *Pneumocystis carinii*, *Candida glabrata*, *Blastomyces dermatitidis*, *Toxoplasma gondii*, and *P. marneffii* may be misidentified as *H. capsulatum*. Less experienced pathologists also may mistake staining artifacts for *H. capsulatum*.

FUNGAL CULTURES

Cultures provide the strongest proof for histoplasmosis but are limited by low sensitivity (10 to 15 percent) in self-limited infections and delayed growth (2 to 4 weeks).[61] In disseminated histoplasmosis, the highest yield is from bone marrow or blood—positive in more than 75 percent of cases.[39,54] In cavitary histoplasmosis, organisms can be found in sputum or bronchoscopy specimens in 60 to 85 percent of cases. Several specimens must be cultured to achieve the highest yield.[61] Cultures usually are negative in patients with mild acute pulmonary, pericardial, or rheumatogic manifestations and need not be performed.[61]

SEROLOGIC TESTS

Serologic tests are very useful but require familiarity with their limitations. Antibodies to *H. capsulatum* measured by immunodiffusion or complement fixation develop in most patients. Limitations of tests for antibodies include a 4 to 8-week delay in diagnosis while antibodies are being produced after acute infection, false-negative results in immunocompromised patients, and false-positive results in patients with blastomycosis, coccidioidomycosis, and paracoccidioidomycosis. Also, antibodies that persist after an earlier episode of histoplasmosis may cause confusion in patients with other diseases, such as malignancy, aspergilloma, or mycobacterial lung disease.

HISTOPLASMIN SKIN TEST

Skin tests are not useful diagnostically because of high background rates of skin test positivity (50 to 80 percent) in endemic areas, false-positive results in patients with other fungal diseases, and false-negative results in patients with disseminated disease.[11] Furthermore, skin tests boost antibody levels, compromising interpretation of serologic tests.

Treatment
ACUTE SYNDROMES

Diffuse Pulmonary
Patients with acute pulmonary histoplasmosis causing hypoxia benefit from antifungal therapy and adjunctive corticosteroid therapy (Table 148-1). Other patients with acute pulmonary histoplasmosis who remain moderately symptomatic for at least a month also may benefit from therapy, but controlled trials have not been conducted establishing efficacy in this situation. Amphotericin B is fungicidal and may induce a more rapid response in severely ill patients. Amphotericin B is preferred as initial therapy in patients who are more severely ill. Azoles or triazoles are fungistatic but are highly effective in patients with milder illnesses.

Mediastinal Granuloma
Patients with obstructive symptoms or fistulas caused by mediastinal granuloma may benefit from antifungal therapy or surgery if the problem is sufficiently bothersome.[40] Antifungal treatment

TABLE 148-1

Indications for Treatment in Patients with Histoplasmosis

Treatment Indicated	Treatment Not Indicated
Acute pulmonary with hypoxia	Acute self-limited syndromes
Acute pulmonary >1 month	Acute pulmonary, mildly ill
Disseminated	Rheumatologic
Chronic pulmonary	Pericarditis
Mediastinal granuloma with obstruction or invasion of adjacent tissue	Fibrosing mediastinitis?
	Histoplasmoma
	Broncholithiasis
	Presumed ocular

or resection of enlarged mediastinal lymph nodes to prevent progression to fibrosing mediastinitis is not indicated, since progression of granulomatous mediastinitis to fibrosing mediastinitis has not been documented and must be rare.[25] Rheumatologic syndromes and pericarditis are noninfectious inflammatory manifestations and respond to anti-inflammatory therapy.[37,59] Antifungal therapy is not indicated unless the bone, joint, or pericardium is the site of disseminated infection.

Chronic Pulmonary

Treatment improves survival, reduces symptoms, promotes radiographic healing, and eradicates *H. capsulatum* from the sputum.[43] Most patients with chronic pulmonary histoplasmosis can be managed without hospitalization and respond well to treatment with itraconazole. Amphotericin B may be needed in patients with more severe respiratory insufficiency to achieve a more rapid response to therapy.

Disseminated

Treatment is indicated in all patients with disseminated disease. The mortality for untreated disseminated histoplasmosis is 80 percent, but it can be reduced to less than 25 percent with therapy.[14,39] Amphotericin B and itraconazole are highly effective therapy even in immunocompromised hosts, inducing a remission in 85 to 90 percent of patients.[8,54,56]

Broncholithiasis

Surgical therapy is required for patients with significant hemoptysis or recurrent pneumonia and for repair of bronchoesophageal fistulas. Antifungal therapy would not be expected to reduce the symptoms, since active infection is uncommon in such cases.

Mediastinal Fibrosis

Antifungal treatment is not believed to improve the outcome of mediastinal fibrosis, but a few patients treated with ketoconazole showed some improvement.[46] Antifungal therapy may be tried in patients with positive serologic tests and elevated sedimentation rates.[46] Although most authorities discourage surgical therapy, improvement after resection of the scar tissue has been reported.[26] Operative mortality is high (about 25 percent), however.

SELECTION OF ANTIFUNGAL AGENTS

Amphotericin B

Amphotericin B may act more rapidly than other antifungal agents. Abatement of fever occurs within 1 week in more than 80 percent of patients with disseminated infection.[39] Tolerability, however, is poor. Liposomal amphotericin B may overcome this limitation and permit more aggressive therapy of patients with severe illnesses. If the drug is used exclusively for treatment of disseminated or chronic pulmonary histoplasmosis, at least 30 mg/kg should be given over 2 to 4 months to adult patients. More commonly, however, treatment is changed to itraconazole after clinical improvement has occurred.

Itraconazole

Itraconazole was successful in 85 to 100 percent of cases with disseminated or chronic pulmonary histoplasmosis,[8,56] compared

TABLE 148-2

Drug Interactions of Azole and Triazole Antifungal Agents That Increase Concentrations of Other Drugs Metabolized by Hepatic Cytochrome P450

Drug	Effect
Terfenadine (Seldane)	
Astemizole (Hismanal)	Ventricular tachycardia
Cisapride (Propulsid)	
Coumadin	Bleeding
Oral hypoglycemic	Hypoglycemia
Digitalis	Digitalis toxicity
Phenytoin	Phenytoin toxicity
Cyclosporine tacrolimus (FK506)	Renal failure
Rifabutin	Uveitis
Triazolam (Halcion)	Sedation
Midazolam (Versed)	Sedation
Quinidine	Tinnitus
Dihydropyridine Ca channel blockers	Edema, hyponatremia

to 56 to 70 percent for ketoconazole.[9] Itraconazole was effective in 85 percent of cases of disseminated histoplasmosis in patients with AIDS. Itraconazole requires an acidic gastric environment for solubilization and should be given with food or cola. Medications that reduce gastric acidity (H_2 antagonists are discouraged, and omeprazole is disallowed) should be avoided (Table 148-2). Blood concentrations should be measured during the second week of therapy 2 to 4 h after a dose, in an effort to reach a concentration above 1 μ/ml and preferably higher (4 to 10 μ/ml).

Itraconazole is eliminated by hepatic metabolism. Hepatic enzyme inducers (rifampin, rifabutin, phenytoin, phenobarbitol) reduce itraconazole concentrations. Treatment failures have occurred in patients receiving rifampin, the most potent of the cytochrome p450 inducers. Rifampin should not be given to patients receiving itraconazole for serious fungal infections. Rifabutin reduces itraconazole concentrations by about 75 percent and should be avoided if possible. If treatment with cytochrome p450 enzyme inducers is essential, itraconazole concentration should be monitored.

Itraconazole impairs hepatic metabolism of many drugs by inhibition of cytochrome p450 enzymes. This interaction causes an increase in blood concentrations of terfenadine (Seldane), astemizole (Hismanal), and cisapride (Propulsid), potentially causing serious ventricular arrhythmias and even death. Such combinations should be strictly avoided. Interactions increasing the blood concentrations and toxicities of phenytoin, coumadin, oral hypoglycemics, digitalis, cyclosporin, and calcium channel blockers also must be recognized so that these treatments can be monitored appropriately.

Ketoconazole

Ketoconazole is effective for treatment of histoplasmosis but appears to be less active than itraconazole. More gastrointestinal upset occurs with ketoconazole than with itraconazole. The pharmacokinetic and drug interaction profiles of ketoconazole and itraconazole are very similar. While ketoconazole is only one-third as expensive as itraconazole, it remains a second choice for oral therapy because of its reduced efficacy and poorer tolerability.

Fluconazole

Fluconazole is less active in vitro than itraconazole for *H. capsulatum* and also appears to be less effective for treatment of histoplasmosis. Fluconazole 200 to 400 mg induced responses in 40 and 75 percent of cases in chronic pulmonary and disseminated histoplasmosis, respectively (Pappas, unpublished report, 1995). Treatment with 800 mg daily induced remission in 74 percent of AIDS patients with mild to moderately severe manifestations of disseminated histoplasmosis, but one-third relapsed during maintenance treatment with 400 mg daily (Wheat, unpublished report, 1995).

Prevention

In two reports, fluconazole did not appear to reduce the occurrence of histoplasmosis,[32] perhaps because of its relative weak activity against *H. capsulatum*. A placebo-controlled study using itraconazole 200 mg daily in persons with AIDS has been completed in four cities with high rates of histoplasmosis (about 10 percent per year). Until the results are known, prophylaxis cannot be supported in view of the lack of beneficial effect on mortality, the potential for drug interactions, toxicity, and the likely pressure for emergence of infection with triazole-resistant fungi, particularly candidiasis.

COCCIDIOIDOMYCOSIS

Coccidioidomycosis is the most serious of the endemic mycoses, often defying aggressive antifungal therapy. Recent outbreaks in southern California have placed large numbers of persons at risk for coccidioidomycosis. Whereas most cases are recognized within the endemic areas of the southwestern United States, increasingly cases are identified in travelers who have visited those areas.

Mycology

Coccidioidomycosis is caused by the pathogenic fungus *Coccidioides immitis*. *C. immitis* is the most virulent of the pathogenic fungi, causing infection upon exposure to only a few conidia and severe disease with larger inocula. *C. immitis* grows as a mold with septate hyphae in the soil and on culture media and as an endosporulating spherule in the tissues of patients. Its arrow shaped arthroconidia are 2.5 to 4 by 3 to 6 μm in size and are the infectious particles found in soil.

C. immitis converts to an endosporulating spherule at 37 to 40°C. Spherules measure 30 to 60 μm in diameter and contain multiple 2- to 5-μm

endospores (Fig. 148-7). Growth on fungal media occurs rapidly (in less than 5 days), and identification may be possible by the tenth day.

Epidemiology

Coccidioidomycosis occurs in a spotty distribution in the southwestern United States, northern Mexico, and Central America (Fig. 148-8). Growth is enhanced by bat and rodent droppings. Climates in the endemic areas are characterized by hot summers, mild winters, and arid conditions. Exposure is heaviest in the late summer and fall, when the soil is dry and conditions are windy—especially after rainy winters.

Workers exposed to soil are at increased risk for coccidioidomycosis. Cases most often are identified in construction or agricultural workers and archaeologists or students doing projects in the desert. However, large windborn outbreaks have exposed people many miles from the desert who had no direct exposure to contaminated soil. Coccidioidomycosis also is a threat to laboratory workers experimenting with live arthroconidia.

Coccidioidomycosis has become a serious opportunistic infection in patients with AIDS in Texas, Arizona, and southern California. In Tucson, coccidioidomycosis was the third most frequently reported opportunistic infection in persons with AIDS, occurring in one-fourth of patients.[1]

Cases often are identified outside the endemic area in travelers who have visited the Southwest, emphasizing the importance of travel history in patients with compatible clinical syndrome. In a recent study of AIDS patients with coccidioidomycosis, nearly half were from nonendemic areas, emphasizing the importance of considering the diagnosis throughout the United States. Disease also may develop outside the endemic region in persons who lived in those areas earlier, presumably through reactivation of clinically dormant foci of infection.

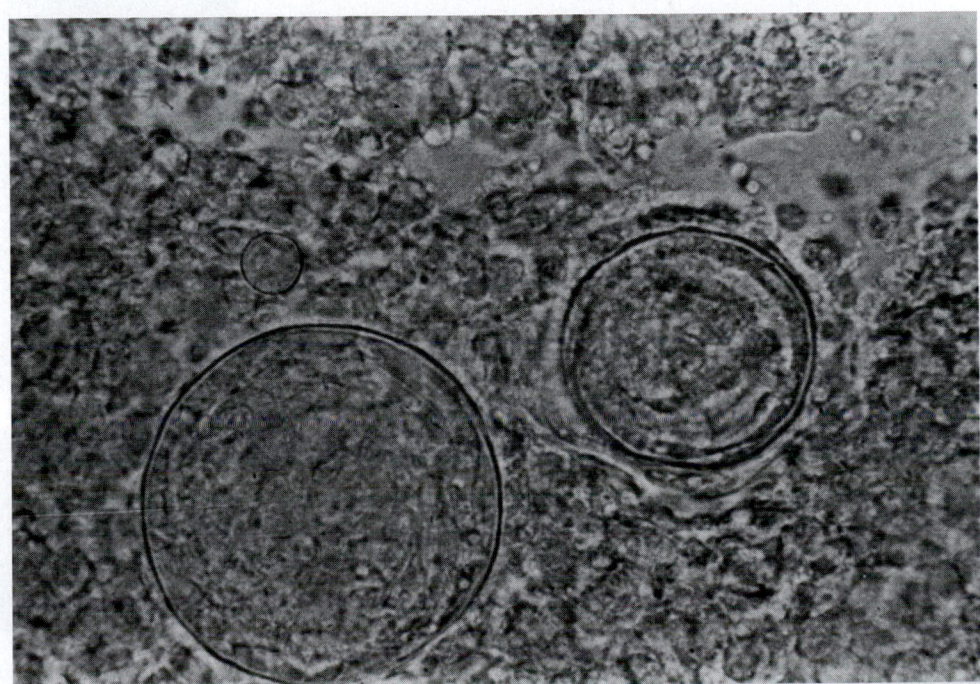

FIGURE 148-7   Fungal stains showing *Coccidiodes immitis* spherules in tissues.

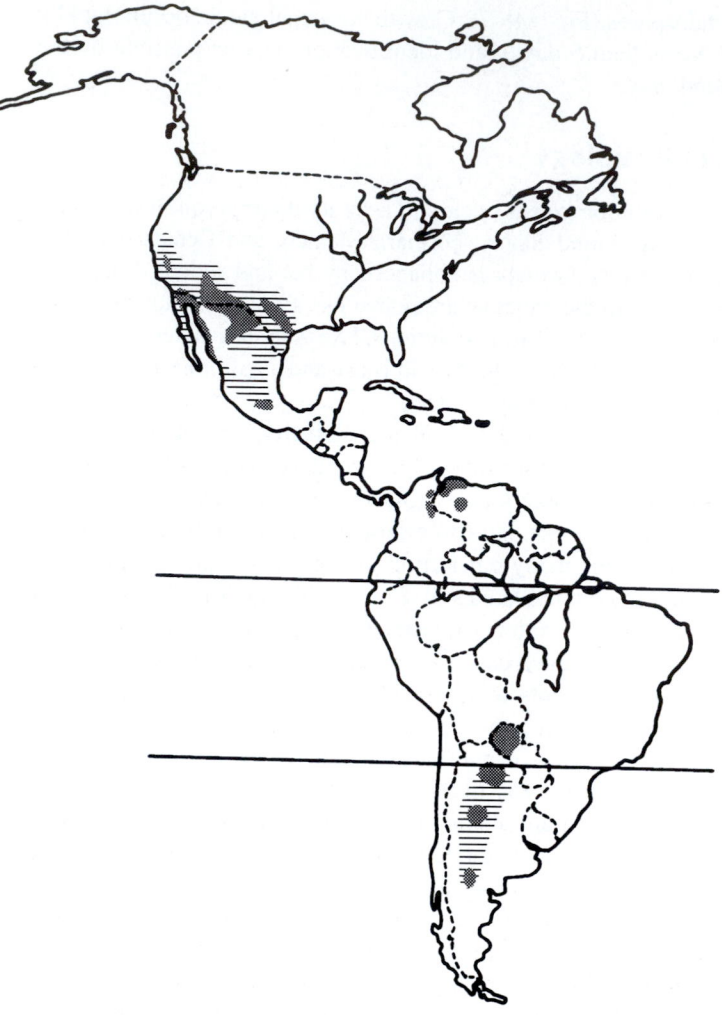

FIGURE 148-8 Endemic distribution of coccidioidomycosis in North, Central, and South America showing the high incidence in the southwestern United States. *(From Rippon,[35] with permission.)*

Pathogenesis and Pathology

Infection occurs following inhalation of arthroconidia of the mycelial phase of the fungus or reactivation of latent infection. Person-to-person transmission or exposure by direct inoculation is rare. Arthroconidia enlarge and form thick-walled spherules, which contain multiple endospores. Spherules rupture releasing endospores, which spread locally and disseminate hematogenously.

Cellular immunity and neutrophils both are engaged in host defense in coccidioidomycosis. Patients with deficient cellular immunity experience severe progressive forms of coccidioidomycosis. Pathologically, coccidioidomycosis is characterized by a pyogranulomatous reaction. In contrast to *H. capsulatum*, *C. immitis* is not an intracellular pathogen. Inflammation is less pronounced in patients with AIDS. The neutrophil response and caseous necrosis may lead to development of large abscesses, which often require surgical drainage. Abscesses also may spontaneously rupture or produce fistulas. Fibrosis may be prominent in the lungs or meninges. As with histoplasmosis, healed lesions frequently calcify. Tissue and blood eosinophilia may be pronounced in coccidioidomycosis.

Clinical Manifestations

About 40 percent of nonimmune persons experience symptoms 1 to 4 weeks after exposure to *C. immitis*, while the others have subclinical infection.[10,28] Pulmonary illness is most common. More than 90 percent of symptomatic patients recover without treatment, while the rest develop chronic pulmonary or extrapulmonary complications. The illness is more severe in immunosuppressed persons, African Americans, and Filipinos.

PRIMARY PULMONARY

Symptoms develop within a few weeks after exposure, depending on the intensity of the inoculum and the immunity of the patient. Flulike symptoms include pleuritic or dull chest pain, nonproductive cough, fever, and malaise. Patients with more extensive pulmonary infection may experience dyspnea or respiratory failure.

Chest radiograms show patchy infiltrates, often with mediastinal adenopathy (Fig. 148-9). Nodular coin lesions (coccidiomas) and thin-walled cavities may follow in 5 percent of patients. Pleural invasion is uncommon (in less than 10 percent) and

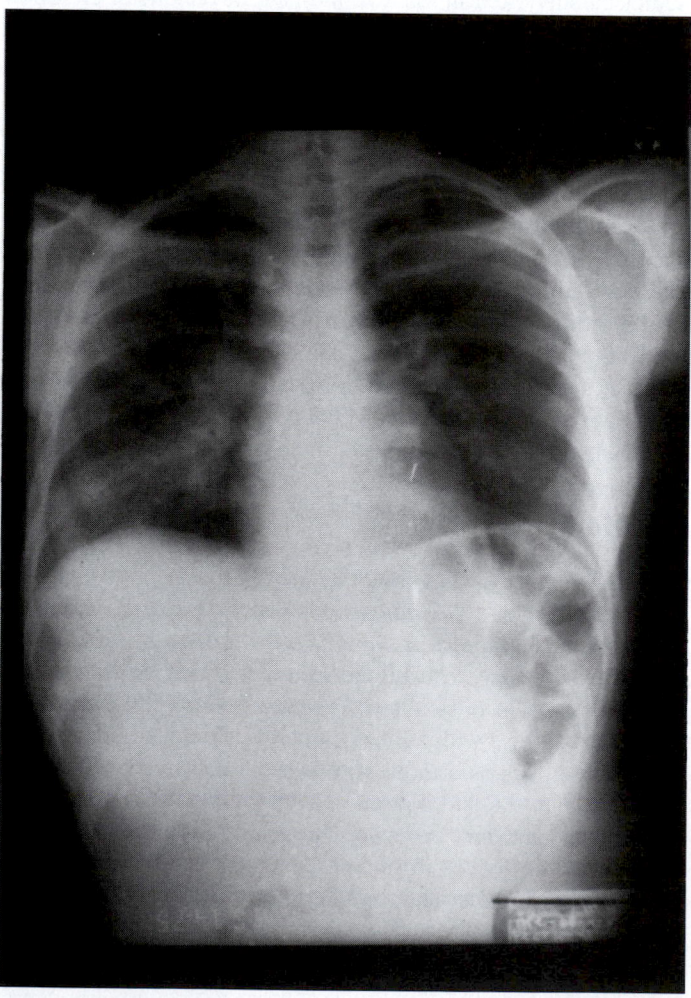

FIGURE 148-9 Chest radiogram showing bilateral hilar lymphadenopathy and a patchy right-lower-lobe infiltrate in a patient with acute pulmonary coccidioidmycosis.

is characterized by pleuric pain, friction rub, and effusion. Pneu-mothorax, bronchopleural fistulas, or empyema may complicate such cases. Pericardial effusions are commonly seen less.[28]

RHEUMATOLOGIC

Women often exhibit erythema nodosum or multiforme as a man-ifestation of primary coccidioidomycosis. This manifestation is similar to that seen in histoplasmosis. Arthralgias or arthritis commonly accompanies the skin lesions. These manifestations resolve without antifungal treatment.

CHRONIC PULMONARY

Chronic fibrocavitary infection with progressive fibrosis and re-traction similar to that seen with histoplasmosis and tuberculo-sis also may be seen in coccidioidomycosis. This manifestation is seen in patients with underlying lung disease and tends to progress without treatment.

DISSEMINATED

Extrapulmonary dissemination occurs in less than 1 percent of per-sons with coccidioidomycosis and typically is diagnosed during the year after exposure.[42] Sites most commonly affected are skin, bone, joints, and meninges (Fig. 148-10). Skin manifestations in-clude papules, pustules, plaques, nod-ules, ulcers, abscesses, and proliferative lesions.[13] Organisms are readily demon-strated in skin lesions. A septic shock syndrome associated with respiratory failure has been described in patients presenting with focal or diffuse pul-monary coccidioidomycosis who later are found to have disseminated disease.

Meningitis is a particularly impor-tant complication because of its fre-quency and poor prognosis.[47] Meningi-tis occurs in up to half of patients with disseminated coccidioidomycosis, of-ten as the sole clinical manifestation of the disease. Patients with meningitis manifest headache, nausea, vomiting, and confusion. Cerebrospinal fluid shows lymphocytic pleocytosis.[13]

Other sites of infection are lymph nodes, liver, peritoneum, kidneys, epi-didymis, prostate, testes, retina, ears, larynx, heart, thyroid, adrenal, pitu-itary, esophagus, and pancreas.[10] Ab-scesses rarely occur in the brain or spinal cord. Brain abscesses may occur in the absence of meningitis or obvious sites of dissemination in other tissues; they are believed to develop as a con-sequence of hematogenous spread rather than direct extension from the meninges.

Pulmonary impairment is common in patients with dissemi-nated coccidiodomycosis. Chest radiographs show diffuse retic-ulonodular infiltrates in most cases, but focal pulmonary lesions, nodules, cavities, adenopathy, and pleural effusions also may be seen.[13] Miliary infiltrates represent hematogenous impairment of the lungs.[12] Diffuse infiltrates appear to be more common in pa-tients with AIDS than in other patient groups, and the prognosis is poor (70 percent mortality).

Diagnosis

Diagnosis of chronic pulmonary or disseminated coccid-ioidomycosis is made from fungal stain and culture. Examina-tion of sputum is appropriate in patients with pulmonary mani-festations. If the sputum examination yields negative results, bronchoscopy, which improves the yield, should be considered.[48] Spherules may be seen in respiratory secretions or tissues (Fig. 148-8). Cultures are usually positive from the above sites, with growth in 3 to 5 days in most patients. Blood cultures are sel-dom positive.[13] Organisms isolated from cultures can be rapidly identified as *C. immitis* with DNA probe technology.

Serologic tests, positive in more than 80 percent of cases, is most valuable for diagnosis of coccidioidomycosis and has been reviewed in detail.[28] Demonstration of elevated levels of anti-bodies to *C. immitis* often is the sole basis for diagnosis in pa-tients with primary pulmonary coccidioidomycosis. The IgM an-

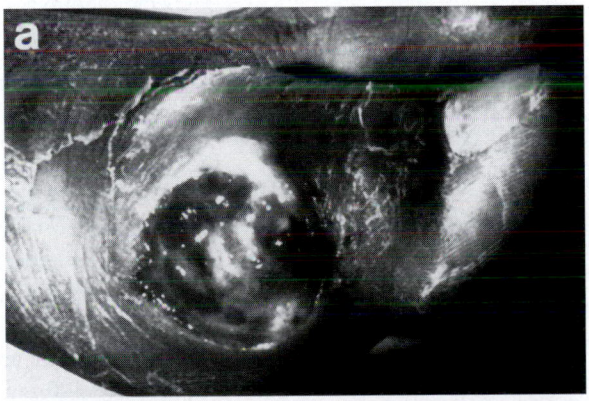
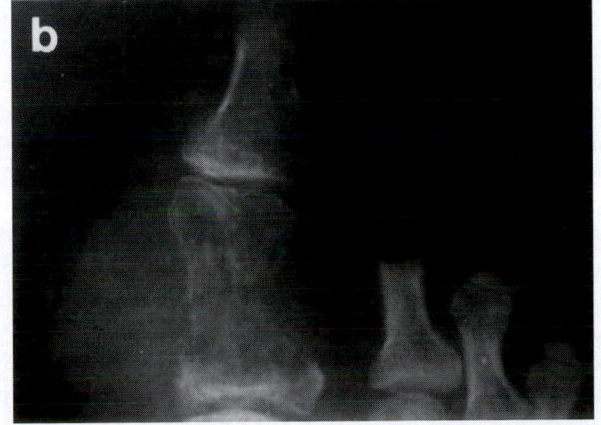
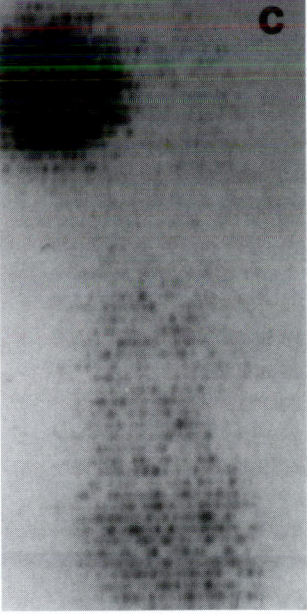

FIGURE 148-10   Skin and bone manifestations of coccidioidomycosis. *A.* A chronic skin ulcer of the great toe. *B.* Erosion of the proximal phalanx of the bone underlying the ulcer. *C.* Increased up-take of gallium by nuclear scan in a patient with disseminated coccidioidomycosis.

tibody response to coccidioidin is first detected from tube precipitation. The IgG response measured by complement fixation follows the IgM response and persists longer. High titers of complement-fixing antibodies at a dilution of 1:16 or greater suggest severe infection and support the need to exclude dissemination. Detection of antibody in cerebrospinal fluid is invaluable for diagnosis of meningitis. Serial testing in patients with primary pulmonary coccidioidomycosis is helpful in monitoring recovery, as rising antibody titers suggest dissemination.

SKIN TEST

Skin testing is very useful for diagnosis of primary pulmonary coccidioidomycosis.[42] Development of positive skin tests precedes development of antibodies by several weeks.[28] Additionally, antibodies remain undetectable in up to 20 percent of patients with self-limited illnesses and in 95 percent of asymptomatic skin test converters.[28] Cross reactions with other mycoses are uncommon, and skin tests do not induce production of antibodies to coccidioidal antigens. The standard reagent should be diluted for use in patients with erythema nodosum, however, as severe reactions may occur.[42]

Treatment

Treatment is less effective in coccidioidomycosis than in other systemic mycoses. Up to one-fourth of patients with disseminated coccidioidomycosis fail therapy, and a similar proportion of responders subsequently relapse. Outcome is worse in patients who have meningitis or chronic pulmonary infection than in those with primary pulmonary or other forms of disseminated disease.[4,15,22,38,44] Outcome also is worse in persons with serious underlying immunosuppression such as AIDS, in whom the mortality reaches 70 percent in the subgroup with diffuse pulmonary impairment.[13]

INDICATIONS FOR TREATMENT

Acute pulmonary or rheumatologic manifestations of coccidioidomycosis usually resolve without treatment, but most other syndromes are progressive and eventually fatal. Therapy is appropriate in patients with disseminated or chronic pulmonary coccidioidomycosis and in those with symptomatic acute pulmonary infection who experience hypoxia or protracted morbidity (longer than 1 to 2 months) or are immunosuppressed. Persons who are seropositive or who previously experienced symptomatic coccidioidomycosis perhaps should receive therapy if they are to undergo intensive immunosuppression such as that required for organ or bone marrow transplantation.[42]

SELECTION OF ANTIFUNGAL AGENTS

Amphotericin B is effective treatment in more than 90 percent of cases.[10,63] Amphotericin B is recommended for initial therapy for patients who are severely ill or have diffuse interstitial

TABLE 148-3

Guidelines for Selection of Therapy for Endemic Mycoses

Infection	Moderately or Severely Ill	Mildly Ill	Maintenance
Histoplasmosis	Amphotericin B	Itraconazole	Itraconazole
Blastomycosis	Amphotericin B	Itraconazole	Itraconazole
Coccidioidomycosis	Amphotericin B	Fluconazole or itraconazole	Fluconazole or itraconazole

infiltrates because of its fungicidal action and more rapid effect (Table 148-3). If it is used as the sole therapy, at least 35 mg/kg is needed to achieve satisfactory and durable responses. Increasingly, however, amphotericin B therapy is being replaced by fluconazole or itraconazole after patients improve clinically.

Ketoconazole was poorly effective (response 28 to 76 percent, with relapse of more than 50 percent in responding patients)[16,21] and also moderately toxic at doses of 400 mg daily or higher used to treat coccidioidomycosis.

Newer triazoles have proved useful for treatment of coccidioidomycosis. Fluconazole induced a clinical response in 79 percent of patients with meningitis,[15] 76 percent with cutaneous and 86 percent with skeletal manifestations of disseminated infection.[4] Response was poorer in patients with chronic pulmonary infection (55 percent).[4] Itraconazole also has been used for treatment of coccidioidomycosis, inducing a response in 57 to 94 percent of patients with chronic pulmonary or disseminated disease.[22,44] Outcome was better in those with skeletal or cutaneous lesions than in those with chronic pulmonary coccidioidomycosis.[44]

Optimal dosages and duration of therapy for fluconazole or itraconazole are unknown. Doses used in trials have ranged from 200 to 400 mg daily for fluconazole[4] and 50 to 400 mg daily for itraconazole.[7,22,44,45] Recognizing the high risk for relapse or progression of coccidioidomycosis with fluconazole (37 percent)[4] and itraconazole (16 to 19 percent),[22,44] prolonged therapy (for more than 1 year) with high daily doses (400 to 800 mg) would seem appropriate. Toxicities may be greater with doses above 400 mg daily, however, especially for itraconazole.

Chronic maintenance therapy is essential for all patients with meningitis or AIDS, and perhaps in others who have relapsed after appropriate therapy or who have persistent foci of chronic infection that cannot be removed surgically. Recurrence or demonstration of active infection at autopsy following treatment supports this approach.[13] Nearly 80 percent of patients treated for coccidioidal meningitis with ketoconazole, fluconazole, or itraconazole relapsed after stopping therapy.[6] Relapse appears to occur more commonly with fluconazole and ketoconazole than with itraconazole.[4,22,44] Fluconazole or itraconazole 400 mg or more daily or amphotericin B 50 mg administered weekly are options, but they have not been prospectively studied for this purpose. Fluconazole is preferred in patients with meningitis because of its cerebrospinal fluid penetration.

COCCIDIOIDAL MENINGITIS

Treatment of coccidioidal meningitis offers a special challenge. Amphotericin B, given intravenously and intrathecally, has been the treatment of choice for meningitis despite its toxicity and incomplete efficacy. The relatively poor response to amphotericin B is partly explained by its poor penetration into the cerebrospinal fluid. Aggressive treatment with high individual doses (1.0 to 1.5 mg) and overall courses (more than 40 mg total) of amphotericin B given intrathecally may improve response (90 percent survival versus 33 percent in historical controls treated less aggressively).[24]

Fluconazole is an attractive alternative to amphotericin B for treatment of coccidioidal meningitis because of its excellent penetration into the cerebrospinal fluid. Eighty percent of patients with coccidioidal meningitis responded to fluconazole treatment, often after failing amphotericin B therapy.[15] Lifelong therapy to prevent recurrence is mandatory for patients with coccidioidal meningitis.

Ketoconazole and itraconazole play a lesser role in treatment of meningitis. Ketoconazole penetrates the cerebrospinal fluid poorly (5 percent of blood level) but was used successfully at doses of 800 to 1200 mg daily in four patients with meningitis.[5] Itraconazole induced a clinical response in four of five patients with meningitis in another report.[45] However, since itraconazole does not achieve detectable concentrations in cerebrospinal fluid, support for its use in meningitis is weak. Fluconazole is superior to intrathecal amphotericin B for chronic maintenance therapy of coccidioidal meningitis.

ADJUNCTIVE SURGICAL THERAPY

Surgical débridement or resection of infected tissue often is necessary as an adjunct to antifungal therapy in coccidioidomycosis. Chronic foci of pulmonary necrosis or cavitation may require resection to prevent progression during therapy or recurrence following therapy. Soft-tissue, joint, or bone abscesses may require drainage or débridement.

Prevention

A study to evaluate fluconazole 200 mg daily for prevention of coccidioidomycosis in patients with AIDS in the southwestern United States could not be completed because of poor accrual. Without supportive clinical studies, prophylaxis cannot be recommended. Efforts to develop an effective vaccine have been unsuccessful. Patients with AIDS or other diseases that impair cellular immunity probably should avoid areas experiencing active outbreaks and the desert during dry and windy periods.

BLASTOMYCOSIS

Blastomycosis is the least common of the endemic mycoses. The lack of good serologic or skin-testing reagents has prevented thorough investigation of the epidemiologic and clinical aspects of blastomycosis. Although its geographic distribution overlaps that of histoplasmosis, its environmental niche is poorly understood.

Mycology

Blastomyces dermatitidis is a thermally dimorphic fungus producing mycelia with 2- to 10-μm dumbbell-shaped conidia at 25°C and doubly refractile broad-based budding yeasts varying in size from 8 to 30 μm at 37°C (Fig. 148-11). Isolation of *B. dermatitidis* in the mycelial form from cultures may occur rapidly or require several weeks of incubation for slow-growing strains.

Epidemiology

The organism may be found in microfoci enriched with animal excreta. Although the epidemiology of blastomycosis is incompletely understood, cases most often occur in the southeastern United States in a distribution overlapping that of *H. capsulatum* (Fig. 148-12). Rare isolations from soil have occurred in samples from areas inhabited by farm animals and from beaver lodges or dams. Decaying organic matter enhances its growth in the environment. Several common source outbreaks have been reported, often in association with outdoor activities such as hunting, camping, or canoeing in wooded or swampy environments.

Pathogenesis and Pathology

Pulmonary disease follows inhalation of conidia and often is accompanied by hematogenous dissemination. Neutrophils are first recruited to sites of infection, but lymphocytes arrive later and lead to pyogranuloma formation. Cellular immunity plays a role in defense against *B. dermatitidis,* but perhaps less than against

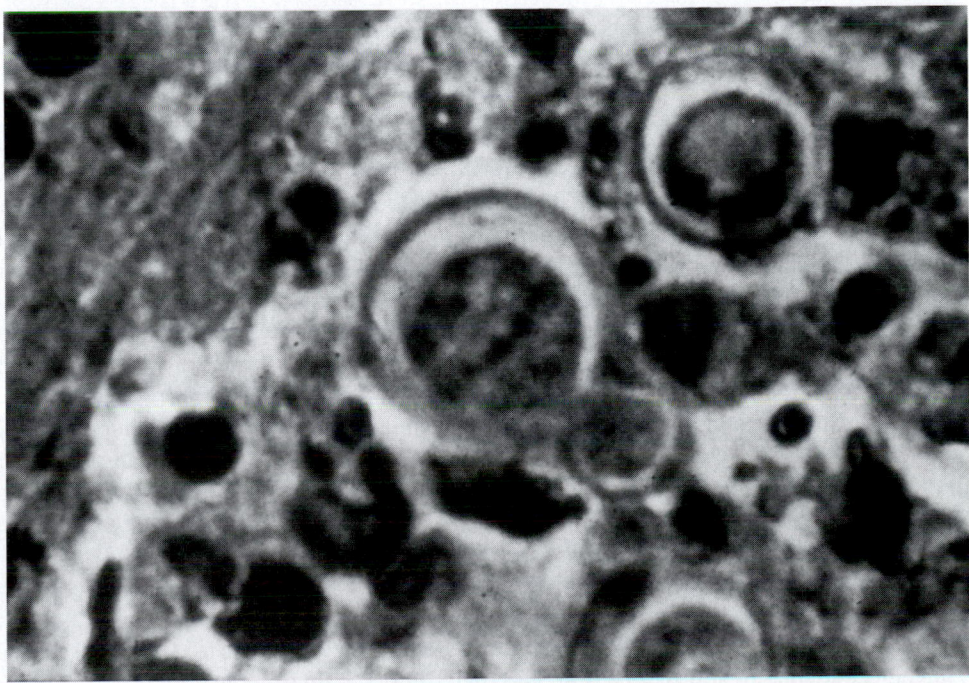

FIGURE 148-11   Fungal stain showing typical double refractile staining of yeast phase of *Blastomyces dermatitidis*.

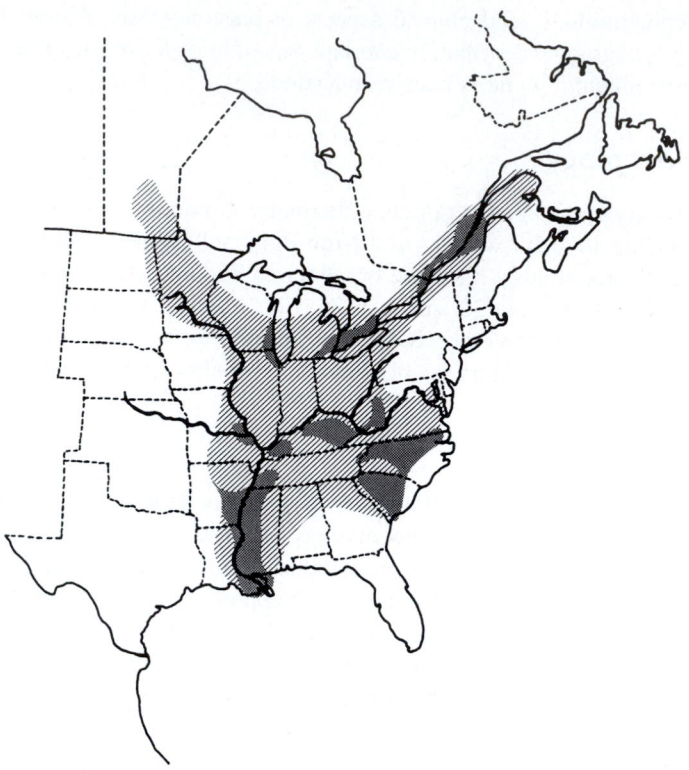

FIGURE 148-12 Endemic distribution of blastomycosis in North America. *(From Rippon,[35] with permission.)*

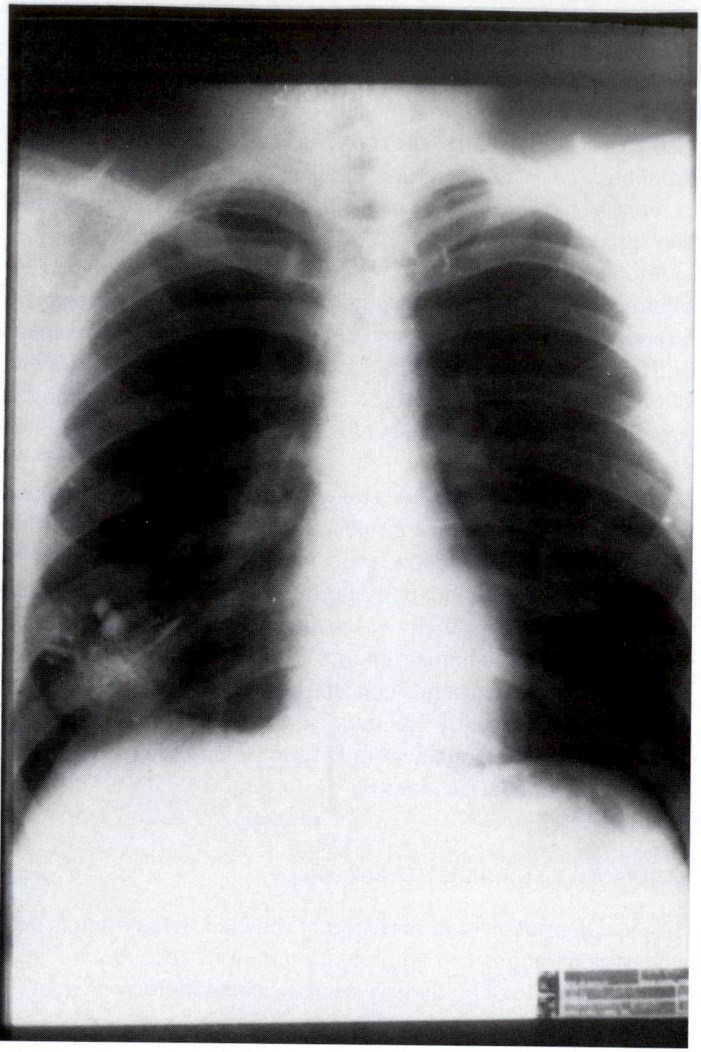

FIGURE 148-13 Chest radiogram showing nodular lower-lobe infiltrate in a patient with pulmonary and disseminated blastomycosis.

other endemic mycoses. Infection is more extensive and outcome is worse in immunosuppressed subjects.

Pathologically, blastomycosis is characterized by granuloma formation with central microabscesses, so-called pyogranuloma, but not by caseation as seen in histoplasmosis or tuberculosis. Histologic changes in the skin may resemble those of squamous cell carcinoma or keratoacanthoma (Fig. 148-13).

Clinical Manifestations

PULMONARY

Patients present with localized pulmonary impairment or with disseminated disease, each occurring in about half of patients.[3,30,31] Presenting symptoms in patients with pulmonary blastomycosis include fever, cough, dyspnea, chest pain, and weight loss of an insidious onset. The course may be self-limited[33] or chronic and progressive.[3] Tracheal and endobronchial invasion also has been seen in patients with pulmonary blastomycosis.

Chest radiographs usually (in 75 percent of cases) show focal alveolar infiltrates in the upper lobes, often nodular in character (Fig. 148-14).[41] Cavities occur in one-third of cases.[41] A minority of patients present with miliary or diffuse infiltrates associated with respiratory failure.[27,41] In contrast to the presentation of histoplasmosis, mediastinal adenopathy and calcification are uncommon (20 percent).[41] Mass lesions may resemble those seen with lung cancer, occurring in about 15 percent of cases.[3,41] Pleural involvement occurs in 20 percent of cases and may invade adjacent bone or soft tissues (Fig. 148-14). Chest CT findings confirm those noted radiographically.[62]

DISSEMINATED

Skin and bone lesions are the most common manifestations of disseminated disease, but many organs may be affected. Cutaneous lesions occur in half of patients with disseminated blastomycosis and may be acquired by hematogenous dissemination or direct inoculation. Typical lesions are painless erythematous nodules, which develop verrucous or ulcerative surfaces (Fig. 148-15); they may be mistaken for skin cancer.[3] Bone and joint lesions occur in less than half of patients with disseminated blastomycosis and are characterized by osteolysis.

CNS impairment manifested as meningitis, brain lesions, or epidural abscesses is relatively common (in at least 15 percent of cases).[3] CNS impairment is more common in immunocompromised patients, occurring in nearly 20 percent of cases (Pappas, unpublished report, 1996). Chronic meningitis is the most common manifestation and may be accompanied by intracranial or epidural abscesses. Isolated intracranial or epidural abscesses occur in 20 to 30 percent of these. Pulmonary affliction or dissemination to skin, bone, or other tissues commonly is found in patients with neurologic manifestations, assisting in diagnosis.

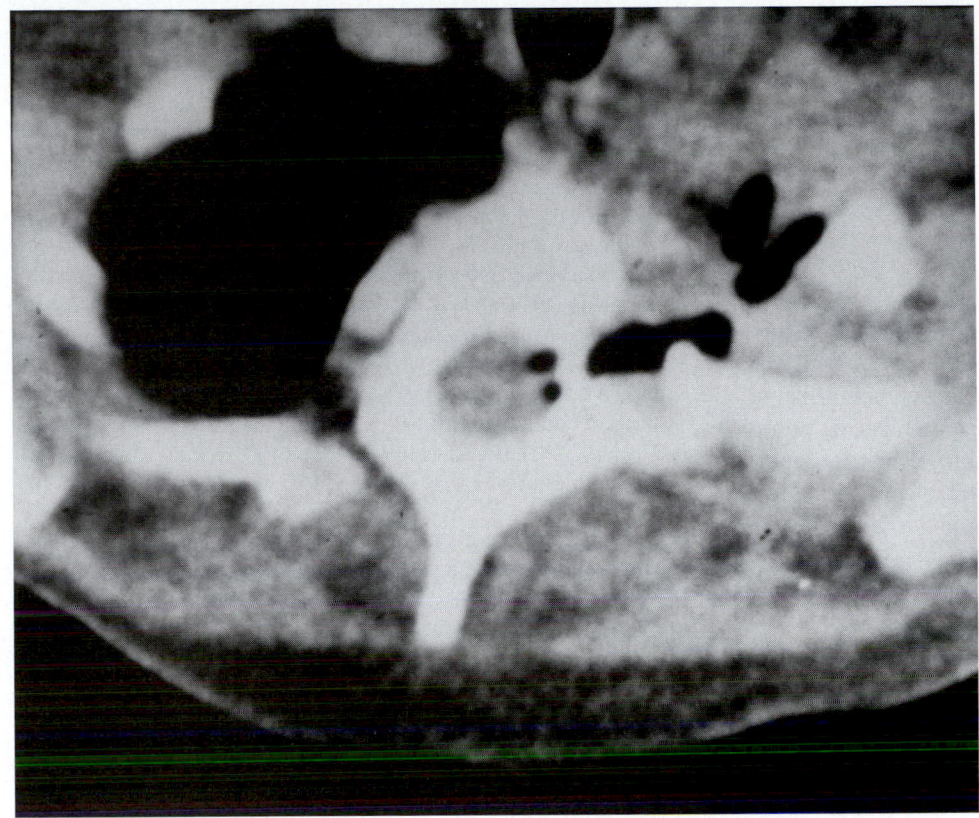

FIGURE 148-14   Chest CT scan showing an upper-lobe infiltrate with cavitation invading into the adjacent vertebral body and epidural space in a patient with chronic pulmonary blastomycosis.

Laryngeal impairment also has been reported frequently and may be mistaken for cancer visually and histologically.[3,34] The larynx may be infected directly from the respiratory route or following hematogenous dissemination.[3] The paranasal sinuses and ears also may be affected.

Genitourinary tract impairment of the kidneys, testes, prostate, or epididymis also is relatively common in blastomycosis.[3] Other sites of dissemination are the spleen, liver, pericardium, eyes, adrenal glands, and thyroid.[30] Patients have presented with clinical findings of septicemia.

Diagnosis

MYCOLOGIC

Diagnosis is based on demonstration of organisms in culture or fungal stain.[3] Cultures are positive in more than 90 percent of patients.[30] *B. dermatitidis* has been isolated most frequently from bronchoscopy specimens, cerebrospinal fluid, or brain, skin, and blood. Of note is that fungal stains have been positive in most cases, providing a more rapid diagnosis.

SEROLOGIC

Tests for antibodies may be falsely negative or falsely positive and are not useful for diagnosis of blastomycosis.[30] Efforts are in progress to improve serologic diagnosis of blastomycosis.

ANTIGEN DETECTION

Diagnosis by antigen detection could be useful in patients with extensive pulmonary or disseminated disease. A cross-reacting antigen may be detected in the *H. capsulatum* antigen assay in most patients with disseminated disease (Wheat, unpublished report, 1996). Specimens of urine or blood may be submitted to the Histoplasmosis Reference Laboratory in Indianapolis for antigen testing.

Treatment

INDICATIONS FOR TREATMENT

First, a decision to treat must be made. Some patients with acute pulmonary blastomycosis after a point-source exposure recover without treatment.[33] Spontaneous recovery may be followed by symptomatic recurrence or extrapulmonary dissemination, however, making long-term follow-up important. Patients with persistent or recurrent

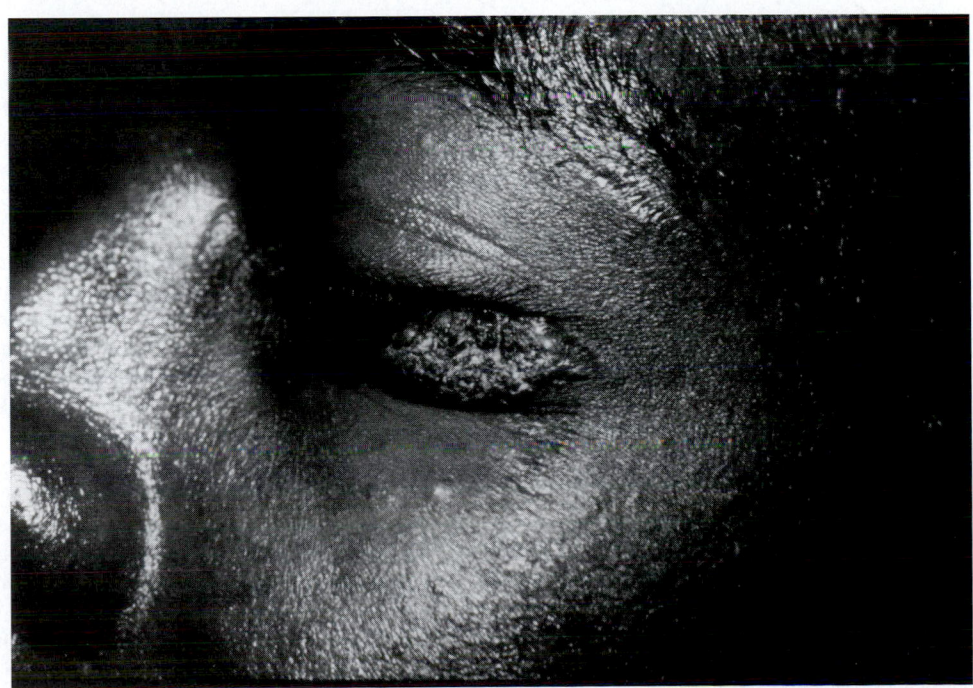

FIGURE 148-15   Hyperkeratotic skin lesion in a patient with disseminated blastomycosis. (*From Wheat,[49] with permission.*)

symptoms after acute infection, chronic pulmonary disease, pleural involvement, or dissemination should be treated.

SELECTION OF ANTIFUNGAL AGENTS

Selection of antifungal agents should be individualized on the basis of illness severity.

Amphotericin B

Amphotericin B is highly effective and is the treatment of choice for patients with severe manifestations or who are immunosuppressed (Table 148-3).[30] In immunocompromised subjects, the response has been better to amphotericin B (71 percent) than to azoles or triazoles (39 percent) (Pappas, unpublished report, 1996). Several studies using amphotericin B for treatment report response rates of 77 to 90 percent in patients receiving at least 1 G.[3]

Itraconazole

Itraconazole is highly effective in treatment of blastomycosis.[8] In a prospective, noncomparative trial in nonimmunocompromised patients with pulmonary or disseminated blastomycosis, itraconazole 200 to 400 mg daily was successful in 90 percent of cases.[8] Whether itraconazole is more effective than ketoconazole remains unknown, since comparative trials have not been reported.

Ketoconazole

Ketoconazole at doses of 400 to 800 mg daily for at least 6 months is reasonably effective, producing responses in more than 80 percent of patients in two studies.[3,9] Relapse occurred within 2 years of completion of therapy in 4 of 58 patients (7 percent) who responded to ketoconazole, however.[9] The outcome treatment with ketoconazole in immunosuppressed patients is relatively poor, discouraging its use in this population.[30,31]

Fluconazole

Fluconazole is less effective in treatment (approximately 65 percent response) of blastomycosis but can be used at doses of 400 to 800 mg daily if itraconazole is contraindicated.[29]

DURATION OF THERAPY

Treatment should be continued until clinical and laboratory findings have normalized and radiographs stabilized to represent chronic residual manifestations of healed infection. Prolonged therapy often is needed in view of the slow response to therapy and significant risk of relapse after treatment is stopped. Lifelong maintenance therapy is essential in all patients with AIDS and may also be appropriate in those who require chronic immunosuppressive therapy or have relapsed after appropriate courses of therapy.

REFERENCES

1. Ampel NM, Dols CL, Galgiani JN: Coccidioidomycosis during human immunodeficiency virus infection: Results of a prospective study in a coccidioidal endemic area. *Am J Med* 94:235–240, 1993.

2. Arrigoni MG, Bernatz PE, Donoghue FE: Broncholithiasis. *J Thorac Cardiovasc Surg* 62:231–237, 1971.

3. Bradsher RW: Blastomycosis. *Clin Infect Dis* 14 (Suppl):S82–S90, 1992.

4. Catanzaro A, Galgiani JN, Levine BE, et al: Fluconazole in the treatment of chronic pulmonary and nonmeningeal disseminated coccidioidomycosis. *Am J Med* 98:249–256, 1995.

5. Craven PC, Graybill JR, Jorgensen JH, et al: High-dose ketoconazole for treatment of fungal infections of the central nervous system. *Ann Intern Med* 98:160–167, 1983.

6. Dewsnup DH, Galgiani JN, Graybill JR, et al: Is it ever safe to stop azole therapy for *Coccidioides immitis* meningitis? *Ann Intern Med* 124:305–310, 1996.

7. Diaz M, Puente R, DeHoyos LA, Cruz S: Itraconazole in the treatment of coccidioidomycosis. *Chest* 100:682–684, 1991.

8. Dismukes WE, Bradsher RW Jr, Cloud GC, et al: Itraconazole therapy for blastomycosis and histoplasmosis. *Am J Med* 93:489–497, 1992.

9. Dismukes WE, Cloud G, Bowles C, et al: Treatment of blastomycosis and histoplasmosis with ketoconazole: Results of a prospective randomized clinical trial. *Ann Intern Med* 103:861–872, 1985.

10. Drutz D, Catanzaro A: Coccidioidomycosis. Parts 1 and 2. *Am Rev Respir Dis* 117:559–585, 727–771, 1978.

11. Edwards LB, Acquaviva FA, Livesay VT, et al: An atlas of sensitivity to tuberculin, PPD-B, and histoplasmin in the United States. *Am Rev Respir Dis* 99 (Suppl):1–132, 1969.

12. Einstein HE, Royce HJ: Coccidioidomycosis: New aspects of epidemiology and therapy. *Clin Infect Dis* 16:349–356, 1993.

13. Fish DG, Ampel NM, Galgiani JN, et al: Coccidioidomycosis during human immunodeficiency virus infection: A review of 77 patients. *Medicine* 69:384–391, 1990.

14. Furcolow ML: Comparison of treated and untreated severe histoplasmosis. *JAMA* 183:121–127, 1963.

15. Galgiani JN, Catanzaro A, Cloud GA, et al: Fluconazole therapy for coccidioidal meningitis. *Ann Intern Med* 119:28–35, 1993.

16. Galgiani JN, Stevens DA, Graybill JR, et al: Ketoconazole therapy of progressive coccidioidomycosis. *Am J Med* 84:603–610, 1988.

17. Gilliland MD, Scott LD, Walker WE: Esophageal obstruction caused by mediastinal histoplasmosis: Beneficial results of operation. *Surgery* 95:59–62, 1984.

18. Goodwin RA, Nickell JA, Des Prez RM: Mediastinal fibrosis complicating healed primary histoplasmosis and tuberculosis. *Medicine (Baltimore)* 51:227–246, 1972.

19. Goodwin RA Jr, Owens FT, Snell JD, et al: Chronic pulmonary histoplasmosis. *Medicine* 55:413–452, 1976.

20. Goodwin RA Jr, Snell JD Jr: The enlarging histoplasmoma: Concept of a tumor-like phenomenon encompassing the tuberculoma and coccidioidoma. *Am Rev Respir Dis* 100:1–12, 1969.

21. Graybill JR, Lundberg D, Donovan W, et al: Treatment of coccidioidomycosis with ketoconazole: Clinical and laboratory studies of 18 patients. *Rev Infect Dis* 2:661–673, 1980.

22. Graybill JR, Stevens DA, Galgiani N, et al: Itraconazole treatment of coccidioidomycosis. *Am J Med* 89:282–290, 1990.

23. Kataria YP, Campbell PB, Burlingham BT: Acute pulmonary histoplasmosis presenting as adult respiratory distress syndrome: Effect of therapy on clinical and laboratory features. *South Med J* 74:534–537, 1981.

24. Labadie EL, Hamilton RH: Survival improvement in coccidioidal meningitis by high-dose intrathecal amphotericin B. *Arch Intern Med* 146:2013–2018 1985.

25. Loyd JE, Tillman BF, Atkinson JB, Des Prez RM: Mediastinal fibrosis complicating histoplasmosis. *Medicine* 67:295–310, 1988.

26. Mathisen DJ, Grillo HC: Clinical manifestation of mediastinal fibrosis and histoplasmosis. *Ann Thorac Surg* 54:1053–1058, 1992.

27. Meyer KC, McManus EJ, Maki DG: Overwhelming pulmonary blastomycosis associated with the adult respiratory distress syndrome. *New Engl J Med* 329:1231–1236, 1993.

28. Pappagianis D, Zimmer BL: Serology of coccidioidomycosis. *Clin Microbiol Rev* 3:247–268, 1990.

29. Pappas PG, Bradsher RW, Chapman SW, et al: Treatment of blastomycosis with fluconazole: A pilot study. *Clin Infect Dis* 20:267–271, 1995.

30. Pappas PG, Pottage JC, Powderly WG, et al: Blastomycosis in patients with the acquired immunodeficiency syndrome. *Ann Intern Med* 116:847–853, 1992.

31. Pappas PG, Threlkeld MG, Bedsole GD, et al: Blastomycosis in immunocompromised patients. *Medicine (Baltimore)* 72:311–325, 1993.

32. Powderly WG, Finkelstein DM, Feinberg J, et al: A randomized trial comparing fluconazole with clotrimazole troches for the prevention of fungal infections in patients with advanced human immunodeficiency virus infection. *New Engl J Med* 332:700–705, 1995.

33. Recht LD, Philips JR, Eckman MR, Sarosi GA: Self-limited blastomycosis: A report of thirteen cases. *Am Rev Respir Dis* 120:1109–1111, 1979.

34. Reder PA, Neel B III: Blastomycosis in otolarynology: Review of a large series. *Laryngoscope* 103:53–58, 1993.

35. Rippon JW: Coccidioidomycosis, in *Medical Mycology: The Pathogenic Fungi and the Pathogenic Actinomycetes,* 3d ed. Philadelphia, WB Saunders, 1988, pp 433–473.

36. Rippon JW: Histoplasmosis (Histoplasmosis capsulati), in *Medical Mycology: The Pathogenic Fungi and the Pathogenic Actinomycetes,* 3d ed. Philadelphia, WB Saunders, 1988, pp 381–423.

37. Rosenthal J, Brandt KD, Wheat LJ, Slama TG: Rheumatologic manifestations of histoplasmosis in the recent Indianapolis epidemic. *Arthritis Rheum* 26:1065–1070, 1983.

38. Sarosi GA, Parker JD, Doto IL, Tosh FE: Chronic pulmonary coccidioidomycosis. *New Engl J Med* 283:325–330, 1970.

39. Sathapatayavongs B, Batteiger BE, Wheat LJ, et al: Clinical and laboratory features of disseminated histoplasmosis during two large urban outbreaks. *Medicine* 62:263–270, 1983.

40. Savides TJ, Gress FG, Wheat LJ, et al: Dysphagia due to mediastinal granulomas: Diagnosis with endoscopic ultrasonography. *Gastroenterology* 109:366–373, 1995.

41. Sheflin JR, Campbell JA, Thompson GP: Pulmonary blastomycosis: Findings on chest radiographs in 63 patients. *Am J Roentgenol* 154:1177–1180, 1990.

42. Stevens DA: Coccidioidomycosis. *New Engl J Med* 332:1077–1082, 1995.

43. Sutliff WD, Andrews CE, Jones E, Terry RT: Histoplasmosis cooperative study: Veterans Administration–Armed Forces Cooperative Study on histoplasmosis. *Am Rev Respir Dis* 89:641–650, 1964.

44. Tucker RM, Denning DW, Arathoon EG, et al: Itraconazole therapy for nonmeningeal coccidioidomyosis: Clinical and laboratory observation. *J Am Acad Dermatol* 23:593–601, 1990.

45. Tucker RM, Denning DW, Dupont B, Stevens DA: Itraconazole therapy for chronic coccidioidal meningitis. *Ann Intern Med* 112:108–112, 1990.

46. Urschel HC Jr, Razzuk MA, Netto GJ, et al: Sclerosing mediastinitis: Improved management with histoplasmosis titer and ketoconazole. *Ann Thorac Surg* 50:215–221, 1990.

47. Vincent T, Galgiani JN, Huppert M, Salkin D: The natural history of coccidioidal meningitis: VA–Armed Forces cooperative studies, 1955–1958. *Clin Infect Dis* 16:247–254, 1993.

48. Wallace JM, Catanzaro A, Moser KM, Harrell JH: Flexible fiberoptic bronchoscopy for diagnosing pulmonary coccidioidomycosis. *Am Rev Respir Dis* 123:286–290, 1980.

49. Wheat J: Endemic mycoses in AIDS: A clinical review. *Clin Microbiol Rev* 8:146–159, 1995.

50. Wheat J: Histoplasmosis and coccidioidomycosis in individuals with AIDS. *Infect Dis Clin North Am* 8:467–482, 1994.

51. Wheat LJ: Histoplasmosis in Indianapolis. *Clin Infect Dis* 14 (Suppl 1):S91–S99, 1992.

52. Wheat J: Histoplasmosis: Recognition and treatment. *Clin Infect Dis* 19 (Suppl 1):S19–S27, 1994.

53. Wheat LJ, Batteiger BE, Sathapatayavongs B: *Histoplasma capsulatum* infections of the central nervous system: A clinical review. *Medicine* 69:244–260, 1990.

54. Wheat LJ, Connolly-Stringfield PA, Baker RL, et al: Disseminated histoplasmosis in the acquired immune deficiency syndrome: Clinical findings, diagnosis and treatment, and review of the literature. *Medicine* 69:361–374, 1990.

55. Wheat LJ, Connolly-Stringfield P, Blair R, et al: Histoplasmosis relapse in patients with AIDS: Detection using *Histoplasma capsulatum* variety *capsulatum* antigen levels. *Ann Intern Med* 115:936–941, 1991.

56. Wheat J, Hafner R, Korzun AH, et al: Itraconazole treatment of disseminated histoplasmosis in patients with the acquired immunodeficiency syndrome. *Am J Med* 98:336–342, 1995.

57. Wheat LJ, Kohler RB, Tewari RP: Diagnosis of disseminated histoplasmosis by detection of *Histoplasma capsulatum* antigen in serum and urine specimens. *New Engl J Med* 314:83–88, 1986.

58. Wheat LJ, Slama TG, Eitzen HE, et al: A large urban outbreak of histoplasmosis: Clinical features. *Ann Intern Med* 94:331–337, 1981.

59. Wheat LJ, Stein L, Corya BC, et al: Pericarditis as a manifestation of histoplasmosis during two large urban outbreaks. *Medicine* 62:110–119, 1983.

60. Wheat LJ, Wass J, Norton J, et al: Cavitary histoplasmosis occurring during two large urban outbreaks: Analysis of clinical, epidemiologic, roentgenograghic, and laboratory features. *Medicine* 63:201–209, 1984.

61. Williams B, Fojtasek M, Connolly-Stringfield P, Wheat J: Diagnosis of histoplasmosis by antigen detection during an outbreak in Indianapolis, Ind. *Arch Pathol Lab Med* 118:1205–1208, 1994.

62. Winer-Muram HT, Beals DH, Cole FH Jr: Blastomycosis of the lung: CT features. *Radiology* 182:829–832, 1992.

63. Winn W: Coccidioidomycosis. *Med Clin North Am* 47:1131–1148, 1963.

CRYPTOCOCCAL INFECTIONS

Mitchell Goldman / L. Joseph Wheat

Cryptococcosis is an illness caused by infection with the encapsulated fungus *Cryptococcus neoformans,* an organism with a worldwide distribution. Inhalation of *C. neoformans* initiates the infection in the lung, with hematogenous dissemination most often into the meninges. Although pulmonary infection may be discovered in the presence of disseminated infection, meningoencephalitis remains the most commonly diagnosed form of cryptococcal infection. In recent years, the incidence of cryptococcosis has risen because of the immunosuppression associated with the acquired immunodeficiency syndrome (AIDS) and the increased use of immunosuppressive medications for other medical conditions.

EPIDEMIOLOGY

Cryptococcal infection can affect people with intact immune systems, although it is diagnosed most often in persons with underlying immune defects. Among those without immunosuppressive disease or therapy, the infection is rare, with an estimated incidence at 0.2 case per million persons per year.[20] Approximately 80 to 90 percent of cases of cryptococcal infection are diagnosed in patients with AIDS.[18] Other patient populations at increased risk for the infection are those with T cell–mediated immune defects such as patients with lymphoreticular malignancy (particularly Hodgkin's disease), pa-

tients requiring chronic corticosteroid therapy, recipients of solid organ transplants, and those with sarcoidosis.[18] The disease also appears to be more frequent in diabetics. Before the AIDS epidemic, 20 to 50 percent of cryptococcal infections were discovered in persons *without* an obvious underlying condition associated with immunosuppression. There appears to be no race-related predilection for cryptococcosis, while the infection has been diagnosed in two to three times as many males as females— an observation that may be explained by inhibition of fungal growth due to estrogens or differential exposure to the organism in the environment.[27]

The fungus *C. neoformans* demonstrates no endemic pattern of distribution.[27] Four serotypes of *C. neoformans* have been described. Serotypes A and D predominate in North America and Europe and grow best in composted bird droppings or rotted vegetation. Serotypes B and C are classified as *C. neoformans* variety *gattii* and are more common in tropical and subtropical regions in association with eucalyptus trees rather than avian excreta. Outbreaks or clusters of cryptococcosis cases are rare. In most cases, a history of exposure to birds or dust is lacking. Person-to-person transmission does not occur, although cryptococcal infection has been reported to be transmitted through tissue transplantation,[6] and cutaneous infection has occurred after direct inoculation.

MICROBIOLOGY

C. neoformans is a yeast that is characterized by its thick polysaccharide capsule. The yeast measures 4 to 6 mm in diameter, but the capsule thickness varies from 1 to more than 30 μm.[27] Organisms are smaller and less well encapsulated in the environment, explaining their ability to reach the terminal airways after inhalation. *C. neoformans* grows readily in fungal media, allowing isolation in less than 48 h and identification with biochemical tests or DNA probes.

PATHOGENESIS

Cryptococcosis is acquired by inhaling aerosols containing the yeast; it rarely occurs as a consequence of direct inoculation. Progressive disease often follows exposure in patients with impaired cellular immunity. In tissue, a mixed macrophage, lymphocyte, and plasma cell response is seen, but inflammation is often minimal in immunodeficient subjects. Granulomas are uncommonly found in the nervous system but may be seen in other tissues.

Macrophages, natural killer cells, and T lymphocytes play the key roles in cellular defense against *C. neoformans*.[22] Inflammatory cytokines (IL-2, IL-12, interferon-γ)[12,32] anmacrophage colony–stimulating factor[33] enhance the antifungal activity of these cellular mechanisms. Humoral immunity complements cellular mechanisms in defense against *C. neoformans*.[30]

CLINICAL FINDINGS

Cryptococcal infection results in self-limited pulmonary disease in most healthy persons. Occasionally, isolated pulmonary cryptococcosis is diagnosed,[23] but meningoencephalitis is the most commonly recognized manifestation of cryptococcosis and the most common cause of death from cryptococcal infection. Hematogenous dissemination to almost any tissue occurs in fewer than 25 percent of cases.

Pulmonary

Isolated pulmonary infection may be identified in nonimmunosuppressed subjects, and saprophytic colonization has been observed in patients with underlying lung disease. There is no distinguishing constellation of signs or symptoms of pulmonary cryptococcosis. Nonimmunocompromised hosts with pulmonary cryptococcal infection develop symptoms in about one-half of cases, while the remaining patients are discovered to have cryptococcosis only after evaluation of an abnormality discovered on routine chest radiographic examination.[45]

In those who are symptomatic, the infection is often indolent, with some combination of dry cough, dull chest discomfort, and low-grade fever reported. Less commonly, night sweats, fatigue, weight loss, or hemoptysis may occur. The majority of isolated pulmonary infections in patients without immunosuppression have been shown to resolve over time without antifungal therapy.[23] Occasionally, a chronic slowly progressive pulmonary infection develops or disseminated infection manifested by meningoencephalitis or other organ involvement may present after apparent abatement or resolution of the pulmonary process.[23]

In contrast to nonimmunocompromised patients, most patients with AIDS and pulmonary cryptococcosis have symptoms of fever and cough.[28] Immunosuppressed patients with pulmonary cryptococcosis commonly (in about 80 percent of cases) develop meningoencephalitis, supporting the need for therapy in these patients.[23] Since most immunocompromised patients receiving a diagnosis of pul-

monary cryptococcosis have concurrent meningoencephalitis,[8,11] the importance of performing a lumbar puncture in immunocompromised patients with cryptococcal pneumonia despite the absence of clinical findings of meningitis should be emphasized. Concurrent pulmonary involvement occurs in one-third of AIDS patients with cryptococcal meningitis and may be severe.[8]

The spectrum of pulmonary involvement ranges widely, although the radiographic pattern can be correlated with the host's immune status. Well-defined nodular (single or multiple) infiltrates or well-defined patchy infiltrates are commonly seen in the normal host[45] and may or may not be associated with symptoms (Fig. 149-1). Diffuse pulmonary disease associated with diffuse interstitial infiltrates, or widespread alveolar consolidation along with respiratory failure, is more commonly seen in AIDS patients or in those who are severely immunodeficient (Fig. 149-2).[19,28,37,45] Diffuse infiltrates in a patient with AIDS may be mistakenly attributed to *Pneumocystis carinii* pneumonia, leading to inappropriate treatment with corticosteroids.[5] The radiographic appearance in patients with less profound cell-mediated immune defects—such as those receiving corticosteroid therapy, transplant recipients, or patients with lymphoreticular malignancy—can vary widely, although most commonly nodular or patchy alveolar infiltrates are seen (Fig. 149-3).[45] Mass lesions are not uncommon and may resemble malignancy. Cavitation is uncommon, and mediastinal adenopathy, pleural effusion, and calcification are rare. These manifestations may be more common in patients with AIDS.[28] Empyema,[31] pneumothorax,[48] and pleural involvement suggesting a Pancoast's tumor[29] have been reported.

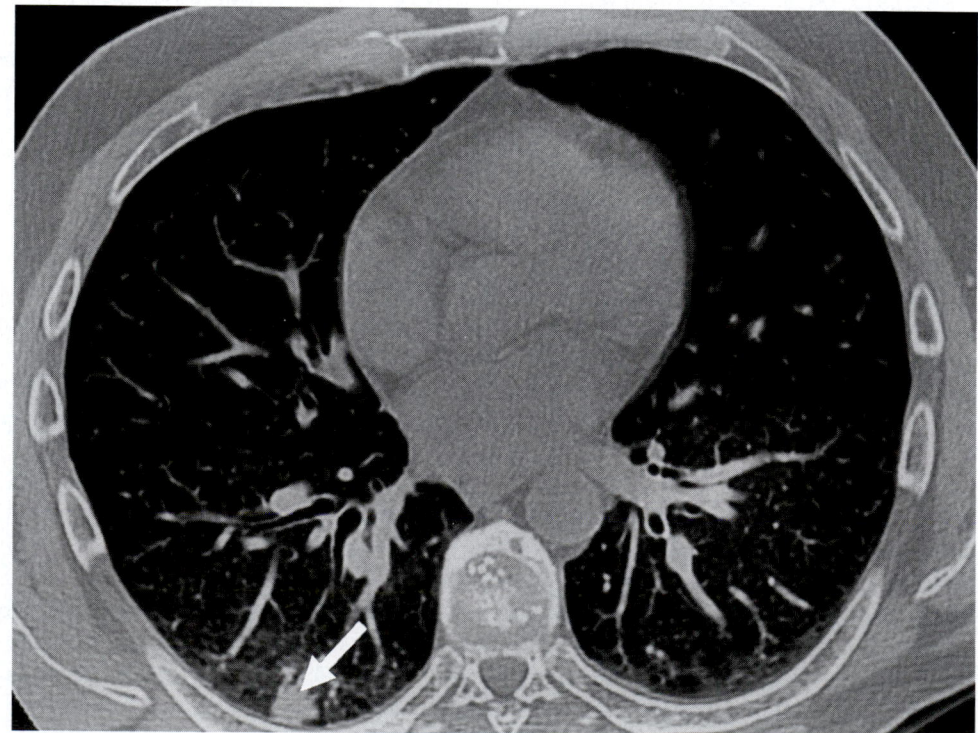

FIGURE 149-1   Chest CT of asymptomatic patient with small right lower-lobe lung nodule (arrow) that revealed *C. neoformans* on fine-needle aspiration of lesion.

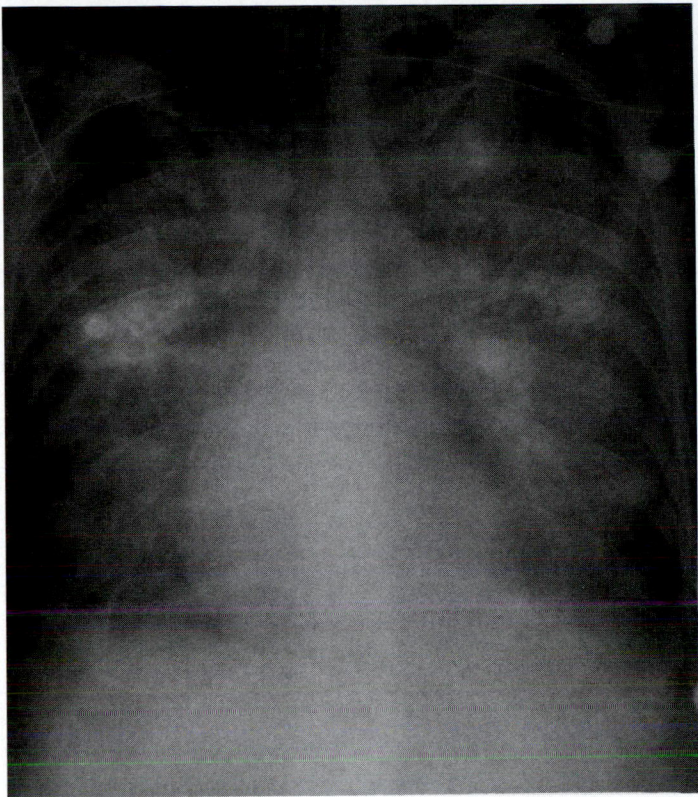

FIGURE 149-2 Chest radiograph of AIDS patient with cryptococcosis presenting as diffuse interstitial infiltrates with respiratory failure.

Meningoencephalitis

Meningoencephalitis is the most common manifestation of cryptococcosis, with 90 percent of cases occurring in patients with AIDS.[40] Typically, diffuse involvement of the cerebral cortex, cerebellum, and brain stem occur concurrently. A gradual onset of symptoms over a few months is typical, but a more rapid onset of symptoms occurs in patients with AIDS or other severe immunodeficiencies. Presenting symptoms include fever, headache, nausea, and vomiting. Less than one-third of patients exhibit meningismus, altered mentation, or focal neurologic abnormalities.[11] Elevated intracranial pressure is common and may cause serious problems, including death from brain-stem herniation.[16,39,52] Focal brain lesions (cryptococcomas) are seen in about 10 percent of cases, either as isolated manifestations or in combination with meningoencephalitis (Fig. 149-4).[1] Imaging procedures more often show meningeal enhancement, hydrocephalus, cerebral edema, or cerebral atrophy.[1]

Other Sites of Dissemination

Extraneural involvement occurs in up to half of patients with AIDS who have cryptococcal meningitis. Hepatosplenomegaly and bone marrow suppression causing pancytopenia are seen most commonly, while lesions in the skin, eyes, bones, or joints each may be seen in about 5 percent. Involvement of the prostate, although infrequently recognized, may be common in patients with AIDS.[25] Other sites of dis-

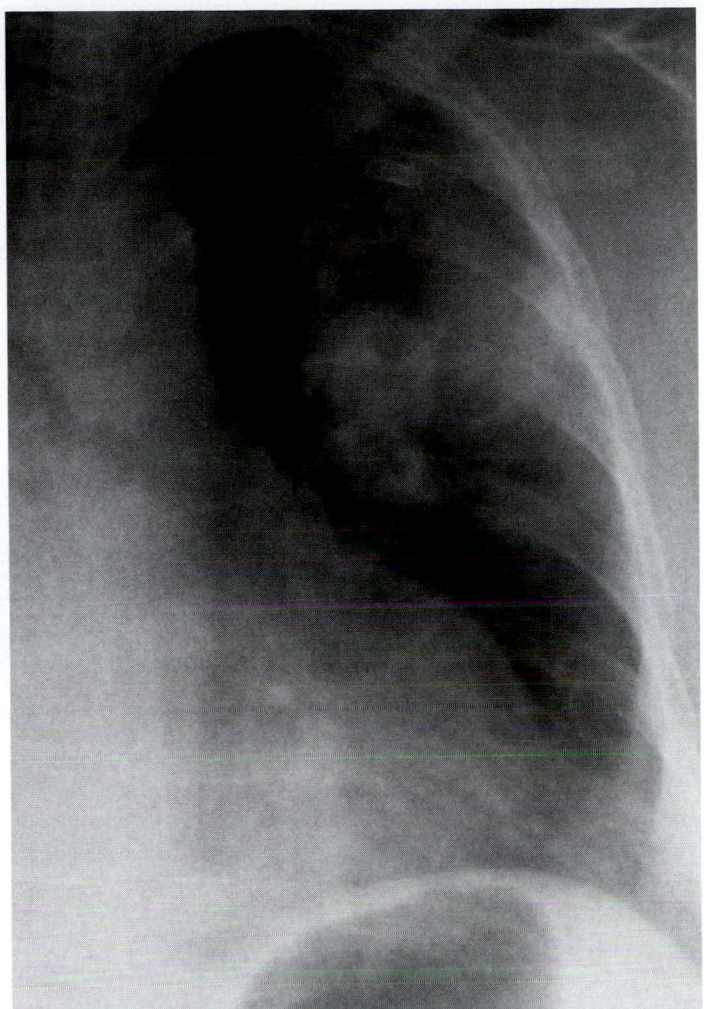

A

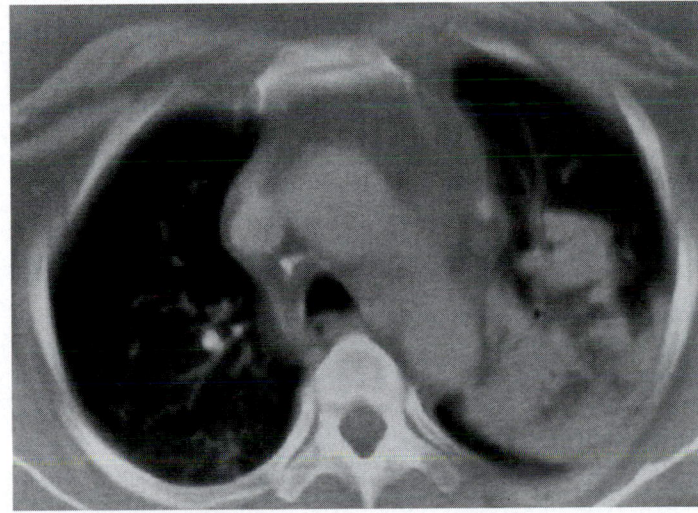

B

FIGURE 149-3 Chest radiograph *(A)* and CT of chest *(B)* reveal a mass lesion along with focal consolidation of the left upper lobe in a renal transplant patient with cryptococcal pneumonia.

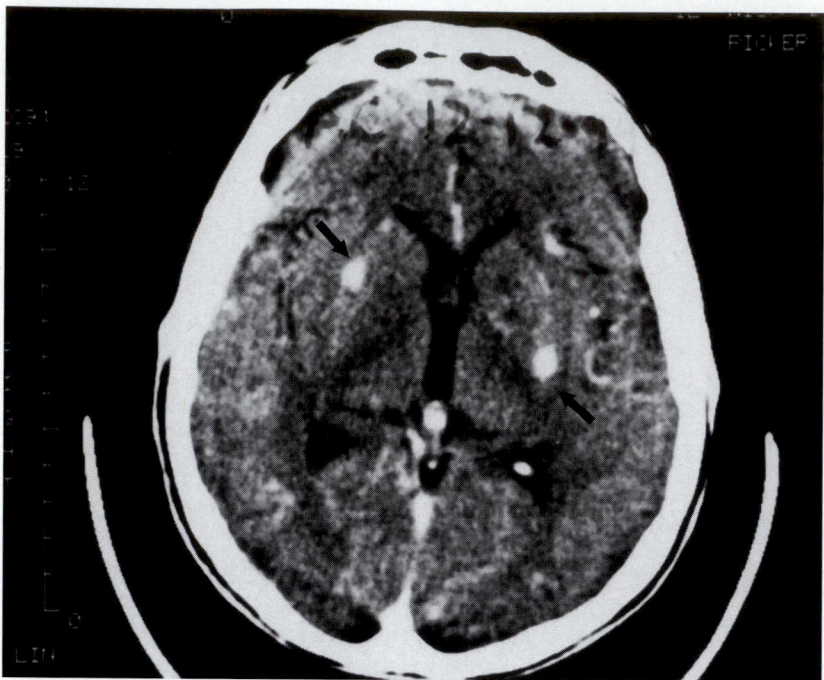

FIGURE 149-4 CT scan of brain in a patient with cryptococcal meningitis revealing lesions consistent with cryptococcomas (arrows).

semination are the heart, pericardium, muscle, gastrointestinal tract, peritoneum, thyroid, larynx, breast, placenta, urinary tract, and organ of Corti.

DIAGNOSIS

Pneumonia

Diagnosis of cryptococcal pneumonia requires isolation of the organism from pulmonary secretions or tissues or visualization in histopathologic specimens. Sputum cultures reveal *C. neoformans* growth in up to 50 percent of cases with proven cryptococcal pneumonia.[23,28] Growth of *C. neoformans* from sputum, however, does not establish a definitive diagnosis, as the organism can be recovered from the sputum of patients with lung disease due to other causes, particularly malignancy or other chronic pulmonary disorders.[43] If nodular or mass lesions are present and accessible, and the patient can safely tolerate the procedure, a fine-needle aspirate of the lesion should be considered for diagnosis. Cytologic examination as well as culture of the biopsied material should be performed. Bronchoalveolar lavage (BAL) may be the procedure of choice for those with interstitial or alveolar infiltrates. Cultures of BAL fluid or lung tissue yield the organism in 50 to 90 percent of cases, while fungal stains are positive less often.[2,8,28] When present, pleural effusions may be positive for *C. neoformans* growth in about 40 percent of cases.[51]

In tissue, *C. neoformans* can be recognized as a globose or oval to lemon-shaped yeast with a polysaccharide capsule. Cryptococci may be difficult to visualize on routine hematoxylin-and-eosin–stained sections, although identification of the organism can be enhanced by the use of appropriate special stains. Cryptococci are uniformly positive with the Gamori methenamine sil-

ver and periodic acid–Schiff stains, as are other fungal organisms. More specific stains for *C. neoformans* include the Mayers mucicarmine stain, which stains the fungal capsule, and the Masson-Fontana melanin stain, which may detect capsule-deficient cryptococci in tissue.[24]

Direct microscopic examination of BAL fluid sediment stained with India ink can help to identify the organism. Cryptococci may also be identified in sputum or pus after treatment with 10 percent sodium hydroxide.[24]

In patients with cryptococcal pneumonia, the serum cryptococcal antigen is usually not detected unless dissemination beyond the lung has occurred. A negative serum cryptococcal test should not be used to exclude *C. neoformans* lung infection, particularly in patients without AIDS. Among AIDS patients with pulmonary cryptococcosis, the serum cryptococcal antigen may be positive in more than 95 percent of cases.[28] Cryptococcal antigen testing also may be detected in lavage fluid[3] and in pleural fluid,[51] although antigen detection from these fluids has not been used routinely for diagnosis of pneumonia. Blood cultures are positive for *C. neoformans* in severely immunocompromised hosts, often with widespread disease or meningitis, but are not found in immunocompetent patients with isolated pulmonary involvement.

It should be emphasized that once a diagnosis of pulmonary cryptococcosis is made, an *evaluation for extrapulmonary dissemination* should be initiated. A serum cryptococcal antigen test should be performed along with fungal blood culture and CSF examination; in men, a urine fungal culture after prostatic massage should be obtained.

Meningoencephalitis

The diagnosis of meningitis can be made initially on detection of cryptococcal polysaccharide antigen in cerebrospinal fluid and confirmed by isolation of the organism from fungal cultures.[10,11] Antigen also can be detected in serum in at least 95 percent of patients with AIDS who have cryptococcal meningitis, often providing a clue to the diagnosis before lumbar puncture is performed. Encapsulated organisms may be seen with India ink staining in 75 percent of cases (Fig. 149-5). *C. neoformans* may be isolated from blood, skin lesions, bone marrow, urine, or other sites in up to two-thirds of patients.[10,46]

The sensitivity for each of these diagnostic techniques is lower in patients without AIDS, making diagnosis more difficult. Occasionally, cisternal puncture or brain biopsy must be performed to establish the diagnosis in such patients. Research to develop DNA probes[44] and polymerase chain reaction methods for rapid diagnosis may yield more sensitive techniques.

TREATMENT

Treatment is indicated in patients with symptomatic pulmonary infections, especially if they are immunocompromised, and in all patients with meningoencephalitis or disseminated infection. Pa-

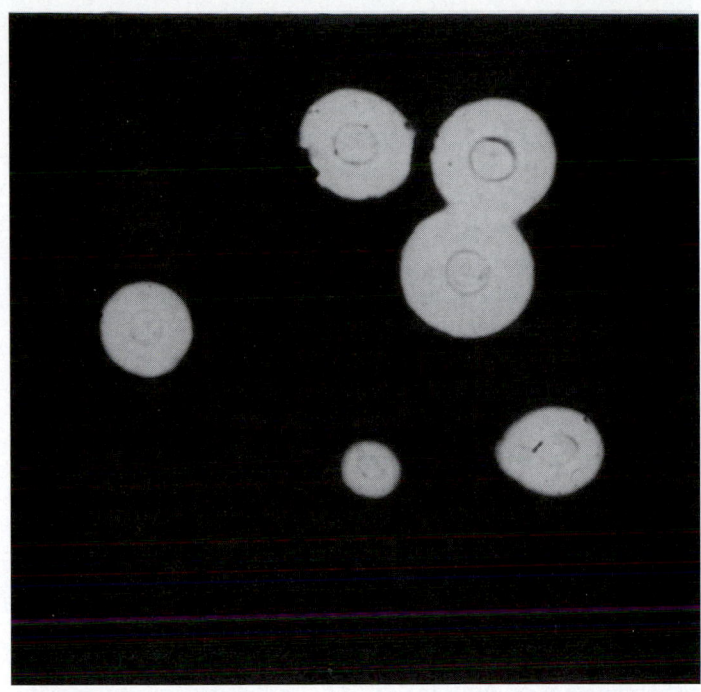

FIGURE 149-5 India ink preparation of cerebrospinal fluid demonstrating *C. neoformans.*

tients with a diagnosis of cryptococcosis at any site should be provided close follow-up for *at least 1 year,* as most relapses occur during this time.

Pulmonary Cryptococcosis

For asymptomatic patients with isolated pulmonary cryptococcal infection and no identifiable underlying immune deficits (see below), antifungal therapy may be withheld for 2 to 3 months as long as close observation is provided and any pulmonary lesions are stable or decreasing in size. As the treatment of pulmonary cryptococcosis has not been the subject of extensive study, recommendations regarding therapy for this form of cryptococcal infection must be inferred from treatment regimens used for meningitis.

Among nonimmunosuppressed symptomatic patients, asymptomatic patients whose disease progresses during observation, or non-AIDS patients with milder degrees of immunosuppression, amphotericin B is the treatment of choice for those who are more severely ill, while oral therapy with fluconazole is appropriate in milder cases or after a clinical and microbiologic response to amphotericin B. Intravenous amphotericin B at a dose of 0.3 to 0.6 mg/kg a day combined with oral 5-flucytosine at a dose of 75 to 100 mg/kg a day (divided into four daily doses) for 3 to 6 weeks can be used to treat cryptococcal pneumonia. The 5-flucytosine dose should be adjusted to keep serum levels less than 100 μg/ml. Alternatively, amphotericin B alone at a dose of 0.5 mg/kg a day or higher can be used for severe infections and in those who cannot take flucytosine. After initial improvement is seen with a regimen containing amphotericin B, completion of ther-

apy with oral fluconazole 400 mg daily is reasonable, with a suggested total duration of therapy of at least 3 months.

Initiating treatment with oral fluconazole at a dose of 400 mg daily can be considered, particularly for nonimmunocompromised patients and those with milder forms of immunosuppression with mild infections, with a suggested duration of at least 3 months. As experience with oral therapy for these conditions is limited, consideration for treatment durations longer than 3 months should be given. In patients with AIDS and cryptococcal pneumonia, disseminated infection and relapse are common, supporting the need for lifelong maintenance therapy after an initial induction therapy once cryptococcal infection is diagnosed. Patients with AIDS and cryptococcal pneumonia should probably receive treatment as outlined for meningitis (see below).

Cryptococcal Meningitis and Disseminated Nonmeningeal Cryptococcosis

INDUCTION THERAPY

In patients with AIDS and cryptococcal meningitis, amphotericin B at doses of about 0.4 mg/kg a day, with or without 5-flucytosine, or fluconazole 200 to 400 mg daily, was associated with a mortality of 15 to 20 percent.[46] A recent study in patients with AIDS compared amphotericin B in higher doses (0.7 mg/kg) with or without 5-flucytosine (100 mg/kg daily) for two weeks, followed by itraconazole or fluconazole, each 400 mg daily, to complete 10 weeks of induction treatment (Charles Van Der Horst and Michael Saag, unpublished report, 1995). Mortality was only 5 percent after 10 weeks of treatment.

Itraconazole seemed to work as well as fluconazole during the next 8 weeks of therapy, despite poor penetration into CSF. Cultures remained positive at the completion of therapy in only 5 percent of cases, representing a superior mycologic response to that observed with fluconazole or amphotericin B (about 0.4 mg/kg per day) in the earlier study (40 to 50 percent positive at 10 weeks).[46] Use of the higher dose of amphotericin B was believed to have accounted for the improved outcome in the more recent study. Others also have shown improved outcome when using higher doses of amphotericin B.[15] Aggressive management of elevated intracranial pressure through removal of large volumes (about 25 ml) of CSF was emphasized during the trial, contributing to its improved outcome.

Addition of 5-flucytosine to amphotericin B did not appear to improve outcome. Studies in patients without AIDS using amphotericin B, however, showed an advantage for combination therapy with 5-flucytosine.[4,17]

Fluconazole might prove to be more effective if higher doses were used. In a small trial, five of six patients responded clinically and all six responded mycologically to fluconazole 800 mg daily.[21] 5-Flucytosine and fluconazole interact synergistically for *C. neoformans.*[34] Of 32 patients treated with fluconazole 400 mg daily and 5-flucytosine 150 mg/kg a day for 10 weeks, 63 percent responded clinically and cultures became negative in more than 80 percent.[26] Ongoing studies are evaluating higher doses of fluconazole (at least 800 mg daily) combined with 5-flucytosine (Robert Larsen, University of Southern California and the California Collaborative Treatment Group, unpublished report).

Liposomal preparations of amphotericin B are less toxic than the standard formulation and may be used at higher dosage. In a study of 18 patients treated with liposomal amphotericin B (AmBisome) 3 mg/kg a day, 78 percent improved clinically and *C. neoformans* was eradicated from the CSF in two-thirds.[14] AmBisome was well tolerated, causing systemic toxicity in less than five percent of patients. Dosage was interrupted for renal impairment in only 2 of 26 subjects (8 percent). In a second study, 86 percent of 21 patients with AIDS treated with amphotericin B lipid complex (Abelcet) had a clinical response, but culture of the CSF became negative in only 42 percent.[47] A randomized, double-blind comparison of AmBisome with amphotericin B is in progress.

Until results of newer trials are available, initial treatment for meningitis and disseminated infection in moderately or severely ill patients should include amphotericin B 0.7 mg/kg daily, perhaps with 5-flucytosine 75 to 100 mg/kg daily. Levels of 5-flucytosine should be monitored and maintained between 50 and 100 μg/ml to reduce toxicity. Responding patients might be switched to oral therapy with fluconazole, 400 to 800 mg daily, to complete a 10-week induction course. Itraconazole 200 mg twice daily is an alternative in patients unable to take fluconazole.

The duration of induction therapy should be 10 weeks in patients with AIDS, who will remain on lifelong maintenance therapy. The duration of therapy for patients without AIDS who have meningitis and are treated with amphotericin B and 5-flucytosine should be at least 6 weeks.[4,17]

Fluconazole, 400 mg to 800 mg daily, perhaps with 5-flucytosine, may be acceptable induction treatment for patients with mild clinical manifestations. Reduced mental status means a poorer outcome and disqualifies patients for oral therapy.[39] Fluconazole has not been evaluated for treatment of meningitis, disseminated nonmeningeal infection, or pulmonary cryptococcosis in non-AIDS patients. Thus, the duration of therapy in this group is unknown. By comparison to studies using azoles for other systemic mycoses, perhaps regimens relying primarily on oral therapy with fluconazole should be continued for 12 to 24 months, based on speed of clinical response and resolution of CSF abnormalities.

MANAGEMENT OF INTRACRANIAL HYPERTENSION

Intracranial hypertension contributes to the early mortality observed in patients with cryptococcal meningitis.[16] Repeated lumbar puncture to remove 25 ml of cerebrospinal fluid produced dramatic improvement in one case.[49] Removal of CSF is appropriate in patients with opening pressures above 180 mm H_2O who are lethargic or confused or manifest cranial nerve palsies, visual impairment, or symptoms of severe headache or vomiting, and in those with pressures above 350 mmH_2O irrespective of symptoms. Acetazolamide may be given to patients whose condition does not improve after removal of CSF. Placement of a ventriculoperitoneal shunt may be useful if other therapies have failed. Corticosteroids also have been used for management of intracranial hypertension; they must be given cautiously, however, since further immune suppression may accelerate the infection.[5]

CHRONIC MAINTENANCE THERAPY

Chronic treatment is required to prevent recurrence in patients with AIDS. In a placebo-controlled trial, cryptococcal infection recurred in 37 percent of patients receiving placebo, compared to only 3 percent of those receiving fluconazole.[7] In a clinical trial, fluconazole 200 mg daily was more effective than amphotericin B 100 mg weekly for prevention of recurrence.[42] Relapse over a median of 9.4 months occurred in 18 percent of patients receiving amphotericin B, compared to only 2 percent receiving fluconazole. A recent trial compared itraconazole and fluconazole, each 200 mg daily. Relapse occurred in 24 percent of patients with itraconazole, compared to 4 percent with fluconazole (Michael Saag, unpublished report, 1995). Fluconazole 200 mg daily is the preferred maintenance treatment. Itraconazole at a dose of 200 mg twice daily or amphotericin B 50 to 100 mg once or twice weekly is an alternative for patients unable to take fluconazole or who have failed fluconazole therapy. The efficacy of itraconazole regimens is incompletely demonstrated.

DEVELOPMENT OF RESISTANCE

Development of resistance to antifungal therapy may be a cause of treatment failure in some cases but has not been fully evaluated. A study of five patients who experienced relapse of cryptococcal meningitis reported no increase in minimum inhibitory concentration (MIC) at relapse as compared to baseline; however, MICs of each strain from relapsed patients were relatively high (20 to 40 μg/ml), perhaps accounting for the treatment failures.[9] Two cases have been reported in which the MIC for fluconazole increased to 25 μg/ml and 64 μg/ml at relapse.[13,36] Prospective studies establishing the frequency of resistance as a cause of treatment failure in cryptococcal meningitis have not been reported. Treatment failure caused by an amphotericin B–resistant strain also has been described.[41] Newer azoles are under development and may overcome problems with resistance to fluconazole, should this emerge as a significant problem.

PREVENTION OF CRYPTOCOCCOSIS IN PATIENTS WITH AIDS

In a retrospective study, patients receiving fluconazole 100 mg daily experienced less cryptococcal meningitis (0.3 percent) than did historical controls (4 percent).[35] In a prospective trial, fluconazole 200 mg daily reduced the occurrence of cryptococcal meningitis from 7.1 to 0.9 percent, as compared to clotrimazole. Prophylaxis also prevented most cases of oropharyngeal and esophageal candidiasis. However, the mortality caused by systemic fungal infection was low and not affected by prophylaxis. Prophylaxis is expensive and may exert selective pressure for mutant strains of fungi that are resistant to fluconazole, including *Candida krusei* and *C. glabrata,* discouraging routine use in uninfected persons.[38,50] Targeted prophylaxis for groups identified to be at unusually high risk merits consideration.

REFERENCES

1. Andreula CF, Burdi N, Carella A: CNS cryptococcosis in AIDS: Spectrum of MR findings. *J Comput Assist Tomogr* 17:438–441, 1993.

2. Batungwanayo JH, Taelman J, Bogaerts S, et al: Pulmonary cryptococcosis associated with HIV-1 infection in Rwanda: A retrospective study of 37 cases. *AIDS* 8:1271–1276, 1994.

3. Baughman RP, Rhodes JC, Dohn MN, et al: Detection of cryptococcal antigen in bronchoalveolar lavage fluid: A prospective study of diagnostic utility. *Am Rev Respir Dis* 145:1226–1229, 1992.

4. Bennett JE, Dismukes WE, Duma RJ, et al: A comparison of amphotericin B alone and combined with flucytosine in the treatment of cryptococcal meningitis. *New Engl J Med* 301:126–131, 1979.

5. Bernstein B, Flomenberg P, Letzer D: Disseminated cryptococcal disease complicating steroid therapy for *Pneumocystis carinii* pneumonia in a patient with AIDS. *South Med J* 87:537–538, 1994.

6. Beyt BE, Waltman SR: Cryptococcal endophthalmitis after corneal transplantation. *New Engl J Med* 298:825–826, 1978.

7. Bozzette SA, Larsen RA, Chiu J, et al, and California Collaborative Treatment Group: A placebo-controlled trial of maintenance therapy with fluconazole after treatment of cryptococcal meningitis in the acquired immunodeficiency syndrome. *New Engl J Med* 324:580–584, 1991.

8. Cameron M, Bartlett JA, Gallis H, Waskin HA: Manifestations of pulmonary cryptococcosis in patients with acquired immunodeficiency syndrome. *Rev Infect Dis* 13:64–67, 1991.

9. Casadevall A, Spitzer ED, Webb D, Rinaldi MG: Susceptibilities of serial *Cryptococcus neoformans* isolates from patients with recurrent cryptococcal meningitis to amphotericin B and fluconazole. *Antimicrob Agents Chemother* 37:1383–1386, 1993.

10. Chuck S, Sande M: Infections with *Cryptococcus neoformans* in the acquired immunodeficiency syndrome. *New Engl J Med* 321:794–799, 1989.

11. Clark RA, Greer D, Atkinson W, et al: Spectrum of *Cryptococcus neoformans* infection in 68 patients infected with human immunodeficiency virus. *Rev Infect Dis* 12:768–776, 1990.

12. Clemons KV, Brummer E, Stevens DA: Cytokine treatment of central nervous system infection: Efficacy of interleukin-12 alone and synergy with conventional antifungal therapy in experimental cryptococcosis. *Antimicrob Agents Chemother* 38:460–464, 1994.

13. Coker RJ, Harris JR: Failure of fluconazole treatment in cryptococcal meningitis despite adequate CSF levels (letter). *J Infect* 23:101–103, 1991.

14. Coker RJ, Viviani M, Gazzard BG, et al: Treatment of cryptococcosis with liposomal amphotericin B (AmBisome) in 23 patients with AIDS. *AIDS* 7:829–835, 1993.

15. De Lalla F, Pellizzer G, Vaglia A, et al: Amphotericin B as primary therapy for cryptococcosis in patients with AIDS: Reliability of relatively high doses administered over a relatively short period. *Clin Infect Dis* 20:263–266, 1995.

16. Denning DW, Armstrong RW, Stevens DA: Elevated cerebrospinal fluid pressures in patients with cryptococcal meningitis and acquired immunodeficiency syndrome. *Am J Med* 91:267–272, 1991.

17. Dismukes WE, Cloud G, Gallis HA, et al, and the National Institute of Allergy and Infectious Diseases Mycoses Study Group: Treatment of cryptococcal meningitis with combination amphotericin B and flucytosine for four as compared with six weeks. *New Engl J Med* 317:334–341, 1987.

18. Dromer F, Mathoulin S, Dupont B, Laporte A, and the French Cryptococcosis Study Group: Epidemiology of cryptococcosis in France: A 9-year survey (1985–1993). *Clin Infect Dis* 23:82–90, 1996.

19. Friedman EP, Miller RF, Severn A, et al: Cryptococcal pneumonia in patients with the acquired immunodeficiency syndrome. *Clin Radiol* 50:756–760, 1995.

20. Friedman GD: The rarity of cryptococcosis in Northern California: The 10-year experience of a large defined population. *Am J Epidemiol* 117:230–234, 1983.

21. Haubrich RH, Haghighat D, Bozzette SA, et al, and the California Collaborative Treatment Group: High-dose fluconazole for treatment of cryptococcosis disease in patients with human immunodeficiency virus infection. *J Infect Dis* 170:238–242, 1994.

22. Huffnagle GB, Yates JL, Lipscomb MF: Immunity to a pulmonary *Cryptococcus neoformans* infection requires both CD4+ and CD8+ T cells. *J Exp Med* 173:793–800, 1991.

23. Kerkering TM, Duma RJ, Shadomy S: The evolution of pulmonary cryptococcosis. *Ann Intern Med* 94:611–616, 1981.

24. Kwon-Chung KJ, Bennett JE: *Medical Mycology*. Philadelphia, Lea & Febiger, 1992.

25. Larsen RA, Bozzette S, McCutchan JA, et al, and the California Treatment Group: Persistent *Cryptococcus neoformans* infection of the prostate after successful treatment of meningitis. *Ann Intern Med* 111:125–128, 1989.

26. Larsen RA, Bozzette SA, Jones BE, et al: Fluconazole combined with flucytosine for treatment of cryptococcal meningitis in patients with AIDS. *Clin Infect Dis* 19:741–745, 1994.

27. Levitz SM: The ecology of *Cryptococcus neoformans* and the epidemiology of cryptococcosis. *Rev Infect Dis* 13:1163–1169, 1991.

28. Meyohas MC, Roux P, Bollens D, et al: Pulmonary cryptococcosis: Localized and disseminated infections in 27 patients with AIDS. *Clin Infect Dis* 21:628–633, 1995.

29. Mitchell DH, Sorrell TC: Pancoast's syndrome due to pulmonary infection with *Cryptococcus neoformans* variety *gattii*. *Clin Infect Dis* 14:1142–1144, 1992.

30. Mukherjee S, Lee SC, Casadevall A: Antibodies to *Cryptococcus neoformans* glucuronoxylomannan enhance antifungal activity of murine macrophages. *Infect Immun* 63:573–579, 1995.

31. Mulanovich VE, Dismukes WE, Markowitz N: Cyptococcal empyema: Case report and review. *Clin Infect Dis* 20:1396–1398, 1995.

32. Murphy JW: Cytokine profiles associated with induction of the anticryptococcal cell-mediated immune response. *Infect Immun* 61:4750–4759, 1993.

33. Nassar F, Brummer E, Stevens DA: Macrophage colony–stimulating factor (M-CSF) induction of enhanced anticryptococcal activity in human monocyte-derived macrophages: Synergy with fluconazole for killing. *Cell Immunol* 164:113–118, 1995.

34. Nguyen MH, Barchiesi F, McGough DA, et al: In vitro evaluation of combination of fluconazole and flucytosine against *Cryptococcus neoformans* var. *neoformans*. *Antimicrob Agents Chemother* 39:1691–1695, 1995.

35. Nightingale SD, Cal SX, Peterson DM, et al: Primary prophylaxis with fluconazole against systemic fungal infections in HIV-positive patients. *AIDS* 6:191–194, 1992.

36. Paugam A, Dupouy-Camet J, Blanche P, et al: Increased fluconazole resistance of *Cryptococcus neoformans* isolated from a patient with AIDS and recurrent meningitis. *Clin Infect Dis* 19:975–976, 1994.

37. Perla EN, Maayan S, Miller SN, et al: Disseminated cryptococcis presenting as the adult respiratory distress syndrome. *NY State J Med* 85:704–706, 1985.

38. Pinner RW, Hajjeh RA, Powderly WG: Prospects for preventing cryptococcosis in persons infected with human immunodeficiency virus. *Clin Infect Dis* 21 (Suppl 1):S103–S107, 1995.

39. Powderly WG: Therapy for cryptococcal meningitis in patients with AIDS. *Clin Infect Dis* 14 (Suppl 1):S54–S59, 1992.

40. Powderly WG: Cryptococcal meningitis and AIDS. *Clin Infect Dis* 17:837–842, 1993.

41. Powderly WG, Keath EJ, Anderson-Sokol M, et al: Amphotericin B–resistant *Cryptococcus neoformans* in a patient with AIDS. *Infect Dis Clin Pract* 1:314–316, 1990.

42. Powderly WG, Saag MS, Cloud GA, et al: A controlled trial of fluconazole or amphotericin B to prevent relapse of cryptococcal meningitis in patients with the acquired immunodeficiency syndrome. *New Engl J Med* 326:793–798, 1992.

43. Randhawa HS, Pal M: Occurrence and significance of *Cryptococcus neoformans* in the respiratory tract of patients with bronchopulmonary disorders. *J Clin Microbiol* 5:5–8, 1977.

44. Rhew DC, Goetz MB, Louie MH: Reversible CD4+ T lymphocyte depletion in a patient who had disseminated histoplasmosis and who was not infected with human immunodeficiency virus. *Clin Infect Dis* 21:702–703, 1995.

45. Rozenbaum R, Gonçalves AJR: Clinical epidemiology study of 171 cases of cryptococcosis. *Clin Infect Dis* 18:369–380, 1994.

46. Saag MS, Powderly WG, Cloud GA, et al: Comparison of amphotericin B with fluconazole in the treatment of acute AIDS-associated cryptococcal meningitis. *New Engl J Med* 326:83–89, 1992.

47. Sharkey PK, Graybill JR, Johnson ES, et al: Amphotericin B lipid complex compared with amphotericin B in the treatment of cryptococcal meningitis in patients with AIDS. *Clin Infect Dis* 22:315–321, 1996.

48. Signs DJ, Wagner DS: Pulmonary cryptococcus presenting as pneumothorax in a patient with AIDS. *Clin Infect Dis* 21:1524–1525, 1995.

49. van Gemert HMA, Vermeulen M: Treatment of impaired consciousness with lumbar punctures in a patient with cryptococcal meningitis and AIDS. *Clin Neurol Neurosurg* 93:257–258, 1991.

50. Wheat LJ, Goldman M: Antifungal prophylaxis in AIDS: Should it be the standard of care? *AIDS Clin Care* 6:27–30, 1994.

51. Young EJ, Hirsh DD, Fainstein V, Williams TW: Pleural effusions due to cryptococcus neoformans: A review of the literature and report of two cases with cryptococcal antigen determinations. *Am Rev Respir Dis* 121:743–747, 1980.

52. Zuger A, Louie E, Holzman RS, et al: Cryptococcal disease in patients with the acquired immunodeficiency syndrome: Diagnostic features and outcome of treatment. *Ann Intern Med* 104:234–240, 1986.

CHAPTER 150

PNEUMOCYSTIS CARINII

Jay Alan Fishman

Despite significant advances in our understanding of the treatment and pathophysiology of *Pneumocystis* infection, *Pneumocystis carinii* remains an important pathogen in the immunocompromised host. Since the original association of this organism with epidemics of "interstitial plasma cell pneumonitis" of young, malnourished children, *P. carinii* has been identified as a cause of pneumonia in a broad range of immunocompromised hosts.[21,33,49,53,57] The apparent incidence of *Pneumocystis* pneumonia has increased with the prolonged survival of immunocompromised patients and with improvements in diagnostic techniques for this pathogen. Particular susceptibility has been noted in patients receiving corticosteroid therapy and in those infected with human immunodeficiency virus (HIV).[27]

HISTORY AND BACKGROUND

The cyst form of *P. carinii* was described in 1909 (Chagas) and 1910 (Carini) as a part of the life cycle of the trypanosome. It was described in 1912 (Delanoe and Delanoe) as a unique organism infecting the lungs of rats. *P. carinii* was not seen in man until 1942 (van der Meer and Brug) and was not associated with human disease until 1952 (Vanek and Jirovec),[53] when it was found in association with "plasma cell interstitial pneumonitis" in malnourished children and neonates. Small epidemics of plasma cell interstitial pneumonitis had been noted in children in orphanages in Europe in the 1930s. In the 1950s, studies of the immune system led to the recognition of congenital immune deficiencies and to the development of immunosuppressive therapies. At that time, *P. carinii* was recognized in patients receiving corticosteroids and chemotherapeutic drugs, and in immunosuppressed rats receiving corticosteroids.[30] The first case of *P. carinii* pneumonia was reported in the United States in 1956.

The increasing incidence of *P. carinii* pneumonia led to epidemiologic and therapeutic studies of the disease by the Centers for Disease Control (CDC) in 1970[46] and in 1974,[58] based on the provision of the sole therapeutic agent available at that time (pentamidine methanesulfonate) by the CDC. Clusters of *P. carinii* have been reported at a variety of clinical oncology centers. However, the development of pyrimethamine and sulfadoxine[47] and of trimethoprim (TMP) and sulfamethoxazole (SMX)[35] for the treatment and prevention of *Pneumocystis* infection greatly reduced the occurrence and the morbidity of the infection. These agents are now generally used in a fixed combination (TMP-SMX, co-trimoxazole). *P. carinii* became the first disease-defining illness associated with AIDS in the 1980s, with more than 200,000 cases of *P. carinii* pneumonia occurring since 1979. Up to 40,000 cases a year would be seen without the use of antibiotic prophylaxis and antiretroviral therapy in the HIV-infected population. Despite improved anti-*Pneumocystis* prophylaxis, 26.7 percent of community-acquired pneumonias in HIV-infected persons are still due to *P. carinii*.[11]

STRUCTURE AND LIFE CYCLE

In humans and animals, three forms of the organism have been identified: trophozoite, cyst, and sporozoite (or "intracystic bodies") (Fig. 150-1). The trophozoite, 2 to 5 μ in diameter, is either round or sickle-shaped and contains a nucleus, mitochondria, and vacuoles; it also includes pseudopodia and filopodia, used in limited motility. The cyst usually measures between 3 and 6 μ in diameter. Its cell wall consists of three layers, and its cytoplasm contains eight small pleomorphic intracystic (oval) bodies (sporozoites). Two other cystic forms have been described, but these are probably intermediates including empty or developing cysts (Fig. 150-1). Many small surface projections

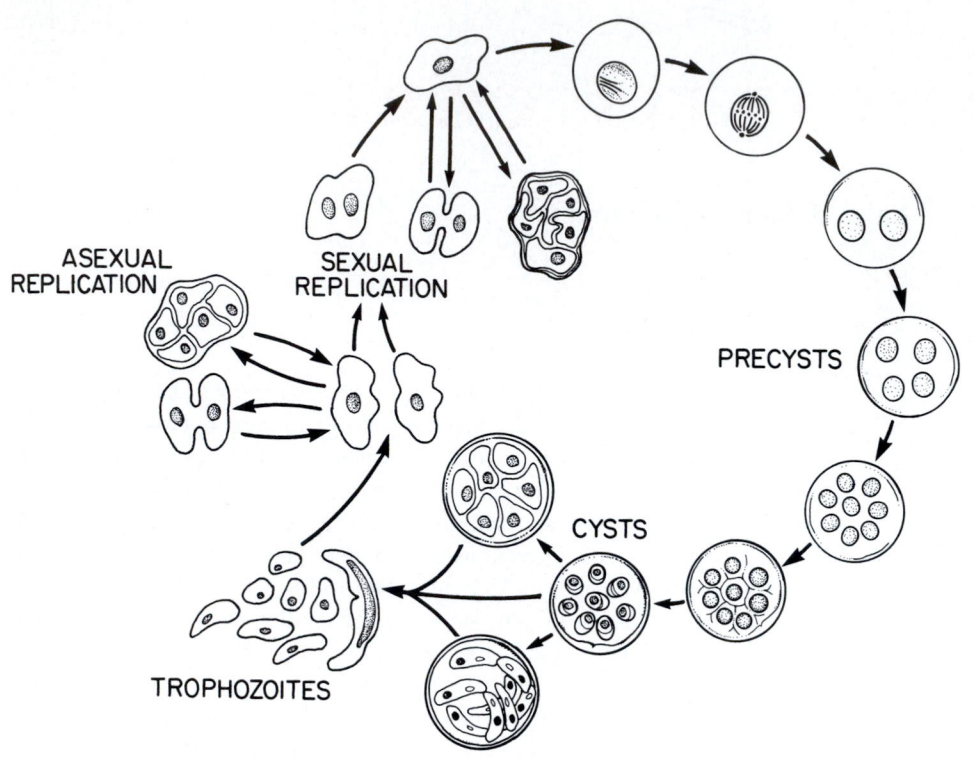

ASEXUAL
REPLICATION

SEXUAL
REPLICATION

PRECYSTS

CYSTS

TROPHOZOITES

FIGURE 150-1 The life cycle of *Pneumocystis carinii.*

("tubular expansions") form a branching network over the surfaces of the cysts and the trophozoites. The role of these projections is unknown.

In the alveolus, *Pneumocystis* are covered with a variety of glycoproteins derived from both the organism and the environment. Specific and nonspecific immunoglobulins, albumin, surfactant proteins, laminin, fibronectin, and other serum and lung proteins coat the surface. The organism itself produces a relatively limited array of surface glycoproteins that share antigenic epitopes; these are 110 to 120 kd, 55 to 60 kd, 40 to 50 kd, and 20 to 27 kd in molecular weight. These, and some minor components, are found on both animal- and human-derived organisms. *P. carinii* from different species share antigenic epitopes in addition to carrying unique epitopes. Of note is that most adult patients with *Pneumocystis* pneumonia carry antibodies to the major epitopes of the organism. The cell wall contains cholesterol but no ergosterol and does not appear to synthesize sterols de novo; this accounts for the lack of susceptibility to many of the antifungal antibiotics. The presence of chitin in the cell wall is controversial. The surface of *P. carinii* is carbohydrate rich with glucose, mannose, and β-1,3-glucan, which may play a role in phagocytosis of the organism by macrophages.[16] The surface also contains carbohydrate-binding moieties, which may play a role in attachment to epithelial or surfactant layers.

The life cycle of *Pneumocystis* is poorly understood (Fig. 150-1).[33] Many of the studies of the life cycle have used organisms derived from infected animals and passaged on a "feeder cell" layer of epithelial or fibroblastoid cells in tissue culture. Continuous growth has not been achieved in this system, and the human-derived organism has not been grown consistently in vitro. Success with axenic or cell-free cultivation of *P. carinii*

has been limited. It is now believed that the sporozoites (daughter forms) emerge from the cyst to develop into trophozoites; some of the trophozoites mature to form cysts and then repeat the cycle. This sequence is far from settled, however, and both sexual and asexual intermediate stages have been postulated. It is likely that some differences exist in *Pneumocystis* growth in different hosts and with different immune defects.

Research on *Pneumocystis* has been hampered by the difficulties encountered in propagating the organism in vitro. Studies have been performed on organisms derived from immunosuppressed rodents, which "spontaneously" develop *P. carinii* pneumonia. Hughes and coworkers have used this model to demonstrate the aerosol transmission of *P. carinii.*[34,35] Cell culture techniques have not yet become useful diagnostically, because of the difficulty in culturing the organism from infected human tissues. *Pneumocystis* is occasionally grown as a "contaminant" in viral cultures of bronchial lavage fluid on a variety of feeder cell lines.

TAXONOMY AND MOLECULAR BIOLOGY

Phylogenetic data support the identification of *P. carinii* with the fungi (*Rhizopoda, Myxomycetes, Zygomycota, Schizosaccharomyces, Neurospora, Candida,* and the red yeasts in various studies), based on conserved mRNA sequences.[14] The presence of separate genes encoding the thymidylate synthase and dihydrofolate reductase of *P. carinii,* the presence of a cyst wall rich in β-glucan that stains with periodic acid–Schiff and silver stains, the poorly developed mitochondria, the absence of typical protozoan intracellular organelles, and the airborne spread of infection all support this taxonomic position.[15,59,61] The neutral lipid fraction of *P. carinii* includes a variety of phytosterols shared by plants and fungi, including *Physarum* species.[23] However, the appearance of the organism with a thick-walled cyst with internal "sporozoites" and ameboid trophozoites, the absence of ergosterol, susceptibility to antibiotics used in the treatment of protozoan infections (pentamidine, atovaquone, sulfamethoxazole), and the existence of "antigenic variation" in the major surface glycoprotein (gp120, gpA, MSG) lend credence to identification with the protozoa.

It is likely that a new phylogenetic category may be needed within the *Ascomycota* for *Pneumocystis.* Unique cell wall components (glucans, phytosterols) and synthetic pathways (e.g., topoisomerases) may participate in the pathogenesis of infection due to *P. carinii* and may provide targets for the development of new antibiotics. Difficulty in ascribing *Pneumocystis* to one or another family may be further complicated by the apparent exchange of membrane lipids and perhaps glycoproteins between *P. carinii* and host cells. This may allow the adaptation of *P. carinii* to the host environment, decrease the effectiveness of the immune response, and enhance survival by decreasing the membrane synthetic demands of the organism.

The existence of different "strains" of *Pneumocystis* have been demonstrated using pulsed-field gel electrophoresis to establish chromosomal patterns. It appears that infections are often clonal, although many strains may coexist in the infected person. Characteristic chromosome patterns have not yet been associated with specific virulence or host characteristics. Characteristic shifts in the telomeric ends of the chromosomes suggest that genetic exchange is ongoing between chromosomes, as occurs in the mechanism of antigenic variation by movement of genetic cassettes noted in the subtelomeric region of the trypanosomes.

P. carinii expresses both unique and some common antigens in different host species. Surface antigens have been characterized at the glycoprotein and molecular levels. The major surface glycoprotein (MSG) represents the main humoral immunogen in the rat model, though other antigens (gp45–55) may have importance in human infection.[19,39,55] Several MSG types (up to three) have been observed simultaneously in single infected humans and animals with monoclonal antibody staining and with genetic characterization. Because some antigens are shared between glycoproteins of differing sizes and between species, it is unclear whether a single organism can express more than one MSG or switch MSG expression during the life cycle. The MSG appears to represent a large family of related genes (more than 30), many of which are located in tandem repeated arrays in the subtelomeric regions and may contribute to the generation of the variety of antigenic types.[55]

Data from a number of laboratories, including our own, suggest that each genomic copy of an MSG includes an upstream highly conserved "expression" site and a unique segment downstream that encodes the differing antigenic characteristics of each clone. The organization of the joining region between the conserved and variant segments contains alternating conserved and variant segments, whose function remains to be determined. It is not yet clear whether the conserved intron-exon structure represents a splicing system related to that of the African trypanosomal variant surface glycoprotein, which allows the serial expression of a variety of antigenic types. No evidence for active "switching" of genotypes has been developed to date (e.g., under selective immune pressure). However, the presence of splicing is suggested by the absence of genomic intergenic regions in the mRNA transcripts encoding cloned MSGs.

EPIDEMIOLOGY OF INFECTION DUE TO *PNEUMOCYSTIS*

Over the past 50 years, *P. carinii* pneumonia has been transformed from a medical curiosity into an important respiratory infection that affects four categories of immunocompromised host: (1) *congenital,* caused by inborn immune defects in antibody-synthesizing capacity and/or in the cellular mechanisms responsible for delayed hypersensitivity; (2) *induced,* by immunosuppressive therapy, especially corticosteroids in the treatment of hematopoietic malignancies; (3) *acquired,* occurring as part of AIDS, often as the identifying opportunistic pathogen in HIV infection; and (4) *nutritionally deficient with epidemic infection,* seen primarily in neonates and infants.

P. carinii causes pneumonia in persons with a wide variety of underlying immune deficiencies (Table 150-1). Studies performed in immunosuppressed animals and clinical experience indicate that a T-cell immune defect is generally needed to initiate *P. carinii* infection.[24] Passive transfer of immune T lymphocytes is protective against *P. carinii* pneumonia in mice, whereas transfer of immune globulin alone is only partly protective.[26] The relative risk of infection with *Pneumocystis* is predictable in most hosts in which this infection occurs. Disease occurring outside the hosts or a timeframe predicted on the basis of the assumed level of immune suppression should suggest an epidemiologic hazard or immune deficiency beyond that known to exist. For example, the risk of *Pneumocystis* pneumonia is greatest in the first 6 months after transplantation, after 3 to 6 months of oral corticosteroid therapy, and during periods of increased immune suppression (for example, during the use of bolus corticosteroids or antilymphocyte therapies for graft rejection).[21] In AIDS, the risk increases with the progressive fall of the CD4-positive lymphocyte counts to below 200 per cubic centimeter or to less than 20 percent of the total lymphocyte pool.[43] The occurrence of *P. carinii* infection in persons not in these categories should suggest exposure to infected persons, other immunosuppressive effects (e.g., coinfection with cytomegalovirus, lymphoma, neutropenia), or, in the HIV-infected person, a rapid progression of viral infection with the accompanying decline in systemic immune function.

The natural reservoir of infection remains unknown. Aerosol transmission of infection has been demonstrated by a number of investigators in animal models, and clusters of infections have developed in clinical settings—for instance, between HIV-infected persons and renal transplant recipients.[12,50,54] *P. carinii* DNA has been detected by the polymerase chain reaction in the air of hospital rooms, bronchoscopy suites, and clinics used by infected subjects. The frequency of infection varies both by institution and by geography. For example, it appears that the incidence of *Pneumocystis* in AIDS patients is much lower in Africa than in the United States. However, this may reflect lim-

TABLE 150-1

Conditions Associated with *Pneumocystis* Pneumonia

Acquired immunodeficiency syndrome (AIDS)
Chemotherapy (especially corticosteroids)
Radiation therapy
Organ transplantation
Prematurity
Malnutrition (protein and calorie)
Malignancies (especially hematopoietic)
Congenital immune deficiency diseases (cellular and/or humoral)
Collagen vascular disease
Hematologic disorders
Cushing's syndrome
Nephrotic syndrome

ited diagnostic capabilities and the morbidity associated with the endemic level of tuberculosis and diarrheal pathogens in Africa, rather than a reduced epidemiologic exposure. The use of polymerase chain reaction (PCR) technology suggests that carriage of *P. carinii* in African AIDS patients is, in fact, common.

The prevalence of infection with *P. carinii* in patients with AIDS has prompted a large effort to develop diagnostic serologic tests that might be applied to the general population. Serologic testing has reinforced the view that subclinical infection is common and that a reactivation of latent infection is often a factor in the pathogenesis of *P. carinii* pneumonia.[44] However, in studies of rats cured of *Pneumocystis* pneumonia by trimethoprimsulfamethoxazole (TMP-SMX), immunosuppression alone does not result in recurrent infection if the animals are maintained in a sterile environment.[2] Recent molecular studies in animals and humans using a variety of genetic probes, including probes for *P. carinii,* ribosomal mRNA internal transcribed spacer regions have suggested that *both reinfection and the reactivation of latent infection are significant factors in the incidence of disease.*

Most people have serologic evidence of exposure by age 4.[44] The rate of identification of organisms in autopsy studies is less than 8 percent. An autopsy series from patients with malignant lymphoma or leukemia demonstrated a 5 percent incidence of identification of pulmonary *P. carinii,* compared with a less than 0.5 percent incidence in immunologically normal subjects. Further, following treatment with TMP-SMX for active infection, immunosuppression in animal models does not result in the reemergence of infection in animals maintained in isolation cages.[2] Thus, while the isolation of patients infected or potentially infected with *P. carinii* from immunologically normal patients (who are likely to be seropositive for *Pneumocystis* antigens) is not essential, uninfected, immunocompromised patients should not be exposed to persons with active *P. carinii* infection.

The incidence of infection relates to the intensity and duration of immune suppression. T-lymphocyte deficiencies are particularly important in predisposing to *P. carinii* infection.[6] Thus, persons with AIDS have a predisposition based on both the progressive decline in the T-cell population and the macrophage defects inherent to HIV infection (see Chapter 152).[22] The correlation with T-lymphocyte numbers is such that the rate of infection nearly doubles with a drop in CD4-positive lymphocyte counts from between 100 and 200 to below 100 per cubic centimeter.

A clear correlation with the circulating viral load in AIDS has not yet been established. However, preliminary data suggest that the incidence of opportunistic infections, in general, appears to decrease with a fall in HIV level below that detectable by currently available PCR (approximately 200 copies per milliliter) or signal amplification virus detection techniques (approximately 500 copies per milliliter). Historically, the rate of *Pneumocystis* pneumonia in AIDS was halved by the use of zidovudine for the duration of the effective antiviral effect of this agent. Similar effects are expected with the newer antiviral agents and combinations, especially those including the antiviral protease inhibitors. The rate of infection appears to double in homosexual males with AIDS when compared with intravenous drug users. Two groups of AIDS patients, those without insurance and intravenous drug abusers, have a significantly lower use of prophylaxis, zidovu-

dine use, and AIDS diagnoses before admission with the initial episode of *Pneumocystis* pneumonia. In the absence of effective prophylaxis, more than 80 percent of AIDS patients are expected to develop *Pneumocystis* pneumonia.

Corticosteroid use, neutropenia, and lung transplantation are also major predisposing factors in the development of infection. However, in most non-AIDS patients, the risk of disease is around 5 to 15 percent, depending on the nature and duration of the immune suppression. In the solid organ transplant recipient, chronic immune suppression that includes corticosteroids is most often associated with *Pneumocystosis* (Fig. 150-2). Bolus corticosteroids and cyclosporine may also contribute to the risk for *Pneumocystis* pneumonia.[29,40] Active infection due to cytomegalovirus (CMV) may also enhance the growth of *Pneumocystis* in any affected population (Figs. 150-3D and 150-5B). Whether CMV directly stimulates the proliferation of *Pneumocystis,* acts systemically as an immunosuppresive agent, or is simply a fellow traveler in the immunocompromised host remains to be settled. The clinical association of CMV with *P. carinii* may reflect similarities in the susceptible hosts or subtle shifts in the alveolar microenvironment.

Clinically apparent infection may emerge during the weaning of immunosuppressive agents. This is consistent with the limited inflammatory response generated by the organism in the susceptible host. Patients with *P. carinii* pneumonia generally have both antibodies and T lymphocytes directed at the organism at the time of presentation. Thus, the assumption has been made that such immunities are not protective, that the correlates of protection (the target antigens) have not yet been identified, that antigenic variation has "switched" the antigens expressed on the surface of the organisms, or that protection rests with the cellular immune control of alveolar macrophage function. In the presence of *P. carinii,* cytokine production and phagocytosis by alveolar macrophages are abnormal.[36] Surfactant proteins A and D, members of the collectin family, are increased during *Pneumocystis* pneumonia in patients and in animal models, while surfactant lipids are reduced. These changes may contribute to diminished uptake of organisms by resident macrophages.

CLINICAL PRESENTATION

The hallmark of infection due to *P. carinii* is the presence of marked hypoxemia, dyspnea, and cough out of proportion to physical or radiologic findings. In the transplant recipient or the person undergoing corticosteroid therapy, *Pneumocystis* pneumonia is generally acute to subacute in development and often masked by other processes, including allograft rejection or infection. In the AIDS patient with first episode of infection, the evolution is more gradual (often 2 to 5 weeks) and constitutional symptoms and weight loss are prominent.[37] Subsequent infections may evolve more rapidly. In the cancer patient receiving chemotherapy or in the organ or bone marrow transplant recipient, the use of corticosteroids, prior lung infection, abnormal pulmonary lymphatics (after heart, lung, or liver transplantation), and neutropenia may contribute to the absence of radiologically apparent disease. The rate of development of clinical infection is exacerbated by the presence of preexisting lung disease or other infections (e.g., CMV, *Legionella,* mycobacteria) (Fig. 150-2) or allograft

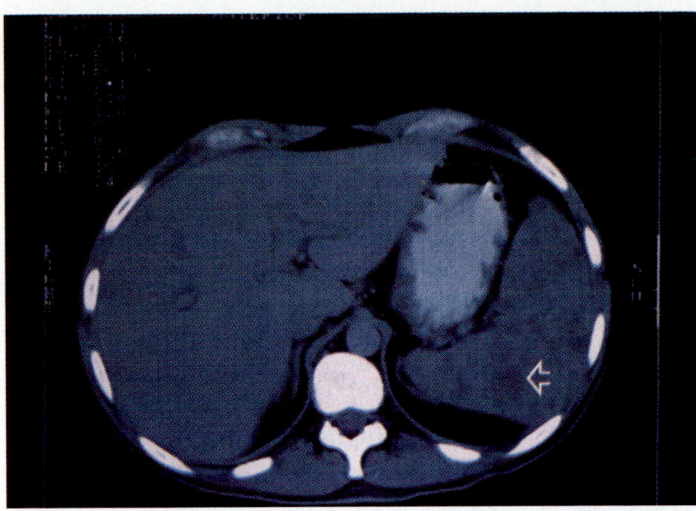

A

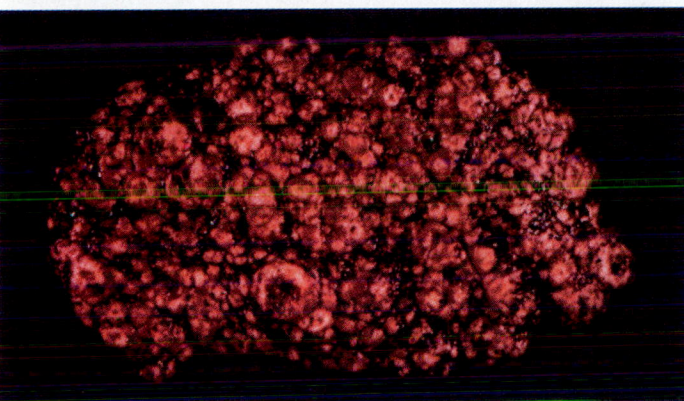

B

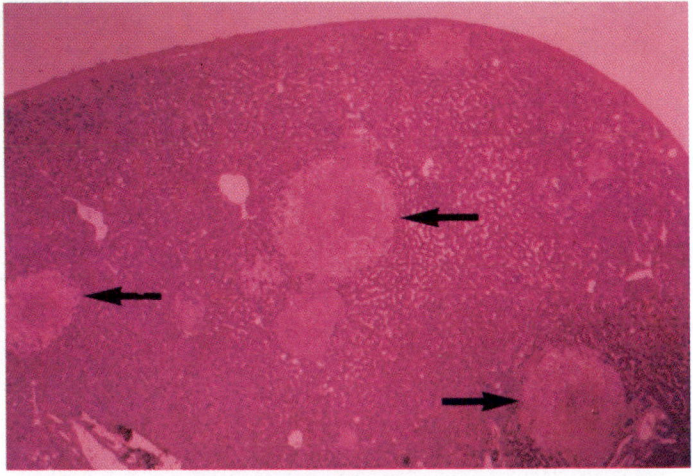

C

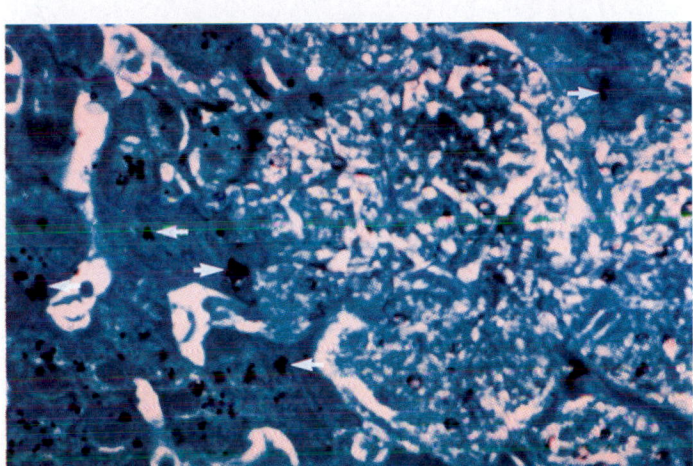

D

FIGURE 150-2 Extrapulmonary pneumocystosis in a patient with AIDS on aerosolized pentamidine prophylaxis presented as a splenic mass lesion with abdominal pain. The computerized body tomographic (CBT) scan reveals a mass lesion *(A)*, seen after splenectomy on gross pathology *(B and C)* and on microscopic examination (silver stain, *D*). *(Courtesy of Dr. J. Davis Allen, Jr., New England Deaconess Hospital.)*

rejection (in lung transplantation recipients). In the organ transplant recipient, *Pneumocystis* pneumonia will occur approximately 2 to 4 months after the initiation of immune suppression or during periods of increased immune suppression (pulsed steroids, antilymphocyte therapies, CMV infection). The incidence of infection varies between institutions and with the prophylactic regimens employed. In patients receiving lung transplants, the rate of asymptomatic isolation of *P. carinii* approaches two-thirds of the total in some series.[28] Of these, up to half are expected to develop symptomatic disease without treatment.

In AIDS patients, the presentation of *Pneumocystis* pneumonia is often complicated by a variety of factors. Prophylaxis with aerosolized pentamidine or with other antibiotics may delay or alter the presentation of disease. Coinfection may accelerate the progression of disease or alter the radiographic pattern; in particular, CMV, *Histoplasma capsulatum, Legionella* species, and mycobacterial species may contribute to the constitutional symptoms, to hypoxemia, and to the locality of pulmonary lesions.

Acute exposure to *Pneumocystis* is rarely documented; in an-

imal models, inoculation of *P. carinii* induces a neutrophilic infiltrate that is rapidly (in 2 to 3 days) replaced with lymphocytes and macrophages. Similarly, in transplant recipients and despite therapy with cyclosporine, *Pneumocystis* induces lymphocyte- and neutrophil-predominant infiltration into the lungs acutely, followed by macrophage infiltration and clearance of organisms. This contrasts with the macrophage- and neutrophil-predominant infiltrates seen in AIDS patients with acute disease. The lymphocytes are primarily T lymphocytes with normal CD4/8 ratios. *Coinfection with CMV and other pathogens will be detected in more than half of Pneumocystis-infected patients.* The nature of the immune suppression will determine the types of other opportunistic pathogens that coinfect the compromised host. Thus, fungal coinfection has increased as cyclosporine has replaced high-dose corticosteroids in transplant recipients. The expected mortality due to *Pneumocystis* pneumonia is increased in patients taking cyclosporine when compared with other imunocompromised hosts.

EXTRAPULMONARY PNEUMOCYSTOSIS

Pneumocystis was known to cause extrapulmonary disease in the pre-AIDS era, but metastatic infection to significant degrees has been observed only in patients with AIDS.[22,48] Few cases of sys-

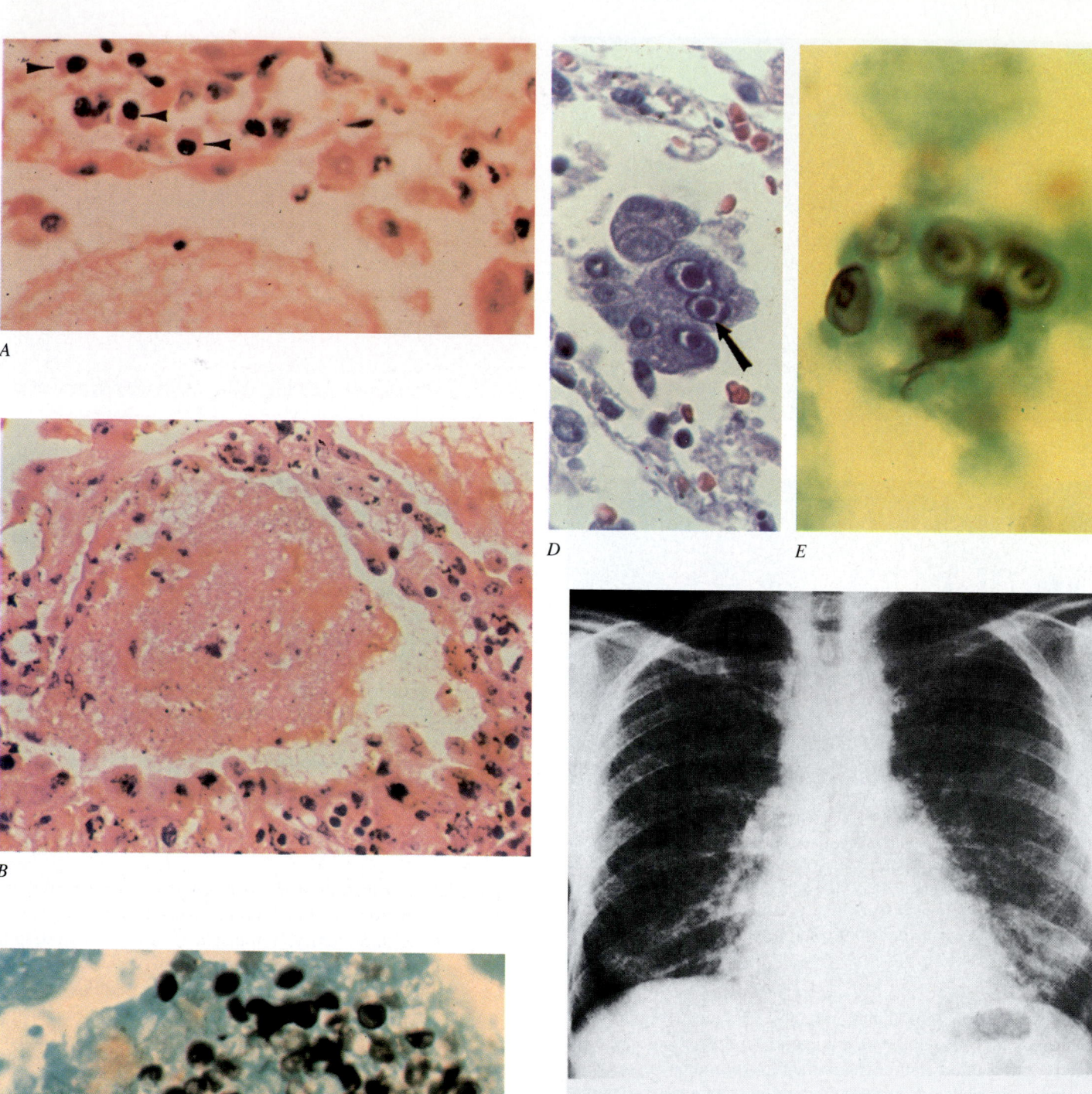

FIGURE 150-3 *Pneumocystis carinii* pneumonia: *A.* Lung of a malnourished infant showing an intra-alveolar foamy exudate and plasma cells (arrowheads) in the interstitium. (H&E stain, ×620.) *B.* Typical alveolar exudative pattern from the lung of an adult with *Pneumocystis* pneumonia after therapy with corticosteroids. Swelling of the alveolar epithelial cells and interstitial edema are seen. Inflammatory response in intersititium is minimal. (H&E stain, ×500.) *C. Pneumocystis* in the form of thick-walled cysts within the foamy exidate. (Displayed by Gomori's methenamine-silver nitrate stain and brilliant green counterstain, ×1250.) *D.* Cytomegalovirus inclusion bodies in alveolar macrophages in a patient with *Pneumocystis* pneumonia. (H&E stain, ×720.) *E. Pneumocystis* cysts in cytologic preparation of induced sputum from an AIDS patient. (Silver stain, ×1250.) *F. Pneumocystis* pneumonitis. Typical chest radiograph showing bilateral, diffuse interstitial infiltrates extending from hilar area.

temic infection due to *P. carinii* have been observed in patients receiving systemic prophylaxis with TMP-SMX, while the diagnosis is occasionally not considered in patients using pentamidine prophylaxis. Pulmonary disease may be minimal or absent in such patients. In our hands, blood samples from up to half of the patients with *Pneumocystis* pneumonia have PCR evidence of circulating DNA from this organism. In addition to the liver and spleen, sites of extrapulmonary disease have included eye, ear, lymph nodes, thymus, skin, mastoids, ascites, GI tract and omentum, pleura, kidney, bone marrow, pancreas, and adrenal glands, and it has been reported as a cause of thromboembolic disease. Vasculitis has been reported due to *P. carinii* as a cause of ischemic necrosis of digits.

The presentation of extrapulmonary infection is generally a mass lesion with accompanying fever, sweats, and malaise. Visual loss may accompany retinal lesions, hepatitis with liver impairment, and ascites and GI tract obstruction with peritoneal and omental lesions. By computed tomographic (CT) scan, many nonenhancing, low-attenuation masses, often with necrosis and/or hemorrhage, may be seen in the liver or spleen (Fig. 150-2). Calcification may occur at the edge of such necrotic lesions during the acute infection, often in the hepatic or renal parenchyma. Histopathology will demonstrate granulomas with giant cells, calcification, or cavities. Distant sites may also contain the same frothy hyaline material seen in the alveoli in pulmonary disease (Fig. 150-3). *P. carinii* will be seen adherent to the blood vessel walls, with myointimal inflammation and thrombosis.

Dual infections may occur with any organism, including mycobacteria, *Histoplasma*, *Legionella*, fungi, or common bacteria. Unless superinfection has occurred or splenic rupture or other life-threatening condition is imminent, systemic treatment of multiple small abscesses due to *Pneumocystis* infection should be adequate without surgical intervention.

RADIOGRAPHY

The Chest Radiograph

The chest radiograph plays a central role in the dignosis of *P. carinii* pneumonia (Figs. 150-4 and 150-5).[20] However, no radiographic pattern is pathognomonic for *Pneumocystis* infection, any more than for the other "atypical" pneumonias—interstitial processes on chest radiograph that present with hypoxemia and fever, but without sputum production. The radiographic pattern depends on the patient's underlying or accompanying disease, the state of immunosuppression, and the duration of infection. Sometimes the chest radiograph is normal despite overt pulmonary disease. More often, the early stage of *P. carinii* pneumonia is manifested by fine, bilateral, perihilar, diffuse infiltrates that progress to an interstitial alveolar butterfly pattern; from the hilar region, the infiltrates spread to the apices or bases. Despite therapy, this pattern is often succeeded in 3 to 5 days by progressive consolidation, the appearance of air bronchograms, and complete opacification of the lung fields.

As in many of the "atypical pneumonias," unusual courses and patterns are seen: nodules, unilateral infiltrates, or even lobar consolidations (Fig. 150-4 and 150-5). Small pleural effusions also occur. Distortions in pattern are commonly produced by prior radiation, drug-induced pulmonary injury, or concurrent infection with other organisms. The patient with recurrent disease may develop chronic interstitial markings, small cysts, or "honeycombing" on chest radiograph. The distribution of cysts in pneumocystosis, when present at all, is more often diffuse, while peripheral or apical bullae are often seen without infection in intravenous drug abusers. Rarely, cavitary disease is seen in the absence of other pathogens; however, *P. carinii* can superinfect fungal or mycobacterial cavities.

The use of aerosolized pentamidine for the therapy and prophylaxis of *Pneumocystis* pneumonia in AIDS has created some new problems in the diagnosis and treatment of pneumocystosis (Fig. 150-5). The disease may present largely or solely in the upper lobes on chest radiograph. Similar disease may be seen without pentamidine use, suggesting a predilection of infection for the upper lobes. Cystic changes are more common in patients undergoing prophylaxis who develop *Pneumocystis* pneumonia. The development of spontaneous pneumothoraces may indicate the recurrence of *P. carinii* in the upper lobes despite ongoing prophylactic therapy. Pneumothorax may also complicate the management of intubated patients with *Pneumocystis* pneumonia; active pneumonia or fibrosis in the upper lobes is usually implicated. Undiagnosed, this complication is responsible for a 50 percent mortality. Dense consolidation of tissues may suggest dual infection, often with a bacterial agent.

In lung transplant patients, rejection and infection often produce abnormal chest radiographs. In the first month, rejection of the transplanted lung will cause radiographic changes in up to 75 percent of patients. These changes include nodular and interstitial infiltrates in the perihilar area and the lower lobes, which may progress to consolidation. These changes may also occur with infection, of which CMV is the most common. CMV may be indistinguishable from organ rejection without biopsy. After the first month, rejection less often yields radiographic changes (about 25 percent), and the radiographic findings of infection are similar to those of other immunocompromised hosts.

Inflammation Imaging

Nuclear medicine scans are generally nonspecific and add little to the diagnosis of pulmonary pneumocystosis. However, a normal scan will generally exclude diffuse pulmonary infection due to *Pneumocystis*. Gallium citrate, technetium, indium-immunoglobulin, white blood cell, and diethylenetriamine pentaacetate (DTPA) scans are abnormal in more than 90 percent of patients with *Pneumocystis* infection. These may be most useful in following the resolution of infection. [67]Gallium scintigraphy can be entirely normal for patients with opportunistic pneumonia with or without AIDS. Conversely, AIDS patients may have abnormal gallium scans in the absence of other infection. Gallium scans often become abnormal before the radiographic appearance of pulmonary disease. Lymph node uptake alone may indicate the condition formerly referred to as AIDS-related complex (ARC), due to HIV infection. Diffuse pulmonary uptake may indicate occult infection in the asymptomatic patient, which would allow early intervention for therapy or prophylaxis. The cost of routine gallium scanning for AIDS patients probably outweighs utility when compared with the judicious use of antivi-

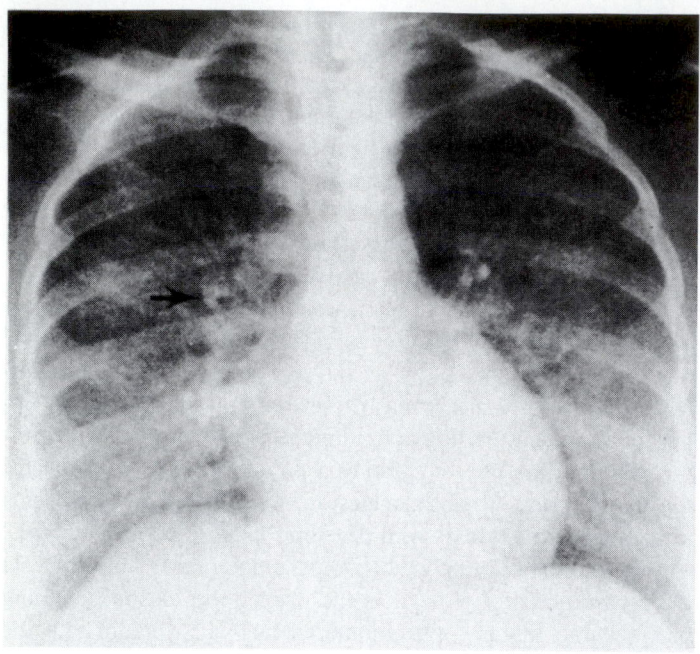

A

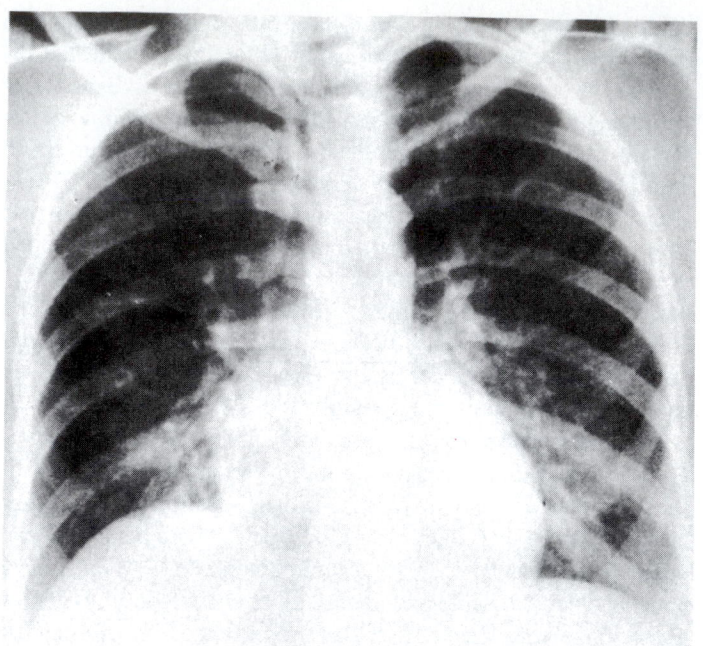

B

FIGURE 150-4 Atypical pattern of *Pneumocystis* with *Mycobacterium avium-intracellulare* in a Haitian woman with AIDS. *A.* Diffuse pulmonary infiltrates before treatment of *Pneumocystis* infection. Arrow indicates small abscess cavity. *B.* After treatment for *Pneumocystis,* many small cavities persist (arrow). *C.* Transbronchial lung biopsy of initial infiltrate reveals *Pneumocystis* cysts. (Silver, ×760.) *D.* Open lung biopsy after therapy for *P. carinii* included areas of pneumonitis atypical for *Pneumocystis* (upper), which contain *M. avium-intracellulare* (arrowheads, lower). (Kinyoun acid-fast stain, ×950.)

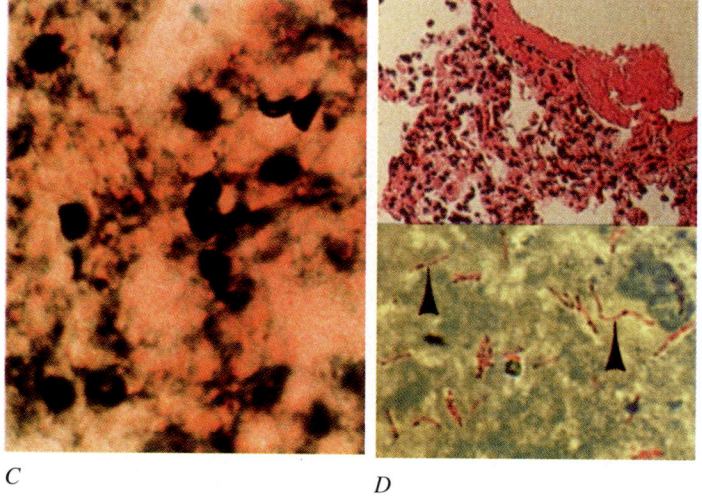

C   *D*

ral or anti-*Pneumocystis* antibiotics based on CD4 cell counts, viral load measurements, or other clinical data. The pattern of lymphoid interstitial pneumonitis (LIP) in children with AIDS is indistinguishable from that of *Pneumocystis* pneumonia.

Some centers make a presumptive diagnosis of *P. carinii* pneumonia in the patient with AIDS when a decrease in diffusing capacity ($D_{L_{CO}}$) is coupled with an abnormal chest radiograph and gallium scan. The clearance of radiolabeled inhaled DTPA is also increased in *P. carinii* pneumonia (as in other pulmonary infections). Although these tests are usually abnormal in *P. carinii* pneumonia, they lack specificity.

Imaging with radiolabeled ([111]indium) human immunoglobulin (IgG) has proved to be a useful adjunct to the diagnosis and treatment of *Pneumocystis* pneumonia, for two reasons. First, the "IgG scan" is more sensitive to inflammatory changes than is the gallium scan. This allows the detection of superimposed focal pulmonary processes due to other pathogens in addition to the diffuse pattern seen in *P. carinii.* This sensitivity also allows the IgG scan to be used to follow the resolution of infection in response to therapy, which has not been possible with gallium. Second, the IgG scan has been useful in detecting unsuspected extrapulmonary foci of infection; this may be important in the management of AIDS patients with disseminated *P. carinii* or other processes. The IgG scan is not useful in the neutropenic patient or the uremic patient with dysfunctional neutrophils.

Other Diagnostic Techniques

The chest CT scan will detect interstitial and micronodular disease not visible on routine chest radiographs. Further, the CT and magnetic resonance imaging (MRI) scans and ultrasound imaging are better suited to the definition of pneumocystomas occurring outside the lung (discussed above; see Fig. 150-2).

LABORATORY FINDINGS

A number of nonspecific indicators of pulmonary processes have been used in the presumptive diagnosis of *Pneumocystis* pneumonia. In general, the patient will have a P_{O_2} less than 60 mmHg and a respiratory alkalosis. The serum lactic dehydrogenase (LDH) enzyme will be elevated in most cases of *Pneumocystis* pneumonia (over 300 IU/ml), with high levels (over 600 to 700 IU/ml) carrying a poor prognosis in the setting of histologically confirmed infection. Lymphoma, other diffuse pneumonias, and LIP

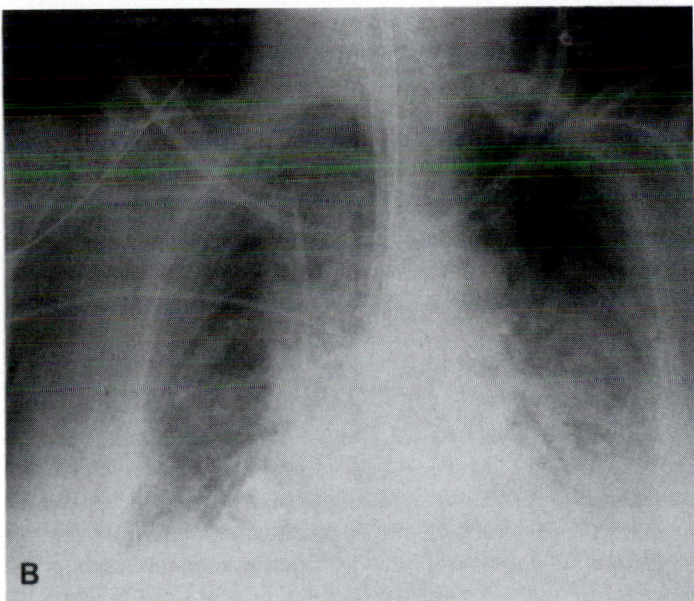

FIGURE 150-5 "Atypical" pneumocystosis. *A.* Upper-lobe pneumonia in an AIDS patient on prophylactic aerosolized pentamidine therapy for a history of *Pneumocystis* pneumonia. The patient had both *P. carinii* and *Legionella pneumophila* infections. *B.* Persistent pulmonary infiltrates in a patient undergoing chemotherapy for non-Hodgkin's lymphoma. Despite 21 days of therapy for *P. carinii*, oxygenation and pulmonary infiltrates failed to improve. An open lung biopsy revealed cytomegalovirus pneumonitis (which responded to therapy with ganciclovir) and drug-induced interstitial fibrosis.

may also raise the LDH level. Respiratory distress and respiratory failure requiring intubation carry a poor prognosis. The marked hypoxemia of *Pneumocystis* pneumonia is accompanied by a $P_{A_{O_2}}$–Pa_{O_2} gradient rise; gradients over 30 mmHg at the start of therapy are associated with a high mortality (and are an indication for the use of adjunctive corticosteroid therapy). Both LDH and the arterial oxygenation gradient will return to normal with successful therapy. Another nonspecific indicator of lung injury in *P. carinii* pneumonia is the angiotensin-converting enzyme (ACE) level (also elevated by smoking and by sarcoidosis, among other causes). While pulmonary function testing may reveal abnormalities in oxygen exchange and compliance in *Pneumocystis* pneumonia, they are not useful diagnostically. Arterial blood gas measurements are helpful in the management of patients with regard to decisions about intubation and the use of corticosteroids as an adjunct to initial antibiotic therapy (see "Therapy," below). Corticosteroids are of greatest use in nonintubated patients with Pa_{O_2} of less than 75 mmHg and greater than 35 mmHg on room air, or a "hypoxemia ratio" ($Pa_{O_2}/F_{I_{O_2}}$) of less than 350 and greater than 75.

SPUTUM EXAMINATION AND HISTOLOGIC DIAGNOSIS

The diagnosis of *P. carinii* pneumonia depends on the identification of characteristic organisms on examination of pulmonary specimens (Table 150-2). The methods used in making the diagnosis have been changed by the use of the induced sputum examination and bronchoscopic alveolar lavage (BAL) without biopsy, and by immunofluorescent staining using monoclonal antibodies to *P. carinii*.[7,38,41,42,56] As a result, the morbidity associated with diagnostic procedures has been reduced and the diagnosis of simultaneous pathogens by these methods is decreased.

The initial step in the diagnosis of *P. carinii* pneumonia is the realization that the patient is at risk for opportunistic infection. The first procedure should be a routine sputum examination for bacterial, mycobacterial, and fungal stains and cultures. Subsequently, the choice of diagnostic test depends on the status of the patient (ability to cooperate with sputum induction), the distribution of pulmonary disease, and the urgency of diagnosis. Given a single procedure, a more invasive test may be preferred. The diagnostic test of choice is the induced sputum examination, coupled with direct immunofluorescent staining for *P. carinii* and for mycobacterial smears and cultures. Some bacteria and fungi may not survive the hypertonic saline used for induction, and the yields for these pathogens do not exceed those of routine sputum samples. Induced sputum may be collected after 20 to 30 minutes of exposure to aerosolized hypertonic saline or water, or after oral hydration. Particularly with AIDS, patients may be significantly dehydrated by the time of clinical presentation.

Before the availability of immunofluorescent antibody staining techniques, smears were prepared from the mucoid, nonpurulent portion of the specimen and stained with Giemsa or Diff-Quik stain (for intracystic bodies or sporozoites and trophozoites; see Fig. 150-6) or with toluidine blue O or silver, which stains the cyst wall. Because cysts represent only 5 to 10 percent of the organism burden, many laboratories prefer the Giemsa to the more complex silver stain, but Giemsa-stained smears are more

TABLE 150-2

Diagnostic Techniques for *P. carinii*

Technique	Yield	Complications	Comments*
Routine sputum	Poor	Rare	Cultures needed
Induced sputum	30–75%	Rare	First choice; excellent in AIDS
Transtracheal aspiration	Fair (with experience)	Common: bleeding, subcutaneous air	Rarely worthwhile
Gallium scan	Nonspecific	Injection site of infected patients	Positive in >95%
Bronchoalveolar lavage (BAL)	>50% (>95% in AIDS)	Bleeding, aspiration fever, bronchospasm	Wedged terminal BAL with immuno-fluorescence
BAL/brushing	As for BAL alone	As for BAL	Not useful for *P. carinii*
BAL/transbronchial biopsy	>90% (all patients)	See BAL; pneumothorax	Impression smears; cultures/pathology
Open lung biopsy	>95% (all patients)	Anesthesia, air leakage, altered respiration, wound infection	"Gold standard" noninfectious/infec tious processes; large sample
Needle aspirate	≤60%	Pneumothorax, bleeding	Best in localized disease

*All samples should be cultured and stained for bacteria (including mycobacteria), fungi, and viruses and examined for protozoa. Optimal procedures will depend on the locally available expertise.

difficult to read. In experienced hands, these stains should detect *P. carinii* in up to 85 percent of AIDS patients and in up to 60 percent of other immunocompromised patients. Proper induction and smearing techniques are critical to success.

The staining method of choice for sputum as BAL specimens is direct immunofluorescent staining with monoclonal antibodies (Fig. 150-6). This method is costly, but significant cost savings may be achieved in terms of specimen preparation and examination time. Rapid staining with immunofluorescent monoclonal antibodies directed against surface antigens of *P. carinii* has a high degree of specificity and a sensitivity for screening of sputum smears. This technique may detect 10 to 15 percent of *Pneumocystis* infections beyond the standard histologic stains (Fig. 150-2). Some of the commercially available antibodies produce high backgrounds and some nonspecific staining; each laboratory must optimize the fluorescent staining technique. Smears may be improved through use of mucolytic agent (Mucomyst, dithiothreitol) just before preparation.

As with PCR testing, the heightened sensitivity of immunofluorescent staining, coupled with the use of either induced sputum or bronchoscopic lavage samples, may detect "infections" that are not of clinical significance. The meaning of a few organisms on smear in a patient with fever and cough may not be clear. Owing to the broad antibacterial spectrum of TMP-SMX, response to therapy is only a partial confirmation of the existence of *P. carinii* pneumonia. AIDS patients will often have residual (dead) organisms in their sputum for many weeks after successful treatment. However, organisms found in the non–AIDS-immunosuppressed patient should suggest disease meriting therapy. Insignificant "colonization" of the respiratory tract before therapy has not been demonstrated; significant numbers of organisms have not been found by BAL in asymptomatic AIDS patients. Of note is that a negative smear does not indicate the absence of *P. carinii*. With use of ribosomal sequence–derived primers on pulmonary specimens, the PCR has more than 98 percent specificity and sensitivity, compared with a 78 percent sensitivity for immunofluorescence on the same samples. Serologic tests are useful only for epidemiologic studies.

The *histopathology* of *Pneumocystis*-infected lung is usually distinctive enough to be diagnostic even when organisms cannot be identified. In the adult, the disease appears to be predominantly alveolar. The airspaces are filled with a foamy eosinophilic exudate and appear honeycombed. The intra-alveolar exudate consists of organisms, large amounts of surface glycoprotein, proteinaceous exudate from the lungs, and debris of macrophages and inflammatory cells. At the same time, the alveolar interstitium is infiltrated by polymorphonuclear leukocytes and lymphocytes (Fig. 150-3). Patchiness in the distribution of disease within the lungs is common. In contrast to the adult disease, *Pneumocystis* pneumonia in malnourished infants has a major interstitial component: the interstitium is filled with fluid, plasma cells, and lymphocytes; these formed elements seem to overflow into the airspaces, which are also filled with a frothy eosinophilic exudate. In both forms, the organisms usually appear intermingled with alveolar macrophages in the alveolar exudate (Fig. 150-3). By light microscopy, trophozoites predominate numerically (in more than 90 percent of the organisms), but cysts are more readily identified.

The earliest indication of disease is the presence of organisms adjacent to the epithelial layer. Cysts or clumps of trophozoites may be seen, with a minimal inflammatory infiltrate. As the number of organisms increases, epithelial injury occurs. The mechanism of alveolar epithelial cell injury is uncertain. The organism preferentially adheres to and injures the surface of type I alveolar epithelial cells, while the adjacent type II cells undergo hyperplasia. Desquamation of alveolar epithelial cells occurs early in the course of disease; denuded basement membrane is occasionally seen. Epithelial injury is followed by mononuclear cell infiltration in the interstitium. Organisms may be seen within vacuolated alveolar macrophages, as well as free in the proteinaceous and cellular debris that fills the airspace (Fig. 150-3).

In AIDS, the interstitial inflammation is less marked than in other adult forms of *Pneumocystis* pueumonia, and greater numbers of both cysts and trophozoites are seen in the alveoli. While HIV-infected alveolar macrophages appear to bind organisms normally, internalization of *P. carinii* may be impaired and clearance of organisms delayed. Many dead macrophages are found in BAL samples from HIV- and *Pneumocystis*-infected lungs. In children with AIDS, the appearance is similar to that of adult AIDS, with the addition of some degree of plasma cell infiltration of the interstitium. Although hyaline membranes may line alveoli, they are not diagnostic of infection with *Pneumocystis,* since oxygen toxicity, alveolar proteinosis, or ARDS can evoke similar changes. These may coexist with *Pneumocystis* infection. In pediatric AIDS, lymphocytic interstitial pneumonitis, without evidence of an infectious origin, and bacterial pneumonia may mimic or coexist with *P. carinii* pneumonia.

The *Pneumocystis* cyst wall is displayed by a variety of staining techniques. Of these, the Gomori methenamine silver nitrate method (which stains organisms brown or black) is most reliable, even though it is susceptible to artifacts and does not stain intracellular bodies (Fig. 150-3). Sporozoites and trophozoites are stained by polychrome stains, particularly the Giemsa stain. The Giemsa, Wright, toluidine blue O, and Grocott's rapid silver stain techniques are most useful in dealing with lung imprints, BAL fluid, and pulmonary aspirates. Rapid polychrome staining (Diff-Quik) and a rapid silver staining technique have proved useful in screening smears (Fig. 150-6). When a silver stain is used, a counter stain such as Gram, Wright, Giemsa, hematoxylin,

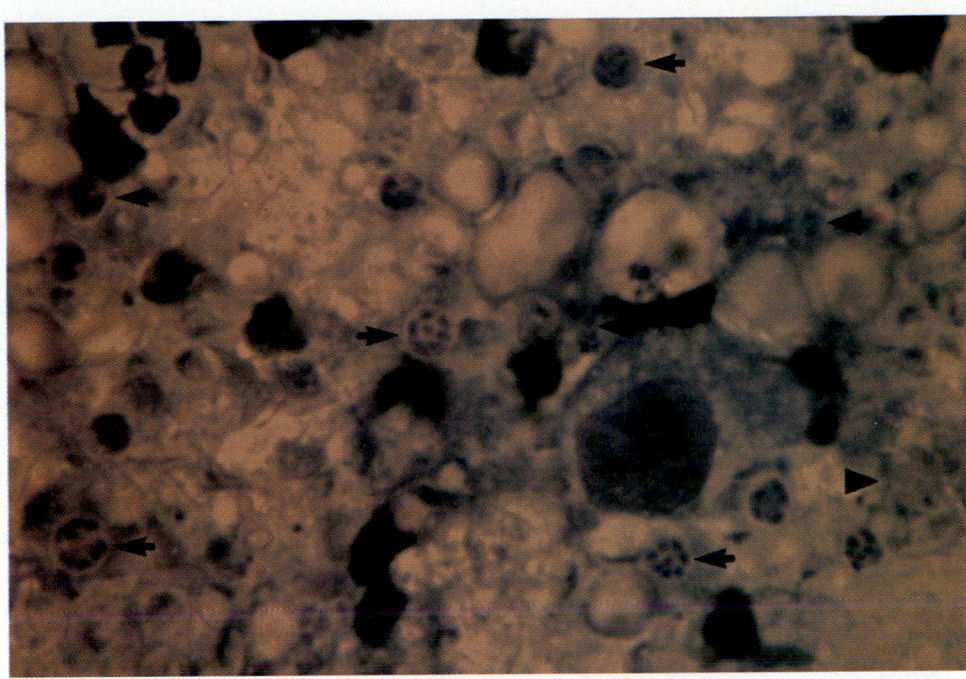

A

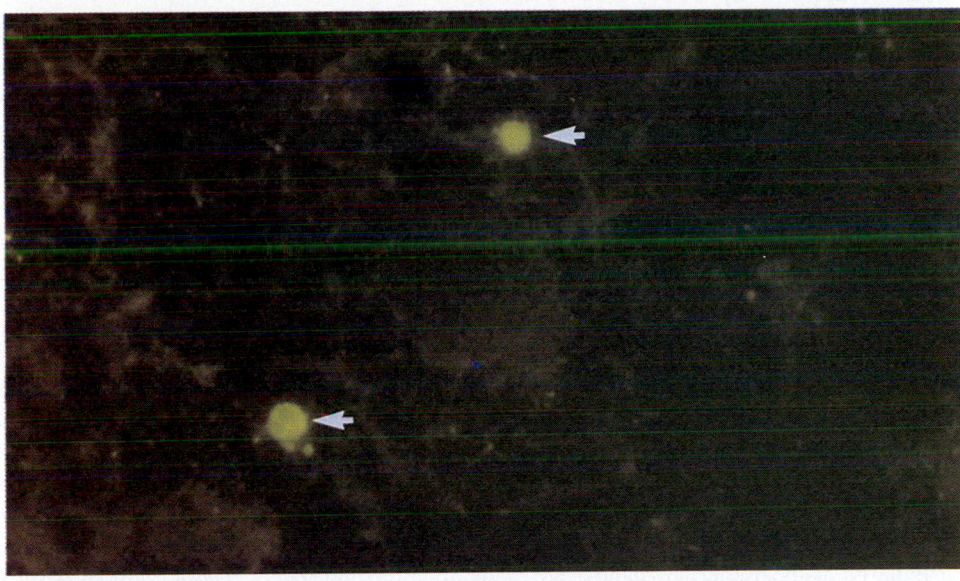

B

FIGURE 150-6   Rapid staining of sputum and biopsy specimens for *P. carinii:* A. Impression smear ("touch preparation") from the cut surface of a human lung biopsy stained with Diff-Quik stain reveals the nuclei of clumped trophozoites (arrowheads) and of the sporozoites within cysts (arrows). B. Human *P. carinii* cysts in an induced sputum specimen that has been stained with fluoresceinated monoclonal antibodies raised to the 116-kd surface antigen of human *P. carinii.*

or trichrome may be required to identify intracystic bodies and to distinguish cysts from red blood cells and yeasts. Up to 97 percent of the organisms are trophozoites. Thus, silver stain substantially underestimates the organism burden.

Even when chest radiography indicates that *P. carinii* pneumonia has cleared, interstitial fibrosis is likely to be found at rebiopsy or autopsy. Unfortunately, the contribution of *Pneumocystis* to the residual fibrosis is often obscured by the tendency of superimposed infection, therapeutic agents, or intervening radiation therapy to elicit inflammatory responses in the interstitium. Subsequent infections are likely to present with more rapid progression to hypoxemia due to persistent restrictive lung disease. In AIDS patients, pulmonary interstitial fibrosis has been observed in up to 27 percent of autopsy and biopsy series, and emphysematous changes are also common. These changes do not appear to be associated with prior *Pneumocystis* infection. A pathogenic role for chronic or recurrent viral (HIV, CMV) infections or immunologic injury has been postulated.

The demonstration of CMV by culture is not helpful in regard to the presence of CMV *disease.* Coinfection due to CMV and *P. carinii* is common, however, and may necessitate treatment for both entities. Nucleic acid diagnostics (hybridization and/or PCR) are used routinely at some centers; the interpretation of positive results remains uncertain because of the high degree of sensitivity of the test. PCR may be best used to determine the risk of *Pneumocystis* infection in patients who might otherwise not receive prophylaxis. Preliminary data support the hypothesis that systemic dissemination is common during infection in AIDS patients (up to 50 percent have *Pneumocystis* DNA in the blood), but it is generally well controlled by resident phagocytes.

INVASIVE DIAGNOSIS OF PNEUMOCYSTOSIS

In the immunocompromised patient with significant pulmonary disease, the inability to make a diagnosis of infection on examination of the induced sputum, or the failure to respond to appropriate therapy, should lead to a more invasive diagnostic procedure: BAL (with biopsies if possible), radiologically guided needle aspiration (for accessible cystic or mass lesions), or open lung biopsy. The choice of the specific test depends on the clinical condition of patient and on the expertise available at the institution (Table 150-2).

Invasive procedures for the diagnosis of *P. carinii* pneumonia fall into several categories: tracheal aspiration, fiberoptic bronchoscopy, transthoracic aspiration, and open lung biopsy. Attempts to avoid the use of invasive procedures by resorting to empiric therapy run a great risk of inappropriate medications and undesirable side effects, as well as delaying effective therapy. Pulmonary specimens obtained by invasive approaches should be processed for bacterial (including mycobacteria, *Nocardia, Actinomyces,* and *Legionella*), fungal, and viral evaluation in addition to making slides for rapid staining with fluorescent antibodies, toluidine blue O, silver, Diff-Quik, Giemsa, or Wright stain. Early diagnosis can be made and therapy initiated on the basis of such smears, especially in AIDS.

Tracheal Aspiration

The yield from this procedure is generally low, and the hazards, particularly in inexperienced hands, are high. In intubated patients, respiratory secretions should be carefully smeared on slides, stained, and examined. If the physician or the microbiology technician has had little experience with *Pneumocystis* smears, and direct imunofluorescence techniques are not available, fiberoptic bronchoscopy or open lung biopsy is indicated for the immunocompromised patient with pulmonary disease, followed by methenamine silver staining of the tissue sections.

Fiberoptic Bronchoscopy

The importance of knowing the success rate of the institution as a basis for selecting the optimal invasive technique is illustrated by published reports of diagnostic yields from fiberoptic bronchoscopy. In proven instances of *P. carinii* pneumonia in non–AIDS-immunocompromised hosts, the reported yields range from 5 to 95 percent.[51] As a rule, institutions with a large experience with *P. carinii* pneumonia are very successful in identi-

fying the organism. Indeed, when bronchial lavage and transbronchial lung biopsies are part of the diagnostic procedure, the success rate exceeds 90 percent. The yield has been even higher in AIDS, and lavage alone (i.e., without biopsy), coupled with immunofluorescent staining of the specimens, will be successful in up to 95 percent of cases.[10,13,32] In these patients, lavage specimens must be gathered from a wedged bronchoscope with at least 50 ml of physiological saline for alveolar washings. Lavages should be performed from the upper lobes if diffuse disease is present. The diagnostic yield in HIV-infected persons with pulmonary symptoms is more than 60 percent: 18 percent with *P. carinii* and another pathogen, 16 percent with *P. carinii* alone, and 25 percent with other infectious causes, including *Histoplasma, Cryptococcus,* mycobacteria, and other bacteria.[3] Trophozoites predominate in bronchial washings, so Giemsa or Diff-Quik staining should be performed routinely to back up other staining methods. In general, lung biopsy is not essential for the diagnosis of *P. carinii* pneumonia in AIDS patients. Patients suspected of harboring multiple pathogens may still benefit from any of the more invasive procedures. Although bleeding from the biopsy site is common (in up to 25 percent of patients), it is rarely life-threatening if the coagulation indices are normal.

Percutaneous Needle Aspiration

High success rates in finding *P. carinii* have also been reported in patients with *P. carinii* pneumonia (up to 60 percent), particularly when aspiration of localized radiologic infiltrates is performed under fluoroscopic guidance. Needle aspiration is also advantageous when a focal process (e.g., abscess) is peripherally located in the lung parenchyma. Pneumothoraces occur in up to one-third of patients as a result of the procedure. In approximately 20 percent of pneumothoraces, insertion of a chest tube will be necessary.

Lung Biopsy

Thoracotomy followed by open lung biopsy affords the most unequivocal avenue for diagnosis. Although the patient may be quite ill by the time this step is taken, in the hands of skilled surgeons, thoracotomy is remarkably safe, even for the intubated patient. This procedure, like the transbronchial biopsy, will provide histologic information that may allow the separation of significant infection of the lower respiratory tract from colonization of the upper respiratory tract by a variety of respiratory pathogens. This information may be critical to therapeutic decision making, as in the use of antiviral agents in the treatment of CMV infection. Thoracoscopic biopsies can often be performed as minimally invasive procedures.

One study has suggested that the use of bronchoscopic evaluation in AIDS patients with pulmonary disease is associated with a lower incidence of death.[4] Coinfections will often go undetected in patients not receiving bronchoscopic evaluation; most such infections are bacterial or fungal. However, other studies suggest that the outcome of hospitalization for AIDS-related pneumonias may not be altered by the use of empiric therapy against *P. carinii* when compared with the use of bronchoscopic evaluation.

Often, accurate diagnosis in the non-AIDS patient may require invasive procedures despite the excellent yields of sputum induction and immunofluorescence (Table 150-2). One element in the choice of procedure depends on the clinical state of the patient: patients who have an uncorrectable coagulopathy are poor candidates for either bronchoscopy with biopsy or open lung biopsy. Patients with atypical presentations or unique epidemiologic exposures have a higher incidence of dual processes or non-*Pneumocystis* infections. Institutions unfamiliar with the proper technique for sampling or handling specimens for the diagnosis of *Pneumocystis* infection should probably use open lung biopsies, which are likely to be more rewarding. Because disease caused by *P. carinii* pneumonia may progress rapidly, the likelihood of success in treatment is greatest at the outset. Therefore, invasive procedures to disclose the organism and any secondary infections should be undertaken early in the course of the disease.

The demonstration of *Pneumocystis* organisms is necessary for diagnosis in the transplant recipient. No more than 15 to 25 percent of pulmonary infiltrates are caused by *P. carinii* in the non-AIDS patient, although regional and underlying disease-specific variations exist. Empiric therapy is more reasonable in the AIDS patient not receiving prophylaxis, as *P. carinii* pneumonia occurs in up to 90 percent of such persons; however, dual infections remain common. Empiric therapy in the transplant recipient may delay specific treatment for other opportunistic pathogens and subject the patient to avoidable toxicities of TMP-SMX or pentamidine. Demonstration of infection due to *P. carinii* should lead to successful treatment, barring superinfection or ARDS.

PROPHYLAXIS AND PROPHYLACTIC STRATEGIES

In the pre-AIDS era, the prevention of *P. carinii* pneumonia was associated with time-limited antibiotic use in the setting of prolonged neutropenia due to cancer chemotherapy. Because many of the chemotherapeutic regimens included corticosteroids, the incidence of *Pneumocystis* pneumonia was predictably high. Prophylactic TMP-SMX was pioneered by Walter Hughes and his colleagues at the St. Jude's Children's Research Hospital for use in children with hematopoietic malignancies and severe combined immunodeficiency (SCID) syndrome.[33,35] This combination agent became the standard for prophylaxis in the AIDS era as well. In AIDS, however, such prophylaxis is lifelong rather than time-limited. Among AIDS patients, more than 60 percent of those cured of *P. carinii* pneumonia will suffer a recurrence within 1 year despite therapy with zidovudine or other antiviral agents. The increased incidence (50 to 60 percent) of side effects due to TMP-SMX in AIDS when compared with patients without AIDS (10 to 20 percent) has led to the development of alternative regimens for prophylaxis against *P. carinii*. The number of prophylactic antibiotics available to be used in AIDS has grown. Among non-AIDS patients, routine prophylaxis should be reserved for centers or patient groups that are known to have a fixed high incidence of disease (i.e., about 3 to 5 percent of susceptible hosts), or for persons with recurrent *Pneumocystis* disease.

The use of appropriate prophylaxis should prevent *Pneumocystis* pneumonia.[52] In AIDS patients and in transplant recipients, the failure to utilize appropriate prophylaxis is generally a reflection of the toxicities associated with the necessary medications or a failure in compliance due to the large number of medications these patients may be expected to consume. Prophylaxis should be maintained in the stable transplant patient for at least 6 months after surgery. In liver and bone marrow transplant recipients with significant graft-versus-host disease or overall poor recovery, prophylaxis is extended to a full year. It should be noted that in transplant centers without a fixed, high incidence of *Pneumocystis* pneumonia, prophylaxis may be reserved for patients in whom chronic, high-level immune suppression, especially with corticosteroids, is needed to maintain graft function. If immune suppression cannot be reduced after a course of treatment for *Pneumocystis* pneumonia, prophylaxis should be maintained indefinitely. In Europe, where immunosuppressive regimens are often less intense, such reductions may not be feasible. Prophylaxis should be reinstituted with increases in immune suppression, including those resulting from pulse steroids or antilymphocyte therapies in transplantation, CMV infection in AIDS or transplantation, treatment of graft-versus-host disease following bone marrow transplantation, new-onset neutropenia, or similar conditions.

In HIV infection, adults and adolescents with CD4+ counts of fewer than 200 cells per cubic millimeter (or 15 to 20 percent of the total lymphocyte number), unexplained fever for more than 2 weeks, a history of oropharyngeal candidiasis, or rapid progression of disease, as measured by rising viral titers or falling CD4+ counts, should receive prophylaxis. Prophylaxis in HIV-infected children is recommended for CD4+ counts of fewer than 1500 cells per cubic millimeter for less than 11 months, fewer than 1000 cells per cubic millimeter between 1 and 5 years, or fewer than 500 cells per cubic millimeter after age 5, and in any child in whom the CD4+ percentage falls to less than 24 percent. The greatest risk for children may be at 3 to 6 months of age, making the identification of the HIV-infected infant critical to survival.

Prophylaxis is needed against many opportunistic infections in AIDS and other compromised patients. In patient infected with CMV or HIV, antiviral therapy is central to the prevention and treatment of *Pneumocystis* pneumonia. Many patients are unable to afford or to comply with complex prophylactic and therapeutic regimens. Very few HIV-infected persons are capable of completing a long-term (36 months) course of any particular agent. The median time to switch of therapies that have begun with either TMP-SMX or dapsone is approximately 2.5 years, with approximately 20 percent of patients requiring several (two or more) changes in prophylactic regimen. Thus, over time, more patients receive less adequate therapies. Prophylaxis has a significant impact on survival, quality of life, and hospitalization frequency. Benefits (about 9 to 12 months' survival) are less marked outside North America, where the incidence of *Pneumocystis* pneumonia is lower.

The need for continued anti-*Pneumocystis* prophylaxis in AIDS patients who recover CD4+ T-cell counts greater than 200 per cubic millimeter during antiviral therapy is not known yet. Functional assays of immune function for such patients are not available. In general, prophylaxis is continued with TMP-SMX, given the protection against bacterial infections at all levels of CD4 counts. This approach may change as more data emerge.

Resistance of *P. carinii* to antibiotics has not been demonstrated despite the apparent clinical failure of antibiotics in some patients. Resistance *may* develop in association with mutations in the dihydropteroatesynthase gene of *P. carinii*. Predictably, the use of prophylaxis both for *P. carinii* and for yeasts and the resultant improved survival of HIV-infected persons have increased the relative frequency of other causes of pulmonary disease in transplant recipients, including both infections (e.g., CMV, azole-resistant fungi, mycobacteria) and noninfectious processes. This shift in the "pattern" of opportunistic infections has been best demonstrated in AIDS patients.[31]

Trimethoprim-sulfamethoxazole (TMP-SMX, co-trimoxazole) is the agent of choice for the prevention of *Pneumocystis* infection in any patient who can tolerate this fixed-combination agent.[18,29] At a dose of one single-strength tablet per day (80 mg TMP and 160 mg SMX), a wide variety of opportunistic infections are prevented, including *P. carinii, Toxoplasma gondii, Listeria monocytogenes, Nocardia asteroides, Isospora belli,* and susceptible bacteria, including pneumococci, *Hemophilus influenzae,* community-acquired staphylococci, and some enteric gram-negative rods. While the protection against *T. gondii* is incomplete in AIDS patients (80 to 90 percent effective) at this dosage (generally a double-strength tablet a day might be used in seropositive persons without a history of *T. gondii* infection), breakthrough infection has not been seen in transplant recipients or in cancer patients. Studies of low- and high-dose regimens for prophylaxis (single- or double-strength TMP-SMX) in HIV-positive subjects suggest no advantage to the higher dose (no disease in either group when compliant) and earlier occurrence of toxicity in the high-dose group.

Drug toxicity is commonly observed even with low-dose regimens, especially in the form of mild bone marrow suppression. Such bone marrow toxicity is notable in combination with other marrow suppressive agents (e.g., azathioprine, ganciclovir, cytoxan, allopurinol), malnutrition, or infection (HIV, mycobacteria, or cytomegalovirus). For *Pneumocystis* prevention, it is equally effective, given the slow replication of the organism, to administer the antibiotics on 3 days a week. Toxicity has been related to serum levels of the sulfa component in AIDS. Some patients will not tolerate any dose of sulfa drugs, owing to significant rash (occasional Stevens-Johnson syndrome), hepatitis (particularly in liver allograft patients), eosinophilic nephritis, or neutropenia. Generally, significant toxicities evolve within the first month of therapy. Hyperkalemia may be observed in the setting of normal renal function as a result of trimethoprim's interfering with the secretion of potassium in the renal distal tubule. This is reversible and more common during therapy than with prophylaxis. In general, neutropenia should not be treated with folate, which has been associated with treatment failures. Both oral and intravenous desensitization regimens will allow the use of TMP-SMX in many patients otherwise intolerant of the combination. Reintroduction of TMP-SMX at reduced dose is often tolerated in persons not severely intolerant of this agent. This is generally preferable to the use of any alternative agent.

Alternative regimens are available for the patient intolerant of TMP-SMX. The use of prophylaxis with aerosolized pentami-

dine isethionate (300 mg every 3 to 4 weeks) was pioneered in AIDS patients and is well tolerated in organ transplant recipients. Pentamidine aerosol prophylaxis is generally effective after the second or third dose administered by experienced personnel with a nebulizer (e.g., Fisons, Respirgard II), producing droplets in the range of 1 to 3 μ. The Fisons nebulizer has also been used with an alternative schedule of five 60-mg doses over 2 weeks, followed by 60 mg every 2 weeks. Because the distribution of drug may not reach the upper lobes, or because the growth of *Pneumocystis* may be favored in the upper lobes, adjusting patient positioning during inhalation may be useful.

Breakthrough infection has been observed in some patients receiving aerosolized and intravenous pentamidine prophylaxis (particularly in the upper lobes). These breakthroughs are in patients receiving primary prophylaxis after transplantation or in AIDS patients who have not yet received two or more doses of antibiotic (i.e., in the first 8 to 10 weeks), in CMV-infected persons, or in secondary prophylaxis after incomplete clearance of infections. In single-lung transplant recipients, prophylactic failures have been observed in the residual (native) lung despite successful protection of the allograft. When breakthrough occurs, diagnosis by noninvasive means is often complicated by reduced organism numbers; biopsy may be required. The use of *intravenous* pentamidine (300 mg every 3 to 4 weeks) for prophylaxis has been successful, with the single exception of disease occurring in transplant patients coinfected with CMV or receiving antilymphocyte globulins for graft rejection, or in AIDS patients with rapidly progressive disease and/or infected with CMV.

Cough and bronchospasm are the common side effects of aerosolized pentamidine therapy; they are generally reversible with bronchodilator therapy. Less often, pneumothorax and hypoglycemia or hyperglycemia are noted. Transient, mild hypoglycemia or nausea is more common after intravenous administration than with the aerosolized method. The use of pentamidine prophylaxis requires the simultaneous administration of a second antibiotic (e.g., quinolone) for antibacterial prophylaxis in transplant recipients—which is not required in patients receiving TMP-SMX.

In general, alternative prophylactic agents have been preferred to pentamidine. In AIDS patients, dapsone (diaminodiphenylsulfone), with or without trimethoprim or pyrimethamine, is in wide use in a variety of combinations. In general, neutropenia (especially in the G6PD-deficient host), hepatitis, and rash are limiting for each of these regimens, and they offer no benefit over low-dose TMP-SMX. Because of a long half-life, dapsone may be administered in doses of 50 to 100 mg per day to 100 mg per week. Breakthrough infection has been observed in AIDS patients at 50 mg per day, but toxicity begins to be limiting at 100 mg a day. Therefore, pyrimethamine is administered weekly (25 or 50 mg) to supplement dapsone in a dose of 50 mg a day. It should be noted that significant excess mortality (almost twofold) occurred in AIDS patients receiving 50 mg a day of dapsone alone in a comparison trial with aerosolized pentamidine for secondary prophylaxis. Trials of dapsone at doses of 100 mg two or three times per week show equivalence to pentamidine therapy; doses of 100 mg per day are equivalent to TMP-SMX therapy. Trimethoprim may replace pyrimethamine in this regimen (100 to 200 mg per day) in patients with creatinine clearances over 15 ml per min. The incidence of intolerance to dapsone—65 to 70 percent—is roughly equivalent to that for TMP-SMX. Up to half of the patients who discontinue prophylactic therapy with either of these agents will be able to tolerate the other drug. This strategy is not recommended for any person with severe allergic reactions, including desquamation to sulfa drugs, persistent bone marrow suppression, G6PD deficiency, or severe hepatitis. Toxicities observed with dapsone are long-lived and may limit utility, especially in liver transplantation recipients.

Fansidar (weekly) has been used successfully to prevent pneumocystosis.[17] Atovaquone (formerly BW566c80) has been approved by the FDA for the treatment of mild to moderate *P. carinii* infections and may be equally useful for prophylaxis because it is well tolerated, undergoes enterohepatic circulation without metabolism, and has a long half-life.[34] The drug has been reformulated as a liquid to improve bioavailability. Large-scale toxicity studies have not been performed in the non–HIV-infected host. In AIDS patients receiving 750 mg orally (three tablets) three times a day, some breakthrough infections have been observed. Rash, nausea, and elevated liver transaminases were occasionally documented. Experience suggests that the bioavailability in AIDS patients is one-half to one-third that in other compromised hosts. Prophylactic doses of reformulated liquid drug in the range of 1000 to 1500 mg a day exceed the MIC in serum for *P. carinii* in transplant recipients, but higher doses

(1500 to 2250 mg a day) may be needed in AIDS patients. The incidence of side effects is quite low in either population. Some patients complain about the flavor and color of atovaquone liquid (which stains clothes), but many find it preferable to aerosolized pentamidine. In small numbers of transplant recipients, interactions of atovaquone with cyclosporine and other toxicities have been insignificant; prospective randomized comparative studies are under way.

Patients receiving prophylaxis for toxoplasmosis (sulfadiazine, triple sulfa, clindamycin/primaquine, atovaquone) generally have also been protected against *P. carinii*. Transplantation recipients receiving quinolone for postoperative prophylaxis will be at the same risk for *Pneumocystis* pneumonia as the general transplant population.

TREATMENT OF *PNEUMOCYSTIS* PNEUMONIA

The incidence of *Pneumocystis* infection in AIDS patients has led to the development of a number of newer options for the treatment of this infection in all susceptible hosts (Table 150-3). Treatment should be initiated as soon as the suspicion of *Pneumocystis* infection is entertained. The short-term use of treatment (48 h) will not impair the diagnosis of infection if, for example, bronchoscopic or laboratory support services are unavailable. It

TABLE 150-3

Treatment of *P. carinii**		
Agent(s)(route)†	*Dose*	*Options†*
Trimethoprim and sulfamethoxazole (TMP-SMX) (IV/PO)	15 mg/kg/day TMP (to 20) 75 mg/kg/day SMX (to 100)	Treat through rash: reduce TMP or SMX by one-half; desensitize; first choice
Pentamidine isethionate (IV)	4 mg/kg/day 300 mg/day max.	Lower dose (2–3 mg/kg) after loading; IM not advised
Dapsone (PO) with TMP (PO/IV)	100 mg/day 15–20 mg/kg/day (900 mg)	Methemoglobinemia, G6PD; *may* be tolerated in sulfadizaine allergy
Clindamycin (IV/PO) and primaquine	450–600 mg q6h 15–30 mg base qd	Methemoglobinemia, diarrhea (pyrimethamine for primaquine)
Trimetrexate (IV) with folinic acid (leucovorin)	30–45 mg/m²/day 80–100 mg/m²day	Leukopenia, anemia, thrombocytopenia; relapse common
Pyrimethamine (PO) with sulfadiazine (PO)	load 50 mg bid x2d, then 25–50 mg qd load 75 mg/kg, then 100 mg/kg/day	Not studied fully Max. 4 gm in two doses; up to 8 g
Piritrexim (IV) with folinic acid	Under study	Like trimetrexate
Atovaquone (PO) suspension	750 mg (PO) tid	Variable absorbance, improved with fatty food; rash, but few side effects

*Adjunctive therapies (see text): Corticosteroids (high dose with rapid tapering), possibly γ-interferon, granulocyte-macrophage colony–stimulating factor.
†Based on clinical judgment of physician; some agents not FDA approved for this indication.

is likely to be more useful clinically to obtain specimens for *P. carinii*, mycobacteria, *Legionella*, fungi, and routine cultures when these can be properly handled by the clinical laboratory. Further, because the pneumonia can be rapidly progressive, early therapy is essential. Treatment of *Pneumocystis* should be successful if a 14- to 21-day course of therapy is tolerated.

The incidence of adverse reactions to antibiotics, necessitating switching of agents, is increased in the organ and marrow transplant recipient, as it is in AIDS patients. In general, side effects in transplantation are related to synergistic drug toxicities. For example, the bone marrow suppression seen in infection with CMV and treatment of this infection with ganciclovir may be further exacerbated with TMP-SMX. Generally, elevations in liver function tests in the liver transplant recipient or depression in the leukocyte count in the marrow recipient due to therapy with TMP-SMX is of concern in the transplant recipient but may be tolerable in other hosts. Nephrotoxicity is common in transplant recipients (both renal and extrarenal) receiving therapy with TMP-SMX, even with adjustment of dosing for renal dysfunction. Thus, while the incidence of intolerance by transplant recipients to one or another agent is somewhat less than the 50 percent seen in AIDS patients, significant toxicity remains a common feature of therapy. As was noted, resistance to antibiotics has not yet been demonstrated by *P. carinii*. Thus, changing antibiotics *other than for toxicity* does not appear to be indicated. While there are patients who appear to "do better" on one agent than another, it is much more common to recognize a second process (infection, tumor, allergy, ARDS) as complicating *Pneumocystis* pneumonia than a "resistant" infection. The chest radiograph is a less reliable indicator of failure than is oxygenation. Adding pentamidine to TMP-SMX offers no advantage over simply switching agents. Indeed, animal experiments suggest the possibility of antagonism between these agents when used in combination. As a rule, patients who need to be switched from co-trimoxazole to pentamide, or vice versa, do not fare as well as those who can be treated for 14 to 21 days with either agent alone. The success rate with either pentamidine or TMP-SMX for initial treatment is around 60 to 80 percent. Adjunctive therapies (see below) may also be more useful than switching agents.

The proper duration of therapy has not been studied but is generally 14 to 21 days in all patients. Residual organisms persist after treatment for a number of months (up to 3), but the role of these organisms in recrudescent or persistent infection is not clear. Following treatment with TMP-SMX, most residual organisms are dead; relapse in the non–AIDS-immunocompromised patient should not be expected *as long as immunosuppression can be reduced* (notably, with steroid therapy).

Trimethoprim-sulfamethoxazole is the agent of choice for the treatment of *Pneumocystis* pneumonia and extrapulmonary disease in all hosts.[8,60] This combination antibiotic has the advantage of excellent tissue penetration, the most rapid clinical response of anti-*Pneumocystis* agents (3 to 4 days), and bioavailability from oral therapy comparable with that of parenteral administration. Survival without intubation and mechanical ventilation appears to be greater with TMP-SMX than with pentamidine (by up to 20 percent). The incidence of some of the side effects is related to serum concentrations and is also greater than with other agents. In part, this is a reflection of the use of

dosage schedules derived for children in adults and in the setting of abnormal renal function. The proper dosing in adults has not been completely studied. Therapy is initiated at 15 to 20 mg/kg per day of the TMP component (100 to 150 mg/kg per day of SMX), divided into three or four doses. Therapy should be initiated intravenously if there is uncertainty about GI function or marked hypoxemia. Peak levels are obtained about 2 h after oral dosing and should approach the range of 100 to 150 μg/ml of SMX (5 to 15 μg/ml TMP). Levels of over 200 μg/ml of SMX are associated with a higher incidence of side effects, especially bone marrow suppression. After a clinical response is observed, the dosing can be reduced to 10 to 15 mg/kg per day, in divided doses.

Therapy can be continued (with adjustments) despite mild side effects (rash, transaminase elevations, neutropenia) tolerable to the patient and physician. Dose reduction will often eliminate toxicity in AIDS patients. Desensitization to TMP-SMX may be used in the patient with mild intolerance. With renal dysfunction, dosing must be reduced; daily dosing is sufficient (3 to 5 mg/kg per day) for a glomerular filtration rate of 10 to 50 ml per min. Renal impairment developing in a patient taking TMP-SMX should prompt a search for urinary eosinophils and an assessment of the need for further therapy with this agent. Nephrotoxicity occurs frequently in the renal transplant recipient on full-dose therapy; this toxicity is both idiosyncratic and dose related. Nephrotoxicity often occurs without demonstrable urinary eosinophils, perhaps as a reflection of the use of corticosteroids for immune suppression. In these patients, interstitial eosinophils may be found on renal biopsy. The transplanted liver is particularly susceptible to TMP-SMX toxicity (eosinophilic infiltrates, hepatocyte necrosis, bilirubinemia) and may be confused with, or complicate treatment for, early rejection or systemic infection. The side effects of TMP-SMX are generally those of sulfa allergy: rash (including Stevens-Johnson syndrome), transaminase elevation, neutropenia, thrombocytopenia, erythema multiforme exudativum, and nephrotoxicity. The bone marrow suppression is marked in patients with underlying hematologic disorders; folinic acid supplementation is rarely useful and should be avoided in patients with acute leukemia.

Dapsone (100 mg orally per day), in place of SMX and in combination with oral TMP (15 mg/kg per day), is an effective alternative therapeutic regimen. Many AIDS patients intolerant of sulfamethoxazole will tolerate dapsone, which is metabolized by the liver (half-life at least 30 h). However, the long half-life and side-effect profile in the non-AIDS patient (hemolysis in G6PD deficiency, rash, hepatitis) may be particularly disadvantageous in the transplant recipient. Manifestations of sulfa and TMP toxicity may be masked by corticosteroids. Similarly, side effects of azathioprine (hepatitis, macrocytic anemia, neutropenia, hepatic veno-occlusive disease) may be accentuated by TMP-SMX. In AIDS, the toxic side effects of TMP-SMX are generally those of the sulfonamide; however, trimethoprim allergy is not uncommon, and allergies to the "carriers" in the various preparations of TMP-SMX (dyes, coatings, filler) have also been reported. Both components of TMP-SMX interfere with folate metabolism. Leukopenia, thrombocytopenia, and anemia caused by co-trimoxazole are generally relieved by folinic acid, whereas drug rash, fever, azotemia, and increased blood levels of transaminases will reverse only when therapy is stopped. Folinic acid should not be used in patients with acute leukemia.

Pentamidine isethionate is the first alternative agent for the treatment of *Pneumocystis* pneumonia. Pentamidine isethionate was first administered intramuscularly during an epidemic of the infantile form of the disease. It decreased mortality from 50 to 3.5 percent of those affected. Subsequently, less dramatic effects were obtained with this agent in older children and adults: survival rates of 25 to 85 percent have been reported following its use. Pentamidine is now judged to be about 70 percent effective. Pentamidine isethionate may be administered either intravenously or intramuscularly, although only the intravenous route is currently recommended. Complications with early therapy occurred in up to 50 percent of patients, notably sterile abscesses at the site of intramuscular injection. Intravenous pentamidine isethionate is given by slow (1- to 2-h) infusion in 5 percent glucose solution as a single dose of 4 mg/kg per day. Evidence exists that lower doses (3 mg/kg per day) are equally effective. Pentamidine achieves therapeutic levels in the lungs slowly (in 5 to 7 days), owing to high levels of extrapulmonary tissue binding. Slow accumulation of pentamidine in pulmonary tissue may account for the delayed onset of activity when compared with TMP-SMX. However, increased serum levels and a long serum half-life and gradual accumulation in the lungs may play a role in the continued therapeutic effect after the cessation of therapy. Because this agent has a long serum half-life (6.4 h) and delayed excretion due to extensive tissue binding (more than 240 h), pentamidine tends to accumulate during therapy. The reduction of symptoms by pentamidine may be due, in part, to suppression of the secretion of tumor necrosis factor by alveolar macrophages as well as to treatment of infection. Pentamidine has largely been supplanted by TMP-SMX for therapy of *Pneumocystis* infection in the non-AIDS patient. But pentamidine continues to be used for infection in patients with adverse reactions to trimethoprim or to sulfonamides.

Idiosyncratic side effects include transient hypoglycemia, pancreatitis, diabetes (after prolonged therapy, with or without prior pancreatitis), pancytopenia, hypotension, and renal dysfunction. These side effects are exacerbated by intravenous administration and in the presence of decreased renal function. Pentamidine should be avoided in pancreas transplant recipients, owing to the potential for islet cell necrosis. New diamidine compounds under development may have significantly superior therapeutic and side-effect profiles when compared to the parent molecule.

Alternative regimens have been developed as a reflection of toxicities observed in AIDS patients treated with either TMP-SMX or pentamidine. Atovaquone (750 mg orally three times a day) has been approved by the FDA for the treatment of mild to moderately severe *Pneumocystis* pneumonia. Atovaquone is a hydroxynapthoquinone and inhibitor of electron transport with a prolonged serum half-life (at least 70 h). Absorption is enhanced by fatty foods and decreased by diarrhea and in AIDS patients. Bioavailability has been improved by reformulation as a liquid form. Comparative trials between atovaquone (tablets) and TMP-SMX suggest that TMP-SMX is the preferred agent in patients who tolerate this therapy. Up to 7 percent of HIV-infected patients develop limiting toxicity on atovaquone (compared to 20 percent for TMP-SMX); however, significantly more patients failed therapy owing to lack of response in the atovaquone group than in the TMP-SMX group. When pentamidine was compared with atovaquone for therapy of mild to moderate infection, lack of response was observed in 29 percent of atovaquone patients and 19 percent of pentamidine patients. However, atovaquone was better tolerated. Like TMP-SMX, atovaquone may *clear P. carinii* from the lungs in patients who complete a course of therapy better than other alternative agents, reducing the rate of relapsed infection.

Trimetrexate (NeuTrexin, US Bioscience, 45 mg/m^2 per day) *with* folinic acid (80 mg/m^2 per day) has been approved for use in moderately severe pneumonia.[1] Trimetrexate is a dihydrofolate reductase inhibitor and is lipid soluble, with a serum half-life up to 34 h. It will produce severe neutropenia in the absence of folinic acid supplementation (which should be continued for 3 to 5 days after cessation of trimetrexate), in some patients with simultaneous infections due to HIV or CMV, or during therapy with antiviral antibiotics. Side effects include fever, rash, leukopenia, and transaminase elevation. Infection relapse in AIDS patients has been somewhat more frequent than with other therapies. The survival rate following therapy in AIDS patients is higher for TMP-SMX than for trimetrexate for moderately severe *Pneumocystis* pneumonia. Piritrexim is pharmacologically similar to trimetrexate but has been most useful in combination with a sulfonamide.

The combination of clindamycin (600 to 900 mg intravenously every 6 to 8 h) and primaquine (15 to 30 mg base per day orally) is effective in mild to moderate infection, with the main side effect being *Clostridium difficile* colitis. Pyrimethamine (50 to 100 mg a day by mouth after 100 to 200-mg load) and sulfadiazine or trisulfapyrimidines (4 to 8 gm a day) are also effective, but require folinic acid (10 mg a day) supplementation. Pyrimethamine will decrease the renal clearance of creatinine without attaining the glomerular filtration rate. The newer macrolides (azithromycin, clarithromycin) have little efficacy alone but appear to enhance the efficacy of sulfamethoxazole. However, this combination provides little benefit over TMP-SMX. The utility of DFMO (α-difluoromethylornithine) has not been established. The presence of the target enzyme in *P. carinii* (ornithine decarboxylase) suggests that efficacy is possible, but it binds the drug less well than the host enzyme. Newer agents under study include the echinocandins (glucan synthase inhibitors), which block formation of cysts, the 8-aminoquinolines, the dicationic substituted bis-benzimidazoles (pentamidine derivatives), isoprinosine, bilobalide (a sesquiterpene from *Gingko biloba* leaves), quinghaosu albendazole, proguanil, terbinafine, guanylhydrazones, and some nonquinolone topoisomerase inhibitors.

Adjunctive therapies to the treatment of *Pneumocystis* pneumonia include corticosteroids and, potentially, colony-stimulating factors. Delayed response to therapy or the inability to reduce immune suppressive therapy may allow progressive disease despite appropriate therapy for *Pneumocystis* pneumonia. Given the risks of nosocomial superinfection associated with intubation for assisted ventilation, the use of adjunctive corticosteroids was developed to prevent the early deterioration of AIDS patients with documented *Pneumocystis* pneumonia.[9,25,45] The use of corticosteroids (prednisone, 40 to 60 mg three or four times a day, orally or intravenously) in the first 72 h after admission may reduce pulmonary inflammation to a degree sufficient to avoid intubation. When studied in AIDS patients, the use of corticosteroids in patients with a P_{AO_2} of 35 to 72 mmHg or with a hypoxemia ratio of 75 to 350 was of significant benefit in terms of preventing deterioration in oxygenation in the first 7 days of therapy, mortality, and the avoidance of intubation (50 percent reduction). After such therapy, the exercise tolerance and survival of patients were also improved. Steroid tapering is necessary to avert relapse of pulmonary inflammation. Patients experience an increase in oral thrush and herpes simplex after 2 to 3 weeks of therapy and tapering. The impact of corticosteroids in the non–AIDS-compromised host and in AIDS patients failing initial therapy appears to be similar. However, the utility of additional steroids in the transplant or cancer patient has not been subjected to a controlled clinical trial.

Cytokines, including γ-interferon, have been shown to reduce the amount of *Pneumocystis* found in animal models of disease without greatly increasing the inflammatory response.[5] The colony-stimulating factors (CSF), including those for the monocyte/macrophage (M-CSF), granulocytes (G-CSF), and granulocyte/macrophage (GM-CSF) lineages, have come into use to supplement immunity in the immunocompromised host. G-CSF has been used successfully in many of our neutropenic cancer and organ transplant recipients without adversely affecting the transplanted organs. GM-CSF has been used with systemic antifungal therapy in patients with acute fungal infections with some success. Preliminary data suggest that M-CSF and GM-CSF may be useful in enhancing the clearance of *P. carinii* by resident alveolar macrophages. Some investigators have endorsed the use of aerosolized pentamidine in addition to standard anti-*Pneumocystis* therapy. Some theoretical advantage may accrue to local administration.

The response to therapy is generally excellent in patients who receive a diagnosis before respiratory failure. The ability to reduce immune suppression or to supplement the immune response (see above) also improves the rapidity of clearance of infection. The failure to observe clinical improvement by days 4 to 5 (TMP-SMX) or 5 to 7 (pentamidine) should suggest the presence of another process: fibrosis, ARDS, dual infection (especially CMV), abscess, bronchial obstruction, drug allergy, carcinoma. Bronchoscopic lavage and biopsy for microbiology and pathology, or chest tomography (CT scan), may be revealing in these patients.

REFERENCES

1. Allegra CJ, Chabner BA, Tuazon CU, et al: Trimetrexate for the treatment of *Pneumocystis carinii* pneumonia in patients with the acquired immunodeficiency syndrome. *New Engl J Med* 317:978–985, 1987.
2. Bartlett MS, Fishman JA, Durkin MM, et al: *Pneumocystis carinii*: Improved models to study efficacy of drugs for treatment or prophylaxis of *Pneumocystis* pneumonia in the rat (*Rattus* spp.). *Exp Parasitol* 70:100–106, 1990.
3. Baughman RP, Dohn MN, Frame PT: The continuing utility of bronchoalveolar lavage to diagnose opportunistic infection in AIDS patients. *Am J Med* 97:515–522, 1994.
4. Beck EJ, French PD, Helbert MH, et al: Improved outcome of *Pneumocystis carinii* pneumonia in AIDS patients: A multifactorial treatment effect. *Int J STD AIDS* 3:182–187, 1992.
5. Beck JM, Liggitt HD, Brunette EN, et al: Reduction in intensity of *Pneumocystis carinii* pneumonia in mice by aerosol administration of gamma interferon. *Infect Immunol* 59:3859–3862, 1991.
6. Beck JM, Warnock ML, Curtis JL, et al: Inflammatory responses to *Pneumocystis carinii* in mice selectively depleted of helper T lymphocytes. *Am J Respir Cell Mol Biol* 5:186–197, 1991.
7. Bigby PD, Margolskee D, Curtis J, et al: Usefulness of induced sputum in diagnosis of pneumonia in patients with acquired immunodeficiency syndrome. *Am Rev Respir Dis* 133:515–518, 1986.
8. Bozzette SA, Finkelstein DM, Spector SA, et al, and NIAID AIDS Clinical Trials Group: A randomized trial of three antipneumocystis agents in patients with advanced human immunodeficiency virus infection. *New Engl J Med* 332:693–699, 1995.
9. Bozzette SA, Sattler FR, Chiu J, et al, and California Collaborative Treatment Group: A controlled trial of early adjunctive treatment with corticosteroids for *Pneumocystis carinii* pneumonia in the acquired immunodeficiency syndrome. *New Engl J Med* 323:1451–1457, 1990.
10. Broaddus C, Dake MD, Stulbarg MS, et al: Bronchoalveolar lavage and transbronchial biopsy for the diagnosis of pulmonary infections in the acquired immunodeficiency syndrome. *Ann Intern Med* 102:747–752, 1985.
11. Burack JH, Hahn JA, Saint-Maurice D, Jacobson MA: Microbiology of community-acquired bacterial pneumonia in persons with and at risk for human immunodeficiency virus type 1 infection. *Arch Intern Med* 154:2589–2596, 1994.
12. Chave J, David S, Wauters J, Francioli P: Transmission of *Pneumocystis carinii* from AIDS patients to other immunosuppressed patients: A cluster of *Pneumocystis carinii* pneumonia in renal transplant recipients. *AIDS* 5:927–932, 1991.
13. Coleman DL, Dodek PM, Luce JM, et al: Diagnostic utility of fiberoptic bronchoscopy in patients with *Pneumocystis carinii* pneumonia and the acquired immune deficiency syndrome. *Am Rev Respir Dis* 128:795–799, 1983.
14. Edman JC, Kovacs JA, Masur H, et al: Ribosomal RNA sequence shows *Pneumocystis carinii* to be a member of the Fungi (letter). *Nature* 334:519–522, 1988.
15. Edman U, Edman JC, Lundgren B, Santi DV: Isolation and expression of the *Pneumocystis carinii* thymidylate synthase gene. *Proc Natl Acad Sci USA* 86:6503–6507, 1989.
16. Ezekowitz RAB, Williams DJ, Koziel H, et al: Uptake of *Pneumocystis carinii* mediated by the macrophage mannose receptor. *Nature* 351:155–158, 1991.
17. Fischl MA, Dickinson GM: Fansider prophylaxis of *Pneumocystis* pneumonia in the acquired immunodeficiency syndrome (letter). *Ann Intern Med* 105:629, 1986.
18. Fischl MA, Dickinson GM, La Voie L: Safety and efficacy of sulfamethoxazole and trimethoprim chemoprophylaxis for *Pneumocystis carinii* pneumonia in AIDS. *JAMA* 259:1185–1189, 1988.
19. Fishman JA: A gene family related to the major antigen gene of *Pneumocystis*. Bristol-Myers Squibb symposium on cell and molecular biology of bacterial–host cell interactions (abstract). Monterrey, CA, February 1993.
20. Fishman JA: Radiologic approaches to *Pneumocystis carinii* infection, in Walzer PD (ed), *Pneumocystis Carinii Pneumonia*. New York, Dekker, 1994, pp 415–436.
21. Fishman JA: *Pneumocystis carinii* and parasitic infections in transplantation. *Infect Dis Clin North Am* 9:1005–1044, 1995.
22. Fishman JA: Case records of the Massachusetts General Hospital. *New Engl J Med* 332:249–257, 1995.

23. Furlong S, Thibault K, Samia J, et al: Lipids characteristic of fungi in *Pneumocystis carinii*. *Antimicrob Agents Chemother* 38: 2534–2540, 1994.

24. Furuta T, Ueda K, Fujiwara K, Yamanouchi K: Cellular and humoral immune responses of mice subclinically infected with *Pneumocystis carinii*. *Infect Immunol* 47:544–548, 1985.

25. Gagnon S, Boota AM, Fischl MA, et al: Corticosteroids as adjunctive therapy for severe *Pneumocytis carinii* pneumonia in the acquired immunodeficiency syndrome: A double-blind, placebo-controlled trial. *New Engl J Med* 323:1444–1450, 1990.

26. Gigliotti F, Hughes WT: Passive immunoprophylaxis with specific monoclonal antibody confers partial protection against *Pneumocystis carinii* pneumonitis in animal models. *J Clin Invest* 81:1666–1668, 1988.

27. Graves DC, McNabb SJN, Ivey MH, Worley MA: Development and characterization of monoclonal antibodies to *Pneumocystis carinii*. *Infect Immunol* 51:125–133, 1986.

28. Gryzan S, Paradis IL, Zeevi A, et al: Unexpectedly high incidence of *Pneumocystis carinii* infection after lung-heart transplantation: Implications for lung defense and allograft survival. *Am Rev Respir Dis* 137:1268–1274, 1988.

29. Hardy AM, Wajszczuk CP, Suffredini AF, et al: *Pneumocystis carinii* pneumonia in renal transplant patients treated with cyclosporin and steroids. *J Infect Dis* 149:143–147, 1984.

30. Hendley JO, Weller TH: Activation and transmission in rats of infection with pneumocystis. *Proc Soc Exp Biol Med* 137:1401–1404, 1971.

31. Hoover DR, Saah AJ, Bacellar H, et al, and Multicenter AIDS Cohort Study: Clinical manifestations of AIDS in the era of *Pneumocystis* prophylaxis. *New Engl J Med* 329:1922–1926, 1993.

32. Hopewell PC: Bronchoalveolar lavage and transbronchial biopsy for the diagnosis of pulmonary infections in the acquired immunodeficiency syndrome. *Ann Intern Med* 102:747–752, 1985.

33. Hughes WT: Pneumocystis Carinii *Pneumonitis*. New York, CRC, 1987.

34. Hughes W, et al: Comparison of atovaquone (566C80) and trimethoprim-sulfamethoxazole to treat *Pneumocystis carinii* pneumonia in patients with AIDS. *New Engl J Med* 328:1521–1527, 1993.

35. Hughes WT, McNabb PC, Makres TD, et al: Efficacy of trimethoprim and sulfamethoxazole in the prevention and treatment of *Pneumocystis carinii* pneumonitis. *Antimicrob Agents Chemother* 5:289–293, 1974.

36. Kandil O, Fishman JA, Koziel H, et al: Human immunodeficiency virus type I infection of human macrophages modulates the cytokine response to *Pneumocystis carinii*. *Infect Immun* 62: 644–650, 1994.

37. Kovacs JA, Hiemenz JW, Macher AM, et al: *Pneumocystis carinii* pneumonia: A comparison between patients with the acquired immunodeficiency syndrome and patients with other immunodeficiencies. *Ann Intern Med* 100:663–671, 1984.

38. Kovacs JA, Ng VL, Masur H, et al: Diagnosis of *Pneumocystis carinii* pneumonia: Improved detection in sputum with use of monoclonal antibodies. *New Engl J Med* 318:589–593, 1988.

39. Kovacs JA, Powell F, Edman JC, et al: Multiple genes encode the major surface glycoprotein of *Pneumocystis carinii*. *J Biol Chem* 268:6034–6040, 1993.

40. Kuller J, First MR, D'Archiardi R, et al: *Pneumocystis carinii* pneumonia in renal transplant recipients. *Am J Nephrol* 2:312–315, 1982.

41. Lim SK, Eveland WC, Porter RJ: Direct fluorescent-antibody method for the diagnosis of *Pneumocystis carinii* pneumonitis from sputa or tracheal aspirates from humans. *Appl Microbiol* 27:144–149, 1974.

42. Masur H, Gill VJ, Ognibene FP, et al: Diagnosis of *Pneumocystis* pneumonia by induced sputum technique in patients without the acquired immunodeficiency syndrome. *Ann Intern Med* 109:755–756, 1988.

43. Masur H, Ognibene FP, Yarchoan R, et al: CD4 counts as predictors of opportunistic pneumonias in human immunodeficiency virus (HIV) infection. *Ann Intern Med* 111:223–231, 1989.

44. Meuwissen JHET, Tauber I, Leeuwenberg ADEM, et al: Parasitologic and serologic observations of infection with *Pneumocystis* in humans. *J Infect Dis* 136:43–49, 1977.

45. Montaner JSG, Lawson LM, Levitt N, et al: Corticosteroids prevent early deterioration in patients with moderately severe *Pneumocystis carinii* pneumonia and the acquired immunodeficiency syndrome (AIDS). *Ann Intern Med* 113:14–20, 1990.

46. Perera DR, Western KA, Johnson HD, et al: *Pneumocystis carinii* pneumonia in a hospital for children: Epidemiologic aspects. *JAMA* 214:1074–1078, 1970.

47. Post C, Fakoughi T, Dutz W, et al: Prophylaxis of epidemic infantile pneumocystosis with a 20:1 sulfadoxine and pyrimethamine combination. *Curr Ther Res* 13:273–279, 1971.

48. Raviglione MC: Extrapulmonary pneumocystosis: The first 50 cases. *Rev Infect Dis* 12:1127–1138, 1990.

49. Robbins JB, DeVita VT, Dutz W: Symposium on *Pneumocystis carinii* infection, in National Cancer Institute (ed), *NCI Monograph No 43*. Washington, DC, 1976.

50. Ruebush TK, Weinstein RA, Baehner RL, et al: An outbreak of *Pneumocystis* pneumonia in children with acute lymphocytic leukemia. *J Dis Child* 132:143–148, 1978.

51. Stover DE, Zaman MB, Hajdu SI, et al: Bronchoalveolar lavage in the diagnosis of diffuse pulmonary infiltrates in the immunosuppressed host. *Ann Intern Med* 101:1–7, 1984.

52. Swartzberg JE, Remington JS: Transplant associated infections, in Bennett JV, Brachman PS (eds), *Hospital Infections*. Boston, Little, Brown, 1979, pp 453–488.

53. Vanek J, Jirovec O: Parasitäre Pneumonie: "Interstitielle" plasmazellen pneumonie der frühgeborenen verursacht durch *Pneumocystis Carinii*. *Zentralbl Bakt* 158:120–127, 1952.

54. Vogel P, Miller CJ, Lowenstine LL, Lackner AA: Evidence of horizontal transmission of *Pneumocystis carinii* pneumonia in simian immunodeficiency virus–infected rhesus macaques. *J Infect Dis* 168:836–843, 1993.

55. Wada M, Katada K, Saito M, et al: cDNA sequence diversity and genomic clusters of major surface glycoprotein genes of *Pneumocystis carinii*. *J Infect Dis* 168:979–985, 1993.

56. Waldron MA, Fishman JA: *Pneumocystis carinii*: Advances in diagnosis. *Clin Microbiol News* 14:161–166, 1992.

57. Walzer PD: Pneumocystis Carinii *Pneumonia*. New York, Dekker, 1994.

58. Walzer PD, Perl DP, Krogstad DJ, et al: *Pneumocystis carinii* pneumonia in the United States: Epidemiologic, diagnostic, and clinical features. *Ann Intern Med* 80:83–93, 1974.

59. Watanabe J, Hori H, Tanabe K, Nakamura Y: Phylogenetic association of *Pneumocystis carinii* with the "Rhizopoda/Myxomycota/Zygomycota group" indicated by comparison of 5S ribosomal RNA sequences. *Mol Biochem Parasitol* 32:163–167, 1989.

60. Wharton JM, Coleman DL, Wofsy CB, et al: Trimethoprim-sulfamethoxazole or pentamidine for *Pneumocystis carinii* pneumonia in the acquired immunodeficiency syndrome. *Ann Intern Med* 105: 37–44, 1986.

61. Ypma-Wong MF, Fonzi WA, Sypherd PS: Fungus-specific translation elongation factor 3 gene present in *Pneumocystis carinii*. *Infect Immun* 60:4140–4145, 1992.

CHAPTER 151

VIRAL INFECTIONS OF THE LUNG AND RESPIRATORY TRACT

Stephen B. Greenberg

GENERAL PRINCIPLES

Epidemiology

The most common illnesses afflicting humans are the respiratory viral infections. In the United States, respiratory infections and influenza are the seventh leading cause of death. More than 500 million acute respiratory illnesses are estimated to occur yearly in this country, accounting for half of all ill-child visits to physicians. The estimated cost of medical care, unnecessary antibiotics, and time lost from work and school is estimated to be more than $7 billion per year.

Many viruses can infect the respiratory tract and produce symptoms and signs of upper or lower respiratory tract infection. In healthy persons, respiratory viral infections produce acute morbidity but little increased mortality. Persons with underlying illness or immunosuppression exhibit increased mortality as well as morbidity after acute lower respiratory viral infections.

To identify the virus causing a respiratory illness, a respiratory tract specimen or acute and convalescent sera must be analyzed in a clinical virology laboratory. Even if a virus is not identified, the most likely candidate can often be deduced from clinical and epidemiologic data. Patient age, time of year, clinical presentation (laryngitis, croup, or pneumonia), and knowledge of community surveillance are useful as aids to narrow the viral cause in a given patient (Table 151-1). Nevertheless, different viruses cause the same respiratory syndromes, making clinical diagnosis a good guess, at best.

Upper respiratory tract viral infections include the common cold, pharyngitis, sinusitis, acute otitis media, and laryngitis. Lower respiratory viral infections include acute laryngotracheobronchitis (croup), influenza, bronchitis, bronchiolitis, and pneumonia. Complications of respiratory virus disease include secondary bacterial infections, Reye's syndrome, Guillain-Barré syndrome, myositis, encephalopathy, myopericarditis, and febrile seizures. Newly described complications associated with well-described respiratory viruses (influenza virus and toxic shock syndrome) and newly described viruses

TABLE 151-1

Respiratory Viral Infections: Clinical Syndromes, Treatment, and Prevention

Virus Group	Clinical Syndromes*					Antiviral Agents†		Approved Vaccine
	Common Cold	Pharyngitis	Croup	Bronchiolitis	Pneumonia	Prophylaxis	Treatment	
Adenoviruses	–	+	–	+	+	N	N	Y
Coronaviruses	++	–	–	–	–	N	N	N
Herpesviruses								
CMV	–	+	–	–	+	Y	Y	N
EBV	–	++	–	–	+	N	N	N
HSV	–	++	–	–	+	Y	Y	N
VZV	–	–	–	–	+	Y	Y	Y
Orthomyxoviruses								
Influenza A, B, C	+	++	+	+	++	Y	Y	Y
Paramyxoviruses								
Measles	–	–	–	–	+	Y	N	Y
Parainfluenza 1, 2, 3	+	++	+++	++	–	N	N	N
Respiratory syncytial	–	+	++	+++	++	N	Y	N
Picornavirus								
Enterovirus	+	–	–	–	–	N	N	N
Rhinovirus	+++	++	+	+	–	Y	N	N

*+++ = most commonly isolated with syndrome; ++ = common isolates; + = uncommon isolates; – = rarely or not identified with clinical syndrome.
†Approved for use or experimental studies demonstrate clinical benefit; Y = yes; N = no.

associated with well-described respiratory syndromes (*Hantavirus*—see Chapter 153—and ARDS) have been reported recently.

The number of viruses accounting for lower respiratory tract infection has been considered to be restricted. Serious virus infections below the larynx are reported predominantly in infants and children and in immunocompromised or high-risk adults.[41] Upper respiratory tract viral infections are associated with a larger number of viruses, chiefly because of the more than 100 types of rhinovirus that can cause the common cold.

Diagnosis

Diagnosis of respiratory viral infections relies on both tissue culture cell techniques and serologic tests.[39] Tissue culture cells are employed for their ability to sustain virus growth and demonstrate cytopathic effects. A combination of tissue culture cell lines is used, much in the same way the bacteriology laboratory uses selective media for detecting specific bacteria. Serologic tests are performed on acute and convalescent sera obtained 2 to 4 weeks apart. Standard tests include complement fixation (CF), neutralization (Nt), hemagglutination-inhibition (HAI), and enzyme-linked immunosorbent assay (ELISA). Tests that measure specific IgM antibodies are available for a few viruses, but most assays detect IgG antibodies. In most test assays, a fourfold or greater rise in serum antibody between acute and convalescent sera is needed to demonstrate recent infection. For some respiratory viruses, culture is superior to serologic methods; for others, serology is most useful for diagnosis (Table 151-2).

Newer diagnostic techniques such as polymerase chain reaction (PCR) will provide rapid identification of specific viral agents. The use of these methods by viral diagnostic laboratories throughout the United States may lead to the institution of specific antiviral therapy more quickly. Diagnostic virology laboratories of the future will also function to monitor nosocomial viral infections as well as look for possible new agents and imported exotic viral infections.

Prevention and Treatment

Although a number of antiviral agents have been approved for use in respiratory viral infections, their clinical utility has been best demonstrated when they have been given as prophylaxis rather than as treatment. For example, amantadine and rimantadine have far superior anti-illness effects when given prophylactically than when begun once influenza symptoms are present.

Prevention of certain respiratory viral infections has depended on vaccine use, and the development of new respiratory virus vaccines is of increasing importance (see Chapter 124). Improved influenza virus vaccines are being tested for widespread utilization. Candidate vaccines for respiratory syncytial virus (RSV) and parainfluenza viruses are a priority research area for the future. Because of the multitude of immunotypes of rhinoviruses, it is unlikely that vaccines will be easily constructed for this group.[7] As more epidemiologic studies are published on the expanded role of coronaviruses in serious respiratory tract infections in both children and adults, this group of respiratory viruses will require additional consideration for vaccine development. Postexposure prophylaxis with immune globulin therapy has not been effective, except in measles and varicella infections.

TABLE 151-2

Modes of Detection for Respiratory Viruses

Virus	Culture	Detection by* Direct Detection	Serology	Comments
Adenoviruses	+	+/−	+	Culture and IF† are preferred methods of diagnosis; significance of isolate must be interpreted in relationship to serotype and clinical findings
Coronaviruses	−	−	+	Diagnosis not routinely available
Enteroviruses	+	−	−	Significance of isolate must be interpreted in relationship to type isolated and clinical findings
EBV	−	−	+	Nonspecific heterophilic antibodies (e.g., Monospot) are most readily available but not reliable in children <4 years old; serology for virus-specific antigens is also available
CMV	+	+/−	+	Culture is most readily available. Rapid diagnostic methods reported include IF, molecular hybridization, and electron microscopy
HSV	+/−	+	+	Culture and IF are both preferred to serology; significance of isolate must be interpreted in relationship to clinical findings
VZV	+/−	+	+	Direct detection by nonspecific (e.g., Tzanck preparation, electron microscopy) and specific (e.g., IF) techniques often superior to culture in speed and sensitivity; FAMA‡ is the most sensitive serologic method; enzyme immunoassay and anticomplement IF also are sufficiently sensitive for most uses.
Orthomyxoviruses (influenza A, B, and C,) Paramyxoviruses (parainfluenza, RSV)	+	+	+	For RSV, direct detection (IF, ELISA) approaches the sensitivity and specificity of viral culture; for influenza and parainfluenza viruses, direct antigen detection is not as available or as sensitive as viral isolation
Rhinovirus	+	−	−	Culture is the only routinely available method for rhinovirus detection

*+ = Available methods using commercially obtainable reagents; − = not routinely available or not consistently reliable.
†IF = immunofluorescence.
‡FAMA = fluorescent antibody to membrane antigen.
SOURCE: Data from Greenberg.[19]

UPPER RESPIRATORY TRACT VIRAL INFECTIONS

The Common Cold

A self-limited, acute coryzal illness has come to be known as the *common cold*. As a leading cause of physician office visits and of absence from work or school, the common cold is caused by one of several families of respiratory viruses. The five most commonly reported virus families retrieved from infected patients are orthomyxovirus (influenza A and B), paramyxovirus (parainfluenza virus and RSV), adenovirus, picornavirus (rhinovirus), and coronavirus. In clinical studies concerning the causes of colds, 25 to 30 percent remain undiagnosed. The frequency of illness episodes relates to the large number of causative viruses and the demonstrated reinfections with certain viruses (e.g., corona viruses).

Epidemics of upper respiratory tract infections occur worldwide, usually in the fall, winter, and spring in temperate climates.

Rhinoviruses are recovered predominantly in early fall and late spring, but are also isolated throughout the rest of the year. Coronaviruses are documented chiefly in winter months. Yearly or biannual community-wide outbreaks of influenza virus, parainfluenza virus, or RSV are also common throughout the world. In the United States, children average six to eight colds each year and adults two to four. An increase in the incidence of colds is associated with the beginning of the school year and indoor crowding. Children are often infected in day-care centers or school and pass the infection to other family members. Prolonged exposure leads to increased secondary attack rates, so that parents and other children in the home are most likely to acquire these infections.

Transmission of these viruses may be secondary to contact with infected secretions or droplet nuclei in the air.[24] Experiments have demonstrated that hand-to-hand transmission of rhinoviruses from contaminated skin can take place.[20] Other human volunteer challenge models have shown the ability to transmit other viruses through large- and small-particle aerosols.

Shedding of common cold viruses is usually short-lived, lasting a few days to a week. Large quantities of rhinovirus are detected in nasal secretions at the time of maximal illness. Asymptomatic infections do occur but are uncommon. Recent studies have suggested that chemical mediators and neurologic reflexes are important in common cold symptomatology, especially secondary to rhinoviruses.

Symptoms of the common cold usually begin 1 to 3 days after infection. In addition to nasal discharge and obstruction, sneezing, sore throat, and cough are commonly experienced.[21] Most cold symptoms last 1 week but not uncommonly can persist for up to 2 weeks. Physical examination rarely provides specific clues to the diagnosis. Most cold diagnoses are self-reported. In persons with hay fever and vasomotor rhinitis, it may be difficult to distinguish an allergic pattern from viral infection.

Rhinoviruses and influenza viruses are readily isolated from nasopharyngeal specimens. Serologic studies will often be needed to document recent infection with parainfluenza virus, RSV, coronavirus, and adenovirus. However, acute and convalescent sera are often not obtained or must be sent off to health department laboratories, delaying serologic diagnosis.

Symptomatic relief of the common cold is currently the only effective approach to treatment. Antibiotics are not effective in the absence of proven secondary bacterial infection. Nasal symptoms can be diminished with decongestants or vasoconstrictors.[22] Cough may be suppressed with codeine or nonsteroidal anti-inflammatory drugs, such as naproxen. Mild fever and sore throat may respond to antipyretics. Most controlled studies have failed to document an anti-illness effect due to vitamin C ingestion.

In experimentally induced and naturally acquired colds, prophylactic administration of recombinant interferon-α was shown to be effective.[22,36] However, interferon was not effective when given therapeutically. The adverse local effects of intranasal interferon have limited the widespread use of recombinant interferon. Interruption of transmission by hand washing or disposable nasal tissues may decrease secondary transmission.

Pharyngitis

Most cases of viral pharyngitis occur in conjunction with other clinical signs and symptoms of colds or influenza. Bacteria, especially group A β-hemolytic streptococci, can also cause pharyngitis that is clinically indistinguishable from viral pharyngitis.[29] In large series of pharyngitis, approximately 30 percent of cases have no identifiable cause. Peak prevalence of pharyngitis is from fall to spring, when most respiratory viral infections occur. Family spread of infection is common, especially in households with young children.

Among the viral causes of pharyngitis, rhinoviruses are probably the single most commonly isolated pathogen. Adenoviruses often cause pharyngitis in combination with conjunctivitis and fever. Herpes simplex virus has been documented as a cause of pharyngitis—especially in susceptible, nonimmune college students. Coronaviruses, influenza viruses, and parainfluenza viruses have been isolated from cases of acute respiratory disease and pharyngitis. Epstein-Barr virus (EBV) and cytomegalovirus (CMV) can cause a mononucleosis syndrome in which

pharyngitis is a prominent clinical feature. During primary infection with HIV, pharyngitis and a mononucleosis-type syndrome have also been reported to occur.

Pharyngeal exudates are not commonly seen with rhinovirus, influenza, parainfluenza, coronavirus, or HIV-related pharyngitis. However, exudates have been documented in cases of adenovirus, herpes simplex virus, and EBV-associated cases. Clinically, these viral causes of exudative pharyngitis are indistinguishable from group A streptococcal, *Mycoplasma pneumoniae,* or *Chlamydia pneumoniae* pharyngitis. The presence or absence of other respiratory signs and symptoms can be helpful in making a presumptive etiologic diagnosis.

Rapid antigen detection tests for group A streptococci are sensitive and specific enough to warrant widespread use. A positive test is sufficient for initiating specific antibiotic treatment; a negative test is an indication for throat culture. If a test is negative in a patient with exudates and fever, a careful examination for unusual and potentially serious bacterial infections (e.g., diphtheria) must be considered.

Specific viral cultures are available for most of the commonly associated respiratory viruses. However, coronaviruses, EBV, and CMV require serologic tests. At the time of pharyngitis secondary to HIV, a serum p24 antigen test may be positive but the screening ELISA or Western blot will be negative. Special cultures are needed to recover diphtheria, *Arcanobacterium hemolyticus, M. pneumoniae,* or *C. pneumoniae.*

Patients with streptococcal pharyngitis should receive penicillin treatment. Mycoplasmal or chlamydial pharyngitis will respond to oral macrolides. Most cases of viral pharyngitis will require symptomatic therapy only. Fluids, analgesics, and bed rest constitute the basic treatment. In one study, a nonsteroidal anti-inflammatory drug relieved pain faster than acetaminophen in children with pharyngitis and tonsillitis.[4] Hospitalization is needed only if life-threatening complications or serious systemic illness is documented.

Routine tonsillectomy is not recommended for children with recurrent pharyngitis. If patients are at risk of rheumatic fever, penicillin prophylaxis is recommended. Vaccines for influenza viruses are recommended for annual use in targeted groups. No vaccine for group A streptococci has been developed, although experiments are under way to test candidate vaccine preparations.

Laryngitis

Laryngitis or hoarseness secondary to laryngeal inflammation occurs in 20 percent of common respiratory viral illnesses, often associated with cough and pharyngitis. The most commonly documented viruses causing laryngitis are influenza viruses, rhinoviruses, adenoviruses, parainfluenza viruses, and RSV. Because of the difficulty in identifying coronaviruses, their importance in causing laryngitis is unclear. In adults with acute laryngitis, *Moraxella (Branhamella) catarrhalis* has been recovered in 50 percent of cases. Laryngitis has also been described in a few cases caused by group A streptococci. Rare cases of laryngitis have been reported to be due to *Mycobacteria tuberculosis,* varicella-zoster virus, *Histoplasma capsulatum,* and *Candida* species.

Treatment is symptomatic in most cases of laryngitis. Resting the voice is advocated. In one controlled trial, there was a faster return of normal voice in erythromycin-treated patients than in those receiving a placebo.[37] The isolation of *M. catarrhalis* was also significantly reduced in the antibiotic-treated group. Studies employing penicillin have failed to demonstrate a clinical benefit for patients with laryngitis.

Hoarseness lasts 10 days to 2 weeks for most patients. If the symptoms persist, laryngoscopic examination is suggested to look for tumors or other chronic conditions.

ACUTE LARYNGOTRACHEOBRONCHITIS (CROUP)

Epidemiology

Laryngotracheobronchitis (croup) is a viral infection of both the upper and lower respiratory tract in young children, associated with dyspnea and inflammation of the subglottic region. Characteristic findings are inspiratory stridor, hoarseness, and cough. Most children have only one episode of croup in a lifetime, but recurrences do occur. Most cases of croup occur in boys during the second year of life.

Parainfluenza virus type 1 is the most commonly documented infectious agent causing croup in the United States and usually occurs in the fall of every other year. Parainfluenza virus type 3, influenza viruses A and B, and RSV are the next most frequently isolated viruses. Cases of croup secondary to RSV usually occur in the first year of life. Outbreaks of croup in the winter and spring are most commonly associated with influenza viruses and less commonly with RSV. Adenoviruses are uncommon causes of croup. Rhinoviruses, enteroviruses, and parainfluenza virus type 4 rarely cause croup. When parainfluenza virus type 1 and influenza viruses occur in epidemics, there are usually concomitant increases in croup cases in the community. With RSV outbreaks, there are no increases in community croup cases.

Pathogenesis

It is unclear why these respiratory viruses are associated with croup in young children, but several possible explanations have been put forth. First, primary infections with parainfluenza viruses may be more likely to infect the lower respiratory tract. Second, the diameter of the larynx and glottis is relatively small in children less than 2 years of age. With decreased airway diameter, there is increased airway resistance. Last, children with croup have higher IgE antibody levels to parainfluenza viruses and demonstrate greater histamine release from leukocytes than do children not having croup. Reinfection with the same type of parainfluenza virus does occur, and this partial immunity may reduce both the likelihood and the severity of croup. This may explain why croup is not common in adults.

Clinical Manifestations

Before the clinical onset of croup, most children have symptoms of upper respiratory infection for 1 to several days. Fever is common, and a nonproductive cough is usual. The child often awakens at night with the distinctive raspy cough, tachypnea, and in-

spiratory stridor. The respiratory rate is usually greater than 40 a minute. On physical examination, rales, rhonchi, or wheezes can be heard or, if late in the course, decreased breath sounds. Children tend to feel better in the morning and worse in the evening. A typical case lasts 3 to 4 days but occasionally up to 2 weeks. During the acute illness, hypoxemia is documented in 80 percent of hospitalized croup patients and hypercapnia in 50 percent.

The differential diagnosis of croup includes foreign-body aspiration, smoke inhalation, angioneurotic edema, and anaphylaxis—all of which are associated with cough, hoarseness, and stridor. Two other infections must be considered in the differential diagnosis of croup: epiglottitis and bacterial tracheitis. Rhinorrhea and laryngitis are not found with epiglottitis. Marked dysphagia and drooling are common with epiglottitis but not croup. A helpful finding on radiographs of the neck is subglottic swelling. Bacterial tracheitis occurs more commonly in older children and is associated with purulent sputum in addition to fever, stridor, and dyspnea. Organisms most commonly identified in bacterial tracheitis are *Staphylococcus aureus,* group A β-hemolytic streptococci, and *Hemophilus influenzae* type b. There is often a rapidly progressive clinical course that responds to antibiotics.

Complications of croup include occasional postintubation subglottic stenosis and, rarely, noncardiogenic pulmonary edema. In most published series of hospitalized cases, mortality has ranged up to 2.7 percent. In long-term follow-up studies, an increase in hyperactivity of the airways has been documented.

Diagnosis

The diagnosis of croup is usually made clinically. Routine laboratory tests are not helpful. A specific virus has been identified in only 30 to 60 percent of cases. Virus cultures are available for parainfluenza viruses, influenza viruses, and RSV in most diagnostic virology laboratories. Because parainfluenza viruses may be shed for weeks, obtaining specimens for virus culture several days into a typical illness may be helpful.[14] Cultures usually become positive in 5 to 10 days but may take as long as 3 weeks. Type-specific serologic rises to parainfluenza viruses may not be found because of cross reactivity with the other parainfluenza viruses.

Prevention and Treatment

Although steam or mist vaporizers are often recommended for use in cases of croup, they are of unproven benefit. Animal experiments suggest that cold dry, cold moist, or dry air may be more effective than warm moist air. Nebulized epinephrine led to clinical improvement in some studies. The use of steroids is more controversial. Some investigators have reported fewer intubations and more rapid clinical improvement in hospitalized croup patients who received two to four doses of dexamethasone (0.3 to 0.6 mg/kg). Antibiotics are not warranted unless a bacterial superinfection is proven.

Since hypoxemia is common, hospitalized patients should have oximetry measurements and supplemental oxygen provided. If the Pa_{CO_2} rises and respiratory failure is imminent, nasotracheal intubation should be performed. Tracheostomy is associated with more complications than nasotracheal intubation and should not be employed.

INFLUENZA

Epidemiology

For several centuries, influenza viruses have caused recurrent epidemics of acute, febrile respiratory illness every winter. A high attack rate during a 1- to 2-month period is characteristic of a community outbreak. Increased school absenteeism and excess mortality are two prominent epidemiologic features of epidemic influenza.

Influenza viruses are members of the Orthomyxoviridae family. Influenza viruses type A and type B are two genera. Influenza virus type C has not been classified and uncommonly induces illness. Antigenic variations in influenza type A and, to a lesser extent, influenza type B account for the yearly epidemics. Influenza type C has not demonstrated antigenic variation. Minor changes in the two external glycoproteins, the hemagglutinin (HA) and neuraminidase (NA), occur frequently and lead to seasonal strain differences. These minor antigenic variations are termed *antigenic drift* and account for the yearly updating of vaccine strains to be employed. Major changes in the HA or NA antigens are associated with pandemic influenza that causes severe disease in susceptible populations.

Yearly epidemics of influenza begin abruptly and last 5 to 6 weeks.[13] Increased numbers of febrile respiratory illnesses in children are often the first indication of an epidemic (Fig. 151-1). Later indicators of influenza in a community are increased school and industrial absenteeism and deaths due to pneumonia.[3] Epidemics occur from December to April in the Northern Hemisphere and from May to September in the Southern Hemisphere.[32] Attack rates during most epidemics are 10 to 20 percent but may be 40 to 50 percent in certain high-risk groups. Two strains of a single subtype or two subtypes have been isolated simultaneously in a single epidemic period. Subtype A may be prevalent in 1 year and subtype B in the next year. There is no easy way to predict which "new" variant will circulate in the next epidemic period, but strains isolated at the end of an epidemic period may "herald" the epidemic virus for the following year.

Worldwide influenza pandemics occur when a new virus emerges for which there is no immunity. Three of the pandemics of the twentieth century (1957, 1968, and 1977) began in China. One hypothesis for this geographic source of pandemics is that, in China, influenza viruses can be isolated throughout the year and the proximity of birds and humans increases the opportunity for recombination of animal and human influenza viruses, leading to new antigenic shifts in HA or NA.

Pathogenesis

Transmission of influenza virus probably occurs by small-particle aerosol. Virus deposited in the lower respiratory tract attaches to and infects columnar epithelial cells. Replication of virus takes 4 to 6 h, so that infection of new, adjacent susceptible cells takes place in a short time. Thus, the incubation period may be as short as 18 h or up to 3 to 4 days.

Infected patients begin shedding virus a day before the onset of illness and continue shedding for 5 to 10 days. Although fever and systemic symptoms are quite common, recovery of influenza virus from blood has been rare. A biopsy of nasal or bronchial epithelium in persons with acute influenza will demonstrate desquamation of the ciliated columnar epithelium. In the rare cases of influenza virus pneumonia, alveolar hemorrhage and hyaline membrane formation are common. At the time of clinical improvement, interferon can be measured in nasal secretion samples.

During the second week of illness, type-specific serum antibodies are detectable. Specific antibodies can be detected by HAI, CF, or ELISA methods. Specific influenza virus antibodies persist for months to years but decline gradually after the acute illness. The primary benefit of anti-HA antibody may be to inhibit infection. Anti-NA antibody appears to reduce illness but not affect infection. Secretory IgA to influenza virus develops after infection and is apparently an important component of protection from reinfection.

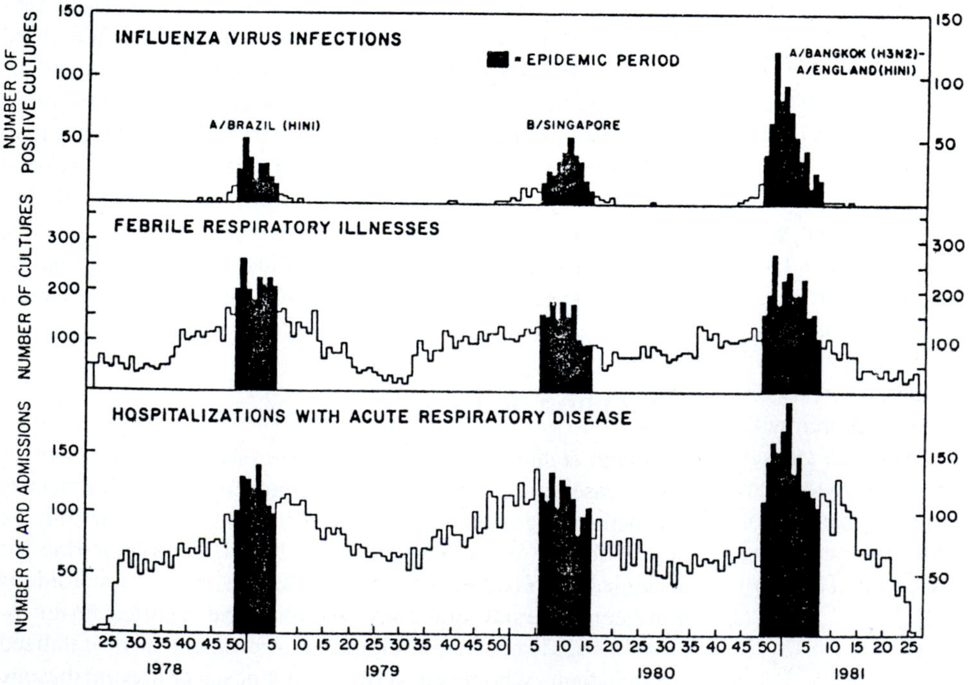

FIGURE 151-1 Number of persons with febrile respiratory illnesses presenting to surveillance sites and number with positive cultures for influenza viruses compared to number of persons hospitalized with acute respiratory disease by week, Harris County, TX, July 1978–June 1981. *(Based on data of Perrotta et al,[32] with permission.)*

Clinical Manifestations

A typical case of influenza is characterized by an abrupt onset of symptoms that include fever, chills, headache, malaise, and myalgias. Dry cough and nasal discharge become progressively worse over a 3- to 5-day period. The cough is usually nonproductive, is associated with substantial chest pain, and persists for weeks after other symptoms may have disappeared. Fever as high as 104°F typically persists for 1 to 3 days and occasionally 1 week. With the disappearance of fever, the systemic symptoms usually resolve. Some studies have suggested that influenza B illness is less severe than influenza A illness. Influenza C infection produces the influenza syndrome rarely, and commonly presents as an afebrile common cold.

Complications from influenza are most common in adults, especially the elderly. Pulmonary complications include primary influenza pneumonia and secondary bacterial pneumonia. Primary influenza pneumonia is uncommon, but is associated with a high mortality. The pneumonia is often bilateral and manifested by severe hypoxia, negative Gram's stain of respiratory secretions, and lack of response to antibiotics. Preexisting cardiovascular disease and pregnancy are two settings in which influenza pneumonia may occur with increased frequency.

Secondary bacterial pneumonia has been described in patients who appear to be recovering from influenza but experience recurrence of fever and worsening of respiratory symptoms 1 to 2 weeks later. On physical exam, there is evidence of pulmonary consolidation. Sputum cultures usually grow *Streptococcus pneumoniae, S. aureus,* or *H. influenzae.* Although *S. pneumoniae* is the most commonly isolated bacterial pathogen, there is increased isolation of *S. aureus* (approximately 20 percent) compared with nonepidemic community-acquired pneumonia series. The elderly and patients with chronic obstructive pulmonary disease (COPD) are at increased risk of pneumonia. Mortality from secondary bacterial pneumonia, however, is lower than in those with primary influenza pneumonia. Most patients recover after appropriate antibiotic therapy.

Other respiratory complications are transient pulmonary function abnormalities, exacerbation of COPD, and croup. Abnormalities in gas exchange and small-airway function are common in influenza infection and may persist for weeks to months after clinical illness. Exacerbation of chronic bronchitis, asthma, and cystic fibrosis has been reported with both influenza virus type A and type B infections. In children, influenza A and occasionally influenza B outbreaks have led to increased cases of croup, but at a lower frequency than with parainfluenza virus infections.

Central nervous system complications occur with both influenza virus type A and type B infections. Influenza A infections have been associated with Guillain-Barré syndrome, transverse myelitis, and encephalitis. Reye's syndrome is a complication of influenza B and occasionally influenza A. It occurs predominantly in children, has a high mortality, and is seen in conjunction with aspirin ingestion. Many other viruses, especially varicella-zoster virus, have been reported in Reye's syndrome, but confirmed influenza B cases are most common. In addition to altered mental status leading to coma, hepatic dys-

function is common. Recovered patients will often have serious neurologic sequelae. With the recommendation that acetaminophen be used in place of aspirin in children with influenza or varicella virus infections, cases of Reye's syndrome have declined.

Less common complications of influenza include myositis, toxic shock syndrome, and myopericarditis. Influenza B has been reported in children with myositis and myoglobinuria. Tender leg muscles and an apparent inability to walk are noted for a few days during the acute illness, with eventual recovery being the rule. Recently, toxic shock syndrome in children and adults has been reported during outbreaks of influenza. Whether there is an association with concurrent pulmonary staphylococcal infection is not yet clear. Rarely, myopericarditis is related to acute influenza A and B infections.

Diagnosis

Influenza viruses can be isolated from respiratory tract specimens. Nasal wash, throat swab, or sputum specimens will yield virus if transported to the laboratory in viral transport medium. Several tissue culture cells sensitive to influenza virus growth are available. Approximately 70 percent of cultures are positive for virus within 72 h of inoculation. Most are positive within 10 days. Rapid diagnostic tests on respiratory secretions are available in research laboratories and provide specific answers within 24 h of receipt of a culture-positive specimen. Specific influenza virus antibody can be detected 2 to 4 weeks after acute illness.[8] Specific antibodies can be detected using HAI, CF, or ELISA techniques. In epidemiologic surveys, combined use of tissue cell cultures and serologic assays documented more influenza virus illnesses than did either method alone.

Prevention and Treatment

Amantadine and rimantadine are available for prophylaxis and treatment of influenza A (not influenza B) infection.[9] In uncomplicated influenza A, both amantadine and rimantadine reduce the duration of clinical signs and symptoms by half. The lower frequency of CNS side effects reported with rimantadine than with amantadine suggests that rimantadine is the preferred antiviral agent, especially in elderly patients. Resistant influenza A isolates have been detected from patients treated with amantadine and rimantadine. The clinical impact of these resistant isolates is yet to be fully defined. Because rimantadine is extensively metabolized, there is significantly less accumulation than with amantadine in the elderly and in patients with renal insufficiency. Therefore, the daily dose of amantadine should be reduced in the elderly and in patients with renal failure. The recommended dose of rimantadine for acute illness is 100 mg once daily for 3 to 5 days.

In selected unvaccinated high-risk patients, daily administration of rimantadine or low-dose amantadine should be considered for prophylaxis. If vaccine is given simultaneously with either amantadine or rimantadine, the antiviral agent can be discontinued 2 weeks after the presumed rise of a specific influenza antibody. The level of protection for amantadine and rimantadine given prophylactically is equivalent to vaccine, or 75 to 90 percent.

Aerosolized ribavirin has had clinical benefit in treating influenza A and B infections in healthy young adults but has not been approved for this indication. Further studies need to define its potential for treating seriously ill, hospitalized influenza patients. Other antivirals need to be developed that have activity against influenza B.

Supportive treatment for acutely ill patients includes adequate fluid intake and bed rest. Fever should be controlled with acetaminophen, not aspirin. Nasal sprays and cold-mist vaporization may provide local relief. Cough suppressants may be useful. Suspected bacterial superinfection requires hospitalization.

Inactivated influenza virus vaccines have been in use for 50 years. The composition of the vaccine is updated yearly and depends on the circulating virus and its variation from the year before (Table 151-3). For at least 15 years, influenza virus vaccine has contained H1N1, H3N2, and B antigens.[5] Children who are eligible for vaccine should receive two doses and adults one dose yearly. When the circulating virus matches a vaccine strain, influenza vaccine has a 75 percent protection rate against illness in healthy persons under 65 years of age. Hospitalizations for pneumonia and influenza are also reduced by 30 to 70 percent in the elderly.

Side effects are minimal with current influenza vaccines. Local reactions at the injection site occur in 25 to 50 percent of recipients within 24 h. In a few cases, these reactions may be severe. Systemic reactions including fever are more common in children than in adults. The excess rate of Guillain-Barré syndrome reported in 1976 during the swine influenza vaccine program has not recurred in any other year.

The targeted groups for influenza virus vaccine include those at increased risk for influenza-related complications and those who can transmit influenza to persons at high risk (Table 151-4).[27,30] In addition, physicians should provide vaccine to any persons who want to reduce the risk of becoming ill with influenza. Vaccination of pregnant women is considered safe at any stage of pregnancy. The severity of influenza in HIV-infected patients does not appear to be different from that in uninfected persons. Recent reports suggest that influenza virus vaccine administration may be associated with transient increases in HIV replication. The clinical significance of this observation has not been determined.

Contraindications to influenza virus vaccine administration include anaphylactic hypersensitivity to eggs or to other components, such as the preservative of the vaccine. Acute febrile illnesses in adults should abate before vaccine is given. However, children with minor illnesses, with or without fever, can be vaccinated without delay.

BRONCHIOLITIS

Epidemiology

Bronchiolitis is characterized by wheezing and other lower respiratory tract symptoms in children less than 2 years of age.[1] RSV accounts for more than half the cases, with parainfluenza viruses, adenoviruses, rhinoviruses, and *M. pneumoniae* accounting for an additional third of cases.[34] Most cases are reported in winter and early spring, when RSV is often prevalent. The attack rate peaks in the first 6 to 8 months of life and declines thereafter. Hospitalizations in the first year of life are often due to bronchiolitis and are more often of boys than girls.

Pathogenesis

The pathogenesis of bronchiolitis results from direct effects of the virus and exaggerated host responses to the infection.[43] The edema and mucous plugging of small airways cause severe lower respiratory symptoms. Leukotrienes and eosinophil cationic protein are detected in increased quantities in secretions from wheezing children. Studies have shown increases in specific IgE antibody to RSV and augmented histamine release in infants with clinical bronchiolitis.[42]

Clinical Manifestations

For several days before the tachypnea and wheezing that characterize bronchiolitis, mild fever and coryza are commonly observed. Nonspecific symptoms such as anorexia and irritability as well as cough usually are also present. Poor oral intake, vomiting, and tachypnea often result in dehydration. Full recovery usually takes 10 to 14 days, with significant improvement in as little as 3 to 4 days.

Hypoxemia is a very common finding in hospitalized infants with bronchiolitis. Hyperinflation and depressed diaphragms are characteristic findings on chest radiographs. It may be impossible to differentiate bronchiolitis from pneumonia, since atelectatic areas may be confused with infiltrates.

Premature infants or infants with serious cardiopulmonary disorders are at increased risk of a complicated course. Apnea is a common complication, especially in RSV-associated bronchiolitis. Recurrent episodes of bronchospasm often occur after bronchiolitis. The full impact of bronchiolitis on pulmonary function in later life has not been defined, but several longitudinal studies reveal small-airway abnormalities that persist for years. The importance of RSV infection occurring early in life versus genetic factors in determining the long-term consequences of bronchiolitis is currently under study.

TABLE 151-3

Recommendations for the Use of Influenza Vaccine

Any person ≥6 months of age at increased risk for complications of influenza
Health-care workers and household members in close contact with persons in high-risk groups
Any person who wishes to reduce the chance of becoming infected with influenza
Two doses 1 month apart in children
One dose in adults

SOURCE: Data from CDC.[5]

TABLE 151-4

Target Groups for Special Influenza Vaccination Programs

Groups at Increased Risk for Influenza-Related Complications

Persons ≥65 years of age

Residents of nursing homes and other chronic-care facilities that house persons of any age with chronic medical conditions

Adults and children with chronic disorders of the pulmonary or cardiovascular systems, including children with asthma

Adults and children who have required regular medical follow-up or hospitalization during the preceding year because of chronic metabolic diseases (including diabetes mellitus), renal dysfunction, hemoglobinopathies, or immunosuppression (including immunosuppression caused by medications)

Children and teenagers (6 months to 18 years of age) who are receiving long-term aspirin therapy and therefore might be at risk for developing Reye's syndrome after influenza

Groups That Can Transmit Influenza to Persons at High Risk

Persons who are clinically or subclinically infected and who care for or live with members of high-risk groups can transmit influenza virus to them. Some persons at high risk (e.g., the elderly, transplant recipients, and persons with AIDS) can have a low antibody response to influenza vaccine. Efforts to protect these members of high-risk groups against influenza might be improved by reducing the likelihood of influenza exposure from their caregivers. Therefore, the following groups should be vaccinated:

Physicians, nurses, and other personnel in both inpatient and outpatient-care settings; employees of nursing homes and chronic-care facilities who have contact with residents

Providers of home care to persons at high risk (e.g., visiting nurses and volunteer workers)

Household members (including children) of persons in high-risk groups.

SOURCE: Data from CDC.[5]

Rarely, acute bronchiolitis due to measles, influenza viruses, or adenoviruses leads to bronchiolitis obliterans, and over weeks to months, patients have repeated bouts of bronchiolitis. The course can be rapidly fatal over several weeks or can develop more slowly. Chronic pulmonary disease develops in most recovering children. No specific therapy appears to be effective.

Diagnosis

Virus isolation from respiratory secretions is helpful in most cases of bronchiolitis. Newer rapid diagnostic tests are available for RSV detection within a few hours. Routine tissue cell culture will isolate respiratory viruses. Because maternal antibody is present in young infants, serum antibody tests are not helpful for a specific diagnosis.

Prevention and Treatment

Since hypoxemia is common with bronchiolitis, oxygen administration and mechanical ventilation are usually required. With RSV bronchiolitis, aerosolized ribavirin has proved useful.[6] Administration of this antiviral agent for 2 to 5 days improves clinical scores and alleviates hypoxemia.[40] Whether bronchodilators are beneficial for bronchiolitis patients remains questionable. Some studies have shown improvement with either aerosolized or parenteral bronchodilators; others have not shown a benefit. Neither corticosteroids nor antibiotics are of benefit in the treatment of bronchiolitis.

PNEUMONIA

Epidemiology

Viral pneumonia occurs in children and adults who are immunocompetent or immunocompromised.[15] Most respiratory viruses have been implicated in cases of pneumonia, but influenza viruses and RSV are particularly common causes.[19] Most cases occur in the winter months, in closed populations, and in patients with cardiac or pulmonary disease.[31] Immunocompromised patients are infected more often with herpesviruses or measles. However, parainfluenza viruses and RSV are being reported with increased frequency in transplant recipients.[35]

In children, RSV, parainfluenza viruses, and influenza A and B are the major causes of viral pneumonia.[26] Schoolchildren and infants in day-care centers are important epidemiologic units for transmission.[12] Approximately 50 percent of viral pneumonias in children less than 3 years of age are caused by RSV.[28] Like bronchiolitis, RSV pneumonia is most commonly reported between 2 and 6 months of age.

In adults, influenza virus types A and B, adenoviruses, parainfluenza viruses, and RSV are the major causes of pneumonia. In hospitalized patients with community-acquired pneumonia, approximately 8 percent of cases are caused by viruses. Mixed infections with bacteria are commonly identified. Of all the cases of community-acquired viral pneumonia in adults, more than 50 percent are due to influenza A. RSV pneumonia is reported less often in adults than in children, but it is being diagnosed more often in the elderly and in transplant recipients.[11] Other common respiratory viruses have been reported to cause pneumonia, but only rarely in adults.

The herpesviruses have also been reported to cause pneumonia in both healthy and immunocompromised adults.[18] Organ transplant patients have particular susceptibility to herpesvirus infections. CMV pneumonia occurs in 25 percent of bone marrow and renal transplant recipients and has a high mortality. Superinfection with bacteria, fungi, and protozoa has been documented in approximately 50 percent of CMV pneumonia patients. The most common secondary pathogen has been *Pneumocystis carinii.*

Factors for dissemination and pneumonitis in herpes simplex virus (HSV) and varicella-zoster infections include bone marrow and organ transplantation, malignancy, chemotherapy, malnutrition, and severe burns. In organ transplant and cancer patients, mortality secondary to HSV and varicella-zoster pneumonitis ranges from 10 to 25 percent. Children with acute leukemia and varicella have a 33 percent incidence of pneumonitis. Pneumonia after herpes zoster occurs at a lower incidence than after varicella. Bacterial superinfection following varicella-zoster pneumonia with long-term lung dysfunction is being described commonly.

Pneumonia secondary to HSV infection has been reported predominantly in immunocompromised hosts.[16] Tracheobronchitis secondary to HSV has been well described, especially in ventilated burn patients. The possible association of HSV infection of the lung and adult respiratory distress syndrome remains controversial and will require further confirmatory studies (Fig. 151-2). Nevertheless, HSV activation may have a role in acute lung injury in ventilated patients.

Less common causes of viral pneumonia include adenoviruses, measles, and the recently described Hantavirus pulmonary syndrome. Adenovirus pneumonia in military recruits is uncommon but serious. Bone marrow transplant patients with adenovirus pneumonia have been reported.[25]

In children with measles, pneumonia is an uncommon complication.[2] Although rarely seen in adults, measles pneumonia has a high mortality, especially during pregnancy. Whether bacterial superinfection is the primary reason for the high mortality with measles pneumonia is unknown. Sixty percent of deaths in infants with measles are secondary to pneumonia. Measles in immunocompromised patients is associated with a high percentage of pneumonia and death. Immunocompromised patients exposed to measles have developed giant-cell pneumonia without the typical rash. Measles encephalitis is another serious complication in immunocompromised hosts.

In the summer of 1993, an outbreak of respiratory illness with a case fatality rate of 76 percent was reported in the southwestern United States.[10] An influenzalike illness, followed by unexplained respiratory failure, was reported in most of the cases. The differential diagnosis of the illness included community-acquired pneumonia and pulmonary edema. Chest radiographs were consistent with noncardiogenic pulmonary edema (Fig. 151-3). Autopsied lung tissue revealed intra-alveolar edema with few neutrophils and no viral inclusions (Fig. 151-4). A previously unknown Hantavirus, Muerto Canyon virus, was isolated from the lungs of these patients and represents the first known cause of human disease by a hemorrhagic fever virus in North America.

Pathogenesis

With the exception of CMV and varicella-zoster virus, viruses causing pneumonia spread from the upper to the lower respiratory tract. The pathologic changes induced in the lung are similar for all viruses.[38] Necrosis and sloughing of epithelium lead to loss of the normal mucosal surface. Mucus production increases, leading to bronchiolar plugging. One week after infection, alveoli fill with fluid and leukocytes. Mononuclear cells are noted in peribronchial areas, and intranuclear inclusions may be seen in alveoli. In measles and parainfluenza virus pneumonia, multinucleated giant cells have been reported.

Recovery from respiratory viral infection relies on both specific and nonspecific host defenses. High concentrations of interferon are detected in the lungs at the time of maximal virus

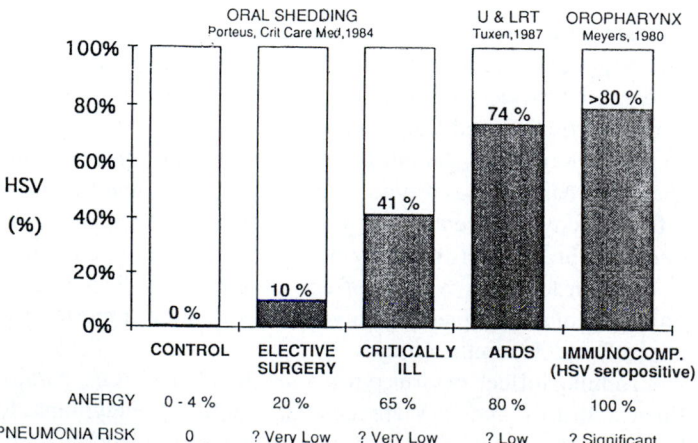

FIGURE 151-2 HSV reactivation rates in different population groups compared with the incidence of anergy in similar population groups and the speculated risk of pulmonary parenchymal invasion. Immunocomp = immunocompromised; U and LRT = upper and lower respiratory tract. (*From Tuxen: Chest 106:32S, 1994.*)

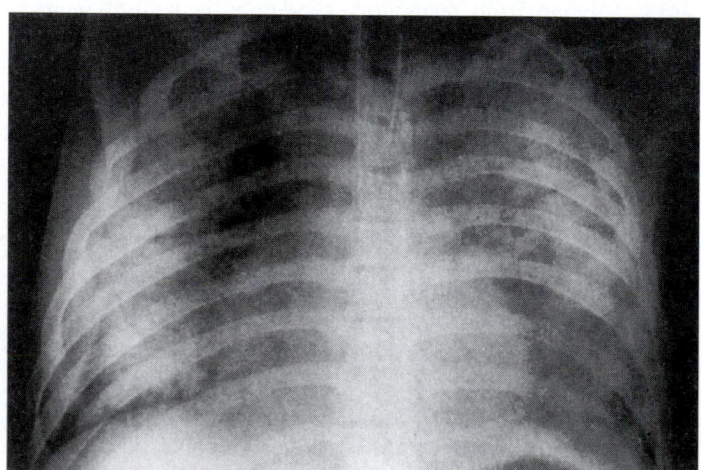

FIGURE 151-3 Chest radiograph showing diffuse interstitial and alveolar infiltrates in a patient with hantavirus infection. (*Based on data of Duchin et al,[10] with permission.*)

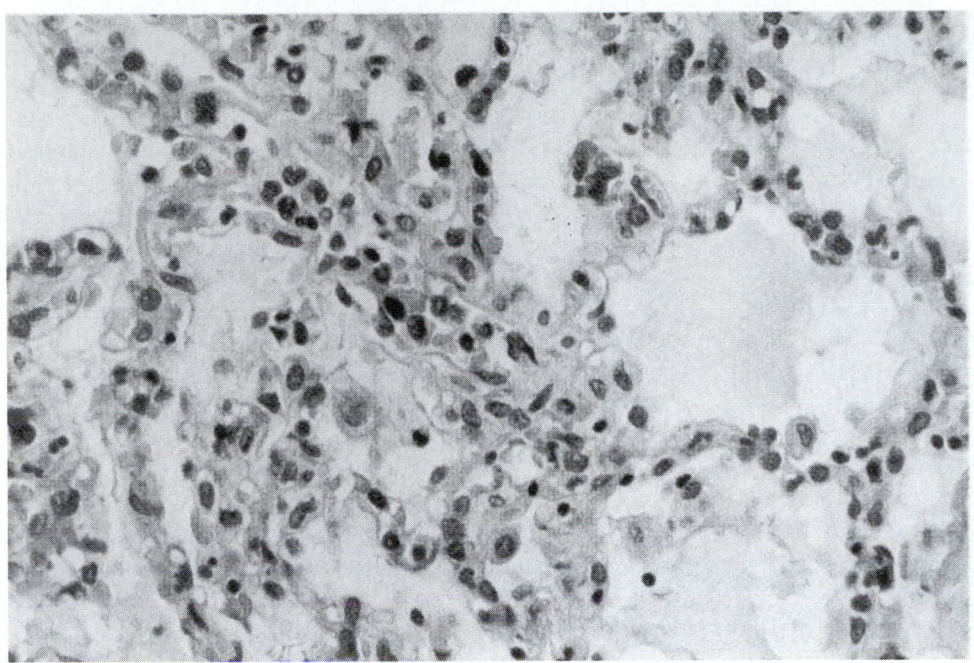

FIGURE 151-4   Hantavirus by tissue. Lung-tissue specimen from a patient with hantavirus-associated interstitial pneumonitis. *(Based on data of Duchin et al,[10] with permission.)*

RSV pneumonia in infants is associated with hypoxia and apnea. Chest radiographs often demonstrate air trapping and multilobar patchy infiltrates (Figs. 151-5 and 151-6). A high percentage of RSV pneumonia patients demonstrate right upper lobe collapse or consolidation. However, no radiographic pattern is specific for this or any other respiratory virus.

Diagnosis

Respiratory viruses are rarely isolated from asymptomatic persons and therefore are considered to be significant if recovered from cultured specimens. The most frequently positive specimens are nasal washes, nasopharyngeal swabs, and throat swabs. Specimens from bronchoscopy secretions or lung biopsy may be useful in diagnosis. Nonrespiratory specimens such as stool, urine, or blood may be sent for virus isolation, but the yield is low and positive results should be interpreted carefully.

There are several rapid tests for viral antigen detection. Immunofluorescent staining or ELISA kits are rapid but not as sensitive as tissue culture systems. PCR techniques and in situ hybridization of tissue specimens are being used in the detection of respiratory viruses. Although there are no commercially available PCR assays for respiratory viruses, this technology is likely to be in place in most viral diagnostic laboratories in the next few years.

concentration. Specific antiviral antibody can be found in the lower respiratory tract secretions by the third day of infection. Cytotoxic T lymphocytes appear at the same time and destroy virus-infected epithelial cells. Thus, the humoral and cell-mediated immune responses are necessary for full recovery from viral pneumonia.

Bacterial superinfection in the lung often occurs after respiratory viral infection. The increased adherence and colonization of gram-positive and -negative bacteria in virus-infected epithelial cells are thought to be due to alterations of host cell surfaces, induction of receptors on exposed surfaces, and changes in the extracellular environment allowing for increased bacterial attachment. Virus-induced suppression of the immune response and alterations in phagocytic function probably contribute to increased bacterial growth and decreased bacterial clearance from the respiratory tract. Virus growth in the lower respiratory tract is associated with altered bactericidal mechanisms of alveolar macrophages and neutrophils. Animal models of viral pneumonia demonstrate reduced lung phagocytic function at a time when bacterial superinfection is likely to develop.

Clinical Manifestations

Infants and children with viral pneumonia usually present with 1 or 2 days of cough and low-grade fever. Young infants may present with minimal fever and apneic spells. Wheezing is found when bronchiolitis is present. Myalgia, anorexia, and malaise in addition to upper respiratory tract symptoms are often reported. Air trapping and perihilar infiltrates are found on chest radiographs. Lobar involvement is seen mainly in older children. Small pleural effusions are uncommon. Peripheral leukocytosis is common. Cultures of blood and sputum should be obtained for diagnosis of bacterial lung infections.

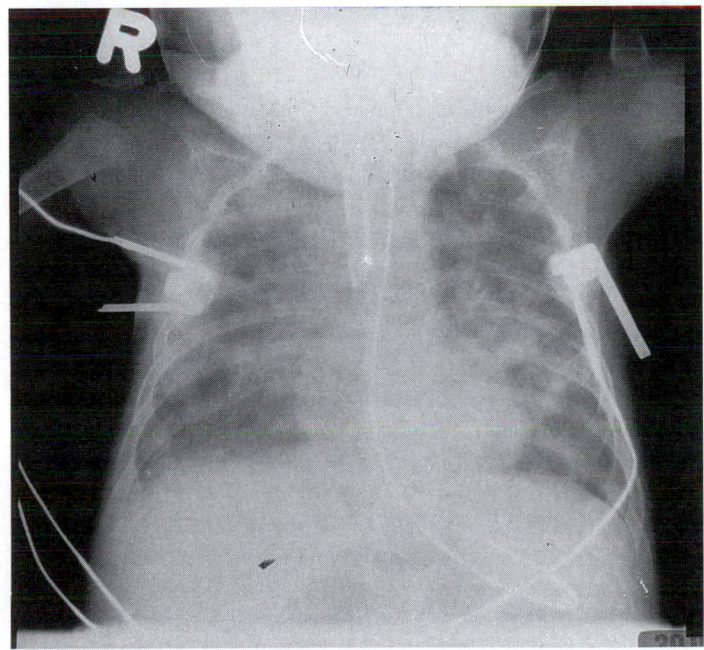

FIGURE 151-5   Premature infant at 3 months of age with respiratory syncytial virus pneumonia. *(Courtesy of Dr. Janet Englund, Baylor College of Medicine.)*

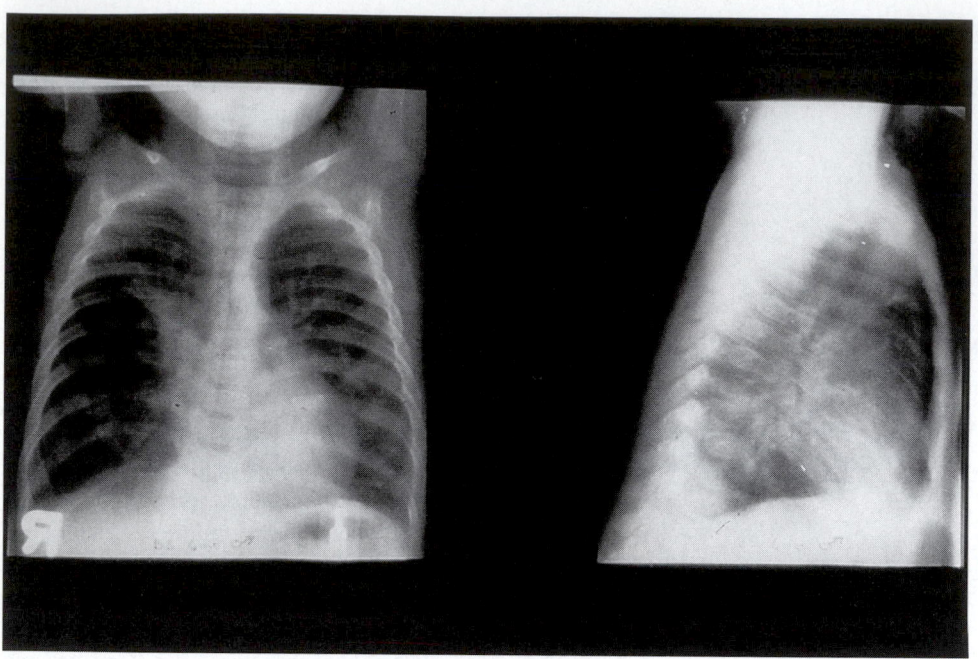

FIGURE 151-6   Chest radiograph (PA and lateral views) of respiratory syncytial virus pneumonia in a 1-year-old child. *(Courtesy of Dr. Janet Englund, Baylor College of Medicine.)*

Standard serologic tests are often available through local or state laboratories. Acute and convalescent sera are needed to demonstrate a significant antibody rise. IgM antibody assays are not routinely available.

Prevention and Treatment

Most antiviral agents approved for respiratory viral infections are not yet approved for viral pneumonia. Ganciclovir therapy for CMV pneumonia has been ineffective.[33] Acyclovir has been given for presumed HSV and varicella pneumonia, but there have been no controlled studies of its effectiveness. An aerosol formulation of ribavirin is approved for severe RSV disease in young children. More rapid resolution of hypoxia and decreased virus shedding were found in ribavirin-treated infants than in the control group.

Amantadine and rimantadine have not been systematically tested in influenza virus pneumonia. Interferon-α has broad antiviral activity against most respiratory viruses, but it has not been very effective in alleviating respiratory virus disease once symptoms have begun.

Employing antibiotics prophylactically in viral pneumonia has not proved effective in preventing bacterial pneumonia. However, when influenza illness is followed by signs and symptoms of pneumonia, antibiotic treatment of the most common bacterial causes is appropriate. If immunocompromised patients are exposed to measles or varicella, immune globulin should be given. Infants born to women with clinical measles should receive immune globulin. Nonimmunocompromised persons exposed to measles can be given live measles vaccine instead of immune globulin to prevent measles infection. No approved antivirals are available for treating measles, although ribavirin has been tried.

NOSOCOMIAL RESPIRATORY VIRAL INFECTIONS

Nosocomial respiratory viral diseases are recognized predominantly in children but are also seen in elderly persons and chronically ill adults (Table 151-5).[17] Increased morbidity, mortality, and hospital costs have been documented as a result of these hospital-acquired infections. Respiratory viruses account for approximately 70 percent of nosocomial viral illnesses.

Outbreaks of nosocomial respiratory viral infections can be detected during seasonal respiratory viral epidemics in the community. Respiratory viruses are introduced to hospitalized patients by infected patients, visitors, or personnel. Transmission occurs through infected hospital staff or patients as well as transfer of virus from hands, aerosols, or fomites. Nosocomial respiratory viral infections can occur in any exposed person, whether at "high risk" or not.

Respiratory Syncytial Virus

The chief cause of nosocomial respiratory viral disease is RSV. Prolonged RSV shedding provides increased opportunity for nosocomial transmission. When RSV is prevalent in the community, one-third of infants admitted to hospitals for other reasons will acquire nosocomial RSV disease. The risk of nosocomial RSV increases with increased lengths of stay. Children with co-morbid conditions, such as congenital heart disease or immunosuppression, are at increased risk of severe nosocomial RSV disease.

During outbreaks of nosocomial RSV, almost half the personnel caring for these children will become ill with tracheobronchitis or influenzalike illness. Loss of work among hospital staff is common. Similar effects on staffs have been reported in nursing home outbreaks of RSV and influenza. Although small-particle aerosol may result in RSV transmission, close contact and direct inoculation onto mucous membranes appear to be the major mode of RSV transmission. Control of nosocomial RSV has been demonstrated after cohorting of sick children and instituting gown and masks for all direct patient care. However, the major infection control measure for interrupting RSV spread continues to be good hand washing.

Influenza

Nosocomial influenza infections are similar in epidemiology to RSV. Community influenza outbreaks are associated with increased nosocomial cases. Personnel can transmit virus to pa-

TABLE 151-5

Epidemiology and Control of Nosocomial Respiratory Viruses

Virus	RSV	Influenza	Parainfluenza	Adenovirus	Rhinovirus
Community pattern	Epidemic winter-spring	Epidemic winter-spring	Type 1, 2: epidemic Type 3: epidemic, endemic	Endemic all year	Endemic all year
Nosocomial spread	++++	++++	+++	+	++
Lower respiratory text disease	++++	++	++	+	?
Suggested mode of spread	Close contact, skin fomite	Close contact, aerosol (?), skin fomite	Close contact (?), skin fomite	Close contact, fecal-oral, skin fomite (?), aerosol	Close contact, skin fomite (?), aerosol
Recommended Control Measures					
Hand washing	+	+	+	+	+
Gowns (pediatrics)	+	+	+	(+)*	(+)
Gloves				±	
Masks		+		±	
Eye-nose goggles	±				
Single room/cohorting†	+	+	+	(+)	(+)
Cohort staff	+	+		(+)	(+)
Limit visitors‡	+	+			
Isolate high-risk	+	+			
Avoid admission of high-risk patients	+	+			

*Parentheses indicate control measures that apply only to neonatal infection.
†Single room with negative air pressure indicated for influenza, possibly adenovirus pneumonia. Cohorting of patients applies when individual isolation is not possible (*see* Table 151-3).
‡Restrict visitors with respiratory symptoms.
SOURCE: Data from Graman and Hall.[17]

tients as well as becoming infected at work. Unlike RSV infection, influenza is thought to be transmitted by small-particle aerosol. Prevention of influenza in hospital personnel can be approached through annual influenza vaccination programs. Health-care workers are candidates to receive vaccine, and it should be offered in the fall of every year.

Chemoprophylaxis with amantadine or rimantadine can be considered during an influenza epidemic for persons who were not recently vaccinated. Outbreaks of influenza A in institutions with high-risk patients should prompt amantadine or rimantadine therapy as soon as possible to reduce virus spread. The drug should be given to all residents of the institution, whether or not they received the most recently approved influenza vaccine. Drug should be given for 2 weeks during an epidemic or for 1 week after the outbreak is concluded. Amantadine or rimantadine can also be offered to unvaccinated staff providing care to high-risk patients. Prophylaxis should be offered to all employees if the outbreak strain of influenza A is not thought to be included in the vaccine.

Other Nosocomial Respiratory Viruses

Parainfluenza viruses are known to be nosocomially transmitted in hospitalized children, in renal transplant units, and in nursing homes. The mode of transmission of parainfluenza viruses is unknown. Use of control precautions similar to those recommended for RSV is currently suggested. No specific antiviral agent or vaccine is available for treatment or prophylaxis of parainfluenza viruses.

Adenoviruses have been reported to be transmitted at eye clinics, inpatient pediatric units, nursing homes, and intensive care units. Hospital personnel have developed pharyngoconjunctival fever when exposed to infected patients. Secondary cases among patients have been few, but if they occur, they can be severe. Transmission probably can occur by fomites, hand-to-hand contact, or small-particle aerosol. Fecal-oral transmission may also occur. Infection control should include isolation of infected patients and case cohorting. Hospital personnel with adenovirus conjunctivitis should have no patient contact until eye drainage has ceased. Gloves should be worn if patient contact is required. Hand washing is important. Whether wearing goggles will reduce self-inoculation is unknown. No specific antivirals are approved for adenovirus. A live attenuated adenovirus vaccine has been used in the military, but it has not been studied for general use.

Rhinoviruses may be associated with nosocomial spread throughout the year. Mode of spread is thought to be by close contact or aerosol. Hand washing is thought to be the major control measure. No antivirals or vaccines are available for use.

REFERENCES

1. Agah R, Cherry JD, Garakian AJ, et al: Respiratory syncytial virus infection rate in personnel caring for children with RSV infections. *Am J Dis Child* 141:695–697, 1987.
2. Atmar RL, Englund JA, Hammill H: Complications of measles during pregnancy. *Clin Infect Dis* 14:217–226, 1992.
3. Barker WH, Mullooly JP: Pneumonia and influenza deaths during epidemics: Implications for prevention. *Arch Intern Med* 142:85–89, 1982.
4. Bertin L, Pons G, d'Athis P, et al: Randomized, double-blind, multicenter controlled trial of ibuprofen versus acetaminophen (paracetamol) and placebo for treatment of symptoms of tonsillitis and pharyngitis in children. *J Pediatr* 119:811–814, 1991.
5. CDC: Prevention and control of influenza. *MMWR Morb Mortal Wkly Rep* 44(RR-3):1–10, 1995.
6. Chanock RM, Parrott RH, Connors M, et al: Serious respiratory tract disease caused by respiratory syncytial virus: Prospects for improved therapy and effective immunization. *Pediatrics* 90:137–143, 1992.
7. Colonno RJ: Virus receptors: The Achilles' heel of human rhinoviruses. *Adv Exp Med Biol* 312:61–70, 1992.
8. Couch RB, Kasel JA: Immunity to influenza in man. *Annu Rev Microbiol* 37:529–549, 1983.
9. Dolin R, Reichman RC, Madore HP, et al: A controlled trial of amantadine and rimantadine in the prophylaxis of influenza A infection. *New Engl J Med* 307:580–584, 1982.
10. Duchin JS, Koster FT, Peters CJ, et al: Hantavirus pulmonary syndrome: A clinical description of 17 patients with a newly recognized disease. *New Engl J Med* 330:949–1005, 1994.
11. Englund JA, Sullivan CJ, Jordan C, et al: Respiratory syncytial virus infection in immunocompromised adults. *Ann Intern Med* 109:203–208, 1988.
12. Frenck RW, Glezen WP: Respiratory tract infections in children in day care. *Semin Pediatr Infect Dis* 1:234–244, 1990.
13. Glezen WP: Serious morbidity and mortality associated with influenza epidemics. *Epidemiol Rev* 4:25–44, 1982.
14. Glezen WP, Frank AL, Taber LH, et al: Parainfluenza virus type 3: Seasonality and risk of infection and reinfection in young children. *J Infect Dis* 150:851–857, 1984.
15. Glezen WP: Viral pneumonia as a cause and result of hospitalization. *J Infect Dis* 147:765–770, 1983.
16. Graham BS, Snell JD Jr: Herpes simplex virus infection of the adult lower respiratory tract. *Medicine (Baltimore)* 62:384–393, 1983.
17. Graman PS, Hall CB: Epidemiology and control of nosocomial viral infections. *Infect Dis Clin North Am* 3:815–841, 1989.
18. Greenberg SB: Respiratory herpesvirus infections: An overview. *Chest* 106:1S–2S, 1994.
19. Greenberg SB: Viral pneumonia. *Infect Dis Clin North Am* 5:603–621, 1991.
20. Gwaltney JM Jr, Moskalski PB, Hendley JO: Hand-to-hand transmission of rhinovirus colds. *Ann Intern Med* 88:463–467, 1978.
21. Gwaltney JM Jr, Phillips CD, Miller RD, et al: Computed tomographic study of the common cold. *New Engl J Med* 330:25–30, 1994.
22. Gwaltney JM Jr: Combined antiviral and antimediator treatment of rhinovirus colds. *J Infect Dis* 166:776–782, 1992.
23. Hayden FG, Gwaltney JM Jr.: Intranasal interferon-α_2 for prevention of rhinovirus infection and illness. *J Infect Dis* 148:543–550, 1983.
24. Hendley JO, Gwaltney JM Jr: Mechanisms of transmission of rhinovirus infections. *Epidemiol Rev* 10:243–258, 1988.
25. Hierholzer JC: Adenoviruses in the immunocompromised host. *Clin Microbiol Rev* 5:262–274, 1992.
26. Hotez PJ, Goldstein B, Ziegler J, et al: Adult respiratory distress syndrome associated with parainfluenza virus type 1 in children. *Pediatr Infect Dis J* 9:750–752, 1990.
27. Keitel WA, Cate TR, Couch RB: Efficacy of sequential annual vaccination with inactivated influenza virus vaccine. *Am J Epidemiol* 127:353–364, 1988.
28. Khamapirad T, Glezen WP: Clinical and radiographic assessment of acute lower respiratory tract disease in infants and children. *Semin Respir Infect* 2:130–144, 1987.
29. McMillian JA, Sandstrom C, Weiner LB, et al: Viral and bacterial organisms associated with acute pharyngitis in a school-aged population. *J Pediatr* 109:747–752, 1986.
30. Mullooly JP, Bennett MD, Hornbrook MC, et al: Influenza vaccination programs for elderly persons: Cost-effectiveness in a health maintenance organization. *Ann Intern Med* 121:947–952, 1994.
31. Oda Y, Katsuda S, Okada Y, et al: Detection of human cytomegalovirus, Epstein-Barr virus, and herpes simplex virus in diffuse interstitial pneumonia by polymerase chain reaction and immunohistochemistry. *Am J Clin Pathol* 102:495–502, 1994.
32. Perrotta DM, Decker M, Glezen WP: Acute respiratory disease hospitalizations as a measure of impact of epidemic influenza. *Am J Epidemiol* 122:468–476, 1985.
33. Reed EC, Bowden RA, Dandliker PS, et al: Treatment of cytomegalovirus pneumonia with ganciclovir and intravenous cytomegalovirus immune globulin in patients with bone marrow transplantation. *Ann Intern Med* 109:783–788, 1988.
34. Ruuskanen O, Ogra PL: Respiratory syncytial virus. *Curr Probl Pediatr* 50–79, 1993.
35. Sable CA, Hayden FG: Orthomyxoviral and paramyxoviral infections in transplant patients. *Infect Dis Clin North Am* 9:987–1003, 1995.
36. Samo TC, Greenberg SB, Couch RB, et al: Efficacy and tolerance of intranasally applied recombinant leukocyte A interferon in normal volunteers. *J Infect Dis* 148:535–542, 1983.
37. Schalen L, Eliasson I, Fex S, et al: Acute laryngitis in adults: Results of erythromycin treatment. *Acta Otolaryngol (Stockh)* 492(Suppl):55–57, 1992.
38. Shanley JD: Mechanisms of injury by viral infections of the lower respiratory tract. *Rev Med Virol* 5:41–50, 1995.
39. Smith TF, Wold AD, Espy MJ, Marshall WF: New developments in the diagnosis of viral diseases. *Infect Dis Clin North Am* 7:183–201, 1993.
40. Taber LH, Knight V, Gilbert BE, et al: Ribavirin aerosol treatment of bronchiolitis due to respiratory syncytial virus infection in infants. *Pediatrics* 72:613–618, 1983.
41. Wallace JM: Pulmonary infections in human immunodeficiency disease: Viral pulmonary infections. *Semin Respir Infect* 8:534–536, 1989.
42. Welliver RC, Ogra PC: Immunology of respiratory viral infections. *Annu Rev Med* 39:147–162, 1988.
43. Wohl MEB: Bronchiolitis. *Pediatr Ann* 15:307–313, 1986.

CHAPTER 152

THE LUNG IN HUMAN IMMUNODEFICIENCY VIRUS INFECTION

Elizabeth A. Rich

HIV BIOLOGY

HIV DISEASE

LUNG-SPECIFIC FEATURES OF HIV INFECTION
Immunologic Considerations
Cell Targets
Viral Determinants
Activation of HIV in the Lung

CONCLUSIONS

The first patients with the acquired immune deficiency syndrome (AIDS) were reported by the Centers for Disease Control and Prevention (CDC) in 1981 in *Morbidity and Mortality Weekly Report*. The etiologic agent of AIDS, the human immunodeficiency virus (HIV), was soon discovered—in 1983.[5,21,32] By December 1995, more than one-half million persons (513,486) with AIDS in the United States had been reported to the CDC; of these, more than 62 percent had died.[9,10] The World Health Organization estimated in 1995 that 18 million adults and 1.5 million children had been infected with HIV, resulting in approximately 4.5 million AIDS cases worldwide.[57] Although current therapies show promise, there is not yet a cure for this still increasing human plague.

The lung is beset by both infectious and noninfectious complications in HIV disease, accounting for a large part of the morbidity and mortality that are associated with AIDS (reviewed in Chapter 135). In attempts to understand the basis for the lung's extraordinary predilection for disease in HIV infection, a large number of pulmonary-related studies have been performed from which current concepts of disease pathogenesis have emerged. Understanding of pulmonary disease associated with HIV requires knowledge of the biology of the virus, the pathogenesis of HIV disease, and the specific features of HIV infection in the lung.

HIV BIOLOGY

HIV is a lentivirus in the Retroviridae family of viruses. All lentiviruses are cytopathic to cells and, as their name implies, cause slow disease progression. Lentiviruses that infect nonhuman primates include the visna virus, which causes encephalitis and pneumonitis in sheep; caprine arthritis virus, which causes chronic arthritis in goats; equine infectious anemia virus in horses; and simian immunodeficiency virus (SIV) of monkeys. HIV infects humans only. HIV-1 is the major cause of AIDS. HIV-2 is found primarily in West African patients and also causes AIDS but may be less pathogenic than HIV-1. HIV, as used in this chapter, will refer to HIV-1.

HIV is a spherical structure composed of a viral coat called the envelope and a core. The core contains the genetic RNA material and viral enzymes, including reverse transcriptase, integrase, and protease (Fig. 152-1).[33] The p24 core protein and viral RNA levels are common measures of extent of HIV replication in the plasma and cells of HIV-infected patients and in experimental systems.

The life cycle of HIV in cells begins with binding of the gp120 protein to the HIV receptor, CD4, on host cells (Fig. 152-2). It is now recognized that another cell surface G protein–coupled receptor is required for fusion and entry of the virus. The fusion receptor preferential for lymphocytotropic viruses is called fusin and has homology to the interleukin 8 (IL-8) receptor.[20] IL-8 is a chemokine (C-X-C family) and is chemotactic for lymphocytes and neutrophils. The fusion factor preferential for macrophage tropic strains is a receptor for other chemokines (C-C family), including RANTES, macrophage inflammatory protein–1α (MIP-1α), and MIP-1β.[4] C-C chemokines are generally chemotactic for lymphocytes and monocytes. These chemokines are potent inhibitors of HIV replication, perhaps by binding to their respective receptors and preventing HIV fusion.[14] The recent discovery of fusin and similar receptors has enormous implications for disease pathogenesis and for new therapeutic options.

Upon entry, HIV undergoes reverse transcription of its RNA into DNA, a process catalyzed by viral reverse transcriptase. The most extensively used antiretroviral agents—including azidothymidine (AZT), deoxycytosine (ddC), deoxyinosine (ddI), and 3TC—are inhibitors of viral reverse transcription. Viral DNA then enters the cell nucleus and is integrated into host chromosomal DNA via viral integrase. In its integrated state, HIV may remain latent for long periods before replication. Replication requires that the integrated DNA be transcribed back into RNA, a process that is extremely intricate.

Unlike many other retroviruses, HIV has several regulatory genes that interact in complex and still incompletely understood ways to accomplish the transcriptional and viral packaging

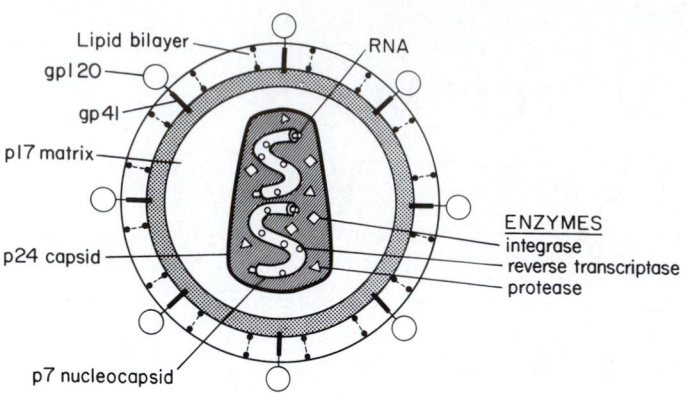

FIGURE 152-1   Structure of HIV. HIV is composed of an envelope and a core. The envelope is a lipid bilayer derived from the host cell membrane and is studded with external viral glycoproteins called gp120 attached to gp41 transmembrane proteins. The core contains the viral proteins p17 (outer core) and p24 (inner core). The cone-shaped p24 structure contains two strands of viral RNA surrounded by the nucleocapsid protein p7. Viral enzymes, including reverse transcriptase, integrase, and protease, also are contained within the core.

processes.[22] These genes include *tat*, *nef*, and *rev*. Before transcription can occur, however, the infected host cell itself must be activated. Numerous stimuli may activate the cell, including antigens, mitogens, and cytokines such as tumor necrosis factor–α (TNF-α) and IL-1. Upon exposure to such stimuli, cell proteins—in particular those from the NFκB/Rel protein family—become activated and bind to specific binding sites in the viral long terminal repeat (LTR). Binding of cellular proteins to the HIV promoter (in the LTR) initiates viral transcription through activation of still another host cell protein, RNA polymerase II, which is required for completion of transcription. Thus, latent HIV DNA is transcribed into RNA only after cellular activation and by usurping cell proteins. This concept is of fundamental importance for understanding the mechanisms of activation of HIV replication in general and in the lung specifically. Furthermore, clinical trials with immune response modifiers such as TNF inhibitors show promise for limiting the overall viral burden in infected persons.

After cellular activation, the viral regulatory genes are transcribed first, and these are short RNAs that leave the nucleus. The *tat* gene in particular functions to accelerate transcription of HIV DNA. The *nef* gene also is expressed early, and although it has both positive and negative influences on transcription in vitro, in vivo *nef* negative mutants are less pathogenic. The *rev* gene product switches the transcriptional process to the longer RNAs that code for the structural proteins of HIV, including those of the envelope and core as well as the viral enzymes. Also present in the longer RNAs are the *vif*, *vpr*, and *vpu* regulatory genes, whose functions are still being discerned but which may be engaged in viral assembly after transcription and in viral infectivity. The precursor protein products of all these genes, as well as complete copies of viral RNA, accumulate in the cytoplasm and then move to the cell surface. Viral particles bud off from the cell membrane, acquiring their envelope lipid bilayer. Viral protease becomes active during this last stage, cutting up the precursor proteins to complete the assembly of core proteins and

enzymes. The protease inhibitors such as saquinavir, ritonavir, and indinavir are directed against the viral protease essential for these assembly and packaging events. In combination with the nucleoside analogs and 3TC, these protease inhibitors are powerful inhibitors of HIV load in infected persons.[15] The long-term impact of this new class of antiretroviral agents, however, remains to be determined.

HIV DISEASE

The typical course of HIV infection begins with an acute HIV syndrome, within 3 to 6 weeks after primary infection, characterized by mononucleosislike symptoms including sore throat, myalgias, and fever (Fig. 152-3).[40] During this acute phase, HIV disseminates widely and seeds the lymphoid organs. HIV RNA and HIV p24 levels are usually high in the plasma during the acute phase of infection. An immune response to HIV is detectable within 1 week to 3 months after primary infection. The symptoms of acute HIV syndrome subside within 1 to several weeks, and infected persons are generally free of symptoms for 8 to 10 years—a condition known as clinical latency. During the

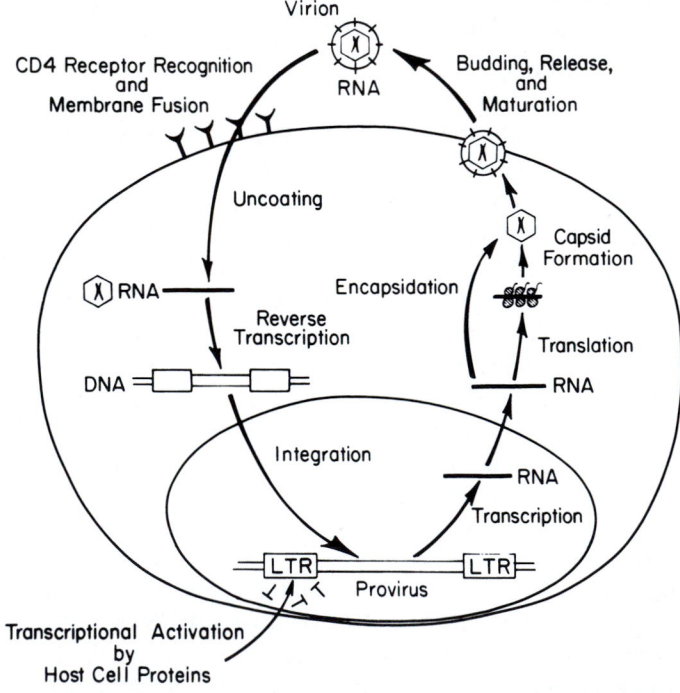

FIGURE 152-2   The HIV replication cycle. Viral gp120 binds to cellular CD4 receptors and to cofactors (fusin and fusinlike molecules), resulting in entry into the cell through fusion with the cell membrane. Virus is uncoated in the cell cytoplasm and is reversely transcribed into DNA. After transport to the nucleus, the viral genome is integrated into host cell chromosomal DNA, where it may remain stable for long periods. The stably integrated provirus is transcribed back into RNA through complex mechanisms first requiring stimulation of the cell that activates cellular proteins such as NFκB, which then enhance transcription upon binding to the viral promoter (in the LTR). Transcription of provirus results in mRNA that is translated to regulatory and then structural proteins and enzymes. Transcripts are packaged into virion particles. Budding from the cell wall where the viral envelope is formed leads to release of progeny virion capable of initiating a new cycle of infection.

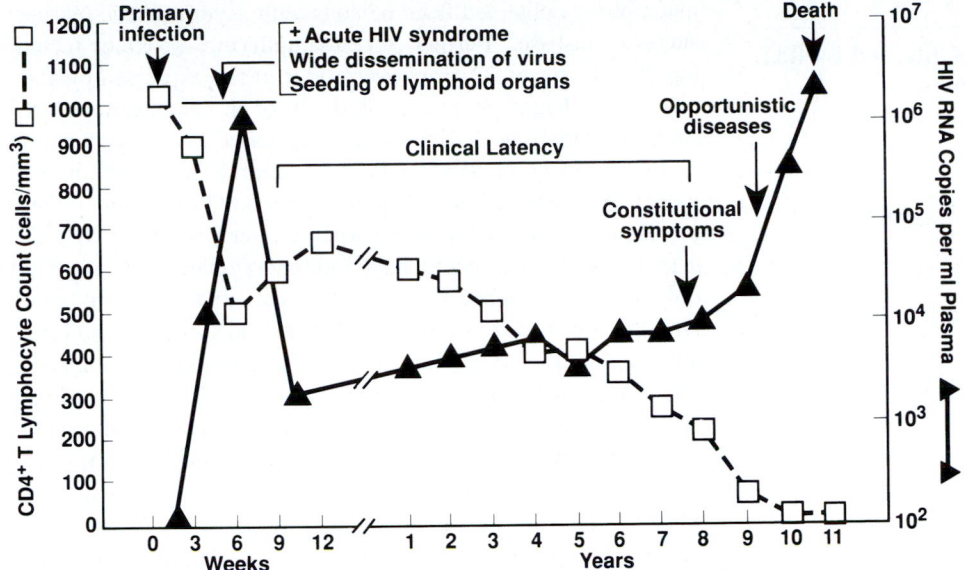

FIGURE 152-3   Natural history of HIV disease. *(Courtesy of Dr. Anthony Fauci.)*

period of clinical latency, plasma viral RNA levels plateau. Nevertheless, active viral transcription is an ongoing, persistent process even during clinical latency.[39] Billions of HIVs are being produced and removed from the blood daily, as CD4 T cells are turned over at an extraordinary rate.[25,54] Furthermore, huge levels of HIV are found in the lymphoid organs in this earlier stage of disease.[39] A small subgroup of patients are long-term nonprogressors with HIV disease and remain in the clinical latency stage for 15 to 20 years.[8,41] Presumably, the virus is also more latent in long-term survivors. Most infected people, however, begin to develop constitutional symptoms sooner. As peripheral CD4 cell numbers decline, plasma HIV RNA levels rise. Opportunistic diseases begin when the number of peripheral CD4 cells decreases to fewer than 100 to 200 cells/mm^3. Death usually occurs within 2 years after onset of opportunistic diseases.

The immune defects in HIV disease correspond in large part to loss of the population of CD4 T helper cells. As early as 1984, 3 years after the first patient with AIDS was described, it was demonstrated that HIV is selectively tropic for CD4$^+$ T helper cells. CD4$^+$ monocytes and dendritic cells also can be infected with HIV.[7,35] Subsequent studies, however, using a variety of techniques—including viral cultures, gene amplification by the polymerase chain reaction (PCR), and in situ hybridization—revealed that the major cell in the blood and lymph nodes harboring HIV in infected persons is the CD4 T lymphocyte and not monocytes or dendritic cells.[48] The level of HIV in CD4 T cells rises with disease progression but is surprisingly low for the degree of immunodeficiency.[19] This is possibly explained by the recent findings of high levels of HIV in lymph nodes. Tissue macrophages from a variety of organs also can be infected with HIV, including the lung, brain, skin, and gastrointestinal tract. Since these mononuclear phagocytes are less susceptible to the cytopathic effects of HIV, the widespread opinion has evolved that macrophages may be the major reservoir of HIV in (non-lymphoid) tissues.

The cellular immune defects resulting from infection of T helper cells include lymphocytopenia, decreased helper-to-

suppressor ratio (less than 1.5:1), cutaneous anergy, and poor in vitro proliferative and cytokine responses of blood lymphocytes to mitogenic and antigenic stimuli. Blood monocytes have decreased antigen-presenting function for T cells. Information regarding effector functions of blood monocytes, including phagocytosis and killing of microorganisms, is controversial.[33] Monokines including TNF and IL-1 are increased in the plasma and cells of some infected persons. Humoral immune abnormalities include hypergammaglobulinemia, with associated autoimmune phenomena (thrombocytopenia, hemolytic anemia, a lupuslike syndrome), and impaired primary, but intact anamnestic, antibody responses. The occurrence of opportunistic infections as CD4 levels decline is due to impaired cellular immune responses. The increased incidence of bacterial infections such as pneumococcosis may be explained by the decreased ability to mount a specific primary antibody response to newly encountered antigens and to loss of T helper cell function.

LUNG-SPECIFIC FEATURES OF HIV INFECTION

Immunologic Considerations

Numerous studies support the general concept that the immune response is compartmentalized and that pulmonary responses often differ from those of blood-derived cells. It is thus imperative to study pulmonary-specific host defenses during HIV infection to understand how infectious and noninfectious complications occur. Only through such understanding will the best therapeutic and preventive options be developed. Longitudinal studies to address the relationships between immunologic/virologic events and development of clinical complications are needed and seriously lacking. Cross-sectional studies of patients at various stages of disease (with and without concurrent opportunistic infections) using bronchoalveolar lavage (BAL) have been the major approach to studies of lung cells in HIV disease. Results of these are summarized in Table 152-1.

Alveolar lymphocytes are increased in number in the lungs of HIV-infected persons during both early and later stages of disease.[23] The increase in alveolar lymphocytes is paradoxical, considering the progressive decline in CD4 lymphocytes in the peripheral blood. Whether the increase in number of alveolar lymphocytes is due to increased recruitment from the blood or in situ proliferation is not known. It is clear, however, that most of the alveolar lymphocytes in HIV-infected people are T cells (CD3$^+$) and that most of the T cells are CD8$^+$. Among the CD8$^+$ T cells, most are D44$^+$ cytotoxic T lymphocytes (CTL) that are class II major histocompatibility complex (MHC) restricted.[3]

TABLE 152-1

Phenotype and Function of Lung Cells Obtained by BAL from HIV-infected Individuals

Alveolar Lymphocytes

Increased number

Predominantly T cells that are CD8$^+$D44$^+$ cytotoxic T lymphocytes (CTL)

CTL activated and specifically cytotoxic for alveolar macrophages expressing HIV antigens (class II MHC restricted)

MHC-unrestricted CTL with natural killer markers present but low in number and variable activity

B lymphocytes polyclonally activated

Alveolar Macrophages

Increased in number

Accessory function for T cells enhanced

Increased expression of markers of activation

Increased production of cytokines (TNF, IL-1, IL-6)

Normal killing of *Toxoplasma gondii* and *Chlamydia psitacci* and normal response to interferon-γ

Phagocytosis of *Staphylococcus aureus* normal

Little known about phagocytosis and killing of more common infectious agents in the lung in HIV disease

Alveolar Neutrophils

Increased during opportunistic infection

Correlate with poor prognosis

These alveolar CTL are specifically cytotoxic for alveolar macrophages expressing HIV antigens[42] and are activated in situ as determined by expression of markers of activation such as the p75 chain of the IL-2 receptor, which is not expressed on resting T cells.[3] The HIV-specific cytotoxic activity of alveolar lymphocytes may be a major mechanism of local host defense against this virus. CTL activity of alveolar lymphocytes, however, decreases with disease progression,[26] suggesting a correlation with development of pulmonary complications.

Also found in the lungs of HIV-infected patients are CD8$^+$ alveolar lymphocytes coexpressing CD56/CD57, which are natural killer cell markers. Cytotoxic activity of these cells, which are MHC unrestricted, is highly variable, so their overall impact on host defense in the lung is not yet clear. B lymphocytes are polyclonally activated in both blood and BAL cells, as evidenced by increased numbers of IgG-releasing cells and IgG levels.[58] The role of mucosal immunity (mucosal B cells, IgA, M cells) in the airways in HIV disease has not been addressed, but this front-line system is probably important in overall host defense in the lung.

Alveolar macrophages also are increased during HIV disease.[3] Perhaps unexpectedly, the immunoregulatory functions of alveolar macrophages from HIV-infected persons are increased. Accessory function for T-cell responses to self antigens and mitogen is enhanced.[53] Expression of markers of activation such as HLA-DR, -DQ, and -DP also is increased, even in alveolar

macrophages obtained from persons with asymptomatic (earlier) stages of disease.[6] Further, T cell–amplifying cytokines including IL-1, IL-6, and TNF are overproduced and expressed by alveolar macrophages either constitutively or in response to stimuli such as lipopolysaccharide.[3,51] The increased accessory function of alveolar macrophages in HIV disease can be attributed, in part, to HIV-1 *tat* gene–induced IL-6 production.[29] Production of these cytokines is enhanced in both earlier and later stages of HIV disease. Thus, alveolar macrophage immunoregulatory functions not only are preserved but also are enhanced, apparently throughout HIV disease. The consequences of increased cytokines, however, although no doubt beneficial to T-cell response, may not be beneficial overall in the lung because these cytokines can activate HIV replication and also may inflict damage to parenchymal cells.

The effector functions of alveolar macrophages in HIV disease on defense against other microbes are less well defined. Murray and coworkers demonstrated that alveolar macrophages of infected patients kill *Toxoplasma gondii* and *Chlamydia psittaci* normally and that killing of *T. gondii* and release of hydrogen peroxide are enhanced normally by interferon-γ.[36] Phagocytosis of *Staphylococcus aureus* by alveolar macrophages from HIV-infected patients with pneumonia is decreased, whereas phagocytosis is enhanced in alveolar macrophages from asymptomatic HIV-infected persons.[37] Surprisingly little, however, is known about phagocytosis or killing of the more common infectious agents associated with HIV disease, including *Pneumocystis carinii*, pneumococcus, and mycobacteria, by alveolar macrophages from HIV-infected persons.

Neutrophils are the other major cell type with antimicrobial functions. Neutrophils are increased in the lungs of HIV-infected patients with concurrent opportunistic infection.[3] Further, the presence of neutrophils obtained by BAL correlates with a poor prognosis.[2]

In summary, there is a CD8$^+$ T-lymphocytic alveolitis and a macrophage alveolitis in HIV disease, and both of these cell populations are activated. The CD8$^+$ cells exert specific cytotoxic activity on HIV antigen–expressing alveolar macrophages, which may help to control local HIV infection. Alveolar macrophages show increased immunoregulatory functions for T-lymphocyte responses to soluble stimuli and normal antimicrobial function for selected infectious targets, but antimicrobial activities for common infectious agents associated with HIV disease are not known. Neutrophils are present during opportunistic infections, but whether their functions are impaired in the lung is not known. One can conclude from the studies amassed that many host defense mechanisms are preserved in the lung during HIV infection and even enhanced but that some of these defenses deteriorate with disease progression. Considering the natural history of the disease in which pulmonary complications become more and more problematic for patients, it is likely that still undetermined defects in host defense mechanisms may emerge that help to explain this extraordinary predilection for lung disorders in HIV disease.

Cell Targets

The diversity of pulmonary complications associated with HIV disease, both infectious and noninfectious, suggests that multiple cell types in the lung are affected by the virus, through either direct infection or indirect injury. HIV has been detected in lung tissue and in bronchoalveolar cells obtained by BAL. Although absolute levels of HIV infection of lung cells vary among studies, some conclusions can be drawn.

HIV mRNA can be detected by in situ hybridization of lung tissue, and levels are particularly high in patients with lymphocytic interstitial pneumonitis.[11] With this technique, the frequency of lung cells expressing active viral mRNA is low. Whether more sensitive assays, such as the reverse transcribed polymerase chain reaction (RT PCR), might reveal more evidence of active viral transcription in the lung has not been examined. Levels of latent HIV (HIV DNA not undergoing active transcription) also have not been determined in lung parenchymal cells. Such studies are difficult because it is not feasible to obtain lung tissue from HIV-infected subjects during asymptomatic stages of disease, and studies of lung tissue from autopsy specimens of patients with lung disease would reflect the impact of a variety of other infectious agents on HIV replication in the lung.

Most studies of HIV load in lung cells have used material obtained by the more feasible method of BAL. Cell-free BAL fluid does not contain free virus. For unseparated bronchoalveolar cells, viral cultures, which determine capacity for transmission of HIV in vitro, are positive in 9 to 59 percent of HIV-infected patients.[12,16,51] By DNA PCR, which detects latent virus, 50 to 86 percent of patients studied harbored HIV in bronchoalveolar cells.[3,13,51] Thus, the proportion of subjects in whom latent HIV DNA is present in their bronchoalveolar cells is higher than that in whom their bronchoalveolar cells readily transmit HIV in culture.

Purified alveolar macrophages were discovered to harbor HIV in 1986.[47] Subsequent studies confirm that alveolar macrophages from HIV-infected patients can carry the virus.[3,51] Alveolar macrophages from 33 to 75 percent of HIV-infected patients with late-stage disease are positive for HIV by viral co-cultures; 47 to 100 percent are positive by HIV DNA PCR. In one study, alveolar macrophages from all HIV-infected subjects were positive for HIV DNA, but in none was HIV antigen or mRNA actively expressed, suggesting that active viral transcription in alveolar macrophages is uncommon.[30] Thus, most patients with later-stage HIV disease carry proviral HIV in their alveolar macrophages, and approximately one-half carry virus in alveolar macrophages that is transmissible to lymphocytes in vitro, but active viral transcription in situ may be quite low. Alveolar macrophages from early-stage HIV disease (CD4 level more than 400 cells per microliter), however, are rarely infected with HIV as determined by viral cultures and DNA PCR.[51] Thus, alveolar macrophages are not reservoirs of HIV at earlier-stage disease but may become reservoirs in later stages of disease.

When alveolar lymphocytes from HIV-infected patients are highly purified, HIV DNA can be detected by PCR in cells from most patients studied.[50] This is a surprising finding that needs to be confirmed. Most alveolar lymphocytes in HIV disease are CD8 T cells, which generally are not infectable with HIV. Thus, the high level of proviral expression may reflect an unusual predilection of HIV infection of CD8 T cells in the lung.

It is difficult to attribute all the known pulmonary complications associated with HIV disease to viral infection of T cells and macrophages because pathologic changes may occur relatively early in the course, before viral burden in such lung cells is high. The pathologic and functional entities associated with HIV disease include emphysema, pulmonary hypertension, nonspecific interstitial pneumonitis, low diffusion capacity, and unexplained dyspnea.[18,56] These pulmonary disorders could be a consequence of infection of mesenchymal or ectodermal cells with HIV or could reflect damage induced by inflammatory cells or by products of HIV. Evidence for lung damage in HIV disease is an increase in alveolocapillary permeability in HIV-infected patients without active opportunistic infection but with a cytotoxic T-lymphocytic alveolitis, suggesting T cell–induced injury to this membrane.[34]

There is precedence for HIV infection of nonimmunologic cells including skin fibroblasts, brain endothelial cells, intestinal epithelial cells, and others.[33] Such infection is generally quite low-grade, but may have important biologic sequelae. Evidence for HIV infection of parenchymal lung cells, however, is scanty. Lung-derived fibroblasts can be productively infected with HIV in vitro.[33] In one study, fibroblasts in the lungs of HIV-infected patients expressed HIV antigens, and HIV mRNA and DNA were detected.[43] Lung-derived epithelial cells also can be infected in vitro.[33] There are no reports to date, however, of HIV infection in vivo of epithelial or endothelial cells of the alveolocapillary membrane. Nevertheless, whether such cells are infected directly or damaged indirectly during HIV disease, it is likely that certain of the physiological and structural abnormalities in the lungs of HIV-infected persons may be attributed to distortion in the integrity of parenchymal cells.

Viral Determinants

Variations in HIV may influence pathogenesis of disease as well as response to therapy. The heterogeneity of HIV strains is at several levels, including serotypic, biologic, and genetic.[33] Serotypic variations in HIV are demonstrated as differences in susceptibility of HIV strains to serum neutralization and to enhancing antibodies. Biologic differences in HIV strains may be at the level of virus replication, latency, cytopathicity, and cell tropism. Regarding cell tropism, there are HIV strains that preferentially infect T cells (T-cell tropic strains) and HIV strains that infect both T cells and macrophages; some of the latter strains infect macrophages to a much greater extent than others (macrophage tropic). Differences in cellular tropism are determined, in part, at the level of entry of virus into the cell and may reflect variations in binding to fusin or fusinlike chemokine receptors on cells. During early stages of disease, viral isolates from the peripheral blood of infected persons may grow more slowly, do not induce syncytia (a cytopathologic marker of infection), and are tropic for monocyte lineage cells.[35] In contrast, progression of HIV infection is associated with the emergence of syncytium-inducing strains that are more T-cell tropic.[33,35]

The genetic structure of HIV determines such differences in biologic activities of various strains. For example, tropism of HIV for T cells and macrophages correlates, in part, with structural differences in HIV gp120 envelope protein, most clearly with the presence of certain residues in a 35–amino acid region within the highly variable principal neutralizing V3 domain of gp120.[33] The V3 loop of gp120 also is a target of both neutralizing antibodies and cytotoxic T cells. It is believed that mutations in the *env* gene encoding this region result in evasion of host immune defenses by HIV, leading to further propagation of the virus. A high rate of mutation of the *pol* gene that codes for reverse transcriptase also confers heterogeneity to the HIV genome. Such mutations result in reverse transcriptases with activity despite large concentrations of nucleoside analogs such as AZT and are therefore the principal reason for development of resistance to these drugs.

The nonsyncytium-forming or relatively noncytopathic, macrophage-tropic strains that predominate in the blood of many HIV-infected persons in early stages of disease also can be found in the lung as well as other tissues, including the brain and salivary glands.[3] Such noncytopathic strains may be found in the lung even once T cell–tropic, syncytium-forming strains are established in the blood at later stages of disease.[49] The pathogenic significance of these strains in the lung, however, may not relate to differences in syncytium formation (which requires membrane fusion), because in one study, differences in the capacity of macrophage and lymphocyte-tropic HIV strains to replicate in alveolar macrophages were not attributable to membrane fusion.[45]

Itescu and colleagues found that HIV strains from bronchoalveolar cells differ from those of blood mononuclear cells in that the V3 domain nucleotide sequences are more homogeneous in the C-terminal region and contain a highly conserved, negatively charged amino acid motif.[28] This V3 C-terminal structure could be important in the capacity of HIV to infect alveolar macrophages. Phylogenetic analyses of the V3 domain nucleotide sequences in blood monocytes and alveolar macrophages further suggest that the strains in alveolar macrophages independently evolved from a presumed ancestral strain that might have originated with strains in blood monocytes. These results lend further credence to the likelihood that the pulmonary complications of HIV disease are dictated, in part, by the microenvironment of the lung. Much more work, however, needs to be done to promote full understanding of HIV heterogeneity in the lung and the consequences of such strain differences on local disease pathogenesis.

Activation of HIV in the Lung

Replication of retroviruses including HIV in cells requires that the cell is activated. The exogenous stimuli capable of activating cells and thus HIV production include antigens, mitogens, and other viruses, including HTLV-1, herpes simplex virus, and cytomegalovirus. Endogenous stimuli that can activate cells and thus HIV include growth and differentiation factors such as IL-1, GM-CSF, M-CSF, and IL-3 and cytokines such as TNF and IL-1. TGF-β, interferon-α, and IL-13 are cytokines that can inhibit HIV replication in vitro. There is increased expression of several cytokines, in particular TNF, during HIV disease as detected in blood, lymph nodes, and other tissue compartments. These cytokines then may, in turn, increase HIV replication through autocrine or paracrine mechanisms. Cellular activation affects HIV replication at several stages in the life cycle of the

virus, including rate and completion of reverse transcription, integration of DNA into the host cell genome, and transcription.[33,44] In general, cytokines activate HIV through transcriptional upregulation.

Given the absolute requirement of cellular activation for HIV replication, it is of extreme importance to fully understand the mechanisms of activation of cells and consequent HIV replication both in vitro and in vivo so that improved therapeutic strategies can be implemented to control the growth of HIV. In the lung, in vitro studies show that alveolar macrophages from healthy HIV-negative subjects are more susceptible to productive infection with HIV than are blood monocytes from the same subjects.[46] Blood monocytes cultured in vitro to allow differentiation are far more susceptible to infection than are freshly isolated monocytes. Thus, the state of differentiation of macrophages may influence the ability of HIV to replicate in these cells. Since alveolar macrophages are chronically exposed to inhaled antigens and particulates, activation of these cells by such agents in situ also may render them more capable of supporting HIV replication than their blood monocyte precursors.

Alveolar macrophages from healthy HIV-negative cigarette smokers are significantly more susceptible to productive infection with HIV in vitro than are alveolar macrophages from healthy nonsmokers (Fig. 152-4).[1] The increased viral production is not due to increased entry or extent of reverse transcription of the virus or to production of several cytokines. Since alveolar macrophages from smokers are morphologically and metabolically activated, it is presumed that their increased capacity to support HIV replication is due, in part, to their state of activation. Although controversial, several epidemiologic studies suggest that smoking may increase the likelihood of HIV infection and the rate of progression of HIV disease once infection takes over.[1] The finding of increased HIV production in alveolar macrophages from smokers provides biologic plausibility to these epidemiologic studies. Case-control, prospective longitu-

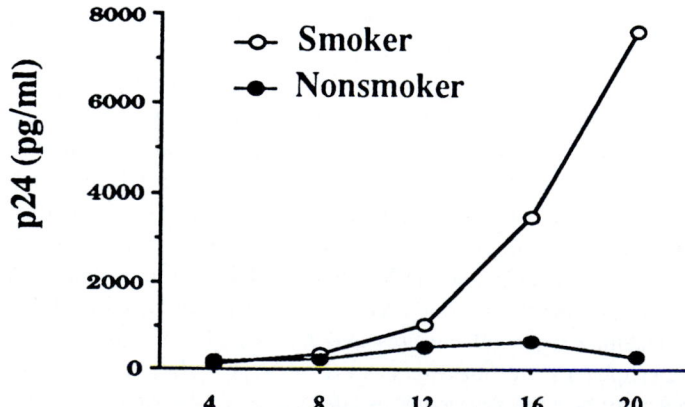

FIGURE 152-4 Kinetics of HIV production by alveolar macrophages from smokers and nonsmokers. Representative experiment shows that alveolar macrophages from a healthy smoker infected with HIV-1 JR-FL strain support higher levels of HIV production than alveolar macrophages from a nonsmoker. Supernatants were collected over 24 h every 4 days after infection for 2 to 3 weeks and p24 gag protein levels determined by ELISA. (*Based on data of Abbud et al,[1] with permission.*)

dinal studies of CD4-matched HIV-infected subjects, however, are needed to firmly establish that smoking enhances progression of HIV disease. Such proof would have obvious clinical implications in further support of smoking cessation in the HIV-infected person.

Given the great frequency of pulmonary and nonpulmonary infectious complications associated with HIV, one of the most important clinical and basic issues to be resolved is whether—and, if so, how—these HIV-associated infections increase the rate of progression of HIV disease. One possibility is that these other infectious agents directly activate HIV. Examples are herpes simplex virus and cytomegalovirus, which increase HIV replication in infected cells. Another possibility is that cytokines are induced by infection of cells with these other pathogens—which, in turn, activate HIV. In support of this hypothesis and as applied to the lung, Israel-Biet and coworkers established that TNF production is increased in alveolar macrophages of HIV-infected patients and that production of this cytokine correlates with presence of lung opportunistic infections and to expression of HIV by these cells.[27]

Recent epidemiologic studies suggest that tuberculosis is a factor in progression of HIV disease. Whalen and colleagues have shown that tuberculosis in an HIV-positive subject is associated with shortened survival compared to CD4-matched HIV-infected controls without tuberculosis.[55] Monocytes from patients with tuberculosis support increased production of HIV after infection in vitro.[52] Monocytes from these patients are activated to produce increased levels of TNF, IL-1, and IL-6 upon stimulation with lipopolysaccharide or purified protein derivative of *Mycobacterium tuberculosis*. As these cytokines activate HIV replication, it is likely that the increases in proinflammatory cytokines contribute to the increased support of HIV production by monocytes from patients with tuberculosis. Mycobacterial antigens induce HIV transcription through the HIV LTR, an effect mediated by TNF.[31] Evidence also suggests that tuberculosis promotes HIV replication in the lung.[38] Further, alveolar macrophages from healthy subjects coinfected with HIV and *M. avium* in vitro show enhanced production of HIV after several days in culture, suggesting that mycobacterial growth may act as an important cofactor for HIV replication in the lung.[17] Thus, both in vitro and in vivo evidence support the possibility that chronic mycobacterial infection may increase the rate of progression of disease through effects on viral replication.

CONCLUSIONS

Much has been learned about HIV biology and HIV disease pathogenesis since the first patients with AIDS were reported over 16 years ago. Clearly, there are unique features in the lung with respect to both the virus and the host response to the virus. HIV strains in alveolar macrophages appear to have evolved independently from blood-derived strains. A T-lymphocytic alveolitis composed of CD8[+] cells that specifically kill alveolar macrophages expressing HIV antigens may be an important host defense to limit replication of HIV in the lung. Nevertheless, these alveolar lymphocytes may themselves be infected with the virus. Alveolar macrophages from HIV-infected subjects harbor the virus, but levels are low and increase during later stages of disease, perhaps indicating loss of protective mechanisms in the lung. Alveolar macrophages are highly activated immunologically even during asymptomatic stages of HIV disease, but the consequences of such activation on HIV replication and injury to the lung are not known. Smoking and pulmonary opportunistic infections probably activate HIV in lung cells. Despite these general conclusions, however, the mechanisms by which pulmonary diseases interact with infected persons are far from completely understood. More basic molecular and cellular studies employing lung cells and lung-derived HIV strains are needed. Prospective longitudinal studies also will be required for us to be able to decipher relationships between HIV replication, host defenses, and development and progression of the pulmonary complications of AIDS.

REFERENCES

1. Abbud RA, Finegan CK, Guay LA, Rich EA: Enhanced production of human immunodeficiency virus type 1 by in vitro–infected alveolar macrophages from otherwise healthy cigarette smokers. *J Infect Dis* 172:859–863, 1995.
2. Agostini C, Zambello R, Trentin L, et al: Prognostic significance of the evaluation of bronchoalveolar lavage populations in patients with HIV-1 infection and pulmonary involvement. *Chest* 100:1601–1606, 1991.
3. Agostini C, Trentin L, Zambello R, Semenzato G: HIV-1 and the lung: Infectivity, pathogenic mechanisms, and cellular immune responses taking place in the lower respiratory tract. *Am Rev Respir Dis* 147:1038–1049, 1993.
4. Alkhatib G, Combadiere C, Broder CC, et al: CC CKR5: A RANTES, MIP-1α, MIP-1β receptor as a fusion cofactor for macrophage-tropic HIV-1. *Science* 272:1955–1958, 1996.
5. Barré-Sinoussi F, Chermann JC, Rey F, et al: Isolation of a T-lymphotropic retrovirus from a patient at risk for acquired immune deficiency syndrome (AIDS). *Science* 220:868–871, 1983.
6. Buhl R, Jaffe HA, Holroyd KJ, et al: Activation of alveolar macrophages in asymptomatic HIV-infected individuals. *J Immunol* 150:1019–1028, 1993.
7. Cameron PU, Lowe MG, Crowe SM, et al: Susceptibility of dendritic cells to HIV-1 infection in vitro. *J Leukoc Biol* 56:257–265, 1994.
8. Cao Y, Qun L, Zhang L, et al: Virologic and immunologic characterization of long-term survivors of human immunodeficiency virus type 1 infection. *New Engl J Med* 332:201–208, 1995.
9. Centers for Disease Control and Prevention: HIV/AIDS Surveillance Report. 7 (no. 2):1–40, 1995.
10. Centers for Disease Control and Prevention: First 500,000 AIDS cases United States. *MMWR* 44:849–853, 1995.
11. Chayt KJ, Harper ME, Marselle LM, et al: Detection of HTLV-III RNA in lungs of patients with AIDS and pulmonary involvement. *JAMA* 256:2356–2359, 1986.
12. Clarke JR, Williamson JD, Mitchell DM: Comparative study of the isolation of human immunodeficiency virus from the lung and peripheral blood of AIDS patients. *J Med Virol* 39:196–199, 1993.
13. Clarke JR, Gates AJ, Coker RJ, et al: HIV-1 proviral DNA copy number in peripheral blood leukocytes and bronchoalveolar lavage cells of AIDS patients. *Clin Exp Immunol* 96:182–186, 1994.
14. Cocchi F, DeVico AL, Garzino-Demo A, et al: Identification of RANTES, MIP-1α, and MIP-1β as the major HIV-suppressive factors produced by CD8[+] T cells. *Science* 270:1811–1815, 1995.

15. Cohen J: Protease inhibitors: A tale of two companies. *Science* 272:1882–1883, 1996.

16. Dean NC, Golden JA, Evans LA, et al: Human immunodeficiency virus recovery from bronchoalveolar lavage fluid in patients with AIDS. *Chest* 93:1176–1179, 1988.

17. Denis M, Ghadirian E: Interaction between *Mycobacterium avium* and human immunodeficiency virus type 1 (HIV-1) in bronchoalveolar macrophages of normal and HIV-1 infected subjects. *Am J Respir Cell Mol Biol* 11:487–495, 1994.

18. Diaz PT, Clanton TL, Pacht ER: Emphysema-like pulmonary disease associated with human immunodeficiency virus infection. *Ann Intern Med* 116:124–128, 1992.

19. Fauci AS: Immunopathogenesis of HIV infection. *J Acquir Immune Defic Syndr* 6:655–662, 1993.

20. Feng Y, Broder CC, Kennedy PE, Berger EA: HIV-1 entry cofactor: Functional cDNA cloning of a seven-transmembrane, G protein–coupled receptor. *Science* 272:872–877, 1996.

21. Gallo RC, Salahuddin SZ, Poovic M, et al: Frequent detection and isolation of cytopathic retroviruses (HTLV-III) from patients with AIDS and at risk for AIDS. *Science* 224:500–503, 1984.

22. Greene WC: The molecular biology of human immunodeficiency virus type 1 infection. *New Engl J Med* 324:308–317, 1991.

23. Guillon J-M, Autran B, Denis M, et al: Human immunodeficiency virus–related lymphocytic alveolitis. *Chest* 94:1264–1270, 1988.

24. Harbison MA, Gillis JM, Pinkston P, et al: Effects of recombinant soluble CD4 (rCD4) on HIV-1 infection of monocyte/macrophages. *J Infect Dis* 161:1–6, 1990.

25. Ho DD, Neumann AU, Perelson AS, et al: Rapid turnover of plasma virions and CD4 lymphocytes in HIV-1 infection. *Nature* 373:123–126, 1995.

26. Hoffenbach A, Langlade-Demoyen P, Dadaglio G, et al: Unusually high frequencies of HIV-specific cytotoxic lymphocytes in humans. *J Immunol* 142:452–462, 1984.

27. Israel-Biet D, Cadranel J, Beldjord K, et al: Tumor necrosis factor production in HIV seropositive subjects. Relationship with lung opportunistic infections and HIV expression in alveolar macrophages. *J Immunol* 147:490–494, 1991.

28. Itescu S, Simonelli PF, Winchester RJ, Ginsberg HS: Human immunodeficiency virus type 1 strains in the lungs of infected individuals evolve independently from those in peripheral blood and are highly conserved in the C-terminal region of the envelope V3 loop. *Proc Natl Acad Sci USA* 91:11378–11382, 1994.

29. Iwamoto GK, Konicek SA, Twigg iHL III: Modulation of accessory cell function and interleukin-6 production by the HIV-1 tat gene. *Am J Respir Cell Mol Biol* 10:580–585, 1994.

30. Lebargy F, Branellec A, Deforges L, et al: HIV-1 in human alveolar macrophages from infected patients is latent in vivo but replicates after in vitro stimulation. *Am J Respir Cell Mol Biol* 10:72–78, 1994.

31. Lederman MM, Georges DL, Kusner DJ, et al: Mycobacterium tuberculosis and its purified protein derivative activate expression of the human immunodeficiency virus. *J Acquir Immune Defic Syndr* 7:727–733, 1994.

32. Levy JA, Hoffman AD, Kramer SM, et al: Isolation of lymphocytopathic retroviruses from San Francisco patients with AIDS. *Science* 225:840–842, 1984.

33. Levy JA: Pathogenesis of human immunodeficiency virus infection. *Microbiol Rev* 57:183–289, 1993.

34. Meignan M, Guillon J-M, Denis M, et al: Increased lung epithelial permeability in HIV-infected patients with isolated cytotoxic T-lymphocytic alveolitis. *Am Rev Respir Dis* 141:1241–1248, 1990.

35. Meltzer MS, Skillman DR, Gomatos PJ, et al: Role of mononuclear phagocytes in the pathogenesis of human immunodeficiency virus infection. *Annu Rev Immunol* 8:169–194, 1990.

36. Murray HW, Gellene RA, Libby DM, et al: Activation of tissue macrophages from AIDS patients: In vitro response of AIDS alveolar macrophages to lymphokines and interferon. *J Immunol* 135:2374–2377, 1985.

37. Musher DM, Watson DA, Nickeson D, et al: The effect of HIV infection on phagocytosis and killing of *Staphylococcus aureus* by human pulmonary alveolar macrophages. *Am J Med Sci* 299:158–163, 1990.

38. Nakata K, Weiden M, Ho D, et al: High genetic variability of HIV-1 in BAL from tuberculous lung. *Am J Respir Crit Care Med* 153:A808, 1996.

39. Pantaleo G, Graziosi C, Demarest JF, et al: HIV infection is active and progressive in lymphoid tissue during the clinically latent stage of disease. *Nature* 362:355–358, 1993.

40. Pantaleo G, Graziosi C, Fauci AS: The immunopathogenesis of human immunodeficiency virus infection. *New Engl J Med* 328:327–335, 1993.

41. Pantaleo G, Menzo S, Vaccarezza M, et al: Studies in subjects with long-term nonprogressive human immunodeficiency virus infection. *New Engl J Med* 332:209–216, 1995.

42. Plata F, Autran B, Martins LP, et al: AIDS virus–specific cytotoxic T lymphocytes in lung disorders. *Nature* 328:348–351, 1987.

43. Plata F, Garcia-Pons F, Ryter A, et al: HIV-1 infection of lung alveolar fibroblasts and macrophages in humans. *AIDS Res Hum Retroviruses* 6:979–985, 1990.

44. Poli G, Pantaleo G, Fauci AS: Immunopathogenesis of human immunodeficiency virus infection. *Clin Infect Dis* 17(Suppl 1):S224–S229, 1993.

45. Potash MJ, Ziera M, Huang Z-B, et al: Virus–cell membrane fusion does not predict efficient infection of alveolar macrophages by human immunodeficiency virus type 1 (HIV-1). *Virology* 188:864–868, 1992.

46. Rich EA, Chen ISY, Zack JA, et al: Increased susceptibility of differentiated mononuclear phagocytes to productive infection with human immunodeficiency virus–1 (HIV-1). *J Clin Invest* 89:176–183, 1992.

47. Salahuddin SZ, Rose RM, Groopman JE, et al: Human T lymphotropic virus type III infection of human alveolar macrophages. *Blood* 68:281–284, 1986.

48. Schnittman SM, Psallidopoulos MC, Lane HC, et al: The reservoir for HIV-1 in human peripheral blood is a T cell that maintains expression of CD4. *Science* 41:305–308, 1989.

49. Schuitemaker H, Koot M, Koostra NA, et al: Biological phenotype of human immunodeficiency virus type 1 clones at different stages of infection: Progression of disease is associated with a shift from monocytotropic to T-cell–tropic virus population. *J Virol* 66:1354–1360, 1992.

50. Semenzato G, Agostini C, Ometto L, et al: CD8+ T lymphocytes in the lung of acquired immunodeficiency syndrome patients harbor human immunodeficiency virus type 1. *Blood* 85:2308–2314, 1995.

51. Sierra-Madero J, Toossi Z, Hom DL, et al: Relationship between load of virus in alveolar macrophages of human immunodeficiency virus–infected persons, production of cytokines and clinical status. *J Infect Dis* 169:18–27, 1994.

52. Toossi Z, Sierra-Madero JG, Blinkhorn RA, et al: Enhanced susceptibility of blood monocytes from patients with pulmonary tuberculosis to productive infection with human immunodeficiency virus type 1. *J Exp Med* 177:1511–1516, 1993.

53. Twigg HL III, Lipscomb MF, Yoffe B, et al: Enhanced accessory cell function by alveolar macrophages from patients infected with human immunodeficiency virus: Potential role for depletion of CD4$^+$ cells in the lung. *Am J Respir Cell Mol Biol* 1:391–400, 1989.

54. Wei X, Ghosh SK, Taylor ME, et al: Viral dynamics in human immunodeficiency virus type 1 infection. *Nature* 373:117–122, 1995.

55. Whalen C, Horsburgh CR, Hom D, et al: Accelerated course of human immunodeficiency virus infection after tuberculosis. *Am J Respir Crit Care Med* 151:129–135, 1995.

56. White DA, Matthay RA: Noninfectious pulmonary complications of infection with the human immunodeficiency virus. *Am Rev Respir Dis* 140:1763–1787, 1989.

57. World Health Organization: The current global situation of the HIV/AIDS pandemic. Geneva, Switzerland, World Health Organization, 1995.

58. Young KR, Rankin JA, Naegel GP, et al: Bronchoalveolar lavage cells and proteins in patients with the acquired immunodeficiency syndrome. *Ann Intern Med* 103:522–533, 1985.

EMERGING INFECTIOUS DISEASES AND HANTAVIRUS PULMONARY SYNDROME

Jay C. Butler / Sherif R. Zaki

An emerging infectious disease may be defined as a disease of infectious origin that appears to have increased in incidence or threatens to increase in the near future.[25] Many factors may contribute to the emergence or reemergence of infectious diseases. New diseases may result from the evolution of microbial pathogens, and previously recognized agents may change with respect to pathogenicity or drug susceptibility. Known diseases may spread to new geographic areas or occur in persons living in previously unpopulated areas. Because most parts of the world may now be reached within 24 h by jet, diseases previously thought to be "exotic" tropical infections may be seen in recent travelers anywhere in the world. New diseases may appear as the result of changes in our indoor and outdoor surroundings that increase exposure to insects, animals, or environmental sources harboring new or unusual infectious agents. Uncommon opportunistic infections may be recognized more frequently because of the growing number of people immunosuppressed by medication and underlying illnesses. Existing diseases that have gone undetected may be recognized because of the occurrence of clusters of cases or the use of new diagnostic methods.

A number of emerging infectious agents involve the respiratory tract (Table 153-1). These microbes present new challenges in the diagnostic evaluation and therapeutic management of patients with evidence of pulmonary infection. Previously unknown respiratory pathogens have become commonplace in a relatively short time. For example, *Legionella pneumophila* and *Chlamydia pneumonia*, two bacterial agents that were unheard

of before 1976, are now known to cause 8 to 17 percent of sporadic (non–outbreak-related) community-acquired pneumonias.[32] However, most cases of respiratory infection occur without an etiologic agent being identified. Even in prospective studies with extensive diagnostic testing of patients hospitalized with community-acquired pneumonia, a cause is identified for only about 50 percent of cases.[32] Mortality records indicate that death due to pneumonia of "unspecified etiology" has increased since 1979 and that this designation has superseded *Pneumocystis carinii* pneumonia (see Chapter 150) as the leading cause of death among persons infected with HIV.[9,41] Some of these pneumonias of undetermined origin may represent disease caused by currently unrecognized pathogens.

Emergence of new microbial strains of previously recognized agents can complicate treatment of common infections. Until recently, *Streptococcus pneumoniae,* the leading cause of community-acquired pneumonia, was exquisitely susceptible to penicillin. However, the prevalence of pneumococcal strains with altered penicillin-binding proteins that impart resistance to β-lactam antibiotics has increased substantially in recent years.[3] Penicillin-resistant pneumococci are often resistant to other antimicrobial agents as well and have raised concerns of an approaching "postantibiotic era."[17]

Hantavirus pulmonary syndrome (HPS) is a newly recognized acute infectious disease with prominent respiratory symptoms and may be viewed as a prototypical emerging infectious disease.[18] This chapter provides a clinical overview of HPS and highlights the critical role of clinicians, pathologists, epidemiologists, and basic scientists in the discovery and elucidation of emerging infectious diseases. Other specific respiratory diseases associated with emerging infectious agents are addressed elsewhere in this volume, including Legionnaires' disease (Chapter 144) and *Bartonella* species (Chapter 157).

HISTORY OF HPS

In May 1993, several cases of acute febrile illness with respiratory failure, shock, and high mortality were identified by physicians in the southwestern United States. Initial microbiologic testing and autopsy findings did not identify the cause of the ill-

TABLE 153-1

Examples of Emerging Respiratory Infections

Disease	Etiologic Agent	Factors Possibly Contributing to Emergence	Recent Trends/Outbreaks
Chlamydial pneumonia, pharyngitis	*Chlamydia pneumoniae*	Increased recognition	Increasingly recognized among patients with community-acquired pneumonia; occasional outbreaks, particularly among college students and otherwise healthy adults[21]
Coccidioidomycosis	*Coccidioides immitis*	Increased population in areas of endemicity, environmental conditions	1990s—Increasing number of cases in southern San Joaqin Valley, Calif.[38] 1994–Large community-wide outbreak after earthquake in Ventura County, Calif.[8]
Diphtheria	*Corynebacterium diphtheriae*	Underutilization of diphtheria toxoid vaccine, crowding and migration due to political instability, inadequate public health infrastructure	1989–94—More than 50-fold increase in cases reported in the new independent states of the former Soviet Union[11]
Drug-resistant pneumococcal pneumonia, sepsis	Drug-resistant strains of *Streptococcus pneumoniae*	Selective pressure of antibiotics, transcontinental spread of resistant strains	1990s—Dramatic increase in drug-resistant strains in the U.S.[3]
Hantavirus pulmonary syndrome	Sin Nombre virus, related Hantaviruses	Increased recognition after epidemic, climatic and ecologic factors	1993—Outbreak in southwestern U.S concurrent with increased deer mouse population after period of unusually cool and wet weather
Hemorrhagic pneumonitis associated with leptospirosis	*Leptospira interrogans*	Climatic and ecologic factors	1995—Outbreak in Nicaragua after unusually heavy rains[7]
Influenza	Influenza A, influenza B viruses	Antigenic drift, genetic reassortment among virus subtypes	20th century—Regional epidemics every few years, three global pandemics (1918, 1957, 1968)[47]
Legionnaires' disease	*Legionella* species	Proliferation of organism in manmade water systems, increased recognition	1990s—Outbreaks associated with exposure to infectious aerosol produced by cooling towers, plumbing systems, whirlpool spas[6,26]
Pneumocystosis	*Pneumocystis carinii*	Increased population of immunocompromised persons	1980s—Sudden increased prevalence associated with AIDS epidemic 1990s—Declining mortality among patients coinfected with HIV, possibly reflecting increased use of chemoprophylaxis[41]
Tuberculosis	*Mycobacterium tuberculosis*	Immigration from areas with high endemicity, increased population of immunocompromised persons, increased transmission in institutional settings, deteriorating public health infrastructure	1980s and '90s—Increasing number of cases in U.S. after decades of declining incidence, emergence of multiple-drug–resistant strains[5]

ness. Affected persons lived in rural areas, but there was no obvious epidemiologic connection between patients. Patient specimens were tested for a wide variety of agents at the Centers for Disease Control and Prevention (CDC).[30] Immunoglobulin (Ig) M and G antibodies against several hantaviruses were detected in the sera of patients by enzyme immunoassay (EIA), suggesting that illness was due to a previously unrecognized but serologically cross-reactive hantavirus. Additionally, antigen was detected in the endothelium of various organs of affected patients by immunohistochemical testing using a monoclonal antibody reactive with conserved hantavirus nucleoprotein epitopes.[48] Hantavirus nucleotide sequences were detected in patient tissue specimens by reverse transcriptase–polymerase chain reaction (RT-PCR).[37] The hantavirus associated with the 1993 outbreak, Sin Nombre virus (SNV; previously called Four Corners virus and Muerto Canyon virus), was determined to be unique by nucleotide sequence analysis of amplified viral genetic material.[37]

Before the 1993 HPS outbreak, all hantaviruses known to cause human disease (Hantaan, Seoul, Puumala, and Dobrava) were associated with hemorrhagic fever with renal syndrome (HFRS), an illness with variable degrees of fever, hemorrhagic manifestations, and acute renal failure, or nephropathia epidemica (NE), a usually benign form of HFRS. HFRS and NE are endemic in Eurasia, but outbreaks of human disease associated with hantavirus infection had not been identified in the Americas. Although primary pulmonary edema can occur and subtle pulmonary radiographic abnormalities may be observed, respiratory symptoms are generally not prominent in HFRS and NE.

As often occurs when a new infectious agent is recognized, the increased frequency of submission and testing of clinical specimens led to recognition of related but previously unknown agents. At least three additional hantaviruses associated with HPS in North America were recognized after the 1993 outbreak. In June 1993, a 58-year-old man in Louisiana died of an acute febrile respiratory illness and shock.[28] Because of the similarity between this patient's illness and that of persons infected with SNV in the ongoing HPS outbreak in the Southwest, tissues collected at autopsy were tested for hantavirus. Hantaviral nucleotide sequences and antigen were identified in the tissue by RT-PCR and immunohistochemical staining. Analysis of the genetic sequences showed the virus to be a novel hantavirus, provisionally named Bayou virus.[35] Other unique hantaviruses causing HPS have been identified in south Florida (Black Creek Canal virus) and in the northeastern United States (New York virus).[22,24,39]

EPIDEMIOLOGY AND TRANSMISSION

In the first 30 months after HPS was recognized, more than 125 cases occurring in at least 24 states were identified. Of cases reported to the CDC, more than 50 percent were fatal; persons with HPS who died and those who survived were similar in age, sex, and race/ethnicity.[4,34] Cases were evenly distributed by sex. Most cases occurred in adults aged 20 to 49 years, and few cases were identified among children or the elderly.[1,4,13,29,34] The reason for the rarity of disease among young children and the elderly is not known, but it may reflect the role of the immune response in the pathophysiology of HPS. Most patients lived in rural areas.[4] Al

though cases have been reported during all months of the year, the peak incidence during the first 2 years of surveillance occurred during the late spring and early summer.[34] As with many other emerging infectious diseases, cases of SNV infection in humans predating the initial 1993 outbreak were recognized after identification of the etiologic agents of HPS. SNV infection has been confirmed by immunohistochemical staining in patients who died of illness compatible with HPS as early as 1978.[49] Serologic evidence of past SNV infection has been identified in a Utah resident who survived an HPS-compatible illness that occurred 1959.[19]

Like other hantaviruses, those causing HPS appear to be maintained in nature by chronic, asymptomatic infection of a specific rodent species. Transmission to humans generally occurs after inhalation of aerosolized rodent excreta or contaminated particulates or, rarely, from the bite of an infected rodent.[45] A survey of rodents for evidence of infection with hantaviruses was conducted as part of the investigation of the 1993 HPS outbreak in the Southwest. The deer mouse (*Peromyscus maniculatus*) was identified as the primary reservoir of SNV.[15] The likely primary rodent reservoirs for other HPS-associated viruses are the rice rat (*Oryzomys palustris*) for Bayou virus,[44] the cotton rat (*Sigmodon hispidus*) for Black Creek Canal virus,[39] and the white-footed deer mouse (*P. leukopus*) for New York virus.[24] The collective ranges of *P. maniculatus, S. hispidus, O. palustris,* and *P. leukopus* cover most of North America, indicating that the potential for HPS transmission exists in any region of the continent. The incubation period for HPS is not known but is presumed to be similar to that of HFRS—4 to 42 days (average, 12 to 16 days).[50]

In a case control study conducted during the 1993 HPS outbreak, activities associated with contracting HPS included cleaning areas of the home used for food storage, cleaning barns and other outbuildings, plowing with hand tools, and animal herding.[50] Each of these activities may result in exposure to aerosolized rodent excreta or airborne contaminated particulates. A greater median number of small rodents were trapped at patients' households than at control households, suggesting that greater domestic rodent infestation increases the risk of transmission. Trapping of rodents in or around the home was also associated with HPS, but not after controlling for the number of rodents captured by investigators at the household—suggesting that trapping was an indication of household rodent infestation rather than an activity directly associated with transmission. No specific household characteristics were associated with transmission of SNV.[14] Self-reported occupation of herder was associated with HPS, although specific herding activities were not.[50] Many of the herders participating in the case-control study were American Indians who expand their herding range during the spring and reoccupy small structures, such as hogans, at "sheep camps" that had been closed during the winter. Anecdotal case reports also suggest that cleaning or inhabiting vacant rodent-infested structures, such as vacation cabins, may constitute a special risk for contracting HPS.[2] Exposure to rodents, generally within the home, has been found in roughly half of reported cases.[4,48]

There is no evidence for person-to-person transmission of HPS. In a survey of 266 health-care workers, clinical laboratory person nel, autopsy technicians, and pathologists caring for HPS patients or processing their body fluids or tissues during the 1993 outbreak, Vitek and colleagues found no evidence of nosocomial transmission of HPS.[46] The occurrence of more than one case of HPS among persons in a household was unusual.[50] When more than one case occurred within a household, illnesses generally developed within days of one another, suggesting exposure to a common source in the environment rather than transmission between family members. Among pregnant women who have survived HPS, transmission of SNV to their newborns has not been detected.[20]

MICROBIOLOGY AND PATHOGENESIS

The etiologic agents of HPS are single-stranded, negative-sense RNA viruses of the family *Bunyaviridae*.[16,22,28,35,39] Virus particles are 70 to 120 nm in diameter. A lipid envelope with glycoprotein spikes surrounds a core consisting of the trisegmented genome and its associated nucleocapsids (Fig. 153-1). Factors contributing to the sudden "emergence" of SNV during the 1993 outbreak are poorly understood. SNV appears to have been present in rodent populations in North America and to have been causing unrecognized HPS for at least a decade before the outbreak.[36,49] The three segments of the SNV genome appear to have evolved in parallel, and there is no evidence indicating RNA segment reassortment with other well-characterized hantaviruses as an explanation for the sudden appearance of a highly pathogenic strain of hantavirus.[16] Climatic factors leading to a sudden increase of the deer mouse population in the Southwest may have played a role in facilitating increased transmission of SNV during the spring and summer of 1993.[13]

Postmortem examination of tissue from HPS victims has routinely revealed serous pleural effusions and heavy edematous lungs. Histopathologic changes characteristic of HPS are mainly seen in the lung and spleen, but the degree of involvement varies among patients.[4,48] In most cases, microscopic examination of the lung reveals mild to moderate interstitial pneumonitis with variable amounts of mononuclear infiltrates in alveolar septa, congestion, septal and alveolar edema, and focal hyaline membranes (Fig. 153-2). In typical cases, neutrophilic infiltrates are scanty and the respiratory epithelium is intact, with no evidence of cellular debris, nuclear fragmentation, or type II pneumocyte hyperplasia. As the disease progresses, proliferation of reparative-type pneumocytes, edematous and fibroblastic thickening of the alveolar septa with airspace disorganization and distortion of the lung architecture, suggestive of diffuse alveolar damage, may be seen, particularly among patients who survive for more than a few days in hospital before death.[48] Large mononuclear cells with the appearance of immunoblasts are

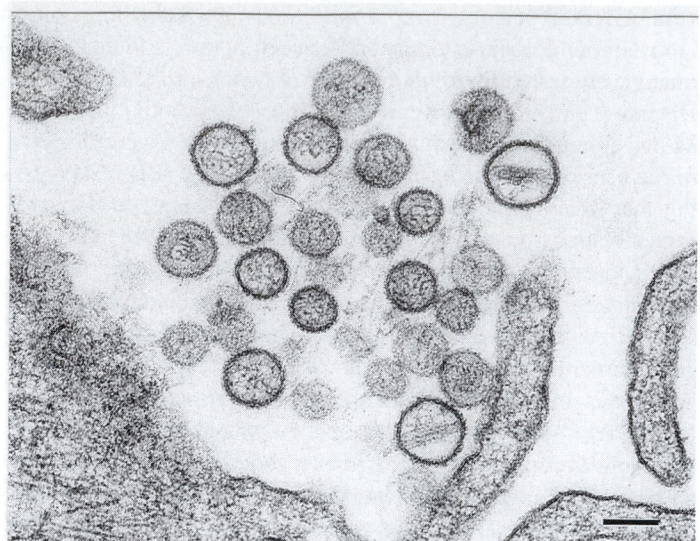

FIGURE 153-1 Electron micrograph of Vero-E6 tissue culture cells showing extracellular Sin Nombre virus particles. The envelope, which contains small surface spikes, surrounds a core containing nucleocapsids arranged in filaments. Scale bar = 100 nm.

found in the lungs, red and periarteriolar white pulp of the spleen, and hepatic portal triads.[18,48]

The site of initial infection and of subsequent viral replication is currently unknown; however, immunohistochemical analysis of tissues with specific antibodies that cross-react with conserved Hantavirus nucleoprotein epitopes indicates that the virus is present in the capillary endothelium of numerous organs.[48] The pathophysiological role of endothelial involvement in the increased vascular permeability, which is the hallmark of this syndrome, remains to be elucidated. Although endothelial cell infection is typical of the hantaviruses, SNV appears to have

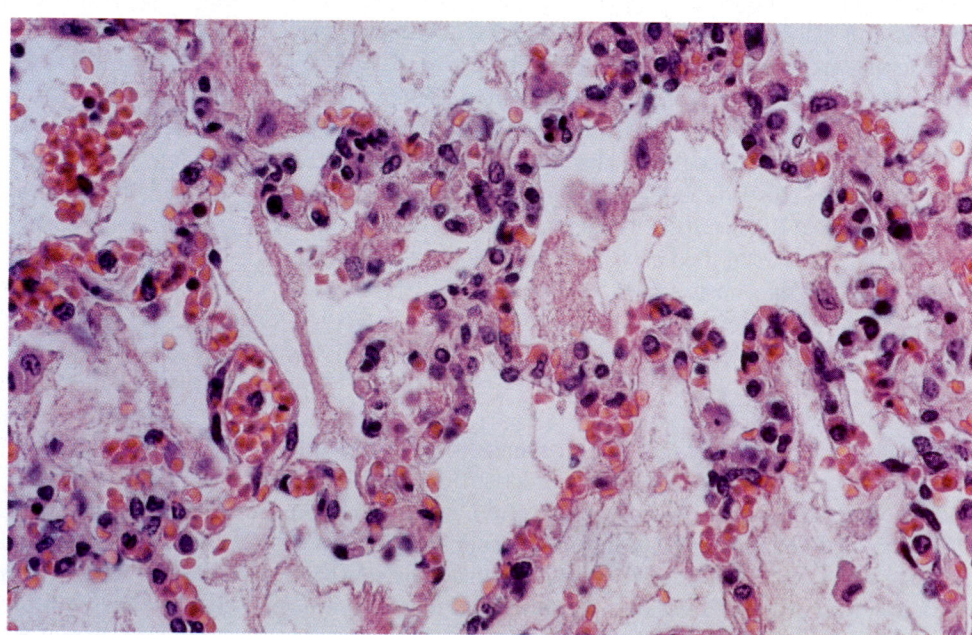

FIGURE 153-2 Photomicrograph showing interstitial pneumonitis and intra-alveolar edema in lung of patient with Hantavirus pulmonary syndrome. The inflammatory infiltrate is predominantly mononuclear. H&E stain, original magnification ×100.

a unique trophism for the pulmonary vasculature, possibly explaining the pronounced respiratory manifestations of HPS. Immunohistologic studies of tissues collected at autopsy of patients who died of HPS provide evidence for extremely high levels of viral antigens in the pulmonary microvasculature and compartmentalization of a selective immune response in the lung (Fig. 153-3). The mononuclear cells within the lung appear to be a mixture of macrophages and CD8 lymphocytes, suggesting that inflammatory cell recruitment in the lungs of HPS patients may occur as a result of specific attraction and adherence of a selective population of inflammatory cells to a specialized activated endothelium.[48]

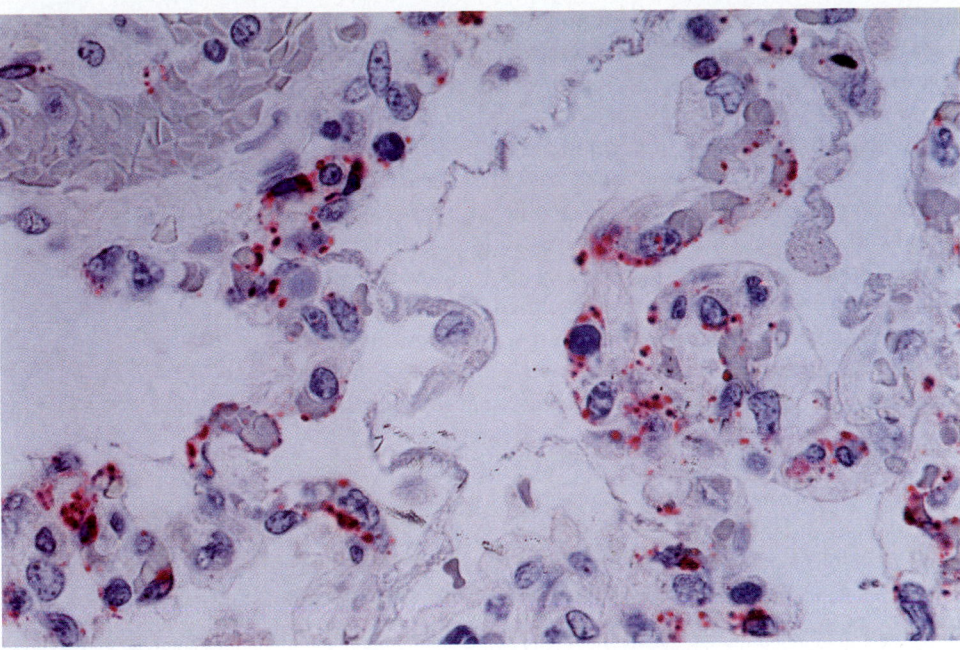

FIGURE 153-3 Prominent endothelial immunostaining of Sin Nombre virus (SNV) antigens in pulmonary microvasculature. Rabbit anti-SNV serum. Original magnification ×158.

CLINICAL MANIFESTATIONS

The course of HPS generally progresses through three distinct clinical phases: prodromal, cardiopulmonary, and convalescent (Table 153-2). Fever is an almost universal feature during the prodrome, and myalgias are also common.[18,48] Early in the course of illness, respiratory symptoms are frequently absent. Distinguishing prodromal-phase HPS from other febrile illnesses, such as influenza or aseptic meningitis, may be difficult; however, sore throat, coryza, and meningismus are unusual in HPS.[18]

Progression to the cardiopulmonary phase is heralded by shock and respiratory distress. Clinical and radiographic dete-

TABLE 153-2

Clinical and Laboratory Characteristics of HPS Associated with Sin Nombre Virus Infection

Phase	Average Duration	Predominant Signs and Symptoms	Common Laboratory Findings	Chest Radiograph
Prodrome	3–6 days	Fever, myalgia, malaise, headache, dizziness, nausea, vomiting, abdominal pain	WBC normal, slight left shift occasionally seen Platelet count normal, declining count may be seen with repeated testing	Generally normal
Cardiopulmonary	5–10 days	Same as prodrome, plus tachypnea, tachycardia, hypotension	Hypoxemia Leukocytosis, frequently with left shift and slight atypical lymphocytosis Thrombocytopenia Hemoconcentration Metabolic acidosis Prolonged PTT Elevated LDH and AST Mild to moderate proteinuria	May be normal initially Rapidly developing interstitial edema, progressing to alveolar infiltrates Normal cardiac silhouette Pleural effusions common
Convalescent	1–2 weeks	Resolution of shock and respiratory distress, diuresis common	Improving oxygenation, often rapid Normalization of laboratory abnormalities Mild anemia occasionally noted	Clearing

NOTE: WBC = peripheral white blood cell count; PTT = partial thromboplastin time; LDH = lactate dehydrogenase; AST = aspartate aminotransferase.

rioration may ensue over a period of hours (Fig. 153-4). Tachypnea may precede the auscultatory finding of rales and abnormalities of the chest radiograph. Leukocytosis may be marked (more than 25,000 cells per cubic millimeter). Fibrinogen levels are generally normal, although disseminated intravascular coagulation has been reported occasionally in HPS.[42] Frank renal failure is not a feature in most cases associated with SNV, and mild creatinine elevations (usually greater than 2.5 mg/dl) occur only in severe cases.[48] Conversely, in the reported cases of HPS associated with Black Creek Canal or Bayou virus, acute renal insufficiency was a prominent characteristic, suggesting that there may be a group of genetically related hantaviruses causing illness somewhat intermediate between HPS and HFRS.[28]

Radiographic abnormalities during the cardiopulmonary phase include prominent interstitial edema, manifested by Kerley's B lines, hilar indistinctness, or peribronchial cuffing, with rapid development of airspace disease in the majority of cases (Fig. 153-4).[27] Certain radiographic findings in patients with HPS, including the early prominence of interstitial edema and the lack of a peripheral distribution of initial airspace disease, are uncommon among patients with adult respiratory distress syndrome (ARDS) and may be useful in distinguishing patients with HPS.[27] Lobar infiltrates, commonly seen in patients with pneumococcal sepsis and pneumonia, have not been observed among patients with HPS.[33]

Patients with HPS often require intubation and mechanical ventilation for progressive hypoxemia during the cardiopulmonary phase. Pa_{O_2}/Fi_{O_2} values become quite low during the cardiopulmonary phase, with nadir values generally less than 100.[31] In some cases, large volumes of clear, proteinaceous fluid are obtained by endotracheal tube suctioning. Bronchoalveolar lavage (BAL) specimens from patients with HPS

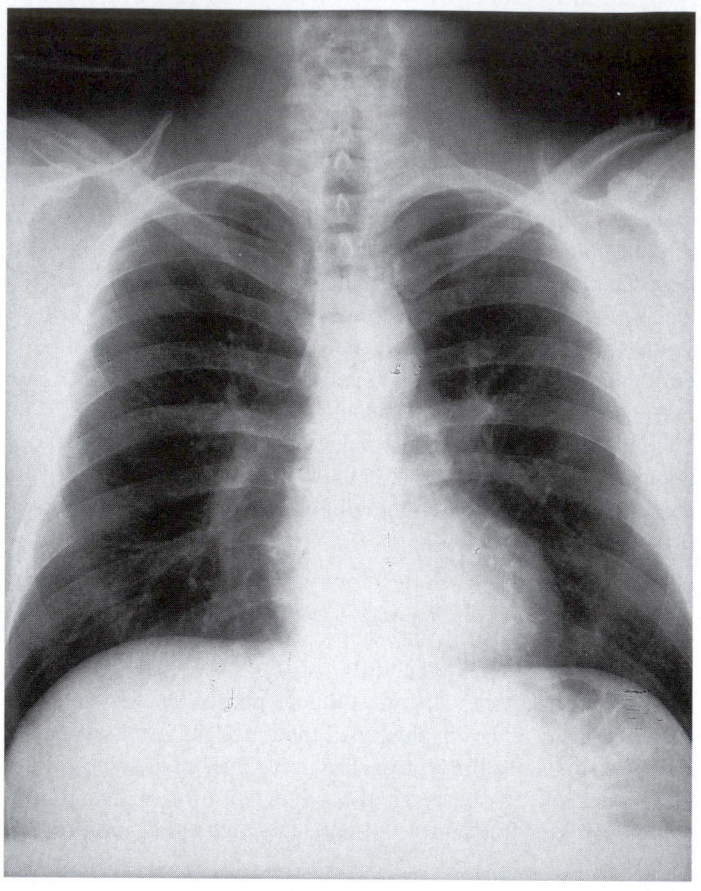

A

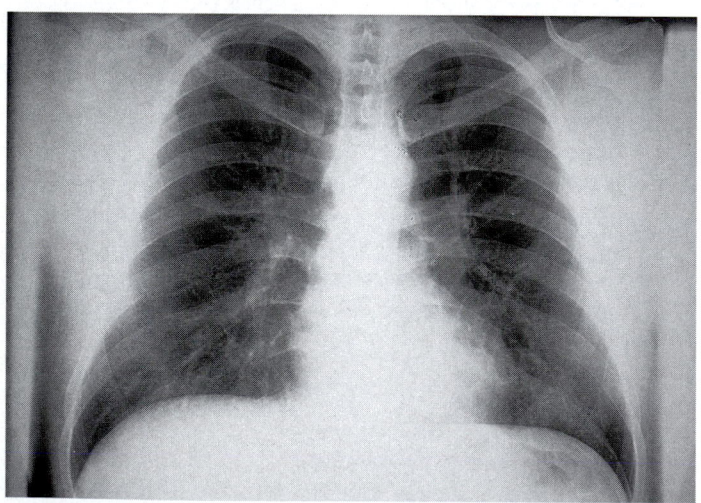

B

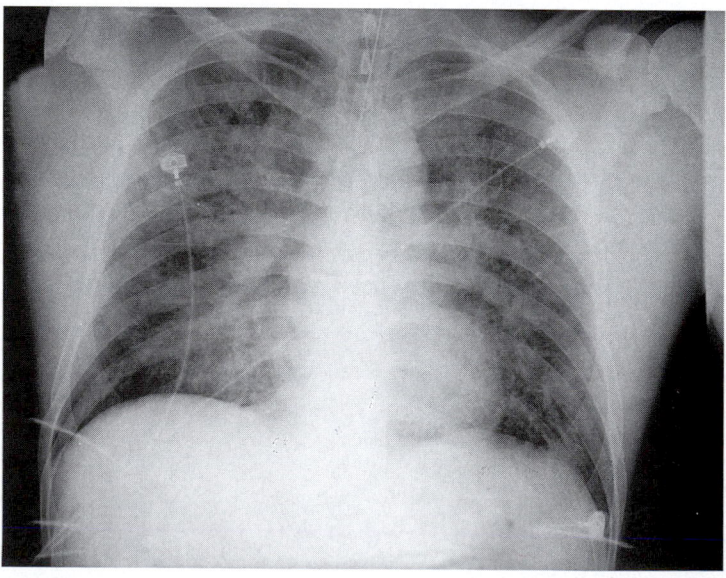

C

FIGURE 153-4   Chest radiographs of a 33-year-old man with Hantavirus pulmonary syndrome. At initial presentation, he reported having experienced several days of progressive headache and myalgia. Temperature was 38.8°C; vital signs were otherwise unremarkable. Transcutaneous capillary oxygen saturation was 94 percent, and the chest radiograph showed no abnormalities *(A)*. On the following morning, he denied having cough or dyspnea. Systolic blood pressure was <90 mm Hg, and the chest radiograph demonstrated subtle perihilar and bibasilar interstitial infiltrates *(B)*. Over the next several hours, respiratory distress developed, necessitating intubation and mechanical ventilation for progressive hypoxemia. A chest radiograph taken late that afternoon showed progression of interstitial infiltrates with hilar indistinctness and prominent peribronchial cuffing *(C)*. The patient died approximately 24 h later.

generally contain few cells but have high protein concentrations.[23] In patients who have had Swan-Ganz catheters inserted, normal or elevated systemic vascular resistance and depressed cardiac output were observed, in contrast to the typical findings in bacterial sepsis (see Chapter 133).[18,31] Initial pulmonary artery wedge pressures were low. Pronounced left ventricular dysfunction demonstrated by transthoracic echocardiography was noted in some cases.[31] Depressed myocardial function and intractable hypotension terminating with cardiac dysrhythmia are the most common cause of death in patients with HPS. Death generally occurs within 1 week after onset of symptoms.[18] Progressive hypotension in spite of adequate arterial oxygenation is common, suggesting that hypotension was not solely the result of hypoxemia.

Progression to the convalescent phase can be remarkably rapid. Apparently moribund patients requiring maximal ventilatory and inotropic support may progress to extubation and withdrawal of vasoactive agents over a period of a few days. Although no data on the long-term sequelae of HPS are currently available, recovery has been apparently complete in patients surviving the cardiopulmonary phase. Serologic testing of persons with minimal or no symptoms suggestive of HPS indicates that clinically mild or asymptomatic infection rarely occurs.[1,43,50]

The diagnosis of HPS should be entertained for any previously healthy person presenting with a febrile prodrome followed by the development of pulmonary compromise and shock. The diagnosis of prodromal HPS solely on the basis of clinical findings is extremely difficult because of the nonspecificity of symptoms. By onset of the cardiopulmonary phase, however, a complete medical evaluation often presents such a characteristic composite of illness history, clinical laboratory findings, and chest radiograph that the diagnosis can be suspected. Data from a study comparing clinical features of patients with HPS and those of patients with other febrile respiratory illnesses during the 1993 outbreak have been used to develop a flow chart to assist in identifying patients with possible HPS (Fig. 153-5).[33] Nevertheless, until evaluation of competing diagnoses is complete, patients should not be assumed to have HPS but, rather, should be treated for reasonable alternative diagnoses.

Laboratory diagnosis of HPS is made by serologic tests detecting hantavirus IgM antibodies in serum or a fourfold or greater rise in hantavirus IgG antibodies, detection of hantavirus antigen in tissue by immunohistochemistry, and amplification of hantaviral nucleotide sequences by RT-PCR. Results of these three diagnostic methods are almost always concordant when adequate material is available for testing.[30,48] Serologic tests for SNV are generally diagnostic at the time of hospital admission and are available at several sites, including many state public health laboratories. Because SNV RNA is present within circulating mononuclear white blood cells of patients with HPS, RT-PCR testing of blood specimens may be a useful diagnostic tool.[23] Only one of three BAL fluid cell pellets from patients with HPS tested by RT-PCR were positive, probably reflecting the low cellularity of the BAL fluid and the endothelial localization of the virus.[23] Isolation of hantaviruses in cell culture has been very difficult and is not practical for diagnosis.

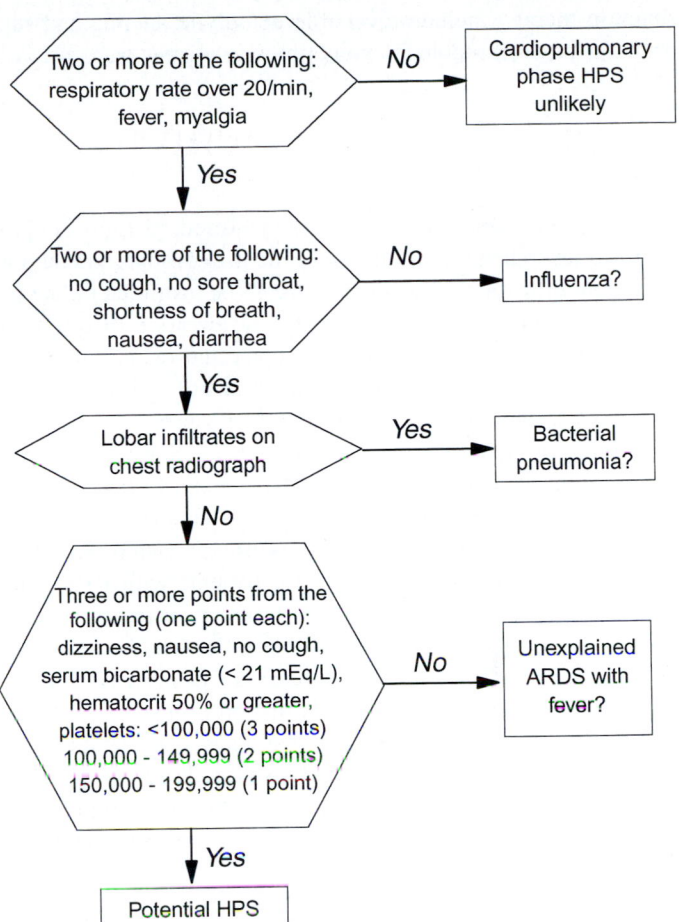

FIGURE 153-5 Flow chart to assist in differentiating patients with HPS from those with influenza, bacteremic pneumococcal pneumonia, and unexplained ARDS with fever, based on multivariate analysis of routinely available clinical data for patients in the southwestern United States during the 1993 HPS outbreak. (*From Moolenaar et al,*[33] *with permission.*)

TREATMENT

The cornerstone of medical management of HPS is close monitoring of patients in an intensive care unit. Hypoxemia and shock should be treated with oxygen administration, intubation, and mechanical ventilation. Inotropic and vasopressor agents should be used as needed. Capillary leak appears to play a central role in pathogenesis; therefore, it seems rational that fluids should be given cautiously if HPS is suspected. Early use of inotropic agents should supplant "pushing" fluids to maintain tissue perfusion. Ribavirin, a nucleoside analog with activity against hantaviruses and previously shown to reduce mortality when administered early during the course of HFRS, was available for intravenous administration to patients with suspected HPS through a nonrandomized, open-label trial conducted for 1 year after the recognition of HPS in 1993. However, the survival rate among HPS patients receiving ribavirin in the open-label trial was similar to that of those not receiving the drug.[12] In the absence of a double-blind, controlled trial, the role of intravenous ribavirin, a drug not currently licensed for use in the United States, remains to be defined. Untoward effects of intravenous ribavirin therapy include reversible hemolytic anemia and suppression of erythropoiesis, sometimes requiring transfusion.[12]

PREVENTION OF DISEASE CAUSED BY NEWLY RECOGNIZED AGENTS

When new infectious syndromes are identified, measures to prevent further transmission through patient isolation and environmental modification or avoidance should be instituted on the basis of available scientific data, with consideration of estimated costs versus benefits. If feasible, contact and respiratory isolation is prudent for patients during outbreaks of serious, possibly infectious respiratory disease of unknown cause.

Before the identification of the hantaviral cause of HPS and the availability of data indicating that person-to-person transmission of HPS was unlikely, respiratory isolation was instituted as early as possible in the course of disease for each patient. Universal precautions are appropriate for patients with HPS; however, respiratory protection may be prudent during procedures likely to aerosolize infected body fluids or tissues. General measures to prevent HPS require avoidance of rodents and their excreta by environmental modifications that prevent entry of rodents in human habitations.[10] A vaccinia-vectored vaccine against Hantaan virus for the prevention of HFRS is under development;[40] however, the efficacy of such a vaccine for the prevention of HPS is unknown and may be limited by the incomplete serologic cross reactivity between Hantaan and SNV.[30]

SPECIAL CONSIDERATIONS FOR SUSPECTED NEW INFECTIOUS DISEASES

Clinicians play an integral role in identifying new infectious diseases. New clinical syndromes and infections associated with previously unknown pathogens are often recognized only after clusters of cases occur. For at least 15 years before the recognition of the syndrome during the 1993 outbreak, cases of HPS occurred in North America.[49] Disease caused by a new agent was probably not suspected in these earlier cases because of the clinical similarity of HPS with the presumed causes of the illnesses. This underscores the importance of vigilance and perseverance in pursuing an etiologic diagnosis in cases of severe illness of unknown origin. Special care should be taken to collect and store specimens for diagnostic testing from patients with evidence of respiratory infection for whom the diagnosis is not apparent on the basis of routinely available tests. Early identification of the hantaviral cause of HPS was based, in part, on the demonstration of changing antibody levels in paired acute- and convalescent-phase serum specimens.[30] Testing of paired specimens was facilitated by the availability of a saved acute-phase serum specimen from a patient surviving the illness. Autopsies should be performed on patients who die of possibly infectious diseases of undetermined origin, and material should be systematically collected and archived.[49] Testing of stored biologic material from patients who died of unexplained illnesses has provided the opportunity to retrospectively confirm cases of illnesses such as HPS and Legionnaires' disease occurring years before the initial recognition of these syndromes.[49]

Recognizing and reporting the initial cases of HPS in 1993 led to a multidisciplinary investigation by clinicians, field epidemiologists and biologists, laboratory researchers, and public health educators that facilitated clinical characterization of HPS, identification of the etiologic agent and the rodent reservoir, and development of prevention and treatment strategies within a period of several weeks. Suspected clusters or outbreaks of cases of infectious diseases of unknown cause should be reported to state health departments and the CDC for assistance with diagnostic testing and the formulation of strategies to prevent additional cases.

REFERENCES

1. Armstrong LR, Bryan RT, Sarisky J, et al: Mild hantaviral disease caused by Sin Nombre virus in a four-year-old child. *Pediatr Infect Dis J* 14:1108–1110, 1995.
2. Armstrong LR, Zaki SR, Goldoft MJ, et al: Hantavirus pulmonary syndrome associated with entering or cleaning rarely used, rodent-infested structures (letter). *J Infect Dis* 172:1166, 1995.
3. Breiman RF, Butler JC, Tenover FC, et al: Emergence of drug-resistant pneumococcal infections in the United States. *JAMA* 271:1831–1835, 1994.
4. Butler JC, Zaki SR, Khabbaz RF, Peters CJ: Hantavirus pulmonary syndrome. *Infect Dis Clin Pract* 4:189-193, 1995.
5. Cantwell MF, Snider DE, Cauthen GM, Onorato IM: Epidemiology of tuberculosis in the United States, 1985 through 1992. *JAMA* 272:535–539, 1994.
6. Centers for Disease Control and Prevention: Legionnaires' disease associated with cooling towers—Massachusetts, Michigan, and Rhode Island, 1993. *MMWR Morb Mortal Wkly Rep* 43:491–499, 1994.
7. Centers for Disease Control and Prevention: Outbreak of acute febrile illness and pulmonary hemorrhage—Nicaragua, 1995. *MMWR Morb Mortal Wkly Rep* 44:841–843, 1995.
8. Centers for Disease Control and Prevention: Coccidioidomycosis following the Northridge earthquake—California, 1994. *MMWR Morb Mortal Wkly Rep* 43:194–195, 1994.
9. Centers for Disease Control and Prevention: Pneumonia and influenza death rates—United States, 1979–94. *MMWR Morb Mortal Wkly Rep* 44:535–537, 1995.
10. Centers for Disease Control and Prevention: Hantavirus infection—Southwestern United States: Interim recommendations for risk reduction. *MMWR Morb Mortal Wkly Rep* 42(RR-11):1–12, 1993.
11. Centers for Disease Control and Prevention: Diphtheria epidemic—New independent states of the former Soviet Union, 1990–1994. *MMWR Morb Mortal Wkly Rep* 44:177–181, 1995.
12. Chapman LE, Mertz G, Khan AS, et al, and the Ribavirin Study Group: Open label intravenous ribavirin for hantavirus pulmonary syndrome, in *Abstracts of the 34th Interscience Conference on Antimicrobial Agents and Chemotherapy, Orlando, Florida, October 4–7, 1994.* Washington, DC, American Society for Microbiology, 1994, p 240. Abstract #H111.
13. Chapman LE, Khabbaz RF: Etiology and epidemiology of the Four Corners hantavirus outbreak. *Infect Agent Dis* 3:234–244, 1994.
14. Childs JE, Krebs JW, Ksiazek TG, et al: A household based case-control study of risk factors associated with hantavirus pulmonary syndrome in the southwestern United States. *Am J Trop Med Hyg* 52:393–397, 1995.
15. Childs JE, Ksiazek TG, Spiropoulou CF, et al: Serologic and genetic identification of *Peromyscus maniculatus* as the primary rodent reservoir for a new hantavirus in the southwestern United States. *J Infect Dis* 169:1271–1280, 1994.

16. Chizhikov VE, Spiropoulou CF, Morzunov SP, et al: Complete genetic characterization and analysis of isolation of Sin Nombre virus. *J Virol* 69:8132–8136, 1995.

17. Cohen ML: Epidemiology of drug resistance: Implications for a post-antimicrobial era. *Science* 257:1050–1055, 1992.

18. Duchin JS, Koster F, Peters CJ, et al, and Hantavirus Study Group: Hantavirus pulmonary syndrome: A clinical description of 17 patients with a newly recognized disease. *New Engl J Med* 330:949–955, 1994.

19. Frampton JW, Lanser S, Nichols CR, Ettestad PJ: Sin Nombre virus infection in 1959. *Lancet* 346:781–782, 1995.

20. Gilson GJ, Maciulla JA, Nevils BG, et al: Hantavirus pulmonary syndrome complicating pregnancy. *Am J Obstet Gynecol* 171:550–554, 1994.

21. Grayston JT, Campbell LA, Kuo C-C, et al: A new respiratory tract pathogen: *Chlamydia pneumoniae* strain TWAR. *J Infect Dis* 161:618–625, 1990.

22. Hjelle B, Krolikowski J, Torrez-Martinez N, et al: Phylogenetically distinct hantavirus implicated in a case of hantavirus pulmonary syndrome in the northeastern United States. *J Med Virol* 46:21–27, 1995.

23. Hjelle B, Spiropoulou CF, Torrez-Martinez N, et al: Detection of Muerto Canyon virus RNA in peripheral blood mononuclear cells from patients with hantavirus pulmonary syndrome. *J Infect Dis* 170:1013–1017, 1994.

24. Hjelle B, Lee S-W, Song W, et al: Molecular linkage of hantavirus pulmonary syndrome to the white-footed mouse, *Peromyscus leucopus*: genetic characterization of the M genome of New York virus. *J Virol* 69:8137–8141, 1995.

25. Institute of Medicine: *Emerging Infections: Microbial Threats to Health in the United States.* Washington, DC, National Academy Press, 1992.

26. Jernigan DB, Hofmann J, Cetron MS, et al: Outbreak of Legionnaires' disease among cruise ship passengers exposed to a contaminated whirlpool spa. *Lancet* 347:494–499, 1996.

27. Ketai LH, Williamson MR, Telepak RJ, et al: Hantavirus pulmonary syndrome (HPS): Radiographic findings in 16 patients. *Radiology* 191:665–668, 1994.

28. Khan AS, Spiropoulou CF, Morzunov S, et al: Fatal illness associated with a new hantavirus in Louisiana. *J Med Virol* 46:281–286, 1995.

29. Khan AS, Ksiazek TG, Zaki SR, et al: Fatal hantavirus pulmonary syndrome in an adolescent. *Pediatrics* 95:276–280, 1995.

30. Ksiazek TG, Peters CJ, Rollin PE, et al: Identification of a new North American hantavirus that causes acute pulmonary insufficiency. *Am J Trop Med Hyg* 52:117–123, 1995.

31. Levy H, Simpson SQ: Hantavirus pulmonary syndrome. *Am J Respir Crit Care Med* 149:1710–1713, 1994.

32. Marrie TJ: Community-acquired pneumonia. *Clin Infect Dis* 18:501–515, 1994.

33. Moolenaar RL, Dalton C, Lipman HB, et al: Clinical features that differentiate hantavirus pulmonary syndrome from three other acute respiratory illnesses. *Clin Infect Dis* 21:643–649, 1995.

34. Moolenaar RL, Breiman RF, Peters CJ: Hantavirus pulmonary syndrome: A clinical review. *Semin Respir Infect.* In press.

35. Morzunov SP, Feldmann H, Spiropoulou CF, et al: A newly recognized virus associated with a fatal case of hantavirus pulmonary syndrome in Louisiana. *J Virol* 69:1980–1983, 1995.

36. Nerurkar VR, Song J-W, Song K-J, et al: Genetic evidence for a hantavirus enzootic in deer mice (*Peromyscus maniculatus*) captured a decade before the recognition of hantavirus pulmonary syndrome. *Virology* 204:563–568, 1994.

37. Nichol ST, Spiropoulou CF, Morzunov S, et al: Genetic identification of a hantavirus associated with an outbreak of acute respiratory illness. *Science* 262:914–917, 1993.

38. Pappagianis D: Marked increase in cases of coccidioidomycosis in California: 1991, 1992, and 1993. *Clin Infect Dis* 19(Suppl 1):S14–S18, 1994.

39. Ravkov EV, Rollin PE, Ksiazek TG, et al: Genetic and serologic analysis of Black Creek Canal virus and its association with human disease and *Sigmodon hispidus* infection. *Virology* 210:482–489, 1995.

40. Schmaljohn CS, Hasty SE, Dalrymple JM: Preparation of candidate vaccinia-vectored vaccines for haemorrhagic fever with renal syndrome. *Vaccine* 10:10–13, 1992.

41. Selik RM, Chu SY, Ward JW: Trends in infectious diseases and cancers among persons dying of HIV infection in the United States from 1987 to 1992. *Ann Intern Med* 123:933–936, 1995.

42. Shefer AM, Tappero JW, Bresee JS, et al: Hantavirus pulmonary syndrome in California: Report of two cases and investigation. *Clin Infect Dis* 19:1105–1109, 1994.

43. Simonsen L, Dalton MJ, Breiman RF, et al: Evaluation of the magnitude of the 1993 hantavirus outbreak in the southwestern United States. *J Infect Dis* 172:729–733, 1995.

44. Torrez-Martinez N, Hjelle B: Enzootic of Bayou hantavirus in rice rats (*Oryzomys palustris*) in 1983 (letter). *Lancet* 346:780–781, 1995.

45. Tsai TF: Hemorrhagic fever with renal syndrome: Mode of transmission to humans. *Lab Animal Sci* 37:428–430, 1987.

46. Vitek CR, Breiman RF, Ksiazek TG, et al: Evidence against person-to-person transmission of hantavirus to health care workers. *Clin Infect Dis* 22:824–826, 1996.

47. Webster R, Bean W, Gorman O, et al: Evolution and ecology of influenza A viruses. *Microbiol Rev* 56:152–179, 1992.

48. Zaki SR, Greer PW, Coffield LM, et al: Hantavirus pulmonary syndrome: Pathogenesis of an emerging infectious disease. *Am J Pathol* 146:552–579, 1995.

49. Zaki SR, Khan AS, Goodman RA, et al: Retrospective diagnosis of hantavirus pulmonary syndrome, 1978–1993: Implications for emerging infectious diseaes. *Arch Pathol Lab Med* 120:134–139, 1996.

50. Zeitz PS, Butler JC, Cheek JE, et al: A case-control study of hantavirus pulmonary syndrome during an outbreak in the southwestern United States. *J Infect Dis* 171:864–870, 1995.

CHAPTER 154

POLIOVIRUS AND OTHER ENTEROVIRUS INFECTIONS

Joseph L. Melnick

This may be the final chapter on poliomyelitis to appear in a textbook. As of this writing, vaccination has eliminated all non–vaccine-related cases reported for the Western Hemisphere. Wild poliovirus has even been eliminated from the environment. Immunization, chiefly by oral poliovirus vaccine (OPV), is protecting more than 500,000 persons a year worldwide from paralysis, and by the beginning of the next century, poliomyelitis may be gone. The postpolio syndrome persists. Furthermore, as long as any poliovirus exists anywhere on the globe, the risk of epidemic polio remains. Other enteroviruses, and viruses of different families, also affect the respiratory tract and cause asymptomatic or minor discomfort, or life-threatening disease.

Sporadic cases of paralytic poliomyelitis have occurred for at least as long as human history has been recorded. From ancient times until the late 1800s, polioviruses were widely distributed in most of the world's populations, surviving in an endemic fashion by continuously infecting susceptible infants newly born into the community.[29] Because most poliovirus infections were subclinical, only rare sporadic cases of poliovirus-caused paralysis were noted. A syndrome retrospectively identifiable as paralytic poliomyelitis—almost always in infants or young children—began to be mentioned in the medical literature in the mid-1700s, but it was not fully recognized and described as a clinical entity until the later part of that century and the first half of the next. In the mid-1800s, outbreaks of paralytic polio began to be seen. For the next century, in urban, industrialized parts of Europe and North America, there followed epidemics that grew more severe, more frequent, and more widespread. Cases of what had been called *infantile paralysis* began to be observed also in adolescents and even in young adults. Large epidemics spread across the United States and Europe in the first half of the twentieth century. In the United States in the summer of 1916, more than 27,000 persons were reported to have been paralyzed, with 6000 deaths. In New York City during this one season, more than 9000 cases and more than 2000 deaths were recorded.

Zamula's description of the times indicates that "the 1916 epidemic caused widespread panic. Thousands fled the city to nearby mountain resorts. Movie theaters were closed, meetings were cancelled, public gatherings were shunned. Children were warned not to drink from water fountains; amusement parks and bathing beaches were off limits. In some towns, visitors from the New York City area were turned away by armed citizens who feared the spread of contagion."[45] Increased public awareness and fear, together with the ongoing developments that had taken place in medical science, led to intensified study of the disease and its control by vaccination, as described below.

CLASSIFICATION AND PROPERTIES

Poliovirus belongs to the enterovirus group, which includes polioviruses, coxsackieviruses, and echoviruses (Table 154-1).[15] These agents, which share a number of clinical, epidemiologic, and ecologic characteristics as well as physical and biochemical properties, are classified as the *Enterovirus* genus of the family Picornaviridae. Poliovirus type 1 is the type species of the genus.

Enteroviruses are transient inhabitants of the human alimentary tract and may be isolated from the throat of the infected person (from just before disease onset to 1 week after onset) or from the lower intestine (from just before onset to several weeks after onset). Healthy carriers are common; they usually excrete virus in the feces for several weeks.

Intratypic differences exist within each enterovirus type, which can be distinguished by use of the recently developed tools of molecular biology: highly strain-specific adsorbed or monoclonal sera, oligonucleotide mapping, and sequencing of the bases of the viral genome. Isolates are identified by type, country (or city), strain number, and year of isolation. Thus, P1/Houston/23/62 designates a type 1 poliovirus strain, number 23, isolated in Houston in 1962.

TABLE 154-1

Taxonomy of Human Enteroviruses

Polioviruses:	*Types 1–3; neurovirulent for monkeys and transgenic mice*
Coxsackieviruses A:	Types A1–A24 and several variants; in infant mice, group A viruses characteristically produce flaccid paralysis as a result of extensive myositis and the infection and destruction of striated muscle throughout the body
Coxsackieviruses B:	Types B1–B6; the disease caused in infant mice by group B viruses is characterized by a widespread infection of the brain and fat pads and a more limited infection of muscle and other tissue; cultured primate cells are highly susceptible to infection
Echoviruses:	31 types; cytopathogenic for cells grown in culture but not for mice; although types were numbered sequentially 1–34, three have been reclassified (echovirus 10 as a reovirus, echovirus 28 as a rhinovirus, and echovirus 34 as a variant of coxsackievirus A24); echovirus 9 is antigenically similar to coxsackievirus A23 but lacks pathogenicity for mice
Enterovirus:	Types 68–71; these later additions would formerly have been classified as either coxsackievirus or echovirus types, but the distinction—based on host susceptibility—has become blurred
Enterovirus type 72:	Hepatitis A virus was provisionally classified here but is now classified as a separate genus within the picornavirus family
Enterovirus:	A number of viruses have been classified as enteroviruses but have not been typed

Among the enteroviruses, polioviruses have proved to be the ones most often producing serious disease in humans. Consequently, poliovirus has been the enterovirus studied in most detail and, in this chapter, will serve as a model. The typical enterovirus is approximately 28 nm in diameter and consists of a capsid shell of 60 subunits, each with four proteins (VP1–VP4) arranged in icosahedral symmetry around a genome made up of a single strand of positive-sense RNA.[33] These polypeptides are cleaved from a larger precursor polyprotein. Radiographic diffraction studies of poliovirus have revealed the three-dimensional molecular structure of the virion. The three largest proteins (VP1–VP3) are similar in core structure; the peptide backbone of the protein loops back on itself, forming a barrel of eight strands held together by hydrogen bonds (the β barrel). Between the β barrel and the amino and carboxyl terminal portions of the protein, the amino acid chain contains a series of loops, which include the chief antigenic sites found on the virion surface; these sites are active in the neutralization of virus infection.

Enteroviruses are stable at acid pH for 1 to 3 h and have a buoyant density in cesium chloride of about 1.34 g/ml.[33] Because the virion has no lipid-containing envelope, it is not affected by lipid solvents such as ether or sodium deoxycholate. The virus is completely inactivated when heated at 55°C for 30 min. In the presence of molar magnesium chloride, poliovirus is protected against thermal inactivation—a property that has been utilized in stabilizing OPV.[14] Enteroviruses replicate in the cytoplasm of the infected cell. In the diagnostic laboratory, virus is cultivated in primary or continuous-line cell cultures from various human or monkey tissues. The typical enterovirus infects only primate cells that contain a specific membrane receptor for the virus on the cell surface.

Poliovirus adsorbs to cells at specific cell receptor sites.[14,33] This is evidenced by the fact that intact poliovirus infects only primate cells in culture, whereas the viral RNA isolated from its surrounding capsid also infects nonprimate cells (rabbit, guinea pig, chick), where only one cycle of multiplication occurs. Multiple cycles of infections are not observed in the nonprimate cells because the progeny of the viral RNA genome now possess protein coats that do not bind to the cells lacking the viral receptors. Usually the entire poliovirus genome, acting as its own mRNA, is translated to form a single large polypeptide that is subsequently cleaved to produce the various viral capsid polypeptides.[33]

CLINICAL PRESENTATIONS

When a person susceptible to infection is exposed to poliovirus, one of the following responses may occur: inapparent infection without symptoms, mild (minor) illness ("abortive poliomyelitis"), aseptic meningitis ("nonparalytic poliomyelitis"), and paralytic poliomyelitis.[3,29] As the infection progresses, one response may merge with a more severe form: a minor illness may be followed by a few symptom-free days and then by a major, severe illness. This biphasic course is more commonly seen in children than in adults. Only about 1 percent of poliovirus infections result in a paralytic illness (Table 154-2).

Asymptomatic Infection By far the most common form of infection is asymptomatic or is marked by no more than minor malaise. The subclinical course is taken by 99 percent of poliovirus infections.

Minor Illness ("Abortive Poliomyelitis") The most common form of disease caused by poliovirus is characterized by fever, malaise, drowsiness, headache, nausea, vomiting, constipation, or sore throat in various combinations. This manifestation has been estimated to occur in 4 to 8 percent of infections. Even during an epidemic, the diagnosis of abortive poliomyelitis cannot be made with assurance on clinical grounds unless virus is isolated or antibody development is measured. Many other viruses may cause the same signs and symptoms, and may circulate during the same seasons as poliovirus.

Aseptic Meningitis or Transient Mild Paresis ("Nonparalytic Poliomyelitis") In addition to the above-described symptoms and signs, the patient has stiffness and pain in the back and neck. Occasionally, there may be mild muscle weakness or transient paralysis. The disease lasts 2 to 10 days, and recovery is almost always complete. About 1 or 2 percent of infections take this

TABLE 154-2

Illnesses Associated with Respiratory Virus Infection

Syndrome	Signs and Symptoms	Typical Viruses
Rhinitis	Nasal obstruction and discharge, sneezing	Rhinoviruses, coronaviruses
Pharyngitis-tonsillitis	Sore throat, pharyngeal erythema, ± tonsillar enlargement, ± exudate, cervical adenitis	Adenoviruses, coxsackievirus, herpes simplex virus, Epstein-Barr virus
Croup	Coryza, hoarseness, inspiratory stridor, expiratory cough	Parainfluenza viruses, influenza viruses, respiratory syncytial virua
Tracheobronchitis	Paroxysmal, nonproductive , cough substernal discomfort	Respiratory syncytial virus, parainfluenza, influenza viruses
Bronchiolitis	Coryza, tachypnea, wheezing, weak cough	Respiratory syncytial virus, parainfluenza virus type 3, adenoviruses
Pneumonia	Cough, fever, headache, malaise lethargy, dyspnea, pulmonary infiltrate	Respiratory syncytial virus, parainfluenza, influenza viruses, adenoviruses

SOURCE: From Cate.[6]

course during epidemics. In a small percentage of cases, meningitis advances to paralysis. It should be noted that a number of other viruses—particularly other members of the enterovirus family—also produce this syndrome.

Paralytic Poliomyelitis   The major illness comprises the manifestations listed above for aseptic meningitis, along with persisting weakness of one or more muscle groups, either skeletal or cranial. It accounts for about 1 percent of poliovirus infections. The onset of paralysis may follow the minor illness after a symptom-free interlude, or it may occur without an antecedent phase of illness. The predominant sign is flaccid paralysis resulting from lower motor neuron damage. Incoordination secondary to brainstem invasion may also occur, and there may be painful spasms of nonparalyzed muscles. The amount of damage varies widely, and the respiratory muscles are not spared. Usually muscle impairment is maximal within a few days after the paralytic phase begins. Maximal recovery usually occurs within 6 months, with residual paralysis lasting much longer, often for life.

Other enteroviruses can, on rare occasions, cause a syndrome difficult or impossible to distinguish on clinical grounds from paralytic polio. As the worldwide drive to eradicate both poliomyelitis and its viruses proceeds and surveillance for cases becomes crucial, recognition of these other paralytogenic agents will be of increasing importance.

The late-onset postpolio syndrome (PPS) consists of muscle weakness, muscle pain, and unaccustomed fatigue.

This has occurred with increasing frequency among former poliomyelitis patients.[39] There are about 300,000 to 600,000 American survivors of the polio epidemics of the 1940s and 1950s who live with some degree of residual disability. In the 1990s, more than one-third of these patients are experiencing the new problems and symptoms of PPS. The age of the patient with PPS is less important as a determinant of onset than the length of time after the acute illness. The incidence peaks at an interval of about 30 to 40 years after the acute poliomyelitis. It seems that PPS results from the neuromuscular disease process initiated at the time of the acute illness. The disease is not caused by a reactivation of the original poliovirus or by a reinfection with a current strain; it develops when the patient's remaining motor units in the central nervous system start to respond poorly to their overuse through many years (Fig. 154-1).[39]

Coxsackieviruses, a large subgroup of the enteroviruses, are divided into groups A and B on the basis of different pathogenic potentials for mice.[14] They produce a variety of illnesses in humans. Herpangina, hand, foot, and mouth disease, and acute hemorrhagic conjunctivitis are caused by certain group A serotypes. Pleurodynia, myocarditis, pericarditis, and meningoencephalitis are caused by group B viruses. In addition to these, a number of group A and B serotypes give rise to aseptic meningitis, respiratory and undifferentiated febrile illnesses, hepatitis, and sometimes paralysis. Generally, paralysis produced by nonpolio enteroviruses is incomplete and reversible. Coxsackie B viruses are the most commonly identified causative agents of viral heart disease.

Echoviruses (**e**nteric **c**ytopathic **h**uman **o**rphan viruses) are grouped together because they infect the human enteric tract and

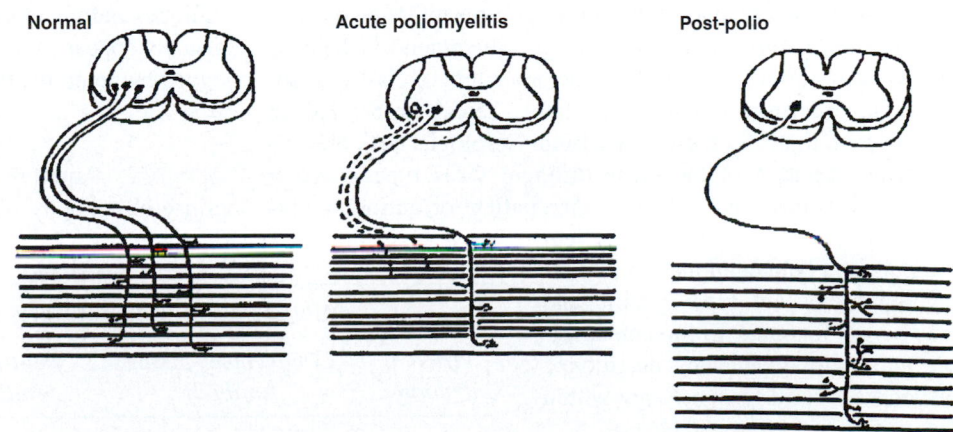

Normal   **Acute poliomyelitis**   **Post-polio**

FIGURE 154-1   Schematic representation of motor units to a muscle. *Normal* represents the 100 to 1000 motor neurons of a muscle and the 5 to 1500 muscle fibers each axon innervates. *Acute poliomyelitis* depicts viral destruction of some of the anterior horn cells with atrophy of denervated muscle fibers. *Postpolio* represents axon sprouting by recovered nerve cells with reinnervation of the orphaned muscle fibers and subsequent hypertrophy. *(Based on data of Smith,[39] with permission.)*

because they can be recovered from humans only by inoculation of certain tissue cultures.[14] More than 30 serotypes are known, but not all cause human illness. Aseptic meningitis, febrile illnesses with or without rash, common colds, and acute hemorrhagic conjunctivitis are among the diseases caused by echoviruses. Some produce disease of the upper respiratory tract.

New enteroviruses that are discovered concurrently are grouped together. Four of these enteroviruses (types 68–71) grow in monkey kidney cultures, and three of them cause human disease. Enterovirus 68 has been isolated from the respiratory tracts of children with bronchiolitis or pneumonia. Enterovirus 70 is the chief cause of acute hemorrhagic conjunctivitis, and enterovirus 71 has been isolated from patients with meningitis, encephalitis, and paralysis resembling poliomyelitis.

Several enteroviruses have been associated with mild illness of the upper respiratory tract, including rhinitis, particularly during the summer and autumn.[6] These include coxsackievirus A2, 10, 21, and 24 and B2 and 5. CA21 virus has caused epidemics of pharyngitis in military recruits. The echoviruses that have been isolated from cases of respiratory illness are types 1, 4, 9, 11, 19, 20, 22, and 25. These viruses most commonly cause outbreaks in young children, in whom pneumonia and bronchiolitis may sometimes occur. The small caliber of an infant's bronchioles makes them easily obstructed by the inflammatory response to respiratory syncytial virus (RSV) infection, producing the syndrome of bronchiolitis. Adults who have small-airway disease secondary to prolonged smoking also tend to have more frequent and severe lower-tract symptoms (cough, sputum, dyspnea) with respiratory viral infections than do normal persons. Secretory immunoglobulins induced by prior infection help prevent reinfection, but the secretory antibody titer decreases more rapidly than the serum antibody level; thus, reinfections occur with respiratory viruses such as parainfluenza or RSV, although residual, partial immunity can reduce disease severity. Impaired cell-mediated immunity has been associated with prolonged shedding of respiratory viruses and with severe viral pneumonia.

DIAGNOSIS

In an individual case, diagnosing an enterovirus infection on clinical grounds is impossible (Table 154-2). The diagnosis depends on laboratory tests (Table 154-3). The procedure of choice is isolation of virus from throat swabs, stools, rectal swabs, and, in aseptic meningitis, cerebrospinal fluid. Serologic tests are impractical—because of the many different virus types—except when a virus has been isolated from a patient or during an outbreak of typical clinical illness. Neutralizing and hemagglutination inhibiting antibodies are type specific and may persist for years. Complement-fixing antibodies give many heterotypic responses, but all responses are within the enterovirus grouping.

If an agent is isolated in tissue culture, it is tested with specifically designed combination pools of antisera against enteroviruses, known as the LBM pools.[15] Determination of the type of virus present depends on neutralization by a single specific combination of antisera. At times, infection with two enteroviruses may occur simultaneously.

The identification of an enterovirus by isolation and neutralization is the standard method, but new assays are becoming increasingly used. The most promising reports have been the application of polymerase chain reaction (PCR).[34] Viral RNA is extracted from the patient specimen by phenol-chloroform-sodium dodocyl sulfate or guanidinium thiocyanade and then treated with reverse transcriptase. After 30 cycles of denaturation, annealing, and extension in the presence of polymerase, the amplified product is detected. PCR is also used for study of genetic changes in the virus.

Cerebrospinal Fluid Changes in Polio   The CSF contains increased numbers of leukocytes—usually 10 to 200 per microliter, seldom more than 500 per microliter. Early in the disease, the ratio of polymorphonuclear cells to lymphocytes is high, but within a few days the ratio is reversed.[3] The total cell count slowly subsides to normal levels. The protein content of the CSF is elevated; the average is about 40 to 50 mg per deciliter, but higher levels may occur and persist for weeks. The glucose content is normal.

Recovery of Virus   For cultivating poliovirus, cultures of human or monkey cells should be used.[21] In contrast to the situation with certain other enteroviruses, poliovirus has rarely been isolated from the CSF. The virus may be recovered from throat swabs taken soon after onset of illness; usually, however, it is recovered from rectal swabs or feces for 1 or 2 months after onset, but in falling concentrations. Poliovirus has been recovered from about 80 percent of patients during the first 2 weeks of illness but in only 25 percent during the third 2-week period. No permanent carriers are known.

In fatal cases, virus tests should include the cervical and lumbar enlargements of the spinal cord, the medulla, and the colon contents. The spinal cord and parts of the brain should be examined histologically. If paralysis lasted 4 to 5 days, it may be difficult to recover the virus from the cord. Specimens should be kept frozen during transit to the laboratory and treated with antibiotics before inoculation of cell cultures. Cytopathic effects usually appear in 3 to 6 days. An isolated virus is identified and typed by neutralization with specific antiserum (Figs. 154-2 and 154-3).

Serology   Paired serum specimens are required in order to show a rise in antibody titer (Table 154-3).[31] Neutralizing antibodies

TABLE 154-3

Interpretation of Laboratory Data in Poliovirus Infection

Virus Infection	Complement-Fixing Antibody	Neutralizing Antibody	Antibody of IgM Class	Interpretation of Infection
−	−	−	−	None
+	−	−	−	Early
+	+	+	+	Current
−	+	+	+	Recent
−	−	+	−	Old

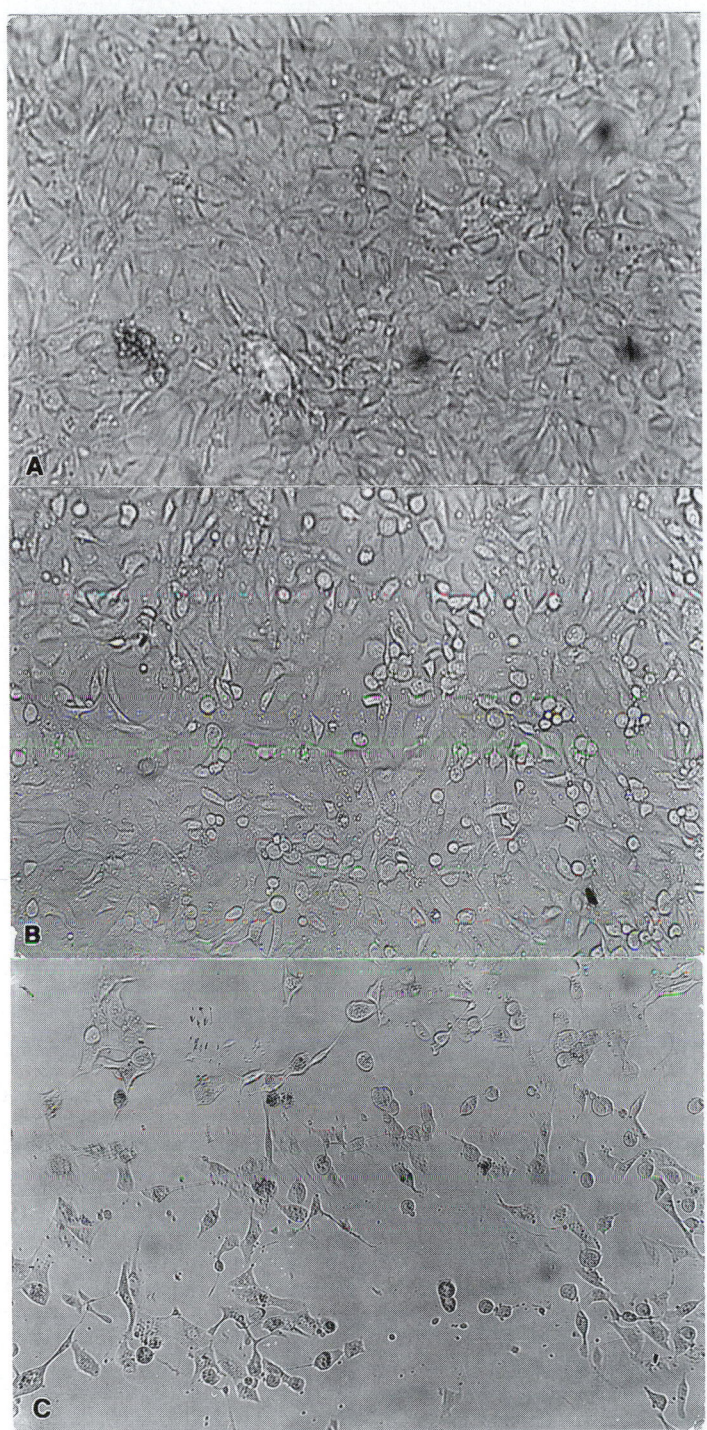

FIGURE 154-2 Unstained living culture of Type I poliovirus in monkey kidney cells. Normal cells (shown in *A*) are also typical of cells exposed to virus neutralized by antibody. Low power of magnification.

appear early, and for polio they are usually already detectable at the time of hospitalization. If the first specimen is taken sufficient early, a rise in titer can be demonstrated during the course of the disease. Only the first infection with a poliovirus produces strictly type-specific complement-fixation responses. Subsequent infections with heterotypic polioviruses recall or induce antibodies mostly against the heat-stable group antigen shared by all three poliovirus types. In Table 154-3 are summarized the vari-

ous combinations of laboratory results that may be obtained. The last column indicates the interpretation in terms of the presence and nature of a poliovirus infection.

Rapid methods, particularly those based on the polymerase chain reaction, have been used for direct detection of poliovirus and other enteroviruses in clinical specimens.[34] These tests hold great promise and are being introduced for use in a routine diagnostic laboratory, where specific primers are used and the product of the reaction is probed immediately with a nonisotopically labeled probe that is virus specific.

PATHOGENESIS AND PATHOLOGY

The portal of entry of the virus is the mouth. Primary multiplication takes place in the oropharynx or the intestine, and for a few days virus may appear in the blood. The virus can be isolated regularly from the throat just before and at the first signs of illness. The incubation period is usually between 7 and 14 days but may range from 3 to 35 days. By 1 week after onset, there is little virus in the throat, but large amounts of virus continue to be excreted in the stools for several weeks, even though humoral antibodies usually develop during the same period.

As the enterovirus travels from the mouth, implantation and multiplication take place in the oropharynx and the small intestine. The incubation period (defined as the time from exposure to onset of disease) is usually between 7 and 14 days, but may range from 2 to 35 days. By 3 to 5 days after exposure, virus can be recovered from blood, throat, and feces. At this time symptoms of the "minor illness" may appear, or the infection may remain asymptomatic. Viremia is present for a few days before the onset of CNS signs in those who develop either "nonparalytic polio" (aseptic meningitis) or the paralytic disease. Antibodies develop early and extinguish the viremia, usually before paralysis appears (discussed further below under "Control Through Vaccination"). However, infectious virus bound to antibody may be detected for a few additional days.[20]

After initial multiplication in the tonsils, the lymph nodes of the neck, Peyer's patches, and the small intestine, poliovirus then spreads by way of the bloodstream to other susceptible tissues, namely other lymph nodes, brown fat, and the CNS. Poliovirus can also spread along axons of peripheral nerves to the CNS, whence it continues to progress along the fibers of the lower motor neurons to invade the spinal cord and parts of the brain. Tonsillectomy or other surgery in the oropharynx increases the risk of CNS impairment at times when polioviruses are prevalent. This may result from virus in the pharynx gaining direct access to cut nerve fibers, or it may be a secondary consequence of the removal of immunologically active lymphoid tissue.

Poliovirus invades only certain types of nerve cells; in the process of its intracellular multiplication, it may damage or completely destroy these cells.[35] The anterior horn cells of the spinal cord are most prominently involved, but in severe cases the intermediate gray ganglia and even the posterior horn and dorsal root ganglia are often affected. Lesions are found as far forward as the hypothalamus and thalamus. In the brain, the reticular formation, the vestibular nuclei, the cerebellar vermis, and the deep cerebellar nuclei are most often affected. The cortex is virtually spared, with the exception of the motor cortex along the precentral gyrus.

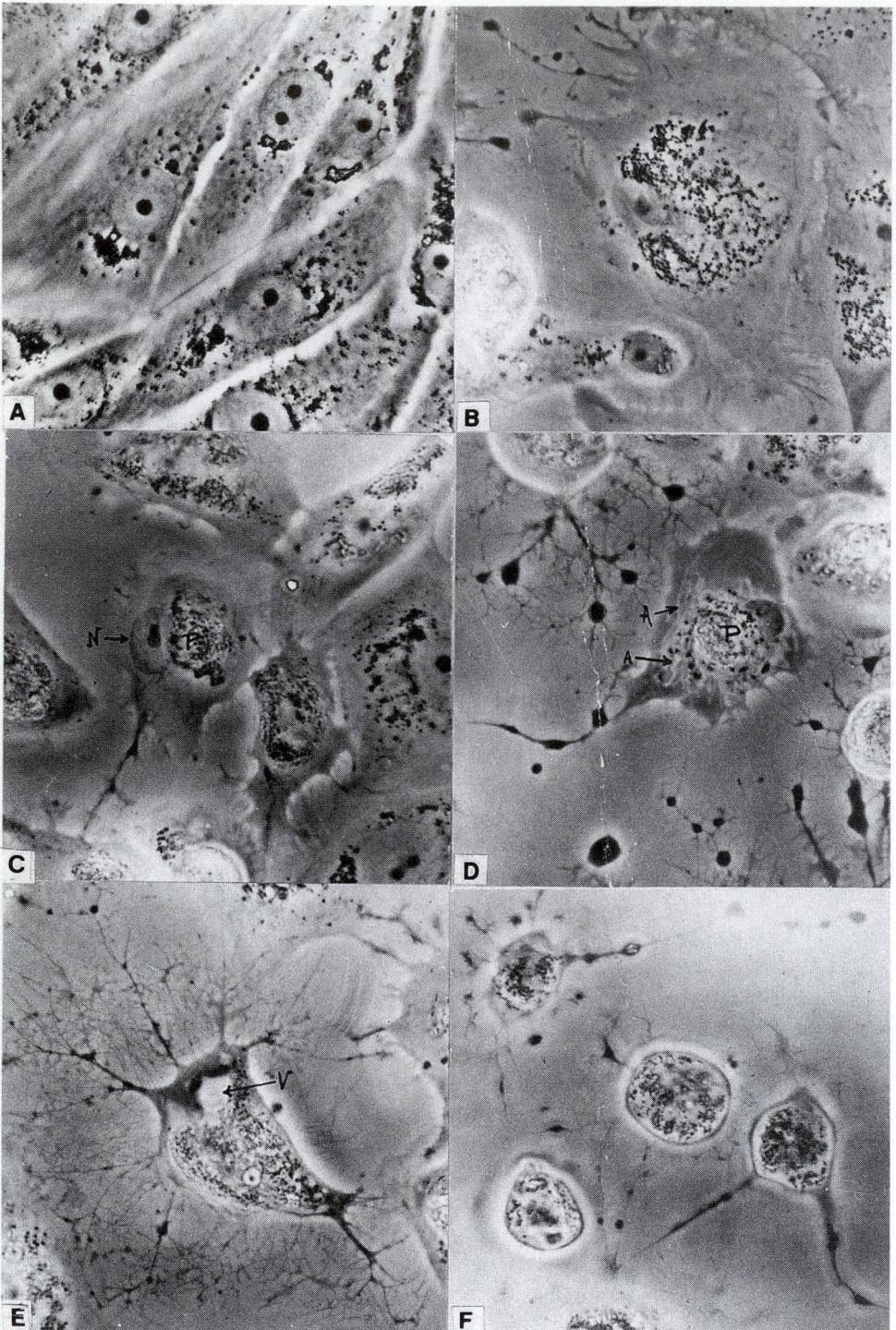

FIGURE 154-3   Unstained living culture of Type I poliovirus in monkey kidney cells. Normal cells (shown in *A*) are also typical of cells exposed to virus neutralized by antibody. High power of magnification.

Hodes[11] has given an excellent discussion of the role the poliovirus plays in respiratory difficulty:

> Respiratory failure resulting from paralysis of the diaphragm and intercostal muscles represents the most serious complication of paralytic poliomyelitis. Aspiration pneumonia, pulmonary edema, myocarditis, paralytic ileus, gastric dilatation and ielus of the bladder may also complicate acute paralytic disease. Poliomyelitis may affect respiration adversely in several ways. Invasion of the motor nerve cells by the virus causes loss of discharge, the basic stimulus which activates striated muscles, including diaphragm, intercostals and accessory muscles of respiration. The degree of weakness produced is proportional to the number of motor cells which have lost their capacity to function. There results partial or complete loss of the ability to produce the rhythmic changes in the thoracic volume which bring about pulmonary ventilation.
>
> Poliomyelitis virus also may injure the neurons in the medulla which control the rate, the rhythm and the integration of respiratory movements. The damaged neurons do not respond in the normal manner to changes in CO_2 concentration, pH and oxygen saturation of arterial blood. Disturbances in the regularity and the depth of respiratory movements result. In poliomyelitis, therefore, respiratory difficulty may arise from interference with the peripheral motor or central control factors of respiration. These may occur singly or in combination of various degrees of severity....
>
> During the course of poliomyelitis, respiratory tract obstruction may result from paralysis of the abductors of the vocal cords. More frequently, it is caused by inability to swallow saliva and mucus as a result of paralysis of the muscles of deglutition. Paralysis of these muscles leads to accumulation of secretions which interfere with the entrance of air into the larynx and which may be aspirated into the trachea, the bronchi or the alveoli. In either case, less effective pulmonary ventilation results. Aspiration of these secretions may lead to atelectasis of portions of the lung and further loss of respiratory function.
>
> Pulmonary edema may occur during the course of severe poliomyelitis, particularly when extensive bulbar disease is present. It probably is due to injury of the medullary autonomic centers which control blood pressure. This injury causes constriction of the systemic vascular bed, resulting in transfer of blood to the

Although flaccid paralysis is the hallmark of poliomyelitis, the virus does not multiply in muscle in vivo. The changes that occur in peripheral nerves and voluntary muscles are secondary to destruction of nerve cells within the CNS. Cells that are not killed, but lose function temporarily, may recover completely within 3 to 4 weeks after onset. Inflammation occurs secondary to the attack on nerve cells.

lungs in sufficient quantity to raise the hydrostatic pressure in the pulmonary capillaries to a degree sufficient to cause edema.

A key determinant of poliovirus infection is the cell receptor, upon which the restricted tropism of the virus depends.[1,30] Molecular clones of the poliovirus receptor have been isolated, and the encoded protein has been identified as a new member of the immunoglobulin family. Transgenic mice have been developed in which the human gene-encoding cellular receptors for poliovirus have been introduced into the mouse genome. The new mice have proved to be susceptible to all three poliovirus types and are being investigated as models for testing OPV lots for neurovirulence, which currently requires the monkey test.

TREATMENT AND PROGRESS

Treatment for polio entails reducing pain and muscle spasm, maintaining respiration and hydration, allaying fear, taking steps to minimize ensuing skeletal deformities, and anticipating and forestalling other indirect effects of the paralysis, some of which are transient and some long-term.[3] When the fever subsides, early mobilization and active exercise are begun. All pharyngeal and bowel discharges are considered infectious and should be disposed of quickly and safely.

Usually, recovery is complete in nonparalytic polio and in patients with mild muscle weakness. In cases of severe paralysis, recovery of muscle function starts soon after the acute phase and may continue for up to 2 years. However, 80 percent of the eventual recovery attained is achieved within 6 months. The extent of muscle recovery is inversely proportional to the extent of nerve cell damage. Some muscles seem to recover completely, whereas others never improve. The case fatality rate is about 4 percent, but in epidemics involving older people it has reached 10 percent.

EPIDEMIOLOGY

Human beings are the only known reservoir of poliovirus infection. At times when a poliovirus is widely prevalent in an area, houseflies become contaminated and may passively distribute virus to food.[43] The significance of flies in transmitting the viruses is not fully understood; in areas of poor sanitation, they may play a more significant role. Polioviruses are often present in urban sewage,[16] which may then serve as a source of direct or indirect transmission through flies or through contaminated water used for drinking, bathing, or irrigation. However, close human contact is the primary avenue of spread. From persons who are infected, whether or not they develop clinical illness, the oropharynx and intestine can yield virus, which is generally shed for as long as 1 or 2 months in stools—but for a much shorter period in oropharyngeal secretions. The usual source of transmission is infectious feces spread by contaminated fingers. Viruses are most readily spread within the family. Poliomyelitis and enteroviral diseases occur year-round in the tropics and during summer and fall in temperate zones. Winter outbreaks are rare.[28]

The disease occurs in all age groups, but children are usually more susceptible than adults because of the acquired immunity of the adult population. In isolated populations (Arctic Eskimo), poliomyelitis has attacked all ages equally. In developing areas, where conditions favor the wide dissemination of virus, poliomyelitis continues to be a disease of infancy. In developed countries before the onset of vaccination, the age distribution shifted so that most patients were over age 5, and 25 percent were over age 15 years.[26] With rising levels of hygiene and sanitation, a similar trend has occurred in developing countries.

Under conditions of poor hygiene and sanitation in warm areas, where almost all children become immune early in life, enteroviruses maintain themselves by continuously infecting a small part of the population. In temperate zones with high levels of hygiene, epidemics have been followed by periods of little spread of virus, until sufficient numbers of susceptible children have grown up to provide a pool for transmission in the area. Warm weather favors the spread of virus by increasing human contacts, the susceptibility of the host, or the dissemination of virus by extrahuman sources. The prevalence of infection is highest among household contacts. When the first case is recognized in a family, all susceptible members of the family are already infected as a result of rapid dissemination of virus.[26]

CONTROL THROUGH VACCINATION

In 1950, Koprowski fed his rodent-adapted type 2 poliovirus to small groups in New York and California. Within the next decade, he and Cox and their associates[5,12] fed millions more throughout the world with the three types of viruses. Others,[18,37] including Sabin[37] in the United States, had also developed attenuated strains, and Chumakov and his associates[8] in the former Soviet Union had fed these to millions more. The results were so striking that a number of countries immediately adapted these strains as the polio vaccines of choice. However, in Berlin, the father of a Cox-vaccinated child developed paralysis and died.[17] Poliovirus with the properties of the Cox strain was isolated from his brain tissue, and the strain was withdrawn. The intracerebral and intraspinal routes were used to further test the Sabin, Koprowski, and Cox strains in monkeys. The results favored the Sabin strains, which were then adopted for use in the United States.[19,25]

Both live[15,36] and killed[38] vaccines are now readily available for polio, but most countries have relied almost entirely on live OPV, the vaccine recommended by the World Health Organization. In 1977, only 5 percent of all children in the world had received the required three doses of OPV in the first years of life, but in 1995 this percentage had increased to 80 percent. By 1995, OPV was preventing at least 500,000 cases of paralytic poliomyelitis each year. Injectable vaccine (Salk)[38] is prepared from virus grown in monkey kidney cultures by formalin inactivation. It is known as IPV. At least four inoculations over a period of 1 to 2 years are recommended in the primary series. Periodic booster immunizations are necessary to maintain immunity. IPV induces humoral antibodies, but upon exposure, virus is still able to multiply in the gut and be transmitted to another susceptible person.

OPV (Sabin)[15,36] contains live attenuated virus grown in primary monkey or human diploid cell cultures. OPV multiplies and infects, and thus immunizes. In the process, infectious progeny of the vaccine virus are disseminated in the community. Although the viruses, particularly types 2 and 3, mutate in the course of their multiplication in vaccinated children, only extremely rare cases (about 1 per 500,000 susceptible children) of paralytic poliomyelitis have occurred in recipients of OPV or their close contacts. Booster vaccinations are important to establish permanent immunity. The poliovaccine induces not only IgM and IgG antibodies in the blood but also secretory IgA antibodies in the intestine, which then becomes resistant to reinfection.[27]

The mutations that occur during replication of OPV have produced, in just a few instances, viral progeny with neurovirulence sufficiently increased to cause paralysis in vaccine recipients and their susceptible contacts. Poliovirus replication is accompanied by an error frequency of about $10^{-3.5}$ per nucleotide incorporated into the nascent poliovirus RNA genome, which consists of about 7400 nucleotides. This error rate suggests that most newly synthesized poliovirus RNA molecules differ in at least one nucleotide from the sequence of the parental template RNA. Thus, every batch of poliovirus is a population of viral genomic sequences that compete for dominance. Any change in growth conditions will alter the relative replicative efficiency of the competing viral sequences. This concept of a dynamic viral population explains the rapid changes of viral phenotype that can occur during manufacture or after application to a vaccinated person. A sensitive measure of reversions from uracil to cytosine at nucleotide 472 of type 3 OPV can be used to predict the result of the expansive and somewhat variable monkey neurovirulence test, the one being used by most manufacturers today.[32]

Other types have similar reversions.[31] Thus, for type 1, a G→A reversion occurs at nucleotide position 480. Lots of type 1 in which the level 480A was 2.7 percent of revertants have passed the monkey neurovirulence test. Thus, the in vitro genetic test that detects 480A is even more sensitive than the monkey test for neurovirulence.[31]

Molecular characterization of poliovirus strains isolated from stool samples of 70 vaccine-associated cases showed that 50 percent of type 2 and 67 percent of type 3 strains had a recombinant genome.[9] This was in contrast to the very low proportion of recombinants among strains serially isolated from healthy OPV vaccinees up to 2 months after vaccination. Most of these strains, from both paralyzed and healthy vaccinees, carried mutations in nucleotide positions that play a role in poliovirus attenuation. It appears that recombination plays a role in the neuropathogenicity of vaccine-derived strains. In some vaccine-associated cases, both recombinant and nonrecombinant strains have been found, indicating that the stool isolates might not always be representative for the etiologic agent of the paralysis. All strains isolated from the spinal cords of vaccine-associated cases lost the attenuated phenotype of the original Sabin strains as tested in transgenic mice carrying the receptor gene and making them sensitive to poliovirus infection.[1,30]

The application of recombinant DNA technology may permit the development of a live poliovirus that cannot mutate to increased neurovirulence. Recombinant viruses have been constructed from parental viruses belonging to different poliovirus serotypes and between virulent and attenuated strains of the same serotype.[4] Sequences in the viral genome that are responsible for an attenuated phenotype have been identified. The type 1 vaccine virus, which is extremely stable genetically, has been used as a vector for type 2 and 3 nucleotide sequences encoding immunogenic regions of their VP1 proteins.[4] The new "chimeric" strains

have the desired biologic characteristics of type 1, but with the added immunogenic properties of type 2 or type 3. Such advances may lead to a more genetically stable type 3 vaccine. It will be difficult to field-test such a new vaccine candidate, as it will be necessary to prove that the new vaccine produces less than one vaccine-associated case per million susceptible recipients.

Circulating serum antibody is not the only source of protection against poliovirus infection. Local or cellular immunity is manifested by protection against intestinal reinfection after recovery from a natural infection or after immunization with OPV. Local or secretory IgA is generally recognized as having an important role in defense against enteroviral infection. The development of serum and secretory antibody responses to OPV and to intramuscular inoculation of IPV has been investigated. The IPV was not very effective in inducing secretory antibody in the respiratory or intestinal tract. It had been hoped that the newer, enhanced-potency IPV would stimulate a more effective secretory antibody response.

In a study[27] on the development of antibody responses to the whole virus and to the subunit virion proteins in humans, infants immunized with enhanced IPV or with OPV were studied for serum and secretory antibody responses to the poliovirus itself and to polypeptides VP1, VP2, and VP3. Both vaccines induce neutralizing IgG and IgG detectable by enzyme immunoassay to the whole virus and to VP1 and VP3 and similarly detected secretory IgA to VP1 and VP2 in the nasopharyngeal secretions without any anti-VP3 response. However, in regard to the neutralizing antibody response in nasopharyngeal secretions, OPV was markedly more effective than the enhanced IPV: 70 percent of the infants developed this response after OPV, as against only 27 percent of those who had received enhanced-potency IPV.

Studies with synthetic peptides that contain neutralizing epitope residues reveal that they are weak immunogens. Thus, when nonliving antigen is required, the use of inactivated whole virus (IPV) is indicated.[38] However, live attenuated virus (OPV) continues to be the vaccine of choice worldwide.[15,36]

VACCINATION POLICY

Trivalent oral poliovaccine is generally used in the United States, where primary immunization begins at 2 months of age, simultaneously with the first diphtheria-tetanus-pertussis inoculation. The second and third doses should be given at 2-month intervals thereafter, and a fourth dose at 18 months of age. The multiple doses are recommended to maximize immunity for all three serotypes. A trivalent vaccine booster is recommended for all children entering elementary school. No further boosters are currently recommended.

An immunization schedule in which IPV is given before the first feeding of OPV would be expected to eliminate the risk of vaccine-associated paralytic poliomyelitis for OPV recipients, and reduce the risk among contacts of OPV recipients and immunocompromised children. In the United States, two doses of enhanced IPV—given at 2 and 4 months of age—are being considered for complete protection against subsequent doses of OPV. The gastrointestinal and mucosal immunity induced by a sequence of IPV-IPV-OPV-OPV given at 2, 4, 6, and 25 months of age has been suggested.[24]

In the 1950s, just before the beginning of vaccination campaigns in the United States, about 21,000 cases of paralytic poliomyelitis occurred annually. Currently, fewer than 10 vaccine-associated cases occur each year. They are the result of back-mutations. No wild virus has been isolated in the United States since 1979, and the disease has almost vanished in all industrialized countries globally, and in all of the Western Hemisphere through the special programs of the Pan American Health Organization. However, there is a continuing global need for adequate vaccination schedules in order to limit the spread of wild viruses. In developing countries, particularly in tropical areas, the usual schedule should be accelerated. Not only should primary immunization begin very early—even at birth—but in particular immunization should be completed early in infancy. In some tropical areas where neither OPV nor IPV was able to eliminate all cases, a combined schedule of OPV and IPV has been used successfully to eradicate the clinical disease in spite of the occurrence of wild viruses in the region.[10,13,40] Denmark[42] has adopted this schedule. The United States is considering a combined schedule.

The global situation has recently been reviewed by the Centers for Disease Control and Prevention.[7]

Since 1988, the global incidence of paralytic polio has decreased substantially, and polio apparently has been completely eliminated from the Western Hemisphere. The number of global polio cases reported in 1993 represents a 33% decrease compared with 1992 and with a 70% decrease compared with 1988. Furthermore, nearly three-quarters of all countries reported zero cases of polio in 1993, and polio-free zones are present or emerging in the Americas, northern, southern, and eastern Africa, the Arabian peninsula, Western and Central Europe, and the Western Pacific. Despite this substantial progress over-all, paralytic polio remains highly endemic throughout the Indian subcontinent, and continues to occur in most countries of sub-Saharan Africa and Asia, including many republics of the former Soviet Union. . . . Lower than optimal levels of routine vaccination coverage, pockets of unvaccinated children within otherwise highly vaccinated populations, crowding, poor sanitation, and suboptimal seroconversion to poliovirus types 1 and 3 following three routine doses of OPV in many tropical and subtropical regions probably contribute to ongoing wild poliovirus transmission in these areas. . . .

In addition to remaining areas of endemic transmission, outbreaks of paralytic polio have recently occurred in several countries 2 or more years after the last previously reported case of polio, despite high levels of routine vaccination coverage. Genotypic comparisons between wild poliovirus strains in the global laboratory network have demonstrated that outbreaks in Oman, Jordan, Malaysia, and the Netherlands occurred as a result of importation of wild poliovirus from polio-endemic countries in the Indian subcontinent. Thus, until polio is eradicated globally, every polio-free country may be at risk for importation of wild poliovirus from remaining polio-endemic reservoirs.

The CDC *Morbidity and Mortality Weekly Report* subsequently stated (on September 29, 1994): "Ongoing surveillance for acute flaccid paralysis cases and for the presence of wild poliovirus must be maintained. International communication and collaboration will continue to be necessary for the rapid detection of importations of wild poliovirus and timely implementation of control efforts."

The results in one area are illustrative of what can be done in that area even when it is subjected to regular importation of wild polio.[10] After the introduction of trivalent OPV, the incidence of paralytic poliomyelitis in Israel declined dramatically. Yet in 1988, an outbreak of 15 cases of type 1 polio occurred, most in fully vaccinated people aged 11 to 35 years. It appeared that the young adult population was not adequately immune against the epidemic virus. All persons up to age 40 years were offered a single dose of OPV. In addition, a new infant vaccination schedule was introduced, based on a combination of three doses of eIPV and three doses of OPV. Since the outbreak, no cases of paralytic poliomyelitis have occurred in Israel, even though the disease remains endemic in neighboring countries and wild polio isolates were detected in sewage in Gaza.

Two studies were conducted to assess the immune status of the population. The immediate antibody response and long-term persistence of neutralizing antibodies were examined in adults vaccinated with OPV in 1988. Four years later, geometric mean titers (GMTs) were lower than the levels immediately after the booster, but all vaccinees had titers of at least 1:64 against the type 1 epidemic strain. In a second study, blood samples were drawn from 65 infants, aged 16 to 20 months, vaccinated with the new combined eIPV/OPV schedule. All had antibody titers of at least 1:64 against the epidemic strain, and GMTs against all poliovirus types were considerably higher than those achieved in schedules based on OPV alone. These findings indicate that the mass vaccination campaigns in 1988 and the new combined vaccination schedule for infants have produced extremely high levels of immunity in the population. As a result, paralytic poliomyelitis has been eradicated as of 1988 from Israel, as it had been from Gaza and the West Bank, where combined IPV/OPV schedules have been used since 1978.[13]

SUMMARY AND CONCLUSIONS

The widespread application of OPV has achieved eradication of poliomyelitis from the Western Hemisphere, and with each passing year the number of cases in the world continues to fall. The global application of the present OPV is fast achieving an interruption of the circulation of wild poliovirus, closing the window during which any newly developed vaccine strains can be properly field-tested. Worldwide eradication may be achieved through the use of the currently available and properly safety-tested vaccines.[44]

This leads to a new question soon to be considered: should we simply *stop* vaccinating for a disease that no longer exists in the world? In the case of smallpox, the answer was clear. No harm was done to those vaccinated and to their healthy contacts. With OPV, one in every 500,000 children receiving their first dose will develop paralysis. The recovered virus from such cases is virulent and has produced devastating paralysis in some healthy contacts. Another factor is the long period during which vaccinees are healthy carriers and remain contagious. It is essential that the contacts of vaccinated children be immunized together with or before immunization of the vaccinated child. In injectable vaccine the virus is inactivated, so healthy carriers cannot be the result. To lessen a potential risk in manufacture, the virulent strains in currently available IPV can be replaced by Sabin's attenuated strains of OPV. At least one manufacturer is already testing such an IPV preparation. Following the eradication of polio by OPV, there should be 1 or 2 years during which only IPV is used. In the absence of intestinal excretion of OPV progeny, poliovirus will disappear.

REFERENCES

1. Abe S, Yoshihiro O, Koike S, et al: Neurovirulence test for oral live poliovaccines using poliovirus-sensitive transgenic mice. *Virology* 206:1075–1083, 1995.

2. Aycock WL, Luther EH: The occurrence of poliomyelitis following tonsillectomy. *New Engl J Med* 200:164–167, 1929.

3. Bodian D, Horstmann DM: Polioviruses, in F. L. Horsfall, I. Tamm (eds), *Viral and rickettsial infections of man,* 4th ed. Philadelphia, JB Lippincott, 1965, pp 430–473.

4. Burke KL, Almond JW, Evans DJ: Antigen chimeras of poliovirus, in Melnick JL (ed), *Progress in Medical Virology,* vol 38. Basel, Karger, 1991, pp 56–68.

5. Cabasso VJ, Jervis GA, Moyer AW, et al: Cumulative testing experience with consecutive lots of oral poliomyelitis vaccine, in *Live Polio Virus Vaccine.* PAHO, 1959, pp 102–134.

6. Cate TR: Respiratory tract infection, in Rotchschild H, Cohen JC (eds), *Virology in medicine.* Oxford University Press, 1986, pp 111–132.

7. Centers for Disease Control and Prevention: Progress toward global eradication of poliomyelitis, 1988–1993. *MMWR Morb Mortal Wkly Rep* 43:499–503, 1994.

8. Chumakov MP, Gagarina AV, Lashkevich VA, et al: Characteristics of live poliovirus vaccine produced in the Institute for Poliomyelitis Research, Academy of Medical Sciences of the USSR, and comparison to Sabin's original vaccine from attenuated poliovirus strains, in *Live Polio Virus Vaccine.* Pan American Health Organization, 1959, pp 140–155.

9. Furione M, Guillot S, Otelea D, et al: Polioviruses with natural recombinant genomes isolated from vaccine-associated paralytic poliomyelitis. *Virology* 196:199–208, 1993.

10. Goldblum N, Gerichter CB, Tulchinsky TH, Melnick JL: Poliomyelitis control in Israel, the West Bank and Gaza Strip: Changing strategies with the goal of eradication in an endemic area. *Bull WHO* 72:783–796, 1994.

11. Hodes HL: Treatment of respiratory difficulty in poliomyelitis, in *Poliomyelitis: Papers and Discussions Presented at the Third International Poliomyelitis Conference.* Philadelphia, JB Lippincott, 1955, pp 91–96.

12. Koprowski HL, Jervis GA, Norton TW: Immune responses in human volunteers upon oral administration of a rodent-adapted strain of poliomyelitis. *Am J Hyg* 55:108–126, 1952.

13. Lasch EE, Abed Y, Abdulla K, et al: Successful results of a program combining live and inactivated poliovirus vaccines to control poliomyelitis in Gaza. *Rev Infect Dis* 6:S467–S470, 1984.

14. Melnick JL: Enteroviruses: Polioviruses, coxsackieviruses, echoviruses, and newer enteroviruses, in Fields BN, Knipe DM, Chanock RM, et al (eds), *Fields Virology,* 2d ed. 1990, pp 549–605.

15. Melnick JL: Live attenuated poliovaccines, in Plotkin SA, Mortimer EA Jr (eds), *Vaccines,* 2d ed. Philadelphia, WB Saunders, 1994, pp 155–204.

16. Melnick JL: Poliomyelitis virus in urban sewage in epidemic and in nonepidemic times. *Am J Hyg* 45:240–253, 1947.

17. Melnick JL: Problems associated with the use of live poliovirus vaccine. *Am J Public Health* 50:1013–1031, 1960.

18. Melnick JL: Variation in poliomyelitis virus on serial passage through tissue culture. *Cold Spring Harb Symp Quant Biol* 18:178–179, 1953.

19. Melnick JL, Brennan JC: Monkey neurovirulence of attenuated poliovirus vaccines being used in field trials, in *Live Polio Virus Vaccine.* Pan American Health Organization, pp 65–101, 1959.

20. Melnick JL, Proctor RO, Ocampo AR, et al: Free and bound virus in serum after administration of oral poliovirus vaccine. *Am J Epidemiol* 84:329–342, 1966.

21. Melnick JL, Wenner HA, Phillips GA: Enteroviruses, in Lennette EH, Schmidt NJ (eds), *Diagnostic Procedures for Viral, Rickettsial, and Clamydial Infections,* 5th ed. Washington, DC, American Public Health Association, pp 471–534, 1979.

22. Melnick JL, Wimberly IL: Lyophilized combination pools of enterovirus equine antisera: New LBM pools prepared from reserves of antisera stored frozen for two decades. *Bull WHO* 63:543–550, 1985.

23. Metcalf TG, Melnick JL, Estes MK: Environmental virology: From detection of virus in sewage and water by isolation to identification by molecular biology—A trip of over 50 years. *Annu Rev Microbiol* 49:461–487, 1995.

24. Modlin JF: Poliomyelitis and poliovirus immunization, in Rotbart HA (ed), *Human Enterovirus Infections.* Washington, DC, American Society for Microbiology, 1995, pp 195–220.

25. Murray R, Kirschstein G, Van Hoosier G, Baron S: Comparative virulence for rhesus monkeys of poliovirus strains used for oral administration, in *Live Polio Virus Vaccine.* Pan American Health Organization, 1959, pp 39–64.

26. Nolan JP, Wilmer BJ, Melnick JL: Poliomyelitis: Its highly invasive nature and narrow stream of infection in a community of high socioeconomic level. *New Engl J Med* 253:945–954, 1955.

27. Ogra PL, Faden HS, Abraham R, et al: Effect of prior immunity on the shedding of virulent revertant virus in feces after oral immunization with live attenuated poliovirus vaccines. *J Infect Dis* 164:191–194, 1991.

28. Paul JR, Riordan JT, Melnick JL: Antibodies to three different antigenic types of poliomyelitis virus in sera from North Alaskan Eskimos. *Am J Hyg* 54:275–285, 1951.

29. Paul JR: *A history of poliomyelitis.* New Haven, Yale University Press, 1971.

30. Ren R, Racaniello VR: Human poliovirus receptor gene expression and poliovirus tissue tropism in transgenic mice. *J Virol* 66:296–304, 1992.

31. Rezapkin GV, Chumakov KM, Lu Z, et al: Microevolution of Sabin 1 strain in vitro and genetic stability of oral poliovirus vaccine. *Virology* 202:370–378, 1994.

32. Rezapkin GV, Norwood LP, Taffs RE, et al: Microevolution of type 3 Sabin strain of poliovirus in cell cultures and its implications for oral poliovirus vaccine quality control. *Virology* 211:377–384, 1995.

33. Rueckert RR: Picornaviridae and their replication, in Fields BN, Knipe DM, Chanock RM, et al (eds), *Fields Virology,* 2d ed. New York, Raven, 1990, pp 507–548.

34. Rotbart HA (ed): *Human Enterovirus Infections.* Washington, DC, American Society for Microbiology, 1995.

35. Sabin AB, Hennessen WA, Winsser J: Studies on variants of poliomyelitis virus: I. Experimental segregation and properties of avirulent variants of three immunologic types. *J Exp Med* 99:551–576, 1954.

36. Sabin AB: Paralytic poliomyelitis: Old dogmas and new perspectives. *Rev Infect Dis* 3:543–564, 1981.

37. Sabin AB: Recent studies and field tests with a live attenuated poliovirus vaccine, in *Live Polio Virus Vaccine.* Pan American Health Organization, 1959, p 33.

39. Smith LK: Current issues in neurological rehabilitation: Part I, in Umphred DA (ed), *Neurological Rehabilitation.* St. Louis,

39. Smith LK: Current issues in neurological rehabilitation: Part I, in Umphred DA (ed), *Neurological Rehabilitation.* St. Louis, Mosby–Year Book, 1990, pp 1–11.

40. Tulchinsky TH, Handsher R, Melnick JL, et al: Immune status to various strains of wild poliovirus among children in Gaza immunized with live attenuated oral vaccine alone compared with a combination of live and inactivated vaccines. *J Vir Dis* 1:3:5–13, 1994.

41. Von Magnus H, Melnick JL: Tonsillectomy in experimental poliovirus. *Am J Hyg* 48:113–119, 1948.

42. Von Magnus H, Petersen I: Vaccination with inactivated poliovirus vaccine and oral poliovirus vaccine in Denmark. *Rev Infect Dis* 6:S471–S474, 1984.

43. Ward R, Melnick JL, Hortsmann DM: Poliomyelitis virus in fly-contaminated food collected at an epidemic. *Science* 101:491–493, 1945.

44. World Health Organization: Poliomyelitis in 1985–1989. *Wkly Epidemiol Rec* 62:273–280, 1987; 64:273–279, 1989; 66:49–53, 70–72, 1991.

45. Zamula E: A new challenge for former polio patients. *FDA Consumer,* June, 1991.

PROTOZOAN INFECTIONS OF THE THORAX

J e f f r e y K . G r i f f i t h s / D a v i d J . W y l e r

Although debilitating and even fatal protozoal infections are among the most prevalent infections worldwide, they rarely involve the lungs and pleura. In temperate climates, protozoal pulmonary infections occur primarily in patients who are immunosuppressed, typically by virtue of infection with the human immunodeficiency virus (HIV) or because they are receiving potent immunosuppressive drugs. Protozoal involvement of thoracic structures generally occurs as a complication of infection at other sites, which leads to signs and symptoms that usually dominate the initial clinical presentation. These complications may require specific therapeutic interventions, which in the case of malaria or amebiasis, for example, can be lifesaving. This chapter reviews the pulmonary complications of important protozoal infections and provides an overview of the systemic features of these infections.

Pulmonary complications or infections with other protozoans, such as free-living amoebae, *Toxoplasma* (toxoplasmosis), *Babesia* (babesiosis), *Cryptosporidium* (cryptosporidiosis), *Leishmania* (leishmaniasis), and *Microsporida* (microsporidiosis) have recently been recognized. In this chapter we will review the etiology, epidemiology, transmission, pathophysiology, clinical features, treatment, and prevention of these diseases. The incidence of pulmonary amebiasis is now matched at many institutions by the incidence of newer emerging infections.

AMEBIASIS

Etiology and Epidemiology

Entamoeba histolytica is the causative agent of amebiasis.[1,2,5,22,23,24,30,44,60] A number of other *Entamoeba* species, such as *E. coli, gingivalis, hartmani,* and *polecki,* are found as commensals in the intestinal tracts of humans and other hosts, but they have rarely if ever been convincingly incriminated in invasive intestinal disease. Liver abscess, and the associated complication of thoracic disease, can be considered exclusively caused by *E. histolytica*. This amoeba is found worldwide, both in humans and in ground waters such as lakes and streams. It has been found throughout North America, Europe, Asia, Africa, Central and South America, the Caribbean, and South and Southeast Asia. Indeed, the clinician should think of the parasite as ubiquitous. As the apocryphal Mexican saying goes, "There are only two kinds of people in the world: Those who know they have amoebas and those who do not."

E. histolytica is the cause of much morbidity and mortality in the developing world, where infection rates of approximately 50 percent are common. Recent epidemics of disease in the developed world have been related to both point-source and multicentric propagative outbreaks in institutions and in specific populations. Risk groups in North America include migrant workers, immigrants, travelers, sexually active male homosexuals, lower socioeconomic groups in the southern United States, and institutionalized groups, such as prisoners, orphans, children in day care centers, and the mentally ill or retarded.[44] Within some of these risk groups, such as practicing male homosexuals and institutionalized persons, carriage rates may exceed 50 percent. In North America the populationwide infection rate is thought to be about 4 to 5 percent. Globally, about 10 percent of the world's population is infected with *E. histolytica,* and about 100,000 deaths per year occur secondary to amebiasis.[44] Persistence of infection in a population is a complex interaction between sanitation, personal hygiene, water and food supplies, socioeconomic status, and crowding.

Environmentally robust cysts are ingested by the human host, and after surviving passage through the stomach, trophozoite forms of the parasite are released in the small intestine. Trophozoites are carried to the ileum and colon, where they reproduce by binary fission. Cysts are formed only in the colon, and it has been theorized that encystation is due to unfavorable colonic conditions that do not support further trophozoite growth. Cysts are able to survive in the environment for weeks to months, whereas trophozoites die rapidly after leaving the body.

Cysts of the parasite are spherical and are 5 to 20 μm in diameter, with a mean of 12 μm, and are found in the fecal stream of infected individuals. Depending on the maturity of the cyst, it contains one to four nuclei, which are identical to the nucleus found in the trophozoite. Trophozoites are the motile replicating form that breach the intestinal barrier and cause invasive disease. Trophozoites are 12 to 60 μm in diameter, with a mean of approximately 25 μm. The circular nucleus contains clumped, or beaded, peripheral nuclear chromatinin and a central prominent karyosome (nucleolus). Only one nucleus is seen in the trophozoite form. The trophozoite cytoplasm contains vacuoles and often has a granular characteristic. Movement is accomplished by the extension of cytoplasmic pseudopods, which differentiate *E. histolytica* from the free-living amoebae *Naegleria* and *Acanthamoeba,* which can also cause invasive disease as discussed below; *E. histolytica* is the only intestinal amoeba that ingests red blood cells, which process, seen in a section or biopsy from tissue, secures the diagnosis. The invasive manifestations of amebiasis include dysentery, liver abscess, and the uncommon extraintestinal infections of the lung, brain, skin, and other more rare sites. Despite the ability of the parasite to do these deeds, the vast majority of individuals with intestinal *E. histolytica* suffer no adverse consequences.

In recent years, much has been written on the biochemical and genetic evidence separating *E. histolytica* into distinct pathogenic and nonpathogenic strains. The former are uniformly found in invasive disease and the latter in asymptomatic individuals. However, about 1 percent of infected, asymptomatic people carry the invasive type of *E. histolytica,* and about 10 percent of this group (1 in 1000 overall) will eventually develop invasive amebiasis. Those who carry the nonpathogenic strains tend to clear the infestation within 1 year. Differentiation into pathogenic and nonpathogenic strains has been accomplished by zymodene analysis, genomic DNA differences, and restriction fragment [polymerase chain reaction (PCR)] techniques. Some have suggested that the pathogenic organisms be reclassified into a new species, *Entamoeba dispar,* but there is no clinically available method to differentiate "*dispar*" isolates from "*histolytica*" isolates. Perhaps diagnostic techniques will improve to the point where noninvasive organisms can be identified and left untreated, but this is not now the case. Current practice is to eradicate the organism when found, as there is no way to differentiate the uncommon invasive strain from its more benign relative. In the absence of symptoms or signs of illness, eradicating the organism from patients in heavily contaminated environments where reinfestation and reinfection are likely is pointless.

Transmission

The organism is classically spread through fecal–oral contamination. Routes of transmission include contaminated food and water, person-to-person contact with cyst passage, and sexual practices that include fecal–oral contact. Person-to-person spread is now considered more important than contaminated food or water in the United States. With very rare exception, the form of the parasite that is responsible for transmission is the cyst. Cases of transmission of amebiasis after colonic irrigation or endoscopy may be the exceptions that prove this rule. Attempts to stop transmission in institutions via mass treatment, or by quarantining cyst passers, have in general failed. In addition to the high-risk groups mentioned earlier, one must note that malnourished individuals and children tend to suffer more acutely than do their well-nourished or older peers.

Pleuropulmonary complications have been estimated to occur in 1 in 1000 patients, and when the liver is involved, the incidence rises substantially to 15 to 20 percent. For unknown reasons men outnumber women by 10- to 15-fold in many published series, and the peak ages for pulmonary amebiasis are between 20 and 40 years. It is unclear if these predilections are real or if they represent reporting bias.

Pathophysiology

Entry into the thorax is most commonly the result of extension of liver disease, such as abscess. Other routes exist, such as hematogenous spread that can lead to metastatic brain, lung, and other abscesses, although the frequency of these pathways is far lower. Amebae that have broached the mucosal barrier are thought to gain entry to the liver via the portal vein. Subsequent liver abscesses can be either purely amebic or mixed bacterial and amebic. Because normal defenses against amoebae are far less efficient than defenses against less complex creatures such as bacteria, these abscesses tend to progress and may extend or rupture into the pleural space or the peritoneum in 10 to 20 percent of cases if not treated. There is some evidence to suggest that extension of amebic infections across the diaphragm via lymphatics may occur.

E. histolytica has a large array of pathogenic properties. It produces a surface lectin that allows it to adhere to mucosal epithelial cells, leukocytes, erythrocytes, submucosal colonic cells, and even bacteria that have galactose-containing lipopolysaccharides. Amoebae only kill cells after direct contact. Once contact has been made, the host cell suffers a marked and sustained elevation of intracellular calcium. In addition, a parasitic saponinlike compound has been identified in parasite granules that may contribute to dissolution of host cell membranes. Proteolytic enzymes are released into the extracellular milieu and may help in dissolving the host. Targeted host cells may also die via induced suicide, that is, apoptosis, and this host-induced suicide process is not inhibitable by the *bcl*-2 gene. The initial host cell response is that of host polymorphonuclear leukocytes; when they are lysed by the amoebae, neutrophil contents contribute to the inflammatory and destructive lesion.

Indeed, host immunity is not very effective in the virginal host. Although individuals cured of invasive amebiasis develop high titres of antibody and appear resistant to *subsequent* infection, the serum responses of the host during *primary* invasive disease do not appear to be helpful. By the end of the first week of illness naive hosts will develop antiamebocidal antibody that will inhibit amebic attachment in vitro, but they will nonetheless have progressive, unremitting disease. Antibody to amoebae appears to act via activation of the classical and alternate complement system—but trophozoites purified from invasive lesions are resistant to complement-mediated lysis. In contrast, trophozoites found in the intestinal lumen are sensitive to complement, perhaps explaining the mechanism by which antibody is able to prevent reinvasion in the experienced host. Thus, the host antibody response is useful in preventing subsequent invasive episodes but is not of much use in the initial event. Similarly, cell-mediated immunity is of some benefit but is not paramount. For example, people with AIDS do not appear to have a higher incidence of invasive amebiasis compared to HIV-seronegative individuals, suggesting that the mucosal immune response is not tightly associated with cellular immunity. Nonetheless, amebic disease can be fulminant in the malnourished, in the very young, in those given steroids, and in pregnant women, in whom cell-mediated responses are blunted. The reader should take away from this discussion a healthy respect for how poor the human immune response is to this pathogen.

CLINICAL PRESENTATIONS OF THORACIC AMEBIASIS

True thoracic disease complicates 7 to 20 percent of hepatic disease and about 2 percent of intestinal disease. Three major forms of pleuropulmonary disease have been well described. Perhaps most common is a *sympathetic* or *neighbor* reaction to an unruptured abscess within the liver. Another common presentation is empyema, after rupture of the liver abscess into the pleural space. Rupture of a liver abscess can also result in the third major presentation, that of parenchymal involvement with abscess, consolidation, or hepatobronchial fistula. Because the major route of invasion into the lung and thorax is the liver, elevation of the right hemidiaphragm is one of the earliest signs of thoracic involvement. Indeed, most thoracic disease is within the right hemithorax, since 80 percent of liver abscesses are located within the right lobe of the liver. Dyspnea (5 percent), cough (10 percent), right hemithorax pain (10 percent), and right shoulder pain (about 30 percent) have been reported in individuals with liver abscess. The pain may be pleuritic or abdominal, and many people with liver abscess will appear to have a predominantly pulmonary disease, with fever, chills, chest pain, cough, and weight loss. Right lower lobe consolidative signs and/or effusion may be present in nearly half of all patients with liver abscess. Figure 155-1 shows typical chest radiograph findings, alveolar space amoebae, and necrotic changes.

Clinical signs helpful to the diagnosis of an amebic liver abscess include pain and tenderness in the right upper quadrant, a palpable liver, and fever; each of these signs is found in about 75 percent of patients. Localized intercostal pain is present between the midaxillary and midclavicular lines on the right in most patients. Hepatobronchial fistula formation may be marked by the presence of foul, "anchovy paste" or "chocolatey" sputum. Approximately half of those with thoracic disease will develop a hepatobronchial fistula, versus about 30 percent who develop an effusion and empyema. Lung abscess occurs in about 14 percent and true consolidation alone in about 10 percent of patients.

Individuals with thoracic disease should *always* be evaluated for possible pericardial infection. The latter can lead to cardiac tamponade and death, congestive heart failure or pericarditis, or simply to a slow unremitting clinical deterioration. Pericardial disease is thought to occur most frequently after rupture of an adjacent abscess, often from the left lobe of the liver, into the pericardium. Pericardial effusions should be seen as a warning of impending rupture. In Mexico City, Ibarra-Perez noted pericardial disease in about 10 percent of patients referred for thoracic complications.[24] In contrast, in Adams and MacLeod's series of more than 5000 patients, it was a complicating factor in just over 1 percent of the patients.[1,2]

Diagnosis of Hepatic and Thoracic Amebiasis

Radiographic and ultrasonic investigations may be very helpful in delineating the architectural confines of the disease, as may computerized tomography. Liver abscess may be confirmed with ultrasound or CT evaluations; most disease is in the right lobe of the liver (about 80 percent), and the abscesses are usually spherical. Differentiation between bacterial, amebic, and mixed bacterial and amebic infections may be difficult. Happily for the diagnostician, serologic tests are usually positive (about 95 percent) in those with invasive disease and negative in those without invasion. The hoary tradition of making the diagnosis by aspiration of the abscess is now rarely needed, given the availability of serologic testing, and is usually needed in only a small percentage of patients. Therapeutic drainage in toxic patients is required in only about 5 percent of individuals.

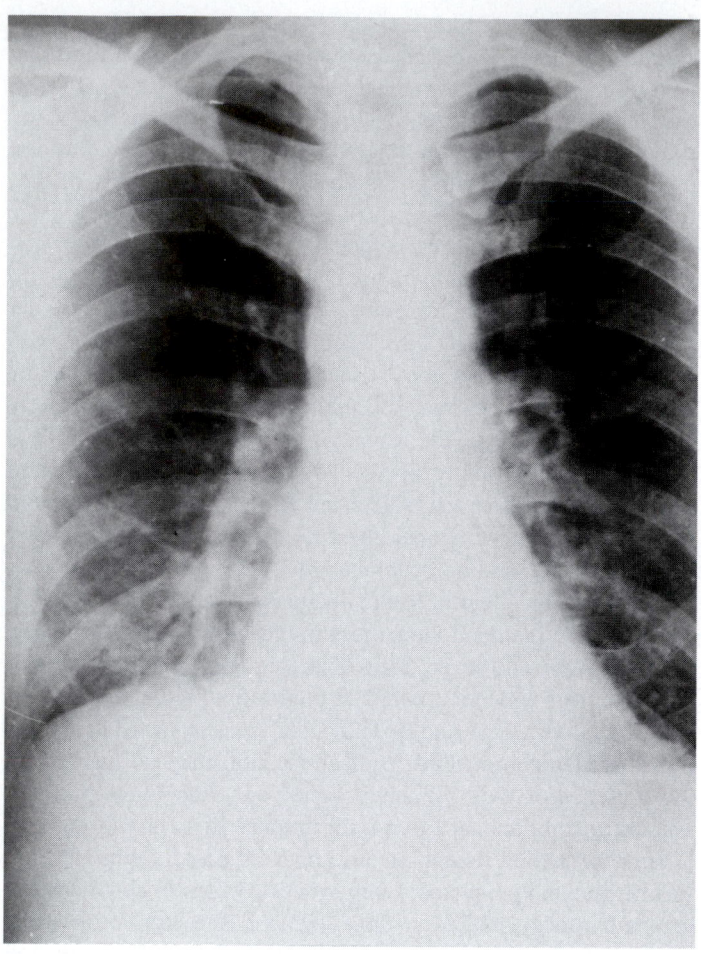

A

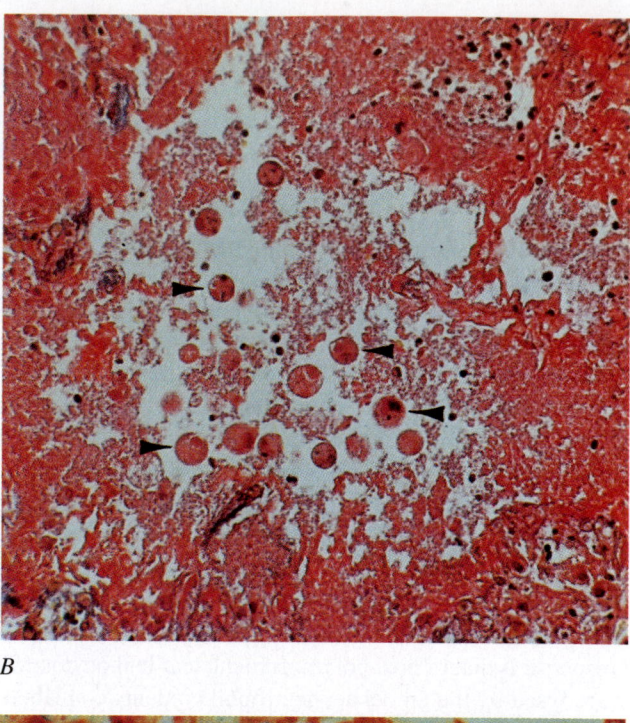

B

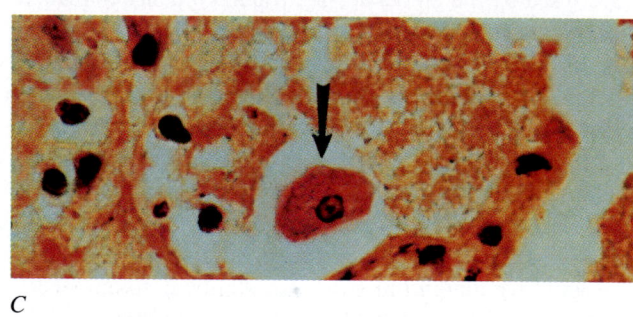

C

FIGURE 155-1 *Entamoeba histolytica* involving the right lung after rupture of a hepatic abscess through the right hemidiaphragm. *A.* Chest radiograph shows elevated right hemidiaphragm, right lower lobe infiltrate, and effusion. *(Courtesy of Armed Forces Institute of Pathology.)*

B. Alveolar spaces are filled with amebic cysts (arrowheads). *(Iron hematoxylin stain, ×300; courtesy of Dr. Y. Gutierrez.) C.* Trophozoites (arrow) and necrotic debris.

Early on, elevation of the right hemidiaphragm is found in more than half the patients. As noted above, atelectasis and a sympathetic reaction may be seen sympathetic to subdiaphragmatic abscess. When present, effusions must be delineated, as they may represent empyema, and aspiration of fluid for diagnostic studies is required. More convincing evidence of extension into the thorax includes overt consolidative changes, abscess, or fistula formation. As noted above, pericardial disease may occur, usually after rupture of an adjacent abscess into the pericardial space, and ultrasonic or CT evaluation of the pericardium is warranted if there is any question of pericardial disease.

Treatment

Treatment for hepatic or pulmonary disease consists of drainage when indicated (toxemia, empyema, pericarditis) and drug therapy. Metronidazole is both inexpensive and effective, given at a dose of 750 mg three times daily orally or by vein for at least 10 days. Iodoquinol (650 mg three times daily orally for 20 days), paromomycin (500 mg four times daily orally), chloroquine, or

diloxanide are used to eliminate parasites from the gut. Very serious complications of abscess, such as rupture into the abdomen with peritonitis, or pericardial disease, can be treated with dehydroemetine. Therapeutic options are outlined in Table 155-1.

FREE-LIVING AMOEBAE: *NAEGLERIA* AND *ACANTHAMOEBA*

Free-living amoebae rarely infect humans, but when they do, the results are devastating, and the outcome is almost always death. Three conditions have been classically associated with these organisms: primary meningoencephalitis due to *Naegleria fowleri*, subacute meningoencephalitis after hematogenous spread of dermal or pulmonary disease with an *Acanthamoeba* species, and keratitis secondary to *Acanthamoeba*. Unlike *E. histolytica*, infection with one of these agents does not appear related to sanitation and hygiene levels, nor is any vector known for these organisms. It appears that transmission to the human occurs after contact with the amoeba in its natural, free-living state. These amoebae are discussed here because the diagnosis of pulmonary

TABLE 155-1

Therapy of Amebiasis with *Entamoeba Histolytica*

Syndrome	Drugs of Choice	Adult Dosage	Pediatric Dosage
Severe intestinal, hepatic, thoracic, or pericardial disease*	Metronidazole	750 mg tid × 10 days of longer (abscess, empyema, etc.)	35–50 mg/kg per day divided into three doses for 10 days
	Tinidazole†	800 mg tid (abscess, empyema, etc.) for at least 5 days; 600 mg po bid may be used for intestinal disease without abscess	50–60 mg/kg per day divided into two or three doses for 3–5 days (maximum dose of 2 g total per day)
Mild to moderate intestinal disease	Metronidazole	750 mg tid × 10 days	35–50 mg/kg per day divided into three doses for 10 days
	Tinidazole	2 g total daily dose for 3 days	50 mg/kg per day divided tid for 3 days; maximum 2 g
Asymptomatic	Iodoquinol‡	650 mg tid × 20 days	30–40 mg/kg per day divided into three doses × 20 days (maximum of 2 g total per day)
	Paromomycin	25–35 mg/kg per day divided into three doses × 7 days	25–35 mg/kg per day divided into three doses × 7 days
	Diloxanide furoate§	500 mg tid × 10 days	20 mg/kg per day divided into three doses × 10 days

*Surgical drainage is often not required for liver abscess but is mandatory in empyema or pericarditis (see accompanying text). Treatment of systemic disease should be followed by treatment with a luminal agent to rid the host of intestinal luminal amebiasis.
†Tinidazole and ornidazole are not marketed in the United States but are available elsewhere. Tinidazole is at least as effective as, and better tolerated than, metronidazole.
‡Dosing of iodoquinol should not be exceeded, as optic neuritis is a complication of therapy. No more than 2 g per day total should be administered.
§In the United States, diloxanide furoate is available through the CDC Drug Service, Centers for Disease Control and Prevention, Atlanta, GA, (404) 639-3670.

disease with *Acanthamoeba* may allow the institution of life-saving therapy before meningoencephalitis begins. *Leptomyxid* species of amoebae behave similarly to *Acanthamoeba* species, have rarely been isolated from humans with granulomatous subacute meningoencephalitis, and should be mentioned in passing as they appear to act identically to *Acanthamoeba*.

Naegleria fowleri is found worldwide in surface waters, in soil, river, and lake waters, and in thermally polluted wastewater sites. Its presence is directly related to temperature, and it thrives up to 45°C. Acquisition of the disease often occurs in children and young adults after swimming in fresh water. In the United States it has been reported most frequently in the southeastern states, probably because of the presence of warm fresh waters. *Naegleria* probably invades the central nervous system after disruption of the olfactory mucosa, penetration of the submucosal nervous plexus and the cribiform plate, and subsequent entrance into the CNS. This disease is acute in onset and rapidly progressive.

In contrast, *Acanthamoeba* species cause CNS infections after hematogenous spread of amoebae from the skin, lungs, or other sites.[51] *Acanthamoeba* species have also been isolated from soil and water from diverse origins. The hosts for these infections also differ: *N. fowleri* infections occur in normal hosts in excellent health, whereas *Acanthamoeba* infections tend to occur in those with AIDS, diabetes mellitus, pregnancy, liver disease, malignancies with or without steroid or chemotherapy treatment, and transplantation. *Acanthamoeba* infections are probably more common than recognized and have been reported from a variety of animal species as well as humans. For example, *A. culbertsoni* was isolated from the lung lesions of a 1-year-old greyhound puppy that was one of several dogs that died of a progressive respiratory and then neurological illness in a kennel.[4] The similarity of this presentation in canines and that of human illness is striking. Despite the small number of reported cases, however, the potential for infection is probably large, as these amoebae have been found in surprising locations. Investigations designed to study respiratory viruses in healthy families found that 38 of 2289 individuals had culturable *Acanthamoeba* species in their pharynx.[59] These results have recently been confirmed by a study in Spain, in which two *Acanthamoeba* isolates were found in the nasal and pharyngeal mucus of 58 children in Madrid.[32] One of the two isolates was found to be highly pathogenic in mice.[32] Eye wash stations, helpful in flushing noxious chemicals from the eye in manufacturing or laboratory settings, have also been found to be contaminated with *Acanthamoeba*; indeed, these amoebae caused persistent pulmonary infections in inoculated mice.[55]

The onset of *Acanthamoeba* disease is insidious, and focal neurological deficits are common. Classically the host response is granulomatous, but if the host is immunosuppressed this may be absent. Usually the primary site in the lungs or skin has been present for weeks to months before the CNS disease becomes apparent. Lesions in the brain spare the leptomeninges except when there are overlying areas of cortical involvement. Cerebral edema is common, as is death from uncal or tonsillar herniations. The necrotizing granulomatous lesions contain perivascular motile trophozoites and cysts. The perivascular nature of the lesions has suggested hematogenous spread. *Acanthamoeba* keratitis is associated with the use of contact lenses and minor corneal trauma and occurs in normal hosts like *N. fowleri* infections do.

Two patients with *Acanthamoeba* meningoencephalitis after bone marrow transplantation were recently described.[3] They presented with fever and nodular pulmonary infiltrates 6 and 9 months after transplantation for leukemia. Both patients had a history of sinusitis and had been treated with steroids. One of the two had painful subcutaneous nodules that ulcerated. Mental obtundation, seizures, and coma occurred, and CT scan findings included hydrocephalus. Cerebrospinal fluid (CSF) findings included low glucose and elevated protein levels and little or no pleocytosis. At autopsy one patient was found to have necrotizing meningoencephalitis, pneumonitis, and adrenalitis, and the second had meningoencephalitis and dermatitis. Thus the clinician should include this amebic disease in the differential diagnosis of nodular pulmonary infiltrates in the immunosuppressed patient.

Diagnosis is made by finding the amoeba in histological samples; unhappily, diagnosis has almost always been at autopsy. Brain, or by extension lung or skin, biopsy is the only way to make the diagnosis during life, as the organism has not been isolated from the CSF of a patient with granulomatous amebic encephalitis. Lumbar puncture is often contraindicated because of the risk of herniation.

At times, culture is the only way to diagnose the infection. A nonnutrient agar overlaid with killed *E. coli* or *Aero-bacter aerogenes* will support the growth of *Acanthamoeba,* often when biopsy material is negative. Cysts and trophozoites can be visualized with Wright, Giemsa, hematoxylin-eosin, and periodic-Schiff stains. Calcofluor white, which is a fluorescent laundry detergent brightener, will also stain the organisms in biopsy specimens.

Treatment of *Acanthamoeba* infections has been dismally poor in cases of meningoencephalitis; cases of keratitis have been more successfully treated. This is likely to be the result of ear-lier recognition of ocular disease, the fact that debridement of the cornea can be undertaken easily, and the ability to achieve high local concentrations of drugs using topical therapy. None of these are true with systemic forms of *Acanthamoeba*. Amphotericin B, neomycin, 5-fluorocytosine, paromomycin, ketoconazole, and miconazole have in vitro activity. In general, each clinical isolate should be tested for sensitivities to these drugs as well as the most effective class, the diamidine group, which includes propamidine and pentamidine. Table 155-2 outlines some of the therapeutic options.

MALARIA

Infection with *Plasmodium falciparum* (falciparum malaria) should be considered a medical emergency because a delay in diagnosis and in the institution of appropriate therapy can result in death. However, because the signs and symptoms of malaria can mimic those of a variety of other diseases, the correct diagnosis may be elusive unless it is considered in any patient with fever who has an appropriate exposure history. Examination of appropriately stained blood smears is the only conclusive way to establish the diagnosis. Smears should be negative on three consecutive days if malaria is to be ruled out.

Symptoms and signs of respiratory disease frequently accompany even uncomplicated falciparum malaria,[20] whereas respiratory failure is an uncommon, potentially fatal complication of infection. Typically, but not exclusively, respiratory failure accompanies other complications such as renal failure and encephalopathy (cerebral malaria)[12,13] and is best understood in the context of an overview of falciparum malaria.

Biology of *Plasmodium falciparum*

Like the other Plasmodium species that infect humans, *P. falciparum* is transmitted primarily by the bites of mosquitoes. Only

TABLE 155-2

Therapy of *Naegleria* or *Acanthamoeba* Infection

Syndrome	Drugs of Choice	Adult Dosage	Pediatric Dosage
Acanthamoeba meningitis, or systemic or disseminated infection, including pneumonia	Usually susceptible to pentamidine, ketoconazole, flucytosine, and to some extent amphotericin B. Disseminated infection has been treated with pentamidine, chlorhexidine, and ketoconazole, followed by itraconazole.*		
Acanthamoeba keratitis	Usually susceptible to chlorhexidine, polyhexamethylene biguandide, propamide, pentamidine, neomycin, diminazine, or combinations thereof.†		
Naegleria meningitis, or systemic or disseminated infection	Amphotericin B. Successful treatment has been effected with amphotericin B, rifampin, and chloramphenicol; amphotericin B, rifampin, and ketoconazole; and amphotericin B alone.‡	1 mg/kg per day iv for an uncertain period	1 mg/kg per day iv for an uncertain period

*Slater CA et al, *New Engl J Med* 331:85, 1994.
†Hay J et al, *Eye*, 8:155, 1994.
‡Drugs for parasitic infections. *The Medical Letter on Drugs and Therapeutics* 37:99–108, 1995.

rarely does infection result from inoculation of infected blood via blood transfusion, contaminated hypodermic needles, organ transplantation from infected donors, or breaches in barriers of maternal–fetal circulation (congenital malaria). Infected mosquitoes inject sporozoites while taking a blood meal. These extracellular-stage parasites rapidly circulate to the liver where they invade hepatocytes and differentiate as tissue schizonts (also called *hepatic exoerythrocytic* forms). After an incubation period of approximately 2 weeks, thousands of extracellular malaria parasites called *merozoites* are released from the tissue schizonts into the circulation. These merozoites rapidly invade erythrocytes wherein they undergo a cycle of asexual reproduction (schizogony) during a 48-h period, growing at a logarithmic rate. The cycle culminates in the rupture of merozoite-laden erythrocytes. The next cycle is initiated when the just-released merozoites invade other erythrocytes. Schizont rupture is associated with the dramatic features of the malarial paroxysm, most notably high fever and rigors.

In addition to the asexual-stage parasites, gametocytes develop from a subpopulation of merozoites, and, when they are ingested by vector mosquitoes, the sexual cycle is initiated and culminates in the formation of infective sporozoites. The gametocytes are not pathogenic and may persist in the circulation even after successful chemotherapeutic eradication of the asexual-stage parasite.

Pathophysiology of Falciparum Malaria

The current perspective on the complications of falciparum malaria emphasizes the role of tissue hypoxia and the deleterious effects of cytokines (particularly tumor necrosis factor) in the pathogenesis of organ dysfunction.[63] The intravascular location of the infection makes virtually every organ susceptible to insult, but the typical targets are the brain, kidneys, lungs, and gastrointestinal tract. Tissue hypoxia develops by at least two identified mechanisms: reduced oxygen-carrying capacity that results from severe hemolytic anemia, and obstruction to microcirculation that results from the adherence of infected erythrocytes to the postcapillary endothelium of the microcirculation.

Hemolysis occurs when schizont-infected erythrocytes rupture, releasing the many merozoites that give rise to the next generation of intraerythrocytic parasites. Additional mechanisms play secondary roles in the pathogenesis of anemia in malaria. Because asexual parasite replication is logarithmic, a rapid rise in parasitemia is possible, as is the ensuing extensive hemolysis. *Plasmodium falciparum* can grow in erythrocytes of all ages, so theoretically there is no limit to the magnitude of parasitemia that can be attained. In contrast, infection with the *Plasmodium* species that cause nonlethal human malaria is restricted to subpopulations of erythrocytes (e.g., young erythrocytes for *P. vivax* and *ovale*), which limits the attainable parasitemia and consequently also morbidity.

Plasmodium falciparum parasites produce adhesion molecules as they mature within the erythrocyte. The adhesion molecules are translocated to, and become inserted in, the erythrocyte plasma membrane, where they mediate binding of the infected cell to the surface of endothelial cells in postcapillary venules. The cytoadherence that results takes place primarily in postcapillary venular beds and physically obstructs the microcirculation.[63] Obstruction to blood flow, combined with the reduced oxygen-carrying capacity from anemia, compromises normal tissue metabolism.

A third and more recently considered component in the pathogenesis is the substantial elaboration of tumor necrosis factor alpha (TNF-α) during the infection. At the time of schizont rupture, parasite and host-cell-derived materials are released into the circulation, which can stimulate macrophages to produce TNF-α. TNF-α, in turn, can up-regulate its own expression in endothelial cells. TNF-α also induces the expression by endothelial cells of intercellular adhesion molecule–1 (ICAM-1) and certain other adhesins that mediate cytoadherence of infected erythrocytes on endothelial cells and can have direct cytotoxic effects. These pathogenic elements converge to damage endothelial integrity leading to adult respiratory distress syndrome (ARDS). Based on limited data, it was originally proposed that fluid overload, noncardiogenic pulmonary edema, and a vaguely defined "allergic reaction" are the three potential mechanisms of this complication. Subsequent hemodynamic studies in patients with this complication, combined with an increased awareness of the importance of microvascular obstruction, support the current view that the complication is a form of ARDS. Nonetheless it is important to distinguish this complication from cardiogenic pulmonary edema that can be precipitated by anemia and fever in patients with underlying cardiac insufficiency (Fig. 155-2).

Respiratory Failure in Falciparum Malaria

Estimates from the 1940s suggested that some form of pulmonary complication occurs in 3 to 10 percent of patients with falciparum malaria.[12] However, noncardiogenic pulmonary edema occurred in only 3 of 3300 cases of falciparum malaria in military personnel stationed in Vietnam in the mid-1960s.[50] This may represent a more contemporary complication rate that could be expected in cases diagnosed rapidly and treated with appropriate antimalarial therapy and adjunctive supportive care.

The potentially dire consequences of delay in the diagnosis and in institution of appropriate management of respiratory insufficiency in patients with falciparum malaria argues for their early admission to an intensive care unit when respiratory symptoms develop. A benign initial clinical presentation should not dissuade this course, especially if reduced oxygen saturation accompanies the respiratory symptoms. Patients may complain initially of nondiagnostic chest tightness and cough, and within hours can be restless, dyspneic, orthopneic, and cyanotic. Noncardiogenic pulmonary edema can develop very suddenly, even after appropriate antimalarial therapy has been instituted and even after parasites are no longer detected on blood smears. An appropriate parasitological response to antimalarial chemotherapy is no assurance that the patient will not develop late pulmonary complications. The late complication may represent cytokine-mediated pathogenic mechanisms.

The risk of developing noncardiogenic pulmonary edema in falciparum malaria is greatest in patients who have developed renal failure, cerebral malaria, or hyperparasitemia (greater than 5 percent infected erythrocytes) or who are pregnant or immediately postpartum. Evidence of disseminated intravascular coag-

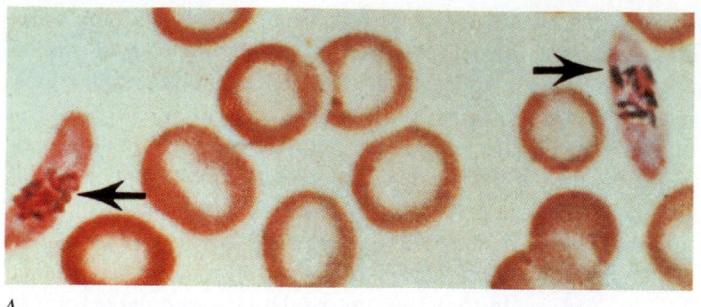

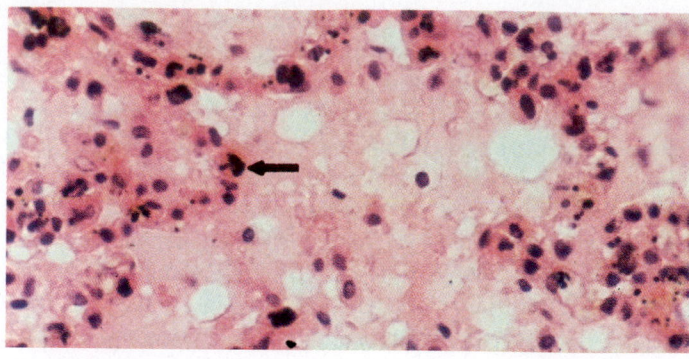

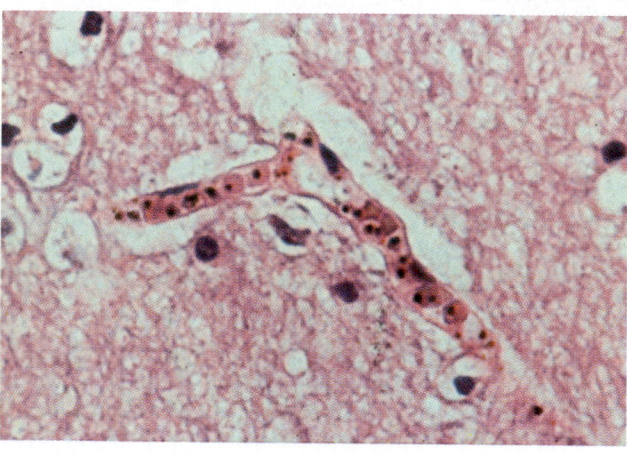

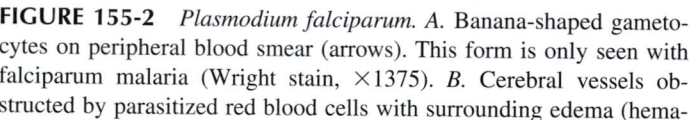

FIGURE 155-2 *Plasmodium falciparum. A.* Banana-shaped gameto-cytes on peripheral blood smear (arrows). This form is only seen with falciparum malaria (Wright stain, ×1375). *B.* Cerebral vessels ob-structed by parasitized red blood cells with surrounding edema (hema-toxylin and eosin stain, ×1375). *C.* Acute pulmonary edema due to pul-monary venular occlusion (organism at arrow; hematoxylin and eosin). *D.* Deposition of malarial pigment (arrows) in vicinity of occluded pul-monary vessels

ulation is a frequent finding.[8,47] The specific therapeutic ap-proaches in malaria, are like those for adult respiratory distress syndrome of other causes. Intravenous quinidine (with continu-ous electrocardiographic monitoring) should be instituted for an-timalarial therapy (see Table 155-3 for therapy). Exchange trans-fusion can achieve the desired rapid reduction in parasitemia and might be lifesaving.[53]

Overall survival of those with pulmonary insufficiency, even with supportive care and parenteral antimalarial chemotherapy, is approximately 25 percent. One potentially useful prognostic indicator is the magnitude of parasitemia at the onset of pul-monary edema. In one series, fatal cases had greater than 30 per-cent parasitemia, whereas survivors had less than 3 percent par-asitemia.[47] Long-term sequelae in survivors have not been assessed systematically.

The therapy for malaria is presented in Table 155-3.

CRYPTOSPORIDIUM PARVUM

Epidemiology and Life Cycle

Cryptosporidium parvum is an ubiquitous organism that appears to be able to infect most if not all mammalian species. Like many other coccidian organisms, *C. parvum* is acquired by ingestion of infectious oocysts in contaminated food and water and has been responsible for major outbreaks of disease in normal and immunosuppressed hosts throughout North America and Europe as well as Africa and other continents. Unlike other coccidians, however, no specific treatment exists for *C. parvum* and it is of-ten lethal in the immunosupressed host. Increasing recognition has been given to its role in infections of the respiratory tract, as well as its well-documented role in diarrhea and wasting in AIDS patients and children. Pneumonia can be the presenting com-plaint in individuals with HIV and cryptosporidiosis, and it is a common though mild complication of intestinal cryptosporidio-sis in the immunocompetent host.

It appears that two species of *Cryptosporidium* infect mam-mals (usually *C. parvum* and, rarely, *C. muris*), whereas other dis-tinct species infect avians (e.g., *C. baileyi*), saurians, or fish; *C. parvum* appears able to cause severe disease in humans and ru-minants such as cattle and sheep. The close ecological association between humans and cattle may foster cross-contamination and sharing of parasites, and many human infections may be zoonotic.

The life cycle of the organism is that of most coccidians. Sporo-zoites are released from the infectious oocysts once they have passed the barrier of the stomach and its acidic milieu. The tissue tropism of the organism appears to be limited to epithelial cells, such as those of the respiratory tree and the intestine, and the ini-tial attachment event is probably mediated by a parasite lectin. These sporozoite forms invade intestinal villus cells and undergo several cycles of asexual replication (schizogony) before micro- and macrogametocytes form and fuse to produce the ookinete, or

TABLE 155-3

Therapy of Malaria with *Plasmodium Falciparum* or Other Species

Syndrome	Drugs of Choice	Adult Dosage	Pediatric Dosage
Chloroquine-resistant *Plasmodium falciparum* (oral therapy)	Quinine sulfate, with one of the following:	650 mg q8h × 3–7 days	25 mg/kg per day divided into three doses for 3–7 days
	Tetracycline	250 mg qid × 7 days	20 mg/kg per day qid × 7 days*
	Pyrimethamine-sulfadoxine†	3 tablets together (500 mg sulfadoxine: 25 mg pyrimethamine per tablet) on the last day of quinine	<1 yr $\frac{1}{4}$ tablet 1–3 yr: $\frac{1}{2}$ tablet 4–8 yr: 1 tablet 9–14 yr: 2 tablets
	Clindamycin (can be used in pregnancy)	900 mg tid × 3–5 days	20–40 mg/k per day tid × 3–5 days
Alternative oral regimens	Mefloquine	1250 mg, administered as 750 mg once followed in 6–8 hours by 500 mg	<45 kgs: 25 mg/kg once
	Halofantrine	500 mg q6h × three doses, repeated in 1 week	<40 kg: 8 mg/kg q6h × three doses, repeated in 1 week
Parenteral therapy	Quinidine gluconate—continuous ECG, glucose, and blood pressure monitoring are required as cardiac conduction abnormalities and hypoglycemia have been reported.	10 mg/kg loading dose (maximum of 600 mg) over 2 h in saline, followed by 0.02 mg/kg per min until oral therapy can be initiated	Same as adult dose
	Quinine dihydrochloride—same cautions as for quinidine.	20 mg/kg loading dose in 5% dextrose water over 4 h, followed by 10 mg/kg over 2–4 h q8h (maximum 1800 mg/d) until oral therapy can be begun.	Same as adult dose
All other malaria, oral therapy	Chloroquine phosphate‡	1 g (600 mg base) then 500 mg 6 h later, then 500 mg at 24 and 48 h	10 mg/kg base, then 5 mg/kg base at 6, 24, and 48 h

Note: Unexplained fever in an individual who has traveled to malarious regions should be pursued as possible malaria. Relapsing malaria caused by *Plasmodium vivax* and *P. ovale* can be prevented by treatment with primaquine phosphate, 15 mg base daily for 14 days or 45 mg base weekly for 8 weeks (0.3 mg base/kg per day × 14 days in children).
*Should be avoided in children under the age of 8. Some clinicians have used doxycycline 100 mg po or iv twice daily instead of tetracycline, but equivalency studies in malaria are lacking.
†Resistance has been confirmed in parts of East Africa, South and Southeast Asia, Pacific islands, and the Amazon basin.
‡Chloroquine-resistant *Plasmodium vivax* has been reported from Indonesia, Papua-New Guinea, India, Myanmar (Burma), and Brazil. A single dose of mefloquine (15 mg/kg) has been used to treat these infections.

fertilized sexual form. The result of this sexual union is a new oocyst, which may be shed in the fecal stream to infect anew. Thus, the organism is acquired and shed in a classic fecal–oral pattern.

The parasite's intracellular location is unique and topologically fascinating. It is intracellular yet extracytoplasmic. The parasite enters the host cell and becomes covered by the host-cell membranes, making it intracellular, yet it does not enter the cytoplasm. At the site of the initial attachment to the host cell, the parasite fuses its membranes with that of the host cell, so that its cytoplasm is separated from that of the host cell by a membrane of dual origin. Thus it remains extracytoplasmic; as it is covered by the host surface membranes, it is intracellular. Other coccidian parasites, such as *Toxoplasma gondii* or the malarial species, fully enter the host and reside in a parasitophorous vac-

uole within the host-cell cytoplasm. This unique location may account for the parasite's striking resistance to therapy that affects other coccidian parasites (discussed below).

The oocyst stage is extremely robust, and it is essentially unaffected by chlorination. Indeed, researchers routinely resuspend fecal samples containing oocysts in dilute bleach to rid the sample of bacteria and other infectious agents, leaving viable intact oocysts behind. Water supplies can (realistically) be rendered free of *C. parvum* oocysts only by filtration, as the oocysts are 3 to 5 μm in size. The estimated cost in the United States of filtering the majority of the country's water supplies to eliminate the risk of cryptosporidiosis transmission is in the range of hundreds of billions of dollars. Unhappily, filtration does not appear to lower the risk to zero.

In a recent epidemic in Las Vegas, a city with an excellent, state-of-the-art filtration and chlorination system, an outbreak of cryptosporidiosis was linked to ingestion of unboiled tap water. Both people with and without HIV infection were infected, despite the inability of researchers to find any *Cryptosporidium* oocysts in samples of water obtained during the epidemic. On an intermittent basis oocysts were found after the investigation in source, filter backwash, and finished water. Of 61 HIV-infected persons who acquired the infection during the first quarter of 1994, 32 were dead by June 30, 1994.[17]

The global epidemiology of this infection is startling and is all the more remarkable given that the infection was essentially unrecognized as a pathogen in humans until 1976, when the first human case was reported. It is now thought to be one of the three most common enteropathogens causing diarrhea in the world.[10] For example, an outbreak of water-borne cryptosporidiosis in Milwaukee during 1993 has been estimated to have caused over 400,000 cases of watery diarrhea.[31] During the early 1980s, persons with AIDS began to present with choleralike diarrhea and wasting after infection with *C. parvum,* prompting its evaluation as a cause of diarrhea in normal and immunosuppressed hosts. Most children throughout the world have been infected by the age of 4, and in these hosts the infection presents as a watery diarrheal illness with cough that persists well beyond that usually seen with viral watery diarrheal illness. Many studies have reported prevalence in fecal samples submitted for analysis to be between 2 and 8 percent, a strikingly high rate for a previously unrecognized pathogen. Transmission in temperate climes is most common during the summer and fall months, as the organism can be killed by freezing of ground waters. Transmission in tropical countries is year-round but more common during the rainy season.

Cryptosporidium parvum is also a significant pathogen of cattle, and, as a major cause of neonatal calf diarrhea, kills about 5 percent of calves in some areas. Household pets such as dogs may also carry the organism on a chronic basis. Many of the described epidemics in the United States and the United Kingdom have been thought to be related to contamination of the water supply by cattle feces. Dairy farmers have been found to be infected by the organism more frequently than their non-dairy-farming peers, as one might predict. Preliminary genetic typing of *C. parvum* isolates obtained from infected humans and calves reveals somewhat different characteristics, and AIDS patients may have illness from either bovine or human isolates. Isolates from AIDS patients given to calves appears to cause more mild disease than isolates from other cattle.

Outbreaks tend to occur in day care centers, institutions, and other relatively closed populations such as family units.[28] Transmission within hospitals is common, and disease in house staff caring for AIDS patients with cryptosporidiosis has been described in the United States. In a Danish hospital, an incontinent psychotic AIDS patient infected at least 18 other AIDS patients (8 of whom died of the disease) after fecally soiling ice in a shared icemaker.

Immunity

Immunity to the parasite is not absolute, even in normal hosts who have had recent infection, as they can become reinfected soon after recovering from the illness. Since this is a disease of the intestinal and respiratory epithelium, it is mucosal immunity that is most relevant to the disease. IgA deficiency has been described as a risk factor for persistent disease, but even in this group it is uncommon. Indeed, AIDS patients with chronic cryptosporidiosis have elevated levels of secretory IgA antibodies in saliva and serum yet are unable to control the infection. In contrast, numerous studies have shown, in both humans and in animal models, that cell-mediated immunity is the critical defense element against the parasite. For example, as AIDS progresses and CD4 helper cell numbers fall, the risk of persistent infection with *C. parvum* increases. Retrospective studies in both the United States and the United Kingdom indicate that a CD4 count of about 180 per cubic microliter is a threshold number, below which recovery from acute infection is distinctly less common than above. Adoptive transfer experiments in murine models tend to support this conclusion. In addition, gamma interferon appears to be a crucial cytokine required for the resolution of infection, without which death occurs in murine models.[57] The immunologic events that occur during acute infection, let alone in infection in AIDS patients, are still poorly characterized overall. Suffice it to say, however, that antibody appears far less important than does cellular immunity.

Pathophysiology of Diarrheal Disease in Cryptosporidiosis

During infection, the architecture of the intestinal villus is altered. The villus becomes short and blunt, contributing to the decreased absorptive capacity of the intestine, and the intestinal crypts may become hyptertrophied. In animal studies of intestinal function, secretory capacity is relatively spared, and absorptive capacity is decreased.[9,41] Localized prostanoid production contributes to the diarrhea by inhibiting Na+ absorption and inducing net chloride secretion. There is some suggestion from animal studies that local tumor necrosis factor production may induce chloride secretion through a paracrine mechanism involving prostaglandin release. One cautionary note is that the much of our understanding of the physiology of cryptosporidiosis is derived from acute infections in immunologically normal animals, not from immunologically deficient animals more akin to humans with AIDS. This is most evident in our current inability to explain the astoundingly profuse diarrhea seen in some AIDS patients, which is most similar to toxin-mediated diarrhea such as cholera.[9] No toxin has ever been isolated from cryptosporidiosis patients or from the organism, though as-yet poorly characterized enterotoxic activities have been described. We are unaware of any physiological studies of pulmonary function during cryptosporidiosis (Fig. 155-3).

Presentations of Intestinal Cryptosporidiosis

As alluded to, intestinal symptoms tend to present in one of two forms. In the first, the naïve host (usually a child) is infected and has an influenzalike illness with mild systemic complaints and watery diarrhea. The illness is usually dismissed by medical workers as a viral diarrhea, although its resolution over several weeks is at the far end of the temporal spectrum for viral diarrhea. Mild malabsorption is common. Disaccharidase enzyme

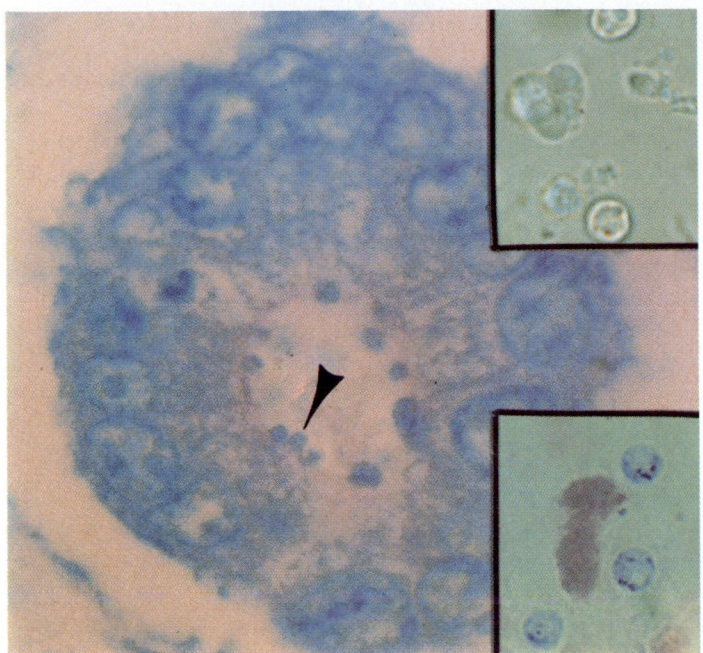

FIGURE 155-3 *Cryptosporidium parvum* infecting an intestinal crypt (arrowhead). Parasites line the apical surface of the epithelial cells and are covered by host membranes. *Insets:* Oocysts isolated from feces: *upper* = organisms isolated after a Sheather's sugar flotation, ×1360; *lower* = Giemsa-Jenner stain, ×1360. (*Courtesy of J. A. Fishman, Massachusetts General Hospital.*)

levels of the intestinal lining decrease during infection, recovering after the infection has resolved. In well-conducted studies performed in West Africa, Guatemala, South America, and South east Asia, cryptosporidiosis is also a predictor of death in malnourished children. These studies can be summarized as suggesting that children with cryptosporidiosis have a death rate approximately two- to fourfold higher than that seen in children with other diarrheal pathogens.[39] It is difficult to tell if the malnutrition these children suffer is a risk factor for acquiring cryptosporidiosis or if the infection is worse in these children given the impaired cellular immunity of malnutrition; it is a classic "chicken or the egg" circumstance (more on the analogies to chickens below . . .).

In the second major form of the disease, it may present as overwhelming fulminant watery diarrhea that is life-threatening. We have cared for individuals who excrete 20 percent of their body weight in diarrheal fluid in a 24-h period, justifying its description as choleralike. Parenteral fluids are lifesaving in this circumstance, and eventual use of parenteral hyperalimentation and fluid replacement is a common fate for the immunosuppressed individual who cannot shake off the illness. Vitamin B12 absorption and D-xylose absorption negatively correlate with the intensity of infection, with intestinal injury in proportion to the number of organisms infecting the intestine.[19] Although data from the Centers for Disease Control and other centers in the United States suggest that about 3 percent of AIDS patients will become infected with cryptosporidiosis during their symptomatic period, in other countries (such as Brazil or Ethiopia) the prevalence rate may be 40 to 50 percent in hospitalized AIDS patients.[28] In Malaysia, 23 percent of intravenous drug users with

AIDS in a drug rehabilitation center had asymptomatic cryptosporidiosis.[27] In this immunosuppressed group the disease is a true scourge. Persistent infection of the biliary and pancreatic ducts can occur, leading to acalculous cholecystitis, obstructive hepatic failure, and pancreatitis. Other immunosuppressed populations, such as those undergoing chemotherapy for malignancies, are similarly at risk.

Respiratory Cryptosporidiosis

The other major manifestation of cryptosporidiosis includes cough and other respiratory symptoms. This is not surprising given the tens or hundreds of billions of oocysts that are excreted by a normal host during infection (to say nothing of the trillions that may be excreted by an AIDS patient with chronic disease) and the ability of the parasite to invade the respiratory tract epithelium. In studies of childhood cryptosporidiosis, cough is one of the most commonly reported symptoms, reported in about one-fifth to one-third of normal children. In 250 Ivoirian children with cryptosporidial diarrhea, 77 percent had profuse diarrhea, 58 percent had fever, and 19 percent had pulmonary symptoms.[29] Pulmonary symptoms are about threefold more frequent in children admitted to hospital with cryptosporidial diarrhea than in children with other intestinal pathogens, based on carefully conducted prospective case-controlled studies.[36] In humans with AIDS, respiratory infection is marked by severe persistent cough and dyspnea.

The major analogous disease is cryptosporidiosis in birds. In avians such as turkeys and chickens, death from respiratory cryptosporidiosis (infected with the related avian species *Cryptosporidium baileyi*) is common. It is unclear why there should be such a high mortality in birds but not in humans. Perhaps the relatively large airways of the human, in contrast to the far narrower avian respiratory tracts, are less prone to occlusion by secretions. Few data in the literature support this or other theories. Many experts in cryptosporidiosis believe that infection of the respiratory tract occurs in most cases of intestinal disease but that it is relatively silent in the absence of other factors. One individual with AIDS and immunosuppressive therapy after allogeneic kidney transplantation has been found to have been infected with *Cryptosporidium baileyi*, with involvement of the trachea, larynx, lungs, and intestines at autopsy.[11]

Respiratory cryptosporidiosis in people with AIDS (as in birds) is manifested by cough, copious tracheal secretions, and dyspnea. In a review from Spain, chronic cough was present in 91 percent, fever in 59 percent, and dyspnea in 64 percent.[7] Although respiratory tract infection was followed by diarrhea in most, the cause of death in most was respiratory in nature. Chest radiographs usually reveal diffuse interstitial infiltrates with bronchial accentuation, which may be difficult to distinguish from other processes, such as *Pneumocystis carinii* pneumonia (PCP). Histologic samples show parasites in the ciliated epithelium and a mononuclear cell infiltrate. Death from respiratory cryptosporidiosis can also occur in individuals with other immunosuppressive conditions, such as malignant lymphoma or bone marrow transplantation.[15] In an immunosuppressed rat model, infection of the respiratory tract leads to respiratory distress, severe weight loss, and enlarged, elastic lungs. Increased mucus production and exfoliative necrosis of the epithelium led to the accumulation of extensive mucocellular exudates in the airways and patchy alveolitis. The scanty data that exist suggest that this is also the case in humans. It would be correct to say, however, that the pathobiology of pulmonary cryptosporidiosis has been far less studied than cryptosporidiosis of the gut.

Respiratory cryptosporidiosis can be the presenting feature of AIDS. In one published report from Copenhagen, 8 of 86 bronchoscopies performed for diagnostic reasons in AIDS patients were positive for *C. parvum* as well as a medley of other (often unsuspected) pathogens.[26] We suspect that if bronchoscopy samples were stained for *C. parvum* on a more routine basis, more cases would be reported in the literature (Fig. 155-4).

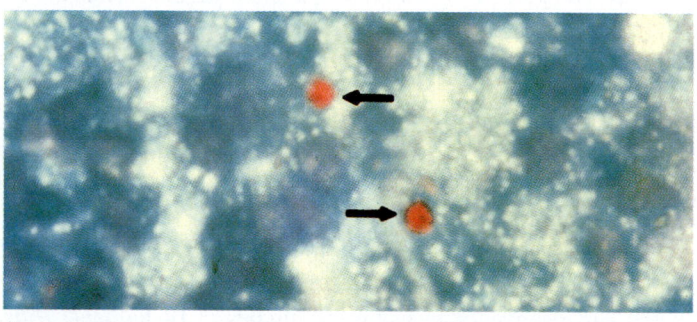

A

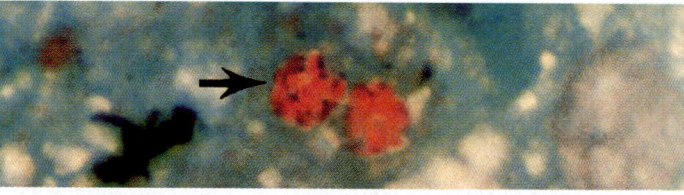

B

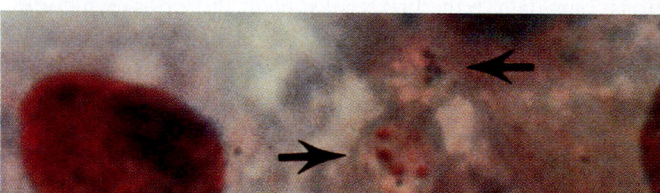

C

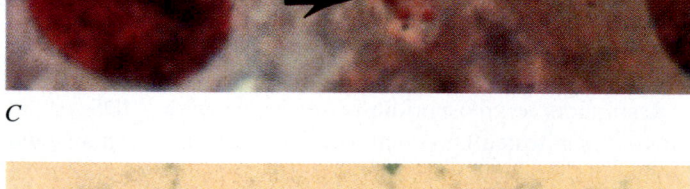

D

FIGURE 155-4 Pulmonary cryptosporidiosis. *A.* Touch preparation from a lung biopsy of a patient with AIDS. Arrows show organisms stained with a modified acid-fast stain (modified cold Kinyoun, MCK), which stains the organisms red (×880). *B.* Same preparation and stain as *A* showing internal red-black dense granules characteristic of the organism. *C.* Same preparation as *A* showing similar morphology using a rapid Giemsa hemacolor stain. *D.* Sputum stained with MCK technique reveals organisms. *(A through D courtesy of Dr. P. Ma.)*

Diagnosis of Respiratory Cryptosporidiosis

The clinician should have a high suspicion of this process in a patient with intestinal cryptosporidiosis. Humans infected with *C. parvum* can have the infection diagnosed by several methods such as biopsy or stool sampling. Biopsies stained with classic hematoxylin and eosin stain should be examined under high oil magnification (×600 to 1200) as the parasites are small and only seen on the epithelial surface and can be mistaken for debris or yeast unless the slide reviewer is attuned to this possibility. Nonetheless the parasites are easily recognized when looked for. The organism can also be detected by performing a modified acid-fast staining of the expectorated sputum, which is classically nonpurulent, or of bronchial brushings or biopsy material obtained at bronchoscopy. The diagnosis of cyptosporidial pneumonia has been made when acid-fast stains have been performed in a quest for tuberculosis. The parasite oocysts are 4 to 5 μm in diameter, avidly acid-fast, and when observed under phase microscopy the oocyst wall may appear somewhat birefringent. A fluorescent monoclonal antibody to the parasite is also commercially available (Meridian Diagnostics, Cincinnati, OH) and can be helpful in confirming the diagnosis. Published series have suggested that the fluorescent antibody is far more sensitive than the acid-fast technique for finding rare parasites in stool samples, although unhappily this is rarely a problem in AIDS patients. Parasite numbers do tend to correlate with the extent of infection and severity of the disease.

Treatment Options

Treatment of cryptosporidiosis is problematic, as no consistently effective drug therapy exists. Paromomycin is an aminocytol (aminoglycoside) type antibiotic that is too toxic for systemic use but has found limited use for specific parasitic infections. It is the most commonly effective agent available, although other agents such as azithromycin and atovoquone have had anectodal success. There is a single case report of inhalation therapy of paromomycin in a case of respiratory infection and hypoxia in a patient with AIDS, which was successful.[38] Because paromomycin is a luminally active agent, it has been shown in animal models to be most successful when used when the flux of diarrhea is not too great.[56] One suspects that this may work to the advantage of the individual given inhaled paromomycin, since the true equivalent of diarrhea of the lung does not exist.

Immunotherapy has been tried with varying degrees of success. One agent has been hyperimmune bovine colostrum administered orally at high doses. Hyperimmune colostrum has antibodies to *C. parvum* of 1 to 100,000 in some preparations, contrasting with titres of about 1 to 1000 in unselected bovine colostrum. This exogenous antibody therapy likely acts by antibody binding to the parasite and blocking successful recognition of the host cell or some other initial event in the invasion process. It has been of help in perhaps half the patients who have received the colostrum, based on our own experience in clinical trials. Nonhyperimmune colostrum is useless. Other immunomodulatory measures, such as placing the patient on antiretroviral drugs if they have AIDS or deferring chemotherapy and allowing the immune system to recover if a malignancy is present, have proved beneficial and at times lifesaving. Malnutrition is characterized by a defect in cell-mediated immunity that normalizes with refeeding. In a study from a nutritional center in Chile, 34 percent of malnourished children had cryptosporidiosis, which spontaneously resolved with nutritional support. Sixty-one percent of these children had respiratory symptoms.[58]

TOXOPLASMOSIS

Etiology and Epidemiology

Toxoplasma gondii is an ubiquitous coccidian parasite that infects all mammals and avians. Its definitive host is the feline (Felidae), be it the house cat or the tiger. Not all *Toxoplasma* infection results in disease, however, and the term *toxoplasmosis* is reserved for those with illness due to the parasite. The parasite persists in the infected host after infection, and thus disease can be either acute or recurrent. The latter is particularly important in the immunosuppressed host, where reactivation can occur as immunity wanes. Pulmonary disease is significant only in the immunosuppressed or congenitally incompetent host.

The life cycle of the parasite is important to understanding its clinical presentations. In its definitive host, the feline, an *intestinal* intraepithelial sexual cycle leads to the passage of oocysts that are 10 to 20 μm in size in the fecal stream. An infected house cat can pass millions of oocysts per day, and the oocysts can persist in the soil for more than a year. They are infectious after sporulation occurs, several days after excretion. In nonfeline hosts such as humans, infection is extraintestinal and asexual. Humans usually acquire the infection by the ingestion of infectious oocysts or by the ingestion of poorly cooked meat that contains cysts filled with the parasite. Vegetables and other crops contaminated with oocysts have also been incriminated in transmission. Human-to-human transmission does not occur except as the result of mother-to-fetus transmission, unless cannibalism is practiced. The ingestion of oocysts or cysts by humans leads to tissue invasion and systemic dissemination of the parasite, as these transmission forms are relatively resistant to stomach acid. Commonly infected mammalian tissues include skeletal and cardiac muscle and brain. Thus steak tartare is an ideal vector for the transmission of this infection. Seropositivity rates in France are high, often over 90 percent of the adult population, in contrast to far lower rates in the United States (3 to 70 percent depending on the region). Infection rates are highest in warm and wet climates with a high density of cats; rates are lowest in high, dry, arid climates with few felines. Congenital infection of the fetus, a major public health problem, almost always occurs as a result of infection during gestation, although rare reports of congenital infection after maternal infection just before conception exist. Other rare modes of transmission include transfusion and organ transplantation.

The invasive active asexual form of *Toxoplasma gondii* is the tachyzoite, which is 3 by 7 μm in size and obligatorily intracellular. The tachyzoite invades host cells, where it multiplies within an intracellular parasitophorous vacuole. Unlike many other intracellular parasites, the tachyzoite can infect nearly any mammalian cell. Eventually the cell lyses, and the motile tachyzoites invade new host cells. In active acute or recurrent disease in immunocompromised humans, this may be the form seen at diagnosis. In the normal host, cysts eventually form, filled with metabolically quiescent bradyzoite parasites. These cysts persist for life, and are 10 to 200 μm in diameter. The bradyzoites can be killed by heating (cooking) above 65°C for 4 min or longer, freezing at −20°C for 24 h or longer with subsequent thawing, or irradiation. Cysts act as a source of infection to the next animal that eats the host or as a source of recrudescent infection should immunity wane.

Immunocompromised people are at great risk of dying from either severe acute or severe recurrent disease. HIV seropositivity or chemotherapy during the treatment of lymphoreticular or hematological malignancy or after organ transplantation are major risk factors. In particular, the receipt of organs from a *Toxoplasma*-seropositive donor by a seronegative recipient has been identified as a major risk. On the basis of experience with cardiac transplantation, it has been theorized that acute infection in the seronegative recipient host is far more dangerous than reactivation of latent disease in the seropositive host. In this latter group, residual antibody may limit disease. Because of the risk of fatal toxoplasmosis in high-risk patients, "baseline" serologic studies for toxoplasmosis are warranted and recommended in those with HIV infection and with lymphomas or leukemias and in patients prior to organ transplantation.

Reactivation of latent disease has been incriminated in many cases of toxoplasmosis in HIV patients. In contrast to the organ transplantation recipient, the HIV-seropositive individual (who has marked dysregulation of both cellular and humoral immunity) who is *Toxoplasma* seropositive (a marker of latent infection) is at much greater risk than the HIV-seropositive, *Toxoplasma*-seronegative person. The estimated risk of an HIV-infected, latently *Toxoplasma*-infected person developing recurrent disease is about 25 to 50 percent. In contrast, the incidence of acute toxoplasmosis in the *Toxoplasma*-seronegative, HIV-seropositive person in the United States is only about 3 percent.

Serologic Testing and Other Diagnostic Methods

Older serologic methods for the detection of *Toxoplasma* antibodies have been replaced in many settings by the availability of enzyme-linked immunosorbent assay (ELISA)-based assays. These include the Sabin-Feldman dye test, the complement fixation test, hemagglutination tests, and the IgM fluorescent antibody test. More modern techniques include ELISA assay methods for both IgG and IgM antibodies, which can assist the clinician in differentiating acute from past exposure. Prior editions of this text, and the references, may be consulted for a thorough description of these largely supplanted techniques. Falling antibody titres in immunocompromised hosts have been associated with active disease, and antibody titres can be unreliable guides in the host with dysregulation of the humoral response, such as with AIDS. In hosts of this nature, a definitive diagnosis rests upon the histological demonstration of parasites or the detection of *Toxoplasma gondii* DNA using molecular techniques. The molecular assays are fundamentally still research tools, and we emphasize that an aggressive attitude toward obtaining biopsy samples is often crucial to the survival of an immunocompromised patient.

In rare instances, body fluids or ground tissues from biopsies can be used to inoculate mice or tissue culture cells to make a diagnosis when serologic methods are unreliable.

CLINICAL SYNDROMES AND DIAGNOSTIC FEATURES

Congenital infection is the result of infection in utero.[49] Central nervous system disease is the major sequela, with chorioretinitis, strabismus, blindness, epilepsy, psychomotor or mental retardation, anemia, encephalitis, pneumonitis, microcephaly, intracranial calcification, hydrocephalus, hepatosplenomegaly, and thrombocytopenia reported. Approximately 1 percent of cases are fatal, about 10 percent are severe, 40 percent are mild, and about 50 percent are asymptomatic in the infantile period. Congenital toxoplasmosis in pregnant women with HIV has been reported to be quite virulent. Infection early in gestation appears to result in increased fetal loss and more severe fetal disease. Recent studies suggest that significant disease such as blindness will occur in a majority of the asymptomatic group with the passage of time, and that anti-*Toxoplasma* drug therapy is indicated.[49] This disease is termed *ocular* or *reactivation toxoplasmosis* and is nearly always the result of congenital infection. Scarring of the retina and underlying choroid occurs, and rupture of cysts later in life may result in new disease.

Acute acquired toxoplasmosis in the immunocompetent host is usually of little long-term concern—80 to 90 percent of these cases are asymptomatic, and asymptomatic cervical lymphadenopathy is the hallmark of this disease. It may be confused with mononucleosis caused by Epstein-Barr virus or cytomegalovirus. Fever, malaise, sore throat, and hepatosplenomegaly are also seen, and the peripheral blood may manifest atypical lymphocytosis. Chorioretinitis may be the most significant long-term problem. Very rarely, acute acquired disease may present with severe dissemination, marked by pneumonitis, hepatitis, encephalitis, polymyositis, or myocarditis. This may be the result of an inadequate host immune response.

Histologically, follicular hyperplasia with cortical and paracortical clusters of epithelioid cells that encroach upon the germinal centers is a classic finding in lymph nodes. Sinus histiocytosis is also seen. In cases of dissemination, pulmonary histologic findings include interstitial pneumonitis with focal necrosis and a mononuclear cell infiltrate. Tachyzoites can be found both within and without host cells, and cysts may also be seen. The latter are only rarely found in the normal host when histologic samples are obtained.

Acute toxoplasmosis in the immunocompromised host is manifested most often by necrotizing encephalitis as a result of brain cyst reactivation. Myocarditis, hepatosplenomegaly, fever, and interstitial pneumonitis are also common, especially if the disease is the result of acute infection and not reactivation of old latent disease. Toxoplasmic encephalitis usually presents subacutely with focal symptoms in about 90 percent of patients. Computerized tomography or magnetic resonance imaging usually shows discrete focal low-density lesions in the brain with ring enhancement with the administration of an enhancing agent. Indeed, focal neurologic deficits with this set of findings in the *Toxoplasma*-seropositive patient should be initially treated as toxoplasma encephalitis, without performance of a brain biopsy. Diffuse encephalitis can occur with toxoplasmosis in this population, though it is uncommon. Pulmonary disease due to toxoplasmosis is being increasingly recognized.

Pulmonary disease in the immunocompromised host with AIDS is usually manifested by prolonged fever, cough, and dyspnea. Rales and a decrease in the percussion note have been observed. Other symptoms and signs of dissemination such as hepatosplenomegaly, headache, myocarditis, and encephalitis may also be present. Blood-borne tachyzoites have been isolated from AIDS patients with this syndrome, supporting the concept of a disseminated disease. Indeed, infection of the bone mar-row, adrenals, lymph nodes, kidneys, and nearly every other organ has been documented in this process. *Toxoplasma* pneumonia may be hard to differentiate from *Pneumocystis carinii* pneumonia, and the two may coexist. The mortality rate in this disease is about one in three. The differential diagnosis in the HIV-seropositive individual includes PCP, disseminated *Mycobacterium tuberculosis,* cryptococcosis, leishmaniasis, coccidioidomycosis, and histoplasmosis. Pulmonary cryptosporidiosis or microsporidiosis is usually far milder and is not associated with fevers of the magnitude seen in *Toxoplasma* pneumonitis. In a thoughtful review of the subject, Pomeroy and Filice[45] have suggested that the term *pulmonary toxoplasmosis* be used to describe those with both apparent and inapparent toxoplasmosis of the lung, and the term *Toxoplasma pneumonia* be reserved for those individuals with clinically apparent disease.

Radiographic patterns include interstitial pneumonia, micronodular infiltrates, nodular densities, cavitation, pleural effusion, and lobar pneumonia. Hilar or mediastinal adenopathy is unusual. Histologically, large numbers of parasites may be seen both free and intracellularly, the latter within epithelial cells or pulmonary macrophages. Hyaline membrane formation, thickened alveolar septae with mononuclear infiltrates, and necrosis due to infarction are found.

Given the large differential diagnosis, bronchoscopy with bronchoalveolar lavage and biopsy are extremely useful in obtaining a secure diagnosis when characteristic CNS disease is lacking or if there is doubt about a single pathogenic process being present. Organisms may be seen within macrophages or other cells, or free in the tissues, and must be differentiated from other intracellular pathogens such as *Leishmania* in the appropriate clinical setting (Figure 155-5). Bronchoalveolar lavage alone will not detect all cases of *Toxoplasma* pneumonitis, and biopsy should be undertaken expeditiously if lavage alone does not reveal the cause of disease.

Pulmonary disease in the immunocompromised host without AIDS is similar to that in AIDS patients with several small differences. In a recent series of 121 patients[25] with organ transplants or underlying malignancies, 23 percent had pulmonary involvement. Most (76 percent) had CNS involvement, and 38 percent had cardiac disease. In the subset that had received transplants, 58 percent had myocarditis. Death or serious morbidity was nearly inevitable if the correct diagnosis was not accomplished (88 of 89 patients).

Therapy is outlined in Table 155-4.

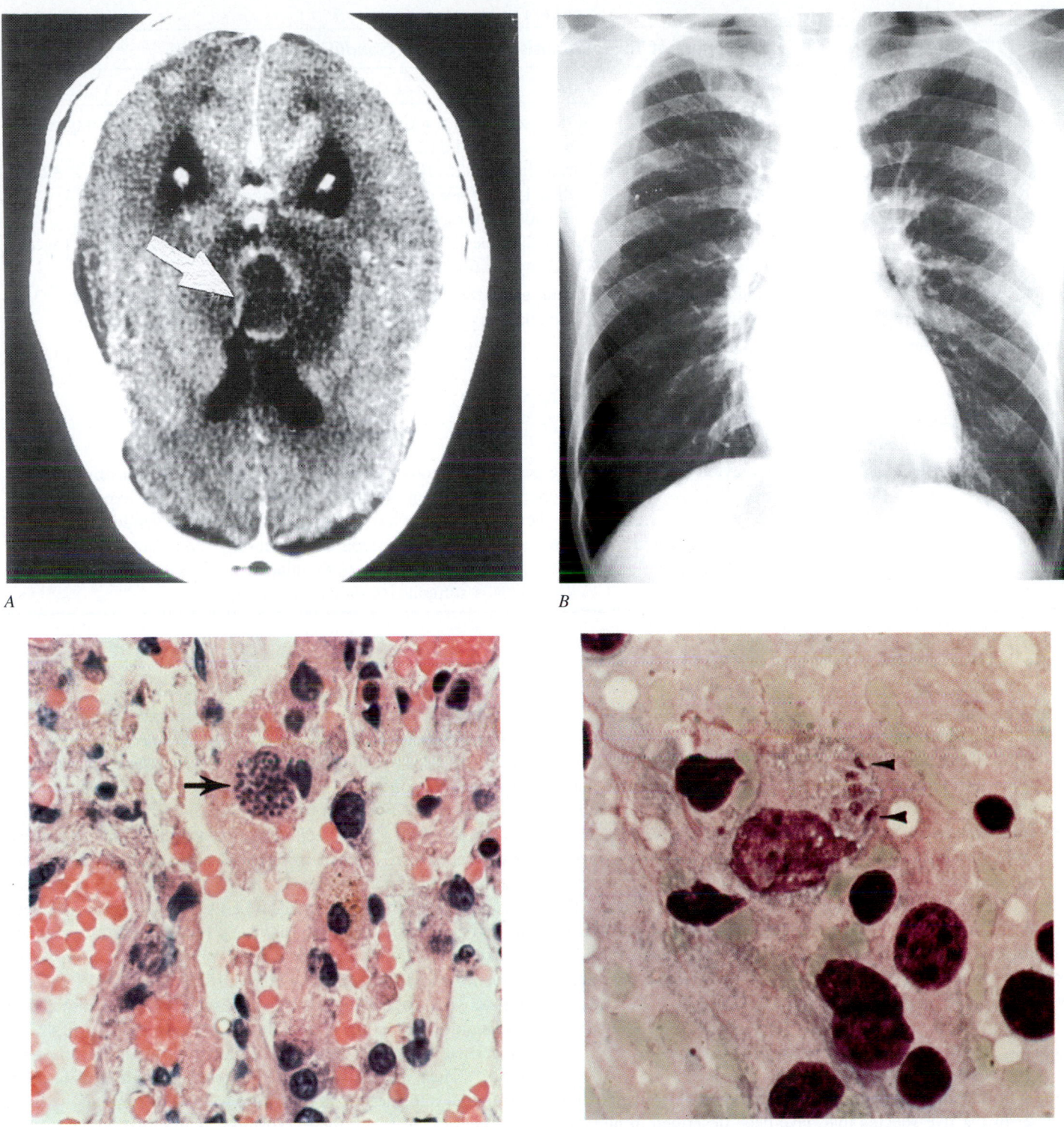

FIGURE 155-5 *Toxoplasma gondii* in brain and lung of a patient with AIDS. *A.* Brain CT scan shows *Toxoplasma* abscess as a contrast-enhancing lesion (arrow). *B.* Chest radiography. Diffuse bilateral infiltrates and hilar adenopathy. *C.* Lung biopsy show, *Toxoplasma* forms (hematoxylin and eosin stain, ×1000). *D.* Impression smear of brain biopsy shows five intracellular tachyzoite (trophozoite) forms (arrowheads; Giemsa stain ×1500). *(C and D are courtesy of Dr. Y. Gutierrez.)*

TABLE 155-4

Therapy of Toxoplasmosis (*Toxoplasma Gondii*)

Syndrome	Drugs of Choice	Dosing
Disseminated disease in AIDS*	Sulfadiazine and pyrimethamine	Sulfadiazine: 1–1.5 g qid × 3–4 weeks (100–200 mg/kg per day × 3–4 weeks in children). Pyrimethamine: 25–100 mg/day × 3–4 weeks (2 mg/kg per day × 3 days, then 1mg/kg per day (maximum 25 mg/day) × 4 weeks. See alternate regimen for dosing pyrimethamine below.
	Pyrimethamine and Clindamycin	Pyrimethamine: 200 mg once, followed by 50–100 mg daily × 4 weeks. Clindamycin: 600 mg iv q 6–8 hours.
Ocular disease	Sulfadiazene and pyrimethamine	Dosing as above. Steroids have been recommended to minimize the chances of retinal inflammation during treatment.
Acute disease in the normal host	No therapy suggested	
Acute disease in the immunocompromised host	Pyrimethamine and sulfadiazine	Dosing as above.
Congenital (in utero) infection		
Maternal treatment	Spiramycin	3–4 g per day for mother until the time of delivery. If transmission to the fetus has been documented before delivery, the expectant mother should be treated with pyrimethamine and sulfadiazine.
Infant treatment	Pyrimethamine and a sulfa drug	Should congenital transmission have occurred, the infant should be treated with pyrimethamine every 2–3 days, and a sulfa drug such as sulfadiazine daily, for 1 year.

*Therapy may need to be continued indefinitely.

MICROSPORIDIOSIS

Microsporidia are a diverse group of obligate intracellular pathogens that form spores. They lack mitochondria and have the small subunit ribosomal structures usually found in prokaryotes, suggesting that they diverged from eukaryotes at a very early evolutionary stage. Historically they have been recognized as important pathogens of bees, silkworms, and fish. Over 100 genera and 1000 species are recognized. In the last decade, Microsporidia have emerged as pathogens of humans with AIDS. Though usually thought of as intestinal pathogens, Microsporidia have been found to cause disseminated disease including pneumonia.[21,61,62]

Transmission and Life Cycle

Details of transmission in humans are quite scanty. Given that a number of the five species that have been described in humans have primarily intestinal manifestations, the suspicion has been that the pathogen is primarily acquired through the ingestion of spores. Pulmonary infections also suggest that aerosol or inhalation transmission is possible. Sexual transmission has also been considered, since spores can be found in the urine in disseminated disease. In laboratory animals such as rabbits, ingestion of urine can efficiently transmit *Encephalitozoon cuniculi*. Vertical transmission to nonhuman species has been documented but not in humans to date.

Supportive epidemiologic information that suggests fecal–oral transmission exists. This includes long-term prospective studies in Brazil, where *C. parvum* and Microsporidia, but not other causes of diarrhea, were significantly more associated with diarrheal disease in HIV-seropositive individuals than in HIV-seronegative controls.[64] Similarly, coinfection has been found in children with AIDS. In a retrospective study from Los Angeles, 60 formalinized stool specimens from patients thought to have cryptosporidiosis or microsporidiosis were retested for the other pathogen: thirty percent had *C. parvum* alone, 42 percent had Microsporidia alone, and 28 percent had both.[14] A serosurvey conducted in Tanzania in HIV-positive and HIV-seronegative patients with diarrhea found the overall seropositivity rate to *Encephalitozoon cuniculi* and *E. hellem* to be 18 percent and 19 percent, respectively, suggesting that microsporidiosis is a common and undiagnosed infection.[18] In addition, microsporidiosis has been diagnosed as a cause of traveler's diarrhea in immunocompetent hosts.[62] Thus, there is suggestive but not conclusive evidence that fecal–oral transmission is important with Microsporidia.

The life cycle of these creatures is fascinating and quite bizarre. The microsporidium spore is environmentally resistant and is able to resist desiccation. Species that infect humans are 1 to 2 μm in diameter and ovoid or piriform in shape. They contain a coiled tubular structure called the *polar filament*. Its length, when uncoiled, may be tens of times longer than the size of the spore. When an appropriate stimulus (a change in pH, shifting ionic concentrations, and so on) occurs, the polar tube everts and forms a long tubule through which the infective sporoplasm is injected into a host cell. It is as if a football or soccer ball suddenly thrust out a 50-foot long tube and speared a hapless nearby host. In the next phase, the injected sporoplasm develops into proliferative stages (meronts) either by binary fission or multiple fission. In the third phase (sporogony), the meronts form sporonts, then sporoblasts, and then spores, without division. The infected host cell swells with all this activity and ruptures. Science fiction, in our view, could be no more creative than this.

Four microsporidial genera have clearly been involved in human disease: *Nosema* (usually pathogens of bees and other insects), *Encephalitozoon* (*E. cuniculi, E. hellem*), *Enterocytozoon bieneusi* (only found in humans to date), and *Pleistophora* (usually a pathogen of fish). *Septata intestinalis* has now been reclassified as *Encephalitozoon intestinalis* and is only found in humans. Several other infections have not been classifiable, although they resembled the genus *Nosema*. *E. cuniculi* has been found in mammals and birds, whereas *E. hellem* has only been found in humans. *Nosema* infections have been described in an immunologically privileged site, the corneum, in normal hosts.

Pathology

In the first autopsy conducted on an AIDS patient with disseminated microsporidiosis, the striking finding was the presence of *E. hellem* in the eyes, urinary tract, and respiratory tract. Numerous organisms were found lining the tracheobronchial tree, suggesting respiratory acquisition of the infection. Gunnarsson and colleagues at the New England Deaconess Hospital in Boston have reviewed a total of 39 cases of disseminated microsporidiosis and found that the respiratory tract involvement was surpassed only by the intestinal and urinary tracts for involvement.[21] Pulmonary microsporidiosis appears to present with bronchiolitis and with infiltrates. Slight fibrosis of the alveolar walls, and intraepithelial infiltration of bronchioli by lymphocytes, has been found. Clusters of spores found in the supranuclear region of bronchial epithelial cells are characteristically seen with *E. bieneusi* infections.

Presentation and Diagnosis

Patients with pulmonary microsporidiosis have presented with dyspnea on exertion, cough, wheezing, small interstitial infiltrates on chest radiographs, small infiltrates, and small pleural effusions. An increased alveolar–arterial oxygen gradient has also been seen.[21,61,62]

Sputa, bronchoalveolar lavage fluid, stool, urine, biopsy samples, and impression smears have all been useful in making the diagnosis. Figure 155-6 shows a pulmonary macrophage (stained with Giemsa) in a sputum sample laden with microsporidial spores, indicating their tiny size. The diagnosis of microsporidiosis is difficult in the typical clinical laboratory. Methods that have proved useful include a modified trichrome stain and fluorescent dye techniques, which take advantage of the fact that the wall of the microsporidial cyst contains chitin and binds the dye. Electron microscopy is the diagnostic gold standard, but its expense makes its routine use impractical.

Treatment

No known drug treats all Microsporidia genera. Albendazole and other benzimidazoles have been used in a variety of settings and

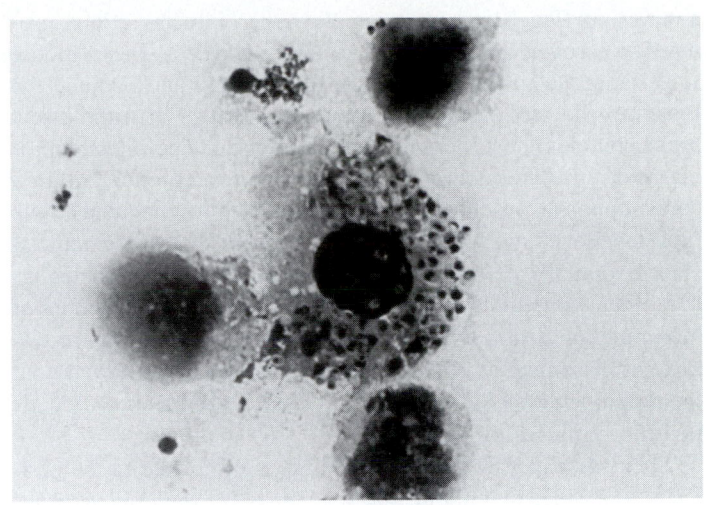

FIGURE 155-6   Pulmonary microsporidiosis. Tiny organisms (~1 μm) within a pulmonary macrophage obtained via bronchoalveolar lavage (Giemsa-Wright stain, ×1000). *(Courtesy of Dr. C. Wanke.)*

appear to be useful in the treatment of *Enterocytozoon bieneusi, Encephalitozoon (Septata) intestinalis,* and other *Encephalitozoon* species.[21,62] We urge the reader to seek the latest literature should a diagnosis of microsporidiosis be entertained, as the field is changing rapidly.

LEISHMANIASIS

Leishmaniasis has emerged as a rare pulmonic infection, usually in the HIV-infected individual or in the organ transplant recipient. *Leishmania* species, protozoa of the order Kinetoplastida, cause distinctive syndromes: cutaneous disease with nonhealing ulcerations ("Aleppo sore," "Delhi boil"), diffuse cutaneous disease, mucosal and facial disease with rather severe disfigurement ("espundia"), and visceral or systemic leishmaniasis ("kala-azar"). These diseases are rare and usually imported into North America or northern Europe; however, there are important foci around the Mediterranean, the Balkans, the Middle East, and northern Africa. In Central and South America leishmaniasis is endemic, as it is in South Asia, China, and the Himalayan countries such as Pakistan and Iran. Leishmaniasis has been reported from every country on the continental Americas except Canada, Chile, and Uruguay; Brazil and Peru are the countries with the highest incidence in South America. Given the expanding HIV pandemic, pulmonary leishmaniasis will be seen more and more frequently. For example, increasing numbers of reports from France, Italy, and Spain describe visceral leishmaniasis in HIV-seropositive individuals.

Leishmania species have a dimorphic life cycle. In mammalian hosts, such as humans, canines, and rodents, the organisms live within macrophages. Canines are an important reservoir host for *Leishmania,* and canine control programs have proved crucial to the elimination of this chronic and debilitating disease. Parasites are ingested by the bite of the insect vector, usually a sandfly of the genus *Lutzomyia* in the Western hemisphere and *Phlebotomus* elsewhere. Within the sandfly, the parasite transforms from the intracellular amastigote form through a series of flagellated intermediate stages into infectious promastigotes over the course of an ensuing week. These motile stages migrate to the proboscis of the sandfly and occlude the lumen of the proboscis. They are then injected when the insect probes the next host, hoping for a blood meal. The injected promastigotes invade mononuclear phagocytes, and, once within a parasitophorous vacuole, transform back into the amastigote (nonflagellar) stage. Amastigotes then replicate by asexual fission. Eventually cell death occurs, and released amastigotes infect other mononuclear phagocytic cells recruited to the area of inflammation. In local disease the lesions are limited, but in visceral or disseminated disease, parasites can be found throughout the reticuloendothelial system. No sexual stage has been identified in *Leishmania* to date.

Speciation of *Leishmania* is of little significance to the clinician, and older taxonomic species names (*L. aethiopica, amazonensis, archibaldi, braziliensis, chagasi, donovani, garnhami, guyanensis, infantum, major, mexicana, panamensis, peruviana, pifanoi, tropica,* and *venezuelensis*) are in flux as modern genetic analysis occurs.

CLINICAL MANIFESTATIONS AND DIAGNOSIS

Disseminated or Visceral Disease (Kala-azar)

In this syndrome, fever and abdominal organomegaly are the rule. Kala-azar is the older but still pleasing term for generalized involvement that includes the spleen, bone marrow, liver, and other organs. The usual incubation period is 3 to 8 months but can be as long as 3 years. Fever, weight loss, pallor, anorexia, anemia, hypergammaglobulinemia, and hepatosplenomegaly are the major consequences. Death is frequently due to concomitant infections, such as tuberculosis, pneumonia, sepsis, or dysentery, or to the effects of the infection itself with malnutrition, cachexia, and progressively severe anemia.

Individuals with HIV typically present with fever, hepatosplenomegaly, and pancytopenia, although atypical presentations occur without all these three findings.[37,40,43] Involvement of the lungs and other thoracic structures, oral mucosa and esophagus, intestine, skin, and bone marrow has been reported. In addition to the other manifestations of disseminated disease, cough and dyspnea are hallmarks of pulmonary leishmaniasis. Chest radiographs usually show a diffuse and subtle interstitial process unless a second pneumonic process is present. It is in this circumstance that the pulmonary physician is most likely to diagnose pulmonary leishmaniasis, via bronchoscopy and detection of parasites within pulmonary macrophages. Leishmaniasis must be differentiated from pulmonary histoplasmosis or other fungal infections and toxoplasmosis. As one might expect, there have been rare cases of pulmonary leishmaniasis diagnosed in people without HIV infection, usually at autopsy. Characteristically, a mild, diffuse interstitial mononuclear cell infiltrate and occasional macrophages with Leishman-Donovan bodies (intracellular parasites) are seen. Note that rapid progression of disease in immunocompetent hosts does also occur. Respiratory distress syndrome, disseminated intravascular coagulation, and hepatic and renal insufficiency with subsequent death have occurred

after antileishmanial therapy was begun for disseminated leishmaniasis. Leishmaniasis has also rarely been seen in organ transplant recipients.[42]

Cutaneous and Mucosal (Localized) Disease

Phrases such as *Delhi boil* and *Aleppo sore* date to colonial times in India and the Middle East and describe cutaneous nonhealing ulcers due to *Leishmania* species. These all refer to localized disease, found at the site of a sandfly bite and inoculation. In general this form of leishmaniasis is not life threatening, and resolution of the ulcer occurs with the development of immunity to the strain of infecting *Leishmania*. Cutaneous disease is far more common than mucosal disease in the Old World.

In contrast, in the New World, mucosal disease is relatively more common and more worrisome and is a major public health hazard in some countries. *Espundia* is a Brazilian word describing mucosal disease. Mucosal disease may include destructive lesions of the oropharynx that prevent the ingestion of foods, and death from inanition may result. In addition, aspiration pneumonia is a common event in the late stages of oronasal destruction.[34,35]

The major therapeutic options in leishmaniasis are outlined in Table 155-5.

BABESIOSIS

Babesiosis is caused by tick-borne parasites of the genus *Babesia*. Clinically this disease most resembles malaria, as the organism is a parasite of erythrocytes. In most people, this is a relatively mild disease. In the splenectomized or otherwise immunosuppressed person, the disease can be fatal.[46] The diagnosis of ARDS due to *Babesia* is just as much an emergency as it is for falciparum malaria, and drug therapy and exchange transfusion are likely to be lifesaving.[6]

Babesiosis in Europe is caused mostly by *B. bovis* and *divergens*; in contrast, most cases in the United States are caused by *B. microti*. In the eastern United States, the tick vector for the infection is the same as the vector for Lyme disease and for ehrlichiosis: *Ixodes daminii*. This tick's natural hosts include mice and deer, and thus babesiosis is a zoonosis.[52] In people who have serologic evidence of Lyme disease (borreliosis caused by *Borrelia burgdorferi*), some 20 to 40 percent also have evidence of babesiosis, and some of ehrlichiosis.[33] As one might expect, babesiosis has also been transmitted by transfusion.[16]

In the normal host, babesiosis is self-limited, and probably of little long-term consequence. Nonetheless it is manifested by fever, myalgias, anorexia, hemolysis, and occasionally jaundice and hemoglobinuria. It is said that a dry cough is not uncommon in babesiosis. The fever of babesiosis is usually not cyclical, as it may be in established malaria caused by a single brood of parasites. Thrombocytopenia is common in moderate to severe disease, as is renal dysfunction. The diagnosis is made by examination of blood smears, which show typical intraerythrocytic ring forms or tetrads of parasites. Malaria and babesiosis are often confused by the inexperienced reviewer of the peripheral blood smear. However, the lack of gametocytes in babesiosis, parasites that fill the erythrocyte in malaria, or malarial pigment help to distinguish *Babesia* from *Plasmodium* parasites.

TABLE 155-5

Therapy of Leishmaniasis and Babesiosis

	Drugs of Choice	Adult dosage	Pediatric Dosage
Leishmaniasis*	Sodium stibogluconate	20 Sb mg/kg per day iv or im × 21–28 days; may need to be repeated or extended	Same as adult dosage
	Meglumine antimonate	20 Sb mg/kg per day iv or im × 21–28 days; may need to be repeated or extended	Same as adult dosage
	Pentamidine	2–4 mg/kg daily or qod IM × 15 doses	Same as adult dosage
	Amphotericin B	0.25–1 mg/kg per day or qod for 4–8 weeks	Same as adult dosage
Babesiosis†	Quinine and Clindamycin	Quinine: 650 mg po tid × 7 days (may be extended)	Quinine: 25 mg/kg per day divided in three doses × 7 days
		Clindamycin: 600 mg iv or po tid × 7 days (may be extended)	Clindamycin: 20–40 mg/kg per day divided in three doses × 7 days

*Other alternatives, such as the following, have been reported but are not commonly used: aminosidine ointment for cutaneous disease; aminosidine and sodium stibogluconate in kala-azar; liposomal encapsulated amphotericin B for multidrug-resistant systemic leishmaniasis; ketoconazole for 8 weeks in cutaneous disease; and recombinant human gamma interferon with antimony, or pentamidine and antimony, in *L. donovani* infections resistant to sodium stibogluconate or meglumine antimonate.

†Exchange transfusion has proved to lifesaving in severely ill patients with high parasitemias (e.g., ≥10% erythrocytes parasitized). Other reportedly useful regimens include atovoquone (750 mg bid) and azithromycin (100 mg po daily) when quinine and clindamycin therapy has failed.

In severe cases, especially in those people with no spleen, the presentation can mimic sepsis and include respiratory failure with ARDS.[6] The mechanism of respiratory embarrassment is unknown, though it acts like ARDS both radiologically and clinically. In endemic areas, evaluation of the cause of the sepsis syndrome should include the review of a blood smear for *Babesia* parasites. The diagnosis is often serendipitously made by hematology laboratory technologists who are performing a manual differential leukocyte count.

Treatment, if warranted, usually consists of clindamycin 600 mg (intravenous or oral, thrice daily) combined with quinine (650 mg thrice daily) for at least 7 days. Therapy may need to be extended in the very ill, immunosuppressed, or splenectomized host. Treatment options are outlined in Table 155-5.

MISCELLANEOUS PROTOZOA

Trichomonads

Trichomonads have been found in sputum, pleural fluid, and lung tissue samples from individuals with pleuropulmonary disease. Although at times they may be contaminants or saprophytes, in a number of cases these infections responded to metronidazole therapy and drainage.[48] *Trichomonas tenax* is an inhabitant of the oropharynx, especially in those with poor oral hygiene. It is the species that has been most frequently associated with disease, in particular pleural effusions and empyema. Most case reports have provided evidence for disease in those at risk for aspiration, such as alcoholics.

Giardia Lamblia

In a case report from 1981, a single patient with cancer and pneumonitis had *G. lamblia* isolated from bronchoalveolar fluid.[54]

REFERENCES

1. Adams EB, MacLeod IN: Invasive amebiasis: I. Amebic dysentery and its complications. *Medicine* 56:315–323, 1977.
2. Adams EB, MacLeod IN: Invasive amebiasis: II. Amebic liver abscess and its complications. *Medicine* 56:325–334, 1977.
3. Anderlini P, Przepiorka D, Luna M, et al: *Acanthamoeba* meningoencephalitis after bone marrow transplantation. *Bone Marrow Transplant* 14:459–461, 1994.
4. Bauer RW, Harrison LR, Watson CW, et al: Isolation of *Acanthamoeba* spp. from a greyhound with pneumonia and granulomatous amebic encephalitis. *J Vet Diag Invest* 5:386–391, 1993.
5. Bookless AS: Thoracic amoebiasis. *J R Army Med Corps* 94:52–60, 1950.
6. Boustani MR, Lepore TJ, Gelfand JA, Lazarus DS: Acute respiratory failure in patients treated for babesiosis (review). *Am J Respir Crit Care Med* 149:1689–1691, 1994.
7. Brea Hernando AJ, Bandres Franco E, Mosquera Lozano JD, et al: Criptosporidiosis pulmonar y SIDA. Presentacion de un caso y revision de la literatura. *An Med Interna* 10:232–236, 1993.
8. Brooks MH, Keil FW, Sheehy TW, et al: Acute pulmonary edema in falciparum malaria: A clinicopathological correlation. *New Engl J Med* 279:732–737, 1968.
9. Clark DP, Sears SL: The pathogenesis of cryptosporidiosis. *Parasitol Today* 12:221–225, 1996.
10. Current WL, Garcia LS: Cryptosporidiosis. *Clin Microbiol Rev* 4:325–358, 1991.
11. Ditrich O, Palkovic L, Sterba J, et al: The first finding of *Cryptosporidium baileyi* in man. *Parasitol Res* 77:44–47, 1991.
12. Feldman RM, Singer C: Noncardiogenic pulmonary edema and pulmonary fibrosis in falciparum malaria. *Rev Infect Dis* 9:134–139, 1987.
13. Gachot B, Wolff M, Nissack G, et al: Acute lung injury complicating imported *Plasmodium falciparum* malaria. *Chest* 108:746–749, 1995.
14. Garcia LS, Shimizu RY, Bruckner DA: Detection of microsporidial spores in fecal specimens from patients diagnosed with cryptosporidiosis. *J Clin Microbiol* 32:1739–1741, 1994.

15. Gentile G, Venditti M, Micozzi A, et al: Cryptosporidiosis in patients with hematologic malignancies. *Rev Infect Dis* 13:842–846, 1991.

16. Gerber MA, Shapiro ED, Krause PJ, et al: The risk of acquiring Lyme disease or babesiosis from a blood transfusion. *J Infect Dis* 170:321–324, 1994.

17. Goldstein ST, Juranek DD, Ravenholt O, et al: Cryptosporidiosis: An outbreak associated with drinking water despite state-of-the-art water treatment. *Ann Intern Med* 124:459–468, 1996.

18. Gomez Morales MA, Atzori C, Ludovisis A, et al: Opportunistic and non-opportunistic parasites in HIV-positive and negative patients with diarrhoea in Tanzania. *Trop Med Parasitol* 46:109–114, 1995.

19. Goodgame RW, Kimball K, Ou CN, et al: Intestinal function and injury in acquired immunodeficiency syndrome-related cryptosporidiosis. *Gastroenterology* 108:1075–1082, 1995.

20. Gozal D: The incidence of pulmonary manifestations during *Plasmodium falciparum* malaria in non-immune subjects. *Trop Med Parasitol* 43:6–8, 1992.

21. Gunnarsson G, Hurlbut D, DeGirolami PC, et al: Multiorgan microsporidiosis: Report of five cases and review. *Clin Infect Dis* 21:37–44, 1995.

22. Herrera-Llerandi R: Thoracic repercussions of amebiasis. *J Thorac Cardiovasc Surg* 52:361–375, 1966.

23. Ibarra-Perez C: Diagnosis and treatment of amebic empyema. Report of eighty-eight cases. *Am J Surg* 134:283–287, 1977.

24. Ibarra-Perez C: Thoracic complications of amebic abscess of the liver. Report of 501 cases. *Chest* 79:672–677, 1981.

25. Israelski D, Remington J: Toxoplasmosis in the non-AIDS immunocompromised host, in Remington J, Schwartz M (eds), *Current Clinical Topics in Infectious Diseases*, vol 13. Boston, Blackwell Scientific Publications, 1993, pp 322–356.

26. Jensen BN, Gerstoft J, Hojlyng N, et al: Pulmonary pathogens in HIV-infected patients. *Scand J Infect Dis* 22:413–420, 1990.

27. Kamel AG, Maning N, Arulmainathan S: Cryptosporidiosis among HIV positive intravenous drugs users in Malaysia. *Southeast Asian J Trop Med Pub Health* 25:650–653, 1994.

28. Keusch GT, Hamer D, Joe A, et al: Cryptosporidia—who is at risk? *Schweizerische Medizinische Wochenschrift* 125:899–908, 1995.

29. Kone M, Penali LK, Enoh S, et al: La cryptosporidiose chez les enfants ivoiriens de Yopougon. *Bull Soc Pathol Exotique* 85:167–169, 1992.

30. Kubitschek KR, Peters J, Nickeson D, et al: Amebiasis presenting as pleuropulmonary disease. *West J Med* 142:203–207, 1985.

31. MacKenzie WR, Hoxie NJ, Proctor ME, et al: A massive outbreak in Milwaukee of Cryptosporidium infection transmitted through the public water supply. *New Engl J Med* 331:161–167, 1994.

32. Madrigal Sesma JM, Santillana Lopez I: Aislamiento de amebas de vida libre en muestras de origen respiratorio. *Revista de Sanidad e Higiene Publica* 63:63–72, 1989.

33. Magnarelli LA, Dumler JS, Anderson JF, et al: Coexistence of antibodies to tick-borne pathogens of babesiosis, ehrlichiosis, and Lyme borreliosis in human sera. *J Clin Microbiol* 33:3054–3057, 1995.

34. Marsden PD, Nonata RR: Mucocutaneous leishmaniasis—a review of clinical aspects. *Rev Soc Bras Med Trop* 9:309–326, 1975.

35. Marsden PD, Sampaior RNR, Rocha R, et al: Mucocutaneous leishmaniasis—an unsolved clinical problem. *Trop Doct* 7:7–11, 1977.

36. Mausezahl D, Egger M, Odermatt P, Tanner M: Klinik und Epidemiologie der Kryptosporidiose bei immunkompetenten Kindern. *Schweizerishce Rundschau fur Medizin Praxis* 80:936–940, 1991.

37. Medrano FJ, Hernandez-Quero J, Jimenez E, et al: Visceral leishmaniasis in HIV-1 infected individuals: A common opportunistic infection in Spain. *AIDS* 6:1499–1503, 1992.

38. Mohri H, Fujita H, Asakur Y, et al: Case report: Inhalation therapy of paromomycin is effective for respiratory infection and hypoxia by Cryptosporidium with AIDS. *Am J Med Sci* 309:60–62, 1995.

39. Molbak K, Hojlyng N, Gottschau A, et al: Cryptosporidiosis in infancy and childhood mortality in Guinea Bissau, west Africa. *BMJ* 307:417–420, 1993.

40. Montalban C, Calleja JL, Erice A, et al: Visceral leishmaniasis in patients infected with human immunodeficiency virus. Co-operative Group for the Study of Leishmaniasis in AIDS. *J Infect* 21:261–270, 1990.

41. Moore R, Tzipori S, Griffiths JK, et al: Temporal changes in permeability and structure of piglet ileum after site-specific infection by *Cryptosporidium parvum*. *Gastroenterology* 108:1030–1039, 1995.

42. Moulin B, Ollier J, Bouchouareb D, et al: Leishmaniasis: A rare cause of unexplained fever in a renal graft recipient. *Nephron* 60:360–362, 1992.

43. Peters BS, Fish D, Golden R, et al: Visceral leishmaniasis in HIV infection and AIDS: Clinical features and response to therapy. *Q J Med* 77:1101–1111, 1990.

44. Petri WA, Ravdin JI: Amebiasis in institutionalized populations, in Ravdin JI (ed), *Amebiasis: Human Infection by Entamoeba histolytica*. New York, Churchill Livingstone, 1988, pp 576–581.

45. Pomeroy C, Filice GA: Pulmonary toxoplasmosis. A review. *Clin Infect Dis* 14:863–870, 1992.

46. Pruthi RK, Marshall WF, Wiltsie JC, Persing DH: Human babesiosis (review). *Mayo Clin Proc* 70:853–862, 1995.

47. Punyagupta S, Srichaikul T, Nitiyanant P, et al: Acute pulmonary insufficiency in falciparum malaria: Summary of 12 cases with evidence of disseminated intravascular coagulation. *Am J Trop Med Hyg* 23:551–559, 1974.

48. Radosavljevic-Asic G, Jovanovic D, Radovanovic D, Tucakovic M: Trichomonas in pleural effusion. *Eur Resp J* 7:1906–1908, 1994.

49. Remington JS, McLeod R, Desmonts G: Toxoplasmosis, in Remington J, Klein JO (eds), *Infectious Diseases of the Fetus and Newborn Infant*, 4th ed. Philadelphia, Saunders, 1995, pp 140–267.

50. Sheehy TW, Reba RC: Complications of falciparum malaria and their treatment. *Ann Intern Med* 66:807–809, 1967.

51. Sotelo-Avila C: *Naegleria* and *Acanthamoeba*. Free-living amebas pathogenic for man. *Perspect Pediatr Pathol* 10:51–85, 1987.

52. Spielman A: The emergence of Lyme disease and human babesiosis in a changing environment (review). *Ann New York Acad Sci* 740:146–156, 1994.

53. Srichaikul T, Leelasiri A, Polvicha P, et al: Exchange transfusion therapy in severe complicated malaria. *Southeast Asian J Trop Med Pub Health* 24 (suppl 1):100–105, 1993.

54. Stevens WJ, Vermeire PA: *Giardia lamblia* in bronchoalveolar lavage fluid. *Thorax* 36:875, 1981.

55. Tyndall RL, Lyle MM, Ironside KS: The presence of free-living amoebae in portable and stationary eye wash stations. *Am Ind Hyg Assoc J* 48:933–934, 1987.

56. Tziproi S, Rand W, Griffiths J, et al: Evaluation of an animal model system for cryptosporidiosis: The therapeutic efficacy of paromomycin and hyperimmune bovine colostrum-immunoglobulin. *Clin Diagn Immunol* 1:450–463, 1994.

57. Tzipori S, Rand W, Theodos C: Evaluation of a two-phase scid mouse model preconditioned with anti-interferon-gamma monoclonal antibody for drug testing against *Cryptosporidium parvum*. *J Infect Dis* 172:1160–1164, 1995.

58. Vidal T, Gamboa C, Henriquez MI, Biolley A: Cryptosporidium: Brote epidemico en un centro de recuperacion nutricional, Temuco. *Revista Medica de Chile* 119:1136–1139, 1991.

59. Wang SS, Feldman HA: Isolation of *Hartmanella* species from human throats. *New Engl J Med* 277:1174–1179, 1967.

60. Wanke C, Butler T, Islam M: Epidemiologic and clinical features of invasive amebiasis in Bangladesh: A case-control comparison with other diarrheal diseases and postmortem findings. *Am J Trop Med Hyg* 38:335–341, 1988.

61. Weber R, Kuster H, Keller R, et al: Pulmonary and intestinal microsporidiosis in a patient with the acquired immunodeficiency syndrome. *Am Rev Respir Dis* 146:1603–1605, 1992.

62. Weber R, Bryan RT, Schwartz DA, Owen RL: Human microsporidial infections (review). *Clin Microbiol Rev* 7:426–461, 1994.

63. White NJ, Ho M: The pathophysiology of malaria. *Adv Parasitol* 31:83–173, 1992.

64. Wuhib T, Silva TM, Newman RD, et al: Cryptosporidial and microsporidial infections in human immunodeficiency virus-infected patients in northeastern Brazil. *J Infect Dis* 170:494–497, 1994.

CHAPTER 156

HELMINTHIC DISEASES OF THE LUNGS

Adel A. F. Mahmoud

Parasitic helminths are a distinct group of infectious agents that are responsible for worldwide morbidity and mortality in humans. People with helminthic infections of the lungs often seek medical advice because of one or more common chest complaints—cough, pain, or breathlessness. They pose a diagnostic challenge, particularly in areas where helminthic infections are not endemic. Other, more common causes of chest complaints have to be excluded, a history of residence in certain geographic locations has to be elicited, and the proper procedures for making the diagnosis of helminthiasis have to be selected.

In humans, worms produce a variety of pulmonary parenchymal and vascular diseases (Table 156-1). Because several stages in the life cycle of the parasite are found in humans, and because pulmonary lesions occur at a particular phase of the life cycle, familiarity with the biologic behavior of the organisms is essential for proper diagnosis and treatment.

BIOLOGY AND IMMUNOLOGY

Biology of Helminths

Worms are multicellular organisms that vary considerably in size, from a few millimeters to several meters.[22] They are among the most developed and elaborate of human parasites. Their parasitic capabilities are such that they often parasitize more than one host

and survive different hostile environments. Despite their relatively large size, the infective stages of worms invade human tissues by ingestion, by penetration of skin, or through the bite of insect vectors. Furthermore, parasitic helminths have developed a myriad of mechanisms by which they can evade the protective mechanisms of the host.

A basic biologic generalization about helminthic infections is that the worms, as a rule, cannot multiply within the mammalian host. This phenomenon is important to the understanding of the dynamics of helminthic infection and of the relationship between the intensity of a particular worm load within the host and its pathologic consequences. However, there are exceptions to this rule. For example, *Strongyloides stercoralis* and *Echinococcus granulosus* can increase their numbers within a host even though the host is not exposed to additional infective forms. This ability of *S. stercoralis* to autoinfect the same subject and cause a hyperinfection syndrome is of considerable clinical significance, especially in immunosuppressed patients, and often proves fatal.[23] A different example is that of echinococcosis, in which dissemination is usually a consequence of leakage or rupture of a hydatid cyst—thereby releasing its contents, which seed sites elsewhere and initiate similar lesions.

Another biologic characteristic of worm infections, particularly those migrating in host tissues such as the lungs, is the association with eosinophilia in the peripheral blood and tissue.[2] When eosinophilia is marked, this association provides a clinically useful sign of a migratory worm infection. The prominent peripheral blood eosinophilia of tissue migratory worm infections contrasts with no eosinophilia in persons in whom the worm infection is confined to the gut lumen or in whom the infection is due to other agents (e.g., viruses or bacteria). The mechanism and specificity of this eosinophilic response depend on the integrity of the *cellular* immune response of the host: sensitized T lymphocytes produce mediators that induce differentiation in the bone marrow or progenitor cells into mature eosinophils; this is done either directly or via other cell products from mononuclear phagocytes. Eosinophilia does not occur in athymic nude mice infected with *Trichinella spiralis* or *Schistosoma mansoni*. Similarly, eosinophilia often does not feature prominently when strongyloidiasis occurs in immunosuppressed persons. Eosinophil production appears to be affected by interleukin 3 (IL-3), GM-CSF, and IL-5. Only IL-5, how-

TABLE 156-1

Pulmonary Parenchymal and Vascular Diseases Produced by Worms

Major Pulmonary Presentation	Infection	Causative Organism	Infective Stage	Pathogenic Stage
Loeffler-like syndrome	Ascariasis	*Ascaris lumbricoides*	Embryonated eggs in soil	Migrating larvae
	Hookworms	*Ancylostoma duodenale, Necator americanus*	Larvae in soil Larvae in soil	Migrating larvae
	Strongyloidiasis	*Strongyloides stercoralis*	Larvae in soil	Migrating rhabditiform larvae
	Hyperinfection with *S. stercoralis*	*S. stercoralis*	Larvae in bowel	Migrating filariform larvae
Pulmonary eosinophilia	Lymphatic filariasis	*Wuchereria bancrofti, Brugia malayi*	Larvae in mosquito	Microfilariae
Space-occupying lesions	Echinococcosis	*Echinococcus granulosus*	Eggs in soil	Hydatid cysts
	Paragonimiasis	*Paragonimus westermani*	Metacercariae	Adult worms
	Schistosomiasis	*Schistosoma mansoni, S. japonicum, S. haematobium*	Cercariae in fresh water	Eggs

ever, is specific for the maturation of eosinophils and basophils.[8] The cytokine interact with eosinophils through a cell surface–specific receptor. It induces a state of metabolic as well as functional activation of eosinophils.[30] In contrast, the specific helminthic antigens responsible for initiating this response are unknown.

Investigations have suggested that the increased eosinophil level that occurs in experimental animals or humans with helminthiasis is related to their biologic role as an integral component of host defenses. In vitro, eosinophils along with antibodies or complement kill the larval forms of several helminths.[3] The killing of parasites is accompanied by a respiratory burst in these cells and evacuation of the contents of their granules onto the surface of the helminth. In vivo, depletion of eosinophils in experimental animals leads to loss of their acquired resistance to infection from several helminths, such as *T. spiralis* and *S. mansoni*.[24] Both oxidative and nonoxidative products of eosinophil granules have been implicated in target killing.

Host-Parasite Relationship in Pulmonary Helminthiases

Human disease caused by pulmonary helminthiases results from various factors. Several classes of helminths reside in human lungs during one or more of their parasitic stages. These include nematodes (roundworms), trematodes (flatworms), and cestodes (segmented worms). The stage of the life cycle that causes human pulmonary disease also varies—e.g., larvae of nematodes, eggs of schistosomes, and adult worms in paragonimiasis. The multiplicity and complex structure of these etiologic agents lead to a heterogeneous set of responses, both immunologic and nonimmunologic.[27] Moreover, disease may result either from the

mechanical presence of worms (space-occupying lesions) and the associated inflammatory responses or as a byproduct of the host immune responses, or both. For example, in echinococcosis, hydatid cysts displace lung tissues, but in pulmonary schistosomiasis, the vascular obstructive lesions are predominantly the outcome of the delayed-hypersensitivity granulomatous response of the host. The understanding of host-parasite relationship in pulmonary helminthiasis is, therefore, based on an appreciation of the heterogeneity of etiologic agents and the corresponding host responses.

An additional and biologically relevant factor concerning helminthic infections and their role in etiology of human disease is the intensity of infection.[2] Since most worms that infect humans cannot increase their population without additional exposure to the infective stages, the worm load largely determines the degree of pathologic sequelae. For example, the number of schistosome eggs reaching the pulmonary circulation is an essential determinant of the severity of the induced disease. Although the number of eggs reaching the lungs may be influenced by several factors, the most important determinant is the number of adult worms in the infected person.

The immune responses of the host often feature prominently in shaping the pathologic consequences of helminthic infection of the lungs. In experimental animals, the degree of tissue injury and host responsiveness to several helminthiases has been shown to be regulated by modulatory antibody, cellular, and cytokine responses.[27]

Whether humans acquire resistance to helminthic infection and whether resistance can be induced have not been settled. Resistance against several helminths occurs in experimental animals after primary infection, and it can be induced by defined antigens.[19]

APPROACH TO THE PATIENT WITH HELMINTHIC INFECTION OF THE LUNGS

As indicated above, the major symptoms and signs of pulmonary disease are common to most etiologic agents, noninfectious as well as infectious. Although helminth infections are, in general, particularly common in temperate and hot areas of the world, some are transmitted in the United States and in other colder and developed areas. A history that the patient has lived overseas or in certain parts of the United States is helpful in alerting the examiner to the possibility of a helminthic infection. The geographic distribution of the major helminthic infections is roughly known. Also, some infections, such as those with *E. granulosus,* are common in sheep-raising countries and in certain sheep-raising areas in the United States. Knowledge of the immunologic status of the patient is valuable in suggesting helminthic infection—e.g., the hyperinfection syndrome caused by *S. stercoralis.*

Eosinophilia in peripheral blood, sputum, or pulmonary tissue is a helpful clue in directing the diagnostic workup. Although increased eosinophil counts do occur in several other pulmonary diseases, the close association with helminthic infections necessitates appropriate diagnostic procedures to determine whether a worm is implicated. Definitive diagnosis of helminthic infections of the lungs requires isolation and identification of diagnostic stages in the life cycle of the parasite that routine examination of appropriate specimens may miss. Therefore, the appropriate laboratory personnel should be alerted to the possibility of a worm infection so that proper samples can be obtained and preserved for special examinations. Serologic testing for helminthiasis is particularly useful in nonendemic areas. It should always be considered an adjunct and important diagnostic procedure.

DISEASES DUE TO NEMATODES (ROUNDWORMS)

Ascariasis, Hookworms, and Strongyloidiasis

Human infections with *Ascaris lumbricoides,* with the hookworms *Ancylostoma duodenale* and *Necator americanus,* and with *S. stercoralis* are among the most prevalent helminthiases worldwide.[29] Transmission also occurs in the southeastern United States.[21]

ETIOLOGY

Human ascariasis (Fig. 156-1) results from ingestion of embryonated *A. lumbricoides* eggs that are contained in feces-contaminated soil. Ingestion of contaminated vegetables and fruits that

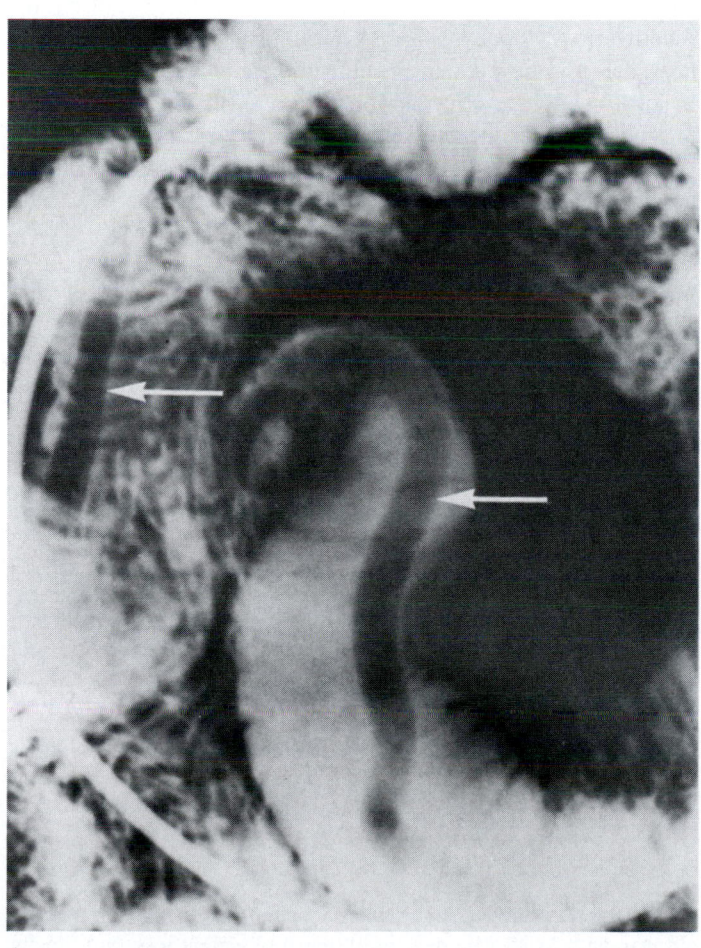

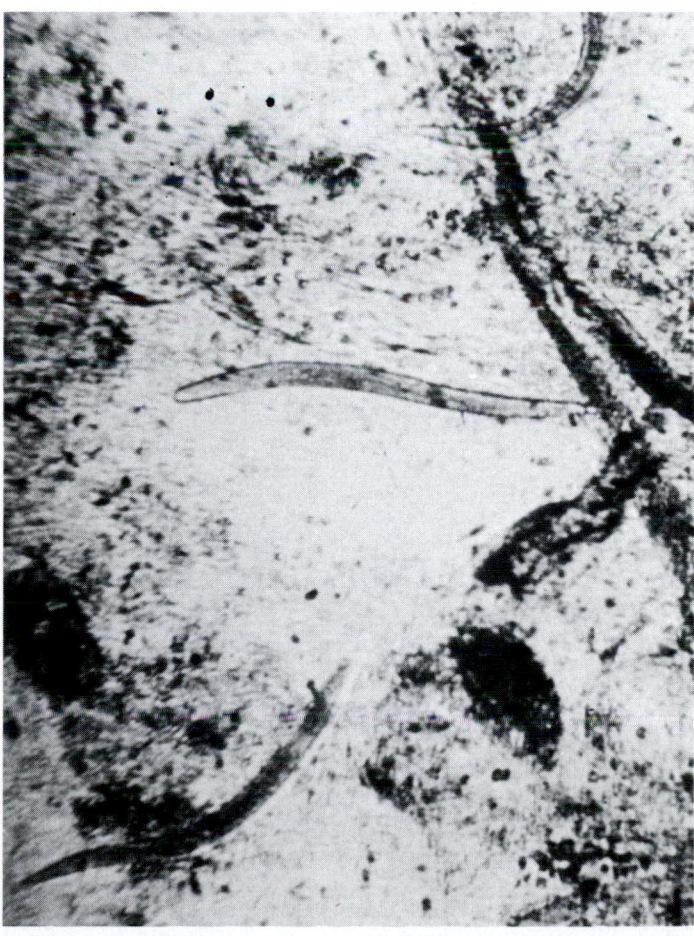

A   *B*

FIGURE 156-1   Nematodes. *A.* Ascariasis. Barium in the small intestine outlines two *Ascaris* worms (arrows). (From Shaba.[30a]). *B. Strongyloides stercoralis.* Rhabditiform larvae. *(Courtesy of Dr. Stanley H. Abadie.)*

have not been properly washed is the most frequent transmission vehicle. *Ascaris* eggs hatch in the gastrointestinal tract, producing larvae that penetrate the gut wall and migrate via venous blood and the right side of the heart to the lungs. Hookworms (*A. duodenale* and *N. americanus*) and *S. stercoralis* infect humans when infective larvae, found in soil, penetrate intact skin. Larvae of hookworms or of *S. stercoralis* travel via the bloodstream to the lungs (Table 156-1). The parasite larvae migrate via pulmonary capillaries into alveolar spaces. They then ascend toward the trachea to be swallowed en route to their final habitat in the small intestine. Although larvae are sometimes found in the sputum of infected persons, more often the eggs (*A. lumbricoides, A. duodenale,* and *N. americanus*) or the larvae (*S. stercoralis*) are found in stools. Passage to the outside environment, where the stool forms develop into stages infective for humans, completes their life cycle.

PATHOGENESIS AND PATHOLOGY

In nematode infections, the most prominent pulmonary pathologic changes occur in persons with ascariasis[21] or with the hyperinfection syndrome of strongyloidiasis.[23] *Ascaris* pneumonia may occur in 1 to 2 weeks after infection. Portions of larvae are seen in the pulmonary parenchyma, surrounded by patchy infiltrate of neutrophils and eosinophils. The alveoli contain a serous exudate; the production of bronchial mucus is increased. Later, migrating larvae are destroyed within aggregates of eosinophils. The nature of the inflammatory process in *Ascaris* pneumonia suggests hypersensitivity. The intensity of the reaction depends on the number of parasite larvae and on previous sensitization. In areas in which transmission of *Ascaris* eggs occurs seasonally, pulmonary reactions are usually more in evidence during these periods.[6]

In *immunocompetent* subjects, pulmonary disease caused by hookworms or *S. stercoralis* is unremarkable. However, infection with *S. stercoralis* can be life-threatening in *immunocompromised* subjects.[7] Filariform larvae seem to develop prematurely in immunocompromised persons and invade the gut wall or the perianal skin. Tissue migration occurs through most body organs, including the lungs. Initially, the pulmonary lesions resemble those of *Ascaris* pneumonia. In some patients, bronchopneumonia and lung abscesses develop. The lungs of fatal cases show intra-alveolar hemorrhages and inflammatory changes.

CLINICAL FEATURES

The major clinical manifestations caused by infection of the lungs with the larval forms of intestinal nematodes resemble those of Loeffler's syndrome; these manifestations occur typically in patients with seasonal or *Ascaris* pneumonia. The symptoms include persistent, irritating, and nonproductive cough, substernal pain, and, in the severely ill, hemoptysis and dyspnea. Eosinophilia is the most consistent laboratory finding. Radiographic signs—e.g., patchy or miliary infiltrate—are sometimes seen.

The onset of the Loeffler-like syndrome caused by intestinal nematodes usually occurs 2 to 3 weeks after infection, coincident with larval migration from the pulmonary circulation to the alveoli.[21] This coincidence was illustrated by the occurrence of the syndrome in a group of students exposed to eggs of the pig roundworm (*A. suum*). Typical symptoms occurred 10 to 15 days later; some of the students developed marked respiratory failure. In locations where transmission of ascariasis is cyclic because of environmental factors, pneumonitis occurs seasonally. Mild symptoms are occasionally encountered in persons with hookworm infection or in immunocompetent subjects who have strongyloidiasis.

The most clinically significant pulmonary syndrome induced by intestinal nematodes is caused by hyperinfection with *S. ster-*

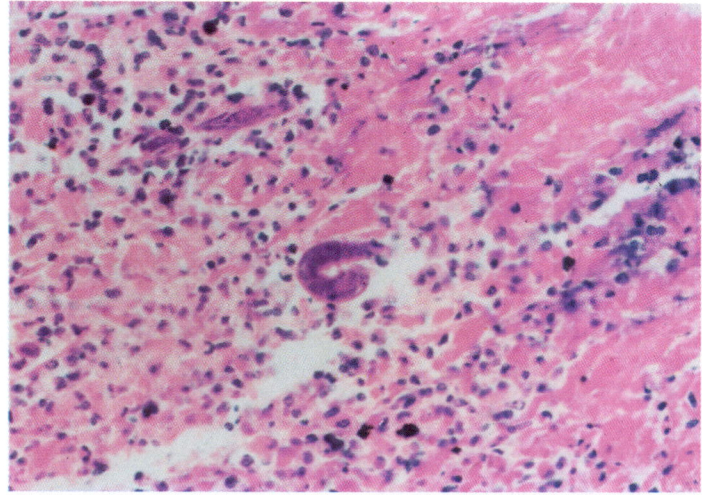

A   *B*

FIGURE 156-2 Strongyloidiasis. *A.* 55-year-old man with chronic lymphocytic leukemia who presented with abdominal discomfort and weight loss. The patient developed progressive pulmonary congestion and edema with dyspnea, fever to 103°, and progressive hypotension before death. Blood cultures revealed *Escherichia coli*. Histologic section of colon at autopsy shows adult *S. stercoralis* in wall. *B.* 24-year-old man with AIDS who developed diarrhea, weight loss, and, finally, shock with *E. coli* bacteremia and strongyloidiasis. The larval form is shown in the jejunum. *(Courtesy of Dr. Jay A. Fishman.)*

coralis (Fig. 156-2). As a rule, the syndrome occurs in patients with compromised cell-mediated immunity, although it is occasionally encountered in normal persons.[23] Immunosuppression is usually caused by neoplastic diseases, such as Hodgkin's, other lymphomas and leukemias, or nonmalignant conditions that are being treated with corticosteroids—e.g., organ transplantation. The sequence of events in immunosuppressed patients indicates that a change has occurred in the reproductive cycle of the parasite: in nonimmunosuppressed subjects, the rhabditiform larvae have to go to the outside world to transform into the infective filariform organisms; in immunosuppressed patients, the change to infective larvae occurs within the host. The organisms penetrate the intestinal mucosa—resulting in massive invasion of almost every organ, including the lungs. The major clinical features include asthma, pulmonary opacities and cavitation, consolidation, and diffuse focal infiltrates.[33] Usually, widespread dissemination of the nematode is accompanied by secondary infection caused by gram-negative organisms carried along with *S. stercoralis*. Eosinophilia is often absent in patients with the *S. stercoralis* hyperinfection syndrome, probably because of defective cell-mediated immunity. The *S. stercoralis* hyperinfection syndrome is often fatal: mortality occurs in up to 77 percent of people with such infections.

MANAGEMENT

Diagnosis of infection with intestinal nematodes that causes a Loeffler-like syndrome can be difficult.[29] Only occasionally is the search for parasite larvae in sputum rewarding. Indeed, not infrequently, definitive diagnosis is delayed for weeks, until the adult worms mature in the small intestine. At this stage, fecal examination will disclose the characteristic eggs of hookworms or *Ascaris* or the larvae of *S. stercoralis*. The management of patients with the pulmonary manifestations of these parasitic worms is nonspecific and symptomatic. Reduction of exposure in areas where transmission of ascariasis is seasonal will decrease the prevalence and severity of clinical presentations. Specific antihelminthic therapy is ineffective during the pulmonary stage but can cure the infection once the parasites reach maturity in the small intestine.

Mebendazole is the drug of choice for treating ascariasis and hookworms. It is given orally, 100 mg per day for 2 to 3 days. Thiabendazole, 25 mg/kg body weight, twice daily for 2 days, is the recommended treatment for intestinal strongyloidiasis. In patients suspected of having the hyperinfection syndrome, early diagnosis, modification of the immunosuppressive therapy, and prompt anti-*Strongyloides* chemotherapy are the important elements in averting a fatal outcome. A high degree of suspicion that strongyloidosis is also present is needed in dealing with pulmonary disease associated with bacteremia in immunosuppressed patients. Most instances of strongyloidiasis in these patients are diagnosed at autopsy or shortly before death. Aggressive efforts at demonstrating *S. stercoralis* larvae entail repeated examination of stools and duodenal aspirates. Sputum and bronchial washings are examined for parasite larvae. Serology may be of help.[4] In these patients, thiabendazole is started as early as possible and continued for 10 to 15 days.

Pulmonary Filariasis (Tropical Pulmonary Eosinophilia)

Persons living in areas endemic for *Wuchereria bancrofti* and *Brugia malayi* may present with an acute or chronic lung disease usually referred to as *tropical pulmonary eosinophilia*.[13] This is still a poorly defined clinical entity. Its main features are a history of residence in filaria-endemic areas, particularly India, chronic nocturnal paroxysmal cough, marked eosinophilia, positive serologic evidence, and a therapeutic response to the administration of diethylcarbamazine.

ETIOLOGY

Human infection with the tissue nematodes *W. bancrofti* or *B. malayi* can cause several amicrofilaremic syndromes, including tropical pulmonary eosinophilia. Infection is transmitted by the bite of several species of mosquitoes, thereby introducing the infective third-stage larvae. These organisms undergo ill-defined maturational stages culminating in the development of adult male and female worms that are usually situated in lymphatic vessels and lymph nodes. Mature worms deposit microfilariae that appear in peripheral circulation, often at maximum numbers at specific times of the day. However, some filariae show no periodicity with respect to the appearance of their microfilariae in peripheral blood. Microfilariae are taken up by mosquitoes during their bites, thereby completing the life cycle of the parasite.

The life span of adult filariae is not known. Nonetheless, serologic or histopathologic evidence of infection can be obtained in the syndrome known collectively as *amicrofilaremic states*, even though larvae cannot be found in the blood. For example, in tropical pulmonary eosinophilia, high concentrations of antifilarial IgG and IgE in serum have been demonstrated despite invariably negative blood examinations for parasites. Also, despite the negative blood examinations, microfilariae have been found in lung and lymph node biopsies, confirming the filarial origin of this syndrome.

PATHOGENESIS AND PATHOLOGY

Patients with pulmonary filariasis *(tropical pulmonary eosinophilia)* show evidence of humoral hyperreactivity manifested as increased serum levels of total IgE and antifiliarial IgG and IgE.[26] The possibility has been raised that these antibodies play a causal role in producing the pulmonary symptoms by inducing clearance of microfilariae and acute IgE-mediated responses, which are manifested clinically as asthma and eosinophilic pulmonary infiltrates. Histopathologically, the earliest lesions are histiocytic infiltrates in the interstitium and alveolar spaces. In established cases, the cell infiltrate consists predominantly of eosinophils, lymphocytes, and histiocytes, and it assumes a nodular configuration.

CLINICAL FEATURES

Young males are predominantly afflicted with tropical pulmonary eosinophilia. The syndrome is characterized by episodes of dry night cough, low-grade fever, and general fatigue. Examination of the chest may reveal coarse rales and rhonchi, along with wheezing.[13] In many patients, pulmonary function tests disclose a restrictive pattern in which vital and total lung capacity and residual volumes are all decreased. Some patients with chronic disease have perfusion impairment. Radiographically, the syndrome may be associated with reticulonodular opacities and increased bronchovascular markings. The sera of these patients usually demonstrate high IgE levels and specific antibodies to the parasite. Eosinophil counts in peripheral blood generally exceed 3000 per cubic millimeter.

MANAGEMENT

Diagnosis is based on the typical clinical, radiographic, functional, and immunologic findings in the setting of an appropriate epidemiology history—i.e., previous residence in a filaria-endemic area. A favorable response to diethylcarbamazine therapy confirms the diagnosis. The drug is usually administered as 5 mg/kg body weight per day in divided doses for 2 to 3 weeks. Recurrences of tropical pulmonary eosinophilia are rare. If they do occur, a second course of antihelminthic chemotherapy is indicated.

DIROFILARIASIS

Another filarial parasite, *Dirofilaria immitis* (dog heartworm), may accidentally be transmitted to humans by the bites of the mosquito intermediate vector (Fig. 156-3). Several cases of dirofilariasis have been reported in the United States.[1] In most, the infection was discovered as a coin lesion on the chest radiograph.

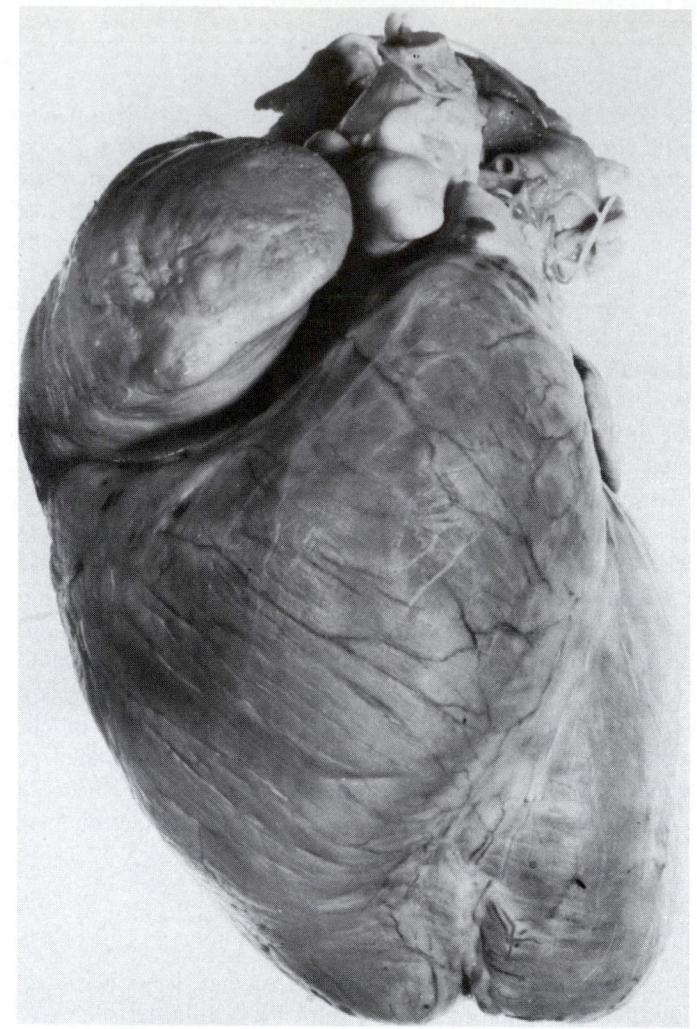

B

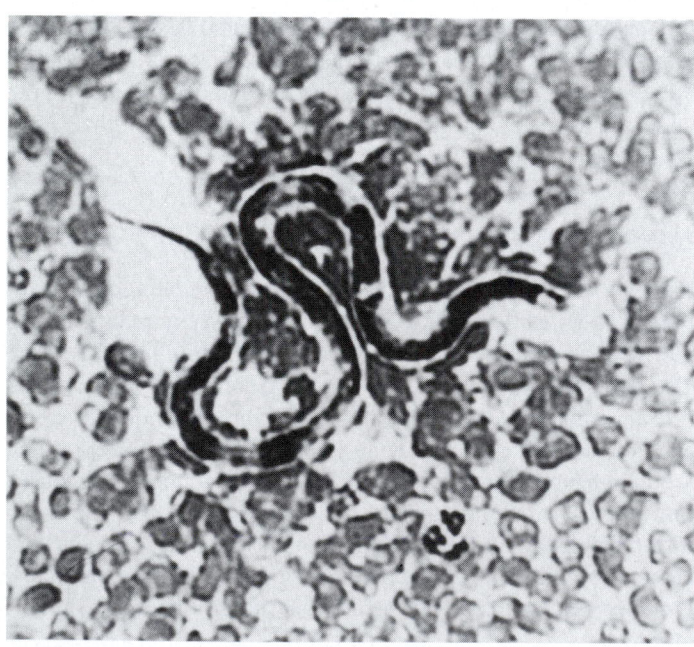

A

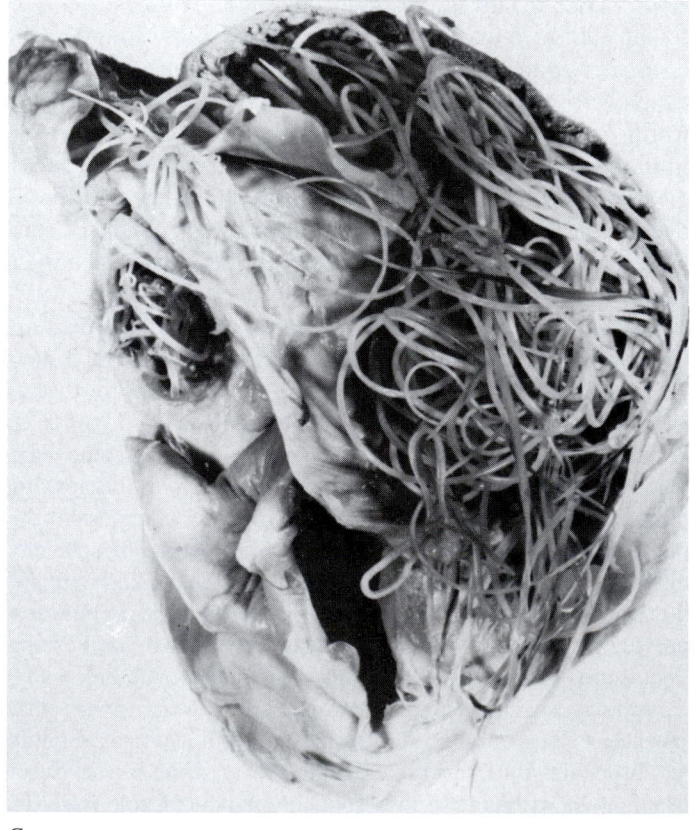

C

FIGURE 156-3 Pulmonary dirofilariasis in the dog. *A.* Microfilaria *(Dirofilaria immitis)* in blood. *B.* Right ventricular hypertrophy due to dirofilariasis. *C.* Heartworms filling the right atrium and protruding through the pulmonary valve. *(Courtesy of Dr. David H. Knight; from Shaba.[30a])*

In some, cough, chest pain, hemoptysis, and eosinophilia were manifested. Definitive diagnosis is usually obtained from microscopic examination of excised lesions.

Toxocariasis (Visceral Larva Migrans)

Toxocariasis is due to human infection with animal parasites (dog or cat ascarids). It is most commonly encountered in children. The invading parasite larvae migrate in human tissues, but cannot mature to adult worms. *Toxocara canis* and *T. cati* are the two recognized etiologic agents of human visceral larva migrans. They both are widely distributed, in both developing and developed countries.[14]

ETIOLOGY

The eggs of *T. canis* and *T. cati* are passed in the stools of dogs and cats, respectively. Transmission to humans occurs by ingestion of embryonated eggs in the soil or by contamination of food.[9] Larvae hatch in the small intestine, penetrate the gut wall, migrate to the liver, and are then carried via systemic veins to the systemic arterial circulation for distribution throughout the body. Larval migration through the host tissues and the associated inflammatory responses are considered responsible for the manifestations of disease. Most of these manifestations relate to liver pathology, eosinophilia, and pulmonary invasion. The concentrations in serum of total and specific immunoglobulins are also increased.

PATHOGENESIS AND PATHOLOGY

It is not clear whether tissue injury results from the invasion of different organs by the parasite larvae or from death and encapsulation of some organisms by an eosinophilic response of the host. The most commonly affected organ is the liver, in which granulomas surround parasite larvae. Similar lesions can be induced in experimental animals (Fig. 156-4). In the few fatal cases of toxocariasis, autopsy revealed that the major pathologic lesions were in the central nervous system.

CLINICAL FEATURES

Toxocariasis is a disease of children 1 to 4 years of age. It is particularly common in those with a history of pica. The two main presenting features relate to the chest and abdomen. Pulmonary complaints, such as cough and wheezing, and pulmonary infiltrates occur in more than one-third of symptomatic children. Peripheral eosinophilia is usually marked and may persist for years. In one study of serologically proven toxocariasis, hepatomegaly was present in 25 percent of patients.

MANAGEMENT

Toxocariasis is a cosmopolitan infection of children. Diagnosis is suspected because of the clinical presentation and serologic evidence of anti-*Toxocara* antibodies. Since the disease is usually benign and self-limiting and since the efficacy of most antihelminthics against *Toxocara* infection is doubtful, no specific therapy is recommended. Corticosteroids may be necessary to

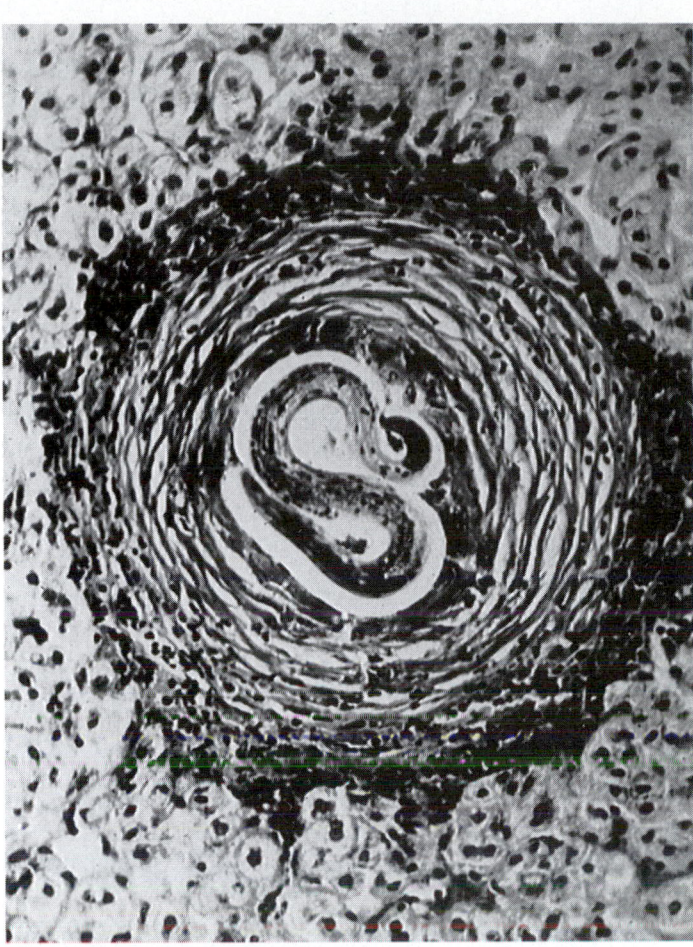

FIGURE 156-4   *Toxocara canis.* Granulomatous response to larvae in the liver. *(Courtesy of the American Society of Pathologists.)*

limit the inflammatory response in patients with extensive disease of the lungs or central nervous system.

RARE NEMATODE INFECTIONS

In severe human *T. spiralis* infection, pneumonitis is accompanied by eosinophilia. The pulmonary syndrome follows the intestinal phase of infection and is usually associated with other allergic manifestations of trichinosis, including periorbital edema, muscle swelling, and weakness.

Anisakiasis in humans results from infection with the larval form of a nematode of marine mammals. The disease has been reported in Japan and Western Europe. Although it is usually manifested as an intestinal eosinophilic disorder, it has also been implicated as the probable cause of cough, eosinophilia, and pleural effusion.

DISEASES DUE TO CESTODES (SEGMENTED WORMS)

Echinococcosis

Human infection with the larval stage of the canine tapeworm *Echinococcus granulosus* is one of the most important helminthic pulmonary diseases. *E. granulosus* is worldwide in distribution;

it occurs most commonly in sheep- and cattle-raising areas, particularly in Australia, South America, the Mediterranean, and some parts of Africa. The infection has also been reported in the United States.

ETIOLOGY

Adult *E. granulosus* worms are found in the intestines of dogs and wolves; they release eggs from their gravid segments that are passed in the feces. Humans acquire the infection by ingesting the eggs; embryos are then released and migrate to the liver, where most cysts in humans are found. Embryos may also migrate to the lungs or other tissues. Once the parasite has lodged in human tissues, it may develop in a space-occupying hydatid cyst. The inner lining of these cysts is a germinal layer capable of producing daughter cysts that may seed other organs upon spontaneous rupture or surgical manipulation of the original cyst (Fig. 156-5).

PATHOGENESIS AND PATHOLOGY

Hydatid cysts are more frequently found in the lungs of children than of adults. In most instances, the slowly enlarging, space-occupying lesion is well tolerated. Cysts in the lungs are usually discovered early in the course of the disease because radiographic examinations of the chest are now so common. Pulmonary cysts are usually solitary, in 72 percent of cases affecting one lobe. The classic unilocular hydatid cyst is usually fertile: cyst contents can

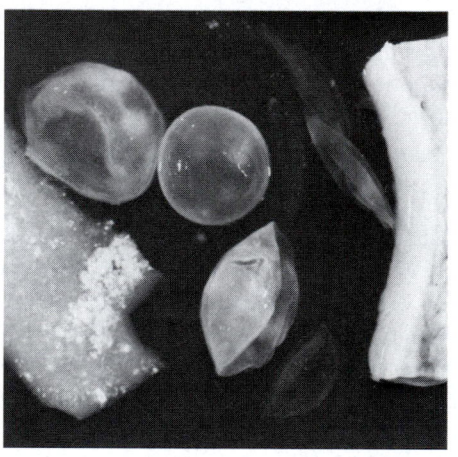

B

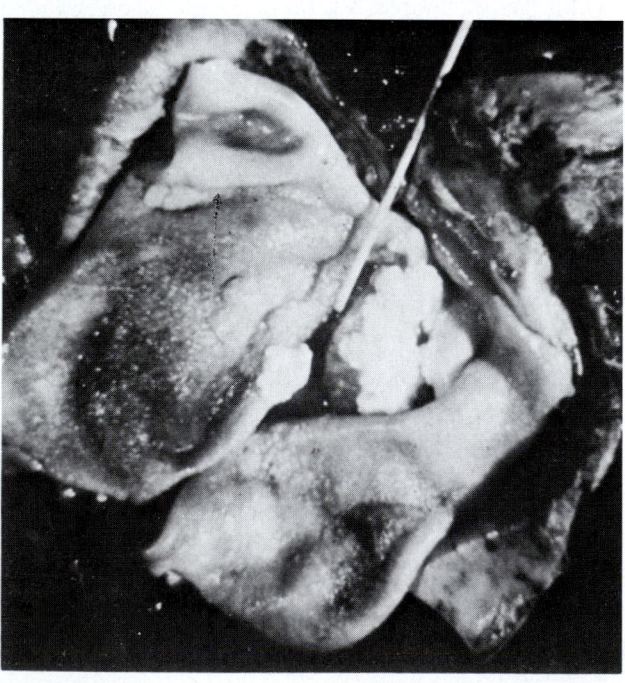

A

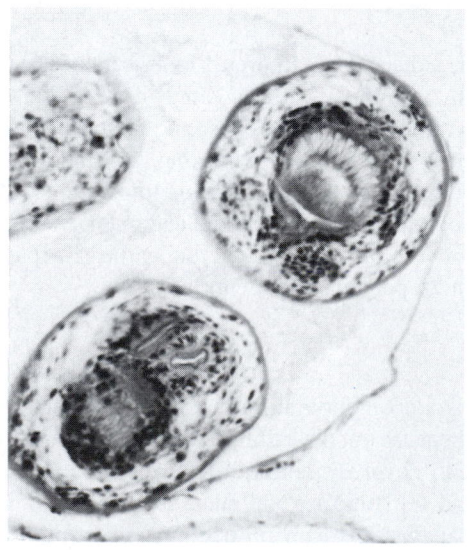

D

FIGURE 156-5 Echinococcosis. *A.* Hydatid cyst in the lung. The glistening membrane constitutes the wall of the cyst. *B.* Hydatid cysts in mesentary. Note similarity to appearance in the lung. *C.* Fragment of liver on the right is lined with *Echinococcus* membrane. Brood capsules are on the left. *D.* Three scoleces of *E. granulosus.* The upper right scolex shows the hooklets of the organism. *(A, courtesy of Dr. Stanley H. Abadie; B to D, courtesy of Dr. Daniel H. Connor, Armed Forces Institute of Pathology.)*

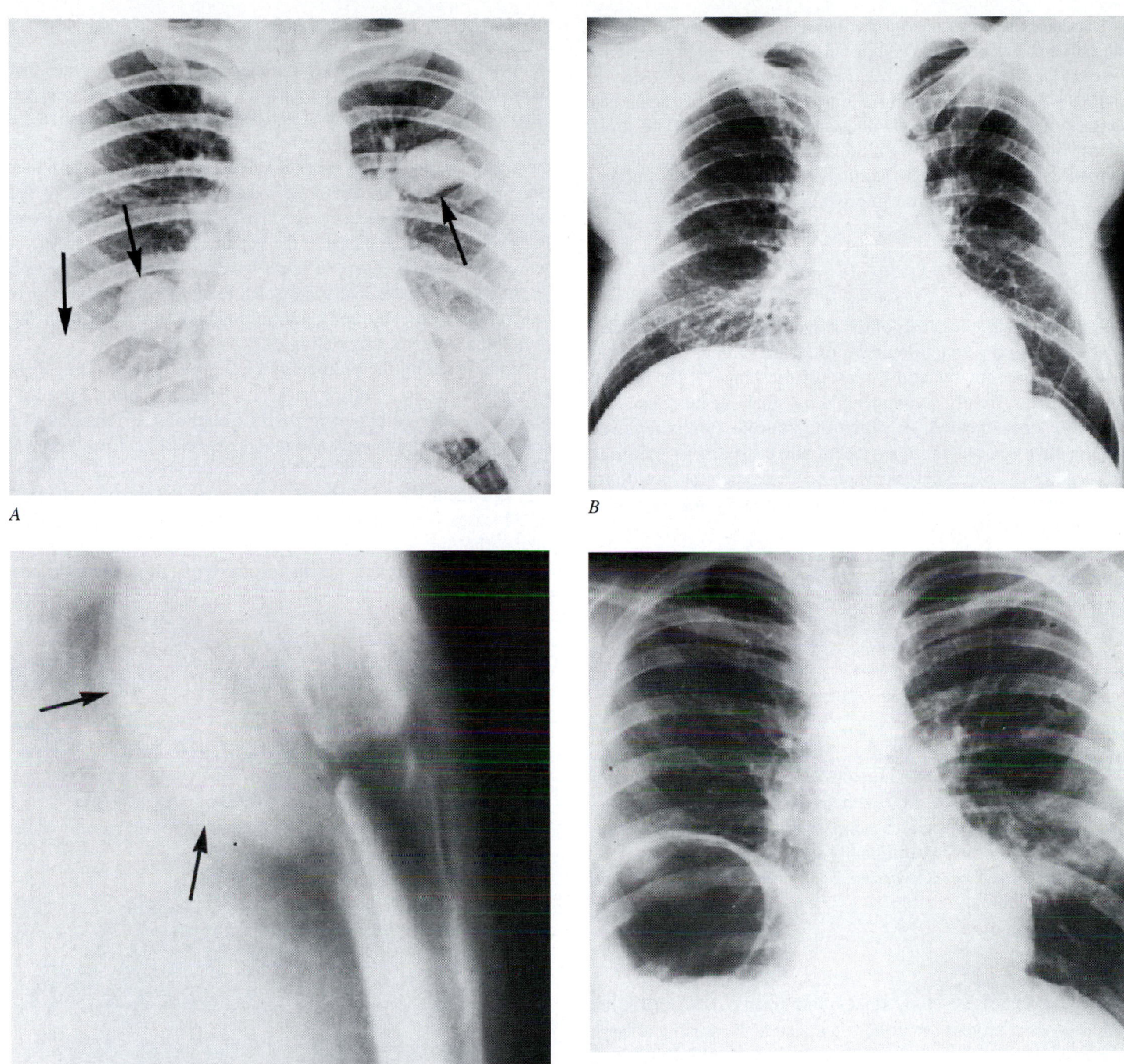

FIGURE 156-6   Echinococcus. *A.* Multiple pulmonary cysts (arrows). *(Courtesy of Dr. Carl Heitz.) B.* Another patient with echinococcus cyst behind the sternum. The retrosternal mass is difficult to discern on the posteroanterior radiograph. *C.* Lateral view. Mass (cyst) is seen (arrows). *D.* Hydatid cyst, right lower lobe. *(Courtesy of Dr. Philip Lerner.)*

seed other sites and start new cysts. The cyst is surrounded early in the course of infection by a granulomatous reaction on the part of the host; later, the inflammatory reaction is succeeded by fibrosis. Rupture of a fertile hydatid cyst may occur through a bronchus, leading to expectoration of scoleces in the sputum. Rupture into the mediastinum or pleural cavity can lead to secondary implantations. The fluid content of a hydatid cyst is believed to be immunogenic, and leakage of the cyst may evoke an anaphy-

lactic response. Although eosinophilia has been reported to accompany hydatid disease of the lung, its frequency is not known.

CLINICAL FEATURES

Hydatid cysts are usually asymptomatic; approximately half of the clinically diagnosed cysts are in the lungs. Most patients with pulmonary hydatid disease are children. In about three-fourths of patients, the cysts are in one lobe.[12] Approximately half of the patients present with cough; smaller fractions present with dyspnea or chest pain. On chest radiography, the lesions vary in diameter from 1 to 20 cm; sometimes the cyst is surrounded by an area of pneumonitis or atelectasis. Less often, a fluid level, "water lily sign" (Fig. 156-6), or calcification is seen. Other diagnostic procedures—e.g., serology[5] and computed tomography[31]—may be useful in improving characterization of the lesions.

MANAGEMENT

In most instances, diagnosis of the hydatid nature of a pulmonary cyst depends on immunologic procedures. Surgery is the treatment of choice for hydatid disease of the lungs.[34] The Barrett procedure is currently recommended for small- or moderate-size cysts; the open method, in which the parasite cyst is removed but the cavity is left draining to the pleural space, is preferred for large cysts. More extensive procedures, such as lobectomy and segmental resection, may not be necessary for most pulmonary hydatid cysts.

There is no satisfactory medical treatment for hydatid disease. This is particularly the case in pulmonary hydatid disease. Albendazole is the current recommended therapeutic agent.

DISEASES DUE TO TREMATODES (FLAT WORMS)

Schistosomiasis

Schistosomal infections of humans represent one of the major endemic helminthiases in Southeast Asia, the Middle East, Africa, the Caribbean, and South America. Five species represent the most common and clinically significant infections: *Schistosoma haematobium, S. mansoni, S. japonicum, S. mekongi,* and *S. intercalatum.*[23]

ETIOLOGY

The schistosomes are blood flukes; in humans, they inhabit the venous system around the urinary bladder or the small and large intestines. Human infection is initiated by penetration of intact skin by the free-living cercariae that are shed by specific freshwater snails. The cercariae change within a few hours into schistosomula, which migrate from the subcutaneous tissues to the lungs and then the liver, where they mature into adult worms. Fecund adult parasites then migrate to their final habitat: the veins around the ureters and urinary bladder (*S. haematobium*) and the mesenteric veins (all other species). Adult worms deposit eggs that are intended to pass through the lumen of ureters or gut to the outside environment in order to complete the life cycle of the parasite. However, some of these ova may be trapped in the host tissues. Other ova may be carried by the venous circulation to the heart and then lungs. In *S. haematobium* infection, schistosome eggs reach the pulmonary circulation via the inferior vena cava. Eggs of the other species reach the systemic circulation after the development of portal hypertension and portosystemic anastomosis.

PATHOGENESIS AND PATHOLOGY

Schistosome eggs reach the pulmonary circulation by routes that depend on the species of the parasite, their final habitat, and the stage of infection. Because *S. haematobium* worms parasitize the vesical plexus, which connects directly with the inferior vena cava, egg seeding to the lungs may occur at any phase of infection. By contrast, the anatomic location of adult worms of the other species in the mesenteric veins does not allow parasite ova to travel through the portal to the hepatic, and subsequently systemic, circulations. Eggs of these species are believed to reach the lungs only in the late stages of infection, after portal hypertension develops and anastomotic channels open between the portal and systemic circulations.

Upon reaching the pulmonary circulation, schistosome eggs usually gather in small arterioles, where they induce the formation of delayed-hypersensitivity granulomas,[32] made up of eosinophils, lymphocytes, and macrophages (Fig. 156-7). In addition, deposition of fibrous tissue causes narrowing, thickening, and occlusion of pulmonary arterioles. In an autopsy study of 32 cases of *S. mansoni* cor pulmonale, two characteristic histopathologic lesions were identified: (1) focal changes related directly to the presence of schistosome eggs; these were located

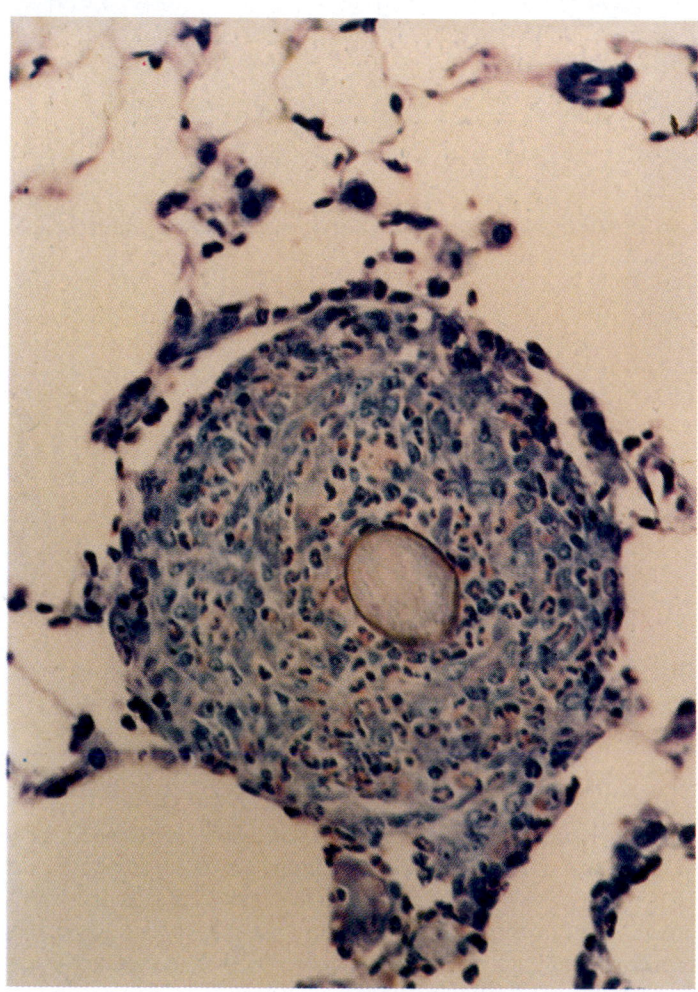

FIGURE 156-7 Schistosomal granuloma. (*Courtesy of Dr. Jay A. Fishman.*)

either within the alveolar tissue or within the pulmonary arteries or arterioles; and (2) plexiform or angiomatoid lesions consisting of several thin-walled and dilated vessels. The most prominent vascular lesions were associated with the focal changes surrounding mature schistosome eggs in the lumen of pulmonary arteries or arterioles. These were accompanied by fibrin deposition and remarkable proliferation of endothelial cells.[28] Fibrosis surrounds most focal lesions. Because of the curtailment of the pulmonary vasculature and the decreased distensibility caused by the perivascular fibrosis, pulmonary hypertension and cor pulmonale ensue. Pulmonary function is predominantly restrictive and is accompanied by a decrease in the diffusing capacity.

CLINICAL FEATURES

It is not clear whether schistosome infection during its early phases in humans is associated with appreciable pulmonary disease. Migration of schistosomula through human lungs is not known to cause detectable symptoms or signs. By contrast, after the onset of oviposition, some ova may reach the lungs, particularly in *S. haematobium* infection. Furthermore, chronic infection with the other schistosome species may be associated with sufficient deposition of eggs in the lungs to cause the development of cor pulmonale.[16] The clinical features and radiographic findings in schistosomal pulmonary hypertension and cor pulmonale are not distinctive. The prevalence of the pulmonary hypertensive syndrome in schistosome-infected patients is not known. In Egypt, 7.5 percent of patients hospitalized with schistosomal hepatomegaly had cor pulmonale; in Brazil, 23 percent of similar patients had pulmonary hypertension (i.e., pulmonary arterial blood pressure higher than 20 mmHg).

MANAGEMENT

Diagnosis of pulmonary disease due to schistosomiasis may be achieved by finding the parasite eggs in urine or stools of persons with suggestive clinical manifestations. However, pulmonary disease may occur several years after infection, and finding parasite ova may be difficult. Under these circumstances, demonstrating the characteristic pathologic changes and ova in tissues or positive serology may settle the diagnosis.[25]

Active schistosome infections are treated with praziquantel, which kills adult worms and stops further destruction of tissue by ova deposition. The drug is administered as a single oral dose of 40 mg/kg body weight for *S. mansoni* and *S. haematobium* infection and in a dose of 20 mg/kg body weight three times a day for *S. japonicum* infection. However, reversal of pathologic lesions in the lungs after antischistosomal chemotherapy has not been documented.

Paragonimiasis

Human infection with species of the lung fluke *Paragonimus* is prevalent in the Far East, Africa, and South and Central America.[10] Infection is maintained in endemic areas through contamination of water sources, with feces or sputum of infected individuals resulting in infection of the intermediate snail and crustacean hosts. Symptomatic paragonimiasis is initially characterized by cough and bloody sputum that may lead to bronchiectasis or lung abscesses.

ETIOLOGY

Human infection with *Paragonimus* is acquired from eating raw or pickled crustacea (freshwater crayfish and crabs) that harbor the infective parasite stage (metacercariae). These forms excyst in the duodenum, penetrate the intestinal wall, and migrate via the diaphragm and pleural cavity to the lungs, where they mature into adult worms ($12 \times 6 \times 5$ mm). Adult *Paragonimus* worms are hermaphroditic; they produce golden-brown eggs, which are coughed up and voided through either sputum or feces. The life cycle of the parasite outside the human host goes through a specific snail intermediate host; metacercariae then encyst on freshwater crustacea.

PATHOGENESIS AND PATHOLOGY

The primary site of infection in humans is the lungs. The worm is also found in the brain in 25 percent of patients and less often in many other tissues. During invasion of the lungs by the maturing adult worms, parasite tunnels in the pulmonary parenchyma can usually be demonstrated, particularly in peripheral areas. The tunnels and parasites are surrounded by a granulocytic reaction made of eosinophils and neutrophils. Charcot-Leyden crystals are often seen. In patients with encysted worms, the parasites are enclosed with cystic lesions that may communicate with each other or with a bronchus. Death of the worms usually leads to collapse of the cyst, disintegration of the parasite, and fibrosis or calcification. The surrounding pulmonary tissue may show evidence of atelectasis, bronchiectasis, or compensatory emphysema. In some patients, secondary infection and lung abscess develop in the cystic lesions surrounding adult parasites. The radiographic changes correspond roughly to the three stages of parasite development within the lungs: (1) on arrival in the lungs, maturing worms are associated with the development of radiographic opacities; (2) these are succeeded by nodules that correspond to the parasite cysts; (3) fibrosis or calcification ensues.

CLINICAL FEATURES

The incubation period between infection and the development of maturing adults in the lungs is 2 to 20 days. Few specific symptoms have been described during this stage. In persons with established infection, the worm load seems to determine the extent of clinical features. Light infection is invariably asymptomatic. In moderate to heavy worm loads, complaint of cough and respiratory discomfort (particularly upon rising in the morning) and rusty, blood-tinged sputum containing parasite eggs, necrotic material, and Charcot-Leyden crystals are common. Frank hemoptysis, sometimes severe, also occurs in patients with pulmonary paragonimiasis.

The chest radiograph is normal in 10 to 20 percent of infected persons. Radiographic signs in the others include infiltrate, cavitation, fibrosis, and pulmonary thickening. The characteristic ring shadow with a crescent corona occurs in some infected persons.[11]

MANAGEMENT

The diagnosis of paragonimiasis is made from detection of the characteristic eggs in the sputum or stools of infected persons. Serologic testing may be helpful in egg-negative cases. The drug of choice for treating paragonimiasis is praziquantel. It is administered orally, 75 mg/kg per day for 2 days.[18] Chemotherapy usually leads to cessation of egg passage in sputum and stools, some clearing of the chest radiograph in almost two-thirds of treated patients, and a decrease in serum IgG antibodies against the parasite.

REFERENCES

1. Adkins RB, Dao AH: Pulmonary dirofilariasis: A diagnostic challenge. *South Med J* 77:372–374, 1984.
2. Anderson RM, May RM: *Infectious Diseases of Humans: Dynamics and Control.* New York, Oxford University Press, 1991, pp 433–606.
3. Butterworth AE, Sturrock RF, Houba V, et al: Eosinophils as mediators of antibody dependent damage to schistosomula. *Nature* 256:727–729, 1975.
4. Conway DJ, Bailey JW, Lindo JF, et al: Serum IgG reactivity with 41-, 31- and 28-kDa larval proteins of *Strongyloides stercoralis* in individuals with strongyloidiasis. *J Infect Dis* 168:784–787, 1993.
5. Force L, Torres JM, Carrillo A, Bass I: Evaluation of eight serological tests in the diagnosis of human echinococcosis and follow-up. *Clin Infect Dis* 15:473–480, 1992.
6. Gelpi AP, Mustafa A: Ascaris pneumonia. *Am J Med* 44:377–389, 1968.
7. Genta RM: Global prevalence of strongyloidiasis: Critical review with epidemiologic insights into the prevention of disseminated diseases. *J Infect Dis* 11:755–767, 1989.
8. Gleich G, Adolphson C, Leiferman K: The biology of the eosinophilic leukocyte. *Annu Rev Med* 43:85–101, 1993.
9. Glickman LT, Magnaual J-F: Zoonotic round worm infection. *Infect Dis Clin North Am* 7:717–732, 1993.
10. Harinasuta T, Bunnag D: Liver, lung and intestinal trematodiasis, in Warren KS, Mahmoud AAF (eds): *Tropical and Geographical Medicine,* 2d ed. New York, McGraw-Hill, 1990, pp 473–489.
11. Im J-G, Whang HY, Kim WS, et al: Pleuropulmonary paragonimiasis: Radiologic findings in 71 patients. *AJR Am J Roentgenol* 159:39–43, 1992.
12. Jerray M, Benzarti M, Garrouch A, et al: Hydatid disease of the lungs: Study of 386 cases. *Am Rev Respir Dis* 146:185–189, 1992.
13. Kazura JW: The filariasis, in Mahmoud AAF (ed), *Parasitic Lung Diseases.* New York: Dekker, 1997, pp 109–124.
14. Kazura JW: Visceral larva migrans and other tissue nematodes, in Mahmoud AAF (ed), *Parasitic Lung Diseases.* New York, Dekker, 1997, pp 125–133.
15. King CH: Cestodes (tapeworm), in Mandell GL, Bennett JE, Dolin R (eds), *Principles and Practice of Infectious Diseases,* 4th ed. New York, Churchill Livingstone, 1995, pp 2544–2553.
16. King CL: Schistosomiasis, in Mahmoud AAF (ed), *Parasitic Lung Diseases.* New York, Dekker, 1997, pp 135–155.
17. Mahmoud AAF: The ecology of eosinophils in schistosomiasis. *J Infect Dis* 145:613–622, 1982.
18. Mahmoud AAF: Praziquantel for the treatment of helminthic infections. *Adv Intern Med* 32:193–206, 1987.
19. Mahmoud AAF: Parasitic protozoa and helminths: Biological and immunological challenges. *Science* 246:1015–1022, 1989.
20. Mahmoud AAF: Eosinophilia, in Warren KS, Mahmoud AAF (eds), *Tropical and Geographical Medicine,* 2d ed. New York, McGraw-Hill, 1990, pp 65–69.
21. Mahmoud AAF: Intestinal nematodes (roundworms), in Mandell GL, Bennett JE, Dolin R (eds), *Principles and Practice of Infectious Diseases,* 4th ed. New York, Churchill Livingstone, 1995, pp 2526–2531.
22. Mahmoud AAF: Diseases due to helminths: Introduction, in Mandell GL, Bennett JE, Dolin R (eds), *Principles and Practice of Infectious Diseases,* 4th ed. New York, Churchill Livingstone, 1995, pp 2525–2526.
23. Mahmoud AAF: Strongyloidiasis. *Clin Infect Dis,* 23:949–953, 1996.
24. Mahmoud AAF, Abel Wahab MF: Schistosomiasis, in Warren KS, Mahmoud AAF (eds), *Tropical and Geographical Medicine,* 2d ed. New York, McGraw-Hill, 1990, pp 458–473.
25. Mahmoud AAF, Warren KS, Peters PA: A role for the eosinophil in acquired resistance to *Schistosoma mansoni* infection as determined by antieosinophil serum. *J Exp Med* 142:805–813, 1975.
26. Ottesen EA: The Wellcome Trust Lecture: Infection and disease in lymphatic filariasis: An immunological perspective. *Parasitology* 104:571–594, 1992.
27. Pearlman E: Pathogenesis and immunity in helminthic infection, in Mahmoud AAF (ed), *Parasitic Lung Diseases.* New York, Dekker, 1997, pp 33–46.
28. Sadigursky M, Andrade ZA: Pulmonary changes in schistosomal cor pulmonale. *Am J Trop Med Hyg* 31:779–784, 1982.
29. Salata R: Intestinal nematodes, in Mahmoud AAF (ed), *Parasitic Lung Diseases.* New York, Dekker, 1997, pp 89–108.
30. Sanderson, C.J: Interleukin-5, eosinophils and disease. *Blood,* 12:3101–3109, 1993.
30a. Shaba JK: Protozoan and metazoan infections, in Fishman AP (ed). *Pulmonary Diseases and Disorders.* New York, McGraw-Hill, 1980, pp 1182–1201.
31. von Sinner WN: New diagnostic signs in hydatid disease: Radiography, ultrasound, CT and MRI correlated to pathology. *Eur J Radiol* 12:150–159, 1991.
32. Warren KS, Domingo ES, Cowan RBT: Granuloma formation around schistosome eggs as a manifestation of delayed hypersensitivity. *Am J Pathol* 51:735–745, 1967.
33. Woodring JH, Halfhill H II, Reed JC: Pulmonary strongyloidiasis: Clinical and imaging features. *AJR Am J Roentgenol* 162:537–542, 1994.
34. Zelik C, Inci I, Toprak M, et al: Surgical treatment of pulmonary hydatidosis in children: Experience in 92 patients. *J Pediatr Surg* 29:392–395, 1994.

CHAPTER 157

ZOONOTIC AND OTHER UNUSUAL BACTERIAL PNEUMONIAS

Arnold N. Weinberg / Howard M. Heller

ZOONOTIC BACTERIAL PNEUMONIAS
Pasteurella multocida **Respiratory Infections**
Pneumonia due to *Yersinia pestis*
Pneumonia due to *Francisella tularensis*
Pneumonia due to *Rhodococcus equi*

ENVIRONMENTAL AND ANIMAL PRODUCT PNEUMONIAS
Anthrax Respiratory Disease
Pneumonia due to *Brucella* **Species**
Pneumonia due to *Burkholderia (Pseudomonas) pseudomallei*
Pulmonary Infections due to *Yersinia enterocolitica*

PNEUMONIAS CAUSED BY OBLIGATE HUMAN COMMENSALS
Neisseria meningitidis
Moraxella (Branhamella) catarrhalis

Many different microorganisms can infect the lungs, but routes of spread are few, clinical presentations overlap, radiologic changes are often nonspecific, and pathophysiological mechanisms are limited. Making a clinical diagnosis of pneumonia is relatively easy; defining the causative agent can be difficult. The search for the specific agent is driven by a number of compelling issues, including the desire to use a specific therapy for a specific pathogen; the potential for progressive respiratory impairment when the wrong antibiotic is used; and epidemiologic concerns in the family, in the hospital community, and in the public at large for isolation and containment.[40]

In the two decades that have passed since the epidemic of acute respiratory disease erupted among delegates to the American Legion Convention in Philadelphia, physicians, microbiologists, and epidemiologists have been better prepared for the challenges of patients with unusual pneumonias.[22] The rapid response leading to the identification of the hantavirus as causing a newly recognized respiratory syndrome is an example of the multidisciplined approach toward recognition of emerging infectious diseases.[16] The increased awareness of investigators and clinicians to the variety of infectious agents capable of causing

respiratory infections is illustrated by the increased frequency of the *clinical* diagnosis of Q fever (due to *Coxiella burnetti*) in addition to retrospective serologic diagnoses.[47] *Chlamydia pneumoniae,* the former "TWAR" agent, has been identified in military and school epidemics and as an important cause of pneumonia in isolated cases.[26] These infectious agents and diseases are covered in detail elsewhere in the text. However, they often appear as part of the differential diagnosis in obscure pneumonia, and illustrate the range of pathogens associated with animals and their environments and acute respiratory outbreaks among young people.

This discussion of *unusual bacterial pneumonias* focuses on a limited number of microorganisms and not on an exhaustive list of possible causative agents. The unique properties of these bacteria exemplify how bacteriology, ecology, epidemiology, and pathogenesis serve as helpful clues to earlier etiologic diagnosis and, therefore, specific therapy (Table 157-1).[60]

ZOONOTIC BACTERIAL PNEUMONIAS

A wide variety of domestic and wild vertebrates are colonized by bacteria capable of producing pneumonia in humans. In this section, four diseases that illustrate the mechanisms for dissemination and the characteristic features of respiratory invasion are described. There are few unique distinguishing clinical features that reveal the causes of these infections. Clues derived from a careful history of immunologic competence, travel, occupation, hobbies, and animal and arthropod contact, however, are invaluable aids to the correct diagnosis and therapy and can be lifesaving.[60]

Pasteurella multocida Respiratory Infections

Pasteurella multocida is a common commensal of the oral cavity of most felines and many dogs and a frequent respiratory pathogen in animals and birds. In the United States, domestic associations are responsible for many cases of cellulitis following cat or dog bites. Respiratory infections are probably underreported, with fewer than 50 cases on record. Sputum isolates, however, are not

TABLE 157-1

An Overview of Zoonotic and Other Unusual Pneumonias

Environmental Niche	Microorganism	Disease	Epidemiologic Associations	Distribution
Live animal contact or via arthropod	Francisella tularensis	Tularemia	Contact with animals, birds, or arthropods	North America, Europe, Asia
	Pasteurella multocida	Pasteurellosis	Feline and dog contact; chronic lung disease	Worldwide
	Rhodococcus equi	Rhodococcus pneumonia	Airborne; contact with soil contaminated with horse, cow, or swine excrement	Worldwide
	Yersinia pestis	Plague	Contact with rodents, fleas; contact with plague pneumonia case	Worldwide, including Asia, southwest U.S.
Soil, stagnant water, and inert animal products	Bacillus anthracis	Inhalation anthrax or wool-sorter's disease	Industrial; use of animal products in hobbies	Worldwide in warmer regions
	Brucella species	Brucellosis	Ingestion or contact with infected animal products	Worldwide
	Burkholderia pseudomallei	Melioidosis	Direct penetrating contact with soil, water	Latitude 20°N to 20°S, especially rural Asia
	Yersinia enterocolitica	Yersiniosis	Ingestion of contaminated foods, water; cirrhosis	Worldwide
Obligate human commensal	Neisseria meningitidis	Meningococcal pneumonia	Airborne, human to human; postviral, nosocomial	Humans worldwide
	Moraxella catarrhalis	Moraxella pneumonia	Aspiration, especially individuals with underlying lung disease	Humans worldwide

infrequent in patients with chronic pulmonary disease. Immunocompromised patients, including those with AIDS, may be prone to infection without traumatic dog or cat exposures.[15]

BACTERIOLOGY

P. multocida is a small gram-negative bipolar-staining coccobacillary organism that resembles *Hemophilus* species and may form pairs and chains. Rapid growth on blood agar and inhibition by MacConkey medium help to separate this microorganism from other common components of the respiratory flora, including *Hemophilus* species. The organism produces a capsule that interferes with phagocytosis. Besides cell envelope endotoxin, no other pathogenic properties have been identified.

ECOLOGY AND EPIDEMIOLOGY

In cats and other felines, the organism resides periodontally in the anterior regions of the mouth. Isolates from dogs are characteristically from the posterior pharynx. Many birds and domestic and wild animals worldwide harbor this organism as a commensal in oral or gastrointestinal areas. *P. multocida* is occasionally found in the secretions of persons with chronic lung disease, especially those with bronchiectasis and with a history of domestic animal contacts. Human-to-human transmission has been documented from mother to newborn infant, resulting in neonatal aspiration pneumonia. The organism can survive in soil and water for more than 3 weeks and in animal carcasses for approximately 2 months. In about half the cases of respiratory disease, no clue to airborne spread exists, but there are usually cats in the local environment.

PATHOGENESIS AND PATHOPHYSIOLOGY

Pathogenic strains have a polysaccharide capsule that inhibits phagocytosis, and they contain endotoxin in the cell envelope. Exotoxins and other pathogenicity-promoting factors have not been identified. Almost all patients who develop respiratory infections have underlying chronic pulmonary disease. Aspiration probably initiates active infection. Necrosis and lung abscess, empyema, septicemia, and transbronchial spread to other lung segments have been described.[58]

CLINICAL AND RADIOLOGIC FEATURES

The clinical features of *P. multocida* respiratory disease include worsening of the patient's baseline respiratory function—especially when high fever, tenacious secretions, and pleural effusions develop. Radiologic changes include lobar, multilobar, or diffuse patchy infiltrates, usually sparing the upper lobes, superimposed on underlying chronic lung disease (Fig. 157-1). Effusions have been noted in approximately 20 percent of cases.[58]

DIAGNOSTIC FEATURES

The diagnosis depends on isolation of the organism from sputum, pleural fluid, or blood. The pathogen can usually be identified with the routine methods of the diagnostic laboratory. The bipolar gram-negative staining bacilli resemble *Brucella* species, *Yersinia pestis*, *Francisella tularensis*, *Burkholdaria* (formerly *Pseudomonas*) *pseudomallei*, and *Hemophilus* species, but the clinical history and bacteriologic characteristics can rapidly clarify the identification.

TREATMENT

Most strains are exquisitely susceptible to penicillin or ampicillin. The third-generation cephalosporins, cefotaxime and ceftriaxone, are as active as penicillin and more potent than earlier-generation relatives. Tetracycline and chloramphenicol are useful when a history of immediate-type allergic reactions precludes use of a β-lactam agent. Oral preparations of cephalosporins and penicillins are not recommended for treating pneumonias due to *P. multocida*. (See Table 157-2 for specific dosages of useful agents.) Fluoroquinolones are very active in vitro, and although they have been used successfully in animals with pasteurella pneumonia, there have been no reports of their use in treating the disease in humans.[43]

Pneumonia due to *Yersinia pestis*

This organism left an indelible mark on humanity long before its late-nineteenth-century isolation and characterization. The cause

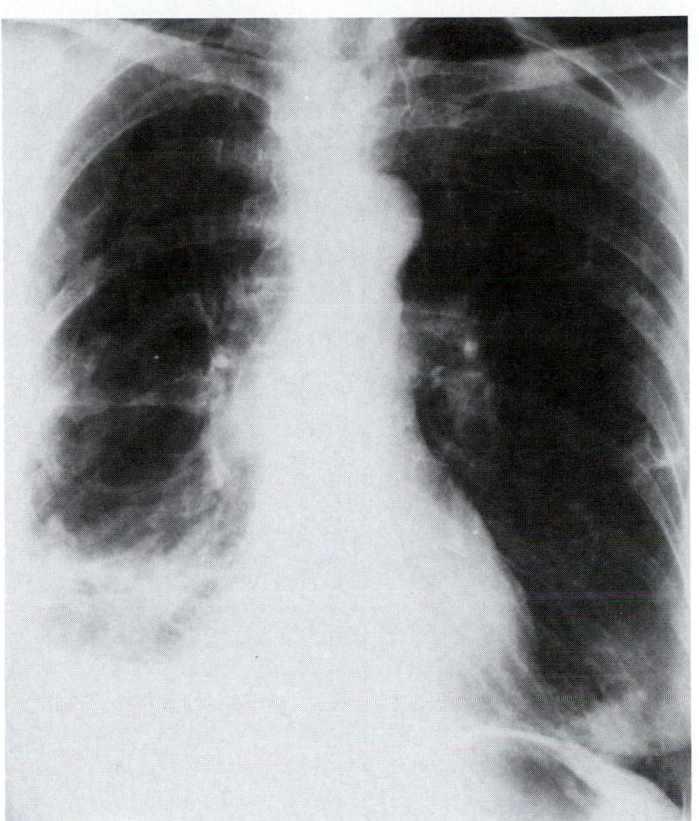

FIGURE 157-1 Bilateral pneumonia due to *Pasteurella multocida* in a 69-year-old woman suffering from chronic obstructive pulmonary disease and a prior right lower lobectomy for carcinoma. Infiltrates disappeared with penicillin therapy.

of three major pandemics from the sixth through the nineteenth centuries, pulmonary disease in a few victims led to aerosol spread to countless others, resulting in acute primary pneumonia and the "black death" of epidemic plague. A contemporary global scare emanated from India's Maharashtra state in 1994, with reports of suspected pneumonic and bubonic plague.[9] No exported cases were documented during rigorous quarantine and airplane surveillance measures, and no travelers to India became ill with a plague syndrome. In the United States, approximately 20 cases of plague are reported yearly, of which 1 in 5 have lung involvement. Early recognition and specific therapy, combined with isolation procedures and appropriately directed prophylaxis of contacts, should help maintain the record of no human-to-human transmission that has pertained since the 1920s.

BACTERIOLOGY

Y. pestis is a bipolar-staining, gram-negative bacillus closely related to *Escherichia coli* and other Enterobacteriaceae. It grows well on blood or MacConkey agar and is identified definitively with differential biochemical tests, agglutination reactions, and direct fluorescent antibody staining.

ECOLOGY AND EPIDEMIOLOGY

In the United States, *Y. pestis* is endemic in rock squirrels, prairie dogs, and other ground animals. Spread among animals occurs

TABLE 157-2

Diagnostic Studies and Treatment Recommendations in Zoonotic Pneumonias

Disease	Gram's Stain Morphology	Culture Methods	Identifying Tests	Therapy Total Dose/Number of Doses*
Anthrax	Large gram-positive bacillus (rarely seen)	BAP, blood cultures	FA	PCN (12–18 mu/6) CL (4–6 g/6) or D (200 mg/2)
Brucellosis	Small gram-negative coccobacillus (rarely seen)	Media enriched with serum, $CO_2 + O_2$	Rise in AA, Prozone	TMP-SMX (480 mg + 2.4 g/3) + SM (1 g/2) D (200 mg/2) + RI (600 mg/1)
Melioidosis	Bipolar staining gram-negative bacillus	BAP, MAC	Morphology, FA, AA	TMP-SMX (640 mg + 3.2 g/4) and ceftazidime (6–9 g/3) or CL (4–6 g/4) + D (200 mg/2)
Pasteurellosis	Small bipolar staining gram-negative bacillus	BAP, CO_2	Inhibited by MAC, biochem. tests	PCN or A (6 mu or 8 g/4) or cefotaxime (6–8 g/4) or CL (3 g/4)
Plague	Enteric bipolar staining gram-negative bacillus	BAP, MAC, enteric media, blood cultures	Biochem. tests, FA, AA	SM (2 g/2) and D (200 mg/2) or CL (4–6 g/4)
Rhodococcus	Gram-positive coccobacilli (slightly acid-fast positive)	BAP	Biochem. tests	E (2 g/4) or CLA (1 g/2) or AZ (500 mg) and CIP (1.5 g/2) and RI (600 mg)
Tularemia	Small gram-negative coccobacillus	Enriched media with cysteine, serum	FA, AA, rarely cultured	SM or gentamicin (2 g/2 or 4.5 mg/kg/3) or CL (3–4 g/4) or D (200 mg/2)
Yersiniosis	Enteric gram-negative bacillus	BAP, MAC, enteric media, blood cultures	Biochem. tests, motility 25°C	A (8 g/4) or 2d or 3d gen. cephalosp. (4–6 g/4) or CL (3 g/4)

*Expressed as million units (mu), grams (g), or milligrams (mg) divided by number of doses in 24 h.

NOTE: BAP = blood agar; MAC = MacConkey agar; FA = fluorescent antibody; AA = agglutin antibody. Antibiotics include A = ampicillin; AZ = azithromycin; CIP = ciprofloxacin; CL = chloramphenicol; CLA = clarithromycin; D = doxycycline; E = erythromycin; PCN = penicillin; RI = rifampin; SM = streptomycin; TMP-SMX = trimethoprim-sulfamethoxazole.

via several species of rodent fleas. Domestic animals that wander outdoors, like cats, can become infected by direct contact with sick rodents or via rodent flea bites. In addition, cats and dogs can inadvertently carry fleas into the home. Occasionally rodent die-offs, called epizootics, occur, and many dead animals can be found with viable organisms in carcasses and in the soil surrounding ground dwellings.

In the United States, spread to humans occurs in the endemic areas west of the Rockies—especially in California, northern Arizona, and New Mexico—when a hungry flea feeds on a susceptible person. Living or working in proximity to local enzootic "hot spots" places certain groups (such as Native Americans, geologists, hikers, veterinarians, and pet owners) at risk. Bubonic and cutaneous plague is usually acquired by contact with infected fleas, but aerosols from ill animals or from carcasses can lead to primary pneumonia, pharyngitis, or conjunctivitis. Several cases of cat-to-human aerosol spread have been associated with respiratory infection or submandibular abscess in pets.[14] The great fear of physicians caring for patients with respiratory infection is the potential for rapid airborne dissemination, especially during coughing and face-to-face contacts.

PATHOGENESIS AND PATHOPHYSIOLOGY

Once the organism gains access to human tissues at 37°C, rapid multiplication occurs with formation of a polysaccharide capsule. The capsule imparts virulence properties that include resisting phagocytosis and persistence of bacteria within nonsensitized monocytes. Virulence factors impacting on the host also include a potent endotoxin and V and W antigens of the cell envelope, which also influence intracellular survival. Bacteremic spread usually follows initial multiplication in regional nodes or at the local flea bite site. Secondary pneumonia involving the well-perfused basal segments can follow. When a person with plague pneumonia coughs, there may be aerosol spread to persons nearby, resulting in primary pneumonia and rapidly developing adult respiratory distress syndrome (ARDS).

CLINICAL AND RADIOLOGIC FEATURES

The clinical presentation of pneumonia depends on the mechanism of spread. In contemporary experience in the United States, cases have all been secondary to bubonic plague, to primary septicemia without an overt skin lesion, or to inhalation of droplets from an infected pet cat.[14,21] The onset of respiratory disease follows after days to a week of a febrile illness, and is ushered in by the gradual onset of cough, dyspnea, and increasing toxicity. A hemorrhagic productive cough, pleurisy, and increasing respiratory distress are additional symptoms. The unique feature in most cases of pneumonia is the epidemiologic association with classic bubonic plague in a person recently in an endemic area or who has had contact with a pet cat ill with respiratory symptoms or a facial abscess. From cases of primary inhalation pneumonia described previously, exposure to an index case may be followed by the rapid development of a fulminating respiratory illness, with dyspnea, cyanosis, and thin, watery sputum that rapidly becomes hemorrhagic.[38] The clinical picture is not unlike that of overwhelming pneumococcal pneumonia, with

marked toxicity and mental torpor associated with progressive cyanosis.[21]

The radiologic features of secondary pneumonia include basal segment nodular to hazy airspace infiltrates, hilar and mediastinal node hypertrophy, and occasionally pleural effusions. In primary pneumonia, infiltrates may be minimal during the first 24 h, followed by progressive airspace disease resembling ARDS or pulmonary edema.[2]

DIAGNOSIS AND DIFFERENTIAL DIAGNOSIS

The presence of characteristic bipolar-staining gram-negative bacilli in sputum supports the diagnosis when epidemiologic factors are suggestive. Cultures of blood, sputum, and lymph node aspirates often yield positive results. Direct fluorescent antibody staining, if available, can provide immediate etiologic confirmation. A passive hemagglutination test can be performed as a confirmatory study on acute and convalescent sera at selected reference laboratories of the Centers for Disease Control and Prevention. Other acute respiratory infections caused by microorganisms that appear as gram-negative bacilli with bipolar staining must be considered, including *F. tularensis* and *P. multocida.*

TREATMENT AND PREVENTION

The combination of streptomycin and tetracycline has been the treatment of choice for serious plague infections. Gentamicin can be substituted for streptomycin if intravenous therapy is necessary or streptomycin is not available. In patients with impaired renal function, chloramphenicol should be used in place of tetracycline. (See Table 157-2 for dosage schedules.)

Persons suspected of having plague pneumonia should be rapidly isolated, and strict contact, respiratory, and conjunctival precautions instituted. Anyone exposed face to face with a coughing patient, including health-care workers, should be given preventive tetracycline, 2 g daily, divided into four doses, for 5 to 10 days. Isolation procedures are continued until productive cough is no longer present or sputum cultures are negative for *Y. pestis.*

A vaccine is available for laboratory workers and others with frequent exposure to the microorganisms or to hyperendemic areas. Careful surveillance of ground rodent populations, posting warnings in endemic regions, watching for die-offs that indicate epizootic spread, and spraying for local flea control may also be effective preventive measures.

Pneumonia due to *Francisella tularensis*

Tularemia is a common animal disease in the United States. The causative agent, *F. tularensis,* is ubiquitous, distributed among many species of wild and domestic animals and birds. Bloodsucking arthropods, especially ticks and deer flies, serve an important role in transmission to humans.[4] As with plague, the major clinical manifestations include skin lesions and swollen or draining regional lymph nodes. Pulmonary impairment occurs secondary to bacteremia or as a primary inhalation or aspiration pneumonia. Approximately 150 human cases are reported in the

United States yearly, but this is probably an underestimate. Pulmonary invasion is seen in 10 to 15 percent of ulceroglandular cases and in more than 50 percent of patients with the typhoidal syndrome in addition to primary inhalation pneumonia.[19]

BACTERIOLOGY

F. tularensis is a fragile-appearing gram-negative coccobacillary organism that grows poorly on artificial media unless fortified with serum and cysteine (or sulfhydryl compounds). The potential for laboratory-acquired inhalation or ingestion-associated disease is great. Most routine laboratories will not attempt to culture the organism, leaving this to special reference centers. Identification is on the basis of morphologic and biochemical determinants, but direct fluorescent staining or agglutination reactions with specific antisera are also useful.

ECOLOGY AND EPIDEMIOLOGY

The organism is associated with more than 100 species of wild and domestic animals and birds, but most clinical cases arise from contact with rabbits, squirrels, or arthropods. Aquatic mammals and their immediate water and mud living environments can also be contaminated with *F. tularensis*.[63] Bloodsucking arthropods, especially ticks and deerflies, act as reservoirs capable of harboring the pathogen for long periods and are responsible for dissemination among wildlife species. Domestic cats represent a potentially increasing problem.[6]

Most human cases are acquired from contact with infected animals during hunting, trapping, and other outdoor pursuits, especially during colder months. In southern areas, or in the summer season in northern latitudes, bloodsucking arthropods, especially ticks and deerflies, constitute a significant mode of spread. Ingestion of contaminated food, animal bites, conjunctival contact, and aerosol dissemination are also important mechanisms for acquiring the pathogen.[52] In recent years, cases secondary to arthropods have been more frequent than those associated with direct animal contact, although domestic cat bites and airborne spread appear to be increasing.[6] Human-to-human transmission is not recognized, in contrast to the significant theoretical potential for spread of pneumonic plague.

PATHOGENESIS AND PATHOPHYSIOLOGY

F. tularensis contains a number of protein and polysaccharide antigens in the cell envelope and an endotoxin component that is similar to endotoxins of other gram-negative microorganisms. Very little is known about other mechanisms of pathogenesis. The organism is capable of remaining viable in reticuloendothelial cells of nonimmune subjects and in macrophages that have not been stimulated by recent exposure to intracellular pathogens. As few as 10 to 50 organisms can initiate disease following cutaneous penetration or by inhalation, but a significant number are required when the challenge is through ingestion of contaminated foods. Local growth usually is followed by regional node suppuration and occasionally bacteremic dissemination to many organs, including the lungs. Rhabdomyolysis of uncertain cause may accompany bacteremia and pneumonia.[32] Ingestion may result in pharyngeal infection, involvement of the gastrointestinal tract, or subclinical disease followed by the typhoidal syndrome. Primary pneumonia follows inhalation of organisms, resulting in numerous areas of inflammation, necrosis, a tendency to granuloma formation, and pleural inflammation.

CLINICAL AND RADIOLOGIC FEATURES

Respiratory disease is heralded by the onset of a nonproductive cough, usually in a febrile patient ill with the ulceroglandular form of tularemia. In the absence of a local chancriform lesion or tender swollen lymph node (bubo), the disease may be dominated by constitutional symptoms, with high fever and shaking chills (typhoidal tularemia).[41] Pneumonia following an inhalation exposure results in cough, dyspnea, and occasionally pleurisy. Respiratory disease can be subtle, and the diagnosis may be apparent only if a chest radiograph is done.

Radiologic changes include evidence of parenchymal and pleural disease, which is often out of proportion to the physical findings. Diffuse areas of bronchopneumonia occur, with hilar node enlargement. Unilateral or bilateral pleural effusions are often noted (Fig. 157-2). Central oval infiltrates, described as characteristic in early reports, are seldom observed today.[45] Lobar airspace disease and lung abscess are unusual additional patterns that have been described.

DIAGNOSIS AND DIFFERENTIAL DIAGNOSIS

Any febrile patient with animal or arthropod exposure in an endemic region, especially presenting with a skin lesion or tender

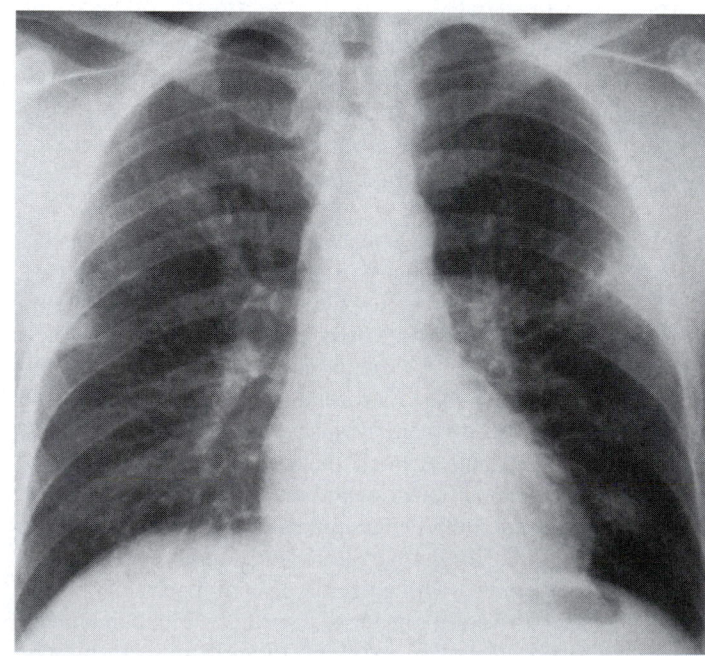

FIGURE 157-2 Patchy nodular and bronchopneumonia, hilar adenopathy, and left pleural effusion due to *Francisella tularensis* in a 38-year-old veterinarian exposed to a cat dying with a respiratory infection. All the findings resolved with tetracycline therapy.

lymph nodes, should be evaluated for tularemia. Respiratory involvement is confirmed by radiologic study. Cough, when present, is usually nonproductive, and blood cultures are seldom positive. Characteristic organisms are rarely seen in pleural fluid or aspirates of suppurating nodes. Direct fluorescent antibody staining of exudates can confirm the diagnosis, but this method is not widely available. Other rapid diagnostic tests—including urine antigen detection, polymerase chain reaction, and a ribosomal probe—are in development. Serologic testing remains the method of choice for confirming a diagnosis. Currently the ELISA and microagglutination methods are preferred to tube agglutination testing. A single convalescent titer of 1:160 or greater is considered highly suspect for active disease, but a fourfold rise in titer between acute and convalescent (1 to 5 weeks) sera is more reliable, since antibodies of the IgM and IgG class can persist for many years after infection.[19] An elevated blood level of creatine phosphokinase is a sign that tularemia-induced rhabdomyolysis is the cause of the acute infection, especially in highly endemic areas.[32] Skin testing can be helpful in diagnosis, but the antigen is not commercially available.

Among the respiratory infections that are confused with tularemia, perplexing diseases, which are also associated with outdoor and animal exposures such as psittacosis and Q fever, are especially important. Legionnaires' disease and mycoplasmal pneumonia can present with similar clinical courses, without diagnostic sputum. Plague, tuberculosis, and systemic fungal infections produce a spectrum of acute to chronic respiratory manifestations that can be confused with pulmonary tularemia.

TREATMENT AND PREVENTION

Streptomycin was the first effective antibiotic for treating all forms of tularemia, and it remains the agent of choice. Gentamicin appears to be equally potent and has the advantage of a broader spectrum of activity if one is initiating treatment when the etiologic diagnosis is less secure. Additionally, it can be given intravenously, and blood levels can be monitored. *Tobramycin, however, appears to be unreliable and therefore should not be substituted.* Recent experience confirms that results of therapy are optimal when an aminoglycoside is chosen early in the clinical illness. Tetracycline and chloramphenicol are useful alternatives when an aminoglycoside is contraindicated, but relapse rates are higher, especially when tetracycline is given for less than 2 weeks. Fluoroquinolones, imipenem, and erythromycin are promising, but their use in the treatment of tularemia has not been extensively evaluated. β-Lactam antibiotics are not effective. The prognosis is excellent with appropriate antimicrobial therapy. (See Table 157-2 for specific dosages.)

Cautious practices are required when one is dealing with animals and their carcasses. Using gloves, cooking wild animal meat thoroughly, and wearing protective clothing and repellants to avoid sucking arthropods are helpful measures. Immunoprophylaxis with a live attenuated strain is in the trial stage and, when available, may be effective in protecting high-risk persons such as hunters, trappers, and selected laboratory personnel, since it induces both cell-mediated and humoral immunity.[51]

Pneumonia due to *Rhodococcus equi*

Rhodococcus equi, formerly known as *Corynbacterium equi*, was first isolated in 1923 by Magnussen when it was identified as a cause of suppurative pneumonia in foals. It was later shown to be a frequent pathogen in horses, cattle, and swine. First described as a pathogen in humans in 1967,[25] it has been most commonly reported as causing pneumonia in immunocompromised hosts, especially those receiving corticosteroid therapy.[55] In recent years, the majority of recognized cases of *R. equi* disease have been in patients infected with the human immunodeficiency virus (Table 157-3).[18,30]

BACTERIOLOGY AND IMMUNOLOGY

Rhodococcus is a pleomorphic gram-positive bacillus in the order Actinomycetales. It grows well on most media aerobically, at 37°C, as mucoid pale-pink or salmon-pink colonies that are usually observed by 48 h after incubation. *R. equi* has a high cell wall mycolic acid content and, as a result, like *Nocardia* species and Mycobacteriaceae, is weakly acid fast. Some strains will ferment glucose, but most will not ferment carbohydrates. Most produce catalase and hydrogen sulfide. β-Lactamase is present in some strains.

R. equi is a facultative intracellular pathogen that survives within macrophages. Prevention of phagosome–lysosome fusion is a major pathogenic mechanism. Humoral response as well as cell-mediated immunity has been demonstrated in animals, but it is unclear how much of a protective role each plays. In equine models, administration of antibody decreases the severity of pneumonia in foals challenged with aerosol inoculation of organisms. Protection was not seen in a murine model when the animals were infected with intravenous inoculation of organisms. In murine models, depletion of both CD4$^+$ T cells and CD8$^+$ T cells impairs the ability to clear the infection. The CD8$^+$ cells appear to play a much more significant role than the CD4$^+$ cells.[39]

EPIDEMIOLOGY

Most of the reported cases occurring in humans without HIV infection have been in patients who had significant contact either with livestock or with soil and environment that were heavily contaminated with livestock waste. In contrast, HIV-related *Rhodococcus* disease appears to occur in patients who do not have any particular environmental exposure history—implying a wide distribution of the organism.[30] There is no geographic endemicity.

TABLE 157-3

Diagnosing *Rhodococcus equi* Respiratory Infection

History of exposure to horses, cattle, or their environment
Immunocompromised host: malignancy, steroids, HIV
Cavitary or nodular infiltrates on radiograph
Gram-positive pleomorphic bacilli
Modified acid fast
Pale-pink or salmon-pink mucoid colonies
Grows rapidly, aerobically on most media
Differential diagnosis includes *Nocardia* species, mycobacteria

PATHOGENESIS AND PATHOPHYSIOLOGY

R. equi usually enters the body by direct inhalation, although soft tissue infections after cutaneous inoculation can occur. It is an intracellular pathogen and causes disease in patients with impaired cell-mediated immunity and defects in phagocytic processing of organisms.

Affected tissue usually shows a necrotizing granulomatous reaction, with histiocytes and macrophages frequently containing bacteria. Unlike lesions infected with *Mycobacterium tuberculosis* and systemic fungi, there is also a prominent infiltration of neutrophils in the affected areas, a characteristic shared with *Actinomyces* species.

CLINICAL AND RADIOLOGIC FEATURES

Patients most frequently complain of indolent symptoms, such as fever, nonproductive cough, and mild dyspnea. Typically there is a paucity of findings on physical examination of the chest, but signs of consolidation and pleural friction rubs may be present. Patients with HIV infection generally present in a manner similar to patients without HIV infection, though pleuritic chest pain may be more common. In HIV-infected patients, *R. equi* infections tend to occur after there has been significant deterioration in their immune systems, with CD4 lymphocyte counts lower than 200 cells/mm^3. Often it is found concurrent with other pulmonary infections. Extrapulmonary dissemination occurs in both HIV-infected and non–HIV-infected patients, but there appears to be a significantly greater rate of recovery of the organism from blood cultures in HIV patients. The central nervous system is a recognized site of metastatic infection, as it is for *Nocardia* species.

The most common radiographic abnormalities are lobar infiltrates, which usually evolve into nodular or cavitating lesions within weeks or months. There is no predilection for involvement of any particular lobe. Pleural effusions are common, occurring in up to 40 percent of HIV patients with pulmonary *R. equi* infection. Significant hilar adenopathy is unusual.

DIAGNOSIS AND DIFFERENTIAL DIAGNOSIS

R. equi can readily be cultured from sputum, bronchial lavage, pleural fluid, or other infected tissue and often from blood. Since the organisms stain as pleomorphic gram-positive bacilli, grow readily on most media, and are usually catalase producers, they can be mistaken for "diphtheroid" or "Coryneform" contaminants unless further testing is done. It is therefore important for the clinician to alert the microbiology laboratory staff if the possibility of *R. equi* is entertained. They are slightly acid fast when stained with Ziehl-Neelsen stain.

Rhodococci share many microbiologic features with *Mycobacteria* and *Nocardia,* and this may account for similarities in the subacute to chronic evolution of the disease. The high mycolic acid content of their cell walls results in their acid-fast staining properties and may also play a role in their similar clinical and pathologic manifestations. *Nocardia* species, *M. tuberculosis,* and nontuberculous mycobacteria should also be considered when acid-fast organisms are found in clinical specimens, especially in immunocompromised patients with nodular or cavitary pneumonia.

Other considerations in the differential diagnosis of nodular or cavitating pulmonary lesions are malignancy, fungal infection such as that from *Cryptococcus neoformans,* anaerobic lung abscess, and necrotizing pneumonia caused by facultative bacteria such as *Staphylococcus aureus* or *Klebsiella pneumoniae.*

TREATMENT

Antibiotic therapy alone is usually adequate to achieve cure. As with mycobacterial infections, multidrug regimens and therapy of 2 to 6 months' duration may be needed. Erythromycin, rifampin, ciprofloxacin and other quinolones, chloramphenicol, sulfonamides, and aminoglycosides are active against most isolates. *R. equi* is an intracellular pathogen that is capable of multiplying in phagocytes. Therefore, antibiotics that are capable of achieving high intracellular levels, such as rifampin or quinolones, but especially erythromycin and the expanded-spectrum macrolides, clarithromycin or azithromycin, are preferred. (See Table 157-2 for specific dosage recommendations.) In some patients, surgical resection of a nodular or cavitating lesion may be necessary to achieve cure.

ENVIRONMENTAL AND ANIMAL PRODUCT PNEUMONIAS

This section focuses on four diseases that are spread to humans predominantly from contact with contaminated soil, water, foods, or animal structural elements. Epidemiologic and ecologic aspects are essential to understanding how humans become infected. The diagnosis usually depends on a careful history. Once alerted, the clinician can request studies that can reveal the cause of these often obscure diseases. It should be apparent that this distinction—an association with environmental contamination and animal products—is somewhat arbitrary. For example, anthrax bacilli can spread directly from animals to humans, and *R. equi* contamination of feces could place it in this group rather than in the group infected via direct animal exposure.

Anthrax Respiratory Disease

Inhalation anthrax was a common enough disease in the nineteenth and early twentieth centuries to be referred to variously as Bradford's disease, after the English town, and woolsorter's disease for the epidemiologic association with the sheep industry. Fortunately, inhalation anthrax has become a rare disease, and reports available in the Western literature number only seven (two in the United States) during the past 25 years and fewer than 50 cases since the early part of the century. An epidemic of anthrax occurred in the area of Sverdlovsk, in the former USSR, in 1979. A recent report attempts to clarify evidence for an inhalation mechanism of this event.[1] The potential exposure of susceptible persons to *Bacillus anthracis* spores argues for including this devastating, usually lethal, disease in this chapter.

BACTERIOLOGY

B. anthracis is a large (red blood cell diameter), square-ended bacillus that stains gram positive and has a tendency to form chains. Growth on sheep blood agar results in dull, sticky, irregularly shaped colonies within 24 h. The organism possesses a polyglutamic acid capsule, produces a complex potent exotoxin, and, under adverse conditions, forms highly refractile, centrally located spores that are very resistant to temperature and moisture extremes. More than a century ago, Louis Pasteur used serial passage at 43°C to develop an effective, safe vaccine for animals, and it is now known that toxin production is mediated by a temperature-sensitive plasmid that is killed at 43°C.

ECOLOGY AND EPIDEMIOLOGY

Anthrax is primarily a disease of herbivores. The resistant spores are present after animals dying of the disease contaminate the soil. Anthrax "hot spots" are found, for example, in milder regions in the United States, like Oklahoma, Texas, and California. The optimal conditions for germination of spores and multiplication of bacilli include alkaline soils containing adequate calcium and low areas that are wet for prolonged periods, termed *incubator areas,* with thick vegetation that produces heat with decay. Periods of extreme drought after a rainy season, flavor spore formation. Animals grazing in these areas can inhale or ingest spores or pick them up on their fur. The cycle is completed when an animal develops the disease and dies, returning organisms to the soil, where they eventually sporulate under adverse conditions.

Inhalation anthrax rarely occurs from contact with live infected animals, and there is no human-to-human transmission. Working in the animal hide industry, being exposed to bone meal fertilizer, and using imported raw wool in home crafts can lead to inhalation of spores and clinical disease in susceptible persons. The unvaccinated person who occasionally enters a goat wool or hide processing plant to do needed repairs is at greatest risk for an inhalation exposure.

PATHOGENESIS AND PATHOPHYSIOLOGY

Inhalation results in activation of bronchial clearing mechanisms and entrapment of spores in hilar and mediastinal nodes, where reversion to vegetative bacilli can occur. The polyglutamic acid capsule is antiphagocytic, and the extracellular microorganisms produce a tripartite protein exotoxin that leads to profound local edema acutely, accompanied by hemorrhage in the mediastinal and hilar areas. Compromise of airflow results. Recent studies have elucidated the mechanism of edema formation. The protective antigen fragment of the toxin is the binding domain, essential for cell penetration by the edema factor portion of the molecule. Edema factor is a potent adenylate cyclase. Activation within mammalian cells stimulates production of cyclic AMP, and the resultant flux of sodium, potassium, and water leads to profound local edema.[36] When this process takes place in hilar and mediastinal nodes and surrounding tissues, profound airway obstruction ensues, with pooling of secretions and, if the patient survives, secondary bacterial pneumonia. The pathogen rarely invades lung tissue, as death from asphyxia occurs rapidly, usually associated with pleural effusions (secondary to lymphatic obstruction) and hemorrhagic septicemic lesions in many organs, including the central nervous system. Typical thoracic pathologic

findings include hemorrhagic mediastinitis with hemorrhagic mediastinal lymphadenopathy.[1]

CLINICAL AND RADIOLOGIC FEATURES

The onset of inhalation anthrax is insidious, usually resembling a nonspecific febrile influenzalike illness. Malaise and muscle aches, mild headache, coryza, pharyngitis, and chest pains have been described as early symptoms. Cough, if present, is usually mild and nonproductive, and fever is low grade. At this stage, it is hardly possible for the physician to entertain a presumptive or possible diagnosis of anthrax unless a history of industrial or craft-related exposure to imported animal hair or hides or to animal products such as bone meal is obtained. A number of the nonspecific features described above may be relevant. Watery nasal discharge can be indicative of nasal or paranasal sinus edema. Cough may represent hilar and mediastinal node swelling, and careful auscultation may reveal prolonged expiration or wheezes. Chest pain may be the first clue that hilar and mediastinal inflammation is present.[42]

Within hours to a few days, the mild complaints abruptly worsen and acute airway obstructive features dominate the clinical picture. Any activity precipitates severe dyspnea, stridor, and wheezing. Impairment of the nervous system (hemorrhagic meningitis) and hypoxemia result in decreasing levels of consciousness. Edema of the pharynx, neck, and anterior chest may develop. Chest pain, fever, and cyanosis are progressive changes. Worsening airway obstruction can lead to intercostal space retraction, and pleural effusions are noted on examination. Death usually occurs within hours to a day once acute respiratory symptoms are present.

Inhalation anthrax is primarily a mediastinitis, and the radiologic features mostly reflect the pathologic findings. Widening of the mediastinum or prominence of hilar nodes is the earliest radiologic finding, sometimes accompanied by pleural effusions. In advanced cases, the mediastinal shadow is greater than 9 cm in width and sharply demarcated from surrounding lung tissue because of absence of airspace consolidation. There may be perihilar and peribronchial streaking associated with edema and hemorrhage.[56]

DIAGNOSTIC FEATURES

A physician alerted to the possibility of inhalation anthrax has few laboratory studies to rely on. Nasal secretions and sputum rarely reveal the characteristic bulky gram-positive bacilli. Half of the reported cases of inhalation disease are complicated by meningitis, and hemorrhagic cerebrospinal fluid with observable organisms will confirm the diagnosis. There are no available data on examination of buffy-coat smears, and therapy must be instituted before blood culture results become available. Unfortunately, the most commonly recognized form of anthrax, the cutaneous chanceriform necrotic lesion, does not usually accompany inhalation cases.

The differential diagnosis includes other causes of acute mediastinitis, such as esophageal perforation. Tuberculosis and histoplasmosis rarely produce acute respiratory failure as part of hilar and mediastinal node involvement. Hantavirus pulmonary syndrome is associated with similar central pulmonary changes, including edema, but should be separable from anthrax by epidemiologic data and absence of mediastinal involvement. Lymphoproliferative diseases, like nodular sclerosing Hodgkin's, evolve at a slower pace. Chest wall and neck edema, associated with acute breathing difficulties, can accompany diphtheria or *Streptococcus pyogenes* pneumonia, and bilateral pleural effusions may be an early manifestation of streptococcal pneumonia. Acute epiglottitis, caused by *Hemophilus influenzae,* is usually a disease of preteen children, and a large epiglottis can be seen by direct examination or a lateral radiograph of the neck.

TREATMENT AND PREVENTION

Intravenously administered penicillin is the treatment of choice. Chloramphenicol or tetracycline is an effective substitute in penicillin-allergic patients. (See Table 157-2 for specific dosage recommendations.) Unfortunately, the lower-airway obstructive manifestations are not reversible once acute respiratory manifestations have developed. Assisted ventilation, drainage of pleural effusions, and use of diuretics are all reasonable support efforts, but they are generally not successful.

Mortality in inhalation anthrax approaches 100 percent of cases, compared to the rarity of death from cutaneous disease. In the animal hide industry, prevention is the cornerstone of dealing with anthrax. Plant workers and others in contact with potentially infected animal products should be immunized with the currently available vaccine. A genetically engineered vaccine based on toxin specificity is in the development stage. Animal products imported from endemic regions of the world (such as the Near East and the Indian subcontinent) are steam sterilized, and modern ventilation is in the workplace. At-risk subjects, then, are people who service these plants, such as ventilation workers and other transients. Bone meal is another vehicle for carrying inert spores. It should be treated by heat sterilization before packaging for use by commercial and home gardeners. Those who import craft yarn from endemic areas are at special risk unless the rules for commercial hide sterilization are also imposed on casual imports.

Pneumonia due to *Brucella* Species

In the approximately 200 cases of brucellosis that are reported yearly in the United States, acute respiratory manifestations are usually insignificant. Brucellosis is often a prolonged and perplexing illness, however, and in chronic cases, pleurisy, hilar adenopathy, and nodular lung lesions are encountered. Exposure to animals or to animal foods or residence in an endemic region is usually present when sought for in the history.

BACTERIOLOGY

Brucellae are small coccobacillary, gram-negative, nonmotile, aerobic, nonencapsulated organisms that are now classified with the alpha-proteobacteria, closely related to *Rochalimaea* and *Bartonella* species. Carbon dioxide is essential for growth of *Brucella abortus,* and all four pathogenic species require growth medium enriched with vitamins and serum. With the aid of a bat-

tery of biochemical, metabolic, and immunologic criteria, brucellae pathogenic for humans can be classified as *B. abortus, B. suis, B. melitensis,* and *B. canis.* In general, the species designation corresponds to the animal usually colonized or diseased.

ECOLOGY AND EPIDEMIOLOGY

Brucella species are distributed worldwide, wherever their natural hosts reside. Infection and disease occur primarily in domestic animals in geographic regions such as the Mediterranean littoral (*B. melitensis*), worldwide except in areas of Europe and Japan (*B. abortus*), in the midwestern United States (*B. suis*), and in North and Latin America (*B. canis*). Spread from one region to another occurs with live animal movements; and when infected animal products are commercially or privately shipped. Rigorous control measures such as herd inspections and vaccination procedures have dramatically reduced enzootic and epizootic disease in many regions.

The epidemiology of brucellosis is intimately related to the association of susceptible persons with infected animals and animal products. Abattoir workers (especially slaughterers) and others in the meat-processing industry, farmers, dairy workers, veterinarians, and bacteriology laboratory technicians account for most cases in the United States and a preponderance of male victims. Also at risk are travelers to endemic regions who eat local foods and people who consume imported goat cheese, sausage, and other unpasteurized edibles from endemic areas. The organisms are usually acquired by ingestion, through skin abrasions and lacerations, or via conjunctival inoculation. Evidence indicates that aerosol spread can be a route in abattoir workers.[31] No human-to-human transmission has been reported.

PATHOGENESIS AND PATHOPHYSIOLOGY

Organisms invade the local reticuloendothelial system and lymph nodes, followed by bacteremic spread to many organs during the following weeks. There is increasing evidence that the aerosol route may be especially efficient as a portal of entry. The distribution of nodular lesions in lung tissue is primarily in basal segments, however, which argues for bacteremia rather than primarily an inhalation mechanism for most cases of pulmonary disease.

A race between bacterial growth and the development of cell-mediated immunity ensues, primarily in lymph nodes and the reticuloendothelial system. As with tuberculosis, the end result is often containment within granulomas that eventually become fibrotic or calcify. Species and strain differences account for the wide variety of tissue reactions encountered, including granulomas, necrosis, and abscess formation. Smooth variants appear to be more virulent than rough forms, and many contain polysaccharide polymers in their superficial envelope that, like true capsules, inhibit phagocytosis and intracellular destruction. Lipopolysaccharide endotoxin is present in the cell envelope and may be responsible for profound metabolic and cardiovascular effects initially and as organisms are killed during therapy. *Brucella* species are able to survive within nonstimulated macrophages and can destroy these cells while escaping host antibodies and physician-directed antibiotic therapy. As macrophages become activated, they develop the capacity to rapidly kill phago-cytosed *Brucella* organisms. The development of host immunity appears to be primarily cell mediated, just as in *M. tuberculosis* disease. Impairment of cell-mediated immunity can lead to activation of latent *Brucella* or to greater susceptibility and severity of a primary infection.

CLINICAL AND RADIOLOGIC FEATURES

The clinical expression of brucellosis is dominated by nonspecific flulike constitutional manifestations, including fever and headache. Nonproductive cough has been described in 10 to 33 percent of cases, but other indicators of respiratory involvement are rarely or poorly described. In one review of 59 cases, dyspnea and pleuritic chest pain were present in 10 percent of the patients.[28] Hoarseness, bronchitis, and, rarely, mucopurulent, purulent, or hemorrhagic sputum have been noted. Only one patient with verified pulmonary invasion was described in a review of 160 acute and subacute cases of brucellosis reported in 1974.[5] Most modern reports lack clinical details and physical findings of respiratory disease.[37]

The most frequent radiologic findings have been perihilar and peribronchial infiltrates or solitary granulomas. Unilateral hilar adenopathy, nodular basilar infiltrates, and pleural effusions occur occasionally.

DIAGNOSTIC FEATURES

During the acute illness or in relapse, blood cultures may be positive—especially if kept for a minimum of 14 days. In the presence of an infiltrate or pleural effusion, material for Gram's stain and culture should be obtained, even though the yield from these studies is small. A positive culture may be obtained from a lymph node or pulmonary granuloma biopsy. In most cases the diagnosis is made from a fourfold rise or a single value of at least 1:160 in the agglutination titer. Occasionally "inhibitory" or blocking antibodies are present in the serum, and a positive titer will be discovered only if the serum is further diluted (so-called prozone phenomenon). The standard tube agglutination test utilizes *B. abortus* as the antigen and will detect antibodies to *B. suis* and *B. melitensis,* but not to *B. canis.* Diagnostic confusion and numerous alternative diagnoses are the rule in cases of brucellosis. Acute disease can be confused with miliary tuberculosis, endocarditis, tularemia, disseminated histoplasmosis, and lymphoproliferative diseases. Subacute and chronic cases must be differentiated from subacute bacterial endocarditis, tuberculosis, histoplasmosis, and other systemic fungal infections and sarcoidosis.

TREATMENT AND PREVENTION

The combination of doxycycline with rifampin for 4 to 6 weeks is the most effective oral antibiotic regimen. Doxycycline combined with streptomycin 1 g daily or with trimethoprim-sulfamethoxazole is also an effective alternative regimen. Fluoroquinolones are active in vitro, but they are associated with an unacceptably high relapse rate. (See Table 157-2 for specific dosage schedules.)

Preventive measures for cattle have been successful utilizing vaccination programs and destruction of diseased animals. Quarantine and inspection activities have diminished the risk of importing infected animals into the United States, and this reduction of disease in cattle has resulted in a decline in human cases. The program for *B. suis* eradication has been ineffective, and human cases of *B. suis* now outnumber those due to *B. abortus.* The efficacy of human vaccines is marginal. Education programs for workers in abattoirs have been aimed at protecting and preventing skin lacerations and eye contamination. Deployment of experienced workers in killing rooms assures that skilled persons immune from subclinical exposures will be the ones active in the most contaminated areas.[31]

Pneumonia due to *Burkholderia (Pseudomonas) pseudomallei*

Melioidosis is primarily an acute necrotizing or, in the later stage, a chronic fibronodular cavitating process indistinguishable from tuberculosis. It is a disease of tropical latitudes, and most cases have been seen in Southeast Asia, associated with rural settings. Infection with *Burkholderia pseudomallei* has been seen almost exclusively in this country after a latent period of months to years in military personnel returning from regions such as Vietnam and in refugees from endemic areas.

BACTERIOLOGY

The organism is an aerobic, bipolar-staining gram-negative bacillus that is motile and lacks a well-defined capsule. Similar to the pseudomonads, *B. pseudomallei* grows well on minimal as well as enriched media, including blood and MacConkey agar, used in most routine laboratories. Typical colonies are distinctive in appearance, rough or wrinkled, and cream to orange in color; they may resemble a flower with folds radiating from a central core. Colonies have the typical musty, fruity odor of the pseudomonads but lack pyocyanin and other pigments that characteristically color the surrounding medium. Identification rests on a battery of biochemical reactions, and confirmation is based on agglutination or fluorescent antibody studies.

ECOLOGY AND EPIDEMIOLOGY

B. pseudomallei occupies an environmental niche that includes moist soils, rice paddies, and other stagnant water in tropical and subtropical regions, approximately subtended by latitude 20° north to 20° south.[3,20] Evidence of subclinical and clinical disease occurs in wild and domestic animal populations, as well as in humans living permanently or transiently in rural endemic areas, especially in Southeast Asia and northeast Australia. As many as 10 to 30 percent of native populations have evidence of prior infection from serologic data. Approximately 1 to 2 percent of healthy American military personnel who served in Southeast Asia have antibodies, and almost 9 percent of soldiers wounded in Vietnam have titers for *B. pseudomallei.* A significant number of the approximately 3 million American soldiers who fought in the region constitute a reservoir of latent disease that, like tuberculosis, can become active even decades later, far removed from an endemic area. Refugees from southeast Asia represent another important group of carriers.

Transmission is mainly by direct contact with contaminated soil or water through minor abrasions or major wounds. Ingestion and inhalation are probably less frequent modes of spread, but common source outbreaks occur in animals and humans.[57] Animal-to-human disease has not been seen, and the only reported human-to-human spread has been associated with Foley catheter contamination and venereal transmission. In endemic regions, lack of previous exposure and debilitating circumstances, including malnutrition and uncontrolled diabetes, may increase susceptibility to infection and disease.

PATHOGENESIS AND PATHOPHYSIOLOGY

There is no information available on the mechanisms of pathogenicity of *B. pseudomallei,* although crude thermolabile cell-free extracts have produced necrotic lesions in experimental animals. The absence of an antiphagocytic capsule and the presence of potent endotoxin have been noted. Acute infections are associated with necrotic lesions containing polymorphonuclear neutrophiles (PMNs) in lung and in other tissues. Chronic infections, especially in the respiratory tract, resemble tuberculosis with granuloma formation, Langhans' or foreign-body giant cells, central caseation necrosis, and occasionally a PMN response in the necrotic area. Activation of latent infection after a period of months to even decades occurs. This "awakening" can be in the wake of influenza and other acute infections, acute stress (trauma, thermal burn, surgery, etc.), and immunosuppressing illnesses or therapies, but spontaneous activation also occurs. The location of dormant microorganisms and the specific molecular events that stimulate recurrent disease are unknown.

An antecedent local infection in an area of broken skin can be followed by acute septicemia in nonimmune subjects. Initial pulmonary lesions occur predominantly in the better-vascularized basal segments, but eventually other areas of the lungs and other tissues are affected. Subacute and chronic disease may result from a subclinical primary focus, often localized in an apical segment, resembling tuberculosis in location and propensity for granuloma formation and cavitation. Subpleural invasion can result in empyema or sympathetic sterile effusions.

CLINICAL AND RADIOLOGIC FEATURES

Primary melioidosis occurs within a few days to 2 weeks of exposure, usually in persons present in or recently from an endemic area. Military personnel with outdoor injuries constitute a potential group for delayed active disease. In the United States, the acute phase of melioidosis is rarely seen. The portal of entry may be present as a small necrotic skin lesion in an area of known trauma, with accompanying cellulitis or lymphangitis. In addition to marked toxicity and high fevers, the respiratory complaints include cough, dyspnea, pleuritic pain, and purulent sputum. Bibasilar rales may be heard, but objective findings are often minimal in the face of severe toxicity. Mortality approaches 75 percent, even when the diagnosis is suspected and appropriate therapy immediately instituted.[57]

Milder types of subacute and chronic pneumonia are usually seen in patients developing clinical illness after leaving an endemic area. In addition to fever, productive cough, and pleuritic pain, many patients experience marked weight loss and a clinical picture resembling tuberculosis or fungal disease. Secondary skin manifestations are rarely seen unless bacteremia ensues. Physical changes are often subtle but can include localized rales, a pleural friction rub, signs of an effusion, and manifestations of disease localized to soft tissues, lymph nodes, bones, or joints.[20]

Radiologic findings reflect the stage of disease present. In acute fulminant infections, airspace disease can be absent or miliary to larger nodular densities seen in basal segments. In subacute and chronic cases, fibronodular or cavitary apical lesions are found.[20]

DIAGNOSTIC FEATURES

Melioidosis should be seriously entertained in any febrile patient with a history of residence in a major endemic region such as Southeast Asia or northeast Australia. If sputum is available, the gram-negative bipolar staining bacilli may be seen, and the organisms can be readily cultured and identified by the routine laboratory. Blood and urine cultures are frequently positive in acute cases. In more indolent infections, biopsy may be necessary. Serologic studies can be helpful in active and recrudescent disease. A specific IgM immunofluorescence test is often positive in recent infections and recrudescent disease. Complement fixation and indirect hemagglutination tests are available and require testing of paired sera over several weeks to confirm active disease.

DIFFERENTIAL DIAGNOSIS

In patients from Southeast Asia, acute fulminating infections with pneumonia may be due to traditional bacteria and viruses, but it may also be caused by infection with *Y. pestis* (plague) and *F. tularensis* (tularemia) (see above).

Chronic forms of melioidosis resemble tuberculosis and fungal infections such as histoplasmosis and blastomycosis. Occupation, travel, and history of respiratory illness should help to clarify the cause. Confirmation usually requires biopsy with special stains and culture, or serologic data.

TREATMENT AND PREVENTION

Recommendations for therapy of acute septicemic melioidosis must be couched in cautious statements. During the Vietnam War, mortality greater than 50 percent occurred, even with use of three-drug regimens in massive doses. In subacute and chronic pneumonias and recrudescent disease, cure rates approach 100 percent. Treatment must be prolonged, and surgical intervention for drainage or removal of cavitary lesions is sometimes necessary to prevent relapse.[35]

Since the mid-1970s, a number of encouraging reports have confirmed the efficacy of trimethoprim-sulfamethoxazole for acute and other forms of respiratory disease. Strains from some geographic areas, however, may be resistant to trimethoprim-sulfamethoxazole. A recent study of clinical isolates from Thailand demonstrated an 81 percent resistance rate among 200 isolates tested.[50]

Ceftazidime in high doses is effective therapy, but first- and second-generation cephalosporins are not.[61] Imipenem, amoxicillin-clavulanate, ampicillin-sulbactam, and ticarcillin-clavulanate have good activity in vitro, but clinical experience with these drugs is limited. *B. pseudomallei* is an intracellular pathogen. When β-lactam antibiotics are used, an antimicrobial that achieves good intracellular levels, such as trimethoprim-sulfamethoxazole, should be administered concurrently.[49] The tetracyclines and chloramphenicol are effective therapy and also are generally used in combination. Kanamycin, but not other aminoglycosides, is active. Fluoroquinolones are not active at levels achievable in serum.

Although contemporary experience is limited and in vitro data must serve as a guide, specific recommendations for acute and chronic infections are outlined in Table 157-2. It should be emphasized that this is a controversial area, dosages are enormous, and drug toxicity can limit the usefulness of many recommended agents. Modifications in these programs must be guided by clinical circumstances and await more definitive studies.

There are no prophylactic antimicrobial studies available, nor has a vaccine been developed. People traveling, living, or working in endemic regions should be advised of this soil- and water-dwelling organism. Care and caution should be used to avoid traumatic injuries, and any wounds contaminated with soil or stagnant water should be assiduously cleaned.

Pulmonary Infections due to *Yersinia enterocolitica*

Most infections caused by *Y. enterocolitica* are in the gastrointestinal tract, resulting in a self-limited gastroenteritis- or appendicitis-mimicking mesenteric and terminal ileum adenitis. Septicemias and involvement of the lungs and other viscera are extremely rare, usually occurring in persons suffering from cirrhosis or who are immunocompromised.

Yersinia belong to the family Enterobacteriaceae. *Y. enterocolitica* is a gram-negative, facultative bacillus that resembles many other enteric microbes. Identification procedures include the ability to grow and exhibit motility at room temperature plus a battery of biochemical and serologic tests. Although occasionally overlooked in stool because it is confused with many other members of the fecal flora, the organism is readily identified in blood and respiratory specimens. Most strains are nonlactose or slow lactose fermenters, causing confusion with *Y. pestis, Salmonella, Shigella,* and several other members of the Enterobacteriaceae family. Cold enrichment techniques and highly selective media, extensively used to identify this organism in fecal specimens, are not necessary in nonfecal material. Various serotypes and biotypes, with distribution in geographically distinct regions, have been described.

Y. enterocolitica has been isolated from a variety of rodents and other wild animals, and from cats and dogs. There is little evidence for direct transmission or for spread among people other than by the fecal–oral route. Most cases occur singly, but epidemics involving families and hundreds of people have been described. Disease is initiated by ingestion of contaminated milk or other food.[8] Most cases of respiratory disease have been reported in immunocompromised hosts, alcoholics, and cirrhotics.

Direct aspiration may be the mechanism for initiation of pulmonary disease, following an initial pharyngeal focus. Bacteremia can complicate pharyngeal disease, although the most likely mechanism entails ulceration of Peyer's patches in the terminal ileum, mesenteric adenitis, and portal bacteremia. Systemic shunting to the lungs can follow, especially in cirrhotics, the group that most frequently develops septicemia. Mechanisms of pathogenesis are not clarified, but strains virulent for animals and causing human disease have plasmid-mediated V and W envelope antigens, temperature-sensitive calcium dependency (as with *Y. pestis*), a factor that enhances cell penetration, and endotoxin. An enterotoxin, similar to stable toxin of *E. coli,* is also produced, but an extragastrointestinal role has not been established for this material. The development of immune-complex manifestations such as erythema nodosum and nonsuppurative polyarthritis may contribute to pathogenicity.

During the past decade, concomitant with greater recognition of this pathogen as a cause of gastroenteritis, cases of pneumonia and lung abscess have been reported. Respiratory infections occur in association with an acute febrile septicemic illness or as a primary respiratory process, with cough, dyspnea, and signs of consolidation. The history is usually vague for gastrointestinal symptoms, animal exposure, or unusual food intake. There may be signs of increasing hepatic failure with ascites or peritonitis in patients with underlying cirrhosis. Radiologic findings include nodular basilar densities consistent with septicemic spread, dependent segment infiltrates suggesting an aspiration mechanism, occasionally with cavitation, and fluffy widespread densities consistent with septic emboli.[12] Immunocompromised patients may be especially prone to severe necrotizing pulmonary infections.[27]

The diagnosis often depends on information obtained from blood or sputum cultures. Entericlike gram-negative bacilli can be seen in sputum. Pharyngeal cultures should be done if signs of local inflammation are present. Suppurating nodes and peritoneal or joint fluids are other sources of material that may contribute to the diagnosis when sputum is not available.

Cases of respiratory infection have responded well to a variety of antibiotics, including ampicillin or second-generation cephalosporins. Third-generation cephalosporins, chloramphenicol, and aminoglycosides are also effective.[24] Underlying diseases influence the outcome, but when pneumonia is the major problem, prognosis is excellent. Treatment is usually continued for a total of 3 to 6 weeks. (See Table 157-2 for dosage details.)

Preventive measures include avoiding rodent or domestic animal contamination of food and water supplies.[8] Opportunities for susceptible persons to come in contact with this zoonotic microorganism may be increasing as well, as immunocompromised people look to natural foods and mineral waters for improved health.

PNEUMONIAS CAUSED BY OBLIGATE HUMAN COMMENSALS

Most bacterial pneumonias are caused by obligate human commensals that are easy to isolate, such as *Streptococcus pneumoniae*. Among the less common causes of pneumonia due to human commensals, *Neisseria meningitidis* (the meningococcus) and *Moraxella* (formerly *Branhamella*) *catarrhalis* stand out as pathogens or opportunists that may escape bacteriologic identification and therefore present problems in diagnosis and therapy.

Neisseria meningitidis

During the influenza viral pandemic of 1918–19, *N. meningitidis* was an important respiratory pathogen. Afterward, few references to the meningococcus appeared in the medical literature on bacterial pneumonias, as reports of meningococcal disease focused on its role in causing meningitis and septicemia. With the advent of improved bacteriologic techniques, more than 100 cases of *N. meningitidis* pneumonia have been reported during the past 15 years—and this is almost certainly a low estimate.[59] It remains to be established whether this is a true increase in incidence or reflects greater awareness on the part of physicians.

BACTERIOLOGY AND IMMUNOLOGY

Neisseria are oxygen-requiring, gram-negative–staining cocci recognized from their characteristic pairing as kidney-shaped diplococci. They are fastidious, succumbing rapidly to the external environment and to dry or cold conditions. Although *Neisseria* can grow on blood agar, optimal conditions include enriched media, such as chocolate agar, and incubation in an atmosphere of 6 percent CO_2 at 35 to 37°C with 50 percent humidity. *N. meningitidis* is distinguishable from other *Neisseria* species that are residents of the oral-respiratory region by sugar-fermentation reactions and by serologic identification, which depends on specific capsular polysaccharides. Isolation and identification of *N. meningitidis* in sputum are facilitated by the use of a selective medium, such as modified Thayer-Martin agar (MTM), which contains antibiotics that suppress more rapidly growing microorganisms. The presence of *Neisseria*-like diplococci in a Gram-stained smear of sputum should provide the impetus to culture the specimen on MTM media as well as on less selective media, such as blood and chocolate agar (Fig. 157-3).

N. meningitidis is a typical gram-negative organism containing a potent lipopolysaccharide endotoxin in the outer membrane layer of the cell envelope. Exterior to this layer is a polysaccharide capsule, by which *N. meningitidis* can be separated into at least 13 chemically defined serogroups. Groups A, B, C, X, Y, Z, and W-135 are currently the most important clinically.

Immunity to meningococci is complex. Bactericidal antibody, present in the newborn, disappears by approximately 6 months of age. During childhood and adolescence, overt disease and subclinical encounters with various capsular strains of *N. meningitidis*, as well as with nonpathogenic *Neisseria* species, lead to stimulation of bacterial antibody. Facilitated by terminal complement components C5 through C8, this can result in immune lysis of organisms. Congenital absence of one or more of the terminal complement components has been associated with recurrent acute meningococcal disease.[13] Antibodies to certain outer membrane proteins and to a variety of envelope antigens of *E. coli* and other commensals cross-react with antigens from *N. meningitidis*. Persons lacking bactericidal or capsular antibody to a specific serogroup are susceptible to colonization and to dis-

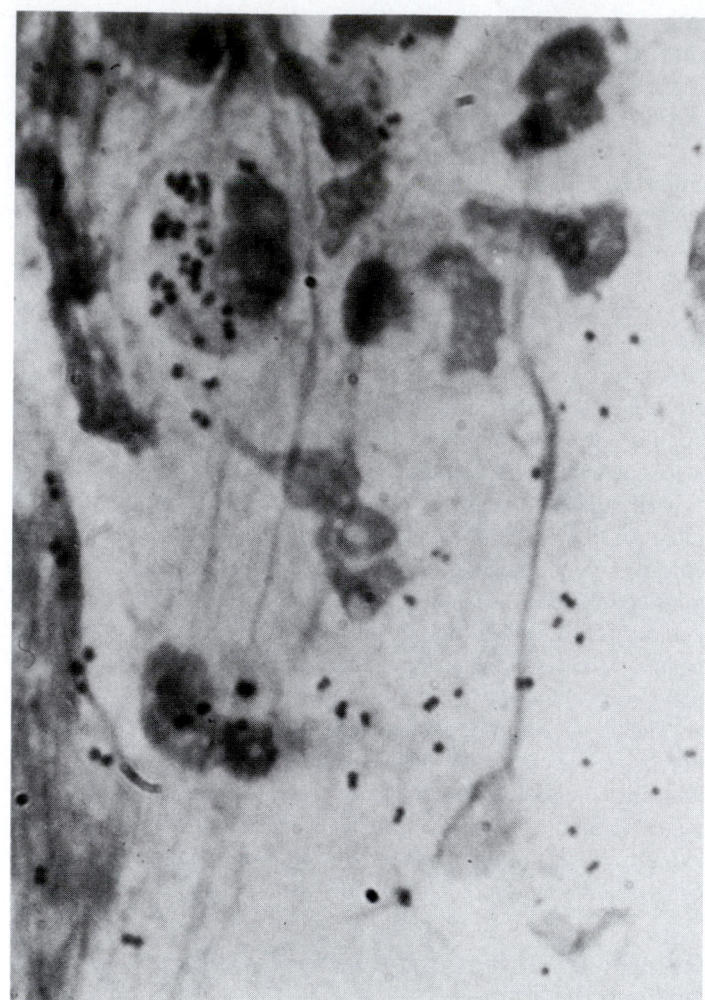

FIGURE 157-3   Gram's stain of expectorated sputum from a patient with proven *Moraxella* pneumonia. In this black-and-white photomicrograph, the distinguishing features include the presence of morphologic kidney-shaped diplococci (gram negative) associated with polymorphonuclear neutrophils. This appearance suggests *Neisseria* or *Moraxella* infection.

ease caused by that serogroup. With increasing age, acquisition of protective antibodies is associated with less likelihood of developing clinical disease.

EPIDEMIOLOGY

Nasopharyngeal carriage of various serogroups of meningococci occurs in approximately 5 to 15 percent of subjects. Convening and crowding large numbers of young persons from widely separated geographic areas, as occurs in the military or in boarding schools, can result in significant and rapid spread of an individual serogroup from a few asymptomatic carriers to many susceptibles. A case of meningococcal disease in a family is often associated with an increased prevalence of meningococcal isolation from relatives with symptoms of upper respiratory infection. In the military, carrier rates can rapidly approach 100 percent, followed by many cases of meningitis, if prophylactic antibiotics and other prevention measures are not undertaken.

Respiratory disease due to meningococci was recognized early in the twentieth century, especially during the influenza pandemic of 1918–1919. In the mid-1970s, outbreaks of serogroup Y meningococcal pneumonia occurred in military installations.[33] Over the past 15 to 20 years, isolated respiratory disease, primarily due to serogroups Y and W-135, has been detected in civilian populations and nosocomially in persons in contact with an index case.[11,17,44] Spread is probably by aerosol droplets during close contact, since drying rapidly kills meningococci. People ill with influenza or adenoviral respiratory infections appear to be more susceptible—as occurs with other respiratory pathogens, such as *S. pneumoniae* and *Staphylococcus aureus*.[64]

PATHOGENESIS AND PATHOPHYSIOLOGY

Initiation of infection begins when an encapsulated strain colonizes the nasopharynx of a person lacking immunity to that serogroup. Attachment to mucosal cells is facilitated by filamentous pili and perhaps by the action of bacterial IgA1 protease.[34] The lower respiratory tract is invaded by aspiration or inhalation of droplet particles. A preceding viral infection can stimulate excessive airway secretions, damage surface epithelial structures, and interfere with clearance of microorganisms. Septicemia, petechial eruptions, meningitis, diffuse intravascular coagulation, and ARDS rarely accompany pneumonia, supporting a postulated aspiration mechanism. Bronchopneumonia, lobar extension, and necrosis and abscess formation are seen. Modern pathologic correlations are lacking, since there are no animal models of meningococcal pneumonia and histopathologic material is essentially nonexistent.

CLINICAL AND RADIOLOGIC FEATURES

The clinical presentation of meningococcal pneumonia resembles that of pneumococcal infection. Productive cough, pleuritic pain, chills, and fever are associated with physical changes of rales with consolidation. In contrast to the picture of pneumococcal disease, pleural rubs and hemoptysis are unusual. Suspicion of meningococcal disease is enhanced if many cases of bacterial pneumonia erupt in closed populations such as military or school groups or among hospital patients.[11] Pharyngitis is often an early complaint.

Radiologic features are nonspecific and include patchy bronchopneumonia and lobar airspace infiltrates, usually located in a lower or right middle lobe, accompanied by an effusion in about 20 percent of cases. Occasionally the radiologic appearance resembles diffuse pulmonary edema or an antecedent viral infection.

DIAGNOSTIC FEATURES

Diagnosis depends on isolation of predominantly *N. meningitidis* from a carefully collected sputum specimen that has characteristic gram-negative diplococci and PMNs on the stained smear (Fig. 157-3). Attention to these criteria is essential, since pathogenic and nonpathogenic *Neisseria* and *Moraxella* species are part of the normal respiratory flora. Invasive procedures, such as transtracheal aspiration, are not necessary if a valid sputum is available, and the Gram's stain appearance prompts culturing the specimen on MTM media. Alternative methods of identification include the capsular swelling technique (Quellung), latex bead coagglutination, and fluorescent antibody staining. Recent purification of all of the major group-specific capsular polysaccharides should lead to expansion of these rapid diagnostic methods. Blood and CSF cultures are rarely positive in meningococcal respiratory disease (Table 157-4).

DIFFERENTIAL DIAGNOSIS

Respiratory infections due to other causes, especially when there are many cases, must be considered in the differential diagnosis.

Viral Pneumonia
Acute respiratory infections affecting a number of people, especially under institutional or crowded circumstances, can be caused by viral agents such as influenza A or B or adenoviruses. Diagnosis is usually confirmed by the epidemiologic and clinical circumstances, a nonspecific sputum examination, absent or interstitial infiltrates radiologically, and paired serologic titers.

Mycoplasmal Pneumonia
The illness is frequently biphasic, with upper respiratory inflammation and headache prominent early symptoms and, occasionally, bullous tympanitis producing severe ear pain. The sputum is often purulent, with a mixture of PMNs and mononuclear cells, but no dominant microorganism is observed. Diagnosis is usually confirmed by a cold agglutinin titer of 1:32 or greater or a rising titer of complement-fixing antibody. When many cases occur in a closed community, they usually erupt over many weeks rather than days to a week.

Pyogenic Pneumonia
Acute bacterial pneumonias often follow in the wake of viral respiratory infections. *S. pneumonia* and *S. aureus* infections are differentiated with microscopic examination, culture of sputum, and the results of blood cultures. In hospitals, especially among immunocompromised patients or patients attached to respirators, a variety of gram-negative microorganisms can produce pneumonia. *H. influenzae* infections can usually be suspected, but *M. catarrhalis* resembles *Neisseria* morphologically and may not respond to penicillin treatment (see below).

Rocky Mountain Spotted Fever
Acute respiratory failure secondary to small-vessel endothelial cell damage or to ARDS can complicate this rickettsial disease. A petechial or morbilliform eruption is usually seen on the ex-

---

TABLE 157-4

Diagnosing Meningococcal Pneumonia

Antecedent viral respiratory infection
Multiple community or hospital respiratory cases
Purulent or frothy sputum
Kidney-shaped gram-negative diplococci on smear (Fig. 157-3)
Culture sputum on modified Thayer-Martin medium
Incubation with CO_2 enrichment

tremities. With meningococcal respiratory disease, a rash is rarely seen.

TREATMENT AND PREVENTION

Low-dose penicillin is effective for most cases, although those complicated by cavitation or empyema should be treated with a minimum of 6 million units daily. Patients allergic to penicillin can be given chloramphenicol. The third-generation cephalosporins also are effective. In contrast to meningitis or meningococcemia, respiratory infections appear to respond uniformly well to treatment.

Meningococci spread via aerosols, so isolation of suspected cases is essential, especially during the first 24 h of treatment. Chemoprophylaxis and immunoprophylaxis have been found effective in epidemics of meningitis, but no data are available for respiratory disease protection. Penicillin, the drug of choice for treating active disease, does not reliably eradicate the carrier state or protect intimately exposed contacts. Probably because of its transport into oral and respiratory tract secretions in high concentrations, rifampin is an effective prophylactic agent. The usual protective dose is 600 mg orally, twice daily for 2 days. Fluoroquinolones such as ciprofloxacin, at a dose of 500 mg twice daily for 5 days, is also effective. Minocycline diffuses into upper respiratory secretions in high concentrations and is a useful alternative to rifampin. Labyrinthitis, a frequent toxic side effect, prevents wider use of this agent, however.

Immunoprophylaxis has been safe and effective when given systematically to large at-risk groups in military installations, schools, day-care centers, or defined communities. A quadrivalent vaccine, containing serogroups A, C, Y, and W-135, is commercially available, and an octavalent preparation is in development. Although group Y and W-135 isolates have commonly been causal, there are no data for efficacy of the vaccine for respiratory infections.[23] Children below the age of 2 years respond poorly to the group C vaccine and unpredictably to the other polysaccharide products. This younger age group remains vulnerable, and protection must be provided, when necessary, with chemoprophylaxis. Immunizing persons with influenza viral vaccines should eliminate some cases of secondary bacterial infections, including those caused by *N. meningitidis*.

Moraxella (Branhamella) catarrhalis

Formerly considered a nonpathogenic respiratory commensal, *M. catarrhalis* has aroused renewed interest as an opportunist and primary pathogen.[7] Resemblance to *Neisseria* on Gram's stain and penicillin resistance of many clinically significant isolates are features that encourage inclusion in this section.

BACTERIOLOGY

Moraxella are gram-negative cocci that pair as kidney-shaped diplococci; hence they cannot be distinguished morphologically from *Neisseria*. The organisms grow well on nonselective media such as sheep blood agar and enriched chocolate agar, especially when supplemented with added CO_2. Growth of *Moraxella* is variable on selective media such as MTM—in contrast to path-

ogenic *Neisseria*, which thrive on that medium. They fail to utilize a variety of sugars. These and other biochemical tests help to distinguish them from *Neisseria*. Many clinical isolates produce β-lactamase and, therefore, are resistant to penicillin.

EPIDEMIOLOGY

A member of the resident microflora of the nasopharynx and pharynx, *M. catarrhalis* can also colonize the mucosa of the genital tract. Among persons with chronic lung disease it can be found, along with other bacteria, in respiratory secretions.[46] The extent of colonization of mucous surfaces in healthy or diseased subjects is not known. There is no evidence for human-to-human transmission, although infections in the hospital setting occur and are probably related to the selective pressures from the various antimicrobials used. In normal children and adults, otitis media, sinusitis, and laryngotracheobronchitis probably result from direct spread from colonized mucosal surfaces. This view is supported by the finding of mixed infections and other commensals, such as *H. influenzae* and mouth anaerobes.

PATHOGENESIS AND PATHOPHYSIOLOGY

In contrast to pathogenic *Neisseria*, *Moraxella* lack antiphagocytic capsules and IgA proteases. They have outer-envelope lipopolysaccharide endotoxin, characteristic of all gram-negative microbes, but no specific pathogenic factors have been described.

The mechanism of initiation of respiratory disease appears to be primarily related to underlying obstruction and chronic inflammation. Aspiration of nasopharyngeal secretions, stimulated by an acute viral upper respiratory infection, is the most common proposed pathophysiological factor. Contributing conditions that are immunocompromising—such as steroid therapy, malignancy, hypogammaglobulinemia, and neutropenia—are present in a large number of patients. Paranasal sinus and ear infections occur predominantly in children, probably because of compromised drainage ducts in anatomically crowded areas. Rarely, *Moraxella* produce primary invasive diseases outside the respiratory tract, including meningitis, endocarditis, septic arthritis, and, in immunocompromised patients, septicemia.[54]

CLINICAL AND RADIOLOGIC FEATURES

Most people who develop respiratory infections are adults with chronic lung disease associated with smoking, industrial exposures, or bronchitis and bronchiectasis.[29] Purulent bronchitis or bronchopneumonia can follow an intercurrent viral infection. Respiratory distress, if present, may be related to the acute process, with bronchospasm and fever superimposed on the chronic underlying disease. Signs of consolidation or pleural fluid may be present, along with persistent obstructive changes. Evidence has been accumulating that normal adults may develop primary laryngitis and children a nonproductive cough as other manifestations of clinical respiratory tract disease, but primary pneumonia is very uncommon at any age in subjects with healthy lungs.[10,62]

The radiologic appearance is influenced by the underlying chronic lung disease. No acute changes may be observed, but usually increased markings are seen superimposed on the findings of obstructive lung disease and fibrosis. Patchy consolidation is often noted. Lobar infiltrates, cavitation, and pleural effusions are distinctly unusual findings and suggest mixed infections or other complications of the underlying disease.[54]

DIAGNOSTIC FEATURES

The unique feature in cases of *M. catarrhalis* respiratory infections is the finding of gram-negative kidney-shaped diplococci associated with PMN exudate cells (Fig. 157-3). Diagnosis depends on careful examination of an adequate expectorated sputum sample and culturing the specimen on nonselective blood and enriched chocolate agar as well as on selective MTM.[48] The use of several media assures that these fastidious organisms will be identified in a crowd of other commensals. Blood cultures should be obtained in cases associated with immunosuppression or malignancy, and pleural effusions aspirated and examined bacteriologically. Transtracheal aspiration rarely adds to the examination of an adequate expectorated sputum. Serologic methods are not available to help verify a pathogenic role for *Moraxella* in mixed infections (Table 157-5).

DIFFERENTIAL DIAGNOSIS

The major diagnostic confusion results from the presence in sputum of *Neisseria* species and other potential pathogens, such as *S. pneumoniae* and *H. influenzae*. In patients with chronic lung disease, mixed infections make it impossible to ascribe pathogenicity to a single organism. Coccobacillary microorganisms, or gram-negative bacilli that demonstrate bipolar staining (e.g., *Brucella, Pasteurella*), can be confused with *M. catarrhalis*.

TREATMENT

As the pathogenic role for *M. catarrhalis* was recognized, it became apparent that many isolates produced β-lactamase and were resistant to penicillin and ampicillin. Numerous treatment failures with penicillins have been described, often with dramatic improvement once an alternative antibiotic was administered. β-Lactamase production is present in approximately 75 percent of isolates from middle ear, sinus, and nasopharyngeal locations in children. In adults with bronchopulmonary disease, the range is broader. From 10 to 100 percent of isolates are penicillin resistant. Of 994 strains randomly collected in Sweden, without regard to clinical significance, 35 percent produced β-lactamase. Therapy should, therefore, be initiated with either a second-generation cephalosporin such as cefuroxime, erythromycin, or

the expanded-spectrum macrolides clarithromycin or azithromycin, the combination of amoxicillin–clavulanic acid (Augmentin), a fluoroquinolone,[53] or trimethoprim-sulfamethoxazole until β-lactamase activity is determined. In vitro testing may appear to demonstrate susceptibility to penicillin, amoxicillin-clavulanate, or first-generation cephalosporins if β-lactamase production is at a low level. However, clinical failures may occur if these drugs are used. Supportive therapy with adequate hydration, bronchodilators, and other measures directed at the underlying respiratory disease is essential for a successful outcome.

REFERENCES

1. Abramova FA, Grinberg LM, Yampolskaya OV, Walker DH: Pathology of inhalational anthrax in 42 cases from the Sverdlovsk outbreak of 1979. *Proc Natl Acad Sci USA* 90:2291–2294, 1993.
2. Alsofrom DJ, Mettler FA, Mann JM: Radiographic manifestations of plague in New Mexico, 1975–1980. *Radiology* 139:561–565, 1981.
3. Barnes PF, Appleman MD, Cosgrove MM: A case of melioidosis originating in North America. *Am Rev Respir Dis* 134:170–171, 1986.
4. Boyce JM: Recent trends in the epidemiology of tularemia in the United States. *CEC News* 131:197–198, 1975.
5. Buchanan TM, Faber LC, Feldman RA: Brucellosis in the United States, 1960–1972. *Medicine* 53:403–413, 1974.
6. Capellan J, Fong IW: Tularemia from a cat bite: Case report and review of feline-associated tularemia. *Clin Infect Dis* 16:472–475, 1993.
7. Catlin BW: *Branhamella catarrhalis:* An organism gaining respect as a pathogen. *Clin Microbiol Rev* 3:293–320, 1990.
8. Centers for Disease Control: Outbreak of *Yersinia enterocolitica*—Washington State. *MMWR* 31:562–564, 1982.
9. Centers for Disease Control: Update: Human Plague—India. *MMWR* 43:722–723, 1994.
10. Claesson BA, Leinonen M: *Moraxella catarrhalis*—An uncommon cause of community-acquired pneumonia in Swedish children. *Scand J Infect Dis* 26:399–402, 1994.
11. Cohen MS, Steere AC, Baltimore R, et al: Possible nosocomial transmission of group Y *Neisseria meningitidis* among oncology patients. *Ann Intern Med* 91:7–12, 1979.
12. Cropp AJ, Gaylord SF, Watanakunakorn C: Case report: Cavitary pneumonia due to *Yersinia enterocolitica* in a healthy man. *Am J Med Sci* 288:130–132, 1984.
13. Densen P: Complement deficiencies and meningococcal disease. *Clin Exp Immunol* 86(Suppl 1):57–62, 1991.
14. Doll JM, Zeitz PS, Ettestad P, et al: Cat-transmitted fatal pneumonic plague in a person who traveled from Colorado to Arizona. *Am J Trop Med Hyg* 51:109–114, 1994.
15. Drabick JJ, Gasser RA Jr, Saunders NB, et al: *Pasteurella multocida* pneumonia in a man with AIDS and nontraumatic feline exposure. *Chest* 103:7–11, 1993.
16. Duchin JS, Koster FT, Peters CJ, et al: Hantavirus pulmonary syndrome: A clinical description of 17 patients with a newly recognized disease. *New Engl J Med* 330:949–955, 1994.
17. Ellenbogen C, Graybill JR, Silva J Jr, Homme PJ: Bacterial pneumonia complicating adenoviral pneumonia. *Am J Med* 56:169–178, 1974.
18. Emmons W, Reichwein B, Winslow DL: *Rhodococcus equi* infection in the patient with AIDS: Literature review and report on an unusual case. *Rev Infect Dis* 13:91–96, 1991.
19. Evans ME, Gregory DW, Schaffner W, McGee ZA: Tularemia: A 30-year experience with 88 cases. *Medicine* 64:251–269, 1985.

TABLE 157-5

Diagnosing *Moraxella* Pneumonia

Underlying chronic lung disease
History of aspiration
Kidney-shaped gram-negative diplococci on smear (Fig. 157-3)
Culture sputum on sheep blood and enriched chocolate media
Culture sputum on selective modified Thayer-Martin medium

20. Everett ED, Nelson RA: Pulmonary melioidosis. *Am Rev Respir Dis* 112:331–340, 1975.

21. Finegold MJ: Pathogenesis of plague: A review of plague deaths in the United States during the last decade. *Am J Med* 45:549–554, 1968.

22. Fraser DW, Tsai TR, Orenstein W, et al: Legionnaires' disease: Description of an epidemic of pneumonia. *New Engl J Med* 297:1189–1197, 1977.

23. Galaid EI, Cherubin CE, Marr JS, et al: Meningococcal disease in New York City, 1973–1978: Recognition of groups Y and W-135 as frequent pathogens. *JAMA* 244:2167–2171, 1980.

24. Gayraud M, Scavizzi MR, Mollaret HH, et al: Antibiotic treatment of *Yersinia enterocolitica* septicemia: A retrospective review of 43 cases. *Clin Infect Dis* 17:405–410, 1993.

25. Golub B, Falk G, Spink WW: Lung abscess due to *Corynebacterium equi:* Report of first human infection. *Ann Intern Med* 66:1174–1177, 1967.

26. Grayston JT, Thorn DH: The chlamydial pneumonias, in Remington J, Swartz M (eds), *Current Clinical Topics in Infectious Diseases,* vol II. Boston, Blackwell Scientific, 1990, pp 1–18.

27. Greene JN, Herndon P, Nadler JP, Sandin RL: Case report: *Yersinia enterocolitica* necrotizing pneumonia in an immunocompromised patient. *Am J Med Sci* 305:171–173, 1993.

28. Greer AE: Pulmonary brucellosis. *Dis Chest* 29:508–519, 1956.

29. Hager H, Verghese A, Alvarez S, Berk S: *Branhamella catarrhalis* respiratory infections. *Rev Infect Dis* 9:1140–1149, 1987.

30. Harvey RL, Sunstrum JC: *Rhodococcus equi* infection in patients with and without human immunodeficiency virus infection. *Rev Infect Dis* 13:139–145, 1991.

31. Kaufman AG, Fox MD, Boyce JM, et al: Airborne spread of brucellosis. *Ann NY Acad Sci* 353:105–114, 1980.

32. Klotz SA, Penn RL, Provenza JM: The unusual presentations of tularemia: Bacteremia, pneumonia, and rhabdomyolysis. *Arch Intern Med* 147:214, 1987.

33. Koppes GM, Ellenbogen C, Bebhart RJ: Group Y meningococcal disease in United States Air Force recruits. *Am J Med* 62:661–666, 1977.

34. Kornfeld SF, Plaut AG: Secretory immunity and the bacterial IgA proteases. *Rev Infect Dis* 3:521–534, 1981.

35. Leelarasamee A, Bovornkitti S: Melioidosis: Review and update. *Rev Infect Dis* 11:413–425, 1989.

36. Leppela SH: Anthrax toxin edema factor: A bacterial adenylate cyclase that increases cyclic AMP concentrations in eukaryotic cells. *Proc Natl Acad Sci USA* 79:3162–3166, 1982.

37. Lulu AR, Araj GF, Khateeb MI, et al: Human brucellosis in Kuwait: A prospective study of 400 cases. *Q J Med* 66:39–54, 1988.

38. Meyer KF: Pneumonic plague. *Bact Rev* 25:249–261, 1961.

39. Nordmann P, Ronco E, Nauciel C: Role of T-lymphocyte subsets in *Rhodococcus equi* infection. *Infect Immunol* 60:2748–2752, 1992.

40. Ortqvist A: Initial investigation and treatment of the patient with severe community-acquired pneumonia. *Semin Respir Infect* 9:166–179, 1994.

41. Penn RL, Kinasewitz GT: Factors associated with a poor outcome in tularemia. *Arch Intern Med* 147:265–268, 1987.

42. Plotkin SA, Brachman PS, Utell M, et al: An epidemic of inhalation anthrax, the first in the twentieth century. *Am J Med* 29:992–1000, 1960.

43. Prescott JF, Yielding KM: *In vitro* susceptibility of selected veterinary bacterial pathogens to ciprofloxacin, enrofloxacin and norfloxacin. *Can J Vet Res* 54:195–197, 1990.

44. Putsch RW, Hamilton JD, Wolinsky E: *Neisseria meningitidis:* A respiratory pathogen? *J Infect Dis* 121:48–54, 1970.

45. Rubin SA: Radiographic spectrum of pleuropulmonary tularemia. *Am J Roentgenol* 131:277–281, 1978.

46. Sarubbi FA, Myers JW, Williams JJ, Shell CG: Respiratory infections caused by *Branhamella catarrhalis:* Selected epidemiologic features. *Am J Med* 88(5A):9S–14S, 1990.

47. Sienko DG, Bartlett PC, McGee HB, et al: Q fever: A call to heighten our index of suspicion. *Arch Intern Med* 148:609–612, 1988.

48. Slevin NJ, Aitken J, Thornley PE: Clinical and microbiological features of *Branhamella catarrhalis* bronchopulmonary infections. *Lancet* 1:782–783, 1984.

49. Sookpranee M, Boonma P, Susaengrat W, et al: Multicenter prospective randomized trial comparing ceftazidime plus co-trimoxazole with chloramphenicol plus doxycycline and co-trimoxazole for treatment of severe melioidosis. *Antimicrob Agents Chemother* 36:158–162, 1992.

50. Sookpranee T, Sookpranee M, Mellencamp MA, Preheim LC: *Pseudomonas pseudomallei,* a common pathogen in Thailand that is resistant to bactericidal effects of many antibiotics. *Antimicrob Agents Chemother* 35:484–489, 1991.

51. Tarnvik A: Nature of protective immunity to *Francisella tularensis.* *Rev Infect Dis* 11:440–451, 1989.

52. Teutsch SM, Martone WJ, Brink EW, et al: Pneumonic tularemia on Martha's Vineyard. *New Engl J Med* 301:826–828, 1979.

53. Thys JP, Jacobs F, Motte S: Quinolones in the treatment of lower respiratory tract infections. *Rev Infect Dis* 11(Suppl 5): S1212–S1219, 1989.

54. Verghese A, Berk SL: *Moraxella (Branhamella) catarrhalis,* in Wallace RJ Jr (ed), *Infectious Disease Clinics of North America,* vol 5. Philadelphia, WB Saunders, 1991, pp 523–538.

55. Verville TD, Huycke MM, Greenfield RA, et al.: *Rhodococcus equi* infections of humans: 12 cases and a review of the literature. *Medicine (Baltimore)* 73:119–132, 1994.

56. Vessal K, Yeganehdoust J, Dutz W, Kohout E: Radiological changes in inhalation anthrax: A report of radiological and pathological correlation in two cases. *Clin Radiol* 26:471–474, 1975.

57. Weber DJ, Douglass LE, Brundage WG, Stallkamp TC: Acute varieties of melioidosis occurring in U.S. soldiers in Vietnam. *Am J Med* 46:234–244, 1969.

58. Weber DJ, Wolfson JS, Swartz MN, Hooper DC: *Pasteurella multocida* infections. *Medicine* 63:133–154, 1984.

59. Weinberg AN: Pneumonia due to *Neisseria meningitidis,* in Weinstein L, Fields BN (eds), *Seminars in Infectious Disease,* vol 6. New York, Thieme-Stratton, 1983, pp 147–158.

60. Weinberg AN, Heller HM: Unusual bacterial pneumonias, in Pennington JE (ed), *Respiratory Infections: Diagnosis and Management,* 3d ed. New York, Raven, 1994, pp 485–513.

61. White NJ, Dance DAB, Chaowagul W, et al: Halving of mortality of severe melioidosis by ceftazidime. *Lancet* 2:698–700, 1989.

62. Wright PW, Wallace RJ Jr, Shepherd JR: A descriptive study of 42 cases of *Branhamella catarrhalis* pneumonia. *Am J Med* 88(5A):2S–8S, 1990.

63. Young LS, Bicknell DS, Archer BG, et al: Tularemia epidemic, Vermont 1968: Forty-seven cases linked to contact with muskrats. *New Engl J Med* 280:1253–1260, 1969.

64. Young LS, LaForce FM, Head JJ, et al: A simultaneous outbreak of meningococcal and influenza infections. *New Engl J Med* 287:5–9, 1972.

CHAPTER 158

THE EPIDEMIOLOGY, TRANSMISSION, AND PREVENTION OF TUBERCULOSIS IN THE UNITED STATES

Ida M. Onorato / Renée Ridzon

Mycobacterium tuberculosis has coexisted with humanity since the days before recorded history, and evidence of tuberculosis or phthisis has been found in the skeletal remains of mummies in both the Old and New Worlds.[23,48] In Europe, tuberculosis rates reached their peak in the late eighteenth and early nineteenth centuries.[23] With the introduction of industrialization and movement of people from the agrarian life of the countryside to the crowded cities, conditions were set for efficient person-to-person spread of the tubercle bacilli. It is estimated that as much as 10 percent of some populations died from tuberculosis, or consumption, as it was known at that time.[23] Presently, the number of deaths caused by tuberculosis worldwide exceed those caused by any other organism,[55] and tuberculosis aptly bears the name of "the Captain of all these Men of Death."[8] It has been estimated that approximately one-third of the world's population is infected with the tubercle bacillus and that there are 8 million new cases and 3 million deaths annually from tuberculosis in the world.[55]

TUBERCULOSIS SURVEILLANCE IN THE UNITED STATES

Tuberculosis is a reportable disease within all health jurisdictions in the United States, and national surveillance began in 1952. From 1953 to 1985, states reported tuberculosis cases in aggregate; no individual case information was collected at the national level. Starting in 1985, each state reported individual anonymous tuberculosis case information to the Centers for Disease Control and Prevention (CDC). According to the CDC case

TABLE 158-1

CDC Case Definition of Tuberculosis

Laboratory criteria for diagnosis:

Isolation of *M. tuberculosis* from a clinical specimen

Or, when a culture has not been or cannot be obtained, demonstration of acid-fast bacilli in a clinical specimen

For cases that lack laboratory confirmation, all elements of the clinical case definition must be met:

A positive tuberculin skin test

Signs and symptoms compatible with tuberculosis, such as an abnormal, unstable (worsening or improving) chest radiograph or clinical evidence of disease

Treatment with two or more antituberculous medications

A completed diagnostic evaluation

definition (see Table 158-1), a case of tuberculosis is confirmed by identification of *M. tuberculosis* from a clinical specimen or, if culture is not available, by demonstration of acid-fast bacilli (AFB) in a clinical specimen. In addition, a case may be defined by the following four criteria: (1) a positive tuberculin skin test; (2) signs and symptoms consistent with tuberculosis, such as worsening or improving chest radiograph or clinical evidence of disease; (3) treatment with two or more antituberculous drugs; and (4) a completed diagnostic evaluation.[17]

EPIDEMIOLOGY OF TUBERCULOSIS

Tuberculosis is a disease of overcrowding and poverty. The story of the epidemiology of tuberculosis in the United States during the first eight decades of the twentieth century is a dynamic one. A convergence of factors such as infection with human immunodeficiency virus (HIV), increased immigration from countries of high tuberculosis incidence, and a fractured public health system set the stage for increased transmission of tuberculosis in the crowded inner-city population, whose access to health care was limited. As a result, during the 1980s and early 1990s, there was a dramatic increase in case numbers and rates of tuberculosis in this country.[10]

The epidemiology of tuberculosis has changed drastically over the last half of the twentieth century. Tuberculosis changed from a disease seen in older populations, with a steadily declining rate, to one of increasing incidence seen in younger, urban populations. In addition, the epidemiology has been changed by drug resistance, HIV, and immigration of foreign-born persons from areas with high rates of tuberculosis. Multiple drug-resistant tuberculosis has emerged as a significant public health threat and clinical challenge. Through efforts fo-

cused on strengthening health departments through increased resources, education of providers, and close follow-up of patients and their contacts, the increasing trend has been reversed.

Incidence in the United States

From 1953 to 1985, there was a steady decline in the number of tuberculosis cases reported in the United States; the average was between 5 and 6.1 percent per year.[50] In 1953, there were 84,304 cases reported (53 cases per 100,000). This number steadily declined until 1985, when 22,201 cases were reported (9.3 cases per 100,000). From 1985 through 1992, annual rates rose, and in 1992 26,673 cases were reported (10.5 cases per 100,000). This represented a 20 percent increase over the 1985 case number. During this time, an estimated 51,700 excess cases were reported.[10] Following intense public health efforts, focused particularly in high-incidence areas, a reversal in the upward trend of cases has occurred. In both 1993 and 1994, total reported cases of tuberculosis declined compared to previous years (Fig. 158-1). During 1995, 22,813 cases of tuberculosis were reported (incidence of 8.7 per 100,000).[19a]

Geographic Distribution

The increase in the number of cases during 1985–1992 was not evenly distributed throughout the United States and was greatest in urban areas. The states of New York, New Jersey, Texas, Florida, and California had the largest increase in case numbers, accounting for 92 percent of the total national increase from 1985 to 1992.[10] In New York, New Jersey, and California, increases in total reported cases were 84 percent, 81 percent, and 54 percent, respectively. (Table 158-2). Cities with populations over 250,000 persons represent 18 percent of the United States population, yet during 1991 these cities reported 44 percent of the nation's total tuberculosis cases.[16]

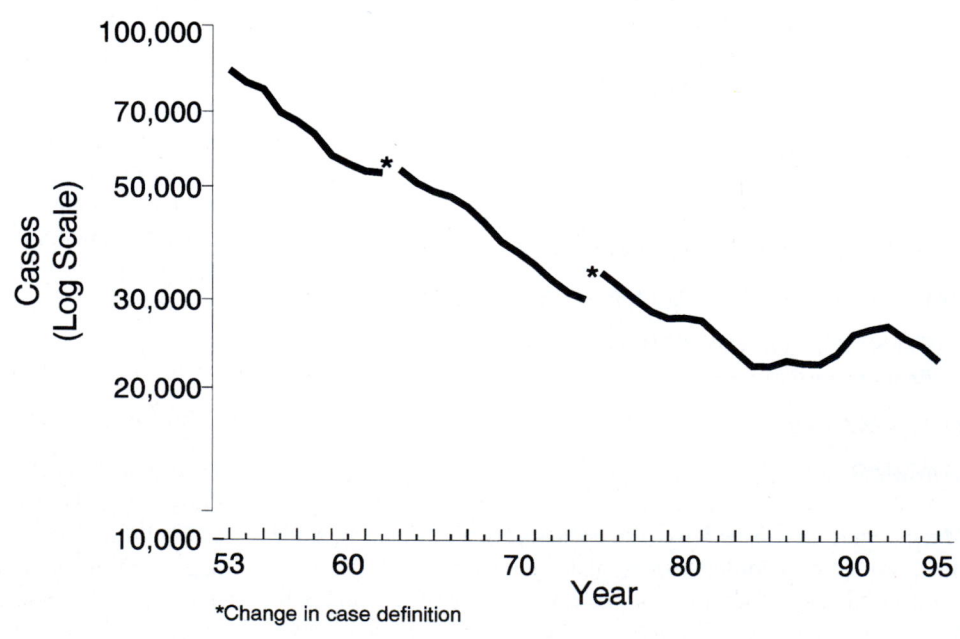

FIGURE 158-1 Reported tuberculosis cases in the United States, 1953–1995.

Race/Ethnicity Distribution

Minority populations have been disproportionally burdened with tuberculosis. Socioeconomic status is probably the most important factor explaining the differences in white and nonwhite populations, and rates of tuberculosis are inversely related to income level (Fig. 158-2). Even while tuberculosis rates in the United States were decreasing prior to 1985, the rate of decrease was less for the nonwhite than the white population. From 1985 through 1992, case numbers in whites continued to decrease, albeit not as sharply, and marked increases in case numbers were observed in minority populations. For example, between 1985 and 1992, cases among non-Hispanic blacks and Hispanics increased 26.8 and 74.5 percent, respectively. As the total number of cases declined between 1992 and 1995, so did numbers in minority populations; except for Asian/Pacific Islanders, and Native Americans, decreases were seen in all minority groups (Table 158-3).[15]

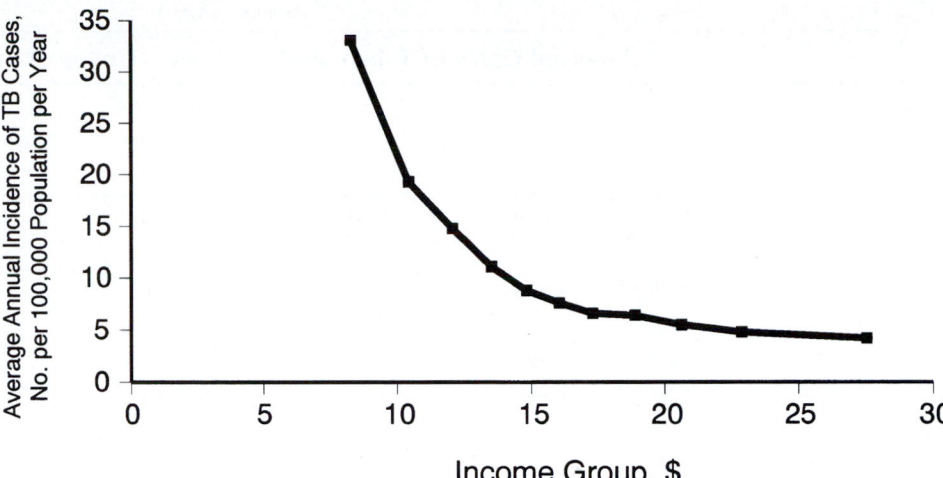

FIGURE 158-2   Seven-year average annual incidence of tuberculosis by income group, United States, 1985–1991.

Age

In the elderly, most tuberculosis is not a result of newly acquired infection but rather is due to reactivation of latent infection acquired earlier in life and reflects prevalence of the disease at the time that infection was transmitted. Tuberculosis in infants and children, on the other hand, serves as a sentinel event of recent infection. By virtue of their young age, infection in children cannot be a remote event. Further, primary tuberculosis may develop within as many as 60 percent of untreated infected infants.[6] As the incidence of tuberculosis declined in the United States, the median age of persons with tuberculosis increased; in 1985, the median age of persons with tuberculosis was 49 years. Nearly one-third of the total cases were in persons 65 years and older.[10] With increasing cases, in 1985, the median age of tuberculosis fell to 43 years, and there were marked increases in cases of tuberculosis in younger groups, especially in medically underserved minority populations. In non-Hispanic blacks and Hispanics, cases in those 25 to 44 years old increased by 63 and 99 percent, respectively. Accordingly, case numbers in young children, who are the likely contacts of 25- to 44-year-old adults, also increased dramatically. For children from birth up to 14 years of age, cases increased 31 and 99 percent among non-Hispanic blacks and Hispanics, respectively. Despite the decline in cases in 1993 and 1994, cases in children under 15 years have not declined appreciably.[14,15]

Place of Birth

Because tuberculosis is highly endemic in some countries of Central and South America, Africa, and Asia, persons who are born in these countries are more likely to have tuberculosis than U.S.-born persons. Place of birth for persons with tuberculosis has been included in reports to CDC since 1986.[46] At that time, 22 percent of cases were in foreign-born persons. The percentage has continued to increase, and in 1994, 32 percent of all cases occurred in foreign-born persons. For the years 1986 to 1993, the rate of tuberculosis in the foreign-born was 3.7 times higher than that in the U.S.-born population (30.6 per 100,000 versus 8.1 per 100,000, respectively). For those less than 15 years old, the rate in the foreign-born was 13.2 times higher than that in the U.S.-born (2.1 per 100,000 versus 27.7 per 100,000, respectively).[46] Of 7627 cases of tuberculosis in foreign-born persons reported in 1994, the greatest number of cases were in persons

TABLE 158-2

Reported Cases of Tuberculosis by State—United States, 1985–1994

State	1985	1992	1995	1985–1992 Change by no. of cases	1985–1992 Change by Percentage	1992–1994 Change by no. of cases	1992–1995 Change by Percentage
New York	2,481	4,574	3,066	+2,093	+84.4	− 938	−33.0
New Jersey	545	984	848	+ 439	+80.6	− 129	−13.8
California	3,491	5,382	4,622	+1,891	+54.2	− 523	−14.1
Texas	1,891	2,510	2,369	+ 619	+32.7	+ 32	− 5.6
Florida	1,425	1,707	1,577	+ 282	+19.8	− 55	− 7.6
Total	22,201	26,673	22,813	+4,472	+20.1	−2,312	−14.5

TABLE 158-3

Reported Cases of Tuberculosis by State—United States, 1985–1994

Race/ Ethnicity	1985	1992	1995	1985–1992 Change by no. of cases	1985–1992 Change by Percentage	1992–1994 Change by no. of cases	1992–1995 Change by Percentage
White non-Hispanic	8,453	7,618	5,950	− 835	− 9.9	−1124	−21.9
Black non-Hispanic	7,592	9,623	7,521	+2,031	+26.8	−1287	−21.8
Hispanic	3,092	5,397	5,074	+2,305	+74.5	− 360	− 5.9
Asian/Pacific Islander	2,530	3,698	3,821	+1,168	+46.2	+ 170	− 3.3
American Indian/ Alaskan Native	397	305	331	− 92	−23.3	+ 35	+ 8.8

born in Mexico (24 percent), the Philippines (14 percent), and Vietnam, (11 percent).[15]

Clinical Site of Tuberculosis

Pulmonary tuberculosis accounts for approximately 80 percent of tuberculosis reported and has the greatest public health impact because of infectiousness.[15,25] Sites of extrapulmonary tuberculosis most commonly reported are disease of the pleura, the lymphatic system and genitourinary tract as well as miliary disease.[25] In children, meningeal and miliary tuberculosis are more common than in adults and account for approximately 20 percent of cases reported in newborns to 4-year-olds.[15]

HIV and Tuberculosis

Infection with HIV is the strongest risk factor known for progression from latent infection with *M. tuberculosis* to active disease.[52] Reactivation rates for those with *M. tuberculosis* and HIV infection have been estimated at 7 to 10 percent year, making the *yearly* risk of reactivation equivalent to the *lifetime* risk of an immunocompetent host.[52] In addition to the increased risk of reactivation of latent infection, persons with HIV infection who become newly infected with *M. tuberculosis* have an increased risk of developing primary disease, often with rapid progression. This has been illustrated in recent outbreaks of multidrug-resistant tuberculosis.[22,24] In persons with HIV infection, cavitary tuberculosis is less common than it is in the immunocompetent host.[4] Extrapulmonary tuberculosis, on the other hand, is more common. In some studies, as many as 40 to 60 percent of patients had extrapulmonary disease, although most had pulmonary disease accompanying extrapulmonary tuberculosis.[49,53] An individual's HIV status does not appear to increase their infectiousness as tuberculosis patients. In a study comparing contacts of tuberculosis patients, 42 percent of contacts of HIV-negative patients were found to have positive tuberculin skin tests, whereas 31 percent of contacts of patients with acquired immunodeficiency syndrome (AIDS) had positive tuberculin skin tests.[11]

The interaction between HIV and tuberculosis is reflected in the epidemiology of both of these diseases. The changing face of tuberculosis epidemiology in the United States was signaled, in 1985, by the reversal of the downward trend of cases and mirrored the epidemiology of reported AIDS cases. Individuals infected with either HIV or tuberculosis were similar with regard to age, racial/ethnic background, and geographic distribution. For example, during 1985 through 1992, persons 25 to 44 years of age accounted for most of the AIDS cases reported as well as the increased number of tuberculosis cases. In the five states with the highest number of reported AIDS cases, increased morbidity due to tuberculosis was most apparent. Tuberculosis case numbers decreased or remained stable in areas of low or intermediate cumulative AIDS incidence; in areas of high cumulative AIDS incidence, case numbers rose sharply. Racial/ethnic groups with the greatest burden of AIDS cases also experienced the sharpest increases in tuberculosis cases, and it has been estimated that HIV-infected individuals accounted for at least 50 percent of the excess cases seen in the United States (Fig. 158-3).[10]

A serologic survey for HIV infection among patients attending tuberculosis clinics found a prevalence of 3.4 percent.[49] However, the range of HIV seroprevalence varied from 0 to 46 percent, and coinfection between *M. tuberculosis* and HIV was most prevalent in the northeastern United States and in non-Hispanic blacks. When national AIDS and tuberculosis registries were matched for the years 1981 through 1991, 5.1 percent of tuberculosis cases were also reported to have AIDS. The highest proportion of tuberculosis cases with AIDS were in New York City (15.1 percent); New York State excluding New York City (8.8 percent); New Jersey (8.4 percent); and Florida (8.0 percent). Since pulmonary tuberculosis was not classified as an AIDS-defining criterion until 1993, this percentage is most likely an underestimate, as the match only included cases already diagnosed with AIDS.[9]

Multidrug-Resistant Tuberculosis

Drug resistance in mycobacteria comes about through random spontaneous mutation.[39] In a large population of bacilli, there

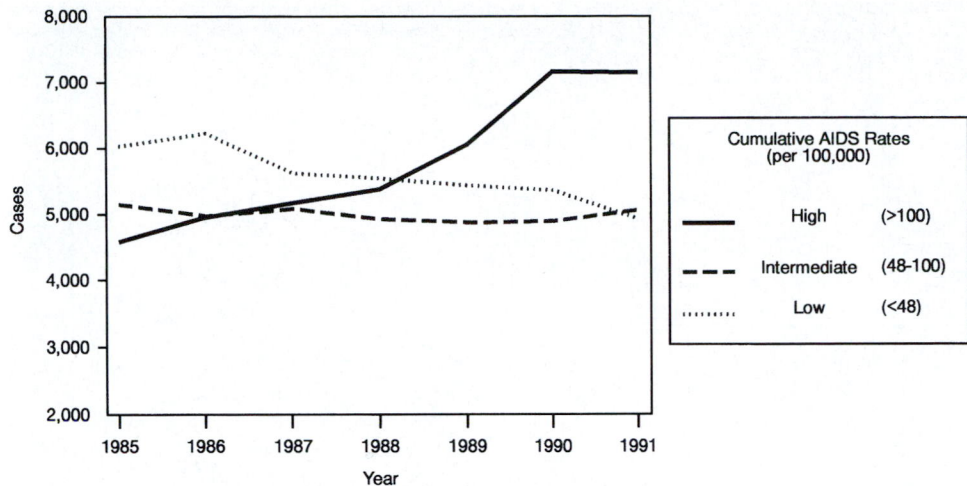

FIGURE 158-3   Tuberculosis cases among U.S. born stratified by cumulative acquired immunodeficiency syndrome (AIDS) rates of reporting by states, United States, 1985–1992.

will be a number of mutants that have resistance to a single antituberculous drug. Upon exposure to a single drug, a small subpopulation of organisms resistant to that drug will be selected and eventually may make up the entire population of infecting organisms. This phenomenon is termed *acquired drug resistance.* Thus, in all treatment of tuberculosis disease, at least two drugs to which the organism is susceptible must be used.[2,39] Each drug reduces the growth of organisms that are resistant to the other agent. Drug-resistant organisms can be transmitted to others directly. Persons with drug-resistant tuberculosis who have no history of prior tuberculosis treatment are said to have primary or initial drug resistance.[2] Drug-resistant tuberculosis has been associated with increased treatment failure, defined as the failure of treatment to produce negative cultures and cure. In trials, treatment failure in patients with drug-resistant disease was 83 times higher than in patients with drug-susceptible tuberculosis, (11.6 versus 0.15 percent, respectively).[47]

Multidrug-resistant tuberculosis (MDR-TB) is generally taken to involve tuberculosis caused by an organism resistant to at least isoniazid *and* rifampin, the cornerstones of tuberculosis therapy. Multidrug-resistant tuberculosis poses problems from both a clinical and public health perspective. It is difficult to treat and generally requires a minimum of 18 to 24 months of therapy; resectional surgery is occasionally needed.[39]

From the public health perspective, management of MDR-TB is challenging. Since acquired drug resistance is a result of prior inadequate therapy,[39] efforts should focus on ensuring patient compliance with treatment regimens for the full duration of therapy. The CDC and the American Thoracic Society recommend that all patients with drug-resistant tuberculosis receive directly observed therapy (DOT).[2] Since it is not known to what level preventive antibiotic therapy for MDR-TB is effective, prevention of transmission of MDR-TB is the only effective preventive measure. Studies have shown that patients with MDR-TB, even when treated with two or more effective agents, remain smear- and culture-positive longer than patients with susceptible tuberculosis,[30,56] perhaps because of decreased potency of medications used for treatment of MDR-TB.

The greatest risk factor for the presence of MDR-TB is a history of prior treatment for tuberculosis.[39] Besides those with such a history, others who are at increased risk for drug resistance include persons from foreign countries and American communities where there are high rates of MDR-TB.[5,32] In a nationwide survey of drug resistance, 18 percent of *M. tuberculosis* isolates from foreign-born persons had resistance to at least one antituberculous medication.[5] Resistance to isoniazid or streptomycin, which are the drugs used most commonly for the treatment of tuberculosis outside of the United States, is seen more frequently in foreign-born persons with tuberculosis.[5] In a study of drug resistance in isolates from tuberculosis patients in New York City, resistance to isoniazid and rifampin was seen in 19 percent of all isolates and in 30 percent isolates from patients with a history of prior treatment.[32]

The etiology of the problem of MDR-TB in the United States appears to be multifactorial. First, increased rates of tuberculosis led to increased patient care needs. Health departments with inadequate resources could not meet the medical needs for all patients.[32] This, in turn, contributed to increased risk of development of resistance, especially in patients in unstable living conditions, such as the homeless and users of injection drugs. Since there are high rates of HIV coinfection in these groups, there were increased rates of reactivation after infection or progression to primary disease.[4,22] There have been eight nosocomial outbreaks of MDR-TB investigated by the CDC, all of which involved patients who were HIV-infected.[40] Common features to the outbreaks that contributed to the transmission included delay in diagnosis, delay in laboratory confirmation and susceptibility results, delay in therapy, and inadequate isolation of patients with infectious tuberculosis.

INTERPERSONAL SPREAD OF TUBERCULOSIS

In 1882, Robert Koch isolated the tubercle bacillus and demonstrated that it is the causative agent of tuberculosis.[3] Tuberculosis is transmitted by airborne spread from person to person via infected respiratory secretions.[51] Inhalation of droplet nuclei containing the tubercle bacillus may result in infection. Respiratory droplets are produced when someone with pulmonary tuberculosis coughs, or, in the case of laryngeal tuberculosis, with speaking or singing. While these respiratory droplets are airborne, water evaporates, leaving small 1- to 5-μm particles called droplet nuclei. Because of their small size, these droplet nuclei may remain suspended in air currents for hours and, when inhaled, may escape the host's upper airway defenses.[51] When these droplet nuclei reach the alveoli, infection may result.

Infectiousness of a tuberculosis patient is dependent on the number of tubercle bacilli expelled into the air. The bacillary load is related to a number of factors, including presence of disease in the lungs, cavity formation, disease in the airways or larynx, presence or induction of cough, failure of the patient to cover the mouth while coughing, and presence of acid-fast bacilli (AFB) on microscopic examination of sputum specimens (Fig. 158-4). The period of infectiousness may be prolonged with inappropriate therapy of tuberculosis.[13] Interpersonal spread of tuberculosis may be enhanced in areas of overcrowding, poor air circulation, or recirculated, unfiltered air. Rates of tuberculous infection in exposed contacts of individuals with active tuberculosis may also be dependent on the duration of exposure. In a study of a student with laryngeal tuberculosis, infection was noted in classroom contacts with as little as 5 h of exposure.[7] In general, tuberculosis is not regarded as highly infectious; of household contacts of sputum AFB-smear positive cases, approximately 30 percent are

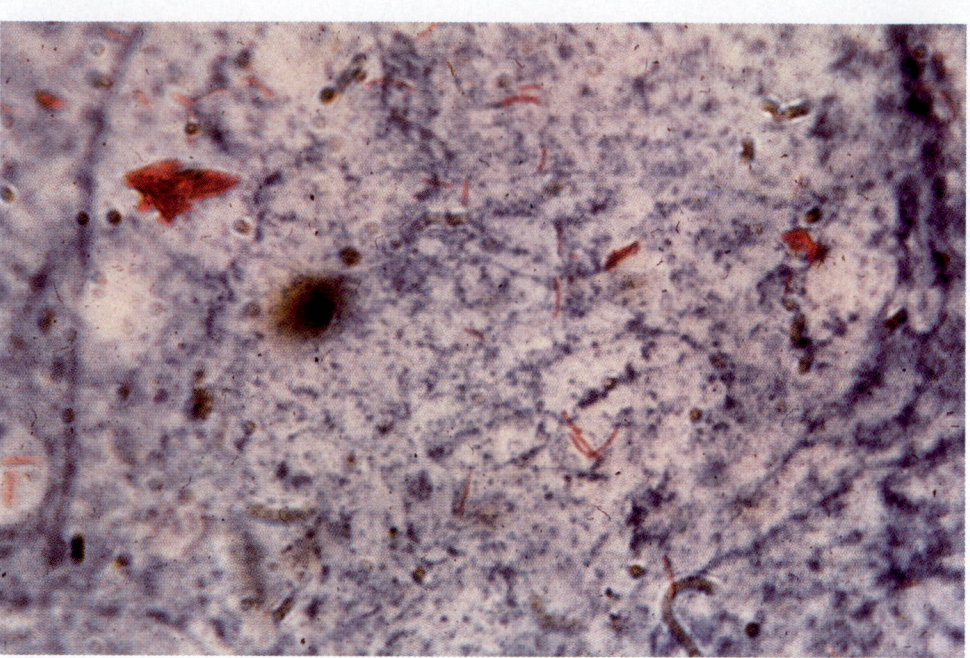

FIGURE 158-4   Photomicrograph of acid-fast bacilli in sputum.

infected.[35] In general, children are far less infectious than adults, because the tubercle bacilli are rare in their endobronchial secretions and they lack the tussive force of adults. As a result, children contribute little to the interpersonal spread of tuberculosis.[54]

Tuberculosis is not transmitted by fomites such as droplets on clothing or other inanimate objects. Transmission of infection has been associated rarely with generation of infectious aerosols from use of water irrigation on draining skin wounds and reciprocating saws used in autopsy rooms.[37,57] In a study that examined the rates of skin test conversion of pulmonary and infectious disease fellows, pulmonary fellows were more likely to convert their tuberculin skin tests than infectious disease fellows (11 versus 2.4 percent, respectively). The increase of skin test conversions was attributed to time spent in contact with patients in intensive care units and performance of invasive procedures such as endotracheal intubation and fiberoptic bronchoscopy.[43]

PREVENTION OF INFECTION

The prompt recognition and appropriate treatment of persons with potentially infectious tuberculosis is the best means of preventing the spread of *M. tuberculosis* infection. Even after appropriate therapy has been instituted, patients with tuberculosis may remain infectious for a period of time. Tuberculosis has been recognized in the past as an occupational hazard for persons caring for tuberculosis patients.[45] With the rise of drug-resistant tuberculosis, the risk of tuberculous infection and disease in health care workers has received attention in the literature. Several nosocomial outbreaks have demonstrated the spread of infection and disease from hospitalized patients to health care workers and other patients.[24,29]

The CDC has issued guidelines[19] for the prevention of transmission of tuberculosis in health care settings. These guidelines call for a hierarchy of control measures. The first level is that of administrative controls; the second, engineering controls; and the third, a respiratory protection program. Administrative controls are designed to reduce the number of persons exposed to a potentially infectious tuberculosis patient. This includes rapid identification, isolation, diagnostic evaluation and treatment of patients likely to have tuberculosis. Hospitalized patients with confirmed or suspected tuberculosis should remain in AFB isolation until three consecutive sputums, obtained on separate days, are AFB smear–negative. Also, to promote effective work practices (such as correct use of respiratory protection), health care workers should be educated about tuberculosis. Engineering controls are used to prevent spread of potentially infectious droplet nuclei. Patients with known or suspected tuberculosis should be placed in a private room that has negative pressure with respect to the hallway and has at least six air changes per hour. Ultraviolet germicidal irradiation is also used in some institutions. Health care workers caring for tuberculosis patients should use personal respiratory protection. To assess for evidence of nosocomial transmission of infection, health care workers should be screened periodically by tuberculin skin testing.[19]

Preventive Therapy

Among immunocompetent hosts, tuberculosis infection acquired in childhood progresses to active disease at some time during life in approximately 10 percent.[21] Risk is highest in the first several years after infection.[26,27] Certain medical conditions (see Table 158-4) increase the risk of disease development. The most important of these is HIV infection. In a study of HIV-infected injecting drug users, the yearly risk of developing tuberculosis was 7 to 10 percent in those with *M. tuberculosis* infection.[52]

Preventive therapy is currently widely used in the United States for the treatment of tuberculous infection to prevent the development of disease. In the absence of active disease, a positive tuberculin skin test indicates latent infection. Preventive therapy is directed at eliminating the small number of tubercle bacilli residing in the body that may cause disease at a later date.

The recommendation for preventive therapy depends not only on the extent of reaction to the tuberculin skin test (i.e., millimeters of induration), but also on the patient's risk factors for developing active tuberculosis.

Isoniazid (INH) as a single agent is used, with some exceptions, as preventive therapy. The drug is given as a single daily dose of 5 to 10 mg/kg, not to exceed 300 mg/day. Hepatotoxity is the most commonly seen adverse effect.[33] When considering the use of INH preventive therapy, the clinician must weigh the immediate risk of INH toxicity during therapy against the lifetime risk of development of active tuberculosis. Because INH hepatotoxicity is age-related,[41] INH preventive therapy is usually offered only to those who are younger than 35 years.[2] However, in those who are at high risk of developing active tuberculosis, preventive therapy is recommended regardless of age. In considering the use of preventive therapy, it is important to first rule out active tuberculosis, so that treatment of active disease with a single agent and potential emergence of resistance can be avoided.[2]

Table 158-4 reviews the CDC and American Thoracic Society recommendations for tuberculin skin test interpretation and the use of preventive therapy.[2] For those considered at highest risk for the development of disease, a 5-mm cutoff is used to define a positive test, and preventive therapy should be administered regardless of age. This includes those who are close contacts of someone with infectious tuberculosis, those with HIV infection, those with known risk factors for HIV infection whose HIV status is unknown but are suspected of having HIV infection, and those with fibrotic lesions on chest radiograph who have received no or inadequate preventive therapy. A 10-mm cutoff is used to define a positive test, and preventive therapy is recommended regardless of age for persons with medical conditions that are reported to increase risk of developing active disease. These include diabetes mellitus, prolonged therapy with corticosteroids, treatment with immunosuppressive therapy, hematologic and reticuloendothelial diseases associated with decreased cellular immunity (e.g., Hodgkin's disease and leukemia), injecting drug users who are known to be HIV-negative, end-stage renal disease, and clinical conditions associated with substantial weight loss or malnutrition. In persons from countries with high tuberculosis incidence, from medically underserved low-income populations, or who are residents of correctional, mental, or extended care facilities, and do not have a medical risk factor mentioned above, a positive tuberculin skin test is defined as in duration ≥ 10 min.

Preventive therapy is recommended for those younger than 35 years. For all other persons without a risk factor for tuberculosis, 15 mm is the recommended cutoff for a positive test, and preventive therapy is recommended for those younger than 35 years. In addition, since recent infection is a risk factor for development of active disease, those who have a conversion of the tuberculin skin test from negative to positive within the preceding 2 years (see Table 158-4) should receive preventive therapy regardless of age.[2]

The recommended duration of preventive therapy is 6 months. For young children, INH is given for 9 months.[1] For those who are HIV-infected or who have a chest radiograph suggestive of old disease and have received either no or inadequate therapy, 12 months of therapy is recommended. Preventive therapy with INH is generally not recommended during pregnancy. However, in pregnant women with HIV infection or recent tuberculin skin test conversion, INH may be administered after the first trimester of pregnancy.[58] In patients who are HIV-seropositive and anergic, some experts recommend preventive therapy, especially if the person is from a high-risk group or geographic area with a high prevalence of *M. tuberculosis* infection.[18]

The efficacy of INH used as preventive therapy has been examined in a number of trials.[26,27] For those who have completed a full course of INH preventive therapy with good compliance,

TABLE 158-4

Recommended Guidelines for Preventive Therapy

Induration of tuberculin skin test	Indication for Preventive Therapy
≥5 mm	HIV infection
	Close contacts of an infectious case
	Chest radiograph consistent with old, healed TB with no or incomplete prior therapy
	Those with a known risk factor for HIV and whose HIV status is unknown
≥10 mm	Diabetes mellitus
	Prolonged therapy with corticosteroids
	Immunosuppressive therapy
	Hematologic/reticuloendothelial diseases that are associate with decreased cellular immunity (i.e., Hodgkin's disease, leukemia)
	Injecting drug user known HIV-negative
	Substantial weight loss or malnutrition
	Foreign-born, from a country with incidence of tuberculosis*
	Medically underserved, low-income population*
	Residents of correctional, mental, or extended-care facilities*
	Infants and children under 4 years of age
≥15 mm	All others without above risk factors*
	Tuberculin skin test conversions†

* Preventive therapy administered to those <35 years.
† Definition of a tuberculin skin test conversion:
    Age < 35 years; increase ≥10 mm within 2 years.
    Age ≥ 35 years; increase ≥15 mm within 2 years.
SOURCE: From American Thoracic Society,[2] with permission.

reduction in rates of tuberculosis as great as 70 percent have been seen.[26,27,38] There is no evidence to suggest that preventive therapy with INH will lead to the development of INH resistance.[26,27] If the infecting organism has primary INH resistance, INH preventive therapy will probably be of little benefit.[26,27] For persons who are contacts of a source case with an isolate that is INH-resistant and rifampin-susceptible, rifampin is recommended as preventive therapy at a dose of 10 mg/kg per day, not to exceed 600 mg/day.[2] There are few data on the use of this agent for preventive therapy in normal hosts; this use is recommended based on animal studies.[42] However, data on its use in chemotherapy of disease is vast. In a group of high school students with infection from a source case with INH-resistant tuberculosis, rifampin preventive therapy was well tolerated.[59]

Preventive therapy for persons infected with bacilli resistant to both INH and rifampin poses a much more difficult question. Because of the difficulty of treatment of MDR-TB and its higher morbidity and mortality, alternative preventive therapy should be considered, especially in persons with a high risk of tuberculosis, such as those who are HIV-seropositive and are felt likely to be infected with MDR-TB. Combinations of pyrazinamide, ethambutol, and a fluoroquinolone are usually used.[2] Limited data show that tolerance to these regimens is poor.[36,44] There are no data on the efficacy of these alternative preventive therapy regimens. Before initiating them, physicians should seek consultation from experts in the treatment and management of MDR-TB.

BCG VACCINE

In 1908 Albert Calmette and Camille Guérin began to subculture a strain *M. tuberculosis* from a cow with tuberculous mastitis. After 13 years and 230 serial subcultures, the strain was no longer virulent in animals, and in 1921 use of bacille Calmette-Guérin (BCG) in humans was begun. This is a live vaccine, and it is the most widely used vaccine in the world today.[28,34] Due to genetic variation of strains and differences in production techniques, not all BCG vaccines are identical.[28] The vaccine does not protect against infection with the tubercle bacilli,[31] and the efficacy of BCG in preventing active disease has ranged from 20 to 80 percent in trials conducted.[28] Explanations for this variability in vaccine efficacy may be related to regional differences in environmental mycobacteria and different strains of BCG used in the trials.[28] Exposure to and infection with environmental mycobacteria may provide cross-protection against tuberculosis, and BCG may add little to that protection.[28] In one meta-analysis of 26 trials, the estimated protective effect of BCG was 50 percent.[20]

Vaccination with BCG usually produces a reaction to the tuberculin skin test, and there is no reliable way to distinguish tuberculin sensitivity caused by vaccination with BCG from natural infection with *M. tuberculosis.*[12] Reactivity wanes over time and, in the absence of infection with *M. tuberculosis,* is not likely to persist over 10 years after vaccination.[12] A diagnosis of *M. tuberculosis* infection should be considered for a BCG-vaccinated person with a positive skin test if any of the following conditions are met: (1) the size of the skin test induration is large, (2) there is history of contact with a person with tuberculosis, (3) there is a family history of tuberculosis, (4) the person's

country of origin has a high prevalence of tuberculosis, or (5) several years have passed between vaccination and tuberculin skin testing.[12] Administration of BCG is not a contraindication to tuberculin skin testing.[12] The consensus in the United States is that tuberculosis control is best accomplished with prompt identification and treatment of persons with infectious tuberculosis, with preventive therapy for persons who have positive tuberculin skin tests. Therefore, because of the low risk for tuberculosis in the general population, wide variability of BCG efficacy, and potential loss of valuable tuberculin skin test information, BCG vaccine is not recommended for general use in the United States.[12] The exception to this is the case of infants and children with negative tuberculin skin tests who are at high risk of exposure to persons with infectious tuberculosis and who cannot be placed on preventive therapy or are continuously exposed to persons with multidrug-resistant tuberculosis.[12]

SUMMARY

After declining throughout the twentieth century, tuberculosis cases in the United States rose in the mid-1980s. These increases were focal, affecting certain geographic areas and populations—namely large urban areas and poor, minority, and medically underserved persons. The increase was attributed to decreased resources to health departments for tuberculosis control, the HIV epidemic, and increased immigration of persons from countries of high tuberculosis incidence. Drug-resistant tuberculosis has emerged as a significant public health problem and has caused explosive outbreaks in populations of persons dually infected with HIV and multidrug-resistant tuberculosis. In the years 1993–1995, tuberculosis incidence in the United States once again declined, due in part to a focused public health effort for control in areas of highest incidence.

Mycobacterium tuberculosis transmission is via an airborne route. Transmission in the health care setting has been documented and may be the result of delayed recognition, incomplete diagnostic evaluation, and inappropriate treatment of cases of pulmonary tuberculosis. Guidelines for the prevention of transmission of tuberculosis in health care facilities call for administrative and engineering control measures and a respiratory protection program for health care workers.

Once infection with *M. tuberculosis* has occurred, preventive therapy with isoniazid has been shown to decrease progress of latent infection to active tuberculosis. Recommendations for preventive therapy depend on the millimeters of induration of the tuberculin skin test and an individual's risk of infection. For those who are likely to have been infected with isoniazid-resistant *M. tuberculosis,* alternative regimens for preventive therapy have been proposed. Because of the low overall incidence of tuberculosis in the United States, and the potential loss of the tuberculin skin test as a valuable screening tool, BCG vaccination is not recommended except in rare circumstances.

REFERENCES

1. American Academy of Pediatrics: Tuberculosis, in Peter G (ed): *1994 Red Book: Report of Committee on Infectious Diseases,* 23d ed. Elk Grove Village, IL, American Academy of Pediatrics, 1994,

pp 480–500.

2. American Thoracic Society: Treatment of tuberculosis and tuberculosis infection in adults and children. *Am J Respir Crit Care Med* 149:1359–1374, 1994.

3. Baldwin ER: Tuberculosis: history and etiology, in Osler W (ed): *Modern Medicine*. Philadelphia, Lea & Febiger, 1925.

4. Barnes PF, Bloch AB, Davidson PT, Snider DE: Tuberculosis in patients with human immunodeficiency virus infection. *New Engl J Med* 324:1644–1650, 1991.

5. Bloch AB, Cauthen GM, Onorato IM, et al: Nationwide survey of drug-resistant tuberculosis in the United States. *JAMA* 271:665–671, 1994.

6. Brailey M: Mortality in tuberculin-positive infants. *Milbank Q* 15:37–47, 1937.

7. Braden CR and an investigative team: Infectiousness of an university student with laryngeal and cavitary tuberculosis. *Clin Infect Dis* 21:1565–1570, 1995.

8. Bunyan J: *The Life and Death of Mr. Badman*. London, Dent, 1928, p 282. (Originally published in 1680.)

9. Burwen DR, Bloch AB, Griffin LD, Ciesielski CA. National trends in the concurrence of tuberculosis and acquired immunodeficiency syndrome. *Arch Intern Med* 155:1281–1286, 1995.

10. Cantwell MF, Snider DE, Cauthen GM, Onorato IM: Epidemiology of tuberculosis in the United States, 1985 through 1992. *JAMA* 272:535–539, 1994.

11. Cauthen GM, Dooley SW, Onorato IM, et al: Transmission of *M. tuberculosis* from tuberculosis patients with HIV infection or AIDS. *Am J Epidemiol* 144:69–77, 1996.

12. Centers for Disease Control: The role of BCG vaccine in the control of tuberculosis in the United States. *Morb Mortal Wkly Rep* 45(No. RR-3):1–18, 1996.

13. Centers for Disease Control: The use of preventive therapy for tuberculous infection in the United States. *Morb Mortal Wkly Rep* 39(No, RR-8):1–12, 1990.

14. Centers for Disease Control: *Reported Tuberculosis in the United States, 1993*. October 1994.

15. Centers for Disease Control: *Reported Tuberculosis in the United States, 1994*. July 1995.

16. Centers for Disease Control: *Tuberculosis Statistics in the United States, 1992*. July 1994.

17. Centers for Disease Control: Case definitions for public health surveillance. *Morb Mortal Wkly Rep* 39(No. RR-13):39–40, 1990.

18. Centers for Disease Control: USPHS/IDSA Guidelines for the prevention of opportunistic infections in persons infected with human immunodeficiency virus: A summary. *Morb Mortal Wkly Rep* 44(RR-8):9–10, 1995.

19. Centers for Disease Control: Guidelines for preventing the transmission of *Mycobacterium tuberculosis* in health-care facilities, 1994. *Morb Mortal Wkly Rep* 43(No. RR-13):57, 1994.

19a. Centers for Disease Control and Prevention: Reported tuberculosis in the United States, 1995. August 1996, p 5

20. Colditz GA, Brewer T, Berkley C, et al: Efficacy of BCG in the prevention of tuberculosis: Meta-analysis of the published literature. *JAMA* 271:698–702, 1994.

21. Comstock GM, Livesay VT, Woolpert SF: The prognosis of positive tuberculin reaction in childhood and adolescence. *Am J Epidemiol* 99:131–138, 1974.

22. Daley CL, Small PM, Schecter GF, et al: An outbreak of tuberculosis with accelerated progression among persons infected with the immunodeficiency virus. *New Engl J Med* 326:231–235, 1992.

23. Dubos R, Dubos J: *The White Plague: Tuberculosis, Man and Society*. New Brunswick, NJ, Rutgers University Press, 1987.

24. Edlin BR, Tokars JI, Grieco MH, et al: An outbreak of multi-drug resistant tuberculosis among hospitalized patients with the acquired immunodeficiency syndrome. *New Engl J Med* 326:1514–1521, 1992.

25. Farer LS, Lowell LM, Meador MP: Extrapulmonary tuberculosis in the United States. *Am J Epidemiol* 109:205–217, 1979.

26. Ferebee SH: Controlled chemoprophylaxis trials in tuberculosis: A general review. *Adv Tuberc Res* 17:28–106, 1969.

27. Ferebee SH, Mount FW, Murray FJ, Livesay VT: A controlled trial of isoniazid prophylaxis in mental institutions. *Am Rev Respir Dis* 88:161–175, 1963.

28. Fine PEM: Variation in protection by BCG: Implications of and for heterologous immunity. *Lancet* 346:1339–1345, 1995.

29. Fischl MA, Uttamchandani RB, Daikos GL, et al: An outbreak of tuberculosis caused by multi-drug-resistant tubercle bacilli among patients with HIV infection. *Ann Intern Med* 117:177–183, 1992.

30. Fischl MA, Daikos MD, Uttamchandani MD, et al. Clinical presentation and outcome of patients with HIV infection and tuberculosis caused by multiple-drug-resistant bacilli. *Ann Intern Med* 117:184–190, 1992.

31. Fok JS, Ho RS, Arora PK, et al: Host-parasite relationships in experimental tuberculosis: V. Lack of hematogenous dissemination of *Mycobacterium tuberculosis* to the lungs in animals vaccinated with bacille Calmette-Guérin. *J Infect Dis* 133:137–144, 1976.

32. Frieden TR, Sterling T, Pablos-Mendez A, et al: The emergence of drug-resistant tuberculosis in New York City. *New Engl J Med* 328:521–526, 1993.

33. Garibaldi RA, Drusin RE, Ferebee SH, Gregg MB: Isoniazid-associated hepatitis. *Am Rev Respir Dis* 106:357–365, 1972.

34. Grange JM, Gibson J, Osborn TW: What is BCG? *Tubercle* 64:129–139, 1983.

35. Grzybowski S, Barnett GD, Styblo K. Contacts of active pulmonary tuberculosis. *Bull Int Union Tuberc* 50:90–106, 1975.

36. Horn DL, Hewlett D, Alfalfa C, et al: Limited tolerance of ofloxacin and pyrazinamide prophylaxis against tuberculosis (letter). *New Engl J Med* 330:1241, 1994.

37. Hutton MD, Stead WW, Cauthen GN, et al: Nosocomial transmission of tuberculosis associated with a draining abscess. *J Infect Dis* 161:286–295, 1990.

38. International Union Against Tuberculosis Committee on Prophylaxis: Efficacy of various durations of isoniazid preventive therapy for tuberculosis: Five years follow-up in the IUAT trial. *Bull WHO* 60:555–564, 1982.

39. Iseman MD: Treatment of Multidrug-resistant tuberculosis. *New Engl J Med* 329:784–791, 1993.

40. Jarvis WR: Nosocomial transmission of multidrug-resistant *Mycobacterium tuberculosis*. *Res Microbiol* 144:117–122, 1993.

41. Kopanoff DE, Snider DE, Caras GJ: Isoniazid related hepatitis. *Am Rev Respir Dis* 117:991–1001, 1978.

42. Lecoeur HF, Truffot-Pernot C, Grosset JH: Experimental short-course preventive therapy of tuberculosis with rifampin and pyrazinamide. *Am Rev Respir Dis* 140:1189–1193, 1989.

43. Malasky C, Jordan T, Potulski F, Reichman LB: Occupational tuberculous infections among pulmonary physicians in training. *Am Rev Respir Dis* 142:505–507, 1990.

44. Meador J, Maxwell R, Weismuller P, et al: Intolerance to pyrazinamide and ofloxacin chemoprophylaxis in a group of young, healthy adults exposed to multi-drug resistant tuberculosis (abstr). *Am J Respir Crit Care Med* 153: A487, 1996.

45. Menzies D, Fanning A, Yuan L, Fitzgerald M: Tuberculosis among health care workers. *N Engl J Med* 332:92–98, 1995.

46. McKenna MT, McCray E, Onorato IM: The epidemiology of tuberculosis among foreign-born persons in the United States, 1986 to 1993. *New Engl J Med* 332:1071–1076, 1995.

47. Mitchison DA, Nunn AJ: Influence of initial drug resistance on the response to short-course chemotherapy of pulmonary tuberculosis. *Am Rev Respir Dis* 133:423–430, 1986.

48. Morell V: Mummy settles TB antiquity debate. *Science* 263:1686–1687, 1994.

49. Onorato IM, McCray E, Field Services Branch: Prevalence of human immunodeficiency virus among patients attending tuberculosis clinics in the United States. *J Infect Dis* 165:87-92, 1992.

50. Reider HL, Cauthen GM, Comstock GW, Snider DE: Epidemiology of tuberculosis in the United States. *Epidemiol Rev* 11:79-98, 1989.

51. Riley RL: Airborne infection. *Am J Med* 57:466–475, 1974.

52. Selwyn PA, Hartel D, Lewis VA, et al: A prospective study of the risk of tuberculosis among intravenous drug users with human immunodeficiency virus infection. *New Engl J Med* 230:545–550, 1989.

53. Small PM, Schecter GF, Goodman PC, et al: Treatment of tuberculosis in patients with advanced human immunodeficiency virus infection. *New Engl J Med* 324:289–294, 1991.

54. Smith MHD, Starke JR, Marquis JR: Tuberculosis and opportunistic mycobacterial infections, in Feigin RD, Cherry JD (eds): *Textbook of Pediatric Infectious Diseases,* 3d ed. Philadelphia, Saunders, 1992, pp 1321–1361.

55. Sudre P, ten Dam G, Kochi A: Tuberculosis: A global overview of the situation today. *Bull WHO* 70:149–159, 1992.

56. Telzak EE, Sepkowitz K, Alpert P, et al: Multidrug resistant tuberculosis in patients without HIV infection. *New Engl J Med* 333:907–911, 1995.

57. Templeton GL, Illing LA, Young L, et al: The risk of transmission of *Mycobacterium tuberculosis* at the bedside during an autopsy. *Ann Intern Med* 122:922–925, 1995.

58. Vallejo JG, Starke JR: Tuberculosis in pregnancy. *Clin Chest Med* 13:693–707, 1992.

59. Villarino M, Ridzon R, Weismuller P, et al: Lack of toxicity of rifampin for tuberculosis preventive therapy (abstr). *Am J Respir Crit Care Med* 151:A553, 1995.

CHAPTER 159

THE MICROBIOLOGY OF THE MYCOBACTERIA

Frits van der Kuyp

LABORATORY WORKERS

COLLECTION AND TRANSPORTATION OF THE SPECIMEN

DIRECT MICROSCOPIC EXAMINATION

CONVENTIONAL CULTURE TECHNIQUES

OTHER TECHNIQUES FOR THE RAPID DIAGNOSIS OF TUBERCULOSIS

DRUG SUSCEPTIBILITY TESTING

SEROLOGIC DIAGNOSIS

CLINICAL IMPLICATIONS

The isolation of *Mycobacterium tuberculosis* is the "gold standard" for the diagnosis of tuberculosis. A positive direct smear for acid-fast bacilli (AFB) in the proper setting may serve as presumptive evidence for tuberculosis but may also represent nontuberculous mycobacteria, known as mycobacteria other than tuberculosis (MOTT). These two groups of mycobacteria are indistinguishable on direct smear—with the exception of *M. kansasii*, which can be suspected from its larger size and banded appearance.

The similarity of MOTT to *M. tuberculosis* is not restricted to the morphology by direct smear. Many organisms in the MOTT category cause disease that is clinically, radiologically, and histopathologically indistinguishable from tuberculosis. The main differences between the two groups are that the MOTT are ubiquitous environmental organisms and not transmitted from person to person. Disease caused by this group of organisms is therefore not infectious and does not require contact investigation. Most patients with progressive pulmonary disease caused by MOTT have preexisting chronic pulmonary disease such as bronchiectasis, pneumoconiosis, or healed tuberculosis or fungal disease. Isoniazid preventive therapy for tuberculosis is very effective; there is more limited experience in the prevention of MOTT disease in AIDS which suggests that improved survivals may be achieved with appropriate prophylaxis. Other differences are the sensitivity patterns to the usual antituberculosis drugs. There are also definite biochemical differences (Table 159-1).

Some MOTT are not pathogenic; moreover, an isolation of even potentially pathogenic MOTT often represents contamination or the presence of a saprophytic relationship or colonization.[22–24] An *M. tuberculosis* isolate, on the other hand, should be considered pathogenic. Rare exceptions include a single isolate from a usually nonsterile site such as sputum, especially when this includes a very low colony count. Such isolates may be the result of cross contamination in the laboratory or during collection or transportation of the specimen.

Because MOTT organisms often appear as colonizers and because of their ubiquitous presence, it is clear that the mere isolation of a specific MOTT organism from a specimen does not necessarily establish the diagnosis of disease caused by that organism. For a specific diagnosis, one has to adhere to stricter criteria than is the case for the diagnosis of tuberculosis (Table 159-2).[18,19] First, there must be pathologic changes present that are consistent with disease caused by the MOTT under consideration. Other reasonable causes of the pathologic findings should be ruled out, and generally one expects evidence of progressive disease with multiple isolates. A single isolate is acceptable in the proper setting—for instance, when found in conjunction with histologic evidence of mycobacterial disease.

LABORATORY WORKERS

Workers in mycobacteriology laboratories should be well trained not only in the technical skills but also in the application of standard safety procedures. Established engineering safeguards to protect workers against infections should be strictly followed, and workers should be carefully examined for the presence of tuberculosis infections and disease before employment and periodically thereafter. Workers who acquire an infection (evidenced by conversion to a positive tuberculin reaction), as well as those with prior infections who meet established criteria, should be offered a course of preventive therapy.

COLLECTION AND TRANSPORTATION OF THE SPECIMEN

Proper collection and transportation of specimens to be examined are critical. Sputum specimens are by far the most frequent specimens submitted for mycobacterial examination. Early-

TABLE 159-1

M. Tuberculosis vs. MOTT: Similarities and Differences

Similarities	Differences
Morphology of organism	Infectiousness
Clinical characteristics	Biochemical findings
Radiologic findings	Molecular genetics
Histopathologic findings	Drug susceptibility
	Pathogenicity
	Response to treatment
	Effectiveness of preventive therapy

morning specimens, collected after awakening, have the highest yield in demonstrating AFB, since they represent secretions accumulated overnight. Early-morning gastric lavage contains pulmonary secretions swallowed during sleep. Sterile water should be used and Na_2CO_3 powder added to the bottle to neutralize gastric acid and protect the bacilli. For ambulatory patients whose sputum specimens are collected in the clinic, as well as for institutionalized patients with scant sputum production, induction with warm aerosolized saline or distilled water is desirable. Because of the increased risk of infection to health-care workers present in the bronchoscopy suite and because of its cost, bronchoscopy strictly for obtaining specimens should be considered only after attempts to obtain proper spontaneously expectorated or induced specimens have failed or after proper initial specimens have been reported negative for AFB and confirmation or exclusion of mycobacterial disease remains essential. Sputum induction facilities and bronchoscopy suites should be equipped with negative airflow, and employees should wear appropriate respirators.

Other specimens submitted for mycobacterial examination are urine, cerebrospinal fluid, joint and pleural fluid, and tissue biopsy specimens. These should be collected in sterile, leak-proof disposable plastic or glass containers produced specifically for this purpose. Likewise, special procedures for collection, transportation, and handling of blood cultures for mycobacterial organisms should be strictly adhered to. Specimens should be transported for processing preferably without delay, but they may be refrigerated to prevent overgrowth with contaminating organisms. A minimum number of three and preferably five sputum specimens should be obtained, because of the fluctuation of the number of bacilli found. Once two initial direct smears are reported to yield a significant number of AFB, one may wish to

TABLE 159-2

Diagnostic Criteria for MOTT Disease

Presence of disease process consistent with disease caused by MOTT under consideration

Other reasonable causes have been ruled out

Presence of progressive disease

Multiple isolates of specific MOTT

stop collecting additional pretreatment specimens in order to limit the risk of infection to health-care workers. To monitor the effectiveness of treatment for pulmonary tuberculosis, additional specimens need to be collected at weekly or two-week intervals until at least two consecutive specimens are reported negative for AFB. A new series of specimens should be collected if there is clinical or radiologic suspicion of treatment failure or reactivation of the disease.

DIRECT MICROSCOPIC EXAMINATION

Direct examination of specimens by means of an acid-fast stain is the first procedure performed on all specimens sent to the mycobacteriology laboratory. The presence of AFB provides supportive evidence of mycobacterial disease many days or weeks before the culture report and final identification of the organism are available. In the proper setting, it may establish the need for isolation and prompt treatment of the patient. The standard acid-fast stain is the Ziehl-Neelsen procedure. The term *acid fast* refers to the fact that dilute acids fail to remove basic dyes such as carbolfuchsin from the mycobacterial cell wall, owing to its lipid-rich complex structure.

The fluorochrome acid-fast stain has replaced the standard Ziehl-Neelsen stain in many laboratories because it is more sensitive, allowing the lab technician to review the slide at lower power, without oil. A larger number of fields can be examined in a much shorter time. A fluorescent microscope is required for the procedure, but most modern laboratories are equipped with this.

Microscopic examination is the most rapid diagnostic method available; it is simple and economical, and it can be performed in any laboratory.[1] Its relatively low sensitivity is a significant limitation, however. More than 10,000 bacilli per milliliter are required for the average technician to demonstrate a positive result. This number may be as low as 1000 bacilli per milliliter using the fluorochrome stain with proper sputum concentration technique. The yield of microscopic examination also correlates with the extent of disease, the presence of cavitation, and the quality of the specimen. It is a good marker for the infectiousness and the response to treatment. A decrease in the number of organisms in sputum specimens during the first few weeks indicates response to treatment. The lack of such a decrease or an increase of the number of AFB suggests either noncompliance with the prescribed treatment regimen or the presence of drug resistance. Drug resistance may evolve as the result of poor patient compliance, a prescribed suboptimal regimen, or—in rare circumstances—poor absorption of the drug (acquired or secondary drug resistance). Primary drug resistance indicates that the patient originally was infected with drug-resistant organisms.

Direct smear negative/culture positive sputum specimens are frequently encountered in pulmonary tuberculosis cases with minimal disease. This phenomenon may sometimes be found even in recent tuberculin converters with no radiologic abnormalities. The reverse may be seen in cases with advanced cavitary lesions with a significant amount of necrotic material. These patients may continue to excrete nonviable AFB for extended periods, sometimes for many months, with negative cultures. Occasionally, direct smear positive/culture negative reports may indicate bacilli with attenuated viability due to suboptimal chemotherapy.

For proper interpretations of the results of bacteriologic tests, it is crucial to consider the quality of the specimen submitted. The presence of elastic fibers in sputum wet mounts with potassium hydroxide indicates tissue necrosis and hence the fact that a proper specimen has been obtained. In spite of its low sensitivity, the direct smear has been employed extensively as the most cost effective diagnostic tool for tuberculosis in developing countries.

CONVENTIONAL CULTURE TECHNIQUES

The traditional culture techniques followed by biochemical tests for the identification of mycobacteria require 4 to 8 weeks or more. Culturing of sputum and other specimens requires concentration of the material. Specimens from nonsterile sites need to be decontaminated. After such processing, specimens should be inoculated into both liquid and solid media. The solid medium may be the BACTEC 460 12B bottle or the Mycobacterium Growth Indicator Tube (MGIT), both of which are manufactured by Becton Dickinson Labs, Cockeysville, MD, or one of the "automated" broth culture media.[11] The latter are liquid media in bottles, whose contents are read out spectrophotometrically for the presence of one or more gases that indicate metabolism of mycobacterial organisms. Solid media can be any combination of egg based (Lowenstein-Jensen, for example) or non–egg based (Middlebrook). The broth and solid media will often be supplemented with antibiotics to further reduce the chance of contamination of the cultures. A biphasic medium, the Septi-check bottle (Becton Dickinson), is also available for isolation of mycobacteria.[21] While it affords good overall recovery of mycobacterial isolates, it does not provide the timeliness that one derives from liquid media such as BACTEC or MGIT.

The broth culture medium provides for a turnaround time of about 10 to 12 days for M. tuberculosis and even less for many of the MOTT organisms. The agar medium requires about 3 to 4 weeks for colonies to be seen macroscopically. The use of a dissecting scope allows for the detection of "microcolonies" on solid media in 10 to 12 days—comparable to the time needed for liquid media.[20]

Once an isolate is recovered in broth or on solid media, identification should proceed as rapidly as possible.[18] The p-nitro-alpha-acetylamino-beta-hydroxy-propiophenone (NAP) test, a gene probe, or high-performance liquid chromatography (HPLC) should be employed. The conventional biochemical confirmation of M. tuberculosis,— i.e., niacin positivity, nitrate positivity, and the presence of an unstable catalase—requires 3 to 4 weeks after isolation. The NAP test requires about 4 to 5 days, gene probes about 2 1/2 h, and HPLC about 5 to 8 h.

OTHER TECHNIQUES FOR THE RAPID DIAGNOSIS OF TUBERCULOSIS

One of the most impressive recent developments has been the use of amplification of nucleic acids directly within the clinical specimen to avoid the delays of culturing. Two examples of currently available techniques for amplification are transcription-mediated amplification, (TMA, Gen-Probe, San Diego, CA) and polymerase chain reaction, (PCR, Roche Molecular Systems, Nutley, NJ).[2,3,6,13,15] These amplification procedures require about 5 to 6 h of processing, and the products are commercially available. The amplification procedures are currently specific for M. tuberculosis complex only. A possible drawback is the fact that nonviable mycobacterial organisms may produce positive results. Moreover, many laboratories are unable to afford the high cost entailed. This is especially true in areas with a low incidence of tuberculosis. A negative test result in the proper setting may negate the need for isolation and specific treatment of the patient. However, the sensitivity of these assays with smear negative specimens has been only about 70 percent.[12]

DNA fingerprinting of mycobacterial DNA allows for the identification of individual strains of M. tuberculosis.[7,9] In addition to its diagnostic value, this procedure has proved to be extremely helpful in epidemiologic investigations to establish a link between cases in outbreaks of tuberculosis in various institutions and other congregate settings. Coupled with amplifications by PCR, this link may alert the clinician to the presence of a specific drug-resistant isolate, allowing for the prompt selection of an effective drug regimen.

DNA fingerprinting is based on analysis of the distribution of specific insertion sequences (e.g., IS6110) within the mycobacterial genome.[10] Individual strains have their own banding pattern (restriction fragment length polymorphism, or RFLP).

DRUG SUSCEPTIBILITY TESTING

A poor therapeutic outcome is likely when chemotherapeutic agents are used to which more than 1 percent of bacilli in a given population demonstrate in vitro resistance. This information is crucial for the selection of appropriate drug combinations in the initial treatment, as well as in the re-treatment, of tuberculosis.

Drug susceptibility tests are performed by comparing the amount of growth in a medium containing various concentrations of the drugs with that in a control medium—i.e., one containing no drugs. The conventional method for susceptibility testing takes up to 4 weeks. This period may be significantly reduced by use of the BACTEC radiometric system.[14]

SEROLOGIC DIAGNOSIS

Mycobacteria are rich in antigens that stimulate the production of antibodies and lymphokines. The development of a satisfactory serologic test should therefore be feasible. Attempts to develop such a test have been based on enzyme-linked immunosorbent assays (ELISA) and radioimmunoassays.[5,8] To date, no test is available that meets criteria for its widespread use based on a high level of sensitivity, specificity, and relative simplicity.[16]

CLINICAL IMPLICATIONS

Robert Koch discovered the tubercle bacillus, M. tuberculosis, in 1882, and although some mycobacterium species other than tuberculosis (MOTT) were recognized within a decade after Koch's discovery, it was not until the second half of the 20th century that the impact of MOTT as a cause of human disease was fully appreciated. Historically, MOTT isolates from human material have been called paratuberculosis, opportunistic, pseudotubercle, unclassified, atypical, nontuberculous, and tuberculoid bacilli.[17] Reported differences between MOTT and *M. tuberculosis* pulmonary disease are that MOTT tend to produce more thin-walled cavities with less pericavitary infiltrate and less frequently cause pleural effusions. The tuberculin skin test in MOTT disease may be entirely nonreactive or produce only small indurations. The clinical spectrum of disease caused by some MOTT has changed since their initial recognition. During the past quarter of a century, for instance, we observed a shift of pulmonary disease caused by *M. avium-intercellulare* complex (MAC) from afflicting predominantly middle-aged and elderly men with preexisting pulmonary disease to disease affecting increasing numbers of women with minor or no prior pulmonary pathology. During the past decade, the great majority of MAC encounters occurred as disseminated disease in patients with AIDS. In addition to MAC, the most frequent MOTT causes of human disease are *M. kansasii, M. marinum, M. fortuitum–M. chelonei* complex, and *M. scrofulaceum* (Table 159–3).[4,22–24]

M. tuberculosis is by far the most frequent cause of mycobacterial disease in the lungs. An organism that grows slowly, is nonpigmented, and is niacin positive is likely to represent *M. tuberculosis*. Further confirmatory tests are necessary, the most recently developed being susceptibility to NAP. Most *M. tuberculosis* isolates are susceptible to the standard antituberculosis drugs.

TABLE 159-3

Genus *Mycobacterium*

Mycobacteria associated with human disease:
  Mycobacterium tuberculosis complex
    M. tuberculosis
    M. bovis
    M. africanum
  Mycobacterium avium complex
    M. avium
    M. intracellulare
  Mycobacterium scrofulaceum
  Mycobacterium kansasii
  Mycobacterium genevense
  Mycobacterium xenopi
  Mycobacterium szulgai
  Mycobacterium malmoense
  Mycobacterium haemophilum
  Mycobacterium marinum
  Mycobacterium ulcerans
  Mycobacterium leprae
  Mycobacterium fortuitum-chelonae complex
    M. fortuitum
    M. chelonae
Usually saprophytic mycobacteria:
  Mycobacterium gordonae
  Mycobacterium terrae complex
  Mycobacterium flavescens
  Mycobacterium smegmatis

M. bovis has been virtually eradicated in the United States and some other industrialized countries by destruction of tuberculin-positive cattle, which can spread the infection through milk. A low-virulence strain, the bacillus of Calmette and Guérin (BCG), is used for immunization against tuberculosis. This strain is occasionally the cause of disseminated disease in persons with certain cancers, to whom it has been administered therapeutically as a nonspecific potentiator of immunity.

The third representative of *M. tuberculosis* complex, *M. africanum,* has characteristics intermediate between *M. tuberculosis* and *M. bovis*.

MAC, consisting of two organisms, *M. avium* and *M. intracellulare,* is by far the most frequent MOTT species associated with human disease. As mentioned earlier, MAC is a frequent cause of fatal disseminated disease in AIDS patients. The components can be separated by DNA probe technique and by seroagglutination. On the basis of glycolipid typing antigens, some 28 seroagglutination types are recognized. Unlike *M. tuberculosis,* all strains of MAC are naturally resistant to standard antituberculosis drugs. MAC is widely distributed in nature and may be found in soil and water and in various birds and mammals.

M. scrofulaceum is sometimes lumped with MAC because of some shared genetic characteristics. The extended complex is then referred to as MAIS complex. *M. scrofulaceum* is a known cause of cervical adenitis in children and very rarely causes pulmonary disease. It has been found in soil, water, and dairy products.

M. kansasii may be suspected in stained smears as large, cross-barred bacilli. Colonies are photochromogenic, developing pigment after exposure to light. Although it can be found in water, an *M. kansasii* isolate is more likely to represent a real pathogen than is the case with most other MOTT. It is the second most frequent cause of human disease among the MOTT; it usually causes pulmonary disease, although other organs may be affected. The disease responds very well to treatment with antituberculosis drugs in spite of some degree of resistance to isoniazid.

M. xenopi is peculiar for its geographic distribution and for the fact that its optimal growth temperature of 42° to 45°C is higher than that for other mycobacteria. Although it is rarely isolated in most parts of the world, its relative frequency is high in southeastern England, in Ontario, Canada, and in Scandinavian countries. It usually affects the lungs, and some outbreaks have been related to contamination of hot-water tanks. The response to drug treatment is variable.

M. marinum and *M. ulcerans* produce skin lesions. More benign lesions are caused by *M. marinum* from abrasions acquired in fishtanks and contaminated swimming pools (swimming pool or fish-tank granuloma). The organism is photochromogenic and is susceptible to rifampin, ethambutol, and amikacin but resistant to isoniazid. *M. ulcerans* causes more severe necrotizing disease and is encountered in tropical areas, primarily in Africa, Australia, and in Mexico. The disease is known as Bairndale ulcer in Australia and as Buruli ulcer in Uganda.

M. haemophilum almost exclusively affects immunosuppressed persons, mostly renal transplant recipients—in whom it causes painful subcutaneous nodules, which may resolve spontaneously or develop suppuration and ulceration. This organism requires hemin or other iron sources for its growth in media.

M. fortuitum-chelonae complex is a group of rapidly growing mycobacteria. *M. chelonae* also known as *M. abscessus,* has been mostly associated with wound abscesses, although occasional reports of this organism as the cause of pulmonary disease have appeared in the literature. *M. fortuitum* is the occasional cause of pulmonary disease. Both organisms are found in the soil. *M. fortuitum* and *M. chelonae* are resistant to the first-line antituberculosis drugs. Isolates of *M. fortuitum* are usually susceptible to amikacin, ciprofloxacin, and sulfonamides, whereas isolates of *M. chelonae* are frequently susceptible to amikacin. Individual strains may be susceptible to other antimicrobial agents.

REFERENCES

1. Baily GVJ, Savic D, Gothi GD, et al: Potential yield of pulmonary tuberculosis cases by direct microscopy of sputum in a district of south India. *Bull World Health Organ* 37:875–892, 1967.

2. Bodmer T, Gurtner A, Schopfer K, Matter L: Screening of respiratory tract specimens for the presence of *Mycobacterium tuberculosis* by using the Gen-Probe Amplified *Mycobacterium Tuberculosis* Direct Test. *J Clin Microbiol* 32:1483–1487, 1994.

3. Clarridge JE III, Shawar RM, Shinnick TM, Pikaytis BB: Large-scale use of polymerase chain reaction for detection of *Mycobacterium tuberculosis* in a routine mycobacteriology laboratory. *J Clin Microbiol* 31:2049–2056, 1993.

4. Davidson PT: The diagnosis and management of disease caused by *M. avium* complex, *M. kansasii,* and other mycobacteria. *Clin Chest Med* 10:431–433, 1989.

5. Daniel TM, Debanne SM: The serodiagnosis of tuberculosis and other mycobacterial diseases by enzyme-linked immunosorbent assay. *Am Rev Respir Dis* 135:1137–1151, 1987.

6. Eisenach KD, Cave D, Bates JH, Crawford JT: Polymerase chain reaction amplification of a repetitive DNA sequence specific for *Mycobacterium tuberculosis. J Infect Dis* 161:977–981, 1990.

7. Ellner PD, Kiehn TE, Cammarata R, Hosmer M: Rapid detection and identification of pathogenic mycobacteria by combining radiometric and nucleic acid probe methods. *J Clin Microbiol* 26:1349–1352, 1988.

8. Good RC: Serologic methods for diagnosing tuberculosis (editorial). *Ann Intern Med* 110:97–98, 1989.

9. Hermans PW, van Soolingen D, Dale JW, et al: Insertion element IS986 from *Mycobacterium tuberculosis*: A useful tool for diagnosis and epidemiology of tuberculosis. *J Clin Microbiol* 28:2051–2058, 1990.

10. Mazurek GH, Cave MD, Eisenach KD, et al: Chrom osomal DNA fingerprint patterns produced with IS6110 as strain-specific markers for epidemiologic study of tuberculosis. *J Clin Microbiol* 29:2030–2033, 1991.

11. Middlebrook G, Reggiardo Z, Tigrett WD: Automatable radiometric detection of growth of *Mycobacterium tuberculosis* in selective media. *Am Rev Respir Dis* 115:1066–1069, 1977.

12. Miller N, Hernandez SG, Cleary TJ: Evaluation of Gen-Probe Amplified *Mycobacterium Tuberculosis* Direct Test and PCR for direct detection of *Mycobacterium tuberculosis* in clinical specimens. *J Clin Microbiol* 32:393–397, 1994.

13. Musial CE, Tice LS, Stockman L, Roberts GD: Identification of mycobacteria from culture by using the Gen-Probe Rapid Diagnostic System for *Mycobacterium avium* complex and *Mycobacterium tuberculosis* complex. *J Clin Microbiol* 26:2120–2123, 1988.

14. Prince DS, Peterson DD, Steiner RM, et al: Infection with *Mycobacterium avium* complex in patients without predisoping conditions. *New Engl J Med* 321:863–868, 1989.

15. Snider DE Jr, Good RC, Kilburn JO, et al: Rapid drug susceptibility testing of *Mycobacterium tuberculosis. Am Rev Respir Dis* 123:402–406, 1981.

16. Steele RA, Daniel TM: Evaluation of the potential role of serodiagnosis of tuberculosis in a clinic in Bolivia by decision analysis. *Am Rev Respir Dis* 143:713–716, 1991.

17. Tenover FC, Crawford JT, Huebner RE, et al: The resurgence of tuberculosis: Is your laboratory ready? *J Clin Microbiol* 31:767–770, 1993.

18. Vestal AL: Procedures for the isolation and identification of mycobacteria. Atlanta, Centers for Disease Control. DHEW publication no. (CDC) 76-82301:97–115, 1975.

19. Wallace RJ Jr, O'Brien R, Glassroth J, et al: Diagnosis and treatment of disease caused by nontuberculous mycobacteria (official statement of the American Thoracic Society). *Am Rev Respir Dis* 142:940–953, 1990.

20. Welch DF, Guruswamy AP, Sides SJ, et al: Timely culture for mycobacteria which utilizes a microcolony method. *J Clin Microbiol* 31:2178–2184, 1993.

21. Whittier PS, Westfall K, Setterquist S, Hopfer RL: Evaluation of the Septi-Chek AFB system in the recovery of mycobacteria. *Eur J Clin Microbiol Infect Dis* 11:915–918, 1992.

22. Wolinsky E: Nontuberculous mycobacteria and associated diseases. *Am Rev Respir Dis* 119:107–159, 1979.

23. Wolinksy E: Mycobacterial diseases other than tuberculosis. *Clin Infect Dis* 15:1–10, 1992.

24. Woods GL, Washington JA 2d: Mycobacteria other than *Mycobacterium tuberculosis*: Review of microbiologic and clinical aspects. *Rev Infect Dis* 9:275–294, 1987.

CHAPTER 160

PATHOGENESIS OF PULMONARY TUBERCULOSIS

Arthur M. Dannenberg, Jr. / Joseph F. Tomashefski, Jr.

INFECTIONS WITH MYCOBACTERIUM TUBERCULOSIS

Overview

The *development of pulmonary tuberculosis* from its onset to its various clinical manifestations is dependent upon a series of interactions or "battles" between the host and the bacillary invader.[16,18,36] 1. An inhaled unit of one to three bacilli is ingested by an alveolar macrophage. Either the bacillus is destroyed before any lesion is produced or it multiplies within the alveolar macrophage, which dies and releases the amplified infectious agent. 2. Many of the bacilli are then ingested by and grow within monocyte/macrophages that have emigrated from the bloodstream. These cells accumulate at the site, forming a microscopic lesion. 3. When the host becomes tuberculin positive, a caseous center develops in this lesion. A lesion with a small caseous center (up to 2 mm in diameter) may enlarge or may heal (or stabilize) before it is detectable by radiography. 4. A larger caseous lesion may also heal or stabilize; or it may enlarge, shedding bacilli into the blood and lymph. 5. Alternatively, a caseous lesion may liquefy and form a cavity (from which the bacilli enter the bronchial tree). In the liquefied caseum, the bacilli will grow *extracellularly* (for the first time), and from the cavity they spread to other parts of the lung and to the environment. In general, each successive battle is won by the host with increasing difficulty. Furthermore, within a given lesion, each battle between the host and bacilli is fought almost independently of the battles occurring in other lesions of the same host.

The *weapons of the host* include *activated macrophages,* which can kill or inhibit ingested tubercle bacilli, [16,18,36] and *cytotoxic cells,* which can directly or indirectly kill *nonactivated* macrophages with actively replicating tubercle bacilli in their cytoplasm.[16,18] The killing of such nonactivated macrophages eliminates the *intracellular* environment that is favorable to bacillary growth and replaces it with the extracellular environment of *solid* caseous (necrotic) tissue that is inhibitory to bacillary growth.

The *weapons of the bacillus* include the ability to multiply logarithmically within nonactivated macrophages (i.e., within monocytes that have recently migrated from the bloodstream into the local site of infection)[16,18,36] and the ability to multiply (sometimes tremendously) in *liquefied* caseous material. When the bacilli multiply extracellularly in the liquefied caseum, the resulting large antigenic load causes more tissue necrosis, erosion of bronchial walls, and cavity formation, followed by spread of bacilli into the airways. The bacillus itself is nontoxic. It damages host tissue by means of the host's own immune response to tuberculin-like products.

Once the first small tuberculous lesion is established, all subsequent battles occur in a host that has developed both *cell-mediated immunity* and *tissue-damaging delayed-type hypersensitivity.* Cell-mediated immunity activates local macrophages so that they can destroy ingested tubercle bacilli. Tissue-damaging delayed-type hypersensitivity enables the host to stop the intracellular growth of tubercle bacilli in nonactivated macrophages. Each of these immune responses is T-lymphocyte dependent.

The control of bacillary multiplication by *both* cell-mediated immunity and tissue-damaging delayed-type hypersensitivity was conclusively proved by correlating bacillary growth curves (Fig. 160-1) with the observed gross pathology and histopathology (Figs. 160-2, 160-3, and 160-4). The growth curves were produced by infecting susceptible and resistant inbred rabbits with aerosolized virulent tubercle bacilli and culturing their lungs for viable bacilli during the course of the resulting disease.[1,36,37] After the tubercle bacillus is inhaled into the alveolar spaces, it is ingested by an alveolar macrophage (Fig. 160-2A). Such macrophages, in genetically resistant rabbits, appear to be more nonspecifically activated and better able to destroy or inhibit tubercle bacilli than those of susceptible rabbits. Therefore, at 7 days after infection, there is a 20- to 30-fold difference in the number of bacilli in the lungs of the two strains of rabbits (Fig. 160-1). Subsequently, the two infections follow a parallel course.

At first, a logarithmic growth phase occurs. This is the stage of symbiosis in which the bacilli multiply freely in accumulating nonactivated macrophages (Fig. 160-2B). Logarithmic growth *stops* at the same time in both rabbit strains (Fig. 160-2C) because each strain has developed comparable levels of tuberculin-sensitivity,[36] which kills nonactivated macrophages in which the bacilli are multiplying. (Susceptible animals develop equivalent tuberculin reactions because 20 to 30 times the number of bacilli secrete[2] larger amounts of antigen(s).

Subsequently, the two growth curves remain on a parallel course (Fig. 160-1), but for different reasons. In the *susceptible rabbits,* bacilli escape from the edge of the caseum and are ingested by *poorly activated* macrophages. Intracellular multiplication of bacilli again occurs (Fig. 160-3A); and, again, the poorly activated macrophages harboring the bacilli are killed by the delayed-type hypersensitivity. As the process is repeated, the local lung tissue is destroyed. This strategy is effective for months, because the total number of viable bacilli in the lung does not increase. In the *resistant rabbits,* bacilli escaping from the edge of the caseum are ingested by the *highly activated macrophages* that have surrounded the caseum (Fig. 160-3B). These activated macrophages inhibit or destroy the bacilli, and would arrest the disease were it not for the process of liquefaction and cavity formation (Fig. 160-4). Liquefaction usually begins about 5 weeks after infection in resistant rabbits, and does not occur in susceptible rabbits. In liquefied caseum, where they cannot be reached by activated macrophages, tubercle bacilli often grow *extracellularly,* sometimes reaching large numbers (see below). All of these principles of pathogenesis, developed in the rabbit model, seem applicable to tuberculosis in human beings. Additional information may be obtained from the classic texts by Canetti,[9] Long,[34] Lurie,[36] Poole and Florey,[45] and Rich.[49]

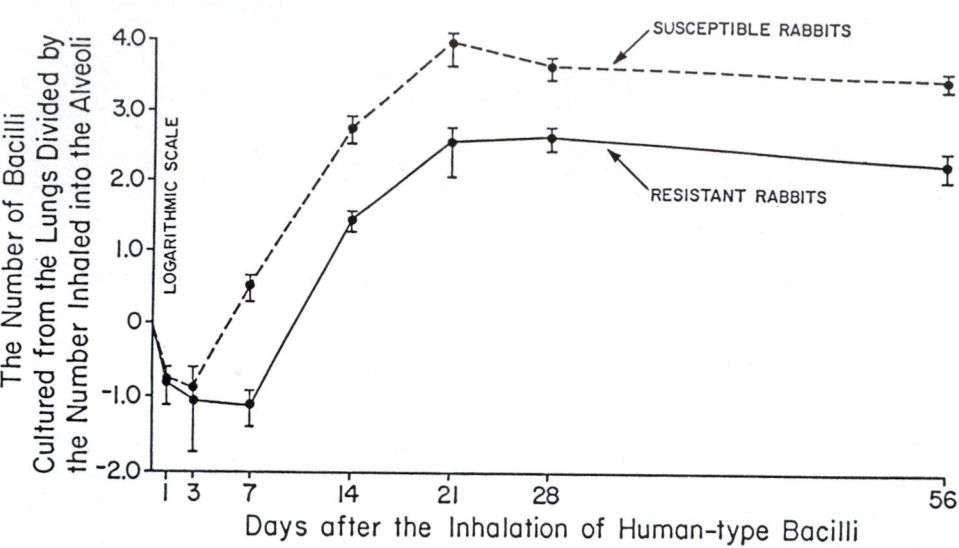

FIGURE 160-1   Changes in the number of virulent human-type tubercle bacilli in the lungs of natively resistant rabbits and natively susceptible rabbits at different intervals after infection by quantitative airborne inhalation. Means and their standard errors are shown. *(Based on data of Lurie et al,[37] with permission.)*

Components of Tuberculous Lesions

Many of the components of the host defense against microorganisms (including the tubercle bacillus) have been identified by immunologists over the past 10 years (Table 160-1). They are reviewed below.

MACROPHAGES, ACTIVATED MACROPHAGES, EPITHELIOID CELLS, AND GIANT CELLS

The term *mononuclear cells* is used to describe the cellular infiltrate of macrophages and lymphocytes. These cells are the major component of tuberculous lesions.

Activated macrophages are rich in lysosomes and mitochondria and the enzymes of these organelles.[15] Certain activated macrophages are highly phagocytic; others are highly microbicidal (because of factors including reactive oxygen and nitrogen intermediates); others are rich in digestive enzymes; others produce cytokines and other secretory products; and still others release or present antigens from the tubercle bacilli within them. The term *activated* is generally used to describe macrophages in which some of these activities are enhanced. Macrophages must be activated before they can destroy tubercle bacilli.[4,15,16,38] Nonactivated macrophages provide a fertile environment for the intracellular growth of tubercle bacilli.

In addition to ingestive and digestive functions, macrophages have *extracellular* functions that are important in tuberculosis.[43] Upon activation, macrophages *secrete* a variety of substances, including elastase, collagenase, plasminogen activator, and lysozyme; clotting factors; interferons, colony-stimulating factors (which enhance monocyte and granulocyte production in the bone marrow); and a variety of cytokines (including various interleukins, chemokines, and factors that stimulate fibroblasts).[35] Such cytokines attract lymphocytes and macrophages to the site, activate them, and cause them to proliferate. Thus, cytokines play a major role in the formation of the tuberculous granuloma and its resolution (see below). *Chemokines* are chemotactic (and activating) cytokines that are produced locally by many cells in sites of inflammation. For example, the chemokine monocyte chemoattractant protein–1 (MCP-1) seems to play a role in macrophage accumulation and activation in tuberculous lesions.

Epithelioid cells are macrophages in various states of activation that are sometimes organized into an epitheliumlike pattern. They have large vesicular (euchromatic) nuclei, suggesting active DNA transcription for synthetic functions. The *mature* epithelioid cells[36] found in tuberculous lesions are often highly activated cells.[15] They are rich in enzymes and microbicidins, and are more effective than immature epithelioid cells in destroying ingested bacilli.[4,15,16,36] Some epithelioid cells are secretory macrophages.

Langhans' giant cells are multinucleated epithelioid cells that have fused together, probably around caseous material. The nuclei are arranged about the periphery of the cell—in contrast to the usual foreign body type, in which the nuclei are scattered throughout the cytoplasm, often in clusters. The presence of Langhans' cells is a sign of chronicity, but they play little role in the pathogenesis of tuberculosis.

Macrophages and lymphocytes entering an established tuberculous lesion do not remain there.[58] Within 10 days, more than 90 percent of them have "turned over" (i.e., they have died or left the lesion via the lymphatics). The rate of both entry and activation of these cells is increased with the development of cell-mediated immunity and delayed-type hypersensitivity. The increased rate of cell entry compensates for the increased rate of cell loss that occurs simultaneously. The local accumulation of large numbers of highly activated macrophages that can destroy or inhibit tubercle bacilli is the mechanism by which the progression of the disease is controlled.

LYMPHOCYTES AND CYTOKINES

T and B lymphocytes (see Table 160-1)[30] provide *immunologic specificity* to the host's cell-mediated immunity and delayed-type hypersensitivity responses to tubercle bacilli, including the "memory" enabling the rapid recall of such immunity. When exposed to the antigen for which they have receptors, these T and B cells respond by clonal proliferation, which greatly increases their number. *Cytokines* are local "hormones," produced by cells participating in inflammatory processes.[30,35]

In tuberculosis, *T lymphocytes* appear to have two main functions: killing poorly activated macrophages (in which the bacilli are multiplying) and producing cytokines that activate macrophages (Table 160-1). *B cells* produce antibodies, and their production is enhanced by differentiation into plasma cells. Plasma cells are frequently found in tuberculous lesions, but their role in these lesions has not yet been determined.

In tuberculous lesions, cytokines are manufactured and released by T lymphocytes that have *specific receptors* for the various antigens of the tubercle bacillus. When exposed to such anti-

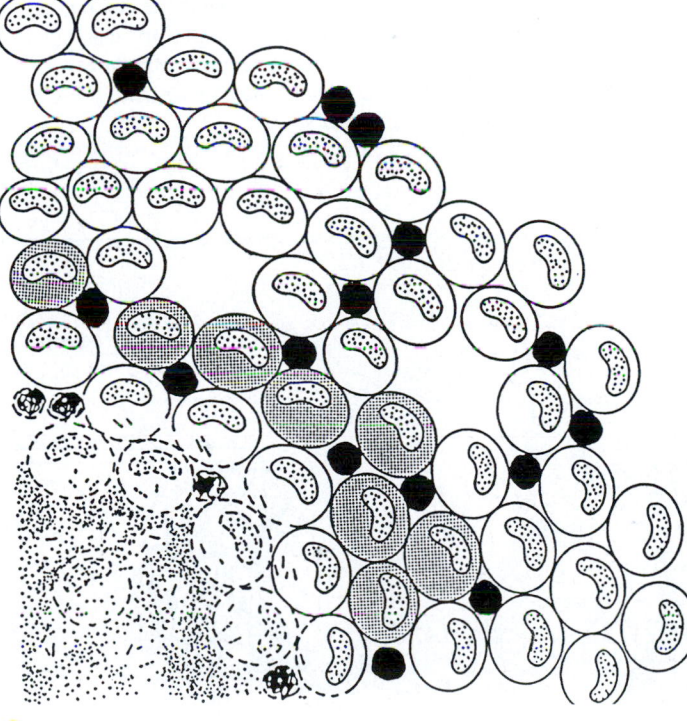

FIGURE 160-2   Early stages in the development of pulmonary tubercles: *A. Stage I.* An alveolar macrophage with two tubercle bacilli in a phagocytic vacuole. The cytoplasm of this macrophage is darkly shaded to depict a high degree of activation—i.e., high levels of lysosomal and oxidative enzymes. *B. Stage II.* An early primary tubercle, in which tubercle bacilli multiply logarithmically within the macrophages that have emigrated from the bloodstream into the developing lesion. The cytoplasm of these macrophages is unshaded to depict the lack of activation. *C. Stage III.* A tubercle (about 3 weeks of age) with a caseous necrotic center and a peripheral accumulation of partly activated macrophages (lightly shaded) and lymphocytes (small dark cells). Dead and dying macrophages are depicted by fragmented cell membranes. Intact and fragmented bacilli are present, both within macrophages and within the caseum. *(Reprinted from Dannenberg and Rook,[18] with permission.)*

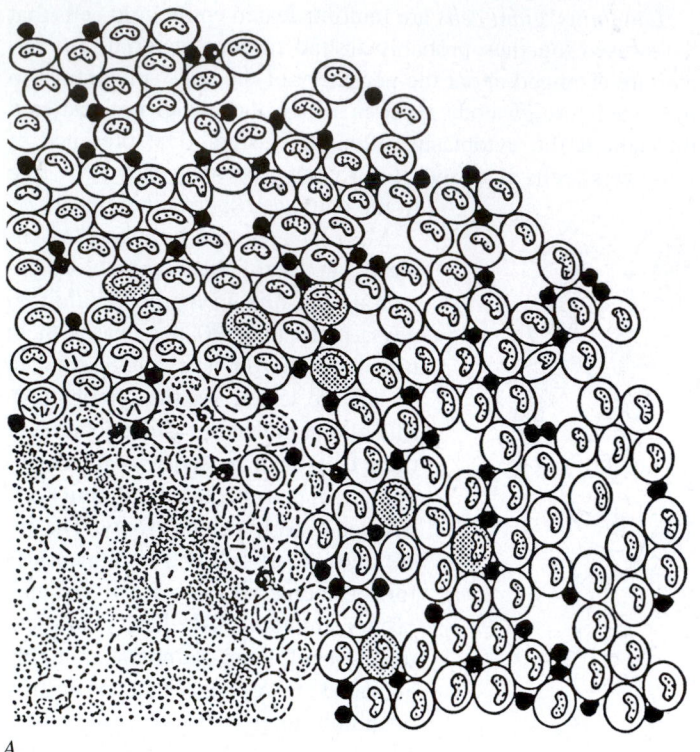

A

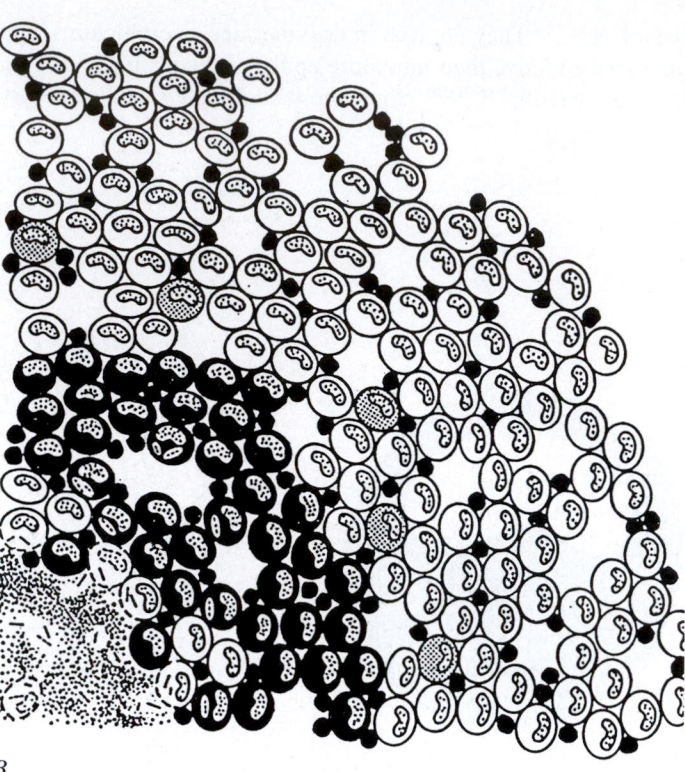

B

FIGURE 160-3 *Stage IV.* Established tubercles: *A.* A progressing tubercle, 4 to 5 weeks of age, like those found in Lurie's *susceptible* rabbits. The caseous center enlarges because nonactivated (unshaded) and partly activated macrophages (lightly shaded) are unable to inhibit intracellular bacillary multiplication. *B.* An arrested tubercle, 4 or 5 weeks of age, like those found in Lurie's *resistant* rabbits. The caseous center remains small because highly activated (competent) macrophages (darkly shaded), which surround the caseum, ingest and destroy or inhibit the bacilli escaping from the edge of the caseum. *(Reprinted from Dannenberg and Rook,[18] with permission.)*

gens, these T cells produce chemotactic cytokines; macrophage-activating factors, such as interferon-γ (IFN-γ)[42] and tumor necrosis factor; interleukin 2 (IL-2), which expands lymphocyte populations; and a variety of other factors. T lymphocytes can be divided into two subsets, Th1 and Th2, on the basis of the cytokines they produce.[41] The *Th1 subset* produces IL-2, which causes T-cell proliferation, as well as IFN-γ and tumor necrosis factor-β (TNF-β), both of which can activate macrophages to inhibit or destroy ingested tubercle bacilli. IL-12 is the major cytokine that specifically expands the Th1 population and up-regulates its functions. Macrophages and natural killer cells (see below) are the main producers of IL-12,[8,22] especially when activated by *M. tuberculosis* and certain other bacteria. Therefore, IL-12 plays a major role in producing the cell-mediated immunity and delayed-type hypersensitivity that control the pathogenesis of tuberculosis.[14,32]

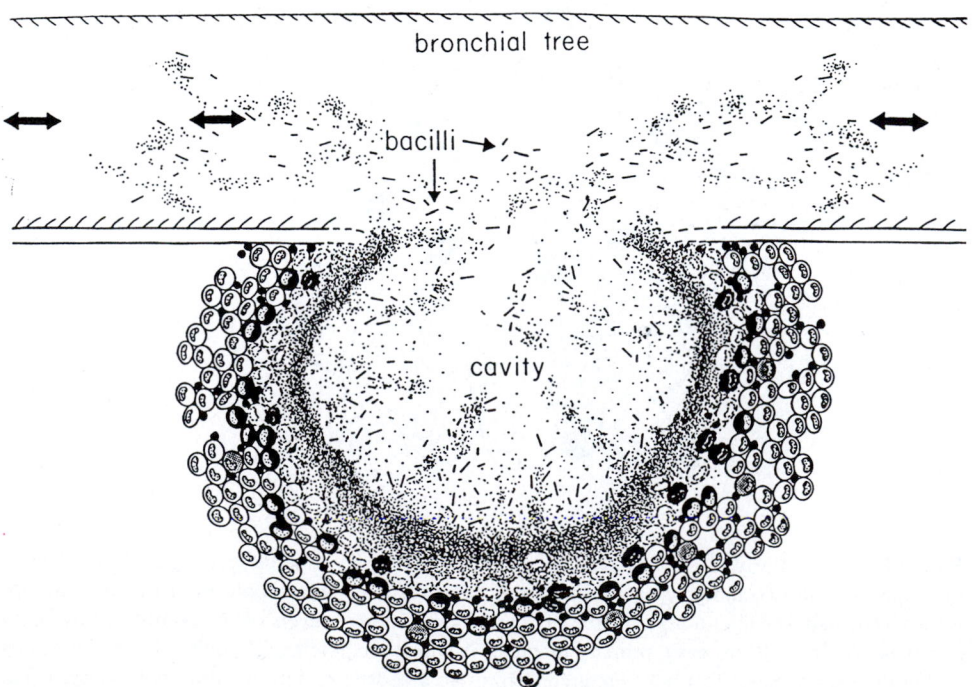

FIGURE 160-4 *Stage V.* Cavitary tuberculosis. A recently formed small cavity is discharging liquefied caseous material into a bronchus. The bacilli in the liquefied caseum are multiplying extracellularly, unreachable by the highly activated macrophages (dark cells) at the periphery. *(Reprinted from Dannenberg and Rook,[18] with permission.)*

TABLE 160-1

Major Cell Types Involved in Specific and Nonspecific Host Defense Reactions Against the Tubercle Bacillus

Macrophages

Nonactivated monocyte/macrophages allow *tubercle bacilli* to multiply within them; *highly activated* macrophages destroy or inhibit tubercle bacilli.

Lymphocytes (T Cells and B Cells)

These cells provide immunologic specificity to the host defense against tubercle bacilli. Antigen-activated T cells (from the thymus) activate macrophages by producing cytokines. Antigen-activated B cells (from the bone marrow) produce antibodies. The T cells have been subdivided in a variety of ways, based on (1) their surface markers (CD4 and CD8 T cells), (2) the cytokines they produce (Th1 and Th2 T cells), and (3) their functions (helper, regulatory, and cytotoxic T cells).

Antigen-Presenting Cells

Dendritic cells (both local and circulating) are the most efficient APCs. Macrophages and B cells also present antigens. Antigens of tubercle bacilli are presented to lymphocytes both locally in the tuberculous lesion and more distally in the draining lymph nodes.

Natural Killer Cells

NK cells (both local and circulating) are important early defense cells against intracellular microorganisms (viruses, bacteria, fungi, and protozoa). In tuberculosis, NK cells kill bacilli-laden macrophages and produce interferon-γ (IFN-γ), which activates macrophages and stimulates a Th1 cytokine immune response.

NATURAL KILLER CELLS AND CYTOTOXIC T LYMPHOCYTES

The killing of *poorly* activated macrophages with replicating tubercle bacilli in the cytoplasm is a major host defense mechanism for preventing the progression of this disease. Natural killer (NK) cells and cytotoxic T lymphocytes (CTL) play important roles in this defense reaction. *Natural killer cells* (which comprise 10 to 15 percent of the blood mononuclear cell population) are cytotoxic cells that have the morphology of large granular lymphocytes but do not express certain T-cell markers.[51] These NK cells are activated by macrophages that contain intracellular bacteria and produce IL-12[14,32] and TNF-α.[51] NK cells, then, produce IFN-γ and other cytokines that nonspecifically activate macrophages *early* during an infection and favor a subsequent Th1-specific immune response over a Th2 response.[57] NK cells can also directly lyse cells in which bacteria (including *M. tuberculosis*) and viruses are multiplying.[51] NK cells, therefore, are important in the *antigen-independent* (nonspecific) host resistance to infection that occurs *early* during an infection, before specific immunity develops.

Antigen-dependent (specific) host resistance is produced by Th1 lymphocytes that activate macrophages and by *cytotoxic T lymphocytes* (CTL) (also often Th1) that kill bacillus-laden macrophages.

ANTIGEN-PRESENTING CELLS AND THE MAJOR HISTOCOMPATIBILITY COMPLEX

In tuberculosis, T cells with *alpha-beta* antigen peptide receptors[30] are the major cells producing the specific immune response. With protein antigens, these T cells require antigen-presenting cells that present a specific peptide in the context of the major histocompatibility complex (MHC).[30] The main antigen-presenting cells for T cells are the dendritic cells in the marginal zones of lymph nodes, whereas the main antigen-presenting cells for B cells are the dendritic cells of the lymphoid follicles. Macrophages and B cells can also present antigens, but they do so less efficiently than dendritic cells. Dendritic cells also circulate in the blood and probably enter the tuberculous lesions.

The main immune response depends, in part, on the affinity of each person's MHC for various processed antigens. Thus, some people produce a strong immune response to the antigens of the tubercle bacillus, while others produce a weaker response.

A population of T cells with *gamma-delta* antigen receptors also exists.[30] Such gamma-delta T cells do not require antigen processing and presentation and may be important in the early phases of the *specific* immune response to tubercle bacilli.

Mycolic acid and lipoarabinomannan are cell wall components of the tubercle bacillus. These lipid and glycolipid antigens have been found to be presented to T cells in association with CD1 surface molecules,[46] rather than in association with major histocompatibility complex class I and II molecules.[30] The presentation of nonpeptide antigens complexed with CD1 molecules has not yet been extensively studied but promises to be extremely important in the control of many microbial infections, including tuberculosis.

TUBERCULOUS GRANULATION TISSUE

Tuberculous granulation tissue is the viable part of tuberculous lesions. It contains young macrophages, activated macrophages (now called *epithelioid cells,* see above), lymphocytes, plasma cells, granulocytes (near areas of necrosis), capillaries, lymphatics, reticular fibers, and, in time, fibroblasts and the collagen and ground substance that they produce. Ill-defined granulomas and areas of caseous necrosis are often present in this granulation tissue, as are small or large numbers of tubercle bacilli, depending on the resistance of the host. Tuberculous hypersensitivity granulomas are induced by a variety of cytokines,[11] including IL-2 and IFN-γ from lymphocytes, IL-1, IL-12, TNFα, MCP-1 and MIP-1 from macrophages. (MCP-1 is monocyte chemoattractant protein-1; MIP-1α is macrophage inflammatory protein-1α.)

DEAD CELLS AND NECROTIC TISSUE

The exact cause of death of bacilli-laden macrophages and nearby tissues is not known. Intact bacilli seem rather nontoxic to macrophages. Caseous necrosis occurs in tuberculous lesions simultaneously with the development of delayed-type hypersensitivity (i.e., with the conversion of the tuberculin test to positive). The relation of caseous necrosis to the immune process is not clearly understood, but several possibilities have been offered (Table 160-2): (1) NK cells and cytotoxic T cells seem to kill bacilli-laden macrophages and may also injure nearby tissues; (2) clotting factors from macrophages, as well as from necrotic cells and tissues, may activate the clotting system, impairing the local blood supply and causing additional tissue injury; (3) reactive oxygen and nitrogen intermediates, produced by (activated) macrophages, may kill cells and tissues (as well as bacilli); (4) certain cytokines produced by T lymphocytes and macrophages (e.g., TNF-α and TNF-β) are probably toxic in certain concentrations; (5) when macrophages are activated, more bacilli are destroyed, and bacillary toxic components (e.g., the "cord factor," trehalose dimycolate) are probably released in greater quantities; (6) antigen-antibody reactions or even aggregated proteins in the necrotic tissues may locally activate the complement system, which may injure cells; (7) hydrolytic enzymes (e.g., proteinases, nucleases, and lipases), released from live and disintegrating macrophages (and granulocytes), may injure tissues directly. However, combinations of these mechanisms are the most likely cause of the tissue damage.[33]

Regardless of the exact mechanisms, it is generally agreed that almost all the cell death and tissue damage found in tuberculosis are due to delayed-type hypersensitivity, either directly or indirectly. In the hamster, which does not develop much delayed-type hypersensitivity, tuberculous lesions show little or no necrosis.[17] This animal, however, is unable to inhibit the intracellular growth of tubercle bacilli, which grow abundantly in its macrophages. (The resulting granulomas progress until the animal succumbs to the disease.) In other words, cytotoxic delayed-type hypersensitivity enables the host to stop bacillary multiplication within (nonactivated) macrophages (Fig. 160-1), but the price of this beneficial effect is damage to host tissue.[16,18]

CASEOUS AREAS

Necrotic tissue in tuberculosis is described as *caseous* because it resembles cheese, being rather homogeneous, yellow-white, and rich in lipids and proteins derived from tubercle bacilli and dead cells. No connective-tissue fibers are found within the caseum, because of hydrolysis by the collagenase and elastase of macrophages (and granulocytes) in the tubercle before caseation occurred. In time, caseous foci may calcify or even ossify. Although bacilli may survive in solid caseous material, these bacilli are usually inhibited by the reduced oxygen tension and reduced pH, as well as by the local accumulation of fatty acids. In contrast, the bacilli readily multiply intracellularly in young, poorly activated macrophages present in the surrounding (still viable) tuberculous granulation tissue.

Whether or not the caseous center will enlarge depends on the ability of macrophages in the surrounding tuberculous granulation tissue to destroy ingested bacilli. Bacilli-laden macrophages are frequently killed (along with nearby tissue) by the delayed-type hypersensitivity reaction to the tuberculin-like products of the bacillus. As discussed above, this defense reaction stops bacillary multiplication.[16,18] However, some of the bacilli escape from the edge of the caseum, where they are ingested by new macrophages. If these new macrophages are poorly activated, they will permit the bacillus to grow intracellularly, and the delayed-type hypersensitivity reaction will again kill the cells and the surrounding tissue. In this case, the caseous center will increase in size, and the lesion will enlarge. If, however, these new macrophages are strongly activated, the ingested bacilli will be inhibited or killed, and the lesion will regress or stabilize.

Activated macrophages cannot penetrate very far into the caseous center, which is avascular with adjacent blood vessels thrombosed. As mentioned above, the caseous center also has a relatively low oxygen tension and pH, and probably contains toxic metabolic products. Finally, the center contains many tuberculin-like bacillary components, which, in high concentrations, seem to be toxic to macrophages. Thus, the host's defenses cannot eliminate tubercle bacilli within solid caseous foci, but (fortunately) such bacilli cannot multiply appreciably within these foci because of the adverse conditions listed above.

LIQUEFIED AREAS

Liquefaction occurs when caseous material softens.[19,36] In contrast to pyogenic abscesses, which liquefy soon af-

---

TABLE 160-2

Causes of Tissue Damage and Caseous Necrosis

Cytotoxic T Cells and Natural Killer Cells
  Involving perforin, apoptosis, and other mechanisms causing cell death
Anoxia
  Produced by thrombosis—macrophages produce clotting factors
Toxic Cell Products
  Reactive oxygen and nitrogen intermediates; certain cytokines, such as tumor necrosis factor (TNF); hydrolytic enzymes; and complement
Toxic Bacillary Products
  Intact tubercle bacilli are nontoxic, but when they are broken down, toxic products, such as "cord factor" (trehalose dimycolate), may be released.
Overview
  Caseous necrosis is initiated by a tissue-damaging delayed-type hypersensitivity reaction to high local concentrations of tuberculinlike bacillary products. Th1-type lymphocytes impart specificity to this reaction.

ter they form, the caseous foci of tuberculosis may not liquefy for months, if ever.

Although the exact cause of liquefaction is not known, the following scenario is consistent with present knowledge (Table 160-3). The antigens of the tubercle bacillus, especially tuberculinlike antigens[61] and perhaps others,[3,14] cause an accumulation of macrophages. Then the proteinases,[19] nucleases,[19] and lipases released from these macrophages liquefy the solid caseous material. The breakdown products of caseous material are osmotically active, so water is absorbed from the surrounding tissues. This liquefied material, rich in nutrients, is an excellent culture medium for tubercle bacilli, which now can grow *extracellularly*.[36] The walls of the bronchial tree are eroded by the host's delayed-type hypersensitivity reaction to the large amounts of tuberculinlike substances produced by these bacilli. The liquefied caseum is discharged into the bronchus, and a cavity forms. Air enters, and its high O_2 content provides an additional stimulus for this extracellular bacillary growth.

HEALING TUBERCULOUS LESIONS

The enlargement of *solid* caseous lesions is usually prevented by (activated) perifocal macrophages.[15,16,18,36] Caseous centers, 0.1 to 3 mm in diameter, may be completely eliminated by these surrounding macrophages, which phagocytize the debris from the perimeter. Slightly larger caseous centers (2 to 8 mm) may be digested by macrophage-derived extracellular and intracellular hydrolytic enzymes and replaced by fibrous tissue. Still larger caseous foci (5 to 20 mm) may undergo fibrous encapsulation and become sequestered within the lung. These larger foci may reactivate many years later if the resistance of the patient becomes lowered or if liquefaction occurs.

The *healing* of small *secondary* tubercles and small foci of *reinfection* employs basically the same mechanisms as healing of the primary focus—namely, the local accumulation and activation of macrophages at the site of infection. However, because the cell-mediated immunity and delayed-type hypersensitivity already exist in the host, macrophage accumulation and activation occur more rapidly and usually limit bacillary growth in the new tubercles soon after they begin.

If many macrophages accumulate and become highly activated, the bacilli are ingested and destroyed. Conversely, if few macrophages accumulate and do not become highly activated, the bacilli will multiply intracellularly, and the lesion will

progress. The interplay of *local* factors determines the fate of the tuberculous lesion.[15,54] Thus, patients with clinical tuberculosis may have progressing and healing lesions within the same lung. In a given lesion, large numbers of actively multiplying bacilli secreting tuberculinlike products are detrimental to the host, whereas large numbers of activated macrophages are beneficial to the host.

PERSISTING VIABLE TUBERCLE BACILLI

After even an inapparent tuberculous infection heals, the lungs may contain one or more small encapsulated, solid or semisolid caseous foci. In such foci, tubercle bacilli may persist in a dormant and nonmetabolizing state, unsusceptible to killing by antimicrobial agents. (Many bacteria, including the tubercle bacillus, have dormancy genes that enable such persistence.[23]) In addition, tubercle bacilli may *possibly* persist within viable macrophages as L forms (i.e., forms without a cell wall). This bacillary persistence is the reason why any infection with virulent tubercle bacilli is potentially dangerous. The bacilli may remain viable in the host for life and cause active disease when resistance is lowered by advanced age, corticosteroids, immunosuppressants, human immunodeficiency virus (HIV), or other factors.

Persistence of viable tubercle bacilli is also the reason why a positive tuberculin reaction is usually maintained for life. Each time the bacillus multiplies in a primary or secondary focus, the immune system is stimulated. Although new secondary foci usually heal as microscopic lesions, sufficient bacillary antigen is almost always produced within them to maintain the tuberculin reaction.

One of the arguments in favor of vaccination with effective bacille Calmette-Guérin (BCG) strains is that the host is safer harboring BCG than harboring virulent tubercle bacilli. Although both the attenuated and the virulent strains increase the resistance of the host to exogenous reinfection, hosts harboring the virulent strain have a greater risk of endogenous progressive infection should their resistance be impaired.

Types of Tuberculous Lesions and Disease

OVERVIEW

In most people, tuberculosis is arrested as a single inapparent primary pulmonary lesion that is sufficient to produce a positive tuberculin reaction but is usually not large enough to be detected in a chest radiograph. Some primary lesions, however, do not heal while they are microscopic but progress to a larger size.

In time, hosts with a primary lesion of any size develop both delayed-type hypersensitivity and cell-mediated immunity, which accelerate tissue reactions to the bacillus. At secondary sites of bacillary lodgment, lymphocytes and macrophages accumulate at a rapid

---

TABLE 160-3

Causes and Results of Liquefaction

Causes
  Delayed-type hypersensitivity to tuberculin-like bacillary products
  Hydrolytic enzymes
    Proteases, DNases and RNases, and probably lipases
Results
  Extracellular (sometimes tremendous) multiplication of the bacilli, often resulting in
    drug-resistant mutants
  Erosion of bronchial walls and cavity formation resulting in spread of
    bacilli through the air passages to other parts of the lung and to other people

rate, causing an *exudative* or a *proliferative* response, depending on the tuberculin sensitivity of the host and on the number of tubercle bacilli, their rate of growth, and the quantity of their tuberculin-like products.

The various types of lesions and types of disease found in pulmonary tuberculosis are listed in Table 160-4. The lesions sometimes change from one type to another or are a composite of several. Also, one type of lesion may coexist in the lung with other types. Furthermore, the disease as a whole may fluctuate between periods of exacerbation and remission.

ROLE OF ALVEOLAR MACROPHAGES IN THE ESTABLISHMENT OF THE INFECTION

A *large* inhaled particle containing more than three tubercle bacilli will not reach the alveolar spaces. It impinges on the walls of the bronchial tree, moves toward the pharynx on the mucociliary escalator, and is subsequently swallowed. The bronchial tree and alimentary canal are relatively resistant to low numbers of tubercle bacilli and do not become infected. However, a *small* inhaled particle containing one to three bacilli can remain suspended in the airstream, and about one-third of such particles reach the alveolar spaces. In the alveolar spaces, the bacillary particle is usually ingested by an alveolar macrophage. Occasionally it is exhaled from the alveolus, and occasionally it drains to lymphoid tissue, where it is usually destroyed. A tuberculous lesion will or will not develop, depending, respectively, on the capacity of the bacillus for intracellular growth or the capacity of the alveolar macrophage to inhibit such growth. Immunocompetent human beings are rather resistant to tuberculosis. Although one inhaled bacillary unit of one to three bacilli may establish the disease, authorities estimate that an average of 20 to more than 200 inhaled units are usually required to do so.

Within an alveolar macrophage, the bacillus may be killed immediately, it may multiply, or it may remain dormant for various periods. If it multiplies, its progeny will eventually kill the original alveolar macrophage, which then releases the bacilli into the alveolar spaces. Tubercle bacilli are highly chemotactic, so they are soon ingested by other alveolar macrophages and by blood-borne monocyte-macrophages that enter the lesion. Newly arrived macrophages are initially *incapable* of limiting the growth of tubercle bacilli. Soon the developing lesion becomes almost entirely composed of these macrophages, many containing multiplying bacilli.

Thus, alveolar macrophages determine whether or not a tuberculous lesion becomes established *but have little effect on its subsequent course.* They usually remain at the periphery of the lesion, far from the more centrally located bacilli (Fig. 160-5A). However, alveolar macrophages (most of which are highly activated cells) may prevent the development of secondary lesions when small numbers of bacilli are discharged into the bronchial tree from sites of progressing disease.

Genetically determined, nonspecific activation of the host's alveolar macrophages determines whether an inhaled bacillary particle fails to establish a primary lesion.[16,18] [*Antigen-specific activation* of macrophages from the bloodstream (via lymphocytes and their cytokines) is also genetically determined.[36]]

THE EARLY PRIMARY LESION

The earliest clinical evidence of a tuberculous lesion somewhere in the body is a positive tuberculin skin test (see Chapter 161). The test becomes positive when the tubercle bacilli in the early primary lesion have multiplied sufficiently to produce a sensitizing antigenic load, in humans usually 1 to 2 months after the bacilli were inhaled. At this time, the lesion is a small tubercle with a caseous center. This center is composed of incompletely autolyzed macrophages and pulmonary tissue, bacillary breakdown products, and dead and live (often dormant) intact bacilli. Surrounding it are the blood-borne macrophages that control the subsequent fate of the lesion (Fig. 160-5A).

Usually, *only one primary lesion* is found in human beings. This is because only small numbers of bacilli are inhaled at one time, 20 to more than 200 bacillary units are usually needed to establish the infection (see above), and once the primary lesion is fully established, the host has sufficient immunity to prevent subsequently developing microscopic lesions from reaching grossly visible size.[36]

ENCAPSULATED CASEOUS OR CALCIFIED NODULES

If the primary lesion reaches 4 to 16 mm in size, it may be detected in the chest radiograph (Fig. 160-5B). In most people, a lesion of this size is arrested and encapsulated by fibrous tissue. Its caseous center may remain caseous, or it may liquefy, calcify, or occasionally ossify. During calcification, fine, dustlike particles or more solid masses of calcium carbonate and calcium phosphate are deposited within caseous material, which make the lesion more visible in the chest radiograph. This encapsulated nodule usually remains inactive for the life of the patient.

PROLIFERATIVE TYPE OF PULMONARY LESION

The proliferative lesion (Fig. 160-6), sometimes called a "hard" tubercle, is

---

TABLE 160-4

Basic Types of Pulmonary Tuberculosis

Types of Lesions
  Encapsulated caseous, liquefied, or calcified nodules
  Proliferative type of pulmonary lesions
  Exudative type of pulmonary lesions
  Cavities
Types of Disease
  Small discrete tubercles of hematogenous origin; focally localized or
    scattered diffusely throughout both lungs (miliary tuberculosis)
  Liquefied caseous lesions with cavity formation and bronchogenic spread
  Progressive, locally destructive lesions

SOURCE: Modified from Rich.[49]

more common when small quantities of bacilli establish secondary lesions in a host with high native resistance to tuberculosis. The cellular infiltrate consists of macrophages, lymphocytes, plasma cells, and fibroblasts. Mature epithelioid cells are common, and Langhans' giant cells occur occasionally. Connective tissue, interspersed among the cells, contributes to the compact nature of this type of lesion. Bacillary multiplication is minimal because of the effective host response.

In human beings, the classic orientation (i.e., a caseous center surrounded by viable tuberculous granulation tissue containing epithelioid cells) is common in young lesions, such as those of miliary tuberculosis. In older lesions, this classic orientation is frequently undiscernible; instead, intact epithelioid and giant cells are intermixed with caseous material and fibrous tissue. Proliferative lesions may become chronic, with some areas undergoing caseous necrosis and other areas undergoing fibrosis. Such lesions may eventually progress and give rise to satellite tubercles that may coalesce, but more commonly they stabilize with encapsulation by collagenous connective tissue that is often hyalinized and sometimes contains calcium deposits.

EXUDATIVE TYPE OF PULMONARY LESION

The exudative lesion (Fig. 160-7A and B) is more frequent in tuberculin-positive hosts when large quantities of bacilli and their tuberculin-like products are present at the local site. Mononuclear cells and some granulocytes accumulate in the alveolar spaces as a rather loose exudate containing variable amounts of fibrin. In this exudate the bacilli multiply readily, especially in a host with weak defenses. These lesions vary from small, loose "soft" tubercles (which are frequently confluent) to small or large areas of tuberculous pneumonia (Fig. 160-7A and B). Caseous necrosis is common. Occasionally, exudative lesions resolve almost completely, leaving only microscopic residues, but, in the absence of antimicrobial agents, they usually progress.

Lesions exhibiting *both* proliferative and exudative features are more common (Fig. 160-7C) than those of un-

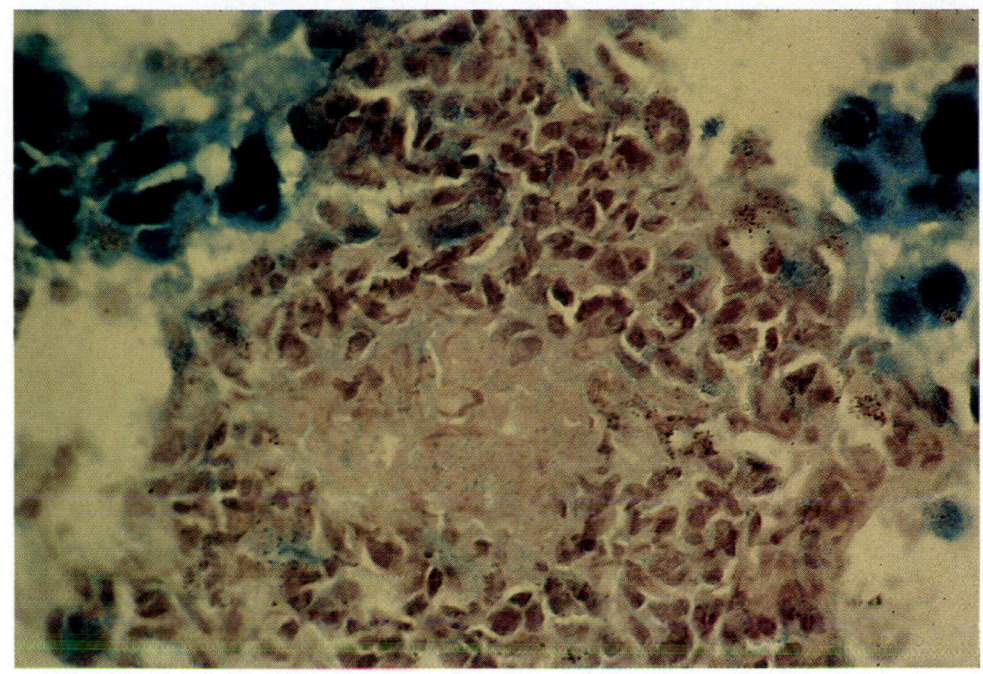

A

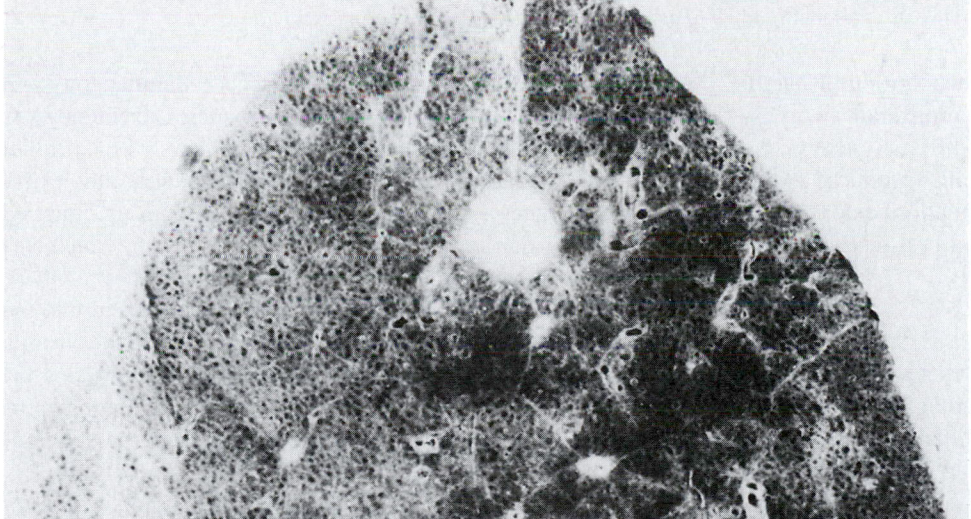

B

FIGURE 160-5 A very early and a very late (arrested) pulmonary tuberculous lesion. *A.* A 10-day lesion, produced in a rabbit by the intravenous injection of BCG.[52] In the small caseous center are disintegrated β-galactosidase–negative macrophages containing more than 10 faintly stained tubercle bacilli. Around the small caseous center are viable young β-galactosidase–negative macrophages from the bloodstream, which control the fate of the tuberculous lesion. Alveolar macrophages, staining *darkly* for β-galactosidase (a marker for macrophage activation), have accumulated in the surrounding alveolar area (rather far from the bacilli in the center). 5-Bromo-4-chloro-3-indolyl–β-D-galactoside, carbol fuchsin & hematoxylin, ×400. *B.* An arrested caseous lesion in the lung of a 40-year-old woman, caused by virulent *M. tuberculosis,* probably inhaled during childhood. This was an incidental finding at necropsy. *(Courtesy of the collection of the late Professors A. R. Rich and W. G. MacCallum, Department of Pathology, Johns Hopkins School of Medicine.)*

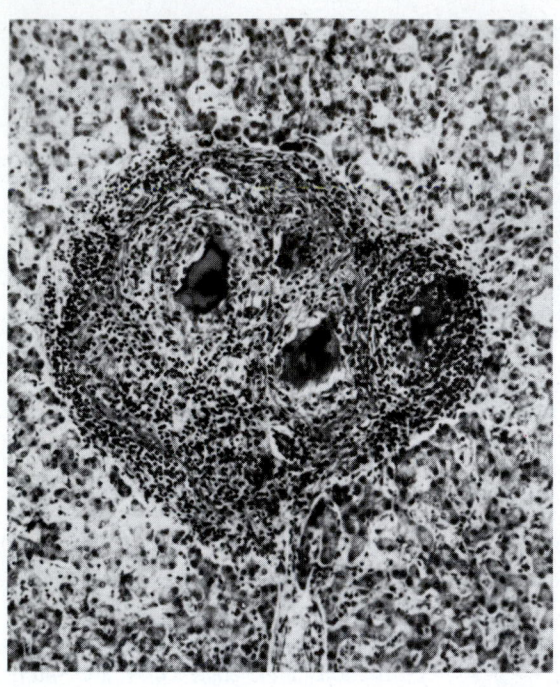

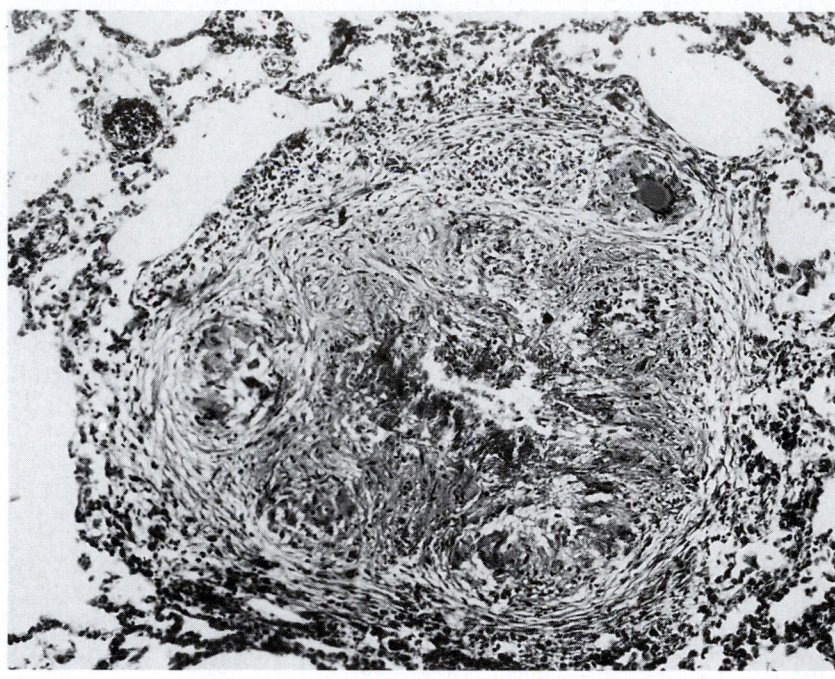

A

B

FIGURE 160-6 Proliferative tuberculous lesions. *A.* A proliferative type of miliary tubercle in the liver of an 8-month-old boy. Parts of four Langhans' giant cells are seen. H&E, ×116. *(Courtesy of the collection of the late Professors A. R. Rich and W. G. MacCallum, Department of Pathology, Johns Hopkins School of Medicine.) B.* A well-encapsulated pulmonary lesion formed from confluent tubercles in a 5-month-old child dying of tuberculous meningitis. The central area of necrosis is surrounded by smaller satellite necrotic areas. One Langhans' giant cell is visible. This was a small proliferative tubercle that exacerbated as the patient became terminally ill. H&E, ×107. *(Courtesy of the collection of the late Professors A. R. Rich and W. G. MacCallum, Department of Pathology, Johns Hopkins School of Medicine.)*

mixed type; each depends on the *local* concentration of bacilli and their tuberculin-like components. Both proliferative and exudative lesions may occur concurrently in different parts of the lung. When large numbers of tubercle bacilli (produced extracellularly during liquefaction and cavity formation) enter the airways, an exudative response can occur even in a resistant host.

MILIARY TUBERCULOSIS

Most tuberculous lesions, particularly those that are progressing, shed at least a few bacilli into the bloodstream from time to time. Bacilli in pulmonary lesions enter local capillaries and venules. Bacilli in the hilar lymph nodes usually drain into the blood via the efferent lymphatics (although a caseous node may occasionally erode a blood vessel or even the adjacent part of the bronchial tree). Wherever they are deposited, the bacilli are usually ingested by macrophages, a microscopic tubercle is created, rapid macrophage activation occurs, the bacilli are destroyed, and the lesion resolves. Occasionally, however, the bacilli are not destroyed, and one or more tubercles form in the lungs, kidney, spleen, liver, bone, testes, ovary, or brain. In the brain, a semisolid or liquefied caseous tubercle near the subarachnoid or ventricular space may rupture and discharge its contents into the cerebrospinal fluid, causing tuberculous meningitis.

Miliary tuberculosis results when a massive dose of tubercle bacilli is discharged from a caseous or liquefied focus into the bloodstream and the resistance of the host is inadequate, as in early infancy, in old age, and in immune-depressed persons of any age. In this type of tuberculosis, many small tubercles of uniform size and hematogenous origin occur simultaneously in the lungs (Fig. 160-8) and/or in the liver, spleen, or kidneys. A miliary tubercle is 2 to 4 mm in diameter, the size of a millet seed (hence the name *miliary*). Bacilli distributed into the extrapulmonary organs usually originate from a caseous or liquefied pulmonary lesion discharging into a pulmonary *vein,* which carries them to the left side of the heart. Relatively few of these bacilli pass through the peripheral capillary bed and return to the lungs. Bacilli distributed into the lungs usually originate from a caseous hilar lymph node that drains the infective particles via the lymphatic trunks into the great systemic veins. Endogenous bacilli that reach the lungs can also originate from any tuberculous lesion elsewhere in the body.

Miliary tubercles may be of two types, depending on the resistance of the host: the compact "hard" tubercle with epithelioid cells and occasional giant cells (i.e., the proliferative type of lesion with or without caseous centers) (Fig. 160-6) and the loosely formed exudative type or "soft" tubercle (Fig. 160-7A). (Both are described in the preceding section.) The exudative type contains more bacilli (Fig. 160-7B), which continue to multiply—at least for a while. This type usually undergoes early and complete caseation and progresses rapidly. Tubercles with mixed hard and soft characteristics are also common (Fig. 160-7C).

LIQUEFIED CASEOUS LESIONS AND CAVITIES; BRONCHOGENIC SPREAD

The liquefaction of caseous foci perpetuates pulmonary tuberculosis among the human population, because it results in cav-

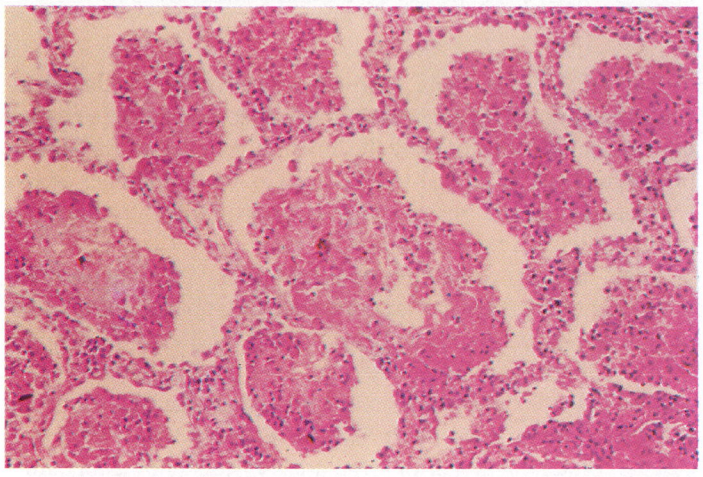

A

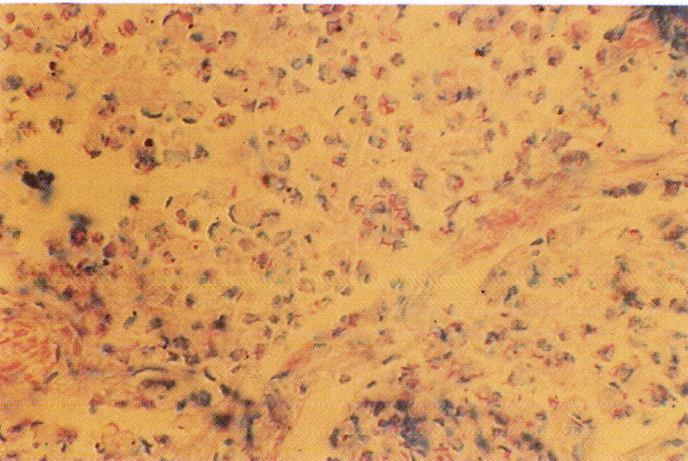

B

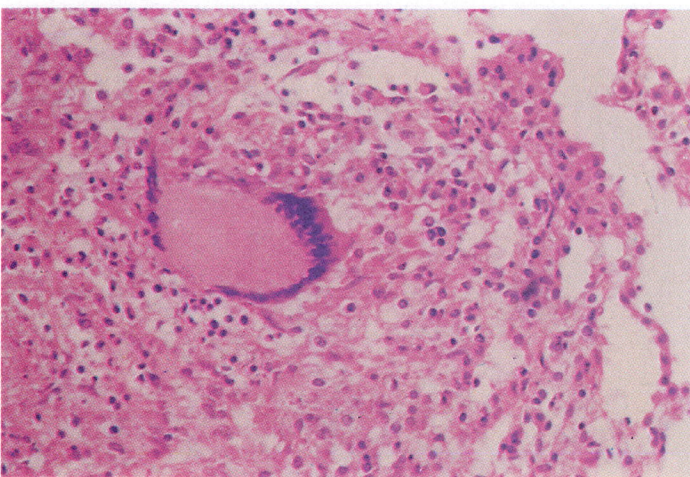

C

FIGURE 160-7 Exudative and proliferative-exudative tuberculous lesions. *A.* An exudative type of tuberculous lesion in the lung of a 47-year-old black man. Depicted is an area of tuberculous pneumonia. A necrotic exudate fills the alveolar spaces, and the alveolar walls are thickened by infiltrating cells. H&E, ×150. *B.* An exudative lesion similar to that in *A,* but stained for tubercle bacilli. Ziehl-Neelsen, counterstained with methylene blue, ×450. *C.* Part of a typical pulmonary tubercle, exhibiting both proliferative and exudative features and a Langhans' giant cell, from a 12-month-old child with miliary tuberculosis. H&E, ×300. *(Courtesy of the collection of the late Professors A. R. Rich and W. G. MacCallum, Department of Pathology, Johns Hopkins School of Medicine.)*

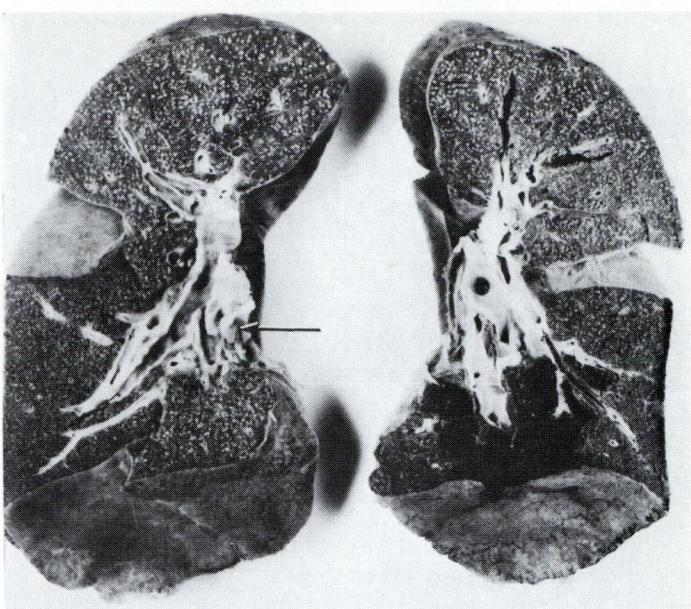

FIGURE 160-8 Miliary tuberculosis of the lung in a 19-year-old man. A caseous lymph node (arrow) can be seen. From caseous plaques (not shown) in the branches of the pulmonary veins, bacilli seeded the general circulation and were carried to other organs in the body. *(Courtesy of the collection of the late Professors A. R. Rich and W. G. MacCallum, Department of Pathology, Johns Hopkins School of Medicine.)*

ity formation. From the cavity the bacilli spread via the bronchial tree to other parts of the lung and to the environment.

Before a caseous focus liquefies, tubercle bacilli mainly multiply intracellularly in poorly activated macrophages. Extracellular bacilli in solid caseous tissue rarely multiply. After a caseous focus liquefies, however, the extracellular bacilli may multiply extensively and exacerbate the disease. As the bacilli reach large numbers within a liquefied or cavitary lesion, the likelihood of mutation increases, so that resistance to one or more of the antimicrobial agents may develop. For this reason, tuberculosis is usually treated with multiple antimicrobial agents (see Chapter 162).

A cavity is formed when a caseous focus ruptures through the wall of a nearby bronchus and discharges its contents into the air passages (Figs. 160-9 and 160-10 *A* and *B*). The walls of most cavities consist of an external zone of collagen (the cavity's capsule, which occasionally is hyalinized) and a caseous (often liquefying) internal zone, where the high oxygen content (from the ambient air) nurtures the growth of bacilli. By coughing, the patient aerosolizes this infectious material, disseminating bacilli to other parts of the lung and to the outside world.

Between the external and internal zones of the cavity wall is an intermediate zone of granulation tissue, rich in capillaries, granulocytes, macrophages, lymphocytes, and fibroblasts. At times, it contains typical tubercles. The three zones are of variable thickness and not clearly demarcated from each other. With newly formed cavities, the *internal* caseous zone is thickest. With older, still-active cavities, the *external* capsule is thickest. Around the capsule, usually between the pleura and the cavity, an area of atelectasis is often present. This atelectatic area may prevent perforation into the pleural spaces.

Erosion of incompletely thrombosed vessels in the intermediate zone leads to hemorrhage into the wall of the cavity (Fig.

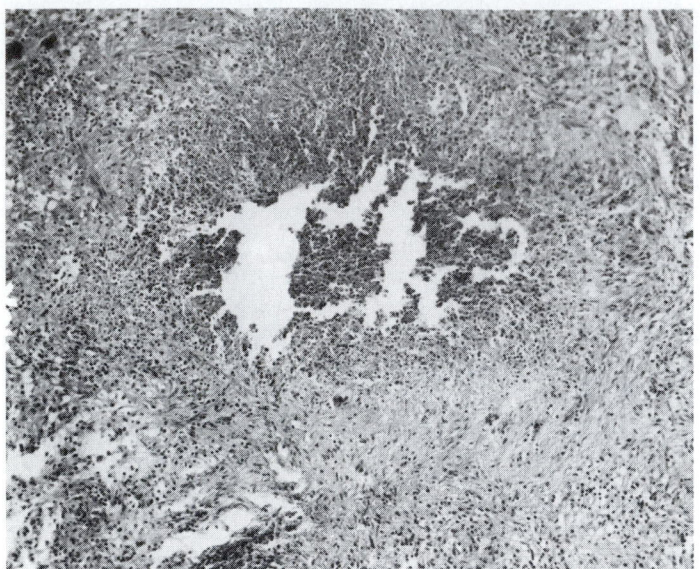

FIGURE 160-9 Early liquefaction in a small tubercle from a 12-month-old child who died of miliary tuberculosis. The lesion is partly surrounded by fibrous tissue. H&E, ×90. *(Courtesy of the collection of the late Professors A. R. Rich and W. G. MacCallum, Department of Pathology, Johns Hopkins School of Medicine.)*

160-11). There, blood may pool and give rise to some hemoptysis. Massive hemoptysis, which is sometimes fatal, is usually due to the leakage or rupture of a blood vessel located in the wall of the cavity or traversing the lumen.

When a liquefied caseous lesion in the lung or hilar lymph node discharges its contents into the air passages, the resulting

lesions range from small, nearby pneumonic foci, to larger areas of pneumonia, to a complete lobar pneumonia. The extent of the disease is determined by the amount of liquefied caseum aspirated into the bronchial tree, as well as by the number of live and dead bacilli and the quantity of tuberculinlike products that this liquefied caseum contains.

Local deposits containing small quantities of bacilli and their components commonly cause scattered compact proliferative-type tubercles or (more rarely) confluent proliferative tubercles with small foci of encapsulated caseous pneumonia (Fig. 160-12). However, local deposits containing large quantities of bacilli and their components cause exudative-type lesions that soon caseate, producing small or large areas of tuberculous pneumonia (Fig. 160-7*A* and *B*).

Cavitary tuberculous lesions may never heal. They may enlarge, shrink, or remain stable. Spontaneous healing results from a gradual collapse of the cavity, progressive fibrosis from without, or obstruction of the bronchocavitary junction followed by absorption of the air within the cavity. Fibrosis is often incomplete, and variable amounts of caseous and fibrocaseous material may remain within the fibrotic lesion. Calcium deposition is common, and occasionally ossification occurs. A "healed" cavity, like a "healed" caseous focus, is seldom completely free of tubercle bacilli, which may persist for years, often in a dormant state.

Since the advent of effective antimicrobial agents, "open healing" of cavities can occur. Successful treatment with antimicrobial agents eliminates most of the bacilli from the cavity. Inflammation then decreases, and much or all of the necrotic contents drains through the still-patent bronchocavitary junction. Such drainage is facilitated if the cavity is located in an upper

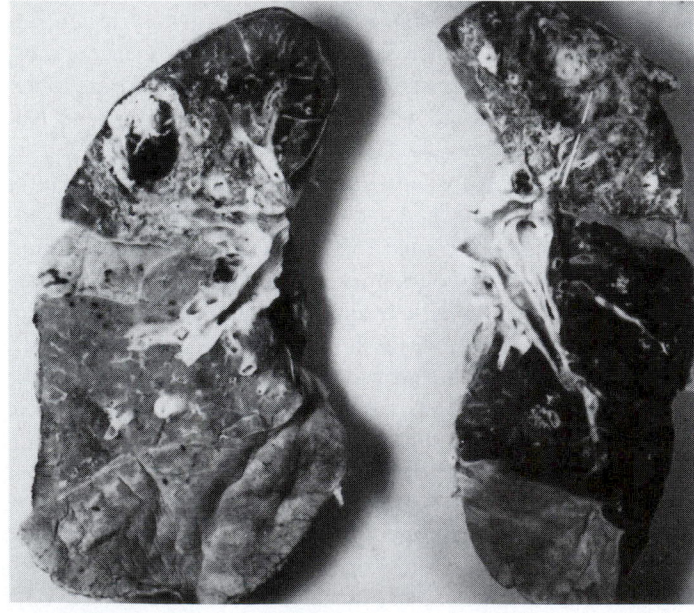

A

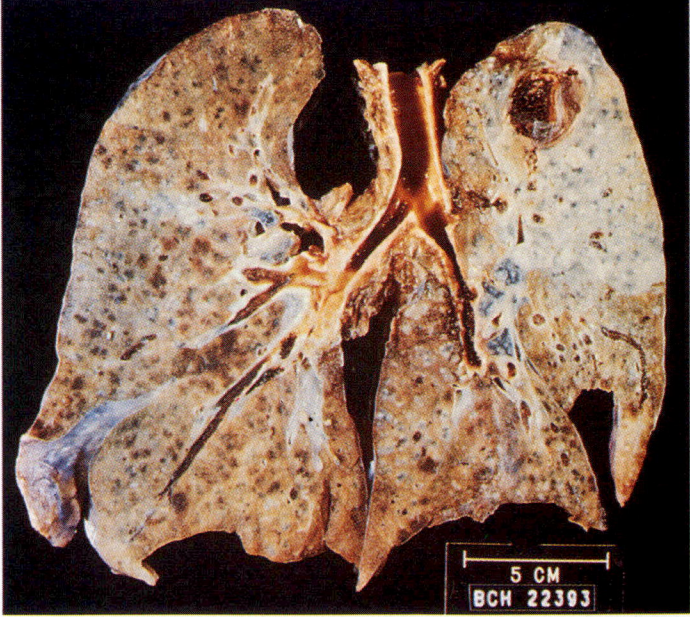

B

FIGURE 160-10 Tuberculous cavities. *A.* Bilateral cavities in the upper lobes in a 39-year-old diabetic woman. Caseous areas surround the cavities. Although infected, the hilar lymph nodes are not markedly enlarged. In the lung on the right, an applicator stick marks the communication between the cavity and the bronchus. *B.* An apical cavity of moderate size in an adult. There is extensive surrounding caseous con-

solidation of pneumonic origin. Several caseous foci are also present in the other lung. The hilar lymph nodes are slate gray in color. They contain a few caseous areas but are only slightly enlarged. *(Courtesy of collection of the late Professors A. R. Rich and W. G. MacCallum, Department of Pathology, Johns Hopkins School of Medicine.)*

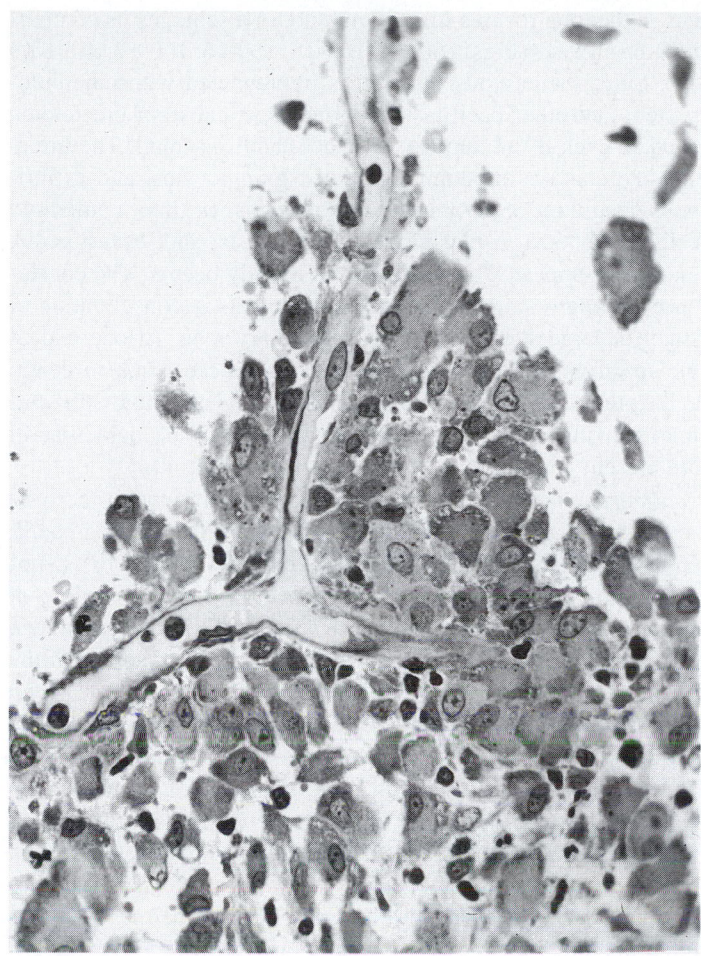

FIGURE 160-11   A small blood vessel extending into the lumen of a cavity in a tuberculous rabbit.[13] Such exposed vessels are the source of blood in the sputum. The inner wall of the cavity contains disintegrating mature epithelioid cells. Glycol methacrylate-embedded tissue section stained with Giemsa. ×400. (*Based on data of Converse et al,[13] with permission.*)

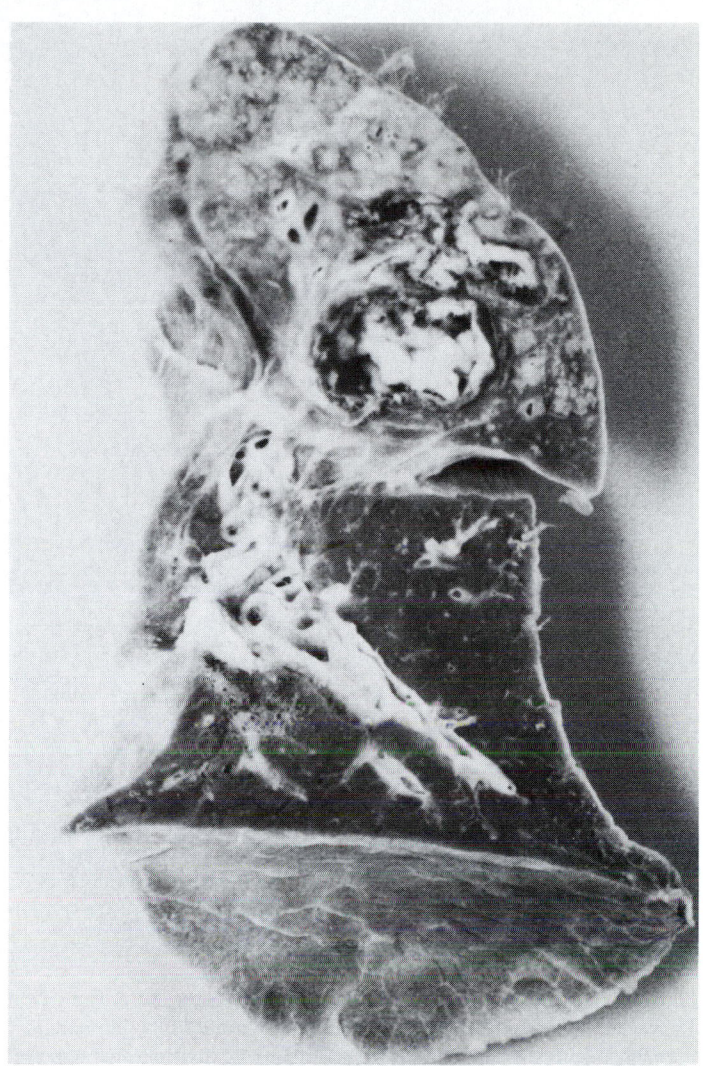

FIGURE 160-12   A cavity in the base of the upper lobe of the left lung of a 17-month-old child. The apical portion was adherent to the chest wall and solidified with confluent "proliferative" tubercles and encapsulated caseous pneumonic foci. (*Courtesy of the collection of the late Professors A. R. Rich and W. G. MacCallum, Department of Pathology, Johns Hopkins School of Medicine.*)

lobe (the usual place). Metaplastic bronchial epithelium (squamous with no cilia) may eventually line the cavity. The "open-healed" cavity may persist as one with a thick or thin fibrotic wall, or as an emphysematous bleb or bulla.

PROGRESSIVE LOCALLY DESTRUCTIVE LESIONS

Tuberculous lesions may progress slowly or rapidly. Slowly progressing caseous or cavitary foci are the most common type of progressive tuberculosis in adults (Fig. 160-10A). These foci have compact walls that contain epithelioid and giant cells and show considerable reparative fibrosis (Fig. 160-13). Progression is intermittent. The advancing edge of the lesion contains fresh tubercles, or fresh or organizing pneumonia in the adjacent alveolar spaces. Encapsulated caseous foci and tubercles, embedded in fibrous tissue, are prominent; hence the term *fibrocaseous* (Fig. 160-6B). Satellite lesions are frequent, and cavitation and extension via the bronchial passages sometimes occur.

Rapidly progressing caseous foci with inconspicuous fibrosis (Figs. 160-14 and 160-15) are often present when host resistance is low. Such lesions grow peripherally as a loose exudate ex-

tending into nearby alveolar spaces. The exudate (which soon becomes necrotic) contains young macrophages, granulocytes, fibrin, erythrocytes, and serum protein. This type of tuberculosis commonly occurs in young children. It is rare in adults, except when they are immunosuppressed or when they aspirate large numbers of bacilli from a cavity.

ADVANCED FIBROCASEOUS TUBERCULOSIS

The most common form of advanced tuberculosis seen in adults is the fibrocaseous type, which may lead to death. In this form of the disease, different lobes of the lung may contain confluent cavities, confluent caseous foci, areas of caseous pneumonia, or combinations of these conditions (Figs. 160-16 and 160-17). Because of the large numbers of bacilli that ascend the bronchial tree and are subsequently swallowed, lesions may occur in the bronchi, trachea, larynx, and intestinal tract—all of which are rather resistant

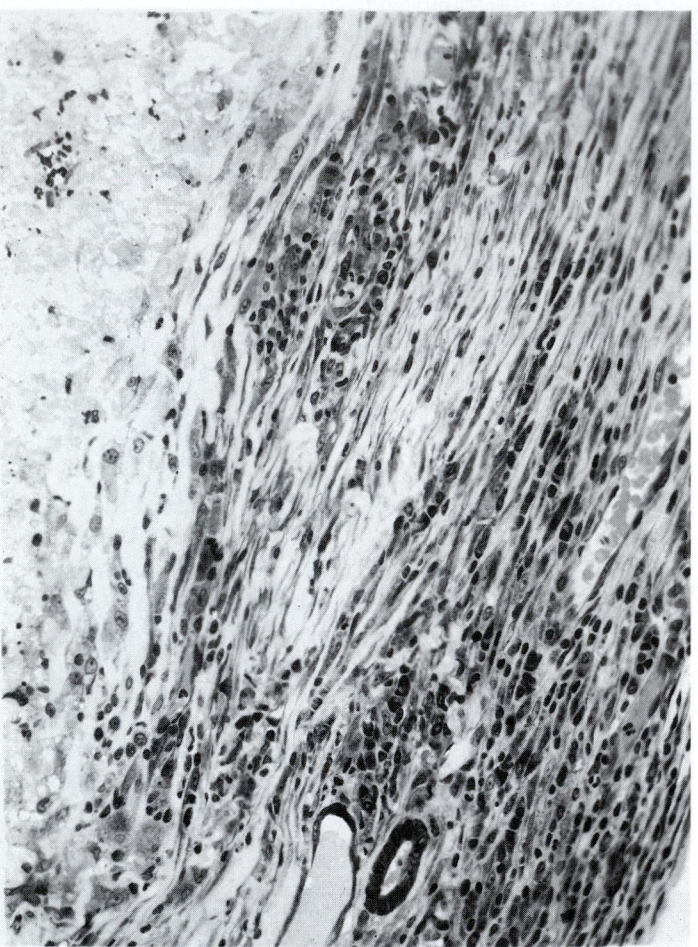

FIGURE 160-13   A portion of a large cavity in the lung of a rabbit 18 weeks after the inhalation of about 5000 virulent tubercle bacilli.[13] A thick fibrous capsule (on the right) surrounds the liquefied caseum. Many fibroblasts are present in the fibrous capsule, along with some macrophages, lymphocytes, and plasma cells. At the bottom of the figure, an oval metaplastic alveolus is seen next to a small blood vessel. Liquefied caseum is shown at the upper left. Glycol methacrylate–embedded tissue sections stained with Giemsa. ×250.

to small numbers of bacilli. The patient whose lungs are shown in Fig. 160-16 had lesions in each of these locations. Figure 160-18 shows an example of tuberculous laryngitis, which rarely occurs with effective chemotherapy. Occasionally, an infected bronchus may undergo cicatricial stenosis and become obstructed, producing atelectasis of the lung distal to that site.

In spite of the extensive fibrocaseous pulmonary disease, the hilar nodes of adults usually show minimal involvement. This is in contrast to childhood tuberculosis, in which large *caseous* hilar nodes often play a major role in the progression of the disease, usually by seeding bacilli into the bloodstream (via efferent lymphatics).

TUBERCULOUS PNEUMONIA AND PLEURISY

Tuberculous pneumonia is an exudative response in the alveolar spaces, caused by the presence of numerous live and dead tubercle bacilli and their antigenic products. Small or extensive areas of pneumonia commonly occur when a liquefied caseous fo-

cus in the lung (or in a hilar lymph node) discharges its contents into the airways (Figs. 160-7A, 160-15, 160-16, 160-17, and 160-19). Since the caseous material is impregnated with tuberculoprotein and other bacillary components, it causes a pneumonic exudate even if the number of intact bacilli is small. The initial exudate contains mononuclear cells, granulocytes, and a fibrinous coagulum of serum and cell proteins. In time, epithelioid cells, lymphocytes, plasma cells, fibroblasts, and, occasionally, giant cells appear. Caseous necrosis usually occurs. The confluence of progressing exudative lesions results in consolidation of small or large segments of the pulmonary lobe. At one end of the spectrum, such tuberculous pneumonia can result in death; at the other end, the pneumonia can undergo resolution with minimal scarring, especially if only small numbers of viable bacilli are present and the lung structure is preserved.

Pleurisy results when subpleural caseous lesions in the lung (or in the hilar lymph nodes) leak or rupture, discharging bacilli and their components into the pleural cavity (Fig. 160-16). (Similarly, *tuberculous pericarditis* can develop from the rupture of such caseous lesions into the pericardial sac.) The pleurisy can take many forms—e.g., mild, uncomplicated roughenings of the pleural surface; large or small numbers of miliary tubercles on this pleural surface; serous effusions (from large or numerous surface lesions); or frank tuberculous empyema. Serous effusions are bacteriologically sterile in more than half of the cases, because they usually are a response to tuberculin-like products released into the pleural cavity. Tuberculous empyema, a purulent exudate in the pleural cavity (frequently superinfected with pyogenic bacteria), was a serious complication before the antimicrobial era.

The type of pleural disease is determined by (1) the number of live and dead bacilli, (2) the quantity of their tuberculin-like products in the caseous material, (3) the level of tuberculin sensitivity of the host, (4) the friction of the roughened visceral pleura against the parietal pleura, (5) the number and types of cells in the exudate, (6) the inherent ability of the host to localize and fibrose new sites of tuberculous infection, and (7) the presence or absence of superinfection with other bacteria.

Tuberculous pleurisy may resolve completely or may heal with fibrosis, focal adhesions, and sometimes calcification. Depending on the amount of exudate in the pleural space, a large or small portion of the lung may collapse. Organization of the exudate and subsequent fibrosis tend to maintain this collapse.

CHILDHOOD TUBERCULOSIS: LYMPHATIC SPREAD AND THE GHON COMPLEX

Tuberculosis in children differs from tuberculosis in adults in several respects: (1) young children, especially infants, usually have lower native and acquired resistance to this disease; (2) their hilar lymph nodes more commonly become enlarged and caseous (Figs. 160-14, 160-19, and 160-20); (3) blood-borne dissemination occurs more readily (Fig. 160-14; see also Fig. 160-8), but still is an exception rather than the rule; (4) calcification of caseous foci is more common; and (5) the primary pulmonary lesion in children is usually subpleural in well-ventilated regions of the lung (Fig. 160-20), whereas such lesions in adults are usually subapical (see below).

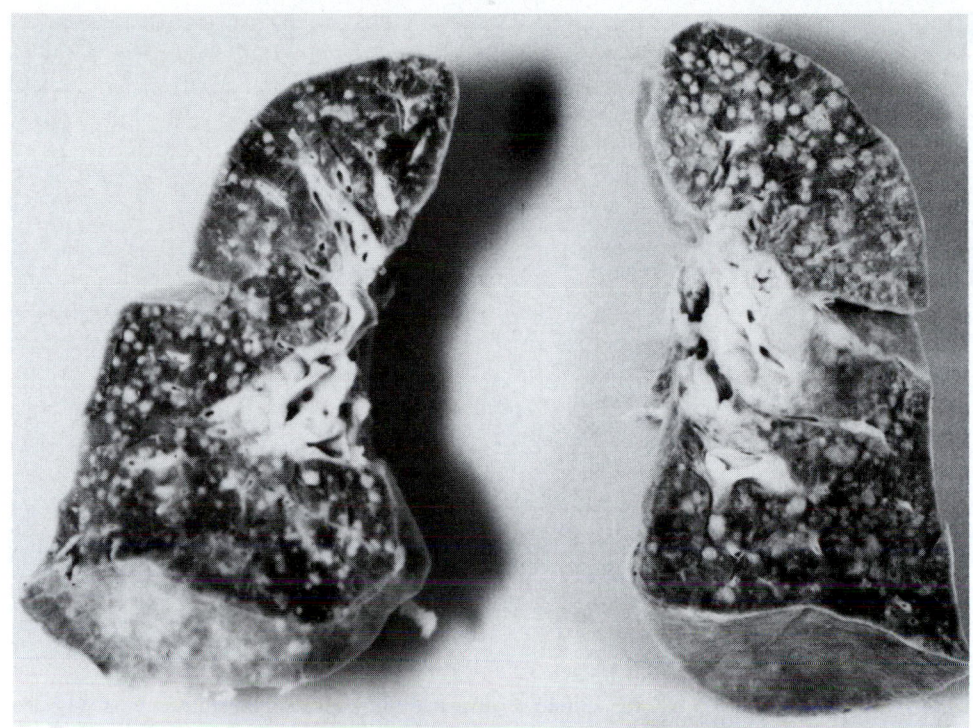

FIGURE 160-14 Rapidly progressing disseminated tuberculosis in an 11-month-old child. Both hematogenous and bronchogenic spread from caseous hilar lymph nodes occurred in the lungs. Most of the caseous foci are hematogenous in origin, but in the lung on the right are areas of caseous pneumonia, caused by two caseous hilar lymph nodes rupturing into bronchi. *(Courtesy of collection of the late Professors A. R. Rich and W. G. MacCallum, Department of Pathology, Johns Hopkins School of Medicine.)*

Tubercle bacilli, either free or within immature macrophages (or granulocytes), spread via the lymphatics from the primary lesion to the hilar lymph nodes, where in children (and in adults with low resistance) the bacilli can cause large caseous lesions. The combination of one or more enlarged caseous hilar node(s) and a tuberculous focus in the lung periphery constitutes a *Ghon complex* (Fig. 160-20).

Sometimes, a tuberculous hilar node obstructs a bronchus by external compression or by extension of the disease process into the bronchial wall. The obstruction causes segmental or lobar collapse and pneumonitis, the so-called *right middle lobe syndrome.* Sometimes such a node ruptures into a bronchus (Figs. 160-14 and 160-19), causing distally focal or diffuse pneumonic lesions. Such lesions can be minimal or extensive, depending on the concentration of bacilli and their antigenic products and on the host's reaction to them. Both situations occur mainly in infants, since older children and adults rarely have extensive involvement of the hilar nodes.

ADULT TUBERCULOSIS: ENDOGENOUS AND EXOGENOUS REINFECTION

As a rule, tuberculosis progresses more slowly in adults than it does in infants, because the resistance of adults is usually higher. Secondary endogenous tuberculous foci of lymphatic or hematogenous origin also occur less often in adults. However, the resistance of immunocompetent adults may be overwhelmed when a liquefied caseous focus ruptures and seeds large numbers of bacilli directly into a bronchus or into a blood or lymphatic vessel of appreciable size.

Reinfection-type or *adult-type* tuberculosis may be caused by either exogenous or endogenous tubercle bacilli. This type of tuberculosis consists of a small to large pulmonary lesion that is most often in the subapical region and is *unaccompanied* by any marked enlargement of the hilar lymph nodes. Adult-type tuberculosis may occur as a *primary* infection in either adults or children with resistance high enough to restrict bacillary multiplication in the hilar nodes.

The active subapical lesion is frequently a localized area of bronchopneumonia containing macrophages, epithelioid cells, lymphocytes, giant cells, and fibroblasts. The lesion usually heals, and fibrosis results in a thickened pleura. Sometimes, a cavity forms either at the time of the initial subapical infection or, more commonly, years later if reactivation of a formerly dormant subapical lesion occurs. Then the disease may progress into one of the more serious types described above.

Why the subapical region of the lungs (Figs. 160-10, 160-16, and 160-17) is a favored site for the onset of adult-type tuberculosis is not known. One possibility is that the high O_2 tension and the low blood and lymph flow aid the exogenous and endogenous bacilli that lodge in that site. The subapical environment must play some role in the local establishment of a lesion, because most exogenous inhaled bacilli deposited elsewhere in the lung are destroyed initially by alveolar macrophages or, during the following weeks, by cell-mediated immunity and by delayed-type hypersensitivity. Another possibility is that during primary infection or reactivation, bits of caseous tissue containing bacilli (probably from the hilar lymph nodes, which drain into the superior vena cava) are preferentially distributed by the bloodstream into the subapical regions.

Exogenous bacilli, giving rise to adult-type tuberculosis, may be inhaled directly into the lung subapical regions, while *endogenous* bacilli are probably carried there by the bloodstream from lesions elsewhere. Endogenous tubercle bacilli usually remain dormant, probably in the hilar nodes or in a subapical region of the lung. They produce adult-type tuberculosis only when the resistance of the host is lowered.

TUBERCULOSIS IN THE IMMUNOCOMPROMISED HOST

In immunocompromised patients (especially in patients with HIV infections), tuberculosis is most often the result of reactivation of a latent focus, but it is sometimes a primary infection.

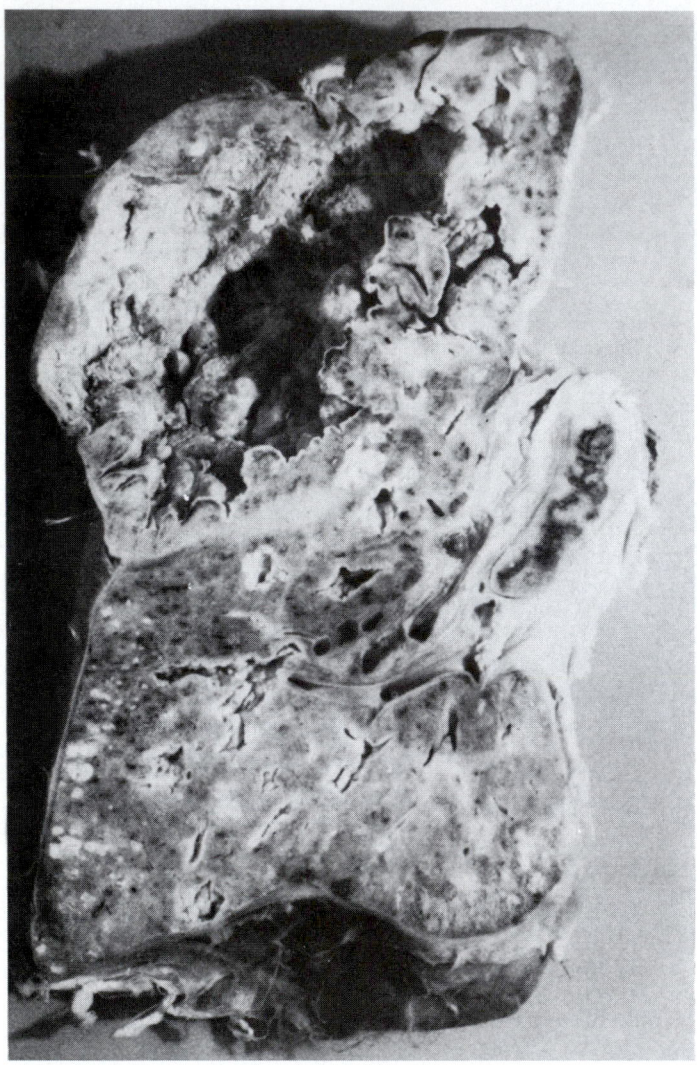

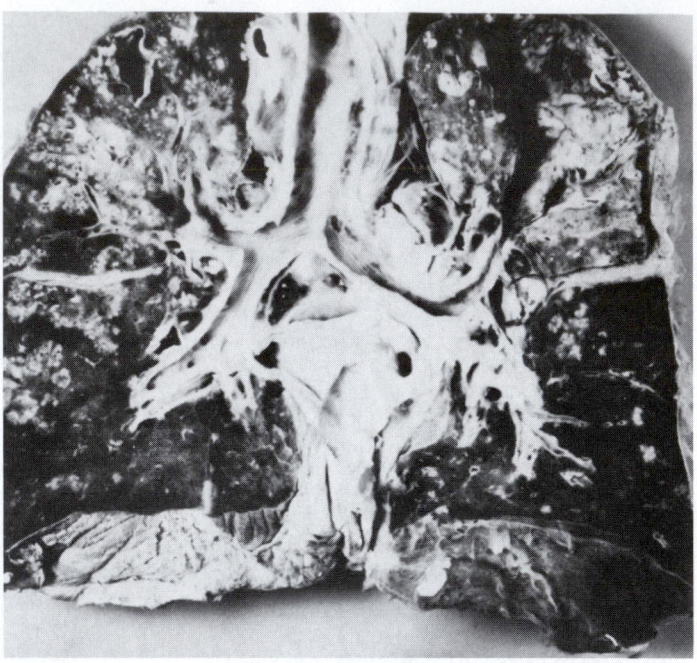

FIGURE 160-16 Advanced fibrocaseous tuberculosis in an 11-year-old girl who died before the advent of the antimicrobial era. The contents of bilateral cavities in the upper lobes have caused areas of caseous bronchopneumonia. Pleural adhesions were present, the fibrous tissue of which is visible on the right. The hilar lymph nodes contain several caseous foci. *(Courtesy of the collection of the late Professors A. R. Rich and W. G. MacCallum, Department of Pathology, Johns Hopkins School of Medicine.)*

FIGURE 160-15 A large, rapidly formed tuberculous cavity in the upper lobe. Caseous pneumonia is present throughout the rest of the lung. Fibrosis is minimal. The hilar node is markedly enlarged and mostly caseous. *(Courtesy of the collection of the late Professors A. R. Rich and W. G. MacCallum, Department of Pathology, Johns Hopkins School of Medicine.)*

In such patients, tuberculosis is usually more severe and rapidly progressive than in immunocompetent patients: mortality is higher, and extrapulmonary involvement is more frequent.[6] In AIDS patients, the disease of reactivation often resembles childhood tuberculosis with hilar adenopathy, frequent lower-lobe involvement, and absence of both cavitation and scar formation (Figs. 160-21 and 160-22).

In all immunosuppressed patients, the morphology of tuberculous lesions reflects poor host resistance. For example, in corticosteroid-treated patients, tuberculous lesions show abundant caseation with little or no encapsulation or granulomatous reaction. Large numbers of bacteria are usually present within the lesions (Figs. 160-23 and 160-24). These changes are morphologically similar to those found experimentally in corticosteroid-treated tuberculous animals.[36]

In patients with AIDS, the histologic pattern of tuberculosis generally correlates with the degree of immunosuppression. In premortem biopsy samples, the granulomas are more prolifera-

tive (and less exudative) than in necropsy-derived tissue. As the peripheral CD4 lymphocytes decrease, the type of necrosis changes from caseous to caseosuppurative (i.e., caseous necrosis containing neutrophils and more undigested nuclear debris) (Fig. 160-22). Also, the number of mycobacteria within lesions increases.[26]

Immune Mechanisms

CELL-MEDIATED IMMUNITY (ACQUIRED CELLULAR RESISTANCE)

In tuberculosis, *cell-mediated immunity* is characterized by an expanded population of antigen-specific Th1 lymphocytes, which, in the presence of the antigen, produce cytokines that activate macrophages (Fig. 160-25). In tuberculosis, *acquired cellular resistance* is characterized by a *local* population of microbicidal macrophages activated by the cytokines of Th1 lymphocytes stimulated by specific antigens (Fig. 160-25).

In the 1960s, Mackaness[38] showed that *acquired cellular resistance,* once produced, was nonspecific. Activated macrophages could destroy or inhibit many types of facultative intracellular bacteria, not just the type that caused their activation. However, once these activated macrophages have disappeared, following the healing of the primary infection, only the *specific* bacterial species could *rapidly* produce them again. This rapid "recall" response is due to the presence of expanded populations of long-lived (i.e., nondividing) recirculating Th1 lymphocytes ("memory" cells) with receptors for the specific antigens.[3] Antigens secreted by tubercle bacilli[2,44] growing in nonactivated

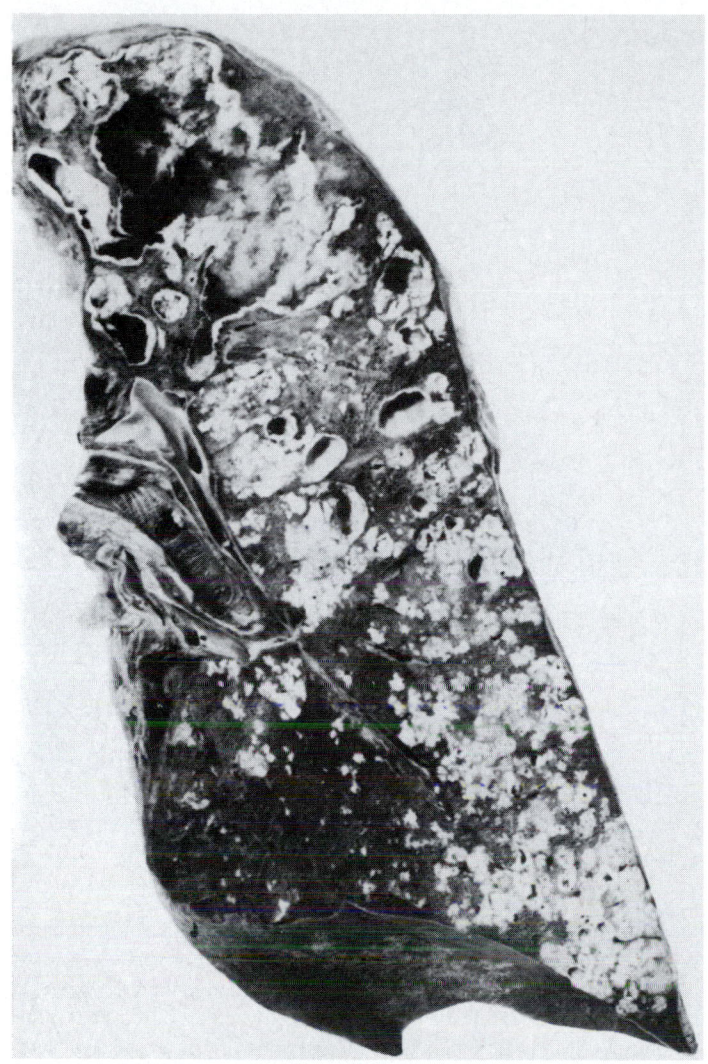

FIGURE 160-17   A large cavity in the upper lobe. Caseous bronchopneumonia is present throughout the lung. *(Courtesy of the collection of the late Professors A. R. Rich and W. G. MacCallum, Department of Pathology, Johns Hopkins School of Medicine.)*

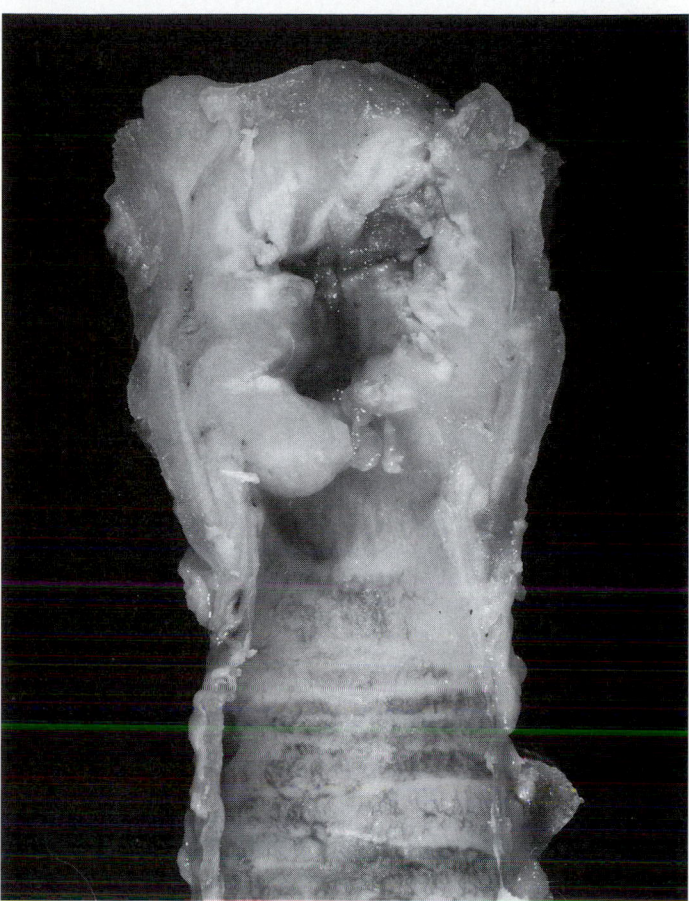

FIGURE 160-18   Tuberculous laryngitis in a rabbit that had inhaled 300 virulent bovine-type tubercle bacilli 33 weeks previously. The lung of this rabbit had 14 lesions, 4 of which had formed cavities. The cavity in the right lower lobe of the lung apparently discharged so many bacilli into the bronchial tree that the larynx became infected. This laryngeal lesion partly obstructed the airway. ×6.3. *(Reprinted from Converse et al,[13] with permission.)*

macrophages stimulate this long-lived, specific Th1 lymphocyte population (in the developing lesion and in its draining lymph nodes) to release IL-2, which autocatalytically further expands and activates these specific Th1 cells, and also to release IFN-γ,[3] which activates macrophages. The rapid accumulation and activation of local macrophages at the site of reinfection usually prevent the progression of new lesions. In other words, the expanded specific Th1 lymphocyte population rapidly produces many activated macrophages at the site of bacillary lodgment.

DELAYED-TYPE HYPERSENSITIVITY

In tuberculosis, delayed-type hypersensitivity (like cell-mediated immunity) is a Th1 lymphocyte response to the antigens of the tubercle bacillus. It plays a major role in the accumulation of lymphocytes and macrophages at the sites where the bacilli are lodged. If there is *too much local antigen,* delayed-type hypersensitivity causes tissue necrosis. (Such necrosis is readily observed in a patient with very high sensitivity to tuberculin [PPD]

when a standard [rather than a reduced] concentration is injected into the skin.) The bacillus itself is nontoxic. In tuberculosis, the bacillus multiplies logarithmically in nonactivated macrophages.[16,18,36] The only way to control bacillary growth is to kill these bacilli-laden macrophages. This is a highly effective defense mechanism because the tubercle bacilli cannot multiply in the *solid* caseous necrotic tissue resulting from such killing.

REACTIONS TO TUBERCULIN

In patients with active, but nonterminal, tuberculosis, the size of the tuberculin reaction is of no prognostic significance. In one study, rabbits with high genetic resistance to tuberculosis developed large tuberculin reactions early during a primary infection, because these rabbits responded to bacillary antigens more efficiently than did genetically susceptible rabbits.[36] The natively *susceptible* rabbits also developed large tuberculin reactions as the infection progressed, because the large number of multiplying bacilli was a strong antigenic stimulus.[36] Because neither the resistance of the host nor the antigenic load of bacilli can be determined in patients, a large tuberculin reaction has no prognostic value. In *inactive* tuberculosis, the size of the tuberculin re-

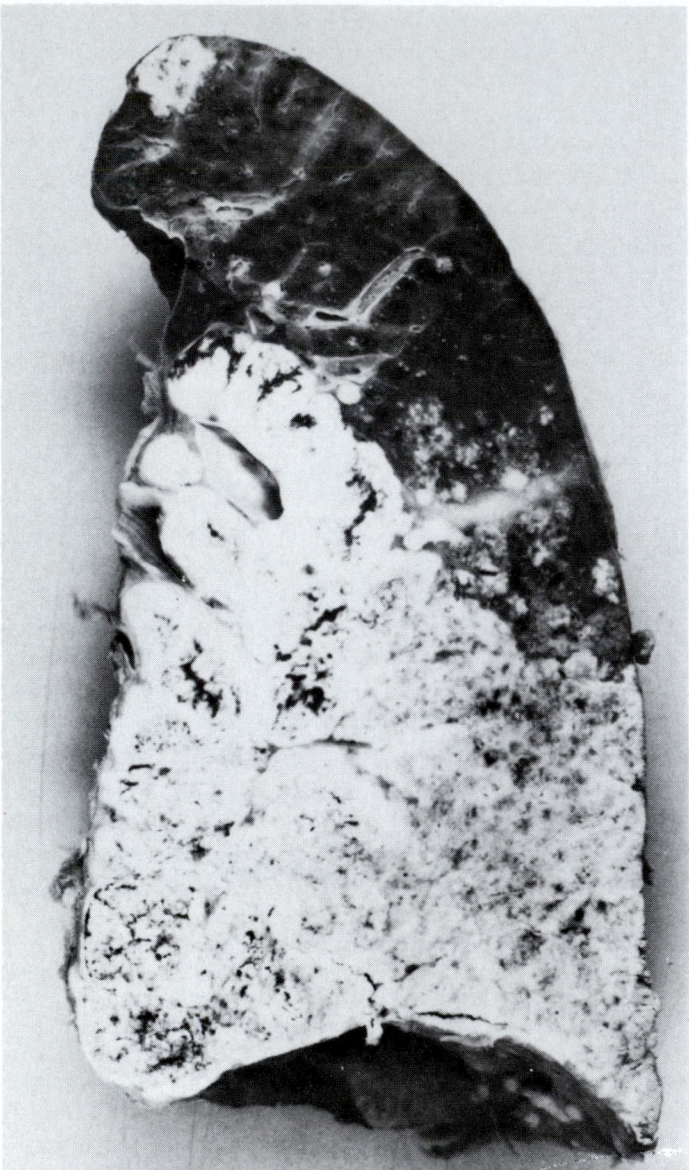

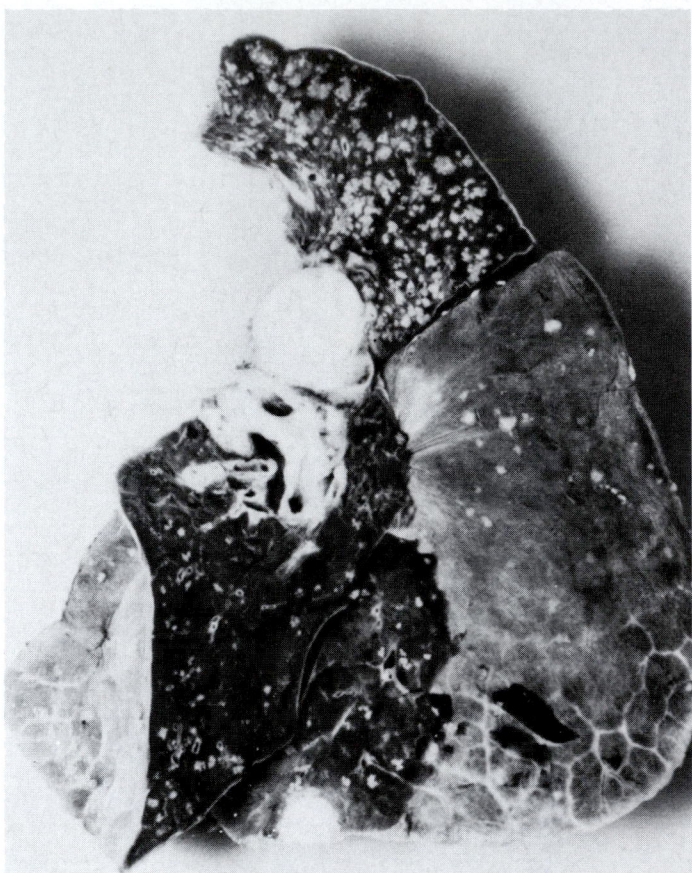

FIGURE 160-20 A progressive Ghon complex in the midportion of the lung from a 6-year-old boy who died of *tuberculous meningitis*. At the lower edge of the specimen is a circumscribed primary subpleural caseous lesion. Near the center is a markedly enlarged caseous hilar lymph node. Many tubercles of hematogenous origin are also present. *(Courtesy of the collection of the late Professors A. R. Rich and W. G. MacCallum, Department of Pathology, Johns Hopkins School of Medicine.)*

FIGURE 160-19 Extensive confluent caseous pneumonia in a 13-month-old child caused by the rupture of a liquefied caseous hilar lymph node into the bronchus supplying the lower lobe. *(Courtesy of the collection of the late Professors A. R. Rich and W. G. MacCallum, Department of Pathology, Johns Hopkins School of Medicine.)*

action seems to be related to the occasional release of virulent bacilli from the focus of infection. A patient frequently releasing such bacilli would have a large tuberculin reaction and perhaps an increased risk of developing active disease. (The tuberculin reaction is discussed in detail in Chapters 158 and 161.)

An immunocompetent patient may have active tuberculosis and yet show a negative tuberculin reaction to first-strength PPD. This situation is common in the terminal stages of the disease but is also present on admission in 20 to 25 percent of patients hospitalized with pulmonary tuberculosis. When they are recovering, such patients again become skin-test positive. One of the possible mechanisms responsible for this anergy may be compartmentalization. Tuberculous lesions may collect most of the antigen-specific T cells, so that few are available to participate

in the dermal tuberculin reaction.[7] *Tuberculin-negative* patients with *active* tuberculosis also have a greater number of immunosuppressor monocytes and lymphocytes in their peripheral blood.[20,27,50] PGE_2,[20] transforming growth factor–beta (TGF-β)[27] and IL-10[27,30,41] produced by such mononuclear cells are partly responsible for the suppressive effect. Soluble IL-2 receptors (sIL-2R) were found to be elevated in the serum of *most* patients with active pulmonary tuberculosis and might suppress tuberculin reactivity in some of the patients with active disease.[56] In fact, sIL-2R may prove to be a useful serologic marker for the progression of this disease.[10]

IMPROVING VACCINES

Epidemiologic studies on various live BCG and *Mycobacterium microti* vaccines have demonstrated that *no correlation* exists between the amount of protection and the amount of tuberculin sensitivity produced by the vaccine. Vaccines causing low tuberculin sensitivity were just as effective in preventing clinical tubercu-

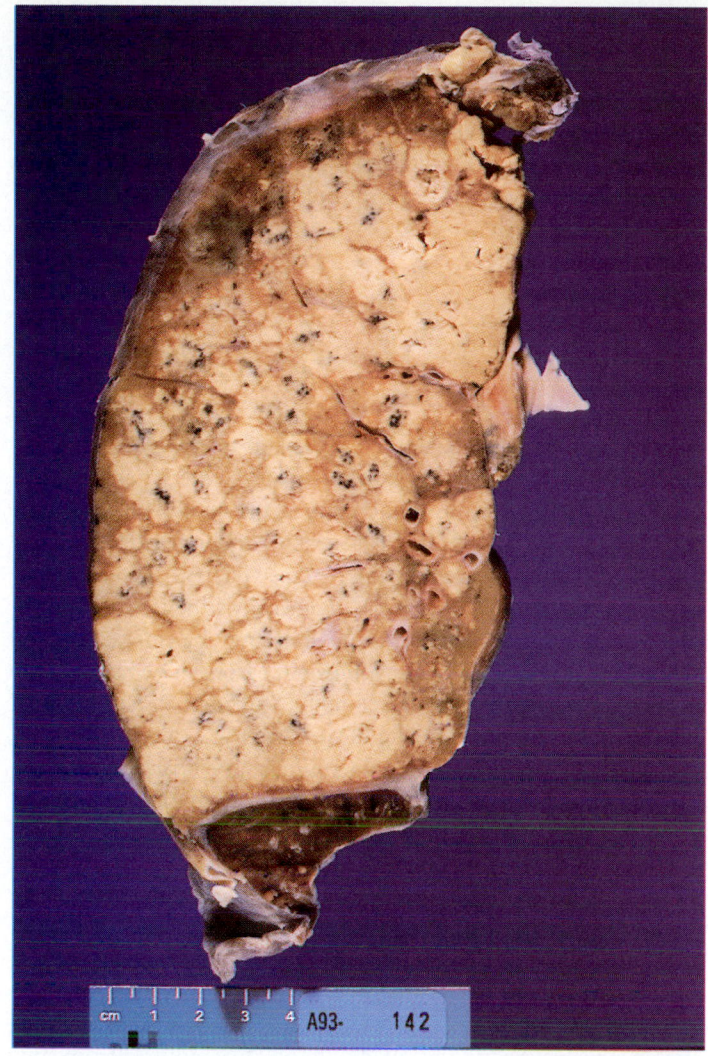

FIGURE 160-21 Confluent, multidrug-resistant tuberculous pneumonia in a patient with AIDS. Lung parenchyma is replaced by pale nodular zones of caseation necrosis.

(PPD) contribute to cell-mediated immunity as well as to delayed-type hypersensitivity. Immunization with an inappropriate vaccine could produce an *improper* balance of delayed-type hypersensitivity and cell-mediated immunity, which might lead to excessive tissue destruction and more rapid liquefaction and cavity formation. Immunotherapy with killed *M. vaccae,* in combination with chemotherapy, has shown promise.[53] Such immunotherapy may prove especially useful in the treatment of multidrug-resistant tuberculosis.

ANTIBODIES AND EXTRACELLULAR FACTORS

In both active and inactive tuberculosis, antibodies to protein, glycolipid, and polysaccharide components of tubercle bacilli are present in the circulation, but their titers have little diagnostic or prognostic value. The passive transfer of such antibodies provides no protection to normal laboratory animals.

Other extracellular factors may be of more benefit to the host than antibodies. Various fatty acids are among the factors inhibiting the growth of the bacillus in the solid caseous centers of tubercles. Transferrin in plasma and lactoferrin in granulocytes withhold iron that is needed for the growth of microorganisms, including tubercle bacilli.[24] The liver is able to lower plasma iron levels by storing increased amounts of iron when the host is invaded by microorganisms.

FACTORS CONTROLLING RESISTANCE TO TUBERCULOSIS

Human beings are *natively* relatively resistant to tuberculosis, to varying degrees.[29,36,49] During adolescence and old age, however, native resistance is somewhat reduced, and during infancy it is markedly reduced. Native resistance in animal models is associated with the rapid local accumulation and activation of macrophages in tuberculous lesions.[36]

losis as those causing high sensitivity.[12] Therefore, an improved vaccine (possibly an altered BCG) that does not convert the tuberculin (PPD) skin test should be possible. Tubercle bacilli contain antigens not present in the tuberculin preparations. The response to stimulation by these other bacillary antigens probably explains the occasional instances in which (1) the host is desensitized to tuberculin but retains resistance to the infection, and (2) the host is effectively immunized with bacillary preparations that have created little or no tuberculin sensitivity. Conversely, a host made sensitive to tuberculin may possess little or no resistance to the infection because other bacillary antigens were removed or inactivated in the preparations used for sensitization. Thus, multiple antigens of the tubercle bacillus in addition to tuberculin

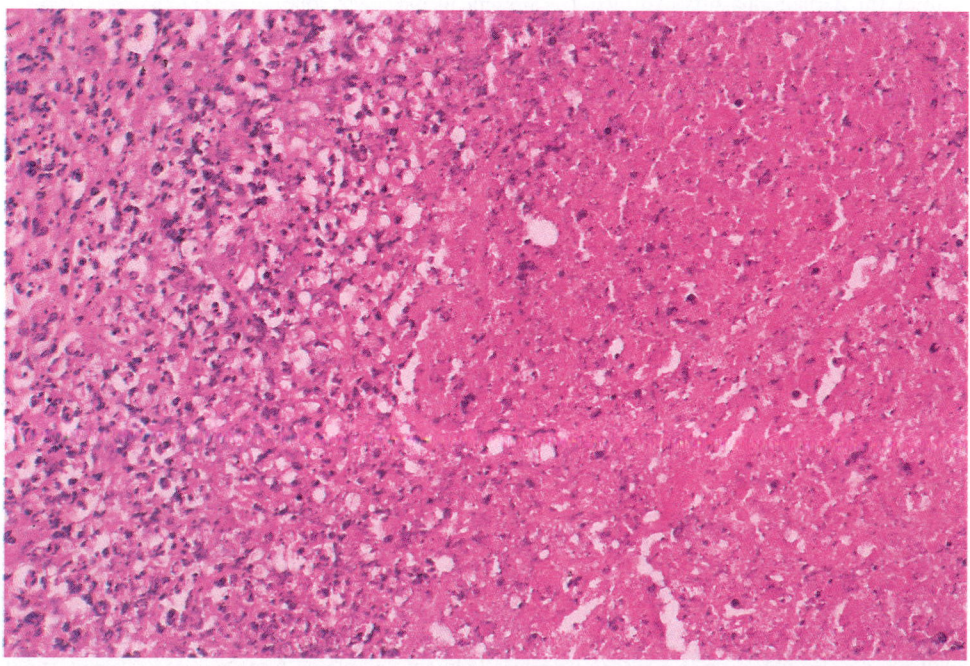

FIGURE 160-22 Caseosuppurative necrosis (right) and poorly organized granulation tissue (left) due to drug-resistant *Mycobacterium tuberculosis* (from the lung of the AIDS patient depicted in Fig. 160-21).

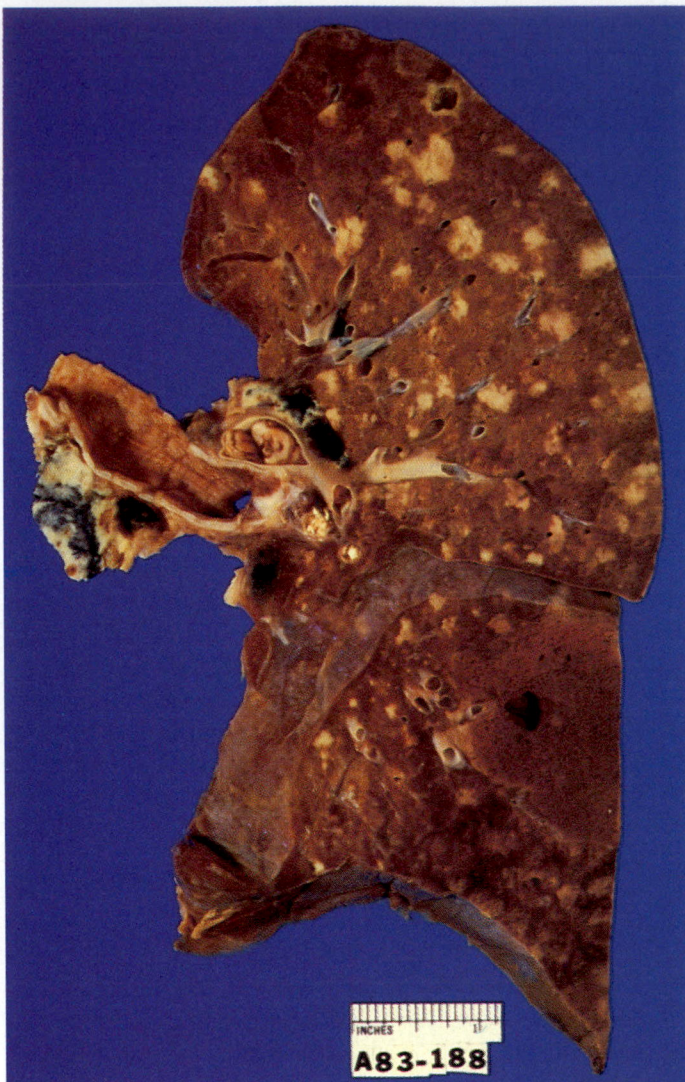

FIGURE 160-23 Progressive miliary tuberculosis and tuberculous pneumonia in the left upper lobe of a 42-year-old woman on corticosteroids for dermatomyositis. An infarct is present in the lower lobe.

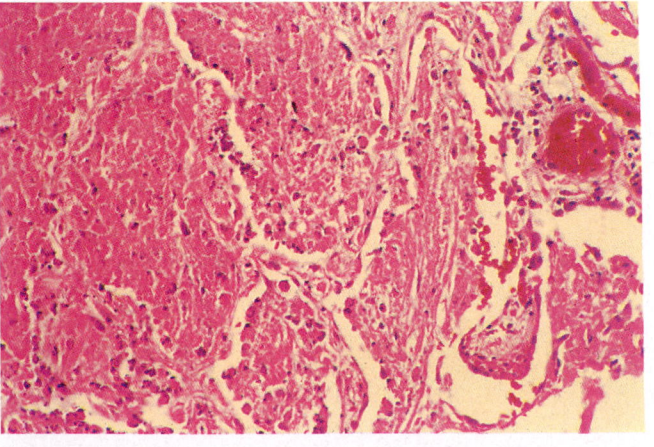

A

B

FIGURE 160-24 Tuberculous lesions in the immunocompromised patient of Fig. 160-23. *A.* An exudative lesion with extensive caseous necrosis, without granuloma formation or Langhans' giant cells. Within adjacent alveoli (right) is an exudate of fibrin and caseous debris. H&E, ×150. *B.* Numerous intracellular and extracellular acid-fast bacilli found at the edge of a necrotic area in the lung of the same patient. Ziehl-Neelsen, counterstained with methylene blue, ×1500.

Both native and acquired resistance to tuberculosis are lowered by immunosuppressive drugs, glucocorticoids, immunosuppressive viruses (e.g., HIV); silicosis, sarcoidosis, uremia, diabetes, alcoholism, and certain neoplastic diseases; gastrectomy; and starvation and other nutritional deficiencies. Conversely, genetic and phenotypic variations in the virulence of the infecting tubercle bacillus would have significant effects on the course of the resulting clinical disease.

INFECTIONS WITH NONTUBERCULOUS MYCOBACTERIA

Overview

Nontuberculous mycobacteria are a well-recognized cause of pulmonary disease (see Chapter 164). Nontuberculous mycobacteria are ubiquitous inhabitants of the natural environment and exist in a variety of animal hosts and nonbiologic reservoirs, including the soil and water. Among these bacteria, the *M. avium* complex (MAC), followed by *M. kansasii,* is the most common cause of pulmonary disease.[60] The lung may be infected by inhalation of nontuberculous mycobacteria from the environment, or it may be infected by dissemination of nontuberculous mycobacteria from a primary site elsewhere, most often in the gastrointestinal tract. Since nontuberculous mycobacteria are organisms of relatively low pathogenicity, saprophytic colonization of the lung must be distinguished from overt pulmonary disease. The repeated recovery of large numbers of *M. avium* complex or *M. kansasii* from the sputum is usually associated with lung disease, but the repeated recovery of other nontuberculous mycobacteria, such as *M. fortuitum* and *M. gordonae,* may represent colonization with no invasive lung disease.[55] The presence of granulomas in lung biopsy specimens, with or without demonstrable acid-fast bacilli (coupled with positive cultures from sputum or bronchial washings), establishes the diagnosis of nontuberculous mycobacteria lung disease in patients in whom the diagnosis could not be made by other criteria.[59]

Chronic Progressive Pulmonary Disease

Nontuberculous mycobacteria typically infect persons with underlying chronic pulmonary conditions, such as pneumoconioses (especially silicosis), emphysematous bullae, chronic obstructive pulmonary disease, cystic fibrosis, prior tuberculosis, malignancies, esophageal disease with chronic aspiration (*M. fortuitum* and *M. chelonei*), and following gastrectomy (*M. xenopi*).[40,60] In these patients, pulmonary infection with nontuberculous mycobacteria resembles reactivation infection with *M. tuberculosis,* both clinically and radiographically.[40]

An increasing number of patients, particularly elderly Caucasian women, with pulmonary nontuberculous mycobacteria infection (usually due to *M. avium* complex) have no discernible predisposing lung disease.[47] In this subgroup of patients, chest radiographs and CT scans differ from those of classic tuberculosis. They have bilateral nodules associated with bronchiectasis, most frequently in the *lower* lungs.[40]

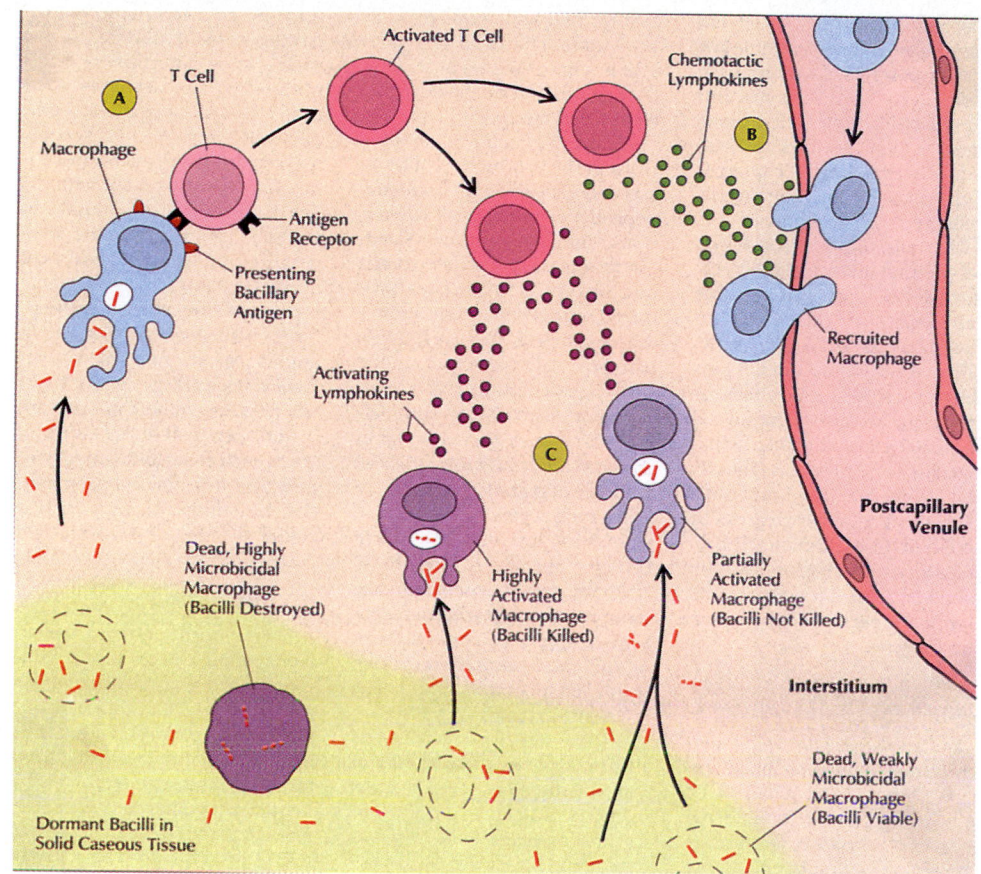

FIGURE 160-25 Activation of macrophages in the tuberculous lesion by means of cell-mediated immunity. *A.* A macrophage ingests tubercle bacilli. Macrophages and dendritic cells present bacillary antigens to T lymphocytes with specific receptors for such antigens. *B.* These lymphocytes proliferate and secrete lymphokines that both recruit monocyte/macrophages from the bloodstream and activate them. *C.* Activated macrophages kill the tubercle bacilli that they ingest, but such activation can be variable, with some macrophages only partly activated and weakly microbicidal and other macrophages highly activated and strongly microbicidal. IFN-γ and TNF-α are major macrophage-activating lymphokines. Chemokines, such as monocyte chemoattractant (activating) protein–1 (MCP-1) (produced by many mononuclear cells within tuberculous lesions), autocatalytically enhance these host defense functions (not illustrated). *(Reprinted from Dannenberg,[16] with permission.)*

host. Exudative granulomatous pneumonia is present in about 10 percent of infections. Acid-fast bacilli are usually sparse within the caseum.[55] When found, *M. kansasii* organisms often appear large and beaded.[55]

Dimorphic mycobacterial granulomas are defined by Reid and Wolinsky as lesions with central suppuration (containing numerous neutrophils) surrounded by noncaseous granulation tissue (containing macrophages and epithelioid cells).[48] Such granulomas are found in about 23 percent of pulmonary nontuberculous mycobacterial infections (Fig. 160-29). Unfortunately, the incidence of dimorphic granulomas in *M. tuberculosis* infections is unknown because numerous neutrophils are often present during the early stages of caseous necrosis (Fig. 160-22) and when large numbers of tubercle bacilli occur during later stages of the disease.[55]

To summarize, the pathology of chronic lung infections produced by the various species of nontuberculous mycobacteria is usually indistinguishable from that produced by *M. tuberculosis.* Histologically, dimorphic granulomas appear to be more common in the nontuberculous mycobacteria group. Nongranulomatous lung disease from nontuberculous mycobacteria may be caused by an aberrant response in immunosuppressed hosts, by saprophytic colonization with such mycobacteria, or simply by a biopsy sampling error.

Histopathologically, nontuberculous mycobacteria infections may show (1) many foamy histiocytes, (2) granulomatous endobronchitis and bronchiolitis, (3) epithelioid granulomas without caseation, (4) nonspecific organizing pneumonia, and (5) interstitial fibrosis without granulomas.[39] Most patients with nonspecific organizing pneumonia or nongranulomatous interstitial fibrosis are immunocompromised.[39] Lung disease caused by nontuberculous mycobacteria usually cannot, however, be differentiated histopathologically from that caused by *M. tuberculosis.*[55] Both nontuberculous mycobacteria and *M. tuberculosis* usually produce caseating granulomas and similar types of cavitation, associated with variable degrees of fibrosis (Figs. 160-26, 160-27, and 160-28). No distinctive histopathologic differences are produced in lesions caused by different species of nontuberculous mycobacteria.[55]

In general, chronic nontuberculous mycobacterial pulmonary disease tends to remain confined within the lung, with little tendency toward lymphatic or hematogenous spread to hilar lymph nodes or to extrathoracic viscera in the immunologically normal

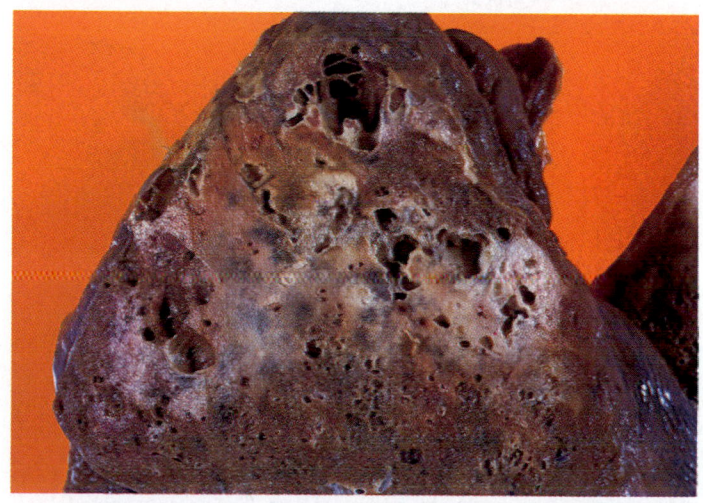

FIGURE 160-26 Chronic cavitary *M. kansasii* infection in the right upper lobe in a 38-year-old alcoholic man. The cavities are surrounded by pale foci of granulomatous pneumonia.

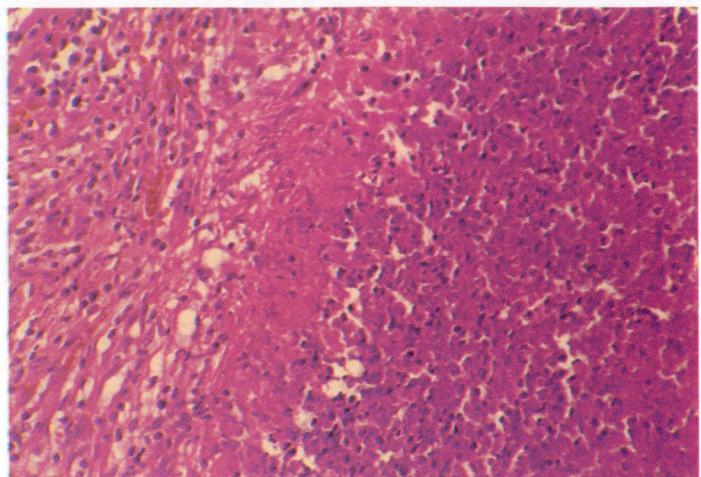

FIGURE 160-29 A dimorphic granuloma produced by *M. fortuitum* in a 24-year-old woman with bronchiectasis. Degenerated neutrophils abound in the necrotic center of the lesion, on the right. Surrounding the necrosis is an area of tuberculous-type granulation tissue (Fig. 160-28). H&E, ×200.

Disseminated Disease

The lung is often affected in disseminated nontuberculous mycobacterial infection, a disorder that has become prevalent in patients with AIDS (see Chapters 163 and 164). But even before the outbreak of AIDS, nontuberculous mycobacteria were known as a cause of disseminated disease, especially in immunocompromised hosts. The organisms producing disseminated disease in patients without AIDS were *M. avium* complex, *M. kansasii,* scotochromogens, and rapid growers, in order of decreasing frequency.[21] In AIDS patients, the preponderant pathogen is *M. avium* complex, although most other species of nontuberculous mycobacteria can also sometimes cause disseminated infection. Disseminated *M. avium* complex disease is found at necropsy in approximately 15 to 24 percent of AIDS patients.[28]

Among non-AIDS patients with disseminated *M. avium* complex infection, the lung was reported to be affected in 65 percent, followed by bone marrow, liver, lymph nodes (46 percent each), and spleen (22 percent).[21] Histologically, disseminated *M. avium* complex disease in non-AIDS patients is usually characterized by poorly formed granulomas containing loose aggregates of mononuclear cells, abundant neutrophils, infrequent epithelioid cells, and focal necrosis. In bone and skin, however, there are often acute and chronic inflammatory areas and abscesses *without* granuloma formation. In most cases, acid-fast bacilli are scarce, but in 20 percent of one large series, tremendous numbers of acid-fast bacilli were seen within macrophages, just as in lepromatous leprosy.[21]

Disseminated *M. avium* complex disease in AIDS patients predominantly affects the reticuloendothelial system, especially the spleen. The portals of entry of *M. avium* complex are thought to be the gastrointestinal and respiratory tracts. Histologically, the lesions at all sites consist of poorly formed granulomas or loose aggregates of striated macrophages, which usually contain numerous acid-fast bacilli (Fig. 160-30). In the small bowel, periodic acid–Schiff–positive macrophages, laden with mycobacteria, histologically resemble those seen in Whipple's disease (Fig.

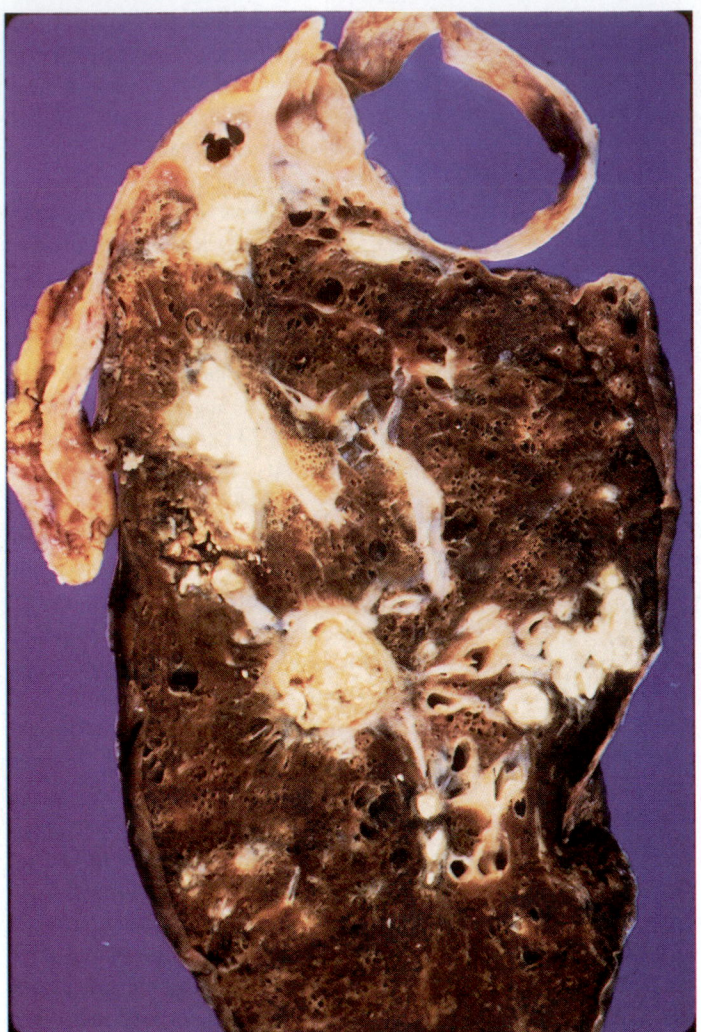

FIGURE 160-27 Resected upper lobe of a 40-year-old man with chronic *M. avium* complex (MAC) disease, showing inspissated fibrocaseous granulomas and early cavitation. An apical fibrobulla and focal areas of centriacinar emphysema are also present.

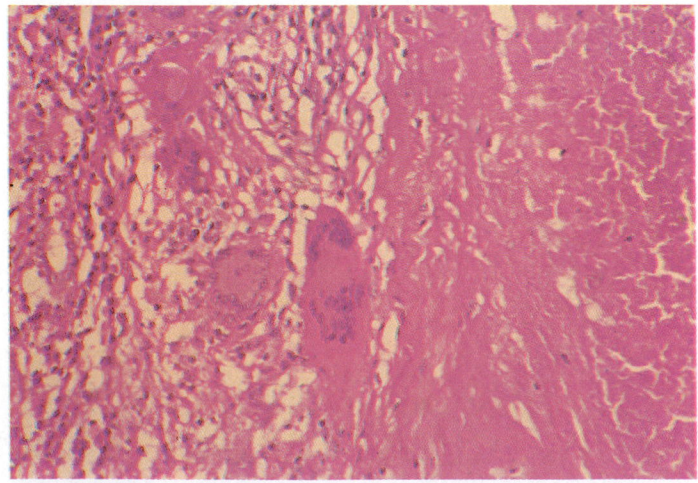

FIGURE 160-28 A fibrocaseous granuloma due to MAC in a 19-year-old woman with a congenital bronchial cyst. The caseous material (on the right) is surrounded by tuberculous-type granulation tissue containing collagen fibers, lymphocytes, macrophages, and several Langhans' giant cells. H&E, ×200.

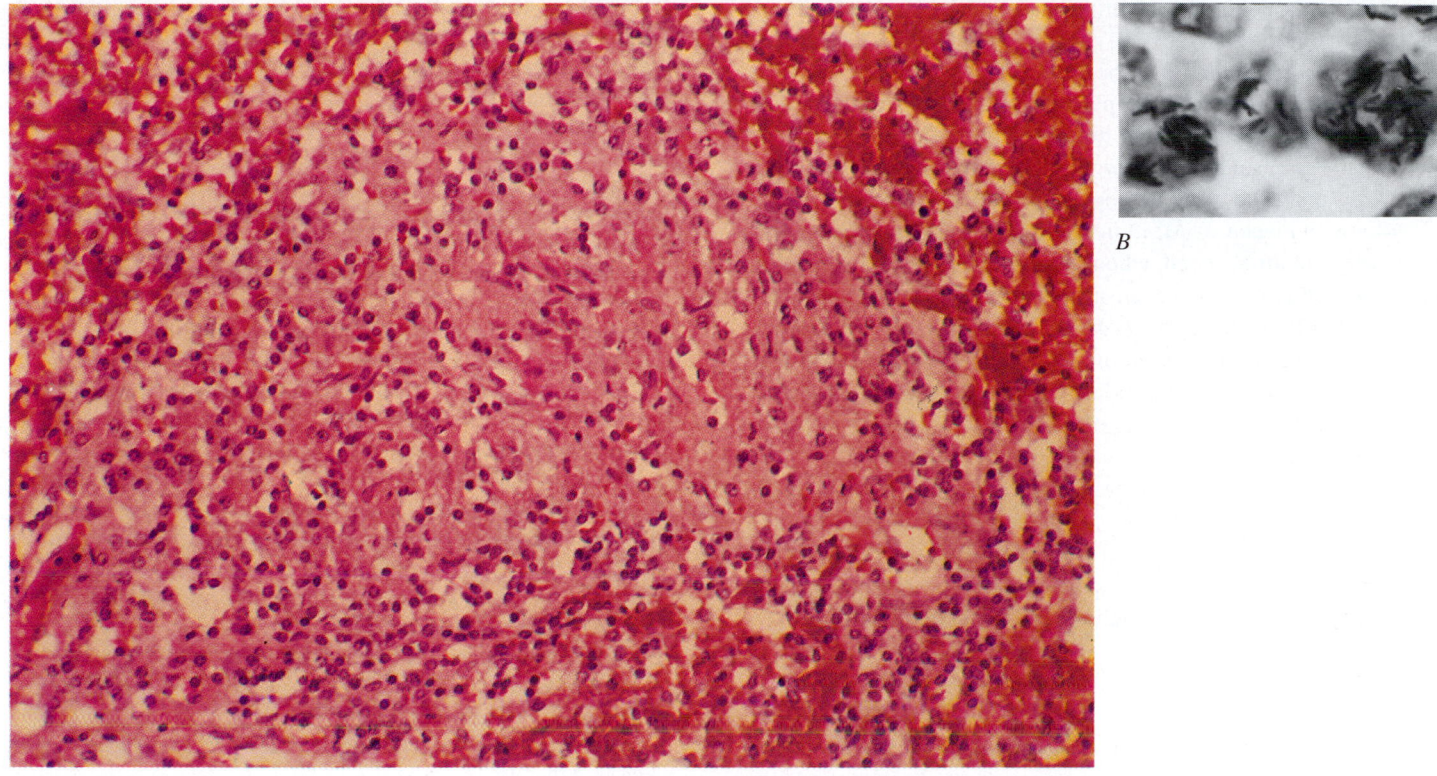

A

FIGURE 160-30   Disseminated infection with MAC in a 30-year-old man with AIDS. *A.* A noncaseating granuloma in the spleen. H&E, ×250. *B.* Macrophages laden with acid-fast bacilli from the same spleen. Ziehl-Neelsen, counterstained with methylene blue, ×1500.

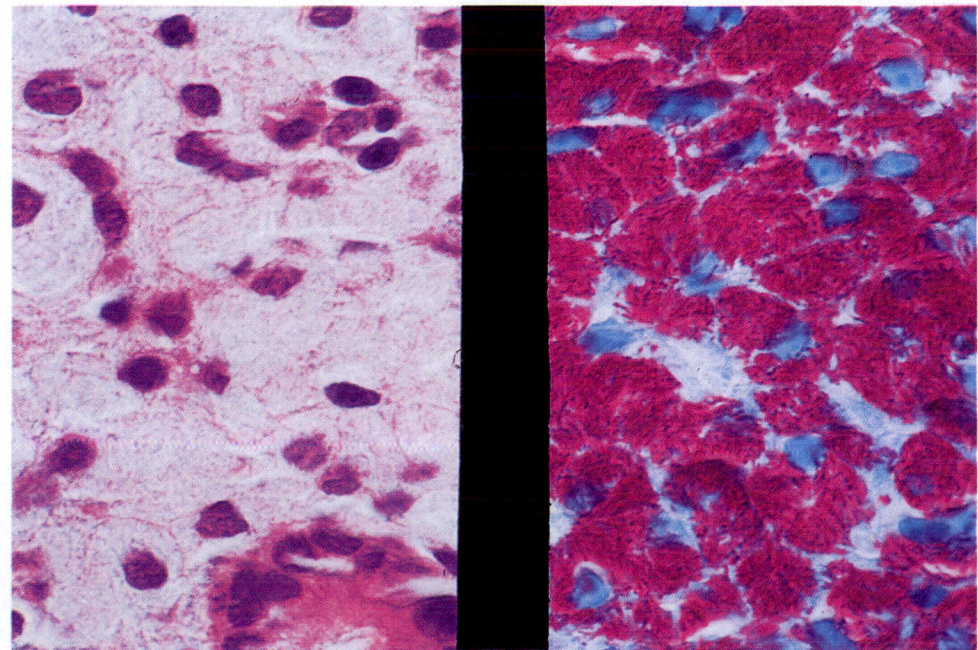

FIGURE 160-31   Disseminated infection with MAC in an AIDS patient. *Left:* Sheets of foamy macrophages laden with acid-fast bacilli in the lamina propria of the small bowel. H&E, ×1000. *Right:* The same cells stained with Ziehl-Neelsen for acid-fast bacilli (counterstained with methylene blue). ×1000.

160-31). In the lungs, however, granulomas or macrophage aggregates are not often seen.[31]

M. avium complex has been cultured from the lung at necropsy in approximately 36 percent of AIDS patients with disseminated *M. avium* complex disease. But clinically significant pulmonary disease due to *M. avium* complex is uncommon and is usually overshadowed by coexistent opportunistic infections. Histologic evidence of *M. avium* complex pulmonary infection is usually minimal, even when lung cultures are positive for *M. avium* complex. However, a *minority* of AIDS patients develop clinically significant *M. avium* complex lung disease with necrotizing granulomas containing variable numbers of acid-fast bacilli. If the disease in their hilar lymph nodes extends into central bronchi, tumorlike masses of granulomatous tissue may obstruct the airways.[31]

Disseminated *M. avium* complex infection in AIDS patients usually occurs when the number of CD4 lymphocytes in the peripheral blood drops below 100 cells/mm^3. Phagocytosis of mycobacteria by macrophages appears to be competent, but the killing of mycobacteria by such macrophages is impaired.[40]

REFERENCES

1. Allison MJ, Zappasodi P, Lurie MB: Host-parasite relationships in natively resistant and susceptible rabbits on quantitative inhalation of tubercle bacilli. *Am Rev Respir Dis* 85:553–569, 1962.
2. Andersen P: The T cell response to secreted antigens of *Mycobacterium tuberculosis. Immunobiology* 191:537–547, 1994.
3. Andersen P, Andersen AB, Sorensen AL, Nagai S: Recall of long-lived immunity to *Mycobacterium tuberculosis* infection in mice. *J Immunol* 154:3359–3372, 1995.
4. Ando M, Dannenberg AM Jr, Sugimoto M, Tepper BS: Histochemical studies relating the activation of macrophages to the intracellular destruction of tubercle bacilli. *Am J Pathol* 86:623–634, 1977.
5. Asnis LA, Gaspari AA: Cutaneous reactions to recombinant cytokine therapy. *J Am Acad Dermatol* 33:393–410, 1995.
6. Barnes PF, Bloch AB, Davidson PT, Snider, DE Jr: Tuberculosis in patients with human immunodeficiency virus infection. *New Engl J Med* 324:1644–1650, 1991.
7. Barnes PF, Mistry SD, Cooper CL, et al: Compartmentalization of a CD4$^+$ T-lymphocyte subpopulation in tuberculous pleuritis. *J Immunol* 142:1114–1119, 1989.
8. Biron CA, Gazzinelli RT: Effects of IL-12 on immune responses to microbial infections: A key mediator in regulating disease outcome. *Curr Opin Immunol* 7:485–496, 1995.
9. Canetti G: *The Tubercle Bacillus in the Pulmonary Lesion of Man.* New York, Springer, 1955.
10. Chan CHS, Lai K-N, Leung JCK, Lai CKW: T-lymphocyte activation in patients with active tuberculosis. *Am Rev Respir Dis* 144:458–460, 1991.
11. Chensue SW, Warmington K, Ruth J, et al: Cytokine responses during mycobacterial and schistosomal antigen-induced pulmonary granuloma formation. *Am J Pathol* 145:1105–1113, 1994.
12. Comstock GW: Identification of an effective vaccine against tuberculosis. *Am Rev Respir Dis* 138:479–480, 1988.
13. Converse PJ, Dannenberg AM Jr, Estep JE, et al: Cavitary tuberculosis produced in rabbits by aerosolized virulent tubercle bacilli. *Infect Immun* 64:4776–4787, 1996.
14. Cooper AM, Flynn JA: The protective immune response to *Mycobacterium tuberculosis. Curr Opin Immunol* 7:512–516, 1995.
15. Dannenberg AM Jr: Cellular hypersensitivity and cellular immunity in the pathogenesis of tuberculosis: Specificity, systemic and local nature, and associated macrophage enzymes. *Bacteriol Rev* 32:85–102, 1968.
16. Dannenberg AM Jr: Immunopathogenesis of pulmonary tuberculosis. *Hosp Pract (Off Ed)* 28:51–58, 1993.
17. Dannenberg AM Jr: Pathogenesis of tuberculosis: Native and acquired resistance in animals and humans, in *Microbiology 1984.* Washington, DC, American Society for Microbiology, 1984.
18. Dannenberg AM Jr, Rook GAW: Pathogenesis of pulmonary tuberculosis: An interplay of tissue-damaging and macrophage-activating immune responses—Dual mechanisms that control bacillary multiplication, in Bloom BR (ed), *Tuberculosis: Pathogenesis, Protection and Control.* Washington, DC, American Society for Microbiology, 1994, chap 27.
19. Dannenberg AM Jr, Sugimoto M: Liquefaction of caseous foci in tuberculosis. *Am Rev Respir Dis* 113:257–259, 1976.
20. Ellner JJ, Wallis RS: Immunologic aspects of mycobacterial infections. *Rev Infect Dis* 11 (Suppl 2):S455–S459, 1989.
21. Farhi DC, Mason UG, Horsburgh CR Jr: Pathologic findings in disseminated *Mycobacterium avium-intracellulare* infection. *Am J Clin Pathol* 85:67–72, 1986.
22. Flynn JAL, Goldstein MM, Triebold KJ, et al: IL-12 increases resistance of BALB/c mice to *Mycobacterium tuberculosis* infection. *J Immunol* 155:2515–2524, 1995.
23. Gangadharam PRJ: Mycobacterial dormancy. *Tubercle Lung Dis* 76:477–479, 1995.
24. Gobin J, Moore CH, Reeve JR Jr, et al: Iron acquisition by *Mycobacterium tuberculosis:* Isolation and characterization of a family of iron-binding exochelins. *Proc Natl Acad Sci USA* 23:92: 5189–5193, 1995.
25. Gumperz JE, Parham P: The enigma of the natural killer cell. *Nature* 378:245–248, 1995.
26. Hill AR, Somasundaram P, Brustein S, et al: Disseminated tuberculosis in the acquired immunodeficiency syndrome era. *Am Rev Respir Dis* 144:1164–1170, 1991.
27. Hirsch CS, Hussain R, Toossi Z, et al: Cross-modulation by transforming growth factor β in human tuberculosis: Suppression of antigen-driven blastogenesis and interferon γ production. *Proc Natl Acad Sci USA* 93:3193–3198, 1996.
28. Horsburgh CR Jr: *Mycobacterium avium* complex infection in the acquired immunodeficiency syndrome. *New Engl J Med* 324:1332–1338, 1991.
29. Ivanyi J: Molecular biology of natural resistance-associated macrophage protein. *Parasitol Today* 10:416–417, 1994.
30. Janeway CA Jr, Travers P: *Immunobiology: The Immune System in Health and Disease.* New York, Garland, 1994.
31. Kalayjian RC, Toossi Z, Tomashefski JF Jr, et al: Pulmonary disease due to infection by *Mycobacterium avium* complex in patients with AIDS. *Clin Infect Dis* 20:1186–1194, 1995.
32. Kaufmann SHE: Immunity to intracellular microbial pathogens. *Immunol Today* 16:338–342, 1995.
33. Laskin DL, Pendino KJ: Macrophages and inflammatory mediators in tissue injury. *Annu Rev Pharmacol Toxicol* 35:655–677, 1995.
34. Long ER: *The Chemistry and Chemotherapy of Tuberculosis,* 3d ed. Baltimore, Williams & Wilkins, 1958.
35. Luger TA, Schwarz T: The role of cytokines and neuroendocrine hormones in cutaneous immunity and inflammation. *Allergy* 50:292–302, 1995.
36. Lurie MB: *Resistance to Tuberculosis: Experimental Studies in Native and Acquired Defense Mechanisms.* Cambridge, MA, Harvard University Press, 1964.
37. Lurie MB, Zappasodi P, Tickner C: On the nature of genetic resistance to tuberculosis in the light of the host-parasite relationship in

natively resistant and susceptible rabbits. *Am Rev Tuberc Pulm Dis* 72:297–323, 1955.

38. Mackaness GB: The immunology of antituberculous immunity. *Am Rev Respir Dis* 97:337–344, 1968.

39. Marchevsky A, Damsker B, Gribetz A, et al: The spectrum of pathology in nontuberculous mycobacterial infections in open-lung biopsy specimens. *Am J Clin Pathol* 78:695–700, 1982.

40. Miller WT Jr: Spectrum of pulmonary nontuberculous mycobacterial infection. *Radiology* 191:343–350, 1994.

41. Mosmann TR, Sad S: The expanding universe of T-cell subsets: Th1, Th2 and more. *Immunol Today* 17:138–146, 1996.

42. Murray HW: Interferon-gamma, the activated macrophage, and host defense against microbial challenge. *Ann Intern Med* 108:595–608, 1988.

43. Nathan CF: Secretory products of macrophages. *J Clin Invest* 79: 319–326, 1987.

44. Pal PG, Horwitz MA: Immunization with extracellular proteins of *Mycobacterium tuberculosis* induces cell-mediated immune responses and substantial protective immunity in a guinea pig model of pulmonary tuberculosis. *Infect Immun* 60:4781–4792, 1994.

45. Poole JCF, Florey HW: Chronic inflammation and tuberculosis, in Florey HW (ed), *General Pathology,* 4th ed. Philadelphia, Saunders, 1970, pp 1183–1224.

46. Porcelli SA, Modlin RL: CD1 and the expanding universe of T-cell antigens. *J Immunol* 155:3709–3710, 1995.

47. Prince D, Peterson DD, Steiner RM, et al: Infection with *Mycobacterium avium* complex in patients without predisposing conditions. *New Engl J Med* 321:863–878, 1989.

48. Reid JD, Wolinsky E: Histopathology of lymphadenitis caused by atypical mycobacteria. *Am Rev Respir Dis* 99:8–12, 1969.

49. Rich AR: *The Pathogenesis of Tuberculosis,* 2d ed. Springfield, IL, Charles C Thomas, 1951.

50. Rohrbach MS, Williams DE: T-lymphocytes and pleural tuberculosis (editorial). *Chest* 89:473–474, 1986.

51. Scott P, Trinchieri G: The role of natural killer cells in host-parasite interactions. *Curr Opin Immunol* 7:34–40, 1995.

52. Shima K, Dannenberg, AM Jr, Ando M, et al: Macrophage accumulation, division, maturation, and digestive and microbicidal capacities in tuberculous lesions: I. Studies involving their incorporation of tritiated thymidine and their content of lysosomal enzymes and bacilli. *Am J Pathol* 67:159–180, 1972.

53. Stanford JL, Stanford CA: Immunotherapy of tuberculosis with *Mycobacterium vaccae* NCTC 11659. *Immunobiology* 191:555–563, 1994.

54. Suga M, Dannenberg AM Jr, Higuchi S: Macrophage functional heterogeneity *in vivo*: Macrolocal and microlocal macrophage activation, identified by double-staining tissue sections of BCG granulomas for pairs of enzymes. *Am J Pathol* 99:305–323, 1980.

55. Tomashefski JF Jr: Tuberculosis and atypical mycobacterial infections, in Saldana M (ed), *Pathology of Pulmonary Disease.* Philadelphia, JB Lippincott, 1994, pp 451–462.

56. Toossi Z, Sedor JR, Lapurga JP, et al: Expression of functional interleukin-2 receptors by peripheral blood monocytes from patients with active pulmonary tuberculosis. *J Clin Invest* 85:1777–1784, 1990.

57. Trinchieri G: Interleukin-12 and interferon-γ. Do they always go together? *Am J Pathol* 147:1534–1538, 1995.

58. Tsuda T, Dannenberg AM Jr, Ando M, et al: Mononuclear cell turnover in chronic inflammation: Studies on tritiated thymidine-labeled cells in blood, tuberculin traps, and dermal BCG lesions of rabbits. *Am J Pathol* 83:255–268, 1976.

59. Wallace RJ Jr, O'Brien R, Glassroth J, et al: Diagnosis and treatment of disease caused by nontuberculous mycobacteria. *Am Rev Respir Dis* 142:940–953, 1990.

60. Wolinsky E: Mycobacterial diseases other than tuberculosis. *Clin Infect Dis* 15:1–12, 1992.

61. Yamamura Y, Ogawa Y, Maeda H, Yamamura Y: Prevention of tuberculous cavity formation by desensitization with tuberculin-active peptide. *Am Rev Respir Dis* 109:594–601, 1974.

CHAPTER 161

SCREENING FOR TUBERCULOSIS AND TUBERCULOSIS INFECTION IN HIGH-RISK POPULATIONS*

Alan B. Bloch

Tuberculosis (TB) is caused by bacteria (*Mycobacterium tuberculosis* complex, which includes *M. tuberculosis, M. bovis,* and *M. africanum*) transmitted from an infectious source to susceptible persons primarily through the air (e.g., by coughing).[1] Most infected persons do not experience clinical illness, but are usually asymptomatic and noninfectious. The only evidence of infection may be a reaction to a tuberculin skin test. Infection can persist for years, however, and infected persons can remain at risk for developing clinical TB, especially if the immune system becomes impaired. The estimated number of persons having latent TB infection in the United States ranges from 10 million to 15 million (CDC, unpublished data).

Because of a higher prevalence of infection or a higher risk of disease for any given prevalence of infection among certain groups, the incidence of TB may be higher among these groups than among the total population. Screening and preventive therapy programs are important for persons in these high-risk groups.

PRIORITY OF SCREENING AMONG TB PREVENTION AND CONTROL ACTIVITIES

Three basic strategies are critical to the prevention and control of TB. The first priority is identifying and completely treating all persons who have active TB.[2,3] The second priority is contact investigation (i.e., finding and evaluating persons who have had contact with TB patients, determining whether they have TB

*Adapted from *Morbidity and Mortality Weekly Report,* 44 (RR-11), 19–34, 1995 (Outline added); Recommendations of the Advisory Council for the Elimination of Tuberculosis; U.S. Department of Health and Human Services, Public Health Service, Centers for Disease Control and Prevention (CDC).

infection or disease, and treating them appropriately).[4] Contact investigations are important for identifying persons who have active TB and infected persons at high risk for developing TB. The third priority is screening populations at high risk for TB to locate persons infected with TB and giving complete therapy to prevent the infection from progressing to active, contagious disease.[3,5] This screening also may identify cases of active disease.

Although screening high-risk populations for TB infection and providing preventive therapy are crucial to achieving the nation's goal of eliminating TB,[6] completion of TB therapy and contact investigation should have priority over screening. Decisions to screen particular groups should be based on local epidemiologic data and made in consultation with local health jurisdictions to ensure appropriate follow-up, evaluation, and management of persons with TB infection or disease. Health-care agencies or other facilities should consult with the local health department before starting a skin testing program, to ensure that adequate provisions are made for the evaluation and treatment of persons whose tuberculin skin test results are positive. Tuberculin skin testing programs that identify infected persons without current disease should be undertaken only if the diagnostic evaluation and a course of prescribed therapy can be initiated and completed.

Because most state and local TB control programs that report high TB morbidity have inadequate resources to screen all persons in high-risk groups and treat persons who are infected, participation of other health-care providers in screening and preventive treatment activities is important. These health-care providers can augment the limited resources of health departments by conducting appropriate screening efforts. This collaboration will necessitate additional efforts to train health-care workers in the administration, reading, and interpretation of the tuberculin skin test and in the appropriate use of preventive therapy. Priorities for screening activities should be determined by assessment of available resources and the probability of infection and disease among groups in the community.

Groups that have the highest priority in all areas of the country include contacts of persons who have suspected or confirmed TB and patients who have been infected with the human immunodeficiency virus (HIV) or are at risk for HIV infection. In particular areas of the country, groups at high risk may also include persons who inject illicit drugs, persons who have certain medical risk factors, foreign-born persons recently arrived from countries with a high incidence or prevalence of TB, and residents of congregate settings where risk for transmitting *M. tuberculosis* is increased (e.g., correctional facilities, long-term care facilities, and homeless shelters). Screening persons in low-risk groups is not likely to be cost-effective and should be discontinued.

HIGH-RISK GROUPS

Based on published reports in the medical literature and CDC surveillance data, the Advisory Council for the Elimination of Tuberculosis recommends that the following groups be screened for TB and TB infection:

1. Close contacts (those sharing the same household or other enclosed environments) of persons known or suspected to have TB.

2. Persons infected with HIV.

3. Persons who inject illicit drugs or other locally identified high-risk substance abusers (e.g., crack cocaine users).

4. Persons who have medical risk factors known to increase the risk for disease if infection occurs (see "Persons with Other Medical Risk Factors").

5. Residents and employees of high-risk congregate settings (e.g., correctional institutions, nursing homes, mental institutions, other long-term residential facilities, and shelters for the homeless).

6. Health-care workers who serve high-risk clients.

7. Foreign-born persons, including children, recently arrived (within 5 years) from countries that have a high TB incidence or prevalence.

8. Some medically underserved, low-income populations.

9. High-risk racial or ethnic minority populations, as defined locally.

10. Infants, children, and adolescents exposed to adults in high-risk categories.

Flexibility is needed in defining high-priority groups for screening. The changing epidemiology of TB indicates that the risk for TB among groups currently considered high priority may decrease over time, and groups currently not identified as at risk subsequently may be considered as high priority. Local public health officials should identify community groups among whom TB and transmission of infection occur. Identification of these groups requires collecting and analyzing data on newly reported cases available as part of TB surveillance (e.g., residence, occupation, race/ethnicity, country of origin, and status of HIV infection, injected-drug use, homelessness, and congregate settings); data not routinely collected and analyzed (e.g., indicators of socioeconomic status); and data from tuberculin screening programs (e.g., at correctional institutions and health-care facilities). These data will enable health departments and other local facilities to target screening and treatment programs to locally defined high-risk populations and areas.

Using surveillance information, local or state TB programs should take the lead in determining groups to be screened. Responsibility for conducting screening will vary, depending on local circumstances. For some groups, the local health department should conduct the screening. For others, the health department should discuss the need for screening with other appropriate persons (e.g., correctional facility staff, hospital infection control officers, and shelter operators) and offer assistance in training, evaluation, and, if necessary and possible, provision of supplies. In some areas, gaining the commitment of private health-care providers and community health centers to screen and provide follow-up for the high-risk patients they serve will be vital.

GENERAL COMMENTS ON SCREENING

Screening persons other than members of high-risk groups is not recommended because screening low-risk persons diverts resources from high-priority activities and because many positive test results in low-risk persons do not represent TB infection. The goal of screening programs must be clearly defined: screening is usually conducted to identify infected persons who are at high risk for disease and who would benefit from preventive therapy or to find persons who have clinical disease and need treatment. Screening programs also can provide epidemiologic data for assessing TB and its trends in a community, data for assessing the value of continued screening, and baseline data to help with assessment if subsequent exposure occurs (e.g., for nursing home residents and employees in some occupations). Screening programs should not be undertaken unless necessary facilities for patient evaluation and treatment are identified and made available and unless patients found to be positive are likely to complete preventive therapy.

To the extent possible, members of high-risk groups and their health-care providers should be active in the design, implementation, and promotion of screening programs.[6–8] Implementation may be enhanced by use of health department or other staff (including trained volunteers) who have linguistic and cultural familiarity with the population at risk.

SCREENING METHODS

Tuberculin skin testing is the standard method for identifying persons infected with *M. tuberculosis*.[1] The Mantoux test (the intracutaneous administration of 5 units of purified protein derivative [PPD] tuberculin) is best for detecting infection. Because they are less specific than the Mantoux test, multiple-puncture devices should not be used to screen high-risk populations.[9]

Screening for disease rather than infection may be more appropriate in some circumstances (e.g., when the tuberculin skin test results may be unreliable, when administering and reading the test or following up infected persons for preventive therapy may be impractical, when the risk for disease is high, or when the consequences of an undiagnosed case may be severe). Chest radiography is the preferred screening method when the objective is to identify persons who have current pulmonary TB and when preventive therapy for infected persons is not the primary goal (e.g., in high-turnover jails or in some homeless shelters). In these screening programs, patients who have signs and symptoms suggesting pulmonary or pleural TB (e.g., cough of more than 2 weeks' duration) should have a standard posteroanterior chest radiograph, regardless of the tuberculin skin test result. Although TB produces certain radiographic abnormalities more frequently than others, almost any form of pulmonary radiographic abnormality may result from TB, especially in immunosuppressed persons.[1]

THE TUBERCULIN SKIN TEXT

A detailed review of the tuberculin skin test has been published recently and is summarized here.[10] Tuberculin skin test results should be evaluated within the context of each patient's epidemiologic and environmental potential for infection.[11]

Sensitivity, Specificity, and Positive Predictive Value of the Tuberculin Skin Test

Although the tuberculin skin test is now the only method for detecting *M. tuberculosis* infection, the test is neither 100 percent sensitive nor 100 percent specific. Sensitivity is a test's ability to correctly identify persons who have a condition (e.g., those infected with *M. tuberculosis*). Specificity is a test's ability to correctly identify persons who do not have a condition. In populations with a high prevalence of infection with nontuberculous mycobacteria or vaccination with bacille Calmette-Guérin (BCG), the specificity of the tuberculin test will be low.

The positive predictive value of the tuberculin test is also variable. Positive predictive value reflects the ability of a positive test to identify persons who have a condition (i.e., the probability that a condition is present when the test is positive). As the prevalence of TB infection in the population decreases, the positive predictive value of the tuberculin test also decreases. The prevalence of infection among the total adult population in the United States is an estimated 5 to 10 percent (CDC, unpublished data). Among populations residing in areas where cross-reactions caused by nontuberculous mycobacteria are common, the positive predictive value of the tuberculin test is low if a cutoff of greater than or equal to 10 mm is used to define a positive test.

Interpreting Tuberculin Skin Test Results

The criteria endorsed by the American Thoracic Society (ATS) and CDC for a positive tuberculin skin test result are intended to increase the likelihood that persons at high risk for TB will be candidates for preventive therapy and that persons having tuberculin reactions not caused by *M. tuberculosis* will not receive unnecessary diagnostic evaluation or treatment.[1,3,4]

For persons who have had recent close contact with a person who has active TB and for those whose chest radiographic findings suggest TB, skin test reactions are likely to represent infection with *M. tuberculosis*. Persons infected with HIV may have a limited ability to respond to tuberculin, even if they are infected with tubercle bacilli. These groups are at high risk for TB. Thus, to ensure that persons infected with TB are evaluated and appropriately treated, the sensitivity provided by a greater than or equal to 5-mm cutoff for a positive test is appropriate for these groups (Table 161-1). Although persons with HIV infection have a decreased ability to respond to tuberculin, some severely immunosuppressed persons infected with tubercle bacilli may still manifest a positive reaction and benefit from tuberculin skin testing.

Other factors (e.g., certain medical conditions or injected-drug use without simultaneous HIV infection) moderately increase the risk for active TB. A reaction of greater than or equal to 10 mm should be considered positive for these groups (Table 161-1). This cutoff is also appropriate for other groups: persons born in countries with a high prevalence or incidence of TB; medically underserved, low-income populations; residents and employees of most correctional institutions and nursing homes; health-care workers in high-risk settings (as defined in CDC guidelines); and, because of the increased risk for severe disease, children less than 4 years of age.

Routine screening is not recommended for populations at low risk for infection with *M. tuberculosis*. If these persons are tested, however, a higher cutoff of greater than or equal to 15 mm is recommended (Table 161-1).

TABLE 161-1

Summary of Interpretation of Tuberculin Skin Test Results

An induration of ≥5 mm is classified as positive in the following:
    Persons who have had recent close contact with persons who have active TB
    Persons who have human immunodeficiency virus (HIV) infection or risk factors for HIV infection but unknown HIV status
    Persons who have fibrotic chest radiographs consistent with healed TB
An induration of ≥10 mm is classified as positive in all persons who do not meet any of the above criteria but who belong to one or more of the following groups having high risk for TB
    Injected-drug users known to be HIV seronegative
    Persons who have other medical conditions that have been reported to increase the risk for progressing from latent TB infection to active TB, including diabetes mellitus, conditions requiring prolonged high-dose corticosteroid therapy and other immunosuppressive therapy (including bone marrow and organ transplantation), chronic renal failure, some hematologic disorders (e.g., leukemias and lymphomas), other specific malignancies (e.g., carcinoma of the head or neck), weight loss of ≥10% below ideal body weight, silicosis, gastrectomy, jejunoileal bypass
    Residents and employees of high-risk congregate settings: prisons and jails, nursing homes and other long-term facilities for the elderly, health-care facilities (including some residential mental health facilities), and homeless shelters
    Foreign-born persons recently arrived (i.e., within the last 5 years) from countries having a high prevalence or incidence of TB
    Some medically underserved, low-income populations, including migrant farm workers and homeless persons
    High-risk racial or ethnic minority populations, as defined locally
    Children <4 years of age or infants, children, and adolescents exposed to adults in high-risk categories
An induration of ≥15 mm is classified as positive in persons who do not meet any of the above criteria

False-Positive Reactions

A small percentage of tuberculin reactions may be caused by errors in administering the test or in reading results. However, false-positive results are more commonly attributable to the presence in tuberculin of antigens shared with other mycobacteria. The potential sources of cross-reactions caused by these antigens are infection with nontuberculous mycobacteria and vaccination with BCG. Distinguishing clearly between reactions caused by infection with *M. tuberculosis* and those caused by other mycobacteria is difficult. The larger the induration, however, the greater is the likelihood that the reaction represents infection with *M. tuberculosis*. Similarly, clearly distinguishing between a tuberculin skin test reaction caused by infection with *M. tuberculosis* and a reaction caused by BCG vaccination is difficult. The probability that a skin test reaction results from infection with *M. tuberculosis* rather than from BCG vaccination increases (1) as the size of the reaction increases, (2) when the patient is a contact of a person who has TB (especially if that person has infected others), (3) when a family history of TB exists or when the patient's country of origin has a high incidence or prevalence of TB, and (4) as the interval between vaccination and tuberculin testing increases (because vaccination-induced reactivity wanes over time and is unlikely to persist for more than 10 years).[12,13] A history of BCG vaccination is not a contraindication to skin testing.

False-Negative Reactions

False-negative tuberculin skin test reactions have many potential causes.[1] Nonresponsiveness to delayed-type hypersensitivity–inducing antigens like tuberculin is common among persons with impaired immunity (e.g., HIV-infected persons). Delayed-type hypersensitivity can be assessed with skin test antigens such as tetanus toxoid, mumps, and *Candida*. Most healthy persons are sensitized to these antigens. However, the scientific basis for anergy testing is tenuous.[14] Most skin test antigens used for anergy testing have no standardization. Thus, anergy testing is usually not part of screening for TB infection.

All HIV-infected persons should be tuberculin tested.[15,16] Those who are tuberculin positive (greater than or equal to 5 mm) should be evaluated for TB disease and placed on appropriate curative or preventive therapy. Preventive therapy should be administered to tuberculin-positive, HIV-infected persons, regardless of age. If they are at high risk for TB, persons failing to react to tuberculin may be evaluated for anergy,[17] although the lack of standardization of anergy testing practices should be considered.

Booster Phenomenon and Two-Step Tuberculin Skin Testing

Periodic use of the tuberculin skin test is valuable for the surveillance of tuberculin-negative persons at risk for exposure to *M. tuberculosis*. Repeated testing of uninfected persons does not sensitize them to tuberculin. However, delayed-type hypersensitivity resulting from mycobacterial infection or BCG vaccination may gradually wane with years. Although subsequent initial skin test results may be negative, the stimulus of a first test may boost or increase the size of the reaction to a second test administered 1 week to 1 year later and thus may suggest an apparent—but false—tuberculin conversion.

Although the booster phenomenon may occur at any age, its frequency increases with age and is highest among persons more than 55 years of age and among persons who have had prior BCG vaccination.[18] When tuberculin skin testing of adults is repeated periodically, as in employee-health or institutional screening programs, an initial two-step approach can reduce the likelihood that a boosted reaction will be misinterpreted as the sign of a recent infection. If the first tuberculin test result is negative, a second 5-tuberculin unit (TU) test should be administered 1 to 3 weeks later. A positive second result probably indicates boosting from a past infection or prior BCG vaccination. Persons having a boosted reaction should be classified as reactors, not converters. If the second result is negative, the person is probably uninfected, and a positive reaction to subsequent tests indicates a true tuberculin skin test conversion (see "Definition of a Tuberculin Skin Test Conversion").

Because of problems with continued cross-reactions with other mycobacteria, the specificity of the tuberculin test is less when serial skin testing is performed than when a single test is administered. Thus, serial skin testing programs tend to overestimate the incidence of new TB infection in the tested population. Because of this potential for overestimation of incidence, serial skin testing programs should be targeted to populations at high risk for continued exposure to infectious TB.

Definition of a Tuberculin Skin Test Conversion

Recent tuberculin skin test converters are considered at high risk. An increase in induration of greater than or equal to 10 mm within a 2-year period is classified as a conversion to a positive test among persons less than 35 years of age. An increase in induration of greater than or equal to 15 mm within a 2-year period is classified as a conversion for persons at least 35 years of age. Regardless of age, for employees in facilities where a person who has TB poses a hazard to many susceptible persons (e.g., health-care facilities, schools, and child-care facilities), an increase of greater than or equal to 10-mm induration should be considered positive.

Tuberculin Testing During Pregnancy

Studies in which the same patients were tested during and after pregnancy have demonstrated that pregnancy has no effect on cutaneous tuberculin hypersensitivity. Tuberculin skin testing is considered valid and safe throughout pregnancy. No teratogenic effects of testing during pregnancy have been documented.[19]

RECOMMENDATIONS FOR SPECIFIC HIGH-RISK GROUPS

Contacts of Persons with Infectious TB

Because the risk for infection and disease is particularly high among close contacts of persons with TB, these persons should be identified promptly (usually within 3 days) and examined soon (usually within 7 days) after identification of the potentially infectious patient.[4,6] State and local health departments should work with local health-care providers to ensure completion of these monitoring activities. Prompt notification of state and local agencies about suspected or newly diagnosed and potentially infectious cases is critical for contact investigation.

Persons with HIV Infection

HIV infection is the strongest risk factor yet identified for the development of TB disease in persons with TB infection.[20–23] All HIV-infected persons should receive a PPD-tuberculin skin test (5-TU, PPD by the Mantoux method).[15,16]

Tuberculin testing for persons infected with HIV should be conducted in settings where HIV-infected persons or those at risk for HIV infection receive care. Administrators should ensure that the recommended screening is implemented and that prompt follow-up, evaluation, and treatment occur. Because tuberculin skin test results are less reliable as CD4+ lymphocyte counts decline, screening should be completed as soon as possible after HIV infection occurs. HIV-infected patients at high risk for continuing exposure to patients who have TB should be screened periodically for TB infection. If they have TB symptoms or are exposed to a patient with pulmonary TB, HIV-infected persons should be evaluated promptly for TB. Because active disease can develop rapidly in HIV-infected persons, the highest priority for contact investigation should be given to persons potentially coinfected with HIV and TB.

Persons Who Inject Drugs

Because they are at high risk for TB and HIV infection, the priority for screening is high for persons who inject illicit drugs.[16,20–22,24,25] Drug treatment programs and other settings that provide care for persons who inject drugs should skin-test injected-drug users. If further evaluation and case management are necessary, adequate referral mechanisms should be in place. Coordination of these activities with local alcohol and other drug abuse treatment programs should be encouraged. Priority should be given to screening in facilities that are able to provide on-site, directly observed preventive therapy for 6 to 12 months to persons who have TB infection (e.g., clients on methadone maintenance treatment programs or residential treatment programs).

Persons with Other Medical Risk Factors

Health-care providers should administer tuberculin tests to all patients who have medical risk factors that substantially increase the risk for TB.[3,22] These patients should be screened in settings where they receive primary or subspecialty care (e.g., infectious disease, immunology, endocrinology, hematology/oncology, nephrology, rheumatology, pulmonology, and gastroenterology) or on admission to a hospital. These medical risk factors include: HIV infection, diabetes mellitus, conditions requiring prolonged high-dose corticosteroid therapy and other immunosuppressive therapy (including bone marrow and organ transplantation), chronic renal failure, some hematologic disorders (e.g., leukemias and lymphomas), other specific malignancies (e.g., carcinoma of the head or neck), weight of greater than or equal to 10 percent below ideal body weight, silicosis, gastrectomy, and jejunoileal bypass.

In addition, persons who have an abnormal chest radiograph showing fibrotic lesions consistent with old, healed TB should be skin tested. Regardless of age, persons who have a positive skin test result and parenchymal lung scarring are at high risk for TB if they have not received TB treatment or preventive therapy.

Residents and Employees of High-Risk Congregate Settings

High-risk environments are settings where persons who have infectious TB are more likely to live, environmental characteristics (e.g., type of ventilation and size) are conducive to transmission, and many susceptible persons at risk for prolonged exposure to potentially infectious patients may be located. These environments include prisons and jails,[26,27] nursing homes and other long-term facilities for the elderly,[28] health-care facilities,[29] homeless shelters,[30] and residential settings for HIV-infected persons.[31] Persons working in these settings should be educated about the risk for transmission, the signs and symptoms of TB, and proper procedures for minimizing the risk for transmitting TB infection. Clients and employees should be tuberculin tested on admission or initial employment.

Residents and Employees of Prisons and Jails

Recommendations for screening, treatment, and prevention in correctional facilities advise that, on entry, all inmates should be screened for TB symptoms with a standardized interview process.[26,27] Persons who have symptoms suggesting pulmonary TB should be immediately isolated and evaluated for active TB. Initial screening of inmates may vary, depending on each inmate's length of stay and on an assessment of the risk for transmission of TB infection in the facility.

In long-term facilities, tuberculin skin test screening of all inmates without a documented positive skin test result should be mandatory. If boosting is common among the population served by the facility, two-step skin testing should be considered. Inmates who have HIV infection and those at risk for HIV infection but whose HIV status is unknown should have a chest radiograph as part of the initial screening, regardless of skin test results.

In short-term facilities serving high-risk populations, tuberculin skin test screening is generally not feasible, but is recommended for inmates who will remain in custody for at least 14 days. Inmates who have HIV infection and those at risk for HIV infection but whose HIV status is unknown should have a chest radiograph as part of initial screening, regardless of skin test status. In some large jails, officials should consider using on-site chest radiography to screen all inmates (short- and long-term) for TB. In short-term facilities serving low-risk populations, screening inmates may be limited to screening for symptoms, provided that arrangements are made with a collaborating facility to receive inmates exhibiting symptoms.

Tuberculin skin test screening also should be mandatory for all correctional staff in short- or long-term facilities. Staff should be informed that if they are immunosuppressed, they should consult a health-care provider for appropriate follow-up and screening for TB.

Medical units within correctional facilities should conduct a thorough risk assessment and follow recommendations for prevention of transmission of TB infection in health-care facilities.[29] Correctional authorities have primary responsibility for implementing these programs, but health departments should assist in program planning and training as well as regulating, advising, monitoring, and evaluating TB control activities in correctional facilities.

Residents and Employees of Nursing Homes/Facilities for the Elderly

Because TB case rates increase with age among all racial and ethnic groups and both sexes, screening for TB in facilities providing long-term care to the elderly is recommended.[28] The incidence of disease is two to seven times higher among nursing home residents in some areas than among demographically similar persons in other settings. Studies indicate that unsuspected transmission of *M. tuberculosis* in nursing homes/facilities presents a risk to residents and workers.[32,33] Residents should be screened for TB infection on admission by use of the two-step skin testing method. Screening with chest radiographs alone is insufficient. Although few residents will be candidates for preventive therapy, baseline test results are essential to interpretation of subsequent tests if an acute exposure occurs. The two-step method also should be used for baseline screening of employees. Testing should be repeated in the event of exposure.

Residents and Workers at Homeless Shelters

Screening to find cases of active TB among the homeless consists of a chest radiograph (and possibly a sputum smear and culture) to determine current disease.[30] Tuberculin skin testing programs identifying infected persons who do not have current disease should be undertaken only if the diagnostic evaluation and course of preventive therapy can be initiated and completed. A special effort should be made to identify homeless persons coinfected with TB and HIV infection and to provide directly observed preventive therapy. Unless a shelter has its own health-care staff, the local government or a government-funded agency should assume responsibility for conducting screening programs for the homeless.

Health-Care Workers

Transmission of *M. tuberculosis* is a recognized risk in health-care facilities.[29] Transmission is most likely to occur from patients who have unrecognized pulmonary or laryngeal TB, who are not on effective anti-TB therapy, and who have not been placed in TB isolation. Recent TB outbreaks in health-care facilities, including outbreaks of multidrug-resistant TB, have created heightened concern about nosocomial transmission. Increases of TB in some geographic areas are related to the high risk for TB among immunosuppressed persons infected with HIV. Transmission of *M. tuberculosis* to HIV-infected persons is of particular concern because, if infected with TB, these persons are at high risk for the rapid development of active TB. Thus, health-care facilities should be particularly alert to the need for preventing transmission of *M. tuberculosis* in settings where persons who have HIV infection receive care or work.

Health administrators and infection control departments in hospitals are responsible for ensuring the implementation of these recommendations. Implementing an effective TB control program requires risk assessment; early identification, isolation, and complete treatment of infectious TB patients; effective engineering controls; an appropriate respiratory protection program; and education, counseling, screening, and evaluation for health-care workers.

The Foreign-Born

TB is a problem among persons who arrive in the United States from countries with a high prevalence or incidence of TB (most countries in Africa, Asia, and Latin America).[34–37] Foreign-born persons at risk include immigrants (documented and undocumented), refugees, and some migrant workers and students. Because disease rates among the foreign-born are highest in the first few years after arrival in the United States, efforts should be made to screen new immigrants. Culturally and linguistically sensitive evaluation and treatment programs should be provided to help ensure a successful treatment outcome. Services should not be denied because of a real or perceived undocumented immigration status.

Other High-Incidence Population Groups

The incidence of TB is closely related to socioeconomic status; higher rates occur among persons in low-income groups.[38] Special control strategies aimed at these low-income groups are needed. In addition, community leaders from high-risk populations and service providers (e.g., health, welfare, and housing) for these groups should be engaged in planning and implementing programs.[8]

Implementation of TB prevention and control efforts among lower socioeconomic groups presents special problems because these groups usually have less access to care, are more likely to have coexisting diseases, lack adequate shelter and transportation, and encounter more obstacles to treatment and health-care delivery. However, screening programs have demonstrated success in reaching these groups.[39,40]

Screening for TB infection among certain occupational groups may occur at the worksite or other community sites. Screening migrant farm workers for TB infection is best conducted near home sites rather than at temporary work locations, so that preventive therapy can be completed more easily for those who are infected.[41] High-risk groups also may be screened whenever they have access to health care.

Persons Who Use Alcohol and Other Noninjected Drugs

Because many persons who use alcohol and other noninjected drugs are members of high-risk groups (e.g., HIV-infected persons, the homeless, residents of correctional facilities, and medically underserved, low-income persons), they should be included in screening activities if they also belong to a high-risk group. Because persons who use alcohol and other noninjected drugs may be at risk for repeated exposure to others who have TB, a risk assessment and, if necessary, screening for TB infection should be administered on admission to a treatment program and on an annual basis, unless these persons are known to be tuberculin positive. Screening is not recommended for persons who use alcohol and other noninjected drugs but who are not members of high-risk groups, because this screening diverts resources from higher-priority activities.

RECOMMENDATIONS FOR SCREENING CHILDREN AND ADOLESCENTS

Although children in high-risk groups or those exposed to adults in high-risk groups may benefit from screening, most children are not members of high-risk groups. Mass or individual screening of children at low risk is not recommended, because screening persons at low risk for TB infection diverts resources from higher-priority activities and identifies few infected children.[42,43] In addition, the reactions in low-risk children are often false positive.

School-based screening for TB infection among children was started in the 1950s when infection and disease rates were higher than at present. The major purpose of school testing is to identify infected children who can be treated before the infection progresses to infectious TB during adolescence or adulthood. Because broad-based school testing entails screening large numbers of low-risk children and because most children who have TB are preschool age, generalized school screening as a public health measure is an ineffective method of detecting or preventing cases of childhood TB and should be discontinued.[43]

Well-conducted contact tracing of infectious cases and refugee or immigration testing are more efficient methods than nonselective school-based testing for detecting children who have TB infection. However, targeted testing of high-risk children should be encouraged and may be conducted in school.[44] Before any testing program for children is implemented, arrangements for evaluation and treatment of children who test positive should be in place.

REPEAT SCREENING OF PERSONS AT CONTINUING RISK FOR EXPOSURE

The need for repeat skin testing should be determined from the likelihood of continued exposure to infectious TB. All tuberculin-negative persons should be retested if they are exposed to an infectious person. In some institutional and group-living environments (e.g., hospitals, prisons, nursing homes, and shelters for the homeless), the risk for exposure is enough to justify repeat testing at regular intervals. The frequency of repeat testing depends on the degree of risk for exposure, as determined by locally generated data. To assist in making these decisions, local facilities should compile and analyze their epidemiologic and programmatic data.

ROLE OF HEALTH DEPARTMENTS

In conjunction with local providers serving high-risk populations, health departments should assist in the development, implementation, and evaluation of TB screening programs appropriate for their communities by participating in specific activities:

Establishing Priorities for Prevention and Control Activities Screening for TB infection should not be given preference over higher-priority activities, especially complete treatment of patients with TB or TB/HIV infection as well as prompt, effective contact investigation.

Determining Priorities for Screening Activities This determination should be made from evaluation of available resources, the probability of infection and disease among groups in the community, and the ability to ensure that persons infected with TB will complete preventive therapy. Groups with the highest screening priorities include contacts of persons suspected or confirmed to have TB and patients having HIV infection.

Reviewing Epidemiologic and Programmatic Data to Identify Additional Groups for Whom Screening Programs Should Be Developed This review includes assessing the incidence, prevalence, and sociodemographic characteristics of persons with TB or TB infection; identifying high-risk groups and settings to determine whether a need for screening is indicated; designing tuberculin screening programs to reach the high-risk groups in communities; and ensuring completion of preventive therapy.

Identifying and Establishing Working Relationships with Persons, Facilities, and Agencies Providing Health-Care Services to High-Risk Populations These service providers should be assisted in the development, implementation, and evaluation of screening programs appropriate to the needs of the community. The decision to initiate a skin testing program for a high-risk group should be based primarily on the ability of the TB control program and health-care providers to provide adequate preventive therapy services (i.e., tuberculin skin testing, reading and interpreting the tests, evaluating persons who have positive results, initiating preventive therapy when appropriate, monitoring patients for adverse reactions, and ensuring that patients complete preventive therapy). To be effective, the plan for evaluation and treatment should be developed before testing begins.

Assisting Health-Care Providers Who Serve High-Risk Groups These providers should be assisted in providing screening services, evaluating data from screening programs to determine program effectiveness, and recommending appropriate future screening activities.

Providing Support for Staff Training Staff should be trained to perform, read, and record results of tuberculin skin tests; evaluate positive tuberculin reactors for clinical TB and preventive therapy; provide preventive therapy and monitor for adherence and adverse drug reactions; and educate clients regarding the need for preventive therapy. The health department or facility may certify staff completing this training.

Identifying Medical Consultants Having Expertise in TB Patient Management These consultants should be able to assist in managing persons who have TB or are suspected to have TB, their contacts, and persons receiving preventive therapy.

Arranging Referrals and Monitoring Upon request, assistance should be provided in making arrangements for referring and monitoring persons who have clinical TB or adverse drug reactions while on preventive therapy.

Reviewing Screening Activities Periodic assessments of screening activities are needed to examine the effectiveness of identifying infected persons and of ensuring that these persons complete preventive therapy.

Evaluating Screening Programs Regular assessments of screening programs are needed to determine their effectiveness. Recommendations for continuing or discontinuing screening programs should be made on the basis of their effectiveness.

REFERENCES

1. American Thoracic Society/CDC: Diagnostic standards and classification of tuberculosis. *Am Rev Respir Dis* 142:725–735, 1990.
2. CDC: Initial therapy for tuberculosis in the era of multidrug resistance: Recommendations of the Advisory Council for the Elimination of Tuberculosis. *MMWR* 42(No. RR-7), 1993.
3. American Thoracic Society/CDC: Treatment of tuberculosis and tuberculosis infection in adults and children. *Am J Respir Crit Care Med* 149:1359–1374, 1994.
4. American Thoracic Society/CDC: Control of tuberculosis in the United States. *Am Rev Respir Dis* 146:1623–1633, 1992.
5. CDC: The use of preventive therapy for tuberculous infection in the United States: Recommendations of the Advisory Committee for Elimination of Tuberculosis. *MMWR* 39 (No. RR-8):9–12, 1990.
6. CDC: A strategic plan for the elimination of tuberculosis in the United States. *MMWR* 38(No. S-3), 1989.
7. CDC: Essential components of a tuberculosis program: Recommendations of the Advisory Council for the Elimination of Tuberculosis. *MMWR* 44(No. RR-11):1–16, 1995.
8. CDC: Prevention and control of tuberculosis in U.S. communities with at-risk minority populations: Recommendations of the Advisory Council for the Elimination of Tuberculosis. *MMWR* 41(No. RR-5):1–11, 1992.
9. Starke JR, Jacobs RF, Jereb J: Resurgence of tuberculosis in children. *J Pediatr* 120:839–855, 1992.
10. Huebner RE, Schein MF, Bass JB Jr: The tuberculin skin test. *Clin Infect Dis* 17:968–975, 1993.
11. Sbarbaro JA: Tuberculin test: A re-emphasis on clinical judgement (editorial). *Am Rev Respir Dis* 132:177–178, 1985.
12. Snider DE Jr: Bacille Calmette-Guérin vaccinations and tuberculin skin tests. *JAMA* 253:3438–3439, 1985.
13. CDC: Use of BCG vaccines in the control of tuberculosis: A joint statement by the ACIP and the Advisory Committee for Elimination of Tuberculosis. *MMWR* 37:663–664, 669–675, 1988.
14. Caiaffa WT, Graham NMH, Galai N, et al: Instability of delayed-type hypersensitivity skin test anergy in human immunodeficiency virus infection. *Arch Intern Med* 155:2111–2117, 1995.
15. CDC: USPHS/IDSA guidelines for the prevention of opportunistic infections in persons infected with human immunodeficiency virus: A summary. *MMWR* 44(No. RR-8), 1995.
16. CDC: Tuberculosis and human immunodeficiency virus infection: Recommendations of the Advisory Committee for the Elimination of Tuberculosis (ACET). *MMWR* 38:236–238, 243–250, 1989.
17. CDC: Purified protein derivative (PPD)–tuberculin anergy and HIV infection: Guidelines for anergy testing and management of anergic persons at risk of tuberculosis. *MMWR* 40 (No. RR-5):27–33, 1991.
18. Sepulveda RL, Ferrer X, Latrach C, Sorensen RU: The influence of Calmette-Guérin bacillus immunization on the booster effect of

tuberculin testing in healthy young adults. *Am Rev Respir Dis* 142:24–28, 1990.

19. Snider D: Pregnancy and tuberculosis. *Chest* 86(Suppl):10S–13S, 1984.

20. Selwyn PA, Hartel D, Lewis VA, et al: A prospective study of the risk of tuberculosis among intravenous drug users with human immunodeficiency virus infection. *New Engl J Med* 320:545–550, 1989.

21. Selwyn PA, Sckell BM, Alcabes P, et al: High risk of active tuberculosis in HIV-infected drug users with cutaneous anergy. *JAMA* 268:504–509, 1992.

22. Rieder HL, Cauthen GM, Comstock GW, Snider DE Jr: Epidemiology of tuberculosis in the United States. *Epidemiol Rev* 11:79–98, 1989.

23. Antonucci G, Girardi E, Raviglione MC, Ippolito G, Gruppo Italiano di Studio Tubercolosi e AIDS (GISTA): Risk factors for tuberculosis in HIV-infected persons: A prospective cohort study. *JAMA* 274:143–148, 1995.

24. Reichman LB, Felton CP, Edsall JR: Drug dependence, a possible new risk factor for tuberculosis disease. *Arch Intern Med* 139:337–339, 1979.

25. Braun MM, Byers RH, Heyward WL, et al: Acquired immunodeficiency syndrome and extrapulmonary tuberculosis in the United States. *Arch Intern Med* 150:1913–1916, 1990.

26. CDC: Prevention and control of tuberculosis in correctional institutions: Recommendations of the Advisory Committee for the Elimination of Tuberculosis. *MMWR* 38:313–320, 325, 1989.

27. CDC: Prevention and control of tuberculosis in correctional facilities: Recommendations of the Advisory Council for the Elimination of Tuberculosis. *MMWR* 45 (No. RR-8), 1996.

28. CDC: Prevention and control of tuberculosis in facilities providing long-term care to the elderly: Recommendations of the Advisory Committee for Elimination of Tuberculosis. *MMWR* 39(No. RR-10):7–20, 1990.

29. CDC: Guidelines for preventing the transmission of *Mycobacterium tuberculosis* in health care facilities, 1994. *MMWR* 43(No. RR-13), 1994.

30. CDC: Prevention and control of tuberculosis among homeless persons: Recommendations of the Advisory Council for the Elimination of Tuberculosis. *MMWR* 41(No. RR-5):13–23, 1992.

31. Daley CL, Small PM, Schecter GF, et al: An outbreak of tuberculosis with accelerated progression among persons infected with the human immunodeficiency virus. *New Engl J Med* 326:231–235, 1992.

32. Stead WW, Lofgren JP, Warren E, Thomas C: Tuberculosis as an endemic and nosocomial infection among the elderly in nursing homes. *New Engl J Med* 312:1483–1487, 1985.

33. Hutton MD, Cauthen GM, Bloch AB: Results of a 29-state survey of tuberculosis in nursing homes and correctional facilities. *Public Health Rep* 108:305–314, 1993.

34. Rieder HL, Cauthen GM, Kelly GD, et al: Tuberculosis in the United States. *JAMA* 262:385–389, 1989.

35. Cantwell MF, Snider DE Jr, Cauthen GM, Onorato IM: Epidemiology of tuberculosis in the United States, 1985 through 1992. *JAMA* 272:535–539, 1994.

36. McKenna MT, McCray E, Onorato I: The epidemiology of tuberculosis among foreign-born persons in the United States, 1986 to 1993. *New Engl J Med* 332:1071–1076, 1995.

37. CDC: Tuberculosis among foreign-born persons entering the United States: Recommendations of the Advisory Committee for Elimination of Tuberculosis. *MMWR* 39(No. RR-18), 1990.

38. Hinman AR, Judd JM, Kolnik JP, Daitch PB: Changing risks in tuberculosis. *Am J Epidemiol* 103:486–497, 1976.

39. Friedman LN, Sullivan GM, Bevilaqua RP, Loscos R: Tuberculosis screening in alcoholics and drug addicts. *Am Rev Respir Dis* 136:1188–1192, 1987.

40. Grzybowski S, Allen EA, Black WA, et al: Inner-city survey for tuberculosis: Evaluation of diagnostic methods. *Am Rev Respir Dis* 135:1311–1315, 1987.

41. CDC: Prevention and control of tuberculosis in migrant farm workers: Recommendations of the Advisory Council for the Elimination of Tuberculosis. *MMWR* 41(No. RR-10), 1992.

42. American Academy of Pediatrics Committee on Infectious Diseases: Screening for tuberculosis in infants and children. *Pediatrics* 93:131–134, 1994.

43. Starke JR: Universal screening for tuberculosis infection: School's out! (editorial). *JAMA* 274:652–653, 1995.

44. Mohle-Boetani JC, Miller B, Halpern M, et al: School-based screening for tuberculous infection: A cost-benefit analysis. *JAMA* 274:613–619, 1995.

CHAPTER 162

CLINICAL PRESENTATION AND TREATMENT OF TUBERCULOSIS

Milton D. Rossman / A. Fusun Oner-Eyuboglu

Tuberculosis (TB) is a disease that has afflicted humankind before and throughout recorded history. Spinal lesions that are highly suggestive or classic for TB have been observed in a skeleton recovered from a grave near Heidelberg that dates from 5000 BC, from a skeleton excavated from the Arene Candide Cave in Liguria, Italy, that dates from 4000 BC, and from similar graves in Denmark and the Jordan Valley. *Mycobacterium tuberculosis* DNA has been recovered from a pre-Columbian mummy from Peru. The earliest records that are consistent with TB are Egyptian wall paintings that depict typical hunchback deformities and correlate with the findings of spinal TB in mummies. The first written description of TB is from India around 700 BC. Hippocrates not only described the disease but also named it *phthisis,* which means to melt or to waste away. Aristotle noted its contagious nature, but it was not until Koch discovered the tuberculous bacillus in 1882 that the causative agent was discovered. Today TB describes an infection in humans that is caused by either *M. tuberculosis* or *M. bovis.* Infections caused by other mycobacteria should be referred to as disease caused by the specific mycobacterium (see Chapters 159, 163, and 164). Despite the discovery of the cause of TB and the development of effective chemotherapy in the 1950s, TB continues to be a major pulmonary pathogen and is the leading cause of death in adults due to infectious disease (see Chapter 158).

The pathogenesis of TB has been reviewed in Chapter 160 and will be only summarized here. Initial infection with *M. tuberculosis* occurs by the airborne route. Since *M. tuberculosis* cannot penetrate mucus, the organism must bypass the mucous barrier by staying suspended in the air until it arrives in the alveolar zone, where no mucus is present.[16,43] Only organisms suspended in droplets between 1 and 10 μm are able to pass to the alveolar zone and avoid being safely eliminated. Although the minimal infecting dose for humans of *M. tuberculosis* is unknown, in rabbits and guinea pigs one to three live organisms may be sufficient.[8,43] These organisms are initially ingested by alveolar macrophages. Since resident alveolar macrophages and nonactivated, recently arrived macrophages cannot kill intracellular *M. tuberculosis*, the organisms initially replicate within macrophages and rapidly increase in number. During this period, before the development of specific immunity, the organisms appear in draining lymph nodes and a bacteremia or hematogenous dissemination occurs.

This initial phase of uninhibited growth of *M. tuberculosis* ends with the development of an immune response to *M. tuberculosis*. At the initial site of infection (primary infection), the organisms are usually completely eliminated. At the disseminated sites, however, the organism is not eliminated but only arrested. It is not known whether the organism is growing very slowly or is actually dormant during this period. Months to years later, for reasons that are not entirely known, the organism again begins to grow more rapidly, resulting in the development of symptomatic TB. Although these sites may be anywhere, they are most frequently in the apices of the lungs, bones, meninges, and kidneys. It is believed that the high tissue tensions of oxygen may be an important factor in the localization and continued growth of *M. tuberculosis* in these locations.

CLINICAL PRESENTATION OF PULMONARY TUBERCULOSIS

Signs and Symptoms

Because *M. tuberculosis* grows relatively slowly, pulmonary TB frequently develops insidiously without any striking clinical evidence of disease. Two major clinical syndromes are recognized. The first occurs with primary infection, and the second occurs with reactivation of latent or dormant foci.

The initial localized infection usually results in few or no clinical symptoms or signs. At the onset of tuberculin hypersensitivity (4 to 6 weeks), mild fever and malaise may develop, and occasionally other hypersensitivity manifestations are noted. Thus, the initial infection with *M. tuberculosis* frequently is clinically insignificant and unrecognized. Only patients with some immunosuppression will probably present with primary TB. This includes children under 1 year old, HIV-positive subjects, and patients on chemotherapy. In most patients, the organism stays dormant either indefinitely or for many years, and when disease occurs, it may be secondary to a decrease in body immunity (Table 162-1).

However, since the disease has a wide spectrum of manifestations, ranging from skin positivity with negative radiographs to far-advanced tuberculosis, a variety of clinical presentations

TABLE 162-1

Populations with Increased Susceptibility to Tuberculosis

Nonspecific decrease in resistance
    Adolescence
    Senescence
    Malnutrition
    Postgastrectomy state
    Uremia
    Diabetes mellitus
Decrease in resistance due to hormonal effects
    Pregnancy
    Therapy with adrenocortical steroids
Decrease in local resistance
    Silicosis
Decrease in specific immunity
    Lymphomas
    Immunosuppressive therapy
    Sarcoidosis
    Live virus vaccination
    HIV infection

also occur. Until pulmonary disease is moderately or far advanced, as shown by changes on the radiograph, symptoms are usually minimal and often attributable to other causes, such as excessive smoking, hard work, pregnancy, a viral infection, and old age.

Symptoms may be divided into two categories, systemic and pulmonary. The systemic symptom most frequently observed is a low-grade fever. As the disease progresses, fevers can be quite marked. The fever characteristically develops in the late afternoon and may not be accompanied by pronounced symptoms. With defervescence, usually during sleep, sweating occurs (night sweats). Other systemic signs of toxemia—such as malaise, irritability, weakness, unusual fatigue, headache, and weight loss—may be present. In some reviews, cough, anorexia, and weight loss were the most common symptoms.[45] With the development of caseation necrosis and concomitant liquefaction of the caseation, the patient will usually notice cough and sputum, often associated with mild hemoptysis. Up to 10 percent of patients with a chronic productive cough may have active TB. Chest pain is often localized and pleuritic. Shortness of breath usually indicates extensive disease, with widespread involvement of the lung and parenchyma or some form of tracheobronchial obstruction, and therefore usually occurs late in the disease.

Physical examination of the chest is often completely normal early in the disease. The principal findings over areas of infiltration are posttussive rales (fine rales detected on deep inspiration, followed by full expiration and a hard cough). These are usually detected in the apexes of the lungs, where reactivation disease is most common. Percussion of the clavicles may reveal dullness as the disease progresses. Other findings will also be present. Allergic manifestations may occur, usually developing at the time of onset of infection. These include erythema nodosum and phlyctenular conjunctivitis. The former is due to circulating immune complexes, with resultant localized vascular damage. Initially, erythema nodosum occurs in the dependent portion of the body and, if the reaction is severe, may be followed by a more disseminated process.

Laboratory Examination

Although routine laboratory examinations (Table 162-2) are rarely helpful in establishing the diagnosis, they may suggest the presence of a chronic inflammatory condition.[39] A mild normochromic normocytic anemia may be present in chronic tuberculosis. The WBC count is often normal, and counts over 20,000/ml would suggest another infectious process; a leukemoid reaction may occasionally occur in miliary TB, but not in TB confined to the chest. Although a "left shift" in the differential WBC count can occur in advanced disease, WBC changes are neither specific nor useful. Other nonspecific tests may be elevated in active TB (sedimentation rate, α_2-globulins, and γ-globulin). Pyuria without bacteria on Gram's stain suggests renal involvement. Liver enzymes (transaminases and alkaline phosphatase) may occasionally be elevated before treatment. However, this finding is usually due to concomitant liver disease secondary to other problems, such as alcoholism, rather than to tuberculous involvement. On rare occasions, the serum sodium is low, owing to inappropriate secretion of antidiuretic hormone. This only occurs in advanced pulmonary TB.

A positive delayed hypersensitivity reaction to tuberculin (as discussed in Chapters 160 and 161) indicates only the occurrence of a prior primary infection and not necessarily clinically active disease.[24] However, very large reactions (greater than 25 mm of induration) are more frequently associated with active TB than smaller reactions. A negative reaction to tuberculin does not rule out the diagnosis, because the patient may be anergic or have specific anergy to tuberculin. Older persons with TB have a lower rate of tuberculin positivity than young adults (67.6 versus 86.2 percent, respectively).[38]

Chest Radiography

Despite the introduction of new techniques for the radiographic evaluation of pulmonary lesions, the simple posteroanterior chest radiograph remains the primary laboratory test for suggesting the diagnosis of pulmonary TB.[15]

Primary Tuberculosis

Typically, primary TB has been a disease of infants and children. In developed countries, however, with the expanding numbers of adults that have never been infected with the tuberculous bacillus, primary TB must also be considered an adult disease (Fig. 162-1. The most common radiographic appearance of primary TB is a normal radiograph. Since the initial infection occurs from infected droplet nuclei that are deposited in the periphery of the lungs in proportion to total ventilation, in primary TB parenchymal involvement can happen in any segment of the lung.[10] The airspace consolidation appears as a homogeneous density with ill-defined borders, and cavitation is rare except in malnourished or other immunocompromised patients. Miliary involvement at the onset is seen in fewer than 3 percent of cases (Fig. 162-2), most commonly in children under 2 years of age. An isolated pleural effusion of mild to moderate degree may be the only manifestation of primary TB (Fig. 162-3).

Hilar or paratracheal lymph node enlargement with or without a parenchymal infiltrate is a characteristic finding in primary tuberculosis. In 15 percent of the cases, bilateral hilar adenopathy may be present and could be confused with sarcoidosis. Usually, the adenopathy is unilateral. Unilateral hilar adenopathy and

TABLE 162-2

Biochemical Abnormalities in 265 Patients with Pulmonary Tuberculosis

Abnormality	Percent of Patients with Abnormality
Anemia	60
Leukocytosis with neutrophilia	40
Lymphopenia	17
Monocytopenia	50
Thrombocytosis	52
Sedimentation rate	80
Increased ferritin	94
Increased B_{12}	57
Abnormal RBC folic acid	17
Increased liver function tests	33
Hyponatremia	43
Hypoalbuminia	72

SOURCE: Adapted from Morris et al.,[47] with permission.

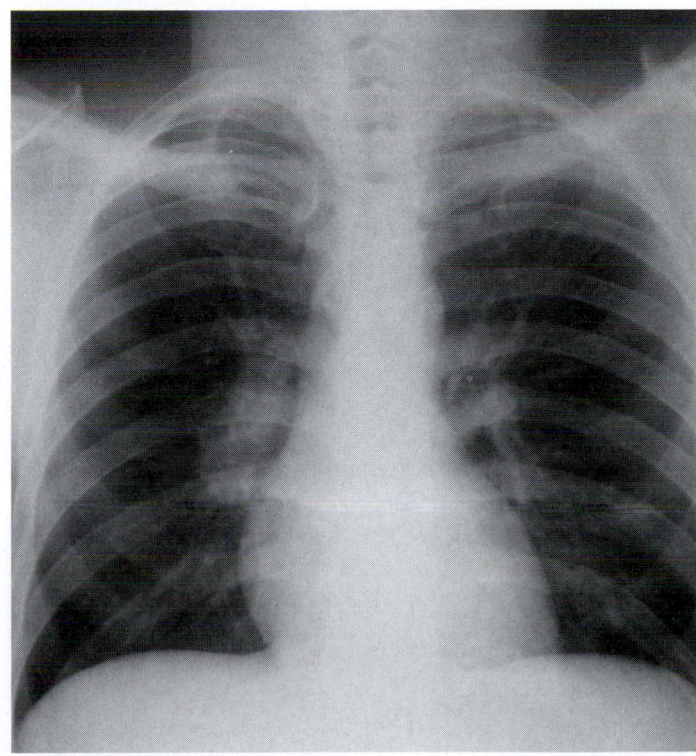

FIGURE 162-1 Chest radiograph of primary TB in a 21-year-old African American. Unilateral right hilar adenopathy is noted.

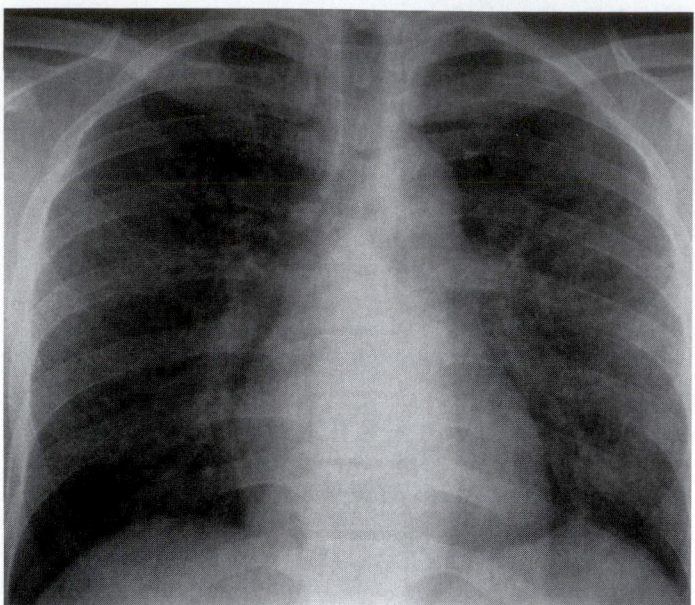

FIGURE 162-2 Chest radiograph demonstrating miliary TB that presented in a 27-year-old Cambodian man with a stiff neck.

unilateral hilar and paratracheal adenopathy are equally common. Massive hilar adenopathy may herald a complicated course. Atelectasis with an obstructive pneumonia may result from bronchial compression by inflamed lymph nodes or from a caseous lymph node that ruptures into a bronchus.

Reactivation Tuberculosis

In 95 percent of localized pulmonary TB, the lesions will be present in the apical or posterior segment of the upper lobes or the superior segment of the lower lobes, although reactivation TB may affect any lung segment. If only the anterior segment of the upper lobe is affected, TB is extremely unlikely.[11] The radiolo-

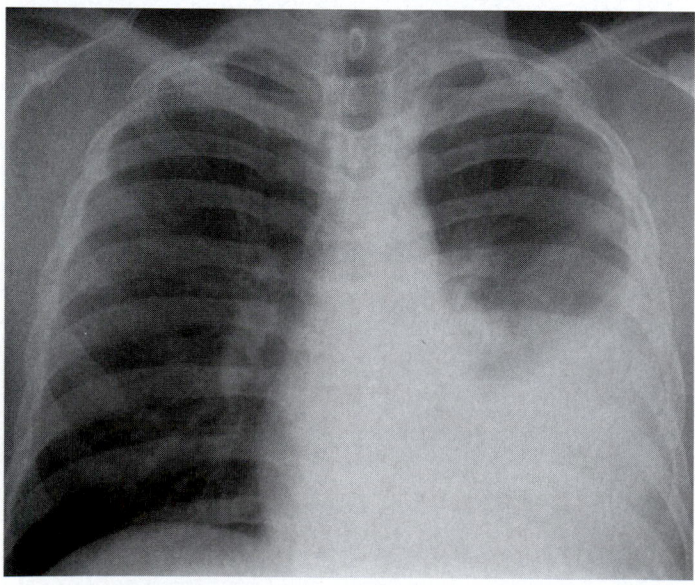

FIGURE 162-3 Tuberculous pleural effusion that presented in a 22-year-old man.

gist should never attempt to describe the activity of a lesion on the basis of its radiographic appearance (see Chapter 160). The documentation of activity is best left to bacteriologic and clinical evaluation. A person with lesions reported as inactive or stable by radiography can have sputum smears and cultures that are positive for *M. tuberculosis* (Fig. 162-4).

The most common pattern of reactivation TB is of a focal air-space consolidation in a patchy or confluent nature. Frequently, linear densities connect to the ipsilateral hilum (Fig. 162-5). Cavitation is common, but lymph node enlargement is rare. Because the lesions are usually chronic, destruction of tissue, fibrosis, calcification, and volume loss are usually present in the affected lung. The combination of patchy pneumonitis, fibrosis, and calcification should always suggest chronic granulomatous disease, usually TB.

Although the cavities that develop in TB usually have a moderately thick wall, a smooth inner surface, and no air–fluid level, thin- or thick-walled cavities, with or without air–fluid levels and little or extensive parenchymal infiltrate, can be observed in TB. Cavitation is frequently associated with endobronchial spread of disease. Radiographically, endobronchial spread appears as multiple small acinar shadows, usually in the superior segment of the lower lobes.

Besides the simple posteroanterior chest radiograph, lordotic films may be useful for demonstrating apical disease. Computed tomography may raise the suspicion of TB when cavitary lesions or multifocal lesions are observed that were not suspected on the plain film. In multidrug-resistant disease, documentation of the extent of disease may be important if surgery is being considered. Currently, magnetic resonance imaging has little role in pulmonary TB.

Diagnosis

The gold standard for the diagnosis of TB is bacteriologic confirmation. It is important to remember that a positive acid-fast smear is not specific for *M. tuberculosis*. Other mycobacteria, both saprophytes and potential pathogens, can be acid-fast. In addition, a negative acid-fast smear should not perplex the clinician, since 50 percent of patients whose cultures are positive will have a negative acid-fast smear. Thus, culture of *M. tuberculosis* is the only absolute way of confirming the diagnosis.

Freshly expectorated sputum is the best sample to stain and culture for *M. tuberculosis*. Sputum samples 24 h old are frequently overgrown with mouth flora and are much less useful. If a patient is not spontaneously producing sputum, induced sputum is the next best specimen for study. It can be obtained by having the patient breathe an aerosol of isotonic or hypertonic saline for 5 to 15 min. If the patient cannot cooperate to give a spontaneous sputum sample, a gastric aspirate to obtain swallowed sputum may be useful. This sample must be obtained in the morning, before the patient arises or eats.

In most patients, the above-mentioned procedures will be successful in providing positive material for culture. Smears of gastric contents for acid-fast bacilli are of limited value and are not recommended, because of the presence of nontuberculous ingested acid-fast bacilli. However, gastric aspiration may be especially useful in the diagnosis of TB in infants, in whom the collection of spontaneous or induced sputum is almost impossi-

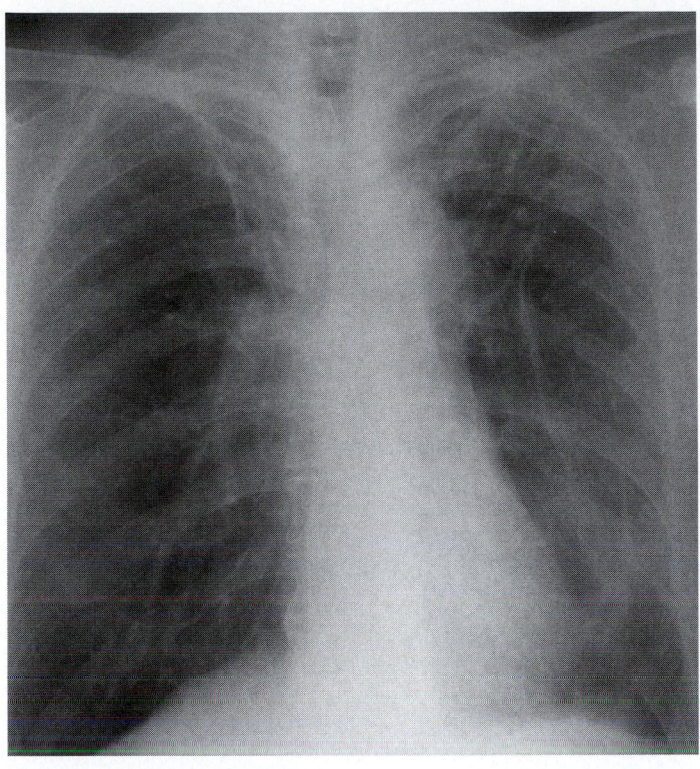

A

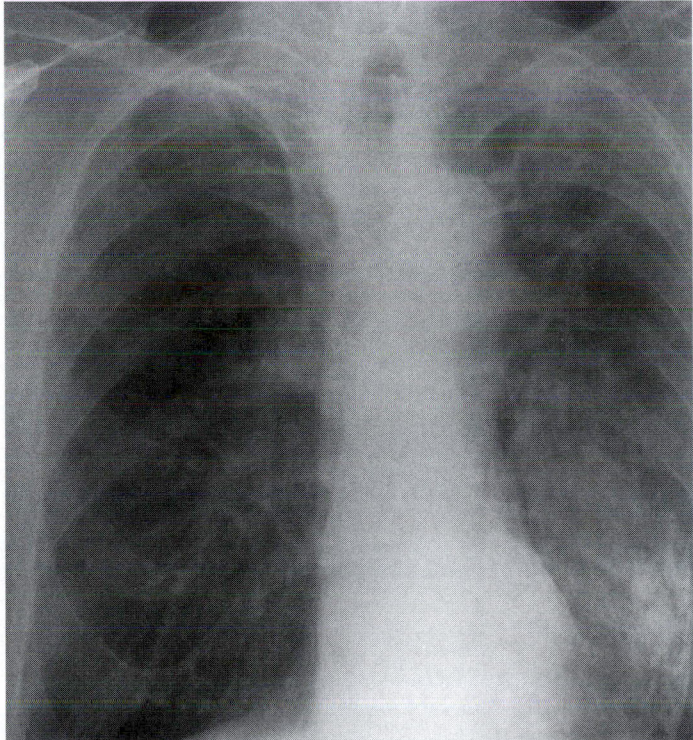

B

FIGURE 162-4   Stable radiographic TB that looks inactive but is smear positive. *A.* Chest radiograph from 8/11/56 demonstrating bilateral upper-lobe retraction and fibrosis. *B.* Chest radiograph from 6/3/75 demonstrating stable bilateral upper-lobe disease with left lower-lobe infiltrate. Patient was thought initially to have stable inactive TB and bacterial pneumonia. Cultures were positive for *M. tuberculosis.* This case illustrates the danger in attempting to equate radiologically stable disease with inactive disease.

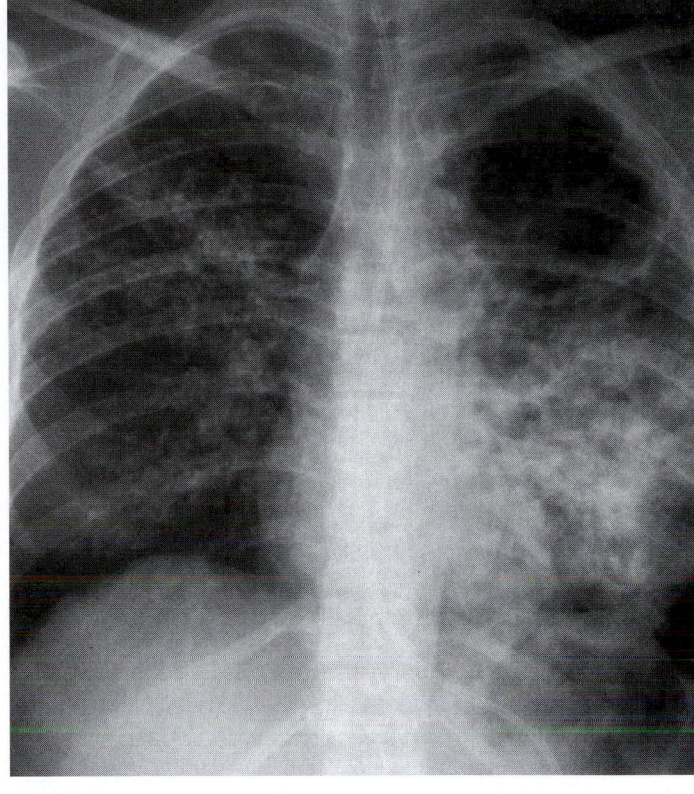

FIGURE 162-5   Chest radiograph of far-advanced cavitary TB in a 27-year-old woman. Large left upper-lobe cavity and endobronchial spread to the left lower lobe and right upper lobe are demonstrated.

ble. In 75 percent of infants with pulmonary TB, the gastric aspirate can be positive.[12] In a few cases, one may have to resort to bronchoscopy. In 41 patients proven to have TB, cultures of specimens, taken during fiberoptic bronchoscopy, were positive in 39 cases.[61] Stainable mycobacteria were seen in 14 of the cases, and in 8 cases granulomas were seen on biopsy. Similar results have been obtained in another study, of 22 patients with proven mycobacterial disease and negative smears before bronchoscopy.[10] The local anesthetics used during fiberoptic bronchoscopy may be lethal to *M. tuberculosis,* so specimens for culture should be obtained with a minimal amount of anesthesia. However, irritation of the bronchial tree during the fiberoptic bronchoscopy procedure will frequently leave the patient with a productive cough. Thus, collection of the postbronchoscopy sputum can be another valuable source of diagnostic material. In nine (13 percent) of the 22 patients mentioned above, the postbronchoscopy sputum was the only source of positive material.

However, obtaining diagnostic culture material is not always possible. In 1994, only 80.2 percent of TB reported to the Centers for Disease Control and Prevention had the diagnosis confirmed by positive cultures. In an additional 1.0 percent of the cases, only the smear was positive. In 11.5 percent of reported cases, both smears and cultures were reported as negative. Thus, in a significant number of cases, the diagnosis of TB was made in the absence of bacteriologic confirmation. In these cases, the diagnosis was made by a combination of a positive skin test, a compatible chest radiograph, and a therapeutic trial.

Newer diagnostic tests may be available soon. Molecular testing for *M. tuberculosis* DNA may eventually replace culture as a diagnostic test for TB. These tests have a sensitivity for TB that is equivalent to culture techniques. Unfortunately, false-positive tests occur too frequently for these tests to replace culture at present. Nevertheless, the ability to get diagnostic results within 6 h of obtaining the specimen makes molecular testing for *M. tuberculosis* DNA an attractive technique for the future.

Differential Diagnosis

Today, TB is a disease most frequently present in persons older than 25. In adults, primary TB is becoming more common and may appear as a lower-lobe pneumonia. Young adults usually present with more symptoms (especially fever and night sweats) than the elderly.[38] Common bacterial pneumonias are usually easily differentiated from TB. The localized alveolar infiltrate on the chest radiograph and the prompt response to antibiotic therapy usually differentiate bacterial pneumonia from TB. When in doubt, treatment for a bacterial pneumonia should be given first and TB therapy withheld until adequate sputums have been obtained and the response to antibiotics determined. Lung abscesses can usually be differentiated from tuberculous cavities by prominent air–fluid level, more common lower-lobe distribution, and clinical findings (associated with seizures, alcoholism, dental caries, etc.).

In the elderly, the major differential diagnosis is usually between TB and carcinoma of the lung (Fig. 162-6). An important concept to remember is that carcinoma may cause a focus of TB to spread; thus, carcinoma of the lung and TB may be present simultaneously. In cases with the simultaneous presentation of carcinoma and TB, the diagnosis of TB frequently is made first, and the diagnosis of carcinoma is delayed for several months. Thus, if radiographic and clinical findings suggest carcinoma but the sputum has acid-fast bacilli, further procedures to diagnose carcinoma may still be indicated. Isolated involvement of the anterior segment of the upper lobe, isolated lower-lobe involvement, or the presence of irregular cavities would suggest carcinoma, and further diagnostic workup may be indicated despite acid-fast bacilli in the sputum smear.

Any type of infectious or granulomatous disease may be radiographically identical to TB. Three broad categories must be distinguished: fungi (histoplasmosis, coccidioidomycosis, and blastomycosis), bacteria (*Burkholderia pseudomallei*), and atypical mycobacteria (mainly *Mycobacterium kansasii* and *M. avium* complex). Culture of the organism from the patient's sputum is the best way to differentiate these diseases, although serum antibody titers to fungi are also valuable.

COMPLICATIONS DUE TO PULMONARY INVOLVEMENT

Pneumothorax

Although a relatively uncommon complication of tuberculous infection, the development of a pneumothorax requires rapid attention. After trauma, TB may be the second most common cause of bilateral pneumothorax in adults.[3] Miliary TB can also rarely present as bilateral spontaneous pneumothorax.

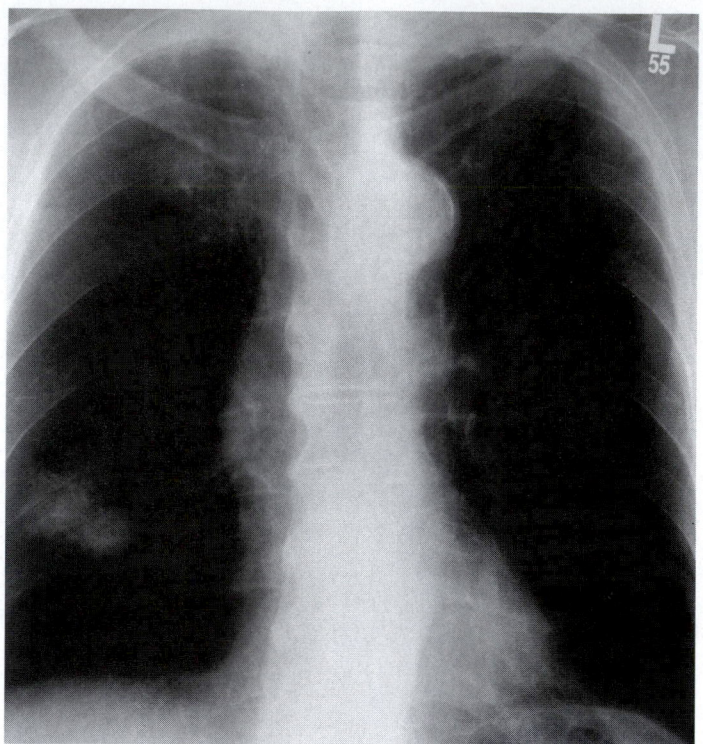

A

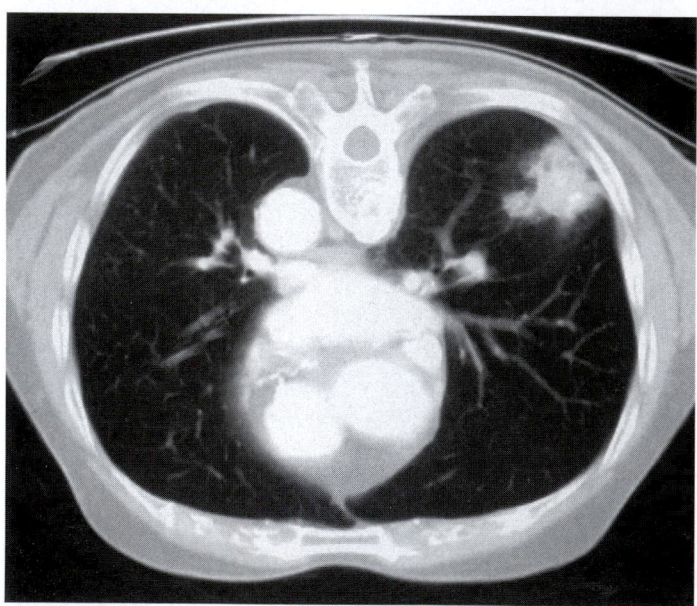

B

FIGURE 162-6   TB presenting as a nodular lesion that could be mistaken for a cancer. A 90-year-old man who presented with a right lower-lobe mass. *A.* Chest radiograph demonstrating right lower-lobe nodule and also right upper-lobe infiltrate. *B.* Chest CT demonstrating right lower-lobe nodules.

Two postulated mechanisms can account for the development of a pneumothorax from TB. A bronchopleural fistula is created with the rupture of a cavity that connects the tracheobronchial tree with the pleural space. Contamination of the pleural space results in spread of the infection to the pleura, with a tendency to produce pleural fibrosis, fibrothorax, and restrictive pulmonary dysfunction. Immediate therapy can prevent this complication. A second mechanism for the development of a pneumothorax from TB is the development of a subpleural bleb. This results from a submucosal bronchiolar lesion, with air trapping in an acinus or subsegment. When such a bleb ruptures into the pleural space, tuberculous infection of the pleural space does not necessarily follow. However, both occurrences should be treated with rapid expansion of the lungs by tube suction to avoid the possibility of further infection and fibrosis of the pleura with trapping of the lung. A bronchopleural fistula may persist after these episodes of pneumothorax and, especially if untreated, often results in mixed empyema because of complication of the tuberculous infection by secondary invaders.

Endobronchial Stenosis

Minor endobronchial disease is a common occurrence in TB. Fiberoptic bronchoscopy demonstrated 136 lesions in 62 patients.[35] Exudative lesions were most common (43.3 percent) and usually healed. Ulcerative lesions, though less common (9.7 percent), also usually healed. However, lesions that already had evidence of scarring (26.5 percent) or appeared bronchoglandular (20.5 percent) often progressed to stenosis. Resected lung specimens will also frequently show either ulceration or stenosis of the draining bronchioles or bronchi. Stenosis of significance only rarely occurs in the major bronchi. At times, it results from involvement of the central lymph nodes draining into the lobar bronchi, with caseation, ulceration, and fibrosis. Since fibrosis due to TB tends to contract and aggravate the stenosis, resection of the affected lung segment may be required after chemotherapy has produced inactivity of the acute inflammatory reaction.

Bronchiectasis

The endobronchial processes in TB may also result in bronchiectasis. Bronchiectasis can be associated with active TB, and sputum cultures should be sent to rule out an active process. In healed TB, the bronchiectasis usually is distal and frequently is in the upper lobes. The so-called dry bronchiectasis (without sputum) often is the result of prior pulmonary TB and may manifest itself chiefly as low-grade hemoptysis. Bronchiectasis can result in life-threatening hemoptysis. Treatment for this complication is either bronchial artery embolization or surgery.

Empyema

Empyema rarely occurs from a primary infection with an associated tuberculous pleural effusion, since tuberculous pleural effusions usually clear with or without treatment. Empyema is more common later in the disease, occurring after a pneumothorax, and is often associated with debility and loss of resistance to infection. It is usually a part of a progressive, extensive parenchymal infection with caseation and cavitation, the presumed sources of pleural contamination. In many cases there is evidence of calcification of the pleura on the chest radiograph, and the process may have existed for many years. Because there is relatively poor penetration of antituberculous medication into the empyema cavity, chemotherapy alone is usually inadequate and may result in the development of drug resistance. Therefore, surgical removal of a calcified loculated empyema is necessary.

For patients with mild symptoms, empyemectomy with lung resection is well tolerated. For chronic debilitated patients with severe symptoms, however, adequate drainage with a thoracostomy should be performed first; definitive surgery can be attempted later, when the patient is in better physical condition.[59]

Late Secondary Infections

If, after treatment of extensive TB, the patient is left with open, healed cavities as well as with areas of bronchiectasis, colonization of these areas can occur with a variety of infectious agents. Usually, colonization by aerobic and anaerobic upper respiratory bacteria results in a chronic productive cough, the syndrome of "wet" bronchiectasis. Other mycobacteria may be recovered during the development of inactivity and were at one time considered to be a sign of healing. However, the presence of other pathogenic mycobacteria does not rule out the possibility of active infection with *M. tuberculosis*.

Mycetoma

Aspergillus species are common in badly damaged lung areas, especially those that are cavitary. In England, a prospective study[5] revealed that 25 percent of clinically healed TB patients who had residual cavities developed positive precipitins to *Aspergillus* species and 11 percent had demonstrable cavitary "balls," presumed to be aspergillomas or "fungus balls." Three years later, these numbers had risen to 34 and 17 percent, respectively. TB continues to be a leading predisposition to the development of mycetoma. The finding of mycetoma does not rule out active TB, since 10 to 15 percent of patients may have active disease. Hemoptysis appears to be the major cause of death in these patients. Because systemic arteries may also feed the mycetoma cavity, bronchial artery embolization is not as effective for hemoptysis due to mycetoma as it is for hemoptysis due to bronchiectasis. Surgery is the best option for patients with significant hemoptysis. For patients who have little pulmonary reserve and may not tolerate surgery, a transthoracic catheter that is placed into the mycetoma cavity may be lifesaving.

Hemorrhage

Mild hemoptysis is very common in acute infection and not infrequently calls the attention of an otherwise unconcerned patient to the presence of serious disease. Young adults may have a higher incidence of hemoptysis than the elderly. Massive hemorrhage and death are dramatic events that occur in advanced cases of TB. Rupture of a mycotic aneurysm of a branch of the pulmonary artery (Rasmussen's aneurysm) has been well publicized as a cause of death; aspergilloma or bronchiectasis may be associated with severe and fatal hemorrhage. However, less well-defined major hemorrhages may also occur.

Resection of the affected area had been the most widely used method of control in the past, and bleeding remains the main reason for surgery in patients today. The introduction of the technique of bronchial artery embolization has decreased the need for surgery and is 98 percent effective in the treatment of hemoptysis due to TB.[9] Unfortunately, many patients die before this can be accomplished, and often (as in the case of aspergillomas) the areas are multiple and do not lend themselves to excisional therapy or bronchial artery embolization.

Hyponatremia

With extensive active disease, two interesting complications have been reported, the syndrome of inappropriate antidiuretic hormone (SIADH) and a reset osmostat.[42] Both manifest themselves by abnormally low serum sodium. However, the former is associated with all of the other clinical and renal abnormalities associated with primary SIADH. A reset osmostat is characterized by decreased serum osmolality without clinical symptoms and the obligatory renal salt wasting found in SIADH. Both conditions disappear with control of the infection; they should be differentiated from each other, however, since SIADH requires metabolic control.

EXTRAPULMONARY MANIFESTATIONS OF TUBERCULOSIS

Extrapulmonary tuberculosis occurs as a result of exposure of superficial mucosal surfaces to infected respiratory secretions; contiguous spread of infection; and lymphohematogenous dissemination, commonly in immunocompromised hosts. Local progression of disseminated foci of infection may be the first sign of underlying immune compromise, such as AIDS (see Chapter 163).

Local oral or gastrointestinal complications of tuberculosis, with oral or abdominal pain, are more common in patients with laryngeal involvement or who come late to medical care. Among the observed lesions are nonhealing oral ulcers of the tongue or mouth; otitis media; gastric and duodenal ulcers, superinfection of preexisting gastrointestinal ulcers, perirectal ascess, or obstructive lesions due to infection and scarring; hoarseness and dysphagia with laryngeal infection. Localized symptoms (e.g., chest pain) may occur in association with extrapulmonary extension of infection by *M. tuberculosis*. Extension of infection or inflammation to the parietal pleura may be associated with pleurisy and fever. Pleural involvement may result in fusion of the visceral and parietal pleural surfaces (e.g., dry pleurisy when adjacent to an old cavity) or in serofibrinous effusion, often in association with primary infection or reactivation disease, and more often on the right side. Tuberculous empyema is uncommon. Granulomas are often seen on biopsy (60 percent), and cultures are generally positive despite negative acid-fast smears of pleural fluid.

Miliary tuberculosis may present with the initial manifestations in any organ system in proportion to blood flow: spleen, liver, lungs, bone marrow, kidneys, adrenal, or the eyes. Symptoms may include splenomegaly or hepatomegaly with abscesses; primary hepatic disease with apparent cholangitis; leukopenia, anemia, thrombocytopenia, myelofibrosis, or leukemoid reactions; Addison's disease; peritonitis; meningitis; choroidal tubercles, or pericarditis. Silent foci may serve as the source of miliary infection from the kidneys, prostate, bones, or deep lymph nodes. Renal infection is generally asymptomatic and temporally distant from the original infection. Patients present with "sterile" pyuria, hematuria, dysuria, and occasionally flank pain.

Renal infection or miliary infection may cause epidymitis, orchitis, or prostatitis, and sexual transmission of infection may occur. Involvement of the fallopian tubes or uterus may cause dysfunctional bleeding, pain, or infertility.

Tuberculous meningitis generally occurs, in the normal host, several weeks into the illness via rupture of a subependymal tubercle (Rich focus) into the subarachnoid space, rather than by direct seeding of the meninges or cerebrospinal fluid during bacteremia. The basal meninges are most commonly involved. Symptoms may reflect vasculitis (aneurysm, thrombosis, hemorrhage), hemiplegia, entrapment of cranial nerves (usually III, IV, VI, and occasionally VII), hydrocephalus, or uncommonly direct brain, meningeal, or spinal seeding with abscesses, transverse myelitits, radiculopathy, or spinal compression from paraspinous fibrosis.

Bone and joint involvement favors weight-bearing joints including the vertebral column (50 percent), hip, and knee. Monoarticular disease favors joints with prior trauma. The presentation includes symptoms of arthritis and osteomyelitis with pain, ofter with fever and weight loss. Vertebral infections initially involve the anterior part of the vertebral body with spread to the intervertebral disc and the adjacent vertebrae. Sinus tracts may occur with presentations distant from the initial bony focus (e.g., with empyema from a lower thoracic infection). Neurologic complications (paraplegia or paresis) are not rare. Joint infections have high white cell counts (25,000 to 100,000), low glucose measurements, rice (fibrin) bodies, and negative smears with positive cultures in the majority. The yields of histologic and mycobacterial studies of synovial biopsies, as for the pleura, are high.

In AIDS, between 30 and 60 percent of patients with tuberculosis have extrapulmonary foci. Only half of those with extrapulmonary disease have identifiable concomitant pulmonary infection. Disseminated disease with multiple foci of involvement is common, including pneumonia, bilateral pleuritis, disseminated intravascular coagulation, omental and abdominal nodal involvement, and abscesses of multiple organs including prostate, liver, spleen, chest and abdominal wall, and pancreas.

Extrapulmonary foci in the immunologically mormal host respond well to standard therapeutic regimens. Maximal, prolonged therapy is reserved for unique foci in the central nervous system or basal ganglia, in joints, or in bones, particularly in the spine.

HISTORY OF THE TREATMENT OF TUBERCULOSIS

In the late 1800s, before chemotherapeutic agents had been discovered, patients with TB were isolated in sanitariums for nutrition and rest. Lung collapse therapy was performed by pneumothorax or various surgical techniques that frequently left patients disfigured for life. In 1946, streptomycin was introduced as an effective antituberculosis drug and initially was used in TB patients by Feldman and Henshaw. However, it quickly became evident that streptomycin monotherapy resulted in relapse and the emergence of drug resistance. PAS, which was also used as monotherapy in 1944, could reduce the emergence of resistance to streptomycin; thus, two-drug therapy was born. In 1953, isoniazid (INH) and pyrazinamide (PZA) were released for therapy, and an era of truly effective chemotherapy began. Following the development of ethanebutol (EMB) in 1964, INH and EMB became the cornerstone of an 18-month treatment regimen. RMP was developed in 1965 and released for use in 1971. In the early 1980s, it was found that RMP and INH reduced the course of therapy to 9 months. Addition of PZA to this regimen shortened the duration of treatment to 6 months. Thus, in the 50 years since the introduction of the first effective drugs for the treatment of TB, the care of these patients has been transformed from long hospitalizations and a lifetime of fear of relapse to a relatively short outpatient treatment regimen and cure. The challenge today is not so much how to treat TB as how to ensure that patients receive the proper treatment. Failure to deliver proper care is the major cause for the development of drug-resistant strains and the fear for the recrudescence of this dreaded malady.

THEORETICAL BASIS FOR EFFECTIVE TREATMENT STRATEGIES

Effective chemotherapy is based on several considerations. The first is that only actively replicating organisms are killed by chemotherapy. In addition, differences in mycobacteria metabolic rate are associated with differences in mycobacteria susceptibility to antituberculosis drugs.[4,21] Four major subpopulations of TB bacilli can be identified.

Group 1   The organisms living extracellularly in pulmonary cavities are metabolically very active and are rapidly and continuously growing in a hyperoxic and neutral-pH environment. These organisms are highly susceptible to streptomycin (SM), INH, and EMB.

Group 2   The organisms living extracellularly in closed caseous lesions are less or only intermittently metabolically active in a hypoxic and neutral-pH environment. This group of organisms is susceptible to rifampin (RMP) and INH.

Group 3   The intracellular organisms that live in the acid, hypoxic environment of macrophages have slow or intermittent growth PZA and RMP are uniquely effective against these organisms, and INH is less effective.

Group 4   Some trapped organisms may become completely dormant and are unaffected by both antimicrobials and cellular immune mechanisms. Such persisting organisms can exist in tissues that healed with fibrosis and encapsulation.

   Effective therapy for these bacterial subpopulations (Table 162-3) has to involve a bactericidal phase, during which most organisms (group 1) are rapidly killed, and a slower sterilizing phase, during which residual susceptible, slowly or intermittently metabolizing organisms (groups 2 and 3) are inhibited or killed.[1]

A second major consideration for effective chemotherapy is the presence of naturally occurring drug-resistant mutants. These mutants develop spontaneously at a rate of 10^{-7} to 10^{-10} mutations per bacterium per generation.[11] Their occurrence is less important in noncavitary pulmonary or extrapulmonary lesions, where bacillary populations are relatively small, whereas in a cavitary environment containing 10^8 to 10^9 bacilli,[6] approximately 10^1 to 10^3 organisms exist that are resistant to any single drug. In addition, the development of resistance to one drug is independent of the development of resistance to any other drug. Therefore, the probability of resistance to two drugs is the product of their individual rates (i.e., $10^{-7} \times 10^{-7} = 1 \times 10^{-14}$)—a negligible number, as such mutants are practically nonexistent among a population of 10^9 organisms. Thus, antituberculosis therapy should always consist of at least two effective antituberculous drugs to prevent the emergence of drug-resistant mycobacteria.

SPECIFIC ANTITUBERCULOSIS DRUGS

First-Line Drugs

Isoniazid   Because of its bactericidal effect and low cost, isoniazid (INH) is the most important drug used for the treatment of TB. INH should be included in all regimens except when a high proportion of INH-resistant organisms are present. INH is the hydrazide of isonicotinic acid, which most probably acts by inhibiting mycolic acid synthesis by mycobacteria.[1,21] For INH to be effective, three things must occur. First, the drug has to be taken up by the organisms. Second, INH needs to be activated by a catalase-peroxidase enzyme within mycobacteria. The *katG* gene, encoding the catalase-peroxidase enzyme of *M. tuberculosis,* has been identified.[23] In some highly INH-resistant isolates, either complete deletion or missense mutations are observed in the *katG* gene. Third, this activated form of INH interferes with mycolic acid synthesis. A second gene, *inhA,* encoding inhA protein active in mycolic acid synthesis, was cloned in 1994.[2] The overexpression of this gene results in a phenotype of low-level INH resistance and cross resistance to ethionamide.

TABLE 162-3

Actions of First-Line Antituberculous Agents

Drugs	Activity
Isoniazid (INH)	Bactericidal against both intracellular and extracellular bacilli
Rifampin (RMP)	Bactericidal against both intracellular and extracellular bacilli; sterilizing against particularly slowly metabolizing organisms
Pyrazinamide (PZA)	Bactericidal against slowly metabolizing intracellular organisms; active at acid pH; good sterilizing activity synergistically with INH and other drugs
Streptomycin (SM)	Bactericidal against extracellular bacilli; active at neutral pH; effective against intracavitary bacilli
Ethambutol (EMB)	Bactericidal against both intracellular and extracellular organisms at 25 mg/kg; bacteriostatic at 15 mg/kg

SOURCE: Haas and Des Prez,[21] with permission.

InhA protein also requires NAD or NADP as a cofactor, which is produced as a result of the interaction of INH with catalase-peroxidase enzyme. Because of these interactions of INH with mycobacteria, a single molecular test to identify INH-resistant organisms is unlikely.

INH has a bactericidal effect for both intra- and extracellular organisms and is well absorbed from the gastrointestinal tract, reaching serum levels equal to those following parenteral administration. The peak serum concentration of 3 to 5 μg/ml occurs 1 to 2 h after a dose of 5 mg/kg. The small molecular size of INH allows widespread distribution. The drug can be detected in serous membranes, caseous foci, cavities, and macrophages. INH is metabolized in the liver by both acetylation and oxidation via the cytochrome P-450 system. The serum half-life is around 3 h in slow acetylators and 1 h in rapid acetylators. The inactive metabolites are excreted in the urine, accounting for 75 to 95 percent of a dose within 24 h. If the serum creatinine levels are higher than 12 mg/dl, these metabolites will accumulate in the body. In renal failure, INH should be administered after dialysis.[18,21] The drug can be given by nasogastric tube, by intramuscular injection, or intravenously if the patient is unconscious.

When INH and phenytoin are administered together, an increase in serum concentrations of phenytoin will be observed, since INH is a noncompetitive inhibitor of diphenylhydantoin (DPH). In such patients, the serum levels of phenytoin should be monitored and a dose reduction may be necessary. In cases of DPH intoxication, the drug should be discontinued for at least a week and then therapy restarted with low doses (100 to 200 mg/day).[18,55] INH may also decrease the threshold for acetaminophen hepatotoxicity.[48]

A major toxic manifestation of INH is peripheral neuritis. Susceptibility is highest in chronic alcoholics, persons with malnutrition, and slow acetylators. Major manifestations are sensory dysfunctions and numbness of the lower extremities. The syndrome is dose related (in 40 percent of patients at doses of 20 mg/kg/day, in 20 percent at 10 mg/kg/day, and in 1 to 2 percent at 5 mg/kg/day). Owing to its pyridoxinelike structure, INH competitively inhibits pyridoxine-requiring reactions. INH-induced depletion of pyridoxine stores[57] can be prevented with pyridoxine 50 mg/day. Unless there is an obvious muscle weakness (i.e., atrophy or fasciculations), the symptoms of peripheral neuritis are reversible within a few weeks after withdrawal of INH and treatment with pyridoxine 100 to 200 mg/day. Autonomic dysfunctions, ataxia, muscle twitching, CNS irritability, depression, acute psychosis, and encephalopathy are other neurologic symptoms that may also occur after INH therapy or overdose. Pyridoxine may terminate all these adverse effects.

The other major side effect of INH is toxic hepatitis. This is related to toxic drug metabolites. After acetylation, INH converts to hydrazine, which may be changed to a toxic agent, acetyl hydrazine. In addition, as RMP inducts the enzymatic conversion of INH to acetyl hydrazine, the hepatotoxic effect is potentiated when these drugs are used together.[4,18,14,57] In the first months of therapy, a mild elevation of transaminase levels may occur in 10 to 20 percent of patients receiving INH. If the enzyme levels rise above three times normal values, the drug should be discontinued. Monthly monitoring of liver enzymes is recom-

mended for all patients on INH therapy. The frequency of tests should be increased in patients who have elevated enzyme levels.[18,40,57] INH causes a hepatocellular type of hypersensitivity reaction, and histology is indistinguishable from that of viral hepatitis.[4,14,18] INH-induced hepatitis is age dependent, occurring in 2 to 3 percent of patients over 50 years of age but seen in less than 1 percent of children. Fatal liver damage may occur in 1 to 2 percent of patients[40,55] with INH hepatitis. This may be asymptomatic until jaundice develops. Before onset of jaundice, patients may suffer from weakness, fatigue, and generalized malaise. Therefore, patients may unknowingly continue taking INH after the onset of drug-induced hepatitis. Patients given INH should be warned about such symptoms and instructed to promptly inform their physician if such symptoms occur.[1,55]

INH and RMP together produce hepatotoxicity more frequently than either drug alone.[4] Risk factors for hepatitis are age greater than 35, slow acetylation, history of cholelithiasis, alcohol use, and preexisting liver disease.[1,40,55] Liver transplantation has been successful in two patients who developed hepatic failure after either INH alone or INH and RMP therapy. Thus, liver transplantation may be a lifesaving therapy.[14]

Rifampin   Rifampin (RMP) is bactericidal against intra- and extracellular bacterial populations. It is a semisynthetic antibiotic that inhibits RNA synthesis by inhibiting DNA-dependent RNA-polymerase enzyme, encoded by the *rpoB* gene. Most strains of *M. tuberculosis* are inhibited in vitro with 0.20 μg/ml. RMP is considered to be a "sterilizing" agent. A standard oral dose of 600 mg/day in an adult may produce serum concentrations of 7 to 10 μg/ml in 1 to 2 h. RMP is metabolized in the liver and excreted in bile.[21] As only 30 percent of the drug is excreted in the urine, dose reduction is not necessary in renal failure. RMP is able to penetrate into caseous foci, serous membranes, and macrophages. RMP does not pass the blood–brain barrier under normal conditions, but inflammation of the meninges causes an increase in penetration. Rifampin penetrates well into tissues and can be detected in urine, tears, sweat, and other body fluids, coloring them to red-orange. Patients should be advised of this harmless discoloration. Although it is a major antituberculosis drug, because it is expensive, its use in therapeutic regimens in developing countries is limited.[1,21] RMP can be given to unconscious patients either by nasogastric tube or by intravenous injection.

In nearly all isolates of *M. tuberculosis* resistant to RMP, a short region of 27 codons in the center of the *rpoB* gene was mutated.[27,58] Most of the these were missense mutations, although small in-frame insertions and deletions also occurred.

Major side effects of RMP are gastrointestinal upset, skin eruptions, and fever. Twenty percent of patients receiving high-dose intermittent RMP (600 to 1200 mg/day) develop an immunologically mediated influenzalike reaction, hemolytic anemia, acute renal failure, and thrombocytopenia. When these syndromes occur, RMP should be discontinued.[1,55]

Another important adverse effect of RMP is its hepatic toxicity. An elevation in serum hepatic enzyme levels occurs in 5 to 10 percent of patients.[20] Usually this resolves spontaneously, and therapy does not need to be altered or interrupted. The clinical presentation of hepatotoxicity varies from transaminase elevations to fatal hepatic necrosis. RMP is also a potent inducer of hepatic microsomal enzymes, resulting in an increased rate of metabolism of a number of drugs and, thus, a rapid elimination and diminished effect of these drugs, which include methadone, coumadin derivatives, glucocorticoids, estrogens, oral hypoglycemic agents, and antiarrhythmic agents.

Several studies have shown that the incidence of hepatitis in regimens containing both INH and RMP is approximately two to four times that of INH alone.[57] Hepatic toxicity due to INH usually occurs after 2 months of therapy. In contrast, in INH and RMP combined therapies, jaundice may occur within the first 2 weeks of therapy and may be fulminant. The reason for this toxic effect was the accelerated production of toxic metabolites of INH due to the stimulation of hepatic microsomal P-450 system by RMP.

There are several reports about renal toxicity due to RMP. The main histologic changes were tubulointerstitial nephritis, interstitial fibrosis, and tubular necrosis. Two patients developed crescentic glomerulonephritis with rapidly progressive renal failure. After discontinuation of RMP and addition of corticosteroids and other immunosuppressive agents, dramatic responses occurred. Further studies are necessary to document the incidence, mechanism, and treatment of RMP nephrotoxicity.[36]

Pyrazinamide   Pyrazinamide (PZA) is a nicotinic acid derivative similar to INH, but it has no cross-resistance with INH. Its bactericidal activity at acid pH makes PZA particularly effective against slowly metabolizing intracellular bacilli. This "sterilizing" property has made PZA an essential component of short-course therapy. Regimens not including PZA require at least 9 months to succeed. This beneficial effect is limited to the first 2 to 3 months of treatment. PZA is absorbed from the gastrointestinal tract and distributed throughout the body, including the central nervous system. PZA is excreted from the kidneys. Serum levels of 30 to 50 μg/ml are achieved with doses of 20 to 25 mg/kg of PZA. It has a minimum inhibitory concentration (MIC) of 15 to 20 μg/ml.[21,29]

Neither the mode of action nor the resistance mechanisms of PZA are clear. Konno and colleagues identified an enzyme, pyrazinamidase, which is toxic to pyrazinoic acid, and suggested that it may be absent in resistant strains.[37] Studies done by Salfinger and colleagues in 1990 showed that pyrazinamidase was not present in all susceptible strains, but it was identified in some resistant strains.[51]

The most adverse reaction of PZA is hepatotoxicity. After 2 months of therapy, 15 percent of patients who receive PZA at a dose of 3000 mg a day (40 to 50 mg/kg) develop liver dysfunctions and 2 to 3 percent develop jaundice.[1] Liver function should be monitored closely, and the treatment should be discontinued if elevations of SGOT levels occur.[13,14] Another common side effect of PZA is hyperuricemia. Occasionally, mild nongouty polyarthralgias occur as a result of inhibition of urate excretion. This complication usually responds to nonsteroidal anti-inflammatory drugs. Clinical gout is rarely seen, and allopurinol therapy is usually indicated. Therapy is not necessary for patients who have only elevated urate levels without symptoms. Other side effects, such as skin rash and gastrointestinal intolerance, are rare.[1,29,51]

Ethambutol   Ethambutol (EMB) is a bacteriostatic agent whose antibacterial effect is limited to *M. tuberculosis*. It has no activity on bacilli in the stationary growth phase. It is a unique butanol derivative that may block a step of cell wall synthesis. Following a 5-mg/kg oral dose, the peak serum level is approximately 4 μg/ml after 2 to 4 h. Serum half-life is approximately 4 h and is prolonged in renal failure.[1,21] EMB may be bactericidal at 25-mg/kg doses, whereas it is bacteriostatic at 15-mg/kg doses. EMB is active against both intra- and extracellular bacilli. Most strains of *M. tuberculosis* are inhibited in vitro by 1 to 5 μg/ml of EMB. Cerebrospinal fluid concentrations are low (1 to 2 μg/ml), even in the presence of meningeal inflammation. It is often added to short-term therapy regimens when there is a concern about primary drug resistance.

The main toxicity of EMB is optic neuritis. This is manifested by central scotoma, decreased red-green color vision, decreased visual activity, and, rarely, concentric concentration of visual fields, leading to gun-barrel vision. This side effect is dose-dependent and largely reversible. Optic neuritis occurs in 3 percent of patients taking 25 mg/kg but in less than 1 percent of patients taking 15 mg/kg. Patients should be questioned concerning visual symptoms, and tests of visual acuity and color vision should be performed. In cases of optic neuritis, the visual function returns after withdrawal of the drug. Like PZA, EMB may cause hyperuricemia and, rarely, gout. Skin rash, drug fever, and gastrointestinal disturbance are other rarely seen side effects.[1,21,51]

Streptomycin   Streptomycin (SM) was the first major antituberculosis drug released. SM acts through inhibition of protein synthesis. It is effective only against extracellular bacterial populations in cavities, where the pH is neutral. SM must be administered parenterally, as it is not absorbed from the gut. Peak serum concentration of 40 μg/ml occurs approximately 1 h after a 15-mg/kg intramuscular dose. Most strains of *M. tuberculosis* are inhibited in vitro at a concentration of 8 μg/ml. SM's half-life is 5 h in blood.

Several mechanisms are responsible for resistance to SM. One of them is a mutation in the *rpsL* gene, encoding the S12 protein. Seventy percent of SM-resistant clinical isolates have modifications of the *rpsL* gene.[28,44] An additional mechanism of resistance found by Kempsell's team in 1992 concerns the *rrs* gene, encoding 16S rRNA.[34] Two conserved regions of this molecule are known to be engaged in SM resistance. Little is known about a third mechanism, a low-level resistance, which is found in about 30 percent of resistant clinical isolates that do not carry modifications of the genes mentioned above. In these strains, permeability or cell wall barrier modifications could be playing a role.

Although SM has good tissue penetration, it can enter the cerebrospinal fluid only in the presence of meningeal inflammation. Its major toxicity is irreversible eighth nerve damage, leading to vestibular dysfunction and, less frequently, deafness. It is a nephrotoxic drug like other aminoglycosides, and the frequency of renal toxicity is increased in patients with preexisting renal diseases or with simultaneous use of other nephrotoxic drugs. Renal and eighth-nerve toxicity increases in patients more than 50 years of age, and SM should be used very cautiously in these patients. Patients should be questioned regarding balance and asked to perform simple tests of vestibular function. In TB treatment, its use is usually limited to 2 months. Although SM itself is relatively inexpensive, the additional cost of needles and syringes increases the effective cost. Although it is routinely given intramuscularly, it can be given safely intravenously.[1,21]

Second-Line Drugs

The second-line drugs include some older drugs that were used early in the treatment of TB; as less toxic regimens became available, however, their routine administration for TB was discontinued.

Para-amino Salicylic Acid   Para-amino salicylic acid (PAS) was the first oral antituberculosis drug that had strong bacteriostatic effect. This effect is potentiated when it is used in conjunction with SM or INH. As the drug is excreted rapidly, high doses are necessary to maintain bacteriostatic activity. The usual oral daily therapeutic dose is approximately 150 mg/kg, and the total dose should not exceed 10 to 12 g/day. The 10- to 12-g/day dosage causes a high rate of adverse gastrointestinal effects, including nausea, vomiting, diarrhea, and epigastric pain. The half-life of PAS is about 1 h and is markedly prolonged in renal failure. PAS is well absorbed orally but does not cross the blood–brain barrier. In 5 to 10 percent of patients, PAS may also cause hypersensitivity reactions and, rarely, hepatitis, hypothyroidism, or hemolytic anemia. Adverse effects may be diminished by beginning therapy with a low dose and gradually increasing to a full dose over 7 to 10 days. To avoid gastrointestinal effects, PAS should be taken after eating. Antacids may also be helpful to reduce these side effects.[1,21]

Ethionamide   Ethionamide has a structure similar to INH but cross-resistance with INH is very rare. A dose of 2.5 μg/ml has a bacteriostatic effect. Ethionamide is well absorbed from gut and metabolized in the liver. Peak serum levels are 15 to 20 mg/ml. The optimum dosage is usually 1 g. It is almost completely and widely distributed in the body compartments. Nausea, vomiting, loss of appetite, and abdominal pain are the most common adverse effects. Serious neurologic reactions include headache, restlessness, diplopia, tremors, and convulsions. It is necessary to increase the dose to the full amount gradually. As it is very irritative for the gastrointestinal tract, a bedtime dose is recommended with an antiemetic and a hypnotic drug. Hepatitis may develop in 1 percent of patients. To monitor hepatotoxicity, monthly hepatic enzyme determination is necessary. In the presence of a fivefold elevation of liver enzyme levels, the drug should be stopped. If well tolerated, ethionamide can be a lifesaving agent in patients with drug-resistant TB.[1,21,29]

Cycloserine   Cycloserine is a bacteriostatic drug. It is an analog of D-alanine and competes with it for incorporation into the cell wall. It is rapidly absorbed from the gut and is distributed to all compartments. Urine excretion accounts for 70 percent of the active form of the drug, as only 30 percent is metabolized. Common side effects include neurologic and psychiatric disturbances ranging from headache, tremor, memory problems, and somno-

lence to psychosis (paranoid, depressive, or catatonic reactions) and seizure. Some patients with depression or anxiety have committed suicide. The usual dose is 15 to 20 mg/kg, with a maximal dosage of 1 g/day. Most of the adverse CNS effects are dose related and disappear when the medication is discontinued. To prevent serious psychic problems, periodic monitoring of mental status and serum drug levels is necessary. To diminish the potential for seizures and convulsions, pyridoxine at doses of 100 to 150 mg/day is helpful. Cycloserine may affect the elimination of phenytoin, especially when taken with INH. Dose reduction of phenytoin is necessary in these cases. In the presence of renal failure, the daily dose of the drug must be reduced.[1,21,29]

Kanamycin   Kanamycin is an aminoglycoside antibiotic that acts on ribosomes, inhibiting protein synthesis. It is an agent that has limited activity against *M. tuberculosis*. The usual dosage is 15 to 30 mg/kg/day, 5 days a week, given intramuscularly with a maximum daily dose of 1 g. For the resistant strains of bacilli, serum concentrations of kanamycin should be in a range of 15 to 20 μg/ml. Ototoxicity is more common with kanamycin than with streptomycin or capreomycin. Hearing loss, tinnitus, and vestibular disturbances are the major symptoms of ototoxicity. Monthly audiometry monitoring is recommended following a baseline audiogram before therapy. Renal toxicity has greatly reduced the use of these aminoglycosides. Nephrotoxicity occurs at the same rate as for capreomycin. Regular, monthly monitoring of serum creatinine and BUN levels is necessary. The frequency of monitoring should be increased in patients who have a history of renal disease. Kanamycin has a cross-resistance with streptomycin and amikacin.

Capreomycin   Capreomycin is chemically distinct from aminoglycosides, but it is likely to have cross-resistance with SM, amikacin, and kanamycin.[2] It has the same therapeutic activity, pharmacology, and toxicity. Daily recommended dosage is 15 to 30 mg/kg by intramuscular injection. Maximum dosage should not exceed 1 g/day. After 2 to 4 months, the drug can be given three times or twice a week until the sputum cultures become negative. It is toxic to the eighth cranial nerve. In many patients (5 to 10 percent), hearing loss develops before vestibular dysfunction. Renal toxicity occurs more frequently than with SM. In elderly patients (over 60 years of age), in the presence of similar susceptibility to capreomycin and amikacin, capreomycin should be the first choice, since older patients seem to have more renal and eighth nerve toxicity with amikacin.[1,21,29]

Amikacin   Amikacin is another aminoglycoside that is bactericidal against several species of mycobacteria in vitro. It has eighth-nerve and renal toxicity, as do the other aminoglycosides. The usual dose is a single intramuscular injection of 15 mg/kg/day for 5 days a week. The same dose can be administered intravenously in 30 min. Average peak serum concentration is 21 μg/ml 1 h after administration of 7.5 mg/kg. The MIC for amikacin is 4 to 8 μg/ml. The major adverse effect is nephrotoxicity, and regular BUN and creatinine monitoring is necessary. If renal insufficiency occurs, the dose and frequency should be reduced. Other side effects are audiovestibular dysfunction and chemical imbalance (low levels of Ca, K, and Mg). Monthly audiogram monitoring is necessary, as for the other aminoglycosides. If a patient receives more than one injectable drug, the frequency of audiograms and kidney function tests should be increased. Monthly serum concentrations of the drugs should be monitored so that the dosage of aminoglycosides can be adjusted. There is cross-resistance to kanamycin and streptomycin.[1,21,29]

Viomycin   Viomycin is chemically different from aminoglycosides but acts like them. In case of SM-resistant tuberculosis, viomycin is used if other alternatives to aminoglycosides are not available. The dosage and duration of therapy are the same as for the other injectable drugs. Viomycin is less likely to show a cross-resistance with SM. To prevent side effects, kidney function should be monitored closely.[29]

Thiacetazone   Thiacetazone is a thiosemicarbazole antibiotic that is not available in the United States because of its severe gastrointestinal, hepatic, bone marrow, and dermatologic toxicity. As it is very cost-effective, it is commonly used in many third-world countries. It is usually used with INH, as its bioactivity is related to INH. It has a bacteriostatic effect and is more toxic than INH. The recommended adult dosage is 150 mg/day or 450 mg twice a week. Commonly, INH 300 mg and thiacetazone 150 mg are combined in a single tablet. Thiacetazone may potentiate the vestibular toxicity of streptomycin. Cutaneous adverse effects may be very severe and may resemble exfoliative dermatitis or Stevens-Johnson syndrome. These reactions frequently occur in AIDS patients. For that reason, its usage is contraindicated in this patient group. There seems to be a better tolerance of this drug in African populations than in Asians.[1,21,29]

POTENTIALLY EFFECTIVE DRUGS IN TUBERCULOSIS TREATMENT

Fluoroquinolones   Fluoroquinolones are broad-spectrum antibacterial agents that act by inhibiting DNA gyrase enzyme. They have activity in vitro against *M. tuberculosis*. There is no cross-resistance between fluoroquinolones and other antituberculosis drugs. The MIC for both ciprofloxacin and ofloxacin is between 0.25 and 2.0 μg/ml, and the predictable serum level for ofloxacin is 8.0 to 11.0 μg/ml. Unless there is the evidence of higher activity of other quinolones, ofloxacin is recommended as the first choice among this family because of its greater bioavailability. In clinical trials, it was given in single (600- to 800-mg) or double (400-mg) daily doses. The dose of ciprofloxacin is 750 mg twice a day or 750 to 1000 mg once a day.[13,49] For more than 7 years, both drugs have been used for multidrug-resistant cases. Administration of quinolones with theophylline increases serum theophylline levels and the risk of adverse effects from theophylline. Ferrous sulfate and antacids with magnesium and aluminum may affect the absorption of quinolones. Further studies are needed to determine the role of fluoroquinolones, including such newer agents as sparfloxacine, lomefloxacine, and levofloxacine.

Rifamycins   Several experimental rifamycins are active against *M. tuberculosis*. Rifabutin, a spiropiperidylrifamycin that is used against *M. avium* infections in AIDS, has 2- to 20-fold greater bactericidal effect against *M. tuberculosis* than rifampin. For that

reason, the possibility exists of using rifabutin as an antituberculosis drug, especially for MDR-TB. As the two drugs have the same mechanism of action and a single-step mutation is responsible for RMP resistance, rifabutin should not be a treatment alternative for RMP-resistant TB. Serum concentration of rifabutin is seven to 10 times lower than that of RMP. Rifabutin has a lower half-life (45 $\pm$ 6 h), and the Cmax:MIC and MBC:MIC ratios are similar to those of RMP. Important advantages of rifabutin are the extensive tissue distribution, higher intracellular penetration, lower enzyme-inducing activity, and no modification of activity when administered under fasting conditions or after a meal.[22,49]

In 520 newly diagnosed TB patients, rifabutin was used instead of RMP, and 150 mg/day of rifabutin was successful for the initial treatment of RMP-susceptible TB.[19,22] The role of rifapentine, P-DEA, CGP-7040, and other rifamycins in the treatment of TB remains to be defined.

New Macrolides   These are semisynthetic derivatives of erythromycin. Currently, they are used against *M. avium-intracellulare*. Azithromycin, roxithromycin, and clarithromycin are thought to have significant activity against *M. tuberculosis*. Further studies are necessary to determine the role of these drugs for patients with TB.[1,55]

Combination of β-Lactam Antibiotics and β-Lactamase Inhibitors   The β-lactam antibiotics have limited activity against mycobacteria, as these organisms produce β-lactamases. In vitro, they have activity against *M. tuberculosis*. But even with the addition of β-lactamase inhibitors, such as sulbactam and clavulonic acid, they do not appear to be clinically effective. Therefore, β-lactams do not have a prominent future in the treatment of TB. However, they may be tried in patients with no other therapeutic option.[1,49]

PRINCIPLES ON STARTING THERAPY

When a decision is made about initiating antituberculosis therapy, physicians should consider the following issues and try to avoid common mistakes (Table 162-4).

1. Tuberculosis should be viewed not only as a disease affecting personal health requiring treatment to cure the patient but also as a disease of public health concerns because of community transmission.
2. Before starting therapy, one should attempt to confirm the diagnosis by sending material to the laboratory for culture.
3. In newly diagnosed TB patients, at least three sputum samples should be sent for culture and drug susceptibility testing before the start of therapy.
4. In smear-negative cases, five or six sputum samples and, if necessary, bronchoalveolar lavage material should be sent for mycobacterial culture.
5. If no other cause can be found in a severely ill, smear-negative, presumed TB patient, antituberculosis therapy should be started immediately.
6. Initial therapy should be with four drugs when the incidence of primary drug resistance is greater than 4 percent.

TABLE 162-4

Common Errors in the Management of Tuberculosis

Addition of a single drug to a failing regimen
Failure to identify preexisting or acquired drug resistance
Chest radiographic findings absent or misinterpreted
Inadequate primary regimen
Failure to identify and address noncompliance
Inappropriate isoniazid preventive therapy

SOURCE: Adapted from Mahmoudi and Iseman,[41] with permission.

7. The emergence of drug resistance is usually due to non-compliance and failure to take all of the drugs (Table 162-4). Resistance is usually to the omitted drug. Directly observed therapy should be considered in all patients.

8. Therapy should never be stopped unless one is certain that the cultures are negative.

CURRENT THERAPY REGIMENS

Before RMP became available, treatment for TB required 18 to 24 months with the drug combination of INH and EMB/PAS. After the introduction of RMP and INH as a drug combination, therapy was successfully shortened from 18 months to 9 months. The duration of therapy was reduced to 6 months after PZA was added to INH and RMP. PZA seems to be the key additional drug in 6-month regimens.

The current therapeutic recommendations for new cases of TB are summarized in Tables 162-5 and 162-6 on the basis of the ATS/CDC recommendations published in 1994.[1] The ATS and CDC currently recommend a 6-month regimen that is based on an initial 2-month "bactericidal phase," consisting of INH and RMP and PZA and either SM or EMB (if the INH resistance possibility is more than 4 percent), and a "continuation phase" of INH and RMP daily or twice weekly for 4 months as an alternative to 9 months of INH and RMP therapy.

The effectiveness of the therapy for TB was demonstrated in a USPHS study that compared a three-drug (INH, RMP, and PZA), 6-month regimen to the standard two-drug (INH and RMP), 9-month regimen. A rapid conversion of sputum in 16 weeks (94.6 versus 89.9 percent) and lower noncompliance rates (16.8 versus 29.2 percent) were observed without any change in relapse rates (3.5 versus 2.8 percent, respectively) 96 weeks after completion of therapy. Additional worldwide studies confirmed the efficacy of 6-month regimens in smear-positive patients.[54] The initial addition of a fourth drug (SM) in smear-positive disease was superior to three drugs.[54] Although PZA is the first choice as

TABLE 162-5

Current Recommendations for Therapy

Four-Month Therapy

   Options 1, 2, and 3 (below, under 6-month therapy) can be administered for 4 months in patients who are not at high risk and have smear-negative, culture-negative pulmonary TB.

Six-Month Therapy

 Option 1

   Eight weeks of daily INH, RMP, and PZA, followed by 16 weeks of INH and RMP daily or two to three times per week.* In areas where the rate of primary INH resistance is not documented to be <4%, EMB and SM should be added to the initial regimen until susceptibility to INH, RMP, and PZA is demonstrated. Continue treatment for at least 6 months and 3 months beyond culture conversion. A TB medical expert should be consulted if the patient is symptomatic or smear culture positive after 3 months.

 Option 2

   Two weeks of daily INH, RMP, PZA, and SM or EMB, followed by 6 weeks (by DOT) of the same drugs twice a week* and subsequently with twice-a-week administration of INH and RMP for 16 weeks (by DOT). A TB medical expert should be consulted if the patient is symptomatic or smear culture positive after 3 months.

 Option 3

   Treat by DOT three times per week with INH, RMP, PZA, and EMB or SM for 6 months.* A TB medical expert should be consulted if the patient is symptomatic or smear culture positive after 3 months.

Nine-Month Therapy

   Nine months of daily INH and RMP or 1 to 2 months of daily INH and RMP, followed by 7 to 8 months of twice-weekly administration. EMB or SM should be added for the first 2 months if INH resistance rate is not documented to be <4%.

HIV-Related Tuberculosis

   Option 1, 2, or 3 can be used for a total of 9 months and at least 6 months beyond culture conversion.* Patients should be followed much more closely, and in the presence of any problem with response to therapy, the evaluation should ensue.

*All regimens administered twice or three times per week should be monitored by DOT for the duration of therapy.
Note: DOT = directly observed therapy.
SOURCE: Adapted from the American Thoracic Society/Centers for Disease Control and Prevention, 1994,[1] with permission.

TABLE 162-6

Recommended Dosage for the Initial Treatment of Tuberculosis in Children* and Adults

	Dosage					
	Daily Dose		Twice-Weekly Dose		Thrice-Weekly Dose	
Drugs	Children	Adults	Children	Adults	Children	Adults
Isoniazid, mg/kg	10–20 Max 300 mg	5 Max 300 mg	20–40 Max 900 mg	15 max Max 900 mg	20–40 Max 900 mg	15 max Max 900 mg
Rifampin, mg/kg	10–20 Max 600 mg	10 Max 600 mg	10–20 Max 600 mg	10 Max 600 mg	10–20 Max 600 mg	10 Max 600 mg
Pyrazinamide, mg/kg	15–30 Max 2 g	15–30 Max 2 g	50–70 Max 4 g	50–70 Max 4 g	50–70 Max 3 g	50–70 Max 3 g
Ethambutol, mg/kg†	15–25	15–25	50	50	25–30	25–30
Streptomycin, mg/kg	20–40 Max 1.0 g	15 Max 1.0 g	25–30 Max 1.5 g	25–30 Max 1.5 g	25–30 Max 1.5 g	25–30 Max 1.5 g

*Children < 12 years of age
†Ethambutol is generally not recommended for children whose visual acuity cannot be monitored (<8 years of age). However, ethambutol should be considered for all children with organisms resistant to other drugs when susceptibility to ethambutol has been demonstrated or susceptibility is likely.
SOURCE: Adapted from the American Thoracic Society/Centers for Disease Control and Prevention, 1994,[1] with permission.

a third drug to add to INH and RMP for short-course therapy, there is no advantage in continuing PZA after the first 2 months of therapy. If the organism is resistant to INH or there is an intolerance to INH, however, INH should be stopped and PZA should be maintained for the entire 6 months. Of interest is that when a good clinical and bacterial response to therapy is observed, whether the initial culture was resistant to either INH and SM did not change the results of 6-month therapy.[46]

In cases in which both INH and PZA cannot be used, EMB and RMP have been recommended for 12 months, although there are not enough data about the efficacy of this approach. A third drug might be necessary to attain adequate success rates. If RMP cannot be used, INH, PZA, and SM may be used daily for 9 months or INH and EMB may be used daily or twice weekly for 18 months.

If INH and RMP cannot be used together because of toxicity, it is wise to use at least three drugs to which the organism is sensitive and continue therapy until culture conversion is documented, followed by at least 12 months of two-drug therapy. The standard 6-month regimen should be extended to 12 months in children with miliary, meningeal, or bone and joint disease.

A 9-month therapy regimen was shown to be very effective against most forms of TB.[19,33,49] In the presence of INH resistance, addition of EMB to the regimen is recommended until culture sensitivity reports are available. If the incidence of primary INH resistance is documented to be greater than 4 percent, EMB at the beginning of therapy is recommended.

Dutt and colleagues observed a very good response in smear- and culture-negative pulmonary TB after 4 months of INH and RMP either daily or twice weekly.[12] A study from Hong Kong showed that the smear- and culture-negative patients responded well to 4 months of either daily or thrice-weekly four-drug therapy.[26] For this group of patients, a treatment period of 4 months

is acceptable. The same regimen can be used for adults who are PPD positive and seem to have an old healed lesion on their chest radiographs or as an alternative regimen to 12 months of preventive INH therapy for PPD-positive, sputum smear– and culture-negative adults.[1]

MONITORING FOR ADVERSE REACTIONS

For evaluation of standard regimens, baseline measurements of a complete blood count, hepatic enzymes, serum bilirubin, and creatinine levels should be obtained. If PZA is used, serum uric acid levels should be monitored. Patients receiving EMB should have both visual acuity measurement and a red-green color perception testing. The baseline tests have two major goals—first, to detect abnormalities that would complicate the regimen and, if necessary, make rearrangements and, second, to monitor the adverse reactions of drugs by means of comparing the baseline measurements with the follow-up results. The same tests should be repeated at monthly examinations. The patients with abnormalities detected on the baseline tests should be evaluated for the cause of this result. If symptoms suggesting drug toxicity occur, appropriate laboratory testing should be performed. Patients should always be informed about the common adverse effects of drugs (Table 162-7) before starting therapy.[1,21]

DURATION OF OBSERVATION AND EVALUATION OF RESPONSE TO TREATMENT

Patients with Positive Pretreatment Sputum

To monitor conversion and to detect the possible emergence of drug resistance, sputum smear and cultures should be obtained

TABLE 162-7

Side Effects of Antituberculosis Drugs

Drugs	Most Common Side Effects	Tests to Detect Side Effects	Remarks
Isoniazid	Peripheral neuritis, hepatotoxicity, hypersensitivity	SGOT, SGPT	Pyrodixine 50 mg as prophylaxis for neuritis; 100–200 mg as treatment
Rifampin	Hepatitis, GI upset (skin eruptions, fever*)	SGOT, SGPT	Orange urine and other body secretions
Pyrazinamide	Hyperuricemia, hepatotoxicity (skin rash, GI irritation*)	Serum uric acid level, SGOT, SGPT	NSAIDS for nongouty polyarthralgias; allopurinol for frank gout
Streptomycin	8th-nerve damage, nephrotoxicity	Vestibular function, audiograms; BUN/creatinine	Use with caution in older patients or those with renal disease
Ethambutol	Optic neuritis (reversible), (hyperuricemia, gout, skin rash, drug fever, GI irritation*)	Red-green color discrimination and visual acuity	Use with caution when eye test is not feasible
Ethionamide	GI intolerance, endocrine disturbances, hepatitis, hypersensitivity	SGOT, SGPT	Consider antiemetics or bedtime dosing
Cycloserine	Neurologic and psychiatric disturbances	Serum levels of drug, regular control of mental status	Pyridoxine
Capreomycin, Kanamycin, Amikacin, Viomycin,	Hearing loss, vestibular damage, renal toxicity, electrolyte disturbances	Audiogram, vestibular examination, BUN/creatinine	Use with caution in older patients or those with renal disease
p-amino-salicylic acid	GI intolerance, hepatitis, hypersensitivity	SGOT, SGPT	Consider antacids or dosing at mealtime
Ciprofloxacin, Ofloxacin	GI intolerance, headache, restlessness, hypersensitivity, drug interactions	Monitoring for drug interactions	Avoid antacids, iron, zinc, and sucralfate, which decrease absorption
Clofazimine	Abdominal pain, skin discoloration (both dose related), photosensitivity		Consider dosing at mealtime; avoid sunlight; efficacy is unproven

*Less common side effects.
SOURCE: From Simone and Dooley,[53] with permission.

monthly or at least after 2, 4, and 6 months of therapy. With INH- and RMP-containing regimens, sputum should convert to negative within 2 months. If smear and culture results continue to be positive after 2 months of therapy, emerging drug resistance and noncompliance should be major concerns. A new drug susceptibility test should be performed immediately. Unless drug resistance is demonstrated, the regimen in use should be continued carefully under direct observation. If drug resistance occurs, at least two new drugs to which the organism is sensitive should be added to the therapy and administered under direct observation. Addition of a single drug to therapy should never be done, since it increases the risk of the rapid development of resistance to the new drug. Bacteriologic culture and sensibility tests should be performed at monthly intervals until the cultures become neg-

ative. Relapse of drug-sensitive infections after adequate INH- and RMP-containing treatment is very infrequent. For patients who have completed a standard regimen and who have had a satisfactory bacteriologic response, follow-up after completion of therapy is not necessary. In contrast, the patient with extensive disease, immunosuppressed patients, the persistence of radiographic findings after therapy, or suspicion of poor patient compliance, are indications for prolonged follow-up.

A chest radiograph before the start of therapy is necessary to compare with one taken after the completion of therapy. Monthly chest radiographs during therapy are helpful but not as essential as sputum examinations. A chest radiograph taken at the end of therapy will also help for comparison with any future films.

Patients with Negative Sputum

In patients with radiographic abnormalities and clinical findings consistent with TB, diagnostic tests should be performed to isolate *M. tuberculosis*. If an alternative diagnosis cannot be established, treatment against TB should be started while culture results are awaited. For this group of patients, clinical evaluation and chest radiographs are the major indicators of response to therapy. If cultures are negative and radiographic changes have not occurred after 3 months of an INH- and RMP-containing regimen, the abnormality is probably due to another disease or a TB fibrotic scar.

Retreatment of Patients Who Have Relapsed

Patients whose sputum is persistently positive after 5 to 6 months of therapy are considered treatment failures. A current sputum specimen should be obtained for the susceptibility testing. While susceptibility results are pending, the original therapy may be continued, or at least three new drugs added to the therapy. Direct supervision of therapy should be implemented if that has not already been done. When the new susceptibility test results are received, a new regimen should be adopted in accordance with the results of the susceptibility tests. Patients who relapse after completing a regimen containing both INH and RMP, and whose organisms were susceptible to the drugs at the outset of treatment, may be restarted on their original therapy, since the organisms are still usually susceptible. In contrast, patients who relapsed after taking a regimen that did not contain both INH and RMP should be assumed to be infected with an organism that is resistant to all previous drugs and managed accordingly.

ADHERENCE AND DIRECTLY OBSERVED THERAPY

Nonadherence to therapy is a major reason for the failure of antituberculosis treatment. To overcome this problem, therapy should be given under direct observation, if possible. A medical or other responsible person should observe as the patient ingests antituberculosis drugs. A health-care worker may observe the patient in the "field" (patient's home, place of work, school, etc.) or in the clinic. Following the daily initial therapy, directly observed therapy (DOT) may be administered during the second phase. DOT is especially useful in alcoholic, drug addictive, or homeless patients, as the risk of nonadherence is very high in these groups. Currently, only 10 to 12 percent of patients in the United States receive DOT.

The effectiveness of DOT was demonstrated in Baltimore by observation of a declining TB case rate, while similar cities that did not use DOT had unchanged or rising TB case rates.[7] In Texas, after initiation of a DOT regimen, a fall in the frequency of primary drug resistance, acquired drug resistance, and relapses with multidrug-resistant organisms was observed. This was in spite of the rising TB case rate and increasing rates of AIDS and homelessness.[63] The cost of including supervision adds only $400 to the cost of unsupervised therapy.[31] The cost of such therapy is insignificant compared to the cost of treatment for hospitalization for advanced TB or multidrug-resistant TB.

TREATMENT OF DRUG-RESISTANT TUBERCULOSIS

Patients can become infected with *Mycobacteria* resistant to drugs in two ways. The first is to become infected with resistant organisms. This is called primary resistance. The second is that the resistant organism develops in TB patients during therapy. This is called secondary resistance. In certain parts of the world, primary resistance rates to INH and SM may exceed 20 to 35 percent. In some Asian populations in the United States, the rate has been reported to be as high as 58 percent.[53] In 1983, the CDC reported that primary resistance was most common for INH (4 percent), SM (3.8 percent), and ethionamide (1.1 percent). The rates for RMP, EMB, kanamycin, cycloserine, capreomycin, and PAS were less than 1 percent.

During the initial phase of treatment with a single drug, most of the susceptible bacilli are destroyed, but the small number of resistant mutants continue to grow and, after 2 weeks to several months, the resistant bacilli outgrow the susceptible bacilli; this is known as the "fall and rise" phenomenon. In a large population, additional mutation can occur, resulting in doubling resistant mutants. Basically, nonadherence to prescribed therapy and the use of inadequate therapy regimens cause the development of drug resistance. The best treatment for drug-resistant TB is to make sure the patient receives adequate treatment initially and prevent the emergence of drug resistance.

Current CDC recommendations are an initial regimen of four drugs when the primary INH-resistant rate in a community is greater than 4 percent. If resistance occurs, the basic principle of managing patients whose organisms are resistant to one or more drugs is the administration of at least two agents that have activity against *M. tuberculosis* strains. Isolated INH resistance is well documented. For patients infected with INH-resistant organisms, INH should be discontinued and PZA should be continued for the entire 6 months of therapy. When INH resistance is discovered during a 9-month regimen, INH should be discontinued. If EMB was given from the beginning of therapy, it should be continued with RMP for a minimum of 12 months. If EMB was not in the regimen, INH should be discontinued, and two new drugs (EMB and PZA) should be added. The regimen can be adjusted when the results of the susceptibility test become available.

Multidrug resistance is defined as the in vitro resistance of a strain of *M. tuberculosis* to two or more antituberculosis drugs. This is a very serious and difficult therapeutic problem. Clinically, the most important pattern of multidrug resistance is resistance to both INH and RMP. Goble and coworkers[17] treated 171 INH-RMP–resistant patients under DOT. At least three new drugs not given previously (one parenteral, two oral), to which TB bacilli were fully susceptible, were added to the regimen. In addition, drugs to which the organisms were at least partly susceptible or drugs previously given for a relatively short time were also added to the regimen. From 171 patients, the sputum cultures of only 87 patients became negative within 1 to 8 months. Despite treatment, 47 percent remained sputum culture positive and 12 percent of patients suffered relapses. Including those who had relapses, 44 percent had unfavorable outcomes. The ATS also recommends giving at least three new drugs to which the organism is susceptible. These regimens usually contain six or seven drugs. When both INH and RMP are ineffective, therapy should continue for 24 months after conversion of cultures to negative, as it may take several months for a patient with multidrug-resistant TB to become culture negative, the total duration of treatment may last well beyond 2 years, and adherence to therapy and drug toxicity become an even greater problem during this period.[30,49]

For patients who are infected with organisms that are resistant to multiple drugs and in whom the preponderance of disease is in one lung or lobe, the therapeutic efficacy of surgery was studied by Iseman and colleagues.[32] Of 99 multidrug-resistant patients, 27 had surgery and 25 remained sputum culture negative for a mean duration of 36 months (combination of surgery and medical therapy).

SURGERY

Surgery is rarely used for treatment of TB. Before the chemotherapeutic era, surgery was used as an adjunct to "resting" of the lungs. Operations such as artificial pneumothorax, artificial pneumoperitoneum, plombage, artificial phrenic nerve paralysis, thoracoplasty, pulmonary resection, cavity drainage, and decortication were performed as important adjunctive treatment for managing cavitary lesions, progressive local diseases, empyemas, and fibrothorax. Today, surgery has a role to cure treatment failures, such as multidrug-resistant TB cases with localized disease (as mentioned above), chronic empyema, bronchopleural fistula, life-threatening hemoptysis unresponsive to arteriographic embolization, and closed pleural space evacuation.

ADJUNCTIVE CORTICOSTEROID THERAPY

Corticosteroids do not play a major role in treatment of TB, but they are useful in some types of diseases. In fulminant miliary disease and obstructive lymphadenopathy, 20 to 30 mg daily prednisone is very helpful to relieve symptoms, improve oxygenation, and abolish fever. Patients with tuberculous meningitis at stages 2 and 3 (uncomplicated cases) seem to benefit from corticosteroid therapy. Prednisone should be begun at 60 to 80 mg daily and gradually be decreased after 1 to 2 weeks. Corticosteroid therapy has been recommended in treatment of pericardial TB to prevent constriction.

REFERENCES

1. American Thoracic Society/Centers for Disease Control and Prevention: Treatment of tuberculosis infection in adults and children. *Am Rev Respir Dis* 149:1359–1374, 1994.
2. Banerjee A, Dubnau E, Quemard A, et al: *InhA*, a gene encoding a target for isoniazid and ethionamide in *Mycobacterium tuberculosis*. *Science* 263:227–230, 1994.
3. Beg MH, Reyazuddin: Bilateral simultaneous pneumothorax—a study of 25 cases. *Indian J Chest Dis Allied Sci* 32:25–27, 1990.
4. Board of the Pittsfield Anti-tuberculosis Association: Standard therapy for tuberculosis 1985. *Chest* 87(Suppl):117S–124S, 1985.
5. British Thoracic and Tuberculosis Association, Research Committee: Aspergilloma and residual tuberculous cavities—the results of a survey. *Tubercle* 51:227–245, 1970.
6. Canetti G: Present aspects of bacterial resistance in tuberculosis. *Am Rev Respir Dis* 92:687–703, 1965.
7. Chaulk CP, Moore-Rice K, Rizzo R, Chaisson RE: Eleven years of community-based directly observed therapy for tuberculosis. *JAMA* 274: 945–951, 1995.
8. Comstock GW, Livesay VT, Woolpert SF: The prognosis of a positive tuberculin reaction in childhood and adolescence. *Am J Epidemiol* 99:131–138, 1974.
9. Cremaschi P, Nascimbene C, Vitulo P, et al: Therapeutic embolization of bronchial artery: A successful treatment in 209 cases of relapse hemoptysis. *Angiology* 44:295–299, 1993.
10. Danek SJ, Bower JS: Diagnosis of pulmonary tuberculosis by flexible fiberoptic bronchoscopy. *Am Rev Respir Dis* 119:677–679, 1979.
11. David HL: Probability distribution of drug-resistant mutants in selected populations of *Mycobacterium tuberculosis. Appl Microbiol* 20:810–814, 1970.
12. Dutt AK, Moers D, Stead WW: Smear- and culture-negative pulmonary tuberculosis: Four-month short-course chemotherapy. *Am Rev Respir Dis* 139:867–870, 1989.
13. Ellner JJ, Hinman AR, Dooley SW, et al: Tuberculosis symposium: Emerging problems and promise. *J Infect Dis* 168:537–551, 1993.
14. Farrell FJ, Keeffe EB, Man KM, et al: Treatment of hepatic failure secondary to hepatitis with liver transplantation. *Dig Dis Sci* 39:2255–2259, 1994.
15. Fraser RG, Paré JAP. *Diagnosis of Diseases of the Chest.* Philadelphia, WB Saunders, 1977, pp 731–764.
16. Glassroth J, Robbins AG, Snider DE. Tuberculosis in the 1980s. *New Engl J Med* 302:1441–1450, 1980.
17. Goble M, Iseman MD, Madsen LA, et al: Treatment of 171 patients with pulmonary tuberculosis resistant to isoniazid and rifampin. *New Engl J Med* 328:527–532, 1993.
18. Goldman LA, Braman SS: Isoniazid: A review with emphasis on adverse effects. *Chest* 62:71–77, 1972.
19. Gonzalez-Montaner LJ, Natal S, Yongchaiyud P, Olliaro P, the Rifabutin Study Group: Rifabutin for the treatment of newly diagnosed pulmonary tuberculosis: A multinational, randomized, comparative study versus rifampicin. *Tubercle Lung Dis* 75:341–347, 1994.
20. Grosset J, Leventis S: Adverse effects of rifampin. *Rev Infect Dis* 5(Suppl 3):S440–S450, 1983.
21. Haas DW, Des Prez RM: Current treatment and management, in Rossman MD, MacGregor RR (eds), *Tuberculosis.* New York, McGraw-Hill, 1995, pp 187–207.
22. Heifets LB, Lindholm-Levy PJ, Flory MA: Bactericidal activity in vitro of various rifamycins against *Mycobacterium avium* and *Mycobacterium tuberculosis. Am Rev Respir Dis* 141:626–630, 1990.
23. Heym B, Zhang Y, Poulet S, et al: Characterization of the *katG* gene encoding a catalase-peroxidase required for the isoniazid susceptibility of *Mycobacterium tuberculosis. J Bacteriol* 175:4255–4259, 1993.
24. Holden M, Dubin MR, Diamond PH: Frequency of negative intermediate-strength tuberculin sensitivity in patients with active tuberculosis. *New Engl J Med* 285:1506–1509, 1971.
25. Hong Kong Chest Service/British Medical Research Council: Controlled trial of 2, 4, and 6 months of pyrazinamide in 6-month, three-times-weekly regimens for smear-positive pulmonary tuberculosis, including an assessment of a combined preparation of isoniazid, rifampin, and pyrazinamide. *Am Rev Respir Dis* 143:700–706, 1991.
26. Hong Kong Chest Service/Tuberculosis Research Centre, Madras/British Medical Research Council: A controlled trial of 3-month, 4-month, and 6-month regimens of chemotherapy for sputum-smear-negative pulmonary tuberculosis. *Am Rev Respir Dis* 139:871–876, 1989.

27. Honore N, Cole ST: Molecular basis of rifampin resistance in *Mycobacterium leprae. Antimicrob Agents Chemother* 37:414–418, 1993.

28. Honore N , Cole ST: Streptomycin resistance in mycobacteria. *Antimicrob Agents Chemother* 38:238–242, 1994.

29. Houston S, Fanning A: Current and potential treatment of tuberculosis. *Drugs* 48:689–708, 1994.

30. Iseman MD: Treatment of multidrug-resistant tuberculosis. *New Engl J Med* 329:784–791, 1993.

31. Iseman MD, Cohn DL, Sbarbaro JA: Directly observed treatment of tuberculosis: We can't afford not to try it. *New Engl J Med* 328:576–578, 1993.

32. Iseman MD, Madsen L, Goble M, Pomerantz M: Surgical intervention in the treatment of pulmonary disease caused by drug-resistant *Mycobacterium tuberculosis. Am Rev Respir Dis* 141:623–625, 1990.

33. Jabes D, Della Bruna C, Rossi R, Olliaro P: Effectiveness of rifabutin alone or in combination with isoniazid in preventive therapy of mouse tuberculosis. *Antimicrob Agents Chemother* 38:2346–2350, 1994.

34. Kempsell KE, Ji YE, Estrada IC, et al: The nucleotide sequence of the promoter, 16S rRNA and spacer region of the ribosomal RNA operon of *Mycobacterium tuberculosis* and comparison with *Mycobacterium leprae* precursor rRNA. *J Gen Microbiol* 138:1717–1727, 1992.

35. Kim YH, Kim HT, Lee KS, et al: Serial fiberoptic bronchoscopic observations of endobronchial tuberculosis before and early after antituberculosis chemotherapy. *Chest* 103:673–677, 1993.

36. Kohler LJ, Gohara AF, Hamilton RW, Reeves RS: Cresentic fibrillary glomerulonephritis associated with intermittent rifampin therapy for pulmonary tuberculosis. *Clin Nephrol* 42:263–265, 1994.

37. Konno K, Feldman FM, McDermott W: Pyrazinamide susceptibility and amidase activity of tubercle bacilli. *Am Rev Respir Dis* 95:461–469, 1967.

38. Korzeniewska-Kosela M, Krysl J, Muller N, et al: Tuberculosis in young adults and the elderly: A prospective comparison study. *Chest* 106:28–32, 1994.

39. MacGregor RR: A year's experience with tuberculosis in a private urban teaching hospital in the postsanatorium era. *Am J Med* 58:221–228, 1975.

40. Maddrey WC, Boitnott JK: Isoniazid hepatitis. *Ann Intern Med* 79:1–12, 1973.

41. Mahmoudi A, Iseman MD: Pitfalls in the care of patients with tuberculosis: Common errors and their association with the acquisition of drug resistance. *JAMA* 270:65–68, 1993.

42. Mayock RL, Goldberg M: Metabolic considerations in disease of the respiratory system, in Duncan GG (ed), *Diseases of Metabolism.* Philadelphia, WB Saunders, 1964, pp 1395–1402.

43. Mayock RL, MacGregor RR: Diagnosis, prevention and early therapy of tuberculosis. *Dis Mon* 22:1–60, 1976.

44. Meier A, Kirschner P, Bange FC, et al: Genetic alterations in streptomycin-resistant *Mycobacterium tuberculosis:* Mapping of mutations conferring resistance. *Antimicrob Agents Chemother* 38:228–233, 1994.

45. Miller WT, MacGregor RR: Tuberculosis: Frequency of unusual radiographic findings. *Am J Roentgenol* 130:867–875, 1978.

46. Mitchinson DA, Nunn AJ: Influence of initial drug resistance on the response to short-course chemotherapy of pulmonary tuberculosis. *Am Rev Respir Dis* 133:423–430, 1986.

47. Morris CD, Bird AR, Nell H: The haematological and biochemical changes in severe pulmonary tuberculosis. *Q J Med* 73:1151–1159, 1989.

48. Murphy R, Richard S, Watkins PB: Severe acetaminophen toxicity in a patient receiving isoniazid. *Ann Intern Med* 113:799–800, 1990.

49. Peloquin CA, Berning SE: Infection caused by *Mycobacterium tuberculosis. Ann Pharmacother* 28:72–84, 1994.

50. Poppius H, Thomander K: Segmentary distribution of cavities: A radiologic study of 500 consecutive cases of cavernous pulmonary tuberculosis. *Ann Med Intern Fenn* 46:113–119, 1957.

51. Salfinger M, Crowle AJ, Reller LB: Pyrazinamide and pyrazinoic acid activity against tuberculosis bacilli in cultured human macrophages and in the BACTEC system. *J Infect Dis* 162:201–207, 1990.

52. Senderovitz T, Viskum K: Corticosteroids and tuberculosis. *Respir Med* 88:561–565, 1994.

53. Simone PM, Dooley SW: The phenomenon of multidrug-resistant tuberculosis, in Rossman MD, MacGregor RR (eds), *Tuberculosis.* New York, McGraw-Hill, 1995, pp 219–311.

54. Singapore Tuberculosis Service/British Medical Research Council: Assessment of a daily combined preparation of isoniazid, rifampin, and pyrazinamide in a controlled trial of three 6-month regimens for smear-positive pulmonary tuberculosis. *Am Rev Respir Dis* 143:707–712, 1991.

55. Smith H: Complications of treatment, in Rossman MD, MacGregor RR (eds), *Tuberculosis.* New York, McGraw-Hill, 1995, pp 209–219.

56. Snider DE, Graczyk J, Bek E, Rogowski J: Supervised six-months treatment of newly diagnosed pulmonary tuberculosis using isoniazid, rifampin, and pyrazinamide with and without streptomycin. *Am Rev Respir Dis* 130:1091–1094, 1984.

57. Steele MA, Burk RF, Des Prez RM: Toxic hepatitis with isoniazid and rifampin. *Chest* 99:465–471, 1991.

58. Telenti A, Imboden P, Marchesi F, et al: Detection of rifampicin-resistance mutations in *Mycobacterium tuberculosis. Lancet* 341:664–665, 1993.

59. Tsubota N, Yoshimura M, Murotani A, et al: Results of surgical treatment for calcified tuberculous empyema: Improved pulmonary function obtained with lung preserving policy. *Tohoku J Exp Med* 171:235–242, 1993.

60. Vallejo JG, Ong LT, Starke JR: Clinical features, diagnosis, and treatment of tuberculosis in infants. *Pediatrics* 94:1–7, 1994.

61. Wallace JM, Deutsch AL, Harrell JH, Moser KM: Bronchoscopy and transbronchial biopsy in evaluation of patients with suspected active tuberculosis. *Am J Med* 70:1189–1194, 1981.

62. Weber AL, Bird KT, Janower WL: Primary tuberculosis in childhood with particular emphasis on changes affecting the tracheobronchial tree. *Am J Roentgenol* 103:123–132, 1968.

63. Weis SE, Slocum PC, Blais FX, et al: The effect of directly observed therapy on the rates of drug resistance and relapse in tuberculosis. *New Engl J Med* 330:1179–1184, 1994.

CHAPTER 163

MYCOBACTERIAL INFECTIONS AND HIV INFECTION

Richard E. Chaisson

Mycobacterial infections are important complications of human immunodeficiency virus (HIV) disease. In the past decade, the emerging HIV pandemic has resulted in dramatic increases in illness caused by mycobacteria. In particular, the HIV epidemic has contributed to resurgent tuberculosis in developed countries, exacerbations of hyperendemic tuberculosis in developing countries, and unprecedented numbers of patients with disseminated *Mycobacterium avium*–complex (MAC) infections. Infections with other nontuberculous mycobacteria, such as *M. kansasii* and *M. hemophilum,* are also associated with HIV infection. The importance of mycobacterial infections in patients with HIV disease can be seen in Fig. 163-1. This figure portrays the incidence of mycobacterial infections in patients with advanced HIV infection (CD4 count under 300) followed at the Johns Hopkins Hospital HIV Clinic. The risk of *M. avium*–complex disease was approximately 20 percent after 3 years, while tuberculosis occurred in approximately 3 percent of patients. In developing countries, tuberculosis is exceedingly common in patients with HIV infection, while *M. avium* complex is more unusual. Fig. 163-2 shows the worldwide prevalence of coinfection with HIV and *M. tuberculosis.* The World Health Organization estimates that at least 6 million adults are infected with both agents. Throughout the world, mycobacterial infections are common complications of HIV-associated immunodeficiency. This chapter will review the clinical and therapeutic aspects of HIV-related mycobacterial infections.

MYCOBACTERIUM TUBERCULOSIS

Epidemiology

The overlap of HIV and *M. tuberculosis* infections has resulted in a number of significant interactions between these two pathogens. Epidemiologic data indicate that HIV infection is increasingly common in populations with a high prevalence of *M. tuberculosis* infection. In the United States, for example, HIV is prevalent in injection drug users, people from racial and ethnic minority groups, and residents of inner cities—populations with historically high rates of tuberculosis. The increased susceptibility of these coinfected persons to developing active tuberculosis contributed to a 20 percent increase in tuberculosis morbidity in the United States between 1985 and 1992.[37] In developing countries, where the prevalence of tuberculosis infection in adults may exceed 50 percent, the spread of HIV has caused sharp increases in tuberculosis case rates. Substantial increases in tuberculosis morbidity have occurred in sub-Saharan African countries, Thailand, and Latin American countries where HIV is prevalent (Fig. 163-2). The World Health Organization estimates that the prevalence of HIV-related tuberculosis cases doubled worldwide between 1990 and 1995 (from 4 percent to more than 8 percent of all cases), and will increase a further 65 percent by the year 2000.[35] As case rates of tuberculosis have increased as a consequence of the HIV epidemic, additional problems have emerged. Outbreaks of tuberculosis in HIV-infected persons in hospitals or other congregate living facilities and multidrug-resistant tuberculosis are problems that have assumed enormous proportions.

Pathogenesis

HIV infection profoundly alters host defenses against *M. tuberculosis* (see Chapter 160). In persons with latent tuberculosis infection, the acquisition of HIV infection produces progressive loss of cell-mediated immunity, which impairs containment of tubercle bacilli. A number of immunologic defects have been noted in patients with HIV and *M. tuberculosis* infections, in-

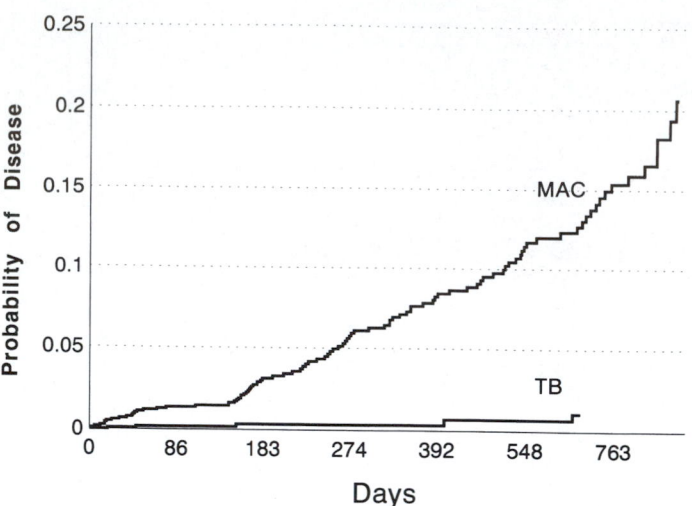

FIGURE 163-1 Incidence of mycobacterial infections in patients with HIV infection and CD4 counts <300/mm³ followed in the Johns Hopkins HIV Clinic Cohort. MAC = *M. avium*–complex; TB = *M. tuberculosis. (From Moore and Chaisson: Ann Intern Med 124, 1996.)*

cluding reductions in CD4 cell levels, impaired T-cell proliferation, decreased cytolytic T-cell responses, deranged intracellular killing, and reduced cytokine elaboration in response to mycobacterial antigen challenge. Patients with latent tuberculosis infection and HIV have a 2 to 10 percent annual risk of developing active tuberculosis.[29,37] The risk of reactivation rises as CD4 cell levels decline.

The early natural history of *M. tuberculosis* infection is also greatly affected by HIV disease. People with HIV infection who acquire new tuberculosis infections have an extraordinarily high rate of progressive, primary tuberculosis. In an outbreak of tuberculosis among HIV-infected residents of a residential facility in San Francisco, 38 percent of susceptible patients developed active pulmonary tuberculosis with an identical strain of *M. tuberculosis* (identified with restriction fragment length polymorphism analysis) within 4 months of exposure to the index case.[14] The rapid progression of tuberculosis infection to tuberculosis disease in persons with HIV infection has resulted in numerous epidemics of tuberculosis in institutions such as hospitals, nursing homes, and prisons, as well as in community settings. Recent molecular epidemiologic studies have shown that approximately 40 percent of tuberculosis cases in urban areas of the United States are epidemiologically clustered, indicating recent transmission and primary disease.[41] In these settings, HIV infection is significantly associated with clustering of tuberculosis cases.

While HIV has a major effect on the natural history of tuberculosis, there is

also evidence that tuberculosis may affect the course of HIV disease. Activation of CD4 lymphocytes by tuberculosis enhances susceptibility to HIV infection in vitro, and HIV-infected CD4 cells stimulated by mycobacterial antigens have enhanced in vitro HIV replication.[43] Cytokine elaboration by lymphocytes and macrophages in patients with tuberculosis and HIV—in particular, tumor necrosis factor and interleukin 1—may up-regulate HIV expression.[47] Preliminary studies indicate that HIV plasma viral load is increased in patients with active tuberculosis and HIV infection. Thus, prevention of tuberculosis in HIV-infected persons may prevent AIDS-related morbidity in addition to tuberculosis. Conversely, the occurrence of tuberculosis in an HIV-infected patient may be a clinical marker of immune system failure rather than a cause of enhanced immunodeficiency.

Clinical Manifestations

The clinical features of tuberculosis in persons with HIV infection may differ considerably from those seen in patients without HIV infection. Nonetheless, like HIV-seronegative patients, most patients with HIV-related tuberculosis have pulmonary impairment. In patients with higher CD4 cell counts (more than 300), tuberculosis may be more typical, involving the lungs predominantly with upper-lobe infiltrates, with or without cavitation. As CD4 cell levels decline, tuberculosis in the HIV-infected patient is more likely to be disseminated, both within the lung and throughout the body.[23] The pulmonary presentation of tuberculosis in these patients may mimic *Pneumocystis carinii* pneumonia, with diffuse interstitial infiltrates or alveolar infiltrates (Fig. 163-3). Hilar adenopathy and lower-lobe infiltrates are found in patients with progressive, primary tuberculosis. In advanced HIV disease, extrapulmonary tuberculosis is more common. Sites of extrapulmonary invasion that are most prevalent are lymph nodes, the urinary tract, meninges, and blood and bone marrow. Mycobacteremia is not unusual, particularly in patients

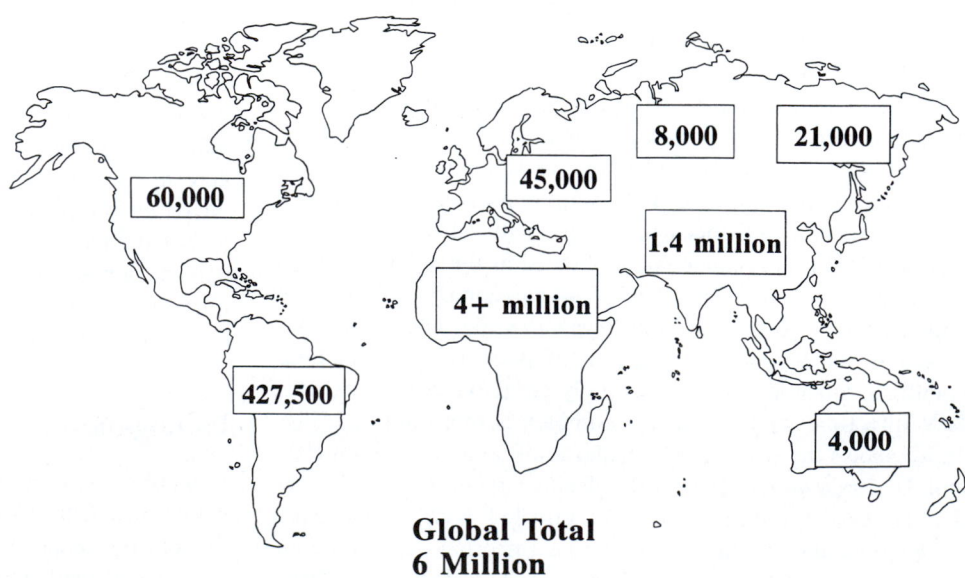

FIGURE 163-2 Global prevalence of infection with both HIV and *M. tuberculosis. (Courtesy of Mario C. Raviglione, M.D., World Health Organization.)*

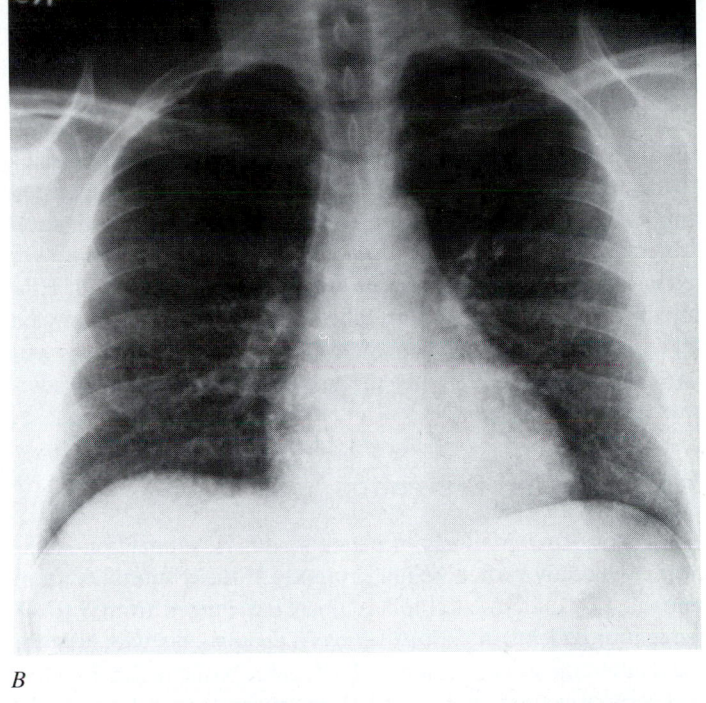

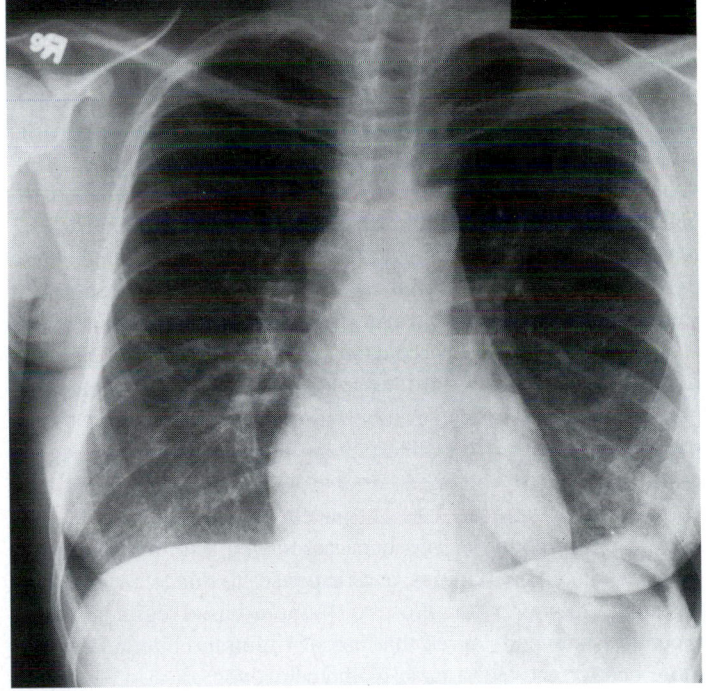

A

B

C

FIGURE 163-3   Chest radiographs from patients with HIV infection and pulmonary tuberculosis. *A.* Right paratrachial adenopathy and right upper-lobe infiltrate in a 43-year-old HIV-seropositive woman with tuberculosis. Needle fragments are also seen in right neck and right lower midlung. *B.* Miliary tuberculosis in a 40-year-old HIV-infected man. *C.* Bilateral lower-lung infiltrates in a 36-year-old HIV-seropositive pregnant woman with an axillary mass. An admission chest radiograph 8 days earlier was normal. The mass and sputum specimens grew *M. tuberculosis.*

with low CD4 cell counts. One study found that mycobacterial blood cultures were positive in 49 percent of HIV-infected tuberculosis patients with CD4 counts at or under 100 per mm³, as opposed to 11 percent for patients with CD4 counts above 100 per mm³.[23]

The diagnosis of tuberculosis in the HIV-infected patient requires a high index of suspicion and the utilization of appropriate diagnostic tests. Acid-fast smears of respiratory secretions or tissue samples are useful, in that positive smears are strongly suggestive of tuberculosis, even in populations where *M. avium* complex is more common. In addition, the sensitivity of acid-fast smears of respiratory secretions is not altered in advanced HIV disease. However, only two-thirds to three-quarters of HIV-infected patients with pulmonary tuberculosis will have a positive acid-fast smear. Rapid diagnostic methods—such as radiometric culture systems, nucleic acid amplification, and other novel techniques—are necessary to establish a timely diagnosis. Both bronchoalveolar lavage and transbronchial biopsy can be of value in diagnosing HIV-related pulmonary tuberculosis, as well as in determining the presence or absence of other

pathogens, such as *P. carinii.* Biopsy is particularly useful for patients with pulmonary nodules or hilar or subcarinal lymphadenopathy; identification of granulomas or caseous necrosis is strongly suggestive of tuberculosis. Because of the moderate sensitivity of acid-fast smears, presumptive therapy for tuberculosis is often necessary after diagnostic studies have been performed and cultures are pending.

As discussed elsewhere, the diagnosis of tuberculosis infection with the purified protein derivative (PPD) skin test is less sensitive in patients with HIV infection than in other populations. Graham and colleagues found that only 14 percent of HIV-infected drug users had a reaction of at least 5 mm induration to PPD, whereas 25 percent of HIV-seronegative drug users had a reaction of at least 10 mm induration.[17] The sensitivity of the tuberculin skin test declines as CD4 cell levels fall in HIV-infected patients. The use of anergy testing in such patients is controversial. Although several studies have demonstrated increased rates of tuberculosis in HIV-infected patients,[2] others have suggested that anergy testing is unstable over time[6] and that reactivation tuberculosis is uncommon in anergic subjects. Tuberculin skin testing can be extremely useful, however, in patients with HIV infection suspected of having tuberculosis. Even with advanced HIV disease, almost half of patients with active tuberculosis will have a positive PPD, giving the test important positive predictive value clinically.

Treatment and Prevention

Treatment of tuberculosis in patients with HIV infection is extremely effective when begun promptly.[40] Early mortality from untreated or undertreated tuberculosis has ranged from 5 to 18 percent of patients in various series. When patients with HIV-related tuberculosis are treated with rifampin-based regimens, clinical responses are similar to those in tuberculosis patients without HIV infection. Several recent studies have indicated that short-course regimens (i.e., 6 months' treatment) are highly successful, with low relapse rates.[10] Moreover, therapy given under direct supervision is associated with better outcomes and longer survival. Regimens for the treatment of tuberculosis in patients with HIV infection are given elsewhere (see Chapter 162). Whereas earlier recommendations stated that HIV-infected tuberculosis patients should be treated for at least 6 months after conversion of cultures to negative, current guidelines recognize the high rate of success with conventional 6-month regimens. It should be emphasized, however, that even with appropriate therapy, between 2 and 5 percent of patients will relapse. For this reason, some clinicians still favor longer courses of treatment for patients with HIV-related tuberculosis. HIV-infected patients successfully treated for tuberculosis may also become exogenously reinfected with new strains of *M. tuberculosis* and develop recurrent disease. Use of thiacetazone in place of rifampin in developing countries has been associated with a high rate of serious cutaneous toxicities, and responses to thiacetazone-based regimens are poorer than those to rifampin-based regimens. Most tuberculosis experts agree that use of rifampin is both safer and more cost-effective than use of thiacetazone.

Resistance to antituberculosis agents is a growing problem that has been exacerbated by the HIV epidemic.[4,15] Although the molecular mechanisms of isoniazid and rifampin resistance were elucidated only recently, the manner in which drug resistance occurs in patients has long been known. Inappropriate exposure to antituberculosis drugs, through patient nonadherence or physician mistake, promotes emergence of innately resistant strains of *M. tuberculosis*.[27] The magnitude of drug-resistant tuberculosis has grown substantially in recent years, particularly in the United States. In New York City, the prevalence of drug resistance in tuberculosis isolates from April 1991 was approximately 33 percent, while multidrug resistance (resistance to isoniazid and ri-

fampin) was detected in 19 percent of isolates. Outbreaks of multidrug-resistant tuberculosis were reported in hospital patients and prison inmates in New York, Florida, and other locations, primarily in HIV-infected subjects. Case fatality rates have approached 80 percent in these outbreaks. Control of multidrug-resistant tuberculosis has required enormous investments in tuberculosis treatment programs and institutional infection control programs. With the emergence of multidrug-resistant tuberculosis, the United States Centers for Disease Control and Prevention and the American Thoracic Society have recommended that the initial treatment of active tuberculosis consist of at least a four-drug regimen, and that therapy be supervised unless adherence to treatment is assured.[1] Treatment of multidrug-resistant tuberculosis is frequently unsuccessful, even in immunocompetent patients, underscoring the importance of prevention of this complication. While recent reports emphasize longer survival of HIV-infected patients with multidrug-resistant tuberculosis, cure rates are still very low.

Several recent reports have documented the emergence of rifampin resistance during therapy for HIV-related tuberculosis. Some cases may be due to patient noncompliance or to inappropriate physician prescribing, while others have been associated with rifabutin prophylaxis against *M. avium*–complex infection. Nonetheless, the risk of developing rifampin resistance appears to be greatly increased in patients with HIV infection. The reasons for this phenomenon are not fully understood, but it has been suggested that malabsorption of medications may play a role.

Prevention of tuberculosis in HIV-infected persons with isoniazid chemoprophylaxis is extremely important. Several studies have demonstrated the effectiveness of isoniazid preventive therapy. Pape and colleagues showed that isoniazid preventive therapy reduced the risk of both tuberculosis and death in HIV-seropositive Haitian adults.[33] The benefit of preventive therapy was apparent only in tuberculin skin test–positive patients, although the number of anergic patients studied was too small for firm conclusions to be drawn. The United States Public Health Service and Infectious Disease Society of America recommend that 1 year of isoniazid preventive therapy be given to PPD-positive (at least 5 mm induration), HIV-seropositive persons who do not have evidence of active tuberculosis.[8] Prophylaxis should also be given to HIV-seropositive persons with a history of a previous positive PPD who are currently anergic to PPD and to persons exposed to an infectious case.

The role of prophylaxis in anergic patients remains controversial. Prospective studies are under way to determine whether preventive therapy is efficacious in anergic subjects. Alternatives to isoniazid prophylaxis are under study also. The combination of rifampin and pyrazinamide, given for 2 months, is extremely effective in the murine model of chronic tuberculosis. One study has suggested that this regimen is active in HIV-infected, PPD-positive adults, and a larger study is still under way. Other alternatives are short courses of rifampin, rifabutin, and the combination of isoniazid and rifampin. For patients infected with or exposed to multidrug-resistant tuberculosis, referral to an expert is recommended. Anecdotal reports suggest that the use of fluoroquinolones (e.g., ciprofloxacin or ofloxacin) with one or more other antituberculosis agents may be protective. The use of Bacillus Calmette-Guérin (BCG) vaccine to prevent tuberculosis in HIV-infected patients is contraindicated. Disseminated BCG infections have been reported in patients with HIV who have received this live vaccine.

Mycobacterium Avium Complex

Epidemiology

Mycobacterium avium–complex infections are an increasingly common complication of HIV disease (Fig. 163-1; see also Chapter 164). Although disseminated M. avium–complex infections were extremely rare before the AIDS epidemic, tens of thousands of cases have occurred in the United States alone among AIDS patients. In addition to causing substantial morbidity in advanced HIV disease, M. avium–complex infections are associated with shortened survival.[11] Because of their frequency, severity, and effect on survival, treatment and prevention of M. avium–complex infections have become increasingly important to physicians caring for patients with HIV infection.

M. avium complex is a common environmental mycobacterium that is distributed throughout the world. The organism is concentrated in soil and water and also has a number of animal reservoirs. The environmental sources responsible for most human infections are not known. Although M. avium complex is found widely in the environment, the incidence of disseminated M. avium complex in patients with HIV disease varies geographically. For example, although more than 15 percent of AIDS patients in the United States will develop M. avium–complex disease, the disease is unusual in African AIDS patients. Within the United States, AIDS patients from some regions have a higher prevalence of M. avium complex than patients from other areas.[20] The reason for these geographic differences in M. avium–complex prevalence is not known, but several possibilities exist.

Environmental concentrations of M. avium complex differ geographically.[25] In the acidic swamps of the southeastern United States, for example, the quantity of M. avium complex in soil, water, and aerosol samples is substantially higher than that in freshwater lakes. Exposure to higher environmental concentrations of M. avium complex may more frequently lead to disease. On the other hand, most environmental M. avium–complex isolates are not linked to human disease. A second possible explanation for geographic variation in M. avium–complex incidence is that some populations of AIDS patients may not survive long enough to be at risk of M. avium–complex disease. In developing countries, for instance, patients with AIDS may succumb to tuberculosis or pyogenic bacterial infections at CD4 cell levels that are sufficient to protect against M. avium complex. Another possibility is that populations of patients with exposure to other mycobacterial infections, such as tuberculosis or BCG, may have acquired immunity to M. avium complex that is protective against disseminated disease, even with severe HIV-induced immunodeficiency. Data discussed below suggest that genetic susceptibility to M. avium–complex infections could underlie population differences in rates of disease caused by the organism. Casting doubt on this hypothesis is the observation that African patients with HIV infections who migrate to Europe have rates of M. avium–complex disease similar to those of European patients.[32]

Finally, it is also possible that lack of diagnostic capabilities or less intense clinical evaluation leads to lower rates of M. avium recovery in some locales. None of these hypotheses has been convincingly proved.

M. avium complex may be acquired from the environment in a number of ways, and the means by which most patients become infected is not known. Studies using molecular epidemiologic techniques have shown that some patients with AIDS and disseminated M. avium complex may have infection with organisms that are found in hospital hot-water supplies or in community water sources.[46] Patients with isolates similar to those found in hospital water supplies presumably acquired the organism from showering. Intensive prospective studies of patients with HIV infection at risk for M. avium complex have failed to establish any connection between environmental exposures and subsequent disease, however. In a study in which numerous environmental sites in the homes and communities of patients with HIV infection were sampled, M. avium was isolated from only one of 528 water samples and one of 397 food samples, but from 43 of 157 (27 percent) soil samples.[49] This study implicates soil rather than water and food as a possible source of infection. The results of the epidemiologic studies of M. avium complex leave considerable uncertainty about risk factors for acquiring infection, and specific recommendations for avoiding exposure cannot be made with confidence.

Pathogenesis

The pathogenesis of M. avium–complex infections in patients with HIV is poorly understood. The M. avium–complex family comprises numerous organisms of varying serotypes from the species M. avium and M. intracellulare. While a large proportion of patients with pulmonary M. avium–complex disease harbor M. intracellulare, most AIDS patients who get disease are infected with M. avium. Both monoclonal and polyclonal infections are known to exist,[3] and the timing of the acquisition of initial infection is unclear. Mallal and coworkers have shown that in Western Australia, a reactive PPD skin test following the initiation of zidovudine indicates subsequent high risk for disseminated M. avium–complex disease.[28] This suggests that latent infections may reactivate as cellular immunodeficiency progresses. Alternatively, ongoing exposure to the organism in the environment may culminate in an effective inoculation late in HIV disease. A positive skin test could be a marker of exposure to the organism, rather than of latent infection.

Several other host factors for disseminated M. avium complex have been identified. The most important predictor of subsequent disseminated M. avium complex is low CD4 lymphocyte count. Several prospective studies have shown that as CD4 counts fall to below $100/mm^3$, the annual incidence of M. avium–complex bacteremia rises substantially.[11] For patients with CD4 counts below $50/mm^3$, the risk of M. avium–complex bacteremia is between 10 and 20 percent per year. Conversely, patients with CD4 counts of at least $100/mm^3$ are very unlikely to develop M. avium–complex disease in the subsequent year. Patients found to have M. avium–complex bacteremia, on the other hand, almost always have CD4 lymphocyte counts below $20/mm^3$. Other immunologic abnormalities that may contribute to the development of *M. avium*–complex disease are impaired intracellular killing of organisms by macrophages, variations in cytokine production (especially interleukin 12), and derangements in antigen presentation to effector cells.

The role of genes in host resistance to *M. avium* complex and other mycobacterial infections in humans is not clear. Studies in mice reveal a gene that confers resistance to mycobacterial infections (*Bcg*) that is associated with enhanced intracellular killing of organisms within macrophages.[45] Stead and colleagues have shown racial differences in susceptibility to tuberculosis that might be genetically mediated.[42] There is some evidence that HLA phenotypes also may be related to susceptibility to mycobacterial infections. The importance of genetic resistance, however, could be negligible in advanced immunodeficiency.

Prior colonization of the respiratory and gastrointestinal tracts increases the risk of disseminated *M. avium* complex significantly, but most patients with *M. avium*–complex bacteremia never show evidence of colonization. Chin and coworkers reported that in patients with CD4 counts under 50/mm³ who were cultured for mycobacteria every 3 months, colonization of the stool increased the risk of disseminated *M. avium*–complex disease sixfold and colonization of the sputum increased the risk more than twofold.[13] Nonetheless, two-thirds of the patients who ultimately developed bacteremia never had evidence of colonization. Thus, screening of stools or sputum cannot be recommended routinely.

After an initial infection is established, seeding of other organs, such as lymph nodes, may ensue. Subsequent dissemination develops when cell-mediated immunity has been ablated by progressive HIV infection. For some time it has been hypothesized that *M. avium*–complex bacteremia is an "overflow" phenomenon, with organisms spilling into the blood from heavily infected organs. Several recent studies suggest that bacteremia precedes dissemination and may be transient. Patients with transient bacteremia have less severe disease and longer survival than patients with sustained bacteremia. With sustained bacteremia there is ongoing seeding of organs and an increasing tissue burden.

Clinical Manifestations

Common symptoms of disseminated *M. avium* complex include fever, sweats, weight loss, diarrhea, and malaise. The onset of illness is usually insidious, and symptoms are often present for many weeks before the diagnosis is established. Accompanying clinical signs and laboratory abnormalities frequently include cachexia and weight loss, hepatosplenomegaly, anemia, neutropenia, and elevation of the alkaline phosphatase. In some patients, *M. avium* complex may be restricted to the lymph nodes, gastrointestinal tract, or lungs. *M. avium*–complex infections of the lungs, including focal pneumonia and endobronchial lesions, may occur with or without bacteremia. Pulmonary impairment may be acute or chronic. Figure 163-4*A* shows the radiographic findings of chronic *M. avium*–complex pulmonary disease in a patient with advanced HIV infection with long-standing bacteremia. Cavitary disease with extensive infiltrates is common in this setting. Figure 163-4*B* is a chest radiograph of a young woman with disseminated *M. avium*–complex disease who presented with a large, bloody, pleural effusion.

The diagnosis of disseminated *M. avium*–complex disease is usually made from isolation of organisms from blood or bone marrow cultures. Patients in whom *M. avium* complex is identified in other tissues should have blood cultures performed to detect disseminated disease. Cultures should be performed with Bactec or another rapid culture assay so that results can be obtained expeditiously. Use of DNA-RNA hybridization probes allows speciation within 1 to 2 days after growth in liquid media. Isolating *M. avium* complex in stool or sputum does not necessarily indicate systemic disease, although patients with positive respiratory or gastrointestinal cultures, as noted above, are at increased risk of disseminated disease subsequently. The diagnosis of *M. avium* complex is suggested by fever, night sweats, and weight loss in a patient with a CD4 count below 50/mm³. The signs and symptoms of *M. avium*–complex disease are extremely nonspecific, however, and empiric diagnosis is subject to a considerable degree of error. In some circumstances, presumptive therapy for the disease may be initiated while cultures are pending, but long-term treatment should be based on isolation of the organism in culture. If blood cultures are unrevealing in a patient with suspected *M. avium*–complex disease, a bone marrow aspirate and biopsy may confirm the diagnosis.

Treatment and Prevention

Treatment of disseminated *M. avium*–complex disease in patients with HIV infection has improved substantially since early in the AIDS epidemic. Early reports noted that standard antimycobacterial agents had minimal activity against this pathogen, although four- or five-drug combination regimens were shown to have moderate to good effect in some studies.[24] Therapy against *M. avium* complex has been advanced considerably by the extended-spectrum macrolides clarithromycin and azithromycin (Table 163-1). These agents have been shown to have superior activity against *M. avium*–complex disease.[9,50] Clarithromycin given alone significantly reduces levels of bacteremia and is associated with clinical improvement. Lower doses of clarithromycin (≤ 1 gm/day total) are better tolerated, with fewer gastrointestinal side effects than with high doses, and are asso-

TABLE 163-1

Regimens for the Treatment of *Mycobacterium avium*–Complex Disease in Patients with HIV Infection

First-line therapy	
Drug	Dosage
Clarithromycin	500 mg twice daily
(Azithromycin)	(600 mg daily)
plus	
Ethambutol	15 mg/kg daily
±Rifabutin	300–450 mg daily
Second-line therapy	
Drug	Dosage
Amikacin	7.5 mg/kg daily
Ciprofloxacin	500–750 mg once or twice daily
(Clofazimine)	(100 mg daily)

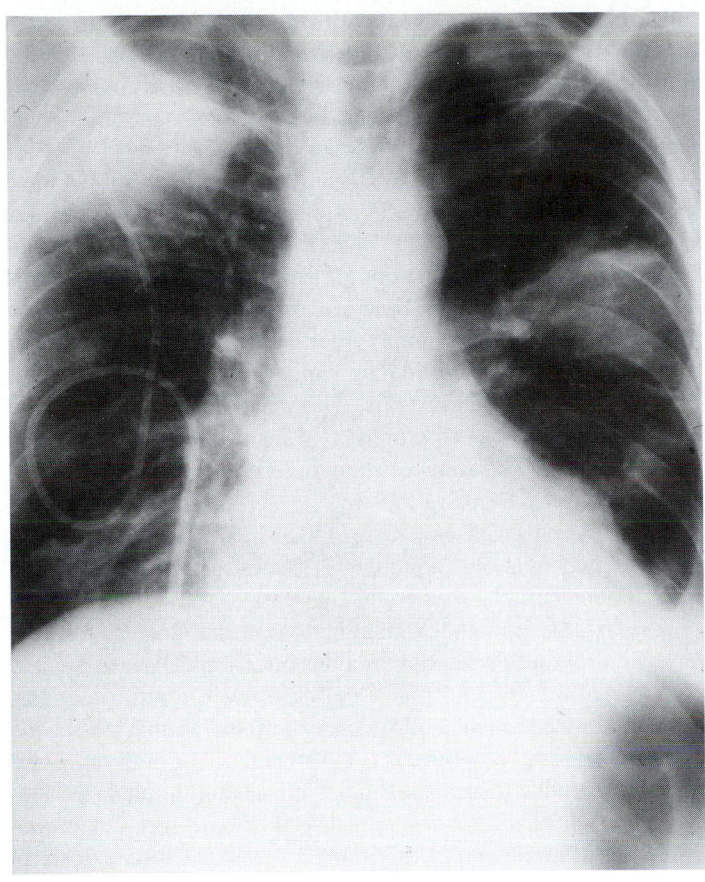

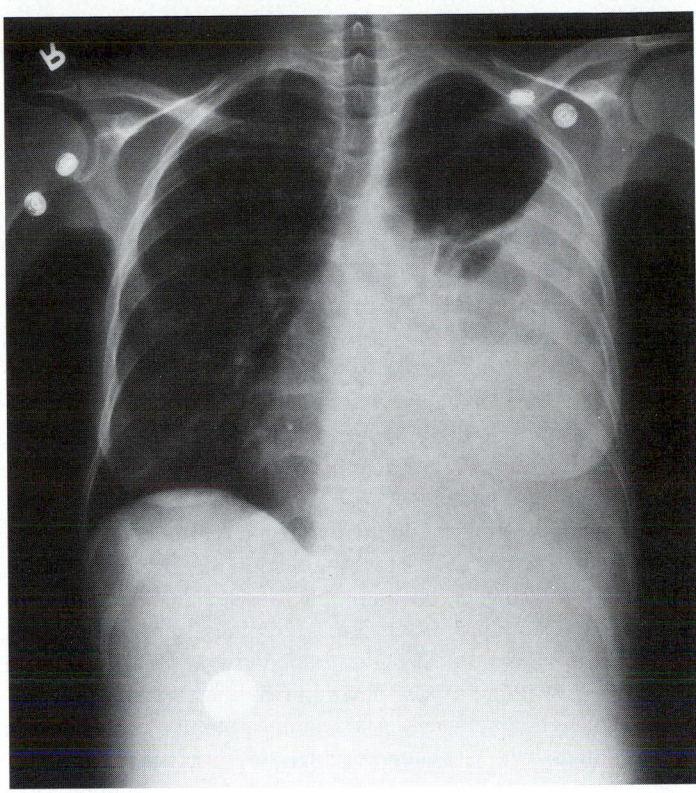

B

A

FIGURE 163-4   Radiographic presentations of *M. avium*–complex pulmonary disease in patients with HIV infection. *A.* Cavitary infiltrates in a 37-year-old man with AIDS and long-standing *M. avium*–complex bacteremia. *B.* Chest radiograph showing a left hemothorax in a 28- year-old woman with disseminated *M. avium*–complex disease, with positive cultures of blood, bloody pleural effusion, and lymph nodes. After three therapeutic thoracenteses, the patient responded to antimy- cobacterial drugs.

ciated with better survival, for unclear reasons. Treatment of *M. avium*–complex bacteremia with clarithromycin alone is associ- ated with emergence of drug-resistant organisms and recrudes- cence of symptoms. The mechanism for development of drug-resistant disease is selection of preexisting, innately macrolide-resistant *M. avium* clones during therapy. Azithromycin also reduces the level of bacteremia, and its use as monotherapy similarly results in emergence of drug-resistant disease. Resistant organisms usually begin to emerge after 2 to 3 months of treat- ment, and most patients will experience relapses with drug-resis- tant isolates after 4 or more months of monotherapy.

Combination therapy for disseminated *M. avium* complex is necessary to prevent the emergence of resistance. Regimens should consist of clarithromycin or azithromycin with at least one other antimycobacterial agent. Combination therapy with clarithromycin and ethambutol is clinically active and prevents relapses with drug-resistant organisms in a large proportion of patients.[9] The addition of clofazimine to this regimen does not improve efficacy and is associated with greater mortality. The use of a three-drug regimen of clarithromycin, rifabutin, and ethambutol is also very effective.[39] The use of clarithromycin and clofazimine results in high rates of relapse with drug-resis- tant organisms. The role of amikacin and ciprofloxacin remains unclear. In general, these agents are reserved for patients failing first-line therapy. The value of these agents in combination with clarithromycin has not been studied, however.

A major limitation to the treatment of *M. avium*–complex dis- ease is the occurrence of adverse reactions. Clarithromycin and azithromycin are associated with dose-related gastrointestinal toxicity, which affects up to one-half of patients. Common com- plaints include abdominal pain, nausea, vomiting, and diarrhea. Dose reduction or drug holiday may alleviate symptoms and per- mit further treatment. Taste and smell perversion occurs in 5 to 15 percent of patients treated with macrolides. Hepatotoxicity and rash are less common. Ethambutol is generally well toler- ated, although gastrointestinal intolerance sometimes occurs. Op- tic neuritis is rare at doses of less than 20 mg/kg daily. Rifabutin, a semisynthetic rifamycin S derivative with activity against *M. avium* complex, may cause nausea, rash, and neutropenia. Discoloration of urine, tears, and sweat is a predictable compli- cation in one-third to one-half of patients. Rifabutin-associated uveitis is common at high doses (450 to 600 mg daily) of the drug, particularly when clarithromycin and fluconazole are used concomitantly.[38] Clearance of rifabutin by P450 cytochromes is inhibited by clarithromycin and fluconazole, resulting in higher serum concentrations of rifabutin.

Currently, routine testing of all *M. avium*–complex isolates for drug susceptibility is not recommended. The value of susceptibility test results in predicting clinical outcomes is apparent only for clarithromycin. Making treatment decisions about patients who appear to be failing therapy is difficult. For a patient who develops symptoms of disseminated *M. avium* complex after an initial response, it is important to rule out other opportunistic diseases with similar signs and symptoms. Blood cultures should be obtained for mycobacteria and held for 4 to 6 weeks, as drug therapy may delay growth. If cultures are positive, testing for clarithromycin susceptibility is reasonable. For the patient known or thought to be failing treatment, at least two new agents should be added or substituted. Azithromycin should not be substituted for clarithromycin, as cross-resistance to these agents is the rule. Recently, interferon-γ has been shown to be active in controlling disseminated *M. avium*–complex infections in patients without HIV.[19] The efficacy of interferon-γ in patients with AIDS is not known.

Because disseminated *M. avium*–complex infection is a predictable late complication of HIV infection that occurs in a large proportion of patients, chemoprophylaxis to prevent disease is desirable. A summary of current guidelines for prevention of *M. avium*–complex infections in patients with HIV is given in Table 163-2. Rifabutin was shown in two placebo-controlled trials to reduce the incidence of *M. avium*–complex bacteremia in AIDS patients with CD4 counts under 200/mm^3 by 50 percent.[31] The 2-year probability of developing *M. avium*–complex bacteremia was approximately 40 percent in placebo recipients and 20 percent in rifabutin recipients. In addition to reducing the risk of bacteremia, the drug was associated with a reduction in signs and symptoms of disseminated *M. avium*–complex disease. Rifabutin was well tolerated in the clinical trials, and relatively few patients experienced treatment-limiting adverse reactions. No survival advantage was demonstrated in these studies, although an analysis of the long-term follow-up showed significantly improved survival associated with rifabutin use. On the basis of the rifabutin trials, the United States Public Health Service recommended that lifelong rifabutin preventive therapy be offered to HIV-infected patients with CD4 counts under 100/mm^3.

Several recent studies have shown that clarithromycin and azithromycin are also effective in preventing *M. avium*–complex bacteremia in patients with advanced HIV infection.[18,34] In addition to reducing the risk of *M. avium*–complex disease, clarithromycin prophylaxis prolongs survival. Among patients who

TABLE 163-2

Guidelines for Prevention of *M. avium*–Complex Disease in Patients with HIV Infection

1. Begin prophylaxis for patients with CD4 counts <75/mm^3.
2. Rule out active tuberculosis by clinical exam and appropriate laboratory studies.
3. Obtain mycobacterial blood culture to rule out subclinical bacteremia.
4. Regimens:　Azithromycin, 1200 mg weekly
   or　Clarithromycin, 500 mg twice daily
   or　Rifabutin, 300 mg daily

SOURCE: Adapted from MMWR.[8]

failed clarithromycin preventive therapy, however, disease with clarithromycin-resistant organisms was found in a substantial proportion. Similarly, azithromycin prophylaxis is also associated with the emergence of disease caused by macrolide-resistant organisms in a small proportion of patients.

Both clarithromycin and azithromycin have been shown to be more efficacious than rifabutin in preventing *M. avium*–complex disease in patients with HIV infection and CD4 cell counts under 100/mm^3. The combination of azithromycin and rifabutin is more effective than either drug alone, while adding rifabutin to clarithromycin does not improve efficacy. Adverse reactions to rifabutin or either macrolide are similarly frequent, while combination therapy is more toxic. The major disadvantage to the use of the macrolides as prophylaxis against *M. avium* complex is the occurrence of drug-resistant disease in a proportion of patients who fail preventive therapy.

Since the publication of the original U.S. Public Health Service recommendations, a number of issues regarding prevention of *M. avium*–complex bacteremia have arisen. First, when should prophylaxis be initiated? Guidelines from the Centers for Disease Control and Prevention and the Infectious Disease Society of America recommend that prophylaxis be offered to patients with HIV infection and a CD4 count of 50 to 75/mm^3.[8] A second concern regarding prophylaxis is the emergence of drug resistance during preventive treatment. Failure of rifabutin prophylaxis does not appear to select for drug-resistant *M. avium*–complex organisms, but several reports of rifamycin-resistant tuberculosis in patients receiving rifabutin have appeared.[48] One would expect, however, that use of rifabutin in persons with latent *M. tuberculosis* infection would be effective in preventing disease, as rifabutin is extremely active against the organism and is of proven value in treating tuberculosis disease.[16,22] It does not appear, therefore, that rifabutin use poses a major risk of drug-resistant tuberculosis. It should be recalled that the use of isoniazid to prevent tuberculosis in patients with latent *M. tuberculosis* infections is not associated with the emergence of drug-resistant disease. To rule out the possibility of active tuberculosis, however, patients treated with rifabutin should be clinically evaluated before starting treatment.

Drug–drug interactions are another concern with *M. avium*–complex prophylaxis. Rifabutin enhances cytochrome P450 enzymes and may increase the clearance of other drugs, including HIV protease inhibitors, macrolides, and ketoconazole. Although fluconazole metabolism is not affected by rifabutin, coadministration of these agents results in a near doubling of rifabutin serum concentrations.[30,44] There have been recent reports of uveitis in patients treated with rifabutin in higher doses, particularly in conjunction with fluconazole.[34] Most cases of rifabutin-associated uveitis have been in patients on higher doses of rifabutin (450 to 600 mg daily) who were also taking clarithromycin or fluconazole. Since the recognition of this complication of rifabutin, the incidence appears to have declined, primarily as a result of reductions in the doses of rifabutin administered. Clarithromycin may cause an increase in serum concentrations of rifabutin, astemizole, and HIV protease inhibitors.

Azithromycin appears to have minimal interactions with drugs metabolized by hepatic cytochromes. Guidelines for prevention of *M. avium*–complex disease in patients with HIV infection are currently in flux. Because prophylaxis against *M. avium* complex reduces disease incidence and prolongs life, this therapy is generally considered standard for patients with CD4 counts under 5/mm³. Clarithromycin 500 mg twice daily or azithromycin 1200 mg weekly is generally preferred as initial therapy, and rifabutin 300 mg daily is an alternative.

OTHER MYCOBACTERIA

Patients with HIV infection are susceptible to a number of other mycobacterial infections, although these are less common than tuberculosis or *M. avium* complex. *M. kansasii* infections generally mimic tuberculosis, occurring in severely immunocompromised HIV-infected patients with cavitary or diffuse pulmonary infiltrates.[26] Patients often have concomitant pulmonary infections, most often *P. carinii* pneumonia. Bacteremia, osteomyelitis, and soft tissue infections are also seen. Without therapy, the disease is generally progressive. Treatment with isoniazid, rifampin, and ethambutol for 12 to 18 months is recommended, and clarithromycin is also active against this organism.

M. genavense causes disseminated disease in advanced immunodeficiency, with bacteremia and other organ involvement.[5] The organism grows poorly in liquid media and cannot be cultured on solid media. It is detectable with amplification of genomic sequences by the polymerase chain reaction, but this is not readily available in most settings. The diagnosis is suggested in HIV-infected patients with an *M. avium* complex–like illness who have weakly positive (low growth index) cultures that cannot be speciated or who have negative cultures but tissue samples showing acid-fast bacilli. Formal studies of treatment for *M. genavense* infections have not been conducted, but anecdotal information suggests that regimens active against *M. avium* complex are also effective for this organism. *M. hemophilum* may cause skin and soft tissue infections in AIDS patients, and case reports of infections with *M. fortuitum*, *M. chelonei*, and *M. xenopi* have appeared.

REFERENCES

1. American Thoracic Society: Treatment and prevention of tuberculosis in adults and children. *Am J Respir Crit Care Med* 149: 1359–1374, 1994.

2. Antonucci G, Girardi E, Raviglione MC, Ippolito G: Risk factors for tuberculosis in HIV-infected persons: A prospective cohort study. *JAMA* 274:143–148, 1995.

3. Arbeit RD, Slutsky A, Barber TW, et al: Genetic diversity among strains of *Mycobacterium avium* causing monoclonal and polyclonal bacteremia in patients with AIDS. *J Infect Dis* 167:1384–1390, 1993.

4. Bloch AB, Cauthen GM, Onorato IM, et al: Nationwide survey of drug-resistant tuberculosis in the United States. *JAMA* 271:665–671, 1994.

5. Böttger EC, Teske A, Kirschner P, et al: Disseminated *Mycobacterium genavense* infection in patients with AIDS. *Lancet* 340:76–80, 1992.

6. Caiaffa WT, Graham NMH, Galai N, et al: Instability of delayed-type hypersensitivity skin test anergy in human immunodeficiency virus infection. *Arch Intern Med* 155:2111–2117, 1995.

7. Cantwell MF, Snider DE Jr, Cauthen GM, Onorato IM: Epidemi-

8. Centers for Disease Control and Prevention: USPHS/IDSA guidelines for the prevention of opportunistic infections in persons infected with human immunodeficiency virus: A summary. *MMWR* 44:1–10, 1995.

9. Chaisson RE, Keiser P, Pierce M, et al: Clarithromycin and ethambutol with or without clofazimine for disseminated *Mycobacterium avium* complex infection in patients with AIDS (in press).

10. Chaisson RE, Clermont HC, Holt E, et al: Six-month intermittent tuberculosis therapy in Haitian patients with and without HIV infection. *Am J Respir Crit Care Med* 154:1034–1038, 1996.

11. Chaisson RE, Moore RD, Richman DD, et al: Incidence and natural history of *Mycobacterium avium*–complex infections in patients with advanced human immunodeficiency virus disease treated with zidovudine. *Am Rev Respir Dis* 146:285–289, 1992.

12. Chaisson RE, Benson CA, Dube MP, et al: Clarithromycin therapy for bacteremic *Mycobacterium avium* complex disease—A randomized, double-blind, dose-ranging study in patients with AIDS. *Ann Intern Med* 121:905–911, 1994.

13. Chin DP, Hopewell PC, Yajko DM, et al: *Mycobacterium avium* complex in the respiratory or gastrointestinal tract and the risk of *M. avium* complex bacteremia in patients with human immunodeficiency virus infection. *J Infect Dis* 169:289–295, 1994.

14. Daley CL, Small PM, Schecter GF, et al: An outbreak of tuberculosis with accelerated progression among persons infected with human immunodeficiency virus: An analysis using restriction-fragment-length polymorphisms. *New Engl J Med* 326:231–235, 1992.

15. Frieden TR, Sterling T, Pablos-Mendez A, et al: The emergence of drug-resistant tuberculosis in New York City. *New Engl J Med* 328:521–526, 1993.

16. Gonzalez-Montaner LJ, Natal S, Yongchaiyud P, Olliaro P: Rifabutin for the treatment of newly-diagnosed pulmonary tuberculosis: A multinational, randomized, comparative study versus rifampicin. *Tuber Lung Dis* 75:341–347, 1994.

17. Graham NMH, Nelson KE, Solomon L, et al: Prevalence of tuberculin positivity and skin test anergy in HIV-1–seropositive and –seronegative intravenous drug users. *JAMA* 267:369–373, 1992.

18. Havlir D, Dube M, Sattler FR, et al: Prophylaxis agaoinst disseminated *Mycobacterium avium* complex with weekly azithromycin, daily cifabutin, or both. California Collaborative Treatment Group. *New Engl J Med* 335: 392–398, 1996.

19. Holland SM, Eisenstein EM, Kuhns DB, et al: Treatment of refractory disseminated nontuberculous mycobacterial infection with interferon gamma: A preliminary report. *New Engl J Med* 330: 1348–1355, 1994.

20. Hoover DR, Graham NMH, Bacellar H, et al: An epidemiologic analysis of *Mycobacterium avium* complex disease in homosexual men infected with human immunodeficiency virus type 1. *Clin Infect Dis* 20:1250–1258, 1995.

21. Horsburgh CR Jr, Metchock B, Gordon SM, et al: Predictors of survival in patients with AIDS and disseminated *Mycobacterium avium* complex disease. *J Infect Dis* 170:573–577, 1994.

22. Jabes D, Della BC, Rossi R, Olliaro P: Effectiveness of rifabutin alone or in combination with isoniazid in preventive therapy of mouse tuberculosis. *Antimicrob Agents Chemother* 38:2346–2350, 1994.

23. Jones BE, Young SM, Antoniskis D, et al: Relationship of the manifestations of tuberculosis to CD4 cell counts in patients with human immunodeficiency virus infection. *Am Rev Respir Dis* 148: 1292–1297, 1994.

24. Kemper CA, Meng T-C, Nussbaum J, et al: Treatment of *Mycobacterium avium* complex bacteremia in AIDS with a four-drug

ology of tuberculosis in the United States, 1985–1992. *JAMA* 272:535–539, 1994.

oral regimen: Rifampin, ethambutol, clofazimine, and ciprofloxacin. *Ann Intern Med* 116:466–472, 1992.

25. Kirschner RA Jr, Parker BC, Falkinham JO III: Epidemiology of infection by nontuberculous mycobacteria: *Mycobacterium avium, Mycobacterium intracellulare,* and *Mycobacterium scrofulaceum* in acid, brown-water swamps of the southeastern United States and their association with environmental variables. *Am Rev Respir Dis* 145:271–275, 1992.

26. Levine B, Chaisson RE: *Mycobacterium kansasii:* A cause of treatable pulmonary disease associated with advanced human immunodeficiency virus (HIV) infection. *Ann Intern Med* 114:861–868, 1991.

27. Mahmoudi A, Iseman MD: Pitfalls in the care of patients with tuberculosis: Common errors and their acquisition of drug resistance. *JAMA* 270:65–68, 1993.

28. Mallal SA, James IR, French MAH: Detection of subclinical *Mycobacterium avium intracellulare* complex infection in immunodeficient HIV-infected patients treated with zidovudine. *AIDS* 8:1263–1269, 1994.

29. Moreno S, Baraia-Etxaburu J, Bouza E, et al: Risk for developing tuberculosis among anergic patients infected with HIV. *Ann Intern Med* 119:194–198, 1993.

30. Narang PK, Trapnell CB, Schoenfelder JR, et al: Fluconazole and enhanced effect of rifabutin prophylaxis. *New Engl J Med* 330:1316–1317, 1994.

31. Nightingale SD, Cameron DW, Gordin FM, et al: Two controlled trials of rifabutin prophylaxis against *Mycobacterium avium* complex infection in AIDS. *New Engl J Med* 329:828–833, 1993.

32. O'Farrell N, Gant V, Bradbeer C, Bateman N: *Mycobacterium avium* infection in Ugandans with AIDS living in London (letter). *Lancet* 343:1639, 1994.

33. Pape JW, Jean SS, Ho JL, et al: Effect of isoniazid prophylaxis on incidence of active tuberculosis and progression of HIV infection. *Lancet* 342:268–272, 1993.

34. Pierce M, Crampton S, Henry D, et al. A randomized trial of clarithromycin as prophylaxis against disseminated *Mycobacterium avium* complex infection in patients with advanced acquired immunodeficiency syndrome. *New Engl J Med* 335:384–391, 1996.

35. Raviglione MC, Snider DE Jr, Kochi A: Global epidemiology of tuberculosis: Morbidity and mortality of a worldwide epidemic. *JAMA* 273:220–226, 1995.

36. Reichman LB, McDonald RJ, Mangura BT: Rifabutin prophylaxis against *Mycobacterium avium* complex infection (letter). *New Engl J Med* 330:437–438, 1994.

37. Selwyn PA, Hartel D, Lewis V, et al: A prospective study of the risk of tuberculosis among intravenous drug users with human immunodeficiency virus infection. *New Engl J Med* 320:545–550, 1989.

38. Shafran SD, Deschênes J, Miller M, et al: Uveitis and pseudojaundice during a regimen of clarithromycin, rifabutin, and ethambutol (letter). *New Engl J Med* 330:438–439, 1994.

39. Shafran SD, Singer J, Zarowny DP, et al: A comparison of two regimens for the treatment of *Mycobacterium avium* complex bacteremia in AIDS: Rifabutin, ethambutol, and clarithromycin versus rifampin, ethambutol, clofazimine, and ciprofloxacin: Canadian HIV Trials Network Protocol 010 Study Group. *New Engl J Med* 335:377–383, 1996.

40. Small PM, Schecter GF, Goodman PC, et al: Treatment of tuberculosis in patients with advanced human immunodeficiency virus infection. *New Engl J Med* 324:289–294, 1991.

41. Small PM, Hopewell PC, Singh SP, et al: The epidemiology of tuberculosis in San Francisco: A population-based study using conventional and molecular methods. *New Engl J Med* 330:1703–1709, 1994.

42. Stead WW, Senner JW, Reddick WT, Lofgren JP: Racial differences in susceptibility to infection by *Mycobacterium tuberculosis. New Engl J Med* 322:422–427, 1990.

43. Toosi Z, Vjecha M, Amir-Tahmasseb M, et al: Enhanced susceptibility of blood monocytes from patients with pulmonary tuberculosis to productive infection with human immunodeficiency virus type 1. *J Exp Med* 177:1511–1516, 1993.

44. Trapnell CB, Narang P, Li R, Lavelle JP: Increased plasma rifabutin levels with concomitant fluconazole therapy in HIV-infected patients. *Ann Intern Med* 124:573–576, 1996.

45. Vidal SM, Malo D, Vogan K, et al: Natural resistance to infection with intracellular parasites: Isolation of a candidate for Bcg. *Cell* 73:469–485, 1993.

46. von Reyn CF, Maslow JN, Barber TW, et al: Persistent colonisation of potable water as a source of *Mycobacterium avium* infection in AIDS. *Lancet* 343:1137–1141, 1994.

47. Wallis RS, Vjecha M, Amir-Tahmasseb M, et al: Influence of tuberculosis on human immunodeficiency virus (HIV-1): Enhanced cytokine expression and elevated β_2-microglobulin in HIV-1–associated tuberculosis. *J Infect Dis* 167:43–48, 1993.

48. Weltman AC, Righi SP, DiFerdinando GT Jr, et al: Rifampicin-resistant *Mycobacterium* tuberculosis (letter). *Lancet* 345:1513, 1995.

49. Yajko DM, Chin DP, Gonzales PC, et al: *Mycobacterium avium* complex in water, food, and soil samples collected from the environment of HIV-infected individuals. *J Acquir Immune Defic Syndr Hum Retrovirol* 9:176–182, 1995.

50. Young LS, Wiviott L, Wu M, et al: Azithromycin for treatment of *Mycobacterium avium-intracellulare* complex infection in patients with AIDS. *Lancet* 338:1107–1109, 1991.

CHAPTER 164

DISEASES DUE TO MYCOBACTERIA OTHER THAN MYCOBACTERIUM TUBERCULOSIS

Paul T. Davidson

Mycobacterium tuberculosis and *M. leprae* are the most common mycobacterial species causing disease in humans. Many other species of mycobacteria have been found and described during the past 100 years. Although very common as environmental inhabitants, these mycobacteria rarely cause disease and do so only under special circumstances. For the most part, they are opportunists and become pathogens only when there has been a considerable breakdown in host defense mechanisms. Some of these mechanisms remain poorly understood. Others have become more apparent as a consequence of the opportunistic association between mycobacterial infection and the acquired immunodeficiency syndrome (AIDS) (see Chapter 163). Diseases with mycobacterial species, such as the avium complex, now occur more frequently and challenge the capabilities of the medical community.

ORGANISM AND DISEASE

The mycobacteria considered in this chapter sometimes cause human disease but are not obligate human parasites as are *M. tuberculosis* and *M. leprae.* They have been isolated from many environmental locations, principally soil and water, studied thoroughly, and carefully speciated.[19]

Microbiology

The microbiology of these organisms is well understood, although taxonomic changes continue to be made periodically. For the most part the organisms are easily isolated and grown under laboratory conditions. To simplify the understanding of these organisms, particularly as applied to clinical circumstances, they often are grouped into complexes of closely related species. The *M. avium* complex, for example, consists of many serotypes, including *M. avium, M. intracellulare,* and *M. scrofulaceum.* Certain species are associated with human disease more often than others and are presumed to be more virulent. Table 164-1 lists the relative virulence of some of the species.

Epidemiology and Pathogenesis

Unfortunately the epidemiology and pathogenesis of disease in humans are less well understood than the microbiology. Presumably human exposure to one or more of these mycobacteria is nearly universal. The route of exposure is uncertain. In some cases direct inoculation is known to result in disease, e.g., puncture wounds and the *M. fortuitum* complex. More commonly, asymptomatic infection occurs via the respiratory or gastrointestinal systems. These infections rarely lead to disease. In fact, it is best to consider the organisms as normal flora in these locations in the absence of clinical disease. Data remain unclear at present in regard to the gastrointestinal tract, although it is likely a common source of disseminated infection with the *M. avium* complex in AIDS.[21] Its presence in stool specimen from these patients may actually reflect enormous numbers of organisms and suggests a pathologic rather than a commensal state.

Attribution of pulmonary disease to these organisms is complicated by the common presence of opportunistic mycobacteria in sputum. For the diagnosis of disease caused by these organisms, not only should the organism be repeatedly isolated, usually in larger numbers, but also an appropriate clinical syndrome should coexist. When the organisms are found in sites that are otherwise sterile, their implication in the pathogenesis of the disease is more likely.

The histology of disease is indistinguishable from that caused by *M. tuberculosis* particularly in the normal host. Even though culture isolates may have certain morphologic differences on acid-fast staining from those of *M. tuberculosis,* differentiation on the basis of tissue staining is unreliable. Disease should be

TABLE 164-1

Relative Virulence of Mycobacteria in Humans

Species	Virulence
M. tuberculosis complex	4+
M. avium complex	3+
M. kansasii	3+
M. marinum	3+
M. szulgai	3+
M. simiae	2+
M. xenopi	2+
M. malmoense	2+
M. genavense	2+
M. fortuitum complex	1+
M. haemophilum	1+
M. gordonae	0
M. terrae	0
Many others	

treated as caused by *M. tuberculosis* until identification of the organism proves otherwise. It is important to bear in mind that the usual histopathologic response may not occur in patients with overwhelming infection and/or severe underlying cellular immune deficiency.

Terminology

An acceptable terminology to apply to both the laboratory and clinical circumstances of these organisms has been difficult to achieve. However, since the term *tuberculosis* refers to the pathophysiology of the disease process, it can, therefore, be used when referring to disease caused by mycobacterial species other than *M. tuberculosis*. A proposed glossary of clinical terminology that applies to mycobacterial disease on this basis is shown in Table 164-2.

Disease caused by *M. tuberculosis* is potentially communicable and is usually transmitted by the airborne route. The means of transmission of other mycobacteria remains uncertain. However, the evidence strongly suggests that transmission from the environment to a susceptible host and not transmission from one host to another is the most likely route. *M. tuberculosis* is therefore a much more important public health concern than the other species. It is also an obligate parasite surviving for long periods only in the living host. The disease it causes is generally more virulent and destructive to the host than are other species. For these reasons, and others, many clinicians prefer to restrict the term tuberculosis to those conditions caused by *M. tuberculosis*. For clinical purposes on this basis, the other mycobacteria as a group are designated *nontuberculous mycobacteria* or *nontuberculosis-causing mycobacteria*. The latter terminology has the advantage of being grammatically correct.

Drug susceptibility studies for mycobacterial species other than *M. tuberculosis* have not been standardized. In vitro, when tested in a manner similar to that used for *M. tuberculosis,* most species show variable resistance to the most common antituberculosis drugs. There is often a poor correlation between the re-

sults of susceptibility testing and the outcome of treatment.[10] Indeed, clinical responses often occur despite laboratory "resistance" of the organism. Therefore, susceptibility studies for these organisms are less useful in directing treatment than for treating *M. tuberculosis*. When susceptibility is demonstrated, that drug or drugs should be included in the treatment regimen, if possible, since response may be better.[11]

Clinical Picture

The spectrum of disease is broad and essentially parallels that of *M. tuberculosis* in the immunocompetent patient. The lungs are the most common site of involvement. Extrapulmonary locations occur and predominate in certain subgroups of patients. Lymphadenopathy is common in children, and disseminated disease is common in patients with AIDS. Clinical manifestations vary according to location and duration of disease. Disease may be localized or widespread, in the lungs or in the body; it may not progress for months or years, or it may progress rapidly. Because the results of treatment are uncertain for some species, the clinician must assess the importance of the disease for the individual patient before deciding whether to treat.

TREATMENT

The approach to treatment varies with the species. Many patients respond to antimycobacterial drug regimens that entail the use of several drugs (see Case 1, Figs. 164-1 to 164-3). Certain antibiotics that are of little use in treating *M. tuberculosis* sometimes give good results in treating diseases produced by these other mycobacteria. Unfortunately, standardized treatment regimens for treating disease caused by these mycobacteria have not been established by controlled clinical trial, largely because the diseases that they cause are relatively uncommon, and each clinic introduces variables and differences in approaches to therapy. Nonetheless, it is possible to generalize about the optimal contemporary treatment of disease caused by the different species.

M. KANSASII

Fortunately this organism is readily killed by rifampin. Response to a three-drug regimen of isoniazid, rifampin, and ethambutol is excellent.[7,13] Isoniazid is given at a dose of 400 to 600 mg daily because of the relative resistance of *M. kansasii* to this drug. The rifampin dose is 600 mg daily, and ethambutol is given at 25mg/kg per day until the sputum is culture negative; the dosage is then decreased to 15mg/kg per day. The total duration of treatment is 18 to 24 months, although good results with 12 months of therapy have been reported.[1] Other drugs usually given in three-drug combinations are effective for retreatment of disease that has become resistant to rifampin; they include ethionamide, cycloserine, streptomycin, capreomycin, and kanamycin.

M. MARINUM

This organism usually causes superficial skin infections following trauma and exposure to infected water (swimming pool granuloma). The disease will often disappear spontaneously. When

TABLE 164-2

A Glossary of Clinical Terminology for Infections and Disease Caused by Members of the Genus *Mycobacterium* in Humans and Animals

Mycobacteriosis: any infection or disease caused by mycobacteria.

I. Tuberculosis: a mycobacteriosis characterized by the formation of tubercles and caseous necrosis in the tissue.

   A. Tuberculosis (prototype variety). Tuberculosis caused by *M. tuberculosis* complex, an obligate parasite transmissible from one human host to another.

   B. Tuberculosis (atypical variety). Tuberculosis caused by mycobacteria other than *M. tuberculosis,* generally saprophytic and transmissible from the environment to a human host; examples include:

1. *M. avium*	6. *M. simiae*
2. *M. kansasii*	7. *M. malmoense*
3. *M. marinum*	8. *M. xenopi*
4. *M. fortuitum complex*	9. *M. ulcerans*
5. *M. szulgai*	

II. Leprosy: a mycobacteriosis caused by *M. leprae* and characterized by the formation of tubercles and lepra cells without caseation in the tissue and affecting chiefly the cooler parts of the body.

Application of above terminology.

I. *Tuberculosis* when used alone always denotes disease caused by *M. tuberculosis.*

II. *Atypical tuberculosis* is a general term that refers to tuberculosis caused by mycobacteria other than *M. tuberculosis.* When the causative species is known, the terminology is: Tuberculosis caused by *M. "species,"* e.g., tuberculosis caused by *M. kansasii;* tuberculosis caused by *M. chelonei;* or tuberculosis caused by *M. avium complex.*

III. Terminology in both I and II may be preceded by organ location or clinical description;

    Pulmonary tuberculosis

    Disseminated tuberculosis caused by *M. tuberculosis*

    Renal tuberculosis caused by *M. kansasii*

IV. Acceptable alternative terminology:

   A. Mycobacteriosis caused by *M. "species"* (particularly useful when the pathologic changes are ambiguous)

   B. Mycobacterial disease caused by *M. "species"*

   C. Atypical tuberculosis caused by *M. "species"*

V. When the causative species is not known, the terminology is tuberculosis, cause to be determined, or of undetermined cause, or mycobacteriosis, cause to be determined, or of undetermined cause

SOURCE: Revised from *Review of Infectious Diseases,* vol 3, no 5, September–October 1981, p 817.

the disease is more prolonged or extensive, treatment with isoniazid and rifampin is often successful. Minocycline or a trimethoprim-sulfa drug is sometimes useful when this approach fails.[8]

M. FORTUITUM COMPLEX

This complex includes *M. chelonei* with two subspecies (*chelonei* and *abscessus*). Soft-tissue abscesses related to trauma or surgery are the most common form of disease. Pulmonary disease is rare. These organisms are resistant to antituberculosis drugs. Some strains are susceptible to tetracyclines, erythromycin and other macrolides, amikacin, sulfonamides, quinolones, or

cephalosporins, but clinical response to these drugs is unpredictable. Surgical debridement or excision and drainage is done when possible. Otherwise, combinations of two or more drugs should be tried based on the susceptibility studies. Treatment must be given for an extended time, usually several months beyond clinical stability.[18]

M. AVIUM COMPLEX

This complex includes the various serovars of *M. avium, M. intracellulare,* and *M. scrofulaceum.* From the clinical standpoint, these organisms are the most important group of opportunistic mycobacteria (see Cases 1 to 3). They commonly cause disease and are difficult to treat. Most strains are resistant to antituberculosis drugs. Despite the resistance to individual drugs, most pulmonary patients respond clinically to treatment with multiple drug combinations (see Case 1). Although successful treatment may prove to be related to the in vitro synergistic effect of the antibiotics against these organisms, susceptibility studies using combinations of antibiotics have not yet been adequately studied to indicate any clinical application.

Pulmonary Disease in Non-AIDS Patients

Pulmonary disease is most commonly caused by these organisms. The spectrum of clinical pulmonary disease is wide, and the long-term prognosis is uncertain, largely because of preexisting underlying conditions, such as chronic obstructive airway disease. In some patients, the value of therapy is also uncertain. A decision to treat is complicated by unpredictability about the effectiveness of the drugs and the frequent occurrence of serious side effects to the multiple drugs that are needed to eradicate the organisms. In most patients with *M. avium* complex pulmonary tuberculosis, the disease is stable and causes few, if any, symptoms. Because of this fact, several months of observation are usually necessary before treatment is undertaken. Should the clinical situation be stable and symptoms be absent or minor, treatment for the mycobacterial infection may not be indicated. However, adequate treatment for underlying conditions, such as obstructive airways disease or bronchiectasis, is continued. Unfortunately, because there is no way to predict which patient will remain clinically stable or for how long, a monitoring program or periodic clinic reassessment and chest radiography are necessary. The interval of reassess-

Case 1

Forty-five-year-old male who had a chronic cough for several months followed by a flulike syndrome with chills, fever, and fatigue. Cavitary changes were noted in the left upper lung which progressed for several weeks, at which time *Mycobacterium avium* was found in his sputum. He was started on multidrug antituberculosis therapy and became consistently sputum culture-negative after 2 months of treatment. His chest radiograph gradually improved. The patient remained asymptomatic more than 7 years after completing therapy. See Figs. 164-1 to 164-3.

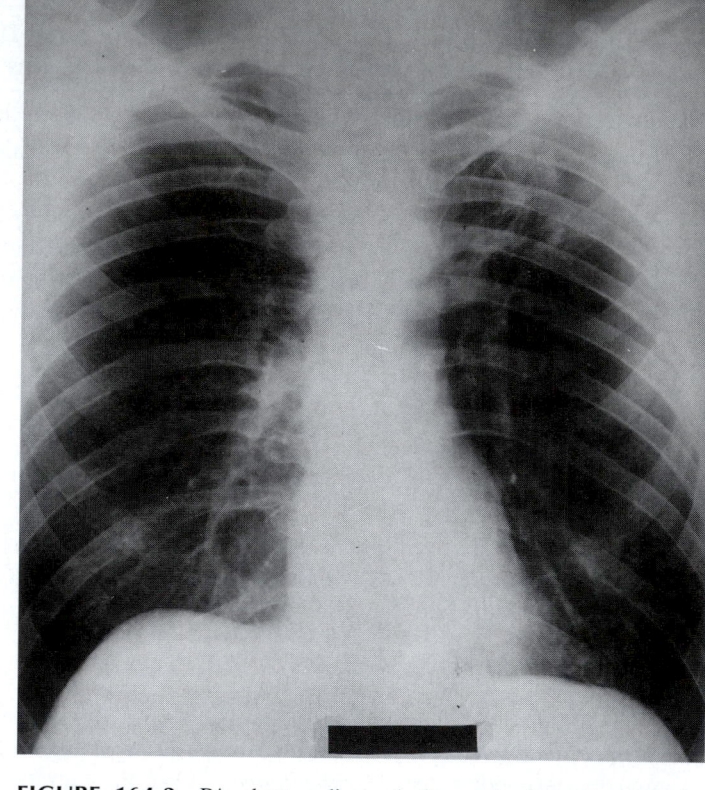

FIGURE 164-2 PA chest radiograph 2 months later showing decreased infiltration.

ment depends on the general condition of the patient; ordinarily it is of the order of every 6 to 12 months.

The typical patient with pulmonary disease caused by *M. avium* complex presents either with new symptoms or for an evaluation of a chronic lung condition. An abnormal chest radiograph compatible with tuberculosis is found. Smears and cultures of sputum are made. Sputum examination may show acid-fast bacilli on smear. Based on the likelihood that *M. tuberculosis* is responsible, the patient is started on conventional antituberculosis drug therapy. However, a therapeutic dilemma appears when the diagnostic reports indicate *M. avium* complex; not infrequently both the clinical and radiographic manifestations of the pulmonary disease improve during the several weeks of treatment before the diagnostic results become available. In these patients, the initial therapy is ordinarily continued. In a few, sputum examinations become negative; most will become stable clinically. In others, symptoms return or worsen despite continued therapy (see Case 2). Those that stabilize or improve should have drug therapy continued for a total of 18 to 24 months. If the disease progresses or

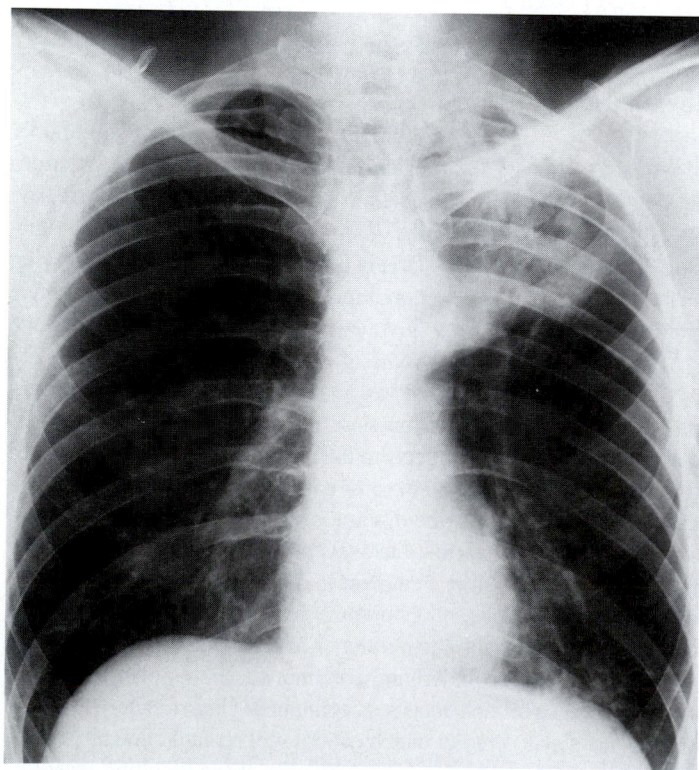

FIGURE 164-1 PA chest radiograph showing exudative infiltrate and probable cavitation in left upper lung.

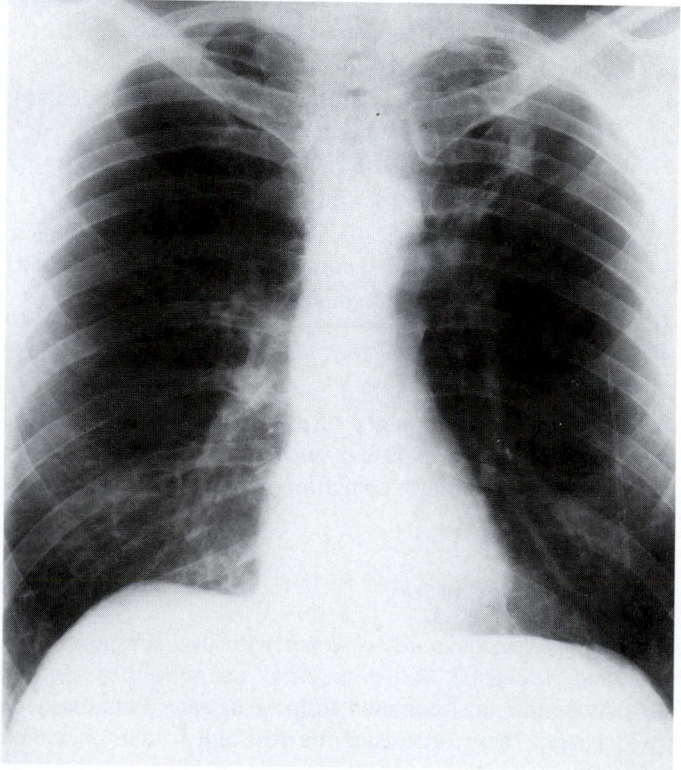

FIGURE 164-3 PA chest radiograph 7 years later showing a stable scar in left upper lung.

Case 2

Forty-seven-year-old male diagnosed with pneumonia 3 1/2 years earlier. *Mycobacterium avium* was also isolated from his sputum at that time. Because of a persistent infiltrate and positive cultures, he received multidrug treatment for 1 1/2 years without response. He was only mildly symptomatic, but the infiltrate progressed, and a right upper lobectomy was done. Postoperatively the cultures were negative, and the patient remained asymptomatic for at least 5 years. Multiple antituberculosis drugs were given before and after surgery. See Figs. 164-4 to 164-6.

if symptoms return after the medications are stopped, a more aggressive form of therapy has to be considered. In some of these patients, reintroduction of the previously used medications will restore clinical stability. This may be a reasonable clinical goal despite the continued presence of organisms in the sputum. In these patients, treatment with a combination of drugs such as rifampin, isoniazid, and ethambutol or azithromycin, rifabutin, and ethambutol for an indefinite time is feasible and often beneficial.

Those patients in whom clinical signs and symptoms return or worsen either during initial therapy or while under observation, as well as those who have extensive disease at the time the diagnosis is first made, are candidates for more aggressive therapy. If the disease is localized and if the patient can tolerate surgery, resection of the involved area is indicated although medications will also be necessary; the results are excellent (see Case 2, Figs. 164-4 to 164-6). As a rule, if the disease is confined to one lobe, a total lobectomy gives a better result than either a segmental, or subseg-

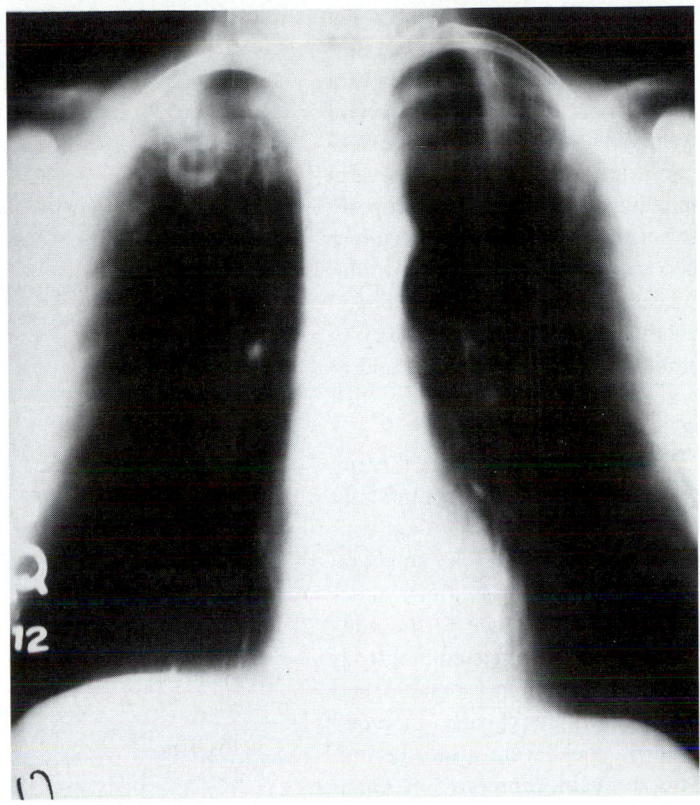

FIGURE 164-5   Tomogram shows thick walled cavity in right upper lobe.

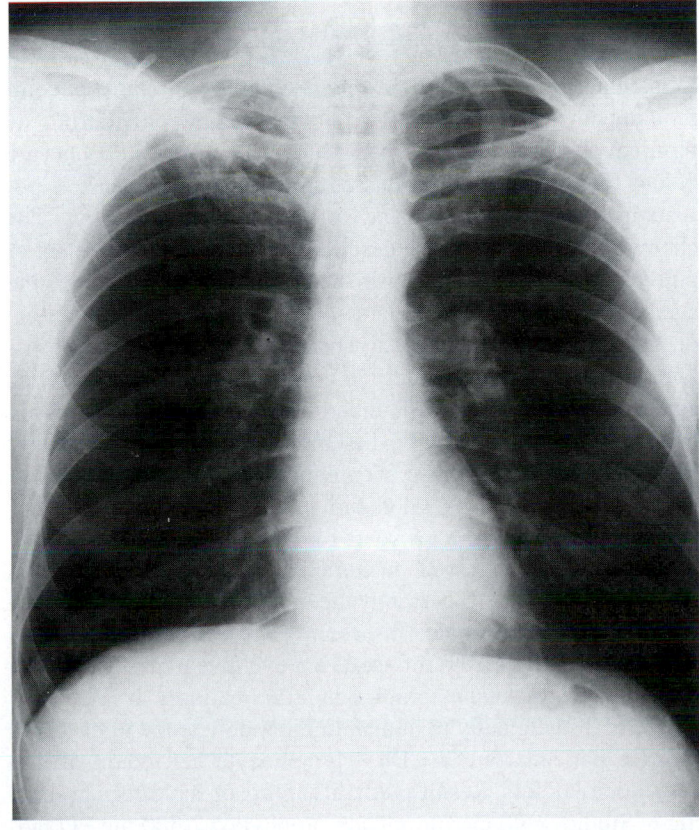

FIGURE 164-4   PA chest radiograph shows chronic right upper lobe infiltrate. Presence of cavity uncertain.

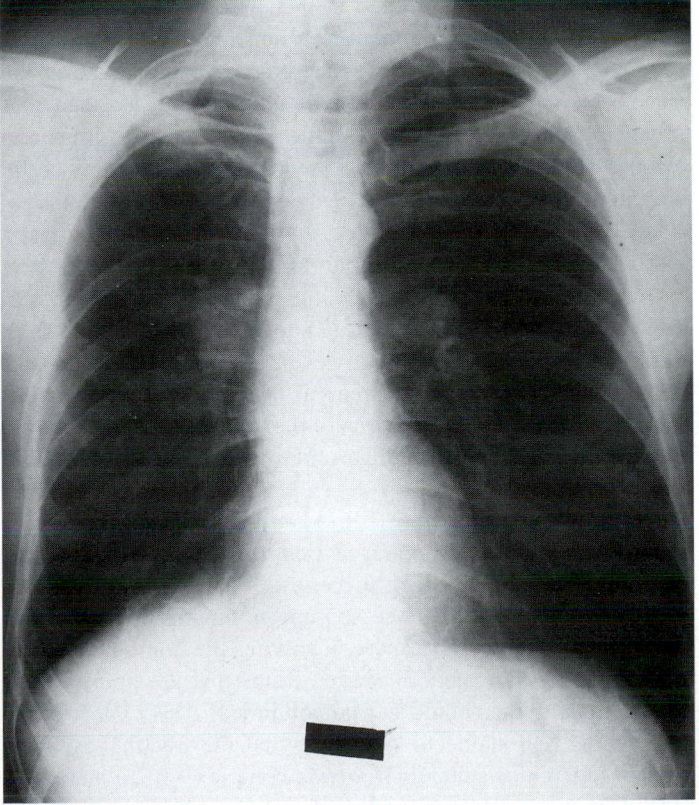

FIGURE 164-6   PA view of the chest 4 months after right upper lobectomy.

mental, resection. Pneumonectomy is indicated in unusual circumstances. The patient should be given antimycobacterial agents for several weeks before surgery; the medications are continued for several months postoperatively. In properly selected patients, the sputum culture becomes negative immediately after successful surgery. If not, prolonged chemotherapy will be necessary to eradicate remaining disease and to prevent serious complications, such as bronchopleural fistula.

More aggressive chemotherapy is necessary for those clinically unstable patients who are not candidates for surgery. The selection of a regimen is partly empirical because drug resistance to the antituberculosis drugs tested in vitro is common. Rifampin, isoniazid, and ethambutol are usually included even if they were used before. Streptomycin, capreomycin, kanamycin, or amikacin is added as well as one or two drugs taken orally, usually azithromycin or clarithromycin, ethionamide and/or clofazimine. Cycloserine is substituted for one of the other drugs if one is not tolerated by the patient. All medications are continued until the sputum culture is negative for 3 to 6 months. The injectable drug is stopped at that time, and the oral drugs continued until the sputum culture is negative for 12 months. At this juncture, it is usually necessary to stop one or more of the drugs because of side effects. The remaining drugs are then continued for another 12 months. Table 164-3 lists the drugs and dosages for treating adults with atypical tuberculosis. Careful and intensive monitoring for drug side effects and toxicity is essential for a successful outcome.

The success rate with multiple drug therapy has varied from 50 to 80 percent.[5,7] Unfortunately, the relapse rate following successful treatment has been high (15 to 25 percent) (see Case 3, and Figs. 164-7 and 164-8). However, relapse rates are considerably lower (less than 5 percent) in patients who have undergone successful surgical excision of the localized lesion. The role of newer agents such as the macrolides in preventing relapse has not yet been assessed.

Aggressive chemotherapy is tried only as a last resort. In general, a minimum of 6 months of treatment is necessary before deciding whether it has been successful. The clinical state of the patient may stabilize, but the sputum cultures remain positive. The approach discussed earlier, involving the continued use of drugs, may be indicated. However, drugs that are poorly tolerated or toxic drugs should not be continued.

It seems reasonable to anticipate that the treatment of pulmonary tuberculosis due to M. avium complex will be more successful as more effective and predictable drugs become available. However, to date the newer agents have offered only limited advantage to the regimens previously used. In vitro susceptibility studies have raised the possibility that rifabutin,[16] clofazimine, the macrolides, and the quinolones may have significant potential.

TABLE 164-3

Dosages of Drugs Used in Treating Adults with Atypical Tuberculosis

Rifampin	600–900 mg per day in a single dose
Isoniazid	300–600 mg per day in a single dose
Ethambutol	25 mg/kg daily in a single dose until cultures are negative for 6 months, then 15 mg/kg daily thereafter
Streptomycin, capreomycin, kanamycin, amikacin	15 mg/kg up to 1 gm, once daily 5 days a week—when cultures are negative or significant toxicity occurs, dosages can be reduced and/or the drug given less frequently
Azithromycin	500–1000 mg per day in a single dose
Clarithromycin	500–750 mg twice daily
Ciprofloxacin	500–750 mg twice daily
Ofloxacin	800 mg per day in a single dose
Clofazimine	100–200 mg per day in a single dose
Rifabutin	300–600 mg per day in a single dose
Ethionamide	500–1000 mg per day usually in divided dose; give highest tolerated dose
Cycloserine	500–1000 mg per day usually in divided doses; give highest tolerated dose

Disseminated Disease in AIDS Patients

Disseminated disease with M. avium complex is relatively common in patients with AIDS. It occurs more commonly during the terminal phase of AIDS when CD4+ lymphocyte cell counts are below 100 cells/microl. In this circumstance, the disease is potentially life-threatening and often requires therapy. The chemotherapeutic approach described above for the treatment of pulmonary disease is effective in some patients. However, the agents are often not well tolerated by AIDS patients. Rifampin or, more recently, rifabutin, an ansamycin closely related to rifampin, has been used widely in combination with a macrolide and/or a quinolone and ethambutol and an aminoglycoside in treating AIDS patients with disseminated M. avium infection.[4] The long-term results have been equivocal, although initial improvement often occurs. Clofazimine, a riminophenazine derivative used for a number of years to treat leprosy, also has good in vitro activity against M. avium complex and, in combination with the other drugs, is currently the treatment of choice for many patients with disseminated disease.

Rifabutin is approved for use as a preventive treatment against disseminated M. avium complex in AIDS patients. It is given at a dose of 300 mg daily to human immunodeficiency virus (HIV) positive patients with a CD4+ lymphocyte cell count of 200 cells/microl or less. Results with this approach have been promising.[14] Studies with clarithromycin prophylaxis (500 mg PO bid) in AIDS patients suggest efficacy, although clarithromycin resistance has been observed. Prophylaxis using a variety of com-

Case 3

Fifty-eight-year-old male with chronic obstructive lung disease. *Mycobacterium avium* was diagnosed following an episode of pneumonia. A right upper lobectomy was done. Initially he did well, but 2 years later *M. avium* was again isolated from his sputum. Several attempts at treatment with multiple drugs were unsuccessful, and his condition gradually deteriorated over the next few years. He died during an attempt to remove the remainder of the right lung. See Figs. 164-7 and 164-8.

binations of antimycobacterial agents, including azithromycin, clofazamine, rifabutin, ethambutol, and clarithromycin, are under study in this population (see Chapter 163).

Other Presentations of *M. Avium* Complex Disease

In children, cervical lymphadenitis caused by *M. avium* complex is best treated by surgical excision. The role of chemotherapy is unclear. Although the disease is usually self-limited in children, surgical excision is needed to establish the diagnosis and affords a better cosmetic result.[17] The role of new agents such as the macrolides has not been established.

When a solitary pulmonary nodule has been surgically removed for diagnostic purposes and is found to be a granuloma caused by *M. avium* complex, i.e., after *M. avium* is isolated, further

chemotherapy is unnecessary. Figure 164-9 summarizes a clinical approach to managing patients with M. avium complex disease.

OTHER SPECIES

Rare instances of disease are caused by other species of mycobacteria. *M. simiae* is a highly drug resistant niacin-positive organism (as is *M. tuberculosis*), which may cause pulmonary disease. Methods of treatment are uncertain, but one reasonable approach is the use of multiple antituberculosis drugs.[2] *M. szulgai* is a rare organism with a drug susceptibility pattern similar to *M. kansasii*. Limited experience suggests that disease caused by this organism responds to regimens that include rifampin.[15] *M. xenopi*, a rare cause of pulmonary disease in the United States, may respond to antituberculosis regimens that consist of two or three of the following drugs: isoniazid, rifampin, and streptomycin.[9]

Other species have been more recently described as causes of disease in humans. *M. malmoense* is primarily a pulmonary pathogen, *M. haemophilum* has been recovered from cutaneous lesions in immune-suppressed patients.[20] *M. genavense* has been repeatedly isolated from patients with AIDS. It may be more common than originally suspected because of its fastidious growth requirements and clinical manifestations similar to *M. avium* complex.[3]

The reader can find additional information regarding the species of mycobacteria discussed in this chapter by referring to a number of published resources (see references 6, 7, and 12).

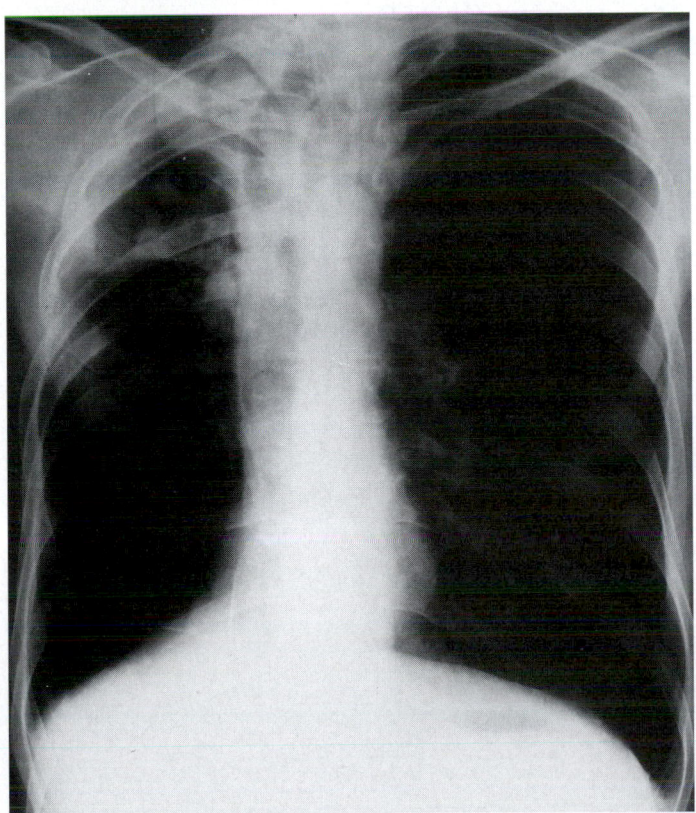

FIGURE 164-7   PA radiograph view of the chest showing extensive bilateral emphysema with cavitary destruction of right upper lobe.

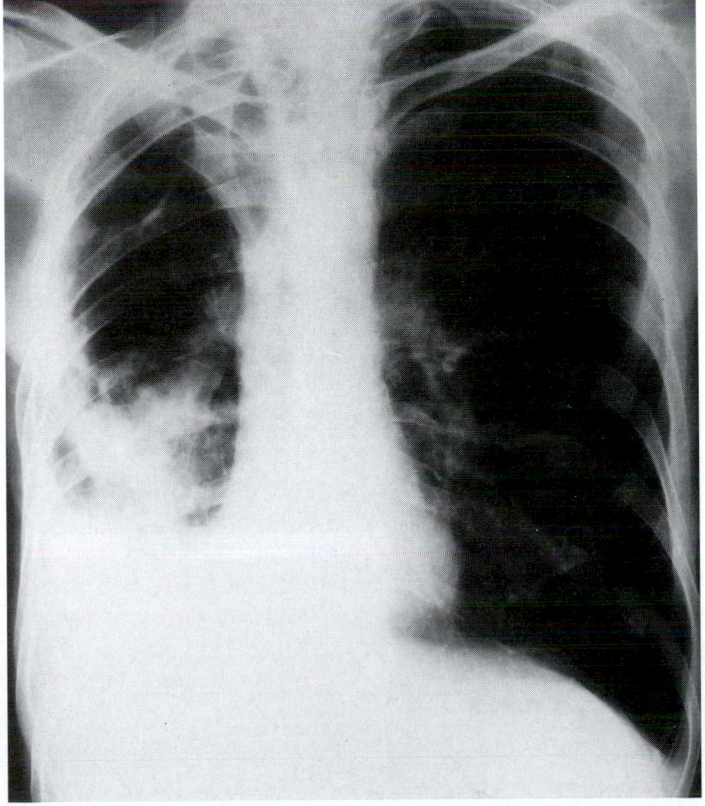

FIGURE 164-8   PA chest radiograph 2 1/2 years later showing pleural involvement and further marked progression of disease and destruction of the right lung.

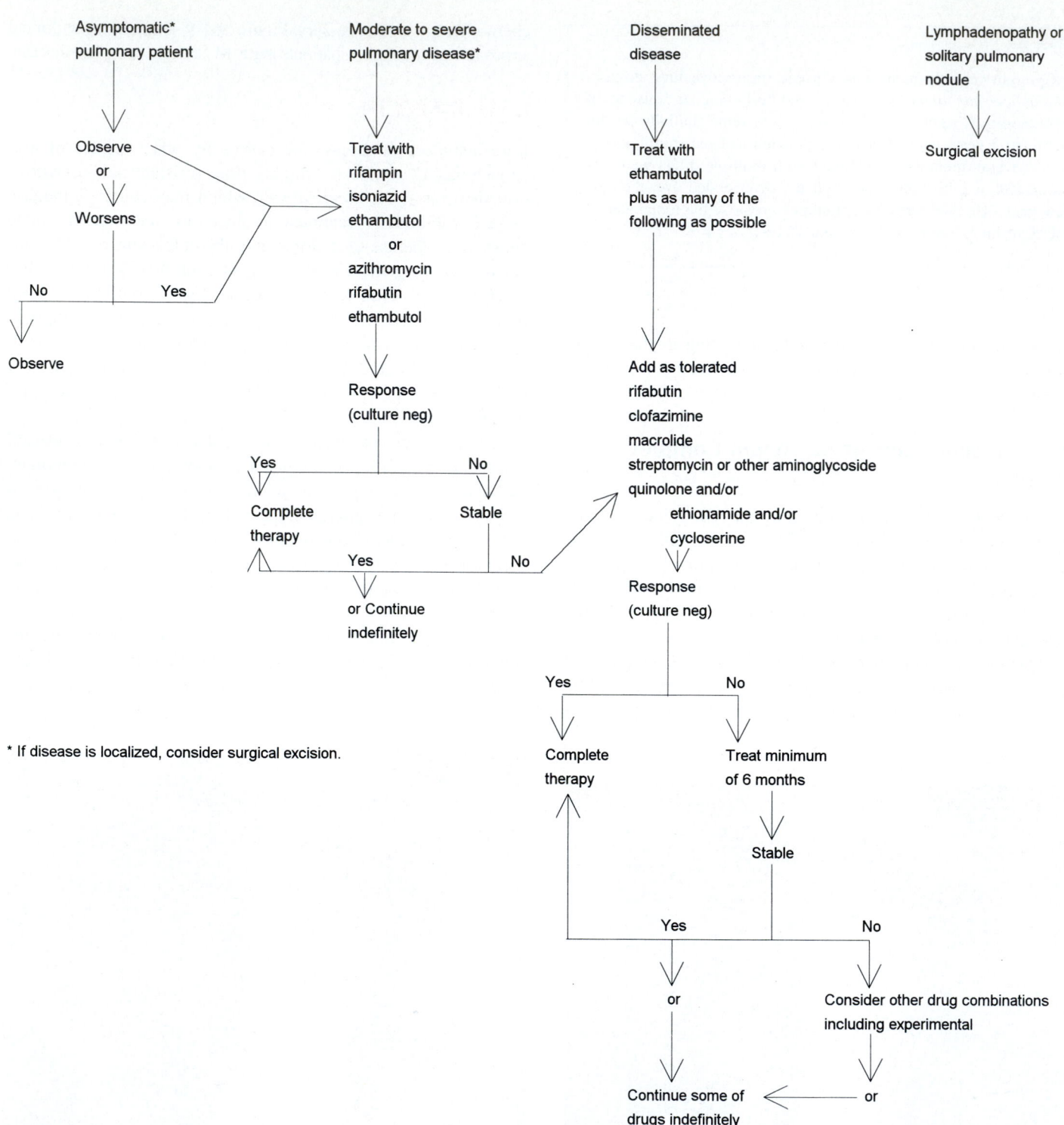

FIGURE 164-9   Management of disease with *M. avium* complex.

REFERENCES

1. Ahn CH, Lowell JR, Ahn SS, et al: Short-course chemotherapy for pulmonary disease caused by Mycobacterium kansasii. *Am Rev Respir Dis* 128:1048–1050, 1983.

2. Bell RC, Higuchi JH, Donovan WN, et al: Mycobacterium simiae. Clinical features and follow-up of twenty-four patients. *Am Rev Resp Dis* 127:35–38, 1983.

3. Bottger EC: Mycobacterium genavense: an emerging pathogen. *Eur J Clin Microbiol Infect Dis* 13:932–936, 1994.

4. Chiu J, Nussbaum J, Bozzette S, et al: Treatment of disseminated Mycobacterium avium complex infection in AIDS with amikacin, ethambutol, rifampin, and ciprofloxacin. *Ann Intern Med* 113:358–361, 1990.

5. Davidson, PT, Khanijo V, Goble M, Moulding T: Treatment of disease due to Mycobacterium intracellulare. *Rev Infect Dis* 3:1052–1059, 1981.

6. Davidson PT: International conference on atypical mycobacteria. *Rev Infect Dis* 134:442–445, 1986.

7. Davidson PT: M. avium complex, M. kansasii, M. fortuitum, and other mycobacteria causing human disease, in Reichman LB, Herschfield ES (eds), *Tuberculosis: A comprehensive international approach.* New York, Dekker, 1993, pp 505–530.

8. Donta ST, Smith PW, Levitz, RE, Quintiliam R: Therapy of Mycobacterium marinum infections. *Arch Intern Med* 146:902–904, 1986.

9. Dornetzhuber V, Martin R, Burjanona B, et al: Pulmonary mycobacteriosis caused by mycobacterium xenopi: Report of a case. *Eur J Respir Dis* 63:293–297, 1982.

10. Etzkorn ET, Aldaronda S, McAllister CK, et al: Medical therapy of Mycobacterium avium-intracellulare pulmonary disease. *Am Rev Respir Dis* 134:442–445, 1986.

11. Horsburgh CR Jr, Mason UG 3d, Heifets LB, et al: Response to therapy of pulmonary Mycobacterium avium-intracellulare infection correlates with results of in vitro susceptibility testing. *Am Rev Respir Dis* 135:418–421, 1987.

12. Iseman MD, Corp RF, O'Brien RJ, et al: Diseases due to Mycobacterium avium-intracellulare. *Chest* 87(Suppl):139–149, 1985.

13. Lillo M, Orengo S, Cernoch P, Harris RL: Pulmonary and disseminated infection due to Mycobacterium kansasii: A decade of experience. *Rev Infect Dis* 12:760–767, 1990.

14. Maddix DS, Tallian KB, Mead PS: Rifabutin: A review with emphasis on its role in the prevention of disseminated Mycobacterium avium complex infection. *Ann Pharmacother* 28:1250–1254, 1994.

15. Maloney JM, Gregg CR, Stephens DS, et al: Infections caused by Mycobacterium szulgai in humans. *Rev Infect Dis* 9:1120–1126, 1987.

16. O'Brien RJ, Geiter LJ, Lyle MA: Rifabutin (ansamycin LM427) for the treatment of pulmonary Mycobacterium avium complex. *Am Rev Respir Dis* 141:821–826, 1990.

17. Taha AM, Davidson PT, Bailey WC: Surgical treatment of atypical mycobacterial lymphadenitis in children. *Pediatr Infect Dis* 4:664–667, 1985.

18. Wallace RJ, O'Brien R, Glassroth J, et al: Diagnosis and treatment of disease caused by nontuberculous mycobacteria. Official statement of the American Thoracic Society. *Am Rev Respir Dis* 142:940–953, 1990.

19. Wayne LG: The atypical mycobacteria: Recognition and disease association. *CRC Crit Rev Microbiol* 12:185–222, 1985.

20. Woods GL, Washington JA 2d: Mycobacteria other than Mycobacterium tuberculosis: Review of microbiologic and clinical aspects. *Rev Infect Dis* 9:275–294, 1987.

21. Yajko DM, Chin DP, Gonzalez PC, et al: Mycobacterium avium complex in water, food, and soil samples collected from the environment of HIV-infected individuals. *J Acquired Immune Defic Syndr Hum Retovirol* 9:176–182, 1995.

PART SEVENTEEN

ACUTE RESPIRATORY FAILURE

CHAPTER 165

RESPIRATORY FAILURE: AN OVERVIEW

Michael A. Grippi

CLASSIFICATION OF RESPIRATORY FAILURE

PATHOPHYSIOLOGY
Hypoxemic Respiratory Failure
Hypercapnic Respiratory Failure
Ventilatory Supply Versus Demand

CATEGORIES OF RESPIRATORY FAILURE
Abnormalities of the Central Nervous System
Abnormalities of the Peripheral Nervous System or
Chest Wall
Abnormalities of the Airways
Abnormalities of the Alveoli

APPROACH TO THE PATIENT

PRINCIPLES OF MANAGEMENT
Triage Decisions
Airway Management
Correction of Hypoxemia and Hypercapnia
Search for an Underlying Cause

**MONITORING PATIENTS WITH ACUTE RESPIRATORY
FAILURE**

COMPLICATIONS OF ACUTE RESPIRATORY FAILURE
Pulmonary
Cardiovascular
Gastrointestinal
Infectious
Renal
Nutritional

PROGNOSIS
Morbidity and Mortality in Acute Hypoxemic
Respiratory Failure
Morbidity and Mortality in Acute Hypercapnic
Respiratory Failure

Respiratory failure is a condition in which the respiratory system fails in one or both of its gas-exchanging functions—i.e., oxygenation of, and carbon dioxide elimination from, mixed venous (pulmonary arterial) blood. Hence, respiratory failure is a syndrome rather than a disease. Many diseases result in respiratory failure, as discussed elsewhere in this volume.

Respiratory failure may be acute or chronic. The clinical presentations of patients with acute and chronic respiratory failure usually are quite different. While acute respiratory failure is characterized by life-threatening derangements in arterial blood gases and acid-base status, the manifestations of chronic respiratory failure are more indolent and may be clinically inapparent.

Although the causes of respiratory failure are diverse, common underlying pathophysiological mechanisms and management strategies merit a general discussion. This chapter begins with a focus on the definition of respiratory failure and underscores distinctions between acute and chronic varieties. Hypoxemic and hypercapnic respiratory failure are described, and the pathophysiological underpinnings of each type are reviewed. The concepts of ventilatory supply and demand are considered before an overview of the many categories of disease that result in respiratory failure. Finally, an approach to clinical evaluation and management is outlined, followed by a summary of complications and comments on prognosis.

CLASSIFICATION OF RESPIRATORY FAILURE

As noted previously, respiratory failure is characterized by inadequate blood oxygenation or carbon dioxide removal. "Adequacy" is defined by tissue requirements for oxygen uptake and carbon dioxide elimination. In the absence of bedside techniques for direct measurement of these metabolic parameters, clinicians must rely on arterial blood gas values.

Respiratory failure may be classified as *hypercapnic* or *hypoxemic* (Fig. 165-1).[42] *Hypercapnic respiratory failure* is defined as an arterial P_{CO_2} (Pa_{CO_2}) greater than 45 mm Hg. *Hypoxemic respiratory failure* is defined as an arterial P_{O_2} (Pa_{O_2}) less than 55 mm Hg when the fraction of oxygen in inspired air (F_{IO_2}) is 0.60 or greater. In many cases, hypercapnic and hypoxemic respiratory failure coexist.

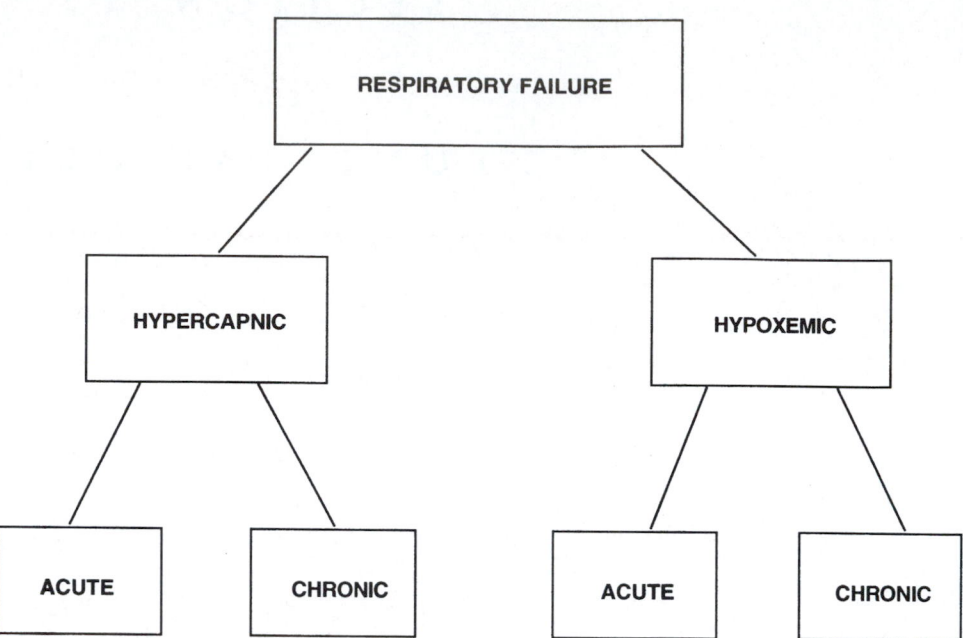

FIGURE 165-1   Classification of respiratory failure. Although depicted as distinct entities, hypercapnic and hypoxemic respiratory failure frequently coexist. Either may be acute or chronic.

Disorders that initially cause hypoxemia may be complicated by respiratory pump failure (see below) and hypercapnia. Conversely, diseases that produce respiratory pump failure are frequently complicated by hypoxemia due to secondary pulmonary parenchymal processes (e.g., pneumonia) or vascular disorders (e.g., pulmonary embolism).

Distinctions between *acute* and *chronic* respiratory failure are summarized in Table 165-1. In general, acute hypercapnic respiratory failure is defined as a Pa_{CO_2} greater than 45 mm Hg with accompanying acidemia (pH less than 7.30).[23] The physiological effect of a sudden increment in Pa_{CO_2} depends on the prevailing level of serum bicarbonate anion. In patients with chronic hypercapnic respiratory failure—e.g., due to chronic obstructive pulmonary disease (COPD)—a long-standing increase in Pa_{CO_2} results in renal "compensation" and an increased serum bicarbonate concentration. A superimposed acute increase in Pa_{CO_2} has a less dramatic effect than does a comparable increase in a patient with a normal bicarbonate level.

Distinction between acute and chronic hypoxemic respiratory failure may not be readily made on the basis of arterial blood gas values.[23] The presence of markers of chronic hypoxemia (e.g., polycythemia or cor pulmonale) provides clues to a long-standing disorder, whereas abrupt changes in mental status suggest an acute event.

It is important to bear in mind that even though the definition of hypoxemic respiratory failure rests on measurement of Pa_{O_2}, the important threat of arterial hypoxemia is inadequate tissue oxygenation, reflected in tissue *oxygen delivery*. Tissue oxygen delivery is determined by the product of cardiac output and blood *oxygen content* (see Chapter 14); the latter, in turn, depends on hemoglobin concentration and oxygen saturation. Therefore, factors that lower cardiac output or hemoglobin concentration, or inhibit dissociation of oxygen from hemoglobin at the tissue level, may promote tissue hypoxia without technically producing respiratory failure.

PATHOPHYSIOLOGY

Respiratory failure can arise from an abnormality in any of the "effector" components of the respiratory system—central nervous system, peripheral nervous system, respiratory muscles and chest wall, airways, or alveoli (Fig. 165-2). A defect in any of the first four components, which constitute the "respiratory pump," may cause coexistent hypercapnia and hypoxemia; at least initially, disorders of the alveoli are more apt to result in hypoxemia.[16]

Hypoxemic Respiratory Failure

As described in Chapters 11, 12, and 13, four pathophysiological mechanisms account for the hypoxemia seen in a wide variety of diseases: alveolar hypoventilation, ventilation-perfusion mis-

TABLE 165-1

Distinctions Between Acute and Chronic Respiratory Failure

Category	Characteristic
Hypercapnic respiratory failure	Pa_{CO_2} >45 mmHg
Acute	Develops in min to h
Chronic	Develops over several days or longer
Hypoxemic respiratory failure	Pa_{O_2} <55 mmHg when $F_{IO_2} \geq 0.60$
Acute	Develops in min to h
Chronic	Develops over several days or longer

match, shunt, and diffusion limitation. Alveolar hypoventilation occurs in neuromuscular disorders that affect the respiratory system. In the absence of underlying pulmonary disease, the hypoxemia accompanying alveolar hypoventilation is characterized by a normal alveolar-arterial oxygen gradient, as defined by Eq. (1):

$$P_{A_{O_2}} - Pa_{O_2} = [P_{I_{O_2}} - Pa_{CO_2}/R] - Pa_{O_2} \tag{1}$$

where

$$
\begin{aligned}
P_{A_{O_2}} &= \text{alveolar } P_{O_2} \\
Pa_{O_2} &= \text{arterial } P_{O_2} \\
P_{I_{O_2}} &= \text{inspired } P_{O_2} \\
Pa_{CO_2} &= \text{arterial } P_{CO_2} \\
R &= \text{respiratory exchange ratio}
\end{aligned}
$$

In contradistinction, disorders in which any of the other three mechanisms are operative are characterized by widening of the alveolar-arterial oxygen gradient, which is normally less than 20 mm Hg. With ventilation-perfusion mismatching, areas of low ventilation relative to perfusion contribute to the hypoxemia. Similarly, with shunt, either intrapulmonary or intracardiac, deoxygenated mixed venous blood bypasses ventilated alveoli, resulting in "venous admixture." Finally, diseases that increase the diffusion pathway for oxygen from the alveolar space to pulmonary capillary impair oxygen transport across the alveolar-capillary membrane.

Although changes in minute and alveolar ventilation can change Pa_{CO_2} considerably, this is not so for Pa_{O_2}. Increases in minute ventilation and, secondarily, in alveolar ventilation modestly increase Pa_{O_2}. Indeed, at a Pa_{O_2} above 55 to 60 mm Hg, the effect of increasing ventilation on oxygen content is minimal, since the oxyhemoglobin dissociation curve is flat in this range.

Hypercapnic Respiratory Failure

At a constant rate of CO_2 production ($\dot{V}_{CO_2}$), Pa_{CO_2} is determined by the level of alveolar ventilation.[17] The relationship between alveolar ventilation, rate of CO_2 production, and Pa_{CO_2} is described by Eq. (2):

$$\dot{V}_A = K \cdot \dot{V}_{CO_2}/Pa_{CO_2} \tag{2}$$

where

$$
\begin{aligned}
\dot{V}_A &= \text{minute alveolar ventilation} \\
K &= \text{a constant} \\
\dot{V}_{CO_2} &= \text{rate of } CO_2 \text{ production}
\end{aligned}
$$

When $\dot{V}_{CO_2}$ is constant, Pa_{CO_2} is determined by $\dot{V}_A$, which, in turn, is dictated by two factors: minute ventilation ($\dot{V}_E$) and the relationship between $\dot{V}_E$ and $\dot{V}_A$. The latter is determined by the proportion of $\dot{V}_E$ that constitutes dead space ventilation—i.e., the dead space to tidal volume ratio (V_D/V_T):

$$\dot{V}_E = K \cdot (\dot{V}_{O_2} \cdot RQ)/(Pa_{CO_2}/[1 - V_D/V_T]) \tag{3}$$

where

$$
\begin{aligned}
\dot{V}_{O_2} &= \text{rate of } O_2 \text{ consumption} \\
RQ &= \text{respiratory quotient (the respiratory exchange ratio in} \\
&\quad \text{the steady state)} \\
V_D &= \text{dead space volume} \\
V_T &= \text{tidal volume}
\end{aligned}
$$

Inspection of the third equation indicates that disorders reducing $\dot{V}_E$ or increasing the proportion of dead space ventilation may result in hypercapnia.[44]

Ventilatory Supply Versus Demand

A useful theoretical construct for understanding the pathophysiological basis for hypercapnic respiratory failure is the relationship between ventilatory supply and ventilatory demand (Fig. 165-3).[24]

Ventilatory supply is the maximal spontaneous ventilation that can be maintained without development of respiratory muscle fatigue; ventilatory supply is also known as *maximal sustainable ventilation* (MSV).

Ventilatory demand is the spontaneous minute ventilation, which, when maintained constant, results in a stable Pa_{CO_2} (assuming a fixed rate of CO_2 production).

Normally, ventilatory supply greatly exceeds ventilatory demand. Hence, major changes in minute ventilatory requirements (e.g., during exercise) may occur without hypercapnia. In lung disease, significant abnormalities may be present before ventilatory demand encroaches on MSV. Consequently, hypercapnia is a late finding. When ventilatory demand exceeds MSV, Pa_{CO_2} increases.

As a general rule, MSV is approximated as one-half the *maximal voluntary ventilation,* or MVV (see Chapter 36). A 70-kg adult has an MVV of about 160 liters per minute, an MSV of 80 liters per minute, and, under basal conditions, a $\dot{V}_E$ of approximately 6 to 7 liters per minute (90 ml/kg/min). Normally, therefore, there is a 10- to 15-fold difference between resting $\dot{V}_E$ and MSV. In disease states, the $\dot{V}_E$ re-

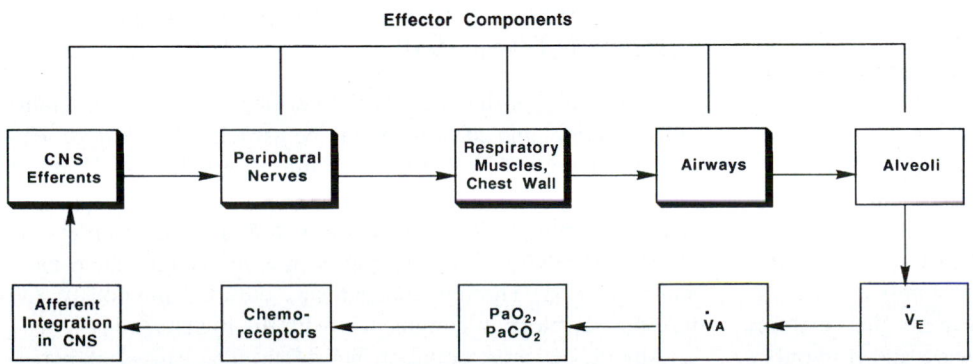

FIGURE 165-2 Functional components of the respiratory system and its controller. Abnormalities in any of the effector components can result in respiratory failure. The central and peripheral nervous systems, respiratory muscles and chest wall, and airways constitute the "respiratory pump" (shaded boxes). Hypercapnia is the hallmark of respiratory pump failure, while hypoxemia constitutes the primary disturbance in alveolar disorders producing respiratory failure. (*From Lanken.*[24])

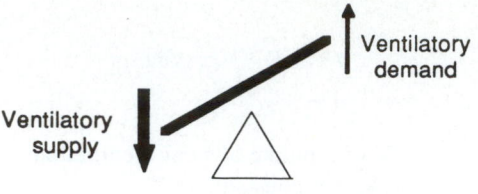

A.   Ventilatory supply exceeds ventilatory demand.

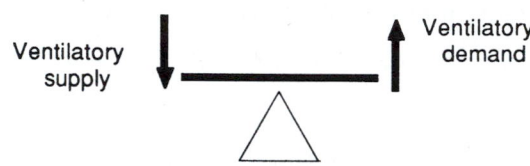

B.   Ventilatory supply equals ventilatory demand.

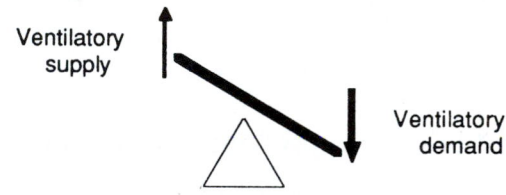

C.   Ventilatory demand exceeds ventilatory supply.

FIGURE 165-3 Relationship between ventilatory supply (maximal sustainable ventilation) and ventilatory demand (overall level of ventilation specified by the CNS controller). Relative size of the arrows indicates levels of supply and demand in each of the three circumstances illustrated. *A.* Normal. Ventilatory supply greatly exceeds ventilatory demand. Physiological "reserve" is maintained. *B.* Ventilatory supply is decreased and ventilatory demand increased (e.g., acute asthma attack). "Borderline" respiratory failure exists. *C.* Ventilatory demand exceeds ventilatory supply (e.g., sepsis in a patient with COPD). Respiratory muscle fatigue develops, and hypercapnic respiratory failure ensues. See text for details. (*From Lanken.*[23])

quirement may approach a markedly reduced MSV. Further reductions in MSV result in ventilatory demand exceeding supply, and hypercapnia occurs.

FACTORS THAT REDUCE VENTILATORY SUPPLY OR INCREASE VENTILATORY DEMAND

Disruption of any component of the efferent arm of the respiratory control system may diminish ventilatory supply (Table 165-2). While a variety of diseases produce specific abnormalities along the efferent pathway (e.g., phrenic nerve and respiratory muscle disorders), some result in respiratory muscle fatigue—the biochemical, cellular, and molecular mechanisms of which remain poorly understood.[1]

As described previously, ventilatory demand can be assessed according to equation 3:

$$\dot{V}_E = K \cdot (\dot{V}_{O_2} \cdot RQ)/(Pa_{CO_2}/[1 - V_D/V_T])$$

Any factor that affects terms on the right-hand side of the equation may result in ventilatory demand exceeding supply. Selected clinical examples are given in Table 165-3.

CATEGORIES OF RESPIRATORY FAILURE

Although many different diseases that cause respiratory failure exist, they may be grouped conveniently according to primary abnormalities in the individual effector components of the respiratory system.[4,21,24]

Abnormalities of the Central Nervous System

A variety of pharmacologic, structural, and metabolic disorders of the CNS are characterized by suppression of the neural drive to breathe.[24] The resultant hypoventilation and hypercapnia may be acute or chronic.

An overdose of a narcotic or other drug with sedative properties is a common cause of respiratory failure. While the most striking clinical picture occurs with an acute overdose, long-standing use of some agents (e.g., methadone) may result in chronic hypercapnia.

"Structural" CNS abnormalities producing hypercapnic respiratory failure include meningoencephalitis, localized tumors or vascular abnormalities of the medulla, and strokes affecting medullary control centers. Usually, respiratory failure is observed in the context of other neurologic findings.

A variety of metabolic derangements may produce hypercapnia through depression of respiratory control centers. Examples include severe myxedema, hepatic failure, and advanced uremia. In addition, elevation of P_{CO_2} in the CNS results in neural depression, further enhancing CO_2 retention. A common clinical setting in which elevation of Pa_{CO_2} is observed is chronic metabolic alkalosis (e.g., due to diuretic use), as detailed in Chapter 15.

Finally, obesity-hypoventilation syndrome is characterized by hypercapnia due to hypoventilation on a central basis. The underlying mechanisms have not yet been elucidated.

Abnormalities of the Peripheral Nervous System or Chest Wall

A wide variety of disorders of the peripheral nerves, neuromuscular junction, and chest wall may be associated with hypercapnic and hypoxemic respiratory failure.[2,12,25,30,34,39,40,51] While the hallmark is an inability to maintain a level of $\dot{V}_E$ appropriate for the rate of CO_2 production, many of these disorders are complicated by impaired expiratory muscle strength, atelectasis, and aspiration. Through mechanisms outlined previously, hypoxemia develops in conjunction with the hypercapnia.

Among the most common neuromuscular causes of hypercapnic respiratory failure are Guillain-Barré syndrome, myasthenia gravis, polymyositis, the muscular dystrophies, and a large number of metabolic muscle disorders. In addition, acute poliomyelitis and traumatic spinal cord injury are associated with hypercapnia. Development of respiratory muscle fatigue[1,12] dur-

TABLE 165-2

Factors That Diminish Ventilatory Supply

Factor	Examples
Decreased respiratory muscle strength	
Muscle fatigue	Recovery from acute respiratory failure, high respiratory rates, increased Pdi/Pdi_{max},* increased inspiratory time
Disuse atrophy	Prolonged mechanical ventilation, following phrenic nerve injury
Malnutrition	Protein-calorie starvation
Electrolyte abnormalities	Low serum phosphate or potassium concentrations
Arterial blood gas abnormalities	Low pH, low Pa_{O_2}, high Pa_{CO_2}
Fatty infiltration of diaphragm	Obesity
Unfavorable alteration in diaphragm length–tension relationship	Flattened domes of diaphragm caused by hyperinflation
Increased muscle energy requirement or decreased substrate supply	
High elastic work of breathing	Low lung or chest wall compliance, high respiratory rate
High resistive work of breathing	Airway obstruction
Reduced diaphragm perfusion	Shock, anemia
Decreased motor neuron function	
Decreased phrenic nerve output	Polyneuropathy, Guillain-Barré syndrome, phrenic nerve transection or injury, poliomyelitis
Decreased neuromuscular transmission	Myasthenia gravis, use of paralyzing agents
Abnormal respiratory mechanics	
Airflow limitation	Bronchospasm, upper-airway obstruction, excessive airway secretions
Loss of lung volume	After lung resection, large pleural effusion
Other restrictive defects	Pain-limited inspiration; tense abdominal distention due to ileus, peritoneal dialysis fluid, or ascites

ing prolonged weaning from mechanical ventilation is a common cause of recurrent hypercapnia in the critical care setting.

Pharmacologic causes of hypercapnia in the intensive care unit are frequently encountered. Use of depolarizing and nondepolarizing paralyzing agents, particularly in conjunction with systemic corticosteroids (e.g., in management of status asthmaticus), cholinergic crisis during therapy of myasthenia gravis, and administration of aminoglycosides to patients with myasthenia are examples.

Primary disorders of the chest wall constitute another important category of neuromuscular respiratory failure. The prototype is severe kyphoscoliosis. Additional examples include flail chest (Chapter 105), extensive thoracoplasty, morbid obesity, and massive abdominal distention due to ascites or distended loops of bowel.

In each of these disorders, a common pathophysiological sequence develops. Because of inadequate activation of inspiratory muscles or limited

thoracic excursion, tidal volume falls. While an increase in respiratory rate compensates initially for the fall in $\dot{V}_E$ (and in $\dot{V}_A$), $\dot{V}_E$ eventually declines. In addition, the sigh mechanism is impaired, which, in conjunction with the low tidal volume, results in atelectasis and reduced lung compliance. Reduced lung compliance produces a further fall in tidal volume and an increase in the elastic work of breathing (Chapter 10). Hence, ventilatory supply becomes limited, while ventilatory demand increases due

TABLE 165-3

Factors That Increase Ventilatory Demand

Factor	Clinical Examples
Increased V_D/V_T	Acute asthma, emphysema, late phase of acute respiratory distress syndrome, pulmonary emboli
Increased $\dot{V}_{O_2}$	Fever, sepsis, trauma, shivering, increased work of breathing, massive obesity
Increased RQ	Excessive carbohydrate feeding
Decreased Pa_{CO_2}	Hypoxemia, metabolic acidosis, anxiety, sepsis, renal failure, hepatic failure

SOURCE: Data from Lanken.[23]

to a rise in V_D/V_T (as a result of atelectasis and other factors noted below). An imbalance between ventilatory supply and demand arises, and hypercapnia ensues. Furthermore, an impaired gag reflex in the setting of bulbar weakness, coupled with impaired cough due to respiratory muscle involvement, may result in aspiration pneumonia and secondary hypoxemia.

In addition to the pathophysiology described, structural abnormalities of the thoracic cage (e.g., severe kyphoscoliosis) are characterized by an increase in the elastic component of the work of breathing. This results in a higher $\dot{V}_{O_2}$ and a higher proportion of total O_2 consumption by the respiratory muscles (normally, less than 5 percent of $\dot{V}_{O_2}$).

Abnormalities of the Airways

Obstructive diseases of the airways—either upper or lower—are common causes of acute and chronic hypercapnia. Examples in the upper airways include acute epiglottitis, aspirated foreign body, tracheal tumor, and narrowing of the trachea or glottis by fibrotic tissue. Disorders of the lower airways include chronic obstructive pulmonary disease, asthma, and advanced cystic fibrosis. The underlying mechanisms are multifaceted and variable. However, several common pathophysiological pathways are operative.

Airway narrowing results in a greater transthoracic pressure gradient requirement for inspiratory airflow. The resistive component of the work of breathing is increased, and the increase is associated with an elevation in $\dot{V}_{O_2}$. In addition, tidal volume falls and dead space ventilation increases. Respiratory muscle fatigue may develop; the consequences of a shallow breathing pattern ensue.

Finally, in some disorders (e.g., acute asthma or an exacerbation of COPD), air trapping and lung hyperinflation occur, resulting in diaphragm flattening and worsening diaphragm mechanics (see Chapters 10 and 44).[10] The overall effect is a growing imbalance between ventilatory supply and demand.[23]

Abnormalities of the Alveoli

Although diseases characterized by diffuse alveolar filling frequently result in hypoxemic respiratory failure, hypercapnia may complicate the picture. Common clinical examples in this category include cardiogenic and noncardiogenic pulmonary edema, diffuse pneumonia, extensive pulmonary hemorrhage, aspiration of stomach contents, and near-drowning.[22]

Diffuse alveolar filling creates a large right-to-left shunt as pulmonary blood flows through nonventilated or poorly ventilated regions of the lung. In addition, coexisting interstitial edema may impair diffusion across the alveolar-capillary membrane, further impairing oxygenation of mixed venous blood.

In extensive, acute pulmonary disease characterized by alveolar filling, ventilatory demand is high because of hypoxemia and increases in V_D/V_T, the elastic work of breathing (due to reduced lung compliance), the resistive work of breathing (due to airway narrowing and increased airway reactivity), and the neural drive to breathe (mediated by pulmonary parenchymal vagal fibers). In conjunction with heightened ventilatory demand, ventilatory supply is reduced because of alveolar flooding, reduced lung elasticity, respiratory muscle fatigue, and, possibly, reduced blood supply to the diaphragm secondary to shock. Once again, the imbalance between ventilatory supply and demand results in hypercapnia.

TABLE 165-4

Changes in Arterial Blood Gases, P_{AO_2}-Pa_{O_2}, and Ventilation in Acute Respiratory Failure

Failed Respiratory System Component	pH	Pa_{CO_2}	Pa_{O_2}	P_{AO_2}-Pa_{O_2}	$\dot{V}_E$	$\dot{V}_A$
Central Nervous System	↓	↑	↓ *	NL or ↑ †	↓	↓
Peripheral Nervous System or Chest Bellows	↓	↑	↓ *	NL or ↑ †	↓	↓
Airways						
In acute asthma						
Early phase (before respiratory failure)	↑	↓	NL	↑	↑	↑
"Crossover point"	NL	NL	NL or ↓	↑	↑	NL
With development of respiratory muscle fatigue	↓	↑	↓	↑	↓ ‡	↓
In COPD						
Non–CO_2 retainer	↓	NL or ↑ §	↓	↑	↑	↓
CO_2 retainer						
Baseline	NL to ↓	↑	↓	↑	NL or ↑	↓
Flare	↓	↑↑	↓↓	↑	NL, ↑ or ↓ ‡	↓
Alveoli						
Before respiratory muscle fatigue develops	↑	↓	↓↓	↑↑	↑	↑
After respiratory muscle fatigue develops	↓	↑	↓↓	↑↑	↓	↓

*Pa_{O_2} may decrease when pneumonia or atelectasis occurs as a complication.
†(P_{AO_2}-Pa_{O_2}) widens when pneumonia or atelectasis occurs as a complication.
‡$\dot{V}_E$ declines when frank respiratory muscle failure occurs.
§Pa_{CO_2} may increase during an exacerbation.
Note: ↑ = increased; ↑↑ = very increased; ↓ = decreased; ↓↓ = very decreased; NL = in normal range.
SOURCE: Data from Lanken.[23]

APPROACH TO THE PATIENT

The diagnosis of acute or chronic respiratory failure begins with clinical suspicion of its presence. Confirmation of the diagnosis is based on arterial blood gas analysis (Table 165-1). Evaluation for an underlying cause must be initiated early, frequently in the presence of concurrent treatment for acute respiratory failure. While the diagnosis of chronic respiratory failure is usually easily established with clinical findings of chronic hypoxemia (with or without findings of hypercapnia), the diagnosis of acute respiratory failure requires more careful analysis.

Signs and symptoms in acute respiratory failure reflect the underlying disease process and associated hypoxemia or acidemia due to hypercapnia. Localized pulmonary findings reflecting the acute causes of hypoxemia (e.g., pneumonia, pulmonary edema, asthma, or COPD) may be readily apparent. Alternatively, the predominant findings may be systemic (e.g., hypotension due to sepsis). The principal manifestations may even be remote from the thorax—e.g., abdominal pain in acute pancreatitis or leg pain due to a long bone fracture—each associated with acute (adult) respiratory distress syndrome (Chapter 167). Frequently, neurologic or cardiovascular symptoms and signs predominate. Neurologic manifestations include restlessness, anxiety, confusion, seizures, or coma. Asterixis may be seen with severe hypercapnia. Common cardiovascular findings include tachycardia and a variety of arrhythmias. Finally, there may be few or no findings other than a complaint of dyspnea, as in some patients with hypoxemia due to pulmonary embolism.

Once respiratory failure is suspected on clinical grounds, arterial blood gas analysis is performed to confirm the diagnosis, to assist in the distinction between acute and chronic forms, to assess the magnitude and metabolic impact, and to help guide management (Table 165-4).

PRINCIPLES OF MANAGEMENT

The principles of management of patients in acute respiratory failure include those that are cause-specific and those that are more general.[5,9,28,46,49] Triage of the patient to the proper clinical setting, airway maintenance, correction of hypoxemia and hypercapnia, and management of the underlying cause are of paramount importance.

Triage Decisions

The first step in management is to determine the appropriate setting for care—admission to a standard inpatient facility or to an intensive or intermediate care unit. Factors that constitute the basis for this decision include the acuity of the respiratory failure; the degree of hypoxemia, hypercapnia, and acidemia; the presence of co-morbid conditions (e.g., cardiac disease or renal insufficiency); and the clinical direction that the patient takes over the first few minutes or hours of observation. At one end of the spectrum is the patient with fulminant hypoxemic respiratory failure, metabolic acidosis, and imminent cardiovascular collapse, who needs emergent intubation, mechanical ventilation, and admission to a critical care unit. At the other end of the spec-

trum is the patient with COPD and chronic, compensated hypercapnic respiratory failure, who requires observation in an intermediate care unit.

Airway Management

Assurance of an adequate airway is key in the patient with acute respiratory distress.[11] Whether emergency intubation is required depends on the clinical circumstances described previously. For patients with chronic respiratory insufficiency, the need for intubation depends on critical arterial blood gas values and the patient's early acute course. When progressive hypoxemia or hypercapnia is observed over the first few minutes or hours of care, intubation and mechanical ventilation are warranted.

Correction of Hypoxemia and Hypercapnia

Once the airway is secured, the clinician must turn attention to the treatment of hypoxemia—the most life-threatening aspect of acute respiratory insufficiency. The goal is to assure adequate oxygen delivery to tissues, generally achieved with a Pa_{O_2} of about 60 mm Hg (assuming an adequate hematocrit and cardiac output). In patients who have coronary or cerebrovascular disease, a slightly higher level of arterial oxygenation may be desirable in order to provide a "buffer" for any sudden, unpredictable changes in gas exchange.

The means by which supplemental oxygen is administered is determined by the clinical circumstances. While some patients may simply require nasal prongs or a face mask to achieve an adequate Pa_{O_2}, others are best treated with controlled-flow oxygen delivered via a Venturi mask—e.g., the patient with COPD and chronic hypercapnia (see Chapters 44 and 172). Generally, if an acceptable level of oxygenation, as judged by arterial blood gases, cannot be attained using a face mask, or if administration of supplemental O_2 causes hypercapnia to worsen significantly (e.g., in some patients with COPD), intubation is required.

While correcting hypoxemia, the clinician must also address any coexisting hypercapnia and respiratory acidosis.[49] Once again, the immediacy of correction depends on the magnitude of the acidosis and its attendant effects (e.g., elevation of serum potassium). A partly compensated respiratory acidosis in a patient with COPD usually constitutes a less urgent clinical circumstance than does profound respiratory acidosis in a patient with a drug overdose.

Search for an Underlying Cause

Finally, as therapy is initiated to correct the hypoxemia, hypercapnia, and acidosis of respiratory failure, a search for the cause of the problem and its management must be undertaken. In some cases, the cause and management are straightforward (e.g., administration of a narcotic antagonist to the patient with a narcotic overdose). In others, a more protracted course may be in store (e.g., long-term ventilator management of fulminant acute respiratory distress syndrome due to sepsis).

In both brief and prolonged cases of respiratory failure, attention to details of management is important in order to minimize the risks of complications of therapy, as discussed below.

MONITORING PATIENTS WITH ACUTE RESPIRATORY FAILURE

Repeated assessment of the patient with incipient or resolving respiratory failure, as well as the patient with frank hypoxemic or hypercapnic failure, is critical in formulating decisions about therapy. Monitoring methods range from routine bedside observations to use of invasive techniques.[48]

For many patients with acute respiratory failure, simple observation of respiratory rate, tidal volume, use of accessory muscles, and presence of paradoxical breathing movements provides evidence of worsening respiratory failure and the need for intubation and mechanical ventilation. The patient with asthma or an acute exacerbation of COPD will frequently manifest rapid, shallow breathing and paradoxical thoracoabdominal breathing movements as respiratory mechanics deteriorate.[40]

Once placed on mechanical ventilation, the patient must be carefully monitored for ventilator-associated complications (see below). In addition, placement of indwelling arterial and venous catheters, patient immobilization, and use of a broad range of pharmacologic agents present additional potential threats to the acutely ill patient.

While many monitoring techniques are routine and may be universally applicable to patients in a critical care setting (e.g., pulse oximetry), others may be of particular importance in selected clinical circumstances. For example, routine assessment of static respiratory system compliance in a mechanically ventilated patient with acute respiratory distress syndrome or pulmonary fibrosis may provide an early warning of barotrauma.[28] In the patient with status asthmaticus requiring mechanical ventilation, development of hypotension due to auto-PEEP,[35] as discussed in Chapters 175 and 176, may signal the need to alter ventilator settings or implement sedation or pharmacologic paralysis.

COMPLICATIONS OF ACUTE RESPIRATORY FAILURE

The respiratory patient in a critical care unit must navigate not only the obstacles presented by the underlying pulmonary process but also the hazards associated with use of mechanical devices and pharmacologic agents. Complications of acute respiratory failure[37] may be broadly categorized as pulmonary, cardiovascular, gastrointestinal, renal, infectious, nutritional, and other (Table 165-5). For details in each of these areas, the reader is referred to chapters elsewhere in this volume.

Pulmonary

Common pulmonary complications of acute respiratory failure include pulmonary emboli, pulmonary barotrauma, pulmonary fibrosis, and complications directly related to use of mechanical devices.[27,37]

Pulmonary emboli have been reported in up to one-fourth of patients with respiratory failure in intensive care units. The diagnosis is difficult in this setting, since patients typically have diffuse underlying lung disease, abnormal gas exchange, and many coexisting potential causes for the clinical, radiographic, and physiological consequences of pulmonary emboli.

Pulmonary barotrauma, identified as the presence of extra-alveolar air in structures that do not normally contain air, may occur in patients receiving mechanical ventilation for a variety of indications. It is particularly common in patients with acute respiratory distress syndrome.[13] Manifestations of barotrauma include pulmonary interstitial emphysema, pneumothorax, pneumomediastinum, pneumoperitoneum, subcutaneous emphysema, tension lung cysts, and subpleural air cysts.[19,37]

Pulmonary fibrosis may follow acute lung injury associated with acute respiratory distress syndrome. In addition, use of high inspired concentrations of oxygen may enhance development of fibrosis in the presence of acute lung injury.

Common device-related complications include those due to pulmonary artery flotation catheters, endotracheal intubation, and tracheotomy.[45]

Cardiovascular

Common cardiovascular complications in patients with acute respiratory failure include hypotension, reduced cardiac output, arrhythmias, pericarditis, and acute myocardial infarction. These complications may be related to the underlying disease process, mechanical ventilation, or use of pulmonary artery flotation catheters.

Gastrointestinal

The major gastrointestinal complications associated with acute respiratory failure are hemorrhage, gastric distention, ileus, diarrhea, and pneumoperitoneum. "Stress" ulceration is extremely common in patients with acute respiratory failure. Associated risk factors include trauma, shock due to a variety of causes, sepsis, renal failure, and liver disease.[37]

Infectious

Nosocomial infections are a frequent complication of acute respiratory failure. Principal among these are pneumonia, sepsis, and urinary tract infections. Each typically occurs with the use of mechanical devices, including endotracheal and tracheotomy tubes, indwelling central venous and pulmonary artery catheters, and urinary bladder catheters.

The incidence of nosocomial pneumonia[3,31,50] in the critically ill may be as high as 70 percent for patients in respiratory units, particularly those with acute respiratory distress syndrome. The need for prolonged mechanical ventilation is a harbinger for development of nosocomial pneumonia.[8] Not unexpectedly, nosocomial pneumonia occurring in the medical intensive care unit is associated with a significantly increased length of stay[37] and higher mortality.

Renal

Acute renal failure and abnormalities in electrolyte and water homeostasis are not uncommon in critically ill patients with acute respiratory failure; the former is observed in approximately 10 to 20 percent of patients in intensive care units. Development of acute renal failure in a patient with acute respiratory failure carries a

TABLE 165-5

Complications of Acute Respiratory Failure

Pulmonary
  Pulmonary emboli
  Pulmonary barotrauma (interstitial emphysema, pneumothorax, subcutaneous emphysema, pneumoperitoneum, tension lung cyst, subpleural air cyst)
  Pulmonary fibrosis
Related to Use of Mechanical Devices
  Complications of mechanical ventilation (infection, arterial desaturation, hypotension, barotrauma, others)
  Complications of insertion and maintenance of pulmonary artery catheter (pneumothorax, air embolism, arrhythmias, infection, thrombosis, pulmonary artery rupture)
  Complications of tracheal intubation
    Related to prolonged intubation attempt (hypoxemic brain injury, cardiac arrest, seizures, others)
    Related to right main bronchus intubation (hypoventilation, pneumothorax, atelectasis)
    Self- or inadvertent extubation
    Endotracheal tube dislodgment
    Endotracheal tube cuff leak
    Injury to pharynx, larynx, trachea
  Complications of tracheotomy (pneumothorax, bleeding, tube dislodgment, tracheoinominate fistula, tracheoesophageal fistula, tracheal stenosis)
Gastrointestinal
  Hemorrhage (including "stress" ulceration)
  Ileus
  Diarrhea
Cardiovascular
  Hypotension
  Arrhythmias
  Decreased cardiac output
  Myocardial infarction
  Pulmonary hypertension
Renal
  Acute renal failure
  Fluid retention
Infectious
  Nosocomial pneumonia
  Bacteremia
  Sepsis
  Paranasal sinusitis
Nutritional
  Complications of underlying malnutrition (decreased respiratory muscle strength, immune suppression, others)
  Complications of enteral feeding (pneumothorax, pleural effusion, sinusitis, aspiration, diarrhea)
  Complications of parenteral feeding (pneumothorax, sepsis, hyperglycemia, hyperosmolar coma, hypophosphatemia, liver function test abnormalities)
  Complications of refeeding (hypercapnia)
Other
  Psychiatric (anxiety, depression, confusion, sleep dysfunction, psychosis)
  Hematologic (anemia, thrombocytopenia)

poor prognosis and a high mortality. The causes of acute renal failure are numerous and include prerenal azotemia and acute tubular necrosis due to hypotension or use of nephrotoxic drugs.[37]

Nutritional

Nutritional complications of acute respiratory failure include the effects of malnutrition on respiratory performance and complications related to the administration of enteral or parenteral nutrition. Complications of enteral nutritional support relate to initial insertion of the catheter (e.g., tracheal or pleural space penetration, pneumomediastinum, pneumothorax, and pleural effusion) and its maintenance (e.g., paranasal sinusitis and aspiration).[41] In addition, vomiting, abdominal distention, and diarrhea are common. Complications of parenteral nutrition are mechanical (e.g., pneumothorax during catheter insertion), infectious (e.g., catheter-related sepsis), or metabolic (e.g., metabolic acidosis, hyperglycemia and hyperosmolar coma, and hypophosphatemia). Hypercapnia, induced by enteral as well as parenteral nutrition, can complicate management of patients who have limited ventilatory reserve.[6]

PROGNOSIS

Interpretation of studies addressing the prognosis of patients with acute respiratory failure is subject to a number of constraints, including marked clinical variability in the patients studied, predominance of studies from intensive care units in large university teaching hospitals, and variability in treatment methods employed over the time span of studies performed. In addition, many studies report only hospital mortality, not long-term survival or quality of life. Finally, findings from large-population studies are difficult to extrapolate to prediction of outcome in a single patient. Nonetheless, several generalizations can be made regarding the prognosis of patients hospitalized with acute respiratory failure.[7,15,18,20,29,33,38,45,47,52,53]

Morbidity and Mortality in Acute Hypoxemic Respiratory Failure

As expected, mortality in hypoxemic respiratory failure depends on the underlying cause.[29] A number of studies have addressed outcome in patients with acute respiratory distress syndrome.

The mortality in acute respiratory distress syndrome does not appear to have changed dramatically over the past 30 years, although several recent investigations have suggested that the rate in certain subpopulations (e.g., patients with sepsis) may be declining.[32] Initial figures indicated a 60 percent overall mortality, while more recent data suggest a rate of approximately 40 percent.[32,53]

Patients who develop sepsis after trauma have a lower mortality than do patients with sepsis that complicates medical disorders. Not surprisingly, younger patients (those under the age of 65 years) have better survival rates than do older patients.[32] It is interesting to note that patients with preexisting lung disease, higher F_{IO_2} or PEEP requirements, or a lower Pa_{O_2} may not necessarily have a poorer chance of survival.

Approximately two-thirds of patients who survive an episode of acute respiratory distress syndrome will manifest some im-

pairment of pulmonary function 1 or more years after recovery.[14] However, most will have only mild or moderate abnormalities. Abnormalities that persist beyond 1 year after recovery are unlikely to resolve thereafter. In most, however, pulmonary function test abnormalities are not associated with clinically significant respiratory impairment.

Morbidity and Mortality in Acute Hypercapnic Respiratory Failure

In general, several parameters presage a higher mortality in patients admitted with hypercapnic respiratory failure: (1) the patient's "physiological reserve," as determined by concurrent cardiopulmonary, renal, hepatic, or neurologic disease and the patient's age; (2) the underlying cause of the acute deterioration; (3) the severity of the respiratory failure, as defined by arterial pH and P_{CO_2}; and (4) development of complications after onset of acute respiratory failure—e.g., sepsis, pneumonia, renal failure, or gastrointestinal bleeding.[53] Cachexia and home confinement before hospitalization may also presage a poorer outcome. These harbingers appear to hold true regardless of whether the patient requires mechanical ventilation.

For patients with COPD and acute respiratory failure, overall mortality has declined from approximately 26 percent to 10 percent when studies over the past 10 to 15 years are compared with older analyses.[53] Not unexpectedly, older patients who are significantly more acidemic, hypotensive, or uremic appear to have a higher mortality.[20] The magnitude of the hypoxemia or hypercapnia at the time of presentation may not reliably foretell mortality.

REFERENCES

1. Aubier M: Respiratory muscles: Working or wasting? *Intensive Care Med* 19:S64–S68, 1993.
2. Barr CW, Claussen G, Thomas D, et al: Primary respiratory failure as the presenting symptom in Lambert-Eaton myasthenic syndrome. *Muscle Nerve* 16:712–715, 1993.
3. Chastre J, Fagon JY: Invasive diagnostic testing should be routinely used to manage ventilated patients with suspected pneumonia. *Am J Respir Crit Care Med* 150:570–574, 1994.
4. Colice GL, Bernat JL: Neurologic disorders and respiration. *Clin Chest Med* 10:521–543, 1989.
5. Corrado A, Gorini M, DePaola E: Alternative techniques for managing acute neuromuscular respiratory failure. *Semin Neurol* 15:84–89, 1995.
6. Covelli HD, Black JW, Olsen MS, Beekman JF: Respiratory failure precipitated by high carbohydrate loads. *Ann Intern Med* 95:579–581, 1981.
7. Crawford SW, Petersen FB: Long-term survival from respiratory failure after marrow transplantation for malignancy. *Am Rev Respir Dis* 145:510–514, 1992.
8. Cunnion KM, Weber DJ, Broadhead WE, et al: Risk factors for nosocomial pneumonia: Comparing adult critical-care populations. *Am J Respir Crit Care Med* 153:158–162, 1996.
9. Curtis JR, Hudson LD: Emergent assessment and management of acute respiratory failure in COPD. *Clin Chest Med* 15:481–500, 1994.
10. Derenne J-P, Fleury B, Pariente R: Acute respiratory failure of chronic obstructive pulmonary disease. *Am Rev Respir Dis* 138:1006–1033, 1988.

11. Einarsson O, Rochester CL, Rosenbaum S: Airway management in respiratory emergencies. *Clin Chest Med* 15:13–34, 1994.

12. Epstein SK: An overview of respiratory muscle function. *Clin Chest Med* 15:619–639, 1994.

13. Gammon RB, Shin MS, Groves RH Jr, et al: Clinical risk factors for pulmonary barotrauma: A multivariate analysis. *Am J Respir Crit Care Med* 152:1235–1240, 1995.

14. Ghio AJ, Elliott CG, Crapo RO, et al: Impairment after adult respiratory distress syndrome: An evaluation based on American Thoracic Society Recommendations. *Am Rev Respir Dis* 139: 1158–1162, 1989.

15. Gracey DR, Naessens JM, Krishan I, Marsh HM: Hospital and posthospital survival in patients mechanically ventilated for more than 29 days. *Chest* 101:211–214, 1992.

16. Greene KE, Peters JI: Pathophysiology of acute respiratory failure. *Clin Chest Med* 15:1–12, 1994.

17. Grippi MA: Distribution of ventilation, in Grippi MA (ed), *Pulmonary Pathophysiology*. Philadelphia, JB Lippincott, 1995, pp 41–53.

18. Hawley PH, Ronco JJ, Guillemi SA, et al: Decreasing frequency but worsening mortality of acute respiratory failure secondary to AIDS-related *Pneumocystis carinii* pneumonia. *Chest* 106:1456–1459, 1994.

19. Jantz MA, Pierson DJ: Pneumothorax and barotrauma. *Clin Chest Med* 15:75–91, 1994.

20. Jeffrey AA, Warren PM, Flenley DC: Acute hypercapnic respiratory failure in patients with chronic obstructive lung disease: Risk factors and use of guidelines for management. *Thorax* 47:34–40, 1992.

21. Kelly BJ, Luce JM: The diagnosis and management of neuromuscular diseases causing respiratory failure. *Chest* 99:1485–1494, 1991.

22. Klepper MS, Guntupalli KK, Interiano B, et al: Postoperative respiratory failure secondary to *Pneumocystis carinii* pneumonia. *Chest* 101:1155–1157, 1992.

23. Lanken PN: Pathophysiology of respiratory failure, in Grippi MA (ed), *Pulmonary Pathophysiology*. Philadelphia, JB Lippincott, 1995, pp 267–280.

24. Lanken PN: Respiratory failure: An overview. In Carlson RW, Geheb MA (eds), *Principles and Practice of Medical Intensive Care*. Philadelphia, WB Saunders, 1993, pp 754–763.

25. Lynn DJ, Woda RP, Mendell JR: Respiratory dysfunction in muscular dystrophy and other myopathies. *Clin Chest Med* 15:661–674, 1994.

26. Manfreda J, Maoy, Litvin W: Morbidity and mortality from chronic obstructive pulmonary disease. *Am Rev Respir Dis* 140:519–526, 1989.

27. Marcy TW, Marini JJ: Respiratory distress in the ventilated patient. *Clin Chest Med* 15:55–73, 1994.

28. Marini JJ: Lung mechanics in the adult respiratory distress syndrome: Recent conceptual advances and implications for management. *Clin Chest Med* 11:673–690, 1990.

29. Matthay MA: The adult respiratory distress syndrome: Definition and prognosis. *Clin Chest Med* 11:575–580, 1990.

30. McParland C, Resch EF, Krishnan B, et al: Inspiratory muscle weakness in chronic heart failure: Role of nutrition and electrolyte status and systemic myopathy. *Am J Respir Crit Care Med* 151:1101–1107, 1995.

31. Meduri GU: Diagnosis and differential diagnosis of ventilator-associated pneumonia. *Clin Chest Med* 16:61–93, 1995.

32. Milberg JA, Davis DR, Steinberg KP, Hudson LD: Improved survival of patients with acute respiratory distress syndrome (ARDS): 1983–1993. *JAMA* 273:306–309, 1995.

33. Montaner JSG, Hawley PH, Ronco JJ, et al: Multisystem organ failure predicts mortality of ICU patients with acute respiratory failure secondary to AIDS-related PCP. *Chest* 102:1823–1828, 1992.

34. Pehrsson K, Nachemson A, Olofson J, et al: Respiratory failure in scoliosis and other thoracic deformities: A survey of patients with home oxygen or ventilator therapy in Sweden. *Spine* 17:714–718, 1992.

35. Pepe PE, Marini JJ: Occult positive end-expiratory pressure in mechanically ventilated patients with airflow obstruction. *Am Rev Respir Dis* 126:166–170, 1982.

36. Peters JU, Bell RC, Prihoda TJ, et al: Clinical determinants of abnormalities in pulmonary functions in survivors of the adult respiratory distress syndrome. *Am Rev Respir Dis* 139:1163–1168, 1989.

37. Pingleton SK: Complications of acute respiratory failure. *Am Rev Respir Dis* 137:1463–1493, 1988.

38. Rieves RD, Bass D, Carter RR, et al: Severe COPD and acute respiratory failure: Correlates for survival at the time of tracheal intubation. *Chest* 104:854–860, 1993.

39. Rochester DF: Respiratory muscles and ventilatory failure: 1993 perspective. *Am J Med Sci* 305:394–402, 1993.

40. Rochester DF, Esau SA: Assessment of ventilatory function in patients with neuromuscular disease. *Clin Chest Med* 15:751–763, 1994.

41. Rouby J-J, Laurent P, Gosnach M, et al: Risk factors and clinical relevance of nosocomial maxillary sinusitis in the critically ill. *Am J Respir Crit Care Med* 150:776–783, 1994.

42. Roussos C, Macklem PT: The respiratory muscles. *New Engl J Med* 307:786–797, 1982.

43. Stauffer JL, Fayter NA, Graves B, et al: Survival following mechanical ventilation for acute respiratory failure in adult men. *Chest* 104:1222–1229, 1993.

44. Selecky PA, Wasserman K, Klein M, Ziment I: A graphic approach to assessing interrelationships among minute ventilation, arterial carbon dioxide tension and ratio of physiologic dead space to tidal volume in patients on respirators. *Am Rev Respir Dis* 117:181–184, 1978.

45. Stauffer JL, Olson DE, Petty TL: Complications and consequences of endotracheal ventilation and tracheotomy. *Am J Med* 70:65–76, 1981.

46. Stoller JK, Kacmarek RM: Ventilatory strategies in the management of the adult respiratory distress syndrome. *Clin Chest Med* 11:755–772, 1990.

47. Swinburne AJ, Fedullo AJ, Bixby K, et al: Respiratory failure in the elderly: Analysis of outcome after treatment with mechanical ventilation. *Arch Intern Med* 153:1657–1662, 1993.

48. Tobin MJ: Respiratory monitoring in the intensive care unit. *Am Rev Respir Dis* 138:1625–1642, 1988.

49. Unterborn JN, Hill NS: Options for mechanical ventilation in neuromuscular diseases. *Clin Chest Med* 15:765–781, 1994.

50. Valles J, Artigas A, Rello J, et al: Continuous aspiration of subglottic secretions in preventing ventilator-associated pneumonia. *Ann Intern Med* 122:179–186, 1995.

51. Vallet B, Fourrier F, Hurtevent JF, et al: Myasthenia gravis and steroid-induced myopathy of the respiratory muscles. *Intensive Care Med* 18:424–426, 1992.

52. Vasilyev S, Schaap RN, Mortensen JD: Hospital survival rates of patients with acute respiratory failure in modern respiratory intensive care units: An international, multicenter, prospective survey. *Chest* 107:1083–1088, 1995.

53. Weiss SM, Hudson LD: Outcome from respiratory failure. *Crit Care Clin* 10:197–215, 1994.

CHAPTER 166

ACUTE RESPIRATORY DISTRESS SYNDROME: PATHOGENESIS

Jean E. Rinaldo / John W. Christman

A brief overview of the sequence of events that occur during the evolution of the acute, or adult, respiratory distress syndrome (ARDS) underscores its remarkable biologic and clinical complexity. Initially, ARDS is characterized by lung edema and hypoxemia. Lung histology shows denudation of epithelial lining cells, swelling of endothelial cells and hyaline membranes, and marked neutrophilic inflammation. If bronchoalveolar lavage is performed at this time, the findings include serum proteins, neutrophils, cytokines, and a variety of other soluble markers of acute neutrophilic inflammation. Concurrent physiological abnormalities include pulmonary hypertension and decreased lung compliance.

The second phase of ARDS is a proliferative one, characterized histologically by increases in type II alveolar epithelial cells and mesenchymal cells, angiogenesis, and resolution of neutrophilic inflammation. Hypoxemia persists but gradually resolves, while lung compliance may transiently worsen because of hypercellularity of the healing lung. Finally, gas exchange improves and, ultimately, near-perfect architectural restoration is observed in most survivors. In some cases, however, the lung appears to heal aberrantly, resulting in interstitial fibrosis and microvascular obliteration; these patients may eventually die.

Since noncardiogenic pulmonary edema and hypoxemia represent the initially described clinical hallmarks of ARDS, it is not surprising that for the first 15 years of investigation, most experimental studies employed physiological approaches based on measurements of lung vascular reactivity, permeability, edema formation, and gas exchange. In the late 1970s, a multicenter, prospective, controlled study of extracorporeal membrane oxygenation (ECMO) challenged the investigative emphasis on physiology. This study was conceived in an era of exuberance about the therapeutic potential of new life-support innovations; it rested on the premise that supporting oxygenation would give edema time to resolve.

The ECMO study remains the only published multicenter, controlled trial of ARDS therapy to date funded by the National Institutes of Health. While the study was a "negative" one, showing no effect of ECMO on mortality, it was important as a large, carefully conceived, and well-funded investigation. The study was the first occasion on which lung histology was critically examined in a large group of patients with ARDS. The observations were stunning.[43] ARDS was shown to involve much more than edema formation. Rather, respiratory failure was accompanied by marked architectural changes appearing to involve virtually all structures and, by implication, all cell types. In fatal cases (90 percent of enrollees), the disorder culminated in the most impressive lung fibrosis ever seen. State-of-the-art life support did not prevent this dire progression. Overnight, ARDS began its metamorphosis from a physiologist's to a biologist's disease. The subsequent federal grant-funding mandate shifted to finding the "cause" of ARDS and exploring the basic biology of acute lung injury and its sequential resolution.[45]

Melding with shifting research questions were simultaneous rapid advances in cell biology, immunology, and molecular genetics. With the concurrent development of a new question and new methods, the early 1980s were characterized by the emergence of the cellular biology of ARDS as one of the dominant themes in funded lung research—a trend that has continued. The result of the research sometimes appears to be a bewildering compendium of reductionist observations in arcane experimental systems whose relevance often seems tenuous. In addition, the concept of ARDS is no longer organ specific; rather, it is now viewed as a multisystem disorder, with a broad base in cell and molecular biologic research. As a consequence, ARDS research is indistinguishable from other investigations of basic biologic processes, including regulation of gene expression, receptor-coupled signaling, inflammation, and apoptosis.

The goal of this chapter is to develop the four conceptual themes that appear important in the pathogenesis of ARDS: lung cellular injury, cytokine networks and cascades, pulmonary vascular dysregulation, and the fibroproliferative response.

LUNG CELLULAR INJURY

All of the clinical and physiological manifestations of ARDS are presumed to arise from injury to lung cells. "Injury" is a nebulous term that may refer to structural damage to cells, cell denudation, ischemic cell death, metabolic dysfunction, or altered functional response. Increasingly, the lines between signaled changes in cellular functional response and cytotoxicity have become blurred. Even cell death can be a signaled response. Nonetheless, "injury" remains a common shorthand term for all these effects. In the following section, the central role of inflammation in triggering cell injury and the biochemical mediators of injury are discussed. Apoptosis, or programmed cell death, which can be viewed as the "ultimate" signaled injury, is also considered. Finally, the most clinically important functional sequelae of injury to cells that line lung capillaries (endothelial cells) and airspaces (epithelial cells) are enumerated.

Role of Inflammation in the Production of Lung Cell Injury

A key concept in the pathogenesis of ARDS is that acute inflammation mediates acute lung injury. Tracing the evolution of this hypothesis is instructive. In 1968, a clinical study of patients undergoing hemodialysis revealed that contact of blood with the dialysis membrane activated complement and initiated transient granulocytopenia.[29] Mild hypoxemia occurred concurrently. Ten years passed before this important observation was linked to ARDS—a link that was ultimately to completely alter the face of ARDS research. Because the "missing" neutrophils were found aggregated in the microvessels of the lung, a critical intuitive leap was made: Pathophysiological changes in ARDS might be similar to changes occurring in hemodialysis, only amplified. In support of this theory, it was noted that trauma, intravascular infusion of air, endotoxin, or fibrin, and pancreatic injury were all associated with ARDS. Each caused neutrophil-dependent lung injury in animals, and all activated complement. Enthusiasm for the hypothesis peaked in 1980 with publication of a study showing a strong correlation between intravascular complement activation and onset of ARDS.[23] Notably, this key observation could not be reproduced in other investigations.

Subsequent clinical studies provided more convincing confirmatory observations. In 1984, investigators reported that peripheral blood neutrophils were activated in patients with ARDS.[21] Bronchoalveolar lavage (BAL), a technique that became popular in the early 1980s, led to the seminal observation that an influx of neutrophils occurred early in the course of ARDS. Pulmonary cell biology came to the forefront at this time, fueled, in part, by dissemination of reliable techniques for culturing endothelial cells. Human studies confirmed similar investigations in animal models, suggesting that activated neutrophils could injure the pulmonary vasculature. The constellation of diverse clinical, animal, and cell culture studies prompted the consensus that activated neutrophils have a central role in the pathogenesis of ARDS.[44]

BAL played an additional important role in the study of ARDS because it was the first tool to allow lung-derived cells from patients with ARDS to be studied directly. Since 1985 there have been repeated observations[18] that the percentage of neutrophils is greatly increased in the cellular fraction of BAL fluid of patients with ARDS, as well as in patients with diffuse, acute lung injury that is not severe enough to meet usual physiological criteria for ARDS. Some studies have correlated the presence of neutrophils in BAL fluid with independent indices of lung injury, such as the ratio of Pa_{O_2} to Fi_{O_2} and lavage fluid total protein concentration. In an important study linking neutrophils in BAL fluid to clinical outcome, a significant correlation between sustained neutrophilic alveolar inflammation and mortality was noted.[54] Thus, neutrophilic inflammation is an early and universal feature of the cellular pathobiology of ARDS. If such inflammation is not reversed, it appears to be statistically associated with and predictive of a fatal outcome.

The neutrophil hypothesis was modified somewhat when it was reported that ARDS also occurs in profoundly neutropenic patients,[39] indicating that there must be neutrophil-independent mediators of injury. Possible culprits abound. The lung contains resident tissue phagocytes—alveolar and interstitial macrophages—which, like neutrophils, release proteolytic enzymes and reactive oxygen species (discussed below). Chemotherapy, which depletes neutrophils, is usually not associated with a decreased number of tissue macrophages, since the half-life of these cells in vivo is much longer; their numbers are not markedly reduced by the relatively brief duration of cytotoxic chemotherapy. Furthermore, there are other mediators of lung vascular permeability in addition to those derived from leukocyte activation. Bacterial exotoxins,[17] vascular permeability factor (also known as vascular endothelial growth factor),[16] and arachidonate-lipoxygenase metabolites are examples of endogenous mediators that could increase vascular permeability in ARDS.

Mediators of Inflammatory Injury

Leukocyte-mediated cytotoxicity to lung cells results from an overwhelming, misdirected chemical assault, utilizing an arsenal normally directed against bacterial pathogens. The major putative mediators of injury are proteases and reactive oxygen species.

PROTEASES

Preformed proteases and other enzymes are stored in the lysosomes of neutrophils, ready for instant release during the degranulation response that is a component of neutrophil activation. Stimulated neutrophils release a variety of proteases, including neutrophil elastase, which can degrade elastin and other structural molecules and cause disruption of normal lung architecture. Several studies have detected elastase and other proteases in abnormal amounts in the BAL fluid of patients with ARDS. The neutrophil elastase from BAL fluid in such patients is strongly correlated with Pa_{O_2}/FI_{O_2}, suggesting that this hallmark physiological abnormality is causally related to neutrophil elastase.[27] Furthermore, plasma elastase levels are markedly increased in patients whose condition progresses to ARDS compared with those whose condition does not progress.[18]

REACTIVE OXYGEN SPECIES

Reactive oxygen species (ROS) is a generic term that usually denotes three highly reactive products formed by reduction of molecular oxygen: superoxide anion (O_2^-), hydrogen peroxide (H_2O_2), and the hydroxyl radical (OH^-) (see Chapter 172). Formation is catalyzed by NADPH oxidase, a membrane-bound enzyme that is activated by a variety of signals, such as bacterial peptides, complement fragments, and immune complexes. NADPH oxidase is found only in cells that are differentiated for pathogen killing—e.g., neutrophils and macrophages. NADPH oxidase is cell membrane bound and causes O_2^- to be released extracellularly. O_2^- is a highly reactive but unstable free radical that is rapidly dismutated (chemically reduced) to H_2O_2, a substance that is more stable in aqueous solution. If reduced iron (Fe^{2+}) is present, a Fenton reaction ensues in which Fe^{2+} reduces H_2O_2 to the most reactive cytotoxic species, OH^-, leaving iron in the Fe^{3+} form. If there is ongoing production of O_2^-, O_2^- reduces Fe^{3+} back to Fe^{2+}, making it available to generate more OH^- from H_2O_2. This electron shuttle system is called the iron-catalyzed Haber-Weiss reaction; as long as iron is present, the reaction allows NADPH oxidase to generate OH^-. The ability of iron chelators to limit tissue injury by O_2^- suggests that this mechanism causes some free radical–mediated injury. Recently, it has been recognized that superoxide can generate other powerful free radicals by interacting with nitric oxide to form peroxynitrite ($ONOO^-$), which is cleaved to form toxic by-products that are as potent oxidizing moieties as is OH^-.[4]

OH^- and products of $ONOO^-$ appear to be the major species causing tissue injury. These potent oxidizing free radicals disrupt membranes by the process of lipid peroxidation. In addition, they oxidize sulfhydryl groups, thereby inactivating any enzymes that are dependent on disulfide bonds, and depolymerize polysaccharide, which can cause interruption of certain cell functions, and cause hydroxylation of nucleotide bases, with nicking of DNA, formation of adducts, and disruption of gene transcription. Neutrophils (and macrophages) are major progenitors of these toxic free radicals, since they all arise from activation of NADPH oxidase during leukocyte activation. It should be added, however, that although NADPH produces the highest molar quantities of O_2^-, it is not the only source. Xanthine oxidase, released from ischemic liver or other tissues, is a potential source of extracellular as well as intracellular O_2^-, which supports the Haber-Weiss reaction generation of OH^- in lung endothelial cells. Xanthine oxidase, which has been implicated in ischemia-

reperfusion tissue injury,[35] can thus produce the entire cascade of reactive oxygen species.

ANTIPROTEASE AND ANTIOXIDANT DEFENSES

The normal lung has protective mechanisms to counter both the elastolytic assault and reactive oxygen species (ROS). α_1-Antiprotease (α-1AP) constitutes a major source of protection against elastase. In ARDS, an overproduction of elastase due to neutrophil influx,[36] inactivation of α-1AP by oxidation,[16] and a resultant imbalance between elastolytic activity and antiprotease activity in airspaces have been proposed. However, the applicability of this concept to the pathogenesis of ARDS has been challenged by observations suggesting that the antiprotease balance in ARDS appears shifted toward active antiprotease.[61] Normal lung cells contain ample antioxidant defense activity in the forms of superoxide dismutase and catalase, which detoxify O_2^- and H_2O_2, respectively.[56] Intracellular glutathione is also a major scavenger of H_2O_2. Glutathione has been reported to be depleted in BAL fluid from patients with ARDS.[40] There is no specific scavenger of hydroxyl radical or $ONOO^-$, but their formation is prevented if O_2^- is effectively scavenged.

Apoptosis

The previous discussion rests on the assumption that inflammatory cell injury results from external chemical attack. However, given the usual effectiveness of biologic mechanisms of homeostasis, the premise that the pericellular milieu becomes lethally toxic is unconvincing. The emerging concept of *apoptosis* modifies the notion of cytotoxicity. Apoptosis, also known as programmed cell death, implies that cells self-destruct in response to a subtle signal, rather than dying from a toxic assault. The signaled "suicide" is effected by regulated changes in gene expression. In a teleologic sense, an advantage of genetically programmed cell suicide is that it blocks replication of cells that may have sustained genotypic injury. Instead, these cells are sacrificed and replaced by replicating healthy cells. Apoptosis manifests morphologic hallmarks, including plasma membrane blebbing, cell volume loss, nuclear condensation, and degradation of DNA at nucleosomal intervals to form a "ladder" electrophoretic pattern. Whether a cell dies by apoptosis is determined by the balance of regulatory molecules that either induce or suppress apoptosis. Some of these molecules, such as P53 (a proapoptotic factor) and BCL-2 (an antiapoptotic factor), have been identified in immune cells.

Extension of the apoptosis concept from immunology and embryology to ARDS is quite recent. In 1991, the cytokine tumor necrosis factor (TNF) was reported to induce apoptosis in normal endothelial cells.[46] More recently, alveolar epithelial cells cultured in vitro were found to release a factor that protects pulmonary artery endothelial cells from apoptosis in response to TNF.[60] This observation suggests that the integrity of the two alveolar cell types injured in ARDS—endothelial and epithelial—are interdependent. No direct study of apoptosis in ARDS has been performed; indeed, clinical studies lag behind basic discoveries. However, for the purposes of facilitating an understanding of the pathophysiology of ARDS, several key concepts have been advanced: (1) cell destruction is not traumatic but is signaled; (2) intercellular communication is an integral component of cell viability, as well as function; and (3) cytokines, the hormones of inflammation (see below), may initiate the programmed death of lung endothelial and endothelial cells, leading to ARDS.

Functional Consequences of Lung Endothelial and Epithelial Injury

Endothelial cells line the vascular lumen. Injury to endothelial cells affects their interactions with circulating leukocytes and may also make capillaries "leaky," promoting pulmonary edema. Epithelial cells line the airspaces along the alveolar-capillary barrier. Injury to these cells permits fluid to enter the airspaces; alveolar flooding may cause the airspaces to collapse because of diminished surface tension. All these findings are physiological hallmarks of ARDS and constitute examples of obvious links between cellular injury and the clinical syndrome.

ENDOTHELIAL INJURY

Whether "injury" to pulmonary vascular lining cells is signaled or trauma induced, it initiates many functional consequences that contribute to ARDS. Two important manifestations are discussed below: altered interactions with circulating inflammatory cells and increased lung microvascular permeability.

Increased Adhesion   Increased vascular "stickiness" for formed elements in the blood causes polymorphonuclear leukocytes to adhere or aggregate in microvessels during hemodialysis, in sepsis, and in ARDS. The stickiness of injured pulmonary microvascular lining cells reflects the surface expression of cellular adhesion molecules (CAM) on surfaces of endothelial cells, leukocytes, and platelets. The existence of these inducible surface glycoproteins has been known for only about 10 years, although many earlier bioassays demonstrated that endothelial cells became stickier in response to endotoxin, oxidants, and cytokines. Identification of the adhesion glycoproteins, like that of many other protein markers of inflammation, was made possible by progress in molecular biology that led to the cloning of related gene families. Between 1983 and 1994, nine specific endothelial and nine leukocyte adhesion molecules were cloned. At present, three families of molecules appear to be involved: the selectins, the integrins, and the immunoglobulin superfamily.

Integrins are located on leukocytes, immunoglobulin superfamily members on endothelial cells, and selectins on both. The structural and functional characteristics of these molecules have been summarized.[3] Normally, there is rapid linear transit of leukocytes through pulmonary capillaries. Before migrating out of vessels, leukocytes must decelerate. During the slowdown phase, leukocytes roll along the vascular wall. This rolling phase is mediated by the *selectins,* which move to the cell surface of endothelial cells after stimulation by cytokines, ROS, or various other proinflammatory signals. Endothelial selectins bind specific carbohydrates on leukocyte cell membranes, and vice versa. Because the tethering is loose, deceleration (rolling) of the leukocytes occurs, rather than tight adherence. After the rolling, the second and third families of CAM are expressed, causing the leukocytes to flatten and to stick firmly at a specific anatomic location, the postcapillary venules; in addition, the leukocytes become activated. The leukocyte-associated *integrins* (CD 11/-a/CD18) and the endothelium-associated *immunoglobulin superfamily* (ICAM-1 and -2, VCAM-1) mediate adhesion and activation steps by mutual binding: Leukocyte integrins bind endothelial ICAMs as ligands on the leukocytes and vice versa. Finally, the cells migrate between endothelial cell junctions and through the basement membrane, following a concentration gradient of chemotactic factors leading toward the alveolar lumen.

Increased Permeability   The existence of altered lung microvascular permeability in ARDS has been inferred from the temporal correlation of lung edema with normal pulmonary arterial occlusion pressure, one of the fundamental physiological criteria commonly examined in clinical studies of ARDS.[5] Measurement of lung microvascular permeability in patients with ARDS has proved difficult, although a few studies using radiolabeled tracers appear to support the existence of altered capillary permeability.[24] The inference is further supported by extensive investigations in animal models of ARDS, particularly the sheep model, in which a cannulated caudal mediastinal lymph duct is considered to produce only lung lymph. If lung lymph is further assumed to represent unaltered endothelial filtrate in the steady state, lung lymph proteins can be measured as an indicator of capillary sieving properties. Such studies suggest alterations in lung microvascular permeability in lung edema induced by intravenous endotoxin and many other ARDS-like experimental insults.[10]

Another experimental approach has been based on studies of the permeability characteristics of cultured endothelial cell monolayers, in which both neutrophil proteases[42] and oxidants[51] cause increased permeability. In vitro studies have led to a *paradigm shift* concerning the nature of altered endothelial permeability. Traditionally, capillary leak was thought to reflect traumatic rents in the capillary basement membrane or areas of denuded endothelium. However, monolayer studies indicate that increased permeability represents another signaled functional property of endothelial cells. Endothelial cells feature an elaborate internal contractile cytoskeleton. Cytokines and ROS signal contraction, which results in a change in endothelial cell shape[51]—which, in turn, alters intercellular junctional geometry. The alteration in geometry decreases sieving by the monolayer of serum proteins that are close to the same molecular radius as the pore. The permeability changes appear to involve receptor-coupled signal transduction. Thus, like apoptotic death, lung microvascular "leakiness" is probably more of a signal response phenomenon than a traumatic event.

EPITHELIAL INJURY

Alveolar type I cells line the alveolar airspaces and make up the major gas exchange surface of the lung; they also constitute a permeability barrier that restricts the flow of water and solutes into airspaces. Alveolar type II cells are progenitors of type I cells and, in addition, perform an important metabolic function in regulating surfactant homeostasis in airspaces. Evidence exists that both cell types are injured in ARDS. Injury to type I cells is suggested primarily by alterations in barrier function (permeability) and in gas exchange. Injury to type II cells is reflected in deranged surfactant function.

Increased Epithelial Permeability   Epithelial injury has been harder to study than endothelial injury because experimental model systems have been much more difficult to establish than for the endothelium. No convenient animal model yields epithelial filtrate, and alveolar epithelial cells rapidly dedifferentiate in tissue culture. Nonetheless, it seems indisputable that two important manifestations of epithelial injury are alveolar flooding and altered surfactant function. Alveolar flooding is inferred from alveolar filling defects and florid pulmonary edema, often found in ARDS, while increased protein in BAL fluid indicates epithelial permeability changes, even in more subtle clinical settings. Although epithelial tight junctions are markedly different from endothelial junctions (under normal conditions, yielding a much more impermanent monolayer), oxidants appear to alter epithelial permeability by mechanisms that are similar to those found for endothelial monolayers.

Surfactant Abnormalities   Surfactant is the complex phospholipid- and protein-containing material that permits unstable, air-filled alveoli to avoid collapse by the lowering of surface tension (see Chapter 7). Surfactant is synthesized and released by alveolar type II cells. Surfactant function in ARDS is abnormal; the surface tension–lowering capability of BAL fluid from patients with ARDS is reduced.[22] Interactions with plasma proteins, oxidation, and inflammatory proteases appear to play a role in altering the biophysical properties of surfactant in ARDS. The dysfunctional surfactant leads to collapse of lung units, pulmonary edema, increased work of breathing, and hypoxemia. Administration of exogenous surfactant markedly diminishes these effects in experimental models. Only recently has it been appreciated that natural surfactant also serves as an important scavenger of reactive oxygen and nitrogen species.[14] This suggests that a significant consequence of alveolar epithelial injury may be the loss of antioxidant defenses associated with surfactant depletion. Conversely, the salutary effects of surfactant installation in patients—even infants—with respiratory distress syndrome may well result, at least in part, from protection against ROS-mediated injury.

CYTOKINE NETWORKS AND CASCADES

The cytokine-mediated "signals" that regulate the functional activities of lung parenchymal cells have been alluded to previously. The roles of cytokines in the orchestration of inflammation in ARDS and sepsis deserve further elaboration. Studies of sepsis syndrome are highly relevant to ARDS because sepsis is the major condition predisposing to ARDS, and acute lung injury is common in sepsis—even though the injury may not be severe enough to meet strict ARDS-defining criteria.

Definition and Action of Cytokines

Cytokines are defined as peptides that permit "signaling cells" to influence the functional activities of target cells. The signaling cells communicate their "request" for a functional response by releasing a soluble cytokine. Since cytokines are usually not stored as preformed molecules, their elaboration requires regulation of release of the cytokine at the level of gene transcription. After release, the cytokine may act locally or at a distant site reached through the circulation. The cytokine binds to a signal-transducing receptor, which may be located on the cell that produced the cytokine (i.e., an autocrine function), on nearby cells (i.e., a paracrine function), or on distant cells (i.e., an endocrine function). Receptor binding of the cytokine is linked to the desired functional response by an array of second-messenger systems. The functional response elicited commonly includes phosphorylation or dephosphorylation of important enzymes, expression of new gene products, or release of mediators.

Cytokines are produced by a variety of immune and nonimmune cells in response to different stimuli, most commonly injury or receptor-mediated activation. Virtually all types of lung cells—including endothelial cells, mesenchymal cells, alveolar macrophages and neutrophils, and epithelial cells—can be stimulated to produce cytokines. Cytokine release tends to occur in a networklike sequence, so that cytokine interactions are complicated and not easily predicted. Cytokines can increase or decrease the production of other cytokines, modulate the expression of their own or other cytokine receptors on target cells, cause paradoxical effects on multiple target cells, and act synergistically with, antagonize, or redundantly duplicate the effects of other cytokines. It is generally assumed that activation of the network at low levels and at sequestered locations brings about the cellular functional changes necessary to perform homeostatic functions—e.g., host defense and wound healing. However, excessive or unregulated systemic release of cytokines is thought to result in both the sepsis syndrome and pulmonary inflammation leading to ARDS. ARDS or its milder variant, *acute lung injury,* is viewed as a pulmonary manifestation of ubiquitous, panendothelial injury brought about by excessive activation of the cytokine network during sepsis.

Cytokine Cascades

The concept of a cytokine "cascade" suggests a defined temporal sequence of cytokine release. Current data implicate four cytokines in ARDS, two of which are produced early in the cascade—tumor necrosis factor–alpha (TNF-α) and interleukin-1β (IL-1β)—and two late in the cascade: interleukin-6 (IL-6) and interleukin-8 (IL-8). TNF-α and IL-1β are "proximal" cytokines; they appear first and seem to initiate a cytokine cascade by stimulating lung cells to produce "distal" or "terminal" cytokines. Distal cytokines, including IL-6 and IL-8, appear to be active in regulating lung inflammation and repair. Key components of the cytokine cascades implicated in ARDS are listed in Table 166-1.

ROLE OF THE PROXIMAL CYTOKINES, TNF-α AND IL-1β, IN ARDS

TNF-α and IL-1β are produced by mononuclear phagocytes in response to gram-negative endotoxin and are found in the systemic circulation early during the course of human sepsis. Infusion of either TNF-α or IL-1β in humans results in a sepsis-like state with pathophysiological features that are indistinguishable from those after infusion of gram-negative endotoxin.

Considerable data link elevated plasma levels of the proximal cytokines with development of clinical ARDS. Plasma TNF-α levels in patients with ARDS and "high-risk" patients who never

TABLE 166-1

Cytokine Cascade in ARDS Associated with Sepsis Syndrome: Key Components

Classification	Examples	Role in Pathogenesis	Comments
Proximal cytokines	TNF-α, IL-1β	Stimulate cytokine production	Infusion results in sepsis-like psysiology;- present in BAL of ARDS patients; not specific for ARDS
Distal cytokines	IL-8	Chemotactic for neutrophil	Not specific for ARDS; levels in BAL correlate with number of neutrophils
Anti-inflammatory cytokines	IL-6, IL-10	Block cytokine production	IL-6 stimulates hepatic production of acute-phase protein; plasma levels correlate with survival in sepsis; no data in ARDS
Soluble cytokine receptors	sTNFR	Block binding of cytokines to receptor	Marked plasma elevation in sepsis; present in BAL of patients with ARDS
Cytokine antagonists	IL-1ra	Block signal transduction of IL-1	Marked plasma elevation in sepsis; no data in ARDS

develop study criteria for ARDS have been investigated. Plasma TNF levels are markedly elevated in the plasma of 75 percent of patients with ARDS, but levels are also increased in half of the at-risk patients, indicating that circulating levels of TNF-α are not specific markers of ARDS.[41] Furthermore, survivors of ARDS seem to have low initial titers, which decline rapidly with time, while plasma levels are higher and remain elevated in non-survivors.[37]

More data linking the proximal cytokines with ARDS have become available from studies employing bronchoalveolar lavage. TNF-α in cell-free BAL fluid is increased in patients with ARDS, as well as in at-risk patients, compared with normal subjects.[26] These findings have been confirmed in a report[57] that demonstrated elevated levels of both TNF-α and IL-1β in BAL fluid in ARDS, which continued to increase further during the evolution of the disorder. These studies suggest that plasma and BAL levels of TNF-α and IL-1β are not specific markers of ARDS, but that persistently elevated cytokine levels in plasma and BAL fluid are a bad prognostic indicator.

Where are the cytokines found in plasma and BAL fluid in ARDS synthesized? Messenger RNA (mRNA) is present only in cells actively transcribing message RNA; therefore, hybridization techniques that identify mRNA in cells provide evidence that those cells are engaged in active synthesis of message for the protein of interest. Using this approach, investigators[58] have detected TNF-α mRNA by in situ hybridization in BAL cells from patients with ARDS, but rarely in BAL cells from normal

volunteers. This suggests that intra-alveolar inflammatory cells (macrophages and neutrophils) may be a source of TNF-α in BAL fluid from patients with ARDS. However, evidence for a causal link between alveolar macrophage-derived cytokines and the pathogenesis of ARDS is still lacking.

ROLE OF THE DISTAL CYTOKINES, IL-8 AND IL-6, IN ARDS

The mechanism by which neutrophils infiltrate the lung is complex and entails the interaction of adhesion molecules on the surface of neutrophils and pulmonary endothelial cells, as discussed previously, as well as anatomic factors that are specifically related to the lung. These factors include (1) a highly branched microvascular network; (2) dispersion forces related to blood flow in pulmonary capillaries; (3) surface deformability of activated neutrophils; and (4) the establishment of a migratory response to gradients of chemotactic agents, such as IL-8, which attract neutrophils toward airspaces. The role of neutrophil chemotactic factors in ARDS is not a new concept, since complement fragments (C5a), arachidonic acid metabolites (LTB$_4$ and PAF), immunoglobulin fragments, and antigen-antibody complexes have been studied for decades. In the past decade, however, molecular cloning has revealed entire new families of previously unknown bioactive peptides, including a group of recently described chemotactic cytokines known as *chemokines.*

IL-8 is a chemokine produced primarily by monocytic phagocytes, as well as a wide variety of other cells, including lymphocytes, fibroblasts, epithelial cells, and endothelial cells, when these cells are stimulated with endotoxin, TNF-α, or IL-1β. IL-8 is a member of a large supergene family of cytokines that functions as a major neutrophil activator and chemotactic protein for neutrophils in humans. All chemokines have a molecular weight between 6 and 10 kD and have four cysteine residues, which form two disulfide bridges important for the molecule's tertiary structure and function. IL-8 is classified as a "CXC" chemokine because the first two cysteine residues (C) are separated by a single amino acid (X). In "CC" chemokines, which include monocyte chemotactic factor–1 (MCP-1), the first two cysteine residues are adjacent. In general, CXC chemokines affect primarily neutrophils, while CC chemokines affect predominantly mononuclear cells.

Just as for the proximal cytokines, evidence for IL-8 involvement in the pathogenesis of ARDS is strong but circumstantial. A number of clinical studies have shown that IL-8 in BAL fluid is statistically correlated with the number of neutrophils in the lavageable airspace. Protein chemotactic activity is increased in BAL fluid of patients with ARDS. This observation preceded techniques in molecular biology that allow the precise measurement of a single protein in a disease process. Molecular cloning of IL-8 in 1987 permitted its measurement in biologic fluids utilizing antibodies made against recombinant IL-8. Subsequently, IL-8 levels were measured in BAL fluid of 12 patients with ARDS, six with severe pneumonia uncomplicated by ARDS, and seven healthy subjects.[13] IL-8 levels in the fluid were elevated in both ARDS and pneumonia, but the level was higher in patients with ARDS. The increased IL-8 in BAL fluid from patients with ARDS correlates with the percentage of neutrophils in the fluid, and the highest measured levels appear to be associated with the highest mortality.[38] These data suggest that elaboration of IL-8 in airspaces is associated with ARDS and may well be involved in pathogenesis.

The other distal cytokine, IL-6, signals very different functional responses in target cells, distinct from those elicited by IL-8. IL-6 is a pyrogen, a lymphocyte activator, a mitogen for fibroblasts, and, like TNF-α and IL-1β, an activator of the hepatic acute phase reaction. Although plasma levels of IL-6 correlate with the severity of sepsis and development of end organ failure, infusion of recombinant IL-6 does not result in the characteristic hemodynamic manifestations of sepsis or lung inflammation. IL-6 can down-regulate the production of TNF-α and IL-1β by stimulated alveolar macrophage, an effect that may be important in the recovery phase of ARDS. IL-6 also regulates fibroblast proliferation and collagen production. Thus, likely roles of IL-6 in ARDS include the "turning off" of initial inflammatory signals, regulation of protein metabolism, and modulation of the evolution of lung repair and fibrosis.

CYTOKINE NETWORKS IN THE DOWN-REGULATION OF INFLAMMATION

It was noted earlier that persistent neutrophilia in BAL fluid portends a fatal outcome. This implies that a critical component of host survival following activation of cytokine cascades is the ability to terminate the cascades. In addition to the mechanism of repression of synthesis of proinflammatory cytokines, several other novel mechanisms of down-regulation have been described to date; many more no doubt await discovery. Important mechanisms by which activity of proinflammatory cytokines is balanced include two types of circulating competitive inhibitors: soluble receptors, of which the soluble TNF receptor (sTNFR) is a prototype, and receptor antagonists, of which the IL-1 receptor antagonist (IL-1ra) is a prototype. Synthesis of cytokines whose functional effects are primarily anti-inflammatory constitutes another kind of control mechanism.
Soluble Cytokine Receptors   The circulating competitive inhibitors described above are released during sepsis and may have important counterregulatory roles in the pathogenesis of ARDS. Types I and II sTNFR have been described. At the nucleotide level, these receptors are highly homologous to the extracellular binding portions of the TNF receptor, suggesting that the same molecule that transduces TNF "signals" when membrane associated can be shed into the circulation, where it competes with membrane-associated receptors and inactivates circulating TNF.

Experimental and clinical data regarding sTNFR are largely limited to patients with sepsis syndrome in general, rather than with ARDS specifically. Since there appears to be substantial variability in sTNFR levels in normal persons, it has been proposed that lower levels may bestow susceptibility to sepsis syndrome.[2] Both soluble TNF-α type I and soluble TNF-α type II receptors are markedly elevated in plasma obtained from critically ill patients[59] or after endotoxin infusion in animals or human volunteers.[50] Sparse data exist regarding the role of sTNFR in ARDS. Soluble types I and II TNF receptors are increased in BAL fluid from patients with ARDS; these receptors may modulate the biologic activity on TNF-α in airspaces.
Endogenous Cytokine Receptor Antagonists   IL-1β has a different natural counterregulatory molecule—a receptor antagonist (IL-1ra). This molecule binds to the receptor, but it does not cause activation of the signal-transducing mechanism; rather, it merely blocks the signal so that circulating IL-1 cannot bind to it. IL-1ra has been isolated from the urine of febrile patients and its bioactivity characterized. It is a relatively weak, but specific, competitor, as it is for binding of the authentic cytokine.[49] The IL-1ra is increased in plasma of both volunteers given endotoxin and critically ill septic patients;[20] in sepsis, levels appear to be higher in survivors than nonsurvivors. To date, there have been no measurements specifically in patients with ARDS.
Anti-inflammatory Cytokines   A third down-regulatory mechanism for cytokines is the transcriptional regulation of other cytokines, whose effects are predominantly anti-inflammatory. A group of "counterinflammatory" cytokines includes interleukin-10 (IL-10), interleukin-4 (IL-4), and, to some extent, IL-6 and transforming growth factor–β (TGF-β); each down-regulates the inflammatory response.[8] IL-10, for example, is released into the circulation during human sepsis and is a potent agent capable of blocking the production of TNF-α, IL-1β, and IL-8 by stimulated mononuclear phagocytes.[33] Although these cytokines have not yet been measured in patients with ARDS, they are potentially part of an intricate system of checks and balances in the inflammatory cascade that can be disturbed or compromised in disease states, including ARDS.

Regulation of Cytokine Transcription by Nuclear Factor Kappa B

One therapeutic strategy to interrupt deleterious cytokine cascades is termination of a single signal, which is critical for induction of transcription of many components of the cascade. Cytokines are not presynthesized or stored for release. For cytokine release, the promoter that turns on transcription of the encoding genes must be activated. Transcriptional activation is usually effected by DNA-binding proteins called transcription factors, which bind in a sequence-specific manner to specific regions of DNA in the cytokine gene's promoter. One very important transcription factor, nuclear factor–kappa-B (NF-κB), appears to have a central role in the cytokine cascade. Binding sequences for NF-κB are found in the promoters of many cytokines thought to be important in the production of acute neutrophilic inflammation, including TNF-α, IL-1β, IL-6, and IL-8.[52]

NF-κB is a heterodimeric protein complex containing two members of the Rel family of transcription factors, termed p50

(NF-κB1) and p65 (RelA). In quiescent cells, the dimer is sequestered in the cytoplasm, complexed to an inhibitor. When the cell receives a signal that requires cytokine synthesis, the inhibitor is phosphorylated and degraded, leaving the dimer free to enter the nucleus to bind specific sites in the cytokine promoters and to initiate transcription of the cytokines. Many levels for autoregulation exist in the cascade of intracellular events that result in activation and translocation of NF-κB. The NF-κB1 transcriptional regulatory system is an important one, since it regulates at a proximal step the production of many of the cytokines implicated in the pathogenesis of sepsis and ARDS. Thus, NF-κB1 is a prime target for future development of prophylactic and therapeutic strategies. The putative sequence of events in NF-κB activation is shown in Fig. 166-1.

A possible link exists between injury by ROS and activation of NF-κB. Stimulation of cells in vitro with H_2O_2 results in activation of NF-κB,[48] while pretreatment of cells with *N*-acetylcysteine, a glutathione precursor, blocks activation of NF-κB by endotoxin.[7] Hence, a mechanism exists by which oxidative stress from inflammation could initiate a self-amplifying systemic inflammatory response. In this scenario, ROS causes the cytoplasmic inhibitor to become dissociated and to be degraded, leading to NF-κB translocation to the nuclei of target cells. This, in turn, induces transcription and release of cytokines, which signal leukocyte activation and generate ROS. If oxidative stress initiates inflammation by activation of NF-κB, ROS scavengers may be capable of blocking activation of cytokine cascades at a proximal step in transcriptional regulation at the same time they directly inhibit ROS-mediated tissue injury.

PULMONARY VASCULAR DYSREGULATION

In the preceding discussion, the correlation between inflammatory mediators and parameters of oxygenation, including Pa_{O_2}/Fi_{O_2}, have been described. Efficient oxygenation is dependent, in large part, on ventilation-perfusion matching. Therefore, the physiological manifestations of ARDS induced by vasomotor dysregulation are important to consider, bearing in mind that the inflammatory cascades discussed in detail in the preceding sections are ultimately responsible for the physiological effects.

Pulmonary Hypertension

An important facet of the pathophysiology of ARDS is the apparent modification of pulmonary vasoconstriction that results in both an overall increase in pulmonary vascular resistance and ventilation-perfusion mismatching. In early clinical investigations of severe ARDS, mild or moderate pulmonary hypertension was often noted. Subsequent investigations of patients who had pulmonary artery catheters inserted confirmed a moderate increase in pulmonary vascular resistance in patients with ARDS. Early experimental observations showed that intravenous infusions of endotoxin caused the almost immediate development of pulmonary hypertension, mediated by thromboxane A_2, a cyclooxygenase product of arachidonic acid.[11] Endothelin, a recently described endothelial cell–derived peptide cytokine that is a potent stimulator of vascular smooth-muscle contraction,[28]

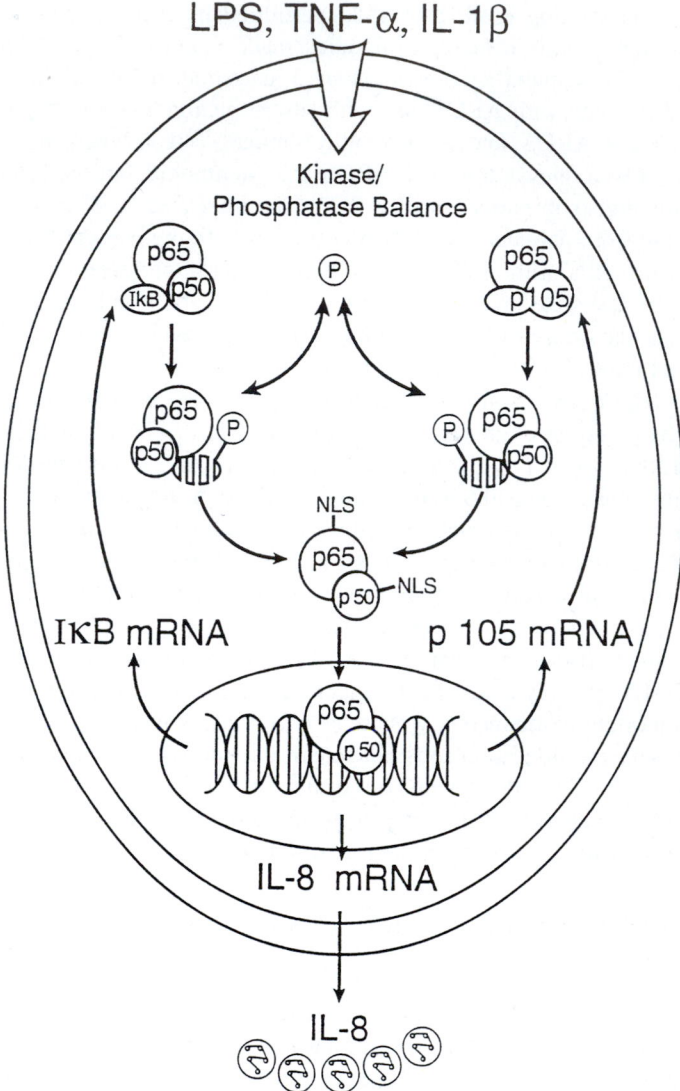

FIGURE 166-1 Activation of nuclear factor κB (NF-κB). Endotoxin (LPS), TNF-α, or IL-1β interacts with cell membrane receptors and initiates signal transduction, which involves the generation of intracellular reactive oxygen species (ROS). ROS either increase phosphokinase activity or decrease phosphatase activity. The NF-κB proteins, p65 and p50, exist as stable cytoplasmic heterodimers attached to an inhibitory protein (I-κB). In activated cells, increased cytoplasmic kinase activity results in phosphorylation of I-κB, which undergoes proteolysis while still attached to the p65 and p50 heterodimers. Degradation of I-κB results in expression of nuclear localization signals (NLS) on p50 and p65 that result in translocation to the nucleus. NF-κB binds to enhancer DNA motifs in the promoter region of cytokine genes, including TNF-α, IL-1β, IL-6, and IL-8. In the illustration, binding to the promoter region of the IL-8 genes results in transcription of IL-8 mRNA. IL-8 mRNA is translated to a biologically active IL-8 protein, which plays a role in the chemotactic recruitment of neutrophils. Since the IκBα gene contains an NF-κB binding sequence, activation of NF-κB is associated with new transcription of κB. Newly synthesized κB can bind to p50 and p65 to stabilize cytoplasmic NF-κB. In addition, the p50 gene, which codes for the precursor protein for p50, contains an NF-κB binding sequence. Activation of NF-κB results in new transcription in the cytoplasm of p105, which also has κB-like inhibitory properties.

may also be involved. Pulmonary hypertension may contribute to right-sided heart failure or, through the phenomenon of ventricular interdependence, to an element of left-sided heart failure.

Ventilation-Perfusion Mismatching

Another important sequela of vasomotor dysregulation in ARDS is ventilation-perfusion mismatching, the major contributing factor to hypoxemia in ARDS. Hypoxic vasoconstriction in the normal lung minimizes arterial hypoxemia when lung units become fluid filled or poorly ventilated (Chapter 12). Regional hypoxia in underventilated alveoli is sensed, and through unknown mechanisms, blood flow is diverted to other areas of the lung. In ARDS, this mechanism appears compromised.

In 1983, Brigham and coworkers showed in a model of acute lung injury that hypoxemia is not correlated with lung water, as had been assumed previously; hypoxemia is related to an inability to restrict blood flow to injured areas of the lung.[11] Blood flow continues to underventilated areas because failure of hypoxic pulmonary vasoconstriction creates shuntlike physiology. Poorly oxygenated blood from unventilated lung regions mixes with normally oxygenated blood in the left heart, lowering mean arterial saturation. Presumably, in ARDS, vasodilating mediators such as nitric oxide (NO), produced by injured endothelium, lead to continued perfusion of poorly ventilated lung regions.

Interest in ventilation-perfusion mismatching in ARDS has been revived because of the observed salutary effects of inhaled NO in patients with ARDS.[47] NO is a potent endogenous vasodilator that is produced by endothelial cells from L-arginine. Therapeutic NO delivered by inhalation is an ideal treatment for ventilation-perfusion mismatching[62] because it is inhaled and is chemically unstable. With inhalation, NO is delivered only to ventilated alveoli, where it dilates contiguous blood vessels, increasing blood flow to ventilated areas and reestablishing a match between perfusion and ventilation. Since it is unstable, NO cannot diffuse in its active form to any other vascular beds. This is advantageous, since such diffusion might cause increased, rather than decreased, venous admixture and consequent hypoxemia, as occurs with other pulmonary vasodilators (e.g., nitroprusside). Unfortunately, NO does not provide benefit to all patients with ARDS. Indeed, much of the vasoconstriction of ARDS is "fixed" as a result of thrombosis, leukocyte aggregation, and the obscure, marked microvascular obliteration that may be seen during the fibroproliferative phase, as described below.

REPAIR: THE FIBROPROLIFERATIVE RESPONSE

Patients who succumb to ARDS are often found at autopsy to have densely fibrotic lungs with marked vascular obliteration. Before death, pathologic processes result in increasingly stiff lungs, which are inefficient in exchange of both oxygen and carbon dioxide. About 15 percent of patients with ARDS ultimately die of respiratory failure, showing progressive hypercapnia, despite a high minute ventilation, and refractory hypoxemia. These anatomic and pathophysiological events suggest a loss of regulation of mesenchymal proliferation or matrix deposition and concomitant failure of neovascularization. In contrast, patients who recover from ARDS commonly experience normalization of

the chest radiograph and lung volumes; hypoxemia resolves and the diffusing capacity improves over the ensuing months, indicating reversal of fibrosis and revascularization of alveoli. Thus, regulation of fibrosis and angiogenesis during the fibroproliferative phase appears to be key variables in determining the outcome of ARDS.

Fibrosis

Following the acute inflammatory phase of lung injury in ARDS, a "fibroproliferative" response, leading to a marked derangement of lung architecture, is seen.[45] Hyperplasia of type II alveolar epithelial cells, fibroblasts, and smooth-muscle cells is observed. When the repair process goes on to resolution, the alveolar microcirculation, interstitial space, and alveolar surfaces are reconstructed. This complex process comprises matrix deposition, cell migration, controlled cell proliferation, and differentiation. In a subset of patients with ARDS, the repair process goes awry. Interstitial mesenchymal cells migrate into airspaces, replicate, and deposit connective-tissue matrix, ultimately obliterating the alveoli. Biopsy samples from these patients show exuberant intra-alveolar and interstitial fibrosis. Biochemical confirmation of excessive deposition of collagen between days 14 and 28 is made in patients with ARDS.[63]

The fibroproliferative phase is one of the most important and least well understood components of the pathogenesis of ARDS. Several reasons may account for this. The fibroproliferative lung is regionally heterogeneous, involves many sequential, cell-cell communicative events, and occurs in cells that are fixed to tissue, rather than circulating in blood or recoverable by lavage. Thus, it is virtually impossible to obtain sufficient tissue samples noninvasively from patients with fibroproliferative ARDS in order to characterize regulation of the events. To circumvent this problem, BAL has been used in the study of lung fibrosis in ARDS.

While it is an imperfect approach to the study of an interstitial process, BAL has some useful features for evaluating the pulmonary interstitium. First, it allows sequential data to be obtained with minimal complications. Second, it allows recovery of alveolar macrophages, cells that have long been thought to be important sources of the cytokines that regulate fibrosis in idiopathic pulmonary fibrosis—a process that fibroproliferative ARDS resembles morphologically. Furthermore, early in the evolution of fibrosis in ARDS, a proteinaceous, fibronectin-rich exudate is found in alveoli; later, the exudate is replaced by dense intra-alveolar fibrosis. Hence, sampling alveolar lining fluid may provide insight into at least the intra-alveolar component of early fibrosis.

In the largest study to date using BAL to study fibrosis in ARDS, investigators examined BAL fluid from 117 patients with ARDS identified prospectively.[15] They measured procollagen III, the N-terminal peptide of the collagen III precursor molecule. Collagen III is the collagen type laid down in early wound healing. Procollagen III was measured on days 3, 7, and 14 of ARDS. Eighty percent of patients with ARDS, but no normal controls, had measurable procollagen III in BAL fluid. The relative risk of death from ARDS was doubled in those who had high procollagen III levels. The study indicates that collagen synthesis probably takes place within lavageable airspaces of most patients with ARDS, and that patients with the most intense intra-alveolar matrix synthesis are at high risk of a fatal outcome. However, these observations shed no light on the mechanisms of dysregulation of the fibrotic process.

Viewing the fibroproliferative phase of ARDS as "wound healing in the lung" may help elucidate underlying mechanisms. Wound healing in more accessible tissues is regulated by the cascades of proximal and distal cytokines, discussed previously, as well as an expanding list of other growth factors. Some, such as platelet-derived growth factor (PDGF), have been identified in bioactive form in BAL fluid from patients with ARDS. Growth factor–like activity in BAL fluid from patients with ARDS has been examined.[53] Three peptides related to PDGF with growth-promoting activity have been described. The same PDGF homologues were previously identified in BAL fluid from patients with pulmonary fibrosis. In experimental models of lung fibrosis, another growth factor—transforming growth factor–α (TGF-α), a potent mitogen and chemotactic factor—has been immunologically co-localized to areas of intra-alveolar fibrosis; it may regulate the early fibrotic response.[31] This growth factor is essential for wound healing in other organs. These two growth factors, PDGF and TGF-α, each have chemotactic and mitogenic bioactivities, making them prime candidates for both attracting mesenchymal cells into the interstitium and stimulating their replication. Undoubtedly, many other growth factors are involved; the timing of their appearance is probably important.

Considerable cell-cell communication exists between epithelial cells and fibroblasts in the regulation of fibrosis.[1] It is likely that epithelial injury plays a role in stimulating fibroblast replication; conversely, mesenchymal replication probably plays a role in initiating reepithelialization. If that is true, complications of therapy—e.g., hyperoxia or alveolar distention—may alter the healing process.[25] By injuring or inhibiting replication of contiguous epithelial or endothelial cells,[34] the lung fibrotic response may be modified.

Apoptosis,[46,60] described previously, may be of particular importance during the resolution phase of ARDS. In addition to its role in acute endothelial injury, apoptosis is important in the regression of cell structures that become redundant during tissue differentiation (e.g., morphogenesis during embryonic development). The healing lung is confronted with such a situation. Hundreds of grams of cellular tissue, comprising billions of viable cells, must vanish as the cellular proliferative lung, containing dense depositions of intra-alveolar fibroblasts, again becomes an air-filled structure with filamentous septae. During embryogenesis, such outmoded structures regress by apoptosis, and it has been proposed that apoptosis in the fibroproliferative phase of ARDS occurs in a similar manner.

Angiogenesis

Angiogenesis is another process essential for normal wound healing. Repair of the injured lung requires reconstitution of the damaged microvasculature. Angiogenesis is a complex process entailing cell migration, replication, and matrix depo-

sition in a highly controlled, but poorly elucidated, sequence. Angiogenesis becomes deranged in angioproliferative diseases, such as psoriasis and rheumatoid arthritis, and in retinal disorders, such as retrolental fibroplasia. Like pulmonary fibrosis, pulmonary angiogenesis is difficult to study in humans, so extrapolation from other models has been necessary. Although repair of the microvasculature is a critical component of recovery from acute lung injury, little is known about its regulation. Some of the same cytokines that regulate acute inflammation, including TNF and the CXC cytokines,[12,30,55] may regulate angiogenesis. Another factor, basic fibroblastic growth factor, is a potent angiogenic factor, but it has mitogenic effects on many cell types.

Vascular endothelial growth factor (VEGF)[19] has generated excitement because of its action as a specific mitogen for endothelial cells, having little effect on epithelial cells or fibroblasts. VEGF binds with high affinity to two receptors on endothelial cells and has been shown to increase vascular permeability, as well as exerting mitogenic effects. Following hyperoxic lung injury, which damages predominantly endothelial cells, alveolar epithelial cells express mRNA for VEGF.[32] In conjunction with other studies denoting a role for alveolar epithelial cells in the intercellular communications in wound healing,[1] this finding suggests that alveolar type II cells in the fibroproliferative phase of ARDS may orchestrate reconstitution of the microvasculature, as well as the interstitium.

CONCLUSION

Pathogenesis of ARDS, from the phase of acute microvascular injury to the phase of repair, raises questions integral to every basic molecular biologic process, as well as physiological processes of permeability and gas exchange. We have barely begun to unravel the pathogenesis of ARDS. An overriding theme gleaned from recent research is that even the most apparently disordered processes—e.g., leaky capillaries, cell death, and fibrosis—are, in fact, signaled events, subject to a high degree of regulation at the levels of gene expression and receptor-modulated signal transduction. Indeed, clinical outcome in ARDS may someday be further improved by knowledge gained through study of basic biologic processes.

REFERENCES

1. Adamson IY, Hedgecock RC, Bowden DH: Epithelial cell-fibroblast interactions in lung injury and repair. *Am J Pathol* 137:385–392, 1990.
2. Aderka D, Engelmann H, Shemer-Avni Y, et al: Variation in serum levels of the soluble TNF receptors among healthy individuals. *Lymphokine Cytokine Res* 11:157–159, 1992.
3. Albelda SM, Smith CW, Ward PA: Adhesion molecules and inflammatory injury. *FASEB J* 8:504–512, 1994.
4. Beckman J, Beckman T, Chen J, et al: Apparent hydroxyl radical production by peroxynitrite: Implications for endothelial injury from nitric oxide and superoxide. *Proc Natl Acad Sci USA* 87:1620–1624, 1990.
5. Bernard GR, Artigas A, Brigham KL, et al: The American-European Consensus Conference on ARDS: Definitions, mechanisms, relevant outcomes, and clinical trial coordination. *Am J Respir Crit Care Med* 149:818–824, 1994.

6. Bhakdi S, Tranum-Jensen J: Damage to mammalian cells by pore-forming bacterial cytolysins. *Prog Allergy* 40:1–43, 1988.

7. Blackwell TS, Holden EP, Blackwell TR, et al: Activation of NF-kB in rat lungs by treatment with endotoxin: Modulation by treatment with *N*-acetylcysteine. *J Immunol* In press.

8. Bogdan C, Nathan C: Modulation of macrophage function by transforming growth factor-beta, interleukin-4, and interleukin-10. *Ann NY Acad Sci* 685:713–739, 1993.

9. Brigham KL: Metabolites of arachidonic acid in experimental lung vascular injury. *Fed Proc* 44:43–45, 1985.

10. Brigham KL, Bowers RE, Haynes J: Increased sheep lung vascular permeability caused by *Escherichia coli* endotoxin. *Circ Res* 45:292–297, 1979.

11. Brigham KL, Kariman K, Harris TR, et al: Correlation of oxygenation with vascular-permeability surface area but not with lung water in humans with acute respiratory failure and pulmonary edema. *J Clin Invest* 72:339–349, 1983.

12. Cao Y, Chen C, Weatherbee JA, et al: gro-β, a-CXC chemokine, is an angiogenesis inhibitor that suppresses the growth of Lewis lung carcinoma in mice. *J Exp Med* 182:2069–2077, 1995.

13. Chollet-Martin S, Montravers P, Gibert C, et al: High levels of interleukin-8 in the blood and alveolar spaces of patients with pneumonia and adult respiratory distress syndrome. *Infect Immun* 61:4553–4559, 1993.

14. Cifuentes J, Oronoz J, Myles C, et al: Interaction of surfactant mixtures with reactive oxygen and nitrogen species. *J Appl Physiol* 78:1800–1805, 1995.

15. Clark JG, Milberg JA, Steinberg KP, Hudson LD: Type III procollagen peptide in the adult respiratory distress syndrome. *Ann Intern Med* 122:17–23, 1995.

16. Cochrane CG, Spragg R, Revak SD: Pathogenesis of the adult respiratory distress syndrome: Evidence of oxidant activity in bronchoalveolar lavage fluid. *J Clin Invest* 71:754–761, 1983.

17. Collins PD, Connolly DT, Williams TJ: Characterization of the increase in vascular permeability induced by vascular permeability factor in vivo. *Br J Pharmacol* 109:195–199, 1993.

18. Donnelly SC, MacGregor I, Zamani A, et al: Plasma elastase levels and the development of the adult respiratory distress syndrome. *Am J Respir Crit Care Med* 151:1428–1433, 1995.

19. Ferrara NK, et al: Molecular and biological properties of the vascular endothelial growth factor family of proteins. *Endocr Res* 13:18–32, 1992.

20. Fischer E, Van Zee KJ, Marano MA, et al: Interleukin-1 receptor antagonist circulates in experimental inflammation and in human disease. *Blood* 79:2196–2200, 1992.

21. Fowler AA, Fisher BJ, Centor RM, Carchman RA: Development of the adult respiratory distress syndrome: Progressive alteration of neutrophil chemotactic and secretory processes. *Am J Pathol* 116:427–435, 1984.

22. Gregory T, Longmore W, Moxley M, et al: Surfactant chemical composition and biophysical activity in acute respiratory distress syndrome. *J Clin Invest* 88:1976–1981, 1991.

23. Hammerschmidt DE, Weaver LJ, Hudson LD, et al: Association of complement activation and elevated plasma-C5a with adult respiratory distress syndrome. *Lancet* 1:947–949, 1980.

24. Harris T, Bernard G, Brigham K, et al: Lung microvascular transport properties measured by multiple indicator dilution methods in patients with adult respiratory distress syndrome. *Am Rev Respir Dis* 141:272–280, 1990.

25. Haschek WM, Reiser KM, Klein-Szanto AJ, et al: Potentiation of butylated hydroxytoluene-induced acute lung damage by oxygen: Cell kinetics and collagen metabolism. *Am Rev Respir Dis* 127:28–34, 1983.

26. Hyers TM, Tricomi SM, Dettenmeier PA, Fowler AA: Tumor necrosis factor levels in serum and bronchoalveolar lavage fluid of patients with the adult respiratory distress syndrome. *Am Rev Respir Dis* 144:268–271, 1991.

27. Idell S, Kucich U, Fein A, et al: Neutrophil elastase-releasing factors in bronchoalveolar lavage from patients with adult respiratory distress syndrome. *Am Rev Respir Dis* 132:1098–1105, 1985.

28. Inoue A, Yangisawa M, Kimura S, et al: The human endothelin family: Three structurally and pharmacologically distinct isopeptides predicted by three separate genes. *Proc Natl Acad Sci USA* 86:2863–2867, 1989.

29. Kaplow LS, Goffinet JA: Profound neutropenia during the early phase of hemodialysis. *JAMA* 203:1135–1137, 1968.

30. Koch A, Polverini PJ, Kunkel SL, et al: Interleukin-8 as a macrophage-derived mediator of angiogenesis. *Science* 258:1798–1801, 1992.

31. Madtes DK, Busby HK, Strandjord TP, Clark JG: Expression of transforming growth factor–alpha and epidermal growth factor receptor is increased following bleomycin-induced lung injury in rats. *Am J Respir Cell Mol Biol* 11:540–541, 1994.

32. Maniscalco W, Watkins R, Finkelstein J, Campbell M: Vascular endothelial growth factor mRNA increases in alveolar epithelial cells during recovery from oxygen injury. *Am J Respir Cell Mol Biol* 13:377–386, 1995.

33. Marchant A, Devière J, Byl B, et al: Interleukin-10 production during septicemia. *Lancet* 343:707–708, 1994.

34. Martin WJ, Kuchel DL: Oxygen-mediated impairment of human pulmonary endothelial cell growth: Evidence for a specific threshold of toxicity. *J Lab Clin Med* 113:412–421, 1989.

35. McCord JM: Oxygen-derived free radicals in post-ischemic tissue injury. *New Engl J Med* 312:1259–1263, 1985.

36. McGuire WW, Spragg RC, Cohen AB, Cochrane CG: Studies on the pathogenesis of the adult respiratory distress syndrome. *J Clin Invest* 69:543–553, 1982.

37. Meduri GU, Headley S, Kohler G, et al: Persistent elevation of inflammatory cytokines predicts a poor outcome in ARDS: Plasma IL-1 beta and IL-6 levels are consistent and efficient predictors of outcome over time. *Chest* 107:1062–1073, 1995.

38. Miller EJ, Cohen AB, Nagao S, et al: Elevated levels of NAP-1/interleukin-8 are present in the airspaces of patients with the adult respiratory distress syndrome and are associated with increased mortality. *Am Rev Respir Dis* 146:427–432, 1992.

39. Ognibene FP, Martin SE, Parker MM, et al: Adult respiratory distress syndrome in patients with severe neutropenia. *New Engl J Med* 315:547–551, 1986.

40. Pacht ER, Timerman AP, Lykens MG, Merola AJ: Deficiency of alveolar fluid glutathione in patients with sepsis and the adult respiratory distress syndrome. *Chest* 100:1397–1403, 1991.

41. Parsons PE, Moore FA, Moore EE, et al: Studies on the role of tumor necrosis factor in adult respiratory distress syndrome. *Am Rev Respir Dis* 146:694–700, 1992.

42. Peterson MW, Stone P, Shasby DM: Cationic neutrophil proteins increase transendothelial albumin movement. *J Appl Physiol* 62:1521–1530, 1987.

43. Pratt PC, Vollmer RT, Shelburne JD, Crapo JD: Pulmonary morphology in a multihospital collaborative extracorporeal membrane oxygenation project. *Am J Pathol* 95:191–214, 1979.

44. Rinaldo JE: Mediation of ARDS by leukocytes: Clinical evidence and implications for therapy. *Chest* 89:590–593, 1986.

45. Rinaldo JE, Rogers RM: Adult respiratory distress syndrome: Changing concepts of lung injury and repair. *New Engl J Med* 306:900–909, 1982.

46. Robaye B, Mosselmans R, Fiers W, et al: Tumor necrosis factor induces apoptosis (programmed cell death) in normal endothelial cells in vitro. *Am J Pathol* 138:447–453, 1991.

47. Rossaint R, Falke KJ, Lopez F, et al: Inhaled nitric oxide for the adult respiratory distress syndrome. *N Engl J Med* 328:399–405, 1993.

48. Schreck R, Albermann K, Baeuerle PA: Nuclear factor κB: An oxidative stress-responsive transcription factor of eukaryotic cells (a review). *Free Radic Res Commun* 17:221–237, 1992.

49. Seckinger P, Williamson K, Balavoine JF, et al: A urine inhibitor of interleukin 1 activity affects both interleukin 1α and 1β but not tumor necrosis factor alpha. *J Immunol* 139:1541–1545, 1987.

50. Shapiro L, Clark BD, Orencole SF, et al: Detection of tumor necrosis factor soluble receptor p55 in blood samples from healthy and endotoxemic humans. *J Infect Dis* 167:1344–1350, 1993.

51. Shasby DM, Lind SE, Shasby SS, et al: Reversible oxidant-induced increases in albumin transfer across cultured endothelium: Alterations in cell shape and calcium homeostasis. *Blood* 65:605–614, 1985.

52. Siebenlist U, Franzoso G, Brown K: Structure, regulation and function of NF-κB. *Annu Rev Cell Biol* 10:405–455, 1994.

53. Snyder LS, Hetz MI, Peterson MS, et al: Acute lung injury: Pathogenesis of intraalveolar fibrosis. *J Clin Invest* 88:663–673, 1991.

54. Steinberg KP, Milberg JA, Martin TR, et al: Evolution of bronchoalveolar cell populations in the adult respiratory distress syndrome. *Am Rev Respir Crit Care Med* 150:113–122, 1994.

55. Streiter RM, Polverine PJ, Kunkel SL, et al: The functional role of the ELR motif in CXC chemokine-mediated angiogenesis. *J Biol Chem* 270:27348–27357, 1995.

56. Summerville FL, Massaro D: Protection from oxygen toxicity with endotoxin: Role of the endogenous antioxidant enzymes of the lung. *J Clin Invest* 65:1104–1110, 1980.

57. Suter PM, Suter S, Girardin E, et al: High bronchoalveolar levels of tumor necrosis factor and its inhibitors, interleukin-1, interferon, and elastase, in patients with adult respiratory distress syndrome after trauma, shock, or sepsis. *Am Rev Respir Dis* 145:1016–1022, 1992.

58. Tran Van Nhieu J, Misset B, Lebargy F, et al: Expression of tumor necrosis factor–alpha gene in alveolar macrophages from patients with the adult respiratory distress syndrome. *Am Rev Respir Dis* 147:1585–1589, 1993.

59. Van Zee KJ, Kohno T, Fischer E, et al: Tumor necrosis factor soluble receptor circulate during experimental and clinical inflammation and can protect against excessive tumor necrosis factor α in vitro and in vivo. *Proc Natl Acad Sci USA* 89:4845–4849, 1992.

60. Wendt CH, Polunovsky VA, Peterson MS, et al: Alveolar epithelial cells regulate the induction of endothelial cell apoptosis. *Am J Physiol (Cell Physiol)* 267:C893–900, 1994.

61. Wewers MD, Herzyk DJ, Gadek JE: Alveolar fluid neutrophil elastase activity in the adult respiratory distress syndrome is complexed to alpha-2-macroglobulin. *J Clin Invest* 82:1260–1274, 1988.

62. Zapol WM, Rimar S, Gillis N, et al: Nitric oxide and the lung. *Am Rev Respir Crit Care Med* 149:1365–1380, 1994.

63. Zapol WM, Trelsted RL, Coffey JW, et al: Pulmonary fibrosis in severe acute respiratory failure. *Am Rev Respir Dis* 119:547–554, 1979.

CHAPTER 167

ACUTE RESPIRATORY DISTRESS SYNDROME: CLINICAL FEATURES, MANAGEMENT, AND OUTCOME

Leonard D. Hudson / Kenneth P. Steinberg

DESCRIPTION AND DEFINITION

Acute respiratory distress syndrome (ARDS) was first described as a clinical syndrome comprising obvious respiratory distress, severe hypoxemia, diffuse infiltrates on chest radiographs, and decreased lung compliance, associated with a variety of underlying medical and surgical conditions.[5] The concept that this syndrome represents acute diffuse lung injury, occurring either directly via the airways (as with aspiration of gastric contents or toxic substances) or indirectly via the bloodstream (as with sepsis or trauma), underlies our understanding of the syndrome. This concept has led to an attempt in some definitions to exclude other causes of the above constellation of findings, such as congestive heart failure or bilateral atelectasis. Other definitions have required inclusion of an underlying risk factor or risk condition that is known to be associated with mechanisms that could lead to ARDS.

Subsequent definitions have included some of the original clinical components (for example, compliance may be excluded) and have attempted to quantify the oxygenation criteria. In 1994, the American-European Consensus Conference on ARDS published a definition agreed on by a group of international ARDS investigators.[8] This group defined ARDS as requiring (1) a $Pa_{O_2}/F_{I_{O_2}}$ ratio of 200 or less, regardless of the presence or level of positive end-expiratory pressure (PEEP); (2) a chest radiograph with bilateral pulmonary infiltrates compatible with pulmonary edema; and (3) no clinical evidence of congestive heart failure or, if a pulmonary artery catheter is in place, a pulmonary artery balloon occlusion (wedge) pressure of 18 mmHg or less. The level of $Pa_{O_2}/F_{I_{O_2}}$ ratio may have to be adjusted for patients at high altitude; in these circumstances, a Pa_{O_2}/PA_{O_2} ratio of less than 0.20 has been used. (For respiratory abbreviations and symbols, see Appendix C.)

A spectrum of acute lung injury exists in which ARDS represents the most severe end. The American-European Consensus Conference on ARDS attempted to define a milder form of injury, which they labeled acute lung injury (ALI).[8] Their definition of ALI was the same as for ARDS except for a less stringent oxygenation criterion, consisting of a $Pa_{O_2}/F_{I_{O_2}}$ ratio of less than 300 (but greater than 200) (Table 167-1). This definition was not based on any previous data, and subsequent studies that have attempted to evaluate these criteria found little difference in the course of patients meeting ALI criteria from that of those meeting the criteria for ARDS.[16] Previous studies had also suggested that the initial severity of the abnormality in oxygenation did not significantly affect mortality if other criteria for the syndrome were present.[47] Thus, although the concept proposed by the Consensus Conference of a less severe form of acute lung injury with

TABLE 167-1

Diagnostic Criteria for Acute Lung Injury (ALI) and ARDS

	Onset	Oxygenation*	Chest Radiograph	PAOP
ALI criteria	Acute	$Pa_{O_2}/F_{I_{O_2}} \leq 300$ mmHg	Bilateral interstitial or alveolar infiltrates	≤ 18 mmHg if measured or no clinical evidence of left atrial hypertension
ARDS criteria	Acute	$Pa_{O_2}/F_{I_{O_2}} \leq 200$ mmHg	Bilateral interstitial or alveolar infiltrates	≤ 18 mmHg if measured or no clinical evidence of left atrial hypertension

*Regardless of level of positive end-expiratory pressure (PEEP).
NOTE: PAOP = pulmonary artery occlusion pressure.
SOURCE: Adapted from Bernard et al.[8]

a milder clinical course and better outcome makes intuitive sense, the current definition does not accurately reflect this concept.

Another attempt to standardize the definition or the comparison of patients with severe acute lung injury is the Lung Injury Score,[41] which grades four parameters on a scale of 0 to 4: $Pa_{O_2}/F_{I_{O_2}}$ ratio, total respiratory compliance, level of PEEP used, and number of quadrants involved on chest radiograph. The composite score is then divided by 4. A score of at least 2.5 is required for severe ALI (equivalent to ARDS). The Lung Injury Score, a modified lung injury score, and the American-European Consensus Conference definition of ARDS identify similar patients when applied to a population with diagnoses that clearly place them at risk for ARDS.[40]

EPIDEMIOLOGY/HOST FACTORS

Patients at Risk for ARDS

A wide variety of conditions have been reported to be associated with ARDS. The underlying risk conditions for ARDS can be divided into two broad groups according to whether their pathophysiological mechanism represents direct or indirect injury to the lung (Table 167-2). *Direct* injuries are those in which a toxic substance directly injures lung epithelium. Examples include aspiration of gastric contents and inhalation of toxic gases. The risk of ARDS is dependent on the toxicity, concentration, and dose of the substance. The *indirect* pathophysiological mechanism of ARDS is more common—via blood-borne systemic inflammatory processes that have been referred to as *malignant systemic inflammation* or *rogue inflammation*.[24] This category consists of inflammatory mechanisms that are usually beneficial but have escaped their usual controls, thereby causing organ injury.

Most of the information regarding conditions that place a patient at risk come from retrospective analyses—series in which ARDS might be identified prospectively but the risk conditions are identified only retrospectively.

Alternatively, information concerning risk is derived from either small series or case reports of a given condition that occurs together with ARDS. Although these reports provide information on the conditions that are associated with ARDS, they do not allow calculation of a true incidence for developing ARDS because the denominator (the size of the population with the given condition of interest) is not known.[20,28]

However, two relatively large studies, one in Seattle and the other in Denver, have examined prospectively the frequency with which each of the carefully defined risk factors for ARDS has been associated with the development of ARDS (Table 167-3).[19,29] These studies suggest that the common conditions with the highest incidence of ARDS include severe sepsis or sepsis syndrome, severe trauma, and aspiration of gastric contents. One of the two series found that pneumonia that was sufficiently severe to warrant admission to the intensive care unit (ICU)—the so-called ICU pneumonia—was associated with ARDS. The discrepancy between the two studies is possibly explained by the difficulty in distinguishing diffuse pulmonary infection from pneumonia associated with sepsis.

Although these prospective studies do indicate the frequency with which ARDS is associated with specific risk factors in these two institutions, other institutions may differ considerably with respect to patient mix and, therefore, in risk conditions for ARDS.

TABLE 167-2

Clinical Disorders Associated with ARDS

Direct Lung Injury	Indirect Lung Injury*
Aspiration of gastric contents	Severe sepsis
Pulmonary contusion	Major trauma
Toxic gas (smoke) inhalation	Multiple long-bone fractures
Near-drowning	Hypovolemic shock
Diffuse pulmonary infection	Hypertransfusion
	Acute pancreatitis
	Drug overdose
	Reperfusion injury
	Post–lung transplantation
	Post–cardiopulmonary bypass

*Due to activation of an acute, systemic inflammatory response with hematogenous delivery of inflammatory mediators to the lung.

TABLE 167-3

Clinical Disorders Associated with ARDS

Disorder	Estimated Incidence (%)
Frequent causes	
Sepsis	
Bacteremia without sepsis syndrome	4
Severe sepsis/sepsis syndrome	35–45
Major trauma	25
Multiple long-bone fractures	5–10
Pulmonary contusion	17–22
Hypertransfusion	5–36
Aspiration of gastric contents	22–36
Less frequent causes	
Drug overdose	5–8
Pancreatitis	
Burn/smoke inhalation	
Near-drowning	
Viral pneumonia	
Irritant gas inhalation	

SOURCE: Data from Fowler et al[19] and Hudson et al.[29]

In North America, sepsis appears to be the most common cause of ARDS, as well as being the risk condition that is associated with the highest incidence of development of ARDS. This may differ considerably in other countries or regions. For example, in tropical countries, malaria and leptospirosis are common causes of ARDS.

SEVERE SEPSIS

Infection was the most frequent cause of ARDS in both of the prospective series. Bacteremia per se, however, does not seem to place a patient at a significant risk for ARDS, whereas the clinical syndrome of severe sepsis does. In the Denver study, the frequency of ARDS in patients with bacteremia (defined as two positive blood cultures growing pathogens) was only 4 percent.[19] In the Seattle study, a syndrome of sepsis was associated with a 10-fold higher incidence of ARDS.[29] The definition of sepsis syndrome used in the Seattle study, the first attempt at defining this syndrome for research purposes, called for two types of evidence.[42] The first is evidence of infection or inflammation; acceptable evidence consisted of two of the following criteria: (1) local infection, (2) positive blood culture, (3) abnormal white blood cell count, and (4) abnormal body temperature. The second (additional) type of evidence consisted of some harmful systemic effect; acceptable as evidence is one of the following: (1) hypotension for more than 2 h, (2) systemic vascular resistance under 800 dynes/s/cm^2, and (3) unexplained metabolic acidosis. These systemic criteria probably reflected inadequate tissue perfusion—which, in turn, implied at least a mild degree of septic shock. A subsequent Consensus Conference definition of severe sepsis was based on the same principles but was less stringent in that it accepted evidence of organ failure other than cardiovascular insufficiency.[10] Presumably, the sepsis syndrome definition adopted in the Seat-

tle study, which reflects inadequate tissue perfusion, would be associated with a higher incidence of ARDS than the definition used in the consensus study. In several intervention trials that used the Consensus Conference definition or similar definitions, the frequency with which ARDS developed in the placebo arms of the trials ranged from 25 to 38 percent.

SEVERE TRAUMA

Severe trauma is a common risk for ARDS. Although the mechanism is thought to be intravascular activation of inflammation, similar to sepsis, the exact mechanisms and the specific markers for injury that are associated with development of ARDS have not been clearly defined. In several series, hemorrhagic shock has been associated with the development of both ARDS and multiple organ failure. However, it is not clear that shock is a prerequisite for developing trauma-associated ARDS. The trauma risks evaluated in the prospective Seattle study were (1) multiple transfusions for purposes of emergency resuscitation (at least 15 units in the 24-h period), (2) multiple fractures (either multiple long-bone fractures or an unstable pelvic fracture), and (3) pulmonary contusion (defined by the appearance of a localized infiltrate on chest radiograph beneath an external manifestation of trauma, such as ecchymosis of the chest wall, that occurred within 6 h after the trauma).[29]

In the Seattle series, multiple transfusions constituted the risk factor associated with the highest incidence of ARDS (25 percent as a single risk, 47 percent when transfusions occurred with another risk, and an overall total of a 37 percent incidence). Whether multiple transfusions reflect the presence of hemorrhagic shock, are a marker of severe injury, or play a mechanistic role in causing ARDS and multiple organ failure is not clear. The same criterion of multiple transfusions also was associated with a high incidence of ARDS—44 percent—for nontrauma patients. Since transfusion practices have changed substantially in trauma patients since these data were collected, however, the associated incidence of ARDS may now be different. Also, in the Seattle study, pulmonary contusion was associated with a 22 percent incidence of ARDS, whereas the criterion of multiple fractures was associated with the lowest incidence: 11 percent.

In the Denver series, less stringent criteria for fractures and transfusions were associated with a lower incidence of ARDS.[19] Thus, fractures, including fracture of a single bone, were associated with only a 5 percent incidence of ARDS. Multiple transfusions, defined as 10 units in 24 h, also carried only a 5 percent incidence.

Sepsis occurring in trauma patients is a significant risk for developing both ARDS and multiple organ failure.[10,29,42] Trauma cohort studies that examined predictors of multiple organ failure identified the following risk factors (among others): age, number of transfusions, hypovolemic shock, injury severity score (ISS) of at least 25. Obviously, several of these factors (including an ISS to grade the global severity of multiple trauma) are interrelated. In a study using multiple logistic regression, age over 55, ISS greater than 25, and transfusion of more than 6 units of blood in 12 h were found to be independent indicators of the development of multiple organ failure.[46]

ASPIRATION OF GASTRIC CONTENTS

Aspiration of gastric contents, defined either as being directly observed by medical personnel or as suctioning gastric contents from the trachea, was associated with an incidence of ARDS of 36 percent in the Denver study and 26 percent in the Seattle study. The combination of aspiration of gastric contents and drug overdose that required intensive care was associated with a higher incidence of ARDS than was aspiration of gastric contents alone, raising the possibility that drug overdose may be associated with other mechanisms for developing ARDS.

OTHER

A wide variety of other associated conditions for ARDS have been reported. Many of these reflect specific infections that could be associated with either a sepsislike syndrome or with diffuse direct pulmonary involvement.[19,29] Others may represent varying mechanisms by which the lung could be diffusely injured as part of an either systemic or localized disease process. These are discussed in more detail in the section below dealing with differential diagnosis. A history of alcohol abuse, when present in combination with some of the other underlying risk factors, particularly sepsis, appears to be associated with a higher incidence of ARDS.[39]

Both prospective studies identifying risk factors were based on data collected in the early 1980s. Newer studies are required to improve our understanding of the epidemiology of ARDS and to improve the reliability of our current information regarding patients at risk.

CLINICAL MANIFESTATIONS

ARDS occurs in the setting of acute severe illness. Clinical manifestations of ARDS reflect the underlying illnesses, the severe pulmonary injury, or the multiple organ failure that may coexist. The clinical manifestations can vary considerably, depending on the underlying disease and the number and type of organs other than the lungs that are failing. A variety of risk factors (see below) have been associated with ALI and ARDS; the most common is severe sepsis or sepsis syndrome; multiple severe trauma also carries a high risk for ARDS. Sepsis and trauma presumably cause acute lung (and other organ) injury by way of inflammatory mediators in the blood that damage both endothelium and epithelium. Leakage of protein-rich fluid from the vascular space initiates the syndrome, resulting in protein-rich pulmonary edema and abnormality of surfactant. The end result is widespread, patchy alveolar edema and areas of atelectasis, primarily in dependent regions of the lungs.[21,33] The fluid-filled lungs and atelectasis cause intrapulmonary shunting, resulting in severe arterial hypoxemia and dyspnea. Other manifestations reflect failure of other organs that are injured by the same initiating mechanisms. Fever and leukocytosis, which can be prominent, are related to the underlying disease or injury, to the intravascular inflammation, or to the marked inflammatory process that occurs in the lungs in ARDS.

Clinical Diagnosis

The diagnosis of ARDS requires a constellation of historical and physical findings, as well as the exclusion of specific processes that mimic ARDS. In most cases, the inciting event is obvious, and the development of respiratory failure can be seen as a direct consequence of that event. In such a setting, very little is generally required to make a clinical diagnosis, and certain principles of supportive therapy can be applied regardless of etiology. Whenever the presentation is less clear, a more thoughtful process may be required to establish the diagnosis.

The development of ARDS is usually rapid, occurring most often within 12 to 48 h of the predisposing event, although it may take up to 5 days.[19,29] Awake patients become anxious, agitated, and dyspneic. Initially, dyspnea may occur only during exertion, but it may progress quickly to severe dyspnea at rest, in association with arterial hypoxemia. Inflammatory changes in the lung lead to a decrease in lung compliance. This stiffening of the lungs leads, in turn, to an increase in the work of breathing, small tidal volumes, and rapid respiratory rate (tachypnea). Initially, patients may be able to compensate and maintain acceptable arterial blood gases, perhaps even generating a respiratory alkalosis. The vast majority of patients deteriorate over several hours, requiring intubation and mechanical ventilation. Mechanical ventilation, however, is not a necessary requirement for the diagnosis of ARDS. A few patients with mild lung injury and normal mentation can avoid intubation, either with high-flow oxygen therapy or with the use of noninvasive respiratory support such as mask continuous positive airway pressure (CPAP). If measured, pulmonary artery occlusion pressure should be less than 18 mmHg, although lung injury can coexist with intravascular volume overload. Total respiratory compliance is often reduced, but this is generally not required for the diagnosis. Regardless of the criteria applied, it is important to recognize that acute pulmonary dysfunction represents a spectrum of severity, with definable ALI and ARDS at the far end.

Laboratory Studies

To date, no laboratory findings have been characterized as pathognomonic for ARDS, but some have been identified as necessary to meet the diagnostic criteria of the syndrome. Usually, the chest radiograph reveals diffuse bilateral infiltrates consistent with pulmonary edema; these infiltrates may be mild or dense, interstitial or alveolar, patchy or confluent. However, they should represent parenchymal disease and not effusions, atelectasis, or masses. Initially, the chest radiograph can be misleading, since there is no distinct pattern to the development of these infiltrates. They may develop quickly and symmetrically, even before arterial hypoxemia, or more gradually and asymmetrically (Figs. 167-1, 167-2, and 167-3). In fact, unilateral ARDS has been seen in patients in whom blood flow to the contralateral lung has been curtailed by pulmonary embolism or unilateral pulmonary artery hypoplasia. Early in the course of ARDS, the chest radiograph may show focal infiltrates that are interpreted at that time as pneumonia or patchy, segmental atelectasis—only to have them progress over a few hours or days to a complete "whiteout." It can also be difficult to distinguish radiographically be-

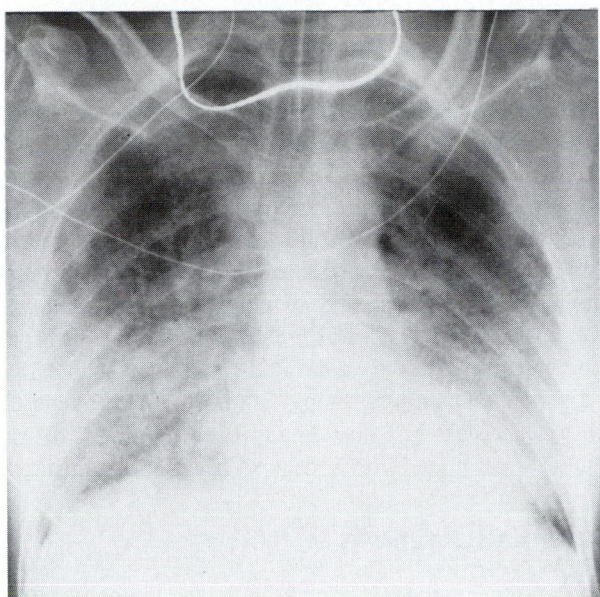

FIGURE 167-1   Influenza pneumonia causing ARDS with delayed reversal in a 47-year-old woman. On admission, bilateral alveolar infiltrates were evident.

tween cardiogenic pulmonary edema and ARDS. Finally, as noted above, the correlation between the radiographic abnormalities and the degree of hypoxemia can vary. In an at-risk patient in the proper clinical setting, these radiographic conundrums should not exclude early ARDS as the cause of the patient's acute deterioration.

Arterial blood gas measurements are markedly abnormal in patients with ARDS. Initially, depending on the acid-base balance associated with the patient's underlying condition, arterial hypoxemia may coexist with respiratory alkalosis. Because of the common use of O_2-enriched inspired air, which, in turn, in-

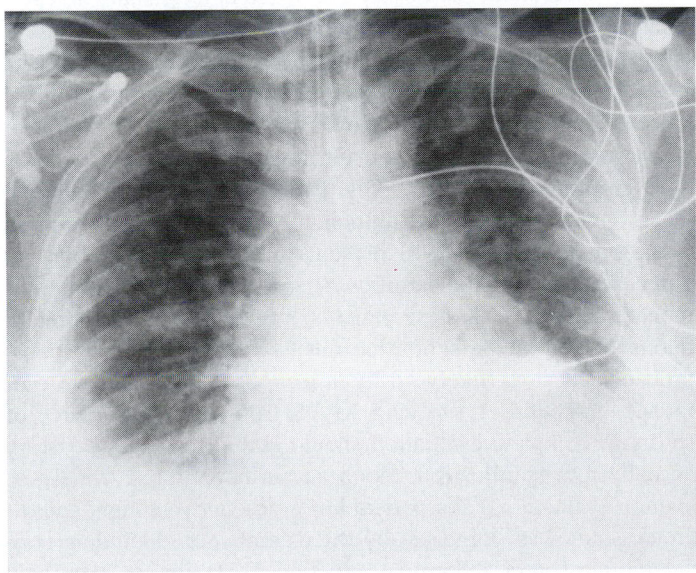

FIGURE 167-3   ARDS with bronchiolitis obliterans caused by Legionnaires' disease in a 50-year-old woman one month after admission. There are nodular infiltrates in both lungs and bilateral chest tubes for pneumothoraxes.

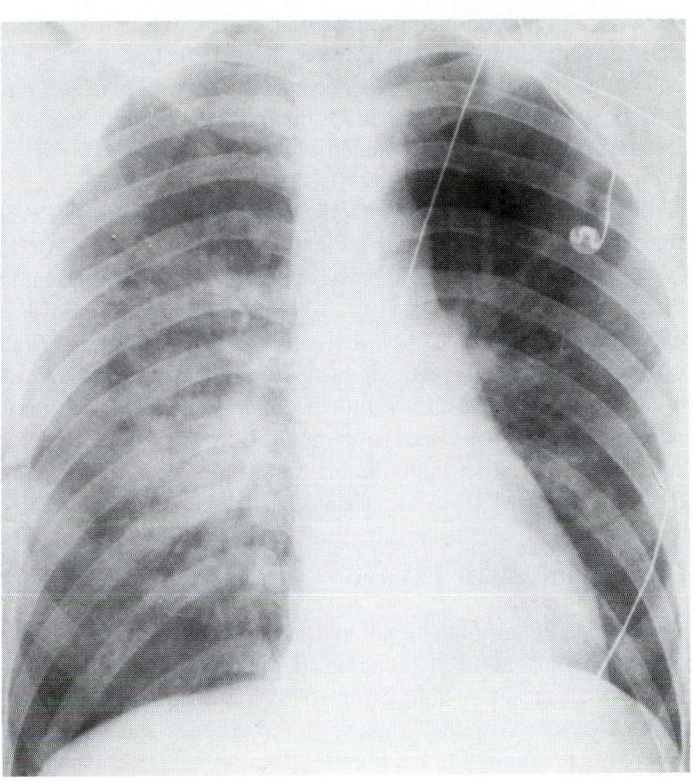

FIGURE 167-2   ARDS accompanied by severe damage to the airways in a 21-year-old woman exposed to smoke in a kitchen fire. On admission, bilateral infiltrates were more marked on the right. There are copious tracheobronchial secretions.

fluences the arterial P_{O_2}, most ARDS definitions describe hypoxemia in terms of the ratio of arterial P_{O_2} to the fraction of O_2 in inspired air (Pa_{O_2}/FI_{O_2} or an arterial to alveolar oxygen ratio (Pa_{O_2}/PA_{O_2}).

CO_2 exchange may be abnormal early on. Because of alveolar hyperventilation, respiratory alkalosis is generally a feature at the onset of ARDS. This reflects the presence of dead-space ($\dot{V}/\dot{Q} = D$) units causing abnormal CO_2 exchange simultaneously with shunt ($\dot{V}/\dot{Q} = O$) units causing arterial hypoxemia. As dead-space ventilation and the work of breathing increase, the ability to effectively clear CO_2 is compromised, and the initial respiratory alkalosis gives way to respiratory acidosis. In later phases of ARDS, abnormalities in oxygenation frequently abate, and despite the increased minute ventilation, respiratory acidosis, resulting from the abnormal CO_2 exchange, may be the predominant abnormality in gas exchange.

Few other laboratory abnormalities have been specifically linked to ARDS. Even though many abnormalities have been identified in ARDS, a diagnostic test for lung injury does not yet exist. Many of the abnormal laboratory tests in patients with ARDS relate to the underlying illness. Because ARDS usually occurs in conjunction with systemic inflammation, abnormalities in the functioning of other organs are frequent. Hematologic abnormalities, including leukocytosis or leukopenia and anemia, are very common. Thrombocytopenia, a reflection of underlying systemic inflammation and endothelial injury, is also common. Full-blown disseminated intravascular coagulation occurs less frequently; usually it is due to sepsis, severe trauma, or head injury. Renal function may be abnormal, owing to decreased renal perfusion or acute tubular necrosis. Liver function test results can be abnormal and show a hepatocellular or cholestatic pattern of injury. These abnormalities, which reflect multiorgan dysfunction, may be entirely related to the underlying systemic inflammation that accompanies ARDS (see Chapter 168).

Other tests indicative of endothelial injury are being explored for their value in identifying patients who are at risk for ARDS or who have ARDS. Among these are levels of von Willebrand's factor or complement in serum. Similarly, although serum levels of acute-phase reactants, such as ceruloplasmin and various cytokines (e.g., TNF, IL-1, IL-6, IL-8), either singly or in combination, increase in the serum of patients at risk for or with ARDS. None of these indicators has yet proved to be of practical clinical use either in predicting the development of ARDS or mortality from ARDS or in guiding diagnosis or management.[24]

Bronchoalveolar Lavage

Many investigators have explored the lungs of ARDS patients for biochemical and cellular abnormalities that might presage onset or outcome of ARDS. Inflammatory mediators such as cytokines, reactive oxygen species, leukotrienes, and activated complement fragments are found in the bronchoalveolar lavage (BAL) fluid of affected patients. Cellular analysis of BAL fluid reveals high neutrophil counts in patients at risk for or with early ARDS. Neutrophils commonly make up more than 60 percent of the total cell population of BAL fluid (normal is under 5 percent). Attempts have been made to relate the concentrations of different types of inflammatory cells to the outcome of ARDS. In general, as ARDS resolves, neutrophils are replaced by alveolar macrophages. It is postulated that although macrophages can certainly contribute to the acute inflammatory process, they also seem to be important in the resolution and healing of lung injury. Among patients with severe sepsis as a risk factor for ARDS, those who eventually die have a sustained alveolar neutrophilia, whereas those who survive manifest a decrease in neutrophils and an increase in macrophages, lending support to the hypothesis that sustained alveolar inflammation contributes to, or is associated with, a poor outcome.[6,50]

One interesting finding in BAL is a marker of pulmonary fibrosis known as procollagen peptide III (PCP-III). Activated lung fibroblasts secrete type III collagen, first as a procollagen, from which a fragment is cleaved to create collagen. PCP-III is the fragment left after creation of type III collagen. In a study of serial bronchoscopies done during the course of ARDS, increased concentrations on PCP-III in BAL correlated very strongly with mortality.[13] The presence of pulmonary fibrosis during ARDS has been shown to correlate with poor outcome, and PCP-III in BAL probably reflects this fibrosis process.[31] This measurement is currently being used experimentally to determine whether high-risk patients might respond to therapies designed to decrease the fibrotic response after lung injury.

Bronchoscopy with BAL is one of the mainstays in the evaluation of patients, immunocompromised or not, who have ARDS of unclear origin. This can be accomplished safely in most patients by experienced operators. Although the composition of BAL fluid is not specific for ARDS, the fluid is analyzed to rule out other acute processes. The presence of high numbers of eosinophils (more than 15 to 20 percent of the total cell count) suggests acute eosinophilic pneumonia. High lymphocyte counts suggest hypersensitivity pneumonitis, sarcoidosis, bronchiolitis obliterans organizing pneumonia (BOOP), and other acute forms of interstitial lung disease. The presence of many erythrocytes, especially in the presence of hemosiderin-laden macrophages, suggests pulmonary hemorrhage. Cultures should be sent for all likely infectious agents, depending on the clinical setting, and cytologic examination should be considered for *Pneumocystis carinii,* malignancy, and viral inclusion bodies. Transbronchial lung biopsies are generally contraindicated in mechanically ventilated patients. Open lung biopsy is rarely of help: generally, if the disease process has not already been identified by careful clinical evaluation and bronchoscopy, it is not diagnostic.

Differential Diagnosis

The differential diagnosis of ARDS includes congestive heart failure, diffuse pulmonary infections (Table 167-4), and many other specific causes of acute respiratory failure associated with parenchymal infiltrates on chest radiograph (Table 167-5). Congestive heart failure, or intravascular volume overload, is an important consideration in the evaluation of these patients. It may, in fact, be the most common alternative diagnosis for ARDS in the ICU. Restoration of circulating blood volume is critical in the management of patients with trauma and sepsis, and the volumes of fluid administered for maintenance of blood pressure and organ perfusion may result in pulmonary edema. As discussed earlier, the chest radiograph, by itself, often cannot distinguish cardiogenic from noncardiogenic pulmonary edema. In these situations, whereby patients are clearly at risk for ARDS, the difficulty in distinguishing between these two processes is evident. To complicate matters further, acute lung injury and volume overload can coexist: the presence of cardiogenic edema does not exclude the possibility of coexistent lung injury and permeability pulmonary edema. When this possibility exists, and if the patient appears clinically capable of tolerating reduction in circulating blood volume, it is reasonable to attempt diuresis. Once the intravascular volume overload has resolved, a more accurate assessment of lung injury can be made.

Even more challenging is the patient for whom no immediate or obvious cause of the pulmonary process can be identified. Occasionally, patients will present to an emergency room or clinic acutely ill with significant hypoxemia and diffuse pulmonary infiltrates. In these patients, a careful search for precipitating causes of the syndrome must be carried out. The most probable cause is likely to be infectious—either diffuse pulmonary infection or evolving ARDS from an occult source of sepsis. A complete evaluation should include a detailed history and physical examination, blood and urine cultures, urinalysis, sputum evaluation if the patient has a productive cough, and directed studies as suggested by the examination, including consideration of intra-abdominal infection. BAL may be extremely helpful in evaluating for viral pneumonia, pneumocystis pneumonia, tuberculosis, *Legionella* species, fungal infection, and other unusual pathogens. *Pneumocystis* pneumonia and tuberculosis should be considered in patients with this presentation, even

TABLE 167-4

Infectious Agents Associated with Diffuse Pulmonary Infiltrates and Respiratory Failure

Bacteria
  Gram-positive
    Staphylococcus aureus
    Streptococcus pneumoniae
  Gram-negative
    Franciscella tularensis
    Legionella species
      L. pneumophila
      L. micdadei
    Pasteurella multocida
    Salmonella species
    Yersinia pestis
  Mycobacterium tuberculosis
  Mycoplasma
    M. pneumoniae
    M. fermentans
  Rickettsia
    Coxiella burnetti
  Chlamydia
    C. psittaci
    C. pneumoniae
Viruses
  Cytomegalovirus (CMV)
  Respiratory syncytial virus (RSV)
  Herpes simplex virus (HSV)
  Varicella zoster virus (VZV)
  Adenovirus
  Influenza virus
  Hantavirus
Fungi
  Histoplasma capsulatum
  Coccidioides immitis
  Cryptococcus neoformans
Parasites
  Pneumocystis carinii
  Toxoplasma gondii
  Strongyloides stercoralis

when no apparent risk for immunosuppression exists. When immunosuppression does exist—as in AIDS, hematologic malignancy, neutropenia, or organ transplantation—the search for the infections noted above, and for other opportunistic infections, becomes a high priority.

Hantavirus pulmonary syndrome (HPS), a viral disease described in 1993, is a unique cause of severe acute respiratory failure. The virus is thought to be transmitted by aerosols of the infected feces and urine of the deer mouse. Signs and symptoms of HPS include fever, hypotension secondary to profound volume depletion from increased vascular permeability and extravascular sequestration of fluids, thrombocytopenia, neutrophilia, increased hematocrit (secondary to volume depletion), and increased concentration of serum LDH. As the illness progresses, dyspnea, pleuritic chest pain, hemoptysis, and diffuse rales develop rapidly. Respiratory failure, due to noncardiogenic

pulmonary edema, is characterized by highly proteinaceous fluid accumulation in the lungs. The chest radiograph reveals diffuse alveolar infiltrates. Autopsy studies have revealed diffuse alveolar damage with edema, hyaline membranes, and a marked, mononuclear, interstitial inflammatory infiltrate. Unlike the case with other causes of ARDS, polymorphonuclear leukocytes are generally not seen.

Because of the unique clinical syndrome, viral origin, and pathology (lack of polymorphonuclear leukocytes), it is not clear that HPS should be considered to be ARDS. HPS is associated with a high mortality. Treatment consists of aggressive supportive care. For these reasons, HPS is similar to ARDS; hence its inclusion in this chapter.

High-altitude pulmonary edema, a type of pulmonary edema associated with pulmonary microvascular leakage of fluid, is not included as a form of ARDS because of its distinctive clinical presentation, course, pathology, and response to therapy.

ARDS may develop as a part of the syndrome of fat embolism after long-bone fractures. Fat embolism syndrome is characterized by changes in mental status, conjunctival and axillary petechiae, anemia and thrombocytopenia, and diffuse lung injury that occurs 24 to 72 h after the injury (Fig. 167-4). Acute lung injury follows long-bone fractures in 5 to 10 percent of patients. Although the pathogenesis has not been clearly elucidated, it is believed to be due to release of toxic free fatty acids from bone marrow fat after trauma. The incidence of full-blown fat embolism syndrome has decreased dramatically in recent years, presumably because fractures are stabilized sooner.

There are many other noninfectious causes of acute respiratory failure associated with diffuse pulmonary infiltrates; most of these are included in Table 167-5. These disease processes are dealt with elsewhere in this book. Some of the entities are chronic or subacute disorders that may mimic ARDS only when they progress unusually fast or are first seen when the disease is far advanced.

Several drug overdoses have been associated with acute lung injury. Again, whether these reactions should be called ARDS is controversial. Many of these drugs also alter consciousness, and concurrent aspiration of gastric contents may be a factor. High doses of heroin and other narcotics (including narcotic antagonists) occasionally cause noncardiogenic pulmonary edema. The etiology of this injury remains unclear, and several hypotheses fail to explain all the observations. Possibilities include hypersensitivity reactions, neurogenic mechanisms, and hypoxia with or without transient left ventricular dysfunction. Regardless of the mechanism and as long as concurrent aspiration did not occur, the prognosis of narcotic-induced pulmonary edema is quite good in response to supportive therapy alone. Diuresis is generally not required, since the process resolves quickly with oxygen therapy and positive-pressure ventilation.

Drug overdoses that can cause acute lung injury also include those from aspirin and tricyclic antidepressants; the mechanisms are likewise unknown. Paraquat causes a very severe form of lung injury. Toxic gases, especially those that are relatively insoluble in water, such as phosgene or oxides of nitrogen, can also cause tremendous lung damage. Many of these gases are present in smoke, especially when plastics are burned, and contribute to the parenchymal injury seen with smoke inhalation.

TABLE 167-5

Noninfectious Causes of Acute Respiratory Failure Associated with Diffuse Pulmonary Infiltrates

Cardiovascular	Congestive heart failure
Drugs/toxins	Paraquat
	Aspirin
	Heroin/narcotics
	Toxic gas inhalation
	Tricyclic antidepressants
	Acute radiation pneumonitis
Idiopathic	Acute eosinophilic pneumonia
	Acute interstitial pneumonitis
	Bronchiolitis obliterans organizing pneumonia*
	Idiopathic interstitial pneumonia
	Rapidly progressive idiopathic pulmonary fibrosis*
	Sarcoidosis*
Immunologic	Acute lupus pneumonitis
	Goodpasture's syndrome
	Idiopathic pulmonary hemosiderosis*
	Hypersensitivity pneumonitis
	Leukoagglutinin reaction
	Pulmonary vasculitis with hemorrhage
Metabolic	Alveolar proteinosis*
Miscellaneous	Fat embolism syndrome
	Amniotic fluid embolism
	High-altitude pulmonary edema
	Neurogenic pulmonary edema
Neoplastic	Lymphangitic carcinomatosis*
	Leukemic infiltration
	Lymphoma

*Usually a subacute or chronic disorder that can progress rapidly or be far advanced on first presentation.

An uncommon but important process to consider is acute eosinophilic pneumonia, which was initially described in 1989. This syndrome apparently differs from other eosinophilic pulmonary disorders and generally presents in previously healthy young adults with no identifiable precipitating cause (although some drugs are associated with eosinophilic pulmonary reactions). These patients often do not have peripheral blood eosinophilia but do have a marked eosinophilia in BAL fluid, generally more than 15 percent of the total white blood cell count. This is an important entity to recognize, since it responds briskly to high-dose corticosteroid therapy.

Other noninfectious diseases that can present with fulminant respiratory failure are hypersensitivity pneumonitis, BOOP, diffuse pulmonary hemorrhage, acute lupus pneumonitis, neurogenic pulmonary edema, and acute leukoagglutinin reactions after blood transfusion. Often the historical details reveal the probable diagnosis. For example, in patients with cancer, severe thrombocytopenia can lead to intrapulmonary hemorrhage. The likelihood of a drug-induced pneumonitis, due to radiation or chemotherapy, also increases in this population. Idiopathic interstitial pneumonia is a complication of bone marrow transplantation.[12] Acute interstitial pneumonitis (AIP) is a designation for the rare patient with classic ARDS, including the pathologic findings, but for whom absolutely no predisposing condition can be found. Some authors claim that AIP corresponds to the disease originally described by Hamman and Rich in 1935;[30] others believe that Hamman-Rich syndrome is a form of rapidly progressive idiopathic pulmonary fibrosis. Both carry a high mortality, and supportive therapy for the two diseases is similar, although most clinicians would treat rapidly progressive idiopathic pulmonary fibrosis with corticosteroids and immunosuppressive agents.

THERAPY

Goals

The therapeutic goals in ARDS are threefold: (1) treatment of the underlying precipitating event, (2) cardiorespiratory support, and (3) specific therapies targeted at the lung injury. It cannot be overemphasized that identification and early, aggressive treatment directed at the inciting cause of ARDS are imperative for resolution of lung injury and respiratory failure. This section deals primarily with the support and treatment of the resultant lung injury. *Supportive therapies* are directed at correction of physiological abnormalities that present a threat to life or organ function, especially hypoxemia and tissue hypoxia, while avoiding complications from the therapeutic interventions. *Specific therapies* are those that have a therapeutic effect in modifying or hastening the resolution of ARDS. Some overlap exists between these categories, since some supportive therapies have theoretical or real effects on lung inflammation. Surfactant replacement is one example of a therapy designed to correct physiological abnormalities that may have anti-inflammatory properties as well. Regardless of some overlap, it is useful to think of new and existing therapies in this light.

Ventilator Management

The strategy of mechanical ventilation for patients with acute lung injury is currently in a state of flux. It is ironic that unprecedented research efforts relating to the use of mechanical ventilation for acute lung injury have resulted in novel strategies

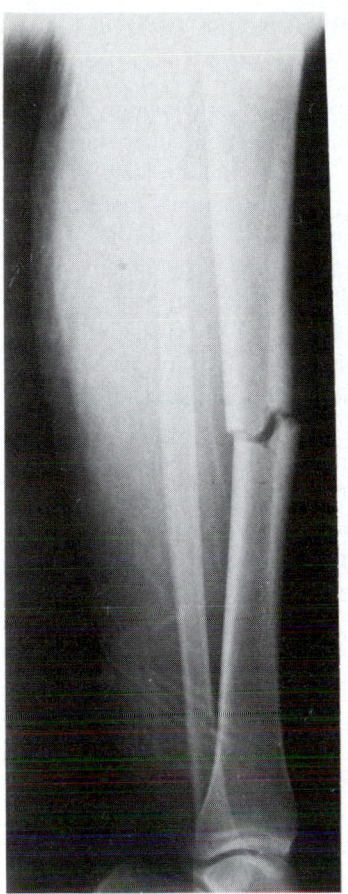
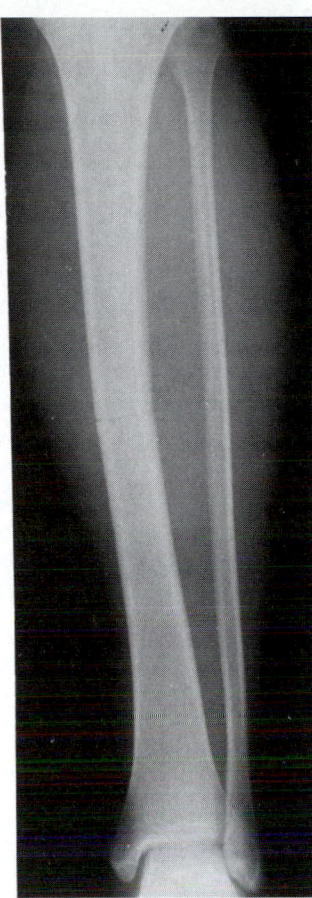

A

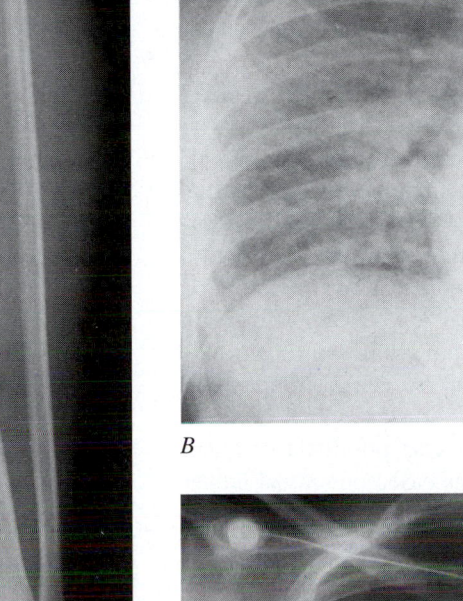

B

FIGURE 167-4   Fat embolism causing acute respiratory distress syndrome (ARDS) with rapid reversal in an 18-year-old woman. *A*. Radiographs of the lower legs showing fractures of both fibulas sustained in a fall from a ladder. Chest radiograph on admission appeared normal. *B*. Eighteen hours after admission, Pa_{O_2} fell to 59 mmHg on 100% O_2 with 10 cm H_2O PEEP. *C*. Four days after admission, pulmonary function had rapidly returned to normal.

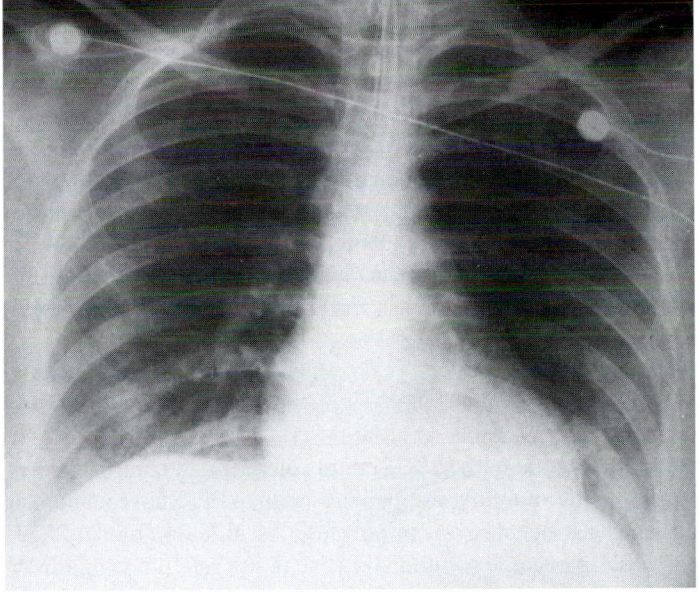

C

that have proved more powerful in theory and in animal models than in randomized, controlled trials in humans.

TRADITIONAL MECHANICAL VENTILATION STRATEGY FOR ALI/ARDS

The original description of ARDS by Ashbaugh and associates in 1967 included the first report of a beneficial physiological response to positive end-expiratory pressure (PEEP)—i.e., significant improvement in Pa_{O_2} shortly after addition of PEEP.[5] The traditional strategy for the use of mechanical ventilation in ARDS was developed shortly after this initial report and remained with only minor modifications until a few years ago. This strategy can be summarized as: (1) volume-cycled ventilation using relatively large tidal volumes (V_T), in the range of 10 to 15 ml/kg body weight; (2) respiratory rate to maintain a normal pH; and (3) PEEP adjusted with respect to Pa_{O_2} and $F_{I_{O_2}}$. In general, the goals have included a value for Pa_{O_2} that would produce an Sa_{O_2} of more than 90 percent at an $F_{I_{O_2}}$ that is considered to be safe or nontoxic.

None of these elements (and few subsequent modifications) were studied in randomized, controlled trials to evaluate outcomes. A study by Bendixen and colleagues is often cited as the basis for using relatively large tidal volumes for most patients receiving mechanical ventilation (not just those in whom acute lung injury is the basis for their acute respiratory failure.[7] This study involved 18 patients, presumably with normal lungs, who underwent surgery (mostly intra-abdominal). Progressive arterial hypoxemia developed during pressure-limited ventilation at peak pressures of 15 to 20 cm H_2O. The patients were then given breaths at 30 cm H_2O and then at 40 cm H_2O peak pressure; the breaths were held for 15 s. With these large sustained breaths, Pa_{O_2} returned to baseline values. The tidal volumes that resulted from these various pressures were not reported. The results of the study were interpreted as showing progressive atelectasis during surgery, which reversed when larger breaths were delivered by the higher pressures—an interpretation that seems entirely reasonable: because microatelectasis had been reported to occur early in ARDS, large V_{TS}, produced by inspired pressures in the range of 10 to 15 cm H_2O, were recommended in the attempt to prevent further atelectasis and to recruit alveoli that were already atelectatic. Moreover, since any degree of acidosis was likely to be harmful, adjusting the respiratory rate to achieve a normal pH also seemed reasonable.

Although the goal set for pressures using PEEP also seemed reasonable, less clear was the level of F_{IO_2} that would not be toxic to the lungs of patients with acute lung injury. Exposure of normal lungs to an F_{IO_2} of 0.8 for more than a few days results in acute lung injury with pulmonary edema that is indistinguishable from that resulting from other causes of ARDS.[43] Whether lower concentrations in O_2 in the inspired air would be clinically toxic in patients with ALI is less certain on several grounds: (1) prior oleic acid–induced lung injury in rabbits significantly attenuates the lethal effects of oxygen as compared to oxygen administered to animals with normal lungs;[49] (2) great species-to-species differences exist in susceptibility to oxygen injury, making assumptions for humans based on animal model data suspect; (3) reluctance, for ethical reasons, on the part of more recent investigators to repeat the studies in the 1960s that entailed exposure to varying levels of F_{IO_2}; and (4) the many clinical variables in patients with acute lung injury that complicate any clinical observations regarding the use of oxygen. Despite these uncertainties, many critical care clinicians are tending to use higher levels of F_{IO_2} than previously: in the 1970s, an F_{IO_2} of 0.4 or less was frequently a stated goal; currently, F_{IO_2} levels of 0.65 or less are accepted as being relatively safe by many experienced clinicians.

MODIFICATIONS AND CHALLENGES

Intermittent mandatory ventilation (IMV) was introduced as a ventilation mode in the 1970s amid considerable controversy regarding its suitability for patients with ALI. Subsequently, it emerged as the most commonly used ventilatory mode. However, it also became common practice to use relatively high IMV rates in patients with ARDS, because of their obvious increase in work of breathing. With this modification, the use of IMV in patients with ALI essentially remained a volume-cycled mode of ventilation using relatively high V_{TS}.

Some investigators advocated high levels of PEEP (25 to 50 cm H_2O or higher), but the trials were uncontrolled. Subsequently, controlled trials were conducted in patients with milder forms of ALI, but the numbers of patients were relatively small. Not only did the studies fail to demonstrate any benefit but some even showed higher rates of complications in patients in whom the level of PEEP was set to minimize the shunt instead of enabling reduction in F_{IO_2}.[23,34] The latter modification has not achieved widespread use, and its application remains limited. On the other hand, a strategy of using the "least PEEP" to achieve the traditional strategy goals stated above, along with the trend toward using higher levels of inspired F_{IO_2}, coupled with the common use of pulmonary artery catheters for hemodynamic monitoring, appears to have led to the fairly widespread adoption of lower levels of PEEP.

THE "NEW" MECHANICAL VENTILATION STRATEGY FOR ALI/ARDS

Since the mid-1980s, animal studies have convincingly demonstrated the potential of mechanical ventilation either starting or propagating acute lung injury.[14,17,18,32,52] High stretch (high tidal volumes accompanied by relatively high peak and plateau pressures) was demonstrated to be associated with injury. At first, the evidence from animal experiments was discounted by many as irrelevant to mechanical ventilation in humans because of the large V_{TS} that were used (30 to 40 ml/kg). It gradually became clear, however, that because much of the lungs of patients with ARDS was edematous, atelectatic, or fibrotic, some of the relatively normal regions of lung were being exposed to high regional tidal volumes, possibly in the range of those used in the animal experiments. This realization was aided by the computed tomographic images of lung in ARDS patients showing patchy rather than diffusely homoeogeneous injury.[21,33]

In addition to high stretch as mechanism of injury, cyclic reopening of atelectatic alveoli emerged as a second mechanism. Acceptance was based on studies that showed partial protection from the injury associated with high stress if PEEP was added, especially PEEP greater than the lower inflection point of the volume-pressure curve.[14,52]

These experiments on animals resulted in the hypothesis that injury from mechanical ventilation in patients with ALI could be prevented or minimized in two ways: avoiding tidal volumes that resulted in plateau pressures that exceeded the upper inflection point of the volume-pressure cure (the point above which a significant percent of alveoli were probably "overdistended") and using a PEEP level slightly above the lower inflection point.[32]

Acceptance of part, or all, of this hypothesis has led to two forms of the new strategy for mechanical ventilation strategy in patients with acute lung injury: the more popular entails the avoidance of high tidal volumes; the second adds the feature of using a level of PEEP above the lower inflection point and limiting tidal volumes. As anticipated, this strategy results in high P_{CO_2} levels and respiratory acidosis. Although hypercapnia was not a desired result of the strategy—greater priority was placed on avoiding lung hyperinflation—it was accepted as a necessary by-product of this strategy (*permissive hypercapnia*).

Whether the primary goal should be to limit the tidal volume or the pressure is debatable. Most seasoned clinicians have suggested that the most practical method is to limit the plateau pressure to less than 35 cm H_2O (or even to less than 30 cm H_2O, in order to avoid injury). This practice allows a range of V_T (generally from 4 to 8 ml/kg) that depends on the compliance of the lungs and chest wall.

The elements of the new strategy for mechanical ventilation of patients with ALI can be summarized as follows:

1. Use pressure-*targeted* ventilation (either pressure- or volume-controlled ventilatory modes can be used with appropriate monitoring), limiting V_T (4 to 8 ml/kg) *and* plateau pressure (less than 35 cm H_2O).

2. Allow P_{CO_2} to increase, if necessary, to meet above objectives.

3. Adjust PEEP for Pa_{O_2}/F_{IO_2} and to keep PEEP above the lower inflection point.

Two uncontrolled series directed attention to a low-stretch, permissive hypercapnia strategy. The first was a retrospective report, and the second was in a prospective but uncontrolled series.[26] Mortality was reported less than predicted by the APACHE rating of illness severity. No lower limit of pH was set, and no adverse effects of respiratory acidosis were reported. These reports undoubtedly resulted in increased use of the permissive hypercapnia approach.

Randomized, controlled trials of elements or all of this new strategy are currently under way. A trial conducted by European centers that compared low-stretch ventilation with conventional ventilation, but without modifying PEEP, was stopped when it became clear that it was unlikely to show benefit of the low-stretch ventilatory strategy. A similar trial, being conducted in the United States by an NIH-sponsored ARDS network of 10 centers, tests only low versus high (conventional) stretch; it also does not include a strategy for PEEP above the lower inflection point. The PEEP levels for both groups are relatively low for the F_{IO_2} used.

The combination of low stretch and PEEP above the lower inflection point—the *open lung approach,* based on 28 patients—showed: (1) the goal of separating plateau pressure between the new and conventional approach was met; (2) the new approach showed significant advantages in improved Pa_{O_2}/F_{IO_2} and fewer deaths due to progressive respiratory failure and a trend toward improved rate of successful weaning; but (3) no difference in mortality.[2] Subsequent experience in the same clinic showed a significant reduction in mortality in the new-approach group.[3] This work at a single center needs confirmation by a multicenter trial both to confirm the results and to demonstrate its applicability to a larger population of ALI patients. One lingering problem is that of determining the lower inflection point or of determining, in some indirect way, that PEEP exceeds the lower inflection point without becoming excessively high.

A major difficulty with this strategy is measuring or estimating the lower inflection point of the volume-pressure curve. Obtaining a volume-pressure curve is difficult and unlikely to be carried out routinely in ICUs. It entails paralyzing the patient and using increments in volume while measuring pressure. Identification of the lower inflection "point" from this curve can be difficult and can vary considerably among observers. It has been stated that the lower inflection point, at V_T of 7 to 8 ml/kg, generally occurs at a pressure of 10 to 15 cm H_2O.[32] Therefore, many have assumed that "moderate" levels of PEEP are likely to exceed this value, especially if lower V_Ts are employed, and that actual measurement of the lower inflection point may not be necessary. However, the only published data from a randomized, controlled trial showing benefit used initial mean PEEP levels of 18 cm H_2O, with the goal of PEEP being 2 cm H_2O above the measured lower inflection point.[2] This suggests that the mean lower inflection point and its range may be considerably higher than previously thought and that PEEP of about 10 cm H_2O or slightly higher cannot be assumed to exceed the lower inflection point.

Fluid Management

Perhaps the predominant clinical feature of ARDS is the presence of noncardiogenic pulmonary edema that is a result of increased vascular permeability. In this type of edema, as well as in hemodynamic pulmonary edema, hydrostatic forces can contribute importantly to an increase in total extravascular lung water (EVLW) (Fig. 167-5). Therefore, decreasing intravascular volume, and thereby pressures, might decrease pulmonary edema and improve pulmonary function. However, limiting fluid administration, or even promoting diuresis, can decrease the circulating volume to the point of compromising cardiac output and blood flow to peripheral organs, particularly if high levels of PEEP are used. Because multiple organ failure is a much more common cause of death in ARDS than is respiratory failure, care must be taken not to compromise organ perfusion. Whether fluid loss improves outcome or is simply a marker of resolving pulmonary vascular injury is unclear. Several clinical studies have confirmed that pulmonary function often improves if EVLW or pulmonary artery wedge pressure can be safely reduced.[37] However, it has yet to be confirmed that this management strategy improves clinical outcomes.

As a rule, the administration of albumin intravenously in the attempt to increase intravascular oncotic pressure and reduce EVLW is not helpful. Albumin traverses the highly permeable alveolar-capillary barrier, thereby increasing the protein content of both. As a result, in alveolar and interstitial fluid, oncotic forces can favor an increase in EVLW. Albumin is also expensive, carries some risk of transmission of infectious agents, and has a very short half-life after administration. For these reasons, the routine use of albumin in patients with ARDS as a means of decreasing EVLW is not recommended.

Pharmacologic Therapy

ARDS has resisted pharmacologic manipulation for nearly 30 years. Nonetheless, novel therapeutic approaches continue to be developed. Some of the important potential therapies, new and old, are considered in the sections that follow. For the sake of expediency, drugs are divided into two categories: those that are

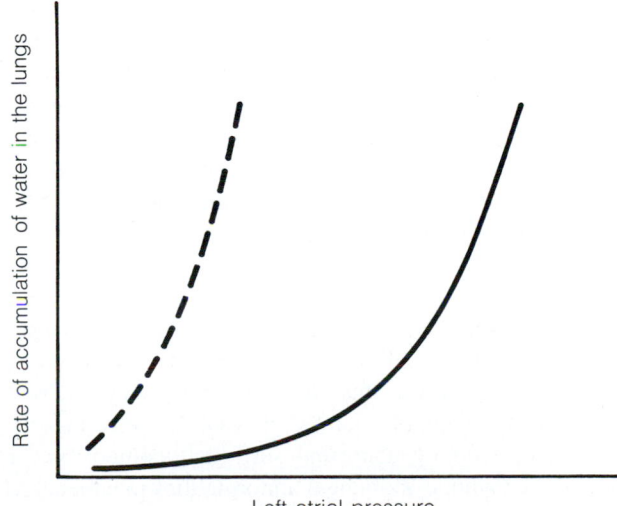

FIGURE 167-5 Hypothetical relationship between left atrial pressure and the rate of accumulation of edema fluid in a normal person (solid line) and in a patient with ARDS (dashed line).

primarily supportive (to correct physiological abnormalities) and those designed to inhibit or reverse acute lung inflammation. These designations are somewhat arbitrary, since several of the drugs, including surfactant, may have overlapping effects. Similarly, inhibiting the inflammatory response might decrease the risks of ventilator-induced lung injury.

DRUGS TO CORRECT PHYSIOLOGICAL ABNORMALITIES

Almitrine

Almitrine is an agent that is administered intravenously to increase respiratory drive and to improve ventilation-perfusion matching, presumably by enhancing hypoxic pulmonary vasoconstriction. When almitrine is administered to patients with ARDS, arterial oxygenation improves and venous admixture decreases. In one study, mean pulmonary artery pressure and cardiac output increased slightly, without significant changes in systemic blood pressure or systemic vascular resistance.[44] No significant adverse effects have been observed during the administration of almitrine. Unfortunately, the effect of the agent is short-lived, and arterial oxygenation returns to baseline shortly after the drug is discontinued. No randomized, controlled trials have been reported concerning the effects of the improvement in oxygenation on survival or the duration of mechanical ventilation.

Nitric Oxide

When inhaled at low concentration, nitric oxide (NO) is a selective pulmonary vasodilator that is limited to ventilated regions of the lungs. The effect reduces intrapulmonary shunting, improves ventilation-perfusion matching, lowers pulmonary artery pressures, and improves arterial oxygenation. When NO is used in conjunction with almitrine, the improvements in gas exchange are greater than those with either agent alone.[45]

Unfortunately, NO is very difficult to administer safely because it requires specialized delivery and monitoring systems. It has been given with success to infants with persistent pulmonary hypertension as well as to adults with pulmonary hypertension. It has also been administered for extended periods to adults with ARDS.[22] In principle, if the improvements in arterial oxygenation brought about by NO enabled a significant reduction in F_{IO_2}, thereby lessening the prospect of pulmonary oxygen toxicity, improvement in survival or a decrease in the duration of mechanical ventilation might be expected. To date, however, there are no data to indicate that the use of NO in ARDS improves survival.

Surfactant

In their landmark article, Ashbaugh and colleagues noted a striking similarity between ARDS and hyaline membrane disease. They went on to postulate that surfactant deficiency might also play a role in the pathophysiology of ARDS.[5] Since that time, ample evidence linking abnormal surfactant composition and function to the pathophysiological abnormalities in patients with ARDS has accumulated.[25] Mechanisms for this include decreased surfactant production due to alveolar type II cell injury, as well as inactivation and destruction of existing or newly formed surfactant.

Several anecdotal reports and small series in the literature describe the successful treatment of ARDS with various surfactant products. Also, two small randomized, controlled trials yielded encouraging results. Subsequently, however, a large trial of surfactant replacement by aerosol indicated that the agent was ineffective against sepsis-induced ARDS.[4] The surfactant product used in this trial was artificial without protein moieties; this deficiency may have contributed to the disappointing results. The possibility has also been raised that aerosolization was inadequate in delivering surfactant to the distal airspaces.

Although other surfactant products and delivery techniques continue to be studied, it appears unlikely that surfactant replacement—so successful in neonatal respiratory distress syndrome—will have dramatic therapeutic effects in ARDS. Unlike neonatal ARDS, surfactant dysfunction is only part of the problem in ARDS—in which it is a result, not the cause, of acute lung injury. On the other hand, surfactant appears to have several anti-inflammatory effects that may enhance its therapeutic effectiveness beyond what was originally hypothesized. Until proven otherwise, surfactant replacement remains experimental and cannot be recommended for the treatment of ARDS.

Perfluorocarbons

The idea of liquid ventilation performed by instilling liquids into the lungs has been around for many years. Perfluorocarbons are liquids that consist primarily of fluorinated carbon chains, are biologically and chemically inert, and are probably free of toxic metabolites; they also have low surface tension and high density. Oxygen and carbon dioxide are highly soluble in these perfluorocarbon liquids. Recent clinical trials with perflubron, one type of perfluorocarbon liquid, have demonstrated the safety and efficacy of a technique called partial liquid ventilation (PLV).[27] This method entails introducing liquid to fill the functional residual capacity and ventilating with tidal volumes of gas. PLV has been reported to improve oxygenation and survival in infants with severe RDS after surfactant replacement and conventional management have failed. Perflubron PLV has also been reported to be safe, to improve pulmonary compliance, and to decrease physiological shunting in patients with ARDS receiving extracorporeal life support. Complications of this therapy include pneumothorax and formation of mucous plugs. A randomized clinical trial is currently under way in patients with ALI and ARDS to determine whether outcomes are also improved by PLV.

DRUGS USED TO SUPPRESS LUNG INFLAMMATION

Corticosteroids

Although corticosteroid therapy has been widely used in the treatment of respiratory failure, recent well-controlled clinical trials have failed to demonstrate any clear benefit either in the early treatment or in the prevention of ARDS.[9] Randomized, controlled trials have also failed to confirm a previous report that suggested a beneficial effect of corticosteroids in sepsis. In fact, in some of these trials, the use of corticosteroids in early ARDS and sepsis was associated with an increased number of deleterious consequences, including prolonged mechanical ventilation, nosocomial infection, and death.

In addition to reducing inflammation, corticosteroids may suppress collagen formation and facilitate collagen breakdown; for this reason, steroids are used in many fibrotic diseases of the lungs. Consequently, corticosteroids may have a beneficial effect on the fibroproliferative stage of ARDS, leading several researchers to attempt treatment of so-called chronic ARDS with high-dose corticosteroids. Several small series have demonstrated a consistently high survival rate.[35] Unfortunately, in addition to being small, these studies were neither randomized nor controlled, so firm conclusions cannot be drawn. A large, multicenter, randomized, controlled trial is now under way to assess the effect of corticosteroids in late-phase ARDS. Unless there are specific indications, generally related to the underlying illness, the routine use of corticosteroids is not currently recommended in patients with ARDS.

Prostaglandins

Prostaglandin E$_1$ (PGE$_1$) is a vasodilator with weak anti-inflammatory properties that has been shown to lower pulmonary artery pressures and increase cardiac output in ARDS. Additionally, it can inhibit platelet aggregation and modulate neutrophil-mediated inflammatory responses. Because the drug is 95 percent metabolized during a single pass through the lung, PGE$_1$ can be a selective pulmonary vasodilator with minimal effects on the systemic vasculature. PGE$_1$ can therefore result in decreased pulmonary hypertension and lung inflammation. Despite earlier reports of improved survival in ARDS patients treated with PGE$_1$, a subsequent multicenter, controlled trial showed no reduction in ARDS severity, duration, or mortality.[11] Cardiac output and oxygen delivery were improved in the treated group. Several patients developed systemic hypotension in response to PGE$_1$ despite its purportedly selective properties.

Another study concerning treatment with PGE$_1$ demonstrated a decrease in arterial oxygenation and an increase in intrapulmonary shunting despite a decrease in pulmonary arterial pressures. In response to the possibility that the failure to find a beneficial effect may have been due to limited access of the drug to inflammatory sites, a small phase II study of liposomal PGE$_1$ was undertaken. This study revealed improved oxygenation, increased lung compliance, and decreased ventilator dependency in the treated group.[1]

Aerosolized prostacyclin (PGI$_2$) has also been reported to improve ventilation-perfusion matching by selectively dilating pulmonary vessels that serve ventilated regions of lung.[51] This improvement was accompanied by decreases in pulmonary arterial pressures, with only minimal effect on systemic blood pressures. The efficacy of PGI$_2$ on gas exchange is similar to that achieved with inhaled NO.[51] A randomized, controlled trial looking at mortality has not yet been undertaken.

Ketoconazole

Ketoconazole is a synthetic imidazole derivative approved for use as an antifungal agent. Ketoconazole is also a potent in vitro inhibitor of several proinflammatory pathways in macrophages. Moreover, it is both a thromboxane synthetase inhibitor and a 5-lipoxygenase inhibitor, thereby blocking the synthesis of prostaglandins and leukotrienes that can promote lung inflammation. Two preliminary studies have suggested that ketocona-zole may be effective in reducing the incidence of ARDS in critically ill surgical patients.[48,53] In high-risk patients, one study showed a decrease in the incidence of ARDS from 31 percent to 6 percent; the decrease in mortality from 42 percent to 31 percent was statistically insignificant.[48] The second study demonstrated a decrease in the incidence of ARDS from 64 percent to 15 percent, accompanied by a significant decrease in mortality, from 39 percent to 15 percent.[53] Although both of these studies on surgical patients included multiple trauma, other causes were also represented. On the basis of these encouraging results, a multicenter trial sponsored by the NIH is being conducted to test whether ketoconazole is effective as a treatment for early ALI and ARDS.

Other Agents

Other modulators of the inflammatory response—including pentoxifylline, lisophylline, ibuprofen, antioxidants, neutrophil elastase inhibitors, and antibodies directed against endotoxin, complement fragments, interleukin-1, and tumor necrosis factor—have recently been studied or are currently being studied. Other cytokine agonists and antagonists, such as an anti–IL-8 antibody, are likely to be studied. So far, none of these therapies can be recommended for the routine treatment of ARDS.

CLINICAL COURSE AND OUTCOME

Pathophysiological Changes

The pathophysiological abnormalities associated with ARDS include impaired gas exchange, altered lung mechanics, and pulmonary vascular changes. Although the course of illness varies in severity from patient to patient, patients are often profoundly hypoxemic during the early, exudative phase of ARDS. Severe pulmonary edema is a common problem during early ARDS as fluid leaves the vascular space through the porous alveolar-capillary membranes. Alveoli become atelectatic and filled with exudate and hyaline membranes, resulting in profound hypoxemia with a high degree of intrapulmonary shunting.[15,31] Patients often require high levels of inspired oxygen during this phase of the illness and can be quite responsive to PEEP therapy.

As ARDS evolves, fibroproliferation becomes a predominant feature, while pulmonary edema tends to resolve as the alveolar epithelial lining is reconstituted. Loss of minute pulmonary vessels leads to increased dead-space ventilation and pulmonary hypertension. Ventilation-perfusion abnormalities cause arterial hypoxemia. The lungs may become fibrotic and very noncompliant. Carbon dioxide elimination may be quite impaired, even while oxygenation is improving. At this time, patients respond less well to the application of PEEP, but they usually require lower concentrations of inspired oxygen. Many patients develop severe fibrotic lung disease and respiratory insufficiency that often end in death. In patients who survive, the lungs undergo remodeling and healing that are accompanied by gradual improvement in lung compliance and reduction in minute ventilation; eventually these patients can therefore resume unassisted ventilation.

Duration and Complications of Mechanical Ventilation

Once a patient develops ARDS, the course is extremely variable, lasting from a few days to several months. Even when the underlying illness or injury resolves and the patient responds readily to supportive therapy, the course usually lasts several days. In contrast, patients with cardiogenic pulmonary edema who respond to therapy experience improvement within a few hours to days.

The mean duration of mechanical ventilation in ARDS is generally 10 to 14 days; approximately 10 to 20 percent of patients remain ventilator dependent for longer than 3 weeks.[38,47] Most patients who die with ARDS do so within the first 2 weeks of their illness.[38,47] Recovery for survivors can take several weeks or longer. In fact, the duration of mechanical ventilation is inversely correlated with survival. The survival rate of patients on mechanical ventilation after 3 weeks of ARDS is very high. In one study, 95 percent of the nonsurvivors had died by 5 weeks and the survival of patients remaining in the hospital after 5 weeks was independent of ventilator status.[47]

One significant complication in patients with ARDS is pulmonary barotrauma with resultant pneumothorax (Figs. 167-6 and 167-7). Although the frequency of barotrauma in mechanically ventilated patients with ARDS has been correlated with the level of peak airway pressure and with the use of large tidal volumes, the frequency is probably related to the severity of the underlying lung injury.[43] The pathogenesis probably involves overdistention of lung regions that have already been structurally weakened by alveolar inflammation. Subsequent rupture of overdistended alveoli leads to the tracking of gas along bronchovascular bundles into the mediastinum. Continued air leakage may result in further soft-tissue dissection into retroperitoneal and subcutaneous tissues, or the accumulated mediastinal emphysema may rupture across the thin mediastinal pleura, causing pneumothorax. In patients on positive-pressure ventilation, immediate placement of a chest tube is essential to avoid the life-threatening complications of a tension pneumothorax. If appropriately treated, barotrauma does not appear to be associated independently with poor outcomes.

Other complications of mechanical ventilation in patients with ARDS are nosocomial pneumonia, sinusitis, and local damage to the airway.[43] Laryngeal injury, when it occurs, usually develops very early in the course and is probably not related to the duration of intubation. The issue of timing and the necessity of tracheostomy are controversial. For patients with prolonged mechanical ventilation, tracheostomy can improve comfort, decrease the risk of sinusitis, and increase the security of the airway. Early tracheostomy probably does not decrease the risk of trauma to the larynx. Because of the use of low-pressure, high-volume cuffs on endotracheal tubes, tracheomalacia, tracheoesophageal fistulas, and erosion into the innominate artery are seen far less frequently now than previously but continue to occur as occasional complications in the ICU.[43]

Fatality Rate

Until recently (see below), fatality rates of ARDS have been reported to be very high, generally in excess of 50 percent; in patients more than 60 years old and in those with sepsis-induced ARDS, fatality rates were reported to be even higher.[36,47] In these reports, factors contributing to mortality were the severity of underlying illness as reflected in the injury severity score in trauma patients, or advanced malignancy, and the presence or development of multiple organ failure. Although the severity of the initial lung injury, measured as an index of gas exchange, such as the Pa_{O_2}/FI_{O_2} ratio or a composite lung injury score, is not indicative of outcome, improvement in Pa_{O_2}/FI_{O_2} ratio over the first 3 days to 1 week is associated with improved survival.[40,47]

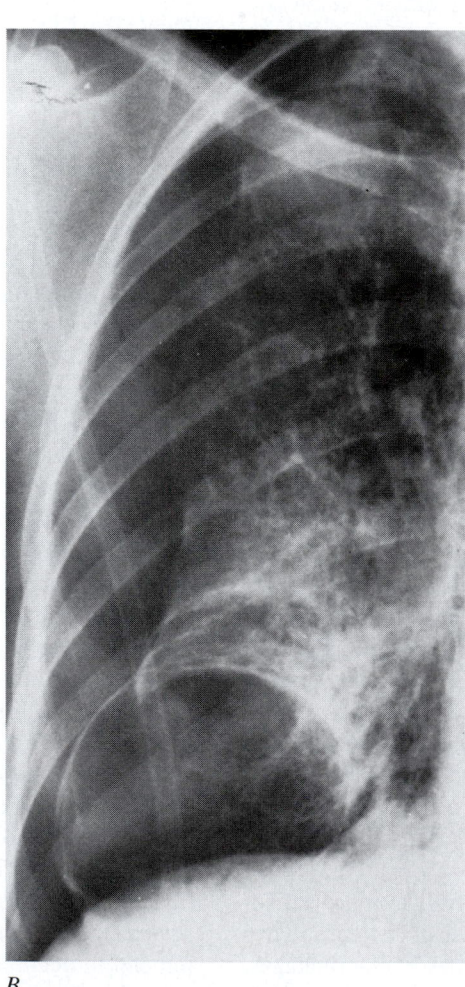

A   *B*

FIGURE 167-6 Subpleural air cysts in a 46-year-old woman with ARDS. *A.* After 4 weeks of mechanical ventilation, subpleural cysts appeared at the base of the lung and grew rapidly. *B.* Two days later, the patient developed a pneumothorax on the right. Note the thin lateral wall of the cyst.

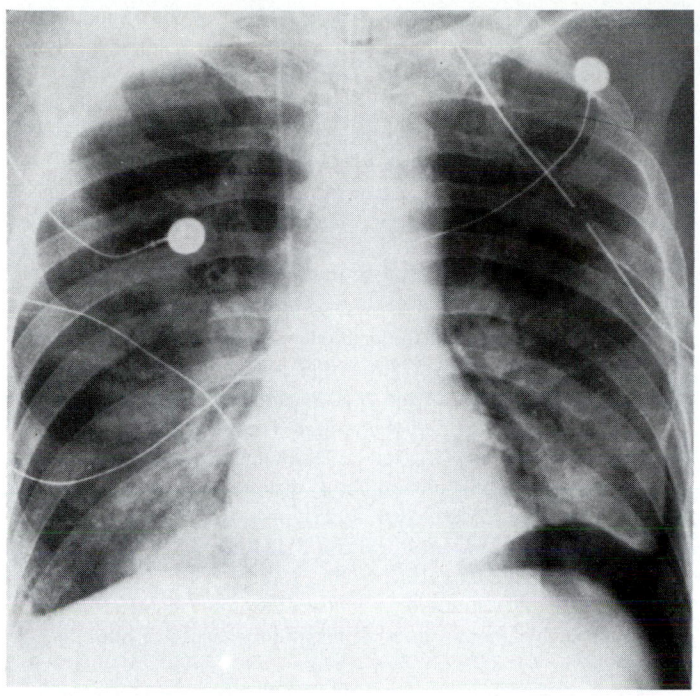

FIGURE 167-7   Pneumomediastinum in a patient with ARDS. An associated pneumothorax on the left has been partly evacuated; its margins are sharply outlined by the opacified left lung.

A recent analysis at one institution of temporal trends in ARDS fatality rates indicates a decrease in fatality rates since 1989, reaching a nadir of 36 percent in 1993.[36] This observation applied to all risk groups but was most notable in patients with sepsis-induced ARDS and in those less than 60 years of age. This improvement was in the face of APACHE-II scores indicating that the severity of illness at the onset of ARDS had not changed in recent years. Other investigators have also reported a reduction in mortality in patients with ARDS enrolled in control or placebo arms of clinical trials.

Causes of Death

One-third of the deaths in ARDS patients are related to the underlying disease or injury—that is, deaths caused by events occurring before the onset of ARDS.[38] Patients who die of their underlying illnesses usually succumb early in the course of ARDS, often within the first 3 days. Only a relatively small percentage of patients—6 to 11 percent of all ARDS patients in two studies—die a respiratory death due to irreversible hypoxemia or refractory respiratory acidosis. The remaining deaths are due to complications that have their onset either coincident with or after the onset of ARDS; these deaths often occur later in the course of ARDS. The most common cause of death in these patients is sepsis and associated multiple organ system failure.

A recent study in our clinic suggests that recent improvements in survival may be due to decreased death from complications of respiratory failure. The proportion of patients dying early from their underlying illness or injury remains unchanged, whereas improvement in survival is seen in patients who survive beyond 3 days. Although most deaths are still due to sepsis and multi-ple organ failure, the actual death rate from these and other complications is declining. Since more patients are surviving prolonged courses of ARDS, these data underline the importance of supportive care and diligence in preventing and treating the complications of acute respiratory failure.

Sequelae

An early impression held by many investigators and clinicians was that pulmonary function in most survivors returned to normal or near-normal levels. Studies of function in ARDS survivors are difficult to perform because they require long-term follow-up and a high degree of patient cooperation. This is further complicated by the fact that many patients do not live in the city where they were hospitalized, since they may have been transported to institutions with the specialized ability to manage patients with ARDS.

Several recent studies have demonstrated that the picture is generally bright.[23,34] Nearly all patients have reached maximal recovery by 6 months after endotracheal extubation, with only a few subjects undergoing further improvement after that time. Thus, 6 months following extubation could be used as a single time point for evaluation of pulmonary function recovery after ARDS. Although pulmonary function markedly improves in most patients during their recovery, approximately half of the patients continue to have some abnormality of pulmonary function at this 6-month point. This abnormality generally consists of either a mild restrictive impairment or, more often, a mild impairment in diffusing capacity; however, more marked abnormalities do occur. These patients who have continuing pulmonary dysfunction are more apt to have had a more severe course of ARDS, identified either from failure of physiological variables to improve several days into the course of ARDS or from the duration of mechanical ventilation.[34] Occasionally, but fortunately rarely, patients continue to have severe pulmonary functional abnormalities and may require long-term home oxygen therapy. Finally, although survivors of ARDS continue to have impairments in overall physical and psychosocial function, these are usually mild, are not perceived by the patients to be related to their pulmonary condition, and are often related to other aspects of their acute injury or illness.[34]

REFERENCES

1. Abraham E, Park YC, Covington P, et al: Liposomal prostaglandin E$_1$ in acute respiratory distress syndrome: A placebo-controlled, randomized, double-blind, multicenter clinical trial. *Crit Care Med* 24:10–15, 1996.
2. Amato MBP, Barbas CSV, Medeiros DM, et al: Beneficial effects of the "open lung approach" with low distending pressures in acute respiratory distress syndrome. *Am J Respir Crit Care Med* 152:1835–1846, 1995.
3. Amato MBP, Barbas CSV, Medeiros D, et al: Improved survival in ARDS: Beneficial effects of a lung protective strategy (abstract). *Am J Respir Crit Care Med* 153:A531, 1996.
4. Anzueto A, Baughman RP, Guntupalli KK, et al: Aerosolized surfactant in adults with sepsis-induced acute respiratory distress syndrome. *New Engl J Med* 334:1417–1421, 1996.

5. Ashbaugh DG, Bigelow DB, Petty TL, Levine BE: Acute respiratory distress in adults. *Lancet* 2:319–323, 1967.

6. Baughman RP, Gunther KL, Rashkin MC, et al: Changes in the inflammatory response of the lung during acute respiratory distress syndrome—Prognostic indicators. *Am J Respir Crit Care Med* 154:76–81, 1996.

7. Bendixen HH, Hedley-Whyte J, Laver MB: Impaired oxygenation in surgical patients during general anesthesia with controlled ventilation. *New Engl J Med* 269:991–997, 1963.

8. Bernard GR, Artigas A, Brigham KL, et al, and the Consensus Committee: The American-European Consensus Conference on ARDS: Definitions, mechanisms, relevant outcomes, and clinical trial coordination. *Am J Respir Crit Care Med* 149:818–824, 1994.

9. Bernard GR, Luce JM, Sprung CL, et al: High-dose corticosteroids in patients with the adult respiratory distress syndrome. *New Engl J Med* 317:1565–1570, 1987.

10. Bone RC, Balk RA, Cerra FB, et al, and the ACCP/SCCM Consensus Conference Committee: Definitions for sepsis and organ failure and guidelines for the use of innovative therapies in sepsis. *Chest* 101:1644–1655, 1992.

11. Bone RC, Slotman G, Maunder R, et al: Randomized double-blind, multicenter study of prostaglandin E$_1$ in patients with adult respiratory distress syndrome. *Chest* 96:114–119, 1989.

12. Clark JG, Hansen JA, Hertz MI, et al: Idiopathic pneumonia syndrome after bone marrow transplantation. *Am Rev Respir Dis* 147:1601–1606, 1993.

13. Clark JG, Milberg JA, Steinberg KP, Hudson LD: Type III procollagen peptide in adult respiratory distress syndrome: Association of elevated peptide levels in lavage with increased risk of death. *Ann Intern Med* 122:17–23, 1995.

14. Corbridge TC, Wood LDH, Crawford GP, et al: Adverse effects of large tidal volumes and low PEEP in canine acid aspiration. *Am Rev Respir Dis* 142:311–315, 1990.

15. Dantzker DR, Brook CJ, DeHart P, et al: Ventilation-perfusion distributions in the adult respiratory distress syndrome. *Am Rev Respir Dis* 120:1039–1052, 1979.

16. Doyle RL, Szaflarski N, Modin GW, et al: Identification of patients with acute lung injury—Predictors of mortality. *Am J Respir Crit Care Med* 152:1818–1824, 1995.

17. Dreyfuss D, Soler P, Basset G, et al: High inflation pressure pulmonary edema: Respective effects of high airway pressure, high tidal volume, and positive end-expiratory pressure. *Am Rev Respir Dis* 137:1159–1164, 1988.

18. Dreyfuss D, Soler P, Saumon G: Mechanical ventilation-induced pulmonary edema: Interaction with previous lung alterations. *Am J Respir Crit Care Med* 151:1568–1575, 1995.

19. Fowler AA, Hamman RF, Good JT, et al: Adult respiratory distress syndrome: Risk with common predispositions. *Ann Intern Med* 98:593–597, 1983.

20. Garber BG, Hébert PC, Yelle J-D, et al: Adult respiratory distress syndrome: A systematic overview of incidence and risk factors. *Crit Care Med* 24:687–695, 1996.

21. Gattinoni L, Mascheroni D, Tomesin A, et al: Morphological response to positive end expiratory pressure in acute respiratory failure: Computerized tomography study. *Intensive Care Med* 12:137–142, 1986.

22. Gerlach H, Pappert D, Lewandowski K, et al: Long-term inhalation with evaluated low doses of nitric oxide for selective improvement of oxygenation in patients with adult respiratory distress syndrome. *Intensive Care Med* 19:443–449, 1993.

23. Ghio AJ, Elliott CG, Crapo RO, et al: Impairment after adult respiratory distress syndrome: An evaluation based on American Thoracic Society recommendations. *Am Rev Respir Dis* 139:1158–1162, 1989.

24. Goodman RB, Strieter RM, Martin DP, et al: Inflammatory cytokines in patients with persistence of the acute respiratory distress syndrome. *Am J Respir Crit Care Med* 154:602–611, 1996.

25. Gregory TJ, Longmore WJ, Moxley MA, et al: Surfactant chemical composition and biophysical activity in acute respiratory distress syndrome. *J Clin Invest* 88:1976–1981, 1991.

26. Hickling KG, Walsh J, Henderson S, et al: Low mortality rate in adult respiratory distress syndrome using low-volume, pressure limited ventilation with permissive hypercapnia: A prospective study. *Crit Care Med* 22:1568–1578, 1994.

27. Hirschl RB, Pranikoff T, Wise C, et al: Initial experience with partial liquid ventilation in adult patients with the acute respiratory distress syndrome. *JAMA* 275:383–389, 1996.

28. Hudson LD: Causes of the adult respiratory distress syndrome—Clinical recognition. *Clin Chest Med* 3:195–212, 1982.

29. Hudson LD, Milberg JA, Anardi D, Maunder RJ: Clinical risks for development of the acute respiratory distress syndrome. *Am J Respir Crit Care Med* 151:293–301, 1995.

30. Katzenstein AA, Myers JL, Mazur MT: Acute interstitial pneumonia. *Am J Surg Pathol* 10:256–267, 1986.

31. Lamy M, Fallat RJ, Koeniger E, et al: Pathologic features and mechanisms of hypoxemia in adult respiratory distress syndrome. *Am Rev Respir Dis* 114:267–284, 1976.

32. Marini JJ: Evolving concepts in the ventilatory management of acute respiratory distress syndrome. *Clin Chest Med* 17:555–575, 1996.

33. Maunder RJ, Shuman WP, McHugh JW, et al: Preservation of normal lung regions in the adult respiratory distress syndrome: Analysis by computed tomography. *JAMA* 255:2463–2465, 1986.

34. McHugh LG, Milberg JA, Whitcomb ME, et al: Recovery of function in survivors of the acute respiratory distress syndrome. *Am J Respir Crit Care Med* 150:90–94, 1994.

35. Meduri GU, Chinn AJ, Leeper KV, et al: Corticosteroid rescue treatment of progressive fibroproliferation in late ARDS: Patterns of response and predictors of outcome. *Chest* 105:1516–1527, 1994.

36. Milberg JA, Davis DA, Steinberg KP, Hudson LD: Improved survival of patients with acute respiratory distress syndrome (ARDS): 1983–1993. *JAMA* 273:306–309, 1995.

37. Mitchell JP, Schuller D, Calandrino FS, Schuster DP: Improved outcome based on fluid management in critically ill patients requiring pulmonary artery catheterization. *Am Rev Respir Dis* 145:990–998, 1992.

38. Montgomery AB, Stager MA, Carrico CJ, Hudson LD: Causes of mortality in patients with the adult respiratory distress syndrome. *Am Rev Respir Dis* 132:485–489, 1985.

39. Moss M, Bucher B, Moore FA, et al: The role of chronic alcohol abuse in the development of acute respiratory distress syndrome in adults. *JAMA* 275:50–54, 1996.

40. Moss M, Goodman PL, Heinig M, et al: Establishing the relative accuracy of three new definitions of the adult respiratory distress syndrome. *Crit Care Med* 23:1629–1637, 1995.

41. Murray JF, Matthay MA, Luce JM, Flick MR: An expanded definition of the adult respiratory distress syndrome. *Am Rev Respir Dis* 138:720–723, 1988.

42. Pepe PE, Potkin RT, Holtman Reus D, et al: Clinical predictors of the adult respiratory distress syndrome. *Am J Surg* 144:124–130, 1982.

43. Pingleton SK: Complications of acute respiratory failure. *Am Rev Respir Dis* 137:1463–1493, 1988.

44. Reyes A, Lopez-Messa JB, Alonso P: Almitrine in acute respiratory failure: Effects on pulmonary gas exchange and circulation. *Chest* 91:388–393, 1987.

45. Rossaint R, Falke KJ, Lopez F, et al: Inhaled nitric oxide for the adult respiratory distress syndrome. *New Engl J Med* 328:399–405, 1993.

46. Sauaia A, Moore FA, Moore EE, et al: Early predictors of postinjury multiple organ failure. *Arch Surg* 129:39–45, 1994.

47. Sloane PJ, Gee MH, Gottlieb JE, et al: A multicenter registry of patients with acute respiratory distress syndrome. *Am Rev Respir Dis* 2:419–426, 1992.

48. Slotman GJ, Burchard KW, D'Arezzo A, Gann DS: Ketoconazole prevents acute respiratory failure in critically ill surgical patients. *J Trauma* 28:648–654, 1988.

49. Smith G, Winter PM, Wheelis RF: Increased normobaric oxygen tolerance of rabbits following oleic acid–induced lung damage. *J Appl Physiol* 35:395–400, 1973.

50. Steinberg KP, Milberg JA, Maunder RJ, et al: Evolution of bronchoalveolar cell populations in the adult respiratory distress syndrome. *Am J Respir Crit Care Med* 150:113–122, 1994.

51. Walmrath D, Schneider T, Schermuly R, et al: Direct comparison of inhaled nitric oxide and aerosolized prostacyclin in acute respiratory distress syndrome. *Am J Respir Crit Care Med* 153:991–996, 1996.

52. Webb HH, Tierney DF: Experimental pulmonary edema due to intermittent positive pressure ventilation with high inflation pressures: Protection by positive end-expiratory pressure. *Am Rev Respir Dis* 110:556–565, 1974.

53. Yu M, Tomasa G: A double-blind, prospective, randomized trial of ketoconazole, a thromboxane synthetase inhibitor, in the prophylaxis of the adult respiratory distress syndrome. *Crit Care Med* 21:1635–1644, 1993.

CHAPTER 168

THE SYSTEMIC INFLAMMATORY RESPONSE SYNDROME AND THE MULTIPLE ORGAN DYSFUNCTION SYNDROME

Clifford S. Deutschman

DEFINITIONS, NATURAL HISTORY, AND EPIDEMIOLOGY
  The "Stress"/SIRS/Sepsis Syndrome/MODS Continuum
  Clinical Patterns of SIRS/MODS
  Epidemiology of SIRS/MODS

PATHOPHYSIOLOGY
  Altered Physiology and Metabolism
  Hypotheses

MANAGEMENT
  Pulmonary Dysfunction
  Perfusion Management
  Rational Use of Inotropes and Vasopressors
  Metabolic Management

CONCLUSION

The systemic inflammatory response syndrome (SIRS) and multiple organ dysfunction syndrome (MODS) are diseases of medical progress. Before the advances in critical care medicine that have characterized the past 3 decades, SIRS and MODS were unknown. However, the ability to treat shock, manage acute renal insufficiency, support pulmonary failure, and even transplant organs such as the liver has unmasked this new syndrome. Indeed, the initial reports of MODS, which was at the time called *sequential system failure* or *multiple system organ failure*[5,26,29,51] heralded the ability to rescue patients from such diverse catastrophic events as ruptured abdominal aortic aneurysms, severe trauma, pancreatitis, multiple transfusion, and progressive infections. Attempts to manage MODS have led, in turn, to a host of important biochemical, metabolic, and physiological discoveries.

This chapter defines the clinical findings that constitute SIRS/MODS and places these disorders in context by relating them to a continuum of clinical abnormalities and syndromes and briefly reviewing the natural history. Several pathogenic hypotheses, management strategies, and intriguing new forms of therapy are examined.

DEFINITIONS, NATURAL HISTORY, AND EPIDEMIOLOGY

The "Stress"/SIRS/Sepsis Syndrome/MODS Continuum

There is a characteristic response to inflammatory stimuli, such as surgery and trauma, that has classically been referred to as *the stress response*.[20] The importance of this response is that it has evolved to facilitate survival and repair. Initially, an orchestrated neural-endocrine-humoral response directs substrate delivery to the most vital organs, the heart and brain. This is accomplished by vasoconstriction, fluid retention, and translocation of intracellular water to the vasculature. In the absence of exogenous support, death will ensue from shock if these endogenous mechanisms are insufficient. Following resuscitation from this initial period of shock, hypermetabolism develops.[16] The driving force behind this second phase is the repair of damaged tissue, and white blood cells are the primary effectors of this process.[15] To support the increased white cell mass, substrate is mobilized from endogenous sources and glucose reserves are rapidly depleted. Because white cells are obligate glucose users, muscle (both skeletal and smooth) is broken down to provide precursors for hepatic gluconeogenesis. In addition, amino acids are used to synthesize structural proteins and enzymes. Energy to support the liver, heart, and other organs is derived from fat and amino acids, since there appears to be a block to the utilization of glucose by tissues other than blood cells and neurons. To allow glucose delivery to avascular wound tissue, there is a generalized capillary recruitment and leak. The amount of fluid in the extracellular compartment, particularly the extravascular matrix, increases dramatically. Continued fluid retention and movement of water out of cells are essential to fill the dilated, leaky vasculature. Vasodilatation is accompanied by an increase in cardiac output, which further facilitates substrate delivery. By the fourth day after injury, neovascularization of damaged tissue has occurred. As substrate delivery to the newly vascularized wound tissue increases sharply, there is a decrease in capillary leak, generalized increases in vascular tone, and mobilization and excretion of the fluid in the matrix. Water also returns to cells, and in most cases the patient recovers uneventfully.

In an unknown percentage of patients, the inflammatory process becomes persistent, progressing to become the SIRS, which is defined by the presence of two or more of the criteria listed in Table 168-1.[11] These findings, however, are almost universally observed after major surgery or trauma and are part of a normal stress response. Therefore, the hallmark of SIRS is persistence of these findings beyond 3 to 5 days.[7] In general, SIRS is associated with a persistent inflammatory source such as a nidus of infection or an undrained hematoma. Such occurrences generally reflect extensive trauma, delayed resuscitation, surgery complicated by extensive, rapid blood loss, or inflammation such as occurs with pancreatitis or aspiration pneumonitis. If a clear source of infection is present, the disorder is classified as sepsis. Further subclassifications of sepsis are detailed in Table 168-2. While SIRS/sepsis may be complicated by hypotension, lactic acidosis, acute lung injury, or oliguria, clear organ dysfunction is not present. When abnormalities of organ function develop, the syndrome is termed MODS.

The organ systems affected in MODS include the pulmonary, hepatic, renal, cardiovascular, hematologic, nervous, gastrointestinal, and immunologic. Defining which abnormalities in individual organs constitute dysfunction, however, is problematic. Although many different criteria have been used, none is universally accepted.[22] Indeed, an ACCP/SCCM Consensus Conference Committee declined to recommend the adoption of any specific definitions.[11] There is a reasonable explanation for this. Just as MODS falls on a continuum of abnormalities, so there is a spectrum of abnormalities in each organ system. The transition from adaptive response to dysfunction may be clinically obscure, and the distinction between SIRS and MODS is often simply semantic. (See Chapters 166 and 167 for detailed descriptions of acute respiratory insufficiency and acute respiratory distress syndrome [ARDS].) Some generally used criteria for organ dysfunction in other systems are detailed in Table 168-3.

While SIRS/MODS was presumed for quite some time to reflect an underlying source of infection, this is no longer believed to be true. SIRS/MODS requires a persistent source of inflammation, but this need not result from the effects of microorganisms. The second key point has to do with the host's role in the inflammatory process. While once thought to be an "innocent bystander" in the "septic" process, it is now clear that the patient—in particular, the patient's im-

mune system—is an important and active participant in SIRS/MODS. (See "Cytokine Hypothesis," below.)

Clinical Patterns of SIRS/MODS

There are two well-defined forms of SIRS/MODS (Fig. 168-1).[7] In either, the development of acute lung injury or ARDS is of key importance to the natural history. ARDS is the earliest manifestation in almost all cases. In the more common form of SIRS/MODS, the lungs are the predominant, and often only, organ system affected until very late in the disease. This primary pulmonary form of MODS is identical to ARDS and, as such, is described in depth elsewhere. It is important to point out, however, that the natural history of patients with this type of MODS is well established. These patients most often will present with a primary pulmonary affliction (pneumonia, aspiration, contusion, near-drowning, COPD exacerbation, hemorrhage, pulmonary embolism), but the disorder may also occur following burns, trauma, or surgery[42] and will progress to meet criteria for ARDS. Pulmonary dysfunction, often accompanied by encephalopathy and a mild coagulopathy, will persist for approximately 2 to 3 weeks. At that time, the patient will either begin to recover or progress to develop fulminant dysfunction in another organ system, most often hepatic, renal, or cardiovascular.[7] A high proportion of these last patients will not survive. The pulmonary origin of this form of SIRS/MODS is diagnostically useful, since the population at risk often can be defined to some extent.

Diagnosis of the second form of SIRS/MODS is the more problematic. While the earliest manifestation of the syndrome remains pulmonary, these patients most often have an inciting source remote from the lung. Thus, this group consists of patients with major trauma (including isolated head injury),

TABLE 168-1

Criteria for the Diagnosis of the Systemic Inflammatory Response Syndrome

Temperature $> 38°C$ or $< 36°C$
Heart rate > 90 beats/min
Respiratory rate > 20 breaths/min or $P_{CO_2} < 32$ mmHg
White count $> 12 \times 10^9$/L or $< 4 \times 10^9$/L or $> 10\%$ immature forms

SOURCE: Adapted from Bone et al.[11]

TABLE 168-2

Subclassifications of Sepsis

Sepsis: Systemic inflammatory response to infection

Severe sepsis: Sepsis associated with organ dysfunction, hypoperfusion, or hypotension (including lactic acidosis, oliguria, altered mental status)

Septic shock: Sepsis-induced hypotension despite adequate fluid resuscitation + presence of perfusion abnormalities. If pressors or inotropes are required to maintain normotension or normal perfusion, the patient is in septic shock.

Sepsis-induced hypotension: Systolic blood pressure < 90 mmHg or a reduction of ≥ 40 mmHg from baseline in the absence of other causes of hypotension

SOURCE: Adapted from Bone et al.[11]

intra-abdominal sepsis, extensive blood loss, pancreatitis, vascular catastrophes such as ruptured or dissecting aneurysms, and a host of other conditions.[7,42] Acute lung injury and ARDS develop early, but dysfunction in other organs soon becomes evident. Most studies have found the liver to be the second organ to become affected.[22] Indeed, if one considers bleeding associated with elevation of the prothrombin time to be an abnormality of the hepatic and not the hematologic system, the liver may well become dysfunctional even in cases classified as primary pulmonary MODS. Gastrointestinal, cardiovascular, and renal dysfunction are equally cited as the third system involved. Patients remain in a pattern of compensated dysfunction for several weeks and then either recover or deteriorate further and die.[7] The diversity of the population at risk makes early diagnosis of the second form of SIRS/MODS difficult. Further, most of these patients undergo some surgical procedure. Development of mild hypoxemia and increased lung water is a normal finding after surgery, and incipient ARDS may therefore go unrecognized. Thus, SIRS/MODS may not be recognized until dysfunction in several organ systems has become well established. This may be an important determinant of poor outcome.

Epidemiology of SIRS/MODS

It is exceedingly difficult to determine the incidence of SIRS/MODS. This primarily reflects the diverse etiology of the syndromes. The epidemiology of primary pulmonary SIRS/MODS—i.e., ARDS—is discussed in Chapters 166 and 167, but the incidence is estimated to be in excess of 150,000 cases a year.[7] With regards to the second, multiorgan form of SIRS/MODS, the most useful data are derived from trauma patients and have recently been reviewed by Regel and associates.[49] Unfortunately, this is a diffuse and heterogeneous group. On the basis of these data, however, the incidence of MODS following trauma severe enough to warrant admission to an ICU appears to be about 14 percent.

Mortality from MODS remains distressingly high. Estimated mortality from ARDS alone is approximately 50 percent.[47] In the study by Regel and colleagues, the involvement of additional organ systems increases the incidence of poor outcome, so the presence of dysfunction in more than three systems virtually assures death.[38,49] Several other studies have reported lower death rates.[3,40] These data clearly reflect the lack of consensus on definitions of organ dysfunction. Other investigations have demonstrated that mortality is also a function of the length of time that patients are in organ failure.

TABLE 168-3

Some Generally Used Criteria for Organ Dysfunction

	Mild	*Severe*
Pulmonary	Hypoxia/hypercarbia requiring assisted ventilation for 3–5 days	ARDS requiring PEEP $\geq$ 10 cm H_2O and $F_{I_{O_2}}$ $\geq$ 0.5
Hepatic	Bilirubin 2–3 mg/dl or other liver function tests > twice normal, PT elevated to twice normal	Jaundice with bilirubin 8–10 mg/dl
Renal	Oliguria (<500 ml/day) or increasing creatinine (2–3 mg/dl)	Dialysis
Gastrointestinal	Intolerance of gastric feeding > 5 days	Stress ulceration with need for transfusion, acalculous cholecystitis
Hematologic	PTT $\geq$ 125% of normal, platelets < 50,000–80,000	DIC
CNS	Confusion	Coma
PNS	Mild sensory neuropathy	Combined motor and sensory deficit
Cardiovascular	Decreased ejection fraction, persistent capillary leak	Hypodynamic state not responsive to pressors

SOURCE: Adapted from Deitch.[22]

PATHOPHYSIOLOGY

Altered Physiology and Metabolism

The major factor limiting the treatment of MODS is lack of a clear understanding of the underlying pathophysiological defect. In fact, if not viewed carefully, the changes associated with SIRS/MODS may simply resemble an extension of those observed after uncomplicated stress. Thus, patients recovering from major surgery have increases in metabolic rate, oxygen consumption, and carbon dioxide production. There is relative glucose intolerance and hyperglycemia. The vasculature is dilated and the cardiac output increases to promote oxygen transport. In fact, there may even be an increase in lactate production, which reflects the overall increase in metabolism and not tissue hypoxia.

Although simple stress and SIRS/MODS have in common altered intermediary metabolism, a hyperdynamic circulation, and systemic signs of inflammation, two important distinctions have been observed uniformly. First is the previously mentioned difference in time course. Whereas postoperative hypermetabolism runs a 5- to 7-day course and resolves with neovascularization, the time course of SIRS/MODS is longer, usually 3 to 4 weeks.[7] The second distinction is in the subtle metabolic and physiological parameters. In simple stress and early SIRS, the increase in metabolic demand can be met by an increase in supply or in oxygen extraction. As the disease progresses toward MODS, however, the ability to extract, and perhaps utilize, oxygen is lost in certain tissue beds.[36] This situation is unstable because demand on the cellular level is increased. Similarly, in simple stress there appears to be a block in the peripheral utilization of glucose.[7]

This glucose intolerance becomes more pronounced in SIRS/MODS, possibly because of a defect in the enzyme pyruvate dehydrogenase, which catalyzes the conversion of pyruvate to acetyl CoA.[7] As a result, the increased metabolic demand of

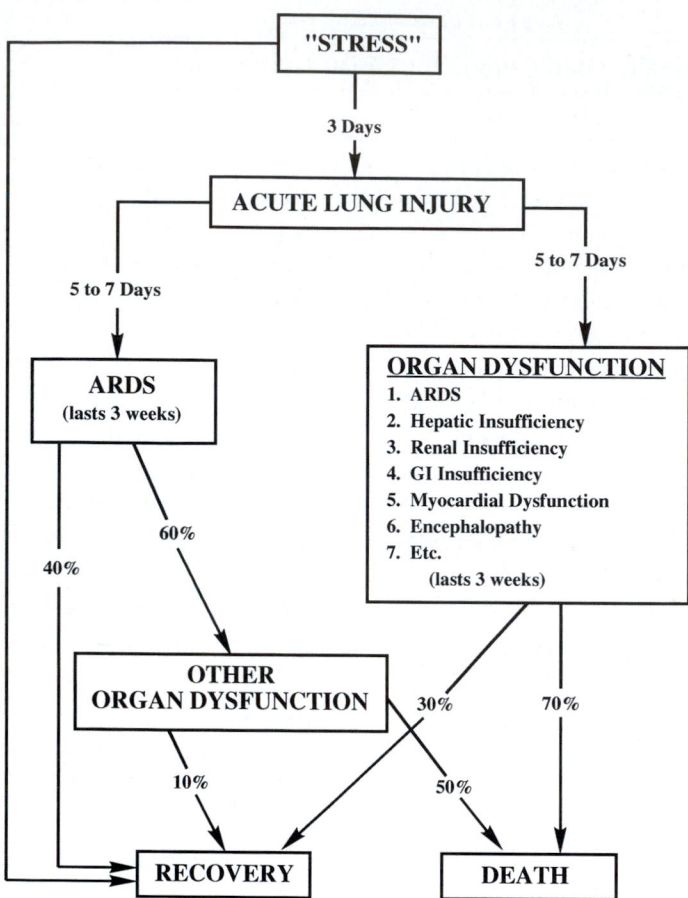

FIGURE 168-1 Diagrammatic representation of the two classic patterns of MODS pathogenesis. Percentages indicate the proportion of patients following the pathway. Patients develop respiratory insufficiency after an initial insult. In some cases (left side of diagram) this persists for 2 to 3 weeks, and the patients then rapidly develop abnormalities of other organ systems. Over the course of the next week, patients either recover or die. In a second group of patients, multiple organ dysfunction rapidly follows the onset of respiratory insufficiency. These abnormalities persist for 2 to 3 weeks. Over the next week, patients then either recover or die.

tissue causes an increase in the activity of the Krebs cycle and in the generation of lactate (aerobic glycolysis). Consequently, serum lactate increases in direct proportion to the increase in pyruvate. If a microcirculatory perfusion deficit develops, increases in lactate exceed increases in pyruvate. These changes in glucose metabolism become progressively less responsive to modulation by insulin. Ultimately, futile cycling of alanine and lactate between the liver and the periphery occurs.

The onset of hepatic dysfunction is heralded by increments in serum lactate, which are disproportionate to the increments in pyruvate. Fat metabolism is markedly altered as well. Stress is characterized by levels of ketosis that are disproportionately low for the degree of starvation.[57] It also elicits an increase in hepatic gluconeogenesis, which, in turn, causes hyperinsulinemia.

Stress is associated with lipolysis, decreased lipogenesis, and increased oxidation of long- and medium-chain triglycerides.[57] In early SIRS/MODS, lipogenesis is decreased further; however,

oxidation of long chain triglycerides by the liver decreases[59] in association with a decrease in expression of key beta-oxidative enzymes.[2,4] Ultimately, this process results in fat intolerance as the liver continues to fail.[16]

In the setting of SIRS/MODS, with significant abnormalities of both glycolysis and beta-oxidation, amino acids become an important fuel source.[16] As oxidation of amino acids increases, urea production does too. Exogenous protein can be an important energy source, but ultimately, hepatic failure compromises ureagenesis and limits this energy source as well.

On the physiological level, vasodilatation and peripheral edema become more pronounced. Cardiac output increases as afterload decreases, but ultimately the heart, too, fails as energy sources are depleted. Renal mechanisms are then called upon to conserve fluid but also to excrete urea. The generalized edema limits the ability to concentrate the urine maximally, thereby leading to two incompatible goals. As a result, the renal excretory system also becomes dysfunctional.

One additional hallmark of progressive SIRS/MODS is a loss of the normal hormonal modulation of cellular processes. Thus, as insulin-mediated glucose uptake decreases, the ability of catecholamines to modulate vascular tone decreases and blood pressure becomes unresponsive to all but the most potent vasopressors; also, glucagon-induced alterations in gluconeogenesis disappear. The mechanisms by which these changes occur are unknown.

A large number of hypotheses have been advanced to explain the pathophysiology of SIRS/MODS. From these have emerged two general concepts concerning etiology: (1) the primary defect is in the microcirculation—along with an overall decrease in peripheral vascular tone, demand and supply at the microcirculatory level are mismatched, resulting in maldistribution of flow—and (2) the defect is primarily one of cellular and, indeed, mitochondrial metabolism. However, all hypotheses invoke a process that "activates" an inflammatory cascade, which, in turn, "mediates" "end-organ responses." In time, these responses become dysfunctional. It is generally accepted that dysfunction in some way results from an inability to meet metabolic demand, because of either inadequate flow or direct metabolic block.

Hypotheses

CYTOKINE HYPOTHESIS

Cytokines are mediators produced and secreted by a number of cells, most notably inflammatory and endothelial cells. These mediators bind to a receptor on the cell membrane and initiate intracellular events, which alter cell behavior. The cell whose behavior is altered may be the same cell that produces the cytokine (autocrine), a nearby cell (paracrine), or a distant cell (endocrine). Cytokines activate a number of intracellular signal transduction pathways.[6,28] The ultimate effect may be direct (activation of a membrane channel or an intracellular protein) or may result from stimulation of gene expression. Cytokines that have been implicated in SIRS/MODS include tumor necrosis factor–α (TNF-α), interleukin-1 (IL-1), IL-6, and interferon-γ (INF-γ).

The behavior of cytokines after simple stress has been well described.[6,28] TNF or IL-1 is produced by inflammatory cells drawn to the site of injury or inflammation and by local endothelial cells. These cytokines are then released into the circulation and affect distant organs. The behavior of TNF-α on the liver serves as a useful paradigm. A 26-kD form of TNF-α is produced by local cells and expressed on the cell surface.[30,41] This form of TNF is, in some unknown way, active in the control of débridement and infection at the local level. Ultimately, however, 26-kD TNF is cleaved by a matrix metalloproteinase to a 17-kD circulating form. The blood carries the 17-kD form from remote organs. The 17-kD form is capable not only of producing vasodilatation, perhaps via a nitric oxide–linked pathway, but also of stimulating other inflammatory and noninflammatory cells. For example, in the liver, TNF stimulates resident macrophages (Kupffer cells) to produce more TNF as well as other cytokines, such as IL-1 and especially IL-6.[6,28] TNF, IL-1, and IL-6 then induce hepatocytes to express the genes for a number of proteins called acute-phase reactants. These secreted proteins have diverse activities that help to control the inflammatory response. Since low levels of TNF (and IL-1) are released from the initial site of inflammation, the process should be self-limited.

In the cytokine theory of MODS, it is hypothesized that overproduction of TNF, IL-1, or IL-6 results in uncontrolled inflammation. The net result is prolonged, uncontrollable vasodilatation and damage to viable organ function by the activated macrophages and other inflammatory cells. In support of this theory,[7,22] high levels of circulating TNF, IL-1, IL-6, and INF-γ have been found in fulminant septic shock, (e.g., as in disseminated meningococcemia).[31,55] Similarly, in animal models in which endotoxin is administered intravenously, serum levels of TNF-α and IL-1 are increased.[9] Studies in animals and human volunteers indicate that TNF-α is probably the most proximal mediator, initiating the expression and release of the other cytokines. TNF-α is cytotoxic to a number of cells, initiating programmed cell death (apoptosis) in culture.[37] Antibodies to TNF-α are protective in lethal endotoxemic and bacteremic animal models,[9,52] while certain intracellular proteins can block TNF-induced apoptosis.[8,53,56] Finally, administration of TNF-α to animals results in a syndrome that mimics septic shock, whereas giving low doses of this cytokine to humans mimics certain metabolic aspects of SIRS. Substantial data indicate, however, that this view of SIRS/MODS is simplistic. In animal models of bacterial peritonitis, neutralizing TNF-α in the serum increases mortality,[25,27] whereas levels of cytokines in the blood of septic patients vary considerably from study to study. Also, clinical trials of anti-TNF in human SIRS have been disappointing.[1] Recent data indicate that serum levels do not reflect tissue levels and that the cell-associated, 26-kD form (and not the 17-kD circulating form) of TNF-α mediates organ injury (L. L. Moldawer, personal communication). Evidence from studies of IL-6 knockout mice indicates that this cytokine is an important component of hepatic regeneration;[19] therefore, it may be protective rather than injurious. Since a host of other mediators and pathways are activated in SIRS, it is reasonable to conclude that cytokines are important mediators of certain aspects of SIRS/MODS but that other factors are at work.

MICROCIRCULATORY HYPOTHESIS

The common link in the microcirculatory hypothesis is that the failure of cells or organs to receive adequate levels of oxygen or some important nutrient or substrate triggers SIRS/MODS. Low flow, as is likely to occur in hypotension or shock, contributes to cellular dysfunction. However, the release of vasoactive mediators and vascular congestion secondary to microthrombi and leukocytes are also held to be important.[22]

Reperfusion of ischemic tissue may be as important a determinant of tissue injury as decreased flow itself.[35] In particular, the generation of oxygen free radicals and peroxidation of membrane lipids following reperfusion may contribute to tissue injury. Sources of free radicals include the conversion of molecular oxygen to superoxide by xanthine oxidase, activated leukocytes, mitochondria, and prostaglandin synthase. The first two are probably the most important.

Circulatory shock, microvascular compromise, and free radical generation are likely to affect the endothelium directly. These cells are active in free radical formation, provide a point of attachment for leukocytes, may be exquisitely sensitive to hypoxia, and not only produce but also are also affected by vasoactive mediators.[44] These interactions provide the link between the cytokine and microvascular hypotheses.[48] Cytokines activate endothelial cells to elaborate other vasoactive substances and to express surface proteins that promote leukocyte adhesion; endothelial cells are also important participants in the formation of microthrombi. In support of the microvascular hypothesis, circulatory shock often occurs before MODS; autopsy data indicate the presence of microvascular injury in patients with MODS; and microthrombi containing platelets, neutrophils, and fibrin are common in MODS. Antibodies to CD18, which block leukocyte adhesion, do occur in circulatory shock and are protective in some forms of ischemia-reperfusion injury;[22,54] they are not protective against liver injury or leukocyte adherence in experimental sepsis.[39,54] The microthrombi, microvascular constriction, and free radicals are valuable in limiting the spread of infection.

GUT HYPOTHESIS

For a long time, the syndrome that is now designated as "SIRS" was believed to be the result of uncontrolled infection, presumably due to endotoxin released by gram-negative bacteria; however, organisms other than gram-negative bacteria have been implicated.[24,58] Moreover, in many patients, neither microorganisms nor a source of bacteria has been identified.[34] It has been proposed that inflammation is due, in part, to bacteria in the gastrointestinal tract (or their associated endotoxins) that translocate to the mesenteric lymph nodes, the liver, and the circulation.[21,22] Various insults have been shown to lead to such translocation of bacteria in endotoxin, and the intestinal barrier is disrupted in many clinical situations that can precede MODS.[12,22,34,43] As a rule, translocation involves a combination of insults, including an alteration in the indigenous GI flora, resulting in bacterial overgrowth, impaired host defenses, and physical disruption of the intestinal barrier.[21,22]

The gut hypothesis overlaps the cytokine and microcirculatory hypotheses. Bacteria or endotoxin activates white cells and induces production of the cytokines. Each can alter the behavior of both endothelial cells and the coagulation system, leading to microvascular aggregation and the production of free radicals, which can create a self-sustaining cycle that culminates in MODS. Exposure to intestinal flora activates hepatic macrophages (Kupffer cells), releases cytokines, and damages hepatic cells, reinforcing the hypothesis that translocated bacteria are important in the pathogenesis of SIRS/MODS.

"TWO-HIT" HYPOTHESIS

A second insult, subsequent to an initial "hit," may be of major importance in the pathogenesis of SIRS/MODS.[22] According to this hypothesis, an initial period of hypotension "primes" the trauma patient for SIRS/MODS, i.e., the initial insult activates other processes that amplify the effects of the initial event, however mild.

Priming could involve activation of white cells or platelets, disruption of the intestinal mucosal barrier, or the induction of free radicals and the enzymes (such as xanthine oxidase) that produce these reactive species. Although this hypothesis overlaps others—such as the cytokine, microcirculatory, and gut hypotheses—animal studies in which a single insult is followed by a second, more severe insult have shown that the first "hit" is actually protective.

CONNECTIONIST HYPOTHESIS

By viewing biologic systems as made up of oscillators, with the oscillations reflecting a continuously changing series of external events, we can regard the loss of either the external stimuli or the ability to respond to these stimuli as pathologic.[14,32] On the basis of this approach and with the application of nonlinear modeling, the transition from SIRS to MODS has been depicted as an erosion in the ability of different organs to communicate with each other,[32] e.g., hepatocellular metabolic pathways, such as gluconeogenesis, respond inadequately to hormonal stimulation in experimental sepsis.[17,23] Similarly, beat-to-beat cardiac variability in human volunteers is lost during experimental endotoxemia.[33] The connectionist hypothesis supplements, rather than substitutes for, the hypotheses presented above.

TRANSCRIPTION HYPOTHESIS

Other hypotheses are being explored. For example, the possibility is being investigated that the seemingly diffuse abnormalities in SIRS and MODS may be related to deficits in hepatic metabolism.[2] In keeping with this hypothesis is the observation that gluconeogenesis, beta-oxidation, and ureagenesis are impaired in septic animals. These alterations are due in part to a decrease in the transcription of genes coding for key enzymes in each pathway. Further, when important transcription factors are examined, it becomes clear that there may be a link between pulmonary and hepatic dysfunction.

MANAGEMENT

Pulmonary Dysfunction

Pulmonary dysfunction most often takes the form of ARDS (see Chapters 166 and 167).

Perfusion Management

On the basis of virtually all the pathogenic theories outlined above, it is clear that inadequate tissue perfusion will potentiate SIRS and may catalyze the progression to MODS. This is especially true for the kidneys, which are sensitive to hypoperfusion even when there is no additional pathology. Moreover, underperfusion of the kidneys will activate the renin-angiotensin-aldosterone system. Since angiotensin II is the major determinant of portal perfusion of the liver[50] and liver dysfunction figures prominently in MODS, disturbances in the renin-angiotensin-aldosterone system may contribute to disturbances in hepatic function. Disturbances in ventilation-perfusion relationships secondary to pulmonary hypoperfusion may contribute to arterial hypoxemia.

Therefore, fluids should be administered liberally to the patient with SIRS/MODS. The assessment of volume of fluids to administer is problematic, however, largely because the function of the end-organs, the best index of adequate perfusion, is already impaired. One practical rule of thumb is to achieve a stroke volume of approximately 1 ml/kg of body weight. If the administration of fluid does not increase stroke volume, cardiac dysfunction is probably present and the administration of additional fluid is not likely to be helpful.

Rational Use of Inotropes and Vasopressors

Animal and clinical studies indicate that SIRS/MODS render the cardiovascular system relatively resistant to the effects of natural and synthetic catecholamines.[13] Therefore, powerful agents are required to achieve any hemodynamic effect. Also, the vasodilatation may represent a compensatory response to a metabolic defect, so induced vasoconstriction may worsen this defect.[18,45,46]

One practical expedient is to treat hypotension when evidence of myocardial ischemia develops, usually at a diastolic blood pressure around 40 mmHg. Norepinephrine is the drug of choice. This agent constricts the somatic (muscle) beds but appears to spare the splanchnic circulation, thereby transferring fluid from the periphery into the central, visceral compartment. Dopamine, long a preferred agent, is no longer advocated, since it is apt to cause maldistribution of flow.

Metabolic Management

As SIRS progresses to MODS, the intrinsic metabolic defect that is associated with the disorder worsens. Although glucose intolerance is apparent very early in the course of the disease, fat intolerance eventually develops. Additionally, there is progressive azotemia as amino acids are increasingly deaminated and their carbon skeletons enter the Krebs cycle. Ultimately, hepatic dysfunction becomes so severe that even this process becomes limited. The intrinsic defect appears to be a decrease in the transcription of genes coding for certain key enzymes in metabolic pathways.[2] Although compensation can occur early in the course of the disorder, ultimately this fails.

To meet caloric needs, most clinics rely on a formula that is relatively hypocaloric and protein rich.[7] Although the blood urea level may rise with this formula, increase in blood urea nitrogen is generally well tolerated in adequately hydrated patients. This tolerance contrasts with the results of overfeeding with fat or glucose. However, if the increase in blood urea nitrogen is a manifestation of uremia rather than an isolated consequence of protein overfeeding, renal dialysis may become necessary.

The administration of exogenous insulin should be avoided. Although insulin may lower serum glucose levels, it does so by driving glucose into fat cells; insulin does not increase glucose oxidation in any tissue. Moreover, even though insulin can block the catabolism of skeletal muscle, its does not have this effect on smooth muscle. Therefore, smooth muscle in the vasculature and the gastrointestinal tract may be mobilized, worsening the vascular and gastrointestinal defects.

CONCLUSION

SIRS/MODS represent a major cause of mortality and morbidity, but the nature of the pathologic defect is unknown. Current treatment is supportive: ventilation, oxygenation, fluids, metabolic support, an intensive search for an excisable or drainable inflammatory site, and avoidance of secondary injury.

REFERENCES

1. Abraham EA, Wunderink R, Silverman H, et al: Efficacy and safety of monoclonal antibody to human tumor necrosis factor a in patients with sepsis syndrome: A randomized, controlled, double-blind, multicenter trial. *JAMA* 273:934–941, 1995.
2. Andrejko KM, Deutschman CS: Altered hepatic gene expression in fecal peritonitis: Changes in transcription of gluconeogenic, b-oxidative and ureagenic genes. *Shock*. In press.
3. Barie PS, Hydo LJ, Fischer E: A prospective comparison of two multiple organ dysfunction/failure scoring systems for prediction of mortality on critical surgical illness. *J Trauma* 37:660–666, 1994.
4. Barke RA, Brady PS, Brady LJ: The effect of peritoneal sepsis on the hepatic gene expression and hepatic mitochondrial long-chain fatty acid oxidation in rats. *Surg Forum* 42:62–65, 1991.
5. Baue AE: Multiple, progressive, or sequential system failure: A syndrome for the 70's. *Arch Surg* 110:779–781, 1975.
6. Baumann H, Gauldie J: The acute phase response. *Immunol Today* 15:74–80, 1994.
7. Beal AL, Cerra FB: Multiple organ failure syndrome in the 1990s: Systemic inflammatory response and organ dysfunction. *JAMA* 271:226–233, 1994.
8. Beg AA, Baltimore D: An essential role for NF-kB in preventing TNF-α induced cell death. *Science* 274:782–784, 1996.
9. Beutler B, Milsark IW, Cerami A: Passive immunization against cachetin/tumor necrosis factor protects mice from lethal effect of endotoxin. *Science* 229:869–871, 1985.
10. Billiar TR, Maddaus MA, West MA, et al: The role of intestinal flora on the interactions between nonparenchymal cells and hepatocytes in coculture. *J Surg Res* 44:397–403, 1988.
11. Bone RC, Balk RA, Cerra FB, et al: Definitions for sepsis and organ failure and guidelines for the use of innovative therapies in sepsis. *Chest* 101:1644–1655, 1992.
12. Border J R, Hassett J, LaDuca J, et al: The gut origin septic states in blunt multiple trauma (ISS = 40) in the ICU. *Ann Surg* 206:427–448, 1987.
13. Breslow MJ, Miller CF, Parker SD, et al: Effect of vasopressors on organ blood flow during endotoxin shock in pigs. *Am J Physiol* 252:H291–H300, 1987.
14. Buchman TG: Physiologic stability and physiologic state. *J Trauma* 41:599–605, 1996.
15. Caldwell MD: Importance of cellular metabolism in the inflammatory response to tissue injury, in Bihari DJ, Cerra FB (eds), *New Horizons: Multiple Organ Failure.* Fullerton, CA, Society of Critical Care Medicine, 1989, pp 37–60.
16. Cerra FB: Hypermetabolism, organ failure and metabolic support. *Surgery* 191:1–14, 1987.
17. Clemens MG, Chaudry IH, Daigneau N, Baue AE: Insulin resistance and depressed gluconeogenic capacity during early hyperglycemic sepsis. *J Trauma* 24:701–708, 1984.
18. Cobb JP, Natason C, Hoffman WD, Parillo JE: N-omega-Amino-L-arginine, an inhibitor of nitric oxide synthase, raises vascular resistance but increases mortality in awake canines challenged with endotoxin. *J Exp Med* 176:1175–1182, 1992.
19. Cressman DE, Greenbaum LE, DeAngelis RA, et al: Liver failure and defective hepatocyte regeneration in interleukin-6–deficient mice. *Science*. In press.
20. Cuthbertson D, Tilstone W: Metabolism during the post injury period. *Adv Clin Chem* 12:1–55, 1977.
21. Deitch EA: Bacterial translocation of the gut flora. *J Trauma* 30(Suppl):S184–S189, 1990.
22. Deitch EA: Multiple organ failure: Pathophysiology and potential future therapy. *Ann Surg* 216:117–134, 1992.
23. Deutschman CS, De Maio A, Clemens MG: Sepsis-induced attenuation of glucagon and 8-BrcAMP modulation of the phospho-*enol*pyruvate carboxykinase gene. *Am J Physiol* 38:R584–R591, 1995.
24. Deutschman CS, Konstantinides FN, Tsai M, et al: Physiology and metabolism in isolated viral septicemia: Further evidence of an organism-independent, host-dependent response. *Arch Surg* 122:21–25, 1987.
25. Echtenacher B, Falk W, Mannel DN, Krammer PH: Requirement for endogenous tumor necrosis factor/cachetin for recovery from experimental peritonitis. *J Immunol* 145:3762–3766, 1990.
26. Eiseman B, Beart R, Norton L: Multiple organ failure. *Surg Gynecol Obstet* 144:323–326, 1977.
27. Eskandari MK, Bolgos G, Miller C, et al: Anti-tumor necrosis factor antibody therapy fails to prevent lethality after cecal ligation and puncture or endotoxemia. *J Immunol* 148:2724–2727, 1992.
28. Fey GH, Hocke GM, Wilson DR, et al: Cytokines and the acute phase response in the liver, in Arias IM, Boyer JL, Fausto N, et al (eds), *The Liver: Biology and Pathobiology.* New York, Raven, 1994, pp 113–143.
29. Fry DE, Pearlstein L, Fulton RL, Polk HC: Multiple system organ failure: The role of uncontrolled infection. *Arch Surg* 115:136–140, 1980.
30. Gearing AJH, Beckett P, Christodoulou M, et al: Matrix metalloproteinases and processing of pro-TNF-α. *J Leukoc Biol* 57:774–777, 1995.
31. Girardin E, Grau GE, Dayer JM, et al: Tumor necrosis factor and interleukin-1 in the serum of children with severe infectious purpura. *New Engl J Med* 319:397–400, 1988.
32. Godin PJ, Buchman TG: Uncoupling of biological oscillators: A complementary hypothesis concerning the pathogenesis of multiple organ dysfunction syndrome. *Crit Care Med* 24:1107–1116, 1996.
33. Godin PJ, Fleisher LA, Eidsath A, et al: Experimental human endotoxemia increases cardiac regularity: Results from a prospective randomized, crossover trial. *Crit Care Med* 24:1117–1124, 1996.

34. Goris RJ, Beokhorst PA, Nuytinck KS: Multiple organ failure: Generalized autodestructive inflammation. *Arch Surg* 120:1109–1115, 1985.

35. Granger DN: Role of xanthine oxidase and granulocytes in ischemia-reperfusion injury. *Am J Physiol* 251:H1269–H1275, 1988.

36. Gutierriz G, Lund N, Bryan-Brown C: Cellular oxygen utilization during multiple organ failure. *Crit Care Clin* 5:271–287, 1989.

37. Hsu H, Shu HB, Pan MG, Goeddel DV: TRADD-TRAF2 and TRADD-FADD interactions define two distinct TNF receptor 1 signal transduction pathways. *Cell* 84:299–308, 1996.

38. Knaus WA, Draper EA, Wagner DP, Zimmerman JE: Prognosis in acute organ-system failure. *Ann Surg* 202:685–693, 1985.

39. Langdale LA, Flaherty LC, Liggitt HD, et al: Neutrophils contribute to hepatic ischemia-reperfusion injury by a CD18 independent mechanism. *J Leukoc Biol* 53:511–517, 1993.

40. Marshall JC, Cook DJ, Christou NV, et al: The multiple organ dysfunction score: A reliable descriptor of complex clinical outcome. *Crit Care Med* 23:1638–1652, 1995.

41. McGeehan GM, Becerer JD, Bast RC Jr, et al: Regulation of tumour necrosis factor–α processing by a metalloproteinase inhibitor. *Nature* 370:558–561, 1994.

42. Meakins JL: Etiology of multiple organ failure. *J Trauma* 30(Suppl):S165–S168, 1990.

43. Meakins JL, Marshall JC: The gastrointestinal tract: The "motor" of MOF. *Arch Surg* 121:197–201, 1986.

44. Osborn L: Leukocyte adhesion to the endothelium in inflammation. *Cell* 62:3–6, 1990.

45. Pastor CM, Payen DM: Effect of modifying nitric oxide pathway on liver circulation in a rabbit endotoxin shock model. *Shock* 2:196–202, 1994.

46. Petros A, Bennett D, Vallance P: Effect of nitric oxide synthase inhibitors on hypotension in patients with septic shock. *Lancet* 338:1557–1558, 1991.

47. Petty TL: ARDS: Refinement of concepts and definition. *Am Rev Respir Dis* 138:724–728, 1988.

48. Pober JS, Cotran RS: Cytokines and endothelial cell biology. *Physiol Rev* 70:427–451, 1990.

49. Regel G, Grotz M, Weltner T, et al: Pattern of organ failure following severe trauma. *World J Surg* 20:422–429, 1996.

50. Reilly PM, MacGowen S, Miyachi M, Bulkley GB: Mesenteric vasoconstriction in cardiogenic shock in pigs. *Gastroenterology* 102:1968–1979, 1992.

51. Tilney NL, Bailey GL, Morgan AP: Sequential system failure after rupture of abdominal aortic aneurysms: An unsolved problem in postoperative care. *Ann Surg* 178:117–122, 1973.

52. Tracey KJ, Fong Y, Hesse DG, et al: Anti-cachectin/TNF monoclonal antibodies prevent septic shock during lethal endotoxemia. *Nature* 330:662–664, 1987.

53. Van Antwerp DJ, Martin SJ, Kafri T, et al: Suppression of TNF-α–induced apoptosis by NF-kB. *Science* 274:787–789, 1996.

54. Vedder NB, Winn RK, Rice CL, Harlan JM: Neutrophil-mediated vascular injury in shock and multiple organ failure. *Prog Clin Biol Res* 299:181–191, 1989.

55. Waage A, Halstensen A, Espevik T: Association between tumour necrosis factor in serum and fatal outcome in patients with meningococcal disease. *Lancet* 1:355–357, 1987.

56. Wang C-Y, Mayo MW, Baldwin AS Jr: TNF and cancer therapy-induced apoptosis: Potentiation by inhibition of NF-kB. *Science* 274:784–787, 1996.

57. Wannemacher RW, Pace JC, Beall FA, et al: Role of the liver in regulation of ketone body production during sepsis. *J Clin Invest* 64:1565–1572, 1979.

58. Wiles JB, Cerra FB, Siegel JH, Border JR: The systemic septic response: Does the organism matter? *Crit Care Med* 8:55–60, 1980.

59. Wolfe RR, Shaw JHF: Glucose and FFA kinetics in sepsis: Role of glucagon and sympathetic nervous system activity. *Am J Physiol* 248:E236–E243, 1985.

CHAPTER 169

RESPIRATORY DISTRESS SYNDROME IN PREMATURE NEWBORN INFANTS

Walker A. Long / Anthony Corbet

Respiratory distress syndrome (RDS) is the most common lung disease of newborn infants. Despite major advances in medical therapy, RDS remains the single most common cause of death and morbidity in the first month of life. Insufficiency of pulmonary surfactant at birth has been firmly established as the cause of this disorder.

This chapter considers the epidemiology, clinical findings, pathology, pathophysiology, and etiology of RDS. Methods of prevention, laboratory evaluation, and relation to bronchopul-

monary dysplasia are reviewed prior to discussion of treatment modalities. The differential diagnosis of respiratory distress in the newborn is then considered. Finally, surfactant replacement therapy in RDS and its adult counterpart, acute adult respiratory distress syndrome (ARDS), is presented.

EPIDEMIOLOGY

The incidence of RDS is about 1 percent of all births worldwide. A strong relationship of RDS with prematurity exists. At a gestational age of 29 weeks the incidence is 60 percent, but this declines progressively to near zero by 39 completed weeks of gestation. At all levels of gestation, the condition is more common in males than females and in white infants than black infants.[31] RDS occurs in a familial pattern; premature infants born to mothers who had a previous infant with RDS are at increased risk. Spontaneous labor provides an important protective effect; at any given gestation, the incidence of RDS is higher for abdominal delivery without labor than for vaginal delivery with labor. Risk for RDS is significantly increased if elective cesarean section is performed prior to completion of 39 weeks gestation.[43]

When corrected for gestation, the incidence of RDS is significantly higher in infants of diabetic mothers, especially if the infant is overnourished and large for gestational age. In recent years, the problem has been less frequent, mainly because medical control of the diabetic state during pregnancy has improved. Infants who are undernourished and small for gestational age at birth may have a decreased incidence of RDS, but this has not been apparent in the less mature infants seen in recent years. Although the incidence of RDS may be lower in pregnancy-induced hypertension, subacute placental abruption, maternal narcotic addiction, and maternal tobacco or cocaine abuse, the incidence of RDS may be increased in these conditions if cesarian section is performed before the onset of labor.[56] Although somewhat controversial, when gestation is carefully controlled, the incidence of RDS is reduced in the presence of prolonged rupture of amniotic membranes (24 to 48 h before birth).

Based on measurements in placental umbilical artery blood samples, at birth, infants with RDS are no more acidemic than control infants without RDS. Hence, it is very unlikely that fetal asphyxia has any role in causing the RDS in premature infants. Furthermore, although the incidence of RDS is higher in second-born twins than in first-born twins, based on the assessment of cord blood samples at birth, acidemia occurs no more frequently in second-born twins.

CLINICAL FINDINGS

The onset of RDS is at birth or in the first few hours of life. Infants with RDS may have the classic signs of labored breathing or respiratory distress: (1) tachypnea, (2) flaring of the alae nasae, (3) expiratory grunting, (4) intercostal recessions, (4) subcostal retractions, and (5) cyanosis in room air. In addition, these infants have signs of prematurity: (1) low birth weight, (2) reduced muscle tone and strength, (3) thin, translucent skin, (4) fine downy hair, (5) smooth soles, (6) small nipples, and (7) immature genitalia. In most cases, an inspired fraction of oxygen (F_{IO_2}) of at least 0.4 is needed to improve the cyanosis, and over the first 24 h, the F_{IO_2} requirement often increases to 1.0. If the infant is very premature or very depressed at birth from the effects of asphyxia or sedation, the need for mechanical ventilation obscures the clinical findings. Larger and stronger infants may have a more delayed and slowly progressive course.

The chest radiograph is characterized by diffuse, fine, reticular-granular densities and reduced lung volume (Fig. 169-1). The radiographic findings reflect widespread microatelectasis, but the degree of atelectasis varies with respiratory muscle strength, chest wall compliance, and applied airway pressure. The blood-gas findings indicate a modest or severe defect in oxygenation, moderate hypercarbia, and mild lactic acidosis. Infants show evidence of general body edema, reduced urine output, poor peripheral perfusion, and systemic hypotension. Many infants require mechanical ventilation. Usually, the disease reaches its maximal intensity at about the age of 72 h. Subsequently, a significant diuresis and steadily improving oxygenation are observed. In uncomplicated cases, infants may breath room air without cyanosis by the age of 1 week.

In many infants the disease is not resolved in 1 week; continued mechanical ventilation and oxygen therapy are necessary. Failure of the respiratory distress to resolve may be due to the development of complications, e.g., an air leak or bronchopulmonary dysplasia. Alternatively, it may be due to other problems, such as episodes of recurrent apnea, chronic pulmonary insufficiency caused by high chest wall compliance, cerebral intraventricular hemorrhage (IVH), systemic bacterial infection, or patent ductus arteriosus (PDA). With modern therapy, it is now unusual for infants to die of RDS; however, some infants die of complications, such as IVH, BPD, or infection.

PATHOPHYSIOLOGY

The respiratory rate is elevated above 60 breaths per minute; although tidal volume is reduced, minute ventilation is increased. The functional residual capacity, as measured by nitrogen washout or helium dilution method, is decreased from normal values of 20 ml/kg to 5 to 10 ml/kg. Low values for lung volume reflect diffuse micro-atelectasis and poorly ventilated lung units; the greater the need for oxygen, the smaller the measured value for lung volume.[51] Static lung compliance, measured by multiple airway occlusions during exhalation, is decreased from normal values of 1 to 2 ml/cmH$_2$O/kg to about 0.5 ml/cmH$_2$O/kg.[16] Measurements of airway resistance suggest a 50 percent increase, probably related to the reduced lung volume. From these measurements, a very short ventilation time constant of 0.05 s in RDS can be calculated. Nitrogen washout curves suggest "fast" and "slow" spaces. Therefore, in some regions of the lung, time constants may be longer.

The alveolar-arterial oxygen gradient and right-to-left shunt estimated in 100% oxygen are very high. Shunt values may be 50 to 90% indicating a very low effective pulmonary blood flow. Right-to-left shunts occur at the ductus arteriosus, at the foramen ovale, and in the large interstitial compartment of the lung. Since the response to supplemental oxygen is good, there must be ventilated lung regions with low ventilation-perfusion ratios.[12] Measurements of the arterial-alveolar nitrogen gradient are increased, but not as much as expected, because hypoxic vasoconstriction limits blood flow to units with low ventilation-perfusion ratios. Because a large part of the lung is collapsed or poorly ventilated, most ventilation is diverted to only a small part of the lung. Measurements of pulmonary blood flow, utilizing methods based on the disappearance of gases that enter ventilated lung, confirm that perfusion of ventilated lung is very low. Hence, measurements of the arterial-alveolar CO$_2$ gradient are high.[26] Although minute ventilation is increased, alveolar ventilation is decreased, and hypercarbia is significant. These findings are consistent with a three-compartment lung model: (1) a compartment with a right-to-left shunt, (2) a ventilated compartment with a low ventilation-perfusion ratio, and (3) a compartment with a high ventilation-perfusion ratio. Comparisons of expected and measured blood-gas values under several conditions suggest that this model is valid.

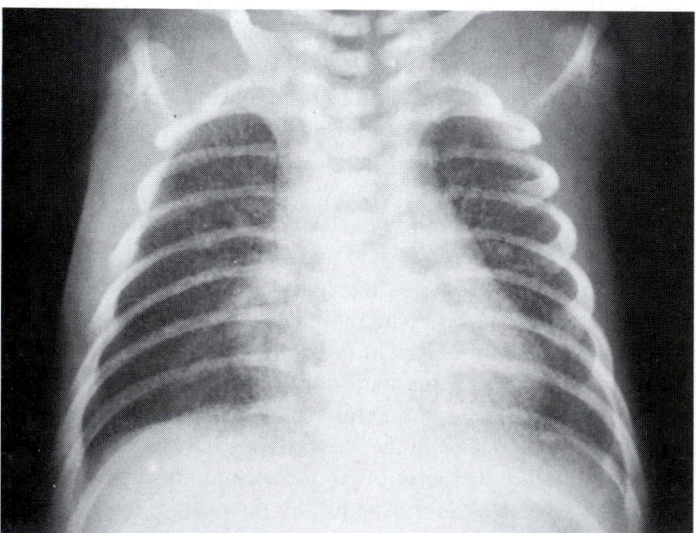

FIGURE 169-1   Neonatal RDS demonstrating the reticular-granular pattern of microatelectasis. (*Courtesy of Dr. Ronald Ablow.*)

PATHOLOGY

In RDS the gross findings at autopsy include diffuse lung atelectasis, congestion, and edema. If the lungs are inflated at autopsy, lung distensibility is found to be greatly reduced. The histology shows diffuse alveolar atelectasis, but the respiratory bronchioles are dilated and lined with hyaline membranes composed of plasma proteins and epithelial debris (Fig. 169-2). These findings reflect significant lung injury. Epithelial injury appears within 30 min of birth, and capillary injury with plasma leakage appears within 3 h of birth. Experimentally, epithelial and endothelial injury may be prevented by timely administration of exogenous surfactant.[46] It would appear that in the face of alveolar atelectasis, the terminal conducting airways are overdistended, either by spontaneous breaths or by mechanical ventilation; this overdistension produces significant lung injury.

ETIOLOGY

RDS results from a developmental insufficiency at birth of pulmonary surfactant in the terminal airspaces. The deficiency causes reduced expansion of alveoli, respiratory bronchiole injury, and surfactant inactivation by plasma proteins. Based on animal experiments, the air spaces of the mature infant have been estimated to contain 75 mg/kg of saturated phosphatidylcholine (SPC); the adult has 10 to 15 mg/kg, and the preterm infant with RDS has only 1 to 10 mg/kg.[32] As RDS resolves, the air space pool approaches that of term infants. Normal newborn infants have five to seven times more surfactant at birth than do adults. Teleologically, the higher levels of surfactant are required to overcome the nonspecific inhibitory effects of the fluid and proteins normally present in the lung at birth. Infants with RDS have more than enough surfactant present in the lungs to line the airways.[6] The problem is that infants with RDS cannot package and export sufficient surfactant to the alveolar surface; hence, SPC cannot function as surfactant (Fig. 169-3). Infants with RDS lack lamellar bodies and have a complete absence of tubular myelin

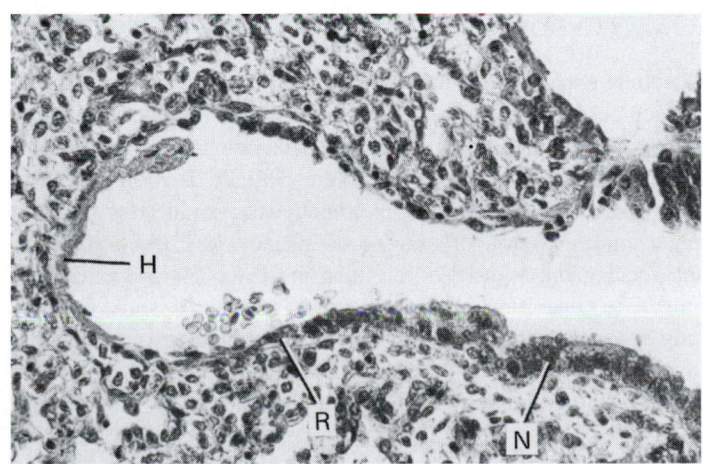

FIGURE 169-2   Neonatal RDS. Photomicrograph of lung. Dilated terminal conducting airway surrounded by atelectatic terminal airspaces. The transition from normal bronchiolar epithelium (N) to necrotic epithelium (R) and hyaline membrane (H) is shown (×190).

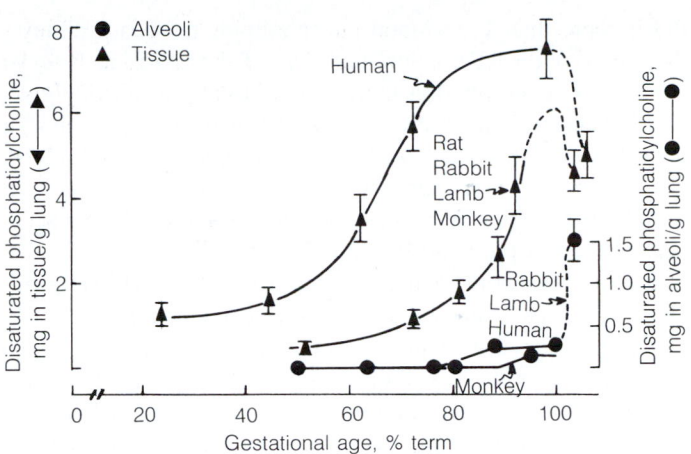

FIGURE 169-3   Accumulation of saturated phosphatidylcholine (SPC) in fetal lungs. The curves show lung tissue and airway accumulation of SPC as a percent of term gestation for humans and several other mammals. SPC accumulates in humans much earlier, consistent with early lung maturation. Theoretically, the amount present is more than enough to form a functional surfactant; however, in RDS, SPC is not appropriately packaged and transported to the epithelial surface. (*From Clements and Tooley.*[6])

in the air spaces.[15] In addition, these infants have a deficiency of immunostained surfactant protein A (SP-A) in the endoplasmic reticulum and in lamellar bodies.[15]

PREVENTION OF RESPIRATORY DISTRESS SYNDROME

The best way to prevent RDS is to prevent premature labor and delivery. The most effective strategies include cervical cerclage, antibiotic treatment of maternal bacteruria, and the liberal use of tocolytics. However, our ability to control premature labor is limited. At present, the more encouraging strategies for reducing the incidence of RDS include prenatal prediction, antenatal treatment with corticosteroids, and prophylactic administration of exogenous surfactant.

Because some fetal lung liquid enters the amniotic cavity by passing through the fetus's nasopharynx, the surfactant system can be assessed before birth by analyzing amniotic fluid samples. Most commonly, SPC or lecithin is measured, and the concentration is standardized to the concentration of sphingomyelin—the *L/S ratio*. In normal pregnancies, values for the L/S ratio increase to 1.0 at 32 weeks and to 2.0 by 35 weeks. In abnormal pregnancies, values are much more variable; the L/S ratio may reach 2.0 as early as 28 weeks, or it may remain at 1.0 until nearly term gestation. The risk for RDS is 100 percent if the L/S ratio is less than 1.0 and is less than 1 percent if the L/S ratio is 2.0 or greater. In diabetic pregnancies, a ratio of 3.0 is observed before the risk is less than 1 percent. In African-American mothers, the risk is very low if the L/S ratio exceeds 1.2. Gestational age should be considered in the evaluation of the L/S ratio; a low L/S ratio carries a lower risk at near-term gestation.

A supplementary test for assessing the risk of RDS is the measurement of phosphatidylglycerol (PG). If the concentration of

PG is more than 1% of total phospholipids (a "positive" test), then the risk for RDS is less than 1%. If the L/S ratio is under 2.0 and PG concentration under 1% of total phosphatidylglycerol (a "negative" test), the risk for RDS is over 80 percent.[24] If the L/S ratio is under 2.0, but the PG is positive, the risk for RDS is very low. Measurement of SP-A and surfactant protein B (SP-B) in amniotic fluid does not improve the predictive accuracy of the L/S ratio and PG concentration.[49]

Less expensive methods for assessing risk of RDS are available. By reducing surface tension, surfactant stabilizes air bubbles. This effect constitutes the basis for a prognostic test which is based upon shaking an aliquot lung fluid to create bubbles and observing the bubbles' stability. In the stable microbubble test, fewer than 5 stable bubbles per square millimeter carries a risk for RDS of 95 percent.[4] Another test, the automated fetal lung maturity test, referred to as *TDx-FLM,* is based on fluorescence polarization. This test measures fluorescence after the introduction of a fluorescent probe and may be as good as the L/S ratio in predicting RDS.[29]

The use of antenatal betamethasone to prevent RDS has been widespread abroad for some time. Recently, an NIH Consensus Development Panel concluded that the evidence for antenatal corticosteroids in premature labor is compelling, that corticosteroid treatment reduces the incidence of RDS and neonatal death by 50 percent, and that corticosteroid treatment greatly reduces the incidence of cerebral IVH.[45] Furthermore, the benefits were apparent for all infants between 24 to 34 weeks gestation, regardless of race or gender. Although the original studies indicated that treatment should be for more than 24 h, the NIH panel concluded that shorter exposures carry benefit. Therefore, the panel recommended that obstetricians use corticosteroids in all patients with premature labor, unless delivery is likely to be immediate. This latter recommendation is an important subpoint, as steroids have not been widely used in the United States because obstetricians have been concerned that they may be unable to delay delivery for a full 24 h. Clear evidence indicates that the effects of prenatal corticosteroids and postnatal exogenous surfactant are additive and that use of both agents improves survival of premature infants.

Several clinical trials of thyrotropin-releasing hormone (TRH) in premature labor have been reported. In the trials, prenatal TRH conferred additional benefit to corticosteroid administration. However, use of prenatal TRH is still considered experimental. Prophylactic administration of exogenous surfactant postnatally has also been shown to reduce the incidence of RDS in small, premature infants at high risk.[30] The effect has been confined to mammalian surfactants and has not been seen with synthetic preparations.

LABORATORY TESTS IN INFANTS WITH RESPIRATORY DISTRESS SYNDROME

Serial arterial blood-gas analyses in infants with RDS show moderate or severe hypoxemia, significant hypercarbia, and mild metabolic acidosis. The L/S ratio, PG concentration, and SP-A levels remain low in tracheal aspirates for 48 h; they increase with recovery.

BRONCHOPULMONARY DYSPLASIA

If RDS fails to resolve by the end of 1 week of life, premature infants may develop bronchopulmonary dysplasia (BPD). In mild BPD, affected infants require supplemental oxygen and have abnormal chest radiographs at age 1 month. In severe BPD, affected infants require supplemental oxygen when they are at full term postconceptional age. The incidence of BPD increases with decreasing gestational age.

BPD is produced by an inflammatory response to the barotrauma or volutrauma of mechanical ventilation and high concentrations of oxygen. In RDS, tracheal aspirates show elevated white blood cell counts and cytokine concentrations on the first day; the values peak at 3 days and then decline to low levels in those who recover. However, in those that develop BPD, levels remain elevated. BPD is a major problem in clinical practice. It contributes significantly to infant mortality, to the number of children with brain injuries, and to the overall expense of hospital care.

TREATMENT OF RESPIRATORY DISTRESS SYNDROME

Thirty years ago the mortality of RDS exceeded 80 percent. Currently, although mortality from RDS depends on gestational age, it is very rare in infants weighing more than 1000 g. This remarkable improvement in outcome is due to a multitude of factors but, in large part, may be ascribed to the introduction of positive airway pressure in the late 1960s and surfactant replacement in the early 1990s.

RESUSCITATION

The mortality of infants with RDS is increased by birth asphyxia; infants who are small for gestational age are often asphyxiated at birth. The latter association may explain why RDS in infants who are small for gestational age is often very severe. It is important to have a skilled resuscitation team present at birth.

LUNG EXPANSION

Adequate expansion of the lungs at birth provides a stimulus for surfactant secretion. It is prudent to intubate all infants under 1000 g birth weight and to provide adequate mechanical ventilation with positive end-expiratory pressure (PEEP) as soon as possible. As discussed below, this approach also provides for prophylactic administration of exogenous surfactant. Early intubation and mechanical ventilation are also indicated for premature infants who make poor respiratory efforts at birth. In some centers, lung expansion is achieved by the early application of nasal continuous positive airway pressure (CPAP), with intubation and exogenous surfactant reserved for those with more severe disease.

THERMAL NEUTRALITY

A minimal infant energy expenditure of 55 cal/kg per day can be achieved by servo-controlling the infant's anterior abdominal temperature at 36.5°C; in very small premature infants this setting may have to be increased to 36.9°C to maintain the rectal temperature at 37°C. Supplying heat is important, because initially it is difficult to provide more than about 30 cal/kg per day, given the restrictions on fluid intake in these infants.

MONITORING

Infants with RDS require close monitoring of blood pressure, arterial blood gases, electrolytes, and calcium, glucose, and bilirubin concentrations.

OXYGEN THERAPY

Oxygen therapy is effective in RDS despite the presence of a large right-to-left shunt. An increase in F_{IO_2} produces: (1) an increase in alveolar P_{O_2} in the ventilated compartment with a low ventilation-perfusion ratio, (2) relief of local hypoxic vasoconstriction, (3) a reduction in right-to-left shunt, and (4) an increase in arterial oxygen saturation.

FLUID AND ELECTROLYTE MANAGEMENT

Since RDS is characterized by pulmonary edema associated with high surface tension and increased permeability, it is usual to restrict fluid intake to 50 to 70 ml/kg per day. A controlled trial has demonstrated improved outcome with fluid restriction.[55] Premature infants have excess extracellular water at birth and are expected to lose 10 percent of body weight in the first week.

It is not necessary to provide sodium for infants in the first 3 days of life; in fact, sodium administration may be harmful. Because infants have very thin skin, insensible water losses may be high, and such losses may result in hypernatremia and brain injury. Infants with RDS should be cared for in a humid environment to reduce insensible water losses. If it is necessary to liberalize fluid intake to treat hypernatremia, hyperglycemia may develop; under these circumstances, a gastric infusion of glucose-free water may be helpful.

Infants with RDS may also develop dangerous hyperkalemia related to insufficiency of the sodium-potassium ATPase protein. The hyperkalemia is exacerbated by renal insufficiency. Potassium should not be provided in the first few days of life. As infants with RDS also have transient hypoparathyroidism, adequate calcium supplementation must be provided.

MINIMAL STIMULATION

Infant manipulations such as heel sticks, diaper changes, and weighings should be avoided, as they may cause dangerous hypoxemia and hypertension in the infant with RDS. Many centers now use both umbilical arterial and venous catheters in managing infants with RDS. Glucose can be infused through the venous catheter and saline through the arterial catheter, which can then be used to monitor the blood glucose. If used properly, an umbilical venous catheter is not associated with increased rates of infection or thrombosis.

ANTIBIOTIC THERAPY

Group B streptococcal infection can mimic or coexist with RDS. As a result, it is prudent to obtain a blood culture and begin ampicillin and gentamicin in all infants with apparent RDS. If cultures are negative and the white blood cell count is normal, antibiotics can be stopped at age 3 days; however, it is common to treat for at least 1 week. If the mother receives antibiotics during labor, interpretation of negative blood cultures in the infant is difficult.

BLOOD PRESSURE SUPPORT

Premature infants with RDS often have a low blood pressure on the first day of life; mean blood pressures of less than 30 mmHg may be injurious to the brain.[37] Occasionally, hypotension is due to hypovolemia, which responds to administration of plasmanate at a dose of 10 to 20 ml/kg. However, echocardiographic studies have shown poor cardiac contractility and low cardiac output in many infants with RDS. Such cardiac dysfunction responds better to a continuous infusion of dopamine at 5 to 15 mcg/kg per minute. Recent evidence suggests that these infants may have relative adrenal insufficiency and respond to therapy with hydrocortisone or dexamethasone.[27] Hypotension should be corrected slowly, since a rapid increase in blood pressure may predispose the infant to IVH.

ALKALI THERAPY

Sodium bicarbonate is used occasionally to correct documented metabolic acidosis, but routine, continuous infusions are not indicated.

CONTINUOUS POSITIVE AIRWAY PRESSURE

Continuous positive airway pressure (CPAP) in the infant may be administered by endotracheal tube, nasopharyngeal tube, long or short nasal prongs, face mask or head box, or negative pressure applied around the chest. Prior to use of mechanical ventilation, use of CPAP was associated with reduced mortality only in infants over 1500 g birth weight. If CPAP is started early, the need for supplemental oxygen and mechanical ventilation is reduced, and survival may be improved. Some centers provide CPAP by nasal prongs to all infants with RDS on admission to the nursery, with the intent of avoiding intubation and mechanical ventilation. This approach may reduce the incidence of BPD, but no randomized trials addressing this issue have been reported. However, since the advent of exogenous surfactant therapy, many centers have abandoned use of CPAP in RDS, except prior to extubation in recovering infants.

CONVENTIONAL MECHANICAL VENTILATION

The present approach is that all infants with established RDS needing an F_{IO_2} of at least 0.5 are intubated and treated with mechanical ventilation and exogenous surfactant. The aim is to correct blood-gas abnormalities, including hypoxemia and hypercarbia, with as little pulmonary injury and circulatory compromise as possible. As the ventilation time constant in RDS is short, the inspiration time should be 0.2 to 0.3 s; long inspiration times are usually unnecessary and may be associated with air leaks. In a condition characterized by microatelectasis, it is appropriate to use generous levels of PEEP (between 4 and 8 cmH$_2$O).

Several controlled trials have established that ventilator respiratory rates of 60 per minute produce less lung injury than rates of 30 per minute; under isocarbic conditions, a faster respiratory rate allows smaller tidal volumes to be used; smaller tidal volumes reduce the risk of overdistension in the terminal conducting airways. The peak inflation pressure (PIP) should be sufficient to visibly move the upper chest. Commonly used levels of PIP are 15 to 30 cmH$_2$O. The arterial P$_{O_2}$ should be maintained between 50 and 70 mmHg by adjusting F$_{IO_2}$. Oxygenation may also be modulated by changes in mean airway pressure, which should be increased with PEEP or PIP. Many clinicians aim for an arterial P$_{CO_2}$ of 45 to 55 mmHg; such "permissive hypercapnia" minimizes use of high PIP associated with high tidal volumes. High tidal volumes, associated with high levels of PIP, produce lung injury.

If the infant breathes asynchronously with the ventilator, a phenomenon which may cause IVH, a number of strategies may be used: (1) The respiratory rate can be increased to 70 or 80 breaths per minute; (2) the ventilator can be set in the assist-control mode; or (3) the infant can be sedated or sedated and pharmacologically paralyzed. When sedation and paralysis are used, because expiratory braking is inhibited, it is prudent to increase the PEEP level to promote maintenance of lung volume. In our experience, only a few infants fail mechanical ventilation and must be treated with high-frequency oscillatory ventilation (HFOV) or extracorporeal membrane oxygenation (ECMO).

CLOSURE OF THE PATENT DUCTUS ARTERIOSUS

In many infants with RDS the ductus arteriosus remains open. Although initially the shunt through a patent ductus arteriosus (PDA) is right to left, by the end of the first day of life the shunt is left to right. Whether the shunt contributes to pulmonary edema on the first day of life is controversial, but by 3 to 4 days of age, when the pulmonary vascular resistance has further decreased, the PDA may cause deterioration and predispose the infant to the development of BPD (especially in infants under 1000 g birth weight).[17] Under these circumstances, treatment with indomethacin is indicated, and, if this fails, surgical ligation should be performed. However, there is only fair agreement from four clinical trials that treatment with indomethacin starting at 3 days of age is helpful in reducing the incidence of BPD.[11]

EXOGENOUS SURFACTANT THERAPY

In infants under 1000 g birth weight, the risk for RDS is very high. Therefore, these infants should be treated prophylactically with exogenous surfactant within 15 to 30 min of birth, after adequate stabilization has been achieved.[9,10] In larger infants, treatment should be more selective and initiated only in those with good evidence for RDS; if possible, "rescue" treatment should

be started by 2 h of age.[47] Use of a mammalian surfactant is currently preferred,[23] although the results with synthetic surfactant have been nearly as good. The usual phospholipid dose of mammalian surfactant is 100 mg/kg. The agent should be instilled directly into the endotracheal tube using bag-tube ventilation to ensure proper distribution; in general, 2 to 3 doses should be instilled at 8- to 12-h intervals until the F$_{IO_2}$ requirement is less than 0.3. Following surfactant instillation, it is customary to continue with mechanical ventilation, but in some centers infants are placed on endotracheal or nasal CPAP in the hope that the incidence of BPD will be reduced.

CORTICOSTEROIDS

There is good evidence that inflammation in RDS starts on the first day of life as a result of lung injury from atelectasis, mechanical ventilation, and administration of supplemental oxygen. Results from two studies suggest that corticosteroid treatment started on the first day reduces the incidence of BPD.[53,57] The findings require further confirmation.

HIGH-FREQUENCY VENTILATION

If an infant with RDS develops pulmonary interstitial emphysema during conventional mechanical ventilation, institution of high-frequency ventilation (HFV) is commonly employed. In a controlled trial, high-frequency jet ventilation (HFJV) using a low-pressure strategy was shown to be more effective than conventional ventilation; a more rapid resolution of pulmonary interstitial emphysema, as well as a modest reduction in the mortality, was noted.[34] In some centers it is common to try high-frequency flow interrupter ventilation (HFIV); in some reports, high-frequency oscillator ventilation (HFOV) appears to be successful. A low-pressure strategy, seeking to "derecruit" the lung, appears to offer the best chance for success in addressing pulmonary interstitial emphysema. Such an approach may improve air leak and allow healing over a period of several days, while still providing an adequate level of oxygenation. In the absence of pulmonary interstitial emphysema, if conventional ventilation for RDS fails and the infant deteriorates with severe hypoxemia, it is reasonable to try HFOV. In this case, a high-pressure strategy is employed to improve recruitment of the lung. In larger infants with RDS who meet ECMO criteria, a controlled trial has demonstrated that at least 50 percent of patients will do well on HFOV and not require ECMO.[5]

OTHER CONDITIONS PRODUCING RESPIRATORY DISTRESS IN THE NEWBORN

RDS can usually be diagnosed accurately on clinical grounds, but several other diseases can mimic or even coexist with RDS.

Transient Tachypnea of the Newborn

The normal fetal lung contains lung liquid (20 ml/kg) produced by chloride pump proteins in the cell membrane of granular pneumocytes. The liquid is progressively cleared from the lung during labor and delivery and during the first 6 h of life; the process is accelerated by high catecholamine levels. Sodium pump proteins in the granular pneumocytes play an important role in liquid clearance, serving to transport the liquid from alveoli to interstitium. From the interstitium, the liquid is cleared into the circulation, either directly by osmotic forces or through the lymphatics. In some infants, clearance is delayed, resulting in respiratory distress, known as transient tachypnea of the newborn (TTN), which lasts for 24 to 48 h after birth. This condition is common in both mature and premature infants, especially if delivery is by cesarian section before the onset of labor. It is also seen commonly in infants of diabetic mothers.

In TTN, the oxygenation defect is mild; the right-to-left shunt is only 20 percent, similar to that seen in normal newborns. The problem is related primarily to poorly ventilated air spaces with low ventilation-perfusion ratios. It is unusual for more than 40 percent oxygen to be required for relief of hypoxemia. The functional residual capacity, measured by helium dilution, is normal, whereas the thoracic gas volume, measured by plethysmography, is increased, indicating the presence of gas trapping from compression of small airways by interstitial fluid. Significant hypercarbia may be present initially, but this resolves before the age of 24 h without the need for mechanical ventilation. The chest radiograph shows hyperinflation due to small-airway obstruction. The radiograph may also show coarse alveolar or interstitial densities and small pleural effusions; these abnormalities clear within 24 h. The condition is benign and not progressive like RDS. Infants need only oxygen therapy, and most tolerate room air by 24 h of age, although tachypnea, without labored breathing, may last for up to 1 week in some cases.

Meconium Aspiration Pneumonia

About 15 percent of deliveries are accompanied by meconium-stained amniotic fluid (MSAF). This complication has a strong association with gestational age; it occurs in only 2 percent of deliveries prior to 37 weeks' gestation, but in 44 percent after 42 weeks' gestation. MSAF appears to be a marker for chronic fetal distress and is frequently associated with fetal malnourishment and high levels of erythropoietin. The relationship with acute fetal distress is much less certain, as many newborns with MSAF have no evidence of depression or acidemia at birth. In MSAF, the meconium may be thin and well dispersed in the amniotic fluid, in which case little harm may result from aspiration. However, in some cases, the meconium is thick and particulate, in which case aspiration may cause meconium aspiration pneumonia (MAP). If acute fetal distress is superimposed on chronic fetal distress in the presence of MSAF with thick meconium, deep fetal gasping may cause meconium aspiration into the upper trachea or, much less commonly, into the mainstem bronchi and more distal airways.

Several studies have shown that MAP may be prevented by obstetric suctioning of the pharynx at the time the fetal head is delivered and while the chest remains compressed by the birth canal. Other studies have shown that tracheal suctioning immediately after birth is also effective in preventing MAP. In many institutions, the occurrence of MAP has virtually disappeared since these procedures have been performed routinely. Tracheal suctioning is important even if meconium is not seen at the lar-

ynx, as meconium is recovered from the trachea in up to 10 percent of cases. However, MAP may occur despite apparently effective endotracheal suctioning at birth. In these cases, the meconium may be aspirated so deeply into the lungs prior to birth that it cannot be recovered by tracheal suctioning. Once aspirated into the lung periphery, meconium causes severe obstruction of the peripheral airways and severe chemical pneumonitis. Infants with MAP have many of the classical signs of respiratory distress, as described for RDS. However, these infants do not have signs of prematurity, and they are hyperinflated rather than hypoinflated. Infants with MAP are mature or postmature; the skin or umbilical cord is usually stained with meconium. Loose skin and subcutaneous wasting (typical of fetal malnourishment) or dry, peeling skin (typical of the postmaturity syndrome) are often observed.

If possible, mechanical ventilation should be avoided in MAP, since the incidence of air leaks is high. Humidified oxygen and gentle chest physical therapy are the best initial treatments. If necessary, peripheral airway function may be improved with nasal or endotracheal CPAP. Bronchial lavage with saline is not helpful and, indeed, may cause deterioration. The traditional indications for mechanical ventilation are an arterial P_{O_2} under 50 mmHg with an F_{IO_2} of 1.0, hypercarbia with a pH less than 7.20, or significant apnea. Since these infants are large and often vigorous, they may fight the ventilator, in which case heavy sedation with or without neuromuscular blockade is warranted. It is imperative to drain any pneumothorax; chest tubes should be carefully positioned so the tips lie anteriorly.

Some evidence suggests that meconium may cause inactivation of surfactant. In a recent report of infants with MAP needing mechanical ventilation, three large doses of mammalian surfactant (each dose, 150 mg/kg) given at 6-h intervals produced a large improvement in oxygenation after the second dose; the number of infants who needed ECMO was significantly reduced.[21] Some infants with MAP may also have persistent pulmonary hypertension, in which case treatment with inhaled nitric oxide (5 to 20 ppm) may be useful.[35] If hypoxemia persists, infants may respond to HFOV. However, since gas trapping is prominent, pulmonary perfusion may be altered by high levels of mean airway pressure, making hypoxemia worse; HFOV may then fail. Infants with severe hypoxemia due to MAP usually respond well to treatment with ECMO, requiring relatively short courses of treatment of only 3 to 4 days.

Neonatal Pneumonia

Newborn infants may develop bacterial pneumonia by three different mechanisms: (1) In the case of Listeria and syphilis, bacteria may spread across the placenta from the mother, causing a transplacental pneumonia. (2) In amnionitis, the bacteria may be aspirated from amniotic fluid, causing postamnionitis pneumonia. The most common organism in this form of pneumonia is the group B Streptococcus, but *Escherichia coli* is also not uncommon. Amnionitis is often a complication of prolonged rupture of amniotic membranes, but amnionitis also occurs with intact membranes and causes preterm labor. The mother may have signs of fever, leukocytosis, tenderness, and cervical discharge. (3) Some infants develop pneumonia after aspirating infected maternal secretions in the birth canal, producing a transcervical pneumonia. This is probably the most common cause of neonatal pneumonia. In these cases, the mother has no signs of illness and no evidence of amnionitis.

Infants with neonatal pneumonia may resemble infants with RDS; for this reason, it is usually recommended that infants with RDS receive antibiotics, at least until cultures reports are available. In neonatal pneumonia, the infant may also have signs of poor systemic perfusion or present with apnea in the first 12 h of life. The blood culture is usually positive, and the white blood cell count may show leukocytosis and an increased number of band forms. Alternatively, the white blood cell count may show neutropenia in severe cases. A lumbar puncture should be performed to evaluate for meningitis, although most clinicians delay this procedure until the infant is more stable. Urinary rapid antigen tests are usually reliable in infants with definite signs of illness, but such tests are not useful screening devices in normal infants. The chest radiograph may show the same reticular-granular appearance as in RDS, or it may show a coarse reticular-nodular pattern. Pleural effusions are often present in infants with pneumonia, but they are uncommon in infants with RDS.

Infants with pneumonia should be treated with large doses of ampicillin for at least 10 days, and gentamicin should be used initially to add synergy. Most cases are treated with conventional mechanical ventilation, but if this fails, HFOV is usually successful. Sometimes the picture may be dominated by pulmonary hypertension, thought to be secondary to thromboxane mediators. In such cases, additional treatment with inhaled nitric oxide (5 to 20 ppm) may be useful.[35] In other cases, myocardial insufficiency (thought to be produced by cytokines) may dominate the picture, and ECMO may be necessary to support the circulation until antibiotics take effect and the heart recovers.

Persistent Pulmonary Hypertension of the Newborn Syndrome

Infants with persistent pulmonary hypertension of the newborn syndrome (PPHNS) are usually mature or postmature infants, but on occasion they may be premature. The lung histology of infants with PPHNS takes one of three forms.

In the hypertrophic type of PPHNS, the muscular tissue of the pulmonary arteries is hypertrophied and extends peripherally to the acini; the hypertrophy causes narrowing of the arteries and high resistance to pulmonary blood flow. This type of PPHNS is thought to be the result of sustained fetal hypertension in the pulmonary circuit, chronic vasoconstriction in chronic fetal distress, or sustained excessive pulmonary blood flow after in utero closure of the ductus arteriosus. Some cases of the last-cited mechanism may be due to maternal ingestion of salicylates or related drugs during pregnancy. In the hypoplastic type of PPHNS, the lungs, including the pulmonary arteries, are underdeveloped, usually as a result of congenital diaphragmatic hernia or prolonged leakage of amniotic fluid. The cross-sectional area of the pulmonary vascular bed is inadequate for normal neonatal pulmonary blood flow.

In the reactive type of PPHNS, lung histology is presumably normal (at least initially), but active vasoconstriction causes pulmonary hypertension. High levels of thromboxane, leukotrienes,

norepinephrine, or other mediators may be responsible for pulmonary vasoconstriction. Streptococcal infections and acute asphyxia at birth are common causes.

In practice, all three mechanisms of PPHNS are often present. For example, in pulmonary hypoplasia, the cross-sectional area of the pulmonary bed is greatly reduced, but secondary pulmonary vascular hypertrophy develops in response to the high pulmonary arterial pressures caused by normal pulmonary blood flow through hypoplastic lungs. These hypertrophic vessels are exceedingly sensitive to comparatively normal levels of vasoconstrictor mediators.

Infants with PPHNS may be depressed at birth and need immediate mechanical ventilation. Alternatively, they may develop progressive respiratory distress with increasing cyanosis, despite administration of supplemental oxygen. In some cases, the onset of respiratory distress is surprisingly delayed. Mild tachypnea may be the only sign until cyanosis develops after about 24 h.

In primary PPHNS, the chest radiograph may show clear or hyperlucent lungs, indicative of oligemia. Alternatively, the lungs may show a modest degree of pulmonary edema, perhaps secondary to birth asphyxia. In secondary PPHNS, the chest radiograph reflects the underlying condition—RDS, MAP, or pneumonia. A very common form of secondary PPHNS is that associated with congenital diaphragmatic hernia and accompanying pulmonary hypoplasia.

In one published series of infants with idiopathic (primary) PPHNS, lung lavage samples showed high levels of leukotriene mediators. Leukotrienes cause pulmonary vasoconstriction and high-permeability pulmonary edema. Experimental evidence suggests that PPHNS may be related to elevated levels of thromboxane; the high pulmonary artery resistance may be reversed with indomethacin. No clinical evidence supports use of this agent. In MAP, it is possible that meconium induces platelet aggregation and thromboxane release. A strong clinical correlation exists between meconium aspiration, transient thrombocytopenia, and PPHNS. Most infants with PPHNS have elevated levels of endothelin, another pulmonary vasoconstrictor.[52] Infants with PPHNS also have reduced urinary levels of nitrite and nitrate; thus, infants with PPHNS may not produce sufficient nitric oxide (NO) to adequately dilate the pulmonary arteries; the reduced NO may be due to reduced expression of nitric oxide synthase in endothelial cells.

Although PPHNS varies in severity, severe cases are life-threatening. Sooner or later, all infants with severe PPHNS develop severe hypoxemia and the need for mechanical ventilation using an F_{IO_2} of 1.0. The echocardiogram shows right-to-left shunting at the level of the ductus arteriosus, the foramen ovale, or both. In addition, dilation of the right ventricle or right atrium, tricuspid regurgitation (the systolic jet indicates the degree of pulmonary hypertension), compression of the left ventricle by the dilated right ventricle, impaired ventricular filling, and decreased systemic cardiac output are seen. Cardiac contractility may be poor, particularly when birth asphyxia or bacterial infection are responsible for PPHNS.

Correction of accompanying hypothermia, hypoglycemia, or hypocalcemia is important in the treatment of PPHNS. If the hematocrit is 65 percent or more, a dilutional exchange transfusion is indicated. Infants with PPHNS should be fluid restricted (70 ml/kg per day) to avoid pulmonary edema. It is also advisable to catheterize both the umbilical artery and vein. Sufficient supplemental oxygen should be given to maintain the arterial P_{O_2} at 90 to 100 mmHg, if possible. Since oxygenation is very labile in this condition, higher target levels of arterial P_{O_2} are recommended, with the caution that BPD may be a serious complication if the clinical course is prolonged. In very severe cases, an arterial P_{O_2} as low as 40 mmHg may be tolerated; if there are concerns about hypoxia, normal blood lactate levels provide considerable assurance. The mean blood pressure should be maintained in the range of 50 to 60 mmHg, as systemic hypotension promotes right-to-left atrial and ductal shunting and severe hypoxemia. Circulatory support should be provided with plasmanate, red blood cells, and dopamine (5 to 15 μg/kg per minute).

The infant should receive mechanical ventilation at rates of 60 to 90 breaths per minute, with the aim of producing a low arterial P_{CO_2} and an arterial pH in the range of 7.55 to 7.60. Continuous infusions of alkali (0.5 meq/kg per hour) can also be used to raise blood pH. Alkalosis often dramatically dilates the pulmonary arteries and improves oxygenation, but there is little evidence that this strategy actually improves the outcome of PPHNS. If respiratory alkalosis cannot be achieved without excessive peak inspiratory pressures, it may be advisable to use HFOV for adequate control of arterial P_{CO_2}; the evidence that HFOV is effective in this situation is sound.

Various drugs have been used as pulmonary artery vasodilators. Dobutamine (5 to 15 μg/kg per minute) may provide some reduction of pulmonary vascular resistance, as well as improved cardiac output. Tolazoline has been a traditional choice, but its propensity to cause systemic hypotension and its long half-life have severely limited its usefulness. Experimentally, tolazoline has produced improved oxygenation after endotracheal instillation. Nitroprusside (1 to 2 μg/kg per minute) provides a more controlled effect on the pulmonary circulation, but it is not specific, and there is no real evidence for its efficacy in this condition. In recent years, inhaled nitric oxide (5 to 20 ppm) has provided very encouraging improvements in oxygenation,[35] and the results of several controlled trials examining the overall outcome are awaited with interest. The great advantage of nitric oxide is that its vasodilatory effects are limited to the pulmonary circulation. Nitric oxide is inhaled into the lungs first and then inactivated by hemoglobin before it can exert systemic effects. Several studies report encouraging effects with use of continuous magnesium sulfate infusions, but experimental evidence suggests that this treatment does not produce specific pulmonary artery dilation. More recently, continuous infusions of adenosine have been shown to cause pulmonary vasodilation without inducing systemic hypotension.[36] Adenosine, like nitric oxide, has a very short half-life.

If the infant with PPHNS has underlying RDS, meconium aspiration pneumonia, or neonatal bacterial pneumonia, exogenous surfactant may be helpful. As a last resort, if the arterial P_{O_2} cannot be maintained above 40 mmHg, most patients will do well with ECMO. The most difficult cases of PPHNS are those associated with congenital diaphragmatic hernia and pulmonary hypoplasia. Over half of those who need ECMO eventually die, usually after ECMO is discontinued; their pulmonary hypoplasia is not consistent with survival.

Postasphyxial Pulmonary Edema

Some mature and postmature infants develop respiratory failure following severe birth asphyxia. These infants may need mechanical ventilation immediately in the delivery room, or they may be resuscitated only to then develop progressive respiratory distress under an oxygen hood after admission to the nursery. Infants with postasphyxial pulmonary edema (PAPE) do not have evidence of prematurity (as in the case of RDS), MAP, or neonatal pneumonia. Instead, infants with PAPE have asphyxia, heart failure, ventricular dysfunction, pulmonary edema, and, sometimes, pulmonary hypertension. Some may develop clinical pulmonary hemorrhage, the most severe form of PAPE. This condition has been reproduced in newborn lambs by clamping the umbilical cord prior to delivery; the lambs show elevated pulmonary capillary pressures and transudation of fluid into the lungs.[1]

Acquired Respiratory Distress Syndrome

Infants with acquired respiratory distress syndrome are thought to have fetal asphyxia prior to birth. They are usually mature infants who have a course similar to that of premature infants with RDS.[20] The chest radiograph resembles RDS with a reticular-granular pattern, but these infants do not have signs of prematurity (as in RDS) or evidence of heart failure or ventricular dysfunction (as in PAPE). Although not proved, these infants are thought to have a mature L/S ratio prior to birth, reflecting a mature surfactant system, but they then develop surfactant inactivation. The infants respond well to conventional mechanical ventilation or HFOV and exogenous surfactant therapy; only a very few with PAPE deteriorate sufficiently to need ECMO.

Congenital Alveolar Proteinosis due to SP-B Deficiency

Severe, fatal RDS has been described in siblings of several families. The lung histology is that of congenital alveolar proteinosis; the alveoli are packed with a proteinaceous material rich in SP-A and surfactant protein C (SP-C). Neither the mRNA for SP-B nor the protein itself can be detected. This defect is due to a mutation in exon 4 of the SP-B gene; a 2-base insertion produces a frameshift signal for termination of translation. Amniotic samples have shown a low L/S ratio at term and the absence of SP-B.[25] To make the diagnosis, tracheal aspirates should be examined for SP-B by ELISA assay or Western Blot, or lung tissue from biopsy or autopsy should be examined by immunostaining. These infants have died even after use of ECMO, but several short-term survivors following lung transplantation have been reported.

SURFACTANT REPLACEMENT THERAPY FOR RESPIRATORY DISTRESS SYNDROME

The earliest attempts to provide surfactant replacement therapy in RDS were not successful because: (1) SPC alone was used, without an additive to accelerate adsorption to the surface; (2)

the small dose used did not account for destruction of surfactant in the airways; and (3) the method of delivery by nebulization was not practical. However, Enhorning and associates[18] showed experimentally that the lung surface active film can be reconstituted by pharyngeal or tracheal deposition of exogenous surfactant at birth. The first successful trial of surfactant replacement in humans was conducted by Fujiwara and colleagues.[22] In this study, marked improvements in oxygenation in infants with RDS were demonstrated (Fig. 169-4).

Several types of exogenous surfactant are available: (1) bovine lung mince lipid extract, enriched with synthetic lipids (Survanta, Abbott Laboratories); (2) porcine lung mince lipid extract, enriched by chromatography (Curosurf, Chiesi Pharmaceuticals); (3) bovine lung lavage lipid extract (Infasurf, Forrest Laboratories; Alveofact, Boeringer Ingelheim); mixtures of synthetic lipids (Exosurf, Glaxo-Wellcome; Pneumactant, Britannia Pharmaceuticals); and (5) mixtures of synthetic lipids and SP-B peptides (KL4 surfactant). Exogenous surfactants are instilled directly into the endotracheal tube and dispersed into the lung by mechanical ventilation or by bag-tube ventilation. Two treatment strategies are used: (1) a prophylactic strategy, in which all infants under 1000 g birth weight, who are considered high risk for RDS, are treated in the delivery room before 15 to 30 min of life; and (2) a rescue strategy, in which larger infants with established RDS are treated as soon as the diagnosis is established.

A large number of randomized controlled trials have established that exogenous surfactant in premature infants markedly reduces the severity of RDS and, as a result, reduces neonatal mortality by approximately 50 percent.[42] This beneficial effect on neonatal survival largely is maintained through 1 year of age.[39] In addition, surfactant reduces the incidence of pulmonary air leak and increases survival of infants without BPD. The latter is an important finding, because BPD increases health care expenditures and contributes to additional late deaths. However, probably because there are more survivors, the overall reduction in BPD is not large after exogenous surfactant, although major reductions in the incidence of BPD have been seen in a few trials (especially those with rescue treatment with Exosurf).[9,39]

In the smallest infants (500 to 699 g birth weight), evidence that surfactant is effective in reducing mortality is not convincing,[54] although analyses of annual mortality statistics suggest that it may have some benefit in infants with a birth weight of 600 g or more. Exogenous surfactant is effective in larger infants with birth weights over 1500 g; in these patients, surfactant therapy is associated with a significant reduction in the incidence of BPD, as well as substantial hospital cost savings. The incidence of RDS is lower in larger infants, but in many centers it is the larger infants who make up most of the population with RDS. Life-saving therapy should not be withheld simply because the incidence of the target disease is low.

The optimal phospholipid dose for mammalian surfactants is thought to be in the range of 100 mg/kg; smaller doses (e.g., 60 mg/kg) are not as effective. In the case of Exosurf, the optimal SPC dose is considered to be 67.5 mg/kg; smaller doses are not as effective, and larger doses add no further benefit. Multiple doses are more effective than a single dose; 4 doses do not improve the results over 2 doses, and 6 doses do not improve the results over 3 doses. Therefore, the appropriate number of doses is 2 or 3 in most cases.[9] There is general agreement that the dosage interval should be 12 h, based on the experimental half-life of surfactant. However, in a few studies the interval was as frequent as every 6 h if the patient did not respond well.[38] When the F_{IO_2} is below 0.3, it is reasonable to discontinue surfactant treatment. Late doses in the setting of low ventilator pressures may cause an unnecessary deterioration during drug administration.

Several controlled trials have established that in small premature infants the prophylactic strategy is superior to the rescue strategy,[33] and that in the rescue strategy, it is better to treat at 2 h of age than at 3 to 6 h of age.[47] These observations are consistent with evidence that lung injury in RDS is present by 3 h of age and that exogenous surfactant treatment may prevent such injury.[46]

The most dramatic effect of surfactant is an improvement in oxygenation, frequently within minutes. The improvement correlates well with improved lung volume and improved static lung compliance, as new air spaces are recruited and effective pulmonary blood flow is increased. Improvements in dynamic compliance have been more difficult to demonstrate. Despite these improvements, there has been concern about other effects.

Surfactant instillation may be associated with a transient reduction in mean blood pressure and cerebral blood flow, followed by transient hypercarbia and an increase in cerebral blood flow. A disturbing cerebroelectric depression[28] and reduced brain oxyhemoglobin may occur.[19] Surprisingly, these phenomena have not been associated with an increased incidence of IVH, except in a few isolated trials. However, although it might be expected from reduced severity of RDS, the overall incidence of IVH has not been reduced by surfactant, except in larger infants with RDS.[9,39] The procedure used for instillation may increase the incidence of IVH and obscure the possible benefits of reduced

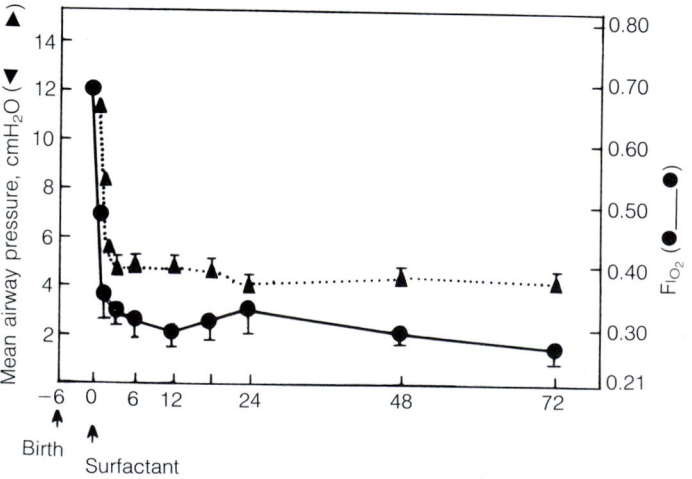

FIGURE 169-4 Response to exogenous surfactant in infants with RDS. Twelve premature infants were treated at 6 h of age with an endotracheal instillation of bovine surfactant, 100 mg/kg. Immediately following treatment, inspired oxygen and mean airway pressure requirements decreased rapidly and remained low through 72 h. [*From Fujiwara T: Surfactant replacement in neonatal RDS, in Robertson B, Van Golde LMG, Batenburg J (eds), Pulmonary Surfactant. Amsterdam, Elsevier, 1984.*]

severity of RDS on the incidence of IVH. In addition, a very rapid response to surfactant may produce a sudden reduction in pulmonary vascular resistance and a large left-to-right shunt at the ductus arteriosus; this shunt may "steal" brain blood flow and further predispose to IVH.

A large left-to-right shunt at the ductus may also increase pulmonary capillary pressures. A meta-analysis has established that the incidence of pulmonary hemorrhage (hemorrhagic pulmonary edema) is increased after exogenous surfactant.[50] Although an increased incidence of symptomatic PDA may also be expected as a result of more prolonged left-to-right shunting at the ductus, symptomatic PDA has not been observed in most surfactant trials, presumably because improved oxygenation encourages ductal closure.

Direct comparisons between synthetic and mammalian surfactants have not suggested any major differences in efficacy. The incidence of pulmonary air leaks is reduced more with mammalian surfactants. Ventilator settings improve more rapidly with mammalian surfactants. However, many studies have shown other trends in favor of mammalian surfactants. In a meta-analysis, the overall mortality appears to be 20 percent lower with mammalian surfactants than with Exosurf[23]; this difference may translate into 1 extra survivor for every 40 infants treated. In an important comparative study, Survanta produced a faster improvement in lung volume and oxygenation over a period of 2 h than did Exosurf; the response to Exosurf occurred more slowly (over 6 h).[13] Others have shown a much faster improvement of static lung compliance with mammalian surfactants. The slower response with Exosurf may be explained by the relative inefficiency of the alcohol additive in speeding adsorption of SPC when compared with SP-B and SP-C in mammalian preparations. Some experimental data suggest that Exosurf may function better at ventilator rates higher than are commonly used in many hospitals.

In animal models, administration of surfactants derived from other species causes production of antibodies. Such antibodies have been demonstrated to cause respiratory failure by cross-reacting with and inhibiting endogenous surfactant in recipient animals. Antibodies against animal-derived surfactants have been demonstrated in infants, but in several studies the levels of antibody were similar in treated and control infants. These findings suggest that the antibody response to endogenous surfactant entering the circulation is a result of lung injury rather than a response to exogenous surfactant. The significance of these findings is not yet apparent, but an increased antibody level may be associated with BPD.

About 15 percent of treated infants do not have an adequate response to surfactant. Such failures may be due to pulmonary complications such as pneumonia, interstitial emphysema, or pulmonary edema secondary to PDA, or to nonpulmonary complications such as IVH (which by itself can cause pulmonary edema). A poor response to surfactant is associated with high risk for development of BPD. Exogenous surfactants which contain high levels of SP-B and SP-C, such as Infasurf and Alveofact, may be more resistant to inactivation by edema fluid and plasma proteins. SP-A is particularly important in protecting against inactivation,[58] but none of the available surfactant preparations contain SP-A.

Economic evaluations have suggested cost savings of 5 to 20 percent per survivor, but some have worried that the increased number of surviving, small, premature infants may increase the overall level of hospital expenditures.[44] More recent analyses indicate that savings in larger infants outweigh costs incurred for smaller infants.[3] Extensive controlled evaluation of infants treated with exogenous surfactant has established that the neurodevelopmental outcome at age 1 to 2 years is similar to that of controls.[8] Most important, surfactant does not increase the absolute number of surviving handicapped children, who might place an increased load on the existing community services.[40]

SURFACTANT REPLACEMENT THERAPY FOR ACUTE ADULT RESPIRATORY DISTRESS SYNDROME

A substantial body of evidence indicates that the surfactant system is dysfunctional in both animal models of acute lung injury and patients with acute adult respiratory distress syndrome (ARDS).[48] The possible role of surfactant dysfunction in ARDS was recognized in the original description of the disorder some 30 years ago. However, whether surfactant replacement can improve the outcome of ARDS remains unclear. Despite encouraging results in two phase II trials of aerosolized synthetic surfactant in patients with sepsis-induced ARDS, a large phase III trial in the same patient population failed to confirm the beneficial effects.[2]

The absence of demonstrable benefit of synthetic surfactant in patients with ARDS, despite multiple reports of life-saving effects in infants with RDS,[40] remains puzzling. Potential explanations include: (1) The hydrophobic proteins of natural surfactant may be required for beneficial effects in ARDS; (2) aerosolizing surfactant may be a suboptimal way of delivering surfactant in ARDS; (3) a type II statistical error might be operative; (4) surfactant dysfunction may be an epiphenomenon in ARDS. The most likely explanation is that hydrophobic proteins are needed in ARDS, since much of the surfactant dysfunction is secondary to nonspecific inhibition by pulmonary edema fluid. Protein-containing surfactants appear to withstand nonspecific inhibitors better than synthetic surfactants. Unfortunately, isolating, purifying, and sterilizing protein-containing surfactants obtained from animal sources is expensive, and the cost of the material per patient with ARDS probably precludes widespread application of animal-derived surfactants in treatment. When third-generation, genetically engineered, peptide-containing surfactants become available, improving the outcome of ARDS with surfactant replacement may finally become a reality.

REFERENCES

1. Adamson TM, Boyd RDH, Hill JR, et al: Effect of asphyxia due to umbilical cord occlusion in the foetal lamb on leakage of liquid from the circulation and on permeability of lung capillaries to albumin. *J Physiol* 207:493–505, 1970.

2. Anzueto A, Baughamn RP, Guntupalli KK, et al: Aerosolized surfactant in sepsis-induced acute respiratory distress syndrome. *New Engl J Med* 334:1418–1421, 1996.

3. Backhouse ME, Mauskopf JA, Jones D, et al: Economic outcomes of synthetic surfactant rescue therapy in infants weighing 1250 grams or more with respiratory distress syndrome: Results from a randomized trial. *PharmacoEconomics* 6:358–369, 1994.

4. Chida S, Fujiwara T: Stable microbubble test for predicting the risk of respiratory distress syndrome: Comparisons with other predictors of fetal lung maturity in amniotic fluid. *Eur J Pediatr* 152:148–151, 1993.

5. Clark RH, Yoder BA, Sell MS: Prospective randomized comparison of high frequency oscillation and conventional ventilation in candidates for extracorporal membrane oxygenation. *J Pediatr* 124:447–454, 1994.

6. Clements JA, Tooley WH: Kinetics of surface active material in the fetal lung, in Hodson, WA (ed), *Development of the Lung*. New York, Dekker, 1977, pp 349–366.

7. Corbet A, Bucciarelli R, Goldman S, et al: Decreased mortality rate among small premature infants treated at birth with a single dose of synthetic surfactant: A multicenter controlled trial. *J Pediatr* 118:277–284, 1991.

8. Corbet A, Long W, Schumacher R, et al: Double blind developmental evaluation at 1 year corrected age of 597 premature infants with birth weights 500–1350 grams enrolled in 3 placebo controlled trials of prophylactic surfactant. *J Pediatr* 126:S5–S12, 1995.

9. Corbet A: Clinical trials of synthetic surfactant in the respiratory distress syndrome of premature infants. *Clin Perinatol* 20:737–760, 1993.

10. Corbet AJ, Bucciarelli R, Goldman SA, et al: Decreased mortality rate among small premature infants treated at birth with a single dose of synthetic surfactant: A multicenter controlled trial. *J Pediatr* 118:277–284, 1991.

11. Corbet A: Medical manipulation of the ductus arteriosus, in Garson A, Bricker JT, Fisher DJ, Neish SR (eds), *The Science and Practice of Pediatric Cardiology*. Philadelphia, Lea and Febiger. In press.

12. Corbet AJS, Ross JA, Beaudry PH, Stern L: Ventilation perfusion relationships as assessed by aA*DN$_2$ in hyaline membrane disease. *J Appl Physiol* 36:74–81, 1974.

13. Cotton RB, Olsson T, Law AB, et al: The physiologic effects of surfactant treatment on gas exchange in newborn premature infants with hyaline membrane disease. *Pediatr Res* 34:495–501, 1993.

14. DeMello DE, Heyman S, Phelps DS, Floros J: Immunogold localization of SP-A in lungs of infants dying of respiratory distress syndrome. *Am J Pathol* 142:1631–1640, 1993.

15. DeMello DE, Chi EY, Doo E, Lagunoff D: Absence of tubular myelin in lungs of infants dying with hyaline membrane disease. *Am J Pathol* 127:131–139, 1987.

16. Dreizzen E, Migdal M, Praud JP, et al: Passive compliance of total respiratory system in preterm newborn infants with respiratory distress syndrome. *J Pediatr* 112:778–781, 1988.

17. Dudell GG, Gersony WM: Patent ductus arteriosus in neonates with severe respiratory disease. *J Pediatr* 104:915–920, 1984.

18. Enhorning G, Grossman G, Robertson B: Tracheal deposition of surfactant before the first breath. *Am Rev Respir Dis* 107:921–927, 1973.

19. Fahnenstich H, Schmidt S, Spaniol S, Kowalewski S: Relative changes in oxyhemoglobin, de-oxyhemoglobin and intracranial blood volume during surfactant replacement therapy in infants with respiratory distress syndrome. *Dev Pharmacol Ther* 17:150–153, 1991.

20. Faix RG, Viscardi RM, DiPietro MA, Nicks JJ: Adult respiratory distress syndrome in full term infants. *Pediatrics* 83:971–976, 1989.

21. Findlay RD, Taeusch HW, Walther FJ: Surfactant replacement therapy for meconium aspiration syndrome. *Pediatrics* 97:48–52, 1996.

22. Fujiwara T, Maeta H, Chida S, et al: Artificial surfactant therapy in hyaline membrane disease. *Lancet* 1:55–59, 1980.

23. Halliday HL: Overview of clinical trials comparing natural and synthetic surfactants. *Biol Neonate* 67(suppl 1):32–47, 1995.

24. Hallman M, Teramo K: Measurement of the lecithin sphingomyelin ratio and phosphatidylglycerol in amniotic fluid: An accurate method for the assessment of fetal lung maturity. *Br J Obstet Gynaecol* 88:806–813, 1981.

25. Hamvas A, Cole FS, deMello DE, et al: Surfactant protein B deficiency: Antenatal diagnosis and prospective treatment with surfactant replacement. *J Pediatr* 125:356–361, 1994.

26. Hansen TN, Corbet AJS, Kenny JD, et al: Effects of oxygen and constant positive pressure breathing on aA*DCO$_2$ in hyaline membrane disease. *Pediatr Res* 13:1167–1171, 1979.

27. Helbock HJ, Insoft RM, Conte FA: Glucocorticoid responsive hypotension in extremely low birth weight newborns. *Pediatrics* 92:715–717, 1993.

28. Hellstrom-Westas L, Bell AH, Skov L, et al: Cerebro-electric depression following surfactant treatment in preterm neonates. *Pediatrics* 89:643–647, 1992.

29. Herbert WNP, Chapman JF, Schnoor MM: Role of the TDx FLM assay in fetal lung maturity. *Am J Obstet Gynecol* 168:808–812, 1993.

30. Hoekstra RE, Jackson JC, Myers TF, et al: Improved neonatal survival following multiple doses of bovine surfactant in very premature neonates at risk for respiratory distress syndrome. *Pediatrics* 88:10–18, 1991.

31. Hulsey TC, Alexander GR, Robillard PY, et al: Hyaline membrane disease: The role of ethnicity and maternal risk factors. *Am J Obstet Gynecol* 168:572–576, 1993.

32. Ikegami M, Ueda T, Absolom D, et al: Changes in exogenous surfactant in ventilated preterm lamb lungs. *Am Rev Respir Dis* 148:837–844, 1993.

33. Kendig JW, Notter RH, Cox C, et al: A comparison of surfactant as immediate prophylaxis and as rescue therapy in newborns of less than 30 weeks gestation. *New Engl J Med* 324:865–871, 1991.

34. Keszler M, Donn SM, Bucciarelli RL, et al: Multicenter controlled trial comparing high frequency jet ventilation and conventional mechanical ventilation in newborn infants with pulmonary interstitial emphysema. *J Pediatr* 119:85–93, 1991.

35. Kinsella JP, Neish SR, Shaffer E, Abman AH: Low dose inhalational nitric oxide in persistent pulmonary hypertension of the newborn. *Lancet* 340:819–820, 1992.

36. Konduri GG, Garcia DC, Kazzi NJ, Shankaran S: Adenosine infusion improves oxygenation in term infants with respiratory failure. *Pediatrics* 97:295–300, 1996.

37. Kopelman AE: Blood pressure and cerebral ischemia in very low birth weight infants. *J Pediatr* 116:1000–1002, 1990.

38. Liechty EA, Donovan E, Purohit D, et al: Reduction of neonatal mortality after multiple doses of bovine surfactant in low birth weight neonates with respiratory distress syndrome. *Pediatrics* 88:19–28, 1991.

39. Long WA, Thompson T, Sundell H, et al: Effects of two doses of a synthetic surfactant on mortality rate and survival without bronchopulmonary dysplasia in 700–1350 gram infants with respiratory distress syndrome. *J Pediatr* 118:595–605, 1991.

40. Long WA, Zucker JZ, Kraybill EN: Symposium on synthetic surfactant II: Perspective and commentary. *J Pediatr* 126:S1–S4, 1995.

41. Mauskopf JA, Backhouse ME, Jones D, et al: Synthetic surfactant for rescue treatment of respiratory distress syndrome in premature infants weighing from 700 to 1350 grams: Impact on hospital resource use and charges. *J Pediatr* 125:94–101, 1995.

42. Mercier CE, Soll RF: Clinical trials of natural surfactant extract in respiratory distress syndrome. *Clin Perinatol* 20:711–735, 1993.

43. Morrison JJ, Rennie JM, Milton PJ: Neonatal respiratory morbidity and mode of delivery at term: Influence of timing of elective cesarian section. *Br J Obstet Gynaecol* 102:101–106, 1995.

44. Mugford M, Piercy J, Chalmers I: Cost implications of different approaches to the prevention of respiratory distress syndrome. *Arch Dis Child* 66:757–764, 1991.

45. NIH Consensus Development Conference Statement: Effect of corticosteroids for fetal maturation on perinatal outcomes. *Am J Obstet Gynecol* 173:246–252, 1995.

46. Nilsson R, Grossman G, Robertson B: Lung surfactant and the pathogenesis of neonatal bronchiolar lesions induced by artificial ventilation. *Pediatr Res* 12:249–255, 1978.

47. OSIRIS Collaborative Group: Early versus delayed neonatal administration of a synthetic surfactant: the judgement of OSIRIS. *Lancet* 340:1363–1369, 1992.

48. Pattishall E, Long WA: Surfactant replacement in adult respiratory distress syndrome, in Fishman AP (ed), *Update: Pulmonary Diseases and Disorders*. New York, McGraw-Hill, 1992, pp 225–236.

49. Pryhuber GS, Hull WM, Fink I, et al: Ontogeny of surfactant proteins A and B in human amniotic fluid as indices of fetal lung maturation. *Pediatr Res* 30:597–605, 1991.

50. Raju TNK, Langenberg P: Pulmonary hemorrhage and exogenous surfactant therapy: A meta-analysis. *J Pediatr* 123:603–610, 1993.

51. Richardson CP, Jung AL: Effects of continuous positive airway pressure on pulmonary function and blood gases of infants with respiratory distress syndrome. *Pediatr Res* 12:771–774, 1978.

52. Rosenberg AA, Kennaugh J, Koppenhafer SL, et al: Elevated immunoreactive endothelin-1 levels in newborn infants with persistent pulmonary hypertension. *J Pediatr* 123:109–114, 1993.

53. Sanders RJ, Cox C, Phelps DL, Sinkin RA: Two doses of early intravenous dexamethasone for prevention of bronchopulmonary dysplasia in babies with respiratory distress syndrome. *Pediatr Res* 36:122–128, 1994.

54. Stevenson D, Walther F, Long W, et al: Controlled trial of a single dose of synthetic surfactant at birth in premature infants weighing 500–699 grams. *J Pediatr* 120:S3–S12, 1992.

55. Tammela KT, Lanning FP, Koivisto ME: The relationship of fluid restriction during the first month of life and the occurrence and severity of bronchopulmonary dysplasia in low birth weight infants: A 1 year radiological follow up. *Eur J Pediatr* 151:367–371, 1992.

56. Tubman TRJ, Rollins MD, Patterson C, Halliday HL: Increased incidence of respiratory distress syndrome in babies of hypertensive mothers. *Arch Dis Child* 66:52–54, 1991.

57. Yeh TF, Torre JA, Rastogi A, et al: Early postnatal dexamethasone therapy in premature infants with severe respiratory distress syndrome: A double blind controlled study. *J Pediatr* 117:273–282, 1990.

58. Yukitake K, Brown CL, Schlueter MA, et al: Surfactant apoprotein A modifies the inhibitory effect of plasma proteins on surfactant activity in vivo. *Pediatr Res* 37:21–25, 1995.

CHAPTER 170

ACUTE RESPIRATORY FAILURE IN THE SURGICAL PATIENT

Robert M. Kotloff

Advances in surgical technique, anesthesia and analgesia, and postoperative supportive care have facilitated application of sophisticated surgical procedures to an expanding spectrum of patients. Emboldened by diminished operative mortality rates, clinicians are increasingly willing to subject older and sicker patients to rigorous but potentially life-saving surgical interventions. In most instances, the success or failure of the surgery is defined not in the operating room but postoperatively, when the adverse effects of surgery may first become apparent and when intercurrent complications may jeopardize the patient's well-being.

The respiratory system is particularly vulnerable to the effects of general anesthesia and surgery, and postoperative respiratory impairment is common. While generally mild and well tolerated in otherwise healthy, young patients, postoperative respiratory compromise may have serious consequences in the elderly and in patients with preexisting lung disease. Potentially devastating postoperative complications—such as pneumonia, aspiration, and acute respiratory distress syndrome (ARDS)—may lead to respiratory failure independent of the patient's presurgical status. Overall, pulmonary complications account for approximately 25 percent of postoperative deaths. This figure is, in fact, conservative, since many patients with respiratory failure can be supported on mechanical ventilation, only to die of other nonrespiratory complications (e.g., sepsis, gastrointestinal bleeding, and multiorgan failure). In addition to their effect on mortality, respiratory complications exact a toll in lengthening intensive care and hospital stay, delaying convalescence, and escalating the cost of care. Therefore, clinicians who provide preoperative evaluation and postoperative care must be familiar with the factors that predispose to pulmonary impairment in the surgical patient. Many of these concepts are considered in Chapter 104. This chapter focuses on the most fulminant of the perioperative respiratory considerations—acute respiratory failure.

IDENTIFICATION OF THE HIGH-RISK PATIENT

In a review of over 7000 patients undergoing various gastrointestinal, urologic, gynecologic, and orthopedic procedures, an incidence of postoperative pulmonary complications of 4.8 percent was noted.[32] Most complications were minor; respiratory failure requiring mechanical ventilation beyond 24 h occurred in only 0.8 percent. However, based on this and other studies, it is clear that risk varies markedly. While risk of postoperative respiratory failure is negligible in the young, healthy nonsmoker undergoing elective knee surgery, it is significant in the elderly patient with underlying chronic obstructive pulmonary disease (COPD) undergoing emergent repair of a thoracoabdominal aortic aneurysm.

Considerable effort has been devoted to objectively defining the factors that affect the risk of postoperative pulmonary complications. Drawing firm conclusions from published studies is problematic because of their methodologic weaknesses, inconsistencies in the definition of postoperative complications, conflicting results, and the retrospective study design frequently em-

TABLE 170-1

Risk Factors for Postoperative Pulmonary Complications

Factors related to the patient
  COPD
  Advanced age
  Extensive (and recent) smoking history
  Obesity
  High physical status category per American Society of
    Anesthesiologists (ASA)
Factors related to the surgery
  Thoracic and upper abdominal procedures
  Emergency surgery
  Prolonged anesthesia time (>3 h)
  Large intraoperative blood transfusion requirements

ployed. Nonetheless, a number of preoperative and operative factors have been identified (Table 170-1). The factors that have been most thoroughly studied in association with postoperative respiratory failure are discussed below.

Type of Operative Procedure

Procedures involving the upper abdomen or thorax carry the greatest risk of postoperative pulmonary complications, including respiratory failure (Table 170-2). In large part, the risk is attributable to the profound derangement in pulmonary mechanics accompanying these procedures (see below). Thoracoabdominal aneurysm repair carries the greatest risk of postoperative respiratory failure.[18,28,41] Given the need for both abdominal and thoracic incisions as well as division of the diaphragm and costal margin, this observation is not surprising. Other procedures with significant risk include abdominal aortic aneurysm repair, upper gastrointestinal surgery, thoracotomy, and open heart surgery. Lower abdominal procedures carry a much smaller risk than those involving the upper abdomen; procedures involving the extremities carry a negligible risk.

In some cases, the surgical approach can be modified to lessen the risk of postoperative pulmonary complications in patients who are marginal operative candidates because of advanced age or comorbid conditions. For example, use of a transverse abdominal incision appears to carry less risk than a vertical mid-

TABLE 170-2

Incidence of Respiratory Failure Following Surgery

Procedure	References	Incidence of Postoperative Respiratory Failure
TAAA repair	[18, 28, 41]	8–33%
AAA repair	[20, 28]	5–24%
Lung resection	[3, 27]	4–15%
CABG	[43]	5–8%
All types[a]	[32]	0.8%

Abbreviations: TAAA = thoracoabdominal aortic aneurysm; AAA = abdominal aortic aneurysm; CABG = coronary artery bypass grafting.
[a]Refers to general survey of gastrointestinal, urologic, gynecologic, and orthopedic procedures.

line incision. Preliminary data suggest that laparoscopic cholecystectomy is associated with a lower incidence of pulmonary complications than the conventional open approach.[37] For thoracic procedures, a median sternotomy or muscle-sparing lateral thoracotomy[24] is better tolerated than the standard posterolateral thoracotomy. However, these approaches provide more limited access to the thorax than does standard thoracotomy. In addition, they are generally inadequate for resection of the left lower lobe or for tumors involving the posterior chest wall, diaphragm, or superior sulcus. Additionally, removal of bulky tumors via the muscle-sparing approach may be problematic. Video-assisted thoracoscopic surgery (VATS) also holds promise as a less morbid thoracic procedure. It has been applied successfully in the performance of pleurodesis, pleural decortication, lung biopsy, pulmonary resection (including lobectomy), and esophagomyotomy.[17] Preliminary data suggest that VATS results in reduced postoperative pain and hospital stay compared with thoracotomy.[17] Whether this procedure carries a diminished risk of postoperative pulmonary complications remains unanswered.

Chronic Obstructive Pulmonary Disease

An association between chronic obstructive pulmonary disease (COPD) and postoperative pulmonary complications is well established. In a study performed in the 1960s, two-thirds of patients with evidence of airflow obstruction had postoperative pulmonary complications, while only approximately 3 percent of those with normal pulmonary function had such complications.[39]

A number of studies performed subsequently have addressed more specifically the association between COPD and postoperative respiratory failure. A 5 percent incidence of postoperative respiratory failure was noted in a group of 134 patients with COPD.[16] Similar to previously reported observations, these episodes were seen exclusively after upper abdominal and thoracic procedures. A preoperative $FEF_{25-75\%}$ of less than 50 percent predicted, in conjunction with a FVC of less than 75 percent predicted, defined a group at high risk for respiratory failure. However, while these indices successfully identified most patients who developed respiratory failure, they were not specific; many patients who met the criteria did not develop respiratory failure.

Three studies have focused exclusively on patients with severe COPD whose pulmonary function placed them in a range once considered "prohibitive" for the performance of surgery. In one study,[50] only 3 of 16 patients with severe airflow obstruction (mean FEV_1, 0.89 L) developed postoperative respiratory failure—each following thoracotomy. In another, only 2 of 42 patients with an FEV_1 between 0.3 and 1 L developed respiratory failure requiring ventilator support for more than 24 h following 53 nonthoracic procedures, including 15 involving the upper abdomen.[31] In both cases, the respiratory failure followed upper abdominal surgery. Finally, in the largest and most recent study,[23] 89 patients with severe COPD (mean FEV_1, 37.8 percent predicted) who underwent 107 consecutive operations were evaluated for the overall incidence of postoperative pulmonary complications. Twenty-nine percent of patients developed respiratory complications; these patients could not be distinguished on the basis of preoperative spirometric values. Six episodes of respiratory failure (a 5.6 percent incidence) were noted, with four terminating in death; these episodes occurred predominantly after cardiac surgery.

Taken in sum, these studies document a relatively low and acceptable incidence of postoperative respiratory failure in patients with COPD. The studies corroborate the observation that patients undergoing thoracic, cardiac, and upper abdominal procedures are at greatest risk; however, the data fall short of establishing whether COPD is an independent risk factor for respiratory failure following these procedures.

This issue is further addressed by studies focusing on outcomes following specific high-risk procedures. In this regard, the risk of postoperative respiratory failure and death in patients with severe COPD undergoing lung resection is significant. A 50 percent incidence of respiratory failure and death was reported in 6 patients with a predicted postresection FEV_1 of less than 40 percent of normal, while there were no deaths and only 2 episodes of transient respiratory failure (a 4 percent incidence) in a group of 47 patients whose predicted lung function exceeded this value.[27] In another study,[30] respiratory failure developed in all 10 patients who had a predicted postoperative FEV_1 of less than 30 percent of normal. There is some evidence that patients who maintain a good performance status in spite of severe COPD fare better after lung resection. An uncomplicated postoperative course was described in 7 of 8 patients with a predicted postresection FEV_1 of less than 30 percent of normal who had a peak oxygen consumption of equal to or greater than 15 ml/kg per minute on formal exercise testing.[29]

The relationship between postoperative respiratory failure and COPD is less clear cut in the setting of other thoracic and abdominal procedures. In one study employing multivariate analysis, COPD was found to be an independent risk factor for respiratory failure following repair of thoracoabdominal aortic aneurysm.[41] Respiratory failure developed in 53 percent of patients with COPD and in only 23 percent of patients without this disorder. The risk of respiratory failure correlated linearly with preoperative spirometry, precluding identification of a particular set of "threshold" values. In contrast, in two other studies of thoracoabdominal aneurysm surgery that employed similar statistical means, COPD was not identified as a significant predictive variable for postoperative respiratory failure.[18,28]

The impact of COPD on outcome following coronary artery bypass grafting (CABG) has also been examined.[6] Compared with a group of matched controls, a significantly higher percentage of patients with COPD required mechanical ventilation in excess of 48 h (18.9 vs. 3.7 percent) or reintubation (13.5 vs. 3.7 percent). In a similar study, a group of patients with moderate to severe lung disease undergoing cardiac surgery had a statistically greater incidence of pulmonary complications and a longer length of stay in the intensive care unit compared with a control group without pulmonary disease.[2] Notably, however, there were no episodes of respiratory failure in either group.

Finally, factors associated with need for prolonged mechanical ventilation following major abdominal vascular surgery, including abdominal aortic aneurysm repair and aortobifemoral bypass grafting, have been investigated.[20] Following these procedures, 24 percent of patients required ventilatory support for more than 24 h. In most cases, extubation was accomplished

immediately postoperatively, but reinstitution of ventilatory support was subsequently necessitated by progressive hypoxemia due to atelectasis. While an extensive smoking history and low preoperative Pa_{O_2} were predictive of prolonged postoperative ventilatory support, the severity of COPD as defined by preoperative spirometry was not. Indeed, no prospective evaluation of patients undergoing abdominal surgery has shown that pulmonary function studies can reliably identify patients at increased risk of serious postoperative pulmonary complications.

Several conclusions can be drawn from this conflicting body of literature. First, the presence of severe COPD appears to affect the outcome of lung resection adversely. For this population of patients, a predicted postoperative FEV_1 of less than 30 to 40 percent of normal defines a group at high risk for respiratory failure. Second, for patients undergoing cardiac procedures, the data suggest that COPD poses an independent risk for postoperative respiratory morbidity; however, further studies are required to better define this risk and its relationship to preoperative lung function. Finally, there are currently no consistent data defining COPD as an independent risk factor for respiratory failure following upper abdominal surgery. In sum, COPD, even when severe, does not in its own right pose a prohibitive risk for postoperative respiratory failure in patients undergoing abdominal and nonresectional thoracic procedures. Acknowledging current uncertainties about the full contribution of COPD to postoperative risk, the presence of significant lung disease should prompt a careful analysis of the necessity of the surgery planned; however, it should not preclude surgery deemed likely to extend patient survival or to markedly improve quality of life.

Patients with COPD scheduled for surgery should undergo a preparatory pulmonary regimen intended to optimize lung function and minimize airway secretions. This regimen typically consists of smoking cessation, institution or intensification of inhaled bronchodilator therapy, and use of oral antibiotics in the presence of purulent secretions or a "loose" cough. Patients should be instructed on the use of incentive spirometry or cough and deep breathing techniques prior to surgery. A short course of oral corticosteroids should be considered in patients who have a significant bronchospastic component to their disease. Such a preparatory regimen is simple and inexpensive and has been shown to have a favorable impact on the incidence of postoperative pulmonary complications.[16] Other than the assurance of strict compliance with the regimen, there is no reason to believe that hospitalization is superior to outpatient preparation of the patient.

Smoking

Smoking has been shown to be a risk factor for postoperative pulmonary complications in general[33,47] and for prolonged ventilatory support in particular.[20,41] Smoking does not appear to be simply a surrogate marker of COPD; rather, it poses risk that is independent of the magnitude of pulmonary impairment. Detrimental effects of smoking include bronchial irritation with resultant excessive airway secretions; impairment in mucociliary clearance; and elevation of carboxyhemoglobin levels, with consequent impaired oxygen uptake and tissue oxygen utilization. While preoperative smoking cessation has been shown to diminish the risk of postoperative pulmonary complications, a minimum of 8 weeks of abstinence is required to achieve this risk reduction.[47]

IMPACT OF ANESTHESIA AND POSTOPERATIVE ANALGESIA ON PULMONARY FUNCTION

The effects of anesthetics on pulmonary function may be considered with regard to the type of intraoperative anesthesia (general versus regional) and use of postoperative analgesia.

General Anesthesia

Use of general anesthetic agents is associated with a number of well-characterized alterations in pulmonary mechanics, gas exchange, and respiratory drive.[33,42] In the controlled environment of the operating room, these physiological derangements are clinically inconsequential and easily overcome by simple adjustments of the ventilator. However, lingering effects of general anesthesia after completion of surgery may impede efforts to extubate the patient or may precipitate respiratory failure in the recovery room.

Administration of general anesthesia, whether by the inhaled or intravenous route, results in an almost immediate loss of diaphragmatic and intercostal muscle tone, a cephalad shift of the diaphragm, and a decrease in the transverse thoracic diameter. These dimensional alterations in thoracic volume result in a 20 percent reduction in functional residual capacity (FRC) and in the development of compressive atelectasis. As demonstrated using computed tomography to image patients during and after general anesthesia,[40] patients develop crescent-shaped areas of atelectasis in dependent areas of lung within 10 min of induction. Atelectatic areas make up approximately 2 to 10 percent of total lung volume and disappear with the application of positive end-expiratory pressure (PEEP). Dependent atelectasis develops after administration of either inhalational or intravenous anesthetics. A notable exception is ketamine, a drug that is unique in its maintenance of respiratory muscle tone. The degree of atelectasis appears unaffected by whether the patient is breathing spontaneously or is mechanically ventilated.

Areas of dependent atelectasis perturb the normal balance of ventilation and perfusion in the lung. Persistent perfusion of nonventilated atelectatic areas results in an increase in the shunt fraction, which may approach 15 percent. The alveolar-arterial oxygen gradient widens. The magnitude of shunt correlates directly with the volume of atelectatic lung and may be further magnified by impairment of hypoxic pulmonary vasoconstriction induced by certain inhalational anesthetics. Elderly patients, those who are obese, and patients with underlying COPD are most likely to develop clinically apparent hypoxemia in response to general anesthesia; the effect may persist into the early postoperative period.

The inhaled anesthetic agents in common usage are respiratory depressants that blunt the response to both hypoxemia and hypercapnia. These agents depress the ventilatory response to CO_2 in a dose-dependent fashion. They have a negligible effect on the hypercapnic response at the low concentrations encountered during emergence from anesthesia. In contrast, hypoxemic drive is markedly attenuated even at very low, subanesthetic concentrations of the volatile agents. As a result of deposition of these agents in muscle and fat, concentrations sufficient to depress hypoxic drive persist for several hours after termination of anesthesia. This can result in significant postoperative respiratory depression in patients who, by virtue of chronic hypercapnia, are dependent upon a hypoxic ventilatory drive to breathe.

Regional Anesthesia

It is common practice for those providing preoperative assessment of high-risk patients to recommend the use of regional (i.e., spinal or epidural) anesthesia, predicated on the impression that this route of administration lessens the adverse impact of anesthesia on the respiratory system. Spinal anesthesia does possess a number of favorable physiological features. In contrast to the effects of general anesthesia, spinal anesthesia preserves diaphragmatic innervation and function. External intercostal muscle paralysis is induced by thoracic levels of spinal anesthesia, but the level is generally two dermatomes below the sensory level because of the lesser sensitivity of motor neurons to the effects of the anesthetic agent. Hypoxic pulmonary vasoconstriction is unaffected by regional anesthesia, and the ventilatory response to CO_2 is unimpaired; indeed, the CO_2 response may be heightened. Despite the ostensibly favorable effects of regional anesthesia on respiratory mechanics and respiratory drive, a clinically significant benefit over general anesthesia has not been demonstrated consistently.[42] While limited available data preclude the drawing of firm conclusions, regional anesthesia should not be viewed as clearly superior to general anesthesia in the compromised patient.

Postoperative Analgesia

Postoperative analgesia is an essential component of the care of the surgical patient. Analgesia is important not only in ensuring patient comfort but also in mitigating the adverse effects of pain on respiratory function. Inadequate pain relief can lead to splinting and patient reluctance to cough and breathe deeply; the end result is promotion of retained secretions, atelectasis, hypoxemia, and possibly pneumonia. For major surgical procedures, particularly those involving the chest and upper abdomen, administration of opiates via the parenteral or epidural route has become the analgesic method of choice. Studies comparing the effect of epidural and parenteral opiates on pulmonary function are conflicting. While most have documented the superior analgesic effect of the epidural route, this has not invariably translated into greater improvement in respiratory mechanics and gas exchange or a lower incidence of postoperative pulmonary complications. This suggests that factors other than pain (see below) contribute significantly to alterations in pulmonary function occurring with thoracic or abdominal surgery. Nonetheless, this should not lead to the false impression that pain control is superfluous; failure to control pain adequately will potentiate postoperative pulmonary dysfunction.

Physicians caring for the postsurgical patient must be aware of the risk of narcotic administration in precipitating life-threatening respiratory depression. The reported incidence of severe respiratory depression with epidural narcotics ranges from 0.09 to 2.3 percent;[35] it is not yet clear whether this differs significantly from the incidence following more conventional routes of administration. Risk factors for respiratory depression following epidural opiates include advanced age, the concomitant administration of systemic opiates or other central nervous system depressants, and extensive surgery. Hydrophilic narcotics (e.g., morphine) have a greater tendency than lipophilic compounds (e.g., fentanyl) to remain in the cerebrospinal fluid and to spread rostrally to the respiratory center located in the floor of the fourth ventricle. When it complicates epidural narcotic administration, respiratory depression almost invariably occurs within the first 24 h. It is typically heralded by increasing sedation due to a combination of central drug effect and CO_2 narcosis. Treatment consists of administration of naloxone in 0.1- to 0.4-mg aliquots. Ventilation should be supported with a face mask and ambu bag, reserving intubation for the failure of naloxone to swiftly rectify the problem.

IMPACT OF SURGERY ON POSTOPERATIVE PULMONARY FUNCTION

Surgery involving the upper abdomen and thorax results in a pronounced impairment in pulmonary function in the postoperative period. The impairment is more severe and prolonged than that due to administration of general anesthesia alone. Typically, upper abdominal and thoracic procedures are associated with a fall in lung volumes, development of atelectasis, and hypoxemia. These adverse effects commonly necessitate short-term administration of low-flow supplemental oxygen, but when severe or accompanied by underlying lung disease, they may precipitate respiratory failure.

Upper Abdominal Surgery

Within 24 h following upper abdominal surgery, vital capacity declines by 50 percent.[11] Although the vital capacity improves with time, marked impairment persists for as long as 7 days after the surgery. In contradistinction, vital capacity falls by only 25 percent following lower abdominal procedures; it returns to normal by the third postoperative day.[11] Underlying these profound changes after upper abdominal surgery is the development of diaphragmatic dysfunction, as reflected in a reduction in transdiaphragmatic pressure with tidal respirations and in a shift from abdominal to rib cage breathing.[12,13]

Two main theories have been proposed to explain the observed impairment in diaphragmatic function. One theory is that there is a primary alteration in diaphragmatic contractility induced by local irritation, inflammation, surgical trauma, or pain. This theory has been rendered improbable with the demonstration that external stimulation of the phrenic nerves produces normal peak transdiaphragmatic pressure in patients recovering from upper abdominal surgery.[12] In other words, in this clinical setting, when maximally stimulated, the diaphragm functions in a normal fashion.

The alternative and currently favored theory proposes that diaphragmatic dysfunction results from diminished phrenic nerve output. The basis for the attenuation in neural drive remains a matter of speculation, although several putative pathways can be rationally eliminated. For example, general anesthesia is known to depress output from the central respiratory centers as well as to inhibit synaptic transmission. However, as noted previously, the effects of general anesthesia on diaphragmatic tone are transient and modest. Additionally, the degree of dysfunction observed after upper abdominal procedures is not seen following general anesthesia for procedures on the lower abdomen and extremities. An inhibitory arc initiated by abdominal nociceptors for pain is unlikely, given that achievement of adequate pain control by epidural opiates fails to consistently improve pulmonary function or to normalize diaphragmatic performance. In contrast, the epidural administration of anesthetic agents such as bupivacaine does ameliorate diaphragmatic dysfunction following upper abdominal surgery. Since these agents produce sympathetic blockade in addition to pain control, it has been argued that visceral sympathetic afferents are responsible for providing an inhibitory signal that downgrades central neural drive and phrenic nerve activity, thereby leading to impaired diaphragmatic function. Supporting the notion of a reflex inhibitory arc mediated by visceral afferents is the demonstration in experimental animals that mechanical gallbladder stimulation strongly inhibits electromyographic activity and motion of the diaphragm.

Cardiac Surgery

Although CABG—the most commonly performed cardiac surgical procedure—has been most intensively scrutinized with respect to its impact on the respiratory system, other related cardiac procedures (e.g., valve replacement) are likely to have similar effects. Lung volumes decrease by approximately 30 percent after CABG; the return to preoperative values may take several months.[1,4,43] Lung function may decline to a greater degree when internal mammary harvesting and grafting are employed.[1] Gas exchange is also impaired after CABG, as evident in the development of hypoxemia and significant widening of the alveolar-arterial oxygen gradient. In 125 patients who had daily room air arterial blood gas determinations prior to and following CABG, Pa_{O_2} fell from approximately 75 mmHg preoperatively to a nadir of 55 mmHg on postoperative day 2. The Pa_{O_2} improved but remained below preoperative values at the end of the first postoperative week.[38] A similar pattern and magnitude of decline in oxygenation have been demonstrated in other studies, with the development of hypoxemia associated with an increase in calculated shunt fraction from 3 percent preoperatively to a peak of 19 percent postoperatively.[43] The increase in shunt fraction is readily accounted for on the basis of atelectasis, which is invariably present postoperatively, especially on the left side.

A number of factors have been implicated in the development of post-CABG pulmonary dysfunction and atelectasis. Alterations in chest wall compliance and motion may result from division of the sternum, harvesting of the internal mammary artery, and traumatic injury to the costovertebral joints and first rib induced by retraction. Intraoperative lung retraction may directly injure the left lower lobe, leading to contusion and atelectasis, and, perhaps, accounting for the predilection for radiographic infiltrates on the left side. An alternative explanation for post-CABG left-lower-lobe atelectasis is intraoperative injury to the left phrenic nerve and consequent diaphragmatic paralysis or paresis. The phrenic nerve courses along the lateral surface of the pericardium and is vulnerable to thermal injury induced by the commonly employed cardioplegic technique of instilling iced slush into the open pericardial sac. Additionally, stretch and ischemic injury to the nerve may occur with sternal retraction, dissection of the internal mammary artery, or prolonged distention of the pericardium. The actual incidence of phrenic nerve dysfunction after CABG is best defined in studies employing electrophysiological techniques rather than nonspecific radiographic methods. Two such studies documented unequivocal evidence of phrenic nerve palsy in 10 percent of patients.[26,49] In one of these studies, less definitive abnormalities were noted in an additional 60 percent, but this finding was ascribed largely to technical difficulties in localizing the postoperative position of the diaphragm for surface electrical recording.[49] These studies suggest that phrenic nerve injury is a definite but uncommon cause of postoperative pulmonary dysfunction.

Finally, cardiopulmonary bypass may contribute to pulmonary impairment after cardiac surgery. The duration of bypass has been linked to the severity of postoperative atelectasis;[49] however, whether this relationship is causal is unclear. It has been hypothesized that the use of cardiopulmonary bypass leads to abnormal surfactant production—possibly due to ischemic, thermal, or toxic injury to the alveolar epithelium—predisposing to the development of atelectasis. More clearly established is the ability of the bypass pump to induce a capillary leak syndrome, marked by extravasation of fluid into the alveolar interstitium and, rarely, into the airspaces. This process is thought to result from exposure of blood to nonendothelial surfaces, resultant activation of complement and other inflammatory cascades, and sequestration of neutrophils within the microvasculature. Except when fulminant ("postperfusion lung"; see below), the extent to which an increase in extravascular water contributes to alterations in lung volumes and gas exchange observed following cardiac surgery has not yet been defined.

Lung Resection

Unique to lung resection surgery is the immediate loss of lung function due to removal of lung parenchyma. The magnitude of the loss can be estimated reliably from preoperative quantitative lung scanning in conjunction with standard spirometry. The impact of lung resection on pulmonary function is further magnified in the perioperative period by other factors. For example, the standard posterolateral thoracotomy incision represents significant chest wall trauma, with rib retraction and resection, and transection of intercostal, latissimus dorsi, trapezius, and serratus anterior muscles. As a result, total respiratory compliance may fall by as much as 75 percent, work of breathing increases, and lung volumes decline dramatically, out of proportion to the surgical loss of functional lung. Following standard thoracotomy and lung resection (either lobectomy or wedge resection), FEV_1 and FVC fall to 25 percent of preoperative values at 1 h and to 30 percent at 24 h. When a more limited, muscle-sparing inci-

sion is used, the impact on pulmonary function is markedly attenuated.[24]

As with cardiac and upper abdominal surgery, atelectasis is frequently present after lung surgery and results in impaired oxygenation. Phrenic nerve activity remains normal and diaphragmatic function during tidal breathing is preserved, although maximal diaphragmatic strength may be reduced.

CAUSES OF POSTOPERATIVE RESPIRATORY FAILURE

The development of acute respiratory failure in the surgical patient should prompt a systematic assessment of the likely causes (Table 170-3). In approaching this life-threatening problem, one must consider the nature and magnitude of preexisting pulmonary disease, type of surgery performed, drugs administered intra- and postoperatively, and predominant derangement in gas exchange (i.e., hypoxemia or hypercapnia). In conjunction with important information derived from the physical examination and chest radiograph, the analysis should readily identify factors responsible for or contributing to respiratory failure. The following discussion focuses on the more common causes of postoperative respiratory failure and highlights features unique to the surgical setting.

Atelectasis

Atelectasis is the most common pulmonary complication encountered in the surgical patient, particularly following thoracic and upper abdominal procedures. As discussed previously, anesthesia and surgical manipulation act in concert to produce regional atelectasis through incompletely defined mechanisms, including diaphragmatic dysfunction and diminished surfactant activity. The atelectasis is typically basilar and segmental in distribution, obscuring the hemidiaphragms radiographically. A distinct and less common cause of postoperative atelectasis is plugging of central airways by retained secretions. This problem is encountered in the surgical patient whose efforts to clear secretions are compromised by depressed consciousness, inadequate pain control, or a weak, ineffective cough. When situated in a

---

TABLE 170-3

Causes of Postoperative Respiratory Failure

Factors extrinsic to the lung
    Depression of central respiratory drive (anesthetics, opioids, sedatives)
    Phrenic nerve injury/diaphragmatic paralysis
    Obstructive sleep apnea
Factors intrinsic to the lung
    Atelectasis
    Pneumonia
    Aspiration
    Acute lung injury (ARDS)
    Volume overload/congestive heart failure
    Pulmonary embolism
    Bronchospasm/COPD

mainstem bronchus, mucous plugs can result in collapse of an entire lung; more distal obstruction leads to lobar collapse. An abrupt termination of the proximal bronchial air shadow and the absence of air bronchograms within the atelectatic portion of lung are clues to the possible presence of mucous plugging.

While often clinically insignificant, postoperative atelectasis may lead to severe hypoxemia and respiratory distress. The magnitude of hypoxemia is dictated by the extent of atelectasis, the presence and severity of underlying lung disease, and the integrity of the hypoxemic pulmonary vasoconstrictive response. Impairment of hypoxemic pulmonary vasoconstriction by vasodilatory drugs, commonly administered to surgical patients for treatment of underlying hypertension or ischemic heart disease, prevents the compensatory diversion of blood flow away from nonventilated areas of lung and magnifies the shunt fraction.

Respiratory distress due to atelectasis usually evolves insidiously over the first several postoperative days. Supplemental oxygen requirements increase in association with worsening basilar infiltrates noted on the chest radiograph. The clinicoradiographic picture may be indistinguishable from that of pneumonia. While fever and leukocytosis suggest infection, these signs are common and nonspecific. When atelectasis is due to central airway occlusion by mucous plugs, hypoxemia and respiratory distress may develop quickly. A chest radiograph obtained immediately after the onset of symptoms may be surprisingly unrevealing if sufficient time has not passed to permit resorption of gas from the air spaces of the nonventilated lung. Careful examination of the patient, however, will reveal an absence of breath sounds over the involved lung, providing an important clue to the presence of central airway obstruction and obviating pursuit of other considerations, such as pulmonary embolism.

Treatment of respiratory failure due to atelectasis is directed toward the combined goals of adequate oxygenation and reexpansion of lung segments. Supplemental oxygen should be titrated to achieve an arterial oxyhemoglobin saturation of at least 90%. Refractory hypoxemia, severe respiratory distress, progressive hypercapnia, or inability of the patient to clear copious airway secretions should prompt immediate intubation and mechanical ventilatory support. This lifesaving intervention permits more efficient delivery of oxygen, secures access for suctioning of the airways, and facilitates performance of bronchoscopy should it be necessary. Moreover, the positive pressure and large tidal volumes delivered by the ventilator are often effective in rapidly reexpanding collapsed lung segments. In less dire circumstances, non-invasive delivery of continuous positive airway pressure (CPAP) via a nasal or face mask may be equally effective.[10]

Fiberoptic bronchoscopy has a limited role in the treatment of serious postoperative atelectasis; its indiscriminate use should be avoided. The immediate use of fiberoptic bronchoscopy does not result in more rapid or complete resolution of acute lobar atelectasis when compared with standard chest physiotherapy, consisting of deep breathing, coughing, suctioning of the intubated patient, aerosolized bronchodilator treatments, chest percussion, and postural drainage.[25] Resolution of atelectasis appears to be dictated not by the treatment modality employed but by radiographic evidence of central airway patency. Both chest physiotherapy and bronchoscopy are highly effective in the absence of

an air bronchogram; the presence of an air bronchogram, indicating that the atelectasis is not due to proximal airway obstruction, is associated with minimal response to either modality. Therefore, simple and standard respiratory therapy techniques applied to either the spontaneously or mechanically ventilated patient form the mainstay of treatment for lobar atelectasis. Fiberoptic bronchoscopy should be reserved for those situations where chest physiotherapy is contraindicated (e.g., chest trauma, immobilized patient), poorly tolerated, or unsuccessful. In these circumstances, the decision to employ bronchoscopy should be tempered by the presence of an air bronchogram.

A number of other measures are commonly employed in the treatment of atelectasis. Judicious use of analgesia is an essential adjunct, permitting the patient to breathe deeply, cough forcefully, and participate comfortably in chest physiotherapy maneuvers. Care must be taken to avoid excessive sedation, which will offset the beneficial effects of pain control. In the setting of marked hypoxemia, attempts should be made to discontinue vasoactive drugs with the potential to influence the pulmonary vascular bed; examples include nitrates, nitroprusside, calcium channel blockers, angiotensin-converting enzyme inhibitors, and hydralazine. Mucolytics, such as N-acetyl cysteine, are commonly administered in an effort to promote clearance of tenacious secretions; however, their efficacy in this setting has not been well documented. Some clinicians and respiratory therapists advocate the use of nasotracheal suctioning of the nonintubated patient with a weak and ineffective cough. However, this technique is associated with considerable discomfort and, in the opinion of the author, is an inefficient and highly transient means of clearing secretions from the tracheobronchial tree.

The important role of prophylactic maneuvers in reducing the incidence and magnitude of postoperative atelectasis in high risk patients should not be overlooked. These techniques are intended to promote periodic full lung expansion. Included are intermittent positive-pressure breathing (IPPB), cough and deep breathing exercises, and incentive spirometry. All three techniques have been shown to be equally efficacious and superior to no therapy in the prevention of postoperative pulmonary complications.[5] However, IPPB has largely been abandoned, due to its expense, the need for specially trained personnel and close patient supervision, and tendency to produce abdominal distention. For maximal benefit, prophylactic measures should be taught and instituted prior to surgery and utilized hourly in the postoperative period. Early ambulation of the postsurgical patient has been found to be as effective as respiratory therapy maneuvers in the prevention of postoperative atelectasis and should be strongly encouraged.

Pneumonia

Pneumonia is the second most common nosocomial infection and the most lethal, with an associated mortality rate of 20 to 50 percent. It represents a principal cause of postoperative respiratory compromise and may precipitate acute respiratory failure as well as complicate respiratory failure in the patient who is ventilator-dependent for other reasons. In epidemiologic surveys, surgery has been identified as an independent risk factor for nosocomial pneumonia. In particular, the risk is greatest following standard thoracic and upper abdominal procedures, where an incidence of 15 to 20 percent has been documented. Lung transplant recipients represent an emerging population with a similarly high risk of postoperative pneumonia. In contrast, the risk of pneumonia is only 5 percent following lower abdominal surgery, and it is even less frequently encountered following procedures remote from the chest and abdomen. Overall, the incidence of nosocomial pneumonia is up to fivefold greater among patients in surgical intensive care units than among patients in medical intensive care units.[7]

Epidemiologic studies have identified a number of other risk factors for nosocomial pneumonia, but these studies fail to fully distinguish those factors that are causally linked from those that are simply surrogate markers.[14,15] Factors reflective of poor preoperative health—including a low serum albumin level, presence of COPD, extensive smoking history, advanced age, protracted preoperative hospital stay, and high status according to the American Society of Anesthesiologists (ASA) preanesthesia classification—have been linked to an excessive risk of pneumonia. A direct relationship between duration of surgery and incidence of postoperative pneumonia has been demonstrated. Other identified risk factors include presence of a nasogastric tube, use of antacids or H_2 blockers for stress ulcer prophylaxis, immunosuppression, impaired consciousness, and witnessed aspiration. Perhaps the most important and consistently identified risk factor is the need for prolonged mechanical ventilatory support. Overall, mechanically ventilated patients have a 3- to 21-fold increased risk of pneumonia compared with non-ventilated patients. Moreover, the risk of pneumonia is linked to the duration of ventilatory support, approximating 1 percent per day on the ventilator.

The microbiologic profile of nosocomial pneumonia is distinctly different from that of community-acquired infection. Gram-negative aerobic bacilli of the Enterobacteriaceae family prevail, collectively accounting for approximately one-third of all infections. Other highly virulent gram-negative rods that are commonly encountered are *Pseudomonas aeruginosa* and *Acinetobacter* species. Of the gram-positive organisms, *Staphylococcus aureus* predominates, while the pneumococcus, the most common bacterial respiratory pathogen in the community setting, plays an insignificant role. Often the pneumonia is polymicrobial; studies employing bronchoscopic culture techniques or postmortem cultures of lung tissue have identified more than one organism in up to 46 percent of cases.

While organisms may reach the lower respiratory tract by several routes, microaspiration of oropharyngeal secretions appears to be the predominant mechanism in the pathogenesis of nosocomial pneumonia. A critical initiating event in this pathway is colonization of the oropharynx with gram-negative aerobic bacilli, a process that characteristically occurs in response to serious illness or surgical stress. Clinically occult aspiration of these virulent organisms is facilitated by a number of iatrogenic measures imposed upon the surgical patient. Paramount among these is the placement of an endotracheal tube, which impairs swallowing, and stents open the glottis, permitting pooling of secretions above the tube cuff. The inflated cuff is an imperfect barrier and allows intermittent seepage of secretions into the lower airways. Prolonged intubation has also been associated with postextubation swallowing dysfunction. Depressed consciousness as a consequence of general anesthesia and postoperative analgesia further contributes to the risk of aspiration.

Attention has recently focused on the stomach as an additional source of bacteria in the development of nosocomial pneumonia. While the acidic milieu of the stomach normally inhibits bacterial growth, the common use of H_2 blockers and antacids as stress ulcer prophylaxis overrides this natural barrier and promotes gastric colonization with gram-negative enteric organisms. Gastroesophageal reflux, a common feature of the critically ill patient, permits bacteria-laden gastric contents to enter the respiratory tract either directly or by first colonizing the oropharynx. This route of migration has been confirmed by recovery of technetium-99m–labeled gastric contents in endobronchial secretions and by the demonstration in some patients that organisms cultured from the airways first appeared in the stomach.[44] Perhaps the most compelling albeit circumstantial evidence derives from several studies that have shown a higher incidence of nosocomial pneumonia in patients receiving H_2 blockers or antacids than in those given sucralfate, a drug that does not result in alkalinization of gastric pH.[9] However, conflicting data abound, and firm conclusions about the role of gastric colonization in the pathogenesis of nosocomial pneumonia await the outcome of larger and more methodologically rigorous studies.

The fate of organisms introduced into the lower respiratory tract is dependent upon the integrity of mechanical and immunologic pulmonary defense mechanisms. Impairment of the mucociliary escalator (e.g., due to recent cigarette smoking or underlying COPD), weak and ineffective cough, and use of immunosuppressive medications (e.g., corticosteroids) favor the proliferation of organisms and the development of pneumonia. It is widely held that postoperative atelectasis predisposes to pneumonia by entrapping bacteria. However, recent data demonstrating a lack of concordance between the degree of atelectasis and the subsequent risk of pneumonia challenge this contention.[21]

The constellation of fever, leukocytosis, purulent sputum, and radiographic infiltrates has traditionally defined the presence of pneumonia. While these diagnostic criteria are reasonably accurate in the previously healthy outpatient, they are notoriously nonspecific in the setting of recent surgery, particularly with prolonged use of mechanical ventilation. In one autopsy series, traditional clinical and radiographic criteria provided the correct antemortem diagnosis in only 70 percent of cases.[15] Alternative etiologies of radiographic infiltrates include atelectasis, pulmonary edema, infarction or hemorrhage due to pulmonary emboli, pulmonary contusion, and chemical pneumonitis. Cultures of sputum and tracheal aspirates are poorly reflective of the bacterial flora of the distal airways, since these specimens are contaminated by colonizing organisms in the oropharynx and upper respiratory tract. In an attempt to enhance diagnostic certainty, bronchoscopic sampling of the distal airways using a sterile sheathed brush or bronchoalveolar lavage has been advocated. While the absence of a "gold standard" for the diagnosis of pneumonia has complicated attempts to define the accuracy of these techniques, rates of false-positive and false-negative results have generally fallen into the range of 30 percent. It is questionable, therefore, whether the performance of bronchoscopy actually contributes significantly to a reduction in the degree of diagnostic uncertainty. These concerns, coupled with the need to perform the procedure prior to institution of antibiotics and to collect and process specimens in a fastidious and standardized fashion, have severely limited the utility and acceptance of currently available bronchoscopic techniques. Despite all of the pitfalls, most clinicians continue to rely on conventional assessment strategies in establishing a diagnosis of pneumonia and in determining the need for therapy.

Empiric treatment of nosocomial pneumonia is broad in spectrum and includes effective coverage of gram-negative organisms (including *Pseudomonas*) and *S. aureus*. The initial choice of antibiotics is influenced by the particular epidemiologic profile and microbiologic susceptibility patterns at a given institution; many intensive care units are currently plagued by highly resistant organisms, such as *Acinetobacter* or methicillin-resistant *Staphylococcus,* which have unusual but predictable susceptibilities.

Preventative strategies intended to diminish the risk of pneumonia are an important consideration in the care of the surgical patient. Prevention begins in the preoperative phase with emphasis on abstinence from cigarette smoking for a minimum of 8 weeks prior to elective surgery. Following surgery, nasogastric and endotracheal tubes should be removed as soon as possible. Postoperative analgesia must be titrated to permit the patient to cough comfortably and vigorously, but excessive sedation impairing protection of the airway and enhancing the risk of aspiration must be avoided.

For the high-risk, ventilator-dependent patient, maintenance of a semierect position has been shown to diminish the magnitude of clinically occult aspiration of gastric contents; whether this simple measure will reduce the risk of pneumonia is unclear. While the use of sucralfate appears to be associated with a lower incidence of gastric colonization and nosocomial pneumonia compared with agents that raise gastric pH, additional corroborating studies are required before a firm recommendation to employ sucralfate preferentially in stress ulcer prophylaxis can be made.

A novel but still investigational approach to pneumonia prevention in the high-risk patient is selective digestive decontamination (SDD). This technique involves the use of topical antibiotics applied to the oropharynx as a paste and to the stomach as a slurry in an attempt to prevent gram-negative colonization of these known bacterial reservoirs. Preliminary data are conflicting, and a definitive reduction in the incidence of pneumonia in the general population of patients in intensive care units has not been demonstrated consistently. However, preoperative SDD targeted to high-risk surgical patients may reduce the risk of postoperative pneumonia. Further studies are necessary to confirm that this laborious technique is indeed beneficial and cost-effective and that it is not accompanied by the frequent emergence of resistant pathogens.

Aspiration of Gastric Contents

In 1946, Mendelson, studying gravid women undergoing general anesthesia, first called attention to the potentially devastating consequences of aspiration of acidic gastric contents. Mendel-son's syndrome, the aspiration of gastric contents, typically occurs when the mechanisms of glottic closure and cough, which normally protect the airway, are compromised.

In the surgical patient, the period of maximal vulnerability for aspiration spans from the induction of general anesthesia to full return of consciousness postoperatively. A number of factors combine to enhance the risk of aspiration during this period. Most important is the blunting of consciousness that accompanies induction and administration of general anesthesia. Insufflation of air into the stomach during induction may cause gastric distention and promote vomiting. Vomiting may also be provoked by noxious stimulation of the posterior oropharynx during intubation or extubation. Reflux of gastric contents is facilitated by medication-induced relaxation of the lower esophageal sphincter, placement of the patient in a supine position, and manipulation of the bowel during abdominal procedures. At the completion of surgery, extubation is commonly performed in the semiconscious patient who, while able to ventilate adequately, may not yet be capable of fully protecting the airway. Furthermore, translaryngeal intubation, even when brief, may cause residual glottic dysfunction for up to 8 h following removal of the tube. While the risk of aspiration diminishes beyond the immediate perioperative period, it remains a concern in the patient receiving narcotic analgesia, which may not only induce vomiting but also depress consciousness.

The risk of aspiration during the immediate perioperative period was delineated in a survey of over 215,000 general anesthetic procedures performed at the Mayo Clinic.[48] Aspiration was defined as the presence of bilious or particulate matter in the airways or the development of a new infiltrate on the immediate postoperative chest radiograph. The overall incidence of aspiration was only 0.03 percent, but the incidence was nearly fourfold higher (0.11 percent) in the setting of emergency surgery. In addition to the use of general anesthesia, other predisposing factors were present in over half of the patients who aspirated. These included gastrointestinal obstruction, swallowing dysfunction, altered sensorium, previous esophageal surgery, and a recent meal. The majority of events occurred during laryngoscopy (in preparation for insertion of the endotracheal tube) and during tracheal extubation. Twenty percent of patients who aspirated required postoperative mechanical ventilation in excess of 6 h; 5 percent died as a direct result of this complication.

Acidic liquid introduced into the airways is rapidly disseminated throughout the bronchial tree and lung parenchyma, producing a chemical pneumonitis within minutes. Injury to the alveolar capillary membrane results in flooding of the interstitium and airspaces with proteinaceous edema fluid. Surfactant levels drop precipitously due to both direct acid denaturation and diminished production, leading to alveolar instability and atelectasis. The magnitude of injury to the lung parenchyma is directly related to the pH and volume of aspirated material. In experimental animals, a pH of less than 2.5 and a volume in excess of 0.4 ml/kg have been defined as critical threshold values for the induction of lung injury; material with a more alkaline pH or of a smaller volume appears to be relatively innocuous. The presence of food particles contributes to lung injury by inducing an inflammatory reaction within the airways; the delayed development of obliterative bronchiolitis and granuloma formation may be observed. Large food particles may also cause airway obstruction and atelectasis. Notably, infection does not play a significant role in the initial lung injury from aspiration of acidic gastric contents, as the low pH serves to maintain relative sterility of the inoculum. However, the development of chemical pneumonitis enhances the risk of subsequent bacterial superinfection.

The diagnosis of aspiration is most firmly established in the setting of witnessed vomiting or recovery of gastric contents from the airways. More often, the diagnosis is suspected circumstantially in a patient with risk factors and a compatible clinicoradiographic picture. Massive aspiration presents in a characteristic fashion, with the development of fever, tachypnea, and diffuse rales within several hours of the event. Wheezing is appreciated in approximately one-third of patients and may be due either to obstruction of airways by particulate matter or, more commonly, to reflex bronchospasm. Hypoxemia is universally present and is sufficiently severe in the majority of patients to mandate use of mechanical ventilation. The initial presence of apnea or shock is a particularly ominous sign encountered in approximately one-quarter of patients; they portend a high risk of subsequent death. Initial radiographic patterns vary, depending upon the volume, causticity, and distribution of the aspirated material. However, three general patterns have been described: (1) extensive bilateral consolidation resembling diffuse pulmonary edema; (2) widespread but discrete patchy infiltrates; and (3) focal consolidation usually localized to one or both lung bases.

The clinical course following massive aspiration is variable, but it typically diverges along one of several pathways. A minority of patients follow a fulminant course marked by refractory hypoxemia and shock, which eventuates in death within several days. More commonly, patients demonstrate progressive radiographic and clinical improvement over the first several days. Although most of these patients will go on to full recovery, a subset demonstrate secondary deterioration due to the development of ARDS or nosocomial pneumonia. The overall mortality rate associated with massive aspiration is approximately 30 percent and exceeds 50 percent in those patients with initial shock or apnea, secondary pneumonia, or ARDS.

The treatment of respiratory failure secondary to aspiration is supportive and is based on mechanical ventilation and use of PEEP to maintain adequate oxygenation in the more severe cases. Bronchoscopy is indicated only when large airway obstruction by particulate matter is suspected on the basis of a localized wheeze or lobar atelectasis. Because acid is disseminated and endogenously neutralized within seconds, large-volume bronchoalveolar lavage is ineffective in attenuating the degree of injury and is not recommended. Studies of the administration of systemic corticosteroids in the treatment of aspiration pneumonitis have been inconclusive and do not currently justify their use. Similarly, use of prophylactic antibiotics is discouraged in the absence of supportive data and because of fear that this practice will preferentially select more highly resistant organisms. Admittedly, it takes tremendous restraint on the part of the clinician to initially withhold antibiotics in a critically ill patient with fever, leukocytosis, and infiltrates immediately following an aspiration event. Reassurance should be derived from the understanding that the immediate insult is chemical and not infectious in nature. However, up to 40 percent of patients will develop a superimposed bacterial pneumonia within several days of the aspiration event, often heralded by a new fever, new or progressive infiltrates, and purulent sputum. Aggressive antibiotic therapy directed toward gram-positive and gram-negative aerobes as well as anaerobic mouth flora is indicated at that time.

The high morbidity and mortality associated with aspiration and the lack of effective therapy once the event has occurred have focused attention on measures to prevent this complication. The most straightforward and widely utilized measure is the convention of overnight fasting prior to elective surgery. However, despite prolonged fasting, up to one-third of patients will maintain a gastric volume in excess of 0.4 ml/kg (approximately 25 to 30 ml in the average adult), and up to three-quarters will have a gastric pH below 2.5—meeting critical thresholds for the potential of inducing severe lung injury (see above). Since administration of H_2 blockers can effectively raise the pH and reduce the volume of gastric contents, some clinicians now advocate their use during the 12 h preceding surgery, often in combination with a prokinetic agent such as metoclopramide or cisapride. Given the exceedingly low incidence of aspiration in the general surgical population undergoing elective procedures, the cost-effectiveness of this approach can be questioned. Unfortunately, there is generally insufficient time to allow these agents to act in the setting of emergency surgery, where the risk of aspiration is highest. In high-risk patients, rapid sequence induction of anesthesia should be employed to shorten the time between loss of consciousness and tracheal intubation. During induction, manual pressure should be applied to the cricoid cartilage (Sellick maneuver) and maintained until the endotracheal tube is in proper position and the cuff is inflated. It is especially important that this maneuver be maintained in the face of emesis; the risk of esophageal rupture in this setting is minimal and is far outweighed by the risk of aspiration. Postoperatively, extubation should be performed only when consciousness and the gag reflex have returned to a level sufficient to permit adequate protection of the airway.

Acute Lung Injury

The hallmark of acute lung injury is the presence of noncardiogenic pulmonary edema resulting from widespread damage to the alveolar capillary membrane. Commonly referred to as acute respiratory distress syndrome (ARDS), this condition is defined clinically by the constellation of hypoxemic respiratory failure, diffuse pulmonary infiltrates, and a normal pulmonary artery occlusion pressure. Acute lung injury represents the end result of a variety of insults that either involve the lung directly (e.g., aspiration of gastric contents) or trigger pulmonary inflammation as part of a systemic process (e.g., sepsis). Many of the risk factors associated with development of acute lung injury are commonly encountered in surgical patients (Table 170-4). In decreasing order of risk, these include sepsis, massive blood transfusion, pulmonary contusion, aspiration of gastric contents, and multiple fractures.[19] Additional precipitants of acute lung injury of particular relevance to the surgical patient, and, in some cases, unique to this population are described in greater detail below.

TABLE 170-4

Incidence of Acute Respiratory Distress Syndrome (ARDS) by Risk Factor

Risk Factor	Incidence of ARDS
Sepsis	41%
Massive transfusions	36%
Pulmonary contusion	22%
Aspiration	22%
Multiple fractures	11%

SOURCE: From Hudson et al.,[19] with permission.

POSTPNEUMONECTOMY PULMONARY EDEMA

Over the past decade, a number of investigators have independently reported the rapid development of pulmonary edema in the remaining lung of some patients following pneumonectomy. Initially attributed to overzealous fluid administration in the operating room, it has since been demonstrated that this complication occurs in the face of a normal pulmonary artery occlusion pressure. In addition, the edema fluid is protein-rich, arguing for pulmonary edema on a permeability rather than a hydrostatic basis. Postmortem studies confirm the universal presence of pathological features of ARDS. The exact mechanism responsible for lung injury after pneumonectomy remains obscure. In a study employing stringent criteria for excluding patients with congestive heart failure or known risk factors for ARDS, the incidence of postpneumonectomy pulmonary edema was 2.6 percent.[45] For unclear reasons, the complication was encountered more frequently following right pneumonectomy. In this study, postpneumonectomy pulmonary edema was uniformly fatal despite aggressive supportive measures.

POSTPERFUSION LUNG

Fulminant noncardiogenic pulmonary edema may rarely complicate use of cardiopulmonary bypass. The risk appears to be greatest when the duration of cardiopulmonary bypass exceeds 150 min. The mechanisms by which cardiopulmonary bypass induces lung injury remain speculative. They may relate in part to accumulation within the pulmonary capillary bed of neutrophils that have been damaged by exposure to foreign surfaces and release proteolytic enzymes and other toxic mediators. Exposure of blood to nonendothelialized surfaces may also cause complement activation, which may contribute to neutrophil sequestration and activation within the lung. In some instances, the acute lung injury may actually represent an idiosyncratic reaction to protamine, used to reverse the effects of heparin at the end of the pump "run." The syndrome evolves gradually, with progressive hypoxemia and pulmonary infiltrates culminating in frank respiratory failure by the third or fourth postoperative day. Pulmonary involvement may occur in isolation or may be accompanied by fever, leukocytosis, renal insufficiency, bleeding diathesis, or transient neurologic impairment. While the natural history remains poorly characterized, it appears that this form of acute lung injury carries a more favorable prognosis than that typically associated with ARDS.

AMIODARONE

Amiodarone-induced pulmonary toxicity usually presents as a subacute illness characterized by cough, dyspnea, fever, and patchy pulmonary infiltrates. The use of amiodarone has more recently been linked to the development of ARDS immediately following cardiac and noncardiac surgery. In most of the reported cases, amiodarone was administered preoperatively for varying periods of time for control of arrhythmias. The majority of patients had no evidence prior to surgery of the more indolent form of amiodarone pulmonary toxicity. Recently, development of ARDS was described in patients whose only exposure to amiodarone occurred in the postoperative period, when the drug was initiated as prophylaxis for atrial arrhythmias following lung resection.[46] In this report, postoperative ARDS developed in 11 percent of patients receiving amiodarone and in only 1.8 percent of untreated patients. Further studies are required to define the specific perioperative factors that act in concert with amiodarone to produce acute lung injury.

TRANSFUSION-RELATED ACUTE LUNG INJURY

The transfusion of blood and blood products has been linked to the development of ARDS in two ways. Epidemiologically, an association between massive blood transfusion (>15 U/24 h) and ARDS has been noted, but it remains unclear whether this link is truly causal or is indirect and reflective only of the critically ill nature of the patient requiring such massive transfusion support.[19] More precisely defined is the induction of acute lung injury by the passive transfer in transfused blood products of donor antibodies directed against recipient leukocytes, a process that has been termed *transfusion-related acute lung injury* (TRALI) or the *leukoagglutinins reaction*. These antibodies, which typically derive from multiparous female donors, result in leukoagglutination and activation of recipient neutrophils within the pulmonary microvasculature, triggering increased capillary permeability and the formation of noncardiogenic pulmonary edema.

A recent study documented 36 cases of TRALI within a 2-year period of observation—an incidence of 0.02 percent per unit and 0.16 percent per patient transfused.[34] Most cases were detected in surgical patients in the immediate postoperative period, a fact that likely reflects the frequent need for transfusions in this setting and the close monitoring of cardiopulmonary function in the postanesthesia recovery area.

The clinical picture is characterized by the abrupt onset of respiratory distress, hypoxemia, and diffuse pulmonary infiltrates within 2 to 4 h of transfusion. Accompanying features include fever, chills, and hypotension; urticaria is present in a minority of patients. Respiratory distress and hypoxemia are of sufficient magnitude to require mechanical ventilatory support in most patients. The reaction tends to be self-limited and is typically characterized by rapid clearing of infiltrates and improved oxygenation within several days. However, a more protracted course of more than 1 week was reported in 17 percent of patients in the series noted above; a mortality rate of 6 percent was attributed to this complication.

When TRALI is suspected, the blood bank should be notified and all units that have been transfused should be assayed for the presence of leukoagglutinating antibodies. Any blood product containing plasma or plasma proteins is capable of inducing this reaction. Indeed, packed red blood cells, which contain only 60 to 100 mL of plasma, are among the more commonly implicated precipitants.

ISCHEMIA-REPERFUSION INJURY

The restoration of blood flow to previously ischemic tissue may, paradoxically, worsen tissue injury. This ischemia-reperfusion effect involves a "two-hit" mechanism. Tissue ischemia leads to formation of xanthine oxidase and its substrate, hypoxanthine, while reperfusion supplies molecular oxygen, which fuels the reaction to produce oxygen free radicals injurious to cells. Neutrophils recruited to the site of ischemia-reperfusion serve as an additional source of oxygen free radicals as well as proteolytic enzymes. Within the lung, ischemia-reperfusion produces diffuse injury to the alveolar epithelium and resultant noncardiogenic pulmonary edema. This mechanism underlies the development of acute lung injury in two important clinical settings: lung transplantation and pulmonary thromboendarterectomy.

Pulmonary edema is a nearly universal feature of the freshly implanted lung allograft, but it is usually mild and self-limited. In approximately 15 percent of cases, however, the allograft is severely injured, with widespread and persistent alveolar edema causing profound hypoxemia and low pulmonary compliance, necessitating mechanical ventilatory support beyond the immediate posttransplant period. This entity, termed *primary graft failure,* is nonimmunologic in nature and is believed to represent an extreme form of ischemia-reperfusion injury. Primary graft failure occurs despite acceptable ischemic times below the perceived safe threshold of 6 h. Injury is manifest exclusively in the allograft, sparing the native lung in cases of single lung transplantation. The presence of unilateral lung injury may create difficulties in postoperative ventilator management. This is particularly true in the presence of underlying COPD, when positive-pressure breaths and PEEP are preferentially applied to the highly compliant emphysematous lung, leading to progressive hyperinflation, mediastinal shift, and potentially catastrophic impairment in gas exchange and hemodynamics. This situation mandates insertion of a double-lumen endotracheal tube, enabling use of independent lung ventilation and selective application of PEEP to the edematous allograft; the native lung is ventilated using low pressures and a prolonged expiratory phase.

Pulmonary thromboendarterectomy is an emerging surgical technique for definitive treatment of chronic thromboembolic pulmonary hypertension. Although operative mortality has decreased dramatically to less than 10 percent, severe reperfusion pulmonary edema continues to complicate the postoperative course in one-third of cases.[8] Reperfusion edema may occur intraoperatively upon restoration of blood flow, but more commonly it evolves over the first several postoperative days. A striking characteristic is the radiographic restriction of edema to those lung zones supplied by previously obstructed vessels. Exacerbating the degree of shunt and hypoxemia associated with this complication is the redistribution of blood from previously well-perfused segments to newly endarterectomized vessels supplying edematous areas of lung—a phenomenon referred to as *pulmonary artery steal.*

TREATMENT AND OUTCOME

A detailed discussion of the management of ARDS is beyond the scope of this chapter but is covered elsewhere in this volume as well as in recent reviews (e.g., Ref. 22). However, several fundamental aspects of care should be underscored. First and foremost, clinical management remains supportive; specific therapies aimed at ameliorating lung injury or accelerating healing are presently lacking. Care largely centers on use of mechanical ventilation, adjusted to maintain adequate gas exchange, while minimizing potentially harmful effects of high concentrations of oxygen and high airway pressures, both of which can induce further acute lung injury. To this end, efforts should be made to reduce the F_{IO_2} to 0.6 or less, accepting an arterial saturation in excess of 90 percent and utilizing PEEP to recruit atelectatic areas of lung and improve oxygenation. A respiratory pattern of small tidal volume (5 to 10 cc/kg) and high respiratory rate is preferred in an attempt to limit airway pressure to less than 45 cmH$_2$O and to minimize overdistention of normal alveolar units. Alternatively, pressure-controlled ventilation can be employed to precisely set the maximal inspiratory pressure. These ventilatory strategies frequently result in hypoventilation and hypercapnia, which are well tolerated unless extreme. In cases of severe respiratory acidosis (pH < 7.25), sodium bicarbonate can be infused intravenously to maintain an acceptable pH.

Continuous sedation should be administered to maintain patient comfort and promote synchronous breathing with the ventilator. Paralysis of the patient is occasionally required in the acute situation of life-threatening hypoxemia or hypercapnia, but prolonged use of neuromuscular blocking agents is discouraged because of the risk of a debilitating myopathy.

Inhaled nitric oxide preferentially vasodilates vessels supplying well-ventilated areas of lung and has been shown in limited studies to reduce shunt fraction and improve oxygenation in patients with severe ARDS. While this technique holds tremendous promise as a supportive therapy in this setting, further studies are required to confirm the efficacy of inhaled nitric oxide. At present, use of the drug is limited to centers participating in clinical trials.

Despite aggressive support, the overall mortality from ARDS approximates 50 percent. The mortality rate is significantly higher in the elderly and in those with concurrent failure of other organ systems. On the other hand, patients with acute lung injury attributable to cardiopulmonary bypass or TRALI tend to have a milder, more limited course and a more favorable prognosis.

Phrenic Nerve Injury and Diaphragmatic Paralysis

Phrenic nerve injury is a well-described complication of CABG, arising chiefly from the use of cold cardioplegic solution in proximity to the nerves. Thermal injury causes both demyelination and axonal degeneration of the phrenics, with resultant slowing of conduction and impaired activation of the diaphragm. As discussed previously, unilateral phrenic nerve injury, typically involving the left phrenic, occurs in approximately 10 percent of patients having CABG. This complication is usually clinically inconsequential except in the marginal patient with significant underlying pulmonary disease. Bilateral phrenic nerve injury is, fortunately, a rare complication following CABG, with an estimated incidence of only 1 to 3 percent. When present, bilateral injury results in marked impairment in pulmonary function and frequently in frank respiratory failure.

Phrenic nerve injury is not restricted to CABG but is also seen in association with other thoracic procedures, including valve replacement, pulmonary thromboendarterectomy, and lung transplantation. In the case of transplantation, topical cardioplegia is not employed, but the hemithorax is typically packed with ice to preserve the allograft during reimplantation. This effect may account for the reversible phrenic nerve dysfunction that has been reported. In some cases, diaphragmatic paralysis is permanent and is likely the result of actual transection of the phrenic nerve.

In the proper setting, bilateral phrenic nerve injury should be suspected when attempts to wean the patient from mechanical ventilation result in progressive hypercapnia or atelectasis. The spontaneously breathing patient will often complain of orthopnea, which may be misinterpreted by the unsuspecting clinician as indicative of congestive heart failure. However, the orthopnea is actually due to further impairment in diaphragmatic function due to loss of gravitational assistance in diaphragm descent. The detection of inspiratory thoracoabdominal paradox—an inward movement of the abdominal wall with concurrent expansion of the thorax—is an important bedside clue to the presence of bilateral diaphragmatic paralysis and is best evoked in the supine position. The chest radiograph may also hold important clues, demonstrating small lung volumes and bibasilar atelectasis (Fig. 170-1); however, these findings are not specific for diaphragm dysfunction following thoracic surgery.

A fundamental understanding of the available diagnostic tests is essential to appreciate their limitations and avoid pitfalls in interpretation. Standard pulmonary function testing, readily available at the bedside in many hospitals, demonstrates marked restriction with concurrent reduction in maximal inspiratory pressure. More informative, however, is the measurement of vital capacity in both erect and supine positions. In the presence of bilateral diaphragmatic dysfunction, the vital capacity should fall by greater than 25 percent with assumption of the supine position. This simple maneuver is limited by the inability of many patients to lie flat due to severe dyspnea.

A more precise physiological assessment of diaphragmatic performance is obtained with measurement of transdiaphragmatic pressure (Pdi) during a maximal inspiratory effort. This requires the transnasal insertion of balloon catheters into the esophagus and stomach and transduction of intraesophageal and intragastric pressures. With diaphragmatic dysfunction, the intercostal and accessory muscles are still capable of generating negative intrathoracic pressure, but the flaccid diaphragm is pulled passively cephalad, leading to a fall in intraabdominal pressure. As a result, Pdi fails to rise normally; in cases of complete paralysis, it approximates zero (Fig. 170-2). Although measurement of Pdi is an invaluable diagnostic tool in this setting, the technique is limited by the need for specialized equipment and expertise that are not widely available outside of academic medical centers.

In cases of unilateral diaphragm paralysis, fluoroscopic inspection readily reveals paradoxical upward movement of the af-

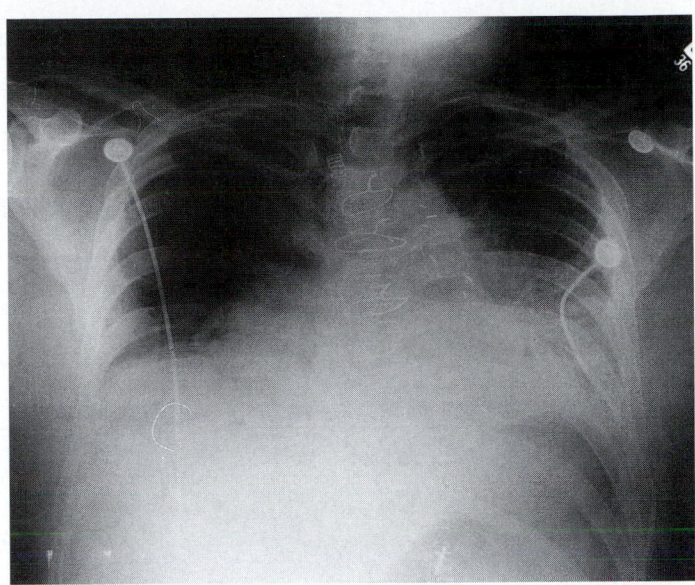

FIGURE 170-1 Chest radiograph of a patient with bilateral diaphragmatic paralysis following coronary artery bypass grafting. Note the small lung volumes and bilateral lower lobe atelectasis. The patient subsequently required reintubation for progressive hypoxemia and hypercapnia and spent several weeks on the ventilator before being successfully weaned.

fected hemidiaphragm with a maximal inspiratory effort ("sniff"). Unfortunately, the situation is more problematic with bilateral dysfunction. In this setting, patients often assume an altered breathing pattern marked by active contraction of the abdominal muscles during expiration, forcing the flaccid hemidiaphragms upward. With subsequent inspiration, the abdominal muscles relax and the hemidiaphragms descend briefly, potentially creating the false impression that they are functional. Because of this, fluoroscopy is confirmatory in only a minority of these patients.

The "gold standard" for confirmation of phrenic nerve injury is electrophysiological testing, although even this methodology is occasionally flawed. The phrenic nerve is stimulated transcutaneously in the neck, and the diaphragmatic electromyogram (EMG) is recorded by surface electrodes placed in the seventh intercostal space at the costochondral junction. Demonstration of a prolonged latency between nerve stimulation and diaphragmatic action potential, consistent with a demyelinating injury, confirms the diagnosis. It is more difficult to interpret the significance of a diminished amplitude of the diaphragmatic EMG in the face of normal latency. This finding could represent either an axonal degenerative neuropathy or failure to properly localize the diaphragm, which is typically shifted caudally in the postoperative patient and therefore away from the surface electrodes. Direct puncture of the diaphragm with a recording electrode may be employed to clarify this issue, but the technique requires a high level of expertise and carries a risk of pneumothorax.

Management of patients with respiratory failure due to phrenic nerve dysfunction is supportive. Continuous mechanical ventilation is typically required early in the course of the injury, but with partial recovery of diaphragmatic function, many patients can be weaned to a schedule of nocturnal support only. In less severe cases, mechanical ventilation can often be provided non-

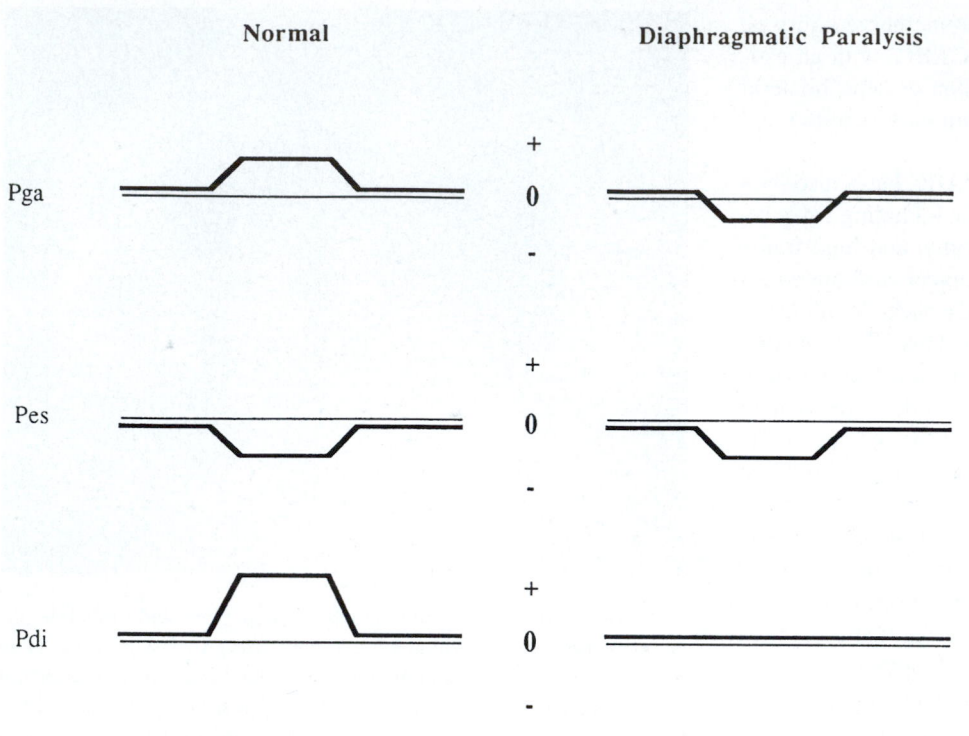

FIGURE 170-2 Schematic depiction of intrathoracic and intraabdominal pressure tracings obtained with esophageal and gastric balloon catheters. With normal diaphragmatic function, the diaphragm descends with inspiration, lowering intraesophageal pressure (Pes) and raising intragastric pressure (Pga). The resulting transdiaphragmatic pressure (Pdi) which is the difference between Pga and Pes, becomes markedly positive. With diaphragmatic paralysis, intercostal and accessory muscles contract to lower Pes, but the flaccid diaphragm is drawn cephalad, producing a fall in Pga. The net result of these offsetting effects is a Pdi that approximates zero.

Unfortunately, little information pointing specifically to a diagnosis of pulmonary embolism is easily gleaned at the bedside. The patient is often dyspneic, and tachypnea and tachycardia are observed on physical examination. However, these features are common in many postoperative patients because of pain and atelectasis. More informative but infrequently detected is evidence of acute cor pulmonale: distended neck veins, a parasternal heave, right-sided third heart sound, and accentuation of the pulmonic component of the second heart sound. An electrocardiogram may also demonstrate evidence of right heart strain, with an "S1Q3T3" pattern or new right bundle branch block. The chest radiograph is most suggestive of pulmonary embolism when it is normal in the face of severe hypoxemia. When it is abnormal, the greatest utility of the chest radiograph is in identifying other causes of hypoxemia such as pneumonia, pneumothorax, or ARDS.

The choice of diagnostic studies is dictated by the urgency of the situation. In the setting of life-threatening hypoxemia or hemodynamic instability, pulmonary angiography provides the most definitive and expeditious means of establishing the diagnosis. Pulmonary angiography also permits the immediate placement of an inferior vena caval filter or performance of catheter embolectomy. In stable patients, a noninvasive approach consisting of lung scanning and lower extremity impedance plethysmography or ultrasonography may be utilized; pulmonary angiography is then reserved for patients who have a nondiagnostic noninvasive evaluation.

While anticoagulation with heparin forms the mainstay of therapy for the otherwise stable patient, the presence of life-threatening hypoxemia, often accompanied by hemodynamic instability, should prompt consideration of alternative interventions. Since additional clot burden could be fatal, insertion of an inferior vena caval filter is generally advised. Certainly this intervention is mandatory when anticoagulation is contraindicated. Thrombolytic therapy should also be considered in the critically ill patient, but its use in the postoperative period is limited by the risk of precipitating bleeding at the site of recent surgery. This risk appears to fall to an acceptable level beyond the seventh postoperative day; the exception is cranial surgery, which contraindicates use of lytic agents for at least 3 months. Finally, embolectomy performed either surgically or by means of specially designed pulmonary artery catheters should be considered in the deteriorating patient for whom lytic therapy is either contraindicated or unsuccessful.

invasively via a tightly fitting nasal mask. Attempts should be made to keep the spontaneously breathing patient in a seated position in order to allow for gravitational assistance of diaphragmatic excursion. Recovery from thermally induced phrenic neuropathy is usually complete but typically protracted, requiring 6 to 12 months in severe cases.

Pulmonary Embolism

An increased risk of pulmonary embolism accompanies a number of surgical procedures, including upper abdominal, neurosurgical, cardiac, major urologic, and lower extremity orthopedic procedures. Other, nonsurgical risk factors that predispose the patient to pulmonary embolism may also be present, including obesity, immobility, and underlying malignancy.

While alterations in gas exchange typify pulmonary embolism, frank hypoxemic respiratory failure is relatively uncommon and suggests massive clot burden. Lesser degrees of clot burden may produce equally devastating physiological impairment in patients with underlying pulmonary disease. In the presence of severe hypoxemia, there is little remaining cardiopulmonary reserve. Failure to establish a correct diagnosis and to intervene swiftly and appropriately can prove lethal.

Obstructive Sleep Apnea

Obstructive sleep apnea (OSA) is a common disorder affecting 2 to 4 percent of the adult population. It is characterized by repetitive upper airway obstruction during sleep, resulting in periodic arterial desaturation, hypercapnia, and arrhythmias. The perioperative period is a particularly precarious time for patients with this disorder, as the use of volatile anesthetics, opioids, and sedatives diminishes the activity of the upper airway musculature and increases the frequency and duration of obstructive apneas. Failure to recognize and appropriately support patients with OSA in the perioperative period has led to serious complications, including respiratory arrest, hypoxemia, confusion, and ventricular arrhythmias.[36] Institution of nasal CPAP immediately after extubation facilitates safe administration of anesthetic, analgesic, and sedative agents, without undue risk of precipitating life-threatening airway obstruction.[36] As many patients with OSA are undiagnosed at the time of surgery, a high index of suspicion is required to heighten vigilance for this complication and to intervene appropriately when upper airway obstruction is observed.

REFERENCES

1. Berrizbeitia LD, Tessler S, Jacobowitz IJ, et al: Effect of sternotomy and coronary bypass surgery on postoperative pulmonary mechanics: Comparison of internal mammary and saphenous vein bypass grafts. *Chest* 96:873–876, 1989.
2. Bevelaqua F, Garritan S, Haas F, et al: Complications after cardiac operations in patients with severe pulmonary impairment. *Ann Thorac Surg* 50:602–606, 1990.
3. Bolliger CT, Jordan P, Soler M, et al: Exercise capacity as a predictor of postoperative complications in lung resection candidates. *Am J Respir Crit Care Med* 151:1472–1480, 1995.
4. Braun SR, Birnbaum ML, Chopra PS: Pre- and postoperative pulmonary function abnormalities in coronary artery revascularization surgery. *Chest* 73:316–320, 1978.
5. Celli BR, Rodriguez KS, Snider GL: A controlled trial of intermittent positive pressure breathing, incentive spirometry, and deep breathing exercises in preventing pulmonary complications after abdominal surgery. *Am Rev Respir Dis* 130:12–15, 1984.
6. Cohen A, Katz M, Katz R, et al: Chronic obstructive pulmonary disease in patients undergoing coronary artery bypass grafting. *J Thorac Cardiovasc Surg* 109:574–581, 1995.
7. Cunnion KM, Weber DJ, Broadhead WE, et al: Risk factors for nosocomial pneumonia: Comparing adult critical care populations. *Am J Respir Crit Care Med* 153:158–162, 1996.
8. Daily PO, Dembitsky WP, Iversen S, et al: Risk factors for pulmonary thromboendarterectomy. *J Thorac Cardiovasc Surg* 99:670–678, 1990.
9. Driks MR, Craven DE, Celli BR, et al: Nosocomial pneumonia in intubated patients given sulcralfate as compared with antacids or histamine type 2 blockers. *New Engl J Med* 317:1376–1382, 1987.
10. Duncan S, Negrin RS, Mihm FG, et al: Nasal continuous positive airway pressure in atelectasis. *Chest* 92:621–624, 1987.
11. Dureuil B, Cantineau JP, Desmonts JM: Effects of upper or lower abdominal surgery on diaphragmatic function. *Br J Anaesth* 59:1230–1235, 1987.
12. Dureuil B, Viires N, Cantineau JP, et al: Diaphragmatic contractility after upper abdominal surgery. *J Appl Physiol* 61:1775–1780, 1986.
13. Ford GT, Whitelaw WA, Rosenal TW, et al: Diaphragm function after upper abdominal surgery in humans. *Am Rev Respir Dis* 127:431–436, 1983.
14. Garibaldi RA, Britt MR, Coleman ML, et al: Risk factors for postoperative pneumonia. *Am J Med* 70:677–680, 1981.
15. George DL: Epidemiology of nosocomial pneumonia in intensive care unit patients. *Clin Chest Med* 16:29–44, 1995.
16. Gracey DR, Divertie MB, Didier EP: Preoperative pulmonary preparation of patients with chronic obstructive pulmonary disease: A prospective study. *Chest* 76:123–129, 1979.
17. Harris RJ, Kavuru MS, Rice TW, Kirby TJ: The diagnostic and therapeutic utility of thoracoscopy: A review. *Chest* 108:828–841, 1995.
18. Hollier LH, Symmonds JB, Pairolero PC, et al: Thoracoabdominal aortic aneurysm repair: Analysis of postoperative morbidity. *Arch Surg* 123:871–875, 1988.
19. Hudson LD, Milberg JA, Anardi D, Maunder RJ: Clinical risks for development of the acute respiratory distress syndrome. *Am J Respir Crit Care Med* 151:293–301, 1995.
20. Jayr C, Matthay MA, Goldstone J, et al: Preoperative and intraoperative factors associated with prolonged mechanical ventilation: A study in patients following major abdominal vascular surgery. *Chest* 103:1231–1236, 1993.
21. Johnson D, Kelm C, To T, et al: Postoperative physical therapy after coronary artery bypass surgery. *Am J Respir Crit Care Med* 152:953–958, 1995.
22. Kollef MH, Schuster DP: The acute respiratory distress syndrome. *New Engl J Med* 332:27–37, 1995.
23. Kroenke K, Lawrence VA, Theroux JF, Tuley MR: Operative risk in patients with severe obstructive pulmonary disease. *Arch Intern Med* 152:967–971, 1992.
24. Lemmer JH, Gomez MN, Symreng T, et al: Limited lateral thoracotomy: Improved postoperative pulmonary function. *Arch Surg* 125:873–877, 1990.
25. Marini JJ, Pierson DJ, Hudson LD: Acute lobar atelectasis: A prospective comparison of fiberoptic bronchoscopy and respiratory therapy. *Am Rev Respir Dis* 119:971–978, 1979.
26. Markand ON, Moorthy SS, Mahomed Y, et al: Postoperative phrenic nerve palsy in patients with open-heart surgery. *Ann Thorac Surg* 39:68–73, 1985.
27. Markos J, Mullan BP, Hillman DR, et al: Preoperative assessment as a predictor of mortality and morbidity after lung resection. *Am Rev Respir Dis* 139:902–910, 1989.
28. Money SR, Rice K, Crockett D, et al: Risk of respiratory failure after repair of thoracoabdominal aortic aneurysms. *Am J Surg* 168:152–155, 1994.
29. Morice RC, Peters EJ, Ryan MB, et al: Exercise testing in the evaluation of patients at high risk for complications from lung resection. *Chest* 101:356–361, 1992.
30. Nakahara K, Ohno K, Hashimoto J, et al: Prediction of postoperative respiratory failure in patients undergoing lung resection for lung cancer. *Ann Thorac Surg* 46:549–552, 1988.
31. Nunn JF, Milledge JS, Chen D, Dore C: Respiratory criteria of fitness for surgery and anaesthesia. *Anaesthesia* 43:543–551, 1988.
32. Pedersen T, Eliasen K, Henriksen E: A prospective study of risk factors and cardiopulmonary complications associated with anaesthesia and surgery: Risk indicators of cardiopulmonary morbidity. *Acta Anaesthesiol Scand* 34:144–155, 1990.
33. Pittet JF, Wiener-Kronish JP: Postoperative complications, in Murray JF (ed): *Pulmonary Complications of Systemic Disease.* New York, Marcel Dekker, 1992, pp 549–586.
34. Popovsky MA, Moore SB: Diagnostic and pathogenetic considerations in transfusion-related acute lung injury. *Transfusion* 25:573–577, 1985.

35. Ready LB: Intraspinal opioid analgesia in the perioperative period. *Anesth Clin North Am* 10:145–159, 1992.

36. Rennotte MT, Baele P, Aubert G, Rodenstein DO: Nasal continuous positive airway pressure in the perioperative management of patients with obstructive sleep apnea submitted to surgery. *Chest* 107:367–374, 1995.

37. Rovina N, Bouros N, Tzanakis N, et al: Effects of laparoscopic cholecystectomy on global respiratory muscle strength. *Am J Respir Crit Care Med* 153:458–461, 1996.

38. Singh NP, Vargas FS, Cukier A, et al: Arterial blood gases after coronary artery bypass surgery. *Chest* 102:1337–1341, 1992.

39. Stein M, Koota GM, Simon M, Frank HA: Pulmonary evaluation of surgical patients. *JAMA* 181:765–770, 1962.

40. Strandberg A, Tokics L, Brismar B, et al: Atelectasis during anaesthesia and in the postoperative period. *Acta Anaesthesiol Scand* 30:154–158, 1986.

41. Svensson LG, Hess KR, Coselli JS, et al: A prospective study of respiratory failure after high-risk surgery on the thoracoabdominal aorta. *J Vasc Surg* 14:271–282, 1991.

42. Sykes LA, Bowe EA: Cardiorespiratory effects of anesthesia. *Clin Chest Med* 14:211–226, 1993.

43. Taggart DP, El-Fiky M, Carter R, et al: Respiratory dysfunction after uncomplicated cardiopulmonary bypass. *Ann Thorac Surg* 56:1123–1128, 1993.

44. Torres A, Serra-Batlles J, Ros E, et al: Pulmonary aspiration of gastric contents in patients receiving mechanical ventilation: The effect of body position. *Ann Intern Med* 116:540–543, 1992.

45. Turnage WS, Lunn JL: Postpneumonectomy pulmonary edema: A retrospective analysis of associated variables. *Chest* 103:1646–1650, 1993.

46. Van Mieghem W, Coolen L, Malysse I, et al: Amiodarone and the development of ARDS after lung surgery. *Chest* 105:1642–1645, 1994.

47. Warner MA, Divertie MB, Tinker JH: Preoperative cessation of smoking and pulmonary complications in coronary artery bypass patients. *Anesthesiology* 60:380–383, 1984.

48. Warner MA, Warner ME, Weber JG: Clinical significance of pulmonary aspiration during the perioperative period. *Anesthesiology* 78:56–62, 1993.

49. Wilcox P, Baile EM, Hards J, et al: Phrenic nerve function and its relationship to atelectasis after coronary artery bypass surgery. *Chest* 93:693–698, 1988.

50. Williams CD, Brenowitz JB: "Prohibitive" lung function and major surgical procedures. *Am J Surg* 132:763–766, 1976.

CHAPTER 171

PUMP FAILURE: THE PATHOGENESIS OF HYPERCAPNIC RESPIRATORY FAILURE IN PATIENTS WITH LUNG AND CHEST WALL DISEASE

Steven G. Kelsen / Gerard Joseph Criner

COMPENSATORY/ADAPTIVE MECHANISMS
    Respiratory Chemosensitivity
    Responses to Heightened Respiratory Load
    Integrated Motor Responses
    Changes in Respiratory Structure

DECOMPENSATING/MALADAPTIVE RESPONSES
    Respiratory Muscle Fatigue
    Rapid, Shallow Breathing
    Undernutrition

SPECIFIC DISEASES
    COPD
    Asthma
    Neuromuscular Diseases
    Kyphoscoliosis

ASSESSMENT OF PATIENTS WITH ABNORMALITIES OF THE VENTILATORY PUMP
    Symptoms
    Physical Findings
    Maximum Static Inspiratory Pressure

TREATMENT
    Abnormalities in Chemosensitivity
    Respiratory Muscle Weakness or Fatigue

The ventilatory pump accomplishes bulk transfer of air to and from the alveoli. Accordingly, diseases that perturb the mechanical properties of any component of the ventilatory pump (i.e., the bony rib cage, the extra- and intrathoracic conducting airways, and the respiratory muscles) may interfere with CO_2 elimination and O_2 uptake. If disturbances in the function of the ventilatory pump are sufficiently severe, alveolar hypoventilation and respiratory acidosis may ensue. Hypercapnic respiratory failure is defined as a steady-state $PaCO_2$ while awake at more than 45 mmHg, the upper limit of normal. This definition is somewhat arbitrary but has proved clinically useful.

Conceptually, diseases that cause hypercapnic respiratory failure do so by deranging respiratory mechanics and lung dead-space volume [e.g., chronic obstructive pulmonary disease (COPD), asthma, or kyphoscoliosis] or by impairing the contractile properties of the respiratory muscles (e.g., neuromuscular disease). Diseases that impair respiratory mechanics increase the elastic or resistive load against which the respiratory muscles must contract. On the other hand, neuromuscular diseases impair the strength or endurance properties of the respiratory muscles and impair their ability to generate swings in intrathoracic pressure sufficient to maintain ventilation.

A variety of compensatory neural mechanisms that sense alterations in blood gas tensions or ventilatory performance elicit increases in the neuromuscular drive to breathe—which, in turn, helps preserve alveolar ventilation. In fact, in most patients, rather marked abnormalities in ventilatory pump performance are required before hypercapnic respiratory failure ensues. Conceptually, the susceptibility to develop CO_2 retention in the setting of lung, chest wall, or respiratory muscle dysfunction, therefore, depends on the balance between the severity of the derangement in ventilatory pump function and the intensity of the respiratory neuromuscular drive to breathe.

This chapter deals with the pathogenic mechanisms at work in the development of CO_2 retention in lung and chest wall diseases. The compensatory/adaptive mechanisms that help preserve ventilation (e.g., respiratory chemosensitivity, motor responses to alterations in the mechanics of breathing, and intrinsic changes in respiratory muscle strength and endurance) and the decompensating/maladaptive responses that predispose to CO_2 retention (e.g., respiratory muscle wasting and fatigue and a rapid, shallow pattern of breathing) will be discussed.

COMPENSATORY/ADAPTIVE MECHANISMS

Respiratory Chemosensitivity

OVERVIEW—REGULATION OF VENTILATION

Hypoxia and hypercapnia stimulate chemoreceptors in the arterial circulation (peripheral chemoreceptors) and ventrolateral medulla (central chemoreceptors) that reflexly increase motor activity to the respiratory skeletal muscles of the chest wall and upper airway.[28,58] Contraction of the muscles of the chest wall (e.g., diaphragm, intercostals, abdominals, and neck muscles) deforms the ventilatory pump and moves air. Contraction of the muscles of the upper airway (genioglossus, alae nasae, posterior arytenoids, pharyngeal dilators, sternohyoid, etc.) increases the caliber of the upper airway and diminishes its susceptibility to collapse during inspiration.

Chemoreceptor-induced increases in inspiratory and expiratory muscle activity, therefore, determine both the magnitude of the swings in intrathoracic pressure and resistance and compliance of the upper airway; are proportional to the severity of abnormalities in blood gas tensions; and represent a feedback control loop that restores blood gas tensions toward normal by enhancing alveolar ventilation. The maintenance of blood gas tensions within a relatively narrow, normal range from neonatal life to senescence attests to the power of this homeostatic mechanism.

Hypoxic and hypercapnic chemical drives to breathe exert the following stereotypic effects on the activity of chest wall and upper-airway muscles.[38] Peak respiratory muscle electrical activity and its rate of rise are increased. For the inspiratory muscles,

these changes in muscle electrical activity increase the rate of change and peak inspiratory intrathoracic pressure, inspiratory airflow, and tidal volume. For the expiratory muscles, increased electrical activity enhances the rate of expiratory airflow. For the upper-airway muscles, the resistance to inspiratory airflow decreases.

Chemosensitivity-induced increases in respiratory activity also affect the timing of respiratory motor activity as reflected in the duration of inspiration (T_I) and expiration (T_E). Hypoxia and hypercapnia lead to decreased T_I and T_E, allowing the frequency of breathing to increase. Reductions in T_E are generally out of proportion to T_I, thereby increasing the fraction of the respiratory cycle spent in inspiration. This partitioning of the respiratory cycle is reflected in the T_I/T_T ratio, where T_T is the total breath cycle duration (i.e., the sum of T_I and T_E).

Hypoxia and hypercapnia differ in their effects on the activity of the inspiratory muscles after the cessation of inspiratory airflow, the so-called postinspiratory inspiratory activity (PIIA). Hypoxia increases PIIA in both chest wall inspiratory muscles and muscles that constrict the laryngeal aperture. Accordingly, hypoxia has a braking effect on the rate of expiratory airflow.[38] As T_E decreases with increasing hypoxic drive, end-expiratory lung volume increases. PIIA-induced increases in lung volume increase the caliber of the intrathoracic airways and the O_2 content of the lung. Hypoxia-induced PIIA affects the load on the respiratory muscles in complex fashion; that is, PIIA reduces inspiratory resistive work of breathing but increases the inspiratory elastic and expiratory resistive work of breathing. It has been suggested, however, that the net effect of hypoxia-induced PIIA is a reduction in overall energy expenditure during breathing. In contrast, hypercapnia diminishes the duration of PIIA.

Indices of Respiratory Motor Output

Ventilation is a well-accepted index of respiratory motor output. Traditionally, ventilation was viewed as the product of tidal volume (V_T) and respiratory rate (which is equal to $60/T_T$). More recently, ventilation has been viewed as the product of separate "drive" and "timing" components.[48] The average rate of inspiratory airflow, V_T/T_I—which reflects the rate of rise of inspiratory muscle activity and intrathoracic pressure—is increased when blood gas tensions are deranged. Accordingly, V_T/T_I has been taken as a reflection of the activity of mechanisms that regulate the drive to breathe. Of note, V_T/T_I may also be increased by excitatory inputs arising from respiratory mechanoreceptor afferents (e.g., vagal irritant receptors) and higher CNS structures engaged in thermoregulation and emotion (i.e., hypothalamic and limbic areas). Conversely, the T_I/T_T ratio has been taken as a reflection of the activity of mechanisms that regulate respiratory timing. The T_I/T_T ratio is strongly affected by afferent input from mechanoreceptors in the lungs, airways, and respiratory muscles, as well as increasing chemical drive. For example, T_I/T_T increases in anesthetized animals when vagal stretch receptors are stimulated by increases in lung volume and is decreased by bronchoconstriction-induced activation of vagal irritant receptors.[20]

In subjects with normal lung function, V_T/T_I and ventilation are accurate reflections of inspiratory muscle electrical activity and the rate of rise of intrathoracic pressure.[48] On the other hand, diseases that adversely affect the mechanical properties of the ventilatory pump (e.g., obstructive lung disease, kyphoscoliosis) interfere with the translation of changes in intrathoracic pressure into ventilation and airflow. Conversely, conditions that impair respiratory muscle contractility (e.g., neuromuscular diseases, respiratory muscle fatigue) interfere with the translation of inspiratory muscle electrical activity into intrathoracic pressure changes. Accordingly, V_T/T_I reflects the intensity of motor outflow to the inspiratory muscles produced by increasing chemical drive only when the mechanical properties of the ventilatory pump and inspiratory muscle strength are normal. When the ventilatory pump function is abnormal, respiratory motor outflow is best assessed from respiratory muscle electrical activity (i.e., diaphragm EMG activity), a complicated measurement largely confined to the research laboratory.

A simpler, clinically useful measurement that reflects the neuromuscular drive to breathe and the driving pressure to inspiratory airflow is the airway occlusion pressure.[2] The occlusion pressure is the pressure generated at the airway opening 100 ms after the onset of an occluded inspiratory effort (i.e., P_{100} or $P_{0.1}$) initiated at end-expiratory lung volume. Since the airway is occluded, the inspiratory muscles contract quasi-isometrically, a condition in which muscle force correlates closely with muscle electrical activity. Measurements are made early in inspiration (100 ms) to prevent behavioral responses elicited in response to airway occlusion from altering the shape/trajectory of the pressure waveform. The lack of flow or volume change during the measurement means that the occlusion pressure is unaffected by abnormalities in the flow-resistive or compliance properties of the ventilatory pump. The occlusion pressure, therefore, has been used to assess the drive to breathe in patients with lung diseases (e.g., COPD and asthma) and chest wall diseases (e.g., kyphoscoliosis) during resting and chemically stimulated breathing.[2] On the other hand, the occlusion pressure depends on the ability of the inspiratory muscles to convert neural activity into force and pressure. Accordingly, like ventilation, occlusion pressure may not reflect respiratory motoneuron activity when the inspiratory muscles are weak (e.g., neuromuscular disease) or fatigued.

HYPOXIC RESPONSE

Under isocapnic conditions, ventilation (or occlusion pressure) increases in curvilinear fashion as P_{O_2} falls.[57] However, hypoxic responses depend importantly on the prevailing level of Pa_{CO_2} (i.e., the O_2–CO_2 interaction). When Pa_{CO_2} is in the hypocapnic range, arterial P_{O_2} must fall considerably (to approximately 55 to 60 mmHg or less) before respiratory activity increases. Hypercapnia profoundly increases the response to hypoxia by shifting the threshold of the response toward higher levels of P_{O_2} and augmenting the change in ventilation elicited for a given reduction in P_{O_2}.

Although the physiological stimulus for the hypoxic response is the Pa_{O_2} of the blood perfusing the peripheral chemoreceptors, for convenience the oxyhemoglobin saturation assessed with a pulse oximeter has been taken as a reflection of the stimulus.[57] Use of the oxyhemoglobin saturation linearizes the relationship between the hypoxic stimulus, ventilation, and occlusion pressure. The intensity of the hypoxic response has been assessed

from the slope of the change in ventilation (or occlusion pressure) relative to the change in O_2 saturation (i.e., $\Delta V_E/\Delta \% O_2$ sat) and from the intercept of the relationship (e.g., ventilation at O_2 saturation of 85 percent).

HYPERCAPNIC RESPONSE

In contrast to the response to hypoxia, the ventilatory and occlusion pressure responses to hypercapnia under iso-oxic conditions are linear over a relatively wide range of Pa_{CO_2} above and below the resting level of 40 mmHg.[57] The intensity of the ventilatory and occlusion pressure response to CO_2 has been assessed from the slope of the relationship of V_E to Pa_{CO_2} (i.e., $\Delta V_E/\Delta Pa_{CO_2}$) and from the intercept of the relationship (i.e., V_E at Pa_{CO_2} 50 mmHg).

The ventilatory response to hypercapnia is strongly affected by the prevailing level of Pa_{O_2} and is heightened as Pa_{O_2} decreases. In fact, hypoxemic and hypercapnic stimuli interact multiplicatively to enhance inspiratory and expiratory motor activity. Worsening hypoxemia enhances the ventilatory response to hypercapnia in accordance with the O_2–CO_2 interaction. The strength of a subject's chemosensitivity to O_2 and CO_2 and, in particular, to the O_2–CO_2 interaction is a powerful feedback mechanism opposing the tendency to retain CO_2 in patients with ventilatory pump dysfunction.

Consequently, treatment of the hypercapnic, hypoxemic patient with supplemental oxygen may decrease V_T/T_I and T_I/T_T and, hence, worsen hypercapnia in accordance with O_2–CO_2 interaction. Increases in Pa_{O_2} in hypoxic, hypercapnic subjects move the O_2 response to the right (less stimulus) and decrease the slope and shift the intercept of the ventilatory response to *hypercapnia* to the right (Fig. 171-1). Shifts in the CO_2 response with increases in the prevailing Pa_{O_2} mean that a higher CO_2 stimulus is required to maintain ventilation at the baseline level. Accordingly, ventilation falls and Pa_{CO_2} rises. The magnitude of the rise in Pa_{CO_2} in COPD patients in acute respiratory failure produced by supplemental oxygen varies widely among subjects as determined by their chemosensitivity (Fig. 171-2).

Of note, hypercapnia induced by supplemental oxygen in patients with COPD is multifactorial and reflects increases in lung dead-space volume as well as reductions in alveolar ventilation.[7] Hypoxemia causes bronchoconstriction via increases in parasympathetic outflow to airway smooth muscle. Accordingly, relief of hypoxemia causes bronchodilation and increased dead-space volume.

ROLE OF BLUNTED CHEMOSENSITIVITY IN DEVELOPMENT OF RESPIRATORY FAILURE

Chemosensitivities to hypoxemia and hypercapnia are hereditofamilial and ethnic traits that vary widely interindividually (Fig. 171-3).[15,35,36,56] In a given subject, responses to hypoxemia and hypercapnia correlate weakly, so that subjects with strong responses to hypercapnia also tend to have strong responses to hypoxia. Respiratory chemosensitivity to both hypoxemia and hypercapnia declines with age.[56] The decline in chemosensitivity with aging may explain why elderly subjects with lung disease (e.g., COPD) or chest wall disease (e.g., kyphoscoliosis) develop

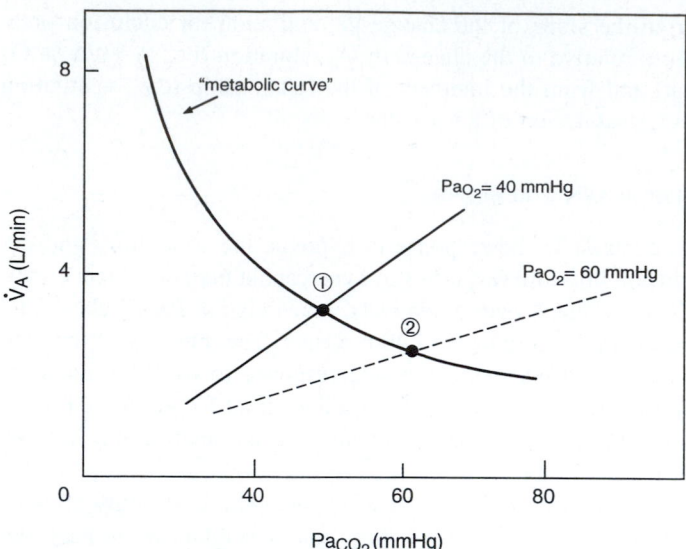

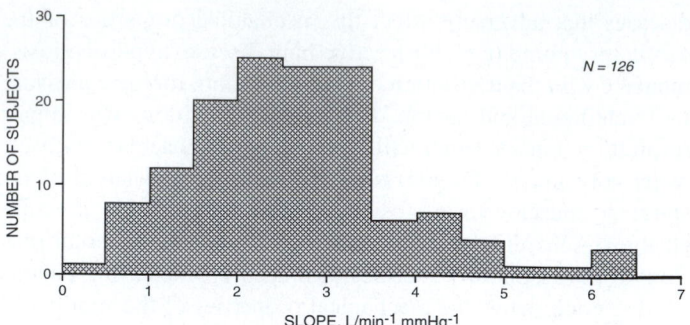

FIGURE 171-3   Variability of the slopes of the ventilatory responses to progressive hypercapnia (i.e., $\dot{V}E/P_{CO_2}$) in a normal population. Shown is the frequency distribution histogram of the slopes in 126 normal South African medical students. Note the considerable interindividual variation in CO_2 responsiveness. In some healthy subjects, the ventilatory response is blunted to less than 1 L/min/mmHg P_{CO_2}. *(Based on data of Irsigler,[35] with permission.)*

FIGURE 171-1   Theoretical effects of supplemental oxygen on the ventilatory response to CO_2 and steady-state arterial P_{CO_2} in subjects with COPD in hypercapnic respiratory failure. Increasing Pa_{O_2} decreases alveolar ventilation and increases Pa_{CO_2} as dictated by effects of oxygen on the CO_2 ventilatory response. The two straight lines represent hypercapnic ventilatory response curves at Pa_{O_2} of 40 and 60 mmHg. As may be seen, increasing Pa_{O_2} produces a downward, rightward shift of the ventilatory response. In contrast, the hyperbolic line intersecting the ventilatory response lines is the metabolic CO_2–ventilation curve, which represents the effect of increasing alveolar ventilation (independent variable) on Pa_{CO_2} (the dependent variable) when CO_2 production is normal ($\sim$200 ml/min). Steady-state alveolar ventilation and Pa_{CO_2} at rest are dictated by intersection of the ventilatory response curves with the metabolic curve (points 1 and 2). Note the increase in Pa_{CO_2} as the ventilatory response with Pa_{O_2} 60 mmHg intersects at a lower alveolar ventilation and higher Pa_{CO_2} (point 2) compared to the higher ventilatory response when Pa_{O_2} was 40 mmHg (point 1).

hypercapnic respiratory failure more frequently than young adults. When chemosensitivity is low, subjects with diseases of the ventilatory pump are predisposed to develop hypercapnic respiratory failure.

In patients with advanced COPD, the severity of airway obstruction required to cause CO_2 retention varies widely from subject to subject (Fig. 171-4).[43] Subjects with the greatest respiratory effort responses to changes in Pa_{CO_2}—as measured by diaphragm EMG, respiratory work of breathing, or occlusion pressure—have arterial Pa_{CO_2} values closer to normal than subjects with blunted responses to CO_2 but the same severity of lung dysfunction.[27,43] Accordingly, when chemosensitivity is low, subjects with diseases of the ventilatory pump are predisposed to develop hypercapnic respiratory failure. However, since CO_2 retention per se may blunt the response to acute hypercapnia, studies in patients in respiratory failure have not been able to determine whether blunted CO_2 responses are a cause or consequence of respiratory failure.

The tendency for chemosensitivity to be inherited has been used in a number of subsequent studies to assess the role of hypoxic and hypercapnic responses in the pathogenesis of CO_2 retention in the setting of obstructive lung disease.[27,37,49] Study of relatives with normal lung function and blood gases has been employed to circumvent the effects of CO_2 retention on respiratory chemosensitivity in patients with COPD.

In general, normal relatives of hypercapnic patients with COPD have lower ventilatory responses to hypoxia and hypercapnia than relatives of eucapnic patients with COPD (Fig. 171-5).[27,49] Among the offspring of COPD patients with equally severe airway obstruction, the slopes of the ventilatory responses to isocapnic hypoxemia and hyperoxic hypercapnia are 30 to 40 percent lower in the offspring of hypercapnic patients than in offspring of eucapnic patients. Similarly, the slopes of the ventilatory and airway occlusion pressure responses to isocapnic hypoxia in the offspring of hypercapnic patients are approximately 40 percent of the values obtained in the offspring of normocapnic patients. In one study, the Pa_{O_2} of COPD patients while in a

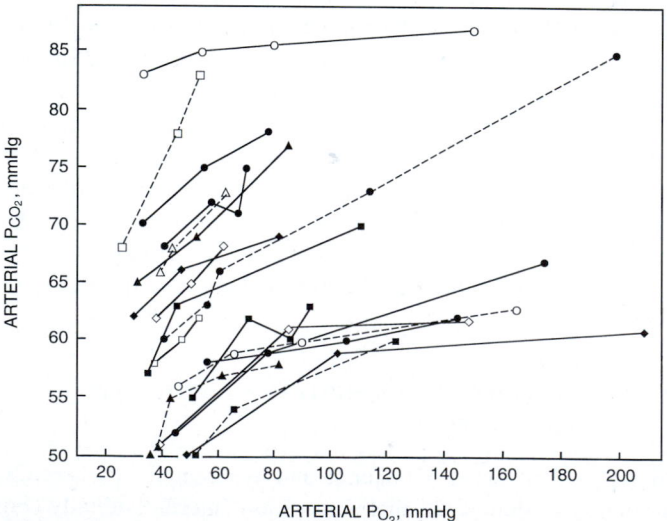

FIGURE 171-2   Effect of supplemental oxygen on steady-state arterial P_{CO_2} in 19 patients in acute respiratory failure from exacerbations of COPD. The point farthest to the left for each patient represents the values breathing room air. Note the considerable interindividual variation in the magnitude of CO_2 elevation in response to increases in arterial P_{O_2}. *(Based on data of Eldridge and Gherman, 1968,[26] with permission.)*

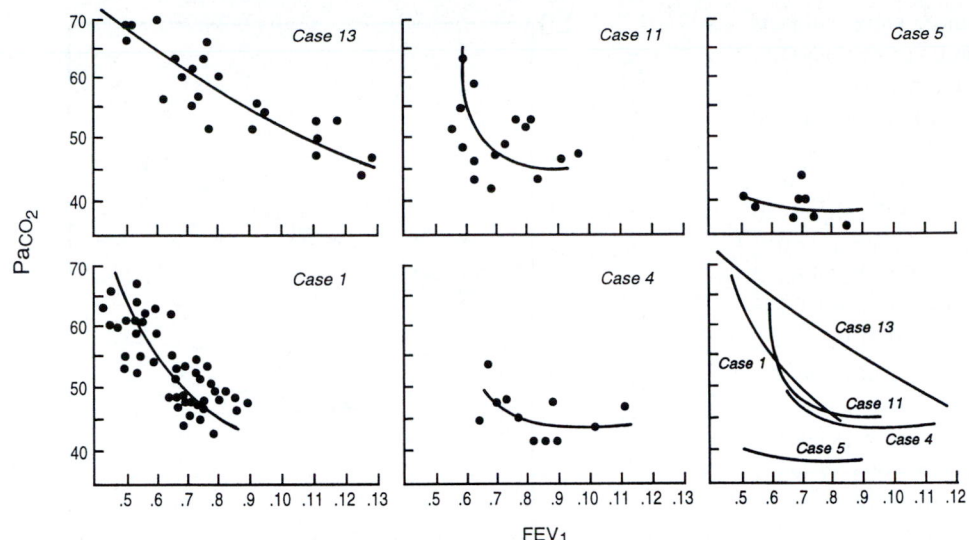

FIGURE 171-4   Results of repeated measurements of arterial P_{CO_2} and FEV_1 (liters) in five patients with advanced COPD. Free-hand curves of the data are shown plotted together in the lower right graph. Note that cases 1, 11, and 13 show marked increases in P_{CO_2}, with relatively small changes in FEV_1, whereas cases 4 and 5 do not. *(Based on data of Lane et al,[43] with permission.)*

stable state and the Pa_{O_2} and Pa_{CO_2} during COPD exacerbations correlated with the hypoxic ventilatory response of their sons.[39] It appears that blunted chemosensitivities to hypoxia and hypercapnia are likely to be premorbid characteristics of hypercapnic patients with COPD, which contribute to the development of respiratory failure.

A number of reports describe patients with asthma and respiratory failure who had blunted ventilatory responses to hypoxia and hypercapnia and whose healthy immediate family members also showed blunted hypoxic and hypercapnic responses.[33,49] Respiratory responses to hypoxia and hypercapnia in patients with asthma who have near-fatal attacks differ from those of asthmatics who did not have near-fatal attacks and age-matched, normal subjects.[40] The slopes of the ventilatory and occlusion pressure responses to hypoxia in the patients with a history of near-fatal asthma are approximately 33 percent of the responses of the asthmatics without near-fatal attacks or normals, which are similar. Hypercapnic responses tend to be lower in the near-fatal asthmatic groups than in the other two groups, but the differences are smaller in magnitude.

Responses to Heightened Respiratory Load

A complex array of mechano- and proprioceptors whose afferents project to respiratory neurons in the brain stem and higher CNS structures provides the respiratory controller with information about the mechanics of breathing and performance of the ventilatory pump.[20,28,64] The sensory receptors providing this afferent feedback and the CNS structures that integrate this feedback into a coordinated respiratory response (see below) are not perfectly understood. However, mechanoreceptors in the intercostal muscles that sense muscle tension and length (Golgi tendon receptors and spindle organs, respectively) and pressure and flow sensors in the lower (vagal irritant receptors) and upper airway (larynx and mouth) clearly play a role in shaping the

neuromuscular response to alterations in the mechanics of breathing.

Diseases of the airways (COPD and asthma) or chest wall (kyphoscoliosis) change the resistance and compliance properties of the ventilatory pump and, hence, stimulate mechanoreceptors in the ventilatory pump. In normal subjects and subjects with COPD, mechanoreceptor afferent inputs increase inspiratory neuromuscular output as reflected in airway occlusion pressure in response to bronchoconstriction or external resistances or elastance.[4,39] Changes in ventilation during acute increases in airway resistance are inversely related to changes in occlusion pressure. Thus, the magnitude of the motor response to increases in respiratory load determines the ventilatory response.

External ventilatory loads that can be consciously detected and alter the intensity of the sensations associated with breathing elicit increases in respiratory effort as reflected by the diaphragm EMG and occlusion pressure. Increases in effort occur abruptly within the first loaded breath and in feed-forward fashion; that is, the experience of the previous breath elicits a response in anticipation that the load will still be present. These responses are eliminated by general anesthesia and dulled if not absent in stages III and IV and REM sleep. The afferent input to the CNS elicited by external ventilatory loads probably arises from spindle and tendon organs in the respiratory muscles that project to the sensorimotor cortex and medullary respiratory neurons. The motor response to external ventilatory loads is thought to be behavioral.

The magnitude of the respiratory motor response to external loads varies widely from subject to subject and may be a hered-

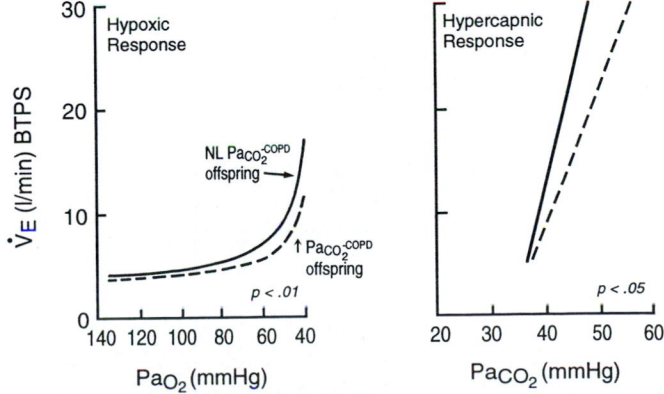

FIGURE 171-5   Mean isocapnic hypoxia and hyperoxic hypercapnic ventilatory response curves of 12 offspring of hypoventilating patients with COPD (solid line) and 10 offspring of eucapnic COPD patients (dashed line). Ventilatory responses to hypoxia and hypercapnia are significantly lower in the offspring of hypercapnic COPD than in offspring of eucapnic COPD patients. *(Based on data of Mountain et al,[49] with permission.)*

itofamilial trait.[37] Of considerable importance, some subjects with COPD demonstrate lesser occlusion pressure responses to acutely applied external resistive loads than age-matched normal subjects (Fig. 171-6).[4,63] It has been suggested that the blunted respiratory motor response to external loads may be a form of sensory adaptation to chronic increases in respiratory resistance. The fact that occlusion pressure responses of COPD subjects to external elastic loads and asthmatic subjects to external resistive loads are normal supports this concept. Of interest, the blunted motor response to external loads in some subjects with COPD may reflect an increase in endogenous opiates within the CNS, since naloxone administration immediately enhances the response.[63]

In subjects with COPD, bronchoconstriction increases airway occlusion pressure in proportion to increases in airway resistance and to a greater extent than with external flow-resistive loads.[73] Bronchoconstriction increases the activity of vagal "irritant" receptors in the airway, which exert an inspiratory augmenting effect on breathing. Irritant receptors may also be excited chemically by inflammatory mediators (e.g., histamine, $PGF_{2\alpha}$) and, in contrast to external loads, elicit simple monosynaptic reflexes not abolished by sleep or anesthesia.[20]

Mechanoreceptor inputs modify the respiratory motor responses to chemical stimuli to breathing. Increases in the elastic or resistive load to inspiration augment inspiratory muscle electrical activity and the airway occlusion pressures to hypoxia and hypercapnia. Subjects with asthma show heightened occlusion pressure responses to hypoxia and hypercapnia for this reason (Fig. 171-7).[39] Increases in the inspiratory neuromuscular

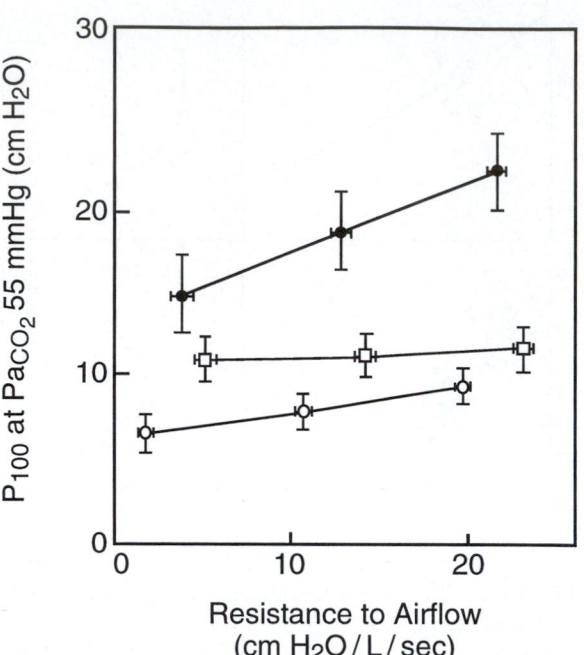

FIGURE 171-7   Occlusion pressure responses to progressive hypercapnia and inspiratory resistive loading in stable asthmatics (●), in COPD patients (△), and in normal subjects (○). Occlusion pressure (P_{100}) was measured at P_{CO_2} 55 mmHg, produced by hyperoxic hypercapnia. Resistance was increased by superimposing inspiratory resistive loads during rebreathing trials. Points farthest to the left are during free rebreathing. Note the greater occlusion pressure values during hypercapnia at any level of resistance in asthmatics than in COPD and normal subjects. *(From Kelsen et al: Am Rev Respir Dis 120:517–527, 1979, with permission.)*

drive to breathe allow ventilation to be maintained in the face of abnormalities in respiratory mechanics. Respiratory motor activity (i.e., occlusion pressure) also tends to be increased when the respiratory muscles are weak. In all likelihood, this reflects the fact that the maintenance of force output by a weakened muscle requires an increase in activation by the CNS.

Increased ventilatory loads also alter the pattern of breathing in load-dependent fashion.[18] Subjects breathing against resistive loads breathe slowly and deeply, with an increase in tidal volume and prolongation of T_I and T_E. In contrast, subjects breathing against elastic loads tend to breathe with smaller tidal volumes and a reduced T_I and T_E; that is, they demonstrate a rapid and shallow pattern of breathing. Slow, deep breathing during resistive loading and rapid, shallow breathing during elastic loading diminish the resistive and elastic work of breathing, respectively. Alterations in breathing pattern when the mechanics of breathing are deranged are believed to be attempts to minimize the work of breathing, muscle tension, or energy expended.

Integrated Motor Responses

Respiratory motor responses to heightened chemical or mechanoreceptor drives to breathe elicit highly coordinated patterns of muscle activity that optimize the mechanical output of the respiratory musculature contracting in concert. These responses may take the following forms: (1) simple reflex-mediated recruitment

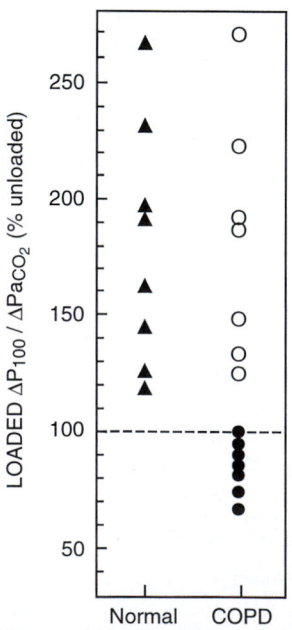

FIGURE 171-6   Effect of external inspiratory resistive load (18 cm $H_2O/L/s$) on the occlusion pressure responses to hypercapnia in normal subjects and patients with stable COPD. Note that ~50% of the COPD subjects show no increase in occlusion pressure in response to acute administration of resistive ventilatory loading. *(Based on data of Santiago et al,[63] with permission.)*

of additional agonists, which exert similar mechanical effects on the chest wall; (2) sequential activation of inspiratory and expiratory muscles, which exert opposing effects on chest wall structures; and (3) complex behavioral acts that use nonrespiratory muscles to effect changes in body posture and expiratory airflow, minimizing dyspnea.

For example, hypercapnia and hypoxia recruit the external intercostal and parasternal muscles during inspiration in a stereotypic rostral-to-caudal direction, and the internal intercostals and triangularis sterni during expiration in the opposite direction.[22,38] Preferential activation of the inspiratory external intercostal and parasternal muscles in the rostral-most interspaces decreases the impedance of the rib cage to rostral movement and, hence, facilitates thoracic expansion. Conversely, recruitment of the expiratory internal intercostals and triangularis sterni in the most caudal interspaces decreases the impedance to caudal movement and facilitates thoracic deflation. In addition, recruitment of the parasternal intercostal muscles facilitates inspiratory pressure as tidal volume increases. The parasternal intercostal muscle fiber length, which is optimum for tension development, is shorter than that of the diaphragm and occurs at higher lung volume. Accordingly, the parasternal muscles become mechanically more effective than the diaphragm as lung volume increases above functional residual capacity (FRC).[22]

Moreover, hypercapnia and hypoxia increase phasic and tonic inspiratory activity in the dilator muscles of the upper airway (e.g., posterior arytenoid, alae nasae, genioglossus). Increases in activity of the dilator muscles of the upper airway decrease the load on the chest wall pumping muscles by decreasing the resistance to inspiratory airflow through the upper airway. Increased activity of these muscles also diminishes the susceptibility of the upper airway to collapse as inspiratory efforts become greater and subpharyngeal pressure becomes more subatmospheric.

In addition, phasic increases in abdominal expiratory muscle electrical activity during expiratory airflow accelerate lung emptying, thereby allowing the time of expiration to decrease. When sufficiently intense, activation of the abdominal muscles reduces end-expiratory lung volume and improves the ability of the diaphragm to generate pressure by favorably affecting its precontraction length, radius of curvature, and alignment with the rib cage. Reductions in end-expiratory lung volume achieved by the expiratory muscles also allow elastic work to be stored in the passive recoil of the chest wall and released suddenly at the onset of inspiration. Sudden release of the recoil pressure of the chest wall thereby "assists" the inspiratory muscles by contributing to the driving pressure to inspiratory airflow. A portion of the inspiratory load is thus assumed by the expiratory muscles.

Finally, hyperinflated, dyspneic patients with COPD often assume a stereotypic body posture that improves diaphragm, neck accessory, and pectoral girdle muscle mechanical advantage.[24] This posture is forward flexion of the trunk, extension of the head and neck, bracing of the pectoral girdle by rounding of the shoulders, and grasping of the thighs with the arms. The effect of this posture is to increase abdominal pressure (thus increasing diaphragm precontraction length and radius of curvature); provide more favorable alignment of the scalenes and sternomastoid with the upper rib cage; and anchor the pectoral gir-

dle muscles, allowing them to apply an inspiratory action on the rib cage. In this posture, transdiaphragmatic pressure is increased and diaphragm and sternomastoid muscle EMG activity is decreased. Patients with advanced COPD also spontaneously adopt pursed-lip breathing to slow expiratory airflow, thus minimizing dynamic airway compression.

EFFECTS OF SLEEP

Responses to chemical stimuli to breathing are powerfully influenced by CNS state (e.g., sleep versus waking).[38,67] Slow-wave and REM sleep depress O_2 and CO_2 chemosensitivity, with greatest depression occurring in REM sleep. While the subject is awake, apnea does not occur in the presence of even marked hypocapnia, and ventilation is largely independent of changes in P_{CO_2}. Rather, ventilation persists even when Pa_{CO_2} is less than about 30 to 35 mmHg. Persistence of ventilation in the setting of hypocapnia (the so-called wakefulness drive to breathe) probably represents the effects on medullary neurons of inputs activated by auditory, visual, and tactile stimuli. In contrast, in the sleeping or anesthetized state, the ventilatory response to CO_2 extrapolates to zero ventilation in the hypocapnic range.[67] In fact, apnea occurs when P_{CO_2} falls only 4 to 6 mmHg below waking eucapnic levels. Sleep-related changes in chemosensitivity, therefore, underlie the recurrent periods of apnea and hyperpnea and exaggerated hypercapnia that occur in some patients with diseases of the lung and chest wall.

The increase in respiratory motor activity induced by derangements in respiratory mechanics is also state dependent; that is, heightened activity in awake subjects is absent in sleeping or anesthetized subjects. REM sleep, in particular, impairs the "load" response and causes collapse of the upper rib cage during inspiration, which adversely affects the level of ventilation as well as its distribution. Descending inhibitory drives to spinal α and spindle γ motoneurons in REM sleep cause atonia of all the respiratory muscles except the diaphragm. Muscle spindle γ efferent activity determines spindle sensitivity by progressively contracting the intrafusal fiber. Accordingly, reductions in muscle spindle γ efferent activity diminish spindle organ sensitivity and interfere with a mechanism for augmenting respiratory muscle spinal α motoneuron activity. The diminished or absent load response during sleep and anesthesia probably explains the exaggerated increases in Pa_{CO_2} that occur during these periods in patients with lung and chest wall disease. In fact, REM sleep is the period in which Pa_{CO_2} is highest and Pa_{O_2} lowest in patients with stable COPD (Fig. 171-8).[42]

Changes in Respiratory Structure

RESPIRATORY MUSCLES

The respiratory muscles are highly plastic and undergo changes in structure, biochemistry, and contractile properties in response to chronic increases in load or changes in precontraction length.[1,44,71] Chronic increases in inspiratory muscle activity enhance their strength and endurance.[44] In animal models, chronic increases in inspiratory load produced by emphysema or inspiratory resistive loading increase diaphragm endurance and the con-

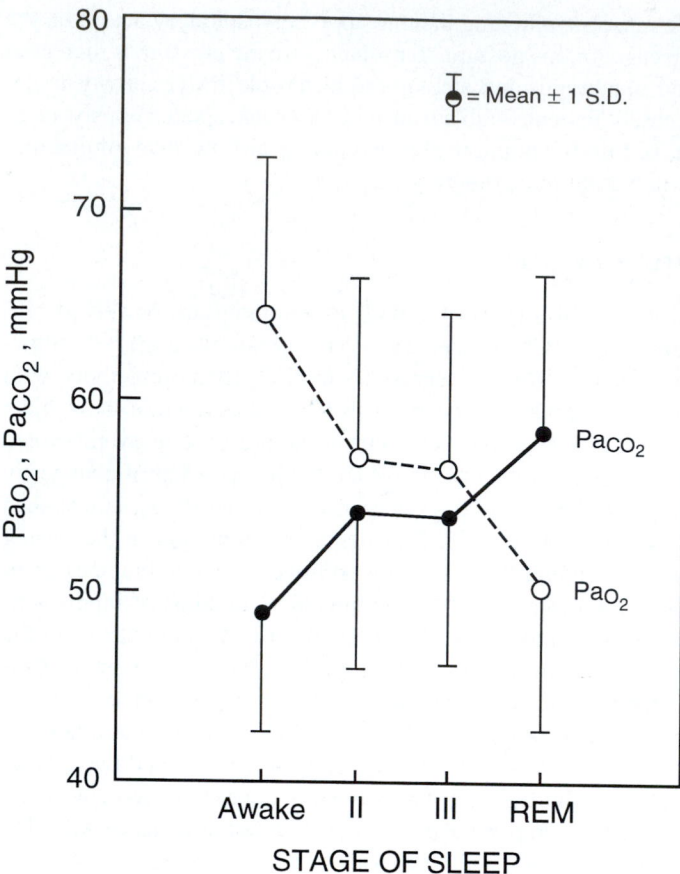

FIGURE 171-8 Changes in steady-state arterial P_{CO_2} during sleep in eight patients with stable COPD. Note that arterial P_{CO_2} increases and arterial P_{O_2} decreases during sleep. Greatest changes occur during rapid eye movement (REM) sleep. For Pa_{CO_2}, average increase is 10 mmHg. *(Based on data of Koo et al,[42] with permission.)*

tent of oxidant enzymes (e.g., succinic dehydrogenase and citrate synthase) essential for high-energy phosphate synthesis. In patients with chronic asthma, inspiratory and expiratory muscle endurance assessed from the time course of the fall in maximum static pressure is about 40 percent greater than in normal controls.[45] The effect of COPD per se on inspiratory muscle endurance has not been assessed. In subjects with COPD, however, daily training with inspiratory resistive ventilatory loads increases inspiratory muscle strength by about 40 percent as reflected by maximum static inspiratory pressure (PImax) over an 8- to 10-week period.[32]

Hyperinflation impairs the force- and pressure-generating ability of the inspiratory muscles by decreasing muscle precontraction length and unfavorably changing muscle alignment with the chest wall.[22] In particular, severe hyperinflation alters diaphragm shape (i.e., flattening) and decreases the zone of apposition with the rib cage. Flattening of the diaphragm displaces the vector of contraction force from a rostral–caudal direction to a medial–lateral direction and diminishes the ability of the diaphragm to increase abdominal pressure. Reductions in the zone of apposition diminish the inflationary effects on the lower rib cage produced by increases in abdominal pressure induced by the diaphragm. In extreme cases of hyperinflation, the diaphragm may exert an expiratory action on the lower rib cage and retract the lower rib cage on inspiration (Hoover's sign).

In part, hyperinflation-induced impairment in the action of the diaphragm is compensated for by adaptive changes in the intrinsic muscle length–tension characteristic. In emphysematous animals, the active and passive length–tension curve of the costal diaphragm is displaced toward shorter lengths, thereby allowing maximum tension to be developed at significantly shorter lengths and higher lung volumes (Fig. 171-9).[55,71] The shift in the length–tension curve appears to be the reverse of normal growth, in which muscle length is increased by addition of sarcomeres in series. A similar adaptation seems to occur in chronically hyperinflated, stable outpatients with COPD.[66]

CHEST WALL ANATOMY

Chronic hyperinflation elicits adaptive changes in the pressure–volume (P–V) characteristic of the passive chest wall. In animal models of emphysema, the static deflation, chest wall P–V curve is shifted up and to the left, so there is a decrease in elastic recoil at any given lung volume.[74] Shifts in the passive P–V curve are accomplished by a structural remodeling of the rigid structures in the chest wall. The length of the sternum and the lengths of the ribs in anteroposterior and transverse dimensions are increased. This displacement of the chest wall P–V curve diminishes the inspiratory elastic work of breathing during hyperinflation and preserves the zone of apposition of the diaphragm. An increase in the zone of apposition of the diaphragm in hyperinflation preserves the appositional force exerted by the diaphragm on the lower rib cage by virtue of changes in abdominal pressure. If present in patients with COPD, the process is reversible, since recent ob-

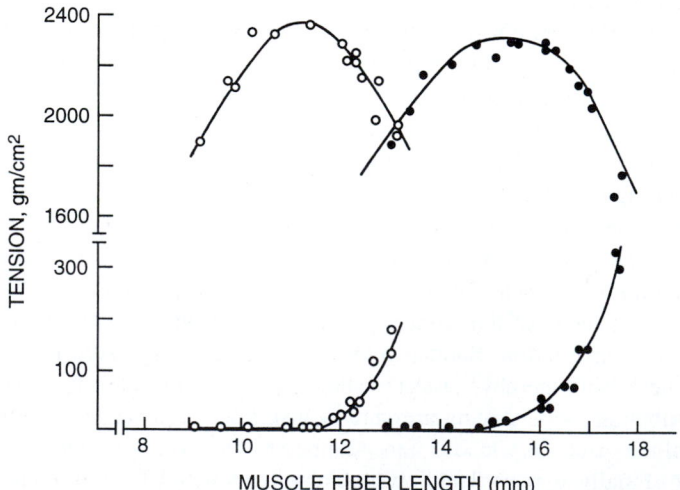

FIGURE 171-9 Active (upper trace) and passive (lower trace) length–tension relationship of costal diaphragm of emphysematous (open circles) and normal hamsters (solid circles), assessed in vitro during electrical stimulation. Note that in emphysematous animals, the L–T curve is displaced toward shorter fiber lengths. This adaptive change in emphysematous animals allows the diaphragm to generate maximal tension (force) at shorter fiber lengths and helps preserve diaphragm contractile performance in the face of considerable hyperinflation. *(From Supinski et al: J Clin Invest 70:978–988, 1982, with permission.)*

servations of the thorax after volume reduction surgery or lung transplantation for COPD indicate that chest wall shape can quickly revert to normal.[69]

DECOMPENSATING/MALADAPTIVE RESPONSES

Respiratory Muscle Fatigue

OVERVIEW/DEFINITION

Studies in the laboratory and in the clinic indicate that the respiratory skeletal muscles, like muscles in the limbs, fatigue under conditions of intense activity, leading to respiratory failure.[12,13,19] Conditions that increase the level of phasic inspiratory muscle activity, or the duty cycle of breathing, or that decrease the maximal pressure-generating capacity of the muscle, make fatigue more likely. For example, derangements in the mechanical properties of the lung or chest wall or increases in ventilatory drive increase inspiratory muscle contractile activity. Of note, increases in ventilatory drive increase both the peak inspiratory pressure and T_I/T_T ratio, the latter by causing greater reductions in the duration of expiration than in that of inspiration.

Decreases in inspiratory muscle strength caused by aging, protein-calorie malnutrition, or electrolyte imbalances predispose to fatigue at any given level of inspiratory impedance or ventilation by decreasing P_{Imax}.[62] Finally, on the basis of data from animal models, reductions in diaphragm blood flow are likely to decrease the level of muscle activity that leads to fatigue.[8]

Respiratory muscle fatigue has been defined as a loss in muscle capacity to develop force or shorten resulting from muscle fiber activity under load and is reversible by rest.[58] In contrast, respiratory muscle weakness has been defined as impairment in the capacity of a fully rested muscle to generate force.

Fatigue is viewed as developing when the muscle is highly active and generating appreciable levels of force. Recovery from fatigue is generally observed over a short time (e.g., minutes to hours). On the other hand, muscle weakness is commonly caused by muscle fiber atrophy, metabolic derangements that impair the ability of actomyosin cross-bridges to generate force (e.g., acidosis or electrolyte abnormalities that affect intracellular calcium flux), or chronic reductions in muscle precontraction length that impose a mechanical disadvantage (e.g., hyperinflation of the thorax and its effects on the inspiratory muscles). Implied in the definition of weakness is the idea that alterations in muscle function are secondary to alterations in muscle structure or lung volume and hence induce changes in muscle function that are more slowly reversible than fatigue (e.g., days to weeks). In the clinical setting, however, the distinction between muscle weakness and fatigue is difficult and not easily accomplished. Moreover, a close association exists between respiratory muscle weakness and respiratory muscle fatigue. In fact, weak muscles are predisposed to fatigue (see below).

Fatigue produces complex effects on muscle mechanical output. Fatigue prolongs contraction and relaxation time and depresses the force generated at a given stimulus frequency and fiber length, and reduces the velocity of shortening against a given load.[59]

TABLE 171-1

Classification of Respiratory Muscle Fatigue

Central
  Refers to decreases in phrenic motor output mediated by spinal or supraspinal mechanisms
Peripheral
  Refers to fatigue occurring at the level of the muscle itself
    Transmission
      Failure of mechanisms operative in muscle excitation ("high-frequency" fatigue)
    Contractile
      Failure of mechanisms involved in excitation–contraction coupling or contractile protein function ("low-frequency" fatigue)

Depending on the cause of the fatigue, depression of force output can occur at primarily subtetanizing frequencies of muscle stimulation (e.g., less than 15 to 20 Hz), a condition called low-frequency fatigue, or at frequencies above 50 Hz, a condition called high-frequency fatigue (Table 171-1, Fig. 171-10).[5] The biochemical and biophysical processes that underlie low-frequency and high-frequency fatigue differ. Muscle force responses to tetanizing frequencies of stimulation (i.e., above 50 Hz) are primarily determined by the processes of neuromuscular transmission and muscle excitation.[47] In contrast, muscle mechanical output at subtetanizing frequencies is determined primarily by the processes of excitation–contraction coupling (e.g., calcium release from the sarcoplasmic reticulum, calcium–troponin interactions), perhaps caused, in part, by oxygen free-radical–induced injury.[3]

Of interest, recovery from high-frequency fatigue is more rapid (minutes) than recovery from low-frequency fatigue (hours) (Fig. 171-11).[5] Moreover, the two forms of fatigue have different physiological consequences. High-frequency fatigue impairs muscle force output under conditions in which the muscle is maximally driven by the CNS (i.e., when muscle strength is being evaluated). Low-frequency fatigue, on the other hand, impairs force generation during resting breathing, when phrenic motor unit discharge rates are typically about 15 Hz. Since low- and high-frequency fatigue reflect impairments occurring at the level of the muscle, they have been termed *peripheral fatigue*.

Performance of strenuous ventilatory tasks may also elicit an additional, qualitatively different response—i.e., a reduction in central motor output and failure of the CNS to fully activate the respiratory muscles.[11] That is, the diaphragm EMG or phrenic neurogram may decrease late in the performance of strenuous respiratory efforts before the point of exhaustion. This reduction in motor activity may limit task performance. The failure of CNS mechanisms to fully activate the muscle near the point of exhaustion has been termed *central fatigue*. The mechanisms underlying central fatigue are poorly understood. It is not clear whether central fatigue represents a behavioral response elicited by the unpleasant sensations present during ventilatory loading or is mediated reflexly, or by changes in brain neurotransmitter levels.

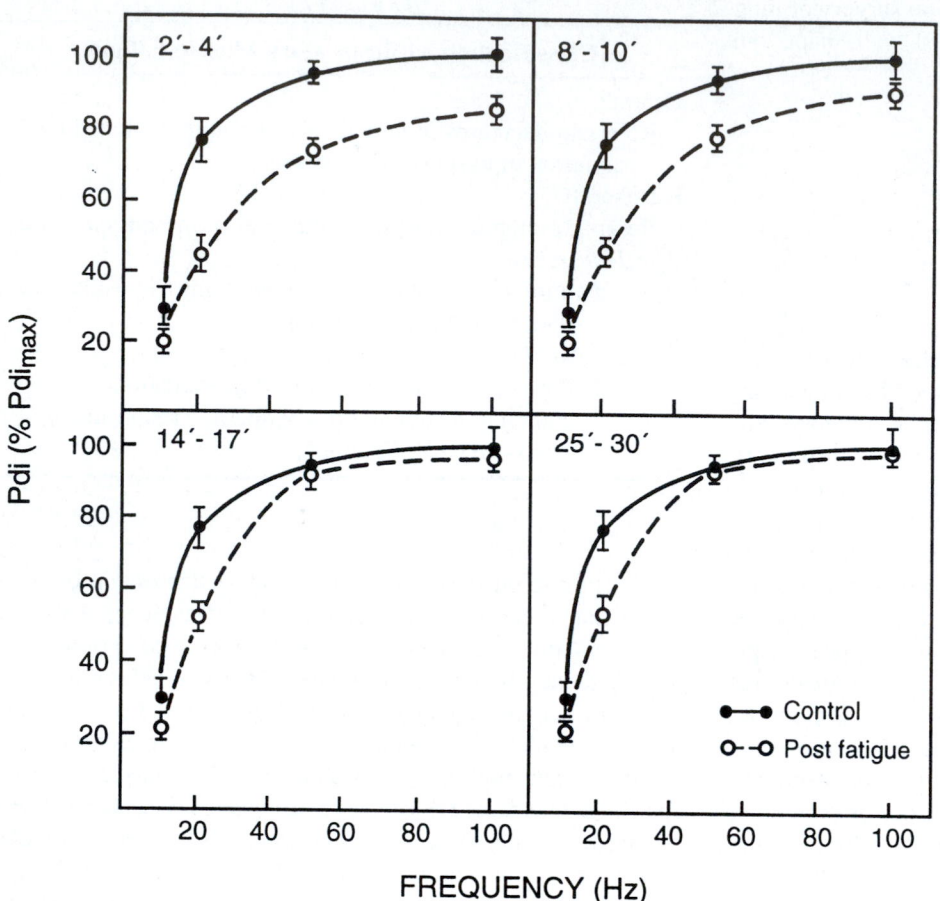

FIGURE 171-10 Force–frequency relationship of the human diaphragm during electrophrenic stimulation showing rate of recovery from high- and low-frequency fatigue. Data obtained in four subjects before and after a period of inspiratory resistive loading to exhaustion. At the point of exhaustion, the subject was unable to generate targeted values of transdiaphragmatic pressure (Pdi). Note the decrease in Pdi in response to low (20 Hz) and high (50 Hz) electrical stimulation immediately after loading, indicating the presence of both high- and low-frequency fatigue. Note also that high-frequency fatigue disappears within 14 to 17 min. In contrast, low-frequency fatigue persists beyond the period of observation (>30 min). *(Based on data of Aubier et al,[5] with permission.)*

DETECTION OF RESPIRATORY MUSCLE FATIGUE

Diaphragm muscle fatigue has been diagnosed in humans from changes in the response of the muscle to electrical stimulation (i.e., the force–frequency relationship), the power spectral content of the EMG, and Pimax.[5,45,50] As will be seen, the force–frequency relationship and EMG power spectrum analyses are complex and require sophisticated electronics and instrumentation. Consequently, their use has been confined to the research laboratory. On the other hand, Pimax is convenient and easily performed at the bedside but suffers from relative nonspecificity.

Electrical Stimulation

The force–frequency relationship represents a way of assessing muscle mechanical output over a wide range of stimulus intensities. Since fatigue shifts the force–frequency curve downward (and possibly to the left), the magnitude of the shift in the force–frequency relationship can be used to assess the severity of low- and high-frequency fatigue and the time course of recovery.

Electrical stimulation of the muscle of interest has several advantages. It allows the muscle to be activated in response to a standard stimulus without the cooperation of the subject. Hence, neurologic deficits, decreased effort, or central fatigue, which may diminish muscle activation, is circumvented and peripheral fatigue can be detected.

A recent development that shows considerable promise is electrophrenic twitch stimulation of the diaphragm (Fig. 171-11).[11] This approach is well tolerated. By combining twitch contraction during breath-holding at end-expiration with superimposed twitches applied during the performance of graded inspiratory efforts, the twitch occlusion technique, diaphragmatic strength (Pdimax) can be calculated.[11] The rationale behind the twitch occlusion pressure is as follows. As a muscle is activated to a progressively greater extent, progressively more motor units are recruited and individual motor units move up their force–frequency curve toward the plateau. Consequently, the magnitude of the superimposed twitch is inversely proportional to the extent of muscle activation (Fig. 171-11). When the muscle is maximally activated—that is, all motor units are recruited and on the flat portion of their force–frequency curve—the superimposed twitch will be undetectable or zero. The twitch occlusion technique is analyzed quantitatively by plotting the magnitude of the volitional contraction on the X axis against the magnitude of the superimposed twitch on the Y axis. When that is extrapolated to the X axis, the maximum pressure output of the muscle is determined. The twitch occlusion technique therefore allows detection of high-frequency fatigue as well as low-frequency fatigue (Fig. 171–12).

The twitch occlusion technique has been used to assess diaphragm function in stable outpatients with COPD and the mechanisms of fatigue in normal subjects during volitional contractions against large external inspiratory resistive loads to exhaustion. The twitch occlusion method demonstrates that the fresh diaphragm can be maximally activated volitionally. However, task performance during prolonged ventilatory loading to exhaustion—that is, the ability to generate a targeted transdiaphragmatic pressure (Pdi)—is in part limited by central fatigue.

EMG Power Spectrum

Fatigue alters the power-EMG spectral content of the raw EMG of the respiratory muscles[50] analyzed by fast Fourier transform (Fig. 171-11). In the fresh diaphragm, the power (or voltage) contained in the EMG waveform reaches a maximum between approximately 85 and 105 Hz, and thereafter declines. (Maxi-

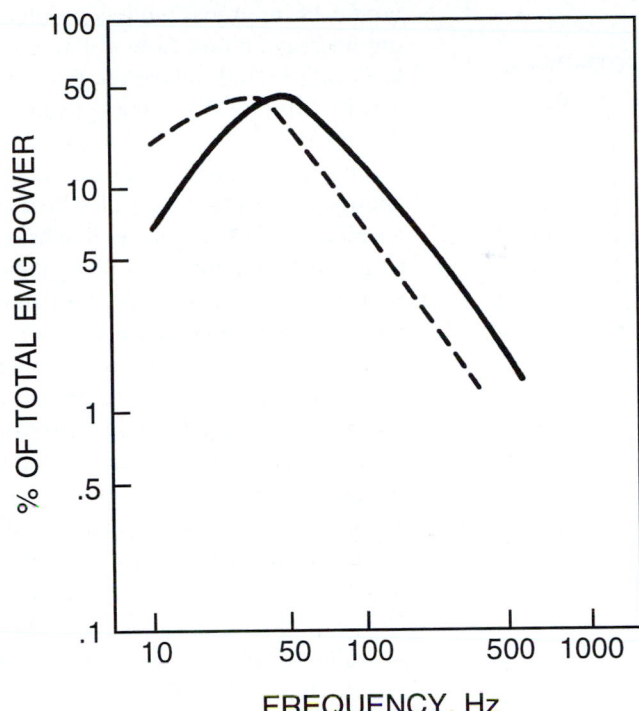

FIGURE 171-11   Schematic representation of the power-spectral density of a respiratory muscle EMG determined by fast Fourier transform. Note the concave appearance of the relationship. Note that fatigue (dashed line) decreases and increases power in the high- and low-frequency domains, respectively, thereby shifting the relationship toward the left. (*Based on data of Moxham et al,[50] with permission.*)

mum power in the EMG of the diaphragm, parasternal intercostal, and sternocleidomastoid occurs at somewhat different frequencies, however.) Fatigue-inducing contractions cause a leftward shift of the power spectral density, so that more of the power in the EMG is contained in a lower-frequency domain. The power-spectral density of the contracting diaphragm changes almost immediately with fatiguing contractions and considerably before the mechanical output of the muscle fails. The diaphragmatic EMG power spectrum can be obtained from the raw EMG of the muscle, recorded from surface electrodes on the chest wall or within the esophagus. It is, therefore, relatively noninvasive and well tolerated. Moreover, the EMG power spectrum, unlike maximal static pressure, can be measured continuously—i.e., breath by breath—and does not require subject cooperation. Accordingly, the EMG power spectrum has proved to be a useful tool to study the pathophysiological mechanisms of human respiratory muscle fatigue. A significant caveat in the use of the power spectrum is the suggestion that it may be unable to detect low-frequency fatigue.[50]

PATHOGENESIS OF RESPIRATORY MUSCLE FATIGUE

Studies designed to examine the pathogenetic mechanisms that lead to respiratory muscle fatigue have largely focused on the diaphragm. The diaphragm has been the primary focus of attention for several reasons. First, it is the major respiratory muscle. Second, anatomic considerations allow the mechanical output of the diaphragm (i.e., transdiaphragmatic pressure) and its EMG,

an index of phrenic motor outflow and fatigue state, to be assessed relatively easily. Finally, the cervical phrenic nerves can be electrically stimulated, thereby allowing the mechanical output of the muscle to be assessed under standard conditions as well as during volitional contractions.

Muscle Activity

In seminal studies, Roussos and Macklem[62] observed that the time of onset of diaphragm fatigue was *not* related to the magnitude of the phasic inspiratory swings in Pdi during loading alone or to Pdimax alone. Rather, the time of onset of mechanical failure of the diaphragm was a unique curvilinear function of the ratio of Pdi generated on each breath over Pdimax (Pdi/Pdimax) (Fig. 171-13). Values of Pdi/Pdimax less than 40 to 50 percent could be maintained indefinitely; values greater than this threshold were associated with progressively more rapid exhaustion. These results made several important points. First, diaphragm fatigue depended on the relative intensity of contraction (i.e., muscle force output as a percentage of its strength). Second, contractions below some critical threshold could be sustained indefinitely and did not lead to fatigue.

Subsequent studies demonstrated that the timing as well as the intensity of diaphragmatic contractions determined the time of onset of mechanical failure of that muscle. Increases in the ratio of the T_I over the T_T increased the rapidity of onset of fatigue at any given Pdi/Pdimax ratio.[12,13,62] That is, increasing the duration of diaphragm contraction relative to the period during which the diaphragm is relaxed, the duty cycle of breathing, predisposes to fatigue. In fact, diaphragm fatigue appears to be largely a function of the product of Pdi/Pdimax times T_I/T_T, which has been termed the diaphragm tension–time index (TTI) (Fig. 171-14). The TTI is, in essence, the integrated area under the pressure waveform over time. The TTI is usually expressed not in absolute terms of pressure per unit time but, rather, in relative terms as a dimensionless value (i.e., as a percentage of the maximum) to reflect the importance of relative changes in pressure and timing of contraction. The TTI determines muscle energy utilization as reflected in the oxygen consumption.

A threshold for the onset of fatigue occurs at a TTI of approximately 15 to 20 percent of maximum (Fig. 171-14). The greater the TTI above this value, the more rapidly fatigue ensues.

Subsequent studies in normal subjects demonstrated that mechanical failure of the inspiratory muscles as pressure generators can be accelerated at a given TTI by increasing the V_T/T_I. Increases in V_T/T_I reflect an increase in the velocity of inspiratory muscle shortening. Since the greater the velocity of shortening and the more rapid actomyosin cross-bridge cycling, the greater the rate of ATP splitting, this is not surprising. Also of interest, respiratory maneuvers associated with high levels of ventilation appear to selectively fatigue the diaphragm, whereas maneuvers that produce high levels of pressure primarily fatigue the intercostal and neck muscles.

Muscle Blood Flow

Diaphragm fatigue may relate, in part, to a compromise of muscle blood flow during intense contractions. The relationship of diaphragm blood flow to muscle contractile activity is complex and depends, like fatigue itself, on both the intensity and timing

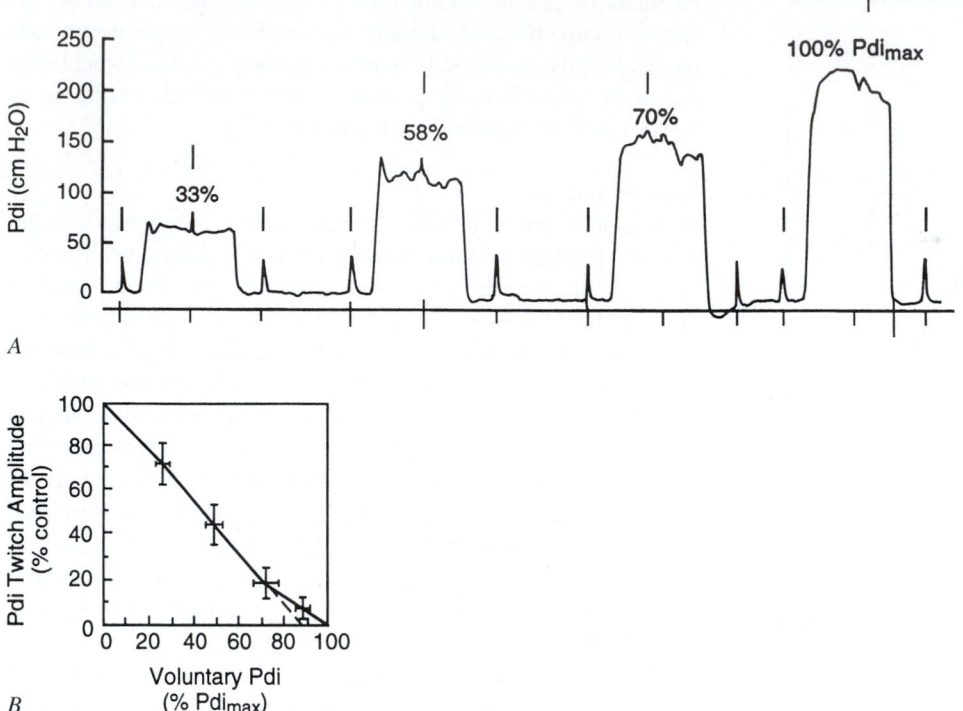

FIGURE 171-12 *A.* Effect of diaphragm contraction intensity as reflected in the transdiaphragmatic pressure (Pdi) on the magnitude of the superimposed twitch contraction. Subject is performing progressively more intense diaphragm contractions. Vertical dotted lines in top panel mark the time at which electrical stimulus is applied to the phrenic nerves. Note that the superimposed twitch Pdi is greatest when the diaphragm is relaxed at FRC and decreases progressively with increasingly intense volitional efforts from 33 to 100% of maximum. *B.* Relationship between the amplitude of the voluntary Pdi and the superimposed twitch contraction. Voluntary Pdi and twitch Pdi normalized as percentage of Pdimax. Note the inverse linear relationship. Maximum static Pdi is calculated as the intercept on the abscissa. *(Based on data of Bellemare and Grassino,[12] with permission.)*

of contractions.[9] The level and pattern of diaphragm activation, therefore, determine not only muscle energy utilization but also the availability of metabolic fuel (i.e., glucose, free fatty acids, and other nutrients).

Contractions of low intensity increase blood flow. In contrast, contractions in excess of 20 to 30 percent of Pdimax mechanically compromise blood flow and cause postcontraction hyperemia. When the diaphragm contracts rhythmically, the T_I/T_T also affects diaphragm blood flow. At Pdi/Pdimax values that compromise blood flow during contraction (i.e., above 20 to 30 percent), blood flow occurs solely during the phase of muscle relaxation. Consequently, increases in the T_I/T_T ratio decrease overall blood flow by encroaching on relaxation time. Diaphragm blood flow is, therefore, a function of the TTI rather than Pdi/Pdi max or the T_I/T_T alone. Blood flow increases up to a TTI of 20 to 30 percent and thereafter falls progressively with further increases in TTI. Compromise of diaphragm blood flow when TTI is greater than 20 to 30 percent of maximum may lead to a condition in which the metabolic needs of the muscle outstrip the availability of energy supply. Alternatively, the importance of blood flow may lie in washing out toxic metabolites (e.g., hydrogen and phosphate ions) from the muscle. The diaphragmatic TTI associated with limitation of blood flow is also a complex function of the level of systemic arterial pressure.[34] Reductions in arterial pressure

produced in animal models by bleeding decrease blood flow at any given level of TTI and reduce the Pdi value at which blood flow is mechanically impeded.

Of considerable importance, diaphragm blood flow may also be a determinant of steady-state diaphragm contractile function in COPD patients in acute respiratory failure.[9] In small numbers of COPD patients, 30 to 50 percent increases in diaphragm blood flow with intravenous dopamine (8 μg/kg/min) caused rapid, approximately 40 percent increases in Pdi during electrophrenic twitch contractions. These findings require confirmation before vasodilator therapy to improve diaphragm function can be advocated. However, they suggest the possibility that diaphragm blood flow may be compromised by intense contractile activity in patients with severe lung disease.

Rapid, Shallow Breathing

Patients with abnormalities in ventilatory pump function breathe rapidly and shallowly in respiratory failure.[6] Respiratory rate is increased and tidal volume is decreased. Reductions in T_I are out of proportion to reductions in T_E, so the duty cycle of breathing, T_I/T_T, is reduced to less than normal values (below 40 percent). Average inspiratory airflow (V_T/T_I) tends to be normal, despite abnormalities in mechanics, because of increases in the neuromuscular drive to breathe as reflected in the airway occlusion pressure. Reductions in T_I have the effect of increasing the dead-space-to-tidal-volume ratio (V_D/V_T) and predisposing to alveolar hypoventilation.

A rapid, shallow pattern of breathing with an abnormally low T_I/T_T ratio and reduced tidal volume is extremely common in patients with COPD during acute exacerbations and tends to improve with improvements in clinical condition. Rapid, shallow breathing appears to cause rather than result from CO_2 retention. It can be produced in COPD patients by histamine-induced bronchoconstriction and reversed by topical airway anesthesia. Subjects with neuromuscular disease in whom the ability to generate inspiratory pressure is impaired require more intense motor outflow to the respiratory muscles to maintain tidal volume. Patients with respiratory muscle weakness also tend to breathe rapidly and shallowly.

The pattern of breathing has been quantified in adults receiving ventilatory support for acute respiratory failure from the ratio of respiratory rate (breaths per minute) divided by tidal volume (liters).[77] This useful parameter has been termed the rapid shallow breathing index (RSBI). It has proved to be an extremely powerful way of assessing weanability in adults with a variety

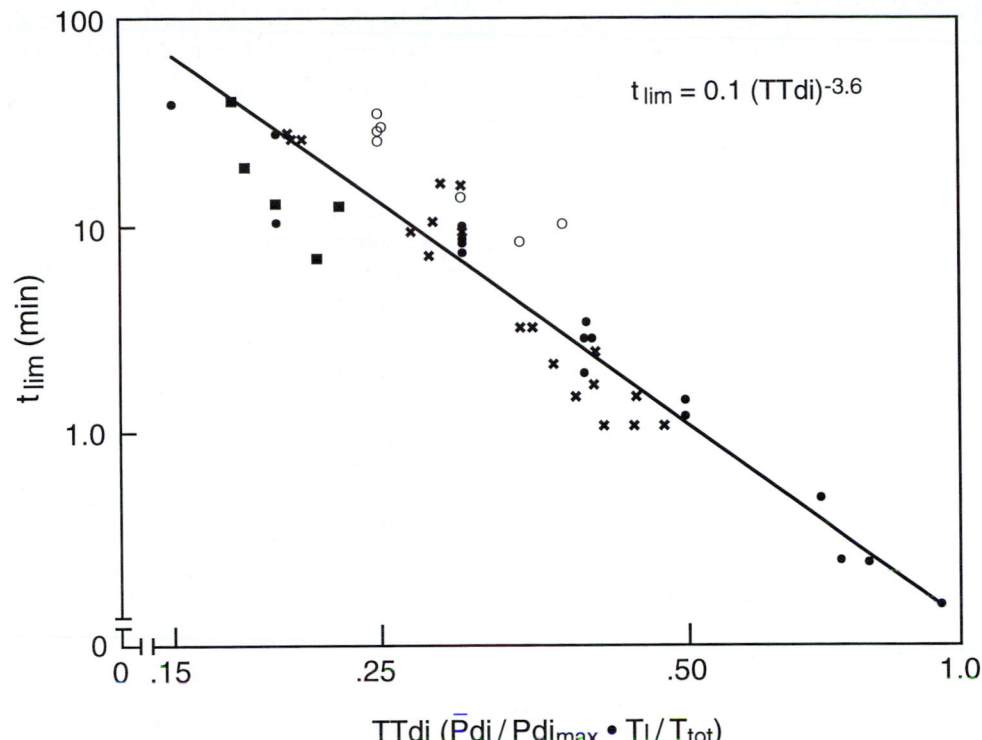

$$t_{lim} = 0.1 \, (TTdi)^{-3.6}$$

FIGURE 171-13   Effect of increasing Pdi/Pdimax (i.e., the ratio of peak inspiratory Pdi) during resistance breathing over maximum static Pdi (ordinate) on the time of onset of mechanical failure of the diaphragm, tlim (abscissa). Data from three normal subjects (shown as separate symbols). Note that progressive increases in Pdi/Pdimax are associated with more rapid onset of diaphragm fatigue. Note also the curvilinear nature of the relationship, with apparent asymptote between 40 and 50% Pdi/Pdimax, which represents a fatigue threshold. *(Based on data of Roussos and Macklem,[62] with permission.)*

of medical and surgical conditions. The greater the value, the more rapid and shallow is the pattern of breathing. Values for the RSBI exceeding 100 are associated with a high probability of failure to wean from mechanical ventilation. The RSBI lends itself to a more general use in patients with disorders of the ventilatory pump not requiring mechanical ventilation.

Rapid, shallow breathing leading to CO_2 retention exerts a number of deleterious effects. First, CO_2 retention decreases Pa_{O_2} and arterial pH. Decreases in Pa_{O_2} result in accordance with the alveolar air equation. In general, a 1-mmHg increase in P_{CO_2} causes a 1.25-mmHg reduction in Pa_{O_2} (assuming a respiratory quotient of 0.8; larger respiratory quotient values are associated with smaller changes in Pa_{O_2}). Second, renal compensation for hypercapnia-induced respiratory acidosis stimulates bicarbonate resorption. Increases in body fluid bicarbonate restore pH toward normal values but blunt the ventilatory response to further increases in CO_2. Third, hypercapnia depresses diaphragm contractility; that is, Pdi is decreased at a given level of diaphragm electrical activity in proportion to the increase in P_{CO_2}.

However, rapid, shallow breathing may also confer beneficial effects to subjects with severe ventilatory pump dysfunction. First, CO_2 retention increases the CO_2 partial-pressure gradient between the alveolus and atmosphere. Accordingly, during hypercapnia the same volume of metabolically produced CO_2 can be excreted at a lower level of alveolar and minute ventilation and oxygen cost of breathing than during eucapnia. As such, CO_2 retention affords a mechanism to diminish the activity level of

the inspiratory muscles and their propensity to fatigue. Normal humans and animal models fatigued by inspiratory resistive loads in the laboratory spontaneously minimize the diaphragm TTI after fatigue by adopting a shallow, rapid pattern of breathing.[54] In fact, a large study of stable outpatients with advanced COPD indicates that the inspiratory muscle TTI is below the fatigue threshold even in markedly hypercapnic (above 60 mmHg) subjects (see below). Second, rapid, shallow breathing minimizes the magnitude of dynamic hyperinflation in patients with severe COPD who breathe on the envelope of the maximum expiratory flow-volume loop; that is, reductions in tidal volume and decreases in the TI/TT ratio diminish the volume to be exhaled and prolong the expiratory time available to reach FRC.

The balance between the beneficial and deleterious effects of CO_2 retention is difficult to define with precision; however, the balance probably is determined by the magnitude and rapidity of the changes in Pa_{CO_2} and pH and their effect on the cardiovascular and central nervous systems. Relatively small (5 to 15 mmHg), changes in Pa_{CO_2}, produced gradually over days to weeks and leaving pH at levels of 7.25 to 7.30, are likely to be well tolerated and, on balance, beneficial. On the other hand, Pa_{CO_2} changes that occur rapidly and reduce pH to less than 7.25 are likely to exert net negative effects. In fact, respiratory acidosis to pH values under 7.25 is life-threatening and generally considered an indication for intubation and mechanical ventilation. Cardiac function and sympathetic regulation of peripheral vascular resistance are impaired at this level of pH. Patients become encephalopathic (i.e., somnolent and unable to care for themselves and control their airway secretions). Obviously, hypercapnia of such magnitude is to be avoided.

PATHOGENSIS OF RAPID, SHALLOW BREATHING

The neurophysiological mechanisms driving the altered pattern of breathing are obscure. Moreover, whether changes in breathing pattern in animal models and humans are reflexly induced or behaviorally mediated, or reflect changes in brain neurotransmitter levels (e.g., endorphins), is unclear. However, chemosensitivity-induced alterations in respiratory activity do *not* appear to be the explanation. Hypoxia- and hypercapnia-induced reductions in TE are disproportionately greater than reductions in TI, so the TI/TT ratio increases. Moreover, VT/TI and the tidal volume increase rather than decrease.

Reflexes originating from mechanoreceptors in the contracting rib cage muscles and diaphragm (i.e., Golgi tendon organs,

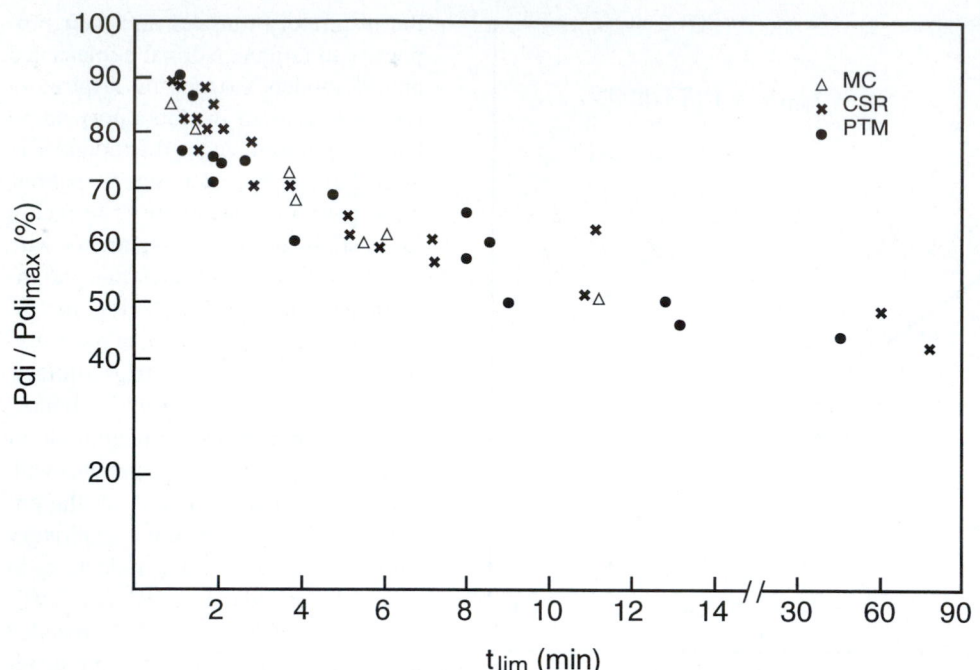

FIGURE 171-14 Relationship between the intensity of diaphragm contractile activity reflected in the diaphragm tension–time index (TTdi)—i.e., the product of Pdi/Pdimax × TI/TT and the time of onset of mechanical failure of the diaphragm, Tlim. The two scales are logarithmic. Data obtained in normal subjects during strenuous volitional contractions during inspiratory resistive ventilatory loading. Note that above approximately 15% TTdi, Tlim decreases progressively with increasing TTdi. These data indicate that a fatigue threshold exists for the human diaphragm above TTdi 15–20% and that above this threshold, diaphragm endurance is a unique function of the TTdi. *(Based on data of Bellemare and Grassino,[13] with permission.)*

sensation of dyspnea can be expressed quantitatively by each of these parameters raised to a power[41]:

$$\text{Dyspnea} = P^{1.3} \times T_I/T_T^{1.14} \times \text{freq}^{-0.97}$$

Increases in intrathoracic pressure required to maintain airflow and tidal volume in patients with abnormalities in ventilatory pump function increase the sense of dyspnea. Given the greater exponential value for P than for the timing variables, it can be seen that the magnitude of the swing in inspiratory pressure is the predominant determinant of dyspnea. Thus, at a given level of minute ventilation and set of respiratory mechanics, the pattern of breathing determines the intensity of breathlessness. When the mechanics of breathing are deranged by COPD or kyphoscoliosis, diminishing peak inspiratory intrathoracic pressure (i.e., tidal volume) and increasing respiratory rate (i.e., a rapid, shallow pattern of breathing) tend to minimize the sense of breathlessness.

At equivalent levels of airway resistance and inspiratory effort, the sense of dyspnea is greater during bronchoconstriction than during external resistive loading, probably because of the activation of vagal irritant receptors.[73] Differences in the intensity of dyspnea at any given level of airway obstruction, therefore, may depend on the site of airway obstruction (i.e., intra- versus extrathoracic). Also, the sense of dyspnea at a given level of peak intrathoracic pressure, TI/TT ratio, and frequency of breathing are increased in the setting of inspiratory muscle fatigue, probably because a greater motor command is required to generate a given level of intrathoracic pressure.[70] Finally, it should be apparent from the above equation that the sense of dyspnea depends on the same variables that determine respiratory muscle fatigability. However, respiratory muscle fatigue, in contrast to dyspnea, does not appear to depend on the pattern in which TTI is developed; that is, whether a given TTI is arrived at by a higher P/Pmax or a higher TI/TT is irrelevant in the development of fatigue, but it *is* important in the generation of respiratory sensations.

Perceptual acuity of the respiratory sensations elicited when the mechanical properties of the ventilatory pump are deranged is a major determinant of the pattern of breathing and tendency to develop CO₂ retention in subjects with COPD. For example, when airway resistance is increased experimentally, COPD subjects who retain CO₂ are those with the greatest perceptual acuity for changes in intrathoracic pressure.[53] That is, spontaneous tidal volume and TI are smallest in COPD subjects with the highest perceptual acuity for changes in intrathoracic pressure.

On the other hand, when airway resistance was increased experimentally by external resistive loads, asthmatics with near-fa-

spindle organs, and type III and type IV endings) probably play a role in shaping the rapid, shallow pattern of breathing. In deeply anesthetized animals, stretch of the intercostal muscles or an increase in diaphragm tension may abruptly terminate inspiration.[64] Activation of vagal irritant receptors in the airway may also produce rapid, shallow breathing.[20] In animal models, rapid, shallow breathing produced acutely by inhalation of allergen or inflammatory mediators (e.g., histamine, bradykinin) can be prevented by vagal blockade. These observations suggest that rapid, shallow breathing in bronchoconstriction may be mediated by vagal sensory endings in the airways.

Finally, changes in the pattern of breathing may represent a behavioral response to minimize the sense of dyspnea. The sense of dyspnea is a complex perceptual construct that is not fully understood but is probably multifactorial.[41,46] In fact, an important determinant of the sense of dyspnea is the magnitude of the CNS motor command to the inspiratory muscles as reflected in the peak inspiratory intrathoracic pressure. Studies indicate that the sense of breathlessness increases for any set of respiratory mechanical conditions with increases in peak inspiratory pressure, the duration of inspiration, or respiratory rate.[41] In particular, the magnitude of the sense of dyspnea depends on inspiratory pressure (P) swings as a percent of maximum (P/Pmax), the duration of inspiration relative to the total breath cycle (TI/TT), and the respiratory rate (freq). However, the relative importance of these three terms is quite different. The peak inspiratory pressure has a far greater effect than the duration of inspiration, which in turn has a greater effect than breathing frequency. The tal attacks experienced less dyspnea at any level of resistance than normal subjects (Fig. 171-15).[40] Accordingly, in patients with COPD the acuity of respiratory perception plays an important role in the pathogenesis of respiratory failure. The mechanism by which respiratory perception contributes to respiratory failure awaits clarification.

Undernutrition

Undernutrition, defined as a body weight less than 90 percent of the ideal, is extremely common in patients with COPD, occurring in about 25 percent of stable outpatients and about 40 percent of hospitalized patients.[17] Undernutrition is an independent risk factor for mortality.[31] For a given level of lung function, undernourished patients with COPD have a greater 5-year mortality than normally nourished subjects. The respiratory muscles, like skeletal muscles in other parts of the body, atrophy under conditions of chronic protein-calorie deficiency.[60] In patients without lung disease, Pimax is significantly smaller in undernourished than in well-nourished subjects.[4] In subjects with COPD at autopsy, the mass (i.e., weight and thickness) of the diaphragm is diminished in undernourished compared to well-nourished patients. Both slow and fast fibers in respiratory muscles (e.g., the diaphragm and intercostals) atrophy in subjects with advanced COPD. In COPD patients, resting Pa_{CO_2} is inversely related to Pimax.[10] The weaker the subject, the greater the Pa_{CO_2}. Reductions in Pimax predispose to inspiratory muscle fatigue by increasing the Pdi/Pdimax ratio and, hence, the TTI during breathing against a given set of lung mechanics. Of practical importance, aggressive nutritional repletion, which increases body weight, augments Pimax and Pdimax.[61] Thus, respiratory muscle wasting and atrophy are reversible in undernourished patients with COPD.

The pathogenesis of body wasting in subjects with chronic diseases like COPD is unclear. However, increases in the work of breathing and respiratory muscle activity increase resting energy expenditure by as much as 50 to 100 percent above normal. In normal subjects in whom basal energy requirements are similarly increased by heavy physical labor (e.g., lumberjacks), caloric intake is increased appropriately to meet metabolic demands and body weight is preserved. Accordingly, the root of the problem in undernourished patients with COPD may be "relative anorexia," so that increases in basal caloric requirements are not accompanied by adequate caloric intake. Undernourished subjects with COPD have higher blood levels of the cachexia factor TNF-α than well-nourished COPD subjects.[29]

SPECIFIC DISEASES

COPD

Patients with advanced COPD develop CO_2 retention because of abnormalities in the gas exchange and mechanical properties of the lung. The relationship between the severity of COPD as reflected by the FEV_1 and steady-state resting P_{CO_2} is curvilinear (Fig. 171-16). In general, Pa_{CO_2} does not increase above normal until the FEV_1 decreases to about 20 to 25 percent of predicted normal values.[43]

The effects of COPD on lung gas exchange are complex. Simply put, increases in lung dead space and abnormalities in ventilation/perfusion relationships impair CO_2 elimination and oxygen uptake. Increases in physiological dead space require greater than normal levels of ventilation and tidal volume to maintain eucapnia. Maintenance of "normal tidal volume" in the setting of increased dead space predisposes to CO_2 retention because of an unfavorable VD/VT. Normally, during resting breathing, ventilation is 4 to 5 L/min, of which alveolar ventilation is approximately 70 to 80 percent. In COPD, abnormalities in lung gas exchange for O_2 and CO_2 (i.e., increased dead-space volume and alveolar–arterial oxygen gradient) require greater than normal

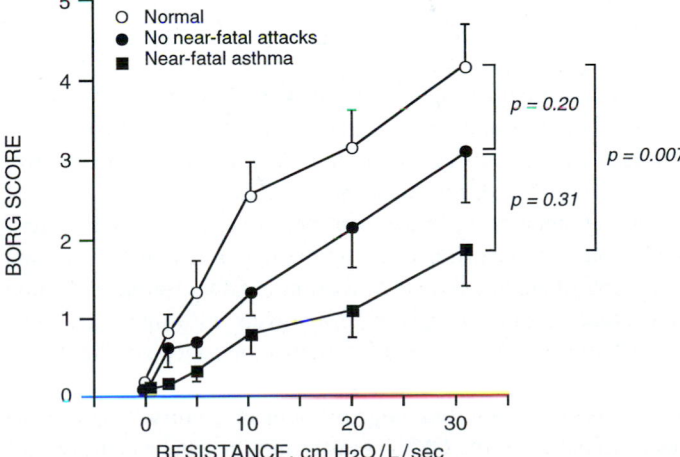

FIGURE 171-15 Severity of dyspnea experienced during breathing against external resistive ventilatory loads in normal subjects, patients with asthma but no near-fatal attacks, and patients with near-fatal asthma. **Y** axis indicates the intensity of dyspnea (i.e., Borg score). Increasing numerical values on the Borg score indicate increasing dyspnea. Note that at any given level of external resistance, dyspnea was significantly less in patients with near-fatal asthma than in the normal group. *(Based on data of Kikuchi et al,[40] with permission.)*

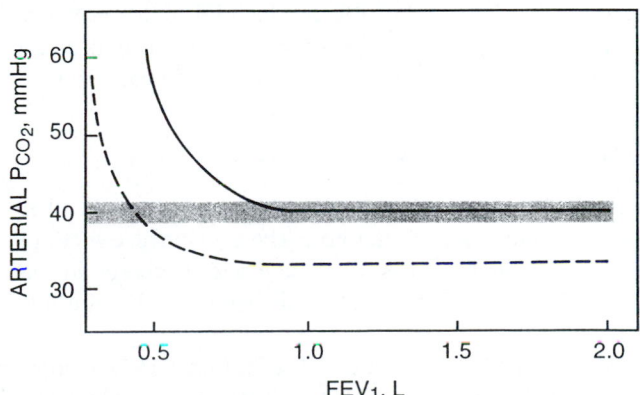

FIGURE 171-16 Relationship between the severity of airway obstruction reflected in the FEV_1 and steady-state arterial P_{CO_2} in COPD and asthma. Shaded area represents normal range of arterial P_{CO_2}. The relationship is curvilinear, so CO_2 retention occurs only after FEV_1 is considerably reduced. The asthmatic curve (dashed line) lies below and to the left of the curve for COPD, indicating that much greater levels of obstruction are necessary before arterial P_{CO_2} rises. *(From Fishman: Pulmonary Diseases and Disorders, 1980, vol 1, p 426, fig 32–7, with permission.)*

levels of ventilation to maintain eucapnia and euoxia. Consequently, in subjects with advanced COPD, minute ventilation is typically two to three times the normal value (i.e., 10 to 15 L/min). Minute ventilation is increased still further in hypoxemia. Increases in ventilation require increases in airflow, tidal volume, and the duty cycle of breathing.

Hyperinflation and heightened airway resistance are common in patients with advanced COPD. Hyperinflation and increases in FRC in patients with COPD are multifactorial. First, emphysema decreases lung (and possibly chest wall) elastic recoil pressure. Second, tonic activation of chest wall inspiratory muscles throughout the respiratory cycle enhances transpulmonary pressure. Third, activation of laryngeal constrictor muscles and pursed-lip breathing during expiration slow the rate of expiratory airflow. Fourth, severely obstructed patients breathing on the envelope of the maximum expiratory flow–volume curve may have insufficient time during expiration to exhale to passively determined FRC.

In advanced COPD, increases in airway resistance and hyperinflation require greater than normal swings in intrathoracic pressure to generate normal levels of airflow and tidal volume. In consequence, the respiratory neuromuscular drive to breathe, peak inspiratory intrathoracic pressure, and the TTI of the inspiratory muscles are increased considerably.[12] Normally, at rest, respiratory muscle oxygen consumption is less than 2 percent of total body oxygen consumption (i.e., about 5 ml/min or less). In contrast, patients with advanced cardiopulmonary disease may have levels of respiratory muscle oxygen uptake greater than 50 percent of total body oxygen uptake (i.e., in excess of 125 ml/min).[23]

In subjects with severe COPD, hyperinflation reduces inspiratory muscle mechanical advantage, which decreases the capacity of the inspiratory muscles to generate pressure (Pmax). Pmax values in COPD patients may be as low as one-third to one-half that of age-matched normal subjects (Fig. 171-17).[65] Moreover, aging- and malnutrition-associated changes in the diaphragm may further impair Pdimax in subjects with COPD.[76] COPD typically becomes disabling in the sixth and seventh decades of life, a period of life at which Pdi falls normally. For example, Pdimax is about 25 percent less in normal men over 65 years of age than in normal men under 35 years of age.[76]

RESPIRATORY MUSCLE FATIGUE IN COPD

Severe COPD is arguably the clinical condition most likely to cause inspiratory muscle fatigue. The combined effects of increases in inspiratory muscle activity and decreases in muscle strength in severe COPD increase the diaphragm TTI during resting breathing in elderly COPD patients considerably above the normal value of 1 to 2 percent.[14] The TTI may, in fact, approach the fatigue threshold (i.e., 15 to 20 percent) in patients with COPD (Fig. 171-18). These and similar data indicate that diaphragm activity is increased in patients with advanced COPD, and that the diaphragm is highly susceptible to fatigue when breathing is increased above spontaneous levels by minor increases in tidal volume or Ti/Tt. The diaphragm TTI is higher in hypercapnic than in eucapnic COPD subjects, but even in hypercapnic subjects it does not exceed the fatigue threshold.[10] Mean TTI, even for hypercapnic subjects, is approximately 10 percent. Therefore, hypercapnia per se does not indicate the pres-

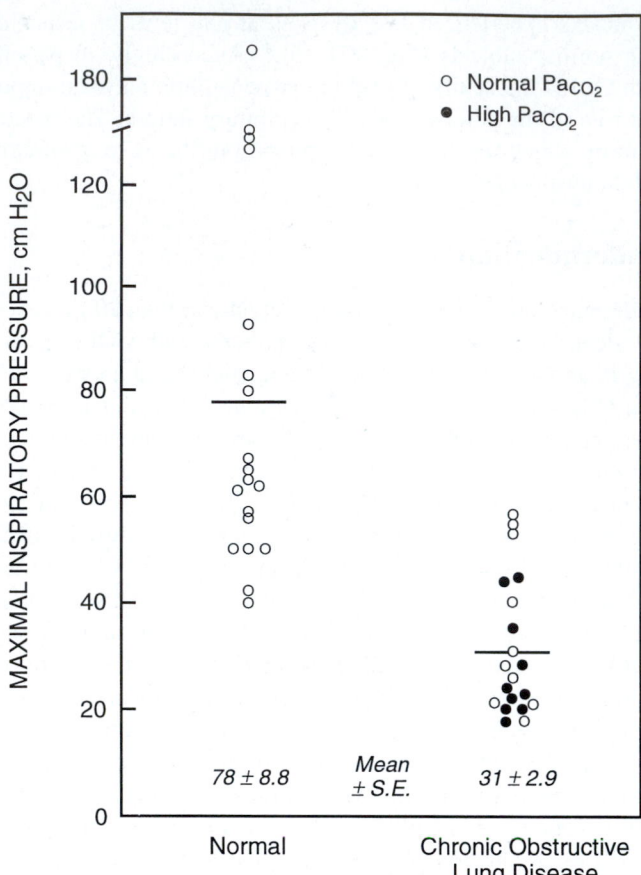

FIGURE 171-17 Inspiratory muscle strength as reflected in the maximum static inspiratory pressure (Pimax) at FRC in subjects with advanced COPD and age-matched normal subjects. Each symbol represents a single subject. Note that in COPD subjects, because of hyperinflation and muscle wasting, Pimax is reduced to approximately 40% of the value in normal subjects. Note the tendency for hypercapnic subjects to have even lower values of Pimax than eucapnic COPD subjects. *(Based on data of Sharp et al,[65] with permission.)*

ence of diaphragm fatigue even in patients with severe COPD. Rather, hypercapnia may be a manifestation of a breathing strategy (i.e., rapid, shallow breathing) that minimizes inspiratory muscle activity and, hence, prevents fatigue.

On the other hand, inspiratory muscle fatigue may be a relatively common occurrence during the hyperpnea of exercise and could contribute to exercise limitation in COPD subjects. A high percentage (about 50 percent) of subjects with moderate to severe COPD demonstrate EMG evidence of scalene or diaphragm EMG (or both) during endurance exercise before the termination of exercise.[62] Of interest, improvement in exercise performance and elimination of the EMG signs of fatigue can be achieved following inspiratory resistance training.

Subjects with COPD in acute respiratory failure requiring mechanical ventilation are more likely to show evidence of inspiratory muscle fatigue. During weaning from mechanical ventilation, diaphragm EMG changes indicative of fatigue precede the increases in Pa_{CO_2}.[19,52] These findings suggest that diaphragm fatigue contributes to ventilator dependence after the onset of hypercapnic respiratory failure in at least some critically ill subjects.

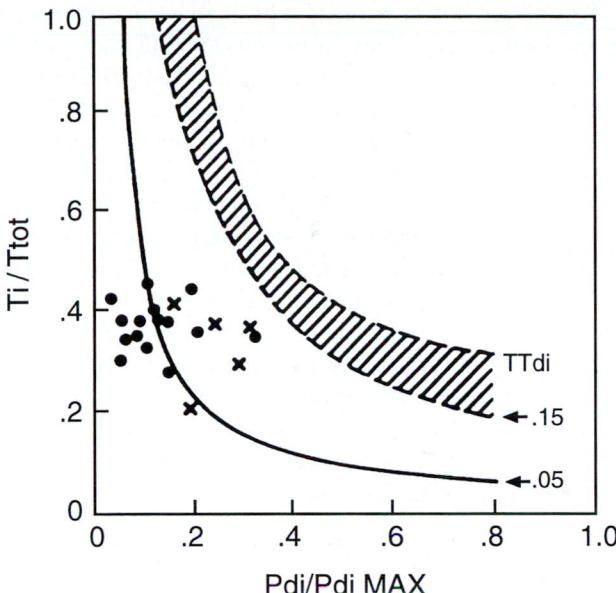

FIGURE 171-18 Diaphragmatic tension–time index in 20 stable outpatients with COPD breathing room air at rest. Each symbol represents a separate COPD subject. Shaded area represents the fatigue threshold in normal subjects. Most COPD subjects breathe well below the fatigue threshold and cluster around .05 TTdi. *(Based on data of Bellemare and Bigland-Ritchie,[11] with permission.)*

In COPD patients being weaned from mechanical ventilation during a bout of acute respiratory failure, the tracheal occlusion pressure is usually greater than 6 cm H_2O and EMG evidence of diaphragm fatigue is present during spontaneous breathing.[52] Patients with persistently elevated tracheal occlusion pressure values (above 6 cm H_2O) and EMG evidence of diaphragm fatigue generally cannot be successfully weaned from mechanical ventilation.[52] In contrast, sternomastoid muscle fatigue is evident in fewer than 10 percent of COPD patients hospitalized for worsening respiratory distress.[25]

In summary, most subjects with stable COPD adopt a pattern of breathing that minimizes the diaphragm TTI and prevents inspiratory muscle fatigue. Behavioral mechanisms may be operative in an attempt to minimize the sensation of dyspnea. On the other hand, inspiratory muscle fatigue contributes to the morbidity of a subgroup of patients with COPD by preventing weaning from mechanical ventilation, and possibly by impairing exercise performance. The reported number of COPD subjects with respiratory muscle fatigue is small, however, and may represent a highly select population. Further studies are needed to define the extent of this problem.

Asthma

The pathophysiology of CO_2 retention appears to be generally similar in patients with asthma and COPD, but the likelihood of developing CO_2 retention is less in asthma than in COPD. That is, the level of expiratory airway obstruction required to produce CO_2 retention in subjects with acute asthma is greater than that required in subjects with COPD (Fig. 171-18). Several possibilities may explain this tendency. First, it appears that inspiratory

drive is higher in patients with asthma than in those with COPD. The airway occlusion pressure is considerably higher at any given level of Pa_{CO_2} in patients with asthma than in normal subjects or patients with COPD.[39] The heightened inspiratory drive in patients with asthma may in part arise from irritant receptors within the airway, which have an augmenting effect on inspiratory motoneuron activity. Furthermore, the inspiratory muscles are stronger, and ventilatory responses to CO_2 and hypoxia are greater, in the younger asthmatic than in COPD subjects. These differences are not simply due to age, as the endurance of the inspiratory and expiratory muscles is greater in asthmatic than in age-matched normal subjects.[45] The increased respiratory muscle endurance in subjects with asthma may be a response to chronic increases in inspiratory muscle load. Finally, greater lung elastic recoil in asthma than in COPD tends to preserve maximal inspiratory airflow.

Neuromuscular Disease

Subjects with neuromuscular disease and weak inspiratory muscles tend to breathe rapidly and shallowly. Despite this breathing pattern, these subjects tend to have hypocapnia at rest, and hyperventilate at any given level of CO_2 during progressive hypercapnia. Increases in ventilation are associated with increases in airway occlusion pressure. Heightened occlusion pressure in the setting of weak inspiratory muscles suggests that the drive to the inspiratory muscles early in inspiration is greater than normal.

The pathogenesis of hypercapnic respiratory failure is very different in patients with neuromuscular disease than in patients with COPD. Patients with neuromuscular disease demonstrate an impaired ability to sigh (i.e., a greater than twofold increase in the tidal volume) because of inspiratory muscle weakness. Inability to sigh decreases lung compliance by interfering with the redistribution of surfactant within the alveolar space. Progressive stiffening of the lung leads to microatelectasis and ultimately lobar atelectasis. Breathing high concentrations of oxygen accelerates this process. In addition, expiratory muscle weakness impairs the cough mechanism and causes retention of secretions.

The best indicators of a tendency to develop CO_2 retention in patients with neuromuscular disease are reductions in inspiratory muscle strength (PImax) and forced vital capacity (FVC). Reductions in PImax and FVC to less than 30 and 25 percent of predicted, respectively, are associated with CO_2 retention. Suffice it to say, hypercapnia is a late manifestation of neuromuscular disease and requires marked impairment in inspiratory and expiratory muscle function. With diaphragm dysfunction, hypercapnia may be more common and occur earlier during sleep (especially REM sleep) than while the subject is awake.

Kyphoscoliosis

Kyphoscoliosis decreases chest wall and lung compliance, presumably as a result of atelectasis and deformation of the lungs (see Chapter 97). The elastic work of breathing is markedly increased.[16] In addition, the mechanical action of the respiratory muscles may be impaired by changes in configuration of the bony structures on which the respiratory muscles insert. Ventilation/perfusion mismatch and increase in the arterial oxygen gradient are common. As expected in patients with diminished respiratory compliance, subjects with kyphoscoliosis breathe rapidly and shallowly. The tendency to develop CO_2 retention is a function of the severity of the restrictive process in kyphoscoliosis, as reflected in the Cobb angles, and is predicted separately for the magnitude of scoliosis and kyphosis.

Hypercapnic respiratory failure tends to develop late in life, even if the severity of the spinal deformity has not changed since childhood; that is, stability of the Cobb angles of kyphosis and scoliosis does not preclude development of hypercapnic respiratory failure. It is not clear why respiratory failure ensues late in life. However, several possibilities exist. Aging adversely affects compliance of the chest wall, leading to an increase in the elastic work of breathing. In addition, aging diminishes respiratory muscle strength. Finally, chemosensitivity to O_2 and CO_2 declines with advancing age, and it seems likely that the subject's ability to compensate for derangements in blood gas tensions is progressively impaired.

ASSESSMENT OF PATIENTS WITH ABNORMALITIES OF THE VENTILATORY PUMP

Symptoms

Dyspnea appears to be an early manifestation of respiratory muscle impairment in neuromuscular disease and typically occurs before the development of CO_2 retention. Breathlessness in the supine position is characteristic of isolated diaphragm dysfunction. In the supine position, the increased hydrostatic pressure imposed by the abdominal viscera represents an increased inertial load on the diaphragm.

Physical Findings

Physical signs of ventilatory pump dysfunction revolve around evidence of accessory respiratory muscle recruitment, abnormal thoracoabdominal movement, and rapid, shallow breathing.

USE OF ACCESSORY MUSCLES

Inspection and palpation demonstrate accessory respiratory muscle use. Intense respiratory efforts are associated with visible activation of the neck accessory muscles, interosseous intercostals, and abdominal expiratory muscles and flaring of the ala nasae.

ABNORMAL THORACOABDOMINAL MOVEMENT

Normally, in the supine position, the anterior abdominal wall displays a prominent outward movement during inspiration. With impaired diaphragm function, as occurs in diaphragm weakness or fatigue, the abdominal wall may move inward on inspiration. This is called *abdominal paradox*. Abdominal paradox reflects cephalad movement of the contracting diaphragm in response to the negative intrathoracic pressure generated by the inspiratory action of the neck and intercostal muscles. Abdominal paradox

may also be present in patients with marked derangements in lung mechanics, in whom inspiratory intrathoracic pressure swings exceed 30 percent of maximum.[75] Abdominal paradox, therefore, is not specific for diaphragm weakness or fatigue.

Abdominal paradox, resulting from ineffectual contractions of the diaphragm, should be distinguished from *pseudo–abdominal paradox*, resulting from strong contractions of the expiratory muscles during expiration, with rapid relaxation during early inspiration. For example, intense contraction of the transverse abdominis muscles causes inward movement of the lateral abdominal wall and outward movement of the anterior abdominal wall during expiration. Subsequent relaxation of the abdominal muscles with the onset of inspiration causes outward movement of the lateral abdominal wall and inward movement of the anterior abdominal wall. Tenseness of the lateral abdominal wall during expiration easily distinguishes *pseudo–* from true *abdominal paradox*.

Maximum Static Inspiratory Pressure

Perhaps the most practical method of assessing the function of the inspiratory muscles contracting in aggregate is from the pressure generated during maximal volitional contractions against an occluded airway at FRC. This parameter is dealt with in greater detail in Chapter 99 on neuromuscular disease. In brief, however, reductions in Pımax indicate inspiratory muscle weakness or high-frequency fatigue. Improvements in Pımax occurring over several hours to several days in a patient with COPD suggest that lung volume is improving toward normal and that the mechanical disadvantage imposed on the inspiratory muscles is disappearing. More rapid improvements (occurring over hours) may indicate resolution of high-frequency fatigue or elimination of the metabolic disturbances (e.g., hypercapnia or hypophosphatemia) that depress inspiratory muscle function. Of note, Pımax does not pinpoint low-frequency fatigue.

Pımax depends on patient cooperation and motivation. With training, however, patients can provide reproducible values. Performance of the maneuver at FRC, where respiratory system recoil is zero, is preferred; that is, at FRC, changes in airway pressure during inspiratory efforts equal the pressure generated by the inspiratory muscles (Pmus).

Maximum static expiratory pressure at FRC (Pemax) has been used in the laboratory setting to assess the endurance properties of the expiratory muscles. The Pemax has not been used extensively in the clinical setting, however, because of the perception that it is more difficult to obtain consistent values than Pımax with breathless subjects.

TREATMENT

Abnormalities in respiratory mechanics and gas exchange are the most important pathogenetic factors in the development of respiratory failure. Accordingly, therapy should be directed toward achieving maximum improvement in airway, lung, and respiratory muscle function. For example, in patients with COPD or asthma, an intensive regimen of bronchodilators (e.g., β_2-adrenergic agonists, anticholinergics, and theophylline) and anti-inflammatory therapy (e.g., corticosteroids) can correct respiratory failure by diminishing airway resistance, FRC, lung dead-space volume, the alveolar–arterial O_2 partial-pressure gradient, and the work of breathing. Improvements in lung function in certain patients with advanced COPD and emphysema may also be accomplished by lung volume reduction surgery (volume reduction pneumectomy) or lung transplantation. Lung volume reduction surgery removes 20 to 30 percent of the most emphysematous regions of lung and appears to improve FRC, FEV_1, ventilatory capacity, inspiratory muscle function, and elastic recoil pressure of the lung. In patients with myasthenia gravis, cholinesterase inhibitors can improve inspiratory muscle strength and vital capacity and reverse atelectasis, which causes hypercapnia.

Abnormalities in Chemosensitivity

Respiratory failure caused by impaired chemosensitivity is difficult to treat, since drug treatments to improve chemosensitivity to hypoxia or hypercapnia are not very effective. Since it was observed that women exhibit alveolar hypoventilation during pregnancy and the luteal phase of the menstrual cycle, progestational agents have been used for many years to treat idiopathic hypoventilation syndromes. In some subjects, medroxyprogesterone acetate, given orally in a dose of 20 mg three times a day, acts centrally to augment the ventilatory responses to hypercapnia and hypoxemia and can improve resting arterial blood gas tensions.[67,72] Medroxyprogesterone is generally well tolerated in women but may produce feminizing side effects in men. The onset of action of the drug is slow. Several weeks may be required before a response is observed. Theophylline, in doses that produce blood levels in the therapeutic range (10 to 15 $\mu g/ml$), also have weak respiratory stimulatory effects, which may contribute to a reduction in Pa_{CO_2} in patients with COPD.[51] Theophylline also produces modest improvements (about 10 to 20 percent) in diaphragm contractile function in this population. Finally, in some patients with hypercapnia, elimination of medications having CNS respiratory depressant effects (e.g., opiate analgesics, benzodiazepine anxiolytics) can lead to improvements in Pa_{CO_2}.

Hypoxemia leading to pulmonary artery hypertension and cor pulmonale may be the most serious complication of chronic hypercapnic respiratory failure. Supplemental oxygen is usually indicated in patients with chronic hypercapnic respiratory failure. Supplemental O_2 may produce exaggerated increases in Pa_{CO_2} in patients with disorders of ventilatory control in whom the ventilatory response to CO_2 is blunted but the O_2 response is preserved.[26] Accordingly, blood gas tensions should be monitored closely when O_2 is applied initially. During sleep, patients with disorders of the control of breathing typically display exaggerated increases in Pa_{CO_2} (e.g., 15 to greater than 30 mmHg) with hypoxemia and severe respiratory acidosis. In these subjects, mechanically assisted ventilation (typically with nasal positive-pressure ventilation), with or without oxygen, may be required during the sleeping period. Nasal positive-pressure ventilation is an effective way of improving blood gas tensions during sleep. In fact, improvements in blood gas tensions achieved by nocturnal mechanical ventilation may carry over to the waking period in these patients, perhaps by preventing nocturnal increases in serum bicarbonate or hypoxic depression of CNS function.

Respiratory Muscle Weakness or Fatigue

The treatment of respiratory muscle weakness depends on pathogenic mechanisms. For example, inspiratory muscle weakness related to the hyperinflation of COPD is best treated by aggressive improvement of airway function. On the other hand, decreases in muscle strength caused by electrolyte abnormalities (e.g., hypophosphatemia) or protein-calorie malnutrition are best dealt with by repletion of the deficits.

The treatment of respiratory muscle fatigue has not been systematically studied. However, several approaches based on theoretical considerations appear to be applicable (Table 171-2). It is clear that diaphragm fatigue is a result of muscle overactivity (i.e., a TTI greater than 20 percent). Accordingly, attempts should be made to decrease the TTI of the inspiratory muscles to values below the fatigue threshold by improving lung mechanics or reducing ventilatory drive. In patients with abnormalities in airway resistance and hyperinflation secondary to severe COPD, this can best be accomplished with bronchodilators and corticosteroids. Reductions in ventilatory drive in hypoxic or febrile patients can be accomplished by administration of oxygen or antipyretics.

Unloading the inspiratory muscles by reducing the TTI may be sufficient to prevent or reverse fatigue and allow the muscle to recover. In some cases, however, respiratory muscle fatigue may be sufficiently advanced so that the muscle must be placed at complete rest. Mechanical ventilation and ventilatory muscle rest are certainly indicated when the pH is less than 7.25 or the patient appears unable to maintain ventilation and stable blood gas tensions. The precise duration of mechanical ventilation to rest the inspiratory muscles in patients with respiratory muscle fatigue is unclear. However, no attempts at weaning should be made until the conditions that initiated fatigue are reversed. Since low-frequency fatigue persists for 24 h or more, it may not be

---

TABLE 171-2

Principles of Therapy for Respiratory Muscle Fatigue

Decrease inspiratory swings in transdiaphragmatic pressure (Pdi)
  Improve the mechanics of breathing (i.e., decrease airway resistance, improve thoracic compliance and static lung volume)
  Decrease ventilatory drive (i.e., relieve hypoxemia, hypercapnia, metabolic acidosis, fever, pulmonary congestion/inflammation, ARDS)
Increase Pdimax
  Correct hyperinflation
  Correct muscle atrophy induced by protein-calorie deficiency
  Correct electrolyte and blood gas abnormalities (i.e., hypoxemia, hypercapnia, hypophosphatemia, hypokalemia, hypocalcemia, hypomagnesemia)
Optimize muscle blood flow and substrate availability
  Correct low cardiac output state (e.g., cardiogenic shock, hypovolemic shock)
  Correct hypoxemia, anemia, hypoglycemia

advisable to wean patients with respiratory muscle fatigue from mechanical ventilation for at least 24 h even if the factors that caused fatigue have been corrected.

REFERENCES

1. Akabas SR, Bazzy AR, DiMaurio S, et al: Metabolic and functional adaptation of the diaphragm to training with resistive loads. *J Appl Physiol* 66:529–535, 1989.
2. Altose MD, McCauley WC, Kelsen SG, et al: Effects of hypercapnia and inspiratory flow-resistive loading on respiratory activity in chronic airways obstruction. *J Clin Invest* 59:500–507, 1977.
3. Anzueto A, Supinski GS, Levine SM, Jenkinson SG: Mechanisms of disease: Are oxygen derived free radicals involved in diaphragmatic dysfunction? *Am J Respir Crit Care Med* 149:1048–1052, 1994.
4. Arora NS, Rochester DF: Respiratory muscle strength and maximal voluntary ventilation in undernourished patients. *Am Rev Respir Dis* 126:5–8, 1982.
5. Aubier M, Farkas A, De Troyer RT, et al: Detection of diaphragmatic fatigue in man by phrenic stimulation. *J Appl Physiol* 50:538–544, 1981.
6. Aubier M, Murciano D, Menu Y, et al: Dopamine effects on diaphragmatic strength during acute respiratory failure in chronic obstructive pulmonary disease. *Ann Intern Med* 110:17–23, 1983.
7. Aubier M, Murciano D, Rournier M, et al: Central respiratory drive in acute respiratory failure of patients with chronic obstructive pulmonary disease. *Am Rev Respir Dis* 122:191–200, 1980.
8. Aubier M, Trippenbach T, Roussos C: Respiratory muscle fatigue during cardiogenic shock. *J Appl Physiol* 51:499–508, 1981.
9. Bark H, Supinski G, Kelsen SG: Relationship of changes in diaphragmatic muscle blood flow to muscle contractile activity. *J Appl Physiol* 62:291–299, 1987.
10. Begin P, Grassino A. Inspiratory muscle dysfunction and chronic hypercapnia in chronic obstructive pulmonary disease. *Am Rev Respir Dis* 143:905–912, 1991.
11. Bellemare F, Bigland-Ritchie B: Central components of diaphragmatic fatigue assessed by phrenic nerve stimulation. *J Appl Physiol* 62:1307–1316, 1987.
12. Bellemare F, Grassino A: Effect of pressure and timing of contraction on human diaphragm fatigue. *J Appl Physiol* 53:1190–1195, 1982.
13. Bellemare F, Grassino A: Evaluation of human diaphragm fatigue. *J Appl Physiol* 53:1196–1206, 1982.
14. Bellemare F, Grassino A: Force reserve of the diaphragm in patients with chronic obstructive pulmonary disease. *J Appl Physiol* 55:8–15, 1983.
15. Beral V, Read DJC: Insensitivity of respiratory centre to carbon dioxide on Enga people of New Guinea. *Lancet* 2:1290–1294, 1971.
16. Bergofsky EH: State of the art: Respiratory failure in disorders of the thoracic cage. *Am Rev Respir Dis* 119:643–669, 1979.
17. Braun SR, Keim NL, Dixon RM, et al: The prevalence and determinants of nutritional changes in chronic obstructive pulmonary disease. *Chest* 86:558–563, 1984.
18. Cherniack NS, Altose, MD: Respiratory responses to ventilatory loading, in Hornbein TF (ed), *Lung Biology in Health and Disease*, vol 17: *Regulation of Breathing*, part II. New York, Dekker, 1981, pp 905–987.
19. Cohen CA, Zagelbaum G, Gross D, et al: Clinical manifestations of inspiratory muscle fatigue. *Am J Med* 73:308–316,1982.
20. Coleridge HM, Coleridge JCG: Reflexes evoked from tracheobronchial tree and lungs, in Cherniack NS, Widdicombe JG (eds), *Handbook of Physiology*, section 3: *The Respiratory System*, vol II: *Control of Breathing*, part 1. Bethesda, MD, American Physiological Society, 1986, pp 395–429.
21. Cunningham DJC, Robbins PA, Wolff CB: Integration of respiratory responses to changes in alveolar partial pressures of CO_2 and O_2 and in arterial pH, in Cherniack NS, Widdicombe JG (eds), *Handbook of Physiology*, section 3: *The Respiratory System*, vol II: *Control of Breathing*, part 2. Bethesda, MD, American Physiological Society, 1986, pp 475–528.
22. De Troyer A, Loring SH: Action of the respiratory muscles, in Macklem PT, Mead J (eds), *Handbook of Physiology*, section 3: *The Respiratory System*, vol III: *Mechanics of Breathing*, part 2. Bethesda, MD, American Physiological Society, 1986, pp 443–461.
23. Donohoe M, Rogers RR, Wilson DO, Pennock BE: Oxygen consumption of the respiratory muscles in normal and in malnourished patients with chronic obstructive pulmonary disease. *Am Rev Respir Dis* 140:385–391, 1989.
24. Druz WS, Sharp JT: Electrical and mechanical activity of the diaphragm accompanying body position in severe chronic obstructive pulmonary disease. *Am Rev Respir Dis* 125:275–280, 1982.
25. Efthimiou J, Fleming J, Spiro SG: Sternomastoid muscle function and fatigue in breathless patients with severe respiratory disease. *Am Rev Respir Dis* 136:1099–1105, 1987.
26. Eldridge F, Gherman C: Studies of oxygen administration in respiratory failure. *Ann Intern Med* 68:569–578, 1968.
27. Fleetham JA, Arnup ME, Anthonisen NR: Familial aspects of ventilatory control in patients with chronic obstructive pulmonary disease. *Am Rev Respir Dis* 129:3–7, 1984.
28. Frazier DT, Revelette WR: Role of phrenic nerve afferents in the control of breathing. *J Appl Physiol* 70:491–496, 1991.
29. Godoy I, Donahoe M, Calhoun WJ, et al: Elevated TNF-α production by peripheral blood monocytes of weight-losing COPD patients. *Am J Respir Crit Care Med* 153:633–637, 1996.
30. Grassino AE, Goldman MD: Respiratory muscle coordination, in Macklem PT, Mead J (eds), *Handbook of Physiology*, section 3: *The Respiratory System*, vol III: *Mechanics of Breathing*, part 2. Bethesda, MD, American Physiological Society, 1986, pp 463–509.
31. Gray-Donald K, Gibbons L, Shapiro SH, et al: Nutritional status and mortality in chronic obstructive pulmonary disease. *Am J Respir Crit Care Med* 153:961–966, 1996.
32. Harver A, Mahler DA, Daubenspeck JA: Targeted inspiratory muscle training improves respiratory muscle function and reduces dyspnea in patients with chronic obstructive pulmonary disease. *Ann Intern Med* 111:117–124, 1989.
33. Hudgel DW, Weil JV: Asthma associated with decreased hypoxic ventilatory drive: A family study. *Ann Intern Med* 80:623–625, 1974.
34. Hussain SNA, Roussos C, Magder S: Effects of tension, duty cycle, and arterial pressure on diaphragmatic blood flow in dogs. *J Appl Physiol* 66:968–976, 1989.
35. Irsigler GB: Carbon dioxide response lines in young adults: The limits of the normal response. *Am Rev Respir Dis* 114:529–536, 1976.
36. Kawakami Y, Tadashi I, Shida A, et al: Familial factors affecting arterial blood gas values and respiratory chemosensitivity in chronic obstructive pulmonary disease. *Am Rev Respir Dis* 125:420–425, 1982.
37. Kawakami Y, Yoskikawa T, Shida A, et al: Control of breathing in young twins. *J Appl Physiol* 52:537–542, 1982.
38. Kelsen SG, Cherniack NS, Jammes Y: Control of motor activity to the respiratory muscles, in Roussos C, Macklem PT (eds), *The Thorax*, part A: *Physiology*. New York, Dekker, 1985, pp 493–529.

39. Kelsen SG, Fleegler B, Altose MD: The respiratory neuromuscular response to hypoxia, hypercapnia, and obstruction to airflow in asthma. *Am Rev Respir Dis* 120:517–527, 1979.

40. Kikuchi Y, Okabe S, Tamura G, et al: Chemosensitivity and perception of dyspnea in patients with a history of near-fatal asthma. *New Engl J Med* 330:1229–1234, 1994.

41. Killian KJ, Summers E, Basalygo M, et al: Effect of frequency on perceived magnitude of added loads to breathing. *J Appl Physiol* 58:1616–1621, 1985.

42. Koo KW, Sax DS, Snider GL: Arterial blood gases and pH during sleep in chronic obstructive pulmonary disease. *Am J Med* 58:663–670, 1975.

43. Lane DJ, Howell JBL, Giblin B: Relation between airways obstruction and CO_2 tension in obstructive airways disease. *Br Med J* 3:707–709, 1968.

44. Leith DE, Bradley M: Ventilatory muscle strength and endurance training. *J Appl Physiol* 41:508–516, 1976.

45. McKenzie DK, Gandevia SC: Strength and endurance of inspiratory, expiratory and limb muscles in asthma. *Am Rev Respir Dis* 134:999–1004, 1986.

46. Manning HL, Schwartzstein RM: Pathophysiology of dyspnea. *New Engl J Med* 333:1547–1553, 1995.

47. Metzger JM, Fitts RH, et al: Fatigue from high- and low-frequency muscle stimulation: Role of sarcolemma action potentials. *Exp Neurol* 93:320–333, 1986.

48. Milic-Emili J, Whitelaw WA, Grassino AE: Measurement and testing of respiratory drive, in Hornbein TF (ed), *Lung Biology in Health and Disease,* vol 17: *Regulation of Breathing,* part II. New York, Dekker, 1981, pp 675–743.

49. Mountain R, Zwillich CW, Weil JV: Hypoventilation in obstructive lung disease: The role of familial factors. *New Engl J Med* 297:521–525, 1978.

50. Moxham J, Edwards RHT, Aubier M, et al: Changes in EMG power spectrum (high-to-low ratio) with force fatigue in humans. *J Appl Physiol* 53:1094–1099, 1982.

51. Murciano D, Auclair MH, Pariente R, Aubier M: A randomized, controlled trial of theophylline in patients with severe chronic obstructive pulmonary disease. *New Engl J Med* 320:1521–1525, 1989.

52. Murciano D, Boczkowski J, Lecocguic Y, et al: Tracheal occlusion pressure: A simple index to monitor respiratory muscle fatigue during acute respiratory failure in patients with chronic obstructive pulmonary disease. *Ann Intern Med* 108:800–805, 1988.

53. Oliven A, Kelsen SG, Deal EC, et al: Respiratory pressure sensation. *Am Rev Respir Dis* 132:1214–1218, 1985.

54. Oliven A, Lohda S, Adams ME, et al: Effect of fatiguing resistive loads on the level and pattern of respiratory activity in awake goats. *Respir Physiol* 73:311–324, 1988.

55. Oliven A, Supinski GS, Kelsen SG: Functional adaptation of diaphragm to chronic hyperinflation in emphysematous hamsters. *J Appl Physiol* 60:225–231, 1986.

56. Patrick JM, Howard A: The influence of age, sex, body size, and lung size on control and patterns of breathing during CO_2 inhalation in caucasians. *Respir Physiol* 16:337–350, 1972.

57. Rebuck AS, Slutsky AS: Measurement of ventilatory response to hypercapnia and hypoxia, in Hornbein TF (ed), *Lung Biology in Health and Disease,* vol 17: *Regulation of Breathing,* part II. New York, Dekker, 1981, pp 745–904.

58. Respiratory Muscle Fatigue Workshop Group: Respiratory muscle fatigue. *Am Rev Respir Dis* 142:474–480, 1990.

59. Road J, Vahi R, Rio PD, Grassino A: In vivo contractile properties of fatigued diaphragm. *J Appl Physiol* 63:471–478, 1987.

60. Rochester DF: Malnutrition and the respiratory muscles. *Clin Chest Med* 7:91–99, 1986.

61. Rogers RM, Donahoe M, Costantino J: Physiologic effects of oral supplemental feeding in malnourished patients with chronic obstructive pulmonary disease. *Am Rev Respir Dis* 146:1511–1517, 1992.

62. Roussos CS, Macklem PT: Inspiratory muscle fatigue, in Macklem PT, Mead J (eds), *Handbook of Physiology,* section 3: *The Respiratory System,* vol III: *Mechanics of Breathing,* part 2. Bethesda, MD, American Physiological Society, 1986, pp 511–527.

63. Santiago TV, Remolina C, Scoles V, Edelman NH: Endorphins and the control of breathing: Ability of naloxone to restore flow-resistive load compensation in chronic obstructive pulmonary disease. *New Engl J Med* 304:1190–1195, 1981.

64. Shannon R: Reflexes from respiratory muscle and costovertebral joints, in Cherniack NS, Widdicombe JG (eds), *Handbook of Physiology,* section 3: *The Respiratory System,* vol II: *Control of Breathing,* part 1. Bethesda, MD, American Physiological Society, 1986, pp 431–447.

65. Sharp JT, van Lith P, Nuchprayoon C, et al: The thorax in chronic obstructive lung disease. *Am J Med* 44:39–46, 1968.

66. Similowski T, Yan S, Gauthier AP: Contractile properties of the human diaphragm during chronic hyperinflation. *New Engl J Med* 325:917–923, 1991.

67. Skatrud JB, Dempsey JA: Relative effectiveness of acetazolamide versus medroxyprogesterone acetate in correction of chronic carbon dioxide retention. *Am Rev Respir Dis* 127:405–412, 1983.

68. Skatrud JB, Dempsey JA: Interaction of sleep state and chemical stimuli in sustaining rhythmic ventilation. *J Appl Physiol* 55:813–822, 1983.

69. Slone RM, Gierada DS: Radiology of pulmonary emphysema and lung volume reduction surgery. *Semin Thoracic Cardiovasc Surg* 8:61–82, 1996.

70. Supinski GS, Clary SJ, Bark H, Kelsen SG: Effect of inspiratory muscle fatigue on perception of effort during loaded breathing. *J Appl Physiol* 62:300–307, 1987.

71. Supinski GS, Kelsen SG: Effect of elastase-induced emphysema on the force-generating ability of the diaphragm. *J Clin Invest* 70:978–988, 1982.

72. Sutton FD, Zwillich CW, Creagh E, et al: Progesterone for outpatient treatment of Pickwickian syndrome. *Ann Intern Med* 83:476–479, 1975.

73. Taguchi O, Kikuchi Y, Hida W, et al: Effects of bronchoconstriction and external resistive loading on the sensation of dyspnea. *J Appl Physiol* 71:2183–2190, 1991.

74. Thomas A, Supinski GS, Kelsen SG: Changes in chest wall structure and elasticity in elastase induced emphysema. *J Appl Physiol* 61:1821–1829, 1986.

75. Tobin MJ, Perez W, Guenther SM, et al: Does rib cage–abdominal paradox signify respiratory muscle fatigue? *J Appl Physiol* 63:851–860, 1987.

76. Tolep K, Higgins N, Muza S, et al: Comparison of diaphragm strength between healthy adult elderly and young men. *Am J Respir Crit Care Med* 152:677–682, 1995.

77. Yang KL, Tobin MJ: A prospective study of indexes predicting the outcome of trials of weaning from mechanical ventilation. *New Engl J Med* 324:1445–1450, 1991.

CHAPTER 172

OXYGEN THERAPY AND PULMONARY OXYGEN TOXICITY

Michael F. Beers

SUMMARY

With the momentous discovery of molecular oxygen by Joseph Priestley in 1775[43] and the subsequent demonstration of respiratory gas exchange by Lavoisier,[14] oxygen inhalation soon became a part of eighteenth-century therapeutic regimens for the treatment of a variety of clinical ailments. While the widespread use of inhaled oxygen initially accelerated, a backlash of criticism grew throughout the nineteenth century regarding its efficacy. The criticism was commensurate with physiological studies demonstrating that, under ambient conditions, the oxygen-carrying capacity of arterial blood was nearly maximal and that further increases in the fraction of inspired O_2 produced no appreciable additional physiological benefit. Furthermore, in 1899, Lorrain-Smith confirmed the early suspicions of Priestley, Lavoisier, and others regarding the potential toxicity of inhaled oxygen with the first description of the pulmonary pathologic alterations associated with excessive oxygen exposure.[34] As a result of these observations, the use of oxygen as a therapeutic modality fell into disrepute.

It was not until the early 1920s that supplemental oxygen breathing was rigorously evaluated. Through pioneering efforts by Meakins, Baruch, and others, the concept of a therapeutic window for oxygen inhalation was established.[36] Many investigators independently demonstrated that a reduction in oxygen availability had serious physiological consequences and that, in pathological states, the detrimental consequences of hypoxia could often be circumvented by administration of oxygen. Thus, oxygen therapy again became a mainstream therapy, but as adjuvant treatment for cardiac and pulmonary diseases which specifically produced hypoxemia and hypoxia.

Over the past 70 years, with the advent of improved oxygen delivery systems, mechanical ventilation, the modern intensive care unit, and long-term home oxygen administration, oxygen has become widely available and frequently prescribed. As with any drug, there are indications for and contraindications to its use.[3] Nevertheless, despite a large clinical experience, huge gaps exist in our understanding, and many uncertainties prevail which continue to inhibit the rational use of oxygen therapy. Consensus conferences and numerous studies have established guidelines and have defined clinical criteria for the proper use of supplemental oxygen,[20,37,39] but in practice oxygen therapy is often currently prescribed without careful evaluation of its potential benefits and side effects and with inadequate supervision.[31] In a retrospective study of 90 consecutive hospitalized patients, O_2 therapy was prescribed inappropriately in 21 percent; monitoring was inadequate in 85.5 percent; and documentation of physiological criteria for termination of therapy was lacking in 88 percent of all patients.[17] Prospective studies have also indicated that only 44 percent of hospitalized patients receiving O_2 do so at the prescribed dosage and flow.[29]

The overall goal of this chapter is to provide the basis for the rational use of inhaled oxygen therapy. The chapter provides a review of the physiology of tissue oxygenation, the current indications and guidelines for acute oxygen therapy, the role of long-term oxygen therapy, and the pathophysiological basis for pulmonary oxygen toxicity associated with its overuse. Because most prescribed oxygen is administered under normobaric conditions, in the discussion that follows, oxygen therapy and its toxic consequences are considered in this setting (i.e., one atmosphere).

TISSUE OXYGENATION

The physiological basis for oxygen therapy has been well documented for over 30 years. Treatment and prevention of hypoxemia are the most common indications for oxygen therapy, the ultimate goal of which is correction or avoidance of tissue hypoxia. In 1965, Chance first demonstrated that a partial pressure of oxygen (P_{O_2}) in mitochondria of 18 mmHg or more is required to generate the high-energy phosphate bonds (as adenosine triphosphate) which are essential for all major cellular biochemical functions.[6] At rest, the average adult male consumes about 225 to 250 ml of oxygen per minute; this rate of consumption may increase as much as tenfold during exercise.[40] Ongoing oxygen utilization in peripheral tissues dictates that there is a very small oxygen reserve which can be quickly consumed within 4 to 6 min of cessation of spontaneous ventilation. A complete understanding of the concepts of oxygen delivery and utilization is required for the careful assessment of the hypoxic patient and implementation of proper therapy.

Oxygen Delivery and Utilization

Transport of oxygen from atmospheric air to tissue mitochondria (the ultimate sites of oxygen utilization) requires the integrated function of the pulmonary, cardiovascular, and hematologic systems. Figure 172-1 demonstrates that under normal conditions, a pronounced drop in P_{O_2} occurs from ambient atmosphere to tissues. The measured basal tissue P_{O_2} (i.e., mixed venous P_{O_2} or $\overline{v}_{O_2}$) is only marginally greater than the threshold value for mitochondrial anaerobic metabolism measured in vitro (as illustrated in Fig. 172-1 by the dashed line at a P_{O_2} of 20 mmHg). The consequence of such a steep gradient of oxygen concentration and of a marginal tissue reserve is that a variety of environmental and pathologic factors can ultimately impact on tissue oxygenation significantly by altering P_{O_2} at one of these other intermediary stages. The result is that tissue hypoxia develops whenever oxygen delivery is inadequate to meet tissue metabolic demands.

Oxygen delivery to the periphery is determined by two major factors: (1) oxygen content of arterial blood and (2) the amount of blood flow, i.e., cardiac output. In particular, total O_2 delivery is calculated by multiplying the cardiac output by arterial O_2 content. Total O_2 delivery (D_{O_2}) can be calculated according to Eq. (1):

$$D_{O_2} = CO \times CaO_2 \times 10 \tag{1}$$

where

D_{O_2} = oxygen delivery, ml/min

CO = cardiac output in L/min

CaO_2 = O_2 content of arterial blood, ml/dl

The oxygen content of arterial blood is a function of the hemoglobin concentration and its degree of saturation with molecular oxygen, plus the fractional amount of oxygen physically

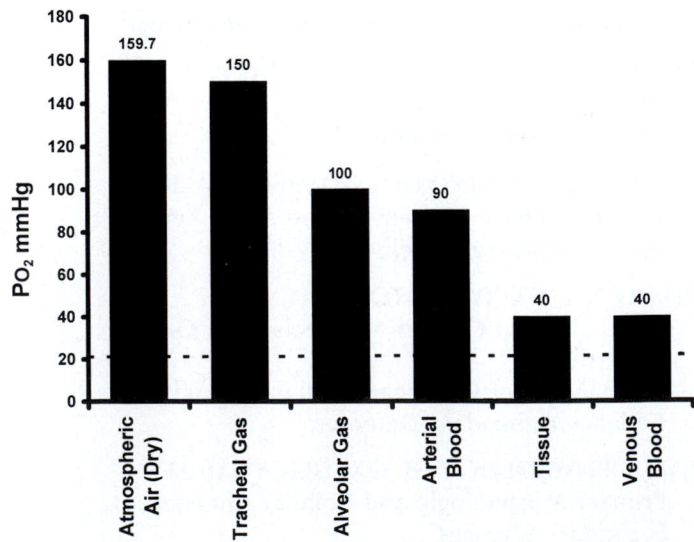

FIGURE 172-1 Graphical representation of sequential steps in the drop in oxygen tension (P_{O_2}) at various stages of oxygen transport from atmosphere to peripheral tissues. Values depicted are calculated using the alveolar gas equation (Appendix D). Dashed line represents the approximate intracellular anaerobic threshold. (*From Caldwell et al.[6]*)

dissolved in solution.[40] The amounts of both the bound and dissolved oxygen are directly related to the oxygen tension in arterial blood (Pa_{O_2}). The percentage of hemoglobin saturated with oxygen is a function of Pa_{O_2}, as described by the classic oxyhemoglobin dissociation curve (see Chapter 14). The amount of oxygen dissolved in solution is a function of the solubility coefficient of oxygen and Pa_{O_2}. Equation (2) describes the contribution of these two components to total arterial oxygen content:

$$Ca_{O_2} = ([Hg] \times 1.34 \times Sa_{O_2}) + (Pa_{O_2} \times 0.0031) \quad (2)$$

where

$[Hg]$ = hemoglobin concentration, gm/dl

1.34 = O_2 carrying capacity of hemoglobin at 37°C, ml/gm hemoglobin

Sa_{O_2} = measured %O_2 saturation of hemoglobin

0.0031 = solubility coefficient for oxygen

Mechanisms of Hypoxia

Aerobic metabolism requires a balance between oxygen delivery (D_{O_2}) and O_2 utilization ($\dot{V}_{O_2}$). As shown in Fig. 172-2, a biphasic relationship between D_{O_2} and $\dot{V}_{O_2}$ has been observed. Under physiological circumstances of normal aerobic metabolism, oxygen transport and oxygen utilization are independent variables. Whereas the amount of O_2 delivered to tissues per unit time defines the upper limit of oxygen available for the body's total metabolic needs, delivery of oxygen under normal circumstances always exceeds peripheral oxygen utilization. In this "supply-independent" region of the graph, oxygen consumption is commensurate with the rate of adenosine 5'-triphosphate (ATP) production and represents a measure of tissue cellular energy requirements. If oxygen delivery falls below a critical threshold (D_{O_2} critical), or if utilization exceeds delivery (e.g., with strenuous exercise), tissues must shift from aerobic to anaerobic metabolism to supply adequate energy for total metabolic needs. When an imbalance arises, excessive lactic acid production ensues, resulting in progressive acidosis, disrupted cellular metabolism, and, potentially, cell death.

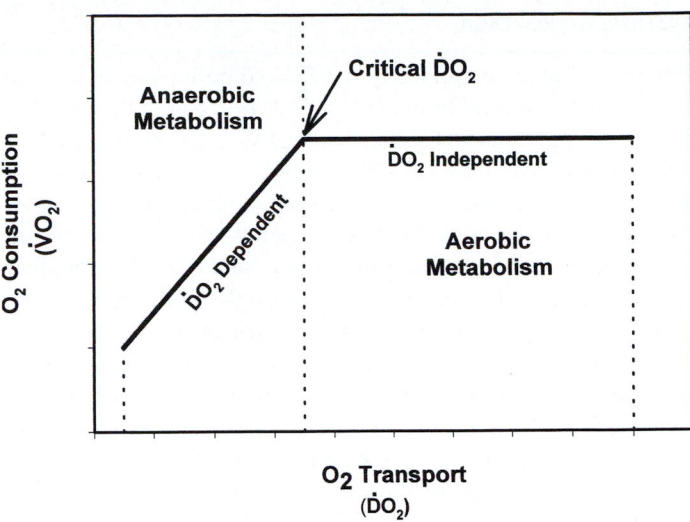

FIGURE 172-2 Relationship between oxygen consumption ($\dot{V}_{O_2}$) and oxygen transport (D_{O_2}). The critical D_{O_2}, indicative of the part of transition from supply-dependent to supply-independent conditions, is denoted by the arrow. Anaerobic metabolism exists under supply-dependent conditions and ensues when O_2 consumption exceeds O_2 supply.

The major causes of tissue hypoxia are listed in Table 172-1. On a mechanistic basis, these can be divided into three broad categories: (1) arterial hypoxemia, (2) reduced oxygen delivery, and (3) excessive or improved tissue utilization.

Maintenance of tissue oxygenation depends on the proper integration of three separate organ systems, including the cardiovascular system, which determines cardiac output and blood flow distribution, the hematologic system, which determines hemoglobin concentration, and the pulmonary system, which determines Pa_{O_2}.[40] Therefore, etiologies of hypoxemia generally represent a failure of proper oxygen loading of the blood (low P_{O_2}), caused primarily by abnormal function of the pulmonary system. However, defects in oxygen transport may result from dysfunction of either the cardiovascular system or the hematologic system. Finally, "misutilization" of delivered oxygen resulting from either defects in cellular metabolism or excessive demand represents another class of disorders characterized by hypoxia. These three categories are further discussed below.

TABLE 172-1

Causes of Tissue Hypoxia

Category	Clinical Correlate	Pa_{O_2}	$\bar{v}_{O_2}$	Cardiac Output
Hypoxemic	See Table 172-2	↓	⟷ or ↓	↓ or ↑ or ⟷
Impaired delivery				
Circulatory (forward flow)	Hypovolemia; heart failure	⟷	↓	↓
Distributive	Sepsis; arterial insufficiency	↓ or ⟷	⟷ or ↓	↑ or ⟷
Defective Blood-O_2 transport	Inherited abnormal hemoglobins			
	Acquired abnormal hemoglobin (CO poisoning)	⟷	⟷ or ↓	↑ or ⟷
	Anemia			

ARTERIAL HYPOXEMIA

Hypoxemia may be defined as a validated deficiency of oxygen tension in the arterial blood.[31,32,40,49] A P_{O_2} below the range of normal for age-matched subjects establishes the presence of arterial hypoxemia. Table 172-2 summarizes the major causes of hypoxemia. Since the driving force for oxygen transport across the alveolar barrier into the blood depends on both the concentration of oxygen in the alveolus ($P_{A_{O_2}}$) and overall respiratory function, arterial hypoxemia can result only from either reduction of the inspired oxygen tension or respiratory dysfunction.

The most common pulmonary causes of hypoxemia include ventilation-perfusion mismatch, true shunt, a diffusion barrier, and, occasionally, a low mixed venous oxygen tension (see Chapters 12, 13). Alveolar hypoventilation, which also results in hypoxemia, acts indirectly through mechanisms which increase alveolar P_{CO_2} and secondarily decrease alveolar P_{O_2}. To a varying degree, most causes of arterial hypoxemia can be improved by administration of supplemental oxygen. However, the magnitude of the response differs, based on the etiology, as discussed in Chapter 165.

REDUCED OXYGEN DELIVERY

In the setting of a normal Pa_{O_2}, tissue hypoxia may result from abnormalities in any of the determinants of oxygen delivery, including circulatory causes, abnormal blood oxygen transport, or maldistribution of blood flow.

Circulatory hypoxia results when fully oxygenated blood is delivered to tissues in insufficient quantity or at an inadequate level to support tissue metabolic needs. Usual etiologies include low cardiac output states, systemic hypovolemia, and arterial insufficiency of peripheral tissues. Compensation is partially effected at the tissue level initially by increased oxygen extraction from blood, resulting in lowering of mixed venous oxygen tension ($\bar{v}_{O_2}$). Thus, a low $\bar{v}_{O_2}$ is the hallmark of circulatory hypoxia. Because Pa_{O_2} may be normal and the hemoglobin normally saturated, oxygen administration is unlikely to be of great help in the majority of these disorders.

Tissue hypoxia may also result from *abnormal blood-oxygen transport,* in which the oxygen-carrying capacity of the blood is reduced, as manifested primarily by a decrease in the total hemoglobin content (i.e., anemia), or secondarily as a consequence of abnormal hemoglobin-O_2 affinity. States of abnormal hemoglobin-O_2 affinity include an inability to bind oxygen or to release oxygen to tissues, e.g., with hemoglobinopathies and low levels of 2,3-diphosphoglycerate, respectively. Acquired defects typically result from the binding of a ligand with stronger affinity for hemoglobin than oxygen, such as carbon monoxide, or a toxic alteration in hemoglobin structure, e.g., with methhemoglobinemia. Under these circumstances, cardiac output is increased as an adaptive response, and $\bar{v}_{O_2}$ is normal or decreased. Although not a primary therapy, oxygen administration may play an adjunctive role. In certain situations, including carbon monoxide poisoning, hyperbaric oxygen therapy may be helpful.

Finally, tissue hypoxia may result from *maldistribution* of a normal or supranormal cardiac output. Examples include microvascular perfusion defects observed in classical septic shock or in the more recently recognized systemic inflammatory response syndrome (SIRS). Maldistribution of perfusion leading to tissue hypoxia has also been described in other situations, such as experimental interleuken-2 therapy. The hallmark of a maldistribution hypoxia is the development of precapillary shunting in peripheral tissues. Thus, cardiac output is normal or increased, and $\bar{v}_{O_2}$ is usually low. Because of the presence of peripheral shunting, supplemental oxygen is usually not effective in increasing local cellular oxygen tension.

CELLULAR CAUSES OF HYPOXIA

Hypoxia may also arise from misutilization of oxygen at the tissue level. Cellular hypoxia results from inhibition of either intracellular enzymes or oxygen carrying molecules involved in intermediary metabolism and energy generation. A classic case is accidental or deliberate exposure to hydrogen cyanide. In hydrogen cyanide poisoning, Pa_{O_2}, hemoglobin concentration, percentage of hemoglobin saturation, and tissue perfusion are normal. However, peripheral utilization of O_2 is impaired as cyanide binds to cytochrome oxidase and inhibits intramitochondrial transport of electrons to molecular oxygen. This event blocks production of ATP via oxidative phosphorylation resulting in a lactic acidosis as anaerobic metabolism is alternatively utilized.

TABLE 172-2

Causes of Arterial Hypoxemia and Response to Oxygen Therapy

Cause	*Clinical Examples*	*Effect of Oxygen Therapy*
Decreased oxygen intake	High altitude	Rapid increase in Pa_{O_2}
Ventilation-perfusion imbalance (high $\dot{V}/\dot{Q}$)	Obstructive airway disease	Moderately rapid increase in Pa_{O_2}
Shunt (low $\dot{V}/\dot{Q}$)	Atrial septal defect; pulmonary arteriovenous fistula	Variable increase in Pa_{O_2} depending on size of shunt
Diffusion defect	Interstitial pneumonitis	Moderately rapid increase in Pa_{O_2}
Alveolar hypoventilation	Chronic obstructive pulmonary disease	Initial response—increase in Pa_{O_2}; late response—variable, depending on whether supplemental O_2 depresses minute ventilation

In addition, oxygen extraction is often impaired, leading to a normal or increased $\bar{v}_{O_2}$. Although oxygen therapy is usually not effective, 100% oxygen is often administered while the patient is treated with specific antedotes.

"Demand hypoxia" results when tissue oxygen utilization is supernormal, exceeding the rate of oxygen delivery. Common causes include maximal exercise and hypermetabolic states, such as thyrotoxicosis. As in circulatory hypoxia, $\bar{v}_{O_2}$ is decreased, but in contrast, cardiac output is normal or, more likely, increased. Because oxygen-carrying capacity is normal, oxygen administration is often ineffective, and definitive treatment requires control of the underlying disorder.

RECOGNITION AND ASSESSMENT OF TISSUE HYPOXIA

The correct use of oxygen therapy requires clinical recognition of tissue hypoxia; careful evaluation of the pathophysiological basis for the hypoxia; understanding of factors which predict those hypoxic patients likely to benefit; and continued assessment of the optimal dosage, balancing benefit against potential toxicity. In most circumstances, tissue hypoxia is not directly measurable, and detection is usually accomplished through a combination of clinical and laboratory parameters. In cases of isolated arterial hypoxemia, awareness of tissue hypoxia is enhanced through inference of abnormal measurements of arterial oxygen saturation.

Clinical Manifestations

Clinical manifestations of hypoxia are highly variable and non-specific and depend on both duration of the hypoxia (acute or chronic) and the individual's fitness.[31,40] Symptoms and signs associated with acute hypoxia are outlined in Table 172-3. They include changes in mental status, dyspnea, tachypnea, respiratory distress, and cardiac arrhythmias. Alterations in mental status range from impaired judgment to confusion or coma. Cyanosis, often considered a hallmark of hypoxia, occurs only when the concentration of reduced hemoglobin in the blood is 1.5 gm/dl or greater. However, this is not a reliable sign, given its absence in anemia and during periods of poor peripheral perfusion.[31]

Laboratory and Other Objective Assessments

Because of the variability of presentation and nonspecificity of the symptoms and signs of hypoxia, the laboratory assessment of the state of tissue oxygenation is desirable. Unfortunately, the current state of the art remains imprecise. Quantification of the degree of oxygenation of individual tissues is difficult. Use of proton nuclear magnetic resonance (NMR) to assess tissue pH, and of phosphorous NMR to assess high-energy phosphate stores, remains experimental. The $\bar{v}_{O_2}$ represents an approximation of mean tissue P_{O_2}, and a level of less than 30 mmHg indicates overall tissue hypoxia. However, measurements of $\bar{v}_{O_2}$ require pulmonary artery catheterization and, therefore, are limited to intensive care settings.

In most clinical situations, direct determinations of Pa_{O_2} or arterial oxygen saturation are the major parameters available to the clinician. These determinations are made either invasively with blood samples obtained from arterial puncture or indwelling arterial catheters or noninvasively by infrared pulse oximetry.[46] Both are useful in excluding arterial hypoxemia; neither directly measures tissue P_{O_2}. Inadequate tissue oxygen delivery is inferred from moderate decreases in Pa_{O_2}, and the inference is usually warranted in acutely ill patients whose Pa_{O_2} is less than 50 mmHg. However, this judgment may be unsubstantiated in patients who are chronically hypoxemic and who have developed compensatory mechanisms. In addition, assumptions about the adequacy of tissue oxygenation may not be warranted in clinical settings in which factors other than arterial hypoxemia are responsible for the development of hypoxia (Table 172-1).

INDICATIONS FOR OXYGEN THERAPY

In every sense, oxygen must be thought of as a drug having a therapeutic window based on the level of use and duration of administration.[3] In addition, the cost of both short-term oxygen therapy for hospitalized patients and long-term therapy for patients with chronic lung disease (in the United States, 800,000 patients at an annual cost of $1.8 million)[41] dictates an understanding regarding its rational administration. Indications for use of supplemental oxygen must be clear. Oxygen should be administered in precise amounts, and patients should be monitored for both efficacy and toxicity of treatment. Despite the facts that the scientific foundation underlying these principles is incomplete and that all-inclusive guidelines have been difficult to develop, the economic implications and requirements for laboratory monitoring have prompted development of recommendations for oxygen therapy. These recommendations allow flexibility for the physician in exercising appropriate

TABLE 172-3

Symptoms and Signs of Acute Hypoxia

System	Symptoms and Signs
Respiratory	Tachypnea, breathlessness, dyspnea, cyanosis
Cardiovascular	Increased cardiac output, palpitations, tachycardia, arrhythmias, hypotension, angina, vasodilatation, diaphoresis, and shock
Central nervous	Headache, impaired judgment, inappropriate behavior, confusion, euphoria, delerium, restlessness, papilledema, seizures, obtundation, coma
Neuromuscular	Weakness, tremor, asterixis, hyperreflexia, incoordination
Metabolic	Sodium and water retention, lactic acidosis

clinical judgment in prescribing oxygen in a cost-effective manner in both the acute and chronic settings.

Short-Term Oxygen Therapy

Recommendations for administration of supplemental oxygen, based upon guidelines of the American College of Chest Physicians and the National Heart, Lung and Blood Institute,[20] as well as other organizations, are compiled in Table 172-4.

TISSUE HYPOXIA ASSOCIATED WITH ARTERIAL HYPOXEMIA

In the acute setting, the most common indication for supplemental oxygen, regardless of the underlying etiology, is arterial hypoxemia. For a normal, middle-aged adult, the usual level of hypoxemia at which oxygen therapy is instituted is a Pa_{O_2} of less than 60 mmHg. Based on the oxyhemoglobin dissociation curve, this value for Pa_{O_2} results in a hemoglobin saturation of about 90%. Because of the sigmoidal shape of the curve at this level of Pa_{O_2}, a further decrease in oxygen tension results in a considerable drop in oxygen saturation.

Ventilation-perfusion mismatch is the most common pathophysiological cause of arterial hypoxemia (see Chapter 12). The magnitude of the response to administration of supplemental O_2 depends upon the range and degree of ventilation-perfusion mismatch within individual lung regions. Therefore, repeated measurement of Pa_{O_2} or Sa_{O_2} should be done to document an effective response to a particular level of $F_{I_{O_2}}$.

Hypoxemia secondary to right to left shunting is often less responsive to O_2 administration. Mixing of shunted and unshunted blood results in a large fall in Pa_{O_2}. When the shunt fraction is greater than 20 to 25 percent, hypoxemia may persist, despite an $F_{I_{O_2}}$ of 1.0.

Finally, alveolar hypoventilation is often easily corrected with supplemental oxygen. However, recognition and correction of the underlying cause and immediate restoration of ventilation are the primary aims of treatment.

Although a Pa_{O_2} of 60 mmHg is a reasonable goal in the initial treatment of arterial hypoxemia, in certain clinical situations the acceptable threshold level may be adjusted upward or downward. For example, in patients with low O_2-carrying capacity (e.g., severe anemia), or in flow-limited states (e.g., acute angina pectoris), increases in Pa_{O_2} beyond 60 mmHg (yielding increases in Sa_{O_2} from 90 to 100%) may result in marginal but potentially important increases in tissue O_2 delivery. Conversely, the "acceptable Pa_{O_2}" may have to be set at a lower level in patients with abnormal control of respiration, such as those with an acquired induced hypoxic ventilatory drive due to chronic carbon dioxide retention.

TISSUE HYPOXIA WITH NORMAL Pa_{O_2}

The efficacy of supplemental oxygen in diseases that cause arterial hypoxemia is well-established. However, in cases where tissue hypoxia may exist without concomittant arterial hypoxemia, treatment should be directed ultimately to correcting the underlying cause. In these cases, Pa_{O_2} is an inadequate index of the need for, or the potential to benefit from, oxygen therapy. When available, alternative indices of tissue oxygenation should be utilized; oxygen therapy should be initiated and modified, based on the indices. Nevertheless, in some disorders, oxygen therapy has often been used even if Pa_{O_2} is not at a substantially depressed level. There is not always a consensus about the proper uses of oxygen in these circumstances.

ACUTE MYOCARDIAL INFARCTION

Hypoxemia is extremely common in acute myocardial infarction. In such patients, oxygen administration is of unquestioned benefit.[44] Data supporting use of oxygen therapy in nonhypoxemic patients with acute myocardial infarction is controversial. Double-blinded studies of the value of oxygen in uncomplicated myocardial infarction demonstrate no significant effects on morbidity or mortality.

INADEQUATE CARDIAC OUTPUT (LOW-FLOW STATES)

Oxygen has been recommended for temporary treatment of inadequate systemic perfusion resulting from cardiac failure. Although this practice seems reasonable, no clinical studies to date have proved the value of oxygen therapy in this setting. Oxygen therapy is utilized in conjunction with inotropic agents and other devices to assist cardiac output as definitive treatment is undertaken.

TRAUMA AND HYPOVOLEMIC SHOCK

Oxygen has been advocated as adjunctive therapy in the setting of acute trauma. The low-flow state induced by acute hemorrhage is best treated by increasing the supply of circulating hemoglobin. However, supplemental oxygen as supportive therapy seems warranted until red blood cells become available for transfusion.

TABLE 172-4

Guidelines for the Institution of Acute Oxygen Therapy

*Accepted Indications**

Acute hypoxemia (Pa_{O_2} < 60 mmHg; Sa_{O_2} < 90%)
Cardiac and respiratory arrest
Hypotension (systolic blood pressure < 100 mmHg)
Low cardiac output and metabolic acidosis (bicarbonate < 18 mmol/L)
Respiratory distress (respiratory rate > 24/min)

Questionable Indications

Uncomplicated myocardial infarction
Dyspnea without hypoxemia
Sickle cell crisis
Angina

---

*From Fulmer and Snider.[20]

NOTE: Pa_{O_2} = partial pressure of arterial oxygen; Sa_{O_2} = arterial oxygen saturation.

CARBON MONOXIDE INTOXICATION

In carbon monoxide poisoning, the Pa_{O_2} is a poor guide to the need for oxygen therapy. Despite a normal or "supranormal" Pa_{O_2}, a state of significant tissue hypoxia exists, as often indicated by a severe metabolic acidosis. Because of the high concentration of carbon-monoxide-bound hemoglobin (carboxyhemoglobin), administration of supplemental oxygen does not increase tissue oxygen delivery. However, administration of pure oxygen markedly shortens the half-life of circulating carbon monoxide (80 min versus 320 min on room air). Thus, oxygen administration for carbon monoxide poisoning constitutes an accepted therapy. Hyperbaric oxygen administration represents the current standard of care for those patients with high carboxyhemoglobin levels and evidence of end-organ ischemia-reperfusion damage.[52]

MISCELLANEOUS DISORDERS

Use of supplemental oxygen as adjuvant therapy in sickle cell crisis, to accelerate resorption of air in pneumothorax, and for relief of dyspnea without hypoxemia remains controversial.

Chronic Oxygen Therapy

In recent years, use of long-term oxygen therapy in the chronically ill patient has increased. In the United States, over 800,000 patients currently receive long-term oxygen therapy; most are patients with arterial hypoxemia.[42,49] Patients with chronic obstructive pulmonary disease (COPD) represent the largest group of patients, and most of the data regarding clinical efficacy of supplemental oxygen come from studies of these patients.[22]

Early studies of oxygen therapy in COPD showed that continuous supplemental oxygen administered for 4 to 8 weeks decreased the hematocrit, improved exercise tolerance, and lowered pulmonary vascular pressures. In the early 1980s, two well-controlled studies demonstrated the value of long-term oxygen administration in patients with chronic hypoxemia due to COPD. Both the Nocturnal Oxygen Therapy Trial (NOTT) and the British Medical Research Council Domiciliary (BMRCD) study documented a significant reduction in mortality in patients receiving supplemental oxygen compared with controls who received no supplemental oxygen.[37,39] Although the treatment groups in the two studies are not directly comparable (patients in NOTT received either continuous or nocturnal oxygen, whereas those in BMRCD received nocturnal oxygen or no supplementation), nocturnal oxygen (>15 h per day) is better than no oxygen; continuous supplemental oxygen imparts the most benefit. The greatest efficacy is seen in patients with polycythemia, pulmonary hypertension, or hypercapnia. Although similar studies in other groups of patients with chronic hypoxemia are not available, extension of the concept of long-term oxygen therapy for patients with resting hypoxemia from a variety of cardiopulmonary diseases, including restrictive lung disease, cystic fibrosis, and chronic cardiac disease, has become widely accepted in clinical practice.

Table 172-5 lists the currently accepted indications for long-term oxygen therapy. In addition to chronic arterial hypoxemia at

---

TABLE 172-5

Indications for Long-Term Oxygen Therapy

Continuous Oxygen

Resting Pa_{O_2} < 55 mmHg or oxygen saturation < 88%

Resting Pa_{O_2} of 56–59 mmHg or oxygen saturation of 89% in the presence of any of the following indicative of cor pulmonale:

   Dependent edema suggesting congestive heart failure

   P pulmonale on the electrocardiogram (P wave greater than 3 min in standard leads II, III, or aVF)

Polycythemia (hematocrit > 56%)

Resting Pa_{O_2} > 59 mmHg or oxygen saturation > 89% reimbursable only with additional documentation justifying the oxygen prescription and a summary of more conservative therapy that has failed

Noncontinuous Oxygen[*]

During exercise: Pa_{O_2} 55 mmHg or oxygen saturation 88% with a low level of exertion

During sleep Pa_{O_2} 55 mmHg or oxygen saturation 88% with associated complications, such as pulmonary hypertension, daytime sommolence, and cardiac arrhythmias

[*]Oxygen flow rate and number of hours per day must be specified.

---

rest, continuous-flow oxygen therapy is indicated for patients with exercise-induced hypoxemia (i.e., exercised-induced arterial desaturation). Current data suggest that supplemental oxygen improves exercise endurance, as assayed by either treadmill walking or bicycle ergometry.[20] However, since ventilatory, rather than circulatory, factors often limit exercise in patients with airflow obstruction, increasing oxygen saturation is not a reliable predictor of improved exercise performance in all patients.

A third group of patients who benefit from chronic oxygen administration are those who develop significant decreases in arterial oxygen during sleep. Included are patients with primary sleep-disordered breathing (e.g., obstructive sleep apnea and obesity hypoventilation syndrome) and patients with primary lung disease who exhibit nocturnal desaturation. In the former group, oxygen therapy may need to be coupled with invasive or noninvasive ventilatory support for treatment of hypercarbia; the latter group can often make use of low-flow oxygen to blunt arterial desaturation.

In all patients, the need for additional supplemental oxygen should be based on measurements of arterial saturation. Certificates of medical necessity can then be completed appropriately. Most data support the notion that strategies for delivery of long-term oxygen should include early follow-up for assessing efficacy, followed by routine reevaluation at 6-month intervals.[10,32]

TECHNIQUES OF OXYGEN ADMINISTRATION

In either the acute or chronic setting, once the need for supplemental oxygen is established, one of several types of delivery devices can be used to supply the patient with O_2-enriched gas. The choice of delivery system is based upon a variety of criteria, including: (1) the degree of hypoxemia, (2) the requirement for precision of delivery, (3) patient comfort, and (4) cost. The devices discussed below are reserved primarily for conscious, awake patients who are capable of protecting their airways. Not included in the discussion are details on the use of endotracheal intubation (Chapter 174) or mechanical ventilation (Chapters 176, 177).

Oxygen Delivery Systems in the Acute Setting

A variety of delivery systems are available for short-term oxygen administration.[30,31,40] The systems vary in complexity, expense, efficiency, and precision of O_2 delivery. Other than anesthetic breathing circuits, virtually all oxygen delivery systems are nonrebreathing (full or partial). In nonrebreathing circuits, the inspiratory gas is not made up of any portion of the exhaled volume, and the only inhaled CO_2 is that which is entrained from ambient room air. Rebreathing is avoided through use of one-way valves to sequester expired gases from inspired gases. In addition, in all these systems, inspired gas mixtures must be presented in sufficient volume and at flows to allow compensation for the high-flow demands often exhibited by critically ill patients.

The major types of oxygen delivery systems are outlined in Fig. 172-3. They can be divided into low-flow and high-flow varieties. Both varieties can deliver humidified, inspired gases; each offers advantages and drawbacks.

LOW-FLOW OXYGEN DEVICES

Low-flow oxygen delivery systems provide a fraction of the patient's minute ventilatory requirement as pure oxygen; the remainder of the ventilatory requirement is fulfilled by addition of another gas, usually entrained room air. Flows supplied through these devices are low (less than 6 L/min), and they cannot deliver constant inspired oxygen concentrations, since small fluctuations in each tidal volume lead to variations in the amount of entrained room air. Consequently, in patients with an abnormal or variable ventilation pattern, there may be marked variation in the fraction of inspired oxygen. Patient-related factors that affect the fractional concentration of inspired oxygen include shallow breathing, which results in entraining less room air and, therefore, a higher concentration of inspired oxygen; deep, hyperpneic breathing, which enhances entraining of more room air; and changes in respiratory frequency, which affect exhalation time and, thereby, produce variable filling of the device's inspiratory reservoir. Therefore, when the delivery of a constant F_{IO_2} is required, e.g., in patients with chronic carbon dioxide retention, low-flow systems should not be used.

Nasal Cannulae

Nasal catheters and cannulae are the most widely used devices for delivering low-flow oxygen. They are simple, inexpensive,

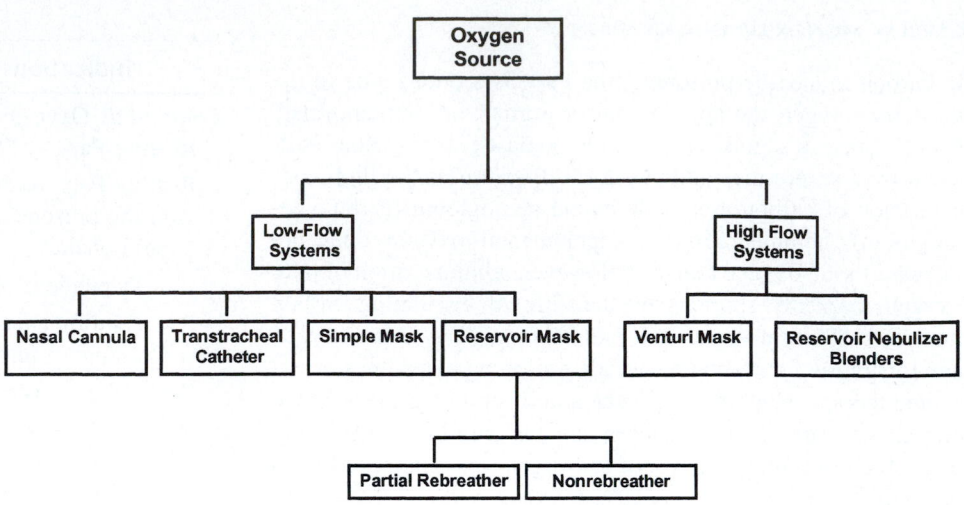

FIGURE 172-3   Commonly utilized oxygen delivery systems. See text for complete descriptions.

easy to use, and well tolerated. As for all low-flow systems, the F_{IO_2} may vary greatly, depending on the oxygen flow, inspiratory flow, and minute ventilation. As Table 172-6 illustrates, with low-flow nasal cannulae set to deliver oxygen to the nasopharynx at flows between 1 and 6 L/min, the F_{IO_2} ranges between 0.24 and 0.44. Flows above 6 L/min do not significantly increase F_{IO_2} above 44 percent; these higher flows may result in drying of mucous membranes.

Oxygen Masks

Simple plastic oxygen masks which cover the nose and mouth are capable of delivering concentrations of oxygen up to 50 to 60%. Depending on mask size, these devices provide a self-contained reservoir of 100 to 200 ml of additional gas, thereby facilitating increases in the achievable fraction of inspired oxygen above 0.44. Simple face masks require a flow of inspired oxygen of 5 to 6 L/min to avoid accumulation of carbon dioxide within the mask.

Conventional oxygen masks suffer from the limitations of all face masks. They interfere with drinking, eating, and expectorating, and they can become displaced, particularly at night as the patient sleeps. In addition, use of face masks increases the risk of aspiration by concealment of vomitus or containment of regurgitant materials. Therefore, when using these devices, the risk-benefit ratio should be considered. As with nasal cannulae, respiratory mucous membrane drying from the inspired gas mixture is possible. Humidification of inspired gas reduces the magnitude of the problem.

Masks with Reservoir Bags

To deliver an F_{IO_2} of greater than 0.6 to patients who do not have artificial airways, a reservoir bag (600 to 1000 cc) can be attached to a simple face mask. A source of continuous oxygen at flow rates of 5 to 8 L/min is needed to ensure adequate distention of the bag and to flush out carbon dioxide from the mask. If there are no one-way valves on the reservoir bag, the apparatus is referred to as a *partial nonrebreathing mask* (Fig. 172-4A). Partial nonrebreathing masks can deliver oxygen in concentrations of 80 to 85%. The true nonrebreathing mask makes use of a one-way valve between the mask and the bag so that the patient can only inhale from the reservoir bag and exhale through separate valves on either side of the mask. A nonrebreathing mask is illustrated in Fig. 172-4B. A very high F_{IO_2} can be achieved when these masks fit tightly against the patient's face. However, tight-fitting molded masks, including those used to deliver continuous positive airway pressure (CPAP), are often uncomfortable and are not suitable for use for more than a few hours.

HIGH-FLOW OXYGEN DELIVERY DEVICES

High-flow oxygen delivery systems maintain the selected F_{IO_2} by incorporating a reservoir whose volume exceeds the patient's anatomic dead space or by delivering oxygen at a very high flow. In quantitative terms, the flow of all high-flow systems exceeds fourfold the patient's actual minute volume; otherwise, entrainment of room air at peak inspiration arises.

Two common clinical indications for use of a high-flow oxygen delivery system are (1) treatment of hypoxic patients who depend on their hypoxic drive to breathe but who require controlled increments in F_{IO_2} and (2) young, vigorous patients with hypoxemia who have an abnormal ventilatory pattern and whose ventilatory requirements may exceed the delivery capabilities of low-flow systems. When a clinical indication exists for a tightly controlled high F_{IO_2}, or when high flows are necessary, a high-flow delivery system should be used.

Jet-Mixing Venturi Masks

Another high-flow oxygen delivery device is the Venturi mask, the operation of which is based on the Venturi modification of the Bernoulli principle of fluid physics for gaseous jet-mixing. As illustrated in Fig. 172-5, as forward flow of inspired gas increases, the lateral pressure adjacent and perpendicular to the vector of flow decreases, resulting in entrainment of gas. In a Venturi mask, a jet of 100% oxygen flows through a fixed constrictive orifice, past open side ports, thereby entraining room air. The flow of jetting gas passing through and then out of the central orifice of the mask increases in velocity, and the resultant pressure drop along the sides of the jet draws room air into the face mask via the side ports. The amount of air entrained and, therefore, the resultant F_{IO_2}, depend on the size of the side ports and flow of oxygen. Since both of these variables are fixed, the resultant O_2-room air mixing ratio is held steady, resulting in a well-controlled, constant F_{IO_2}. Exhalation occurs through valved exhalation ports. Table 172-6 lists the range of F_{IO_2} obtainable through adjustments in the amount of entrained room air and oxygen flow (i.e., the "entrainment ratio"). The masks currently in use deliver gas with a F_{IO_2} between 0.24 and 0.50.

Since the Venturi mask reliably provides an accurate F_{IO_2} up to 0.50, it is an ideal device for use in treatment of hypoxemia in patients with COPD and chronic respiratory failure characterized by a blunted hypercarbic respiratory drive. Although the F_{IO_2} usually can be regulated precisely, technical factors can alter the value. For example, water drops may clog the oxygen injector device, resulting in changes in gas flow. In addition, development of back pressure by occluded exhalation ports may lead to decreases in the volume of entrained room air and a resultant increase in F_{IO_2}.

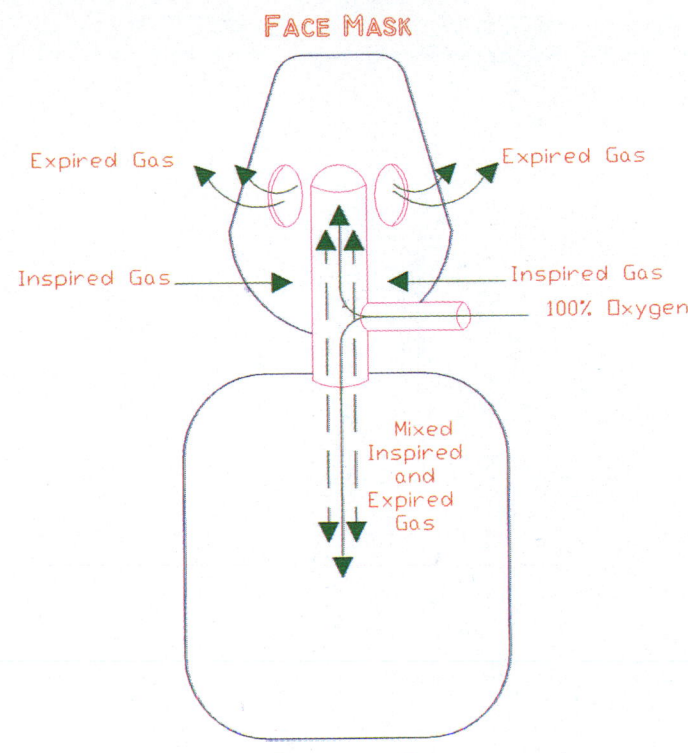

FIGURE 172-4 Mask-reservoir bag systems, illustrating airflows with partial rebreathing (A) and nonrebreathing (B) masks. Arrows indicate direction of airflow. See text for details. (Modified from Block ER, Oxygen therapy, in Fishman AP (ed), Pulmonary Diseases and Disorders, 2d ed. New York, McGraw-Hill, 1988, p 2325.)

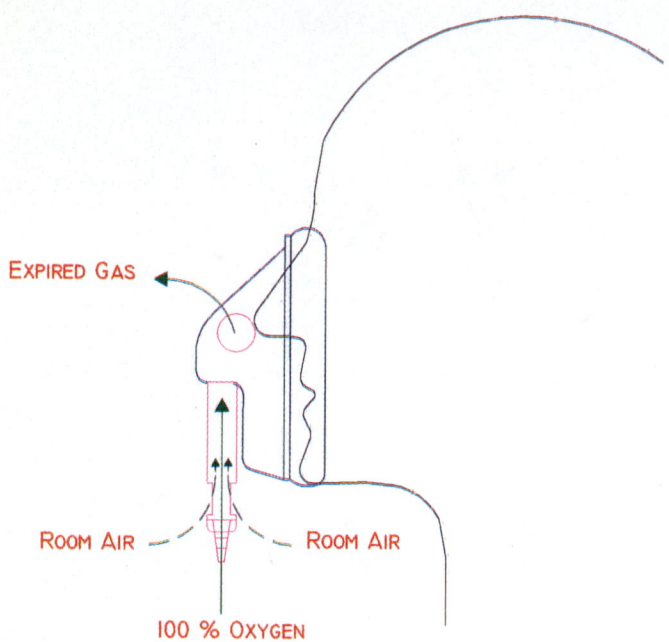

EXPIRED GAS

ROOM AIR   ROOM AIR

100 % OXYGEN

FIGURE 172-5   Venturi mask. Arrows denote direction of airflow. See text for details.

Other High-Flow Systems

Reservoir nebulizers and humidifiers are used to provide supplemental oxygen or highly humidified gas (including room air).[31,40] Provision of high humidification is often important as adjuvant management of increased airway secretions. Usually, this delivery system is combined with T-tubes or tracheostomy collars, and, therefore, its use is limited to patients with artificial airways. However, such delivery systems have also been used in combination with aerosol masks, face tents, and CPAP masks. If high-flow rates (in excess of 40 L/min) are supplied, they can usually provide a constant and predictable F_{IO_2}.

Air-oxygen blenders consist of precision metering devices that convert high-pressure wall sources of compressed air and oxygen (at 50 to 70 psi) to usable, predictable flows of up to 100 L/min at an F_{IO_2} ranging from 0.21 to 1.0. These devices also require pressure-reduction valves and an inlet pressure monitor to ensure consistency of F_{IO_2} against minor fluctuations in wall pressure. Although they provide a predictable F_{IO_2}, the devices have some disadvantages. They are noisy and require specialized personnel to set up and monitor the instrumentation.

Long-Term Oxygen Delivery Systems

A variety of modes of oxygen delivery and oxygen administration devices are available for use in the home and other chronic care settings.[42,49] Gas supplies for long-term oxygen therapy include oxygen concentrators and compressed gas or liquid oxygen sources. Most patients requiring a stationary source of supplemental oxygen use oxygen concentrators. Because the concentrators weigh about 35 lb and require wall current, their use is limited as a fixed source of oxygen. Unless patients are immobile or confined to bed, both stationary and mobile oxygen delivery systems should be employed. Both compressed gas and liquid oxygen portable systems are available, but the liquid system containers are easier to refill than high-pressure cylinders.

TABLE 172-6

Approximate Fraction of Inspired Oxygen with Low- and High-Flow Oxygen Devices*

100% O_2 Flow (L/min)	F_{IO_2}, %
Low-flow systems	
Nasal cannulae	
1	24
2	28
3	32
4	36
5	40
6	44
Transtracheal	
0.5–4	24–40
Oxygen mask	
5–6	40
6–7	50
7–8	60
Mask with reservoir bag	
6	60
7	70
8	80
9	90
10	>99
Nonrebreathing	
4–10	
0.60–1.00	
High-flow systems	
Venturi masks†	
3 (80)	0.24
6 (68)	0.28
9 (50)	0.40
12 (50)	0.40
15 (41)	0.50

* Values listed in this table are approximations based on numerous published reports and modified from Block ER: Oxygen therapy, in Fishman AP (ed), *Pulmonary Diseases and Disorders*, 2d ed. New York, McGraw-Hill, 1988, p 2324.
†Numbers in parentheses indicate total flow of entrained room air in the Venturi mixture.
NOTE: F_{IO_2} = approximate fraction of inspired oxygen.

The major disadvantages of liquid oxygen are higher cost and the requirement for pressure-relief venting.

The delivery devices for long-term oxygen therapy include most of the low-flow devices described previously. Most patients who receive chronic oxygen use nasal cannulae and flow oxygen rates of 2 to 4 L/min.

To improve the efficiency of oxygen delivery, limit the need for repetitive home delivery, and limit cost, a number of devices have been designed to "conserve" home oxygen. These include reservoir nasal cannulae, electronic demand devices, and transtracheal catheters.

The reservoir nasal cannulae has a pouch that stores 20 ml of extra oxygen during expiration and delivers the oxygen as a bolus at the onset of the next inspiration. Electronic demand devices, triggered by the onset of inspiration, deliver a pulse of oxygen early in the breath. Both types of devices are prone to failure.

Transtracheal catheters improve oxygen delivery by bypassing the anatomic dead space of the upper airway, using the upper airway as an oxygen reservoir during inspiration and expiration.[7,8,21,25] Transtracheal oxygen is delivered directly into the trachea via a hollow catheter implanted surgically under local anesthesia or inserted percutaneously using the Seldinger technique. Transtracheal catheters have been shown in numerous studies to effect reductions in total oxygen usage of 50 to 75 percent. Other advantages of transtracheal oxygen systems include their inconspicuousness, lack of nasal or facial irritation due to oxygen flow, and infrequency of catheter displacement during sleep. Disadvantages include an increased incidence of infection, development of potentially fatal "mucus balls," and catheter breakage which necessitates replacement.

PULMONARY OXYGEN TOXICITY

The potential adverse effects of exposure to increased oxygen tensions at one atmosphere can be divided into two groups: (1) alterations of normal physiological functions and (2) oxygen-mediated tissue damage.[3,13]

Physiological changes to high concentrations of oxygen involve perturbations of both pulmonary and extrapulmonary homeostasis and are easily correctable, if recognized promptly. Extrapulmonary physiological effects of hyperoxia include suppression of erythropoiesis, systemic vasoconstriction, and depression of cardiac output; these effects are usually clinically insignificant. In contrast, the pulmonary physiological effects of hyperoxia include depression of hypoxic ventilatory drive, pulmonary vasodilation, and absorption atelectasis; each is clinically relevant.

In addition to the adverse physiological effects, oxygen in high concentrations is cytotoxic. Whereas all respiring cells are potentially susceptible to the toxicity derived of hyperoxia, the major clinical adverse effects are related to lung damage.

Molecular and Cellular Mechanisms of Oxygen Toxicity

The molecular and cellular bases for tissue injury in oxygen toxicity are thought to be mediated biochemically by reactive free radicals, the formation of which directly depends on oxygen concentration.[13,16,33] Since oxygen concentration is directly proportional to partial pressure, breathing 100% O_2 at an altitude of 5000 ft (0.8 ata), 80% O_2 at sea level (1 ata), or 40% O_2 in a hyperbaric chamber (2 ata) for the same duration results in a similar toxicity profile.[9]

Aerobic cells utilize oxygen both as a metabolic substrate for the generation of ATP via the electron transport chain and as a cofactor in intermediary metabolism involving oxidation or hydroxylation of various substrates. Molecular oxygen (O_2), per se, is relatively nonreactive and nontoxic. However, modification of molecular oxygen by addition of electrons (e^-) can result in formation of highly reactive free radicals. The consequences of the sequential addition of single electrons to molecular oxygen are illustrated in the following reaction:

$$O_2 \xrightarrow{e^-} O_2^{\cdot-} \xrightarrow{e^- + 2H} H_2O_2 \xrightarrow{e^-} OH^\cdot \xrightarrow{e^- + H} H_2O \qquad (3)$$

Superoxide anion ($O_2^{\cdot-}$), hydrogen peroxide (H_2O_2), and hydroxyl radical ($OH^\cdot$) represent 1-, 2-, and 3-electron reduction products of oxygen, respectively.[4,19,33] Singlet oxygen (O_{2*}), a potent electrophile, is also generated as a byproduct of oxygen-dependent metabolism. During normal cellular metabolism, almost all molecular oxygen is completely converted to water, and the enzymes responsible for the reduction reactions (e.g., cytochrome oxidase, cytochrome P-450, dopamine-β-hydroxylase) release few or no O_2 intermediates. However, under certain conditions, these cellular enzymes, as well as others, can be misutilized by serving as incomplete electron donors (i.e., fewer than four electrons) to molecular oxygen, generating and releasing the reactive O_2 intermediates shown in Eq. (3) above.

Figure 172-6 depicts general mechanisms responsible for generation of toxic metabolites of oxygen reduction. $O_2^{\cdot-}$ (reaction 1) and H_2O_2 (reaction 2) are each generated by both enzymatic and nonenzymatic processes. Although both molecular species may have direct toxic effects, their interaction via the Haber-Weiss cycle, in the presence of metal ions (typically, Fe^{3+}), may generate hydroxyl radicals (reaction 3) which represent the most highly reactive and potentially dangerous of the O_2-derived products.

Superoxide has also clearly been shown to interact with other molecular species, e.g., nitric oxide (NO), to produce the free radical, peroxynitrite (ONOO),[-27] as illustrated in reaction 4 in Fig. 172-6. The second-order rate constant for the reaction of NO and $O_2^{\cdot-}$ to form peroxynitrite is 6.7×10^9 $M^{-1}s^{-1}$. This represents a reaction rate which is three times faster than the clearance of superoxide by superoxide dismutase.

Mechanisms of Pulmonary Cellular Toxicity

It is likely that in the lung most of the aforementioned generalized mechanisms and metabolic intermediates are operative. Hyperoxia has been shown to stimulate increases in oxygen radical production in whole rat lungs, lung mitochondria, lung microsomes, lung nuclear membranes, and in cultured pulmonary en-

$$[1] \quad O_2 + A^{2+} \longrightarrow O_2^{\cdot-} + A^{3+}$$

$$[2] \quad O_2 + H_2A \longrightarrow H_2O_2 + A$$

$$[3] \quad O_2^{\cdot-} + H_2O_2 \xrightarrow{Fe^{3+}} OH^\cdot + OH^- + O_2$$

$$[4] \quad O_2^{\cdot-} + NO \longrightarrow ONOO^-$$

FIGURE 172-6 Generation of free radicals. Mechanisms for generation of toxic species of oxygen include: (1) superoxide anion (O_2^-) generation by 1-electron reduction of molecular oxygen (O_2) through a variety of electron donors (A^{2+}); (2) hydrogen peroxide (H_2O_2) generation by 2-electron reduction of molecular oxygen, usually via enzymatic catalysis; (3) interaction of superoxide and hydrogen peroxide in the presence of metals which generate hydroxyl radical; and (4) production of peroxynitrite by diffusion-limited reaction of superoxide and NO.

dothelial cells, providing important support for the free radical hypothesis.[18,50] Likewise, peroxynitrite formation has been detected in cultured cells in some animal models of acute lung injury, as well as in infants with bronchopulmonary dysplasia.[28]

Mitochondria appear to be the major subcellular source of $O_2^{.-}$ which is produced by the oxidation of ubisemiquinone as part of the normal mitochondrial electron transport chain and by autooxidation of NADH dehydrogenase.[3,33] Additional $O_2^{.-}$ is generated by (1) the endoplasmic reticulum (and microsomes), through the autooxidation of flavins (e.g., cytochrome P-450) or other components, as well as during turnover of NADPH-cytochrome c reductase, and (2) plasma membranes, by autooxidation of cytochromes and during prostaglandin synthesis. H_2O_2 is produced at most of the aforementioned sites by the dismutation of $O_2^{.-}$ and via oxidase activity (e.g., urate oxidase) in peroxisomes. HO· is generated where concentrations of $O_2^{.-}$ and H_2O_2 are greatest, i.e., near their production sites. Because peroxynitrite is generated by a diffusion-limited reaction, it may be formed as physiological pH at any cellular sites which contain significant amounts of NO and $O_2^{.-}$.

The biochemical alterations produced by modification of cellular components by oxygen radicals and peroxynitrite are depicted in Table 172-7. Lipid peroxidation and protein oxidation are thought to represent important mechanisms of direct O_2 radical toxicity. Lipids containing unsaturated fatty acids are particularly susceptible to injury. Lipid hydroperoxides produced as intermediates are extremely toxic and can propagate the peroxidation process in an autocatalytic manner. Proteins are inactivated by reaction of radicals with sulfhydryl groups, through cross-linkage of proteins or oxidation of constituent amino acids.

Destruction of lipid and protein results in damage to cellular and organellar membranes, inactivation of key enzymes, and disruption of cellular transport mechanisms. In addition, DNA, pyridine nucleotides, and complex carbohydrates are susceptible to oxidative processes, leading to mutagenesis, growth inhibition, and alteration of intermediary metabolism. Peroxynitrite is a powerful oxidant and, as such, has been shown to oxidize many cellular components. Of particular interest is its interaction with proteins, resulting in oxidation of sulfydryl groups and formation of nitrotyrosine residues.[27]

Cellular Antioxidant Defenses

The half-life and tissue levels of most reactive oxygen species are low, in part due to an elaborate network of cellular antioxidant defenses.[3] Antioxidant mechanisms include any cellular process which: (1) prevents formation of free radicals, (2) converts oxidants to less reactive species, (3) "compartmentalizes" reactive species away from important cellular structures, or (4) initiates repair of molecular injury by free radicals.

Cellular oxygen radical defenses are classified into three basic categories: (1) enzymatic scavenging systems, which directly catalyze removal of free radicals; (2) enzyme-cofactor systems, which utilize a recyclable (renewable) intermediate to remove or prevent formation of O_2 radicals; and (3) nonenzymatic free radical scavengers, which rereduce O_2 radicals or quench radical-producing reactions.

The major enzymatic O_2 radical scavenger in the lungs is superoxide dismutase (SOD).[19] SOD is a metalloprotein present in three distinct forms, each of which has a metallic cofactor. Copper-zinc SOD is a dimeric protein which is predominantly cytosolic; manganese SOD is found mainly in mitochondria. Copper SOD, a tetrameric peptide, has been isolated from plasma. All forms of SOD catalyze the dismutation of $O_2^{.-}$ to H_2O_2 at very high rates. Hydrogen peroxide is subsequently removed enzymatically by either the glutathione (GSH) redox cycle (see below) or by catalase.

The glutathione redox cycle is the most important cellular scavenger of H_2O_2. It represents a unique system which utilizes multiple enzymes and a renewable, low-molecular-weight scavenger. Glutathione peroxidase removes both H_2O_2 and lipid peroxides at the expense of GSH oxidation. GSH is regenerated by glutathione reductase, utilizing NADPH as a cofactor.

Low-molecular-weight, nonenzymatic free radical scavengers include ascorbic acid (vitamin C), α-tocopherol (vitamin E), and β-carotene (vitamin A). These nonrecyclable compounds are derived from extrinsic (dietary) sources.

TABLE 172-7

Biochemical Alterations and Cellular Dysfunction from Free Radical Damage

Cell Component	Cellular Manifestation
Oxygen radicals	
Lipids	Damage to cell and organelle membranes
Lipid peroxidation	
Surfactant	Altered lung mechanics
Eicosanoids	Changes in cellular metabolism and intracellular signaling
Proteins	Inactivation of enzymes and transport proteins; altered cellular and intercellular permeability
Nucleic acids	Inhibition of cell growth and division
Pyridine nucleotides	Altered intermediary metabolism
Complex carbohydrates	Altered recognition of macromolecules
Peroxynitrite	
Proteins	
Nitrotyrosine formation	Inactivation of enzymes and transport proteins
Sulfhydryl group oxidation	
Nucleic acids	Cell death
8-nitroguanine formation	
Lipid peroxidation	Cell and organelle membrane damage

PATHOPHYSIOLOGY OF OXYGEN TOXICITY

The toxic effects of oxygen on the lung occur when free radical production during hyperoxic exposure overwhelms intrinsic antioxidant defenses. Excess free radicals interact with cellular components, resulting in cytotoxic events which produce a characteristic cascade of biochemical, cellular, morphologic, and physiological changes. The biochemical reactions, in turn, result in a sequence of characteristic cellular and morphologic changes.[11]

Primary Morphologic and Cellular Changes

Based primarily on data from animal models and some limited human studies, four basic phases constitute the development of oxygen toxicity in lung tissue.[11] The first three phases—initiation, inflammation, and destruction—occur during exposure to both lethal and sublethal doses of hyperoxia. The fourth phase—proliferation and fibrosis—occurs if there is reexposure to sublethal oxygen levels. If lethal exposure persists, ongoing tissue destruction and death are observed.

INITIATION PHASE

The initiation phase of oxygen toxicity comprises the first few hours and continues throughout the duration of exposure. Initiation follows short-term exposure to lethal doses of O_2 and occurs over longer periods, with sublethal hyperoxia. In each setting, the initiation phase is associated with enhanced rates of oxygen radical formation; however, there is no significant evidence of morphologic injury. Decreased rates of protein synthesis, alterations in tracheobronchial clearance of particulates, and changes in endothelial cell function have been described.

INFLAMMATORY PHASE

The earliest morphologic changes in the lung in response to hyperoxia occur as a consequence of primary cellular damage. They involve subtle changes in endothelial cell structure, resulting in pericapillary accumulation of fluid. Increased leakage from the pulmonary microcirculation via disruptions in the endothelial lining follows,[23] along with accumulation of proteinaceous fluid, formation of hyaline membranes, and an influx of inflammatory blood cell elements with release of mediators.[2] This combination of events gives rise to a pathologic picture resembling noncardiogenic pulmonary edema, including morphologic characteristics of diffuse alveolar damage—a process frequently associated with acute respiratory distress syndrome (ARDS) and other forms of lung injury (see Chapter 166).

DESTRUCTION PHASE

Overt cellular destruction begins shortly after the inflammatory phase. The earliest evidence for impending cellular destruction appears at the ultrastructural level. Observed changes in lung epithelial and endothelial cells include membrane damage, vacuolarization of cytoplasm, mitochondrial swelling, and nuclear degeneration. Soon thereafter, frank cell death is seen, and exposure of the basement membrane occurs.

PROLIFERATION AND FIBROSIS PHASE

If exposure to toxic levels of O_2 is terminated, a subacute or chronic stage, termed the *proliferative phase*, develops. The cellular proliferative response blunts the destructive phase and may enhance survival. Proliferation of type II pneumocytes occurs as alveolar remodeling takes place. In addition, an influx and proliferation of interstitial cells (fibroblasts, monocytes, and macrophages) appears to be mediated by both cytokine and autocrine factors; collagen deposition is seen as well. In baboons, lung histology and function have been shown to return to normal within 6 months of recovery from severe oxygen toxicity.[12] However, in other settings, the end result may, instead, be varying degrees of fibrosis or emphysema. The regulating factors remain to be defined.

In the aggregate, the pathophysiological and morphologic changes associated with hyperoxic stress are similar to other forms of diffuse alveolar damage. An initial inflammatory response (exudative phase) is followed by fibrosis and repair (proliferative phase), a sequence not dissimilar from other forms of ARDS.

Secondary Changes

The cellular changes which occur in response to toxic O_2 exposure also produce secondary changes in lung function. The increased capillary permeability which occurs with cellular damage results in decreased lung compliance, an increased alveolar-arterial oxygen gradient, and a decreased carbon monoxide diffusing capacity. Hyperoxia has also been reported to alter the pulmonary surfactant system. Alveolar surfactant material recovered from animals exposed to hyperoxic conditions exhibits markedly decreased surface tension-lowering capabilities.[26] One potential explanation appears to be inactivation of the biophysical activity of surfactant by serum proteins which leak into the alveolar space.

CLINICAL SYNDROMES OF OXYGEN TOXICITY

The scenario of clinical events following exposure to hyperoxic environments is summarized in Table 172-8.

Acute Toxicity: Tracheobronchitis and Acute Respiratory Distress Syndrome (ARDS)

Normal volunteers exposed to 100% O_2 experience symptoms within 12 to 24 h. The earliest manifestations represent effects on the tracheobronchial mucosa and include substernal chest pain and nonproductive cough.[38] Measurements of tracheobronchial function show decreased particle clearance as early as 6 h after the start of exposure to 100% O_2.[45] Systemic symptoms, including malaise, nausea, anorexia, and headache may be seen.

The onset of acute pulmonary oxygen toxicity usually follows an asymptomatic period during which no physiological changes are seen. In nine male subjects who breathed 100% O_2 for 6 to 12 h, no abnormalities were noted in the alveolar-arterial oxygen gradient, pulmonary artery pressure, vascular resistance, cardiac output, pulmonary extravascular lung water, or chest radio-

TABLE 172-8

Sequence of Pulmonary Changes during Hyperoxic Exposure in Humans

F_{IO_2} at 1 atm	Exposure Duration	Manifestation
1.0	>12 h	Decreased tracheobronchial clearance, decreased forced vital capacity, cough, chest pain
	>24 h	Altered endothelial function
	>36 h	Increased alveolar-arterial oxygen gradient, decreased carbon monoxide diffusing capacity
	>48 h	Increasing alveolar permeability, pulmonary edema, surfactant inactivation
	>60 h	Adult respiratory distress syndrome
0.6	7 days	Mild chest discomfort without changes in lung mechanics, possible changes in morphometry
0.24–0.28	Months	Subclinical pathologic changes, no clinical toxicity documented

graph.[52] By 24 h, the vital capacity has been shown to decrease significantly; at 48 h of exposure to 98% oxygen, decrements in static compliance and carbon monoxide diffusing capacity are seen.[5,24,33] In patients with irreversible brain damage given 100% O_2, the alveolar-arterial gradient increased precipitously after 40 to 60 h.[1] The longest voluntary exposure to 100% O_2 reported is 110 h; the subject developed severe dyspnea, a marked decrease in pulmonary function, and acute respiratory failure.

Chronic Pulmonary Syndromes

Although not well understood in humans, the subacute and chronic phases of oxygen toxicity are well documented in animals and appear to be related to dose and duration of exposure. The best known clinical syndrome of chronic pulmonary oxygen toxicity occurs in newborns receiving oxygen for treatment of neonatal respiratory distress syndrome. Persistent morphologic changes with healing may produce the chronic disorder bronchopulmonary dysplasia.[3] The effects of long-term exposure of adults to inspired oxygen concentrations of 60 to 100% are less clear, although morphometric changes after 13 days of exposure in brain-dead patients have been described. Data on longer exposures, including exposure to lower levels of inspired oxygen, are unavailable.

DIAGNOSIS

Pulmonary oxygen toxicity develops insidiously after a variable lag period during which the biochemical and cellular changes previously described occur. Early clinical detection of oxygen toxicity during this lag period is impossible, and tests to identify biochemical changes (e.g., lipid peroxidation) would improve diagnostic accuracy. However, such tests are currently unavailable for clinical use. Although reversible (early) physiological, anatomic, and biochemical changes can be detected following short exposure to hyperoxia, humans can tolerate 100% oxygen at sea level for 24 h without serious pulmonary injury. Currently, the diagnosis of oxygen poisoning depends on a nonspecific symptom complex or abnormal pulmonary function in the proper clinical setting.

SYMPTOMS AND SIGNS

Development of chest pain, tachypnea, or cough in a patient breathing elevated concentrations of oxygen should alert the clinician to the possibility of oxygen toxicity. There may be no better index of oxygen toxicity than the individual's subjective symptom of retrosternal chest pain.[38] Unfortunately, in critically ill patients requiring mechanical ventilation or who have altered mental status, detection of subjective complaints is difficult or impossible. On physical examination, the presence of crackles suggestive of interstitial or alveolar edema may be noted as a nonspecific finding.

PULMONARY FUNCTION TESTS

Decreases in vital capacity, pulmonary compliance, or carbon monoxide diffusing capacity, as well as a widening of the alveolar-arterial oxygen gradient, have been observed during hyperoxic exposures.[5,24] Monitoring serial changes in vital capacity has been proposed as a means of detecting and following injury from oxygen exposure. However, the practicality and cost-effectiveness of such testing remains unsubstantiated.

RADIOGRAPHIC CHANGES

The chest radiographic findings of increased interstitial markings or alveolar filling are similar to those found in other causes of diffuse alveolar damage; the findings are nonspecific and are insensitive as early markers.

Potentiation of Oxygen Toxicity

Susceptibility of cells or organisms to oxygen toxicity can be modified by factors other than intrinsic cellular antioxidant mechanisms. Many therapeutic drugs act synergistically with hyperoxia, accelerating free radical production and worsening oxygen toxicity. Bleomycin has been shown to increase lung injury and fibrosis through enhanced production of $O_2^{\cdot-}$.[35] Potentiation of oxygen toxicity by disulfiram occurs through inhibition of cytosolic superoxide dismutase by diethyldithiocarbamate, which is produced in vivo from the conversion (reduction) of disulfiram.[3] The metabolism of nitrofurantoin and paraquat result in production of superoxide or hydroxyl radicals, and O_2 has been shown to increase their cytotoxicity.[47] Variability of dietary intake can also modify oxygen tolerance. Protein malnutrition, as well as dietary deficiency of any of the antioxidant quenchers, may alter the response to hyperoxia.[15] Protein deficiency is thought to potentiate toxicity from hyperoxia due to a lack of sulfur-containing amino acids which are crucial for glutathione synthesis. The adverse effects of vitamin A and vitamin E deficiencies are also well described.

Prevention and Therapy

As with other drugs, oxygen should be administered judiciously, in doses designed to achieve therapeutic efficacy with limited toxicity.[3] Because early detection of O_2 toxicity has remained elusive and specific therapy is lacking, avoidance of pulmonary toxicity during oxygen therapy remains the cornerstone of management. The best approach is to monitor the efficacy of the inspired oxygen concentration and to adhere to guidelines to use doses that have not been found to be associated with major side effects.

The primary therapeutic goal associated with use of supplemental oxygen is assurance of adequate tissue oxygenation without use of toxic levels of F_{IO_2}. A significant obstacle in achieving this goal centers around monitoring the efficacy of oxygen therapy and assessing the adequacy of tissue oxygenation. As noted previously, in most clinical settings, exclusion of arterial hypoxemia as a cause of tissue hypoxia and quantitation of the response to supplemental oxygen administration through measurement of Pa_{O_2} are the mainstays of monitoring. In recent years, substitution of continuous, cutaneous, infrared pulse oximetry has become standard.[46]

Extrapolations about the state of tissue oxygenation from measurement of $\bar{v}_{O_2}$ using an indwelling pulmonary artery catheter can be used in the critical care setting. Transcutaneous estimations of tissue P_{O_2} and, hence, intracellular oxygen sufficiency, remain experimental. Based upon general consensus, the following guidelines can be offered regarding oxygen administration at 1 atmosphere.

Oxygen in concentrations up to 100% can be administered during cardiopulmonary resuscitation and in the transport and initial management of critically ill patients. In patients who are not on mechanical ventilation, evidence of respiratory depression should be monitored. If needed, an F_{IO_2} of 1.0 can be used for up to 24 h without significant lung injury. During this period, management should be directed toward improving pulmonary gas exchange, optimizing oxygen delivery, and limiting tissue metabolic demands so that inspired O_2 concentration can be decreased to the lowest possible levels.

Oxygen at an F_{IO_2} 0.5 or less can be administered safely to most patients for weeks, although factors specific to individual patients (e.g., prior bleomycin use) may dictate a lower tolerance. The maximal safe duration for oxygen exposures between an F_{IO_2} of 0.5 and 1.0 is less certain, although these concentrations probably can be tolerated longer than 24 h. The upper safe limit of F_{IO_2} for chronic O_2 therapy in the ambulatory setting is largely undefined.

SUMMARY

The ability to provide supplemental oxygen is a powerful tool in the management of the critically ill patient, but it represents a double-edged sword. Commensurate with initiation of its use for management of patients with hypoxia, a careful assessment for the underlying etiology and for specific therapeutic measures aimed at reversal of the pathophysiological events should be undertaken. The proper prescription of oxygen is based upon general principles that are applied to the administration of any other drug. Knowledge of the various techniques of oxygen administration, establishment of clear therapeutic endpoints, monitoring of the efficacy of treatment, and awareness of the potential toxicity of oxygen are required.

REFERENCES

1. Barber RE, Lee J, Hamilton WK: Oxygen toxicity in man: A prospective study in patients with irreversible brain damage. *New Eng J Med* 283:1478–1484, 1970.
2. Barry B, Crapo JD: Patterns of accumulation of platelets and neutrophils in rat lungs during exposure to 100% and 85% oxygen. *Am Rev Resp Dis* 132:548–555, 1985.
3. Beers MF, Fisher AB: Oxygen toxicity, in Carlson RW, Geheb MA (eds), *The Principles and Practice of Medical Intensive Care.* Philadelphia, Saunders, 1992, chap 86.
4. Boveris A, Oshino N, Chance B: The cellular production of hydrogen peroxide. *Biochem J* 128:617–630, 1972.
5. Caldwell PRB, Lee WL, Schildkraut HS, Archibald ER: Changes in lung volume, diffusing capacity, and blood gases in men breathing oxygen. *J Appl Physiol* 21:1477–1483, 1966.
6. Chance B: Reactions of oxygen with the respiratory chain in cells and tissues. *Gen Physiol* 49:163–178, 1965.
7. Christopher K, Spofford BT, Petrun MD, et al: A program of transtracheal oxygen delivery: Assessment of safety and efficacy. *Ann Int Med* 802–808, 1987.
8. Christopher K, Spofford BT, Brannin P, Petty T: Transtracheal oxygen delivery. *JAMA* 256:494–497, 1986.
9. Comroe JH, Dripps RD, Dumke PR, Deming M: Oxygen toxicity. The effects of inhalation of high concentrations of oxygen on normal men at sea level and at a simulated altitude of 18,000 feet. *JAMA* 128:710–717, 1945.
10. Cottrell JJ, Openbrier D, Lave JR, et al: Home oxygen therapy: A comparison of a 2- vs 6-month reevaluation. *Chest* 107:358–361, 1995.
11. Crapo JD: Morphological changes in pulmonary oxygen toxicity. *Ann Rev Physiol* 48:721–731, 1986.
12. De los Santos R, Seidenfeld JJ, Anzueto A: One hundred percent oxygen lung injury in adult baboons. *Am Rev Resp Dis* 136:657–661, 1987.
13. Denke SM, Fanburg BL: Normobaric oxygen toxicity of the lung. *New Engl J Med* 303:76–86, 1980.
14. Duveen DI: Lavoisier, in *Readings from Scientific American. Scientific Genius and Creativity.* New York, Freeman, 1982, pp 35–39.
15. Fanburg BL, Deneke SM: Protein deficiency potentiates oxygen toxicity. *Exp Lung Res* 14:911–919, 1988.
16. Fisher AB: Molecular mechanisms of pulmonary oxygen toxicity. *Appl Cardiovasc Pathophysiol* 3:121–127, 1989.
17. Fitzgerald JM, Baynham R, Powles ACP: Use of oxygen therapy for adult patients outside the critical care areas of a university hospital. *Lancet* 1:983, 1988.

18. Freeman BA, Crapo JD: Hyperoxia increases oxygen radical production in rat lungs and lung mitochondria. *J Biol Chem* 256:10986–10992, 1981.

19. Fridovich IA: Superoxide dismutases. *Ann Rev Biochem* 44: 147–159, 1975.

20. Fulmer JD, Snider GL: ACCP-NHLBI national conference on oxygen therapy. *Chest* 86:234–247, 1984.

21. Gibson RL, Comer PB, Beckham RW, McGraw CP: Actual tracheal oxygen concentrations with commonly used oxygen equipment. *Anesthesiology* 44:71–73, 1976.

22. Hanaford M, Kraft M, Make BJ: Long-term oxygen therapy in patients with chronic obstructive pulmonary disease. *Sem Resp Med* 14:496–514, 1993.

23. Hansen-Flaschen JH, Lanken PN, Pietra GG, et al: Effect of 100% O_2 on passage of uncharged dextrans from blood to lung lymph. *Am J Physiol* 60:1797–1809, 1986.

24. Harabin AL, Homer LD, Weathersby PK, Flynn ET: An analysis of decrements in vital capacity as an index of pulmonary oxygen toxicity. *J Appl Physiol* 63:1130–1135, 1987.

25. Hoffman LA, Dauber JH, Ferson PF, et al: Patient response to transtracheal oxygen delivery. *Am Rev Resp Dis* 135:153–156, 1987.

26. Holm BA, Notter RH, Matalon S: Pulmonary physiological and surfactant changes during injury and recovery from hyperoxia. *J Appl Physiol* 59(5):1402–1409, 1985.

27. Ischiropoulous H, Beckman JS, Crow JP, et al: Detection of peroxinitrite. *Methods: A Comparison to Methods in Enzymology* 7:109–115, 1995.

28. Ischiropoulous H, Al-Mehdi AB, Fisher AB: Reactive species in rat lung injury: contribution of peroxinitrite. *Am J Physiol. Lung Cell Mol Physiol* L158–L164, 1995.

29. Jeffrey AA, Ray S, Douglas NJ: Accuracy of inpatient oxygen administration. *Thorax* 44:1036–1037, 1989.

30. Kacmarek RM, Stoller JK (eds): *Current Respiratory Care.* Toronto, Decker, 1988.

31. Leach RM, Bateman NT: Acute oxygen therapy. *Br J Hosp Med* 49:637–644, 1993.

32. Levi-Valensi P, Weitzenbaum E, Pedinelli JL, et al: Three month follow-up of arterial blood gas determinations in candidates for long term oxygen therapy. *Am Rev Resp Dis* 133:547–551, 1986.

33. Lodato RF: Oxygen toxicity. *Crit Care Clin* 6:749–765, 1990.

34. Lorrain-Smith J: The pathological effects due to increase of oxygen tension in the air breathed. *J Physiol* 24:19–35, 1899.

35. Martin WJ II, Kachel DL: Bleomycin-induced pulmonary endothelial injury: Evidence for the role of iron catalyzed toxic oxygen-derived species. *J Lab Clin Med* 110:153–158, 1987.

36. Meakins J: Observations on the gases in human arterial blood in certain pathological pulmonary conditions, and their treatment with oxygen. *J Pathol Bacteriol* 24:79–90, 1921.

37. Medical Research Council Working Party: Long-term domiciliary oxygen therapy in chronic hypoxic cor pulmonale complicating chronic bronchitis and emphysema. *Lancet* 1:681–686, 1981.

38. Montgomery AB, Luce JM, Murray JF: Retrosternal pain is an early indicator of oxygen toxicity. *Am Rev Resp Dis* 139:1548–1550, 1989.

39. Nocturnal Oxygen Therapy Trial Group: Continuous or nocturnal oxygen therapy in hypoxemic chronic obstructive lung disease. A clinical trial. *Ann Intern Med* 93:391–398, 1980.

40. O'Connor BS, Vender JS: Oxygen therapy. *Crit Care Clin* 11:67–78, 1995.

41. O'Donohue WJ, Plummer AL: Magnitude of usage and cost of home oxygen therapy in the United States. *Chest* 107:301–302, 1995.

42. Pethy TL: Home oxygen therapy. *Mayo Clin Proc* 62:841–847, 1987.

43. Priestley J: Experiments and observations on different kinds of air, vol 2. London, J Johnson (printer), 1775.

44. Rawles JM, Kenmura ACF: Controlled trial of oxygen in uncomplicated myocardial infarction. *Br Med J* 1:1121–1124, 1976.

45. Sackner MA, Landa J, Hirsch J, Zapata A: Pulmonary effects of oxygen breathing: 6 hour study in normal men. *Ann Intern Med* 82:40–43, 1975.

46. Schnapp LM, Cohen NH: Pulse oximetry: Uses and abuses. *Chest* 98:1244–1250, 1990.

47. Shibutani K, Komatsu T, Hubal K, et al: Critical level of oxygen delivery in anesthetized man. *Crit Care Med* 11:640–646, 1983.

48. Smith LL: Mechanism of paraquat toxicity in lung and its relevance to treatment. *Hum Toxicol* 6:31–36, 1987.

49. Tarpey SP, Celli BR: Long-term oxygen therapy. *N Engl J Med* 333:710–714, 1995.

50. Turrens JF, Freeman BA, Crapo JD: Hyperoxia increases H_2O_2 release by lung mitochondria and microsomes. *Arch Biochem Biophys* 217:411–421, 1982.

51. Van de Water JN, Kagey KS, Miller IT, et al: Response of the lung to 6 to 12 hours of 100 percent oxygen inhalation in normal man. *New Engl J Med* 283:621–626, 1970.

52. Youngberg T, Myers RAM, Piantadosi CA: Use of hyberbaric oxygen in carbon monoxide, cyanide, and sulfide intoxication, in Camporesi EM, Barker AC (eds), *Hyperbaric Oxygen Therapy: A Critical Review.* Bethesda, MD, Undersea and Hyperbaric Medical Society, 1991, pp 23–53.

CHAPTER 173

PULMONARY PHARMACOTHERAPY

Scott Manaker / Karen J. Tietze / Eric T. Wittbrodt

BRONCHODILATORS
  Beta-adrenergic Agonists
  Anticholinergics
  Methylxanthines
  Magnesium Sulfate
  Inhaled Diuretics

ANTI-INFLAMMATORY AGENTS
  Corticosteroids
  Corticosteroid-Sparing Agents
  Mast Cell Stabilizers
  Leukotriene Antagonists and Inhibitors

MUCOKINETIC AGENTS
  Dornase Alpha
  N-Acetylcysteine
  Iodinated Agents
  Sodium Bicarbonate
  Guaifenesin

PHYSIOLOGICAL REPLACEMENTS
  Alpha$_1$-Antitrypsin
  Pulmonary Surfactant

RESPIRATORY STIMULANTS
  Acetazolamide
  Almitrine
  Methylxanthines
  Doxapram
  Medroxyprogesterone
  Protriptyline

A wide spectrum of therapeutic agents are currently employed in the treatment of respiratory disorders, including obstructive lung diseases. This chapter reviews the rationale for, and clinical use of, these agents in current clinical practice. A brief discussion of potentially useful therapeutic drug strategies for the future is also provided.

BRONCHODILATORS

Pharmacologic management of obstructive airway diseases is based heavily upon bronchodilation produced by beta-adrenergic agonists, muscarinic antagonists, and methylxanthines. These three classes of agents are often used in combination. In addition, magnesium and inhaled diuretics may ultimately prove to be effective bronchodilators suitable for clinical use.

Beta-adrenergic Agonists

The beta-adrenergic agonists mimic the actions of norepinephrine at neuroeffector and synaptic junctions. Norepinephrine is the major neurotransmitter in the sympathetic nervous system; therefore, this class of drugs is referred to as *adrenergic agonists,* or *sympathomimetics.* Adrenergic receptor stimulation catalyzes the conversion of adenosine triphosphate (ATP) to cyclic-3'5'-adenosine monophosphate (cAMP) by activating adenyl cyclase, a cofactor in the production of cAMP. The increase in cAMP triggers the intracellular events that mediate pulmonary and extrapulmonary responses. The two major types of adrenergic receptors are the alpha and beta receptors; at least two alpha and two beta receptor subtypes have been identified. The beta-adrenergic agonists (Table 173-1) are indicated in the treatment of bronchospasm associated with acute and chronic asthma, bronchitis, emphysema, exercise, and other obstructive pulmonary diseases. Selection of a specific agent and route of administration depends on underlying patient risk factors and the receptor specificity of the drug.

PHARMACOLOGY

Adrenergic receptor stimulation produces a wide range of responses, depending on the effector organ and the specific receptor. Although bronchial smooth-muscle relaxation results from beta$_2$-adrenergic receptor stimulation, none of the currently marketed agonists are completely specific for beta$_2$-adrenergic receptors; many of the agents have significant alpha- and/or beta$_1$-adrenergic agonist activity.

The alpha-adrenergic receptor is generally associated with constrictor/contractor responses, including constriction of arteries and veins and contraction of the uterus, radial and sphincter muscles of the iris, and urinary bladder and stomach sphincters. Beta$_1$-adrenergic receptor stimulation increases heart rate, atrial and ventricular contractility, and cardiac conduction velocity. Effects from beta$_2$-adrenergic receptor stimulation include relaxation of bronchial and uterine smooth muscle, dilatation of ar-

TABLE 173-1

Adrenergic Agonists

Agent	Receptor Activity			Duration, h	Inhaled		Dosage Forms Injection	Oral		
	Alpha	Beta₁	Beta₂		MDI	Neb		IR	SR	Syrup
Catecholamines										
Ephedrine	+	+	+	Short			X	X		X
Epinephrine	+	+	+	Very short	X	X	X			
Isoproterenol		+	+	Short	X	X	X	X*		X
Isoetharine		+	+	Short	X	X				
Bitolterol	±	+++		Short	X	X				
Resorcinols										
Metaproterenol		+	++	Short	X	X		X		X
Terbutaline		±	+++	Short	X		X	X		
Saligenins										
Albuterol		±	+++	Short†	X‡	X		X	X	X
Salmeterol		±	+++	Long	X					
Other										
Pirbuterol		±	+++	Short	X					

Duration: short = 2 to 6 h; long = 8 to 12 h.
*Sublingual tablets.
†Longer duration of action with sustained-release oral dosage form.
‡Albuterol marketed as a powder for inhalation.
MDI = metered dose inhaler; Neb = solution for nebulization; IR = immediate release; SR = sustained release; X = marketed dosage formulation; ± = minimal effect; + = mild effect; ++ = considerable effect; +++ = major effect.

teries and veins, and several metabolic effects, including glycogenolysis, gluconeogenesis, and induction of hepatic pancreatic beta cell secretion.

STRUCTURE-ACTIVITY RELATIONSHIPS

The parent compound for the adrenergic agonists, phenylethylamine (Fig. 173-1), consists of a benzene ring and an ethylamine side chain. Substituents can be added to the alpha or the beta carbons of the ethylamine side chain, to the terminal amine group, or to one or more of the carbons in the aromatic ring.

The basic chemical structures of the adrenergic agonists include the catecholamines, the resorcinols, the saligenins, and the pyridines (Fig. 173-1). The catecholamines, epinephrine and ephedrine, with hydroxyls at positions 3 and 4 of the aromatic ring and a small methyl group on the terminal amine, were the first adrenergic agonists to be marketed. Epinephrine and ephedrine are short-acting drugs with alpha-, beta₁-, and beta₂-adrenergic receptor activity. Bitolterol, an inactive prodrug, was created in an attempt to produce a long-acting beta₂-receptor-selective drug. However, bitolterol acts only slightly longer than the other short-acting catecholamines (4 to 6 h versus 2 to 3 h) and is not considered a long-acting drug. The resorcinols (metaproterenol and terbutaline) have hydroxyls at positions 3 and 5 of the aromatic ring. Terbutaline, with a large substituent on the terminal amine, is selective for beta₂-adrenergic receptors. The saligenins (albuterol and salmeterol) have a hydroxyl at position 4, various carbon moieties on position 3 of the aromatic ring, and large substituents on the terminal

amine. These large substituents confer a longer duration of action and beta₂-adrenergic receptor specificity, particularly for salmeterol. Salmeterol's long side chain results in increased lipophilicity, protecting the structure from metabolism by catechol-o-methyl transferase and allowing the compound to bind both to the beta-receptor and to an adjacent exo-receptor site. The exo-receptor binding site anchors the drug close to the beta-receptor, further prolonging its action. Pirbuterol differs from all other adrenergic agonists in that the aromatic ring is a pyridine, instead of a benzene.

DRUG DELIVERY

The beta-adrenergic agonists may be administered systemically or by inhalation; however, not all drugs are marketed in every dosage form. Systemic dosage forms include oral, subcutaneous, and intravenous preparations. Systemic administration decreases the beta₂-adrenergic receptor selectivity of the drug due to exposure to various metabolic enzymes, including catechol-o-methyl transferase, monoamine oxidase, and sulfatase. These enzymes change the chemical structure of the drug, decreasing the beta₂-adrenergic receptor selectivity and increasing the risk of side effects. The oral route of administration is generally reserved for patients who cannot successfully use metered-dose inhalers (e.g., children or the elderly). Sustained-release, oral dosage forms may be useful in controlling nocturnal symptoms of asthma, although not as effectively as the long-acting, inhaled adrenergic agonists.[5] The subcutaneous route is generally reserved for patients too dyspneic to inhale the drug, and parenteral

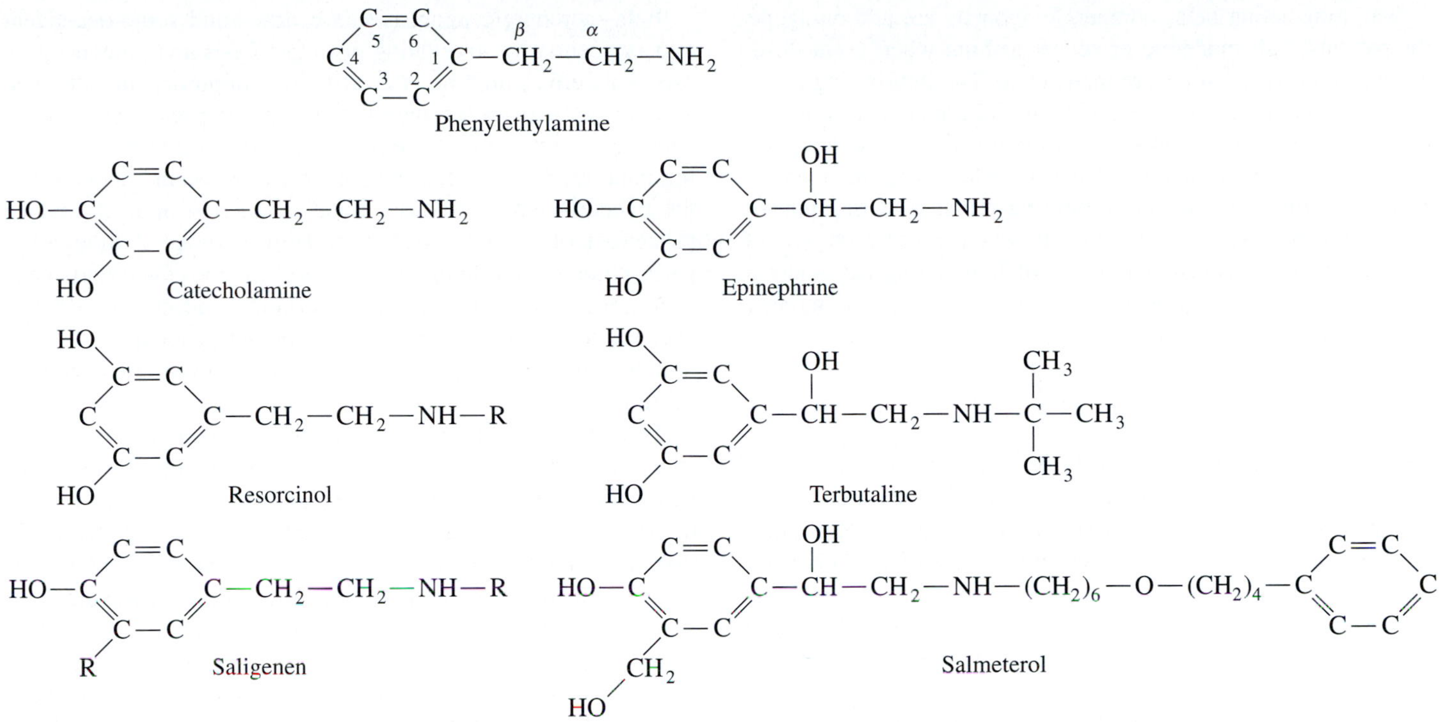

FIGURE 173-1   Structures of adrenergic agonists.

drug administration is generally employed for pediatric patients.

The preferred route of beta-adrenergic agonist administration is by inhalation. Local application of small amounts of drug directly to the airways decreases the amount available for systemic absorption, minimizing systemic side effects. Inhaled beta-adrenergic agonists are available in several dosage forms, including wet aerosols, aerosols from metered-dose inhalers, and dry powder forms. Most commonly, wet aerosols are delivered by jet or ultrasonic nebulizer, whereas metered-dose inhalers are primarily marketed as "press and breathe" devices. Historically, nebulized drug delivery was standard practice for children, emergency treatment of asthma exacerbations, hospitalized patients, and severely obstructed patients. However, nebulized drug delivery is labor-intensive; significant cost savings can be realized, without sacrificing efficacy, by using metered-dose inhalers coupled with spacer devices.[4] Patients too dyspneic or tachypneic to control their inspiratory flow to coordinate the devices respond best to nebulized drug delivery.

Drug delivery by metered-dose inhaler is highly dependent on administration technique. Less than 10 percent of the dose is delivered to the lung using optimal inhalation technique; the rest of the drug is deposited in the mouth. Spacer devices eliminate the split-second timing necessary with proper metered dose inhaler technique and decrease the amount of drug deposited in the oropharynx (an important factor with inhaled corticosteroids); however, they do not provide a therapeutic advantage over correct use of a metered dose inhaler alone.[12]

CLINICAL USE

The beta$_2$-adrenergic agonists are considered first-line drugs in the treatment of both asthma and chronic obstructive pulmonary disease. In asthma, the short acting inhaled beta$_2$-adrenergic ag-

onists are preferred for treating acute symptoms and for preventing exercise-induced bronchospasm. The subcutaneous route of administration is generally reserved for patents unresponsive to frequent, high-dose, inhaled beta$_2$-adrenergic agonists; uncooperative patients; or patients too severely dyspneic to inhale the dose. Subcutaneous or parenteral administration should not be used in patients with angina or a recent history of myocardial infarction. Oral adrenergic agonists may be appropriate for children too young to cooperate with inhaled drug administration; sustained-release, oral adrenergic agonists decrease nocturnal symptoms, but they are less effective than long-acting beta$_2$-adrenergic agonists.

Although the indications for beta$_2$-adrenergic agonists in chronic obstructive pulmonary disease are less well defined, beta$_2$-adrenergic agonists provide modest symptomatic relief and improvement in pulmonary function. Standard doses of inhaled beta$_2$-adrenergic agonists appear as effective as inhaled anticholinergic drugs for relief of acute exacerbations of chronic obstructive pulmonary disease. The value of subcutaneous drugs, of high-dose, short-acting agents, or of long-acting inhaled drugs in the management of chronic obstructive pulmonary disease has not been determined.

The intensity and duration of response to beta$_2$-adrenergic agonists is dose- and frequency-dependent. For patients with asthma, higher doses result in incrementally greater bronchodilation. The dose-response relationships are less well defined for chronic obstructive pulmonary disease. The dose-response curve in asthma led to the development of intensive inhaled beta$_2$-adrenergic agonist drug regimens for the treatment of severe, acute exacerbations. Typically, the nebulized drug is administered every 20 min for three to six doses; some patients respond better to continuous nebulized drug delivery. These regimens are generally well tolerated, although cardiac stimulation is common.

The long-acting beta$_2$-adrenergic agonists are add-on agents for patients with moderate or severe asthma when usual doses of inhaled corticosteroids are inadequate. The long-acting beta$_2$-adrenergic agonists are also considered alternate add-on agents for patients with symptoms of nocturnal asthma. The long-acting beta$_2$-adrenergic agonists have no role in the treatment of acute symptoms; all patients should have a short-acting inhaler and should be instructed on how and when to use each type of beta$_2$-adrenergic agonist. The value of long-acting beta$_2$-adrenergic agonists in the treatment of chronic obstructive pulmonary disease remains undefined.

TOLERANCE

Tolerance, or receptor subsensitivity, is defined as a decreased response to receptor stimulation. Although tolerance to the nonbronchodilator effects of beta-adrenergic agonists, including tremor, tachycardia, prolongation of the QT_C interval on the electrocardiogram, hypoglycemia, hypokalemia, and vasodilator response, has been demonstrated, data on tolerance to the bronchodilator effects of beta-adrenergic agonists are limited and conflicting.[18] Differences in study design, including severity of illness, duration of treatment, lack of run-in periods, dose, and use of concomitant disease-modifying drugs, such as corticosteroids, make comparison of individual studies difficult.

The risk of tolerance to the bronchodilating or antibronchoconstrictor effects of the beta$_2$-adrenergic agonists may depend on the duration of action of the drug. Tolerance to the long-acting drugs may make patients less responsive to short-acting beta$_2$-adrenergic agonists during an acute attack or may mask inadequate control of inflammation. Although the mechanism for tolerance to the long-acting drugs has not been precisely identified, one hypothesis is that prolonged drug-receptor interaction may induce receptor down-regulation. In vitro data support this hypothesis; however, the same data suggest that receptor affinity is increased, potentially compensating for the receptor down-regulation.[39] Concomitant disease-modifying drug therapy (e.g., corticosteroids) may also modify the development of tolerance by modulating adrenoceptor function. More data are needed to clarify the issue of tolerance to both the short-acting and long-acting beta$_2$-adrenergic agonists.

SAFETY

The beta$_2$-selective adrenergic agonists are first-line agents in the management of obstructive airway diseases. The beta$_2$-selective adrenergic agonists produce less cardiovascular toxicity than do the nonselective agents, but beta$_2$-selectivity does not protect from all adverse events. Biochemical abnormalities associated with the beta$_2$-adrenergic agonists include hyperglycemia, hyperinsulinemia, lipolysis, hypokalemia, hypomagnesemia, and lactic acidosis.[19] These side effects are most pronounced with parenteral and oral drug administration; they are minimal with usual doses of inhaled agents. Furthermore, the biochemical abnormalities are more pronounced in drug-naive normal volunteers than in asthmatic patients, suggesting that tolerance develops following chronic drug administration.

Beta$_2$-adrenergic agonists cause dose- and route-dependent hyperglycemia by stimulating glycogenolysis and gluconeogenesis. This effect may be clinically most important in asthmatic patients with diabetes mellitus or during pregnancy. Beta$_2$-adrenergic agonists increase plasma insulin by directly stimulating pancreatic islet cells; indirect increases occur secondary to the hyperglycemic response. Beta$_2$-adrenergic agonists induce the release of free fatty acids from adipose tissue. Although hyperinsulinemia and high concentrations of free fatty acids have been linked with cardiovascular morbidity and mortality, tolerance minimizes these effects. Beta$_2$-adrenergic receptor stimulation also induces muscle glycogenolysis, increasing lactate production.

The beta$_2$-adrenergic agonists induce hypokalemia by directly stimulating the uptake of potassium into skeletal muscle cells. Fenoterol, a selective beta$_2$-adrenergic agonist not marketed in the United States, has a greater tendency to induce hypokalemia than salbutamol or terbutaline.[53] Beta$_2$-adrenergic receptor stimulation induces the cellular uptake of magnesium; hypomagnesemia may induce arrhythmias or worsen symptoms of coronary artery disease. Other adverse beta$_2$-adrenergic agonist effects include: (1) an increased baseline tremor by creating an imbalance in fast- and slow-twitch muscle groups; (2) tachycardia by direct chronotropy and through reflex peripheral vasodilatation and decreased venous return; and (3) central nervous symptoms, such as appetite suppression, headache, nausea, and sleep disturbances. The nervousness reported by many patients is probably a response to the peripheral tremors rather than a result of direct stimulation of the central nervous system.

Beta-adrenergic agonist use has increased coincident with the increase in asthma morbidity and mortality in the United States and other countries. This observation has promoted interest in the possible relationship between asthma mortality and use of these agents. The first link between the beta-adrenergic agonists and an increase in asthma morbidity and mortality was made during the 1960s when the newly marketed nonselective beta-adrenergic agonist, isoproterenol, was associated with an increase in asthma morbidity and mortality in the United Kingdom. Although never conclusively proved, the increase in asthma morbidity and mortality was blamed partly on the lipolytic effect of the drug, which increases the potential for myocardial ischemia, and partly on the high-dose formulation.[47] A second link between the beta-adrenergic agonists and increased morbidity and mortality from asthma was made in the 1970s when fenoterol was linked to an increased death rate in New Zealand. Although never conclusively proved, part of the increased mortality was attributed to the hypokalemic effect of fenoterol.

Interest in the association between regular use of short-acting and long-acting beta-adrenergic agonists and asthma morbidity and mortality was heightened by several reports that use of multiple fenoterol or albuterol inhalers per month was associated with an increased risk of death. A subsequent meta-analysis of case-control studies reported only a very weak, although statistically significant, relationship between the use of nebulized beta-agonists and death from asthma.[37] Although this weak relationship was more likely in adults than in adolescents, data from large, well-designed trials are needed to assess accurately the risk of death associated with long-acting beta-adrenergic agonists. Although currently available data do not support an association between the use of short-acting beta-adrenergic agonist and an increased risk of death,[11] deaths have been reported in patients who unsuccessfully used a long-acting beta-agonist to treat acute symptoms of asthma.

Anticholinergics

Atropine and other anticholinergic alkaloids from plant extracts have been used for thousands of years to relieve respiratory symptoms in humans with airway diseases. Atropine, a prototypic anticholinergic antagonist, is nonselective for the five different molecular forms of muscarinic receptors described to date. Historically, clinical use of atropine and atropinelike agents has been limited by anticholinergic side effects, including dry mouth and skin, tachycardia, and meiosis; higher doses produce difficulties in speaking, swallowing, urinating, and mentating, as well as other neurologic side effects. Therapeutic doses of atropine invariably produce side effects, and patients with glaucoma and bladder outlet obstruction are quite sensitive to these effects.

PHARMACOLOGY

In an effort to avoid systemic side effects, a series of quaternary ammonium congeners of atropine were developed, ultimately leading to the identification of ipratropium bromide. Like other quaternary ammonium compounds, ipratropium bromide is poorly absorbed and does not cross the blood-brain barrier, markedly reducing the potential for systemic side effects. Upon inhalation, what little ipratropium bromide is absorbed is rapidly excreted. Initially approved for clinical use in Europe in 1974, approval was delayed in Canada until 1981 and in the United States until 1987. Ipratropium bromide is available by both metered-dose inhaler and nebulizer solution.

Inhalation of ipratropium bromide produces bronchodilation in seconds to minutes, with a peak effect after 1 to 2 h; bronchodilation may be seen even in normal volunteers without evidence of obstructive lung disease. Ipratropium bromide completely reverses bronchoconstriction induced by methacholine or other cholinergic agonists and partially relieves bronchospasm induced by a broad spectrum of common bronchoconstrictor stimuli, including beta-adrenergic antagonists, histamine, serotonin, exercise, and cold air.

CLINICAL USE

The current literature contains over 1000 studies investigating the effects of ipratropium bromide and other anticholinergic compounds upon human airways. Although many double-blind, placebo-controlled crossover trials have been performed, comparison of individual trials is complicated by differences in patient populations, small group size, and the dosing and administration sequences of various drugs.[17,32]

Ipratropium bromide is most efficacious in patients with chronic obstructive pulmonary disease, including emphysema and chronic bronchitis. In such patients, ipratropium bromide is equally or more effective than beta-adrenergic agonists in increasing forced expiratory volume in 1 second (FEV_1) and in re-

ducing airway resistance; many patients demonstrate bronchodilation in response to the anticholinergics but not to beta-adrenergic agonists. This observation demonstrates that many patients with chronic obstructive pulmonary disease who fail to respond to beta-adrenergic agonist administration have bronchospasm attributable to heightened cholinergic tone rather than fixed airway disease. Chronic ipratropium bromide inhalation does not lead to development of tolerance or tachyphylaxis.

The combination of ipratropium bromide (or other anticholinergics) with beta-adrenergic agonists produces greater improvement in FEV_1 and specific conductance than does administration of either agent alone. In addition, case reports of patients with bronchitis suggest that ipratropium bromide inhalation may reduce oral glucocorticoid requirements. However, most large-scale studies of patients with chronic obstructive pulmonary disease demonstrate that the addition of oral steroids does not increase maximal flow over that achieved by the administration of a beta-adrenergic agonist with inhaled ipratropium bromide. Because of its greater efficacy and longer duration of action than beta-adrenergic agonists, ipratropium bromide is considered to be appropriate initial bronchodilator therapy for patients with chronic obstructive pulmonary disease.

In contrast, ipratropium bromide is less effective than beta-adrenergic agonists in the treatment of asthma. Ipratropium bromide does produce bronchodilation in atopic and nonatopic asthmatics. Although ipratropium bromide has a longer duration of action, greater bronchodilation can be achieved in asthmatics with a beta-adrenergic agonist than with ipratropium. In combination studies employing submaximal dosages, the combination of ipratropium bromide with a beta-adrenergic agonist produces greater bronchodilation than either agent alone. Similarly, a combination of ipratropium bromide with inhaled corticosteroids or inhaled disodium cromolyn produces greater bronchodilation than either agent alone. Furthermore, the inhalation of a submaximal dose of ipratropium bromide substantially improves the bronchodilation achieved with either systemic theophylline administration or the combination of systemic theophylline administration and an inhaled beta-adrenergic agonist. Some asthmatics may gain more relief of bronchospasm from inhalation of ipratropium bromide than from beta-adrenergic agonists. However, this unusual response requires an empiric trial of ipratropium bromide and should be reserved only for patients whose moderate to severe asthma is difficult to control. For patients presenting in acute status asthmaticus, ipratropium bromide should be used only to supplement beta-adrenergic agonist therapy.

After optimal bronchodilation is achieved with maximal doses of beta-adrenergic agonists, the addition of submaximal doses of ipratropium bromide produces additional bronchodilation. Most studies in patients with asthma or chronic obstructive pulmonary disease show increased bronchodilator efficacy with the combination of anticholinergics and beta-adrenergic agonists, although submaximal doses of each agent are usually employed. This combination of submaximal doses of ipratropium bromide and beta-adrenergic agonists may provide superior bronchodilation, fewer side effects, and greater compliance. Also, the rapid bronchodilation achieved with beta-adrenergic agonists and the prolonged action of ipratropium bromide may lead to substantial symptomatic relief from bronchospasm. These observations have resulted in the development of metered-dose inhalers combining fixed doses of ipratropium bromide and various beta-adrenergic agonists.

SAFETY

Ipratropium bromide inhalation is remarkably free of side effects. Up to 10 percent of patients may experience mild cough, although generally this is not severe enough to prompt discontinuation of the medication. Some patients (fewer than 6 percent) experience dry mouth and dysgeusia, but ipratropium bromide inhalation produces no change in heart rate, urinary flow, intraocular pressure, or pupillary size or accommodation. Ipratropium has no effect on pulmonary hemodynamics, ventilation-perfusion matching, or oxyhemoglobin saturation.

Although systemic administration of muscarinic anticholinergics decreases mucus formation, suprisingly, ipratropium bromide has little effect on respiratory secretions. Ipratropium bromide inhalation produces a clinically insignificant decrease in mucus viscosity and does not change mucus transport or ciliary beat frequency. Small reductions or no change in mucus clearance have been reported in normal volunteers, asthmatics, and patients with chronic bronchitis. Although no change in sputum volume has been reported with ipratropium bromide inhalation, some patients with severe bronchorrhea note a decreased volume of respiratory secretions after administration of aerosolized atropine.

Although isolated case reports of elevated plasma levels of hepatic transaminses or paradoxical decrements in pulmonary function have been reported, ipratropium bromide inhalation has gained wide clinical acceptance with few reported toxicities. No drug interactions have been reported between ipratropium bromide and either beta-adrenergic agonists or methylxanthines.

Methylxanthines

Theophylline and aminophylline, the ethylenediamine salt of theophylline, are used to treat asthma and the obstructive component of chronic obstructive pulmonary disease. Other pulmonary diseases for which theophylline may have a role include obstructive sleep apnea, apnea of prematurity, and airway obstruction secondary to pulmonary edema.

Potentially beneficial therapeutic effects of theophylline include bronchial smooth-muscle relaxation, enhanced mucociliary transport, inhibition of mediator release, suppression of permeability edema, decreased pulmonary hypertension, increased right ventricular ejection fraction, improved diaphragmatic contractility, and central stimulation of ventilation. Although bronchial smooth-muscle relaxation is most likely responsible for the majority of theophylline's beneficial therapeutic effects in the treatment of obstructive lung disease, the anti-inflammatory and diaphragmatic effects may contribute to the overall efficacy of the drug.

PHARMACOLOGY

Despite having been marketed and studied for several decades, the precise cellular mechanism of theophylline's bronchodilat-

ing action is unknown. Several cellular mechanisms have been proposed, including phosphodiesterase inhibition, adenosine antagonism, and catecholamine release. Cyclic 3′,5′-adenosine monophosphate and cyclic 3′,5′-guanosine monophosphate are cyclic nucleotides that regulate cellular activity influencing smooth-muscle tone, mediator secretion, and activation of inflammatory cells. The cyclic nucleotides are broken down by numerous phosphodiesterases. Theophylline is a nonselective and weak phosphodiesterase inhibitor, but bronchodilation via phosphodiesterase inhibition does not occur at usual therapeutic ranges. However, phosphodiesterase inhibition may account for some of the anti-inflammatory effects observed with theophylline.

Adenosine inhibits norepinephrine release from autonomic nerve endings and inhibits release of neurotransmitters in the central nervous system. Although therapeutic concentrations of theophylline block adenosine receptors, enprofylline, a 3-propylxanthine, is a more potent bronchodilator with very little adenosine-blocking activity.[31] Therefore, it is unlikely that theophylline bronchodilates via adenosine antagonism. However, many of the extrapulmonary effects associated with theophylline, including cardiac stimulation, anxiety, tremors, seizures, diuresis, gastric secretion, and free fatty acid release have been attributed to adenosine antagonism.

Theophylline may act by stimulating adrenomedullary secretion of catecholamines. Plasma catecholamines may contribute to the early bronchodilatory effects of the drug or may influence mediator release from mast cells, basophils, or epithelial cells. However, asthmatics are unable to sustain elevated levels of circulating catecholamines during continuous theophylline infusion. Other proposed mechanisms for bronchodilation from theophylline include prostaglandin antagonism and mobilization of intracellular calcium. However, although methylxanthines block the constricting effects of prostaglandins E_2 and $F_{2\text{-alpha}}$ on smooth muscle in vitro, this effect is probably mediated through antagonism of other bronchoconstricting mediators.

Anti-inflammatory Effects

Anti-inflammatory actions attributed to theophylline include inhibition of neutrophil and mononuclear cell migration, leukotriene B_4 generation, T-cell proliferation, and lymphokine production; increased activity and number of suppresser T cells; and stabilization or inactivation of macrophages and platelets.[48] Low theophylline doses appear to inhibit the late-phase cellular response to antigen. The anti-inflammatory effect of theophylline appears to be qualitatively different than that of corticosteroids, resulting from the selective inhibition of phosphodiesterase IV at low serum theophylline concentrations. In a recent trial, cromolyn sodium and oral theophylline were equally effective in attenuating the airway response to inhaled histamine in allergic asthmatics. Although there has been a great deal of interest in the immunomodulatory effect of the methylxanthines, the clinical relevance of this effect remains unknown.

Diaphragmatic Effects

Theophylline increases diaphragmatic strength and contractility, actions potentially mediated by transmembrane calcium movement. Most data are from in vitro studies or from normal volunteers; results from controlled clinical trials in patients with chronic obstructive pulmonary disease are limited and conflicting. Initial studies in patients with chronic obstructive pulmonary disease reported that theophylline significantly increased diaphragmatic strength or increased ventilatory endurance. Subsequent clinical trials have failed to replicate these effects, and study design differences, including drug dose, treatment duration, and severity of illness make direct comparisons difficult. However, theophylline may be potentially most beneficial in patients with hypoxic and hypercapnic chronic obstructive pulmonary disease when dosed to midtherapeutic plasma concentrations.

STRUCTURE-ACTIVITY RELATIONSHIPS

Theophylline and aminophylline are 1,3-dimethylxanthines. Other methylxanthines, including theobromine (3,7-dimethylxanthine) and caffeine (1,3,7-trimethylxanthine), differ in the positions of the methyl substituents on the xanthine molecule. N-1 substituents are important for adenosine antagonism, whereas N-3 substituents augment bronchodilator activity. Substituents at N-7 decrease bronchodilator potency; substituents at N-9 decrease the potency of the xanthine. The investigational methylxanthine, enprofylline, a potent bronchodilator without adenosine antagonism, has a propyl substituent at N-3.

CLINICAL USE

For bronchodilation, the target theophylline serum concentration is generally accepted as 10 to 20 mg/dl. The therapeutic range for other effects (e.g., anti-inflammatory properties, enhanced diaphragm capability, respiratory stimulation) may be different, prompting interest in a lower (5 to 15 mg/dl) target range. Approximately 50 percent of maximal bronchodilation is achieved at a serum level of 10 mg/dl, with only an additional 17 percent increase at 20 mg/dl. Although published data support a steep, linear relationship between bronchodilation and serum concentrations, bronchodilatation at low serum theophylline concentrations has been demonstrated only in a limited number of patients.

There are no definitive answers regarding the precise clinical role of theophylline. However, some less controversial indications include severe bronchodilator-dependent chronic obstructive pulmonary disease; severe, systemic, corticosteroid-dependent asthma; nocturnal asthma uncontrolled with adrenergic agonists; and acute, severe asthma progressing to respiratory failure.[25]

SAFETY

Adverse effects associated with theophylline include nausea, vomiting, diarrhea, irritability, insomnia, supraventricular tachycardia, ventricular arrhythmias, and seizures. In patients with serum theophylline levels between 10 mg/dl and 20 mg/dl, no differences were found in the duration of hospital stay or the rate and extent of improvement in peak expiratory flows. However, there was significantly more toxicity with higher serum levels. Although the risk of adverse effects increases at serum concentrations greater than 20 mg/dl, patients also may experience se-

rious adverse effects within the usual therapeutic range. Because of this narrow therapeutic index, emphasis should be placed on achieving the midtherapeutic range for serum theophylline levels (10 to 15 mg/dl), while accepting a broader range (5 to 20 mg/dl) as appropriate.

Magnesium Sulfate

Magnesium, a physiological antagonist to calcium, exerts smooth-muscle effects by altering calcium flux. By blocking calcium entry into smooth-muscle cells, magnesium relaxes muscle fibers. In addition, magnesium may block calcium-dependent mast cell degranulation and mediator release, as well as acetylcholine release at the neuromuscular junction.

Case reports describe the benefit of intravenous magnesium sulfate in patients with acute, life-threatening asthma refractory to nebulized beta-agonists, parenteral corticosteroids, and parenteral terbutaline. The largest trial to date evaluated the use of intravenous magnesium in 135 adults with acute asthma and a FEV_1 less than 75 percent of predicted.[3] Patients were randomized upon presentation to the emergency room to receive either 2 g of magnesium sulfate intravenously over 20 min or placebo; standard therapy with nebulized albuterol and, in some patients, intravenous bronchodilator therapy was also provided. Magnesium administration demonstrated no overall beneficial effect, although in a retrospective analysis, the rate of hospital admissions for patients with severe asthma (FEV_1 less than 25 percent predicted) was reduced significantly in the treatment group. Although some investigators have hypothesized that local drug delivery via nebulization might be beneficial, nebulized magnesium does not affect FEV_1 following methacholine challenge in stable asthmatics. More information is needed to better define the subgroup of asthmatics who might benefit from magnesium sulfate therapy.

Inhaled Diuretics

Furosemide inhibits release of chloride into the bronchial lumen through blockade of ion transport in epithelial cells; in addition, it may attenuate the sensory nerve response to irritant substances. Amiloride and acetazolamide have been reported to prevent bronchoconstriction through unknown mechanisms. In vitro data suggest that furosemide blocks release of histamine and leukotrienes. Furosemide decreases neutrophil chemotaxis following administration of nebulized distilled water, perhaps by inhibiting the release of neutrophil chemotactic factor.

Furosemide is the most extensively studied inhaled diuretic in placebo-controlled trials. Inhaled furosemide significantly blunts the bronchoconstrictive response to cold air in atopic asthmatics, but it significantly slows airway rewarming.[16] In children with exercise-induced asthma, inhaled furosemide is effective at preventing bronchoconstriction; and in asthmatic and normal children, inhaled furosemide decreases the concentration of inhaled acetic acid necessary to induce cough. However, human studies have not demonstrated a salutary effect following administration of other bronchoconstrictive substances, including ultrasonically nebulized distilled water, sodium metabisulfite, adenosine monophosphate, lysine-aspirin, or hypertonic saline.

Inhaled furosemide has no role in the treatment of exacerbations of acute asthma. Furosemide may be useful in the prevention of asthma provoked by exercise and some irritating substances, but additional information is needed before the use of inhaled diuretics can be recommended.

Inhaled diuretics improve sputum rheology and clearance in cystic fibrosis by antagonizing sodium absorption from airway epithelial cells, thus decreasing sputum viscosity. However, the beneficial effects of amiloride on mucus clearance in cystic fibrosis patients are not associated with increased sputum water content;[49] the drug's mechanism of action in this disorder remains undefined. No patients appear to experience adverse effects from inhaled diuretic therapy. Therefore, amiloride warrants further study as an adjunct to standard therapies for cystic fibrosis (antibiotics, mucokinetic agents, physiotherapy).

ANTI-INFLAMMATORY AGENTS

Modern pharmacotherapy of asthma includes relief of bronchoconstriction and suppression of airway inflammation. Whereas corticosteroids are the mainstay of current anti-inflammatory regimens, other agents in clinical use include mast cell stabilizers, leukitriene receptor antagonists, and synthetic inhibitors of leukotrienes. Finally, the inherent toxicities of systemic corticosteroids have spurred clinical investigation of other potential immunosuppressive agents with an improved side effect profile for relief of airway inflammation.

Corticosteroids

Corticosteroids are cortisol-like drugs that influence metabolic pathways and have an anti-inflammatory effect. By reducing airway inflammation, corticosteroids are clearly useful in the management of asthma and may be efficacious in chronic obstructive pulmonary disease.

PHARMACOLOGY

Glucocorticoids (i.e., cortisol) are produced by the adrenal cortex via the hypothalamic-pituitary axis in response to physical and emotional distress. Although the usual daily secretion of cortisol is approximately 10 to 20 mg, as much as 400 to 500 mg per day can be secreted during periods of severe stress. Corticosteroids are derived from cholesterol and are highly protein bound. At the cellular level, circulating corticosteroid diffuses across the cell membrane to a specific cytoplasmic glucocorticoid receptor. The corticosteroid-receptor complex undergoes a conformational change that exposes the DNA-binding region of the receptor. This "activated" corticosteroid-receptor complex enters the nucleus of the cell and binds to specific glucocorticoid-responsive genes. Although the cellular mechanisms are incompletely understood, corticosteroids stimulate the transcription and creation of certain proteins, such as lipocortin-1, and inhibit DNA transcription, resulting in decreased cytokine production. The clinical effects of corticosteroids are delayed for several hours following administration, reflecting the time needed to create new proteins or inhibit cytokine production. Leukocytes, mucous glands, and blood vessels are glucocorticoid targets (Table 173-2).

The inhaled glucocorticoids differ in potency, lipophilicity, relative receptor binding affinity, and pharmacokinetics. Since glucocorticoid preparations delivered by metered-dose inhalers are marketed and prescribed in relatively equipotent doses, potency may be the least important differentiating characteristic. However, lipophilicity and relative receptor binding affinity are important discriminants among the inhaled corticosteroids. These characteristics determine the rate of receptor association and dissociation and the amount of drug absorbed systemically following inhalation. Fluticasone propionate is the most lipophilic among the agents marketed for inhalation; beclomethasone, budesonide, triamcinolone acetonide, and flunisolide follow in descending order of lipophilicity. The relative receptor binding affinity and steroid-receptor complex half-life parallel the lipophilicity profile, with fluticasone propionate having the greatest binding affinity and longest steroid-receptor complex half-life. All corticosteroids undergo hepatic metabolism. Orally administered drugs, including drug swallowed after inhalation, undergo significant first-pass metabolism. Oral bioavailability parallels the lipophilicity profile, with fluticasone propionate having the lowest oral bioavailability.

CLINICAL USE

Inhaled or systemic corticosteroids have become cornerstones of therapy in the treatment of asthma. However, the role of glucocorticoid therapy in chronic obstructive pulmonary disease remains controversial.

Asthma

The role of airway inflammation in asthma is well established, and high-dose systemic (parenteral or oral) corticosteroids have become standard therapy for patients experiencing severe acute exacerbations of asthma. Parenteral administration of corticosteroids is often used preferentially due to the inability of some patients to swallow medications while in respiratory distress or because of lack of oral access after intubation. Oral corticosteroids are as effective as parental corticosteroids in the treatment of acute asthma.[28] Early placebo-controlled studies demonstrated significant benefit from corticosteroid administration in patients with acute severe asthma, with improvements in FEV_1 documented even after a single dose. Dose-ranging studies of intravenous corticosteroids have not established a minimum effective dose, although as little as 120 mg/d of methylprednisolone (in divided doses administered every 6 h) is effective in asthmatic adults having an acute exacerbation.[34] The time to initial response, as evidenced by augmentation of FEV_1 in conjunction with bronchodilator administration, begins as early as 1 h after corticosteroid administration; maximal response is achieved in 8 to 12 h. Parenteral corticosteroid therapy is usually maintained for 24 to 72 h, with subsequent conversion to oral prednisone at 60 mg daily when the FEV_1 reaches a threshold of 50 percent of predicted normal. This dose may be maintained for 2 to 7 days, followed by gradual tapering of the dose over 1 to 3 weeks. Parenteral methylprednisolone is emerging as the corticosteroid of choice, due to its lower mineralocorticoid and greater glucocorticoid effects than hydrocortisone.

TABLE 173-2

Antiinflammatory Mechanisms of Corticosteroids

Effect	Mechanism
Leukocyte trafficking	
↓ Circulating basophils, eosinophils, monocytes, lymphocytes	Inhibition of release factors that stimulate granulocytopoiesis; eosinophil sequestration in tissues
↑ Circulating neutrophils	Marrow neutrophilpoiesis
↓ Mucosal mast cells	Inhibition of release of mast cell growth factors (IL-3, GM-CSF)
↓ Inflammatory cell infiltration	Inhibition of release of chemoattractants; inhibition of release of endothelial-activating cytokines (TNF, IL-1)
Leukocyte function	
↑ β-adrenergic receptor synthesis, affinity, and coupling to adenyl cyclase	
↓ Degranulation of macrophages, basophils, and rodent (but not human) mast cells	For monocytes, ↓ complement receptor number and activity
↓ Release of arachidonic acid metabolites and PAF	Lipocortin synthesis
↓ Cytokine release	
↓ T-lymphocyte proliferation and activation	↓ IL-2 production
Prevention of priming	
—Neutrophils and monocytes to IFN-2	
—Eosinophils to GM-CSF	
Mucus secretion	
↓ Basal and secretagogue (i.e., histamine, leukotriene, PAF, prostanoid)-induced mucus	
Vasculature	Inhibition of chemoattractant and/or endothelial-activating mediator production/release
Vasoconstriction	
Vascular permeability	

↓ = Decrease; ↑ = Increase; PAF = platelet activating factor; IFN-2 = interferon -2; GM-CSF = granulocyte-monocyte colony stimulating factor; IL-3 = interleukin 3; TNF = tumor necrosis factor; IL-1 = interleukin 1; IL-2 = interleukin 2. *(From Cypcar D, Busse WW: Steroid resistant asthma. J Allergy Clin Immunol 92: 362–372, 1993, with permission.)*

Inhaled corticosteroids offer direct delivery to the lung with reduced risk of systemic effects. Fluticasone is a recently approved, high-potency inhaled corticosteroid which undergoes extensive first-pass hepatic metabolism, decreasing the presence of circulating active drug. Budesonide is less potent than fluticasone, followed by flunisolide, beclomethasone, and triamcinolone. Inhaled corticosteroids are superior to placebo in improving peak flows, FEV_1, and FVC and in reducing symptoms of asthma. To achieve the same effect as higher potency agents, the lower potency agents are given in higher doses; adverse effects are more likely to occur. Fluticasone appears more effective than equipotent doses of beclomethasone in reducing diurnal variation in symptoms and in reducing bronchodilator use. Escalating doses of fluticasone provide excellent control of asthma, with negligible adrenal suppression. The lack of systemic effects from fluticasone allow much higher doses to be used, providing greater therapeutic benefit. A linear dose-response curve for fluticasone has been demonstrated for improvement in peak flows, subjective symptom improvement, and reduction in bronchodilator use.[10] Fluticasone offers significant advantages over previously marketed inhaled corticosteroids and will likely assume an important niche in chronic asthma management.

Older studies have confirmed the effectiveness of lower-potency inhaled corticosteroids. Inhaled corticosteroids significantly decrease bronchial responsiveness to provocative substances when compared to beta$_2$-adrenergic agonists or theophylline. Significant disease improvement with use of inhaled corticosteroids has been reported in children, without concurrent suppression of growth or increased incidence of infections. Twice-daily regimens of inhaled corticosteroids are as effective as four-times daily regimens, provided equal daily doses are given. Gradual improvement in flows and symptoms occurs after initiation of inhaled corticosteroid therapy.

High-dose inhaled corticosteroids have been studied in asthma in an attempt to reduce symptoms, improve spirometry, and avoid reliance on systemic corticosteroids for adequate control. Newer inhaled corticosteroids which are less systemically bioavailable (e.g., fluticasone and beclomethasone) lack systemic effects at lower doses. Inhaled fluticasone and beclomethasone at high doses allow discontinuation of oral prednisone in the vast ma-

Oral corticosteroid therapy is seldom indicated for chronic stable asthma due to the advent of inhaled corticosteroids. However, some studies have demonstrated a reduced need for parenteral rescue therapy in patients who receive oral prednisone as compared with those who receive placebo. Oral therapy is maintained at the lowest dose possible to sustain control of symptoms and optimize peak expiratory flow in conjunction with inhaled beta$_2$-adrenergic agonists. Hydrocortisone, methylprednisolone, or prednisone are most commonly used. Unlike prednisone, the first two agents do not require hepatic metabolism for therapeutic activity and are preferred in patients with significant liver disease.

jority of previously steroid-dependent patients.[40] Very high doses of inhaled fluticasone (2000 mg daily) significantly reduce airway hyperresponsiveness to methacholine challenge. However, these higher doses have been associated with a significant increase in local adverse effects.

Chronic Obstructive Pulmonary Disease

The mechanism underlying the beneficial effects of corticosteroids in chronic obstructive pulmonary disease (COPD) is not fully known but may arise from their effects on phosphodiesterase activity in vivo. The resultant increase in cyclic 3',5'-adenosine monophosphate may be responsible for augmentation of inhaled beta-adrenergic agonist effects, such as increased mucus mobilization and bronchodilation.[43]

Placebo-controlled trials of corticosteroids in flares of COPD offer conflicting data. Studies of patients with chronic bronchitis suffering acute, severe airway obstruction who received methylprednisolone every 6 h for 72 h, in addition to standard care with methylxanthines, bronchodilators, and antibiotics, showed improvement in FEV_1 and increased bronchodilator responses compared with placebo-treated patients. However, similar studies employing a single dose of systemic corticosteroids reveal no significant improvement in FEV_1, forced vital capacity (FVC), or hospital admission rates. Since a short duration of administration may limit the benefit, repeated administration of intravenous corticosteroids may be necessary when given adjunctively to treat acute flares of chronic obstructive pulmonary disease. Although systemic corticosteroids may reduce the risk of relapse, the role of high-dose systemic corticosteroids for acute flares of chronic obstructive pulmonary disease remains unclear.

Oral corticosteroids for chronic management of chronic obstructive pulmonary disease significantly improve mean FEV_1 or FVC in most patients. However, up to one-third of patients studied experience marked increases in these values after steroid treatment.[2] Patients with steroid-responsive chronic obstructive pulmonary disease have significant symptom resolution after bronchodilator administration, suggesting coexisting asthma. In such patients, alternate-day oral corticosteroid regimens are as effective as daily regimens. Oral corticosteroids do not improve exercise tolerance in stable patients with chronic obstructive pulmonary disease, as measured by minute ventilation, oxygen consumption, and heart rate achieved during maximal exercise. In summary, although a minority of patients with stable chronic obstructive pulmonary disease may benefit from systemic corticosteroids, further information is required before definitive treatment recommendations can be made.

The relative safety of inhaled corticosteroids in asthmatics prompted studies examining their use in patients with chronic obstructive pulmonary disease. One large-scale, long-term ($2\frac{1}{2}$ years) randomized trial revealed a significant improvement in mean FEV_1, reduced airway hyperresponsiveness, and fewer treatment withdrawals in patients receiving beclomethasone compared with those receiving ipratropium bromide or placebo.[29] Young (age, <40 years) atopic nonsmokers were most likely to have steroid-responsive disease. Smaller studies have revealed that inhaled corticosteroids significantly increase FEV_1 in some

patients; a positive bronchodilator response may be a useful screening technique for isolating those patients with chronic obstructive pulmonary disease who are steroid-responsive. A trial of inhaled corticosteroids appears to be the safest method for assessing benefit in chronic obstructive pulmonary disease.

SAFETY

Short-term use (less than 14 days) of systemic corticosteroids is associated with mild glucose intolerance, fluid retention which may progress to edema and hypertension, proximal muscle weakness (especially with large parenteral doses), and mood alteration. Long-term systemic corticosteroids prolong the short-term effects; in addition, peptic ulcer disease, cataracts, increased risk of infection, and impaired wound healing occur. Truncal obesity, hirsutism, acne, moon-shaped facies, striae, and ecchymoses contribute to a cushingoid appearance. Disruption of bone metabolism predisposes patients to osteoporosis and resultant vertebral and long-bone fractures; inhibition of long-bone growth is the major complication in children who receive systemic corticosteroids. Suppression of the hypothalamic-pituitary-adrenal axis diminishes body cortisol stores, which, in turn, reduces the capacity of the body to confront stress, such as trauma, surgery, or infection.

Inhaled corticosteroids are less systemically bioavailable due to poor absorption from the tracheobronchial tree. The most common adverse effect is local irritation of the oropharynx, cough, and bronchospasm. Dysphonia may arise from vocal cord myopathy induced by the presence of corticosteroid in the oropharynx. Thrush is easily avoided by rinsing the mouth after each use of a corticosteroid inhaler, using a spacer device to decrease deposition of drug particles in the mouth, and keeping the inhaler mouthpiece clean. Newer inhaled corticosteroids, such as fluticasone, undergo extensive first-pass metabolism to inactive substances, thereby decreasing concentrations of active drug and the potential for systemic adverse effects. Long-term studies of inhaled corticosteroids have not documented significant adrenal suppression.

STEROID RESISTANCE

Patients with asthma who are unresponsive to usually sufficient doses of corticosteroids are described as *steroid-resistant*. Steroid resistance has been formally defined by a smaller than 15 percent increase in FEV_1 after 7 days of oral prednisolone administered at a dose of 20 mg daily in bronchodilator-responsive asthmatics.[7] Steroid resistance must be distinguished from steroid dependency, which is usually defined as the need for systemic corticosteroids for maintaining control of asthma.

Steroid resistance may involve reduced metabolism of oral corticosteroids to the active compound or accelerated drug clearance. An impaired cellular response to corticosteroids has been observed in steroid-resistant asthmatics, and altered receptor binding or the presence of antilipocortin antibodies may contribute to the phenomenon. Steroid-resistant asthmatics may be appropriate candidates for empiric therapy with corticosteroid-sparing agents.

Corticosteroid-Sparing Agents

Systemic corticosteroid therapy is often required for the treatment of severe airflow obstruction, although the chronic use of these agents often results in numerous side effects. Among the most serious of these side effects is osteopenia, with resultant skeletal fractures. In addition, diabetes mellitus, hypertension, obesity, cataracts, myopathy, and neuropsychiatric disturbances may occur with systemic corticosteroid administration. Therefore, many anti-inflammatory agents have been evaluated in an effort to identify alternatives to systemic corticosteroid therapy.[22,36]

TROLEANDOMYCIN

Since the 1960s, anecdotal clinical observations have suggested that the macrolide antibiotic troleandomycin might reduce the need for corticosteroids in patients with severe, steroid-dependent asthma, without producing a deterioration in airflow or increase in symptoms. However, results from double-blind, randomized trials are mixed. One large study in which patients were followed for 2 years found no difference in systemic corticosteroid requirements between patients treated with troleandomycin or placebo.

The steroid-sparing mechanism of troleandomycin is unknown. Usual doses of corticosteroids combined with troleandomycin produce cushingoid facies and cytopenias, suggesting a decrease in steroid metabolism. Studies in both adults and children have demonstrated that troleandomycin reduces methylprednisolone clearance by approximately 60 percent, with little effect on prednisolone clearance. Troleandomycin also reduces theophylline metabolism.

Troleandomycin is not a benign drug. Because of its effects on corticosteroid metabolism, patients experience increased complications of systemic corticosteroids, including flushing, cushingoid appearance, weight gain, and increased rates of osteoporosis; rash and urticaria have been anecdotally reported. Some patients develop elevated hepatic transaminases, nausea, and vomiting; one case of troleandomycin-associated hepatitis has been reported.

To date, the weight of evidence suggests that troleandomycin has little or no clinical effect at relieving airway obstruction or inflammation independent of its effects on corticosteroid metabolism. Since significant complications may occur, troleandomycin has little role in the current therapy of severe, steroid-dependent asthma.

METHOTREXATE

From initial observations in patients with rheumatoid arthritis and coexistent asthma, methotrexate therapy appeared to ameliorate both asthmatic and arthritic symptoms. These observations prompted a series of case reports in which *oral* administration of up to 15 mg of methotrexate per week improved symptoms and allowed significant decreases in oral corticosteroid dosages in adults and children with severe asthma. A number of mechanisms have been proposed for these reductions in oral corticosteroid requirements. Methotrexate decreases neutrophil chemotaxis to leukotrone B_4 (LTB$_4$) and the 5_a compo-

nent of complement (C5$_a$), decreases interleukin-1 synthesis, and may also inhibit antigen expression by activated macrophages. Finally, histamine release by basophils is reduced in the presence of methotrexate. Methotrexate has no significant drug interactions with systemic corticosteroids or theophylline.

These initial clinical observations and laboratory studies formed the basis for multiple randomized, double-blind, placebo-controlled clinical trials performed in the past decade. Some studies have reported that methotrexate administration allows reductions in oral steroid dosage by 30 to 50 percent compared to placebo, but most studies report no significant difference between corticosteroid dosage during methotrexate therapy or placebo administration. All these clinical trials enrolled only small numbers of patients, with little to no run-in time for optimization of medical therapy and minimization of systemic corticosteroid administration. Also, maximal inhalation therapy with both bronchodilators and steroids may not have been used in all patients.

The clinical trials of methotrexate administration in severe, steroid-dependent asthmatics reveal numerous side effects. Weekly administration of methotrexate commonly produced nausea, rash, elevated liver enzyme levels, stomatitis, diarrhea, headache, and alopecia. Investigators have raised numerous concerns that long-term administration of methotrexate to steroid-dependent asthmatics may ultimately produce hepatic cirrhosis, bone marrow suppression, and pulmonary toxicity (interstitial pneumonitis). Furthermore, fatal infectious complications have been reported in steroid-dependent asthmatics receiving methotrexate, including development of *Pneumocystis carinii* pneumonia and disseminated varicella-zoster infection.

Currently, no clear documentation exists of the clinical efficacy of methotrexate administration in severe, steroid-dependent asthma. Similarly, there is no consensus of opinion advocating the use of methotrexate in this setting. Methotrexate administration has significant side effects, including potentially fatal complications. Concerns regarding the long-term toxicity of chronic methotrexate in asthmatics have been incompletely addressed. At this time, prudency argues for limiting methotrexate administration in severe, steroid-dependent asthmatics to empiric trials in individual patients or to investigations in large-scale, controlled clinical trials.

CYCLOSPORINE

Cyclosporine inhibits lymphokine synthesis, thereby blocking the activation of T cells, and is used widely in organ transplantation. Multiple studies in the past decade have attempted to define the role of this agent in a wide variety of inflammatory diseases, including asthma. Cyclosporine has no significant drug interactions with beta-adrenergic agonists, corticosteroids, or theophylline, making it particularly attractive as an anti-inflammatory agent for use in asthma.

Case reports and small open-label series in steroid-dependent asthmatics have noted that the addition of cyclosporine to treatment regimens allows a marked reduction in oral corticosteroid dosages. In a double-blind, placebo-controlled study, cyclosporine increased peak expiratory flow and FEV$_1$, reduced exacerbations of airway obstruction, or reduced oral prednisolone dosage by over 60 percent.[30]

Hypertrichosis, hypertension, and reversible nephrotoxicity are associated with cyclosporine administration, as well as a large number of nonspecific side effects. This side effect profile may limit widespread use of cyclosporine, which shows great promise as an anti-inflammatory agent for the treatment of asthma. Additional studies are required to confirm the efficacy of cyclosporine in the treatment of asthma, as well as to define its role as a steroid-sparing adjunct or an independent immunosuppressant.

GOLD

Gold salts have been used for medicinal purposes for centuries. In asthmatics, parenteral administration of gold salts has been sporadically reported in Europe since the 1930s and in Japan since the 1960s. To date, little understanding exists of the putative immunomodulatory mechanisms of gold upon airway inflammation. Based upon the efficacy of gold salt administration in patients with rheumatoid arthritis, several small trials and case series have reported beneficial effects of gold salts, such as decreased bronchial hyperreactivity in mild asthmatics not receiving corticosteroids. In severe, steroid-dependent asthmatics, several studies have noted clinical improvements in some patients treated with gold, although only one trial has demonstrated a statistically significant reduction in oral steroid dosage and a modest improvement in FEV_1.

Parenteral gold salt administration, usually through intramuscular injection, has a broad spectrum of side effects and toxicities: pulmonary fibrosis, exfoliative dermatitis, and bone marrow suppression; nephrotoxicity, dermatitis, stomatis, and proteinuria have caused up to 40 percent of patients to drop out of clinical studies. Oral auranofin is associated with less severe and less frequent side effects that include diarrhea, rash, and stomatitis. At this time, there is no clear demonstration that gold administration improves pulmonary function, reduces flares of obstructive airway disease, or reduces the need for systemic corticosteroid therapy. Therefore, use of gold salts in obstructive airway disease should be restricted to well-designed, controlled clinical trials.

OTHER AGENTS

The search continues for anti-inflammatory agents with potential efficacy in asthma. A broad spectrum of agents have been touted, including pooled immunoglobulins, azathioprine, colchicine, dapsone, hydroxychloroquine, ketotifen, and nonsteroidal antiinflammatory agents.[22,36] The original studies purporting the efficacy of these agents comprise mainly anecdotal reports or small case series. A few controlled trials report modest reductions in systemic steroid requirements. However, the interpretations of these trials are complicated by the small numbers of patients enrolled; significant drop-out rates; little or no improvement demonstrated in pulmonary function; and short run-in times, with little opportunity to achieve an optimal therapeutic regimen.

Mast Cell Stabilizers

Cromolyn sodium and nedocromil exert anti-inflammatory actions by stabilizing mast cells. This blockade of mast cell degranulation prevents inflammatory mediator release, partially responsible for the bronchoconstriction and epithelial injury characteristic of asthma.

CROMOLYN SODIUM

Cromolyn sodium was the first mast cell stabilizer to be approved for clinical use in asthma and is widely employed in pediatric asthmatics.

Pharmacology

Cromolyn sodium is a potent inhibitor of inflammatory responses. Cromolyn sodium diminishes early phase reactions in asthma by blocking the release of intracellular calcium and inhibiting the enzymes responsible for mast cell degranulation; cromolyn reduces late phase reactions in asthma by inhibiting production of the enzymes necessary for superoxide generation. Cromolyn sodium may also exhibit tachykinin antagonism, accounting for some of its anti-inflammatory properties. In vitro, cromolyn sodium potentially inhibits the activation of inflammatory cells, antibody-induced granulocyte cytotoxicity, IgE production by atopic cells, and monocyte IgG production.

Clinical Use

Cromolyn sodium is indicated for the management of asthma in children and in atopic young adults. Early, large-scale clinical trials demonstrated cromolyn sodium, alone or in combination with beta$_2$-adrenergic agonists, improves exercise tolerance, enhances sleep quality, reduces asthma exacerbations, and facilitates patient acceptance of therapy. Patients diagnosed with asthma prior to the age of 4 years, patients less than 17 years of age, and patients with long-term asthma (>5 years) may experience maximal benefit from cromolyn sodium therapy. Cromolyn sodium significantly improves seasonal allergic asthma symptoms and reduces bronchial hyperresponsiveness after direct challenge with histamine or acetylcholine. Long-term use of cromolyn sodium (at least 12 weeks) four times daily is recommended for effective control of chronic bronchial hyperresponsiveness, while a shorter treatment duration (up to 6 weeks) usually suffices for control of seasonal allergic attacks.

Cromolyn sodium prophylaxes against exercise-induced asthma in children as efficaciously as beta$_2$-agonists. Premedication with cromolyn sodium, inhaled beta$_2$-adrenergic agonist, or both, 15 to 30 min prior to vigorous exercise is recommended for children and adults.

Studies comparing inhaled corticosteroids and cromolyn sodium have focused on efficacy. In asthmatic children randomized to treatment with inhaled corticosteroids or cromolyn sodium, reduced nocturnal symptoms were noted in the steroid-treated group.[42] In contrast, cromolyn sodium was as equally efficacious as inhaled triamcinolone acetonide in improving peak expiratory flows, symptoms, FEV_1, and methacholine sensitivity.[45]

Similarly, studies comparing cromolyn sodium with inhaled beclomethasone in adults with atopic asthma have yielded mixed results. Some, but not all, studies demonstrate beclomethasone and cromolyn sodium inhalation are equally effective in improving peak expiratory flow and reducing symptoms. Bronchial hyperresponsiveness to inhaled hypertonic saline, but not methacholine, was significantly reduced by cromolyn sodium in other studies. A randomized placebo-controlled comparison of the effects of theophylline and cromolyn sodium in adult patients with asthma showed no difference in diminishing early- and late-phase reactions to allergen challenge and no difference in blunting bronchial hyperresponsiveness induced by inhaled histamine.[21]

Cromolyn sodium is a useful adjunct to bronchodilators in adults with atopic asthma; it may provide added benefit when administered in conjunction with inhaled corticosteroids.

Safety

Cromolyn sodium causes few adverse effects, even after long-term use. Its efficacy in preventing childhood asthma symptoms and its safety record make cromolyn sodium a first-line agent, in conjunction with beta$_2$-adrenergic agonists, in management of asthma in children.

NEDOCROMIL

Nedocromil also stabilizes mast cells in the bronchial mucosa, but it has a broader anti-inflammatory spectrum than cromolyn sodium. Nedocromil blocks activation of eosinophils and neutrophils, further reducing inflammation. Dose-dependent inhibition of IL-4-induced IgE and IgG production has been demonstrated in vitro.

Nedocromil is useful prophylactically against asthma exacerbations but not therapeutically for acute bronchospasm. Adult asthmatics randomized to either theophylline or nedocromil showed no difference in symptoms or pulmonary function after several weeks of therapy.[9] Nedocromil delays the late-phase response to methacholine and allergen challenges in stable asthmatics and has no effect on the magnitude of bronchoconstriction.

The similar pharmacology of cromolyn sodium and nedocromil have prompted direct comparisons of the two agents in asthmatics. Nedocromil appears to be more effective as a bronchodilator-sparing agent than cromolyn sodium in adults but provides a similar level of protection against exercise-induced asthma in children. Lack of long-term experience with nedocromil relegates it to second-line status as an adjunct to bronchodilators in the management of asthma.

Leukotriene Antagonists and Inhibitors

The leukotriene antagonists and inhibitors are the first new class of asthma drugs to be developed in several decades. Advances in the understanding of the inflammatory pathogenesis of asthma and the role of leukotrienes as inflammatory mediators has generated great interest in the development of, and the therapeutic potential for, these drugs.

Leukotrienes are synthesized from arachidonic acid, a fatty acid stored in phospholipids of cell walls. Numerous stimuli, including IgE receptor activation, antigen-antibody interactions, and activation of phospholipase A$_2$, induce the release of arachidonic acid from phospholipids. Arachidonic acid is converted to a variety of products via several unrelated pathways; the 5-lipoxygenase pathway is the pathway of importance in asthma (Fig. 173-2). Leukotriene A$_4$ (LTA$_4$) is metabolized by two different pathways to either the nonpeptide LTB$_4$ or the cysteinyl leukotrienes (LTC$_4$, LTD$_4$, and LTE$_4$). LTB$_4$ recruits and activates inflammatory cells but has no effect on bronchial tone or reactivity. The cysteinyl leukotrienes stimulate smooth-muscle contraction, increase vascular permeability, and enhance bronchial hyperresponsiveness; thus they have a major role in the pathogenesis of asthma.

Leukotriene action may be inhibited by either selective receptor blockade or interference with synthesis. LTB$_4$ and LTD$_4$ receptor antagonists are under development. However, most clinical experience has been with the LTD$_4$ receptor antagonists, since LTC$_4$, LTD$_4$, and LTE$_4$ interact with a common LTD$_4$ receptor. The first-generation LTD$_4$ receptor antagonists had little clinical efficacy, but the second-generation LTD$_4$ receptor antagonists are highly potent and selective. Zafirlukast, a short-acting oral agent, and montelukast, a long-acting oral agent, are in active clinical trials. Other oral, parenteral, and inhaled receptor antagonists are under investigation. Furthermore, inhibition of 5-lipoxygenase (5-LO) reduces the generation of all leukotrienes, and numerous 5-LO inhibitors are under investigation.

Long-term efficacy and safety data are not available. However, data from controlled trials 4 to 6 weeks long suggest that LTD$_4$ receptor antagonists and 5-LO inhibitors are well tolerated.[24,46] Although there is no information regarding comparative efficacy of the leukotriene inhibitors and other anti-inflammatory drugs, and despite limited data on long-term safety and efficacy, the leukotriene antagonists and inhibitors show promise in the management of chronic moderate asthma and, possibly, in exercise-induced asthma.

MUCOKINETIC AGENTS

Chronic sputum production or inspissated airway secretions plague most patients with obstructive lung disease. Some mucokinetic agents are effective in promoting the clearance of obstructed airways.

Dornase Alpha

Purulent, viscous secretions contribute to airway obstruction and chronic pulmonary infections in patients with cystic fibrosis, chronic bronchitis, and bronchiectasis. High concentrations of mucus contribute to the increased viscosity of bronchial secretions in these conditions. Polymorphonuclear leukocytes recruited to ward off chronic pulmonary infections eventually degenerate, releasing DNA into the extracellular environment. Although human deoxyribonuclease I (DNAse, recombinant human deoxyribonuclease, rhDNAse) metabolizes DNA liberated from airway leukocytes, the high concentration of DNA released in these chronic conditions overwhelms the endogenous ability of the lungs to clear the DNA. Exogenous administration of DNAse assists in the clearance of airway DNA by reducing mucus viscosity, increasing mucus clearance, diminishing airway obstruction, and preventing recurrent pulmonary infections.

Results of randomized clinical trials of nebulized DNAse as short-term adjunctive therapy in patients with cystic fibrosis demonstrate modest dose-dependent improvement in pulmonary function and reduction in symptoms.[15] Placebo-controlled investigations of DNAse in adults with chronic bronchitis or

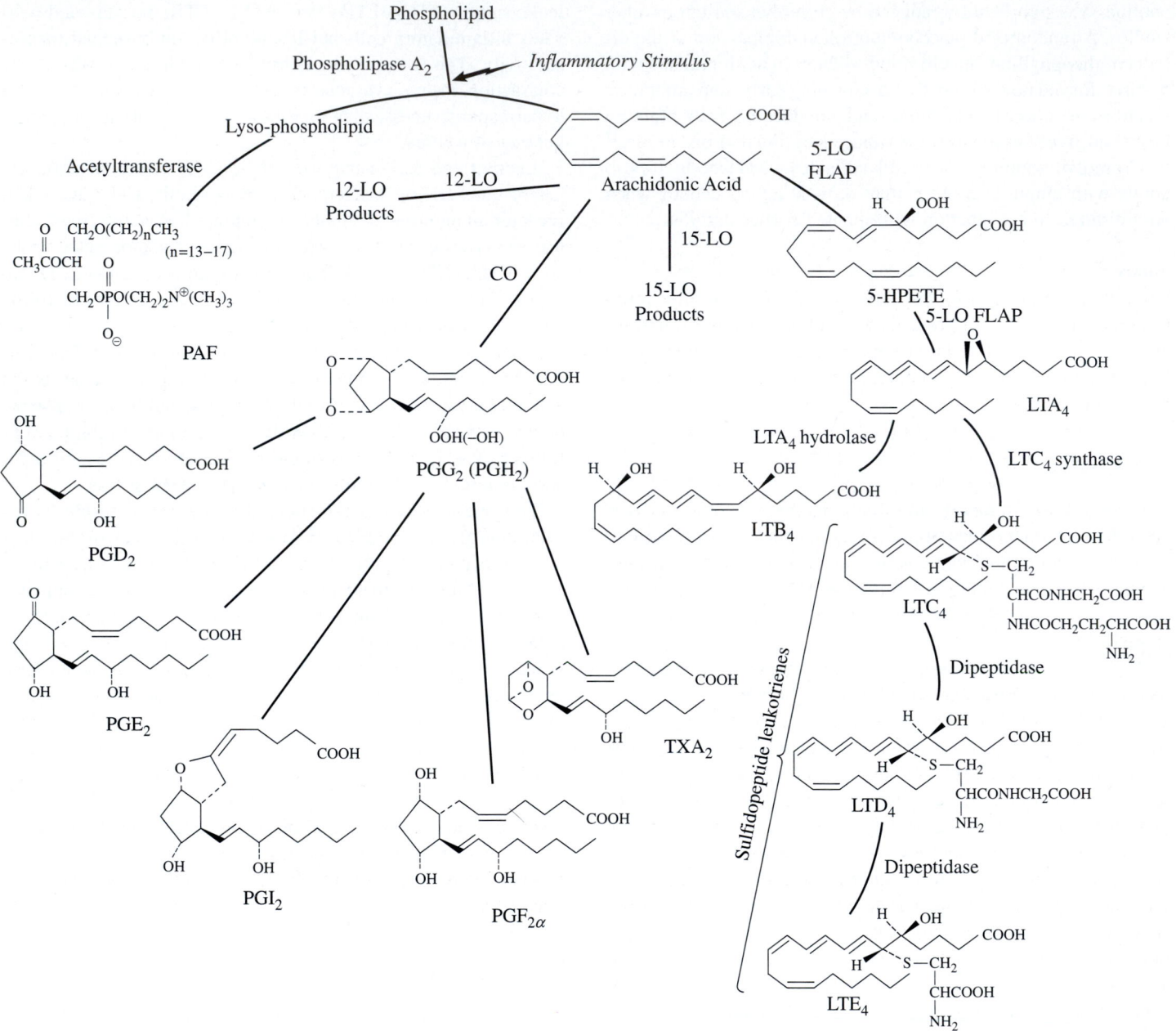

FIGURE 173-2 Formation of platelet-activating factor, and cyclooxygenase and 5-lipoxygenase products of arachidonic acid. CO = cyclooxygenase; FLAP = 5-lipoxygenase-activating protein; HPETE = hydroperoxyeicosatetraenoic acid; LO = lipoxygenase; LT = leukotriene; PAF = platelet-activating factor; PG = prostaglandin; and TX = thromboxane. *(From Henderson W Jr: Role of leukotrienes in asthma.* Ann Allergy Asthma Immunol 274, 1994.)

bronchiectasias not due to cystic fibrosis reveal prolonged antibiotic therapy requirements, no enhancement of pulmonary function, and no improvement in quality of life. Nebulized DNAse provides modest clinical benefit in patients with cystic fibrosis, and its use as a mucokinetic agent in other patients without cystic fibrosis is not supported by published studies.

N-Acetylcysteine

N-acetylcysteine (NAC) lyses disulfide bonds in mucus proteins, reducing airway mucus viscosity. Increased mobilization of mucus and decreased inspissation with use of inhaled NAC has been reported in patients with asthma or chronic obstructive pulmonary disease. However, randomized placebo-controlled trials in chronic obstructive pulmonary disease have demonstrated no objective benefit of NAC treatment.[20]

Due to the in vivo conversion of NAC to the potent antioxidants, glutathione and cysteine, recent investigations have focused on NAC as an immunomodulator. Since antioxidant formation is distinct from the local mucolytic effect, oral NAC has been investigated in most studies. Unfortunately, intravenous NAC in patients with acute lung injury or the acute (adult) respiratory distress syndrome offers no significant reduction in mortality or disease progression.

Although inhaled or nebulized NAC is an effective mucolytic agent, its immune-modulating antioxidant effects are poorly defined. NAC has limited clinical importance in treatment of either chronic obstructive pulmonary disease or acute lung injury.

Iodinated Agents

Some iodinated compounds have mucolytic-expectorant properties. When ingested, iodide is liberated and stored in secretory glands of the tracheobronchial tree. Upon stimulation by coughing or inhalation of irritant substances, iodide promotes secretion of respiratory tract fluid and mucoproteins and augments ciliary activity. Increased mucus mobilization and decreased mucus viscosity result.

The National Mucolytic Study randomized patients with stable chronic bronchitis to receive either iodinated glycerol or placebo daily.[41] Patients who received iodinated glycerol reported significant improvement in cough frequency and chest discomfort. The findings were confirmed in smaller subsequent trials. Adverse events appear to be infrequent, although thyroid dysfunction may be induced by the iodine load and has been reported after long-term use in elderly patients with chronic obstructive pulmonary disease. Clinicians should use iodinated compounds with caution in elderly patients or in patients with preexisting thyroid dysfunction.

Sodium Bicarbonate

Sodium bicarbonate solutions (2 to 7.5%) are frequently used as vehicles for bronchodilators and N-acetylcysteine. By raising the pH of the respiratory tract fluids, aerosolized sodium bicarbonate weakens the saccharide structure of airway mucus, increasing its susceptibility to proteases and promoting its removal through enhanced ciliary activity. These effects are additive when used with N-acetylcysteine and cause reduction in mucous viscosity. Local irritation from hypertonic sodium bicarbonate solutions may occur; cough and bronchospasm have been observed in some patients. Therefore, bronchodilators should be given prior to sodium bicarbonate aerosols.

Guaifenesin

Mobilization of respiratory secretions is useful with chronic bronchitis and other chronic respiratory conditions. Guaifenesin remains the only agent approved by the FDA as an expectorant, based upon a single placebo-controlled trial in patients with chronic bronchitis; guaifenesin significantly reduced sputum volume and improved sputum quality.[14] These patients also experienced subjective relief of respiratory congestion, and no adverse effects were reported, but the purported antitussive properties of guaifenesin have not been substantiated in well-controlled studies.

PHYSIOLOGICAL REPLACEMENTS

The past decade has seen birth of replacement therapy for lung disease. Replacement therapy comprises a novel class of agents to replace deficient, or to augment existing, endogenous substances. To date, replacement therapy has been employed only in adults with α_1-antitrypsin deficiency or neonates with respiratory distress syndrome. However, clinical studies of replacement therapy are underway in patients with a wide spectrum of obstructive and other lung diseases.

Alpha$_1$-Antitrypsin

Alpha$_1$-antitrypsin is a glycoprotein synthesized and secreted by hepatocytes. A protease inhibitor, α_1-antitrypsin blocks the actions of neutrophil-derived elastase in the lung. Inherited deficiency of a$_1$-antitrypsin promotes the development of emphysema in adulthood, and tobacco smoking rapidly accelerates the clinical presentation and severity of emphysema.

PHARMACOLOGY

Attempts to increase endogenous production of α_1-antitrypsin by hormonal manipulations are largely ineffective, and liver transplantation can lead to restoration of serum α_1-antitrypsin levels according to donor phenotype. Since 1988, α_1-antitrypsin replacement therapy has been available for intravenous administration as a purified product from pooled human plasma.

Recombinant α_1-antitrypsin has been produced. However, the recombinant form lacks carbohydrate side chains, resulting in rapid renal excretion. Nonetheless, recombinant α_1-antitrypsin may be efficacious when directly administered by aerosol.

CLINICAL USE

Weekly or monthly intravenous infusion of α_1-antitrypsin to deficient patients increases α_1-antitrypsin levels in serum and bronchoalveolar lavage specimens. Such infusions concomitantly restore antielastase activity in serum and alveolar lining fluid.[23] Numerous case reports and small series dispute whether α_1-antitrypsin replacement reduces the accelerated rate of decline in pulmonary function associated with α_1-antitrypsin-deficiency. It remains unclear if the national registry for α_1-antitrypsin deficient patients will ultimately produce data to assess the therapeutic efficacy of a$_1$-antitrypsin replacement therapy, since a randomized clinical trial to demonstrate efficacy on pulmonary function or mortality is not feasible.

In patients with cystic fibrosis, elastase activity within the lung is increased due to chronic inflammation. Intravenous augmentation with α_1-antitrypsin has no effect on elastase activity in the lungs of these patients. Aerosolized α_1-antitrypsin supplementation in patients with cystic fibrosis reduces, but does not abolish, elastase activity in the lung.[33] The clinical significance of this finding is unknown.

Despite the lack of efficacy data, α_1-antitrypsin replacement therapy is recommended for patients with α_1-antitrypsin deficiency who are older than 18 years of age, who have abnormal pulmonary function tests, and whose serum α_1-antitrypsin level is less than 11 mmol. Replacement therapy for α_1-antitrypsin-deficient patients is not recommended after lung transplantation.

SIDE EFFECTS

α_1-antitrypsin replacement therapy is remarkably nontoxic, and current preparations have few side effects other than mild fever. Repeated administration of α_1-antitrypsin does not shorten the serum half-life, suggesting that α_1-antitrypsin antibodies do not develop, even in patients with complete deficiency.

Pulmonary Surfactant

The administration of pulmonary surfactant to premature infants with, or at risk for, respiratory distress syndrome has become the standard of care in recent years.[26] Surfactant administration decreases mortality from respiratory distress syndrome by 30 to 40 percent and reduces morbidity due to pneumothoraces, interstitial emphysema, bronchopulmonary dysplasia, and intraventricular hemorrhage (see Chapter 7).

Endogenous pulmonary surfactant is an emulsion of phospholipids, cholesterol, and apoproteins that reduces surface tension within alveoli. Natural surfactant is commercially available and is prepared from lung tissue or lavages from a variety of species. Synthetic surfactant is available from a number of commercial sources, although the optimal composition of the material remains to be determined.

In adults, the promise of pulmonary surfactant in the treatment of lung disease derives from a spectrum of biologic activities, in addition to its fundamental role in reducing surface tension.[26] Pulmonary surfactants reduce oxygen toxicity by scavenging free radicals, and the surfactants may be cytoprotective for alveolar cell surfaces. Pulmonary surfactants suppress mediator release by inflammatory cells and may deactivate inflammatory mediators upon release. In vitro studies indicate that surfactant suppresses lymphocyte mitogenic responses, leading to a decrease in inflammatory cell influx. Pulmonary surfactant has both antibacterial and antiviral properties which are mediated by an increase in alveolar macrophage phagocytosis. Surfactant may promote airway clearance by changing the physical properties of mucus, as well as by increasing ciliary beat frequency. Finally, pulmonary surfactant may directly relax airway smooth muscle. This spectrum of putative biologic activities may directly interrupt the pathogensis of airway inflammation, chronic infection, and bronchoconstriction seen in most obstructive lung diseases.

Limited clinical data are available to document the effects of pulmonary surfactant in adults. In anecdotal case reports and small patient series, surfactant administration to patients with respiratory failure has produced occasional increases in Pa_{O_2}, although usually no change in radiographic, physiological, or respiratory findings were reported. However, in two large, double-blind, randomized, placebo-controlled trials, administration of synthetic surfactant for 5 days yielded no demonstrable physiological benefit and no significant decrease in mortality rate measured at 30 days.[1]

Pulmonary surfactant has potential promise for the treatment of obstructive pulmonary diseases, including cystic fibrosis, asthma, and chronic bronchitis. However, few clinical data documenting physiologic efficacy or therapeutic benefit currently exist, and further studies of surfactant administration in adults with obstructive lung disease are necessary.

RESPIRATORY STIMULANTS

Respiratory stimulants are a group of pharmacologically unrelated agents used to treat diverse pathophysiological conditions, including obstructive or central sleep apnea, chronic obstructive pulmonary disease, postanesthesia respiratory depression, and acute mountain sickness.

Acetazolamide

Acetazolamide is a noncompetitive inhibitor of carbonic anhydrase that induces a weak diuresis and mild metabolic acidosis. Currently, acetazolamide is approved for the prophylaxis of acute mountain sickness and is under investigation for the treatment of obstructive sleep apnea. It is sometimes used to treat patients with chronic hypercapnia and drug-induced or compensatory metabolic alkalosis. Acetazolamide may have both indirect and direct respiratory stimulant properties. The increased hydrogen concentration indirectly stimulates respiration via peripheral and medullary chemoreceptor stimulation.[50] Acetazolamide may directly stimulate respiration by increasing cerebral blood flow through mechanisms unrelated to the metabolic acidosis.

Prophylactic acetazolamide decreases the frequency of acute mountain sickness by about 30 to 50 percent.[27] Side effects, such as somnolence, paresthesias, and gastrointestinal distress, are common. Although the precise mechanisms are unknown, acetazolamide lowers baseline resting Pa_{CO_2} and raises alveolar and minute ventilations and Pa_{O_2}, without altering respiratory chemosensitivity to carbon dioxide. Acetazolamide may also relieve symptoms and improve arterial oxygenation in established acute mountain sickness.

Data regarding the efficacy of acetazolamide in sleep apnea are derived from short-term, uncontrolled trials in small numbers of patients. Acetazolamide does not relieve apnea completely, but it may improve symptoms in patients with mild obstructive sleep apnea. Unfortunately, acetazolamide may convert central sleep apnea to obstructive sleep apnea and worsen hypoxemia in patients with central or mixed sleep apnea. Long-term safety and efficacy data are unavailable.

Almitrine

Almitrine bismesylate is a peripheral chemoreceptor agonist with no central respiratory stimulant effect. Almitrine stimulates peripheral chemoreceptors in the carotid body and improves ventilation-perfusion matching by redistributing perfusion away from poorly ventilated areas. Although marketed in Europe, almitrine bismesylate is not available in the United States. Long-term controlled trials suggest that almitrine bismesylate increases Pa_{O_2} in the range of 5 to 13 mmHg.[52] However, toxicities and side effects include right ventricular strain from increased pulmonary artery pressures, peripheral neuropathy, weight loss during long-term therapy, and diuretic activity.

Methylxanthines

Aminophylline and theophylline are methylxanthine bronchodilators which augment the central ventilatory response to hypoxia. The methylxanthines have been used to treat apnea of prematurity and infants with periodic breathing, but they are less useful in the treatment of obstructive sleep apnea. Although aminophylline reduces central apnea and the central component of mixed apneas, it has no effect on obstructive apnea, and it may increase upper airway occlusion during sleep.[13]

Doxapram

Doxapram is a short-acting, parenterally administered peripheral chemoreceptor agonist and central respiratory stimulant.[6] Doxapram has been approved for postanesthesia respiratory depression or apnea, drug-induced central nervous system respiratory depression, and for short-term use as a respiratory stimulant in acute respiratory insufficiency superimposed on chronic pulmonary disease. Case reports describe the use of doxapram as a respiratory stimulant in chronic obstructive pulmonary disease complicated by acute respiratory failure.

Medroxyprogesterone

Medroxyprogesterone is a gestational respiratory stimulant. Although its mechanism of action is unclear, medroxyprogesterone increases minute ventilation and produces hypocapnia in normal subjects. However, it does not improve breathing disturbances during sleep in normocapnic patients with obstructive sleep apnea.[8] Definitive data regarding the role of medroxyprogesterone in hypercapnic patients are unavailable.

Protriptyline

Protriptyline is a tricyclic antidepressant which is cited frequently as an effective respiratory stimulant in patients with obstructive sleep apnea. The mechanism of action may include suppression of rapid eye movement (REM) sleep and increased tone in the upper airway muscles. However, a randomized, double-blind, placebo-controlled study demonstrated that a 14-day course of protriptyline had no significant effect on symptoms or obstructive events.[51] Protriptyline is contraindicated in patients with glaucoma or prostatic hypertrophy, and anticholinergic side effects limit its usefulness.

REFERENCES

1. Anzueto A, Baughman RP, Guntapalli KK, et al: Aerosolized surfactant in adults with sepsis-induced acute respiratory distress syndrome. *New Engl J Med* 334:1417–1421, 1996.
2. Blair GP, Light RW: Treatment of chronic obstructive pulmonary disease with corticosteroids. *Chest* 86:524–528, 1984.
3. Bloch H, Silverman R, Mancherje N, et al: Intravenous magnesium sulfate as an adjunct in the treatment of acute asthma. *Chest* 107:1576–1581, 1995.
4. Bowton DL, Goldsmith WM, Haponik EF: Substitution of metered-dose inhalers for hand-held nebulizers. Success and cost savings in a large, acute-care hospital. *Chest* 101:305–308, 1993.
5. Brambilla C, Chastang C, Georges D, et al: Salmeterol compared with slow-release terbutaline in nocturnal asthma. *Allergy* 49:421–426, 1994.
6. Burki NK: Ventilatory effects of doxapram in conscious human subjects. *Chest* 85:600–604, 1984.
7. Carmichael J, Paterson IC, Diaz P, et al: Corticosteroid resistance in chronic asthma. *Br Med J* 282:1419–1422, 1981.
8. Cook WR, Benich JJ, Wooten SA: Indices of severity of obstructive sleep apnea syndrome do not change during medroxyprogesterone acetate therapy. *Chest* 96:262–266, 1989.
9. Crimi E, Violante B, Pellegrino R, Brusasco V: Clinical aspects of allergic disease. Effect of multiple doses of nedocromil sodium given after allergen inhalation in asthma. *J Allergy Clin Immunol* 92:777–783, 1993.
10. Dahl R, Lundback B, Malo J-L, et al: A dose-ranging study of fluticasone propionate in adult patients with moderate asthma. *Chest* 104:1352–1358, 1993.
11. Devoy MAB, Fuller RW, Palmer JBD: Are there any detrimental effects of the use of inhaled long-acting β2-agonists in the treatment of asthma? *Chest* 107:1116–1124, 1995.
12. Epstein SW, Parsons JE, Corey PN, et al: A comparison of three means of pressurized aerosol inhaler use. *Am Rev Respir Dis* 128:253–255, 1983.
13. Espinoza H, Antic R, Thornton AT, McEvoy RD: The effects of aminophylline on sleep and sleep-disordered breathing in patients with obstructive sleep apnea syndrome. *Am Rev Respir Dis* 136:80–84, 1987.
14. Federal Register: Cold, cough, allergy, bronchodilator and anti-asthmatic drug products for over-the-counter human use: Expectorant drug products for over-the-counter human use. Final monograph. *Federal Register* 54:8494–8509, 1989.
15. Fuchs HJ, Borowitz DS, Christiansen DH, et al: Effect of aerosolized recombinant human DNase on exacerbations of respiratory symptoms and on pulmonary function in patients with cystic fibrosis. *New Engl J Med* 331:637–642, 1994.
16. Gilbert IA, Lenner KA, Nelson JA, et al: Inhaled furosemide attenuates hyperpnea-induced obstruction and intra-airway thermal gradients. *J Appl Physiol* 76(1):409–415, 1994.
17. Gross NJ: Medical intelligence: Ipratropium bromide. *New Engl J Med* 319:485–494, 1988.
18. Grove A, Lipworth BJ: Tolerance with B2-adrenoceptor agonists: Time for reappraisal. *Br J Clin Pharmac* 39:109–118, 1995.
19. Haffner CA, Kendall MJ: Metabolic effects of B2-agonists. *J Clin Pharm Ther* 17:155–164, 1992.
20. Hansen NCG, Skriver A, Brorsen-Riis L, et al: Orally administered N-acetylcysteine may improve general well-being in patients with mild chronic bronchitis. *Respir Med* 88:531–535, 1994.
21. Hendeles L, Harman E, Huang D, et al: Theophylline attenuation of airway responses to allergen: Comparison with cromolyn metered-dose inhaler. *J Allergy Clin Immunol* 95:505–514, 1995.
22. Hill JM, Tattersfield AE: Corticosteroid sparing agents in asthma. *Thorax* 50:577–582, 1995.
23. Hubbard RC, Sellers S, Czerski RN, et al: Biochemical efficacy and safety of monthly augmentation therapy for α1-antitrypsin deficiency. *JAMA* 260:1259–1264, 1988.
24. Israel E, Rubin P, Kemp JP, et al: The effect of inhibition of 5-lipoxygenase by zileuton in mild-to-moderate asthma. *Ann Intern Med* 119:1059–1066, 1993.
25. Jenne JW. What role for theophylline? *Thorax* 49:97–100, 1994.
26. Jobe AH. Pulmonary surfactant therapy. *New Eng J Med* 328:861–868, 1993.
27. Johnson TS, Rock PB: Acute mountain sickness. *New Engl J Med* 319:841–845, 1988.
28. Jonssen S, Kjartansson G, Gislason D, Helgason H: Comparison of the oral and intravenous routes for treating asthma with methylprednisolone and theophylline. *Chest* 94:723–726, 1988.
29. Kerstjens HAM, Brand PLP, Hughes MD, et al: A comparison of bronchodilator therapy with or without inhaled corticosteroid therapy for obstructive airways disease. *New Engl J Med* 327:1413–1419, 1992.

30. Lock SH, Kay AB, Barnes NC: Double-blind, placebo-controlled study of cyclosporin A as a corticosteroid-sparing agent in corticosteroid-dependent asthma. *Am J Respir Crit Care Med* 153:509–514, 1996.

31. Lunell F, Svedmyr N, Andersson K-E, et al: Effects of enprofylline, a xanthine lacking adenosine receptor antagonism in patients with chronic obstructive lung disease. *Eur J Clin Pharmacol* 22:395, 1982.

32. Mann KV, Leon AL, Tietze KJ: Use of ipratropium bromide in obstructive lung disease. *Clin Pharm* 7(9):570–580, 1988.

33. McElvaney NG, Hubbard RC, Birrer P, et al: Aerosol α1-antitrypsin treatment for cystic fibrosis. *Lancet* 337:392–394, 1991.

34. McFadden Jr ER: Dosages of corticosteroids in asthma. *Am Rev Respir Dis* 147:1306–1310, 1993.

35. Mochizuki H, Shimizu T, Morikawa A, Kuroume T: Inhaled diuretics attenuate acid-induced cough in children with asthma. *Chest* 107:413–417, 1995.

36. Moss RB: Alternative pharmacotherapies for steroid-dependent asthma. *Chest* 107:817–825, 1995.

37. Mullen M, Mullen B, Carey M: The association between β-agonist use and death from asthma. *JAMA* 270:1842–1845, 1993.

38. Nierop G, Gijzel WP, Zwinderman AH, Dijkman, JH: Auranofin in the treatment of steroid dependent asthma: A double blind study. *Thorax* 47:349–354, 1992.

39. Nishikawa M, Mak JCW, Barnes PJ: Selective B$_2$-agonists, salbutamol,salmeterol, and formoterol down regulate B$_2$-adrenoceptors. *Am J Respir Crit Care Med* 149:A483, 1994.

40. Noonan M, Chervinsky P, Busse WW, et al: Fluticasone propionate reduces oral prednisone use while it improves asthma control and quality of life. *Am J Resp Crit Care Med* 152:1467–1473, 1995.

41. Petty TL: The national mucolytic study. Results of a randomized, double-blind placebo-controlled study of iodinated glycerol in chronic obstructive bronchitis. *Chest* 97:75–83, 1990.

42. Price JF, Weller PM: Comparison of fluticasone proprionate and sodium cromoglycate for the treatment of childhood asthma. *Respir Med* 89:362–368, 1989.

43. Sahn SA: Corticosteroids in chronic bronchitis and pulmonary emphysema. *Chest* 73:3, 1978.

44. Schluchter MD, Barker AF, Crystal RG, et al: A registry of patients with severe deficiency of alpha$_1$-antitrypsin: Design and methods. *Chest* 106:1223–1232, 1994.

45. Shapiro GG, Sharpe M, DeRouen TA, et al: *J Allergy Clin Immunol* 88:742–748, 1991.

46. Spector SL, Smith LJ, Glass M: Effects of 6 weeks of therapy with oral doses of ICI 204, 219, a leukotriene D4 receptor antagonist, in subjects with bronchial asthma. *Am J Respir Crit Care Med* 150:618–623, 1994.

47. Speizer FE, Doll R, Heaf P, et al: Investigation into use of drugs preceding death from asthma. *Br Med J* 1:339–343, 1968.

48. Szefler SJ, Bender BF, Jusko WJ, et al: Evolving role of theophylline for treatment of chronic childhood asthma. *J Pediatr* 127:176–185, 1995.

49. Tomkiewicz RP, App EP, Zayas JG, et al: Amiloride inhalation therapy in cystic fibrosis. *Am Rev Respir Dis* 148:1002–1007, 1993.

50. White DP, Zwillich CW, Pickett CP, et al: Central sleep apnea. *Arch Intern Med* 142:1816–1819, 1982.

51. Whyte DK, Gould GA, Airlie MAA, et al: Role of protriptyline and acetazolamide in the sleep apnea/hypoapnea syndrome. *Sleep* 11:463–472, 1988.

52. Winkelmann BR, Kullmer TH, Kneissl DG, et al: Low-dose almitrine bismesylate in the treatment of hypoxemia due to chronic obstructive pulmonary disease. *Chest* 105:1383–1391, 1994.

53. Wong CS, Pavard ID, Williams J, et al: Bronchodilator, cardiovascular, and hypokalemic effects of fenoterol, salbutamol, and terbutaline in asthma. *Lancet* 336:1396–1399, 1990.

CHAPTER 174

INTUBATION AND UPPER AIRWAY MANAGEMENT

C. William Hanson III

HISTORY

UPPER AIRWAY ANATOMY

UPPER AIRWAY MANAGEMENT
   Techniques and Equipment
   Tracheal Intubation

CONCLUSION

The evolution of methods to manage the airway is a fascinating part of the history of medicine. A variety of unusual devices have been used through the ages to resuscitate patients or to permit surgical procedures. The development of modern approaches to deliver medical gases and to reliably protect the airway from gastric contents during a procedure is one of the prerequisites for modern surgery, and new techniques in airway management continue to be developed.

HISTORY

The first known use of positive-pressure ventilation as a medical intervention dates back to the sixteenth century, as acknowledged in the following quotation from Vesalius' *de Humani Corporis Fabrica*:

> But that life may in a manner of speaking be restored to the animal, an opening must be attempted in the trunk of the trachea, into which a tube of reed or cane should be put; you will then blow into this, so that the lung may rise again and the animal take in air. Indeed with the slight breath in the case of the living animal, the lung will swell to the full extent of the thoracic cavity, and the heart become strong . . . for when the lung, long flaccid, has collapsed, the beat of the heart and arteries appears wavy, creepy, twisting; but when the lung is inflated at intervals, the motion of the heart and arteries does not stop. . . .

Vesalius subsequently resuscitated a Spanish nobleman by experimentally inflating his lungs through the trachea, which resulted in the resumption of cardiac activity—and nearly in Vesalius' death at the hands of the Inquisitors. Vesalius was viewed as a heretic by his peers, one of whom described him as "an impious madman who is poisoning all of Europe with his vaporings." Vesalius was actually an excellent anatomist and was able to disprove many of the inaccurate but cherished teachings of Galen, which had been accepted as absolute truth for 13 cen-

turies. Vesalius escaped the Inquisition, but he was condemned to a pilgrimage to the Holy Land and died in a shipwreck.[29]

Undoubtedly because of the lack of an enthusiastic response to Vesalius' findings, a 100-year hiatus preceded the next attempt at endotracheal ventilation. In 1667, Robert Hooke of London kept a dog alive by intermittently insufflating air into its trachea with a set of bellows.[16] (Hooke, one of the most prominent mathematicians of his time and one of the first to recommend the use of a balance spring in a watch, was also a geologist and a paleontologist.) After another century had passed, John Fothergill, one of the founders of the British Humane Society, described successful mouth-to-mouth resuscitation of a "dead" man in 1744.[12]

Negative-pressure ventilation was the focus of research in mechanical ventilation during the nineteenth and early twentieth centuries because of concerns over development of emphysema and tension pneumothorax—complications of this technique recognized as early as 1827. Iron lungs, tank ventilators, cuirass ventilators, and a variety of strange and wonderful differential pressure chambers and boxes were developed in the United States and Europe. These devices were powered by hand, water, steam, or electricity and, in some cases, by the patient himself.

Positive-pressure ventilation was a component of the resuscitation strategy of the Dutch Humane society, which advocated mouth-to-mouth ventilation in conjunction with external thoracic and abdominal compression.[13] In 1776, John Hunter described an apparatus that blew fresh air into the lungs with one set of bellows and sucked "bad" air out with a second set.[17]

It was not until the end of the nineteenth century, during a surge in the evolution of thoracic surgery, that tracheal intubation and positive-pressure ventilation through a cuffed endotracheal tube gained acceptance as a component of medical care. An American surgeon, Joseph O'Dwyer, designed a series of metal tubes to be inserted between the vocal cords of children afflicted with diphtheria.[31] Rudolph Matas of New Orleans described O'Dwyer's devices when he spoke of the method of "intralaryngeal intubation" and "insufflation."[26,27] He stated that the "procedure that promises the most benefit in preventing pulmonary collapse in operations is . . . the rhythmic maintenance of artificial respiration by a tube in the glottis." Following O'Dwyer's death in 1898, a German surgeon, Franz Kuhn, in the early part of the twentieth century, described techniques for oral and nasal intubation using flexible metal tubes introduced into the trachea with the assistance of the index finger of the left hand.[22] The airway was sealed with a flange above the larynx and gauze packing, the airway having been anesthetized with topical cocaine before intubation.

The laryngoscope was created in 1895 by Alfred Kirstein in Berlin,[14] but his "autoscope" was never widely accepted. Chevalier Jackson, in 1913, created a U-shaped laryngoscope, still used today in endoscopy performed by otorhinolaryngologists but never accepted by anesthesiologists.[18] In 1913, Janeway described an endotracheal tube with a removable cuff, as well as an anesthesia ventilator and a battery-powered laryngoscope.[18] Others—including Dorrance,[8] Elsberg,[11] and two Germans, Läwen and Sievers,[23]—published descriptions of methods for tracheal intubation and positive-pressure ventilation between 1900 and 1920.

The most influential figure in the history of endotracheal intubation is Sir Ivan Magill,[37] who, with Stanley Rowbotham, performed anesthesia on Royal Army casualties during World War I, including those with disfiguring facial injuries. These patients were often intubated nasally to allow freer access to the face by the surgeon. Magill created the Magill forceps (which is still used to facilitate nasal intubation), semirigid endotracheal tubes fashioned from mineralized rubber, and the Magill circuit—an L-shaped laryngoscope. Magill also described the "sniffing position."

Arthur Guedel, an American contemporary of Magill, refined the cuffed endotracheal tube and, through extensive experimentation on animal tracheas, determined that the best position for the cuff was just below the vocal cords. He popularized use of the cuffed endotracheal tube by publicly anesthetizing his pet dog, Airway, and then immersing the animal in a tank of water. Subsequently, the animal awoke, shook itself off, and left the arena.[5]

The laryngoscope blades commonly used today were invented in the 1940s by Robert Miller, a clinician from Texas, and Robert Macintosh, a professor from Oxford. The Miller blade represented an advance over similar straight blades developed earlier. It was designed to pick up the epiglottis and expose the cords.[28] The curved Macintosh blade departed from previous models and was designed for insertion between the epiglottis and tongue. Although there are many variants of the two blades available today, each having different angulation and incorporating prisms or fiberoptic bundles, the Miller and the Macintosh blades remain mainstays in the anesthesiologist's armamentarium. By the early 1940s, the first departments of anesthesiology were being formed, and the skills required for upper-airway management and endotracheal intubation became widely disseminated throughout the United States and Great Britain.

UPPER AIRWAY ANATOMY

Two functional conduits lie between the trachea and the atmosphere: the oropharynx and the nasopharynx. These conduits join at the level of the base of the skull to form the hypopharynx. The oropharynx contains the tongue, uvula, tonsils, and teeth. The nasopharynx is separated from the oropharynx by the soft palate, which is a freely mobile structure, and the adenoids or nasopharyngeal tonsils. The hypopharynx includes the vallecula, which is the space posterior to the tongue and anterior to the epiglottis, and the openings to the esophagus and the trachea. The adult epiglottis is typically crescentic; it is reasonably stiff and thin. Because of its ligamentous attachments, the adult epiglottis can be elevated indirectly with a curved laryngoscope blade applied to the base of the tongue. The U-shaped infant epiglottis is longer and floppier; therefore, a straight blade is typically required to directly lift it during endotracheal intubation (Fig. 174-1).

The adult and the infant airways differ in several other respects. The narrowest portion of the adult airway is the rima glottidis, the area between the vocal cords. On the other hand, the narrowest portion of the infant's airway is the cricoid. The infant larynx is also more cephalad than the adult's, and the infant cords are angled; the adult cords are perpendicular to the airway.[10]

In an awake patient, with the head in the neutral position (rather than in a flexed or extended position), air moves freely through both the oropharynx and nasopharynx. This is also true during sleep in most normal subjects. Abnormalities in any of the components of the upper airway may impede respiratory airflow during the awake state or selectively during sleep (snoring). A directed history and physical examination should be performed before any procedure on the airway.

A history of nasal polyps or nasal septal deviation mandates caution before nasotracheal intubation, passage of a fiberoptic

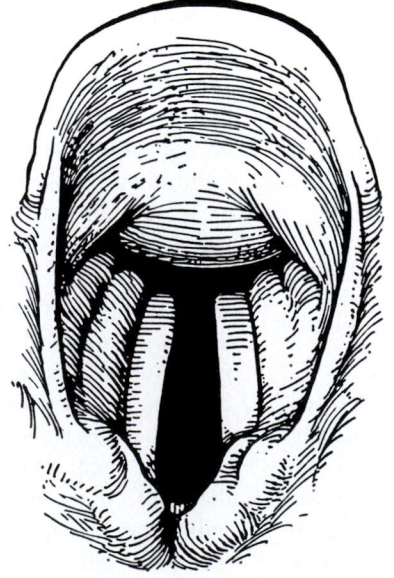
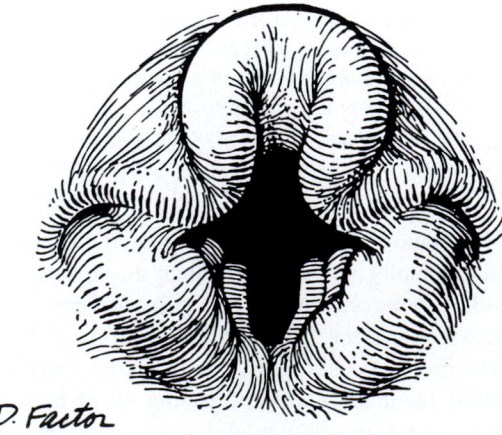

D. Factor

FIGURE 174-1 Comparative anatomy of adult and infant airways. (*Courtesy of Barash P et al (eds.), Philadelphia, Lippincott, Clinical Anesthesia, 1989, p 544, D. Factor, illustrator.*)

scope, or a nasal airway. The patient's spouse is usually the best source of information about snoring, which is a general finding common to many upper airway abnormalities, including nasal obstructions and tissue redundancy in the oropharynx and hypopharynx. A change in voice suggests abnormalities of the vocal cords and warrants evaluation.

The physical examination of the airway begins with conversation with the patient. Hoarseness, stridor, tachypnea, and coughing are all indicative of potential upper airway problems. The examination can then be pursued systematically, beginning with the nasopharynx. The patient's ability to breathe through a single nostril (when the mouth is closed and the other nostril occluded) indicates the relative patency of that passage. Some asymmetry between the two sides often exists, and instrumentation should be performed on the more patent side, whenever possible.

Assessment of mouth aperture is an important component of the examination. The ability to open the mouth is limited with temporomandibular joint disease. Fibrosis of the temporalis muscle (e.g., from radiation) may restrict mandibular mobility. Fractures of the mandible result in limited ability to open the mouth, which disappears with anesthesia when the limitation is caused by pain. Some fractures functionally affect the mobility of the jaw, irrespective of anesthetic state. An inability to open the mouth more than 40 mm is considered significant.

The patient's dentition should also be evaluated. Protruding maxillary incisors, or "buck teeth," interfere with direct laryngoscopy by restricting the angle to which the laryngoscope blade can be flattened. Caps and other dental prostheses are fragile and are easily damaged during laryngoscopy. The laryngoscope can become lodged in gaps between the maxillary teeth. Severe dental caries or periodontal disease make it easier to dislodge teeth during instrumentation of the airway. The edentulous patient often has an atrophic mandible and a large tongue and is difficult to ventilate by mask because of poor mask fit. Intubation of the trachea becomes difficult because the tongue is no longer constrained by the teeth and interferes with visualization of the larynx.

Abnormalities of the tongue, hard palate, tonsillar pillars, and hypopharyngeal structures can also impede or prevent intubation. The tongue is normally small and flexible enough to be displaced by a laryngoscope blade during visualization of the vocal cords. The tongue is enlarged in patients with obesity, angioedema, states of impaired lymphatic drainage (e.g., after surgical procedures or trauma to the neck), and certain neoplasms. Burns, scars, or radiation of the submandibular soft tissue prevent displacement of the tongue into this space during laryngoscopy. Similarly, in patients with small jaws ("receding chins"), it is difficult to displace or flatten the tongue during laryngoscopy, making intubation difficult. A hyomental distance (i.e., the distance from the hyoid bone to tip of the mandible) of less than 6 cm is indicative of potential difficulties with intubation.

The cleft or high-arched palate is one of a variety of congenital abnormalities of the facial bones. Others are Treacher Collins, Pierre Robin, Klippel-Feil, Goldenhar's, Beckwith-Wiedemann, and Cruzon's syndromes and the mucopolysaccharidoses. Patients with these disorders are difficult or impossible to intubate with use of standard approaches.[34] Enlarged tonsils, intraoral and hypopharyngeal tumors, and

cysts also interfere both with laryngoscopy and with ventilation by mask. The epiglottis may be infiltrated, inflamed, floppy, or enlarged by fat. The retropharyngeal and lateral pharyngeal spaces are continuous with the mediastinum and, therefore, are subject to expansion by processes affecting this structure (e.g., formation of edema, blood, pus, emphysema). Patients with epiglottitis and parapharyngeal swelling often exhibit a characteristic posture, sitting upright in the sniffing position; drooling is often present.

The preferred position for visualization of the cords is the sniffing position (Fig. 174-2). The position may be unsuitable for some patients, and it may be impossible to achieve for others. The normal range for flexion and extension of the neck ranges from 90° to 165°. Patients with cervical osteophytes or ankylosing spondylitis[33] are often fixed in an anteroflexed head position and, therefore, are difficult to intubate. Halo fixation imposes similar constraints. Rheumatoid arthritis affects the cervical spine of 25 to 90 percent of patients, many of whom are asymptomatic.[20] Normal aging results in as much as a 20 percent reduction in mobility of the C-spine mobility by the age of 75 years.[2] Injuries to the cervical spine, or the presence of a cervical collar, also impair the ability of the laryngoscopist to position the head. Patients with short, muscular necks have limited neck mobility, as well as redundant soft tissue in the mouth and submandibular space.

A variety of other anatomic features can complicate airway management, including large breasts or a barrel chest, which interfere with the excursion of the butt of the laryngoscope blade. The oral and pharyngeal mucosae are swollen and bleed easily during pregnancy; when compounded by a diminished functional residual capacity and increased volume of acidic gastric contents, this makes intubation of the gravid patient quite hazardous.

The Mallampati scale is a tool commonly used to objectively characterize the airway.[25] The ability to visualize the faucial pillars, soft palate, and base of the uvula is used to predict the degree of difficulty in laryngeal exposure. A careful examination of the airway, with attention to difficulties with prior procedures and the physical features previously described (Table 174-1), permits adequate preparation for instrumentation of the difficult airway.

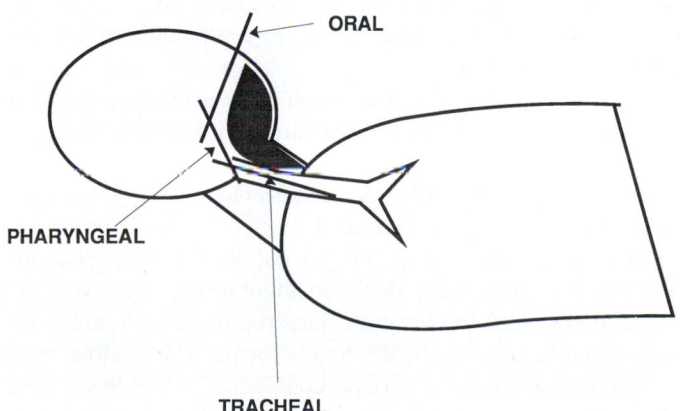

FIGURE 174-2 The sniffing position with the oral, pharyngeal, and tracheal axes.

TABLE 174-1

Mallampati Scale for Characterizing the Airway

Class I
　Soft palate, fauces, uvula, and tonsillar pillars visible
Class II
　Soft palate, fauces, and uvula visible
Class III
　Soft palate and base of uvula visible
Class IV
　Soft palate only visible

UPPER AIRWAY MANAGEMENT

Airway management is well suited to an algorithmic approach. The American Society of Anesthesiologists has developed a somewhat complex airway algorithm. The Advanced Trauma Life Support program includes an airway algorithm, and a number of other problem-specific algorithms have been published. The first decision branch point in an algorithm typically applies to the need for endotracheal intubation, since short-term respiratory insufficiency can often be managed noninvasively.

Factors that must be considered in the care of the patient with respiratory compromise include level of consciousness, clinical context (e.g., perioperative, emergency), anticipated duration of respiratory problem, risk of gastric aspiration, patency of the airway, concurrent medical problems, and anticipated ease of noninvasive versus invasive airway management.

If neurologic depression is due to central nervous system injury, noninvasive management is often inappropriate, owing to the potential for hypercarbia or hypoxia and exacerbation of the primary injury. Conversely, sedation or obtundation secondary to drugs or seizure is often brief, and temporizing measures are appropriate.

Several factors differentiate elective perioperative airway management from emergency care. During surgery, an anesthesiologist or anesthetist is constantly present, the patient is properly prepared (i.e., the stomach is empty and a mucosal drying agent has been administered), and the environment is designed to facilitate airway management (e.g., availability of suction, ventilator, etc.). In contrast, in an emergency, the setting is usually less than optimal, airway management is usually only a component of the care rendered to the patient, and definitive intervention is appropriate in order to allow care providers to concentrate on other problems.

Quickly reversible processes, such as an asthmatic attack or some cases of pulmonary edema, are appropriately managed without intubation. In other instances, as with a blunt injury to the chest, the initial problem can be expected to worsen, and conservative management is warranted.

The volume and acidity of the patient's gastric contents must be considered in any decision about airway management. Aspiration of solid food can be catastrophic, as can large volumes of acidic, enzymatically active gastric fluid. Most studies have indicated that aspirated contents with pH lower than 2.5 or volume greater than 0.5 to 1.0 cc/kg are likely to cause lung damage. The lung damage is manifested by loss of ciliated and nonciliated epithelial cells in the trachea, destruction

of types I and II pneumocytes, surfactant depletion, and increased vascular permeability.[39] Pain and narcotics can alter gastric emptying or change gastric pH—as can a number of disease states, such as intestinal obstruction, diabetic gastroparesis, and obesity. Unless the patient has fasted for more than 8 h and is not subject to the aforementioned confounding factors, a full stomach should be presumed, and airway management handled accordingly.

The patient's coexisting medical issues must be considered in the management of respiratory failure. For example, endotracheal intubation can be a dangerous stress to the patient with coronary artery disease, yet it is performed more safely with preparation than under emergency circumstances. For the patient with Fournier's gangrene (infection of the scrotum and perineum) who requires frequent trips to the operating room for debridement, maintenance of intubation and sedation between trips is appropriate—rather than subjecting the patient to numerous laryngoscopies and intubations. Intubation and mechanical ventilation can prevent aspiration or atelectasis in a patient with hepatic coma awaiting liver transplantation, improving the likelihood of a successful procedure.

Some degree of airway obstruction can be managed without intubation by head positioning and use of oral and nasal airways or positive-airway pressure by mask. A rolled towel or small pillow placed behind the neck or occiput reproduces the sniffing position. Oral and nasal airways alleviate airway obstruction due to redundant airway soft tissue or muscle relaxation. The application of positive pressure to the mouth and nose (mask continuous positive airway pressure, or "mask CPAP") stents open the soft tissue of the airway. For this reason, mask CPAP is frequently used in the management of obstructive sleep apnea, as described in chapter 102. These measures can be used as short-term, temporizing alternatives to intubation in the spontaneously breathing patient in the intensive-care or surgical setting. In the operating room, however, anesthesia is frequently administered with positive pressure by mask. True ventilation by mask is readily accomplished in the anatomically normal patient, whereas features such as a beard, a flat or sharp nose, and sunken cheeks (in the edentulous patient) can make mask-assisted ventilation difficult or impossible.

Indications for intubation of the trachea can be classified in a variety of ways (Table 174-2). Broadly, they fall into the realms of respiratory failure, airway protection, hemodynamic instabil-

TABLE 174-2

Indications for Intubation of the Trachea

Ventilatory failure
　Cardiac arrest, primary lung disease, neuromuscular
　disease or weakness
Airway obstruction
　Primary airway process, neurogenic obstruction
Airway protection
　Upper airway bleeding or injury (burn), central nervous
　system depression
Pulmonary toilet
　Inability to manage secretions

ity, and perioperative management. If intubation is indicated, the clinician must decide on the route and technique.

Techniques and Equipment

Although expertise in intubation is a function of experience, several principles are generally applicable in any approach to airway management. The first applies to correct head positioning, which facilitates mask management, oral or nasotracheal intubation, and fiberoptic examination of the airway. Incorrect positioning can impede these procedures.

The sniffing position, alluded to previously, describes the head extended on the neck with the neck flexed on the thorax (Fig. 174-2). In this position, the hypopharynx is at its maximal circumference and the tongue farthest from the posterior pharyngeal wall. Anterior displacement of the jaw can be accomplished by pulling it forward or by placing pressure on the angle of the mandible (the jaw thrust maneuver). This serves to further open up the retrolingual space. Grasping the tongue with gauze or an instrument and pulling it forward accomplish the same end. This position is appropriate for spontaneous respiration because it limits soft tissue obstruction to airflow. Nasotracheal intubation is easiest in the sniffing position, because the tip of the endotracheal tube is best aligned with the larynx and least likely to be deflected by the walls of the pharynx. Nasal and oral fiberoptic procedures are easier in this position as well, with the oral, pharyngeal, and tracheal axes well aligned (Fig. 174-3). The sniffing position is modified by additional head extension and flattening of the back of the tongue with the laryngoscope blade during oral intubation.

A second general principle in airway management is that saliva and blood interfere with mask ventilation, direct airway visualization, and fiberoptic procedures. Pretreatment with an antisialogogue, such as atropine, glycopyrrolate, or scopolamine, when time permits, significantly diminishes saliva production. Suction must be available before initiation of any elective procedure, and suction equipment should be available on any emergency cart for clearing secretions and use in the event of regurgitation. A large-bore suction tip, such as the Yankauer tonsil suction tip, is commonly used; suction should be maximal in order to clear thick, viscous oral secretions.

A third general principle of airway management refers to preparation of the patient and the airway. Small, titrated doses of sedatives, topical anesthesia, and vasoconstrictor agents markedly alter the ease with which awake procedures—such as fiberoptic, nasotracheal, and oral intubation—are performed. Narcotics are more likely than other agents to obtund the cough reflex. Topical cocaine has anesthetic and vasoconstrictor properties, but because of its classification as a controlled agent, the combination of lidocaine and phenylephrine is often used as an alternative. The light source of the laryngoscope or fiberoptic scope should be checked before instrumentation and, with the latter, the focus adjusted. Finally, it is essential to have a backup plan for airway management if the primary plan goes awry.

Perhaps the most important principle of airway management is that a source of oxygen and a means of ventilation should be available whenever possible. This implies that the pressure in oxygen tanks should be checked, as should proximity to a wall oxygen source. A self-inflating resuscitation bag provides a means of ventilation in the absence of a compressed gas source, but it provides gas only with ambient oxygen tension; bags used for most anesthesia circuits require a gas source for inflation.

AIRWAYS

A large variety of nasal and oral airways designed for children and adults of different sizes are available (Fig. 174-4). Nasal airways are generally made of flexible rubber and have a beveled tip, which permits transit through narrow nasal passages. Oral

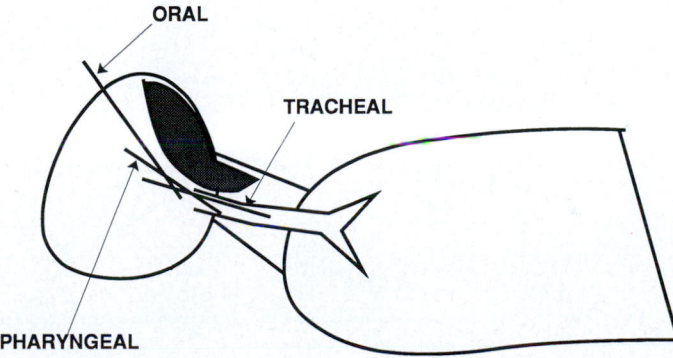

FIGURE 174-3 The sniffing position modified by additional head extension for oral intubation, with alignment of the oral, pharyngeal, and tracheal axes.

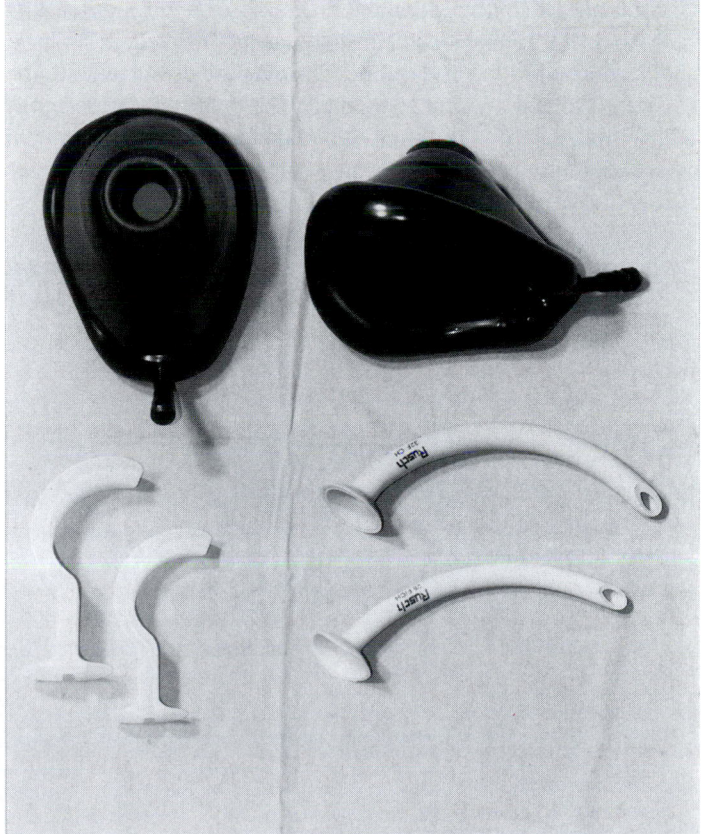

FIGURE 174-4 Oral and nasal airways and face masks.

airways are curved to lie over and behind the tongue. Some are fashioned with slots for ready passage of a suction catheter, whereas others have a central channel designed to accommodate a fiberoptic scope. Binasal airways are designed to fit in a ventilation circuit, permitting ventilation without endotracheal intubation in anesthetized patients.

RESUSCITATION BAGS

Resuscitation bags are available in many styles (Fig. 174-5) and are designed with several common features. They are self-inflating and, therefore, can be used without a pressurized gas source. An internal flap valve system directs inflowing gas to the patient or reservoir, permitting application of positive pressure by mask or endotracheal tube and venting exhaled gas to the atmosphere. Many bags are equipped with oxygen reservoirs. Inspired oxygen concentration is ordinarily limited to 40 to 60% when oxygen inflow is 10 L/min and bag reinflation is rapid, since room air is entrained with each breath. The addition of an oxygen reservoir permits administration of oxygen concentrations between 75 and 90% at flows of 10 to 15 L/min. Some bags are equipped with adjustable valves for application of positive end-expiratory pressure.

MASKS

While there is a large variety of masks (Fig. 174-4), they all have three features in common: a body, a seal, and a connector.[9] The body is usually made of malleable or moldable material and is adjustable to differing facial anatomy. The body of some masks is made of clear plastic to allow diagnosis of regurgitation. The seal is usually a cushioned rim that can be inflated or deflated and is attached to the body, although some are detachable. Some seals are flanged and not cushioned. The connector is designed with a universal fitting (22-mm internal diameter) for attachment to any ventilating circuit; many are equipped with retaining straps

for attachment to mask straps, which pass behind the patient's head, freeing the hand of the operator.

LARYNGEAL MASK AIRWAYS

The laryngeal mask airway (Fig. 174-6) is analogous to the facial mask: It has a compliant cuff that is applied to the dorsal surface of the larynx, isolating the airway from the mouth and esophagus. The laryngeal mask airway came into common intraoperative usage in the early 1990s.[1,32] Although its most extensive use has been in surgical patients, the device has also been used for awake fiberoptic bronchoscopy,[4] in the intensive care unit,[3] and in emergency resuscitation.[24] The airway is inserted by mouth into the hypopharynx, and its correct position is verified by chest auscultation.

Tracheal Intubation

Four approaches are commonly used in tracheal cannulation: nasal, oral, laryngeal, and tracheal. The first two are noninvasive, whereas the last two require surgical incisions.

Nasal intubation can be done blindly or with the assistance of a laryngoscope and forceps. The blind technique, when performed by a skilled operator, allows rapid control of the airway in an awake patient with minimal obtundation of protective airway reflexes. This technique is widely used by paramedics in prehospital patient care; it is a component of many difficult airway algorithms and an integral part of algorithms employed in Advanced Trauma Life Support. The nasal passages should be examined for patency, septal deviation, and the presence of polyps. If the patient is able to cooperate, the larger nasal passage should be selected by alternately occluding each nostril and choosing the one with better airflow. A topical anesthetic and vasoconstrictor agents should be sprayed in the nostril or applied with cotton pledgets. The anesthetic should also be sprayed into the back of the mouth to anesthetize the hypopharynx.

An appropriate-size tube (6 to 7 mm for women, 7 to 8 mm for men) should then be selected and lubricated. Lubrication eases

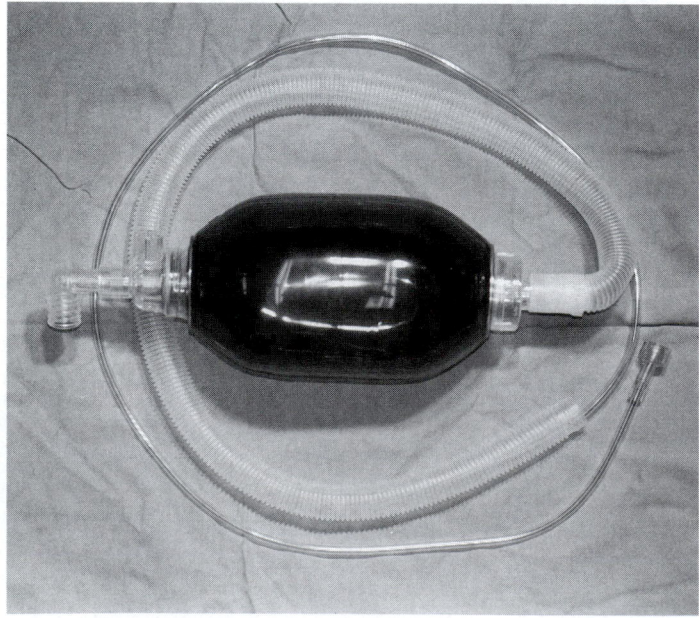

FIGURE 174-5   Self-inflating resuscitation bag.

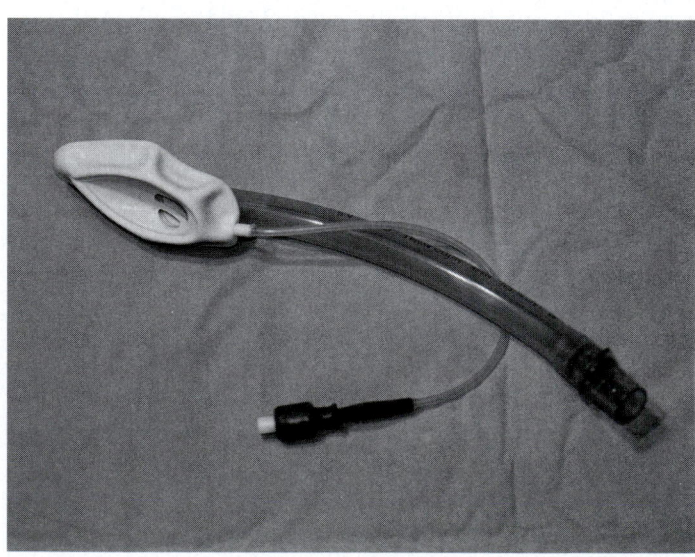

FIGURE 174-6   The laryngeal mask airway.

passage of the tube and prevents abrasion of the nasal mucosa, making bleeding less likely. The patient is placed in the sniffing position, and the tube is placed in the nostril and advanced with slow, firm pressure. The natural curve of the tube is oriented so that the tip initially points toward the occiput and curves in a caudad direction as it advances. If the procedure is done blindly in an awake patient, the operator should listen for breath sounds as the tip approaches the cords. A whistle attachment (Bamm, Great Plains Ballistics) is available to enhance the operator's ability to hear breath sounds (Fig. 174-7). With correct timing, the tube is passed into the airway on inspiration. Slight rotation of the tube at the nose can be used to correct for lateral misalignment. One endotracheal tube (Endotrol, Mallinckrodt) has been modified to allow the operator to anteroflex the tip of the tube with a "trigger" at the connector (Fig. 174-8). This is especially effective in patients with anteriorly positioned cords or in patients who cannot assume the sniffing position (e.g., because of the presence of a cervical collar).

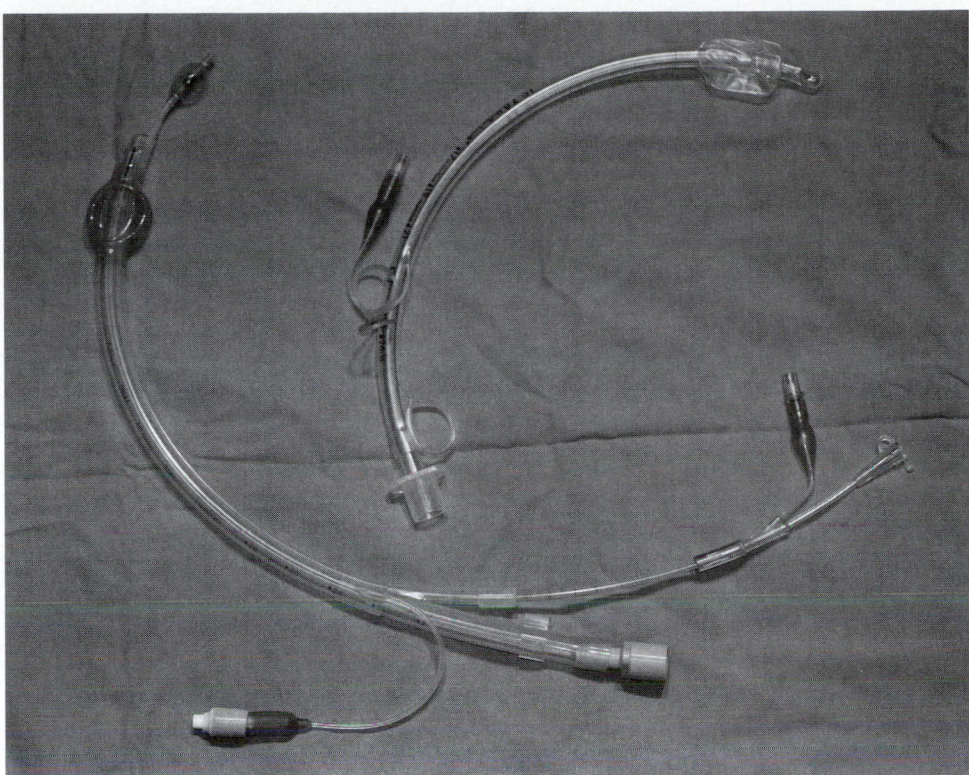

FIGURE 174-8   Endotracheal tube modified with a "trigger" permitting anteroflexion of the tip of the tube during blind nasal intubation. Univent tube for lung isolation (see text).

When the procedure is performed in an anesthetized patient, the endotracheal tube is passed into the hypopharynx above the cords; laryngoscopy is performed and the tube is advanced into the trachea under direct visualization. A Magill forceps (Fig. 174-9) is often used to grasp the tube and to direct the tip between the cords. Care must be taken to avoid grasping the tube with the cuff, which is easily perforated.

Correct tube position can be verified by a number of methods. Audible or palpable air passage (in the spontaneously breathing patient), a visible vapor trail within the tube, and auscultatory evidence of breath sounds over the lung fields are standard approaches. End-tidal capnometry showing phasic variation in the level of carbon dioxide is the "gold standard," a method that has become more feasible in nonsurgical settings since the development of portable and disposable devices.

Extensive literature exists regarding the pros and cons of nasal versus oral intubation in the intensive-care environment. Nasal intubation is associated

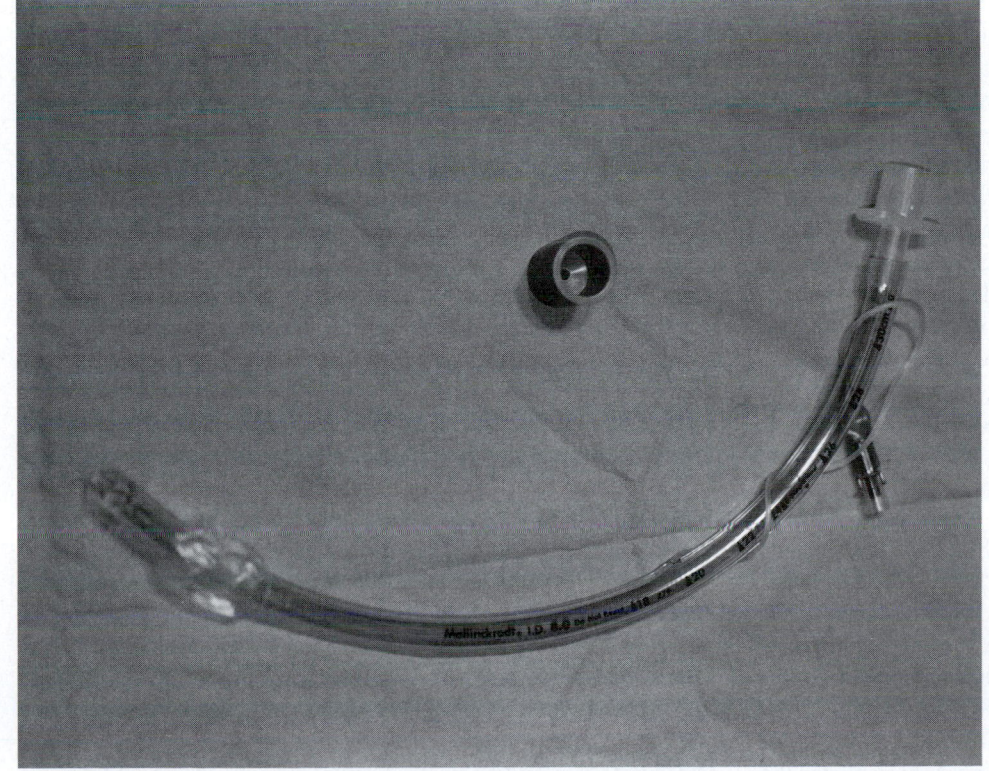

FIGURE 174-7   Standard endotracheal tube with whistle tip attachment to amplify breath sounds during blind nasal intubation.

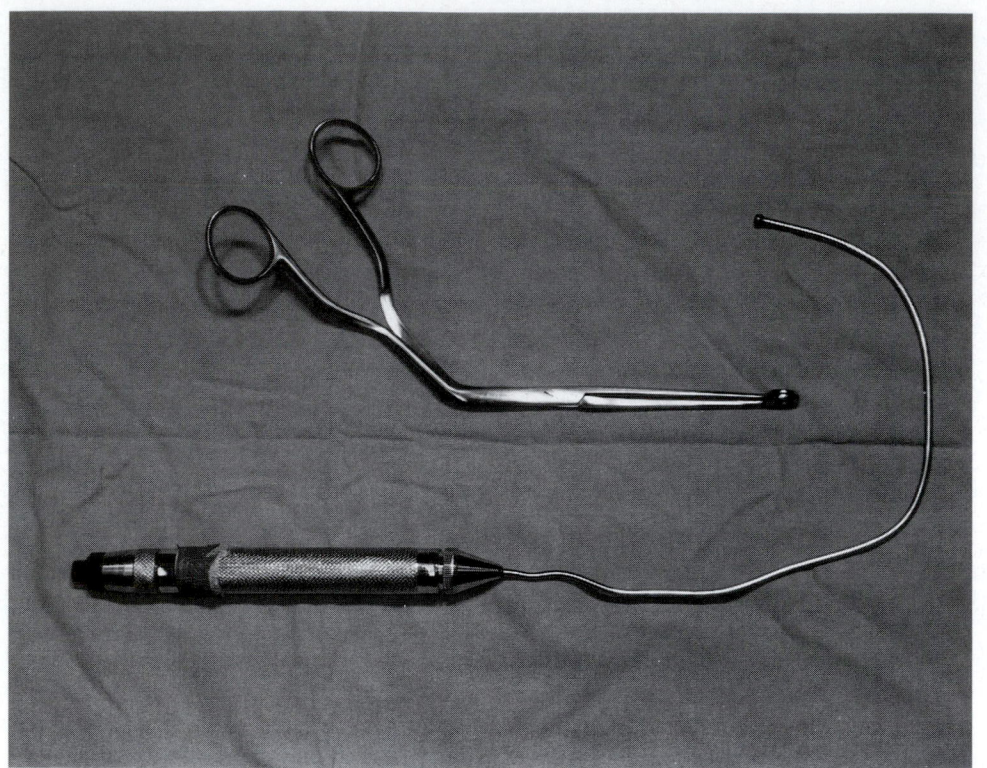

FIGURE 174-9 Magill forceps (see text) and light wand for transillumination of the trachea during blind oral intubation.

with a higher incidence of bleeding.[35] There is a minimal (less than 10 cc) increase in equipment dead space with nasotracheal tubes. However, no significant difference in resistance to airflow is associated with nasotracheal intubation.[21] Although the literature is conflicting on the incidence of sinusitis and pneumonia with nasotracheal and orotracheal intubations, a recent prospective, randomized trial showed no difference between the two routes.[15]

Direct laryngoscopy with orotracheal intubation is far and away the most common method of securing the airway. With the patient's head in the sniffing position, a Macintosh or Miller blade (Fig. 174-10) is inserted into the right side of the mouth with the left hand (regardless of the handedness of the operator). While anatomic considerations may give one blade an advantage over the other (the Miller blade is better with an anatomically anterior larynx), most operators become familiar with one blade and use it preferentially. The blades of both instruments are flanged to keep the tongue to the left side of the oropharynx, out of the visual field. Larger adult blades (Macintosh #4 or Miller #3) are used for patients with long mandibles, whereas shorter blades (Macintosh #3 or Miller #2) are used in patients with average-size anatomy. Smaller blades are used for children. The right hand is used to pull upper and lower lips out of the way, so that these structures are not caught and injured between the blade and the teeth. The tip of the laryngoscope blade is advanced along the tongue until the epiglottis is visible. If the Macintosh blade is used, it should be advanced between the tongue and the epiglottis, whereas with the Miller blade, the epiglottis should be directly elevated. The vocal cords should be visible immediately below the epiglottis. Most infants are in-

tubated with a Miller blade. The shape, length, and pliancy of the infant epiglottis make direct elevation necessary in order to view the vocal cords.

Some patients are difficult to intubate because of anatomic considerations, and a number of alternative approaches have evolved. These include fiberoptic laryngoscopy, in which the trachea is entered with the bronchoscope and an endotracheal tube advanced over the bronchoscope into the airway. A flexible light wand (Fig. 174-9) can be used to transilluminate and, thereby, identify the airway; an endotracheal tube can then be advanced into the airway using the wand as a stylet.[38] Retrograde techniques entail percutaneous cannulation of the trachea in the neck and retrograde passage of a wire or catheter into the oropharynx. The wire is grasped and secured to an endotracheal tube and used to guide its passage back into the trachea. Percutaneous cricothyrotomy kits are available for emergency access to the airway, and there are even percutaneous tracheostomy kits. The

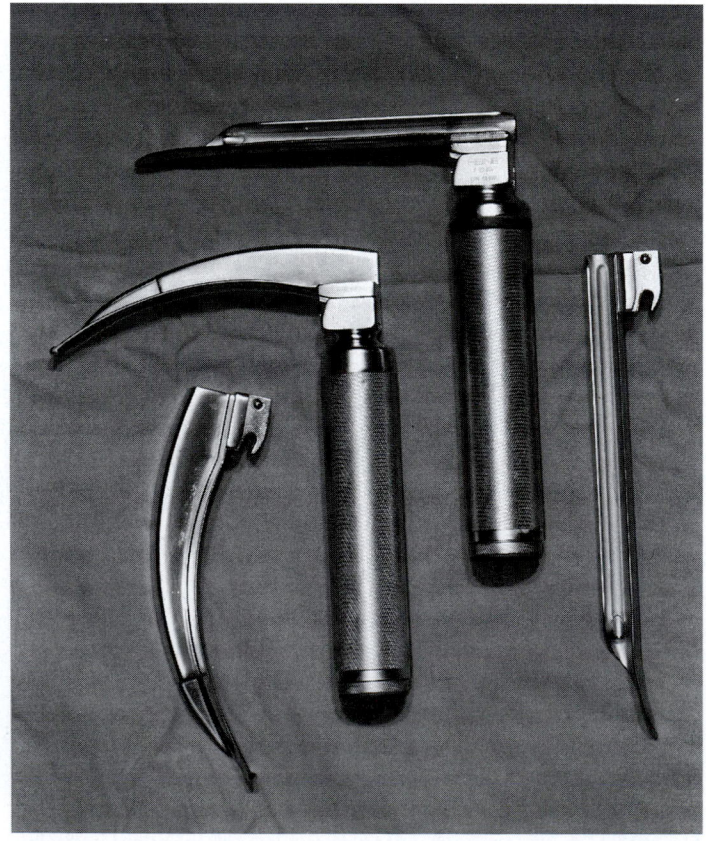

FIGURE 174-10 Macintosh and Miller blades.

manual on Advanced Cardiac Life Support[36] describes percutaneous jet ventilation through the cricothyroid membrane using a needle or intravenous catheter as a component of emergency airway management. The esophageal obturator airway was once widely used in field management of patients with respiratory compromise, but it has largely disappeared from use as paramedics have become trained in endotracheal intubation.

The anatomic features of the "difficult" airway are listed in Table 174-3. While a full discussion of the management of the potentially problematic airway is beyond the scope of this chapter, preparation can prevent catastrophe. The first question to be asked is whether the anatomy predicts difficulty limited to intubation alone, or problems with both ventilation and intubation. An anteriorly placed larynx is suggestive of the former, whereas obesity is more likely indicative of the latter—a more alarming circumstance. The next question is whether airway management is actually necessary: Can the procedure to be performed be done under regional, rather than general, anesthesia? When general anesthesia is required, a plan should be designed with an "escape route." Awake intubation, with sedation and topical airway anesthesia, is an excellent alternative. Direct laryngoscopy and

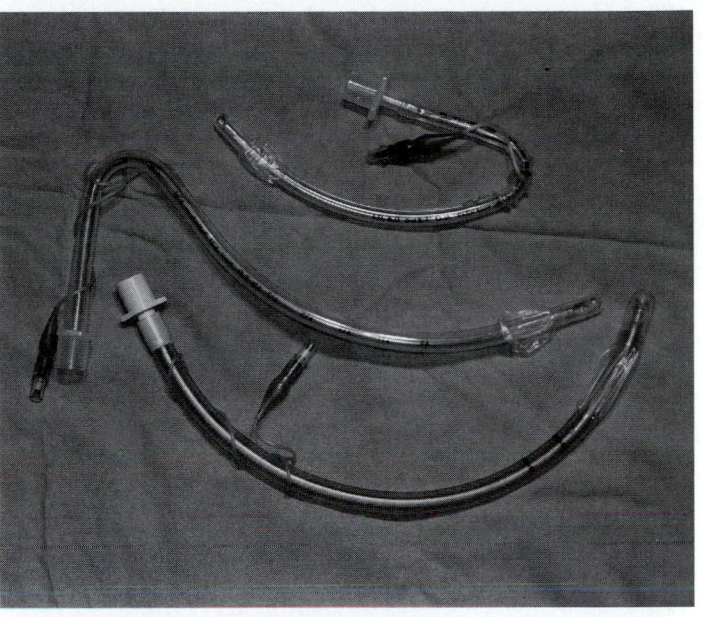

FIGURE 174-11   Oral and nasal preshaped tubes (RAE tubes). Anode, wire-wrapped tubes to prevent kinking.

fiberoptic bronchoscopy are equally appropriate for cooperative patients.

If difficulty with airway management is encountered unexpectedly in an already anesthetized patient, it is essential to ensure ventilation and oxygenation by mask or, if necessary, one of the invasive approaches described in the preceding paragraph. The establishment of reliable ventilation allows time for alternative approaches, including abandonment of the procedure (allowing the patient to awaken) or tracheostomy.

Reusable red rubber single-lumen tubes with separate cuffs were used as recently as the mid-1970s, and red rubber double-lumen tubes were in common use 5 to 10 years ago. Disposable tubes are now widely available; a host of design modifications have been made to make the tubes safer and to accommodate different surgical procedures. The cuff of the adult tube has been changed from a low-volume, noncompliant cuff to a higher-volume, very compliant cuff; as a consequence, the incidence of tracheal stenosis has declined.[6] Pediatric tubes are generally uncuffed because children are more vulnerable than adults to the development of subglottic stenosis due to tube contact with the trachea. Uncuffed tubes also maximize the cross-sectional area of the tube. Oral and nasal RAE tubes (Fig. 174-11) are preconfigured to permit facial and oral surgery without interference from the proximal portion of the endotracheal tube. There are a variety of special tubes for laser surgery. These tubes are less likely to burn when contacted by the laser beam. Reinforced or anode tubes have an embedded wire or nylon filament spiral in the wall of the tube that prevents kinking or collapse due to external pressure (Fig. 174-11). The Hi-Lo Jet endotracheal tube (Mallinckrodt) has four lumina—one for entrained gas, another for jet ventilation, a third for cuff inflation, and a fourth for pressure monitoring. However, endotracheal tube connectors (Fig. 174-7) have been designed to serve the same purpose and eliminate the need for a change in endotracheal tube.

TABLE 174-3

Indicators of a Potentially Difficult Airway

Poor mouth opening
Temporomandibular joint disease
Mandibular fracture
Dental problems
"Buck" anterior teeth
Caries
Dental hardware (caps, dentures)
Gaps
Abnormalities of the tongue
Large (e.g., in obesity)
Swollen
   Edema (surgical)
   Angioedema (allergic)
Fixed
   Scarring (radiation)
   Tumor
Presence of other intraoral structures
Tumors
Enlarged tonsils
Small jaw
"Anterior larynx"
Decreased neck mobility
Cervical disease or injury
   Suspected fracture
   Rheumatoid arthritis
   Ankylosing spondylitis
Increased age (presence of cervical osteophytes)
Congenital syndromes
Cleft palate
Treacher Collins
Pierre Robin
Klippel-Feil

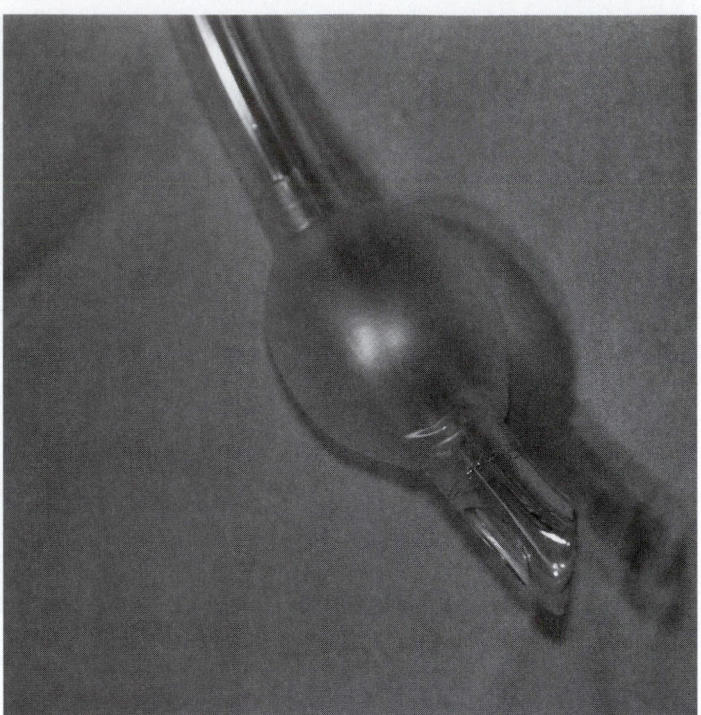

FIGURE 174-12 Endotracheal tube tip with Murphy eye and bevel (see text).

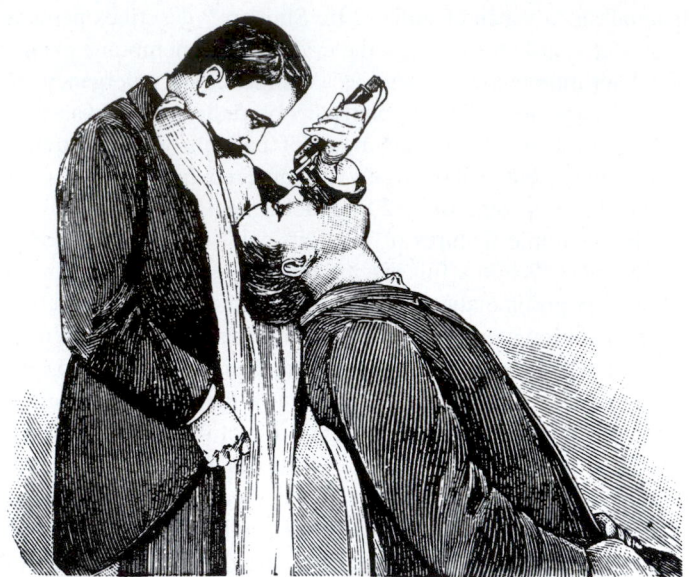

FIGURE 174-14 Earlier diagnostic airway intervention. *(From Kirstein: Archiv Laryngol Rhinol 3:156–164, 1895. Courtesy of Cushing/Whitney Medical Library.)*

All single-lumen tubes have a 15-mm outer diameter connector that fits any standard ventilation device. Most tubes also have a radiopaque stripe permitting tube localization on chest radiographs. The tip of the tube is beveled (Fig. 174-12); the bevel faces the left because endotracheal tubes are generally inserted from the right by right-handed operators. The extra hole opposite the bevel on many tubes is the "Murphy eye,"[30] a design that permits suctioning or antegrade gas flow if the bevel is occluded.

Disposable double-lumen endotracheal tubes are now available. The Carlens and White tubes used in the past were equipped with a carinal hook for correct tube placement. These tubes have largely been abandoned in favor of the Robertshaw design, which has a tracheal and bronchial cuff and no hook. The tube is available in four adult sizes (#35, #37, #39, #41 French) in both right-sided and left-sided designs (Fig. 174-13). The right-sided tube has an oblique bronchial cuff to accommodate takeoff of the right upper-lobe orifice. Correct placement of a double-lumen tube has become easier with development of bronchoscopes small enough to pass through the narrow tube lumina. An alternative to the double-lumen tube, the Univent tube, was introduced in 1982. It has a self-contained endobronchial blocker. The tube is inserted in the standard fashion, and the endobronchial blocker is then advanced, blindly or under direct vision, into the right or left main bronchus. A central lumen in the endobronchial blocker allows its inflation or deflation (Fig. 174-8).

CONCLUSION

Although some of the skills of airway management developed by the early pioneers may be lost to current practitioners (Fig. 174-14), advances in equipment, pharmacology, and product standards have largely eliminated equipment incompatibilities and problems associated with airway management during the era of cyclopropane or ether anesthesia. These advances have made new surgical procedures possible.

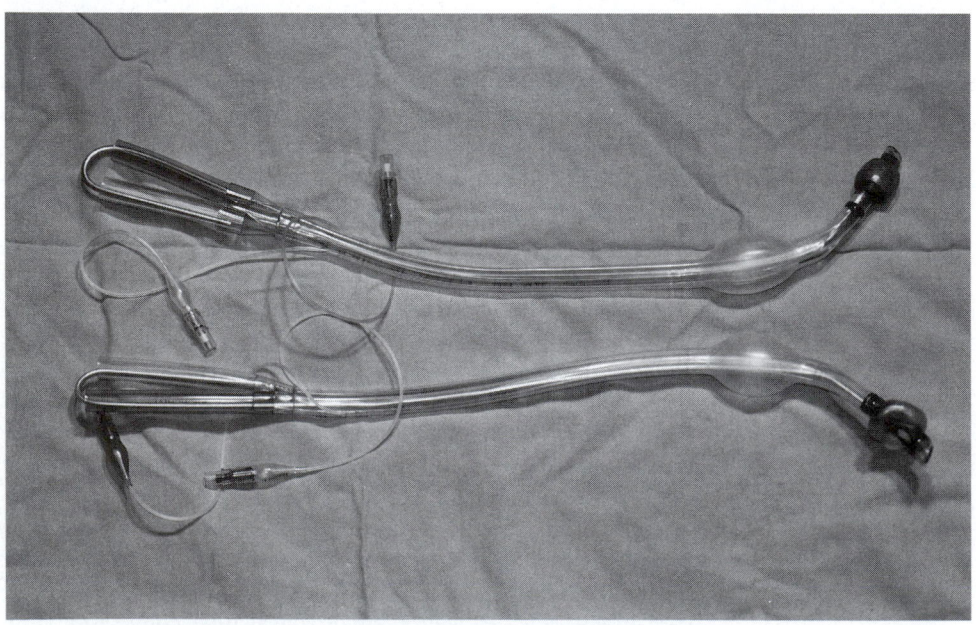

FIGURE 174-13 Right- and left-sided double-lumen endotracheal tubes. Note oblique bronchial cuff on the right-sided tube to accommodate right upper-lobe bronchial orifice.

REFERENCES

1. Asai T, Morris S: The laryngeal mask airway: Its features, effects and role. *Can J Anaesth* 41:930–960, 1994.

2. Brechner VL: Unusual problems in the management of airways: I. Flexion-extension mobility of the cervical vertebrae. *Anesth Analg* 47:362–373, 1968.

3. Brimacombe J, Berry A, Verghese C: The laryngeal mask airway in critical care medicine. *Intensive Care Med* 21:361–364, 1995.

4. Brimacombe J, Tucker P, Simons S: The laryngeal mask airway for awake diagnostic bronchoscopy. A retrospective study of 200 consecutive patients. *Eur J Anaesth* 12:357–361, 1995.

5. Calverlay RK: Arthur E. Guedel (1883–1956), in Rupreht J, van Lieburg MJ, Lee JA, Erdmann W (eds), *Anaesthesia Essays on Its History.* Berlin, Springer, 1985, pp 49–53.

6. Ching NP, Ayres SM, Paegle RP, et al: The contribution of cuff volume and pressure in tracheostomy tube damage. *J Thorac Cardiovasc Surg* 62:402–410, 1971.

7. Depoix JP, Malbezin S, Videcoq M, et al: Oral intubation v. nasal intubation in adult cardiac surgery. *Br J Anaesth* 59:167–169, 1987.

8. Dorrance GM: On the treatment of traumatic injuries of the lungs and pleurae, with the presentation of a new intratracheal tube for use in artificial respiration. *Surg Gynecol Obstet* 11:160–187, 1910.

9. Dorsch JA, Dorsch SE: Face masks and airways, in *Understanding Anesthesia Equipment,* 2d ed. Baltimore, Williams & Wilkins, 1984.

10. Eckenhoff JE: Some anatomic considerations of the infant larynx influencing endotracheal intubation. *Anesthesiology* 12:401–410, 1951.

11. Elsberg CA: The value of continuous intratracheal insufflation of air (Meltzer) in thoracic surgery: With description of an apparatus. *Med Rec* 77:493, 1910.

12. Fothergill J: A case published in the last volume of *Medical Essays* of recovery of a man dead in appearance, by distending the lungs with air, in Lettsam JC (ed), *The Works of John Fothergill MD.* London, C Dilly, 1784.

13. Herholdt JD, Rafn CG: An attempt at an historical survey of life-saving measures for drowning persons and information on the best means by which they can again be brought back to life. Printed at Tikiob Booksellers with M. Seest, Copenhagen, 1796. Reedited by Henning Poulsen; English translation by DW Hannah and A Rousing, 1960. *Scand Soc Anaesth.*

14. Hirsch NP, Smith GB, Hirsch PO: Alfred Kirstein, pioneer of direct laryngoscopy. *Anaesthesia* 41:42–45, 1982.

15. Holzapfel L, Chevret S, Madinier G, et al: Influence of long-term oro- or nasotracheal intubation on nosocomial maxillary sinusitis and pneumonia: Results of a prospective, randomized, clinical trial. *Crit Care Med* 21:1132–1138, 1993.

16. Hooke R: Account of an experiment, made by R. Hooke, of preserving animals alive by blowing through their lungs with bellows. *Philosophical Transactions of the Royal Society of London* 2:539–540, 1667.

17. Hunter J: Proposals for the recovery of people apparently drowned. *Philos Trans R Soc Lond* 1776:66, 1776.

18. Jackson C: The technique of insertion of intratracheal insufflation tubes. *Surg Gynecol Obstet* 17:507, 1913.

19. Janeway HH: An apparatus for intratracheal insufflation. *Ann Surg* 56:328–332, 1912.

20. Jenkins LC, McGraw RW: Anaesthetic management of the patient with rheumatoid arthritis. *Can Anaesth Soc J* 16:407–415, 1969.

21. Kil HK, Bishop MJ: Head position and oral vs nasal route as factors determining endotracheal tube resistance. *Chest* 105:1794–1797, 1994.

22. Kuhn F: Nasotracheal intubation (translated), in Faulconer A, Keys TE (eds), *Foundations of Anesthesiology,* Springfield, IL, Charles C Thomas, 1965, pp 677–680.

23. Läwen A, Sievers R: Zur Praktischen Anwendung der instrumentellen kunstlichen Respiration am Menschen. *MMW* 57:2221, 1910.

24. Leach A, Alexander CA, Stone B: The laryngeal mask airway in cardiopulmonary resuscitation in a district general hospital: A preliminary communication. *Resuscitation* 25:245–248, 1993.

25. Mallampati SR, Gatt SP, Gugino LD, et al: A clinical sign to predict difficult tracheal intubation: A prospective study. *Can Anaesth Soc J* 32:429–434, 1985.

26. Matas R: Intralaryngeal insufflation, for the relief of acute surgical pneumothorax: Its history, and methods with a description of the latest devices for this purpose. *JAMA* 34:1371–1375, 1900.

27. Matas R: Artificial respiration by direct intralaryngeal intubation with a modified O'Dwyer tube and a new graduated air-pump, in its applications to medical and surgical practice. *Am Med* 3:97, 1902.

28. Miller RA: A new laryngoscope. *Anesthesiology* 2:317–320, 1941.

29. Morch ET: History of mechanical ventilation, in Kirby RR, Banner MJ, Downs JB (eds), *Clinical Applications of Ventilatory Support.* New York, Churchill Livingstone, 1990.

30. Murphy FJ: Two improved intratracheal catheters. *Anesth Analg* 20:102–105, 1941.

31. Mushin WW, Rendall-Baker L: *The Principles of Thoracic Anesthesia Past and Present,* Springfield, IL, Charles C Thomas, 1953, pp 44–45.

32. Pennant JH, White PF: The laryngeal mask airway: Its uses in anesthesiology. *Anesthesiology* 80:706–707, 1994.

33. Sinclair JR, Mason RA: Ankylosing spondylitis: The case for awake intubation. *Anaesthesia* 39:3–11, 1984.

34. Smith DW: *Recognizable Patterns of Human Malformation,* 3d ed. Philadelphia, WB Saunders, 1987.

35. Smith JE, Grewal MS: Cardiovascular effects of nasotracheal intubation. *Anaesthesia* 46:683–686, 1991.

36. *Textbook of Advanced Cardiac Life Support.* American Heart Association, 1994, pp 211–213.

37. Thomas KB: Sir Ivan Whiteside Magill, KCVO, DSc, MB, BCh, BAO, FRCS, FFARCS (Hon), FFARCSI (Hon), DA: A review of his publications and other references to his life and work. *Anaesthesia* 33:628–634, 1978.

38. Weis FR, Hatton MN: Intubation by use of the light wand: Experience in 253 patients. *J Oral Maxillofac Surg* 47:577–580, 1989.

39. Wynne JW, Ramphal R, Hood CI: Tracheal mucosal damage after aspiration: A scanning electron microscope study. *Am Rev Respir Dis* 124:728–732, 1981.

HEMODYNAMIC AND RESPIRATORY MONITORING IN ACUTE RESPIRATORY FAILURE

Jonathan Gottlieb

PRINCIPLES AND CONSIDERATIONS OF MONITORING
Normal Range
Sampling Frequency
Cutoff Criteria and Alarms
Cost-Effectiveness Aspects of Monitoring

VITAL SIGNS
Temperature
Heart Rate
Respiratory Rate
Blood Pressure

MONITORING CIRCULATORY FUNCTION
Central Venous Pressure
Pulmonary Artery and Pulmonary Artery Occlusion Pressure Measurement
Cardiac Output

MONITORING RESPIRATORY FUNCTION
Mechanics
Compliance, Resistance, Pressure, and Flow
Lung Volume
Gas Exchange

INTEGRATED SYSTEMS MONITORING
Oxygen Indices
Lactate
Gastric Intramucosal pH

To monitor is to watch or observe, usually for a special purpose. The connotation of anxiously watching derives from the Latin *monere,* "to warn." In another variation on the definition, monitoring implies checking, regulating, and controlling. Patients are monitored in intensive care units for one major purpose: to identify signs of illness before symptoms become debilitating or illness reaches an advanced stage; the goal is to provide therapeutic intervention to halt the progression of the illness. Sometimes the obverse is emphasized: we monitor to assure ourselves that

no indication of serious illness is present. An example of such monitoring includes much "routine" postoperative or "step-down" cardiac monitoring, usually performed more for reassurance than to identify and correct specific cardiac arrhythmias. In these instances, the prevalence of serious illness is much lower than in a special care unit devoted to the care of patients with trauma, acute myocardial infarction, or septic shock, for example. These conditions frequently manifest abnormalities detectable by monitoring that lead to therapeutic intervention.

Too often, monitoring is performed out of tradition or conformity. Patients with conditions associated with a low likelihood of short-term progression or with little benefit from therapeutic intervention will generally not profit from monitoring. For example, the patient with asymptomatic trigeminy without other evidence of cardiac disease or systemic illness is not likely to benefit from continuous electrocardiographic monitoring. Nevertheless, such patients may be extensively monitored out of misplaced medical or legal concerns.

Current approaches to monitoring combine both diagnostic and screening aspects. Monitoring entails the application of tests or procedures, usually in a repetitive or continuous fashion, to identify a signal that either suggests or defines a diagnosis. Thus, paroxysmal atrial tachycardia, intracranial hypertension, respiratory acidosis, oliguria, and other "diagnoses" may be reached through the acquisition of monitored data. Unlike the more common use of diagnostic tests, however, monitoring is seldom employed in response to a specific complaint and is seldom directed at focused hypothesis testing (to "rule out" pulmonary embolism, for instance). Rather, monitoring entails the notion of continuous screening in a population with a high probability of an important finding. In this regard, the value of monitoring must be assessed with respect to the benefits and costs associated with identifying or missing, correctly or mistakenly, the monitored data. Unfortunately, most monitoring has yet to be assessed in this manner. Absence of standard definitions, local variations in practice, difficulty in carrying out prospective randomized trials in critically ill patients, and our indiscriminate attraction to new technology and information all conspire to impede the rational evaluation of monitoring in the critical care setting.

Hemodynamic and respiratory monitoring in acute respiratory failure may be considered special applications of a more generalized approach to hemodynamic and respiratory monitoring in critical care. This chapter addresses advanced monitoring considerations in patients with acute respiratory failure, with an emphasis on interpretation of data in light of physiological mechanisms. Special consideration is given to interpretation of data from combined systems monitoring for two main reasons. First, pathophysiological interactions between the pulmonary and cardiovascular systems in acute respiratory failure present a challenge to interpretation of data from either system. Second, acute respiratory failure often accompanies injury to other systems. For a discussion of basic techniques and complications of procedures that accompany monitoring, the reader is referred to other chapters in the text.

PRINCIPLES AND CONSIDERATIONS OF MONITORING

Inherent to the concept of clinical monitoring is that an accepted standard or normal range exists for the parameters measured. Not only must the frequency of the measurements be specified, but the acceptable variance outside the normal range must be set prospectively and alarms set accordingly. The discussion below addresses these aspects of monitoring and highlights related cost-effectiveness issues.

Normal Range

Standard statistical concepts of normality are universally, but sometimes fallaciously, applied to clinical data. For example, a range of data that encompasses two standard deviations (95 percent of the data) on either side of the mean is frequently used to define what is normal. However, there is no a priori reason to base the definition of what is normal upon this statistical definition. An alternative approach to defining normality might incorporate consideration of consequences to the patient. For example, recent data suggest that more than 5 percent of the American population is above ideal body weight. Hence, the concept of "normal" weight should be considered more narrowly to identify patients whose weight may pose health risks.

Based, in part, on this concept of consequences, many laboratories have established a list of "critical values" for certain tests, any of which may trigger an emergency call to the nursing staff or physician. The magnitude of the measurement that defines such critical value depends more on the life-threatening consequences of the abnormality (for example, a hemoglobin of 4.0 g/dl) than on the value relative to the mean of a group of hemoglobin values.

For the purposes of critical care monitoring, normal ranges are often established on an individual basis. Critical care nurses often set a higher threshold for a heart rate alarm in a young trauma patient who manifests prolonged and refractory sinus tachycardia than for one in an elderly patient with myocardial ischemia. The same value of serum potassium that may be treated

as normal in a patient recovering from renal failure may prompt supplementation in a patient taking digoxin and having ventricular arrhythmias.

Sampling Frequency

The advent of sophisticated electronic analog and digital technology has fostered the practice of regular acquisition and storage of large amounts of clinical data. Temperature, pulse, respiratory rate, and blood pressure may all be sampled at nearly continuous frequencies, and thousands of data points may be digitally stored for subsequent recall and analysis. In general, the frequency of data sampling should depend, in part, on the coefficient of variation of the data normalized for time and weighted by the clinical significance of the variation in the data. For example, serum bilirubin is an important indicator of bilirubin metabolism and may suggest hepatic dysfunction or hemolysis; it may also provide important clues to prognosis in multisystem organ dysfunction accompanying acute respiratory failure. Because the bilirubin level seldom fluctuates substantially over a 6- to 12-h period, however, the practice of monitoring bilirubin generally includes sampling no more often than daily.

In practice, sampling frequency is often dictated by technologic availability. Continuous electrocardiographic monitoring provides a continuous display of the pulse in almost all monitored hospitalized patients, although many patients without significant cardiac arrhythmias benefit little from this "value added" information. Indiscriminate use of high sampling frequency may create dilemmas for the clinician. With the wide availability of transcutaneous oxygen monitoring, the interpretation of transient desaturation may be open to questions of interpretation. Was the observation a result of a mucous plug, a transient fall in cardiac output, redistribution of ventilation and perfusion with positioning, pulmonary embolism, or technical artifact? It was perhaps the uncertain interpretation of such data in one report that led to therapeutic intervention in only 26 percent of patients who desaturated to less than 85 percent by continuous pulse oximetry.[3]

Discretionary sampling frequency provides other clinical conundrums, as in the systematic overweighting of abnormal results. For example, a normal routine arterial blood gas result is likely to be followed by the next "scheduled" blood gas. However, an abnormal result will usually precipitate supplemental tests soon after the first, resulting in greater documentation of the abnormal than of the normal condition. Any archiving strategy that employs blind averaging may unintentionally overweight the contribution of abnormal values.

Cutoff Criteria and Alarms

Clinicians usually rely on the upper limit of the range of temperature, or "Tmax," to make therapeutic decisions, but they do not generally consider the extremes of the ranges of pulse (except, perhaps, in a patient with atrioventricular nodal disease or sick sinus syndrome) in daily decisions. The "Pmax" is not a part of the intensivist's lexicon. Except in the case of certain cardiac arrhythmias, trends of pulse rate, or area under the time–pulse curve, are of greater significance than are maximal values in indicating pain, anxiety, or adequacy of stroke volume. Thresholds for clinical action (cutoff or alarm values) may be viewed in the context of sensitivity and specificity in reflecting a disease or physiological state, and with regard to the consequences of classifying a result as a true or false positive or as a true or false negative.

With the ideal monitoring device, a threshold alarm would be selected that separates all important events from unimportant events, such as normal blood pressure from hypo- or hypertension; only true positives and true negatives would be identified. In reality, however, technical and other issues make such perfect discrimination unattainable. More commonly, a threshold is selected that is biased toward the identification of more true positives (and more false positives) or toward more true negatives (and more false negatives). Where the threshold is optimally set will depend on the likelihood of the event and the consequences of a misclassification (Fig. 175-1).

For example, an end-tidal carbon dioxide monitor may be used in a patient who is hyperventilated for increased intracranial pressure. Because the consequences of rising Pa_{CO_2} may be devastating, the clinician should be prepared to respond to several "false alarms" for every real instance of an increase in Pa_{CO_2}. In order to catch all the instances of hypercarbia, the threshold should be set at a low level (high sensitivity, low specificity). In contrast, the highly agitated patient who continually triggers the rate alarm because of muscle tremor would benefit from a higher rate alarm threshold, in the absence of suspected or known tachyarrhythmias (low sensitivity, high specificity).

The situation becomes slightly more complex when one considers monitoring that substitutes for the "gold standard" measurement. Examples include transcutaneous measurements of gas exchange in place of arterial blood gas analysis, and pulmonary arterial wedge pressure in place of left ventricular end-diastolic volume. In both of these examples, the data provided by the monitor are surrogates for the data that would accrue from the gold standard. Using Bayes' approach to determining the meaning of an event that triggers an alarm or crosses a threshold, the monitoring procedure could be evaluated in terms of its likelihood of representing a true event (predictive value positive), likelihood of signaling a nonevent (false alarm rate), likelihood of silence representing the absence of a true event (predictive value negative or reassurance rate), and likelihood of silence erroneously representing a true event ("lulled into a false sense of security" rate). Such an analysis would be of greater use to clinicians than simple correlation coefficients between surrogate and gold-standard data, since it would describe the *direction* as well as the *magnitude* of the discrepancy (Fig. 175-2).

Cost-Effectiveness Aspects of Monitoring

In addition to intensive nursing care, monitoring is the defining activity in critical care units. With the exception of cardiac monitoring in the peri-infarction period, however, there are few data to support the effectiveness of monitoring in critical care units in relation to cost or outcome. Clinical trials to evaluate monitoring efficacy face formidable design obstacles: 1. Patients would have to be stratified by demographics, health status, etiology of acute illness, and severity of illness. 2. Therapy and procedures would have to be standardized. 3. Meaningful outcome measures would have to be selected among survival to hospital discharge, functional status at some point after discharge, cost of care (including acquisition cost, labor cost of maintaining and using monitors, other marginal costs associated with monitoring), or others. 4. The likely small impact of monitoring in the overall course of critical illness will necessitate large and costly trials. For example, an estimated sample size of 500,000 to 1,900,000 would be required to detect a significant decrease in morbidity using pulse oximetry during operative procedures.[29] 5. Where local standards of care include an assumed level of monitoring, resistance to "blinding" of clinicians to patient physiological data would be expected.

Counterbalancing these problems, recent economic pressures may encourage the careful evaluation of current and future monitoring devices and procedures. Although it may not be feasible in most instances to study the question of whether or not to monitor, it is feasible to study alternative methods of monitoring with respect to cost, effectiveness, or outcome. Taking standard practice as a baseline, new technology should be evaluated for its acquisition cost, maintenance costs, and ability to replace or eliminate other testing or otherwise improve outcome or clinical care. Too often, technologic innovations supplement, rather than supplant, older procedures.

Pulse oximetry provides an instructive example of the difficulties in quantifying the benefits of monitoring. Using the data from insurance files for anesthesiologists in the mid-1980s, a number of authors provided quantitative analyses. In one such retrospective analysis, it was estimated that one-third of all claims related to respiratory gas exchange.[4] Furthermore, it was estimated that more than 90 percent of all injuries related to respiratory gases could have been prevented with proper use and interpretation of pulse oximetry and capnography.[44] Thus, both common sense and several retrospective analyses suggest that

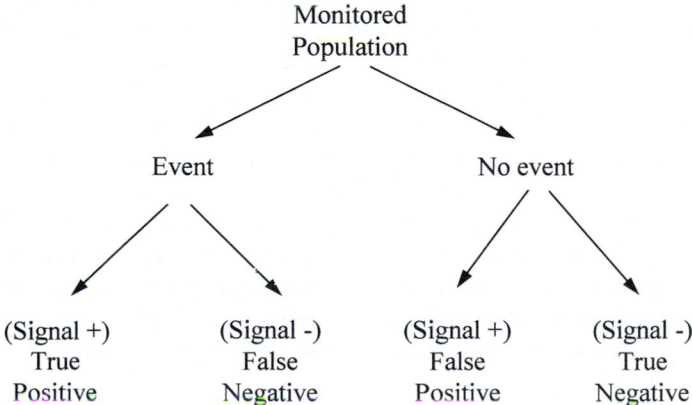

FIGURE 175-1   When a monitor sounds an alarm, the clinician's task is to interpret the signal with respect to the likelihood that it represents a true alarm (true positive/[true positive + false positive]). This likelihood is analogous to the predictive value positive of a diagnostic test result. The complement is the false alarm rate (false positive/[true positive + false positive]). Similarly, absence of an alarm signal may provide appropriate reassurance (true negative/[true negative + false negative]), analogous to the predictive value negative of a test result, or it may represent a false sense of security, in the sense that the clinician is misled by a silent monitor. This likelihood may be calculated as false negative/(false negative + true negative).

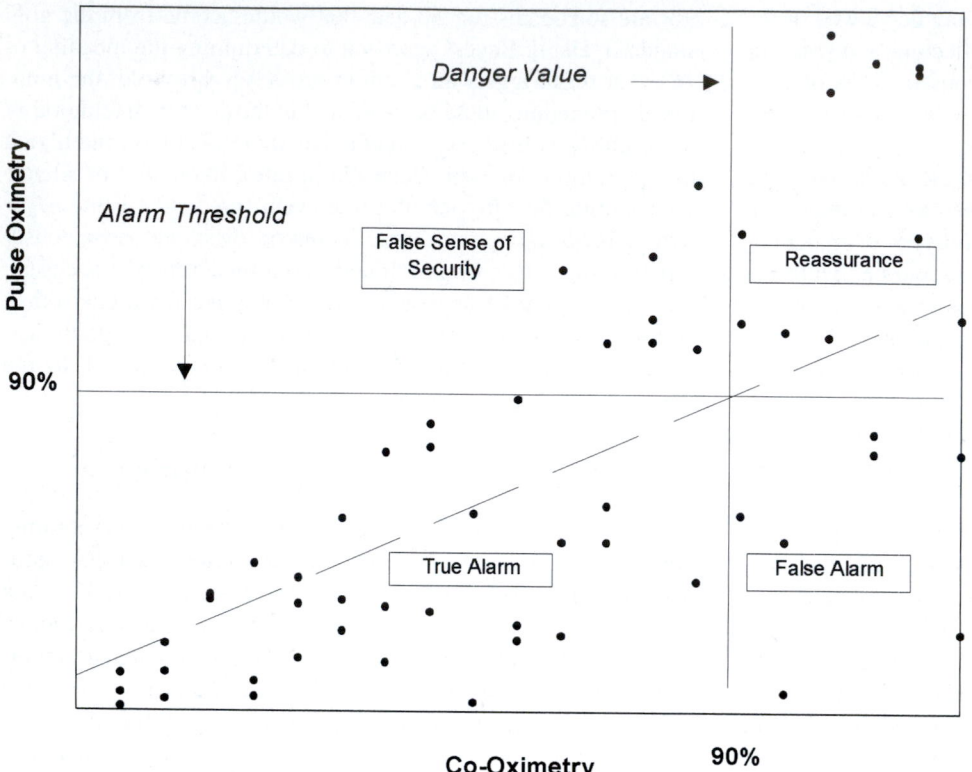

FIGURE 175-2 Monitor result versus gold standard. In this example, representing a range of pulse oximetry measurements, values for co-oximetry below 90% (solid vertical line) are clinically important and reflect a danger threshold; the monitor alarm is accordingly set at the alarm threshold (solid horizontal line). Upper right and lower left quadrants represent reassurance rate of 56% [true negative/(true negative + false negative)] and true alarm rate of 80% [true positive/(true positive + false positive)] areas, respectively. Upper left and lower right quadrants represent false sense of security rate of 44% (false negative/true negative + false negative) and false alarm rate of 20% (false positive/true positive + false positive) values, respectively. Sensitivity is 50% and specificity 67% at a threshold value of 90% saturation. Portrayal of monitor performance in this manner adds additional information to the usual analyses of correlation coefficient ($r = 0.59$, $p < 0.0001$).

monitoring of respiratory gas exchange may significantly reduce complications and improve outcome.

Unfortunately, demonstration of such benefit is elusive in concurrent or prospective investigations. A Canadian study of more than 35,000 patients over a 15-month period failed to demonstrate a significant relationship between use of pulse oximetry and capnography and patient morbidity or mortality.[6] A study of almost 15,000 consecutive ICU admissions failed to demonstrate a reduction in mortality associated with the use of invasive hemodynamic monitoring.[35]

Assuming that pulse oximetry and other standard monitoring does confer some benefit, it is possible to estimate the marginal costs associated with monitoring. Using previously published data[8] suggesting that for every 8000 to 80,000 patients monitored with pulse oximetry, one death would be averted, investigators calculated a cost of $50,000 to $450,000 for each life saved.[34] This figure is of the same order of magnitude as for other interventions, such as antihypertensive therapy. Other cost analyses may take into account savings when one procedure (e.g., pulse oximetry) replaces another (arterial blood gas sampling), or malpractice costs avoided in terms of reduced awards and premiums. Unfortunately, clear evidence of the effectiveness of critical care monitoring is difficult to obtain.

VITAL SIGNS

The value of routine monitoring of vital signs has been amply demonstrated over many years of clinical practice. While the technology for monitoring vital signs has evolved, the basic techniques of recording temperature, heart rate, respiratory rate, and blood pressure provide fundamental information that is critical in assessing patients in a critical care setting.

Temperature

Recent studies of normal temperature have produced results that are at odds with common practice.[24] In one study of normal ambulatory volunteers, the mean oral temperature was 36.8°C (98.2°F), rather than the traditionally cited 37.0°. Moreover, there was a mean daily amplitude of variability of 0.5°C (0.9°F). As many as two-thirds of all critically ill patients demonstrate temperature abnormalities in either direction on admission.[19] Fever may signal not only infection but also hyperthyroidism and a variety of disorders of temperature control, including drug-induced alterations in metabolism, neuroleptic malignant syndrome from centrally acting drugs, malignant hyperthermia, and environmental heat stroke.

Core temperatures below 35°C occur in 3 percent of all ICU admissions in the United States and may carry a mortality of greater than 50 percent, in part because of the association of hypothermia with alcohol use, diabetes mellitus, advanced age, and other underlying conditions. However, many glass thermometers do not record temperatures below 96°F, resulting in an underrecognition and underreporting of the condition. The traditionally cool operating room environment (17 to 21°C) has resulted in comfortable surgeons but hypothermic patients; recent evidence suggests that such hypothermia may be deleterious to certain groups of patients.[22]

Mercury glass thermometers also display the disadvantages of fragility, long equilibration time (3 min), and the need for special thermometers to record low temperatures. Thermistors are frequently used to measure temperature at a variety of sites, as they may be fashioned into probes that will accommodate placement in peripheral catheters, as well as in oral or rectal probes. Composed of oxides of nickel, cobalt, or manganese, thermistors display a drop in resistance with increasing temperature and typically have a time constant well under 90 s. The inherent nonlinearity of the thermistor response can be overcome with additional fixed resistors.

Selection of temperature measurement site can affect the accuracy of the results. Using pulmonary artery thermistor temperature as a gold standard,[37] rectal temperatures agree with pulmonary artery temperature most often. Tympanic membrane temperature correlates less well but is significantly better than axillary measurement, which typically ranges from 1.5 to 2°C below core temperature. Tympanic membrane temperature should not be taken as a substitute for core temperature before otoscopic inspection of the auditory canal has been performed. Oral temperatures may reflect core temperature reasonably well, although more than half of such recorded temperatures may underestimate rectal values by 0.5 to 1.0°C. Tachypnea is a well-recognized cause of falsely low sublingual temperatures.[42]

Temperature has been used to "correct" arterial blood gases measured at 37°C when the patient is hyper- or hypothermic. There appears little justification for this practice. For example, the arterial P_{O_2} of a hypothermic patient measured at 37°C may overestimate the P_{O_2} at patient temperature by a considerable amount, but interpretation is problematic. "Normal"—that is, physiologically appropriate values for pH, P_{O_2} and P_{CO_2}—varies as a function of temperature. Attempts to bring these values in a hypo- or hyperthermic patient into ranges appropriate for a patient at 37°C may not produce the intended outcome.

Normally, peripheral skin temperature is several degrees lower than core temperature. Extreme differences between core and peripheral skin temperature may indicate severe impairment of cardiac output or regional perfusion. Exploiting this direct relationship between peripheral perfusion and skin temperature, some investigators have noted a mortality of 67 percent in adults with toe temperatures below 27°C for 3 h or more.[17] Average temperatures over the first week are elevated to 37.8°C in patients with adult respiratory distress syndrome (ARDS), and survivors have significantly higher temperatures than nonsurvivors by 0.5°C.[41]

Heart Rate

Heart rate is readily and redundantly measured in all patients in critical care units. As a nonspecific sign of neurohumoral stress, tachycardia may signal a variety of disorders, from pain or anxiety to shock. In intubated patients who are sedated and paralyzed, tachycardia may be the first and only sign of serious illness, such as pneumothorax, acidosis, or hemorrhage. In these patients, heart rate, along with blood pressure, is an essential sign of the adequacy of analgesic and sedative therapy. In addition, accurate determinations of heart rate are important because the heart rate is used to calculate many derived indices of cardiovascular function.

Algorithms accompanying computer-assisted data acquisition of blood pressure and electrocardiograms (ECGs) derive a heart rate based on a continuously moving frame that calculates the rate over a given duration, typically several seconds. Low signal voltage or high detection threshold can produce an erroneously low heart rate on ECG monitoring; abnormally elevated T waves or limb tremor have been reported to trigger falsely elevated values. Pressure-derived estimates of heart rate are less problematic, and newer "intelligent" arrhythmia detection devices have improved accuracy of the ECG-determined heart rate.

ECG monitoring, which has been studied more extensively than any other monitoring technique with respect to patient outcome, clearly decreases morbidity and mortality from acute myocardial infarction,[20] provided appropriate action is taken on receipt of the data. One of the likely reasons for the success of ECG monitoring in patients with acute myocardial infarction is the extremely high prevalence of rate or rhythm disturbances, coupled with the dire consequences of undetected events, in light of the efficacy of current arrhythmia therapy. Thus, the patient with acute myocardial infarction presents the need for continuous monitoring and the selection of a low threshold for alarm.

In patients admitted to a noncardiac ICU, the value of sophisticated arrhythmia monitoring is uncertain, although atrial and ventricular tachycardia may occur in 25 percent of general ICU patients. However, the prognostic significance of such arrhythmias is unclear, as is the need for or response to treatment.

One potentially valuable use of heart rate trend analysis is the simple differentiation of sinus tachycardia from a reentrant tachycardia—as might occur during weaning from mechanical ventilation, for example. Sinus tachycardia will be displayed as a gradually increasing heart rate, whereas a supraventricular tachycardia is revealed as a "step-up" in the heart rate trend (Fig. 175-3). The treatment of one tachycardia is clearly different from that of the other; outcome differences have not been investigated. Patients with ARDS generally show tachycardia, with initial rates of about 110—which fall gradually to 100 over the first week.[41]

Respiratory Rate

In spontaneously breathing patients, respiratory rate has been increasingly recognized as an important indicator of respiratory status and prognosis. The measurement is difficult to make, in part because of deficiency in clinical skill and in part because of a lack of patient cooperation. Clinical staff may record a respiratory rate based on observation that is at odds with monitored data more than one-third of the time; however, impedance monitors may show inaccuracies when compared to other measures. Given the importance of measuring respiratory rate, it is worth emphasizing two points. First, sufficient time (1 min or more)

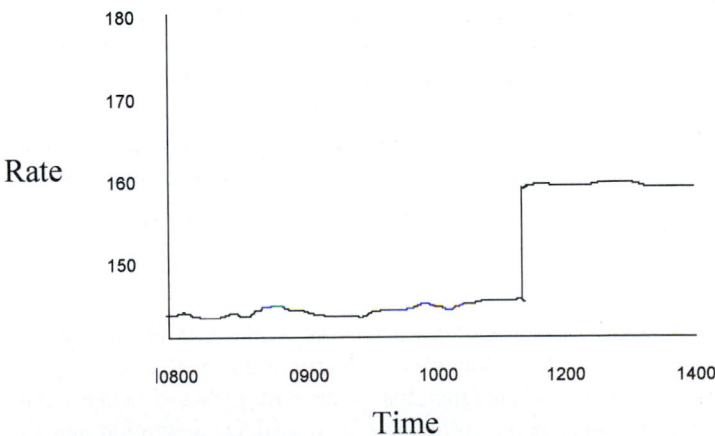

FIGURE 175-3   Continuous trend display of heart rate (vertical axis) over time (horizontal axis). Several minutes earlier than 1200, sudden rapid increase in rate strongly suggests reentrant supraventricular tachycardia, rather than sinus tachycardia. Therapy should be directed at resolving the mechanism of reentry, rather than at causes of sinus tachycardia.

must be allotted to sample the respiratory frequency. Second, because of the requirement for patient cooperation, it is helpful to distract the patient from the activity of being observed. This can be accomplished by observing the patient from a distance, such as outside the room, or by observing the respiratory rate while appearing to take the pulse or auscultate the heart.

Despite careful measurement of the respiratory rate, observation provides only a "snapshot." It is helpful to obtain a trend of respiratory rate over time to gauge the response to weaning, fluid therapy, or other activities. For more than 30 years, the transthoracic electrical impedance change with respiration has been measured as an indicator of respiratory rate. As the distance between electrodes increases with respiration, the resistance changes. Typically recorded from ECG surface electrodes, these changes reflect not only phasic changes of rate but also quantitative changes indicative of tidal volume. However, because of shifts in body position, changes in compliance, and other factors, accurate estimation of tidal volume is not practical using impedance from ECG electrode signals. They are inadequate to detect apnea and may overestimate or underestimate respiratory rate. These discrepancies are usually readily ascertained by glancing at the patient. The main advantages of the method are its universal availability, continuous application, minimal patient discomfort, and low acquisition and maintenance cost.

Although respiratory rate has long been recognized as an important vital sign in its own right, it has recently received greater attention and more careful study, particularly as it relates to successful weaning from mechanical ventilation. In particular, several authors have noted that a rapid respiratory rate (f), in the presence of a low tidal volume (V_T), portends unsuccessful weaning. A ratio of f/V_T greater than 100 breaths/min/L is associated with a 95 percent weaning trial failure rate; a ratio of less than 100 accompanies successful weaning trials in 80 percent of patients.[49]

Blood Pressure

Measurement of blood pressure may be accomplished by a wide variety of methods, both invasive and noninvasive. As an indicator of acute catastrophe (e.g., malignant hypertensive crisis, septic shock), as well as a guide to preventive medicine (ambulatory blood pressure measurement for hypertension), blood pressure determination has benefited from a great deal of technical innovation over the years. Many of the principles fundamental to arterial pressure measurement also apply to measurements of other vascular and fluid pressures.

INVASIVE BLOOD PRESSURE MEASUREMENT

Conversion of vascular pressure into a meaningful display requires a system that includes a pressure transducer, a device producing an electrical signal that varies with pressure changes. An understanding of the principles of transducer operation and of pressure waveform generation are important prerequisites to the interpretation of blood pressure measurements.

Typically, pressure transducers operate by allowing a low-compliance diaphragm to undergo deformation in response to a pressure change across the diaphragm. As the diaphragm bends, it results in lengthening (increasing resistance) of a resistor across its convex surface and a shortening (decreasing resistance) across

its concave surface. When a small current is passed through this arrangement of resistors (Wheatstone bridge), the output voltage varies with change in resistance induced by deformation of the resistors. Modern transducers employ silicon semiconductor technology to create a very small silicon-bonded integrated circuit that functions as a Wheatstone bridge.

Electrical calibration is achieved by unbalancing the Wheatstone bridge with a known voltage; referencing of the transducer to atmospheric pressure is achieved by adjustment of the resistances to the bridge so that no current is produced. Calibration of the display of the amplified signal entails the application of a manometer-referenced pressure signal, with adjustment of the display to reflect the magnitude of the input pressure. Most transducers are manufactured with a constant sensitivity of 50 mv/10 mmHg, thereby facilitating the interchangeability of different transducers with a critical care unit's electronic monitors.

Dynamic pressure measurements such as arterial pressure invoke an additional transducer specification: frequency response. Fortunately, the electronic frequency response of most transducer–preamplifier systems exceeds the fastest physiological frequencies by a factor of 5 to 50, a capability far in excess of that required to accurately reproduce an input signal. A source of considerable concern, however, is the magnification and diminution of the aortic pressure as it travels down the arterial tree and into the fluid-filled catheter connected to the transducer. A number of factors—including length and diameter of the tube, density of the fluid, compliance of the tube walls, and proximity of the catheter tip to the site of wave reflection—may interact to produce a pressure wave at the measurement site that is of significantly different contour from that of the aortic arch. Typically, as the pressure wave moves from the arch to a peripheral artery, high-frequency components (such as the dicrotic notch) are attenuated, whereas peak systolic pressures are exaggerated. A practical observation of these phenomena is that radial or dorsalis pedis peak systolic pressures commonly exceed brachial or aortic pressures, and peripheral diastolic pressures frequently fall below central diastolic pressures. For this reason, mean arterial pressure remains a more constant value across sites of measurement.

Two factors that depend on the physical characteristics of the transducer, tubing, and catheter are the *resonant frequency* and the *damping coefficient*. As the resonant frequency of the system approaches frequencies in the physiological range, the potential for "ringing" is increased, as indicated by exaggeration of the magnitude of the systolic and diastolic peaks (Fig. 175-4). Just as blow-

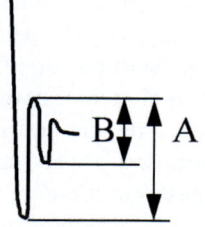

FIGURE 175-4   Ringing of arterial pressure tracking. Release of flush valve causes a sudden fall in pressure and ringing. Ratio of height of B to A is used to calculate a damping ratio. For details, see text.

ing across an air-filled tube produces the loudest tone at the resonant frequency, so may a component of a physiological wave be magnified in amplitude within a catheter-transducer system at its resonant frequency. Unfortunately, small-diameter catheters tend to have lower resonant frequencies, as described by the equation:

$$\text{Resonant frequency} = \frac{1}{2\pi} \sqrt{\frac{\pi D^2 \times \Delta P}{4pL \times \Delta V}} \qquad (1)$$

where

$$
\begin{aligned}
D &= \text{diameter} \\
L &= \text{length} \\
p &= \text{density of liquid} \\
\text{and } \Delta P/\Delta V &= \text{compliance}
\end{aligned}
$$

Practically speaking, long (6 to 8 feet) and narrow extension tubing can increase apparent peak systolic pressure by more than 30 percent.

Opposing the resonant properties that tend to artifactually elevate transient pressures, resistive forces tend to decrease the velocity of the mass of fluid in the catheter, resulting in damping. Like resonance, damping is indirectly proportional to tubing diameter. Thus, increased damping with small-diameter tubing tends to moderate the increased resonance. The damping coefficient ranges from 1.0 (no resonance, static pressures only reflected) to near 0 (no damping of resonant oscillations). In practical terms, a damping coefficient of 0.6 to 0.7 produces the most useful waveforms, with little overshoot and accurate reproduction of waveform transients.

Much has been written about the "fast-flush" technique of assessing the resonant and damping characteristics of a catheter and tubing system (Fig. 175-5). This simple maneuver is useful for detecting undesirable characteristics of such a system as an aid to interpretation of displayed waveforms. The technique consists of opening the system to the pressurized container of flush solution, producing a sustained square wave with an amplitude corresponding to about 300 mmHg. When the valve is released, the pressure abruptly falls. An overdamped system is revealed as a gradual return of pressure to baseline, whereas an underdamped system demonstrates prolonged "ringing" (Fig. 175-5).

NONINVASIVE BLOOD PRESSURE MEASUREMENT

Automated devices that measure and record at regular intervals have expanded the use of noninvasive blood pressure devices in the ICU. Although different devices all have in common an inflatable cuff placed around the arm, the methods of signal detection vary considerably from one device to another. Indeed, the absence of standardization makes interpretation of a particular blood pressure reading dependent, in part, on the method used to obtain it.

When disparate pressures are obtained from a patient with both an intra-arterial catheter and a noninvasive cuff, a question frequently asked is, "Which pressure is correct?" In fact, the two methods measure different phenomena. Arterial cannulation provides information about pressure within the vessel, regardless of flow. In contrast, indirect manometry depends on a technique to detect flow within a vessel as an approximation of pressure. Generalizations are difficult to make, because several confounding

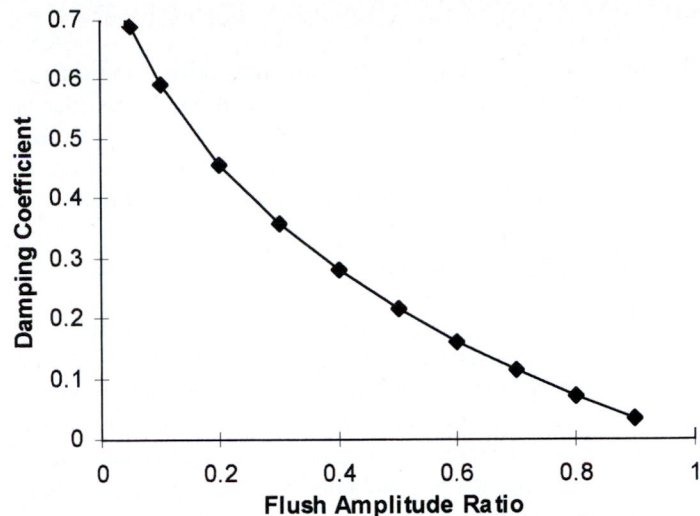

FIGURE 175-5   Fast-flush technique is performed by releasing valve to pressurized flush solution. Ratio of amplitude of pressure oscillations (ratio of B to A in Fig. 175-4) may be used to estimate damping coefficient, according to graphical relationship shown. Coefficients in the range of 0.5–0.7 (amplitude ratios less than 0.2) provide optimal frequency response characteristics for physiological pressure monitoring.

forces are at work. For example, in a moderately underdamped catheter system, peripheral intra-arterial pressures will overestimate peak systolic pressure (see above) and therefore may result in higher systolic pressures than noninvasive measurements in the same patient. Overdamped catheter systems may show the opposite relationship. In addition, shock states may be associated with reduced peripheral flow, leading to an underestimation of the central pressure by noninvasive methods.

Although many methods are used to detect blood flow as surrounding pressure is lowered in the occluded artery, three account for most practical applications. The auscultative method relies on the presence of Korotkov sounds to signal systolic pressure (initial appearance of sound, phase I) and diastole (muffling in phase IV or absence in phase V of sound). Care must be taken to provide a cuff of appropriate width and circumference and to position the stethoscope over the brachial artery. The oscillometric method has become quite popular in many ICUs, as demonstrated by the widely used Dinamap. The technique requires the inflation of the cuff to a pressure sufficient to extinguish pressure oscillations within the cuff. As the cuff pressure falls, oscillations are detected at a point that approximates systolic pressure. Mean arterial pressure correlates with the cuff pressure at which the oscillations reach a maximum.

Diastolic pressure is less directly measured by the oscillometric method; it can be calculated from the systolic and mean arterial pressures. Blood flow may be detected by palpation of the radial or brachial artery (lower systolic pressure than by auscultation), ultrasonic detection (useful for patients in shock or in obese patients), or photoelectric methods (susceptible to erroneously low readings from reduced flow in the extremities). A recent application of pulse oximetry technique exploits the time difference between ear and finger sensors in arrival of the pulse wave to calculate changes in local blood volume and pulse transit time. Following initial calibration, an accurate determination of systolic and diastolic pressure can be obtained.

MONITORING CIRCULATORY FUNCTION

Monitoring of circulatory function assumes critical importance for a wide variety of acutely ill patients with cardiovascular or noncardiovascular disorders. The methods used in measuring central venous pressure, pulmonary artery and pulmonary artery occlusion pressures, and cardiac output are described below.

Central Venous Pressure

In past years, central venous pressure (CVP) was measured by use of a column of water in series with a catheter in the internal jugular or subclavian vein. Current practice employs a transducer–catheter system from which a continuous waveform may be displayed. The major indication for placement of a central venous catheter is vascular access, including frequent blood sampling, parenteral hyperalimentation, long-term vascular access, administration of certain medications (e.g., potassium, chemotherapy), and access for placement of other devices, such as a pacemaker, pulmonary artery flotation catheter, and dialysis catheter. CVP has been shown to be an unreliable substitute for left ventricular filling pressure. However, measurement of CVP can provide several important clinical clues.

A low CVP (normal, 0 to 7 mmHg) usually indicates reduced central blood volume. Rapid administration of 500 cm^3 of saline normally causes a 2 to 4 mmHg rise in CVP, which returns to baseline over 15 min; failure of the CVP to increase or to rapidly return to baseline suggests significant reduction in circulating volume, increased vascular compliance, or elevated unstressed volume. In addition, as a reflection of right atrial or right ventricular end-diastolic pressure, the CVP reflects right ventricular preload. Thus, an elevated CVP may suggest right ventricular volume excess or failure. Measurement of CVP is also helpful in calculating systemic vascular resistance (SVR), as CVP is the pressure at the outflow portion of the circuit:

$$SVR = \frac{\text{mean arterial pressure } (P_{inflow}) - CVP \ (P_{outflow})}{\text{cardiac output (flow)}} \qquad (2)$$

Finally, the CVP is a useful indication of the "back pressure" to venous return, an important determinant of cardiac output, because the gradient between mean systemic pressure and CVP is the driving pressure for venous return.

An elevated CVP, on the other hand, may be an ambiguous sign of the circulatory state. For example, elevations of right ventricular end-diastolic pressure may result from a variety of conditions (e.g., pulmonary embolism, right ventricular infarction, cor pulmonale from emphysema, left ventricular failure), each requiring a different diagnostic and therapeutic approach. An elevated CVP may occur in the presence of systemic hypertension or hypotension, relative hypervolemia, or hypervolemia. Clearly, other sources of information must be used to interpret an elevated CVP.

The effect of positive end-expiratory pressure (PEEP) on CVP interpretation remains a subject of investigation and debate. Increased alveolar pressure at end-expiration may be transmitted to the pressure surrounding the intrathoracic structures by an amount that approximates one-half of the PEEP, when chest wall and lung compliance are approximately equal. Thus, a PEEP of 10 cmH$_2$O may result in an increase of up to 5 cmH$_2$O (about 3 mmHg) in CVP. However, the transmural CVP may change little or, because of the decreased venous return to the thorax, may even be reduced. A helpful rule of thumb is to subtract no more than one-half of the PEEP from the measured CVP; in disease states characterized by decreased lung compliance (e.g., ARDS, pulmonary edema), the effect may be even smaller. Some authors have advocated temporary discontinuation of PEEP in order to measure accurate intravascular pressures, but this is infrequently performed in practice owing to the potential deleterious effects of discontinuing PEEP and the concern about obtaining measurements under conditions that do not reflect treatment conditions.

Although a detailed discussion of catheter insertion techniques is beyond the scope of this text, a brief guide to success and complication rates is presented in Table 175-1. In general, the internal jugular approach is preferred for its relative safety from serious complications, high initial success rate, and ease of access for pulmonary artery catheter placement. Securing the catheter may be awkward in patients with unusual neck anatomy or in those with a tracheotomy.

Pulmonary Artery and Pulmonary Artery Occlusion Pressure Measurement

The pulmonary artery catheter includes a proximal port, located approximately 30 cm from the tip, through which right atrial

TABLE 175-1

Comparison of Subclavian, Internal Jugular, and Femoral Routes of Central Venous Catheterization

	Initial Success Rate	Complications	Suitability for Use for PAC Insertion
Subclavian	80–95%	1–2% arterial puncture 1–5% pneumothorax	Good; supraclavicular approach
Internal jugular	90–99%	1–2% carotid puncture <1% pneumothorax	Very good; may be difficult to secure
Femoral	90–100%	Perception of high rates of infection or thrombosis	Difficult; requires special femoral PAC

NOTE: PAC = pulmonary artery catheter.

pressure can be monitored, and a distal port at the catheter tip, which is used to monitor pulmonary artery or pulmonary artery occlusion pressure. The same caveats that apply to measurement of arterial pressure also apply to the pulmonary artery. In addition, lack of catheter fixation distally in the artery, coupled with beat-to-beat movement of the heart and great vessels, may produce exaggerated ringing of the pulmonary artery signal. This catheter "whip" or "fling" may result in exaggeration of the magnitude of systolic pressure; diastolic pressure may be falsely depressed by an equivalent amount. Catheter fling is usually superimposed as a high-frequency, 5- to 10-mmHg oscillation on the waveform. Solutions to the problem are not readily available. Certainly, the practice of increasing the damping of the system by adding an air bubble is to be avoided, as the "cosmetic" improvement to the waveform display does not merit the loss of appropriate damping and the sacrifice of accurate mean pressure readings. Commercial damping devices are available, but these have not found widespread use in practice.

Pulmonary artery diastolic pressure may be assumed to reflect left ventricular end-diastolic pressure (LVEDP) as a function of left ventricular volume and left ventricular compliance. This assumption requires that several conditions be met. 1. The time constant for emptying of the pulmonary artery (PA) must be sufficiently short for PA diastolic pressure to approach LVEDP. 2. A continuous column of blood must be present between the distal PA catheter port and the area of interest, such as the left ventricle. 3. The intraluminal pressure must reflect volume and transmural pressure, rather than altered compliance or altered surrounding pressure. 4. There must be no flow between the measurement site and the left ventricle. Unfortunately, clinical conditions may negate these assumptions in practice.

A gradient of less than 4 mmHg between PA diastolic pressure (PAD) and pulmonary artery occlusion pressure (PAOP) is common in the absence of significant pulmonary disease. In situations where pulmonary vascular resistance is elevated (e.g., emphysema, interstitial lung disease, pulmonary embolism or other pulmonary vascular disease), the time constant for emptying of the pulmonary vascular bed is increased, so that equilibration between PAD and PAOP does not occur during diastole. The gradient between PAD and PAOP may be as much as 20 to 30 mmHg, leading to the erroneous conclusion that left ventricular end-diastolic volume is elevated when, in fact, it may be significantly less than adequate for optimum cardiac output. This situation may be exaggerated in the presence of tachycardia, making reliance on PAD to estimate the PAOP unwise.

A less common problem occurs when the catheter lodges in a branch of the pulmonary artery supplying lung tissue in a zone 1 or zone 2 condition. Because of gravitational effects on the distribution of pulmonary blood flow, pulmonary artery pressure at the highest portions of the lung may be eclipsed by alveolar pressure (West's zone 1) or may be affected by alveolar pressure superseding pulmonary venous pressure as the effective outflow pressure. In either circumstance, the rise and fall of alveolar pressure cause a rise and fall in PAOP of similar magnitude in zone 1 or zone 2 conditions. Fortunately, increased blood flow to zone 3 areas (relative to zones 1 and 2) usually carries the catheter into those regions. Moreover, the gravitational effects described above are generally irrelevant in critically ill patients, because

the supine position reduces the variation in vertical height of the lung. Nevertheless, high-PEEP or low-flow states may precipitate this situation, causing zone 1 or 2 conditions in the anterior portion of the chest (supine position). Clues include PA catheter pressures that rise and fall with a magnitude similar to that of airway pressure. A cross-table lateral chest radiograph can be used to verify that the catheter is in a dependent portion of the lung.

Even in the absence of pulmonary hypertension or tachycardia, and in the presence of a catheter placed in a zone 3 segment of the pulmonary artery, measured PAOP may result in overestimation of left ventricular volume. Myocardial ischemia, ventricular hypertrophy, impingement of the ventricular septum on the left ventricular cavity due to right ventricular distention, and use of catecholamines such as dopamine, norepinephrine, or epinephrine may all decrease left ventricular compliance, resulting in a higher left ventricular transmural pressure and PAOP for any given left ventricular volume. Although the PAOP is, in this case, "accurate," assumptions about the left ventricular volume are not. Increase in surrounding pressure of the left ventricle due to PEEP, for example, can also result in an increase in measured PAOP. In this situation, as in pericardial disease, the PAOP does not accurately reflect transmural pressure. An attempt to measure surrounding pleural pressure may be made with an esophageal balloon, but this is not frequently undertaken in clinical practice.

Overestimation of LVEDP may occur when flow occurs downstream from the balloon occlusion, but proximal to the left ventricle. Pulmonary venous anastomoses and mitral stenosis may each produce a pressure gradient between the catheter tip and left ventricle owing to interposed blood flow. Therefore, the requirement for an uninterrupted static column of blood between the catheter and left ventricle is not met.

"Overwedging" may turn the catheter so that the distal opening is directed against an arterial wall. Incomplete occlusion may produce a waveform that mimics a tracing of pulmonary artery occlusion pressure but results in overestimation due to artifact. This can be minimized by inflating the balloon slowly (3 s) and by observing the tracing as air is introduced into the balloon. Frequently, only 1 cm^3 of air (rather than the maximum 1.5 cm^3) is needed to obtain occlusion.

At least two conditions may result in a PAOP that is less than the true LVEDP. The first is a measurement artifact from an underdamped tracing. The absolute values of both the zenith of systolic and nadir of diastolic pressures exceed the absolute values of true systolic and diastolic pressures because of resonance (see above). Even in the presence of an optimally damped system, however, PAOP can underestimate LVEDP when LVEDP continues to rise after mitral closure, as in aortic insufficiency (Table 175-2).

Several procedures or observations have been recommended to assure optimal conditions for interpretation of the PAOP.[30] 1. The catheter tubing system should be checked with the fast-flush technique for optimal damping. 2. PAOP must be less than mean pulmonary artery pressure. 3. Aspirated blood from the wedged catheter tip should have an O_2 saturation that approaches (or even exceeds) that of arterial blood. 4. A cross-table lateral radiograph may be used to ascertain that the catheter tip is in a dependent (zone 3) portion of the lung. 5. The balloon should be inflated slowly, using the lowest volume of air sufficient to

TABLE 175-2

Sources of Error in Wedge Pressure and Pulmonary Diastolic Pressure Interpretation

Artifact	Mechanism	Comment
Wedge pressure overestimates left ventricular end-diastolic volume	Flow through a resistance downstream from site of measurement	Mitral stenosis, pulmonary venous anastomosis, pulmonary venous hypertension
	Decreased compliance of left ventricle	Ischemia, left ventricular hypertrophy, catecholamines, pericardial disease, right ventricular interdependence due to distended right ventricle
	Increased pressure surrounding left ventricle	Positive end-expiratory pressure; subtract no more than $\frac{1}{2}$ PEEP
	Interrupted column of blood between catheter and left ventricle	Zone 1 or 2 conditions exist, so that alveolar pressure is the effective back pressure to pulmonary artery; observe for equal airway and PA catheter pressure swings with inspiration
	Catheter is "overwedged" from balloon overdistension	Use smallest volume of air to inflate balloon
PA diastolic overestimates left ventricular end-diastolic volume	All of the above	
	Increased time constant for emptying of pulmonary circulation	Insufficient time for equilibration of PA diastolic and wedge pressure, particularly with tachycardia and pulmonary hypertension
Wedge pressure underestimates left ventricular end-diastolic volume	Closure of mitral valve before end diastole	Aortic insufficiency
PA diastolic underestimates left ventricular end-diastolic volume	Underdamped system	Overestimation of PA systolic and underestimation of PA diastolic

obtain a wedge tracing. 6. Large v waves during balloon occlusion, resulting from mitral insufficiency, may sometimes be distinguished from PA systolic waves in an incompletely wedged catheter by a shift in timing between peak pressure waves and T waves on a simultaneously obtained ECG.

In practice, PEEP is seldom discontinued during measurement of PAOP, because of the potential deleterious effects of removing PEEP and because of the concern that alterations in volume distribution accompanying discontinuation of PEEP may obfuscate interpretation of the data. In one experimental model of acute lung injury, PAOP measurements with PEEP present were found to correlate better than measurements made off PEEP when the true left atrial transmural pressure was relatively high; low filling pressures resulted in greater accuracy with the measurement of PAOP off PEEP.[5]

Monitoring PAOP is often done in patients with ARDS. For any given degree of endothelial or epithelial barrier damage, increased hydrostatic pressure favors increased interstitial and alveolar edema. Thus, recent recommendations emphasize minimizing PAOP.[38] At the other extreme, decreased left ventricular filling may hamper organ perfusion and oxygen delivery in a patient who may benefit from increased levels of oxygen delivery. In light of conflicting data regarding nonsurgical patients with acute lung injury, it appears reasonable to strive to maintain a PAOP as low as possible that permits adequate organ perfusion as determined by blood pressure, urine output, mentation, signs of skin perfusion, and lactate and mixed venous O_2 levels.

Cardiac Output

A variety of methods are available for measuring cardiac output, including thermodilution, dye dilution, Fick, continuous, and bioimpedance techniques. Each is discussed below.

THERMODILUTION

Although indicator dilution techniques have been used to measure blood flow for almost a century, the development of small thermistors has permitted routine measurement of cardiac output using temperature as the indicator. Determination of cardiac output frequently guides treatment decisions regarding fluid administration and titration of inotropic, vasopressor, and afterload-reducing agents. Incorporation of cardiac output values into calculation of vascular resistance may be valuable in differentiating cardiogenic shock from other hypotensive states. In acute respiratory failure, cardiac output may be used to titrate PEEP, to calculate the magnitude of physiological shunt, or to monitor oxygen delivery.

The thermodilution method of determining cardiac output was described more than 40 years ago,[10] but it did not become widely used in clinical medicine until the 1970s. Temperature is used as the trace indicator, with coolth (as opposed to warmth) introduced in the form of cooled saline or dextrose in water. Following injection of a bolus of coolth, a thermistor located several millimeters from the catheter tip records the passage of the bolus as a time–temperature curve. In general, the smaller the area under the curve, the larger is the cardiac output. Calculation of the cardiac output is performed by a dedicated microprocessor using an algorithm based on the Stewart-Hamilton equation:

$$\dot{Q}T = \frac{V_i \times (T_b - T_i) \times K_1 \times K_2}{T_b\,(t)\,dt} \qquad (3)$$

where

$\dot{Q}T$ = cardiac output in milliliter per minute
V_i = volume of injectate
T_b = temperature of blood
T_i = temperature of injectate
K_1 = a factor to take into account specific heat of blood and injectate
K_2 = a factor that takes into account transit time
$T_b\,(t)\,dt$ = the change in blood temperature over time

As can be seen from this equation, a small area under the time–temperature curve represents a large cardiac output, and vice-versa. Tricuspid or pulmonic regurgitation may cause recirculation of the cooled solution, producing a large area under the curve and an erroneously low calculation of cardiac output; severe tricuspid regurgitation may overestimate output. An atrial septal defect or other right-to-left shunt can result in loss of cooled solution at the thermistor and an erroneously elevated calculated output.

Under carefully controlled conditions in the experimental laboratory, thermodilution cardiac output values lie within 10 percent of true output measured with a variety of gold standards. In the critical care unit, the accuracy of thermodilution cardiac output may be considerably less. Some of the loss of accuracy may result from technical problems associated with incorrect computation constants, faulty temperature sensing of injectate, or poor bolus injection technique; other sources of error of interpretation are right-to-left or left-to-right shunts and tricuspid regurgitation. Some of the source of error has to do with sampling frequency in light of inherent variability and ventilator effects.

Three determinations of cardiac output may have only an 89 percent likelihood of obtaining a result that lies within 10 percent of the true value, and six determinations may be necessary to achieve a 90 percent chance of obtaining a result that lies within 5 percent of the true value.[23]

In patients with acute respiratory failure on mechanical ventilation, another potential source of unwanted variation in thermodilution cardiac output is partly under operator control. Several investigators have demonstrated a 40 percent variability (20 percent greater or lower than the mean) in thermodilution cardiac output in a given patient, depending on the point in the respiratory cycle when the bolus is injected. To reduce variability, it may be prudent to perform injection of the bolus at end-expiration, particularly when one is attempting to evaluate the change in cardiac output over time in response to an intervention.

ARDS imposes an altered pulmonary circulation on the distribution of cardiac output. The consistently observed consequence is that increases in cardiac output are accompanied by increases in shunt fraction. Proposed mechanisms include impaired hypoxic pulmonary vasoconstriction leading to overperfusion of underventilated units and, less likely, increased interstitial and alveolar edema from increased perfusion. The increased red blood cell transit time that accompanies increased cardiac output may also prevent equilibration of venous blood P_{O_2} with alveolar P_{O_2}.[15]

PEEP is well known to affect cardiac output by a variety of mechanisms. In the presence of adequate cardiovascular volume, the increase in surrounding pressure may decrease left ventricular transmural pressure, decrease effective afterload, and augment cardiac output. With high intra-alveolar pressures and high lung volume from PEEP, increased pulmonary vascular transmural pressure may result in increased resistance—which, in turn, increases right ventricular afterload and impedes ejection fraction. At the same time, elevated right ventricular end-diastolic pressure may cause leftward displacement of the intraventricular septum, decreasing left ventricular compliance and impeding filling. Additionally, increased intrathoracic pressure decreases the gradient for venous return to the right atrium, thereby decreasing cardiac output. Finally, PEEP may be associated with decreased coronary blood flow and, perhaps, the release of cardiodepressor substances from the lungs. Clearly, the effects of PEEP on cardiac output in the patient with acute respiratory failure will depend on intravascular volume, pulmonary vascular resistance, lung compliance, and other factors. In general, the fall in cardiac output with modest levels of PEEP can be overcome with modest volume resuscitation.

DYE DILUTION

Dye dilution and Fick techniques are similar to thermodilution, except that instead of temperature, dye and oxygen, respectively, are used as the indicators. Indocyanine green dye is injected into the right atrium, and blood is slowly and steadily withdrawn from a distal systemic artery. The concentration of dye is plotted over time, yielding a curve that looks similar to a thermodilution curve. A computer is used to adjust for recirculated dye, whose appearance signals the end of data acquisition. From a knowledge of quantity of dye injected and the area under the curve, cardiac output can be calculated. This method is seldom employed clinically because of the need for special equipment and the inconvenience of arterial sampling.

FICK CARDIAC OUTPUT

The Fick method is more than 100 years old. It is based on measurement of oxygen consumption, arterial oxygen content, and venous oxygen content. Where cardiac output is the dependent variable, an accurate determination of oxygen consumption is desirable. This is usually accomplished by collecting expired gas in a 60-L Douglas bag or sampling with a metabolic oxygen analyzer. Arterial and venous oxygen contents are measured from blood samples obtained from a systemic artery and from the pulmonary artery through the pulmonary artery catheter tip. The general Fick equation is used to calculate cardiac output:

$$\dot{Q} = \frac{V_{O_2}}{Ca_{O_2} - Cv_{O_2}} \quad (4)$$

where

$$\dot{Q} = \text{cardiac output in liters per minute}$$

Alternatively, if there is confidence in the thermodilution cardiac output, oxygen consumption can be calculated. This is the genesis of many "automated" hemodynamic profiles that are provided by physiological monitoring equipment. In acute respiratory failure, the Fick determination of cardiac output is limited primarily by technical inaccuracies in measurement of oxygen consumption that occur when the inspired oxygen fraction ($F_{I_{O_2}}$) exceeds 0.6.[25,47] Some investigators have found that commercially available metabolic monitors are capable of measuring an oxygen consumption within 6 percent of the true oxygen consumption—an accuracy that is preserved even in the presence of high PEEP. Hour-to-hour or day-to-day changes in oxygen consumption may be as great as 30 percent, necessitating the repeated measurement of this variable in order to maintain a current estimate of cardiac output by the Fick method.

CONTINUOUS CARDIAC OUTPUT

Recently developed modifications to the pulmonary artery catheter permit the measurement of cardiac output continuously, using constant detection of temperature changes. One method employs a coil heated to 44°C upstream from the thermistor. Cardiac output is calculated from a knowledge of heat applied to the coil and detected by the thermistor. In most experimental situations, there has been good correlation between bolus injection and continuous thermodilution methods (correlation coefficients of about 0.9).[43] Others have noted interference produced by intravenous infusions of cool solutions, and a response time that renders the method too slow to serve as an instantaneous monitor.[12] Advantages cited include near-continuous availability of cardiac output and derived parameters, such as systemic vascular resistance,[31] and reduced errors from manual bolus injection.

BIOIMPEDANCE

For more than 25 years, thoracic electrical bioimpedance (TEB) has been used to calculate cardiac output. The principle entails the ascribing of changes in bioimpedance to changes in aortic volume with each cardiac ejection and, from assumptions about the predicted geometry of the aorta, calculating a stroke volume. The technique has not gained widespread acceptance because of uncertainty about accuracy, reproducibility, and sources of error. Whereas one study of 50 patients yielded a correlation coefficient of only 0.24 between thermodilution and TEB,[36] a more recent study of 68 critically ill patients found a correlation coefficient of 0.74—a value judged by the authors to be acceptable in light of the noninvasive and continuous nature of the method.[40] Large studies in patients with acute respiratory failure are not available, and questions about the effect of changes in lung water on the accuracy of the method remain unanswered.

RIGHT VENTRICULAR EJECTION FRACTION

Based upon the dye dilution techniques discussed previously, the rate of disappearance of dye from the right ventricle could be used to calculate a right ventricular ejection fraction. Substituting thermodilution for Evans blue dye, new pulmonary artery catheters are available that measure right ventricular ejection fraction continuously. Potential confounding problems include tricuspid regurgitation and arrhythmias, particularly atrial fibrillation. Although this catheter has been found to be valuable in the operating room to monitor right ventricular ischemia, or in the cardiac surgery ICU to detect cardiac tamponade, it has not been well studied in the setting of acute respiratory failure, and its routine use cannot be recommended. In one small study of surgical patients with ARDS, sepsis, and shock, the additional information from the right ventricular end-diastolic volume did not alter management in 43 of 46 instances.[50]

MONITORING RESPIRATORY FUNCTION

A number of measurements of respiratory function are routinely employed in critically ill patients. The techniques address not only the mechanical properties of the respiratory system or lung–mechanical ventilator unit but also aspects of gas exchange. Commonly employed methods are considered below.

Mechanics

For the patient in acute respiratory failure, monitoring respiratory function requires assessment of both the patient and mechanical ventilator function. In some instances, the ventilator facilitates or impedes the measurement of patient respiratory function. In others, it is the ventilator interaction with the patient that must be monitored. Nevertheless, basic principles of respiratory mechanics are applicable to spontaneously breathing and mechanically ventilated patients alike. Most measurements of mechanics can be described in terms of time, volume, flow, pressure, compliance, and resistance (Table 175-3).

Compliance, Resistance, Pressure, and Flow

One of the hallmarks of ARDS is a reduced respiratory system compliance that results from inflammation and edema of the interstitium and alveoli. Normally about 100 ml/cmH$_2$O, respiratory compliance frequently falls to 25 ml/cmH$_2$O in patients with acute lung injury. Accurate measurement depends on accurate measurement of change in volume and change in static pressure. Determination of tidal volume is accomplished by integrating the area under a flow–time curve, where flow is measured with a pneumotachograph or ultrasonic flowmeter incorporated into the ventilator circuit. Change in pressure may be more problematic from the point of view of end-expiratory pressure.

When intrinsic PEEP is present, end-expiratory pressure measured at the trachea may underestimate alveolar pressure, as resistance between the alveolus and trachea results in slowly emptying areas of lung at low flows. Underestimation of end-expiratory pressure results in an overestimation of the change in pressure and an underestimation of the compliance. Measurement of intrinsic PEEP by occluding the expiratory port at end-expiration may provide some estimate of intrinsic PEEP. Usual practice dictates that end-inspiratory pressure be taken as plateau pressure during a 0.5- to 1.0-s inspiratory hold. More accurate measurement of plateau pressure would be obtained by noting the pressure at the point of zero flow, but this capability is generally not present in ventilators in common use. Dynamic compliance reflects the total impedance to volume change of the respiratory system; it includes compliance and resistive components.

Airway resistance may be modestly elevated in ARDS. It is calculated by measuring the difference between the peak inspiratory and plateau pressures, and dividing that difference by the flow. As described above, more accurate determination would be obtained by substituting the pressure at zero flow for both the peak inspiratory and plateau pressures. PEEP may improve compliance up to a maximum; subsequent increases in PEEP may be limited by decreasing compliance, fall in cardiac output, or excessive plateau pressure.

Airway pressure is, perhaps, among the most important measurements to make during mechanical ventilation because of barotrauma and the deleterious effects of high airway pressures on cardiac output. From the above discussion, it is clear that peak inspiratory pressure reflects both compliance and resistive fac-

tors and, therefore, also depends on tidal volume and flow. Barotrauma has been correlated with peak inspiratory pressure, plateau, and mean airway pressures, depending on the particular study. In mechanically ventilated patients with obstructive airway disease, particularly asthma, deleterious effects of hyperinflation may correlate better with lung volume at end-inspiration above functional residual capacity (FRC) than with any particular pressure.[48] Recent attention has been paid to the possible causal link between high lung volumes (reflected by high plateau pressures) and lung injury,[26,46] prompting new enthusiasm for controlled hypercapnic ventilation.[45]

In patients with acute respiratory failure, routine monitoring of positive inspiratory pressure, intrinsic PEEP, plateau pressure, and mean airway pressure is recommended in order to identify potential sources of error in compliance measurements and potential causes of barotrauma, lung injury, or decreased cardiac output. In the absence of elevated plateau or mean airway pressures, high peak inspiratory pressure, particularly in the presence of high inspiratory flow, is probably of no great concern. However, a source of increased resistance should be sought, such as a kinked or obstructed endotracheal tube or airway narrowing. Furthermore, extremely high peak inspiratory pressures (greater than 60 cmH$_2$O) may place the patient at risk of barotrauma,[21] perhaps because such elevations are frequently accompanied by high mean airway pressures as well (Fig. 175-6).

Lung Volume

Other than tidal volume and several other spirometrically derived subdivisions of lung volumes and capacities above residual volume (or FRC), lung volume is difficult to measure in patients with acute respiratory failure. Closed-circuit indicator-dilution techniques using an insoluble indicator and open circuit techniques using radioactive or inert gases have been used, largely in research applications. Although not readily available from commercial sources, a device that is accurate under varying conditions of mechanical ventilation using sulfur hexafluoride as the

---

TABLE 175-3

Basic Components of Mechanics and Their Relationships

Variable	Units	Relationship to Other Variables	Clinical Examples
Time (T)	s		1/frequency, inspiratory time
Volume (V)	L		Tidal volume
Flow (Q)	L/s	Volume/Time	Airflow, cardiac output
Pressure (P)	cm H$_2$O	$\Delta V/\Delta C$, $Q \cdot R$	PIP, P$_{plat}$, PEEP, MAP
Compliance (C$_{stat}$)	L/cm H$_2$O	$\Delta V/\Delta P$, where $\Delta P = (P_{plat} - P_{end\ exp})$	Respiratory system compliance
Dynamic compliance (C$_{dyn}$)	L/cm H$_2$O	$\Delta V/\Delta P$, where $\Delta P = (PIP - P_{end\ exp})$	
Resistance (R)	cm H$_2$O/L/s	$(PIP - P_{plat})/Q$	Airway resistance
Work (W)	joules	$V \cdot P$	Work of breathing

NOTE: P$_{plat}$ = plateau pressure; PIP = peak inspiratory pressure; PEEP = positive end-expiratory pressure; MAP = mean airway pressure.

Airway Pressure

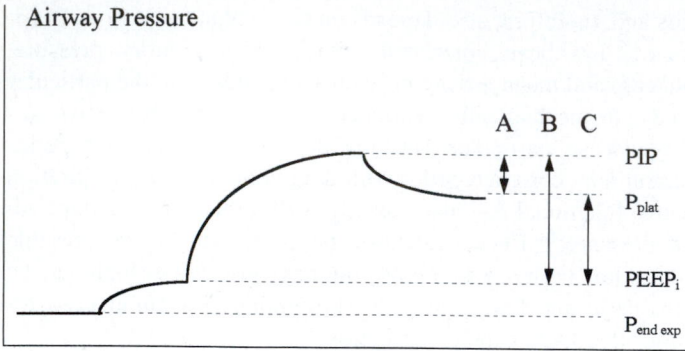

Time

FIGURE 175-6   Airway pressure versus time. The pressure difference indicated by arrow "A" represents the peak inspiratory pressure–plateau pressure gradient (PIP − P_{plat}). When this pressure gradient is divided by flow, resistance may be calculated. Pressure difference "B" represents the peak inspiratory pressure–end-expiratory pressure gradient, corrected for intrinsic PEEP (PEEPi) by occlusion at end-expiration. This quantity may be divided into tidal volume to yield dynamic compliance. Pressure difference "C" represents the plateau pressure–end-expiratory pressure gradient ($P_{plat} − P_{end\ exp}$) corrected for intrinsic PEEP; it is divided into tidal volume to calculate static compliance. Use of ventilator-measured end-expiratory pressure ($P_{end\ exp}$) would yield a falsely low compliance.

tracer gas may be constructed economically.[9] FRC has been shown to be reduced in ARDS and may be restored toward normal by application of PEEP.

Gas Exchange

Abnormal oxygenation is the hallmark of acute lung injury and ARDS, so that monitoring of oxygenation is a primary means of judging progress or failure in management. The time course of oxygenation in patients with ARDS has been shown to be of prognostic significance. Initially indistinguishable on the basis of the F_{IO_2} requirement or Pa_{O_2}/F_{IO_2}, survivors show significant increases in both Pa_{O_2} and the ratio within the first week after diagnosis.[41]

ELECTRODES

The oxygen electrode in common use consists of a modification of the electrode developed by Clark in 1956. It is constructed of a platinum wire tip surrounded by glass. Covered by a membrane permeable to oxygen, this electrode is capable of responding in a linear fashion to oxygen in gaseous or liquid phase from 1 to 100 percent, with less than a 1 percent error. Blood gas samples drawn from a peripheral artery are used to deliver an arterial source for oxygen measurement, as are venous samples for mixed venous calculations.

In contrast, the CO_2 electrode commonly used to measure blood gases is a modified pH electrode; CO_2 diffuses through a membrane into an aqueous solution surrounding the electrode, which measures pH and calculates P_{CO_2} by use of the Henderson-Hasselbalch equation.

PULSE OXIMETRY

Advances in pulse oximetry have revolutionized the monitoring of oxygen tension, providing a noninvasive, continuous estimate of arterial oxygen saturation.[18] As discussed above, this technique has not replaced arterial blood gas analysis in the ICU, but it has replaced it in some ambulatory settings. Light-emitting diodes emit light that passes through perfused tissue in the digit, earlobe, or other location, and a receiving photodiode receives the frequencies of light that have not been absorbed by the tissue. As oxygenated hemoglobin absorbs more infrared light and less red light than deoxygenated hemoglobin, a value for saturation can be calculated from reflected light measurement. With pulse oximetry, the reduction in intensity of light at the photodetector with each pulse is due to increased volume from arterial blood; the technique uses the change in absorbance of the two wavelengths to calculate arterial saturation. Pulse oximetry does not detect carboxyhemoglobin or methemoglobin, either of which may cause a falsely depressed pulse oximetry measurement of oxygen saturation.

In addition to carboxyhemoglobin and methemoglobin, falsely low saturation by pulse oximetry may be seen with methylene blue, fingernail polish (particularly of blue hues), onychomycosis, and severe anemia. In the patient with acute respiratory failure, pulse oximetry may be inaccurate owing to peripheral vasoconstriction from shock states or use of vasopressors. Hypotension without vasoconstriction[39] and hyperbilirubinemia are not important sources of inaccuracy.

TRANSCUTANEOUS MEASUREMENT

Using a modified Clark electrode, transcutaneous oxygen (TcO_2) electrodes can be placed against skin warmed to 41°C. The heat increases blood flow to the cutaneous capillaries, in effect "arterializing" the capillaries. Under careful conditions in neonates, TcO_2 can provide a reliable estimate of P_{O_2}. In adults, correlation of TcO_2 with arterial Pa_{O_2} depends on several factors, including age, cardiac output, local perfusion, skin thickness, and disease states (e.g., diabetes mellitus). These factors may result in up to a 10-fold variation in slope of a plot of TcO_2 versus Pa_{O_2}. Although some authors have found that transcutaneous CO_2 electrodes more reliably reflect arterial Pa_{CO_2},[32] regional differences in peripheral perfusion accompanying acute respiratory failure and ARDS make routine use of these devices unwise.

CAPNOGRAPHY

Capnography refers to the detection of CO_2 in expired gas. Common methods employ either mainstream or sidestream sampling of expired gas. Mainstream sampling utilizes a detector in line with the main expiratory circuit. Advantages include rapid response time and large diameter, thereby minimizing resistance. Drawbacks include the need to manipulate the expiratory circuit directly for cleaning. Sidestream sampling does not interfere with the main breathing circuit and may be used with a nasal cannula in spontaneously breathing patients. Disadvantages include slow response time and a tendency for the small sampling port to become obstructed with secretions.

The primary utility of capnography lies in the detection and confirmation of pulmonary ventilation during endotracheal tube placement, and in the monitoring of change in pulmonary blood flow that accompanies embolism, thromboembolism, or cardiac arrest. In those conditions, decreased pulmonary perfusion results in decreased clearance of CO_2 from the circulation, with an increase in the gradient between end-tidal P_{CO_2} and Pa_{CO_2}. Attempts to use end-tidal P_{CO_2} as a surrogate for Pa_{CO_2} may be quite successful in the spontaneously breathing, or even mechanically ventilated, healthy patient. For this reason, capnography may be a valuable aid in the head-injured patient to prevent unwanted hypoventilation. In situations of cardiovascular instability or lung injury, however, alterations in the distribution of pulmonary blood flow and dead-space ventilation negate the usefulness of capnography as a monitor of Pa_{CO_2}. Initial suggestions that the gradient between end-tidal P_{CO_2} and Pa_{CO_2} would be minimized at optimal levels of PEEP have not been confirmed.[2]

INTEGRATED SYSTEMS MONITORING

Acute respiratory failure may be viewed as a multisystem disorder, so that monitoring of integrated systems may be necessary to understand the subtleties of manifestations. In fact, it is difficult to separate the cardiovascular and respiratory systems when monitoring effects of therapeutic maneuvers in ARDS. The following measurements and calculations assess the roles of the lungs in gas exchange, the cardiovascular system in delivery of oxygen, and the peripheral tissues in distribution and consumption of oxygen.

Oxygen Indices

Several "oxygen indices" constitute useful measures of the gas exchange and oxygen delivery functions of the lungs and cardiovascular systems. These include shunt, alveolar–arterial O_2 gradient, alveolar–arterial P_{O_2} (PA_{O_2}–Pa_{O_2}), O_2 transport, and mixed venous O_2.

SHUNT

In the two-compartment model of the lung, units are ether ideally perfused and ventilated or perfused but not ventilated. Mixed venous blood, which perfuses unventilated units, is shunted past the gas-exchanging units, much as an intracardiac right-to-left shunt bypasses the lungs. In reality, the lung is made up of units with a wide distribution of ventilation and perfusion, only some of which represent shunt. In the absence of a convenient way to measure this ventilation–perfusion distribution, shunt fraction is calculated as a way of following the flow-weighted average ventilation–perfusion ratio of the lung. If total flow (Qt) equals the sum of the shunted flow (Qs) and nonshunted flow (Qns), the oxygen contents of arterial, venous, and capillary blood may be represented as follows:

$$Ca_{O_2} \times Qt = (Cv_{O_2} \times Qs) + (Cc_{O_2} \times Qns) \qquad (5)$$

Substituting $Qt - Qs$ for Qns,

$$Ca_{O_2} \times Qt = (Cv_{O_2} \times Qs) + [Cc_{O_2} \times (Qt - Qs)] \qquad (6)$$

Isolating terms,

$$\frac{Qs}{Qt} = \frac{Cc_{O_2} - Ca_{O_2}}{Cc_{O_2} - Cv_{O_2}} \qquad (7)$$

Pa_{O_2} is used to calculate arterial content, Pv_{O_2} to calculate venous content, and alveolar P_{O_2} from the alveolar air equation to calculate capillary content. Used in this way, the shunt fraction may be helpful in monitoring trends in a given patient with respiratory failure over time, but only if the $F_{I_{O_2}}$ and venous P_{O_2} remain constant and only if the $F_{I_{O_2}}$ is high. Under these conditions, the contribution of units with low ventilation–perfusion ratio is minimized by high $F_{I_{O_2}}$. However, breathing 100 percent oxygen may actually induce a shunt by promoting absorption atelectasis. Furthermore, decreases in cardiac output may lower venous P_{O_2}, thereby decreasing the calculated shunt, while actual shunt fraction may also decrease from lower cardiac output, as described above. In this light, shunt fraction is best thought of as a snapshot of the health of the lung regarding oxygenation, but only for a given cardiac output, venous P_{O_2}, and $F_{I_{O_2}}$.

ALVEOLAR–ARTERIAL OXYGEN GRADIENT AND ALVEOLAR–ARTERIAL P_{O_2} RATIO

Unlike the shunt fraction, the PA_{O_2}–Pa_{O_2} may fluctuate in a biphasic manner with $F_{I_{O_2}}$, depending on the degree of actual shunt fraction and $F_{I_{O_2}}$. Increasing $F_{I_{O_2}}$ may decrease PA_{O_2}–Pa_{O_2} in lung regions with variable ventilation–perfusion ratios, whereas PA_{O_2}–Pa_{O_2} will increase greatly with increasing $F_{I_{O_2}}$ in the presence of true shunt. Because the response of the measurement to changing $F_{I_{O_2}}$ is unpredictable, it is of little use in patients with acute respiratory failure.

In order to account for the change with $F_{I_{O_2}}$, either the alveolar–arterial P_{O_2} ratio or the ratio of Pa_{O_2} to $F_{I_{O_2}}$ has been used to reflect the state of lung oxygenating ability for a given $F_{I_{O_2}}$. Both of these measurements show less fluctuation with $F_{I_{O_2}}$ than does PA_{O_2}–Pa_{O_2}, but both are susceptible to $F_{I_{O_2}}$-related changes, depending on the degree of ventilation–perfusion imbalance, as opposed to true shunt. The higher the degree of shunt, the more the ratios are influenced by $F_{I_{O_2}}$. Although lacking in physiological soundness, the two ratios are used commonly in clinical research studies to describe the oxygenation ability of the lung in acute respiratory failure.

OXYGEN TRANSPORT

Few areas of pathophysiology in critical care have received as much attention in recent years as the value of monitoring and intervening in oxygen delivery in patients with acute respiratory failure. Although a comprehensive review is outside of the scope of this chapter, monitoring considerations are discussed. Oxygen transport (T_{O_2}) may be calculated as the product of cardiac output and arterial oxygen content; normal values are in the range of 500 to 600 ml/min/m². Considerable controversy exists regarding the relationship between delivery of oxygen and the dependency of consumption upon that delivery, as well as the wisdom of augmenting delivery beyond normal levels.

More than 15 years ago in a group of patients with ARDS, oxygen uptake was shown to depend on delivery.[7] Since then, dozens of studies of the relationship have been performed, with conflicting results. Some of the differences may be explained by the methods used to calculate oxygen delivery and consumption. For example, use of thermodilution cardiac output to measure both delivery ($\dot{Q}T \times Ca_{O_2}$) and consumption [$\dot{Q}T \times (Ca_{O_2} - Cv_{O_2})$] may lead to mathematical coupling, whereby variations in cardiac output are plotted on both axes, yielding a spurious relationship between the desired variables.[33] When oxygen consumption is measured by respiratory gases independent of delivery, no such dependent relationship is found.[13]

Therapy aimed at increasing oxygen delivery beyond normal levels has had mixed results, perhaps because of different patient populations or different strategies of attempting to prevent, as opposed to reverse, low oxygen consumption. Improved survival in some studies of surgical patients must be tempered with the increased mortality in medical patients in whom oxygen delivery was increased.[1,14] It would seem reasonable to monitor oxygen delivery and consumption independently and to attempt to correct significantly reduced oxygen delivery. Appropriate surgical patients may benefit from preventive augmentation of oxygen delivery to supranormal levels. Clearly, more study is needed to resolve these important issues.

MIXED VENOUS OXYGEN SATURATION

Widespread availability of pulmonary catheters that include reflectance oximetry capabilities has led to the routine use of the catheters in many critical care centers. The principle behind the continuous monitoring of mixed venous oxygen saturation is straightforward, as indicated by the following relationship:

$$S\bar{v}_{O_2} = Sa_{O_2} - \frac{\dot{V}_{O_2}}{\dot{Q}T} \qquad (8)$$

where

$$S\bar{v}_{O_2} \text{ and } Sa_{O_2} = O_2 \text{ saturations of mixed venous and}$$
$$\text{peripheral arterial blood, respectively}$$
$$\dot{V}_{O_2} = \text{oxygen uptake}$$
$$\dot{Q}T = \text{cardiac output}$$

Equation (8) is based on the assumption that the contribution to oxygen content of dissolved oxygen is negligible, and that arterial and venous hemoglobin levels are equal. Any reduction in mixed venous oxygen saturation must come from a reduction in arterial oxygen saturation, an increase in oxygen consumption, or a decrease in cardiac output. Unfortunately, several of these variables may change simultaneously, often with unpredictable results. For example, a decrease in oxygen consumption accompanying some septic states may balance a reduced delivery, leading to no change in the mixed venous oxygen saturation. As an "early warning" sign that some aspect of the oxygen delivery and consumption equation is out of balance, the mixed venous oxygen saturation may be of some use. Its lack of specificity and low sensitivity limit its usefulness, however.[16]

Lactate

Originally believed to be a sensitive and specific marker of tissue hypoxia, serum lactate may fail to be detected in elevated systemic concentrations despite severe local ischemia. In addi-

tion, it may appear in greatly elevated levels from decreased hepatic clearance, without evidence of anaerobic metabolism. However, many authors have noted the poor prognostic significance of a lactate level that is more than 10 times higher than the upper limit of normal. In the absence of liver disease, an elevated lactate may suggest inadequate tissue perfusion, despite apparently adequate measures of cardiac output, prompting a search for ischemic tissue or attempts at augmentation of oxygen delivery. The cost-effectiveness of lactate determinations is unclear, as is the effect of monitoring levels on patient outcome.[28]

Gastric Intramucosal pH

A common objection to the use of blood lactate and mixed venous oxygen saturation determinations is that blood from hypoxic tissues may be diluted by blood draining normally perfused organs, thereby masking signs of oxygen deficiency. Gastric tonometry has been proposed as a method to detect intramucosal pH—which, in turn, is directly proportional to splanchnic perfusion. The method says little about states of perfusion of other tissues, but it has been used to assess the local balance between oxygen delivery and consumption.

The technique requires insertion into the stomach of a fluid-filled balloon attached to a nasogastric tube. Equilibration of tissue P_{CO_2} with viscus gas occurs, and the CO_2 passes through the semipermeable balloon wall. Fluid within the balloon is withdrawn and analyzed with a P_{CO_2} electrode, and the tissue pH is calculated from the measured P_{CO_2} and measured arterial bicarbonate with the Henderson-Hasselbalch equation.

Gastric tonometry has demonstrated significant correlations with other measures of splanchnic perfusion,[27] and augmentation of oxygen delivery guided by measurement of gastric mucosal pH has resulted in significant improvements in survival. As a prognostic factor, gastric tonometry may be as useful as, or superior to, APACHE II scores, hemodynamic or oxygen transport variables, or arterial lactate.

Enthusiasm should be tempered by some of the known limitations of gastric tonometry, including falsely low mucosal pH when arterial bicarbonate is low, as from a non–anion gap acidosis, and decreased clearance of P_{CO_2} from low blood flow. Nevertheless, gastric tonometry remains a promising tool to monitor the oxygenation of a regional tissue bed.[11]

REFERENCES

1. Bishop MH, Shoemaker WC, Appel PL, et al: Prospective, randomized trial of survivor values of cardiac index, oxygen delivery, and oxygen consumption as resuscitation endpoints in severe trauma. *J Trauma* 38:780–787, 1995.
2. Blanch L, Fernandez R, Benito S: Effect of PEEP on the arterial minus end-tidal carbon dioxide gradient. *Chest* 92:451–454, 1987.
3. Bowton DL, Scuderi PE, Harris L, Haponik EF: Pulse oximetry monitoring outside the intensive care unit: Progress or problem? *Ann Intern Med* 115:450–454, 1991.
4. Caplan RA, Posner KL, Ward RJ, Cheney FW: Adverse respiratory events in anesthesia: A closed claims analysis. *Anesthesiology* 72:828–833, 1990.
5. Carter RS, Snyder JV, Pinsky MR: LV filling pressure during PEEP measured by nadir wedge pressure after airway disconnection. *Am J Physiol* 249:H770–H776, 1985.

6. Cohen MM, Duncan PG, Tweed WA, et al: The Canadian four-centre study of anaesthetic outcomes. *Can J Anaesth* 39:420–429, 1992.

7. Danek S, Lynch JP, Weg JG, Dantzker DR: The dependence of oxygen uptake on oxygen delivery in the adult respiratory distress syndrome. *Am Rev Respir Dis* 122:387–395, 1980.

8. Duncan PG, Cohen MM: Pulse oximetry and capnography in anesthetic practice: An epidemiological approach. *Can J Anaes* 38:619–625, 1991.

9. East TD, Wortelboer PJM, van Ark E, et al: Automated sulfur hexafluoride washout functional residual capacity measurement system for any mode of mechanical ventilation as well as spontaneous respiration. *Crit Care Med* 18:84–91, 1990.

10. Fegler G: Measurement of cardiac output in anaesthetized animals by a thermo-dilution method. *Q J Exp Physiol* 39:153–164, 1954.

11. Gutierrez G, Clark C, Brown SD, et al: Effect of dobutamine on oxygen consumption and gastric mucosal pH in septic patients. *Am J Respir Crit Care Med* 150:324–329 1994.

12. Haller M, Zollner C, Briegel J, Forst H: Evaluation of a new continuous thermodilution cardiac output monitor in critically ill patients: A prospective criterion standard study. *Crit Care Med* 23:860–866, 1995.

13. Hanique G, Dugernier T, Laterre PF, et al: Significance of pathologic oxygen supply dependency in critically ill patients: Comparison between measured and calculated methods. *Intensive Care Med* 20:12–18, 1994.

14. Hayes MA, Timmins AC, Yau EH, et al: Elevation of systemic oxygen delivery in the treatment of critically ill patients. *New Engl J Med* 330:1717–1722, 1994.

15. Hoel BL: Some aspects of the clinical use of thermodilution in measuring cardiac output. *Scand J Clin Lab Invest* 38:383–388, 1978.

16. Jastremski MS, Chelluri L, Beney KM, Bailly RT: Analysis of the effects of continuous on-line monitoring of mixed venous oxygen saturation on patient outcome and cost-effectiveness. *Crit Care Med* 17:148–153, 1989.

17. Joly HR, Weil MH: Temperature of the great toe as an indication of the severity of shock. *Circulation* 39:131–138, 1969.

18. Kelleher JF: Pulse oximetry. *J Clin Monit* 5:37–62, 1989.

19. Kholoussy AM, Sufian S, Pavlides C, Matsumoto T: Central peripheral temperature gradient: Its value and limitations in the management of critically ill surgical patients. *Am J Surg* 140:609–612, 1980.

20. Killip T, Kimball JT: A survey of the coronary care unit: Concept and results. *Prog Cardiovasc Dis* 11:45–52, 1968.

21. Kolobow T, Moretti MP, Fumagalli R, et al: Severe impairment in lung function induced by high peak airway pressure during mechanical ventilation. *Am Rev Respir Dis* 135:312–315, 1987.

22. Kurz A, Sessler DI, Lenhardt R: Perioperative normothermia to reduce the incidence of surgical wound infection and shorten hospitalization. *New Engl J Med* 334:1209–1215, 1996.

23. Lemaire F: Hypoxemia in adult respiratory distress syndrome, in Artigas A, Lemaire F, Suter P, Zapol W (eds), *Adult Respiratory Distress Syndrome.* New York, Churchill Livingstone, 1992 pp 37–63.

24. Mackowiak PA, Wasserman SS, Levine MM: A critical appraisal of 98.6°F, the upper limit of the normal body temperature, and other legacies of Carl Reinhold August Wunderlich. *JAMA* 268:1578–1580, 1992.

25. Makita K, Ninn JF, Royston B: Evaluation of metabolic measuring instruments for use in critically ill patients. *Crit Care Med* 18:638–644, 1990.

26. Marini JJ: Lung mechanics in the adult respiratory distress syndrome—Recent conceptual advances and implications for management. *Clin Chest Med* 11:673–690, 1990.

27. Maynard N, Bihari D, Beale R, et al: Assessment of splanchnic oxygenation by gastric tonometry in patients with acute circulatory failure. *JAMA* 270:1203–1210, 1993.

28. Mizrock BA, Falk JL: Lactic acid in critical illness. *Crit Care Med* 20:80–93, 1992.

29. Moller JT, Johannessen NW, Espersen K, et al: Randomized evaluation of pulse oximetry in 20,802 patients: II. Perioperative events and postoperative complications. *Anesthesiology* 78:445–453, 1993.

30. Morris AH, Chapman RH, Gardner RM: Frequency of wedge pressure errors in the ICU. *Crit Care Med* 13:705–708, 1985.

31. O'Dwyer JP, King JE, Wood CE, et al: Continuous measurement of systemic vascular resistance. *Anesthesia* 49:587–590, 1994.

32. Palmisano BW, Severinghaus JW: Transcutaneous PCO_2 and PO_2: A multicenter study of accuracy. *J Clin Monit* 6:189–195, 1990.

33. Phang PT, Cunningham KF, Ronco JJ, et al: Mathematical coupling explains dependence of oxygen consumption on oxygen delivery in ARDS. *Am J Respir Crit Care Med* 150:318–323, 1994.

34. Polk SL, Roizen MF: Cost–benefit analysis in monitoring, in Blitt C, Hines R (eds), *Monitoring in Anesthesia and Critical Care Medicine.* New York, Churchill Livingstone, 1995.

35. Saarela E, Kari A, Nikki P, et al: Current practice regarding invasive monitoring in intensive care units in Finland: A nationwide study of the uses of arterial, pulmonary artery and central venous catheters and their effect on outcome. *Intensive Care Med* 17:264–271, 1991.

36. Sageman WS, Amundson DE: Thoracic electrical bioimpedance measurement of cardiac output in postaortocoronary bypass patients. *Crit Care Med* 21:1139–1142, 1993.

37. Schmitz T, Bair N, Falk M, Levine C: A comparison of five methods of temperature measurement in febrile intensive care patients. *Am J Crit Care* 4:286–292, 1995.

38. Schuster DP: Fluid management in ARDS: "Keep them dry" or does it matter? *Intensive Care Med* 21:101–103, 1995.

39. Severinghaus JW, Spellman MJ Jr: Pulse oximeter failure thresholds in hypotension and ischemia. *Anesthesiology* 73:532–537, 1990.

40. Shoemaker WC, Wo CC, Bishop MH, et al: Multicenter trial of a new thoracic electrical bioimpedance device for cardiac output estimation. *Crit Care Med* 22:1907–1912, 1994.

41 Sloane PJ, Gee MH, Gottlieb JE, et al: A multicenter registry of patients with acute respiratory distress syndrome. *Am Rev Respir Dis* 146:419–426, 1992.

42. Tandberg D, Sklar D: Effect of tachypnea on the estimation of body temperature by an oral thermometer. *New Engl J Med* 308:945–946, 1983.

43. Thrush D, Downs JB, Smith RA: Continuous thermodilution cardiac output: Agreement with Fick and bolus thermodilution methods. *J Cardiothorac Vasc Anesth* 9:399–404, 1995.

44. Tinker JH, Dull DL, Caplan RA, et al: Role of monitoring devices in prevention of anesthesia mishaps: A closed claims analysis. *Anesthesiology* 71:541–546, 1989.

45. Tsuno K, Miura K, Takeya M, et al: Histopathologic pulmonary changes from mechanical ventilation at high peak airway pressures. *Am Rev Respir Dis* 143:1115–1120, 1991.

46. Tuxen DV: Permissive hypercapnic ventilation. *Am J Respir Crit Care Med* 150:870–874, 1994.

47. Westenskow DR, Cutler CA, Wallace WD: Instrumentation for monitoring gas exchange and metabolic rate in critically ill patients. *Crit Care Med* 12:183–187, 1984.

48. Williams TJ, Tuxen DV, Scheinkestel CD, et al: Risk factors for morbidity in mechanically ventilated patients with acute severe asthma. *Am Rev Respir Dis* 146:607–615, 1992.

49. Yank K, Tobin MJ: A prospective study of predicting outcome of trials of weaning from mechanical ventilation. *New Engl J Med* 324:1445–1450, 1991.

50. Yu M, Takiguchi S, Takanishi D, et al: Evaluation of the clinical usefulness of thermodilution volumetric catheters. *Crit Care Med* 23:681–686, 1995.

CHAPTER 176

MECHANICAL VENTILATION: CONVENTIONAL MODES AND SETTINGS

Martin J. Tobin

The historical evolution of mechanical ventilation is rich and is built on advances in many fields, including endeavors by anatomists, chemists, explorers, physiologists, and clinicians.[8] In 1543, Vesalius demonstrated that positive pressure ventilation could be used to resuscitate a dying animal. Bellows ventilation was advocated by various lay bodies in the resuscitation of near-drowning victims late in the eighteenth century, but in 1827 Leroy demonstrated that overzealous bellows inflation could result in pneumothoraces. Official bodies such as the French Academy condemned the technique, and, thus, early in its infancy, positive-pressure ventilation was banned from use. Around this time, negative-pressure ventilators began to be developed, and they were popularized later in the nineteenth century as a panacea for a wide variety of ailments. The first negative-pressure ventilator to achieve widespread use in clinical practice was the Drinker respirator, developed in 1928. This was later simplified and improved by Emerson and was the mainstay of ventilator assistance until the 1950s.

The modern era of mechanical ventilation began in Copenhagen on August 25, 1952, when Ibsen, an anesthetist, was called to see a 12-year-old girl with acute poliomyelitis who was drowning in her own secretions. During the preceding 3 weeks, 31 patients with bulbar poliomyelitis had been treated with negative-pressure respirators, and 27 had died. Ibsen advised an immediate tracheostomy and the use of positive-pressure ventilation with manual positive pressure from a rubber bag, as was customary in the operating room at that time. Hundreds of medical students worked in relays delivering bag ventilation during the epidemic, and shortly thereafter machines were introduced to deliver positive-pressure ventilation. Over the following 40 years, ventilators changed enormously in appearance, becoming more sophisticated and versatile and having enhanced capabilities for monitoring and alarming. In the wake of these advances, however, a constellation of complications due to mechanical ventilation has been recognized.

OBJECTIVES OF MECHANICAL VENTILATION

The objectives of mechanical ventilation are listed in Table 176-1.[51] In isolation, hypoxemia of mild to moderate severity can be managed by the administration of oxygen through a face mask. With more severe hypoxemia due to shunt or ventilation–perfusion ($\dot{V}/\dot{Q}$) mismatching, it is difficult to guarantee the delivery of a high fractional inspired oxygen concentration (F$_{ICO_2}$) through a face mask. Moreover, these patients are also commonly in considerable distress, so that intubation helps by ensuring delivery of the required F$_{IO_2}$, while positive-pressure ventilation helps by recruiting collapsed lung units leading to improved matching of ventilation and perfusion.

Acute progressive respiratory acidosis is a major indication for mechanical ventilation, although simpler measures can some-

TABLE 176-1

Objectives of Mechanical Ventilation

Improve pulmonary gas exchange
   Reverse hypoxemia
   Relieve acute respiratory acidosis
Relieve respiratory distress
   Decrease oxygen cost of breathing
   Reverse respiratory muscle fatigue
Alter pressure–volume relationships
   Prevent or reverse atelectasis
   Improve lung compliance
   Prevent further lung injury
Permit lung and airway healing
Avoid complications

SOURCE: From Tobin,[51] with permission.

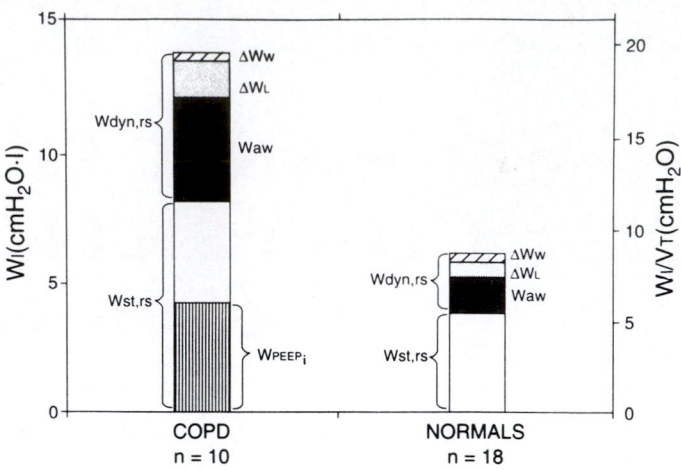

FIGURE 176-1 Partitioning of inspiratory work done on the respiratory system in 10 patients with COPD and 18 normal, anesthetized, paralyzed patients. The values on the right ordinate represent total inspiratory work (W_I), and those on the left ordinate represent W_I normalized for tidal volume (V_T). Total inspiratory work (W_I) in patients with COPD was more than double that in normal subjects. Increased total static work of the respiratory system ($W_{st,rs}$) was due almost totally to work of intrinsic positive end-expiratory pressure (W_{PEEP_i}). Increased total dynamic work of the respiratory system ($W_{dyn,rs}$) was due to increases in airway resistive work (W_{aw}) and work secondary to viscoelastic behavior and time-constant inhomogeneities in the lung (ΔW_L). Viscoelastic work of the chest wall (ΔW_w) was similar in the two groups. *(From Coussa et al,[10] with permission.)*

times reverse the process. For example, in a series of 61 patients with acute severe asthma and hypercapnia (mean Pa_{CO_2} of 54 mmHg and pH of 7.28), all but 5 responded to standard bronchodilator therapy and did not require mechanical ventilation.[43] If severe respiratory depression is expected to persist for some time (e.g., with certain drug overdoses), intubation and mechanical ventilation should be instituted without delay.

A substantial proportion of patients who require (and benefit from) mechanical ventilation have relatively normal arterial blood gases but have clinical signs of increased work of breathing—nasal flaring, vigorous activity of the sternomastoid muscles, tracheal tug, recession of the suprasternal, supraclavicular, and intercostal spaces, paradoxical motion of the abdomen, and pulsus paradoxus. These patients are described as "tiring out" and are at risk of developing respiratory muscle fatigue. Depending on the nature of the underlying disease, work of breathing may be increased as a result of increased airway resistance, increased stiffness of the lungs or chest wall, or the presence of a threshold inspiratory load due to auto- or intrinsic end-expiratory pressure ($PEEP_i$) (Fig. 176-1).[10]

Increased respiratory work increases the O_2 cost of breathing to as much as 50% of total O_2 consumption. In such circumstances, mechanical ventilation decreases the work of breathing and allows precious O_2 stores to be rerouted to other vulnerable tissue beds. In patients with atelectasis or acute lung injury, breathing occurs on the low, flat portion of the pressure–volume curve. By shifting tidal ventilation to the steep, compliant portion of the pressure–volume curve, mechanical ventilation can decrease the work of breathing (Fig. 176-2).[29]

That mechanical ventilation can cause quite dramatic complications such as a pneumothorax and hypotension has been recognized for a long time, but there is a growing awareness that subtle injuries may be more common and hazardous. As a result, the previously unquestioned goals and targets of mechanical ventilation are being reappraised.[47] Reversal of respiratory acidosis and attainment of a normal pH are no longer considered primary targets. Many authorities are more concerned about the risk of alveolar injury and recommend avoiding high inflation pressures, even if this results in considerable respiratory acidosis.

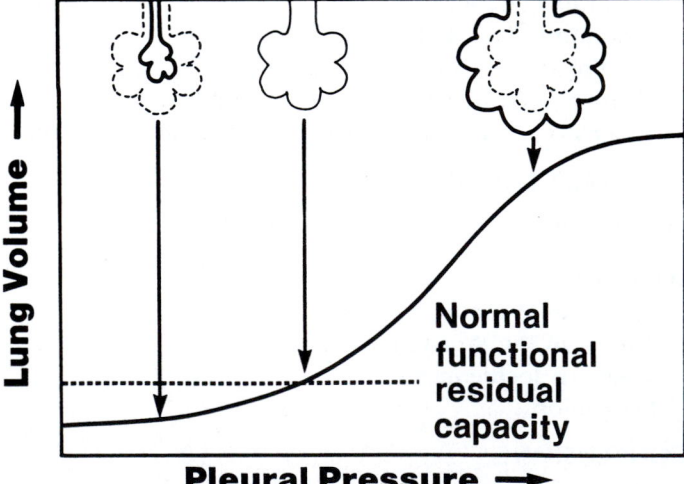

FIGURE 176-2 Lung volume in relation to pleural pressure during mechanical ventilation. Normally, a tidal breath begins at functional residual capacity (FRC), which lies on the steep portion of the pressure–volume curve of the lung. A collapsed airway or alveolus (shown on left of figure) results in a low FRC (on the low, flat portion of the curve) where a large change in pleural pressure is required for even a small change in volume. In this situation, PEEP shifts the end-expiratory lung volume to the steep portion of the curve (shown on right of figure); however, PEEP may also cause a normal alveolus to move to the upper, flat portion of the curve, with consequent overdistension and risk of alveolar rupture. *(From Tobin: Essentials of Critical Care Medicine. New York, Churchill Livingstone, 1989, p 279, with permission.)*

CLASSIFICATION OF MECHANICAL VENTILATION

Some of the terminology used to describe features of mechanical ventilators has been vague and contradictory, leading to considerable confusion. A new comprehensive classification of ventilators[7] has been proposed; the section in this classification dealing with the control and phase variables has greatest relevance for clinicians (Table 176-2). A *control variable* is one that the ventilator manipulates to produce inspiration; it remains constant with changes in the patient's pulmonary mechanics. For a ventilator to be classified as a *pressure controller,* the pressure waveform needs to be unaffected by changes in the patient's resistance and compliance. Although the term *volume control* is commonly used, few ventilators provide volume control in the strict sense, as this requires direct measurement of volume (displacement of a piston or bellows); more often, volume is obtained by integration of the measured flow signal. A ventilator is considered a *flow controller* when volume does not change with alterations in the patient's mechanics, and flow, rather than volume, is measured directly. A ventilator is considered a *time controller* when both pressure and volume waveforms are substantially altered by changes in pulmonary mechanics; in this case, the ventilator controls only the inspiratory and expiratory times. Pressure, volume, and flow are interrelated, so that only one variable can be controlled or predetermined at a point in time (the independent variable), and the other two become dependent variables. For each control variable there are a limited number

TABLE 176-2

Classification of Mechanical Ventilation

Variable Type	Examples
Control variables	
Pressure	Rectangular
Volume	Ramp
	Sinusoidal
Flow	Sinusoidal
	Rectangular
	Ascending ramp
	Descending ramp
	Exponential decay
Time	
Phase variables	
Trigger	Pressure
	Time
	Flow
	Volume
Limit	Peak inspiratory pressure
	Peak inspiratory flow
	Delivered volume
Cycle	Time
	Pressure
	Flow
Baseline	PEEP

For definition of control variable and phase variable, and other details of this classification, please see text.

of waveforms, which can be grouped into four basic categories: rectangular, exponential, ramp, and sinusoidal.

All ventilators monitor one or more of the following four variables: pressure, volume, flow, and time, which are used in deriving the phase variables (Table 176-2). The most common *trigger variables* are pressure and time; flow is a recent addition. The labels *limit* and *cycle* are commonly misused, even by manufacturers. A *limit variable* is allowed to rise no higher than some preset value; that is, the value cannot be exceeded during inspiration. The *cycle variable* terminates inspiration. Although tidal volume is set on most modern ventilators, these ventilators are not truly volume-cycled. Instead, the devices regulate the inspiratory time necessary to achieve the selected tidal volume with the set inspiratory flow, making them time-cycled. Pressure is the only *baseline variable* that is commonly set.

PHYSICAL BASIS OF MECHANICAL VENTILATION

The operational capabilities of every ventilator depend on a pneumatic system, which consists of the mechanical components that regulate gas delivery to the patient.[28] The pneumatic system is powered by a pressurized gas source, which delivers air and 100% oxygen to the ventilator at 50 psi. To avoid harm to the patient and to minimize wear on the components, this initial pressure is immediately decreased to a working pressure. A proportioning valve blends air and oxygen in the pneumatic system to achieve a specific F_{IO_2}. A variety of flow-control mechanisms are used to regulate inspiratory flow and to manipulate its waveform. In addition to delivering gas to the patient, the ventilator is also responsible for humidifying, warming, and filtering the inspired gas. When the patient exhales, gas flows through the expiratory limb of the circuit, passing through a filter and exhalation valve into the atmosphere. The exhalation valve, which is closed during inspiration, is responsible for regulating the level of PEEP. Modern ventilators usually incorporate a microprocessor that controls the inspiratory and expiratory valves; the microprocessor also controls information that is monitored, displayed, and used in the alarm settings. In the event of a pneumatic failure, an antiasphyxia valve opens on the inspiratory limb, permitting the patient to breathe room air. In the event of electrical or pneumatic failure, some ventilators open both the inspiratory and expiratory valves so that gas flows through the circuit.

MODES OF MECHANICAL VENTILATION

The term *mode* refers to the relationship among various breath types (e.g., mandatory, assisted, supported, spontaneous), as well as inspiratory phase variables.

Controlled Mechanical Ventilation

In controlled mechanical ventilation, the ventilator delivers all breaths at a preset rate, and the patient cannot trigger the machine. In the volume-targeted mode, the breaths have a preset volume—so-called volume-controlled ventilation. When the breaths are pressure-limited and time-cycled, the mode is termed *pressure-controlled* ventilation (Chapter 177). Use of volume-controlled ventilation is largely restricted to patients who are apneic as a result of brain damage, sedation, or paralysis.

Assist-Control Ventilation

In the assist-control (AC) mode, the ventilator delivers a breath either when triggered by the patient's inspiratory effort (either pressure- or flow-triggered) or independently, if such an effort does not occur within a preselected time period. All breaths are delivered under positive pressure by the machine, but unlike controlled mechanical ventilation, the patient's triggering effort can exceed the preset rate. If the patient's spontaneous rate drops below the preset back-up rate, controlled ventilation is provided. The pressure to achieve the set tidal volume may be provided solely by the machine or, in part, by the patient. By design, delivered tidal volume is not influenced by patient effort. The more the patient contributes, the less pressure is provided by the machine, and ventilator-generated pressure bears an inverse relationship with patient-generated pressure.[53] The ventilator cycles off when the preset tidal volume is reached, and machine inspiratory time may be shorter or longer than the patient's intrinsic (neural) inspiratory time.[53] If the set tidal volume is reached before the end of neural inspiratory time, the machine cycles off while the patient's inspiratory effort continues. If the patient's inspiratory effort ceases before the set tidal volume is reached, the machine increases pressure to provide continued inspiratory flow. The amount of active work performed by a patient ventilated in the AC mode is critically dependent on the trigger sensitivity and inspiratory flow settings. Even when these settings are selected appropriately, patients actively perform about one-third of the work performed by the ventilator during passive conditions.[37]

Intermittent Mandatory Ventilation

With intermittent mandatory ventilation (IMV), the patient receives periodic positive-pressure breaths from the ventilator at a preset volume and rate, but the patient can also breathe spontaneously between these mandatory breaths.[46] The original design consisted of a continuous gas flow system connected in parallel to the inspiratory limb of the ventilator circuit. The ventilator was set in the control mode. The patient could also take spontaneous breaths from the continuous flow circuit. With this system, no attempt was made to synchronize the delivery of ventilator breaths with the patient's own inspiratory rhythm. This perceived problem led to the introduction of synchronized intermittent mandatory ventilation (SIMV). This was achieved by the incorporation of a patient-triggered demand valve, which functions essentially like assist-control during windows of time set by the manufacturer (usually as a function of the set respiratory rate) (Fig. 176-3). If the patient makes an inspiratory effort while the window is open, a synchronized breath is delivered. If no effort occurs by the time the window closes, the ventilator delivers a controlled positive-pressure breath. In earlier generations of ventilators that provided SIMV, patients had to create considerable negative pressure to open the demand valve, resulting in a twofold or greater increase in the work of breathing compared with the continuous-flow IMV systems. Modern micro-

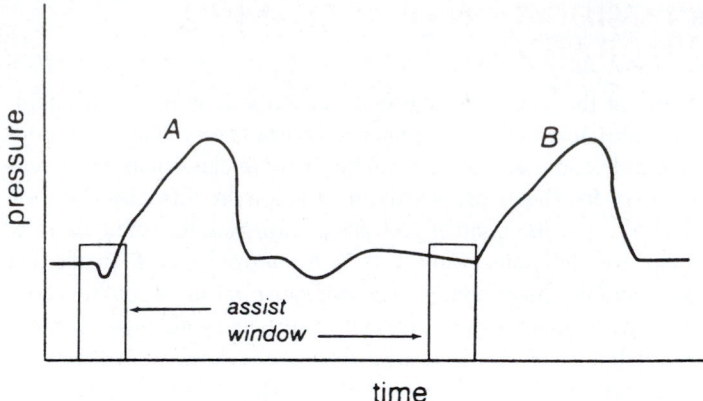

FIGURE 176-3 Synchronization of intermittent mandatory ventilation (IMV) through use of an assist window. If the patient makes an effort during a window of time, the ventilator senses this effort and delivers a breath in synchrony with the patient's effort (A). If no effort is made while the window is open, a controlled breath is delivered (B). *(From Kacmarek and Hess,[28] with permission.)*

processor-based ventilators use a proportional valve that regulates flow under feedback control of pressure, and imposed work is comparable to that with a continuous-flow system.[46]

IMV has a number of advantages over controlled mechanical ventilation. In a retrospective study of 292 patients, ventilator-induced barotrauma was less with IMV (7 percent) than with controlled ventilation (22 percent), despite higher peak airway pressures and PEEP in the IMV group.[41] In patients with normal left-ventricular function, cardiac output was 27 percent higher with IMV than with controlled mechanical ventilation, but in patients with poor left-ventricular function, cardiac output was 19 percent lower with IMV than with controlled ventilation.[40] The more negative intrathoracic pressure during IMV enhances venous return, which presumably accounts for the increased cardiac output in patients with normal left-ventricular function. However, negative intrathoracic pressure also increases left-ventricular afterload, and this effect dominates in patients with poor cardiac reserve, accounting for the reduction in cardiac output in this group.

Comparisons between IMV and AC ventilation are more limited. In a group of 40 patients with acute respiratory failure, cardiac output was 6 percent higher during IMV set at a mandatory rate of 7 breaths per minute (total respiratory rate 34 breaths per minute) compared with AC ventilation at a rate of 15 breaths per minute.[22] Although this difference in cardiac output is within the variability of the thermodilution technique, a trial of IMV is appropriate in patients who exhibit hemodynamic compromise during AC ventilation. Three groups of investigators demonstrated less respiratory alkalosis with IMV than with AC ventilation,[11,22,24] but the differences were small and of questionable clinical significance (Table 176-3). In one of the studies,[24] the higher $PaCO_2$ during IMV was shown to result from a higher rate of CO_2 production, presumably reflecting increased patient work. In the other study in which CO_2 production was measured, no change was seen,[22] and the increase in $PaCO_2$ during IMV was attributed to increased dead-space ventilation, since minute ventilation did not change.

TABLE 176-3

Respiratory Alkalosis in Intermittent Mandatory Ventilation and Assist-Control Ventilation

pH		Pa_{CO_2} (mmHg)		$\dot{V}_{CO_2}$ (ml/min)		Ventilator Rate (breaths per minute)		
IMV	AC	IMV	AC	IMV	AC	IMV	AC	Author
7.41	7.45	43.0	38.0	222	221	7	15	Groeger[22]
7.48	7.51	29.7	28.6	323	301	1/2 AC rate	na*	Hudson[24]
7.42	7.45	40.7	37.9	—	—	4	21	Culpepper[11]

*na = not available.

One of the main objectives of mechanical ventilation is to alleviate discomfort secondary to increased respiratory work. However, patients may have difficulty in adapting to the intermittent nature of ventilator assistance with IMV. In the past, it was assumed that during IMV, the degree of respiratory muscle rest was proportional to the level of machine assistance during IMV. However, recent studies indicate that inspiratory effort is equivalent for spontaneous and assisted breaths during IMV[25,38] (Fig. 176-4). Indeed, the tension–time index for both the spontaneous and assisted breaths is above the threshold associated with respiratory muscle fatigue at IMV rates of 14 breaths per minute or less.[38] At a moderate level of machine assistance, i.e., where the ventilator accounts for 20 to 50 percent of the total ventilation, electromyographic activity of the diaphragm and sternomastoid muscles is equivalent for assisted and spontaneous breaths.[25] These findings suggest that respiratory center output is preprogrammed and that it does not adjust to breath-to-breath changes in load as

occur during IMV. As a result, IMV may contribute to the development of respiratory muscle fatigue or prevent its recovery.

Pressure Support Ventilation

Pressure support (PS) ventilation is patient-triggered, like AC ventilation and IMV, but differs in that it is pressure-targeted and flow-cycled.[6] The physician sets a level of pressure that augments every spontaneous effort, and the patient can alter respiratory frequency, inspiratory time, and tidal volume. Tidal volume is determined by the pressure setting, the patient's effort, and pulmonary mechanics, in contrast to AC ventilation and IMV, where a guaranteed volume is delivered. The lack of guaranteed ventilator assistance in the absence of patient effort can result in apnea in patients with unstable respiratory center output; some ventilators include safety features against this problem, but others (e.g., Siemens Servo 900C) do not. With volume-targeted ventilation, the inspiratory flow setting is a crucial determinant of patient work. There is no flow setting with PS ventilation, although the initial peak flow determines the speed of pressurization and the initial pressure ramp profile. The speed of pressurization was previously fixed and specific for a given ventilator, although this variable can be set on several of the newer ventilators.[6] Cycling to exhalation is triggered by a

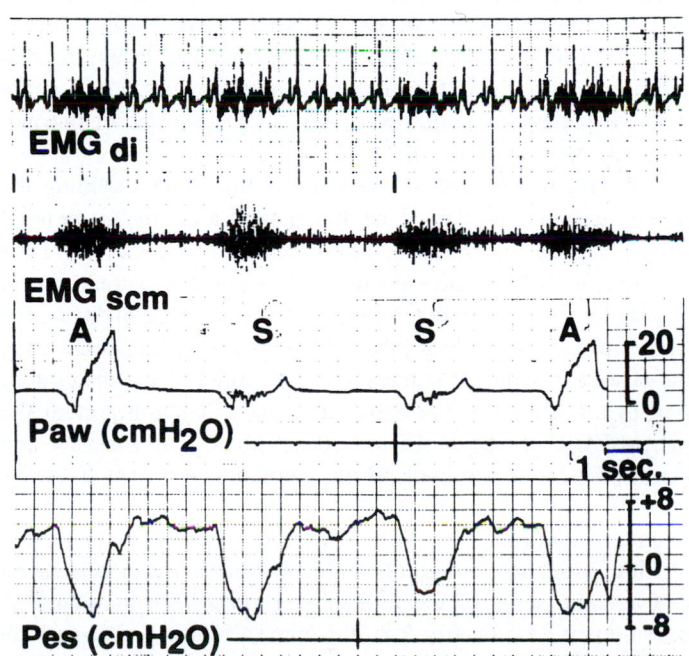

FIGURE 176-4   Electromyograms of the diaphragm (EMGdi) and sternocleidomastoid muscles (EMGscm) in a patient receiving synchronized intermittent mandatory ventilation. Similar intensity and duration of electrical activity during assisted (A) and spontaneous (S) cycles are demonstrated. P_{aw} = airway pressure; P_{es} = esophageal pressure. *(From Imsand et al,[25] with permission.)*

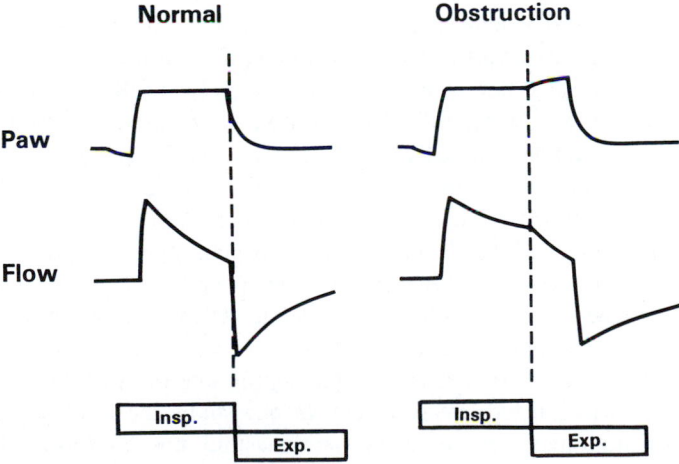

FIGURE 176-5   Airway pressure (P_{aw}) and inspiratory (Insp.) and expiratory (Exp.) flow during pressure support ventilation in patients with normal and obstructed airways. Patient effort triggers the ventilator to deliver a preset pressure, and inspiratory assistance continues until the flow rate falls to 25 percent of the peak inspiratory flow. In patients with airway obstruction who have a prolonged time constant, more time is required for flow to decrease to this threshold value, so that neural expiration commences before the termination of mechanical inflation. The resulting activation of the expiratory muscles hastens the fall in flow, but it also results in dysynchrony between the patient's neuromuscular activity and the mechanical phase of the ventilator—so-called fighting the ventilator.

decrease in inspiratory flow to a preset level, such as 5 L/min or 25 percent of the peak inspiratory flow, depending on the manufacturer's algorithm (Fig. 176-5). Inspiratory assistance can also be terminated by a small increase in pressure (1 to 3 cm H_2O) above the preset level, resulting from expiratory effort.[6] If there is a leak in the system, neither of these mechanisms are effective, and the patient is at risk of overinflation; inclusion of a time limit for inspiration prevents this hazard. Alteration in the flow rate criterion for termination of inspiratory assistance is likely to influence the degree of inspiratory muscle unloading and expiratory muscle loading, although systematic studies investigating these precise interrelationships have not been conducted.

Intermittent positive-pressure breathing (IPPB) is another patient-triggered, pressure-limited mode that was widely used in the 1960s. It differs from PS ventilation in several aspects. A constant level of pressure during inspiration is sought with PS ventilation but not with IPPB. The end of inspiration is flow-cycled with PS ventilation, whereas it is pressure-cycled with IPPB. During PS ventilation, the ventilator responds to an increase in patient effort by increasing flow, but this is not possible with IPPB, since there is no servo control of airway pressure. In seven healthy subjects, inspiratory work was three times higher during IPPB compared with PS ventilation.[35] In addition, the high impeding-flow characteristics of the circuit, combined with the cycling mechanism, can increase expiratory work with IPPB.[35]

Several investigators have shown that PS ventilation is very effective in decreasing the work of inspiration. However, the degree of inspiratory muscle unloading is variable, with a coefficient of variation of up to 96 percent among patients.[27] PS ventilation does not decrease $PEEP_i$ in patients with chronic obstructive pulmonary disease (COPD).[27] Thus, at a PS of 20 cm H_2O, $PEEP_i$ may account for approximately two-thirds of total inspiratory effort.[27] The algorithm used to terminate inspiratory assistance during PS ventilation, namely, a fall in inspiratory flow to a threshold value, can lead to excessive expiratory effort in patients with COPD. Patients with a prolonged time constant require more time for flow to fall to this threshold, and, consequently, mechanical inflation may persist into neural expiration (Fig. 176-5). To counteract such neural–mechanical dysynchrony, patients may activate their expiratory muscles at a time when the ventilator is still inflating the thorax, causing the patient to "fight the ventilator."[27]

There is no consensus as to the appropriate level of PS ventilation for an individual patient. In one study, the level of PS that minimized activity of the sternomastoid muscles was associated with reversal of electromyographic evidence of excessive diaphragmatic stress.[6] More common, the level of PS is titrated to achieve a decrease in respiratory frequency and an increase in tidal volume. However, there is a considerable discrepancy among studies as to the preferred target or "optimal" level of PS. This is partly due to the lack of information on the desirable level of inspiratory work in ventilator-supported patients. As such, the thresholds of the reference values are arbitrary. Moreover, analysis has been performed in a post hoc manner and probably overestimates the usefulness of any of the titration techniques. Furthermore, assessment has been confined to inspiratory effort. Titration of the level of PS to achieve a low respiratory frequency

will generally result in inspiratory muscle unloading, but activity of the expiratory muscles may increase *pari passu* causing the patient to fight the ventilator. Hence, this selection of the optimal level of PS is quite complex.[27]

VENTILATOR SETTINGS

Ventilator settings are based on the patient's size and clinical condition. Determination of the settings is a dynamic process, based upon a patient's physiological response, rather than on a fixed set of numbers. The settings require repeated readjustment over the period of ventilator dependency, and such an iterative process requires careful respiratory monitoring.

Trigger Sensitivity

Most mechanical ventilators employ pressure triggering, whereby a decrease in circuit pressure is required to initiate ventilator assistance. It is difficult to employ a trigger setting more sensitive than −1 to −2 cm H_2O without causing the ventilator to autocycle, but if the setting is less sensitive, work of breathing increases significantly. The actual change in airway pressure with ventilator triggering is usually quite different than the set sensitivity and can be divided into two phases.[45]

The *trigger phase* refers to the time from the commencement of patient effort to the onset of flow delivery; airway pressure at this point is the true or measured (as opposed to set) trigger sensitivity. Trigger phase duration is a function of a patient's respiratory drive (i.e., the change in pressure relative to the change in time, dP/dt) and the degree of dynamic hyperinflation (*vide infra*).[53] In patients with a low respiratory drive, and in those with increased elastic recoil due to dynamic hyperinflation, triggering of the ventilator does not occur until late in the inspiratory time. As a result, the ventilator largely cycles out of phase with the patient's respiratory rhythm, defeating one of the major goals of assisted ventilation.[53]

The *post-trigger phase* refers to the time from attaining the true trigger sensitivity until the maximal decrease in airway pressure; this phase is related to an insufficient initial gas flow. The location of the pressure-sensing site within the patient circuit does not influence the magnitude of the pressure drop during the trigger phase, but it does affect the decrease in pressure during the post-trigger phase. If the sensor is located on the inspiratory port of the ventilator (as opposed to the exhalation port or the patient Y), a smaller gradient between the circuit pressure and target pressure is fed back to the ventilator, resulting in an inadequate flow delivery and an increase in the work necessary to sustain inspiration.[45]

Flow triggering (sometimes termed *flow-by*) was introduced to overcome some of the problems of pressure triggering.[23] A base flow of gas (usually 5 to 20 L/min) is delivered during both the expiratory and inspiratory phases of the respiratory cycle. In the absence of inspiratory effort, gas exiting through the expiratory port of the ventilator is equal to the inspiratory base flow. In the presence of patient effort, gas enters the patient's lungs and is diverted from the exhalation port. The difference between inspiratory and expiratory base flow is sensed electronically and initiates a switch in the ventilator cycle; sensitivity is usually set at 2 L/min. The trigger phase is considerably less with flow-triggering than with pressure triggering.[45] In the post-trigger phase, a flow-triggered system may be more responsive to a patient's ventilatory demand than a pressure-triggered system.[45] As a result, work of inspiration is less with flow triggering than with pressure triggering.

Triggering of the ventilator is more difficult in patients with airflow limitation and dynamic hyperinflation, where the end-expiratory lung volume exceeds the relaxation volume of the respiratory system. In this case, the patient must first generate sufficient pressure to offset the elastic recoil associated with hyperinflation and then overcome the sensitivity threshold. As a result, the patient may make two or more efforts before successfully triggering the ventilator; the patient's intrinsic respiratory rate exceeds that of the ventilator (Fig. 176-6). During unsuccessful triggering attempts there is little or no inflation; hence, lung volume, and, therefore, elastic recoil, continue to decline.[53] Accordingly, the patient is in a better position to trigger the ventilator with the next effort. Nontriggering is more common in patients who have a preceding large tidal volume, short expiratory time, and high expiratory resistance or airflow limitation (all of which lead to an increase in elastic recoil) and who make small inspiratory efforts.

Excessive ventilator cycling may also occur where the machine rate exceeds the patient's intrinsic rate as a result of double triggering of the ventilator by a single inspiratory effort. This can occur during PS ventilation in patients who have a short mechanical time constant (low resistance, low compliance) and a relatively long spontaneous inspiratory time, especially when the cycling-off threshold is based on a variable flow (e.g., 25 percent of the peak inspiratory flow). As patient effort increases, peak flow increases and the cycling-off threshold is met at a higher flow; consequently, the duration of pressure support is shorter. With the loss of pressure, inspiratory muscle effort alone is not sufficient to sustain elastic recoil, so that flow becomes expiratory and elastic recoil decreases. In patients with a prolonged neural inspiratory time, a point is reached where inspiratory muscle pressure exceeds recoil pressure; this results in a negative airway pressure and retriggering of pressure support.[53] Double triggering may also occur during AC ventilation if the inspiratory time set on the machine is much shorter than the patient's intrinsic inspiratory time.

Tidal Volume

A tidal volume of 10 to 15 ml/kg has been the standard recommendation for mechanical ventilation for several years. This value has been challenged by convincing studies in experimental animals indicating that alveolar overdistension can produce endothelial, epithelial, and basement-membrane injuries that are associated with increased microvascular permeability and lung rupture. To minimize this risk, one ideally would like to monitor alveolar volume; however, currently this is not feasible. A reasonable substitute is to monitor peak alveolar pressure as estimated from the plateau pressure, which is measured in a relaxed patient by briefly occluding the ventilator circuit at end-inspiration. The incidence of ventilator-induced lung injury increases markedly when plateau pressure is high. Although data are incomplete, there is a growing tendency to lower delivered tidal volume to 5 to 7 ml/kg (or less) to achieve a plateau pressure no higher than 35 cm H_2O[47]; this range is based on the reasonable notion that total lung capacity should not be exceeded. Since use of small tidal volumes may lead to an increase in Pa_{CO_2}, the strategy is termed *permissive hypercapnia* or *controlled hypoventilation*. When using this approach, it is important to focus on the pH rather than the Pa_{CO_2}. If the pH falls below 7.20, some physicians recommend administration of intravenous bicarbonate; however, this is of unproved benefit and is subject of controversy. In patients with severe asthma requiring mechanical ventilation, uncontrolled studies suggest that permissive hypercapnia results in lower mortality than does conventional ventilation; the same may be true for patients with the acute respiratory distress syndrome (ARDS).

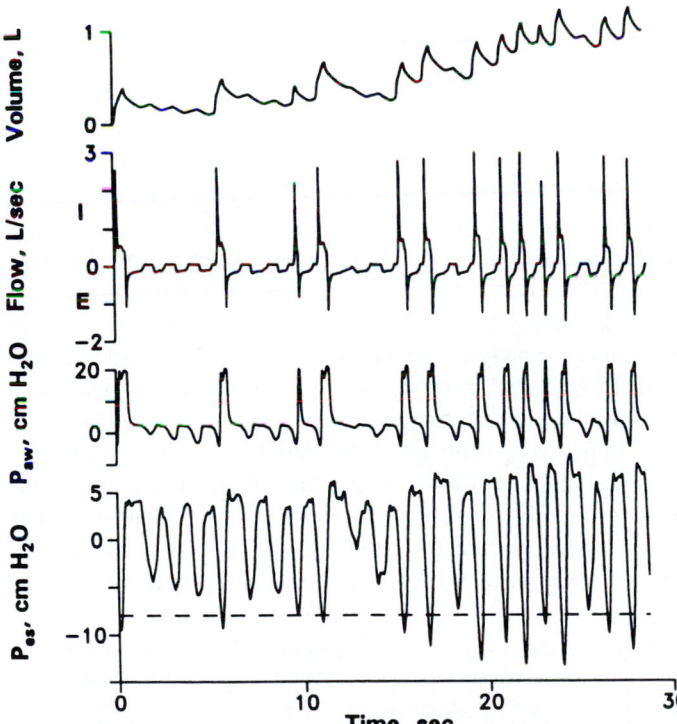

FIGURE 176-6 Recordings of tidal volume, inspiratory (I) and expiratory (E) flow, airway pressure (P_{aw}), and esophageal pressure (P_{es}) in a patient with chronic obstructive pulmonary disease receiving pressure support ventilation. Approximately half of the patient's inspiratory efforts do not succeed in triggering the ventilator. Triggering occurs only when the patient generates P_{es} more negative than -8 cmH$_2$O (indicated by the interrupted horizontal line), a pressure equal in magnitude to the opposing elastic recoil pressure. Expiratory flow exhibits a biphasic pattern, with momentary braking signalling ineffective inspiratory effort. Thus, monitoring of expiratory flow provides a more accurate measurement of the patient's intrinsic respiratory rate than does the number of machine cycles displayed on the bedside monitor. *(From Tobin and Jubran: Schweiz Med Wochenschr 124:2138, 1994, with permission.)*

Respiratory Rate

Correct setting of the ventilator rate depends on the mode of ventilation employed. With AC ventilation, the ventilator supplies a breath in response to each patient effort. With this mode, physicians commonly pay little attention to the machine rate, which may be set much lower than the patient's spontaneous rate. This results in two problems: (1) If the patient has a sudden decrease in respiratory center output, a low machine rate results in serious hypoventilation. (2) A large discrepancy between the patient's spontaneous rate and the machine's back-up rate results in a respiratory cycle with an inverse inspiratory-to-expiratory time (I:E) ratio.[23] This arises because inspiratory time (Ti) on the machine remains fixed at the initial setting and does not change in response to increases in the patient's spontaneous rate (Fig. 176-7). For example, if the machine rate is initially set at 12 breaths per minute (i.e., T_{TOT} of 5 s) and Ti at 1.65 s (either set directly or indirectly as a consequence of the volume and flow settings), then Te will be 3.35 s and the I:E ratio will be 1:2. If the patient's spontaneous respiratory rate is increased to 25 breaths per minute, T_{TOT} will be 2.4 s; since Ti remains fixed at 1.65 s, Te will be 0.75 s and the I:E ratio will be 2:1. Such inverse-ratio ventilation is very uncomfortable, and patients may require increased sedation or even neuromuscular blockade. Based on these issues, during AC ventilation the back-up rate should be set at approximately 4 breaths less than the patient's spontaneous rate. With IMV, the ventilator or mandatory rate is initially set high and then gradually reduced according to patient tolerance. Unfortunately, titration is often based on data from arterial blood gases, and even a small number of ventilator breaths will result in acceptable values for Pa_{O_2} and Pa_{CO_2} but will achieve little or no respiratory muscle rest in patients with increased work of breathing. In ventilator-dependent patients, work of breathing at IMV rates of 14 breaths per minute or less may be sufficient to induce respiratory muscle fatigue.[38] With PS ventilation, the ventilator rate is not set.

Inspiratory Flow Rate

In most patients receiving AC ventilation or IMV, the initial (default) inspiratory flow is 60 L/min; with AC ventilation using certain ventilators (e.g., Siemens Servo 900C), however, such a flow cannot be attained without increasing tidal volume

beyond desirable levels. In patients with COPD, increasing the flow to 100 L/min produces better gas exchange, as reflected by decreases of greater than 20% in venous admixture ($\dot{Q}s/\dot{Q}t$) and VD/VT, probably as a result of more complete emptying of gas-trapped regions due to an increase in expiratory time.[9] A high inspiratory flow setting is also needed in patients with increased respiratory drive. Otherwise, the delivered flow may be insufficient to meet a patient's ventilatory requirements, and the patient will strain against his or her own pulmonary impedance and that of the ventilator, with a consequent increase in the work of breathing.[37]

An excessive flow setting should be avoided, however, since studies in healthy subjects demonstrate that increasing the inspiratory flow setting causes an immediate increase in respiratory frequency and respiratory drive. Although respiratory discomfort results from both excessive and inadequate flow settings, discomfort is 7 times greater when flow is set at 30% less than a healthy subject's preferred level than when set at 300% above the preferred level.[36] When adjusting the flow and trigger sensitivity, it is helpful to examine the contour of the airway pressure waveform (Fig. 176-8). Ideally, the waveform should show a smooth rise and convex appearance during inspiration. In contrast, a prolonged negative phase, with excessive scalloping of the tracing, indicates unsatisfactory sensitivity and flow settings.

Fractional Inspired Oxygen Concentration ($F_{I_{O_2}}$)

Correction of hypoxemia and its prevention are major goals in ventilator-supported patients. Many predictive equations have been published to aid in the selection of an appropriate $F_{I_{O_2}}$, but none is sufficiently accurate to substitute for a trial-and-error approach. Initially, $F_{I_{O_2}}$ is set at a high value, often 1.0, to ensure adequate oxygenation. Thereafter, the lowest $F_{I_{O_2}}$ that achieves satisfactory arterial oxygenation should be selected. The usual target is a Pa_{O_2} of 60 mmHg or an arterial saturation (Sa_{O_2}) of 90%; higher values do not substantially enhance tissue oxygenation. Although it is customary to wait 30 min to assess the response to a change in $F_{I_{O_2}}$, the effect is usually well defined within 10 min. When using arterial blood samples to assess oxygenation, a target of 90% for Sa_{O_2} is appropriate, but if pulse

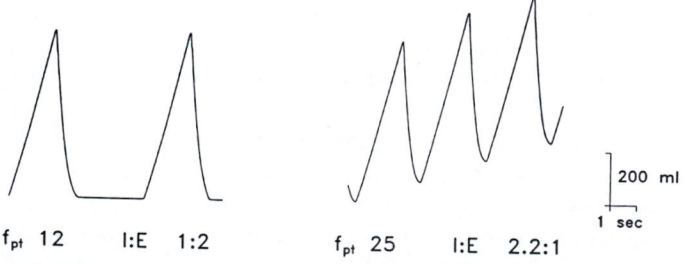

f_{pt} 12   I:E   1:2   f_{pt} 25   I:E   2.2:1

200 ml

1 sec

FIGURE 176-7   Effect of interaction between a patient's respiratory rate and the ventilator back-up rate on inspiratory time–expiratory time ratio (I:E) during assist-control ventilation. Ventilator back-up rate is 12 breaths per minute and inspiratory time (Ti) 1.65 s. *Left panel.* If the patient's intrinsic respiratory (f_{pt}) rate is also 12 breaths per minute, the total respiratory cycle time (T_{TOT}) is 5.0 s, the expiratory time (Te) is 3.35 s, and the I:E ratio is 1:2. *Right panel.* If the patient's respiratory rate increases to 25 breaths per minute, the new T_{TOT} is 2.4 s, Te is 0.75 s, and I:E is 1:0.45 (or, as more conventionally noted, 2.2:1).

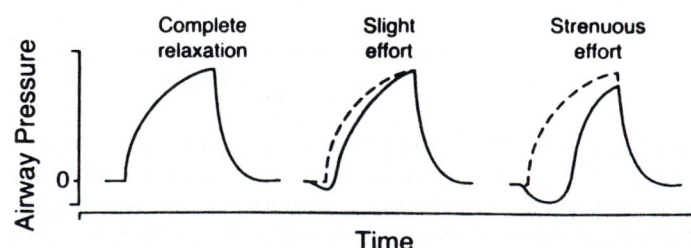

Complete relaxation   Slight effort   Strenuous effort

Airway Pressure

0

Time

FIGURE 176-8   Airway-pressure waveforms recorded during assist-control ventilation. The tracings represent changes in airway pressure during inspiration in a completely relaxed patient, and in patients making slight (center tracing) and strenuous efforts (tracing on right) to breathe. The distance between the dashed line (representing controlled ventilation) and the solid line (representing spontaneous breathing) is proportional to the patient's work of breathing. (*From Tobin,*[51] *with permission.*)

oximetry is employed, this target may result in values for Pa_{O_2} as low as 41 mmHg.[27] In white patients, a target of 92% for Sp_{O_2} indicates satisfactory oxygenation. In black patients, however, this target may still result in significant hypoxemia. Although a higher target value of 95% avoids hypoxemia in black patients, some will have values for Pa_{O_2} approaching 200 mmHg. If the patient is receiving a high $F_{I_{O_2}}$ to achieve this Sp_{O_2} target, oxygen toxicity may result.[27]

In experimental animals, hyperoxia produces diffuse alveolar damage, with histologic changes that are indistinguishable from ARDS due to any other cause.[33] No diagnostic tests distinguish O_2-induced injury from progression of the underlying disease. Thus, the possibility of O_2 toxicity should be considered in any patient receiving an $F_{I_{O_2}}$ of more than 0.50 to 0.60 for 24 to 48 h or longer. Healthy human subjects who inhale 100% O_2 develop acute tracheobronchitis, manifested as substernal discomfort, cough, sore throat, nasal congestion, eye and ear discomfort, paresthesias, and fatigue.[33] Symptoms begin within 4 h; bronchoscopic features of tracheal inflammation are evident after 6 h. Retrosternal discomfort also occurs with an $F_{I_{O_2}}$ of 0.75 but not with an $F_{I_{O_2}}$ of 0.50. Hyperoxia causes absorption atelectasis in lung units with low $\dot{V}_A/\dot{Q}$ ratios, because the rate of absorption of O_2 from the alveoli into the bloodstream is faster than the rate of replenishment from inspired gas.[33] This results in a small shunt (approximately 3%) in healthy elderly subjects and requires only about 6 min to develop.

A decrease in vital capacity is probably the best indicator of O_2 toxicity. In several studies of healthy volunteers breathing 50% O_2 over 7 to 28 days, little, if any, change in vital capacity was observed.[33] When healthy subjects breathed 100% O_2, a decrease in static lung compliance was observed within 3 h. This decrease resolved readily with deep breathing, suggesting that the decreased compliance was due to absorption atelectasis, rather than direct toxicity. Exposure of healthy subjects to 100% O_2 for as long as 4 days resulted in only modest reductions in vital capacity, and gas exchange function returned to normal with air breathing.[33]

Overall, studies in humans reveal much less parenchymal injury than has been observed in experimental animals. It has been suggested the risk of O_2 toxicity might be greater in patients who have coexisting lung injury, but, ironically, indirect data suggest that patients with ARDS may have a reduced risk of O_2 toxicity.[33] Exuded plasma proteins and intraalveolar hemorrhage provide a medium that is rich in antioxidant enzyme capacity and helps to protect against O_2 toxicity.[33] Death in experimental animals exposed to prolonged hyperoxia is usually attributed to acute lung injury. However, several investigators have reported a terminal course characterized by severe cardiac embarrassment associated with focal areas of myocardial necrosis on microscopy.[33]

In the face of potential O_2 toxicity, the only possible clinical strategy is to reduce the $F_{I_{O_2}}$ to the lowest level compatible with adequate systemic oxygenation. Thus, excess O_2 demand should be minimized, and measures to enhance systemic oxygenation should be optimized. Although excessive O_2 administration should be avoided, there is more to fear from severe hypoxemia than from the potential damage that might result from hyperoxia.

Positive End-Expiratory Pressure (PEEP)

Although PEEP was employed prior to the 1930s, it was not until 1967, with the report of its use in ARDS, that PEEP became a major component of modern therapy in the intensive care unit. Ashbaugh and coworkers[1] initially reported 12 patients with ARDS and later expanded the series to 21 patients. Of 14 patients treated with 7 to 10 cmH_2O of PEEP 10 (68 percent) survived; only 2 of the 7 (29 percent) patients who did not receive PEEP survived. Although this study was not randomized or controlled, subsequent favorable experience with PEEP in patients with ARDS indicates that performance of such a study would be unethical.

The term *PEEP* signifies that pressure in the airway is elevated above that of the atmosphere at the completion of expiration; it implies nothing about airway pressure during inspiration, and, by convention, it refers to patients receiving mechanical ventilation. In spontaneously breathing patients, the equivalent state is expiratory positive airway pressure (EPAP). However, since a spontaneously breathing patient must decrease respiratory system pressure below atmosphere to inspire (with a consequent large increase in inspiratory work), application of EPAP has no clinical utility. Instead, continuous positive airway pressure (CPAP) is employed, where airway pressure remains positive during inspiration and expiration. A number of other acronyms were introduced to describe the combination of PEEP with various modes of mechanical ventilation, but they are no longer in common use.

EFFECTS OF PEEP

The beneficial effects of PEEP include improvement in arterial oxygenation, improvement in lung compliance, alleviation of the excessive work of breathing due to $PEEP_i$ in patients with airflow limitation, and, perhaps, a decrease in lung injury resulting from repeated alveolar collapse and reopening. The principal beneficial effect of PEEP is an increase in Pa_{O_2}, which permits a decrease in $F_{I_{O_2}}$ and a reduction in the risk of O_2 toxicity. The major mechanism for the increase in Pa_{O_2} with PEEP is an increase in end-expiratory lung volume (Table 176-4). Patients with ARDS develop alveolar instability and collapse. Consequently, functional residual capacity falls below closing volume, and small airways close during tidal breathing, leading to intrapulmonary shunt and hypoxemia. PEEP increases end-inspiratory lung volume by distending lung units that are already open, preventing collapse of unstable alveoli at end-expiration, recruiting

---

TABLE 176-4

Mechanisms of Increased Pa_{O_2} with PEEP

Increase in end-expiratory lung volume
    Distension of patent lung units
    Recruitment of collapsed lung units
    Redistribution of fluid within the lung
Decrease in shunt
    Increase in end-expiratory lung volume
    Decrease in cardiac output

collapsed lung units, and redistributing liquid within the lung.[12,21,30,34] The decrease in $\dot{V}/\dot{Q}$ with PEEP is proportional to alveolar recruitment.[21] Previously, the decrease in $\dot{V}/\dot{Q}$ was thought to be secondary to a decrease in cardiac output occurring with PEEP.[13] The improvement in Pa_{O_2} was considered an epiphenomenon, reflecting decreased blood flow through diseased regions rather than improved gas exchange capacity. However, in a study in which dopamine was used to prevent the expected decrease in cardiac output in eight patients with acute respiratory failure treated with PEEP, a level of PEEP of 17 cm H_2O caused Pa_{O_2} to increase from 74 to 178 mmHg, and $\dot{V}/\dot{Q}$ decreased from 30 to 13 percent[39]—clear evidence that the decrease in $\dot{V}/\dot{Q}$ with PEEP cannot be explained by a decrease in cardiac output.

Three distinct patterns of response to PEEP in different regions of the lung in patients with ARDS have been described.[8] A linear increase in gas volume with increasing PEEP is the most common pattern (57 percent of regions). This pattern implies greater inflation of lung units that are already open, rather than recruitment of additional units. A biphasic increase in gas volume with increasing pressure is found in 31 percent of regions. Inflation of these regions is signalled by an inflection point (P_{flex}) on the pressure–volume curve, which denotes pulmonary units that are recruited only after a "critical" level of PEEP is exceeded. The remaining 12 percent of regions show no increase in gas volume in response to increasing pressure, presumably because of diffuse consolidation or intraalveolar edema.[18]

When PEEP was increased from 3 to 13 cmH$_2$O in patients with acute respiratory failure, 66 percent of the eventual increase in lung volume was complete within the first breath, and 90 percent within five breaths[30] (Fig. 176-9). The immediate increase in volume was attributed to distension of already open alveoli, whereas the delayed increase in volume was attributed to mechanisms requiring a longer time to overcome forces responsible for collapsing alveoli. These forces might include surfactant-mediated changes in surface tension, stress relaxation of viscoelastic elements of the lung and chest wall, and recruitment of alveoli that remain collapsed after a single inflation.

At one time PEEP was thought to decrease extravascular lung water by "pushing" alveolar fluid back into the circulation. On the contrary, PEEP can actually increase lung water. As alveoli expand with application of PEEP, the interstitial pressure in the extraalveolar space decreases, leading to an increase in transmural pressure across the vessel wall. If intravascular pressures remain the same or increase, the filtration of fluid across the vessel wall increases causing an increase in pulmonary edema; if PEEP causes a decrease in cardiac output and vascular pressures, lung water does not change in pulmonary edema. The beneficial action of PEEP in pulmonary edema is due to the redistribution of edema fluid from the alveolar space into the perivascular cuffs. In dogs with oleic acid–induced pulmonary edema, 13 cmH$_2$O of PEEP decreased $\dot{V}_A/\dot{Q}$ from 48 to 6 percent; the reduction was accompanied by a decrease in the proportion of flooded alveoli from 78 to 22 percent and no change in total lung water.[34] This redistribution of lung water, in association with an increase in end-expiratory lung volume, is the major mechanism underlying the increase in Pa_{O_2} with PEEP.

Lung weight is increased approximately twofold in patients with ARDS,[21] and the hydrostatic pressure generated at any given height of a vertically oriented lung increases progressively toward the bases.[18] This increased hydrostatic pressure is a major determinant of lung collapse, which is more common in the dependent regions. PEEP recruits lung volume mainly by acting as a counterforce against this superimposed hydrostatic pressure, and the required level of PEEP is equivalent to the inflection point on a pressure–volume curve.[18] Repeated collapse and reopening of lung units may induce shear forces that induce lung damage. By increasing PEEP progressively from 0 to 20 cmH$_2$O and measuring recruitment at both end-inspiration (plateau-pressure-induced) and end-expiration (PEEP-induced), the amount of lung tissue that reopens and collapses during each respiratory cycle has been quantitated[20] (Fig. 176-10). As PEEP is increased, the difference in recruitment between end inspiration and end expiration progressively decreases. This difference is not significant at PEEP of 15 cmH$_2$O or higher, indicating that the lung is completely open throughout the respiratory cycle at this level of PEEP.

The degree of lung injury with ARDS varies considerably among patients. Also, within the same patient, the injury is not diffuse and homogeneous, as originally believed. Instead, lesions are nonhomogeneous in distribution, and some normally inflated lung is present in patients with even the

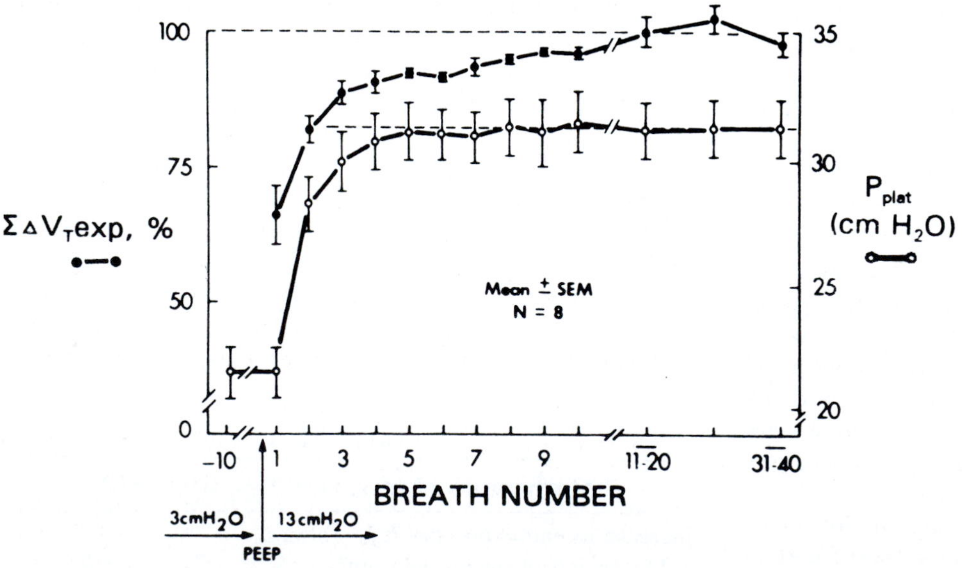

FIGURE 176-9 Increase in lung volume with an increase in PEEP from 3 to 13 cmH$_2$O (vertical arrow) in eight patients with acute respiratory failure. The cumulative net loss of expired tidal volume ($\Sigma\Delta V_{Texp}$) was assumed to reflect the net gain in lung volume. Sixty-six percent of the eventual increase in lung volume (703 ml) was complete within the first breath. End-inspiratory occlusion pressure (P_{plat}) reached a plateau within 4 to 5 breaths after the increase in PEEP. (Modified from Katz et al,[30] with permission.)

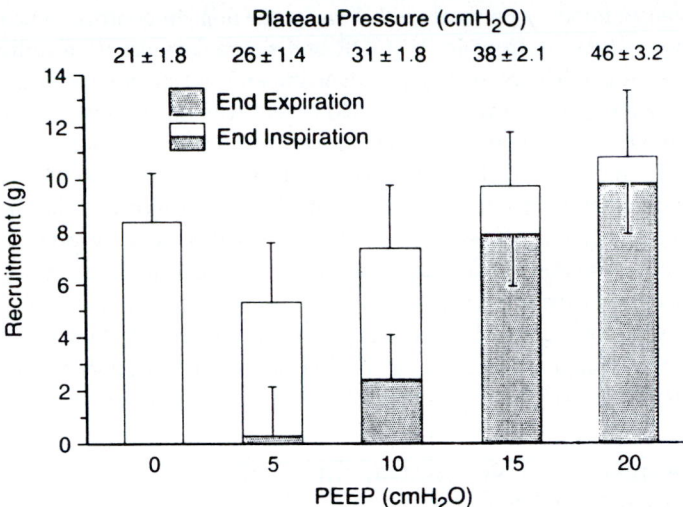

FIGURE 176-10   Lung recruitment, in terms of volume of gas (g), with application of PEEP. Recruitment of lung tissue at end-inspiration (plateau-pressure-induced, the uppermost extent of each column) and end-expiration (PEEP-induced, shaded column) is shown as PEEP is increased from 0 to 20 cmH_2O. Recruitment at end-expiration increases with PEEP, and recruitment at end-inspiration does not vary with PEEP or plateau pressure. The difference between recruitment at end-inspiration and recruitment at end-expiration (open portion of each column) represents reopening-collapsing lung tissue. The difference is not significant at PEEP of 15 and 20 cmH_2O. Bars represent ± standard error. *(From Gattinoni et al,[20] with permission.)*

most severe disease.[21] The inflection point, which is thought to signify the pressure required to open collapsed lung units (see above), varies from about 3 cmH_2O in nondependent regions to approximately 13 cmH_2O in dependent regions[18] and from 6 to 22 cmH_2O among patients with ARDS. This inter- and intra-patient variability makes it difficult to recommend an ideal level of PEEP, since the level that prevents reopening and collapse of lung units in dependent regions may cause overdistension and volutrauma in nondependent regions.

In spontaneously breathing patients, CPAP decreases inspiratory work by shifting tidal breathing to the steep portion of the pressure–volume curve (Fig. 176-2). In 16 patients who were being weaned from mechanical ventilation, an increase in effective lung compliance and a decrease in inspiratory work were noted when CPAP was employed.[29] The level of CPAP that achieved the maximum increase in compliance varied among patients: 6 cmH_2O in 44 percent of the patients, 12 cmH_2O in 25 percent of the patients, and 18 cmH_2O in 31 percent of the patients. Compared with breathing through a T-tube circuit, the level of CPAP that achieved maximum compliance produced a 37 percent decrease in inspiratory work per minute. The decrease in inspiratory work may also have resulted in part from recruitment of the expiratory muscles, which force lung volume below passive relaxation volume. At the onset of the subsequent inspiration, elastic and gravitational energies stored in the respiratory system are converted into kinetic energy, causing inspiratory pressure generation. In this way, the expiratory muscles share in the work of inspiration.

The presence of $PEEP_i$ increases the effort required to trigger the ventilator (see above) (Fig. 176-6). The addition of external

PEEP can be helpful in this setting in patients with airflow limitation because in order to trigger the ventilator, alveolar pressure needs to be decreased only below the level of external PEEP, rather than below zero. This may seem paradoxical: External PEEP, which is used commonly to induce hyperinflation in patients with microatelectasis, is used to decrease the work of breathing induced by hyperinflation. The paradox can be explained by considering the analogy of a waterfall, where the height of the waterfall represents the critical closing pressure of airways (Fig. 176-11).[50] This counteracting effect of external PEEP operates only in the setting of airflow limitation. If $PEEP_i$ results from expiratory muscle activity, the addition of external PEEP constitutes a hindrance and adds to the work of expiration.

OPTIMAL PEEP

Two schools of thought exist with regard to the goals of PEEP. Most physicians consider PEEP a supportive modality that improves oxygenation and assists a patient through an episode of hypoxemia. In effect, PEEP "buys time" for the lungs to heal naturally or as a result of other therapy. Other physicians believe that PEEP fundamentally reverses the primary pathophysiological processes and that improvement in oxygenation is a desirable, but secondary, gain. If cardiac output decreases disproportionally more than Pa_{O_2} increases, PEEP results in an overall decrease in delivery of O_2 to tissues. Thus, "best PEEP" has been defined as the level that achieves maximum O_2 delivery.[48]

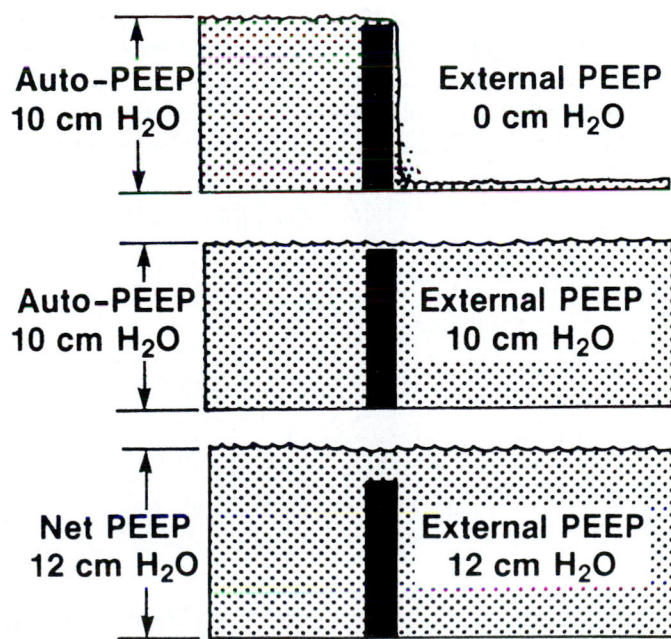

FIGURE 176-11   Effect of external PEEP ("downstream pressure") on $PEEP_i$ ("upstream pressure") during expiration, as demonstrated by the analogy of a waterfall over a dam (indicated by the solid block). Elevation of downstream pressure with external PEEP has no influence on either expiratory flow or upstream pressure ($PEEP_i$) until the downstream pressure is equal to the critical closing pressure. When downstream pressure exceeds the critical closing pressure, the pressure upstream increases and hyperinflation is exacerbated. *(From Tobin and Lodato,[50] with permission.)*

Since measurement of O_2 delivery is invasive, alternative measures of the optimal level of PEEP for a particular patient have been sought. Suter and colleagues[48] reasoned that an optimal level of PEEP would cause tidal ventilation to occur on the steep portion of the patient's pressure–volume curve (highest compliance), and a decrease in cardiac output would occur when the lung is overdistended (as reflected by a decrease in compliance). In a study of 15 patients with acute respiratory failure, the level of PEEP that produced maximum O_2 delivery also achieved the maximal increase in thoracic static compliance.

INFLUENCE OF PEEP ON PULMONARY ARTERY OCCLUSION PRESSURE

Clinical assessment of preload and hemodynamic performance is difficult in patients receiving high levels of PEEP, and a pulmonary artery catheter is often inserted in such patients. However, when PEEP exceeds 5 cmH2O, pulmonary artery occlusion pressure (PAOP) tends to overestimate true transmural left atrial pressure. In the presence of PEEP, alveolar pressure may exceed pulmonary venous pressure (i.e., West zones 1 and 2 will prevail), and PAOP will reflect alveolar pressure, rather than downstream left atrial pressure. To determine in which functional zone the catheter is located, inspection of the changes in pulmonary artery pressure and PAOP during positive-pressure inspiration is helpful.[49]

If the catheter is in zone 1 or 2, the increase in PAOP exceeds the increase in pulmonary artery systolic pressure during inspiration (Fig. 176-12). This arises for three reasons: (1) In zones 1 and 2, PAOP and alveolar pressure increase by similar amounts during positive-pressure inspiration. (2) Pulmonary artery pressure "senses" pleural pressure as the surrounding pressure. (3) Alveolar pressure increases more than pleural pressure during positive-pressure inflation as a result of the obligatory increase in

transpulmonary pressure with lung expansion. In contrast, when the catheter is in zone 3, PAOP and pulmonary artery systolic pressure will increase by equivalent amounts during positive-pressure inspiration (Fig. 176-12). However, even under zone 3 conditions, PAOP may still overestimate true transmural left atrial pressure because PEEP increases pericardial pressure. Recently, measurement of PAOP during the first 1 to 3 s following disconnection of the ventilator—the so-called nadir PAOP or pop-off wedge pressure—was demonstrated to provide an accurate reflection of the transmural left atrial pressure immediately before the disconnection.[44] This relationship holds true for levels of PEEP of at least 15 cmH2O. The physiological reason that nadir PAOP reflects the transmural PAOP on PEEP is not clear.

Noninvasive Ventilation in Acute Respiratory Failure

In the early 1960s, isolated reports in the literature described the delivery of mechanical ventilation through a mouthpiece instead of an endotracheal tube. However, this approach did not initially gain popularity. Interest in noninvasive positive-pressure ventilation (NIPPV) was rekindled in the 1980s with the general acceptance that such ventilation could be lifesaving in patients with certain forms of chronic respiratory failure and with the introduction of more comfortable nasal masks for CPAP in patients with obstructive sleep apnea. Substitution of a mask for an endotracheal tube has considerable appeal for a variety of reasons: (1) It is more comfortable; (2) there is less need for sedation, with enhanced patient alertness and ability to communicate; (3) use of a mask avoids the complications of endotracheal or tracheostomy tubes, such as airway trauma, sinusitis, and pneumonia; (4) airway defenses are maintained, and speech and swallowing permitted; and (5) the patient has a greater sense of control and independence than when intubated.[16,42] Reports on use of NIPPV in patients with acute respiratory failure have included primarily patients with COPD. NIPPV has also been employed in an uncontrolled fashion to treat acute respiratory failure in postoperative patients and in those with cardiac failure, pneumonia, cystic fibrosis, chest wall disorders, and obstructive sleep apnea.[16] Three recently published prospective controlled studies report a beneficial effect of NIPPV in patients with acute respiratory failure (Table 176-5).

In a study of patients with an acute exacerbation of COPD (Pa_{O_2} less than 56 mmHg and Pa_{CO_2} greater than 45 mmHg),[2] Bott and coworkers randomized 60 patients to standard therapy versus standard therapy plus volume-cycled NIPPV delivered by a nasal mask. Four patients assigned to NIPPV did not actually use it, and when they were eliminated from the analysis, mortality was shown to have been re-

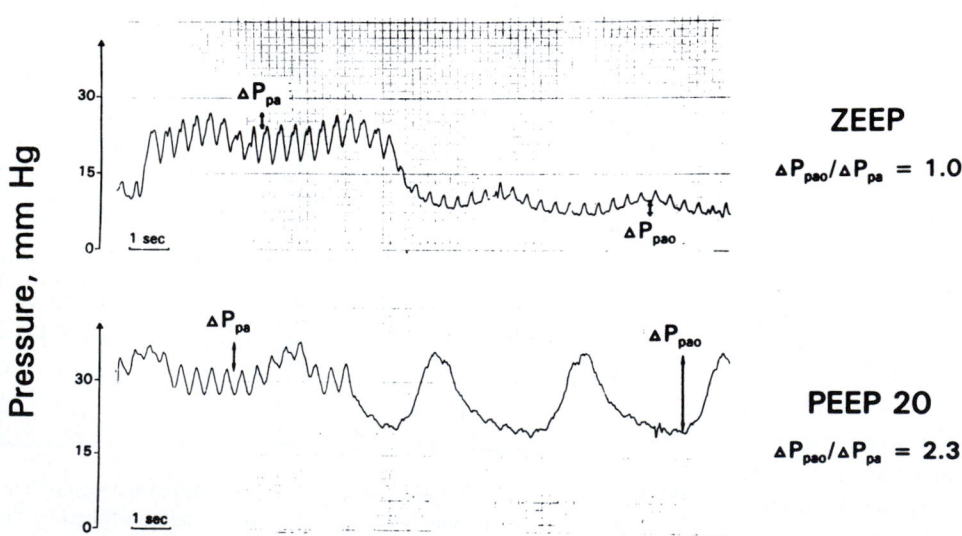

FIGURE 176-12 Pulmonary artery pressure tracings before and after inflation of balloon to obtain pulmonary artery occlusion pressure (P_{pao}). *Upper panel.* The catheter is in zone 3, and positive-pressure inspiration produces equivalent increases in systolic pulmonary artery pressure, P_{pa} (ΔP_{pa}) and P_{pao} (ΔP_{pao}). *Lower panel.* The catheter is in either zone 1 or 2, and the increase in P_{pao} with positive-pressure inspiration is 2.3 times greater than the increase in P_{pa} (see text for details). ZEEP = zero end-expiratory pressure. *(From Teboul et al,[49] with permission.)*

TABLE 176-5

Three Prospective Controlled Studies of Noninvasive Positive-Pressure Ventilation

	Bott[2]		Kramer[31]		Brochard[3]	
	Control	*NIPPV*	*Control*	*NIPPV*	*Control*	*NIPPV*
Number of patients	30	30	15	16	42	43
Intubated, n (%)	0	0	11 (73)	5 (31)	31 (74)	11 (26)
Mortality, n (%)	9 (30)	3 (10)	2 (13)	1 (6)	12 (29)	4 (9)

duced significantly with use of NIPPV (1/26 versus 9/30). However, the difference was not statistically significant when analyzed on an "intention-to-treat" basis.

In another study conducted by Kramer and colleagues,[31] 31 patients with acute respiratory failure (74 percent of whom had COPD) were randomized to NIPPV plus standard therapy versus standard therapy alone. The patient's primary physician considered that intubation was needed in 73 percent of the control group versus 31 percent of the NIPPV group; for analytical purposes, control patients who were judged to need intubation remained in this subgroup even if they refused intubation.

Finally, in a study performed by Brochard and coworkers,[3] out of 275 patients admitted to an intensive care unit with an acute exacerbation of COPD, 85 patients (31 percent) were selected who met objective criteria for a comparison of NIPPV versus standard therapy. Patients in the NIPPV group had a lower rate of intubation (26 percent) than the control group (74 percent). In addition, the NIPPV group had a lower rate of complications (16 versus 48 percent), shorter hospital stay (23 versus 35 days), and lower in-hospital mortality (9 versus 29 percent). The mortality rates in patients treated with NIPPV were quite similar in the three studies: 6 percent,[31] 9 percent,[3] and 10 percent,[2] and intubation rates were similar in two studies: 26 percent[3] and 31 percent.[31] In the study by Kramer and colleagues[31] a mortality rate of 13 percent was described in the control group—a rate that is strikingly lower than the 30 percent reported in the study by Bott and colleagues[2]—but the difference was attributed to the infrequency with which British physicians employ intubation and mechanical ventilation. This explanation, however, cannot account for the equally high mortality (29 percent) in the control group of the study by Brochard and coworkers,[3] since 74 percent of these patients were intubated, an intubation rate comparable to the rate of 73 percent in the study by Kramer and colleagues.[31]

Controlled and uncontrolled investigations have shown that NIPPV is successful in approximately 70 percent of patients with acute respiratory failure. We still do not have firm indications for its use, but patients should have objective evidence of acute respiratory distress on physical examination or acute respiratory acidosis. Patients need to be able to cooperate and follow instructions. NIPPV should be avoided in patients with a respiratory arrest, those who are unstable (e.g., have hypotension or uncontrolled arrhythmias), patients with a high risk of aspiration (e.g., those who are obtunded or have swallowing problems), and patients who have excessive respiratory secretions. Success appears more likely if NIPPV is used early, rather than later, in the

progression of acute respiratory failure—for example, when respiratory frequency first exceeds 30 breaths per minute and pH falls below 7.35.[2,3] The optimal settings and duration of use of NIPPV have not been defined. NIPPV is generally used for about 7 h per day,[2,3] although in one study the technique was used for 20 of the first 24 h of care.[31] When PS is employed as a mode of NIPPV, it is prudent to begin with a low setting and to gradually increase to approximately 6 to 10 cmH_2O over the first hour, reaching 10 to 15 cmH_2O by 24 h; a maximum setting of 20 cmH_2O should be established.

Patients who do well with NIPPV typically show considerable improvement within the first hour of therapy, as indicated by a decrease in respiratory frequency,[3] a fall in Pa_{CO_2}, and an increase in pH.[2] If respiratory frequency is not significantly decreased after the first hour of therapy, intubation and conventional mechanical ventilation should be considered. Most patients are completely weaned off NIPPV after 3 to 6 days,[31] although some patients may require it for as long as 23 days.[31] The decision to stop NIPPV is based on clinical judgment; an advantage of NIPPV is that it is easy to reinstitute if ventilatory failure recurs.

Patients with severe COPD usually exhibit $PEEP_i$ (Figs. 176-1, 176-6). Conventional modes of mechanical ventilation, such as PS ventilation, help to diminish the overall work of breathing, but they do not reduce the level of $PEEP_i$.[27] CPAP counterbalances the threshold inspiratory load associated with $PEEP_i$ in patients with airflow limitation, and delivery of CPAP through a nose or face mask has been shown to decrease markedly inspiratory effort in patients with COPD. Conceivably, if CPAP is added to NIPPV, the success rate of NIPPV may be even greater than that reported.

NIPPV has a number of limitations. About 20 to 25 percent of patients cannot adapt to its use, mainly because of discomfort from the mask.[42] Trauma to the face is a significant problem, and the likelihood of skin ulceration, especially over the bridge of the nose, makes it difficult to use NIPPV continuously for more than 1 to 2 days.[16] The mask needs to be carefully selected and applied to minimize discomfort. With nasal masks, a better fit is generally achieved using smaller sizes; the ideal mask fits closely along the lateral contour of the nose. An excessive leak at the bridge of the nose causes intolerance as a result of air blowing into the patient's eyes. Some leak is to be expected, and excessive pressure to eliminate all leaks is inadvisable. If patients complain of excessive nasal dryness, humidification should be added; rhinorrhea can be reduced by use of ipratropium bromide nasal drops; nasal blockage may respond to ephedrine nasal drops.[16] A chin strap can be used when there is a large leak through the mouth.

Other limitations of NIPPV include lack of direct access to the patient's airway. Consequently, when secretions are copious, mucous plugging and atelectasis may develop. Aerophagia and gastric distension can occur, especially in patients who breathe out of synchrony with the ventilator.[6] If these problems are suspected, a nasogastric tube should be inserted.

ANCILLARY THERAPY

The plumbing of the ventilator circuit needs to be repeatedly evaluated by a knowledgeable person. Several potential components in the circuit, such as the humidifier or expiratory valve, can increase the work of breathing or predispose the patient to barotrauma. Adequate humidification and suctioning are required to prevent secretions from blocking the tracheal tube. In addition to other general aspects of care, bronchodilator therapy and the regular changes in the patient's body position should be considered.

Bronchodilator aerosols are widely used in ventilator-dependent patients. The efficiency of aerosol delivery to the lower respiratory tract depends on several factors that are not of concern in ambulatory patients (Fig. 176-13). Until recently, nebulizers were routinely employed in mechanically ventilated patients, because metered-dose inhalers (MDIs) were considered ineffective due to aerosol impaction in the ventilator circuit and endotracheal tube. Recent studies have established the efficacy of MDI-delivered bronchodilators in mechanically ventilated patients, provided proper technique of administration is employed.[15] A special adaptor is required to connect the MDI canister to the ventilator circuit, and several different devices have become commercially available. Efficacy differs considerably among these devices, and aerosol delivery is much higher using an in-line, chamber device than an elbow adapter.[15]

As in the case of nonintubated patients, several key steps must be followed to achieve maximal aerosol delivery. Because of concerns with aerosol deposition in the endotracheal tube and ventilator circuit, bronchodilator dosage in mechanically ventilated patients is commonly increased much above the usual 2 to 4 puffs used in nonintubated patients. However, when the technique of administration is carefully controlled, maximal bronchodilation is achieved in patients with COPD with as few as 4 puffs of a sympathomimetic aerosol.[14] MDIs offer several advantages over nebulizers, including ease of administration, decreased cost, reliability of dosing, and freedom from contamination.

In patients with ARDS, alterations in posture can markedly influence gas exchange. A substantial increase in Pa_{O_2} occurs in about half of patients when they are turned from the supine to prone position.[19] However, the degree of improvement and response among patients is variable, and some patients actually experience a fall in Pa_{O_2}. Alterations in gas exchange may be due to changes in regional lung inflation, redistribution of ventilation, or redistribution of perfusion.[19] Studies have shown that the increase in Pa_{O_2} in the prone position is due to a decrease in shunt fraction rather than to changes in cardiac output, regional diaphragmatic movement, distribution of regional perfusion, or to the increase in FRC that occurs in that posture. Thus, the alteration in gas exchange must be primarily related to changes in regional ventilation.

In the supine position, the gravitational gradient in pleural pressure is increased, so that pleural pressure is *positive* in dependent regions. Consequently, large areas of the lung are below closing volume, and there is little, if any, ventilation of the dependent dorsal regions. Therefore, in the supine position, regional ventilation decreases along a vertical axis from ventral, nondependent regions, to dorsal, dependent regions. On turning to the prone position, regional ventilation decreases from dorsal to ventral regions, but the gravitational gradient in pleural pressure is smaller, so that the rate of decrease in regional ventilation is less than in the supine posture.[19] In other words, regional ventilation is more homogenous in the prone posture. Achievement of a more even distribution of ventilation appears to be a major factor responsible for better oxygenation.

MONITORING AND COMPLICATIONS

Several devices can be used to monitor pulmonary gas exchange, respiratory neuromuscular function, respiratory mechanics, and patient–ventilator interaction. Use of the derived information permits the physician to better tailor ventilator settings to an individual patient's requirements with the promise of enhancing patient comfort. Monitoring of key variables helps to minimize the risk of iatrogenic complications and alerts the physician to the likelihood of an impending catastrophe, allowing sufficient time for the institution of lifesaving measures. A full discussion of monitoring modalities is outside the scope of this chapter.

Patients receiving mechanical ventilation are at risk for numerous complications, including oxygen toxicity, volutrauma and air leaks, decreased cardiac output, and endotracheal-tube complications. These problems are discussed elsewhere in this text (Chapters 167 and 168).

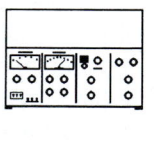

Ventilator Related

Mode of ventilation
Tidal volume
Respiratory rate
Duty cycle
Inspiratory waveform
Breath triggering mechanism

Drug Related

Dose
Timing of MDI actuation
Aerosol particle size

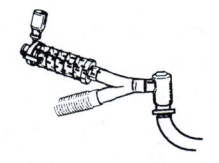

Circuit Related

Type of spacer or adapter used
Position of spacer in circuit
Endotracheal tube size
Inhaled gas humidity
Inhaled gas density/viscosity

Patient Related

Severity of airway obstruction
Mechanism of airway obstruction
Presence of dynamic hyperinflation

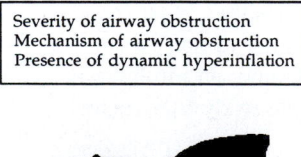

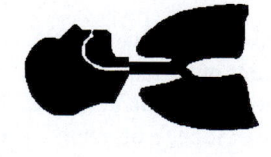

FIGURE 176-13 Factors influencing lower respiratory tract deposition of aerosol delivered by a metered-dose inhaler (MDI) in mechanically ventilated patients. With dry air in the circuit, approximately 30 percent of the dose is delivered to the major airways if the MDI is actuated into a cylindrical spacer; deposition decreases to about 16 percent if inspired gas is humidified. *(From Dhand and Tobin,[15] with permission.)*

WEANING

In the strict literal sense, *weaning* means a slow, gradual decrease in the amount of ventilator support. More commonly, the term is used in a broader sense to refer to all methods of discontinuing mechanical ventilation. In most instances of mechanical ventilation, weaning is quite straightforward, and patients can resume spontaneous breathing with little or no difficulty. About 20 to 30 percent of patients fail initial attempts at discontinuing mechanical ventilation,[17] and these difficult-to-wean patients account for a disproportionate consumption of health-care resources.

Causes of Weaning Failure

Weaning failure most commonly results from respiratory muscle dysfunction; it may also result from problems with oxygenation and psychological difficulties. Respiratory muscle dysfunction results from an imbalance between respiratory neuromuscular capacity and the mechanical load on the respiratory system. Hypoxemia is less commonly a primary cause of weaning failure, partly because weaning is not attempted in patients who appear to be susceptible to the development of hypoxemia. The factor about which we know the least is psychological problems, which may significantly aggravate difficulties in weaning in a substantial number of patients.

Timing of the Weaning Process

One of the major challenges for the clinician in mechanical ventilation is deciding on the best time to wean the patient from the ventilator. On the one hand, if the physician is too conservative and postpones weaning onset, the patient is placed at an increased risk of life-threatening, ventilator-induced complications. On the other hand, if weaning is begun prematurely, the patient may suffer severe cardiopulmonary or psychological decompensation—significant clinical setbacks.

The first prerequisite for initiation of weaning is that the disease process that precipitated the need for mechanical ventilation has resolved sufficiently so that the patient has a reasonable chance of sustaining spontaneous ventilation. Although careful clinical assessment is necessary in deciding when to wean a patient, such assessment alone is not sufficient. Indeed, studies have shown that experienced clinicians frequently err in their predictions. Accordingly, functional tests are helpful in determining a patient's readiness for weaning (Table 176-6).

In general, discontinuation of mechanical ventilation is not even contemplated in a patient with cardiopulmonary instability or persistent hypoxemia (e.g., a Pa_{O_2} less than 55 mmHg with an Fi_{O_2} of 0.40 or higher). However, many patients fail attempts at weaning despite satisfactory oxygenation. A minute ventilation of less than 10 L/min, indicating acceptable ventilatory requirements, is one of the standard criteria used to predict successful weaning. In most studies, however, minute ventilation has been found to be only slightly better than chance in predicting outcome. The second standard predictor of weaning outcome is maximal inspiratory pressure, which assesses global inspiratory muscle strength. Again, in most systematic studies,

---

TABLE 176-6

Variables Used to Predict Weaning Success

Measures of gas exchange
  $Pa_{O_2} \geq 60$ mmHg with $Fi_{O_2} \leq 0.35$
  Alveolar–arterial oxygen gradient < 350 mmHg
  $Pa_{O_2}/Fi_{O_2} > 200$
Measures of ventilatory pump function
  Maximum negative inspiratory pressure < -30 cmH$_2$O
  Minute ventilation < 10 L/min
  Frequency to tidal volume ratio (f/VT) < 100 breaths per
    min per liter

---

maximal inspiratory pressure is very inaccurate in predicting weaning outcome. Thus, neither minute ventilation nor maximal inspiratory pressure are helpful in deciding whether a patient is ready to undergo a weaning trial. Despite the limitations of these measurements, they are useful in a patient who has already failed a weaning trial, in that they provide information on the reason that the patient has failed.

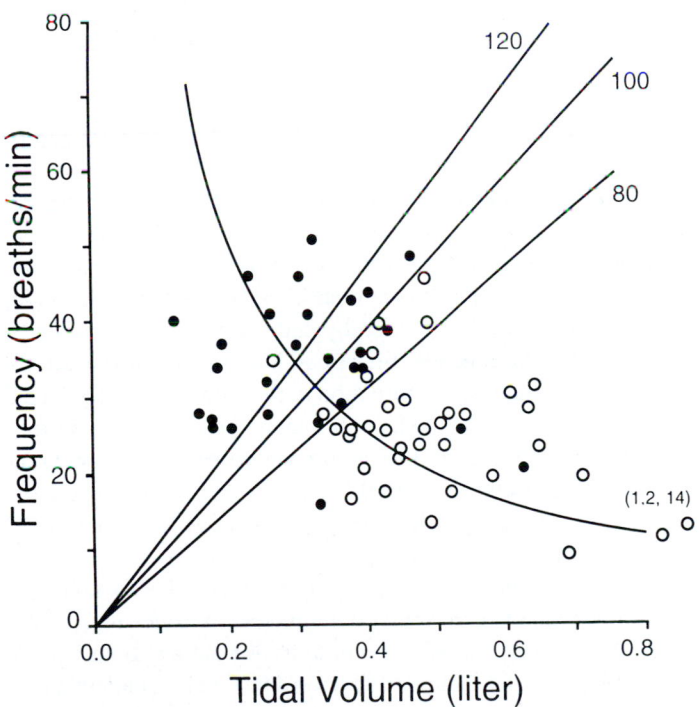

FIGURE 176-14   Isopleths for the ratio of respiratory frequency to tidal volume (f/VT), each representing different degrees of rapid shallow breathing. Patients who fell to the left of the 100 breaths per minute per liter isopleth had a 95 percent likelihood of failing a weaning trial, whereas patients who fell to the right of this isopleth had an 80 percent likelihood of a successful weaning outcome. The hyperbola represents a minute ventilation of 10 L/min, a criterion commonly used to predict weaning outcome; clearly this criterion was of little value in discriminating between patients who were successfully weaned (open circles) and those who failed weaning (solid circles). Values for one patient (VT = 1.2 L, f = 14 breaths per minute) lay outside the graph. *(From Yang and Tobin,[52] with permission.)*

Checking for the absence of rapid, shallow breathing is more helpful in deciding when to attempt weaning. Rapid, shallow breathing can be quantitated as the respiratory frequency–tidal volume ratio (f/Vт); a value less than 100 breaths per minute per liter suggests that rapid shallow breathing is absent and that weaning is likely to be successful (Fig. 176-14).[52] As in the case of any diagnostic test, f/Vт is not a perfect discriminator, and the physician should not feel overly constrained by the threshold value. Instead, the measurement needs to be interpreted in the context of careful clinical assessment.

Weaning Techniques

IMV and PS ventilation are now the most popular methods of weaning. When using IMV for weaning, the mandatory rate from the ventilator is reduced in steps of 1 to 3 breaths per minute, and an arterial blood gas is obtained approximately 30 min following each rate change. Unfortunately, titrating the number of breaths from the ventilator in accordance with the results of arterial blood gases can result in a false sense of security. As little as 2 to 3 positive-pressure breaths per minute can achieve acceptable blood gases, but these values provide no information regarding the patient's work of breathing, which may be excessive. As already discussed, at IMV rates of 14 breaths per minute or less, patient inspiratory efforts are increased to a level likely to cause respiratory muscle fatigue. Furthermore, this occurs not only with the intervening spontaneous breaths but also with ventilator-assisted breaths. Consequently, use of IMV may actually contribute to the development of respiratory muscle fatigue or prevent its recovery.

When PS ventilation is used for weaning, the level of pressure is reduced gradually, in decrements of 3 to 6 cmH$_2$O, and is titrated on the basis of respiratory frequency. Several investigators have shown that PS ventilation can be used to counteract the work of breathing imposed by endotracheal tube and ventilator circuit. Consequently, the notion has arisen that if a patient can sustain spontaneous ventilation at this "compensatory level" of pressure support, he or she will tolerate extubation. The problem with this strategy is that a compensatory level of pressure support varies between 3 to 14 cmH$_2$O[5]; there is no reliable method for accurately determining the required level in an individual patient.

The oldest method of weaning is to undertake spontaneous breathing trials of increasing duration, several times daily. Typically, the approach begins with brief trials (lasting about 5 min), which are gradually increased in accordance with a patient's performance, as assessed by bedside clinical examination. The optimal period of rest between trials has not been defined, but it is commonly as little as 1 to 3 h. When the patient is able to sustain spontaneous ventilation for some fixed time, such as 1 to 2 h, extubation is performed. Having the patient breathe through the ventilator circuit can minimize financial costs, since a T-tube circuit is not needed. However, since this method usually results in a marked increase in the work of breathing, supplying an air–oxygen mixture through a T-tube circuit is usually preferred.

Another method of weaning is to employ a single daily trial of spontaneous breathing through a T-tube circuit. The trial is conducted while the physician is in the intensive care unit. If the patient can sustain spontaneous ventilation for 30 to 60 min without undue distress, he or she is extubated. If the patient develops signs of distress on physical examination, the trial is stopped, and mechanical ventilation is reinstituted. To allow the respiratory muscles to recover from excessive stress, the patient is rested for approximately 24 h with a high level of ventilator assistance, e.g., assist-control ventilation.[32] The patient is reassessed the following morning to see if he or she is ready for another trial of spontaneous breathing.

Two rigorously controlled, prospective studies were recently performed to compare the relative efficacy of different weaning strategies in a subgroup of ventilator-dependent patients who were considered difficult to wean.[4,17] In both studies, IMV was found to delay the weaning process. In one study, a single daily trial of spontaneous breathing was found to achieve a twofold increase in the rate of successful weaning and extubation compared with pressure support (Fig. 176-15).[17] In the second study, pressure support was found to result in faster weaning than T-tube trials.[4] The different outcomes in the studies are probably due to the specific criteria employed at different stages of the weaning process.

A weaning strategy based on a once-daily trial of spontaneous breathing simplifies patient management. In a recent study of more than 500 patients who had received mechanical ventilation for about 7 days, two-thirds were extubated following the first trial of spontaneous breathing.[17] These patients were never truly "weaned" in the strict, literal sense of the term. This observation highlights issues related to IMV and PS weaning methods, in which ventilator settings are adjusted repeatedly and each adjustment is usually followed by a measurement of arterial blood gases. A single daily trial also involves much less personnel time than

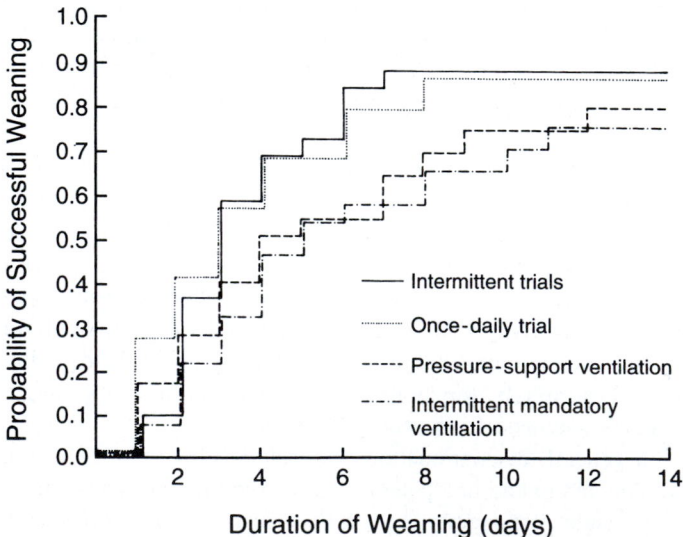

FIGURE 176-15 Kaplan-Meier curves of the probability of successful weaning with intermittent mandatory ventilation, pressure support ventilation, intermittent trials of spontaneous breathing, and a once-daily trial of spontaneous breathing. After adjustment for baseline characteristics in a Cox proportional-hazards model, the rate of successful weaning with a once-daily trial of spontaneous breathing was 2.83 times higher than that with intermittent mandatory ventilation ($P < 0.006$) and 2.05 times higher than that with pressure support ventilation ($P < 0.04$). (*From Esteban et al,*[17] *with permission.*)

the traditional approach of multiple trials of spontaneous breathing performed several times a day. One of the implied goals with all weaning techniques is the reconditioning of respiratory muscles, which may have atrophied or weakened during the period of mechanical ventilation. Based on indirect data, a single daily trial of spontaneous breathing, alternating with a prolonged rest period, should be the most effective method of reconditioning.[17]

Extubation

Patients who can sustain spontaneous ventilation without distress may have difficulty following extubation due to upper airway obstruction, inability to protect the upper airway, or inability to clear secretions. In contrast to the many parameters that have been introduced to predict the outcome of a weaning trial, indices that reliably predict the likelihood of complications following extubation have not been developed. Instead, evaluation consists of clinical assessment of factors such as the patient's level of consciousness, volume of secretions, and ability to cough.

CONCLUSION

Advances in biomedical engineering have resulted in better ventilators and have enhanced our capabilities in patient monitoring. The goals and complications of mechanical ventilation are now better defined. Mechanical ventilation saves lives, but it can result in serious complications. Hence, mechanical ventilation should be discontinued at the earliest possible time.

REFERENCES

1. Ashbaugh DG, Petty TL, Bigelow DB, Harris TM: Continuous positive-pressure breathing (CPPB) in adult respiratory distress syndrome. *J Thorac Cardiovasc Surg* 57:31–39, 1969.
2. Bott J, Carroll MP, Conway JH, et al: Randomised controlled trial of nasal ventilation in acute ventilatory failure due to chronic obstructive airways disease. *Lancet* 341:1555–1557, 1993.
3. Brochard L, Mancebo J, Wysocki M, et al: Noninvasive ventilation for acute exacerbations of chronic obstructive pulmonary disease. *New Engl J Med* 333:817–822, 1995.
4. Brochard L, Rauss A, Benito S, et al: Comparison of three methods of gradual withdrawal from ventilatory support during weaning from mechanical ventilation. *Am J Respir Crit Care Med* 150:896–903, 1994.
5. Brochard L, Rua F, Lorino H, et al: Inspiratory pressure support compensates for the additional work of breathing caused by the endotracheal tube. *Anesthesiology* 75:739–745, 1991.
6. Brochard L: Pressure support ventilation, in Tobin MJ (ed), *Principles and Practice of Mechanical Ventilation*. New York, McGraw-Hill, 1994, pp 239–257.
7. Chatburn RL: Classification of mechanical ventilators, in Tobin MJ (ed), *Principles and Practice of Mechanical Ventilation*. New York, McGraw-Hill, 1994, pp 36–64.
8. Colice GL: Historical perspective on the development of mechanical ventilation, in Tobin MJ (ed), *Principles and Practice of Mechanical Ventilation*. New York, McGraw-Hill, 1994, pp 1–35.
9. Connors AF Jr, McCaffree DR, Gray BA: Effect of inspiratory flow rate on gas exchange during mechanical ventilation. *Am Rev Respir Dis* 124:537–543, 1981.
10. Coussa ML, Guerin C, Eissa NT, et al: Partitioning of work of breathing in mechanically ventilated COPD patients. *J Appl Physiol* 75:1711–1719, 1993.
11. Culpepper JA, Rinaldo JE, Rogers RM: Effect of mechanical ventilator mode on tendency towards respiratory alkalosis. *Am Rev Respir Dis* 132:1075–1077, 1985.
12. Daly BDT, Edmonds CH, Norman JC: In vivo alveolar morphometries with positive end expiratory pressure. *Surg Forum* 24:217–219, 1973.
13. Dantzker DR, Lynch JP, Weg JG: Depression of cardiac output is a mechanism of shunt reduction in the therapy of acute respiratory failure. *Chest* 77:636–642, 1980.
14. Dhand R, Duarte AG, Jubran A, et al: Dose response to bronchodilator delivered by metered-dose inhaler in ventilator-supported patients. *Am J Respir Crit Care Med* 154:388–393, 1996.
15. Dhand R, Tobin MJ: Bronchodilator delivery with metered-dose inhalers in mechanically ventilated patients. *Eur Respir J* 9:585–595, 1996.
16. Elliott M, Moxham J: Non-invasive mechanical ventilation by nasal or face mask, in Tobin MJ (ed), *Principles and Practice of Mechanical Ventilation*. New York, McGraw-Hill, 1994, pp 427–453.
17. Esteban A, Frutos F, Tobin MJ, et al: A comparison of four methods of weaning patients from mechanical ventilation. *New Engl J Med* 332:345–350, 1995.
18. Gattinoni L, D'Andrea L, Pelosi P, et al: Regional effects and mechanism of positive end-expiratory pressure in early adult respiratory distress syndrome. *JAMA* 269:2122–2127, 1993.
19. Gattinoni L, Pelosi P, Valenza F, Macheroni D: Patient positioning in acute respiratory failure, in Tobin MJ (ed), *Principles and Practice of Mechanical Ventilation*. New York, McGraw-Hill, 1994, pp 1007–1076.
20. Gattinoni L, Pelosi P, Crotti S, Valenza F: Effects of positive end-expiratory pressure on regional distribution of tidal volume and recruitment in adult respiratory distress syndrome. *Am J Respir Crit Care Med* 152:1807–1814, 1995.
21. Gattinoni L, Pesenti A, Bombino M, et al: Relationships between lung computed tomographic density, gas exchange, and PEEP in acute respiratory failure. *Anesthesiology* 69:824–832, 1988.
22. Groeger JS, Levinson MR, Carlon GC: Assist control versus synchronized intermittent mandatory ventilation during acute respiratory failure. *Crit Care Med* 17:607–612, 1989.
23. Hubmayr RD: Setting the ventilator, in Tobin MJ (ed), *Principles and Practice of Mechanical Ventilation*. New York, McGraw-Hill, 1994, pp 191–206.
24. Hudson LD, Hurlow RS, Craig KC, Pierson DJ: Does intermittent mandatory ventilation correct respiratory alkalosis in patients receiving assisted mechanical ventilation? *Am Rev Respir Dis* 132:1071–1074, 1985.
25. Imsand C, Feihl F, Perret C, Fitting JW: Regulation of inspiratory neuromuscular output during synchronized intermittent mechanical ventilation. *Anesthesiology* 80:13–22, 1994.
26. Jubran A, Tobin MJ: Reliability of pulse oximetry in titrating supplemental oxygen therapy in ventilator-dependent patients. *Chest* 90:1420–1425, 1990.
27. Jubran A, Van de Graaff WB, Tobin MJ: Variability of patient-ventilator interaction with pressure support ventilation in patients with chronic obstructive pulmonary disease. *Am J Respir Crit Care Med* 152:129–136, 1995.
28. Kacmarek RM, Hess D: Basic principles of ventilator machinery, in Tobin MJ (ed), *Principles and Practice of Mechanical Ventilation*. New York, McGraw-Hill, 1994, pp 65–110.
29. Katz JA, Marks JD: Inspiratory work with and without continuous positive airway pressure in patients with acute respiratory failure. *Anesthesiology* 63:598–607, 1985.

30. Katz JA, Ozanne GM, Zinn SE, Fairley HB: Time course and mechanisms of lung-volume increase with PEEP in acute pulmonary failure. *Anesthesiology* 54:9–16, 1981.

31. Kramer N, Meyer TJ, Meharg J, et al: Randomized, prospective trial of noninvasive positive pressure ventilation in acute respiratory failure. *Am J Respir Crit Care Med* 151:1799–1806, 1995.

32. Laghi F, D'Alfonso N, Tobin MJ: Pattern of recovery from diaphragmatic fatigue over 24 hours. *J Appl Physiol* 79:539–546, 1995.

33. Lodato RF: Oxygen toxicity, in Tobin MJ (ed), *Principles and Practice of Mechanical Ventilation.* New York, McGraw-Hill, 1994, pp 837–855.

34. Malo J, Ali J, Wood LDH: How does positive end-expiratory pressure reduce intrapulmonary shunt in canine pulmonary edema? *J Appl Physiol* 57:1002–1010, 1984.

35. Mancebo J, Isabey D, Lorino H, et al: Comparative effects of pressure support ventilation and intermittent positive pressure breathing (IPPB) in nonintubated healthy subjects. *Eur Respir J* 8:1901–1909, 1995.

36. Manning HL, Molinary EJ, Leiter JC: Effect of inspiratory flow rate on respiratory sensation and pattern of breathing. *Am J Respir Crit Care Med* 151:751–757, 1995.

37. Marini JJ, Capps JS, Culver BH: The inspiratory work of breathing during assisted mechanical ventilation. *Chest* 87:612–618, 1985.

38. Marini JJ, Smith TC, Lamb VJ: External work output and force generation during synchronized intermittent mechanical ventilation. *Am Rev Respir Dis* 138:1169–1179, 1988.

39. Matamis D, Lemaire F, Harf A, et al: Redistribution of pulmonary blood flow induced by positive end-expiratory pressure and dopamine infusion in acute respiratory failure. *Am Rev Respir Dis* 129:39–44, 1984.

40. Mathru M, Rao TLK, El-Etr AA, Pifarre R: Hemodynamic response to changes in ventilatory patterns in patients with normal and poor left ventricular reserve. *Crit Care Med* 10:423–426, 1982.

41. Mathru M, Rao TLK, Venus B: Ventilator-induced barotrauma in controlled mechanical ventilation versus intermittent mandatory ventilation. *Crit Care Med* 11:359–361, 1983.

42. Meyer TJ, Hill NS: Noninvasive positive pressure ventilation to treat respiratory failure. *Ann Intern Med* 120:760–770, 1994.

43. Mountain RD, Sahn SA: Clinical features and outcome in patients with acute asthma presenting with hypercapnia. *Am Rev Respir Dis* 138:535–539, 1988.

44. Pinsky M, Vincent JL, De Smet JM: Estimating left ventricular filling pressure during positive end-expiratory pressure in humans. *Am Rev Respir Dis* 143:25–31, 1991.

45. Sassoon CSH, Gruer SE: Characteristics of the ventilator pressure and flow-trigger variables. *Intensive Care Med* 21:159–168, 1995.

46. Sassoon CSH: Intermittent mandatory ventilation, in Tobin MJ (ed), *Principles and Practice of Mechanical Ventilation.* New York, McGraw-Hill, 1994, pp 221–237.

47. Slutsky AS, ACCP Consensus Conference: Mechanical ventilation. *Chest* 104:1833–1859, 1993.

48. Suter PM, Fairley HB, Isenberg MD: Optimum end-expiratory airway pressure in patients with acute pulmonary failure. *New Engl J Med* 292:284–289, 1975.

49. Teboul JL, Besbes M, Andrivet P, et al: A bedside index assessing the reliability of pulmonary artery occlusion pressure measurements during mechanical ventilation with positive end-expiratory pressure. *J Crit Care* 7:22–29, 1992.

50. Tobin MJ, Lodato RF: Editorial: PEEP, auto-PEEP, and waterfalls. *Chest* 96:449–451, 1989.

51. Tobin MJ: Mechanical ventilation. *New Engl J Med* 330: 1056–1061, 1994.

52. Yang KL, Tobin MJ: A prospective study of indexes predicting the outcome of trials of weaning from mechanical ventilation. *New Engl J Med* 324:1445–1450, 1991.

53. Younes M: Interactions between patients and ventilators, in Roussos C (ed), *The Thorax*, 2d ed. New York, Dekker, 1995, pp 2367–2420.

CHAPTER 177

MECHANICAL VENTILATION: PHYSIOLOGICAL CONSIDERATIONS AND NEWER VENTILATORY TECHNIQUES

John J. Marini

CONCEPTUAL ADVANCES IN MECHANICAL VENTILATION
Acute Airflow Obstruction
Acute Lung Injury
Cardiovascular Compromise and Shock
Work of Breathing During Mechanical Ventilation

NEWER MODES OF VENTILATORY SUPPORT
High-Frequency Ventilation
Airway Pressure Release Ventilation and Biphasic Airway Pressure
"Combination" Modes: Volume Support and Volume-Assured Pressure Support
Proportional-Assist Ventilation

ADJUNCTS TO MECHANICAL VENTILATION
Permissive Hypercapnia
Extrapulmonary Gas Exchange
Tracheal Gas Insufflation

OPTIONS TO ENHANCE OXYGENATION
Independent (Differential) Lung Ventilation
Inverse-Ratio Ventilation
Prone Positioning
Partial Liquid Ventilation

Mechanical ventilation is initiated when effective gas exchange cannot be accomplished at an acceptable energy cost. Recent advances in our knowledge of ventilatory failure and recovery, barotrauma, and the processes of acute lung injury and repair influence the execution of ventilatory support and underscore the need for expedient machine withdrawal. Furthermore, technologic innovations now enable the clinician to monitor patient–ventilator interactions closely and to undertake well-reasoned ventilatory approaches that depart from conventional practice guidelines. This chapter complements Chapter 176 on conventional modes of mechanical ventilation. Key management strategies based on physiological principles are outlined, and alternative approaches that have evolved from our improved understanding of respiratory failure are discussed.

CONCEPTUAL ADVANCES IN MECHANICAL VENTILATION

Mechanical ventilation is usually required for severe airflow obstruction, neuromuscular weakness, acute lung injury, or cardiovascular compromise. The objectives of maximizing patient comfort, minimizing adverse patient–machine interactions, and effecting timely withdrawal of ventilator support are common to each. Significant new information is available to help guide clinical decision-making in four major problem areas that have dominated the recent medical literature on mechanical ventilatory support: management of acute airflow obstruction, avoidance of ventilator-induced lung injury, weaning from mechanical ventilation, and noninvasive ventilation. The first two areas are discussed below; the latter two are covered in Chapter 176.

Acute Airflow Obstruction

Awareness of the importance of dynamic hyperinflation in everyday clinical practice has been a recent development. Dynamic hyperinflation results whenever insufficient expiratory time prevents the chest from decompressing to its resting "equilibrium" volume at the end of tidal exhalation without (or despite) muscular effort. End-expiratory alveolar pressure then exceeds the pressure at the airway opening, and flow continues throughout expiration until interrupted by the next inflation cycle. *Auto-PEEP* (positive end-expiratory pressure), the positive difference between alveolar pressure and the set airway pressure at end-exhalation that characterizes dynamic hyperinflation, is a function of the expiratory resistance to airflow, compliance of the respiratory system, time allowed for expiration, and volume from which exhalation begins.

The consequences of dynamic hyperinflation are linked to associated changes in lung volume and pleural pressure. During exacerbations of asthma and chronic airflow obstruction, *mean* pleural pressure is often lower than normal in patients making spontaneous breathing efforts, despite air trapping. Thus, dynamic hyperinflation does not necessarily imply high mean intrathoracic (intrapleural) pressure or impaired venous return. Active expiratory muscle contraction may keep intrapleural pressure positive until the very end of exhalation, producing positive intrapleural and alveolar pressures without commensurate dynamic hyperinflation or its consequences.[43] At high levels of ventilation, substantial expiratory resistance may arise in the ventilator circuitry, particularly in the endotracheal tube and exhalation valve.[5] Although recent technical innovations have reduced imposed resistance, circuits are still imperfect. Efforts to offset tube and valve resistance by temporarily dropping central airway pressure or controlling carinal pressure during both phases of the ventilatory cycle are currently under preliminary testing.[21] Although auto-PEEP has been noted in other conditions and can occur whenever minute ventilation is high enough, dynamic hyperinflation most commonly occurs during severe airflow obstruction. In this setting, expiratory resistance is often several times greater than inspiratory resistance, especially at end-exhalation. Expiratory resistance is often so high that expiratory flow limitation occurs during tidal exhalation.

Auto-PEEP may exist *without dynamic hyperinflation* when end-expiratory airflow is driven by the expiratory muscles, and *without flow limitation* during tidal breathing, despite airway disease. Commonly, however, auto-PEEP is associated with both dynamic hyperventilation and tidal flow limitation. Dynamic hyperinflation disproportional to *measurable* auto-PEEP routinely occurs in patients with such severe airflow obstruction that airways serving the most compromised areas seal *completely* during the course of exhalation.[29] Undoubtedly, such "ball valving" at least partly accounts for extreme overinflation that cannot be explained by the recorded levels of auto-PEEP during status asthmaticus and exacerbations of chronic obstructive pulmonary disease (COPD) (Fig. 177-1).[29] Closure of this type in severe airflow obstruction probably occurs most extensively in the dependent regions of the lung. Thus, although the clinician measures only one value that averages the contributions from all open airways, auto-PEEP levels vary widely throughout the lung with "diffuse" obstructive disease.

The pathophysiological consequences of auto-PEEP and the response to added end-expiratory pressure depend on the classification category.[35] Whether or not dynamic hyperinflation causes hemodynamically important elevations of mean intrathoracic pressure depends on the activity of the patient's ventilatory muscles.

CONSEQUENCES OF AUTO-PEEP

In very unusual circumstances, auto-PEEP and dynamic hyperinflation can be used with therapeutic intent (see "Inverse-Ratio Ventilation," below). Much more commonly, however, auto-PEEP develops inadvertently, with potentially unfortunate re-

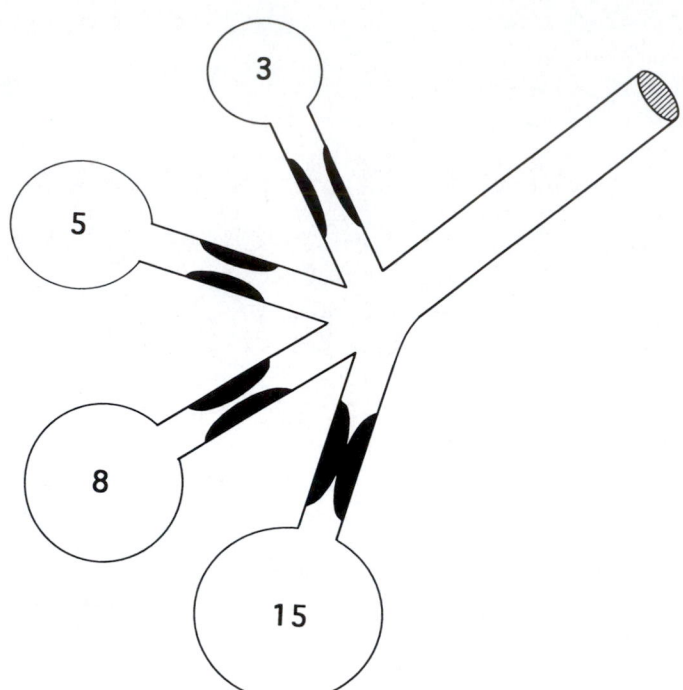

FIGURE 177-1 Variability of the auto-PEEP effect. At the end of exhalation, lung units in different regions develop variable degrees of hyperinflation and auto-PEEP, depending on regional time constants for ventilation. Some lung units may seal completely at end-exhalation. (*From Marini and Wheeler,* [39a] *with permission.*)

sults. Apart from the risk of barotrauma, the lung distention caused by auto-PEEP has two primary adverse consequences: cardiovascular sequelae and increased work of breathing.

Cardiovascular Sequelae

Hemodynamic consequences first brought the auto-PEEP phenomenon to clinical attention.[46] Alveolar overdistention increases right ventricular afterload, and when inflation occurs passively, mean pleural pressure rises, creating a back pressure to venous return. Although the latter effect generally predominates, the increase of right ventricular afterload associated with hyperinflation can prove significant in the setting of a restricted pulmonary vascular bed and preexisting cor pulmonale. Both the preload and afterload effects of dynamic hyperinflation tend to reduce left ventricular filling and impair cardiac output. Simultaneously, pressures measured with a pulmonary artery catheter rise as a consequence of increases in the intrapleural pressure that surrounds the heart. *Transmural* wedge pressure often declines as auto-PEEP develops under passive conditions.[46]

Alterations in the loading conditions of the heart partly explain why hypotension often develops when a spontaneously breathing patient with air-trapping is sedated, intubated, and mechanically ventilated. Mean intrathoracic pressure rises as forceful ventilatory efforts end. (Hemodynamic compromise is much less likely to occur when spontaneous ventilatory efforts continue following intubation, even when these efforts are machine assisted.) Vigorous spontaneous breathing reduces mean intrathoracic pressure and elevates intra-abdominal pressure during the exhalation phase, thereby maintaining the pressure difference driving venous return. Cardiac output is sustained at a relatively high level because of stress and the added work of breathing. Moreover, the reduced intrathoracic pressure accentuates the tendency to form pulmonary edema—a factor of importance in patients already predisposed to congestive heart failure. In patients with severe airflow obstruction, spontaneous breathing increases oxygen consumption and cardiac output demands and predisposes to pulmonary congestion.

The potential for auto-PEEP to depress cardiac output must be considered when pulseless electrical activity (*electromechanical dissociation*) occurs during cardiopulmonary resuscitation. The inability to detect an arterial pulse may be due to gas-trapping and impeded venous return, rather than irreversible myocardial compromise. In the resuscitation of patients with COPD or asthma, an apnea test of 10 to 20 s should be conducted soon after coordinated cardiac electrical activity is noted.

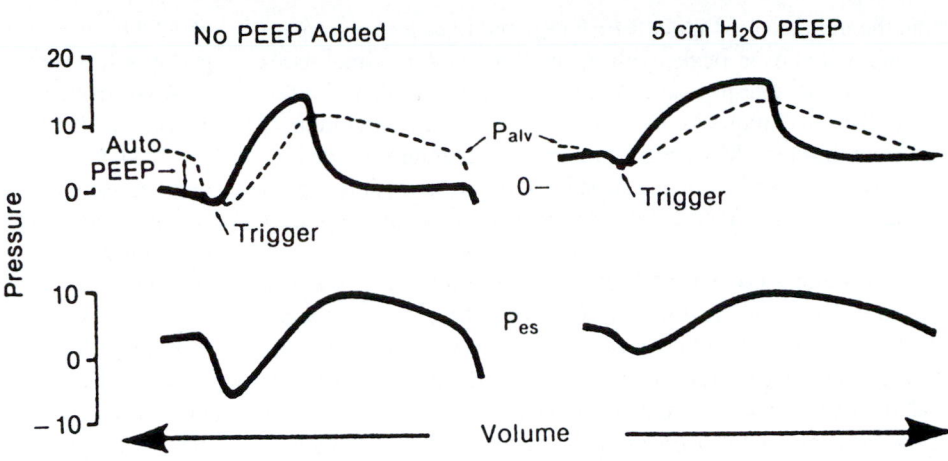

FIGURE 177-2   Influence of dynamic hyperinflation on breathing effort and improvement by addition of PEEP. As a positive end-expiratory alveolar pressure (P_{alv}), auto-PEEP presents an inspiratory threshold load to inspiration that must be overcome by inspiratory effort, reflected by esophageal pressure (P_{es}). The addition of PEEP at a level that is less than the original auto-PEEP in a patient with dynamic airway collapse reduces the triggering threshold and work of breathing.

Work of Breathing

Dynamic hyperinflation increases the oxygen demands on the respiratory muscles during spontaneous ventilation and boosts the ventilating pressures required during machine-assisted breathing. When attempting to initiate a breath, the patient with dynamic hyperinflation encounters an inspiratory threshold load—an expiratory pressure that must be counterbalanced before inspiration can be initiated. During machine-assisted cycles, therefore, auto-PEEP depresses the *effective* triggering sensitivity,[56] and during spontaneous cycles, auto-PEEP adds a "residual elastic" component to the "tidal elastic" and "frictional" components of the work of breathing (Fig. 177-2).

Hyperinflation also compromises the ventilatory pump in accomplishing this increased workload. Operating from a hyperinflated position, the acutely foreshortened inspiratory muscle fibers are preloaded insufficiently to generate maximal tension. The hyperexpanded rib cage recoils inward throughout the tidal breath, opposing inflation, rather than springing outward, as it normally does to aid in lung expansion. Horizontally oriented ribs lose their normal "pump lever" and "bucket handle" actions, further compromising the effectiveness of muscle contraction. Over time, remodeling of the diaphragmatic muscle fibers helps to restore effective preload, but this process occurs slowly. Moreover, the flattened diaphragm is geometrically disadvantaged. Finally, hyperinflation narrows or obliterates the "zone of apposition" with the chest wall that normally helps to expand the lower ribs during inspiration. For all these reasons, dynamic hyperinflation can unbalance a tenuous workload–work capacity relationship.

MEASUREMENT OF AUTO-PEEP

During *passive* ventilation at moderate ventilating frequencies (fewer than about 16 breaths per minute), auto-PEEP can be measured as the difference between end-expiratory airway occlusion pressure (*total PEEP*) and the set level of PEEP.[44] It can also be assessed by observing the positive airway pressure required at the onset of inspiration to bring expiratory flow to zero and to initiate inspiratory flow.[50] These two techniques are likely to give somewhat different results, however, with the latter underestimating the former.[47] (Neither technique samples the often large gas compartment trapped behind sealed airways.) A useful method for end-expiratory port occlusion uses an interposed diverting valve and the ventilator's automatic closure of the expiratory valve at inflation onset as the timing mechanism. Total PEEP is measured during the machine's inspiratory interval as flow is diverted to atmosphere while the respiratory system is temporarily sealed.

Undetected auto-PEEP may cause overestimation of the pressure difference required for tidal inflation and, therefore, underestimation of the true compliance of the respiratory system. Under these conditions, compliance is, perhaps, best judged by dividing the difference in end-inspiratory plateau pressures observed at two different tidal volumes during passive inflation into the tidal volume difference. With effective compliance accurately measured, auto-PEEP can be estimated as the difference between the end-inspiratory static plateau pressure and the quantity (V_T/C) + PEEP, where V_T is tidal volume and C is effective compliance. Operationally, plateau pressure is recorded during a single cycle of volume-controlled ventilation at the usual ventilating frequency. (The end-inspiratory pause should not be applied for more than a single cycle.) Frequency is then drastically reduced (to two or three breaths per minute) for approximately 15 s, after which plateau pressure is remeasured. (The machine's apnea intervention window may need to be temporarily readjusted beforehand.) The difference between the plateau pressures is the auto-PEEP.

A similar technique to estimate auto-PEEP is to first measure the additional, dynamically trapped volume in excess of V_T that is released when a single tidal inflation is delayed by 20 to 30 s and then to divide the measured "dynamically trapped volume" by compliance, as determined by the method just described. Finally, when auto-PEEP results from dynamic airway compression, the increment of added PEEP required to cause an increase in lung volume or peak cycling pressure is sometimes considered to be the pressure required to counterbalance auto-PEEP. This technique is invalid, however, when expiration is not flow limited. Moreover, the applied pressure needed to counterbalance the critical pressure approximates only 75 to 85 percent of the auto-PEEP determined by expiratory port occlusion.

An important point for the clinician to remember is that the pressure of most interest in gauging hyperinflation is not auto-PEEP itself but, rather, the end-*inspiratory* alveolar pressure relative to pleural pressure. This is particularly true when many sealed airways (e.g., in status asthmaticus) result in invalidation of the measured auto-PEEP as an estimator of lung distention.[29] The end-inspiratory plateau pressure, interpreted with the compliance of the chest wall in mind, is more clinically relevant and an easier number to follow.

During spontaneous breathing, auto-PEEP cannot be easily measured, but it can be estimated as the esophageal pressure deflection required to initiate inspiration. This estimate, however, is influenced by expiratory muscular activity, as well as dynamic hyperinflation.[32] Changes in the end-expiratory volume associated with dynamic hyperinflation can be monitored by impedance plethysmography.

INFLUENCE OF PEEP ON DYNAMIC HYPERINFLATION AND AUTO-PEEP

Hyperinflation may or may not worsen as PEEP is deliberately added to auto-PEEP, depending on the mechanism for auto-PEEP generation.[35] PEEP added to a dynamically hyperinflated patient *without* expiratory muscle activity or flow limitation causes lung volume to rise further, exacerbating the workload and compromising the pump. For some patients, however, PEEP or continuous positive airway pressure (CPAP) offers a counterspring against which the expiratory muscles may store elastic energy for release during early inspiration, allowing "work sharing" between the inspiratory and expiratory muscle groups. Assuming that minute ventilation does not change, this work-sharing mechanism is rendered ineffective in the presence of tidal flow limitation, as expiratory effort exacerbates the obstruction, rather than assisting deflation. In this setting, adding an amount of PEEP that is less than the original level of auto-PEEP narrows the difference between end-expiratory airway and alveolar pressures, increasing alveolar pressure little, if at all. PEEP added downstream of the flow limitation site, therefore, reduces the inspiratory threshold, improves triggering sensitivity, and partly alleviates the ventilatory workload.[56] In addition, it is possible that the addition of PEEP will prevent collapse of the more central airways and help reduce dyspnea in this way. PEEP that counterbalances auto-PEEP allows pressure support to more effectively boost tidal volume.

As a rule, the addition of PEEP does *not* reduce chest wall dimensions or improve muscle fiber preload. It should be noted, however, that the function of the extradiaphragmatic muscles, which are particularly important in hyperinflation, may not be as vulnerable as the diaphragm to small volume increments. Furthermore, even when the expiratory flow is limited, the impact

of CPAP on muscle *coordination* or on the synchrony of triggering effort with ventilator assistance may be beneficial.

Apart from helping to rebalance the ratio of workload to work capability, PEEP has no proven therapeutic effect in airflow obstruction. PEEP could, however, beneficially affect the *distribution* of ventilation or reestablish airway patency as it counterbalances auto-PEEP. This would help to explain why peak inflation pressures occasionally fall as low levels of PEEP are applied at a constant tidal volume. Until better evidence is gathered, however, PEEP would seem to have little place in the treatment of paralyzed patients with airflow obstruction.

In a passively ventilated patient, the effect of PEEP on lung and chest wall volumes can be accurately assessed by observation of the peak dynamic or static airway pressures. Failure of these pressures to rise in response to adding PEEP indicates dynamic airway compression, flow limitation, and a potentially beneficial action. Although this technique is less precise during spontaneously triggered breathing cycles, it nonetheless helps to "titrate" PEEP in patients receiving assist-control ventilation or synchronized intermittent mandatory ventilation (SIMV) (Chapter 176).

Acute Lung Injury

Although all regions of the lung may be injured diffusely, the radiographic and mechanical manifestations of acute lung injury are not homogeneously distributed.[19] In the acute respiratory distress syndrome (ARDS), three distinct alveolar populations can be identified: alveoli with relatively normal inflation properties, consolidated units that are uninflatable, and units that are atelectatic and potentially recruitable. Alveoli in the last two categories tend to be located disproportionately in dependent lung regions.[45] Even though the volumes of the chest wall and infiltrated lung may be little different from those of the normal healthy subject, the *aerated* compartment in ARDS may occupy only one-third (or less) of the total volume. These important observations, in conjunction with studies documenting ventilator-induced lung injury and knowledge about the mechanisms of ventilation and gas exchange, have inspired new strategies for mechanical ventilation.

GAS EXCHANGE

The mechanically heterogeneously injured lung challenges the physician to support its principal function—oxygen and CO_2 exchange—without inflicting further damage. Many innovative methods recently introduced to clinical practice were devised after collection of physiological laboratory data or in response to fortuitous clinical observations.

O₂ Exchange

Experiments in animals and observations in human infants and adult patients have demonstrated two relationships of clinical value in formulating a ventilatory strategy to optimize O_2 exchange in diffuse lung injury. First, the number of open units is a joint function of tidal volume and PEEP (Fig. 177-3).[36] Whatever the tidal volume employed, a certain *minimal* lung volume must be maintained to avoid the impaired gas exchange and lung compliance consequent to permanent or tidally phasic derecruit-

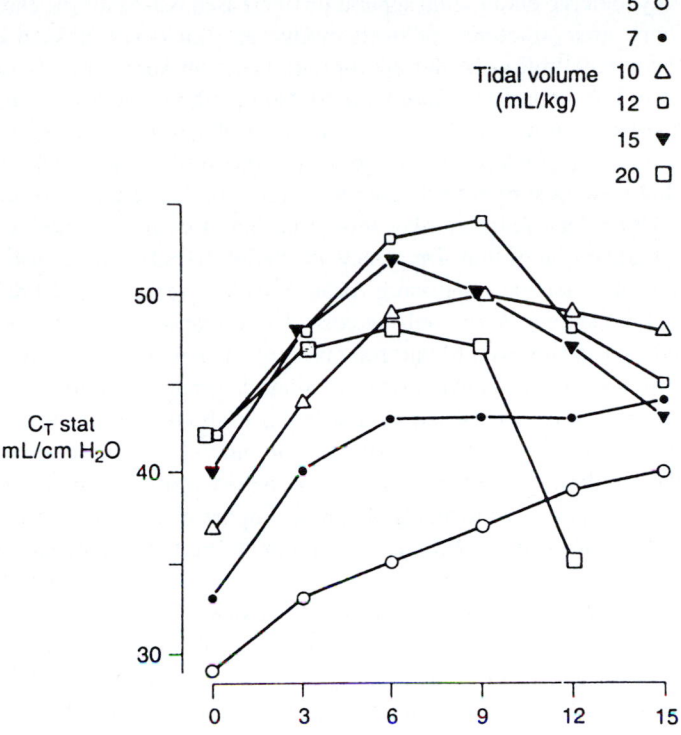

Tidal volume (mL/kg)	
5	○
7	●
10	△
12	□
15	▼
20	◻

FIGURE 177-3 Relationship of respiratory system compliance to PEEP level (horizontal axis, cmH_2O) for small and large tidal volumes. Note that static thoracic compliance (C_{Tstat}) is a joint function of both variables. Higher levels of PEEP are required to maximize compliance when small tidal volumes are used. (*From Suter, Fairley, Eisenberg: Chest 73:158–162, 1978, with permission.*)

ment of unstable alveoli. Second, once this minimally acceptable end-expiratory lung volume has been assured, arterial oxygenation appears to relate directly to average lung volume, which is reflected under conditions of passive inflation by mean airway and mean alveolar pressures.[37] In clinical practice, the slope of the curve relating pulmonary O_2 exchange to mean alveolar pressure varies greatly; oxygenation is strikingly responsive to increasing lung volume in some patients and quite refractory in others. These basic concepts seem to hold during forms of mechanical ventilation that range from conventional support to high-frequency oscillation.[8]

Elevating end-expiratory pressure by applying PEEP or CPAP is the most widely utilized technique for raising mean alveolar pressure. Apart from maintaining lung recruitment, PEEP appears to improve arterial O_2 tension by redistributing lung water and ventilation. Furthermore, when PEEP impairs cardiac output, shunt fraction tends to fall proportionately, improving Pa_{O_2} but compromising O_2 delivery. While an elevated end-expiratory lung

volume can be assured by the deliberate application of PEEP or CPAP, it can also develop (intentionally or inadvertently) as a consequence of dynamic hyperinflation. During passive ventilation, mean airway pressure can be increased by elevation of end-expiratory alveolar pressure or by extension of the inspiratory time fraction, T_I/T_T, where T_I is inspiratory time and T_T is total respiratory cycle time (inspiratory time plus expiratory time).[37] As already noted, the volume-recruiting effect of PEEP is often opposed by expiratory muscle action, a strategy that reduces the inspiratory workload by the work-sharing mechanism during vigorous breathing. Unfortunately, work sharing in this fashion subverts the clinician's attempt to raise end-expiratory lung volume—accounting, in part, for the improvement in Pa_{O_2} often seen following muscle paralysis (Fig. 177-4). Extreme prolongation of T_I/T_T (e.g., with inverse-ratio ventilation; see below) has been suggested as a more effective method of supporting oxygen exchange, but relatively few objective data supporting this contention have been gathered (see below).[31]

CO_2 Exchange

During ventilation with conventional tidal volumes, CO_2 elimination is a direct function of alveolar ventilation. However, high-frequency ventilation (HFV) eliminates CO_2 at tidal volumes much smaller than what was once regarded as the ventilatory "dead space" of a breath of standard size.[9] In animals with extensive collateral ventilation, even an unpulsed, continuous high flow of gas introduced deep into the trachea can provide a substantial portion of the alveolar ventilation needed to maintain homeostasis. Effective CO_2 elimination can be maintained indefinitely in experimental animals and human neonates when a bias flow of gas is augmented by very-high-frequency vibration of the chest wall[14] or gas column.

At conventional frequencies, the precise contour of the inspiratory flow waveform does not influence CO_2 elimination in normal lungs. Evidence from many sources indicates, however, that slowing the rate of gas flow at end-inspiration may improve the

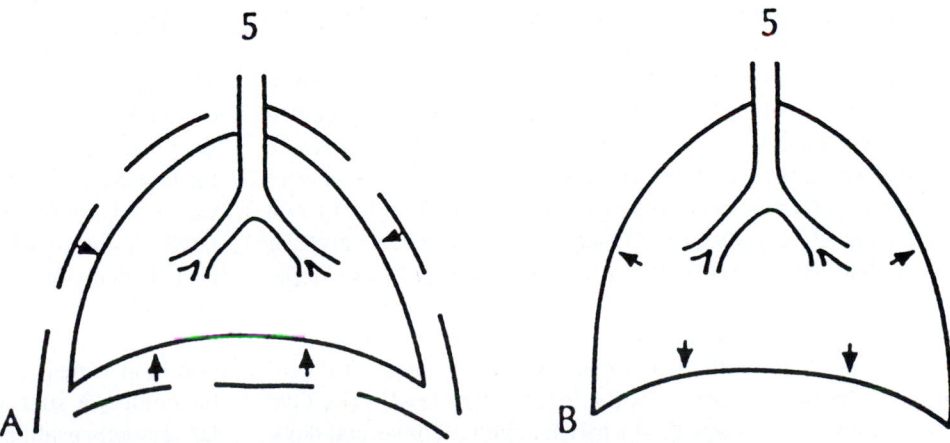

FIGURE 177-4 Effect of expiratory muscle activity on lung volume recruitment by PEEP. *A.* During vigorous active breathing, 5 cmH_2O applied PEEP is opposed by continued activity of expiratory muscles at end-expiration. *B.* After relaxation has been achieved, end-expiratory lung volume increases to the equilibrium value that corresponds to the end-expiratory airway pressure (5 cmH_2O). This is often accompanied by improved arterial oxygenation. [*From Marini, in Cherniack (ed), Chronic Obstructive Pulmonary Disease, Philadelphia, WB Saunders, 1991, page 495, with permission.*]

ventilatory efficiency of lungs with impaired gas exchange. End-inspiratory flow deceleration can be accomplished by adding an end-inspiratory hold (pause), by linearly decelerating flow delivery during volume-preset ventilation,[48] or by using pressure-preset ventilation. Such techniques are currently receiving increased attention in the care of patients with ARDS.

VENTILATOR-INDUCED LUNG DAMAGE

Ventilator-induced tissue damage poses a life-threatening problem for patients with diffuse lung injury. Certain radiographically evident types of alveolar rupture (e.g., pneumothorax) are well-known and feared complications of mechanical ventilation. Until recently, several forms of ventilator-related barotrauma previously reported in infants were not seen in adults. It is now known, however, that interstitial emphysema and tension gas cysts commonly occur in ventilated adult patients with ARDS, and airway changes suggestive of bronchopulmonary dysplasia[51] and systemic gas embolism can occur as well. Perhaps more important, experimental evidence now strongly indicates that high pressures applied for brief periods can injure the endothelial and epithelial membranes of a normal lung, enabling proteinaceous edema to enter the alveolar space.[13] Such observations, in conjunction with the recently acquired knowledge that the mechanical abnormalities of the diffusely injured lung are not homogeneously distributed, raise the possibility that alveolar damage may be perpetuated or extended by the same treatment intended to allow healing.

Unquestionably, barotrauma is a multifactorial process, with underlying disease, secretion retention, patient age, and duration of ventilation playing pivotal roles.[18] Because of the wide range of airway pressures that may accompany radiographic barotrauma, some investigators have cogently argued that disease itself—not overdistention—is the primary cause.[18] No absolutely safe plateau pressure has yet been identified; pneumothorax can occur even during HFV in susceptible patients. Although the safe upper limit of pressure exposure undoubtedly varies from person to person, limiting tidal transalveolar ("transpulmonary") pressures to approximately 30 cmH$_2$O (or to an inspiratory plateau pressure of 35 cmH$_2$O in patients with a normal chest wall) seems a defensible approach that is adequately supported by experimental data. Indeed, this was the recommendation of a joint North American–European consensus conference on mechanical ventilation sponsored by the American College of Chest Physicians.[55] Subsequent work suggests that extensive alveolar overdistention may occur at considerably lower pressures in patients with ARDS.[52]

Neonatal bronchopulmonary dysplasia and endobronchial damage in adults with ARDS can be demonstrated after prolonged exposures to pressures that exceed this level. Peak tidal alveolar pressures as low as 30 cmH$_2$O, applied for several days, can produce diffuse alveolar damage in experimental animals. Because some alveoli remain normally compliant, a natural upper limit for transalveolar pressure is immediately suggested by the healthy lung's pressure–volume relationship. Tidal transpulmonary (transalveolar) pressures higher than those corresponding to total lung capacity (approximately 30 to 35 cmH$_2$O) subject normal alveoli to excessive stress; unusually fragile alveoli

may undergo endothelial separation, increased permeability, capillary stress fractures, or overt rupture at even lower pressures. Precise definition of the appropriate tidal pressure range is of great importance, as more than 30,000 breathing cycles may be applied each day to the airway of a critically ill patient.

Exactly *which* pressure—peak dynamic, peak static, mean, or other—is most relevant to the risk of lung rupture remains somewhat unclear. All may play some role. The first multicenter cooperative trial of high-frequency oscillation (HFO) in neonates[23] indicates that peak pressure, peak alveolar pressure, and tidal volume cannot be the only factors of importance;[8] a similar incidence and severity of barotrauma were encountered in the HFO group as in the conventional ventilation group, despite much lower peak pressures and tidal volumes in the former.[8,23] Whatever the pressure characteristics of the individual breathing cycle, the duration and frequency of pressure exposure ("total mechanical stress") are likely to prove important risk factors for tissue injury. Once epithelial disruption or overt alveolar rupture has occurred, the mean transalveolar pressure may be an important determinant of the *extent* of gas leakage.

It is widely believed that the provision of high-pressure excursions during the tidal cycle gives rise to disproportionately high shearing forces among collapsed units exposed to the amplified stresses of interdependence, and that the combination of high cycling pressure with inadequate PEEP must be avoided in order to prevent hemorrhagic lung damage.[36] In fact, at least one controlled trial conducted in a single center demonstrated improved lung function and better survival when an attempt to prevent this combination was made.[3] Some investigators have questioned whether large tidal volumes alone, independent of high peak transalveolar pressure or insufficient end-expiratory pressure to prevent collapse, could lead to alveolar injury. Although this is an intriguing and plausible hypothesis, a separate contribution of tidal volume has not been unequivocally demonstrated. Prospective, controlled, randomized multicenter studies of ventilatory pattern and outcome are currently under way.

Cardiovascular Compromise and Shock

The work of breathing contributes negligibly to total body O$_2$ consumption in the quietly breathing, healthy subject. However, the breathing workload of ventilatory failure can add greatly to the burden imposed on a compromised cardiovascular system.[30] Conversely, impaired cardiovascular performance can precipitate failure of the ventilatory pump by depriving the respiratory muscles of adequate O$_2$ delivery.[4] It has been estimated that the work of breathing increases by an average of 25 percent when patients with acute respiratory failure are removed from ventilator support.[16] In some patients, the oxygen consumption is doubled. The magnitude of such workloads helps to explain the cardiovascular decompensation experienced during weaning attempts by some patients with simultaneous chronic airflow obstruction and cardiovascular disease. As already noted, abrupt transitions between fully supported and spontaneous breathing promote increases in left ventricular afterload, myocardial ischemia, and translocation of blood volume into the thorax, contributing to ventilatory decompensation and hypoxemia. Desaturation of mixed venous blood resulting from disproportionate oxygen consumption relative to oxygen delivery can add to hypoxemia in patients with ventilation–perfusion mismatching or intrapulmonary or intracardiac right-to-left shunts. Increased right atrial pressure resulting from right ventricular decompensation may cause venous blood to shunt through a patent foramen ovale.

In experimental cardiogenic shock, the ventilatory pump can fail despite intense neural stimulation,[4] justifying early mechanical support in patients with compromised cardiovascular function who face substantial breathing workloads. Ventilator support should be withdrawn cautiously from patients in this category, and only after fluid imbalance and ischemia have been corrected. Pharmacologic interventions to reduce ischemia, vascular congestion, or left ventricular afterload can be useful in carefully selected patients.

Under passive conditions, increased mean airway pressure (e.g., due to PEEP or inverse-ratio ventilation) causes the lung to expand and intrapleural pressures to rise. High levels of PEEP elevate pulmonary vascular pressures, impede venous return, and functionally stiffen the left ventricle through ventricular interdependence.

Work of Breathing During Mechanical Ventilation

Dyspnea, breathing rhythm dyssynchrony, and high cycling pressures may result from adverse interactions between the patient and ventilator. The total transpulmonary pressure change required per breath is a value fixed by the inspiratory flow rate, inspiratory resistance, respiratory system compliance, tidal volume, auto-PEEP (if any), and the pattern of chest inflation. Although the machine is often capable of generating all necessary pressure, the patient and ventilator virtually always work together to accomplish the ventilatory task during patient-triggered, machine-aided cycles. The primary factors influencing the patient's contribution during volume-cycled mechanical ventilation are ventilatory drive, machine flow setting, and respiratory muscle strength.[38] (A debilitated patient cannot produce or sustain a large amount of ventilatory power, limiting the work he or she can do.) It follows that absolute values of work performed by the patient correlate poorly with effort relative to capability or with the relative loads of different subjects.

Ventilatory drive is influenced by the minute ventilation requirement, triggering sensitivity (the sum of the set pressure threshold and any imposed by auto-PEEP), and sensation of breathlessness. In theory, if the machine delivers gas flow exactly as fast as the patient demands it, proximal airway pressure remains at the level of PEEP, and the machine performs no mechanical work on the respiratory system. Conversely, if the patient relaxes immediately and completely after triggering the ventilator, almost the entire breathing workload can be accomplished by the machine (Fig. 177-5). Because the patient's greatest de-

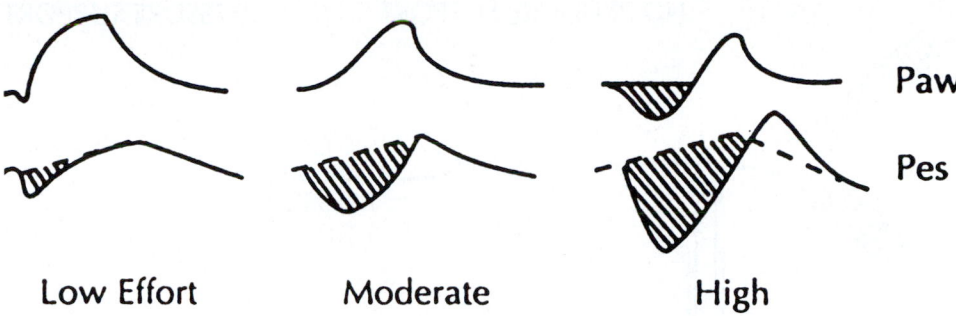

Low Effort   Moderate   High

FIGURE 177-5   Airway (P_{aw}) and esophageal (P_{es}) pressures recorded during low, moderate, and high efforts during flow-controlled, volume-cycled assisted ventilation. The dashed line superimposed on the tracing of P_{es} is the trajectory expected for passive inflation, and the shaded region between the passive and active P_{es} curves reflects the patient's inspiratory work of breathing. Note the reciprocal relationship between patient effort and airway pressure and the fact that the patient works against the impedance of the machine circuitry (shaded P_{aw}) during the first portion of the ventilatory cycle.

mand for flow occurs in the very first part of the machine cycle, it makes sense to employ a decelerating, rather than constant, flow delivery profile for the same tidal volume and inspiratory time setting. Pressure control is inherently flow decelerating; in volume-cycled ventilation, a linearly decelerating profile can be selected.[48] A dyspneic patient helped intermittently by the ventilator (e.g., during SIMV) may exert very similar effort for adjacent spontaneous and machine-aided breaths at the same overall level of machine support.[39] Patients experiencing dyspnea do not adapt breathing effort quickly in response to intermittent unloading of the breathing cycle.

The work of breathing has not been extensively studied during pressure-preset ventilation, but similar principles are likely to apply.[10] Pressure-supported ventilation allows the patient to control breathing cycle timing and depth. Such a *flow-cycled* mode of ventilation might be more comfortable and result in less patient work than a comparable level of flow-preset, *volume-cycled* ventilation. Few objective data exist, however, to confirm or refute this contention. In a study of weaning in which pressure support was compared with SIMV in the same patients, no differences in anxiety or dyspnea were detected.[26] Individual patient preference may well vary with ventilation requirement, machine performance, and chest impedance.

Modern ventilator valving systems provide efficient gas delivery. CPAP is often associated with little additional work cost attributable to the valving or flow capacity of the system. However, no matter how perfectly a gas delivery system maintains the set level of end-expiratory pressure in the external circuit, the patient must contend with endotracheal (ET) tube resistance during each spontaneous breathing cycle (Fig. 177-6). ET tube resistance can be considerably higher in vivo than what is measured in vitro before tube insertion. Secretions, kinks, or impingement of the ET tube on the mucosal surface of the trachea can decrease the tube's effective diameter. Monitoring systems that track flow and pressure simultaneously can often help to detect such problems.[25]

Inspiratory resistive work imposed by the ET tube may be offset by an appropriately selected level of pressure support. The effectiveness of a fixed level of pressure support tends to dete-

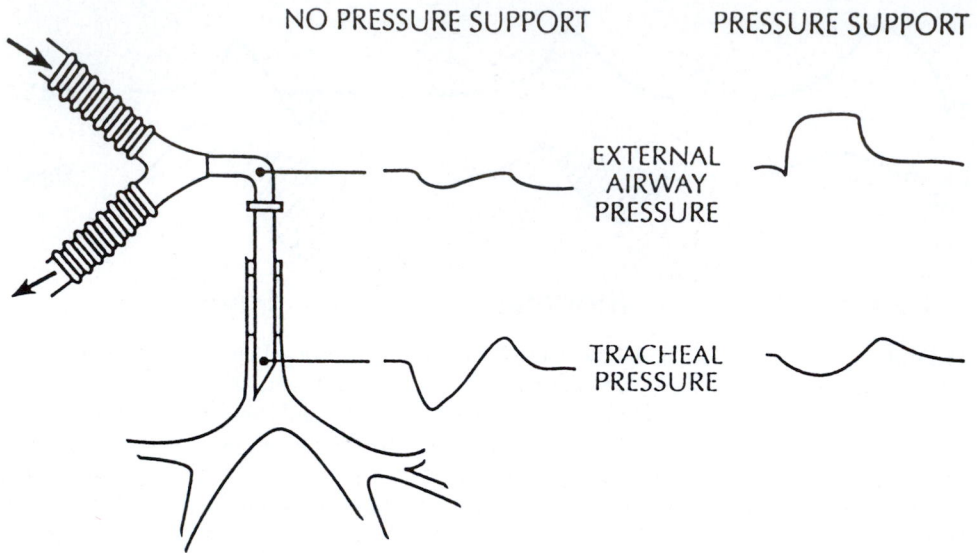

NO PRESSURE SUPPORT   PRESSURE SUPPORT

EXTERNAL AIRWAY PRESSURE

TRACHEAL PRESSURE

FIGURE 177-6   Impact of pressure support on the impedance of the endotracheal tube. However effectively continuous positive airway pressure may be supplied, the patient must draw fresh gas through the endotracheal tube during spontaneous inspiration and overcome the expiratory resistance of the endotracheal tube by passive recoil or active expiratory effort. Adding pressure support helps to overcome the inspiratory workload, but it does nothing to aid the patient in overcoming the expiratory resistance. To minimize work, controlling circuit pressure at the tracheal level during both phases of ventilation is theoretically desirable.

riorate as the ventilatory requirement increases. This occurs, in part, because most machines do not provide sufficient flow at higher breathing frequencies and because the percentage of work borne by the patient increases with the vigor of the breathing effort. A single value of airway pressure cannot provide the same percentage of support across a broad range of minute ventilatory requirements.

However efficient pressure support may be for dealing with inspiratory tube resistance, *expiratory* resistance across the tube and exhalation valve must be overcome by elastic energy stored during inspiration or by expiratory muscle effort. Control of the tracheal pressure during both phases of the ventilatory cycle can be accomplished by sensing or estimating circuit pressure at the carinal end of the endotracheal tube. At least one approach to this problem—automatic tube compensation—is in the advanced stages of clinical testing.[21]

NEWER MODES OF VENTILATORY SUPPORT

Increased awareness of the hazards of positive-pressure ventilation, the importance of patient–ventilator interactions, and the escalating costs of inpatient care have stimulated the development of new strategies and modes for supporting machine-dependent patients (Table 177-1). In the following discussion, newer modes of ventilatory support and gas exchange are described briefly and reviewed in the context of their physiological rationale, potential clinical indications and importance, and shortcomings. With few exceptions, however, indications for use of these methods and their efficacy and safety remain clinically uncertain. In the vast majority of patients requiring mechanical ventilatory support, the standard modes described in Chapter 176 are employed.

High-Frequency Ventilation

At very high ventilating frequencies, effective CO_2 elimination can be accomplished with tidal volumes smaller than the calculated anatomic dead space.[58] The theoretical advantage of such HFV is in lowering peak cycling pressures and reducing tidal lung excursions, two cycle characteristics that may be causally related to barotrauma. Two basic mechanisms appear to account for alveolar ventilation during HFV: convective and nonconvective gas flow. Two basic types of HFV devices are available: jet ventilators and oscillators.[58] The primary mechanism by which HFV achieves ventilation varies with the specific mode of HFV in use and with the frequency range employed. At these high frequencies, acceleration and deceleration (inertance) play crucial roles in distributing fresh gas within the lung.[9]

JET VENTILATION

The primary high-frequency option currently used in adults—jet ventilation—phasically directs a high-velocity stream of humidified gas high into the ET tube at rapid frequencies, entraining additional fresh gas during each insufflation.[9] To achieve the same level of alveolar ventilation, the *total* ventilation provided by the jet—injected and entrained—usually averages several

TABLE 177-1

Established and Newer Modes of Mechanical Ventilation

Established Modes of Mechanical Ventilation	New or Clinically Unproven Modes of Mechanical Ventilation
Assist/control	High-frequency ventilation (HFV)
Volume controlled	Jet
Pressure controlled	Oscillation
Synchronized intermittent mandatory ventilation (SIMV)	Inverse-ratio ventilation
	Airway pressure release
Continuous positive airway pressure (CPAP)*	Biphasic positive airway pressure
	Self-adjusting "combination" modes
Pressure support (PSV)	Volume-assured pressure support
	Volume support
	Proportional-assist ventilation

*Technically, CPAP is a machine setting rather than a mode.

times that of a closed system. The system remains open—i.e., there are no circuit valves to open and close. Jets pulsed at frequencies of 100 to 600 cycles per minute generate very low pressures in the central airway, where the average pressure remains approximately at the set level of CPAP. Tidal volume and effective alveolar ventilation are determined primarily by the pressure driving the jet and by the inspiratory time fraction (duty cycle). In these high ranges, variations in cycling frequency do not markedly affect alveolar ventilation. In fact, beyond a certain threshold range, the Pa_{CO_2} may rise, rather than fall, as frequency increases. In the lower part of the jet frequency range (100 to 200 cycles per minute), HFV appears to accomplish alveolar ventilation primarily by convective gas flow, as in conventional ventilation. Alveolar pressures during high-frequency jet ventilation (HFJV) commonly exceed those measured in the central airway. Mean alveolar pressures may approach those of conventional techniques that provide similar levels of alveolar ventilation.

To this point, HFJV has been disappointing in the care of critically ill adults. Many patients cannot be ventilated successfully with HFJV, and in most, oxygen exchange does not improve until mean alveolar pressures rise significantly. For all its problems, HFJV may yet play a useful role in the acute setting as an adjunctive method to complement bulk flow methods and to improve the efficiency of alveolar ventilation. Intriguing reports suggest that when large tidal volume breaths or periodic recruiting maneuvers are combined with HFV, these techniques may improve oxygenation and recruit atelectatic lung units more effectively than conventional techniques.[8,36] These contentions, however, require further confirmation. Current indications for HFJV include bronchoscopy, upper-airway surgery, and selective cases of bronchopleural fistulas. Although exceptional responses may occur, on the basis of current evidence, HFJV does not appear to be a reliable "salvage" mode for ARDS and should be used only with caution in severe airflow obstruction.

HIGH-FREQUENCY OSCILLATION

High-frequency oscillation has been used primarily in infants; until recently, no machines appropriate for adult use were commercially available. Oscillation is based on a different approach than HFJV: The airway gas column is caused to vibrate at frequencies that far exceed those in HFJV in a semiclosed system. Fresh gas is directed across the external breathing circuit. Oscillatory vibrations facilitate gas exchange, largely by nonconvective mechanisms (e.g., through facilitated diffusion). Chest wall vibration, a crude analog of HFO, enhances CO_2 elimination when added to tracheal gas insufflation.[14]

In a multicenter cooperative trial of oscillation in the infant respiratory distress syndrome, the mortality and incidence of barotrauma with HFO proved similar to those in a control group.[23] There have been important questions raised, however, regarding entry criteria and timing in this study, as well as the precise way in which the study was implemented.[8] Indeed, subsequent work has strongly indicated potential clinical benefit,[11] and HFO is firmly entrenched as a preferred treatment option in neonatal intensive care. Although future employment of HFO as a free-standing mode for adult use remains in doubt, it may still hold promise if used in combination with periodic recruiting

breaths (relatively high pressure applied for 15 to 30 s) and enough mean airway pressure to maintain appropriate lung volume.[8]

Airway Pressure Release Ventilation and Biphasic Airway Pressure

Airway pressure release ventilation (APRV) is a form of partial ventilatory support originally intended to lessen the work required to ventilate patients during a primary crisis of oxygenation.[57] APRV elevates mean airway pressure by maintaining a moderately high level of CPAP. Periodically, the airway rapidly depressurizes during a tidal deflation cycle, exhausting waste gas from the functional expiratory reserve before replacing it with fresh gas as CPAP rebuilds to the baseline level. The release pattern is repeated at a frequency selected by the clinician. Using some machines, the clinician can select the *proportion* of cycles during which release occurs, rather than the *absolute frequency* of system decompression. The ventilatory support provided by APRV is a function of driving pressure (the difference between CPAP and the pressure to which airway pressure falls), the duration and frequency of release cycles, and the impedance of the thorax. Synchronization of the release cycle to occur during exhalation may be important to maximize ventilatory efficiency.

This mode and its close relatives, intermittent mandatory pressure release ventilation and biphasic airway pressure (BIPAP), are analogous to SIMV in that most individual tidal cycles are not assisted by circuit decompression. However, these modes operate with a higher resting pressure and *reduce*, rather than raise, airway pressure during machine release cycles. In BIPAP, the patient breathes spontaneously for substantial periods around each of two levels of CPAP. BIPAP may exhibit a time dependence—improving oxygenation gradually over hours to days. [BIPAP is quite distinct from bilevel CPAP (commercially known as Bi-PAP), a mode in which the CPAP is varied with *each triggered cycle* between two levels. Commercial Bi-PAP can be thought of as a combination of CPAP (the lower level) and pressure support (the difference between the higher and lower levels). Commercial Bi-PAP is generally intended for intermittent ventilatory assistance and, therefore, is usually implemented at relatively low pressure levels using a noninvasive nasal or oral mask appliance.]

Although the airway pressure profile generated by the machine during APRV and BIPAP closely resembles that of inverse-ratio ventilation (see below), the key difference is that APRV and related techniques allow spontaneous breathing, thereby lowering the peak and mean alveolar pressures associated with a given level of ventilatory support. Allowing spontaneous breathing has an undeniable benefit in helping to promote venous return and obviating deep sedation and muscle relaxants. Furthermore, spontaneous breathing is often more efficient than passive inflation in achieving alveolar ventilation and optimal ventilation–perfusion matching. The potential for alveolar overdistention and barotrauma may also be reduced, as peak *airway* pressure is limited to the CPAP applied. It should be noted, however, that a vigorously breathing subject may intermittently be subjected to *transpulmonary* inflation pressures considerably higher than the set level of CPAP, as peak stretching pressure is the algebraic difference (absolute sum) of CPAP and intrapleural pressure. Nonetheless, if protective stretch reflexes are intact and regional ball-valve gas-trapping can be avoided, the risk of barotrauma with this mode should remain relatively low.

Airway pressure release methods pose potential problems. In order to build the pressure difference needed to assist ventilation significantly, CPAP must first be raised to a moderately high level. If chest compliance is high, the respiratory muscles will be disadvantaged by the resulting hyperinflation, promoting the sensation of dyspnea that APRV is designed to relieve. (In ARDS, however, the change in *chest wall* volume may be very modest.) Furthermore, as the number and duration of release cycles increase, mean airway pressure falls—a change often associated with hypoxemia. This, in turn, may generate the need for a compensatory increase in CPAP. Circuits must be carefully designed with valves that function properly; otherwise, an excessive breathing workload may result.

APRV has been successfully implemented in postoperative patients and those with mild to moderate lung disease; it may eventually prove to have application in the management of more severe forms of acute respiratory failure as well. APRV was designed to assist patients with moderate respiratory failure. Whether APRV will prove helpful for patients with extreme weakness, very high breathing workloads, or conditions in which release cycles are relatively ineffectual in achieving ventilation (e.g., severe airflow obstruction) remains open to question.

"Combination" Modes: Volume Support and Volume-Assured Pressure Support

Some newer forms of assisted ventilation continuously regulate the applied pressure or supplement flow, as necessary, to achieve a targeted minute ventilation or tidal volume. Volume support, for example, monitors the tidal volume and ventilation rate achieved over several cycles, compares them to the targeted values, and varies the applied pressure accordingly. Failure to achieve the targeted minute ventilation or tidal volume is met by additional pressure support until the desired ventilation rate is achieved or the tidal volume exceeds 150 percent of the desired minimum value. Should minimum minute ventilation and minimum tidal volume be exceeded, pressure support is reduced.

Volume-assured pressure-support ventilation[2] and augmented minute volume[33] represent other approaches to accomplishing the dual objectives of allowing patient control of cycling rhythm and guaranteeing an appropriate tidal volume (Fig. 177-7). In these modes, a flow generator operating in

parallel with pressure support intervenes to complete the task of delivering the targeted tidal volume if the level of applied pressure support is insufficient to achieve it. A consequence, however, is that the ventilator determines the patient's flow pattern and may extend the inspiratory time. For many purposes, volume-support and volume-assured pressure-support ventilation represent advances over conventional pressure support, but each has shortcomings that preclude them from consideration as ideal methods for partial ventilatory support.

Proportional-Assist Ventilation

A form of ventilatory support that has recently been developed and clinically tested has the potential to overcome many of the coordination problems of other partial ventilatory support modes. With proportional-assist ventilation (PAV), the ventilator is set to function essentially as an "auxiliary muscle" whose vigor is patient controlled, but whose power is clinician adjusted to offset flow-resistive or elastic pressure breathing requirements.[59] Pressure assistance by the machine is proportional to a variable combination of the inspired volume (the elastic assist) and the inspiratory flow rate (the resistive or frictional assist). Proportionality is accomplished by monitoring flow and volume (integrated flow), the two key components of the simplified equation

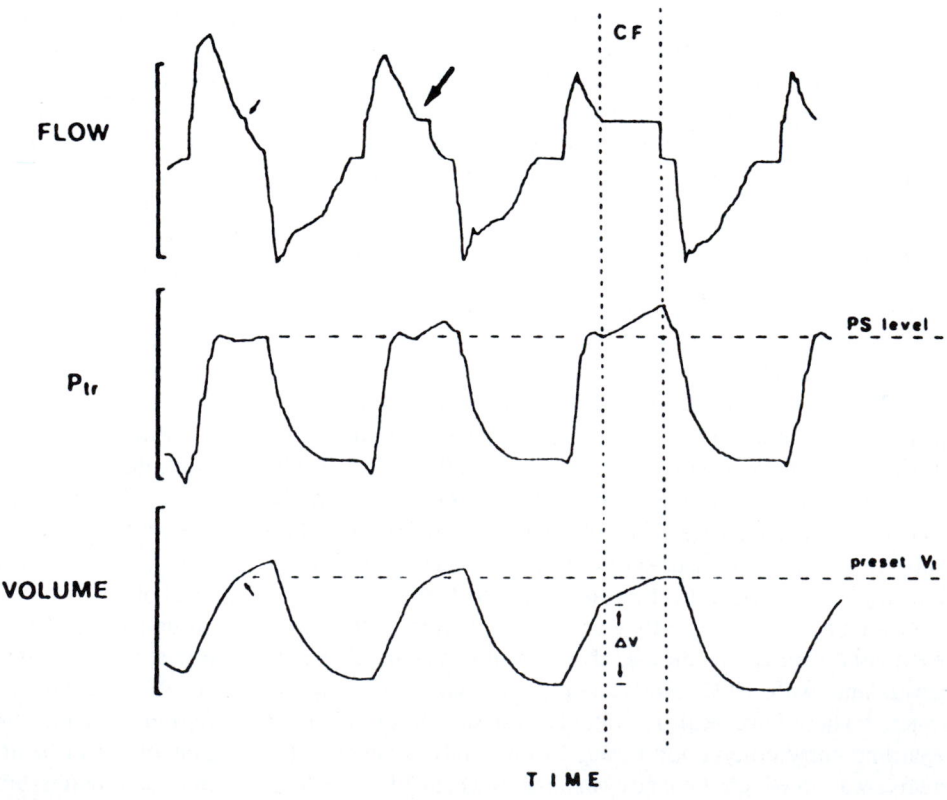

FIGURE 177-7 Tracings of flow, airway pressure (P_{tr}), and tidal volume during volume-assured pressure-support ventilation. In the first breath of the series, the preset tidal volume is accomplished in the requisite time. As the patient's inspiratory effort declines, however, the constant flow generator that guarantees the preset tidal volume is activated (large arrow) on subsequent cycles. (*Based on data of Amato et al,[2] with permission.*)

of motion of the respiratory system that describes the inspiratory pressure (P) across the respiratory system: $P = VR + (\int \dot{V} dt)/C$, where $\dot{V}$ is flow, and R and C are resistance and compliance of the respiratory system, respectively.

PAV is intuitively attractive in that it yields to the patient's own neuromuscular control mechanisms and is guided by the equation of motion of the respiratory system in synchronizing the ventilator's output with the patient's continuously changing needs. Tidal volume and flow are fully controlled by the patient, while the "gain factors" that determine the elastic and flow-resistive assist proportions become the independent variables. (Although superficially similar, this control algorithm differs from other proposed approaches to amplify patient effort that set tidal volume or flow targets.) Thus, the machine acts to amplify the patient's own efforts: When the patient pulls harder, the machine boosts its output; as the patient relaxes, the machine cuts back in parallel. In theory, the clinician can offset any desired fraction of the frictional or elastic workload by adjusting the appropriate gain settings. Across a very wide range of gain combinations, a "runaway" condition (positive feedback) cannot occur. Reflexes that normally prevent lung overdistention might also prevent barotrauma during PAV-assisted breathing.

No mode of partial support is without drawbacks, and PAV is no exception. Because tidal volumes and flow rates are controlled by the natural breathing rhythm, they vary continuously, and PAV requires backup in case the patient ceases ventilatory efforts. Moreover, like pressure support, PAV does not offset auto-PEEP. As with any form of mechanical ventilation, pressure, apnea, and hypoventilation alarms must be set appropriately. Despite these reservations, PAV has the clear potential for providing appropriate ventilatory support in a variety of clinical settings, ranging from acute lung injury to gradual machine withdrawal.

ADJUNCTS TO MECHANICAL VENTILATION

Although usually effective in supporting gas exchange, conventional methods are not invariably successful. Moreover, the cyclic application of pressure to the airway accounts for the great majority of adverse consequences resulting from mechanical ventilation. The common intent of adjuncts for ventilation and oxygenation (Table 177-2) is to improve the lung's gas-transfer functions without the need to distend it or interfere with the breathing rhythm.

Permissive Hypercapnia

The clinician who employs permissive hypercapnia assigns higher priority to avoiding injurious airway pressure than to maintaining normal levels of ventilation.[12,15,22] Allowing Pa_{CO_2} to rise above its baseline value is, perhaps, the simplest approach to reducing the ventilatory workload, the hazards of high pressure, and the total number of machine cycles needed per minute. As Pa_{CO_2} rises, each exhaled breath of a given volume eliminates more CO_2 than during normocapnia. With a reduced ventilation requirement, smaller tidal volumes can be delivered, lowering the peak and mean inflation pressures and reducing the work of breathing. Because ventilatory power varies as $(\dot{V}_E)^2$, small reductions in $\dot{V}_E$ help spare effort and transpulmonary pres-

sure. If the concomitant fall in mean alveolar pressure causes an unacceptable reduction in arterial oxygenation, adding PEEP or extending the inspiratory time fraction may restore it to an appropriate level. Gradual increases in Pa_{CO_2} are accompanied by small shifts in intracellular pH and are generally well tolerated, even to very high concentrations of Pa_{CO_2}. Except in severe status asthmaticus, Pa_{CO_2} seldom needs to exceed 75 mmHg in order to keep ventilating pressures within acceptable bounds.

Despite its relative safety, permissive hypercapnia is not without hazard (Table 177-3). The potent vasodilating effects of CO_2 may increase intracranial pressure or produce hypotension in a patient being treated with a β-adrenergic blocking drug. Pulmonary artery pressure often rises as pH falls. (Inhaled nitric oxide counteracts this effect.) Caution must be exercised, therefore, in patients with head injury, intracranial bleeding, hypertension, cardiovascular instability, coexisting hypoxemia, adrenergic insufficiency or blockade, or extreme pulmonary hypertension. Abrupt reductions in ventilation will cause pH to fall, unless infused buffer augments the serum bicarbonate concentration. Normalization of pH at a higher level of Pa_{CO_2} usually blunts ventilatory drive. Deep sedation, with or without paralysis, is almost invariably required as Pa_{CO_2} rises to a new plateau. Attempts to

---

TABLE 177-2

Adjuncts to Mechanical Ventilation

Nitric oxide/inhaled prostacyclin
Vibration of airway or chest wall
Tracheal gas insufflation
Partial liquid ventilation
Extracorporeal membrane oxygenation (ECMO)
Extracorporeal CO_2 removal ($ECCO_2R$)
Intravenacaval gas exchange (IVOX)
Permissive hypercapnia
Prone positioning

TABLE 177-3

Consequences of Hypercapnia

System	Effect*
Respiratory	Reduced alveolar P_{O_2}
	Rightward shift of oxyhemoglobin curve
	Impaired diaphragm function
	Pulmonary vasoconstriction
	Worsened ventilation–perfusion mismatching
Renal	Enhanced bicarbonate reabsorption
CNS	Cerebral vasodilation
	Increased intracranial pressure
	Depressed consciousness
	Biochemical changes
Cardiovascular	Reduced cardiac contractility†
	Stimulation of sympathoadrenal axis
	Lower systemic vascular resistance

*Most effects wane with time as cellular and extracellular pH readjust.
†Only if not offset by adrenergic compensation.

gradually restore normocapnia are made as clinical status improves.

Lung protective stategies incorporating permissive hypercapnia have been reported to reduce the mortality during status asthmaticus[12] and ARDS,[22] but many clinicians do not view these contentions as proven. Although currently considered unconventional, permissive hypercapnia during the acute phase of illness may eventually prove to be an essential component of a strategy designed to limit pressure-related barotrauma, or "volutrauma," or to wean tenuous patients more quickly from mechanical ventilation.

Extrapulmonary Gas Exchange

Recognition of the spectrum and severity of barotraumatic injury has also stimulated interest in adjunctive techniques designed to reduce the lung's exposure to pressure and volume. Support for the gas-exchanging functions of the lung can be provided by extracorporeal circuits that expose a fraction of the total systemic blood flow to fresh gas across thin, semipermeable, artificial membranes.

EXTRACORPOREAL MEMBRANE OXYGENATION

The first extracorporeal circuits for gas exchange used a venoarterial bypass intended primarily to accomplish oxygen transfer in support of acute lung injury (e.g., ARDS). To significantly affect arterial oxygenation, a large fraction of the total cardiac output must be diverted, because it is not possible to oxygen-load hemoglobin to supranormal values at ambient pressures.

Extracorporeal membrane oxygenation (ECMO) allows major reductions of supplemental oxygen and inflation pressure, but it requires extensive resource commitment and technical support. The dismal results of venoarterial ECMO in an NIH-sponsored trial of this technique in very severe ARDS led to its virtual abandonment in adult patients treated in North America.[60] Sepsis and bleeding were major causes of morbidity. It is now believed that healing of the injured lung may have been delayed or prevented by the ischemia of pulmonary bypass, perhaps in combination with the continuation of conventional, high-pressure ventilatory support.

Even though ECMO apparently failed as a salvage technique for adults, in experienced hands, 80 percent or more of neonates with the infant respiratory distress syndrome treated with a strategy incorporating ECMO may now survive. Despite recent technical improvements in cannulas, insertion techniques, and membranes, the hazards and expense of these methods remain formidable. Whether or not ECMO deserves to be reevaluated as a support technique for *adults* will depend, in part, on the success or failure of less aggressive new modes of ventilation in achieving the same clinical objectives.

EXTRACORPOREAL CO_2 REMOVAL

The experience with venovenous extracorporeal CO_2 removal (ECCO$_2$R) has been significantly different from that of ECMO.[20] The primary objective of ECCO$_2$R is to rest the lungs. Here, a highly efficient membrane clears almost all CO_2 from a much smaller blood flow than ECMO requires—approximately 25 percent of the total cardiac output. The normal CO_2 gradient across the lungs is only about 5 mmHg, and the CO_2 dissociation curve is nearly linear. Total depletion of CO_2 from the diverted venous stream improves its CO_2 elimination eight-fold over that in a similar undiverted stream flowing through a healthy lung. Unlike ECMO, ECCO$_2$R directs all venous return, diverted and undiverted, through the lung, where most oxygen exchange continues to occur. With ECCO$_2$R, circulating volume can easily and quickly be adjusted by ultrafiltration. ECCO$_2$R is extremely effective in reducing the lung's exposure to injurious airway pressures. As currently implemented, only a small number of pressure-controlled ventilator cycles, used in conjunction with CPAP, and a low continuous flow of O_2 are required.

Techniques for implementing ECCO$_2$R have improved substantially in recent years, with percutaneous techniques for femoral catheter insertion routine in several centers. Although the potential for overt circuit disruption and air embolism is always present, the lower-pressure venovenous circuit poses less of an immediate threat than does venoarterial ECMO. Because systemic anticoagulation is required, the long-term morbidity relates primarily to bleeding complications. Regional heparinization of the membrane lung has been successfully implemented, so this major drawback may soon be removed. ECCO$_2$R can provide the extended support for gas exchange required by patients whose lungs heal slowly. In skilled hands, ECCO$_2$R can be conducted for many weeks, with a successful outcome. This capability may be important to survival in the most severe cases, because prolonged periods of lung rest may be required to achieve healing.

Early studies strongly suggested that ECCO$_2$R could significantly improve survival in patients with acute lung injury. However, a recent randomized trial conducted in a single center failed to demonstrate a significant benefit from a strategy that included ECCO$_2$R,[41] and animal models of acute respiratory failure have produced conflicting results. Although an encouraging clinical experience with ECCO$_2$R has accumulated in well-selected patients in experienced centers, the technique has not been proved to be more effective than optimized conventional management.

INTRAVENOUS GAS EXCHANGE

A large-diameter venacaval catheter composed of numerous hollow fibers can accomplish substantial O_2 and CO_2 exchange intravenously, external to the native lungs. When the filament pack of the intravenous gas exchange (IVOX) catheter is unfurled, many thin-gauge, heparin-bonded hollow fibers fill the lumen of the vena cava without substantially impeding flow. As oxygen is drawn through these fibers and past venous blood en route to the right heart, gas exchange takes place across the gas-permeable walls of each filament. In an intact, 80-kg, hypoxemic, hypercarbic subject, the device is capable of delivering up to 170 ml of O_2 per minute and of removing up to 140 ml of CO_2 per minute. Performance varies, however, with size of the catheter, venous gas tensions, and blood flow. Hypercarbia enhances CO_2 removal. Although systemic anticoagulation during IVOX is recommended, the covalently bonded heparin coating of the catheters now available renders their surfaces less thrombogenic than those of earlier prototypes. Although animal studies indicated excellent tolerance and efficiency, the results of the first large-scale clinical studies have been disappointing. If successful, intracaval gas exchange may prove to be an important adjunct to the supportive care of patients with crises of either oxygenation or ventilation.[40] Apart from reducing the overall requirement for ventilatory pressure in the most seriously ill patients with respiratory failure, such techniques could, theoretically, provide weaning assistance or, perhaps, obviate mechanical ventilation in selected cases.

Tracheal Gas Insufflation

Tracheal gas insufflation (TGI) is a technique in which the anatomic dead space of the upper airway can be reduced or effectively bypassed by continuous or phasic injection of fresh gas near the carina.[6] Experimentation with techniques related to TGI has been undertaken for decades. In recent years, a number of investigators have explored the use of TGI as an adjunct to or replacement for conventional bulk flow ventilation.[6,7,27,42,49]

In concept, the efficiency of low tidal volume and low inflation pressure breaths is substantially improved by washing out the anatomic dead space proximal to and slightly beyond the site of fresh gas injection, improving the efficacy of alveolar ventilation (Fig. 177-8). Most benefit from TGI is seen with modest flows of fresh gas and appears to be greatest when the anatomic component exceeds the alveolar component of the physiological dead space. TGI is most effective in the presence of a very high preexisting Pa_{CO_2}.[42] Rather extensive experimental evidence and some encouraging, but limited, clinical experience[6,49] strongly suggest the potential clinical utility of this technique, both for breaths that are powered by positive pressure and for those that occur during spontaneous breathing. Chest wall vibration may enhance the effectiveness of TGI.[14] For the present, however, the technique clearly remains experimental, with significant problems yet to be solved regarding humidification, pressure relief, and mucosal protection before recommendations can be made for widespread clinical use.

Selective expiratory gas insufflation is probably the preferred method of accomplishing TGI because it offers similar efficacy and is less hazardous than continuous TGI.[7,49] The modified "reverse thrust" catheter may address problems related to humidification, mucosal trauma, and auto-PEEP.[27] Specially designed ET tubes conduct the fresh gas stream to the carinal level without interfering with suctioning and protect the mucosa without interfering with ventilation. TGI bears special promise in permissive hypercapnia.

OPTIONS TO ENHANCE OXYGENATION

Certain techniques for improving transpulmonary oxygen exchange (e.g., diuresis, transfusion) that do not require ventilatory manipulation are routinely applied by many clinicians when it is appropriate to do so. Other methods (e.g., administration of nitric oxide or aerosolized prostacyclin) have been introduced to attack the problem pharmacologically. Still another category of adjuncts to improve oxygen exchange modifies the distribution rather than the levels of airway pressures and distending forces.

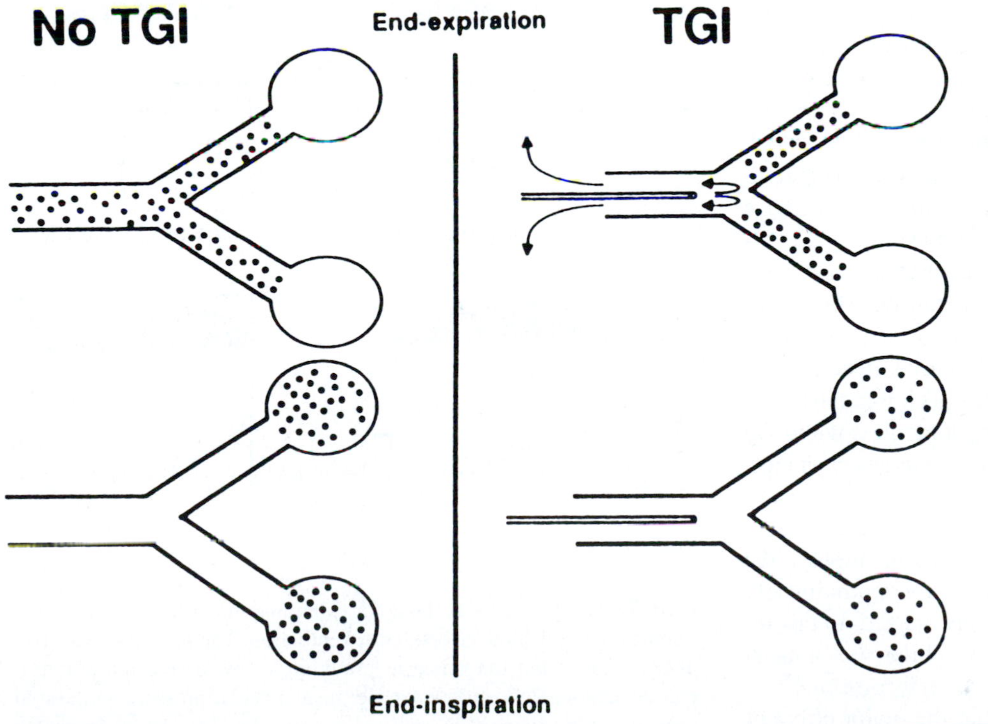

Independent (Differential) Lung Ventilation

When a common pressure is applied to lungs with markedly different inflation characteristics, appropriate pulmonary gas exchange is often difficult to achieve. If PEEP is applied, for example, the more distensible lung may overinflate, while the less distensible lung—still underinflated—receives a disproportionate share of the total blood flow. Aspiration, contusion, bronchopulmonary fistulas, lobar pneumonia, and unilateral lung transplantation sometimes present very challenging therapeutic problems related to the asymmetry of lung pathology.

Differential or independent lung ventilation (ILV) physically separates the ventilation to each lung with a cuffed, double-lumen ET tube. With establishment of two independent breathing cir-

No TGI   **End-expiration**   **TGI**

End-inspiration

FIGURE 177-8 Concept of tracheal gas insufflation (TGI). At the end of normal exhalation, the central airway is filled with CO_2-rich alveolar gas, symbolized as black dots. The application of TGI during expiration substitutes fresh gas, thereby improving ventilatory efficacy.

cuits, the levels of ventilation, inspired oxygen, and end-expiratory pressure appropriate to each lung can be individually adjusted, improving oxygen and CO_2 exchange. Even diffuse, apparently symmetric lung injury has been reported to respond well to ILV used in conjunction with lateral decubitus positioning of the patient.[5] Under these circumstances, a higher level of PEEP is applied to the lower lung, expanding it sufficiently to divert a significant fraction of the dependent blood flow to the well-distended upper lung. Synchronizing the inspiratory cycles of the two ventilators, once thought indispensable, is now believed optional.

Several potential problems should be considered before ILV is begun. Double-lumen tubes usually require fiberoptic bronchoscopy for correct placement. Slippage can result in occlusion of a major bronchus or failure of lung isolation. Current double-lumen tubes that securely cannulate the left main bronchus greatly facilitate this positioning process by their relative ease of insertion and stability of placement. Because they are partitioned, such tubes are unusually bulky, but they have a lower total cross-sectional lumen than a single tube of the same external diameter. Secretion retention or increased breathing workload may, therefore, pose a serious problem for some patients. Nasal intubation is not feasible, and deep sedation is invariably required. Despite these difficulties, ILV is a valuable option for selected problems that otherwise pose insurmountable management difficulties.

Inverse-Ratio Ventilation

More than a quarter century ago, it was first suggested—and it was later convincingly shown—that the oxygenation problems of infant respiratory distress syndrome might be addressed with a ventilatory strategy that extends the inspiratory period (duty cycle) beyond 50 percent of total cycle time (Fig. 177-9). Enthusiastic but largely anecdotal reports or uncontrolled studies appeared in the literature. The exact mechanism by which inverse-ratio ventilation (IRV) improves oxygen exchange remains somewhat unclear, but several plausible mechanisms have been proposed: (1) mean alveolar pressure and average lung volume rise as the pressurized inspiratory phase lengthens and auto-PEEP develops; (2) prolongation of the time during which end-inspiratory alveolar pressure is applied improves collateral ventilation and provides traction adequate to recruit alveolar units that otherwise tend to remain collapsed; and (3) lower mean and end-inspiratory flows are achieved, enabling lung units with long ventilatory time constants to participate actively in gas exchange. This effect has been documented in both animal and human studies; slowing end-inspiratory flow by using a decelerating waveform[48] or adding an end-inspiratory pause tends to improve the ventilatory efficiency of conventional methods by approximately 10 to 20 percent, even when T_I/T_T remains unchanged. In this respect, IRV is quite unlike PEEP, which for a similar rise in mean airway pressure tends to *accentuate* dead-space formation.[34]

The best available evidence suggests that the major effect of IRV on arterial oxygenation (and on cardiac output) is mediated by increasing average lung volume, as reflected under passive conditions by mean airway pressure.[34,37] However, there often

appears to be a substantial delay (perhaps hours) between the time at which IRV is applied or adjusted and the maximal benefit to Pa_{O_2}, suggesting the importance of sustained traction to alveolar recruitment.

In most reports, IRV has been implemented using a pressure-preset, time-cycled waveform (pressure-controlled IRV, or PC-IRV) in deeply sedated, paralyzed subjects. Pressure-preset ventilation effectively limits the risk of alveolar overdistention, but sacrifices control over the volume delivered with each tidal breath. Minute ventilation is a complex and often unpredictable function of pressure, frequency, and impedance. IRV also can be implemented with a volume-cycled algorithm (VC-IRV) that employs a slow, constant flow, a rapid, constant flow with an end-inspiratory pause, or a linearly decelerating flow waveform.[34,48]

VC-IRV can be implemented with most ventilators currently in use. Volume presetting affords control over tidal volume and minute ventilation, but it poses potential problems of its own.[34,48] Alveolar pressure is not controlled; therefore, changes in frequency, flow settings, or pause time can dramatically alter the peak and mean alveolar pressures. Setting appropriate alarms and maintaining rigid control of the ventilatory rhythm are mandatory whenever volume-cycled ventilation is applied at inspiratory duty cycles that exceed 0.5. The occasional patient with unusually subdued ventilatory drive and low ventilation requirements tolerates PC-IRV without the need to obliterate the endogenous breathing rhythm, particularly when the duty cycle is modestly extended

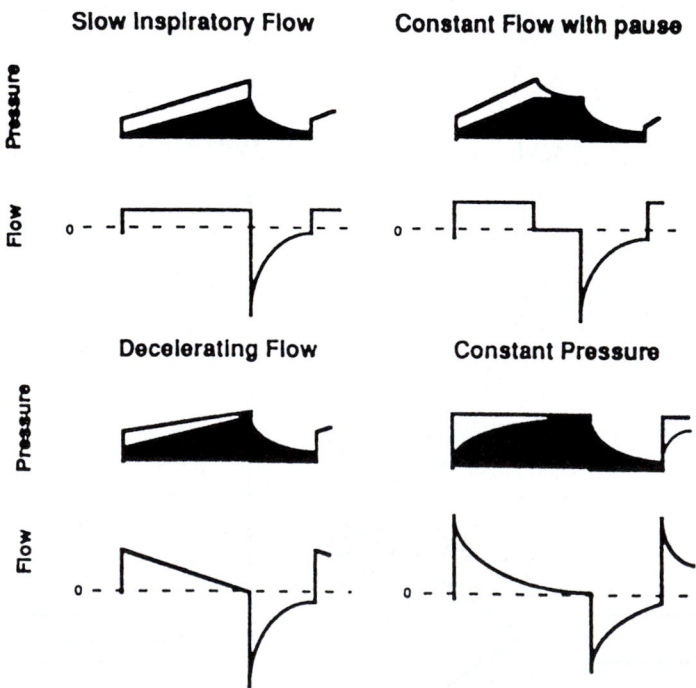

FIGURE 177-9 Four methods for extending the inspiratory time fraction or accomplishing inverse ratio ventilation. The primary benefits of inverse-ratio extension relate to providing a low or negligible rate of end-inspiratory flow and increasing mean alveolar pressure, without increasing peak alveolar distending pressure. Each goal can be accomplished with a variety of flow profiles in either the flow-controlled or pressure-controlled modes. *(From Marini et al, in Ventilatory Failure. Berlin, Springer-Verlag, 1991, pp 269–292, with permission.)*

(inspiratory-to-expiratory time ratio 2:1 or less). Spontaneous efforts cannot be allowed during VC-IRV, however, because increases in breathing frequency can dramatically raise peak and mean alveolar pressures in uncontrolled fashion. For the most seriously ill patients, therefore, PC-IRV may be the safer alternative. For both modes, close observation and monitoring of pressures and flows are essential.

Inverse ratios ranging from 1:1 to 4:1 have been successfully utilized in the clinical setting. However, to achieve the benefits of extending the inspiratory time fraction, it may not always be necessary to invert the inspiratory-to-expiratory ratio. Routine use of ratios greater than 3:1 should be discouraged until better evidence of clinical safety and efficacy is available. Moreover, provided that adequate end-expiratory alveolar pressure is maintained, there appears to be little advantage, and considerable danger, in extending the ratio beyond 2:1. At more extreme inversion ratios, hemodynamic tolerance declines and the potential for barotrauma increases significantly.

Maintenance of a certain minimum end-expiratory alveolar pressure (total PEEP—i.e., the sum of applied PEEP and auto-PEEP—in the range of 7 to 15 cmH$_2$O) is required *early* in the course of ARDS to prevent widespread alveolar collapse (Fig. 177-10).[36] At lower total PEEP levels, a distinct inflection point is frequently observed on the pressure–volume relationship of the respiratory system. Sufficient total PEEP ablates the inflection, which tends to disappear without PEEP later in the clinical course. Although auto-PEEP values in the suggested range can be generated by dynamic hyperinflation alone at very high inspiratory-to-expiratory ratios, PEEP is usually required at ratios of 2:1 or less in patients with acute lung injury, who have low lung compliance. During IRV, therefore, end-expiratory stop-flow pressures may be as important to monitor as are peak and mean alveolar pressures.

Careful comparisons have not shown a striking advantage of IRV over conventional-ratio ventilation in adult patients.[31] IRV has been criticized as dangerous and unnecessary,[54] but it may well prove advantageous if used cautiously and with appropriate attention to keeping alveolar pressures within acceptable limits. Smaller tidal volumes and higher Pa$_{CO_2}$ concentrations (permissive hypercapnia) may be required to maintain adequate control of peak, mean, and end-expiratory alveolar pressures.

Prone Positioning

A growing interest in therapeutic positioning has been stimulated by the observation that many patients with ARDS experience sig-

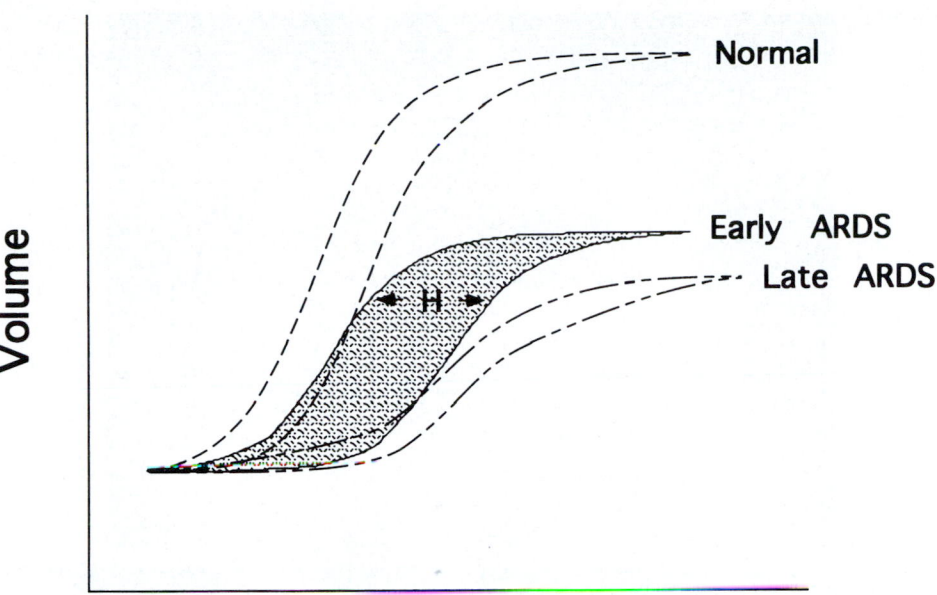

FIGURE 177-10   Static pressure–volume relationships for the normal lung and for early and late ARDS. Inspiratory pressures required to distend the lung are generally higher than those on the deflation limb. This hysteresis (H) is exaggerated in the early phase of ARDS because of inspiratory recruitment of lung volume. Sharp inflection and deflection zones appear on the inflation limb of the pressure–volume curve owing to widespread recruitment and overdistention, respectively. The tendency for hysteresis diminishes in the late stage of ARDS, whereas total lung compliance may decline further. (*From Marini and Wheeler,* [39a] *with permission.*)

nificantly improved pulmonary gas exchange when turned prone.[44] Recruitment of dorsal lung units with improved ventilation–perfusion matching seems to best explain this benefit,[1] and computed tomographic images in ARDS are quite consistent with this interpretation. Although most benefit is observed within minutes, delayed improvement of gas exchange may take hours to develop fully;[44] quite often, the benefit begins to wane after several hours. Some responders to prone positioning continue to maintain better gas exchange when turned back to the supine position.[44]

The prone position improves oxygen exchange in 50 to 70 percent of patients treated in the early phase of ARDS, allowing the physician to reduce both F$_{IO_2}$ and PEEP. Although hemodynamic parameters tend to remain unchanged, hypotension, desaturation, and arrhythmias may occur in the transition from the supine to the prone position. These problems generally do not persist and can be minimized by use of sedation, prior airway suctioning, and 100 percent inspired oxygen during the maneuver. Continuous arterial pressure monitoring, electrocardiography, and pulse oximetry are advisable. Attention must also be given to preserving the position and patency of intravascular lines and ET tubes during the turning process. Although the optimal frequency of supine-to-prone conversions is not clear, in current practice, most experienced centers "flip" patients once or twice daily. It seems reasonable to assign the relative duration in each position in proportion to the gas exchange response (equal times if no important gas exchange difference is observed).

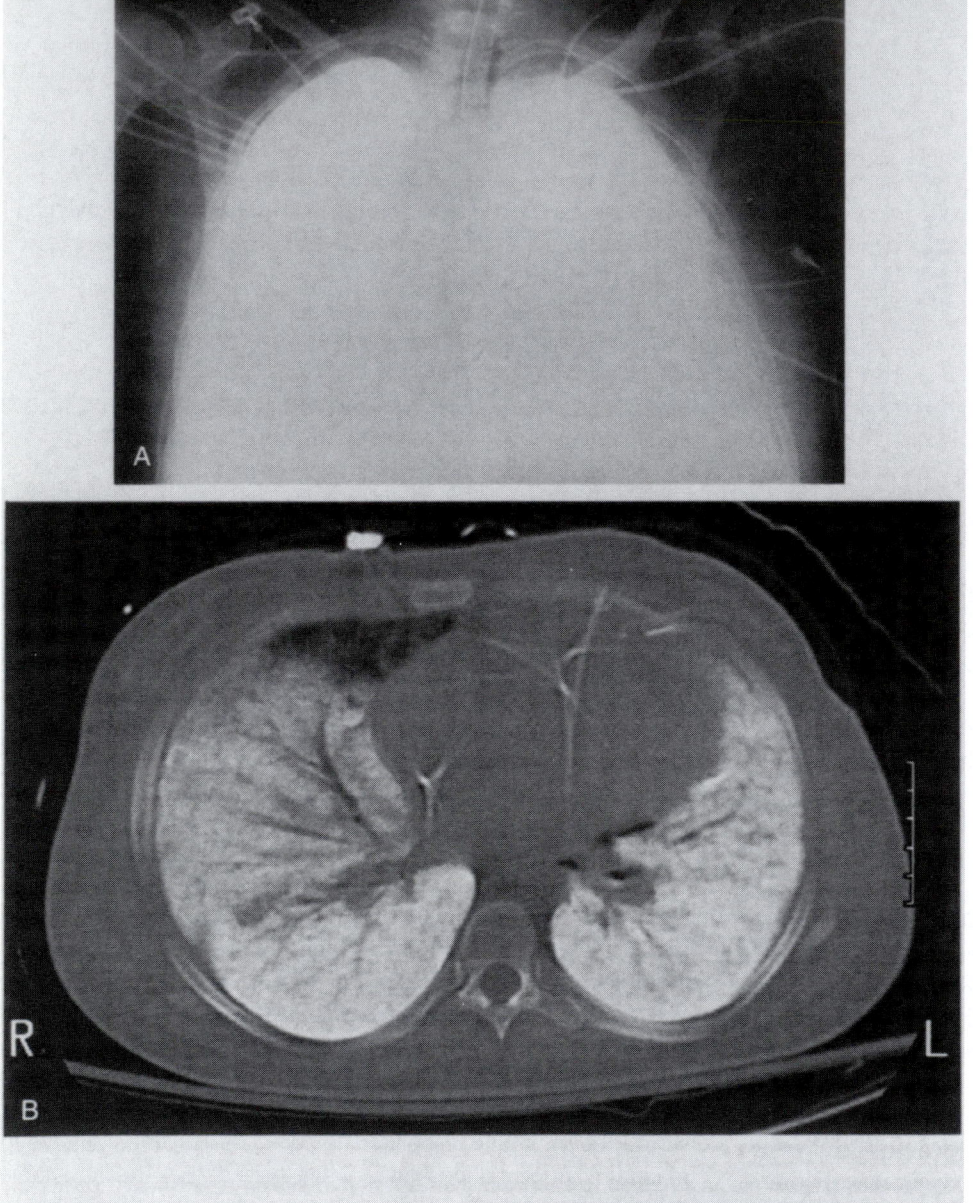

FIGURE 177-11 Chest radiograph (*A*) and computed tomographic scan (*B*) in a patient with ARDS treated with partial liquid ventilation. The extreme radiodensity of the perfluoro chemical tends to impair imaging assessment. (*Data based on Marini,[36] with permission.*)

Partial Liquid Ventilation

An exciting new approach to the problem of recruiting collapsed lung units is to fill the units with a gas-exchanging liquid perfluorocarbon (PFC).[17,24,28,53] Although feasible in the laboratory, full liquid breathing would be exceedingly difficult to implement in the clinical setting with current technology. *Partial* liquid ventilation, however, is quite feasible.[17,24] In partial liquid ventilation, routine tidal gas ventilation is performed with a conventional ventilator in conjunction with a PFC that partly or completely fills the functional residual capacity, thereby serving

the function of PEEP. PFCs dissolve generous volumes of O_2 and CO_2, distribute easily throughout the lung, and gravitate to the lung regions most at risk for airway closure and alveolar collapse.[53] PFCs are not absorbed into the bloodstream in significant amounts. Considerable laboratory and clinical research has been conducted in the use of perfluoro-octyl bromide (perflubron) for such purposes. This PFC is clear but radiopaque (Fig. 177-11), environmentally innocuous, and nonhistotoxic. It is eliminated by evaporation over a period of hours to days.

With a density twice that of water, perflubron gravitates to the most dependent lung regions and lowers the interfacial tension that normally exists between air and surfactant-depleted alveoli. Unlike endogenous or exogenous surfactants, the surface tension–lowering effect of perflubron is not inhibited by proteinaceous exudates. Moreover, secretions and debris lodged in distal airways and alveoli float on the dense PFC, being transported to the central airway during exhalation. These secretions can then be aspirated. Perflubron might find application as a lavage fluid, as it both preserves gas exchange more effectively than saline and, theoretically, tends to recover alveolar debris more effectively. A substantial proportion of blood flowing to dependent regions is redirected to better-ventilated nondependent sectors. PFC-filled alveoli are opened and, perhaps, protected against infection and lung damage. Although PFCs are physiologically exciting and intriguing as a clinical intervention, their final place in the management of ARDS remains unclear. The risks, indications, doses, and appropriate methods for implementing partial liquid ventilation have yet to be fully elucidated.

REFERENCES

1. Albert RK: One good turn . . . *Intensive Care Med* 20:247–248, 1994.
2. Amato MBP, Barbas CSV, Bonassa J, et al: Volume-assured pressure support ventilation (VAPSV): A new approach for reducing muscle workload during acute respiratory failure. *Chest* 102:1225–1234, 1992.
3. Amato MBP, Barbas CSV, Medeiros D, et al: Improved survival in ARDS: Beneficial effects of a lung protective strategy (abstract). *Am J Respir Crit Care Med* 153:A531, 1996.

4. Aubier M, Trippenbach T, Roussos C: Respiratory muscle fatigue during cardiogenic shock. *J Appl Physiol* 51:499–508, 1981.

5. Banner MJ, Blanch PB, Kirby RR: Imposed work of breathing and methods of triggering a demand flow, continuous positive airway pressure system. *Crit Care Med* 21:183–190, 1993.

6. Belghith M, Fierobe L, Brunet F, et al: Is tracheal gas insufflation an alternative to extrapulmonary gas exchangers in severe ARDS? *Chest* 107:1416–1419, 1995.

7. Burke WC, Nahum A, Ravenscraft SA, et al: Modes of tracheal gas insufflation: Comparison of continuous phase specific gas injection in normal dogs. *Am Rev Respir Dis* 148:562–568, 1993.

8. Bryan AC, Froese AB: Reflections on the HIFI trial. *Pediatrics* 87:565–567, 1991.

9. Chang HK, Harf A: High-frequency ventilation: A review. *Respir Physiol* 57:135–152, 1984.

10. Cinnella G, Conti G, Lofaso F, et al: Effects of assisted ventilation on the work of breathing: Volume-controlled versus pressure-controlled ventilation. *Am J Respir Crit Care Med* 153:1025–1033, 1996.

11. Clark RH, Gerstman DR, Null DM, deLemos RA: Prospective randomized trial of high frequency oscillatory and conventional ventilation in respiratory distress syndrome. *Pediatrics* 89:5–12, 1992.

12. Darioli R, Perret C: Mechanical controlled hypoventilation in status asthmaticus. *Am Rev Respir Dis* 129:385–387, 1984.

13. Dreyfuss D, Saumon G: Role of tidal volume, FRC, and end-inspiratory volume in the development of pulmonary edema following mechanical ventilation. *Am Rev Respir Dis* 148:1194–1203, 1993.

14. Eckmann DM, Gavriely N: Chest vibration redistributes intra-airway CO_2 during tracheal insufflation in ventilatory failure. *Crit Care Med* 24:451–457, 1996.

15. Feihl F, Perret C: Permissive hypercapnia: How permissive should we be? *Am J Respir Crit Care Med* 150:1722–1737, 1994.

16. Field S, Kelly SM, Macklem PT: The oxygen cost of breathing in patients with cardiorespiratory disease. *Am Rev Respir Dis* 126:9–13, 1982.

17. Fuhrman BP, Paczan PR, DeFrancisis M: Perfluorocarbon-associated gas exchange. *Crit Care Med* 19:712–722, 1991.

18. Gammon RB, Shin MS, Groves RH Jr, et al: Clinical risk factors for pulmonary barotrauma: A multivariate analysis. *Am J Respir Crit Care Med* 152:1235–1240, 1995.

19. Gattinoni L, Pesenti A, Bombino M: Relationships between lung computed tomographic density, gas exchange and PEEP in acute respiratory failure. *Anesthesiology* 69:824–832, 1988.

20. Gattinoni L, Pesenti A, Mascheroni D, et al: Low frequency positive pressure ventilation with extracorporeal CO_2 removal in severe acute respiratory failure. *JAMA* 256:881–886, 1986.

21. Guttmann J, Eberhard J, Fabry B, et al: Continuous calculation of intratracheal pressure in tracheally intubated patients. *Anesthesiology* 79:503–513, 1993.

22. Hickling KG, Henderson SJ, Jackson R: Low mortality associated with permissive hypercapnia in severe adult respiratory distress syndrome. *Intensive Care Med* 16:372–377, 1990.

23. The HIFI Study Group: High-frequency oscillatory ventilation compared with conventional mechanical ventilation in the treatment of respiratory failure in preterm infants. *New Engl J Med* 320:88–93, 1989.

24. Hirschl RB, Pranikoff T, Wise C, et al: Initial experience with partial liquid ventilation in adult patients with the acute respiratory distress syndrome. *JAMA* 275:383–389, 1996.

25. Jubran A, Tobin MJ: Use of flow-volume curves in detecting secretions in ventilator-dependent patients. *Am J Respir Crit Care Med* 150:766–769, 1994.

26. Knebel AR, Janson-Bjerklie SL, Malley JD, et al: Comparison of

27. Kolobow T, Powers T, Mandava S, et al: Intratracheal pulmonary ventilation (ITPV): Control of positive end-expiratory pressure at the level of the carina through the use of a novel ITPV catheter design. *Anesth Analg* 78:455–461, 1994.

28. Leach CL, Greenspan JS, Rubenstein SD, et al: Partial liquid ventilation with perflubron in premature infants with severe respiratory distress syndrome. *New Engl J Med* 335:761–767, 1996.

29. Leatherman J, Ravenscraft S: Low measured auto-positive end-expiratory pressure during mechanical ventilation of patients with severe asthma: Hidden auto-positive end-expiratory pressure. *Crit Care Med* 24:541–546, 1996.

30. Lemaire F, Teboul JL, Cinotti L, et al: Acute left ventricular dysfunction during unsuccessful weaning from mechanical ventilation. *Anesthesiology* 69:171–179, 1988.

31. Lessard MR, Guérot E, Loroin H, et al: Effects of pressure controlled with different I:E ratios versus volume-controlled ventilation on respiratory mechanics, gas exchange, and hemodynamics in patients with adult respiratory distress syndrome. *Anesthesiology* 80:983–991, 1994.

32. Lessard MR, Lofaso F, Brochard L: Expiratory muscle activity increases intrinsic positive end-expiratory pressure independently of dynamic hyperinflation in mechanically ventilated patients. *Am J Respir Crit Care Med* 151:562–569, 1995.

33. MacIntyre NR, Gropper C, Westfall T: Combining pressure-limiting and volume-cycling features in a patient-interactive mechanical breath. *Crit Care Med* 22:353–357, 1994.

34. Marcy TW, Marini JJ: Inverse ratio ventilation in ARDS: Rationale and implementation. *Chest* 100:494–504, 1990.

35. Marini JJ: Should PEEP be used in airflow obstruction? *Am Rev Respir Dis* 140:1–3, 1989.

36. Marini JJ: Evolving concepts in the ventilatory management of ARDS. *Clin Chest Med* 17:555–575, 1996.

37. Marini JJ, Ravenscraft SA: Mean airway pressure: Physiological determinants and clinical importance. Part 1: Physiological determinants and measurements. *Crit Care Med* 20:1461–1472, 1992. Part 2: Clinical implications. *Crit Care Med* 20:1604–1616, 1992.

38. Marini JJ, Rodriguez RM, Lamb VJ: The inspiratory workload of patient-initiated mechanical ventilation. *Am Rev Respir Dis* 134:902–909, 1986.

39. Marini JJ, Smith TC, Lamb VJ: External work output and force generation during synchronized intermittent mechanical ventilation: Effect of machine assistance on breathing effort. *Am Rev Respir Dis* 138:1169–1179, 1988.

39a. Marini JJ, Wheeler AW: *Critical Care Medicine—the Essentials*, 2d ed. Baltimore, Williams & Wilkins, 1997.

40. Mira JP, Brunet F, Belghith M, et al: Reduction of ventilator settings allowed by intravenous oxygenator (IVOX) in ARDS patients. *Intensive Care Med* 21:11–17, 1995.

41. Morris AH, Wallace CJ, Menlove RL, et al: Randomized clinical trial of pressure-controlled inverse ratio ventilation and extracorporeal CO_2 removal for adult respiratory distress syndrome. *Am J Respir Crit Care Med* 149:295–305, 1994.

42. Nahum A, Shapiro RS, Ravenscraft SA, et al: Efficacy of expiratory tracheal gas insufflation in a canine model of lung injury. *Am J Respir Crit Care Med* 152:489–495, 1995.

43. Ninane V, Yernault JC, de Troyer A: Intrinsic PEEP in patients with chronic obstructive pulmonary disease: Role of expiratory muscles. *Am Rev Respir Dis* 148:1037–1042, 1993.

44. Pappert D, Rossaint R, Slama K, et al: Influence of positioning on ventilation-perfusion relationships in severe adult respiratory distress syndrome. *Chest* 106:1511–1516, 1994.

breathing comfort during weaning with two ventilatory modes. *Am J Respir Crit Care Med* 149:14–18, 1994.

45. Pelosi P, D'Andrea L, Vitale G, et al: Vertical gradient of regional lung inflation in adult respiratory distress syndrome. *Am J Respir Crit Care Med* 149:8–13, 1994.

46. Pepe PE, Marini JJ: Occult positive end-expiratory pressure in mechanically ventilated patients with airflow obstruction. *Am Rev Respir Dis* 126:166–170, 1982.

47. Petrof BJ, Legare M, Goldberg P, et al: Continuous positive airway pressure reduces work of breathing and dyspnea during weaning from mechanical ventilation in severe chronic obstructive pulmonary disease. *Am Rev Respir Dis* 141:281–289, 1990.

48. Ravenscraft SA, Burke WC, Marini JJ: Volume cycled decelerating flow: An alternative form of mechanical ventilation. *Chest* 101:1342–1351, 1992.

49. Ravenscraft SA, Shapiro RS, Nahum A, et al: Tracheal gas insufflation: Catheter effectiveness determined by expiratory flush volume. *Am J Respir Crit Care Med* 153:1817–1824, 1996.

50. Rossi A, Gottfried SB, Zocchi L, et al: Measurement of static compliance of the total respiratory system in patients with acute respiratory failure during mechanical ventilation: The effect of intrinsic positive end-expiratory pressure. *Am Rev Respir Dis* 131:672–677, 1985.

51. Rouby JJ, Lherm T, de Lasale E, et al: Histologic aspects of pulmonary barotrauma in critically ill patients with acute respiratory failure. *Intensive Care Med* 19:383–389, 1993.

52. Roupie E, Dambrosio M, Servillo G, et al: Titration of tidal volume and induced hypercapnia in acute respiratory distress syndrome. *Am J Respir Crit Care Med* 152:121–128, 1995.

53. Slutsky, AS: *Mechanical ventilation. American College of Chest Physicians'* Concensus Conference. *Chest* 104:1833–1859, 1993.

54. Shanholtz C, Brower R: Should inverse ratio ventilation be used in adult respiratory distress syndrome? *Am J Respir Crit Care Med* 149:1354–1358, 1994.

55. Slutsky AS: Mechanical ventilation. American College of Chest Physicians' Consensus Conference. *Chest* 104:1833–1859, 1993.

56. Smith TC, Marini JJ: Impact of PEEP on lung mechanics and work of breathing in severe airflow obstruction: The effect of PEEP on auto-PEEP. *J Appl Physiol* 65:1488–1499, 1988.

57. Stock MC, Downs JB, Frolichter DA: Airway pressure release ventilation. *Crit Care Med* 15:462–466, 1987.

58. Villar J, Winston B, Slutsky AS: Non-conventional techniques of ventilatory support. *Crit Care Clin* 6:579–603, 1990.

59. Younes M: Proportional assist ventilation: A new approach to ventilatory support. *Am Rev Respir Dis* 145:114–120, 1991.

60. Zapol WM, Snider MT, Hill JD: Extracorporeal membrane oxygenation in severe acute respiratory failure. *JAMA* 242:2193–2196, 1979.

CHAPTER 178

NUTRITION IN ACUTE RESPIRATORY FAILURE

Susan K. Pingleton

Nutrition is an important aspect of care in all critically ill patients, particularly those with acute respiratory failure, since poor nutrition adversely affects respiration and can increase morbidity and mortality in the intensive care unit. Adverse effects of malnutrition on lung function include diminished respiratory muscle strength, altered ventilatory capacity, and impaired immune function. Repletion of nutritional status or refeeding results in improvement of respiratory functional status and may be important in improving outcome.

Nutritional management of patients with acute respiratory failure is complicated, since many diseases may result in this syndrome. To facilitate presentation of this topic, acute respiratory failure will be classified according to the patient's nutritional status and the presence or absence of hypermetabolism. Each category defines a specific, characteristic metabolic alteration for which nutritional goals and support differ. *Nutritional status* is defined as whether malnutrition is present; *hypermetabolism* is the degree of excess metabolic activity in a disease state. Clinical prototypes based on this nutritional classification of acute respiratory failure include the patient with severe chronic obstructive pulmonary disease (COPD) who is malnourished but not hypermetabolic and the septic patient with acute respiratory distress syndrome (ARDS) who is generally well nourished but extremely hypermetabolic (Table 178-1). This chapter focuses on the nutritional pathophysiology, goals of treatment, and support of these two general, but diverse, kinds of patients with acute respiratory failure. Nutritional assessment, methods of nutrient delivery, monitoring of nutritional therapy, and complications of nutritional support are discussed. Utilizing this nutritional classification of acute respiratory failure, general principles of nutrition can be applied to respiratory failure resulting from other diseases.

OVERVIEW OF EFFECTS OF MALNUTRITION

Before considering malnutrition in relation to specific pulmonary disorders, including COPD and ARDS, a review of the impact of starvation on intermediary metabolism and of the adverse respiratory effects of malnutrition is warranted.

Effects of Starvation on Intermediary Metabolism

Potential energy sources for fasting humans include glycogen, protein, and fat (Fig. 178-1). Glycogen stores are limited and are totally expended within the first 1 to 3 days of fasting. Body protein represents a large potential energy source, but since each molecule of protein serves specific nonfuel functions, including structural, functional, and enzymatic, prolonged survival depends on protein conservation. Thus, adaptation to starvation involves mechanisms by which fat and fat-derived fuels become the major energy sources, glucose utilization is reduced, and protein is conserved.

In simple starvation or undernutrition, fat and protein are consumed, but the loss of protein is minimized by reducing its use

TABLE 178-1

Nutritional Classification of Acute Respiratory Failure

Malnutrition

> Prototype: severe chronic obstructive pulmonary disease (COPD)

Hypermetabolism

> Prototype: septic acute respiratory distress syndrome (ARDS)

as a source of energy. Nitrogen loss is modified by mobilization of fat; enhanced fat oxidation is the principal source of energy in starvation. However, some protein wasting does occur, despite the availability of fat; protein wasting becomes markedly accelerated when fat stores are used up. For example, when body weight drops to less than 80 percent of ideal body weight, in the spontaneously breathing patient with COPD, protein catabolism occurs.

In critical illness, protein catabolism occurs to provide energy. With inadequate caloric intake, energy sources in critically ill patients are derived from protein breakdown and gluconeogenesis. Of the various protein "pools" available, muscle protein is particularly susceptible to catabolism as a fuel source. Inspiratory and expiratory respiratory muscles, primarily the diaphragm and intercostals, as skeletal muscles, are susceptible to this catabolic effect. Although the diaphragm, as the principal respiratory muscle, has been the focus of most investigation, the considerations below are generally valid for all respiratory muscles. It is important to note that few, if any, data exist based on direct examination of respiratory muscle function and malnutrition in critically ill, mechanically ventilated patients.

Adverse Respiratory Effects of Malnutrition

Malnutrition reduces diaphragmatic muscle mass in health and disease (Table 178-2).[2] In necropsy studies, body weight and diaphragmatic muscle mass were reduced to 70 percent and 60 percent of normal in underweight patients dying from a variety of diseases.[2] Animal studies confirm the loss of diaphragmatic strength in prolonged and acute nutritional deprivation. Respiratory muscle function is also impaired in poorly nourished hu-

mans. When malnourished patients without lung disease were studied, respiratory muscle strength, maximal voluntary ventilation, and vital capacity were reduced by 37 percent, 41 percent, and 63 percent, respectively.[3] Respiratory muscle strength in patients without systemic disease is also decreased. Maximal inspiratory pressures are lower in malnourished postoperative patients compared with normally nourished patients. Similar findings have been reported in patients with anorexia nervosa, a relatively pure model of malnutrition without systemic disease. Transdiaphragmatic pressure, as measured using phrenic nerve stimulation, is markedly diminished in patients with anorexia nervosa prior to institution of enteral nutritional support.[41]

Malnutrition also affects ventilatory drive. The interaction of nutrition and ventilatory drive appears to be a direct function of the influence of nutrition on metabolic rate. In general, conditions that reduce metabolic rate reduce ventilatory drive. A decrease in metabolic rate occurs with starvation. A parallel fall in metabolic rate and hypoxic ventilatory response has been documented in humans.[4] A 58 percent reduction in the ventilatory response to hypoxia was found in volunteers placed on a balanced diet of 550 kcal per day for 10 days. The ventilatory response returned to normal with refeeding. Ventilatory response is also affected by dietary constituents. After a 7-day, protein-free diet, a blunted ventilatory response to carbon dioxide has been observed.[6]

Consequences of decreased respiratory strength and decreased ventilatory drive may include impaired cough and, hence, increased risk for atelectasis and pneumonia in spontaneously breathing patients with respiratory disease. Decreased respiratory muscle strength and drive may also prolong the duration of mechanical ventilation in patients who, otherwise, are candidates for weaning. Thus, the potential for adverse outcome is present in patients who are malnourished from their disease, as well as in patients with respiratory disease who develop malnutrition as a consequence of other intercurrent diseases.

Malnutrition also alters immune function. Protein-calorie malnutrition is one of the most frequent causes of acquired immunodeficiency in humans. Chemotaxis and opsonic function and phagocytic function usually remain normal or are mildly depressed, and intracellular killing is decreased.[45] The thymus, spleen, and lymph nodes become markedly atrophic, and lymphocyte numbers may decrease. Although immunoglobulin levels remain normal or are slightly increased, antibody responses may be depressed. Consequences of altered immune function may include increased respiratory infections, such as pneumonia.

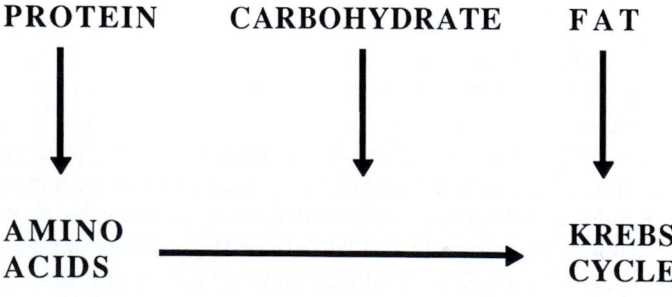

PROTEIN CARBOHYDRATE FAT

AMINO ACIDS → KREBS CYCLE

FIGURE 178-1 Substrate metabolism in starvation. Initial energy sources are glycogen stores, which are rapidly depleted. Fat is then used as energy. Protein is catabolized for energy after fat stores are depleted.

TABLE 178-2

Adverse Effects of Malnutrition on Respiratory Function

Decreased respiratory muscle strength
Altered ventilatory drive
Impaired immunologic function

MALNUTRITION IN COPD

The effect of nutritional status on respiratory muscle function in patients with chronic obstructive lung disease is controversial. In COPD, primary abnormalities of decreased inspiratory pressure and increased work of breathing are found. Inspiratory muscle weakness, as assessed by maximal inspiratory pressure, results from the mechanical disadvantage at which inspiratory muscles are placed due to hyperinflation and, perhaps, generalized muscle weakness. Controversy exists as to the additive role of undernutrition in causing the measured inspiratory muscle weakness. Patients with cystic fibrosis (CF) who had both hyperinflation and malnutrition were compared with asthmatics who had hyperinflation but no malnutrition, with patients with anorexia nervosa who had malnutrition but no hyperinflation, and with control patients who had neither.[52] Peak inspiratory pressure in hyperinflated patients with CF was decreased, as were pressures in patients with anorexia nervosa. With normalization for lung volume, however, there was no difference in inspiratory strength in the CF group. These data suggest that hyperinflation may be a major cause of diminished respiratory muscle weakness in COPD. In contrast, studies of renutrition in COPD and CF in which improved muscle strength was documented suggest that malnutrition is an important cause of diminished muscle strength.[55]

In addition to diminished muscle mass and hyperinflation, a number of other nutritional factors can alter diaphragmatic strength in patients with COPD as well as other respiratory diseases. Mineral and electrolyte deficiencies impair respiratory muscle function. Hypophosphatemia reduces diaphragmatic contractile strength, as measured by transdiaphragmatic pressures in mechanically ventilated patients with acute respiratory failure.[7] Hypocalcemia and hypomagnesemia are also associated with decreased diaphragmatic function. Improvement in diaphragmatic strength has been demonstrated in hypomagnesemic patients following magnesium repletion.

Frequency of Malnutrition in COPD

A substantial proportion of patients with COPD is malnourished. The incidence depends largely on disease severity, which can be assessed in several ways. As many as 25 percent of outpatients with COPD may be malnourished, and almost 50 percent of patients with COPD admitted to the hospital have evidence of malnutrition. The incidence of malnutrition in critically ill patients with COPD and acute respiratory failure is 60 percent.[23] When disease severity is assessed by degree of pulmonary function and gas exchange abnormalities, patients with chronic hypoxemia, or those with normoxemia but with severe airflow obstruction (FEV_1 < 35 percent), demonstrate a 50 percent incidence of malnutrition. An incidence of 25 percent is found in patients with moderate airflow obstruction.[44]

Poor nutritional status may adversely affect respiratory function in patients with lung disease who are spontaneously breathing, as well as those who are mechanically ventilated, by impairing respiratory muscle function, ventilatory drive, or pulmonary defense mechanism. As noted previously, adverse effects of malnutrition occur independent of the presence or absence of primary lung disease. However, adverse effects of malnutrition may be additive in some patients with acute respiratory failure, including those with respiratory failure due to COPD.

In COPD, primary abnormalities of decreased inspiratory pressure and increased work of breathing are found. As noted previously, inspiratory muscle weakness, as assessed by maximal inspiratory pressure, also results from both the mechanical disadvantage at which inspiratory muscles are placed due to hyperinflation and generalized muscle weakness.[32] In COPD, inspiratory muscle weakness must be severe for hypercapnia to occur. In patients with myopathy, hypercapnia occurs when inspiratory pressures are less than one-third of normal. However, hypercapnia is found in the majority of patients with COPD when inspiratory pressures are only less than one-half of normal.[43] Thus, hypercapnia occurs with much less respiratory muscle weakness when other mechanical abnormalities that increase the work of breathing are present. Indeed, malnutrition may further compromise already reduced lung function. Dyspnea may worsen in the spontaneously breathing patient with COPD. Hypercapnic respiratory failure may be precipitated and weaning from mechanical ventilation made more difficult in the malnourished patient with COPD compared with the normally nourished patient with COPD.

Effect of Renutrition on Malnutrition in COPD

Nutritional repletion can improve diminished respiratory muscle strength in some patients. A 37 percent increase in maximal inspiratory pressure and a 12 percent increase in body cell mass were found in 21 of 29 hospitalized patients given parenteral nutrition for 2 to 4 weeks.[27] Short-term oral refeeding in malnourished patients with COPD can also improve respiratory muscle function, although the improvement appears to depend on the presence of weight gain. When 6 ambulatory patients with COPD were given oral nutritional repletion for 2 weeks, body weight increased by 6 percent and transdiaphragmatic pressure increased by 41 percent.[55] In contrast, 8 weeks of nutritional supplementation in 21 malnourished patients with COPD produced no change in weight and no change in respiratory muscle function.[33]

Intensive, nocturnal, nasoenterally administered nutrition in patients with COPD and CF can result in weight gain and improved respiratory muscle and pulmonary function.[53] Renutrition has also been found to improve diaphragmatic contractility in a more "pure" model of malnutrition, that of anorexia nervosa.[41] After 1 month of enteral nutrition (weight gain of 15 percent), stimulated transdiaphragmatic pressure was increased from 16 ± 5 cmH$_2$O to 23 ± 7 cmH$_2$O, documenting improved diaphragmatic function with renutrition. With long-term, nocturnal enteral feeding, patients with CF were found to have improved pulmonary function tests in conjunction with significant weight gain.

The mechanisms of improved muscle performance with renutrition are not clear. In animal and human studies, chronic hypocaloric dieting produces changes in skeletal muscle that may be important in the genesis of muscle dysfunction. In addition to protein catabolism, these changes include depletion of glycolytic and oxidative enzymes, reduction in high-energy phosphate stores, and increases in intracellular calcium. Severe malnutrition depresses muscle glycolytic activity, reducing the availability of energy from glycolysis during muscle contraction. Succinate dehydrogenase, phosphofructokinase, and hydroxy-acyl-CoA-dehydrogenase are reduced in skeletal muscle homogenates of malnourished rats.

Energy stores are also decreased in severe malnutrition. A fall in creatine phosphate level has been reported in a 2-day fasting rat model; the fall is associated with a loss of total muscle creatinine. In addition to the decrease in energy-related phosphorus reserves reported in this study, calculated free adenosine 5′-diphosphate (ADP) rose, suggesting deficient oxidative phosphorylation. The findings suggest that reduced levels of glycolytic and oxidative enzymes, such as phosphofructokinase and succinate dehydrogenase, may limit substrate flux through glycolytic and oxidative pathways.

The electrophysiological properties of muscle can also be altered by modification of cell membrane properties that decrease sodium-potassium pump activity, alter ionic permeability, and create an imbalance in the intracellular electrolyte composition. Therefore, alterations in muscle contractile and endurance properties are not simply a result of changes in the amount of lean tissue. Indeed, studies of renutrition in hypocaloric dieting and fasting individuals, and severe starvation of patients with anorexia nervosa, document improvement in muscle performance at a time when significant changes in body composition cannot be detected. Changes in intracellular electrolytes may be responsible for the early improvement in muscle contractile and endurance properties noted with renutrition.

MALNUTRITION IN ARDS

Malnutrition in ARDS is an important area for consideration. In general, the topic can be reviewed with respect to the effect that the hypercatabolic state that characterizes ARDS has on intermediary metabolism, and the role of hypermetabolism in ARDS.

Effects of Hypermetabolism on Intermediary Metabolism

The critically ill patient faces multiple metabolic stresses, such as sepsis, the systemic inflammatory response syndrome (SIRS), or injury, which markedly increase energy demands. A global acceleration of metabolism occurs in patients with burns, trauma, or sepsis. Thus, critical illness and injury may precipitate metabolic changes that lead to severe and disabling nutritional derangements. These processes are collectively referred to as the *metabolic response to injury* or the *stress response.*

The characteristic metabolic alterations that accompany the response to injury or severe infection have been well described in a variety of patients. In general, patients frequently demonstrate a measured energy expenditure that is greater than predicted in the setting of metabolic stresses such as burns, major surgery, or sepsis. Changes in carbohydrate, fat, and protein metabolism not normally seen in simple starvation are reported in patients with metabolic stress (Fig. 178-2). Increased glucocorticoid and glucagon levels stimulate gluconeogenesis at the expense of lean body tissues, predominantly skeletal muscle. Pro-

tein synthesis is increased, although the rate of catabolism is also accelerated. There is net protein loss, which is manifested as high urinary nitrogen excretion and low serum visceral protein concentrations. Ineffective peripheral utilization of glucose occurs, manifested by an elevated plasma glucose, despite normal or elevated levels of insulin. Fatty acids are utilized increasingly for fuel. The magnitude of these abnormalities is directly proportional to the extent of injury.

The metabolic states that follow injury are described as the *ebb* and *flow* phases.[35] The ebb phase, a phase of initial metabolic dormancy, is characterized by decreased oxygen consumption, inadequate circulation, fluid imbalances, and cellular shock. It lasts 24 to 36 h and gives way to a metabolic peak, or flow phase—a hyperdynamic phase in which substrates are mobilized for energy production. The flow phase is characterized by increased cellular activity and hormonal stimulation. Metabolic rate increases, body temperature rises, and nitrogen loss accelerates. Clinical signs of hypermetabolism include increased cardiac output, tachycardia, bounding peripheral pulses, and a widened pulse pressure. In hypermetabolic patients, both the cardiac index and oxygen consumption are proportional to the severity of illness. Hypermetabolic patients are generally febrile; an increase in body temperature is associated with an increase in metabolic rate of approximately 10 percent per degree above 37°C. Hypermetabolic patients clearly have increased metabolic expenditure and, therefore, increased energy (caloric) needs.

One of the hallmark features of the stress response is protein catabolism, with increased urinary nitrogen loss and muscle wasting (i.e., a hypercatabolic state). The starved patient loses approximately 75 g of muscle protein per day, or about 200 to 300 g of muscle tissue daily. The stressed patient loses considerably more. As much as 250 g of muscle protein, or 750 to 1000 g of muscle mass, may be lost each day. With an increase in protein catabolism, energy needs are met by deamination of amino acids, which provide carbon skeltons for glucose production at sites of gluconeogenesis, such as the liver. Skeletal muscle is the predominant reservoir of amino acids mobilized to the liver. The net loss of amino acids from muscle is due to an increased rate of

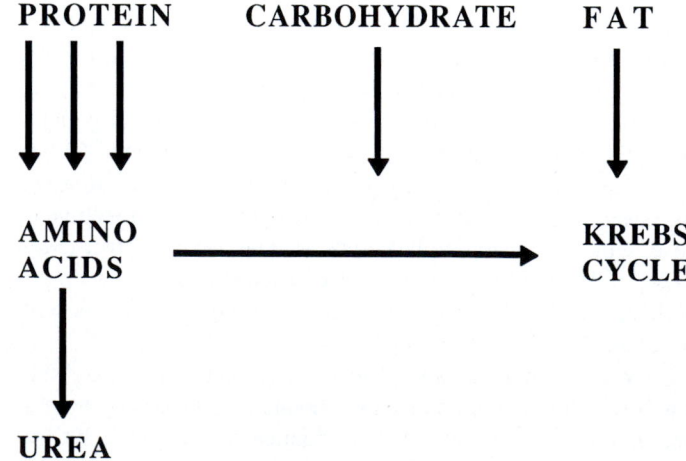

FIGURE 178-2 Substrate metabolism in hypermetabolism. Protein is preferentially catabolized for energy.

muscle protein breakdown and a decreased rate of synthesis. Protein breakdown is similar to other responses to injury in that the intensity of nitrogen loss is proportional to the severity of injury.

The hypermetabolic stress response results in increased energy needs. Up-regulation of metabolism in the stressed patient is at least partly regulated by hormonal and inflammatory mediators. Inadequate insulin levels and elevated levels of glucagon, glucocorticoids, and catecholamines generate glucose at the expense of nitrogen stores (i.e., protein catabolism occurs). Hyperglycemia and insulin resistance follow. The hypothalamic–pituitary axis is stimulated. Growth hormone augments the insulin response to glucose mobilization and use of fat stores and improves nitrogen balance. In addition to the alterations in hormonally mediated processes, multiple inflammatory mediators—including cytokines, such as tumor necrosis factor (TNF), and interleukins (II), such as IL-1, IL-2, IL-6, and IL-8—promote hypermetabolism.

Hypermetabolism in ARDS

Although patients with ARDS may be hypermetabolic during any phase of their illness, hypermetabolism in ARDS is most commonly associated with infection, especially sepsis. When ARDS is a component of multiple system organ failure (MSOF) syndrome, clinical symptoms and signs of hypermetabolism are common.[13] Following onset of ARDS, patients follow one of several clinical patterns.[38]

The favorable clinical course of ARDS is characterized by resolution of hypermetabolism and respiratory failure within 7 to 10 days and the absence of events that predispose to further injury. Resolution of ARDS occurs over several weeks, and the patient survives, albeit with some abnormalities of pulmonary function.

The unfavorable course of ARDS is characterized by death after a prolonged period of respiratory insufficiency. Death is frequently due to MSOF, in which hypermetabolism and infection are common. Less frequently, death occurs after a rapidly progressive downhill course marked by decreasing lung compliance and worsening hypoxemia. Such patients are often not hypermetabolic. Thus, although not well studied, hypermetabolism may be associated with the onset or evolution of ARDS. The duration of hypermetabolism most commonly depends on the cause and the likelihood of successful treatment. During the course of ARDS, hypermetabolism is most often due to infection (i.e., sepsis). Recently, a fibroproliferative response in the later stages of ARDS has been described that is associated with manifestations of hypermetabolism that mimic infection, but in which infectious agents cannot be identified.[38]

NUTRITIONAL ASSESSMENT

The primary function of nutritional assessment is identification of altered nutritional status, most commonly, malnutrition. Such identification warrants a clinical decision—namely, the need to provide nutritional repletion through a variety of routes. Only when hypermetabolism, with its associated protein breakdown, continues unabated for a prolonged period, or is extremely intense for a relatively short period, will techniques of nutritional assessment reveal abnormalities. Therefore, the clinical utility of nutritional assessment resides largely in those patients who, upon admission to the intensive care unit, are suspected of malnutrition. Nutritional assessment techniques are much less helpful during the course of a critical illness with acute respiratory failure.

Assessment of malnutrition in critically ill patients includes evaluation of clinical, anthropometric, chemical, and immunologic parameters that reflect altered body composition.[21] Currently no one, readily available test is both sensitive and specific for malnutrition in critically ill patients. All tests suffer from significant limitations, and any clinical application has to be considered in the light of the limitations.

Loss of body weight is a universal accompaniment of protein-calorie malnutrition (PCM) and provides a readily accessible indication of altered nutritional status. Weight loss in excess of 10 percent of ideal body weight (IBW) suggests malnutrition. Unfortunately, many critically ill patients are edematous, and measured weight does not reflect the real body cell mass.

Hepatic secretory proteins, such as albumin, transferrin, retinol-binding protein, and prealbumin, are markers of visceral protein stores and are used in nutritional assessment. Hepatic protein production, however, is influenced by numerous factors in addition to nutritional status, including hepatic dysfunction, protein-losing states, and acute infection or inflammation. The frequent coexistence of these conditions in patients in the intensive care unit limits use of these proteins as markers of nutritional deficiency or the effectiveness of nutritional support.

Anthropometry involves measurement of skinfold thickness, body circumferences, and skeletal breadths to divide the body into compartments of fat, muscle tissue, and skeletal mass. The primary advantages of anthropometry over more complex body composition measurements include its simplicity, safety, cost, and widespread application. However, although techniques of measurement are standardized, interpretation of results remains controversial and of limited value in the critical care setting.

The *creatinine-height index* is a theoretic estimate of lean body mass derived from measurement of the 24-h urinary creatinine excretion, which is compared to standard values based on height. Factors that influence creatinine excretion and, therefore, complicate the interpretation of this index include age, diet, exercise, stress, and renal disease.

Cellular immunity or *delayed cutaneous hypersensitivity* are commonly tested by assessing recall to skin-test antigens, such as Candida, mumps, Trichophyton, and streptokinase-streptodornase (SKSD). Depression of cellular immunity has been associated consistently with malnutrition; nutritional repletion is associated with improved immunocompetence. In patients in the intensive care unit, the utility of skin testing is limited by multiple factors, such as sepsis, malignancy, radiotherapy, chemotherapy, burns, and other immunocompromising conditions. Technical application and interpretation of skin tests in this patient population remain difficult.

Multiparameter nutritional indexes have been proposed in an attempt to overcome the difficulties with sensitivity and specificity of single tests of nutritional assessment. The prognostic nutritional index (PNI) is a mathematical formula that combines measurements of serum albumin, triceps skinfold thickness, transferrin levels, and measurement of delayed hypersensitivity skin testing.[11] The PNI may predict major morbidity in surgical patients, but its utility in the intensive care unit and in medical patients is less well evaluated.

Muscle function tests have been used as a marker of nutritional status. Clinical investigations have focused on assessment of the abductor pollici, handgrip dynamometry, and respiratory muscle strength.[27,36] In malnourished patients, changes in twitch characteristics of the abductor pollici occur with stimulation of the ulnar nerve. The lack of technical expertise and the need for specialized equipment limit widespread clinical application. Handgrip dynamometry can predict postoperative complications. Respiratory muscle strength, as assessed by maximal mouth or transdiaphragmatic pressures; endurance, as assessed by maximal voluntary ventilation; and vital capacity measurements are reduced in malnourished patients.[3] Limitations of these techniques in the critical care setting are multiple, and they include the need for an awake, alert patient. Metabolic factors, such as hypercapnia, hypoxia, use of medications, and intrinsic muscle diseases also complicate interpretation.

Newer, more sophisticated methods of nutritional assessment currently being evaluated include nuclear magnetic resonance, whole-body conductance and impedance, and neutron activation. Little data exist regarding the utility of these methods with patients in the intensive care unit.

In summary, multiple tests and combinations of tests are available to assess nutritional status. No simple recommendation may be given regarding the "best" test for nutritional assessment. Use of any of these methods may be appropriate, providing the limitations are clearly understood. Although not studied specifically in the intensive care unit, clinical assessment of nutritional status, including measured weight loss (>10 percent of IBW) and physical findings of weight loss, may be as reliable indicators of malnutrition as are more complex tests of nutritional assessment.[8]

General indications for nutritional support in any critically ill patient include inadequate or absent oral intake, presence of malnutrition, or anticipated prolonged clinical course. In patients with acute respiratory failure, the presence or absence of mechanical ventilation is often the first factor considered in the assessment of nutritional support. Nonintubated patients who do not require mechanical ventilation (invasive or noninvasive) are more able to maintain spontaneous oral intake, although this aspect of care needs to be monitored carefully. Nutritional support in these patients may require only appropriate nutritional supplementation to ensure adequate nutritional intake. As discussed previously, mechanically ventilated patients with acute respiratory failure may be considered with regard to two general categories of nutritional status: malnourished or hypermetabolic.

The diagnosis of malnutrition in a ventilated patient with acute respiratory failure mandates nutritional support to prevent further adverse effects of the malnutrition (see above). Obviously, if the respiratory failure is thought to be self-limited, e.g., due to a sedative drug overdose, aggressive nutritional support is not indicated. Malnutrition can be diagnosed upon admission to the intensive care unit, or less commonly, after a prolonged course of hypermetabolic illness. In either circumstance, evaluation or reevaluation of the patient's nutritional status, as well as the need for ongoing nutritional support, is necessary.

Hypermetabolic patients, e.g., septic patients with ARDS, are also candidates for nutritional support. In this setting, the nutritional goal is not correction of malnutrition but rather curtailment of protein catabolism and protein losses. Note that complete reversal of protein catabolism in a severely hypermetabolic patient is probably not possible. The aim is to minimize excessive protein losses while providing maintenance levels of substrates within the constraints of organ disposal mechanisms (e.g., with hepatic or renal insufficiency).

NUTRITIONAL SUPPORT: DETERMINATION OF REQUIREMENTS

General nutritional goals include attaining and maintaining energy (calorie) requirements and nitrogen balance (Table 178-3). Energy balance is achieved when sufficient calories are provided to equal energy expenditure. Positive nitrogen balance occurs when protein is supplied (intake) at a rate to balance the protein catabolic rate (output). Adequate vitamins and minerals must be administered. Fluid intake should be appropriate for the clinical circumstances.

Energy Needs

To avoid nutritional depletion, total calories in an amount that approximates total energy expenditure should be provided. *Total energy expenditure* (TEE) is the amount of energy in calories consumed in a 24-h period, which can be measured directly by heat loss or indirectly by gas exchange (oxygen consumption and carbon dioxide production); 4 kcal of energy are expended for each liter of oxygen consumed. A patient's TEE is the sum of *resting energy expenditure* (REE) and energy expenditure which is dietary-induced, due to cold thermogenesis, and due to activity or stress. In the critically ill patient, the contributions of diet and cold thermogenesis to TEE are small and are generally disregarded for clinical purposes.

HARRIS-BENEDICT EQUATION

Several methods exist for estimating the TEE or caloric requirements of patients with respiratory disease. Levels of energy expenditure can be estimated, calculated using formulas or nomograms, or determined by measurements of energy expenditure (Table 178-4). In mechanically ventilated patients with respiratory disease, a guideline of 25 kcal/kg per day has been suggested.[18]

TABLE 178-3

General Goals of Nutritional Support

Preserve lean body (muscle) mass
    Assure adequate, but not excessive, energy (calorie) stores
    Create positive nitrogen balance
Provide adequate vitamins, minerals, fat
Provide appropriate fluids

TABLE 178-4

Determination of Daily Energy Expenditure in Acute Respiratory Failure

Estimation
    25 kcal/kg per day
Calculation
    Resting energy expenditure (Harris-Benedict)
Measurement
    Indirect calorimetry
    Pulmonary artery catheter measurements

An estimate of basal metabolic rate based on REE can be obtained using the *Harris-Benedict equation,* which relates energy expenditure to sex, weight (in kilograms, W), height (in centimeters, H), and age (in years, A).

$$REE \text{ (males)} = 66.47 + 13.75 \text{ (W)} + 5.0 \text{ (H)} - 6.76 \text{ (A)} \quad (1)$$

$$REE \text{ (females)} = 655.1 + 9.56 \text{ (W)} + 1.7 \text{ (H)} - 4.68 \text{ (A)} \quad (2)$$

A "stress factor" or percent increase in energy requirement based on the severity of the patient's illness is then added to this determination:

$$TEE = REE + \text{stress factor} \quad (3)$$

Thus, TEE equals REE plus the stress factor. Stress factors are based on estimated metabolic needs over and above resting needs and vary with respect to body temperature, degree of physical activity, and extent of injury.[35] Most critically ill patients with respiratory disease have an average stress factor of 1.2. Severely nutritionally depleted or starved patients with COPD may have a smaller stress factor or no stress factor at all if they are receiving totally controlled ventilation. Severely hypermetabolic patients with acute respiratory failure may have an increased stress factor of 1.2 to 1.4 during the period of hypermetabolism. The utility of the Harris-Benedict equation in clinical practice is controversial. Caloric needs may be inaccurate; overestimation of caloric requirements has been noted. However, application of the equation remains a relatively simple method of estimating caloric requirements, especially in critically ill patients.

DIRECT MEASUREMENT

The most accurate method of determination of energy requirements is indirect measurement of actual energy expenditure using a metabolic cart. Caloric requirements are determined by measuring the rate of oxygen consumption, with each liter of oxygen consumed representing approximately 4 to 5 kcal. Metabolic carts can be used to measure oxygen consumption in both mechanically ventilated and spontaneously breathing patients, but they are expensive and require technical expertise. Unfortunately, the stringent conditions that must be imposed during study periods are not the usual conditions under which critical care is delivered. Also, although indirect calorimetry may accurately reflect energy requirements over the 30 to 60 min of measurement, it is difficult to know how to extrapolate the determination to a 2-h time frame.

Energy expenditure can also be measured using a pulmonary artery catheter by assessing the rate of oxygen consumption from the measured cardiac output (using thermodilution techniques) and the O_2 content difference between arterial and mixed venous blood.[34]

CALORIC REQUIREMENTS IN COPD

Energy requirements in patients with COPD follow general guidelines, with several caveats. Malnourished, spontaneously breathing patients with COPD have increased resting energy requirements; the values are approximately 15 percent above those predicted by the Harris-Benedict equation, representing a far greater energy requirement than that of malnourished patients without COPD.[54] This finding is due to the increased energy needs of the ventilatory muscles.[20] The energy cost of the respiratory muscles can be approximated from assessment of the severity of lung hyperinflation. Energy requirements in COPD depend on whether the patient is breathing spontaneously or is mechanically ventilated. Calculation of nutritional requirements in the spontaneously breathing patient with COPD should also consider the limitations that such patients have in augmenting caloric intake due to early satiety, anorexia, bloating, and fatigue.

SUMMARY

When calculating, estimating, or measuring total daily energy needs, remember that the goal is provision of the appropriate number of calories, not underfeeding or overfeeding. Whether nutritional intake is spontaneous, supplemented, or completely controlled, physicians caring for the patient with acute respiratory failure should determine the appropriate daily caloric requirement. Underfeeding over a long period or during hypermetabolic states risks the adverse effects of malnutrition on respiratory function. Overfeeding risks metabolic complications, especially nutrition-related hypercapnia (see below).

Substrate Mix

Once total energy requirements are determined, the substrate mix must be considered, i.e., the percentage of total calories supplied as carbohydrate, fat, and protein. Protein (nitrogen) requirements in the patient with pulmonary disease are not significantly different from those in patients without lung disease. Optimal support establishes neutral or positive nitrogen balance, depending on the need for protein repletion. In the critically ill patient with acute respiratory failure, protein balance can be accomplished by giving 1 to 3 (generally, 1.5 to 2.0) g of protein per kg per day.[18] Generally, this amounts to approximately 20 percent of total calories administered as protein. In patients with acute respiratory failure, higher levels of protein may increase the work of breathing, resulting in further patient fatigue; protein intake may need to be temporarily reduced. Protein admnistration has been shown to increase minute ventilation, oxygen consumption, and the ventilatory response to hypoxia and hypercapnia.[6] However, a prolonged lack of dietary protein contributes to nutritional deficiency.

The most appropriate carbohydrate–fat substrate mix for patients with COPD is complicated and controversial. Determination of the precise substrate mix is largely an issue for patients with respiratory disease who are in the intensive care unit, where nutritional support is totally controlled and adverse sequelae theoretically more likely. Spontaneous oral intake is less problematic, except in those instances when intake is supplemented by prepared oral formulations.

Although the critically ill patient with respiratory failure does use lipids preferentially as a fuel source, glucose oxidation is not impaired, and lipid infusion probably does not change the pattern of fuel oxidation.[14] Thus, in theory, there is no metabolic reason to choose one fuel over another. Glucose and lipids provide no benefit over one another in the "sparing" effect of proteins. However, clear disadvantages of carbohydrate administration exist. Hyperglycemia, especially in diabetics or patients receiving glucocorticoid therapy, can be exacerbated by administration of fluids with a high dextrose concentration. Elevated blood glucose can negatively affect humoral immune function and potentiate the growth of *Candida albicans*. Use of increased amounts of insulin can result in sodium and fluid retention, which may be especially undesirable in patients with cardiac or renal dysfunction. Excess administered glucose is not oxidized but rather is stored as body fat. This can result in increased fat deposition in the liver, as well as in nutrition-associated hypercapnia.

Fat calories may be supplied during nutritional support to provide essential fatty acids. Intravenously administered lipids, even when given slowly, may cause hemodynamic changes in injured lungs,[51] although the clinical significance of these changes may be small. Lipids, especially long-chain triglycerides, can impair reticuloendothelial clearance functions, even when hypertriglyceridemia is absent. Hepatic steatosis is significantly influenced by the proportion of fat calories, as well as glucose calories, in excess of caloric needs. Despite the many disadvantages of intravenous lipids, fats in enteral feeding formulations are well tolerated and are associated with few adverse effects.

While recommendations for an appropriate substrate mix of carbohydrates and fats vary, generally, a mixture of carbohydrates to provide 60 to 70 percent of caloric needs, along with fats to provide 20 to 30 percent of caloric needs, is recommended (Table 178-5).

NUTRITIONAL IMMUNOAUGMENTATION

Recently, alterations in the composition of nutrient formulations have been suggested as a means to promote immune system function, especially in the hypermetabolic patient. The formulation components may be varied in relation not to specific nutrient needs but with respect to constituents that augment the immune system. Several specific nutrients have been studied: glutamine, arginine, and omega-3 fatty acids.[37]

Glutamine is a conditionally essential amino acid that is required because of its increased utilization during stress. It is normally synthesized and stored in skeletal muscle and is a major fuel for the intestine and replicating cells involved in host defense. During critical illness, glutamine is released from skeletal muscle in large amounts, causing tissue levels to fall. When increased release is not corrected by increased uptake, a nega-

TABLE 178-5

Nutritional Recommendation for Acute Respiratory Failure

Determination of daily energy requirements (total calories)
Substrate mix
  Protein
    20 percent of total calories
    1 to 2 gm/kg per day
  Carbohydrates
    60 to 70 percent
  Fat
    20 to 30 percent

tive balance for this amino acid ensues. Glutamine supplementation can reestablish depleted stores. Glutamine may have an important clinical role in maintaining the integrity of the intestinal mucosa and in preventing mucosal atrophy.[50,56] Glutamine may, therefore, attenuate the consequences of intestinal atrophy, which include bacterial translocation to mesenteric lymph nodes and an increase in the risk of infection.[56] Recently, glutamine has been shown to improve intestinal epithelial permeability in enterally fed patients compared with those receiving total parenteral nutrition.[25]

Arginine is another amino acid that has received considerable attention. It is hypothesized that arginine enhances the depressed immune response in injury, surgical trauma, and stress. In studies in experimental animals, arginine supplementation has been shown to result in improved immune cell response.[28]

Finally, omega-3 fatty acids may possess anti-inflammatory properties.[37] Clinical evaluation of these nutrition constituents, either separately or in various combinations, has just begun.[28]

MONITORING NUTRITIONAL SUPPORT

Monitoring nutritional support in patients with acute respiratory failure is important in determining whether the goals of positive energy and nitrogen balance are being met. Positive energy balance can be assessed several ways.[18] Serial monitoring of body weight (over days to weeks) is an important and useful method of assessing the adequacy of caloric support. Unfortunately, fluid shifts in acutely ill patients complicate assessment of tissue accretion or depletion. However, in the critically ill patient, weight loss, in the absence of diuresis, strongly suggests inadequate caloric support.

Nitrogen balance should be assessed in any patient receiving nutritional support. Nitrogen balance is expressed in the formulas

$$\text{Nitrogen}_{\text{balance}} = \text{nitrogen (gms)}_{\text{intake}} - \text{nitrogen (gms)}_{\text{output}} \quad (4)$$

$$\text{Nitrogen}_{\text{balance}} = \frac{\text{protein (gms)}_{\text{intake}}}{6.25} - \text{nitrogen (gms)}_{\text{output}} \quad (5)$$

Urinary nitrogen is measured as 24-h urine urea nitrogen excretion (UUN). Urine urea nitrogen generally makes up about 80 percent of total urinary nitrogen losses. Therefore, multiplication of the measured UUN by 1.25 approximates urinary nitrogen losses. Unfortunately, UUN is not accurate in renal failure when the creatinine clearance is less than 20 ml/min. Measurement of total urinary nitrogen is now possible in many hospital laboratories. Assessment of nitrogen balance should be measured initially after stabilization of nutritional support and weekly thereafter in patients without renal failure.

ROUTE OF NUTRIENT DELIVERY

Nutritional support can be administered systemically as total parenteral nutrition (TPN) or enterally. Although TPN remains an important route of nutrient delivery in critically ill patients who are unable to tolerate enteral nutrition, recent data suggest the importance of using enteral nutrition in patients who have a functioning gastrointestinal tract.

Enteral nutrition restores intestinal integrity and preserves the barrier function of the gut. In animal models of stress, enteral nutrition reduces gut atrophy and maintains the gut mucosa. Direct contact of the gut with nutrients preserves enteral mucosal integrity. Enteral feedings correct the pH balance of the gut and help reduce bacterial overgrowth. Enteral nutrition also reduces gastrointestinal bleeding.[42] Early enteral feeding may enhance motility by minimizing the delay in gastric emptying.

Multiple randomized trials have indicated that in the intensive care unit, early enteral feeding following onset of illness (within 3 days) is safe, efficient, cost-effective, and associated with improved outcome.[1,10,31] Unfortunately, some patients with acute respiratory failure may not have a functioning gastrointestinal tract. In these instances, TPN should be administered to provide nutritional support. Some experts continue enteral nutrition during TPN, even at a markedly reduced infusion rate, if at all possible, to allow some enteral feeding contact with the gastrointestinal tract.[18]

COMPLICATIONS OF NUTRITIONAL SUPPORT

Multiple complications are associated with enteral and parenteral nutrition and are of importance to the patient with respiratory disease (Table 178-6). Complications can be generally classified as mechanical, infectious, gastrointestinal, and metabolic in origin.[9] Although such complications are a concern to all patients requiring enteral nutrition, patients with respiratory disease are particularly susceptible to the adverse sequelae of pulmonary aspiration and the metabolic complication of nutrition-related hypercapnia. The discussion below focuses on complications related to enteral nutrition—the initial modality of nutritional support for most patients with "uncomplicated" acute respiratory failure.

Mechanical

Mechanical complications of enteral feeding relate to the size and position of the feeding tube and include inadvertent nasotracheal passage, clogging, and obstruction of the tube.[29] Adverse pleuropulmonary sequelae that can potentially worsen respiratory disease include pneumothorax, pneumomediastinum, and subcutaneous emphysema; death also may occur. A common

TABLE 178-6
Complications of Enteral Nutrition

Mechanical
   Inadvertent tracheal intubation
   Clogging or obstruction of tube
   Aspiration of enteral feeding
Gastrointestinal
   Vomiting
   Abdominal distention
   Diarrhea
Metabolic
   Hyperglycemia
   Hypophosphatemia
   Hypercapnia

practice in these patients is the use of a wire stylet to assist passage of the flexible feeding tube. Neurologically impaired or pharmacologically sedated patients are at high risk. Radiographic confirmation of tube placement is essential.

Aspiration-Related

Aspiration of enteral feeding has the potential for significant adverse sequelae in patients with respiratory disease. Large-volume aspiration of enteral feedings can precipitate or worsen respiratory failure; small-volume aspiration can cause nosocomial pneumonia with the potential for sepsis. The frequency of aspiration is difficult to determine, since the incidence reported with gastric intubation with feeding tubes varies widely, ranging from 0.8 percent to 77 percent.[12,24,29] In a review of 253 hospitalized patients treated with enteral nutritional support, only 2 patients (0.8 percent) were diagnosed as having aspiration pneumonia.[12] When aspiration was detected by glucose-positive endotracheal secretions, aspiration was diagnosed in 21 percent of mechanically ventilated patients.[29] Likewise, 77 percent of tracheally intubated patients were found to have aspirated, as determined by the presence of methylene blue in tracheal secretions.[24] It is difficult to draw general conclusions from these studies about the effect of feeding tubes, since the studies differ in populations studied, study design, methods used to diagnose aspiration, and size of the feeding tubes.

Multiple factors may affect the frequency and severity of aspiration. Clearly, the presence of an endotracheal tube and the type of endotracheal tube influence the incidence of aspiration. Other risk factors for aspiration include a reduced level of consciousness and consequent compromised glottic closure, the presence of an artificial airway, and ileus or gastroparesis.[40]

Small-bore feeding tubes are generally recommended as a means of decreasing gastroesophageal reflux and, ultimately, aspiration. Data supporting this recommendation are controversial. No aspiration of tube feedings (as determined using methylene blue) was found in 30 ventilated patients who had small-bore (8F) feeding tubes.[12] In contrast, tube size was not a significant variable in witnessed aspiration or aspiration pneumonia occurring in hospitalized patients.[39] Recent data suggest that feeding tube size may also be an unimportant variable in reflux. When reflux was assessed in normal subjects using gastroesophageal scintiscanning, no difference was found between large-bore (14F) and small-bore (8F) nasogastric feeding tubes.[22] These findings suggest that other factors may be more important in reflux, e.g., the position of the patient.

In early work, normal volunteers with nasogastric tubes were studied in the supine postion, at elevations of 10°, 30°, and 45°, and in the upright position. After a large volume of acid was instilled into the stomach, aspiration, as detected by a fall in esophageal pH, occurred only in the supine position. The importance of patient position has been confirmed by more recent studies using scintiscanning of tracheal secretions following isotopic labeling of enteral nutrition.[49] Radioactive counts and, therefore, aspiration, were four times higher in the supine than in the semirecumbent position. Duration of time in the supine position is also important. Aspiration increased 65 percent from 1 to 6 h after placement of the patient in the supine position.[49]

Clinical documentation of aspiration is difficult. Recent studies suggest that detection by glucose determinations of tracheal secretions may be misleading.[30] Prevention of aspiration of gastric contents should be addressed by minimizing the mechanical factors contributing to regurgitation, such as low head placement and improper tube positioning. Gastric residuals should be checked frequently, especially in patients who are at risk for slowed gastric emptying.

Gastrointestinal

Gastrointestinal complications of enteral feeding include vomiting, abdominal distention, and diarrhea. Alterations in gastrointestinal motility occur primarily in the critically ill patient with acute respiratory failure.[51] Clinical manifestations of altered motility include ileus and diarrhea. Decreased bowel sounds and abdominal distention may occur in as many as 50 percent of mechanically ventilated patients.[17] Causes of ileus include electrolyte abnormalities, such as hypokalemia; narcotic drugs, such as morphine, which reduce intestinal motility; and enteral alimentation. Early, aggressive correction of electrolyte abnormalities, reduction of narcotics, and gastrointestinal suction will decrease the morbidity from progressive bowel dilation. Withholding enteral feeding in the presence of abdominal pain or distention, or in the absence of bowel sounds, is controversial. Jejunal tube feeding may result in less abdominal distention than feeding through the gastric route.

The incidence of diarrhea in patients with acute respiratory failure may approach 50 percent.[17] Causes include infection, especially due to *Clostridium* species, and drugs, such as antacids or cimetidine. Diarrhea is frequent in mechanically ventilated patients receiving enteral nutrition, although the precise cause is unknown. In addition to the known causes of diarrhea, such as infection and antibiotics, severe diarrhea in enterally fed patients may also be a symptom of deranged metabolism; that is, the luminal absorptive capacity may be affected by hypotension and reduced mesenteric circulation, toxemia, or the cellular derangements associated with multiple organ failure. Hypoalbuminemia associated with volume expansion and severe catabo-

lism has also been noted in conjunction with diarrhea in critically ill patients.

Multiple adverse effects ensue from diarrhea in patients with acute respiratory failure. Patient discomfort and embarrassment add to the distress of conscious patients. Fecal incontinence in unconscious patients adds to the problems of skin care and allows bowel organisms to contaminate the skin and surrounding areas. The loss of nutrients, water, and electrolytes is obvious, but difficult to measure. Cost of care is increased as a consequence of an increase in required nursing time. Treatment centers first around removal or correction of any known causes. Clostridial infection should always be ruled out. Although fiber provided in the enteral feeding may increase stool bulk and decrease diarrhea in non-seriously ill patients with respiratory disease, it does not appear to decrease diarrhea in critically ill patients.

Metabolic

Metabolic complications of nutritional support include electrolyte abnormalities. Hyperglycemia and hypophosphatemia are common.[26] Hypophosphatemia can worsen or precipitate acute respiratory failure.[7] Periodic evaluation of electrolyte levels should be undertaken in all patients fed enterally.

Nutrition-associated hypercapnia is an important metabolic complication in patients with acute respiratory failure treated with either TPN or enteral nutrition. Nutrition-associated increases in carbon dioxide production can produce hypercapnia.[46] Clinical sequelae include worsening of dyspnea and exercise tolerance, precipitation of acute respiratory failure, and delayed weaning from mechanical ventilation.[15,16] Hypercapnia results from increased CO_2 production for two reasons: (1) Glucose combustion causes more carbon dioxide production ($\dot{V}_{CO_2}$) than combustion of lipid, in that an isocaloric substitution of all lipid for all glucose calories results in a 22 percent reduction in $\dot{V}_{CO_2}$.[46] (2) More important, excess glucose calories result in lipogenesis and a markedly increased respiratory quotient (RQ). The RQ of glucose is 1.0; the RQ of fat is 0.7. However, the RQ of lipogenesis or fat production is approximately 8.0, reflecting proportionally greater CO_2 production relative to oxygen consumption with lipogenesis. In normal individuals, hypercapnia is avoided by increasing ventilation. Patients with compromised ventilatory status, such as those with COPD or a fixed minute ventilation due to weak respiratory muscles, may not be able to increase ventilation appropriately.[15,16]

The cause of nutrition-related hypercapnia is generally thought to be excess carbohydrate (CHO) or glucose calories. Some confusion has existed, however, as to whether the hypercapnia relates to an excess proportion of CHO in the nutritional regimen, or simply an excess of total glucose calories. Prior data suggest that the elevated $\dot{V}_{CO_2}$ and hypercapnia are due to simple excess in total calories.

In a study of surgical patients, a 62 percent increase in $\dot{V}_{CO_2}$ was found to precipitate respiratory distress.[5] Total daily calories were 2.25 times the REE. In another study,[15] acute respiratory failure was precipitated following administartion of TPN in three elderly patients with COPD. Total calories were greater than 2200 per day in all. More recent data confirm an increase in $\dot{V}_{CO_2}$ production with stepwise increases in total calories.[48] Carbon dioxide production increased in ten mechanically ventilated patients receiving nutritional regimens of 1.0, 1.5, and 2.0 times the REE using a mixture of 60 percent carbohydrate and 20 percent fat. $\dot{V}_{CO_2}$ was significantly increased at 1.5 and 2.0 times the REE compared to baseline. In contrast, when ten additional patients were given isocaloric regimens that contained 40 percent, 60 percent, or 75 percent of total calories as carbohydrates, $\dot{V}_{CO_2}$ was not different.[48] These data suggest that *total* calories more clearly influence $\dot{V}_{CO_2}$ production than does *percentage* of carbohydrate calories when total calories are not excessive.

Quantitation of carbon dioxide production is accomplished by indirect calorimetry or by analyzing a timed collection of expired air. The problem of excessive CO_2 production caused by feeding can be avoided by identifying patients at risk, especially those with respiratory disease; excessive total calories should be avoided.

Enteral formulations with altered carbohydrate–fat ratios have been developed and promoted especially for patients with COPD. These formulations commonly have lower carbohydrate and higher fat concentrations. Data on CO_2 production from isocaloric nutritional regimens in COPD are limited. Eight postoperative patients received isocaloric regimens (1.5 $\times$ REE) of either 100 percent glucose or 50 percent glucose and 50 percent fat.[19] $\dot{V}_{CO_2}$ increased in both nutritional regimens compared to basal values, although it was 11 percent higher with glucose alone, compared with glucose and lipid. In a study of exercise gas exchange in normals, $\dot{V}_{CO_2}$ decreased from 290 ml/min to 240 ml/min with a low carbohydrate (10%) concentration.[47] However, despite this decrease, mean minute ventilation was not different during rest or exercise, suggesting that numerical decreases in $\dot{V}_{CO_2}$ as a result of use of a proportion of carbohydrate calories may not have practical significance in decreasing minute ventilation. There appears to be little value in COPD in using special enteral formulations that decrease carbohydrate calories when total calories are appropriate.

SUMMARY

Nutritional management of patients with acute respiratory failure requires recognition of the differing metabolic states of malnutrition and hypermetabolism. Starvation can result in malnutrition and adverse effects on respiratory muscle strength, ventilatory drive, and immune defense mechanisms. General nutritional goals include preservation of lean body mass by providing adequate energy sources and positive nitrogen balance. The general nutritional prescription for both malnutrition and hypermetabolism includes a substrate mix of 20 percent protein, 60 to 70 percent carbohydrate, and 20 to 30 percent fat (by calories). Positive nitrogen balance is difficult to attain in hypermetabolic patients in whom energy requirements are increased compared to starved patients. Enteral nutrition should be the mode of initial nutrient delivery unless the gastrointestinal tract is non-functional. Monitoring of nutritional support is essential. Complications of nutritional support are multiple.

REFERENCES

1. Adams S, Dellinger EP, Wertz MJ, et al: Enteral versus parenteral nutritional support following laparotomy for trauma: A randomized prospective trial. *J Trauma* 26:882–886, 1986.
2. Arora NS, Rochester DF: Effect of body weight and muscularity on human diaphragm muscle mass, thickness and area. *J Appl Physiol* 52:64–70, 1982.
3. Arora NS, Rochester DF: Respiratory muscle strength and maximal voluntary ventilation in undernourished patients. *Am Rev Respir Dis* 126:5–8, 1982.
4. Askanazi J, Rosenbaum SH, Hyman AI, et al.: Effects of parenteral nutrition on ventilatory drive. *Anesthesiology* 53(suppl 1):185, 1980.
5. Askanazi J, Rosenbaum SH, Hyman AI, et al.: Respiratory changes induced by the large glucose loads of total parenteral nutrition. *JAMA* 243:1444–1447, 1980.
6. Askanazi J, Weissman C, La Sala PA, et al: Effect of protein intake on ventilatory drive. *Anesthesiology* 60:106–110, 1984.
7. Aubier M, Murciano D, Lecoguic Y, et al: Effect of hypophosphatemia on diaphragmatic contractility in patients with acute respiratory failure. *N Engl J Med* 313:420–424, 1985.
8. Baker JP, Detsky AS, Wesson D, et al: Nutritional assessment: A comparison of clinical judgment and objective measurements. *N Engl J Med* 306:969–972, 1982.
9. Bernard EA, Weser E: Complications and prevention, in Rombeau JL, Caldwell MD (eds), *Enteral and Tube Feeding*. Philadelphia, Saunders, 1984, pp 542–570.
10. Bower RH, Talamini MA, Sax HC, et al: Postoperative enteral vs parenteral nutrition: A randomized controlled trial. *Arch Surg* 104:1040–1045, 1986.
11. Buzby GP, Mullen JL, Hobbs CL, et al: Prognostic nutritional index in gastrointestinal surgery. *Am J Surg* 139:160–167, 1980.
12. Cataldi-Betcher EL, Seltzer MH, Slocum BA, Jones KW: Complications occurring during enteral nutrition support: A prospective study. *J Parenter Enteral Nutr* 7:546–552, 1983.
13. Cerra FB: Hypermetabolism, organ failure, and metabolic support. *Surgery* 101:1–14, 1987.
14. Cohen FJ: Glucose vs lipid calories. in Zaloga GP (ed), *Nutrition in Critical Care*. St. Louis, Mosby-Year Book, 1994, pp 169–183.
15. Covelli HD, Black JW, Olsen MS, Bechman JF: Respiratory failure precipitated by high carbohydrate loads. *Ann Intern Med* 95:579–581, 1981.
16. Dark DS, Pingleton SK, Kerby GR: Hypercapnia during weaning: A complication of nutritional support. *Chest* 88:141–143, 1985.
17. Dark DS, Pingleton SK: Nonhemorrhagic gastrointestinal complications in acute respiratory failure. *Crit Care Med* 17:755–758, 1989.
18. DeBiasse MA, Wilmore DW: What is optimal nutritional support? *New Horizons* 2:122–130, 1994.
19. Delafosse B, Bouffard Y, Viale JP, et al: Respiratory changes induced by parenteral nutrition in postoperative patients undergoing inspiratory pressure support ventilation. *Anesthesiology* 66:393–396, 1987.
20. Donahoe M, Rogers RM, Wilson DO, et al: Oxygen consumption of the respiratory muscles in normal and malnourished patients with chronic obstructive pulmonary disease. *Am Rev Respir* 149:385–391, 1989.

21. Donahoe M, Rogers RM: Nutritional assessment and support in chronic obstructive lung disease. *Clin Chest Med* 11:487–504, 1990.

22. Dotson R, Robinson R, Pingleton SK: The effect of nasogastric tube size on gastroesophageal reflux. *Am J Respir Crit Care Med* 149:1659–1662, 1994.

23. Driver AG, McAlevy MT, Smith JL: Nutritional assessment of patients with chronic obstructive pulmonary disease and respiratory failure. *Chest* 82:568–571, 1982.

24. Elpern EH, Jacobs ER, Bone RC: Incidence of aspiration in tracheally intubated adults. *Heart Lung* 16:527–531, 1987.

25. Hadfield RJ, Sindari DG, Houldsworth PE, Evan TM: The effect of enteral nutrition and total parenteral nutrition on gut permeability in critical illness. *Am J Respir Crit Care Med* 152:1545–1548, 1995.

26. Heymsfield SB, Erbland M, Casper K, et al: Enteral nutritional support: Metabolic, cardiovascular, and pulmonary interrelations. *Clin Chest Med* 7:41–69, 1986.

27. Kelly SM, Rosa A, Field S, et al: Inspiratory muscle strength and body composition in patients receiving total parenteral nutrition therapy. *Am Rev Respir Dis* 130:33–37, 1984.

28. Kemen M, Senkal M, Haman HH, et al: Early postoperative enteral nutrition with arginine-omega-3 fatty acids and ribonucleic acid-supplemented versus placebo in cancer patients. *Crit Care Med* 23:652–659, 1995.

29. Kingston GW, Phang PT, Leathley MJ: Increased incidence of nosocomial pneumonia in mechanically ventilated patients with subclinical aspiration. *Am J Surg* 161:589–592, 1991.

30. Kinsey GC, Murray MJ, Swensen SJ, Miles JM: Glucose content of tracheal aspirates: Implications for the detection of tube feeding aspiration. *Crit Care Med* 22:1524–1525, 1994.

31. Kudsk KA, Croce MA, Fabian TC, et al: Enteral vs parenteral feeding: Effects on septic morbidity after blunt and penetrating abdominal trauma. *Ann Surg* 215:503–510, 1992.

32. Lands L, Desmond KJ, Demizio D, et al: The effects of nutritional status and hyperinflation on respiratory muscle strength in children and young adults. *Am Rev Respir Dis* 141:1506–1509, 1990.

33. Lewis MI, Belman MJ, Dorr-Uyemural L: Nutritional supplementation in ambulatory patients with COPD. *Amer Rev Respir Dis* 125:1062–1068, 1987.

34. Liggett SB, St John RE, Lefrak SS: Determination of resting energy expenditure utilizing the thermodilution pulmonary artery catheter. *Chest* 91:562–566, 1987.

35. Long CL, Schaffel N, Geiger JW, et al: Metabolic response to injury and illness: Estimation of protein needs from indirect calorimetry and nitrogen balance. *J Parenter Enteral Nutr* 3:452–457, 1979.

36. Lopes JM, Russell DM, Witwell J: Skeletal muscle function in malnutrition. *Am J Clin Nutr* 36:602–610, 1982.

37. Lowry SF, Thompson WA: Nutritional modification of inflammatory mediator production. *New Horizons* 2:164–171, 1994.

38. Meduri GU, Eltorky M, Winer-Muran HJ: The fibroproliferative phase of late ARDS. *Semin Respir Infect* 10:154–175, 1995.

39. Metheny NA, Eisenberg P, Spies M: Aspiration pneumonia in patients fed through nasoenteral tubes. *Heart Lung* 15:256–261, 1986.

40. Mullan H, Robenoff RA, Robenoff R: Risk of pulmonary aspiration among patients receiving enteral nutrition support. *J Parenter Enteral Nutr* 16:160–164, 1992.

41. Murciano D, Armengauk MH, Rigaud D, et al: Diaphragmatic function in severely malnourished patients with anorexia nervosa. *Am J Respir Crit Care Med* 150:1569–1574, 1994.

42. Pingleton SK, Hadzima SK: Enteral alimentation and gastrointestinal bleeding in mechanically ventilated patients. *Crit Care Med* 11:13–17, 1983.

43. Rochester DF, Braun NMT: Determinants of maximal inspiratory pressure in chronic obstructive pulmonary disease. *Am Rev Respir Dis* 132:42–47, 1985.

44. Rochester DF, Esau SA: Malnutrition and the respiratory system. *Chest* 85:411–415, 1984.

45. Shizgal HM: Nutrition and immune function. *Surg Ann* 12:12–29, 1981.

46. Silberman H, Silberman AW: Parenteral nutrition, biochemistry, and respiratory gas exchange. *J Parenter Enteral Nutr* 10:151–154, 1986.

47. Sue DY, Chung MM, Grosvenor M, Wasserman K: Effect of altering the proportions of dietary fat and carbohydrate on exercise gas exchange in normal subjects. *Am Rev Respir Dis* 139:1430–1434, 1989.

48. Talpers SS, Romberger DJ, Bunce SB, Pingleton SK: Nutritionally associated increased carbon dioxide production. Excess total calories vs high proportion of carbohydrate calories. *Chest* 102:551–555, 1992.

49. Torres A, Serra-Batlles J, Rose E, et al: Pulmonary aspiration of gastric contents in patients receiving mechanical ventilation: The effect of body position. *Ann Intern Med* 116:540–543, 1992.

50. Van der Hulst RR, van Kreel BB, von Meyenfeldt MM, et al: Glutamine and the preservation of gut integrity. *Lancet* 341:1363–1365, 1993.

51. Venus B, Smith RA, Patel C, et al: Hemodynamic and gas exchange alterations during Intralipid infusion in patients with adult respiratory distress syndrome. *Chest* 95:1278–1281, 1989.

52. Weiner P, Suo J, Fernandez E, Cherniack RM: The effect of hyperinflation on respiratory muscle strength and efficiency in healthy subjects and patients with asthma. *Am Rev Respir Dis* 141:1501–1505, 1990.

53. Whittaker JS, Ryan CF, Buckley PA, Rood JD: The effects of refeeding on peripheral and respiratory muscle function in malnourished COPD patients. *Am Rev Respir Dis* 142:283–288, 1990.

54. Wilson DO, Rogers RM, Pennock B: Metabolic rate and weight loss in obstructive lung disease. *J Parenter Enteral Nutr* 14:7–11, 1990.

55. Wilson DO, Rogers RM, Sander MH, et al: Nutritional intervention in malnourished patients with emphysema. *Am Rev Respir Dis* 134:672–677, 1986.

56. Zhang W, Frankel WL, Bain L, et al: Glutamine reduces bacterial translocation after small bowel transplantation in cyclosporine-treated rats. *J Surg Res* 58:159–164, 1995.

CHAPTER 179

TREATMENT OF AGITATION AND DISTRESS IN MECHANICALLY VENTILATED PATIENTS

John Hansen-Flaschen

At the time of intubation, patients in respiratory failure lose independent control of most ordinary activities and many bodily functions. Movement is restricted by invasive hardware and protective restraints. Communication is stifled by impairment of laryngeal function. Constant lighting and noise turn night to day, while delirium clouds memory and distorts perception. In this stressful environment, various invasive procedures are performed, often with little warning or explanation, and all privacy is lost.

What do patients actually experience under the extraordinary circumstances of mechanical ventilation for acute respiratory failure? Observations from the bedside provide only limited insight into this question. The experience of most patients undergoing mechanical ventilation is discernible only by asking them simple yes-or-no questions or by observing their behavior. From these limited cues, clinicians suspect that many critically ill patients are uncomfortable and frightened.

This suspicion is supported by the published recollections of intensive care unit (ICU) survivors.[6,25,46,54] Even some patients who appear unconscious throughout an acute illness are subsequently able to describe much of their experience, including strong emotional responses to actual events considered unremarkable at the time by their caregivers.[32] Others are plagued by vivid recollections of hallucinations or dreams that bear no apparent relationship to their actual experience in the ICU. Still other survivors recall nothing of their experience in an ICU: Even persistent questioning may uncover only fragmented memories of occasional conversations or events.

Concern for the experience of patients undergoing mechanical ventilation has led to widespread, routine use of sedating medications in ICUs.[13,21,59] In fact, benzodiazepines and opioids rank among the medications most commonly used in the treatment of critically ill patients. Yet the scientific basis for this practice remains remarkably limited. Research has been restrained by a lack of validated outcome measures to assess the effect of treatment on patient agitation or distress,[20,22] and by practical difficulties in blinding investigators to drugs of different appearance or pharmacokinetic behavior. In part because of these methodologic difficulties, most randomized, comparative studies to date have shown no convincing difference in efficacy between treatment arms. As a result, current practice derives primarily from extrapolation of drug efficacy information obtained in other, more controlled settings, and from consideration of the pharmacokinetics, adverse effects, and comparative costs of available drugs.[20] This chapter presents an empiric approach to the assessment and pharmacologic treatment of agitation and distress in mechanically ventilated patients that is consistent with current scientific knowledge.

INDICATIONS FOR SEDATING MEDICATIONS

Sedating drugs are psychoactive medications that exert a calming effect on thought or behavior. A variety of sedating drugs are available to improve the comfort and safety of patients who require mechanical ventilation for acute respiratory failure.[34] Medications commonly used for these purposes include benzodiazepines, opioids, neuroleptic agents, and intravenous anesthetics (Table 179-1). Given in low to moderate doses, all these drugs can improve the tolerance of critically ill patients for endotracheal intubation and mechanical ventilation without subduing consciousness. When administered in high doses or in combination, sedating drugs induce progressive obtundation that can extend to surgical anesthesia. With the exception of the neuroleptic agents, all sedating drugs currently in use also have the potential to suppress or stop respiration. However, because mechanically ventilated patients are relatively protected from this life-threatening complication, sedating drugs can be administered safely, even to the most acutely ill patients in respiratory failure.

Indications for the use of sedating drugs during mechanical ventilation can be grouped into several categories (Table 179-2). These drugs are used to (1) control agitation, (2) alleviate distress, (3) provide anesthesia for pharmacologic paralysis, and (4) provide analgesia or anesthesia for bedside procedures and special situations. This chapter focuses on the first three of these indications. The specialized treatment of acute pain in critically ill postoperative patients and trauma victims is not discussed.

Agitation

In the ICU, *agitation* is defined as excessive or detrimental motor activity associated with internal tension. Repetitive, nonproductive movement is the hallmark of agitated behavior. In contrast to tremors, seizures, and myoclonic movements, agitation is volitional and often, although not invariably, purposeless. Sometimes the purpose of agitated movement is readily apparent, as in repeated efforts at self-extubation. At other times, the purpose may be difficult to discern; for example, a mechanically ventilated patient who is trying to signal the onset of pleuritic chest pain behaves much the same as a ventilated patient who is dodging demons in a delirious hallucination.[12]

A mildly agitated patient might be described as vaguely uneasy or "fidgety." Ordinary movements may be increased in frequency as if the person cannot quite find a comfortable position to rest, or an extremity is moved back and forth for no apparent reason. Mild, intermittent agitation does not necessarily require pharmacologic treatment. Indeed, mildly excessive motor activity may benefit some critically ill patients by reducing disuse muscle atrophy and decreasing the risk of thromboembolism.

TABLE 179-1

Recommended Sedating Drugs*

Benzodiazepines
  Diazepam (Valium)
  Lorazepam (Ativan)
  Midazolam (Versed)

Neuroleptic agents
  Haloperidol (Haldol)

Opioid analgesics
  Morphine
  Fentanyl

Intravenous anesthetics
  Propofol (Diprivan)

*Administered intravenously for ventilator-dependent, critically ill patients.

At the other extreme, severe agitation threatens the life of mechanically ventilated patients. Not only is the placement of vascular catheters and access tubes endangered by the motion, but respiratory and cardiovascular life support can be severely compromised as well. Unnecessary exertion can promote respiratory and metabolic acidosis by increasing the production of carbon dioxide and lactic acid. Even minor motor activity can cause transient, potentially severe hypoxemia in patients with severe acute lung injury who have large intrapulmonary shunts. Excessive respiratory efforts can cause additional problems. Rapid, erratic breathing efforts can also cause hypotension by increasing intrathoracic pressure throughout the respiratory cycle, thereby interfering with venous return. For these reasons, severe agitation must be treated aggressively.

Agitation is not a primary disturbance but, rather, is a secondary behavioral response to some physical or emotional distress. Understandably, many patients in respiratory failure respond to the initial sensations of intubation and mechanical ventilation with agitated behavior. However, agitation that de-

TABLE 179-2

Indications for Sedating Drugs in the Treatment of Mechanically Ventilated Patients

Control patient *agitation*

Alleviate patient *distress,* particularly:
  Pain
  Anxiety
  Delirium
  Dyspnea

Provide *anesthesia* for neuromuscular blockade

Provide *sedation* or *analgesia* for procedures and special situations, including:
  Endotracheal intubation
  Bedside procedures, such as cardioversion and percutaneous tracheostomy
  Diagnostic imaging studies, such as CT and MR
  Alcohol or sedative drug withdrawal
  Acute brain injury associated with increased intracranial pressure
  Terminal withdrawal of mechanical ventilation

velops in a ventilator-dependent patient who was previously calm and alert suggests that a new form of distress has developed. In most instances, time is available to determine the likely cause of agitation before steps are taken to suppress the excessive motor activity. Identifying the type and origin of distress underlying agitation is the key to appropriate treatment.

Distress

Distress is a global term for suffering, strain, or misery affecting the body or the mind. Distress is thought to underlie most, if not all, episodes of patient agitation in the ICU. The relief of distress is an important indication for the use of sedating drugs, even in patients who do not manifest excessive motor activity. The term is particularly useful in the care of mechanically ventilated patients in whom it is often easier to discern that distress is present than to determine the precise nature of the distress. Nevertheless, it is important to make the distinction, whenever possible, because different types of distress are best treated differently.

Although virtually any sensory impairment or psychological abnormality can be found in the ICU, four types of distress appear to be particularly common during the acute phase of respiratory intensive care: pain, dyspnea, anxiety, and delirium. Each may exist in isolation, or two or more types of distress may coexist and feed on one another. All four types can cause agitation; all four respond to psychoactive medications.

Pain

Pain is an unpleasant physical and emotional sensation associated with a potentially harmful stimulus or an actual tissue injury. Pain is subjective and personal. Unless it can be inferred from the circumstances, a person's pain is inapparent to observers until it is communicated by language or behavior. Because language and behavior are both severely restrained by intensive care, pain is probably underappreciated in this setting. Accordingly, intensivists should frequently consider the possibility of pain in critically ill patients.

In the ICU, it is often appropriate to assume that pain is present and to treat accordingly. Pain is an expected consequence of many of the conditions that give rise to the need for intensive care. Surgery, trauma, and surface burns all cause severe pain—as do many life-threatening medical illnesses, such as myocardial infarction, pancreatitis, and pneumonia with pleurisy. Thus, when a patient arrives in the ICU during or after a pain-provoking event, recognition of the pain is often as straightforward as remembering to think of it.

The unanticipated onset of new pain often signals development of a major new complication. In acute respiratory failure, agitation may be the only apparent manifestation of pain. Therefore, it is important to examine systematically for medical causes of pain and areas of tenderness whenever a previously restful patient becomes agitated without apparent explanation. Pneumothorax, ischemic bowel, embolization of a peripheral artery, and intracranial bleeding are examples of pain-producing complications of intensive care that may first manifest as restlessness or agitation in a critically ill patient who is cognitively impaired.

Even more obvious causes of acute pain can escape detection if they are not considered specifically. For example, more than a few elderly men have been treated inappropriately with sedatives and paralyzing drugs for severe agitation caused by pain from overdistension of the bladder after administration of a diuretic.

The most memorable sources of pain for many critically ill patients are far less dramatic. Survivors often relate that they suffered most not from the pain of major problems or surgical procedures but from the discomfort associated with routine nursing tasks or the presence of invasive hardware.[25,46] Examples include pain from the pressure of an endotracheal tube against the nares, the constriction caused by tape wrapped around a forearm that has become edematous, and pain at a chest tube site exacerbated by coughing. Some patients identify endotracheal suctioning as a particularly uncomfortable experience associated with mechanical ventilation.[25,30] If recognized, many such sources of pain or discomfort can be alleviated without the use of medication by simple adjustment of bedside procedures or paraphernalia.

Not only is pain underrecognized in the ICU but also it is often undertreated—even when recognized. Treatment may be withheld deliberately for fear of exacerbating hypotension or masking evolution of a possible acute abdomen. More often, perhaps, the pain of a silent patient fails to register as a priority to clinicians in the context of other serious problems that also require attention. Pain should be no less a priority and no less treatable in the ICU than it is in the operating theater or postanesthesia recovery unit, where it is always treated.

Dyspnea

Contrary to a common misperception, dyspnea is often not relieved by the restoration of adequate arterial blood gases during mechanical ventilation for acute respiratory failure.[31,37] The reasons for this are incompletely understood. One potentially reversible cause is a lack of coordination between mechanically assisted respiration and the breathing efforts of the patient.

The central respiratory control center sets not only the rate but also the depth of spontaneous breaths and the dynamic characteristics of the force generated by respiratory muscles during inspiratory and expiratory efforts. If the patient's spontaneous breathing pattern differs in certain ways from the set pattern of the ventilator, a sensation of air hunger frequently results. Delay in the onset of airflow at the initiation of a spontaneous inspiratory effort and an insufficient airflow during the inspiration are two common problems that appear to be particularly important in this regard.

When confronted by an uncommunicative patient who is agitated for unclear reasons, the physician can test for the presence of a reversible cause of dyspnea by empiric readjustment of the ventilator. Sometimes, agitated behavior stops abruptly when the inspiratory flow is reset above a threshold value that corresponds to the patient's spontaneous inspiratory flow. To reduce resistance at the onset of inspiration, the inspiratory trigger pressure should be set as low as possible and water should be drained from the ventilator tubing. Occasionally, patients appear more comfortable if the tidal volume is reduced. Alternative modes of ventilation, such as pressure support, may relieve dyspnea in other instances (see Chapters 176 and 177).

Dyspnea is also commonly experienced during weaning from prolonged mechanical ventilation.[11] Anxiety during intermittent mandatory ventilation or pressure support ventilation has been shown to be closely associated with dyspnea.[31] In fact, anxiety may often be the most apparent outward manifestation of dyspnea during weaning from mechanical ventilation. Mild dyspnea and anxiety may be unavoidable as patients who have weak respiratory muscles are retrained during weaning trials to sustain spontaneous respiration. Sedation probably helps some patients through. Increasingly severe dyspnea experienced during weaning is generally an indication to restore a higher level of ventilatory support.

Anxiety

Anxiety is a third major form of distress in the ICU. *Anxiety* is defined as a diffuse and unpleasant emotion of apprehension that is not associated with a specific threat. *Fear* is distinguished from anxiety by a defined external threat or danger. Anxiety and fear are both alerting signals that warn of impending peril, whether real or imagined. In the ICU, the overriding apprehension is the fear of death. Helplessness, dependency, and the inability to predict upcoming events all contribute to anxiety during mechanical ventilation, as do pain, dyspnea, and the disturbed perceptions associated with delirium.[7,41]

Anxiety and fear provoke a multifaceted response. Neuroendocrine and autonomic manifestations of apprehension include a host of disagreeable somatic sensations, such as nausea, palpitations, headache, dyspnea, and a perception of weakness. Anxious patients frequently experience difficulty sleeping, and some frightened patients actually try to remain awake for fear that they will die in their sleep. In addition to somatic sensations, anxiety can cause objective changes in bodily functions. Cardiovascular and respiratory responses to anxiety include sweating, tachycardia, tachypnea, and systolic hypertension. Skeletal muscle function is also affected. Some patients respond to anxiety with a generalized increase in muscle tone; others develop twitches or complex repetitious movements, such as clenching and opening a hand or kicking a bedrail. Uncoordinated motion is often increased as well. In the grip of profound anxiety or fear, even cognitively intact persons sometimes develop an uncontrollable urge to headlong flight: No effort at reassurance can prevent these patients from struggling to break free of their hospital bed.

Anxiety can also produce confusion and distortions of perception. Anxious patients lose the ability to concentrate and to recognize associations or context. They tend to focus attention on certain sensations or events to the exclusion of others, so that perspective and judgment may become severely impaired. Distorted perceptions and selective attention can amplify certain fears and bring about a further increase in overall anxiety.

Anxiety is sometimes difficult to detect at the bedside of a patient in respiratory failure. When asked, many patients admit that they are anxious or fearful, but others may be genuinely unaware of their anxiety. When an agitated patient is not clearly dyspneic or in pain, it may be reasonable to assume that anxiety is contributing to the agitation.

Delirium

Organic brain syndromes are commonly present during mechanical ventilation for acute and chronic respiratory failure.[29,41] Disorders of cognition can cause agitation, and they can greatly complicate assessment and management of the patient who is uncomfortable or agitated for some other reason. Consultation with a psychiatrist may be necessary to sort out the origin and nature of organic mental disturbances that come to light in the ICU, particularly if preexisting psychopathology is suspected. However, intensive care specialists should be able to recognize the most common organic mental syndrome in an acute illness or injury, which is delirium.

Delirium is defined as an acute, reversible disturbance of consciousness and cognitive function that fluctuates in severity.[9,12] Delirium is characterized by defective perception, reduced short-term memory, confusion, disorientation, and hallucinations that are often predominantly visual. The ability to think clearly and to process information is disturbed, and reasoning is impaired. Disorientation, spotty loss of memory, and distorted perceptions often give rise to anxiety or fear that does not respond to simple reassurance.

The cognitive impairment of a delirious patient typically fluctuates and may take on a diurnal pattern. Delirium is often most severe in the evening and early morning hours. During the day, periods of clouded consciousness may be interrupted by intervals of unexpected lucidity. Psychomotor activity can also vary markedly. The patient may be lethargic or nearly unresponsive at one point and then dangerously hyperactive later on. Autonomic disturbances such as cardiac arrhythmias, flushing, diaphoresis, and nausea sometimes accompany the periods of agitation as well.

The causes of delirium during mechanical ventilation for respiratory failure are protean. They include neurologic injuries, neoplastic syndromes, severe cardiovascular, hematologic, and respiratory disorders, endocrine and metabolic disturbances, and a variety of toxins. Drugs used in the treatment of critically ill patients can cause or exacerbate delirium as well. Epidemiologic studies point to narcotics, benzodiazepines, and anticholinergic drugs, in particular.[17,38] Like adverse drug effects, delirium associated with severe acid-base abnormalities or metabolic disturbances can resolve rapidly after the underlying cause is addressed.

Other potentially reversible causes of delirium may be less apparent. Intermittent partial seizure activity can be difficult to detect unless prolonged or repeated electroencephalography is performed. Drug withdrawal is a common cause of delirium that may not be immediately apparent in nonverbal patients in the ICU. The possibility of drug or alcohol withdrawal should be considered whenever delirium appears abruptly during the first 2 or 3 days of hospitalization.

Sleeplessness is a common contributing factor to the development of delirium in the ICU.[53] Total deprivation of sleep for several days can actually cause a mild form of delirium characterized by irritability, lapses of memory, suspiciousness, "waking dreams," and an impairment of cognitive performance. Several short-term polysomnographic studies have suggested that prolonged total deprivation of sleep occurs uncommonly in the

ICU; more commonly observed is a severe fragmentation and depatterning of sleep. Whether disruption of the normal sleep pattern causes delirium by itself is uncertain; however, the sleep disturbances experienced in the ICU almost certainly facilitate the onset and enhance the severity of the cognitive impairment and hallucinations that are precipitated by other causes.

ASSESSMENT OF PATIENT AGITATION AND DISTRESS

No research instrument has yet been validated for assessment of agitation or distress in critically ill adults who require intubation and mechanical ventilation. Nevertheless, clinicians can obtain useful information by observing their patients and by asking those who are capable of answering a few simple questions. Basic assessment of agitation and distress should become a routine component of the bedside evaluation of ventilator-dependent patients, replacing the interval history that is appropriate for other hospitalized patients who are able to talk.

Assessment begins by observing the patient's spontaneous behavior. Because even severe agitation may be intermittent, this component of the assessment is best performed by nurses who enter and leave the patient's room frequently. In addition to excessive or detrimental movement, the patient is observed for increased muscle tone and for facial expressions suggestive of distress. A semiquantitative scale of the severity of agitation can be useful to facilitate communication and flow sheet documentation. The scale presented in Fig. 179-1 has served this purpose for more than 3 years at the Hospital of the University of Pennsylvania.

Assessment continues by verifying that the patient can see, hear, understand, and respond appropriately to simple questions. Because critically ill patients are often separated from their eyeglasses or hearing aids, a special effort may be needed to communicate with them. Vision, hearing, and the ability to respond can all be confirmed by asking a single question: "Show me that you understand by blinking your eyes this many times [show two or three fingers]." An awake patient who does not respond appropriately to such commands—despite adequate hearing, vision, and muscle strength—is likely to be delirious or otherwise neurologically impaired.

Responsive patients should then be asked about their comfort with direct questions that intubated patients can answer by shaking their head or by some other unambiguous movement: "Do you have any pain now?" "Are you short of breath now?" "Do you feel anxious now?" "Do you still feel nauseated?"

Questions are expressed in the present tense because many critically ill patients experience short-term memory deficits that preclude meaningful answers about their experiences in the recent past. Affirmative responses are followed, when appropriate, with additional questions that can be answered by movement or gesture—e.g., "Point to where you feel the pain."

Quantitation of distress is often useful in planning and monitoring a therapeutic response. Research conducted in a variety of settings, including the ICU, has demonstrated the utility of visual analog scales for measuring the intensity of subjective experiences, such as pain, anxiety, and dyspnea.[18,31,57] Although analog scales appear preferable to fixed-interval scales for research, use of simple numeric scales often facilitates communication with intubated patients while still providing adequate information for clinical purposes. Analog and numeric scales are illustrated in Fig. 179-2.

An instrument called the confusion assessment method (CAM) has been validated for the diagnosis of delirium in hospitalized patients.[27,28,38] Scoring of the CAM instrument requires conversational responses by the subject to questions. Some mechanically ventilated patients can provide interpretable answers to these questions by mouthing words or writing on a clipboard.[65] Unfortunately, CAM has not been adapted to most ventilator-de-

P	Paralyzed	Neuromuscular blocking agent in effect.
0	Calm	Movements are appropriate and coordinated and do not interfere with treatment.
1	Mild	Movements are occasionally inappropriate or excessive. Muscle tone may be increased.
2	Moderate	Patient is fidgety or changes body position frequently. Vascular access and tubes are not threatened. Ventilation is not compromised.
3	Severe	Patient poses immediate threat to self or staff. Excessive movements repeatedly threaten vascular access and tubes, cause frequent episodes of hypoxemia, or repeatedly trigger peak pressure alarm on ventilator

FIGURE 179-1   Semiquantitative scale for recording the severity of patient agitation.

A. Visual Analog Scale (VAS)

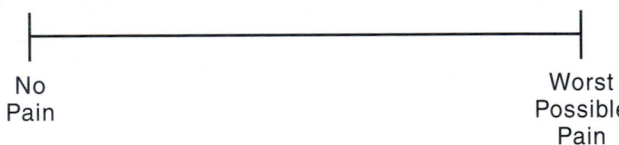

No Pain   Worst Possible Pain

B. Numeric Intensity Scale

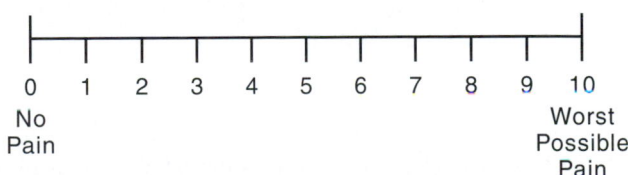

0   1   2   3   4   5   6   7   8   9   10
No   Worst
Pain   Possible
                                      Pain

FIGURE 179-2   Examples of scales for measuring the intensity of patient distress. Dyspnea or anxiety can be substituted for pain. *A.* On a 10-cm visual analog pain scale, a mark is placed to indicate the severity of pain. Pain is then measured by the distance in millimeters from the "No Pain" end to the mark. *B.* Use of a numeric intensity scale facilitates communication with a physically restrained, mechanically ventilated patient who can answer only with a head nod or other simple gesture.

pendent patients, who can answer only yes or no. Nevertheless, a subjective impression of delirium in critically ill patients can often be obtained by asking carefully crafted yes-or-no questions and by observing patient behavior over time. The clinician should look for evidence of the key features in the CAM diagnostic protocol: acute change in mental status with a fluctuating course, inattention, disorganized thinking, and altered level of consciousness. Delirium can probably be assumed in most critically ill patients who are agitated and uncommunicative, provided that their hearing and vision are known to be adequate.

DRUGS FOR AGITATION AND DISTRESS

Four types of drugs are currently used, singly or in combination, to treat patient agitation and distress during mechanical ventilation for respiratory failure: opioids, benzodiazepines, neuroleptic drugs, and intravenous anesthetic agents (Table 179-2). These types of drugs differ considerably in pharmacologic properties; however, all share the effect of depressing the central nervous system (CNS) in a dose-dependent fashion. Mildly sedating doses reduce motor activity and calm the patient. Higher doses cause progressive dissociation from the environment and, ultimately, induce coma.

Opioid Analgesics

The *opioids* are a group of compounds that bind preferentially to the six known opioid receptors in the central nervous system. The opioid agonists relieve the pain associated with noxious stimuli, and they cause sedation.[34,63,64] In contrast to the nonsteroidal analgesics, opioids provide pain relief that is dose related and does not exhibit a ceiling effect. Increasing doses of an opioid analgesic produce tranquillity, progressive sedation, mental clouding, stupor, respiratory depression, and, finally, surgical anesthesia; however, the dose required to achieve and sustain these desired effects varies considerably from one person to another. Although opioids have some anxiolytic effect—primarily because they relieve pain and other forms of discomfort— they should not be prescribed primarily for anxiolysis because benzodiazepines are more effective for this purpose. Also, in contrast to benzodiazepines, opioids do not reliably produce amnesia at commonly used analgesic doses. Opioids have minimal, if any, effect on intracranial hemodynamics or pressure.[43]

In addition to their analgesic and sedating properties, all opioid agonists exhibit other effects of considerable importance to patients in respiratory failure.[8]

RESPIRATORY EFFECTS

Opioids depress respiration in a dose-related fashion by reducing the responsiveness of the brain-stem respiratory centers to carbon dioxide. Respiratory arrest can result, especially in patients who have limited respiratory reserve. Opioids suppress the cough reflex, even at low doses. At high doses, these drugs rarely cause permeability pulmonary edema (see Chapter 85). Morphine occasionally increases bronchospasm in asthmatic patients by causing histamine release. When anesthetic doses of fentanyl are given rapidly, rigidity of the respiratory muscles sometimes

occurs, with the result that ventilation becomes difficult. This effect is reversed by naloxone or a neuromuscular blocker.

CARDIOVASCULAR EFFECTS

At therapeutic doses, the opioids reduce systemic vascular resistance and cause pooling of blood in the periphery. The consequent reduction in venous blood return to the heart may be beneficial to patients in left heart failure, but it can also cause significant hypotension in patients who are volume depleted. Severe hypotension is particularly likely to occur in the setting of cor pulmonale or when an opioid is combined with a benzodiazepine. Opioid-induced hypotension is usually transient and generally responds to volume replacement.

EFFECTS ON ENERGY EXPENDITURE

Therapeutic doses of morphine can reduce oxygen demand and energy expenditure in critically ill patients by 20 percent or more.[51] Whether this represents a specific effect of opioids or a nonspecific effect of sedation is uncertain.

GASTROINTESTINAL EFFECTS

Opioids decrease motility of the stomach and the intestines. Gastric emptying and digestion are delayed, thereby increasing the likelihood of gastroesophageal reflux, ileus, and constipation. Morphine constricts the sphincter of Oddi and can cause paradoxical exacerbation of biliary colic. Opioids can also cause nausea and vomiting.

GENITOURINARY EFFECTS

Opioids inhibit the urinary voiding reflex and increase the tone of the external sphincter. As a consequence, catheterization of the bladder may be required, particularly for elderly men.

OTHER EFFECTS

Opioids can cause pruritus and flushing of the skin. Miosis is a common effect. Occasionally, opioids produce delirium.

Morphine, the time-honored opioid for relief of pain, is one of the most commonly used drugs in North American ICUs. Morphine is reliable and inexpensive, and it is available in a variety of dosing forms for parenteral, enteral, and short- or long-acting oral administration. After intravenous bolus injection, the peak effect occurs within 20 min, and the duration of action is usually 2 to 4 h. When given rapidly in large doses, morphine causes release of histamine and secondarily increases plasma catecholamines. These effects can induce hypotension, tachycardia, flushing, and pruritus and exacerbate preexisting bronchospasm. Morphine is metabolized in the liver, and the metabolites are excreted in the urine. One of the hepatic metabolites, morphine-6-glucuronide, is more active than morphine. Consequently, the effects of morphine can be prolonged considerably in patients who have hepatic or renal insufficiency or poor perfusion of either organ.[45]

Fentanyl is a synthetic opioid whose action is more rapid to peak effect (5 to 15 min) and shorter in duration of action (30 to 60 min) than morphine after single intravenous bolus injection.[40] This distinction is lost after prolonged administration, because fentanyl is a highly lipid-soluble drug that accumulates in fat and then "leeches out" after administration is discontinued. Fentanyl is comparable in cost to morphine for intravenous administration. It is not distributed for clinical use in enteral or oral dosage forms, although it is available in a long-acting transdermal formulation. Fentanyl causes considerably less histamine release than morphine. Consequently, fentanyl may be preferable to morphine for patients who have a mean arterial pressure less than 60 mmHg or right heart failure. Also, in contrast to morphine, fentanyl does not produce active metabolites to accumulate in renal insufficiency. For that reason, fentanyl may be preferable to morphine in patients who have a serum creatinine greater than 2 mg/dl or are acutely oliguric.

Two synthetic opioids, *alfentanil* and *sufentanil,* are available for parenteral use in the United States. These are highly lipid-soluble drugs with rapid onset and cessation of effect. They are widely used for anesthesia. However, because both alfentanil and sufentanil are considerably more expensive than morphine or fentanyl, they have not gained wide acceptance outside the operating room.

Benzodiazepines

The *benzodiazepines* are a group of structurally related compounds that exert similar effects on the central nervous system. These effects include sedation, reduction of anxiety, hypnosis, muscle relaxation, anticonvulsant activity, and amnesia. Increasing doses cause progressive drowsiness. If given alone, however, benzodiazepines do not produce true surgical anesthesia, even at exceedingly high doses. These drugs do not relieve pain, and they do not potentiate the analgesic effects of opioids, although their anxiolytic and amnestic properties may improve tolerance to pain somewhat.[34,64]

The therapeutic-to-toxic ratio for the benzodiazepines is exceptionally high; even massive doses are rarely fatal unless the benzodiazepine is combined with other psychoactive drugs. Rapid intravenous administration can cause transient respiratory depression, hypotension, or tachycardia. These adverse effects occur more frequently, and to a greater extent, when benzodiazepines are combined with an opioid or neuromuscular blocking agent.

The most important adverse effects of the benzodiazepines are neuropsychiatric.[19] At low or moderate doses, benzodiazepines sometimes exert a disinhibiting effect on the central nervous system that can give rise to a paradoxical increase in anxiety, irritability, or agitation. This effect may be observed transiently as the dose is increased. Distorted perceptions, including mistaken perceptions of sexual abuse,[15] have been noted after benzodiazepine sedation for procedures. In other acutely ill patients, benzodiazepine administration is closely associated with the onset of delirium.[38] Physical dependence can occur after continuous, prolonged administration of benzodiazepines in high doses.

Of the many benzodiazepines that are currently available, diazepam, lorazepam, and midazolam are preferred for use during mechanical ventilation for respiratory failure.

Diazepam is the least expensive benzodiazepine available for intravenous administration. After a single bolus injection, diazepam has a duration of action of 40 to 95 min.[4] However, because this highly lipid-soluble drug accumulates in fat and because active, slowly cleared metabolites are formed, full recovery may require 5 to 7 days or longer after prolonged infusion, particularly in critically ill patients who have impaired hepatic or renal function. Because of its cost advantage, diazepam is an appropriate choice for patients who require sedation for 2 weeks or longer, such as those needing mechanical ventilation for severe adult respiratory distress syndrome (ARDS) or Guillain-Barré syndrome. For long-term use in the ICU, diazepam is generally given by intermittent injection. Like midazolam, diazepam commonly causes phlebitis or local thrombosis after repeated injection into a peripheral vein.

Lorazepam is has a slower onset of action (15 to 30 min) than diazepam. The duration of action is approximately 6 to 8 h after single intravenous bolus injection. This drug is less lipid soluble than the others and has no active metabolites. The elimination half-life is not measurably prolonged after single injection in elderly patients or those with renal insufficiency. Although lorazepam can be given safely by continuous intravenous infusion, there are several reasons to favor intermittent intravenous injection for routine use in the ICU.[10,47] Lorazepam sometimes precipitates in the bag or tubing when administered by continuous infusion. Large volumes of fluid are required for continuous infusion, averaging 1.2 L per 24 h in one study of patients in an ICU.[47] Also, limited experience suggests that considerably lower total doses may be required to maintain adequate sedation when lorazepam is given intermittently, rather than continuously. Therefore, intermittent injection is usually less expensive.

Midazolam, the most lipid-soluble benzodiazepine, has a more rapid onset of sedation (1 to 5 min) and a shorter duration of sedative effect (30 to 120 min) after single intravenous bolus injection than lorazepam. Nevertheless, the total time to achieve adequate sedation in the ICU is generally similar for the two drugs.[47] Midazolam and its active metabolites, the hydroxymidazolams, can accumulate in critically ill patients; consequently, there is considerable variation among critically ill patients in the time to awakening after a continuous infusion of midazolam.[44,47] In published studies of prolonged sedation in ICUs, midazolam has generally been given by continuous infusion, rather than by intermittent injection.[2,4,10,26,47,50] Like lorazepam, midazolam requires large volumes of fluid for continuous infusion (e.g., 1 to 1.5 L per 24 h).

The relative cost of intravenous benzodiazepines varies considerably at different hospitals. A rough cost comparison can be made at an individual hospital by assuming that the ratio in milligrams of midazolam to lorazepam required to maintain an equivalent level of sedation during an average course of therapy in the ICU is approximately 4:1 if lorazepam is given by continuous infusion[47] or 9:1 if it is given by intermittent injection.[10]

Neuroleptic Drugs

Neuroleptic drugs differ substantially from other sedating drugs in pharmacologic effects and therapeutic applications. In the ICU, these drugs are particularly useful for the treatment of agitation associated with delirium. The neuroleptic agents decrease spontaneous motor activity, reduce initiative, and diminish aggressive or impulsive behavior. These drugs have minimal amnestic and no analgesic effects. Many neuroleptic drugs cause drowsiness initially, but sedation is a comparatively minor effect until exceedingly high blood levels are achieved. Thus, critically ill, delirious patients who respond to neuroleptic agents appear relatively indifferent to their emotions and their environment while they remain awake and continue to withdraw from painful stimuli. The neuroleptics provide several additional benefits in the ICU: To some extent, they protect against catecholamine-induced cardiac arrhythymias; they decrease intracranial pressure; and they effectively reduce nausea and vomiting.

Of the many neuroleptic drugs available today, the butyrophenone *haloperidol* is most commonly used in the ICU.[1,49,42,60] Compared with other psychoactive agents, this drug has little adverse effect on cardiovascular function in the supine position, and it causes essentially no respiratory depression. Haloperidol does not interact with most other drugs used in the ICU, and it is relatively inexpensive.

After intravenous administration, the therapeutic effects of haloperidol appear after 10 to 15 min, and the peak effect is observed after to 40 to 60 min. The half-life for elimination of haloperidol is 10 to 19 h in healthy subjects. Haloperidol is metabolized in the liver and then excreted in the urine. The drug can be used safely in multiple organ failure, although metabolism may be delayed in patients who have severe hepatic dysfunction.

Haloperidol causes three types of adverse effects of particular importance in the ICU: extrapyramidal reactions, the neuroleptic malignant syndrome, and torsade de pointes.

Extrapyramidal reactions may be less common when haloperidol is given intravenously than when it is given orally, particularly if it is given concomitantly with a benzodiazepine.[42,52] Nevertheless, important extrapyramidal reactions do sometimes occur in the ICU, particularly acute dystonia, akathisia, and akinesia. *Dystonia* manifests most commonly as spasm of the tongue, jaw, neck, or shoulder muscles. Spasm of the jaw muscles is especially disconcerting in the ICU, since the airway can be occluded abruptly. *Akathisia* refers to the sensation by the patient of a compelling need to remain in constant motion. Patients often respond to this sensation with repetitive, purposeless motions of the head or extremities. Akathisia can be difficult to distinguish from the agitated behavior haloperidol is intended to treat. *Akinesia* is a generalized slowing of volitional movement accompanied by increased muscle tone that can resemble parkinsonism.

The neuroleptic malignant syndrome is an uncommon, life-threatening drug reaction that resembles a severe form of parkinsonism.[48] Younger men appear to be at higher risk. Patients develop diffuse muscle spasms that can cause metabolic acidosis or myoglobinuria. Catatonia, stupor, autonomic instability, and persistent fever are also frequently observed. This reaction can occur at any time during use of a neuroleptic drug and may persist for days after the offending drug is stopped.

A third serious complication of intravenous haloperidol is dysmorphic ventricular tachycardia, also known as torsade de pointes.[66] This potentially life-threatening dysrhythmia is typically, although not invariably, preceded by progressive widening of the Q–Tc interval and postpause extrasystoles noted on the electrocardiogram. The incidence is unknown, but it is likely to be uncommon. Women and patients with preexisting prolonged Q–Tc intervals may be at higher risk.

Anesthetic Agents

Of the many general anesthetics that have been tested for use as sedating drugs in the ICU, only one, *propofol,* is currently widely used for this purpose.[2,26,55] Propofol is a CNS depressant that is unlike any other available for clinical use. This alkyl phenol has one of the highest lipid–aqueous partition ratios of all known substances. Consequently, propofol is delivered intravenously as an oil-in-water emulsion in 10 percent Intralipid (Diprivan). Because of its high lipid solubility, the anesthetic effects of the drug are exceptionally rapid in onset and offset. After a bolus injection, propofol at 2 mg/kg causes unconsciousness within one pass of the circulation from the injection site to the brain. During continuous infusion, the CNS depressant effect of propofol can be titrated rapidly from mild sedation to surgical anesthesia. At lower doses, propofol does not have analgesic or amnestic properties, but it may have anxiolytic effects. Recovery occurs reliably within minutes after continuous infusion of the drug for 2 weeks or longer, even in patients who have hepatic or renal dysfunction. Fifteen to 30 min after infusion is discontinued, most recipients are alert and interactive again.

Propofol may be more likely to cause hypotension than are the opioids or benzodiazepines. Rapid injection of a full loading dose of propofol sometimes causes precipitous hypotension in critically ill patients.[26] Consequently, the drug should be loaded by continuous infusion at a rate that is increased in stepwise fashion. During continuous infusion, a 5 to 15 percent reduction in mean arterial blood pressure is not uncommon, but it is generally tolerated.

The lipid vehicle Intralipid can cause a measurable increase in intrapulmonary shunting when a large dose is infused rapidly into patients who have ARDS (e.g., 500 ml of 20 percent emulsion over 6 h). This effect has not been observed clinically during continuous infusions of propofol. Therapeutic doses of propofol do sometimes cause severe hypercholesterolemia. For that reason, blood cholesterol should be monitored at 48- to 72-h intervals during prolonged infusions. Also, the lipid calorie content of the formulation is often sufficient to warrant adjustment of the prescription for total parenteral nutrition during a continuous infusion of the drug.[35] Propofol requires a dedicated intravenous line and special precautions to protect against sepsis associated with rapid bacterial growth in the lipid base.[5] Isolated case reports suggest that propofol may increase the risk of seizures or opisthotonus.[62]

Because propofol is expensive compared with other available intravenous sedating drugs, many intensivists reserve this drug for short-term use in special situations. The infusion rate and, hence, the cost can be controlled by combining propofol with an opioid or a benzodiazepine at the expense of a longer recovery time after sedation is discontinued.

NEUROMUSCULAR BLOCKING DRUGS

Neuromuscular blocking agents are used in the ICU to achieve rapid control of life-threatening acute agitation and to facilitate mechanical ventilation in patients who have severe acute lung injury or severe asthma.[61,64] By quieting agitation, these drugs can appear to relieve a patient's distress; however, they have no known beneficial effect on discomfort, anxiety, or disordered cognition. Indeed, muscle relaxants generally add to the fear and suffering experienced by patients unless they are used together with anesthetic doses of one or more sedating drugs.

Two types of neuromuscular blocking drugs are currently available: the depolarizing and the nondepolarizing or competitive blocking agents. Only the latter are used to sustain muscle relaxation during mechanical ventilation. Of the many nondepolarizing drugs currently available, pancuronium, vecuronium, atracurium, and cisatracurium are most commonly used in ICUs today. All nondepolarizing muscle relaxants work by the same mechanism: They bind competitively to the end-plates of neuromuscular junctions and block access of acetylcholine to its receptors.[24]

Pancuronium and *vecuronium* are aminosteroids structurally related to curare. Pancuronium exerts a vagolytic action that can sometimes cause tachycardia and hypertension after bolus injection. Pancuronium also causes histamine release, resulting occasionally in clinically significant hypotension. Vecuronium does not cause histamine release and is not associated with important adverse cardiovascular effects. Pancuronium and vecuronium are cleared primarily by hepatic metabolism. In contrast, *atracurium,* a benzylisoquinoline, is degraded spontaneously to inactive metabolites in the blood at a rate that is unaffected by kidney, liver, or cardiovascular dysfunction. Like pancuronium, atracurium can cause histamine release. The *cis*-isomer of atracurium, *cisatracurium,* does not cause this problem and is now available commercially. Of the four muscle relaxants commonly used in ICUs, pancuronium is the least expensive. Cisatracurium is generally less expensive than the other two per 24 h of continuous infusion.

Other than the cardiovascular effects mentioned above, single doses of neuromuscular blocking drugs are remarkably free of adverse pharmacologic effects when administered short term in the controlled environment of the operating room. However, other serious complications become apparent when these drugs are given by repeated injection or prolonged, continuous infusion in the ICU. In this setting, disconnection of a paralyzed patient from the ventilator can cause cardiopulmonary arrest within seconds if unobserved. Paralyzed patients do not adjust their respiratory rate to changing needs, so frequent arterial blood gas measurements are needed to avoid severe respiratory acidosis or alkalosis. Paralyzed patients cannot cough or swallow to clear and protect their airway. Patients treated with muscle relaxants are prone to corneal abrasions because they are unable to blink, and to hypothermia because they are unable to shiver. Immobilization gives rise to pressure sores or contractures unless the patient is repositioned frequently and joints are appropriately splinted. Improper handling can cause hyperextension injuries and nerve compression damage.

Yet another complication of prolonged neuromuscular relaxation has come into focus only in the past several years: Some patients fail to regain muscle strength for hours to many days after muscle relaxants are discontinued.[23,56] As a consequence, weaning from mechanical ventilation may be significantly delayed.

Two mechanisms are recognized for prolonged weakness after sustained pharmacologic paralysis. The first is delayed recovery from neuromuscular blockade. Pancuronium, vecuronium, and other aminosteroid blocking agents are normally cleared from the circulation within several hours, primarily by the liver. However, in the presence of renal failure (creatinine clearance less than 30 ml/min), functionally active 3-hydroxy metabolites of these drugs accumulate and persist in the blood. As a result, neuromuscular blockade may continue for as long as 7 days after drug administration is stopped. Delayed reversal of neuromuscular blockade can be prevented by avoiding aminosteroid blocking drugs in favor of benzylisoquinoline agents, such as atracurium or cisatracurium, in patients who have renal failure. These muscle relaxants are degraded spontaneously to inactive metabolites in the blood at a rate that is unaffected by kidney, liver, or cardiovascular dysfunction.

A second mechanism of prolonged muscle weakness after neuromuscular blockade is postulated from several case reports and retrospective clinical series reporting a dramatic complication of treatment for asthma-induced respiratory failure.[23,33,56] Several days or longer after the onset of mechanical ventilation for severe asthma, some patients are found to have symmetric muscle weakness associated with prominent atrophy and necrosis of skeletal muscle. In the most severe instances, flaccid quadriplegia occurs, sparing only the muscles of the face.

The common feature in most of these patients is repeated or continuous administration of a nondepolarizing neuromuscular blocking agent in combination with moderate to high doses of a corticosteroid. Early case reports and small clinical series suggested that this complication was associated exclusively with the aminosteroid muscle relaxants pancuronium and vecuronium. More recent reports have also implicated benzylisoquinoline agents, such as atracurium.[33] Rather than the choice of drug, the duration of neuromuscular blockade appears to be the most important indicator of persistent muscle weakness. In one series, only 6 percent of patients who received a paralyzing drug for less than 24 h developed mild weakness, whereas 85 percent of those who were paralyzed for more than 72 h remained weak—some profoundly so.[33]

The mechanism of muscle injury following combined use of neuromuscular blocking drugs and corticosteroids is uncertain; however, experiments on rats suggest that denervation of skeletal muscle unleashes or greatly amplifies a previously unappreciated acute form of corticosteroid-induced myopathy, possibly by increasing the number of corticosteroid receptors in the affected muscle.[39] Muscle biopsies from experimental rats and from affected humans show a selective loss of thick (myosin) filaments not observed in other forms of acute muscle injury, thereby further supporting a distinct mechanism for this apparent adverse drug interraction.[3] Both rats and humans recover muscle function over weeks after denervation is reversed.

Given the frequency and severity of complications associated with prolonged neuromuscular blockade, physicians must weigh the hazards against the potential benefits of muscle relaxation when treating patients in respiratory failure.

PHARMACOLOGIC APPROACH TO TREATMENT OF AGITATION AND DISTRESS

Mild agitation need not be treated with drugs in every instance. Reassurance or other nonpharmacologic interventions sometimes suffice to reduce agitated behavior.[16] Depending on the severity of cardiovascular or pulmonary dysfunction, some motor activity may even be beneficial if it reduces muscle atrophy or diminishes the risk of thromboembolism. At the other extreme, acute, severe agitation requires immediate attention to prevent physical injury or decannulation of essential catheters and access tubes.

Whether manifest or presumed, patient distress should be treated aggressively. There is rarely, if ever, a compelling reason to delay treatment of a mechanically ventilated patient for pain or severe dyspnea beyond the several minutes required to complete an initial evaluation of the problem.

Acute, Severe Agitation

If a quick, directed examination does not reveal an immediately correctable cause for life-threatening agitation—such as a ruptured endotracheal tube balloon, tension pneumothorax, or a distended bladder—fentanyl may be administered at a dose of 0.05 to 0.1 mg by intravenous bolus every 2 to 5 min, up to 0.4 mg or more, while one is monitoring for hypotension. If alcohol, benzodiazepine, or barbiturate withdrawal is the suspected cause, lorazepam should be considered (1- to 2-mg boluses, repeated at 10- to 15-min intervals, to a total of 10 mg or more, as needed). Alternatively, or if either of these drugs fails, the patient should be paralyzed with an intravenous injection of pancuronium, 0.1 mg/kg. If the patient was conscious beforehand, the paralyzing agent should be followed as soon as possible by bolus loading doses of an opioid and a benzodiazepine at doses sufficient to induce analgesia, deep sedation, and amnesia (e.g., fentanyl, 0.3 to 0.4 mg, and lorazepam, 3 to 6 mg). The patient should then be thoroughly reassessed to identify the problem that precipitated the agitation.

Neuromuscular blockade should be continued beyond the duration of action of an initial bolus of pancuronium only if the patient does not tolerate return of muscle activity despite deep sedation. Some patients in severe respiratory failure, particularly those with acute asthma or severe ARDS, require continued paralysis to maintain adequate ventilation and oxygenation. In patients with normal renal function, a continuous infusion of pancuronium should be used to continue neuromuscular blockade beyond several hours. To avoid prolonged neuromuscular blockade associated with the accumulation of an active pancuronium metabolite (see above), cisatracurium can be substituted if the patient is acutely oliguric or if the serum creatinine exceeds 2.0 mg/dl.

Prevention of the complications of paralysis requires particular vigilance of highly skilled nurses, respiratory therapists, and other allied health personnel.[14] The muscle relaxant should be administered at the lowest dose that achieves the therapeutic goal; in many instances, complete paralysis is not necessary. Overdose can be avoided by use of a peripheral nerve stimulator to monitor the degree of junctional blockade.[14] In all cases, and particularly when a corticosteroid is administered concomitantly, neuromuscular blockade should be discontinued as soon as possible—ideally within 24 h—to minimize the likelihood of prolonged muscle weakness. Many intensivists recommend withdrawal of pharmacologic paralysis once every 24 h (a "drug holiday"), whenever possible, to allow a complete physical examination, including assessment of the level of sedation, and to determine whether paralysis is still necessary.

Intravenous infusion of propofol is another alternative for control of acute, moderate to severe agitation, particularly in patients who are expected to require mechanical ventilation for only a few days or when rapid recovery from sedation is required (Table 179-3).[2,26,50] Initially, because of its unusually short onset of action after a bolus dose, it was hoped that propofol would enable physicians to obtain rapid control of severe agitation without resorting to neuromuscular blockade. Unfortunately, bolus loading of propofol was found to cause unacceptable hypotension in critically ill patients. Because propofol must be loaded by controlled infusion, the time required for initial control of agitation is similar to that of benzodiazepines and opioids. Instead, the chief advantage of this expensive, short-acting sedative is its rapid offset of action. With propofol, the depth of hypnosis can be increased temporarily to produce a brief period of anesthesia for an uncomfortable procedure, or decreased temporarily to allow for a complete neurologic examination. Even after 1 to 2 weeks, a patient receiving propofol can be awakened within 30 to 60 min before extubation.

An infusion of propofol is initiated at a rate of 0.3 mg/kg/h. The infusion rate is then increased by 0.3 to 0.6 mg/kg/h until the therapeutic effect is achieved. Maintenance infusion rates typically range between 1 and 6 mg/kg/h. Addition of an opioid infusion generally permits reduction of the dose of propofol and, hence, the total cost of sedation.

The serum cholesterol is monitored every 24 to 72 h. The lipid content in the intravenously administered hyperalimentation is adjusted for the load of lipid in the propofol vehicle. The unused portion of propofol and the tubing are replaced every 12 h to reduce the risk of infection.

Regardless of which drug or drugs are used, hypotension often complicates aggressive pharmacologic treatment of severe agitation during respiratory failure. The effect of drug-induced peripheral vasodilation on blood pressure is amplified in patients who have intravascular volume depletion. Hypotension usually responds to volume replacement—supplemented, if necessary, by intravenous phenylephrine.

Moderate, Sustained Agitation

To treat moderate agitation, a single sedating drug—an opioid, a benzodiazepine, or a neuroleptic agent—should be given in-

---

TABLE 179-3

Propofol and Fentanyl for Agitation

Loading doses
   Give fentanyl 0.025- to 0.10-mg IV bolus, then start a propofol infusion at 0.3 mg/kg/h; increase the propofol infusion rate by 0.3–0.6 mg/kg/h at 5-min intervals to therapeutic effect.

Infusion doses
   Continue propofol infusion at the final loading infusion rate, typically 0.6–6 mg/kg/h; start fentanyl infusion at 0.05 mg/hr; adjust propofol infusion rate to maintain desired level of sedation.

travenously. A loading dose is administered and titrated to effect by administration of repeated bolus injections at intervals appropriate to the onset of action of the drug. A maintenance dose rate is established only after adequate control of agitation is achieved. There is no absolute upper limit to the dose of sedating drugs for mechanically ventilated patients. Indeed, huge doses (10 to 50 times usual) are sometimes needed to quell agitation, particularly for patients who have developed tolerance to sedating drugs or alcohol. However, the likelihood of adverse effects does tend to increase with increasing dose. For that reason, addition of a second and, sometimes, a third sedating drug may be appropriate in refractory cases to increase sedation while limiting the dose of any one drug.

Agitation often occurs as sedating drugs are withdrawn in anticipation of weaning. The cause is unclear; however, development of drug dependency may be the cause in some instances. If agitation is severe, the patient should be reloaded with the sedating drug, and then the dose should be tapered at a slower rate.

The choice of drug therapy for persistent, moderately severe agitation is based on the assumption that agitation represents an outward manifestation of distress. Accordingly, the choice should be directed at alleviating the form of distress that is thought to be underlying the agitation. Other important considerations in drug selection are adverse effects, pharmacokinetics, and cost. Recommendations for sedation of agitated patients with various forms of distress are summarized below.

Opioids for Pain, Dyspnea, or Agitation

Epidural anesthesia or analgesia is often the treatment of choice for localized, self-limited pain associated with surgery, trauma, or burns, provided that the patient is not agitated and remains sufficiently responsive to report paresthesias or early symptoms of intravascular injection. Other local approaches to pain control are sometimes appropriate in the ICU as well.[58] Intravenously administered opioids should be used for most diffuse or persistent types of pain, and for patients who are too agitated or delirious to cooperate with local forms of pain control.

Opioid analgesics should *not* be given subcutaneously or intramuscularly to critically ill patients, unless intravenous access is temporarily unobtainable, because the injections themselves are painful, absorption is particularly unpredictable in this setting, and relief of discomfort is unnecessarily delayed. Bolus intravenous administration is appropriate to provide analgesia for painful procedures, such as placement of a chest tube. Otherwise, systemic opioids should generally be given by continuous intravenous infusion in the ICU, to avoid lapses in pain control common to intermittent opioid dosing regimens. Fentanyl is preferable to morphine for patients with renal insufficiency, systemic hypotension, or right ventricular failure. Lower maintenance doses are used for patients in hepatic failure.

A continuous infusion of morphine or fentanyl should be initiated by administration of an adequate loading dose (Table 179-4). The tendency is to give too little medication too slowly. Larger boluses (e.g., morphine, 5 mg, or fentanyl, 0.1 mg) can be given more safely to patients in respiratory failure than to other patients, provided that the ventilator is set to sustain adequate ventilation in the event of respiratory depression. Boluses

---

TABLE 179-4

Opioids for Pain, Dyspnea, or Agitation

Morphine

  Loading dose

    2–10-mg IV bolus; repeat every 15 min to therapeutic effect.

  Infusion dose

    Start by infusing $\frac{1}{4}$ the loading dose per hour, typically 1–4 mg/h; infusions of 50 mg/h or more can be given if necessary to treat refractory pain or agitation.

Fentanyl

  Loading dose

    0.025–0.1-mg IV bolus; repeat every 2–5 min to therapeutic effect.

  Infusion dose

    Start by infusing $\frac{1}{4}$ the loading dose per hour, typically 0.025–0.125 mg/h; infusions of 1.0 mg/h or more can be given if necessary to treat refractory pain or agitation.

---

are repeated at 5- to 10-min intervals, guided by a visual analog or numeric pain scale, until pain is relieved. Transient hypotension can be treated with an infusion fluid or a vasopressor, such as phenylephrine.

Once appropriate analgesia is achieved, a continuous infusion is begun at an hourly rate that replaces one-half of the loading dose during the expected half-life for elimination of the drug. The patient is monitored for the common adverse effects of opioid analgesia—i.e., nausea and vomiting, delayed gastric emptying and reduced intestinal motility, pruritus, and flushing, urinary retention, and physical dependency. Morphine has an elimination half-life of approximately 2 h, so the initial hourly infusion rate is set at about one-fourth of the loading dose (commonly 1 to 4 mg per hour). In healthy adults, the half-life for elimination of fentanyl varies with the duration of infusion, from approximately 1 h after an initial injection to a plateau of approximately 6 h after 8 h of infusion. In the ICU, maintenance infusion rates for fentanyl commonly fall between 0.025 and 0.125 mg per hour.

The goal of continuous intravenous analgesia is to achieve and sustain a blood level of opioid that equals or exceeds the minimum effective analgesic concentration (MEAC) for the drug.[63] The dose of opioid required to sustain the MEAC cannot be determined by measurement of blood levels, but it can be found empirically by repeated patient assessment with a visual analog or numeric pain scale. Alternatively, a patient-controlled infusion pump can be employed to maintain appropriate opioid dosing for mechanically ventilated patients who are sufficiently awake and alert.[58] Indeed, this patient-friendly analgesic technique is probably underutilized in most ICUs.

The pharmacologic treatment of dyspnea experienced during mechanical ventilation has not been studied systematically. Limited published experience in other settings suggests that opioids may be more effective than benzodiazepines for the relief of breathlessness.[57] Opioid infusions for dyspnea are initiated and maintained as described above for the control of pain.

Benzodiazepines for Anxiety or Agitation

In patients mechanically ventilated for acute respiratory failure, anxiety that does not respond to nonpharmacologic measures[16] should be treated with a benzodiazepine administered intravenously (Table 179-5). Agitation attributable to anxiety should also be treated with a benzodiazepine if reassurance alone does not suffice. Because the anxiolytic efficacy and adverse effects of the commonly used intravenous benzodiazepines are similar, selection should be based primarily on pharmacokinetic considerations and cost. Monitoring is required for the common adverse effects of benzodiazepines, including hypotension, dysarthria, paradoxical excitation, delirium, and physical dependency.

Lorazepam is recommended when the anticipated duration of parenteral sedation is expected to be less than 5 days. Treatment is initiated with a bolus loading dose (0.5 to 2 mg), repeated every 15 min if necessary, to control anxiety or agitation. Sedation is maintained with intermittent injections of 1 to 3 mg every 4 to 12 h. If more than 12 mg per day of lorazepam is needed, one should consider adding a continuous infusion of fentanyl or morphine instead of further increasing the dose of lorazepam to control the total cost of sedation.

A continuous infusion of midazolam can be used instead of lorazepam for short- or intermediate-term sedation, although the total cost of sedation is likely to be greater.[10] Midazolam can be given by patient-controlled infusion.[36] The control offered patients by self-administration of a benzodiazepine may, in itself, help to limit anxiety under certain circumstances, such as prolonged, difficult weaning from mechanical ventilation.

Diazepam is considerably less expensive than either lorazepam or midazolam. However, because sedation may persist for many days after a prolonged infusion, diazepam is recommended primarily for mechanically ventilated patients who are expected to require intravenous sedation for long-term sedation—longer than 2 weeks. To avoid delay of weaning from mechanical ventilation, diazepam should be discontinued or replaced with a shorter-acting drug 5 days or more before return of full awareness is desired.

The minimum duration of continuous treatment associated with development of benzodiazepine dependence in critically ill patients is unknown because drug withdrawal symptoms are particularly difficult to distinguish from other causes of irritability, anxiety, and restlessness in this patient group. Lower doses are used for maintenance in patients with hepatic failure. Many patients recovering from a critical illness who have received a benzodiazepine continuously for longer than 2 or 3 weeks appear more comfortable if the dose is tapered, rather than withdrawn abruptly. In some instances, tapering should continue after discharge from the hospital.

Neuroleptic Drugs and Benzodiazepines for Agitated Delirium

No published scientific study has shown that any psychotropic drug restores normal cognitive function or alertness to patients with critical illnesses who are acutely delirious. However, neuroleptic drugs do appear to calm agitated delirium in many instances. Because of its favorable hemodynamic and respiratory profile, haloperidol is commonly used for this purpose in the ICU.[42,49,52,60] Benzodiazepines can have a similar calming effect on patients who are agitated and delirious, particularly when delirium results from withdrawal of alcohol or some other sedating substance.

To treat agitated delirium not associated with alcohol or sedative withdrawal, 5 mg of haloperidol may be administered by intravenous bolus injection (2 mg for patients more than 65 years old) (Table 179-6). Additional intravenous doses of 2 to 10 mg may be administered every 20 min at an injection rate not exceeding 5 mg a minute until agitation is controlled. During haloperidol loading, the Q–Tc interval on the electrocardiogram should be monitored continuously,

---

TABLE 179-5

Benzodiazepines for Anxiety, Agitation, or Delirium

Lorazepam
  Loading dose
    0.5–2-mg IV, administered at a maximum rate of 2 mg/min; repeat every 15 min to therapeutic effect.
  Maintenence by intermittent injection
    1–3-mg IV every 4–12 h.
  Maintenence by infusion
    Start with 1 mg/h; increase infusion rate as needed in *continuous* increments of 1 mg/h after 1-mg boluses; to reduce cost, consider adding an infusion of morphine or fentanyl if more than 3 mg/h is needed.

Midazolam
  Loading dose
    1–2-mg IV bolus; repeat every 5 min to therapeutic effect.
  Maintenance dose
    Start with 1–4 mg/h; to reduce cost, consider adding an infusion of morphine or fentanyl if more than 5 mg/h is needed.

Diazepam
  Loading dose
    5–10-mg IV, administered at a maximum rate of 5 mg/min; repeat every 5 min to therapeutic effect.
  Maintenance dose
    Start by giving 2–10 mg as a bolus every 2–4 h; over the next 3 days, the injection interval can be increased to 8–12 h; adjust downward for liver failure.
  Discontinuation
    After prolonged use, recovery from diazepam sedation may require 5–7 days or more; when the anticipated duration of further treatment is less than 5 days, discontinue diazepam and substitute lorazepam if needed.

TABLE 179-6

Haloperidol for Agitated Delirium

Loading dose

5-mg IV bolus (2 mg for patients >65 years old); give an additional
2–10 mg every 20 min at a maximum rate of 5 mg/min until the
patient is calm.

Maintenance dose

Give $\frac{1}{4}$ the total loading dose of haloperidol by intermittent injection at
6-h intervals for the first 24–48 h; then decrease the dose by 25–50%
per day; if more than 20 mg haloperidol is given per day, add
lorazepam.

---

and the loading regimen should be discontinued if the interval exceeds 480 ms,[66] to reduce the risk of torsade de pointes. The patient should also be monitored for development of extrapyramidal side effects (dystonia, especially in the muscles of the face and neck, and akathisia), torsade de pointes, and the neuroleptic malignant syndrome. If trismus or other forms of acute dystonia occur, benzotropine, 1 to 2 mg, may be administered intravenously and repeated every 12 h if necessary. Other extrapyramidal reactions can be treated with diphenylhydramine, 25 to 50 mg intravenously, repeated every 6 h, if needed. Akathisia responds poorly to either of these drugs but may abate after administration of a benzodiazepine.

No upper limit has been defined for a loading dose of haloperidol. Quantities in excess of 400 mg per 24 h have been given without apparent adverse effect,[60] although the efficacy of such high doses is uncertain. Addition of lorazepam should be considered if more than 20 mg of haloperidol is needed in 24 h.

Control of agitated delirium is maintained by giving one-fourth the total loading dose of haloperidol every 6 h by intermittent intravenous injection for the first 24 to 48 h. The dose is then decreased by 25 to 50 percent per day, as tolerated. Haloperidol can also be given by continuous infusion.[49]

Benzodiazepines are preferred for the treatment of delirium associated with alcohol or sedative withdrawal because they are effective for the prevention and treatment of withdrawal seizures, whereas haloperidol and most other neuroleptic drugs probably lower the seizure threshold. Many benzodiazepines have been used for this purpose. The choice of drug is not as important as appropriate dosing. For moderate or severe agitation associated with alcohol or drug withdrawal, unusually large doses of benzodiazepines are often required initially (e.g., lorazepam 6 to 12 mg). Once control of agitation is achieved, the dose can often be reduced by 25 percent or more each day thereafter.

SUMMARY

Sedating drugs are widely used to control agitation and alleviate distress experienced by patients who are mechanically ventilated for acute deterioration in respiratory status. Treatment is facilitated by a systematic approach to bedside evaluation aimed at gauging the severity of agitation and the nature and severity of the patient's distress. Agitation need not be treated unless excessive movement endangers health or safety. On the other hand, patient distress should always be addressed. If phar-

macologic therapy is indicated, one or more sedating drugs are chosen in accordance with the type or types of distress experienced by the patient and with consideration of the pharmacokinetics, risk of adverse reactions, and cost of the available drugs. Sedating drugs are given intravenously to critically ill patients at doses adjusted to frequent reassessment of the patient. Nondepolarizing, neuromuscular blocking agents are given, if necessary, to control life-threatening agitation or to facilitate mechanical ventilation in severe asthma or severe, acute lung injury. Neuromuscular blocking drugs should be discontinued as soon as possible, particularly in patients concomitantly receiving corticosteroids, in order to minimize the risk of prolonged muscle weakness.

REFERENCES

1. Adams F: Emergency intravenous sedation of the delirious, medically ill patient. *J Clin Psychiatry* 29(suppl):22–26, 1988.
2. Aitkenhead A, Pepperman M, Willatts S, et al: Comparison of propofol and midazolam in critically ill patients. *Lancet* 2:704–709, 1989.
3. Al-Lozi M, Pestronk A, Yee W, et al: Rapidly evolving myopathy with myosin-deficient muscle fibers. *Ann Neurol* 35:273–279, 1994.
4. Ariano R, Kassum D, Aronson K: Comparison of sedative recovery time after midazolam versus diazepam administration. *Crit Care Med* 22:1492–1496, 1994.
5. Bennett S, McNeil M, Bland L, et al: Postoperative infections traced to contamination of an intravenous anesthetic, propofol. *New Engl J Med* 333:147–154, 1995.
6. Bergbom-Engberg I, Haljamäe H: Assessment of patients' experience of discomforts during respirator therapy. *Crit Care Med* 17:1068–1072, 1989.
7. Bone R, Hayden W, Levine R, et al: Recognition, assessment, and treatment of anxiety in the critical care patient. *Dis Mon* 41:293–360, 1995.
8. Buck M, Blumer J: Opioids and other analgesics: Adverse effects in the intensive care unit. *Crit Care Clin* 7:615–637, 1991.
9. Cameron D, Thomas T, Mulvihill M, Bronheim H: Delirium: A test of the *Diagnostic and Statistical Manual III* criteria on medical inpatients. *J Am Geriatr Soc* 35:1007–1010, 1987.
10. Cernaianu A, DelRossi A, Flum D, et al: Lorazepam and midazolam in the intensive care unit: A randomized, prospective, multicenter study of hemodynamics, oxygen transport, efficacy, and cost. *Crit Care Med* 24:222–228, 1996.
11. Criner G, Tzouanakis A, Kreimer D: Overview of improving tolerance of long-term mechanical ventilation. *Crit Care Clin* 10:845–866, 1994.
12. Crippen D: Stress, agitation and brain failure in critical care medicine. *Crit Care Nurs Q* 15:52–74, 1992.
13. Dasta J, Fuhrman T, McCandles C: Patterns of prescribing and administering drugs for agitation and pain in a surgical intensive care unit. *Crit Care Med* 22:974–980, 1994.
14. Dulin P, Williams C: Monitoring and preventive care of the paralyzed patient in respiratory failure. *Crit Care Clin* 10:815–843, 1994.

15. Dundee J: Fantasies during sedation with intravenous midazolam or diazepam. *Med Leg J* 58:29–34, 1990.

16. Fontaine D: Nonpharmacologic management of patient distress during mechanical ventilation. *Crit Care Clin* 10:695–708, 1994.

17. Francis J, Martin D, Kapoor W: A prospective study of delirium in hospitalized elderly. *JAMA* 263:1097–1101, 1990.

18. Gift A: Visual analogue scales: Measurement of subjective phenomena. *Nurs Res* 38:286–288, 1989.

19. Gudex C: Adverse effects of benzodiazepines. *Soc Sci Med* 33:587–596, 1991.

20. Hansen-Flaschen J: Improving patient tolerance of mechanical ventilation: Challenges ahead. *Crit Care Clin* 10:659–672, 1994.

21. Hansen-Flaschen J, Brazinsky S, Basile C, Lanken PN: Use of sedating drugs and neuromuscular blocking agents in patients requiring mechanical ventilation for respiratory failure: A national survey. *JAMA* 266:2870–2875, 1991.

22. Hansen-Flaschen J, Cowen J, Polomano R: Beyond the Ramsay Scale: The need for validated measures of sedating drug efficacy in the ICU. *Crit Care Med* 22:732–733, 1994.

23. Hansen-Flaschen J, Cowen J, Raps E: Neuromuscular blockade in the intensive care unit: More than we bargained for. *Am Rev Respir Dis* 147:234–236, 1993.

24. Hanson C: Pharmacology of neuromuscular blocking agents in the intensive care unit. *Crit Care Clin* 10:779–797, 1994.

25. Hayden W: Life and near death in the intensive care unit: A personal experience. *Crit Care Clin* 10:651–658, 1994.

26. Higgins T, Yared J, Estafanous F, et al: Propofol versus midazolam for intensive care unit sedation after coronary artery bypass grafting. *Crit Care Med* 22:1415–1423, 1994.

27. Inouye S, van Dyck C, Alessi C, et al: Clarifying confusion: The confusion assessment method: A new method for detection of delirium. *Ann Intern Med* 113:941–948, 1990.

28. Inouye S, Viscoli C, Horwitz R, et al: A predictive model for delirium in hospitalized elderly medical patients based on admission characteristics. *Ann Intern Med* 119:484–491, 1993.

29. Isaac L, Hungerpiller J, Criner G: Neuropsychologic deficits in chronic ventilator dependent patients. *Chest* 96(suppl):255S, 1989.

30. King S: The tracheotomized patient: Tracheal toilet and speech. *Clin Pulm Med* 1:365–368, 1994.

31. Knebel A, Janson-Bjerklie S, Malley J, et al: Comparison of breathing comfort during weaning with two ventilatory modes. *Am J Respir Crit Care Med* 149:14–18, 1994.

32. Lawrence M: What do ICU patients remember after being unconscious? *Am J Crit Care* 4:227–232, 1995.

33. Leatherman J, Fluegel W, David W, et al: Muscle weakness in mechanically ventilated patients with severe asthma. *Am J Respir Crit Care Med* 153:1686–1690, 1996.

34. Levine R: Pharmacology of intravenous sedatives and opioids in critically ill patients. *Crit Care Clin* 10:709–731, 1994.

35. Lindholm M: Critically ill patients and fat emulsions. *Minerva Anestesiol* 58:875–879, 1992.

36. Loper K, Ready B, Brody M: Patient-controlled anxiolysis with midazolam. *Anesth Analg* 67:1118–1119, 1988.

37. Lush M, Janson-Bjerklie S, Carrieri V, Lovejoy N: Dyspnea in the ventilator-assisted patient. *Heart Lung* 17:528–535, 1988.

38. Marcantonio E, Juarez G, Goldman L, et al: The relationship of postoperative delirium with psychoactive medications. *JAMA* 272:1518–1522, 1994.

39. Massa R, Carpenter S, Holland P, Karpati G: Loss and renewal of thick myofilaments in glucocorticoid-treated rat soleus after denervation and reinnervation. *Muscle Nerve* 15:1290–1298, 1992.

40. Mather L: Clinical pharmacokinetics of fentanyl and its newer derivatives. *Clin Pharmacokinet* 8:422–446, 1983.

41. McCartney J, Boland R: Anxiety and delirium in the intensive care unit. *Crit Care Clin* 10:673–680, 1994.

42. Menza M: Controlled study of extrapyramidal reactions in the management of delirious, medically ill patients: Intravenous haloperidol versus intravenous haloperidol plus benzodiazepines. *Heart Lung* 17:238–241, 1988.

43. Mirski M, Muffelman B, Ulatowski J, Hanley D: Sedation for the critically ill neurologic patient. *Crit Care Med* 23:2038–2053, 1995.

44. Oldenhof H, de Jong M, Steenhoek A, Janknegt R: Clinical pharmacokinetics of midazolam in intensive care patients, a wide interpatient variability? *Clin Pharmacol Ther* 43:263–269, 1988.

45. Osborne R, Joel S, Slevin M: Morphine intoxication in renal failure: The role of morphine-6-glucuronide. *Br Med J* 292:1548–1549, 1986.

46. Parker M, Schubert W, Shelhamer J, Parrillo J: Perceptions of a critically ill patient experiencing paralysis in an ICU. *Crit Care Med* 12:69–71, 1984.

47. Pohlman A, Simpson K, Hall J: Continuous intravenous infusion of lorazepam versus midazolam for sedation during mechanical ventilatory support: A prospective, randomized study. *Crit Care Med* 22:1241–1247, 1994.

48. Rampertaap M: Neuroleptic malignant syndrome. *South Med J* 79:331–336, 1986.

49. Riker R, Fraser G, Cox P: Continuous infusion of haloperidol controls agitation in critically ill patients. *Crit Care Med* 22:433–440, 1994.

50. Ronan K, Gallagher T, George B, Hamby B: Comparison of propofol and midazolam for sedation in intensive care unit patients. *Crit Care Med* 23:286–293, 1995.

51. Rouby J, Eurin B, Glaser P, et al: Hemodynamic and metabolic effects of morphine in the critically ill. *Circulation* 64:53–59, 1981.

52. Sanders K, Minnema A, Murray G: Low incidence of extrapyramidal symptoms in treatment of delirium with intravenous haloperidol and lorazepam in the intensive care unit. *J Intensive Care Med* 4:201–204, 1989.

53. Schwab R: Disturbances of sleep in the intensive care unit. *Crit Care Clin* 10:681–695, 1994.

54. Seltzer R: *Raising the Dead: A Doctor's Encounter with His Own Mortality.* New York, Viking, 1994.

55. Shepherd M: Criteria for use of propofol in critically ill adults. *Am J Hosp Pharm* 51:111–113, 1994.

56. Sladen R: Neuromuscular blocking agents in the intensive care unit: A two-edged sword. *Crit Care Med* 23:423–428, 1995.

57. Stark R: Dyspnoea: Assessment and pharmacological manipulation. *Eur Respir J* 1:280–287, 1987

58. Stevens D, Edwards W: Management of pain in mechanically ventilated patients. *Crit Care Clin* 10:767–778, 1994.

59. Sun X, Quinn T, Weissman C: Patterns of sedation and analgesia in the postoperative ICU patient. *Chest* 101:1625–1632, 1992.

60. Tesar G, Murray G, Cassem N: Use of high-dose intravenous haloperidol in the treatment of agitated cardiac patients. *Clin Psychopharmacol* 5:344–347, 1985.

61. Topulos G: Neuromuscular blockade in adult intensive care. *New Horizons* 1:447–462, 1993.

62. Valente J, Anderson G, Branson R, et al: Disadvantages of prolonged propofol sedation in the critical care unit. *Crit Care Med* 22:710–712, 1994.

63. Veselis R: Intravenous narcotics in the ICU. *Crit Care Clin* 6:295–313, 1990.

64. Wheeler A: Sedation, analgesia, and paralysis in the intensive care unit. *Chest* 104:566–577, 1993.

65. Williams M: An algorithm for selecting a communication technique with intubated patients. *Dimens Crit Care Nurs* 11:222–229, 1992.

66. Wilt J, Minnema A, Johnson R, Rosenblum A: Torsade de pointes associated with the use of intravenous haloperidol. *Ann Intern Med* 119:391–394, 1993.

CHAPTER 180

DECISION MAKING IN THE INTENSIVE CARE UNIT

Mark A. Kelley

The care of the critically ill patient is a complex interplay of science, health-care economics, ethics, and the art of medicine. In the intensive care unit (ICU), the health-care team utilizes costly technology to rescue patients from the extremes of illness. This struggle places emotional strain on patients, their families, and health-care professionals, as they balance the desire for cure with concerns for dignity, comfort, and patient autonomy. In this difficult scenario, the physician must provide facts to patients and their families about the severity of illness and prognosis. This chapter includes a description of the objective information available on the outcome of critically ill patients.

Critical care in the United States utilizes expensive health-care technology. Recently, general health costs have escalated to approximately 14 percent of the U.S. gross national product, and critical care accounts for as much as 10 percent of this value. Whether this investment in critical care results in improved health for the nation has been questioned, as has whether most patients even desire this type of treatment. Consequently, considerable research has been performed in defining the prognosis of critically ill patients, both through historical case series and through objectively derived predictive instruments.

This chapter covers three specific areas. The first section describes the prognosis of patients with the most common conditions found in the medical ICU, such as respiratory failure and sepsis. The second section provides an overview of the outcome instruments that have been developed to predict mortality in the ICU. The third section discusses social issues in critical care, such as expectations of patients and their families, advanced directives, and stratification of critically ill patients by resource utilization.

OUTCOMES OF MEDICAL CONDITIONS COMMONLY SEEN IN THE INTENSIVE CARE UNIT

Since ICUs were organized in the 1960s, many case series have delineated the outcomes of critically ill patients with specific primary diagnoses. Critical care originally focused on two major conditions: respiratory failure requiring mechanical ventilation and acute myocardial infarction with arrhythmia monitoring. However, outcomes in other disorders were soon described: acute respiratory distress syndrome (ARDS), sepsis, and multiorgan failure. While prognosis in such patients has been widely studied, most case studies have been poorly controlled for severity of illness, patient selection, and treatment variability. With these caveats in mind, the following discussion centers on the major diagnoses in the ICU and their prognosis.

Respiratory Failure

Acute respiratory failure (ARF) has been one of the most widely studied critical conditions. Studies have focused on three disorders: chronic obstructive pulmonary disease, status asthmaticus, and ARDS.

CHRONIC OBSTRUCTIVE PULMONARY DISEASE

ARF in chronic obstructive pulmonary disease (COPD) has often been defined using different criteria, but the most common criterion is the presence of an arterial CO_2 tension (Pa_{CO_2}) exceeding 50 mmHg. These historical data have not controlled for advances in therapy, such as more effective antibiotics and ventilator care, or for social issues, such as advanced directives, which may exclude patients from the ICU. And none of the studies have been controlled for other contributory illnesses.

With these limitations, pooled statistics show that before 1974, patients with COPD and ARF had a hospital mortality of 26 percent. Since 1975, the figure has decreased to 10 percent. Patients who require mechanical ventilation have a higher mortality, ranging from 20 to 60 percent.

Several investigators have examined both the acute and long-term prognosis of patients with COPD who are hospitalized for ARF. In a small series of patients with COPD and repetitive episodes of ARF, hospital survival was 70 percent after the first episode, 57 percent after the second episode, and 33 percent after the third episode.[18] Prognosis was particularly poor for patients with short intervals between each episode. Another series showed that hospital survival was 94 percent with the first episode, but that the 2-year survival of such patients was only 28 percent.[32] In a third series of patients with COPD treated with mechanical ventilation for ARF, 80 percent survived the episode, but 1-year survival was only 38 percent.[33] In this study, the premorbid severity of COPD and overall mortality were correlated.

These statistics were confirmed in a subsequent report of a 5-year experience with mechanical ventilation for ARF from all causes.[47] Fifty percent of patients survived to hospital discharge, but only 30 percent were alive 1 year after hospitalization. Combining these data with those from 10 previously reported series indicated that hospital survival in ARF is 43 percent; 1-year survival is 30 percent. The authors concluded that survival is related to younger age and respiratory failure associated with COPD or the postoperative state, and that prognosis is worse in patients who are resuscitated after a cardiopulmonary arrest. Overall survival was affected by age and the underlying cause of the respiratory failure, but not by the duration of mechanical ventilation.

A recent prospective study of 17,440 patients in ICUs has shed more light on the outcome of patients with COPD and ARF.[44] In this series, patients had a hospital survival of 76 percent, but a 1-year survival of 41 percent. After control for disease severity, the need for mechanical ventilation did not influence outcome. Hospital mortality was more closely associated with multiorgan failure than with the degree of respiratory failure or previous pulmonary function. However, mortality at 180 days was significantly related to prior pulmonary function.

Based on these observations, a reasonable conclusion is that patients with COPD who are admitted to the ICU for ARF appear to have a hospital survival that exceeds 70 percent. Hospital survival for such patients is influenced by the overall severity of illness, rather than the degree of respiratory failure, whether acute or chronic. However, survival for this group at 2 years is less than 50 percent, and is influenced by the severity of COPD.

STATUS ASTHMATICUS

The overall mortality of asthma in the United States appears to be rising.[19] Historical series have reported mortality ranging from 10 to 38 percent in patients with status asthmaticus treated with mechanical ventilation.[52] Two reports have suggested a better prognosis under these circumstances. In a group of 60 patients with status asthmaticus and hypercapnia, only five patients required mechanical ventilation; none died.[37] This observational study challenged the notion that hypercapnia in status asthmaticus requires mechanical ventilation and also signaled that aggressive use of bronchodilators may rescue these patients from modest respiratory failure.

In a series of 64 patients with status asthmaticus, mechanical ventilation was required in 30 percent of 80 episodes of acute respiratory failure.[4] There were no deaths, which may reflect the conservative use of mechanical ventilation, consequent diminished incidence of barotrauma, and aggressive use of bronchodilators.

Despite this glimmer of optimism, patients with near-fatal asthma, when followed prospectively, have an alarming mortality. At 1-year follow-up, the mortality of such patients is 10 percent; at 3 years, 14 percent; and at 6 years, as much as 25 percent.[31] Anoxia and prehospital asphyxiation are typical presentations. The statistics emphasize that the critically ill patient with asthma may require special follow-up after discharge in order to prevent recurrence of near-fatal asthma.

ACUTE RESPIRATORY DISTRESS SYNDROME (ARDS)

Acute respiratory distress syndrome (ARDS), a common cause of hypoxic respiratory failure, is often triggered by conditions such as sepsis, shock, and transfusion of blood products (see Chapter 166). ARDS has become more prevalent because of advances in ventilatory support, treatment of infections, and use of cardiopulmonary resuscitation.

An early hypothesis was that patients with ARDS might have an improved outcome if their ventilatory failure could be corrected. This led to a randomized, controlled study of extracorporeal membrane oxygenation to prevent death from hypoxia. The results of this study demonstrated that such intervention did not improve survival.[3]

After more experience with ARDS, it became clear that mortality is related not simply to respiratory failure but also to infection and failure of other organs, especially the liver, kidney, and central nervous system.[36] Study of ARDS has provided new insight into the interaction of organ systems in critical illness, and described the role of infection as an important cause of mortality in critically ill patients.

The outcome of ARDS has varied over time.[51] Petty and colleagues reported a mortality in ARDS of 60 percent in the years 1967 through 1981. Since then, however, published death rates have ranged from 32 to 47 percent. More recent reports have noted improved mortalities of 30 to 35 percent. More closely regulated treatment of ARDS and improved antibiotic therapy may be responsible for the improvement.[51]

Several factors appear to influence the outcome of patients with ARDS. The degree of organ failure and mortality in ARDS are strongly correlated.[45] Failure of two or more organs (brain, liver, lung, heart, kidney) increases mortality to approximately 80 percent. Failure of three or more organs raises the overall mortality from ARDS to 90 percent. Age also may correlate with prognosis, since for patients over 65 years of age the mortality is 66 percent; for patients under age 65, the mortality is 47 percent.[48]

The degree of hypoxemia in ARDS has been studied as a prognostic indicator.[21] The initial ratio of $Pa_{O_2}/F_{I_{O_2}}$ has only a modest correlation with ultimate survival. A much better correlation has been found between the combination of APACHE III score (see below) and primary ICU diagnosis and treatment location before admission to the ICU. This suggests that initial hypoxemia is simply a marker of the severity of the ARDS, and that the ultimate outcome is influenced by other factors.

Despite severe physiological and pathologic derangement in ARDS, survivors may have remarkable recovery of pulmonary function. Several reports suggest that patients are left with only modest respiratory function abnormalities.[14,17] Many patients have only a reduced diffusing capacity, or a slight fall in oxygen during exercise. Some have impairment due to restrictive lung disease. Severe abnormalities are unusual in the survivors of ARDS, however, and the functional outcome is good when patients are tested about a year after recovery. These findings lend considerable hope for supporting such patients through even the most severe respiratory failure.

Sepsis and the Systemic Inflammatory Response Syndrome

Infection and its complications frequently accompany critical illness. Bacteremia in hospitalized patients has an overall mortality of 20 to 30 percent.[6] The most common sources of infection are the urinary tract, respiratory tract, and indwelling devices, such as intravenous catheters. Urologic sepsis generally has a lower mortality than other types.

Advanced treatment strategies in areas like oncology and surgery have magnified the role of infection as a complication in hospitalized patients. Although many patients in ICUs present with signs and symptoms suggestive of sepsis (e.g., hypotension, fever), infection is not always documented. In 1992, a consensus conference developed the concept of "systemic inflammatory response syndrome" (SIRS).[1] The diagnosis of SIRS is based on a unified set of criteria to describe patients with a "sepsislike syndrome," which may or may not be caused by infection.[6] Other causes of SIRS are such conditions as pancreatitis, trauma, liver failure, and ARDS.

The new concept of SIRS has been subjected to only a limited number of prospective studies. In a series of nearly 4000 ICU patients in ICUs, 68 percent met the criteria for SIRS.[41] Among this group, 26 percent developed sepsis, 18 percent severe sepsis, and 4 percent septic shock. The hospital mortalities for the groups were 7 percent for SIRS, 16 percent for sepsis, 20 percent for severe sepsis, and 46 percent for septic shock. Similar results were found in a prospective study of 12,000 admissions to 170 ICUs in France.[6] Sepsis occurred in 9 percent of ICU admissions, and severe sepsis occurred in 6.3 percent. The 28-day mortality of patients with severe sepsis was 56 percent. In these reports, mortality increased with progressive multiorgan failure, coagulation disorders, and shock. The studies confirm that SIRS is common in critically ill patients and that it often progresses to sepsis and septic shock.

Nontraumatic Coma

Patients with nontraumatic coma are frequently admitted to critical care units. As a result of prospective studies,[26,27] there is considerable information about the prognosis of such patients. Patients without brain-stem function within the first 12 h of the onset of coma have little chance for meaningful neurologic recovery. Observations must be made in the absence of CNS depressant drugs or status epilepticus. Prognosis is independent of the cause of nontraumatic coma, but nontraumatic coma is frequently encountered in patients who have been the victims of cerebral hypoxia after cardiopulmonary resuscitation.

Malignancy

Patients with malignancy may require advanced procedures or therapies that result in the need for intensive care. Cancer victims who enter the ICU for reasons other than postoperative care have a 50 percent hospital mortality. The need for mechanical ventilation increases this figure to 70 percent.[43] Patients with leukemia who require mechanical ventilation have a mortality of 80 percent.[39] Bone marrow transplant recipients who require ventilatory support are particularly vulnerable, with a hospital mortality exceeding 95 percent.[11] Even if patients with malignancy recover from their critical illness, their prognosis is poor. The mean survival of these patients after ICU entry is only 5 months.[43]

Cardiopulmonary Resuscitation

The outcome of cardiopulmonary resuscitation (CPR) has been a subject of debate for more than 3 decades. Reported success rates range from 3 to 27 percent. Rates have been influenced by the setting in which the CPR is performed (in hospital versus out of hospital), age of the patients, and underlying diseases. A recent review summarized the reported experience of more than 26,000 patients who underwent in-hospital resuscitation.[42] The data suggest that while a third of hospitalized patients may be successfully resuscitated, fewer than half of this group will be discharged from the hospital alive. The long-term outcome of discharged patients appears to be favorable, since nearly three-quarters survive 1 year.

These summary statistics denote some other important prognostic factors. Patients with ventricular tachycardia or ventricular fibrillation have a better survival than those with asystole or electromechanical disassociation. Other favorable indicators are witnessed arrest, arrest in an emergency room or coronary care unit, respiratory arrest, short duration of CPR, and absence of comorbidity. Therefore, it appears that underlying disease, premorbid conditions, and the circumstances of the arrest are important determinants of outcome in CPR.

Age

Controversy exists over whether age is an independent predictor of mortality in critically ill patients. Approximately half of all patients in the United States who are admitted to the ICU are over 65 years of age. The percentages are much lower in other Western countries. Past reports suggested a correlation between increasing age and hospital mortality. However, more recent investigations using prognostic scoring systems have found that age is a weak variable in portending the likelihood of death.[8] More predictive power rests with such factors as underlying disease, previous functional status, and the number of failing organs. Nonetheless, older age is associated with a greater likelihood of disease and poor functional status, but no large studies have compared patients in different age groups with similar disease severity.

Two other elements in relation to patient age have been studied: utilization of ICU resources and cost and quality of life. While about 10 percent of critically ill patients consume about 50 percent of ICU costs, the costs are not disproportionately attributable to elderly patients. The functional assessment of quality of life in the elderly has yielded mixed results. Some studies suggest that there is no difference in functional outcome between elderly and young patients, while others suggest that the elderly are more impaired after critical care.[8] The studies have not been stratified for severity of illness, making comparisons between the two age groups difficult.

Acquired Immune Deficiency Syndrome

Treatment of complications of AIDS, especially respiratory failure due to *Pneumocystis carinii* pneumonia (PCP), has become increasingly common in the ICU. In a recent prospective study of 1550 patients with HIV infection admitted to ICUs, 54 percent of admissions were for respiratory failure, most of them due to PCP.[12] The hospital mortality for the entire group was 51 percent, while the death rates for respiratory failure and mechanical ventilation were 63 and 79 percent, respectively. These figures are very similar to those in another recent report, in which the mortality from severe PCP was 76 percent.[49]

SEVERITY OF ILLNESS SCORING SYSTEMS AND MORTALITY PREDICTION

The complexity of critically ill patients has exposed the limitations of historical methods of prognostication, such as case studies and clinical judgment. From the time of Socrates, physicians have accurately predicted outcome in patients at the extreme ends of the spectrum of disease severity. For example, even inexperienced clinicians can predict the high likelihood of death in a patient with multiple organ failure and shock. Similarly, these clinicians can correctly judge that patients admitted to the ICU only for arrhythmia monitoring have an excellent prognosis.

The challenge is that most patients entering the ICU fall somewhere in between these extremes of prognosis. Therefore, the outcome of most patients cannot be accurately assessed by application of clinical judgment. For example, a patient presenting with sepsis and hypotension might have a predicted mortality ranging from 15 to 40 percent, depending on underlying diseases, source of the infection, and other organ system disorders.

A number of compelling reasons exist for defining the severity of disease and the prognosis in all patients in the ICU. Assessing the quality of ICU care is difficult without some means to compare the severity of disease among ICUs. In an era of public accountability, critical-care physicians must ensure that their patients are provided the best possible care. Objectively measuring disease severity and prognosis allows rational description of patients in the ICU and lays the foundation for quality assessment. In addition, utilization of a severity scoring system provides a stable platform for research in ICU therapeutics and economics. Previous studies of critical illnesses have been hampered by difficulties in comparing severity of illness in patients in different ICUs. An objective scoring system stratifies patients by disease severity, permitting measurement of therapeutic effects and economic consequences. Finally, severity scoring systems may be useful in clinical decision making, especially in mapping the trajectory of the patient's critical illness.

This section provides a brief overview of the methodology of scoring systems and describes the three most commonly used and validated instruments.

Methods Employed in Developing Severity-Scoring Systems

Severity-scoring systems utilized in critical-care settings assign numeric values to various degrees of illness. The scores are then applied in a mathematical formula to calculate predicted mortality. To a great extent, the ultimate importance of the severity score is its power to predict mortality. Two characteristics are essential in judging predictive instruments: discrimination and calibration.

Discrimination is the accuracy of a given prediction. For example, if a scoring instrument predicts a mortality of 90 percent for a certain group of patients, discrimination is perfect if the observed mortality is 90 percent.

Calibration describes the accuracy of prediction over a wide range of predicted mortalities. In the example used above, an instrument is well calibrated if its predictive accuracy is excellent at mortalities of 90, 50, and 20 percent.

As noted previously, the time-honored method of outcome prediction has been clinical judgment provided by expert clinicians. As discussed, this judgment tends to be highly discriminate at the extremes of prognosis (e.g., 10 percent mortality and 90 percent mortality). Prediction by clinical judgment tends to be poorly calibrated, however, since its accuracy is erratic in the intermediate ranges of mortality.

The characteristics of discrimination and calibration are depicted in Fig. 180-1. A predictive instrument with perfect calibration and discrimination has predicted mortalities identical to observed mortalities over the complete range of mortality prediction. This corresponds to the line of identity seen on the graph. A poorly calibrated instrument has wide variability around the line of identity, while an instrument with better calibration has less variability around the line. Therefore, the ideal prediction instrument strives to reduce variability and to come as close to the line of identity as possible.

The methods used in developing ICU severity-scoring systems consist of several steps. The first step is to assess a representative patient population from a variety of ICUs. The key clinical characteristics of these patients are then analyzed statistically with multivariate analysis and logistic regression methods. The variables with the most discriminatory power for predicting mortality are then tested and validated on another patient population.

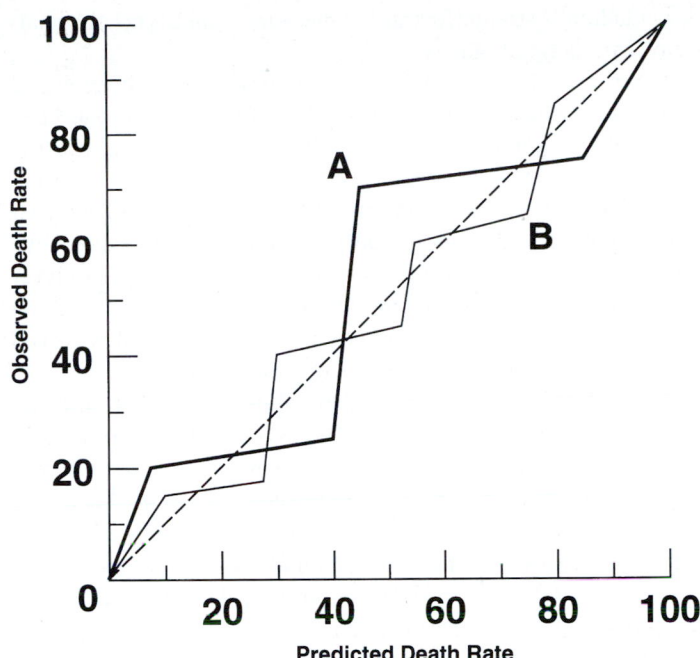

FIGURE 180-1   Calibration curves for two hypothetical scoring instruments. Perfect calibration is described by the line of identity. Instrument A has a wide variation around the identity line. Instrument B has less variability and therefore is better calibrated across the range of death rates. *(Data from Cowen and Kelley.*[10]*)*

Based on this process, the severity-scoring system and mortality prediction algorithms are derived.

Several important features are common among outcome instruments. They should measure an outcome of clinical significance. Most severity-scoring systems in critical care have focused on hospital mortality, but there is increasing interest in mortality beyond hospitalization and functional status. These instruments should also be easy to use. Data collection on critically ill patients can be time-consuming and costly. Therefore, outcome instruments have focused on data that are simple to record and reproduce. Finally, these instruments have limitations to their application. Notably, they cannot accurately predict outcome for populations not included in their derivation data sets. For example, ICU severity-scoring systems are not applicable to all hospitalized patients. It is important to understand these limitations so that outcome instruments are not misused.

Acute Physiology, Age, and Chronic Health Evaluation Scoring System

The Acute Physiology, Age, and Chronic Health Evaluation (APACHE) scoring system has two versions (II and III), which are widely used in the United States and have been reviewed fairly recently.[10] APACHE II was derived from studies in 13 hospitals, based on approximately 6000 patients. This instrument assigns points for age, underlying disease, and several other elements of chronic health status; it adds points for physiological variables measured in the first 24 h of ICU admission. The total severity score is entered into a logistic regression equation, which provides a predicted mortality.

APACHE II has excellent calibration and discrimination, but it has several flaws. The first is that the instrument is not as accurate when applied to patients in the ICU who are transferred from other inpatient facilities. The mortality of these patients is generally underestimated by APACHE II as a result of an effect known as "lead time bias." The second flaw is that the derivation database is not powerful enough to allow stratification of patients by certain disease categories, such as liver failure, respiratory failure, etc. Therefore, APACHE II cannot accurately predict outcome for any specific patient subgroup.

The updated version of APACHE II, called APACHE III, has addressed these problems. APACHE III was derived from 40 representative hospitals and more than 17,000 patients. This instrument includes many of the variables in APACHE II but adds prior treatment location and the disease requiring admission to the ICU.[20] APACHE III also updates prognosis daily, based on newly measured physiological variables.

The APACHE instruments have been published widely and studied internationally. Their discrimination and calibration have been well validated; the flaws in older versions have been addressed and corrected. However, the APACHE scores require a great deal of data collection and an investment in expensive proprietary computer technology. In addition, it remains unclear whether specific disease subgroups can be assessed, even with the expanded APACHE III database.

Simplified Acute Physiological Score

The simplified acute physiological score (SAPS) was developed to reduce the amount of data required by APACHE. SAPS concentrates on physiological variables, as well as such elements as the type of admission and underlying diseases, to provide a summary score after 24 h of ICU admission. SAPS II uses 17 variables: 12 physiological variables, age, type of admission, and three underlying disease variables (AIDS, metastatic cancer, hematologic malignancy). The scoring system was derived from 8500 patients and validated on a sample of 4500 patients.[24] The model provides a score that is entered into a mathematical formula whose solution provides a predicted hospital mortality. SAPS II does not require a principal ICU diagnosis, which is mandated with APACHE III. Based on the published data, SAPS II has excellent discrimination and calibration.[7]

Mortality Prediction Model

Like SAPS, the mortality prediction model (MPM) was developed to simplify severity scoring in critically ill patients. MPM was originally developed in one hospital, but its second version (MPM II) had a derivation database of 12,610 patients from many hospitals.[25] MPM requires that patients be placed in categoric classifications that correspond to certain scores. The categories consist of several physiological assessments, chronic diagnoses, acute diagnoses, and other characteristics, such as type of admission, age, CPR, and use of mechanical ventilation. The total score is derived from 15 easily obtainable variables.

The MPM score is determined immediately upon ICU admission (MPM 0), but it can be updated after 24 h (MPM 24). The update contains five of the admission variables and eight additional variables, such as arterial blood gases, creatinine, prothrombin time, urine output, etc. Like SAPS II, MPM II has excellent calibration and discrimination.[7] MPM 0 utilizes measurements made immediately upon ICU admission. This measurement time may define a patient population that is different from that assessed 24 h after treatment and after the evolution of other diagnoses. Only the MPM 24 can be compared to SAPS and APACHE, since all three instruments use measurements performed within the first 24 h of admission.

USE OF SEVERITY SCORES IN THE INTENSIVE CARE UNIT

The development of reliable severity scoring systems in critical care has opened the field to a wide range of opportunities in health-care management and research. In addition, severity-scoring systems can be considered with regard to their implication in resource allocation, quality management, and clinical decision making.

Allocation of Resources

The allocation of ICU resources is grounded in the fundamental principle of fairness, which itself has several potential interpretations.[34] The first is the concept of *equality,* which implies that all patients are entitled to the same access and level of ICU care. The second interpretation is the principle of *equity,* whereby a patient's level of care does not jeopardize that of others. A third concept, *utilitarianism,* places the overall benefit of society above that of the individual. The final application of fairness is *distribution according to medical need,* regardless of social issues (see Chapter 181).

In the United States, medical need has traditionally dictated allocation of critical care resources. Recently, outcomes and outcome prediction in critical care have raised the issue of medical suitability. This concept dictates that outcome of care, as well as medical need, should be used to assess application of ICU resources. The critical-care community has summarized these issues in a consensus statement on triage of critically ill patients.[46] The guiding principles in this statement are patient advocacy, equitable distribution of care, and provision of care on the basis of expected benefit.

Outcome instruments have been useful in the management of hospital resources. Severity scores have been used to identify patients who no longer need intensive nursing and who can be placed in lower-cost settings. Physician and nursing staffs can be assessed in relation to ICU severity, and appropriate adjustments made. These analyses may extend beyond the hospital walls to include a regional approach to critical care. Like trauma patients, critically ill patients may be triaged by severity of illness, so that the most complex cases are treated in larger ICUs.

Quality Management

Because of the rising costs of health care, patients and their insurers have sought methods to compare the value of choosing certain providers. This "health-care value" has been defined conceptually as quality divided by cost. While the economic side of this equation is straightforward to measure, quantifying the quality of care is more elusive.

In critical care, severity-scoring instruments have been useful in several examples of assessing quality of ICU care, as has been reviewed.[40] Some uncontrolled studies using predictive scoring instruments suggest that patient outcome is better in ICUs staffed by trained intensivists.[5,28] Interhospital comparisons of hospital mortality have been widely published since several states have mandated outcome measurements in all hospitals. In the Cleveland metropolitan area, all critically ill patients are assessed using the APACHE III system to compare predicted and observed mortality and to link these results to hospital costs.

Pennsylvania and New York also publish outcome results according to hospital and provider. Pennsylvania uses a proprietary predictive instrument called Medisgroup, which, unlike most predictive instruments, has not been published and has not been subjected to peer review scrutiny. The developers of Medisgroup claim that it works well for all hospitalized patients, including those in the ICU. However, the validity of the published statistics provided by this instrument has recently been challenged, at least for the diagnosis of pneumonia.[29]

Institutional comparisons with predictive instruments may be misleading. Two studies using APACHE II demonstrated that previous patient treatment location can influence the accuracy of APACHE II. In the first report, APACHE II underestimated mortality in an ICU that accepted transfers from other institutions.[13] In the second study, APACHE II underestimated mortality for patients previously treated in the hospital, but it overestimated mortality for patients admitted from the emergency room.[15] As previously described, this phenomenon, called lead-time bias, has been adjusted in APACHE III. However, this example demonstrates that even a well-designed instrument such as APACHE II can have unanticipated problems, making institutional comparisons challenging.

Controversies abound concerning the accuracy and relevance of measuring quality of care. Critical care has several advantages in the assessment of quality of care: (1) the patient population in ICUs is well defined, and the provision of care is well circumscribed; (2) there is substantial evidence that the degree of illness in the ICU is the major determinant of patients' hospital mortality; (3) these instruments have considerable power to risk-adjust ICU populations and to permit evaluation of ICU effectiveness and efficiency. Therefore, severity-scoring systems provide a foundation for assessing quality of critical care.

Clinical Decision Making

Severity-scoring systems can be helpful in predicting outcome across the entire range of prognosis. However, in assessment of an individual patient in the ICU, only the extremes of probability are of practical importance. For purpose of triage, patients who are clearly terminal, or who do not require intensive care, are useful to identify. For such assessment, clinical judgment, often based on historical case series, is as accurate as any outcome instrument. Patients in between these extremes of prognosis are usually eligible for critical care.

A concept of continuous prognostication has been introduced into the APACHE III instrument. With this technology, disease severity and prognosis can be continuously updated to plot the trajectory of the patient's illness.[20] This updated severity score may have more predictive power than that obtained in the first 24 h of ICU admission.[50] The implication is that continuous monitoring of disease severity may assist in critical decisions, such as limiting or withdrawing therapy. This idea has evolved into the concept of "potentially ineffective care" that categorizes patients with a poor prognosis who consume an inordinate amount of resources.[16]

The challenge is that there may be a substantial disparity in how health-care workers use prognostic information compared to patients and their families. In Canada, one survey demonstrated that health-care workers could not even agree among themselves on criteria for withdrawing life support.[9] Two studies have documented that do-not-resuscitate orders are increasingly common in ICUs.[2,23] However, one of these reports indicated that patients and their families did not always participate in this process.[2]

The recently published Study to Understand Prognoses and Preferences for Outcomes and Risks of Treatment (SUPPORT) examined how communicating continuously updated prognosis in the ICU influences clinical decision making.[22] The study consisted of an observational period that, in addition to measuring prognosis, demonstrated significant differences in the outcome expectations of health-care workers, patients, and families. The intervention component of the study attempted to bridge the communication gap by sharing the updated prognoses and establishing better methods of communication among the health-care providers, patients, and families. Surprisingly, the study showed that this intervention had no measurable effect on clinical decision making. The ICU teams continued to emphasize the technologic quest for cure, rather than concentrating on the patients' desire to avoid suffering and prolonged, painful dying. The investigators concluded that, at least in the five tertiary academic centers studied, critical-care providers appear to be insensitive to the needs and expectations of patients.

SUPPORT underscores the need for better communication in the ICU with patients and their families. Health-care professionals, in general, may need more training in communication skills and in understanding the social and cultural diversity that characterizes the American population. Finally, SUPPORT suggests that patients may have limited and more realistic expectations of high technology than do the critical-care physicians who foster it. Therefore, severity-scoring systems should be used to facilitate doctor-patient communication, rather than supplant it.

REFERENCES

1. American College of Chest Physicians/Society of Critical Care Medicine Consensus Conference: Definitions for sepsis and organ failure and guidelines for the use of innovative therapies in sepsis. *Crit Care Med* 20:864–875, 1992.
2. Asch DA, Hansen-Flaschen J, Lanken PN: Decisions to limit or continue life-sustaining treatment by critical care physicians in the United States: Conflicts between physicians' practices and patients' wishes. *Am J Respir Crit Care Med* 151:288–292, 1995.
3. Bartlett RH, Morris AH, Fairley HB, et al: A prospective study of acute hypoxic respiratory failure. *Chest* 89:684–689, 1986.
4. Braman SS, Kaemmerlen JT: Intensive care of status asthmaticus: A 10-year experience. *JAMA* 264:366–368, 1990.
5. Brown JJ, Sullivan G: Effect on ICU mortality of a full-time critical care specialist. *Chest* 96:127–129, 1989.
6. Brun-Buisson C, Doyon F, Carlet J, et al: Incidence, risk factors, and outcome of severe sepsis and septic shock in adults: A multicenter prospective study in intensive care units. *JAMA* 274:968–974, 1995.
7. Castella X, Artigas A, Bion J, Kari A, The European/North American Severity Study Group: A comparison of severity of illness scoring systems for intensive care unit patients: Results of a multicenter, multinational study. *Crit Care Med* 23:1327–1335, 1995.
8. Chelluri L, Grenvik A, Silverman M: Intensive care for critically ill elderly: Mortality, costs, and quality of life. *Arch Intern Med* 155:1013–1022, 1995.
9. Cook DJ, Guyatt GH, Jaeschke R, et al: Determinants in Canadian health care workers of the decision to withdraw life support from the critically ill. *JAMA* 273:703–708, 1995.
10. Cowen JS, Kelley, MA: Predicting intensive care unit outcome: Errors and bias in using predictive scoring systems. *Crit Care Clin* 10:53–72, 1994.
11. Crawford SW, Petersen FB: Long-term survival from respiratory failure after marrow transplantation for malignancy. *Am Rev Respir Dis* 145:510–514, 1992.
12. DePalo VA, Millstein BH, Mayo PH, et al: Outcome of intensive care in patients with HIV infection. *Chest* 107:506–510, 1995.
13. Dragsted L, Jorgensen J, Jensen NH, et al: Interhospital comparisons of patient outcome from intensive care: Importance of lead-time bias. *Crit Care Med* 17:418–422, 1989.
14. Elliott CG: Pulmonary sequelae in survivors of the adult respiratory distress syndrome. *Clin Chest Med* 11:789–800, 1990.
15. Escarce JJ, Kelley MA: Admission source to the medical intensive care unit predicts hospital death independent of APACHE II score. *JAMA* 264:2389–2394, 1990.
16. Esserman L, Belkora J, Lenert L: Potentially ineffective care: A new outcome to assess the limits of critical care. *JAMA* 274:1544–1551, 1995.
17. Ghio AJ, Elliott CG, Grapo RO, et al: Impairment after adult respiratory distress syndrome: An evaluation based on American Thoracic Society recommendations. *Am Rev Respir Dis* 139:1158–1162, 1989.
18. Gottlieb LS, Balchum OH: Course of chronic obstructive pulmonary disease following first onset of respiratory failure. *Chest* 63:5–8, 1973.
19. Jackson R, Sears MR, Beaglehole R, Rea HH: International trends in asthma mortality: 1970 to 1985. *Chest* 94:914–918, 1988.
20. Knaus WA, Wagner DP, Draper EA, et al: The APACHE III prognostic system: Risk prediction of hospital mortality for critically ill hospitalized adults. *Chest* 100:1619–1636, 1991.
21. Knaus WA, Sun X, Hakim RB, Wagner DP: Evaluation of definitions for adult respiratory distress syndrome. *Am J Respir Crit Care Med* 150:311–317, 1994.
22. Knaus WA: The SUPPORT Principal Investigators: A controlled trial to improve care for seriously ill hospitalized patients: The Study to Understand Prognoses and Preferences for Outcomes and Risks of Treatments (SUPPORT). *JAMA* 274:1591–1598, 1995.
23. Jayes RL, Zimmerman JE, Wagner DP, et al: Do-not-resuscitate orders in intensive care units: Current practices and recent changes. *JAMA* 270:2213–2217, 1993.
24. Le Gall J-R, Lemeshow S, Saulnier F: A new simplified acute physiology score (SAPS II) based on a European/North American multicenter study. *JAMA* 270:2957–2963, 1993.

25. Lemeshow S, Teres D, Klar J, et al: Mortality probability models (MPM II) based on an international cohort of intensive care unit patients. *JAMA* 270:2478–2486, 1993.

26. Levy DE, Plum F: Outcome prediction in comatose patients: Significance of reflex eye movement analysis (letter). *J Neurol Neurosug Psychiatry* 51:318, 1988.

27. Levy DE, Bates D, Caronna JJ, et al: Prognosis in nontraumatic coma. *Ann Intern Med* 94:293–301, 1981.

28. Li TC, Phillips M, et al: On-site physician staffing in a community hospital intensive care unit: Impact on test and procedure use and on patient outcome. *JAMA* 252:2023–2027, 1984.

29. Localio AR, Hamory BH, Sharp TJ, et al: Comparing hospital mortality in adult patients with pneumonia: A case study of statistical methods in a managed care program. *Ann Intern Med* 122:125–132, 1995.

30. Mansel JK, Stogner SW, Petrini MF, Norman JR: Mechanical ventilation in patients with acute severe asthma. *Am J Med* 89:42–48, 1990.

31. Marquette CH, Saulnier F, Leroy O, et al: Long-term prognosis of near-fatal asthma. *Am Rev Respir Dis* 146:76–81, 1992.

32. Martin TR, Lewis SW, Albert RK: The prognosis of patients with chronic obstructive pulmonary disease after hospitalization for acute respiratory failure. *Chest* 82:310–314, 1982.

33. Menzies R, Gibbons W, Goldberg P: Determinants of weaning and survival among patients with COPD who require mechanical ventilation for acute respiratory failure. *Chest* 95:398–405, 1989.

34. Miller DH: The rationing of intensive care. *Crit Care Clin* 10:135–143, 1994.

35. Molfino NA, Nannini LJ, Rebuck AS, Slutsky AS: The fatality-prone asthmatic patient: Follow-up study after near-fatal attacks. *Chest* 101:621–623, 1992.

36. Montgomery AB, Stager MA, Carrico CJ, Hudson LD: Causes of mortality in patients with the adult respiratory distress syndrome. *Am Rev Respir Dis* 132:485–489, 1985.

37. Mountain RD, Sahn SA: Clinical features and outcome in patients with acute asthma presenting with hypercapnia. *Am Rev Respir Dis* 138:535–539, 1988.

38. Peters JI, Bell RC, Prihoda TJ, et al: Clinical determinants of abnormalities in pulmonary functions in survivors of the adult respiratory distress syndrome. *Am Rev Respir Dis* 139:1163–1168, 1989.

39. Peters SG, Meadows JA III, Gracey DR: Outcome of respiratory failure in hematologic malignancy. *Chest* 94:99–102, 1988.

40. Rafkin HS, Hoyt JW: Objective data and quality assurance programs: Current and future trends. *Crit Care Clin* 10:157–177, 1994.

41. Rangel-Frausto MS, Pittet D, Costigan M, et al: The natural history of the systemic inflammatory response syndrome (SIRS): A prospective study. *JAMA* 273:117–123, 1995.

42. Saklayen M, Liss H, Markert R: In-hospital cardiopulmonary resuscitation survival in one hospital and a review of the literature. *Medicine* 74:163–175, 1995.

43. Schapira DV, Studnicki J, Bradham DD, et al: Intensive care, survival, and expense of treating critically ill cancer patients. *JAMA* 269:783–786, 1993.

44. Seneff MG, Wagner DP, Wagner RP, et al: Hospital and 1-year survival of patients admitted to intensive care units with acute exacerbation of chronic obstructive pulmonary disease. *JAMA* 274:1852–1856, 1995.

45. Sloane PJ, Gee MH, Gottlieb JE, et al: A multicenter registry of patients with acute respiratory distress syndrome. *Am Rev Respir Dis* 146:419–426, 1992.

46. Society of Critical Care Medicine: Consensus statement on the triage of critically ill patients. *JAMA* 271:1200–1203, 1994.

47. Stauffer JL, Fayter NA, Graves B, et al: Survival following mechanical ventilation for acute respiratory failure in adult men. *Chest* 104:1222–1229, 1993.

48. Suchyta MR, Clemmer TP, Elliott CG, et al: The adult respiratory distress syndrome: A report of survival and modifying factors. *Chest* 101:1074–1079, 1992.

49. Wachter RM, Luce JM, Safrin S, et al: Cost and outcome of intensive care for patients with AIDS, pneumocystis carinii pneumonia, and severe respiratory failure. *JAMA* 273:230–234, 1995.

50. Wagner DP, Knaus WA, Harrell FE, et al: Daily prognostic estimates for critically ill adults in intensive care units: Results from a prospective, multicenter, inception cohort analysis. *Crit Care Med* 22:1359–1372, 1994.

51. Weiss SM, Hudson LD: Outcome from respiratory failure: Predicting intensive care unit outcome. *Crit Care Clin* 10:197–215, 1994.

52. Westerman DE, Benatar SR, Potgieter PD, Ferguson AD: Identification of the high-risk asthmatic patient: Experience with 39 patients undergoing ventilation for status asthmaticus. *Am J Med* 66:565–572, 1979.

CHAPTER 181

ETHICS IN THE INTENSIVE CARE UNIT

Paul N. Lanken

Two seemingly paradoxical paradigms of contemporary medicine characterize patient care in the modern intensive care unit (ICU). In one, the ICU defines the setting in which depersonalized, "high-tech" medicine is practiced. In the other, the ICU represents a health care delivery site in which the deeply humanistic concerns of bioethics are evident on a day-to-day basis. *Ethics,* in simple terms, is the discipline that concerns itself with defining the right action for the right reasons. *Bioethics* generically refers to the ethics encompassing health care and health care professionals as well as basic biological and physical scientific research relevant to human health and disease.

Many ethical dilemmas in the ICU share common themes. For example, advanced technology and a high level of professional intervention in the ICU can keep patients alive for prolonged periods. However, this same capacity for delivering life-sustaining care often fails to achieve what patients really want and what has been the traditional goal of critical care medicine: restoration of patients to sufficiently good health to permit them to leave the ICU. Ethical dilemmas that characterize critical care medicine often arise from this interface between the ability to prolong life by expensive and sometimes scarce technology and an inability to cure the patient. The relevant ethical question often is whether the technology is being used wisely, i.e., whether the patient's life *should* be prolonged. The question becomes even more complex for practitioners and patients' families when different ethical principles suggest conflicting answers.

Although the practice of critical care medicine encompasses a broad range of bioethical issues, several are particularly common, including end-of-life decision making, medical futility, resource allocation, and "do not resuscitate"(DRN) orders. These issues are among the most challenging to ICU practitioners and constitute the focus of this chapter.

FUNDAMENTAL PRINCIPLES OF BIOETHICS

Three fundamental principles of bioethics are particularly relevant in the ICU: (1) beneficence, (2) respect for patient autonomy, and (3) justice.[4] Ethical dilemmas in the ICU arise when two or more of these principles are in conflict. To resolve the conflict, health care providers must violate one or more ethical principles in determining which is the overriding one. Potential conflicts among bioethical principles are illustrated in Fig. 181-1.

Also shown in the figure are the moral entities that relate to each principle. The principle of beneficence primarily involves physicians, nurses, other health care providers, and health care institutions, all of which are moral agents, having inherent values and moral responsibilities. Respect for patient autonomy relates to patients, their families, and surrogate decision makers or proxies—i e , individuals who speak on behalf of those patients who lack the capacity to make medical care decisions.

In Fig. 181-1, *justice* refers to fairness in the distribution of limited resources, i.e., *distributive justice.* This principle is usually discussed in terms of two levels of applicability. First, on the level of *macroallocation* of resources, distributive justice entails governmental and institutional decisions on the relative importance of funding health care among a number of social goods and services (e.g., education and defense). *Macroallocation* also refers to the distribution of health care resources among various regions and communities—e.g., funding for Medicare, Medic-

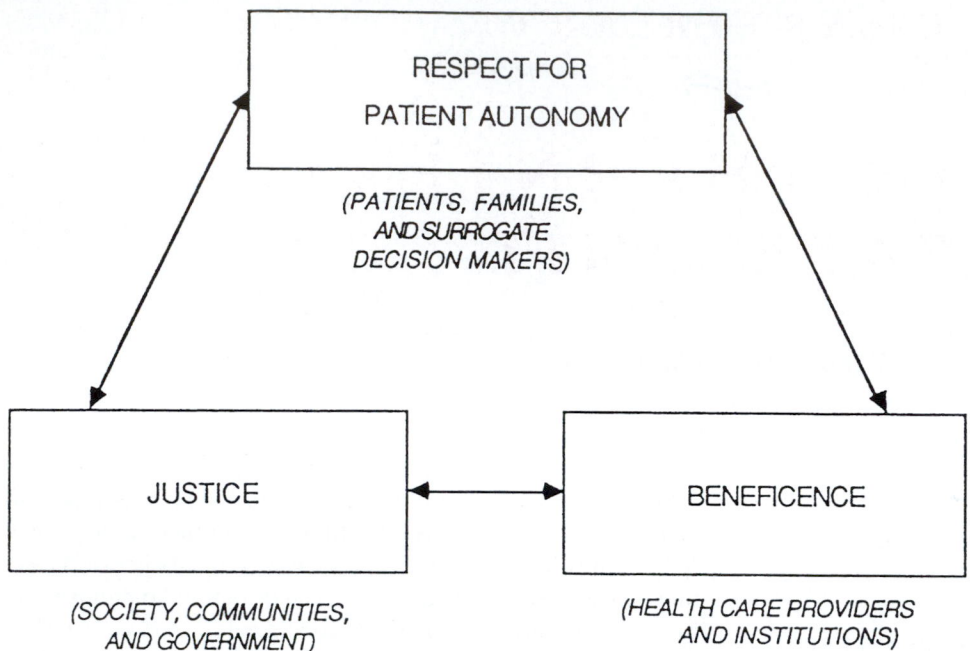

RESPECT FOR
PATIENT AUTONOMY

(PATIENTS, FAMILIES,
AND SURROGATE
DECISION MAKERS)

JUSTICE   BENEFICENCE

(SOCIETY, COMMUNITIES,   (HEALTH CARE PROVIDERS
AND GOVERNMENT)   AND INSTITUTIONS)

FIGURE 181-1   Three basic ethical principles and related moral agents commonly involved in ICU ethical dilemmas: respect for patient autonomy, beneficence, and justice. Opposing arrows represent potential conflicts between principles.

aid, and the Veterans Administration health care system. Second, on the level of *microallocation* of resources, *distributive justice* refers to decision making about an individual patient or resource allocation within an individual ICU, hospital, or local health care system. These three important bioethical principles are developed further below.

Beneficence

The principle of *beneficence* refers to the traditional aim of medicine and nursing to provide services that benefit the patient. Beneficence may be broadly interpreted to include the principle of *nonmaleficence*—i.e., doing no harm to the patient. The Hippocratic maxim *primum non nocere,* which can be translated as "First of all do no harm," reflects the fundamental importance of this principle for physicians. These two principles—beneficence and nonmaleficence—commonly conflict when the patient suffers pain as a consequence of receiving beneficial care, e.g., discomfort of suctioning while intubated. The bioethical conflict can be resolved when it can reasonably be concluded that the discomfort of suctioning is more than balanced by its beneficial effects.

In the Hippocratic tradition of beneficence and nonmaleficence, physicians had not only the responsibility but also the authority to determine what was best for their patients. This has evolved to the more contemporary notion, especially prominent in the United States, that the patient, rather than the physician, determines what is best for the patient. The physician's role has evolved from the traditional authoritarian model to that of someone whose role is to educate the patient about appropriate choices and to make recommendations. In this interpretation, the principles of beneficence and nonmaleficence are congruent with the principle of respect for patient autonomy.

Respect for Patient Autonomy

The principle of *respect for patient autonomy* is embodied by the legal concept of *self-determination:* A competent adult has a right to determine what will be done to his or her body. This principle also relates closely to the legal principle of an individual's right to privacy. According to these principles, the patient has the right to decide whether or not to undergo medical interventions. The principle of respect for autonomy is also the basis for informed consent.[2] Except in emergency circumstances, a competent adult must give informed consent prior to receiving medical care, especially that which involves potentially hazardous interventions. Under emergency conditions—i.e., when the patient's life, limb, or other vital functions are at risk without the intervention—consent is presumed. In the United States, there is a widespread societal and professional consensus that health care providers should not only respect a patient's autonomy but also enhance it through shared medical decision making.[19]

Distributive Justice

In the context of the ICU, the principle of justice refers to the principle of distributive justice. As alluded to previously, this principle pertains to defining fairness in allocating resources among individuals when not all can receive the resources. Aristotle stated the concept of distributive justice as the "principle of formal justice," according to which equals should be treated equally and unequals unequally.[4,26] Although it appears rather straightforward, this formulation cannot be applied easily, because reasonable criteria need to be identified in judging whether two individuals are equal or unequal. When applied to distributive justice, various ethical theories define different values as the most relevant criterion, as described below.

EGALITARIAN THEORY

The *egalitarian theory* of justice holds that individuals have equal intrinsic worth and that therefore distributions should not be made based on perceptions of individuals' different social worth. One egalitarian strategy for fair allocation of health care resources is that patients having the same medical need should have the same medical resources. An example of this is health care funding in the United States for patients with end-stage renal disease (ESRD), all of whose medical expenses are covered by Medicare. Another egalitarian approach holds that each person should have an equal chance of receiving a scarce resource. Examples include dialysis centers that, prior to Medicare funding, held lotteries to determine who would receive chronic dialysis, and centers that took applicants on a "first come, first served" basis. The latter practice can be considered equivalent to a "natural lottery," although nonuniform access to the health care system by poor (uninsured) and wealthy patients may have made it a biased one.

UTILITARIAN THEORY

Other theories of ethics are based on different criteria. The *utilitarian* theory of justice is centered on the principle of utility and contends that a fair decision should maximize utility as its consequence. For example, the maxim "The greatest good for the greatest number" reflects utilitarianism. According to this theory, a country with limited health care resources could justify disproportionate spending on public health interventions benefiting many citizens, rather than on critical care beds that benefit relatively few. In the United States, prior to universal Medicare coverage for chronic dialysis, some centers based treatment access on perceived social worth—a utilitarian schema. Patients were prioritized according to whether they were employed, their type of employment, family status, and other measures of perceived social worth.[26] Not unexpectedly, successful dialysis candidates resembled the white, male, middle-class constituents of the anonymous "selection committees." When this approach was publicized, it was criticized as unfair and discriminatory, and public outcry was the impetus for universal Medicare funding for patients with ESRD.

LIBERTARIAN THEORY

Another approach to distributive justice, the *libertarian* view, holds that health care resources should be allocated according to one's resources and ability to pay for them. Private health insurance in the United States is an example of the libertarian view.

DEONTOLOGICAL THEORIES

Deontological, or duty-based, theories of justice are based on rules that define ethical behavior. One influential deontological theory, Rawls theory, relates to social institutions in general.[9,26] From Rawls' theory were derived the concepts of provision of fair, decent, minimum healthcare benefits for all, and fair, equal opportunity.[21] The latter concept supports provision of *more than an equal share* of resources to those who are disadvantaged in order to promote a basic level of societal functioning. On this basis, health care resources should be allocated according to need of the individual patient in order to preserve or restore a basic level of functioning.

Another deontological principle that affects the distribution of limited resources is the so-called rule of rescue.[13] This principle refers to the duty of society to expend resources to save an identified individual's life if society has the means to do so. The rule underlies well-publicized rescue efforts for individuals whose lives are in danger. Equally predictable but unidentifiable (i.e., anonymous) statistical deaths are not accorded the same moral obligation. Emphasis on the practice of "rescue-type" medicine in the United States, including the burgeoning of ICUs, has been heavily influenced by the rule of rescue.

RELATIONSHIP BETWEEN HEALTH CARE LAW AND ETHICS

Ethical behavior and legal requirements may not be exactly congruous. For example, traditional application of the law to health care providers has been viewed as a type of "minimal morality." States *require* that practitioners providing medical or nursing care be licensed. In contrast, the professional ethics of these practitioners represents ideal professional behavior: Care *should* always be provided in accord with the principle of beneficence. For many clinical issues, the relationship between ethical and legal viewpoints is more complex.

The legality of what health care professionals do may change, depending on external circumstances. For example, health care law may vary considerably over time between two different jurisdictions. Similarly, what is regarded as ethical or unethical behavior for physicians may change. As an example, consider active euthanasia by physicians. Although this is a controversial issue, the practice of euthanasia is considered unethical by all major American professional medical societies. Furthermore, according to state law, it is illegal in the United States. However, euthanasia administered by physicians may become both ethical and legal in the future.

A good example of the complexity of bioethics is the issue of active euthanasia in the Netherlands. On the one hand, it can be viewed as illegal because of a statute against it. On the other, euthanasia can be viewed as ethical for physicians to perform if it is done in accord with an agreed-upon process. As these considerations highlight, bioethics should be viewed by health care providers not as a concrete body of knowledge but rather as a continually evolving field, not unlike clinical medicine.

PRINCIPLES REGARDING END-OF-LIFE ISSUES IN THE INTENSIVE CARE UNIT

During the last two decades a broad societal consensus has developed regarding the ethics of withholding or withdrawing life-sustaining therapies or life support.[20] This consensus was catalyzed, for the most part, by precedent-setting judicial decisions, such as the 1972 Spence decision in the District of Columbia on informed consent,[8] the 1976 New Jersey Supreme Court decision regarding Karen Ann Quinlan,[12] and the 1984 California Supreme Court decision regarding Bartling.[3] Based on these and related decisions, this consensus has been established, which underscores a number of general principles guiding health care professionals in making decisions related to withholding and withdrawing life-sustaining therapy. These principles are discussed in this and subsequent sections.

Principle 1: Informed adults with decision-making capacity can forgo any life-sustaining medical therapy, even if the action results in their death.

The key words and phrases in Principle 1 are *adult, informed,* and *decision-making capacity.* The principle applies only to adults, since children generally lack the personal autonomy required by legal or ethical standards. An adult must have appropriate information, provided in an understandable format, in order to arrive at an informed decision. In addition, he or she must have sufficient mental capacity to evaluate the specific decision being considered. Assessment of the adequacy of decision-making capacity is described below.

Principle 2: Forgoing life-sustaining therapy includes not only the withholding of such therapy as cardiopulmonary resuscitation but also its withdrawal. Life-sustaining therapies include mechanical ventilation, nutrition, and hydration. There is no significant ethical or legal difference between withholding and withdrawing life-sustaining therapy.

Controversy over the moral distinctions between actions and omissions leading to a patient's death ended when consensus developed that withdrawing care is ethically equivalent to withholding care.[20] Likewise, in general, there are no legal distinctions between withholding and withdrawing.

The legal issue of whether medically provided food and water constitutes medical care was decided when the U.S. Supreme Court deemed it so in its 1990 decision on Nancy Cruzan.[7] This decision established the legal right to refuse any medical care by competent adults or by appropriate surrogate decision makers acting in accord with the patient's previously expressed preferences or values.

Principle 3: Surrogate decision makers should make decisions to forgo life-sustaining therapy on behalf of patients who have lost decision-making capacity as long as the decisions are based on knowledge of what the patient would have wanted under similar circumstances. In the absence of such knowledge, decisions should be based on the patient's best interests.

Surrogate decision makers are commonly one or more members of the patient's immediate family. However, others may serve in this role under a number of circumstances. When a patient has legally designated someone as health care proxy by means of a durable power of attorney for health care, the designee must be the surrogate decision maker, even if he or she is not a member of the patient's family. When the patient has not arranged for a valid durable power of attorney but has otherwise identified someone as health care proxy, either in writing or verbally, his or her choice should be respected. Finally, when the patient has not designated a health care proxy or where state statutes do not specify a formal legal hierarchy that determines the order of selection of a surrogate, the presumption is that a close family member who knows the patient well should be the surrogate decision maker. In these circumstances, the patient's attending physician, as an advocate for protecting the patient's interests, has the responsibility for evaluating the appropriateness of a surrogate decision maker.

Two ethical and legal standards guide the decisions of a surrogate decision maker: (1) the *substituted judgment standard* and (2) the *best interests standard.*

Under the substituted judgment standard, the surrogate decision maker expresses what the patient would have preferred under the circumstances. The decision maker must have knowledge either about the preferences of the patient, as expressed orally or in writing in an advanced directive (e.g., a living will), or about the patient's values and life goals, from which valid inferences can be made.

Under the best interests standard, such knowledge is lacking, and the surrogate decision maker must weigh the *benefits* of life-sustaining therapy against its *burdens;* the decision is based on the outcome of the balance. For example, the benefits of life,

chance of survival, and chance of full recovery are weighed against the burdens of pain, additional suffering, and eventual quality of life.

Principle 4: When in doubt about a patient's preferences, health care providers should err on the side of sustaining life.

The essence of Principle 4 may be obvious. Less obvious is a corollary to the principle: Health care providers who work to sustain a patient's life should be willing to stop life-sustaining therapy if it is later determined that the patient would not have wanted it or that it was not in his or her best interests. Consistent with this principle is the concept of a therapeutic trial of life support: Certain life-sustaining therapy may be started, despite uncertainty about its effectiveness, in order to determine whether the therapy will benefit the patient. This approach has additional rationale since, once therapy is under way, the decision to continue it or not can be made by an objective assessment, rather than a "prediction," of its effectiveness. For example, the question often arises whether a patient with acute respiratory failure complicating severe chronic obstructive pulmonary disease, once intubated and ventilated, can be successfully weaned from mechanical ventilation. In many cases, the question can be resolved only by a time-limited therapeutic trial of assisted ventilation. In certain instances, it can be agreed before the therapeutic trial that the ventilator will be withdrawn and the patient allowed to die if extubation or progress toward extubation is not made after a finite period. Such a therapeutic trial is preferable to not attempting potentially efficacious therapy because of uncertainty or because of the patient's fear that once such therapy is started, it would be continued indefinitely, even against his or her preferences.

Principle 5: As long as the patient or surrogate decision maker has given informed consent, it is appropriate to provide medication to relieve pain and other suffering, such as dyspnea, even if the medication has the potential to hasten the patient's death.

Administering medication to relieve pain and suffering should not be confused with active euthanasia or assisted suicide. When acting in accord with this principle, the health care provider's intention is to relieve pain and suffering. This follows from the principle of beneficence. By contrast, the intention of the health care provider in performing active euthanasia or assisted suicide is to *cause* the patient's death. Withdrawal of mechanical ventilation to allow patients to die from disease is ethically and legally distinct from active euthanasia or assisted suicide. However, referral in the past to such withdrawal as *passive euthanasia* has been misleading. Since this term may be confused with active euthanasia, its use should be avoided when referring to acts of withholding or withdrawing life support.

Principle 6: It is inappropriate to force physicians or other health care providers to comply with a patient's request to forgo life-sustaining therapy if compliance violates the health care provider's personal moral values. Under these circumstances, responsibility for care of the patient should be transferred to another provider who can respect the patient's request.

This principle affirms individual values and acknowledges the pluralistic nature of society, especially in the United States. Although the principle respects the right of the health care provider to act in accord with personal values, despite conflict with the patient's preferences, it continues to support the patient's autonomy. There may be difficulty in implementing this principle if the health care provider who is in conflict with the patient is uncooperative. For example, if the attending physician refuses to comply with the patient's or family's request to withdraw life support because of his or her personal values, the family may have to assert themselves in having that physician transfer the patient to another, more supportive, physician, as described below.

ETHICS RELATED TO FUTILE MEDICAL CARE

The issue of a patient's family demanding continuation of what health care providers judge as futile care remains controversial. While some suggest that there are limits to the respect for patient autonomy and that there is no ethical "right" to receive useless or futile care,[1,22] others argue that the definition of medical futility is so subjective that use of the term, and decision making based upon it, are unjustified.[16,25]

Principle 7: Health care professionals are not obligated to provide medical care that they judge as futile, even if requested by the patient or family. Futile life support can be limited without consent of the patient or surrogate decision maker.

Although Principle 7 lacks the strong consensus that supports the six preceding ethical principles, limiting life-sustaining therapy that has been judged futile has, in one form or another, already been incorporated into clinical practice.[2,8] One may ask whether the term *futile life support* is inherently contradictory. If an intervention supports life, how can it be futile?

One should make a distinction between *physiological futility* and *medical futility*. An intervention that is judged to be *physiologically futile* is one that is not expected to or does not achieve the relevant physiological function as an end point. For example, cardiopulmonary resuscitation (CPR) is judged to be physiologically futile whenever health care providers stop an unsuccessful resuscitation. The CPR has failed in its goal of restoring the circulation. In the same sense, CPR is regarded as physiologically futile in a patient with refractory septic shock who has a cardiac arrest, despite use of maximal vasopressor therapy for persistent hypotension. Under these circumstances—a cardiac arrest occurring despite maximal medical therapy—the conclusion that CPR would have virtually no chance of being successful appears reasonable. Cardiopulmonary resuscitation would not only prolong the patient's dying but could also potentially harm the patient physically. Prolonging dying is not one of the goals of medicine and, under these circumstances, CPR would violate the principle of nonmaleficence (see above). Forcing health care providers to perform CPR with virtually no prospect of success violates the ethical integrity of the medical profession.

Although there is modest consensus about physiological futility, medical futility is more difficult to define. Some have suggested that an intervention can be judged to be medically futile if reasoning and experience indicate that the intervention would have a high likelihood of failing to result in "meaningful survival." In applying this definition, the key words are *high likelihood*, which acknowledges the uncertainties inherent in clinical decision making, and *meaningful survival*. Meaningful survival signifies that survival has a quality and duration that are of value

to the particular individual. Importantly, *quality of life* refers to the *patient's* point of view, not that of the health care provider. As an extension of this definition, some organizations of critical care specialists have recommended that survival of patients with permanent loss of consciousness, such as those in a persistent vegetative state, should be regarded as meaningless.[1] Using this criterion, life-sustaining intervention for such patients is medically futile and therefore not obligatory. Because application of the concepts of physiological or medical futility as the basis for withholding or withdrawing life-sustaining intervention can be misapplied due to their subjective definitions, appropriate guidelines and safeguards for their application should be incorporated within a health care institution's written policies. Furthermore, appropriate resources, such as institutional ethics committees or consulting bioethicists, should be available to provide consultations to clinicians and families. In contrast to the legacy of high-level, important court decisions affirming a patient's right to forgo life-sustaining therapy, case law on use of physiological or medical futility as the basis for withdrawal of life support is quite limited and, at present, inconclusive.

ETHICAL PRINCIPLES RELATED TO MICROALLOCATION OF ICU RESOURCES

As noted above, microallocation includes the process of admitting patients who are competing for a limited number of ICU beds or of providing specific scarce resources to patients within the ICU—e.g., use of extracorporeal life support (ECLS). Microallocation encompasses concepts of both triage and rationing. *Triage* is the system of prioritizing patients according to severity of illness and, under some circumstances (e.g., in combat or in disasters with mass casualties), according to the degree of benefit accrued to the patient by access to medical care; it entails consideration of the impact of caring for one patient on the system's capacity to care for others.[1] In the broad sense, *rationing* is an economic term that refers to the process of deciding among competing goals when resources are limited. In a narrow sense, rationing implies depriving some patients of beneficial care when not all can receive that care; an example is the use of waiting lists for solid organ transplants.

In contrast to the constant lack of sufficient numbers of solid organs for transplantation, ICU bed shortages seem to occur intermittently. Furthermore, in the face of *persistent* excess demand, ICU shortages can be addressed by spending more money to open more ICU beds, whereas the same does not hold for the scarcity of solid organs.

Compared to the obvious impact of an insufficient supply of solid organs on mortality, the impact on patient outcomes of situations when ICU demand exceeds ICU supply is unclear. This may be due to the presence of some flexibility in ICU supply and demand compared to the circumstances of shortage of solid organs. Flexibility of supply arises from using "intermediate care" units for patients who do not necessarily need critical care but who still require monitoring and more care than provided on a general inpatient unit. There is also flexibility in demand, since patients who normally would be admitted to an ICU postoperatively can be held in postanesthesia care units. During severe ICU bed shortages, elective surgical cases can be canceled. Finally, emergency departments may be able to function for short periods in a similar holding capacity in response to ICU bed shortages.

The following principles are derived from fundamental legal and ethical principles[4,26] and can serve as guides to making microallocation decisions in the ICU, despite the lack of an explicit societal consensus in how to allocate care and expensive health care resources.

Principle 8: Each individual's life is equally valuable.

This principle affirms two fundamental concepts: (1) All individuals are equal and (2) all human life is valuable. The principle reflects the egalitarian concept that all individuals are equal because of their same intrinsic worth, which arises from humanity and their human dignity. On this basis, each individual should receive respect and equal treatment. According to this principle, access to ICU resources and other services should not be prioritized according to perceptions of relative social worth among individuals. Patients should not be regarded as more or less valuable to society by virtue of their social class, employment status, or family status.

The principle has its roots in legal principles derived from concepts of due process in the Constitution of the United States. Although there is no legal right to health care in general for citizens of the United States, there is a legal obligation for health care providers to administer care in emergency situations. Because care in the ICU is similar to emergency care from the perspective of the need to address urgent and often life-threatening medical needs, one could argue that for patients in need, ICU care is as much a right as emergency care. Although this remains an unresolved legal issue, external accrediting and state regulatory bodies hold health care institutions accountable to have resources available to meet the medical needs of their patients.

Principle 9: Vulnerable members of the community should be protected.

This principle reiterates Principle 8 that all members of the community should be treated as having equal value. However, Principle 9 goes beyond a simple sense of equality by highlighting that additional safeguards should be taken to ensure that society's vulnerable members are treated fairly.

One of these safeguards is protection against potential tyranny of the majority. For example, consider a policy in which the majority of subscribers of a health maintenance organization (HMO) decide to not fund beneficial critical care for premature infants or the elderly in order to make money available for other health care purposes. Such a policy would adversely affect these vulnerable groups, whether or not the majority's motives were judged to be altruistic (e.g., improving public health programs) or self-serving (e.g., providing free cosmetic surgery).

Historical justifications for this precaution reflect past events when society has restricted access to education, employment, or health care for certain vulnerable groups, such as the poor, the handicapped, or ethnic and racial minorities. Out of respect for the principle of fair equality of opportunity,[9,21,26] there is an egalitarian duty to provide extra (not equal) resources to those who are disabled or disadvantaged as a means of helping them function effectively in society. For example, education of handicapped children is supplemented by access to additional resources; the supplementation provides the handicapped with a fair equality of opportunity to achieve a basic level of education. The same rationale justifies provision of additional health care resources, such as critical care, to patients in greater need, rather than provision of each person with an equal amount, irrespective of need.

Current legal protections for certain vulnerable groups in the United States also reflect this principle. For example, as potential subjects in clinical research, children and other persons with absent or limited autonomy, such as the mentally retarded or prisoners, are accorded extra protection.

Principle 10: Access to intensive care should be based on the patient's medical need and the potential benefit of such care; judgments about whether a benefit is worthwhile should reflect not only the values of the patient and health care providers but also the values of the community.

This principle affirms that decisions to admit and care for patients in the ICU should be primarily based on *medical* appropriateness. In general, this principle holds that patients with the same degree of medical need should be treated the same. However, the principle also recognizes that different medical interventions can be used for the same medical need and have a range of potential benefits from minimally (marginally) beneficial to clearly beneficial. On this basis, patients should receive critical care only when they have sufficient medical need and when critical care provides a sufficient degree of potential benefit.

Evaluating the value of receiving critical care is a complicated process that incorporates three points of view: those of the health care provider, the patient, and the community. The health care provider's professional knowledge is required for assessing the patient's medical needs, deciding which interventions can meet those needs, and predicting the likelihood of success. In addition, although medical benefit denotes how well an intervention meets the patient's needs, only the patient can determine if the potential benefit of an intervention has sufficient personal value to justify receiving it. Finally, the community and health care institution—the parties ultimately paying for the resources—have a legitimate role in deciding whether the potential benefit of a certain intervention has sufficient value to society to make it worth the financial cost. For example, the question of whether a marginally beneficial therapy should be covered by a health care plan needs a societal perspective that extends beyond medical expertise and patient opinion. Denial of care because of very low potential benefit should reflect the community's values and priorities for using its resources.

Communities and their health care institutions may place different values on the same services. For example, a position may be held that patients in states of permanent unconsciousness should be restricted from care in the ICU. Another position may hold sanctity of life above all other considerations. A health care system, its members, and its providers might decide not to provide critical care for all patients with irreversibly fatal diseases when death is imminent. In a financially closed system, such as one with full capitation or a global budget, money saved by such a decision could fund a comprehensive hospice home care program for the same category of patients. Involvement of health care providers in decision making provides a safeguard from the tyranny of the majority of the community, whereby vulnerable members are treated unfairly by denying reimbursement for clearly beneficial therapies.

Principle 11: Although health care providers have a primary obligation to benefit their patients, this duty has limits when it unfairly compromises the availability of resources for others.

The primary moral duty of health care providers is to promote their patients' best interests. This responsibility is derived from the principles of beneficence and fidelity and constitutes the core of the physician-patient relationship. In a physician-patient relationship, the physician has a *fiduciary responsibility* to his or her patients. Under this responsibility, physicians are obligated to put their patients' interests above their own and those of others when providing medical care. The fiduciary obligation for physicians was established because of marked inequalities of medical knowledge and experience between health care providers and patients. This obligation also recognizes the patient's vulnerability and dependency on the health care provider due to sickness and disability.

In a closed system in which physicians put their patients' interests foremost without regard for limited resources, a situation arises that some have likened to the "tragedy of the commons."[10,11] In this analogy, each herdsman is only motivated by self-interest and keeps adding cows to a common grazing area. Overgrazing eventually results in tragic consequences for the cows. Likewise, if health care providers spend limited health care resources on their own patients, the resources will eventually be depleted. The result is unavailability of certain resources for anyone. From these considerations arises the need for limits on the physician's duty. However, limitations cause an inherent tension for physicians between duty to patients and obligation to support a system whose availability of resources could be compromised by unchecked promotion of patient interests (e.g., by expending resources in the pursuit of expensive minimal benefits).

Even though health care providers should practice cost-effective medicine whenever possible—i.e., they should select the less costly of two therapies with equivalent effectiveness—in the absence of a closed system and explicit limits, providers are not obligated to withhold beneficial care from patients solely because of personal concerns over cost.

Allocation rules for the ICU should not be made at the level of the individual practitioner but rather at the institutional level. An individual physician may not be free of subjective biases about issues that constitute worthy bases for allocation decisions. Decision making on an institutional basis provides additional safeguards that the process is fair, since institutional policy making is an explicit process that has built-in mechanisms for review and public scrutiny.

SPECIFIC ETHICAL CONSIDERATIONS IN THE ICU

Principles 1 through 11 can be illustrated more fully when applied to a number of important ethical questions commonly arising in the ICU.

Can intubated patients in the ICU really express their preferences?

Although communication may be a difficult and slow process, selected patients receiving mechanical ventilation may be quite lucid, especially when not receiving sedation. At these times, it is not uncommon for health care professionals to communicate with the patient verbally and for the patient to write responses or questions. When the patient cannot write (e.g., due to neuromuscular weakness) more creative means of communication can be tried. Examples include having the patient blink in response to yes or no questions and creating controlled leaks around the tracheal cuff to allow patients to phonate during the inspiratory phase of mechanical ventilation.

Should one assume that patients in the ICU are capable of valid decision making?

Under ordinary circumstances in medical practice, one should presume that adult patients have adequate decision-making capacity. In fact, by law, an adult is presumed competent until judged by a court to be incompetent. However, one could argue that a critically ill patient in an ICU generally lacks decision-making capacity. Many factors may compromise the decision-making capacity of a critically ill patient: effects of the underlying disease; use of sedatives, narcotics, and other mind-altering medications; sleep deprivation; pain; anxiety; disorientation; and fear. Adopting this point of view, health care providers should carefully assess the patient's decision-making capacity, relying on his or her communication, as discussed below.

What if the family or surrogate decision maker of a critically ill, incapacitated patient overrides the patient's previously known preferences regarding life-sustaining therapy?

In general, according to the principle of respect for patient autonomy, the patient's preferences should guide therapy, even if these preferences are opposed by the patient's family or surrogate decision maker. However, if the patient's surrogate has a valid durable power of attorney over the patient's health care decisions, the surrogate can legally exercise control over decisions—although it would be quite unusual for the person holding a durable power of attorney to ignore a patient's preferences. Regardless of the legal status of the surrogate, in the event of a conflict, the recommended first step for health care providers is discussion of differences directly with the surrogate. If needed, a request for informal or formal consultation from the hospital's ethics committee or bioethicist can be taken as the next step. In these circumstances, the principle of beneficence and the health care provider's fiduciary relationship with the patient obligate the health care provider to act as the patient's advocate. Only in rare instances should the conflict have to be resolved in a court of law.

What if health care providers do not agree with the patient's or surrogate's preferences regarding life support?

When there is disagreement between health care providers and patients or their surrogates regarding life support, physicians and nurses have little choice except to transfer care to other health care professionals. (This assumes, of course, that the decisions are made by an informed patient with adequate decision making capacity or by a surrogate who has a valid durable power of attorney.) A classic example of this type of conflict is refusal of blood products on religious grounds by a Jehovah's Witness despite the presence of life-threatening gastrointestinal bleeding. In this case, health care providers must respect the patient's legal and ethical right to refuse the blood, even if such action results in the patient's death. When conflicting bioethical principles arise (Fig. 181-1), respect for patient autonomy overrides beneficence. Under different circumstances—e.g., if the patient is a child of a Jehovah's Witness and is a minor—health care providers can regularly obtain a court order to give blood products, despite the parents' opposition.

When preferences are expressed by a surrogate decision maker who lacks a valid durable power of attorney, the strength of the surrogate's directives is less compelling. If the patient's health care providers are concerned that the surrogate may not be acting in the patient's best interests, they should seek consultation to resolve the conflict, as outlined previously.

When might a "slow code" or "Hollywood code" be ethically acceptable?

A "slow code" occurs when health care providers perform CPR with less than the usual intensity; the intent of such an approach is to allow the patient to die. The premise is that resuscitating the patient is inappropriate. A "Hollywood code" carries the same meaning as "slow code" but includes the pretense that the code is genuine. The deception in both of these practices makes them morally problematic and ethically unacceptable. These practices may be employed when CPR is considered futile for patients in hospitals that do not have policies allowing DNR orders on the basis of physiological futility. One way to discourage these types of codes is for institutions to give physicians authority to use professional judgment in not providing futile care.

If CPR or other life-sustaining therapy is judged to be futile, what should health care providers do? Can they be forced to provide futile care?

When health care providers judge that CPR or other life support is futile, they should discuss this with the patient (if possible) or the patient's surrogate decision maker. Sometimes the surrogate or family agrees with the physician's judgment that limitation of life support is appropriate; some families may be thankful and relieved that the physician has taken responsibility for the decision to withhold or stop the intervention. If the surrogate opposes withholding CPR or other interventions that are judged futile, attempts to reach agreement through further discussion and consultation with the ethics committee should be made. If these efforts are unsuccessful, attempts should be made to transfer the patient to another physician in the same or another institution for provision of the particular intervention in question. However, patients for whom judgments of futility apply are often too unstable to be moved to another institution. Ultimately, if the patient cannot be transferred and if it is allowed by hospital policy, the physician should write a DNR order on the basis of futility and should inform the surrogate. If such DNR orders are not permitted by hospital policy and if the patient cannot be transferred to another hospital, the physician faces a number of alternatives: (1) acquiescence and provision of futile care, (2) resignation from the case by transferring care to another physician in the same institution, or (3) procurement of a court order to limit therapy on the basis of futility.

Is the current system of "first come, first served" regarding ICU admissions fair? Which patients should be discharged from a full ICU in order to make room for other patients?

Whether the admissions policy of an ICU is fair or unfair can be assessed by first considering the policy in relation to the basic principle of distributive justice: equals should be treated equally and unequals treated unequally. If admission is granted solely on the basis of whether a patient's severity of illness meets a threshold, and if critical care can provide more than minimal potential benefit, the patient should be admitted to an available bed. This practice constitutes an example of "equals being treated equally," where the overriding criteria for equality or inequality are a sufficient degree of medical need and the potential for deriving benefit. If policies limit admissions to the ICU based solely on gender, race, ethnicity, or age—even if a patient meets thresholds for severity of illness and derivation of potential benefit—equals are being treated unequally and the decision is considered unfair.

If patients do not meet the thresholds for degree of illness or derivation of potential benefit, they should not be admitted, even if requested by the patient or his or her family. This scenario is an example of unequals (i.e., those with lower medical needs) being treated unequally (e.g., not being admitted to the ICU), where a sufficient degree of illness or derivation of potential benefit are the determinative criteria. These same considerations should govern not only decisions to admit patients to the ICU but also decisions to continue care in the ICU.

What are the alternatives when a critically ill patient needs admission to a full ICU? Providers could refuse to admit the patient, irrespective of the relative degrees of illness among the new and old patients, assuming all existing ICU patients meet the criteria of sufficient medical need and derivation of potential benefit. This decision is consistent with the "first come, first served" rule, discussed previously. The waiting patient could be admitted to another ICU in the same hospital or stabilized and transferred to another hospital where an ICU bed is available. Alternatively, providers could transfer the least sick patient in the full ICU to another ICU in the same hospital or to an intermediate care unit in order to make room for the new patient (assuming the new patient is clinically more in need than the transferred patient). Resources in the intermediate care unit might need to be increased temporarily to care for the transferred patient adequately. In addition, one could discharge the ICU patient with the poorest prognosis in order to make room for the new patient (assuming the new patient had a better prognosis than the one discharged). Unless differences in prognoses are striking, deciding on the relative benefits of critical care among patients is subject to bias and value judgments—problematic issues from an ethics standpoint.

Currently available objective estimates of outcome in an ICU may improve decision making regarding resource allocation by decreasing subjectivity[5,14,17] (see Chapter 180). However, these estimates are problematic when used in this regard. Estimated risk of death assumes that the patient has received critical care; hence, a low predicted risk of death would not constitute firm grounds in *excluding* a patient from the ICU. It is clear that objective determination about who would do well in an intermediate care unit instead of an ICU would be useful in making these kinds of triage decisions. In addition, it is not clear how accurate the current generation of objective prognostic systems are in comparing relative risks of survival. For example, is a predicted mortality risk of 40 percent significantly different from a 50 percent risk? Finally, even if these systems predict mortality risks greater than 90 percent, it is unlikely that families of critically ill patients would accept a 5 or 10 percent chance of survival as futile.

When should an individual patient's consumption of scarce or expensive resources be limited?

When a provided resource meets a patient's medical needs, the resource should be limited only if the patient is consuming a *disproportionate share;* that is, if continued consumption would threaten availability for others. For example, a patient who has persistent variceal hemorrhage, despite all possible therapeutic attempts, may require an almost continuous infusion of blood products to prevent death from exsanguination. When availability of the blood bank's supply of that type of blood product may be compromised, it is appropriate to stop transfusions. Some would argue that there is an *obligation* to do so. Such a decision by clinicians and appropriate consultants should be communicated to the family (since the patient is likely to be encephalopathic under these circumstances). However, deciding on the point at which a patient's share of a resource is disproportionate may be difficult.

With regard to consumption of limited or expensive resources, physicians face an ethical dilemma between two conflicting professional roles: (1) as patient advocate, keeping the patient alive in accord with the principles of beneficence and respect for autonomy, and (2) as steward of a health care system's limited resources. Few guidelines exist that address the tension created by these dual roles.[18] Although the limited resource in the example provided above was blood, the same argument could apply to health care costs. Money is as limited a resource as tangible medical products and interventions in a large health care system that is financially closed. In a closed system, money spent on behalf of one patient decreases funds available for other patients. One important future ethical challenge for health care providers in the ICU is integration of these roles as financial resources become even more constrained.[15]

"DO NOT RESUSCITATE" (DNR) ORDERS IN THE INTENSIVE CARE UNIT

End-of-life decisions play a prominent role in the management of patients in intensive care units. For critically ill patients, DNR orders are common, and the majority of patients dying in intensive care units have DNR orders at the time of their death.[23,24] Clinicians practicing critical care must be familiar with the details of DNR decision making.

When to Discuss Withholding or Withdrawing Life-Sustaining Therapy

Ideally, a patient's preferences for withholding or withdrawing life support should have been discussed with his or her primary health care provider well before admission to an ICU. If done properly, the provider should have incorporated use of life support into the patient's overall plan for medical care, in accord with the patient's life goals and values. At the time of this discussion, the patient should have been encouraged to prepare a written advance directive and to designate a surrogate decision maker or durable power of attorney. Preferences for degrees of medical interventions under various scenarios should have been discussed in the context of particular medical problems. For example, in the case of a patient with severe lung disease who has needed mechanical ventilation previously, what are the patient's preferences regarding likely situations? Does the patient want to be intubated again if clinically indicated? What should be done if the patient cannot be weaned after 1 week or after 2 or more weeks?

After a patient is admitted to an ICU, the patient, a family member, surrogate decision maker, or health care provider may initiate discussions about life support. If the patient has an advance directive, its meaning and applicability should be explored to clarify why the patient was admitted to the ICU. If the advance directive simply indicates that life support should be withdrawn when there is no reasonable hope for meaningful recovery (a common phrase in many living wills), the patient's interpretation of "reasonable" and "meaningful recovery" must be understood before appropriate recommendations are offered regarding continuation or discontinuation of life support.

However, if the patient has not written an advance directive (which is the case in the vast majority of admissions), he or she may have talked to family or friends about preferences regarding life support (e.g., a preference "not to be kept alive by machines"). Alternatively, even if the patient has not expressed anything specifically about life support, family or close friends might agree about what the patient's preferences would be, based on their knowledge of his or her life goals and values.

In circumstances in which a patient's prognosis is very poor and provision of CPR or other interventions would be futile or highly burdensome, the attending physician should initiate end-of-life discussions with the patient's family or surrogate decision maker.

Assessment of a Patient's Decision-Making Capacity

Competency should be distinguished from decision-making *capacity.* An adult is legally competent until a court of law decides otherwise; children, as minors (unless emancipated by parenthood or marriage), lack legal competency. In contrast, decision-making *capacity* refers to a patient's functional ability as determined by the patient's attending physician. Many legally competent patients lack adequate decision-making capacity when critically ill or heavily sedated. Conversely, a patient who is legally incompetent may retain some decision-making capacity, e.g., a teenager who has opinions about his or her medical care.

A patient has adequate decision-making capacity in relation to a specific decision when the patient demonstrates all of the following: (1) comprehension, (2) comparative judgment, and (3) communication. The patient should understand information about his or her medical condition, its prognosis, and treatment alternatives, including having no treatment at all. The patient should also be able to judge and compare the medical alternatives and outcomes relative to personal values and life goals. Finally, the patient should be able to communicate preferences consistently. One should specify the context of the assessment for decision-making capacity since, in some cases, patients may have adequate capacity for certain decisions but not for others.

The attending physician is responsible for assessing the patient's decision-making capacity. The process includes review of the patient's medical history, performance of mental status examinations, and consultation with the patient's nurses and family. If doubt or conflict arises about the determination, additional information should be obtained, e.g., by requesting a psychiatric consultation.

Identification and Role of Surrogate Decision Makers

As is often the case, when a patient in the ICU lacks decision-making capacity, the physician commonly turns to a surrogate decision maker. The choice of proxy may be legally mandated in states that have established a legal hierarchy, e.g., spouse first, parents next, etc. Another legal mandate is an individual having a valid durable power of attorney for health care decisions. In the absence of a legal directive, if the patient has informally designated someone as surrogate decision maker, that choice should be followed with some exceptions. In most cases, the surrogate decision maker will be a close family member. An appropriate surrogate should be willing to serve in that role and to accept responsibility for making the patient's decisions, preferably based on knowledge of the patient's preferences, values, and life goals. This knowledge allows the surrogate to act on the basis of a substituted judgment, i.e., what the patient would have wanted under the circumstances.

In unusual cases, no individual who knows the patient or who is willing to serve as a surrogate decision maker can be identified. In such circumstances, it is desirable to find a relatively neutral party (generally not a hospital employee) to act as surrogate—e.g., the chairperson of a hospital's ethics committee. If this is not possible, prior to their implementation, DNR decisions should be reviewed by knowledgeable health care providers who are not involved in the case. The aim of the review is to ensure that the process of determination of DNR status is sound, i.e., is based on a best interests standard or futility judgment.

Deciding on the DNR Order

A DNR order actually consists of much more than a proscription of CPR. In many hospitals, it refers to withholding or withdrawing one or more life-sustaining therapies. For a patient in the ICU, these therapies may include antiarrhythmic drugs (chemical cardioversion), intubation, mechanical ventilation, dialysis, blood products, intravenous pressors, antibiotics, and parenteral and enteral nutrition.

How should limitation of certain therapy be decided? One approach is to define the goals of therapy that are applicable to the patient. Once these goals are established, one can decide which therapies are compatible with them. In some institutions, DNR orders have been classified into three levels, each with a different goal of treatment (Table 181-1).

TABLE 181-1

Do Not Resuscitate (DNR) Orders: Levels of Intervention and Associated Therapeutic Goals

Level	Interventions	Goals of Therapy
A	All therapies except CPR	Patient is to receive all medically indicated therapies to preserve life and restore function, including those to *prevent* cardiac or respiratory arrest. However, if patient suffers cardiopulmonary arrest, *no* resuscitative efforts will be made unless specified in advance (e.g., only drug therapy permitted). Patient will not be intubated or mechanically ventilated. Restrictions may be temporarily suspended during general anesthesia or other invasive procedures if agreed upon previously. "No ICU transfer" may be specified.
B	No additional therapy and no CPR	Therapy already under way to be continued as medically indicated, but in general, no additional treatment given except for patient comfort. Goal is maintenance of status quo while discussions evolve or prognosis becomes more certain. If cardiac or pulmonary arrest occurs, no resuscitative efforts to be made.
C	Palliation Only	Treatment limited to nursing care and therapy whose goal is comfort. Treatment for relief of pain or dyspnea may be used even if the treatment worsens cardiac or respiratory function. All life-sustaining interventions, including artificially provided food and water, will be discontinued unless exceptions agreed upon (e.g., continued mechanical ventilation).

As a first step in the decision-making process, health care providers should meet with the patient's family or surrogate decision maker to inform them about the current medical situation, review the goals of therapy, and reassess the appropriateness of the level of current treatment in relation to the goals. The discussion should include the patient unless he or she lacks decision-making capacity. Attendance should include the attending physician, the patient's primary care physician (if applicable), consultants (when relevant for explanations and discussions of prognosis), house staff, and one or more ICU nurses and respiratory therapists caring for the patient. These meetings promote open communication among parties, help all to feel involved in the decision-making process, and facilitate understanding and acceptance of the results. "Family meetings," in which families have the opportunity to grieve while making DNR decisions, have become a way of life in the practice of critical care medicine.

Carrying Out the DNR Order

After deciding on the limits of therapy, the attending physician should document the meeting's discussion in the medical record and the justification for the DNR order. The DNR order should be written in a clearly identifiable location in the record as well as communicated orally to other health care providers. Details of the policies vary among institutions. For example, in New York State, the signature of a capable patient or surrogate decision maker is required to write a DNR order. If a patient is to be removed from mechanical ventilation, the order is carried out by the patient's nurse and respiratory therapist. In this case, intravenous narcotics are titrated to sedate the patient and control dyspnea. After the desired level of sedation has been achieved, the patient is extubated. This may be done by a physician, nurse, or respiratory therapist. If a staff member is uncomfortable with removal of life support, he or she should be given the option of not participating. Ultimately, the physician who writes the DNR order must be prepared to extubate or remove the patient from the ventilator if need be.

Resolution of Conflicts

If communication during the decision-making process is good, conflicts occur infrequently. However, if communication is poor among physicians and nurses, conflicts are common. Conflicts may also occur between the patient's family and the health care team. Conflicts may arise when one party favors forgoing life support and the other does not—for example, if the family wants full critical care continued despite pessimism about the patient's recovery on the part of the health care team. Alternatively, a family may wish to stop life support while the attending physician is reluctant to do so.

Resolution of conflicts begins with open communication among all parties. It may be helpful to consult with the hospital's ethics committee. The conflict may be resolved in several ways, e.g., by reviewing hospital policy, identifying legal myths or real limits, or getting all parties around the same table for discussion. Rarely should conflicts have to be referred for judicial

review. If the situation reaches an impasse, it may be more prudent to transfer the patient to another hospital or another attending physician than to go to court.

CONCLUSION

In today's critical care environment, death in the ICU usually occurs after life-sustaining therapy is halted. Many ethical considerations in the ICU arise from the frequency and complexity of this process. Health care providers face ethical dilemmas in which decisions violate one or more ethical principles in order to respect an overriding ethical principle. Weighing ethical principles in limiting life support is supported by a broad ethical, legal, and professional consensus. As a general rule, the overriding principle is respect for patient autonomy; hospital policies regarding DNR orders should reflect this. Despite well-written policies, conflicts still occur, and other resources—e.g., ethics committees or consulting bioethicists—are frequently helpful in their resolution. Only in very rare cases should a conflict have to be resolved in court.

REFERENCES

1. American Thoracic Society: Withholding and withdrawing life-sustaining therapy. *Am Rev Respir Dis* 144:726–731, 1991.
2. Asch DA, Hansen-Flaschen JH, Lanken PN: Decisions to limit or continue life-sustaining treatment in the United States: Conflicts between physicians' practices and patients' wishes. *Am J Respir Crit Care Med* 151:288–292, 1995.
3. *Bartling* v. *Superior Court, California Court of Appeal, Second District,* 163 Cal., App.3d 186, 209 Cal.Rptr. 220, 1984.
4. Beauchamp TL, Childress JF: *Principles of Biomedical Ethics,* 4th ed. New York, Oxford University Press, 1994.
5. Bone RC, LeGall JR, Lemeshow S, Saulnier F: A new simplified acute physiology score (SAPS II) based on a European/North American multicenter study. *JAMA* 270:2957–2963, 1993.
6. *Canterbury* v. *Spence, United States Court of Appeals, District of Columbia Circuit,* 464 F 2d 772, 1972.
7. *Cruzan* v. *Director, Missouri Dept. of Health,* 110 S. Ct 284 (1990).
8. Curtis JR, Park DR, Krone MR, Pearlman RA: Use of the medical futility rationale in do-not-attempt-resuscitation orders. *JAMA* 273:124–128, 1995.
9. Daniels N: *Just Health Care.* Cambridge, England, Cambridge University Press, 1985.
10. Hardin G: The tragedy of the commons. *Science* 162:1243–1248, 1968.
11. Hiatt HH: Protecting the medical commons: Who is responsible? *New Engl J Med* 293:235–241, 1975.
12. *In re Quinlan,* 70 N.E. 10, 355 A2d 647, *cert denied* 429 US 922 (1976).
13. Jonsen A: Bentham in a box: Technology assessment and health care allocation. *Law Med Health Care.* 14:172–174, 1986.
14. Knaus WA, Wagner DP, Draper EA, et al: The APACHE III prognostic system: Risk prediction of hospital mortality for critically ill hospitalized adults. *Chest* 100:1619–1636, 1991.
15. Lanken PN: Critical care medicine at a new crossroads: The intersection of economics and ethics in the intensive care unit. *Am J Respir Crit Care Med* 149:3–5, 1994.
16. Lantos JD, Singer PA, Walker PM, et al: The illusion of futility in clinical practice. *Am J Med* 87:81–84, l989.

17. Lemeshow S, Teres D, Avrunin JS, et al: Mortality probability models (MPM II) based on an international cohort of intensive care unit patients. *JAMA* 270:2478–2486, 1993.

18. Morrein EH: *Balancing Act: The New Medcial Ethics of Medicine's New Economics.* Washington, DC, Georgetown University Press, 1995.

19. President's Commission for the Study of Ethical Problems in Medicine and Biomedical and Behavioral Research: Making health care decisions: The ethical and legal implications of informed consent in the patient-practitioner relationship. Washington, DC, U.S. Government Printing Office, l982, Vol I.

20. President's Commission for the Study of Ethical Problems in Medicine and Biomedical and Behavioral Research: Deciding to forego life-sustaining treatment: Ethical, medical and legal issues in treatment decisions. Washington, DC: U.S. Government Printing Office, 1983.

21. Rawls J: *A Theory of Justice.* Cambridge, MA, Harvard University Press, 1971.

22. Schneiderman LJ, Jecker NS, Jonsen AR: Medical futility: Its meaning and ethical implications. *Ann Intern Med* 112:949–954, 1990.

23. Smedira NG, Evans BH, Grais LS, et al: Withholding and withdrawal of life support from the critically ill. *New Engl J Med* 322:309–315, 1990.

24. Teres D: Trends from the United States with end of life decisions in the intensive care unit. *Intens Care Med* 19:316–322, 1993.

25. Waisel DB, Truog RD: The cardiopulmonary resuscitation-not-indicated order: Futility revisited. *Ann Intern Med* 122:304–308, 1995.

26. Winslow, GR: *Triage and Justice.* Berkeley, CA. University of California Press, 1982.

CHAPTER 182

PREVENTION AND CONTROL
OF LUNG DISEASE

Suzanne S. Hurd / Claude Lenfant

CHRONIC OBSTRUCTIVE PULMONARY DISEASE

ASTHMA

TUBERCULOSIS

NEONATAL PULMONARY DISEASES

CARDIOPULMONARY DISORDERS OF SLEEP

CONCLUSION

As one reviews the emergence and evolution of the interest in prevention and control of lung disease in the United States, it appears that the publication of the Surgeon General's report on smoking and health[15] was truly a decisive moment. In the ensuing years, pulmonary scientists and clinicians began to recognize the importance of research on prevention. A task force group was asked to develop a blueprint for action; their report was printed in 1978[14] and was considered an important companion piece to the first task force report that set the stage for the implementation of a national basic and clinical research program in pulmonary biology and medicine.[13] Since then, prevention has become an integral part of the national pulmonary research program in the United States. Later, in 1992, another panel was convened to update the 1978 report. Its report, "Task Force on Research and Education for the Prevention and Control of Respiratory Diseases,"[16] created a new impetus for additional research and will serve as a blueprint for action well into the next century.

This chapter focuses on some of the prevention and control approaches that have been taken or are being developed, especially for some pulmonary diseases. Lung cancer, pneumonia, infectious diseases (including acquired immunodeficiency syndrome, or AIDS) and most occupational and environmental lung diseases are not included in this chapter. However, approaches for disease prevention that are described may indeed be adaptable to the prevention of many other lung diseases.

Although today research on prevention and control of lung diseases is lagging behind basic and clinical research on pathogenesis, diagnosis, and treatment, some accomplishments are already evident. It appears that they can be attributed to the development of formal curricula at medical schools throughout the country to improve the teaching of preventive pulmonary medicine at all levels of medical education and to promote research related to the prevention of pulmonary diseases.

Why are prevention and control programs of high priority? The answer is that many respiratory diseases, perhaps more than any other types of disease, are more easily prevented than cured. Chronic obstructive pulmonary disease (COPD), primarily caused by cigarette smoking, is the most prevalent of all lung diseases and may also play a contributory role in the development and exacerbation of other respiratory conditions. Tuberculosis is making a comeback in the United States and other western countries, concomitant with the onset of the AIDS epidemic. Asthma prevalence appears to be on the increase in this country and around the world and, although asthma is usually not a fatal condition, the relatively high rate of mortality among asthmatics in the large inner city and rural areas in the United States is of concern. Respiratory diseases cause 30 percent of all deaths in term infants in the United States and even more worldwide, yet many of these diseases are preventable through immunization programs, improved nutrition, adequate prenatal care, and the application of existing technologies.

A common thread in all pulmonary disorders is that once the disease process has been initiated, the behavior of the patient and that of the family or caregiver may be an important factor in management of the disease. For many pulmonary diseases, whether the patient is a young child with cystic fibrosis or asthma or an elderly individual with COPD or asthma, patients themselves must take action to control the disease. Taking medications, avoiding tobacco smoke and allergens, engaging in regular physical activity, doing breathing exercises, or using postural drainage are daily routines for most pulmonary patients. Motivating the patient to perform these tasks and to continue to perform them over a long period of time must be an important goal of a health care program. How to implement effective measures in a cost-containment mode remains a problem. Yet researchers, especially those with expertise in behavioral medicine and health education, working in concert with pulmonary physicians, are making important contributions in understanding how best to implement prevention programs. Some of the results they are providing are presented in this chapter.

Primary prevention programs focus on measures to reduce susceptibility within the population. For example, COPD could be prevented with effective tobacco control measures (29 percent of the adults in the United States are cigarette smokers); tuberculosis, once effectively eliminated in western countries, could again be prevented through active involvement of the health care community in advocating control measures similar to those introduced in these countries in the early 1900s; respiratory distress syndrome, apnea of prematurity, and bronchopulmonary dysplasia are predominantly the result of premature births, which can be reduced markedly by good prenatal care, prevention of teenage pregnancy, and maternal avoidance of drugs; and identification of risk factors for asthma is the first step toward developing effective strategies for the primary prevention of this common disease.

Once lung diseases occur, secondary prevention measures are important to reduce morbidity and mortality. These include, for example, assessment of disease etiology and differential diagnosis and evaluation of severity levels as well as initiation of appropriate medical care, proper nutrition, patient or parent health education programs, and education of health care personnel, school and day-care workers, workplace personnel, and the general public. Therapeutic approaches, such as surfactant replacement therapy, have been shown to markedly reduce both morbidity and mortality among premature infants. Aggressive monitoring, health education programs, and therapeutic approaches for patients with asthma have been shown to be effective means of reducing hospitalizations and emergency room visits. Patients themselves, including young children, can prevent the onset of attacks by recognizing their early signs. Tertiary treatments for lung diseases are supportive, including avoidance of hypoxemia, good nutrition, bronchodilation, and respiratory therapy.

The major theme of this chapter is recent accomplishments and future research directions in primary and secondary prevention.

CHRONIC OBSTRUCTIVE PULMONARY DISEASE

The fourth leading cause of death, and one that is on the increase, is COPD, which affects approximately 11 percent of the population in the United States. As more women begin to smoke cigarettes, COPD will continue to impact significantly on the health care system. Yet, this disease is preventable. It is not the intent of this chapter to examine the pathogenetic mechanisms by which cigarette smoking, the most important and best-documented risk factor, leads to COPD or the methodologies for smoking cessation and prevention. These topics have been covered elsewhere,[17] as well as in Chapter 45 of this volume. However, it is valuable to explore the role of early detection, monitoring, and health education programs both for the patient and the physician in our efforts to prevent this chronic lung disease.

Of particular interest are the first results from a large multi-center investigation, the Lung Health Study, that focused on the early course and prognosis of COPD in subjects recruited from the general population.[1] This 12-center study included 5887 subjects who were current smokers and who had an $FEV_1/FVC\%$ less than 70 percent but were otherwise in good health. Patients with any previous history of heart or lung disease, including asthma, were excluded. The results were encouraging in that patients who quit smoking had a slight improvement in FEV_1 over the initial years of the 5-year study, with a very small decline bringing them back to near preenrollment levels of ventilatory function. By contrast, those who continued to smoke had a much more rapid decline of lung function. On a discouraging note, aggressive and intensive (therefore expensive) smoking cessation programs were required, yet only 40 percent of patients in the special care group had stopped smoking at some point in the 5-year intervention program. The study has proven, however, that large groups can be screened for early COPD and that aggressive smoking cessation intervention can have a major impact on the progression of disease.

An interesting finding from the Lung Health Study was that deaths from lung cancer exceeded those from heart attack and stroke and all other causes; no patient died of COPD during the 5-year follow-up because of the mild degree of airflow obstruction present at enrollment. The investigators concluded that the presence of airflow obstruction can be a powerful marker for risk of death from other common causes.

Because COPD is common, costly, preventable, and readily detectable, it is an appropriate target for primary, secondary, and tertiary preventive strategies. All health care organizations should have systems in place to identify smokers and to target them for regular smoking cessation messages and efforts. Special emphasis should be given to current smokers during pregnancy, those with established COPD, and patients following a cardiovascular event.

Individuals deficient in alpha-1 protease inhibitor are at increased risk for the development of COPD, and treatment with human plasma alpha-1 protease inhibitor has been demonstrated to increase the biochemical levels of this substance in both the blood and the lung. However, data are not yet available to show whether or not replacement therapy alters the rate of development of COPD in these patients.

In spite of the intensive research effort in COPD, virtually all the fundamental questions remain. For example, who is at greatest risk? What techniques will detect COPD in its early stages? What are the pathogenetic features? What are the optimal forms of treatment? However, these uncertainties should not obscure the recognition that COPD occurs primarily because of cigarette smoking in the susceptible person, that it typically begins long before symptoms appear, that it is largely irreversible, that smoking cessation is almost always beneficial in terms of slowing the deterioration of lung function in susceptible smokers, and that efforts at getting people to stop smoking can work.

ASTHMA

Asthma is an extremely prevalent disorder (Chapter 47), affecting over 10 million people of all ages, of both genders, and of all ethnic backgrounds. Medical care—including emergency room visits, hospitalizations, and medications—costs over $2.65 billion annually. The prevalence of asthma increased 60 percent from 1979 to 1989. Although mortality is relatively low, at about 4000 deaths per year in this country, tragically, many of these deaths occur in otherwise healthy adolescents and young adults. Data from several sources suggest that many asthma deaths may be preventable.[8,16]

These observations emphasize the importance of preventing asthma and its complications. To date, however, we have less knowledge about how to prevent the onset of asthma than about how to manage and control it on a day-to-day basis and how to treat it in the hope of preventing its progression to irreversible airflow obstruction with consequent disability. However, primary prevention of asthma is a goal that should be achievable. Identification of risk factors for asthma is the first step toward development of an effective strategy to meet this goal.

Population-based studies confirm an association between asthma and atopy. Allergen exposure increases nonspecific airway responsiveness in people with asthma and in those with hay fever but without asthma. This suggests that the effects of inhaled allergens on the airways are at least partly responsible for the association between asthma and atopy. It may be that asthma and atopy are distinct but genetically linked, or that these conditions frequently coexist because they are caused by the same underlying cellular or biochemical defects. In any event, the data suggest that prevention of atopy should translate into a reduction in the occurrence or severity of asthma.[16] Atopy appears to result from both genetic and environmental factors, some of which are potentially amenable to modifications that may help prevent atopy or at least help prevent its severe manifestations.

Familial aggregation of asthma has been noted for many years. Children of parents with hay fever, eczema, or asthma appear to be more likely than the general population to develop the same condition as their parents rather than a dissimilar allergic condition. This has led to the suggestion that predispositions to atopy and asthma may be inherited as independent genetic traits. Investigators[7] recently mapped bronchial hyperresponsiveness to a region of the chromosome (5q) previously reported as one site for a major locus regulating serum total IgE. This area of the chromosome is rich in a number of proinflammatory regulator cytokines that are potentially important in asthma and allergy. While this research is still in very preliminary stages, genetic studies on allergy and asthma should eventually lead to the identification of basic immunologic and pathophysiologic mechanisms that are important in these disorders. These approaches may also lead to new specific therapies or methodologies for presymptomatic diagnosis and disease prevention.

Environmental control measures to reduce exposure to indoor and outdoor allergens and air pollutants should be applied as much as possible as a means to prevent asthma exacerbations and reduce the need for pharmacologic treatment. Among the wide variety of indoor allergens are domestic (house dust) mites, animal allergens, cockroach allergens, and fungi; these remain a major focus for primary prevention programs. Indoor allergens have increased in developed countries where homes have been carpeted, heated, cooled, and humidified and where outdoor ventilation has been reduced to make the homes energy-efficient. The result is in an ideal habitat not only for domestic mites, cockroaches, and other insects but also for molds and bacteria. Reducing exposure to domestic mites, especially for infants, appears to be a highly promising preventive measure.

Cats, dogs, and rodents release allergens in secretions (saliva), excretions (urine and feces), and dander, which are well documented causes of asthma exacerbations. Removal of such animals from the home is important; at a minimum, animals should be kept out of the sleeping area. If a cat is present in the home and cannot be removed, washing it weekly appears to reduce the allergen load.[5]

An important measure is to avoid passive and active cigarette smoking; all patients with asthma should be advised not to smoke. Because passive smoking increases the risk of allergic sensitization in children and the frequency and severity of respiratory symptoms, parents of children with asthma should be advised to not smoke and not to allow smoking in rooms used by their children.

Several other areas are being examined as potential means to prevent asthma. However, data remain controversial and further studies are required. For example, many investigators believe that the influence of respiratory infections in early life on the risk of developing asthma may be relevant to the primary prevention of asthma, especially with more and more infants and young children in day-care centers. Others are exploring exposure to antigenic biological agents that contaminate indoor air: mold, dampness, NO_2 from gas stoves, and residential wood burning have been reported to be associated with an increased prevalence of asthma.[16]

Despite the probable pathophysiological importance of exposure to agents in indoor air, the feasibility and effectiveness of reducing such exposure for the purpose of primary asthma prevention in the population at large are likely to be quite limited and possibly not cost-effective. However, identification of susceptible subgroups on the basis of family history, genetic markers, or umbilical cord blood total IgE level might allow environmental change to be made by persons most likely to benefit from such preventive measures.

Much has been written about air pollution and asthma.[8,10,16] While results from several studies suggest that air pollution may aggravate existing asthma, it appears that exposure to current ambient pollution levels does not have an etiologic role in the development of asthma. It does appear that controlled exposure to ambient or near-ambient levels of ozone, nitrogen dioxide, and sulfuric acid aerosol during exercise causes an increase in the nonspecific airway responsiveness of healthy subjects.

It has been estimated that 2 percent of cases of asthma in the United States are caused by occupational exposures. Although the list of materials implicated as causing occupational asthma is large, it appears that IgE-mediated hypersensitivity to a specific workplace antigen is an important underlying mechanism.[5] Most agents can be classified into plant proteins (e.g., flour, cotton dust); inorganic chemicals (e.g., platinum salts, stainless steel fumes); or organic chemicals (e.g., antibiotics, formaldehyde).[8]

In summary, although some advances have been made in understanding asthma prevention in relation to passive smoking and occupational asthma, primary prevention is as yet an area of unproved benefit; much more work remains to be done. The major emphasis to date has been on secondary prevention of asthma, with goals to prevent exacerbations of asthma in those who already have the condition and to avoid deterioration in lung function or death from this chronic lung disease. In this regard much work is under way, thanks to two programs: the National Asthma Education and Prevention Program and the Global Initiative for Asthma conducted in collaboration with the World Health Organization. Publications from these two programs, which have been widely distributed,[8,9,11] describe a six-part asthma management program: (1) education of patients to develop a partnership in asthma management; (2) assessment and monitoring of asthma severity, with both symptom reports and measurements of lung function; (3) avoidance or control of asthma triggers; (4) establishment of individual medication plans for long-term management; (5) establishment of individual plans for managing exacerbations; and (6) provision of regular follow-up care.

The goals of a successful asthma management program include (1) achievement and maintenance of control of symptoms; (2) prevention of asthma exacerbations; (3) maintenance of pulmonary function as close to normal levels as possible; (4) maintenance of normal activity levels, including exercise; (5) avoidance of adverse effects from asthma medications; (6) prevention of development of irreversible airflow limitation; and (7) prevention of asthma mortality. Medication plans, based on disease classification, are described by a stepwise approach to pharmacological therapy; medications are recommended for both the reversal and prevention of symptoms and airflow limitation.

Several evaluation projects are under way in the United States and many other countries to explore approaches to implementation of successful asthma management programs in children and adults in large urban, small village, and rural settings; to examine their effectiveness in reduction of asthma morbidity and mortality; and to gain a better appreciation of methods to ultimately prevent the onset of this disease.

TUBERCULOSIS

In the years following World War II, stringent public health measures and the development of new drugs led to a considerable reduction in the incidence and prevalence of tuberculosis in most western countries, including the United States. However, the appearance of widespread human immunodeficiency virus (HIV) infection has increased tuberculosis rates worldwide. Once again, tuberculosis control programs and programs to assure patient compliance to prescribed regimens must be implemented to fight this disease. Problems caused by the entry of drug-resistant strains pose a special challenge, as does the burden of attempting to reach the large numbers of victims who are poor, elderly, malnourished, poorly housed, homeless, or alcoholic. Prevalence rates of active tuberculosis for homeless persons are estimated to be 150 to 300 times greater than those for the general population.[2]

A broad array of tuberculosis prevention methods have been recommended by the Centers for Disease Control and Prevention (CDC).[14] Because crowding and poor ventilation enhance the spread of tuberculosis, improvement in housing conditions is the best prevention, but it is also the most complex and least likely to happen. The CDC recommends that homeless patients with newly diagnosed active tuberculosis be placed in settings that allow full supervision of initial treatment, so as to avoid the possibility of infecting others, such as peers or shelter staff members. However, it must also be recognized that transmission of tuberculosis in shelters is well documented, and that the longer individuals stay in the shelter system, the more likely they will be to have a positive skin test.[2]

Compliance with treatment regimens is a particularly difficult problem for homeless patients. A study from Portland, Oregon, in 1987[2] reported that of 62 individuals who initiated a thera-

peutic regimen, 31 completed therapy. However, the investigators ascribed this degree of compliance to a particularly effective outreach worker. A study in a hospital-based clinic in Central Harlem showed that 89 percent of a group of over 200 patients with tuberculosis were lost to follow-up before completing therapy.[2] Thus, with problems of stolen medications, long waiting times in clinics, and more immediate concerns of the daily battle to obtain food, clothing, and shelter, compliance is, not surprisingly, worse in the homeless population.

Some approaches that appear to be meeting with success in completing a prescribed treatment program include the placement of medical teams in shelters to provide care and compliance with therapy. Patients can be treated in shelter clinics after hospital discharge with a reasonable degree of success. Cooperation between local shelters and health departments is key to tracking patients and should help to prevent the reevaluation of already diagnosed patients.

Here again, the implementation of comprehensive tuberculosis education programs for the medical school curriculum should focus on methods to prevent tuberculosis in children and adults through a variety of target groups, including medical students, residents, faculty, community physicians, and health department clinics.

NEONATAL PULMONARY DISEASES

Respiratory disease will remain a major health problem for children in the United States until effective prenatal and child care programs are developed for all mothers and children. It has been effectively demonstrated and well documented that prevention of teenage pregnancy, cessation of smoking and drug use, immunization, improved nutrition, and adequate prenatal care would have a major impact on the prevention of respiratory distress syndrome (RDS) and bronchopulmonary dysplasia (BPD).[16]

Research continues on effective methods to reach high-risk groups, where innovative application of behavioral science techniques is urgently needed to try to decrease the frequency of premature births and improve the quality of pregnancies so that the incidence of neonatal infection and lung injury is reduced. For example, smoking cessation programs should be given high priority as part of routine prenatal care; although effective programs are available, their adoption by health care providers has been very slow.

Neonatal group B streptococcal infections can be prevented by programs designed to improve access to and cooperation with prenatal care programs. Emphasis should be given to detection of maternal cervical infections and colonization with group B streptococcus. Early detection and effective treatment of the mother would have dramatic effects on the frequency of neonatal disease.

Secondary prevention focuses on prevention of RDS in premature infants, such as enhancement of surfactant production through administration of prenatal glucocorticoids administered to the mother several days prior to delivery. A review of the data available led an NIH consensus panel to conclude that "Antenatal corticosteroid therapy is indicated for women at risk of premature delivery with few exceptions and will result in a substantial decrease in neonatal morbidity and mortality, as well as substantial savings in health care costs. The use of antenatal corticosteroids for fetal maturation is a rare example of a technology that yields substantial cost savings in addition to improving health."[6]

Prevention of RDS will result in a substantial reduction in BPD. Secondary prevention of BPD is based on judicious use of the therapy needed to support infants who develop RDS. There is still considerable controversy, however, as to the most appropriate strategy for the use of oxygen and positive pressure ventilation in this population. Current research on an animal model of BPD may provide important clues that will be helpful in the design of strategies for prevention and management of this chronic lung disease.

CARDIOPULMONARY DISORDERS OF SLEEP

It is estimated that 40 million Americans are chronically affected by various sleep disorders. Sleep apnea, estimated to occur in about 10 million people, strikes men and women of all races, ages, socioeconomic strata, and ethnicity. However, it appears to occur less frequently in women prior to menopause, and it may be more common in African Americans than in Caucasians. The potential consequences include hypertension, stroke, cognitive impairment, neuropsychiatric problems, and injuries due to accidents. Effective prevention programs are a goal, with work under way to develop diagnostic tools for identification of the site of airway obstruction during sleep and ambulatory monitoring of oxygenation and heart rate. Identification of risk factors, markers, predictors, and antecedents of disease, particularly in the early phases, should lead to better ambulatory screening tools, which will be required before progress can be made toward prevention of common sleep disorders.[18]

Several abnormalities of control of breathing are problems in infants and children, including obstructive sleep apnea of prematurity and sudden infant death syndrome (SIDS). Because, at the present time, there is no way to prevent or detect the underlying abnormalities in control of breathing associated with obstructive sleep apnea, the focus of primary prevention is on the education of parents and health care providers to recognize obstructive sleep apnea and obtain sleep histories.

CONCLUSION

Prevention and control of respiratory disease and illness has been a focus of national health programs for decades, and considerable progress has been made through efforts of physicians, health education specialists, and behavioral scientists working in unison to accomplish shared goals. However, much work remains to be done—work that will require a coordinated effort by research scientists, practicing physicians, and the public to accomplish the ultimate goal of better pulmonary health for all.

REFERENCES

1. Anthonisen NR, Connett JE, Altose MD, et al: Effects of smoking interventions and the use of inhaled anticholinergic bronchodilator on the rate of decline of FEV_1: The Lung Health Study. *JAMA* 272:1497–1505, 1994.
2. Brickner PW, Scharer LL, McAdam JM: Tuberculosis in homeless populations, in Reichman LB, Hershfield ES (eds): *Tuberculosis: A Comprehensive International Approach.* New York, Marcel Dekker, 1993, pp 433–354.
3. Centers for Disease Control: Tuberculosis control among homeless populations. *MMWR* 36:257–260, 1987.
4. Chan-Yeung M, Malo JL: Table of the major inducers of occupational asthma, in Bernstein IL et al (eds): *Asthma in the Workplace.* New York, Marcel Dekker, 1993, pp 595–623.
5. De Blay F, Chapman MD, Platts-Mills TA: Airborne cat allergen (Fel d l): Environmental control with the cat in situ. *Am Rev Respir Dis* 143:1334–1339, 1991.
6. Effect of corticosteroids for fetal maturation on perinatal outcomes: NIH Consensus Development Panel. *JAMA* 273:413–417, 1995.
7. Gadek JE, Klein HG, Holland PV, Crystal RG: Replacement therapy of alpha-1 antitrypsin deficiency: Reversal of protease-antiprotease imbalance within the alveolar structures of PiZZ subjects. *J Clin Invest* 68:1158–1165, 1981.
8. *Global Strategy for Asthma Management and Prevention.* Bethesda, MD, National Heart, Lung, and Blood Institute, National Institutes of Health, NIH pub no 95-3659, 1995.
9. *Guidelines for the Diagnosis and Management of Asthma.* Bethesda, MD, National Heart, Lung, and Blood Institute, National Institutes of Health, NIH pub no 91-3042, 1991.
10. Imai M, Katsumi Y, Kitagawa M: Mortality from asthma and chronic bronchitis associated with changes in sulfur oxides air pollution. *Arch Environ Health* 41:29–35, 1986.
11. *International Consensus Report on Diagnosis and Management of Asthma.* Bethesda, MD, National Heart, Lung, and Blood Institute, National Institutes of Health, NIH pub no 92-3091, 1992.
12. Postma DS, Bleecker ET, Amelung PJ, et al: Genetic susceptibility to asthma: Bronchial hyperresponsiveness coinherited with a major gene for atopy. *New Eng J Med* 333:894–900, 1995.
13. *Respiratory Diseases: Task Force Report on Problems, Research Approaches, Needs.* Bethesda, MD, National Heart, Lung, and Blood Institute, National Institutes of Health, NIH pub 73–432, 1973.
14. *Respiratory Diseases: Task Force Report on Prevention, Control and Education.* Bethesda, MD, National Heart, Lung, and Blood Institute, National Institutes of Health, NIH pub no 77–1248, 1977.
15. *Smoking and Health: Report of the Advisory Committee to the Surgeon General of the Public Health Service.* Washington, DC, U.S. Public Health Service, DHEW pub no 1103, 1964.
16. Buist AS, Becker MH (eds): Task Force on Research and Education for the Prevention and Control of Respiratory Diseases. *Chest* 102(suppl): 215S–301S 1992.
17. *The Health Consequences of Smoking: Chronic Obstructive Lung Disease: A Report of the Surgeon General.* Washington, DC, U.S. Department of Health and Human Services, 1984.
18. *Wake Up America: A National Sleep Alert: A Report of the National Commission on Sleep Disorders Research.* Bethesda, MD, DHHS, NHLBI, National Center for Sleep Disorders Research, 1994.

NOTES

NOTES

NOTES

NOTES

NOTES

NOTES

NOTES

NOTES

APPENDIXES

RESPIRATORY QUESTIONNAIRE

Name _____ Social Security no. _____ Date _____

Plant _____ Sex _____ Date of birth _____ Age _____

Questionnaire administered by _____

I. Occupational history: Please list entire work history, starting with present job and going back to first job. (Use extra sheet if necessary.)

Industry (or company) and location	From	To	Specific job

	Yes	No	Number of years
A. Have you ever worked in a dusty job?			
1. In a mine?			
2. In a quarry?			
3. In a foundry?			
4. In a pottery?			
5. In a cotton, flax, or hemp mill?			
6. With asbestos?			
7. In a brick plant?			
8. As a sandblaster?			
9. In the manufacture of glass, ceramics, or abrasives?			
10. In other dusty jobs? Specify_____			
B. Have your ever worked with chemicals?			
1. Solvents? Specify_____			
2. Acids? Specify_____			
3. Lead?			
4. Plastics? Specify_____			
5. TDI?			

	Yes	No

II. Previous illnesses

   A. Have you ever had any of the following problems?

      1. Asthma? . . . .

      2. Emphysema? . . . .

      3. Chronic bronchitis? . . . .

      4. Pneumonia? . . . .

      5. Tuberculosis? . . . .

      6. Pleurisy? . . . .

      7. Heart trouble of any type? . . . .

   B. Have you ever had surgery on your chest or lungs? . . . .

      If yes, specify._____

      _____

   C. Chest x-rays

      Last one (date) _____

      Ever abnormal? . . . .

   D. Tuberculosis skin test

      Last one (date) _____

      Positive? . . . .

III. Symptoms

   A. Cough

      1. Do you usually cough first thing in the morning? . . . .

      2. Do you usually cough at other times during the day or night? . . . .

Skip 3 to 6 if answer
to 1 and 2 is "no."
Answer if "yes."

      3. Do you cough on most days for as much as 3 months
         of the year? . . . .

      4. For how many years have you had this cough?

         Less than 2 years _____

         2 to 5 years _____

         5 years or more_____

      5. Do you cough more on any particular day of the week? . . . .

         If yes, which day?_____

      6. Do you cough during any particular season of the year? . . . .

         If yes, which season? _____

   B. Sputum

      1. Do you usually bring up phlegm, sputum, or mucus from your
         chest first thing in the morning? . . . .

      2. Do you usually bring up phlegm, sputum, or mucus from your
         chest at other times of the day or night? . . . .

Skip 3 and 4 if answer
to 1 and 2 is "no."
Answer if "yes."

      3. Do you bring up phlegm, sputum, or mucus from your chest on
         most days for as much as 3 months of the year? . . . .

      4. For how many years have you raised phlegm, sputum, or mucus
         from your chest?

         Less than 2 years _____

         2 to 5 years _____

         5 years or more_____

   C. Wheezing

      1. Does your breathing ever sound wheezy? . . . .

      2. Have you ever had attacks of shortness of breath
         with wheezing? . . . .

      3. Have you ever had a feeling of tightness in your chest? . . . .

Skip 4 to 6 if answer
to 1, 2, and 3 is "no."
Answer if "yes."

      4. At what age did wheezing first occur?_____

      5. How frequently does wheezing occur?

         Daily _____

         Nightly _____

         A few times per week_____

	Yes	No

A few times per month _____

A few times per year _____

6. Is it worse on any particular day of the week?
What day? _____

D. Breathlessness

1. Do you get short of breath when walking on level ground? . . . .

2. Do you get short of breath while walking up stairs? . . . .

3. How many flights of stairs can you climb up without stopping?

1 to 2? _____

2 to 3? _____

More than 3? _____

E. Hemoptysis

1. Have you ever coughed up blood from your chest? If yes, when
was the last time this happened? _____ . . . .

IV. Smoking

A. Smoking (currently)

1. Do you now smoke regularly (cigarettes, pipe, cigars)? . . . .

Skip 2 to 6 if answer to 1 is "no." Answer if "yes."

2. How old were you when you started smoking?
_____

3. For how many years have you smoked regularly?
_____

4. How many cigarettes do you now smoke each day?
_____

5. How much pipe tobacco do you now smoke each week?
_____

6. How many cigars do you now smoke each day?
_____

B. Smoking (formerly)

1. Have you ever smoked regularly? . . . .

Skip 2 to 7 if answer to 1 is "no." Answer if "yes."

2. How old were you when you started smoking regularly?
_____

3. For how many years did you smoke regularly?
_____

4. When did you quit smoking?
Month _____
Year _____

5. How many cigarettes did you usually smoke per day?
_____

6. How much pipe tobacco did you usually smoke per week?
_____

7. How many cigars did you usually smoke per day?
_____

V. Additional comments

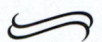

NORMAL VALUES

TYPICAL VALUES FOR A 20-YEAR-OLD SEATED MAN*

Ventilation (BTPS)

Tidal volume, L	0.6
Frequency, breaths/min	12
Minute volume, L/min	7.2
Respiratory dead space, ml	150
Alveolar ventilation, L/min	5.4

Lung Volumes and Capacities (BTPS)

Inspiratory capacity (IC), L	3.0
Expiratory reserve volume (ERV), L	1.9
Vital capacity (VC), L	4.9
Residual volume (RV), L	1.4
Functional residual capacity (FRC), L	3.2
Total lung capacity (TLC), L	6.3
Residual volume/total lung capacity $\times 100$ (RV/TLC,%)	22

Mechanics of Breathing

Forced vital capacity (FVC), L	4.9
Forced expiratory volume, first second (FEV_1), L	4.0
Maximum voluntary ventilation (MVV), L/min	170
Forced expiratory volume in 1 s/forced vital capacity $\times$ 100% (FEV_1/FVC,%)	83
Forced expiratory volume in 3 s/forced vital capacity $\times$ 100% (FEV_3/FVC,%)	97
Forced expiratory flow during middle half of FVC (FEF_{25-75}), L/s	4.7
Forced inspiratory flow at the middle of FIVC (FIF_{50}), L/s	5.0
Static compliance of the lungs (Cst, L), L/cm H_2O	0.2
Compliance of lungs and thoracic cage, L/cm H_2O	0.1
Airway resistance at FRC (Raw), cm H_2O/L/s	1.5
Pulmonary resistance at FRC, cm H_2O/L/s	2.0
Airway conductance at FRC (Gaw), L/s/cm H_2O	0.66
Specific conductance (Gaw/V_L)	0.22
Work of quiet breathing, (kg · m)/min	0.5
Maximum work of breathing, (kg · m)/breath	10
Maximum inspiratory pressure, mmHg	−75
Maximum expiratory pressure, mmHg	120

Distribution of Inspired Gas

Single-breath N_2 test (ΔN_2 from 750 to 1250 ml in expired gas), % N_2	<1.5
Alveolar N_2 after 7 min of breathing O_2, % N_2	<2.5
Closing volume (CV), ml	400
CV/VC $\times$ 100%	8
Closing capacity (CC), ml	1900

*Height = 165 cm; weight = 64 kg; body surface area = 1.7 m².

CC/TLC $\times$ 100%	30
Slope of phase III in single-breath N_2 test, % N_2/L	<2

Gas Exchange

O_2 consumption at rest (STPD), ml/min	240
CO_2 output at rest (STPD), ml/min	192
Respiratory exchange ratio (R), CO_2 output/O_2 uptake	0.8

ALVEOLAR GAS

$P_{A_{O_2}}$, mmHg	105
$P_{A_{CO_2}}$, mmHg	40

ARTERIAL BLOOD

Pa_{O_2}, mmHg	95
Sa_{O_2}, %	98
pH	7.41
Pa_{CO_2}, mmHg	40
Pa_{O_2}, while breathing 100% O_2, mmHg	640

Alveolar Ventilation

Alveolar ventilation, L/min	4.2
Physiological dead space/tidal volume $\times$ 100 (V_D/V_T, %)	<30
Alveolar-arterial P_{O_2}, P(A-a)$_{O_2}$, mmHg	<10

Diffusing Capacity

Diffusing capacity at rest for CO, single-breath ($DL_{CO_{sb}}$), ml CO/min/mmHg	29
Diffusing capacity per unit alveolar volume (DL/VA)	4.8

Control of Ventilation

Ventilatory response to hypercapnia, L/min/per Δ Pa_{CO_2} mmHg	>0.5
Ventilatory response to hypoxia, L/min per ΔS_{O_2} (%)	>0.2
Arterial blood P_{O_2} during moderate exercise, mmHg	95

Pulmonary Hemodynamics

Pulmonary blood flow (cardiac output), L/min	5.4
Pulmonary artery pressure, systolic/diastolic, mmHg	25/8
Pulmonary capillary blood volume, ml	100
Pulmonary "capillary" blood pressure (wedge), mmHg	<10

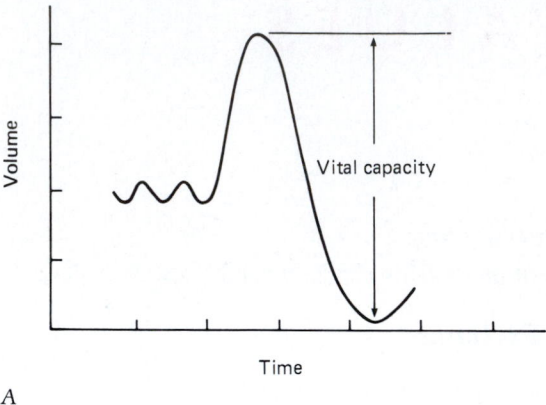

A

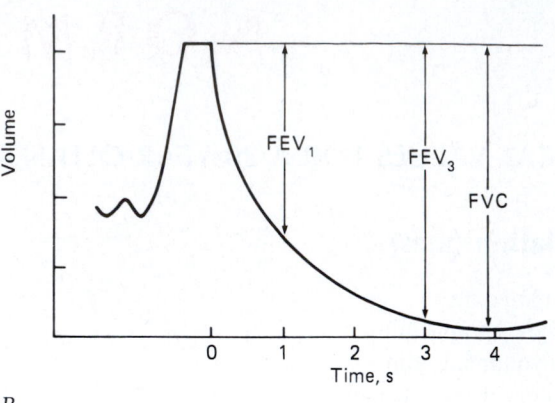

B

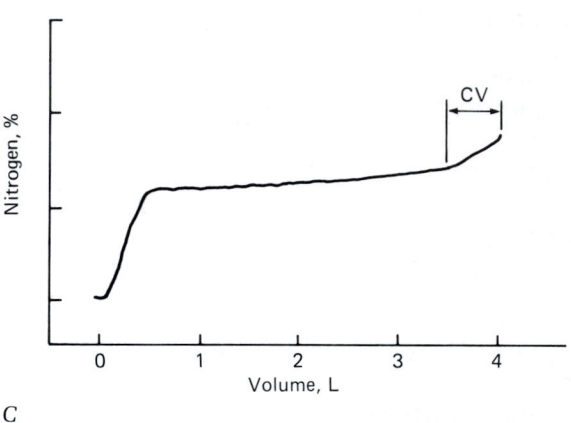

C

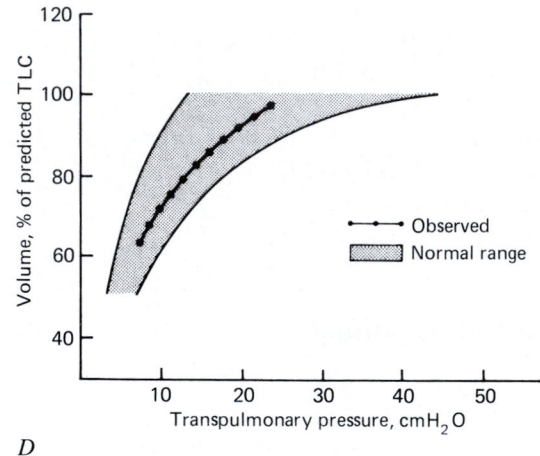

D

Figure B-1. Representative tracings and graphs commonly used in assessing pulmonary function. *A.* Lung volumes (vital capacity). *B.* Mechanics of breathing (forced expiratory volumes). *C.* Distribution of inspired gas (closing volumes). *D.* Mechanics of breathing (compliance of lungs).

APPENDIX C

TERMS AND SYMBOLS IN RESPIRATORY PHYSIOLOGY

GENERAL SYMBOLS

P	Partial pressure in blood or gas.
	P_{O_2} = partial pressure of O_2
$\overline{X}$	A bar over the symbol indicates a mean value.
	$\overline{P}$ = mean pressure, as distinct from instantaneous pressure
$\dot{X}$	A time derivative (rate) is indicated by a dot above the symbol.
	$\dot{V}_{O_2}$ = O_2 consumption per minute
	$\dot{V}_{CO_2}$ = CO_2 production per minute
% X	Percent sign preceding a symbol indicates percentage of the predicted normal value.
X/Y%	Percent sign following a symbol indicates a ratio function with the ratio expressed as a percentage. Both components of the ratio must be designated.
	FEV_1/FVC, % = $100 \times FEV_1/FVC$
XA, Xa	A small capital letter or a lower-case letter on the same line following a primary symbol is a qualifier to further define the primary symbol. Alternatively, subscript letters may be used.
	$XA = X_A$, $Xa = X_a$
$P_{E_{CO_2}}$	Additional qualifiers of the primary symbol may be identified as shown.

GAS PHASE SYMBOLS

PRIMARY SYMBOLS

V	Volume of gas.
$\dot{V}$	Flow of gas.
F	Fractional concentration of a gas.

Qualifying Symbols

I	Inspired.
	V_I = inspired volume
E	Expired.
	V_E = expired volume
A	Alveolar.
	V_A = alveolar volume
	$\dot{V}_A$ = alveolar ventilation per minute
T	Tidal.
	V_T = tidal volume
D	Dead space.
	V_D = volume of dead space
	$\dot{V}_D$ = dead-space ventilation per minute
B	Barometric.
	P_B = barometric pressure
STPD	Standard conditions: temperature 0°C, pressure 760 mmHg, and dry (0 mmHg water vapor).
BTPS	Body conditions: body temperature and ambient pressure, saturated with water vapor at these conditions.
ATPD	Ambient temperature and pressure, dry.
ATPS	Ambient temperature and pressure, saturated with water vapor at these conditions.

an	Anatomic.
p	Physiological.
f	Respiratory frequency, per minute.
max	Maximum.
t	Time.

BLOOD PHASE SYMBOLS

Primary Symbols

Q   Volume of blood.

$\dot{Q}$ Blood flow.

                $\dot{Q}$ = cardiac output, L/min

C   Concentration in the blood phase.

                C_{N_2} = concentration of N_2 in blood, ml of N_2 per 100 ml of blood

S   Saturation in the blood phase.

                S_{O_2} = saturation of hemoglobin with O_2, percent

Qualifying Symbols

a   Arterial.

                Ca_{O_2} = concentration of O_2 in arterial blood, ml of O_2 per 100 ml of blood

c   Capillary.

                Cc_{O_2} = concentration of O_2 in capillary blood, ml of O_2 per 100 ml of blood

c'   Pulmonary end-capillary.

                Pc'_{CO_2} = partial pressure of CO_2 in end-capillary blood, mmHg

v   Venous.

                Cv_{O_2} = concentration of O_2 in venous blood, ml of O_2 per 100 ml of blood

$\bar{v}$ Mixed venous.

                $C\bar{v}_{O_2}$ = concentration of O_2 in mixed venous blood, ml of O_2 per 100 ml of blood

VENTILATION AND LUNG MECHANICS TESTS AND SYMBOLS

Static Lung Volumes*

PRIMARY COMPARTMENTS

RV	Residual volume. Volume of air remaining in the lungs after maximum expiration.
CV	Closing volume. Volume of air expired from the onset of airways closure to residual volume. May be expressed as a fraction of VC: CV/VC,%.
ERV	Expiratory reserve volume. Maximum volume of air expired from the resting end-expiratory level.
V_T	Tidal volume. Volume of air inspired or expired with each breath during quiet breathing. When tidal volume is used in gas-exchange formulations, this symbol is used. When indicating a subdivision of lung volumes, the symbol TV may be used.
IRV	Inspiratory reserve volume. Maximum volume of air inspired from the end-tidal inspiratory level.

Lung Capacities†

IC	Inspiratory capacity. The sum of IRV and TV.
IVC	Inspiratory vital capacity. Maximum volume of air inspired from the point of maximum expiration.
VC	Vital capacity. Maximum volume of air expired from the point of maximum inspiration.
FRC	Functional residual capacity. Sum of RV and ERV. FRC is the volume of air remaining in the lungs at the resting end-expiratory position.
TLC	Total lung capacity. Volume of air in the lungs after maximum inspiration. Also, the sum of all volume compartments of the lungs.
RV/TLC,%	Residual volume to total lung capacity ratio, expressed as a percentage.
CC	Closing capacity. Closing volume plus residual volume, may be expressed as a ratio of TLC: CC/TLC,%.

*Expressed at BTPS.
†Combinations of volumes for practical purposes.

Forced Respiratory Maneuvers During Spirometry*

FVC	Forced vital capacity. The maximum volume of air forcibly expired from total lung capacity.
FIVC	Forced inspiratory vital capacity. Maximum volume of air forcibly inspired starting from residual volume.
FEV_t	Timed forced expiratory volume. Volume of air expired in a specified time in the course of the forced vital capacity maneuver.

FEV_1 = volume of air expired during the first second of the FVC

FEV_t/FVC, %	Ratio of time forced expiratory volume to forced vital capacity, expressed as a percentage.
FEF_x	Forced expiratory flow, related to some portion of the FVC curve. Modifiers refer to the amount of the FVC that has been expired at the time of measurement.
$FEF_{200-1200}$	Forced expiratory flow between 200 and 1200 ml of the FVC (formerly called the maximum expiratory flow rate).
FEF_{25-75}	Forced expiratory flow during middle half of the FVC (formerly called the maximum midexpiratory flow rate).
PEF	Peak expiratory flow. Highest value for expiratory flow.
$\dot{V}max_x$	Maximum flow when x percent of the FVC has been expired.

$\dot{V}max_{75}$ = flow (instantaneous) when 75 percent of the FVC has been expired

FIF_x	Forced inspiratory flow. As in the case of the FEF, appropriate modifiers designate the volume at which flow is being measured. Unless otherwise specified, the volume qualifiers indicate the volume inspired from RV at the point of measurement.

FIF_{25-75} = forced inspiratory flow during the middle half of the FIVC

$I\dot{V}max_x$	Maximum inspiratory flow (instantaneous) when x percent of the FIVC has been inspired.
MVV	Maximum voluntary ventilation. Volume of air exhaled during maximum breathing efforts within a specified time period. Formerly called maximum breathing capacity. If breathing frequency is set by the examiner, it is indicated by the qualifier.

MVV_{60} = MVV at a breathing frequency of 60 per minute

Measurements Related to Ventilation

$\dot{V}_E$	Expired volume per minute (BTPS).
$\dot{V}_I$	Inspired volume per minute (BTPS).
$\dot{V}_{CO_2}$	Carbon dioxide production per minute (STPD).
$\dot{V}_{O_2}$	Oxygen consumption per minute (STPD).
R	Respiratory exchange ratio, the ratio of CO_2 output to O_2 intake in the lungs.
$\dot{V}_A$	Alveolar ventilation per minute (BTPS).
$\dot{V}_D$	Ventilation per minute of the physiological dead space (BTPS) defined by the equation

$$\dot{V}_D = \dot{V}_E \frac{Pa_{CO_2} - P_{E_{CO_2}}}{Pa_{CO_2} - P_{I_{CO_2}}}$$

V_D	Volume of the physiological dead space, calculated as $\dot{V}_D/f$.
$\dot{V}_{D_{an}}$	Ventilation per minute of the anatomic dead space, that portion of the conducting airway in which no significant gas exchange occurs (BTPS).
$V_{D_{an}}$	Volume of the anatomic dead space (BTPS).

Mechanics of Breathing†

PRESSURE TERMS

Paw	Pressure at any point along the airways.
Pao	Pressure at the airway opening.
Ppl	Pleural pressure.
P_A	Alveolar pressure.
Pbs	Pressure at the body surface.
Pes	Esophageal pressure: used to estimate Ppl.
P_A–Pbs	Transthoracic pressure.
P_A–Ppl	Transpulmonary pressure.
Ppl–Pbs	Pressure difference across the chest wall.
Paw–Ppl	Transbronchial pressure, estimated as difference between airway and pleural pressures.

*All values at BTPS.
†All pressures expressed relative to ambient pressure unless otherwise specified.

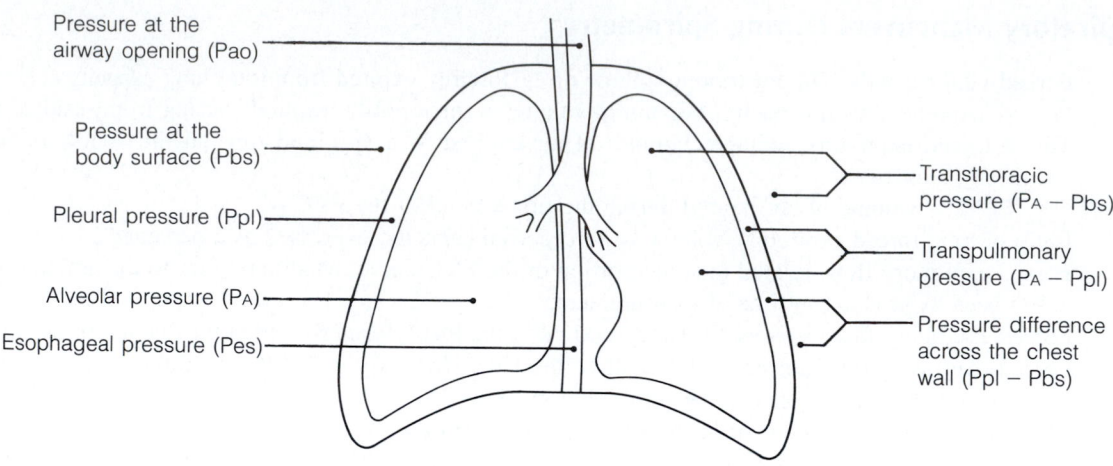

FLOW-PRESSURE RELATIONSHIPS*

R	General symbol for frictional resistance, defined as the ratio of pressure difference to flow.
Raw	Airway resistance, calculated from pressure difference between airway opening (Pao) and alveoli (PA) divided by the airflow, cm H_2O/L/s.
R_L	Total pulmonary resistance, measured by relating flow-dependent transpulmonary pressure to airflow at the mouth.
Rti	Tissue resistance (viscous resistance of lung tissue), calculated as difference between R_L and Raw.
Rus	Resistance of the airways on the upstream (alveolar) side of the point in the airways where intraluminal pressure equals Ppl, i.e., equal pressure point. Measured during a forced expiration.
Rds	Resistance of the airways on the downstream (mouth) side of the point in the airways where intraluminal pressure equals Ppl, i.e., equal pressure point. Measured during a forced expiration.
Gaw	Airway conductance, reciprocal of Raw.
Gaw/V_L	Specific conductance, airway conductance, expressed per liter of lung volume at which Gaw is measured.
$\dot{W}$	Rate of work or power. Expressed either in kpm/min or J/s (watt).

VOLUME-PRESSURE RELATIONSHIPS

C	General symbol for compliance of the lungs, chest wall, or total respiratory system. Volume change per unit change in applied pressure. For the lungs, the applied pressure is the pressure difference across the lungs, or transpulmonary pressure, Pao–Ppl; for the chest wall, the applied pressure is the transthoracic pressure, Ppl–Pbs; for the entire respiratory system, the applied pressure is Pao–Pbs.
Cdyn	Dynamic compliance. Value for compliance determined at time of zero gas flow at the mouth during uninterrupted breathing. The respiratory frequency appears as a qualifier.
	$Cdyn_{40}$ = dynamic compliance at a respiratory frequency of 40 per minute
Cst	Static compliance, value for compliance determined on the basis of measurements made during a period of zero airflow.
C/V_L	Specific compliance. Compliance divided by the lung volume at which it is determined, usually FRC.
Pst	Static pulmonary pressure at a specified lung volume.
	Pst_{TLC} = static recoil pressure of the lung measured at TLC (maximum recoil pressure)
W	Mechanical work of breathing.

DIFFUSING CAPACITY TESTS AND SYMBOLS

DL_x, D_x	Diffusing capacity of the lung expressed as volume (STPD) of gas (x) uptake per minute per unit alveolar-capillary pressure difference for the gas used. A modifier can be used to designate the technique:
	$DL_{CO/sb}$ = single-breath CO diffusing capacity
	$DL_{CO/ss}$ = steady-state CO diffusing capacity
DM	Diffusing capacity of the alveolar-capillary membrane (STPD).

*Unless otherwise specified, all resistance measurements assumed to be made at FRC.

θ	Reaction rate coefficient for red blood cells. Determined as the volume of gas (STPD) that will combine per minute with 1 unit volume of blood per unit of gas tension. If the specific gas is not stated, θ is assumed to refer to CO and is a function of existing O_2 tension.
Vc	Capillary blood volume. This should be Qc for consistency with other symbols, but Vc is entrenched in the literature. In the equation that follows for $1/D_L$, Vc represents the effective pulmonary capillary blood volume, i.e., capillary blood volume in intimate association with alveolar gas.
$1/D_L$	Total resistance to diffusion, including resistance to diffusion of test gas across the alveolar-capillary membrane, through plasma in the capillary, and across the red blood cell membrane ($1/D_M$), the resistance to diffusion with the red cell arising from the chemical reaction of the test gas and hemoglobin ($1/\theta Vc$), according to the formulation $$\frac{1}{D_L} = \frac{1}{D_M} + \frac{1}{\theta Vc}$$
D_L/V_A	Diffusing capacity per unit of alveolar volume. D_L is expressed STPD, and V_A is expressed in liters, BTPS.

BLOOD GAS SYMBOLS

Symbols for these values are readily composed by combining general symbols. Some examples include the following.

Pa_{CO_2}	Arterial CO_2 tension, mmHg.
Sa_{O_2}	Arterial O_2 saturation, percent.
Cc'_{O_2}	Oxygen content of pulmonary end-capillary blood, ml of O_2 per 100 ml of blood.
$PA_{O_2} - Pa_{O_2}$ $P(A\text{-}a)_{O_2}$	Alveolar-arterial difference in the partial pressure of O_2, mmHg.
$Ca_{O_2} - C\bar{v}_{O_2}$	O_2 content difference between arterial and mixed venous blood (arteriovenous O_2 difference), ml of O_2 per 100 ml of blood.

PULMONARY SHUNT SYMBOLS

$\dot{Q}s$	Flow of blood via shunts. This is usually determined as percent of cardiac output ($\dot{Q}$) while breathing 100% O_2, according to the equation $$\frac{\dot{Q}s}{\dot{Q}} = \frac{Cc'-Ca}{Cc'-C\bar{v}},$$ where $$\frac{\dot{Q}s}{\dot{Q}} = \text{"anatomic" venous admixture}$$ and $$Cc'_{O_2} = O_2 \text{ content of end-capillary blood}$$ $$Ca_{O_2} = O_2 \text{ content of arterial blood}$$ $$C\bar{v}_{O_2} = O_2 \text{ content of mixed venous blood}$$

INDEX

Index

Page numbers followed by *f* indicate figures; page numbers followed by *t* indicate tables.

A

A-60477, and mast cells, 295
Abdominal aortic aneurysm surgery, respiratory failure and, *2590t*
Abdominal distension, from enteral nutrition, 2736
Abdominal motion analysis, in neuromuscular diseases, 1570
Abdominal paradox, 2622
Abdominal respiratory muscles, 68. *See also* Respiratory muscle(s)
Abdominal surgery, upper, and respiratory failure, 2593
ABPA. *See* Aspergillosis, allergic bronchopulmonary
Abscesses
  Bezold's, 1982
  brain, from arteriovenous malformations, pulmonary, 1380, *1383f*
  hepatic
    amebic, 2181, *2182f*, 2379, 2380
    pleural effusions, 1420
  intraabdominal, and pleural effusions, 1420, *1421f*
  lung. *See* Lung abscess
  peritonsillar (quinsy), 1974
  subperiosteal, frontal (Pott's puffy tumor), 1978
  subphrenic, pleural effusions, 1420
Acanthamoeba, 2382–2384
  treatment of, *2384t*
Acanthosis nigricans, 411
Acclimatization, ventilatory, *967f–969f*, 967–969
Acetaldehyde, inhalation injury, 991
Acetazolamide, 2649, 2658
  for mountain sickness, 2658
  for sleep apnea, 1627, 2658
Acetylcholine
  carotid body, 165
  and sleep, 1602
  vasodilating effects, *1241f*, 1248
Achalasia, 1217, *1219f*, 1521
  imaging, *478f*
Acid, renal excretion of, 209, *210f*
Acid anhydrides, asthma from, 921–922
Acid-base balance, 207–210, *208t*
  alternative concepts of, 212–213
  bicarbonate reclamation, 208–209, *209f*
  kidney role in, 207–208
  renal acid excretion, 209, *210f*
  respiratory contribution to, 210–211
Acid-base disturbances, 211–219, *561t. See also individual disorders*

adaptation to, 174
approach to patient with, 213–218
  nomograms, 214, *214f*
classification, *561t*
mixed, 217–218
  case illustration, 219
Acid-base nomogram, 214, *214f*
Acid hydrolases, 293
Acid maltase deficiency, 1579
Acidosis. *See also* Metabolic acidosis; Respiratory acidosis
  dyspnea and, 368
  and pulmonary hypertension, 1265
Acinetobacter
  pneumonia
    neonatal, 1998
    nosocomial, 1922, 2218, *2219t*, *2220t*, 2596
    treatment, *2224t*
  sputum examination, 1930
Acinic cell tumors (Fechner tumors), of lung, 1839
Acinus, anatomy, 24
Acne, drug-induced, 402
Acquired immunodeficiency syndrome. *See* Human immunodeficiency virus (HIV) disease
Acrolein
  inhalation injury, 991
  in tobacco, 679
Acromegaly, and lung cancer, *1842t*, 1845–1846
  biology, 1846
  diagnosis, 1846
  treatment, 1846
Acrosclerosis, 414
Actinic keratoses, 401
Actinomycin D
  pulmonary disorders from, *1005t*, 1008
  and radiation therapy, 1106
Actinomycosis, 2257–2259
  aspiration pneumonia, 1921, *1921f*
  clinical manifestations, 2257–2258, *2258f*, *2259f*
  cutaneous manifestations, 398, 404
  cytopathology, 493
  diagnosis, 2258–2259, *2259f*
  epidemiology and pathogenesis, 2257
  lung infections, *2015t*
  mediastinitis, *2037t*
  therapy, 2259
Acute respiratory distress syndrome (ARDS). *See* Adult respiratory distress syndrome (ARDS)

Adaptation, 226–228
  optimizing, 227–228
Adefovir, 2110
Adenocarcinoma, *1820t. See also* Lung cancer, non–small cell
  cytopathology, *501f*, 501–502
  epidemiology of, 1708
  pathology of, 1741, 1743–1746, *1744f*, *1745f*
  prognostic variables for, 1756
  as solitary nodule, 1728
  well-differentiated fetal, 1748
Adenoid cystic carcinoma, *1820t*, 1839. *See also* Lung cancer, non–small cell
  pathology, 1754, *1755f*
Adenoma, mucous gland, 1833
Adenomatous (bronchioalveolar) hyperplasia, 1746
Adenomatous polyposis, familial, colonic, 1700
Adenosine, pulmonary toxicity, 1022
Adenosine deaminase (ADA) deficiency, 2171
Adenosquamous carcinoma, *1740t*, *1820t. See also* Lung cancer, non–small cell
  pathology, 1747–1748
Adenoviruses
  after bone marrow transplantation, 2147
  bronchiolitis from, 833, *835f*, 2340–2341
  bronchitis from, 1985
  common cold from, 1973, *2334t*, 2335
  cutaneous manifestations, 398
  cytopathology, 496
  diagnosis, *2335t*
  laryngitis from, 1975, 2336–2337
  nosocomial infections from, 2345, *2345t*
  pleural effusions from, 1419
  pneumonia from, 2342
    differential diagnosis of, 2427
  respiratory infections from, *2334t*
  in severe combined immunodeficiency, 2171
  vaccine, *1963t*, 1964–1965
Adenylyl cyclase, and airway smooth cells, 110
Adhesion molecules, and asthma, 730
Adrenal metastases, lung cancer, non–small cell, 1769–1770, *1770f*
Adrenergic agonists, beta. *See* Beta-adrenergic agonists
Adrenergic antagonists, beta. *See* Beta-adrenergic antagonists
Adrenocorticotropic hormone (ACTH), ectopic, 1844–1845, *1845f*
  and lung cancer, *1842t*, 1844–1845

ISBN 0-07-911167-X

ISBN 0-07-021180-9